CLINICAL
ANESTHESIA

CLINICAL ANESTHESIA

Fourth Edition

Edited by

Paul G. Barash, MD

Professor, Department of Anesthesiology
Yale University School of Medicine
Attending Anesthesiologist
Yale–New Haven Hospital
New Haven, Connecticut

Bruce F. Cullen, MD

Professor, Department of Anesthesiology
University of Washington School of Medicine
Anesthesiologist-in-Chief
Harborview Medical Center
Seattle, Washington

Robert K. Stoelting, MD

Professor and Chair, Department of Anesthesia
Indiana University School of Medicine
Indianapolis, Indiana

LIPPINCOTT WILLIAMS & WILKINS
A **Wolters Kluwer** Company
Philadelphia • Baltimore • New York • London
Buenos Aires • Hong Kong • Sydney • Tokyo

Acquisitions Editor: R. Craig Percy
Developmental Editor: Tanya Lazar
Supervising Editor: Mary Ann McLaughlin
Production Manager: Toni Ann Scaramuzzo
Production Editor: Mary McDonald/P. M. Gordon Associates
Compositor: The PRD Group, Inc.
Printer/Binder: Courier Westford
Cover Designer: Christine Jenny

© 2001 by LIPPINCOTT WILLIAMS & WILKINS
530 Walnut Street
Philadelphia, PA 19106 USA
LWW.com

Copyright © 1997 by Lippincott–Raven Publishers.
Copyright © 1992, 1989 by J. B. Lippincott Company.

Printed in the USA

Library of Congress Cataloging-in-Publication Data

Clinical anesthesia / edited by Paul G. Barash, Bruce F. Cullen, Robert K. Stoelting.—
   4th ed.
      p. ; cm.
   Includes bibliographical references and index.
   ISBN 0–7817–2268–3
   1. Anesthesiology. 2. Anesthesia. I. Barash, Paul G. II. Cullen, Bruce F. III. Stoelting,
Robert K.
   [DNLM: 1. Anesthesia. 2. Anesthesiology. 3. Anesthetics. WO 200 C6398 2000]
RD81.C58 2000
617.9′6—dc21
                                                                        00–037065

Care has been taken to confirm the accuracy of the information presented and to describe generally accepted practices. However, the authors, editors, and publisher are not responsible for errors or omissions or for any consequences from application of the information in this book and make no warranty, expressed or implied, with respect to the currency, completeness, or accuracy of the contents of the publication. Application of this information in a particular situation remains the professional responsibility of the practitioner.

The authors, editors, and publisher have exerted every effort to ensure that drug selection and dosage set forth in this text are in accordance with current recommendations and practice at the time of publication. However, in view of ongoing research, changes in government regulations, and the constant flow of information relating to drug therapy and drug reactions, the reader is urged to check the package insert for each drug for any change in indications and dosage and for added warnings and precautions. This is particularly important when the recommended agent is a new or infrequently employed drug.

Some drugs and medical devices presented in this publication have Food and Drug Administration (FDA) clearance for limited use in restricted research settings. It is the responsibility of health care providers to ascertain the FDA status of each drug or device planned for use in their clinical practice.

10 9 8 7 6 5 4 3 2

To All Students of Anesthesiology

CONTRIBUTING AUTHORS

Stephen E. Abram, MD
Professor and Chair
Department of Anesthesiology
University of New Mexico School of Medicine
Albuquerque, New Mexico

J. Jeffrey Andrews, MD
Professor and Vice-Chair for Clinical Development
Department of Anesthesiology
University of Alabama School of Medicine
Birmingham, Alabama

Douglas R. Bacon, MD
Associate Professor
Department of Anesthesiology
Mayo Clinic
Rochester, Minnesota

Audrée A. Bendo, MD
Associate Professor
Department of Anesthesiology
SUNY Health Science Center at Brooklyn
Brooklyn, New York

Christopher M. Bernards, MD
Associate Professor
Department of Anesthesiology
University of Washington School of Medicine
Seattle, Washington

Arnold J. Berry, MD, MPH
Professor
Department of Anesthesiology
Emory University School of Medicine
Atlanta, Georgia

Frederic A. Berry, MD
Professor of Anesthesiology and Pediatrics
Department of Anesthesiology
University of Virginia Health Sciences Center
Charlottesville, Virginia

David R. Bevan, MD
Professor and Head
Department of Anaesthesia
University of British Columbia Faculty of Medicine
Vancouver, British Columbia

W. Chase Boyd, MD
Assistant Professor
Department of Anesthesiology
Cornell University–New York Hospital
New York, New York

Barbara W. Brandom, MD
Professor
University of Pittsburgh School of Medicine
Children's Hospital of Pittsburgh
Department of Anesthesiology
Pittsburgh, Pennsylvania

Russell C. Brockwell, MD
Assistant Professor
Department of Anesthesiology
University of Alabama School of Medicine
Birmingham, Alabama

Morris Brown, MD
Professor of Anesthesiology
Wayne State University School of Medicine
Chairman
Department of Anesthesiology
Henry Ford Hospital
Detroit, Michigan

F. Peter Buckley, MD
Associate Professor
Department of Anesthesiology
University of Washington School of Medicine
Medical Director
Pain and Toxicity Program
Fred Hutchinson Cancer Research Center
Seattle, Washington

Rod K. Calverley*
Clinical Professor of Anesthesiology
University of California, San Diego, School of Medicine
La Jolla, California

Levon M. Capan, MD
Associate Professor
New York University School of Medicine
New York, New York

Barbara A. Castro, MD
Assistant Professor of Anesthesiology and Clinical
   Pediatrics
University of Virginia School of Medicine
Charlottesville, Virginia

Frederick W. Cheney, MD
Professor and Chair
Department of Anesthesiology
University of Washington School of Medicine
Seattle, Washington

Jen W. Chiu, MBBS, MMed, DEAA
Associate Consultant
Department of Anesthesiology
K Women's and Children's Hospital
Singapore

Barbara A. Coda, MD
Assistant Professor
Department of Anesthesiology
University of Washington School of Medicine
Harborview Medical Center
Seattle, Washington

---

* Deceased.

Edmond Cohen, MD
Associate Professor of Anesthesiology
Director of Thoracic Anesthesia
Mount Sinai School of Medicine of New York University
New York, New York

James E. Cottrell, MD
Professor and Chairman
Department of Anesthesiology
SUNY Health Science Center at Brooklyn
Brooklyn, New York

Joseph P. Cravero, MD
Assistant Professor of Anesthesiology and Pediatrics
Department of Anesthesiology
Dartmouth Medical School
Hanover, New Hampshire

Anthony J. Cunningham, MD
Professor
Department of Anaesthesia
Beaumont Hospital
Dublin, Ireland

Tina Desai, MD
Instructor
Department of Surgery
University of Chicago Pritzker School of Medicine
Chicago, Illinois

Stephen F. Dierdorf, MD
Professor
Department of Anesthesiology
Indiana University School of Medicine
Indianapolis, Indiana

François Donati, MD
Professor and Chair
Department of Anaesthesia
University of Montreal
Montreal, Quebec

Noreen Dowd, MD
Professorial Unit
Beaumont Hospital
Dublin, Ireland

John C. Drummond, MD, FRCPC
Professor and Chair
Department of Anesthesiology
University of California, San Diego, School of Medicine
La Jolla, California

Thomas J. Ebert, MD, PhD
Professor
Department of Anesthesiology
Medical College of Wisconsin
Milwaukee, Wisconsin

Jan Ehrenwerth, MD
Professor
Department of Anesthesiology
Yale University School of Medicine
New Haven, Connecticut

John H. Eichhorn, MD
Professor and Chair
Department of Anesthesiology
University of Mississippi School of Medicine and Medical Center
Jackson, Mississippi

James B. Eisenkraft, MD
Professor of Anesthesiology
Director of Anesthesia Research
Mt. Sinai School of Medicine of New York University
New York, New York

John E. Ellis, MD
Associate Professor
Department of Anesthesia and Critical Care
University of Chicago Pritzker School of Medicine
Chicago, Illinois

Alex S. Evers, MD
Professor and Chair
Department of Anesthesiology
Washington University School of Medicine
St. Louis, Missouri

Lynne R. Ferrari, MD
Associate Professor
Department of Anesthesiology
Harvard Medical School
Medical Director of Perioperative Services
Children's Hospital
Boston, Massachusetts

Mieczyslaw Finster, MD
Professor of Anesthesiology, Obstetrics, and Gynecology
Department of Anesthesiology
Columbia University
College of Physicians and Surgeons
New York, New York

Leonard L. Firestone, MD
Safar Professor and Chair
Department of Anesthesiology and Critical Care Medicine
University of Pittsburgh School of Medicine
Pittsburgh, Pennsylvania

Susan Firestone, MD
Associate Professor
Department of Anesthesiology and Critical Care Medicine
University of Pittsburgh School of Medicine
Pittsburgh, Pennsylvania

Lee A. Fleisher, MD
Associate Professor
Department of Anesthesiology and Critical Care
Johns Hopkins University School of Medicine
Baltimore, Maryland

Jeffrey E. Fletcher, PhD
Vice President, Scientific Affairs
Trinity Communications
Conshohocken, Pennsylvania

Simon Gelman, MD, PhD
Professor and Chair
Department of Anesthesiology, Perioperative and Pain
   Medicine
Harvard Medical School
Brigham and Women's Hospital
Boston, Massachusetts

Hugh C. Gilbert, MD
Associate Professor
Department of Anesthesiology
Northwestern University Medical School
Evanston Hospital
Evanston, Illinois

Alexander W. Gotta, MD
Professor of Anesthesiology
Department of Anesthesiology
SUNY Health Science Center at Brooklyn
Brooklyn, New York

George J. Graf, MD
Assistant Clinical Professor
Department of Anesthesiology
UCLA School of Medicine
Attending
Departments of Internal Medicine and Anesthesiology
Cedars Sinai Medical Center
Los Angeles, California

John Hartung, PhD
Associate Professor
Department of Anesthesiology
SUNY Health Science Center at Brooklyn
Brooklyn, New York

Simon C. Hillier, MB, ChB, FRCA
Associate Professor
Department of Anesthesiology
Indiana University School of Medicine
Riley Hospital for Children
Indianapolis, Indiana

Peter S. Hodgson, MD
The Daniel Moore/D. Bridenbaugh Fellow in Regional Anes-
   thesia
Virginia Mason Medical Center
Seattle, Washington

Terese T. Horlocker, MD
Assistant Professor
Department of Anesthesiology
Mayo Clinic
Rochester, Minnesota

Robert J. Hudson, MD, FRCPC
Professor of Anesthesia
University of Manitoba Faculty of Medicine
St. Boniface General Hospital
Winnipeg, Manitoba

Anthony D. Ivankovich, MD
Professor and Chair
Department of Anesthesiology
Rush Medical College
Rush-Presbyterian-St. Luke's Medical Center
Chicago, Illinois

Joel O. Johnson, MD
Department of Anesthesiology and Perioperative Medicine
University of Missouri, Columbia
Columbia, Missouri

Ira S. Kass, PhD
Professor of Anesthesiology and Physiology and
   Pharmacology
Department of Anesthesiology
SUNY Health Science Center at Brooklyn
Brooklyn, New York

Jonathan D. Katz, MD
Associate Clinical Professor
Department of Anesthesiology
Yale University School of Medicine
Attending Anesthesiologist
St. Vincent's Medical Center
Bridgeport, Connecticut

Donald A. Kroll, MD, PhD
Professor
Department of Anesthesiology
UT Memphis College of Medicine
Chief of Anesthesiology
Memphis Veterans Affairs Medical Center
Memphis, Tennessee

Carol L. Lake, MD
Professor and Chair
Department of Anesthesiology
Associate Dean for Continuing Medical Education
University of Louisville
Louisville, Kentucky

Charles E. Laurito, MD
Medical Director, Center for Pain Management
   and Rehabilitation Medicine
University of Illinois at Chicago
Chicago, Illinois

Noel W. Lawson, MD
Professor and Chair
Department of Anesthesiology and Perioperative Medicine
University of Missouri School of Medicine, Columbia
Columbia, Missouri

Serle K. Levin, MD
Assistant Professor
Department of Anesthesiology
Cornell University–New York Hospital
New York, New York

Jerrold H. Levy, MD
Professor
Department of Anesthesiology
Emory University School of Medicine
Atlanta, Georgia

J. Lance Lichtor, MD
Professor
Department of Anesthesia and Critical Care
University of Chicago Pritzker School of Medicine
Chicago, Illinois

Spencer S. Liu, MD
Staff Anesthesiologist
Virginia Mason Medical Center
Seattle, Washington

Timothy R. Lubenow, MD
Associate Professor
Department of Anesthesiology
Rush Medical College
Rush-Presbyterian-St. Luke's Hospital
    Medical Center
Chicago, Illinois

Srinivas Mantha, MD
Associate Professor
Department of Anesthesiology in Intensive Care
Nizam's Institute of Medical Sciences
Hyderabad, India

Kenneth Martay, MD
Acting Assistant Professor
Department of Anesthesiology
University of Washington School of Medicine
Seattle, Washington

John T. Martin, MD
Professor Emeritus
Department of Anesthesiology
Medical College of Ohio at Toledo
Toledo, Ohio

Mali Mathru, MD
Professor
Department of Anesthesiology
The University of Texas Medical Branch
Galveston, Texas

Robert J. McCarthy, Pharm D
Associate Professor
Department of Anesthesiology
Rush Medical College
Rush-Presbyterian-St. Luke's Medical Center
Chicago, Illinois

Kathryn E. McGoldrick, MD
Professor
Department of Anesthesiology
Yale University School of Medicine
New Haven, Connecticut

Roger S. Mecca, MD
Executive Director, Surgical Services
Danbury Hospital
Danbury, Connecticut

Sanford M. Miller, MD
Assistant Professor of Clinical Anesthesiology
New York University School of Medicine
New York, New York

Terri G. Monk, MD
Professor
Department of Anesthesiology
University of Florida College of Medicine
Gainesville, Florida

John R. Moyers, MD
Professor
Department of Anesthesia
University of Iowa College of Medicine
Iowa City, Iowa

Michael F. Mulroy, MD
Staff Anesthesiologist
Virginia Mason Medical Center
Seattle, Washington

Stanley Muravchick, MD, PhD
Professor
Department of Anesthesia
University of Pennsylvania School of Medicine
Philadelphia, Pennsylvania

Glenn S. Murphy, MD
Associate Professor
Department of Anesthesiology
Northwestern University Medical School
Evanston Hospital
Evanston, Illinois

Phillip S. Mushlin, MD, PhD
Associate Professor
Department of Anesthesiology, Perioperative and Pain
    Medicine
Harvard Medical School
Brigham and Women's Hospital
Boston, Massachusetts

George Mychaskiw II, DO
Associate Professor of Anesthesiology, Surgery, and
    Physiology
Director, Cardiac Anesthesiology
University of Mississippi School of Medicine and Medical
    Center
Jackson, Mississippi

Steven M. Neustein, MD
Assistant Professor of Anesthesiology
Mount Sinai School of Medicine of New York University
New York, New York

David A. O'Gorman, MD, FFARCSI
Fellow in Obstetric Anesthesiology
St. Luke's-Roosevelt Hospital Center
Columbia University College of Physicians and Surgeons
New York, New York

Charles W. Otto, MD
Professor
Department of Anesthesiology
University of Arizona College of Medicine
Tucson, Arizona

Nathan Leon Pace, MD
Professor
Department of Anesthesiology
University of Utah School of Medicine
Salt Lake City, Utah

Charise T. Petrovitch, MD
Chair
Department of Anesthesia
Providence Hospital
Washington, DC

Karen L. Posner, PhD
Research Associate Professor
Department of Anesthesiology
University of Washington School of Medicine
Seattle, Washington

Donald S. Prough, MD
Professor and Chair
Department of Anesthesiology
The University of Texas Medical Branch
Galveston, Texas

Linda Jo Rice, MD
Director, Pediatric Pain Service
All Children's Hospital
St. Petersburg, Florida

Michael F. Roizen, MD
Professor and Chair
Department of Anesthesia and Critical Care
University of Chicago Pritzker School of Medicine
Chicago, Illinois

Stanley H. Rosenbaum, MD
Department of Anesthesiology
Yale University School of Medicine
New Haven, Connecticut

Henry Rosenberg, MD
Professor
Department of Anesthesiology
Jefferson Medical College
Thomas Jefferson University
Philadelphia, Pennsylvania

William H. Rosenblatt, MD
Department of Anesthesiology
Yale University School of Medicine
New Haven, Connecticut

Carl Rosow, MD, PhD
Associate Professor
Department of Anesthesia and Critical Care
Harvard Medical School
Massachusetts General Hospital
Boston, Massachusetts

Peter T. Rothstein, MD
Professor of Clinical Anesthesiology and Clinical
    Pediatrics
Columbia University College of Physicians and Surgeons
New York, New York

Alan C. Santos, MD
Associate Director of Anesthesiology
St. Luke's-Roosevelt Hospital Center
Columbia University College of Physicians and Surgeons
New York, New York

Christian R. Schlicht, DO
Assistant Professor
Department of Anesthesiology
University of New Mexico School of Medicine
Albuquerque, New Mexico

Phillip G. Schmid III, MD
Associate
Department of Anesthesia
University of Iowa College of Medicine
Iowa City, Iowa

Jeffrey J. Schwartz, MD
Associate Clinical Professor
Department of Anesthesiology
Yale University School of Medicine
New Haven, Connecticut

M. Christine Stock, MD
Associate Professor
Department of Anesthesiology
Emory University School of Medicine
Atlanta, Georgia

Colleen A. Sullivan, MD
Clinical Professor
Department of Anesthesiology
SUNY Health Science Center at Brooklyn
Brooklyn, New York

Stephen J. Thomas, MD
Professor and Vice Chair
Department of Anesthesiology
Cornell University–New York Hospital
New York, New York

Judith A. Toski, BA
Resident
Department of Emergency Medicine
SUNY Buffalo School of Medicine
Buffalo, New York

Kenneth J. Tuman, MD
Professor and Vice Chair
Department of Anesthesiology
Rush Medical College
Rush-Presbyterian-St. Luke's Medical Center
Chicago, Illinois

Gary Tzeng, MD
Attending Staff Anesthesiologist
Lincoln Park Anesthesia and Pain Management
Chicago, Illinois

Jeffrey S. Vender, MD
Professor and Associate Chair
Department of Anesthesiology
Northwestern University Medical School
Evanston Hospital
Evanston, Illinois

Carla M. Vincent, MD
Associate
Department of Anesthesia
University of Iowa College of Medicine
Iowa City, Iowa

Mark A. Warner, MD
Professor
Department of Anesthesiology
Mayo Clinic
Rochester, Minnesota

Denise J. Wedel, MD
Professor
Department of Anesthesiology
Mayo Clinic
Rochester, Minnesota

B. Craig Weldon, MD
Assistant Professor of Anesthesiology and Pediatrics
Department of Anesthesiology
University of Florida College of Medicine
Gainesville, Florida

Paul F. White, PhD, MD
Professor
Department of Anesthesiology and Pain Management
University of Texas Southwestern Medical Center
Dallas, Texas

James R. Zaidan, MD, MBA
Professor
Department of Anesthesiology
Emory University School of Medicine
Atlanta, Georgia

PREFACE

The twelve years since the publication of the first edition of *Clinical Anesthesia* have witnessed some of the most significant advances our specialty has ever seen. In 1989, the term "managed care" was a new phrase in the health-care lexicon. In contrast, both the medical *and* economic considerations now play an important role in the care of all patients. The mortality rate from all anesthetic causes has plummeted, and operating rooms are now considered among the safest sites in the hospital. Anesthesiologists are pioneers in maintaining a safe environment for our patients, and the techniques we have used are now being emulated and adopted by initiatives from the federal government and other medical specialties. In addition, anesthesiologists are now "perioperative physicians" supervising care in a variety of locations from preoperative evaluation clinics, to intensive care units and pain clinics, and to operating room sites as varied as the cardiac OR and a physician's office. Finally, both critical care and pain are now recognized subspecialties of anesthesiology, pediatric anesthesia is now recognized for fellowship status, and certification can be achieved for transesophageal echocardiography.

It is with this background of vast change that we have undertaken the editorial process for the fourth edition of *Clinical Anesthesia.* New paradigms for OR management and cost containment are highlighted. Our safety and that of our patients is extensively reviewed with particular emphasis on latex allergy. Recent developments are enhancing our understanding of the mechanism of action of anesthetics, and this research has important implications for the creation of new anesthetic agents. The preanesthetic clinic is becoming a major focus of activity, since it serves as an important gateway to the OR. Efficient, medically appropriate, and cost-effective care is covered extensively. With the rapid proliferation of new drugs, publicity about medical errors related to drug administration, and public concern about herbal preparations, the addition of an entirely new chapter on drug interactions and anesthesia is timely. Newer monitoring techniques, including transesophageal echocardiography and transcranial Doppler, are discussed in several chapters including those on neuroanesthesia, cardiac anesthesia, and monitoring. Minimally invasive surgery presents challenges to the anesthesiologist and enhances our ability to contribute significantly to the care of the patient. Here again, in addition to a chapter specifically focused on minimally invasive surgical procedures, a number of contributors have emphasized the critical issues for patient management in their individual chapters. With an increasing number of patients in the geriatric age group, even relatively noncomplex surgical procedures pose a significant anesthetic challenge. The geriatrics chapter has been considerably revised to reflect this concern. As trauma continues to be a leading cause of mortality and morbidity in the United States, the updated chapter on anesthesia for trauma provides an excellent review of the many new methods for treatment of trauma patients. The extensive use of conscious sedation protocols not only in the OR but throughout the hospital has placed the anesthesiologist in a leadership role for our peers. The relevant chapter serves to prepare us to enter these discussions with a broad base of information. Recently, no area in anesthesiology has garnered more attention and controversy than office-based anesthesia. The complexities of administering an anesthetic in this environment are reviewed by national leaders in this field. In addition to these subjects, each of the other chapters has been extensively revised for the current edition, with emphasis on up-to-date information and relevance to contemporary anesthetic clinical care.

The hallmark of *Clinical Anesthesia* is the presentation of concepts in a crisp and clinically useful manner. Clinical options are prioritized by the contributors, each of whom is a recognized expert within the scope of his/her chapter. As editors, we have eliminated duplication among chapters and have presented an integrated approach to the specialty of anesthesiology. On occasion, however, redundancy and even disagreement in approaches to patient management have been kept because they also reflect the realities of the practice of anesthesiology.

We hope that you, the reader, will benefit from this new edition, and we trust that it will improve your understanding of the field and your clinical care of patients. We welcome your comments and suggestions as to how we may continue to make *Clinical Anesthesia*—and its companion handbook, review book, and CD-ROM—as useful as possible to clinicians, residents, and students.

Finally, we wish to express our gratitude to the individual contributors whose hard work and dedication expedited the development and production of this edition. We also acknowledge the support of our administrative assistants, Gail Norup, Karen Rutherford, and Deanna Walker, each of whom gave unselfishly of her time to facilitate the editorial process. Thanks to our colleagues at Lippincott Williams & Wilkins who continually demonstrate their commitment to excellence in medical publishing: Craig Percy, Executive Editor; Tanya Lazar, Developmental Editor; Andrea Allison-Williams, Administrative Assistant; and Mary McDonald and Peggy Gordon at P.M. Gordon Associates for making the final stages of production a joy.

Paul G. Barash, M.D.
Bruce F. Cullen, M.D.
Robert K. Stoelting, M.D.

CONTENTS

CLINICAL
ANESTHESIA

ONE

INTRODUCTION TO ANESTHESIA PRACTICE

Clinical Anesthesia (4/e), edited by
Paul G. Barash, Bruce F. Cullen, and
Robert K. Stoelting. Lippincott Williams &
Wilkins, Philadelphia, © 2001.

CHAPTER 1

THE HISTORY OF ANESTHESIOLOGY

JUDITH A. TOSKI, DOUGLAS R. BACON, AND
ROD K. CALVERLEY*

The sixteenth of October 1846 marked the start of a silent revolution in medicine. William T. G. Morton provided anesthesia to a patient named Edward Gilbert Abbott, administering diethyl ether prior to the surgical removal of a vascular lesion from the side of Mr. Abbott's neck. The pain that this patient would otherwise have suffered was thus laid mute. October 16, 1846, has obvious importance to historians of medicine, but it is also pertinent to anesthesia providers. It is the inauguration of a specialty that is driven to relieve pain. In the operating room, battlefield, delivery suite, and pain clinic, countless patients have benefited from the attentions of the anesthesia care team whose members trace their origins to this momentous event. A firm understanding of the historical aspects of the development of anesthetic technique and technology—and an appreciation for the diverse personalities involved in the evolution of anesthesiology as a specialty—reveals that the practice of relieving pain is more than a technical skill. It is an art.

THE EARLY HISTORY OF ANESTHESIOLOGY

"Prehistory"

Pain control during surgery was not always as centrally important as it is today. The Roman writer Celsius encouraged "pitilessness" as an essential characteristic of the surgeon, an attitude that prevailed for centuries. Although some surgeons confessed that they found elements of their work intensely disturbing, most became inured to their patients' agony. Medical students emulated their teachers, usually omitting any appraisal of the patient's distress while taking notes of the operations that they witnessed. Even the authors of leading surgical texts often ignored surgical pain as a topic of discussion. Just before the advent of anesthesia, Robert Liston's 1842 edition of *Elements of Surgery* contained detailed descriptions of elective and emergency procedures on the extremities, head and neck, breast, and genitals, but neglected a significant discussion of any form of analgesia. In Liston's time, as in the countless ages before, pain was considered primarily a symptom of importance.[1]

Prior to the introduction of anesthesia with diethyl ether, many surgeons like Liston held that pain was, and would always be, an inevitable consequence of surgery. Despite this sentiment, many different agents were used to achieve anesthesia. Dioscorides, a physician from the first century A.D., commented upon mandragora, a drug prepared from the bark and leaves of the mandrake plant. He stated that the plant substance could be boiled in wine and strained, and used "in the case of persons . . . about to be cut or cauterized, when they wish to produce anesthesia."[2] Mandragora was still being used to anesthetize patients as late as the 17th century.

From the 9th to the 13th centuries, the soporific sponge was a dominant mode of providing pain relief during surgery. Mandrake leaves, along with black nightshade, poppies, and other herbs, were boiled together and cooked onto a sponge. The sponge was then reconstituted in hot water, and placed under the patient's nose prior to surgery. Prepared as indicated by published reports of the time, the sponge generally contained morphine and scopolamine in varying amounts—drugs used in modern anesthesia.[3] In addition to using the "sleeping sponge," Europeans attempted to relieve pain by hypnosis, by the ingestion of alcohol, herbs, and extracts of botanical preparations, and by the topical application of pressure or ice.

In the 11th century, the anesthetic effects of cold water and ice were being discovered. In the middle of the 17th century, Marco Aurelio Severino described "refrigeration anesthesia"; placing snow in parallel lines across the incisional plane, he was able to render a surgical site insensate within minutes. The technique never became popular, probably because of the challenge of maintaining stores of snow year-round.[4]

Diethyl ether had been known for centuries prior to its first public use in surgical anesthesia. It may have been compounded first by an 8th-century Arabian philosopher Jabir ibn Hayyam, or possibly by Raymond Lully, a 13th-century European alchemist. But diethyl ether was certainly known in the 16th century, both to Valerius Cordus and Paracelsus, who prepared it by distilling sulfuric acid (oil of vitriol) with fortified wine to produce an *oleum vitrioli dulce* (sweet oil of vitriol). Paracelsus (1493–1541) observed that it caused chickens to fall asleep and awaken unharmed. He must have been aware of its analgesic qualities, because he reported that it could be recommended for use in painful illnesses. There is, however, no record that his suggestion was followed.

For three centuries thereafter, this simple compound remained a therapeutic agent with only occasional use. Some of its properties were examined by distinguished British scientists, including Robert Boyle, Isaac Newton, and Michael Faraday, but without sustained interest. Its only routine application came as an inexpensive recreational drug among the poor of Britain and Ireland, who sometimes drank an ounce or two of ether when taxes made gin prohibitively expensive. An American variation of this practice was conducted by groups of students who held ether-soaked towels to their faces at nocturnal "ether frolics."

Like ether, nitrous oxide was known for its ability to induce lightheadedness and was often inhaled by those seeking a thrill. It was not used as frequently as was ether because it was more complex to prepare and awkward to store. It was produced by heating ammonium nitrate in the presence of iron filings. The evolved gas was passed through water to eliminate toxic oxides of nitrogen before being stored. Nitrous oxide was first prepared in 1773 by Joseph Priestley, an English clergyman and scientist, who ranks among the great pioneers of chemistry. During his years of study, Priestley prepared and examined several gases, including nitrous oxide, ammonia, sulfur dioxide, oxygen, carbon monoxide, and carbon dioxide.

At the end of the 18th century in England, there was a strong interest in the supposed salubrious effects of mineral waters and healthful gases. This led to the development of spas, which were sought out by people of society. Particular waters and gases were believed to prevent and treat disease. A dedicated interest in the potential use of gases as remedies for scurvy, tuberculosis, and other diseases led Thomas Beddoes to open his Pneumatic Institute close to the small spa of Hotwells, in the city of Bristol, where he hired Humphry Davy in 1798 to conduct research projects.

---

* Deceased.

Humphry Davy (1778–1829) was a young man of ability and drive. He performed a brilliant series of investigations of several gases but focused much of his attention on nitrous oxide, which he and his associates inhaled through face masks designed for the Institute by James Watt, the distinguished inventor of the steam engine. Davy used this equipment to measure the rate of uptake of nitrous oxide and its effect on respiration and other central nervous system actions. These results were combined with research on the physical properties of the gas in *Nitrous Oxide*, a 580-page book published in 1800. This impressive treatise is now best remembered for a few incidental observations: Davy's comments that nitrous oxide transiently relieved a severe headache, obliterated a minor headache, and briefly quenched an aggravating toothache. The most frequently quoted passage was a casual entry: "As nitrous oxide in its extensive operation appears capable of destroying physical pain, it may probably be used with advantage during surgical operations in which no great effusion of blood takes place."[5] Although Davy did not pursue this prophecy, perhaps because he was set on a career in basic research, he did coin the persisting sobriquet for nitrous oxide, "laughing gas."

Another lost opportunity to discover anesthesia occurred two decades before the demonstration of ether in Boston. An English physician searched intentionally in 1823 and 1824 for an inhaled anesthetic to relieve the pain of surgery. Henry Hill Hickman might have succeeded if he had used nitrous oxide or ether, but the mice and dogs he studied inhaled high concentrations of carbon dioxide. Carbon dioxide has some anesthetic properties, as shown by the absence of response to an incision in the animals of Hickman's study, but it is not an appropriate clinical anesthetic. Hickman's concept was magnificent; his choice of agent, regrettable. This seminal work was ignored both by surgeons and by the scientists of the Royal Society.

Almost Discovery: Clarke, Long, and Wells

William E. Clarke may have given the first ether anesthetic in Rochester, New York, in January 1842. From techniques learned as a chemistry student in 1839, Clarke entertained his companions with nitrous oxide and ether. Lyman reported that "Clarke diligently propagated this convivial method among his fellow students. Emboldened by these experiences, in January 1842, having returned to Rochester, he administered ether, from a towel, to a young woman named Hobbie, and one of her teeth was then extracted without pain by a dentist named Elijah Pope."[6] A second indirect reference to Clarke's anesthetic suggested that it was believed that her unconsciousness was due to hysteria. Clarke was advised to conduct no further anesthetic experiments.[7]

There is no doubt that two months later, on March 30, 1842, Crawford Williamson Long (1815–1878) administered ether with a towel for surgical anesthesia in Jefferson, Georgia. His patient, James M. Venable, was a young man who was already familiar with ether's exhilarating effects, for he reported in a certificate that he had previously inhaled it frequently and was fond of its use. Venable had two small tumors on his neck but refused to have them excised because he dreaded the cut of the knife. Knowing that Venable was familiar with ether's action, Dr. Long proposed that ether might alleviate pain and gained his patient's consent to proceed. After inhaling ether from the towel, Venable reported that he was unaware of the removal of the tumor.[8] In determining the first fee for anesthesia and surgery, Long settled on a charge of $2.00.

As a rural physician with a very limited surgical practice, Crawford Long had few opportunities to give ether anesthesia, but he did conduct the first comparative trial of an anesthetic. He wished to prove that insensibility to pain was caused by ether and was not simply a reflection of the individual's pain threshold or the result of self-hypnosis. When ether was withheld during amputation of the second of two toes, his patient reported great pain and strenuously proclaimed a preference for ether.

For Long to gain an unrivaled position as the discoverer of anesthesia, all that remained was for him to present his historic work in the medical literature. Long, however, remained silent until 1849, when ether anesthesia was already well known. He explained that he practiced in an isolated environment and had few opportunities for surgical or dental procedures. From our perspective it is difficult to understand why he was so reluctant to publish. This remarkable man might have changed the course of the history of medicine, but, because of his failure to publish, the public introduction of anesthesia was achieved by more assured and bolder persons.

In contrast to the limited opportunities for surgery presented to rural practitioners in the mid-19th century, urban dentists regularly met patients who refused restorative treatment for fear of the pain inflicted by the procedure. From a dentist's perspective, pain was not so much life-threatening as it was livelihood-threatening. A few dentists searched for new techniques of effective pain relief. Pasteur's yet-to-be-delivered aphorism, that chance only favors the prepared mind, would have provided an apt description of one of these men, Horace Wells (1815–1848), of Hartford, Connecticut. Wells recognized what others had ignored, the analgesic potential of nitrous oxide.

Horace Wells' great moment of discovery came on December 10, 1844, when he attended a lecture-exhibition by an itinerant "scientist," Gardner Quincy Colton, who prepared nitrous oxide and encouraged members of the audience to inhale the gas. Wells observed that a young man, Samuel Cooley (later, Colonel Cooley of the Connecticut militia), was unaware that he had injured his leg while under the influence of nitrous oxide. Sensing that nitrous oxide might also relieve the pain of dental procedures, Wells contacted Colton and boldly proposed an experiment in which Wells was to be the subject. The following day, Colton gave Wells nitrous oxide before a fellow dentist, William Riggs, extracted a tooth.[9] When Wells awoke, he declared that he had not felt any pain and termed the experiment a success. Colton taught Wells to prepare nitrous oxide, which the dentist administered with success in his practice. His apparatus probably resembled that used by Colton. The patient placed a wooden tube in his mouth through which he rebreathed nitrous oxide from a small bag filled with the gas.

A few weeks later, in January 1845, Wells attempted a public demonstration in Boston at the Harvard Medical School. He had planned to anesthetize a patient for an amputation, but, when the patient refused surgery, a dental anesthetic for a medical student was substituted. Wells, perhaps influenced by a large and openly critical audience, began the extraction without an adequate level of anesthesia, and the trial was judged a failure.

The exact circumstances of Wells' lack of success are not known. His less than enthusiastic patient may have refused to breathe the anesthetic. Alternatively, Wells might have lost part of his small supply of nitrous oxide, which might have happened if the patient involuntarily removed his lips from the mouthpiece or if his nostrils were not held shut. It might have been that Wells did not know that nitrous oxide lacks sufficient potency to serve predictably as an anesthetic without supplementation. In any event, the student cried out, and Wells was jeered by his audience. No one offered Wells even conditional encouragement or recognized that, even though Wells' presentation had been flawed, nitrous oxide might become a valuable therapeutic advance.

The disappointment disturbed Wells deeply, and, although he continued to use nitrous oxide in his dental practice for some time, his life became unsettled. While profoundly distressed, Wells committed suicide in 1848. Wells was an important pioneer of anesthesia, for he was the first person to recognize the anesthetic qualities of nitrous oxide, the only 19th-century drug still in routine use.

W. T. G. Morton and October 16, 1846

A second New Englander, William Thomas Green Morton (1819–1868), briefly shared a dental practice with Horace Wells in Hartford. Wells' daybook shows that he gave Morton a course of instruction in anesthesia, but Morton apparently moved to Boston without paying for his lessons. In Boston, Morton continued his interest in anesthesia and, after learning from Charles Jackson that ether dropped on the skin provided analgesia, began experiments with inhaled ether. The diethyl ether that Morton used would prove to be much more versatile than nitrous oxide.

Before the invention of the hollow needle and an awareness of aseptic technique, the only class of potential anesthetics that could offer a prompt, profound, and temporary action were the inhaled drugs. Of the available drugs, ether was a superb first choice. Bottles of liquid ether were easily transported, and the volatility of the drug permitted effective inhalation. The concentrations required for surgical anesthesia were so low that patients did not become hypoxic when breathing air. It also possessed what would later be recognized as a unique property among all inhaled anesthetics: the quality of providing surgical anesthesia without causing respiratory or cardiovascular depression. These properties, combined with a slow rate of induction, gave the patient a great margin of safety when physicians were attempting to master the new art of administering an inhaled anesthetic.[10]

After anesthetizing a pet dog, Morton became confident of his skills and anesthetized patients in his dental office. Encouraged by that success, Morton gained an invitation to give a public demonstration in the Bullfinch amphitheater of the Massachusetts General Hospital. William Morton's demonstration of ether caught the world's attention in part because it took place in a public arena, the surgical amphitheater of a public institution, the Massachusetts General Hospital. Surgical amphitheaters, and the charitable hospitals of which they were a part, were then a relatively recent addition to American medical teaching.

On Friday, October 16, 1846, William T. Morton secured permission to provide an anesthetic to Edward Gilbert Abbott before the surgeon, John Collins Warren, excised a vascular lesion from the left side of Abbott's neck. Morton was late in arriving, so Warren was at the point of proceeding when Morton entered. The dentist had been obliged to wait for an instrument-maker to complete his inhaler (Fig. 1-1). It consisted of a large glass bulb containing a sponge soaked with colored ether and a spout, which was to be placed in the patient's mouth. An opening on the opposite side of the bulb allowed air to enter and to be drawn over the ether-soaked sponge with each breath.

The conversations of that morning were not accurately recorded; however, popular accounts state that the surgeon responded testily to Morton's apology for his tardy arrival by remarking, "Sir, your patient is ready." Morton directed his attention to his patient and first conducted a very abbreviated preoperative evaluation. He inquired, "Are you afraid?" Abbott responded that he was not and took the inhaler in his mouth. After a few minutes, Morton is said to have turned to the surgeon to respond, "Sir, your patient is ready." Gilbert Abbott later reported that he was aware of the surgery but had experienced no pain. At the moment that the procedure ended, Warren turned to his audience and announced, "Gentlemen, this is no humbug."[11] Oliver Wendell Holmes soon suggested the term *anaesthesia* to describe this state of temporary insensibility.

What would be recognized as America's greatest contribution to 19th-century medicine had been realized, but the immediate prospect was clouded by subterfuge and argument. Some weeks passed before Morton admitted that the active component of the colored fluid, which he had called "Letheon," was the familiar drug, diethyl ether. Morton, Wells, Jackson, and their supporters soon became caught up in a contentious, protracted, and fruitless debate over priority for the discovery, popularly termed "the ether controversy." In short, Morton had applied for a patent for Letheon, and when it was granted, tried to receive royalties for the use of ether as an anesthetic. Eventually, the matter came before the U.S. Congress where the House of Representatives voted to grant Morton a large sum of money for the discovery; however, the Senate quashed the deal.

When the details of Morton's anesthetic technique became public knowledge, the information was transmitted by train, stagecoach, and coastal vessels to other North American cities, and by ship to the world. Anesthetics were performed in Britain, France, Russia, South Africa, Australia, and other countries almost as soon as surgeons heard the welcome news of the extraordinary discovery. Even though surgery could now be performed with "pain put to sleep," the frequency of operations did not rise rapidly. Several years would pass before anesthesia was even universally recommended.

A "Blessing" to Obstetrics

James Young Simpson, a successful obstetrician of Edinburgh, Scotland, had been among the first to use ether for the relief of the pain of labor. He became dissatisfied with ether and sought a more pleasant, rapid-acting anesthetic. He and his junior associates conducted a bold search for a new inhaled anesthetic by inhaling samples of several volatile chemicals collected for Simpson by British apothecaries. David Waldie suggested chloroform, which had first been prepared in 1831.

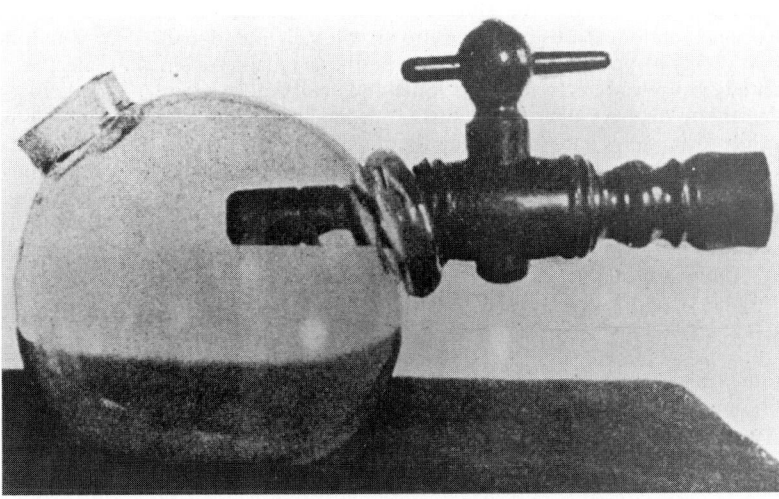

Figure 1-1. Morton's ether inhaler (1846).

Simpson and his friends inhaled it at a dinner party in Simpson's home on the evening of November 4, 1847. They promptly fell unconscious. They awoke delighted at their success. Simpson quickly set about encouraging the use of chloroform. Within 2 weeks, he had dispatched his first account of its use to *The Lancet.* Although Simpson introduced chloroform with celerity, boldness, and enthusiasm and was later to become a vocal defender of the use of anesthesia for women in labor, he gave few anesthetics himself. His goal was simply to improve a patient's comfort during his operative or obstetric activities.

The relief of obstetrical pain had significant social ramifications, particularly in the 19th century, and made anesthesia during delivery a controversial subject. Simpson himself argued against the prevailing view that relieving the pain of childbirth was contrary to God's will. The pain of the parturient was perceived as both a component of punishment, and a means of atonement for Original Sin. Less than a year after administering the first anesthesia during childbirth, Simpson addressed these concerns in a pamphlet entitled "Answers to the Religious Objections Advanced Against the Employment of Anaesthetic Agents in Midwifery and Surgery and Obstetrics." In this work, Simpson recognized the Book of Genesis as being the root of this sentiment, and noted that God promised to relieve the descendants of Adam and Eve of the curse. Additionally, Simpson asserted that labor pain is a result of scientific and anatomic causes, and not the result of religious condemnation. He stated that the upright position humans assumed necessitated strong pelvic muscles to support the abdominal contents. As a result, he argued, the uterus necessarily developed strong musculature—with such great contractile power that it caused pain—to overcome the resistance of the pelvic floor.[12]

The response to Simpson's assertions was variable. While he was criticized for these ideas by fellow physician Samuel Ashwell in an editorial published in *The Lancet,* many other physicians commented favorably, including some who had opposed obstetric anesthesia for medical reasons. All in all, Simpson's pamphlet probably did not have much impact in terms of changing the prevailing viewpoints about pain control during labor, but he did articulate many concepts that his contemporaries were debating at the time.[13] But it was John Snow (1813–1858), an English contemporary of the Scottish Simpson, who achieved fame as an obstetric anesthetist by treating Queen Victoria.

Queen Victoria's consort, Prince Albert, interviewed John Snow before he was called to Buckingham Palace, at the request of the Queen's obstetrician, to give chloroform for the Queen's last two deliveries. During the monarch's labor, Snow gave analgesic doses of chloroform on a folded handkerchief, a technique that was soon termed *chloroform à la reine.* Victoria abhorred the pain of labor and enjoyed the relief that chloroform provided. She wrote in her journal, "Dr. Snow gave that blessed chloroform and the effect was soothing, quieting, and delightful beyond measure."[14] After the Queen, as head of the Church of England, endorsed obstetric anesthesia, the religious debate over the appropriateness of the use of anesthesia in labor terminated abruptly. Four years later, Snow was to give a second anesthetic to the Queen, who was again determined to have chloroform. Snow's daybook states that by the time he arrived, Prince Albert had begun the anesthetic and had given his wife "a little chloroform." This may be the only time in history that a Queen had a Prince as her anesthetist. Both monarch and consort were fortunate that there was no complication of their anesthetic adventure.

John Snow: The First Anesthesiologist

John Snow (Fig. 1-2) was already a respected physician who had presented papers on physiologic subjects when the news of ether anesthesia reached England in December 1846. He took an interest in anesthetic practice and was soon invited to work with many of the leading surgeons of the day. He was not only

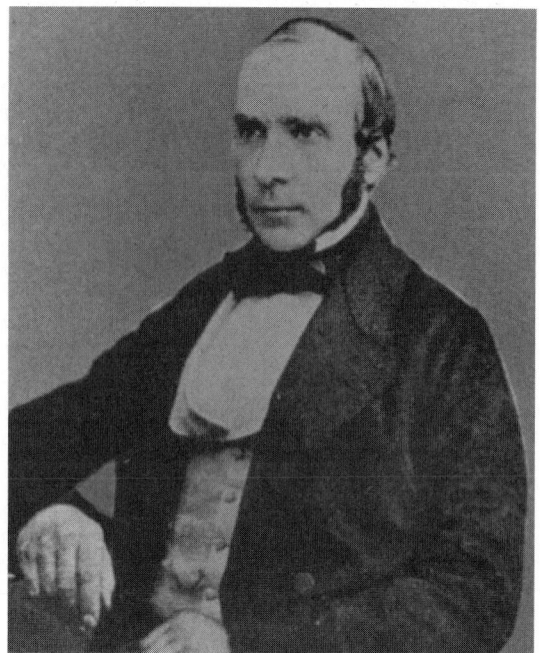

Figure 1-2. John Snow, the first anesthesiologist.

facile at providing anesthesia but was also a remarkably keen observer. His innovative description of the stages or degrees of ether anesthesia based on the patient's responsiveness was not improved upon for 70 years.

In addition to developing a stronger understanding of aspects of anesthetic physiology, Snow also promoted the development of the anesthesia apparatus. He soon realized the inadequacies of ether inhalers into which the patient rebreathed through a mouthpiece. After practicing anesthesia for only 2 weeks, Snow designed the first of his series of ingenious ether inhalers.[15] His best-known apparatus featured unidirectional valves within a malleable, well-fitting mask of his own design, which closely resembles the form of a modern face mask (Fig. 1-3). The face piece was connected to the vaporizer (Fig. 1-4) by a breathing tube, which Snow deliberately designed to be wider than the human trachea so that even rapid respirations would not be impeded. A metal coil within the vaporizer ensured that the patient's inspired breath was drawn over a large surface area to promote the uptake of ether. The device also incorporated a warm water bath to maintain the volatility of the agent. Snow did not attempt to capitalize on his creativity; he closed his account of its preparation with the generous observation, "There is no restriction respecting the making of it."[16]

The following year, John Snow introduced a chloroform inhaler; he had recognized the versatility of the new agent and came to prefer it in his practice. At the same time, he initiated what was to become an extraordinary series of experiments that were remarkable in both their scope and in the manner in which they anticipated sophisticated research performed a century later. Snow realized that successful anesthetics must not only abolish pain but also prevent movement. He anesthetized several species of animals with varying concentrations of ether and chloroform to determine the concentration required to prevent movement in response to a sharp stimulus. Despite the limitations of the technology of 1848, this element of his work anticipated the modern concept of minimum alveolar concentration (MAC).[17] Snow assessed the anesthetic action of a large number of potential anesthetics, and, although he did not find any to rival chloroform or ether, he determined a relationship between solubility, vapor pressure, and anesthetic potency that was not fully appreciated until after World War II when Charles

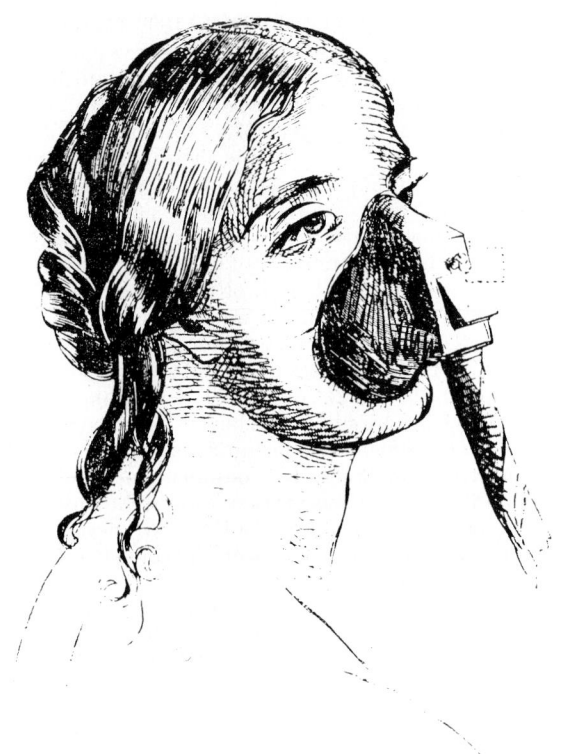

Figure 1-3. John Snow's face mask (1847). The expiratory valve can be tilted to the side to allow the patient to breathe air.

Suckling employed Snow's principles in creating halothane. He also fabricated an experimental closed-circuit device in which the subject (Snow himself) breathed oxygen while the exhaled carbon dioxide was absorbed by potassium hydroxide. Snow published two remarkable books, *On the Inhalation of the Vapour of Ether* (1847) and *On Chloroform and Other Anaesthetics* (1858), which was almost completed when he died of a stroke at the age of 45.

Snow's investigations were not confined to anesthesia. His memory is also respected by specialists in infectious and tropical diseases for his proof, through an epidemiologic study in 1854, that cholera was transmitted by water. At that time, before the development of microbiology by Louis Pasteur and Robert Koch, most physicians in North America and Europe attributed the mysterious recurring epidemics of cholera to the contagion of "fecalized air." For many years, however, Snow had believed

that because the disease affected the gastrointestinal tract, the causative agent must be ingested rather than inhaled. In 1854, he found an opportunity to prove his thesis when cholera visited his section of London and caused the deaths of more than 500 people near his residence. Snow determined that the water supply for these persons had been the Broad Street pump. He prepared what would come to be appreciated as the first epidemiologic survey to prove his contention. With that information, he was able to encourage the parish authorities to remove the pump handle so that residents were obliged to find other sources of water. The prompt end of this already-resolving epidemic was attributed to his action.

Nineteenth-Century British Anesthesia—After John Snow

Throughout the second half of the 19th century, other compounds were examined for their anesthetic potential, but these random searches uniformly ended in failure. The pattern of fortuitous discovery that brought nitrous oxide, diethyl ether, and chloroform forward between 1844 and 1847 continued for decades. The next inhaled anesthetics to be used routinely, ethyl chloride and ethylene, were also discovered as a result of unexpected observations. Ethyl chloride and ethylene were first formulated in the 18th century, and had been examined as anesthetics in Germany soon after the discovery of ether's action; but they were ignored for decades. Ethyl chloride retained some use as a topical anesthetic and counterirritant. It was so volatile that the skin transiently "froze" after ethyl chloride was sprayed upon it. Its rediscovery as an anesthetic came in 1894, when a Swedish dentist sprayed ethyl chloride into a patient's mouth to "freeze" a dental abscess. Carlson was surprised to discover that his patient suddenly lost consciousness. Ethyl chloride became a commonly employed inhaled anesthetic in several countries.

Joseph Clover (1825–1882) became the leading anaesthetist* of London after the death of John Snow in 1858. Clover was a talented clinician and facile inventor, but he never performed research or wrote to the extent achieved by Snow. If he had written a text, he might be better remembered, but most physicians have little knowledge of Clover beyond identifying the

---

* Nineteenth-century "anesthetists" in America became 20th-century "anesthesiologists," but their British and Canadian counterparts (unchallenged by competition from nurses) remained "anaesthetists." The author of this chapter has adhered to this distinction.

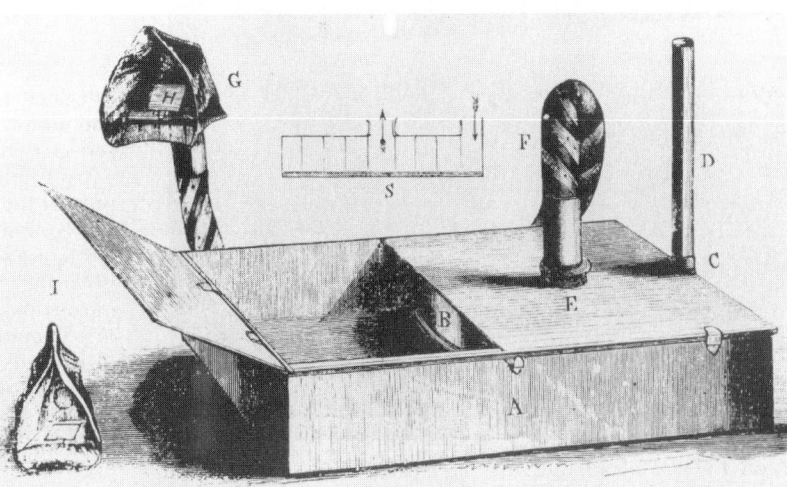

Figure 1-4. John Snow's ether inhaler (1847). The ether chamber (B) contained a spiral coil so that the air entering through the brass tube (D) was saturated by ether before ascending the flexible tube (F) to the face mask (G). The ether chamber rested in a bath of warm water (A).

familiar photograph in which he is seen anesthetizing a seated man while palpating his patient's pulse (Fig. 1-5).

This photograph deserves our attention because it introduces important qualities of the man who maintained the advancement of anesthesia from 1860 until 1880. Clinicians now accept Clover's monitoring of the pulse as a simple routine of prudent practice, but in Clover's time this was a contentious issue. Prominent Scottish surgeons scorned Clover's emphasis on the action of chloroform on the heart. Baron Lister and others preferred that senior medical students give anesthetics and urged them to "strictly carry out certain simple instructions, among which is that of never touching the pulse, in order that their attention may not be distracted from the respiration."[18] Lister also counseled, "it appears that preliminary examination of the chest, often considered indispensable, is quite unnecessary, and more likely to induce the dreaded syncope, by alarming the patients, than to avert it."[19] Little progress in anesthesia could come from such reactionary statements. In contrast, Clover had observed the effect of chloroform on animals and urged other anesthetists to monitor the pulse at all times and to discontinue the anesthetic temporarily if any irregularity or weakness was observed in the strength of the pulse. He earned a loyal following among London surgeons, who accepted him as a dedicated specialist.

Clover was the first anaesthetist to administer chloroform in known concentrations through the Clover bag. This unique device rests over his shoulder in Figure 1-5. He obtained a 4.5% concentration of chloroform in air by pumping a measured volume of air with a bellows through a warmed evaporating vessel containing a known volume of liquid chloroform. The apparatus featured inspiratory and expiratory valves of ivory supported by springs. A flap valve in the face mask permitted

the dilution of the anesthetic with air. In 1868, Clover reported no deaths among 1802 anesthetics using his device, but he later reviewed a later fatality in searching detail. He attributed the death to an unrecognized error in calculating the volume of air diluting the chloroform.[20] After 1870, Clover favored a nitrous oxide–ether sequence. The portable anesthesia machines that he designed were in popular use for decades after his death.

In addition to his work with anesthetic agents, Clover was very facile in managing the airway. He was the first Englishman to urge the now universal practice of thrusting the patient's jaw forward to overcome obstruction of the upper airway by the tongue. Despite the limitation of working before the first tracheal tube was used in anesthesia, Clover published a landmark case report in 1877. His patient had a tumor of the mouth that obstructed the airway completely, despite the jaw thrust maneuver, once the anesthetic was begun. Clover averted disaster by inserting a small curved cannula of his design through the cricothyroid membrane. He continued anesthesia *via* the cannula until the tumor was excised. Clover, the model of the prepared anesthesiologist, remarked, "I have never used the cannula before although it has been my companion at some thousands of anaesthetic cases."[21]

Every element of Clover's records and his published accounts reflect a consistent dedication to patient safety coupled with a prudent ability to anticipate potential difficulties and to prepare an effective response beforehand. In that way, his manner was very much like that of his successor, the first English anaesthetist to be knighted, Sir Frederick Hewitt.

Frederick Hewitt (1857–1916) gained the first of his London hospital anesthesia appointments in 1884. He earned a reputation as a superb and inventive clinician and came to be considered the leading British practitioner of the next 30 years. Hewitt engineered modifications of portable ether and nitrous oxide inhalers and, recognizing that nitrous oxide and air formed a hypoxic mixture, designed the first anesthetic apparatus to deliver oxygen and nitrous oxide in variable proportions. He also was influential in ensuring that anesthesia was taught in all British medical schools. His book, *Anaesthetics and Their Administration,* which first appeared in 1893 and continued through five editions, is considered the first true textbook of anesthesia. In 1908, Hewitt developed an important appliance that would assist all anesthesiologists in managing an obstructed upper airway. He called his oral device an "air-way restorer," thus beginning the practice of inserting an airway to help ventilation during an anesthetic.

Late Nineteenth-Century Anesthesia in America

American clinicians of the second half of the 19th century failed to achieve the lasting recognition gained by their British colleagues. Several factors contributed to this disparity. Snow, Clover, and Hewitt were unique men of genius who had no peers in America. Ether remained the dominant anesthetic in America, where the provision of anesthesia was often a service relegated to medical students, junior house officers, nurses, and nonprofessionals. The subordinate status of anesthesia was reflected in American art. Thomas Eakins' great studies, "The Gross Clinic" of 1876 and "The Agnew Clinic" of 1889, both present the surgeon as the focus of attention, whereas the person administering the anesthetic is seen among the supporting figures.

During this period, however, Americans led the revival of nitrous oxide. Gardner Q. Colton, the "professor" who had first demonstrated the use of nitrous oxide to Horace Wells, developed the Colton Dental Association after he returned from the California gold rush. In several eastern cities he opened offices equipped with nitrous oxide generators and, perhaps profiting from Wells' unhappy experience, larger breathing bags of 30-L capacity. By 1869, his advertisements carried the intriguing slogan "31½ Miles Long." Colton had asked each

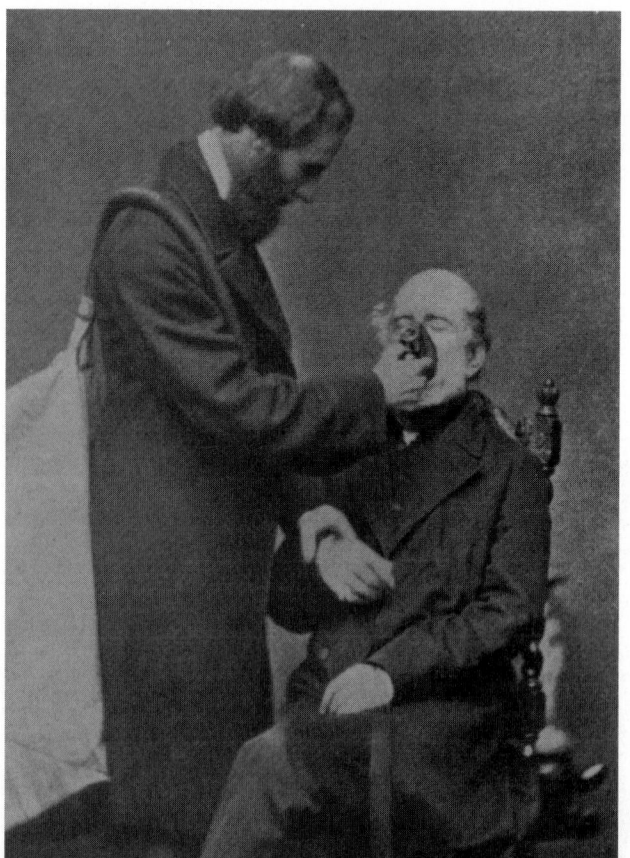

Figure 1-5. Joseph Clover anesthetizing a patient with chloroform and air passing through a flexible tube from a Clover bag.

patient to sign his name to a scroll, which then contained the names of 55,000 patients who had experienced painless extractions of teeth without hazard. He proposed that if this great number of patients were to march past in single file, the line would be extended for 31½ miles.[22]

Colton gave brief exposures of nitrous oxide undiluted with air or oxygen, which raised concern that the gas was acting as an asphyxiant. The following year a Chicago surgeon, Edmund Andrews, experimented with an oxygen–nitrous oxide mixture and proved that nitrous oxide does not cause anesthesia by depriving the brain of oxygen. Although the oxygen–nitrous oxide mixture was safer, he identified a handicap to its use that was unique to that time when patients were attended in their homes. The large bag was conspicuous and awkward to carry whenever Andrews walked along busy streets. He observed that, "In city practice, among the higher classes, however, this is no obstacle as the bag can always be taken in a carriage, without attracting attention."[23] Four years later, Andrews was delighted to report the availability of liquefied nitrous oxide compressed under 750 lb of pressure, which allowed a supply sufficient for three patients to be carried in a single cylinder. Despite Andrews' early enthusiasm, few American surgeons relied on nitrous oxide until it was used in combination with regional anesthesia, the last great contribution to anesthetic practice achieved in the late 19th century.

The Discovery of Regional Anesthesia in the Nineteenth Century

Cocaine, an extract of the coca leaf, was the first effective local anesthetic. Its property of numbing mucous membranes and exposed tissues had been known for centuries in Peru, where folk surgeons performing trephinations of the skull chewed coca leaves and allowed their saliva to fall onto the surfaces of the wound. This was a unique situation in anesthesia; there are no other instances in which both the operator and his patient routinely shared the effects of the same drug. After Albert Niemann refined the active alkaloid and named it *cocaine,* it was used in experiments by a few investigators. It was noted that cocaine provided topical anesthesia and even produced local insensibility when injected, but these observations were not applied in clinical practice before 1884, when the significance of the action of cocaine was realized by Carl Koller, a Viennese surgical intern.

Carl Koller (1857–1944) appreciated what others had failed to recognize because of his past experience and his ambition to practice ophthalmology at a time when many operations on the eye were still being performed without anesthesia. Almost four decades after the discovery of ether, general anesthesia by mask had several limitations for ophthalmic surgery. The anesthetized patient could not cooperate with his surgeon. The anesthesiologist's apparatus interfered with surgical access. At that time, many surgical incisions on the eye were not closed, as fine sutures were not yet available. The high incidence of vomiting following the administration of chloroform or ether threatened the extrusion of the internal contents of the globe, with the risk of irrevocable blindness.

While a medical student, Koller had worked in a Vienna laboratory in a search for a topical ophthalmic anesthetic to overcome the limitations of general anesthesia. Unfortunately, the suspensions of morphine, chloral hydrate, and other drugs that he had used had been ineffectual.

In 1884, Koller's friend, Sigmund Freud, became interested in the cerebral-stimulating effects of cocaine and gave him a small sample in an envelope, which he placed in his pocket. When the envelope leaked, a few grains of cocaine stuck to Koller's finger, which he casually licked with his tongue. It became numb. At that moment, Koller realized that he had found the object of his search. He dashed to the laboratory and made a suspension of cocaine crystals. He and Gustav Gartner, a laboratory associate, observed its anesthetic effect on the eyes of a frog, a rabbit, and a dog before they dropped the solution onto their own corneas. To their amazement, their eyes were insensitive to the touch of a pin.[24]

As an intern, Carl Koller could not afford to attend a Congress of German Ophthalmologists in Heidelberg on September 15, 1884; but, after a friend read his article, a revolution in ophthalmic surgery and other surgical disciplines was initiated. Within the next year, more than 100 articles supporting the use of cocaine appeared in European and American medical journals. Despite this gratifying success, Koller was not able to pursue his goal of gaining a residency position in Vienna. After a duel provoked by an anti-Semitic slur, Koller left Austria and, after studying briefly in Holland and Britain, immigrated in 1888 to New York, where he practiced ophthalmology for the remainder of his career.

American surgeons quickly developed new applications for cocaine. Its efficacy in anesthetizing the nose, mouth, larynx, trachea, rectum, and urethra was described in October 1884. The next month, the first reports of its subcutaneous injection were published. In December 1884, two young surgeons, William Halsted and Richard Hall, described blocks of the sensory nerves of the face and arm. Halsted even performed a brachial plexus block but did so under direct vision while the patient received an inhaled anesthetic. Unfortunately, self-experimentation with cocaine was hazardous, as both surgeons became addicted. Addiction was an ill-understood but frequent problem in the late 19th century, especially when cocaine and morphine were present in many patent medicines.

Other local anesthetic techniques were attempted before the end of the 19th century. The term *spinal anesthesia* was coined in 1885 by Leonard Corning, a neurologist who had observed Hall and Halsted. Corning wanted to assess the action of cocaine as a specific therapy for neurologic problems. After first assessing its action in a dog, producing a blockade of rapid onset that was confined to the animal's rear legs, he administered cocaine to a man "addicted to masturbation." Corning administered one dose without effect, then after a second dose, the patient's legs "felt sleepy." The man had impaired sensibility in his lower extremity after about twenty minutes. He left Corning's office "none the worse for the experience."[25] Although Corning does not refer to the escape of cerebrospinal fluid (CSF) in either case, it is likely that the dog had a spinal anesthetic and that the man had an epidural anesthetic. No therapeutic benefit was described, but Corning closed his account and his attention to the subject by suggesting that cocainization might in time be "a substitute for etherization in genito-urinary or other branches of surgery."[26]

Two other authors, August Bier and Theodor Tuffier, described authentic spinal anesthesia, with mention of cerebrospinal fluid, injection of cocaine, and an appropriately short onset of action. In a comparative review of the original articles by Bier, Tuffier, and Corning, it was concluded that Corning's injection was extradural, and Bier merited the credit for introducing spinal anesthesia.[25]

INTO THE TWENTIETH CENTURY
Spinal Anesthesia

Fourteen years passed before spinal anesthesia was performed for surgery. In the interval, Heinrich Quincke of Kiel, Germany, described his technique of lumbar puncture. He proposed that it was most safely performed at the level of the third or fourth lumbar interspace, because an entry at that level would be below the termination of the spinal cord. Quincke's technique was used in Kiel for the first deliberate cocainization of the spinal cord in 1899 by a surgical colleague, August Bier. Six patients received small doses of cocaine intrathecally, but, because some cried out during surgery while others vomited and experienced headaches, Bier considered it necessary to conduct a clinical experiment.

Professor Bier permitted his assistant, Dr. Hildebrandt, to perform a lumbar puncture, but, after the needle penetrated the dura, Hildebrandt could not fit the syringe to the needle and a large volume of the professor's spinal fluid escaped. They were at the point of abandoning the study when Hildebrandt volunteered to be the subject of a second attempt. They had an astonishing success. Twenty-three minutes later, Bier noted: "A strong blow with an iron hammer against the tibia was not felt as pain. After 25 minutes: Strong pressure and pulling on a testicle were not painful."[27] They celebrated their success with wine and cigars. That night, both developed violent headaches, which they attributed at first to their celebration. Bier's headache was relieved after 9 days of bedrest. The house officer did not have the luxury of continued rest. Bier postulated that their headaches were due to the loss of large volumes of CSF and urged that this be avoided if possible. The high incidence of complications following lumbar puncture with wide-bore needles and the toxic reactions attributed to cocaine explain his later loss of interest in spinal anesthesia.

Surgeons in several other countries soon practiced spinal anesthesia. Many of their observations are still relevant. The first series from France of 125 cases was published by Theodor Tuffier, who later counseled that the solution should not be injected before CSF was seen. The first American report was by Rudolph Matas of New Orleans, whose first patient developed postanesthetic meningismus, a then-frequent complication that was overcome in part by the use of hermetically sealed sterile solutions recommended by E. W. Lee of Philadelphia and sterile gloves as advocated by Halsted. During 1899, Dudley Tait and Guidlo Caglieri of San Francisco performed experimental studies in animals and therapeutic spinals for orthopedic patients. They encouraged the use of fine needles to lessen the escape of CSF and urged that the skin and deeper tissues be infiltrated beforehand with local anesthesia, as had been urged earlier by William Halsted and the foremost advocate of infiltration anesthesia, Carl Ludwig Schleich of Berlin. An early American specialist in anesthesia, Ormond Goldan, published an anesthesia record appropriate for recording the course of "intraspinal cocainization" in 1900. In the same year, Heinrich Braun learned of a newly described extract of the adrenal gland, epinephrine, which he used to prolong the action of local anesthetics with great success. Braun developed several new nerve blocks, coined the term *conduction anesthesia,* and is remembered by European writers as the "father of conduction anesthesia." Braun was the first person to use procaine, which, along with stovaine, was one of the first synthetic local anesthetics produced to reduce the toxicity of cocaine. Further advances in spinal anesthesia followed the introduction of these and other synthetic local anesthetics.

Before 1907, several anesthesiologists were disappointed to observe that their spinal anesthetics were incomplete. Most believed that the drug spread solely by local diffusion before this phenomenon was investigated by Arthur Barker, a London surgeon.[28] Barker constructed a glass tube shaped to follow the curves of the human spine and used it to demonstrate the limited spread of colored solutions that he had injected through a T-piece in the lumbar region. Barker applied this observation to use solutions of stovaine made hyperbaric by the addition of 5% glucose, which worked in a more predictable fashion. After the injection was complete, Barker placed his patient's head on pillows to contain the anesthetic below the nipple line. Lincoln Sise acknowledged Barker's work in 1935 when he introduced the use of hyperbaric solutions of pontocaine. John Adriani advanced the concept further in 1946 when he used a hyperbaric solution to produce "saddle block," or perineal anesthesia. Adriani's patients remained seated after injection as the drug descended to the sacral nerves.

Tait, Jonnesco, and other early masters of spinal anesthesia

used a cervical approach for thyroidectomy and thoracic procedures, but this radical approach was supplanted in 1928 by the lumbar injection of hypobaric solutions of "light" nupercaine by G. P. Pitkin. Although hypobaric solutions are now usually limited to patients in the jackknife position, their former use for thoracic procedures demanded skill and precise timing. The enthusiasts of hypobaric anesthesia devised formulas to attempt to predict the time in seconds needed for a warmed solution of hypobaric nupercaine to spread in patients of varying size from its site of injection in the lumbar area to the level of the fourth thoracic dermatome.

The recurring problem of inadequate duration of single-injection spinal anesthesia led a Philadelphia surgeon, William Lemmon, to report an apparatus for continuous spinal anesthesia in 1940.[29] Lemmon began with the patient in the lateral position. The spinal tap was performed with a malleable silver needle, which was left in position. As the patient was turned supine, the needle was positioned through a hole in the mattress and table. Additional injections of local anesthetic could be performed as required. Malleable silver needles also found a less cumbersome and more common application in 1942 when Waldo Edwards and Robert Hingson encouraged the use of Lemmon's needles for continuous caudal anesthesia in obstetrics. In 1944 Edward Tuohy of the Mayo Clinic introduced two important modifications of the continuous spinal techniques. He developed the now-familiar Tuohy needle as a means of improving the ease of passage of lacquered silk ureteral catheters through which he injected incremental doses of local anesthetic.[30]

Epidural Anesthesia

In 1949, Martinez Curbelo of Havana, Cuba, used Tuohy's needle and a ureteral catheter to perform the first continuous epidural anesthetic. Silk and gum elastic catheters were difficult to sterilize and sometimes caused dural infections before being superseded by disposable plastics. Yet, deliberate single-injection peridural anesthesia had been practiced occasionally for decades before continuous techniques brought it greater popularity. At the beginning of the 20th century, two French clinicians experimented independently with caudal anesthesia. The neurologist Jean Athanase Sicard applied the technique for a nonsurgical purpose, the relief of back pain. Fernand Cathelin used caudal anesthesia as a less dangerous alternative to spinal anesthesia for hernia repairs. He also demonstrated that the epidural space terminated in the neck by injecting a solution of India ink into the caudal canal of a dog. The lumbar approach was first used solely for multiple paravertebral nerve blocks before the Pagés–Dogliotti single-injection technique became accepted. As they worked separately, the technique carries the names of both men. Captain Fidel Pagés prepared an elegant demonstration of segmental single-injection peridural anesthesia in 1921, but died soon after his paper appeared in a Spanish military journal.[31] Ten years later, Achille M. Dogliotti of Turin, Italy, wrote a classic study that made the epidural technique well known.[32] Whereas Pagés used a tactile approach to identify the epidural space, Dogliotti identified it by the loss-of-resistance technique still being currently taught.

Twentieth-Century Regional Anesthesia

Surgery on the extremities lent itself to other regional anesthesia techniques. At first, they were combined with general anesthesia. In 1902, Harvey Cushing coined the phrase "regional anesthesia" for his technique of blocking either the brachial or sciatic plexus under direct vision during general anesthesia to reduce anesthesia requirements and provide postoperative pain relief.[33] Fifteen years before his publication, a similar approach had been energetically advanced to reduce the stress and shock of surgery by George Crile, another dedicated advocate of regional and infiltration techniques during general anesthesia.

An intravenous regional technique with procaine was reported in 1908 by August Bier, the surgeon who had pioneered spinal anesthesia. Bier injected procaine into a vein of the upper limb between two tourniquets. Even though the technique is termed the *Bier block*, it was not used for many decades until it was reintroduced 55 years later by Mackinnon Holmes, who modified the technique by exsanguination before applying a single proximal cuff. Holmes used lidocaine, the very successful amide local anesthetic synthesized in 1943 by Lofgren and Lundquist of Sweden.

Several investigators achieved upper extremity anesthesia by percutaneous injections of the brachial plexus. In 1911, based on his intimate knowledge of the anatomy of the axillary area, Hirschel promoted a "blind" axillary injection. In the same year, Kulenkampff described a supraclavicular approach in which the operator sought out paresthesias of the plexus while keeping the needle at a point superficial to the first rib and the pleura. The risk of pneumothorax with Kulenkampff's approach led Mulley to attempt blocks more proximally by a lateral paravertebral approach, the precursor of what is now popularly known as the Winnie block.

Heinrich Braun wrote the earliest textbook of local anesthesia, which appeared in its first English translation in 1914. After 1922, Gaston Labat's *Regional Anesthesia* dominated the American market. Labat migrated from France to the Mayo Clinic, where he served briefly before taking a permanent position at the Bellevue Hospital in New York, where he worked with Hippolite Wertheim. They formed the first American Society for Regional Anesthesia. After Labat's death, Emery A. Rovenstine was recruited to Bellevue to continue Labat's work. Rovenstein created the first American clinic for the treatment of chronic pain, where he and his associates refined techniques of lytic and therapeutic injections, and used the American Society of Regional Anesthesia to further knowledge of pain management across the United States.[34]

The development of the multidisciplinary pain clinic was one of many contributions to anesthesiology made by John J. Bonica, a renowned teacher of regional techniques. During his periods of military, civilian, and university service at the University of Washington, John Bonica formulated a series of improvements in the management of patients with chronic pain. His classic text, *The Management of Pain,* now in its third edition, is regarded as a classic of the literature of anesthesia.

THE QUEST FOR SAFETY IN ANESTHESIOLOGY

In many ways, the history of late 19th and 20th century anesthesiology is the quest for safer anesthetic agents and methods. The introduction of sophisticated monitoring is critical to the increase in patient safety during this time period. The advances in technology, including components of the anesthesia machine, which produced more accurate and thus safer anesthetics, have obsessed those in the specialty. In addition, the development and widespread use of better patient monitors, such as the electrocardiograph (ECG), arterial blood gas analyzer, and pulse oximeter, has reduced the morbidity and mortality of surgical procedures—and thus allowed patients with critical illnesses to safely undergo potentially life-saving procedures. Endotracheal intubation largely replaced mask ventilation, thereby permitting the anesthesiologist to attend to other aspects of patient care during general anesthesia. Progress in the realm of intraoperative pain control during the late 19th and 20th centuries therefore enhanced the quality of patient care and promoted the development of surgical techniques.

Critical to increasing patient safety was the development of a machine capable of delivering a calibrated amount of gas and volatile anesthetic. In the late 19th century freestanding anesthesia machines were manufactured in the United States and Europe. Three American dentist-entrepreneurs, Samuel S. White, Charles Teter, and Jay Heidbrink, developed the first series of U.S. instruments to use compressed cylinders of nitrous oxide and oxygen. Before 1900 the S. S. White Company modified Hewitt's apparatus and marketed its continuous-flow machine, which was refined by Teter in 1903. Heidbrink added reducing valves in 1912. In the same year other important developments were initiated by physicians. Water-bubble flow meters, introduced by Frederick Cotton and Walter Boothby of Harvard University, allowed the proportion of gases and their flow rate to be approximated. The Cotton and Boothby apparatus was transformed into a practical portable machine by James Tayloe Gwathmey of New York, who demonstrated it at a 1912 Medical Congress in London. The Gwathmey machine caught the attention of a London anesthetist, Henry E. G. "Cockie" Boyle, who acknowledged his debt to the American when he incorporated Gwathmey's concepts in the first of the series of "Boyle" machines that were marketed by Coxeter and British Oxygen Corporation. During the same period in Lubeck, Germany, Heinrich Draeger and his son, Bernhaard, adapted compressed-gas technology, which they had originally developed for mine rescue apparatus, to manufacture ether and chloroform–oxygen machines.

In the years after World War I, several U.S. manufacturers continued to bring forward widely admired anesthesia machines. Some companies were founded by dentists, including Heidbrink and Teter. Karl Connell and Elmer Gatch were surgeons. Richard von Foregger was an engineer who was exceptionally receptive to clinicians' suggestions for additional features for his machines. Elmer McKesson became one of the country's first specialists in anesthesiology in 1910 and developed a series of gas machines. In an era of inflammable anesthetics, McKesson carried nonflammable nitrous oxide anesthesia to its therapeutic limit by performing inductions with 100% nitrous oxide and thereafter adding small volumes of oxygen. If the resultant cyanosis became too profound, McKesson depressed a valve on his machine that flushed a small volume of oxygen into the circuit. Even though his techniques of primary and secondary saturation with nitrous oxide are no longer used, the oxygen flush valve is part of McKesson's legacy.

Carbon dioxide absorbance is important to the anesthetic machine. Initially, because it allows rebreathing of gas, it minimized loss of flammable gases into the room and the risk of explosion. Nowadays, it permits decreased utilization of anesthetic and reduced cost. The first use of carbon dioxide absorbers in anesthesia came in 1906 from the work of Franz Kuhn, a German surgeon. His use of canisters developed for mine rescues by Draeger was a bold innovation, but his circuit had unfortunate limitations—exceptionally narrow breathing tubes and a large dead space, which might explain its very limited use. Kuhn's device was ignored. A few years later, the first American machine with a carbon dioxide absorber was independently fabricated by Dennis Jackson.

In 1915, Jackson, a pharmacologist, developed an early technique of carbon dioxide absorption that permitted the use of a closed anesthesia circuit. He used solutions of sodium and calcium hydroxide to absorb carbon dioxide. As his laboratory was located in an area of St. Louis, Missouri, heavily laden with coal smoke, Jackson reported that the apparatus allowed him the first breaths of absolutely fresh air he had ever enjoyed in that city. The complexity of Jackson's apparatus limited its use in hospital practice, but his pioneering work in this field encouraged Ralph Waters to introduce a simpler device using soda lime granules 9 years later. Waters positioned a soda lime canister between a face mask and an adjacent breathing bag to which was attached the fresh gas flow. As long as the mask was held against the face, only small volumes of fresh gas flow were required and no valves were needed.[35]

When Waters made his first "to-and-fro" device, he was attempting to develop a specialist practice in anesthesia in Sioux City, Iowa, and had achieved limited financial success. Waters believed that his device had advantages for both the clinician and the patient. Economy of operation was an important advance at a time when private patients and insurance companies were reluctant to pay not only for a specialist's services but even for the drugs and supplies he had purchased. Waters estimated that his new canister would reduce his costs for gases and soda lime to less than $.50 per hour. This portable apparatus could be easily carried to the patient's home and, in residential or hospital settings, prevented the pollution of the operating environment with the malodorous and explosive vapors of ethylene. He even noted that the canister conserved body heat and humidified inspired gases.

An awkward element of Waters' device was the position of the canister close to the patient's face. Brian Sword overcame this limitation in 1930 with a freestanding machine with unidirectional valves to create a circle system and an in-circuit carbon dioxide absorber (Fig. 1-6).[36] James Elam and his co-workers at the Roswell Park Cancer Institute in Buffalo, New York, further refined the carbon dioxide absorber, maximizing the amount of carbon dioxide removed with a minimum of resistance for breathing.[37] Thus, the circle system introduced by Sword in the 1930s remains the most popular North American anesthesia circuit.

Alternative Circuits

A valveless device, the Ayre's T-piece, has found wide application in the management of intubated patients. Phillip Ayre practiced anesthesia in England when the limitations of equipment for pediatric patients produced what he describe as "a protracted

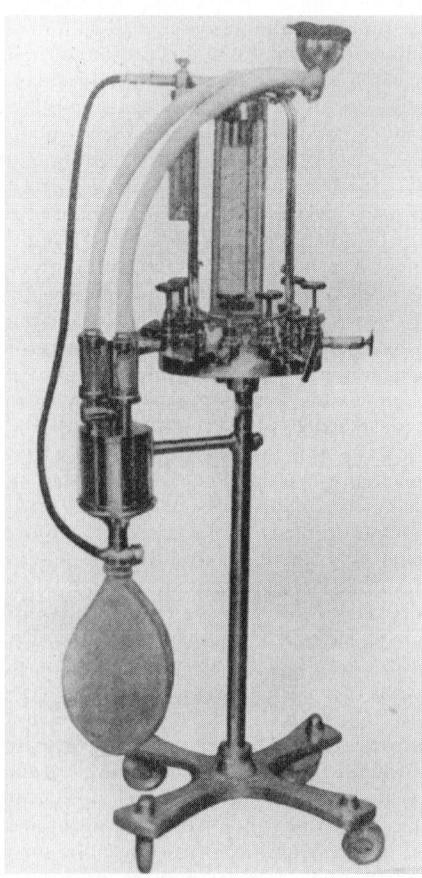

Figure 1-6. Brian Sword's closed-circle anesthesia machine (1930).

and sanguine battle between surgeon and anaesthetist, with the poor unfortunate baby as the battlefield."[38] In 1937, Ayre introduced his valveless T-piece to reduce the effort of breathing in neurosurgical patients. The T-piece soon became particularly popular for cleft palate repairs, as the surgeon had free access to the mouth. Positive pressure ventilation could be achieved when the anesthetist obstructed the expiratory limb. In time, this ingenious, lightweight, nonrebreathing device evolved through more than 100 modifications for a variety of special situations. A significant alteration was Gordon Jackson Rees' circuit, which permitted improved control of ventilation by substituting a breathing bag on the outflow limb.[39]

An alternative method to reduce the amount of equipment near the patient is provided by the coaxial circuit of the Bain–Spoerel apparatus.[40] This lightweight tube-within-a-tube has served very well in many circumstances since its Canadian innovators described it in 1972. However, the Bain–Spoerel circuit was not the first application of coaxial technology in anesthesia. A few 19th-century inhalers, including Hewitt's 1890 chloroform apparatus, used a tube-within-a-tube to lead air into the vaporizer and then back within a smaller tube to the patient.

A more recent precursor of the modern coaxial circuit was created during World War II by Richard Salt and Edgar Pask for tests undertaken by the Royal Air Force of types of life jackets. Many pilots who had survived "ditching" in the frigid North Sea succumbed to hypothermia and drowned after losing consciousness because the life jacket failed to keep the airman's head above water. To simulate an unconscious victim, Dr. Pask was anesthetized with ether *via* a nasal tracheal tube. The unresponsive physician was then lowered into a swimming pool to become the passive subject as a series of life jackets were tested. Even though the tubing of the breathing circuit was many yards long, rebreathing was prevented by the circuit's coaxial design and by the position of the exhalation valve above the surface of the water. This design overcame the risk of pulmonary barotrauma even when the jacket failed and Pask sank to the bottom of the pool. Once the studies were completed, the coaxial circuit passed from use until its utility was recognized by Drs. Bain and Spoerel.

Flow Meters

As closed and semiclosed circuits became practical, gas flow could be measured with greater accuracy. Bubble flow meters were replaced with dry bobbins or ball-bearing flow meters, which, although they did not leak fluids, could cause inaccurate measurements if they adhered to the glass column. In 1910, M. Neu had been the first to apply rotameters in anesthesia for the administration of nitrous oxide and oxygen, but his machine was not a commercial success, perhaps because of the great cost of nitrous oxide in Germany at that time. Rotameters designed for use in German industry were first employed in Britain in 1937 by Richard Salt; but as World War II approached, the English were denied access to these sophisticated flow meters. After World War II rotameters became regularly employed in British anesthesia machines, although most American equipment still featured nonrotating floats. The now universal practice of displaying gas flow in liters per minute was not a uniform part of all American machines until more than a decade after World War II. Some anesthesiologists still in practice learned to calculate gas flows in the cumbersome proportions of gallons per hour.

Vaporizers

Uncalibrated glass vaporizers could be used with confidence for ether but were inadequate for more potent agents. Skilled practitioners gave chloroform with safety, but their success was dependent upon clinical expertise based upon subjective observations that were difficult to teach to neophytes. The art of a smooth induction with a potent anesthetic was a great challenge, particularly if the inspired concentration could not be determined with accuracy. This limitation was particularly true of chloroform, as an excessive rate of administration produced a lethal cardiac depression. Even the clinical introduction of halothane after 1956 might have been similarly thwarted except for a fortunate coincidence: the prior development of calibrated vaporizers. Two types of calibrated vaporizers designed for other anesthetics had become available in the half-decade before halothane was marketed. The prompt acceptance of halothane was in part due to an ability to provide it in carefully titrated concentrations.

The Copper Kettle was the first temperature-compensated, accurate vaporizer. It had been developed by Lucien Morris at the University of Wisconsin in response to Ralph Waters' plan to test chloroform by giving it in controlled concentrations.[41] Morris achieved this goal by passing a metered flow of oxygen through a vaporizer chamber that contained a porex disk to separate the oxygen into minute bubbles. The gas became fully saturated with anesthetic vapor as it percolated through the liquid. The concentration of the anesthetic inspired by the patient could be calculated by knowing the vapor pressure of the liquid anesthetic, the volume of oxygen flowing through the liquid, and the total volume of gases from all sources entering the anesthesia circuit. Although experimental models of Morris' vaporizer used a water bath to maintain stability, the excellent thermal conductivity of copper was substituted in later models. When first marketed, the Copper Kettle did not feature a mechanism to indicate changes in the temperature (and vapor pressure) of the liquid. Shuh-Hsun Ngai proposed the incorporation of a thermometer, a suggestion that was later added to all vaporizers of that class.[42]

Copper Kettle (Foregger Company) and Vernitrol (Ohio Medical Products) vaporizers were universal vaporizers—a property that remained a distinct advantage as new anesthetics were marketed. Universal vaporizers could be charged with any anesthetic liquid, and, provided that its vapor pressure and temperature were known, the inspired concentration could be calculated quickly. This feature gave an unanticipated advantage to American investigators. They were not dependent on the construction of new agent-specific vaporizers.

When halothane was first marketed in Britain, an effective temperature-compensated, agent-specific vaporizer had recently been placed in clinical use. It had been developed for domiciliary obstetric use as many British women were then delivered at home by midwives who required a safe, portable vaporizer with which to provide known concentrations of an inhaled analgesic. The TECOTA (TEmperature COmpensated Trichloroethylene Air) vaporizer had been created by engineers who had been frustrated by a giant corporation's unresponsiveness to their proposals and had formed a new company, Cyprane Limited. The TECOTA featured a bimetallic strip composed of brass and a nickel–steel alloy, two metals with different coefficients of expansion. As the anesthetic vapor cooled, the strip bent to move away from the orifice, thereby permitting more fresh gas to enter the vaporizing chamber. This maintained a constant inspired concentration despite changes in temperature and vapor pressure. After their TECOTA vaporizer was accepted by the Central Midwives Board, their company soon gained a much greater success by adapting their technologic advance to create the "Fluotec," the first of a series of agent-specific "tec" vaporizers for use in the operating room. All major manufacturers now offer a similar instrument.

Ventilators

Mechanical ventilators are now an integral part of the anesthesia machine. Patients are ventilated during general anesthesia by electrical or gas-powered devices that are simple to control yet sophisticated in their function. The history of mechanical

positive pressure ventilation began with attempts to resuscitate victims of drowning by a bellows attached to a mask or tracheal tube. These experiments found little role in anesthetic care for many years. At the beginning of the 20th century, however, several modalities were explored before intermittent positive pressure machines evolved.

A series of artificial environments were created in response to the frustration experienced by thoracic surgeons who found that the lung collapsed when they incised the pleura. Between 1900 and 1910, continuous positive or negative pressure devices were created to maintain inflation of the lungs of a spontaneously breathing patient once the chest was opened. Brauer (1904) and Murphy (1905) placed the patient's head and neck in a box in which positive pressure was continually maintained. Sauerbruch (1904) created a negative pressure operating chamber encompassing both the surgical team and the patient's body and from which only the patient's head projected.

In 1907, the first intermittent positive pressure device, the Draeger "Pulmotor," was developed to rhythmically inflate the lungs. This instrument and later American models such as the E & J Resuscitator were used almost exclusively by firefighters and mine rescue workers. There are accounts that before 1940 in some American communities, surgeons occasionally called the fire department to assist in the ventilation of patients who had stopped breathing while in the operating room. At that time many hospitals lacked any resuscitation equipment.

A few European medical workers had an early interest in rhythmic inflation of the lungs. In 1934 a Swedish team developed the "Spiropulsator," which C. Crafoord later modified for use during cyclopropane anesthesia.[43] Its action was controlled by a magnetic control valve called the flasher, a type first used to provide intermittent gas flow for the lights of navigational buoys. When Trier Morch, a Danish anesthesiologist, could not obtain a Spiropulsator during World War II, he fabricated the Morch "Respirator," which used a piston pump to rhythmically deliver a fixed volume of gas to the patient. After World War II a motorcycle engineer in Britain developed the comparable prototype of the Blease "Pulmoflator" in which an electric motor provided compressed air to inflate the patient's lungs. In those days, when purpose-built miniature motors were unavailable, mechanics adapted automotive parts such as windshield blade motors and other devices for use in their early models.[44]

A major stimulus to the development of ventilators came as a consequence of a devastating epidemic of poliomyelitis that struck Copenhagen, Denmark, in 1952. As scores of patients were admitted, the only effective ventilatory support that could be provided patients with bulbar paralysis was continuous manual ventilation *via* a tracheostomy employing devices such as Waters' "to-and-fro" circuit. This succeeded only through the dedicated efforts of hundreds of volunteers. Medical students served in relays to ventilate paralyzed patients. The Copenhagen crisis stimulated a broad European interest in the development of portable ventilators in anticipation of another epidemic of poliomyelitis.

At this time, the common practice in North American hospitals was to place polio patients with respiratory involvement in "iron lungs," metal cylinders that encased the body below the neck. Inspiration was caused by intermittent negative pressure created by an electric motor acting on a piston-like device occupying the foot of the chamber. During an epidemic, scores of iron lungs might be operated continuously in a single large room.

Some early American ventilators were adaptations of respiratory-assist machines originally designed for the delivery of aerosolized drugs for respiratory therapy. Two types employed the Bennett or Bird "flow-sensitive" valves. The Bennett valve was designed during World War II when a team of physiologists at the University of Southern California encountered difficulties in separating inspiration from expiration in an experimental apparatus designed to provide positive pressure breathing for aviators at high-altitude. An engineer, Ray Bennett, visited their laboratory, observed their problem, and resolved it with a mechanical flow-sensitive automatic valve. A second valving mechanism was later designed by an aeronautical engineer, Forrest Bird.

The use of the Bird and Bennett valves gained an anesthetic application when the gas flow from the valve was directed into a rigid plastic jar containing a breathing bag or bellows as part of an anesthesia circuit. These "bag-in-bottle" devices mimicked the action of the clinician's hand as the gas flow compressed the bag, thereby providing positive pressure inspiration. Passive exhalation was promoted by the descent of a weight on the bag or bellows. The functions of the components of some of the first ventilators to use these principles could be examined with ease through the plastic housing, whereas they are now concealed within the interior of the instrument. As a result, it is now possible to operate the ventilator of an anesthesia machine for years without becoming aware of the principles that direct its action and protect against malfunction.

Anesthesia Machine and Equipment Monitors

The introduction of safety features was coordinated by the American National Standards Institute (ANSI) Committee Z79, which was sponsored from 1956 until 1983 by the American Society of Anesthesiologists. Since 1983, representatives from industry, government, and health care professions have met on Committee Z79 of the American Society for Testing and Materials. They establish voluntary goals that may become accepted national standards for the safety of anesthesia equipment.

Ralph Tovell voiced the first call for standards during World War II while he was the U.S. Army Consultant in Anesthesiology for Europe. Tovell found that, as there were four different dimensions for connectors, tubes, masks, and breathing bags, supplies dispatched to field hospitals might not match their anesthesia machines. As Tovell observed, "When a sudden need for accessory equipment arose, nurses and corpsmen were likely to respond to it by bringing parts that would not fit."[45] Although Tovell's reports did not gain an immediate response, after the war Vincent Collins and Hamilton Davis took up his concern and formed the ANSI Committee Z79. One of the committee's most active members, Leslie Rendell-Baker, wrote an account of the committee's domestic and international achievements.[46] He reported that Ralph Tovell, encouraged all manufacturers to select the now uniform orifice of 22 mm for all adult and pediatric face masks and to make every tracheal tube connector 15 mm in diameter. For the first time, a Z79-designed mask-tube elbow adapter would fit every mask and tracheal tube connector.

Other advances were introduced by the Z79 Committee. Tracheal tubes of nontoxic plastic bear a Z79 or IT (Implantation Tested) mark. The committee also mandated touch identification of oxygen flow control at Roderick Calverley's suggestion, which reduced the risk that the wrong gas would be selected before internal mechanical controls prevented the selection of an hypoxic mixture.[47] Pin indexing reduced the hazard of attaching a wrong cylinder in the place of oxygen. Diameter indexing of connectors prevented similar errors in high-pressure tubing. For many years, however, errors committed in reassembling hospital oxygen supply lines led to a series of tragedies before polarographic oxygen analyzers were added to the inspiratory limb of the anesthesia circuit.

Patient Monitors

Safer machines assured the clinician that an appropriate gas mixture was delivered to the patient. Other monitors were required to provide an early warning of acute physiologic deterio-

ration before a patient suffered irrevocable damage. Every anesthesiologist who has remained in practice during the past 30 years has witnessed a great series of advances in monitoring with the advent of clinically employable forms of electrocardiography, arterial blood gas analysis, anesthetic gas analysis, computer-processed electroencephalography, and pulse oximetry.

Two American surgeons, George W. Crile and Harvey Cushing, developed a strong interest in measuring blood pressure during anesthesia. Both men wrote thorough and detailed examinations of blood pressure monitoring; however, Cushing's contribution is better remembered because he was the first American to apply the Riva Rocci cuff, which he saw while visiting Italy. Cushing introduced the concept in 1902 and had blood pressure measurements recorded on anesthesia records.[48] These improved records were an advance over the first recordings of the patient's pulse that Cushing and a colleague at Harvard Medical School, Charles Codman, had initiated in 1894 in an attempt to assess the course of the anesthetics they administered as students.

Anesthesiologists began to auscultate blood pressure after 1905 when Nicholai Korotkoff, a surgeon-in-training in St. Petersburg, Russia, gave an abbreviated report of the sounds that he heard distal to the Riva Rocci cuff as it was deflated. Although his one-paragraph account does not explain why he came to listen over a normal vessel (a novel approach now used universally for the clinical measurement of blood pressure), it may be that his commitment to vascular surgery caused him to auscultate before incising a mass that might be vascular and would, therefore, produce a bruit. Perhaps he happened to have his stethoscope positioned over a vessel as a cuff was deflated and fortuitously heard sounds never appreciated before. Cuffs and stethoscopes are now often replaced by automated blood pressure devices, which first appeared in 1936 and which operate on an oscillometric principle. The development of inexpensive microprocessors has promoted the routine use of these automatic cuffs in clinical settings.

The first precordial stethoscope was believed to have been used by S. Griffith Davis at Johns Hopkins University.[49] He adapted a technique developed by Harvey Cushing in a laboratory in which dogs with surgically induced valvular lesions had stethoscopes attached to their chest wall so that medical students might listen to bruits characteristic of a specific malformation. Davis' technique was forgotten but was rehabilitated by Dr. Robert Smith, an energetic pioneer of pediatric anesthesiology in Boston. A Canadian contemporary, Albert Codesmith, of the Hospital for Sick Children, Toronto, became frustrated by the repeated dislodging of the chest piece under the surgical drapes and fabricated his first esophageal stethoscope from urethral catheters and Penrose drains. His brief report heralded its clinical role as a monitor of both normal and adventitious respiratory and cardiac sounds.[50] An additional benefit was that the stethoscope could protect against the risk of disconnection of a paralyzed patient from the anesthesia circuit. In the era before audible alarms, the patient's survival depended upon the anesthesiologist's recognition of the sudden disappearance of breath sounds.

Electrocardiography, Pulse Oximetry, and Carbon Dioxide Measurement

Clinical electrocardiography began with Willem Einthoven's application of the string galvanometer in 1903. Within two decades, Thomas Lewis had described its role in the diagnosis of disturbances of cardiac rhythm, while James Herrick and Harold Pardee first drew attention to the changes produced by myocardial ischemia. After 1928, cathode ray oscilloscopes were available, but the risk of explosion owing to the presence of inflammable anesthetics forestalled the introduction of the electrocardiogram into routine anesthetic practice until after World War II. At that time the small screen of the heavily shielded "bullet" oscilloscope displayed only 3 seconds of data, but that information was highly prized. In some hospitals, priorities were established to determine where this expensive monitor was to be used. When an assistant was dispatched to bring the "bullet scope," everyone knew that a major anesthetic enterprise was about to begin.

Pulse oximetry, the optical measurement of oxygen saturation in tissues, is one of the more recent additions to the anesthesiologist's array of routine monitors. Severinghaus states, "Pulse oximetry is arguably the most important technological advance ever made in monitoring the well-being and safety of patients during anesthesia, recovery, and critical care."[51] Although research in this area began in 1932, its first practical application came during World War II. An American physiologist, Glen Millikan, responded to a request from British colleagues in aviation research. Millikan set about preparing a series of devices to improve the supply of oxygen that was provided to pilots flying at high altitude in unpressurized aircraft. To monitor oxygen delivery and to prevent the pilot from succumbing to an unrecognized failure of his oxygen supply, Millikan created an oxygen sensing monitor worn on the pilot's earlobe, and coined the name *oximeter* to describe its action. Before his tragic death in a climbing accident in 1947, Millikan had begun to assess anesthetic applications of oximetry.

For the next three decades, oximetry was rarely used by anesthesiologists, and then primarily in research studies such as those of Faulconer and Pender. Refinements of oximetry by a Japanese engineer, Takuo Aoyagi, led to the development of pulse oximetry. As Severinghaus recounted the episode, Aoyagi had attempted to eliminate the changes in a signal caused by pulsatile variations when he realized that this fluctuation could be used to measure both the pulse and oxygen saturation. Severinghaus observed that this was "a classic example of the adage that 'one man's noise is another man's signal.' "[52]

Although pulse oximetry gives second-by-second data about oxygen saturation, anesthesiologists have recognized a need for breath-by-breath measurement of respiratory and anesthetic gases. After 1954, infrared absorption techniques gave immediate displays of the exhaled concentration of carbon dioxide. Clinicians quickly learned to relate abnormal concentrations of carbon dioxide to threatening situations such as the inappropriate placement of a tracheal tube in the esophagus, abrupt alterations in pulmonary blood flow, and other factors. More recently, infrared analysis has been perfected to enable breath-by-breath measurement of anesthetic gases as well. This technology has largely replaced mass spectrometry, which initially had only industrial applications before Albert Faulconer of the Mayo Clinic first used it to monitor the concentration of an exhaled anesthetic in 1954.

Tracheal Intubation in Anesthesia

The development of techniques and instruments for intubation ranks among the major advances in the history of anesthesiology. The first tracheal tubes were developed for the resuscitation of drowning victims, but were not used in anesthesia until 1878. Although John Snow and others had already anesthetized patients by means of a tracheostomy, the first use of elective oral intubation for an anesthetic was undertaken by a Scottish surgeon, William Macewan. He had practiced passing flexible metal tubes through the larynx of a cadaver before attempting the maneuver on an awake patient with an oral tumor at the Glasgow Royal Infirmary, on July 5, 1878.[53] Because topical anesthesia was not yet known, the experience must have demanded fortitude on the part of Macewan's patient. Once the tube was correctly positioned, an assistant began a chloroform–air anesthetic *via* the tube. Once anesthetized, the patient soon stopped coughing. Macewan abandoned the practice following an unusual fatality. His last patient had been intubated while awake but the tube was removed before the anesthetic could begin. The patient later died while receiving chloroform by mask.

Although there was a sporadic interest in tracheal anesthesia in Edinburgh and other European centers after Macewan, a contemporary American surgeon is remembered for his extraordinary dedication to the advancement of tracheal intubation. Joseph O'Dwyer had witnessed the distressing death by asphyxiation of children with diphtheria and sought an alternative to the mutilation of a hasty tracheotomy. In 1885, O'Dwyer designed a series of metal laryngeal tubes, which he inserted blindly between the vocal cords of children suffering a diphtheritic crisis. Colleagues applauded his humanitarian efforts. Three years later, O'Dwyer designed a second rigid tube with a conical tip that occluded the larynx so effectively that it could be used for artificial ventilation when applied with the bellows and T-piece tube of George Fell's apparatus.[54] The Fell–O'Dwyer apparatus was used during thoracic surgery by Rudolph Matas of New Orleans, who was so pleased with it that he predicted, "The procedure that promises the most benefit in preventing pulmonary collapse in operations on the chest is . . . the rhythmical maintenance of artificial respiration by a tube in the glottis directly connected with a bellows."[54] For several decades, this principle would be transiently rediscovered by other surgeons before Matas' prophecy was fully realized.

After O'Dwyer's death, the outstanding pioneer of tracheal intubation was Franz Kuhn, a surgeon of Kassel, Germany. From 1900 until 1912, Kuhn wrote a series of fine papers and a classic monograph, "*Die perorale Intubation*," which were not well known in his lifetime but have since become widely appreciated.[55] His work might have had a more profound impact if it had been translated into English. Kuhn described techniques of oral and nasal intubation that he performed with flexible metal tubes composed of coiled tubing similar to those now used for the spout of metal gasoline cans. After applying cocaine to the airway, Kuhn introduced his tube over a curved metal stylet that he directed toward the larynx with his left index finger (Fig. 1-7). While he was aware of the subglottic cuffs that had been used briefly by Victor Eisenmenger, Kuhn preferred to seal the larynx by positioning a supralaryngeal flange near the tube's tip before packing the pharynx with gauze. Kuhn even monitored the patient's breath sounds continuously through a monaural earpiece connected to an extension of the tracheal

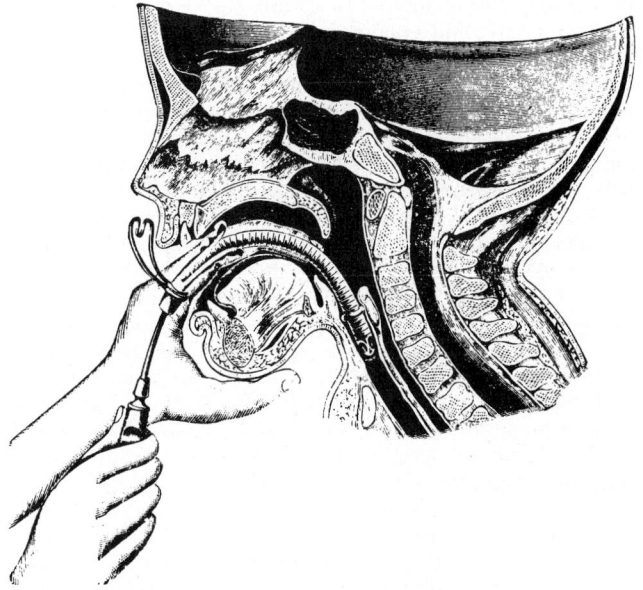

Figure 1-7. Kuhn's endotracheal tube. The tube and introducer were guided to the trachea by the fingers of the operator's left hand.

tube by a narrow tube. His writings reflect a mastery of intubation techniques unequaled for many years.

Intubation of the trachea by palpation was an uncertain and sometimes traumatic act. Even though the use of a mirror for indirect laryngoscopy antedated Macewan's intubations, the technique could not be adapted for use in anesthesia. For some years, surgeons even believed that it would be anatomically impossible to visualize the vocal cords directly. This misapprehension was overcome in 1895 by Alfred Kirstein in Berlin who devised the first direct-vision laryngoscope.[56] Kirstein was motivated by a friend's report that a patient's trachea had been accidentally intubated during esophagoscopy. Kirstein promptly fabricated a hand-held instrument that at first resembled a shortened cylindrical esophagoscope. He soon substituted a semicircular blade that opened inferiorly. Kirstein could now examine the larynx while standing behind his seated patient, whose head had been placed in an attitude approximating the "sniffing position" later recommended by Ivan Magill. Although Alfred Kristin's "autoscope" was not used by anesthesiologists, it was the forerunner of all modern laryngoscopes. Endoscopy was refined by Chevalier Jackson in Philadelphia, who designed a U-shaped laryngoscope by adding a hand grip that was parallel to the blade. The Jackson blade has remained a standard instrument for endoscopists but was not favored by anesthesiologists. Two laryngoscopes that closely resembled modern L-shaped instruments were designed in 1910 and 1913 by two American surgeons, Henry Janeway and George Dorrance, but neither instrument achieved lasting use despite their excellent designs.

Anesthesiologist Inspired Laryngoscopes

Early practitioners of intubation of the trachea were frustrated by laryngoscopes that were cumbersome, ill designed for the prevention of dental injury, and offered only a very limited view of the larynx. Before the introduction of muscle relaxants, intubation of the trachea was often a severe challenge. It was in that period, however, that two blades were invented that became the classic models of the straight and curved laryngoscope. Robert Miller of San Antonio, Texas, and Robert Macintosh of Oxford University created two blades that have maintained lasting popularity. Both laryngoscopes appeared within an interval of 2 years. In 1941, Miller brought forward a slender, straight blade with a slight curve near the tip to ease the passage of the tube through the larynx. Although Miller's blade was a refinement, the technique of its use was identical to that of earlier models as the epiglottis was lifted to expose the larynx.[57]

The Macintosh blade, which passes in front of the epiglottis, was invented as an incidental result of a tonsillectomy, an operation that was then performed without intubation. Sir Robert Macintosh later described the circumstances of its discovery in an appreciation of the career of his technician, Mr. Richard Salt, who constructed the blade. As Sir Robert recalled, "A Boyle-Davis gag, a size larger than intended, was inserted for tonsillectomy, and when the mouth was fully opened the cords came into view. This was a surprise since conventional laryngoscopy, at that depth of anaesthesia, would have been impossible in those pre-relaxant days. Within a matter of hours, Salt had modified the blade of the Davis gag and attached a laryngoscope handle to it; and streamlined (after testing several models), the end result came into widespread use."[58] Sir Robert's observation of widespread use was an understatement; more than 800,000 Macintosh blades have been produced, and many special-purpose versions have been marketed.

These clever innovations may have failed to capture wide attention because intubating laryngoscopes lacked a wide market at a time when there were fewer than 100 anesthesiologists active in the United States. Many of those practitioners never attempted intubation throughout their career. Even after 1940, in some hospitals laryngologists were routinely called to intubate

surgical patients while the attending anesthesiologist confined his attention to the anesthetic. In time, however, all anesthesiologists would learn the skills of atraumatic nasal and oral intubation by using the instruments and techniques developed by a few British and North American specialists.

The most distinguished pioneer of tracheal intubation was a self-trained British anaesthetist, Ivan (later, Sir Ivan) Magill.[59] In 1919, when serving in the Royal Army as a general medical officer, Magill was assigned to a military hospital near London. Although he had only a medical student's training in anesthesia, Magill was obliged to accept an assignment to the anesthesia service, where he was joined by another neophyte, Stanley Rowbotham.[60] They attended casualties disfigured by severe facial injuries who underwent repeated restorative operations. These procedures would be successful only if the surgeon, Harold Gillies, had unrestricted access to the face and airway. Some patients were formidable challenges, but both men became extraordinarily adept. Because they learned from fortuitous observations, they soon extended the scope of tracheal anesthesia.

Magill and Rowbotham's expertise with blind nasal intubation began after they learned to soften semirigid insufflation tubes that they passed through a nostril. Even though they originally planned to position the tips of the tubes only in the posterior pharynx, the slender tubes occasionally entered the trachea. Stimulated by this chance experience, they developed techniques of deliberate nasotracheal intubation. In 1920, Magill devised an aid to manipulating the catheter tip, the Magill angulated forceps, which are still manufactured according to his original design of 75 years ago.

After entering civilian practice, Magill set out to develop a wide-bore tube that would resist kinking but could be curved into a form resembling the contours of the upper airway. While in a hardware store, he found mineralized red rubber tubing which he cut, beveled, and smoothed to produce tubes that clinicians in all countries would come to call "Magill tubes." His tubes remained the universal standard for more than 40 years until rubber products were supplanted by inert plastics. Magill also rediscovered the advantage of applying cocaine to the nasal mucosa, a technique that he employed in developing his mastery of awake blind nasal intubation.

Magill's success in performing awake blind nasal intubation of the trachea excited the curiosity of other anaesthetists. Magill shared his principles at meetings attended by the few specialists in anesthesia, but few colleagues ever matched his control of the airway until muscle relaxants were introduced. Throughout much of his distinguished career, he continued to create new devices. Magill's innovations included tracheal tubes for children, an L-shaped laryngoscope, a tracheoscope, and a wire-tipped endobronchial tube for thoracic surgery.

In 1926, unaware of the prior work of Eisenmenger and Dorrance, Arthur Guedel began a series of experiments that led to the introduction of the cuffed tube.* His goal was to combine the safety of tracheal anesthesia with the safety and economy of the closed-circuit technique, recently refined by his close friend, Ralph Waters.[61] Guedel transformed the basement of his Indianapolis home into a laboratory, where he subjected each step of the preparation and application of his cuffs to a vigorous review.[62] He fashioned cuffs from the rubber of dental dams, condoms, and surgical gloves that were glued

---

* Guedel never recorded how he came to create his black rubber airway, but the event that precipitated the design of its most popular successor, the Berman airway, is known. In 1948, Robert Berman was shocked to observe a safety pin resting in his patient's pharynx as he removed a Guedel airway. He realized that the pin must have been dislodged from within the airway and so set about bivalving other airways to find other foreign bodies hidden from view. In response, he designed an open-sided airway that could be cleaned under direct vision. A friend fabricated the Berman airway from cellulose acetate butyrate and so created the first molded plastic anesthesia device.

onto the outer wall of tubes. Using animal tracheas donated by the family butcher as his model, he considered whether the cuff should be positioned above, below, or at the level of the vocal cords. He recommended that the cuff be positioned just below the vocal cords to seal the airway and to prevent an accumulation of fluid below the cords but above the cuff. Ralph Waters later recommended that cuffs be constructed of two layers of soft rubber cemented together. These detachable cuffs were first manufactured by Waters' children, who sold them to the Foregger Company.

Guedel sought ways to show the safety and utility of the cuffed tube. He first filled the mouth of an anesthetized and intubated patient with water and showed that the cuff sealed the airway. Even though this exhibition was successful, he searched for a more dramatic technique to capture the attention of those unfamiliar with the advantages of intubation. He reasoned that if the cuff prevented water from entering the trachea of an intubated patient, it should also prevent an animal from drowning, even if it were submerged under water. To encourage physicians attending a medical convention to use tracheal techniques, Guedel prepared the first of several "dunked dog" demonstrations (Fig. 1-8). An anesthetized and intubated dog, Guedel's own pet, "Airway," was immersed in an aquarium. After the demonstration was completed, the anesthetic was discontinued before the animal was removed from the water. Airway awoke promptly, shook water over the onlookers, saluted a post, then trotted from the hall to the applause of the audience. By this novel demonstration, the cuffed tube gained wider use.

Endobronchial Tubes—The Next Step

Talented observers may recognize a therapeutic opportunity when presented with what at first appears to be a frustrating complication. After a patient experienced an accidental endobronchial intubation, Ralph Waters reasoned that a very long cuffed tube could be used to ventilate the dependent lung while the upper lung was being resected.[63] On learning of his friend's success with intentional one-lung anesthesia, Arthur Guedel proposed an important modification for chest surgery, the double-cuffed single-lumen tube, which was introduced by Emery Rovenstine. These tubes were easily positioned, an advantage over bronchial blockers that had to be inserted by a skilled bronchoscopist.

Following World War II, several double-cuffed single-lumen tubes were used for thoracic surgery, but after 1953, these were supplanted by double-lumen endobronchial tubes. The double-lumen tube currently most popular was designed by Frank Rob-

ertshaw of Manchester, England, and is prepared in both right- and left-sided versions. Robertshaw tubes were first manufactured from mineralized red rubber but are now made of extruded plastic, a technique refined by David Sheridan. Sheridan was also the first person to embed centimeter markings along the side of tracheal tubes, a safety feature that reduced the risk of the tube's being incorrectly positioned.

New Devices for Airway Management

Conventional laryngoscopes proved inadequate for some patients with a "difficult airway." Two decades ago, if frustrated in intubating a patient whose airway was unexpectedly found to be difficult to visualize, clinicians fervently prayed for an instrument that would resolve their difficulty by permitting them to "look around the corner" or "create a space where no space exists." A few clinicians credit harrowing experiences as their incentive for invention. The challenge of reintubating a patient hemorrhaging into the tissues of the neck following carotid endarterectomy led Cedric Bainton to devise the four-sided Bainton blade that "creates a space" by displacing edematous tissue to provide a direct view of previously obscured vocal cords. Roger Bullard desired a device to "look around the corner" when frustrated in attempts to visualize the larynx of a patient with Pierre-Robin syndrome. In response, he developed the Bullard laryngoscope, whose fiberoptic bundles lie beside a curved blade. The passage of flexible fiberoptic bronchoscopes has been aided by "intubating airways" such as those designed by Berman, Ovassapian, Augustine, Williams, Luomanen, and Patil. Patients requiring continuous oxygen administration during fiberoptic bronchoscopy may breathe through the Patil face mask, which features a separate orifice through which the scope is advanced. The Patil face mask is only one of an extensive series of aides to intubation created by the innovative "Vijay" Patil.

Dr. A. I. J. "Archie" Brain is respected by all clinician-inventors for his perseverance in creating the laryngeal mask airway (LMA). Dr. Brain first recognized the principle of the LMA in 1981 when, like many British clinicians, he provided dental anesthesia *via* a Goldman nasal mask. However, unlike any before him, he realized that just as the dental mask could be fitted closely about the nose, a comparable mask attached to a wide-bore tube might be positioned around the larynx. He not only conceived of this radical departure in airway management, which he first described in 1983,[64] but also spent years in single-handedly fabricating and testing scores of incremental modifications. Scores of Brain's prototypes are displayed in the Royal Berkshire Hospital, Reading, England, where they provide

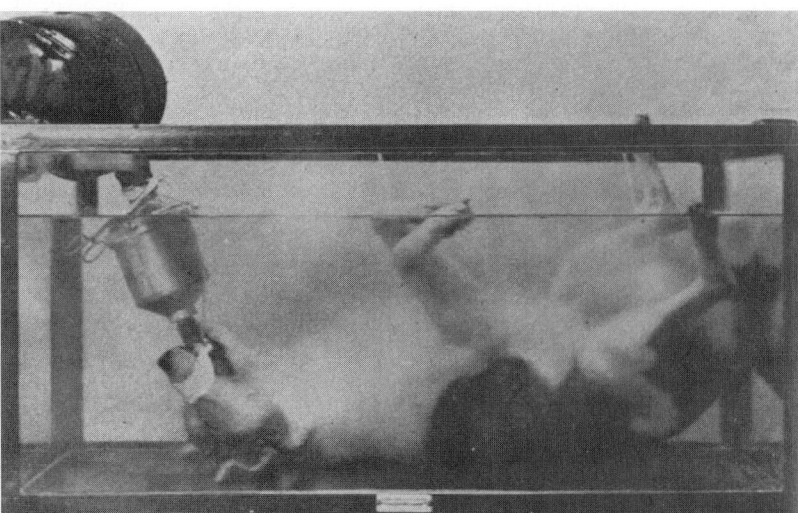

Figure 1-8. "The dunked dog." Arthur Guedel demonstrated the safety of endotracheal intubation with a cuffed tube by submerging his anesthetized pet, Airway, in an aquarium while the animal breathed an ethylene–oxygen anesthetic through an underwater Waters' "to-and-fro" anesthesia circuit.

a detailed record of the evolution of the LMA. He fabricated his first models from Magill tubes and Goldman masks, then refined their shape by performing postmortem studies of the hypopharynx to determine the form of cuff that would be most functional. Before silicone rubber was selected, Brain had even mastered the technique of forming masks from liquid latex. Every detail of the LMA—the number and position of the aperture bars, the shape and the size of the masks—required repeated modification. Every clinician who has studied the Reading collection of LMA prototypes has gained a profound appreciation for Dr. Brain's achievement.

The Evolution of Inhaled Anesthetics During the Twentieth Century

As the mechanisms to deliver drugs were refined, entirely new classes of medications were also developed, with the intention of providing safer, more pleasant pain control. Ether and chloroform, the cornerstones of effective anesthesia for decades, were perceived as imperfect drugs. Ether was unpleasant to inhale; chloroform was shown to have serious toxic effects on the liver and heart. Both gases were volatile and were challenging to store and administer. Ethylene gas was the first alternative to ether and chloroform, but it too had major disadvantages. The rediscovery of ethylene in 1923 also came from an unlikely observation. After it was learned that ethylene gas had been used in Chicago greenhouses to inhibit the opening of carnation buds, it was speculated that a gas that put flowers to sleep might also have an anesthetic action on humans. Arno Luckhardt was the first to publish a clinical study in February 1923. Within a month, two other independent studies were presented, by Isabella Herb in Chicago and W. Easson Brown in Toronto. Ethylene was not a successful anesthetic because high concentrations were required and it was explosive. An additional significant shortcoming was a particularly unpleasant smell, which could only be partially disguised by the use of oil of orange or a cheap perfume. When cyclopropane was introduced, ethylene was abandoned.

There was a fortuitous element in the discovery of cyclopropane's anesthetic action in 1929.[65] W. Easson Brown and Velyien Henderson had previously shown that propylene had desirable properties as an anesthetic when freshly prepared; but after storage in a steel cylinder, it deteriorated to create a toxic material that produced nausea and cardiac irregularities in humans. Henderson, a professor of pharmacology at the University of Toronto, suggested to a chemist, George Lucas, that the toxic product be identified. After Lucas identified cyclopropane among the chemicals in the tank, the chemist prepared a sample in low concentration with oxygen and administered it to two kittens. The animals fell asleep quietly and recovered rapidly. Lucas saw that, rather than being a toxic contaminant, cyclopropane was a very potent anesthetic. After its effects in other animals were studied and cyclopropane proved to be stable after storage, human experimentation began.

Henderson was the first volunteer; Lucas followed. They then arranged a public demonstration in which Frederick Banting, already a Nobel laureate for his discovery of insulin, was anesthetized before a group of physicians. Despite this promising beginning, further research was abruptly halted for an illogical reason. The professor of surgery argued that since there had been three anesthetic deaths in Toronto attributed to ethyl chloride, no clinical trials of cyclopropane would be allowed despite its apparent safety. Rather than abandon the study, Velyien Henderson encouraged an American friend, Ralph Waters, to use cyclopropane at the University of Wisconsin. The Wisconsin group investigated the drug thoroughly and reported their clinical success in 1933. The slow pace of their research was due to the paucity of funding during the Great Depression.

By coincidence, external interference also frustrated the clinical trials of the first anesthetic to be created deliberately from a pharmacologist's knowledge of structure–activity relationships. In 1930, Chauncey Leake and MeiYu Chen performed successful laboratory trials of vinethene (divinyl ether) but were thwarted in its further development by a professor of surgery in San Francisco. Ironically, Canadians, who had lost cyclopropane to Wisconsin, learned of vinethene from Leake and Chen in California and conducted the first human study in 1932 at the University of Alberta, Edmonton.

All potent anesthetics of this period were explosive save for chloroform, whose hepatic and cardiac toxicity limited its use in America. Anesthetic explosions remained a rare but devastating risk to both anesthesiologist and patient. To reduce the danger of explosion during the incendiary days of World War II, British anaesthetists turned to trichloroethylene. This noninflammable anesthetic found limited application in America, as it decomposed to release phosgene when warmed in the presence of soda lime. By the end of World War II, however, another class of noninflammable anesthetics was prepared for laboratory trials. Ten years later, fluorinated hydrocarbons revolutionized inhalation anesthesia.

Fluorinated Anesthetics

Fluorine, the lightest and most reactive halogen, forms exceptionally stable bonds. These bonds, although sometimes created with explosive force, resist separation by chemical or thermal means. For that reason, many early attempts to fluorinate hydrocarbons in a controlled manner were frustrated by the marked chemical activity of fluorine. In 1930, the first commercial application of fluorine chemistry was made in the production of a refrigerant, Freon. This was followed by the first attempt to prepare a fluorinated anesthetic, by Harold Booth and E. May Bixby in 1932. Although their drug, monochlorodifluoromethane, was devoid of anesthetic action, as were all other drugs produced by other investigators during that decade, their report accurately forecasts future developments. It began, "A survey of the properties of 166 known gases suggested that the best possibility of finding a new noncombustible anesthetic gas lay in the field of organic fluoride compounds. Fluorine substitution for other halogens lowers the boiling point, increases stability, and generally decreases toxicity."[66]

The secret demands of the Manhattan Project for refined uranium-235 were the next impetus to an improved understanding of fluorine chemistry. Researchers learned that uranium might be refined through the creation of an intermediate compound, uranium hexafluoride. Part of this project was undertaken by Earl McBee of Purdue University, who had a longstanding interest in the fluorination of hydrocarbons. McBee also held a grant from the Mallinckrodt Chemical Works, a manufacturer of ether and cyclopropane, to prepare new fluorinated compounds, which were to be tested as anesthetics. By 1945, the Purdue team had created small amounts of 46 fluorinated ethanes, propanes, butanes, and an ether.

The value of these chemicals might not have been appreciated, however, if Mallinckrodt had not also provided financial support for pharmacology research at Vanderbilt University. At that time, the Vanderbilt anesthesia department was unique in that its first chairperson was a pharmacologist, Benjamin Robbins, who could assess the drugs more effectively than could any other anesthesiologist of that period. Robbins tested McBee's compounds in mice and selected the most promising for evaluation in dogs. Although none of these compounds found a place as an anesthetic, Robbins' conclusions on the effects of fluorination, bromination, and chlorination in his landmark report of 1946 encouraged later studies that would prove to be successful.[67]

A team at the University of Maryland under Professor of Pharmacology John C. Krantz, Jr., investigated the anesthetic properties of dozens of hydrocarbons over a period of several years, but only one, ethyl vinyl ether, entered clinical use in 1947. Because it was inflammable, Krantz requested that it be fluorinated. In response, Julius Shukys prepared several fluorinated analogs. One of these, trifluorethyl vinyl ether, or fluroxene, became the first fluorinated anesthetic. Fluroxene was marketed from 1954 until 1974. As the drug was marginally inflammable, fluroxene had already been supplanted by more potent agents when it was withdrawn as a consequence of the delayed discovery of the action of a metabolite that was toxic to lower animals. Fluroxene is important not only for its historical interest as the first fluorinated anesthetic but also as a reminder of the importance of the continual surveillance of a drug's action—a process in which all clinicians play a significant role each day.[68]

While American researchers were conducting a rather random search for new anesthetics, a team of British chemists applied a more direct approach. In 1951, Charles Suckling, a chemist of Imperial Chemical Industries who already had an expert understanding of fluorination, was asked to create a new anesthetic. Suckling began by asking clinicians to describe the properties of an ideal anesthetic. He learned from this inquiry that his search must consider several limiting factors, including the volatility, inflammability, stability, and potency of the compounds. Within 2 years, Charles Suckling created halothane. As a reflection of the planning that he had carried out beforehand, halothane was the sixth compound synthesized.

The limited number of chemicals produced for testing reflected Suckling's expert knowledge of the pharmacology of halogens and his ability to appreciate important physical relationships that apply to all anesthetics. His achievement was an extension of a principle that had been recognized in 1939 by his superior, James Ferguson, which Ferguson later learned had first been considered by John Snow in 1848. The principle was to relate the opioid actions of known anesthetics along a thermodynamic scale—the ratio of the partial pressure producing anesthesia over the saturated vapor pressure of the drug at the temperature of the experiment. The resulting ratios fall within a very narrow range, as opposed to the more than 200-fold variations seen when anesthetics are graphed by the inspired concentration required for anesthesia.[69]

Suckling first determined that halothane had an anesthetic action by anesthetizing meal worms and houseflies before he forwarded it to a pharmacologist, James Raventos, along with an accurate prediction, based on Ferguson's principles, of the concentration that would be required for anesthesia in higher animals. After Raventos completed a favorable review, halothane was offered to Michael Johnstone, a respected anesthetist of Manchester, England, who recognized its great advantages over the other anesthetics available in 1956.

Halothane was followed in 1960 by methoxyflurane, an anesthetic that was popular until 1970. At that time, a dose-related nephrotoxicity following protracted methoxyflurane anesthesia was found to be caused by inorganic fluoride, released by the enzymatic cleavage of a monofluoro-carbon bond. As a consequence and because of a persisting concern that rare cases of hepatitis following anesthesia might be due to a metabolite of halothane, the search for newer inhaled anesthetics focused on the resistance of the molecule to metabolic degradation.

Two fluorinated liquid anesthetics, enflurane and its isomer isoflurane, were results of the search for increased stability. They were synthesized by Ross Terrell in 1963 and 1965, respectively. Because enflurane was easier to create, it preceded isoflurane. Its application was restricted after it was shown to be a marked cardiovascular depressant and to have some convulsant properties. Isoflurane was nearly abandoned because of difficulties in its purification, but after this problem was overcome by Louise Speers, a series of successful trials was published in 1971. The release of isoflurane for clinical use was delayed again for more than half a decade by calls for repeated testing in lower animals, owing to an unfounded concern that the drug might be a carcinogen. As a consequence, isoflurane was more thoroughly assessed before being offered to anesthesiologists than any other

drug heretofore used in anesthesia. The era when an anesthetic could be introduced following a single fortuitous observation has given way to a cautious program of assessment and reassessment before a new inhaled agent, such as desflurane or sevoflurane, is advocated in routine practice.

Intravenous Anesthetics

A firm understanding of the circulation, along with adequate intravenous (iv) access, was necessary before drugs could be administered directly into a patient's bloodstream. Both of these aspects were firmly in place well before an appropriate iv anesthetic was devised. In 1909, a German, Ludwig Burkhardt, produced surgical anesthesia by intravenous injections of chloroform and ether. Seven years later, Elisabeth Bredenfeld of Switzerland reported the use of intravenous morphine and scopolamine. Those trials failed to show an improvement over inhaled techniques. None of the drugs had an action that was both prompt and sufficiently abbreviated.

The first barbiturate, barbital, was synthesized in 1903 by Fischer and von Mering. Phenobarbital and all other successors of barbital had very protracted action and found little use in anesthesia. After 1929, oral pentobarbital was used as a sedative before surgery, but when it was given in anesthetic concentrations, long periods of unconsciousness followed. The first short-acting oxybarbiturate was hexobarbital (Evipal), used clinically in 1932. Hexobarbital was enthusiastically received in Britain and America because its abbreviated induction time was unrivaled by any other technique. A London anesthetist, Ronald Jarman, found that it had a dramatic advantage over inhalation inductions for minor procedures. Jarman developed the "falling arm" sign. Immediately before induction, the patient was instructed to raise one arm above him while Jarman injected hexobarbital into a vein of the opposite forearm. As soon as the upraised arm fell, indicating the onset of hypnosis, the surgeon began. Although this technique is now known to be hazardous, it was welcomed in 1933. Patients were also pleased by the barbiturates, because the onset of their action was so abrupt that many awoke unable to believe they had been anesthetized.*

Even though hexobarbital's prompt action had a dramatic effect on the conduct of anesthesia, it was soon replaced by two thiobarbiturates. In 1932, Donalee Tabern and Ernest H. Volwiler of the Abbott Company synthesized thiopental (Pentothal) and thiamylal (Surital). The sulfated barbiturates proved to be more satisfactory, potent, and rapid-acting than were their oxybarbiturate analogs. Thiopental was first administered to a patient at the University of Wisconsin in March 1934, but the successful introduction of thiopental into clinical practice was

---

* Soon after Evipal was introduced, Robert Macintosh administered it to Sir William Morris, the manufacturer of the Morris Garages (MG) automobiles. Macintosh secured a result that later changed the course of anesthesia.[70] When Morris awoke, he glanced at his watch and inquired as to why the operation had been postponed. On learning that his surgery was completed, he was amazed by this "magic experience," which he contrasted with his vivid recollections of the terror of undergoing a mask induction as a child in a dentist's office. So impressed was Morris (later, Viscount Nuffield) with the quality of anesthetic he had received and the potential for further discovery, that he insisted, over the objections of Oxford's medical establishment, on endowing a department of anesthesia for the university as a precondition of his support for a postgraduate medical center. In 1937, Sir Robert Macintosh became Oxford's first professor of anesthesiology and led the growth of the first university department in Europe from the first fully endowed Chair of Anaesthesia in the world. Fifty years later, on July 24, 1987, when the Nuffield Department of Anaesthetics celebrated its Golden Jubilee, Sir Robert greeted alumni who had returned from scores of countries. Morris' "magic experience" of barbiturate anesthesia had led to a result beyond his imagining—the creation of one of the world's most distinguished anesthesia centers.

due to John S. Lundy and his colleagues at the Mayo Clinic, who began their intensive and protracted assessments of thiopental during June 1934.

When first introduced, thiopental was often given in repeated increments as the primary anesthetic for protracted procedures. Its hazards came to be appreciated over time. At first, depression of respiration was monitored by the simple expedient of observing the motion of a wisp of cotton placed over the nose. Only a few skilled practitioners were prepared to pass a tracheal tube if the patient stopped breathing. Such practitioners realized that thiopental without supplementation did not suppress airway reflexes, and they therefore encouraged the prophylactic provision of topical anesthesia of the airway beforehand. The cardiovascular effects of thiobarbiturates were widely appreciated only when the powerful vasodilating effect of thiopental caused fatalities among burned civilian and military casualties in World War II. In response, fluid replacement was used more aggressively and thiopental administered with greater caution.

Muscle Relaxants

Many anesthesiologists regard the introduction of curare as being among the most important advances in anesthesia since the discovery of ether's action in 1846. Anesthesiologists who practiced before muscle relaxants came into use recall the terror they felt when a premature attempt to intubate the trachea under cyclopropane caused persisting laryngospasm. Before 1942, abdominal relaxation was possible only if the patient tolerated high concentrations of an inhaled anesthetic, which might bring profound respiratory depression and protracted recovery. Curare and the drugs that followed transformed anesthesia profoundly. Before this time, tracheal anesthesia was an art reserved for the expert; now it became a skill that all anesthesiologists could acquire. Because intubation of the trachea could now be taught in a deliberate manner, a neophyte could fail on a first attempt without compromising the safety of the patient. For the first time, abdominal relaxation could be attained when curare was supplemented by light planes of inhaled anesthetics or by a combination of intravenous agents providing "balanced anesthesia." New frontiers opened. A sedated and paralyzed patient could now undergo the major physiologic trespasses of cardiopulmonary bypass and deliberate hypothermia, and might receive long-term respiratory support after surgery.

The curares are alkaloids prepared from plants native to equatorial rain forests. The refinement of the harmless sap of several species of vines into toxins that were lethal only when injected was an extraordinary triumph introduced by paleopharmacologists in loincloths. Their discovery was the more remarkable because it was independently repeated on three separate continents—South America, Africa, and Asia. These jungle tribes also developed nearly identical methods of delivering the toxin by darts, which, after being dipped in curare, maintained their potency indefinitely until they were propelled through blowpipes to strike the flesh of monkeys and other animals of the treetops.

Curare was used in surgery in 1912, but the report was ignored for decades. Arthur Lawen, a physiologist/physician of Leipzig, used curare in his laboratory before boldly producing abdominal relaxation at a light level of anesthesia in a surgical patient. His report, written in German, was not appreciated for decades, nor could it have been until his fellow clinicians learned the skills of intubation of the trachea and controlled ventilation of the lungs.[71]

Curare remained a curiosity of laboratory practice until 1938 when Richard and Ruth Gill returned to New York from South America. They had collected 11.9 kg of crude curare near their Ecuadorian ranch for the Merck Company. Their motivation was a mixture of personal and altruistic goals. Some months before, while on an earlier visit to the United States, Richard

Gill had been told by Dr. Walter Freeman that he had multiple sclerosis. Freeman mentioned that there was a possibility that curare might have a therapeutic role in the management of spastic disorders. When the Gills returned to the United States with their supply of crude curare, they were initially disappointed to learn that Merck's researchers had lost interest, but they were later able to share the curare with E. R. Squibb & Co. Squibb scientists soon offered a semirefined curare to two groups of American anesthesiologists, who assessed its action but soon abandoned their studies when it caused total respiratory paralysis in two patients and the death of laboratory animals.

Curare first entered clinical medicine through the actions of psychiatrists. In 1939, A. R. McIntyre refined a portion of Gill's curare. A. E. Bennett of Omaha, Nebraska, initially injected it into children with spastic disorders. After observing no persisting benefit, he administered it to patients about to receive metrazol, a precursor to electroconvulsive therapy. Because it eliminated seizure-induced fractures, they termed it a "shock absorber." By 1941, other psychiatrists followed this practice and, when they found that the action of curare was protracted, occasionally used neostigmine as an antidote.

Some months later, Harold Griffith, the chief anesthetist of the Montreal Homeopathic Hospital, learned of Bennett's successful use of curare and resolved to apply it in anesthesia. As Griffith was already a master of tracheal intubation, he was much better prepared than were most of his contemporaries to attend to potential complications. On January 23, 1942, Griffith and his resident, Enid Johnson, anesthetized and intubated the trachea of a young man before injecting curare early in the course of his appendectomy. Satisfactory abdominal relaxation was obtained as the surgery proceeded without incident. Griffith and Johnson's report of the successful use of curare in the 25 patients of their series launched a revolution in anesthetic care.[72]

The successful use of curare prompted other studies that led to the introduction of other nondepolarizing and depolarizing relaxants. By 1948, gallamine and decamethonium had been synthesized. Metubine, a curare "rediscovered" in the 1970s, was used clinically in the same year. Succinylcholine was prepared by the Nobel laureate Daniel Bovet in 1949 and was in wide international use before historians noted that the drug had been synthesized and tested long beforehand. In 1906, Hunt and Taveaux prepared succinylcholine among a series of choline esters, which they had injected into rabbits to observe their cardiac effects. If their rabbits had not been previously paralyzed with curare, the depolarizing action of succinylcholine might have been known decades earlier.

Research in relaxants was rekindled in 1960, when researchers became aware of the action of maloetine, a relaxant from the Congo basin. It was remarkable in that it had a steroidal nucleus. Investigations of maloetine led to pancuronium and vecuronium. As these drugs provided new avenues for investigation, the pace of muscle relaxant research has accelerated.

Drugs After 1945

During the first decades following World War II, other classes of drugs were developed. Anesthesiologists learned a new vocabulary as words were coined to describe the actions of novel compounds. "Lytic cocktails," "dissociative anesthesia," and "neuroleptanalgesia" became common expressions. Intravenous mixtures concocted from a succession of analgesics and anxiolytics produced a state of euphoria, tranquility, and indifference when provided with care, or profound respiratory depression when presented carelessly. In 1966, the neologism "dissociative anesthesia" was created by Guenter Corrsen and Edward Domino to describe the trance-like state of profound analgesia produced by ketamine. "Neuroleptanalgesia" was coined by a Belgian anesthesiologist, Juan de Castro, who performed the first clinical investigations of combinations of tranquilizers and opioids, synthesized under the direction of Paul Janssen.

Although many pharmacologists are remembered for the introduction of a single drug, Paul Janssen has brought more than 70 agents forward from among 70,000 chemicals created in his laboratory since 1953. His products have had profound effects on disciplines as disparate as parasitology and psychiatry. The pace of productive innovation in Janssen's research laboratory has been astonishing. Chemical R4263 (fentanyl), synthesized in 1960, was followed only a year later by R4749 (droperidol). Although the fixed combination (Innovar) in which they were introduced, is now less popular, Janssen's opioids, sufentanil and alfentanil, have come into common use.

Several induction agents have been brought forward to challenge the preeminence of thiopental. Of these only propofol has found great success. After its synthesis by Imperial Chemical Industries as ICI 35 868, it was first employed in clinical trials in 1977. Investigators found that it produced hypnosis quickly with minimal excitation and that patients awoke promptly once the drug was discontinued. Regrettably, cremaphor, the solvent with which it was formulated, was unsatisfactory. Once propofol was reformulated with egg lecithin, glycerol, and soybean oil, the drug gained great success. As it entered clinical practice in Britain almost coincidentally with the introduction of the LMA, it was soon noted that propofol suppressed pharyngeal reflexes to a degree that permitted the insertion of the LMA without a need for either muscle relaxants or potent inhaled anesthetics.

THE EVOLUTION OF PROFESSIONAL ANESTHESIOLOGY

Anesthesiology evolved slowly as a medical specialty in the United States in part because of the presence of a second group of anesthesia care providers, nurse anesthetists. During the late 19th century, small communities were often served by a single physician, who assigned a nurse to "drop" ether under his direction. In larger towns, doctors practiced independently and did not welcome being placed in what they perceived to be the subordinate role of anesthetist while their competitors enhanced their surgical reputations and collected the larger fees. Many American surgeons recalled the simple techniques they had practiced as junior house officers and regarded anesthesia as a technical craft that could be left to anyone. Some hospitals preferred to pay a salary to an anesthesia nurse while gaining a profit from the fees charged for that person's services. The most compelling argument to be advanced in favor of nurse anesthesia was that of skill: a trained nurse who administered anesthetics every working day was to be preferred to a physician who gave anesthesia only rarely.

Before the beginning of the 20th century, Mary Botsford and Isabella Herb were among the first Americans to become specialists in anesthesia. Both women were highly regarded as clinicians and also were influential in the formation of specialty societies. Dr. Mary Botsford is believed to have been the first woman to establish a practice as a specialist in anesthesia. In 1897, she became the anesthesiologist at a children's hospital in San Francisco. Following her example, several other Californian female physicians entered the specialty. Botsford later received the first academic appointment in anesthesia in the western United States when she became Clinical Professor of Anesthesia at the University of California, San Francisco. Botsford also served as the president of the Associated Anesthetists of the United States and Canada.

One of the first physicians to actually declare himself a "specialist in anesthesia" was Sydney Ormond Goldan of New York, who published seven articles in 1900, including an early description of the use of cocaine for spinal anesthesia. After studying Goldan's early career, Raymond Fink recognized in him some of the qualities of many modern anesthesiologists: "He was

brimful of enthusiasm for anesthesia, an excellent communicator and a prolific writer, a gadgeteer and the owner of several patents of anesthesia equipment."[73] At a time when many surgeons considered that spinal anesthesia did away with their need for an anesthesiologist, Goldan was particularly bold in his written opinions. He called for equality between surgeon and anesthesiologist and was among the first to state that the anesthesiologist had a right to establish and collect his own fee. Goldan regarded the anesthesiologist as being more important than the surgeon to the welfare of the patient. His forthright pronouncements may not have been well received, for he was not listed among the nine founding members of the Long Island Society of Anesthetists when the nation's first specialty society was founded on October 6, 1905, with annual dues of $1.00.

Since the training of physician anesthetists around the turn of the century lacked uniformity, many prominent surgeons preferred nurse anesthetists and directed the training of the most able candidates they could recruit. The Mayo brothers' personal anesthetist was Alice Magaw. George W. Crile relied on the skills of Agatha Hodgins. During World War I, Agatha Hodgins, Geraldine Gerrard, Ann Penland, and Sophie Gran were among the more than 100 nurse anesthetists who attended thousands of American and Allied casualties in France. On their return to the United States, many developed schools of nurse anesthesia.[74] Physician anesthetists sought to obtain respect among their surgical colleagues by organizing professional societies and improving the quality of training.

Organized Anesthesiology

After 1911, the annual fee rose to $3.00 when the Long Island Society became the New York Society of Anesthetists. Although the new organization still carried a local title, it drew members from several states and had a membership of 70 physicians in 1915. A second society with roots in the Midwest became the short-lived American Association of Anesthetists, which, by 1915, became the Interstate Association of Anesthetists. Almost all of the approximately 100 professional anesthesiologists in America belonged to both societies.

One of the most noteworthy figures in the struggle to professionalize anesthesiology was Francis Hoffer McMechan. McMechan had been a practicing anesthesiologist in Cincinnati until 1911, when he suffered a severe first attack of rheumatoid arthritis, which was to leave him confined to a wheelchair, and forced his retirement from the operating room in 1915. McMechan had been in practice only fifteen years, but he had written eighteen clinical articles in this short time. A prolific researcher and writer, McMechan did not permit his crippling disease to sideline his career. Instead of pursuing goals in clinical medicine, he applied his talents to establishing anesthesiology societies.[75]

McMechan supported himself and his devoted wife through editing the *Quarterly Supplement* from 1914 until August 1922, when he became editor of the first journal devoted to anesthesia, *Current Researches in Anesthesia and Analgesia,* the precursor of *Anesthesia and Analgesia,* the oldest journal of the specialty. As well as fostering the organization of the International Anesthesia Research Society (IARS) in 1925, Francis and his wife Laurette McMechan became overseas ambassadors of American anesthesia. Since Laurette was French, it was understandable that McMechan combined his own ideas about anesthesiology with concepts from abroad.[76]

In 1926, McMechan held the Congress of Anesthetists in a joint conference with the Section on Anaesthetics of the British Medical Association. Subsequently, he traveled throughout Europe, giving lectures and networking physicians in the field. Upon his final return to America, he was gravely ill and was confined to bed for two years. His hard work and constant travel paid dividends, however: in 1929, the IARS, which McMechan founded in 1922, had members not only from North America, but from several European countries, Japan, India, Argentina, and Brazil.[77]

In the 1930s, McMechan expanded his mission from organizing anesthesiologists to promoting the academic aspects of the specialty. In 1931, work began on what would become the International College of Anesthetists. This body began to award fellowships in 1935. For the first time, physicians were recognized as specialists in anesthesiology. The certification qualifications were universal, and fellows were recognized as specialists in several countries. Although the criteria for certification were not strict, the College was a success in raising the standards of anesthesia practice in many nations. In 1939, McMechan finally succumbed to illness, and the anesthesia world lost their tireless leader.

Other Americans participated in the promotion of organized anesthesiology. Ralph Waters participated in the evolving anesthesia society; his greatest contribution to the specialty was raising its academic standards. After completing his internship in 1913, he entered medical practice in Sioux City, Iowa, where he gradually limited his practice to anesthesia. His personal experience and extensive reading were supplemented by the only postgraduate training available, a 1-month course conducted in Ohio by E. I. McKesson. At that time, the custom of becoming a self-proclaimed specialist in medicine and surgery was not uncommon. Waters, who was frustrated by low standards and who would eventually have a great influence on establishing both anesthesia residency training and the formal examination process, recalled that before 1920, "The requirements for specialization in many midwestern hospitals consisted of the possession of sufficient audacity to attempt a procedure and persuasive power adequate to gain the consent of the patient or his family."[78]

In an effort to improve anesthetic care, Waters regularly corresponded with Dennis Jackson and other scientists. In 1925, he relocated to Kansas City with a goal of gaining an academic post at the University of Kansas, but the professor of surgery failed to support his proposal. The larger city did allow him to initiate his freestanding outpatient surgical facility, "The Downtown Surgical Clinic," which featured one of the first postanesthetic recovery rooms. In 1927, Erwin Schmidt, professor of surgery at the University of Wisconsin's medical school, encouraged Dean Charles Bardeen to recruit Waters.

In accepting the first American academic position in anesthesia, Waters described four objectives that have been since adopted by many other academic departments. His goals were as follows: "(1) to provide the best possible service to patients of the institution; (2) to teach what is known of the principles of Anesthesiology to all candidates for their medical degree; (3) to help long-term graduate students not only to gain a fundamental knowledge of the subject and to master the art of administration, but also to learn as much as possible of the effective methods of teaching; (4) to accompany these efforts with the encouragement of as much cooperative investigation as is consistent with achieving the first objectives."[79]

Ralph Waters' personal and professional qualities impressed talented young men and women who sought residency posts in his department. He encouraged residents to initiate research interests in which they collaborated with two pharmacologists whom Waters had known previously, Arthur Loevenhart and Chauncey Leake, as well as others with whom he became associated in Madison. Clinical concerns were also investigated. As an example, anesthesia records were coded onto punch cards to form a data base that was used to analyze departmental activities. Morbidity and mortality meetings, now a requirement of all training programs, also originated in Madison. They were attended by members of the department and distinguished visitors from other centers. As a consequence of their critical reviews of the conduct of anesthesia, responsibility for an operative tragedy gradually passed from the patient to the physician. In more casual times, a practitioner could complain, "The patient died because he did not take a good anesthetic." Alternatively, the death might be attributed to a mysterious force such as "status lymphaticus," of which Arthur Guedel, a master of sardonic humor, observed, "Certainly status lymphaticus is at times a great help to the anesthetist. When he has a fatality under anesthesia with no other cleansing explanation he is glad to recognize the condition as an entity."[79] Through the instruction received from Ralph Waters and his colleagues, anesthesiologists in training learned to accept responsibility for their actions by realizing that the fault often was the responsibility of the provider and not the patient who was denied a voice in the clinical debate.

The University of Wisconsin became a regular destination for other specialists. In 1929, Ralph Waters helped organize the Anesthesia "Travel Club," whose members were leading American or Canadian teachers of anesthesia. Each year one member was the host for a group of 20 to 40 anesthesiologists who gathered for a program of informal discussions. There were demonstrations of promising innovations for the operating room and laboratory, which were all subjected to what is remembered as a "high-spirited, energetic, critical review." Even during the lean years of the Depression, international guests also visited. For Geoffrey Kaye of Australia, Torsten Gordth of Sweden, Robert Macintosh and Michael Nosworthy of England, and scores of others, Waters' department was their "mecca of anesthesia." It soon became the model for other academic departments in Europe, South America, and Asia.

Ralph Waters trained 60 residents during the 22 years he was the "chief." From 1937 onward, the alumni, who declared themselves the "Aqualumni" in his honor, returned annually for a professional and social reunion. Thirty-four "Aqualumni" took academic positions, and, of these, 14 became chairpersons of departments of anesthesia. They maintained Waters' professional principles and encouraged teaching careers for many of their own graduates. Sixty-five years after Waters arrived in Madison, more than 80 chairpersons or former chairpersons of academic departments could trace their professional lineage back to Ralph Waters. A great majority of the departments of anesthesia with residency programs in the United States have faculty members who were trained in a department led by a professional "descendant" of Ralph Waters.[80] His enduring legacy was once recognized by the dean who had recruited him in 1927, Charles Bardeen, who observed, "Ralph Waters was the first person the University hired to put people to sleep, but, instead, he awakened a world-wide interest in anesthesia."

Waters also had an important role in establishing organized anesthesia. He energetically supported the growth of physician anesthesia organizations. He supported Paul Wood's drive to give the pre-eminent New York Society of Anesthetists a title reflecting its national role. In 1936, the American Society of Anesthetists was formed from the New York Society in an effort to show the American Medical Association (AMA) that a national anesthesia society favored certification of specialists in the field. Combined with the American Society of Regional Anesthesia, whose president was Emery Rovenstine, the American Board of Anesthesiology (ABA) was organized as a subordinate board to the American Board of Surgery. With McMechan's death in 1939, the AMA favored independence for the ABA largely through the efforts of John Lundy. In 1940, independence was granted.

A few years later, the officers of the American Society of Anesthetists were challenged by Dr. M. J. Seifert, who wrote, "An Anesthetist is a technician and an Anesthesiologist is the specific authority on anesthesia and anesthetics. I cannot understand why you do not term yourselves the American Society of Anesthesiologists."[81] Ralph Waters was declared the first president of the newly named ASA in 1945. In that year, when World War II ended, 739 (37%) of 1977 ASA members were in the armed forces. In the same year, the ASA's first Distinguished Service Award (DSA) was presented to Paul M. Wood for his tireless service to the specialty, one element of which can be examined today in the extensive archives preserved in the Society's Wood Library Museum at ASA headquarters, Park Ridge, Illinois.[82]

After World War II, specialties within the realm of anesthesiology began to thrive. Kathleen Belton was a superb pediatric specialist. In 1948, while working in Montreal, Belton and her colleague, Digby Leigh, wrote the classic text, *Pediatric Anesthesia.* At the same time, a second pediatric anesthesiologist, Margot Deming, was the Director of Anesthesia at the Children's Hospital of Philadelphia. Pediatric anesthesia also figured in the career of Doreen Vermeulen-Cranch, who had earlier initiated thoracic anesthesia in The Netherlands and pioneered hypothermic anesthesia. Obstetric anesthesia also figured prominently in the career of Virginia Apgar. After encountering severe financial and professional frustrations during her training and while serving as Director of the Division of Anesthesia at Columbia University, Apgar turned to obstetric anesthesia in 1949. She dedicated the next decade of her multifaceted career to the care of mothers and their infants.[83]

THE SCOPE OF
MODERN ANESTHESIOLOGY

This overview of the development of anesthesiology could be extended almost indefinitely by an exploration of each subspecialty area, but an assessment of our current roles can be seen by a personal survey of the areas in which anesthesiologists serve in hospitals, clinics, and laboratories. The operating room and obstetric delivery suite remain the central interest of most specialists. Aside from being the location where the techniques described in this chapter find regular application, service in these areas brings us into regular contact with new advances in pharmacology and bioengineering.

After surgery, patients are transported to the postanesthesia care unit or recovery room, an area that is now considered the anesthesiologist's "ward." Fifty years ago, patients were carried directly from the operating room to a surgical ward to be attended only by a junior nurse. That person lacked both the skills and equipment to intervene when complications occurred. After the experiences of World War II taught the value of centralized care, physicians and nurses created recovery rooms, which were soon mandated for all major hospitals. By 1960 the evolution of critical care progressed through the use of mechanical ventilators. Patients who required many days of intensive medical and nursing management were cared for in a curtained corner of the recovery room. In time, curtains drawn about one or two beds gave way to fixed partitions and the relocation of those areas to form intensive care units. The principles of resuscitative and supportive care established by anesthesiologists transformed critical care medicine.

The future of anesthesiology is a bright one. The safer drugs that once revolutionized the care of patients undergoing surgery are constantly being improved upon. The role of the anesthesiologist continues to broaden, as physicians with backgrounds in the specialty have developed clinics for chronic pain control and outpatient surgery. Anesthesia practice will continue to increase in scope, both inside and outside of the operating suite, such that anesthesiologists will become an integral part of the entire perioperative experience.

REFERENCES

1. Duncum BM: The Development of Inhalation Anaesthesia, p 86. London, Oxford University Press, 1947
2. Dioscorides: On mandragora. In: *Dioscorides Opera Libra.* Quoted in Bergman N: The Genesis of Surgical Anesthesia, p 11. Park Ridge, Illinois, Wood Library-Museum, 1998
3. Infusino M, Viole O'Neill Y, Calmes S: Hog beans, poppies, and mandrake leaves—A test of the efficacy of the soporific sponge. In: The History of Anaesthesia p 31. London, Parthenon Publishing Group, 1989
4. Bacon, DR: Regional anesthesia and chronic pain therapy: A history. In Brown DL (ed): Regional Anesthesia and Analgesia, p 11. Philadelphia, WB Saunders, 1996
5. Davy H: Researches Chemical and Philosophical Chiefly Concerning Nitrous Oxide or Dephlogisticated Nitrous Air, and Its Respiration, p 533. London, J Johnson, 1800
6. Lyman HM: Artificial Anaesthesia and Anaesthetics, p 6. New York, William Wood, 1881
7. Steston JB: William E. Clarke and the discovery of anesthesia. In Fink BR, Morris L, Stephen CR (eds): The History of Anesthesia: Third International Symposium Proceedings. Park Ridge, Illinois, Wood Library-Museum, 1992
8. Long CW: An account of the first use of sulphuric ether by inhalation as an anaesthetic in surgical operations. South Med Surg J 5:705, 1849
9. Smith GB, Hirsch NP: Gardner Quincy Colton: Pioneer of nitrous oxide anesthesia. Anesth Analg 72:382, 1991
10. Greene NM: A consideration of factors in the discovery of anesthesia and their effects on its development. Anesthesiology 35:515, 1971
11. Duncum BM: The Development of Inhalation Anaesthesia, p 110. London, Oxford University Press, 1947
12. Caton D: What a Blessing She Had Chloroform, p 103. New Haven, Connecticut, Yale University Press, 1999
13. Caton D: What a Blessing She Had Chloroform, p 106. New Haven, Connecticut, Yale University Press, 1999
14. Journal of Queen Victoria. In Strauss MB (ed): Familiar Medical Quotations, p 17. Boston, Little, Brown, 1968
15. Calverley RK: An early ether vaporizer designed by John Snow, a Treasure of the Wood Library-Museum of Anesthesiology. In Fink BR, Morris LE, Stephen CR (eds): The History of Anesthesia, p 91. Park Ridge, Illinois, Wood Library-Museum, 1992
16. Snow J: On the Inhalation of the Vapour of Ether, p 23 (reprinted by the Wood Library-Museum). London, J Churchill, 1847
17. Snow J: On Chloroform and Other Anesthetics, p 58 (reprinted by the Wood Library-Museum). London, J Churchill, 1858
18. Duncum BM: The Development of Inhalation Anaesthesia, p 540. London, Oxford University Press, 1947
19. Duncum BM: The Development of Inhalation Anaesthesia, p 538. London, Oxford University Press, 1947
20. Calverley RK: J. T. Clover: A giant of Victorian anaesthesia. In Rupreht J, van Lieburg MJ, Lee JA, Erdmann W (eds): Anaesthesia: Essays on Its History, p 21. Berlin, Springer-Verlag, 1985
21. Clover JT: Laryngotomy in chloroform anesthesia. Br Med J 1:132, 1877
22. Colton Dental Association (advertisement from the Public Ledger and Transcript, Philadelphia, December 4, 1869, Reynolds Historical Library, University of Alabama in Birmingham)
23. Andrews E: The oxygen mixture, a new anaesthetic combination. Chicago Medical Examiner 9:656, 1868
24. Becker HK: Carl Koller and cocaine. Psychoanal Q 32:332, 1963
25. Marx G: The first spinal anesthesia: Who deserves the laurels? Regional Anesth 19:429, 1994
26. Corning JL: Spinal anaesthesia and local medication of the cord. NY Med J 42:485, 1885
27. Bier AKG: Experiments in cocainization of the spinal cord, 1899. In Faulconer A, Keys TE (trans): Foundations of Anesthesiology, p 854. Springfield, Illinois, Charles C Thomas, 1965
28. Lee JA: Arthur Edward James Barker, 1850–1916: British pioneer of regional anaesthesia. Anaesthesia 34:885, 1979
29. Lemmon WT: A method for continuous spinal anesthesia: A preliminary report. Ann Surg 111:141, 1940
30. Tuohy EB: Continuous spinal anesthesia: Its usefulness and technic involved. Anesthesiology 5:142, 1944
31. Pagés F: Metameric anesthesia, 1921. In Faulconer A, Keys TE (trans): Foundations of Anesthesiology, p 927. Springfield, Illinois, Charles C Thomas, 1965
32. Fink BR: History of local anesthesia. In Cousins MJ, Bridenbaugh PO (eds): Neural Blockade, p 12. Philadelphia, JB Lippincott, 1980
33. Cushing H: On the avoidance of shock in major amputations by cocainization of large nerve trunks preliminary to their division: With observations on blood-pressure changes in surgical cases. Ann Surg 36:321, 1902
34. Bacon DR, Darwish H: Emery Rovenstine and regional anesthesia. Regional Anesth 22:273, 1997

35. Waters RM: Clinical scope and utility of carbon dioxide filtration in inhalation anesthesia. Curr Res Anesth Analg 3:20, 1923

36. Sword BC: The closed circle method of administration of gas anesthesia. Curr Res Anesth Analg 9:198, 1930

37. Sands RP, Bacon DR: An inventive mind: The career of James O. Elam, M.D. (1918–1995). Anesthesiology 88:1107, 1998

38. Obituary of T. Philip Ayre. Br Med J 280:125, 1980

39. Rees GJ: Anaesthesia in the newborn. Br Med J 2:1419, 1950

40. Bain JA, Spoerel WE: A stream-lined anaesthetic system. Can Anaesth Soc J 19:426, 1972

41. Morris LE: A new vaporizer for liquid anesthetic agents. Anesthesiology 13:587, 1952

42. Sands R, Bacon DR: The copper kettle: A historical perspective. J Clin Anesth 8:528, 1996

43. Shephard DAE: Harvey Cushing and anaesthesia. Can Anaesth Soc J 12:431, 1965

44. Mushin WW, Rendell-Baker L: Thoracic Anaesthesia Past and Present (reprinted by the Wood Library Museum, 1991). Springfield, Illinois, Charles C Thomas, 1953

45. Tovell RM: Problems in supply of anesthetic gases in the European theater of operations. Anesthesiology 8:303, 1947

46. Rendell-Baker L: History of standards for anesthesia equipment. In Rupreht J, van Lieburg MJ, Lee JA, Erdmann W (eds): Anaesthesia: Essays on Its History, p 161. Berlin, Springer-Verlag, 1985

47. Calverley RK: A safety feature for anaesthesia machines: Touch identification of oxygen flow control. Can Anaesth Soc J 18:225, 1971

48. Cushing H: On the avoidance of shock in major amputations by cocainization of large nerve trunks preliminary to their division: With observations on blood-pressure changes in surgical cases. Ann Surg 36:321, 1902

49. Shephard DAE: Harvey Cushing and anaesthesia. Can Anaesth Soc J 12:431, 1965

50. Codesmith A: An endo-esophageal stethoscope. Anesthesiology 15:566, 1954

51. Severinghaus JC, Honda Y: Pulse oximetry. Int Anesthesiol Clin 25:212, 1987

52. Severinghaus JC, Honda Y: Pulse oximetry. Int Anesthesiol Clin 25:206, 1987

53. Macewan W: Clinical observations on the introduction of tracheal tubes by the mouth instead of performing tracheotomy or laryngotomy. Br Med J 2:122, 163, 1880

54. Mushin WW, Rendell-Baker L: Thoracic Anaesthesia Past and Present, p 44 (reprinted by the Wood Library Museum, 1991). Springfield, Illinois, Charles C Thomas, 1953

55. Kuhn F: Nasotracheal intubation (trans): In Faulconer A, Keys TE (eds): Foundations of Anesthesiology, p 677. Springfield, Illinois, Charles C Thomas, 1965

56. Hirsch NP, Smith GB, Hirsch PO: Alfred Kirstein, pioneer of direct laryngoscopy. Anaesthesia 41:42, 1986

57. Miller RA: A new laryngoscope. Anesthesiology 2:317, 1941

58. Macintosh RR: Richard Salt of Oxford, anaesthetic technician extraordinary. Anaesthesia 31:855, 1976

59. Thomas KB: Sir Ivan Whiteside Magill, KCVO, DSc, MB, BCh, BAO, FRCS, FFARCS (Hon), FFARCSI (Hon), DA: A review of his publications and other references to his life and work. Anaesthesia 33:628, 1978

60. Condon HA, Gilchrist E: Stanley Rowbotham, twentieth century pioneer anaesthetist. Anaesthesia 41:46, 1986

61. Calverley RK: Arthur E Guedel (1883–1956). In Rupreht J, van Lieburg MJ, Lee JA, Erdmann W (eds): Anaesthesia: Essays on Its History, p 49. Berlin, Springer-Verlag, 1985

62. Calverley RK: Classical file. Surv Anesth 28:70, 1984

63. Gale JW, Waters RM: Closed endobronchial anesthesia in thoracic surgery: Preliminary report. Curr Res Anesth Analg 11:283, 1932

64. Brain AIJ: The laryngeal mask: A new concept in airway management. Br J Anaesth 55:801, 1983

65. Lucas GHW: The discovery of cyclopropane. Curr Res Anesth Analg 40:15, 1961

66. Calverley RK: Fluorinated anesthetics: I. The early years. Surv Anesth 29:170, 1986

67. Robbins BH: Preliminary studies of the anesthetic activity of the fluorinated hydrocarbons. J Pharmacol Exp Ther 86:197, 1946

68. Calverley RK: Fluorinated anesthetics: II. Fluroxene. Surv Anesth 30:126, 1987

69. Suckling CW: Some chemical and physical factors in the development of Fluothane. Br J Anaesth 29:466, 1957

70. Macintosh RR: Modern anaesthesia, with special reference to the chair of anaesthetics in Oxford. In Rupreht J, van Lieburg MJ, Lee JA, Erdmann W (eds): Anaesthesia: Essays on Its History, p 352. Berlin, Springer-Verlag, 1985

71. Knoefel PK: Felice Fontana: Life and Works, p 284. Trento, Societa de Studi Trentini, 1985

72. Griffith HR, Johnson GE: The use of curare in general anesthesia. Anesthesiology 3:418, 1942

73. Fink BR: Leaves and needles: The introduction of surgical local anesthesia. Anesthesiology 63:77, 1985

74. Bankert M: Watchful Care: A History of America's Nurse Anesthetists. New York, Continuum, 1989

75. Bacon DR: The promise of one great anesthesia society. Anesthesiology 80:929, 1994.

76. Seldon TH: Francis Hoeffer McMechan. In Volpitto PP, Vandam LD (eds): Genesis of American Anesthesiology, p 5. Springfield, Illinois, Charles C Thomas, 1982

77. Bacon DR: The world federation of societies of anesthesiologists: McMechan's final legacy? Anesth Analg 84:1131, 1997

78. Waters RM: Pioneering in anesthesiology. Postgrad Med 4:265, 1968

79. Guedel AE: Inhalation Anesthesia: A Fundamental Guide, p 129. New York, Macmillan, 1937

80. Bacon DR, Ament R: Ralph Waters and the beginnings of academic anesthesiology in the United States: The Wisconsin template. J Clin Anesth 7:534, 1995.

81. Little DM Jr, Betcher AM: The Diamond Jubilee 1905-1980, p 8. Park Ridge, Illinois, American Society of Anesthesiologists, 1980

82. Bamforth BJ, Siebecker KL: Ralph M. Waters. In Volpitto PP, Vandam LD (eds): Genesis of American Anesthesiology, p 51. Springfield, Illinois, Charles C Thomas, 1982

83. Calmes SH: Development of the Apgar Score. In Rupreht J, van Lieburgh MJ, Lee JA, Erdmann W (eds): Anaesthesia: Essays on Its History, p 45. Berlin, Springer-Verlag, 1985

Clinical Anesthesia (4/e), edited by
Paul G. Barash, Bruce F. Cullen, and
Robert K. Stoelting. Lippincott Williams &
Wilkins, Philadelphia, © 2001.

CHAPTER 2

PRACTICE MANAGEMENT

GEORGE MYCHASKIW II AND JOHN H. EICHHORN

The enormous changes in the practice of medicine that accelerated in the late 1990s are continuing in 2000. These changes have been occurring so quickly that treatises on practice management require constant updating. As a result, issues related to the mechanics, details, and finances of practice are demanding more attention and effort than at any previous time. Further, anesthesiologists traditionally have been little involved in the management of many components of practice that are beyond the strictly medical elements of applied physiology and pharmacology, pathophysiology, and therapeutics. This was, perhaps, somewhat understandable because anesthesiologists traditionally spent the vast majority of their time in a hospital operating room (OR) and thus were usually free of the concerns of running an office and managing a busy office-based practice. Very little formal teaching of or training in practice management of any kind occurred in anesthesiology residency programs. Word-of-mouth handing down of what was mostly folklore was often all an anesthesiology resident had to go on after completing training and beginning practice. Interestingly in this regard, the Anesthesiology Residency Review Committee of the Accreditation Council on Graduate Medical Education now requires that the didactic curricula of anesthesiology residencies include material on practice management. Today, most residency programs offer at least a cursory introduction to issues of practice management, but these can be insufficient to prepare satisfactorily the resident being graduated for the real business challenges of the practice of anesthesiology.

This chapter presents a wide variety of topics that, until very recently, were not in anesthesiology textbooks. Several basic components of the administrative, organizational, and financial aspects of anesthesiology practice are outlined. Included is mention of some of the issues associated with practice arrangements in the modern environment increasingly dominated by managed care. Although many of these issues are undergoing almost constant change, it is important to understand the basic vocabulary and principles of this dynamic field. Lack of understanding of these issues may put anesthesiologists at a disadvantage when attempting to forge practice arrangements and, particularly, lobby for a fair fraction of the fully capitated prospective payment health care dollar.

COMPONENTS COMMON TO ALL ANESTHESIOLOGY PRACTICES

Basic Operational Understandings

Practice arrangements and their implications for anesthesiology personnel are perceived as increasingly more important as medical care administration and reimbursement receive more scrutiny and emphasis. Certain basic underpinnings, albeit only a few, are very unlikely to face fundamental challenge. The American Society of Anesthesiologists (ASA) for many years has provided resource material to its members regarding practice in general and arrangements for its execution. These are updated regularly by the ASA through its committees and then its House of Delegates. Although these documents contain broad-brush generalities that must be interpreted in each individual's situa-

tion, they nonetheless stand as a solid foundation on which anesthesiology practice is based. In the past, many anesthesiologists were unaware of the existence of these resources and discovered them only when referred to them during an appeal to the ASA for help in resolving some significant practice problem. Prospective familiarity with these principles likely will help avoid some of the problems leading to calls for help. Further, many anesthesiologists do not know that, if members of the ASA, they receive copies of these and many related documents annually, because they are reprinted in the back of the ASA Directory of Members. A separate compilation of these and often very helpful related documents can be purchased.[1] The current atmosphere in American medicine, which creates the impression that "all of a sudden all the rules and understandings are changing," makes it virtually mandatory that anesthesiologists be familiar with the fundamental background of their profession. The ASA Guidelines for the Ethical Practice of Anesthesiology includes sections on the principles of medical ethics; the definition of medical direction of nonphysician personnel (including the specific statement that an anesthesiologist engaged in medical direction should not personally be administering another anesthetic); the anesthesiologist's relationship to patients and other physicians; the anesthesiologist's duties, responsibilities, and relationship to the hospital; and the anesthesiologist's relationship to nurse anesthetists and other nonphysician personnel. Further, the ASA publishes The Organization of an Anesthesia Department, and states through it that the ASA "has adopted a Statement of Policy, which contains principles that the Society urges its members to consider in structuring their own individual medical practices." This document has sections on physician responsibilities for medical care and on medicoadministrative organization and responsibilities. The ASA has been particularly proactive in helping its members keep up with rapidly changing areas of managed care and practice management, and now sponsors regular conferences specifically devoted to these issues. Additionally, practice management is becoming a regular feature of ASA regional refresher courses and of the annual meeting's refresher courses. In the past, some (probably many) anesthesiology residents finishing training felt unprepared, in a business and organizational sense, to enter the job market and had to learn through a self-taught crash course during negotiations for a position, sometimes to their detriment. Reference to the considerable body of material created and presented by the ASA (see also the section on Practice Arrangements) is a good starting point to help young anesthesiologists during residency to prepare for the increasing rigors of starting a career in the practice of anesthesiology.

The Internet

As of the advent of the year 2000, the Internet has become an important feature of many people's lives. Specifically, through the World Wide Web, more information is readily accessible to essentially any person at any location than at any other time in history. Anesthesiologists are no exception to this phenomenon, and, in fact, may utilize this means of information exchange more than other practitioners. Most anesthesiology societies now have Web locations, as do most journals. Several journals that exist only on the Internet are now in existence, and more are being rapidly developed. Electronic bulletin boards allow anesthesiology practitioners from around the world to immediately exchange ideas on diverse topics, both medical and administrative. Additionally, the body of medical literature is readily accessible to any practitioner, and it is reasonable to assume that practitioners may be held to a higher standard regarding knowledge of the latest published data, which may affect anesthesia practice. Even a superficial overview of the Internet and anesthesiology practice is far outside the scope of this chapter. A modern anesthesiology practice, however, cannot reasonably exist without an Internet connection. Numerous resources are available for further information on the Internet and anesthesiology, including books and journals dedicated specifically to this topic. The "gasnet" (www.gasnet.org) is one World Wide Web site that is particularly helpful. The Web site of the ASA (www.asahq.org) is also a good starting point, as is the site of the Anesthesia Patient Safety Foundation (www.apsf.org).

The Credentialing Process and Clinical Privileges

The system of credentialing a health care professional and granting clinical privileges is motivated by a fundamental assumption that appropriate education, training, and experience, along with the absence of excessive numbers of poor patient outcomes, increase the chances that the individual will deliver acceptable-quality care. As a result, the systems have received considerably increased emphasis in recent years. The process of credentialing health care professionals has been the focus of considerable public attention (particularly in the mass media), in part the result of very rare incidents of untrained persons (impostors) infiltrating the health care system and sometimes harming patients. The more common situation, however, involves health professionals who exaggerate past experience and credentials or fail to disclose adverse past experiences. There has been some justified publicity concerning physicians who lost their licenses sequentially in several states and simply moved on each time to start practice elsewhere (which should be much, much more difficult now).

The patient–physician relationship also has changed radically, with a concomitant increase in suspicion directed toward the medical profession. There is now a pervasive public perception that physicians are inadequately policed, particularly by their own professional organizations and hospitals. Intense public and political pressure has been brought to bear on various law-making bodies, regulatory and licensing agencies, and health care institution administrations to discover and purge both (1) fraudulent, criminal, and deviant health care providers, and (2) incompetent or simply poor-quality practitioners whose histories show sufficient poor patient outcomes to attract attention, usually through malpractice suits. Identifying and avoiding or correcting an incompetent practitioner is the goal. Verification of appropriate education, training, and experience on the part of a candidate for a position rendering anesthesia care assumes special importance in light of the legal doctrine of *vicarious liability,* which can be described as follows: if an individual, group, or institution hires an anesthesia provider or even simply approves of that person (*e.g.,* by granting clinical privileges through a hospital medical staff), those involved in the decision may later be held liable in the courts, along with the individual, for the individual's actions. This would be especially true if it were later discovered that the offending practitioner's past adverse outcomes had not been adequately investigated during the credentialing process.

Out of these various long-standing concerns has arisen the sometimes cumbersome process of obtaining state licenses to practice and of obtaining hospital privileges. It is somewhat analogous to passing through screening and metal detection devices at airports, which is tolerated by the individual in the interest of the safety of all. The stringent credentialing process is intended both to protect patients and to safeguard the integrity of the medical profession. Recently, central credentialing systems have been developed, including those affiliated with the American Medical Association, American Osteopathic Association, and the Federation of State Medical Boards. Perhaps one credentialing entity will become a virtual "universal metal detector" to make the process simpler while maintaining stringent standards and verification mechanisms. At this time, however, these have yet to be fully developed or universally accepted, and the current cumbersome system remains in force in most instances.

There are checklists of the requirements for the granting of medical staff privileges by hospitals.[2,3] In addition, the National Practitioner Data Bank and reporting system administered by the U.S. government now has several years' worth of information in it. This data bank is a central repository of licensing and credentials information about physicians. Many adverse situations involving a physician—particularly instances of substance abuse, malpractice litigation, or the revocation, suspension, or limitation of that physician's license to practice medicine or to hold hospital privileges—must be reported (*via* the state board of medical registration/licensure) to the National Practitioner Data Bank. It is a statutory requirement that all applications for hospital staff privileges be cross-checked against this national data bank. The potential medicolegal liability on the part of a facility's medical staff, and the anesthesiology group in particular, for failing to do so is staggering. The Data Bank, however, is not a complete substitute for direct documentation and background checking. Often, practitioners reach negotiated solutions following medical staff problems, thereby avoiding the mandatory reporting. That is, a suspect physician may be given the option to resign medical staff privileges and avoid Data Bank reporting, rather than undergo full involuntary privilege revocation.

The documentation for the credentialing process for each anesthesia practitioner must be complete. Privileges to administer anesthesia must be officially granted and delineated in writing.[1,2] This can be straightforward (and there are good models offered by the ASA[4]); or it can be more complex to accommodate institutional needs to identify practitioners qualified to practice in designated anesthesia subspecialty areas such as cardiac, infant/pediatric, obstetric, intensive care, or pain management. Specific documentation of the process of granting or renewing clinical privileges is required and, unlike some other records, the documentation is protected as confidential peer review information under the Federal Health Care Quality Improvement Act of 1986. A related 1988 U.S. Supreme Court decision questioning this confidentiality involved a case that occurred in 1981. The 1986 federal law is constructed so that it still applies now, even in light of the 1988 decision.

Verification of credentials and experience is mandatory. Because of another type of legal case, some examples of which have been highly publicized, medical practitioners may be hesitant to give an honest evaluation (or any evaluation at all) of individuals known to them who are seeking a professional position elsewhere. Obviously, someone writing a reference for a current or former co-worker should be honest. Sticking to clearly documentable facts is advisable. Stating a fact that is in the public record (such as a malpractice case lost at trial) should not justify an objection from the subject of the reference. Whether omitting such a fact is dishonest on the part of the reference writer is more of a gray area. Including positive opinions and enthusiastic recommendations, of course, is no problem. Some fear that including facts that may be perceived as negative (*e.g.,* the lost malpractice case or personal problems such as a history of treatment for substance abuse) and negative opinions will provoke retaliatory lawsuits (such as for libel, defamation of character, or loss of livelihood) from the subject. As a result, many reference writers in these questionable situations confine their written material to brief, simple facts such as dates employed and position held.

Because there should be no hesitation for a reference writer to include positive opinions, receipt of a reference that includes nothing more than dates worked and position held should be a suggestion that there may be more to the story. Receipt of such a reference about a person applying for a position should always lead to a telephone call to the writer. A telephone call may be advisable in all cases, independent of whatever the written reference contains. Frequently, pertinent questions over the telephone can elicit more candid information. In rare instances, there may be dishonesty through omission by the reference giver even at this level. This may involve an applicant who an individual, a department or group, or an institution would like to see leave. The subject may have poor-quality practice, but there may also be reluctance by the reference giver(s) to approach licensing or disciplinary authorities (because of the unpleasantness and also out of concern about retaliatory legal action). This type of ''sandbagging'' is fortunately infrequent. The best way to avoid it is to telephone an independent observer or source (such as a former employer or associate who no longer has a personal stake in the applicant's success) when any question exists. Because the ultimate goal is optimum patient care, the subjects applying for positions generally should not object to such calls being made. Discovery of a history of unsafe practices and/or habits or of causing preventable anesthesia morbidity or mortality should elicit careful evaluation as to whether the applicant can be appropriately assigned, trained, and/or supervised to be maximally safe in the proposed new environment.

In all cases, new personnel in an anesthesia practice environment must be given a thorough orientation and checkout. Policy, procedures, and equipment may be unfamiliar to even the most thoroughly trained, experienced, and safe practitioner. This may occasionally seem tedious, but it is both sound and critically important safety policy. Being in the midst of a crisis situation caused by unfamiliarity with a new setting is not the optimal orientation session.

After the initial granting of clinical privileges to practice anesthesia, anesthesiologists must periodically renew their privileges within the institution or facility (*e.g.*, annually or every other year). There are moral, ethical, and societal obligations on the part of the privilege-granting entity to take this process seriously. State licensing bodies often become aware of problems with health professionals very late in the evolution of the difficulties. An anesthesia provider's peers in the hospital or facility are much more likely to notice untoward developments as they first appear. However, privilege renewals are often essentially automatic and receive little of the necessary attention. Judicious checking of renewal applications and awareness of relevant peer review information is absolutely necessary. The physicians or administrators responsible for evaluating staff members and reviewing their practices and privileges may be justifiably concerned about retaliatory legal action by a staff member who is censured or denied privilege renewal. Accordingly, such evaluating groups must be thoroughly objective (totally eliminating any hint of political or financial motives) and must have documentation that the staff person in question is in fact practicing below the standard of care. Court decisions have found liability by a hospital, its medical staff group, or both when the incompetence of a staff member was known or should have been known and was not acted upon.[3]

A major issue in the granting of clinical privileges, especially in procedure-oriented specialties such as anesthesiology, is whether it is reasonable to continue the common practice of ''blanket'' privileges. This process in effect authorizes the practitioner to attempt any treatment or procedure normally considered within the purview of the applicant's medical specialty. These considerations may have profound political and economic implications within medicine, such as which type of surgeon should be doing carotid endarterectomies or lumbar diskectomies. More important, however, is whether the practitioner being evaluated is qualified to do everything traditionally associated with the specialty. Specifically, should the granting of privileges to practice anesthesia automatically approve the practitioner to handle pediatric cardiac cases, critically ill newborns (such as a day-old infant with a large diaphragmatic hernia), ablative pain therapy (such as an alcohol celiac plexus block under fluoroscopy), high-risk obstetric cases, and so forth? This question raises the issue of procedure-specific or limited privileges. The quality assurance (QA) and risk management considerations in this question are weighty if inexperienced or insufficiently qualified practitioners are allowed or even expected, because of peer or scheduling pressures, to undertake major challenges for which they are not prepared. The likelihood of complications will be higher, and the difficulty of defending the practitioner against a malpractice claim in the event of catastrophe will be significantly increased.

There is no clear answer to the question of procedure-specific credentialing and granting of privileges. Ignoring issues regarding qualifications to undertake complex and challenging procedures has clear negative potential. On the other hand, stringent procedure-specific credentialing is impractical in smaller groups, and in larger groups encourages many small ''fiefdoms,'' with a consequent further atrophy of the clinical skills outside of the practitioner's specific areas. Each anesthesia department or group needs to address these issues. At the very least, the common practice of every applicant for privileges (new or renewal) checking off every line on the printed list of anesthesia procedures should be reviewed. Additionally, board certification is now essentially a standard of quality assurance of the minimum skills required for the consultant practice of anesthesiology. Subspecialty boards, such as those in pain management, critical care, and transesophageal echocardiography further objectify the credentialing process. This will become even more significant in the year 2000, when newly issued board certification by the American Board of Anesthesiology will become time-limited and subject to periodic testing and recertification. Finally, the Joint Commission on the Accreditation of Healthcare Organizations (JCAHO) mandates a minimum of 150 hours of AMA category 1 continuing medical education every three years for anesthesiologists. Documentation of meeting this standard again acts as a quality assurance mechanism for the individual practitioner, while providing another objective credentialing measurement.

Medical Staff Participation and Relationships

All medical care facilities and practice settings depend on their medical staffs, of course, for daily activities of the delivery of health care; but, very importantly, they also depend on those staffs to provide administrative structure and support. Medical staff activities are increasingly important in achieving favorable accreditation status (*e.g.*, from the JCAHO) and in meeting a wide variety of governmental regulations and reviews. Principal medical staff activities involve sometimes time-consuming efforts, such as duties as a staff officer or committee member. Anesthesiologists should be participants in—in fact, should play a significant role in—credentialing, peer review, tissue review, transfusion review, OR management, and medical direction of same-day surgery units, postanesthesia care units (PACUs), intensive care units (ICUs), and pain management units. Also, it is very important that anesthesiology personnel be involved in fund-raising activities, benefits, community outreach projects sponsored by the facility, and social events of the facility staff.

The role these and related activities play in anesthesia practice management may not be obvious at first glance, but this is a reflection of the unfortunate fact that, all too often, anesthesiologists have chosen to have very little or no involvement in such efforts. Of course, there are exceptions in specific settings.

However, it is an unmistakable reality that anesthesiologists as a group have a reputation for lack of involvement in medical staff and facility issues due to lack of interest. In fact, anesthesiology personnel are all too often perceived as the ones who slip in and out of the facility anonymously (dressed very casually or even in the pajama-like comfort of scrub suits) and virtually unnoticed. This is an unfortunate state of affairs, and it is starting to come back to haunt those who have not been involved, or even noticed. Anesthesiology personnel sometimes respond that the demands for anesthesiology service are so great that they simply never have the time or the opportunity to become involved. If this is really true, it is likely that more providers of anesthesia care are needed.

In any case, anesthesiologists simply must make the time to be involved in medical staff affairs, both in health care facilities and as part of the organization, administration, and governance of the comparatively large multispecialty physician groups that provide entities with which managed care organizations (MCOs) and health care facilities can negotiate for physician services. The types and styles of these organizations vary widely and are discussed extensively below. The point here is simple. If anesthesiologists are not involved and not perceived as interested, dedicated "team players," they will be shut out of critical negotiations and decisions. Although the most obvious instance in which others will make decisions for anesthesiologists is the distribution of capitated fee income collected by a central "umbrella" organization, there are many such situations; and anesthesiologists will have to comply with the resulting mandates. In the most basic terms, absence from the bargaining table and/or being seen as not involved in the welfare of the large group virtually ensure that anesthesiologists will not receive their "fair share of the pie."

Similarly, involvement with a facility, a medical staff, or a multispecialty group goes beyond formal organized governance and committee activity. Collegial relationships with physicians of other specialties and with administrators are central to maintenance of a recognized position and avoidance of the situation of exclusion described above. Being readily available for formal and informal consults, particularly regarding preoperative patient workup and the maximally efficient and certain way to get surgeons' patients to the OR in a timely, expedient manner, is extremely important. No one individual can be everywhere all the time, but an anesthesiology group or department should strive to be always responsive to any request for help from physicians or administrators. It often appears that anesthesiologists underappreciate just how great a positive impact a relatively simple involvement (starting an intravenous line for a pediatrician, helping an internist manage an ICU ventilator, or helping a facility administrator unclog a jammed recovery room) may have. Unfortunately, anesthesiologists in a great many locations have a negative stereotype to overcome and must work to maintain the perception that they deserve an equal voice regarding the impact of the current changes in the health care system.

Establishing Standards of Practice and Understanding the Standard of Care

Given all the current and future changes in the anesthesiology practice environment, it is more important than ever that anesthesiologists genuinely understand what is expected of them in their clinical practice. The increasing frequency of "production pressure,"[5] with the tacit (or even explicit) directive to anesthesia personnel to "go fast" no matter what and to "do more with less," creates situations in which anesthesiologists may conclude that they must cut corners and compromise maximally safe care just to stay in business. This type of pressure has become even greater with the implementation of more and more protocols or parameters for practice, some from professional societies such as the ASA and some mandated by or developed in conjunction with purchasers of health care (insurance com-

panies or MCOs). Many of these protocols are devised to fast-track patients through the medical care system, especially when an elective procedure is involved, in as absolutely little time as possible, thus minimizing costs. Do these fast-track protocols constitute standards of care that health care providers are mandated to implement? What are the implications of doing so? Of not doing so?

To better understand answers to such questions, it is important to have a basic background in the concept of the *standard of care*. Anesthesiology personnel are fortunate in this regard because for at least a decade American anesthesiology has been recognized as one of the significant leaders in establishing practice standards intended to maximize the quality of patient care and help guide personnel at times of difficult decisions, including the risk–benefit and cost–benefit decisions of specific practices. Another important component of this issue is the unique legal system in the United States, in which the potential liability implications of most decisions must be considered. Businesses, groups, and individuals have had their entire public existences destroyed by staggering legal settlements and judgments allowed by the U.S. legal system. Major attempts at reform of this system have occurred and will continue to occur. However, although a very positive restructuring of the tort liability system could alleviate some of the catecholamine-generating "sword over the head" mentality exhibited by some physicians, it will not relieve anesthesiology personnel of the responsibility to provide maximally safe care for their patients. Integration of systems and protocols to help maximize the quality of patient care, whether from formal standards or not, is an important component of managing an anesthesiology practice.

The *standard of care* is the conduct and skill of a prudent practitioner that can be expected by a reasonable patient. This is a very important medicolegal concept because a bad medical result due to failure to meet the standard of care is malpractice. Extensive discussions have attempted to establish exactly the applicable standard of care. Courts have traditionally relied on medical experts knowledgeable about the point in question to give opinions as to what is the standard of care and if it has been met in an individual case. This type of standard is somewhat different from the standards promulgated by various standard-setting bodies regarding, for example, the color of gas hoses connected to an anesthesia machine or the inability to open two vaporizers on that machine simultaneously. However, ignoring the equipment standards and tolerating an unsafe situation is a violation of the standard of care. Promulgated standards, such as the various safety codes and anesthesia machine specifications, rapidly become the standard of care because patients (through their attorneys, in the case of an untoward event) expect the published standards to be observed by the prudent practitioner.

Understanding the concept of the standard of care is the key to integrating the numerous standards, guidelines, practice parameters, and suggested protocols applicable to American anesthesiology practice in the unfortunately necessary constant undercurrent of concern about potential legal liability. Ultimately, the standard of care is what a jury says it is. However, it is possible to anticipate, at least in part, what knowledge and actions will be expected. There are two main sources of information as to exactly what is the expected standard of care. Traditionally, the beliefs offered by expert witnesses in medical liability lawsuits regarding what was being done in real life (*de facto* standards of care) were the main input juries had in deciding what was reasonable to expect from the defendant. The resulting problem is well known: except in the most egregious cases, it is usually possible for the lawyers to find experts who will support each of the two opposing sides, making the process more subjective than objective. (Because of this, there are even official ASA Guidelines for Expert Witness Qualifications and Testimony.[6]) Of course, there can be legitimate differences of opinion among thoughtful, insightful experts, but even in these cases the jury still must decide who is more believable, looks better, or sounds better. The second, much more objective, source for defining certain component parts of the standard of care has developed over the past decade or so in anesthesiology. It is the published standards of care, guidelines, practice parameters, and protocols now becoming more common. These serve as hard evidence of what can be reasonably expected of practitioners and can make it easier for a jury evaluating whether a malpractice defendant failed to meet the applicable standard of care. Several types of documents exist and have differing implications.

Anesthesiology may be the medical specialty most involved with published standards of care. It has been suggested that the nature of anesthesia practice (having certain central critical functions relatively clearly defined and common to all situations and having an emphasis on technology) makes it the most amenable of all the fields of medicine to the use of published standards. The original intraoperative monitoring standards[7] are a classic example. The ASA first adopted its own set of basic intraoperative monitoring standards in 1986 and has modified them several times (Table 2-1). This document includes clear specifications for the presence of personnel during an anesthetic episode and for continual evaluation of oxygenation, ventilation, circulation, and temperature. The rationale for these monitoring standards is simple; it was felt that functionally mandating certain behaviors oriented toward providing the maximum possible warning of threatening developments during an anesthetic should help minimize intraoperative catastrophic patient injury. These ASA monitoring standards very quickly became part of the accepted standard of care in anesthesia practice. This means they are important to practice management because they have profound medicolegal implications: a catastrophic accident occurring while the standards are being actively ignored is very difficult to defend in the consequent malpractice suit, whereas an accident that occurs during well-documented full compliance with the standards will automatically have a strong defense because the standard of care was being met. Several states in the United States have made compliance with these ASA standards mandatory under state regulations or even statutes. Various malpractice insurance companies offer discounts on malpractice insurance policy premiums for compliance with these standards, something quite natural to insurers because they are familiar with the idea of managing known risks to help minimize financial loss to the company. The ASA monitoring standards have been widely emulated in other medical specialties and even in fields outside of medicine. Although there are definite parallels in these other efforts (such as in obstetrics and gynecology), no other group has pursued the same degree of definition.

Many of the same management questions that led to the intraoperative monitoring standards have close parallels in the immediate preoperative and postoperative periods in the PACU. With many of the same elements of thinking, the ASA has adopted Basic Standards for Preanesthesia Care (Table 2-2) and Standards for Postanesthesia Care (Table 2-3). For the latter, there was consideration of and collaboration with the very detailed standards of practice for PACU care published by the American Society of Post Anesthesia Nurses (another good example of the sources of standards of care).

A slightly different situation exists with regard to the standards for conduct of anesthesia in obstetrics. These standards were originally passed by the ASA in 1988, in the same manner as the other ASA standards, but the ASA membership eventually questioned whether they reflected a realistic and desirable standard of care. Accordingly, the obstetric anesthesia standards were downgraded in 1990 to guidelines (Table 2-4), specifically to remove the mandatory nature of the document. Because there was no agreement as to what should be prescribed as the standard of care, the medicolegal imperative of published standards has been temporarily set aside. From a management

perspective, this makes the guidelines no less valuable, because the intent of optimizing care through the avoidance of complications is no less operative. However, in the event of the need to defend against a malpractice claim in this area, it is clear from this sequence of events that the exact standard of care is debatable and not yet finally established. A new ASA document, Practice Guidelines for Obstetrical Anesthesia, of a new type with more detail and specificity as well as an emphasis on the meta-analytic approach was published in 1999.[8]

The newest type of related document is the practice parameter. This has some of the same elements as a standard of practice but is more intended to guide judgment, largely through algorithms with some element of guidelines, in addition to directing the details of specific procedures as would a formal standard. A good example of a set of practice parameters came some years ago from the cardiologists and addressed the indications for cardiac catheterization. Beyond the details of the minimum standards for carrying out the procedure, these practice parameters set forth algorithms and guidelines for helping to determine under what circumstances and with what timing to perform it. Understandably, purchasers of health care (insurance companies and MCOs) with a strong desire to limit the costs of medical care have great interest in practice parameters as potential vehicles for helping to eliminate "unnecessary" procedures and limit even the necessary ones.

The ASA has been very active in creating and publishing practice parameters. The first published parameter concerned the use of pulmonary artery (PA) catheters.[9] It considered the clinical effectiveness of PA catheters, public policy issues (costs and concerns of patients and providers), and recommendations (indications and practice settings). The next month, the ASA Difficult Airway Algorithm was published.[10] This thoughtful document synthesized a strategy summarized in a decision tree diagram for dealing acutely with airway problems. It has great clinical value, and it is reasonable to anticipate that it will be used to help many patients. However, all these documents are readily noticed by plaintiffs' lawyers, the difficult airway parameter from the ASA being an excellent example. An important and so-far undecided question is whether guidelines and practice parameters from recognized entities such as the ASA *define* the standard of care. There is no simple answer. This will be decided over time by practitioners' actions, debates in the literature, mandates from malpractice insurers, and, of course, court decisions. Some guidelines, such as the FDA preanesthetic apparatus checkout, are accepted as the standard of care. There will be debate among experts, but the practitioner must make the decision as to how to apply practice parameters such as those from the ASA. Practitioners have incorrectly assumed that they *must* do everything specified. This is clearly not true, yet there is a valid concern that these will someday be held up as defining the standard of care. Accordingly, prudent attention within the bounds of reason to the principles outlined in guidelines and parameters will put the practitioner in at least a reasonably defensible position, whereas radical deviation from them should be based on obvious exigencies of the situation at that moment or clear, defensible alternative beliefs (with documentation).

The ASA has many other task forces charged with the development of practice parameters. Several aspects of pain management, transesophageal echocardiography, policies for sedation by nonanesthesia personnel, preoperative fasting, and others have been published and will likely have at least the same impact as those noted above.

On the other hand, practice protocols, such as those for the fast-track management of coronary artery bypass graft patients, that are handed down by MCOs or health insurance companies are a different matter. Even though the desired implication is that practitioners must observe (or at least strongly consider) them, they do not have the same implications in defining the standard of care as the other documents. Practitioners must avoid getting trapped. It may well not be a valid legal defense

Table 2-1. AMERICAN SOCIETY OF ANESTHESIOLOGISTS STANDARDS FOR BASIC ANESTHETIC MONITORING

These Standards apply to all anesthesia care, although, in emergency circumstances, appropriate life support measures take precedence. These standards may be exceeded at any time based on the judgment of the responsible anesthesiologist. They are intended to encourage quality patient care, but observing them cannot guarantee any specific patient outcome. They are subject to revision from time to time, as warranted by the evolution of technology and practice. They apply to all general anesthetics, regional anesthetics, and monitored anesthesia care. This set of standards addresses only the issue of basic anesthetic monitoring, which is one component of anesthesia care. In certain rare or unusual circumstances, (1) some of these methods of monitoring may be clinically impractical, and (2) appropriate use of the described monitoring methods may fail to detect untoward clinical developments. Brief interruptions of continual† monitoring may be unavoidable. Under extenuating circumstances, the responsible anesthesiologist may waive the requirements marked with an asterisk (*); it is recommended that when this is done, it should be so stated (including the reasons) in a note in the patient's medical record. These standards are not intended for application to the care of the obstetrical patient in labor or in the conduct of pain management.

STANDARD I

Qualified anesthesia personnel shall be present in the room throughout the conduct of all general anesthetics, regional anesthetics, and monitored anesthesia care.

Objective

Because of the rapid changes in patient status during anesthesia, qualified anesthesia personnel shall be continuously present to monitor the patient and provide anesthesia care. In the event there is a direct known hazard, *e.g.,* radiation, to the anesthesia personnel which might require intermittent remote observation of the patient, some provision for monitoring the patient must be made. In the event that an emergency requires the temporary absence of the person primarily responsible for the anesthetic, the best judgment of the anesthesiologist will be exercised in comparing the emergency with the anesthetized patient's condition and in the selection of the person left responsible for the anesthetic during the temporary absence.

STANDARD II

During all anesthetics, the patient's oxygenation, ventilation, circulation, and temperature shall be continually evaluated.

OXYGENATION

Objective

To ensure adequate oxygen concentration in the inspired gas and the blood during all anesthetics.

Methods

1. Inspired gas: During every administration of general anesthesia using an anesthesia machine, the concentration of oxygen in the patient breathing system shall be measured by an oxygen analyzer with a low oxygen concentration limit alarm in use.*
2. Blood oxygenation: During all anesthetics, a quantitative method of assessing oxygenation such as pulse oximetry shall be employed.* Adequate illumination and exposure of the patient are necessary to assess color.*

VENTILATION

Objective

To ensure adequate ventilation of the patient during all anesthetics.

Methods

1. Every patient receiving general anesthesia shall have the adequacy of ventilation continually evaluated. Qualitative clinical signs such as chest excursion, observation of the reservoir breathing bag, and auscultation of breath sounds are useful. Continual monitoring for the presence of expired carbon dioxide shall be performed unless invalidated by the nature of the patient, procedure, or equipment. Quantitative monitoring of the volume of expired gas is strongly encouraged.*
2. When an endotracheal tube or laryngeal mask is inserted, its correct positioning must be verified by clinical assessment and by identification of carbon dioxide in the expired gas. Continual end-tidal carbon dioxide analysis, in use from the time of endotracheal tube/laryngeal mask placement, until extubation/removal or initiating transfer to a postoperative care location, shall be performed using a quantitative method such as capnography, capnometry or mass spectroscopy.*
3. When ventilation is controlled by a mechanical ventilator, there shall be in continuous use a device that is capable of detecting disconnection of components of the breathing system. The device must give an audible signal when its alarm threshold is exceeded.
4. During regional anesthesia and monitored anesthesia care, the adequacy of ventilation shall be evaluated, at least, by continual observation of qualitative clinical signs.

CIRCULATION

Objective

To ensure the adequacy of the patient's circulatory function during all anesthetics.

Methods

1. Every patient receiving anesthesia shall have the electrocardiogram continuously displayed from the beginning of anesthesia until preparing to leave the anesthetizing location.*
2. Every patient receiving anesthesia shall have arterial blood pressure and heart rate determined and evaluated at least every 5 minutes.*
3. Every patient receiving general anesthesia shall have, in addition to the above, circulatory function continually evaluated by at least one of the following: palpation of a pulse, auscultation of heart sounds, monitoring of a tracing of intra-arterial pressure, ultrasound peripheral pulse monitoring, or pulse plethysmography or oximetry.

BODY TEMPERATURE

Objective

To aid in the maintenance of appropriate body temperature during all anesthetics.

Methods

Every patient receiving anesthesia shall have temperature monitored when clinically significant changes in body temperature are intended, anticipated, or suspected.

---

† Note that *continual* is defined as "repeated regularly and frequently in steady rapid succession," whereas *continuous* means "prolonged without any interruption at any time."

Approved by House of Delegates on October 21, 1986 and last amended on October 21, 1998. (Effective July 1, 1999.)
Reprinted with permission of the American Society of Anesthesiologists, 515 Busse Highway, Park Ridge, Illinois 60068-3189.

Table 2-2. AMERICAN SOCIETY OF ANESTHESIOLOGISTS BASIC STANDARDS FOR PREANESTHESIA CARE

These Standards apply to all patients who receive anesthesia or monitored anesthesia care. Under unusual circumstances, *e.g.*, extreme emergencies, these standards may be modified. When this is the case, the circumstances shall be documented in the patient's record.

Standard I: An anesthesiologist shall be responsible for determining the medical status of the patient, developing a plan of anesthesia care, and acquainting the patient or the responsible adult with the proposed plan.

The development of an appropriate plan of anesthesia care is based upon:

1. Reviewing the medical record.
2. Interviewing and examining the patient to:
   a. Discuss the medical history, previous anesthetic experiences, and drug therapy.
   b. Assess those aspects of the physical condition that might affect decisions regarding perioperative risk and management.
3. Obtaining and/or reviewing tests and consultations necessary to the conduct of anesthesia.
4. Determining the appropriate prescription of preoperative medications as necessary to the conduct of anesthesia.

The responsible anesthesiologist shall verify that the above has been properly performed and documented in the patient's record.

Approved by House of Delegates on October 14, 1987.
Reprinted with permission of the American Society of Anesthesiologists, 515 Busse Highway, Park Ridge, Illinois 60068-3189.

to justify action or the lack of action because of a company protocol. Difficult as it may be to reconcile with the payer, the practitioner still is subject to the classic definitions of standard of care.

The other type of standards associated with medical care are those of the JCAHO, the best-known medical care quality regulatory agency. As noted earlier, these standards were for many years concerned largely with structure (*e.g.*, gas tanks chained down) and process (*e.g.*, documentation complete), but in recent years they have been expanded to include reviews of the outcome of care. JCAHO standards also focus on credentialing and privileges, verification that anesthesia services are of uniform quality throughout an institution, the qualifications of the director of the service, continuing education, and basic guidelines for anesthesia care (need for preoperative and postoperative evaluations, documentation, and so forth). Full JCAHO accreditation of a health care facility is usually for 3 years. Even the best hospitals and facilities receive some citations of problems or deficiencies that are expected to be corrected, and an interim report of efforts to do so is required. If there are enough problems, accreditation can be conditional for 1 year, with a complete reinspection at that time. Preparing for JCAHO inspections involves a great deal of work, but because the standards usually do promote high-quality care, the majority of this work is highly constructive and of benefit to the institution and its medical staff.

Another type of regulatory agency is the peer review organization. Professional standards review organizations (PSROs) were established in 1972 as utilization review/QA overseers of the care of federally subsidized patients (Medicare and Medicaid). Despite their efforts to deal with quality of care, these groups were seen by all involved as primarily interested in cost containment. Various negative factors led to the PSROs' being replaced in 1984 with the peer review organization (PRO).[11] There is a PRO in each state, many being associated with a state medical association. The objectives of a PRO include 14 goals related

to hospital admissions (*e.g.*, to shift care to an outpatient basis as much as possible) and 5 related to quality of care (*e.g.*, to reduce avoidable deaths and avoidable complications). The PROs comprise full-time support staff and physician reviewers paid as consultants or directors. Ideally, PRO monitoring will discover suboptimal care, and this will lead to specific recommendations for improvement in quality. There is a perception that quality of care efforts are hampered by the lack of realistic objectives and also that these PRO groups, like others before them, will largely or entirely function to limit the cost of health care services.

The practice management implications have become clear. Aside from the as-yet unrealized potential for quality improvement efforts and the occasional denial of payment for a procedure, the most likely interaction between the local PRO and anesthesiology personnel will involve a request for perioperative admission of a patient whose care is mandated to be outpatient surgery. If the anesthesiologist feels, for example, that either (1) preoperative admission for treatment to optimize cardiac, pulmonary, diabetic, or other medical status or (2) postoperative admission for monitoring of labile situations such as uncontrolled hypertension will reduce clear anesthetic risks for the patient, an application to the PRO for approval of admission must be made and vigorously supported. All too often, however, such issues surface a day or so before the scheduled procedure in a preanesthesia screening clinic or even in a preoperative holding area outside the OR on the day of surgery. This will continue to occur until anesthesia providers educate their constituent surgeon community as to what types of associated medical conditions may disqualify a proposed patient from the outpatient (ambulatory) surgical schedule. If adequate notice is given by the surgeon, such as at the time an elective case is booked for the OR, the patient can be seen far enough in advance by an anesthesiologist to allow appropriate planning.

In the circumstance in which the first knowledge of a questionable patient comes 1 or 2 days before surgery, the anesthesiologist can try to have the procedure postponed, if possible, or can undertake the time-consuming task of multiple telephone calls to get the surgeon's agreement, get PRO approval, and make the necessary arrangements. Because neither alternative is particularly attractive, especially from administrative and reimbursement perspectives, there may be a strong temptation to "let it slide" and try to deal with the patient as an outpatient even though this may be questionable. In almost all cases, it is likely that there would be no adverse result. However, the patient would be exposed to an avoidable risk. Both because of the workings of probability and because of the inevitable tendency to let sicker and sicker patients slip by as lax practitioners repeatedly "get away with it" and are lulled into a false sense of security, sooner or later there will be an unfortunate outcome or some preventable major morbidity or even mortality.

The situation is worsened when the first contact with a questionable ambulatory patient is preoperatively on the day of surgery. There may be intense pressure from the patient, the surgeon, or the OR administrator and staff to proceed with a case for which the anesthesia practitioner believes the patient is poorly prepared. The arguments made regarding patient inconvenience and anxiety are valid. However, they should not outweigh the best medical interests of the patient. Although this is a point in favor of screening all outpatients before the day of surgery, the anesthesiologist facing this situation on the day of operation should state clearly to all concerned the reasons for postponing the surgery, stressing the issue of avoidable risk and standards of care, and then help with alternative arrangements (including, if necessary, dealing with the PRO).

Potential liability exposure is the other side of the standard of care issue. Particularly regarding questions of postoperative admission of ambulatory patients who have been unstable in some worrisome manner, it is an extremely poor defense against a malpractice claim to state that the patient was discharged home, only later to suffer a complication because the PRO deemed that operative procedure outpatient and not inpatient surgery. As bureaucratically annoying as it may be, it is a prudent management strategy to admit the patient if there is any legitimate question, thus minimizing the chance for complications, and later haggle with the PRO or directly with the involved third-party payer.

Policy and Procedure

Management of an anesthesiology practice involves business, organizational, and clinical issues. One important organizational point that is often overlooked is the need for a complete policy and procedure manual. Such a compilation of documents is necessary for all practices, from the largest departments covering multiple hospitals to a single-room outpatient facility with one anesthesia provider. Contemplation of this compilation of documents may evoke a collective groan from anesthesiology personnel, and maintaining this manual may be misperceived as a bureaucratic chore. Quite the contrary, such a manual can be extraordinarily valuable, as, for example, when it provides crucial information during an emergency. Some suggestions

for the content of this compendium exist, but, at minimum, organizational and procedural elements must be included.

The organizational elements that should be present include a chart of organization and responsibilities that is not just a call schedule but a clear explanation of who is responsible for what functions of the department and when, with attendant details such as expectations for the practitioner's presence within the institution at designated hours, telephone availability, pager availability, the maximum permissible distance from the institution, and so forth. Experience suggests it is especially important for there to be an absolutely clear specification of the availability of qualified anesthesiology personnel for emergency cesarean section, particularly in practice arrangements in which there are several people on call covering multiple locations. Sadly, these issues often are only considered after a disaster has occurred that involved miscommunication and the mistaken belief by one or more people that someone else would take care of a problem.

The organizational component of the policy and procedure manual should also include a clear explanation of the orientation and checkout procedure for new personnel, continuing medical requirements and opportunities, the mechanisms for

---

Table 2-3. AMERICAN SOCIETY OF ANESTHESIOLOGISTS STANDARDS FOR POSTANESTHESIA CARE

These Standards apply to postanesthesia care in all locations. These Standards may be exceeded based on the judgment of the responsible anesthesiologist. They are intended to encourage quality patient care, but cannot guarantee any specific patient outcome. They are subject to revision from time to time as warranted by the evolution of technology and practice. Under extenuating circumstances, the responsible anesthesiologist may waive the requirements marked with an asterisk (*); it is recommended that when this is done, it should be so stated (including the reasons) in a note in the patient's medical record.

STANDARD I

All patients who have received general anesthesia, regional anesthesia, or monitored anesthesia care shall receive appropriate postanesthesia management.[1]

1. A Postanesthesia Care Unit (PACU) or an area which provides equivalent postanesthesia care shall be available to receive patients after anesthesia care. All patients who receive anesthesia care shall be admitted to the PACU or its equivalent except by specific order of the anesthesiologist responsible for the patient's care.
2. The medical aspects of care in the PACU shall be governed by policies and procedures which have been reviewed and approved by the Department of Anesthesiology.
3. The design, equipment, and staffing of the PACU shall meet requirements of the facility's accrediting and licensing bodies.

STANDARD II

A patient transported to the PACU shall be accompanied by a member of the anesthesia care team who is knowledgeable about the patient's condition. The patient shall be continually evaluated and treated during transport with monitoring and support appropriate to the patient's condition.

STANDARD III

Upon arrival in the PACU, the patient shall be re-evaluated and a verbal report provided to the responsible PACU nurse by the member of the anesthesia care team who accompanies the patient.

1. The patient's status on arrival in the PACU shall be documented.

2. Information concerning the preoperative condition and the surgical/anesthetic course shall be transmitted to the PACU nurse.
3. The member of the Anesthesia Care Team shall remain in the PACU until the PACU nurse accepts responsibility for the nursing care of the patient.

STANDARD IV

The patient's condition shall be evaluated continually in the PACU.

1. The patient shall be observed and monitored by methods appropriate to the patient's medical condition. Particular attention should be given to monitoring oxygenation, ventilation, circulation, and temperature. During recovery from all anesthetics, a quantitative method of assessing oxygenation such as pulse oximetry shall be employed in the initial phase of recovery.* This is not intended for application during the recovery of the obstetrical patient in whom regional anesthesia was used for labor and vaginal delivery.
2. An accurate written report of the PACU period shall be maintained. Use of an appropriate PACU scoring system is encouraged for each patient on admission, at appropriate intervals prior to discharge and at the time of discharge.
3. General medical supervision and coordination of patient care in the PACU should be the responsibility of an anesthesiologist.
4. There shall be a policy to assure the availability in the facility of a physician capable of managing complications and providing cardiopulmonary resuscitation for patients in the PACU.

STANDARD V

A physician is responsible for the discharge of the patient from the PACU.

1. When discharge criteria are used, they must be approved by the Department of Anesthesiology and the medical staff. They may vary depending upon whether the patient is discharged to a hospital room, to the Intensive Care Unit, to a short stay unit, or home.
2. In the absence of the physician responsible for the discharge, the PACU nurse shall determine that the patient meets the discharge criteria. The name of the physician accepting responsibility for discharge shall be noted on the record.

---

[1] Refer to Standards of Post Anesthesia Nursing Practice 1992, published by ASPAN, for issues of nursing care.
Approved by House of Delegates on October 12, 1988 and last amended on October 19, 1994.
Reprinted with permission of the American Society of Anesthesiologists, 515 Busse Highway, Park Ridge, Illinois 60068-3189.

Table 2-4. AMERICAN SOCIETY OF ANESTHESIOLOGISTS GUIDELINES FOR REGIONAL ANESTHESIA IN OBSTETRICS

These guidelines apply to the use of regional anesthesia or analgesia in which local anesthetics are administered to the parturient during labor and delivery. They are intended to encourage quality patient care but cannot guarantee any specific patient outcome. Because the availability of anesthesia resources may vary, members are responsible for interpreting and establishing the guidelines for their own institutions and practices. These guidelines are subject to revision from time to time as warranted by the evolution of technology and practice.

GUIDELINE I

Regional anesthesia should be initiated and maintained only in locations in which appropriate resuscitation equipment and drugs are immediately available to manage procedurally related problems.

Resuscitation equipment should include, but is not limited to: sources of oxygen and suction, equipment to maintain an airway and perform endotracheal intubation, a means to provide positive-pressure ventilation, and drugs and equipment for cardiopulmonary resuscitation.

GUIDELINE II

Regional anesthesia should be initiated by a physician with appropriate privileges and maintained by or under the medical direction[1] of such an individual.

Physicians should be approved through the institutional credentialing process to initiate and direct the maintenance of obstetric anesthesia and to manage procedurally related complications.

GUIDELINE III

Regional anesthesia should not be administered until: (1) the patient has been examined by a qualified individual and (2) the maternal and fetal status and progress of labor have been evaluated by a physician with privileges in obstetrics who is readily available to supervise the labor and manage any obstetric complications that may arise.

Under circumstances defined by department protocol, qualified personnel may perform the initial pelvic examination. The physician responsible for the patient's obstetrical care should be informed of her status so that a decision can be made regarding present risk and further management.

GUIDELINE IV

An intravenous infusion should be established before the initiation of regional anesthesia and maintained throughout the duration of the regional anesthetic.

GUIDELINE V

Regional anesthesia for labor and/or vaginal delivery requires that the parturient's vital signs and the fetal heart rate be monitored and documented by a qualified individual. Additional monitoring appropriate to the clinical condition of the parturient and the fetus should be employed when indicated. When extensive regional blockade is administered for complicated vaginal delivery, the standards for basic anesthetic monitoring[3] should be applied.

GUIDELINE VI

Regional anesthesia for cesarean delivery requires that the standards for basic anesthetic monitoring[3] be applied and that a physician with privileges in obstetrics be immediately available.

GUIDELINE VII

Qualified personnel, other than the anesthesiologist attending the mother, should be immediately available to assume responsibility for resuscitation of the newborn.[2]

The primary responsibility of the anesthesiologist is to provide care to the mother. If the anesthesiologist is also requested to provide brief assistance in the care of the newborn, the benefit to the child must be compared to the risk to the mother.

GUIDELINE VIII

A physician with appropriate privileges should remain readily available during the regional anesthetic to manage anesthetic complications until the patient's postanesthesia condition is satisfactory and stable.

GUIDELINE IX

All patients recovering from regional anesthesia should receive appropriate postanesthesia care. Following cesarean delivery and/or extensive regional blockade, the standards for postanesthesia care[4] should be applied.

1. A postanesthesia care unit (PACU) should be available to receive patients. The design, equipment, and staffing should meet requirements of the facility's accrediting and licensing bodies.
2. When a site other than the PACU is used, equivalent postanesthesia care should be provided.

GUIDELINE X

There should be a policy to assure the availability in the facility of a physician to manage complications and to provide cardiopulmonary resuscitation for patients receiving postanesthesia care.

[1] The Anesthesia Care Team (approved by ASA House of Delegates 10/6/82 and last amended 10/25/95).
[2] Guidelines for Prenatal Care (American Academy of Pediatrics and American College of Obstetricians and Gynecologists, 1988).
[3] Standards for Basic Anesthetic Monitoring (approved by ASA House of Delegates 10/21/86 and last amended 10/23/96).
[4] Standards for Postanesthesia Care (approved by ASA House of Delegates 10/12/88 and last amended 10/19/94).
Approved by House of Delegates on October 12, 1988 and last amended on October 30, 1991.
Reprinted with permission of the American Society of Anesthesiologists, 515 Busse Highway, Park Ridge, Illinois 60068-3189.

evaluating personnel and for communicating this evaluation to them, disaster plans (or reference to a separate disaster manual or protocol), QA activities of the department, and the format for statistical record keeping (number of procedures, types of anesthetics given, types of patients anesthetized, number and types of invasive monitoring procedures, number and type of responses to emergency calls, and the like).

The procedural component of the policy and procedure manual should give both handy practice tips and specific outlines of proposed courses of action for particular circumstances; it also should store little-used but valuable information. Reference should be made to the statements, guidelines, and standards appearing in the back of the ASA's Directory of Members as well as to ASA practice parameters. Also included should be references to or specific protocols for the areas mentioned in the JCAHO standards: preanesthetic evaluation, immediate preinduction re-evaluation, safety of the patient during the anesthetic period, release of the patient from any PACU, recording of all pertinent events during anesthesia, recording of postanesthesia visits, guidelines defining the role of anesthesia services in hospital infection control, and guidelines for safe use of general anesthetic agents. Other appropriate topics include the following:

1. Recommendations for preanesthesia apparatus checkout, such as from the U.S. Food and Drug Administration (FDA)[13] (see Appendixes, Chapter 22)
2. Guidelines for minimal monitoring and duration of stay of an infant, child, or adult in the PACU
3. Procedures for transporting patients to/from the OR, PACU, or ICU
4. Policy on ambulatory surgical patients—e.g., screening, use of regional anesthesia, discharge home criteria
5. Policy on evaluation and processing of same-day admissions

6. Policy on recovery room admission and discharge
7. Policy on ICU admission and discharge
8. Policy on physicians responsible for writing orders in recovery room and ICU
9. Policy on informed consent and its documentation
10. Policy on the use of patients in clinical research
11. Guidelines for the support of cadaver organ donors and its termination
12. Guidelines on environmental safety, including pollution with trace gases and electrical equipment inspection, maintenance, and hazard prevention
13. Procedure for change of personnel during an anesthetic
14. Procedure for the introduction of new equipment, drugs, or clinical practices
15. Procedure for epidural and spinal narcotic administration and subsequent patient monitoring (e.g., type, minimum time, nursing units)
16. Procedure for initial treatment of cardiac or respiratory arrest
17. Policy for handling patient's refusal of blood or blood products, including the mechanism to obtain a court order to transfuse
18. Procedure for the management of malignant hyperthermia
19. Procedure for the induction and maintenance of barbiturate coma
20. Procedure for the evaluation of suspected pseudocholinesterase deficiency
21. Protocol for responding to an adverse anesthetic event

Individual departments may add to the above suggestions as dictated by their specific needs. A thorough, carefully conceived policy and procedure manual is a valuable tool. The manual should be reviewed and updated as needed but at least annually, with a particularly thorough review preceding each JCAHO inspection. Each member of a group or department should review the manual at least annually and sign off in a log indicating familiarity with current policies and procedures.

Meetings and Case Discussion

There must be regularly scheduled departmental or group meetings. Although didactic lectures and continuing education meetings are valuable and necessary, there also must be regular opportunities for open clinical discussion about interesting cases and problem cases. Also, the JCAHO requires that there be at least monthly meetings at which risk management and QA activities are documented and reported. Whether these meetings are called case conferences, morbidity and mortality conferences, or deaths and complications, the entire department or group should gather for an interchange of ideas. More recently these gatherings have been called QA meetings. An open review of departmental statistics should be done, including all complications, even those that may appear trivial. Unusual patterns of small events may point toward a larger or systematic problem, especially if they are more frequently associated with one individual practitioner.

A problem case presented at the departmental meeting might be an overt accident, a near accident (critical incident), or an untoward outcome of unknown origin. Honest but constructive discussion, even of an anesthetist's technical deficiencies or lack of knowledge, should take place in the spirit of peer review. The classic question "What would you do differently next time?" is a good way to start the discussion. There may be situations in which inviting the surgeon or the internist involved in a specific case would be advantageous. The opportunity for each type of provider to hear the perspective of another discipline is not only inherently educational, but also can promote communication and cooperation in future potential problem cases.

Records of these meetings must be kept for accreditation purposes, but the enshrining of overly detailed minutes (potentially subject to discovery by a plaintiff's attorney at a later date) may inhibit true educational and corrective interchanges about untoward events. In the circumstance of discussion of a case that seems likely to provoke litigation, it is appropriate to be certain that the meeting is classified as official "peer review" and possibly even invite the hospital attorney or legal counsel from the relevant malpractice insurance carrier.

Support Staff

There is a fundamental need for support staff in every anesthesia practice. Even independent practitioners rely in some measure on facilities, equipment, and services provided by the organization maintaining the anesthetizing location. In large, well-organized departments, reliance on support staff is often very great. The need for adequate staff and the inadvisability of scrimping on critical support personnel to cut costs is obvious. What is often overlooked, however, is a process analogous to that of credentialing and privileges for anesthesiologists, although at a slightly different level. The people expected to provide clinical anesthesia practice support must be qualified and must at all times understand what they are expected to do and how to do it. It is singularly unfortunate to realize only after an anesthesia catastrophe has occurred that basic details of simple work assignments, such as the changing of carbon dioxide absorbent, were routinely ignored. This indicates the need for supervision and monitoring of the support staff by the involved practitioners. Further, such support personnel are favorite targets of cost-cutting administrators who do not understand the function of anesthesia technicians or their equivalent. In the modern era, administrators seem driven almost exclusively by the "bottom line" and cannot appreciate the connection between valuable workers such as these and the "revenue stream." Even though it is obvious to all who work in an OR that the anesthesia support personnel make it possible for there to be patients flowing through the OR, it is their responsibility to convince the facility's fiscal administrator that elimination of such positions is genuinely false economy because of the attendant loss in efficiency, particularly in turning over the room between surgeries. Further, it is also false economy to reduce the number of personnel below that genuinely needed to retrieve, clean, sort, disassemble, sterilize, reassemble, store, and distribute the tools of daily anesthesia practice. Inadequate attention to all these steps truly creates "an accident waiting to happen." When there is threatened loss of budget funding from a health care facility for the salaries of needed anesthesia support personnel, the practitioners involved must not simply stand by and see the necessary functions thrown into a "hit-or-miss" status by a few remaining heavily overburdened workers. Vigorous defense (or initiation of and agitation for new positions if the staff is inadequate) by the anesthesia practitioners should be undertaken, always with the realization that it may be necessary in some circumstances for them to supplement the budget from the facility with some of their practice income to guarantee an adequate complement of competent workers.

Business and organizational issues in the management of an anesthesia practice are also critically dependent on the existence of a sufficient number of appropriately trained support staff. One frequently overlooked issue that contributes to the negative impression generated by some anesthesiology practices centers on being certain there is someone available to answer the telephone at all times during the hours surgeons, other physicians, and OR scheduling desks are likely to telephone. This seemingly trivial component of practice management is important to the success of an anesthesiology practice as a business whose principal customers are the surgeons. Certainly there is a commercial server–client relationship both with the patient and the purchaser of health care; however, the uniquely symbiotic nature of the relationship between surgeons and anesthesiologists is such that availability even for simple "just wanted to let you know" telephone calls is genuinely important. The person who answers the telephone is the representative of the practice to the world and must take that responsibility seriously. From a management standpoint, significant impact on the success of the practice as a business often hinges on such details. Further, anesthesiologists should always have permanent personal electronic pagers to facilitate communications from other members of the department or group and from support personnel. This may sound intrusive, but the unusual position of anesthesiologists in the spectrum of physicians mandates this feature of managing an anesthesiology practice. Anesthesiology personnel should have no hesitation about spending their own practice income to do so. The symbolism is obvious.

Anesthesia Equipment and Equipment Maintenance

Problems with anesthesia equipment have been discussed for some time.[14,15] However, compared to human error, overt equipment failure very rarely causes intraoperative critical incidents[16] or deaths resulting from anesthesia care.[17] Aside from the obvious human errors involving misuse of or unfamiliarity with the equipment, when the rare equipment failure does occur, it appears often that correct maintenance and servicing of the apparatus has not been done. These issues become the focus of anesthesia practice management efforts because there can often be confusion or even disputes about precisely who is responsible for maintaining the anesthesia equipment—the facility or the practitioners who use it and collect practice income from that activity. In many cases, the facility assumes the responsibility. In situations in which that is not true, however, it is necessary for the practitioners to venture into usually unfamiliar territory.

Programs for anesthesia equipment maintenance and service have been outlined.[18–20] A distinction is made between failure due to progressive deterioration of equipment, which should be preventable because it is observable and should provoke appropriate action, and catastrophic failure, which often practically cannot be predicted. Preventive maintenance for mechanical parts is critical and involves periodic performance checks every 4–6 months. Also, an annual safety inspection of each anesthetizing location and the equipment itself is necessary. For equipment service, an excellent mechanism is a relatively elaborate cross-reference system to identify both the device needing service and also the mechanism to secure the needed maintenance or repair.

Equipment handling principles are straightforward. Before purchase, it must be verified that a proposed piece of equipment meets all applicable standards, which will usually be true when dealing with recognized major manufacturers. On arrival, electrical equipment must be checked for absence of hazard (especially leakage of current) and compliance with applicable electrical standards. Complex equipment such as anesthesia machines and ventilators should be assembled and checked out by a representative from the manufacturer or manufacturer's agent. There are potential adverse medicolegal implications when relatively untrained personnel certify a particular piece of equipment as functioning within specification, even if they do it perfectly. It is also very important to involve the manufacturer's representative in pre- and in-service training for those who will use the new equipment. On arrival, a sheet or section in the master equipment log must be created with the make, model, serial number, and in-house identification for each piece of capital equipment. This not only allows immediate identification of any equipment involved in a future recall or product alert, but also serves as the permanent repository of the record of every problem, problem resolution, maintenance, and servicing occurring until that particular equipment is scrapped. This log must be kept up-to-date at all times. There have been rare but frightening examples of potentially lethal problems with anesthesia machines leading to product alert notices requiring immediate identification of certain equipment and its service status.

Who should maintain and service major anesthesia equipment has been widely debated. There are significant management implications. Equipment setup and checkout have been mentioned. After that, some groups or departments rely on factory service representatives for all attention to equipment, others engage independent service contractors, and still other (often larger) departments have access to personnel (either engineers and/or technicians) in their facility. Needs and resources differ. The single underlying principle is clear: the person(s) doing preventive maintenance and service must be qualified. Anesthesia practitioners may wonder how they can assess these qualifications. The best way is to unhesitatingly ask pertinent questions about the education, training, and experience of those involved, including asking for references and speaking to supervisors and managers responsible for those doing the work. Whether an engineering technician who spent a week at a course at a factory can perform the most complex repairs depends on a variety of factors, which can be investigated by the practitioners ultimately using the equipment in the care of patients. Failure to be involved in this oversight manner exposes the practice to increased liability in the event of an untoward outcome associated with improperly maintained or serviced equipment.

Determining when anesthesia equipment becomes obsolete and should be replaced is another question that is difficult to answer. Replacement of obsolete anesthesia machines and monitoring equipment is a key element of a risk modification program. Ten years is often cited as an estimated useful life for an anesthesia machine, but although an ASA statement repeats that idea, it also notes that the ASA promulgated a Policy for Assessing Obsolescence in 1989 that does not subscribe to any specific time interval. Anesthesia machines considerably more than 10 years old do not meet certain of the safety standards now in force for new machines (such as vaporizer lockout, fresh gas ratio protection, and automatic enabling of the oxygen analyzer) and, unless extensively retrofitted, do not incorporate the new technology that advanced very rapidly during the 1980s, much of it directly related to the effort to prevent untoward incidents. Further, it appears that this technology will continue to advance, particularly due to the adoption of anesthesia workstation standards by the European Economic Union that are expected to affect anesthesia machine design worldwide. Note that some anesthesia equipment manufacturers, anxious to minimize their own potential liability, have refused to support (with parts and service) some of the oldest of their pieces (particularly gas machines) still in use. This disowning of equipment by its own manufacturer is a very strong message to practitioners that such equipment must be replaced as soon as possible.

Should a piece of equipment fail, it must be removed from service and a replacement substituted. Groups, departments, and facilities are obligated to have sufficient backup equipment to cover any reasonable incidence of failure. The equipment removed from service must be clearly marked with a prominent label (so it is not returned into service by a well-meaning technician or practitioner) containing the date, time, person discovering, and the details of the problem. The responsible personnel must be notified so they can remove the equipment, make an entry in the log, and initiate the repair. As indicated in the protocol for response to an adverse event, a piece of equipment involved or suspected in an anesthesia accident must be immediately sequestered and not touched by anybody—particularly not by any equipment service personnel. If a severe accident occurred, it may be necessary for the equipment in question to be inspected at a later time by a group consisting of qualified representatives of the manufacturer, the service personnel, the plaintiff's attorney, the insurance companies involved, and the practitioner's defense attorney. The equipment should thus be impounded following an adverse event and treated similarly to any object in a forensic "chain of evidence," with careful documentation of parties in contact with and responsible for securing the equipment in question following such an event. Also, major equipment problems may, in some circumstances, reflect a pattern of failure due to a design or manufacturing fault. These problems should be reported to the FDA's Medical Device Problem Reporting system *via* the Device Experience Network (telephone 800-638-6725).[21] This system accepts voluntary reports from users and requires reports from manufacturers when there is knowledge of a medical device being involved in a serious incident. Whether or not filing such a report will have a positive impact in subsequent litigation is impossible to know, but it is a worthwhile practice management point that needs to be considered in the unlikely but important instance of a relevant event.

Malpractice Insurance

All practitioners need liability insurance coverage specific for the specialty and role in which they are practicing. Premium rates depend on specialty, subspecialty, and whether the insured performs procedures that the insurance company's experience suggests may be more likely to result in a malpractice lawsuit. It is absolutely critical that applicants for medical liability insurance be completely honest in informing the insurer what duties and procedures they perform. Failure to do so, either from carelessness or from a foolishly misguided desire to reduce the resulting premium, may well result in retrospective denial of insurance coverage in the event of an untoward outcome from an activity the insurer did not know the insured engaged in.

Proof of adequate insurance coverage is usually required to secure or renew privileges to practice at a health care facility. The facility may specify certain minimum policy limits to limit its liability exposure. It is difficult to suggest specific dollar amounts for policy limits because the details of practice vary so much among situations and locations. The malpractice crisis of the 1980s has eased significantly for anesthesiologists, largely due to the decrease in number and severity of malpractice claims resulting from anesthesia catastrophes as anesthesia care in the United States became safer.[22–24] The exact analysis of this phenomenon can be debated, but it is a simple fact that malpractice insurance premiums for anesthesiologists have not been increased at the same rate as for other specialties over the past several years and, in many cases, have actually decreased. This does not mitigate the need for adequate coverage, however. In the late 1990s, coverage limits of $1 million/$3 million would seem the minimum advisable. This specification usually means that the insurer will cover up to $1 million liability per claim and up to $3 million per year, but this terminology is not necessarily universal. Therefore, anesthesiology personnel must be absolutely certain what they are buying when they apply for malpractice insurance. In parts of the United States known for a pattern of exorbitant settlements and jury verdicts, liability coverage limits of $2 million/$5 million may be prudent and well worth the moderate additional cost. An additional feature in this regard is the potential to employ "umbrella" liability coverage above the limits of the base policy, as noted below.

The fundamental mechanism of medical malpractice insurance has changed significantly in recent years because of the need for insurance companies to have better ways to predict what their losses (amounts paid in settlements and judgments) might be. Traditionally, medical liability insurance was sold on an "occurrence" basis, meaning that if the insurance policy was in force at the time of the occurrence of an incident resulting in a claim, whenever that claim might be filed, the practitioner would be covered. Occurrence insurance was somewhat more expensive than the alternative "claims made" policies,

but was seen as worth it by some practitioners. These policies created some open-ended exposure for the insurer that sometimes led to unexpected large losses, even some large enough to threaten the existence of the insurance company. As a result, medical malpractice insurers have converted almost exclusively to claims-made insurance, which covers claims that are filed while the insurance is in force. Premium rates for the first year a physician is in practice are relatively low because there is less likelihood of a claim coming in (a majority of malpractice suits are filed 1–3 years after the event in question). The premiums usually increase yearly for the first 5 years and then the policy is considered mature. The issue comes when the physician later, for whatever reason, must change insurance companies (*e.g.,* because of relocation to another state). If the physician simply discontinues the policy and a claim is filed the next year, there will be no insurance coverage. Therefore, the physician must secure "tail coverage," sometimes for a minimum number of years (*e.g.,* 5) or sometimes indefinitely to guarantee liability insurance protection for claims filed after the physician is no longer primarily covered by the insurance policy. It may be possible in some circumstances to purchase tail coverage from a different insurer than was involved with the primary policy, but by far the most common thing done is to simply extend the existing insurance coverage for the period of the tail. This very often yields a bill for the entire tail coverage premium, which can be quite sizable, potentially staggering a physician who simply wants to move to another state where his existing insurance company is not licensed to do business. The issue of how to pay this premium is appropriately the subject of management attention and effort within the anesthesia practice. Individual situations will vary widely, but it is reasonable for anesthesiologists organized into a fiscal entity to consider this issue at the time of the inception of the group, rather than facing the potentially difficult question of how to treat one individual later. Other strategies have occasionally been employed when insuring the tail period, including converting the previous policy to part-time status for a period of years, and purchasing "nose" coverage from the new insurer—that is, paying an initial higher yearly premium with the new insurer, who then will cover claims that may occur during the tail period.

Another component to the liability insurance situation is consideration of the advisability of purchasing yet another type of insurance called "umbrella coverage," which is activated at the time of the need to pay a claim that exceeds the limits of coverage on the standard malpractice liability insurance policy. Because such an enormous claim is extremely unlikely, many practitioners are tempted to forgo the modest cost of such insurance coverage in the name of economy. As before, it is easy to see that this is potentially a very false economy—if there is a huge claim. Practitioners should consult with their financial managers, but it is likely that it would be considered wise management to purchase umbrella liability insurance coverage.

Medical malpractice insurers are becoming increasingly active in trying to prevent incidents that will lead to insurance claims. They often sponsor risk-management seminars to teach practices and techniques to lessen the chances of liability claims and, in some cases, suggest (or even mandate) specific practices, such as strict observation of the ASA Standards for Basic Anesthetic Monitoring. In return for attendance at such events and/or the signing of contracts stating that the practitioner will follow certain guidelines or standards, the insurer often gives a discount on the liability insurance premium. Clearly, it is sound practice management strategy for practitioners to participate maximally in such programs. Likewise, some insurers make coverage conditional on the consistent implementation of certain strategies such as minimal monitoring, stipulating that the practitioner will not be covered if it is found that the guidelines were being ignored at the time of an untoward event. Again, it is obviously wise from a practice management standpoint to cooperate fully with such stipulations.

Response to an Adverse Event

In spite of the decreased incidence of anesthesia catastrophes, even with the very best of practice, it is likely that each anesthesiologist at least once in his or her professional life will be involved in a major anesthesia accident. (See "What to Do When Sued," Chapter 5.) Precisely because such an event is rare, very few are prepared for it. It is probable that the involved personnel will have no relevant past experience regarding what to do. Although an obvious resource is another anesthetist who has had some exposure or experience, one of these may not be available either. Various authors have discussed what to do in that event.[25-27] Cooper *et al* have thoughtfully presented the appropriate immediate response to an accident in a straightforward, logical, compact format[28] that should periodically be reviewed by all anesthesiology practitioners and should be included in all anesthesia policy and procedure manuals. Unfortunately, however, the principal personnel involved in a significant untoward event may react with such surprise or shock as to temporarily lose sight of logic. At the moment of recognition that a major anesthetic complication has occurred or is occurring, help must be called. A sufficient number of people to deal with the situation must be assembled on site as quickly as possible. For example, in the unlikely but still possible event that an esophageal intubation goes unrecognized long enough to cause a cardiac arrest, the immediate need is for enough skilled personnel to conduct the resuscitative efforts, including making the correct diagnosis and replacing the tube into the trachea. Whether the anesthesiologist apparently responsible for the complication should direct the immediate remedial efforts will depend on the person and the situation. In such a circumstance, it would seem wise for a senior or supervising anesthesiologist quickly to evaluate the scenario and make a decision. This person becomes the incident supervisor and has responsibility for helping prevent continuation or recurrence of the incident, for investigating the incident, and for ensuring documentation while the original and helping anesthesiologists focus on caring for the patient. As noted, involved equipment must be sequestered and not touched.

If the accident is not fatal, continuing care of the patient is critical. Measures may be instituted to help limit damage from brain hypoxia. Consultants may be helpful and should be called without hesitation. If not already involved, the chief of anesthesiology must be notified as well as the facility administrator, risk manager, and the anesthesiologist's insurance company. These latter are critical to allow consideration of immediate efforts to limit later financial loss. (Likewise, there are often provisions in medical malpractice insurance policies that might limit or even deny insurance coverage if the company is not notified of any reportable event immediately.) If there is an involved surgeon of record, he or she probably will first notify the family, but the anesthesiologist and others (risk manager, insurance loss control officer, or even legal counsel) might appropriately be included at the outset. Full disclosure of facts as they are best known—with no confessions, opinions, speculation, or placing of blame—is the best presentation. Any attempt to conceal or shade the truth will later only confound an already difficult situation. Obviously, comfort and support should be offered, including, if appropriate, the services of facility personnel such as clergy, social workers, and counselors.

The primary anesthesia provider and any others involved must document relevant information. Never change any existing entries in the medical record. Write an amendment note if needed with careful explanation of why amendment is necessary, particularly stressing explanations of professional judgments involved. State only facts as they are known. Make no judgments about causes or responsibility and do not "point fingers." The same guidelines hold true for the filing of the incident report in the facility, which should be done as soon as is practical. Further, all discussions with the patient or family should be carefully documented in the medical record. Also, it is likely that it will be recommended at that time that the involved clinical personnel sit down as soon as practical and write out their own personal notes, which will include opinions and impressions as well as maximally detailed accounts of the events as they unfolded. These personal notes are not part of the medical record or the facility files. If written while the involved person is still in the facility, these notes should be taken out of the facility that same day and, in all circumstances, given immediately to each involved person's attorney, even if this is not the defense attorney secured by the malpractice insurance company. This strategy guarantees that the notes are attorney–client work product, and thus not subject to forced discovery (revelation) by other parties to the case.

Follow-up after the immediate handling of the incident will involve the primary anesthesiologist but should again be directed by a senior supervisor, who may or may not be the same person as the incident supervisor. The follow-up supervisor verifies the adequacy and coordination of ongoing care of the patient and facilitates communication among all involved, especially with the risk manager. Lastly, it is necessary to verify that adequate post-event documentation is taking place.

Of course, it is expected that such an adverse event will be discussed in the applicable morbidity and mortality meeting. This is good and appropriate. It is necessary, however, to coordinate this activity with the involved risk manager and attorney so as to be completely certain that the contents and conclusions of the discussion are clearly considered peer review activity, and thus are shielded from discovery by the plaintiffs' attorney.

Unpleasant as it is to contemplate, it is better to have a plan and execute it in the event of an accident causing injury to a patient. Vigorous immediate intervention may improve the outcome for all concerned.

OPERATING ROOM MANAGEMENT

One of the significant issues for anesthesiologists raised by the many recent changes in the organization of the health care system is that of the most effective, most appropriate role for anesthesiologists. Anesthesiologists are becoming increasingly involved in and oriented to expanded roles beyond exclusive attention to what is and will always be the mainstay of their practice, administering anesthetics for surgery. One of these expanded roles is into OR management. The complexity and demands of organizing a modern operating suite will no longer allow the comparatively casual approach seen in some institutions in the past, in which things were taken care of in reasonable time, but with little attention paid to whether the first case of the day started at 7:30 A.M. or 7:50 A.M., how long it took to assemble the special instruments, or whether there was a brief delay in transporting a patient from the preoperative staging area so that the appropriate paperwork could be completed by the one overworked nurse. The current urgent drive for efficiency, cost control, and cost reduction clearly will not tolerate obvious inefficiency and wastefulness. A cooperative approach to these issues by all involved clearly is desirable. However, it has been demonstrated in real life and taught in management courses that strong leadership is necessary in the efforts to achieve maximum efficiency and cost reduction. Representatives of the key constituent groups—anesthesiologists, surgeons, OR nurses and techs, and (in some cases) professional administrators/managers—clearly can debate the question of who is best qualified to be a leader in a given OR environment. Many OR suites have looked to anesthesiologists to head, or at least be key players on, the leadership team. Of course, the different groups have different perspectives. It is clear, however, that anesthesiologists of necessity see and deal with the "big picture" as much as or more than the others on the team. This ability to achieve an overview is the main reason anesthesiologists are almost uniquely qualified to provide leadership in an OR.

In the past, as noted above, some anesthesiologists have avoided involvement in administrative and leadership roles in their work environment, the OR in particular, for a variety of reasons. This has contributed to the sometimes negative perception of anesthesiologists among other health care professionals and workers as well as facility administrators. Such abdication of responsibility has always been unfortunate and inappropriate. However, now, with all the pressures on the health care delivery system, it is overtly dysfunctional. Anesthesiologists who have not done so must step forward and actively seek involvement at the highest possible level in management of the OR(s) in which they practice. Clinical anesthesiologists can very profitably apply their unique insights into the process of OR function and significantly help meet the demands for efficiency and cost reduction while still maintaining high-quality patient care. The associated recognition and appreciation from the other constituent groups will emphasize the value and contributions of anesthesiologists as concerned physicians genuinely interested in the welfare of the entire institution, far beyond their own personal incomes. Failure to be involved not only further aggravates the negative image of anesthesiologists as simply greedy technicians rather than involved physicians practicing medicine, but also likely will contribute to accelerated loss of practice autonomy and the associated reimbursement.

An OR suite is a mini-society with various constituent groups, societal dynamics, and tensions determining the tone, pace, and flow of events. The key groups are the anesthesia providers, the surgeons, the OR staff (which usually comprises nursing, scrub techs, and support personnel), and professional administrators, who usually do not share backgrounds with any of the other three groups. As difficult as it may occasionally seem, it is possible and important for these groups not only to get along, but also to work constructively together to create a friendly, efficient work environment that promotes high-quality patient care. It is difficult to outline anything more than the broadest of general points regarding OR management because there is an extremely wide spectrum of OR types, from the largest inner-city teaching hospitals to the smallest freestanding ambulatory surgery specialty centers, with each particular facility having its own needs and characteristics.

Organization

Because both the anesthesia and surgical components of the OR milieu usually involve physicians who are not employees of the institution, there usually is not one central authority to which all the personnel involved must answer. Even when the physicians are employees, they report through their chiefs of service to the chief of the medical staff, who likely is not the hospital administrator. Therefore, even before considering the relationships between anesthesiologists and surgeons, it must be recognized that there is a natural division between the physicians and the OR staff. In this environment, anesthesia providers often find themselves trying to balance the needs of both the OR staff and the surgeons with what is possible and desirable from an anesthesia standpoint. This balancing act is a significant part of the art of anesthesia practice.

Anesthesia practitioners and surgeons have a symbiotic relationship. Without surgeons, there is no need for anesthesia services and without anesthesia providers, surgeons cannot work. In most circumstances, both groups recognize this and also the common goals of having surgery performed in an expeditious, safe manner. One of the biggest organizational sticking points can involve the age-old question "Who is in charge of the OR?" Sometimes, there can be no real answer because the interrelationships in the OR environment are so many and so complex. If there is a professional OR manager whose sole job it is to be an organizer, this person may have enough authority to

be genuinely recognized as in charge. Further, some institutions have a position that carries the title Medical Director of the OR. The implications to surgeons of an anesthesiologist in that position and vice versa are potentially contentious enough so that some institutions have simply abandoned that title. There does need to be some dispute-resolving and policy-setting authority from the physician perspective, however. If there is no medical director with authority to make relevant decisions and make these decisions stick, the physician authority usually resides with the Operating Room Committee. When there are major policy and financial decisions to be made, this committee becomes a microcosm political system with lobbying and campaigning for votes. No matter what it is called or how it is structured, there will be a forum for this type of activity in every OR in which standard tactics of diplomacy and negotiation will be carried out regularly.

Lines of authority parallel lines of responsibility. Who has hire/fire power over whom and who pays whom will determine a great deal about the organization of an individual OR. A classic example involves perfusionists for cardiac surgery. In some circumstances, they are employed by the hospital; in others, by the cardiac surgeons; in a few, by the anesthesiologists; and occasionally, by no one in that they function as completely independent contractors. The organizational implications of each of the above scenarios are relatively clear as they relate to standard issues such as work and call schedules, policy and procedures for bypass operations, equipment purchases, and so forth. Each institution develops its own tradition, often by trial and error, or by default based on the availability of various resources, including the perfusionists themselves. In some cases, the system that evolves never works well or does and then deteriorates over time. At such a juncture, one of the constituent components of the OR environment that has been out of power steps forward and offers to take (or seizes) control of the perfusionists. Then the cycle begins anew, under new management, and the process starts again. This is essentially healthy because an OR that has no cycles or problems and runs like a finely tuned machine because of a very strong central authority often is an unappealing workplace. There is significant intensity and consequent stress working in an OR simply because of the nature of surgery and its implications for the human condition. This is little appreciated by outsiders, but is also underappreciated by those who work there because to them it becomes routine and even boring—until they stop and reflect for a moment. Therefore, an effort to create a maximally collegial work environment will pay many significant dividends for all involved.

Other issues involving lines of responsibility can greatly affect the daily functioning of the OR. Very often, the OR staff are hospital/facility employees. Often, it is perceived that the hospital is more concerned with limiting the cost of salaries than providing as many personnel as the OR supervisor, surgeons, and anesthesia providers feel are necessary. The topic of adequate nursing and technical support staffing frequently is a never-ending discussion with the hospital administration. If there are genuine issues that cannot be resolved, it is not unreasonable in the appropriate settings for the anesthesiologists, for example, to contribute some of their practice income to hire the additional anesthesia technicians that have been needed. Likewise, surgeons who feel limited by the availability of scrub techs and/or nurses can get together and fund positions of this type from their practice income. This spirit of support and cooperation for the ultimate benefit of all would be both refreshing and most productive.

A central issue for the anesthesia providers in an OR is who among them will be the primary organizational person to interact with the OR. In situations in which all the anesthesia providers are independent contractors, there may be a titular chief of anesthesia who, by default, becomes the contact person. Larger groups or departments that function as a single entity and make their own assignments of personnel often have a clinical director whose job it is to be the contact person with the system and constitute the voice of the anesthesia department on OR organizational matters. Usually there is one anesthesia person supervising the schedule or ''running the board'' daily in the OR for the group. One of the virtues of this person being the clinical director (as opposed to rotating this responsibility among all the anesthesiologists) is that he or she likely has a better day-to-day perspective on the resources and demands related to both anesthesia and OR services. An additional benefit is that a comparative level of consistency in the application of policies, particularly regarding the scheduling of cases, can be more easily applied. One of the most frustrating things to both surgeons and OR staff is inconsistency and unpredictability of decision-making from the anesthesia department. A patient who may be deemed unacceptable for surgery by Anesthesiologist X running the schedule on Monday might well be considered, in exactly the same condition, a routine preop by Anesthesiologist Y on Tuesday. Some of this type of occurrence is unavoidable in a group, but the more there is, the more difficult OR life becomes for the surgeons and the OR staff. Without stifling individual practice styles and philosophies, some measure of consistency applied to similar situations, whether through a clinical director or not, will facilitate OR function considerably.

The availability of the tools of anesthesia administration is another component of OR organization. Usually, the anesthesia service staffs, maintains, and runs an anesthesia work room that contains all the supplies and equipment unique to anesthesia practice, which most often are chosen and ordered by the anesthesia providers and paid for either by the hospital/facility budget or by the practice revenue. There must be coordination with the OR staff as to who will be responsible for the routine equipment not necessarily unique to anesthesia, such as syringes and needles, intravenous fluids, and pulmonary artery catheters. An important goal is the avoidance of duplication and waste. Decisions as to what brands of supplies to buy and regarding major equipment purchases for the anesthesia side of the OR may be the subject of negotiations between the anesthesiologists and the facility administration, but may also reside with the physician members of the Operating Room Committee or its equivalent.

Scheduling Cases

Anesthesiologists need to be involved in the scheduling of OR cases in their institution or facility. In some circumstances, the ''booking office'' and the associated clerical personnel will reside within the department of anesthesiology. More often, however, this function will be part of the OR staff's responsibility, most likely under the direct control of the OR supervisor, who is usually a nurse. In this case, there needs to be a clear mechanism for input from the anesthesia providers to the case scheduling process, both on a daily basis and from the policy management aspect. This is important even in situations in which all the anesthesia providers are independent contractors and not really associated in any way. In such situations, the titular chief of anesthesia should be the one to coordinate schedules to guarantee after-hours coverage and to help plan for program changes, such as the addition of a new group of surgeons to the hospital staff.

When there is an anesthesia department that functions as a cohesive unit, its chairman, clinical director, or appointed representative will be the person who meets with the OR supervisor and surgeons as necessary to establish policies regarding the scheduling of OR cases. There are as many different ways to do this as there are operating suites. Most hospitals and facilities have evolved traditions that attempt to meet the needs of their operating suites. Despite this, OR scheduling remains universally one of the most difficult areas in medical practice.

Acknowledging that it will be impossible to fully satisfy everyone, the anesthesia department should attempt to smooth the process as much as possible. First, the anesthesia department should listen sympathetically to the surgeons' desires and matching them to the OR staff's abilities to provide rooms, equipment, and personnel. Second, the anesthesia department should attempt to establish a schedule of anesthesia services and coverage to mesh realistically with the other two groups.

Regarding scheduling, surgeons are basically divided into two groups: the large majority who want first-in-the-morning operating time for elective cases, and the others—those who will operate essentially any time they can get their cases scheduled and do not understand why the OR cannot run full-tilt 24 hours a day 7 days a week. Neither group can be fully accommodated, and therein lies the need for extensive compromise. Anesthesiologists who approach these disparate desires calmly and with as little confrontation as possible will facilitate the compromise process considerably. There will always be some element of politics involved in these decisions, particularly if the OR uses block time (preassigned guaranteed time for a surgeon or a surgical service to book or post cases before a cutoff time a day or so ahead of the day in question) instead of open scheduling (first-come, first-served for all ORs), and the goal of the anesthesia department should be to appear as neutral as possible while being realistic about what can be accomplished in light of the number of rooms open and the length of the operating day.

Even in small operating suites, case scheduling will be greatly facilitated by some type of computerized scheduling system. Computerized scheduling is simpler and much faster than using a large ledger book. Juggling cases from room to room and trying various possibilities is much simpler on a computer than mass erasing and rewriting of hand entries. Conflicts of personnel or equipment can be instantly identified. Also, most systems of this type will produce reports and statistics automatically. One extremely valuable component of many such programs is automatic assignment of projected case duration based on historical precedent. Suppose Dr. X or service Y has an 8-hour block on a given day and wants to book (or post) four cases. The scheduling program determines what procedures are to be done (such as by CPT-4 code), looks back at past examples of how long that surgeon or service took to do such cases, and then automatically assigns a projected length for each of the cases booked. If the computer concludes that the first three cases will consume the entire available block of time, it will not accept the fourth case into that room's schedule on that day. Once the surgeons' initial resistance is overcome and they get in the habit of either making more realistic time estimates or accepting those from the computer, the scheduling process will become much smoother and far fewer midafternoon disputes will arise between the anesthesia and OR staffs about whether the last case scheduled can actually be done.

In general, there are a great many contributing variables in the scheduling process. The nature of the institution and the patient population served has a great impact. An ambulatory surgery center in an upscale suburban neighborhood doing mostly cosmetic surgery can schedule OR cases of fairly predictable length and complexity well in advance and be relatively certain that the vast majority of patients will appear in appropriate condition, ready to go, at the appointed day and hour. But a large inner-city teaching hospital serving a largely indigent population and receiving mostly acute problems and trauma patients will find it very difficult to schedule the OR much more than a day in advance, if that. In the latter circumstance, maximal cooperation and flexibility from the anesthesiology department (within the limitations of available resources) is mandatory in trying to accommodate the surgeons' requests and the OR staff's ability to do cases. These are two extreme examples from opposite ends of the spectrum. Most situations fall somewhere in between. In all circumstances, however, open communication and honest discussion among the three principal groups involved in OR scheduling about realistic requests and realistic estimates of what is possible will be the key to the smoothest possible functioning of the OR. It is very important to attempt to overcome the "us versus them" attitudes often seen in the OR. Surgeons may be perceived by anesthesia providers as having totally unrealistic expectations or demands for operating time. Anesthesiologists may be perceived by surgeons as arbitrarily canceling or refusing to do cases in an attempt to avoid work. This contentious atmosphere need not prevail. If each of the three groups (plus administrators where applicable) involved in OR scheduling tries hard to understand the positions and thinking of the other two and realizes that all need to be working together toward a common goal—safe, efficient, expedient patient care—then the OR working environment need not be the most difficult in the hospital.

Scheduling Personnel

Except in unusual circumstances, scheduling anesthesia providers is a continual juggling act. Even with independent contractors who make themselves available on lists at various hospitals and depend on surgeons (or OR staff acting at the direction of surgeons) to contact them directly regarding availability and consequent scheduling, there are time conflicts and, conversely, unwanted idle time. When departments or groups accept responsibility for providing anesthesia services for an OR suite, they then have to make sure that there are enough providers to staff the rooms scheduled on any given day. Ideally, a department or group would hire enough people so that there would always be more providers available beyond the minimum needed to run regular rooms during the day and cover the call schedule. In reality, however, this usually does not happen (at least not for long) because it is clearly financially disadvantageous for all to have too many people with no clinical activity. Therefore, there is usually an attempt to have just the right number of providers available, which may work well until someone is out with a family problem or an extended illness. In academic departments, anesthesia attending faculty and residents may be assigned nonclinical time intended for research, teaching, and administration. These people may provide a buffer to help deal with day-to-day variations in the number of people available to work in the OR, but repeated pulling of personnel away from their academic time to provide clinical service quickly undermines the academic programs of a teaching department and also leads to resignations that eventually eliminate that buffer. Accordingly, those responsible for scheduling anesthesia personnel ideally need to anticipate both reasonable needs and available personnel far enough in advance (at least 6 months) to hire accordingly. Doing this, however, has become increasingly difficult. With the sudden major realignments of large segments of the health care system and the advent of managed care systems and the consequent bidding for contracts to care for patients, it may be totally impossible to anticipate the patient load of an OR 6 months hence. There is no easy answer to this and no significant suggestions other than acknowledgment that in all these new arrangements, negotiations, and machinations, data confer power. MCOs must, of necessity, predict OR utilization rates for the groups they cover to allow reasonable negotiating of prospective payments. A great deal of actuarial effort goes into these predictions, and it is reasonable to hope for some degree of accuracy. Therefore, if a health care facility or an organized group of physicians obtains a contract to provide surgery and anesthesia services, it is likely that some reasonable prediction of the need for personnel can be generated.

Again, there are as many different types of situations as there are places to have them. Each operating suite evolves its own system. There needs to be very close coordination between the responsible anesthesia person and the OR supervisor as to how many ORs can be used on any given day and how late in the afternoon or evening they can be open. Inevitably, some cases take much longer than planned and emergency or add-on cases are booked/posted during the day, leading to the need to run more rooms than anticipated at the end of the afternoon and into the evening. The anesthesiology personnel who are thus stuck staying late, whether or not they are being paid overtime, may accept such a situation as a matter of course occasionally, but not routinely. These practitioners become exhausted and also resentful of being abused in general and of the time away from their outside lives. If the practice environment is such that there almost always are rooms that run significantly late, it is likely a worthwhile investment to have additional anesthesia personnel on late call who come in fresh at noon or 1 P.M. with the intention of giving lunch breaks and then staying that evening until all the scheduled cases from the day are finished and there has been a good start on the add-ons, which will then be completed by the anesthesia call personnel.

Scheduling after-hours anesthesia coverage is similarly difficult. In this consideration, the variation among facilities is greater still. Whether or not anesthesia residents, nurse anesthetists, and attending staff need to take in-hospital calls overnight depends on the nature of the institution and workload. Major referral centers for high-risk obstetrics and trauma, for example, need primary providers in-house 24 hours a day and, if these are residents and/or nurse anesthetists, also the attending staff to supervise them. In other settings, primary providers may be in-house with the attending staff taking call from home or both may take calls from home (assuming this is close enough to guarantee arrival in the OR within some agreed-upon interval, such as 30 minutes in the case of a stat cesarean section). The number of people needed on call is always a question. Should the call team be staffed for the minimum, average, or maximum expected load? Often the easiest answer to this is to anticipate an average load and acknowledge that there will be some idle time unused and other instances when the need will outstrip the available personnel. Of course, if that circumstance becomes commonplace rather than unusual, the number of personnel on call needs to be increased.

There are important medicolegal concerns related to this issue. In a small community hospital, for example, if there are three anesthesiologists on staff who do their own cases with no nurse anesthetists involved, they likely will agree that each will cover every third weekend, with the other two being off call and not obligated to the OR. If that one anesthesiologist is administering an anesthetic and cannot safely leave the room and another emergency patient comes into the OR suite with a major acute problem, what should happen? If the other two anesthesiologists are legitimately unavailable and unreachable, should the anesthesiologist in the OR leave the anesthetized patient with, for example, a circulating nurse to watch the monitors and ventilator to tend to the emergency patient in the OR next door? There is no easy answer and, obviously, those on the scene at the time must assess the relative risks and benefits and make hard choices. This example only serves to illustrate the difficulties of trying to provide call coverage to deal with all possible contingencies in the OR.

A related scheduling question is whether anesthesiology personnel who have worked overnight while on call should work in the OR the following day. Again, the individual practice environment will largely dictate the answer. If call almost never means a long night's work, leaving residual fatigue and stress in the morning, it is reasonable for a provider to be scheduled in the OR the following day with the understanding that on the rare occasion when there has been all-night activity, that practitioner will be dismissed as early as possible. Alternatively, if the calls usually do involve extensive night work, there should be no assignment for the next morning. In the rare circumstance that the provider does sleep the night, then he or she is an unexpected extra helper the next day for as long as needed. Common sense and reason guide this thinking. In the same vein, even if there is no indication that fatigue played a role, should an anesthesia catastrophe occur with a practitioner who was up all the previous night, the defense of the resultant malpractice suit may be difficult.

PRACTICE ARRANGEMENTS
The "Job Market" for Anesthesiologists

In the mid-1990s, for the first time, turmoil and uncertainty faced residents finishing anesthesiology training. The long-standing belief that there would be desirable, suitable practice opportunities for the considerable number of residents being graduated yearly finally came to an end. Three main factors contributed to this situation.

A main cause was the number of residents being trained compared to the number of practice opportunity openings. Before about 1993, with the exception of a very few of the most popular cities, finishing residents could first decide where they wanted to live and then seek an anesthesiology practice to join or simply start one themselves. Although a maldistribution of anesthesiologists in the United States existed (and still exists, with underserved rural and core-city areas that may never have had physician anesthesia services), the routine desirable jobs in urban, suburban, and midsize-town private practice groups or facilities began to dry up, particularly starting in 1994. In part, they were simply filled with anesthesiologists who had finished training recently enough to have no intention or desire to move or cut back their practice.

The second significant contributing factor was the proposal in 1993 by the U.S. administration to radically restructure American health care delivery. Although this proposal was eventually abandoned as too radical, it introduced an element of uncertainty that persisted long after it had been dismissed. This element of uncertainty led anesthesiologists and facilities to adopt a "wait and see" attitude about hiring new anesthesiologists, especially in 1994, thus further sharply reducing the number of practice opportunities open that year. (For the first time in recent memory, the Placement Service function at the annual meeting of the ASA was cancelled in October 1994 due to lack of interest from locations seeking to hire or add anesthesiologists. This has subsequently been re-instituted on a smaller scale, and is now more of a computerized journal classified ad section.)

The third major factor is related to the first two. It is the marketplace forces that have been and continue to induce significant changes in the U.S. health care system independent of any government proposal for change. Put as simply as possible, the business community, employers who provide health care insurance for their employees, and government entities that fund programs such as Medicare and Medicaid have stated that it is impossible for them to continue to fund the rapidly increasing expenditures necessary to provide health care coverage. As a result, an entire new industry, managed care, has appeared. The managed care concept is built on the idea that traditional fee-for-service health care has no incentive for health care providers, principally physicians, to limit expenditures. In fact, physicians, health care workers, and health care facilities were financially rewarded the more health care was "consumed" or rendered to patients. Accordingly, MCOs came into being, saying to business and government that a new administrative layer was needed to control (reduce) what physicians and health care facilities spend. This management of care by outside, independent reviewers and decision-makers who determine what care can and should be rendered to the patient is intended to replace the traditional fee-for-service indemnity system (bills submitted by physicians based on what they decide is necessary that are then paid after the fact by a health plan or insurance company) and thereby significantly reduce the cost for health care to employers and governments. Because one of the main

themes of managed care plans is that there will be much less surgery in the future, there has been an impact on the plans of groups and facilities to add new anesthesiologists. Thus, in a very short period of time, the job market for anesthesiologists underwent a radical change. Discussions occurred both within and outside organized anesthesiology about components of this situation,[29-31] but, predictably, no definitive answers are possible. By 1998 the situation had reversed somewhat, as medical students could rapidly read that changing conditions of 1994 and simply stopped choosing anesthesiology as a career. Rapidly, residency programs were faced with a dearth of applicants and many of even the most prominent programs in the nation were unable to fill their allocated resident slots. At the time of this writing the situation seems to be returning, at least somewhat, to conditions similar to the late 1980s with an overall shortage of practitioners and multiple attractive job offers for each resident graduated. The situation is evolving and fluid, but there will always be surgery, no matter what health system changes take place. Moreover, anesthesiologists do more than just OR anesthesia (increasingly so in the future). Therefore, it is appropriate to consider the multitude of issues concerning practice arrangements in anesthesiology.

Types of Practice

With the "alphabet soup" of new practice arrangements for physicians (IPA, PPO, PHO, MCO, MSO, HMO) and the rapidly evolving forces of the health care marketplace, as well as the intermittent appearance of major governmental initiatives to institute radical reform of the health care system, it is difficult to outline the details of all the possible types of opportunities for anesthesiologists. Rather, it is reasonable to provide basic background information and also suggestions of sources of further information.

At least into the first decade of the 21st century, residents finishing anesthesiology training will still need to choose among three fundamental possibilities: academic practice in a teaching hospital environment; a practice exclusively of patient care in the private practice marketplace; and a practice exclusively of patient care as an employee of a health care system, organization, or facility.

Teaching hospitals with anesthesiology residency programs constitute only a very small fraction of the total number of institutions and facilities requiring anesthesia services. These academic departments tend to be among the largest, but the aggregate fraction in academic practices out of the entire anesthesiologist population is also small. It is interesting, however, that most residents finishing their training have almost exclusively been exposed only to academic anesthesiology. Accordingly, finishing residents in the past often were comparatively unprepared to evaluate and enter the anesthesiology job market. As noted, the Anesthesiology Residency Review Committee now requires teaching of job acquisition skills and practice management as part of the residency didactic curriculum.

Specialty certification by the American Board of Anesthesiology (ABA) is likely the goal of most anesthesia residency graduates. Some finishing residents who know they are eventually headed for private practice have started their attending careers as junior faculty. This allows them to obtain some supervisory experience and offers them the opportunity to prepare for the ABA examinations in the nurturing, protected academic environment with which they are familiar. Most, however, do not become junior faculty; they accept practice positions immediately. But such newly trained residents should take into account the need to become ABA-certified and build into their new practice arrangements the stipulation that there will be time and consideration given toward this goal. The hectic and unsettling time of embarking on a new career, possibly moving one's home and family, and getting acclimated to a new professional and financial environment may inhibit optimum performance on the examinations. The possibilities to avoid this disruption may be comparatively limited, but awareness of the problem can help. At the very least, it may lead to the forging of arrangements that will maximize the probability of success.

Academic Practice

For those who choose to stay in academic practice, the first question is whether to consider staying at one's training institution. On the one hand, "the devil you know is better than the devil you don't know." On the other hand, however, fear of the unknown should not inhibit investigation of all possibilities. Aside from obvious personal preferences such as area of the country, size of city, and climate, a number of specific characteristics of academic anesthesia departments can be used as screening questions.

How big is the department? Junior faculty can get lost in very big departments and be treated as little better than glorified senior residents. On the other hand, the availability of subspecialty service opportunities and significant research and educational resources can make large departments extremely attractive. In smaller academic departments, there may be fewer resources, but the likelihood of being quickly accepted as a valued, contributing member of the teaching faculty (and research team, if appropriate) may be higher. In very small departments, the number of expectations, projects, and involvements could potentially be overwhelming. Additionally, a small department may lack a dedicated research infrastructure, so it may be necessary for the faculty in this situation to collaborate with other, larger departments to accomplish meaningful work.

What exactly is expected of junior faculty? If teaching one resident class every other week is standard, the candidate must enthusiastically accept that assignment and the attendant preparation work and time up front. Likewise, if it is expected that junior faculty will, by definition, be actively involved in publishable research, specific plans for projects to which the candidate is amenable must be made. In such situations, clear stipulations about startup research funding and nonclinical time to carry out the projects should be obtained. Particularly important is determining what the expectation is concerning outside funding—it can be a rude shock to realize that projects will suddenly halt after, for example, 2 years if extramural funding has not been secured.

What are the prospects for advancement? Most new junior faculty directly out of residency start with medical school appointments as instructors unless there is something else in their background that immediately qualifies them as assistant professors. It is wise to understand from the beginning what it takes in that department and medical school to facilitate academic advancement. There may be more than one track; the tenure track, for example, is usually dependent on published research whereas the clinical or teacher track relies more heavily on one's value in patient care and as a clinical educator. The criteria for promotion may be clearly spelled out by the institution—number of papers needed, involvement and recognition at various levels, grants submitted and funded, and so on—or the system may be less rigid and depend more heavily on the department chairman's evaluation and recommendation. In either case, careful inquiry before accepting the position can avert later surprise and disappointment.

How much does it pay? Traditionally, academic anesthesiologists have not earned as much as those in private practice—in return for the advantage of more predictable (and maybe less strenuous) schedules, continued intellectual stimulation, and the intangible rewards of academic success. As is clear from this chapter, there is now great activity and attention concerning reimbursement of anesthesiologists, and it is difficult to predict future income for any anesthesiology practice situation. However, all of the forces influencing payment for anesthesia care may significantly diminish the traditional income differential between academic and private practice. This is not a small issue. Anesthesiologists justifiably can expect to live reasonably well. Income is also a valid consideration both because anesthesiologists are frequently at least 30 years old when they finish training and are thus starting well behind their age-mates in lifetime earnings and because most physicians have substantial educational loans to repay when finishing residency. The compensation arrangements in academic practice vary widely in structure. In some cases, a faculty member is exclusively an employee of the institution, which bills and collects or negotiates group contracts for the patient care rendered by the faculty member, and then pays a negotiated amount (either an absolute dollar figure or a floating amount based on volume and/or collections) that constitutes the faculty person's entire income. Under other arrangements, the faculty members themselves can bill and collect or negotiate contracts for their clinical work. Some institutions have a (comparatively small) academic salary from the medical school for being on the faculty, but many do not; and, of these, some channel variable amounts of money into the academic practice (so-called Part A payments) in recognition of teaching and administration. This salary from the medical school, if extant, is then supplemented significantly by the practice income. Usually, the faculty will be members of some type of group or practice plan (either for the anesthesia department alone or the entire faculty as a whole) that bills and collects or negotiates contracts and then distributes the practice income to the faculty under an arrangement that must be examined by the candidate. An important corollary issue is that of the source of the salaries of the department's primary anesthesia providers—residents and, in some cases, nurse anesthetists. Although the hospital usually pays for at least some of these, arrangements vary, and it is important to ascertain whether the faculty practice income is also expected to cover the cost of the primary providers.

Private Practice in the Marketplace

As noted, some residents finish their anesthesia training never having seen a private practice anesthesia setting or even talked to an anesthesiologist who has been in private practice. These candidates are ill-equipped to seek a position in the private practice marketplace. Obviously, rotations to a private practice hospital in the third year of anesthesia residency could help greatly in this regard, but not all residency programs offer such opportunities. In that case, the finishing resident who is certain about going into private practice must find educational opportunities on career development and mentors from the private sector.

Armed with as much information as possible, one fundamental initial choice is between independent individual practice and a position with a group (either a sole proprietorship, partnership, or corporation) that functions as a single financial entity. Independent practice may become increasingly less viable in many locations because of the need to be able to bid for contracts with managed care entities. However, where it is possible, it usually first involves attempting to secure clinical privileges at a number of hospitals or facilities in the area in which one chooses to live. This may not always be easy, and this issue has been the subject of many (frequently unsuccessful) antitrust suits over recent years (see Antitrust Considerations). Then the anesthesiologist makes it known to the respective surgeon communities that he or she is available to render anesthesia services and waits until there is a request for his or her services. The anesthesiologist obtains the requisite financial information from the patient and then either individually bills and collects for services rendered or employs a service to do billing and collection for a percentage fee [which will vary depending on the circumstances, especially the volume of business; for billing (without scheduling services) it would be unlikely to be more than 7% or, at the most, 8% of actual collections]. How much of the needed equipment and supplies will be provided by the hospital or facility and how much by the independent anesthesiologist varies widely. If an anesthesiologist spends considerable time in one operating suite, he or she may purchase an anesthesia machine exclusively for his or her own use and move it from room to room as needed. It is likely to be impractical to move a fully equipped anesthesia machine from hospital to hospital on a day-to-day basis. Among the features of this style of practice are the collegiality and relationships of a genuine private practice based on referrals and also the ability to decide independently how much time one wants to be available to work. The downside is the potential unpredictability of the demand for service and the time needed to establish referral patterns and obtain bookings sufficient to generate a livable income.

Acknowledging that the issues presented above may at some times render components of these suggestions moot, it is reasonable for the finishing resident to know that when seeking a position with a private group, the applicant should search for potential practice opportunities through word of mouth, recruiting letters sent to the training program supervisor, journal advertisements, and placement services (either commercial or professional, such as that provided at the ASA annual meeting). Some of the screening questions are the same as for an academic position, but there must be even more emphasis on the exact details of clinical expectations and financial arrangements. Some residents finish residency and even more so fellowship training very highly skilled in complex, difficult anesthesia procedures. They can be surprised to find that in some private practice group situations, the juniormost anesthesiologist must wait some time, perhaps even years, before being eligible to do, for example, open heart anesthesia and in the meantime will mostly be assigned more routine or less challenging anesthetics. Of course, this is not always the circumstance, but the applicant needs to investigate thoroughly to be certain that the opportunity satisfies the desire for professional challenge.

Financial arrangements in private group practices vary. Some groups are loose organizational alliances of independent practitioners who bill and collect separately and rotate clinical assignments and call for mutual convenience. Many groups act also as a fiscal entity, and there are many possible variations on this theme. In many circumstances in the past, new junior members started out as functional employees of the group for a probationary interval before being considered for full membership or partnership. This is not a classic employment situation because it is intended to be temporary as a prelude to full financial participation in the group. However, there have been enough instances of established groups abusing this arrangement that the ASA includes in its fundamental Statement of Policy the proviso: "Exploitation of anesthesiologists by other anesthesiologists is improper."[1] This goes on to say that after a reasonable trial period, income should reflect services rendered. Unfortunately, these statements have very little meaning or impact on groups in the marketplace today. Some groups have a history of demanding excessively long trial periods during which the junior anesthesiologist's income is artificially low and then denying partnership and terminating the relationship to go on to employ a new probationer and start the cycle over again. Accordingly, new junior staff attempting to join groups should try to have such an arrangement spelled out carefully in the agreement drafted by an expert representing the anesthesiologist. Another variation of this, in an attempt to disguise the fundamentally unethical nature of the practice, is to employ anesthesiologists on a fixed salary with the false incentive of no night or weekend call. This is disingenuous, as the vast majority of income is generated during routine scheduled day work, for which the anesthesiologist-employee is poorly compensated. Yet another usurious scheme is for a group to employ an anesthesiologist for a period of years at a low salary and then require a further cash outlay to purchase partnership in the corporation. As the cash outlay can be quite substantial, it is frequently borrowed from the corporation, leading to a sophisticated form of indentured servitude. Sadly, when the job market conditions are poor as they were a few years ago, the tendency is for there to be less likelihood of securing a prospective commitment of partnership at a specified future time. This is especially true in the more desirable areas of California and the Northeast United States where stories of abuse of junior partners are rife. Whether this should substantially affect an applicant's interest in or willingness to accept a position is a highly individual matter that must be evaluated by each applicant.

Private Practice as an Employee

There has been some trend toward anesthesiologists becoming permanent employees of any one of various fiscal entities. The key difference is that there is no intention or hope of achieving an equity position (share of ownership, usually of a partnership, thus becoming a full partner). Hospitals, outpatient surgery centers, multidisciplinary clinics, other facilities tied to a specific location where surgery is performed, physician groups that have umbrella fiscal entities specifically created to serve as the employer of physicians, and even surgeons may seek to hire anesthesiologists as permanent employees. The common thread in this system is that these fiscal entities see the anesthesiologists as additional ways of generating profits. Again, these employees are rarely paid a salary that is commensurate with their production of receivables. That is, the fiscal entity will pay a salary substantially below collections generated. These arrangements are particularly favored by many large managed care organizations that view anesthesiologists simply as expensive burdens that prevent hospitals from realizing maximum profit. Some anesthesiologists have predicted that this trend will continue to grow, and that eventually most physicians in the support specialties of anesthesiology, radiology, pathology, and emergency medicine will be outright permanent employees of an organized entity of some type. Although some current information might suggest this, it is impossible to speculate on the future in this regard. Other anesthesiologists believe that the future is extraordinarily bright and that anesthesiology will expand its role, predicting that anesthesiologists will increasingly assume positions of central authority, making decisions about hiring physicians of other specialties.

Negotiating for a position as a permanent employee is somewhat simpler and more straightforward than it is in marketplace private practice. It parallels the usual understandings that apply to most regular employer–employee situations: job description, role expectations, working conditions, hours, pay, and benefits. The idea of anesthesiologists functionally becoming shift workers disturbs many in the profession. On the other hand, the major upheaval in the health care delivery system is promoting reorganization that, until very recently, was unheard of. Again, the complex nature and multiple levels of such considerations make it a personal issue that must be carefully evaluated by each individual.

Billing and Collecting

In practices in which anesthesiologists are directly involved with the financial management, they need to understand as much as possible about the complex world of health care reimbursement. This not-small task has been made easier by the ASA, which has added a significant component to its Washington, D.C., office by adding a practice management coordinator to the staff. One of the associated assignments is helping ASA members understand and work with the sometimes confusing and convoluted issues of effective billing for anesthesiologists' services.

There continue to be proposals for significant changes in billing for anesthesiology care. However, the basics have changed only slightly in recent years. It is important to understand that many of the most contentious issues, such as the reimbursement for medical direction of nurse anesthetists, apply almost exclusively to Medicare and, in some states, Medicaid. Thus, the fraction of the patient population covered by these payers is important in any consideration. Different practice situations have different arrangements regarding the financial relationships between anesthesiologists and nurse anesthetists, and this can affect the impact of the rules regarding the ability of nurse anesthetists to bill for their services independently. The nurses may be employees of a hospital, of the anesthesiologists who medically direct them, or of no one in that they are independent contractors billing separately. As of 1998, the Health Care Financing Administration (HCFA) mandated that an anesthesia care team of a nurse anesthetist medically directed by an anesthesiologist could bill as a team no more than 100% of the fee that would apply if the anesthesiologist did the case alone. The implications of this change are complex and variable among anesthesiology practices, particularly because there is another trend—for health care facilities that traditionally had employed nurse anesthetists to seek to shift total financial responsibility for them to the anesthesiologist practice group. In the late 1990s there was also a suggestion from HCFA that CRNAs be allowed to bill for practice without anesthesiologist supervision as independent contractors. Such care would thus be under the medical direction of the surgeon, rather than the anesthesiologist. Obviously, this has caused much consternation among various parties, including the ASA membership, with vigorous lobbying efforts from all sides. At the time of this writing, it appears that the matter has been tabled, but is likely to become active at some future date. Further, the implications of all this for billing payers other than Medicare and Medicaid are exceedingly complex. Obviously, careful consideration of these issues and seeking out advice from knowledgeable resources is critical to fiscal stability in modern anesthesiology practice.

There has been significant consideration of the mechanism of billing for anesthesiology. There have been many suggestions that so-called schedule fees (a single predetermined fee for an anesthetic, independent of its length or complexity) will become more common. Further, there is pressure from some quarters to bundle together all the physicians' fees for one procedure into a single global fee that would pay the surgeon, anesthesiologist, radiologist, pathologist, and so on for one case, such as a laparoscopic cholecystectomy. Further, all of this concern about billing for specific procedures will become irrelevant in systems with prospective capitated payments for large populations of patients, in which each group of involved physicians in a system would receive a fixed amount per enrolled member per month (PMPM) and agree, except in the most unusual circumstances, to provide whatever care is needed by that population for that prospective payment. These are intended to be large-scale operations involving at least tens of thousands of people ("covered lives") in each organization.

At least for the moment, there is still some utility in some places for the traditional method of billing for anesthesiology services. In this system, each anesthetic generates a value of so many units, which represent effort and time. A conversion factor translates the value of a unit into dollars. Each anesthetic has a base value number of units (*e.g.,* 8 for a cholecystectomy) and then the time taken for the anesthetic is divided into units, usually 15 minutes per unit. In some practice settings, it may be allowed to add modifiers, such as extra units for complex patients with multiple problems as reflected by an ASA physical status classification of 3–5 or for insertion of an arterial or pulmonary artery catheter. The sum is the total billing unit value. Determining the base value for an anesthetic in units depends on full and correct understanding of what operation was done. Although this sounds easy, it is the most difficult component of traditional anesthesia billing. The process of determining the procedure done is known as coding because the procedure name listed on the anesthesia record is assigned an identifying code number from the universally used CPT-4 coding book. This code is then translated through the ASA Relative Value Guide, which assigns a base unit value to the type of procedure identified by the CPT-4 code. In the past, some anesthesiologists failed to understand the importance of correct coding to the success of the billing process. Placing this task in the hands of someone unfamiliar with the system and with surgical terminology can easily lead to incorrect coding. This can fail to capture charges and income to which the anesthesiologist is entitled or, worse, can systematically overcharge the payers, which will bring sanctions, penalties and, in certain cases, criminal prosecution. In 2000, the prevailing official attitude is that there are no simple, innocent coding errors. All upcoding is considered to be *prima facie* evidence of fraud and subject to severe disciplinary and legal action. All practices should have detailed compliance programs in place to ensure correct coding for services rendered.[32] Outside expert help (such as from a health care law firm that specializes in compliance programs) is highly desirable for the process of formulating and implementing a compliance plan.

Once the information has been secured, a mechanism must be employed to generate the actual bill and communicate it to the payer (on paper, on disk, or directly computer-to-computer). The potential arrangements for doing this vary widely. Ultimately, the entity actually submitting the bill will verify that it has been paid (posting of receipts) and may or may not actually handle the incoming money. Very often, anesthesia practices or individuals who use a billing service will arrange that the payments go directly to a bank lockbox, which is a post office box (better individual than shared, even if more expensive) to which the payments come and then go directly into a bank account. This system avoids the situation of having the people who generate the bill actually handle the incoming receipts, a practice that has led to theft and fraud. Eventual decisions about how hard to try to collect from payers who deny coverage and then from patients directly will depend on the circumstances.

Anesthesia billing and collecting are among the most complex challenges in the medical reimbursement field. The experience of many people over the years has suggested that it often is well advised to deal with an entity that is not only well experienced in anesthesia billing, but also does anesthesia billing exclusively or as a large fraction of its efforts. It is very difficult for an anesthesiologist or a family member to do billing and collecting on the side. This has led to inefficient and inadequate efforts in many cases, illustrating the value of paying a reasonable fee to a professional who will devote great time and energy to the endeavor.

Antitrust Considerations

Although it is true that there are many potential antitrust implications of business arrangements involving anesthesiologists—particularly with all the realignments, consolidations, mergers, and contracts associated with the advent of managed care—it is also true that the applicable statutes and regulations are poorly understood. Contrary to popular belief, the antitrust laws do not involve the rights of individuals to engage in business. Rather, the laws are concerned solely with the preservation of competition within a defined marketplace and the rights of the consumer, independent of whether any one vendor or provider of service is involved. This misunderstanding has been the source of confusion. When an anesthesiologist has been excluded from a particular hospital's staff or anesthesia group and then sues based on an alleged antitrust violation, the anesthesiologist loses virtually automatically. This is because there is still significant competition in the relevant marketplace and competition in that market is not threatened by the exclusion of one physician from one staff.

In essence, if there are *several* hospitals offering relatively similar services to an immediate community (the market), denial of privileges to one physician by one hospital is not anticompetitive. If, on the other hand, there is only *one* hospital in a smaller market, then the same act, the same set of circumstances, would be seen very differently. In that case, there would be a limitation of competition because the hospital dominates and, in fact, may control the market for hospital services. Exclusion of one physician, then, would limit access by the consumers to alternative competing services and hence would likely be judged an antitrust violation.

The Sherman Antitrust Act is a federal law more than 100 years old. Section 1 deals with contracts, combinations, conspiracy, and restraint of trade. By definition, two or more separate economic entities must be involved in an agreement that is challenged as illegal for this section to apply. Section 2 prohibits monopolies or conspiracy to create a monopoly, and it is possible that this could apply to a single economic entity that has illegally gained domination of a market. Consideration of possible monopolistic domination of a market involves a situation in which a single entity controls at least 50% of the business in that market. The stakes are high in that the antitrust legislation provides for triple damages if a lawsuit is successful. The U.S. Department of Justice and the Federal Trade Commission are keenly interested in the current rapid evolution in the health care industry, and thus are actively involved in evaluating situations of possible antitrust violations. There are two ways to judge violations. Under the *per se* rule, which is applied relatively rarely, conduct that is obviously limiting competition in a market is automatically illegal. The other type of violation is based on the rule of reason, which involves a careful analysis of the market and the state of competition. The majority of complaints against physicians are judged by this rule. The more competitors there are in a market, the less likely that any one act is anticompetitive.

In the current era of rapidly evolving managed care arrangements, the antitrust laws are important. If physicians (individuals or groups) who normally would be competitors because they are separate economic entities meet and agree on the prices they will charge or the terms they will seek in a managed care contract, that can be anticompetitive, monopolistic, and hence possibly illegal. Note that sharing a common office and common billing service alone is not enough to constitute a true group. If, on the other hand, the same physicians join in a true economic partnership to form a new group (total integration) that is a single economic entity (and meets certain other criteria) that will set prices and negotiate contracts, that is perfectly legal. The other criteria are critical. There must be capital investment and also risk sharing (if there is a profit or loss, it is distributed among the group members)—*i.e.*, total integration into a genuine partnership. This issue is very important in considering the drive for new organizations to put together networks of physicians that then seek contracts with major employers to provide medical care. Sometimes, hospitals or clinics attempt to form a network comprising all the members of the medical staff so that the resulting entity can bid globally for total care contracts. Any network is a joint venture of independent practitioners. If the participating physicians of one specialty in a network are separate economic entities and the network advertises one price for their services, this would seem to suggest an antitrust violation (horizontal price fixing). In the past, if a network involved fewer than 20% of one type of medical specialist in a market, that was called a "safe harbor," meaning that it was permissible for nonpartners to get together and negotiate prices. The federal government has tried to encourage formation of such networks to help reduce health care costs and, as a result, announced in late 1994 some relevant exceptions to the application of these rules. As long as the network is nonexclusive (other non-network physicians of a given specialty are free to practice in the same facilities and compete for the same patients), the network can comprise up to 30% of the physicians

of one specialty in a market. Note specifically that this does not allow a local specialty society in a big city to serve as a bargaining agent on fees for its members, because it is very likely that more than 30% of the specialists in an area will be members of the society. The only real exception to this provision is in thinly populated rural areas where there may be just one physician network. In such cases (which are, so far, rare because the major managed care and network activity has occurred in heavily populated urban areas), there is no limit on how many of one specialty can become network members and have the network negotiate fees, as long as the network is nonexclusive.

Clearly, these issues are very complex. Relevant legislation, regulations, and court actions all happen rapidly and often. Mergers among anesthesiology groups in a market area for the purposes of both efficiency and strength in negotiating fees have been very popular as a response to the rapidly changing marketplace. A list of questions must be answered to determine if such a merger would have anticompetitive implications. Although compendia of relevant information are available to anesthesiologists,[33,34] they cannot substitute for expert advice and help. Obviously, anesthesiologists contemplating a merger or facing any one of a great number of other new situations in the modern health care arena must secure assistance from professional advisors, usually attorneys, whose job it is to be aware of the most recent developments, how they apply, and how best to forge agreements in formal contracts. Anesthesiologists hoping to find reputable advisors can start their search with word-of-mouth referrals from colleagues who have used such services. Local or state medical societies frequently know of attorneys who specialize in this area. Finally, the ASA Washington, D.C., office has compiled a state-by-state list of advisors who have worked successfully with anesthesiologists in the past.

Exclusive Service Contracts

Until recently, one of the larger issues faced by anesthesiologists seeking to define practice arrangements was whether an exclusive contract with a health care facility to provide anesthesia services was desirable. An exclusive contract states that anesthesiologists seeking to practice at a given facility must be members of the group holding the exclusive contract and, usually, that members of the group will practice nowhere else. A hospital may want to give an exclusive contract in return for a guarantee of coverage as part of the contract. Also, the hospital may believe that such a contract can help ensure the quality of practitioner because the contract can contain credentialing and performance criteria. It is important to understand that the hospital likely will exercise a degree of control over the anesthesiologists with such a contract in force, such as requiring them to participate as providers in any contracts the hospital makes with third-party payers and also tying hospital privileges to the existence of the contract (the so-called "clean sweep provision" that bypasses any due process of the medical staff should the hospital terminate the contract). Certain of these types of provisions constitute *economic credentialing*, which is defined as the use of economic criteria unrelated to the quality of care or professional competency of physicians in granting or renewing hospital privileges (such as the acceptance of below-market fees associated with a hospital-negotiated care contract or even requiring financial contributions in some form to the hospital). The ASA has issued a statement condemning economic credentialing.[36] The anesthesiologists involved may accept such an exclusive services contract to guarantee that they alone will get the business from the surgeons on staff at that hospital, and hence the resulting income. There may be other considerations on both sides, and these have been outlined in an extensive relevant ASA publication that also includes a sample contract for information purposes only.[32] Although many exclusive contracts with anesthesiology groups are in force, the sentiment in the relevant literature, particularly from the ASA, is against them. As has been stated, it is critical that anesthesiologists faced with important practice management decisions such as whether to enter into an exclusive contract must seek outside advice and counsel. There are a great many nuances to these issues,[33] and anesthesiologists are at risk attempting to negotiate such complex matters alone, just as patients would be at risk if a contract attorney attempted to induce general anesthesia.

Denial of hospital privileges as a result of the existence of an exclusive contract with the anesthesiologists in place at the facility has been the source of many lawsuits, including the well-known Louisiana case of *Hyde v. Jefferson Parish*. In that case, the court found for the defendant anesthesiologists and the hospital, saying that there was no antitrust violation because there was no real adverse effect on competition as far as patients were concerned because there were several other hospitals within the market to which they could go, and therefore they could exercise their rights to take advantage of competition in the relevant market. Thus, existence of an exclusive contract only in the rare setting where anticompetitive effects on patients can be proved might lead to a legitimate antitrust claim by a physician denied privileges.

Managed Care and New Practice Arrangements

As noted, managed care systems for health care delivery fundamentally exist as a mechanism to control and then reduce health care costs by having independent reviewers and decision-makers who are not the physicians rendering the care limit the health care services delivered to large groups of patients. These ideas represent a huge change for American physicians. These changes appear inescapable, not necessarily because of government initiatives, but because of marketplace forces that result from the business community and government entities simply refusing to continue to pay ever-increasing sums for health care. The degree of penetration of managed care into market areas around the country is highly variable. Areas such as Minneapolis, San Diego, eastern Massachusetts, and several other northern cities were the first to become mature managed care markets with a significant majority of the population enrolled in one or another managed care health plan. Other parts of the country with very sparsely populated areas such as sections of the deep South and the far West will be the last to experience the managed care revolution. The impact in these areas is difficult to predict because the organizers of managed care may not be able to enroll enough people to make it worth the effort to create and operate a system. An MCO attempts to secure health care provision contracts with employers who provide health plan coverage and with government agencies (*e.g.,* Medicaid) responsible for the health care of large populations. Each worker or covered head of a household may have dependents covered by the plan. Each person covered is referred to as a *covered life.* An MCO probably needs contracts for at least 10,000 covered lives and preferably many more to make a legitimate entry into the marketplace. The MCO then enrolls physicians or physician groups and hospitals as providers and contracts to send its enrolled patients (the covered lives) to the health care providers under contract. The central issue is finances. The MCO seeks to enroll covered lives by offering the lowest prices possible. In turn, it seeks to contract with providers (individuals and facilities) for the lowest possible fees for medical care in return for sending large volumes of patient business to those providers.

In the initial stages of the evolution of a managed care marketplace, the MCOs usually seek contracts with providers based on discounted fee-for-service arrangements. This preserves the basic traditional idea of production-based physician reimbursement (do more, bill more) but the price of each act of services is lower (the providers are induced to give deep discounts with the promise of significant volumes of patients) and, also, the MCO gatekeeper primary care physicians and the MCO reviewers are strongly encouraged to limit complex and costly services

as much as possible. There are other features intermittently along the way, such as global fees and negotiated fee schedules (agreed-upon single prices for individual procedures, independent of length or complexity). Further, another element is introduced to encourage the providers, both gatekeepers and specialists, to reduce costs. In an application of the concept of risk-sharing (spend too much for patient care and lose income), this usually is initially manifest in the form of "withholds," the practice of the MCO holding back a fraction of the agreed-upon payment to the providers (*e.g.,* 10 or 15%) and keeping this money until the end of the fiscal year. At that time, if there is any money left in the risk pool or withhold account after all the (partial) provider fees and MCO expenses are paid, it is distributed to the providers in proportion to their degree of participation during the year. This is a clever and powerful incentive to providers to reduce health care expenses. It is not as powerful as the stage of full risk-sharing, however. As the managed care marketplace matures and MCOs grow and succeed, the existing organizations and, especially, any new ones, shift to prospective capitated payments for providers.

This eventual reimbursement arrangement constitutes an entirely new world to the providers, involving prospective capitated payments for large populations of patients, in which each group of providers in the MCO receives a fixed amount per enrolled covered life per month (PMPM) and agrees, except in the most unusual circumstances, to provide whatever care is needed by that population for that prospective payment. The most unusual circumstances involve "carve-out" arrangements in which specific very costly and unusual conditions or procedures (such as the birth of a child with disastrous multiple congenital anomalies) are covered separately on a discounted fee-for-service basis. With full capitation, the entire financial underpinning of American medical care does a complete about-face from the traditional rewards for doing more to new rewards for doing less. Some managed care contracts contain other features intended to protect the providers against unexpected overutilization by patients that would stretch the providers beyond the bounds of the original contract with the MCO. The provisions setting the boundaries are called "risk corridors," and the "stop-loss clauses" add some discounted fee-for-service payment for the excess care beyond the risk corridor (capitated contract limit). Providers who were used to getting paid more for doing more suddenly find themselves getting paid a fixed amount no matter how much or how little they do with regard to a specified population—hence the perceived incentive to do, and consequently spend, less. If the providers render too much care within the defined boundary of the contract, they essentially will be working for free, the ultimate in risk-sharing. There are clearly potential internal conflicts in such a system,[37] and how patients react to this potential radical change in attitude on the part of physicians has not yet been fully established and may well eventually play a significant role in how managed care evolves.

Health care providers (physicians, health care workers, and facilities), in turn, are allying themselves in a wide variety of organizations to create strength and desirable resources to present to the MCOs in contract negotiations. Some of these alliances have been formed very quickly, almost in a panic, because of fears by providers that they might get left out of the managed care marketplace and thus deprived of major sources of income or, someday, any income at all. Management service organizations (MSOs) are joint venture network arrangements that do not involve true economic integration among the practitioners, but merely offer common services to physicians who may, as a loosely organized informal group, elect to seek MCO contracts. Preferred provider organizations (PPOs) are network arrangements of otherwise economically independent physicians who form a new corporate entity to seek managed care contracts in which there are significant financial incentives to patients to use the network providers and financial penalties for going to out-of-network providers. Physician–hospital organizations

(PHOs) are similar entities but involve understandings between groups of physicians and a hospital so that a large package or bundle of services can be constructed as essentially one-stop points of care. Independent practice associations (IPAs) are like PPOs but are specifically oriented toward capitated contracts for covered lives with significant risk-sharing by the providers. Groups (or clinics) without walls are collections of practitioners who fully integrate economically into a single fiscal entity (true partnership) and then compete for MCO contracts on the basis of risk-sharing incentives among the partners. Fully integrated groups or health maintenance organizations (HMOs) house the group of partner provider physicians and associated support staff at a single location for the convenience of patients, a big selling point when they seek MCO contracts.

The questions anesthesiologists face when addressing this alphabet soup of organizations are many and complex,[35] even more complex than those faced by office-based primary care or specialty physicians, because of the interdependent relation-ships with health care facilities as practice locations and with surgeons. The era of solo independent practitioners may be ending in many locations. Small groups of anesthesiologists may find themselves at a competitive disadvantage unless they become part of a vertically integrated (multispecialty) or hori-zontally integrated (with other anesthesiologists) organization. An extensive compendium of relevant information has been prepared by the ASA.[33] Because it appears likely that at least most, if not all, anesthesiologists in the United States will be affected by managed care, the central themes of this compen-dium and other publications[38,39] are very important. Negotia-tions with MCOs require expert advice, probably even more so than the traditional exclusive contracts with hospitals noted above. Before any negotiation can even be considered, the MCO must provide significant amounts of information about the cov-ered patient population. The projected health care utilization pattern of a large group of white-collar workers (and their families) from major upscale employers in an urban area will be

---

Table 2-5. TYPES OF DATA AN ANESTHESIOLOGY GROUP SHOULD TRACK AND MAINTAIN CONCERNING ITS OWN PRACTICE

Types of Data the Anesthesiology Group's Computer System Should Track

- ◆ Transaction-based system (track each case and charge as separate record)
  - Track individual charges by CPT-4 code
  - Track individual payments by payer
- ◆ Track all data elements on an interrelated basis
  - By place of service
  - By charge, broken down
    -by number of units (time and base)
    -by ASA modifiers
    -by number of lines
  - By CPT-4 code
  - By payer
  - By payment code (full payment, discount, write-off, or refund)
  - By diagnosis (ICD-9 code)
  - By surgeon
  - By anesthesiologist
  - By anesthesia care team provider
  - By start and stop times
  - By age
  - By gender
  - By employer
  - By ZIP code

Type of Information to Generate From These Data

- ◆ Aggregate number of cases per year for the group
- ◆ Total number of cases per year for each provider within the group
  - Number of cases performed by anesthesiologists
  - Number of cases performed by the anesthesia care team
- ◆ Average number of units per case (as one measure of intensity per case)
- ◆ Average number of units per CPT-4 code
- ◆ Average time units per case and per CPT-4 code
  - Group should be able to calculate time units per individual surgeon
- ◆ Average line charge per case
- ◆ Charges per case by CPT-4 code
- ◆ Payments per case by payer
- ◆ Patient mix
  - Percent traditional indemnity
  - Percent managed care (broken down by each MCO for which services are provided)
  - Percent self-pay
  - Percent Medicare
  - Percent Medicaid
- ◆ Collection rate for each population served
- ◆ Overall collection rate
- ◆ Costs per unit (total costs, excluding compensation ÷ total units) (costs include liability insur-ance, rent, collection costs, and legal and accounting fees)
- ◆ Compensation costs per unit (total compensation ÷ total units) for MCO populations, utiliza-tion patterns by age, gender, and diagnosis

---

Reprinted with permission from American Society of Anesthesiologists: Managed Care Reimburse-ment Mechanisms: A Guide for Anesthesiologists. Park Ridge, IL, ASA, 1994.

quite different from that of a rural Medicaid population. Specific demographics and past utilization histories are absolutely mandatory for each proposed population to be covered, and this information should go directly to the advising experts for evaluation, whether the proposed negotiation is for discounted fee-for-service, a fee schedule, global bundled fees, or full capitation.

Significant questions have also been raised about the reimbursement implications for anesthesiologists of the managed care revolution. Again, the ASA has assembled a great deal of relevant information, the understanding of which is essential to successful negotiations.[33,40] Table 2-5 is a list of information an anesthesia practice should have about its activities, and Table 2-6 is a sample "capitation checklist." Initial consideration of a capitated contract should involve an attempt to take all the data about the existing practice and the proposed MCO-covered

population and translate back from the proposed capitated rate to income figures that would correlate with the existing practice structure, to allow a comparison and an understanding of the relationship of the projected work to projected income. It is, of course, impossible to suggest dollar values for capitated rates for anesthesiology care because details and conditions vary so widely. One ASA publication[40] used examples, purely for illustrative purposes, involving $2.50 or $4.00 PMPM, but there have been unconfirmed reports of capitated rates as low as $0.75 PMPM. Discounted fee-for-service arrangements are easier for anesthesiologists to understand because these are directly referable to existing fee structures. Reports of groups instituting 10–50% discounts off the starting point of 80% of usual and customary reimbursement in various practice circumstances have been circulated at national meetings of anesthesiologists.

Table 2-6. CAPITATION CHECKLIST

Utilization

- Total number of MCO members
- Stability of MCO population over last 5 years
- Target populations of MCO marketing
- Benefit plan: member copayment or cost-sharing

- Channeling of patients to facility or alternative MCO facilities
- Historical frequency of surgical procedures
  - Admissions per thousand

Analysis/Demographics of MCO Population

- Age
- Gender
- Occupation
- Employment status

- Income level
- Breakout by payer group
- New patients or conversion of existing patients

Other Providers

- How are primary care physicians compensated?
- How are other specialists compensated?
- How is hospital or facility compensated?

- Are any of the surgeons MCO employees?
- Relative speed of surgeons under contract with the MCO
- Frequency of updates adding or deleting MCO surgeons

Compensation

- Comparison to fee-for-service
- Risk corridors or stop/loss provisions
- Timing of payment
- Timeframe for adding or deleting members

- Compensation for uncovered services withholds
- Ability to audit MCO enrollment numbers and MCO process for adding or deleting members

MCO Solvency and History

- Ownership of MCO
- Solvency of MCO
  - Audited financial statement
  - Financial summary for previous years (at least 3 to 5 years)

- Management of MCO
- List of management and medical director(s)
- Prior history in dealings with specialists

Scope of Services Covered

- All anesthesia services?
- Financial incentives for other providers to cease performing certain procedures (e.g., insertion of lines)
- Complexity and/or length of particular cases (e.g., cardiac)

- Difficulty of treating certain patients (e.g., chronic pain)
- Non-operating room procedures
- Carve-outs? (e.g., obstetric, cardiac, acute, and chronic pain management call)

Administrative Obligations

- Utilization review
- Quality assurance
- Nature and frequency of reports required

- Nature of case documentation required
- Cost of monitoring MCO experience
- Any counterbalancing cost-effectiveness or efficiency

Sources of Data

- HCFA Medicare utilization
- State health department
- Medicaid
- Worker's compensation
- State employee programs
- Private sector
- Blue Cross/Blue Shield

- Private insurers
- Large local employers
- MCO filings with state insurance health departments
- American Hospital Association
- Hospitals
- Other MCOs

Although it seems likely that average income for anesthesiologists will decrease from past levels under all managed care systems, it also appears that anesthesiologists will continue to have very comfortable incomes, still among the higher figures for all physicians.

Expansion into Perioperative Medicine, Hospital Care, and Hyperbaric Medicine

As the role of the anesthesiologist changes, in part due to the realities of workforce statistics and to the potential for decreased clinical workloads due to the success of managed care health systems, new opportunities should be explored. One set of ideas that has been circulating for some time has led to serious suggestions that the name of the profession of anesthesiology be changed to "perioperative medicine and pain management." This suggestion illustrates that one prospective significant anesthesiology practice management strategy can be more formal organization of responsibilities for patients in the pre- and postoperative periods.

Many anesthesiologists now function at least some of the time in preoperative screening clinics because of the great fraction of OR patients who do not spend the night before surgery in the hospital or who do not come to a hospital at all. In such settings, these anesthesiologists frequently assume a role analogous to that of a primary care physician, planning and executing a work-up of one or more significant medical or surgical problems before the patient can reasonably be expected to undergo surgery. More formalized arrangements of this type would involve the creation of designated perioperative clinics operated and staffed by anesthesiologists. Ophthalmologists and orthopedists, for example, would no longer need to try to manage their surgical patients' medical problems themselves or send their patients proposed for surgery to an internist or other primary care provider for "preop clearance." The anesthesiologist would assume that role at the same time the patient is undergoing preoperative evaluation for anesthesia care.

Likewise, this concept would be excellent for the postoperative period. An anesthesiologist, completely free of OR or other duties, could not only make at least twice-daily rounds on patients after surgery and provide exceedingly comprehensive pain management service, but also could follow the surgical progress and make virtually continuous reports (likely *via* e-mail) to the surgeon's office or alphanumeric pocket communicator. Surgeons would have a much better handle on their patients' progress while having more time to tend to other new patients in the office or OR. The utilization review and fast-track protocol administrators would have a contact person who is not tied up in an OR or office continuously available. Patients would receive much more physician attention and perceive this as actually a significant improvement in their care. Equivalent outpatient or recuperative center services could easily be established. In this regard, some anesthesiologists function as hospitalists for the care of both surgical and medical patients. A fundamental aspect of the practice of anesthesiology is the management of acute problems in the hospital setting. It is logical that anesthesiologists would be among the physicians best suited to provide primary care for patients in the hospital setting. Although the comfort level of anesthesiologists varies in the fields of internal medicine and pediatrics, it is likely that this trend will continue among those interested and competent in hospital care.

Finally, anesthesiologists are becoming increasingly involved in the practice of hyperbaric medicine and wound care. This is likely related to the familiarity of anesthesiologists with concepts of gas laws and physics, along with their constant presence in the hospital. The treatment of various medical conditions by the application of oxygen under increased pressure, usually 2–3 atmospheres absolute, is one of the most rapidly growing hospital services. Anesthesiologists are among the leaders of this field,

with unlimited opportunities for clinical care, teaching, and research. Again, even a brief discussion is outside the scope of this chapter and interested readers are referred to the Undersea and Hyperbaric Medical Society (www.umhs.org).

Creative exploration of new opportunities involving these and other ideas will open new avenues for anesthesiology (or whatever it is eventually called) practice.

CONCLUSION

Practice management in anesthesiology today is more complex and more important than ever before. Attention to details that previously either did not exist or were deemed unimportant can likely make the difference between success and failure in anesthesiology practice.

Outlined here are basic descriptions and understandings of many different administrative, organizational, and financial components and factors in the practice of anesthesiology. Ongoing significant changes in the health care system will provide a continuing array of challenges. Application of the principles presented here will allow anesthesiologists to creatively extrapolate from these basics to their own individual circumstances and forge ahead.

REFERENCES

1. Manual for Anesthesia Department Organization and Management. Park Ridge, IL, American Society of Anesthesiologists, 1995
2. Gilbert B: Relating quality assurance to credentials and privileges. In Chapman-Cliburn G (ed): Risk Management and Quality Assurance: Issues and Interactions, p 79–83. Chicago, Joint Commission on the Accreditation of Hospitals, 1986
3. Peters JD, Fineberg KS, Kroll DA et al: Anesthesiology and the Law. Ann Arbor, MI, Health Administration Press, 1983
4. Manual for Anesthesia Department Organization and Management, p 27–50. Park Ridge, IL, American Society of Anesthesiologists, 1995
5. Gaba DM, Howard SK, Jump B: Production pressure in the work environment. Anesthesiology 81:488, 1994
6. American Society of Anesthesiologists: 2000 Directory of Members, p 483. Park Ridge, IL, ASA, 1999
7. Eichhorn JH, Cooper JB, Cullen DJ et al: Anesthesia practice standards at Harvard: A review. J Clin Anesth 1:56, 1988
8. Hawkins JL (Chair) et al: Practice guidelines for obstetrical anesthesia. Anesthesiology 90:600, 1999
9. Practice guidelines for pulmonary artery catheterization. Anesthesiology 78:380, 1993
10. Practice guidelines for management of the difficult airway. Anesthesiology 78:597, 1993
11. Dans PE, Weiner JP, Otter SE: Peer review organizations: Promises and potential pitfalls. N Engl J Med 313:1131, 1985
12. American Society of Anesthesiologists: Peer Review in Anesthesiology, 1991, p 109–134. Park Ridge, IL, ASA, 1991
13. Eichhorn JH: Anesthesia equipment: Checkout and quality assurance. In Ehrenwerth J and Eisenkraft JB (eds.): Anesthesia Equipment: Principles and Applications, p 473–491. St. Louis, Mosby-Yearbook, 1992
14. Spooner RB, Kirby RR: Equipment-related anesthetic incidents. In Pierce EC, Cooper JB (eds): Analysis of Anesthetic Mishaps. International Anesthesiology Clinics 22:133, 1984
15. Cooper JB, Newbower RS, Kitz RJ: An analysis of major errors and equipment failures in anesthesia management: Considerations for prevention and detection. Anesthesiology 60:34, 1984
16. Cooper JB, Newbower RS, Long CD et al: Preventable anesthesia mishaps: A study of human factors. Anesthesiology 49:399, 1978
17. Lunn JN, Mushin WW: Mortality Associated with Anaesthesia. London, Nuffield Provincial Hospitals Trust, 1982
18. Duberman S, Wald A: An integrated quality control program for anesthesia equipment. In Chapman-Cliburn G (ed): Risk Management and Quality Assurance: Issues and Interactions, p 105–112. Chicago, Joint Commission on the Accreditation of Hospitals, 1986
19. Pierce EC: Risk modification in anesthesiology. In Chapman-Cliburn G (ed): Risk Management and Quality Assurance: Issues and Interactions. Chicago, Joint Commission on Accreditation of Hospitals, 1986

20. American Society of Anesthesiologists: Manual for Anesthesia Department Organization and Management, p 13–15. Park Ridge, IL, ASA, 1995
21. HHS Publication No. (FDA) 85-4196. Food and Drug Administration, Center for Devices and Radiologic Health, Rockville, MD 20857, p 10
22. Eichhorn JH: Influence of practice standards on anesthesia outcome. In Desmonts JM (ed): Outcome After Anesthesia and Surgery. Bailliere's Clinical Anaesthesiology—International Practice and Research 6:663, 1992
23. Eichhorn JH: Prevention of intraoperative anesthesia accidents and related severe injury through safety monitoring. Anesthesiology 70: 572, 1989
24. Keats AS: Anesthesia mortality in perspective. Anesth Analg 71: 113, 1990
25. Bacon AK: Death on the table: Some thoughts on how to handle an anaesthetic-related death. Anaesthesia 44:245, 1989
26. Runciman WB, Webb RK, Klepper ID et al: Crisis management: Validation of an algorithm by analysis of 2000 incident reports. Anaesth Intensive Care 21:579, 1993
27. Davies JM, Webb RK: Adverse events in anaesthesia: The wrong drug. Can J Anaesth 41:83, 1994
28. Cooper JB, Cullen DJ, Eichhorn JH et al: Administrative guidelines for response to an adverse anesthesia event. J Clin Anesth 5:79, 1993
29. Grogono AW: Medical student recruitment: Match results for anesthesiology, 1990–94. ASA Newsletter 58:25, 1994
30. Weiner JP: Forecasting the effects of health reform on U.S. physician workforce requirements. JAMA 272:222, 1994
31. Cullen BF: Anesthesia workforce requirements: Are there too many anesthesiologists? ASA Newsletter 58:27, 1994
32. American Society of Anesthesiologists: Practice Management: Compliance with Medicare and Other Payor Billing Requirements. Park Ridge, IL, ASA, 1997
33. American Society of Anesthesiologists: Practice Management: Practice Perspective for Survival in the Managed Care Marketplace. Park Ridge, IL, ASA, 1994
34. American Society of Anesthesiologists: Contracting Issues: A Primer for Anesthesiologists. Park Ridge, IL, ASA, 1999
35. American Society of Anesthesiologists: Practice Management: Managed Care Contracting. Park Ridge, IL, ASA, 1996
36. American Society of Anesthesiologists: Manual for Anesthesia Department Organization and Management, p 9. Park Ridge, IL, ASA, 1995
37. Rodin MA: Conflicts in managed care. N Eng J Med 332:604, 1995
38. Hetrick WD: Health care reform: Implications for the anesthesiologist. Adv Anesth 12:1, 1995
39. American Society of Anesthesiologists: Health System Reform Survival Guide. Park Ridge, IL, ASA, 1993
40. American Society of Anesthesiologists: Managed Care Reimbursement Mechanisms: A Guide for Anesthesiologists. Park Ridge, IL, ASA, 1994

Clinical Anesthesia (4/e), edited by
Paul G. Barash, Bruce F. Cullen, and
Robert K. Stoelting. Lippincott Williams &
Wilkins, Philadelphia, © 2001.

CHAPTER 3

EXPERIMENTAL DESIGN AND STATISTICS

NATHAN LEON PACE

INTRODUCTION

Medical journals are replete with numbers. These include weights, lengths, pressures, volumes, flows, concentrations, counts, temperatures, rates, currents, energies, and forces. For five decades, anesthesia journals have exhorted the researcher to collect, analyze, and interpret these numbers more carefully. The analysis and interpretation of these numbers require the use of statistical techniques; the design of the experiment to acquire these numbers is also part of statistical competence. The need for these statistical techniques is mandated by the nature of our universe, which is both orderly and random at the same time. For example, the anesthesiologist knows that halothane has a dose-response pharmacology—increasing concentrations produce greater effects: a sufficiently high concentration will anesthetize the patient; even higher concentrations will kill. Yet, for any individual patient, only a guess can be made in advance as to the necessary concentration to produce anesthesia. If everything were known about the function of the body, it is possible that the necessary anesthetizing concentration could be predicted. Instead, one must rely on the minimum alveolar anesthetic concentration (MAC), which characterizes the response to halothane for a group of patients. It allows only an initial guess as to the amount required for any individual patient.

Probability and statistics have been formulated to solve concrete problems, such as betting on cards, understanding biologic inheritance, and improving food processing. Studies in anesthesia have even inspired new statistics; the National Halothane Study prompted new advances in the analysis of frequency tables. The development of statistical techniques is manifest in the increasing use of more sophisticated research designs and statistical tests in anesthesia research.

If a physician is to be a practitioner of scientific medicine, he or she must read the language of science in order to be able to independently assess and interpret the scientific report; and, without exception, the language of the medical report is increasingly statistical. Readers of the anesthesia literature, whether in a community hospital or a university environment, cannot and should not totally depend on the editors of journals to banish all errors of statistical analysis and interpretation. In addition there are regularly questions about simple statistics in examinations required for anesthesiologists. Finally, certain statistical methods have everyday applications in clinical medicine. This chapter briefly scans some elements of experimental design and statistical analysis; it does not provide the systematic review.

DESIGN OF RESEARCH STUDIES

The scientific investigator should view himself or herself as an experimenter and not merely as a naturalist. The naturalist goes out into the field ready to capture and report the numbers that flit into view; this is a worthy activity, typified by the case report. Case reports engender interest, suspicion, doubt, wonder, and, one hopes, the desire to experiment; however, the case report is not sufficient evidence to advance scientific medicine. The experimenter attempts to constrain and control, as much as possible, the environment in which he or she collects numbers to test a hypothesis.

In undertaking a research project, the investigator is implicitly accepting the philosophical concept that the results in a group of patients can be applied to an individual patient. Especially as applied to the therapy of disease, this idea has engendered controversy for centuries. On the one side is the contention that the individuality of each person demands that the therapy of disease be unique. Proponents would argue as follows: "The probabilities and results of a research report may not apply to an individual patient. For the individual patient, a treatment is either a failure or a success. A patient cannot be four-fifths alive, but is either alive or dead. Treatment should be individualized to each patient. Any type of therapy which might be possibly and plausibly beneficial should be allowed."

More persuasive is the argument adopted by proponents of scientific medicine: "No therapeutic agent can be employed with discrimination unless the general efficacy of the agent has been confirmed in analogous cases. Although each patient is distinct and therapy should be adapted to the circumstances, the most likely therapy to benefit a patient will be that which is supported by experimental evidence." The hope for the generalizability of medical research results impels the publication of medical journals.

Sampling

Two words of great importance to statisticians are *population* and *sample*. In statistical language, each has a specialized meaning. Instead of referring only to the count of individuals in a geographic or political region, population refers to any target group of things (animate or inanimate) in which there is interest. For anesthesia researchers, a typical target population might be mothers in the first stage of labor, for example, or head trauma victims undergoing craniotomy. A target population could also be cell cultures, isolated organ preparations, or hospital bills. A sample is a subset of the target population. Samples are taken because of the impossibility of observing the entire population; it is generally not affordable, convenient, or practical to examine more than a relatively small fraction of the population. Nevertheless, the researcher wishes to generalize from the results of the small sample group to the entire population.

Although the subjects of a population are alike in at least one way, these population members are generally quite diverse in other ways. Since the researcher can work only with a subset of the population, he or she hopes that the sample of subjects in the experiment is representative of the population's diversity. Head-injury patients can have open or closed wounds, a variety of coexisting diseases, and normal or increased intracranial pressure. These subgroups within a population are called *strata*. Often the researcher wishes to increase the sameness or homogeneity of the target population by further restricting it to just a few strata; perhaps only closed and not open head injuries will be included. Restricting the target population to eliminate too much diversity must be balanced against the desire to have the results be applicable to the broadest possible population of patients.

The best hope for a representative sample of the population would be realized if every subject in the population had the same chance of being in the experiment; this is called *random sampling*. If there are several strata of importance, random sampling from each stratum would be appropriate. Unfortunately, in most clinical anesthesia studies researchers are limited to using those patients who happen to show up at their hospitals; this is called *convenience sampling*. Convenience sampling is also subject to the nuances of the surgical schedule, the goodwill of the referring physician and attending surgeon, and the willingness of the patient to cooperate. At best, the convenience sample is representative of patients at that institution, with no assurance that these patients are similar to those elsewhere. Convenience sampling is also the rule in studying new anesthetic drugs in volunteers; such studies are typically performed on healthy, young students.

The researcher must define the conditions to which the sample members will be exposed. Particularly in clinical research, one must decide whether these conditions should be rigidly standardized or whether the experimental circumstances should be adjusted or individualized to the patient. In anesthetic drug research, should a fixed dose be given to all members of the sample or should the dose be adjusted to produce an effect or to achieve a specific end point? Standardizing the treatment groups by fixed doses simplifies the research work. There are risks to this standardization, however: (1) A fixed dose may produce excessive numbers of side effects in some patients; (2) a fixed dose may be therapeutically insufficient in others; and (3) a treatment standardized for an experimental protocol may be so artificial that it has no broad clinical relevance, even if demonstrated to be superior.

Control Groups

Even if a researcher is studying just one experimental group, the results of the experiment are usually not interpreted solely in terms of that one group but are also contrasted and compared with other experimental groups. Examining the effects of a new drug on blood pressure during anesthetic induction is important, but what is more important is comparing those results with the effects of one or more standard drugs commonly used in the same situation. Where can the researcher obtain these comparative data? There are several possibilities: (1) Each patient could receive the standard drug under identical experimental circumstances at another time; (2) another group of patients receiving the standard drug could be studied simultaneously; (3) a group of patients could have been studied previously with the standard drug under similar circumstances; and (4) literature reports of the effects of the drug under related but not necessarily identical circumstances could be used. Under the first two possibilities the control group is contemporaneous—either *self-control* (cross-over) or *parallel control* group. The second two possibilities are examples of the use of *historical controls*.

Because historical controls already exist, they are convenient and seemingly cheap to use. Unfortunately, the history of medicine is littered with the debris of therapies enthusiastically accepted on the basis of comparison with past experience but later found to be worthless. A classic example was operative ligation of the internal mammary artery for the treatment of angina pectoris. There is now firm empirical evidence that studies using historical controls usually show a favorable outcome for a new therapy, whereas studies with concurrent controls, *i.e.*, parallel control group or self-control, less often reveal a benefit. Nothing seems to increase the enthusiasm for a new treatment as much as the omission of a concurrent control group. If the outcome with an old treatment is not studied simultaneously with the outcome of a new treatment, one cannot know if any differences in results are a consequence of the two treatments, or of unsuspected and unknowable differences between the patients, or of other changes over time in the general medical environment. One possible exception would be in studying a disease that is uniformly fatal (100% mortality) over a very short time.

Random Allocation of Treatment Groups

Having accepted the necessity of an experiment with a control group, the question arises as to the method by which each subject should be assigned to the predetermined experimental groups. Should it depend on the whim of the investigator, the day of the week, the preference of a referring physician, the wish of the patient, the assignment of the previous subject, the availability of a study drug, a hospital chart number, or some other arbitrary criterion? All such methods have been used and are still used, but all can ruin the purity and usefulness of the experiment. It is important to remember the purpose for sampling: by exposing a small number of subjects from the target population to the various experimental conditions, one hopes to make conclusions about the entire population. Thus, the experimental groups should be as similar as possible to each other in reflecting the target population; if the groups are different, this introduces a bias into the experiment. Although randomly allocating subjects of a sample to one or another of the experimental groups requires additional work, this principle prevents selection bias by the researcher, minimizes (but cannot always prevent) the possibility that important differences exist among the experimental groups, and disarms the critics' complaints about research methods. Random allocation is most commonly accomplished by computer-generated random numbers.

Blinding

Blinding refers to the masking from the view of patient and experimenter the experimental group to which the subject has been or will be assigned. In clinical trials, the necessity for blinding starts even before a patient is enrolled in the research study. There is good evidence that, if the process of random allocation is accessible to view, the referring physicians, the research team members, or both are tempted to manipulate the entrance of specific patients into the study to influence their assignment to a specific treatment group; they do so having formed a personal opinion about the relative merits of the treatment groups and desiring to get the "best" for someone they favor. This creates bias in the experimental groups.

Each subject should remain, if possible, ignorant of the assigned treatment group after entrance into the research protocol. The patient's expectation of improvement, a placebo effect, is a real and useful part of clinical care. But when studying a new treatment, one must ensure that the fame or infamy of the treatments does not induce a bias in outcome by changing patient expectations. Such a study, in which the subject is unaware of the treatment given, is called *single blind*. A researcher's knowledge of the treatment assignment can bias his or her ability to administer the research protocol and to observe and record data faithfully; this is true for clinical, animal, and *in vitro* research. If the treatment group is known, those who observe data cannot trust themselves to record the data impartially and dispassionately. A *double-blind* study, in which both subject and data collector are ignorant of the treatment group, is the best way to test a new therapy.

Types of Research Design

Ultimately, research design consists of choosing what subjects to study, what experimental conditions and constraints to enforce, and which observations to collect at what intervals. A few key features in this research design largely determine the strength of scientific inference on the collected data. These key features allow the classification of research reports (Table 3-1). This classification reveals the variety of experimental approaches and indicates strengths and weaknesses of the same design applied to many research problems.

The first distinction is between *longitudinal* and *cross-sectional*

Table 3-1. CLASSIFICATION OF BIOMEDICAL RESEARCH REPORTS

I. Longitudinal studies
  A. Prospective (cohort) studies
    1. Studies of deliberate intervention
      a. Concurrent controls
      b. Historical controls
    2. Observational studies
  B. Retrospective (case-control) studies
II. Cross-sectional studies

studies. The former's object is the study of changes over time, whereas the latter describes a phenomenon at a certain point in time. For example, reporting the frequency with which certain drugs are used during anesthesia is a cross-sectional study, whereas investigating the hemodynamics of different drugs during anesthesia is a longitudinal one.

Longitudinal studies are next classified by the method with which the research subjects are selected. These methods for choosing research subjects can be either *prospective* or *retrospective;* these two approaches are also known as *cohort* (prospective) or *case-control* (retrospective). A prospective study assembles groups of subjects by some input characteristic that is thought to change an output characteristic; a typical input characteristic would be the primary drug used for anesthetic induction, *e.g.,* alfentanil or sufentanil. A retrospective study gathers subjects by an output characteristic; an output characteristic is the status of the subject after an event, *e.g.,* the occurrence of a myocardial infarction. A prospective (cohort) study would be one in which a group of patients undergoing heart surgery was divided in two groups, given two different anesthetic inductions (alfentanil or sufentanil), and followed for the development of a perioperative myocardial infarction. In a retrospective (case-control) study, patients who suffered a perioperative myocardial infarction would be identified from hospital records; a group of subjects of similar age, gender, and disease who did not suffer a perioperative myocardial infarction also would be chosen, and the two groups would then be compared for the relative use of the two anesthetic induction drugs (alfentanil or sufentanil). Retrospective studies are a primary tool of epidemiology. A case-control study can often identify an association between an input and output characteristic, but the causal link or relationship between the two is more difficult to specify.

Prospective studies are further divided into those in which the investigator performs a deliberate intervention and those in which the investigator merely observes. In a study of *deliberate intervention*, the investigator would choose several anesthetic maintenance techniques and compare the incidence of postoperative nausea and vomiting. If it was performed as an *observational study*, the investigator would observe a group of patients receiving anesthetics chosen at the discretion of each patient's attending anesthesiologist and compare the incidence of postoperative nausea and vomiting among the anesthetics used. Obviously, in this example of an observational study, there has been an intervention; an anesthetic has been given. The crucial distinction is whether the investigator controlled the intervention. An observational study may reveal differences among treatment groups, but whether such differences are the consequence of the treatments or of other differences among the patients receiving the treatments will remain obscure.

Studies of deliberate intervention are further subdivided into those with concurrent controls and those with historical controls. Concurrent controls are either a simultaneous parallel control group or a self-control study; historical controls include previous studies and literature reports. A *randomized controlled trial* is thus a longitudinal, prospective study of deliberate intervention with concurrent controls.

Although most of this discussion about experimental design has focused on human experimentation, the same principles apply and should be followed in animal experimentation. The randomized, controlled clinical trial is the most potent scientific tool for evaluating medical treatment; randomization into treatment groups is relied upon to equally weight the subjects of the treatment groups for baseline attributes that might predispose or protect the subjects from the outcome of interest.

Hypothesis Formulation

Whether the research subjects are tissue preparations, animals, or people, the researcher is constantly faced with finding both similarities and differences among the diversities of a group of subjects. The researcher starts the work with some intuitive feel for the phenomenon to be studied. Whether stated explicitly or not, this is the *biologic hypothesis;* it is a statement of experimental expectations to be accomplished by the use of experimental tools, instruments, or methods accessible to the research team. An example would be the hope that isoflurane would produce less myocardial ischemia than fentanyl; the experimental method might be the electrocardiographic determination of ST segment changes. The biologic hypothesis of the researcher becomes a *statistical hypothesis* during research planning. The researcher measures quantities that can vary—variables such as heart rate or temperature or ST segment change. In a statistical hypothesis, statements are made about the relationship among parameters of one or more populations. A *parameter* is a number describing a variable of a population; Greek letters are used to denote parameters. The statistical hypothesis can be established in a somewhat rote fashion for every research project, regardless of the methods, materials, or goals.

The most frequently used method of setting up the algebraic formulation of the statistical hypothesis is to create two mutually exclusive statements about some parameters determined from the study population (Table 3-2); estimates for the values for these parameters are acquired by sampling data. In the hypothetical example comparing isoflurane and fentanyl, ϕ_1 and ϕ_2 would represent the ST segment changes with isoflurane and with fentanyl. The *null hypothesis* is the hypothesis of no difference of ST segment changes between isoflurane and fentanyl. The *alternative hypothesis* is usually nondirectional, *i.e.,* either $\phi_1 < \phi_2$ or $\phi_1 > \phi_2$; this is known as a two-tail alternative hypothesis. This is a more conservative alternative hypothesis than assuming that the inequality can only be either $<$ or $>$.

Logic of Proof

One particular decision strategy is used almost universally to choose between the null and alternative hypothesis. The decision strategy is similar to a method of indirect proof used in mathematics called *reductio ad absurdum*. If a theorem cannot be proved directly, assume that it is not true; show that the falsity of this theorem will lead to contradictions and absurdities; thus, reject the original assumption of the falseness of the theorem. For statistics, the approach is to assume that the null hypothesis is true even if the goal of the experiment is to show that there is a difference. One examines the consequences of this assumption by examining the actual sample numbers obtained for the variable(s) of interest. This is done by calculat-

Table 3-2. ALGEBRAIC STATEMENT OF STATISTICAL HYPOTHESES

H_0: $\phi_1 = \phi_2$ (null hypothesis)
H_a: $\phi_1 \neq \phi_2$ (alternative hypothesis)
ϕ_1 = Parameter estimated from sample of first population
ϕ_2 = Parameter estimated from sample of second population

Table 3-3. ERRORS IN HYPOTHESIS TESTING: THE TWO-WAY TRUTH TABLE

		REALITY (POPULATION PARAMETERS)	
		Conditions 1 and 2 equivalent	Conditions 1 and 2 not equivalent
CONCLUSION FROM OBSERVATIONS (SAMPLE STATISTICS)	Conditions 1 and 2 equivalent*	Correct conclusion	False-negative Type II error (beta error)
	Condition 1 and 2 not equivalent†	False-positive Type I error (alpha error)	Correct conclusion

* Do not reject null hypothesis: Condition 1 = Condition 2.
† Reject null hypothesis: Condition 1 ≠ Condition 2.

ing what are called *sample test statistics;* sample test statistics are calculated from the sample numbers. Associated with a sample test statistic is a *probability*. One also chooses the *level of significance;* the level of significance is the probability level considered too low to warrant support of the null hypothesis being tested. If sample values are sufficiently unlikely to have occurred by chance (*i.e.,* the probability of the sample test statistic is less than the chosen level of significance), the null hypothesis is rejected; otherwise the null hypothesis is not rejected.

Because the statistics deal with probabilities, not certainties, there is a chance that the decision concerning the null hypothesis is erroneous. These errors are best displayed in table form (Table 3-3); Condition 1 and Condition 2 could be different drugs, two doses of the same drug, or different patient groups. Of the four possible outcomes, two are clearly undesirable. The error of wrongly rejecting the null hypothesis (false positive) is called the *Type I* or *alpha error*. The experimenter should choose a probability value for alpha before collecting data; the experimenter decides how cautious to be about falsely claiming a difference. The most common choice for the value of alpha is 0.05. What are the consequences of choosing an alpha of 0.05? Assuming that there is, in fact, no difference between the two conditions and that the experiment is to be repeated 20 times, then during one of these experimental replications (5% of 20) a mistaken conclusion that there is a difference would be made. The probability of a Type I error depends on just two factors: the chosen level of significance and the existence or nonexistence of a difference between the two experimental conditions. The smaller the chosen alpha, the smaller will be the risk of a Type I error.

The error of failing to reject a false null hypothesis (false negative) is called a *Type II* or *beta error*. The power of a test is 1 minus beta. The probability of a Type II error depends on four factors. Unfortunately, the smaller the alpha, the greater the chance of a false-negative conclusion; this fact keeps the experimenter from automatically choosing a very small alpha. Second, the more variability there is in the populations being compared, the greater the chance of a Type II error. This is analogous to listening to a noisy radio broadcast; the more static there is, the harder it will be to discriminate between words. Next, increasing the number of subjects will lower the probability of a Type II error. The fourth and most important factor is the magnitude of the difference between the two experimental conditions. The probability of a Type II error goes from very high, when there is only a small difference, to extremely low, when the two conditions produce large differences in population parameters.

Sample Size Calculations

Discussion of hypothesis testing by statisticians has always included mention of both Type I and Type II errors, but research-

ers have typically ignored the latter error in experimental design. The practical importance of worrying about Type II errors reached the consciousness of the medical research community about 20 years ago. Some controlled clinical trials that claimed to find no advantage of new therapies compared with standard therapies lacked sufficient statistical power to discriminate between the experimental groups and would have missed an important therapeutic improvement. There are four options for decreasing Type II error (increasing statistical power): (1) Raise alpha, (2) reduce population variability, (3) make the sample bigger, and (4) make the difference between the conditions greater. Under most circumstances, only the sample size can be varied. Sample size planning has become an important part of research design for controlled clinical trials. Some published research still fails the test of adequate sample size planning.

Implications

The elements of good experimental design—random sampling, control groups, random allocation, blinding, and sample size planning—are not mere theoretical concerns; they have a solid empirical basis. This is illustrated by two controversies.

The best anesthetic to minimize perioperative myocardial ischemia and infarction and to lower perioperative mortality in patients undergoing coronary artery bypass grafting (CABG) remains a continuing disputation. After an assertion was made in the 1980s that isoflurane fosters myocardial ischemia, two randomized controlled trials provided conflicting reports about isoflurane's danger or lack thereof. In one study (1989) of about 1000 patients, approximately equal numbers were anesthetized with enflurane, halothane, isoflurane, or sufentanil; in-hospital mortality was low (1–2%) and roughly equivalent among the four groups. In another study (1990) of about 1200 patients, approximately equal numbers were anesthetized with enflurane or isoflurane; in-hospital mortality was significantly higher in those receiving isoflurane (2.1%) compared to those receiving enflurane (0.3%). Is isoflurane safe? Which study should be believed? Many comparisons can be made between the two studies, but one of the most pertinent concerns experimental design. While both studies claimed to use random allocation of treatment groups, the 1990 report actually alternated the anesthetic used in all operating rooms between enflurane and isoflurane every week. This is an example of pseudo random allocation. The 1989 report did indeed randomly allocate patients to their anesthetic group; in fact, to eliminate a misallocation of the four anesthetics among the patients of the four surgeons participating in the research, random allocation was stratified (performed separately) by surgeon. Greater weight should be given to the study design with true random allocation. This experimental design is less likely to be afflicted with biases in patient selection.

Pulse oximetry has helped revolutionize monitoring in the operating room and is now a standard of care in many countries. Yet it was adopted without a prior demonstration of an improvement—by its routine use—of patient outcome. Finally a multicenter, randomized controlled trial was completed and published. More than 20,000 adult patients were randomly divided into two groups: in 10,000 pulse oximetry was applied in the operating room and the post anesthesia care unit; no pulse oximetry monitoring was used for the other 10,000. There were approximately equal numbers of deaths, cardiac arrests, myocardial infarctions, strokes, and all other serious morbidity in the two groups. Editorial comment about this study has focused on the near impossibility of studying the effect of improved monitoring on anesthetic mortality and serious morbidity. Why is there such an impossibility? Anesthesia is now so safe that it may require 500,000 to millions of patients to detect improvement—that is, to have sufficient statistical power to distinguish outcome differences. There are no resources (money, personnel, interest) to perform such large studies.

STATISTICAL TESTING

Statistics is a method for working with *sets* of numbers, a set being a group of objects. Statistics involves the description of number sets, the comparison of number sets with theoretical models, comparison between number sets, and comparison of recently acquired number sets with those from the past. A typical scientific hypothesis asks which of two methods, X and Y, is better. A statistical hypothesis is formulated concerning the sets of numbers collected for X and Y. Statistics provides methods for deciding if the values of set X are different from the values of set Y. Statistical methods are necessary because there are sources of variation in any data set, including random biologic variation and measurement error. These errors in the data cause difficulties in avoiding bias and in being precise. Bias keeps the true value from being known and fosters incorrect decisions; precision deals with the problem of the data scatter and with quantifying the uncertainty about the value in the population from which a sample is drawn. These statistical methods are relatively independent of the particular field of study. Regardless of whether the numbers in sets X and Y are systolic pressures, body weights, or serum chlorides, the approach for comparing sets X and Y is usually the same.

Data Structure

Data collected in an experiment include the defining characteristics of the experiment and the values of events or attributes that vary over time or conditions. The former are called *explanatory variables* and the latter are called *response variables*. The researcher records his or her observations on data sheets or case record forms, which may be one to many pages in length, and assembles them together for statistical analysis. Variables such as gender, age, and doses of accompanying drugs reflect the variability of the experimental subjects. Explanatory variables, it is hoped, explain the systematic variations in the response variables. In a sense, the response variables are dependent on the explanatory variables.

Response variables are also called *dependent variables*. Response variables reflect the primary properties of experimental interest in the subjects. Research in anesthesiology is particularly likely to have repeated measurement variables, *i.e.*, a particular measurement recorded more than once for each individual. Some variables can be both explanatory and response; these are called *intermediate response variables*. Suppose an experiment is conducted comparing electrocardiographic and myocardial responses between five doses of an opioid. One might analyze how ST segments depended on the dose of opioids; here, maximum ST segment depression is a response variable. Maximum ST segment depression might also be used as an explanatory variable to address the more subtle question of the extent to which the effect of an opioid dose on postoperative myocardial infarction can be accounted for by ST segment changes.

The mathematical characteristics of the possible values of a variable fit into five classifications (Table 3-4). Properly assigning a variable to the correct data type is essential for choosing the correct statistical technique. For *interval variables*, there is equal distance between successive intervals; the difference between 15 and 10 is the same as the difference between 25 and 20. *Discrete interval data* can have only integer values, *e.g.*, ages in years, number of live children, or papers rejected by a journal. *Continuous interval data* are measured on a continuum and can be a decimal fraction; for example, blood pressure can be described as accurately as desired, *e.g.*, 136, 136.1, or 136.14 mm Hg. The same statistical techniques are used for discrete and continuous data.

Categorical variables are derived by putting observations into two or more discrete categories; for statistical analysis, numeric values are assigned as labels to the categories. *Dichotomous data* allow only two possible values, *e.g.*, male versus female. *Ordinal data* have three or more categories that can logically be ranked or ordered; however, the ranking or ordering of the variable indicates only relative and not absolute differences between values; there is not necessarily the same difference between American Society of Anesthesiologists Physical Status score I and II as there is between III and IV. Although ordinal data are often treated as interval data in choosing a statistical technique, such analysis may be suspect; alternative techniques for ordinal data are available. *Nominal variables* are placed into categories that have no logical ordering. The eye colors blue, hazel, and brown might be assigned the numbers 1, 2, and 3, but it is nonsense to say that blue < hazel < brown.

Descriptive Statistics

A typical hypothetical data set could be $A = (29, 32, 27, 28, 26, 27, 28, 29, 30, 32, 35, 31)$, representing a sample of ages

Table 3-4. DATA TYPES

Data Types	Definition	Examples
INTERVAL		
Discrete	Data measured with an integer-only scale	Age, parity
Continuous	Data measured with a constant scale interval	Blood pressure, temperature
CATEGORICAL		
Dichotomous	Binary data	Mortality, gender
Nominal	Qualitative data that cannot be ordered or ranked	Eye color, drug category
Ordinal	Data ordered, ranked, or measured without a constant scale interval	ASA physical status score, pain score

(the variable) of 12 residents in an anesthesia training program (the population). Although the results of a particular experiment might be presented by repeatedly showing the entire set of numbers, there are concise ways of summarizing the information content of the set A into a few numbers. These numbers are called *sample* or *summary statistics;* summary statistics are calculated using the numbers of the sample. By convention, the symbols of summary statistics are Roman letters. The two summary statistics most frequently used for interval variables are the *central location* and the *variability,* but there are other summary statistics. Other data types have analogous summary statistics.

Although the first purpose of descriptive statistics is to describe the sample of numbers obtained, there is also the desire to use the summary statistics from the sample to characterize the population from which the sample was obtained. For example, what can be said about the age of all anesthesia residents from the information in set A? The population also has measures of central location and variability called the parameters of the population; as previously mentioned, population parameters are denoted by Greek letters. Usually, the population parameters cannot be directly calculated, because data from all population members cannot be obtained. The beauty of properly chosen summary statistics is that they are the best possible estimators of the population parameters.

These sampling statistics can be used in conjunction with a theoretical probability distribution to provide additional descriptions of the sample and its population. A theoretical probability distribution is an algebraic equation, $f(x)$, which gives a theoretical percentage distribution of x. Each value of x has a probability of occurrence given by $f(x)$. This probability may be expressed as a percentage: $100 \times f(x)$. If $f(x)$ is summed or integrated for all possible values of x, the percentage must total 100% and the probability must total 1.0. The most important probability distribution is the *normal* or *gaussian function.* There are two parameters (population mean and population variance) in the equation of the normal function which are denoted μ and σ^2. The normal equation can be plotted and produces the familiar bell-shaped curve. Why are the mathematical properties of this curve so important to biostatistics? First, it has been empirically noted that when a biologic variable is sampled repeatedly, the pattern of the numbers plotted as a histogram resembles the normal curve; thus, most biologic data are said to follow or to obey a normal distribution. Second, if it is reasonable to assume that a sample is from a normal population, the mathematical properties of the normal equation can be used with the sampling statistic estimators of the population parameters to describe the sample and the population. Third, a mathematical theorem (the Central Limit Theorem) allows the use of the assumption of normality for certain purposes, even if the population is not normally distributed.

Central Location

The three most common summary statistics of central location for interval variables are the arithmetic *mean,* the *median,* and the *mode.* The mean is merely the average of the numbers in the data set. Statistical formulas use a summation notation that considerably reduces the ink needed to print mathematical equations. The summary notation for the arithmetic mean is given below:

$$\bar{x} = \Sigma \, x_i / n \qquad (3\text{-}1)$$

Capital sigma (Σ) is the summation operator; its purpose is to add up all values of x from x_1 to x_n; the sum is then divided by the count of individuals (n) in the sample. Being a summary statistic of the sample, the arithmetic mean is denoted by the Roman letter $\bar{x}$. If all values in the population could be obtained, then the population mean (μ) could be calculated similarly.

Because all values of the population cannot be obtained, the sample mean is used.*

The median is the middlemost number or the number that divides the sample into two equal parts. The median is obtained by first ranking the sample values from lowest to highest and then counting up halfway. The concept of ranking is used in nonparametric statistics. A virtue of the median is that it is hardly affected by a few extremely high or low values. The mode is the most popular number of a sample, *i.e.,* the number that occurs most frequently. A sample may have ties for the most common value and be bi- or polymodal; these modes may be widely separated or adjacent. The raw data should be inspected for this unusual appearance. The mode is always mentioned in discussions of descriptive statistics but is rarely used in statistical practice.

Spread or Variability

Any set of interval data has variability unless all the numbers are identical. The range of ages from lowest to highest expresses the largest difference within set A. This spread, diversity, and variability can also be expressed in a concise manner. Variability is specified by calculating the *deviation* or *deviate* of each individual x_i from the center (mean) of all the x_i's. The *sum of squared deviates* is always positive unless all set values are identical. This sum is then divided by the number of individual measurements. The result is the *averaged squared deviations;* the average squared deviation is ubiquitous in statistics.

The concept of describing the spread of a set of numbers by calculating the average distance from each number to the center of the numbers applies to both a sample and a population; this average squared distance is called the *variance.* The population variance is a parameter and is represented by σ^2. As with the population mean, the population variance is not usually known and cannot be calculated. Just as the sample mean is used in place of the population mean, the sample variance is used in place of the population variance. The sample variance, s^2, is

$$s^2 = \Sigma \, (x_i - \bar{x})^2 / (n - 1) \qquad (3\text{-}2)$$

Statistical theory demonstrates that if the divisor in the formula for s^2 is $n - 1$ rather than n, the sample variance is an unbiased estimator of the population variance. While the variance is used extensively in statistical calculations, the units of variance are squared units of the original observations. The square root of the variance has the same units as the original observations; the square roots of the sample and population variances are called the *sample* and *population standard deviations,* s and σ, respectively.

It was previously mentioned that most biologic observations appear to come from populations with normal or gaussian distributions. By accepting this assumption of a normal distribution, further meaning can be given to the sample summary statistics that have been calculated. This involves the use of the expression $\bar{x} \pm k \times s$, where $k = 1, 2, 3$, etc. If the population from which the sample is taken is unimodal and roughly symmetric, then

$\bar{x} \pm 1 \times s$ encompasses roughly 68% of the sample and population members;

$\bar{x} \pm 2 \times s$ encompasses roughly 95% of the sample and population members;

$\bar{x} \pm 3 \times s$ encompasses roughly 99% of the sample and population members.

In our example of hypothetical resident age, $\bar{x}$ and s are 29.5 and 2.6; calculating the three intervals, $29.5 \pm 1 \times 2.6$ includes 10 of 12 observations, $29.5 \pm 2 \times 2.6$ includes 11 of 12 observa-

---

* Statisticians describe the sample mean as the unbiased, consistent, minimum variance, sufficient estimator of the population mean; thus, $x = \mu$, where μ is the population mean.

tions, and 29.5 ± 3 × 2.6 includes all 12 values. The s usually gives a fairly good approximation of the spread of the sample data.

Confidence Intervals

A confidence interval describes how likely it is that the population parameter is estimated by any particular sample statistic such as the mean.* Confidence intervals are a range of the following form: summary statistic ± (confidence factor) × (precision factor).

The *precision factor* is derived from the sample itself, whereas the *confidence factor* is taken from a theoretical probability distribution and also depends on the specified confidence level chosen. For a sample of interval data taken from a normally distributed population for which confidence intervals are to be chosen for μ, the precision factor is called the *standard error of the mean* (SE) and is obtained by dividing s by the square root of the sample size:

$$SE = \frac{s}{\sqrt{n}} = \sqrt{\Sigma\,(x_i - \bar{x})^2 / n(n-1)} \qquad (3\text{-}3)$$

The confidence factors are the same as those used for the dispersion or spread of the sample and are obtained from the normal distribution. The confidence interval is read as follows:

$\bar{x} \pm 1 \times$ SE has roughly a 68% chance of containing the population mean;

$\bar{x} \pm 2 \times$ SE has roughly a 95% chance of containing the population mean;

$\bar{x} \pm 3 \times$ SE has roughly a 99% chance of containing the population mean.

For Sample A the SE is ~0.8; there is a 95% chance that 29.5 ± 1.6 years will include the mean age of the anesthesia residents in the population sampled. The coefficients given above for confidence intervals are not exact; the 95% interval should use the coefficient 1.96. But 1, 2, and 3 are easier to remember and use. These confidence intervals are also calculated, assuming that the population σ is known. In actuality, s was substituted for σ. Strictly speaking, when σ is not known, the confidence factors should be taken from the *t distribution*, another theoretical probability distribution. These coefficients will be larger than those used above. This is usually ignored if the sample size is reasonable, for example, $n > 25$. Even when the sample size is only five or greater, the use of the coefficients 1, 2, and 3 is simple and sufficiently accurate for quick mental calculations of parameter confidence intervals.

Almost all research reports include the use of SE, regardless of the probability distribution of the populations sampled. This use is a consequence of the Central Limit Theorem—one of the most remarkable theorems in all of mathematics. The Central Limit Theorem states that the SE can always be used, if the sample size is sufficiently large, to specify confidence intervals on the population mean. These confidence intervals are calculated as described above. This is true even if the population distribution is so different from normal that s cannot be used to characterize the dispersion of the population members. Only rough guidelines can be given for the necessary size of n; for interval data, certainly, $n = 25$ and above is large enough and $n = 4$ and below is too small.

Although the SE is discussed along with other descriptive statistics, it is really an inferential statistic. SE and s are mentioned together because of their similarities of computation and because of the confusion of their use in research reports.

This use is most often of the form "mean ± number"; some confusion results from the failure of the author to specify whether the number after the ± sign is the one or the other. More important, the choice between using s and using SE has become controversial; because SE is always less than s, it has been argued that authors seek to deceive by using SE to make the data look better than they really are. The choice is actually simple. When describing the spread, scatter, or dispersion of the sample, use s; when describing the precision with which the population center is known, use the SE.

Proportions

Categorical binary data, also called *enumeration data*, provide counts of subject responses. Given a sample T of n subjects of whom x have a certain characteristic (*e.g.*, death, female sex), a ratio of responders to the number of subjects can be easily calculated as $p = x/n$; this can also be expressed as a percentage, $100 \times p$. The ratio p is a descriptive or summary statistic of the sample T. Assume that $n = 15$ subjects and $x = 10$ deaths for sample T; then $p = 10/15 = 0.67$ and $100 \times p = 67\%$. It should be clear that p is a measure of central location of sample T in the same way that $\bar{x}$ was a measure of central location for sample A. In the population from which the sample T is taken, the ratio of responders to total subjects is a population parameter, denoted π; π is the measure of central location for the population. This population parameter, π is not related to the geometry constant pi ($\pi = 3.1415...$). As with other data types, π is usually not known but must be estimated from the sample. The sample ratio p is the best estimate of π.

The probability of binary data is provided by the *binomial distribution*, another theoretical probability distribution. This distribution calculates the chance of x occurrences in a sample of n subjects from a population with an occurrence rate of π:

$$f(x) = \left(\frac{n!}{(x!\,(n-x)!)}\right) \times \pi^x \times (1-\pi)^{(n-x)} \qquad (3\text{-}4)$$

If the π of a population is known, then the probability of the observed response rate p is easily calculated. For example, if there are 10 deaths in 15 subjects and the population death rate is 50% ($\pi = 0.5$), then the probability is $15!/(10! \times (15-10)!) \times (0.5^{10}) \times (1-0.5)^{(15-10)} = 0.09$. This would be expressed as follows: If the population death rate was 50%, then in a sample of 15 individuals, there would be about a 9% chance of finding 10 deaths.

Since the population π is not generally known, the experimenter usually wishes to estimate π by the sample statistic p and to specify with what confidence π is known. If the sample is sufficiently large ($n \times p \geq 5$ and $n \times (1-p) \geq 5$), advantage is taken of the Central Limit Theorem to derive a standard error analogous to that derived for interval data:

$$SE = \left(p \times \frac{(1-p)}{n}\right)^{0.5} \qquad (3\text{-}5)$$

This sample standard error is exactly analogous to the sample standard error of the mean for interval data, except that it is a standard error of the proportion. Just as a 95% confidence limit of the mean was calculated, so may a confidence limit on the proportion be obtained. Using the data of 10 deaths in 15 subjects, the summary statistic $p = 10/15 = 0.67$. Since $15 \times 0.67 = 10$ and $15 \times (1-0.67) = 5$, then n is sufficiently large. The sample standard error is $(0.67 \times (1-0.67)/15)^{0.5} = 0.12$. The 95% confidence interval on π will be $p \pm 2 \times SE = 0.67 \pm 2 \times 0.12 = 0.67 \pm 0.24$.

Thus, the best guess of the population death rate is 67%, and there is a 95% certainty that in the population sampled the death rate is in the range of 43–91%. The approximate nature of this calculation is reflected by the exact 95% confidence interval (36–86%) derived for these data from the bino-

---

*The technical definition of confidence interval is more rigorous. A 95% confidence interval implies that if the estimation procedure were done over and over again, then 95 of each 100 confidence intervals would be expected to contain the true value of the mean.

mial equation. Larger n's and p's closer to 0.5 will make the approximate and exact confidence intervals closer to identical. The reader can use this simple equation when authors do not calculate confidence intervals on rates and proportions.

Inferential Statistics

There are two major areas of statistical inference: the estimation of parameters and the testing of hypotheses. The use of the SE to create confidence intervals is an example of *parameter estimation*. The testing of hypotheses or *significance testing* is the main focus of inferential statistics. Hypothesis testing allows the experimenter to use data from the sample to make inferences about the population. Statisticians have created formulas that use the values of the samples to calculate test statistics. Statisticians have also explored the properties of various theoretical probability distributions. Depending on the assumptions about how data are collected, the appropriate theoretical probability distribution is chosen as the source of critical values to accept or reject the null hypothesis; if the value of the test statistic calculated from the sample(s) is greater than the critical value, the null hypothesis is rejected. The critical value is chosen from the appropriate probability distribution after the magnitude of the Type I error is specified.

There are parameters within the equation that generate any particular theoretical probability distribution; for the normal probability distribution, the parameters are μ and σ^2. For the normal distribution, each set of values for μ and σ^2 will generate a different shape for the bell-like normal curve. All theoretical probability equations contain one or more parameters and can also be plotted as curves; these parameters may be discrete (integer only) or continuous. Each value or combination of values for these parameters will create a different curve for the probability distribution being used. Thus, each theoretical probability distribution is actually a family of probability curves. Some additional parameters of theoretical probability distributions have been given the special name *degrees of freedom*, and are represented by the letters m, n, p, and s.

Associated with the formula for computing a test statistic is a rule for assigning integer values to the one or more parameters called degrees of freedom. The number of degrees of freedom and the value for each degree of freedom depend on (1) the number of subjects, (2) the number of experimental groups, (3) the specifics of the statistical hypothesis, and (4) the type of statistical test. The correct curve of the theoretical probability distribution from which to obtain a critical value for comparison with the value of the test statistic is obtained with the values of one or more degrees of freedom.

To accept or reject the null hypothesis, the following steps are performed: (1) Confirm that experimental data conform to the assumptions of the intended statistical test; (2) choose a significance level (alpha); (3) calculate the test statistic; (4) determine the degree(s) of freedom; (5) find the critical value for the chosen alpha and the degree(s) of freedom from the appropriate theoretical probability distribution; (6) if the test statistic exceeds the critical value, reject the null hypothesis; (7) if the test statistic does not exceed the critical value, do not reject the null hypothesis. There are general guidelines that relate the variable type and the experimental design to the choice of statistical test (Table 3-5).

Interval Data

Parametric statistics are the usual choice in the analysis of interval data, both discrete and continuous. The purpose of such analysis is to test the hypothesis of a difference between population means. The population means are unknown and are estimated by the sample means. A typical example would be the comparison of the mean heart rates of patients receiving and not receiving atropine. Parametric test statistics have been developed by using the properties of the normal probability distribution and two related theoretical probability distributions, the t and the F distribution. In using such parametric methods, the assumption is made that the sample or samples is/are drawn from population(s) with a normal distribution. The parametric test statistics that have been created for interval data all have the form of a ratio. In general terms, the numerator of this ratio is the variability of the means of the samples; the denominator of this ratio is the variability among all the members of the samples. These variabilities are similar to the variances developed for descriptive statistics. The test statistic is thus a ratio of variabilities or variances. All parametric test statistics are used in the same fashion; if the test statistic ratio becomes large, the null hypothesis of no difference is rejected. The critical values against which to compare the test statistic are taken from tables of the three relevant probability distributions.

By definition, in hypothesis testing, at least one of the population means is unknown, but the population variance(s) may or may not be known. Parametric statistics can be divided into two groups according to whether or not the population variances are known. If the population variance is known, the test statistic used is called the z score; critical values are obtained from the normal distribution. In most biomedical applications, the population variance is rarely known and the z score is little used.

t Test

An important advance in statistical inference came early in the 20th century with the creation of *Student's t test statistic* and the *t distribution*, which allowed the testing of hypotheses when the population variance is not known. The most common use of Student's t test is to compare the mean values of two populations. This use is further subdivided by a particular aspect of experimental design. If each subject has two measurements taken, for example, one before and one after a drug, then one sample or *paired t test* procedure is used; each control measurement taken before drug administration is paired with a measurement in the same patient after drug administration. Of course, this is a self-control experiment. This pairing of measurements in the same patient reduces variability and increases statistical power. There are two target populations in such an experiment: subjects before and subjects after the study drug. The difference d_i of each pair of values is calculated and the average $\bar{d}$ is calculated. In the formula for Student's t statistic, the numera-

Table 3-5. WHEN TO USE WHAT

Variable Type	One-Sample Tests	Two-Sample Tests	Multiple-Sample Tests
Dichotomous or nominal	Binomial distribution	Chi-square test	Chi-square test
Ordinal	Chi-square test	Chi-square test, nonparametric tests	Chi-square test, nonparametric tests
Continuous or discrete	z distribution or t distribution	Unpaired t test, paired t test, nonparametric tests	Analysis of variance, nonparametric analysis of variance

tor is $\bar{d}$, whereas the denominator is the standard error of $\bar{d}$ (SE_d):

$$t \text{ test statistic} = \frac{\bar{d}}{SE_d} \tag{3-6}$$

All t statistics are created in this way; the numerator is the difference of two means, whereas the denominator is the standard error of the two means. If the difference between the two means is large compared with their variability, then the null hypothesis of no difference is rejected. The critical values for the t statistic are taken from the t probability distribution. The t distribution is symmetric and bell-shaped but more spread out than the normal distribution. The t distribution has a single integer parameter; for a paired t test, the value of this single degree of freedom is the sample size minus one. There can be some confusion about the use of the letter t. It refers both to the value of the test statistic calculated by the formula and to the critical value from the theoretical probability distribution. The critical t value is determined by looking in a t table after a significance level is chosen and the degree of freedom is computed.

More commonly, measurements are taken on two separate groups of subjects. For example, one group receives blood pressure treatment, whereas no treatment is given to a control group. The number of subjects in each group might or might not be identical; regardless of this, in no sense is an individual measurement in the first group matched or paired with a specific measurement in the second group. An *unpaired* or *two-sample t test* is used to compare the means of the two groups. The numerator of the t statistic is ($\bar{x} - \bar{y}$). The denominator is a weighted average of the SEs of each sample. The degree of freedom for an unpaired t test is calculated as the sum of the subjects of the two groups minus two. As with the paired t test, if the t ratio becomes large, the null hypothesis is rejected.

Multiple Comparisons and Analysis of Variance

Experiments in anesthesia, whether they are with humans or with animals, may not be limited to one or two groups of data for each variable. It is very common to follow a variable longitudinally; heart rate, for example, might be measured five times before and during anesthetic induction. These are also called repeated measurement experiments; the experimenter will wish to compare changes between the initial heart rate measurement and those obtained during induction. The experimental design might also include several groups receiving different induction drugs, *e.g.*, comparing heart rate across groups immediately after laryngoscopy. Researchers have commonly handled these analysis problems with the t test. If heart rate is collected five times, these collection times could be labeled *A, B, C, D,* and *E*. Then *A* could be compared with *B, C, D,* and *E; B* could be compared with *C, D,* and *E;* and so forth. The total of possible pairings is ten; thus, ten paired t tests could be calculated for all the possible pairings of *A, B, C, D,* and *E*. A similar approach can be used for comparing more than two groups for unpaired data.

The use of t tests in this fashion is inappropriate. In testing a statistical hypothesis, the experimenter sets the level of Type I error; this is usually chosen to be 0.05. When using many t tests, as in the example above, the chosen error rate for performing all these t tests is much higher than 0.05, even though the Type I error is set at 0.05 for each individual comparison. In fact, the Type I error rate for all t tests simultaneously, *i.e.*, the chance of finding at least one of the multiple t test statistics significant merely by chance, is given by the formula $\alpha = 1 - 0.95^k$. If 13 t tests are performed, the real error rate is 49%. Applying t tests over and over again to all the possible pairings of a variable will misleadingly identify statistical significance when there is, in fact, none.

The most versatile approach for handling comparisons of means among more than two groups is called *analysis of variance* and is frequently cited by the acronym ANOVA. Analysis of variance consists of rules for creating test statistics on means when there are more than two groups. These test statistics are called *F ratios*, after Ronald Fisher; the critical values for the *F* test statistic are taken from the *F* theoretical probability distribution that Fisher derived.

Suppose that data for three groups are obtained. What can be said about the mean values of the three target populations? The *F* test is actually asking several questions simultaneously: Is group 1 different from group 2, is group 2 different from group 3, and is group 1 different from group 3? As with the t test, the *F* test statistic is a ratio; in general terms, the numerator expresses the variability of the mean values of the three groups, whereas the denominator expresses the average variability or difference of each sample value from the mean of all sample values. The formulas to create the test statistic are computationally elegant but are rather hard to appreciate intuitively. The *F* statistic has two degrees of freedom, denoted *m* and *n;* the value of *m* is a function of the number of experimental groups; the value for *n* is a function of the number of subjects in all experimental groups. The analysis of multigroup data is not necessarily finished after the ANOVAs are calculated. If the null hypothesis is rejected and it is accepted that there are differences among the groups tested, how can it be decided where the differences are? A variety of techniques are available to make what are called multiple comparisons after the ANOVA test is performed.

Robustness and Nonparametric Tests

Most statistical tests depend on certain assumptions about the nature of the distribution of values in the underlying populations from which experimental samples are taken. For the parametric statistics, *i.e.*, t tests and analysis of variance, it is assumed that the populations follow the normal distribution. However, for some data, experience or historical reasons suggest that these assumptions of a normal distribution do not hold; some examples include proportions, percentages, and response times. What should the experimenter do if he or she fears that the data are not normally distributed?

The experimenter might choose to ignore the problem of non-normal data and inhomogeneity of variance, hoping that everything will work out. Such insouciance is actually a very practical and reasonable approach to the problem. Parametric statistics are called "robust" statistics; they stand up to much adversity. To a statistician, robustness implies that the magnitude of Type I errors is not seriously affected by ill-conditioned data. Parametric statistics are sufficiently robust that the accuracy of decisions reached by means of t tests and analysis of variance remains very credible, even for moderately severe departures from the assumptions.

Another possibility would be to use statistics that do not require any assumptions about probability distributions of the populations. Such statistics are known as *nonparametric tests;* they can be used whenever there is very serious concern about the shape of the data. Nonparametric statistics are also the tests of choice for ordinal data. The basic concept behind nonparametric statistics is the ability to rank or order the observations; nonparametric tests are also called *order statistics*.

Most nonparametric statistics still require the use of theoretical probability distributions; the critical values that must be exceeded by the test statistic are taken from the binomial, normal, and chi-square distributions, depending on the nonparametric test being used. The *nonparametric sign test, Mann-Whitney rank sum test,* and *Kruskal-Wallis one-way analysis of variance* are analogous to the paired t test, unpaired t test, and one-way analysis of variance, respectively. The currently available nonparametric tests are not used more commonly because they do not adapt well to complex statistical models and because they are less able than parametric tests to distinguish between the null and alternative hypotheses if the data are, in fact, normally distributed.

Contingency Tables

In a hypothetical experiment comparing performance on an examination, about 83% of the anesthesia faculty passed, whereas less than 38% of anesthesia residents passed. Is this difference real? This question is also stated as whether there is a dependency or association between the rows and the columns of the 2 × 2 (2 rows and 2 columns) contingency table. A variety of statistical techniques allow us to compare this pass/fail rate in the underlying populations of all anesthesia faculty and all anesthesia residents. The *chi-square test* offers the advantage of being computationally simpler; it can also analyze contingency tables with more than two rows and two columns. The chi-square test statistic is a sum of ratios. For each cell of the contingency table, the observed value has been recorded. Using the assumption that there is no association between the rows and the columns, the expected value for each cell is the row total multiplied by the column total divided by the total number of subjects. For each cell, the squared difference between the observed and expected value divided by the expected value expresses the variability of the observed value away from the expected value. The test statistic is the sum of these difference ratios:

$$X^2_{(df)} = \Sigma \frac{(|\text{observed} - \text{expected}| - 0.5)^2}{\text{expected}} \qquad (3\text{-}7)$$

If the difference between observed and expected cell values grows larger, it is more likely that there is an association between the rows and columns. This equation can be used to calculate a chi-square statistic for any size contingency table. The critical values used with the chi-square test statistic are from the χ^2 or chi-square continuous theoretical probability distribution with its associated degree of freedom. The value of this degree of freedom is the product of the number of rows minus 1 times the number of columns minus 1. For 2 × 2 tables, the value for the degree of freedom is always 1. The smallest expected cell value should be at least 5 or the test statistic will be biased. For 2 × 2 contingency tables, the counts within the four cells are usually labeled a, b, c, and d with n equaling the sum of the counts of the four cells; there is a simpler formula for the calculation of the chi-square test statistic of 2 × 2 contingency tables:

$$X^2_1 = \frac{(|a \times d - b \times c| - n/2)^2 \times n}{(a + b)(a + c)(b + d)(c + d)} \qquad (3\text{-}8)$$

Interpretation of Results

Scientific studies do not end with the statistical test. The experimenter must submit an opinion as to the generalizability of his or her work to the rest of the world. Even if there is a statistically significant difference, the experimenter must decide if this difference is medically or physiologically important. Statistical significance does not always equate with biologic relevance. The questions an experimenter should ask about the interpretation of results are highly dependent on the specifics of the experiment. First, even small, clinically unimportant differences between groups can be detected if the sample size is sufficiently large. On the other hand, if the sample size is small, one must always worry that identified or unidentified confounding variables may explain any difference; as the sample size decreases, randomization is less successful in assuring homogenous groups. Second, if the experimental groups are given three or more doses of a drug, do the results suggest a steadily increasing or decreasing dose–response relationship? Suppose the observed effect for an intermediate dose is either much higher or much lower than that for both the highest and lowest dose;

a dose–response relationship may exist, but some skepticism about the experimental methods is warranted. Third, for clinical studies comparing different drugs, devices, and operations on patient outcome, are the patients, clinical care, and studied therapies sufficiently similar to those provided at other locations to be of interest to a wide group of practitioners? This is the distinction between *efficacy*—does it work under the best (research) circumstances—and *effectiveness*—does it work under the typical circumstances of routine clinical care. Finally, in comparing alternative therapies, the confidence that a claim for a superior therapy is true depends on the study design. The strength of the evidence concerning efficacy will be least for an anecdotal case report; next in importance will be a retrospective study, then a prospective series of patients compared with historical controls, and finally a randomized, controlled clinical trial. The greatest strength for a therapeutic claim is a series of randomized, controlled clinical trials confirming the same hypothesis.

READING JOURNAL ARTICLES

Tens of hundreds of thousands of words are written each year in journal articles relevant to anesthesia. No one can read them all. How should the clinician determine which articles are useful? All that is possible is to learn to rapidly skip over most articles and concentrate on the few selected for their importance to the reader. Those few should be chosen according to their relevance and credibility. Relevance is determined by the specifics of one's anesthetic practice. Credibility is a function of the merits of the research methods, the experimental design, and the statistical analysis; the more proficient one's statistical skills, the more rapidly one can accept or reject the credibility of a research article.

Guidelines

Six easily remembered appraisal criteria for clinical studies can be fashioned from the words WHY, HOW, WHO, WHAT, HOW MANY, and SO WHAT: (1) WHY: Is the biologic hypothesis clearly stated? (2) HOW: What is the research design? (3) WHO: Is the target population clearly defined? (4) WHAT: How was the therapy administered and the data collected? (5) HOW MANY: Are the test statistics convincing? (6) SO WHAT: Is it clinically relevant to my patients? Although the statistical knowledge of most physicians is limited, these skills of critical appraisal of the literature can be learned and can tremendously increase the efficiency and benefit of journal reading.

The Evidenced-Based Medicine Working Group—a group of mainly Canadian physicians and statisticians from McMaster University, Ontario, Canada—has been organized to de-emphasize a foundation of unsystematic clinical experience, clinical intuition, and pathophysiologic rationale as the basis for medical decision and to teach the systematic evaluation of published evidence. Since 1993 members of this group have published more than 20 detailed articles—all titled "Users' Guides to the Medical Literature"—in *JAMA*, the *Journal of the American Medical Association*. Specific topics have ranged from "How to Use an Article About Therapy or Prevention" to "How to Use an Article About Disease Probability for Differential Diagnosis." While some elements of probabilistic reasoning and statistical testing are included, a greater emphasis is on an appreciation of experimental design.

Statistical Resources

Accompanying the exponential growth of medical information since World War II has been the creation of a wealth of biostatistical knowledge. Textbooks with expositions of basic, intermediate, and advanced statistics abound; several introductory texts are listed in the Bibliography. There are new journals of bio-

Table 3-6. LOW-FREQUENCY EVENTS: PROBABILITY THAT A SAMPLE OF 23 WILL HAVE ZERO COMPLICATIONS

If the long-run complication rate is:	Then the probability of observing zero complications in 23 patients is:
1 in 10,000	99.8%
1 in 1000	97.7%
1 in 200	89.1%
1 in 100	79.4%
1 in 50	62.8%
1 in 23	36.0%

medical statistics, including *Controlled Clinical Trials, Statistics in Medicine,* and *Statistical Methods in Medical Research,* whose audiences are both statisticians and biomedical researchers. Some medical journals, *e.g.,* the *British Medical Journal,* regularly publish expositions of both basic and newer advanced statistical methods. Extensive internet resources can be linked from the home page of the long established American Statistical Association (http://www.amstat.org) and at the StatLib (http://lib.stat.cmu.edu) of Carnegie Mellon University including electronic textbooks of basic statistical methods, online statistical calculators, standard datasets, reviews of statistical software, and so on.

Examples of Statistics Applied to Journal Reading

Zero Numerators. During the last two decades anesthesiologists have become more involved with the postoperative management of analgesia using a variety of new drug delivery routes and methods. However, benefits and risks must be weighed in the balance for all therapies, new or old. The strikingly impressive analgesia of neuraxial opioids for most patients is matched by a delayed respiratory depression in a very few patients. Reviews of published reports suggest that current techniques produce an acceptably low complication rate (1 in 1000 or less). There is a continuing onslaught of new reports touting new variations of drug, dosing, route, and adjuvant therapies. How much evidence is necessary before acceptance is given? The answer will, of course, depend on practicality, efficacy, and safety.

Suppose research findings claim that the direct injection of morphine into the cisterna magna of 23 patients produced total postoperative analgesia without apneic episodes. Is this sufficient evidence concerning the safety of this difficult technique? Should this technique be immediately introduced into clinical practice?

Physicians tend to ignore the size of the denominators on which rates are based and focus on numerators. Perhaps a zero numerator carries weight in that it falsely suggests that an event

is impossible. A zero numerator does not mean there is no risk. In fact, in a small sample it is not unusual to find no complications even if the actual rate of complications is clinically important. If, for example, only 1 in 50 patients suffers apnea, there is still about a 40% chance of not observing an apneic episode in 23 patients (Table 3-6). If none of n patients shows the event about which we are concerned, the upper 95% confidence limit of a $0/n$ rate is approximately $3/n$; from a sample with 23 patients having no complications, the best estimate of the population complication rate is 0%, but it might be as high as 13% (Table 3-7). Thus, anesthesiologists should not accept this hypothetical report of 23 patients as sufficient safety evidence to start cisterna magna injections.

Confidence Interval on Difference of Means. Clinical anesthesia research reports often focus on extending the duration of drug effect. Consider, for example, prolongation of post-Cesarean epidural analgesia. Twenty parturients were randomly divided into two groups after surgery; 50 μg sufentanil was given to all patients, 10 with 300 μg epinephrine, 10 without epinephrine. Analgesia without epinephrine lasted 266.7 ± 80.2 minutes, but 348.7 ± 77.8 minutes with epinephrine (mean ± s). This was statistically significant. Unfortunately, the epinephrine group had more pruritus and nausea. Is the difference in duration sufficient to accept more side effects in the epinephrine group?

One approach to this question focuses on the magnitude of benefit from epinephrine and the precision with which it is known; one calculates the confidence intervals on the differences of the means. The best estimate of the true difference between the groups is $(\bar{x}_1 - \bar{x}_2)$. The difference in duration of analgesia is $348.7 - 266.7 = 82$ minutes.

The 95% confidence interval for the difference of means is approximately

$$\bar{x}_1 - \bar{x}_2 - 2 \times SE_{diff} \text{ to } \bar{x}_1 - \bar{x}_2 + 2 \times SE_{diff} \qquad (3\text{-}9)$$

Using the values for n_1, n_2, s_1, and s_2, then SE_{diff} and s are defined by

$$SE_{diff} = s \times \sqrt{\left(\frac{1}{n_1} + \frac{1}{n_2}\right)} \qquad (3\text{-}10)$$

Table 3-7. CONFIDENCE INTERVALS AND LOW-FREQUENCY EVENTS: LONG-RUN RISK RULED OUT BY 0/n (UPPER BOUND OF 95% CONFIDENCE INTERVAL)

Sample rate of:	Rules out any long-run (population) rate higher than:
0 in 10,000	$3/10,000 = 0.03\%$ (0.03%)*
0 in 1000	$3/1000 = 0.3\%$ (0.3%)
0 in 100	$3/100 = 3\%$ (3%)
0 in 50	$3/50 = 6\%$ (6%)
0 in 23	$3/23 = 13\%$ (12%)
0 in 10	$3/10 = 30\%$ (26%)

* Exact results derived by solving $(1 - \text{maximum rate})^n = 0.05$.

$$s = \sqrt{\frac{(n_1 - 1) \times s_1^2 + (n_2 - 1) \times s_2^2}{n_1 + n_2 - 2}} \qquad (3.11)$$

The 95% confidence interval of the difference in means is 11 to 153 minutes. The precision of the estimate of the difference is obviously poor. Considering the increased risk of pruritus and nausea, an anesthesiologist might well decide that the benefit is not sufficiently characterized to warrant a change. Statisticians have encouraged journal authors to cite results with appropriate confidence intervals. This advice has not been widely followed. However, the mathematics is rather simple with an electronic calculator and can be reckoned by the journal reader.

CONCLUSION

One intent of this chapter is to present the scope of support that the discipline of statistics can provide to anesthesia research. Although an intuitive understanding of certain basic principles is emphasized, these basic principles are not necessarily simple and have been developed by statisticians with great mathematical rigor. Academic anesthesia needs more workers to immerse themselves in these statistical fundamentals. Having done so, these statistically knowledgeable academic anesthesiologists will be prepared to improve their own research projects, to assist their colleagues in research, to efficiently seek consultation from the professional statistician, to strengthen the editorial review of journal articles, and to expound to the clinical reader the whys and wherefores of statistics. The clinical reader also needs to expend his or her own effort to acquire some basic statistical skills. Journals are increasingly difficult to understand without some basic statistical understanding. Some clinical problems can be best understood with a perspective based on probability. Finally understanding principles of experimental design can prevent premature acceptances of new therapies from faulty studies.

BIBLIOGRAPHY

Altman D: Practical Statistics for Medical Research. Dordrecht, Kluwer Academic Publishers Group, 1999

Altman D (ed): Statistics with Confidence, 2nd ed. London, BMJ Publishing Group, 2000

Dawson-Saunders B, Trapp RG: Basic & Clinical Biostatistics, 2nd ed. Norwalk, Appleton & Lange, 1994

Glantz SA: Primer of Biostatistics, 4th ed. New York, McGraw-Hill, 1996

Clinical Anesthesia (4/e), edited by
Paul G. Barash, Bruce F. Cullen, and
Robert K. Stoelting. Lippincott Williams &
Wilkins, Philadelphia, © 2001.

CHAPTER 4

HAZARDS OF WORKING IN THE OPERATING ROOM

ARNOLD J. BERRY AND JONATHAN D. KATZ

Anesthesia personnel spend long hours, in fact, most of their waking days, in an environment filled with many potential hazards—the operating room. This setting is unique among workplaces owing to potential exposure to chemical vapors, ionizing radiation, and infectious agents while the anesthesia team is subject to heightened levels of psychological stress engendered by the high-stakes nature of the practice. Although such physical hazards as explosions from flammable anesthetic agents are no longer a concern, occupational illnesses, such as alcohol and drug abuse, are now well recognized as significant within the anesthesia community. Some hazards, such as exposure to trace levels of waste anesthetic gases, have been extensively studied, whereas others, like suicide, have been recognized but not adequately pursued. Only within the past few decades have epidemiologic surveys been conducted to assess the health of anesthesia personnel. In general, the potential health risks to those working in the operating room may be significant, but with awareness of the problems and the use of proper precautions, they are not formidable.

PHYSICAL HAZARDS

Anesthetic Gases

Although the inhalation anesthetics diethyl ether, nitrous oxide, and chloroform were first used in the 1840s, the biologic effects of occupational exposure to anesthetic agents were not investigated until the 1960s. Reports on the effects of chronic environmental exposure to anesthetics have included epidemiologic surveys, *in vitro* studies, cellular research, and studies in laboratory animals and humans. Areas addressed include fertility and spontaneous abortion; incidence of congenital malformations; mortality rate; incidence of cancer, hematopoietic diseases, liver disease, and neurologic disease; and psychomotor and behavioral changes produced by anesthetic exposure.

Anesthetic Levels in the Operating Room

Early investigators established that significant levels of ether were present in the operating room when the open drop technique was used, but the first report of occupational exposure to modern anesthetics was by Linde and Bruce in 1969.[1] They sampled air at various distances from the pop-off valve of anesthesia machines and noted an average concentration of halothane of 10 parts per million (ppm) and of nitrous oxide of 130 ppm.* End-expired air samples taken from 24 anesthesiologists after work revealed 0 to 12 ppm of halothane. Others reported similar levels of halothane around semiclosed and nonrebreathing circuits and showed that the environmental levels could be reduced significantly with the use of scavenging equipment.[2]

Specific anesthetic techniques such as inhalation induction in pediatric patients are associated with higher levels of waste gas exposure.[3] Dosimeters worn by anesthetists recorded 532 ppm/hr (time-weighted average) of nitrous oxide after cases using an inhalation induction, compared with 219 ppm/ hr with intravenous inductions. Although appropriate operating

room ventilation and machine scavenging was used, the nitrous oxide levels in all cases were higher than expected. In spite of the characteristic odors of volatile anesthetics, smell is not a reliable method for detecting trace levels of halothane in operating room air. Only 50% of volunteers could detect 33 ppm of halothane by smell, and 75% could not detect 15 ppm.[4]

The waste anesthetic concentrations in operating rooms where routine scavenging is performed are less than those noted before the 1960s and are often less than those found in the only studies conducted to assess the effects of occupational exposure. This raises the questions of whether chronic exposure to these low levels of waste anesthetic gases actually constitutes a significant occupational hazard and whether results from studies performed in "unscavenged" operating rooms are applicable to current practice.

Epidemiologic Studies

Epidemiologic surveys were among the first studies to suggest the possibility of a hazard resulting from trace levels of anesthetics. Although epidemiologic studies may be useful in assessing problems of this type, they have the potential for errors associated with the collection of data and their interpretation. In his review of the potential of trace anesthetic gases to produce disease, Ferstandig outlined the design strategies necessary for valid epidemiologic studies.[5] First, there should be an appropriate control group for the cohort being studied. Second, the use of questionnaires to obtain personal medical information may be misleading because individuals may knowingly or unknowingly give incorrect information. The use of medical records provides more reliable data. Third, retrospective epidemiologic studies rely on recorded or remembered data. In prospective studies, the anticipated, significant information can be collected temporally. Fourth, cause-and-effect relationships cannot be documented by epidemiologic data unless all other possible etiologies can be ruled out or other lines of evidence are used for substantiation. Fifth, most epidemiologic studies use a p of 0.05 for determination of statistical significance. Walts *et al*, in reviewing one epidemiologic study, argued that this level of statistical significance is too high.[6] Because a false-positive conclusion may have profound implications, even a p level of 0.01 may be too large for epidemiologic data. Sixth, percentage increases in the incidence of disease are sometimes reported. Large changes in percentage may imply clinical significance, even when the findings are not statistically significant. Few epidemiologic studies on the effects of occupational exposure to waste anesthetic gases fulfill these criteria.

Reproductive Outcome. One of the largest studies to assess the effects of trace anesthetics on reproductive outcome was conducted by an Ad Hoc Committee of the American Society of Anesthesiologists (ASA).[7] Questionnaires were sent to 49,585 operating room personnel who had potential exposure to waste anesthetic gases (members of the ASA, the American Association of Nurse Anesthetists, the Association of Operating Room Nurses, and the Association of Operating Room Technicians). A nonexposed group of 23,911 from the American Academy of Pediatrics and the American Nurses' Association served as controls. The Committee concluded that there was an increased risk of spontaneous abortion and congenital abnormalities in children of women who worked in the operating room and

---

* Parts per million is a volume-per-volume unit of measurement; 10,000 ppm equals 1%.

an increased risk of congenital abnormalities in offspring of unexposed wives of male operating room personnel. Several reviews have identified inconsistencies in the data used to compare exposed and unexposed groups and make within-group comparisons. Expected levels of anesthetic exposure did not correlate with reproductive outcome.[5,6]

A Swedish study clearly demonstrates the inaccuracies encountered when surveys rely on data obtained from mailed questionnaires.[8] Women working at one hospital were surveyed to determine the relationship between anesthetic exposure and spontaneous abortion rate and the confounding effects of age, smoking habits, and work site during the first trimester of pregnancy. All spontaneous abortions in the exposed group were accurately documented in the responses to the questionnaire, but a review of hospital records revealed that one third of spontaneous abortions went unreported in the unexposed group. When verified data were analyzed, there was no statistically significant difference between reproductive outcome in the exposed and nonexposed groups.

The ASA commissioned a group of epidemiologists and biostatisticians to evaluate the many epidemiologic surveys that had been published in the literature to provide an assessment of the conflicting data.[9] The group used the relative risk (the ratio of the rate of disease among those exposed to that found in those not exposed) as a measure of the strength of the association between exposure to the operating room environment and several disease processes. In considering studies on spontaneous abortion and congenital abnormalities in offspring of anesthesia personnel, the data from all but five studies were excluded from analysis because of errors in study design or statistical analysis.[7,8,10,11,12] The relative risks of spontaneous abortion for female physicians and female nurses working in the operating room were 1.4 and 1.3, respectively (a relative risk of 1.3 represents a 30% increase in risk when compared with the risk of the control population). The increased relative risk for congenital abnormalities was of borderline statistical significance for exposed physicians only. In considering these findings, Mazze and Lecky[13] noted that the epidemiologic studies assessing the association of cigarette smoking and lung cancer have established a value for relative risk of 8 to 12 for men in the United States. The high relative risks found in smoking studies contrast with the values of less than 2 in most of the well designed reproductive studies among those working in the operating room environment. Relative risks of less than 2 to 3 may occur solely from incorrect classification of subjects. Although Buring et al[9] found a statistically significant relative risk of spontaneous abortion and congenital abnormalities in women working in the operating room, the relative risk was small compared with other, better documented environmental hazards. They also point out that duration and level of anesthetic exposure were not measured in any of the studies and that other factors, such as stress, infections, and radiation exposure, were not considered.

More recent studies have also suggested that there is a slightly greater risk of adverse reproductive outcomes in women occupationally exposed to anesthetics. Using a case-control study design and data obtained from a national register, Hemminki et al noted a small but not significant increase [odds ratio (OR) = 1.2] in spontaneous abortion in female nurses with anesthetic exposures.[14] Another study, using a postal survey of female resident physicians, demonstrated that the overall rate of spontaneous abortion was not increased compared to female partners of male residents.[15] When the data were assessed by specialty, women in anesthesia residencies had a higher rate than those in specialties without anesthetic exposure.

Because some personnel working in dental operatories have exposure to nitrous oxide, the dental literature has also addressed these issues. One pertinent study used data collected via telephone interviews with 418 female dental assistants to assess the effect of nitrous oxide exposure on fertility.[16] Fecund-ability* was significantly reduced in women with 5 or more hours of exposure to unscavenged nitrous oxide per week. In another study of 7000 female dental assistants, questionnaires were used to determine rates of spontaneous abortion.[17] There was an increased rate [relative risk (RR) = 2.6, adjusted for age, smoking, and number of amalgams prepared per week] of spontaneous abortion among women who worked for 3 or more hours per week in offices not using scavenging devices for nitrous oxide. These findings must be viewed with caution because the estimates of nitrous oxide exposure were based solely on respondents' reports, and measurements of nitrous oxide concentrations in the work space were not performed. Therefore, dose–effect relationships cannot be confirmed. It is important to note that in both studies of female dental assistants, use of nitrous oxide in offices with scavenging devices was not associated with an increased risk for adverse reproductive outcomes.[16,17]

A meta-analysis of 19 epidemiologic studies, which included hospital workers, dental assistants, and veterinarians and veterinary assistants, demonstrated an increased risk of spontaneous abortion (RR = 1.48; 95% confidence interval, 1.40–1.58) in women with occupational exposure to anesthetic gases.[18] Additional analysis demonstrated that the relative risk of 1.48 corresponded to an increased absolute risk of abortion of 6.2%. Stratification by job category indicated that the relative risk was greatest for veterinarians (RR = 2.45) followed by dental assistants (RR = 1.89) and hospital workers (RR = 1.30). When the meta-analysis was confined to the five studies[17,19,20,21,22] that controlled for several nonoccupational confounding variables, had appropriate control groups, and had sufficient response rate, the relative risk for spontaneous abortion was 1.90 (95% confidence interval, 1.72–2.09). The author notes that the routine use of scavenging devices has been implemented since the time that most of the studies in this analysis were performed and that there was no risk of spontaneous abortion in studies of personnel that worked in scavenged environments.

Retrospective surveys of large numbers of women who worked during pregnancy indicate that negative reproductive outcomes may be related to job-associated conditions other than exposure to trace anesthetic gases. In a Canadian study, the ratio of observed to expected late spontaneous abortions (16 to 28 weeks) was increased in operating room nurses as well as radiology technicians and employees in agriculture and horticulture.[23] Analysis of the data from health workers demonstrated an increased risk of abortion associated with specific work requirements and conditions: lifting heavy weights more than 15 times a day, other physical effort, working 46 or more hours a week, and changing shift work.

Although many of the existing epidemiologic studies have potential flaws in design, the evidence taken as a whole suggests that there is a slight increase in the relative risk of spontaneous abortion and congenital abnormalities in offspring for female physicians working in the operating room.[24] Whether this is attributable to anesthetic exposure cannot be definitely determined from this type of investigation. Well designed surveys of large numbers of personnel and appropriate control groups are necessary to link trace anesthetic exposures to adverse reproductive outcomes. The routine use of scavenging techniques has generally lowered environmental anesthetic levels in the operating room and may make it more difficult to prove any adverse effects using epidemiologic data.

Mortality and Nonreproductive Diseases. One of the first surveys enumerating causes of death among anesthesiologists was reported by Bruce et al in 1968.[25] The authors compared the death rates of members of the ASA from 1947 to 1966 with those for American men and male policyholders of a large

---

* The ability to conceive, which is measured by the time to pregnancy during periods of unprotected sexual intercourse.

insurance company. There was a higher death rate among male anesthesiologists from malignancies of the lymphoid and reticuloendothelial tissues and from suicide, but a lower death rate from lung cancer and coronary artery disease.

In a subsequent prospective study, Bruce et al compared the causes of death in ASA members during the years 1967 to 1971 with those of men insured by one company.[26] The overall death rate for ASA members was lower than for the controls, and contrary to the previous results, there was no increase in death rates from malignancies of lymphoid and reticuloendothelial tissues. The authors concluded that their data provided no evidence to support the speculation that lymphoid malignancies were an occupational hazard for anesthesiologists.

The national study conducted by the ASA found no differences in cancer rates between men exposed and those not exposed to trace concentrations of anesthetic gases.[7] For women who responded to the survey, there was an approximately 1.3-fold to 2-fold increase in the occurrence of cancer in the exposed group, resulting predominantly from an increase in leukemia and lymphoma. The analysis of Buring et al of these data confirmed an increase in relative risk of cancer in exposed women (1.4) but attributed the increase solely to cervical cancer (2.8).[9] They also noted that the ASA study did not assess the effect of confounding variables, such as sexual history or smoking, that may have contributed to the findings. It is doubtful that the carcinogenic effect of anesthetics would be sex related, and the conflicting results for men and women, especially in light of the low statistical significance of the data, cast doubt that anesthetics were the causative agents.

The data from the ASA survey showed a statistical increase in hepatic disease for female anesthesiologists, female nurse anesthetists, and male anesthesiologists, but not for other exposed groups.[7] Again, it is difficult to explain why male anesthetists did not experience the same consequences from exposure to trace anesthetic gases as their female nurse anesthetist counterparts. Although the investigators tried to exclude infectious hepatitis as a cause of hepatic disease, hepatitis B is asymptomatic in approximately 50% of infected people. At the time that this survey was conducted, the serum markers to identify hepatitis B had not been elucidated. From the information collected for this study, it cannot be determined whether the hepatic disease was caused by anesthetic exposure or by hepatitis B or another viral infection acquired from frequent exposure to blood.

In a survey of mortality among British physicians from 1951 to 1971, the overall mortality rate and incidence of death caused by ischemic heart disease, chronic bronchitis, and lung cancer were lower for anesthesiologists than the average for all medical specialists.[27] There was a slightly increased risk of other cancers (107% of expected) because of cancer of the pancreas in anesthesiologists. These mortality data were confirmed when applied to members of the ASA in a survey published in 1979.[28] ASA membership lists from 1954, 1959, 1967, and 1976 were obtained, so that the population studied included those exposed both to older anesthetics and to halogenated volatile agents. Mortality from all causes in anesthesiologists remained below that of the general population since 1954. Specifically, there was no evidence for an increased rate of cancer or hepatic or renal disease.

The most recent mortality study of anesthesiologists, sponsored by the ASA, was performed by Domino et al.[29] The mortality risks of a cohort of 40,242 anesthesiologists were compared to a matched cohort of internists using data on cause of death from the National Death Index covering the period from 1976 to 1996. There was no difference between the two groups in overall mortality risk or mortality due to cancer or heart disease.

Epidemiologic studies are useful tools for attempting to identify adverse effects of the operating room environment, including exposure to many substances, of which waste anesthetic gases comprise but one factor. The data from epidemiologic surveys can, at best, suggest relationships but can never prove cause-and-effect associations between exposure to some condition or substance and a disease process. There are shortcomings in many surveys that attempt to assess the effects of waste anesthetic gases, and these have resulted in conflicting conclusions. Overall, there appears to be some evidence that the operating room environment produces a slight increase in the rate of spontaneous abortion and cancer in female anesthesiologists and nurses.[9] There is also a statistically significant increase in liver disease in both men and women, but this is consistent with the proven risk of infectious hepatitis among operating room personnel (see section on Infection Hazards, later). Overall mortality rates for anesthesiologists appear lower than for the general population and for other medical specialists.

Laboratory Studies

Concurrent with the epidemiologic studies, investigators have been active in the laboratory, assessing the effects of anesthetic agents on cell, tissue, and animal models. It is hoped that this work will provide the scientific evidence linking anesthetics to the adverse effects that have been suggested by epidemiologic surveys.

Cellular Effects. At clinically useful concentrations, volatile anesthetics interfere with cell division in a reversible manner, possibly because of a reduction in oxygen uptake by mitochondria. There have been no cellular studies to indicate that trace levels of volatile anesthetics have a similar effect.

Nitrous oxide administered in clinically useful concentrations affects hematopoietic and neural cells. After exposure to 0.8 atmospheres (atm) of nitrous oxide for 30 minutes, liver methionine synthetase activity decreased by more than 50% in mice.[30] Although 0.05 atm of nitrous oxide did not affect methionine synthetase activity after 4 hours, exposure to 1100 ppm for 8 to 22 days produced a significant reduction in enzyme activity. Nitrous oxide oxidizes the cobalt atom of vitamin B_{12} from an active to inactive state, which inhibits methionine synthetase. This prevents the conversion of methyltetrahydrofolate to tetrahydrofolate, which is required for DNA synthesis.[30] Inhibition of methionine synthetase in people exposed to high concentrations of nitrous oxide may result in anemia and polyneuropathy, but chronic exposure to trace levels does not appear to produce these effects.[31,32]

Many studies have been performed in animals to assess the carcinogenicity of anesthetics. A preliminary study suggested that isoflurane produced hepatic neoplasia when administered to mice during gestation and early life,[33] but a subsequent, well controlled study failed to reproduce these results.[34] Other studies in mice and rats found no carcinogenic effect of halothane, nitrous oxide, or enflurane.[35,36] In an attempt to simulate environmental exposure to waste anesthetics, rats were exposed to low levels of halothane and nitrous oxide for 7 hours per day, 5 days per week, for 104 weeks.[35] This degree of exposure produced no effect on body weight, behavior, survival, or incidence of tumors.

Several investigators have used the popular Ames bacterial assay system for studying the mutagenicity of anesthetics. This assay is rapid, inexpensive, and has a high true-positive rate when compared with *in vivo* tests. Halothane, enflurane, methoxyflurane, isoflurane, and urine from patients anesthetized with these agents were not mutagenic using this assay.[37,38] Urine from people working in scavenged or unscavenged operating rooms was also negative for mutagens.[39]

There have been reports of structural changes in cells brought about by prolonged exposure of animals to subclinical levels of anesthetics. Chang and Katz reviewed a series of relevant studies from their laboratory.[40] Exposure to halothane, 10 to 500 ppm, for 4 to 8 weeks produced ultrastructural changes in hepatic, renal, and neuronal tissue. Changes included degeneration of the mitochondria, endoplasmic reticulum, and bile canaliculi in hepatocytes. The extent of the changes cannot be ascertained from these reports, and because control animals were not used, the effects of tissue preparation and other factors are unknown. It is also possible that the ultrastructural changes were reversible and resulted from the administration of the xenobiotic. There is no proof that there is a relationship between anesthetic exposure, cellular ultrastructural changes, and functional abnormalities.

Reproductive Outcome.   Because of the suggestion from epidemiologic data that occupational exposure to waste anesthetic gases resulted in an increase in spontaneous abortion and congenital abnormalities, numerous studies have been performed in laboratory animals to assess reproductive outcome. One study exposed male and female rats, for 60 days before mating, to concentrations of halothane and nitrous oxide similar to those found in unscavenged operating rooms.[41] Exposed females had decreased ovulation and implantation efficiency, especially in the groups receiving higher concentrations of anesthetics. There were no major teratologic effects. Chromosomal aberrations were observed in both bone marrow and spermatogonial cells in the male rats.

Prolonged exposure of pregnant rats to 1000 ppm nitrous oxide resulted in smaller litter size, increased frequency of fetal resorption, and reduced fetal crown-rump measurements.[42] Lower concentrations of nitrous oxide had no effect on reproductive outcome. Similarly, daily exposure of mice to 4000 ppm isoflurane before and during pregnancy produced no adverse effect on their litters.[43]

Most animal experiments fail to demonstrate alterations in female or male fertility or reproduction with exposure to subanesthetic concentrations of the currently used anesthetic agents. It is important to realize that data from laboratory investigations in animals may not be directly applicable to humans. Although it is easy to measure and quantify the levels of anesthetic in the operating room air, it is harder to measure and assess the effect of other possible factors, such as stress, alterations in working schedule, and fatigue.

Effects of Trace Anesthetic Levels on Psychomotor Skills

Several studies have been conducted to attempt to clarify whether low concentrations of anesthetics alter the psychomotor skills required for providing high-quality care. Student volunteers were exposed to 500 ppm nitrous oxide with or without 15 ppm halothane in air for 4 hours and were then given tests of perceptual, cognitive, and motor skills.[44] After exposure to halothane and nitrous oxide, their performance was impaired on 4 of 12 tests; exposure to nitrous oxide alone produced decreased performance on only 1 test. A subsequent study by the same investigators assessed the effect of nitrous oxide (500, 50, or 25 ppm) alone or with halothane (10, 1.0, or 0.5 ppm) by using psychomotor tests.[45] After exposure to the highest concentrations of nitrous oxide and halothane, subjects' performance declined on 4 of the 7 tests. Interestingly, there was a decrease in ability in 6 of 7 tests after exposure to the same level of nitrous oxide alone. Exposure to the lowest concentrations studied, 25 ppm nitrous oxide and 0.5 ppm halothane, produced no effects as measured by this battery of tests.

Other investigators, using similar protocols, have found no effect on psychomotor test performance after exposure to trace concentrations of halothane or nitrous oxide.[46] The reason for differences in outcome between studies is unclear, but Bruce, one of the original investigators, has attributed the psychological effects of low levels of anesthetics to unusual sensitivity in the group of paid volunteers used in the study.[47]

Recommendations of the National Institute for Occupational Safety and Health

In 1970, Congress created the National Institute for Occupational Safety and Health (NIOSH), the federal agency responsible for ensuring that workers have a safe and healthful working environment. The agency was to meet these goals through the conduct and funding of research, through education of employers and employees about occupational illnesses, and through establishing occupational health standards. A second federal agency, the Occupational Safety and Health Administration (OSHA), was responsible for enacting job health standards, investigating work sites to detect violation of standards, and enforcing the standards by citing violators.[48,49] In 1977, NIOSH published a criteria document that recommended that waste anesthetic exposure should not exceed 2 ppm (1-hour ceiling) of halogenated anesthetic agents when used alone, or 0.5 ppm of a halogenated agent and 25 ppm of nitrous oxide (time-weighted average during use).[50] In addition, it stated that operating room employees should be advised of the potential harmful effects of anesthetics. The guidelines proposed that annual medical and occupational histories be obtained from all personnel and that any abnormal outcomes of pregnancies should be documented. The publication also included information on scavenging procedures and equipment and methods for monitoring concentrations of waste anesthetic gases in the air. The 1977 NIOSH criteria document[50] has not been adopted by OSHA, which currently does not have a standard for nitrous oxide. Some states, however, have instituted regulations calling for routine measurement of ambient nitrous oxide in operating rooms and have mandated that levels not exceed an arbitrary maximum.

It is interesting to examine the rationale given for the selection of NIOSH's standards for waste anesthetic gases. According to the criteria document, "Based on the available health information a safe level of exposure to the halogenated agents cannot be defined. Since a safe level of occupational exposure to halogenated anesthetic agents cannot be established by either animal or human investigations, NIOSH recommends that exposure be controlled to levels no greater than the lowest level detectable using the sampling and analysis techniques recommended by NIOSH in this document."[50] Based on this, the recommendations for halogenated agents were set for 2 ppm. The recommendations for nitrous oxide were based on the studies of Bruce *et al*, who noted that after exposure to levels of 25 ppm nitrous oxide with 0.5 ppm halothane, there was no impairment of subjects' performance on psychomotor tests.[45]

In 1994, NIOSH published an alert to warn health care personnel that exposure to nitrous oxide may produce "harmful effects."[51] In this document, NIOSH recommends the following to reduce nitrous oxide exposure: (1) monitoring the air in operating rooms; (2) implementation of appropriate engineering controls, work practices, and equipment maintenance procedures; and (3) institution of a worker education program.

In view of the conflicting scientific data, it is reasonable to ask what is an acceptable exposure level for waste anesthetic gases. Although it may be difficult to be certain of a threshold concentration below which chronic exposure is "safe," it is prudent to institute measures that reduce waste anesthetic levels in the operating room environment without compromising patient safety. Methods for reducing and monitoring waste gases in the operating room have been suggested.[52] Through the use of scavenging equipment, equipment maintenance procedures, altered anesthetic work practices, and efficient operating room ventilation systems, the environmental anesthetic concentration can be reduced to minimal levels. Monitors to detect leaks in the high- and low-pressure systems of anesthetic machines, contamination due to faulty anesthetic technique, and scavenging system malfunction should be incorporated in programs to ensure reduced occupational exposure. Environmental levels of anesthetics can be measured using instantaneously collected samples, continuous air monitoring, or time-weighted averages.[52]

With appropriate care, environmental levels of anesthetics in the operating room can be reduced to comply with those suggested by NIOSH. In a survey conducted in Ontario hospitals, the level of exposure to halogenated anesthetics was within the published standard, but nitrous oxide concentrations exceeded 25 ppm in many operating rooms.[53] When improved scavenging devices and routine equipment maintenance were instituted, nitrous oxide levels were reduced. A similar situation was documented through a survey of operating rooms in four Glasgow hospitals.[54]

Anesthetic Levels in the Postanesthesia Care Unit

As patients awaken from general anesthesia, waste anesthetic gases are released into the postanesthesia care unit (PACU). Early investigators reported less than 0.6 ppm halothane[55] and 10–34 ppm nitrous oxide[56] in grab samples taken from the area of the patients' breathing zone in the PACU. In a 1998 study, the time-weighted average concentrations for isoflurane, desflurane, and nitrous oxide were 1.1 ppm, 2.1 ppm, and 29 ppm, respectively, in the breathing zone of PACU nurses.[57] Half of the patients were intubated on arrival in the PACU, suggesting that they were still partially anesthetized and hence exhaling a greater concentration of anesthetic gases than were awake patients. In contrast, other investigators reported time-weighted nitrous oxide levels less than 2.0 ppm from two PACUs.[58] In these institutions, nitrous oxide was routinely discontinued at the end of surgery, approximately 5 minutes before the patient left the operating room, and there was adequate ventilation in the PACUs. This suggests that turning off anesthetics in the operating room can minimize levels of waste anesthetic gases in the PACU, particularly if the PACU is well ventilated.[59]

Chemicals

Methylmethacrylate

Methylmethacrylate is commonly used to cement prostheses to bone or to repair bone defects. The cardiovascular effects of methylmethacrylate in patients have been thoroughly studied and reviewed, but there are fewer data on the effects of occupational exposure. Factory workers exposed to methylmethacrylate complained of respiratory, cutaneous, and genitourinary problems after exposure to levels lower than the 8-hour, time-weighted average allowable exposure of 100 ppm established by OSHA.[60] When the Ames test was used to assess the mutagenic potential of methylmethacrylate, it was found that the compound was toxic; and when it was incubated with a rat liver enzyme metabolizing system, mutagenesis was induced.

When methylmethacrylate is prepared for use in the operating room, concentrations up to 90 ppm have been measured during the period required for polymerization. Use of commercially available scavenging devices for venting methylmethacrylate vapor decreased peak concentrations of the vapor by 75%.

Allergic Reactions

In addition to concerns about toxic effects of methylmethacrylate vapor and waste anesthetic gases, allergic reactions to these substances have been reported. Occupational asthma after exposure to methylmethacrylate in orthopedic operating rooms has been described.[61] One anesthesiologist experienced asthma 8 to 12 hours after administering enflurane to his patients.[62]

Halothane. A thoroughly documented case report of an anesthesiologist in whom recurrent hepatitis developed after exposure to and challenge with halothane was interpreted to indicate that halothane was a sensitizing agent in some individuals.[63] Repeated bouts of hepatitis in this anesthesiologist were attributed to hypersensitivity reactions rather than to a direct toxic effect of halothane.

Latex Sensitivity. Latex in surgical and examination gloves has become a common source of allergic reactions among operating room personnel.[64,65] Approximately 70% of adverse reactions to latex reported to the Food and Drug Administration's (FDA) MedWatch database involve health care workers.[66] The prevalence of latex sensitivity among anesthesiologists is estimated to be 12.5%[67] to 15.8%.[68]

Latex is a complex substance composed of polyisoprenes, lipids, phospholipids, and proteins. A number of additional substances, including preservatives, accelerators, antioxidants, vulcanizing compounds, and lubricating agents (such as cornstarch), are added in the manufacture of the final product. The protein content of latex is responsible for the vast majority of generalized allergic reactions to latex-containing surgical gloves. These reactions are exacerbated by the presence of glove powder such as cornstarch or talc. Latex particles adhere to glove powder and when aerosolized during the donning or removal of gloves, can be spread to room surfaces and to the mucosa and respiratory system of personnel.

Irritant or contact dermatitis accounts for approximately 80% of reactions from latex-containing gloves (Table 4-1). In the study reported by Brown *et al*, 24% of anesthesia personnel were found to manifest evidence of contact dermatitis.[67] True allergic reactions present clinically as T-cell–mediated contact dermatitis (Type IV) or as an IgE-mediated anaphylactic reaction.

Anesthesiologists who believe that they are allergic to latex should take immediate steps to assess this possibility.[64] To help make the diagnosis, a careful clinical history should be obtained

Table 4-1. TYPES OF REACTIONS TO LATEX GLOVES

Reaction	Signs/Symptoms	Cause	Management
Irritant contact dermatitis	Scaling, drying, cracking of skin	Direct skin irritation by gloves, powder, soaps	Identify reaction, avoid irritant, possible use of glove liner, use of alternative product
Type IV—Delayed hypersensitivity	Itching, blistering, crusting (delayed 6–72 hours)	Chemical additives used in manufacturing, (such as accelerators)	Identify offending chemical, possible use of alternative product without chemical additive, possible use of glove liner
Type I—Immediate hypersensitivity (A) Localized contact urticaria	Itching, hives in area of contact with latex (immediate)	Proteins found in latex	Identify reaction. Avoid latex-containing products. Use of nonlatex or powder-free low-protein gloves by co-workers
(B) Generalized reaction	Runny nose, swollen eyes, generalized rash or hives, bronchospasm, anaphylaxis		Anaphylaxis protocol

Modified with permission from Witt SF: Hazard Information Bulletin, OSHA, 1998.

to try to correlate latex exposure with allergic symptoms. The laboratory evaluation for latex allergy, involving both *in vitro* and *in vivo* tests, has been outlined by Warshaw.[69] Once the diagnosis of latex allergy has been established, the affected anesthesiologist must avoid all direct contact with latex-containing products. It is also important that co-workers wear powderless, low latex-allergen gloves to limit the levels of ambient latex allergens. Prevention of exposure to latex protein is the best strategy for avoiding latex allergy because sensitivity cannot be reversed.[64]

Radiation

Oncogenesis, teratogenesis, and long-term genetic effects can occur with sufficiently high exposure to radiation. Regulatory agencies consider two classes medical personnel: those who are only occasionally exposed to radiation (*i.e.*, anesthesia personnel) and radiation workers whose normal duties require them to be in areas with large potential exposure.[70] The nonoccupational limit of exposure is set at less than 500 mrem per year.

There exist numerous situations in which anesthesia personnel may experience radiation exposure. Diagnostic radiographs are taken in the operating room, PACU, and intensive care units. Fluoroscopy is utilized during many surgical procedures. Frequently, patients undergoing diagnostic or therapeutic procedures such as angiography, angioplasty, biliary dilation, extracorporeal shock wave lithotripsy, or radiation therapy require care by anesthesiologists. Anesthesia personnel may also be exposed to radionuclides given to patients for diagnostic procedures or for therapy. Strategies that can be used to reduce exposure to radiation include use of personal protective equipment, such as lead aprons and shields, and maintaining a position as far as possible from the source of radiation.

Technologic advances in imaging equipment and radiation handling have reduced the risk of exposure to significant doses of radiation. McGowan *et al* assessed radiation exposure of anesthesia personnel working in an orthopedic operating room where image intensifiers were commonly used.[71] Since all dosimeter readings were below detectable limits, the authors concluded that anesthesia personnel are at minimal risk for radiation exposure.

Radiation exposure should be monitored with film badges or pocket dosimeters in anesthesia personnel at risk. Educational programs on the effects of radiation and techniques for preventing exposure are important parts of radiation safety programs.

Noise Pollution

A potential health hazard that is virtually uncontrolled in the modern hospital and specifically in the operating room is noise pollution.[72] Noise pollution is quantified by determining both the intensity of the sound in decibels (dB) and the duration of the exposure. The National Institute for Occupational Safety and Health has established a maximum level for safe noise exposure of 90 dB for 8 hours.[73] Furthermore, each increase in noise of 5 dB halves the permissible exposure time, so that 100 dB is acceptable for just 2 hours per day. The maximum allowable exposure in an industrial setting is 115 dB.

The noise level in many operating rooms is surprisingly close to what constitutes a health hazard.[74] In one study it was 77.3 dB.[75] Ventilators, suction equipment, music, and conversation produce background noise at a level of 75 to 90 dB. Superimposed on this are such sporadic and unexpected noises as dropped equipment, surgical saws and drills, and monitor alarms. Resultant noise levels frequently exceed those of a freeway and even of a rock-and-roll band.

Excessive levels of noise can have an adverse influence on the anesthesiologist's capacity to perform his or her chores. Noise can interfere with an anesthesiologist's ability to discern conversational speech[74] and even to hear auditory alarms.[76] Mental efficiency and short-term memory are diminished by exposure to excess noise.[75] The complex psychomotor tasks associated with anesthesiology, such as monitoring and vigilance, are particularly sensitive to the adverse influences of noise pollution.[77]

There also are chronic ramifications of long-term exposure to excessive noise in the workplace. At the very least, noise pollution is an important factor in decreased worker productivity. At higher noise levels, workers are likely to show signs of irritability and demonstrate evidence of stress, such as elevated blood pressure. Ultimately, hearing loss ensues. In a sample of anesthesiologists less than 55 years of age, median hearing threshold was worse than for the general population, and the hearing deficits in the higher frequencies were significant enough to interfere with detection of some equipment alarms.[76] The specific cause of the anesthesiologists' hearing loss could not be determined from the study data.

Conversely, music can provide beneficial effects as a different kind of "background noise." Music proved advantageous as a supplement to sedation for awake patients during surgery.[78] Self-selected background music contributed to reduced autonomic responses in a group of surgeons and improved performance during a stressful nonsurgical laboratory task.[79] The beneficial effects were less pronounced when the music was chosen by a third party. Unfortunately, the latter situation more frequently exists for the anesthesiologist.[80]

Human Factors

The work performed by an anesthesiologist is intricate and includes a number of complex tasks. A large body of research has evolved with the goal of applying high-technology solutions to assist the anesthesiologist in managing this demanding workload. Less attention has been given to using human factor technology to improve our workplace and ensure patient safety. The greatest source of patient morbidity and mortality remains human error.[81]

A number of human factor problems potentially exist in the operating room. These include issues specific to the nature of our workload, as well as team and organizational difficulties. The design and positioning of our equipment can serve as a deterrent to the successful completion of all of our obligatory tasks. Most modern anesthesia machines are direct descendants of Boyle's original apparatus—an apparatus that has undergone progressive embellishment with additional monitors and alarms. Unfortunately, this evolutionary development has not resulted in an optimal product by ergonomic standards. For example, the placement of anesthesia monitors in many operating rooms redirects the anesthesiologist's attention away from the patient. Indeed, nearly half of the anesthesiologist's time is spent performing tasks that are away from the patient–surgeon field and not directly related to patient care.[82,83] This was illustrated in a study by Weinger *et al*, who demonstrated that insertion and monitoring of a transesophageal echocardiograph added significantly to the anesthesiologist's workload while diverting attention away from other patient-specific tasks.[84] Conversely, automated record keeping devices permit an increase in direct patient care activities by reducing time spent on record keeping.

Many tasks that are routinely performed by anesthesiologists involve the ability to respond to critical incidents and to sustain complex monitoring tasks, such as maintaining vigilance; these tasks are vulnerable to the distractions created by poor equipment design or placement. *Vigilance* is "the ability to detect changes in a stimulus during prolonged monitoring tasks when the subject has no prior knowledge of whether or when any

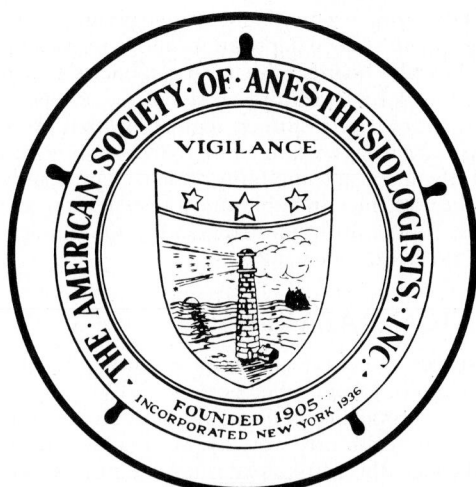

Figure 4-1. Official Seal of the American Society of Anesthesiologists. "VIGILANCE" has always been recognized as the most critical of the anesthesiologist's tasks.

changes might occur."[85] According to Gaba *et al,* "Vigilance is thus a necessary, but not sufficient condition for averting [anesthetic] accidents."[86] The seal of the American Society of Anesthesiologists bears as its only motto, "Vigilance" (Fig. 4-1), and the official motto of the Australian Society of Anaesthetists is "*Vigila et Ventila.*" These mottoes serve as formal recognition of the critical importance of this function.

Several components of the vigilance task deserve attention. First, it is important to recognize that this particular function may be repetitive and monotonous. The task does not fully occupy the anesthesiologist's mental activity, but neither does it leave him or her free to perform other mental functions. Finally, the task is complex, requiring visual attention as well as manual dexterity.

Vigilance tasks are generally performed at the level of 90% accuracy.[87] In a setting where the stakes are as high as that of anesthesia, this leaves an unacceptable margin of error. In fact, human error, in part resulting from lapses in attention, accounts for a large proportion of the estimated 2000 preventable deaths and serious injuries resulting from anesthetic mishaps in the United States annually.[88]

In addition to poor equipment design, a number of other factors at work in the operating room environment serve to diminish the ability of the anesthesiologist to perform multiple tasks that demand cognitive skills.[85] Obvious factors are sleep loss and fatigue. Several studies have documented the deleterious effect of sleep loss and fatigue on work efficiency.[89] In addition, sleep deprivation has detrimental effects on cognitive tasks such as monitoring and accurate clinical decision making.[90,91] Subsequent to a period of sleep deprivation, performance does not return to normal levels until a 24-hour period of rest and recovery has occurred. An interesting phenomenon is the "end-spurt," in which previously deteriorated performance shows improvement when the subject realizes that the task is 90% completed. The converse undoubtedly also occurs, a "let-down" with additional deterioration in performance when the procedure is unexpectedly prolonged.

Any factor that entails the expenditure of excessive energy to perform a given task contributes to fatigue and produces a predictable decrement in performance. Even the most trivial aspect of an operator's performance plays a significant role over the course of time. For example, if the anesthesiologist must make frequent, rapid changes in observation from a dim, distant screen to a bright, nearby one, the continuous muscular activity required for pupil dilation and constriction and lens accommodation promotes fatigue.

Excessive energy expenditure need not be entirely physical. As more functions are monitored in the operating room and more data are processed during the course of a surgical procedure, increasingly larger amounts of mental work are expended. The mental work varies directly with the difficulty encountered in extracting the information from the monitors and displays competing for the anesthesiologist's attention.

Poor design in the monitor displays and the various other sources of information input can adversely affect the anesthesiologist's ability to perform necessary tasks. Engineering details, such as signal frequency and strength, as well as the mode of presentation of the input, significantly influence the operator's performance. For example, if the signal rate is slow, observers tend to produce more false-positive alarms. On the other hand, when confronted with a fast event rate, especially when the signal is of low intensity, the observer tends toward more frequent false-negative findings. Interestingly, monitoring complex displays and the need to "time-share" attention among several vigilance tasks are not associated with a performance decrement.

Even the alarms that have been developed with the specific goal of supplementing the task of vigilance have considerable drawbacks.[92] In a report by Wallace *et al,* 7% of anesthesiologists worked with monitors whose alarm intensities were lower than their detectable threshold.[76] In general, alarms are nonspecific (the same alarm being triggered by as many as 12 different faults) and can be a source of frustration and confusion. They are also susceptible to artifacts and transients (true readings of no significance), and frequent false-positive alarms can distract the observer from more clinically significant information. One depiction of a commercial airline accident, with more than 150 fatalities, describes all three officers in the cockpit completely immersed in concern over a flashing light that indicated the landing gear was still down, a trivial concern at the time. In contrast, the altimeter, which indicated that the aircraft was losing altitude, went unnoticed until too late. Analogous situations occur in the operating room; therefore, it is not unusual for frequently distractive alarms to be deactivated.

Noise may have a detrimental influence on the anesthesiologist working at multiple tasks. The average noise level of 77 dB found in operating rooms has been shown to reduce mental efficiency and short-term memory in anesthesia residents.[75] In general, intrusive noises, such as loud talking, excessive clanging of instruments, and "broadband" noise, are associated with decrements in performance. On the other hand, certain types of background music produce the least effect on vigilance.[93]

Some studies suggest that exposure to low concentrations of waste anesthetic gases may adversely affect the performance of anesthesiologists;[94] however, others have failed to corroborate these findings.[95]

There are team and organizational issues that can adversely affect the ability of the anesthesiologist to perform well. "Production pressure," as a result of increased competition in the health care industry, can engender an environment in which issues of safety are superseded by those of productivity.[96] Production pressure has been associated with the commission of errors resulting from haste and/or deliberate deviations from known safe practices.

Problems with communication among team members can ultimately play a significant role in patient safety. The potential for disaster as a result of poor communication has been well illustrated in a number of airline catastrophes. The possibility for miscommunication and resultant accident is heightened in the operating room where, in contrast to the structure inherent in an airline crew, there is an absence of a well-defined hierarchical structure and borders of expertise and responsibility overlap.[97]

The application of simulation technology has proved very

useful in the study of human performance issues in anesthesiology.[98,99] Much, however, remains to be done in bringing human factor research to the anesthesiologist's work environment.[100]

Work Hours and Night Call

Sleep deprivation and accompanying fatigue are ubiquitous components of many anesthesiologists' life style. For practicing anesthesiologists, 10- to 12-hour workdays are not unusual. Emergency and on-call coverage is usually tacked onto the end of one of these days, resulting in a 24- to 32-hour shift. The average work week was 56 hours in Gravenstein's study of the work patterns of anesthesia providers.[101] Seventy-four percent of the study respondents reported that they had worked without a break for longer periods than they thought was safe. An error in anesthetic management was attributed to fatigue by 64% of the study participants.

The duration of the work week for anesthesiology residents is in general 10 hours longer than that reported among fully trained practitioners.[101,102] However, the work week of a typical anesthesiology resident is shorter than that of residents in other medical specialties (74 hours) and is within current recommendations.[103]

Long hours of work and night call are especially challenging for the aging anesthesiologist. Older individuals are particularly sensitive to disturbances of the sleep-wake cycle and are in general better suited to phase advances (morning work) than phase delays (nocturnal work).[104] Demands associated with night call have been identified as the most stressful aspect of practice,[105] and are most frequently cited as an impetus toward retirement.[106]

Several studies have substantiated the claim that fatigue or continuous wakefulness has a deleterious effect on many physical and cognitive functions. Even simple tasks, such as driving a car, are demonstrably impaired as a result of sleep deprivation among residents in anesthesiology.[107] The performance of more complex cognitive tasks such as monitoring and vigilance are disturbed to a greater extent.[108] What is particularly troubling is the suggestion that this deterioration in psychomotor functioning may contribute directly to anesthetic mishaps. A survey conducted by Gaba et al revealed that 54% of respondents felt that fatigue was a contributing factor in errors they had committed in clinical management.[96] In another survey of serious anesthetic-related accidents, fatigue was one of the two major sources of human error (confusion involving anesthetic equipment was the other).[109] Together, these two sources of error accounted for more than 96% of the lethal or near-lethal human errors reported. Similarly, in an analysis of critical incidents by Cooper et al, fatigue was among the most frequently reported factors associated with anesthetic mishaps and was a contributing factor in 70% of potentially serious anesthetic events.[110]

An additional area of concern is the potential effect of sleep deprivation and chronic fatigue on health and psychosocial adjustment.[111] Work schedules that disrupt circadian rhythms are associated with impaired health, emotional problems, and a decline in performance. The sleep loss pattern experienced by anesthesiologists who take night call is complex and includes elements of each of the three general classes of sleep deprivation: total, partial, and selective sleep deprivation. Selective sleep deprivation resulting from frequent interruptions is most disruptive to the important components of sleep, including slow wave sleep (associated with "body repair") and rapid eye movement sleep ("mind repair"). Indicators of psychosocial distress, including irritability, displaced anger, depression, and anxiety have all been identified in house officers suffering from sleep deprivation.[112]

National attention was focused on the problem of fatigue by the well-publicized Libby Zion case.[113] A large portion of this claim hinged on the allegation that fatal, avoidable mistakes were made by exhausted, unsupervised house officers. A number of medical organizations and state legislatures have identified the problem of sleep deprivation among physicians. Several medical specialty boards have ratified policies that limit the number of work hours for their resident physicians, and some state legislatures have instituted regulations that prohibit resident physicians from working more than 24 consecutive hours. However, the medical community remains significantly behind other industries, most notably the transportation and airline industries, in identifying and regulating work practices that condone excessively long shifts.[114]

INFECTION HAZARDS

Anesthesia personnel are at risk for acquiring infections both from patients and from other personnel.[65] Viral infections reflecting their prevalence in the community are the most significant threat to health care workers. Most commonly, these are spread through the respiratory route—a mechanism that is, unfortunately, the most difficult to control effectively with environmental alterations (Table 4-2). Immunity against some viral pathogens can be provided through vaccination.[115] Bloodborne pathogens such as hepatitis and human immunodeficiency virus cause serious infections, but transmission can be prevented with mechanical barriers blocking portals of entry or, in the case of hepatitis B, by producing immunity by vaccination. Current recommendations from the Centers for Disease Control (CDC) for pre-employment screening, infection control practices, vaccination, postexposure treatment, and work restrictions for infected personnel should be consulted for specific information related to each pathogen.[65,116]

Respiratory Viruses

Respiratory viruses, which are responsible for many community-acquired infections, are usually transmitted by two routes. Small-particle aerosols produced by coughing, sneezing, or talking may propel viruses over large distances. The influenza and measles viruses are spread in this way. The second mechanism requires close person-to-person contact. Transmission can occur when large droplets produced by coughing or sneezing contaminate the donor's hands or an inanimate surface, whereupon the virus is transferred to the oral, nasal, or conjunctival mucous membranes of a susceptible person by self-inoculation. Rhinovirus and respiratory syncytial virus (RSV) are spread by this process.

Influenza Viruses

Since influenza viruses are easily transmitted, community epidemics of influenza are common, with large outbreaks occurring annually. Acutely ill patients shed virus through small-particle aerosols by coughing or sneezing for as long as 5 days after the onset of symptoms. Respiratory isolation precautions can be used for the duration of the clinical illness in an attempt to prevent spread to susceptible individuals. Because of their contact with nasopharyngeal secretions, anesthesiologists may play a role in the spread of influenza virus in hospitals.

Table 4-2. FACTORS INVOLVED IN THE SUCCESSFUL TRANSMISSION OF INFECTIOUS AGENTS, BACTERIA, AND VIRUSES

1. A source of infectious particles, usually from patients or personnel who are carriers
2. The stability of the pathogen in the physical environment
3. The number of infectious particles in the vehicle of transmission
4. The infectivity of the agent
5. The appropriate vector or medium for transmission
6. A portal of entry in a susceptible host

Influenza rarely produces significant morbidity in healthy health care workers, but may result in high rates of absenteeism. Hospital staff, especially those who care for patients in high-risk groups, should be immunized annually with the inactivated (killed virus) influenza virus vaccine.[116,117] Antigenic variation of influenza viruses occurs over time, so that new viral strains (usually two Type A and one Type B) are selected for inclusion in each year's vaccine. Vaccination programs for personnel should be conducted in October or November, because the number of cases of influenza in the community begins to increase in December. During hospital outbreaks of influenza A, the antiviral agents amantadine and rimantadine are reasonably effective in preventing influenza A infection in unvaccinated hospital personnel and, if administered within 48 hours of the onset of illness, can reduce the duration and severity of illness. Another class of drugs, neuraminidase inhibitors, has been shown to be effective in preventing and treating both influenza A and B in clinical trials.[118]

Because of possible morbidity to hospitalized patients and to hospital personnel, it is recommended that during community influenza epidemics, hospitals should consider limiting elective admissions and surgery. If surgery is necessary in a patient with influenza, data from an animal model suggest that general anesthesia results in no increase in respiratory morbidity.[119]

Respiratory Syncytial Virus

Respiratory syncytial virus (RSV) is the most important cause of serious lower respiratory tract disease in infants and young children worldwide.[120] During periods when RSV is prevalent in the community (usually late November through May in the United States), many hospitalized infants and children may carry the virus. Large numbers of virus are present in respiratory secretions of infected children, and viable virus can be recovered for up to 6 hours on contaminated environmental surfaces. Infection of susceptible people occurs by self-inoculation when RSV in secretions is transferred to the hands, which then contact the mucous membranes of the eyes or nose. Although most children have been exposed to respiratory syncytial virus early in life, immunity is not permanent and reinfection is common.

Respiratory syncytial virus is shed for approximately 7 days after infection. Hospitalized patients with the virus should be isolated in a single room or in a unit with other infected patients (contact isolation procedures[121]), but during seasonal outbreaks large numbers of patients may make isolation impractical. Careful hand washing between contacts with patients and the use of gowns, gloves, masks, and goggles have all been shown to reduce RSV infection in hospital personnel.[122]

Herpes Viruses

Varicella-zoster virus (VZV), herpes simplex virus Types 1 and 2, and cytomegalovirus (CMV) are members of the Herpetoviridine family. Close personal contact is required for transmission of all the herpes viruses except for VZV, which is spread by direct contact or small-particle aerosols. After primary infection with herpes viruses, the organism becomes latent and may reactivate at a later time. Most people in the United States have been infected with all of the herpes viruses by middle age. Therefore, nosocomial transmission is uncommon except in the pediatric population and in immunosuppressed patients.

Varicella-Zoster Virus

Varicella-zoster virus produces both chickenpox and herpes zoster (shingles). Although the primary infection (chickenpox) is usually uncomplicated in healthy children, VZV infection in adults may be associated with major morbidity or death. Infection during pregnancy may result in fetal death or, rarely, in congenital defects. Health care workers with active VZV infec-

tion may transmit the virus to other personnel or to immunocompromised patients.

After the primary infection, VZV remains latent in dorsal root or extramedullary cranial ganglia. Herpes zoster results from reactivation of the VZV infection and produces a painful vesicular rash in the innervated dermatome. Anesthesiologists working in pain clinics may be exposed to VZV when caring for patients who have discomfort from herpes zoster.

Varicella-zoster virus is highly contagious, especially from patients with chickenpox or disseminated zoster. The CDC estimates that the period of communicability begins 1 to 2 days before the onset of the rash and ends when all the lesions are crusted, usually 4 to 6 days after the rash appears.[123] Since VZV may be spread through airborne transmission, respiratory isolation should be used for patients with chickenpox or disseminated herpes zoster.[121] Use of gloves to avoid contact with vesicular fluid is adequate to prevent VZV spread from patients with localized herpes zoster.

Most adults in the United States have protective antibodies to VZV and are immune to new infection. One survey of hospital health care workers found that all of those aged 36 years and older had VZV antibodies, whereas 7.5% of those younger were susceptible.[124] Anesthesia personnel should be questioned about prior VZV infection, and those with a negative or unknown history of such infection should be serologically tested.[65] All employees with negative titers should be restricted from caring for patients with active VZV infection and should consider immunization with live, attenuated varicella vaccine. Susceptible personnel with a significant exposure to people with VZV infection are candidates for varicella zoster immune globulin (VZIG), which is most effective when administered within 96 hours after exposure. Because VZIG can prolong the incubation period of the virus, susceptible hospital personnel with significant VZV exposure should not have direct patient contact from the 10th to the 21st day after exposure.[123] Personnel without VZV immunity should be reassigned to alternative locations so that they do not care for patients who have active VZV infections.

Herpes Simplex

Herpes simplex infection is quite common in adults. After viral entry through the mucous membranes of the mouth, the primary infection with herpes simplex virus Type 1 is usually clinically inapparent but may involve severe oral lesions, fever, and adenopathy. In healthy people, the primary infection subsides and the virus persists in a latent state within the sensory nerve ganglion innervating the site of infection. Any of several mechanisms can reactivate the virus to produce recurrent infection, which manifests in the vicinity of the primary lesion.

A second herpes simplex virus, Type 2, is usually associated with infections below the waist and is spread by sexual contact. Newborns may become infected with herpes simplex virus Type 2 during vaginal delivery from the mother's genital infection.

Herpes simplex virus Type 1 is probably spread by self-inoculation after contact with contaminated oral secretions. Asymptomatic individuals can unknowingly transmit herpes simplex virus Type 1, because the virus has been isolated from oral secretions of 5% of some populations. The fingers of health care personnel may be inoculated by direct contact with body fluids carrying either herpes simplex virus Type 1 or 2.

Herpetic Whitlow. Herpetic infection of the finger, herpetic paronychia or herpetic whitlow, is an occupational hazard for anesthesia personnel.[125] The infection usually begins at the portal of viral entry, a site on the distal finger where the integrity of the skin has been broken. Initially, there is itching and pain at the site of infection, followed by the appearance of a vesicle surrounded by erythema. There may be associated constitutional symptoms such as fever, malaise, and lymphadenopathy. Satellite vesicles appear near the primary lesion over several days. Within 3 weeks, the throbbing pain lessens, and the lesions

Table 4-3. PREVENTION OF OCCUPATIONALLY ACQUIRED INFECTIONS[65, 121]

Infectious Agent	Preventive Measures*
Cytomegalovirus	Standard precautions
Hepatitis B	Vaccine; hepatitis B immune globulin, standard precautions
Hepatitis C	Standard precautions
Herpes simplex	Standard precautions; contact precautions if disseminated disease
Human immunodeficiency virus	Postexposure prophylactic antiretrovirals; standard precautions
Influenza	Vaccine; prophylactic antiretrovirals; droplet precautions
Measles	Vaccine; airborne precautions
Rubella	Vaccine; droplet precautions
Tuberculosis	Airborne precautions; isoniazid ± ethambutol for PPD conversion
Varicella-zoster	Vaccine; varicella-zoster immune globulin; airborne and contact precautions; standard precautions if localized disease

* Isolation Precautions outlined in Table 4-4.

begin to heal. A diagnosis of herpes simplex infection can be made by demonstrating multinucleated giant epithelial cells or nuclear inclusion bodies in smears (Tzanck's technique) taken from a vesicle. Although the process may resemble a bacterial paronychia, treatment should be conservative and surgical drainage is not indicated.

To prevent herpes simplex virus infections of the hands, anesthesia personnel should wear gloves when in contact with patients' oral secretions such as during endotracheal intubation and extubation, pharyngeal suctioning, and insertion of nasogastric tubes.[126] Personnel with herpes simplex infections of the

fingers or hands should not contact patients until their lesions are healed.[65] Treatment with acyclovir, an antiviral drug that inhibits replication of herpes simplex virus Types 1 and 2, may shorten the course of primary cutaneous viral infection.

Cytomegalovirus

Cytomegalovirus (CMV) infection commonly occurs during childhood, and antibodies to CMV develop in most individuals after the initial infection, which may be clinically inapparent. After this, there are intermittent periods of virus excretion even in the presence of high levels of circulating antibody. Transmission of CMV probably occurs through close contact with an individual excreting the virus or through contact with contaminated saliva or urine. It is unlikely that aerosols or small droplets play a role in CMV transmission.

Primary or recurrent CMV infection during pregnancy results in fetal infection in up to 2.5% of occurrences. Congenital CMV syndrome may be found in up to 10% of infected infants. Thus, although CMV infection usually does not result in morbidity in healthy adults, it may have significant sequelae in pregnant women. CMV infection can also be deadly in immunocompromised patients, such as those undergoing bone marrow transplantation.

The two major reservoirs of CMV infection within the hospital include infected infants and immunocompromised patients, such as those who have undergone organ transplants or those on oncology units. Studies of employees at a pediatric hospital indicate that personnel with patient care responsibilities have no greater risk of CMV infection than do personnel who have no patient contact.[127] It appears that routine infection control procedures, such as hand washing after patient contact and use of gloves to avoid touching body fluids, are sufficient to prevent CMV infection in health care workers (Tables 4-3 and 4-4).[65] Pregnant personnel should be made aware of the risks associated with CMV infection during pregnancy and of appropriate infection control precautions to be used when caring for high-

Table 4-4. HOSPITAL ISOLATION PRECAUTIONS[121]

STANDARD PRECAUTIONS
These are to be used for the care of all patients regardless of their diagnosis or presumed infection status.
Standard precautions should be used in conjunction with other forms of isolation precautions (see below) for the care of specific patients.

1. *Hand washing*
   After touching blood, body fluids, or contaminated items even if gloves are worn.
2. *Gloves*
   Wear gloves when touching blood, body fluids, or contaminated items.
   Change gloves between tasks on the same patient when there is likely to be a high concentration of organisms.
   Remove gloves after use, before touching noncontaminated items and environmental surfaces.
3. *Mask, eye protection, face shield*
   Use during procedures likely to generate splashes of blood or body fluids that may contaminate face or mucous membranes.
4. *Gown*
   Use during procedures likely to generate splashes of blood or body fluids that may contaminate clothing or arms.
5. *Patient-care equipment*
   Handle soiled equipment in a manner that prevents skin, mucous membrane, clothing, or environmental contamination.
6. *Environmental control*
   Contaminated environmental surfaces should routinely be cleaned and/or disinfected.
7. *Linen*
   Soiled linen should be handled in a manner that prevents contamination of personnel, other patients, and environmental surfaces.
8. *Occupational health and bloodborne pathogens*
   Use care to prevent injuries when using or disposing of needles and sharp devices.
   Contaminated needles should not be recapped or manipulated by using both hands. If recapping is necessary for the procedure being performed, a one-handed scoop technique or mechanical device for holding the needle sheath should be used.
   Contaminated needles should not be removed from disposable syringes by hand.
   Do not break or bend contaminated needles before disposal.
   After use, disposable syringes and needles and other sharp devices should be placed in appropriate puncture-resistant containers located as close as practical to the area in which the items were used.
   Mouthpieces, resuscitation bags, or other ventilation devices should be available for use as an alternative to mouth-to-mouth ventilation.
9. *Patient placement*
   Private rooms should be used for patients who are likely to contaminate the environment.

(continued)

Table 4-4. HOSPITAL ISOLATION PRECAUTIONS[121] (*continued*)

TRANSMISSION-BASED PRECAUTIONS

These should be used along with Standard Precautions for patients known or suspected to be infected or colonized with highly transmissible pathogens requiring additional precautions.

Airborne Precautions

These should be used for patients known or suspected to be infected with microorganisms transmitted by airborne droplet nuclei (particles 5 μm or smaller in size) that can be dispersed over large distances by air currents.

1. *Patient placement*
   The patient should be placed in a private room with (1) documented negative air pressure relative to surrounding areas, (2) 6 to 12 air changes per hour, (3) discharge of air outdoors or monitored high-efficiency filtration of room air before the air is circulated to other areas in the hospital.
   The door to the room should be kept closed and the patient should remain in the room.
2. *Respiratory protection*
   Respiratory protection should be worn when entering the room of a patient with known or suspected infectious pulmonary tuberculosis. Susceptible personnel should not enter the room of patients known or suspected to have measles or varicella if other immune caregivers are available. If susceptible persons must enter the room of a patient known or suspected to have measles or varicella, they should wear respiratory protection. Persons immune to measles or varicella need not wear respiratory protection.
3. *Patient transport*
   Patients should be transported from the isolation room only for essential purposes. When transport is necessary, a surgical mask should be placed on the patient to prevent dispersal of droplet nuclei.
4. *Patients with tuberculosis*
   Current CDC guidelines should be consulted for additional precautions.[177]

Droplet Precautions

These should be used for patients known or suspected to be infected with microorganisms transmitted by large-particle droplets (particles larger than 5 μm) that can be generated during coughing, sneezing, talking, or by performing certain procedures.

1. *Patient placement*
   The patient should be placed in a private room.
2. *Respiratory protection*
   Personnel should wear a mask when working within 3 feet of the patient.
3. *Patient transport*
   Patients should be transported from the isolation room only for essential purposes. When transport is necessary, a surgical mask should be placed on the patient to prevent dispersal of droplets.

Contact Precautions

These should be used for patients known or suspected to be infected or colonized with epidemiologically important microorganisms transmitted by direct contact with the patient or indirect contact with environmental surfaces or patient-care items.

1. *Patient placement*
   The patient should be placed in a private room.
2. *Gloves and hand washing*
   In addition to wearing gloves as outlined under Standard Precautions, gloves (nonsterile) should be worn when entering the patient's room.
   Gloves should be changed after contacting infective material that may contain high concentrations of microorganisms.
   Gloves should be removed before leaving the patient's environment and hands should be washed immediately with an antimicrobial agent or a waterless antiseptic agent.
   After removal of gloves and hand washing, care should be taken so that contaminated environmental surfaces should not be touched to avoid transfer of microorganisms to other patients.
3. *Gown*
   In addition to wearing a gown as outlined under Standard Precautions, a gown (nonsterile) should be worn when entering the room when it is anticipated that clothing will have contact with the patient, environmental surfaces, or contaminated items or if the patient is incontinent or has diarrhea, an ileostomy, a colostomy, or wound drainage not contained by a dressing.
   The gown should be removed before leaving the patient's environment.
   Clothing should not contact potentially contaminated surfaces after removal of the gown.
4. *Patient transport*
   The patient should be transported from the room for only essential purposes.
   If it is necessary to transport the patient, precautions should be maintained to minimize the risk of transmission of microorganisms to other patients and contamination of environmental surfaces or equipment.
5. *Patient-care equipment*
   Dedicate the use of noncritical patient-care equipment (*e.g.*, blood pressure cuffs) to a single patient to avoid transmission of microorganisms to another patient. If use of common equipment is unavoidable, then items should be adequately cleaned or disinfected before use on another patient.
6. *Additional precautions for preventing spread of vancomycin resistance*
   Current CDC guidelines should be consulted.[243]

risk patients. There is no evidence to indicate that it is necessary to reassign pregnant women from patient care areas in which they may have contact with CMV-positive patients.

Rubella

Outbreaks of rubella, or German measles, in hospital personnel have resulted in significant loss in employee working time, employee morbidity, and cost to the hospital. Although most adults in the United States are immune to rubella, up to 20% of women of child-bearing age are still susceptible. Rubella infection during the first trimester of pregnancy is associated with congenital malformations or fetal death.

Rubella is transmitted by contact with nasopharyngeal droplets from infected individuals. Patients are most contagious while the rash is erupting but can transmit the virus from 1 week before to 5 to 7 days after the onset of the rash. Droplet precautions should be used to prevent transmission (Table 4-4).[65]

Ensuring immunity at the time of employment should prevent nosocomial transmission of rubella to personnel. Immunity can be documented by evidence of prior vaccination with live rubella vaccine or serologic confirmation. It has been shown that history is a poor indicator of immunity. A live, attenuated rubella virus vaccine is available to produce immunity in susceptible personnel.[115,128] For individuals without confirmed immunity, routine serologic testing for antibody prior to vaccination is usually not cost-effective. Many state or local health departments mandate rubella immunity for all health care personnel, and local regulations should be consulted.

Measles (Rubeola)

Measles virus is highly transmissible both by large droplets and by the airborne route. Since the introduction of the measles vaccine in the United States in 1963, the incidence of the disease has decreased significantly. After a resurgence in the disease from 1989 to 1991, vaccination programs in preschool-aged children and implementation of programs for a second vaccine dose have successfully eliminated indigenous cases of measles in the United States. Importation of measles from other countries continues to occur.

Health care workers are at increased risk for acquiring measles (13 times that of the general population) and transmitting the virus to co-workers and patients. The CDC recommends that medical personnel have adequate immunity to measles, as documented by one of the following: evidence of two doses of live measles vaccine, a record of physician-diagnosed measles, or serologic evidence of measles immunity (Table 4-3).[65] Susceptible personnel born in or after 1957 should receive two doses of the live measles vaccine at the time of employment.[128]

Viral Hepatitis

Although many viruses may produce hepatitis, the most common are Type A or infectious hepatitis, Type B (HBV) or serum hepatitis, and Type C (HCV), which is responsible for most cases of parenterally transmitted non-A, non-B hepatitis (NANBH) in the United States. Delta hepatitis, caused by an incomplete virus, occurs only in people infected with HBV. Outbreaks of an enterically transmitted NANBH (hepatitis E) have been reported from outside the United States and are usually caused by contaminated water. The greatest risks of occupational transmission to anesthesia personnel are associated with HBV and HCV.

Hepatitis A

About 20–40% of viral hepatitis in adults in the United States is caused by the Type A virus, a picornavirus containing RNA. Hepatitis A is usually a self-limited illness, and no chronic carrier state exists. Spread is predominantly by the fecal–oral route,

either by person-to-person contact or by ingestion of contaminated food or water. Outbreaks are usually found in institutions or other closed groups where there has been a breakdown in normal sanitary conditions. Hospital personnel do not appear to be at increased risk for hepatitis A.

Occasional hospital outbreaks of hepatitis A have occurred when patients were admitted during the prodromal stage of the infection. The use of gloves and meticulous hand washing during contact with feces or contaminated linens or clothing should be adequate to prevent viral spread to hospital personnel. Personnel exposed to patients with hepatitis A should receive immune globulin within 2 weeks of the exposure to reduce the likelihood of infection.[129,130] Immune globulin provides protection against hepatitis A through passive transfer of antibodies and is used for postexposure prophylaxis. Hepatitis A vaccine is prepared from inactivated virus and is not routinely recommended for health care personnel except for those that may be working in countries with high hepatitis A endemicity.[115,130]

Hepatitis B

Hepatitis B is a significant occupational hazard for nonimmune anesthesiologists and other medical personnel who have frequent contact with blood and blood products. The prevalence* of hepatitis B in the general population of the United States is 3–5%, and the carrier rate is 0.2–0.9% based on serologic screening. Serosurveys including more than 2400 anesthesia personnel conducted in the United States and several other countries demonstrated a mean prevalence of HBV serologic markers of 17.8% (range, 3.2–48.6%).[131] The range of seropositive findings in anesthesia personnel in various locations probably reflects the prevalence of HBV carriers in the referral population for the area. Within the United States, the prevalence of hepatitis B markers in anesthesia personnel varied from 19% in one multicenter study[132] to 49% in the anesthesia department of an inner-city hospital.[133]

Acute HBV infection usually resolves without significant hepatic damage. Less than 1% of acutely infected patients will have fulminant hepatitis. The remaining 10% of infected people become chronic carriers of HBV (i.e., serologic evidence demonstrated for more than 6 months). Within 2 years, half of the chronic carriers resolve their infection without significant hepatic impairment. Chronic active hepatitis, which may progress to cirrhosis, is found most commonly in those individuals with chronic viral infection for more than 2 years. Although prior estimates suggested that occupationally acquired HBV resulted in the death of 250 medical personnel each year, the implementation of routine vaccination and use of universal precautions have significantly reduced the risk of HBV infection (90% decline from 1985 to 1994) and its sequelae.[65]

The diagnosis and classification of the stage of HBV infection can be made on the basis of serologic testing. Antibody to the surface antigen (anti-HBs) appears with resolution of the acute infection and confers lasting immunity against subsequent HBV infections. Chronic HBV carriers are likely to have hepatitis B surface antigen (HBsAg) and antibody to the core antigen (anti-HBc) present in serum samples.

Hepatitis B virus transmission in the community takes place through sexual contact, close personal contact (as occurs in institutions), shared use of needles and syringes for intravenous drug use, and perinatally from infected mother to newborn. Anesthesia personnel are at risk for occupationally acquired HBV infection as a result of accidental percutaneous or mucosal contact with blood or body fluids from infected patients. Patient groups with a high prevalence of HBV carriers include immigrants from endemic areas, users of illicit parenteral drugs, homosexual men, and patients on hemodialysis.[129] Carriers are

_____

* The prevalence is the proportion of people who have or have had the condition at the time of the survey.

frequently not identified during hospitalization because the clinical history and routine preoperative laboratory tests may be insufficient for diagnosis. Percutaneous exposure (usually an accidental needle stick) to blood carrying HBV (e-antigen–positive individuals) may result in infection in up to 30% of occurrences. HBV can be found in saliva, but the rate of transmission is less after mucosal contact with infected oral secretions than after percutaneous exposures to blood. HBV is a hardy virus that may be infectious for at least 1 week in dried blood on environmental surfaces.[134]

Hepatitis B Vaccines. Use of hepatitis B vaccine is the primary strategy to prevent occupational transmission of HBV to anesthesia personnel and other health care workers at increased risk.[129] Administration of three doses of vaccine in the deltoid muscle results in the production of protective antibodies (anti-HBs) in more than 90% of healthy hospital workers. Hepatitis B vaccines now available in the United States are composed of HBsAg that has been produced by recombinant technology. Hospitals or anesthesia departments should have policies for educating, screening, and counseling personnel about their risk of acquiring HBV infection and should make vaccination available for susceptible personnel.[129,135]

To ensure adequate postvaccination immunity, serologic testing of vaccinees for anti-HBs should take place within 6 months after the last dose of vaccine. Protective antibodies may develop in nonresponders with additional vaccine doses.[136] Vaccine-induced antibodies decline over time, with maximum titers after vaccination correlating directly with duration of antibody persistence.[136] The CDC states that for vaccinated adults with normal immune status, routine booster doses are not necessary for at least 7 years after vaccination.[129] Surveillance programs are continuing to assess the need for booster doses after longer intervals.

When susceptible, nonvaccinated anesthesia personnel have documented exposure to a contaminated needle or to blood from an HBsAg-positive patient, postexposure prophylaxis with HBV hyperimmune globulin and initiation of HBV vaccine series is recommended.[129,137] HBV hyperimmune globulin (HBIG) is prepared from human plasma that contains a high anti-HBs titer and provides temporary, passive immunity.

Hepatitis C

The hepatitis C virus (HCV) is the etiology of most cases of parenterally transmitted NANBH and is a leading cause of chronic liver disease in the United States.[138] Antibodies to HCV (anti-HCV) can be detected in most patients with hepatitis C, but its presence does not correlate with resolution of the infection or progression of the hepatitis.[139] Immunity against HCV infection is not conferred by anti-HCV. Seropositivity for hepatitis C RNA using polymerase chain reaction is a marker of chronic HCV infection and can be used to identify individuals with potential to transmit the infection.[140]

Sporadic parenteral transmission of NANBH accounts for 20–40% of all reported cases of acute viral hepatitis in the United States. CDC surveillance demonstrates that only about 6% of cases of NANBH are attributed to blood transfusions, whereas 42% are associated with intravenous drug use. Only 2% occur in health care workers from occupational exposure.[141] The prevalence of anti-HCV in the United States is estimated to be 1.8% (3.9 million persons) with 74% (2.7 million persons) positive for HCV RNA.[142]

People infected with HCV have a high rate of chronic hepatitis. Up to 60% of HCV-infected patients will have biopsy-proven chronic hepatitis, with many progressing to cirrhosis. HCV RNA can still be detected in more than 75% of patients after resolution of hepatitis C.[139] Interferon-aIIb has been an effective treatment for chronic hepatitis C, but unfortunately many patients relapse on discontinuation of the therapy. Combination therapy with interferon and ribavirin is more effective than treatment with interferon alone.[143,144]

Like HBV, HCV is transmitted through blood and sexual contact, but the rate of HCV infection through routine personal contact is not high. The risk of hepatitis C after a HCV-infected needle stick exposure appears to be about 2–4%.[145,146] This rate of transmission is significantly less than that for HBV, possibly owing to a lower viral titer in the blood of carriers. There is no effective postexposure prophylaxis available to prevent HCV infection, and use of immune globulin is no longer recommended.[145,147] Interferon treatment begun during the early course of HCV infection is more effective than during chronic infection,[148] but the drug has not been tested for efficacy for postexposure prophylaxis. Personnel who have had a percutaneous or mucosal exposure to anti-HCV-positive blood should have serologic testing and counseling at the time of the exposure and at 6 months.[145]

Pathogenic Human Retroviruses

The agent that produces acquired immunodeficiency syndrome (AIDS) is the Type 1 human immunodeficiency virus (HIV-1), one of several pathogenic human retroviruses.[149] HIV-1 (HIV) is a member of the human T-cell lymphotrophic viruses (HTLV) and was initially designated as HTLV-III. HTLV-I was the first human retrovirus to be discovered and has been documented as a cause of adult T-cell leukemia/lymphoma and a chronic degenerative neurologic disease, tropical spastic paraparesis. HTLV-I has been found in intravenous drug users and female prostitutes in the United States and has been identified and is tested for in the U.S. blood supply. Serologic studies indicate that the virus is endemic in parts of Japan, the Caribbean, and Africa.

Human T-cell lymphotrophic virus II (HTLV-II) is similar to HTLV-I, and initial serologic testing often failed to differentiate the two viruses. HTLV-II is prevalent in intravenous drug users in the United States and Europe. HTLV-II has not been specifically linked with any disease, but the virus has been isolated from some patients with hairy cell leukemia. Transmission of HTLV-I/II appears to be through blood or during sexual intercourse. Occupational transmission to health care workers has not been studied, but because it is a bloodborne infection, this cannot be ruled out.

A second virus, HIV-2, produces an AIDS-like syndrome in parts of western Africa. The epidemiologic pattern of HIV-2 spread is predominantly through heterosexual activity, with almost equal numbers of infected men and women. The only reported cases of HIV-2 infection in the United States have been in patients who came from, or had contact with residents of Africa.

HIV Infection and AIDS

Current estimates suggest that 600,000 to 900,000 people in the United States are infected with HIV. The initial infection presents clinically as a mononucleosis-like syndrome with lymphadenopathy and rash. Although the patient then enters an asymptomatic period, monocyte-macrophage cells serve as a reservoir for the virus throughout the body, and CD4+ T cells harbor the virus in the blood. Infection results in a serum antibody that may be detected by the enzyme-linked immunosorbent assay (ELISA) and is confirmed using the more specific Western blot test. Based on studies of homosexual men, AIDS develops in half of infected persons within 8 years of infection. During this phase of the disease, there is an increase in viral titer and impaired host immunity, resulting in opportunistic infections and malignancies.[150] According to CDC data, from 1981 through June 1999 there have been 711,344 cases of AIDS in the United States.[151] The recent decline in the annual number of new cases of AIDS has been attributed to the effect of new antiretroviral treatments for HIV infection.

Human immunodeficiency virus is spread by sexual contact, perinatally from infected mother to neonate, and through infected blood (transfusion or shared needles) and blood products.[152] Investigation of AIDS patients with no recognized risk factors indicates no evidence for additional modes of transmission. Although the virus can be found in saliva, tears, and urine, these body fluids have not been implicated in viral transmission.[152] Groups of adults that account for the highest percentage of AIDS cases include homosexual/bisexual males, intravenous drug users, heterosexuals with a history of contact with an HIV-infected person, or individuals receiving an infected blood transfusion, blood component, or tissue.

All HIV-infected patients may not be identified as such by their initial or presenting diagnosis. Six percent of patients cared for in one urban hospital emergency department had HIV infection, with 63% of those being unrecognized.[153] Serologic testing of patients at 20 acute care hospitals in 15 U.S. cities indicated an overall rate of HIV seroprevalence of 4.7% and a range of 0.2–14.2%.[154]

Risk of Occupational Human Immunodeficiency Virus Infection. Although there are several modes of transmission for HIV infection in the community, the most important source for occupational transmission of HIV to health care workers is blood contact.[155] Prospective studies by the CDC[156,157] and the National Institutes of Health[158] demonstrated that the rate of seroconversion in prospectively followed health care workers sustaining a percutaneous exposure (needle stick injury) to HIV-infected blood was 0.3%.[157,158,159] Although no infections occurred after cutaneous or mucous membrane exposures in these studies, the rate of transmission of HIV after mucous membrane exposure is estimated to be 0.09%.[160] Through June 1999, the CDC had documented HIV seroconversion in 55 health care workers after occupational exposure.[151] Forty-nine of the infected health care workers had percutaneous exposure. A search of the worldwide literature provided reports of 94 health care workers with occupationally acquired HIV infection through September 1997.[161]

A case-control study has demonstrated that specific factors are associated with an increased rate of HIV transmission after a percutaneous injury.[162] Increased risk was associated with a deep injury, visible blood on the device producing the injury, a procedure in which the needle was placed in an artery or vein, and terminal illness (death from AIDS within 2 months) in the source patient. Therefore, the risk of occupational HIV transmission is greatest after a deep injury with a blood-filled, large-gauge, hollow-bore needle used on a patient in the terminal phase of AIDS.

The occupational risk of HIV infection is a function of the annual number of blood exposures, the rate of HIV transmission with each exposure to infected blood, and the prevalence of HIV infection in the specific patient population. Based on values for these variables taken from the literature, Buergler *et al* calculated a 1-year risk of HIV infection for anesthesiologists to be between 0.001 and 0.129%.[163] Greene *et al* prospectively collected data on 138 contaminated percutaneous injuries to anesthesia personnel.[164] The rate of contaminated percutaneous injuries per year per full time equivalent anesthesia worker was 0.42, and the average annual risk of HIV and HCV infection was estimated to be 0.0016% and 0.015%, respectively. Based on these infection rates, it was estimated that occupational exposures would result in 0.56 HIV infections and 5.18 HCV infections per year in anesthesia personnel.

Anesthesia personnel are frequently exposed to blood and body fluids during invasive procedures such as insertion of vascular catheters, arterial punctures, and endotracheal intubation.[164,165] Although many exposures are mucocutaneous and can be prevented by the use of gloves and protective clothing, these barriers do not prevent percutaneous exposures such as needle stick injuries, which carry a greater risk for pathogen transmission. Thirty-two percent of a sample of anesthesiologists reported a contaminated needle stick injury during the prior year.[166] Because of the tasks they perform, anesthesia personnel are likely to use and be injured by large-bore, hollow needles

such as IV catheter stylets and needles on syringes.[164,167] Because these needles carry a larger volume of blood and possibly a greater viral inoculum when contaminated, they are associated with a higher risk of pathogen transmission.[168] Needleless or protected needled safety devices are becoming available and should be considered to replace standard devices to reduce the risk of needle stick injuries.[135,169] Although safety devices usually are more expensive than a comparable needled item, they may be more cost-effective when the cost of needle stick injury investigation and medical care for infected personnel is considered. Percutaneous injuries have now been accepted as a significant occupational risk for health care workers and several states have passed legislation requiring the use of available needleless or safety needled devices. OSHA has issued a revised directive (CPL 2-2.44D) to its compliance officers that updates enforcement procedures for its Bloodborne Pathogen Standard.[135] The new directive emphasizes the use of safety devices to help reduce the risk of needlesticks and other sharps injuries.

Postexposure Treatment and Prophylactic Antiretroviral Therapy. When personnel have been exposed to patients' blood or body fluids, the incident should immediately be reported to the employee health service or the appropriate individual within the institution. Based on the nature of the injury, the exposed worker and the source individual may be tested for serologic evidence of HIV, HBV, and HCV infection.[170] Current local laws must be consulted to determine policies for testing the source patient. Confidentiality should be maintained at all times. When the source patient is found to be HIV-positive, the employee should be retested periodically for HIV antibodies for a minimum of 6 months after exposure, although most infected people are expected to undergo seroconversion within the first 6 to 12 weeks after exposure. During this period, the exposed employee should follow CDC recommendations for preventing transmission of HIV to family members and patients.[170]

Zidovudine is effective in reducing the rate of transmission of HIV from infected mother to newborn[171] and after a percutaneous occupational exposure to HIV-infected blood.[162] The CDC has published an algorithm for postexposure prophylaxis for health care workers who have incurred a percutaneous injury.[170] The use of specific antiretroviral agents is based on the type of exposure and source patient. Since protocols for chemoprophylaxis are likely to change with additional research and the introduction of new antiretroviral drugs, the most current recommendations should be consulted prior to instituting postexposure prophylactic therapy.

Occupational Safety and Health Administration Standards, Universal Precautions, and Isolation Precautions

The CDC formulated recommendations, or Universal Precautions, for preventing transmission of bloodborne infections (including HIV, HBV, and HCV) to health care workers.[172] The guidelines are based on the epidemiology of HBV as a worst-case model for transmission of bloodborne infections and current knowledge of the epidemiology of HIV and HCV. Because some carriers of bloodborne viruses are not identified, Universal Precautions were recommended for use during all patient contact. Although exposure to blood carries the greatest risk of occupationally related transmission of HIV, HBV, and HCV, it was recognized that universal precautions should also be applied to semen, vaginal secretions, human tissues, and the following body fluids: cerebrospinal, synovial, pleural, peritoneal, pericardial, and amniotic. Subsequently, the CDC synthesized the major features of Universal Precautions into Standard Precautions, a single set of precautions that should be applied to all patients (Table 4-4).[121] Standard Precautions were included in a set of Isolation Precautions which contain guidelines (Airborne Precautions, Droplet Precautions, and Contact Precautions) to reduce the risk of transmission of bloodborne and other pathogens in hospitals.[121]

Standard Precautions recommends use of gloves when a health care worker contacts mucous membranes and oral fluids, such as during endotracheal intubation and pharyngeal suctioning. The selection of specific barriers or personal protective equipment should be commensurate with the task being performed. Gloves may be all that is necessary during insertion of a peripheral intravenous catheter, whereas gloves, gown, mask, and face shield may be required during endotracheal intubation in a patient with hematemesis. Gloves should be removed after they become contaminated to prevent dissemination of blood or body fluids to equipment or personal items. Waterless antiseptics should be available to permit anesthesia personnel to wash their hands after glove removal without leaving the operating room.

Because needlestick injuries are a frequent cause of blood exposure,[164] recommendations for safe needle handling are included in Standard Precautions. Many injuries occur during recapping of contaminated needles; therefore, if recapping is necessary, a one-handed technique should be used.

There is now direct evidence that implementation of Universal Precautions decreases the number of exposure incidents that result in worker contact with patient blood and body fluids.[173] Observational and postal surveys indicate that in many instances Universal Precautions are not being followed.[166] Anesthesiologists were more likely to comply with Universal Precautions if they thought they were caring for an HIV-infected patient. Because all infected patients cannot be identified by the routine preoperative information, the selective application of Universal Precautions is inappropriate.

The Occupational Safety and Health Administration has promulgated standards to protect employees from occupational exposure to bloodborne pathogens.[135] Employers subject to OSHA must comply with these federal regulations. The Standard requires that there must be an Exposure Control Plan specifically detailing the methods that the employer is providing to reduce employees' risk of exposure. The employer must evaluate engineering controls such as needleless devices to eliminate hazards. Work practice controls are encouraged to reduce blood exposures by altering the manner in which personnel perform tasks (*e.g.,* an instrument rather than fingers should be used to handle needles). The employer must furnish appropriate personal protective equipment (*e.g.,* gloves, gowns) in various sizes to permit employees to comply with Universal Precautions. The HBV vaccine must be offered at no charge to personnel. A mechanism for postexposure treatment and follow-up must be provided. An annual educational program should inform employees of their risk for bloodborne infection and the resources available to prevent blood exposures.

Creutzfeldt-Jakob Disease

Creutzfeldt-Jakob disease, caused by a proteinaceous infectious agent, or prion, may be unsuspected in patients presenting with dementia.[174] The disease has been transmitted to patients by contaminated biologic products. The risk of transmission to hospital personnel is unknown because surveillance is complicated by the long period from the time of infection until the onset of symptoms. Universal precautions should be used to prevent contact with spinal fluid, blood, or tissue specimens.[175] Careful hand washing is essential. The prion is difficult to eradicate from equipment, but the use of steam sterilization with or without sodium hydroxide is effective.[175]

Tuberculosis

The incidence of tuberculosis in the United States has declined since 1992, reversing the increase in reported cases that had begun in 1986.[176] Although most individuals infected with tuberculosis are treated on an outpatient basis, undiagnosed patients may be hospitalized for the work-up of pulmonary pathology. Hospital personnel are especially at risk for infection from unrecognized cases.[177,178,179] Groups with a higher prevalence of tuberculosis include (1) personal contacts of people with active tuberculosis; (2) people from countries with a high prevalence of tuberculosis; and (3) alcoholics, homeless people, and intravenous drug users.[177]

Mycobacterium tuberculosis is transmitted through viable bacilli carried on airborne particles, 1–5 μm in size, by coughing, speaking, or sneezing. Respiratory isolation should be used for hospitalized patients suspected of having tuberculosis until they are confirmed as nontransmitters by sputum examination that demonstrates no bacilli.[177,180] Appropriate chemotherapy is the most effective means to prevent spread of tuberculous infection. Elective surgery should be postponed until infected patients have had an adequate course of chemotherapy. If surgery is required, filters should be used on the anesthetic breathing circuit for patients with tuberculosis.[177,181]

Several hospital outbreaks of multidrug-resistant *M. tuberculosis* infection have been reported.[179,182] Mortality associated with these outbreaks is high. Factors responsible for nosocomial transmission include delayed diagnosis of tuberculosis so that multiple patients and personnel were exposed, and delayed recognition of drug resistance resulting in inadequate initial drug therapy.

Effective prevention of spread to health care workers requires early identification of infected patients and immediate initiation of respiratory isolation (negative-pressure rooms with air vented outside; see Table 4-4).[177,181] Patients must remain in isolation until adequate treatment is documented. If patients with tuberculosis must leave their rooms, they should wear face masks to prevent spread of organisms into the air. Health care workers should wear respiratory protective devices when they enter an isolation room or when performing procedures that may induce coughing, such as endotracheal intubation or tracheal suctioning.[177] The CDC recommends that respiratory protective devices worn to protect against *M. tuberculosis* should be able to filter 95% of particles 1 mm in size at flow rates of 50 liters per minute and should fit the face with a leakage rate around the seal of less than 10% documented by fit-testing.[177] High-efficiency particulate air respirators (classified as N95) are NIOSH-approved devices that meet the CDC criteria for respiratory protective devices against *M. tuberculosis*.[183]

Routine periodic screening of employees for tuberculosis should be included as part of a hospital's employee health policy with the frequency of screening dependent on the prevalence of infected patients in the hospitalized population. When a new conversion is detected by skin testing, a history of exposure should be sought to determine the source patient. Treatment or preventive therapy is based on the drug-susceptibility pattern of the *M. tuberculosis* in the source patient, if known. Personnel who have been exposed to a patient with active tuberculosis should be followed by skin testing.

Viruses in Laser Plumes

The laser is commonly being used for vaporizing carcinomatous and viral tumors. Use of lasers is associated with several hazards, both to patients and to operating room personnel. Risks include thermal burns, eye injuries, electrical hazards, and fires and explosions. In addition, there is now evidence that the laser plumes resulting from tissue vaporization contain toxic chemicals such as formaldehyde. Clinical and laboratory studies have demonstrated that when the carbon dioxide laser is used to treat verrucae (papilloma and warts), intact viral DNA could be recovered from the plume.[184] Scientists at the Center for Devices and Radiological Health used an *in vitro* model to demonstrate that viable viruses can be found in plumes produced by both carbon dioxide and argon laser vaporization of a virus-loaded culture plate.[185] Another model indicated that viable viruses were carried on larger particles that traveled less than 100 mm from the site being vaporized.[186]

A case report describes laryngeal papillomatosis in a surgeon who had used a laser to remove anogenital condylomas from several patients.[187] Although DNA analysis of the surgeon's papillomas revealed a viral type similar to that of the condylomas, proof of transmission is lacking.

To protect operating room personnel from exposure to the viral and chemical content of the laser plume, it is recommended that the nozzle from a smoke evacuator be held as close as possible to the tissue being vaporized. This will effectively remove the particulate material in the plume by trapping it in the filter of the evacuator. In addition, operating room personnel working in the vicinity of the laser plume should wear gloves, goggles, and high-efficiency filter masks.[165]

EMOTIONAL CONSIDERATIONS

Stress

Among the potential health hazards of working in the operating room, stress is well recognized.[188] However, there is very little objective information specifically directed toward understanding the nature of job-related stress among anesthesiologists. Stress is a nonspecific response to any change, demand, pressure, challenge, threat, or trauma.[189] There are three distinct components of the stress process: the initiating stressors, the psychological filters that process and evaluate the stressors, and the coping mechanisms that are employed in an attempt to control the stressful situation.

Stress on the job is unavoidable and, to a certain degree, desirable. A moderate, manageable level of stress is the fuel necessary for individual achievement. What distresses individual A may be pleasurable to individual B, or even to individual A in a different circumstance. Hans Seyle, one of the pioneering scientists in the modern study of stress, described a beneficial effect resulting from mild, brief, and controllable episodes of stress: "The absence of stress is death."[190] On the other hand, extreme degrees of stress can be associated with disorders of the psychological homeostatic mechanism and consequently may lead to physical or mental disease. Exactly how an individual responds to a particular stressor is the product of a series of factors, including age, gender, experience, pre-existing personality style, available defense and coping mechanisms, support systems, and concomitant events (such as sleep deprivation).[190]

A number of circumstances that classically define a stressful workplace are characteristic of the practice of anesthesiology. There is a background of chronic, low-level stress punctuated by intermittent episodes of extreme stress. The demands are externally paced, usually out of the anesthesiologist's control. Habituation to the demands is difficult, and perturbations are intermittently but continuously inserted into the system. Finally, failure to meet the demands imposed by the workplace produces grave consequences.

Certain stressors are specific to the practice of anesthesiology. Night call is consistently reported as one of the most stressful elements, especially among older anesthesiologists.[106] Concerns about liability, production pressure, economic uncertainty, and interpersonal relations are other frequently cited stressors.[105]

It is not surprising that the process of inducing anesthesia engenders a great deal of stress in the practitioner. Although this observation is self-evident to any anesthesiologist, documentation is limited to demonstrations of changes in heart rate and blood pressure in the anesthesiologist during induction.[191] Individual observations included cardiac dysrhythmias (premature ventricular contractions), ischemic changes on the electrocardiogram, and elevation of the blood pressure to a maximum of 193/137 mm Hg. The level of training and degree of experience play a role in determining the amount of stress perceived by an anesthesiologist. It has been shown that an inverse relationship exists between the duration of clinical experience and the level of anxiety and hemodynamic changes occurring in the anesthesiologist during the induction of anesthesia.[192]

Interpersonal relationships impose a unique set of demands that may serve as stressors to the anesthesiologist. In most locations within a hospital or clinic setting (e.g., radiology department), direct responsibility for a patient is temporarily transferred to the consulting physician. In contrast, the operating room is an arena where two coequal physicians simultaneously share ultimate responsibility for the well-being of a patient. To many anesthesiologists and surgeons, the overlapping of realms of responsibility produce the highest degree of stress in their clinical practices.

Several studies have focused on personality characteristics, some identifiable before entrance to medical school, that are predictive of subsequent behavior and performance as clinicians.[193,194,195] Prominent among traits predictive of maladaptive responses to stress is the obsessive-compulsive, dependent character structure. These individuals typically manifest pessimism, passivity, self-doubt, and feelings of insecurity. Commonly they respond to stress by internalizing anger and becoming hypochondriacal and depressed. In work reported by Vaillant et al, undergraduate students who demonstrated these characteristics were more likely to have their medical careers disrupted by alcoholism or drug abuse, psychiatric illness, and marital disturbances.[193] McDonald et al have applied some of these considerations in an attempt to identify psychological attributes that may be of value in the selection process for anesthesiology residents.[195] They found a modest correlation of performance on the California Psychological Inventory with some measures of success in an anesthesiology residency.

Stress on the job may produce either an improvement or a decrement in job performance. Only when the magnitude of the stress exceeds the individual's threshold do his or her defenses become exaggerated and inappropriate. It is this situation that gives rise to maladaptive behavior and the personal and professional deterioration that can lead to disorders such as drug addiction, professional burnout, and suicide.

Substance Use, Abuse, and Dependence

Illicit drug use remains one of our society's major afflictions. It is estimated that 20 million Americans are drug users, with some 5 million addicted.

Epidemiology

The abuse of drugs by physicians continues to attract considerable media attention and notoriety.[196] However, recognition of the problem of substance dependence among physicians is not new. In the first edition of *The Principles and Practice of Medicine*, edited by Sir William Osler and published in 1892, it is stated: "The habit [morphia] is particularly prevalent among women and physicians who use the hypodermic syringe for the alleviation of pain, as in neuralgia or sciatica."[197] Two years later, Mattison commented: "It is a fact striking though sad that more cases of morphinism are met with among medical men than in all other professions combined."[198]

Whether substance abuse is more prevalent among physicians than the general population is a subject worthy of debate. There is a large body of literature that attempts to support the notion that drug problems are more frequent among physicians.[199] The data from which this conclusion has been drawn are notoriously difficult to accurately collect and to interpret. In her extensive review of the English-language literature, Brewster finally concluded, "No one really knows how many practicing physicians are having problems with alcohol and other drugs."[200] More recently, Hughes et al did identify alcohol, minor opiates, and benzodiazepine tranquilizers as substances of more frequent abuse among physicians than in the general population.[201] In many cases the drugs were self-prescribed and were considered by the physician to be "self-treatment." On the other hand, physicians were less likely to be current users of illicit substances than their age and gender peers.

Reliable documentation suggests that substance abuse is a significant problem among anesthesiologists.[202,203] In Domino's report, "drug-related deaths" was one category in which the risk of death among anesthesiologists was significantly greater than among the control group of internists.[29] In the view of many observers, addiction represents the primary occupational hazard for the specialty of anesthesiology. This conclusion is supported by a number of studies that examine the problem from various vantage points. One of the most easily accessed and frequently quoted sources of information on drug abuse comes from statistics on the number of individuals who are in drug treatment programs. However, there are major flaws inherent in this system of data collection. Before a physician is entered into any treatment program, he or she must first recognize that he or she has a drug problem. Unfortunately, denial is typically the first and most tenaciously maintained defense mechanism for the physician–substance abuser.

Even after recognizing that a drug-related problem exists, physicians are less likely than the population in general to seek professional assistance.[204] Again, denial plays a major role in this reluctance to undergo counseling or therapy. Medical students learn early in their education to use denial mechanisms to enable them to endure long, sleepless nights and the personal shortcomings that inevitably must be faced in clinical medicine. These well-developed denial mechanisms encourage the physician–addict to conclude that his or her problem is minor and that self-treatment is possible. Physicians typically enter programs for treatment only after they have reached the end stages of their illness.

With these caveats in mind, it is still informative to look at the statistics pertaining to the number of anesthesiologists who are involved in treatment programs for drug-related illness. Probably the most extensive experience comes from the Medical Association of Georgia Disabled Doctors' Program.[205] Their study population includes 1000 disabled physicians, 920 of whom were treated for chemical dependency. One hundred and twenty-one of these patients were anesthesiologists (12%), although anesthesia accounts for just 3.9% of the American physician population. Even more troubling is the fact that anesthesia residents constitute 33.7% of the resident population in their treatment group, despite their representation as only 4.6% of the American resident population. Anesthesia residents have a 7.4-fold excess representation in this treatment population.

Another approach to uncovering the prevalence of substance abuse among anesthesiologists is the directed survey. As with the statistics drawn from the drug treatment programs, there are major weaknesses inherent in this form of data collection. Most obvious is the willingness of the respondent to detail honestly and completely his or her experience in an area as sensitive as drug abuse.

One of the most extensive surveys was conducted by Ward et al.[206] They reported on the results of a questionnaire completed by 247 American anesthesia training programs. Sixty-four percent of the respondents identified at least one of their personnel as an abuser of drugs. In 10 programs (4%), there were 5 or more such individuals identified during the 10-year study period (1970–1980). The overall incidence of suspected abuse was 1.3%, and confirmed abuse was 1.1%. The two most favored substances for abuse were reported to be meperidine and fentanyl, with a definite tendency toward the latter in the most recent half-decade of the study. This preference had previously been observed by Talbott et al, who had treated 105 fentanyl addicts among the 125 anesthesiologists admitted to their facility at the time.[205]

Similar results have been obtained by Menk et al[207] and Gravenstein et al[208] in American training programs and by Weeks et al in Australia.[209] In the study by Gravenstein et al, 76% of the academic department chairs who responded to a survey reported that one or more of their staff had been affected by substance abuse during the period of study (1974–1979). Because of the significance of this problem in anesthesia training programs, the Accreditation Council for Graduate Medical Education's Special Requirements for Anesthesiology require that each residency program "must have a written policy and an educational program regarding substance abuse."[103]

Substance Dependence as a Disease

What accounts for this disproportionately high incidence of substance dependence among anesthesiologists? To answer this, it is best to view substance dependence as a psychosocial, biogenetic disease.[210] As such, the addiction (1) is a primary condition (not a symptom), (2) is associated with specific anatomic and physiologic changes, (3) has a set of recognizable signs and symptoms, (4) has a predictable, progressive course (if left untreated), and (5) has established etiologies (Table 4-5).

It is important to recognize that the causative factors in this disease process involve genetics as well as the environment. The disease results from a dynamic interplay between a susceptible host and a "favorable" environment. Vulnerability in the host is an important factor. What constitutes an instigating exposure to a drug in one person may have absolutely no effect on another. Unfortunately, there is no good predictive tool to identify the susceptible individual until he or she gets the disease.

There are causative factors specific to the specialty of anesthesiology. These include job stress, an orientation toward self-medication, lack of external recognition and self-respect, the availability of addicting drugs, and a susceptible premorbid personality.[211]

Self-prescription is commonly seen as a prelude to more extensive substance abuse and dependence.[201] Similarly, recreational use of drugs may proceed to drug dependence, with the drug used for recreation usually becoming the primary drug of dependence. Of concern is the recreational use of drugs among younger physicians and medical students and the choice of more potent drugs with enhanced potential for addiction, such as cocaine and the synthetic opioids, fentanyl and sufentanil.[212]

The general public's image of the anesthesiologist frequently falls short of that of other physicians. In a report from Australia, only 66% of the patients knew that anesthesiologists needed medical qualifications, and fewer than 10% could remember their anesthesiologist's name.[213] It is even more distressing when co-workers in the medical field fail to recognize the special skills and contributions of anesthesiologists. In another study from Australia, only 83% of hospital nurses knew that anesthesiologists had to be medically qualified.[214]

Positive reinforcement and a sense of "a job well done" are important components of job satisfaction. It is more difficult for the anesthesiologist than the surgeon to achieve recognition from patients and medical colleagues for a successful outcome. The Rodney Dangerfield syndrome, "I don't get no respect," has been cited by several authors as an instigating factor in drug experimentation.[211]

Anesthesiologists work in a climate in which large quantities of powerful psychoactive drugs are freely available. From the experience of the U.S. Army in Vietnam, it is apparent that when there is easy access to narcotics, alcohol use declines in favor of use of opiates.[215] As each new synthetic opioid becomes available for clinical use, it also becomes the drug of choice of abusing anesthesiologists. Currently, fentanyl and sufentanil are seen most frequently as the abused drug.

Because availability of drugs does play a role in the onset of this disease, it is logical that programs that better audit the distribution of drugs within the operating room setting should be a valuable preventive measure. Detailed protocols have been

---

Table 4-5. DSM-IV CRITERIA FOR SUBSTANCE-RELATED DISORDERS

CRITERIA FOR SUBSTANCE DEPENDENCE

A maladaptive pattern of substance use, leading to clinically significant impairment or distress, as manifested by three (or more) of the following, occurring at any time in the same 12-month period:

1. Tolerance, as defined by either of the following:
   a. a need for markedly increased amounts of the substance to achieve intoxication or desired effect
   b. markedly diminished effect with continued use of the same amount of the substance
2. Withdrawal, as manifested by either of the following:
   a. the characteristic withdrawal syndrome for the substance
   b. the same (or a closely related) substance is taken to relieve or avoid withdrawal symptoms
3. The substance is often taken in larger amounts or over a longer period than was intended
4. There is a persistent desire or unsuccessful efforts to cut down or control substance use
5. A great deal of time is spent in activities necessary to obtain the substance (*e.g.*, visiting multiple doctors or driving long distances), use the substance (*e.g.*, chain-smoking), or recover from its effects
6. Important social, occupational, or recreational activities are given up or reduced because of the substance use
7. The substance use is continued despite knowledge of having a persistent or recurrent physical or psychological problem that is likely to have been caused or exacerbated by the substance (*e.g.*, current cocaine use despite recognition of cocaine-induced depression, or continued drinking despite recognition that an ulcer was made worse by alcohol consumption)

Specify if:

With Physiological Dependence: evidence of tolerance or withdrawal (*i.e.*, either Item 1 or 2 is present)
Without Physiological Dependence: no evidence of tolerance or withdrawal (*i.e.*, neither Item 1 nor 2 is present)

Course specifiers:

Early Full Remission
Early Partial Remission
Sustained Full Remission
Sustained Partial Remission
On Agonist Therapy
In a Controlled Environment

CRITERIA FOR SUBSTANCE ABUSE

A. A maladaptive pattern of substance use leading to clinically significant impairment or distress, as manifested by one (or more) of the following, occurring within a 12-month period:
   1. Recurrent substance use resulting in a failure to fulfill major role obligations at work, school, or home (*e.g.*, repeated absences or poor work performance related to substance use; substance-related absences, suspensions, or expulsions from school; neglect of children or household)
   2. Recurrent substance use in situations in which it is physically hazardous (*e.g.*, driving an automobile or operating a machine when impaired by substance use)
   3. Recurrent substance-related legal problems (*e.g.*, arrests for substance-related disorderly conduct)
   4. Continued substance use despite having persistent or recurrent social or interpersonal problems caused or exacerbated by the effects of the substance (*e.g.*, arguments with spouse about consequences of intoxication, physical fights)
B. The symptoms have never met the criteria for Substance Dependence for this class of substance.

---

published for better controlling the distribution of these medications.[216] Talbott *et al* acknowledge that the strategies advocated within the anesthesia community are better than those of our colleagues in other medical specialties.[205] However, these are mostly limited to academic centers and require wider dissemination to be effective.

There is an apparent link between behavior before entering medical school and subsequent development of substance abuse.[217] At least one study examining personality profiles of anesthesiologists revealed a disturbingly high proportion with a predisposition toward maladaptive behavior.[218] Talbott *et al* have observed that many of the anesthesia residents in their treatment program specifically chose the specialty of anesthesiology because of the known availability of powerful drugs.[205] Residency selection committees should consider screening for personality disorders as an important part of the admissions process.

The consequences of substance abuse are ultimately devastating to the practicing anesthesiologist. If left untreated, substance dependence is a fatal illness. There are 100 deaths per year among U.S. physicians that are the direct result of chemical dependency.[219] Domino reported relative risks of 2.75 for drug-related deaths and 1.78 for HIV-related deaths among anesthesiologists compared to internists.[29] In the study reported by Ward *et al*, among the 334 confirmed drug abusers, 27 died of "drug overdose," and in another 3, "abuse was discovered at death."[206] Gravenstein *et al* reported 7 deaths among 44 confirmed drug abusers.[208] Menk *et al* reported 14 drug-related deaths (18%) among the 79 drug abusers who had been re-enrolled in their anesthesiology residencies after treatment.[207]

Intentional or inadvertent drug-related death is, of course, only one of the potential consequences of substance abuse (Table 4-6). More common is a gradual and inexorable deterioration in professional, family, and social relationships. The substance abuser becomes increasingly withdrawn and isolated, first in his or her personal life, and ultimately in his or her professional life. Every attempt is made to maintain a facade of normality at work, because discovery means isolation from the source of the abused drug. When professional conduct is finally impaired such that it is apparent to the physician's colleagues, the disease is approaching its end stage.

In addition to the health hazards of substance dependence,

there are significant legal considerations.[202] Each state has laws that detail the necessary steps for handling the drug-abusing physician. Most states have established Impaired Professionals Programs and require reporting such physicians to the licensing board, so-called "snitch laws." In many cases disciplinary action and even criminal penalties can be imposed on people who knowingly fail to report an impaired physician. Disciplinary action taken against an impaired physician must also be reported to the National Practitioner Data Bank to be in compliance with federal law.

An interesting debate exists regarding the issue of compulsory drug testing of physicians.[220] Random drug testing protocols have already been established in various high-risk industries (nuclear, aviation) and the military. Although many agree that this is a step in the right direction, questions remain about the legality and effectiveness of this approach. Institution of such programs in hospitals is limited.

A very aggressive program of detection and intervention is critical if careers and lives are to be saved.[221] If left untreated, less than 30% of addicted physicians will be practicing in 10 years and some 10% will have died from their disease. On the other hand, physicians are usually highly motivated, and high rehabilitation rates can be expected. Anesthesiologists appear to have a recovery rate approximating that of other physicians.[222] In the report of Ward et al, approximately 55% of the confirmed substance abusers underwent rehabilitation, and half of these were offered re-employment in their original departments.[206]

Controversy remains about the most appropriate career path for the recovering addicted anesthesiologist. Before the reports by Talbott et al[205] and Ward et al,[206] recovering addicts were discouraged from continuing their careers in anesthesiology. However, these and other encouraging reports during the 1980s provided optimism that these individuals could be successfully rehabilitated and safely returned to their practice of anesthesiol-

Table 4-6. SIGNS OF SUBSTANCE ABUSE AND DEPENDENCE

WHAT TO LOOK FOR OUTSIDE THE HOSPITAL

1. Addiction is a disease of loneliness and isolation. Addicts quickly withdraw from family, friends, and leisure activities.
2. Addicts have unusual changes in behavior, including wide mood swings, periods of depression, anger, and irritability alternating with periods of euphoria.
3. Unexplained overspending, legal problems, gambling, extramarital affairs, and increased problems at work are commonly seen in addicts.
4. An obvious physical sign of alcoholism is the frequent smell of alcohol on the breath.
5. Domestic strife, fights, and arguments may increase in number and intensity.
6. Sexual drive may significantly decrease.
7. Children may develop behavioral problems.
8. Some addicts frequently change jobs over a period of several years in an attempt to find a "geographic cure" for their disease, or to hide it from co-workers.
9. Addicts need to be near their drug source. For a health care professional, this means long hours at the hospital, even when off duty. For alcoholics, it means calling in sick to work. Alcoholics may disappear without any explanation to bars or hiding places to drink secretly.
10. Addicts may suddenly develop the habit of locking themselves in the bathroom or other rooms while they are using drugs.
11. Addicts frequently hide pills, syringes, or alcohol bottles around the house.
12. Persons who inject drugs may leave bloody swabs and syringes containing blood-tinged liquid in conspicuous places.
13. Addicts may display evidence of withdrawal, especially diaphoresis (sweating) and tremors.
14. Narcotic addicts often have pinpoint pupils.
15. Weight loss and pale skin are also common signs of addiction.
16. Addicts may be seen injecting drugs.
17. Tragically, some addicts are found comatose or dead before any of these signs have been recognized by others.

WHAT TO LOOK FOR INSIDE THE HOSPITAL

1. Addicts sign out ever-increasing quantities of narcotics.
2. Addicts frequently have unusual changes in behavior, such as wide mood swings, periods of depression, anger, and irritability alternating with periods of euphoria.
3. Charting becomes increasingly sloppy and unreadable.
4. Addicts often sign out narcotics in inappropriately high doses for the operation being performed.
5. They refuse lunch and coffee relief.
6. Addicts like to work alone in order to use anesthetic techniques without narcotics, falsify records, and divert drugs for personal use.
7. They volunteer for extra cases, often where large amounts of narcotics are available (e.g., cardiac cases).
8. They frequently relieve others.
9. They're often at the hospital when off duty, staying close to their drug supply to prevent withdrawal.
10. They volunteer frequently for extra call.
11. They're often difficult to find between cases, taking short naps after using.
12. Addicted anesthesia personnel may insist on personally administering narcotics in the recovery room.
13. Addicts make frequent requests for bathroom relief. This is usually where they use drugs.
14. Addicts may wear long-sleeved gowns to hide needle tracks and also to combat the subjective feeling of cold they experience when using narcotics.
15. Narcotic addicts often have pinpoint pupils.
16. An addict's patients may come into the recovery room complaining of pain out of proportion to the amount of narcotic charted on the anesthesia records.
17. Weight loss and pale skin are also commons signs of addiction.
18. Addicts may be seen injecting drugs.
19. Untreated addicts are found comatose.
20. Undetected addicts are found dead.

Adapted from Farley WJ, Arnold WP: VIDEOTAPE: Unmasking addiction: Chemical Dependency in Anesthesiology. Produced by Davids Productions, Parsippany, NJ, funded by Janssen Pharmaceutica, Piscataway, New Jersey, 1991.
Reprinted with permission from American Society of Anesthesiologists: Task Force on Chemical Dependence of the Committee on Occupational Health of Operating Room Personnel: Chemical Dependence in Anesthesiologists: What you need to know when you need to know it. American Society of Anesthesiologists. Park Ridge, Illinois, 1998.

Table 4-7. POLICY STATEMENT OF THE AMERICAN BOARD OF ANESTHESIOLOGY (ABA)

The Americans with Disabilities Act (ADA) protects individuals with a history of alcoholism or substance abuse who are not currently abusing alcohol or using drugs illegally. The ABA supports the intent of the ADA.

The ABA will admit qualified applicants and candidates with a history of alcoholism to its examination system and to examination if, in response to its inquiries, the ABA receives acceptable documentation that they do not currently pose a direct threat to the health and safety of others.

The ABA will admit qualified applicants and candidates with a history of illegal use of drugs to its examination system and to examination if, in response to its inquiries, the ABA receives acceptable documentation that they are not currently engaged in the illegal use of drugs.

After a candidate with a history of alcoholism or illegal use of drugs satisfies the examination requirements for certification, the ABA will determine whether it should defer awarding its certification to the candidate for a period of time to avoid certifying a candidate who poses a direct threat to the health and safety of others. If the ABA determines that deferral of the candidate's certification is appropriate because the candidate does currently pose a threat to the health and safety of others, the ABA will assess the specific circumstances of the candidate's history of alcoholism or illegal use of drugs to determine when the candidate should write the Board to request issuance of its certification.

Reprinted with permission from Booklet of Information, Board Policies 6.01: Alcoholism and Substance Abuse. Raleigh, North Carolina, American Board of Anesthesiology, December, 1998.

ogy. In contrast, a subsequent report by Menk and colleagues casts doubt on the advisability of addicted anesthesiologists' re-entering the field.[207] Among 79 opioid-dependent anesthesiology residents, there was a 66% (52 of 79) failure rate for successful rehabilitation and return to practice. Even more discouraging, there were 14 suicide or overdose deaths among those 79 returning trainees. Their conclusion is that redirection into another specialty is the safer course after rehabilitation. Others have questioned these conclusions based on concerns regarding the study design.[223]

Because of the contradictory data, no firm recommendations can be made about re-entry into the practice of anesthesia after treatment. Each state has laws or regulations that dictate the circumstances under which a physician recovering from substance abuse can return to practice. Federal laws, such as the Americans with Disabilities Act, impose additional considerations for this difficult decision. The ASA has published a sample chemical dependency policy for departments of anesthesiology.[221] This document describes the process of re-entry and provides a model for a re-entry contract that can be used when a recovering anesthesiologist is considered ready to come back into practice. The American Board of Anesthesiology has established a policy for candidates with a history of alcoholism or illegal use of drugs (Table 4-7).[224]

Impairment

Substance abuse probably accounts for some 85% of the cases of impairment* among physicians.[225] Other factors that may lead to impairment include physical or mental illness and deterioration owing to the aging process. Some authorities include unwillingness or inability to keep up with current literature and techniques as a form of disability.

Data regarding the prevalence of these disabling disorders are more difficult to obtain than are those on drug abuse. Statistics derived from the admitting diagnoses to various psychiatric facilities indicate that close to 1% of those admitted are physicians. In the order of increasing frequency, admission is required for organic psychoses, personality disorders, schizophrenia, neuroses, and affective disorders, particularly depression.[226]

It is not surprising that depression should figure prominently among the personality characteristics of emotionally impaired physicians. Indeed, many of the personality traits that are adaptive and ensure success in the physician's world may also serve

as risk factors for depression when exaggerated. These character traits include self-sacrifice, competitiveness, achievement orientation, denial of feelings, and intellectualization of emotions. Two studies on alcoholic physicians provide some insight into this link between achievement orientation and emotional disturbance. Bissell and Jones reported that more than half of their group of alcoholic physicians graduated in the upper third of their medical school class, 23% were in the upper tenth, and only 5% were in the lower third of their class.[227] Similarly, a report on alcohol use in medical school demonstrated better than average academic performance among those students identified as alcohol abusers.[228] Alcohol abuse clearly does not enhance the learning process. Rather, alcohol abuse is a manifestation of psychological disturbance resulting from excessive degrees of stress among some students who are determined to have flawless records.

It is difficult to identify and appropriately respond to the dilemma of the impaired or unsafe anesthesiologist.[229] Fortunately, in recent years, most state legislatures and medical societies have formally recognized this problem and have formed committees and enacted laws that address the impaired physician. These programs are usually therapeutic and nonpunitive in nature. Ideally, the committees provide a nonthreatening environment for identification and intervention for the impaired physician. Only in cases in which a real risk to the public welfare exists and the involved physician is unwilling voluntarily to suspend practice and accept assistance is the license suspension power of the State Board of Medical Examiners exercised.[230]

Suicide

Perhaps one of the most alarming of the occupationally associated hazards for anesthesiologists is the high rate of suicide.[25,26,28,29,231] The incidence is 3 to 4 times the suicide rate expected among a contemporary, otherwise comparable socioeconomic group and exceeds that of all but one or two other medical specialties.[232] A report from England identified five deaths from suicide over a 5-year period in anesthesiology training programs.[233] Their ratio of 1 suicide per 500 residents compares unfavorably with the approximately 1 suicide per 12,000 in the general U.S. population and 1 suicide in 4000 for physicians per year.[234]

Why should there be such a high rate of suicide among anesthesiologists? A partial explanation lies with the high degree of stress that is an integral part of the job. The relationship between generalized stress and suicide is not direct. But, clearly, in susceptible people, feelings of inability to cope resulting from overwhelming stress may give way to despair and suicide ideation.

Extensive personality profiles have been collected from sui-

---

* An impaired physician is defined as one "whose performance as a professional person and as a practitioner of the healing arts is impaired because of alcoholism, drug abuse, mental illness, senility, or disabling disease."

cide-susceptible individuals; these indicate characteristics such as high anxiety, insecurity, low self-esteem, impulsiveness, and poor self-control. It is disturbing to note that in Reeve's study of personality traits of a sample of anesthesiologists, some 20% manifested psychological profiles that reflected a predisposition to behavioral disintegration and attempted suicide when placed under extremes of stress.[194] His study raises the discomfiting notion that "premorbid"personality characteristics that exist before entering specialty training are not being identified in the admissions process.[235]

One specific type of stress—that resulting from a malpractice lawsuit—may have a direct causative association with suicide among physicians in general and anesthesiologists in particular. An anecdotal report described, in tragic detail, the emotional deterioration and ultimate suicide of an experienced and previously healthy physician involved in a malpractice suit.[236] One study specifically identified the anesthesiologist involved in a lawsuit as being at particularly high risk for suicide.[237] In this report, 4 of 185 anesthesiologists being sued attempted or committed suicide.

Another potential etiologic basis for the observed high suicide rate is the high incidence of drug abuse found among anesthesia personnel. Physicians who are impaired and whose privileges to practice medicine are removed by the licensing authority are at heightened risk for attempting suicide. Crawshaw *et al* reported 8 successful and 2 near-miss suicide attempts among 43 physicians placed on probation for drug-related disability.[238] Other occupational factors that may contribute to the high incidence of suicide include isolation and lack of colleagues' support at work, and the ready access to various means of carrying out the act of suicide.

The Aging Anesthesiologist

Little research has been directed toward the challenges faced by older anesthesiologists. This is in contrast to the situation in most other industries where strict attention is paid to the competence and well-being of older workers. For example, commercial pilots are required to take regular medical examinations and conform to policies regarding hours of work. Frequently, they are subject to contractual age limitations.

There are no age-specific conditions placed on state medical licensure or on the practice of anesthesiology. The American Board of Anesthesiologists has only recently established a recertification examination for those out of residency more than 10 years. In most cases, the decision to limit practice or retire remains at the discretion of the individual anesthesiologist based upon his or her self-evaluation.

As a result of the smaller residency class sizes observed in recent years, the mean age of the anesthesiology workforce is increasing. Approximately one-half of U.S. anesthesiologists were trained before 1980,[239] and 49% of anesthesiologists are aged 45 and older.[240] Several physiologic changes frequently associated with aging have the potential of affecting an individual's ability to practice anesthesiology, including decrements in hearing, vision, short-term memory, strength, and endurance. These potential sources of impairment are often compensated by other advantages conferred by advancing age, including the experience acquired by a lifelong practice of the specialty.

One area of particular difficulty for anesthesiologists is maintaining the stamina required for long work shifts and night call. Older workers have been shown to have a reduced amplitude and a tendency toward morningness in their circadian cycles.[104] Superimposed upon this propensity to sleep disturbance, the demands of night call and associated sleep deprivation are particularly difficult for older anesthesiologists. Night call is considered one of the most stressful aspects of practice and the most frequently cited reason for retirement among older anesthesiologists.[241]

Aging among anesthesiologists raises interesting legal issues.

A number of federal laws potentially impact the decision of the aging anesthesiologist and his or her colleagues to continue to work and at what pace. These include the Age Discrimination Act, Title VII of the Civil Rights Act ("Equal Pay Act"), the Medical and Family Leave Act, the Fair Labor Standards Act, and the Employee Retirement Income Security Act (ERISA). An anesthesiologist's decision to retire must fit within the complex framework of federal and state laws and regulations. Anesthesiologists tend to retire at a younger age than do many other specialists.[106,242] Future research should address issues regarding older anesthesiologists.

REFERENCES

1. Linde HW, Bruce DL: Occupational exposure of anesthetists to halothane, nitrous oxide and radiation. Anesthesiology 30:363, 1969
2. Whitcher CE, Cohen EN, Trudell JR: Chronic exposure to anesthetic gases in the operating room. Anesthesiology 35:348, 1971
3. Wood C, Ewan A, Goresky G, Sheppard S: Exposure of operating room personnel to nitrous oxide during paediatric anaesthesia. Can J Anaesth 39:682, 1992
4. Flemming DC, Johnstone RE: Recognition thresholds for diethyl ether and halothane. Anesthesiology 46:68, 1977
5. Ferstandig LL: Trace concentrations of anesthetic gases: A critical review of their disease potential. Anesth Analg 57:328, 1978
6. Walts LF, Forsythe AB, Moore JG: Critique: Occupational disease among operating room personnel. Anesthesiology 42:608, 1975
7. American Society of Anesthesiologists Ad Hoc Committee on the Effect of Trace Anesthetics on the Health of Operating Room Personnel: Occupational disease among operating room personnel: A national study. Anesthesiology 41:321, 1974
8. Axelsson G, Rylander R: Exposure to anaesthetic gases and spontaneous abortion: Response bias in a postal questionnaire study. Int J Epidemiol 11:250, 1982
9. Buring JE, Hennekens CH, Mayrent SL et al: Health experiences of operating room personnel. Anesthesiology 62:325, 1985
10. Cohen EN, Bellville JW, Brown BW: Anesthesia, pregnancy, and miscarriage: A study of operating room nurses and anesthetists. Anesthesiology 35:343, 1971
11. Knill-Jones RP, Moir DD, Rodrigues LV et al: Anaesthetic practice and pregnancy: Controlled survey of women anaesthetists in the United Kingdom. Lancet 2:1326, 1972
12. Rosenberg P, Kirves A: Miscarriages among operating theatre staff. Acta Anaesthesiol Scand 53(suppl):37, 1973
13. Mazze RI, Lecky JH: The health of operating room personnel. Anesthesiology 62:226, 1985
14. Hemminki K, Kyyrönen P, Lindbohm ML: Spontaneous abortions and malformations in the offspring of nurses exposed to anesthetic gases, cytostatic drugs, and other potential hazards in hospitals, based on registered information of outcome. J Epidemiol Community Health 39:141, 1985
15. Klebanoff MA, Shiono PH, Rhoads GG: Spontaneous and induced abortion among resident physicians. JAMA 265:2821, 1991
16. Rowland AS, Baird D, Weinberg CR et al: Reduced fertility among women employed as dental assistants exposed to high levels of nitrous oxide. N Engl J Med 327:993, 1992
17. Rowland AS, Baird DD, Shore DL et al: Nitrous oxide and spontaneous abortion in female dental assistants. Am J Epidemiol 141:531, 1995
18. Boivin JF: Risk of spontaneous abortion in women occupationally exposed to anaesthetic gases: A meta-analysis. Occup Environ Med 54:541, 1997
19. Cohen EN, Gift HG, Brown BW et al: Occupational disease in dentistry and chronic exposure to trace anesthetic gases. J Am Dent Assoc 101:21, 1980
20. Guirguis SS, Pelmear PL, Roy ML, Wong L: Health effects associated with exposure to anaesthetic gases in Ontario hospital personnel. Br J Ind Med 47:490, 1990
21. Heidam LZ: Spontaneous abortions among dental assistants, factory workers, painters, and gardening workers: A follow up study. J Epidemiol Community Health 38:149, 1984
22. Saurel-Cubizolles MJ, Hays M, Estryn-Behar M: Work in operating rooms and pregnancy outcome among nurses. Int Arch Occup Environ Health 66:235, 1994

23. McDonald AD, McDonald JC, Armstrong B et al: Fetal death and work in pregnancy. Br J Ind Med 45:148, 1988

24. Ebi KL, Rice SA: Reproductive and developmental toxicity of anesthetics in humans. In Rice SA, Fish KJ (eds.): Anesthetic Toxicity, Raven Press, New York, 1994

25. Bruce DL, Eide KA, Linde HW et al: Causes of death among anesthesiologists: A 20-year survey. Anesthesiology 29:565, 1968

26. Bruce DL, Eide KA, Smith NJ et al: A prospective survey of anesthesiologist mortality, 1967–1971. Anesthesiology 41:71, 1974

27. Doll R, Peto R: Mortality among doctors in different occupations. Br Med J 1:1433, 1977

28. Lew EA: Mortality experience among anesthesiologists, 1954–1976. Anesthesiology 51:195, 1979

29. Domino K, Alexander BH, Nagahama SI et al: Mortality of anesthesiologists compared to internists. Anesthesiology 91:A1164, 1999

30. Nunn JF, Sharer N: Inhibition of methionine synthetase by trace concentrations of nitrous oxide. Br J Anaesth 53:1099, 1981

31. Koblin DD, Watson JE, Deady JE et al: Inactivation of methionine synthetase by nitrous oxide in mice. Anesthesiology 54:318, 1981

32. Nunn JF, Sharer N: Serum methionine and hepatic enzyme activity in anaesthetists exposed to nitrous oxide. Br J Anaesth 54:593, 1982

33. Corbett TH: Cancer and congenital anomalies associated with anesthetics. Ann NY Acad Sci 271:58, 1976

34. Eger EI, White AE, Brown CL et al: A test of the carcinogenicity of enflurane, isoflurane, halothane, methoxyflurane and nitrous oxide in mice. Anesth Analg 57:678, 1978

35. Coate WB, Ulland BM, Lewis TR: Chronic exposure to low concentrations of halothane-nitrous oxide: Lack of carcinogenic effect in the rat. Anesthesiology 50:306, 1979

36. Baden JM, Egbert B, Mazze RI: Carcinogen bioassay of enflurane in mice. Anesthesiology 56:9, 1982

37. Baden JM, Brinkenhoff M, Wharton RS et al: Mutagenicity of volatile anesthetics: Halothane. Anesthesiology 45:311, 1976

38. Baden JM, Kelley M, Wharton RS et al: Mutagenicity of halogenated ether anesthetics. Anesthesiology 46:346, 1977

39. Baden JM, Kelley M, Cheung A et al: Lack of mutagens in urines of operating room personnel. Anesthesiology 53:195, 1980

40. Chang LW, Katz J: Pathologic effects of chronic halothane inhalation: An overview. Anesthesiology 45:640, 1976

41. Coate WB, Kapp RW, Lewis TR: Chronic exposure to low concentrations of halothane–nitrous oxide: Reproductive and cytogenetic effects in the rat. Anesthesiology 50:310, 1979

42. Vieura E, Cleaton-Jones P, Austin JC et al: Effects of low concentrations of nitrous oxide on rat fetuses. Anesth Analg 59:175, 1980

43. Mazze RI: Fertility, reproduction and postnatal survival in mice chronically exposed to isoflurane. Anesthesiology 63:663, 1985

44. Bruce DL, Bach MJ, Arbit J: Trace anesthetic effects on perceptual, cognitive and motor skills. Anesthesiology 40:453, 1974

45. Bruce DL, Bach MJ: Effects of trace anaesthetic gases on behavioural performance of volunteers. Br J Anaesth 48:871, 1976

46. Smith G, Shirley AW: A review of the effects of trace concentrations of anaesthetics on performance. Br J Anaesth 50:701, 1978

47. Bruce DL, Stanley TH: Research replication may be subject specific. (letter) Anesth Analg 62:617, 1983

48. Mazze RI: Waste anesthetic gases and the regulatory agencies. Anesthesiology 52:248, 1980

49. Geraci CL: Operating room pollution: Governmental perspectives and guidelines. Anesth Analg 56:775, 1977

50. National Institute for Occupational Safety and Health (NIOSH): Criteria for a Recommended Standard . . . Occupational Exposure to Waste Anesthetic Gases and Vapors. Department of Health, Education, and Welfare (NIOSH) Publication No. 77–140. Cincinnati, Ohio

51. NIOSH Alert: Request for assistance in controlling exposures to nitrous oxide during anesthetic administration. DHHS (NIOSH) Publication No. 94–100, 1994

52. Task Force on Trace Anesthetic Gases of the Committee on Occupational Health of Operating Room Personnel: Information for Management in Anesthetizing Areas and the Postanesthesia Care Unit (PACU). American Society of Anesthesiologists, Park Ridge, Illinois, 1999

53. Rajhans GS, Brown DA, Whaley DA et al: Evaluation of occupational exposure to waste anesthetic gases in Ontario hospitals. Ann Occup Hyg 33:27, 1989

54. Gray WM: Occupational exposure to nitrous oxide in four hospitals. Anaesthesia 44:511, 1989

55. Bruce DL, Linde HW: Halothane content in recovery room air. Anesthesiology 16:517, 1972

56. Berner O: Concentration and elimination of anaesthetic gases in recovery rooms. Acta Anaesthesiol Scand 22:55, 1978

57. Sessler DI, Badgwell JM: Exposure of postoperative nurses to exhaled anesthetic gases. Anesth Analg 87:1083, 1998

58. McGregor DG, Senjem DH, Mazze RI: Trace nitrous oxide levels in the postanesthesia care unit. Anesth Analg 89:472, 1999

59. American Institute of Architects Academy of Architecture for Health, US Department of Health and Human Services. 1996–1997 Guidelines for design and construction of hospital and health care facilities. The American Institute of Architects Press, Washington, DC, 1996

60. Cromer J, Kronoveter K: A Study of Methylmethacrylate Exposure and Employee Health. Department of Health, Education, and Welfare (NIOSH) Publication No. 77–119. Washington DC, U.S. Government Printing Office, 1976

61. Lee CM: Unusual reaction to methyl methacrylate monomer. Anesth Analg 63:371, 1984

62. Schwettmann RS, Casterline CL: Delayed asthmatic response following occupational exposure to enflurane. Anesthesiology 44:166, 1976

63. Klatskin G, Kimberg DV: Recurrent hepatitis attributable to halothane sensitization in an anesthetist. N Engl J Med 280:515, 1969

64. Task Force on Latex Sensitivity of the Committee on Occupational Health of Operating Room Personnel: Natural Rubber Latex Allergy: Considerations for Anesthesiologists. American Society of Anesthesiologists. Park Ridge, Illinois, 1999

65. Bolyard EA, Tablan OC, Williams WW et al: The Hospital Infection Control Practices Advisory Committee: Guideline for infection control in health care personnel, 1998. Am J Infect Control 26:289, 1998

66. FDA mandatory reporting database. October 1997

67. Brown RH, Schauble JF, Hamilton RG: Prevalence of latex allergy among anesthesiologists. Anesthesiology 89:292, 1998

68. Konrad C, Fieber T, Gerber H: The prevalence of latex sensitivity among anesthesiology staff. Anesth Analg 84:629, 1997

69. Warshaw DM: Latex allergy. J Am Acad Dermatol 39:1, 1998

70. National Council on Radiation Protection and Measurements: Radiation Protection for Medical and Allied Health Personnel. Report No. 48. Washington DC, 1977

71. McGowan C, Heaton B, Stephenson RN: Occupational x-ray exposure of anaesthetists. Br J Anaesth 76: 868, 1996

72. Grumet GW: Pandemonium in the modern hospital. N Engl J Med 328:433, 1993

73. NIOSH recommendations for occupational safety and health standard. MMWR 37(suppl 5–7):1, 1988

74. Hodge B, Thompson JF: Noise pollution in the operating theatre. Lancet 335:891, 1990

75. Murthy VSSN, Malhotra SK, Bala I, Raghunathan M: Detrimental effects of noise on anaesthetists. Can J Anaesth 42:608, 1995

76. Wallace MS, Ashman MN, Matjasko MJ: Hearing acuity of anesthesiologists and alarm detection. Anesthesiology 81:13, 1994

77. Eschenbrenner AJ: Effects of intermittent noise on the performance of a complex psychomotor task. Human Factors 16:59, 1971

78. Koch ME, Kain Z, Ayoub C, Rosenbaum SH: The sedative and analgesic sparing effect of music. Anesthesiology 89:300, 1998

79. Allen K, Blascovich J: Effects of music on cardiovascular reactivity among surgeons. JAMA 272:882, 1994

80. Weinger M: Cardiovascular reactivity among surgeons: Not music to everyone's ears. JAMA 273:1090, 1995

81. Gaba D: Human error in anesthetic mishaps. Int Anesthesiol Clin 27:137, 1989

82. Drui AB, Behm RJ, Martin WE: Predesign investigation of the anesthesia operational environment. Anesth Analg 52:584, 1973

83. Weinger MB, Herndon OW, Zornow MH et al: An objective methodology for task analysis and workload assessment in anesthesia providers. Anesthesiology 80:77, 1994

84. Weinger MB, Herndon OW, Gaba DM: The effect of electronic record keeping and transesophageal echocardiography on task distribution, workload, and vigilance during cardiac anesthesia. Anesthesiology 87:144, 1997

85. Weinger M, Englund C: Ergonomic and human factors affecting anesthetic vigilance and monitoring performance in the operating room environment. Anesthesiology 73:995, 1990

86. Gaba DM, Maxwell M, DeAnda A: Anesthetic mishaps: Breaking the chain of accident evolution. Anesthesiology 66:670, 1987

87. Paget NS, Lambert TF, Sridhar K: Factors affecting an anaesthetist's work: Some findings on vigilance and performance. Anaesth Intensive Care 9:359, 1981

88. Cooper JB, Newbower RS, Kitz RJ: An analysis of major errors and equipment failures in anesthesia management: Considerations for prevention and detection. Anesthesiology 60:34, 1984

89. Krueger GP: Sustained work, fatigue, sleep loss and performance: A review of the issues. Work & Stress 3:129, 1989

90. Geer R, Jobes D, Gilfor J et al: Reduced psychomotor vigilance in anesthesia residents after 24 hour call. Anesthesiology 83:A1008, 1995

91. Denisco RA, Drummond JN, Gravenstein JS: The effect of fatigue on the performance of a simulated anesthetic monitoring task. J Clin Monit 3:22, 1987

92. Stanford LM, McIntyre JWR, Nelson TM, Hogan JT: Affective responses to commercial and experimental auditory alarm signals for anesthesia delivery and physiological monitoring equipment. Int J Clin Monit Comput 5:111, 1988

93. Wolf RH, Weiner FF: Effects of four noise conditions on arithmetic performance. Percept Mot Skills 35:928, 1972

94. Bruce DL, Bach MJ: Psychological studies of human performance as affected by traces of enflurane and nitrous oxide. Anesthesiology 42:194, 1975

95. Kortilla K, Pfaffli P, Linnoila M et al: Operating room nurses' psychomotor and driving skills after occupational exposure to halothane and nitrous oxide. Acta Anaesthesiol Scand 22:33, 1978

96. Gaba DM, Howard SK, Jump B: Production pressure in the work environment. Anesthesiology 81:488, 1994

97. Helmreich RL, Schaefer HG: Team performance in the operating room. In Hillsdale BM (ed.): Human Error in Medicine, p 225. New Jersey, Lawrence Erlbaum Associates, 1994

98. Gaba DM, DeAnda A: A comprehensive anesthesia simulation environment: Re-creating the operating room for research and training. Anesthesiology 69:387, 1988

99. Gaba DM, Howard SK, Flanagan B et al: Assessment of clinical performance during simulated crises using both technical and behavioral ratings. Anesthesiology 89:8, 1998

100. Schaefer HG, Helmreich RL: The importance of human factors in the operating room. Anesthesiology 80:479, 1994

101. Gravenstein JS, Cooper JB, Orkin FK: Work and rest cycles in anesthesia practice. Anesthesiology 72:737, 1990

102. Berry AJ, Hall JR: Work hours of residents in seven anesthesiology training programs. Anesth Analg 76:96, 1993

103. Accreditation Council for Graduate Medical Education: Revision of the General Requirements of the Essentials of Accredited Residences in Graduate Medical Education. July 1992

104. Reilly T, Waterhouse J, Atkinson G: Aging, rhythms of physical performance, and adjustment to changes in the sleep-activity cycle. Occupational and Environmental Medicine 54: 812, 1997

105. Travis KW, Mihevc NT, Orkin FK: Aging and stress in anesthetic practice. Anesth Analg 84(suppl):21, 1997

106. Katz JD: Factors leading to retirement among anesthesiologists. Anesthesiology 87:A1013, 1997

107. Geer RT, Jobes DR, Tew JD Jr. et al: Incidence of automobile accidents involving anesthesia residents after on-call duty cycles. Anesthesiology 87:A938, 1997

108. Parker JBR: The effects of fatigue on physician performance: An underestimated cause of physician impairment and increased patient risk. Can J Anaesth 34:489, 1987

109. McDonald JS, Peterson S: Lethal errors in anesthesiology. Anesthesiology 63:A497, 1985

110. Cooper JB, Newbower RS, Long CD et al: Preventable anesthesia mishaps: A study of human factors. Anesthesiology 49:399, 1978

111. McCall TB: The impact of long working hours on resident physicians. N Engl J Med 318:775, 1988

112. Friedman RC, Kornfield DS, Bigger TJ: Psychosocial problems associated with sleep deprivation in interns. J Med Ed 48:436, 1973

113. McCall TB: The Libby Zion case: One step forward or two steps backward? N Engl J Med 318:771, 1988

114. Mitler MM, Carskadon MA, Czeisler CA et al: Catastrophes, sleep and public policy: Consensus report. Sleep 11:100, 1988

115. Centers for Disease Control and Prevention: Immunization of health-care workers: Recommendations of the Advisory Committee on Immunization Practices (ACIP) and the Hospital Infection Control Practices Advisory Committee (HICPAC). MMWR 46(no. RR-18):1, 1997

116. Centers for Disease Control and Prevention: Prevention and control of influenza: Recommendations of the Advisory Committee on Immunization Practices (ACIP). MMWR 46(no. RR-9):1, 1997

117. Wilde JA, McMillian JA, Serwint J et al: Effectiveness of influenza vaccine in health care professionals: A randomized trial. JAMA 281:908, 1999

118. Monto AS, Robinson DP, Herlocher ML et al: Zanamivir in the prevention of influenza among health adults: A randomized controlled trial. JAMA 282:31, 1999

119. Tait AR, DuBoulay PM, Knight PR: Alterations in the course of and histopathologic response to influenza virus infections produced by enflurane, halothane, and diethyl ether anesthesia in ferrets. Anesth Analg 67:671, 1988

120. Simoes EAF: Respiratory syncytial virus infection. Lancet 354: 847, 1999

121. Garner JS: Hospital Infection Control Practices Advisory Committee: Guidelines for isolation precautions in hospitals. Infect Control Hosp Epidemiol 17:56, 1996

122. Agah R, Cherry JD, Garakian AJ, Chapin M: Respiratory syncytial virus (RSV) infection rate in personnel caring for children with RSV infections: Routine isolation procedure vs routine procedure supplemented by use of mask and goggles. Am J Dis Child 141:695, 1989

123. Centers for Disease Control and Prevention: Prevention of varicella: Recommendations of the Immunization Practices Advisory Committee (ACIP). MMWR 45(no. RR-11):1, 1996

124. McKinney WP, Horowitz MM, Battiola RJ: Susceptibility of hospital-based health care personnel to varicella-zoster virus infections. Am J Infect Control 17:26, 1989

125. Juel-Jensen BE: Herpetic whitlow: An occupational risk. Anaesthesia 28:324, 1973

126. DeYoung GG, Harrison AW, Shapley JM: Herpes simplex cross infection in the operating room. Can Anaesth Soc J 15:394, 1968

127. Balcarek KB, Bagley R, Cloud GA, Pass RF: Cytomegalovirus infection among employees of a children's hospital: No evidence for increased risk associated with patient care. JAMA 263:840, 1990

128. Centers for Disease Control and Prevention: Measles, mumps, and rubella—Vaccine use and strategies for elimination of measles, rubella, and congenital rubella syndrome and control of mumps: Recommendations of the Immunization Practices Advisory Committee (ACIP). MMWR 47(no. RR-8):1, 1998

129. Centers for Disease Control and Prevention: Protection against viral hepatitis: Recommendations of the Immunization Practices Advisory Committee (ACIP). MMWR 39(no. RR-2):1, 1990

130. Centers for Disease Control and Prevention: Protection of hepatitis A through active or passive immunization: Recommendations of the Immunization Practices Advisory Committee (ACIP). MMWR 45(no. RR-15):1, 1996

131. Berry AJ, Greene ES: The risk of needlestick injuries and needlestick-transmitted diseases in the practice of anesthesiology. Anesthesiology 77:1007, 1992

132. Berry AJ, Isaacson IJ, Kane MA et al: A multicenter study of the prevalence of hepatitis B viral serologic markers in anesthesia personnel. Anesth Analg 63:738, 1984

133. Fyman PN, Hartung J, Weinberg S, Stackhouse J: Prevalence of hepatitis B markers in the anesthesia staff in a large inner city hospital. Anesth Analg 63:433, 1984

134. Bond WW, Favero MS, Peterson NJ et al: Survival of hepatitis B virus after drying and storage for one week. Lancet 1:550, 1981

135. Department of Labor, Occupational Safety and Health Administration: Occupational exposure to bloodborne pathogens: Final rule (29 CFR Part 1910. 1030). Federal Register 56:64004, 1991

136. Hadler SC, Francis DP, Maynard JE et al: Long-term immunogenicity and efficacy of hepatitis B vaccine in homosexual men. N Engl J Med 315:209, 1986

137. Gerberding JL: Management of occupational exposures to bloodborne viruses. N Engl J Med 332:444, 1995

138. Alter MJ: Hepatitis C: A sleeping giant? Am J Med 91(suppl 3B):112S, 1991

139. Alter MJ, Margolis HS, Krawczynski K et al: The natural history of community-acquired hepatitis C in the United States. N Engl J Med 327:1899, 1992

140. Dore GJ, Kaldor JM, McCaughan GW: Systematic review of role of polymerase chain reaction in defining infectiousness among people infected with hepatitis C virus. Br Med J 315:333, 1997

141. Alter MJ, Hadler SC, Judson FN et al: Risk factors for acute non-A, non-B hepatitis in the United States and association with hepatitis C virus infection. JAMA 264:2231, 1990

142. Alter MJ, Kruszon-Moran D, Nainan OV et al: The prevalence of hepatitis C virus infection in the United States, 1988 through 1994. N Engl J Med 341:556, 1999

143. McHutchison JG, Gordon SC, Schiff ER et al: Interferon alfa-2b alone or in combination with ribavirin as initial treatment for chronic hepatitis C. N Engl J Med 339:1485, 1998

144. Centers for Disease Control and Prevention: Recommendations for prevention and control of hepatitis C virus (HCV) infection and HCV-related chronic disease. MMWR 47(no. RR-19):1, 1998

145. Centers for Disease Control and Prevention: Recommendations for follow-up of health-care workers after occupational exposure to hepatitis C virus. MMWR 46:603, 1997

146. Lanphear BP, Linnemann CC, Cannon CG et al: Hepatitis C virus infection in health care workers: Risk of exposure and infection. Infect Control Hosp Epidemiol 15:745, 1994

147. Krawczynski K, Alter MJ, Taknersley DL et al: Effect of immune globulin on the prevention of experimental hepatitis C virus infection. J Infect Dis 173:822, 1996

148. Camma C, Almasio P, Craxi A: Interferon as treatment for acute hepatitis C. A meta-analysis. Dig Dis Sci 41:1248, 1996

149. Gallo RC, Salahuddin SZ, Popovic M et al: Frequent detection and isolation of cytopathic retroviruses (HTLV-III) from patients with AIDS and at risk of AIDS. Science 224:500, 1984

150. Baltimore D, Feinberg MB: HIV revealed: Toward a natural history of the infection. N Engl J Med 321:1673, 1989

151. Centers for Disease Control and Prevention: HIV/AIDS surveillance report. Vol. 11, 1999

152. Lifson AR: Do alternate modes for transmission of human immunodeficiency virus exist? A review. JAMA 259:1353, 1988

153. Kelen GD, DiGiovanna T, Bisson L et al: Human immunodeficiency virus infection in emergency department patients: Epidemiology, clinical presentations, and risk to health care workers: The Johns Hopkins experience. JAMA 262:516, 1989

154. Janssen RS, St. Louis ME, Satten GA et al: HIV infection among patients in the U.S. acute care hospitals: Strategies for the counseling and testing of hospital patients. N Engl J Med 327:445, 1992

155. Centers for Disease Control and Prevention: Guidelines for prevention of transmission of human immunodeficiency virus and hepatitis B virus to health-care and public-safety workers. MMWR 38(no. S-6):1, 1989

156. Marcus R, CDC Cooperative Needlestick Surveillance Group: Surveillance of health care workers exposed to blood from patients infected with the human immunodeficiency virus. N Engl J Med 319:1118, 1988

157. Tokars JI, Marcus R, Culver DH et al: Surveillance of HIV infection and zidovudine use among health care workers after occupational exposure to HIV-infected blood. Ann Intern Med 118:913, 1993

158. Henderson DK, Fahey BJ, Willy M et al: Risk for occupational transmission of human immunodeficiency virus type I (HIV-1) associated with clinical exposures: A prospective evaluation. Ann Intern Med 113:740, 1990

159. Gerberding JL: Incidence and prevalence of human immunodeficiency virus, hepatitis B virus, hepatitis C virus, and cytomegalovirus among health care personnel at risk for blood exposure: Final report from a longitudinal study. J Infect Dis 170:1410, 1994

160. Ippolito G, Puro V, De Carli G, Italian Study Group on Occupational Risk of HIV Infection: The risk of occupational human immunodeficiency virus infection in health care workers: Italian multicenter study. Arch Intern Med 153:1451, 1993

161. Ippolito G, Puro V, Heptonstall J et al: Occupational human immunodeficiency virus infection in health care workers: Worldwide cases through September 1997. Clin Infect Dis 28:365, 1999

162. Cardo DM, Culver DH, Clesielski CA et al: A case-control study of HIV seroconversion in health care workers after percutaneous exposure. N Engl J Med 337:1485, 1997

163. Buergler JM, Kim R, Thisted RA et al: Risk of human immunodeficiency virus in surgeons, anesthesiologists, and medical students. Anesth Analg 75:118, 1992

164. Greene ES, Berry AJ, Jagger J et al: Multicenter study of contaminated percutaneous injuries in anesthesia personnel. Anesthesiology 89:1362, 1998

165. Task Force on Infection Control of the Committee on Occupational Health of Operating Room Personnel: Recommendations for Infection Control for the Practice of Anesthesiology, 2nd ed. American Society of Anesthesiologists. Park Ridge, Illinois, 1998

166. Tait AR, Tuttle DB: Prevention of occupational transmission of human immunodeficiency virus and hepatitis B virus among anesthesiologists: A survey of anesthesiology practice. Anesth Analg 79:623, 1994

167. Greene ES, Berry AJ, Arnold WP, Jagger J: Percutaneous injuries in anesthesia personnel. Anesth Analg 83:273, 1996

168. Berry AJ: Are some types of needles more likely to transmit HIV to health care workers? (letter) Am J Infect Control 21:216, 1993

169. Culver J: Preventing transmission of blood-borne pathogens: A compelling argument for effective device-selection strategies. Am J Infect Control 25:430, 1997

170. Centers for Disease Control and Prevention: Public Health Service guidelines for management of health-care worker exposures to HIV and recommendations for postexposure prophylaxis. MMWR 47(no. RR-7):1, 1998

171. Centers for Disease Control and Prevention: Public Health Service task force recommendations for the use of antiretroviral drugs in pregnant women infected with HIV-1 for maternal health and for reducing perinatal HIV-1 transmission in the United States. MMWR 47(no. RR-2):2, 1998

172. Centers for Disease Control and Prevention: Update: Universal precautions for prevention of transmission of human immunodeficiency virus, hepatitis B virus, and other bloodborne pathogens in health-care settings. MMWR 37:377, 1988

173. Wong ES, Stotka JL, Chinchilli VM et al: Are universal precautions effective in reducing the number of occupational exposures among health care workers? A prospective study of physicians on a medical service. JAMA 265:1123, 1991

174. Johnson RT, Gibbs CJ: Creutzfeldt-Jakob disease and related transmissible spongiform encephalopathies. N Engl J Med 339:1994, 1998

175. Steelman VMC: Creutzfeld-Jakob disease: Recommendations for infection control. Am J Infect Control 22:312, 1994

176. Centers for Disease Control and Prevention: Progress toward the elimination of tuberculosis–United States, 1998. MMWR 48:732, 1999

177. Centers for Disease Control and Prevention: Guidelines for preventing the transmission of *Mycobacterium tuberculosis* in health care facilities, 1994. MMWR 43(no. RR-13):1, 1994

178. Cocchiarella LA, Cohen RA, Conroy L, Wurtz R: Positive tuberculin skin test reactions among house staff at a public hospital in the era of resurgent tuberculosis. Am J Infect Control 24:7, 1996

179. Menzies D, Fanning A, Yuan L, Fitzgerald M: Tuberculosis among health care workers. N Engl J Med 332:92, 1995

180. Centers for Disease Control and Prevention: Guidelines for preventing the transmission of tuberculosis in health-care settings, with special focus on HIV-related issues. MMWR 39(no. RR-17): 1, 1990

181. Tait AR: Occupational transmission of tuberculosis: Implications for anesthesiologists. Anesth Analg 85:444, 1997

182. Jereb JA, Klevens RM, Privett TD et al: Tuberculosis in health care workers at a hospital with an outbreak of multidrug-resistant *Mycobacterium tuberculosis*. Arch Intern Med 155:854, 1995

183. United States Department of Health and Human Services: 42 CRF Part 84: Respiratory protective devices; proposed rule. Federal Register 59:26849, 1994

184. Garden JM, O'Banion MK, Shelnitz LS et al: Papillomavirus in the vapor of carbon dioxide laser-treated verrucae. JAMA 259:1199, 1988

185. Center for Devices and Radiological Health: Center scientists conduct study for viable viruses in common laser plumes. Medical Devices Bulletin 8:3, 1994

186. Matchette LS, Faaland RW, Royston DD et al: In vitro production of viable bacteriophage in carbon dioxide and argon laser plumes. Lasers Surg Med 11:380, 1991

187. Hallmo P, Naess O: Laryngeal papillomatosis with human papilloma virus DNA contracted by a laser surgeon. Eur Arch Otorhinolaryngol 248:425, 1991

188. Seely HF: The practice of anaesthesia—A stressor for the middle-aged? Anaesthesia 51:571, 1996

189. Jackson SH: The role of stress in anaesthetists' health and well-being. Acta Anaesthesiol Scand 43:583, 1999

190. Seyle H: The Stress of Life. New York, McGraw-Hill, 1984

191. Azar I, Sophie S, Lear E: The cardiovascular response of anesthesiologists during induction of anesthesia. Anesthesiology 63:A75, 1985

192. Pinnock CA, Elling AE, Eastley RJ et al: Anxiety levels in junior anaesthetists during early training. Anaesthesia 41:258, 1986

193. Vaillant GE, Brighton JR, McArthur C: Physicians' use of mood-altering drugs. N Engl J Med 282:365, 1970

194. Reeve PE: Personality characteristics of a sample of anaesthetists. Anaesthesia 35:559; 1980

195. McDonald JS, Lingam RP, Gupta B *et al:* Psychologic testing as an aid to selection of residents in anesthesiology. Anesth Analg 78:542, 1994

196. Hamilton B: Dangerous practice: MDs try to heal selves. New York Post. New York, 1999, p 4

197. Osler W: The Principles and Practice of Medicine, p 1005. New York, D. Appleton & Co., 1892

198. Mattison JB: Morphinism in medical men. JAMA 23:186, 1894

199. Keeve JP: Physicians at risk: Some epidemiologic considerations of alcoholism, drug abuse and suicide. J Occup Med 26:503, 1984

200. Brewster JM: Prevalence of alcohol and other drug problems among physicians. JAMA 255:1913, 1986

201. Hughes PH, Brandenburg N, Baldwin DC *et al:* Prevalence of substance use among US physicians. JAMA 267:2333, 1992

202. Silverstein JH, Silva DA, Iberti TJ: Opioid addiction in anesthesiology. Anesthesiology 79:354, 1993

203. Lutsky I, Hopwood M, Abram SE *et al:* Use of psychoactive substances in three medical specialties: Anaesthesia, medicine and surgery. Report of investigation. Can J Anaesth 41:561, 1994

204. Talbott GD: Elements of the impaired physician program. J Med Assoc Ga 73:747, 1984

205. Talbott DG, Gallegos KV, Wilson PO *et al:* The Medical Association of Georgia's impaired physicians program review of the first 1000 physicians: Analysis of specialty. JAMA 257:2927, 1987

206. Ward CG, Ward GC, Saidman LJ: Drug abuse in anesthesia training programs. JAMA 250:922, 1983

207. Menk EJ, Baumgarten RK, Kingsley CP *et al:* Success of reentry into anesthesiology training programs by residents with a history of substance abuse. JAMA 263:3060, 1990

208. Gravenstein JS, Kory WP, Marks RG: Drug abuse by anesthesia personnel. Anesth Analg 62:467, 1983

209. Weeks AM, Buckland MR, Morgan EB *et al:* Chemical dependence in anaesthetic registrars in Australia and New Zealand. Anaesth Intensive Care 21:151, 1993

210. Talbott GD: Alcoholism and other drug addictions: A primary disease entity. J Med Assoc Ga 75:490, 1986

211. Farley WJ, Talbott GD: Anesthesiology and addiction. Anesth Analg 62:465, 1983

212. McAuliffe WE, Rohman M, Santangelo S *et al:* Psychoactive drug use among practicing physicians and medical students. N Engl J Med 315:805, 1986

213. Burrow BJ: The patient's view of the anaesthetist in an Australian teaching hospital. Anaesth Intensive Care 10:20, 1982

214. Salmon NS: The role of the anaesthetist as seen by nurses in training. Anaesthesia 38:801, 1983

215. Goodwin DW, Davis DH, Robins LN: Drinking amid abundant illicit drugs: The Vietnam case. Arch Gen Psychiatry 32:230, 1975

216. Klein RL, Stevens WC, Kingston HGG: Controlled substance dispensing and accountability in United States anesthesiology residency programs. Anesthesiology 77:806, 1992

217. Moore RD: Youthful precursors of alcohol abuse in physicians. Am J Med 88:332, 1990

218. Reeve PE: Personality characteristics of a sample of anaesthetists. Anaesthesia 335:559, 1980

219. Centrella M: Physician addiction and impairment—Current thinking. Addiction Disease 13:91, 1994

220. Scott M, Fisher KS: The evolving legal context for drug testing programs. Anesthesiology 73:1022, 1990

221. Task Force on Chemical Dependence of the Committee on Occupational Health of Operating Room Personnel: Chemical Dependence in Anesthesiologists: What you need to know when you need to know it. American Society of Anesthesiologists. Park Ridge, Illinois, 1998

222. Spiegelman GS, Saunders L, Mazze RI: Addiction and anesthesiology. Anesthesiology 60:335, 1984

223. Matsumura JS: Substance abuse and anesthesiology training. JAMA 264:2741, 1990

224. American Board of Anesthesiology: Booklet of Information. Raleigh, North Carolina, American Board of Anesthesiology, 1998

225. Canavan DJ: The impaired physician program: The subject of impairment. J Med Soc NJ 80:47, 1983

226. Duffy JC, Litin EM: Psychiatric morbidity of physicians. JAMA 189:989, 1984

227. Bissell L, Jones R: The alcoholic physician: A survey. Am J Psychiatry 133:1142, 1976

228. Clark DC, Eckenfels EJ, Daugherty SR *et al:* Alcohol-use patterns through medical school. JAMA 257:2921, 1987

229. Atkinson RS: The problem of the unsafe anaesthetist. Br J Anaesth 73:29, 1994

230. Canavan DI: The impaired physicians program. J Med Soc NJ 79:980, 1982

231. Carpenter LM, Swerdlow AJ, Fear NT: Mortality of doctors in different specialties: Findings from a cohort of 20,000 NHS hospital consultants. Occup Environ Med 54:388, 1996

232. DeSole DE, Singer P, Aronson S: Suicide and role strain among physicians. Int J Soc Psychiatry 15:294, 1969

233. Helliwel PJ: Suicides amongst anaesthetists-in-training. Anaesthesia 38:1097, 1983

234. Council on Scientific Affairs: Results and implication of the AMA-APA physicians mortality project: Stage II. JAMA 257:2949, 1987

235. Springman SR, Berry AJ, Cascorbi HF *et al:* What attributes do we want in anesthesia residents? Anesthesiology 65:107, 1986

236. Wohl S: Death by malpractice. JAMA 255:1927, 1986

237. Birmingham PK, Ward RJ: A high risk suicide group: The anesthesiologist involved in litigation. Am J Psychiatry 142:1225, 1985

238. Crawshaw R, Bruce JA, Eraker PL *et al:* An epidemic of suicide among physicians on probation. JAMA 243:1915, 1980

239. Roback G, Randolph L, Seidman B: Physician characteristics and distribution in the US. Chicago, American Medical Association, 1994

240. Anonymous: ASA at a glance. Newsletter of the American Society of Anesthesiologists 62:26, 1998

241. Katz JD, Kain ZN: Factors leading to retirement among anesthesiologists: A national survey. Anesthesiology 89:A1341, 1998

242. Grauer H, Campbell NM: The aging physician and retirement. Can J Psychiatry 28:552, 1983

243. Hospital Infection Control Practices Advisory Committee. Recommendations for preventing the spread of vancomycin resistance. Am J Infect Control 23:87, 1995

Clinical Anesthesia (4/e), edited by
Paul G. Barash, Bruce F. Cullen, and
Robert K. Stoelting. Lippincott Williams &
Wilkins, Philadelphia, © 2001.

CHAPTER 5

PROFESSIONAL LIABILITY, RISK MANAGEMENT, AND QUALITY IMPROVEMENT

KAREN L. POSNER, FREDERICK W. CHENEY,
AND DONALD A. KROLL

In anesthesia, as in other areas of life, everything does not always go as planned. Undesirable outcomes occur regardless of the quality of care provided. The legal aspects of medical practice have become increasingly important as the American public has turned to the courts for economic redress when their expectations of medical treatment are not met. Payers such as Medicare are increasingly depending on accreditation through bodies such as the Joint Commission on Accreditation of Healthcare Organizations (JCAHO) to ensure that mechanisms are in place to deliver quality care to all patients. An anesthesia risk management program can work in conjunction with a program for quality improvement to minimize the liability risk of practice while assuring the highest quality of care for patients.

This chapter provides background for the practitioner about how the legal system handles malpractice claims and the role of risk management activity in minimizing and managing liability exposure. An introduction to the concepts of quality improvement (formerly called quality assurance) extends the discussion to the broader arena of quality of care in anesthesia practice.

PROFESSIONAL LIABILITY

This section addresses the basic concepts of medical liability. A more detailed discussion of the steps of the lawsuit process and appropriate actions for physicians to take when sued is available from the American Society of Anesthesiologists (ASA).[1]

Tort System

Although physicians may become involved in the criminal law system in a professional capacity, they more commonly become involved in the legal system of civil laws. Civil law is broadly divided into *contract law* and *tort law*. A tort may be loosely defined as a civil wrongdoing, and negligence is one type of tort. The majority of medical malpractice lawsuits are pursued on the basis of negligence theories, but there are occasional cases in which contract law theories are used. *Malpractice* actually refers to any professional misconduct, but its use in legal terms typically refers to professional negligence.

To be successful in a malpractice suit, the patient-plaintiff must prove four things:

1. Duty: that the anesthesiologist owed the patient a duty;
2. Breach of duty: that the anesthesiologist failed to fulfill his or her duty;
3. Causation: that a reasonably close causal relation exists between the anesthesiologist's acts and the resultant injury; and
4. Damages: that actual damage resulted because of a breach of the standard of care.

Failure to prove any one of these four elements will result in a decision for the defendant-anesthesiologist.

Duty

As a physician, the anesthesiologist establishes a duty to the patient when a doctor–patient relationship exists. When the patient is seen preoperatively, and the anesthesiologist agrees to provide anesthesia care for the patient, a duty to the patient has been established. In the most general terms, the duty the anesthesiologist owes to the patient is to adhere to the *standard of care* for the treatment of the patient. Because it is virtually impossible to delineate specific standards for all aspects of medical practice and all eventualities, the courts have created the concept of the *reasonable and prudent* physician. For all specialties, there is a national standard, which has displaced the local standard.

There are certain general duties that all physicians have to their patients, and breaching these duties may also serve as the basis for a lawsuit. One of these general duties is that of obtaining informed consent for a procedure. Consent may be written, verbal, or implied. Oral consent is just as valid, albeit harder to prove years after the fact, as written consent. Implied consent for anesthesia care may be present in circumstances in which the patient is unconscious or unable, for any reason, to give his or her consent, but where it is presumed that any reasonable and prudent patient would give consent if able.

Although there are exceptions to the requirement that consent be obtained, as a general rule, anesthesiologists should be sure to obtain consent whenever possible. Failure to do so could, in theory, expose the anesthesiologist to possible prosecution for battery.

The requirement that the consent be *informed* is somewhat more opaque. The guideline is determining whether the patient received a fair and reasonable account of the proposed procedures and the risks inherent in these procedures. The duty to disclose risks is not limitless, but it does extend to those risks that are reasonably likely in any patient under the circumstances and to those that are reasonably likely in particular patients because of their condition. For example, it would be prudent to inform the patient of possible sore throat or dental damage associated with tracheal intubation, but not about an unlikely complication such as vocal cord paralysis.

Breach of Duty

In a malpractice action, expert witnesses will review the medical records of the case and determine whether the anesthesiologist acted in a reasonable and prudent manner in the specific situation and fulfilled his or her duty to the patient. If they find that the anesthesiologist either did something that should not have been done or failed to do something that should have been done, then the duty to adhere to the standard of care has been breached. Therefore, the second requirement for a successful suit will have been met.

Causation

Judges and juries are interested in determining whether the breach of duty was the *proximate cause* of the injury. If the odds are better than even that the breach of duty led, however circuitously, to the injury, then this requirement is met.

There are two common tests employed to establish causation. The first is the "*but for*" test, and the second is the *substantial factor* test. If the injury would not have occurred "but for" the action of the defendant-anesthesiologist, or if the act of the anesthesiologist was a substantial factor in the injury despite other causes, then proximate cause is established.

Although the burden of proof of causation ordinarily falls on the patient-plaintiff, it may, under special circumstances, be shifted to the physician-defendant under the doctrine of *res ipsa loquitur* (literally, "the thing speaks for itself"). Applying this doctrine requires proving that:

1. The injury is of a kind that typically would not occur in the absence of negligence.
2. The injury must be caused by something under the exclusive control of the anesthesiologist.
3. The injury must not be attributable to any contribution on the part of the patient.
4. The evidence for the explanation of events must be more accessible to the anesthesiologist than to the patient.

Because anesthesiologists render patients insensible to their surroundings and unable to protect themselves from injury, this doctrine may be invoked in anesthesia malpractice cases. All that needs to be proved is that the injury typically would not occur in the absence of negligence; the anesthesiologist is then put in the position of having to prove that he or she was not negligent.

Damages

The law allows for three different types of damages. *General damages* are those such as pain and suffering that directly result from the injury. *Special damages* are those actual damages that are a consequence of the injury, such as medical expenses, lost income, and funeral expenses. *Punitive damages* are intended to punish the physician for negligence that was reckless, wanton, fraudulent, or willful. Punitive damages are exceedingly rare in medical malpractice cases. More likely in the case of gross negligence is a loss of the license to practice, or in extreme cases, criminal charges may be brought against the physician. Determining the dollar amount of damages is the job of the jury, and the determination is usually based on some assessment of the plaintiff's condition versus the condition he or she would have been in had there been no negligence. Plaintiffs' attorneys generally charge a percentage of the damages, and will, therefore, seek to maximize the award given.

Standard of Care

Because medical malpractice usually involves issues beyond the comprehension of lay jurors and judges, the court establishes the standard of care in a particular case by the testimony of *expert witnesses*. These witnesses differ from factual witnesses mainly in that they may give opinions. The trial court judge has sole discretion in determining whether a witness may be qualified as an expert. Although any licensed physician may be an expert, information will be sought regarding the witness's education and training, the nature and scope of the person's practice, memberships and affiliations, and publications. The purpose in gathering this information is not only to establish the qualifications of the witness to provide expert testimony, but also to determine the weight to be given to that testimony by the jury. In many cases the success of a suit depends primarily on the stature and believability of the expert witnesses.

In certain circumstances, the standard of care may also be determined from published societal guidelines, written policies of a hospital or department, or textbooks and monographs. Some medical specialty societies have carefully avoided applying the term "standards" to their guidelines, in the hope that no binding behavior or mandatory practices have been created. In 1986 the ASA, for the first time, published "Standards for Basic Intra-operative Monitoring" (now entitled "Standards for Basic Anesthetic Monitoring"). These standards have been updated several times since their initial adoption and are more binding than guidelines. The essential difference between standards and guidelines is that guidelines *should* be adhered to and standards *must* be adhered to. Currently, the ASA also publishes standards on preanesthesia care and postanesthesia care, as well as guidelines for a variety of anesthesia-related activities.[2]

Causes of Suits

The principal cause of suits against anesthesiologists is patient injury. In a nationwide analysis of 1002 lawsuits against anesthesiologists conducted by the ASA Committee on Professional Liability, the leading injuries for which suits were filed were death (37%), nerve damage (15%), and brain damage (12%).[3] The causes of death and brain damage were predominantly problems in airway management, such as inadequate ventilation, difficult intubation, and esophageal intubation. Nerve damage, especially to the ulnar nerve, often occurs despite apparently adequate positioning.[4,5] Spinal cord injury was the most common cause of nerve damage claims against anesthesiologists in the 1990s.[4]

Because death and brain damage are high-cost injuries, anesthesia practice is clearly a high-risk endeavor. Anesthesiologists use complex equipment, which can fail or be used incorrectly,[6] and potent drugs, with which mistakes in dose or labeling can have disastrous consequences. Vigilance, which is the highest priority in anesthesia practice, is often difficult to maintain at all times of the day and night through long, tedious surgical procedures. The anesthesiologist is more likely to be the target of a suit if an untoward outcome occurs because the physician–patient relationship is usually tenuous at best. The patient rarely chooses the anesthesiologist, the preoperative visit is brief, and the anesthesiologist who sees the patient preoperatively may not actually anesthetize the patient. Communication between anesthesiologists and surgeons about complications is often lacking and the tendency is for the surgeon to "blame anesthesia."

Supervision of nurse anesthetists is another endeavor that puts the anesthesiologist in a high-risk category. The more nurse anesthetists supervised by any one anesthesiologist, the greater the exposure to the possibility of patient injury. Some professional liability insurance companies specify a staffing ratio of 1:2 or 1:3 and charge higher rates for supervision of more than this number. Anesthesiologists are liable not only for the nurse anesthetists they employ but also for those they supervise who are employed by the hospital.

Because anesthesiologists are involved in the care of patients undergoing high-risk surgical procedures, they are often sued along with the surgeon in the case of an adverse outcome. This may occur even if the outcome was in no way related to the anesthetic care.

What to Do When Sued

A lawsuit begins when the patient-plaintiff's attorney files a complaint and demand for jury trial with the court. The anesthesiologist is then served with the complaint and a summons requiring an answer to the complaint. Until this happens, no lawsuit has been filed. Insurance carriers must be notified immediately after the receipt of the complaint. The anesthesiologist will need assistance in answering the complaint, and there is a time limit placed on the response.

Specific actions at this point include the following:

1. Do not discuss the case with anyone, including colleagues who may have been involved, operating room personnel, or friends.
2. Never alter any records.

3. Gather together all pertinent records, including a copy of the anesthetic record, billing statements, and correspondence concerning the case.
4. Make notes recording all events recalled about the case.
5. Cooperate fully with the attorney provided by the insurer.

The first task the anesthesiologist must perform with an attorney is to prepare an answer to the complaint. The complaint contains certain facts and allegations with which the defense may either agree or disagree. Defense attorneys rely on the frank and totally candid observations of the physician in preparing an answer to the complaint. Physicians should be willing to educate their attorneys about the medical facts of the case, although most medical malpractice attorneys will be knowledgeable and medically sophisticated.

The next phase of the malpractice suit is called *discovery*. The purpose of discovery is the gathering of facts and clarification of issues in advance of the trial. Another purpose of discovery is to assess or harass the defendant to determine how good a witness he or she will make. This occurs at several points in the discovery process, and by several mechanisms.

The anesthesiologist will, in all likelihood, receive a written interrogatory, which will request factual information. The interrogatory should be answered in writing, in consultation with the defense attorney, because carelessly or inadvertently misstated facts can become troublesome later.

Depositions are a second mechanism of discovery. The defendant-anesthesiologist will be deposed as a fact witness, and depositions will be obtained from other anesthesiologists who will act as expert witnesses. The defendant-anesthesiologist may be asked to suggest other anesthesiologists who will review the medical records. A nationally recognized expert in the area in question who is not a personal friend but agrees with the defense position may be very valuable.

The plaintiff's attorney, not the defense attorney, will depose the anesthesiologist. Most often, the arrangements for the deposition will be made amicably by both sides, and the deposition will occur at a place and time convenient for the anesthesiologist, typically in the defense attorney's office. As a general rule, it is best that physicians avoid having the deposition taken in their own offices, because the plaintiff's attorney will carefully note such things as the medical books on the shelves, the diplomas on the walls, and the general state of disarray of the office. Information may thus be provided that the plaintiff's attorney may use against the anesthesiologist. A second reason to avoid pleasant and familiar surroundings is that the physician will tend to lower his or her guard if comfortable and fall prey to certain common traps in deposition. *Despite the apparent informality of the deposition, the anesthesiologist must be constantly aware that what is said during the deposition carries as much weight as what would be said in court.*

It is important to be factually prepared for the deposition. A review of notes, the anesthetic record, and the medical record is necessary. The physician should dress conservatively and professionally because appearance and image are very important. The opposition is assessing the physician to see how he or she will appear to a jury. Answers to questions should be brief and concise. Being evasive or hostile is not helpful. Answer only the question asked, and do not volunteer information. Occasionally, physicians will be asked leading questions that are impossible to answer without qualifications. In this case, the physician may qualify his or her answer but should avoid giving lengthy opinion answers. The defendant-anesthesiologist is being deposed as a witness of facts, not opinions. Experts may give opinions, but the defendant should try to avoid doing so. Physicians should not admit that there are any "definitive" or "authoritative" textbooks on which they rely in their practice, as doing so may make them responsible for everything that is said in the book, whether they agree with it or not. Do not try to be humorous or make a joke, as these efforts do not translate well on paper.

Court reporters will record exactly what is said, so it is important to speak clearly.

There will be depositions from expert witnesses, both for the plaintiff and for the defense. The anesthesiologist should work with his or her attorney to suggest questions and rebuttals. The better educated the attorney is about the medical facts, the reasons the anesthesiologist did what was done, and the alternative approaches, the better able he or she will be to conduct these expert depositions.

If there is some merit in the case but the damages are minimal, or if proof will be difficult, there will probably be a settlement offer. There is a high cost incurred by both plaintiffs and defendants in pursuing a malpractice claim up through a jury trial. Unless there is a strong probability of a large dollar award, reputable plaintiffs' attorneys are not likely to pursue the claim. Thus, even if physicians believe that they are totally innocent of any wrongdoing, they should not be offended or angered about settling of the case: this is solely a matter of money, not medicine.

If a settlement is not reached during the discovery phase, a trial will occur. Only about 1 in 20 malpractice cases ever reaches the point of a jury trial, because both plaintiffs' and defendants' attorneys are aware of the strengths of the case, and it usually becomes clear during discovery whether the suit will be successful. Only those cases in which both sides feel they can win, and which are likely to have significant financial impact, will proceed to trial.

The discussion of deposition testimony also applies to testimony in court, but there are a few additional points to consider during the trial. The members of the jury will not be as sophisticated medically as the attorneys who deposed the anesthesiologist during discovery. A tendency to overuse specific medical terms should be corrected by learning to explain answers in lay terms for the benefit of the jury. Do not underestimate the intelligence of the jury, however, because talking down to them will create an unfavorable impression. If the answer to a question is not known, avoid guessing. If specific facts cannot be remembered, say so. Nobody expects total recall of events that may have occurred years before.

The defendant-physician should be present during the trial, even when not testifying, and should dress conservatively, neatly, and professionally. Displays of anger, remorse, relief, or hostility will hurt the physician in court. When giving testimony, the anesthesiologist must give clear answers to all questions asked. The physician should be able to give his or her testimony without using notes or documents. When it is necessary to refer to the medical record, it will be admitted into evidence. The anesthesiologist's goal is to convince the jury that he or she behaved in this case as any other competent and prudent anesthesiologist would have behaved.

It is important to keep in mind that *proof* in a malpractice case means only "more likely than not." The patient-plaintiff must "prove" the four elements of negligence, not to absolute certainty, but only to a probability greater than 50%. On the positive side, this means that the defendant-anesthesiologist must only show that his or her actions were, more likely than not, within an acceptable standard of care.

RISK MANAGEMENT AND QUALITY IMPROVEMENT

Risk management and quality improvement programs work hand-in-hand in minimizing liability exposure while maximizing quality of patient care. Although the functions of these programs vary from one institution to another, they overlap in their focus on patient safety. They can generally be distinguished by their basic difference in orientation. A hospital risk management program is broadly oriented toward reducing the liability exposure of the organization. This includes not only professional liability (and therefore patient safety) but also contracts, employee safety, public safety, and any other liability exposure of the institution. Quality improvement programs have as their main goal the continuous maintenance and improvement of the quality of patient care and may be broader in their patient safety focus than strictly risk management.

Risk Management

Those aspects of risk management that are most directly relevant to the liability exposure of the anesthesiologist include prevention of patient injury, adherence to standards of care, documentation, and patient relations.

The key factors in the prevention of patient injury are vigilance, up-to-date knowledge, and adequate monitoring.[7] Physiologic monitoring of cardiopulmonary function, combined with monitoring of equipment function, might be expected to reduce anesthetic injury to a minimum. This was the rationale for the adoption of the ASA Standards for Basic Anesthetic Monitoring (see Table 2-1 on page 30).[2]

These standards call for measurement of arterial blood pressure, pulse, electrocardiogram, and pulse oximeter for all anesthetics. For all general anesthetics an oxygen analyzer with a low-limit alarm system is mandated. When a tracheal tube or laryngeal mask airway is placed, correct positioning in the trachea must be verified by detection of expired carbon dioxide. Continual monitoring for the presence of expired CO_2 is required unless invalidated by the nature of the patient, procedure, or equipment. When a mechanical ventilator is in use during general anesthesia, a disconnect alarm must be utilized.

The ASA Directory of Members should be reviewed yearly for any changes in ASA Standards of Practice. It would also be reasonable to review the ASA Guidelines and Statements published in the same directory. It should be noted that, although membership in the ASA is not required for the practice of anesthesiology, expert witnesses will, with virtual certainty, hold any practitioner to the ASA standards. It is also possible that, as a risk management strategy, a professional liability insurer or hospital may hold an individual anesthesiologist to standards higher than those promulgated by the ASA.

Another risk management tool is the use of checklists prior to each case, or at least daily, in an attempt to reduce equipment-related mishaps.[6,8–10] A 1994 Food and Drug Administration (FDA) checklist,[10] while overly complex, contains the basic elements of what needs to be checked.

A regular schedule of equipment maintenance and procedures to follow whenever equipment malfunction is suspected of contributing to patient injury should be established. If equipment malfunction is suspected to have contributed to a complication, the device should be impounded and examined concurrently by the representatives of the hospital, the anesthesiologist, and the manufacturer.

Although it may seem obvious, qualified anesthesia personnel should be in continuous attendance during the conduct of all anesthetics. The only exceptions should be those that lay people (*i.e.*, judge and jury) can understand, such as radiation hazards or an unexpected life-threatening emergency elsewhere. Even then, provisions should be made for monitoring the patient adequately. Adequate supervision of nurse anesthetists and residents is also important, as is good communication with surgeons when adverse anesthetic outcomes occur.

Informed consent should be documented with a general consent, which should include a statement to the effect that, ''I understand that all anesthetics involve risks of complications, serious injury, or, rarely, death from both known and unknown causes.'' In addition, there should be a note in the patient's record that the risks of anesthesia and alternatives were discussed, and that the patient accepted the proposed anesthetic plan. A brief documentation in the record that the common complications of the proposed technique were discussed is helpful. If it is necessary to change the agreed-on anesthesia plan

significantly after the patient is premedicated or anesthetized, the reasons for the change should be documented in the record.

Good records can form a strong defense if they are adequate and can be disastrous if inadequate. The anesthesia record itself should be as accurate, complete, and neat as possible. The use of automated anesthesia records may be helpful in the defense of malpractice cases.[11] In addition to vital signs every 5 minutes, special attention should be paid to ensure that the patient's ASA classification, the monitors utilized, fluids administered, and doses and times of all administered drugs are accurately charted. Because the principal causes of hypoxic brain damage and death during anesthesia are related to ventilation and/or oxygenation, all respiratory variables that are monitored should be documented accurately. It is important to note when there is a change of anesthesia personnel during the conduct of a case. Sloppy, inaccurate anesthesia records, enlarged and placed before a jury, can be damaging to the defense.

If a critical incident occurs during the conduct of an anesthetic, the anesthesiologist should document, in narrative form, in the patient's progress notes, what happened, which drugs were used, the time sequence, and who was present. A catastrophic intra-anesthetic event cannot be summarized adequately in a small amount of space on the usual anesthesia record. The critical incident note should be written as soon as possible. The report should be as consistent as possible with concurrent records, such as the anesthesia, operating room, recovery room, and cardiac arrest records. If significant inconsistencies exist, they should be explained. Records should never be altered after the fact. If an error is made in recordkeeping, a line should be drawn through the error, leaving it legible, and the correction should be initialed and timed. Litigation is a lengthy process, and a court appearance to explain the incident to a jury may be years away, when memories have faded.

In the event of a sudden, unexpected intra-anesthetic cardiac arrest for which there is no readily apparent explanation, blood and urine should be obtained and screened for drugs that may interact adversely with drugs used for anesthesia.

If anesthetic complications occur, the anesthesiologist should be honest with both the patient and family about the cause. Whenever an anesthetic complication becomes apparent postoperatively, appropriate consultation should be obtained quickly, and the departmental or institutional risk management group should be notified. If the complication is apt to lead to prolonged hospitalization or permanent injury, the liability insurance carrier should be notified. The patient should be followed closely while in the hospital, with telephone follow-up, if indicated, after discharge. Also, the anesthesiologist and surgeon should be consistent in their explanations to the patient or the patient's family as to the cause of any complication.

Jehovah's Witnesses and Other Treatment Obligations

It is important to recognize that patients have well-established rights, and that among these is the right to refuse specific treatments because of religious beliefs. In the case of Jehovah's Witnesses, the treatment refused is the administration of blood or blood products. This is a central part of their religious beliefs, which hold that the faithful will be forbidden the pleasures of the afterlife if they receive blood or blood products. Thus, for them to receive a transfusion is a mortal sin, and many Jehovah's Witnesses would actually rather die in grace, as they see it, than live with no possibility of salvation. Anesthesiologists recognize and respect these beliefs but are also cognizant that these convictions may conflict with the physicians' personal, religious, or ethical codes.

Minor children of Jehovah's Witness parents represent a special group for consideration. Although the U.S. Supreme Court has upheld the right of an adult to become a martyr by refusing treatments based on religious convictions, no court has extended to parents the right to martyr their children.[12] Obtaining a proper court order is of critical importance in the care of a minor child of Jehovah's Witness parents when the parents refuse to authorize a blood transfusion.

As a general rule, physicians are not obligated to treat all patients who apply for treatment in elective situations. It is well within the rights of a physician to decline to care for any patient who wishes to place burdensome constraints on the physician or unacceptably to limit the physician's ability to provide optimal care. When presented with the opportunity to provide elective care for a Jehovah's Witness, the physician may decline to provide any care or may limit, by mutual consent with the patient, his or her obligation to adhere to the patient's religious beliefs. If such an agreement is reached, it must be documented clearly in the medical record, and it is desirable to have the patient co-sign the note. Not all Jehovah's Witnesses have identical beliefs regarding blood transfusions or which methods of blood preservation or sequestration will be allowed. Some patients will not allow any blood that has left the body to be reinfused. Yet others will accept autotransfusion if their blood remains in constant contact with the body (*via* tubing). Therefore, it is important to reach a clear understanding of which techniques for blood preservation are to be used and to document this plan in the record.

Emergency medical care imposes greater constraints on the treating physician, as there is no opportunity to decline the care of a patient with an immediately life-threatening condition. If the patient is an adult and is conscious and mentally competent, then he or she has the right to refuse blood transfusion. The exceptions to patients' rights in this regard include pregnant women and adults who are the sole support of minor children. In these circumstances, the interests of the fetus in surviving may supersede the rights of the mother, as may the interests of the state in not being obligated to provide for the welfare of dependent children.[12] In either case, obtaining a court order is the best plan if time permits. If the problem concerns blood products and there is insufficient time to obtain a court order, pregnant women should be given a transfusion to save the life of the fetus, but parents of minor children should not receive transfusions against their wishes unless the dependency of the children is obvious.

When the patient is a minor, it is important to ascertain the true wishes of the parents. Some parents know that a court order can be obtained and view this as a relief from the onerous burden of having to decide whether they are willing to let their child die. However, some parents are adamant that blood not be given, and there have been cases in which children have been ostracized by their parents and religious community for having received a court-ordered transfusion. Reaching an understanding about the consequences for the child who receives a court-ordered transfusion is therefore vital for the determination of what risks will be taken before ordering a transfusion.

The procedure for obtaining a court order may vary, depending on the specific state laws. Typically, an order may be obtained over the telephone. This call initiates the issue of a written order, which will arrive several days later. Although not a totally automatic procedure, it would be very rare for a judge to deny this order for a minor.

National Practitioner Data Bank

It is usually the obligation of the hospital risk management department to make reports to the National Practitioner Data Bank (NPDB), a nationwide information system that theoretically would allow licensing boards and hospitals a means of detecting adverse information about physicians.[13] Simply moving into another state would no longer provide safe haven for incompetent physicians.

The NPDB requires input from four sources: medical malpractice payments, license actions by medical boards, clinical privilege actions taken by hospitals, and membership actions taken by societies if the society has formal peer review mechanisms. There has been a great deal of effort to establish a minimum reporting dollar value below which no report is necessary, but to date, any payment made on behalf of a physician in response to a written complaint or claim must be reported. Settlements made by cancellation of bills or settlements made on verbal complaints are not considered a reportable payment.

Once a report has been submitted, the physician is notified and has 60 days from the date the data bank processed the report to dispute the input. At this time, the reporting entity may correct the form or void it. Failing that, the physician has the option of putting a brief statement in the file or appealing to the U.S. Secretary of Health and Human Services, who may also either correct or void the form. Once it is entered, there is no means of purging the form.

Requiring legitimate inquirers to have an identification number protects the security of the data bank. Hospitals are required to query the data bank at the time a physician initially requests staff privileges and at 2-year intervals, but they may query at any time. State licensing boards also may make a query, and any health care entity that provides patient care may query as long as the entity has a formal peer review process. A plaintiff's attorney may query the data bank only when there is evidence that a hospital failed to make a mandatory query and the claim is made against the hospital. A practitioner may make a query about his or her file at any time. The existence of the NPDB reporting requirements has made physicians reluctant to allow settlement of nuisance suits because it will cause their names to be added to the data bank.

QUALITY IMPROVEMENT IN ANESTHESIA PRACTICE

Quality is a concept that has continued to elude precise definition in medical practice. However, it is generally accepted that attention to quality will improve patient safety and satisfaction with anesthesia care. The field of quality assurance or quality improvement is continually evolving, as is the terminology used to describe such efforts. The term "quality assurance" is rapidly going out of fashion, being replaced by "quality improvement" in an effort to emphasize a change in underlying philosophy. Although quality improvement programs in anesthesia are generally guided by requirements of the JCAHO, they are basically oriented toward improvement of the structure, process, and outcome of health care delivery programs.

The JCAHO annually updates its quality improvement requirements. Recent years have seen major changes in the type of quality improvement activities required by the JCAHO, with a shift in orientation (and underlying philosophy) from quality assurance to quality improvement.[14] As this focus undergoes transition, further changes in JCAHO requirements may be expected. This can prove to be frustrating to the practitioner and hospital. It may seem that as soon as a quality improvement program meets JCAHO requirements, these requirements change.

An understanding of the fundamental principles of quality improvement may clarify the relationship between the continually evolving JCAHO requirements and mandated quality improvement activities. This section provides an introduction to the basic concepts of quality improvement in anesthesia and some issues to be considered in the implementation of quality improvement programs.

Structure, Process, and Outcome: The Building Blocks of Quality

Although quality of care is difficult to define, it is generally accepted that it is composed of three components: structure, process, and outcome.[15] *Structure* refers to the setting in which care was provided, *e.g.*, personnel and facilities used to provide health care services and the manner in which they are organized. This includes the qualifications and licensing of personnel, ratio of practitioners to patients, standards for the facilities and equipment used to provide care, and the organizational structure within which care is delivered. The *process* of care includes the sequence and coordination of patient care activities, *i.e.*, what was actually done. Was a preanesthetic evaluation performed and documented? Was the patient continuously attended and monitored throughout the anesthetic? *Outcome* of care refers to changes in health status of the patient following the delivery of medical care. A quality improvement program focuses on measuring and improving these basic components of care.

From Quality Assurance to Quality Improvement

Continuous quality improvement (CQI) differs from traditional quality assurance (QA) programs in its basic orientation.[16,17] QA programs typically set as their goal the identification of outliers, known euphemistically as "bad apples." Problems, often assumed to stem from operator error, were addressed at the operator level. However, QA programs lacked a method to resolve problems beyond documentation and assignment of blame and an insistence on eliminating errors. CQI, however, takes a systems approach. The operator is just one part of a complex system. An important underlying premise is that poor results may be due to either random or systematic error. Random errors are inherently difficult to prevent and programs focused in this direction are misguided. System errors, however, should be controllable and strategies to minimize them should be within reach. CQI is basically the process of continually evaluating anesthesia practice to identify systematic problems (opportunities for improvement) and implementing strategies to prevent their occurrence.

A CQI program may focus on undesirable outcomes as a way to identify opportunities for improvement in the structure and process of care. The focus is not on blame but rather on identification of the causes of undesirable outcomes. Instead of asking which practitioners have the highest patient mortality rates, a CQI program may focus on the relationship between the process of care and patient mortality. What proportion of deaths was related to the patient's disease process or debilitated condition? Are these patients being appropriately evaluated for anesthesia and surgery? Were there any controllable causes, such as a lack of hands during resuscitation? The latter may lead to a modification of personnel resources (structure) or assignments (process) to be sure that adequate personnel are available at all times.

Formally, the process of CQI involves the identification of opportunities for improvement through the continual assessment of important aspects of care. Peer review and input are critical to this process. It is a process that is instituted from the bottom up, by those who are actually involved in the process to be improved, rather from the top down by administrators. Identification of opportunities for improvement may be carried out by various means, from brainstorming sessions focusing on a systematic evaluation of care activities to the careful measurement of indicators of quality (such as morbidity and mortality). In any event, once areas are identified for improvement, their current status is measured and documented. This may involve measurement of outcomes, such as delayed recovery from anesthesia or peripheral nerve injury. Then the process of care leading to these problems is analyzed. If a change is identified that should lead to improvement, it is implemented. After an appropriate time period, the status is then measured again to determine whether improvement actually resulted. Attention may then be directed to continuing to improve this process or turning to a different process to target for improvement.

An extension of the CQI method is total quality management (TQM). A TQM program would extend beyond patient care to apply CQI methods to all aspects of the patient care delivery system. This would include such things as billing and housekeeping, for example. With expectation of continuing changes in the structure and financing of health care in the United States, CQI programs in anesthesia can be incorporated into TQM of the entire hospital system to maintain the quality of patient care as practice changes are implemented in response to a changing environment.

Difficulty of Outcome Measurement in Anesthesia

Improvement in quality of care is often measured by a reduction in the rate of adverse outcomes. However, adverse outcomes are relatively rare in anesthesia, making measurement of improvement difficult. For example, if an institution lowers its mortality rate of surgery patients from 1 in 1000 to 0.5 in 1000, this difference may not be statistically significant. Many adverse outcomes in anesthesia are even more rare.

To complement outcome measurement, anesthesia CQI programs can focus on critical incidents and sentinel events. *Critical incidents* are events that cause, or had the potential to cause, patient injury if not noticed and corrected in a timely manner. For example, a partial disconnect of the breathing circuit may be corrected before patient injury occurs, but yet has the potential for causing hypoxic brain injury or death. Critical incidents are more common than adverse outcomes. Measurement of the occurrence rate of important critical incidents may serve as a proxy measure for rare outcomes in anesthesia in a CQI program designed to improve patient safety and prevent injury.

Sentinel events are single, isolated events that may indicate a systemic problem. A sentinel event may be a significant or alarming critical incident that did not result in patient injury, such as a syringe swap and administration of a potentially lethal dose of medication that was noted and treated promptly, avoiding catastrophe. Or a sentinel event may be an unexpected significant patient injury such as intraoperative death. In either case, a CQI program may investigate sentinel events in an attempt to uncover systemic problems in the delivery of care that can be corrected. For example, a syringe swap may be analyzed for confusing or unclear labeling of medications or unnecessary medications routinely stocked on the anesthesia cart, setting the scene for unintended mix-up. In the case of death, all aspects of the patient's hospital course from selection for surgery to anesthetic management may be analyzed to determine if similar deaths can be prevented by a change in the care delivery system.

JCAHO Requirements for Quality Improvement

JCAHO requirements for quality improvement activities are updated on an annual basis. These requirements are described in detail in the JCAHO Comprehensive Accreditation Manual for Hospitals.[14] A current copy of this manual should be available in every hospital.

In general, a hospital must adopt a method for systematically assessing and improving important functions and processes of care and their outcomes in a cyclical fashion. The general outline for this CQI cycle is the design of a process or function, measurement of performance, assessment of performance measures through statistical analysis or comparison with other data sources, and improvement of the process or function. Then the cycle repeats. The JCAHO accreditation manual provides specific standards that must be met, with examples of appropriate measures of performance. The goal of this cycle of design, measurement, assessment, and improvement of performance of important functions and processes is to improve patient outcomes.

Anesthesia care is one important function of the care of patients and is defined as follows: "The administration to an individual in any setting, for any purpose, by any route (general, spinal, or other) of major regional anesthesia or sedation (with or without analgesia) for which there is a reasonable expectation that, in the manner used, the analgesia or sedation will result in the loss of protective reflexes."[14] It is important that policies and procedures for administration of anesthesia be consistent in all locations within the organization. Specific JCAHO standards address preanesthetic assessment and planning, informed consent, intraoperative monitoring, and postanesthesia recovery.

The current JCAHO performance measurement requirement calls for hospitals to choose specific indicators from approved measurement systems. An indicator is "a tool used to measure, over time, the performance of functions, processes, and outcomes of an organization."[14] An example of an anesthesia indicator is in-hospital mortality of patients within two days following a procedure involving anesthesia administration, measured as a proportion of all patients receiving surgical anesthesia. Hospitals must collect data on the selected indicators for comparison with other similar hospitals. It is anticipated that by the year 2001, JCAHO will require hospitals to select measures that monitor 35% of patients (or 12 indicators, whichever is less). Exceptions will be made for small hospitals.

Measuring Quality: Approaches to Data Collection

There are various methods in use for collection of CQI data in anesthesia. These include retrospective records review as well as self-reporting by providers of care. Checklists are sometimes used. Important considerations include compliance with reporting requirements, standardization of definitions, and appropriate sampling.

Retrospective records review usually involves a random sample of anesthesia records. The actual review may be done by an anesthesia provider or by a trained medical records specialist. Explicit definitions of quality indicators would be provided, such as "hypotension = blood pressure <80% of baseline for 5 minutes or more." Such "indicators" of possible quality problems and opportunities for improvement are restricted to data that are normally included in the anesthesia record for every patient. Records review is an especially appropriate technique for gathering data on adequacy of documentation.

For collection of data on events or outcomes that may not normally be charted, a self-reporting system may be used. This is an especially good mechanism for tracking critical incidents and sentinel events. For example, a syringe swap that was noted and corrected before drug administration is a critical incident that would not normally be included in an anesthetic record but could be reported by an anesthesia provider in a self-report system. Many self-report systems provide a checklist of events and outcomes that is completed by the provider for each anesthetic. Other systems provide general guidelines of critical incident reporting without specific check-off items.[18,19] The relevant clinical information is then obtained from the practitioner by quality improvement personnel.

Whatever system is used, it is important that it be in compliance with current JCAHO standards. Standardized definitions must be provided. For example, hypotension may be defined as an absolute measurement (systolic blood pressure <70 mm Hg) or relative (<80% baseline). The latter approach may detect fewer false positives and thereby enhance the relevance of data collection to quality improvement. In general, definitions that take into account the context of care (patient status, type of anesthetic) while maintaining explicit criteria for inclusion in the CQI system will most clearly reflect quality issues (rather than, for example, complications related purely to patient physical condition). For example, blood loss and replacement of 8 units would be considered excessive and indic-

ative of a problem during a knee arthroscopy but would be considered minimal during a liver transplant. A strict definition of "excessive blood loss = >5 units" would identify both cases as quality issues where it would only be appropriate for the arthroscopy. Contextualization of definitions will help avoid the frustration of providers when presented with data that otherwise may be irrelevant to improving the process of anesthesia care.

Peer Review

Peer review, which refers to the review of cases by members of one's specialty, is an integral part of quality improvement programs. Peer review is commonly integrated into a quality improvement program in the context of the morbidity and mortality conference. This provides a forum for review of case management by all members of the department, integrating an educational component into the quality improvement process as differing knowledge bases and clinical experiences are shared. Peer review can provide a mechanism to analyze the structure and process of care and opportunities for improvement.

Peer review can also be incorporated into the analysis of critical incidents, sentinel events, and trends in measured outcomes of care. Peer review has the distinct advantage of credibility and an aura of fairness in a democratic system. Although personal bias in clinical care may be recognized, adherence to the "reasonable man" principle provides a basis for analysis that reflects generally accepted principles of care. It provides a basis for analysis of trends and incidents, suggesting hypotheses for their causes and changes in the system that might improve the structure, process, and outcome of care.

However, peer review is subject to bias that may not be recognized by the participants. This is a tendency of anesthesiologists to judge care as less than appropriate if severe patient injury occurs.[20] In a study of anesthesiologists presented with identical case scenarios with differing outcomes, they were more likely to judge the care as appropriate if the injury was temporary and to judge care as less than appropriate if the injury was permanent. In conducting peer review for a CQI system, this tendency toward assessments biased by case outcome should be recognized and resisted. Careful attention to the process of care and opportunities for improvement should be made regardless of the extent of patient injury. Critical incidents resulting in no injury should be as carefully analyzed for opportunities for improvement in the structure and process of care as incidents with adverse outcomes.

Even though anesthesiologists may be biased in their assessment of case management by outcome, they exhibit only moderate levels of general agreement in their assessments.[21,22] When reviewing identical case histories, different anesthesiologists may not always agree on whether the care was appropriate. Although this disagreement may be due to differences in individually held standards and practices, it must be recognized in any analysis of case management for a CQI program. Incorporation of multiple anesthesiologists into the process of case review will compensate for this lack of agreement. Although a consensus may not be reached, decisions will not be subject to the variability of individual judgments. Incorporation of multiple peer reviewers will compensate for differences in assessments and strengthen the process by improving reliability.[22]

The Future of Quality Improvement: A Multidisciplinary Focus

JCAHO is moving toward a focus on the patient's hospital course in a multidisciplinary emphasis rather than departmental quality improvement programs. The shift in emphasis is toward an analysis of the entirety of each patient's care as the process to be improved. Each department's role is just one part of this process, and the care provided by various departments is often not the relevant unit of analysis. This shift in focus may require movement from departmental peer reliance on standing committees to increased use of *ad hoc* study groups. Comparison of outcomes of care across institutions with adjustments for case mix has long been the goal but has proven to difficult to implement.

REFERENCES

1. Kroll DA: Professional Liability and the Anesthesiologist. Park Ridge, Illinois, American Society of Anesthesiologists, 1992
2. American Society of Anesthesiologists: 2000 Directory of Members. Park Ridge, Illinois, American Society of Anesthesiologists, p. 477, 2000
3. Cheney, FW, Posner K, Caplan RA, Ward RJ: Standard of care and anesthesia liability. JAMA 261:1559, 1989
4. Cheney FW, Domino KB, Caplan RA *et al:* Nerve injury associated with anesthesia. A closed claims analysis. Anesthesiology 90:1062, 1990
5. Warner MA, Martin JT: Ulnar neuropathy: Incidence, outcome and risk factors in sedated or anesthetized patients. Anesthesiology 81:1332, 1994
6. Caplan RA, Vistica MF, Posner KL *et al:* Adverse anesthetic outcomes arising from gas delivery equipment. A closed claims analysis. Anesthesiology 87:741, 1997
7. Gaba DM, Maxwell M, DeAnda A: Anesthetic mishaps: Breaking the chain of accident evolution. Anesthesiology 66:670, 1987
8. Petty C: The Anesthesia Machine, p 213. New York, Churchill, Livingstone, 1987
9. Spooner RM, Kirby RR: Equipment-related anesthetic incidents. Int Anesthesiol Clin 22:133, 1984
10. Food and Drug Administration: Anesthesia Apparatus Checkout Recommendations, 1993. Rockville, Maryland, Food and Drug Administration, 1994
11. Kroll DA: The medicolegal aspects of automated anaesthesia records. Balliere's Clin Aneasthesiol 4:237, 1990
12. Benson KT: The Jehovah's Witness patient: Considerations for the anesthesiologist. Anesth Analg 69:647, 1989
13. Baldwin LM, Hart LG, Oshel RE *et al:* Hospital peer review and the National Practitioner Data Bank: Clinical privileges action reports. JAMA 282:349, 1999
14. Joint Commission of Accreditation of Healthcare Organizations: Comprehensive Accreditation Manual for Hospitals. Oakbrook Terrace, Illinois, Joint Commission on Accreditation of Healthcare Organizations, 1999
15. Donabedian A: The quality of care: How can it be assessed? JAMA 260:1743, 1998
16. Deming WE: Out of the Crisis. Cambridge, Massachusetts, Massachusetts Institute of Technology, 1986
17. Juran JM: Juran on Planning for Quality. New York, Free Press, 1989
18. Posner KL, Kendall-Gallagher D, Wright IH *et al:* Linking process and outcome of care in a continuous quality improvement program for anesthesia services. Am J Med Quality 9:129, 1994
19. Posner KL, Freund PR: Trends in quality of anesthesia care associated with changing staffing patterns, productivity, and concurrency of case supervision in a teaching hospital. Anesthesiology 91:839, 1999
20. Caplan RA, Posner KL, Cheney FW: Effect of outcome on physician judgments of appropriateness of care. JAMA 265:1957, 1991
21. Posner KL, Sampson PD, Caplan RA *et al:* Measuring interrater reliability among multiple raters: An example of methods for nominal data. Stat Med 9:1103, 1990
22. Posner KL, Caplan RA, Cheney FW: Variation in expert opinion in medical malpractice review. Anesthesiology 85:1049, 1996

Clinical Anesthesia (4/e), edited by
Paul G. Barash, Bruce F. Cullen, and
Robert K. Stoelting. Lippincott Williams &
Wilkins, Philadelphia, © 2001.

CHAPTER 6

VALUE-BASED ANESTHESIA PRACTICE, RESOURCE UTILIZATION, AND OPERATING ROOM MANAGEMENT

KENNETH J. TUMAN AND ANTHONY D. IVANKOVICH

INTRODUCTION

Value-based anesthesia management defines the relationship between the costs of anesthetic management strategies and the value of this care as reflected by perioperative outcomes. Implicit in this concept of appraising costs and outcomes is identification of those anesthetic management paradigms associated with the best achievable outcome at a reasonable cost, acknowledging that economic resources are limited.[1] Although the relationships between patient outcome and health care costs are complex, it is generally accepted that most cost–benefit relationships have a diminishing slope, with additional investment of resources generally resulting in only marginal increments of improvement and perhaps even declines in outcome when over-investment of resources results in more harmful (iatrogenic) than beneficial effects.[2] The slope of this relationship depends on the efficiency with which anesthesia services are provided (Fig. 6-1). Efficiency can be defined either as operational efficiency or allocative efficiency, both of which are concerned with improving the use of available resources. Operational efficiency addresses the question of how to meet some predefined objective at the least cost. Allocative efficiency considers the higher level question of maximizing the benefit to society, given that resources are finite and that not all desirable objectives can be met. The latter issue is often a central feature of the argument between providing ''adequate and acceptable care'' and the ''best possible'' care. Indeed, efficiency ultimately defines value in anesthesia management and involves assessment of the relationship between all costs (direct and indirect) and outcomes for all potential alternative utilizations of resources.[1] This chapter identifies considerations involved in the decision-making processes that define cost-effective, quality anesthetic care and efficient management of expensive resources, especially in the OR environment.

IMPETUS FOR ASSESSING COST-EFFECTIVENESS OF ANESTHESIA MANAGEMENT

One of the greatest dilemmas in modern medicine is how to continue to improve or maintain the quality of health care while maintaining a reasonable expenditure of resources. A generation ago, the U.S. spent less than 5% of its Gross Domestic Product (GDP) on health care. Health care costs currently account for more than 14% of the GDP[3] and, as a result of five consecutive double-digit annual increases, more than $1 trillion was spent in the U.S. on health care in 1998. Factors affecting the increase in health care expenditures include an increase in population number with a shift in population age and severity of illness, medical inflation in excess of the economy-wide inflation, and advanced (expensive) technologic innovation. In addition, the greatest contributor to the rising costs of health care may be the administration of health care delivery, estimated to account for upwards of 30–40% of recent increases in health care costs.[4] Such staggering statistics have shifted the focus of health care delivery away from solely considering clinical risk versus clinical benefit. As a result, all physicians, including anesthesiologists, are mandated to make cost-conscious decisions that balance the needs and priorities of patients (risks and benefits) with limited available resources.[5]

Outcomes data are exceedingly important but usually limited or unavailable, and cost, patient satisfaction, and provider access are often key measures in the evaluation of health care providers. Costs, however, must be considered without losing sight of quality. It is unavoidable that physicians must include economic considerations in clinical decision-making, and when presented with more than one option for patient assessment or therapeutic intervention, they should not choose the more expensive alternative unless there is compelling evidence that it is associated with greater value. In other words, quality that increases cost should be pursued only to the extent that the benefit exceeds that obtainable from other established medical practices. This is most difficult for interventions that differ little in benefit but significantly in cost.[6]

Anesthesiologists are not immune to the overall directive to conserve health care dollars, especially since it is recognized that expenditures influenced (directly and indirectly) by anesthesia providers represent 3–5% of the total health care costs of the U.S.[7] More and more frequently, anesthesiologists are confronted with difficult decisions about which patients are appropriate for outpatient surgical procedures, what preanesthetic evaluations are actually requisite, what anesthetic drugs or techniques are most cost-effective, what advances in (usually high-cost) monitoring technology are really necessary to equip operating rooms (ORs), and what is the most efficient method of matching personnel resources with elective surgical caseload. To deliver value-based anesthesia services, anesthesiologists must consider not only the goals of the planned intervention, but also the expectations of all customers of their services (patients, surgeons, facility administrators) as well as the costs associated with the anticipated care, because cost awareness is necessary for cost containment, especially in the low-cost provider contracted care scenario. The diversity of factors contributing to costs of anesthesia mandates the need for an organized approach to accurately assess total costs and benefits.[7,8]

The assessment of the value basis of anesthesia management includes not only the technology and procedures utilized by anesthesiologists, but also their important role in administrative and organizational support for health care delivery. In the current market, in which insurers increasingly identify and contract for services with a provider unit that receives a single, prospectively determined, and often discounted payment covering all costs (and professional fees), anesthesiologists are compelled to define the value of their services. In this regard, the value basis of anesthesia services includes assessment of the functions of the anesthesiologist as a perioperative physician and a manager in the OR. Anesthesiologists provide value-based services by defining appropriate preoperative testing and evaluation; optimizing intraoperative management with selection of drugs,

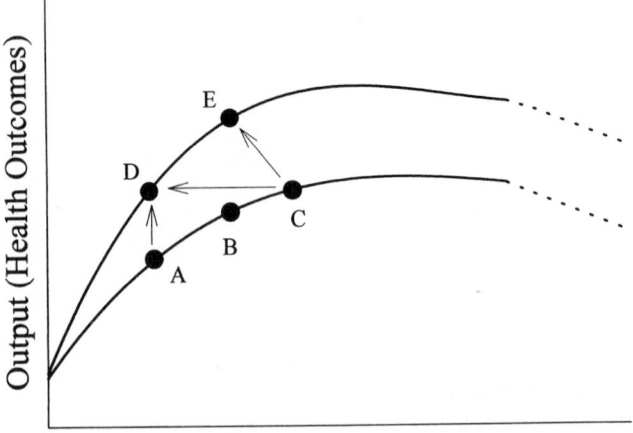

Figure 6-1. Investing additional resources in a health system yields progressively smaller incremental gains in benefits (health outcomes), especially as the system operates along the flatter portion of the curve (A→B→C). A more efficient relationship between costs and health outcomes allows greater benefits for a given cost input (A→D) or similar (C→D) aggregate benefits as well as possibly improved outcome (C→E) at a lower overall cost. When overinvestment of resources occurs, no additional benefits may occur and complications related to additional interventions may actually reduce overall benefit (dashed portion of curve).

techniques, and monitors to balance outcome, patient satisfaction, and facility efficiency with costs; and by participating in postoperative recovery processes and other services outside the OR. Value-based anesthesia management also includes facilitating the efficient use of ORs, recovery areas, and other institutionally based resources. Anesthesiologists are probably the most knowledgeable physicians for provision of administrative and organizational support of these various perioperative activities.

LINKING COST CONTAINMENT AND OUTCOMES

Modeling delivery of health care as a system is a useful approach to understanding the concepts involved in balancing cost-containment and outcome preservation. The attributes of such a system include the input (*i.e.,* the patient with a surgical problem requiring perioperative anesthetic and analgesic management), resources used to manage patients, processes employed in the diagnostic and therapeutic care of patients (including hospital support systems), outcomes that allow measurement of effectiveness and costs of the resources and processes utilized, the environment (including providers and government legislation that create the operating boundaries), and a feedback/evaluation loop for analyzing, troubleshooting, and correcting the identified problems (Fig. 6-2). The amount of input to the system (patients), as well as their acuity and case mix, are important effectors because of the influence on the intensity of services provided to meet the current high expectations of health care. In such a system, the resources include physicians, nurses, laboratory and support personnel, and administrators, as well as diagnostic and therapeutic devices, including drugs, devices, equipment, maintenance procedures, and information systems. Processes include not only the process of diagnostics and therapy, but also the process of access to a health facility. All pertinent outcomes (*e.g.,* morbidity, mortality, costs, length of postoperative stay, duration of recuperative period) must be considered in concert with patient characteristics and practice setting.

The Science of Outcomes Assessment

The capacity to evaluate outcomes and costs, and strategically employ these measures, is integral to maintenance and improvement of cost-effectiveness and ultimately to the determination of value in health care. In the context of anesthetic care, *outcome* refers to the end result of the patient encounter and is considered an essential component of the classic triad (structure, process, outcome) used to evaluate quality of care (see Fig. 6-2). *Process* refers to the ways in which medical resources (structure) are utilized. The assumption behind structure and process evaluation to ensure quality and value is that if these variables are satisfactory, good patient care will follow. This assumption is not always valid: a pulse oximeter may be present and properly used in the OR, yet brain damage may still occur if there is inability to intubate and ventilate. Poor correlation can occasionally exist between processes and outcome so that properly conducted studies to validate and evaluate the effects of process variables on outcome variables are crucial to define value in anesthesia services. In this context, inferences about the benefits of a specific choice of anesthetic management based on differences in intermediate ''process'' variables are generally not as important as those based on differences in real outcome measures. For example, when seeking to identify patterns of care triggered by cost containment that may adversely affect quality of care, evaluation of anesthetic management paradigms using a surrogate endpoint such as hemodynamic stability is much less useful than the assessment of rates and etiologies for unscheduled admissions to treat (or rule out) complications such as myocardial infarction, prolonged postanesthesia care unit (PACU) stays, and other outcomes. Furthermore, funding and reimbursement for certain procedures (*e.g.* chronic pain therapy) may be increasingly restricted or determined by evaluation of quality and assessment of value using outcome data.

Outcome measures are typically defined as those changes, either favorable or adverse, that occur in actual or potential health status after prior or concurrent care.[9] Concepts of health status include not only physical and physiologic parameters (such as death, cardiac arrest, perioperative myocardial infarction, dural puncture headache, or duration of intensive care unit [ICU] or PACU stay), but also psychosocial functions (such as patient satisfaction and duration of disruption of productive and social life). Anesthesiologists have focused on physical and physiologic outcome events, but it is being increasingly recognized that patient satisfaction is a legitimate measure upon which anesthesia management can be valued. Improved quality of care and better patient satisfaction can be achieved by reducing the incidence of common, relatively minor, non–life-threatening adverse events related to anesthesia.[10,11] This is particularly important in ambulatory surgical procedures where the occurrence of minor adverse events leads to patient dissatisfaction.[12] While it is important to focus efforts to avoid such adverse clinical outcomes to improve patient care, it must be acknowledged that other factors, such as the friendliness of a facility staff, may be equally if not more important than some clinical outcomes.[13] A reduction in serious adverse anesthetic outcomes has a variable economic impact on overall costs, depending on different assumptions regarding case mix, the added expense of improving perioperative care and/or preventing complications, the frequency of occurrence of adverse complications, and the relative overall costs of the uncomplicated surgical procedure.[14] Nonetheless, focusing on reduction of minor but frequent perioperative anesthesia-related incidents, events, and complications can be economically beneficial, since these are significant predictors of postanesthesia care utilization in terms of PACU length of stay.[15]

Even when published studies provide data to evaluate outcome effects of new therapies or interventions, determination of relative clinical utility remains difficult. Statistical power, sample size requirements, and related analytic issues are often

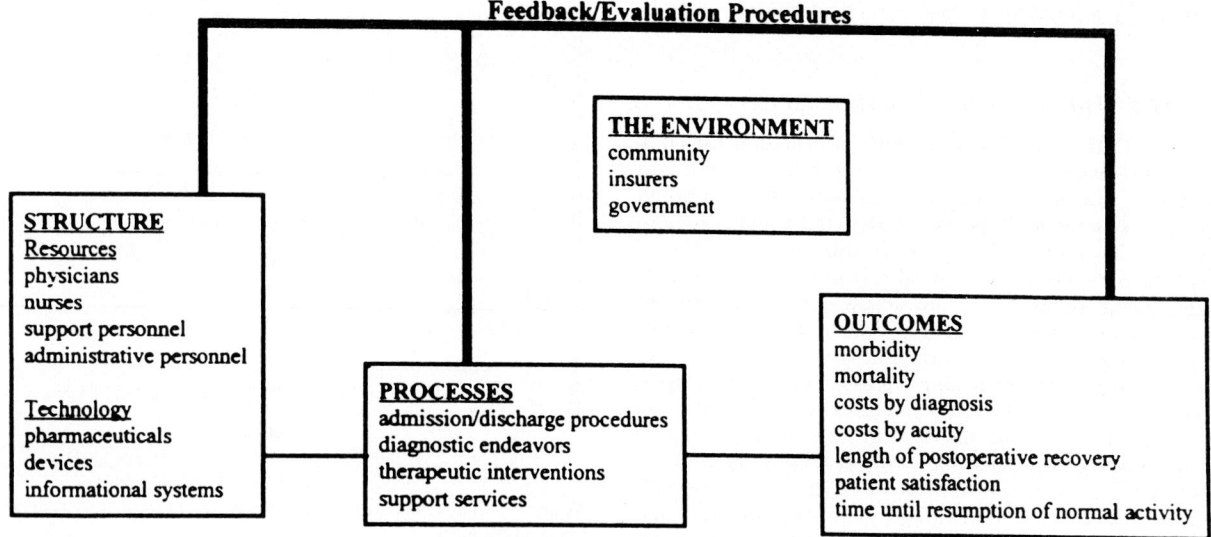

Figure 6-2. Key elements for assessing quality and value in health care.

confusing and sometimes make it difficult to place study results in proper perspective. What may appear to be a large clinically important difference may not be statistically significant if a study sample size is small, whereas less meaningful clinical differences may be highly statistically significant if the sample size is large enough. Special caution must be exercised when interpreting clinical differences that are reported as a relative risk reduction or relative change. For example, if intervention A is associated with a 25% actual reduction in the incidence of a complication (*e.g.*, 0.5 to 0.25) and intervention B is associated with a 1% actual reduction in the incidence of another complication (*e.g.*, 0.02 to 0.01), both could still be described as producing the same relative improvement (50%) despite different clinical utility. This has profound importance for the assessment of cost-effectiveness. A specified anesthetic or antiemetic might need to be administered to just four patients to prevent one episode of nausea and vomiting (hypothetical intervention A), whereas 100 or more costly spinal needles might be needed to prevent one case of post–dural puncture headache (hypothetical intervention B). Calculation of the "number needed to treat" is an important concept when examining cost differences between clinical alternatives.[16]

Anesthesiology is a medical specialty well suited to the application of service attributes as measures of outcome. Some attributes that can be measured to assess value include reliability, satisfaction, ability to handle unusual situations, ability to remedy failures, and cost consistent with service. A number of important characteristics and factors determine the validity and usefulness of outcome measures in assessing value in health care. Ideally, outcomes should reliably reflect the quality of care of the provider and should have limited dependence on correction for severity of illness. Outcome measures should also have construct validity, adequate statistical power, and be uniformly defined, observed, and recorded.[17] Outcome measures such as unadjusted complications and mortality have inherent limitations as direct reflections of provider quality of care. The "failure to rescue" rate (rate of death after complications) has been proposed as a further refined measure of quality of care that focuses on how complications are handled by the provider and de-emphasizes the cause of the complication (which is typically highly related to patient characteristics). Generally there are poor correlations between severity-adjusted death rates and severity-adjusted complication rates, and the rate of failure to rescue can be used to identify differences in quality of care among providers. For example, a reduced failure to rescue from complications has been associated with a higher percentage of board-certified anesthesiologists in a health facility[18] as well as the presence of an anesthesiologist compared to other physician providers of medical direction for anesthesia services.[19]

The value of any outcome rather than another in a given clinical situation may differ markedly according to the needs and preferences of a given patient. For example, evidence of prolonged intense sympathetic block may be a positive outcome for patients with reflex sympathetic dystrophy, but a negative outcome with respect to the postoperative course after a herniorrhaphy performed under lumbar epidural anesthesia. A specific type of substantial negative outcome is a "sentinel event," which is an unusual or unexpected outcome that should not occur under prevailing conditions of care. Sentinel events are often used to detect potential defects in the process or structure of care.

Anesthesia-related outcomes must specify which outcome of what process at what time is being examined. Specification of the process being employed must be explicit if causal relationships between any given outcome and process variable are to be critically evaluated. The salience of whether outcome is related to process cannot be overstated. Absent this relationship, the study of outcome is not useful as a guide for improving the value of anesthetic care. When adverse outcomes are poorly linked to specific anesthetic practices in given clinical circumstances, this only underscores the need for additional rigorous research to establish the causal link of process to outcome using techniques such as well-controlled clinical trials. Although such trials are accepted as the ideal methodology for evaluating a given therapy or process of care, this may be nearly impossible because of sample size requirements and statistical power limitations when the outcome of interest occurs at a low rate.[16] Nonetheless, with sufficiently large populations, variations in outcome can often be attributed to structure and process. Risk stratification organizes a multitude of patient variables to control for structure changes when determining how process affects outcome. The use of observational databases may be the only practical method of linking process to outcome when the outcome in question is rare. Although analysis of observational data can never prove causation as strongly as can randomized trials, reproducible strong associations between process and outcome may be sufficient to guide clinical practice in many instances. The widespread collection of computerized data combined with powerful analytic programs has facilitated outcome assessment for departmental quality improvement and increasingly for evaluation by health care purchasers and the public.

Evaluating Outcomes in Clinical Practice

There are two main sources of outcome information for clinicians: data published in the literature and data collected and analyzed from practice experience. Computerized information management systems are important tools to track outcomes and analyze the cost and benefits of specific aspects of health care delivery.[20] Effective electronic clinical information systems facilitate data analysis by allowing ready access to large amounts of data for queries and trend reports. Practitioners can readily apply statistical process control principles to evaluate outcomes in their individual practice settings. This is particularly important because published data may not exist regarding the outcome effects of a particular medical process or because published data may not be applicable to the practitioners' practice environment. As such, use of control charts and cause-and-effect diagrams can assist in defining variation in outcomes and formulating scientifically valid conclusions to facilitate improvement in outcome.

Cause-and-effect diagrams track the events in a process and allow them to be related to various outcomes. Figure 6-3 illustrates the use of such a diagram to outline the analysis of factors contributing to postoperative nausea and vomiting in a surgicenter setting. Data would be collected and managed in a computerized database. The flow chart and respective database then serve as a substrate for improvement of outcome by identifying sources of variability and then indicating where better control needs to be applied. The departmental database should ideally track as many of the factors identified in the flow diagram as possible.

Outcomes related to the adverse event can be tracked over time and examined to determine overall frequencies of events and control limits. If there is significant variability in the frequency or severity of an outcome (such as postoperative nausea and vomiting) by individual clinicians, adjusted for surgical case mix and patient characteristics, the cause-and-effect database can be used to identify variations within the process of care provided by an individual anesthesiologist (drugs, technique, *etc.*) to several patients. This approach helps reduce the bias entered by analysis of a single case, and provides more insight into the overall process of clinical care.

Control charts are a practical tool for assessing the impact on outcome of observed variation in the process being monitored.[21] Control charts graph the frequency of the outcome of interest on the *y*-axis versus time intervals on the *x*-axis (Fig. 6-4). A horizontal line indicates the mean of the observed measured values while dotted horizontal lines above and below the mean depict the upper and lower control limits (usually 2 or 3 standard deviations above or below the mean value). Use of nar-

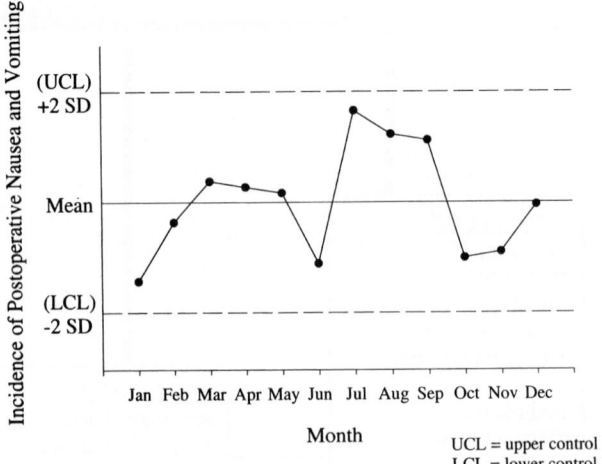

Figure 6-4. Statistical control chart for incidence of postoperative nausea and vomiting.

rower control limits incurs the risk of a Type I statistical error (concluding that a process of care yields results out of control range) while use of wider limits may be associated with a Type II error (concluding that the process results in outcomes within control when it does not).

A fundamental application of statistical control charting in individual practice settings is improvement of a health care process to optimize outcomes. This requires an understanding of the process, defining, measuring, and analyzing process indicators, and implementing changes in the process to subsequently measure as an improved outcome. Intermeshed with process improvement are the concepts of quality health care and outcomes management. The principles of continuous quality improvement promoted by Deming,[22] which profoundly influenced Japan's post-World War II manufacturing rebirth, are being applied in the health care industry. Deming's approach focused on statistical approaches to quality assessment and management by evaluating variation in outcome measures that are considered meaningful. Variation can arise either from common or from special causes. Common cause variation reflects the aggregate sum of small variations inherent to the process and determines the limits and capabilities of current operation.[21] For example, length of PACU or ICU stay can be summarized for a given diagnosis over some time period (*e.g.*, monthly, quarterly). This defines an average length of recovery time that is inherent for treating a specific condition, as well as its standard deviation. If the average duration for recovery is deemed excessive, independent of the monitoring period (*e.g.*, monthly, quarterly), common causes of variation require identification and analysis to reduce this variability. Large variability, suggested by a large standard deviation, is readily identifiable. In contrast, a large change in the complication rates between time periods may indicate special cause variations, which are not a continual part of the process. A large increase in the incidence of emergency reintubation or an unexpected frequency of negative-pressure pulmonary edema in the immediate recovery period might indicate problems with the processes of emergence from anesthesia such as variations in pharmacologic reversal of neuromuscular blockade or premature extubation in the OR. These types of problems can be resolved by addressing their specific etiologies rather than the overall process of care delivery itself. If the data outliers indicate a change toward worse outcome, this should prompt evaluation of the various processes defined in the cause-and-effect diagram in order to improve outcome. If the outliers indicate a change for the better, this also suggests that the variation in the process resulting in the beneficial

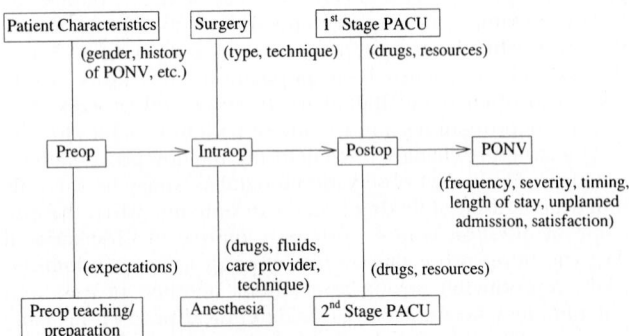

Figure 6-3. Cause-and-effect diagram for postoperative nausea and vomiting (PONV).

outcome should be identified and incorporated more broadly into clinical practice.

It is important to recognize that interventions to alter processes of care may also be indicated even if all data points fall within the upper and lower control limits (special cause variation has been eliminated and the system is in stable statistical control). For example, an outpatient facility may have a stable frequency of postoperative nausea and vomiting with little variation but the mean occurrence rate is increased. This may indicate poor quality relative to comparable external benchmark data, thus initiating an evaluation of processes of care to reduce the frequency of that adverse outcome to levels achievable in other similar practice settings.[23] The source of such benchmarking data may be from published scientific studies, unpublished data obtained from other comparable practice settings, or from national databases that evaluate the outcome(s) in question and define a broader basis for outcomes benchmarking. The determination of whether published data apply to an individual clinician's practice setting requires a careful, organized, evaluative approach.[24,25,26,27,28] While the use of statistical control charts is not the only method for individual practitioners to evaluate the quality of the services they provide, they do encourage continual assessment of outcomes and emphasize the importance of comparing performance over time (both internally and to potentially changing external standards). Continuous collection of outcome data, with results of performance information on quality improvement efforts reported to health care personnel in economic terms, can also be useful to highlight the relative value of various interventions and to promote practitioner involvement in outcomes management.

The context sensitivity of outcome measurements is exceedingly important. Responses to anesthetic management (such as effects on pulmonary function or the stimulation of nausea and vomiting) will differ, depending on whether they are measured one hour, one day, or three days afterwards. Although true for all health care outcomes, it is especially relevant for anesthesiology-related outcomes to note that the longer the period of observation, the weaker the connection between the observed outcomes and the processes of care. The plausible link between process and outcome is threatened significantly as the assessment period expands. The further one gets from direct and short-term outcome measurements, the less useful these measurements are for drawing valid conclusions about causality. Some complications related to anesthesia care, however, may not occur for a significant period of time. For example, a case of non-A, non-B hepatitis resulting from an "unnecessary" transfusion would go undetected in most hospital reviews, since the patient would probably be discharged before the condition was diagnosed. On the other hand, evaluation of nausea and vomiting in the ambulatory recovery area alone may be inadequate to determine the effects of anesthetic management unless further evaluations are made during the 24-hour period after patient discharge.[29] Specification of the point in time at which outcome is measured is a prerequisite for the validity of that measurement.

Another major consideration that characterizes outcome data is specification of its value content. This means that outcome must be examined for its relative value to whom, for what purpose, at what time, and under what circumstances. Anesthetic interventions may have considerable value for certain subsets of patients with highly specific indications or characteristics, but little or no value (even negative value) when applied to other subsets of patients. The main consideration is that the value of a given outcome must be defined and, where possible, quantified in relation to a specific purpose. If this is not done, the tendency is to overgeneralize and invalidly attribute outcome value to applications where it may not be warranted. Generalization about the beneficial effects (or lack thereof) of one anesthetic technique compared to another without due consideration to the specifics of time and circumstances can

lead to incorrect conclusions. For example, it may be that regional anesthesia *per se* is not any more beneficial to outcome in high-risk patients compared to general anesthesia, but that the use of regional techniques extended into the postoperative period for analgesia is beneficial compared to general anesthesia followed by "routine" parenteral pain control.[30]

The value or importance of a given anesthesia-related outcome also depends on whether it is viewed from the perspective of the primary customer or a secondary customer (Table 6-1). When considering nausea and vomiting after outpatient surgery, the patient can be considered a primary customer and the significance of this adverse outcome relates to the severity and frequency of its occurrence and the delay it causes in resumption of daily activities. In this situation, the health care facility is, by contrast, a secondary customer of anesthesia services and the outcomes relevant to nausea and vomiting include the rate of unanticipated admissions, patient satisfaction, the timing of onset of nausea and vomiting (and the subsequent impact on discharge time if vomiting occurs prior to discharge versus after discharge), as well as personnel costs and drug costs involved in managing this adverse event. Although anesthetic management relating to prophylaxis and/or treatment of postoperative nausea and vomiting varies among providers, the process of evaluating customer requirements and balancing those needs to achieve a high degree of satisfaction for all customers is essential to optimize the value of the medical services provided by anesthesiologists. Similarly, the context sensitivity of outcomes related to the establishment and use of an anesthesia preoperative evaluation clinic (APEC) depends on the viewpoint of the customer primarily affected by this service (Table 6-1). In this instance, the health care facility and surgical staff may be considered the primary customers, who consider the impact of this service on outcomes such as OR efficiencies, frequency of cancellations or delays, and reduction in preoperative testing costs as well as the frequency of need for additional medical specialist consultation (important in a capitated payment system).[31,32] Conversely, outcomes applicable to the patient (a secondary customer of these services) would include degree of satisfaction and other factors such as efficacy of preoperative education.

Application of Outcome Data to Manage Costs: Defining Effectiveness and Efficiency

Generalizability of outcome data can be described by the concepts of efficacy and effectiveness.[33] *Efficacy* reflects the beneficial effects of a process of medical care as measured by the outcome achieved in a specific population of patients. *Effectiveness* is defined as the outcome likely to be observed when that process of care is applied into wider clinical practice. Further distinctions must be made among evaluations of efficacy (can it work?), effectiveness (does it work?), and efficiency (is it worth it?). As described, an intervention can be efficacious but not effective, especially if there are difficulties transferring its application from the research setting to actual medical practice. The homogeneity often sought in well-controlled trials in an effort to validly link outcome with process can be at odds with the heterogeneity of the broader base of anesthetic practice. Equally importantly, an intervention can be effective but not efficient if there are other alternative interventions that achieve the same outcome at lower overall cost.

The slope of the overall cost-benefit curve (see Fig. 6-1) becomes more favorable if components of increasing expenditures that have minimal or no incremental benefit (flat slopes) or result in more harm than benefit (negative slopes) are eliminated. In addition to redistribution of resources from services with some benefit to services with greater benefit relative to cost, a more complicated approach to improving the composite cost–benefit relationship involves improving efficiency by altering processes of care to selectively eliminate more costly services

Table 6-1. IMPORTANT OUTCOMES AND VALUES FOR PRIMARY AND SECONDARY CUSTOMERS

POSTOPERATIVE NAUSEA/VOMITING (PONV)

Primary Customers

Patients

Important Outcomes
- Frequency of PONV
- Severity of PONV
- Delay in resumption of daily activities

Values
- Recovery without nausea or vomiting is highly valued by patients, regardless of the cost

Secondary Customers

Health care facility/Payers
Surgeons

Important Outcomes
- Unanticipated admission
- Timing of onset of PONV
- Impact on discharge time
- Personnel and drug costs related to therapy of PONV
- Patient satisfaction

Values
- Cost is highly valued by the health care facility and by payers, but probably not by surgeons
- Patient satisfaction is highly valued by both surgeons and the health care facility

PREOPERATIVE EVALUATION CLINIC

Primary Customers

Health care facility/Payers
Surgeons

Important Outcomes
- Operating room efficiency
- Frequency of case cancellation or delay
- Cost of preoperative tests
- Frequency and cost of specialist consultations

Values
- Health care facilities and payers value potential reduction in costs of:
  - Case cancellation or delay
  - Preoperative tests
  - Specialist consultations
- Surgeons value:
  - Reduced uncertainty regarding the preoperative requirements of anesthesiologists
  - Reduced likelihood of case cancellation or delay

Secondary Customers

Patients

Important Outcomes
- Patient satisfaction
- Patient education

Values
- Convenience
- Assurance that health care providers know about the patient's medical history and physical condition helping to ensure that upcoming surgery will be safe
- Opportunity to receive information and to ask questions regarding upcoming surgery

and replace them with less costly interventions of equal benefit. In the macroeconomic view, total costs equal the product of unit costs times quantity. The reduction of total health care costs must consider both of these factors, as illustrated by the case of laparoscopic cholecystectomy. The use of laparoscopic techniques has significantly shortened the time required for postoperative recuperation after cholecystectomy. Reduced length of hospital stay and better outcomes with less pain and disability allowing a more rapid return to function appear to be a classic example of improved efficiency (lower costs and better outcomes). However, in the macroeconomic view, aggregate cost savings have not been realized because, with the advent of laparoscopic techniques, the rates of cholecystectomy have dramatically increased as a result of the greater desirability of this procedure among patients and a lower threshold among surgeons for removing gallstones from mildly or intermittently symptomatic patients. In one health maintenance organization (HMO), the cholecystectomy rate increased by almost 60% over a 5-year period, and even though the average cost per cholecystectomy decreased by 25%, the total cost for all cholecystectomies increased by 11% because of the increase in surgical volume.[34] This example illustrates the complex nature of defining efficiency and cost saving, including the necessity of defining whether the basis of the analysis is microeconomic or macroeconomic. In addition, it highlights the need for physicians (including anesthesiologists) to balance the perspective of needs of individual patients with the overall needs of the population served by the health care system.

Strategies to contain costs may be applied by the health care system itself or by the individual health provider unit. Third-party payers have aggressively developed strategies to contain costs. The use of prospective payments and implementation of diagnosis-related groups (DRGs) have been adopted to manage care by reducing hospital utilization and limiting total allowable charges. Implementation of utilization review procedures, applying incentives to increase efficiency, and restricting resource accessibility are all tactics employed to contain costs, although resource constraints do not address the process or cost-effectiveness of care. Public insurers can mandate resource restriction, but private insurers do not have that mandate and therefore restrict what they will pay for a service, compelling provider units to contain costs to accommodate reduced charges. Providers generally apply cost-containment maneuvers that either restrain resource utilization or increase the cost-effectiveness and efficiency of various processes (Table 6-2). Examples of such strategies include shifting or optimizing case mix (*e.g.*, redistribution of specialized care to improve cost-

Table 6-2. STRATEGIES FOR COST CONTAINMENT

- Shifting or optimizing case mix
- Restraining or optimizing resource utilization
- Optimizing technology application *via* technology assessment
- Improving technology acquisition and maintenance procedures
- Utilization review, including outcome management and total quality improvement

effectiveness) and restraint or optimization of resource utilization by physicians. Limiting the availability of staff, beds, new programs, and technology may be used to contain costs and/or enhance revenues by increasing efficiency. Optimizing resource utilization by anesthesiologists involves their active participation in policymaking, protocols, and patient management, not only in the OR, but in the pre- and postoperative arenas as well. This requires physician education regarding the direct and variable costs of patient care and a method of providing feedback about performance.[35] Such information is essential for physicians to analyze the effectiveness of changes in the processes of care as well as the impact of technology assessment to ensure that technology is being used wisely and effectively. Providers not only desire to use the most reliable and proven technologies, but also wish to maintain a competitive edge by employing the latest technologies to improve outcome.

Maintenance of cost-effectiveness while simultaneously introducing new technologies is a continual dilemma for anesthesiology and critical care, by virtue of the heavy deployment of technology. A number of experts have emphasized the need for technology assessment before widespread use.[36,37] Such assessment must evaluate the technology's feasibility, efficacy, effectiveness, and economic impact. Information derived from such assessment can be utilized to improve technology acquisition and maintenance procedures, which should also help reduce costs. Establishment of technology assessment committees within institutions can be helpful in this regard by setting priorities, reviewing and recommending equipment requests, avoiding duplicative technologies, and reviewing feasibility, efficacy, and effectiveness data. Eventually, decisions must be made with regard to the economic impact of technology or health care interventions, which requires an understanding of basic methods of economic evaluation.

METHODS OF CLINICAL ECONOMIC ANALYSIS

Although current data to help the clinician decide on the best way to spend the health care dollar are limited, a few basic analytic techniques can help in the assessment of the clinical economic effects of various testing paradigms, drugs, devices and monitors, organizational systems, and other services. These include the use of cost-minimization, cost–benefit, cost-effectiveness, or cost–utility analysis (Table 6-3) and examination of outcome data that are needed to perform these analyses.[38,39] In discussing cost analyses, a brief review of terminology is warranted. *Variable costs* are those costs that change as a function of the volume of services provided. Examples of variable costs in the OR and PACU include those for supplies, drugs, and supplemental nursing services. *Fixed costs* are the ongoing costs of providing service, which are unrelated to volume and include items such as the salary of an OR manager and the costs of capital equipment such as OR and PACU monitors. Variable costs are much more responsive to cost-containment strategies; the challenge is to limit these variable costs without adversely affecting quality and outcome. In addition to classifying costs as fixed versus variable, the concept of direct versus indirect cost allocation is important. *Direct costs* can be explicitly quantitated and unambiguously attributed to the service rendered, whereas *indirect costs* are those of goods and services subsidiary to the primary service. Indirect costs are related to the consequences of the primary service and are frequently difficult to identify and quantitate, but include items such as increased turnover time of ORs, increased PACU time, unanticipated hospital admissions, and costs of drugs to treat side effects as well as time and resources lost from productive or consumptive activities. Finally, the differences between costs and charges must be acknowledged, recognizing that charges are often not a useful surrogate indicator of resource costs incurred with application of a specified health care intervention. Although charges are often used as proxies for cost, and cost-to-charge ratios are frequently applied to convert charges to costs, these conversion factors vary from institution to institution and even within an institution. The cost-to-charge ratio typically varies widely between service areas such as laboratory testing (traditionally small cost-to-charge ratios), pharmacy services, or the OR (commonly large cost-to-charge ratios). Cost center shifting is common in hospitals and can make it difficult to identify true costs of a service (such as the OR), since charges are often not distributed evenly and may even reflect costs of services in other areas of the hospital where reimbursement does not exist or is inadequate to cover cost. The methods of cost shifting in

Table 6-3. COMMON METHODS OF MEDICAL ECONOMIC ANALYSIS

Types of Economic Analysis	Appropriate Application	Limitations
COST MINIMIZATION ANALYSIS— identifies least costly of equally effective alternatives	Selecting among equally effective alternatives	Identical clinical effectiveness is not common, even in same/similar patients
COST–BENEFIT ANALYSIS— compares effectiveness in monetary units, assigning monetary value to outcomes ("willingness to pay")	Selecting intervention with greatest net benefit or best cost–benefit ratio when comparing regimens with different objectives or outcomes	Difficult to assign monetary value of life or health status
COST-EFFECTIVENESS ANALYSIS— unidimensionally evaluates incremental gain in benefit derived from additional cost, measuring effectiveness in physical units (e.g., life years gained), resulting in cost-effectiveness ratios to compare regimens	Selecting among regimens with different clinical effectiveness, when all regimens can be assessed using same outcome marker(s) of effectiveness	Not applicable to all types of interventions; regimens generally not comparable by cost-effectiveness analysis across disease processes
COST–UTILITY ANALYSIS— Multidimensionally evaluates effects of interventions on both quality and quality of life and measures effectiveness in terms of quality-adjusted units, as quality-adjusted life-years (QALY)	Aggregating multiple outcomes into a single adjusted measure of effectiveness; allows comparison of effectiveness of interventions in different medical fields	Difficult to compare utility across individuals; preference for health status varies with medical condition

place at any time in a given institution determine if any hospital unit (such as the OR) appears as a revenue generator or a revenue loser. For example, in a managed care or fixed (global) reimbursement environment, if radiology and laboratory services are attributed to the OR, these common elements of preoperative testing no longer represent a source of revenue; rather, such preoperative testing will be solely regarded as a cost attributable to anesthesia and OR services.

Cost-minimization analysis does not consider indirect costs and is the least useful analytic technique because it assumes identical consequences of each intervention. Historically, cost-minimization analysis has been the first-pass technique applied, because it is the easiest to perform and implementation does not require considerations other than absolute acquisition costs or other direct costs. However, the limitation of such analysis alone is illustrated by the distorted conclusions it might provide (*e.g.*, ketamine and morphine would be preferable to propofol and fentanyl for outpatient surgery). Variations in case mix (type of surgical procedure and patient condition) are generally not assessed when using "cost per case" to compare direct costs among anesthesia providers. Adjustments for case mix that account for type and duration of surgical procedure as well as patient demographics can be applied to define a "cost per unit" which allows a fairer comparison of direct costs among individual providers, anesthesia groups, and health care facilities.[40] However, when considering overall surgical costs for commonly performed low-to-moderate risk surgical procedures, severity of coexisting medical disease has less impact on resource consumption than the consequences of surgical decisions and techniques (*e.g.* the cost of a specific orthopedic joint prosthesis selected by the surgeon).[41]

Traditional cost–benefit analysis uses simple economic values, comparing dollar differences between competing costs with the economic values of benefits. The central feature of cost–benefit analysis is the translation of outcome quantities into dollar values. Although this concept is appealing, there are major practical limitations in placing monetary values on theoretic benefits to patients. For example, a healthy patient undergoing a brief surgical procedure probably places less value on avoidance of nausea than a patient undergoing intensive chemotherapy.

Cost-effectiveness analysis relates monetary costs to attributes of health benefits (effectiveness). Effectiveness is not valued in monetary terms, and a decision-maker, not the cost-effectiveness analyst, must make value judgments. A summary of the important elements of cost-effectiveness analyses is shown in Table 6-4. Effectiveness can be defined by whether an intervention does more good than harm, highlighting the role of outcome measurement as a major management tool in determining cost-effectiveness. Cost-effectiveness cannot be judged without a fundamental understanding of clinical effectiveness. It is essential to define a threshold of acceptability for clinical effectiveness because low-cost/low-effectiveness (low-quality) regimens may reflect the same quantitative cost-effectiveness ratios as regimens characterized by higher costs and higher effectiveness (high quality). The cost differential between interventions divided by the differential clinical unit change translates to the "value" by which the intervention is measured. Even if interventions are associated with additional costs, they may be cost-effective and represent greater value if improvement in outcome is adequate to decrease unit costs. The importance of considering indirect cost in overall cost-effectiveness analysis is exemplified by the scenario where greater pharmacy preparation time and administration costs for one drug with a low acquisition cost could (depending on the differential between direct and indirect costs) result in reduced cost-effectiveness than another drug of equal safety, effectiveness, and spectrum of activity but greater acquisition cost.

Classic cost-effectiveness analysis calculates net costs as the aggregate of direct medical and health care costs—including costs of hospitalization, physician time, medications, laboratory and other ancillary services, costs associated with adverse side effects of an intervention, and costs of treating diseases that would not have occurred if the patient had not lived longer as a result of the original intervention—then subtracts the cost savings in health care, rehabilitation, and custodial costs due to prevention or alleviation of disease. The cost-effectiveness ratio is then calculated as the net cost of one intervention versus another placed over the denominator of their respective outcome differences. Most calculations of net costs do not include lost wages due to missed time from work, despite the fact that loss of productivity may have profound financial consequences for individuals and society (*e.g.*, the difference of returning to work 5 days sooner because of application of a newer intervention such as laparoscopic cholecystectomy). Costs are generally adjusted to account for the difference between present and future monetary values, and discounting of future costs is commonly applied not only to account for inflation, but also to account for the fact that dollars not currently spent can be invested to yield a larger number of real dollars in the future. Because of controversy over the appropriate rate for discounting, most cost-effectiveness analyses test a range of discount rates.

Cost–utility analysis relates economic costs to utility units, which aggregate multiple outcomes into a single adjusted measure of effectiveness and represent the health improvement attributable to the intervention—*e.g.*, dollars spent per quality-adjusted life year (QALY) gained. QALYs represent the number of years of life expected, multiplied by a fraction representing the decrement in quality of life because of less than perfect health. For example, 2 years of life rated as 85% of perfect health translates to 1.7 QALYs. The use of QALYs as a measure of outcome permits comparison of the effectiveness of interventions in different medical fields.

A significant fraction of the published literature on the cost-effectiveness of medical technology utilizes decision analysis as the basis of comparison for various alternative clinical interventions (see Fig. 6-5). Decision analysis focuses on alternative interventions for a given clinical problem and their consequences, subsequent actions required, the consequences of these actions, and so on, until specific definable outcomes are achieved.[42] Probabilities are assigned to the consequences of the interventions, and costs are identified for each of the alternatives. Decision analysis is most useful in comparing interventions A and B, when studies directly comparing A to B are not available or when using data from studies comparing A to C and data from studies comparing B to C (or D). Because it is often difficult to compare studies of varying methodology, statistical methods such as meta-analysis may be required to permit pooling of data from multiple studies. Decision analysis requires explicit identification and stipulation of all possible clinical events that may occur. Each outcome is assigned a quantitative value to allow comparison with other possible outcomes (*e.g.*, survival, intermediate states of health, and morbidity). The values for the probabilities and the outcomes are typically based on estimates from the literature or expert consensus. Sensitivity analysis can be applied to the decision model to determine

---

Table 6-4. COMPONENTS OF COST-EFFECTIVENESS (UTILITY) ANALYSIS

- Identification of all clinical strategies and alternative interventions
- Stipulation of the target population
- Determination of *all* costs for each intervention
- Determination of *all* benefits for each intervention
- Application of discounting if extended time frames of analysis
- Calculations of cost-effectiveness (utility) ratios
- Testing stability of predictions with sensitivity analysis

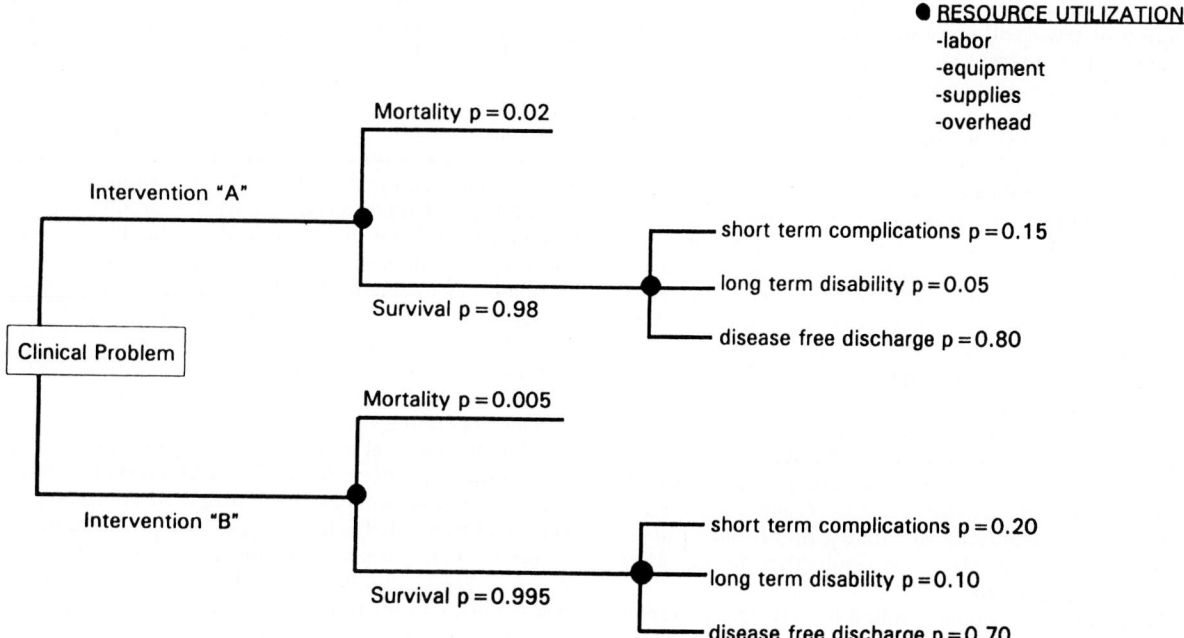

Figure 6-5. Example of decision analysis that can be used to assess cost-effectiveness.

its stability as the underlying parameters are varied singly or simultaneously, allowing application of such models to specific clinical environments. Decision analysis and subsequent application of sensitivity analysis can thus be used to calculate and then evaluate the cost-effectiveness ratios for all alternatives to address a clinical problem. For example, decision analysis has been applied to determine cost-effectiveness ratios for ondansetron, droperidol, and metoclopramide for the prevention of postoperative nausea and vomiting and suggests that the relative cost-effectiveness of prophylactic use of each of these drugs depends significantly on the expected pretreatment incidence of vomiting.[43] The relative cost-effectiveness of these and other drugs depends on the chosen measurement end points; it has been suggested that unplanned hospital admissions after outpatient surgery, patient satisfaction, and duration of recovery period are potentially more crucial outcome measures than the incidence of vomiting alone when assessing the relative economic value of various choices for antiemetic prophylaxis or therapy.[44]

When evaluating these types of economic analyses, direct benefits and costs are the easiest factors to quantitate. Short- or long-term survival or reduction of hospital or overall direct costs can be examined as markers of benefit. In contrast, a specified technology or health care intervention may have certain indirect benefits, which are often difficult to measure. For example, better coagulation monitoring or the use of drugs such as aprotinin may mean less blood product usage and less hepatitis in the future, but it is profoundly difficult to quantitate the avoidance of future morbidity. Therefore, potential reduction of future morbidity and improvement in quality of life are rarely evaluated as indirect benefits of health care interventions. Indirect costs are just as difficult to measure as indirect benefits. When a monitor or test is used to obtain physiologic data that prompt the performance of multiple additional tests and interventions, it is often unknown how to figure in these costs. This difficulty is faced when assessing nearly every technology and testing protocol in the current high-tech practice of medicine. Preanesthetic evaluation, intraoperative management, and postoperative care are three major areas of practice of anesthesiology where clinical economic analysis can be applied to assess value.

COST-EFFECTIVE PREOPERATIVE PRACTICES

The historical practice of routine preoperative hospital admission of even medically stable patients before major operations, including cardiac, thoracic, joint replacement, and major abdominal or urologic procedures, has been with replaced with the contemporary practice of "a.m. admission" processes. This has reduced costs without any demonstrable adverse effect on surgical or anesthetic outcome.[45] Other preoperative practices have been modified because of cost and efficiency concerns. For example, the cost-effectiveness of preoperative autologous blood donation has been examined both for cardiac and for several types of major noncardiac surgery.[46,47,48] Decision analyses utilizing a large number of clinical variables have determined that the cost of autologous blood donation may vary from $40,000 to over $23 million per QALY saved, with the differences between autologous blood collections and transfusion requirements explaining the majority of the variation in cost-effectiveness among the surgical procedures studied.[46,47,48] These types of analyses have altered clinical practice by demonstrating that the collection and processing of a large number of autologous units for operations with low transfusion requirements can make preoperative autologous blood donation far less cost-effective than allogeneic transfusions.[48] The cost per year of life saved (QALY) by preoperative autologous blood donation is several-fold greater than the cost-effectiveness (utility) estimates of many other common and accepted medical practices such as coronary revascularization to treat three-vessel or left-main coronary disease ($6,000/QALY) or screening for cervical cancer every 4 years ($11,000/QALY).[47]

Laboratory testing is a common aspect of both inpatient and outpatient preoperative assessment as well as postoperative care of the critically ill surgical patient. It has been estimated that several billion dollars are spent in North America on preoperative testing (and the subsequent follow-up evaluations initiated secondary to that testing) and that a sizable portion of these costs could be saved by the selective ordering of tests based on patient history or findings of the physical exam.[49] Relatively few abnormalities are unsuspected after a thorough preanesthetic visit, and even then, these abnormalities alter perioperative management in only a very small fraction of cases.[49,50] Nonselective ordering of tests neither results in beneficial changes in perioperative care nor serves as an effective screen for detection of unsuspected disease, and most clinicians currently agree that many preoperative tests can be safely eliminated by ordering only those based on specific abnormalities in the history and physical exam.[49,51]

Extra testing not indicated by history or physical findings bears not only additional direct cost, but also potential extra indirect costs in the form of greater liability risks if abnormalities detected on preoperative screening are not pursued. In addition, assuming that the results of laboratory results are independent of one another, the more tests ordered, the greater likelihood that abnormal results will appear. For example, assuming specificity for laboratory testing of 97%, if 6 tests are ordered, there is almost a 20% chance $[100 \times (0.97)^6]$ that at least one of the tests will be abnormal. Such abnormalities can often generate hidden preoperative costs in addition to the cost of the screening tests themselves. Selective preoperative testing is necessary to reduce direct costs and potentially improve the efficiency of OR schedules by eliminating the need to pursue falsely positive or slightly abnormal results that do not affect perioperative management.

Anesthesiologists are uniquely suited to perform or oversee preoperative evaluative processes because of their knowledge and experience in the effects of perioperative interventions on patient physiology (*e.g.*, the hemodynamic effects of spinal or epidural anesthesia compared to general anesthesia in patients with critical aortic stenosis). Although a primary care physician may understand optimal health status for daily life, this may not represent an optimal preoperative condition. Involvement of anesthesiologists in preoperative assessment maximizes the appropriate application of individualized diagnostic and therapeutic regimens according to the patient's condition and the surgical and anesthetic requirements, thus optimizing cost-effectiveness by reducing the incidence of either too much or too little preoperative evaluation and preparation. Perioperative evaluation and management under the guidance of an anesthesiologist may not have the lowest direct cost, but it may be more cost-effective than ordering tests nonselectively or experiencing unnecessary and costly OR delays related to suboptimal preoperative preparation that could have been avoided by consulting with an anesthesiologist.

The Anesthesia Preoperative Evaluation Clinic: A Model for Value-Based Anesthesia Practice

An anesthesia preoperative evaluation clinic (APEC) which provides near-complete perioperative medical assessment for complex patients can result in impressive institutional savings, despite start-up and operating expenses, because of more focused use of diagnostic testing and medical consultation as well as subsequent improvements in OR efficiency.[31,32] When the anesthesiologist takes the leading role in determining the appropriateness of the patient for anesthesia and surgery, OR utilization and efficiency can be improved by reducing the number of unanticipated delays related to inadequate preoperative evaluation. Delays and cancellations in the OR adversely impact optimal OR utilization and efficiency, and create financial problems related to lost revenues unbalanced by matching reduced costs. When an operating suite is not utilized efficiently, costs may actually increase because personnel costs can increase for work conducted after regularly scheduled hours. Inadequate preoperative preparation can result in inefficiencies in the OR even when patients arrive at the appropriate time prior to surgery. The optimal timing of ambulatory preoperative assessment is dependent on the individual facility. Completion of preoperative assessments in a very early time frame may not reduce OR cancellation rates compared to completion more proximate to the date of scheduled surgery, although it may provide greater flexibility in scheduling surgery by resulting in a pool of patients to fill slots of OR time that would otherwise be underutilized.[52] Conversely, strict adherence to protocols that define time-based performance criteria for completion of specific preoperative processes can help anticipate problems that are likely to result in a cancellation on the day of surgery, potentially allowing time for correction of the problem and avoiding cancellation. Typically, inadequate preoperative preparation for the OR is manifest by the detection during the immediate preanesthesia assessment of medical problems that require additional evaluation and management, thereby delaying elective surgery; however, other nonmedical issues as simple as incomplete financial information also can create significant delays in the OR. Such nonmedical issues may seem less relevant, but they are important factors that must be considered in developing an effective, efficient operating room management scheme.

While the medical evaluation of the patient prior to anesthesia and surgery, with reduction of wasted resources by eliminating unnecessary preoperative testing and consultations, is the central element of effective preoperative preparation, other key elements in the process include centralized reporting of all important preoperative information (diagnostic and laboratory test results, consult reports, admission and financial information) as well as patient and family education regarding anesthesia and the perioperative experience. The APEC model is an effective means for anesthesiologists to be more active in perioperative medicine, enhance the value of their services, and potentially improve patient satisfaction secondary to streamlining of the preoperative process. In addition, patient anxiety may be reduced because of more in-depth patient education than that feasible when the anesthesiologist first encounters an ambulatory patient immediately prior to surgery.

The concepts utilized by an APEC generally require selective modification to fit the individual characteristics of each health care facility. Depending on resources and needs, prespecified criteria vary with respect to which patients are formally processed through an APEC, based upon clinical guidelines for preoperative assessment. All patients should generally undergo some form of minimal preoperative screening with central collection of important medical and administrative data early enough prior to elective surgery so that the OR schedule can be adjusted to avoid an unfilled OR due to inadequate preoperative patient preparation. Finally, in the context of overall OR management, a successful preoperative preparatory process provides the mechanism for all important information to be available to the appropriate members of the OR team. For example, not only would the anesthesiologist scheduled to attend to the patient intraoperatively be made aware of the specific preanesthesia evaluation prior to the day of surgery, but the surgeon would also be notified in a timely manner of any special recommendations that might impact scheduling for subsequent management (*e.g.*, if the anesthesiologist recommended overnight intensive monitoring in a high-risk orthopedic patient). Efficient OR management also mandates that requirements for any special equipment or medical device be communicated to the responsible staff well in advance of the scheduled procedure, to avoid delays related to unavailability of specialized surgical instruments, prostheses or implants, or other special equipment.

EFFECTIVE RESOURCE UTILIZATION IN THE OPERATING ROOM
Anesthetic Drugs and Supplies

Anesthesia drug expenses represent a small fraction of total perioperative costs, but the large number of doses administered contributes to substantial aggregate costs. In the aggregate, cost savings associated with prudent drug selection can be substantial. If just $20 were saved in every anesthetic delivered in the U.S., about $500 million of direct costs would be saved annually. Total annual world expenditure for inhaled anesthetics (excluding nitrous oxide) has been estimated to be $450 million.[53] Uniformly reducing fresh gas flows from 5 to 2.5 L/min would save approximately $100 million annually in the U.S. and about $225 million worldwide.[53,54] This example illustrates how relatively simple measures can have significant impact on cost reduction without markedly impairing styles of clinical practice. Cost-saving measures such as this generate relatively little controversy, are easy to implement, and apply to large numbers of cases. However, anesthesiologists are more frequently confronted with choices between modes of anesthesia care that produce similar acceptable outcomes but at different levels of cost-effectiveness. The decisions involved in making these choices are significantly more complicated and contentious than resolving to conserve resources by reducing fresh gas flows while delivering the same inhalation anesthetics.

When considering the costs of anesthetic drugs and other technologies, a number of variables must be evaluated when comparing "expensive" drugs to apparently cheaper alternatives (Table 6-5). The costs of anesthetic drugs include the cost of the drug itself as well as adjuvant agents, equipment and supplies (*e.g.*, infusion devices or special vaporizers), and the amount of drug wastage that occurs during typical use. In addition, there are other indirect costs associated with a given anesthetic drug that can be difficult to quantitate and are frequently not considered. These include the indirect cost of drug preparation and setup time (which may prolong OR turnover time) as well as the costs of extended PACU stay or additional drug therapy to treat postoperative side effects. Controversy exists over the relative impact of anesthetic drug choices on such indirect costs, intangible costs, or future health care costs.[55]

Direct costs of anesthetic drugs and supplies typically constitute a very small fraction of total perioperative costs; however, they are frequently questioned by health facility administrators, and justification for the use of more expensive drugs generally requires examining the total cost of a therapeutic strategy rather than only drug acquisition costs.[56,57] For example, induction agents such as propofol may have greater initial acquisition costs than alternatives but can potentially save overall hospital costs when used appropriately for outpatient surgery and when patient care protocols allow for less intense and shorter-duration nursing care with fewer complications and earlier dismissal of patients. Conversely, propofol infusions utilized for long, major operations in patients who require postoperative hospitalization may not provide for earlier ambulation and discharge and may not be as cost-effective in this situation as alternative anesthetics. The impact of shorter-acting drugs and those with fewer side effects on overall costs is context sensitive. During long surgical procedures, such drugs may not offer significant advantages over older, less expensive longer-acting

counterparts.[14,58] Under these circumstances, simply promoting cost consciousness using education can reduce total expenditures for a given category of drugs,[59] although long-acting neuromuscular blocking drugs may be associated with residual neuromuscular blockade and longer postoperative recovery time.[60] The greater direct costs of an anesthetic agent must be balanced against the direct and indirect costs of alternative anesthetics that may be associated with a greater frequency of side effects such as postoperative nausea and vomiting. In a fast-paced ambulatory setting, rapid-acting drugs with decreased side effect profiles may theoretically improve OR efficiency by decreasing times between short surgical procedures and reducing facility discharge time (especially when "fast-tracking" with bypass of phase I recovery is feasible).[61] This is particularly important at the end of the workday to reduce recovery room personnel costs.

Many alternative drug choices are available to anesthesiologists, and drugs in the same therapeutic class commonly have widely differing costs. The acquisition costs may vary 40- or 50-fold in any anesthetic pharmacologic category, and it is estimated that the 10 highest expenditure drugs may account for more than 80% of anesthetic drug expenses at many institutions.[62] Surveys indicate that physicians are interested in reducing the cost of drug therapy, but they desire more knowledge of relative acquisition costs and other cost information to make more informed drug selection decisions.[63] Selection and utilization of older but nonetheless effective opioids and muscle relaxants may be associated with considerable savings, especially during longer operations.[64] Such savings may, however, be offset by other costs if there is unanticipated or unplanned prolongation of recovery from anesthesia or requirement of pharmacologic therapy for reversal of prolonged drug effects (or side effects) associated with the use of longer-acting agents.[65] Although newer, typically shorter-duration and more specific-acting drugs are often very useful in short- to intermediate-duration procedures, the marginal benefit of their use may be reduced in longer operations, especially in healthy patients. There is little doubt that newer and more "expensive" drugs are often easier to use, but there are essentially no data to support or refute the hypothesis that most patients would have an equally satisfactory experience when older, less expensive drugs are titrated to effect based on an understanding of pharmacokinetics, pharmacodynamics, and perioperative physiology. It is the bias of many experienced clinicians that prompt awakening can be achieved with a variety of general anesthetics, if they are utilized optimally by experienced clinicians and not compared in a rigid, artificial study protocol. Similarity of awakening times, however, does not necessarily translate to other aspects of recovery profiles.

Disciplined application of pharmacoeconomic and pharmacoepidemiologic principles is required to define the relative value of new drugs. This not only necessitates evaluation of efficacy and side effects, but also involves assessment of parameters such

Table 6-5. REPRESENTATIVE COSTS OF ANESTHESIA DRUGS AND MONITORS

Direct Costs	Indirect Costs
Acquisition of drug or monitor	Rescue therapy for complications
Adjuvant agents or required materials	Delay in resumption of normal activities (lost productivity)
Drug or material wastage	Extended PACU, ICU, or hospital stay (especially if complications)
Consumable equipment and supplies for drug delivery or application of monitoring	Excess operating room or facility turnover time (drug preparation/ drug recovery and preparation/initiation of monitors)
Monitors and other capital equipment	Drug and equipment storage, preparation and setup, including labor
Labor related to insertion and use of monitors (*e.g.*, PAC, SSEP, TEE)	Maintenance and repair of monitoring and drug delivery equipment, including labor
	Drug- or monitoring-related complications

PAC, pulmonary artery catheter; SSEP, somatosensory-evoked potentials; TEE, transesophageal echocardiography as the time until resumption of normal physical or mental activity as well as other measures of outcome. Studies evaluating recovery-related productivity losses are important because these losses, like direct health care expenditures, have an economic impact on society. Even if prevention of a postoperative side effect (such as nausea and vomiting by an expensive antiemetic or a particular anesthetic drug) costs more than the medical costs of treatment of this problem, the preventive approach might be far more economically favorable when the potential economic losses of patients are considered. Such analyses are complex and difficult to perform, and the value of a given intervention will vary among patients in relation to their underlying condition, the anticipated surgical procedure, and the postoperative care requirements.

Beyond drug costs, there is significant potential for cost savings associated with reduction of waste in disposable equipment and materials. Examination of clinical practice patterns to eliminate wasteful and unnecessary practices can result in sizable cost savings without any compromise in quality of medical care. For example, use of computerized tracking methods for continuous monitoring of OR supplies and ongoing evaluation of prepackaged, customized surgical supply packs (permitting nurses to alter preference lists as surgeons' preferences evolve) can result in large savings (more than 60% related to decreased wastage of disposable items such as sutures).[66] Another method that has been demonstrated to be successful in reducing costs has been implementation of the requirement that users provide a justification for the more costly choice among several alternatives for disposable supplies or pharmaceuticals (*e.g.*, neuromuscular blocking drugs).[67,68] Behavior modification programs based on education of staff about costs and general guidelines for equipment and drug utilization have reported variable long-term success.[62,66] This success may be enhanced not only by frequent reinforcement, but also by making clinicians cognizant of the concept of opportunity costs: with limited resources, those utilized for one commodity cannot be used for others that might produce potentially greater benefits.

The concept of opportunity costs is illustrated by data comparing the aggregate annual cost savings of using ionic (versus nonionic) contrast in low-risk patients.[6] The $3.5 million savings per year associated with use of only ionic contrast could alternatively be used to fund breast cancer screening to save 450 female life years (35 deaths), cervical cancer screening to save 2600 female life years (100 deaths), or cholesterol management to prevent 13 sudden deaths, 105 myocardial infarctions, and 250 cardiac events.[6] In the prospective payer market, opportunity costs are an important focus when deciding how to spend limited resources. Rather than abandoning new and useful technology (*e.g.*, drugs, devices) that has improved the current quality of anesthesia care, methods should be focused on eliminating wastage and unnecessary use of valuable but limited resources. In economic terms, it is conceptually useful to relate the cost of the latest unit of health service produced (the marginal cost) to the price that consumers are willing to pay for it (the marginal price). The theoretical point where marginal cost equals marginal price defines the level of service at which clinicians should begin the process of trimming waste and eliminating interventions that cost more than they are worth (valued).

Anesthetic Techniques: Cost Considerations

Value-based anesthesia management, when applied to the choice of anesthetic techniques, requires balancing the benefits and risks of these techniques against the total costs resulting from these choices. When assessing choices for anesthetic techniques, value can be attributed either to similar outcomes at lower total cost (both direct and indirect) or to better outcomes even if total costs are higher. Occasionally, anesthesiologists are able to utilize anesthetic techniques by which improved outcomes can be achieved at lower total cost, but this is less common. Despite general agreement about the definable end points used to quantitate the concept of increased value, the process of deriving value-based decisions regarding choice of anesthetic technique remains complex.

Certain conditions surrounding the planned surgical intervention often supersede cost considerations and predetermine the choice of anesthesia. For example, patient requests (desire to be awake versus asleep) and patient conditions (hypovolemia, severe coagulopathy), as well as provider skill, surgical requirements, and technology available may determine or limit the potential choices for anesthesia. Despite these limiting conditions, many surgeries are possible with two or more different techniques. Although there are a number of potential choices of techniques, the most common are general anesthesia, regional anesthesia (peripheral nerve block, central neuraxial or intravenous regional with or without sedation), combined general-regional anesthesia, local anesthesia with sedation, sedation alone, or local anesthesia alone. The last two choices are utilized only for minor or very limited procedures and are associated with apparent economy,[69] especially when local anesthesia alone is feasible.

Commonly, the choice is between general and regional techniques, especially when the surgical procedure is suitable for either technique. Examples of surgical procedures that can be readily accomplished with either regional or general techniques include lower or upper extremity orthopedic and vascular procedures, genitourinary procedures, and herniorrhaphies. Assessment of the value of specific anesthetic management strategies for such procedures is often difficult and requires analysis of the impact of a given technique on total costs, outcome, and perioperative efficiency. In addition, patients, payers, administrators, surgeons, and anesthesiologists may value alternative outcomes differently.

Currently, data on total costs of alternative anesthetic techniques are not widely available. Some data on total charges are obtainable, but as noted above, much caution must be exercised in the application of charge data. Analysis of some of the available cost data suggests that regional anesthesia may be more economical with regard to direct costs than general anesthesia.[70] However, more data are necessary before firm conclusions can be derived about the impact of anesthetic technique on total costs (including intraoperative, postoperative, and morbidity costs). Systematic evaluation of direct costs of various anesthetic techniques (drugs, equipment, and services) has not been conducted, and these costs may differ widely among institutions. In addition, indirect costs such as out-of-hospital costs (*e.g.*, recovery time at home away from work) or expenses of treating complications related to provision of a given anesthetic technique are largely unquantified. These gaps in our current knowledge are compounded by the likelihood that total costs and benefits may be substantially different for a given anesthetic technique applied to different surgical populations. For example, although several benefits have been attributed to epidural anesthesia and analgesia, and it appears that some of these positive effects may be attributable to postoperative influences after major operative procedures in high-risk patients,[30,71,72,73] actual cost analyses are either rudimentary or absent.

Unfortunately, anesthesia outcome data are currently incomplete; therefore, many comparisons of anesthetic techniques remain somewhat controversial. Few studies have quantitated outcome characteristics that reflect the value patients may place on their anesthetic and surgical experience. Such attributes as "patient satisfaction" or "time until resumption of normal activities" are difficult to measure and have not been commonly reported, although determination of the value of a specific anesthetic technique requires assessment of how these techniques affect patient experiences (*e.g.*, nausea potentially resulting from general anesthesia and headaches potentially resulting from spinal or epidural anesthesia). In addition, the impact of anesthetic technique on the duration or requirement for postanesthesia monitoring, the overall efficiency of perioperative care, staffing requirements, and the cost of complications must be assessed. Accounting for both direct costs (*e.g.*, equipment and material costs, drug costs, labor costs) and indirect costs (*e.g.*, costs of rescue therapy to treat complications, labor and facility costs generated because of prolonged or complicated postoperative recovery) will enable anesthesiologists to determine the relative value of different anesthetic techniques in a given practice setting. The relative value of a specific intervention will vary in different clinical settings and be affected by patient characteristics, surgical considerations, and health facility constraints. Even the impact of an intervention such as forced air warming on net total perioperative costs depends on patient and surgical characteristics and institutional factors related to cost accounting.[74] Since most OR costs are fixed or semivariable[57] the reduction of time involved in postanesthesia recovery by maintaining core normothermia[74,75] may not decrease overall costs unless the aggregate time in the OR or recovery room is reduced sufficiently to decrease staffing or actually allow additional cases to be performed without increasing personnel costs. The influence of various anesthetic interventions on outcomes, perioperative efficiency, and total cost is an important area in which anesthesiologists can define value to patients, surgical colleagues, payers, and health facilities.

Costs of Monitoring

The costs of monitoring include the cost of the anesthesiologist, monitors, consumable items, OR time, maintenance costs, and the costs of complications (see Table 6-5). Capital equipment used for monitoring, assuming a long operational period and a high degree of utilization, generally does not contribute to significant cost on a per-case or per-hour basis. On the other hand, the costs of consumable items as well as the cost of operating time during the placement of invasive monitors can be significant, especially if no other patient-related activity is simultaneously occurring.

Clinical and economic guidelines have been proposed for evaluation of technology (such as monitoring equipment) prior to adoption and implementation.[76] Application of such an analysis requires inclusion of all relevant outcomes and incremental costs of alternative technologies, appropriate discounting of costs and clinical outcomes, and performance of sensitivity analyses. This approach has been criticized, but such guidelines provide a preliminary methodology for systematic economic comparison of various technologies. Such types of analyses have been applied to determine the cost per QALY of applying mechanical ventilation in the elderly (older than 85 years)[77] as well as in patients with various types of cancers.[78]

The magnitude of the problems of evaluating high-cost technology is exemplified by the pulmonary artery (PA) catheter. More than $2 billion is spent annually in the U.S. on hospital charges for the catheter and introducer sheath, sterile setup, transducers, and disposable thermodilution cardiac output supplies; physician charges for insertion of the catheter; and lab charges for mixed venous blood gas tension analyses. Despite the paucity of prospective, randomized trials suggesting beneficial outcome effects with use of the PA catheter to achieve specific therapeutic goals, application of this technology is widespread.[79,80,81] Although the economic issues associated with the routine use of PA catheters are obviously important, the analysis is extremely complex. Application of cost-utility analysis and sensitivity analysis techniques to evaluate the economic impact of PA catheterization in patients undergoing coronary artery revascularization suggests that cost-effectiveness would be less than $50,000 per QALY if PA catheterization reduced mortality

by ≥0.2%, even if the incremental cost of PA catheterization were as high as $500 compared to central venous catheterization alone.[82] Although this compares favorably with some other accepted technologies (albeit in this theoretical derivation, the cost per QALY was greater than the estimated cost-effectiveness of three-vessel CABG surgery itself[46]), the sample size requirements (200,000) would be prohibitively large to test the hypothesis of such an effect of PA catheterization on mortality in a randomized clinical trial.[82]

Superficial analysis might suggest tremendous cost savings if significant numbers of patients with good ventricular function underwent CABG surgery without routine use of a PA catheter. In at least two studies, more than 1200 patients (68%) did not receive routine PA catheter monitoring,[83,84] which conservatively translates into more than $750,000 of direct cost savings in those studies alone. If one half of nearly 400,000 patients undergoing CABG annually in the U.S. did not routinely receive a PA catheter, this would represent approximately $150 million of direct cost reduction each year. However, the indirect costs of use and, if not used, the indirect costs of failure to provide optimal cardiopulmonary support must be assessed. For example, if invasive monitoring helps prolong the life of terminally ill patients, it will be associated with enormous increases in direct costs and may provide limited benefit. On the other hand, if patients who would have died or suffered life-threatening complications can be spared because of precisely titrated care made possible by invasive monitoring, then the benefit is enormous. The direct costs of using PA catheters may therefore be trivial compared with the potential indirect savings. Although the "conservative" approach of selectively using invasive monitors is encouraged in the current medicoeconomic climate, such conservatism may represent a false economy both fiscally and in terms of outcome in certain patients. Practice parameters that guide physicians to the proper use of such technology may not only improve quality of care, but also help decrease costs by reducing unnecessary variability and suboptimal application of technology in clinical practice.[79,80,81,85]

The pulse oximeter is another example of technology that has found widespread use because of the belief that it contributes to better patient outcome. In contrast to the PA catheter, however, simple amortization of the acquisition and maintenance costs (estimated at $3500 and $500, respectively) of a pulse oximeter with a finger probe reused in a single OR for 2000 patients over 2 years yields a cost of approximately $2 per patient. Although the specific cost per case will vary depending on the purchase price, maintenance costs, and utilization rate, the estimated cost per patient of the pulse oximeter is orders of magnitude less than the cost of a PA catheter. Analogous to the PA catheter, there are as yet no prospective controlled investigations that have conclusively demonstrated in a scientific manner that pulse oximetry itself actually makes a difference in morbidity and mortality. A randomized multicenter trial of pulse oximetry in Denmark, which involved 20,802 patients divided into two groups, did not demonstrate an effect of that monitoring on actual morbidity and mortality, except for a decreased incidence of intraoperative myocardial ischemia.[86] For the most serious postoperative complications, anesthesia-related death and myocardial infarction, with incidences of 0.034% and 0.15%, respectively, the sample size requirement to achieve a statistical power of 90% in the latter study would have been more than 1 million and 500,000, respectively. To effectively assess the utility of pulse oximetry, outcome studies would need sample populations many-fold larger than used in the Danish study, would have to include a significantly greater proportion of patients at risk for adverse outcomes (*e.g.*, ASA status III and IV, age over 60 years), and are unlikely to be conducted.

In the absence of such outcome studies, the decision to incorporate pulse oximetry as an ASA standard for basic intraoperative (as well as postanesthesia care unit) monitoring has been motivated primarily by evidence that pulse oximetry is superior to clinical judgment in providing early warning of hypoxic events and because retrospective review of anesthetic management associated with adverse events indicates that a large fraction of negative outcomes could be prevented by application of this technology. Significantly fewer patients have experienced "recovery room impact events" such as hypotension or dysrhythmias after pulse oximetry was introduced into the OR.[87] Another study found 11 major anesthesia-related mishaps in an analysis of more than 1 million anesthetics delivered to ASA I and II patients.[88] In this study eight anesthetic-related accidents involving inadequate ventilation or oxygenation and five deaths occurred during the 9.5 years before routine use of pulse oximetry and only one accident and no deaths occurred during the 3 years after use of pulse oximetry. Other evidence also suggests that pulse oximetry is associated with a reduction in anesthetic-related complications and unanticipated ICU admissions, primarily those related to the need to rule out myocardial infarction,[89] possibly because pulse oximetry facilitates early identification of hypoxemic, hypotensive, or low-perfusion states before subsequent ischemic changes become manifest or persist long enough to be of concern. This postulate is consistent with the Danish multicenter study demonstrating that angina or ECG ischemia occur in significantly fewer patients monitored with pulse oximetry than in a control group not monitored with pulse oximetry.[86] Although the marginal cost of additional ICU time has not been quantified,[89] a tremendous cost savings associated with the use of pulse oximetry is apparent even if we consider only the reduction in the rate of ICU admissions to rule out myocardial events.

Another retrospective analysis of the benefits of pulse oximetry, by the Closed Claims Project of the Professional Liability Committee of the ASA, determined that of 348 "preventable" injuries or deaths, "pulse oximetry . . . would have been efficacious in preventing injury in 138 cases."[90] In contrast, monitors other than pulse oximetry or capnometry (*e.g.*, the PA catheter or automated blood pressure devices) were considered potentially preventative in just 7% of the preventable injuries or deaths. The findings of the Closed Claims Project and those of other studies previously cited[87,88,89] have considerable economic consequences; that is, if use of pulse oximetry is associated with reduction of preventable injury or death, not only will the indirect cost savings to patients and their families be great (especially in the case of permanently disabling injury), but the direct cost savings will also be substantial. Based on closed claims data, the median total cost of settlement or judgment was 11 times greater for injuries judged preventable by additional monitoring ($250,000) compared with those judged not preventable ($22,500).[90] This reduction in the cost of adverse outcomes has been recognized by medical liability insurance underwriters, so that the "liability insurance relativity factor," an industry index of relative risk, subsequently decreased significantly for the specialty of anesthesiology.

Although there is still no published cost–benefit analysis of pulse oximetry, the type of data reviewed above strongly suggest that pulse oximetry improves the safety and outcome of anesthesia care and is probably cost-effective in this manner. Because of the low incidence of critical events and the presence of confounding factors such as other changes in technology, new drugs, and an overall increased awareness of risk management issues with an emphasis on increased vigilance, it will probably never be scientifically proved that pulse oximetry is an independent factor improving safety and outcome after anesthesia. Nonetheless, the weight of evidence supports the contention that the widespread application of pulse oximetry during anesthesia is associated with fewer cases of serious anesthesia-related morbidity and mortality and subsequently with significant cost savings. In contrast, widespread reduction in liability costs have not been attributed to devices such as the PA catheter; to the

contrary, complications associated with the insertion and use of this monitor may occasionally increase costs.[79,80,81]

OPERATING ROOM MANAGEMENT

Operating room management is an activity that is vital to the successful function of health facilities; it is also an activity in which anesthesiologists should participate because of their extensive knowledge and experience in the multiple aspects of the perioperative process. Anesthesiologists, acting in the role of physician-managers, can add significant value to the overall OR process by improving efficiencies in resource utilization and simultaneously, quality of care. Effective OR management requires examination of a process that begins when a surgical procedure is scheduled and encompasses examination and consideration of outcomes, cost-effectiveness, and customer satisfaction (Table 6-6). Construction of the daily OR schedule must be based on the optimum combination of supply and demand of limited and expensive resources (personnel, equipment, drugs, supplies) that contribute substantially to the overall cost of surgical services. Modifications of customary processes are often necessary to improve OR efficiency. For example, one approach to increase OR efficiency and potentially reduce costs in a large facility is the institution of "staggered" start times in alternating ORs for initial cases of the day. For the anesthesiologist responsible for more than one patient simultaneously, staggered start times minimize starting delays related to attending to more than one patient at time, a scenario that otherwise frequently occurs with simultaneously scheduled anesthetic inductions. This approach can be effective when staffing is flexible so that some OR and recovery room nurses can start at later times and split shifts. Such staggered staffing can also secondarily improve staff morale and enhance nursing coverage over broader ranges of hours without incurring extra costs. If preoperative or postoperative facility space is limited and it is occupied at or above capacity, staggered start times can also reduce delays related to patient "bottlenecks" in the preoperative holding area and/or the PACU.

Effective OR management must address preadmission processing, preoperative assessment, OR scheduling, patient intake on the day of surgery, postanesthesia care (including PACU, ICU, and pain management) as well as coordination of nonsurgical support services (radiology, laboratory, clinical instrumentation, housekeeping, and transport [Fig. 6-6]). While the OR plays an essential role in most surgical services, all upstream and downstream activities must be integrated into a coordinated management approach. This is illustrated by the observation

---

Table 6-6. EXAMPLES OF ACTIVITIES INVOLVED IN OPERATING ROOM (OR) MANAGEMENT

ANALYSES
- Incidence and cause of delays, including availability of surgeons, anesthesia personnel, OR staff, ancillary services.
- OR turnaround times, with components and root-cause analyses
- OR scheduling block utilization (by surgeon, time of day, overall)
- OR cancellations (frequency and causes)
- OR scheduling/capacity analysis
- Materials management

SCHEDULING TO OPTIMIZE EFFICIENCY/CUSTOMER SATISFACTION
- Case length forecasting
- Case conflict checks (surgeon, special staff, and equipment availability)
- Allocation and release of block time assignments
- Scheduling of preoperative processing and evaluation
- Scheduling of OR and PACU personnel to optimize staffing with surgical case load

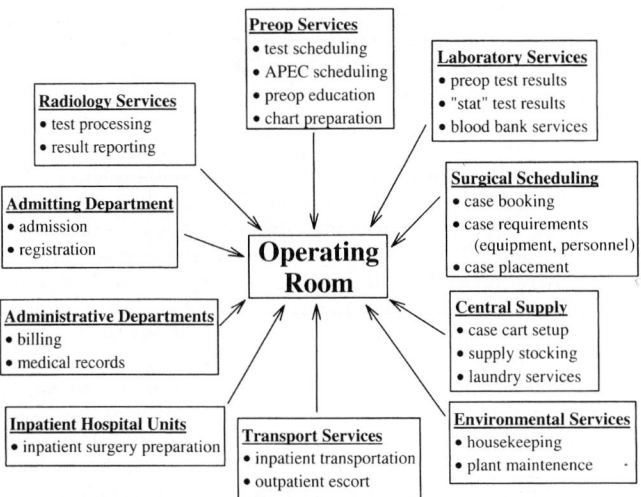

Figure 6-6. Multidisciplinary input into operating room processes.

that nearly 50% of delays in PACU discharge of greater than 30 minutes, which can result in a backup of OR cases, occur in association with nonmedical factors (lack of bed availability, transport delays, unavailability of outpatient's escort to go home, unavailability of physician to write discharge orders/prescriptions, and so on).[91] Because of the multifaceted nature of surgical services, effective coordination of the various components requires clearly defined reporting structures and rules of governance, as well as a well-functioning information management system. A well-managed OR can minimize unplanned delays that increase costs and create dissatisfaction among all OR users (patients, nurses, physicians).

Besides improved preoperative preparation in advance of patient arrival,[32] improvements in OR efficiency can be achieved by analyzing OR data for causes of delays, devising strategies for minimizing the common types of delays and subsequently measuring delay data to determine if improvements are achieved and maintained.[92] Successful implementation of such an approach requires personal accountability and multidisciplinary teamwork aimed at streamlining procedures with parallel rather than serial task performance (*e.g.*, bringing patients into the OR for anesthetic preparation while OR nurses perform tasks simultaneously, rather than waiting until nursing tasks are completed).

Collection of accurate, minimally biased data to assess the etiology of delays is essential to developing process improvement plans. It may not be possible to exclude all bias from data collected by OR personnel, especially if data are self-reported as in the case of nursing delays. It is conceivable that more accurate data and improved efficiency can be obtained with the use of electronic patient tracking devices that monitor patient location as they move through the health facility.[93,94] Such real-

time patient tracking information may be used to make frequent, continual adjustments to OR and personnel assignments to avoid delays and optimize efficient allocation of resources. The problem of collecting accurate data is compounded by inconsistent definitions of various OR times. Definitions of start time and turnover time vary according to individual perspectives (see Table 6-7), and the specific definition of these events must be considered when developing process improvement plans.[95] The Association of Anesthesia Clinical Directors has developed a glossary of procedural times to help promote application of a common language for these terms.[96]

Operating room utilization as a measure of efficiency can be defined as the time the OR is being used (set-up, occupied by patient, clean-up) divided by the length of time that OR is available with regular staffing. Other definitions of OR utilization that do not include set-up and clean-up time (raw utilization) results in lower percentage utilization for blocks of OR time with many cases and frequent room turnovers. Operating room utilization rates >70% are generally considered acceptable, with lower rates reflecting the need for management interventions to improve OR scheduling or other process improvement measures. Optimization of OR utilization requires consideration of variables such as average case duration, average patient waiting time for surgery, number of hours in each OR block time, number of blocks assigned to a surgeon/surgical group, and the specific scheduling strategy applied. Although OR utilization is used as a means to assess global OR efficiency, it may not reflect the impact of certain OR activities that contribute to inefficiency. An example of this occurs when a slow surgeon with long operating times fills his or her assigned block time, which will be reflected in a high rate of OR utilization despite contributing to inefficient use of overall OR time. The importance to cost reductions of shortening operative times cannot be overemphasized, since OR time has a large variable cost component and contributes one-third or more of total OR costs.[57]

Achievement of efficiency in OR use must incorporate consideration of the satisfaction of all customers of the facility. A common problem encountered in developing an efficient OR scheduling algorithm is the difficulty in matching OR availability with the needs of surgeons' non-OR schedules (*e.g.*, clinic practice, OR time at other surgical facility). This commonly results in surgical requests for scheduling in a horizontal fashion, typically resulting in multiple, overlapping requests for early start times. While some flexibility is required on the part of surgeons, use of a more vertical system of arranging cases can lead to improved efficiency, with significant conservation of resources, depending upon the economic structure within an OR facility. When large economic benefits can accrue by applying this strategy, an effective physician-manager may be required to persuade some surgeons to schedule clinic hours in the morning in order to reduce competition for early OR start times and facilitate vertical OR scheduling.

Computer simulation suggests that OR utilization can be max-

Table 6-7. VARIABLE DEFINITIONS OF OPERATING ROOM TIMES*

Perspective	Start Time	Turnover Time
OR nurses	OR "ready" time	Interval when OR unoccupied
Anesthesiologists	Induction time	Interval between PACU report and subsequent patient induction
Surgeons	Incision time	Interval between wound closure/dressing applied and subsequent patient incision
Association of Anesthesia Clinical Directors[96]	Patient OR entry	Interval between patient OR departure and subsequent patient OR entry

* As defined by Glenn DM, Macario A: Management of the operating room: A new practice opportunity for anesthesiologists. Anesth Clin N.A. 17:365, 1999.

imized by allocating block time for elective cases based on expected total hours of elective cases and scheduling patients into the first available date when open block time is available.[97] Implementing such a strategy requires flexibility on the part of the patient and the operating surgeon. It has been proposed that large increases in OR utilization can theoretically be realized by increasing the time patients wait prior to the scheduled date of surgery, although the larger the number of ORs available, the less prolongation of surgical wait time necessary to achieve improved scheduling efficiency.[97] To maximize OR utilization, as many add-on elective cases must be scheduled into any unused OR time slots. Although a variety of algorithms can be used to schedule such add-on cases,[98] all approaches can be constrained by equipment, personnel, and facility limitations, especially when there is overlapping need for specialized but limited resources. For example, although a particular OR can accommodate the addition of a 4-hour add-on elective case, if that case requires the use of extracorporeal circulation, but all cardiopulmonary bypass machines are in use, that case cannot be scheduled as desired. All scheduling strategies aimed at increasing OR utilization must also consider the availability of ORs for urgent or emergent cases and specific mechanisms to schedule surgeons who do not have block time.

In order to more accurately access and correct any sources of inefficiency, the discrete individual functional events that occur as a patient is processed through the OR must be identified. Once these individual steps are identified (see Table 6-8), process analysis can be applied to individual patients to identify on a case-by-case basis at which step the delay occurred. Mean and median values for the time required for each step can be evaluated over time using process control methods. Both internal and external benchmarks can be applied for comparison. When a pattern of avoidable causes for delays is identified, efforts can be focused on individual steps in a process to improve performance. Examination of rates and causes for cancellation rates, for example, can be used to identify a list of common factors contributing to case cancellations, some of which may be easily correctable (*e.g.,* better preoperative patient education regarding NPO status). Whenever avoidable and potentially correctable problems are identified, administrative expertise and intervention in the relevant discipline are required without losing sight of the multidisciplinary/multifaceted nature of these complex processes (Fig. 6-6). These analyses must account for known differences that exist in benchmark data for individual types of surgery. For example, complex orthopedic, neurosurgical, and cardiothoracic procedures consistently require longer periods of time for anesthetic induction, establishment of monitoring, and patient positioning than other types

of operative procedures.[92,99] Use of information systems to track perioperative outcomes and process quality assurance data can be effective in improving outcomes and reducing costs when clinicians are provided regular, personal feedback derived from these systems.[100]

Anesthesia-controlled time typically represents a small fraction (10–20%) of the total case time,[14,92] the remainder (>80%) being surgeon- and nurse-controlled. Actual data for average operating time for a particular surgeon, actual average room turnover time (clean-up and set-up), and actual average anesthesia preparation and positioning times all vary according to the complexity of a particular operative procedure. Incorporation of actual data for these various processes will result in a more accurate prediction for efficient scheduling of OR resources. Avoidance of underutilization or overutilization will permit the maximum number of operations during regular working hours and minimize variable and semi-fixed costs. In the short term, variability in clinical practice can influence an individual surgeon's OR utilization, so that examination of relatively long epochs of block time usage may be more appropriate than evaluation of shorter epochs. Application of time series analysis indicates that the average of twelve successive 4-week periods of total hours of elective cases can be used to reliably predict the OR staffing required to complete a surgical groups' elective caseload during regular scheduled OR hours or to allocate to appropriate hours of block time to minimize OR labor costs.[101,102] Indeed, improving the accuracy of OR scheduling based upon realistic surgical times may have greater positive impact on OR efficiency than OR personnel performance improvements. Inaccurately scheduled OR time contributes to inefficient OR utilization either by leading to gaps of time where ORs are not used or by delaying subsequent procedures with increased staffing costs incurred after regular hours which could be avoided by more appropriate scheduling of cases. In the broader perspective, the cost to a facility resulting from a 30-minute delay in the arrival of the surgeon overshadows the direct costs associated with a 2-hour infusion of propofol.[103]

The relative contribution of reductions in OR turnover time to overall cost savings depends on several interrelated factors. The most significant portion of operating costs is related to fixed personnel costs. If actual turnover time reduction were 30 minutes per day per OR, that may not be sufficient to permit addition of another revenue-producing case to be scheduled during the usual 8-hour shift.[14,99] Furthermore, if OR staffing is flexible, and partially driven by scheduled caseload, then the relative contribution of OR turnover time can achieve greater economic potential. Operating rooms with more frequent turnovers and greater numbers of short-duration cases yield a greater aggregate time and cost savings because extra cases are more likely to be scheduled in this scenario. Whenever high fixed costs exist, adjusting or shifting fixed costs to match patient consumption is necessary to maintain efficiency.

Although using more accurate length of case information to improve scheduling accuracy, reducing variability in OR turnover times, and eliminating day-to-day variation in the number of hours of add-on cases can all improve OR utilization, computer analysis suggests that the most effective strategy to maximize OR utilization may be to select the days that elective cases are to be performed in order to best match OR caseload with staffing of OR personnel.[104]

Another important component of OR management is materials management. Common objectives of efficient materials management are reduction in standing inventory of equipment and supplies as well as standardization of equipment, drugs, and supplies to avoid duplication, consolidate purchasing, and take advantage of volume pricing. Active involvement of physicians to compare and evaluate products of various vendors is essential so that informed decisions can be made about relative equivalency of products. In addition, effective contractual negotiations can often be successful in identifying the most favorable ar-

Table 6-8. PROCESSES IN PATIENT FLOW THROUGH THE OPERATING ROOMS

- Health facility registration if same day/ambulatory patient
- Transport to preoperative holding area
- Preanesthesia preparation by anesthesia team (including immediate preprocedural assessment of medical condition and lab evaluation)
- Transport of patient into OR
- Anesthesia induction, including insertion of additional catheters and monitoring devices
- Patient positioning and sterile preparation
- Operative procedure
- Intraoperative diagnostic procedures (*e.g.,* obtaining fluoroscopy, intraoperative ultrasound)
- Anesthesia emergence
- Transfer out of OR area to PACU or ICU
- Report of patient status to subsequent care provider
- PACU stay
- Transfer from PACU to hospital room or home

rangement for cost reductions when multiple suppliers are offered the opportunity to negotiate lower prices for their product in a competitive bidding procedure.

POSTOPERATIVE ANESTHETIC AND CRITICAL CARE MANAGEMENT

The value of the anesthesiologist as an effective manager to arrange the OR schedule to improve efficiency of OR utilization lies not only in the impact on OR costs, but also in a profound influence on PACU costs at the end of the day. The impact of different temporal distributions of PACU admissions on costs is also determined by patient-to-nurse ratios, peak numbers of patients, and peak admission times. For example, if peak admission rates occur only early in the day, reduction in discharge times may not substantially affect the peak number of patients and subsequently have less direct impact on personnel costs. In contrast, if admission rates are distributed more evenly and continue into the afternoon, peak numbers of patients would decrease, and depending on the patient-to-nurse ratio, the staffing requirements may be reduced. The impact of reducing discharge time on personnel costs will depend not only on the temporal distribution of PACU admissions, but also on the management paradigms employed to distribute nursing personnel in a dynamic environment.

As competition for contracted health care becomes progressively more intense and focused not only on comparisons of the performance of doctors, hospitals, and other health care providers, but also on overall costs, anesthesiologists are confronted with the responsibility of defining the impact of anesthetic management on the efficiency and the overall cost of recovery after surgery. The economic impact of newer anesthetic drugs possessing pharmacokinetic and pharmacodynamic properties resulting in less complicated and more rapid recovery requires systematic investigation, considering overall costs and outcomes, in order to develop evidenced-based practice guidelines and protocols, and ultimately reduce costs (Fig. 6-7). When direct cost analysis indicates that a given alternative to patient care is more expensive than another, failure to quantitate or consider indirect cost savings may result in failure of government and third-party payers to fund that alternative unless an outcome benefit can be demonstrated compared to a "cheaper" alternative. Earlier return of patients to functional status after anesthesia and surgery can save societal costs and should be considered when evaluating overall costs.[105]

Strategies for Cost-Effective Postoperative Management

Evaluation of strategies to improve cost-effectiveness of perianesthetic management has consistently demonstrated that per-

sonnel costs represent the predominant fraction of overall expenditures. Computer simulations using published times to discharge with "fast recovery" drugs predict that use of such drugs would decrease PACU costs primarily if administered in ORs running later each day so that earlier discharge from the PACU would result in less PACU personnel utilization (assuming that the PACU would then close after a single patient was discharged).[106] If use of less expensive drugs is associated with the need for more prolonged postoperative nursing care owing to slower recovery or the need to manage more side effects, there will be a variable increase in the overall costs depending on whether staffing is semi-fixed or more flexible and whether the recovery room is at full occupancy.[106] In the latter instance, prolonged recovery room stay can have negative effects on upstream events, causing back-up of patient flow through the OR and markedly increasing cost. If the recovery room is not at full patient capacity and staffing of nurses is semi-fixed, there may be minimal impact on overall costs of even a 30-minute longer average time until recovery room discharge. Under these circumstances nonselective use of "fast recovery" drugs would probably not substantially diminish PACU costs compared to arranging an OR schedule to optimize admission patterns and reduce the amount of PACU personnel costs, especially at the end of the regular workday.[106] Conversely, if fast-tracking recovery protocols are not employed, even though awakening from anesthesia may be faster with newer, more expensive drugs, actual discharge from the ambulatory facility may not be quicker and overall costs will not be reduced.[106,107] This is analogous to the role of anesthetic management to facilitate fast-tracking of cardiac surgical patients with reduced costs, improved resource utilization, and preserved outcomes.[108,109] Improved resource utilization in all settings, whether involving complex in-patient procedures or relatively "simple" ambulatory procedures, requires a multidisciplinary team approach.

Assessment of high-volume, high-cost medical activities such as CABG surgery must include measures of several distinct aspects of quality: necessity, appropriateness, effectiveness, satisfaction, and efficiency. We can measure the impact of anesthetic and critical care of CABG patients on some of these characteristics. Most techniques currently employed to anesthetize patients for CABG surgery are "effective" in producing the basic elements of general anesthesia: unconsciousness, muscular relaxation, and attenuation of reflex responses to noxious surgical stimuli. Although choice of anesthetic agent *per se* has not been demonstrated to critically influence cardiac or noncardiac outcome after CABG surgery,[110,111] anesthesiologists are being asked to make decisions about anesthetic management based in part on evaluation of customer satisfaction and the overall efficiency of care during and especially after an operation such as the CABG procedure. Outcomes research can facilitate development of practice guidelines to streamline perioperative management and make the recovery process as efficient as possible.

It has been suggested that ICU stays can be shortened if ventilator time is reduced and extubation is performed within a few hours after CABG surgery in awake, stable patients who have acceptable cardiopulmonary status and minimal chest tube drainage. Although anesthetic management with or without the use of more expensive drugs can allow early extubation (1–4 hours postoperatively) after cardiac surgery,[112] this alone will not reduce overall costs unless the overall recovery program (clinical pathway) allows extubated patients to move to the next phase of recovery in an expedited manner compared to patients who are extubated later (10–12 hours).[108] Intraoperative clinical process variables as well as intraoperative and postoperative morbidity overshadow the effect of preoperative risk factors as key determinants of the feasibility of early extubation and ICU length of stay.[113,114] Coordinating early extubation with other aspects of hospitalization for CABG surgery is necessary to improve the efficiency of postoperative processes and to maximize the cost savings of this approach. If there is no impact of anes-

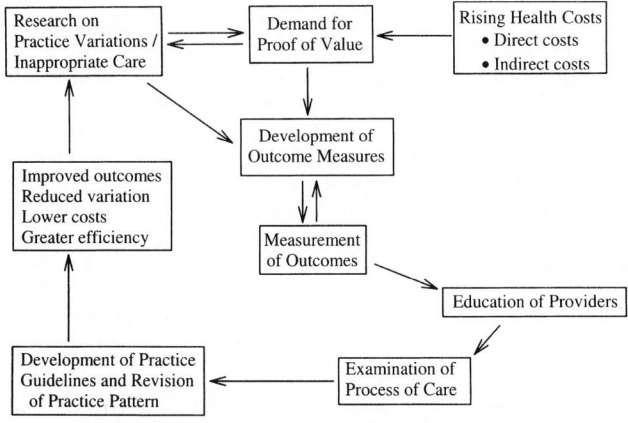

Figure 6-7. Use of outcome data to improve efficiency and reduce costs.

thetic drug on ultimate outcome after cardiac surgery, it may be cost-effective to use longer-acting anesthetic drugs with lower acquisitions costs (compared with more costly, short-acting drugs) if recovery from anesthesia and tracheal extubation can be achieved within a time frame that does not interfere with the overall efficiency of fast-track recovery pathways.[112] As with other expensive and lengthy procedures, drug costs and turn-around time have less impact on overall costs of the CABG procedure compared to shorter-duration, less costly procedures. Other factors, such as the feasibility of using a cardiac surgery recovery area rather than a standard ICU for postoperative recovery, will result in significantly larger cost reductions. Furthermore, modifications of anesthetic and surgical technique to permit myocardial revascularization without extracorporeal circulation may reduce the need for transfusion, OR time, and length of ICU and hospital stay. The latter factors contribute the greatest fraction of total hospital cost for the CABG procedure. Therefore, while the use of additional pharmaceuticals or special equipment to accomplish coronary artery surgery without cardiopulmonary bypass may potentially increase total OR costs (even after considering the costs avoided by not using a cardiopulmonary bypass device), these additional costs are likely to be offset by the overall hospital cost reduction associated with this approach. This example underscores the importance of considering overall costs and illustrates how modifications of clinical practice can be cost-effective even when portions of direct costs increase.

Clinical pathways are based on an organized team approach to patient management and typically are developed by a multidisciplinary group composed of physicians, nurses, pharmacists, administrators, and others who are involved in the patient's experience. These instruments serve as management plans that outline goals for patients and are generally based upon "best practice" experience, clinical practice consensus, and evidence from the scientific literature. They define the ideal sequence and timing of interventions to achieve the prespecified goals with optimal efficiency. Clinical pathways address the variability in practice by standardizing practice in the individual health care setting according to an agreed-upon common regime of clinical interventions. Every detail is important to the success of a clinical pathway, so that all aspects of care can be coordinated to increase efficiency and achieve optimal outcome with expeditious patient discharge. Rapid discharge is important not only for hospitalized patients, but also for patients undergoing ambulatory surgical procedures. Most current clinical pathways are "vertically" directed toward accomplishment of specific goals in a timely fashion. The role of the anesthesiologist is key in many critical pathways so that emergence from anesthesia is prompt and so that intensive physiologic support can be discontinued as expeditiously as possible. This typically facilitates movement of the patient to the next successive goal(s) of the recovery phase. Adequate perioperative analgesia can also facilitate recovery and enhance early mobilization, ambulation, and rehabilitation with the goal of resuming normal activity. The clinical pathway concept applied to perioperative anesthetic patient management with standardization of system management, drugs, and equipment as well as incorporating fast-tracking and phase I recovery bypass options have been shown to be effective in containing costs, enhancing process efficiency, and improving patient outcomes in ambulatory orthopedic surgery.[115]

Recovery after Ambulatory Surgery

Provision of analgesia and avoidance of side effects such as postoperative nausea and vomiting are especially critical in ambulatory surgery so that patients can be promptly discharged home. Postoperative analgesia must be provided and must be effective as soon as possible upon emergence from the OR. Failure to accomplish this can lengthen duration of stay in the PACU, delay home discharge in the ambulatory setting, and result in customer dissatisfaction. In this sense, the customer is not only the patient, but also the facility, which must manage patients efficiently to be competitive in the health delivery market. Judicious use of preoperative and intraoperative analgesics (opioid and nonopioid), application of local anesthetics to the surgical site and regional anesthesia all can facilitate an efficient recovery and high levels of customer satisfaction. Although substantial variability exists among patients' rating of preferences for anesthesia outcomes, avoiding nausea and vomiting appears to be a high priority for most patients, who would be willing to spend more to avoid that outcome compared to some other adverse events.[11] Such information can be applied to guide the choice of anesthetic drugs to provide the greatest value and achieve the highest level of customer satisfaction. This information also highlights that value is context sensitive. The anesthesiologist may place greater value on the intraoperative aspects of managing a complex patient and lesser importance on postoperative nausea after a challenging operative procedure. However, not addressing this issue will potentially result in a failure to meet an important customer expectation (minimal nausea and pain). Even though the anesthesiologist may place greater importance on other aspects of care in this scenario, the value of the anesthesiologist as viewed by the patient (customer) will be diminished unless such expectations are realized. The context sensitivity of values depends on the individual perspective of each customer of anesthesia services, as reflected by the examples illustrated in Table 6-1. The characteristics of a product or service that customers perceive as contributing to value are dynamic, and successful strategies to maintain and continually improve the value of anesthesiology services requires anticipation of future needs of customers that will change perceptions of value.

New drugs or techniques that are associated with less frequent or less severe side effects, prompter recovery, and decreased mean times to discharge may permit total nursing hours to be adjusted downward. Significant cost savings without any change in outcomes can be achieved by avoiding routine admission to first-stage postanesthesia care units and using selective admission to phase II recovery units based upon whether the patient meets specific criteria in the OR at the end of the surgical procedure. If patients meet discharge criteria typically used at the end of a PACU stay, they could be transferred from the OR directly to a less labor-intensive second-stage recovery unit, reducing both postoperative time until discharge and costs. In addition to achieving appropriate physiologic status (satisfactory motor strength and mental status with acceptable vital signs and oxygen saturation while breathing room air), anesthetic management that facilitates bypass of phase I PACU must also be focused on emergence from surgery with no vomiting and minimal pain or nausea. Under these circumstances, use of drugs with greater acquisition costs that have better recovery profiles than drugs with less direct cost can be associated with reduced overall costs and improved customer satisfaction. If the same or a better outcome cannot be achieved with a less expensive drug, the more expensive drug is more cost-effective because it decreases overall unit cost. Maximal cost savings by using drugs with favorable recovery profiles are unlikely to be realized—despite reductions of PACU discharge times or reductions in the peak numbers of patients in the PACU—unless nursing personnel can be shifted, depending on patient load, from one area of perioperative patient care to another (ambulatory admitting, ambulatory Phase I or Phase II recovery). Such a flexible core-staffing model is based on a dynamic distribution of resources, improving the efficiency of personnel utilization. Other methods of decreasing costs involve increasing patient-to-nurse ratios whenever possible, directly decreasing personnel requirements. Such an alternative is feasible if patients awaken promptly and have less complicated recovery profiles (*e.g.*, less nausea and vomiting), necessitating less intense nursing interventions. Elimination or modification of predefined requirements for a minimum number of nurses to staff a recovery area (regardless of whether even a single uncomplicated patient is present) can also reduce costs. Since personnel costs represent a major fraction of PACU costs, less expensive teams of personnel headed by a staff nurse can be utilized in the recovery setting with preservation of quality care. This is especially feasible when greater numbers of patients leave an operating room ready or near-ready for immediate phase II recovery. Because of institutional variability, decision analysis and sensitivity analysis can be useful to determine how various assumptions in nursing staffing and recovery room capacity would affect overall costs when comparing anesthetic techniques with different recovery and side-effect profiles.[56]

Cost Issues in the ICU

Outside of the OR, anesthesiologists who practice in the ICU work in a setting that is a major contributor to escalating health care expenditures. Critical care units account for nearly one-fifth of total hospital costs and one-twelfth of the total U.S. health care.[116] ICU patients constitute the minority of all surgical patients but consume almost half of all surgical resources. The disproportionate share of health care resources devoted to the critically ill is related to the high labor intensity and technologic dependence of ICU care. The magnitude of resources consumed has created intense interest in cost analysis in the ICU. Anesthesiologists practicing critical care medicine in an ICU may be able to demonstrate the value of their services by documenting optimization of processes of care, improved patient outcomes and reduced consumption of resources.[117,118]

Restricting ICU admissions as a method to reduce costs is difficult since, in most cases, it is not possible to accurately predict nonsurvivors from survivors on admission to the ICU, despite the development of many severity-of-illness scoring systems. Nonetheless, some data suggest that ICU bed availability reductions, either by design or demand, can result in fewer patients' being admitted for monitoring alone, with a shift in patient acuity to a higher level but no change in mortality.[119,120] Unfortunately, unlike some inpatient services, such as various elective surgical procedures that can be shifted to the outpatient setting, most critical care is usually inelastic and can be provided only in the ICU environment.

Currently, it is an easier endeavor to diminish charges in the ICU than to restrict admissions. Selective, rather than routine, ordering of so-called "screening" tests is one means of reducing costs. Deletion of standing orders for such tests as blood gases, glucose, electrolytes, complete blood count with differential, ECGs, and chest x-rays can make a large impact on cost reduction, usually with no increase in ICU morbidity rate, length of stay, or cost of medications.[121] For example, in the patient who has cardiopulmonary stability, the use of standing orders for arterial blood gas tension analysis (e.g., beginning of nursing shifts, after every ventilator change) is probably not cost-effective. Replacement of frequent blood gas tension analyses with monitoring using capnometry and oximetry may be more cost-effective, but this requires implementation of formal and standardized guidelines for the most efficient use of such noninvasive monitoring.[122] As with preoperative and intraoperative management, the utility of eliminating "small ticket items" can be great when the cumulative number of these items is large.

Just as routine preoperative testing is inefficient and wasteful of costly resources, routine ordering of postoperative tests must also be avoided, especially when this behavior results from the perceived need to have test results be part of a potential medicolegal record rather than of practical patient value. Similar principles should guide the postoperative use of diagnostic technology such as echocardiography, electroencephalography, and PA catheterization. Such diagnostic technology should be used only if it might change a diagnostic or treatment strategy. Tests with high sensitivity work best for confirming a suspected diagnosis, and those with high specificity are best for excluding a diagnosis. When two technologies have equal diagnostic accuracy, consideration should be given to using the one with the lower cost if patient risks are the same. All of this requires familiarity with the cost, sensitivity, and specificity of the various diagnostic and monitoring technologies we utilize. Teaching these concepts and use of probabilistic reasoning is more effective than simple cost-containment education in improving the efficiency of clinical decisions such as test ordering.[123] Published estimates of sensitivity and specificity cannot be trusted blindly, because a given test or monitor may be very sensitive and moderately specific in one hospital but moderately sensitive and very specific in another, depending on the patient population and how the test or monitor is used. Implementation of practice guidelines and information management systems based on these considerations should help achieve substantial and significant reductions in diagnostic testing of hospitalized patients without adverse effects on quality of care as measured by clinical outcome.[121]

The most difficult issue in containing ICU costs is not that of reducing expenditures on diagnostic testing or monitoring, but involves identification of nonsurvivors as early as possible after ICU entry. This requires dynamic evaluation and has potential for cost containment with little if any change in outcome. Although most physicians, patients, and families want to avoid ordering more and more tests and performing more and more procedures in attempts to "fix something" without changing the outcome of patients who are destined to be nonsurvivors, identification of nonsurvivors remains a difficult process. The application of high levels of technology to patients who are hopelessly ill with essentially no chance of meaningful recovery is being challenged not only by health care economists, but by the public as well. Debate on the use of futile and/or inappropriate intensive care has intensified in the last few years, and many believe that minimizing futile care is one of the first necessary steps in health care reform.[124] Although the savings from reduced use of futile care may be modest,[125] cost savings from reducing inappropriate care may be substantial.[126,127] Inappropriate expectations of medical care sometimes motivate excessive use of diagnostic and therapeutic modalities in the ICU. The course of action dictated by comparing costs with benefits inevitably involves compromise and requires adjustment of expectations of physicians, patients, and those who fund critical care. Alternative methods of patient management such as intensive home care may more cost-effectively bring hospital-level intervention to some patients in their homes or as outpatients. Provision of intravenous nutrition, ventilator support, dialysis, and management of heart failure (e.g., chronic infusions of inotropes) at home with avoidance of long-term hospitalization may not only allow greater patient comfort, but also potentially contribute to large cost savings, especially in patients who require prolonged support but have irreversible disease processes. Significant progress in reducing costs of managing ventilator-dependent patients has already been documented, including the use of step-down, intermediate care units, and general medical floors with lower staff-to-patient ratios and less overhead costs, without changing eventual outcome.[128]

CONCLUSIONS

Value-based anesthesia management focuses on patient needs and expectations to optimize efficiency of care for individual patients. This is a dynamic process that requires the proactive involvement of anesthesiologists in multiple aspects of preoperative, intraoperative, and postoperative care. Intelligent cost-containment measures require efficient use of existing resources and selectivity in perioperative testing, drug choices, and monitoring (Table 6-9). This can be done only with sufficient knowledge of medical economic analysis and data that

Table 6-9. APPROACHES TO ACHIEVE VALUE-BASED ANESTHESIA MANAGEMENT

- Focus on costs, not changes
- Consider all costs (direct and indirect) for all clinical alternatives
- Identify all potential benefits and risks for all clinical alternatives
- Evaluate *allocative* efficiency as well as *operational* efficiency
- Adopt clinical strategies that eliminate ineffective diagnostic and therapeutic procedures (*e.g.,* apply selective discipline in ordering tests and consultations)
- Reduce use of high-cost strategies whose advantage over lower-cost strategies is debatable
- Apply all available cost-effectiveness data to define *value* of anesthesia services and clinical strategies
- Develop clinician-generated practice guidelines with an emphasis on real outcomes
- Assume a proactive role in OR, ICU, and facility management
- Eliminate administrative waste

define the necessary amount of testing and monitoring for effective patient care and eliminate excessive use of technology unless there is compelling evidence that more expensive alternatives are of greater benefit. Indirect costs or benefits of patient management paradigms must be considered: the economic impact of parameters such as the delay in the resumption of normal activities after anesthesia and surgery can be substantial. In addition, both allocative and operational efficiency must be addressed. Reducing length of stay in the ambulatory care unit after hernia surgery is just as important as reducing the length of stay after CABG surgery.

Eliminating waste and increasing flexibility in the administrative aspects of perioperative care are also essential to provide value-based anesthesia services. Replacing rigid protocols such as the requirement of a minimal designated time in a Phase I recovery area (with protocols that apply physiologic end points for discharge criteria) may be required to definitively demonstrate the potential impact of newer, shorter-acting drugs on overall costs. Application of disciplined logic must replace the use of standardized protocols. Practice parameters, based on outcome data that define what really works for patients, can facilitate informed medical decisions but should not mandate individual patient care.

The increasing application of global payment methodologies has created an environment that encourages collaborative economic efficiency. In this regard, a multidisciplinary approach to improving preoperative patient preparation, reducing turnaround time between surgical cases, optimizing OR utilization, and reducing duration of recovery time will help control direct costs as well as lessen overhead costs. Such improvements in efficiency with institutional cost savings have the secondary benefit of making a practice setting more competitive in the medical marketplace. Operating room management is important for successful function of health facilities and is an activity in which anesthesiologists should participate because of their knowledge and experience in the multiple aspects of the perioperative process. As cost constraints on every aspect of health care delivery become more stringently imposed, establishment of a value-based practice of anesthesia requires that the anesthesiologist act pivotally as the perioperative physician with the broadest knowledge and expertise linking the preoperative, intraoperative, and postoperative phases of patient care.

REFERENCES

1. Orkin FK: Moving toward value-based anesthesia care. J Clin Anesth 5:91, 1993
2. Fisher ES, Welch HG: Avoiding the unintended consequences of growth in medical care. JAMA 281:446, 1999
3. Health, United States, 1998: Socioeconomic Status and Health Chartbook. Hyattsville, MD, U.S. Dept of Health and Human Services, 1998. U.S. Dept of Health and Human Services publication PHS 98-1232
4. Levit KR, Lazenby HC, Cowan CA et al: National health expenditures, 1990. Health Care Finan Rev 13:29, 1991
5. Tuman KJ, Ivankovich AD: High cost, high tech medicine—are we getting our money's worth? J Clin Anesth 5:168, 1993
6. Eddy DM: Applying cost-effectiveness analysis: The inside story. JAMA 268:2575, 1992
7. Johnstone RE, Martinec CL: Costs of anesthesia. Anesth Analg 76:840, 1993
8. Broadway PJ, Jones JG: A method of costing anaesthetic practice. Anaesthesia 50:56, 1995
9. Donabedian A: Explorations in Quality Assessment and Monitoring. Vol 3. The Methods and Findings of Quality Assessment and Monitoring: An Illustrated Analysis. Ann Arbor, MI, Health Administration Press, 1985
10. Macario A, Weinger M, Truong P, Lee M: Which clinical anesthesia outcomes are both common and important to avoid? The perspective of a panel of expert anesthesiologists. Anesth Analg 88:1085, 1999
11. Macario A, Weinger M, Carney S, Kim A: Which clinical anesthesia outcomes are important to avoid? The perspective of patients. Anesth Analg 89:652, 1999
12. Tong D, Chung F, Wong D: Predictive factors in global and anesthesia satisfaction in ambulatory surgical patients. Anesthesiology 87:856, 1997
13. Tarazi E, Philip B: Friendliness of OR staff is top determinant of patient satisfaction with outpatient surgery. Am J Anesth 25:154, 1998
14. Dexter F, Tinker JH: The cost efficacy of hypothetically eliminating adverse anesthetic outcomes from high-risk, but neither low- nor moderate-risk, surgical operations. Anesth Analg 81:939, 1995
15. Bothner U, Georgieff M, Schwilk B: The impact of minor perioperative anesthesia-related incidents, events, and complications on postanesthesia care unit utilization. Anesth Analg 89:506, 1999
16. Davidson RA: Does it work or not? Clinical vs. statistical significance. Chest 106:932, 1994
17. Silber JH: Using Outcomes Analysis to Assess Quality of Care: Applications for Cardiovascular Surgery. In Tuman KJ (ed.): Outcome Measurements in Cardiovascular Medicine, p 1. Philadelphia, Lippincott Williams & Wilkins, 1999
18. Silber JH, Williams SV, Krakauer H, Schwartz JS: Hospital and patient characteristics associated with death after surgery: A study of adverse occurrence and failure to rescue. Med Care 30:615, 1992
19. Silber JH, Kennedy SK, Koziol LF et al: Do nurse anesthetists need medical direction by anesthesiologists? Anesthesiology 89(3):A1184, 1998
20. Lubarsky DA, Sanderson IC, Gilbert WC et al: Using an information management system as a cost containment tool: Description and validation. Anesthesiology 86:1161, 1997
21. Lagasse RS, Steinberg ES, Katz RI, Saubermann AJ: Defining quality of perioperative care by statistical process control of adverse outcomes. Anesthesiology 82:1181, 1995
22. Deming WE: Out of the Crisis. Cambridge, MA, MIT, Center for Advanced Engineering Study, 1986
23. Camp RC: Benchmarking: The search for industry best practices that lead to superior performance. Milwaukee, American Society for Quality Control Press, 1989
24. Drummond MF, Richardson WS, O'Brien BJ et al (for the Evidence-Based Medicine Working Group): Users' Guides to the Medical Literature. XIII: How to use an article on economic analysis of clinical practice. A: Are the results of the study valid? JAMA 277:1552, 1997
25. O'Brien BJ, Heyland D, Richardson WS et al (for the Evidence-Based Medicine Working Group): Users' Guides to the Medical Literature. XIII: How to use an article on economic analysis of clinical practice. B: What are the results and will they help me in caring for my patients? JAMA 277:1802, 1997
26. Richardson WS, Detsky AS (for the Evidence-Based Medicine Working Group): Users' Guides to the Medical Literature. VII: How to use a clinical decision analysis. A: Are the results of the study valid? JAMA 273:1292, 1995
27. Richardson WS, Detsky AS (for the Evidence-Based Medicine Working Group): Users' Guides to the Medical Literature. VII: How to use a clinical decision analysis. B: What are the results and will they help me in caring for my patients? JAMA 273:1610, 1995
28. Guyatt GH, Sackett DL, Cook DJ (for the Evidence-Based Medicine

Working Group): Users' Guide to the Medical Literature. II: How to use an article about therapy or prevention. B: What were the results and will they help me in caring for my patient? JAMA 271:59, 1994

29. Tang J, Watcha MF, White PF: A comparison of costs and efficacy of ondansetron and droperidol as prophylactic antiemetic therapy for elective outpatient gynecologic procedures. Anesth Analg 83:304, 1996

30. Liu S, Carpenter RL, Neal JM: Epidural anesthesia and analgesia: Their role in postoperative outcome. Anesthesiology 82:1474, 1995

31. Pollard JB, Zboray AL, Mazze RI: Economic benefits attributed to opening a preoperative evaluation clinic for outpatients. Anesth Analg 83:407, 1996

32. Fischer SP: Development and effectiveness of an anesthesia preoperative evaluation clinic in a teaching hospital. Anesthesiology 85:196, 1996

33. Brook RH, Lohr KN: Efficacy, effectiveness, variations and quality: Boundary-crossing research. Med Care 23:710, 1985

34. Legorretta AP, Silber JH, Costantino GN et al: Increased cholecystectomy rate after the introduction of laparoscopic cholecystectomy. JAMA 270:1429, 1993

35. Cummings KM, Frisof KB, Long MJ et al: The effect of price information on physicians' test ordering behavior: Ordering of diagnostic tests. Med Care 20:293, 1982

36. Donabedian A: The assessment of technology and quality. J Tech Assess Health Care 4:487, 1988

37. Sibbald WJ, Escaf M, Calvin JE: How can new technology be introduced, evaluated, and financed in critical care? Clin Chem 8:1604, 1990

38. Eisenberg JM: Clinical economics: A guide to the economic analysis of clinical practices. JAMA 262:2879, 1989

39. Detsky AS, Naglie IG: A clinician's guide to cost-effectiveness analysis. Ann Intern Med 113:147, 1990

40. Dexter F, Lubarsky DA, Gilbert BC, Thompson C: A method to compare costs of drugs and supplies among anesthesia providers. A simple statistical method to reduce variations in cost due to variations in casemix. Anesthesiology 88:1350, 1998

41. Macario A, Vitez TS, Dunn B, et al: Hospital costs and severity of illness in three types of elective surgery. Anesthesiology 86:92, 1997

42. Kassirer JP, Moskow AJ, Lau J, Pauker SG: Decision analysis: A progress report. Ann Intern Med 106:275, 1987

43. Wachta MF, Smith I: Cost-effectiveness analysis of antiemetic therapy for ambulatory surgery. J Clin Anesth 6:370, 1994

44. Fisher DM: Surrogate endpoints: Are they meaningful? Anesthesiology 81:795, 1994

45. Boothe P, Finegan BA: Changing the admission process for elective surgery: An economic analysis. Can J Anaesth 42:391, 1995

46. Birkmeyer JD, AuBuchon JP, Littenberg B et al: Cost-effectiveness of preoperative autologous blood donation in CABG. Ann Thorac Surg 57:161, 1994

47. Birkmeyer JD, Goodnough LT, AuBuchon JP et al: The cost-effectiveness of preoperative autologous blood donation for total hip and knee replacement. Transfusion 33:544, 1993

48. Etchason J, Petz L, Keeler E et al: The cost effectiveness of preoperative autologous blood donations. N Engl J Med 332:719, 1995

49. Narr BJ, Hansen TR, Warner MA: Preoperative laboratory testing in healthy Mayo patients: Cost effective elimination of tests and unchanged outcomes. Mayo Clinic Proc 66:155, 1991

50. Perez A, Planello J, Bacardaz VC et al: Value of routine preoperative tests: A multicentre study in four general hospitals. Br J Anaesth 74:250, 1995

51. Kaplan EB, Sheiner LB, Boeckmann AJ et al: The usefulness of preoperative laboratory screening. JAMA 253:3576, 1985

52. Pollard JB, Olson L: Early outpatient preoperative anesthesia assessment: Does it help to reduce operating room cancellations? Anesth Analg 89:502, 1999

53. Lampotang S, Nyland ME, Gravenstein N: The cost of wasted anesthetic gases (abstract). Anesth Analg 72:S151, 1991

54. Baum JA: Low flow anaesthesia: The sensible and judicious use of inhalation anaesthetics. Acta Anaesthiol Scand 111:264, 1997

55. Vitez TS: Principles of cost analysis. J Clin Anesth 6:357, 1994

56. Watcha MF, White PF: Economics of anesthetic practice. Anesthesiology 86:1170, 1997

57. Macario A, Vitez T, Dunn B, McDonald T: Where are the costs in perioperative care? Analysis of hospital costs and charges for inpatient surgical care. Anesthesiology 83:1138, 1995

58. Lubarsky D, Glass PSA, Ginsberg B et al: The successful implementation of pharmaceutical practice guidelines. Anesthesiology 86:1145, 1997

59. Lin YC, Miller SR: The impact of price labeling of muscle relaxants on cost consciousness among anesthesiologists. J Clin Anesth 10:401, 1998

60. Ballantyne J, Chang Y: The impact of choice of muscle relaxant on postoperative recovery time: A retrospective study. Anesth Analg 85:476, 1997

61. Lubarsky DA: Fast track in the postanesthesia care unit: Unlimited possibilities? J Clin Anesth 8:70S, 1996

62. Johnstone R, Jozefczyk KG: Costs of anesthetic drugs: Experiences with a cost education trial. Anesth Analg 78:766, 1994

63. Barclay LP, Hatton RC, Doering PL, Shands JW: Physicians' perceptions and knowledge of drug costs: Results of a survey. Formulary 30:268, 1995

64. Szocik JF, Learned DW: Impact of a cost containment program on the use of volatile anesthetics and neuromuscular blocking drugs. J Clin Anesth 6:378, 1994

65. Caldwell JE: The problem with long acting muscle relaxants? They cost more! Anesth Analg 85:476, 1997

66. Rosenblatt WH, Silverman DG: Cost-effective use of operating room supplies based on the REMEDY database of recovered unused materials. J Clin Anesth 6:400, 1994

67. Blakely M, Artman M: Reducing cost in a teaching hospital by requiring justification for the use of vecuronium bromide. Am J Hosp Pharm 54:2422, 1994

68. Narbone RF, McCarthy RJ, Tuman KJ et al: Selectivity in drug utilization: Impact on anesthetic drug costs. Anesth Analg 80:S341, 1995

69. van Sickels JE, Tiner BD: Cost of a genioplasty under deep intravenous sedation in a private office vs. general anesthesia in an outpatient surgical center. J Oral Maxillofac Surg 50:687, 1992

70. Becker KE Jr, Carrithers J: Practical methods of cost containment in anesthesia and surgery. J Clin Anesth 6:388, 1994

71. Ballantyne JC, Carr DB, deFerranti S et al: The comparative effects of postoperative analgesic therapies on pulmonary outcome: Cumulative meta-analyses of randomized, controlled trials. Anesth Analg 86:598, 1998

72. Liu SS, Carpenter RL, Mackey DC et al: Effects of perioperative analgesic technique on rate of recovery after colon surgery. Anesthesiology 83:757, 1995

73. Gottschalk A, Smith DS, Jobes DR et al: Preemptive epidural analgesia and recovery from radical prostatectomy: a randomized controlled trial. JAMA 279:1076, 1998

74. Fleisher LA, Metzger SE, Lam J, Harris A: Perioperative cost-finding analysis of the routine use of intraoperative forced-air warming during general anesthesia. Anesthesiology 88:1357, 1998

75. Lenhardt R, Marker E, Goll V et al: Mild intraoperative hypothermia prolongs postanesthetic recovery. Anesthesiology 87:1318, 1997

76. Laupacis A, Feeny D, Detsky AS et al: How attractive does a new technology have to be to warrant adoption and utilization? Tentative guidelines for using clinical and economic evaluations. Can Med Assoc J 146:473, 1992

77. Cohen IL, Lambrinos J, Fein IA: Mechanical ventilation for the elderly patient in intensive care. JAMA 269:1025, 1993

78. Schapira DV, Studnicki J, Bradham DD: Intensive care, survival, and expense of treating critically ill cancer patients. JAMA 269:783, 1993

79. American Society of Anesthesiologists Task Force on Pulmonary Artery Catheterization: Practice guidelines for pulmonary artery catheterization. Anesthesiology 78:380, 1993

80. Pulmonary Artery Catheter Consensus Conference Participants: Pulmonary artery catheter consensus conference: consensus statement. Crit Care Med 25:910, 1997

81. Mueller HS, Chatterjee K, Davis KB et al: Present use of bedside right heart catheterization in patients with cardiac disease. J Am Coll Cardiol 27:840, 1998

82. Spackman TN: A theoretical evaluation of cost-effectiveness of pulmonary artery catheters in patients undergoing coronary artery surgery. J Cardiothorac Vasc Anesth 8:487, 1994

83. Bashein G, Johnson PW, Davis KB, Ivey TD: Elective CABG without pulmonary artery catheter monitoring. Anesthesiology 63:451, 1985

84. Tuman KJ, McCarthy RJ, Spiess BD et al: Effect of pulmonary artery catheterization on outcome in patients undergoing coronary artery surgery. Anesthesiology 70:199, 1989

85. Shomaker TS: Practice policies in anesthesia: A foretaste of practice in the 21st century. Anesth Analg 80:388, 1995

86. Moller JT, Johannessen NW, Espersen K et al: Randomized evaluation of pulse oximetry in 20,802 patients. Anesthesiology 78: 445, 1993

87. Cooper J, Cullen DJ, Nemeskal AR et al: Effects of information feedback and pulse oximetry on the incidence of anesthesia complications. Anesthesiology 67:686, 1987

88. Eichhorn JH: Prevention of intraoperative anesthesia accidents and related severe injury through safety monitoring. Anesthesiology 70:572, 1989

89. Cullen DJ, Nemeskal AR, Cooper JB et al: Effect of pulse oximetry, age, and ASA physical status on the frequency of patients admitted unexpectedly to a postoperative intensive care unit and the severity of their anesthesia-related complications. Anesth Analg 74:181, 1992

90. Tinker J, Dull DL, Caplan RA et al: Role of monitoring devices in prevention of anesthetic mishaps: Closed claims analysis. Anesthesiology 71:541, 1989

91. Chung F: Recovery pattern and home readiness after ambulatory surgery. Anesth Analg 80:896, 1995

92. Overdyk FJ, Harvey SC, Fishman RL, Shippey F: Successful strategies for improving operating room efficiency at academic institutions. Anesth Analg 86:896, 1998

93. Overdyk F, Haynes G, Arvanitis P, Simms. Patient data in a watchband: An idea whose time has come. Anesthesiology 85:S3, 1996

94. DeRiso B, Cantees K, Watkins WD: The operating rooms: Cost center management in a managed care environment. Int Anesth Clin 33:133, 1995

95. Glenn DM, Macario A: Management of the operating room: A new practice opportunity for anesthesiologists. Anesth Clin N.A. 17:365, 1999

96. Association of Anesthesia Clinical Directors Procedural Times Glossary: Surgical Services Management 3:11, 1997

97. Dexter F, Macario A, Traub RD et al: An operating room scheduling strategy to maximize the use of operating room block time: Computer simulation of patient scheduling and survey of patients' preferences for surgical waiting time. Anesth Analg 89:7, 1999

98. Dexter F, Macario A, Traub RD: Which algorithm for scheduling add-on elective cases maximizes operating room utilization? Use of bin packing algorithms and fuzzy constraints in operating room management. Anesthesiology 91:1491, 1999

99. Mazzei WJ: Operating room start times and turnover times in a university hospital. J Clin Anesth 6:405, 1994

100. McNitt JD, Bode ET, Nelson RE: Long-term pharmaceutical cost reduction using a data management system. Anesth Analg 87: 837, 1998

101. Dexter F, Macario A, Quian F, Traub RD: Forecasting surgical groups' total hours of elective cases for allocation of block time. Application of time series analysis to operating room management. Anesthesiology 91:1501, 1999

102. Strum DP, Vargas LG, May JH: Surgical subspecialty block utilization and capacity planning: a minimal cost analysis model. Anesthesiology 90:1176, 1999

103. Broadway P, Jones JG. A method of costing anaesthetic practice. Anaesthesia 50:56, 1995

104. Dexter F, Macario A, Lubarsky DA, Burns DD: Statistical method to evaluate management strategies to decrease variability in operating room utilization: Application of linear statistical modeling and Monte Carlo simulation to operating room management. Anesthesiology 91:262, 1999

105. Enlund M, Kobosko P, Rhodin A: A cost–benefit evaluation of using propofol and alfentanil for short gynaecological procedures. Acta Anaesth Scand 40:416, 1996

106. Dexter F, Tinker J: Analysis of strategies to decrease postanesthesia care unit costs. Anesthesiology 82:94, 1995

107. Boldt J, Jaun N, Kumle B et al: Economic considerations in the use of new anesthetics: A comparison of propofol, sevoflurane, desflurane and isoflurane. Anesth Analg 86:504, 1998

108. Cheng DCH, Karski J, Peniston C et al: Early tracheal extubation after coronary artery bypass graft surgery reduces costs and improves resource use. A prospective, randomized, controlled trial. Anesthesiology 85:1300, 1996

109. Cheng DCH, Karski J, Peniston C et al: Morbidity outcome in early versus conventional tracheal extubation after coronary artery bypass grafting: A prospective randomized controlled trial. J Thorac Cardiovasc Surg 112:755, 1996

110. Slogoff S, Keats AS: Randomized trial of primary anesthetic agents on outcome of coronary artery bypass operations. Anesthesiology 70:179, 1989

111. Tuman KJ, McCarthy RJ, Spiess BD et al: Does choice of anesthetic agent significantly affect outcome after coronary artery surgery? Anesthesiology 70:189, 1989

112. Butterworth J, James R, Prielipp RC et al: Do shorter-acting neuromuscular blocking drugs or opioids associate with reduced intensive care unit or hospital length of stay after coronary artery bypass grafting? Anesthesiology 88:1437, 1998

113. London MJ, Shroyer AL, Coll JR et al: Early extubation following cardiac surgery in a veterans population. Anesthesiology 88: 1447, 1998

114. Wong DT, Cheng DCH, Kustra R et al: Risk factors of delayed extubation, prolonged length of stay in the intensive care unit, and mortality in patients undergoing coronary artery bypass graft with fast-track cardiac anesthesia: A new cardiac risk score. Anesthesiology 91:936, 1999

115. Williams BA, DeRiso BM, Figallo CM et al: Benchmarking the perioperative process. III: Effects of regional anesthesia clinical pathway techniques on process efficiency and recovery profiles in ambulatory orthopedic surgery. J Clin Anesth 10:570, 1998

116. Jacobs P, Noseworthy TW: National estimates of intensive care utilization and costs: Canada and the U.S. Crit Care Med 17: 1282, 1990

117. Hanson CW, Deutschman C, Anderson HL et al: Effects of an organized critical care service on outcomes and resource utilization: A cohort study. Crit Care Med 27:270, 1999

118. Provonost P, Jenckes M, Dorman T et al: Organizational characteristics of intensive care units related to outcomes of abdominal aortic surgery. JAMA 281:1310, 1999

119. Selker HP, Griffith JL, Dorey FJ et al: How do physicians adapt when the coronary care unit is full? JAMA 257:1181, 1987

120. Singer DE, Carr PL, Mulley AG et al: Rationing intensive care physician responses to a resource shortage. N Engl J Med 309: 1155, 1983

121. Roberts DE, Bell DD, Ostryzniuk T et al: Eliminating needless testing in intensive care–an information based team management approach. Crit Care Med 21:1452, 1993

122. Inman KJ, Sibbald WJ, Rutledge FS et al: Does implementing pulse oximetry in a critical care unit result in substantial arterial blood gas savings? Chest 104:542, 1993

123. Davidoff F, Goodspeed R, Clive J: Changing test ordering behavior: A randomized controlled trial comparing probabilistic reasoning with cost-containment education. Med Care 27:45, 1989

124. Lundberg GD: American health care system management objectives: The aura of inevitability becomes incarnate. JAMA 269: 2554, 1993

125. Emanuel EJ, Emanuel LL: The economics of dying: The illusion of cost savings at the end of life. N Engl J Med 330:540, 1994

126. Murphy DJ, Povar GJ, Pawlson LG: Setting limits in clinical medicine. Arch Intern Med 154:505, 1994

127. Murphy DJ, Matchar DB: Life-sustaining therapy: A model for appropriate use. JAMA 264:2103, 1990

128. Bone RC, Balk RA: Noninvasive respiratory care unit. A cost-effective solution for the future. Chest 93:390, 1988

TWO

BASIC PRINCIPLES OF ANESTHESIA PRACTICE

Clinical Anesthesia (4/e), edited by
Paul G. Barash, Bruce F. Cullen, and
Robert K. Stoelting. Lippincott Williams &
Wilkins, Philadelphia, © 2001.

CHAPTER 7

CELLULAR AND MOLECULAR MECHANISMS OF ANESTHESIA

ALEX S. EVERS

INTRODUCTION

The introduction of general anesthetics into clinical practice 150 years ago stands as one of the seminal innovations of medicine. This single discovery facilitated the development of modern surgery and spawned the specialty of anesthesiology. Despite the importance of general anesthetics and despite over 100 years of active research, the molecular mechanisms responsible for anesthetic action remain one of the unsolved mysteries of pharmacology.

Why have mechanisms of anesthesia been so difficult to elucidate? Anesthetics, as a class of drugs, are challenging to study for three major reasons:

1. Anesthesia, by definition, is a change in the responses of an *intact animal* to external stimuli. It has proved very difficult to definitively link anesthetic effects observed *in vitro* to the anesthetic state observed and defined *in vivo*.
2. There are no apparent structure–activity relationships among anesthetics; a wide variety of structurally unrelated compounds, ranging from steroids to elemental xenon, are capable of producing clinical anesthesia. It is thus unclear whether there are many mechanisms of anesthesia or, as the unitary theory of anesthesia (see Chemical Nature of Anesthetic Targets) suggests, a single mechanism.
3. Anesthetics work at very high concentrations in comparison to drugs, neurotransmitters, and hormones that act at specific receptors. This implies that if anesthetics do act by binding to specific receptor sites, they must bind with very low affinity and probably stay bound to the receptor for very short periods of time. Low-affinity binding is much more difficult to observe and characterize than high-affinity binding.

Despite these difficulties, molecular and genetic tools are now available that should allow for major insights into anesthetic mechanisms to occur in the next decade. The aim of this chapter is to provide a conceptual framework for the reader to catalog current knowledge and integrate future developments about mechanisms of anesthesia. Five specific questions will be addressed in this chapter:

1. What is anesthesia and how do we measure it?
2. What is the anatomic site of anesthetic action in the central nervous system?
3. What are the cellular neurophysiologic mechanisms of anesthesia (*e.g.,* effects on synaptic function *versus* effects on action potential generation) and do anesthetic effects on ion channels and neuromodulatory chemical second messenger systems underlie these mechanisms?
4. What are the molecular targets of anesthetics?
5. How are the molecular and cellular effects of anesthetics linked to the behavioral effects of anesthetics observed *in vivo*?

WHAT IS ANESTHESIA?

General anesthesia can broadly be defined as a drug-induced reversible depression of the central nervous system resulting in the loss of response to and perception of all external stimuli. Unfortunately, such a broad definition is inadequate for two reasons. First, the definition is not actually broad enough. Anesthesia is not simply a deafferented state; amnesia and unconsciousness are important aspects of the anesthetic state. Second, the definition is too broad, as all general anesthetics do not produce equal depression of all sensory modalities. For example, barbiturates are considered to be anesthetics, but they are not particularly effective analgesics. These conflicting problems with definition, can be bypassed by a practical definition of the anesthetic state as a collection of "component" changes in behavior or perception. The components of the anesthetic state include unconsciousness, amnesia, analgesia, immobility, and attenuation of autonomic responses to noxious stimulation.

Regardless of which definition of anesthesia is used, it is clear that anesthesia is always defined by drug-induced changes in behavior or perception. As such, anesthesia can only be defined and measured in the intact organism. Changes in behavior such as unconsciousness or amnesia can be intuitively understood in higher organisms such as mammals, but become increasingly difficult to define as one descends the phylogenetic tree. Thus, while it is known that anesthetics have effects on organisms ranging from worms[1] to man, it is difficult to map with certainty the effects of anesthetics observed in lower organisms to any of our behavioral definitions of anesthesia. This contributes to the difficulty of using simple organisms as models in which to study the molecular mechanisms of anesthesia. Similarly, any cellular or molecular effects of anesthetics observed in higher organisms can be extremely difficult to link with the constellation of behaviors that constitute the anesthetic state. The absence of a simple and concise definition of anesthesia is clearly one of the stumbling blocks to elucidating the mechanisms of anesthesia at a molecular and cellular level.

HOW IS ANESTHESIA MEASURED?

In order to study the pharmacology of anesthetic action, it is absolutely essential that there be a quantitative measurement of anesthetic potency. To this end, Eger and colleagues have defined the concept of MAC, or minimum alveolar concentration. MAC is defined as the alveolar partial pressure of a gas at which 50% of humans will not respond to a surgical incision.[2] In animals, MAC is defined as the alveolar partial pressure of a gas at which 50% of animals will not respond to a noxious stimulus, such as tail clamp,[3] or at which they lose their righting reflex. The use of MAC as a measure of anesthetic potency has two major advantages. First, it is an extremely reproducible measurement that is remarkably constant over a wide range of species.[2] Second, the use of end-tidal gas concentration provides an index of the "free" concentration of drug required to produce anesthesia, since there should be an equilibrium between end-tidal gas concentration and free concentration in plasma. There are also several important limitations to the MAC concept, particularly when trying to relate MAC values to anesthetic potency observed *in vitro*. First, the end point in a MAC determination is quantal: a subject is either anesthetized or unanesthetized; it cannot be partially anesthetized. Furthermore, MAC represents the average response of a whole population of subjects rather than the response of a single subject. The quantal nature of the MAC measurement makes it very difficult to compare MAC measurements to concentration–response curves obtained *in vitro*, where the graded response of a single preparation is measured as a function of anesthetic concentration. The second limitation of MAC measurements is that they can only be directly applied to anesthetic gases. Parenteral anesthetics (barbiturates, neurosteroids, propofol) cannot be assigned a MAC value, making it difficult to compare the potency of parenteral and volatile anesthetics. A MAC equivalent for parental anesthetics is the free concentration of the drug in plasma required to prevent response to a noxious stimulus in 50% of subjects; this value has been estimated for several parenteral anesthetics.[4] The third limitation of MAC is that it is highly dependent on the anesthetic end point used to define it. For example, if loss of response to a verbal command is used as an anesthetic end point, the MAC values obtained (MAC$_{awake}$) will be much lower than classic MAC values based on response to a noxious stimulus. Indeed, it is likely that each behavioral component of the anesthetic state will have a different MAC value. Despite its limitations, MAC remains the most robust measurement and the standard for determining the potency of volatile anesthetics.

The foregoing discussion of MAC brings forth an important and somewhat controversial question. What drug concentration should be measured when determining anesthetic potency? When measuring potency of intravenous anesthetics, the answer to this question is relatively simple. One would like to relate the free concentration of the drug at its site of action (the biophase) to the drug's effect. It is, of course, not practical to measure the drug's concentration in the extracellular fluid of the brain, so free concentration in plasma is used as an approximation of the biophase concentration. This allows one to compare the concentration of drug required to produce anesthesia in humans to the concentrations required to produce specific effects *in vitro*. With the volatile anesthetics, potency is defined by MAC, which is measured in units of partial pressure. Since the partial pressure of a dissolved gas is directly proportional to the free concentration of that gas in a liquid, alveolar partial pressures are accurate reporters of the free anesthetic concentrations in plasma and in brain tissue. However, as one lowers temperature, anesthetic gases become much more soluble in plasma; at a given anesthetic partial pressure the free concentration of anesthetic will markedly increase as one lowers temperature. Thus, anesthetic potency increases significantly as one lowers temperature if potency is defined using MAC values.[5] Most of this apparent increase in potency is due to increased anesthetic solubility; anesthetic potency increases only slightly at lower temperatures, if potency is defined using free concentrations of anesthetic.[6] This issue becomes important in *in vitro* studies of anesthetic mechanisms where experiments are carried out at a variety of temperatures. Anesthetic partial pressures that are considered clinically relevant at room temperature (25°C) are approximately half the partial pressures needed to produce anesthesia at body temperature (37°C). In contrast, the free anesthetic concentrations that should be considered clinically relevant show only small variation with temperature.

WHERE IN THE CENTRAL NERVOUS SYSTEM DO ANESTHETICS WORK?

In principle, general anesthesia could result from interruption of nervous system activity at myriad levels. Plausible targets include peripheral sensory receptors, spinal cord, brain stem, and cerebral cortex. Of these potential sites, only peripheral sensory receptors can be eliminated as an important site of anesthetic action. Animal studies have shown that fluorinated volatile anes-

thetics have no effect on cutaneous mechanosensors in cats[7] and can even sensitize nociceptors in monkeys.[8] Furthermore, selective perfusion studies in dogs have shown that MAC for isoflurane is unaffected by the presence or absence of isoflurane at the site of noxious stimulation, provided that the central nervous system is perfused with blood containing isoflurane.[9]

Spinal Cord

It is clear that anesthetic actions at the spinal cord cannot explain either amnesia or unconsciousness. However, several lines of evidence indicate that the spinal cord is probably the site at which anesthetics act to inhibit purposeful responses to noxious stimulation. This is, of course, the end point used in most measurements of anesthetic potency. Rampil and colleagues have shown that MAC values for fluorinated volatile anesthetics are unaffected in the rat by either decerebration[10] or cervical spinal cord transection.[11] Antognini and colleagues have used the strategy of isolating the cerebral circulation of goats to explore the contribution of brain and spinal cord to the determination of MAC. They found that when isoflurane is administered only to the brain, MAC is 2.9%, whereas when it is administered to the entire body, MAC is 1.2%.[12] Surprisingly, when isoflurane was preferentially administered to the body and not to the brain, isoflurane MAC was reduced to 0.8%.[13] The actions of volatile anesthetics in the spinal cord are mediated, at least in part, by direct effects on the excitability of spinal motor neurons. This has been demonstrated in rats,[14] goats,[15] and humans[16] by showing that volatile anesthetics depress the amplitude of the F wave in evoked potential measurements (F-wave amplitude correlates with motor neuron excitability). These provocative results suggest not only that anesthetic actions at the spinal cord underlie the determination of MAC, but that anesthetic actions on the brain may actually sensitize the cord to noxious stimuli. The plausibility of the spinal cord as a locus for anesthetic effect is also supported by several electrophysiologic studies showing inhibition of excitatory synaptic transmission in the spinal cord.[17-20]

Reticular Activating System

It has long been speculated that the reticular activating system, a diffuse collection of brain stem neurons involved in arousal behavior, is involved in the effects of general anesthetics on consciousness. Evidence to support this notion came from early whole animal experiments showing that electrical stimulation of the reticular activating system could induce arousal behavior in anesthetized animals.[21] A role for the brain stem in anesthetic action is supported by studies examining somatosensory evoked potentials. Generally, these studies show that anesthetics produce increased latency and decreased amplitude of cortical potentials, indicating that anesthetics inhibit information transfer through the brain stem.[22] In contrast, studies using brain stem auditory evoked potentials have shown variable effects ranging from depression to enhancement of information transfer through the reticular formation.[23-25] While there is evidence that the reticular formation of the brain stem is a locus for anesthetic effects, it cannot be the only anatomic site of anesthetic action for two reasons. First, as discussed above, the brain stem is not even required for anesthetics to inhibit responsiveness to noxious stimuli. Second, the reticular formation can be largely ablated without eliminating awareness.[26]

Cerebral Cortex

The cerebral cortex is the major site for integration, storage, and retrieval of information. As such, it is a likely site at which anesthetics might interfere with complex functions like memory and awareness. Anesthetics clearly alter cortical electrical activity, as evidenced by the consistent changes in surface EEG patterns recorded during anesthesia. Anesthetic effects on patterns of cortical electrical activity vary widely among anesthetics,[27] providing an initial suggestion that all anesthetics are not likely to act through identical mechanisms. *In vitro* electrophysiologic studies examining anesthetic effects on different cortical regions support the notion that anesthetics can differentially alter neuronal function in various cortical preparations. For example, volatile anesthetics have been shown to inhibit excitatory transmission at some synapses in the olfactory cortex[28] but not at others.[29] Similarly, whereas volatile anesthetics inhibit excitatory transmission in the dentate gyrus of the hippocampus,[30] these same drugs can actually enhance excitatory transmission at other synapses in the hippocampus.[31] Anesthetics also produce a variety of effects on inhibitory transmission in the cortex. A variety of parenteral and inhalation anesthetics have been shown to enhance inhibitory transmission in olfactory cortex[29] and in the hippocampus.[32] Conversely, volatile anesthetics have also been reported to depress inhibitory transmission in hippocampus.[33] One area of the brain that has been postulated as a potential site of anesthetic action is the thalamus. The thalamus is important in relaying sensory modalities and motor information to the cortex *via* thalamocortical pathways. There is a developing body of evidence that inhalational anesthetics can depress the excitability of thalamic neurons, thus blocking thalamocortical communication.[34] This is a potential mechanism for anesthetic-induced loss of consciousness.

Summary

Anesthetics are able to produce effects on a variety of anatomic structures in the CNS, including spinal cord, brain stem, and cerebral cortex. Whereas certain anesthetic effects may be attributable to specific anatomic locations (*e.g.,* purposeful response to noxious stimulation maps to the spinal cord), there is no basis for identifying a single anatomic site responsible for anesthesia. It is plausible that this difficulty in identifying a site for anesthesia results from the fact that various components of the anesthetic state are being produced by anesthetic effects in different regions of the CNS. Nevertheless, the difficulty in identifying a common anatomic site for anesthesia has led investigators to look for other unifying principles in anesthetic action. Specifically, attention has been focused on identifying common cellular or molecular anesthetic targets that may have a wide anatomic distribution, explaining the ability of anesthetic to affect nervous system function in an anatomically diffuse manner.

HOW DO ANESTHETICS INTERFERE WITH THE ELECTROPHYSIOLOGIC FUNCTION OF THE NERVOUS SYSTEM?

In the simplest terms anesthetics inhibit or "turn off" vital central nervous system functions. They must do this by acting at specific physiologic "switches." A great deal of investigative effort has been devoted to identifying these switches. In principle, there are several ways in which the CNS could be switched off:

1. By depressing those neurons or pattern generators that subserve a pacemaker function in the CNS.
2. By reducing neuronal excitability; either by changing resting membrane potential or by interfering with the processes involved in generating an action potential.
3. By reducing communication between neurons; specifically, by either inhibiting excitatory synaptic transmission or enhancing inhibitory synaptic transmission.

Pattern Generators

There is limited information concerning the effects of anesthetics on pattern-generating neuronal circuits in the CNS, but it is likely that clinical concentrations of anesthetics do have significant effects on these circuits. The simplest evidence for this is the observation that most anesthetics exert profound effects on respiratory rate and rhythm, strongly suggesting an effect on respiratory pattern generators in the brain stem. Experimental evidence from invertebrate studies suggests that volatile anesthetics can selectively inhibit the spontaneous firing of specific neurons. As shown in Figure 7-1, halothane (1.0 MAC) completely inhibits spontaneous action potential generation by one neuron in the right parietal ganglion of the great pond snail while producing no observable effect on the firing frequency of adjacent neurons.[35]

Neuronal Excitability

The ability of a neuron to generate an action potential is determined by three parameters: resting membrane potential, the threshold potential for action potential generation, and the function of voltage-gated sodium channels. There is strong evidence that anesthetics can hyperpolarize (create a more negative resting membrane potential) both spinal motor neurons and cortical neurons,[36,37] and this ability of anesthetics to hyperpolarize neurons correlates with anesthetic potency. In general, the increase in resting membrane potential produced by anesthetics is small in magnitude and is unlikely to have an effect on axonal *propagation* of an action potential. Small changes in resting potential may, however, inhibit the *initiation* of an action potential either at a postsynaptic site or in a spontaneously firing neuron. Indeed, hyperpolarization is responsible for the inhibition of spontaneous action potential generation shown

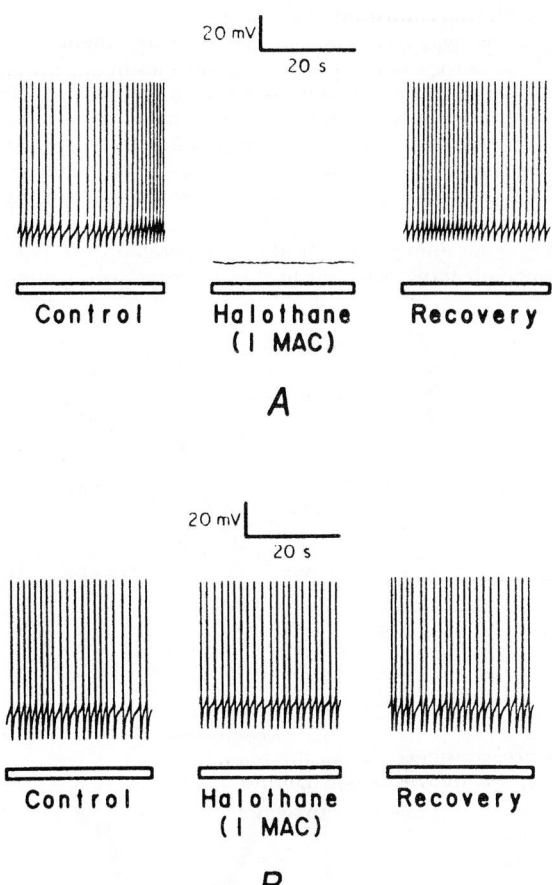

Figure 7-1. Selectivity of volatile anesthetic inhibition of neuronal automaticity. Halothane (1 MAC) reversibly inhibits the spontaneous firing activity of a neuron from the parietal ganglion of *Lymnaea stagnalis* (*Panel A*). The same concentration of halothane has no effect on the firing activity of an adjacent, and apparently identical, neuron (*Panel B*). Note that in Panel *A*, halothane markedly reduces resting membrane potential in addition to inhibiting firing. (Reprinted with permission from Franks NP, Lieb WR: Mechanisms of general anesthesia. Environ Health Perspect 87:204, 1990.)

in Figure 7-1. Recent evidence also indicates that isoflurane hyperpolarizes thalamic neurons, leading to an inhibition of tonic firing of action potentials.[34] There is no evidence indicating that anesthetics alter the threshold potential of a neuron for action potential generation. Similarly, most evidence indicates that clinically relevant concentrations of anesthetics do not alter the function of the voltage-gated channels involved in action potential generation.[38] A possible exception to this is the recent work of Duch showing that clinical concentrations of fluorinated inhalational anesthetics suppress voltage-elicited currents in rat brain sodium channels expressed in a mammalian cell line.[39]

Consistent with the evidence that anesthetics do not have major effects on voltage-gated channels, most experimental evidence indicates that clinically relevant concentrations of anesthetics do not inhibit axonal propagation of action potentials. This was first shown in a classic paper by Larabee and Posternak, in which they demonstrated that concentrations of ether and chloroform that completely block synaptic transmission in mammalian sympathetic ganglia have no effect on presynaptic action potential amplitude.[40] Similar results have been obtained with fluorinated volatile anesthetics in several mammalian brain preparations.[28,30] For completeness, it should be noted that clinical concentrations of general anesthetics have been shown to produce modest depression of action potential amplitude in unmyelinated CNS fibers.[41] In principle, this small amount of action potential depression could lead to reduced synaptic neurotransmitter release.

Synaptic Function

It is widely believed that anesthetic action results from effects on chemical synapses in the CNS rather than on axonal conduction. General anesthetics have been shown to inhibit excitatory synaptic transmission in a variety of preparations, including sympathetic ganglia,[40] olfactory cortex,[28] hippocampus,[30] and spinal cord.[19] The anesthetic concentrations required to inhibit excitatory synaptic transmission in these preparations are one-fifth to one-tenth those required to inhibit axonal conduction. In contrast, there is also experimental evidence showing that anesthetics have no effect on excitatory synaptic function and that they can, in an agent- and synapse-specific manner, *enhance* excitatory transmission.[31] In a similar fashion, general anesthetics have been shown to both enhance and depress inhibitory synaptic transition in various preparations. In a classic paper in 1975, Nicoll showed that barbiturates enhanced inhibitory synaptic transmission by prolonging the decay of the GABAergic inhibitory postsynaptic current.[42] Enhancement of inhibitory transmission has also been observed with many other general anesthetics including halothane[29] and neurosteroids.[43] Although anesthetic enhancement of inhibitory currents has received a great deal of attention as a potential mechanism of anesthesia,[4] it is important to note that there is also a large body of experimentation showing that clinical concentrations of general anesthetics can depress inhibitory postsynaptic potentials in hippocampus[33,44,45] and in spinal cord.[20] Anesthetics do appear to have preferential effects on synapses, but there is a great deal of heterogeneity in the manner in which anesthetic agents affect different synapses. This is not surprising given the large variation in synaptic structure, function (*i.e.*, efficacy), and chemistry (neurotransmitters, modulators) extant in the nervous system.

Presynaptic Effects

The effects of anesthetics on synaptic function may result from actions affecting a number of cellular processes. Anesthetics could alter presynaptic neurotransmitter release by affecting transmitter synthesis, storage, or secretion.[46] Current evidence suggests that anesthetics can inhibit the release of both excitatory transmitters[47,48] and inhibitory transmitters.[49] For example, a study by Perousansky and colleagues conducted in mouse hippocampal slices showed that halothane inhibited excitatory postsynaptic potentials elicited by presynaptic electrical stimulation, but not those elicited by direct application of glutamate. This indicates that halothane must be acting to prevent the release of excitatory neurotransmitter.[50] There have also been some reports that general anesthetics can enhance the release of the inhibitory neurotransmitter GABA.[51,52] The effects of anes-

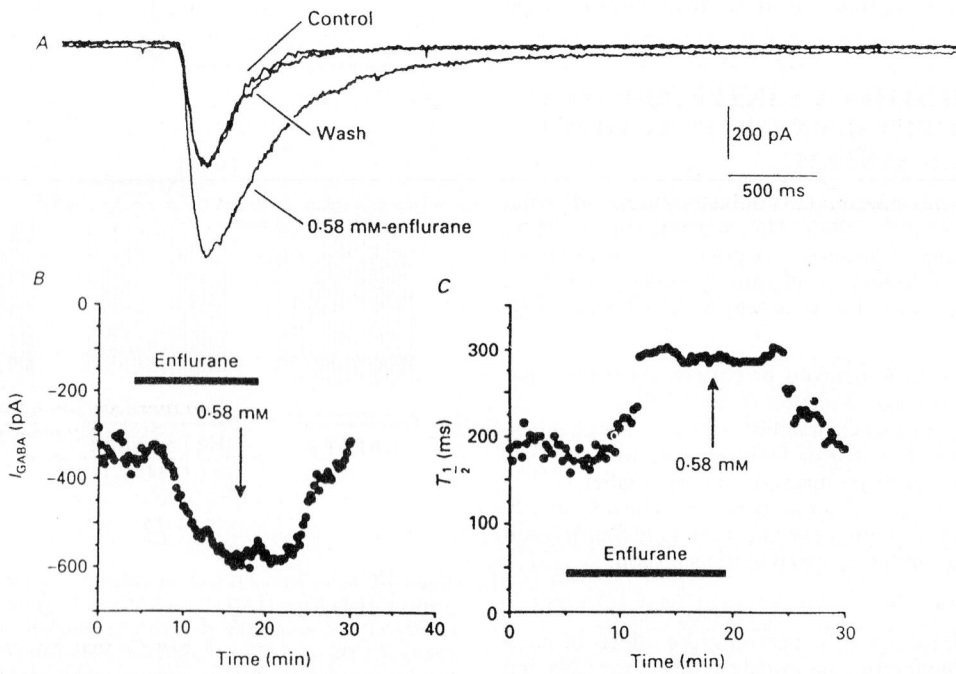

Figure 7-2. Enflurane potentiates the ability of GABA to activate a chloride current in cultured rat hippocampal cells. This potentiation is rapidly reversed by removal of enflurane (wash) (*Panel A*). Enflurane increases both the amplitude of the current (*Panel B*) and the time ($\tau_{1/2}$) it takes for the current to decay (*Panel C*). (Reproduced with permission from Jones MV, Brooks PA, Harrison L: Enhancement of γ-aminobutyric acid-activated Cl⁻ currents in cultured rat hippocampal neurones by three volatile anaesthetics. J Physiol 449:289, 1992.)

thetics on neurotransmitter release do not appear to be mediated by reduced neurotransmitter synthesis or storage, but rather by a direct effect on the process of neurosecretion. Although it is difficult to dissect the mechanism for reduced neurosecretion in intact CNS preparations, work in neuroendocrine cells suggests that anesthetics inhibit neurosecretion by inhibiting the entry of calcium into the cell rather than by depressing the calcium-dependent stimulation of the secretory process.[53–55] More recent work, using genetic approaches in lower organisms, implicates the proteins involved in vesicle release (syntaxin, synaptobrevein, SNAP-25) as potential sites of presynaptic anesthetic action.[56]

Postsynaptic Effects

Anesthetics can also affect synaptic function by altering the postsynaptic response to released neurotransmitter. The effects of general anesthetics on excitatory neurotransmitter action vary depending on neurotransmitter type, anesthetic agent, and preparation. Richards and Smaje examined the effects of several anesthetic agents on the response of olfactory cortical neurons to application of glutamate, the major excitatory neurotransmitter in the CNS.[57] They found that while pentobarbital, diethylether, methoxyflurane, and alphaxalone depressed the electrical response to glutamate, halothane was without effect. In contrast, when acetylcholine was applied to the same olfactory cortical preparation, halothane and methoxyflurane stimulated the electrical response whereas pentobarbital had no effect; only alphaxalone depressed the electrical response to acetylcholine.[58] The effects of anesthetics on neuronal responses to inhibitory neurotransmitters are more consistent. A wide variety of anesthetics, including barbiturates, etomidate, neurosteroids, propofol, and the fluorinated volatile anesthetics, have been shown to enhance the electrical response to exogenously applied GABA (for a review, see Tanelian et al[59]). For example, Figure 7-2 illustrates the ability of enflurane to increase both the amplitude and the duration of the electrical response elicited by application of GABA to hippocampal neurons.[60]

Summary

Attempts to identify a physiologic "switch" at which anesthetics act have suffered from their own success. Anesthetics produce a variety of effects on many physiologic processes that might logically contribute to the anesthetic state, including neuronal automaticity, neuronal excitability, and synaptic function. It is generally thought that the synapse is the most likely target of anesthetic action. Existing evidence indicates that even at this one target, anesthetics produce various effects, including presynaptic inhibition of neurotransmitter release, inhibition of excitatory neurotransmitter effect, and enhancement of inhibitory neurotransmitter effect. Furthermore, the effects of anesthetics on synaptic function differ among various anesthetic agents, neurotransmitters, and neuronal preparations.

ANESTHETIC ACTIONS ON ION CHANNELS

All of the various effects of anesthetics described in the previous section are likely to result from the actions of anesthetics on the machinery used to generate neuronal electrical activity: ion channels, pumps, and transporters. With the advent of patch clamp techniques in the early 1980s, it became possible to examine the function of specific kinds of ion channels and even to look at the currents resulting from single ion channel proteins. It was attractive to think that anesthetic effects on a small number of ion channels might help to explain the complex physiologic effects of anesthetics that we have already described. Accordingly, during the 1980s and 1990s a major effort was directed at describing the effects of anesthetics on the various kinds of ion channels. The following section summarizes and distills this effort. For the purposes of this discussion, ion channels are cataloged according to the stimuli to which they respond by opening or closing (*i.e.,* their mechanism of gating).

Anesthetic Effects on Voltage-Dependent Ion Channels

A variety of ion channels can sense a change in membrane potential and respond by either opening or closing their pore. These channels include voltage-dependent sodium, potassium, and calcium channels, all of which share significant structural homologies. Voltage-dependent sodium and potassium channels are largely involved in generating and shaping action potentials. The effects of anesthetics on these channels have been extensively studied by Haydon and colleagues in the squid giant axon.[38,61] These studies show that sodium channels and potassium channels are remarkably insensitive to volatile anesthetics. For example, 50% inhibition of the peak sodium channel current required halothane concentrations 8 times those required to produce anesthesia. The delayed rectifier potassium channel was even less sensitive, requiring halothane concentrations more than 20 times those required to produce anesthesia. Similar results have been obtained in a mammalian cell line (GH$_3$ pituitary cells) where both sodium and potassium currents were inhibited by halothane only at concentrations greater than 5 times those required to produce anesthesia.[62] A recent study by Rehberg and colleagues challenged the notion that voltage-dependent sodium channels are insensitive to anesthetics. They expressed a rat brain IIA sodium channel in a mammalian cell line, and showed that clinically relevant concentrations of a variety of inhalational anesthetics suppressed voltage-elicited sodium currents.[39] The minimal effect of anesthetics on voltage-dependent sodium and potassium channels that is generally observed is consistent with the observation that anesthetics do not substantively interfere with action potential generation or axonal conduction. The ability of anesthetics to suppress sodium currents in some systems leaves open the possibility that action potential generation or propagation could mediate some anesthetic effects.

Voltage-dependent calcium channels (VDCC) serve to couple electrical activity to specific cellular functions. In the nervous system, VDCCs located at presynaptic terminals respond to action potentials by opening. This allows calcium to enter the cell, activating calcium-dependent secretion of neurotransmitter into the synaptic cleft. There are at least six types of calcium channels (designated L, N, P, Q, R, and T) identified on the basis of electrophysiologic properties and a larger number based on molecular biologic studies.[63] N-, P-, Q-, and R-type channels, as well as some of the untitled channels, are preferentially expressed in the nervous system and are thought to play a major role in synaptic transmission. L-type calcium channels, although expressed in brain, play a predominant role in excitation–contraction coupling in cardiac, skeletal, and smooth muscle and are thought to be less important in synaptic transmission. The effects of anesthetics on L- and T-type currents have been well characterized,[62,64,65] and there are some reports concerning the effects of anesthetics on N- and P-type currents.[66–68] As a general rule, these studies have shown that volatile anesthetics inhibit VDCCs (50% reduction in current) at concentrations two to five times those required to produce anesthesia in humans. This makes VDCCs more sensitive to anesthetics than are voltage-dependent sodium or potassium channels, but suggests that there is less than 20% inhibition of calcium current at clinical concentrations of anesthetics (Fig. 7-3). There have, however, been reports of VDCCs that are extremely sensitive to anesthetics. Takenoshita and Steinbach reported a T-type calcium current in dorsal root ganglion neurons that was inhibited by subanesthetic concentrations of halothane.[69] Additionally, ffrench-Mullen and colleagues have reported a VDCC of unspecified type in guinea pig hippocampus that is inhibited

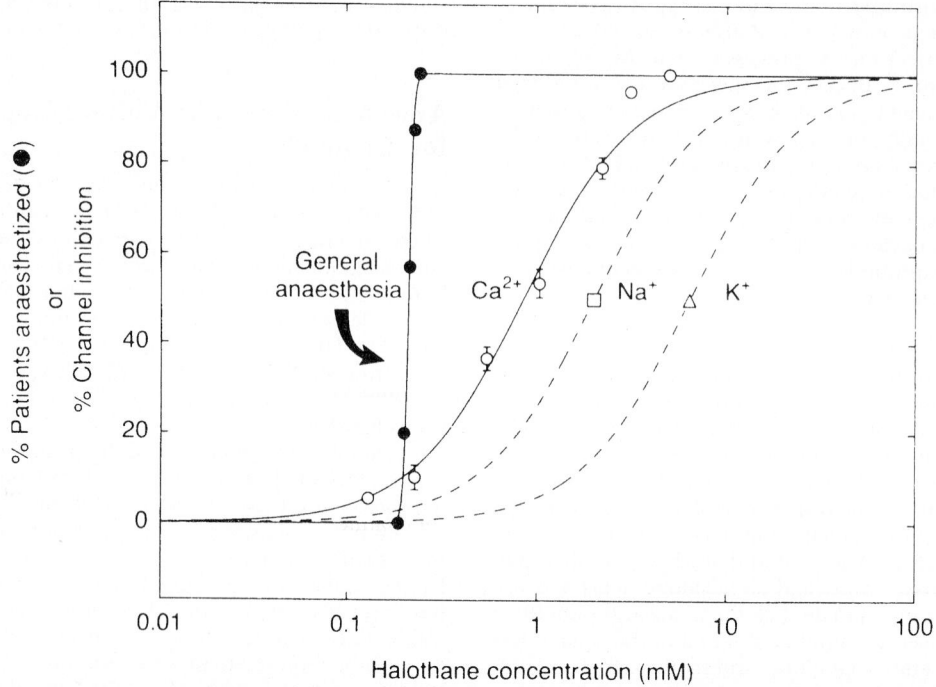

Figure 7-3. Halothane inhibition of voltage-dependent Ca^{2+}, Na^+, and K^+ currents. The Ca^{2+} channels are L-type channels from GH_3 cells, and the Na^+ and K^+ channels are from the squid giant axon. The closed circles show the concentrations of halothane required to anesthetize humans. Note that the Ca^{2+} currents are inhibited about 20% by clinical concentrations of halothane whereas the Na^+ and K^+ currents are not inhibited at all. (Reproduced by permission from Franks NP, Lieb WR: Molecular and cellular mechanisms of anesthesia. Nature 367:607, 1994, Macmillan Magazines Ltd.)

by pentobarbital at concentrations identical to those required to produce anesthesia.[70]

Summary

Existing evidence suggests that VDCCs are modestly sensitive to anesthetics, but there is likely to be significant heterogeneity in the anesthetic sensitivity of specific channel types and subtypes. It is attractive to hypothesize that anesthetic effects on VDCCs could explain the observed inhibition of neurotransmitter release that occurs at some synapses with some anesthetics. Additional experimental data will be required to establish whether anesthetic-sensitive VDCCs are localized to specific synapses at which anesthetics have been shown to inhibit neurotransmitter release.[19]

Anesthetic Effects on Ligand-Gated Ion Channels

Fast excitatory and inhibitory neurotransmission is mediated by the actions of ligand-gated ion channels. Synaptically released glutamate or GABA diffuse across the synaptic cleft and bind to channel proteins that are opened as a consequence of neurotransmitter release. The channel proteins that bind GABA (GABA_A receptors) are members of a superfamily of structurally related ligand-gated ion channel proteins that includes nicotinic acetylcholine receptors, glycine receptors, and 5-HT_3 receptors.[71] Based on the structure of the nicotinic acetylcholine receptor, each ligand-gated channel is thought to be composed of five nonidentical subunits. The glutamate receptors also comprise a family, each receptor thought to be a tetrameric protein composed of structurally related subunits.[72] The ligand-gated ion channels provide a logical target for anesthetic action, because selective effects on these channels could inhibit fast excitatory synaptic transmission and/or facilitate fast inhibitory synaptic transmission. The effects of anesthetic agents on ligand-gated ion channels are thoroughly cataloged in a recent review

by Krasowski and Harrison.[73] The following section provides a brief summary of this body of work.

Glutamate-Activated Ion Channels

Glutamate-activated ion channels have been classified, based on selective agonists, into three categories: AMPA receptors, kainate receptors, and NMDA receptors. Molecular biologic studies indicate that a large number of structurally distinct glutamate receptor subunits can be used to form each of the three categories of glutamate receptors.[74] This structural heterogeneity is probably reflected in functional heterogeneity within each category of glutamate receptor. AMPA and kainate receptors are relatively nonselective cation channels involved in fast excitatory synaptic transmission, whereas NMDA channels are somewhat selective for calcium and are involved in long-term modulation of synaptic responses (long-term potentiation) and glutamate-mediated neurotoxicity. Studies from the early 1980s in mouse and rat brain preparations showed that AMPA- and kainate-activated currents are insensitive to clinical concentrations of halothane,[75] enflurane,[76] and the neurosteroid 3-α-OH-DHP.[77] In contrast, kainate- and AMPA-activated currents were shown to be more sensitive to barbiturates; in rat hippocampal neurons, 50 μM pentobarbital (pentobarbital produces anesthesia at approximately 50 μM) inhibited kainate and AMPA responses by 50%.[77] More recent studies using cloned and expressed glutamate receptor subunits show that submaximal agonist responses of GluR3 (AMPA-type) receptors are inhibited by fluorinated volatile anesthetics whereas agonist responses of GluR6 (kainate-type) receptors are enhanced.[78] In contrast both GluR3 and GluR6 receptors are inhibited by pentobarbital. The directionally opposite effects of the volatile anesthetics on different glutamate receptor subtypes may explain the earlier inconclusive effects observed in tissue, where multiple subunit types are expressed. The directionally opposite effects of the volatile anesthetics on GluR3- and GluR6-containing receptors have also been used as a strategy to identify critical sites on the molecules involved in anesthetic effect. By producing GluR3/GluR6 receptor chimeras (receptors made up of various combinations of sections of the GluR3 and GluR6 receptors) and screening for volatile anesthetic effect, specific areas of the protein required for volatile anesthetic potentiation of GluR6 have been identified. Subsequent site-directed mutagenesis studies have identified a specific glycine residue (Gly-819) as critical for volatile anesthetic action on GluR6-containing receptors.[79]

NMDA-activated currents also appear to be insensitive to most anesthetics. Electrophysiologic studies show virtually no effects of clinical concentrations of volatile anesthetics,[75,76] neurosteroids, or barbiturates[77] on NMDA-activated currents. It should be noted that there is some evidence from flux studies that volatile anesthetics may inhibit NMDA-activated channels. A study in rat brain microvesicles showed that anesthetic concentrations (0.2–0.3 mM) of halothane and enflurane inhibited NMDA-activated calcium flux by 50%.[80] In contrast to other anesthetics, ketamine is a potent and selective inhibitor of NMDA-activated currents. Ketamine stereoselectively inhibits NMDA currents by binding to the phencyclidine site on the NMDA receptor protein.[81–83] The anesthetic effects of ketamine in intact animals show the same stereoselectivity as that observed in vitro,[84] suggesting that the NMDA receptor may be the principal molecular target for the anesthetic actions of ketamine. Two other recent findings suggest that NMDA receptors may be an important target for specific anesthetic agents. These studies show that N_2O[85,86] and xenon[87] are potent and selective inhibitors of NMDA-activated currents. This is illustrated in Figure 7-4, showing that N_2O inhibits NMDA-elicited, but not GABA-elicited, currents in hippocampal neurons.

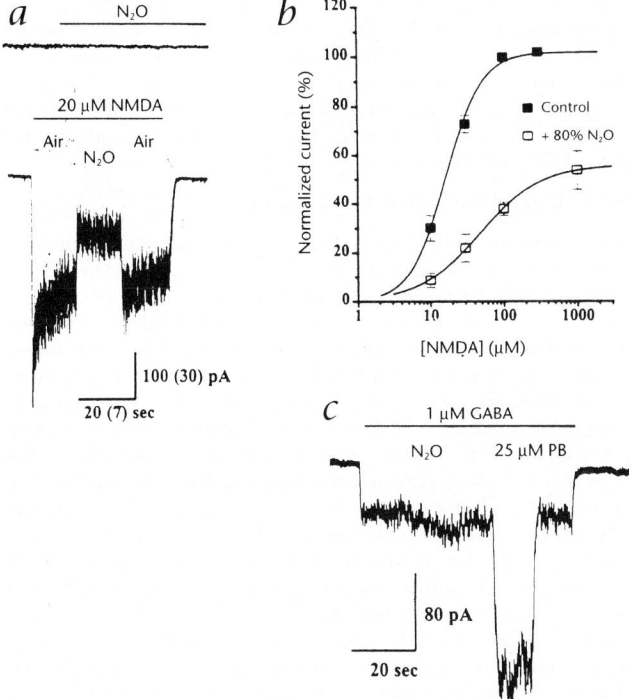

Figure 7-4. Nitrous oxide inhibits NMDA-elicited, but not GABA-elicited, currents in rat hippocampal neurons. *Panel A:* 80% N_2O has no effect on holding current (upper trace), but inhibits the current elicited by NMDA. *Panel B:* N_2O causes a rightward and downward shift of the NMDA concentration–response curve, indicating a mixed competitive/noncompetitive antagonism. *Panel C:* 80% N_2O has little effect on GABA-elicited currents. In contrast, an equipotent anesthetic concentration of pentobarbital markedly enhances the GABA-elicited current. (Reproduced with permission from Jevtovic-Todorovic V, Todorovic SM, Mennerick S *et al:* Nitrous oxide (laughing gas) is an NMDA antagonist, neuroprotectant, and neurotoxin. Nature Medicine 4:460, 1998.)

GABA-Activated Ion Channels

GABA is the most important inhibitory neurotransmitter in the mammalian central nervous system. GABA-activated ion channels ($GABA_A$ receptors) mediate the postsynaptic response to synaptically released GABA by selectively allowing chloride ions to enter, and thereby hyperpolarize, neurons. $GABA_A$ receptors are multisubunit proteins consisting of various combinations of α, β, γ, δ, and ϵ subunits, and there are many subtypes of each of these subunits. The function of $GABA_A$ receptors is modulated by a wide variety of pharmacologic agents including convulsants, anticonvulsants, sedatives, anxiolytics, and anesthetics.[88] The effects of these various drugs on $GABA_A$ receptor function varies across brain regions and cell types. The following section briefly reviews the effects of anesthetics on $GABA_A$ receptor function.

Barbiturates, anesthetic steroids, benzodiazepines, propofol, etomidate, and the volatile anesthetics all modulate $GABA_A$ receptor function.[60,88–91] These drugs produce three kinds of effects on the electrophysiologic behavior of the $GABA_A$ receptor channels: potentiation, direct-gating, and inhibition. *Potentiation* refers to the ability of anesthetics to markedly increase the current elicited by low concentrations of GABA, but to produce no increase in the current elicited by a maximally effective concentration of GABA.[75,92] Potentiation is illustrated in Figure 7-5, showing the effects of halothane on currents elicited by a range of GABA concentrations in dissociated cortical neurons. Anesthetic potentiation of $GABA_A$ currents generally occurs at concentrations of anesthetics within the clinical range. *Direct gating* refers to the ability of anesthetics to activate $GABA_A$ channels in the absence of GABA. Generally, direct gating of $GABA_A$ currents occurs at anesthetic concentrations higher than those used clinically, but the concentration–response curves for potentiation and for direct gating can overlap. It is not known whether direct gating of $GABA_A$ channels is either required for or contributes to the effects of anesthetics on GABA-mediated inhibitory synaptic transmission *in vivo*. In the case of anesthetic steroids, there is strong evidence indicating that potentiation, rather than direct gating of $GABA_A$ currents, is required for producing anesthesia.[93] Anesthetics can also inhibit GABA-activated currents. *Inhibition* refers to the ability of anesthetics to prevent GABA from initiating current flow through $GABA_A$ channels, and has generally been observed at high concentrations of both GABA and anesthetic.[94,95] Inhibition of $GABA_A$ channels may help to explain why volatile anesthetics have, in some cases, been observed to inhibit rather than facilitate inhibitory synaptic transmission.[33]

The effects of anesthetics have also been observed on the function of single $GABA_A$ channels. These studies show that barbiturates,[89] propofol,[91] and volatile anesthetics[96] do not alter the conductance (rate at which ions traverse the open channel) of the channel, but that they increase the frequency with which the channel opens and/or the average length of time that the channel remains open. Collectively, the whole cell and single channel data are most consistent with the idea that clinical concentrations of anesthetics produce a change in the conformation of $GABA_A$ receptors that increases the affinity of the receptor for GABA. This is consistent with the ability of anesthetics to increase the duration of inhibitory postsynaptic potentials (IPSPs), since higher affinity binding of GABA would slow the dissociation of GABA from postsynaptic $GABA_A$ channels. It would not be expected that anesthetics would increase the amplitude of a GABAergic IPSP, since synaptically released GABA probably reaches very high concentrations in the synapse. Higher concentrations of anesthetics can produce additional effects, either directly activating or inhibiting $GABA_A$ channels. Consistent with these ideas, a study by Banks and Pearce showed that isoflurane and enflurane simultaneously increased the duration and decreased the amplitude of GABAergic inhibitory postsynaptic currents in hippocampal slices.[97]

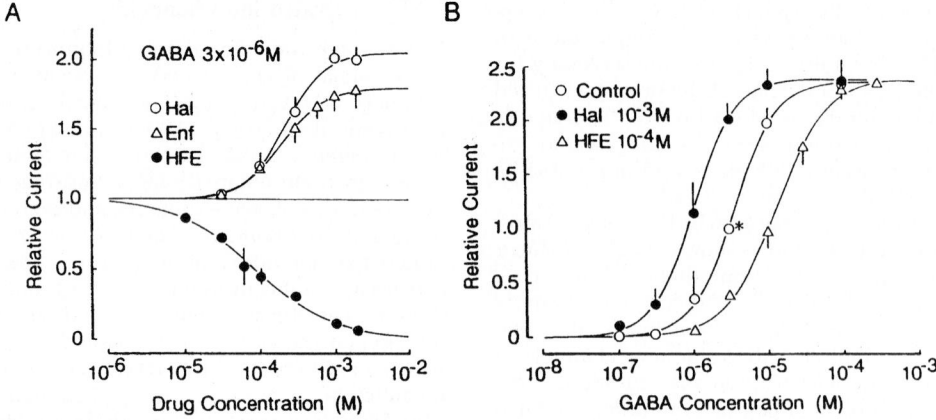

Figure 7-5. The effects of halothane (Hal), enflurane (Enf), and fluorothyl (HFE) on GABA-activated chloride currents in dissociated rat CNS neurons. *Panel A:* Clinical concentrations of halothane and enflurane potentiate the ability of GABA to elicit a chloride current. The convulsant fluorothyl antagonizes the effects of GABA. *Panel B:* GABA causes a concentration-dependent activation of a chloride current. Halothane shifts the GABA concentration–response curve to the left (increases the apparent affinity of the channel for GABA) whereas fluorothyl shifts the curve to the right (decreases the apparent affinity of the channel for GABA). (Reproduced with permission from Wakamori M, Ikemoto Y, Akaike N: Effects of two volatile anesthetics and a volatile convulsant on the excitatory and inhibitory amino acid responses in dissociated CNS neurons of the rat. J Neurophysiol 66:2014, 1991.)

Despite the similar effects of many anesthetics on GABA_A receptor function, there is significant evidence that the various anesthetics do not act by binding to a single common binding site on the channel protein. First, even anesthetics that directly activate the channel probably do not bind to the GABA binding site. This is most clearly demonstrated by molecular biologic studies in which the GABA binding site is eliminated from the channel protein but pentobarbital can still activate the channel.[98] Direct radioligand binding studies have demonstrated that benzodiazepines bind to the GABA_A receptor at nanomolar concentrations and that other anesthetics can modulate binding, but do not bind directly to the benzodiazepine site.[59,88] A series of more complex studies examining the interactions between barbiturates, anesthetic steroids, and benzodiazepines indicate that these three classes of drugs cannot be acting at the same sites.[88] The actions of anesthetics on GABA_A receptors are further complicated by the observation that steroid anesthetics can produce different effects on GABA_A receptors in different brain regions.[99] This suggests the possibility that the specific subunit composition of a GABA_A receptor may encode pharmacologic selectivity. This is well illustrated by benzodiazepine sensitivity, which requires the presence of the $\gamma 2$ subunit subtype.[100] Similarly, sensitivity to etomidate has been shown to require the presence of a $\beta 2$ or $\beta 3$ subunit.[101] More recently, it has been shown that the presence of a δ or ϵ subunit in a GABA_A receptor confers insensitivity to the potentiating effects of some anesthetics.[102,103]

Interestingly, GABA_A receptors composed of ρ-type subunits (referred to as GABA_C receptors) have been shown to be inhibited rather than potentiated by volatile anesthetics.[104] This property has been exploited, using molecular biologic techniques, by constructing chimeric receptors composed of part of the ρ receptor coupled to part of an α, β, or glycine receptor subunit. By screening these chimeras for anesthetic sensitivity, regions of the α, β, and glycine subunits responsible for anesthetic sensitivity have been identified. Based on the results of these chimeric studies, site-directed mutagenesis studies were performed to identify the specific amino acids responsible for conferring anesthetic sensitivity. These studies revealed two critical amino acids, near the extracellular regions of transmembrane domains 2 and 3 (TM2, TM3) on the glycine and GABA_A receptors, that are required for volatile anesthetic potentiation of agonist effect.[105] It is not yet clear if these amino acids represent a volatile anesthetic binding site, or whether they are sites critical to transducing anesthetic-induced conformational changes in the receptor molecule. Interestingly, one of the amino acids shown to be critical to volatile anesthetic effect (TM3 site) has also been shown to be required (in the β_2/β_3 subunit) for the potentiating effects of etomidate.[106] In contrast, the TM2 and TM3 sites do not appear to be required for the actions of propofol, barbiturates, or neurosteroids.[107] Interestingly, a distinct amino acid in the TM3 region of the β_1 subunit of the GABA_A receptor has been shown to selectively modulate the ability of propofol to potentiate GABA agonist effects.[107] Collectively, these molecular biologic data provide strong evidence that there are multiple unique binding sites for anesthetics on the GABA_A receptor protein.

Other Ligand-Activated Ion Channels

Other members of the ligand-gated receptor superfamily include the nicotinic acetylcholine receptors (muscle and neuronal types), glycine receptors, and 5-HT_3 receptors. A large body of work has gone into examining the effects of anesthetics on nicotinic acetylcholine receptors. The muscle type of nicotinic receptor has been shown to be inhibited by anesthetic concentrations in the clinical range[108] and to be desensitized by higher concentrations of anesthetics.[109] The muscle nicotinic receptor is an interesting model to study because of its abundance and the wealth of knowledge about its structure. It is, however, not expressed in the central nervous system and hence not involved in the mechanism of anesthesia. There is a neuronal type of nicotinic receptor, which is widely expressed in the nervous system, and might plausibly be involved in anesthetic mechanisms. Older studies looking at neuronal nicotinic receptors in molluscan neurons[110] and in bovine chromaffin cells[111] indicate that these channels are inhibited by clinical concentrations of volatile anesthetics. More recent studies using cloned and expressed neuronal nicotinic receptor subunits have shown a high degree of subunit and anesthetic selectivity. Acetylcholine-elicited currents are inhibited, in receptors composed of various combinations of α_2, α_4, β_2, and β_4 subunits, by *subanesthetic* concentrations of halothane[112] or isoflurane.[113] In contrast, these receptors are relatively insensitive to propofol. Most interestingly, receptors composed of α_7 subunits are completely insensitive to both isoflurane and propofol.[113] The sensitivity of neuronal nicotinic receptors to subanesthetic concentrations of the volatile anesthetics makes it unlikely that these receptors are involved in producing unconsciousness or loss of response to noxious stimuli; it is conceivable that neuronal nicotinic receptors may be involved in other anesthetics effects, such as analgesia.[114]

Glycine is an important inhibitory neurotransmitter, particularly in the spinal cord and brain stem. The glycine receptor is a member of the ligand-activated channel superfamily that, like the GABA$_A$ receptor, is a chloride-selective ion channel. A large number of studies have shown that clinical concentrations of volatile anesthetics potentiate glycine-activated currents in intact neurons[75] and in cloned glycine receptors expressed in oocytes.[115,116] The volatile anesthetics appear to produce their potentiating effect by increasing the affinity of the receptor for glycine.[116] Propofol,[91] alphaxalone, and pentobarbital also potentiate glycine-activated currents, whereas etomidate and ketamine do not.[115] Potentiation of glycine receptor function may contribute to the anesthetic action of volatile anesthetics and some parenteral anesthetics. 5-HT$_3$ receptors are also members of the genetically related superfamily of ligand-gated receptor channels. Clinical concentrations of volatile anesthetics potentiate currents activated by 5-hydroxytryptamine in intact cells[117] and in cloned receptors expressed in oocytes.[118] In contrast, thiopental inhibits 5-HT$_3$ receptor currents[117] and propofol is without effect on these receptor channels.[118] 5-HT$_3$ receptors may play some role in the anesthetic state produced by volatile anesthetics, and may also contribute to some unpleasant anesthetic side effects such as nausea and vomiting.

Summary

Several ligand-gated ion channels are modulated by clinical concentrations of anesthetics. Ketamine, N$_2$O, and xenon inhibit NMDA-type glutamate receptors, and this effect of the anesthetics may play a major role in their mechanism of action. There is a large body of evidence showing that clinical concentrations of many anesthetics potentiate GABA-activated currents in the central nervous system. This suggests that GABA$_A$ receptors are a probable molecular target of anesthetics. Other members of the ligand-activated ion channel family, including glycine receptors, neuronal nicotinic receptors, and 5-HT$_3$ receptors, are also affected by clinical concentrations of anesthetics and remain plausible anesthetic targets.

Anesthetic Effects on Second Messenger-Activated Ion Channels

Ion channels can be activated by ligands present in the cytoplasm as well as by ligands present in the extracellular space. The intracellular ligands that activate these channels are generally chemical second messengers, including cyclic nucleotides, Ca^{2+} ions, inositol phosphates, and ATP. The structure of second messenger-activated ion channels is not as well understood as that of the voltage- or ligand-activated channels, and there is little information about anesthetic effects on these channels.

One type of second messenger-activated channel, the calcium-dependent channels, has been shown to be inhibited by clinical concentrations of anesthetics.[119] These large conductance potassium channels open in response to increases in cytoplasmic Ca^{2+} concentration and are important in modulating the shape and frequency of action potentials in the central nervous system. While a wide variety of anesthetics inhibit channel opening, this would tend to excite neurons, and is thus unlikely to be important in the depressant effects of anesthetics. Anesthetic effects on these channels may contribute to the excitatory effects of low concentrations of anesthetics and to the convulsant properties of some anesthetic agents. Several other potassium-selective ion channels are also activated by second messengers, including ATP-activated channels and channels activated by muscarinic acetylcholine receptors, but the effects of anesthetics on these channels has not been delineated.

There is potassium-selective channel (referred to as I$_{K(an)}$), found in snail neurons, that has many of the properties of a second messenger-activated channel and that is activated by clinical concentrations of volatile anesthetics.[110,120,121] I$_{K(AN)}$ shares many biophysical properties with a second messenger-activated

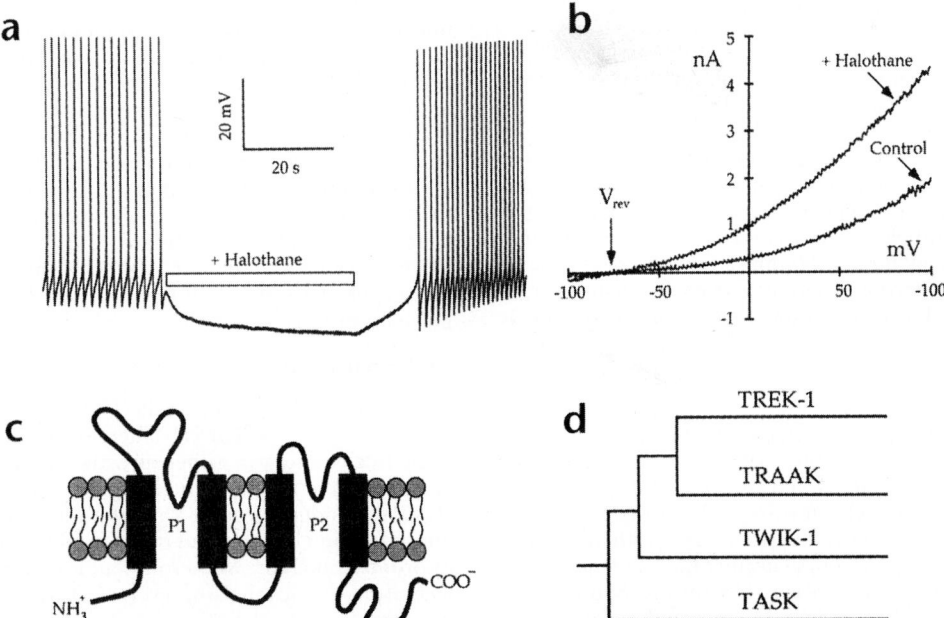

Figure 7-6. Volatile anesthetics activate background K$^+$ channels. *Panel A:* Halothane reversibly hyperpolarizes a pacemaker neuron from *Lymnaea stagnalis* (the pond snail) by activating I$_{Kan}$. *Panel B:* Halothane (300 μM) activates human recombinant TREK-1 channels expressed in COS cells. The figure shows current–voltage relationships with reversal potential (V_{rev}) of −88 mV, indicative of a K$^+$ channel. *Panel C:* Predicted structure of a typical subunit of the mammalian background K$^+$ channels. Note the four transmembrane spanning segments (in black) and the two pore-forming domains (P1 and P2). Some but not all of these 2P/4TM K$^+$ channels are activated by volatile anesthetics. *Panel D:* Phylogenetic tree for the 2P/4TM family. (Reproduced with permission from Franks NP, Lieb WR: Background K$^+$ channels: An important target for anesthetics? Nature Neurosci 2:395, 1999.)

potassium channel found in *Aplysia* neurons that is referred to as the S channel. Recent work by Spencer Yost and colleagues has shown that the S channel is also activated by clinical concentrations of volatile anesthetics.[122] The importance of volatile anesthetic activation of second messenger-activated potassium channels in invertebrates has now become apparent with the discovery of a large family of so-called "background potassium channels" in mammals. These mammalian potassium channels have a unique structure with two pore-forming domains in tandem plus four transmembrane segments (2P/4TM; Fig. 7-6C).[123] TOK1, a member of this family, was first shown by Yost and colleagues to be activated by volatile anesthetics.[124] The laboratory of Michel Lazdunski has studied the effects of a variety of volatile anesthetics on several members of the 2P/4TM family. They found that TREK-1 channels were activated by clinical concentrations of chloroform, diethyl ether, halothane, and isoflurane (Fig. 7-6B). In contrast, closely related TRAAK channels were insensitive to all the volatile anesthetics, and TASK channels were activated by halothane and isoflurane, inhibited by diethyl ether, and unaffected by chloroform. These authors went on to show that the C-terminal regions of TASK and TREK-1 contained amino acids essential for anesthetic actions on TASK and TREK-1 channels.[125] Activation of background K^+ channels in mammalian vertebrates could be an important mechanism through which anesthetics regulate neuronal resting membrane potential and thereby excitability; this effect could plausibly be a significant contributor to some components of the anesthetic state.

Summary

Second messenger-activated ion channels are a plausible target for anesthetic action. Recent evidence suggests that members of the 2P/4TM family of background potassium channels are likely to be important in producing some components of the anesthetic state.

ANESTHETIC EFFECTS ON CHEMICAL SECOND MESSENGER GENERATION AND EFFECT

As discussed above, anesthetics alter the function of at least several types of ion channels. This panoply of effects could be efficiently explained by an anesthetic effect on either the synthesis or the actions of a single modulatory substance that acts on all of the affected channels. A variety of substances, referred to as second messengers, are known to modulate the function of ion channels. These second messengers alter channel function either by directly binding to the channel protein or by changing the phosphorylation state of the channel. This section briefly reviews current knowledge of anesthetic effects on chemical second messengers.

Calcium

Calcium ions are among the most important intracellular chemical second messengers. Cytoplasmic Ca^{2+} concentration ($[Ca^{2+}]_i$) is tightly regulated at ~ 100 nM and can be rapidly elevated by release of Ca^{2+} from intracellular stores or by influx of extracellular Ca^{2+}. It has long been hypothesized that anesthetics might increase resting $[Ca^{2+}]_i$, thereby activating Ca^{2+}-dependent potassium channels and hyperpolarizing neurons. Studies in a variety of preparations have now shown that while volatile anesthetics can transiently increase resting $[Ca^{2+}]_i$ by releasing Ca^{2+} from intracellular stores,[126,127] clinical concentrations of anesthetics produce little, if any, sustained effect on resting $[Ca^{2+}]_i$.[55,128–130] Additionally, anesthetics generally inhibit rather than enhance receptor- or depolarization-stimulated increases in $[Ca^{2+}]_i$. It is thus highly unlikely that elevations in resting $[Ca^{2+}]_i$ make a significant contribution to the mechanism of anesthesia.

G-Proteins

The actions of most cell surface receptors are transduced *via* intracellular GTP-binding proteins (G-proteins), which when activated can stimulate a variety of effector molecules including ion channels, adenylyl cyclase, and phospholipase C. The G-proteins are a family of proteins, which show specificity both in terms of the receptors to which they couple and the effectors that they activate. G-proteins would provide an attractive target for anesthetic action, because their actions at proximal steps in a number of signaling cascades could explain the promiscuous molecular effects of anesthetics. There have been several studies indicating that volatile anesthetics[131,132] and barbiturates[133] can interfere with G-protein function in the brain. Unfortunately, the anesthetic concentrations used in these studies were significantly higher than those used clinically. Studies using clinical concentrations of halothane have failed to show any effect on G-protein function in either rat brain slices[134] or clonal pituitary cells.[55] There is no compelling evidence at the current time to suggest that G-proteins are an important target of anesthetic action in the central nervous system.

Inositol Phosphates

A variety of cell surface receptors act *via* G-proteins to activate a phosphatidylinositol-specific phospholipase C. This enzyme produces two important messenger molecules—inositol trisphosphate (IP_3) and diacylglycerol (DAG). IP_3 activates an intracellular, ligand-activated calcium channel (the IP_3 receptor) which allows release of Ca^{2+} from intracellular stores. DAG binds to and activates protein kinase C. There is evidence from two systems that clinical concentrations of halothane do not affect phospholipase C activity. In rat brain slices[133] and in clonal pituitary cells,[55] clinical concentrations of halothane have no effect on either basal or agonist-stimulated accumulation of inositol phosphates. This indicates that the activity of phospholipase C is not affected by halothane and therefore that the rates of production of both IP_3 and DAG are unaffected by halothane. Interestingly, studies using a human neuroblastoma cell line have shown that volatile anesthetics (halothane and isoflurane) *increase* basal and agonist-stimulated concentrations of IP_3 without affecting total inositol phosphate accumulation.[135] This suggests that while the anesthetics do not affect phospholipase C activity, they may inhibit the breakdown of IP_3. Indeed, there is some evidence that halothane can inhibit inositol 1,4,5-trisphosphatase, the major enzyme involved in IP_3 degradation.[136] In pituitary cells, there is also evidence showing that halothane does not alter the *actions* of IP_3; changes in $[Ca^{2+}]_i$ resulting from receptor-stimulated IP_3 generation were completely unaffected by clinical concentrations of halothane.[55] In summary, current evidence does not suggest a major role for second messengers derived from the phosphatidylinositol system in the mechanism of anesthesia.

Cyclic Nucleotides

Cyclic AMP (cAMP) and cyclic GMP (cGMP) are important second messengers that can alter ion channel function. The cyclic nucleotides can either directly bind to channel proteins or can activate specific protein kinases (cAMP-dependent and cGMP-dependent protein kinase) which can selectively phosphorylate ion channels and other proteins, leading to changes in protein function. Numerous studies have examined the effects of anesthetics on tissue levels of cAMP and cGMP. Although the results of these studies have been somewhat variable, the general trend is to show increased levels of cAMP and decreased levels of cGMP in brain.[137,138] In contrast, studies done in brain slices show minimal effect of clinical concentrations of halothane on basal or agonist-stimulated cyclic nucleotide concentrations.[134] One exception to this is a recent study examining the effects of halothane on NMDA-stimulated changes in nitric oxide and cGMP generation in rat cerebellar slices. This study showed that halothane inhibited NMDA-induced increases in cGMP, but not nitric oxide.[139] This suggests that halothane may affect the ability of nitric oxide to stimulate guanylate cyclase activity. Overall, most of the alterations in cyclic nucleotide levels observed *in vivo* probably reflect anesthetic-induced changes in neuronal activity rather than direct effects on the enzymatic machinery involved in synthesizing and metabolizing cAMP and cGMP. Current evidence does not indicate that cyclic nucleotide generation or metabolism plays a significant role in the mechanism of anesthetic action.

Protein Kinases and Phosphatases

Phosphorylation is the most important known mechanism for regulation of ion channel function. There are many protein kinases, each of which can phosphorylate specific sites on specific ion channels, producing dramatic changes in channel function. There are also a variety of protein phosphatases, which can selectively remove phosphate groups from specific sites on specific ion channels, reversing the effects of the protein kinases. The balance between the activity of protein kinases and protein phosphatases determines the phosphorylation state of specific sites on channel proteins and thus determines the functional state of those channels. It is entirely plausible that anesthetics could produce their effects on the function of ion channels (and other proteins) *via* an action on specific protein kinases or phosphatases. Unfortunately, there is a surprising paucity of data concerning the effects of anesthetics on protein kinases and phosphatases. There is some information concerning the effects of anesthetics on protein kinase C (PKC). This kinase is of particular interest, since it is activated by lipids (DAG, phosphatidylserine, arachidonic acid) and thus may contain hydrophobic sites at which anesthetics might interact. Studies by Slater and colleagues have shown that several anesthetics inhibit purified brain PKC, and that they act *via* an effect on the regulatory (lipid-binding) subunit rather than the catalytic subunit.[140] A conflicting study showed that halothane and propofol *stimulate* purified brain PKC under most assay conditions and cause only modest inhibition under any conditions.[141] Subsequent studies have shown that halothane has two distinct actions on brain PKC: stimulation of PKC activity and potentiation of activation-induced PKC translocation and downregulation.[142] These competing effects may, in part, explain the dissimilar results obtained in various studies examining the effects of volatile anesthetics on PKC activity. It should also be appreciated that PKC purified from animal tissue is a mixture of at least several subtypes (including α, β_1, β_2, and γ) and that studies with the purified isotypes will be required to understand the effects of anesthetics on the biologic activity of PKC. To date, there is limited information available on the actions of anesthetics on protein phosphatase activity. In summary, inhalational anesthetics can affect the activity of protein kinase C in a complex fashion. The importance of this effect to mechanisms of anesthetic action is not known.

Nitric Oxide

Nitric oxide is an important chemical second messenger generated from L-arginine by the enzyme nitric oxide synthase (NOS). Nitric oxide acts by stimulating the enzyme guanalyl cyclase to produce cGMP, and is known to play an important role as an endothelial-derived vasodilator and as a neuromodulator. Studies from the early 1990s showed that systemic administration of the NOS inhibitor, L-NAME, reduced the MAC for halothane by approximately 30%.[143] Subsequent studies showed that an inhibitor specific for neuronal NOS produced a similar MAC-sparing effect for both isoflurane and halothane.[144] In both studies NOS inhibition did not produce anesthesia on its own and produced a maximal MAC reduction of 30–40%. A subsequent study examined the effects of NOS inhibitors on isoflurane MAC in mice lacking the gene for neuronal NOS. These animals were found to have the same MAC for isoflurane as

control mice. The control mice did show a reduction of MAC following administration of a NOS inhibitor while the "neuronal NOS knockout" mice did not.[145] These data indicate that while the nitric oxide pathway can modulate the response to anesthetics, it is not essential to anesthetic action.

WHAT IS THE CHEMICAL NATURE OF ANESTHETIC TARGET SITES?

The Meyer-Overton Rule

Almost 100 years ago, Meyer and Overton independently observed that the potency of gases as anesthetics was strongly correlated with their solubility in olive oil (Fig. 7-7).[146,147] This observation has significantly influenced thinking about anesthetic mechanisms in two ways. First, since a wide variety of structurally unrelated compounds obey the Meyer-Overton rule, it has been reasoned that all anesthetics are likely to act at the same molecular site. This idea is referred to as the *Unitary Theory of Anesthesia*. Second, it has been argued that since solubility in a specific solvent strongly correlates with anesthetic potency, the solvent showing the strongest correlation between anesthetic solubility and potency is likely to most closely mimic the chemical and physical properties of the anesthetic target site in the CNS. Based on this reasoning, it has been assumed that the anesthetic target site is hydrophobic in nature.

The Meyer-Overton correlation suffers from two limitations: (1) it only applies to gases and volatile liquids, since olive oil/gas partition coefficients cannot be determined for liquid anesthetics; (2) olive oil is a poorly characterized mixture of oils. To circumvent these limitations, attempts have been made to correlate anesthetic potency with water/solvent partition coefficients. To date, the best correlation that has been demonstrated is between the anesthetic potency of a compound and its octanol/water partition coefficient. This correlation holds

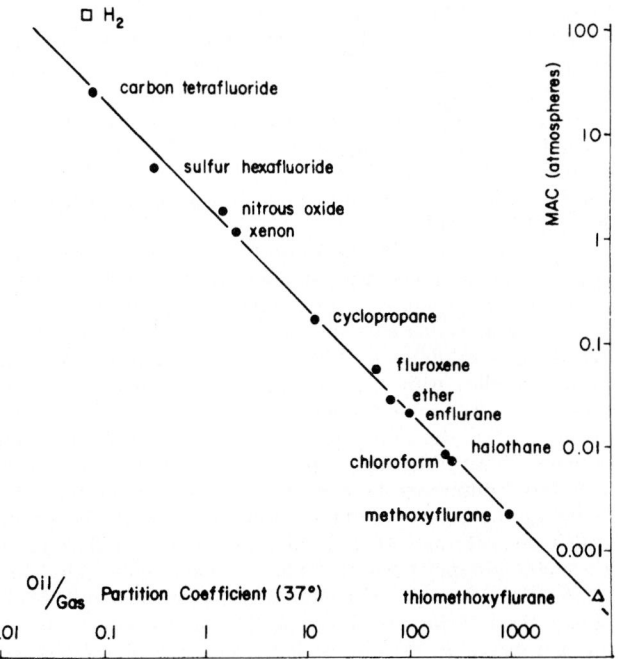

Figure 7-7. The Meyer-Overton rule. There is a linear relationship (on a log–log scale) between the oil/gas partition coefficient and the anesthetic potency (MAC) of a number of gases. The correlation between lipid solubility and MAC extends over a 70,000-fold difference in anesthetic potency. (Reproduced with permission from Tanfiuji Y, Eger EI, Terrell RC: Some characteristics of an exceptionally potent inhaled anesthetic: thiomethoxyflurane. Anesth Analg 56:387, 1977.)

for a variety of classes of anesthetics and spans a 10,000-fold range of anesthetic potencies.[148] The properties of the solvent octanol suggest that the anesthetic site is likely to be amphipathic, having both polar and nonpolar characteristics.

Exceptions to the Meyer-Overton Rule

Halogenated compounds exist that are structurally similar to the inhaled anesthetics, and are convulsants rather than anesthetics.[149] There are also convulsant barbiturates[150] and neurosteroids.[151] One convulsant compound, fluorothyl (hexafluorodiethylether) has been shown to cause seizures in 50% of mice at 0.12 vol%, but to produce anesthesia at higher concentrations (EC_{50} = 1.22 vol%).[152] The concentration of fluorothyl required to produce anesthesia is approximately predicted by the Meyer-Overton rule. In contrast, several polyhalogenated alkanes have been identified that are convulsants, but that do not produce anesthesia. Based on the olive oil/gas partition coefficients of these compounds, anesthesia should have been achieved within the range of concentrations studied.[153] The end point used to determine the anesthetic effect of these compounds was movement in response to a noxious stimulus (MAC). Interestingly, some of these polyhalogenated compounds do produce amnesia in animals.[154] These compounds are thus referred to as *nonimmobilizers* rather than as nonanesthetics. Several polyhalogenated alkanes have also been identified that anesthetize mice, but only at concentrations 10 times those predicted by their oil/gas partition coefficients[153]; these compounds are referred to as *transitional* compounds. The nonimmobilizers and transitional compounds have been proposed as a "litmus test" for the relevance of anesthetic effects observed *in vitro* to those observed in the whole animal.

In several homologous series of anesthetics, anesthetic potency increases with increasing chain length until a certain critical chain length is reached. Beyond this critical chain length, compounds are unable to produce anesthesia, even at the highest attainable concentrations. In the series of *n*-alkanols, for example, anesthetic potency increases from methanol through dodecanol; all longer alkanols are unable to produce anesthesia.[155] This phenomenon is referred to as the *cutoff effect*. Cutoff effects have been described for several homologous series of anesthetics including *n*-alkanes, *n*-alkanols, cycloalkanemethanols,[156] and perfluoroalkanes.[157] While the anesthetic potency in each of these homologous series of anesthetics shows a cutoff, a corresponding cutoff in octanol/water or oil/gas partition coefficients has not been demonstrated. Therefore, compounds above the cutoff represent a deviation from the Meyer-Overton rule.

A final deviation from the Meyer-Overton rule is the observation that enantiomers of anesthetics differ in their potency as anesthetics. Enantiomers (mirror-image compounds) are a class of stereoisomers that have identical physical properties, including identical solubility in solvents such as octanol or olive oil. Animal studies with the enantiomers of barbiturate anesthetics,[158,159] ketamine,[84] neurosteroids,[93] etomidate,[160] and isoflurane[161] all show enantioselective differences in anesthetic potency. These differences in potency range in magnitude from a >10-fold difference between the enantiomers of etomidate or the neurosteroids to a 60% difference between the enantiomers of isoflurane. It is argued that a *major* difference in anesthetic potency between a pair of enantiomers could only be explained by a protein binding site (see Protein Theories of Anesthesia); this appears to be the case for etomidate and the neurosteroids. Enantiomeric pairs of anesthetics have also been used to study anesthetic actions on ion channels. It is argued that if an anesthetic effect on an ion channel contributes to the anesthetic state, the effect on the ion channel should show the same enantioselectivity as is observed in whole animal anesthetic potency. Early studies showed that the (+)-isomer of isoflurane is 1.5–2 times more potent than the (−)-isomer in eliciting an anesthetic-activated potassium current, in potenti-

ating $GABA_A$ currents, and in inhibiting the current mediated by a neuronal nicotinic acetylcholine receptor.[95,110] In contrast, the stereoisomers of isoflurane are equipotent in their effects on a voltage-activated potassium current and in their effects on lipid phase-transition temperature.[110] Studies with the neurosteroids[93] and etomidate[160] show that these anesthetics exert enantioselective effects on $GABA_A$ currents that parallel the enantioselective effects observed for anesthetic potency.

The exceptions to the Meyer-Overton rule do not obviate the importance of the rule. They do, however, indicate that the properties of a solvent such as octanol describe some, but not all, of the properties of an anesthetic binding site. Compounds that deviate from the Meyer-Overton rule suggest that anesthetic target site(s) are also defined by other properties including size and shape.

In defining the molecular target(s) of anesthetic molecules one must be able to account both for the Meyer-Overton rule and for the well-defined exceptions to this rule. It has sometimes been suggested that a correct molecular mechanism of anesthesia should also be able to account for pressure reversal. *Pressure reversal* is a phenomenon whereby the concentration of a given anesthetic needed to produce anesthesia is greatly increased if the anesthetic is administered to an animal under hyperbaric conditions. The idea that pressure reversal is a useful tool for elucidating mechanisms of anesthesia is based on the assumption that pressure reverses the specific physicochemical actions of the anesthetic that are responsible for producing anesthesia; that is to say, pressure and anesthetics act on the same molecular targets. There is now evidence that pressure reverses anesthesia by producing excitation that physiologically counteracts anesthetic depression, rather than by acting as an anesthetic antagonist at the anesthetic site of action.[162] Therefore, in the following discussion of molecular targets of anesthesia, pressure reversal will not be further discussed.

Lipid *vs.* Protein Targets

Anesthetics might interact with several possible molecular targets to produce their effects on the *function* of ion channels and other proteins. Anesthetics might dissolve in the *lipid* bilayer, causing physicochemical changes in membrane structure that alter the ability of embedded membrane proteins to undergo conformational changes important for their function. Alternatively, anesthetics could bind directly to *proteins* (either ion channel proteins or modulatory proteins), thus either (1) interfering with binding of a ligand (*e.g.*, a neurotransmitter, a substrate, a second messenger molecule) or (2) altering the ability of the protein to undergo conformational changes important for its function. The following section summarizes the arguments for and against lipid theories and protein theories of anesthesia.

Lipid Theories of Anesthesia

The elucidation of the Meyer-Overton rule suggested that anesthetics interact with a hydrophobic target. To investigators in the early part of the 20th century, the most logical hydrophobic target was a lipid. In its simplest incarnation, the lipid theory of anesthesia postulates that anesthetics dissolve in the lipid bilayers of biological membranes and produce anesthesia when they reach a critical concentration in the membrane. Consistent with this hypothesis, the membrane/gas partition coefficients of anesthetic gases in pure lipid bilayers correlate strongly with anesthetic potency.[163] This simple theory can account for anesthetics that obey the Meyer-Overton rule, but cannot account for anesthetics that deviate from this rule. For example, the cutoff effect cannot be explained by this theory since compounds above the cutoff can achieve membrane concentrations equal to those of compounds below the cutoff.[164] Similarly, enantioselectivity cannot be explained by this theory. Most importantly, this simplest version of the lipid theory does not explain how the presence of the anesthetic in the membrane is translated into an effect on the function of the embedded proteins.

Membrane Perturbation

More sophisticated versions of the lipid theory require that the anesthetic molecules dissolved in the lipid bilayer cause a change or perturbation in one or more physical properties of the membrane. According to this theory, anesthesia is a function of both the concentration of anesthetic in the membrane and the effectiveness of that anesthetic as a perturbant. This potentially could explain deviations from the Meyer-Overton rule, since nonanesthetics could achieve high concentrations in the membrane, but might not be effective perturbants. In examining this theory it is important to explicitly define the perturbation caused by an anesthetic. One can then test the relevance of a specific perturbation to the mechanism of anesthesia by measuring the perturbation caused by various compounds (anesthetics and nonanesthetics) and correlating perturbation with anesthetic potency. The specific perturbations of membrane structure that have been proposed to be causally related to the anesthetic state are briefly explored in the following section.

Membrane Expansion. Anesthetics dissolved in membranes do increase membrane volume. This occurs both because the anesthetic molecules occupy space and, in principle, because they produce changes in lipid packing and/or protein folding. The *critical volume hypothesis* is an attempt to correlate changes in membrane volume with anesthesia. This hypothesis predicts that anesthesia occurs when anesthetic dissolved in the membrane produces a critical change in membrane volume. Changes in membrane volume could compress ion channels and thus alter their function. Alternatively, increases in membrane thickness could alter neuronal excitability by changing the potential gradient across the plasma membrane.[165] Several studies have shown that anesthetics can produce changes in membrane volume.[166] However, the amount of expansion caused by clinical concentrations of anesthetics is probably very small. One study of erythrocyte membranes showed that halothane (0.27 mM = 1.0 MAC) expanded the membranes by only 0.1%.[167] Another study of erythrocyte membranes showed that both anesthetics and nonanesthetics (long-chain *n*-alkanols above the anesthetic cutoff) produced similar degrees of membrane expansion.[168] While clinical concentrations of anesthetics clearly produce membrane expansion, the small magnitude of anesthetic-induced membrane expansion, coupled with the inability of this theory to account for the cutoff effect, makes it unlikely that membrane expansion is the correct mechanism of anesthesia. A recent study by Cantor revisits this topic.[169] Based on thermodynamic modeling, he argues that anesthetics in biologic membranes preferentially distribute to the interface between lipid and aqueous phases. This distribution results in increased lateral pressure, which could alter the function of membrane-embedded ion channels. His calculations also suggest that nonimmobilizers should not show the same interfacial distribution. There is some experimental evidence showing that anesthetics, but not nonimmobilizers, do preferentially distribute to the lipid/aqueous interface in a membrane.[170] The relationship between these recent observations and anesthetic effects on protein function remains to be determined.

Membrane Disordering. Studies using nuclear magnetic resonance (NMR) spectroscopy[171] and electron spin resonance (ESR) spectroscopy[172] have shown that a variety of anesthetics can disorder the packing of phospholipids in lipid bilayers and in biological membranes. The decrease in membrane order (often referred to as an increase in membrane fluidity) can, in principle, alter the function of ion channels embedded in the lipid bilayer. The ability of anesthetics to fluidize lipid bilayers does show a modest correlation with anesthetic potency.[173] Membrane disordering can also account for the cutoff effect. Studies on synaptic membranes have shown that anesthetic alkanols

(octanol, decanol, dodecanol) fluidize membranes, whereas nonanesthetic alkanols have either no effect on fluidity (tetradecanol) or a rigidifying effect (hexadecanol, octadecanol) on the membranes.[174] Unfortunately, the degree of fluidization produced by clinical concentrations of anesthetics is quite small.[173] While it is unclear how much fluidization would be required to affect ion channel function, anesthetics produce changes in membrane fluidity that can be mimicked by changes in temperature of less than 1°C. Clearly, a 1°C increase in temperature does not cause anesthesia, or even increase anesthetic potency. It is highly unlikely that changes in the fluidity of bulk membrane lipid are responsible for general anesthesia.

Lipid Phase Transitions. Another lipid perturbation that has been proposed to account for general anesthesia is a change in lipid phase-transition behavior. In its original version this theory proposed that anesthetics promote a transition of the lipids in neuronal membranes between a solid (gel) phase and a liquid-crystalline phase. Indeed, in pure lipid systems clinical concentrations of anesthetics do decrease the temperature at which such a transition occurs.[175] A second version of this theory, the *lateral phase-separation theory,* proposed that anesthetics *prevent* phase transitions between the liquid-crystalline and the gel phase.[176] According to this theory, liquid-crystalline to gel phase transition is required for normal ion channel function; inhibition of this phase transition causes anesthesia. There is little evidence to support the phase-transition theories. Anesthetic-induced phase changes have not been observed in biologic membranes, lipid phase transitions are not known to be required for normal ion channel function, and the changes in phase-transition temperature observed in pure lipid systems are less than 1°C.

Protein Theories of Anesthesia

The Meyer-Overton rule could also be explained by the direct interaction of anesthetics with hydrophobic sites on proteins. There are three types of hydrophobic sites on proteins with which anesthetics might interact:

1. Hydrophobic amino acids comprise the core of water-soluble proteins. Anesthetics could bind in hydrophobic pockets that are fortuitously present in the protein core.
2. Hydrophobic amino acids also form the lining of binding sites for hydrophobic ligands. For example, there are hydrophobic pockets in which fatty acids tightly bind on proteins such as albumin and the low–molecular-weight fatty acid–binding proteins. Anesthetics could compete with endogenous ligands for binding to such sites on either water-soluble or membrane proteins.
3. Hydrophobic amino acids are major constituents of the α-helices which form the membrane-spanning regions of membrane proteins; hydrophobic amino acid side chains form the protein surface that faces the membrane lipid. Anesthetic molecules could interact with the hydrophobic surface of these membrane proteins, disrupting normal lipid–protein interactions and possibly directly affecting protein conformation. This last possibility would involve the interaction of many anesthetic molecules with each membrane protein molecule and would probably be a nonselective interaction between anesthetic molecules and *all* membrane proteins.

Direct interactions of anesthetic molecules with proteins would not only satisfy the Meyer-Overton rule, but would also provide the simplest explanation for compounds that deviate from this rule. Any protein binding site is likely to be defined by properties such as size and shape in addition to its solvent properties. Limitations in size and shape could reduce the binding affinity of compounds beyond the cutoff, thus explaining their lack of anesthetic effect. Enantioselectivity is also most easily explained by a direct binding of anesthetic molecules to defined sites on proteins; a protein binding site of defined dimensions could readily distinguish between enantiomers on the basis of their different shape. Protein binding sites for anesthetics could also explain the convulsant effects of some polyhalogenated alkanes. Different compounds binding (in slightly different ways) to the same binding pocket can produce different effects on protein conformation and hence on protein function. For example, there are three kinds of compounds that can bind at the benzodiazepine binding site on the GABA$_A$ channel: *agonists,* which potentiate GABA effects and produce sedation and anxiolysis; *inverse-agonists,* which promote channel closure and produce convulsant effects; and *antagonists,* which produce no effect on their own but can competitively block the effects of agonists and inverse-agonists. By analogy, polyhalogenated alkanes could be inverse-agonists, binding at the same protein sites at which halogenated alkane anesthetics are agonists. The evidence for direct interactions between anesthetics and proteins is briefly reviewed in the following section.

Evidence for Anesthetic Binding to Proteins

One of the initial approaches to probing anesthetic interactions with proteins was to observe the effects of anesthetics on the function of a protein and to try to make inferences about binding from the functional behavior. It is entirely reasonable to assume that direct anesthetic–protein interactions are responsible for functional effects of anesthetics on purified water-soluble proteins, since no lipid or membrane is present in the preparations studied. Firefly luciferase is a water-soluble, light-emitting protein, which is inhibited by a wide variety of anesthetic molecules. Numerous studies have extensively characterized anesthetic inhibition of firefly luciferase activity, and have revealed the following[177,178]:

1. Anesthetics inhibit firefly luciferase activity at concentrations very similar to those required to produce clinical anesthesia.
2. The potency of anesthetics as inhibitors of firefly luciferase activity correlates strongly with their potency as anesthetics, in keeping with the Meyer-Overton rule.
3. Halothane inhibition of luciferase activity is competitive with respect to the substrate D-luciferin.
4. Inhibition of firefly luciferase activity shows a cutoff in anesthetic potency for both *n*-alkanes and *n*-alkanols.

Based on these studies it can be inferred that a wide variety of anesthetics can bind in the luciferin-binding pocket of firefly luciferase. The fact that anesthetic inhibition of luciferase activity is consistent with the Meyer-Overton rule, occurs at clinical anesthetic concentrations, and explains the cutoff effect suggests that the luciferin-binding pocket may have physical and chemical characteristics similar to those of a putative anesthetic binding site in the CNS.

More direct approaches to studying anesthetic binding to proteins have included NMR spectroscopy and photoaffinity labeling. Based on early studies by Wishnia and Pinder, it was suspected that anesthetics could bind to several fatty acid–binding proteins, including β-lactoglobulin and bovine serum albumin (BSA).[179,180] ^{19}F-NMR spectroscopic studies confirmed[181] this, and demonstrated that isoflurane binds to approximately three saturable binding sites on BSA. Isoflurane binding is eliminated by co-incubation with oleic acid, suggesting that isoflurane binds to the fatty acid–binding sites on albumin. Other anesthetics, including halothane, methoxyflurane, sevoflurane, and octanol, compete with isoflurane for binding to BSA.[182] The studies with BSA provide direct evidence that a variety of anesthetics can compete for binding to the same site on a protein. Using this BSA model, it was subsequently shown that anesthetic binding sites could be identified and characterized using a photoaffinity labeling technique. The anesthetic halothane contains a carbon–bromine bond. This bond can be broken by ultraviolet light generating a free radical. That free radical allows the

anesthetic to permanently (covalently) label the anesthetic binding site. Eckenhoff and colleagues used ^{14}C-labeled halothane to photoaffinity-label anesthetic binding sites on BSA,[183] and obtained results virtually identical to those obtained using NMR spectroscopy. Eckenhoff subsequently has identified the specific amino acids that are photoaffinity-labeled by [^{14}C]halothane.[184] NMR and photoaffinity-labeling techniques have also been applied to several other proteins. For example, saturable binding of halothane to the luciferin-binding site on firefly luciferase has been directly confirmed using NMR and photoaffinity-labeling techniques.[185] Both NMR and photoaffinity-labeling techniques are also being applied to membrane proteins. At the current time these techniques can only be applied to purified proteins available in relatively large quantity. The muscle-type nicotinic acetylcholine receptor is one of the few membrane proteins that can be purified in large quantity. Eckenhoff has used photoaffinity labeling to show that halothane binds to this protein. The pattern of photoaffinity labeling is complex, suggesting multiple binding sites.[186] Most recently, Miller and colleagues have developed a general anesthetic that is an analog of octanol and functions as a photoaffinity label. This compound, 3-diazyrinyloctanol, also binds to specific sites on the nicotinic acetylcholine receptor.[187]

Although NMR and photoaffinity techniques can provide extensive information about anesthetic binding sites on proteins, they cannot reveal the details of the three-dimensional structure of these sites. X-Ray diffraction crystallography can provide this kind of three-dimensional detail and has been used to study anesthetic interactions with a small number of proteins. To date, it has been difficult to crystallize membrane proteins; thus, these studies have been limited to water-soluble proteins. In 1965, Schoenborn and colleagues first used X-ray diffraction techniques to examine the interactions of several anesthetics with crystalline myoglobin.[188,189] These studies demonstrated that at a partial pressure of 2.5 atm (xenon MAC = 1 atm), a single molecule of xenon binds to a specific pocket in the hydrophobic core of the myoglobin molecule. The anesthetics cyclopropane and dichloromethane also bind in this pocket, but larger anesthetics do not. It should be noted that xenon occupies a small empty space in the hydrophobic core of myoglobin and that even dichloromethane is a tight fit in this space. These data provided a clear demonstration that anesthetic molecules can bind in the hydrophobic core of a water-soluble protein and that the size of the hydrophobic binding pocket can account for a cutoff in the size of anesthetic molecules that can bind in that pocket. However, myoglobin cannot bind most anesthetic molecules (because of their size) and is therefore not a good model for the actual anesthetic binding site(s) in the central nervous system.

X-Ray diffraction has also been used to demonstrate that a single molecule of halothane binds in a hydrophobic pocket deep within the enzyme adenylate kinase.[190] Halothane binding was localized to the binding site for the adenine moiety of AMP (adenine monophosphate), a substrate for adenylate kinase. Consistent with this finding, halothane was found to inhibit adenylate kinase in a manner that is competitive with respect to AMP. Unfortunately, halothane binding to adenylate kinase only occurs at concentrations well beyond the clinically useful range. Recently, firefly luciferase has been crystallized in the presence and absence of the anesthetic bromoform. X-Ray diffraction studies of these crystals showed that the anesthetic does bind in the luciferin-binding pocket, as had been inferred from functional studies. Interestingly, two molecules of bromoform bind in the luciferin pocket—one that is likely to compete directly with luciferin for binding and one that is not.[191] The binding data with firefly luciferase and adenylate kinase are of particular interest because they demonstrate that anesthetics can bind to endogenous ligand binding sites and there can be a strong correlation between anesthetic binding to a protein site and anesthetic inhibition of protein function.

A recent approach to studying anesthetic interactions with proteins has been to employ site-directed mutagenesis of known anesthetic targets, coupled with molecular modeling to make predictions about the location and structure of anesthetic binding sites. For example, Adron Harris and colleagues have used this approach to predict the location and structure of the alcohol binding site on $GABA_A$ and glycine receptors.[192] A related approach has been to develop model proteins to define the structural requirements for an anesthetic binding site. Using this approach, Johansson has shown that a four-α-helix bundle with a hydrophobic core can bind volatile anesthetics at concentrations (K_D) similar to those required to produce anesthesia.[193]

Summary

There is unequivocal evidence from studies using water-soluble proteins that anesthetics can bind to hydrophobic pockets on proteins. Functional and binding studies with firefly luciferase demonstrate that anesthetics can bind to a protein site at clinically relevant concentrations in a manner that can account for the Meyer-Overton rule and deviations from it. Evidence that direct anesthetic–protein binding interactions may be responsible for anesthetic effects on ion channels in the CNS remains indirect; stereoselectivity currently offers the strongest indirect argument.

Overall, current evidence strongly indicates protein rather than lipid as the molecular target for anesthetic action. While it seems likely that the long-standing controversy between lipid and protein theories of anesthesia is behind us, this leaves numerous unanswered questions about the details of anesthetic–protein interactions. Important questions that remain to be answered include:

1. What is the stoichiometry of anesthetic binding to a protein? (*i.e.*, Do many anesthetic molecules interact with a single protein molecule or only a few?)
2. Do anesthetics compete with endogenous ligands for binding to hydrophobic pockets on protein targets or do they bind to fortuitous cavities in the protein?
3. Do all anesthetics bind to the same pocket on a protein or are there multiple hydrophobic pockets for different anesthetics?
4. How many proteins have hydrophobic pockets in which anesthetics can bind at clinically used concentrations?

HOW ARE THE EFFECTS OF ANESTHETICS ON MOLECULAR TARGETS LINKED TO ANESTHESIA IN THE INTACT ORGANISM?

In previous sections it has been shown that anesthetics affect the function of a number of ion channels and signaling proteins, probably *via* direct anesthetic–protein interactions. It is unclear which, if any, of these effects of anesthetics on protein function are necessary and/or sufficient to produce anesthesia in an intact organism. A number of approaches have been employed to try to link anesthetic effects observed at a molecular level to anesthesia in intact animals. These approaches and their pitfalls are briefly explored in the following section.

Pharmacologic Approaches

An experimental paradigm frequently used to study anesthetic mechanisms is to administer a drug thought to act specifically at a putative anesthetic target (*e.g.*, a receptor agonist or antagonist, an ion channel activator or antagonist), then determine whether the drug has either increased or decreased the animal's sensitivity to a given anesthetic. The underlying assumption is that if a change in anesthetic sensitivity is observed, then the anesthetic is likely to act *via* an action on the specific target of the administered drug. This is a largely flawed strategy that has

nonetheless produced a huge literature. The drugs used to modulate anesthetic sensitivity usually have their own direct effects on central nervous system excitability and thus *indirectly* affect anesthetic requirements. For example, while α_2-adrenergic agonists decrease halothane MAC,[194] they are profound CNS depressants in their own right and produce anesthesia by mechanisms distinct from those used by volatile anesthetics. Thus, the ''MAC-sparing'' effects of α_2-agonists provide little insight into how halothane works. A more useful pharmacologic strategy would be to identify drugs that have no effect on CNS excitability but prevent the effects of given anesthetics. Currently, however, there are no such anesthetic antagonists. Development of specific antagonists for anesthetic agents would provide a major tool for linking anesthetic effects at the molecular level to anesthesia in the intact organism, and might also be of significant clinical utility.

An alternative pharmacologic approach is to develop ''litmus tests'' for the relevance of anesthetic effects observed *in vitro*. One such test takes advantage of compounds that are nonanesthetic despite the predictions of the Meyer-Overton rule. It is argued that ''a site affected by these nonanesthetic compounds is unlikely to be relevant to the production of anesthesia.''[153] A similar argument uses stereoselectivity as the discriminator and argues that a site that does not show the same stereoselectivity as that observed for whole animal anesthesia is unlikely to be relevant to the production of anesthesia.[195] Although these tests may be useful, they are very dependent on the assumption that anesthesia is produced *via* drug action at a *single* site. For example, a nonanesthetic might depress CNS excitability *via* its actions on an important anesthetic target site while simultaneously producing counterbalancing excitatory effects at a second site. In this case the ''litmus test'' would incorrectly eliminate the anesthetic site as irrelevant to whole animal anesthesia. This example is quite plausible given the convulsant effects of many of the nonanesthetic polyhalogenated hydrocarbons.

Summary

Pharmacologic approaches to studying anesthetic mechanism are plagued by issues of pharmacologic and physiologic nonselectivity. Development of selective anesthetic antagonists offers one clear pharmacologic path to link molecular effects of anesthetics to anesthetic action in the intact organism.

Genetic Approaches

An alternative approach to studying the relationship between anesthetic effects observed *in vitro* and whole animal anesthesia is to alter the structure of putative anesthetic targets and determine how this affects whole animal anesthetic sensitivity. Genetic techniques provide the most reliable and versatile methods for changing the structure of putative anesthetic targets. There are genetically determined differences in the sensitivity of individual humans and animals to anesthetics. Selective breeding on the basis of sensitivity to anesthetics can be used to develop strains of animals that differ in their anesthetic sensitivity. In principle, identification of the genetic loci responsible for inter-strain differences in anesthetic sensitivity should provide insight into the molecular targets of anesthetics. Koblin and colleagues have successfully used this strategy to breed two strains of mice (HI and LO) that differ in their sensitivity to N_2O by almost 1.0 atm.[196] A similar strategy has been used to breed mice that have differential sensitivity to the hypnotic effects of the benzodiazepine, diazepam. The two strains of mice (DR and DS) show some modest, but consistent, differences in their sensitivity to volatile anesthetics.[197]

Although the development of the HI/LO and DS/DR strains of mice demonstrates that there is a genetic basis for anesthetic sensitivity, there are several reasons why it is unlikely that this approach will result in identification of genetic loci responsible for anesthetic sensitivity:

1. As with the pharmacologic approach, it is unclear whether the various strains of mice differ in their level of CNS excitability rather than in their response to specific anesthetic agents. This is illustrated by the fact that HI mice have been shown to be more sensitive to a variety of convulsants (including picrotoxin, strychnine, and fluorothyl) than are LO mice,[198] suggesting that HI mice may simply have greater CNS excitability than LO mice.
2. The differences in anesthetic sensitivity between these strains are likely to be polygenic, making it difficult to map the responsible genetic loci. This point is illustrated by cross-breeding studies that were performed between HI and LO mice.[199] If a single gene were responsible for N₂O sensitivity, cross-breeding HI and LO should produce a Mendelian distribution of offspring with HI, LO, and intermediate sensitivity to N₂O. The experimental result showed that all animals had intermediate sensitivity, indicating that N₂O sensitivity is determined by multiple genes.
3. The strains have been developed from a nonuniform genetic background, increasing the complexity of localizing the genes responsible for differential anesthetic sensitivity.
4. Mice and other mammals have a relatively long gestation period, making it difficult to screen large numbers of animals and breed over multiple generations.

Genes responsible for polygenic traits such as anesthetic sensitivity can, in principle, be more easily identified in simpler species, such as the microscopic worm *Caenorhabditis elegans*. This is because of the short breeding time of *C. elegans*, the ability to examine large numbers of worms, the extensive genetic information available (the *C. elegans* genome has now been completely sequenced), and the large number of genetic tools available for studies in *C. elegans*. Studies of anesthetic sensitivity in lower organisms are, however, complicated by the difficulty of assigning appropriate anesthetic end points (see What Is Anesthesia?). Crowder and colleagues have identified behavioral end points in *C. elegans* (mating, coordinated movement, chemotaxis) that are inhibited by volatile anesthetic concentrations similar to human MAC values.[200] Using these behavioral end points and quantitative population genetic techniques, Crowder has identified one major locus and five minor loci responsible for variable sensitivity to halothane.[201] None of these loci affects behavior in the absence of halothane, suggesting that these loci code for targets and/or downstream effectors of halothane in *C. elegans*. Sequencing and identification of these loci is one way in which novel volatile anesthetic targets are likely to be identified.

Anesthetic effects in simple organisms such as *C. elegans* or *Drosophila melanogaster* (the fruit fly) can also be studied using other genetic techniques. For example, a large number of known single gene mutations have been characterized in these species. Crowder has screened many of the behavioral mutants of *C. elegans* for sensitivity to isoflurane and identified the syntaxin gene and several related genes (synaptobrevin, SNAP-25) as potentially important in the anesthetic response. The products of these genes are proteins involved in the process of docking and release of synaptic vesicles. Various mutations in the syntaxin gene produce a 33-fold range of sensitivities to isoflurane.[56] These data indicate that volatile anesthetics may interfere with neurotransmitter release, suggesting a presynaptic mechanism of anesthesia.

One can also administer mutagenic agents to *C. elegans* or *D. melanogaster* and screen the resulting organisms for volatile anesthetic sensitivity. This potentially increases the likelihood of finding novel genes encoding anesthetic sensitivity. Nash and colleagues have used this approach in fruit flies. As an anesthetic end point, flies were considered to be anesthetized when they fell from their perches in a vertically oriented cylinder.[202] Using this end point, four halothane-resistant strains were identified. Two of these strains had abnormal behavior in the absence of

anesthetics, but the other two (Har63 and Har56) were phenotypically indistinguishable from normal fruit flies. Interestingly, Har56 and Har63 produced resistance to some volatile anesthetics but not others. For example, Har63 flies were resistant to halothane, enflurane, and isoflurane, but showed increased sensitivity to diethyl ether.[203] The anesthetic response of the mutant flies was also dependent on the anesthetic end point used. When Har63 flies were assayed for their response to a noxious stimulus (a focused beam of light), they were found to be resistant to enflurane, isoflurane, and desflurane, but had *increased* sensitivity to halothane and diethyl ether.[203]

Morgan and Sedensky have mutagenized *C. elegans* and screened for anesthetic sensitivity using immobility as an anesthetic end point. The anesthetic concentrations required to produce immobility in *C. elegans* are significantly higher than those required to produce anesthesia in higher animals, but the rank-order potency of various inhalational anesthetics is consistent with the Meyer-Overton rule. When worms were chemically mutagenized and screened for halothane sensitivity, two hypersensitive strains, unc-79 and unc-80, were identified.[1] These strains had increased sensitivity to anesthetics with olive oil/gas partition coefficients greater than that of halothane (chloroform, methoxyflurane, thiomethoxyflurane), but not to less lipophilic agents (enflurane, isoflurane, diethyl ether).[204] In a subsequent study, two additional kinds of mutations were identified by screening for alterations in sensitivity to enflurane, isoflurane, and diethyl ether.[205] One class of mutant worms showed increased sensitivity to isoflurane and enflurane, but not to halothane or diethyl ether. A second class of mutant worms showed increased sensitivity to all inhalation anesthetics tested. In total, Morgan and Sedensky have now identified eight genes that affect sensitivity to volatile anesthetics. They have sequenced and identified two of these genes. The first, unc-1, has been identified as a homolog of stomatin, an integral membrane protein thought to regulate an associated ion channel.[206] The second gene, referred to as GAS-1, encodes a mitochondrial protein involved in the respiratory chain.[207] The manner in which these proteins mediate or modulate the immobilizing effects of anesthetics is not understood.

The studies in *Drosophila* and *C. elegans* make two important points. First, the fact that mutations have been isolated that alter sensitivity to some, but not all, anesthetics argues that the mutations are not simply affecting CNS excitability. Second, the mutations isolated from these two species provide evidence against the unitary theory of anesthesia: Mutations that differentially affect sensitivity to various anesthetic agents suggest that different anesthetics may act at different targets. Mutations that differentially affect anesthetic sensitivity depending on the anesthetic end point used suggest that the various components of the anesthetic state may be caused by anesthetic actions at different targets.

Summary

Overall, genetic studies in lower organisms provide a powerful tool for determining which genes and gene products are important in producing anesthesia in an intact organism. It should be remembered that the anesthetic end points used in lower organisms are always subject to question, and it remains possible that the anesthetic targets identified in these animals are unrelated to targets responsible for anesthesia in higher organisms.

A final genetic technique useful in studying anesthetic mechanisms is the use of transgenic or gene "knockout" technology. This approach can be used to produce animals lacking or overexpressing a putative anesthetic target. Limbird and colleagues have successfully used this approach to introduce a nonfunctional α₂ₐ receptor in mice; these mice lost the hypnotic response to dexmedetomidine,[208] showing that the anesthetic effects of α₂-agonists are mediated by the α₂ₐ receptor. In studies aimed at defining the role of GABA_A receptor subunits in producing anesthesia, mice have been generated that lack the α₆ and β₃

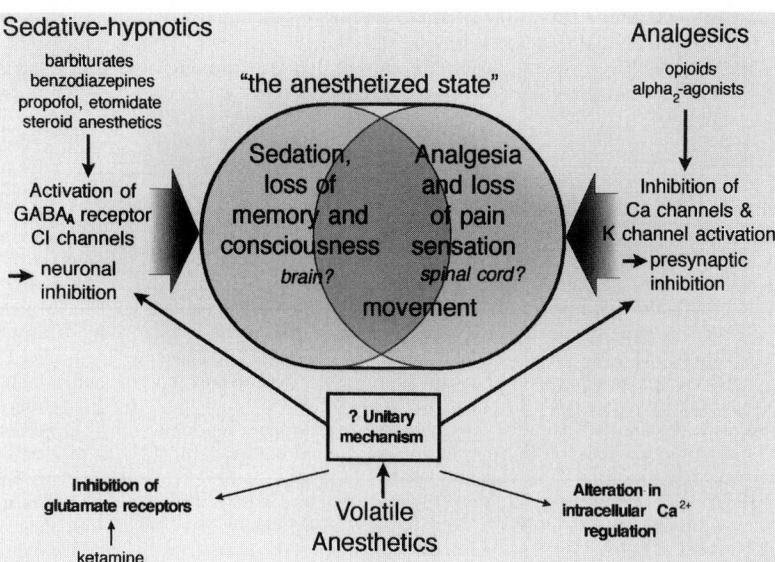

Figure 7-8. A multisite model for anesthesia. The model proposes that presynaptic inhibition (Ca^{2+} channel inhibition, K^+ channel activation) is responsible for analgesic effects, whereas postsynaptic $GABA_A$ receptor activation is responsible for sedation and amnesia. As indicated by the overlapping circles, the behavioral effects of Ca^{2+} channel inhibition and $GABA_A$ receptor activation are not mutually exclusive. The model suggests that some anesthetic agents predominantly affect Ca^{2+} and K^+ channels, other anesthetic agents predominantly affect $GABA_A$ receptors, and volatile anesthetics affect both. As illustrated at the bottom of the model, inhibition of glutamate receptor function is an alternative pathway by which ketamine and perhaps the volatile anesthetics produce anesthesia. (Reproduced with permission from Pancrazio JJ, Lynch C: Snails, spiders, and stereospecificity—Is there a role for calcium channels in anesthetic mechanisms? Anesthesiology 81:3, 1994.)

subunits. Knockout of the α_6 receptor had no effect on sensitivity to barbiturates or volatile anesthetics.[209] Interestingly, mice lacking the β_3 subunit had normal sensitivity to barbiturates, enflurane, and halothane using righting reflex as an end point, but were less sensitive than strain-matched controls to halothane and enflurane when tail-clamp response was used as the anesthetic end point. The β_3 knockout mice also showed significantly shorter sleep times in response to etomidate and midazolam (but not pentobarbital) than did strain-matched controls.[210] It is likely that transgenic and knockout techniques will increasingly be used to test the role of anesthetic targets identified *in vitro* to anesthesia in the intact organism.

CONCLUSIONS

In this chapter evidence has been reviewed concerning the anatomic, physiologic, and molecular loci of anesthetic action. It is clear that anesthetic actions cannot be localized to a specific anatomic site in the central nervous system; indeed, there is some suggestion that different components of the anesthetic state may be mediated by actions at disparate anatomic sites. The actions of anesthetics also cannot be localized to a specific physiologic process. While there is consensus that anesthetics preferentially affect synaptic function as opposed to action potential propagation, the effects of anesthetics are dependent on the agent and synapse studied and can affect presynaptic and/or postsynaptic function. At a molecular level, anesthetics show some selectivity, but still affect the function of multiple ion channels and signaling proteins. Although it is likely that these effects are mediated *via* direct protein–anesthetic interactions, it appears that there are numerous proteins that can directly interact with anesthetics. All of these data suggest that the unitary theory of anesthesia is incorrect and that there are at least several molecular mechanisms of anesthesia.

In keeping with the idea that anesthesia can be produced in a variety of ways, Pancrazio and Lynch have suggested that different anesthetic targets may mediate different components of the anesthetic state.[211] As illustrated in Figure 7-8, they suggest that the analgesic effects of opiates, α_2-agonists, and volatile anesthetics are mediated *via* inhibition of calcium currents and/or activation of potassium currents. Sedation and amnesia, they propose, are mediated by potentiation or activation of $GABA_A$ receptors. In this model, anesthetic states can also be produced by totally independent mechanisms such as the inhibition of glutamate receptors by ketamine. Although there may be many more important anesthetics targets than those suggested by Pancrazio and Lynch, their proposal illustrates the idea that different molecular targets may mediate the various components of the anesthetic state, and that volatile anesthetics are complete anesthetics because they can interact with several of these molecular targets.

Although the precise molecular interactions responsible for producing anesthesia have not been fully elucidated, it has become clear that anesthetics do act *via* selective effects on specific molecular targets. The technologic revolutions in molecular biology, genetics, and cell physiology make it likely that the next decade will provide the answers to the century-old pharmacologic puzzle of the molecular mechanism of anesthesia.

REFERENCES

1. Sedensky MM, Meneely PM: Genetic analysis of halothane sensitivity in *Caenorhabditis elegans*. Science 236:952, 1987
2. Quasha AL, Eger EI, Tinker JH: Determination and applications of MAC. Anesthesiology 53:315, 1980
3. White PF, Johnston RR, Eger E II: Determination of anesthetic requirement in rats. Anesthesiology 40:52, 1974
4. Franks NP, Lieb WR: Molecular and cellular mechanisms of general anesthesia. Nature 367:607, 1994
5. Eger EII, Saidman LJ, Branstater B: Temperature dependence of halothane and cyclopropane anesthesia in dogs: Correlation with some theories of anesthetic action. Anesthesiology 26:764, 1965
6. Cherkin A, Catchpool JF: Temperature dependence of anesthesia in goldfish. Science 144:1460, 1964
7. de Jong RH, Nace RA: Nerve impulse conduction and cutaneous receptor responses during general anesthesia. Anesthesiology 28:851, 1967
8. Campbell JN, Raja SN, Meyer RA: Halothane sensitizes cutaneous nociceptors in monkeys. J Neurophysiol 52:762, 1984
9. Antognini JF, Kien ND: Potency (minimum alveolar anesthetic concentrations) of isoflurane is independent of peripheral anesthetic effects. Anesth Anal 81:69, 1995
10. Rampil IJ, Mason P, Singh H: Anesthetic potency (MAC) is independent of forebrain structures in the rat. Anesthesiology 78:707, 1993
11. Rampil IJ: Anesthetic potency is not altered after hypothermic spinal cord transection in rats. Anesthesiology 80:606, 1994
12. Antognini JF, Schwartz K: Exaggerated anesthetic requirements in the preferentially anesthetized brain. Anesthesiology 79:1244, 1993
13. Borges M, Antognini JF: Does the brain influence somatic responses to noxious stimuli during isoflurane anesthesia? Anesthesiology 81:1511, 1994

14. Rampil IJ, King BS: Volatile anesthetics depress spinal motor neurons. Anesthesiology 85:129, 1996
15. Antognini JF, Carstens E, Buzin V: Isoflurane depresses motoneuron excitability by a direct spinal action: An F-wave study. Anesth Analg 88:681, 1999
16. Zhou HH, Mehta M, Leis AA: Spinal cord motoneuron excitability during isoflurane and nitrous oxide anesthesia. Anesthesiology 86:302, 1997
17. Zorychta E, Esplin DW, Capek R: Action of halothane on transmitter release in the spinal monosynaptic pathway. Fed Proc Am Soc Exp Biol 34:2999, 1975
18. Fujiwara N, Higashi H, Fujita S: Mechanism of halothane action on synaptic transmission in motoneurons of the newborn rat spinal cord in vitro. J Physiol 412:155, 1988
19. Kullman DM, Martin RL, Redman SJ: Reduction by general anaesthetics of group Ia excitatory postsynaptic potentials and currents in the cat spinal cord. J Physiol (Lond) 412:277, 1989
20. Takenoshita M, Takahashi T: Mechanisms of halothane action on synaptic transmission in motoneurons of the newborn rat spinal cord in vitro. Brain Res 402:303, 1987
21. French JD, Verzeano M, Magoun HW: A neural basis for the anesthetic state. Arch Neurol Psychiatry 69:519, 1953
22. Angel A: Central neuronal pathways and the process of anaesthesia. Br J Anaesth 71:148, 1993
23. Mori K, Winters WD: Neural background of sleep and anesthesia. Int Anesthesiol Clin 13:67, 1975
24. Darbinjan TM, Golovchinsky VB, Plehotinka SI: The effects of anesthetics on reticular and cortical activity. Anesthesiology 34:219, 1971
25. Thornton C, Heneghan CPH, James MFM, Jones JG: Effects of halothane or enflurane with controlled ventilation on auditory evoked potentials. Br J Anaesth 56:315, 1984
26. Feldman SM, Waller HJ: Dissociation of electrocortical activation and behavioral arousal. Nature 196:1320, 1962
27. Frost EAM: Electroencephalography and evoked potential monitoring. In Saidman LJ, Smith NT (eds): Monitoring in Anesthesia, 3d ed, p 203. Boston, Butterworth-Heinemann, 1993.
28. Richards CD, Russell WJ, Smaje JC: The action of ether and methoxyflurane on synaptic transmission in isolated preparations of the mammalian cortex. J Physiol (Lond) 248:121, 1975
29. Nicoll RA: The effects of anesthetics on synaptic excitation and inhibition in the olfactory bulb. J Physiol (Lond) 223:803, 1972
30. Richards CD, White AN: The actions of volatile anaesthetics on synaptic transmission in the dentate gyrus. J Physiol (Lond) 252:241, 1975
31. MacIver MB, Roth SH: Inhalational anaesthetics exhibit pathway-specific and differential actions on hippocampal synaptic responses in vitro. Br J Anaesth 60:680, 1988
32. Gage PW, Robertson B: Prolongation of inhibitory postsynaptic currents by pentobarbitone, halothane and ketamine in CA1 pyramidal cells in rat hippocampus. Br J Pharmacol 85:675, 1985
33. Fujiwara M, Higashi H, Nishi S et al: Changes in spontaneous firing patterns of rat hippocampal neurones induced by volatile anaesthetics. J Physiol (Lond) 402:155, 1988
34. Ries CR, Puil E: Mechanism of anesthesia revealed by shunting actions of isoflurane on thalamocortical neurons. J Neurophysiol 81:1795, 1999
35. Franks NP, Lieb WR: Mechanisms of general anesthesia. Environ Health Perspect 87:199, 1990
36. Madison DV, Nicoll RA: General anesthetics hyperpolarize neurons in the vertebrate central nervous system. Science 217:1055, 1982
37. MacIver MB, Kendig JJ: Anesthetic effects on resting membrane potential are voltage-dependent and agent-specific. Anesthesiology 74:83, 1991
38. Haydon DA, Urban BW: The effects of some inhalation anesthetics on the sodium current of the squid giant axon. J Physiol 341:429, 1983
39. Rehberg B, Xiao YH, Duch DS: Central nervous system sodium channels are significantly suppressed at clinical concentrations of volatile anesthetics. Anesthesiology 84:1223, 1996
40. Larrabee MG, Posternak JM: Selective action of anesthetics on synapses and axons in mammalian sympathetic ganglia. J Neurophysiol 15:91, 1952
41. Berg-Johnsen J, Langmoen IA: The effect of isoflurane on unmyelinated and myelinated fibres in the rat brain. Acta Physiol Scand 127:87, 1986
42. Nicoll RA, Eccles JC, Oshima T, Rubia F: Prolongation of inhibitory postsynaptic potentials by barbiturates. Nature 258:625, 1975
43. Harrison NL, Vicini S, Barker JL: A steroid anesthetic prolongs inhibitory postsynaptic currents in cultured rat hippocampal neurons. J Neurosci 7:604, 1987
44. Yoshimura M, Higashi H, Fujita S, Shimoji K: Selective depression of hippocampal inhibitory postsynaptic potentials and spontaneous firing by volatile anesthetics. Brain Res 340:363, 1985
45. Mui P, Puil E: Isoflurane-induced impairment of synaptic transmission in hippocampal neurons. Exp Brain Res 75:354, 1989
46. Griffiths R, Norman RI: Effects of anaesthetics on uptake, synthesis and release of transmitters. Br J Anaesth 71:96, 1993
47. Minchin MCW: The effect of anaesthetics on the uptake and release of gamma-aminobutyrate and d-aspartate in rat brain slices. Br J Pharmacol 73:681, 1981
48. MacIver MB, Mikulec AA, Amagasu SM, Monroe FA: Volatile anesthetics depress glutamate transmission via presynaptic actions. Anesthesiology 85:823, 1996
49. Kendall TJG, Minchin MCW: The effects of anaesthetics on the uptake and release of neurotransmitters in thalamic slices. Br J Pharmacol 75:219, 1982
50. Perouansky M, Barnaov D, Salman M, Yaari Y: Effects of halothane on glutamate receptor-mediated excitatory post-synaptic currents: A patch-clamp study in adult mouse hippocampal slices. Anesthesiology 83:109, 1995
51. Collins GGS: Release of endogenous amino acid neurotransmitter candidates from rat olfactory cortex slices: Possible regulatory mechanisms and the effects of pentobarbitone. Brain Res 190:517, 1980
52. Murugaiah KD, Hemmings HC Jr: Effects of intravenous general anesthetics on [3H]GABA release from rat cortical synaptosomes. Anesthesiology 89:919, 1998
53. Pocock G, Richards CD: The action of pentobarbitone on stimulus-secretion coupling in adrenal chromaffin cells. Br J Pharmacol 90:71, 1987
54. Pocock G, Richards CD: The action of volatile anaesthetics on stimulus-secretion coupling in bovine adrenal chromaffin cells. Br J Pharmacol 95:209, 1988
55. Stern RC, Herrington J, Lingle CJ, Evers AS: The action of halothane on stimulus-secretion coupling in clonal (GH$_3$) pituitary cells. J Neurosci 11:2217, 1991
56. van Swinderen B, Saifee O, Shebester L et al: A neomorphic syntaxin mutation blocks volatile-anesthetic action in Caenorhabditis elegans. Proc Natl Acad Sci USA 96:2479, 1999
57. Richards CD, Smaje JC: Anaesthetics depress the sensitivity of cortical neurones to L-glutamate. Br J Pharmacol 58:347, 1976
58. Smaje JC: General anaesthetics and the acetylcholine-sensitivity of cortical neurones. Br J Pharmacol 58:359, 1976
59. Tanelian DL, Kosek P, Mody I, MacIver MB: The role of the GABA$_A$ receptor/chloride channel complex in anesthesia. Anesthesiology 78:757, 1993
60. Jones MV, Brooks PA, Harrison NL: Enhancements of gamma-aminobutyric acid-activated Cl$^-$ currents in cultured rat hippocampal neurones by three volatile anesthetics. J Physiol 449:279, 1992
61. Haydon DA, Urban BW: The actions of some general anaesthetics on the potassium current of the squid giant axon. J Physiol 373:311, 1986
62. Herrington J, Stern RC, Evers AS, Lingle CJ: Halothane inhibits two components of calcium current in clonal (GH$_3$) pituitary cells. J Neurosci 11:2226, 1991
63. Varadi G, Mori Y, Mikala G, Schwartz A: Molecular determinants of calcium channel function and drug action. Trends Pharmacol Sci 16:43, 1995
64. Eskinder H, Rusch NJ, Supan FD et al: The effects of volatile anesthetics on L-type and T-type calcium channel currents in canine cardiac Purkinje cells. Anesthesiology 74:919, 1991
65. Terrar DA: Structure and function of calcium channels and the actions of anaesthetics. Br J Anaesth 71:39, 1993
66. Hall AC, Lieb WR, Franks NP: Insensitivity of P-type calcium channels to inhalational and intravenous general anesthetics. Anesthesiology 81:117, 1994
67. Study RE: Isoflurane inhibits multiple voltage-gated calcium currents in hippocampal pyramidal neurons. Anesthesiology 81:104, 1994
68. Gundersen CB, Umbach JA, Swartz BE: Barbiturates depress currents through human brain calcium channels studied in Xenopus oocytes. J Pharmacol Exp Ther 247:824, 1988

69. Takenoshita M, Steinbach JH: Halothane blocks low-voltage-activated calcium current in rat sensory neurons. J Neurosci 11: 1404, 1991

70. ffrench-Mullen JMH, Barker JL, Rogawski MA: Calcium current block by (−)-pentobarbital, phenobarbital, and CHEB but not (+)-pentobarbital in acutely isolated hippocampal CA1 neurons: Comparison with effects on GABA-activated Cl⁻ current. J Neurosci 13:3211, 1993

71. Schofield PR, Darlison NG, Fujita N et al: Sequence and functional expression of a GABA$_A$ receptor shows a ligand-gated receptor super-family. Nature 328:221, 1987

72. Rosenmund C, Stern-Bach Y, Stevens CF: The tetrameric structure of a glutamate receptor channel. Science 280:1596, 1998

73. Krasowski MD, Harrison NL: General anaesthetic actions on ligand-gated ion channels. Cell Molec Life Sci 55:1278, 1999

74. Seeburg PH: The TiPS/TINS lecture: The molecular biology of mammalian glutamate receptor channels. Trends Pharmacol Sci 14:297, 1993

75. Wakamori M, Ikemoto Y, Akaike N: Effects of two volatile anesthetics and a volatile convulsant on the excitatory and inhibitory amino acid responses in dissociated CNS neurons of the rat. J Neurophysiol 66:2014, 1991

76. Lin L, Chen LL, Harris RA: Enflurane inhibits NMDA, AMPA and kainate-induced currents in Xenopus oocytes expressing mouse and human brain mRNA. FASEB J 7:479, 1992

77. Weight FF, Lovinger DM, White G, Peoples RW: Alcohol and anesthetic actions on excitatory amino acid-activated ion channels. Ann N Y Acad Sci 625:97, 1991

78. Dildy-Mayfield JE, Eger EI 2nd, Harris RA: Anesthetics produce subunit-selective actions on glutamate receptors. J Pharmacol Exp Ther 276:1058, 1996

79. Minami K, Wick MJ, Stern-Bach Y et al: Sites of volatile anesthetic action on kainate (glutamate receptor 6) receptors. J Biol Chem 273:8248, 1998

80. Aronstam RS, Martin DC, Dennison RL: Volatile anesthetics inhibit NMDA-stimulated ⁴⁵Ca uptake by rat brain microvesicles. Neurochem Res 19:1515, 1994

81. Lodge D, Anis NA, Burton NR: Effects of optical isomers of ketamine on excitation of cat and rat spinal neurons by amino acids and acetylcholine. Neurosci Lett 29:281, 1982

82. Anis NA, Berry SC, Burton NR, Lodge D: The dissociative anesthetics ketamine and phencyclidine selectively reduce excitation of central mammalian neurons by N-methyl aspartate. Br J Pharmacol 79:565, 1983

83. Zeilhofer HU, Swandulla D, Geisslinger G, Brune K: Differential effects of ketamine enantiomers on NMDA receptor currents in cultured neurons. Eur J Pharmacol 213:155, 1992

84. Ryder S, Way WL, Trevor AJ: Comparative pharmacology of the optical isomers of ketamine in mice. Eur J Pharmacol 49:15, 1978

85. Mennerick S, Jevtovic-Todorovic V, Todorovic SM et al: Effect of nitrous oxide on excitatory and inhibitory synaptic transmission in hippocampal cultures. J Neuroscience 18:9716, 1998

86. Jevtovic-Todorovic V, Todorovic SM, Mennerick S et al: Nitrous oxide (laughing gas) is an NMDA antagonist, neuroprotectant and neurotoxin. Nature Med 4:460, 1998

87. Franks NP, Dickinson R, de Sousa SL et al: How does xenon produce anaesthesia? [letter]. Nature 396:324, 1998

88. Macdonald RL, Olsen RW: GABA$_A$ receptor channels. Ann Rev Neurosci 17:569, 1994

89. Macdonald RL, Rogers CJ, Twyman RE: Barbiturate regulation of kinetic properties of the GABA$_A$ receptor channels of mouse spinal neurones in culture. J Physiol 417:483, 1989

90. Barker JL, Harrison NL, Lange GD, Owen DG: Potentiation of gamma-aminobutyric-acid-activated chloride conductance by a steroid anesthetic in cultured rat spinal neurons. J Physiol 386: 485, 1987

91. Hales TH, Lambert JJ: Modulation of the GABA$_A$ receptor by propofol. Br J Pharmacol 93:84P, 1988

92. Parker I, Gundersen CB, Miledi RJ: Actions of pentobarbital on rat brain receptors expressed in Xenopus oocytes. J Neurosci 6: 2290, 1986

93. Wittmer LL, Hu Y, Kalkbrenner M et al: Enantioselectivity of steroid-induced gamma-aminobutyric acid A receptor modulation and anesthesia. Mol Pharmacol 50:1581, 1996

94. Nakahiro M, Yeh JZ, Brunner E, Narahashi T: General anesthetics modulate GABA receptor channel complex in rat dorsal root ganglion neurons. FASEB J 3:1850, 1989

95. Hall AC, Lieb WR, Franks NP: Stereoselective and non-stereoselective actions of isoflurane on the GABA$_A$ receptor. Br J Pharmacol 112:906, 1994

96. Yeh JZ, Quandt FN, Tanguy J et al: General anesthetic action on gamma-aminobutyric acid-activated channels. Ann N Y Acad Sci 625:155, 1991

97. Banks MI, Pearce RA: Dual actions of volatile anesthetics on GABA(A) IPSCs: Dissociation of blocking and prolonging effects. Anesthesiology 90:120, 1999

98. Weiss DS, Amin J: GABA$_A$ receptors need two homologous domains of the beta subunit for activation by GABA but not by pentobarbital. Nature 366:565, 1993

99. Sapp DW, Witte U, Turner DM et al: Regional variation in steroid anesthetic modulation of [³⁵S]TBPS binding to gamma-aminobutyric acid receptors in rat brain. J Pharmacol Exp Ther 262:801, 1992

100. Pritchett DB, Sontheimer H, Shivers BD: Importance of a novel GABA$_A$ receptor subunit for benzodiazepine pharmacology. Nature 338:582, 1989

101. Hill-Venning C, Belelli D, Peters JA, Lambert JJ: Subunit-dependent interaction of the general anaesthetic etomidate with the gamma-aminobutyric acid type A receptor. Br J Pharmacol 120: 749, 1997

102. Zhu WJ, Wang JF, Krueger KE, Vicini S: Subunit inhibits neurosteroid modulation of GABA$_A$ receptors. J Neurosci 16:6648, 1996

103. Davies PA, Hanna MC, Hales TG, Kirkness EF: Insensitivity to anaesthetic agents conferred by a class of GABA$_A$ subunit. Nature 385:820, 1997

104. Mihic SJ, Harris RA: Inhibition of rho1 receptor GABAergic currents by alcohols and volatile anesthetics. J Pharmacol Exp Ther 277:411, 1996

105. Mihic SJ, Ye Q, Wick MJ et al: Sites of alcohol and volatile anaesthetic action on GABA(A) and glycine receptors. Nature 389: 385, 1997

106. Belelli D, Lambert JJ, Peters JA et al: The interaction of the general anesthetic etomidate with the gamma-aminobutyric acid type A receptor is influenced by a single amino acid. Proc Natl Acad Sci USA 94:11031, 1997

107. Krasowski MD, Koltchine VV, Rick CE et al: Propofol and other intravenous anesthetics have sites of action on the gamma-aminobutyric acid type A receptor distinct from that for isoflurane. Molec Pharmacol 53:530, 1998

108. Dilger JP, Vidal AM, Mody HI, Liu Y: Evidence for direct actions of general anesthetics on an ion channel protein. A new look at a unified mode of action. Anesthesiology 81:431, 1994

109. Firestone LL, Sauter JF, Braswell LM, Miller KW: Actions of general anesthetics on acetylcholine receptor-rich membranes from Torpedo californica. Anesthesiology 64:694, 1986

110. Franks NP, Lieb WR: Stereospecific effects of inhalational general anesthetic optical isomers on nerve ion channels. Science 254: 427, 1991

111. Charlesworth P, Richards CD: Anaesthetic modulation of nicotinic ion channel kinetics in bovine chromaffin cells. Br J Pharmacol 114:909, 1995

112. Violet JM, Downie DL, Nakisa RC et al: Differential sensitivities of mammalian neuronal and muscle nicotinic acetylcholine receptors to general anesthetics. Anesthesiology 86:866, 1997

113. Flood P, Ramirez-Latorre J, Role L: Alpha 4 beta 2 neuronal nicotinic acetylcholine receptors in the central nervous system are inhibited by isoflurane and propofol, but alpha 7-type nicotinic acetylcholine receptors are unaffected. Anesthesiology 86:859, 1997

114. Evers AS, Steinbach JH: Supersensitive sites in the central nervous system: anesthetics block brain nicotinic receptors. Anesthesiology 86:760, 1997

115. Mascia MP, Machu TK, Harris RA: Enhancement of homomeric glycine receptor function by long-chain alcohols and anaesthetics. Br J Pharmacol 119:1331, 1996

116. Downie DL, Hall AC, Lieb WR, Franks NP: Effects of inhalational general anaesthetics on native glycine receptors in rat medullary neurones and recombinant glycine receptors in Xenopus oocytes. Br J Pharmacol 118:493, 1996

117. Jenkins A, Franks NP, Lieb WR: Actions of general anaesthetics on 5-HT3 receptors in N1E-115 neuroblastoma cells. Br J Pharmacol 117:1507, 1996

118. Machu TK, Harris RA: Alcohols and anesthetics enhance the func-

tion of 5-hydroxytryptamine$_3$ receptors expressed in *Xenopus laevis* oocytes. J Pharmacol Exp Ther 271:898, 1994

119. Pancrazio JJ, Park WK, Lynch C: Inhalational anesthetic actions on voltage-gated ion currents of bovine adrenal chromaffin cells. Mol Pharmacol 43:783, 1993

120. Franks NP, Lieb WR: Volatile general anaesthetics activate a novel neuronal K$^+$ current. Nature 333:662, 1988

121. Lopes CM, Franks NP, Lieb WR: Actions of general anaesthetics and arachidonic pathway inhibitors on K$^+$ currents activated by volatile anaesthetics and FMRFamide in molluscan neurones. Br J Pharmacol 125:309, 1998

122. Winegar BD, Yost CS: Volatile anesthetics directly activate baseline S K$^+$ channels in aplysia neurons. Brain Res 807:255, 1998

123. Franks NP, Lieb WR: Background K$^+$ channels: An important target for volatile anesthetics?[news]. Nature Neurosci 2:395, 1999

124. Gray AT, Winegar BD, Leonoudakis DJ et al: TOK1 is a volatile anesthetic stimulated K$^+$ channel. Anesthesiology 88:1076, 1998

125. Patel AJ, Honore E, Lesage F et al: Inhalational anesthetics activate two-pore-domain background K$^+$ channels. Nature Neurosci 2:422, 1999

126. Hossain MD, Evers AS: Volatile anesthetic-induced efflux of calcium from IP$_3$-gated stores in clonal (GH$_3$) pituitary cells. Anesthesiology 80:1379, 1994

127. Sill CJ, Uhl C, Eskuri S et al: Halothane inhibits agonist-induced inositol phosphate and Ca^{2+} signaling in A7r5 cultured vascular smooth cells. Mol Pharmacol 40:1006, 1991

128. Daniell LC, Harris RA: Neuronal intracellular calcium concentrations are altered by anesthetics: Relationship to membrane fluidization. J Pharmacol Exp Ther 245:1, 1988

129. Kress HG, Muller J, Eisert A et al: Effects of volatile anesthetics on cytoplasmic calcium signaling and transmitter release in a neural cell line. Anesthesiology 74:309, 1991

130. Puil E, Elbeheiry H, Baimbridge KG: Anesthetic effects on glutamate-stimulated increases in intraneuronal calcium. J Pharmacol Exp Ther 255:955, 1990

131. Dennison RL, Anthony BL, Narayanan TK, Aronstam RS: Effects of halothane on high affinity agonist binding and guanine nucleotide sensitivity of muscarinic acetylcholine receptors from brainstem of rat. Neuropharmacology 26:1201, 1987

132. Baumgartner MK, Dennison RL, Narayanan TK, Aronstam RS: Halothane disruption of alpha-2-adrenergic receptor-mediated inhibition of adenylate cyclase and receptor G-protein coupling in rat brain. Biochem Pharmacol 39:223, 1990

133. Robinson-White AJ, Muldoon SM, Elson L, Collado-Escobar DM: Evidence that barbiturates inhibit antigen-induced responses through interactions with a GTP-binding protein in rat basophilic leukemia (RBL-2) cells. Anesthesiology 72:996, 1990

134. Bazil C, Minneman K: Effects of clinically effective concentrations of halothane on adrenergic and cholinergic synapses in rat brain *in vitro*. J Pharmacol Exp Ther 248:143, 1989

135. Smart D, Smith G, Lambert DG: Halothane and isoflurane enhance basal and carbachol-stimulated inositol (1,4,5) triphosphate formation in SH-SY5y human neuroblastoma cells. Biochem Pharmacol 47:939, 1994

136. Foster PS, Claudianos C, Gesini E, Hopkinson KC: Inositol 1,4,5-trisphosphate phosphatase deficiency and malignant hyperpyrexia in swine. Lancet II:124, 1989

137. Nahrwold ML, Lust WD, Passonneau JV: Halothane-induced alterations of cyclic nucleotide concentrations in three regions of the mouse nervous system. Anesthesiology 47:423, 1977

138. Triner L, Vulliemoz Y, Verosky M, Woo S: Action of volatile anesthetics on cyclic nucleotides in brain. Anesthesci 2:229, 1980

139. Rengesamy A, Pajewski TN, Johns RA: Inhalational anesthetic effects on rat cerebellar nitric oxide and cyclic guanosine monophosphate production. Anesthesiology 86:689, 1997

140. Slater S, Cox KJA, Lombardi JV et al: Inhibition of protein kinase C by alcohols and anesthetics. Nature 364:82, 1993

141. Hemmings HC, Adamo AIB: Effects of halothane and propofol on purified brain protein kinase C activation. Anesthesiology 81:147, 1994

142. Hemming HC, Adamo AIB: Effect of halothane on conventional protein kinase C translocation and down regulation in rat cerebrocortical synaptosomes. Br J Anaesth 78:189, 1997

143. Johns RA, Moscicki JC, DiFazio CA: Nitric oxide synthase inhibitor dose-dependently and reversibly reduces the threshold for halothane anesthesia. A role for nitric oxide in mediating consciousness? Anesthesiology 77:779, 1992

144. Pajewski TN, DiFazio CA, Moscicki JC, Johns RA: Nitric oxide synthase inhibitors, 7-nitro indazole and nitro D-L-arginine methyl ester, dose dependently reduce the threshold for isoflurane anesthesia. Anesthesiology 85:1111, 1996

145. Ichinose F, Huang PL, Zapol WM: Effects of targeted neuronal nitric oxide synthase gene disruption and nitro-L-arginine methyl ester on the threshold for isoflurane anesthesia. Anesthesiology 83:101, 1995

146. Overton CE: Studies of Narcosis, 1st ed. London, Chapman and Hall, 1991.

147. Meyer H: Theorie der alkoholnarkose. Arch Exp Pathol Pharmakol 42:109, 1899

148. Franks NP, Lieb WR: Where do general anaesthetics act? Nature 274:339, 1978

149. Larsen ER: Fluorine Compounds in Anesthesiology. 1960:1.

150. Andrews PR, Jones JG, Pulton DB: Convulsant, anticonvulsant and anesthetic barbiturates. *In vivo* activities of oxo- and thiobarbiturates related to pentobarbitone. Eur J Pharmacol 79:61, 1982

151. Paul SM, Purdy RH: Neuroactive steroids. FASEB J 6:2311, 1992

152. Koblin D, Eger EI, Johnson B et al: Are convulsant gases also anesthetics? Anesth Analg 60:464, 1981

153. Koblin DD, Chortkoff BS, Laster MJ et al: Polyhalogenated and perfluorinated compounds that disobey the Meyer-Overton hypothesis. Anesth Analg 79:1043, 1994

154. Kandel L, Chortkoff BS, Sonner J et al: Nonanesthetics can suppress learning. Anesth Analg 82:321, 1996

155. Alifimoff JK, Firestone LL, Miller KW: Anaesthetic potencies of primary alkanols: Implications for the molecular dimensions of the anaesthetic site. Br J Pharmacol 96:9, 1989

156. Raines DE, Korten SE, Hill WAG, Miller KW: Anesthetic cutoff in cycloalkanemethanols—A test of current theories. Anesthesiology 78:918, 1993

157. Liu J, Laster MJ, Koblin DD et al: A cutoff in potency exists in the perfluoroalkanes. Anesth Analg 79:238, 1994

158. Andrews PR, Mark LC: Structural specificity of barbiturates and related drugs. Anesthesiology 57:314, 1982

159. Richter JA, Holtman JR: Barbiturates: Their *in vivo* effects and potential biochemical mechanisms. Prog Neurobiol 18:275, 1982

160. Tomlin SL, Jenkins A, Lieb WR, Franks NP: Stereoselective effects of etomidate optical isomers on gamma-aminobutyric acid type A receptors and animals. Anesthesiology 88:708, 1998

161. Lysko GS, Robinson JL, Casto R, Ferrone RA: The stereospecific effects of isoflurane isomers *in vivo*. Eur J Pharmacol 263:25, 1994

162. Kendig JJ, Grossman Y, MacIver MB: Pressure reversal of anesthesia: A synaptic mechanism. Br J Anaesth 60:806, 1988

163. Smith RA, Porter EG, Miller KW: The solubility of anesthetic gases in lipid bilayers. Biochim Biophys Acta 645:327, 1981

164. Franks NP, Lieb WR: Partitioning of long chain alcohols into lipid bilayers: Implications for mechanisms of general anesthesia. Proc Natl Acad Sci USA 83:5116, 1986

165. Elliot JR, Haydon DA, Hendry BM, Needham D: Inactivation of the sodium current in squid giant axons by hydrocarbons. Biophys J 48:617, 1985

166. Seeman P: The membrane actions of anesthetics and tranquilizers. Pharmacol Rev 24:583, 1972

167. Franks NP: Is membrane expansion relevant to anaesthesia? Nature 292:248, 1981

168. Bull MH, Brailsford JD, Bull BS: Erythrocyte membrane expansion due to volatile anesthetics, the 1-alkanols, and benzyl alcohol. Anesthesiology 57:399, 1982

169. Cantor RS: The lateral pressure profile in membranes: A physical mechanism of general anesthesia. Biochemistry 36:2339, 1997

170. North C, Cafiso DS: Contrasting membrane localization and behavior of halogenated cyclobutanes that follow or violate the Meyer-Overton hypothesis of general anesthetic potency. Biophys J 72:1754, 1997

171. Metcalfe JC, Seeman P, Burgen ASV: The proton relaxation of benzyl alcohol in erythrocyte membranes. Mol Pharmacol 4:87, 1967

172. Miller KW, Pang KY: General anaesthetics can selectively perturb lipid bilayer membranes. Nature 263:253, 1976

173. Pang K-YY, Braswell LM, Chang L et al: The perturbation of lipid bilayers by general anesthetics: A quantitative test of the disordered lipid hypothesis. Mol Pharmacol 18:84, 1980

174. Miller KW, Firestone LL, Alifimoff JK, Streicher P: Nonanesthetic alcohols dissolve in synaptic membranes without perturbing their lipids. Proc Natl Acad Sci USA 86:1084, 1989

175. Mountcastle DB, Biltonen RL, Halsey MJ: Effect of anesthetics and pressure on the thermotropic behavior of multilamellar dipalmitoylphosphatidylcholine liposomes. Proc Natl Acad Sci USA 75: 4906, 1978

176. Trudell JR: A unitary theory of anesthesia based on lateral phase separations in nerve membranes. Anesthesiology 46:5, 1977

177. Franks NP, Lieb WR: Do general anaesthetics act by competitive binding to specific receptors. Nature 310:599, 1984

178. Franks NP, Lieb WR: Mapping of general anaesthetic target sites provides a molecular basis for cutoff effects. Nature 316:149, 1985

179. Wishnia A, Pinder TW: Hydrophobic interactions in proteins. The alkane binding site of β-lactoglobulins A and B. Biochemistry 5: 1534, 1966

180. Wishnia A, Pinder T: Hydrophobic interactions in proteins: Conformation changes in bovine serum albumin below pH 5. Biochemistry 3:1377, 1964

181. Dubois BW, Evers AS: An ^{19}F-NMR spin–spin relaxation (T_2) method for characterizing volatile anesthetic binding to proteins. Analysis of isoflurane binding to serum albumin. Biochemistry 31: 7069, 1992

182. Dubois BW, Cherian SF, Evers AS: Volatile anesthetics compete for common binding sites on bovine serum albumin: A ^{19}F-NMR study. Proc Natl Acad Sci USA 90:6478, 1993

183. Eckenhoff RG, Shuman H: Halothane binding to soluble proteins determined by photoaffinity labeling. Anesthesiology 79:96, 1993

184. Eckenhoff RG: Amino acid resolution of halothane binding sites in serum albumin. J Biol Chem 271:15521, 1996

185. Burris KE, Dubois BW, Evers AS: Direct observation of saturable halothane binding to firefly luciferase: A photoaffinity labeling and ^{19}F-NMR study. Anesthesiology 79:A700, 1993

186. Eckenhoff RG: An inhalational anesthetic binding domain in the nicotinic acetylcholine receptor. Proc Natl Acad Sci USA 93: 2807, 1996

187. Hussain SS, Forman SA, Kloczewiak MA et al: Synthesis and properties of 3-(2-hydroxyethyl)-3-n-pentyldiazirine, a photoactivable general anesthetic. J Med Chem 42:3300, 1999

188. Schoenborn BP, Watson HC, Kendrew JC: Binding of xenon to sperm whale myoglobin. Nature 207:28, 1965

189. Schoenborn BP: Binding of cyclopropane to sperm whale myoglobin. Nature 14:1120, 1967

190. Sachsenheimer W, Pai EF, Schulz GE, Schirmer RH: Halothane binds in the adenine specific niche of crystalline adenylate kinase. FEBS Lett 79:310, 1977

191. Franks NP, Jenkins A, Conti E et al: Structural basis for the inhibition of firefly luciferase by a general anesthetic. Biophysical J 75:2205, 1998

192. Wick MJ, Mihic SJ, Ueno S et al: Mutations of γ-aminobutyric acid and glycine receptors change alcohol cutoff: Evidence for an alcohol receptor? Proc Natl Acad Sci USA 95:6504, 1998

193. Johansson JS, Gibney BR, Rabanal F et al: A designed cavity in the hydrophobic core of a four-alpha-helix bundle improves volatile anesthetic binding affinity. Biochemistry 37:1421, 1998

194. Segal IS, Vickery RG, Walton JK et al: Dexmedetomidine diminishes halothane anesthetic requirements in rats through a postsynaptic alpha-2 adrenergic receptor. Anesthesiology 69:818, 1988

195. Moody EJ, Harris BD, Skolnick P: The potential for safer anaesthesia using stereoselective anaesthetics. Trends Pharmacol Sci 15: 387, 1994

196. Koblin DD, Dong DE, Deady JE, Eger EI: Selective breeding alters murine resistance to nitrous oxide without alteration in synaptic membrane lipid composition. Anesthesiology 52:401, 1980

197. McCrae AF, Gallaher EJ, Winter PM, Firestone LL: Volatile anesthetic requirements differ in mice selectively bred for sensitivity or resistance to diazepam—Implications for the site of anesthesia. Anesth Analg 76:1313, 1993

198. Koblin DD, O'Connor B, Deady JE, Eger EI: Potencies of convulsant drugs in mice selectively bred for resistance and susceptibility to nitrous oxide anesthesia. Anesthesiology 56:25, 1982

199. Koblin DD, Eger EI: Cross-mating of mice selectively bred for resistance and susceptibility to nitrous oxide: Potencies of nitrous oxide in the offspring. Anesth Analg 60:646, 1981

200. Crowder CM, Shebester LD, Schedl T: Behavioral effects of volatile anesthetics in *Caenorhabditis elegans*. Anesthesiology 85:901, 1996

201. van Swinderen B, Shook DR, Ebert RH et al: Quantitative trait loci controlling halothane sensitivity in *Caenorhabditis elegans*. Proc Natl Acad Sci USA 94:8232, 1997

202. Krishnan KS, Nash HA: A genetic study of the anesthetic response: Mutants of *Drosophila melanogaster* altered in sensitivity to halothane. Proc Natl Acad Sci USA 87:8632, 1990

203. Campbell DB, Nash HA: Use of *Drosophila* mutants to distinguish among volatile general anesthetics. Proc Natl Acad Sci USA 91: 2135, 1994

204. Morgan PG, Sedensky MM, Meneely PM, Cascorbi HF: The effect of two genes on anesthetic responses in the nematode *Caenorhabditis elegans*. Anesthesiology 69:246, 1988

205. Morgan PG, Sedensky MM: Mutations conferring new patterns of sensitivity to volatile anesthetics in *Caenorhabditis elegans*. Anesthesiology 81:888, 1994

206. Rajaram S, Sedensky MM, Morgan PG: Unc-1: A stomatin homologue controls sensitivity to volatile anesthetics in *Caenorhabditis elegans*. Proc Natl Acad Sci USA 95:8761, 1998

207. Kayser EB, Morgan PG, Sedensky MM: GAS-1: A mitochondrial protein controls sensitivity to volatile anesthetics in the nematode *Caenorhabditis elegans*. Anesthesiology 90:545, 1999

208. Lakhlani PP, MacMillan LB, Guo TZ et al: Substitution of a mutant alpha2a-adrenergic receptor via "hit and run" gene targeting reveals the role of this subtype in sedative, analgesic and anesthetic-sparing responses in vivo. Proc Natl Acad Sci USA 94:9950, 1997

209. Homanics GE, Ferguson C, Quinlan JJ et al: Gene knockout of the alpha6 subunit of the gamma-aminobutyric acid type A receptor: Lack of effect on responses to ethanol, pentobarbital, and general anesthetics. Mol Pharmacol 51:588, 1997

210. Quinlan JJ, Homanics GE, Firestone LL: Anesthesia sensitivity in mice that lack the beta3 subunit of the gamma-aminobutyric acid type A receptor. Anesthesiology 88:775, 1998

211. Lynch C, Pancrazio JJ: Snails, spiders and stereospecificity—Is there a role for calcium channels in anesthetic mechanisms? Anesthesiology 81:1, 1994

Clinical Anesthesia (4/e), edited by
Paul G. Barash, Bruce F. Cullen, and
Robert K. Stoelting. Lippincott Williams &
Wilkins, Philadelphia, © 2001.

CHAPTER 8

ELECTRICAL SAFETY

JAN EHRENWERTH

The myriad of electrical and electronic devices in the modern operating room greatly improve patient care and safety. However, these devices also subject both the patient and operating room personnel to increased risks. To reduce the risk of electrical shock, most operating rooms have electrical systems that incorporate special safety features. It is incumbent upon the anesthesiologist to have a thorough understanding of the basic principles of electricity and an appreciation of the concepts of electrical safety applicable to the operating room environment.

PRINCIPLES OF ELECTRICITY

A basic principle of electricity is known as *Ohm's law*, which is represented by the equation:

$$E = I \times R$$

where E is electromotive force (in volts), I is current (in amperes), and R is resistance (in ohms). Ohm's law forms the basis for the physiologic equation BP = CO × SVR; that is, blood pressure (BP) is equal to the cardiac output (CO) times the systemic vascular resistance (SVR). In this case, the blood pressure of the vascular system is analogous to voltage, the cardiac output to current, and systemic vascular resistance to the forces opposing the flow of electrons. Electrical power is measured in watts. Wattage (W) is the product of the voltage (E) and the current (I), as defined by the formula:

$$W = E \times I$$

The amount of electrical work done is measured in watts per unit of time. The watt-second (a joule, J) is a common designation for electrical energy expended in doing work. The energy produced by a defibrillator is measured in watt-seconds (or joules), and the kilowatt-hour is frequently used to measure larger quantities of electrical energy. For example, electrical utility companies charge their customers on the basis of kilowatt-hours of electricity consumed.

Wattage can be thought of as a measure not only of work done but also of heat produced in any electrical circuit. Substituting Ohm's law in the formula

$$W = E \times I$$
$$W = (I \times R) \times I$$
$$W = I^2 \times R$$

Thus, wattage is equal to the square of the current I^2 (amperage) times the resistance R. Using these formulas, it is possible to calculate the number of amperes and the resistance of a given device if the wattage and the voltage are known. For example, a 60-watt light bulb operating on a household 120-volt circuit would require 0.5 amperes of current for operation. Rearranging the formula so that

$$I = W/E$$

we have

$$I = (60 \text{ watts}) / (120 \text{ volts})$$
$$I = 0.5 \text{ ampere}$$

Using this in Ohm's law

$$R = E/I$$

the resistance can be calculated to be 240 ohms:

$$R = (120 \text{ volts}) / (0.5 \text{ ampere})$$
$$R = 240 \text{ ohms}$$

It is obvious from the previous discussion that 1 volt of electromotive force (EMF) flowing through a 1-ohm resistance will generate 1 ampere of current. Similarly, 1 ampere of current induced by 1 volt of electromotive force will generate 1 watt of power.

Direct and Alternating Currents

Any substance that permits the flow of electrons is called a *conductor*. Current is characterized by electrons flowing through a conductor. If the electron flow is always in the same direction, it is referred to as *direct current* (DC). However, if the electron flow reverses direction at a regular interval, it is termed *alternating current* (AC). Either of these types of current can be pulsed or continuous in nature.[1]

The previous discussion of Ohm's law is accurate when applied to DC circuits. However, when dealing with AC circuits, the situation is more complex because the flow of the current is opposed by a more complicated form of resistance, known as *impedance*.

Impedance

Impedance, designated by the letter Z, is defined as the sum of the forces that oppose electron movement in an AC circuit. Impedance consists of resistance (ohms) but also takes capacitance and inductance into account. In actuality, when referring to AC circuits, Ohm's law is defined as

$$E = I \times Z$$

An *insulator* is a substance that opposes the flow of electrons. Therefore, an insulator has a high impedance to electron flow, whereas a conductor has a low impedance to electron flow.

In AC circuits the capacitance and inductance can be important factors in determining the total impedance. Both capacitance and inductance are influenced by the frequency (cycles per second or hertz, Hz) at which the AC current reverses direction. The impedance is directly proportional to the frequency (f) times the inductance (IND):

$$Z \propto (f \times \text{IND})$$

and the impedance is inversely proportional to the product of the frequency (f) and the capacitance (CAP):

$$Z \propto 1 / (f \times \text{CAP})$$

As the AC current increases in frequency, the net effect of both capacitance and inductance increases. However, because impedance and capacitance are inversely related, total impedance decreases as the product of the frequency and the capacitance increases. Thus, as frequency increases, impedance falls and more current is allowed to pass.[2]

Capacitance

A *capacitor* consists of any two parallel conductors that are separated by an insulator (Fig. 8-1). A capacitor has the ability to store charge. *Capacitance* is the measure of that substance's ability to store charge. In a DC circuit the capacitor plates are charged by a voltage source (*i.e.,* a battery) and there is only a momentary current flow. The circuit is not completed and no further current can flow unless a resistance is connected between the two plates and the capacitor is discharged.[3]

In contrast to DC circuits, a capacitor in an AC circuit permits current flow even when the circuit is not completed by a resistance. This is due to the nature of AC circuits, in which the current flow is constantly being reversed. Because current flow results from the movement of electrons, the capacitor plates are alternately charged—first positive and then negative with every reversal of the AC current direction—resulting in an effective current flow as far as the remainder of the circuit is concerned, even though the circuit is not completed.[4]

Because the effect of capacitance on impedance varies directly with the AC frequency (Hz), the greater the AC frequency, the lower the impedance. Therefore, high-frequency currents (0.5–2 million Hz), such as those used by electrosurgical units (ESUs), will cause a marked decrease in impedance. For example, a 20-million–ohm impedance in a 60-Hz AC circuit will be reduced to just a few hundred ohms when the frequency is increased to 1 million Hz.[5]

Electrical devices use capacitors for various beneficial purposes. There is, however, a phenomenon known as *stray capacitance*—capacitance that was not designed into the system but is incidental to the construction of the equipment.[6] All AC-operated equipment produces stray capacitance. An ordinary power cord, for example, consisting of two insulated wires running next to each other will generate significant capacitance simply by being plugged into a 120-volt circuit, even though the piece of equipment is not turned on. Another example of stray capacitance is found in electric motors. The circuit wiring in electric motors generates stray capacitance to the metal housing of the motor.[7] The clinical importance of capacitance will be emphasized later in the chapter.

Inductance

Whenever electrons flow in a wire, a magnetic field is induced around the wire. If the wire is coiled repeatedly around an iron core, as in a transformer, the magnetic field can be very strong. *Inductance* is a property of AC circuits in which an opposing EMF can be electromagnetically generated in the circuit. The net effect of inductance is to increase impedance. Because the effect of inductance on impedance is also dependent on AC frequency, increases in frequency will increase the total impedance. Therefore, the total impedance of a coil will be much greater than its simple resistance.[4]

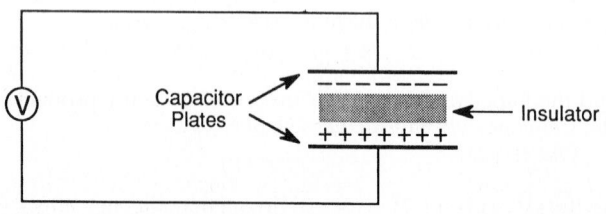

Figure 8-1. A capacitor consists of two parallel conductors separated by an insulator. The capacitor is capable of storing charge supplied by a voltage source.

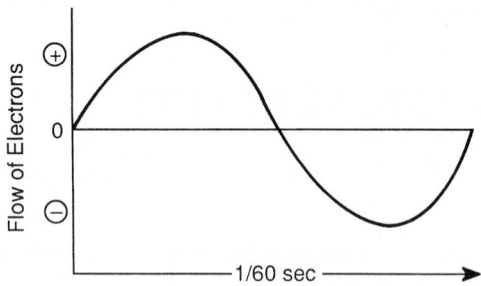

Figure 8-2. Sine wave flow of electrons in a 60-Hz alternating current.

ELECTRICAL SHOCK HAZARDS
Alternating and Direct Currents

Whenever an individual contacts an external source of electricity, an electrical shock is possible. An electrical current can stimulate skeletal muscle cells to contract, and thus can be used therapeutically in devices such as pacemakers or defibrillators. However, casual contact with an electrical current, whether AC or DC, can lead to injury or death. Although it takes approximately three times as much DC as AC to cause ventricular fibrillation,[3] this by no means renders DC harmless. Devices such as an automobile battery or a DC defibrillator can be sources of direct current shocks.

In the United States, utility companies supply electrical energy in the form of alternating currents of 120 volts at a frequency of 60 Hz.* The 60 Hz refers to the number of times in 1 second that the current reverses its direction of flow.[8] Both the voltage and current waveforms form a sinusoidal pattern (Fig. 8-2).

To have the completed circuit necessary for current flow, a closed loop must exist and a voltage source must drive the current through the impedance. If current is to flow in the electrical circuit, there has to be a *voltage differential,* or a drop in the driving pressure across the impedance. According to Ohm's law, if the resistance is held constant, then the greater the current flow, the larger the voltage drop must be.[9]

The power company attempts to maintain the line voltage constant at 120 volts. Therefore, by Ohm's law the current flow is inversely proportional to the impedance. A typical power cord consists of two conductors. One designated as "hot" carries the current to the impedance; the other is neutral, and it returns the current to the source. The potential difference between the two is effectively 120 volts (Fig. 8-3). The amount of current flowing through a given device is frequently referred to as the "load." The load of the circuit is dependent on the impedance. A very high impedance circuit allows only a small current to flow and thus has a small load. A very low impedance circuit will draw a large current and is said to be a large load. A "short circuit" occurs when there is a zero impedance load with a very high current flow.[10]

Source of Shocks

To practice electrical safety it is important for the anesthesiologist to understand the basic principles of electricity and be aware of how electrical accidents can occur. Electrical accidents or shocks occur when a person becomes part of or completes an electrical circuit. To receive a shock, one must contact the

---

* The 120 volts of EMF and 1 ampere of current are the effective voltage and amperage in an AC circuit. This is also referred to as "RMS" (root-mean-square). It takes 1.414 amperes of peak amperage in the sinusoidal curve to give an effective amperage of 1 ampere. Similarly, it takes 170 volts (120 × 1.414) at the peak of the AC curve to get an effective voltage of 120 volts.[8]

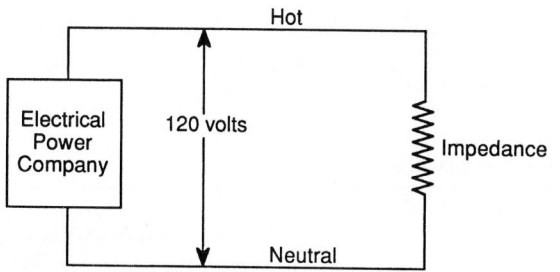

Figure 8-3. A typical AC circuit where there is a potential difference of 120 volts between the hot and neutral sides of the circuit. The current flows through a resistance, which in AC circuits is more accurately referred to as impedance, and then returns to the electrical power company.

electrical circuit at two points, and there must be a voltage source that causes the current to flow through an individual (Fig. 8-4).

When an individual contacts a source of electricity, damage occurs in one of two ways. First, the electrical current can disrupt the normal electrical function of cells. Depending on its magnitude, the current can contract muscles, alter brain function, paralyze respiration, or disrupt normal heart function, leading to ventricular fibrillation. The second mechanism involves the dissipation of electrical energy throughout the body's tissues. An electrical current passing through any resistance raises the temperature of that substance. If enough thermal energy is released, the temperature will rise sufficiently to produce a burn. Accidents involving household currents usually do not result in severe burns. However, in accidents involving very high voltages (*i.e.,* power transmission lines), severe burns are common.

The severity of an electrical shock is determined by the amount of current (number of amperes) and the duration of the current flow. For the purposes of this discussion, electrical shocks are divided into two categories. *Macroshock* refers to large amounts of current flowing through a person, which can cause harm or death. *Microshock* refers to very small amounts of current and applies only to the electrically susceptible patient. This is an individual who has an external conduit that is in direct contact with the heart. This can be a pacing wire or a saline-filled catheter such as a central venous or pulmonary artery

catheter. In the case of the electrically susceptible patient, even minute amounts of current (microshock) may cause ventricular fibrillation.

Table 8-1 shows the effects typically produced by various currents following a 1-second contact with a 60-Hz current. When an individual contacts a 120-volt household current, the severity of the shock will depend on his or her skin resistance, the duration of the contact, and the current density. Skin resistance can vary from a few thousand to 1 million ohms. If a person with a skin resistance of 1000 ohms contacts a 120-volt circuit, he or she would receive 120 milliamperes (mA) of current, which would probably be lethal. However, if that same person's skin resistance is 100,000 ohms, the current flow would be 1.2 mA, which would barely be perceptible.

$$I = E/R = (120 \text{ volts}) / (1000 \text{ ohms}) = 120 \text{ mA}$$

$$I = E/R = (120 \text{ volts}) / (100,000 \text{ ohms}) = 1.2 \text{ mA}$$

The longer an individual is in contact with the electrical source, the more dire the consequences because more energy will be released and more tissue damaged. Also, there will be a greater chance of ventricular fibrillation from excitation of the heart during the vulnerable period of the electrocardiogram (ECG) cycle.

Current density is a way of expressing the amount of current that is applied per unit area of tissue. The diffusion of current in the body tends to be in all directions. The greater the current or the smaller the area to which it is applied, the higher the current density. In relation to the heart, a current of 100 mA (100,000 μA) is generally required to produce ventricular fibrillation when applied to the surface of the body. However, only 100 μA (0.1 mA) is required to produce ventricular fibrillation when that minute current is applied directly to the myocardium through an instrument having a very small contact area, such as a pacing wire electrode. In this case, the current density is 1000-fold greater when applied directly to the heart; therefore, only 1/1000 of the energy is required to cause ventricular fibrillation. In this case, the electrically susceptible patient can be electrocuted with currents well below 1 mA, which is the threshold of perception for humans. The frequency at which the current reverses is also an important factor in determining the amount of current an individual can safely contact. Utility companies in the United States produce electricity at a fre-

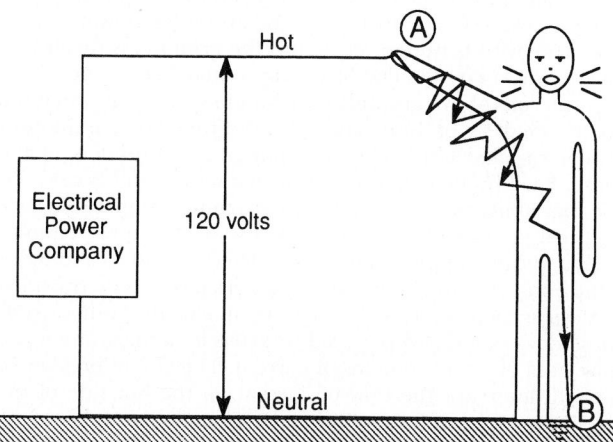

Figure 8-4. An individual can complete an electric circuit and receive a shock by coming in contact with the hot side of the circuit (point *A*). This is because he or she is standing on the ground (point *B*) and the contact point *A* and the ground point *B* provide the two contact points necessary for a completed circuit. The severity of the shock that the individual receives is dependent upon his or her skin resistance.

Table 8-1. EFFECTS OF 60-HZ CURRENT ON AN AVERAGE HUMAN FOR A 1-SECOND CONTACT

Current	Effect
MACROSHOCK	
1 mA (0.001 A)	Threshold of perception
5 mA (0.005 A)	Accepted as maximum harmless current intensity
10–20 mA (0.01–0.02 A)	"Let-go" current before sustained muscle contraction
50 mA (0.05 A)	Pain, possible fainting, mechanical injury; heart and respiratory functions continue
100–300 mA (0.1–0.3 A)	Ventricular fibrillation will start, but respiratory center remains intact
6000 mA (6 A)	Sustained myocardial contraction, followed by normal heart rhythm; temporary respiratory paralysis; burns if current density is high
MICROSHOCK	
100 μA (0.1 mA)	Ventricular fibrillation
10 μA (0.01 mA)	Recommended maximum 60 Hz leakage current

A = amperes; mA = milliamperes; μA = microamperes.

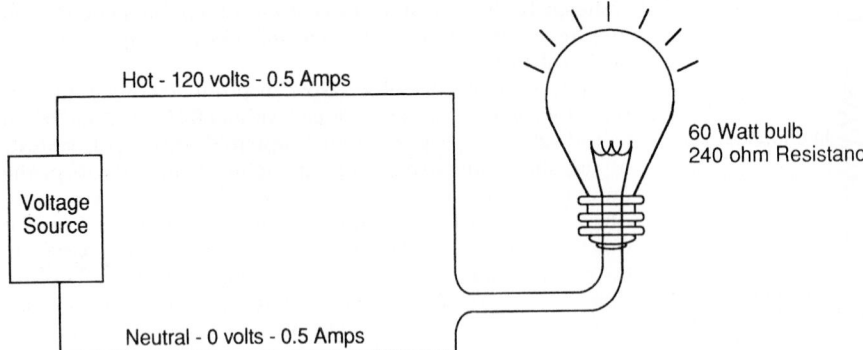

Hot - 120 volts - 0.5 Amps

Voltage Source

60 Watt bulb
240 ohm Resistance

Neutral - 0 volts - 0.5 Amps

Figure 8-5. A 60-watt light bulb has an internal resistance of 240 ohms and draws 0.5 ampere of current. The voltage drop in the circuit is from 120 in the hot wire to 0 in the neutral wire, but the current is 0.5 ampere in both the hot and neutral wires.

quency of 60 Hz. They use 60 Hz because higher frequencies cause greater power loss through transmission lines and lower frequencies cause a detectable flicker from light sources.[11] The "let-go" current is defined as that current above which sustained muscular contraction occurs and at which an individual would be unable to let go of an energized wire. The let-go current for a 60-Hz AC power is 10–20 mA,[10,12,13] whereas at a frequency of 1 million Hz, up to 3 amperes (3000 mA) is generally considered safe.[3] It should be noted that very high frequency currents do not excite contractile tissue; consequently, they do not cause cardiac arrhythmias.

It can be seen that Ohm's law governs the flow of electricity. For a completed circuit to exist, there must be a closed loop with a driving pressure to force a current through a resistance. Just as in the cardiovascular system there must be a blood pressure to drive the cardiac output through the peripheral resistance. Figure 8-5 illustrates that a hot wire carrying a 120-volt pressure through the resistance of a 60-watt light bulb produces a current flow of 0.5 ampere. The voltage in the neutral wire is approximately 0 volts, while the current in the neutral wire remains at 0.5 ampere. This correlates with our cardiovascular analogy, where a mean blood pressure decrease of 80 mm Hg between the aortic root and the right atrium forces a cardiac output of 6 L·min^{-1} through a systemic vascular resistance of 13.3 resistance units. However, the flow (in this case, the cardiac output, or in the case of the electrical model, the current) is still the same everywhere in the circuit. That is, the cardiac output on the arterial side is the same as the cardiac output on the venous side.

Grounding

To fully understand electrical shock hazards and their prevention, one must have a thorough knowledge of the concepts of grounding. These concepts of grounding probably constitute the most confusing aspects of electrical safety because the same term is used to describe several different principles. In electrical terminology, grounding is applied to two separate concepts. The first is the grounding of electrical *power,* and the second is the grounding of electrical *equipment.* Thus, the concepts that (1) power can be grounded or ungrounded and that (2) power can supply electrical devices that are themselves grounded or ungrounded are not mutually exclusive. It is vital to understand this point as the basis of electrical safety (Table 8-2). Whereas

Table 8-2. DIFFERENCES BETWEEN POWER AND EQUIPMENT GROUNDING IN THE HOME AND THE OPERATING ROOM

	Power	Equipment
Home	+	±
Operating room	−	+

+, grounded; −, ungrounded; ±, may or may not be grounded.

electrical *power* is grounded in the home, it is usually ungrounded in the operating room. In the home, electrical *equipment* may be grounded or ungrounded, but it should always be grounded in the operating room.

ELECTRICAL POWER: GROUNDED

Electrical utilities universally provide power that is grounded (by convention, the earth–ground potential is zero, and all voltages represent a difference between potentials). That is, one of the wires supplying the power to a home is intentionally connected to the earth. The utility companies do this as a safety measure to prevent electrical charges from building up in their wiring during electrical storms. This also prevents the very high voltages used in transmitting power by the utility from entering the home in the event of an equipment failure in their high-voltage system.[3]

The power enters the typical home via two wires. These two wires are attached to the main fuse or the circuit breaker box at the service entrance. The "hot" wire supplies power to the "hot" distribution strip. The neutral wire is connected to the neutral distribution strip and to a service entrance ground (*i.e.,* a pipe buried in the earth) (Fig. 8-6). From the fuse box, three wires leave to supply the electrical outlets in the house. In the United States, the "hot" wire is color-coded black and carries a voltage 120 volts above ground potential. The second wire is the neutral wire color-coded white; the third wire is the ground wire, which is either color-coded green or is uninsulated (bare wire). The ground and the neutral wires are attached at the same point in the circuit breaker box and then further connected to a cold-water pipe (Figs. 8-7 and 8-8). Thus, this grounded power system is also referred to as a neutral grounded power system. The black wire is not connected to the ground, as this would create a short circuit. The black wire is attached to the "hot" (*i.e.,* 120 volts above ground) distribution strip upon which the circuit breakers or fuses are located. From here, numerous branch circuits supply electrical power to the outlets in the house. Each branch circuit is protected by a circuit breaker or fuse that limits current to a specific maximum amperage. Most electrical circuits in the house are 15- or 20-ampere circuits. These typically supply power to the electrical outlets and lights in the house. Several higher amperage circuits are also provided for devices such as an electric stove or an electric clothes dryer. These devices are also powered by 240-volt circuits, which can draw from 30 to 50 amperes of current. The circuit breaker or fuse will interrupt the flow of current on the hot side of the line in the event of a short circuit or if the demand placed on that circuit is too high. For example, a 15-ampere branch circuit will be capable of supporting 1800 watts of power.

$$W = E \times I$$
$$W = 120 \text{ volts} \times 15 \text{ amperes}$$
$$W = 1800 \text{ watts}$$

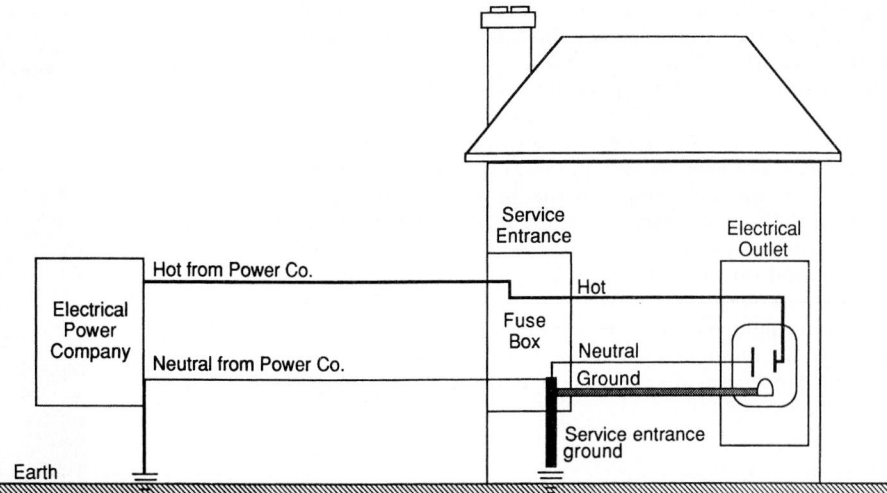

Figure 8-6. In a neutral grounded power system, the electric company supplies two lines to the typical home. The neutral is connected to ground by the power company and again connected to a service entrance ground when it enters the fuse box. Both the neutral and ground wires are connected together in the fuse box at the neutral bus bar, which is also attached to the service entrance ground.

Therefore, if two 1500-watt hair dryers were simultaneously plugged into one outlet, the load would be too great for a 15-ampere circuit, and the circuit breaker would open (trip) or the fuse would melt. This is done to prevent the supply wires in the circuit from melting and starting a fire. The amperage of the circuit breaker on the branch circuit is determined by the thickness of the wire that it supplies. If a 20-ampere breaker is used with wire rated for only 15 amperes, the wire could melt and start a fire before the circuit breaker would trip. It is important to note that a 15-ampere circuit breaker does not protect an individual from lethal shocks. The 15 amperes of current that would trip the circuit breaker far exceeds the 100–200 mA that will produce ventricular fibrillation.

The wires that leave the circuit breaker supply the electrical outlets and lighting for the rest of the house. In older homes the electrical cable consists of two wires, a hot and a neutral, which supply power to the electrical outlets (Fig. 8-9). In newer homes, a third wire has been added to the electrical cable (Fig. 8-10). This third wire is either green or uninsulated (bare) and serves as a ground wire for the power receptacle (Fig. 8-11). On one end, the ground wire is attached to the electrical outlet

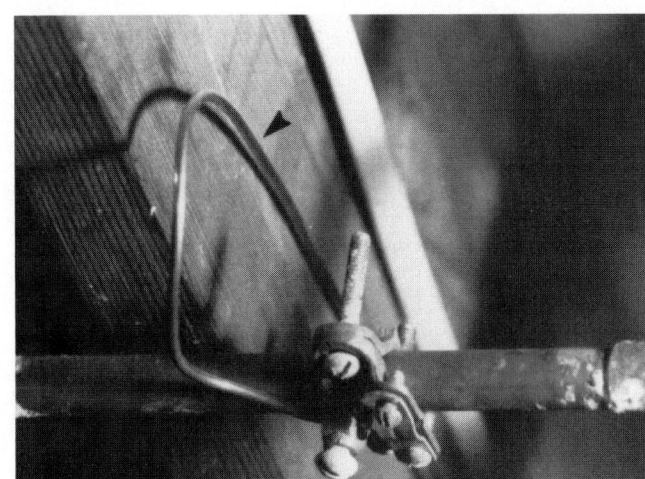

Figure 8-8. The arrowhead indicates the ground wire from the fuse box attached to a cold-water pipe.

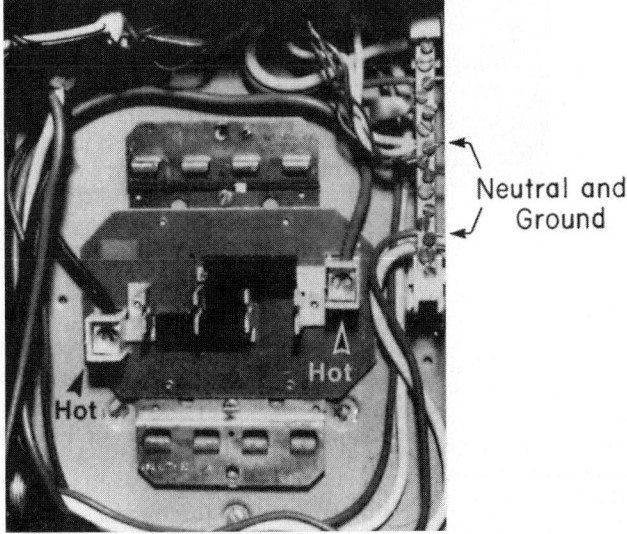

Figure 8-7. Inside a fuse box with the circuit breakers removed. The arrowheads indicate the hot wires energizing the strips where the circuit breakers are located. The arrows point to the neutral bus bar where the neutral and ground wires are connected.

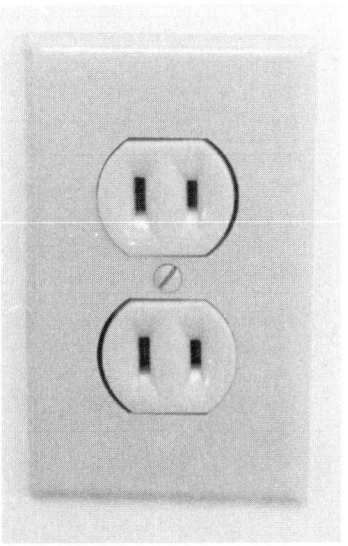

Figure 8-9. An older style electrical outlet consisting of just two wires (a hot and a neutral). There is no ground wire.

(Fig. 8-12); on the other, it is connected to the neutral distribution strip in the circuit breaker box along with the neutral (white) wires (Fig. 8-13).

It should be realized that in both the old and new situations, the power is grounded. That is, a 120-volt potential exists between the hot (black) and the neutral (white) wire and between the hot wire and ground. In this case, the ground is the earth (Fig. 8-14). In modern home construction, there is still a 120-volt potential difference between the hot (black) and the neutral (white) wire as well as a 120-volt difference between the equipment ground wire (which is the third wire), and between the hot wire and earth (Fig. 8-15).

A 60-watt light bulb can be used as an example to further illustrate this point. Normally, the hot and neutral wires are connected to the two wires of the light bulb socket, and throwing

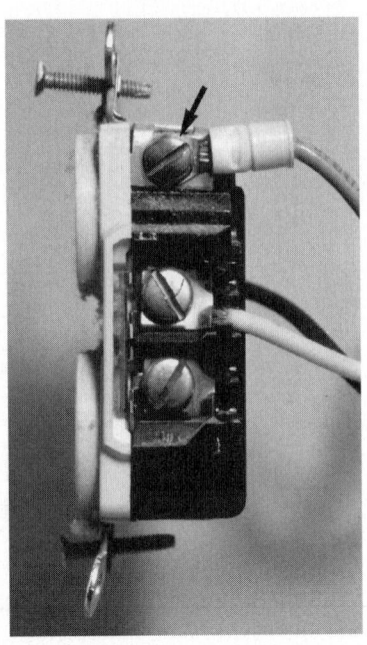

Figure 8-12. Detail of modern electrical power receptacle. The arrow points to the ground wire, which is attached to the grounding screw on the power receptacle.

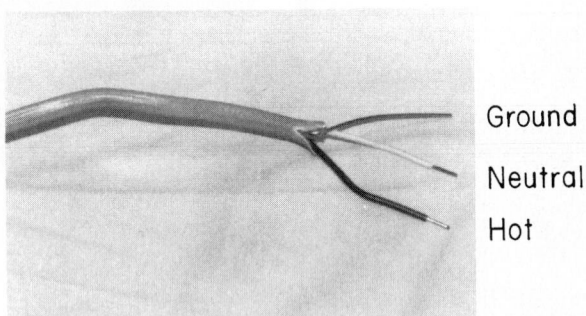

Figure 8-10. Modern electrical cable in which a third, or ground, wire has been added.

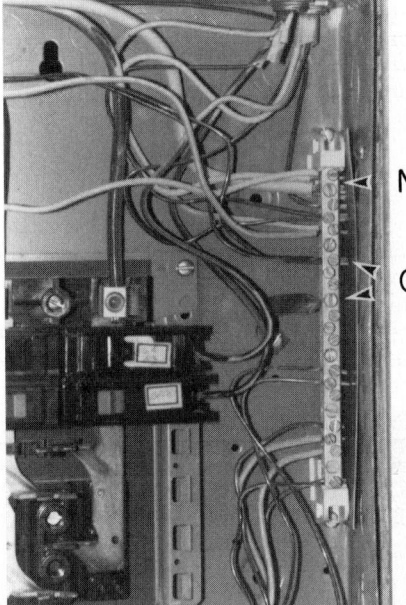

Figure 8-13. The ground wires from the power outlet are run to the neutral bus bar, where they are connected with the neutral wires (arrowheads).

Figure 8-11. Modern electrical outlet in which the ground wire is present. The arrowhead points to the part of the receptacle where the ground wire connects.

the switch will illuminate the bulb (Fig. 8-16). Similarly, if the hot wire is connected to one side of the bulb socket and the other wire from the light bulb is connected to the equipment ground wire, the bulb will still illuminate. If there is no equipment ground wire, the bulb will still light if the second wire is connected to any grounded metallic object such as a water pipe or a faucet. This illustrates the fact that the 120-volt potential difference exists not only between the hot and the neutral wires but also between the hot wire and any grounded object. Thus, in a grounded power system, the current will flow between the hot wire and any conductor with an earth ground.

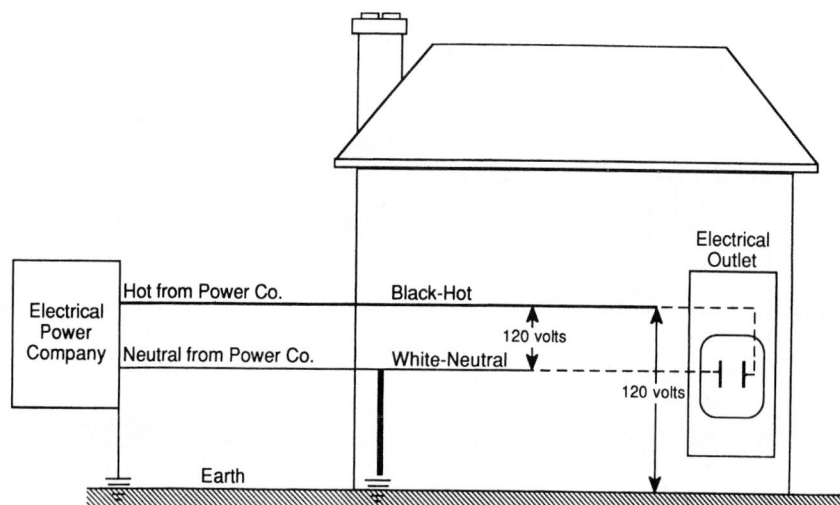

Figure 8-14. Diagram of a house with older style wiring that does not contain a ground wire. A 120-volt potential difference exists between the hot and the neutral wire as well as between the hot wire and earth.

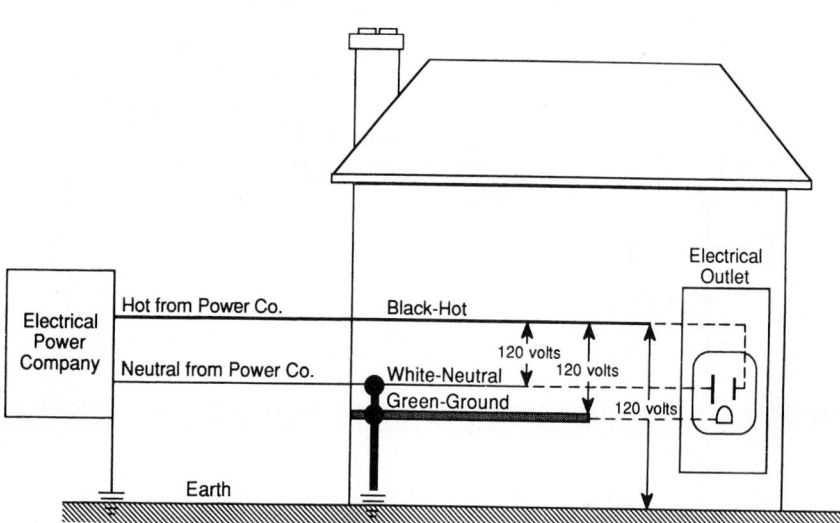

Figure 8-15. Diagram of a house with modern wiring in which the third, or ground, wire has been added. The 120-volt potential difference exists between the hot and neutral wires, the hot and the ground wires, and the hot wire and the earth.

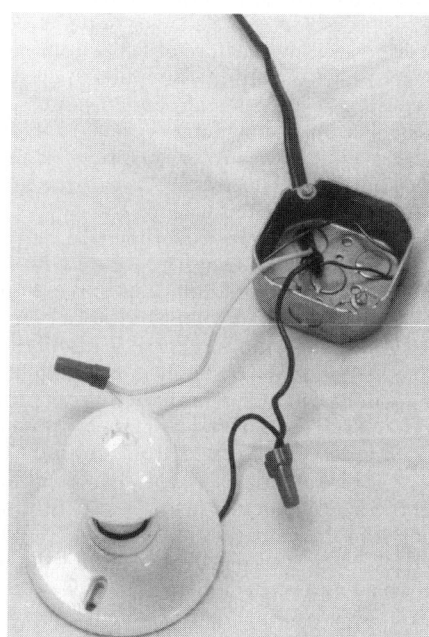

Figure 8-16. A simple light bulb circuit in which the hot and neutral wires are connected with the corresponding wires from the light bulb fixture.

As previously stated, current flow requires a closed loop with a source of voltage. For an individual to receive an electric shock, he or she must contact the loop at two points. Because we may be standing on ground or be in contact with an object that is referenced to ground, only one additional contact point is necessary to complete the circuit and thus receive an electrical shock. This is an unfortunate and inherently dangerous consequence of grounded power systems. Modern wiring systems have added the third wire, the equipment ground wire, as a safety measure to reduce the severity of a potential electrical shock. This is accomplished by providing an alternate, low-resistance pathway through which the current can flow to ground.

Over time the insulation covering wires may deteriorate. It is then possible for a bare, hot wire to contact the metal case or frame of an electrical device. The case would then become energized and constitute a shock hazard to someone coming in contact with it. Figure 8-17 illustrates a typical short circuit, where the individual has come in contact with the hot case of an instrument. This illustrates the type of wiring found in older homes. There is no ground wire in the electrical outlet, nor is the electrical apparatus equipped with a ground wire. Here, the individual completes the circuit and receives a severe shock. Figure 8-18 illustrates a similar example, except that now the equipment ground wire is part of the electrical distribution system. In this example, the equipment ground wire provides a pathway of low impedance through which the current can

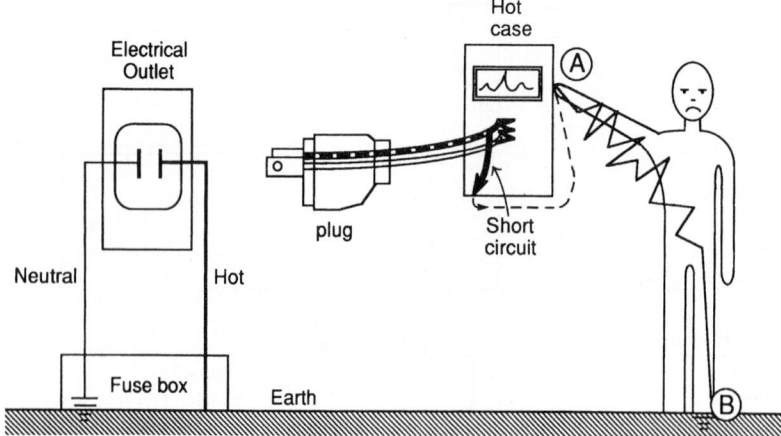

Figure 8-17. When a faulty piece of equipment without an equipment ground wire is plugged into an electrical outlet not containing a ground wire, the case of the instrument will become hot. An individual touching the hot case (point *A*) will receive a shock because he or she is standing on the earth (point *B*) and completes the circuit. The current (dashed line) will flow from the instrument through the individual touching the hot case.

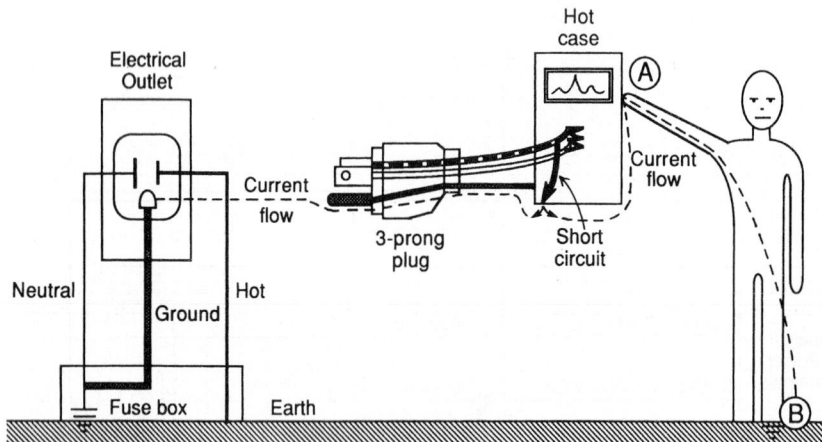

Figure 8-18. When a faulty piece of equipment containing an equipment ground wire is properly connected to an electrical outlet with a grounding connection, the current (*dashed line*) will preferentially flow down the low-resistance ground wire. An individual touching the case (point *A*) while standing on the ground (point *B*) will still complete the circuit; however, only a small part of the current will go through the individual.

travel; therefore, most of the current would travel through the ground wire. In this case, the person may get a shock, but it is unlikely to be fatal.

The electrical power supplied to homes is always grounded. A 120-volt potential always exists between the hot conductor and ground or earth. The third or equipment ground wire used in modern electrical wiring systems does not normally have current flowing through it. In the event of a short circuit, an electrical device with a three-prong plug (*i.e.,* a ground wire connected to its case) will conduct the majority of the short circuited or "fault" current through the ground wire and away from the individual. This provides a significant safety benefit to someone accidentally contacting the defective device. If a large enough fault current exists, the ground wire also will provide a means to complete the short circuit back to the circuit breaker or fuse, and this will either melt the fuse or trip the circuit breaker. Thus, in a grounded power system, it is possible to have either grounded or ungrounded equipment, depending upon when the wiring was installed and whether the electrical device is equipped with a three-prong plug containing a ground wire. Obviously, attempts to bypass the safety system of the equipment ground should be avoided. Devices such as a "cheater plug" (Fig. 8-19) should never be used because they defeat the safety feature of the equipment ground wire.

ELECTRICAL POWER: UNGROUNDED

Numerous electronic devices, together with power cords and puddles of saline solutions on the floor, make the operating

room an electrically hazardous environment for both patients and personnel. Bruner *et al*[14] found that 40% of electrical accidents in hospitals occurred in the operating room. The complexity of electrical equipment in the modern operating room demands that electrical safety be a factor of paramount importance. To provide an extra measure of safety from gross electrical shock (macroshock), the power supplied to most operating rooms is ungrounded. In this ungrounded power system, the current is isolated from ground potential. The 120-volt potential difference exists only between the two wires of the isolated power system, but no circuit exists between the ground and either of the isolated power lines.

Supplying ungrounded power to the operating room requires the use of an *isolation transformer* (Fig. 8-20). This device uses electromagnetic induction to induce a current in the ungrounded or secondary winding of the transformer from energy supplied to the primary winding. There is no direct electrical connection between the power supplied by the utility company on the primary side and the power induced by the transformer on the ungrounded or secondary side. Thus, the power supplied to the operating room is isolated from ground (Fig. 8-21). Because the 120-volt potential exists only between the two wires of the isolated circuit, neither wire is hot or neutral with reference to ground. In this case, they are simply referred to as line 1 and line 2 (Fig. 8-22). Using the example of the light bulb, if one connects the two wires of the bulb socket to the two wires of the isolated power system, the light will illuminate. However, if one connects one of the wires to one side of the isolated power and the other wire to ground, the light will not illuminate. If the wires of the isolated power system are connected, the

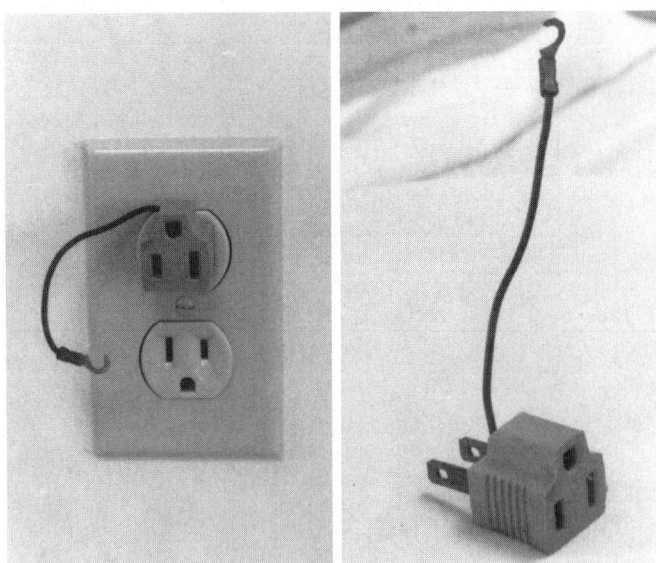

Figure 8-19. *Right:* A "cheater plug" that converts a three-prong power cord to a two-prong cord. *Left:* The wire attached to the cheater plug is rarely connected to the screw in the middle of the outlet. This totally defeats the purpose of the equipment ground wire.

short circuit will trip the circuit breaker. In comparing the two systems, the standard grounded power has a direct connection to ground, whereas the isolated system imposes a very high impedance to any current flow to ground. The added safety of this system can be seen in Figure 8-23. In this case, a person has come in contact with one side of the isolated power system (point *A*). Because standing on ground (point *B*) does not constitute a part of the isolated circuit, the individual does not complete the loop and will not receive a shock. This is because the ground is part of the primary circuit (*solid lines*), and the person is contacting only one side of the isolated secondary circuit (*cross-hatched lines*). The person does not complete either circuit (*i.e.,* have two contact points); therefore, this situation does not pose an electric shock hazard. Of course, if the person

contacts both lines of the isolated power system (an unlikely event), he or she would receive a shock.

If a faulty electrical appliance with an intact equipment ground wire is plugged into a standard household outlet, and the home wiring has a properly connected ground wire, then the amount of electrical current that will flow through the individual is considerably less than what will flow through the low-resistance ground wire. Here, an individual would be fairly well protected from a serious shock. However, if that ground wire were broken, the individual might receive a lethal shock. No shock would occur if the same faulty piece of equipment were plugged into the isolated power system, even if the equipment ground wire were broken. Thus, the isolated power system provides a significant amount of protection from macroshock.

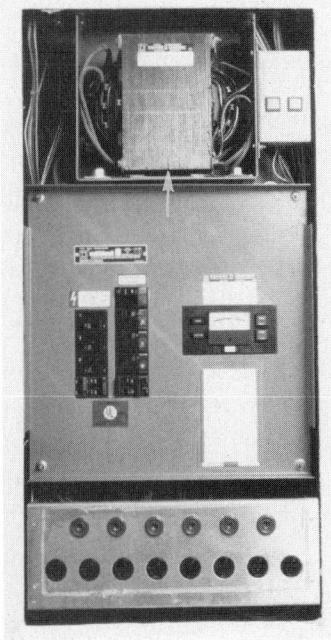
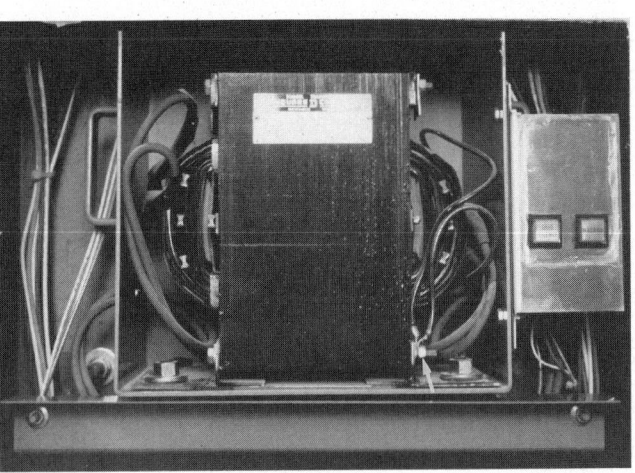

A   B

Figure 8-20. (*A*) Isolated power panel showing circuit breakers, LIM, and isolation transformer (arrow). (*B*) Detail of an isolation transformer with the attached warning lights. The arrow points to ground wire connection on the primary side of the transformer. Note that no similar connection exists on the secondary side of the transformer.

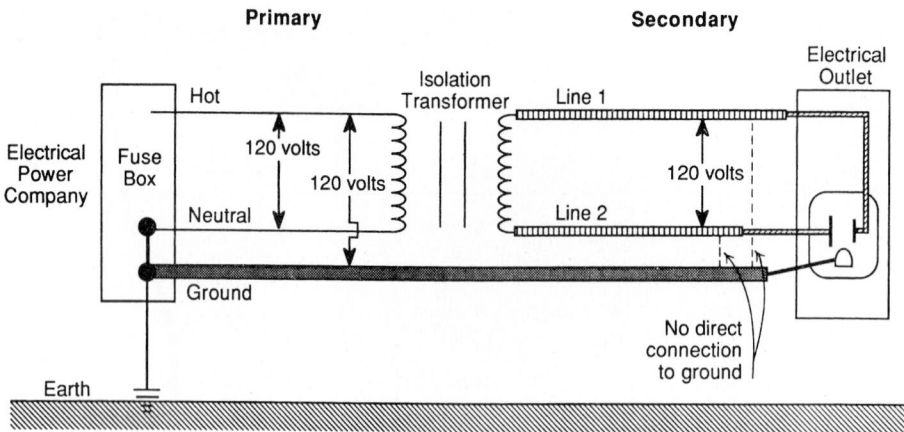

Figure 8-21. In the operating room, the isolation transformer converts the grounded power on the primary side to an ungrounded power system on the secondary side of the transformer. A 120-volt potential difference exists between line 1 and line 2. There is no direct connection from the power on the secondary side to ground. The equipment ground wire, however, is still present.

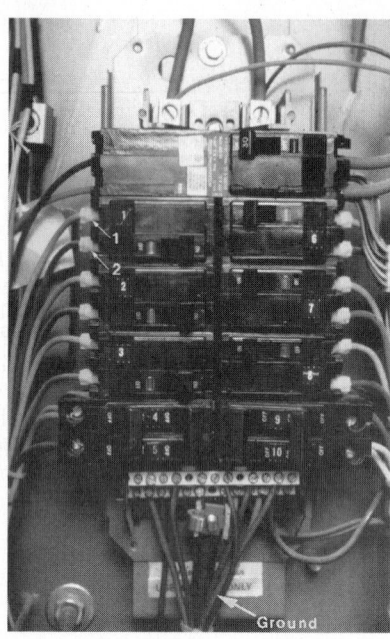

Figure 8-22. Detail of the inside of a circuit breaker box in an isolated power system. The bottom arrow points to ground wires meeting at the common ground terminal. Arrows 1 and 2 indicate lines 1 and 2 from the isolated power circuit breaker. Neither line 1 nor line 2 is connected to the same terminals as the ground wires. This is in marked contrast to Figure 8-13, where the neutral and ground wires are attached at the same point.

Another feature of the isolated power system is that the faulty piece of equipment, even though it may be partially short-circuited, will not usually trip the circuit breaker. This is an important feature because the faulty piece of equipment may be part of a life-support system for a patient. It is important to note that even though the power is isolated from ground, the case or frame of all electrical equipment is still connected to an equipment ground. The third wire (equipment ground wire) is necessary for a total electrical safety program.

Figure 8-24 illustrates a scenario involving a faulty piece of equipment connected to the isolated power system. This does not represent a hazard; it merely converts the isolated power back to a grounded power system as exists outside the operating room. In fact, a *second* fault is necessary to create a hazard.

The previous discussion assumes that the isolated power system is perfectly isolated from ground. Actually, perfect isolation is impossible to achieve. All AC-operated power systems and electrical devices manifest some degree of capacitance. As previously discussed, electrical power cords, wires, and electrical motors exhibit capacitive coupling to the ground wire and metal conduits, and "leak" small amounts of current to ground (Fig. 8-25). This so-called *leakage current* partially ungrounds the isolated power system. This does not usually amount to more than a few milliamperes in an operating room. So an individual coming in contact with one side of the isolated power system would receive only a very small shock (1–2 mA). Although this amount of current would be perceptible, it would not be dangerous.

THE LINE ISOLATION MONITOR

The line isolation monitor (LIM) is a device that continuously monitors the integrity of an isolated power system. If a faulty

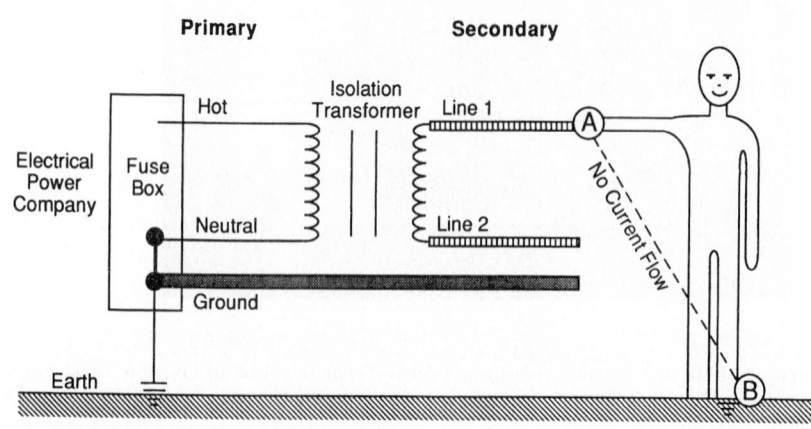

Figure 8-23. A safety feature of the isolated power system is illustrated. An individual contacting one side of the isolated power system (point *A*) and standing on the ground (point *B*) will not receive a shock. In this instance, the individual is not contacting the circuit at two points and thus is not completing the circuit. Point *A* (cross-hatched lines) is part of the isolated power system, and point *B* is part of the primary or grounded side of the circuit. (solid lines).

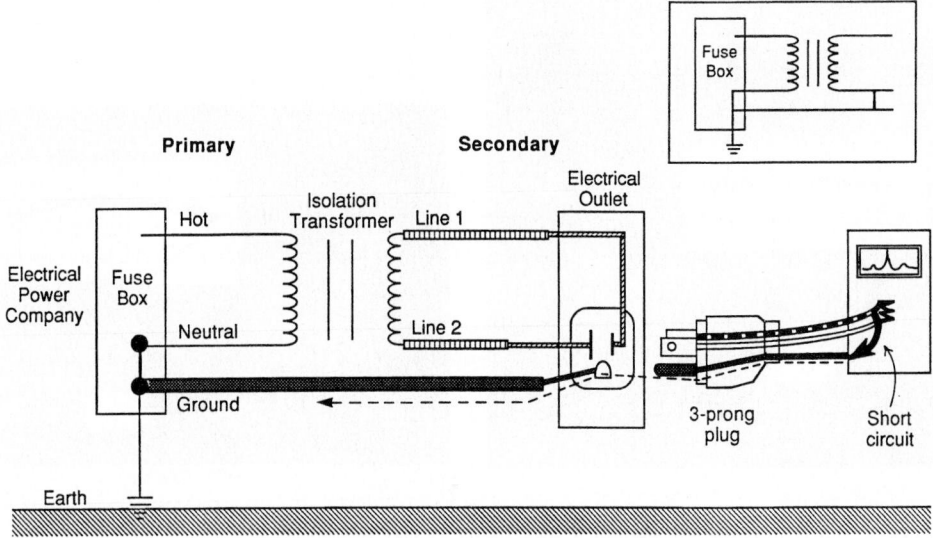

Figure 8-24. A faulty piece of equipment plugged into the isolated power system does not present a shock hazard. It merely converts the isolated power system into a grounded power system. The figure insert illustrates that the isolated power system is now identical to the grounded power system. The dashed line indicates current flow in the ground wire.

piece of equipment is connected to the isolated power system, this will, in effect, change the system back to a conventional grounded system. Also, the faulty piece of equipment will continue to function normally. Therefore, it is essential that a warning system be in place to alert the personnel that the power is no longer ungrounded. The LIM continuously monitors the isolated power to ensure that it is indeed isolated from ground, and the device has a meter that displays a continuous indication of the integrity of the system (Fig. 8-26). The LIM is actually measuring the impedance to ground of each side of the isolated power system. As previously discussed, with perfect isolation, impedance would be infinitely high and there would be no current flow in the event of a first fault situation ($Z = E/I$; if $I = 0$, then $Z = \infty$). Because all AC wiring and all AC-operated electrical devices have some capacitance, small leakage currents are present that partially degrade the isolation of the system. The meter of the LIM will indicate (in milliamperes) the total amount of leakage in the system resulting from capacitance, electrical wiring, and any devices plugged into the isolated power system.

The reading on the LIM meter does not mean that current is actually flowing; rather, it indicates how much current would

flow in the event of a first fault. The LIM is set to alarm at 2 or 5 mA, depending on the age and brand of the system. Once this preset limit is exceeded, visual and audible alarms are triggered to indicate that the isolation from ground has been degraded beyond a predetermined limit (Fig. 8-27). This does not necessarily mean that there is a hazardous situation, but rather that the system is no longer totally isolated from ground. It would require a second fault to create a dangerous situation.

For example, if the LIM were set to alarm at 2 mA, using Ohm's law, the impedance for either side of the isolated power system would be 60,000 ohms:

$$Z = E/I$$

$$Z = (120 \text{ volts}) / (0.002 \text{ amperes})$$

$$Z = 60,000 \text{ ohms}$$

Therefore, if either side of the isolated power system had less than 60,000 ohms impedance to ground, the LIM would trigger an alarm. This might occur in two situations. In the first, a faulty piece of equipment is plugged into the isolated power system. In this case, a true fault to ground exists from one line to ground. Now the system would be converted to the equivalent

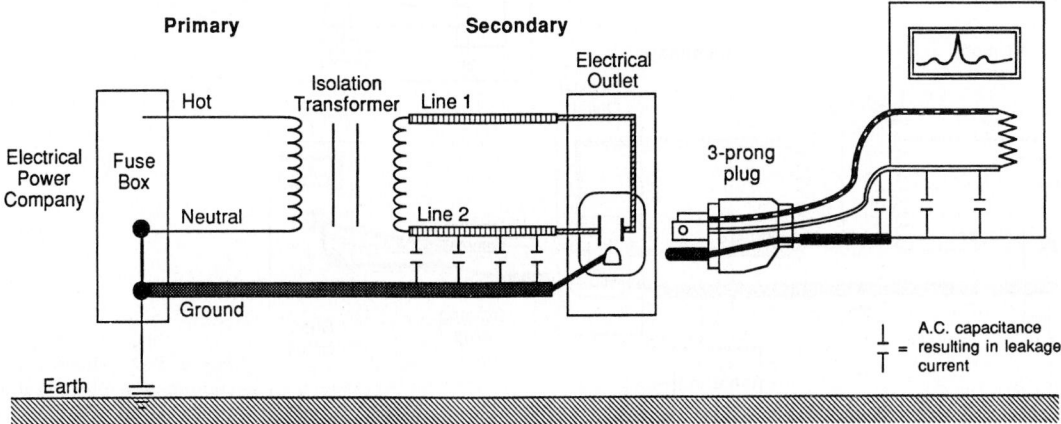

Figure 8-25. The capacitance that exists in AC power lines and AC-operated equipment results in small "leakage currents" that partially degrade the isolated power system.

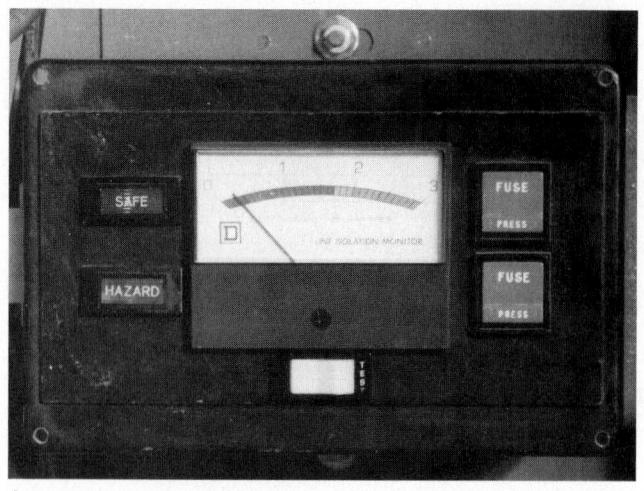
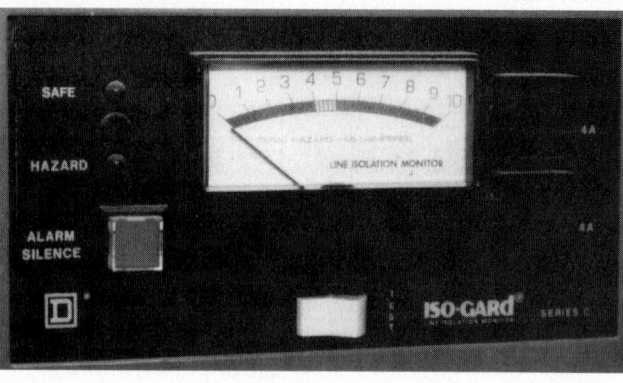

A   B

Figure 8-26. The meter of the line isolation monitor is calibrated in milliamperes. If the isolation of the power system is degraded such that >2 mA (5 mA in newer systems) of current could flow, the hazard light will illuminate and a warning buzzer will sound. Note the button for testing the hazard warning system. (*A*) Older line isolation monitor that will trigger an alarm at 2 mA. (*B*) Newer line isolation monitor that will trigger an alarm at 5 mA.

of a grounded power system. This faulty piece of equipment should be removed and serviced as soon as possible. However, this piece of equipment could still be used safely if it were essential for the care of the patient. It should be remembered, however, that continuing to use this faulty piece of equipment would create the potential for a serious electrical shock. This would occur if a second faulty piece of equipment were simultaneously connected to the isolated power system.

The second situation involves connecting many perfectly normal pieces of equipment to the isolated power system. Although each piece of equipment has only a small amount of leakage current, if the total leakage exceeds 2 mA, the LIM will trigger an alarm. Assume that in the same operating room there are 30 electrical devices, each having 100 μA of leakage current. The total leakage current (30 $\times$ 100 μA) would be 3 mA. The impedance to ground would still be 40,000 ohms (120/0.003). The LIM alarm would sound because the 2-mA set point was violated. However, the system is still safe and represents a state significantly different from that in the first situation. For this reason, the newer LIMs are set to alarm at 5 mA instead of 2 mA.

The newest LIMs are referred to as third-generation monitors. The first-generation monitor, or static LIM, was unable to detect balanced faults (*i.e.,* a situation in which there are equal faults to ground from both line 1 and line 2). The second-generation, or dynamic LIM, did not have this problem but could interfere with physiologic monitoring. Both of these monitors would trigger an alarm at 2 mA, which led to annoying "false" alarms. The third-generation LIM corrects the problems of its predecessors and has the alarm threshold set at 5 mA.[15] Proper functioning of the LIM is dependent on having both intact equipment ground wires as well as its own connection to ground. First- and second-generation LIMs could not detect the loss of the LIM ground connection. The third-generation LIM can detect this loss of ground to the monitor. In this case the LIM alarm would sound and the red hazard light would illuminate, but the LIM meter would read zero. This condition will alert the staff that the LIM needs to be repaired. However, the LIM still cannot detect broken equipment ground wires. An example of the third-generation LIM is the *Iso-Gard* made by the Square D Company (Monroe, NC).

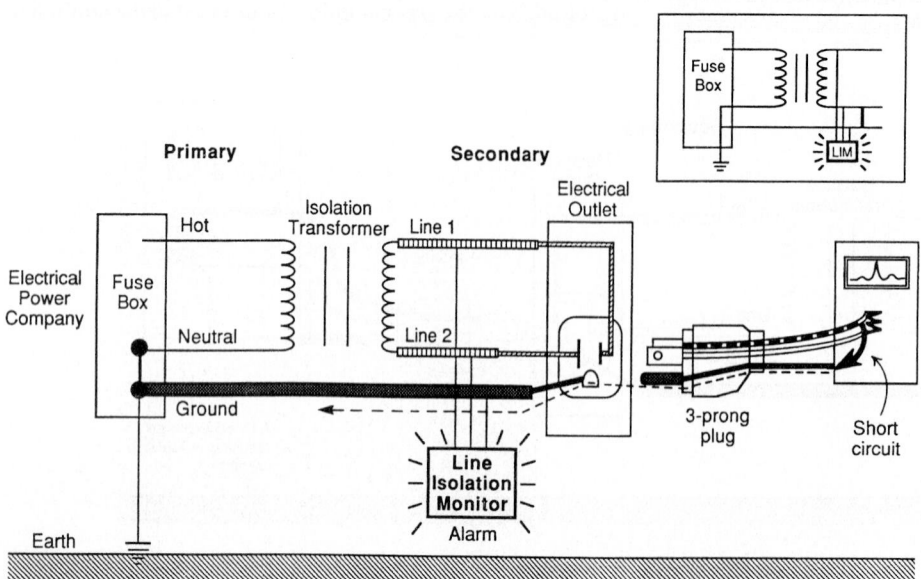

Figure 8-27. When a faulty piece of equipment is plugged into the isolated power system, it will markedly decrease the impedance from line 1 or line 2 to ground. This will be detected by the LIM, which will sound an alarm.

The equipment ground wire is again an important part of the safety system. If this wire is broken, a faulty piece of equipment that is plugged into an outlet would operate normally, but the LIM would not alarm. A second fault could therefore cause a shock, without any alarm from the LIM. Also, in the event of a second fault, the equipment ground wire provides a low-resistance path to ground for most of the fault current (Fig. 8-24). The LIM will only be able to register leakage currents from pieces of equipment that are connected to the isolated power system and have intact ground wires.

If the line isolation monitor alarm is triggered, the first thing to do is to check the gauge to determine if it is a true fault. The other possibility is that too many pieces of electrical equipment have been plugged in and the 2-mA limit has been exceeded. If the gauge is between 2 and 5 mA, it is probable that too much electrical equipment has been plugged in. If the gauge reads >5 mA, most likely there is a faulty piece of equipment present in the operating room. The next step is to identify the faulty equipment, which is done by unplugging each piece of equipment until the alarm ceases. If the faulty piece of equipment is not of a life-support nature, it should be removed from the operating room. If it is a vital piece of life-support equipment, it can be safely used. However, it must be remembered that the protection of the isolated power system and the line isolation monitor is no longer operative. Therefore, if possible, no other electrical equipment should be connected during the remainder of the case, or until the faulty piece of equipment can be safely removed.

GROUND FAULT CIRCUIT INTERRUPTER

The ground fault circuit interrupter (GFCI) is another popular device used to prevent individuals from receiving an electrical shock in a grounded power system. Electrical codes for most new construction require that a GFCI circuit be present in potentially hazardous (*e.g.*, wet) areas such as bathrooms, kitchens, or outdoor electrical outlets. The GFCI may be installed as an individual power outlet (Fig. 8-28) or may be a special circuit breaker to which all the individual protected outlets are connected at a single point. The special GFCI circuit breaker is located in the main fuse/circuit breaker box and can be distinguished by its red test button (Fig. 8-29). As Figure 8-5 demonstrates, the current flowing in both the hot and neutral wires is usually equal. The GFCI monitors both sides of the circuit for the equality of current flow; if a difference is detected, the power is immediately interrupted. If an individual should contact a faulty piece of equipment such that current flowed through the individual, an imbalance between the two sides of the circuit would be created, which would be detected by the GFCI. Because the GFCI can detect very small current differences (in the range of 5 mA), the GFCI will open the circuit in a few milliseconds, thereby interrupting the current flow before a significant shock occurs. Thus, the GFCI provides a high level of protection at a very modest cost.

The disadvantage of using a GFCI in the operating room is that it interrupts the power without warning. A defective piece of equipment could no longer be used, which might be a problem if it were of a life-support nature, whereas if the same faulty piece of equipment were plugged into an isolated power system, the LIM would alarm, but the equipment could still be used.

MICROSHOCK

As previously discussed, macroshock involves relatively large amounts of current applied to the surface of the body. The current is conducted through all the tissues in proportion to their conductivity and area in a plane perpendicular to the current. Consequently, the "density" of the current (amperes per meter squared) that reaches the heart is considerably less

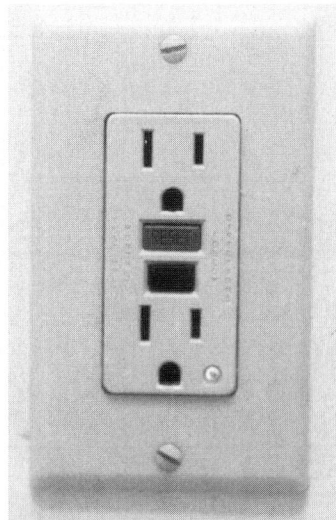

Figure 8-28. A ground fault circuit interrupter (GFCI) electrical outlet with integrated test and reset buttons.

than what is applied to the body surface. However, an electrically susceptible patient (*i.e.*, one who has a direct, external connection to the heart) may be at risk from very small currents; this is called *microshock*.[16] The catheter orifice or electrical wire with a very small surface area in contact with the heart produces a relatively large current density at the heart.[17] Stated another way, even very small amounts of current applied directly to the myocardium will cause ventricular fibrillation. Microshock is a particularly difficult problem because of the insidious nature of the hazard.

In the electrically susceptible patient ventricular fibrillation can be produced by a current that is below the threshold of human perception. The exact amount of current necessary to cause ventricular fibrillation in this type of patient is unknown. Whalen *et al*[18] were able to produce fibrillation with 20 μA of current applied directly to the myocardium of dogs. Raftery *et al*[19] produced fibrillation with 80 μA of current in some patients. Hull[20] used data obtained by Watson *et al*[21] to show that 50% of patients would fibrillate at currents of 200 μA. Because 1000 μA (1 mA) is generally regarded as the threshold of human perception with 60-Hz AC, the electrically susceptible patient can be electrocuted with one tenth the normally perceptible currents. This is not only of academic interest but also of practical concern because many cases of ventricular fibrillation from microshock have been reported.[22–27]

The stray capacitance that is part of any AC-powered electrical

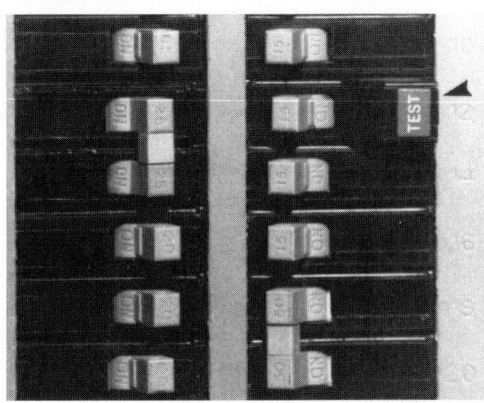

Figure 8-29. Special GFCI circuit breaker. The arrowhead points to the distinguishing red test button.

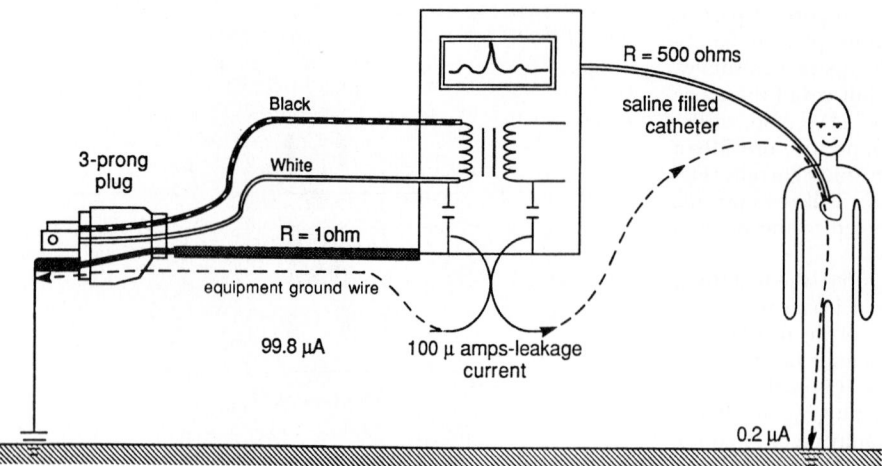

Figure 8-30. The electrically susceptible patient is protected from microshock by the presence of an intact equipment ground wire. The equipment ground wire provides a low-impedance path in which the majority of the leakage current (dashed lines) can flow.

instrument may result in significant amounts of charge buildup on the case of the instrument. If an individual simultaneously touches the case of an instrument where this has occurred and the electrically susceptible patient, he or she may unknowingly cause a discharge to the patient that results in ventricular fibrillation. Once again, the equipment ground wire constitutes the major source of protection against microshock for the electrically susceptible patient. In this case, the equipment ground wire provides a low-resistance path by which most of the leakage current is dissipated instead of stored as a charge.

Figure 8-30 illustrates a situation involving a patient with a saline-filled catheter in the heart with a resistance of ~500 ohms. The ground wire with a resistance of 1 ohm is connected to the instrument case. A leakage current of 100 μA will divide according to the relative resistances of the two paths. In this case, 99.8 μA will flow through the equipment ground wire, and only 0.2 μA will flow through the fluid-filled catheter. This extremely small current does not endanger the patient. If, however, the equipment ground wire were broken, the electrically susceptible patient would be at great risk because all 100 μA of leakage current could flow through the catheter and cause ventricular fibrillation (Fig. 8-31).

Modern patient monitors incorporate another mechanism to reduce the risk of microshock for electrically susceptible patients. This mechanism involves electrically isolating all direct patient connections from the power supply of the monitor by placing a very high impedance between the patient and any device. This limits the amount of internal leakage through the patient connection to a very small value. Currently the standard

is <10 μA. For instance, the output of an ECG monitor's power supply is electrically isolated from the patient by placing a very high impedance between the monitor and the patient's ECG leads.[6,28] Isolation techniques are designed to inhibit hazardous electrical pathways between the patient and the monitor while allowing the passage of the physiologic signal.

An intact equipment ground wire is probably the most important factor in preventing microshock. There are, however, other things that the anesthesiologist can do to reduce the incidence of microshock. One should never simultaneously touch an electrical device and a saline-filled central catheter or external pacing wires. Whenever one is handling a central catheter or pacing wires, it is best to insulate oneself by wearing rubber gloves. Also, one should never let any external current source, such as a nerve stimulator, come into contact with the catheter or wires. Finally, one should be alert to potential sources of energy that can be transmitted to the patient. Even stray radiofrequency current from the ESU can (with the right conditions) be a source of microshock.[29]

It must be remembered that the LIM is not designed to provide protection from microshock. The microampere currents involved in microshock are far below the LIM threshold of protection. In addition, the LIM does not register the leakage of individual monitors, but rather indicates the status of the total system. The LIM reading indicates the total amount of leakage current resulting from the entire capacitance of the system. This is the amount of current that would flow to ground in the event of a first-fault situation.

The essence of electrical safety is a thorough understanding

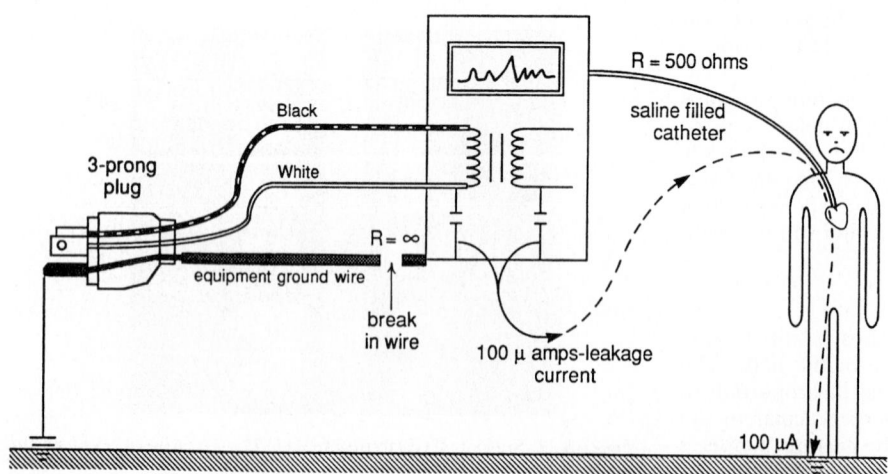

Figure 8-31. A broken equipment ground wire results in a significant hazard to the electrically susceptible patient. In this case, the entire leakage current can be conducted to the heart and may result in ventricular fibrillation.

of all the principles of grounding. According to Bruner, "Grounding is neither safe nor unsafe. Its significance is dependent on what is grounded and in what context."[9] The objective of electrical safety is to make it difficult for electrical current to pass through people. For this reason, both the patient and the anesthesiologist should be isolated from ground as much as possible. That is, their resistance to current flow should be as high as is technologically feasible. In the inherently unsafe electrical environment of an operating room, several measures can be taken to help protect against contacting hazardous current flows. First, the grounded power provided by the utility company can be converted to ungrounded power by means of an isolation transformer. The LIM will continuously monitor the status of this isolation from ground, and warn that the isolation of the power (from ground) has been lost in the event that a defective piece of equipment is plugged into one of the isolated circuit outlets. In addition, the shock that an individual could receive from a faulty piece of equipment is determined by the capacitance of the system and is limited to a few milliamperes. Second, all equipment plugged into the isolated power system has an equipment ground wire that is attached to the case of the instrument. This equipment ground wire provides an alternative low-resistance pathway enabling potentially dangerous currents to flow to ground. Thus, the patient and the anesthesiologist should be as insulated from ground as possible and all electrical equipment should be grounded.

The equipment ground wire serves three functions. First, it provides a low-resistance path for fault currents to reduce the risk of macroshock. Second, it dissipates leakage currents that are potentially harmful to the electrically susceptible patient. Third, it provides information to the LIM on the status of the ungrounded power system. If the equipment ground wire is broken, a significant factor in the prevention of electrical shock is lost. Additionally, the isolated power system will appear safer than it actually is, because the LIM is unable to detect broken equipment ground wires.

Because power cord plugs and receptacles are subjected to greater abuse in the hospital than in the home, the Underwriters Laboratories (Melville, NY) has issued a strict specification for special "hospital grade" plugs and receptacles (Fig. 8-32). The plugs and receptacles that conform to this specification are marked by a green dot.[30] The hospital-grade plug is one that can be visually inspected or easily disassembled to ensure the integrity of the ground wire connection. Molded opaque plugs are not acceptable. Edwards reported that of 3000 non–hospital-grade receptacles installed in a new hospital building, 1800 (60%) were defective after 3 years.[31] When 2000 of the non–hospital-grade receptacles were replaced with ones of hospital grade, no failures occurred after 18 months of use.

ELECTROSURGERY

On that fateful October day in 1926 when Dr. Harvey W. Cushing first used an electrosurgical machine invented by Professor William T. Bovie to resect a brain tumor, the course of modern surgery and anesthesia was forever altered.[32] The ubiquitous use of electrosurgery attests to the success of Professor Bovie's invention. However, this technology was not adopted without a cost. The widespread use of electrocautery has, at the very least, hastened the elimination of explosive anesthetic agents from the operating room. In addition, as every anesthesiologist is aware, few things in the operating room are immune to interference from the "Bovie." The high-frequency electrical energy generated by the electrosurgery unit (ESU) interferes with everything from the ECG signal to cardiac output computers, pulse oximeters, and even implanted cardiac pacemakers.[33]

The ESU operates by generating very high frequency currents (radiofrequency range) of anywhere from 500,000 to 1 million Hz. Heat is generated whenever a current passes through a resistance. The amount of heat (H) produced is proportional to the square of the current and inversely proportional to the area through which the current passes ($H = I^2/A$).[34] By concentrating the energy at the tip of the "Bovie pencil," the surgeon can produce either a cut or a coagulation at any given spot. This very high frequency current behaves differently from the

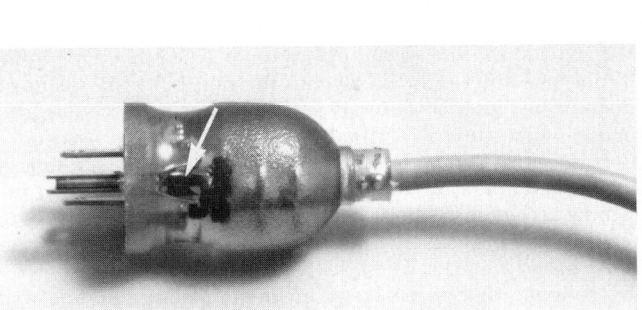
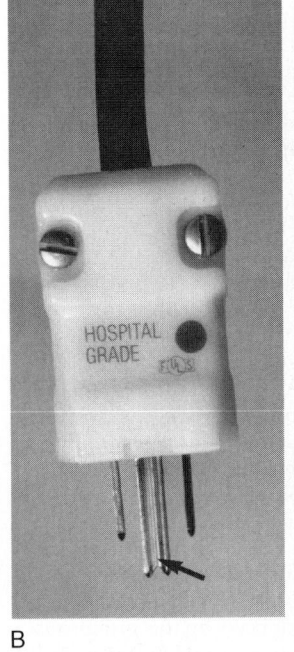
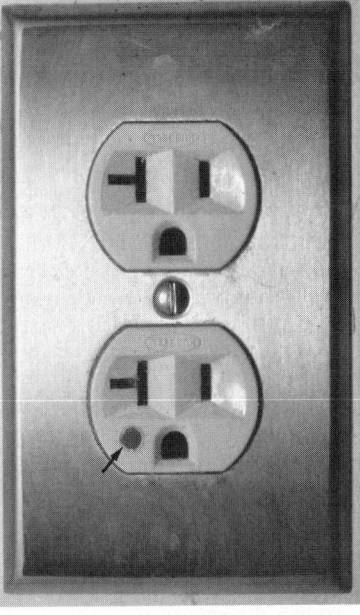

A   B   C

Figure 8-32. (*A*) A hospital-grade plug that can be visually inspected. The arrow points to the equipment ground wire whose integrity can be readily verified. (*B*) A hospital-grade plug that can be easily disassembled for inspection. Note that the prong for the ground wire (arrow) is longer than the hot or neutral prong, so that it is the first to enter the receptacle. (*C*) The arrow points to the green dot denoting a hospital-grade power outlet.

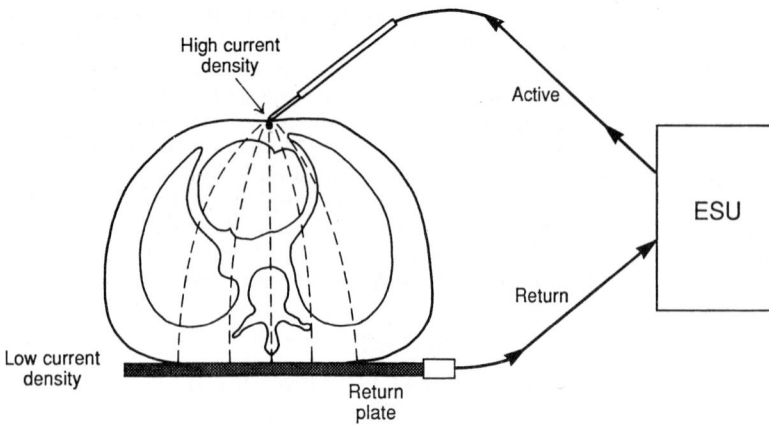

Figure 8-33. A properly applied ESU return plate. The current density at the return plate is low, resulting in no danger to the patient.

standard 60-Hz AC current and can pass directly across the precordium without causing ventricular fibrillation.[34] This is because high-frequency currents have a low tissue penetration and do not excite contractile cells.

The large amount of energy generated by the ESU can pose other problems to the operator and the patient. Dr. Cushing became aware of one such problem. He wrote, "Once the operator received a shock which passed through a metal retractor to his arm and out by a wire from his headlight, which was unpleasant to say the least."[35] The ESU cannot be safely operated unless the energy is properly routed from the ESU through the patient and back to the unit. Ideally, the current generated by the active electrode is concentrated at the ESU tip constituting a very small surface area. This energy has a high current density and is able to generate enough heat to produce a therapeutic cut or coagulation. The energy then passes through the patient to a dispersive electrode of large surface area that returns the energy safely to the ESU (Fig. 8-33).

One unfortunate quirk in terminology concerns the return (dispersive) plate of the ESU. This plate, often incorrectly referred to as a "ground plate," is actually a dispersive electrode of large surface area that safely returns the generated energy to the ESU via a low current density pathway. When inquiring whether the dispersive electrode has been attached to the patient, operating room personnel frequently ask, "Is the patient grounded?" Because the aim of electrical safety is to isolate the patient from ground, this expression is worse than erroneous; it can lead to confusion. Because the area of the return plate is large, the current density is low; therefore, no harmful heat is generated and no tissue destruction occurs. In a properly functioning system, the only tissue effect is at the site of the active electrode that is held by the surgeon.

Problems can arise if the electrosurgical return plate is improperly applied to the patient or if the cord connecting the return plate to the ESU is damaged or broken. In these instances, the high-frequency current generated by the ESU will seek an alternate return pathway. Anything attached to the patient, such as ECG leads or a temperature probe, can provide this alternate return pathway. The current density at the ECG pad will be considerably higher than normal because its surface area is much less than that of the ESU return plate. This may result in a serious burn at this alternate return site. Similarly, a burn may occur at the site of the ESU return plate if it is not properly applied to the patient or if it becomes partially dislodged during the operation (Fig. 8-34). That this is not merely a theoretical possibility is evidenced by the numerous case reports involving patients who have received ESU burns.[36-41]

The original ESUs were manufactured with the power supply connected directly to ground by the equipment ground wire. These devices made it extremely easy for ESU current to return by alternate pathways. The ESU would continue to operate normally even without the return plate connected to the patient. In most modern ESUs the power supply is isolated from ground to protect the patient from burns. It was hoped that by isolating the return pathway from ground, the only route for current flow would be via the return electrode. Theoretically, this would eliminate alternate return pathways and greatly reduce the incidence of burns.[5] However, Mitchell found two situations in which the current could return via alternate pathways, even with the isolated ESU circuit.[42] If the return plate were left either on top of an uninsulated ESU cabinet or in contact with the bottom of the operating room table, then the ESU could operate fairly normally and the current would return via alternate pathways. It will be recalled that the impedance is inversely proportional to the capacitance times the current frequency. The ESU operates at 500,000 to >1,000,000 Hz, which greatly enhances the effect of capacitive coupling and causes a marked reduction in impedance. Therefore, even with isolated ESUs, the decrease in impedance allows the current to return to the ESU by alternate pathways. In addition, the isolated ESU does not protect the patient from burns if the return electrode does not make proper contact with the patient. Although the isolated ESU does provide additional patient safety, it is by no means foolproof protection against the patient receiving a burn.

Preventing patient burns from the ESU is the responsibility of all professional staff in the operating room. Not only the circulating nurse, but also the surgeon and the anesthesiologist must be aware of proper techniques and be vigilant to potential problems. The most important factor is the proper application of the return plate. It is essential that the return plate have the appropriate amount of electrolyte gel and an intact return wire. Reusable return plates must be properly cleaned after each use, and disposable plates must be checked to ensure that the electrolyte has not dried out during storage. In addition, it is prudent to place the return plate as close as possible to the site of the operation. Electrocardiographic pads should be placed as far from the site of the operation as is feasible. Operating room personnel must be alert to the possibility that pools of flammable "prep" solutions such as ether and acetone can ignite when the ESU is used. If the ESU must be used on a patient with a demand pacemaker, the return electrode should be located below the thorax, and preparations for treating potential arrhythmias should be available, including a magnet to convert the pacemaker to a fixed rate, a defibrillator, and an external pacemaker. The ESU has also caused other problems in patients with pacemakers, including reprogramming and microshock.[43,44] If the surgeon requests higher than normal power settings on the ESU, this should alert both the circulating nurse and the anesthesiologist to a potential problem. The return plate and cable must be immediately inspected to ensure that it is functioning and properly positioned. If this does not correct the problem, the return plate should be replaced. If

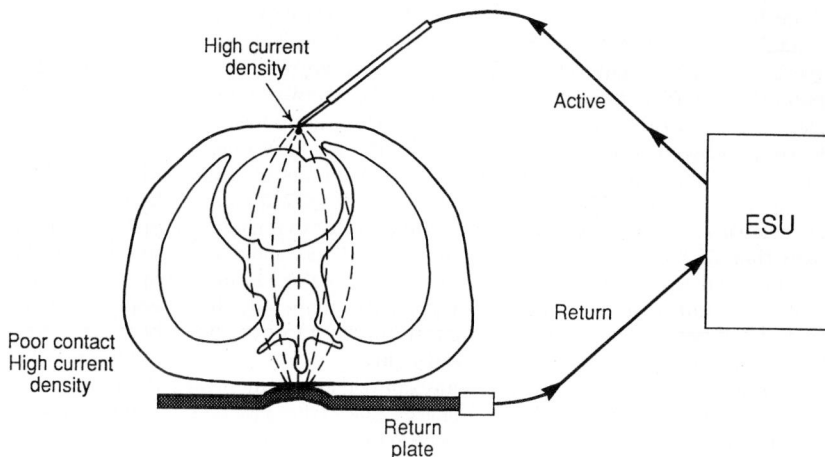

Figure 8-34. An improperly applied ESU return plate. Poor contact with the return plate results in a high current density and a possible burn to the patient.

the problem remains, the entire ESU should be taken out of service. Finally, an ESU that is dropped or damaged must be removed immediately from the operating room and thoroughly tested by a qualified biomedical engineer. Following these simple safety steps will prevent most patient burns from the ESU.

The previous discussion concerned only *unipolar* ESUs. There is a second type of ESU, in which the current passes only between the two blades of a pair of forceps. This type of device is referred to as a *bipolar* ESU. Because the active and return electrodes are the two blades of the forceps, it is not necessary to attach another dispersive electrode to the patient, unless a unipolar ESU is also being used. The bipolar ESU generates considerably less power than the unipolar and is mainly used for ophthalmic and neurologic surgery.[2]

In 1980 Mirowski *et al*[45] reported the first human implantation of a device to treat intractable ventricular tachyarrhythmias. This device, known as the automatic implantable cardioverter-defibrillator (AICD), is capable of sensing ventricular tachycardia (VT) and ventricular fibrillation (VF) and then automatically defibrillating the patient. Since 1980 thousands of patients have received AICD implants.[46,47] Because some of these patients may now present for noncardiac surgery, it is important that the anesthesiologist be aware of potential problems.[48] The use of a unipolar ESU may cause electrical interference that could be interpreted by the AICD as a ventricular tachyarrhythmia. This would trigger a defibrillation pulse to be delivered to the patient and would likely cause an actual episode of VT or VF. The patient with an AICD is also at risk for VF during electroconvulsive therapy.[48] In both cases, the AICD should be disabled by placing a magnet over the device. Although most AICDs can be disabled with a magnet, some require a special device or specific magnet to shut it off. Therefore, it is best to consult with someone experienced with the device before starting surgery. The device can be reactivated by reversing the process. Also, an external defibrillator and a noninvasive pacemaker must be in the operating room whenever a patient with an AICD is anesthetized.

Electrical safety in the operating room is a matter of combining common sense with some basic principles of electricity. Once operating room personnel understand the importance of safe electrical practice, they are able to develop a heightened awareness to potential problems. All electrical equipment must undergo routine maintenance, service, and inspection to ensure that it conforms to designated electrical safety standards. Records of these test results must be kept for future inspection because human error can easily compound electrical hazards. Starmer *et al*[49] cited one case concerning a newly constructed laboratory where the ground wire was not attached to a receptacle. In another study Albisser *et al*[50] found a 14% (198/1424) incidence of improperly or incorrectly wired outlets. Further-

more, potentially hazardous situations should be recognized and corrected before they become a problem. For instance, electrical power cords are frequently placed on the floor where they can be crushed by various carts or the anesthesia machine. These cords could be located overhead or placed in an area of low traffic flow. Multiple-plug extension boxes should not be left on the floor where they can come in contact with electrolyte solutions. These could easily be mounted on a cart or the anesthesia machine. Pieces of equipment that have been damaged or have obvious defects in the power cord must not be used until they have been properly repaired. If everyone is aware of what constitutes a potential hazard, dangerous situations can be prevented with minimal effort.

Sparks generated by the ESU may provide the ignition source for a fire with resulting burns to the patient and operating room personnel. This is a particular risk when the ESU is used in an oxygen-enriched environment as may be present in the patient's airway or in close proximity to the patient's face. Most plastics such as tracheal tubes and components of the anesthetic breathing system that would not burn in room air will ignite in the presence of oxygen and/or nitrous oxide. Tenting of the drapes to allow dispersion of any accumulated oxygen and/or its dilution by room air or use of a circle anesthesia breathing system with minimal to no leak of gases around the anesthesia mask will decrease the risk of ignition from a spark generated by a nearby ESU.

Conductive Flooring

Conductive flooring was mandated for operating rooms where flammable anesthetic agents were being administered. The conductive floor was specified to have a resistance of between 25,000 and 1 million ohms. This would minimize the buildup of static charges that could cause a flammable anesthetic agent to ignite. The standards have been changed to eliminate the necessity for conductive flooring in anesthetizing areas where flammable agents are no longer used.

ENVIRONMENTAL HAZARDS

There are a number of potential hazards in the operating room that are of concern to the anesthesiologist. There is the potential for electrical shock not only to the patient, but also to operating room personnel. In addition, cables and power cords to electrical equipment and monitoring devices can become hazardous. Finally, all operating room personnel should have a plan of what to do in the event of a power failure.

In today's operating room, there are literally dozens of pieces of electrical equipment. It is not uncommon to have numerous power cords lying on the floor, where they are vulnerable to damage. If the insulation on the power cable becomes damaged, it is fairly easy for the hot wire to come in contact with a piece of metal equipment. If the operating room did not have isolated power, that piece of equipment would become energized and a potential electrical shock hazard.[51] Having isolated power minimizes the risk to the patient and operating room personnel. Clearly, getting electrical power cords off the floor is desirable. This can be accomplished by having electrical outlets in the ceiling or by having ceiling-mounted articulated arms that contain electrical outlets. Also, the use of multi-outlet extension boxes that sit on the floor can be hazardous. These can be contaminated with fluids, which could easily trip the circuit breaker. In one case, it apparently tripped the main circuit breaker for the entire operating room, resulting in a loss of all electrical power except for the overhead lights.[52]

Modern monitoring devices have many safety features incorporated into them. Virtually all of them have isolated the patient input from the power supply of the device. This was an important feature that was lacking from the original ECG monitors. In the early days, patients could actually become part of the electrical circuit of the monitor. There have been relatively few problems with patients and monitoring devices since the advent of isolated inputs. However, between 1985 and 1994, the Food and Drug Administration (FDA) received approximately 24 reports where infants and children had received an electrical shock including five children who died by electrocution.[53,54] These electrical accidents occurred because the electrode lead wires from either an ECG monitor or an apnea monitor were plugged directly into a 120-volt electrical outlet instead of the appropriate patient cable. In 1997, the FDA issued a new performance standard for electrode lead wires and patient cables. The new standard requires that the exposed male connector pins from the electrode lead wires must be eliminated. Therefore, the lead wires must have female connections and the connector pins must be housed in a protected patient cable (Fig. 8-35). This effectively eliminates the possibility of the patient being connected directly to an alternating current source since there are no exposed connector pins on the lead wires.

All health care facilities are required to have a source of emergency power. This generally consists of one or more electrical generators. These generators are configured to start up automatically and provide power to the facility within a few seconds after detecting the loss of power from the utility company. The facility is required to test these generators on a regular basis. However, not all health care facilities test them under actual load. There are numerous anecdotal reports of generators not functioning properly during an actual power failure. If the generators are not tested under actual load, it is possible that many years will pass before a real power outage puts a severe demand on the generator. If the facility has several generators and one of them fails, the increased demand on the others may be enough to cause them to fail in rapid succession.

Other situations may also cause unexpected power outages. In our facility, a construction crew was remodeling an existing operating room. They accidentally caused a short circuit in the power supply when they were working on an electrical panel. This caused the ground fault circuit interrupter (GFCI) in the basement to trip, thus shutting off power to a whole section of the operating room. Consequently, several operating rooms were suddenly without power at crucial junctures in surgery. The operating room personnel were waiting for the emergency generators to come on. Obviously, this was not going to happen because there was no interruption of power from the electrical utility. It took approximately 20–30 minutes until the source of the problem could be identified and corrected.

It is vitally important that each operating room have a contingency plan for a power failure. In most cases, the emergency generator will take over, but that is not always going to happen. There should be a supply of battery-operated light sources available in each operating room. A laryngoscope can serve as a readily available source of light that allows one to find flashlights and other pieces of equipment. The operating room's overhead lights should also be connected to some sort of battery-operated lighting system. A supply of battery-operated monitoring devices and pneumatically powered ventilators and anesthesia machines would enable life-support functions to continue. The cost of these contingencies is relatively small but the benefits can be incomparably great in an emergency.

ELECTROMAGNETIC INTERFERENCE (EMI)

Rapid advances in technology have led to an explosion in the number of wireless communication devices in the marketplace. These devices include cellular telephones, cordless telephones, walkie-talkies, and even wireless Internet access devices. All of these devices have something in common: they emit electromagnetic interference (EMI). This most commonly manifests itself when traveling on airplanes. Most airlines require that these devices be turned off when the plane is taking off or landing or, in some cases, during the entire flight. There is concern that the EMI emitted by these devices may interfere with the plane's navigation and communication equipment.

In recent years, the number of people who own these devices has increased exponentially. Indeed, in some hospitals, they form a vital link in the regular or emergency communication system. It is not uncommon for physicians, nurses, paramedics, and other personnel to have their own cellular telephones. In addition, patients and visitors may also have cellular telephones and other types of communication devices. Hospital maintenance and security personnel frequently have walkie-talkie–type radios and some hospitals have even instituted an in-house cellular telephone network that augments or replaces the paging system. There has been concern that the EMI emitted by these devices may interfere with implanted pacemakers or various types of monitoring devices in critical care areas.

Several studies have been done to find out if cellular telephones cause problems with cardiac pacemakers. One study by Hayes et al looked at 980 patients with five different types of cellular telephones.[55] They conducted more than 5000 tests and found that in more than 20% of the cases they could detect some interference from the cellular telephone. Patients were symptomatic in 7.2% of the cases, and clinically significant interference occurred in 6.6% of the cases. When the telephone was held in the normal position over the ear, clinically significant interference was not detected. In fact, the interference that caused clinical symptoms occurred only if the telephone was directly over the pacemaker. Other studies have demonstrated changes such as erroneous sensing and pacer inhibition.[56,57] Again, these occurred only when the telephone was close to the pacemaker. The changes were temporary, and the pacemaker

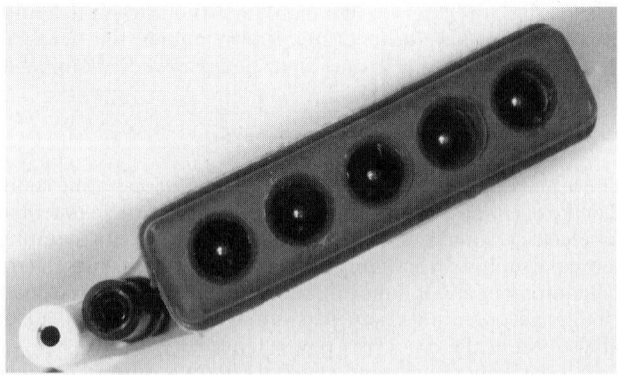

Figure 8-35. The current standard for patient lead wires (*left*) requires a female connector. The patient cable (*right*) has shielded connector pins that the lead wires plug into.

reverted to normal when the cellular telephone was moved to a safe distance. Currently, the FDA guidelines are that the cellular telephones be kept at least 6 inches from the pacemaker. Therefore, the cellular telephone should not be carried in the shirt pocket, which is adjacent to the pacemaker.

Automatic implantable cardioverter-defibrillators (AICDs) comprise another group of devices of concern to biomedical engineers. Fetter *et al* conducted a study of 41 patients who had AICDs.[58] They had a 0% incidence of oversensing and concluded that the cellular telephones did not interfere with the AICDs that they tested. They did, however, recommend keeping the cellular telephone at least 6 inches from the device.

Electromagnetic interference extends well beyond that of cellular telephones. Walkie-talkies, which are frequently used by hospital maintenance and security personnel, paging systems, police radios, and even televisions all emit EMI, which could potentially interfere with medical devices of any nature. Although there are many anecdotal reports, the scientific data on this problem are scanty. Reports of interference include ventilator and infusion pumps that have been shut down or reprogrammed, interference with ECG monitors, and even an electronic wheelchair that was accidentally started because of EMI. It is a difficult problem to study because there are many different types of devices that emit EMI and a vast array of medical equipment that has the potential to interact with these devices. Even though a device may seem "safe" in the medical environment, if two or three cellular telephones or walkie-talkies are brought together in the same area at the same time, there may be unanticipated problems or interference.

Any time a cellular telephone is turned on, it is actually communicating with the cellular network, even though a call is not in progress. Therefore, the potential to interfere with devices exists. The Emergency Care Research Institute (ECRI) reported in the October 1999 issue of *Health Devices* that walkie-talkies were far more likely to cause problems with medical devices than cellular telephones.[59] This is because they operate on a lower frequency than cellular telephones and have a higher power output. The ECRI recommends that cellular telephones be maintained at a distance of 1 meter from medical devices while walkie-talkies be kept at a distance of 6–8 meters.

Many hospitals have made restrictive policies on the use of cellular telephones, particularly in critical care areas.[60] These policies are supported by little scientific documentation and are nearly impossible to enforce. The ubiquitous presence of cellular telephones carried by hospital personnel and visitors makes enforcing a ban virtually impossible. Even when people try to comply with the ban, failure is nearly inevitable because the general public is usually unaware that a cellular telephone in the standby mode is still communicating with the tower and generating EMI.

The real solution is to "harden" devices against electromagnetic interference. This is difficult to do because of the many different frequencies on which these devices operate. Education of medical personnel is essential. When working in an operating room or critical care area, all personnel must be alert to the fact that electronic devices and pacemakers can be interfered with by EMI. Creating a restrictive policy would certainly irritate personnel and visitors, and in some cases, may actually compromise emergency communications.[61]

CONSTRUCTION OF NEW OPERATING ROOMS

A final area of electrical safety that concerns the anesthesiologist is the design of new operating room facilities or the remodeling of older ones. Frequently, an anesthesiologist is asked to consult with hospital administrators and architects in designing new or remodeling older operating rooms. In the past a strict electrical code was enforced because of the use of flammable anesthetic agents. This code included a requirement for isolated power

systems and LIMs. The National Fire Protection Association (NFPA) revised its standard for health care facilities in 1984 (NFPA 99-1984). These standards do not require isolated power systems or LIMs in areas designated for use of nonflammable anesthetic agents only.[62,63] Although not mandatory, NFPA standards are usually adopted by local authorities when revising their electrical codes.

This change in the standard creates a dilemma. The NFPA 99–Standard for Health Care Facilities,1990 Edition, mandates that "wet location patient care areas be provided with special protection against electrical shock." Section 3-4.1.2.6 further states that "this special protection shall be provided by a power distribution system that inherently limits the possible ground fault current due to a first fault to a low value, without interrupting the power supply; or by a power distribution system in which the power supply is interrupted if the ground fault current does, in fact, exceed a value of 6 milliamperes."

The decision of whether to install isolated power hinges on two factors. The first is whether or not the operating room is considered a wet location, and, if so, whether an interruptible power supply is tolerable. Where power interruption is tolerable, a GFCI is permitted as the protective means. However, the Standard also states that "the use of an isolated power system (IPS) shall be permitted as a protective means capable of limiting ground fault current without power interruption."

Most people who have worked in an operating room would attest to its being a wet location. The presence of blood, body fluids, and saline solutions spilled on the floor all contribute to making this a wet environment. The cytoscopy suite serves as a good example.

Once the premise that the operating room is a wet location is accepted, it must be determined whether a GFCI can provide the means of protection. The argument against using GFCIs in the operating room is illustrated by the following example. Assume that during an open heart procedure the cardiopulmonary bypass pump and the patient monitors are plugged into outlets on the same branch circuit. Also assume that during bypass, the circulating nurse now plugs in a faulty headlight. If there is a GFCI protecting the circuit, the fault will be detected and the GFCI will interrupt all power to the pump and the monitors. This undoubtedly would cause a great deal of confusion and consternation among the operating room personnel, and may place the patient at risk for injury. The pump would have to be manually operated while the problem was being resolved. In addition, the GFCI could not be reset (and power restored) until the headlight was identified as the cause of the fault and unplugged from the outlet. However, if the operating room were protected with an isolated power system and LIM, the same scenario would cause the LIM to alarm, but the pump and patient monitors would continue to operate normally. There would be no interruption of power, and the problem could be resolved without risk to the patient.

It should be realized that a GFCI is an active system. That is, a potentially hazardous current is already flowing and must be actively interrupted, whereas the isolated power system (with LIM) is designed to be safe during a first-fault situation. Thus, it is a passive system because no mechanical action is required to activate the protection.[64]

It is likely that hospital administrators may want to eliminate isolated power systems in new operating room construction as a cost-saving measure. Others,[64–66] however, have advocated the retention of isolated power systems. Not to do this would be a short-sighted, foolhardy measure. This is especially true because the cost of adding isolated power is estimated to be 1% of the cost of constructing an operating room.[64] Although not perfect,[67] the isolated power system and LIM do provide both the patient and operating room personnel with a significant amount of protection in an electrically hazardous environment. The value of the isolated power system is illustrated in a report by Day in 1994.[68] He reported four instances of electrical shock to operating room personnel in a 1-year period. The operating suite had been renovated and the isolated power system removed, and it was not until the operating room personnel received a shock that a problem was discovered.

Anesthesiologists need to be aware of this cost-saving attitude and strongly encourage that new operating rooms be constructed with isolated power systems. The relatively small cost savings that the alternative would represent do not justify the elimination of such a useful safety system, and the use of GFCIs is not practical in the operating room environment.

Electrical safety should be the concern of everyone in the operating room. Accidents can be prevented only if proper installation and maintenance of the appropriate safety equipment in the operating room have occurred and the operating room personnel understand the concepts of electrical safety and are vigilant in their efforts to detect new hazards.[69]

REFERENCES

1. Bruner JMR: Hazards of electrical apparatus. Anesthesiology 28:396, 1967
2. Hull CJ: Electrical hazards in monitoring. Int Anesthesiol Clin 19:177, 1981
3. Leonard PF, Gould AB: Dynamics of electrical hazards of particular concern to operating-room personnel. Surgical Clin North Am 45:817, 1965
4. Miller F: College Physics, 2nd ed, p 457. New York, Harcourt Brace and World, 1967
5. Uyttendaele K, Grobstein S, Svetz P: Monitoring instrumentation—isolated inputs, electrosurgery filtering, burns protection: What does it mean? Acta Anaesthesiol Belg 29:317, 1978
6. Leonard PF: Characteristics of electrical hazards. Anesth Analg 51:797, 1972
7. Taylor KW, Desmond J: Electrical hazards in the operating room, with special reference to electrosurgery. Can J Surg 13:362, 1970
8. Leonard PF: Apparatus and appliances: Current thinking. III. Alternating current, the isolation transformer, and the differential-transformer pressure transducer. Anesth Analg 45:814, 1966
9. Bruner JMR: Fundamental concepts of electrical safety. In Hershey SG (ed): ASA Refresher Courses in Anesthesiology, p 11. Philadelphia, JB Lippincott, 1974
10. Harpell TR: Electrical shock hazards in the hospital environment: Their causes and cures. Can Hosp 47:48, 1970
11. Buczko GB, McKay WPS: Electrical safety in the operating room. Can J Anaesth 34:315, 1987
12. Wald A: Electrical safety in medicine. In Skalak R, Chien S (eds): Handbook of Bioengineering, p 34.1. New York, McGraw-Hill, 1987
13. Dalziel CF, Massoglia FP: Let-go currents and voltages. AIEE Trans 75:49, 1956
14. Bruner JMR, Aronow S, Cavicchi RV: Electrical incidents in a large hospital: A 42 month register. JAAMI 6:222, 1972
15. Bernstein MS: Isolated power and line isolation monitors. Biomed Instrum Technol 24:221, 1990
16. Weinberg DI, Artley JL, Whalen RE, McIntosh HD: Electric shock hazards in cardiac catheterization. Circ Res 11:1004, 1962
17. Starmer CF, Whalen RE: Current density and electrically induced ventricular fibrillation. Med Instrum 7:158, 1973
18. Whalen RE, Starmer CF, McIntosh HD: Electrical hazards associated with cardiac pacemaking. Ann NY Acad Sci III:922, 1964
19. Raftery EB, Green HL, Yacoub MH: Disturbances of heart rhythm produced by 50-Hz leakage currents in human subjects. Cardiovasc Res 9:263, 1975
20. Hull CJ: Electrocution hazards in the operating theatre. Br J Anaesth 50:647, 1978
21. Watson AB, Wright JS, Loughman J: Electrical thresholds for ventricular fibrillation in man. Med J Aust 1:1179, 1973
22. Furman S, Schwedel JB, Robinson G, Hurwitt ES: Use of an intracardiac pacemaker in the control of heart block. Surgery 49:98, 1961
23. Noordijk JA, Oey FJI, Tebra W: Myocardial electrodes and the danger of ventricular fibrillation. Lancet 1:975, 1961
24. Pengelly LD, Klassen GA: Myocardial electrodes and the danger of ventricular fibrillation. Lancet 1:1234, 1961
25. Rowe GG, Zarnstorff WC: Ventricular fibrillation during selective angiocardiography. JAMA 192:947, 1965
26. Hopps JA, Roy OS: Electrical hazards in cardiac diagnosis and treatment. Med Electr Biol Eng 1:133, 1963
27. Mody SM, Richings M: Ventricular fibrillation resulting from electrocution during cardiac catheterization. Lancet 2:698, 1962
28. Leeming MN: Protection of the electrically susceptible patient: A discussion of systems and methods. Anesthesiology 38:370, 1973
29. McNulty SE, Cooper M, Staudt S: Transmitted radiofrequency current through a flow directed pulmonary artery catheter. Anesth Analg 78:587, 1994
30. Cromwell L, Weibell FJ, Pfeiffer EA: Biomedical Instrumentation and Measurements, 2nd ed, p 430. Englewood Cliffs, NJ: Prentice-Hall, 1980
31. Edwards NK: Specialized electrical grounding needs. Clin Perinatol 3:367, 1976
32. Goldwyn RM: Bovie: The man and the machine. Ann Plast Surg 2:135, 1979
33. Lichter I, Borrie J, Miller WM: Radio-frequency hazards with cardiac pacemakers. Br Med J 1:1513, 1965
34. Dornette WHL: An electrically safe surgical environment. Arch Surg 107:567, 1973
35. Cushing H: Electro-surgery as an aid to the removal of intracranial tumors: With a preliminary note on a new surgical-current generator by W.T. Bovie. Surg Gynecol Obstet 47:751, 1928
36. Meathe EA: Electrical safety for patients and anesthetists. In Saidman LJ, Smith NT (eds): Monitoring in Anesthesia, 2nd ed, p 497. Boston, Butterworth, 1984
37. Rolly G: Two cases of burns caused by misuse of coagulation unit and monitoring. Acta Anaesthesiol Belg 29:313, 1978
38. Parker EO: Electrosurgical burn at the site of an esophageal temperature probe. Anesthesiology 61:93, 1984
39. Schneider AJL, Apple HP, Braun RT: Electrosurgical burns at skin temperature probes. Anesthesiology 47:72, 1977
40. Bloch EC, Burton LW: Electrosurgical burn while using a battery-operated doppler monitor. Anesth Analg 58:339, 1979
41. Becker CM, Malhotra IV, Hedley-Whyte J: The distribution of radiofrequency current and burns. Anesthesiology 38:106, 1973
42. Mitchell JP: The isolated circuit diathermy. Ann R Coll Surg Engl 61:287, 1979
43. Titel JH, El Etr AA: Fibrillation resulting from pacemaker electrodes and electrocautery during surgery. Anesthesiology 29:845, 1968
44. Domino KB, Smith TC: Electrocautery-induced reprogramming of a pacemaker using a precordial magnet. Anesth Analg 62:609, 1983
45. Mirowski M, Reid PR, Mower MM et al: Termination of malignant ventricular arrhythmias with an implanted automatic defibrillator in human beings. N Engl J Med 303:322, 1980
46. Crozier IG, Ward DE: Automatic implantable defibrillators. Br J Hosp Med 40:136, 1988
47. Elefteriades JA, Biblo LA, Batsford WP et al: Evolving patterns in the surgical treatment of malignant ventricular tachyarrhythmias. Ann Thorac Surg 49:94, 1990
48. Carr CME, Whiteley SM: The automatic implantable cardioverter-defibrillator. Anaesthesia 46:737, 1991
49. Starmer CF, McIntosh HD, Whalen RE: Electrical hazards and cardiovascular function. N Engl J Med 284:181, 1971
50. Albisser AM, Parson ID, Pask BA: A survey of the grounding systems in several large hospitals. Med Instrum 7:297, 1973
51. McLaughlin AJ, Campkin NT: Electrical safety: A reminder (letter). Anaesthesia 53:608, 1998
52. Nixon MC, Ghurye M: Electrical failure in theatre—A consequence of complacency? Anaesthesia 52(1):88, 1997
53. Medical Devices; Establishment of a Performance Standard for Electrode Lead Wires and Patient Cables, Federal Register: May 9, 1997; 62:90, 25477-25498
54. Emergency Care Research Institute: FDA establishes performance standards for electrode lead wires. Health Devices 27:34, 1998
55. Hayes DL, Wang PJ, Reynolds DW et al: Interference with cardiac pacemakers by cellular telephones. N Engl J Med 336:1473, 1997
56. Schlegel RE, Grant FH, Raman S, Reynolds D: Electromagnetic compatibility study of the in-vitro interaction of wireless phones with cardiac pacemakers. Biomed Instrum Technol 32:645, 1998
57. Chen WH, Lau CP, Leung SK et al: Interference of cellular phones with implanted permanent pacemakers. Clin Cardiol 19:881, 1996
58. Fetter JG, Ivans V, Benditt DG, Collins J: Digital cellular telephone interaction with implantable cardioverter-defibrillators. J Am Coll Cardiol 21:623, 1998
59. Emergency Care Research Institute: Cell phones and walkie-talkies:

Is it time to relax your restrictive policies? Health Devices 28: 409, 1999

60. Adler D, Margulies L, Mahler Y, Israeli A: Measurements of electromagnetic fields radiated from communication equipment and of environmental electromagnetic noise: Impact on the use of communication equipment within the hospital. Biomed Instrum Technol 32(6):581, 1998

61. Schwartz JJ, Ehrenwerth J: Electrical safety: In Lake CL, Hines RH, Blitt C (eds): Clinical Monitoring: Practical Applications for Anesthesia and Critical Care, ch 5. Philadelphia: WB Saunders, 2000

62. Kermit E, Staewen WS: Isolated power systems: Historical perspective and update on regulations. Biomed Tech Today 1:86, 1986

63. National Fire Protection Association: National electric code (ANSI/NFPA 70-1984). Quincy, MA, National Fire Protection Association, 1984

64. Bruner JMR, Leonard PF: Electricity, Safety and the Patient, p 300. Chicago, Year Book Medical Publishers, 1989

65. Matjasko MJ, Ashman MN: All you need to know about electrical safety in the operating room. In Barash PG, Deutsch S, Tinker J (eds): ASA Refresher Courses in Anesthesiology, vol 18, p 251. Philadelphia, JB Lippincott, 1980

66. Lennon RL, Leonard PF: A hitherto unreported virtue of the isolated power system (letter). Anesth Analg 66:1049, 1987

67. Gilbert TB, Shaffer M, Matthews M: Electrical shock by dislodged spark gap in bipolar electrosurgical device. Anesth Analg 73:355, 1991

68. Day FJ: Electrical safety revisited: A new wrinkle. Anesthesiology 80:220, 1994

69. Litt L, Ehrenwerth J: Electrical safety in the operating room: Important old wine, disguised new bottles. Anesth Analg 78:417, 1994

Clinical Anesthesia (4/e), edited by
Paul G. Barash, Bruce F. Cullen, and
Robert K. Stoelting. Lippincott Williams &
Wilkins, Philadelphia, © 2001.

CHAPTER 9

ACID–BASE, FLUIDS, AND ELECTROLYTES

DONALD S. PROUGH AND MALI MATHRU

As a consequence of underlying diseases and of therapeutic manipulations, surgical patients may develop potentially harmful disorders of acid–base equilibrium, intravascular and extravascular volume, and serum electrolytes. Precise perioperative management of acid-base status, fluids, and electrolytes may limit surgical morbidity and mortality.

ACID–BASE INTERPRETATION AND TREATMENT

Treatment of acid–base disturbances may be required preoperatively or during the course of anesthesia to limit the complications of metabolic alkalosis, metabolic acidosis, respiratory alkalosis, or respiratory acidosis. Following is a review of the pathogenesis, major complications, physiologic compensatory mechanisms, and treatment of the four simple acid–base disorders.

Overview of Acid–Base Equilibrium

The conventional approach to describing acid–base equilibrium is the *Henderson-Hasselbach* equation:

$$p\text{H} = 6.1 + \log \frac{[\text{HCO}_3^-]}{0.03 \times \text{Paco}_2} \qquad (9\text{-}1)$$

where 6.1 is the pK_a of carbonic acid and 0.03 is the solubility coefficient in blood of carbon dioxide (CO_2). Conventional acid–base terminology defines acid–base disturbances as *metabolic* (those in which the bicarbonate concentration [HCO_3^-] is primarily increased or decreased) and *respiratory* (those in which Paco$_2$ is primarily increased or decreased).

The term used to define the acidity or alkalinity of solutions or blood, *p*H, is the negative logarithm of the hydrogen ion concentration ([H$^+$]). An alternative to the Henderson-Hasselbach equation is the simpler Henderson equation:

$$[\text{H}^+] = \frac{24 \times \text{Paco}_2}{[\text{HCO}_3^-]} \qquad (9\text{-}2)$$

This equation clearly expresses the relationship between the three major variables measured or calculated in blood gas samples. Conversion of *p*H to [H$^+$] can be accomplished by knowing that the [H$^+$] is 40 mmol · l^{-1} at a *p*H of 7.4; that an increase in *p*H of 0.10 *p*H units reduces [H$^+$] to 0.8 times the starting [H$^+$] concentration; that a decrease in *p*H of 0.10 *p*H units increases the [H$^+$] by a factor of 1.25; and that small changes (*i.e.*, <0.05 *p*H units) produce approximately a 1.0 mmol · l^{-1} increase in [H$^+$] for each 0.01 decrease in *p*H or a decrease in [H$^+$] of 1.0 mmol · l^{-1} per 0.01 increase in *p*H.

An alternative approach to acid-base interpretation, proposed by Stewart[1] and reviewed by Eicker,[2] distinguishes between the independent variables and dependent variables that define *p*H. From this perspective, the independent variables are Paco$_2$, the strong (*i.e.*, highly dissociated) ion difference (SID), and the concentration of proteins, which usually are not strong ions. The strong ions, important because they are present in large concentrations, include sodium (Na$^+$), potassium (K$^+$), chloride (Cl$^-$), and lactate. The SID, calculated as (Na$^+$ + K$^+$ − Cl$^-$), under normal circumstances is approximately 42 mEq · l^{-1}. By using a series of equations, the acid–base status can be accurately described using these concepts. However, this review does not utilize the Stewart approach because there is little evidence that the clinical interpretation or treatment of common acid–base disturbances is handicapped by the simpler constructs of the conventional Henderson-Hasselbach or Henderson equations.

Metabolic Alkalosis

Metabolic alkalosis, usually characterized by an alkalemic *p*H (>7.45) and hyperbicarbonatemia (>27.0 mEq · l^{-1}), occurs frequently in hospitalized patients. In critically ill patients, severe metabolic alkalosis is associated with increased mortality.[3] Factors that generate metabolic alkalosis include, among others, nasogastric suction and diuretic administration (Table 9-1).[4] The maintenance of metabolic alkalosis is dependent upon a continued stimulus, such as renal hypoperfusion, hypokalemia, or hypochloremia, for the reabsorption of [HCO_3^-] from the distal renal tubules. Potassium depletion generates metabolic alkalosis in part by increasing the exit of bicarbonate from proximal tubular cells into the circulation.[5] Chloride depletion, even in the absence of volume depletion, may impair bicarbonate secretion by decreasing delivery of chloride to the collecting duct and by inducing potassium depletion.[6]

Metabolic alkalosis exerts multiple physiologic effects. Metabolic alkalosis is associated with a decrease in serum potassium and in ionized calcium.[7] Hypokalemia and alkalemia may precipitate primary ventricular dysrhythmias and may potentiate the toxicity of digoxin. Metabolic alkalosis may also generate compensatory hypoventilation (hypercarbia), sometimes of considerable magnitude (Table 9-2).[8] To the extent that Paco$_2$ is increased, Pao$_2$ will be reciprocally decreased but is easily corrected by oxygen administration. Alkalemia also increases bronchial tone and, through a combination of increased bronchial tone and decreased ventilatory effort, may help to produce atelectasis. A leftward shift in the oxyhemoglobin dissociation curve may reduce the availability of oxygen to tissues, as may alkalemia-induced decreased cardiac output.

In the absence of arterial blood gases, serum electrolytes and a history of major risk factors, such as vomiting, nasogastric suction, or chronic diuretic use, can suggest metabolic alkalosis. Because the vast majority of CO_2 carried in the blood is carried as bicarbonate, the measurement of total CO_2 (usually abbreviated on electrolyte reports as CO_2) should be about 1.0 mEq · l^{-1} greater than [HCO_3^-] calculated on simultaneously obtained arterial blood gases. Therefore, a normal calculated [HCO_3^-] on an arterial blood gas sample should be about 24 mEq and a normal "CO_2" on the serum electrolytes should be approximately 25. If either measurement exceeds normal by >4.0 mEq · l^{-1}, either the patient has a primary metabolic alkalosis or

Table 9-1. GENERATION AND MAINTENANCE OF METABOLIC ALKALOSIS

Generation	Example	Maintenance
I. Loss of acid from extracellular space		
A. Loss of gastric fluid	Vomiting; nasogastric drainage	↓ effective arterial volume (EAV)
B. Loss of acid into urine; continued Na$^+$ deliver to the distal tubule in presence of hyperaldosteronism	1. Primary aldosteronism	1. K$^+$ depletion + aldosterone excess
	2. Diuretic administration	2. ↓ EAV + K$^+$ depletion
II. Excessive HCO$_3^-$ loads		
A. Absolute		
1. HCO$_3^-$	NaHCO$_3$ administration	↓ EAV
2. Metabolic conversion of salts of organic acid anions to HCO$_3^-$	Lactate, acetate, citrate administration	↓ EAV
B. Relative		
1. Alkaline loads in renal failure	Alkali administration to patients with renal failure	Renal failure
III. Post-hypercapnic state	Abrupt correction of chronic hypercapnia	↓ EAV

has conserved bicarbonate in response to chronic hypercarbia. Recognition of hyperbicarbonatemia on the preoperative serum electrolytes justifies arterial blood gas analysis and should alert the anesthesiologist to the possibility that the patient is hypovolemic or hypokalemic.

Confirmation of metabolic alkalosis should serve as a warning to avoid adding iatrogenic respiratory alkalosis to metabolic alkalosis, since that may produce cardiovascular depression, dysrhythmias, and the other complications of severe alkalemia. Table 9-3 is an example of the effects of hyperventilation added to chronic metabolic alkalosis secondary to diuretic administration. The expected effects on pH and [HCO$_3^-$] of acutely and chronically decreasing or increasing Paco$_2$ are illustrated in Table 9-4.

In general, treatment of metabolic alkalosis can be divided into etiologic and nonetiologic therapy. Etiologic therapy consists of measures such as expansion of intravascular volume to increase renal perfusion or the administration of potassium to reverse hypokalemia. For a patient with metabolic alkalosis, 0.9% saline might be preferable to lactated Ringer's solution for intraoperative fluid administration, because lactate provides additional substrate for generation of bicarbonate and administration of 0.9% saline tends to increase serum [Cl$^-$] and decrease serum [HCO$_3^-$].[9] Theoretically, hypoproteinemia can cause a mild metabolic alkalosis.[10–12] However, [HCO$_3^-$] elevations secondary to hypoproteinemia are unlikely to be clinically important. Nonetiologic therapy includes the administration of [H$^+$] (in the form of ammonium chloride, arginine hydrochloride, or 0.1 N hydrochloric acid), the administration of acetazo-

lamide (a carbonic anhydrase inhibitor that causes renal bicarbonate wasting), or acid dialysis.[13] Of these, in an acute situation associated with high risk secondary to metabolic alkalosis, 0.1 N hydrochloric acid most rapidly corrects metabolic alkalosis. However, dilute hydrochloric acid must be given into a central vein; peripheral infusion will cause severe tissue damage.

Metabolic Acidosis

Metabolic acidosis, usually characterized by an acidemic pH (<7.35) and hypobicarbonatemia (<21 mEq · l^{-1}), occurs as a consequence of the buffering by bicarbonate of endogenous or exogenous acid loads or as a consequence of abnormal external loss of bicarbonate. Extracellular volume contains 350 mmol of bicarbonate buffer. Glomerular filtration of plasma volume necessitates reabsorption of 4500 mmol of bicarbonate daily, of which 85% is reabsorbed in the proximal tubule, 10% in the thick ascending limb, and the remainder is titrated by proton secretion in the collecting duct.[14] Approximately 70 mmol of acid metabolites are produced, buffered, and excreted daily; these include about 25 mmol of sulfuric acid from amino acid metabolism, 40 mmol of organic acids, plus phosphoric and other acids.[14]

Table 9-2. RULES OF THUMB FOR RESPIRATORY COMPENSATION IN RESPONSE TO METABOLIC ALKALOSIS AND METABOLIC ACIDOSIS

Metabolic alkalosis
1. Paco$_2$ increases approximately 0.5 to 0.6 mm Hg for each 1.0 mEq · l^{-1} increase in [HCO$_3^-$]
2. The last two digits of the pH should equal the [HCO$_3^-$] + 15
Metabolic acidosis
1. Paco$_2$ = [HCO$_3^-$] × 1.5 + 8.
2. The last two digits of the pH equal [HCO$_3^-$] + 15.

Table 9-3. METABOLIC ALKALOSIS PLUS HYPERVENTILATION

	Normal	Chronic Diuretic Administration	Intraoperative Hyperventilation
BLOOD GASES			
PH	7.40	7.47	7.62
Paco$_2$ (mm Hg)	40	45	30
[HCO$_3^-$] (mEq · l^{-1})	24	32	29
ELECTROLYTES			
"CO$_2$" (mEg · l^{-1})	25	33	30

Note: Respiratory alkalosis, produced by an inappropriately high minute ventilation, has been added to the previously compensated metabolic alkalosis induced by chronic diuretic administration.

Table 9-4. RULES OF THUMB FOR [HCO$_3^-$] AND pH CHANGES IN RESPONSE TO ACUTE AND CHRONIC CHANGES IN Pa$_{CO_2}$

Decreased Pa$_{CO_2}$
1. pH increases 0.10 for every 10 mm Hg decrease in Pa$_{CO_2}$.
2. [HCO$_3^-$] decreases 2 mEq·l^{-1} for every 10 mm Hg decrease in Pa$_{CO_2}$.
3. pH will nearly normalize if hypocarbia is sustained.
4. [HCO$_3^-$] will decrease 5 to 6 mEq·l^{-1} for each chronic 10 mm Hg ↓ in Pa$_{CO_2}$*.

Increased Pa$_{CO_2}$
1. pH will decrease 0.05 for every acute Pa$_{CO_2}$ increase of 10 mm Hg.
2. [HCO$_3^-$] will increase 1.0 mEq·l^{-1} for every Pa$_{CO_2}$ increase of 10 mm Hg.
3. pH will return toward normal if hypercarbia is sustained.
4. [HCO$_3^-$] will increase 4 mEq·l^{-1} for each chronic 10 mm Hg ↑ Pa$_{CO_2}$.

* Note: Hospitalized patients rarely develop chronic compensation for hypocarbia because of stimuli that enhance distal tubular reabsorption of sodium.

Two types of metabolic acidosis may be distinguished, based upon whether the calculated anion gap is normal or increased (Table 9-5).[15] The anion gap (Na$^+$ − [Cl$^-$] + [HCO$_3^-$]) is normal (<13 mEq·l^{-1}) in situations, such as diarrhea, biliary drainage, and renal tubular acidosis, in which bicarbonate is lost externally. Metabolic acidosis associated with a high anion gap (>13 mEq·l^{-1}) is attributed to excess production of lactic acid or ketoacids, increased retention of waste products (such as sulfate and phosphate) that are inadequately excreted in uremic states, and ingestion of toxic quantities of substances such as aspirin, ethylene glycol, and methanol.

The term *anion gap* refers to the fact that we commonly measure more of the cationic than of the anionic components in the serum. The commonly measured cation concentration [Na$^+$] usually exceeds by approximately 9.0 to 13.0 mEq·l^{-1} the total concentration of the anions, [Cl$^-$] + [HCO$_3^-$]. The anion gap remains normal in hyperchloremic acidosis, such as that associated with renal or gastrointestinal loss of bicarbonate or with perioperative infusion of 15 ml·kg^{-1}·hr^{-1} of 0.9% saline.[16] In contrast, lactic acidosis or ketoacidosis increases the anion gap because bicarbonate ions are used to buffer hydrogen ions from the excess production of metabolic acids, while serum [HCO$_3^-$] is displaced by the associated anion.

If pH is sufficiently reduced, myocardial contractility may be reduced,[17] pulmonary vascular resistance may increase,[18] systemic vascular resistance may decrease,[19] and there may be an impaired response of the cardiovascular system to endogenous or exogenous catecholamines.[20] It is particularly important to note that compensatory hyperventilation normally occurs in response to metabolic acidosis.[21] Failure of a patient to appropri-

Table 9-5. DIFFERENTIAL DIAGNOSIS OF METABOLIC ACIDOSIS

Elevated Anion Gap	Normal Anion Gap
Three Diseases	
1. Uremia	1. Renal tubular acidosis
2. Ketoacidosis	2. Diarrhea
3. Lactic acidosis	3. Carbonic anhydrase inhibition
Toxins	4. Ureteral diversions
1. Methanol	5. Early renal failure
2. Ethylene glycol	6. Hydronephrosis
3. Salicylates	7. HCl administration
4. Paraldehyde	8. Saline administration

ately hyperventilate in response to metabolic acidosis is physiologically equivalent to respiratory acidosis and represents a severe disturbance. If a patient with metabolic acidosis requires mechanical ventilation, every attempt should be made to maintain an appropriate level of ventilatory compensation until the primary process can be corrected (see Table 9-2). Table 9-6 illustrates failure to maintain compensatory hyperventilation.

The anesthetic implications of metabolic acidosis are proportional to the severity of the underlying process. Although a patient with hyperchloremic metabolic acidosis may be relatively healthy, those with lactic acidosis, ketoacidosis, uremia, or toxic ingestions will be chronically or acutely ill. Occasionally, on physical examination, metabolic acidosis may be suspected because a patient exhibits obvious hyperpnea. The serum electrolytes will demonstrate a decreased "CO$_2$." Arterial blood gases are indicated if a metabolic acidosis is suspected. Perioperative assessment of the patient should determine whether the patient has ongoing evidence of hypovolemia or hypoperfusion, whether renal function is abnormal, and whether there is pulmonary pathology likely to interfere with intraoperative gas exchange. If shock is the etiology, direct arterial pressure monitoring and, occasionally, pulmonary arterial catheterization may be indicated. Intraoperatively, one should be concerned about the possibility of exaggerated hypotensive responses to drugs and positive pressure ventilation. As noted earlier, sudden cessation of ventilatory compensation for the metabolic acidosis may be devastating. The previous degree of compensatory hyperventilation should be maintained during anesthesia, capnography employed to monitor end-tidal CO$_2$, and arterial blood gases obtained to document the adequacy of intraoperative ventilation and pH maintenance. Consideration also should be given to the composition of intravenous fluids. Assuming that Pa$_{CO_2}$ remains constant, balanced salt solutions containing bicarbonate or bicarbonate substrate (*e.g.*, lactate) will generally increase pH and solutions containing high concentrations of chloride (*e.g.*, 0.9% saline) will generally decrease pH.[9,16]

The treatment of metabolic acidosis consists of the treatment of the primary pathophysiologic process (hypoperfusion, hypoxia), and if pH is severely decreased, administration of NaHCO$_3^-$. A commonly employed calculation of an initial dose of NaHCO$_3$ is:

NaHCO$_3$ (mEq·l^{-1})

$$= \frac{\text{Wt (kg)} \times 0.3 \times (24 \text{ mEq·l}^{-1} - \text{actual HCO}_3^-)}{2} \quad (9\text{-}3)$$

where 0.3 is the assumed distribution space for bicarbonate and 24 mEq·l^{-1} is the normal value for [HCO$_3^-$] on arterial blood gas determination. The calculation markedly underestimates dosage in severe metabolic acidosis.

If [HCO$_3^-$] is infused, arterial blood gases should be measured again after approximately five minutes. In infants and children, an appropriate initial dose is 1.0 to 2.0 mEq·kg^{-1} of body weight. Hyperventilation, though an important compensatory response to metabolic acidosis, is not definitive therapy for metabolic acidosis.

One continuing controversy is the use of NaHCO$_3$ to treat acidemia induced by lactic acidosis. Although the best treatment is restoration of adequate tissue oxygenation, the conventional approach, if pH is <7.25, has been to administer NaHCO$_3$. However, few data support that strategy. In experimental animals, administration of NaHCO$_3$ transiently increases mean arterial blood pressure while increasing pH[22]; however, intracellular pH does not improve. Moreover, there is no substantial difference between NaHCO$_3$, Carbicarb (a combination of sodium carbonate and NaHCO$_3$), and equimolar sodium chloride.[22] This suggests that the primary effect on hemodynamics may be due to the administration of a hypertonic salt solution.

In critically ill patients with lactic acidosis, there were no important differences between the effects of 0.9 M NaHCO$_3$

Table 9-6. FAILURE TO MAINTAIN APPROPRIATE VENTILATORY COMPENSATION FOR METABOLIC ACIDOSIS

		Spontaneous Ventilation		Mechanical Ventilation
Arterial	pH	7.29		7.13
Blood gases	Pa_{CO_2} (mm Hg)	29	→→→→→→→→	49
	$[HCO_3^-]$ (mEq·l⁻¹)	14		16

Note: In the presence of metabolic acidosis, an otherwise innocuous increase in Pa_{CO_2} may create a life-threatening decrease in pH.

and 0.9 M sodium chloride.[23] The effects on cardiac output and arterial pressure were similar, despite increases in pH, $[HCO_3^-]$, and Pa_{CO_2} after receiving sodium bicarbonate. Importantly, $NaHCO_3$ did not improve the cardiovascular response to catecholamines and actually reduced plasma ionized calcium.[23] Several studies have demonstrated that bicarbonate therapy is safe in critically ill patients and in perioperative patients.[24-26] Although many clinicians continue to administer $NaHCO_3$ to patients with persistent lactic acidosis and ongoing deterioration,[27] no study has demonstrated improved outcome. In addition, neither Carbicarb[26] nor dichloroacetate[28] improved clinical outcome. The buffer THAM (tris-hydroxymethyl aminomethane) is effective at reducing $[H^+]$ and does not generate CO_2 as a byproduct of buffering[29]; however, there is no generally accepted indication for THAM.

Respiratory Alkalosis

Respiratory alkalosis, usually characterized by an alkalemic pH (>7.45) and always characterized by hypocarbia ($Pa_{CO_2} \leq 35$ mm Hg), describes an increase in minute ventilation to a level greater than that required to excrete the metabolic production of CO_2. Because respiratory alkalosis may be a sign of pain, anxiety, hypoxemia, central nervous system disease, or systemic sepsis, the development of spontaneous respiratory alkalosis in a previously normocarbic patient requires prompt evaluation.

Respiratory alkalosis, like metabolic alkalosis, may produce hypokalemia, hypocalcemia, cardiac dysrhythmias, bronchoconstriction, and hypotension, and may potentiate the toxicity of digoxin. In addition, acute changes in Pa_{CO_2} alter cerebral blood flow, normally approximately 50 ml·100 g⁻¹·min⁻¹ at a Pa_{CO_2} of 40 mm Hg. Doubling minute ventilation reduces Pa_{CO_2} to 20 mm Hg and halves cerebral blood flow. Conversely, if minute ventilation is halved, Pa_{CO_2} will double and cerebral blood flow will also double. If minute ventilation and Pa_{CO_2} are maintained at abnormally high or low levels for 8 to 24 hours, cerebral blood flow will return toward previous levels, associated with a return of cerebrospinal fluid $[HCO_3^-]$ toward normal.[30,31] Subsequent changes in Pa_{CO_2}, after accommodation of the cerebrospinal fluid $[HCO_3^-]$ and pH levels to chronic hypocapnia or hypercapnia, will again acutely change cerebral blood flow.

Preoperative recognition of chronic hyperventilation necessitates maintenance intraoperatively of a similar Pa_{CO_2}. Acute hyperventilation may be useful in neurosurgical procedures to reduce brain bulk and to control intracranial pressure (ICP) during emergent surgery for patients with acute closed head trauma. In those situations, intraoperative monitoring of arterial blood gases, correlated with capnography, will document adequate reduction of Pa_{CO_2}. Acute profound hypocapnia (<20 mm Hg) may produce EEG evidence of cerebral ischemia.

Respiratory Acidosis

Respiratory acidosis, usually characterized by a low pH (<7.35) and always characterized by hypercarbia ($Pa_{CO_2} \geq 45$ mm Hg), occurs when minute ventilation is insufficient to eliminate CO_2

production without an increased capillary–alveolar CO_2 gradient. Respiratory acidosis may be either acute, without compensation by renal $[HCO_3^-]$ retention, or chronic, with $[HCO_3^-]$ retention offsetting the decrease in pH (Table 9-4). Respiratory acidosis occurs because of a decrease in minute alveolar ventilation ($\dot{V}_A$), an increase in production of carbon dioxide ($\dot{V}_{CO_2}$) or both, from the equation:

$$Pa_{CO_2} = K \frac{\dot{V}_{CO_2}}{\dot{V}_A} \qquad (9\text{-}4)$$

where K is a constant. (Of course, rebreathing of exhaled, carbon dioxide–containing gas may also increase Pa_{CO_2}.) A reduction in $\dot{V}_A$ may be due to an overall decrease in minute ventilation ($\dot{V}_E$) or to an increase in the amount of wasted ventilation ($\dot{V}_D$), according to the equation:

$$\dot{V}_A = \dot{V}_E - \dot{V}_D \qquad (9\text{-}5)$$

Decreases in $\dot{V}_E$ may occur because of central ventilatory depression by drugs or central nervous system injury, because of increased work of breathing, or because of airway obstruction or neuromuscular dysfunction. Increases in $\dot{V}_D$ occur with chronic obstructive pulmonary disease, pulmonary embolism, and most acute forms of respiratory failure. $\dot{V}_{CO_2}$ may be increased by sepsis, high-glucose parenteral feeding, or fever.

Patients with chronic hypercarbia due to intrinsic pulmonary disease require careful preoperative evaluation. The ventilatory restriction imposed by upper abdominal or thoracic surgery may be a particular risk to patients who chronically are unable to excrete $\dot{V}_{CO_2}$ at a normal Pa_{CO_2}. Administration of narcotics and sedatives, even in small doses, may cause hazardous ventilatory depression. Preoperative evaluation should consider direct arterial pressure monitoring and frequent intraoperative blood gas determinations, as well as postoperative pain management. Intraoperatively, a patient with chronic hypercapnia should be ventilated to maintain a normal pH. An abrupt increase in minute ventilation may result in profound alkalemia, and the associated complications, since the chronic elevation in $[HCO_3^-]$ will persist as Pa_{CO_2} is abruptly reduced (analogous to the addition of hyperventilation to metabolic alkalosis described in Table 9-3). Postoperatively, prophylactic ventilatory support may be required for selected patients with chronic hypercarbia. Epidural opioid administration represents one potential alternative that may provide adequate postoperative analgesia without undue depression of ventilatory drive.

The treatment of respiratory acidosis depends upon whether the process is acute or chronic. Acute respiratory acidosis may require mechanical ventilation unless a simple etiologic factor (e.g., opioid overdosage or residual muscular blockade) can be treated quickly. Bicarbonate administration is rarely indicated unless severe metabolic acidosis is also present or unless mechanical ventilation is ineffective in reducing acute hypercarbia. In contrast, chronic respiratory acidosis is rarely managed with ventilation. Rather, efforts are made to improve pulmonary function to permit more effective elimination of carbon dioxide.

PRACTICAL APPROACH TO ACID–BASE INTERPRETATION

Rapid interpretation of a patient's acid–base status involves the integration of three sets of data: arterial blood gases, electrolytes, and history. The following stepwise approach facilitates interpretation (Table 9-7).

Usually, most of the acid–base picture can be assessed before initiating therapy; however, some data require immediate attention. Respiratory acidosis with a pH <7.1 suggests the need for tracheal intubation and ventilatory support while a metabolic acidosis with a similar pH suggests the need for appropriate etiologic intervention and, perhaps, alkalinizing therapy. Life-threatening alkalemia, rarely encountered, is often the consequence of the addition of inappropriate hyperventilation to underlying metabolic alkalosis.

The next problem is to define the primary acid–base disturbance. Is the patient acidemic (pH <7.35) or alkalemic (pH >7.45)? The pH status will usually indicate the primary process: that is, acidosis produces acidemia; alkalosis produces alkalemia. (Note that the suffix "-osis" indicates a primary process that, if unopposed, will produce the corresponding pH change. The suffix "-emia" refers to the pH. A compensatory process is not considered an "-osis.") Of course, a patient may have mixed "-oses," that is, more than one primary process.

Next, one asks whether or not the entire arterial blood gas picture is consistent with a simple acute respiratory alkalosis or acidosis. Table 9-4 lists the rules of pH change associated with acute hyperventilation and the secondary [HCO_3^-] changes. For example, a patient with an acute drop in $Paco_2$ to 30 mm Hg would have a pH increase of 0.10 units to a pH of 7.50 and a calculated [HCO_3^-] of 22. An acute increase in $Paco_2$ (Table 9-4) results in an acute increase in [HCO_3^-] of about 1 mmol for every increase of 10 mm Hg in $Paco_2$ due to intracellular buffering of hydrogen ions and transcellular exchange of chloride for bicarbonate.[14]

If the changes in $Paco_2$, pH and [HCO_3^-] are not consistent with a simple acute respiratory disturbance, a chronic respiratory problem ($\geq$24 hours) should be considered. The rules for a chronic respiratory disturbance are also listed in Table 9-4. Note that the pH becomes nearly normal as the body compensates. For example, if a patient chronically hypoventilates to a $Paco_2$ of 60 mm Hg (*i.e.*, increases $Paco_2$ by 20 mm Hg), the [HCO_3^-] level should increase by 8 mEq $\cdot$ l^{-1}; the arterial blood gases should show a $Paco_2$ of 60 mm Hg, a pH of 7.35, and a [HCO_3^-] of 32 mEq $\cdot$ l^{-1}. An episode of acute hypoventilation of this magnitude would have yielded a pH of 7.30 with a [HCO_3^-] of 26 mEq $\cdot$ l^{-1}. The history will often provide clues as to whether the respiratory changes are acute or chronic. If neither an acute respiratory change nor a chronic compensatory change can describe the entire blood gas picture, then one must assume that a primary metabolic disturbance is also present.

Table 9-2 characterizes the usual compensatory responses that should occur in response to metabolic disturbances. Note

Table 9-7. SEQUENTIAL APPROACH TO ACID-BASE INTERPRETATION

1. Is the pH life-threatening, requiring immediate intervention?
2. Is the pH acidemic or alkalemic?
3. Could the entire arterial blood gas picture represent only an acute increase or decrease in $Paco_2$?
4. If the answer to question #3 is "No," is there evidence of a chronic respiratory disturbance or of an acute metabolic disturbance?
5. Are appropriate compensatory changes present?
6. Is an anion gap present?
7. Do the clinical data fit the acid-base picture?

Table 9-8. HYPOBICARBONATEMIA AND HYPERCHLOREMIC ACIDOSIS DURING PROLONGED SURGERY

Arterial blood gases	pH	7.38
	$Paco_2$	32 mm Hg
	[HCO_3^-]	17 mEq $\cdot$ l^{-1}
Electrolytes	Na^+	140 mEq $\cdot$ l^{-1}
	Cl^-	112 mEq $\cdot$ l^{-1}
	CO_2	18 mEq $\cdot$ l^{-1}
	Anion Gap	10 mEq $\cdot$ l^{-1}

that respiratory compensation for metabolic disturbances occurs more rapidly than metabolic compensation for respiratory disturbances. Several general rules describe compensation. First, overcompensation is rare. Second, inadequate or excessive compensation suggests an additional primary disturbance. Third, a metabolic acidosis associated with an increased anion gap is never compensatory. Finally, the rules-of-thumb only approximate the logarithmic relationship between pH and [H^+]. The more the pH deviates from 7.40, the less accurate the rules become.

The next question, whether an anion gap is present, should be assessed even if the arterial blood gases appear straightforward. The simultaneous occurrence of metabolic alkalosis and metabolic acidosis (as a consequence of pathophysiology producing a high anion gap) may result in an unremarkable pH and [HCO_3^-]; the combined abnormality may only be appreciated by examining the anion gap.[32] Metabolic acidoses associated with a high anion gap require specific treatments, thus necessitating a correct diagnosis. This is particularly important in managing hyperchloremic metabolic acidosis after administration of large volumes of 0.9% saline perioperatively or even in critically ill patients.[33] In these circumstances, no anion gap would be expected and no specific treatment of metabolic acidosis would be required.[9,34]

The final question is whether the clinical data are consistent with the arterial blood gas data. Failure to consider clinical status also may lead to serious errors in blood gas interpretation.

Examples

The foregoing has summarized an approach that simplifies interpretation. The following two hypothetical cases will be approached using the algorithm and rules just discussed.

Example 1

A 65-year-old female has undergone 12 hours of an expected 16-hour radical neck dissection and flap construction. The estimated blood loss is 1000 ml. She has received three units of packed red blood cells and 9 l of 0.9 % saline. Her blood pressure and heart rate have remained stable while anesthetized with 0.5% to 1.0% isoflurane in 70 : 30 nitrous oxide and oxygen. Urinary output is adequate. Arterial blood gas levels are shown in Table 9-8.

The step-by-step interpretation is as follows:

1. The pH is not life-threatening.
2. The pH is <7.40 but is not frankly acidemic.
3. The arterial blood gases cannot be adequately explained by acute hypocarbia. The predicted pH would be 7.48 and the predicted [HCO_3^-] would be 22 mEq $\cdot$ l^{-1} (Table 9-4).
4. A metabolic acidosis appears to be present.
5. The question of compensation is not pertinent during general anesthesia, given that $Paco_2$ is established by mechanical ventilation. However, if this represented spontaneous hypocarbia, it would suggest slight overcompensa-

Table 9-9. EVALUATION OF HYPERCHLOREMIC ACIDOSIS

	Urinary Solutes			
	NH₄⁺	Cl⁻	A⁻	Na⁺
Gi tract HCO₃⁻ loss	↑ (a)	↓ (b)	↔	↓ (c)
Generated/ingested organic acids	↑ (a)	↔	↑ (d)	↓ (e)
HCl intake or equivalent*	↑ (a)	↑ (f)	↔	↑ (e)
Inadequate renal HCO₃⁻	↓ (g)	↔	↔	↔
Renal HCO₃⁻ loss	↓ (g)	↔	↔	↔

* NH_4Cl, chloride salts of amino acids or dilutional acidosis; ↔ designates normal: (a) NH_4^+ > 1 mmol/kg daily; (b) Fe_{Cl} < 1 mmol/kg daily. FE = fractional excretion of a solute. Urinary unmeasured anion concentration (sum of urinary K^+, NH_4^+, and Na^+ less Cl^-) estimates sum of urinary sulphate and organic anion concentrations.
(Reproduced with permission from Gluck SL: Acid–base. Lancet 352:474, 1998.)

tion (Table 9-2) and should prompt a search for a reason for primary respiratory alkalosis.

6. During prolonged anesthesia and surgery, one might assume the presence of lactic acidosis and provide additional fluid therapy or otherwise attempt to improve perfusion. However, serum electrolytes reveal (Table 9-8) a normal anion gap, indicating that the metabolic acidosis is probably the result of dilution of the extracellular volume with a high-chloride fluid.[9,16] A random urine sample could help confirm this etiology of hyperchloremic acidosis (Table 9-9).[14] Hyperchloremic acidosis secondary to infusion of high-chloride fluid requires no treatment.

7. The arterial blood gases and serum electrolytes are compatible with the clinical picture.

Example 2

A 35-year-old male, three days after appendectomy, develops nausea with recurrent emesis persisting for 48 hours. An arterial blood gas reveals the results shown in the middle column of Table 9-10.

1. The pH of 7.50 requires no immediate intervention.
2. The pH is alkalemic, suggesting a primary alkalosis.
3. An acute $Paco_2$ of 46 mm Hg would yield a pH of approximately 7.37; therefore, this is not simply an acute ventilatory disturbance.
4. The patient has a primary metabolic alkalosis, as suggested by the $[HCO_3^-]$ of 35 mEq·l⁻¹.
5. The limits of respiratory compensation for metabolic alka-

losis are wide and difficult to predict for individual patients. The rules of thumb, summarized in Table 9-2, suggest that $[HCO_3^-]$ + 15 should equal the last two digits of the pH and that the $Paco_2$ should increase 5–6 mm Hg for every 10 mEq·l⁻¹ change in serum $[HCO_3^-]$, that is, pH = 7.50 and $Paco_2$ = 46 mm Hg.
6. The anion gap is 12 mEq·l⁻¹.
7. The diagnosis of a primary metabolic alkalosis with compensatory hypoventilation is consistent with the history of recurrent vomiting. Consider how the arterial blood gases would change if vomiting were sufficiently severe to produce hypovolemic shock and lactic acidosis (third column, Table 9-10).

This sequence illustrates the important concept that the final pH, $Paco_2$, and $[HCO_3^-]$ represent the result of all of the vectors operating on acid–base status. Complex, or "triple disturbances," can only be interpreted using a thorough, stepwise approach.

FLUID MANAGEMENT

Physiology

Body Fluid Compartments

Accurate replacement of fluid deficits necessitates an understanding of the distribution spaces of water, sodium, and colloid. Total body water (TBW), the distribution volume of sodium-free water, approximates 60% of total body weight. TBW includes intracellular volume (ICV), which constitutes 40% of total body weight, and extracellular volume (ECV), which constitutes 20% of body weight. Plasma volume (PV) equals about one fifth of ECV, the remainder of which is interstitial fluid (IF). Red cell volume, approximately 2 liters, is part of ICV.

The ECV contains most of total body sodium, with equal sodium concentrations ($[Na^+]$) in the PV and IF. Plasma $[Na^+]$ is approximately 140 mEq·l⁻¹. The predominant intracellular cation, potassium, has an intracellular concentration ($[K^+]$) approximating 150 mEq·l⁻¹. Albumin, the most important oncotically active constituent of ECV, is unequally distributed in PV (~4 g·dl⁻¹) and IF (~1 g·dl⁻¹). The IF concentration of albumin varies greatly among tissues. ECV is the distribution volume both for crystalloid solutions in which $[Na^+]$ is approximately 140 mEq·l⁻¹ and for colloid.

Distribution of Infused Fluids

Conventionally, clinical prediction of plasma volume expansion (PVE) after fluid infusion assumes that body fluid spaces are static. Kinetic analysis of PVE replaces the static assumption with a dynamic description. As an example of the static approach, assume that a 70-kg patient has suffered an acute blood loss of 2000 ml, approximately 40% of the predicted 5-l blood volume. The formula describing the effects of replacement with

Table 9-10. METABOLIC ALKALOSIS SECONDARY TO NAUSEA AND VOMITING WITH SUBSEQUENT LACTIC ACIDOSIS SECONDARY TO HYPOVOLEMIA

		Normal	Metabolic Alkalosis	Metabolic Acidosis
Blood gases	pH	7.40	7.50	7.40
	$Paco_2$ (mm Hg)	40	46	40
	$[HCO_3^-]$ (mEq·l⁻¹)	24	35	24
Serum electrolytes	Na^+ (mEq·l⁻¹)	140	140	140
	Cl^{-1} (mEq·l⁻¹)	105	94	94
	CO_2 (mEq·l⁻¹)	25	36	25
	Anion gap (mEq·l⁻¹)	10	10	21

5% dextrose in water (D5W), lactated Ringer's solution, or 5% or 25% human serum albumin is as follows:

$$\text{Expected PV increment} = \frac{\text{volume infused} \times \text{normal PV}}{\text{distribution volume}} \quad (9\text{-}6)$$

Rearranging the equation yields the following:

Volume infused

$$= \frac{\text{expected PV increment} \times \text{distribution volume}}{\text{normal PV}} \quad (9\text{-}7)$$

To restore blood volume using D5W:

$$28\,l = \frac{2\,l \times 42\,l}{3\,l} \quad (9\text{-}8)$$

where 2 l is the desired PV increment, 42 l is the TBW in a 70-kg person, and 3 l is the normal estimated PV.

To restore blood volume using lactated Ringer's solution:

$$0.3\,l = \frac{2\,l \times 14\,l}{3\,l} \quad (9\text{-}9)$$

where 14 l is the ECV in a 70-kg person.

If 5% albumin, which exerts colloid osmotic pressure similar to plasma, were infused, the infused volume initially would remain in the PV, perhaps attracting additional interstitial fluid intravascularly. Twenty-five percent human serum albumin, a concentrated colloid, expands PV by approximately 400 ml for each 100 ml infused.

However, in kinetic terms, these analyses are simplistic. Infused fluid does not simply equilibrate throughout an assumed distribution volume, but is added to a highly regulated system that maintains intravascular, interstitial, and intracellular volume within narrow limits. Excess fluid is excreted whereas hypovolemia initiates several powerful compensatory mechanisms, including transcapillary refill and intense sodium and water conservation. The purpose of applying kinetic models to intravenous fluid therapy is to allow clinicians to predict more accurately the time course of volume changes produced by infusions of fluids of various compositions in patients with a variety of pathophysiologic abnormalities. Kinetic analysis permits estimation of peak volume expansion and rates of clearance of infused fluid and complements analysis of "pharmacodynamic" effects, such as changes in cardiac output or cardiac filling pressures.

Because infused fluid does not introduce a novel substance that can be measured, the effects of fluid infusion must be inferred from changes in variables such as albumin or hemoglobin concentration [Hb]. In addition, fluids usually are given not as rapid boluses but as infusions over longer time intervals, thereby producing more complicated decay curves than those in conventional pharmacokinetic analysis. To further complicate the comparison, fluid infusion acutely changes the volumes of distribution of infused fluid and may alter clearance mechanisms (*e.g.*, glomerular filtration and tubular reabsorption) as well as neuroendocrine factors such as antidiuretic hormone (ADH), atrial natriuretic peptide (ANP), and aldosterone.

A practical physiologic tracer should permit frequent measurements in order to define more completely the clearance curves. Svensen and Hahn[35] evaluated three endogenous tracers—blood water concentration, serum albumin concentration, and [Hb]—in volunteers who received infusions of acetated Ringer's solution, 6% dextran 70, or 7.5% saline. Although much less tedious than blood water calculations, [Hb] provided similar estimates of volumes of distribution and elimination rate constants.

Figure 9-1 illustrates the conceptual model used by Svensén and Hahn.[35] The top of the figure illustrates a one-compartment model, while the bottom shows a two-compartment model. After infusing the test fluids, Svensén and Hahn fitted the results to one-volume- and two-volume-of-fluid-space (VOFS) models. Each of the two VOFS models is based on physiologic and

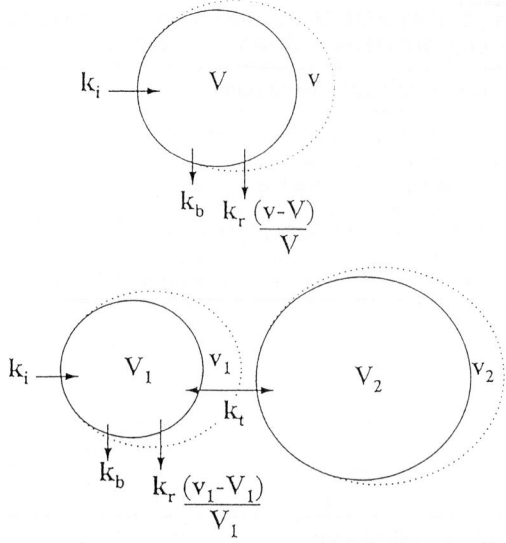

Figure 9-1. Schematic drawing of the kinetic model used to calculate the size of the body fluid spaces expanded by intravenous infusions of fluid in humans. Data are fitted to a one-volume- or two-volume-of-fluid-space (VOFS) model. The assumptions underlying the one-compartment VOFS model (*top*) are as follows: (1) During fluid infusion, fluid enters an expandable space of volume v at a constant rate k_i; (2) the expandable fluid space has a target volume V, which the body strives to maintain; (3) volume v changes by fluid being eliminated from the fluid space at a basal rate, k_b (perspiration and basal diuresis), and at a controlled rate. The controlled rate is proportional by a constant k_r to the relative deviation of v from the target volume V. The assumptions behind the two-compartment VOFS model (*bottom*) are similar: (1) During fluid infusion, fluid enters an expandable space of volume v_1 at a constant rate k_i; (2) there is a secondary expandable fluid space of volume v_2 exchanging fluid with the primary fluid space; (3) volume v_1 changes through exchange with the secondary fluid space and as a result of fluid being eliminated from the primary fluid space at a basal rate, k_b (perspiration and basal diuresis), and at a controlled rate; (4) the primary and secondary fluid spaces have target volumes V_1 and V_2 which the system strives to maintain by acting on the controlled elimination mechanism, k_r, which is proportional to the relative deviation from the target volume of the primary fluid space, and by acting on the fluid exchange mechanism; (5) the net rate of fluid exchange between the two spaces is proportional to the difference in relative deviations from the target volumes by a constant k_t. (Reprinted with permission from Svensén C, Hahn RG: Volume kinetics of Ringer solution, dextran 70, and hypertonic saline in male volunteers. Anesthesiology 87:204, 1997.)

mathematical assumptions (Table 9-11).[36] The two-compartment VOFS model is most likely to be superior to the one-compartment model when urinary excretion in response to infusion is small.[37]

Figure 9-2 shows the mean plasma volume dilution curves obtained with the infusion of Ringer's solution or dextran 70. All dextran infusions were consistent with a one-VOFS model, suggesting that the colloid infusion remained in the PV. Hypertonic crystalloid, like isotonic crystalloid, is associated in individual instances with a mixture of one- and two-VOFS models.

Using this approach, the effects of common physiologic and pharmacologic influences can be examined in experimental animals or humans. As an example, the influence of acute hypovolemia on PVE has been defined experimentally and clinically. In chronically instrumented, splenectomized, unanesthetized sheep, hemorrhage of 300 ml (~12 % of blood volume), plasma transfilling consisted of approximately two-thirds of shed blood volume within 3 hours.[38] In fact, at 3 hours after the end of hemorrhage, PVE was similar to that in animals that had received 25 ml · kg[-1] of 0.9% saline over 20 minutes beginning immediately after the termination of hemorrhage. In conscious

Table 9-11. PHYSIOLOGIC AND MATHEMATICAL ASSUMPTIONS FOR ONE- AND TWO-VOLUME-OF-FLUID-SPACE MODELS

One-Compartment VOFS Assumptions	Two-Compartment VOFS Assumptions
1. During fluid infusion, fluid enters an expandable space of Volume v at a constant rate k_i 2. The expandable fluid space has a target volume V, which the body strives to maintain 3. Volume v changes by fluid being eliminated from the fluid space at a basal rate, k_b (perspiration and basal diuresis), and at a controlled rate. The controlled rate is proportional by a constant k_r to the relative deviation of v from the target volume V	1. During fluid infusion, fluid enters an expandable space of volume v_1 at a constant rate k_i 2. There is a secondary expandable fluid space of volume v_2 exchanging fluid with the primary fluid space 3. Volume v_1 changes through exchange with the secondary fluid space and as a result of fluid being eliminated from the primary fluid space at a basal rate, k_b (perspiration and basal diuresis), and at a controlled rate 4. The primary and secondary fluid spaces have target volumes V_1 and V_2 which the system strives to maintain by acting on the controlled elimination mechanism k_r, which is proportional to the relative deviation from the target volume of the primary, and by acting on the fluid exchange mechanism 5. The net rate of fluid exchange between the two spaces is proportional to the difference in relative deviations from the target volumes by a constant k_t

VOFS, volume-of-fluid-space.

volunteers given $25 \: ml \cdot kg^{-1}$ of acetated Ringer's solution over 30 minutes under conditions of normovolemia or after removal of 450 or 900 ml of blood, plasma dilution (closely related to volume expansion) 50 to 100 minutes after beginning the infusion was greatest after 900 ml of hemorrhage, less after 450 ml of hemorrhage, and least in the absence of hemorrhage.[39] Plasma transfilling appears to contribute substantially to the expansion of plasma volume by intravenous fluids given after hemorrhage, although these observations must be confirmed in anesthetized animals and humans.

Regulation of Extracellular Fluid Volume

Total body water content is regulated by the intake and output of water. Water intake includes ingested liquids plus an average of 750 ml ingested in solid food and 350 ml that is generated metabolically.[40] Insensible losses are normally 1 l per day and GI losses are 100 to 150 ml per day. Thirst, the primary mechanism of controlling water intake, is triggered by an increase in body fluid tonicity or by a decrease in extracellular volume.[41]

Reabsorption of filtered water and sodium is enhanced by changes mediated by the hormonal factors antidiuretic hor-

mone (ADH), atrial natriuretic peptide (ANP), and aldosterone. Renal water handling has three important components: (1) delivery of tubular fluid to the diluting segments of the nephron; (2) separation of solute and water in the diluting segment; and (3) variable reabsorption of water in the collecting ducts.[41] In the descending loop of Henle, water is reabsorbed while solute is retained to achieve a final osmolality of tubular fluid of $\sim1200 \: mOsm \cdot kg^{-1}$ (Fig. 9-3). This concentrated fluid is then diluted by the active reabsorption of electrolytes in the ascending limb of the loop of Henle and in the distal tubule, both of which are relatively impermeable to water.[41] As fluid exits the distal tubule and enters the collecting duct, osmolality is $\sim50 \: mOsm \cdot kg^{-1}$. Within the collecting duct, water reabsorption is modulated by ADH (also called vasopressin). Vasopressin binds to V_2 receptors along the basolateral membrane of the collecting duct cells,[42] then stimulates the synthesis and insertion of the aquaporin-2 water channel into the luminal membrane of collecting duct cells.[42-44]

Plasma hypotonicity suppresses ADH release, resulting in excretion of dilute urine. Hypertonicity stimulates ADH secretion, which increases the permeability of the collecting duct to water

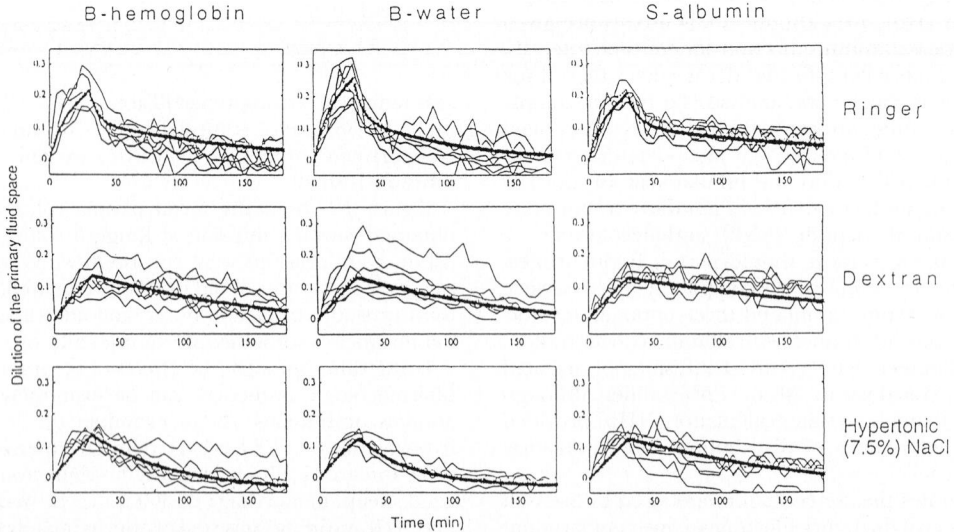

Figure 9-2. Kinetic curves obtained after infusion in adult male volunteers of $25 \: ml \cdot kg^{-1}$ of acetated Ringer's solution (Ringer) or $5 \: ml \cdot kg^{-1}$ of dextran 70 over 30 min. Dilution of plasma volume is calculated from changes in hemoglobin (B-hemoglobin) concentration, blood water (B-water) concentration, and serum albumin (S-albumin) concentration. (Reprinted with permission from Svensén C, Hahn RG: Volume kinetics of Ringer solution, dextran 70, and hypertonic saline in male volunteers. Anesthesiology 87:204, 1997.)

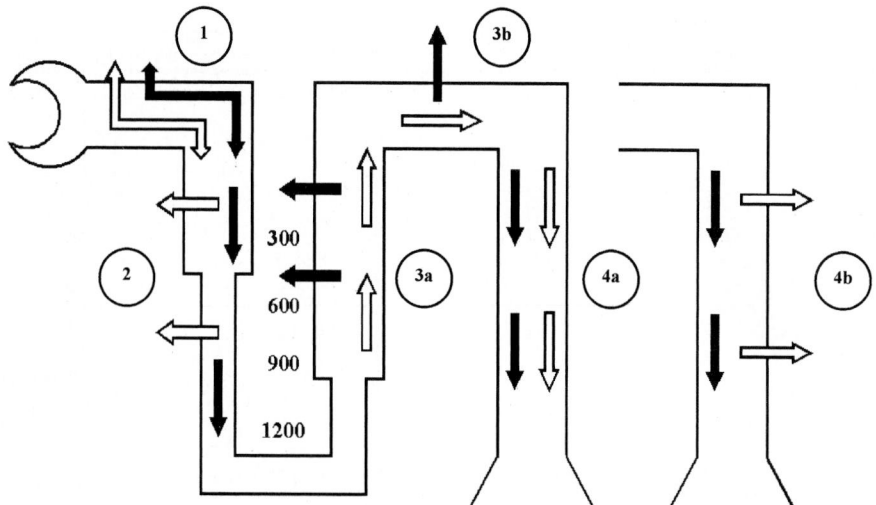

Figure 9-3. Renal filtration, reabsorption, and excretion of water. *Open arrows* represent water and *solid arrows* represent electrolytes. Water and electrolytes are filtered by the glomerulus. In the proximal tubule (1), water and electrolytes are absorbed isotonically. In the descending loop of Henle (2), water is absorbed to achieve osmotic equilibrium with the interstitium while electrolytes are retained. The numbers (300, 600, 900, and 1200) between the descending and ascending limbs represent the osmolality of the interstitium in $mOsm \cdot kg^{-1}$. The delivery of solute and fluid to the distal nephron is a function of proximal tubular reabsorption; as proximal tubular reabsorption increases, delivery of solute to the medullary (3a) and cortical (3b) diluting sites decreases. In the diluting sites, electrolyte-free water is generated through selective reabsorption of electrolytes while water is retained in the tubular lumen, generating a dilute tubular fluid. In the absence of vasopressin, the collecting duct (4a) remains relatively impermeable to water and a dilute urine is excreted. When vasopressin acts on the collecting ducts (4b), water is reabsorbed from these vasopressin-responsive nephron segments, allowing the excretion of a concentrated urine. (Reprinted with permission from Fried LF, Palevsky PM: Hyponatremia and hypernatremia. In Saklayen MG (ed): The Medical Clinics of North America. Renal Disease, p 585. Philadelphia, WB Saunders, 1997.)

and enhances water reabsorption. In response to changing plasma $[Na^+]$, changing secretion of ADH can vary urinary osmolality from 50 to 1200 $mOsm \cdot kg^{-1}$ and urinary volume from 0.4 to 20 $l \cdot day^{-1}$ (Fig. 9-4). Other factors that stimulate ADH secretion, though none as powerfully as plasma tonicity, include hypotension, hypovolemia, and nonosmotic stimuli such as nausea, pain, and medications, including opiates.[41]

Two powerful hormonal systems regulate total body sodium. The natriuretic peptides—atrial natriuretic peptide (ANP), brain natriuretic peptide, and C-type natriuretic peptide—defend against sodium overload,[45] and the renin–angiotensin-aldosterone axis defends against sodium depletion and hypovolemia. ANP, released from the cardiac atria in response to increased atrial stretch, exerts vasodilatory effects and increases the renal excretion of sodium and water.[46,47] ANP secretion is decreased during hypovolemia. Even in patients with chronic renal insufficiency, infusion of ANP in low, nonhypotensive doses increases sodium excretion and augments urinary losses of retained solutes.[48]

Aldosterone is the final common pathway in a complex response to decreased effective arterial volume, whether decreased effective arterial volume is true or relative (edematous states or hypoalbuminemia). In this pathway, decreased stretch in the baroreceptors of the aortic arch and carotid body and stretch receptors in the great veins, pulmonary vasculature, and atria result in increased sympathetic tone. Increased sympathetic tone, in combination with decreased renal perfusion, leads to renin release and formation of angiotensin I from angiotensinogen.[49] Angiotensin-converting enzyme (ACE) converts angiotensin I to angiotensin II, which stimulates the adrenal cortex to synthesize and release aldosterone.[50] Acting primarily in the distal tubules, high concentrations of aldosterone cause sodium reabsorption[50] (Fig. 9-5) and may reduce urinary excretion of sodium nearly to zero. Intrarenal physical factors are also important in regulating sodium balance. Sodium loading decreases colloid osmotic pressure, thereby increasing the glomerular filtration rate (GFR), decreasing net sodium reab-

sorption, and increasing distal sodium delivery, which, in turn, suppresses renin secretion.[50]

Renal adaptation to hypovolemia (and decreased cardiac output) occurs through three primary mechanisms: a reduction in renal blood flow (RBF), a reduction in GFR, and increased tubular reabsorption of sodium and water.[51] Renal perfusion during acute hypovolemia is determined by the balance between renal vasoconstrictive factors (the renal sympathetic nerves, angiotensin II, and catecholamines) and vasodilatory mechanisms (intrinsic renal autoregulation and the renal vasodilatory effects of prostaglandins).[52] Although RBF autoregulates (remains constant over a wide range of perfusion pressures), autoregulation may be impaired or lost during severe, acute hypovolemia.[53] Renal sympathetic stimulation with secretion of α-adrenergic catecholamines and angiotensin II increases renal vascular resistance. Intrarenal vasodilator prostaglandins antagonize vasoconstrictor hormones and maintain RBF during hypovolemia. This protective effect is reduced by nonsteroidal anti-inflammatory drugs.[54]

Fluid Replacement Therapy

Maintenance Requirements for Water, Sodium and Potassium

In healthy adults, sufficient water is required to balance gastrointestinal losses of 100–200 $ml \cdot day^{-1}$, insensible losses of 500–1000 $ml \cdot day^{-1}$ (half of which is respiratory and half cutaneous), and urinary losses of 1000 $ml \cdot day^{-1}$. Two simple formulas are used interchangeably to estimate maintenance water requirements (Table 9-12). Urinary losses exceeding 1000 $ml \cdot day^{-1}$ may represent an appropriate physiologic response to ECV expansion or an inability to conserve salt or water.

Daily requirements for sodium and potassium are approximately 75 $mEq \cdot l^{-1}$ and 40 $mEq \cdot l^{-1}$, respectively, although wider ranges of sodium intake than potassium intake are physiologically tolerated because renal sodium conservation and excretion

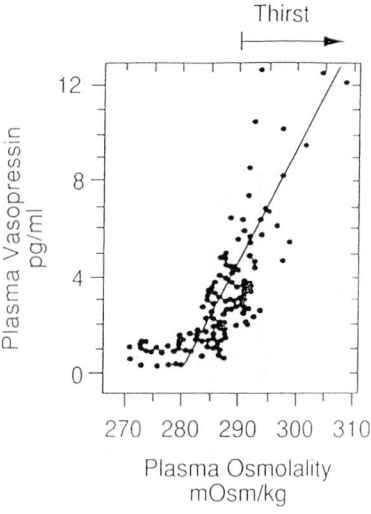

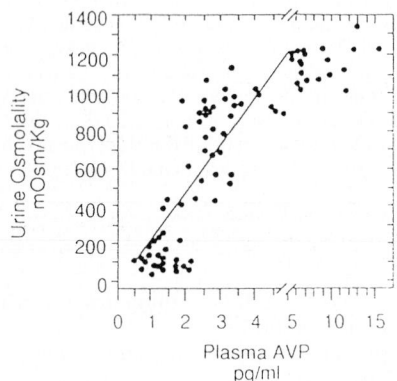

Figure 9-4. *Top:* Relationship between plasma osmolality and plasma vasopressin (AVP; also referred to as ADH). *Bottom:* Relationship between plasma AVP and urinary osmolality. (Reprinted with permission from Ober KP: Endocrine crisis: Diabetes insipidus. Crit Care Clin 7:109, 1991.

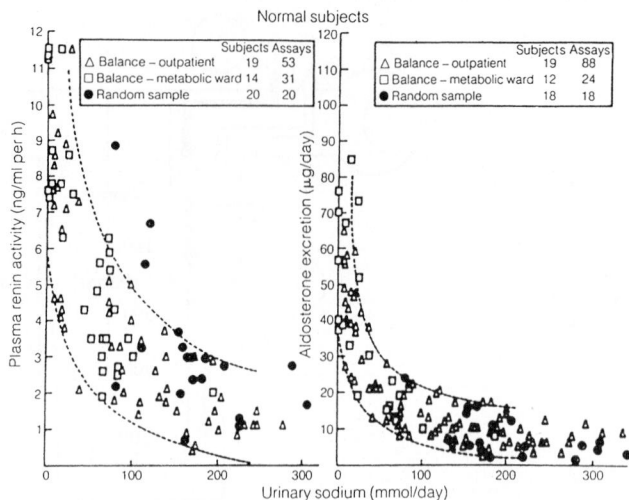

Figure 9-5. Mean urinary sodium excretion for given ranges of plasma renin activity and urinary aldosterone excretion in humans. Aldosterone exerts a regulatory effect on urinary sodium excretion even at low levels of secretory activity and relatively high levels of sodium excretion. (Reprinted with permission from Laragh JH: The endocrine control of blood volume, blood pressure and sodium balance: Atrial hormone and renin system interactions. J Hypertens 4(suppl 2):S143, 1986.)

are more efficient than potassium conservation and excretion. Therefore, healthy, 70-kg adults require 2500 ml · day^{-1} of water containing a [Na$^+$] of 30 mEq · l^{-1} and a [K$^+$] of 15–20 mEq · l^{-1}. Intraoperatively, fluids containing sodium-free water (*i.e.*, [Na$^+$] < 130 mEq · l^{-1}) are rarely used in adults because of the necessity for replacing isotonic losses and the risk of postoperative hyponatremia.

Dextrose

Traditionally, glucose-containing intravenous fluids have been given in an effort to prevent hypoglycemia and limit protein catabolism. However, owing to the hyperglycemic response associated with surgical stress, only infants and patients receiving insulin or drugs that interfere with glucose synthesis are at risk for hypoglycemia. Iatrogenic hyperglycemia can limit the effectiveness of fluid resuscitation by inducing an osmotic diuresis and, in animals, may aggravate ischemic neurologic injury.[55] Although associated with worse outcome in both ischemic[56] (Table 9-13) and traumatic[57] brain injury in humans, hyperglycemia may also constitute a hormonally mediated response to more severe injury.[58]

Surgical Fluid Requirements

Water and Electrolyte Composition of Fluid Losses. Surgical patients require replacement of PV and ECV losses secondary to wound or burn edema, ascites, and gastrointestinal secretions. Wound and burn edema and ascitic fluid are protein-rich and contain electrolytes in concentrations similar to plasma. Although gastrointestinal secretions vary greatly in composition (Table 9-14), the composition of replacement fluid need not be closely matched if ECV is adequate and renal and cardiovascular function are normal. Substantial loss of gastrointestinal fluids requires more accurate replacement of electrolytes (*i.e.*, potassium, magnesium, phosphate). If cardiovascular or renal function is impaired, more precise replacement may require frequent assessment of serum electrolytes. Chronic gastric losses may produce hypochloremic metabolic alkalosis that can be corrected with 0.9% saline; chronic diarrhea may produce hyperchloremic metabolic acidosis that may be prevented or corrected by infusion of fluid containing bicarbonate or bicarbonate substrate (*e.g.,* lactate).

Fluid Shifts During Surgery. Replacement of intraoperative fluid losses must compensate for the acute reduction of functional ECV that accompanies trauma, hemorrhage, and tissue manipulation. For example, otherwise healthy subjects who received no intraoperative sodium while undergoing gastric or gallbladder surgery demonstrated a decline in ECV of nearly 2 liters and a 13% decline in GFR.[59] In contrast, patients who received lactated Ringer's solution maintained ECV and increased GFR by 10%. No data describe changes in PV, IF, and ICV during acute, unresuscitated shock in humans. Patients studied during the first 10 days after resuscitation from massive trauma demonstrated a 55% increase in IF volume (Fig. 9-6).[60] Because of the reduction of colloid osmotic pressure in traumatized patients, the ratio of IF to blood volume was increased, in some patients exceeding 5:1.[60] Based on static assumptions

Table 9-12. MAINTENANCE WATER REQUIREMENTS

Weight (kg)	ml · kg^{-1} · h^{-1}	ml · kg^{-1} · day^{-1}
1–10	4	100
11–20	2	50
21–n	1	20

Table 9-13. INFLUENCE OF MEAN PLASMA GLUCOSE (DAYS 3 TO 7) ON
3-MONTH GLASGOW OUTCOME SCALE (GOS) SCORE IN SAH

Outcome	Glu ≤ 120 mg·dl⁻¹		Glu > 120 mg·dl⁻¹		
	No	*%*	*No*	*%*	*p*
No. of cases	179		322		
GOS score					
Good recovery	132	73.7	160	49.7	<0.0001
Moderate disability	13	7.7	44	13.7	
Severe disability	14	7.8	33	10.2	
Persistent vegetative state	1	0.6	8	2.5	
Death	12	*6.7*	67	*20.8*	<0.0001
Lost to follow-up	7	3.9	10	3.1	

GOS = Glasgow Outcome Score; SAH = subarachnoid hemorrhage.
(Reproduced with permission from Lanzino G, Kassell NF, Germanson T *et al:* Plasma glucose levels and outcome after aneurysmal subarachnoid hemorrhage. J Neurosurg 79:885, 1993.)

regarding the distribution volumes of infused fluids, such patients would require much larger volumes of crystalloids than healthy patients in order to achieve a specific amount of intravascular volume expansion. However, insufficient data are available to confirm that assessment.

Based on these considerations, guidelines have been developed for replacement of fluid losses during surgical procedures. The simplest formula provides, in addition to maintenance fluids and replacement of estimated blood loss, 4 ml·kg⁻¹·hr⁻¹ for procedures involving minimal trauma, 6 ml·kg⁻¹·hr⁻¹ for those involving moderate trauma, and 8 ml·kg⁻¹·hr⁻¹ for those involving extreme trauma.

Mobilization of Expanded Interstitial Fluid

An important corollary of IF expansion is the mobilization and return of accumulated fluid to the ECV and the PV, colloquially termed "deresuscitation." In most patients, mobilization occurs on approximately the third postoperative day. If the cardiovascular system and kidneys cannot effectively transport and excrete mobilized fluid, hypervolemia and pulmonary edema may occur.

Fluid Requirements During Labor and Cesarean Section

Labor is energy-intensive. Prolonged labor without caloric intake may lead to maternal and fetal hypoglycemia, ketosis, and lactic acidosis. In parturients randomized to receive no dextrose, 1% dextrose, or 5% dextrose, administration of dextrose-free solution resulted in umbilical artery hypoglycemia, 1% dextrose maintained euglycemia in both the mother and neonate, and 5% dextrose was associated with neonatal hypoglycemia.[61] Based on these clinical studies, glucose should be given during labor in a dose of 1–2 g·hr⁻¹ (equivalent to 100–200 ml of a 1% dextrose solution), should not exceed 6 g·hr⁻¹, and should be considered especially in patients receiving regional anesthesia without epinephrine (which tends to increase serum glucose).

Aggressive preload augmentation before epidural anesthesia during labor is probably unnecessary because continuous infusion of low doses of local anesthetic agents produces gradual sympathectomy and vasodilation. Furthermore, rapid volume expansion may inhibit uterine activity and, in some high-risk parturients, may precipitate hypervolemia and pulmonary edema. However, preload augmentation and increased cardiac diastolic volume may enhance renal and placental perfusion by stimulating secretion of ANP.[62]

In contrast to epidural anesthesia administered for labor, spinal anesthesia and, to a lesser extent, epidural anesthesia for cesarean section typically causes maternal hypotension. To prevent hypotension, large volumes of crystalloid solutions (10–20 ml·kg⁻¹) are conventionally infused before regional anesthesia. However, hypotension occurred in 55% of patients receiving crystalloid (20 ml·kg⁻¹) preloading, despite left uterine displacement, in comparison to 71% of patients not receiving preloading.[63] In contrast, preloading with 5% albumin solution in Ringer's lactate (15 ml·kg⁻¹) avoided hypotension in comparison to a 30% incidence in a crystalloid group preloaded with crystalloid[64]; the clinical and biochemical status of the infants of mothers receiving albumin was superior. Because most clinical studies evaluated the relative efficacy of crystalloid or colloid solutions used for preloading in terms of blood pressure rather than cardiac output, systemic oxygen transport, or uteroplacental flow, further research defining the effects of preload on maternal and fetal outcome is required.

Colloids, Crystalloids, and Hypertonic Solutions

Physiology and Pharmacology

Osmotically active particles attract water across semipermeable membranes until equilibrium is attained. The *osmolarity* of a solution refers to the number of osmotically active particles per

Table 9-14. AVERAGE VOLUMES AND ELECTROLYTE COMPOSITION OF GASTROINTESTINAL SECRETIONS

Source	Volume (ml·day⁻¹)	Na⁺ (mEq·l⁻¹)	K⁺ (mEq·l⁻¹)	Cl⁻ (mEq·l⁻¹)	HCO₃⁻ (mEq·l⁻¹)
Gastric	1500	60	10	130	—
Ileal	3000	140	5	104	30
Pancreatic	400	140	5	75	115
Biliary	400	140	5	100	35

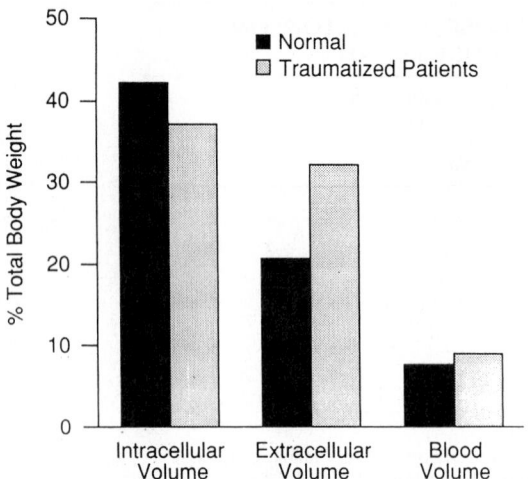

Figure 9-6. In comparison with normal individuals, patients recently subjected to severe trauma (fluid and blood requirements exceeding an average of 21 liters on the day of admission) have a slight decrease in intracellular volume (as percentage of body weight) and an increase in extracellular volume and blood volume. (Data redrawn with permission from Böck JC, Barker BC, Clinton AG *et al:* Post-traumatic changes in, and effect of colloid osmotic pressure on the distribution of body water. Ann Surg 210:395, 1989.)

liter of solvent; *osmolality,* a measurement of the number of osmotically active particles per *kilogram,* can be estimated as follows:

$$\text{Osmolality} = ([Na^+] \times 2) + (\text{glucose}/18) + (\text{BUN}/2.3) \quad (9\text{-}10)$$

where osmolality is expressed in millimoles per kilogram ($mmol \cdot kg^{-1}$), $[Na^+]$ is expressed in milliequivalents per liter ($mEq \cdot ll^{-1}$), serum glucose is expressed in milligrams per deciliter ($mg \cdot dl^{-1}$), and BUN is blood urea nitrogen expressed in $mg \cdot dl^{-1}$. Sugars, alcohols, and radiographic dyes increase measured osmolality, generating an increased "osmolal gap" between the measured and calculated values.

A hyperosmolar state occurs whenever the concentration of osmotically active particles is high. Both uremia (increased BUN) and hypernatremia (increased serum sodium) increase serum osmolality. However, because urea distributes throughout TBW, an increase in BUN does not cause *hypertonicity.* Sodium, largely restricted to the ECV, causes hypertonicity, that is, osmotically mediated redistribution of water from ICV to ECV. The term "tonicity" is also used colloquially to compare the osmotic pressure of a parenteral solution to that of plasma.

Although osmotically active particles in blood represent only a small proportion of plasma proteins, those particles are essential in determining the equilibrium of fluid between the interstitial and plasma compartments of ECV. The reflection coefficient (σ) describes the permeability of capillary membranes to individual solutes, with 0 representing free permeability and 1.0 representing complete impermeability. The reflection coefficient for albumin ranges from 0.6 to 0.9 in various capillary beds. Because capillary protein concentrations exceed interstitial concentrations, the osmotic pressure exerted by plasma proteins (termed *colloid osmotic pressure* or *oncotic pressure*) is higher than interstitial oncotic pressure and tends to preserve PV. The filtration rate of fluid from the capillaries into the interstitial space is the net result of a combination of forces, including the gradient from intravascular to interstitial colloid osmotic pressures and the hydrostatic gradient between intravascular and interstitial pressures. The net fluid filtration at any point within a systemic or pulmonary capillary is represented by Starling's law of capillary filtration, as expressed in the equation:

$$Q = kA[(P_c - P_i) + \sigma(\pi_i + \pi_c)] \quad (9\text{-}11)$$

where Q is fluid filtration, k is the capillary filtration coefficient (conductivity of water), A is the area of the capillary membrane, P_c is capillary hydrostatic pressure, P_i is interstitial hydrostatic pressure, σ is the reflection coefficient for albumin, π_i is interstitial colloid osmotic pressure, and π_c is capillary colloid osmotic pressure.

The IF volume is determined by the relative rates of capillary filtration and lymphatic drainage. P_c, the most powerful factor promoting fluid filtration, is determined by capillary flow, arterial resistance, venous resistance, and venous pressure.[65] If capillary filtration increases, the rates of water and sodium filtration usually exceed protein filtration, resulting in preservation of π_c, dilution of π_i, and preservation of the oncotic pressure gradient, the most powerful factor opposing fluid filtration. When coupled with increased lymphatic drainage, preservation of the oncotic pressure gradient limits the accumulation of IF. If P_c increases at a time when lymphatic drainage is maximal, then IF accumulates, forming edema. In chronic edematous states, IF pressure is reduced by enhanced lymphatic drainage through dilated lymphatic vessels.[66] Increased fluid filtration also dilutes the proteoglycan matrix in the IF, increasing capillary permeability; dehydration of the interstitium reduces vascular permeability.[65]

Clinical Implications of Choices Between Alternative Fluids

If membrane permeability is intact, colloids such as albumin or hydroxyethyl starch preferentially expand PV rather than IF volume. Concentrated colloid-containing solutions (*e.g.,* 25% albumin) may exert sufficient oncotic pressure to translocate substantial volumes of IF into the PV. PV expansion unaccompanied by IF expansion offers apparent advantages: lower fluid requirements, less peripheral and pulmonary edema accumulation, and reduced concern about the cardiopulmonary consequences of later fluid mobilization.

However, exhaustive research has failed to establish the superiority of either colloid-containing or crystalloid-containing fluids (Table 9-15). Systematic reviews of available comparisons of colloid versus crystalloid[67] and albumin *versus* crystalloid[68] suggest increased mortality associated with colloid use. Other reviews suggest that crystalloid may be superior in multiply traumatized patients.[69,70]

Much of the debate has centered on the relative risk of pulmonary edema. Crystalloid infusion can increase P_c and reduce π_c. Colloid can also produce increases, often of greater duration,

Table 9-15. ADVANTAGES AND DISADVANTAGES OF COLLOID VS. CRYSTALLOID INTRAVENOUS FLUIDS

Solution	Advantages	Disadvantages
Colloid	Smaller infused volume	Greater cost
	Prolonged increase in plasma volume	Coagulopathy (dextran > HES)
	Greater peripheral edema	Pulmonary edema (capillary leak states)
	Less cerebral edema	Decreased GFR
		Osmotic diuresis (low molecular weight dextran)
Crystalloid	Lower cost	Transient hemodynamic improvement
	Greater urinary flow	Peripheral edema (protein dilution)
	Replaces interstitial fluid	Pulmonary edema (protein dilution plus high PAOP)

HES = hydroxyethyl starch; GFR = glomerular filtration rate; PAOP = pulmonary arterial occlusion pressure.

in P_c. Moreover, in sepsis or the adult respiratory distress syndrome, increased microvascular permeability decreases the gradient between π_c and π_i. If the oncotic pressure gradient is decreased, minimal increases in hydrostatic pressure can produce clinically important pulmonary edema. After experimentally increasing microvascular permeability, Pearl *et al* found no differences between increases in extravascular lung water induced by colloid or crystalloid.[71] In contrast, albumin therapy slowed extrapulmonary edema accumulation in sheep with sepsis produced by cecal ligation and puncture.[72]

Hypoproteinemia in critically ill patients has been associated with the development of pulmonary edema[73] and with increased mortality,[74] although either crystalloid or colloid administration may precipitate pulmonary edema in patients who have heart failure. In surgical patients at risk for the development of pulmonary edema, pulmonary arterial catheterization may facilitate management. Pulmonary arterial occlusion pressure (PAOP) should be maintained at the lowest level compatible with adequate systemic perfusion. Theoretically, hemodynamic monitoring coupled with volume expansion with colloid (to preserve π_c) should minimize edema formation. However, Virgilio *et al* found no correlation in surgical patients between intrapulmonary shunt fraction (Q_s/Q_t) and the π_c–PAOP gradient.[75]

Although hydroxyethyl starch, the most commonly used synthetic colloid, is less expensive than albumin, large doses produce laboratory evidence of coagulopathy.[76] Nevertheless, 6.0% hydroxyethyl starch, used in recommended volumes (10–15 $ml \cdot kg^{-1}$), was not associated with clinically important coagulopathy in patients undergoing abdominal aneurysm repair,[77] major abdominal surgery,[78] or cardiac surgery.[79] Recently, a new hydroxyethyl starch formulation has been introduced that contains a different mix of molecular sizes and is dissolved in a base consisting of a balanced salt solution rather than 0.9% saline. Proposed advantages of the new formulation include less risk of inducing coagulopathy and of hyperchloremic metabolic acidosis.[80]

Implications of Crystalloid and Colloid Infusions on Intracranial Pressure

Because the cerebral capillary membrane, the blood–brain barrier, is highly impermeable to protein, clinicians have assumed that administration of colloid-containing solutions should increase ICP less than crystalloid solutions. In anesthetized rabbits, plasmapheresis to reduce plasma osmolality by 13 $mOsm \cdot kg^{-1}$ (baseline value = 295 $mOsm \cdot kg^{-1}$) increased cortical water content and ICP; reducing colloid osmotic pressure from 20 to 7 mm Hg produced no significant change in either variable.[81] Of course, because a reduction of 13 $mOsm \cdot kg^{-1}$ is equivalent to a reduction in osmotic pressure that is nearly 20-fold greater, the most important message of this report may simply be that much greater changes in osmotic pressure are possible as a consequence of changing serum sodium concentration than as a consequence of changing protein concentration. Similar independence of brain water and ICP from colloid osmotic pressure has been demonstrated with prolonged hypoalbuminemia[82] and in animals after forebrain ischemia[83] and focal cryogenic injury.[84] In contrast, after fluid percussion brain injury, increasing colloid oncotic pressure with hetastarch reduced brain water in comparison to infusion of 0.9% saline (Fig. 9-7).[85]

Hypertonic Fluid Administration

An ideal alternative to conventional crystalloid and colloid fluids would be inexpensive, would produce minimal peripheral or pulmonary edema, would generate sustained hemodynamic effects, and would be effective even if administered in small volumes. Hypertonic, hypernatremic solutions appear to fulfill some of these criteria (Table 9-16).

Although for more than 75 years investigators have studied the physiologic effects of infusing hypertonic solutions,[86] the

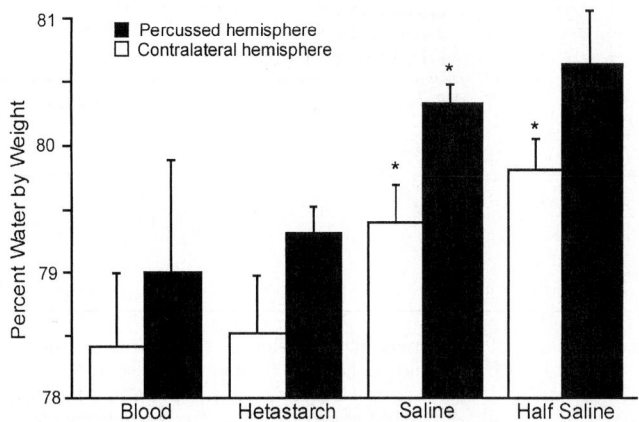

Figure 9-7. The percentage of water content (mean ± SD; wet–dry method) of the percussed (*right*) hemisphere and in the contralateral (*left*) hemisphere in animals that underwent isovolemic exchange with whole blood, hetastarch, normal saline, or half-normal saline. Within each group, the water content of the percussed hemisphere was greater than the water content of the contralateral hemisphere. *$P < 0.05$ versus the corresponding hemisphere in the whole blood and hetastarch groups. (Reproduced with permission from Drummond JC, Patel PM, Cole DJ, Kelly PJ: The effect of the reduction of colloid oncotic pressure, with and without reduction of osmolality, on post-traumatic cerebral edema. Anesthesiology 88:993, 1998.)

current enthusiasm was stimulated by the work of Velasco *et al*, who successfully used small volumes (6.0 $ml \cdot kg^{-1}$) of 7.5% hypertonic saline (HS) as the sole resuscitative measure in dogs after severe hemorrhage.[87] The mechanism by which HS solutions improve hemodynamics is through PV expansion.[88] Experimental evidence *in vivo* suggests that resuscitation with HS/HES (7.2% NaCl + 10% HES) may improve microvascular perfusion by attenuating leukocyte–endothelial interactions.[89] Although hyperosmotic saline solutions (usually 250–300 $mEq \cdot l^{-1}$ sodium) have been used clinically for many years for burn resuscitation, studies in animals[90] and humans[91] suggest limited value for that purpose.

Hypertonic solutions exert favorable effects on cerebral hemodynamics, in part because of the reciprocal relationship between plasma osmolality and brain water.[81] ICP increases during resuscitation from hemorrhagic shock with lactated Ringer's solution but remains unchanged if 7.5% saline is infused in a sufficient volume to comparably improve systemic hemodynamics.[92] In hemorrhaged rats subjected to mechanical brain injury, brain water content is lower in uninjured brain (but similar in injured brain) after resuscitation with a hyperosmotic solution.[93] In dogs with intracranial mass lesions, hypertonic solutions may also restore regional cerebral blood flow better than slightly hypotonic solutions.[92] If fluid resuscitation continues after immediate stabilization, differences between fluids of varying tonicity become negligible.[94] Moreover, delayed increases in ICP have been reported after hypertonic resuscitation from hypovolemic shock accompanied by an intracranial mass lesion (Fig. 9-8).[95]

To address concerns about central nervous system dysfunction due to hypertonicity and hypernatremia associated with HS, Wisner and associates demonstrated, using high-energy phosphate nuclear magnetic resonance spectroscopy, a decreased intracellular *p*H after HS resuscitation compared with lactated Ringer's solution.[96] However, this decrease was not attributable to anaerobic glycolysis, but to concentration of intracellular hydrogen ions in dehydrated cells.[96] In humans resuscitated with HS, acute increases in serum sodium to 155–160 $mEq \cdot l^{-1}$ produced no apparent harm.[97,98] Central pontine myelinolysis, which follows rapid correction of severe, chronic hyponatremia,[99] has not been observed in clinical trials of hypertonic resuscitation.

Table 9-16. HYPERTONIC RESUSCITATION FLUIDS: ADVANTAGES AND DISADVANTAGES

Solution	Advantages	Disadvantages
Hypertonic crystalloid	Inexpensive Promotes urinary flow Small initial volume Improved myocardial contractility? Arteriolar dilation Reduced peripheral edema Lower intracranial pressure	Hypertonicity Subdural hemorrhage Transient effect
Hypertonic crystalloid plus Colloid (in comparison to Hypertonic crystalloid alone)	Sustained hemodynamic response Reduced subsequent volume requirements	Added expense Coagulopathy (dextran > HES) Osmotic diuresis Impaired crossmatch (dextran) Hypertonicity

HES = hydroxyethyl starch.
(Reproduced with permission from Prough DS, Johnston WE: Fluid resuscitation in septic shock: No solution yet. Anesth Analg 69:699, 1989.)

Unfortunately, systemic hemodynamic improvement produced by hypertonic resuscitation is short-lived. After initial improvement, both cerebral blood flow and cardiac output rapidly decline after single-dose resuscitation of hypovolemic dogs with either 0.8% or 7.2% saline.[92] Strategies to prolong the therapeutic effects beyond 30–60 minutes include continued infusion of hypertonic saline, subsequent infusion of blood or conventional fluids, or addition of colloid to hypertonic resuscitation. In hemorrhaged animals, adding 6.0% dextran 70 to 7.5% saline increased the duration of hemodynamic improvement when compared with equal volumes of hypertonic saline, sodium bicarbonate, or sodium chloride/sodium acetate.[100] Vassar et al evaluated the effects of 250 ml of 7.5% sodium chloride with and without 6% and 12% dextran 70 for the prehospital resuscitation of hypotensive trauma patients.[97] Addition of dextran did not improve the blood pressure changes associated with administration of hypertonic saline alone. A small subgroup of patients with Glasgow Coma Scale scores <8, but without severe anatomic injury seemed to benefit most from hypertonic resuscitation.[97] Mattox et al reported improved survival in traumatized patients initially resuscitated with 7.5% saline and requiring surgery.[98]

The least encouraging observations regarding hyperosmotic resuscitation involve models of uncontrolled hemorrhage,[101] in which restoration of blood pressure increases bleeding and may adversely affect mortality.[101] In urban trauma patients, Bickell et al have reported that immediate, prehospital resuscitation does not improve mortality in comparison to resuscitation initiated only after arrival at the hospital.[102]

The clinical efficacy of hypertonic resuscitation in comparison to conventional fluids remains unclear because many preclinical studies have compared the effects of single boluses of experimental and control fluids. In contrast, clinical fluid resuscitation continues until no additional fluid is required. An attempt to simulate clinical resuscitation necessitates a choice among a variety of possible goals of resuscitation. Comparison of two or more resuscitation regimens that alter more than one variable may generate misleading conclusions. For example, because hypertonic fluids reduce systemic vascular resistance, systolic ventricular ejection may improve, leading to decreased PAOP; theoretically, therefore, more fluid would be necessary to restore a filling pressure similar to that produced by a colloid solution.

More physiologically sophisticated goals, also based on invasive monitoring, have been proposed. Oxygen delivery ($\dot{D}o_2$), a theoretically attractive end point for resuscitation, combines in a single term cardiac index (CI) and arterial oxygen content (Pao$_2$) according to the equation:

$$\dot{D}o_2 = CI \times Cao_2 \times 10 \qquad (9\text{-}12)$$

where the factor 10 corrects Paco$_2$, usually measured in ml O$_2 \cdot$ dl^{-1}, to ml $\cdot$ l^{-1}. However, because non-blood–containing fluid resuscitation both increases cardiac output and decreases

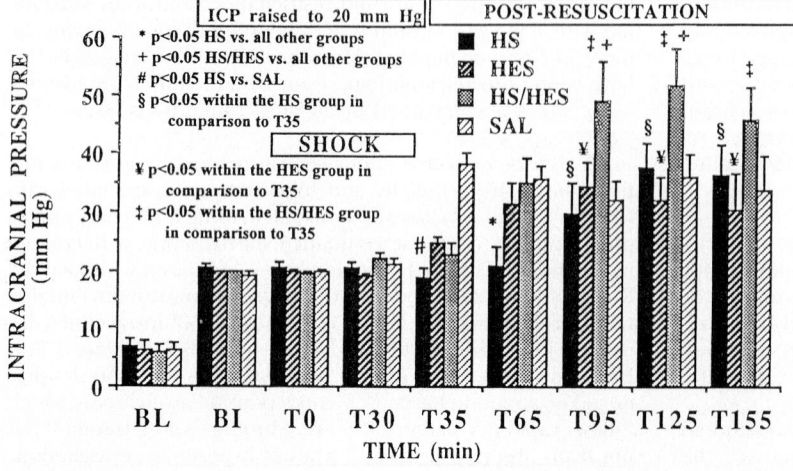

Figure 9-8. Response of intracranial pressure after resuscitation from hemorrhage shock with 0.8% saline (SAL), hypertonic 7.2% saline (HS), 20% hydroxyethyl starch (HES), or hyperoncotic hydroxyethyl starch (HS/HES). Intracranial hypertension induced by inflation of a subdural balloon accompanied hemorrhage. BL = baseline; BI = balloon inflation; T0 = initiation of hemorrhage; T30 = end of hemorrhage and initiation of resuscitation; T35 = end of resuscitation; T65, T95, T125, and T155 = 30, 60, 90, and 120 minutes, respectively, after resuscitation. (Reproduced with permission from Prough DS, Whitley JM, Taylor CL et al: Rebound intracranial hypertension in dogs after resuscitation with hypertonic solutions from hemorrhagic shock accompanied by an intracranial mass lesion. J Neurosurg Anesth 11:102, 1999).

hemoglobin concentration, the application of $\dot{D}o_2$ as a goal poses practical difficulties. Despite the straightforward arithmetic implications of simultaneous increases in cardiac output and decreases in $Paco_2$, many clinicians attempt to increase cardiac output (whether or not it is directly measured) as a goal during rapid volume expansion.

Will clinicians routinely use hypertonic or combination hypertonic/hyperoncotic fluids for resuscitation in the future? Pending further preclinical work, the theoretical advantages of such fluids appear most attractive in the acute resuscitation of hypovolemic patients who have decreased intracranial compliance.[103]

Fluid Status: Assessment and Monitoring

Assessment of Hypovolemia and Tissue Hypoperfusion

For most surgical patients, conventional clinical assessment of the adequacy of intravascular volume is appropriate. For high-risk patients, goal-directed hemodynamic management may be superior.

Conventional Clinical Assessment. Clinical quantification of blood volume and ECV begins with recognition of deficit-generating settings, such as bowel obstruction, preoperative bowel preparation, chronic diuretic use, sepsis, burns, and trauma. Physical signs that suggest hypovolemia include oliguria, supine hypotension, and a positive tilt test. Oliguria implies hypovolemia, although hypovolemic patients may be nonoliguric and normovolemic patients may be oliguric because of renal failure or stress-induced endocrine responses.[104] Supine hypotension implies a blood volume deficit exceeding 30%, although arterial blood pressure within the normal range could represent relative hypotension in an elderly or chronically hypertensive patient.

In the *tilt test*, a positive response is defined as an increase in heart rate by ≥ 20 beats $\cdot$ min^{-1} and a decrease in systolic blood pressure by ≥ 20 mm Hg when the subject assumes the upright position. However, young, healthy subjects can withstand acute loss of 20% of blood volume while exhibiting only postural tachycardia and variable postural hypotension. In contrast, orthostasis may occur in 20% to 30% of elderly patients despite normal blood volume.[105] In volunteers, withdrawal of 500 ml of blood[106] was associated with a greater increase in heart rate on standing than before blood withdrawal but no significant difference in the response of blood pressure or cardiac index. Orthostatic changes in filling pressure, assessed before and after fluid infusion, may represent a more sensitive test of the adequacy of circulating blood volume.[107]

Laboratory evidence that suggests hypovolemia or ECV depletion includes azotemia, low urinary sodium, metabolic alkalosis, and metabolic acidosis. Hematocrit is virtually unchanged by acute hemorrhage until fluids are administered or until fluid shifts from the interstitial to the intravascular space. BUN, normally 8–20 mg $\cdot$ dl^{-1}, is increased by hypovolemia, high protein intake, gastrointestinal bleeding, or accelerated catabolism and decreased by severe hepatic dysfunction. Serum creatinine (SCr), a product of muscle catabolism, may be misleadingly low in elderly adults, females, and debilitated or malnourished patients. In contrast, in muscular or acutely catabolic patients, SCr may exceed the normal range (0.5–1.5 mg $\cdot$ dl^{-1}) because of more rapid muscle breakdown. A ratio of BUN:SCr exceeding the normal range (10–20) suggests dehydration. In prerenal oliguria, enhanced sodium reabsorption should reduce urinary [Na$^+$] to ≤ 20 mEq $\cdot$ l^{-1} and enhanced water reabsorption should increase urinary concentration (*i.e.,* urinary osmolality >400; urine/plasma creatinine ratio >40:1). However, the sensitivity and specificity of measurements of urinary variables may be misleading. Although hypovolemia does not generate metabolic alkalosis, ECV depletion is a potent stimulus for the maintenance of metabolic alkalosis. Severe hypovolemia may result in systemic hypoperfusion and lactic acidosis.

Intraoperative Clinical Assessment. Visual estimation, the simplest technique for quantifying intraoperative blood loss, assesses the amount of blood absorbed by gauze squares and laparotomy pads and adds an estimate of blood accumulation on the floor and surgical drapes and in suction containers. Both surgeons and anesthesia providers tend to underestimate losses.

Assessment of the adequacy of intraoperative fluid resuscitation integrates multiple clinical variables, including heart rate, blood pressure, urinary output, arterial oxygenation, and pH. Tachycardia is an insensitive, nonspecific indicator of hypovolemia. In patients receiving potent inhalational agents, maintenance of a satisfactory blood pressure implies adequate intravascular volume. Preservation of blood pressure, accompanied by a CVP of 6–12 mm Hg, more strongly suggests adequate replacement. During profound hypovolemia, indirect measurements of blood pressure may significantly underestimate true blood pressure. In patients undergoing extensive procedures, direct arterial pressure measurements are more accurate than indirect techniques and provide convenient access for obtaining arterial blood samples. An additional advantage of direct arterial pressure monitoring may be recognition of increased systolic blood pressure variation accompanying positive pressure ventilation in the presence of hypovolemia.[108–111]

Urinary output usually declines precipitously during moderate to severe hypovolemia. Therefore, in the absence of glycosuria or diuretic administration, a urinary output of 0.5–1.0 ml $\cdot$ kg^{-1} $\cdot$ hr^{-1} during anesthesia suggests adequate renal perfusion. Arterial pH may decrease only when tissue hypoperfusion becomes severe. Cardiac output can be normal despite severely reduced regional blood flow. Mixed venous hemoglobin desaturation, a specific indicator of poor systemic perfusion, reflects average perfusion in multiple organs and cannot supplant regional monitors such as urinary output.

Oxygen Delivery as a Goal of Management. No intraoperative monitor is sufficiently sensitive or specific to detect hypoperfusion in all patients. Moreover, acute renal failure, hepatic failure, and sepsis may result from unrecognized, subclinical tissue hypoperfusion. In high-risk surgical patients, average cardiac output and $\dot{D}o_2$ are greater in those who survive than in those who succumb.[112,113] One key variable that has been associated with survival is a $\dot{D}o_2 \geq 600$ ml $O_2 \cdot m^{-2} \cdot min^{-1}$ (equivalent to a CI of 3.0 l $\cdot m^{-2} \cdot min^{-1}$, a hemoglobin concentration of 14 g $\cdot$ dl^{-1}, and 98% oxyhemoglobin saturation). Boyd *et al* randomized 107 patients to conventional treatment or fluid plus dopexamine to maintain oxygen delivery ≥ 600 ml $O_2 \cdot m^{-2} \cdot min^{-1}$ and demonstrated a decrease in mortality and in the number of complications in the patients managed at the higher level of oxygen delivery.[114] Based on these results, the authors calculated that the cost of obtaining a survivor was 31% lower in the protocol group.[115] Wilson *et al* randomized 138 patients undergoing major elective surgery into three groups.[116] One group received routine perioperative care; one received fluid and dopexamine preoperatively, intraoperatively, and postoperatively to maintain oxygen delivery ≥ 600 ml $O_2 \cdot m^{-2} \cdot min^{-1}$; and the third received fluid plus epinephrine preoperatively, intraoperatively, and postoperatively to achieve the same end points. In the two groups in which oxygen delivery was supported, only 3 of 92 died, compared to 8 of 46 control patients. However, the complication rate was significantly lower in the dopexamine group than in the epinephrine group. In contrast, Hayes *et al*, who randomized 109 patients to conventional treatment, or oxygen delivery ≥ 600 ml $O_2 \cdot m^{-2} \cdot min^{-1}$, using a combination of volume and dobutamine, demonstrated an increase in mortality in the treatment group maintained at the higher levels. They speculated that aggressive elevations in $\dot{D}o_2$ actually may have been harmful.[117] At present, available data are consistent with two inferences. First, there is no apparent benefit for patients other than surgical patients.[118] Second, outcome may be strongly influenced by the choice of inotropic agents. One possibility is that dopexamine is associated with fewer complications because it better preserves splanchnic perfusion and is associated with reduced secretion of vasoactive hormones during major abdominal surgery.[119]

ELECTROLYTES

Sodium

Physiologic Role

Increases or decreases in total body sodium, the principal extracellular cation and solute, tend to increase or decrease ECV and PV. Disorders of sodium concentration—hyponatremia and hypernatremia—usually result from relative excesses or deficits, respectively, of water. Sodium also is essential for generation of action potentials in neurologic and cardiac tissue.

Regulation of the quantity and concentration of sodium is accomplished primarily by the endocrine and renal systems (Table 9-17). *Total body sodium* is controlled by secretion of aldosterone and ANP. *Sodium concentration* is primarily regulated by ADH, which is secreted in response to increased osmolality or decreased blood pressure. ADH stimulates renal reabsorption of water, diluting plasma [Na^+]; inadequate ADH secretion results in renal free water excretion, which, in the absence of adequate water intake, results in hypernatremia.

Hyponatremia

Hyponatremia ([Na^+] < 130 mEq · l^{-1}) indicates that body fluids are diluted by an excess of water relative to total solute. The majority of hyponatremic, hospitalized patients have normal or increased quantities of total body sodium. Usually, hyponatremia results from impaired urinary diluting capacity although the causes of the impairment are diverse.

Hyponatremia is the most common electrolyte disturbance in hospitalized patients.[120] The most common clinical circumstances associated with hyponatremia are the postoperative state (30% of patients), followed by acute intracranial disease (17%), malignant disease (17%), medications (9%), and pneumonia (5%).[120] Although hyponatremia is associated with a 7- to 60-fold increase in mortality,[120,121] it is unclear whether the increased mortality is a direct effect of hyponatremia or whether hyponatremia simply serves as a secondary marker of severe systemic disease.[41]

The signs and symptoms of hyponatremia depend on both the rate and severity of the decrease in plasma [Na^+]. Symptoms that can accompany severe hyponatremia ([Na^+] < 120 mEq · l^{-1}) include loss of appetite, nausea, vomiting, cramps, weakness, altered level of consciousness, coma, and seizures.

Acute central nervous system (CNS) manifestations relate to brain overhydration. Because the blood–brain barrier is poorly

Table 9-17. REGULATION OF ELECTROLYTES

Electrolyte	Regulated by
Sodium	Aldosterone
	ANP
	[Na^+] altered by ADH
Potassium	Aldosterone
	Epinephrine
	Insulin
	Intrinsic renal mechanisms
Calcium	PTH
	Vitamin D
Phosphorus	Primarily renal mechanisms
	Minor: PTH
Magnesium	Primarily renal mechanisms
	Minor: PTH, vitamin D

ANP = atrial natriuretic peptide; [Na^+] = sodium concentration; ADH = antidiuretic hormone; PTH = parathyroid hormone.

permeable to sodium but freely permeable to water, a decrease in plasma [Na^+] promptly increases both extracellular and intracellular brain water. Compensatory responses to cerebral edema include bulk movement of interstitial fluid into the cerebrospinal fluid and loss of intracellular solutes,[122] including potassium and organic osmolytes (previously termed "idiogenic osmoles") such as taurine, phosphocreatine, myoinositol, glutamine, and glutamate.[123] Because the brain rapidly compensates for changes in osmolality, the symptoms are considerably more severe in acute than in chronic hyponatremia. The symptoms of chronic hyponatremia probably relate to depletion of brain electrolytes. Once brain volume has compensated for hyponatremia, rapid correction may lead to abrupt brain dehydration.

Hyponatremia is classified as true hyponatremia or pseudohyponatremia. Pseudohyponatremia was diagnosed in severely hyperproteinemic or hyperlipidemic patients when flame photometry, now an archaic technique, was used to measure plasma [Na^+]. Because hyperproteinemia or hyperlipidemia displaced water from plasma, plasma [Na^+] measurements were artifactually depressed. The current analytic method, direct potentiometry, directly measures [Na^+][41] and is uninfluenced by nonaqueous components.

True hyponatremia may be associated with normal, high, or low serum osmolality. In turn, hyponatremia with hypo-osmolality is associated with a high, low, or normal total body sodium and PV. Hyponatremia ([Na^+] < 135 mEq · l^{-1}) with a normal or high serum osmolality results from the presence of a nonsodium solute, such as glucose or mannitol, which does not diffuse freely across cell membranes (Fig. 9-9). The resulting osmotic gradient results in dilutional hyponatremia. For instance, plasma [Na^+] decreases approximately 1.6 mEq · l^{-1} for each 100 mg · dl^{-1} rise in glucose concentration.[124] In anesthesia practice, a common cause of hyponatremia associated with a normal osmolality is the absorption of large volumes of sodium-free irrigating solutions (containing mannitol, glycerine, or sorbitol as the solute) during transurethral resection of the prostate.[125] These solutes cause a dilutional hyponatremia that is responsible for the clinical features of the *TURP syndrome*[126,127] (see Chapter 36). Neurologic symptoms are minimal if mannitol is employed because the agent does not cross the blood–brain barrier and is excreted with water in the urine. In contrast, as glycine or sorbitol is metabolized, hyposmolality will gradually develop and cerebral edema may appear as a late complication.[125] A discrepancy exceeding 10 mOsm · kg^{-1} between measured and calculated osmolality suggests either factitious hyponatremia or the presence of a nonsodium solute.

True hyponatremia with a normal or elevated serum osmolality may occur in renal insufficiency. BUN, included in the calculation of total osmolality, distributes throughout both ECV and ICV. Calculation of *effective* osmolality (2[Na^+] + glucose/18) demonstrates true hypotonicity.

Hyponatremia with hyposmolality (Fig. 9-9) is evaluated by assessing BUN, SCr, total body sodium content, urinary osmolality, and urinary [Na^+]. Hyponatremia with increased total body sodium is characteristic of edematous states—congestive heart failure, cirrhosis, nephrosis, and renal failure. Aquaporin 2, the vasopressin-regulated water channel, is upregulated in experimental congestive heart failure[128] and cirrhosis[129] and decreased by chronic vasopressin stimulation.[130] In patients with renal insufficiency, reduced urinary diluting capacity can lead to hyponatremia if excess free water is given.

The underlying mechanism of hypovolemic hyponatremia is ongoing oral or intravenous intake of hypotonic fluid during secretion of ADH in response to volume contraction.[131] Angiotensin II also decreases free water generation.[41] Thiazide diuretics, unlike loop diuretics, promote hypovolemic hyponatremia by interfering with urinary dilution in the distal tubule.[131] Hypovolemic hyponatremia associated with a urinary [Na^+] > 20 mmol · l^{-1} suggests mineralocorticoid deficiency, especially if serum [K^+], BUN, and SCr are increased.[131]

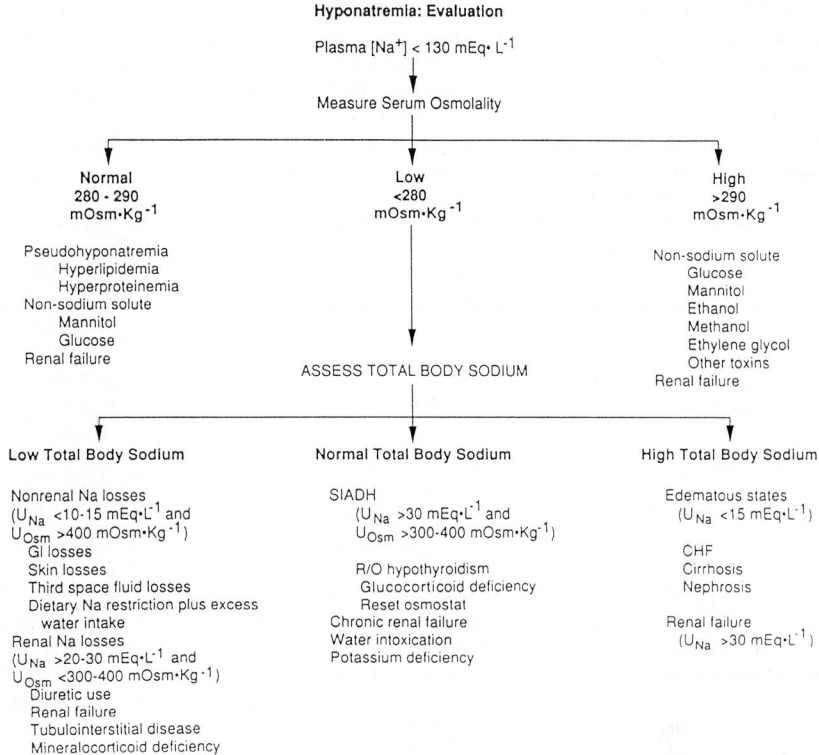

Figure 9-9. Algorithm by which hyponatremia can be evaluated.

The cerebral salt-wasting syndrome is an often severe, symptomatic salt-losing diathesis that appears to be mediated by brain natriuretic peptide[132] and is independent of the syndrome of inappropriate antidiuretic hormone (SIADH); patients at risk include those with cerebral lesions due to trauma, subarachnoid hemorrhage, tumors, and infection.[133–136]

Euvolemic hyponatremia is most commonly associated with nonosmotic vasopressin secretion, such as glucocorticoid deficiency, hypothyroidism, thiazide-induced hyponatremia, SIADH, and the reset osmostat syndrome.[41] Total body sodium and ECV are relatively normal and edema is rarely evident. SIADH may be idiopathic but also is associated with diseases of the central nervous system and with pulmonary disease (Table 9-18). Euvolemic hyponatremia is usually associated with exogenous ADH administration, pharmacologic potentiation of ADH action, drugs that mimic the action of ADH in the renal tubules or excessive ectopic ADH secretion. Tissues from some small-cell lung cancers, duodenal cancers, and pancreatic cancers increase ADH production in response to osmotic stimulation.[137]

The occasional postoperative occurrence of hyponatremia, mental status changes, and seizures has been attributed conventionally to intravenous administration of hypotonic fluids and inappropriate secretion of ADH. However, ADH is only one of many factors, including drugs, intravenous fluid administration, and renal function, that influence perioperative water balance.[138] At least 4.0% of postoperative patients develop plasma $[Na^+] < 130$ mEq $\cdot$ l^{-1}.[139] Although neurologic manifestations usually do not accompany postoperative hyponatremia, signs of hypervolemia are occasionally present.[139] Smaller patients change plasma $[Na^+]$ more in response to similar volumes of hypotonic fluids. In an editorial accompanying a report[140] of apparent postoperative SIADH in a 30-kg, 10-year-old-girl, Arieff[141] suggested that children receive no sodium-free water perioperatively. Women may be particularly vulnerable because estrogens stimulate and androgens suppress ADH release.[142,143] In extreme cases, administration of hypotonic fluids to young, healthy, female surgical patients has resulted in severe neurologic symptoms and death secondary to transtentorial hernia-

tion.[144] However, in experimental animals, hyponatremia produced greater brain swelling in males than females.[145]

Postoperative hyponatremia can develop, even with infusion of isotonic fluids, if ADH is persistently increased.[146] Steele *et al*[146] studied 22 women (mean age 42 years) undergoing uncomplicated gynecologic surgery. Twenty-four hours after surgery, mean plasma $[Na^+]$ had decreased from 140 ± 1 mEq $\cdot$ l^{-1} to

Table 9-18. CAUSES OF THE SYNDROME OF INAPPROPRIATE SECRETION OF ANTIDIURETIC HORMONE (SIADH)

Neoplasms	Pulmonary diseases
Bronchogenic carcinoma	Tuberculosis
Pancreatic carcinoma	Pneumonia
Carcinoma of the duodenum	Bronchiectasis
Prostate carcinoma	Aspergillosis
Thymoma	Cystic fibrosis
Lymphoma	Positive pressure ventilation
Mesothelioma	Medications
Central nervous system diseases	Opiates
Head trauma	Chlorpropamide
Subdural hematoma	Carbamazepine
Subarachnoid hemorrhage	Phenothiazines
Cerebrovascular accident	Tricyclic antidepressants
Meningitis	Clofibrate
Encephalitis	Vincristine
Brain abscess	Cyclophosphamide
Hydrocephalus	Oxytocin
Brain tumors	Miscellaneous
Guillain-Barré	General surgery
Acute intermittent porphyria	Pain
Delirium tremens	Nausea
	Psychosis

(Reprinted with permission from Fried LF, Palevsky PM: Hyponatremia and hypernatremia. In Saklayen MG (ed): The Medical Clinics of North America. Renal Disease, p 585. Philadelphia, WB Saunders, 1997.)

136 ± 0.5 mEq·l⁻¹.[146] Although the patients retained sodium perioperatively, they retained proportionately more water (an average of 1.1 l of electrolyte-free water). In a subsequent letter to the editor, Ayus and Arieff[147] stated that of 158 patients studied because of perioperative hyponatremic encephalopathy, none had received isotonic saline; the authors advised against routine perioperative use of hypotonic fluids. Careful postoperative attention to fluid and electrolyte balance may minimize the occurrence of symptomatic hyponatremia.

If both [Na⁺] and measured osmolality are below the normal range, hyponatremia is further evaluated by first assessing volume status using physical findings and laboratory data. In hypovolemic patients or edematous patients, the ratio of BUN to SCr should be >20:1. Urinary [Na⁺] is generally <15 mEq·l⁻¹ in edematous states and volume depletion and >20 mEq·l⁻¹ in hyponatremia secondary to renal salt wasting or renal failure with water retention.

The criteria for the diagnosis of SIADH include hypotonic hyponatremia, urinary osmolality >100–150 mmol·kg⁻¹, absence of extracellular volume depletion, normal thyroid and adrenal function, and normal cardiac, hepatic, and renal function.[41] Urinary [Na⁺] should be >30 mEq·l⁻¹ unless fluids have been restricted. Arieff[141] has argued that the diagnosis of SIADH may be inaccurately applied to postoperative patients because they are frequently functionally hypovolemic. Therefore, ADH secretion, by definition, would be "appropriate."

Treatment of hyponatremia associated with a normal or high serum osmolality requires reduction of the elevated concentrations of the responsible solute. Uremic patients are treated by free-water restriction or dialysis. Treatment of edematous (hypervolemic) patients necessitates restriction of both sodium and water (Fig. 9-10). Therapy is directed toward improving cardiac output and renal perfusion and using diuretics to inhibit sodium reabsorption. In hypovolemic, hyponatremic patients, blood volume must be restored, usually by infusion of 0.9% saline, and excessive sodium losses must be curtailed. Correction of hypovolemia usually results in removal of the stimulus for ADH release, accompanied by a rapid water diuresis.

The cornerstone of SIADH management is free-water restriction and elimination of precipitating causes. Water restriction, sufficient to decrease TBW by 0.5–1.0 l per day, decreases ECV even if excessive ADH secretion continues. The resultant reduction in GFR enhances proximal tubular reabsorption of salt and water, thereby decreasing free-water generation, and stimulates aldosterone secretion. As long as free-water losses (*i.e.*, renal, skin, gastrointestinal) exceed free-water intake, serum [Na⁺] will increase. During treatment of hyponatremia, increases in

plasma [Na⁺] are determined not only by the composition of the infused fluid, but also, to a major degree, by the rate of renal free-water excretion.[148] Free-water excretion can be increased by administering furosemide.

To calculate the net water loss necessary to increase [Na⁺] in hyponatremia, use the following equation:

$$\text{Current [Na}^+] \times \text{current TBW} = \text{desired [Na}^+] \times \text{desired TBW}$$

$$(9\text{-}13)$$

where TBW is total body water, usually approximately $0.6 \times$ total body weight (kg).[131]

Neurologic symptoms or profound hyponatremia ([Na⁺] < 115–120 mEq·l⁻¹) requires more aggressive therapy. Hypertonic (3%) saline is most clearly indicated in patients who have seizures or patients who acutely develop symptoms of water intoxication secondary to intravenous fluid administration. In such cases, 3% saline may be administered at a rate of 1–2 ml·kg⁻¹·hr⁻¹ to increase plasma [Na⁺] by 1–2 mEq·l⁻¹·hr⁻¹; however, this treatment should not continue for more than a few hours. Treatment of 25 hyponatremic children in this fashion promptly terminated seizures and resulted in no delayed neurologic sequelae.[149] Three percent saline may only transiently increase plasma [Na⁺] because ECV expansion results in increased urinary sodium excretion. Even 29.2% sodium chloride has been used safely in a dose of 50 ml in acute symptomatic hyponatremia.[150] Intravenous furosemide, combined with quantitative replacement of urinary sodium losses with 0.9% or 3.0% saline, can rapidly increase plasma [Na⁺], in part by increasing free-water clearance.

The rate of treatment of hyponatremia continues to generate controversy, extending from "too fast, too soon" to "too slow, too late." Although delayed correction may result in neurologic injury, inappropriately rapid correction may result in abrupt brain dehydration (Fig. 9-11) or permanent neurologic sequelae (*i.e.*, central pontine myelinolysis or the osmotic demyelination syndrome),[99,151,152] cerebral hemorrhage, or congestive heart failure. The symptoms of the osmotic demyelination syndrome vary from mild (transient behavioral disturbances or seizures) to severe (including pseudobulbar palsy and quadriparesis).[122,152] Within 3 to 4 weeks of the clinical onset of the syndrome, areas of demyelination are apparent on magnetic resonance imaging.[153]

The principal determinants of neurologic injury appear to be the magnitude and chronicity of hyponatremia and the rate of correction. The osmotic demyelination syndrome is more likely when hyponatremia has persisted >48 hours.[154] Experi-

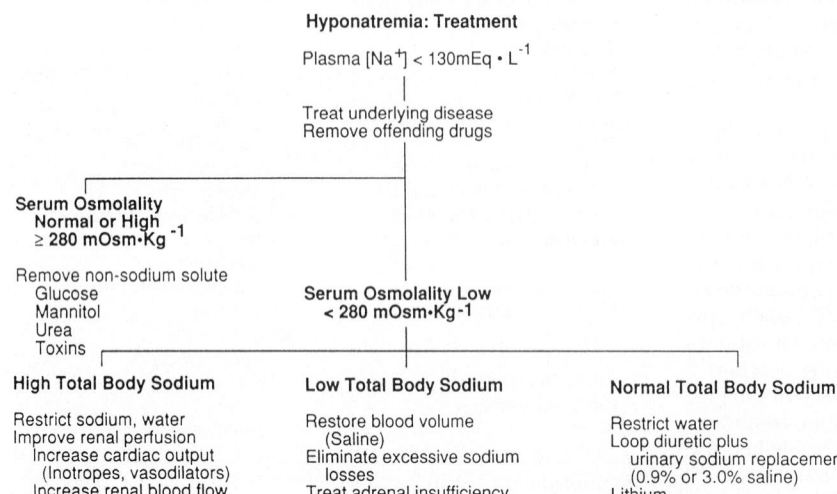

Hyponatremia: Treatment

Plasma [Na⁺] < 130mEq · L⁻¹

Treat underlying disease
Remove offending drugs

Serum Osmolality Normal or High ≥ 280 mOsm·Kg⁻¹

Remove non-sodium solute
  Glucose
  Mannitol
  Urea
  Toxins

Serum Osmolality Low < 280 mOsm·Kg⁻¹

High Total Body Sodium

Restrict sodium, water
Improve renal perfusion
  Increase cardiac output
  (Inotropes, vasodilators)
  Increase renal blood flow
  (Dopamine)

Low Total Body Sodium

Restore blood volume
  (Saline)
Eliminate excessive sodium
  losses
Treat adrenal insufficiency

Normal Total Body Sodium

Restrict water
Loop diuretic plus
  urinary sodium replacement
  (0.9% or 3.0% saline)
Lithium
Demeclocycline
Hemodialysis
Thyroid hormone replacement

Figure 9-10. Hyponatremia is treated according to the etiology of the disturbance, the level of serum osmolality, and a clinical estimation of total body sodium.

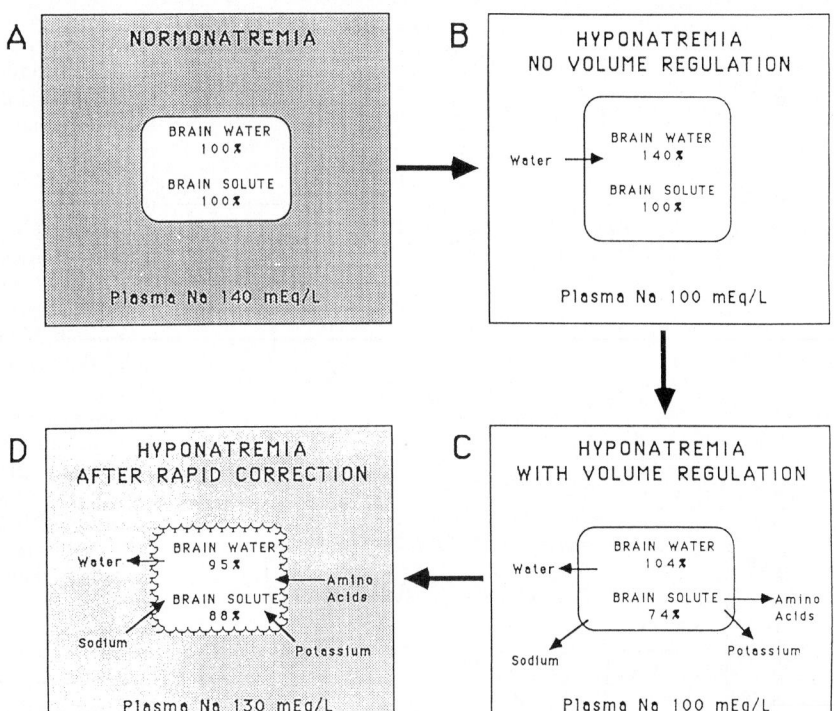

Figure 9-11. Brain water and solute in concentrations in hyponatremia. If normal plasma sodium (Na) (*A*) suddenly decreased, the increase in brain water theoretically would be proportional to the decrease in plasma Na (*B*). However, because of adaptive loss of cerebral intracellular solute, cerebral edema is minimized in chronic hyponatremia (*C*). Once adaptation has occurred, a rapid return of plasma Na concentration toward a normal level results in brain dehydration (*D*). (Reprinted with permission from Sterns RH: Vignettes in clinical pathophysiology. Neurological deterioration following treatment for hyponatremia. Am J Kidney Dis 13:434, 1989.)

mental demyelinating lesions are not observed if the rate of correction is <2.5 mEq · l⁻¹ · hr⁻¹ or if the magnitude of correction is limited to <25 mEq in 24 hours.[155] Most patients in whom the osmotic demyelination syndrome is fatal have undergone correction of plasma [Na⁺] of more than 20 mEq · l⁻¹ · day⁻¹.[152] Other risk factors for the development of this lesion include alcoholism, poor nutritional status, liver disease, burns, and hypokalemia.[156]

The clinician faces formidable difficulties in predicting the rate at which plasma [Na⁺] will increase. During treatment of hyponatremia, increases in plasma [Na⁺] are determined not only by the composition of the infused fluid, but also, to a major degree, by the rate of renal free water excretion.[148] The expected change in plasma [Na⁺] resulting from 1 liter of selected infusate can be estimated using the following equation[157]:

$$\Delta[\text{Na}^+]_s = \frac{[\text{Na}^+]_{\text{inf}} - [\text{Na}^+]_s}{\text{TBW} + 1} \qquad (9\text{-}14)$$

where $\Delta[\text{Na}^+]_s$ is the change in the patient's serum sodium, $[\text{Na}^+]_{\text{inf}}$ is the sodium concentration of the infusate, $[\text{Na}^+]_s$ is the patient's serum sodium concentration, TBW is the patient's estimated total body water in liters, and 1 is a factor added to take into account the volume of infusate.

Treatment should be interrupted or slowed when symptoms improve. Frequent determinations of [Na⁺] are important to prevent correction at a rate of >10 mEq · l⁻¹ over 24 hours.[154] Initially, plasma [Na⁺] may be increased by 1–2 mEq · l⁻¹ · hr⁻¹; however, plasma [Na⁺] should not be increased more than 10 mEq · l⁻¹ in 24 hours or 25 mEq · l⁻¹ in 48 hours.[120,158–162] Another proposed sequence for treating symptomatic hyponatremia is to increase [Na⁺] promptly by about 10 mmol, then to proceed more slowly. The rationale is that cerebral water is increased by approximately 10% in chronic hyponatremia.[131] Hypernatremia should be avoided. Once the plasma [Na⁺] exceeds 120–125 mEq · l⁻¹, water restriction alone is usually sufficient to normalize [Na⁺]. As acute hyponatremia is corrected, CNS signs and symptoms usually improve within 24 hours, although 96 hours may be necessary for maximal recovery.

Because lithium, the first drug used to antagonize ADH, is neurotoxic and has unpredictable effects, demeclocycline is now the drug of choice for patients who require long-term pharmacologic therapy.[131] Up to 50% of patients receiving lithium develop nephrogenic diabetes insipidus (NDI), probably because Aquaporin 2 is downregulated.[163] Although better tolerated than lithium, demeclocycline may induce nephrotoxicity, a particular concern in patients with hepatic dysfunction. Hemodialysis is occasionally necessary in severely hyponatremic patients who cannot be adequately managed with drugs or hypertonic saline. Once hyponatremia has improved, careful fluid restriction is necessary to avoid recurrence of hyponatremia. In the future, vasopressin receptor antagonists may be used to treat hyponatremia.[164]

Hypernatremia

Hypernatremia ([Na⁺] >150 mEq · l⁻¹) indicates an absolute or relative water deficit. Normally, minimal increases in tonicity or sodium stimulate thirst and ADH secretion. Severe, persistent hypernatremia occurs only in patients who cannot respond to thirst by voluntary ingestion of fluid—obtunded patients, anesthetized patients, and infants.

Hypernatremia produces neurologic symptoms (including stupor, coma, and seizures), hypovolemia, renal insufficiency (occasionally progressing to renal failure), and decreased urinary concentrating ability.[165,166] Because hypernatremia frequently results from diabetes insipidus (DI) or osmotically induced losses of sodium and water, many patients are hypovolemic or bear the stigmata of renal disease. Postoperative neurosurgical patients who have undergone pituitary surgery are at particular risk of developing transient or prolonged DI.[167] Polyuria may be present for only a few days within the first week after surgery, may be permanent, or may demonstrate a triphasic sequence: early DI, return of urinary concentrating ability, then recurrent DI.

The clinical consequences of hypernatremia are most serious at the extremes of age and when hypernatremia develops abruptly. Geriatric patients are at increased risk of hypernatremia because of decreased renal concentrating ability and thirst, although the responsiveness of osmoreceptors to hypernatremia is maintained during normal aging.[168,169] Brain shrinkage may damage delicate cerebral vessels, leading to subdural hematoma, subcortical parenchymal hemorrhage, subarach-

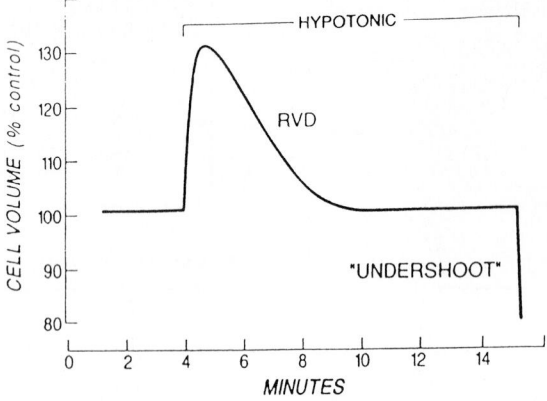

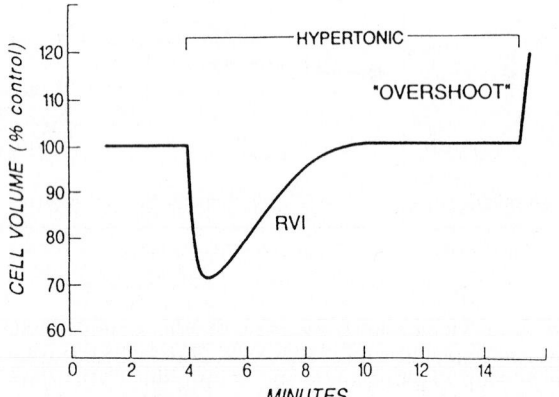

Figure 9-12. Activation of mechanisms regulating cell volume in response to acute osmotic stress. Regulatory volume decrease and regulatory volume increase refer to compensatory losses and gains of solutes. Although the course of these regulatory volume decreases and increases varies with the type of cell and experimental conditions, typically the responses occur over a period of minutes. Returning volume-regulated cells to normotonic conditions causes shrinkage or swelling. (Reprinted with permission from McManus ML, Churchwill KB, Strange K: Regulation of cell volume in health and disease. N Engl J Med 333:1260, 1995.)

noid hemorrhage, and venous thrombosis. Polyuria may cause bladder distention, hydronephrosis, and permanent renal damage. At the cellular level, restoration of cell volume occurs remarkably quickly after tonicity is altered (Fig. 9-12).[170] Although the mortality of hypernatremia is 40–55%, it is unclear whether hypernatremia is the cause or a marker of severe associated disease.[41]

Surprisingly, if plasma [Na$^+$] is initially normal, moderate acute increases do not appear to precipitate central pontine myelinolysis. However, larger accidental increases in plasma [Na$^+$] have produced severe consequences in children. In a 12-year-old diabetic child who accidentally received 500 ml of 5.0% saline during treatment for diabetic ketoacidosis (DKA), plasma [Na$^+$] acutely increased to 172 mEq · l^{-1}; subsequent cranial computed tomography showed many subcortical hemorrhages, and the child suffered brain death.[171] In experimental animals, acute hypernatremia (acute increase from 146 to 170 mEq · l^{-1}) caused neuronal damage at 24 hours, suggestive of early central pontine myelinolysis.[172]

By definition, hypernatremia indicates an absolute or relative water deficit and is always associated with hypertonicity. Hypernatremia can be generated by hypotonic fluid loss, as in burns, GI losses, diuretic therapy, osmotic diuresis, renal disease, mineralocorticoid excess or deficiency, and iatrogenic causes; or it can be generated by isolated water loss, as in DI (Fig. 9-13). The acquired form of NDI is more common and usually less severe than the congenital form. As chronic renal failure advances, most patients have defective concentrating ability, resulting in resistance to ADH associated with hypotonic urine.[173]

Isolated sodium gain is uncommon but occurs in patients who receive large quantities of sodium, such as treatment of metabolic acidosis with 8.4% sodium bicarbonate, in which [Na$^+$] is approximately 1000 mEq · l^{-1}, or perioperative or pre-hospital treatment with hypertonic saline resuscitation solutions. Because hypovolemia accompanies most pathologic water loss, signs of hypoperfusion also may be present. In many patients, before the development of hypernatremia, an increased volume of hypotonic urine suggests an abnormality in water balance.[174]

The TBW deficit can be estimated from the plasma [Na$^+$] using the equation:

$$\text{TBW deficit} = 0.6 \times \text{body weight (kg)} \times [([Na^+] - 140)/140]$$

$$(9-15)$$

where 140 is the middle of the normal range for [Na$^+$].

Hypernatremia: Evaluation

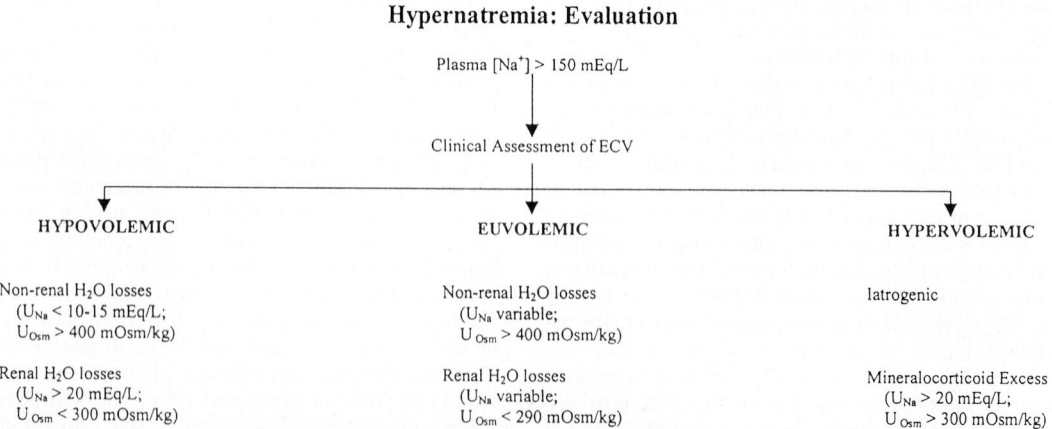

Figure 9-13. Severe hypernatremia is evaluated by first assessing extracellular volume (ECV) to separate patients into hypovolemic, euvolemic, and hypervolemic groups. Next, potential etiologic factors are diagnostically assessed. [Na$^+$], serum sodium concentration; U$_{Na}$, urinary sodium concentration; U$_{Osm}$, urinary osmolality.

Hypernatremic patients can be separated into three groups, based on clinical assessment of ECV (see Fig. 9-13). The plasma [Na⁺] does not reflect total body sodium, which must be estimated based on signs of the adequacy of ECV. In polyuric, hypernatremic patients, the next differential diagnostic decision is between solute diuresis and DI. Measurement of urinary sodium and osmolality can help to differentiate the various causes. A urinary osmolality of <150 mOsm $\cdot$ kg^{-1} in the setting of hypertonicity and polyuria is diagnostic of DI.

Treatment of hypernatremia produced by water loss consists of repletion of water as well of associated deficits in total body sodium and other electrolytes (Table 9-19). Common errors in treating hypernatremia include excessively rapid correction as well as failing to appreciate the magnitude of the water deficit and failing to account for ongoing maintenance requirements and continued fluid losses in planning therapy.

Hypernatremia must be corrected slowly because of the risk of neurologic sequelae such as seizures or cerebral edema (Fig. 9-14).[175] At the cellular level, restoration of cell volume occurs remarkably quickly after tonicity is altered; as a consequence, acute treatment of hypertonicity may result in overshooting the original, normotonic cell volume.[170,176,177] The water deficit should be replaced over 24–48 hours, and the plasma [Na⁺] should not be reduced by more than $1–2$ mEq $\cdot$ l^{-1} $\cdot$ hr^{-1}. Reversible underlying causes should be treated. Hypovolemia should be corrected promptly with 0.9% saline. Although the [Na⁺] of 0.9% saline is 154 mEq $\cdot$ l^{-1}, the solution is effective in treating the volume deficit and will reduce [Na⁺] if it is >154 mEq $\cdot$ l^{-1}. Once hypovolemia is corrected, water can be replaced orally or with intravenous hypotonic fluids, depending on the ability of the patient to tolerate oral hydration. In the occasional sodium-overloaded patient, sodium excretion can be accelerated using loop diuretics or dialysis.

The management of hypernatremia secondary to DI varies according to whether the etiology is central or nephrogenic (see Table 9-19). The two most suitable agents for correcting central DI (an ADH deficiency syndrome) are desmopressin (DDAVP) and aqueous vasopressin. DDAVP, given subcutaneously in a dose of $1–4$ μg or intranasally in a dose of $5–20$ μg every 12 to 24 hours, is effective in the vast majority of patients. DDAVP lacks the vasoconstrictor effects of vasopressin and is less likely to produce abdominal cramping.[178–181] Incomplete ADH deficits (partial DI) often are effectively managed with pharmacologic agents that stimulate ADH release or enhance the renal response to ADH. Chlorpropamide, which potentiates the renal effects of vasopressin, and carbamazepine, which enhances vasopressin secretion, have been used to treat partial central DI, but are associated with clinically important side effects. In NDI, urinary water losses can be decreased by using

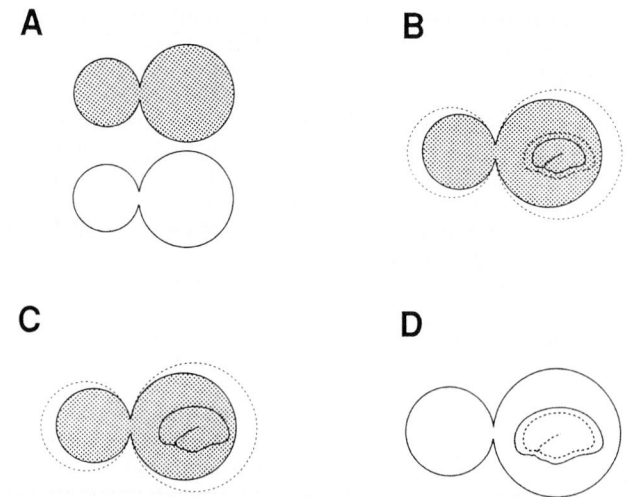

Figure 9-14. (A) The concentration of sodium is reflected in the intensity of the stippling: the upper figure, representing extracellular volume (smaller circle) and intracellular volume (larger circle), is more heavily stippled; that is, serum sodium is higher. (B) In response to an acute increase in serum sodium resulting from water loss, both intracellular and extracellular volume substantially decrease. The brain (schematically illustrated) shrinks in proportion to the reduction in intracellular volume in other tissues. (C) However, owing to the production of idiogenic osmoles, the brain rapidly restores its intracellular volume, despite the persistent reduction in intracellular volume in other tissues and in extracellular volume. (D) With excessively rapid correction of hypernatremia (the reduction in serum sodium is reflected in the decrease in the intensity of stippling), the brain expands to greater than its original size. The resulting increase in cerebral edema and intracranial pressure can cause severe neurologic damage. (Modified with permission from Feig PU: Hypernatremia and hypertonic syndromes. Med Clin North Am 65:271, 1981.)

salt and water restriction or thiazide diuretics to induce extracellular volume contraction, thereby enhancing fluid reabsorption in the proximal tubules. If less filtrate passes through into the collecting ducts, less water will be excreted.

Potassium

Physiologic Role

The intracellular potassium concentration ([K⁺]) is normally 150 mEq $\cdot$ l^{-1} while the extracellular concentration is only 3.5–5.0 mEq $\cdot$ l^{-1}. Serum [K⁺] is about 0.5 mEq $\cdot$ l^{-1} higher than plasma [K⁺] owing to cell lysis during clotting. Total body potassium in a 70-kg adult is approximately 4256 mEq, of which 4200 mEq is intracellular; of the 56 mEq in the ECV, only 12 mEq is located in the PV. Potassium plays an important role in cell membrane physiology, especially in maintaining resting membrane potentials and in generating action potentials in the central nervous system and heart.

Potassium is actively transported into cells by a Na/K ATPase pump, which maintains an intracellular potassium concentration [K⁺] that is at least 30-fold greater than extracellular [K⁺]. The ratio of intracellular to extracellular potassium contributes to the resting potential difference across cell membranes and therefore to the integrity of cardiac and neuromuscular transmission. The primary mechanism that maintains potassium inside cells is the negative voltage created by the transport of three sodium ions out of the cell for every two potassium ions transported in (Fig. 9-15).[182] Both insulin and catecholamines promote sodium entry and potassium exit.[183,184] In contrast, α adrenergic agonists impair cellular potassium uptake.[185] Metabolic acidosis tends to shift potassium out of cells, while metabolic alkalosis favors movement into cells.

Table 9-19. HYPERNATREMIA: ACUTE TREATMENT

Sodium Depletion (Hypovolemia)
Hypovolemia correction (0.9% saline)
Hypernatremia correction (hypotonic fluids)

Sodium Overload (Hypervolemia)
Enhance sodium removal (loop diuretics, dialysis)
Replace water deficit (hypotonic fluids)

Normal Total Body Sodium (Euvolemia)
Replace water deficit (hypotonic fluids)
Control diabetes insipidus
Central diabetes insipidus:
  DDAVP, 10–20 μg intranasally; 2–4 μg sc
  Aqueous vasopressin, 5 U q 2–4 hours im or sc
Nephrogenic diabetes insipidus:
  Restrict sodium, water intake
  Thiazide diuretics

The usual potassium intake is between 50 and 150 mEq $\cdot$ day^{-1}. Most is excreted in the urine, with some fecal elimination. Freely filtered at the glomerulus, 85–90% of potassium is reabsorbed in the proximal convoluted tubule and loop of Henle. The remaining 10–15% reaches the distal convoluted tubule, which is the major site at which potassium excretion is regulated. Excretion of potassium ions is a function of open potassium channels and the electrical driving force in the cortical collecting duct.[182] As sodium reabsorption increases, the electrical driving force opposing reabsorption of potassium is increased. Aldosterone increases sodium reabsorption through promoting a more open configuration of the epithelial sodium channel[186]; potassium-sparing diuretics (amiloride and triamterene) and trimethroprim block the epithelial sodium channel, thereby increasing potassium reabsorption.[187]

Assuming a plasma $[K^+]$ of 4.0 mEq $\cdot$ l^{-1} and a normal GFR of 180 l $\cdot$ day^{-1}, 720 mEq of potassium is filtered daily. Most is reabsorbed; usually, only the amount ingested is lost. As long as GFR is >8 ml $\cdot$ min^{-1}, dietary potassium intake, unless greater than normal, can be excreted. Four factors that favor K^+ excretion are alkalemia, increased aldosterone activity, increased delivery of Na^+ to the distal tubule and collecting duct, and increased urinary flow to these segments. Potassium secretion into the distal convoluted tubules and cortical collecting ducts is increased by aldosterone, hyperkalemia, high urinary flow rates, and the presence in luminal fluid of nonreabsorbable anions such as carbenicillin, phosphates, and sulfates.[188,189] Additional potassium is reabsorbed from the medullary collecting ducts as part of a recycling loop.[190] Within the distal nephron, a magnesium-dependent Na/K ATPase enzyme plays a critical role in potassium reabsorption.[191] Magnesium depletion impairs the activity of the enzyme, leading to renal potassium wasting. The two most important regulators of potassium secretion are the plasma $[K^+]$ and aldosterone, although there is some evidence to suggest the involvement of an enteric reflex mediated by a potassium-rich meal and of the central nervous system.[192]

Hypokalemia

Uncommon among healthy persons, hypokalemia ($[K^+] < 3.0$ mEq $\cdot$ l^{-1}) is a frequent complication of treatment with diuretic drugs and occasionally complicates other diseases and treatment regimens (Table 9-20).[185] Hypokalemia ($[K^+] < 3.0$ mEq $\cdot$ l^{-1}) causes muscle weakness and, when severe, may even cause paralysis. With chronic potassium loss, the ratio of intracellular to extracellular $[K^+]$ remains relatively stable; in contrast, acute redistribution of potassium from the extracellular to the intracellular space substantially changes resting membrane potentials.

Cardiac rhythm disturbances are among the most dangerous complications of potassium deficiency. Acute hypokalemia causes hyperpolarization of the cardiac cell and may lead to ventricular escape activity, re-entrant phenomena, ectopic tachycardias, and delayed conduction. Surprisingly, a prospective clinical study demonstrated that preoperative chronic hypokalemia ap-

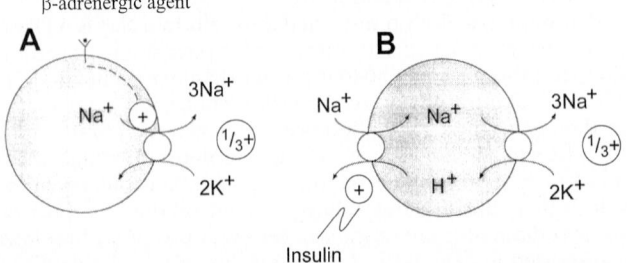

Figure 9-15. Hormones shifting potassium into cells. Major hormones involved are: (*A*) insulin and (*B*) β_2-adrenergic agents. (Reproduced with permission from Halperin ML, Kamel KS: Potassium. Lancet 352:135, 1998.)

Table 9-20. CAUSES OF RENAL POTASSIUM LOSS

Drugs	Bicarbonaturia
Diuretics	Distal renal tubular acidosis
Thiazide diuretics	Treatment of proximal renal tubular acidosis
Loop diuretics	Correction phase of metabolic alkalosis
Osmotic diuretics	Magnesium deficiency
Antibiotics	Other less common causes
Penicillin and penicillin analogues	Cisplatin
Amphotericin B	Carbonic anhydrase inhibitors
Aminoglycosides	Leukemia
Hormones	Diuretic phase of acute tubular necrosis
Aldosterone	Intrinsic renal transport defects
Glucocorticoid-excess states	Barter's syndrome
	Gitelman's syndrome

(Modified with permission from Weiner ID, Wingo CS: Hypokalemia consequences, causes, and correction. J Am Soc Nephrol 8:1179, 1997.)

parently does not increase the incidence of intraoperative dysrhythmias.[193] In patients taking digoxin, hypokalemia increases toxicity by increasing myocardial digoxin binding and pharmacologic effectiveness. Hypokalemia contributes to systemic hypertension, especially when combined with a high-sodium diet.[194] In diabetic patients, hypokalemia impairs insulin secretion and end-organ sensitivity to insulin, thereby worsening hyperglycemia.[195]

Potassium depletion also induces defects in renal concentrating ability, resulting in polyuria and a reduction in GFR.[196] Potassium replacement improves GFR, although the concentrating deficit may not improve for several months after treatment. If hypokalemia is sufficiently prolonged, chronic renal interstitial damage may occur.

The plasma $[K^+]$ poorly reflects total body potassium; hypokalemia may occur with normal, low, or high total body potassium stores. As a general rule, a chronic decrement of 1.0 mEq $\cdot$ l^{-1} in the plasma $[K^+]$ corresponds to a total body deficit of approximately 200–300 mEq. In uncomplicated hypokalemia, the potassium deficit exceeds 300 mEq if plasma $[K^+]$ is <3.0 mEq $\cdot$ l^{-1} and 700 mEq if plasma $[K^+]$ is <2.0 mEq $\cdot$ l^{-1}.

Hypokalemia may result from acute redistribution of potassium from the extracellular to intracellular space, in which case total body potassium will be normal, or from chronic depletion of total body potassium. Redistribution of potassium into cells occurs when the activity of the Na/K ATPase pump is acutely increased by extracellular hyperkalemia or increased intracellular concentrations of sodium, as well as by insulin, carbohydrate loading (which stimulates release of endogenous insulin), β_2 agonists, and aldosterone. Both metabolic and respiratory alkaloses lead to decreases in plasma $[K^+]$.[197]

Causes of chronic hypokalemia include those etiologies associated with renal potassium conservation (extrarenal potassium losses; low urinary $[K^+]$) and those with renal potassium wasting (Fig. 9-16).[182] A low urinary $[K^+]$ suggests inadequate dietary intake or extrarenal depletion (in the absence of recent diuretic use). Diuretic-induced urinary potassium losses are frequently associated with hypokalemia, secondary to increased aldosterone secretion, alkalemia, and increased renal tubular flow. Aldosterone does not cause renal potassium wasting unless sodium ions are present; that is, aldosterone primarily controls sodium reabsorption, not potassium excretion. Renal tubular damage due to nephrotoxins such as aminoglycosides or amphotericin B may also cause renal potassium wasting.

Initial evaluation of hypokalemia includes a medical history (*e.g.* diarrhea, vomiting, diuretic or laxative use), physical examination (*e.g.*, hypertension, cushingoid features, edema), measurement of serum electrolytes (*e.g.*, magnesium), arterial *p*H assessment, and evaluation of the ECG. Measurement of 24-hour urinary excretion of sodium and potassium may distinguish extrarenal from renal causes. Magnesium deficiency, associated with aminoglycoside and cisplatin therapy, can generate hypokalemia that is resistant to replacement therapy. A stress response and release of catecholamines causes the majority of trauma patients to develop hypokalemia that returns to normal within 24 hours without specific therapy.[185] Plasma renin and aldosterone levels may be helpful in the differential diagnosis. Characteristic electrocardiographic changes associated with hypokalemia include flat or inverted T waves, prominent U waves, and ST segment depression.

The treatment of hypokalemia consists of potassium repletion, correction of alkalemia, and removal of offending drugs (Table 9-21). Hypokalemia secondary only to acute redistribution may not require treatment. The need for potassium replacement therapy in mild to moderate hypokalemia (3–3.5 mEq · l^{-1}) without clear symptoms has been questioned.[198] If total body potassium is decreased, oral potassium supplementation is preferable to intravenous replacement. Potassium is usually replaced as the chloride salt because coexisting chloride deficiency may limit the ability of the kidney to conserve potassium.

Potassium repletion must be performed cautiously (usually at a rate of ≤10–20 mEq · hr^{-1}) since the absolute deficit is unpredictable. The plasma [K$^+$] and the ECG must be monitored during rapid repletion (10–20 mEq · hr^{-1}) to avoid hyperkalemic complications.[185,199] The plasma [K$^+$] and ECG should be monitored to detect inadvertent hyperkalemia. Particular care should be taken in patients who have concurrent acidemia, type IV renal tubular acidosis, diabetes mellitus, or in those patients receiving nonsteroidal anti-inflammatory agents, ACE inhibitors, or beta blockers, all of which delay movement of extracellular potassium into cells.

However, in patients with life-threatening dysrhythmias secondary to hyperkalemia, serum [K$^+$] must be rapidly increased. Assuming that PV in a 70-kg adult is 3.0 l, administration of 6.0 mEq · l^{-1} of potassium in 1.0 min will increase serum [K$^+$] by

Table 9-21. HYPOKALEMIA: TREATMENT

Correct Precipitating Factors

Increased *p*H
Decreased [Mg^{2+}]
Drugs

Mild Hypokalemia ([K$^+$] > 2.0 mEq · l^{-1})
Intravenous KCl infusion ≤ 10 mEq · hr^{-1}

Severe Hypokalemia ([K$^+$] ≤ 2.0 mEq · l^{-1}, paralysis or ECG changes)
Intravenous KCl infusion ≤ 40 mEq · hr^{-1}
Continuous ECG monitoring
If life-threatening, 5–6 mEq bolus

no more than 2.0 mEq · l^{-1} because redistribution into interstitial fluid will decrease the quantity remaining in.[182]

Hypokalemia associated with hyperaldosteronemia (*e.g.* primary aldosteronism, Cushing's syndrome) usually responds favorably to reduced sodium intake and increased potassium intake. Hypomagnesemia, if present, aggravates the effects of hypokalemia, impairs potassium conservation, and should be treated. Potassium supplements or potassium-sparing diuretics should be given cautiously to patients who have diabetes mellitus or renal insufficiency, both of which limit compensation for acute hyperkalemia. In patients who are both acidemic and hypokalemic, such as those who have diabetic ketoacidosis, potassium administration should precede correction of acidosis to avoid a precipitous decrease in plasma [K$^+$] as *p*H increases.

In patients with normal serum potassium accompanied by symptoms of potassium depletion (*e.g.* muscle fatigue), history of potassium loss or insufficient intake, or in patients in whom potassium depletion may be of special threat (*e.g.* patients on diuretics, digitalis, or β_2 agonists), muscle biopsy with measurement of muscle potassium concentration may be a useful procedure to detect and quantify potassium depletion. Quantification of muscle potassium concentration is a useful tool for monitoring therapy.[200]

Hyperkalemia

The most lethal manifestations of hyperkalemia ([K$^+$] > 5.0 mEq · l^{-1}) involve the cardiac conducting system and include dysrhythmias, conduction abnormalities, and cardiac arrest. In anesthesia practice, the classic example of hyperkalemic cardiac toxicity is associated with the administration of succinylcholine to paraplegic, quadriplegic,[201] or severely burned[202,203] patients. If plasma [K$^+$] is <6.0 mEq · l^{-1}, cardiac effects are negligible. As the concentration increases further, the electrocardiogram shows tall, peaked T waves, especially in the precordial leads. With further increases, the PR interval becomes prolonged, followed by a decrease in the amplitude of the P wave. Finally, the QRS complex widens into a pattern resembling a sine wave, as a prelude to cardiac standstill (Fig. 9-17).[204] Hyperkalemic cardiotoxicity is enhanced by hyponatremia, hypocalcemia, or acidosis. Because progression to fatal cardiotoxicity is unpredictable and often swift, the presence of hyperkalemic ECG changes mandates immediate therapy. The life-threatening cardiac effects usually require more urgent treatment than do other manifestations of hyperkalemia. However, ascending muscle weakness appears when plasma [K$^+$] approaches 7.0 mEq · l^{-1}, and may progress to flaccid paralysis, inability to phonate, and respiratory arrest.

Hyperkalemia may occur with normal, high, or low total body potassium stores. A deficiency of aldosterone, a major regulator of potassium excretion, leads to hyperkalemia in adrenal insufficiency and hyporeninemic hypoaldosteronism, a state associated with diabetes mellitus, renal insufficiency, and advanced age. Because the kidneys excrete potassium, severe renal insuf-

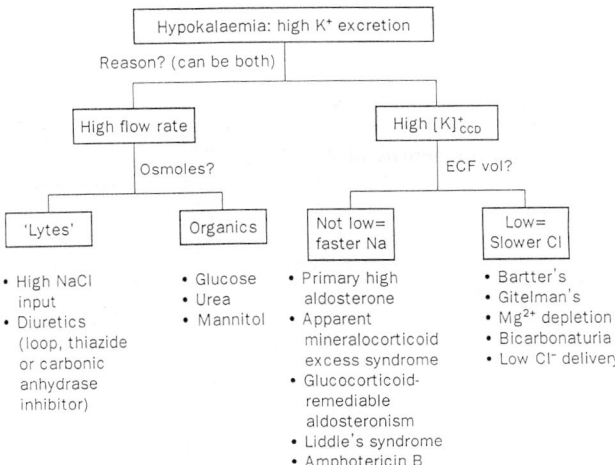

Figure 9-16. Approach to the patient with hypokalemia. Causes for excessive excretion of potassium (>15 mmol · day^{-1}) despite hypokalemia are too high a flow rate in the cortical collecting duct [(CCD), left limb] and/or too high a concentration of potassium [K$^+$] in the lumen of the CCD (right limb). Both flow rate and CCD [K$^+$] should be evaluated. Final considerations are shown by bullet symbols. A relatively slower Cl$^-$ reabsorption in CCD is suggested by high plasma renin activity and NaCl wasting despite low extracellular fluid volume; the converse applies for relatively faster Na$^+$ reabsorption. (Reproduced with permission from Halperin ML, Kamel KS: Potassium. Lancet 352:135, 1998.)

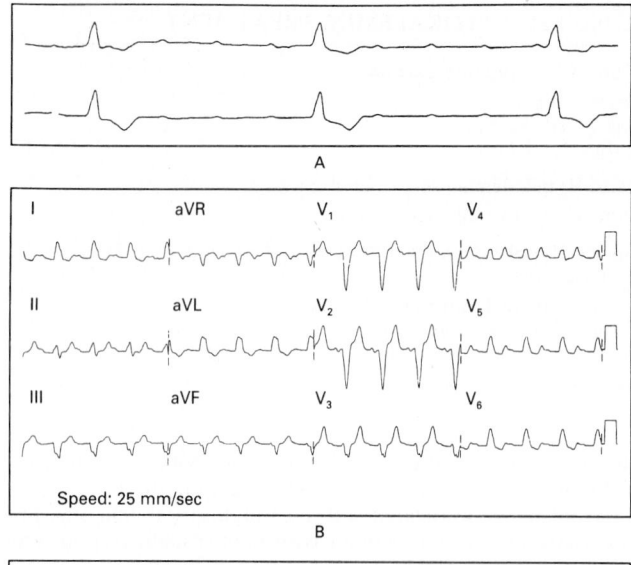

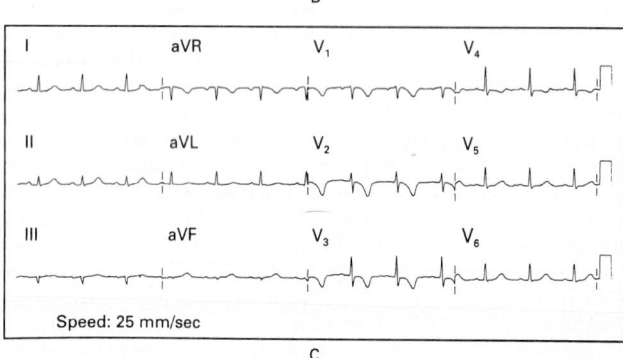

Figure 9-17. Electrocardiographic changes due to hyperkalemia occurring in a 42-year-old woman undergoing placement of an arteriovenous fistula for permanent hemodialysis access to treat end-stage renal disease. During dissection of the brachial artery under local anesthesia, her cardiac rhythm converted from normal sinus rhythm to complete heart block with ventricular escape (approximately 25 beats per minute) (A). Two ampules of calcium gluconate (9.2 mEq) were administered intravenously. An electrocardiogram revealed sinus tachycardia with profound prolongation of the QRS interval (left-bundle-branch morphology), first-degree atrioventricular block, and ''peaked'' T waves (B). The serum potassium concentration was 8.6 mmol $\cdot$ l^{-1}. After reduction of the serum potassium concentration, the electrocardiogram showed sinus rhythm with normalization of the PR and QRS intervals. Anteroseptal ST wave and T wave changes were noted on subsequent electrocardiograms (C). A cardiac exercise imaging study did not show ischemia. (Reprinted with permission from Kuvin JT: Electrocardiographic changes of hyperkalemia. N Engl J Med 338:662, 1998.)

ficiency commonly causes hyperkalemia. Patients with chronic renal insufficiency can maintain normal plasma [K$^+$] despite markedly decreased GFR because urinary potassium excretion depends on tubular secretion rather than glomerular filtration if GFR exceeds 8 ml $\cdot$ min^{-1}.

Drugs are now the most common cause of hyperkalemia.[205] Drugs that may limit potassium excretion include nonsteroidal anti-inflammatory drugs, ACE inhibitors, cyclosporin, and potassium-sparing diuretics such as triamterene. Drug effects most commonly occur in patients with other factors that predispose to hyperkalemia, such as diabetes mellitus, renal insufficiency, advanced age, or hyporeninemic hypoaldosteronism. ACE inhibitors are particularly likely to produce hyperkalemia in patients who have renal insufficiency[206] or severe congestive heart failure.[207]

In patients who have normal total body potassium, hyperkalemia may accompany a sudden shift of potassium from the

ICV to the ECV because of acidemia, increased catabolism, or rhabdomyolysis. Metabolic acidosis and respiratory acidosis tend to cause an increase in plasma [K$^+$]. However, organic acidoses (*i.e.* lactic acidosis, ketoacidosis) have little effect on [K$^+$], whereas mineral acids cause significant cellular shifts. In response to increased hydrogen ion activity because of addition of acids, potassium will increase if the anion remains in the extracellular volume.[182] Neither lactate nor ketoacids remain in the extracellular fluid. Therefore, hyperkalemia in these circumstances reflects tissue injury or lack of insulin.[182]

Pseudohyperkalemia, which occurs when potassium is released from cells in blood collection tubes, can be diagnosed by comparing serum and plasma [K$^+$] levels from the same blood sample. Hyperkalemia usually accompanies malignant hyperthermia.

The most important aspects of diagnosis are a medical history, emphasizing recent drug therapy, and assessment of renal function. The ECG may provide the first suggestion of hyperkalemia in some patients. Despite the familiar effects of hyperkalemia on cardiac conduction and rhythm, the ECG is an insensitive and nonspecific method of detecting hyperkalemia.[208] If hyponatremia is also present, adrenal function should be evaluated.

The treatment of hyperkalemia is aimed at eliminating the cause, reversing membrane hyperexcitability, and removing potassium from the body (Fig. 9-18).[182] Emergent management of hyperkalemia is listed in detail in Table 9-22. Mineralocorticoid deficiency can be treated with 9-α-fludrocortisone (0.025–0.10 mg $\cdot$ day^{-1}). Hyperkalemia secondary to digitalis intoxication may be resistant to therapy because attempts to shift potassium from the ECV to the ICV are often ineffective. In this situation, use of digoxin-specific antibodies has been successful.

Membrane hyperexcitability can be antagonized by translocating potassium from the ECV to the ICV, removing excess potassium, or (transiently) by infusing calcium chloride to depress the membrane threshold potential. Pending definitive treatment, rapid infusion of calcium chloride (1 g of CaCl$_2$ over 3 minutes, or two to three ampules of 10% calcium gluconate over 5 minutes) may stabilize cardiac rhythm (see Fig. 9-17).

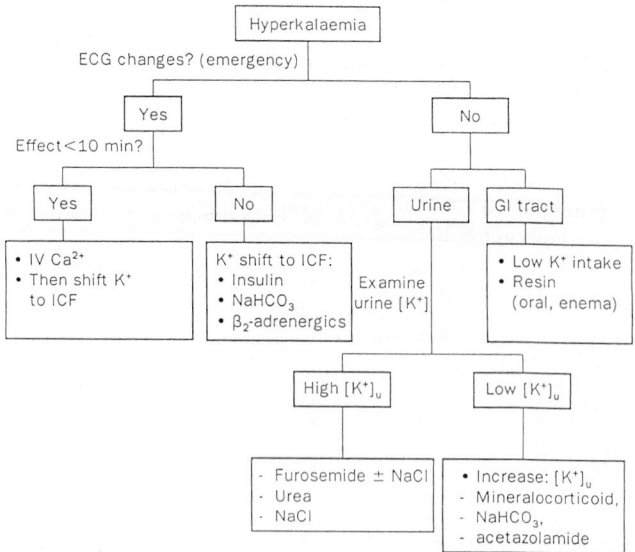

Figure 9-18. Treatment of patient with hyperkalemia. If an emergency is present (usually cardiac), intravenous Ca^{2+} must be given. This treatment should act promptly. Efforts are also taken to shift potassium into cells with insulin with or without NaHCO$_3$. Longer term strategies are to limit intake of potassium, prevent its absorption in the gastrointestinal tract, and promote its excretion; the latter includes measuring urine [K$^+$] and flow rate to decide leverage for therapy. (Reproduced with permission from Halperin ML, Kamel KS: Potassium. Lancet 352: 135, 1998.)

Table 9-22. SEVERE HYPERKALEMIA:* TREATMENT

Reverse membrane effects
 Calcium (10 ml of 10% calcium chloride IV over 10 min)
Transfer extracellular [K⁺] into cells
 Glucose and insulin (D10W + 5–10 U regular insulin per
  25–50 g glucose)
 Sodium bicarbonate (50 to 100 mEq over 5–10 min)
 β_2 agonists
Remove potassium from body
 Diuretics, proximal or loop
 Potassium-exchange resins (sodium polystyrene sulfonate)
 Hemodialysis
Monitor ECG and serum [K⁺] level

---

* Potassium concentration ([K⁺]) > 7.0 mEq·l⁻¹ or electrocardiographic (ECG) changes.

Calcium should be given cautiously if digitalis intoxication is likely. Acute alkalinization using sodium bicarbonate (50–100 mEq over 5-10 minutes in a 70-kg adult) transiently promotes movement of potassium from the ECV to the ICV. Bicarbonate can be administered even if pH exceeds 7.40; however, it should not be administered to patients with congestive cardiac failure or hypernatremia. Insulin, in a dose-dependent fashion, causes cellular uptake of potassium by increasing the activity of the Na/K ATPase pump. Insulin increases cellular uptake of potassium *best* when high insulin levels are achieved by intravenous injection of 5–10 U of regular insulin,[209] accompanied by 50 ml of 50% glucose. β_2-Adrenergic drugs also increase potassium uptake by skeletal muscle and reduce plasma [K⁺],[210] an action that may explain hypokalemia with severe, acute illness. β_2 agonists have been used to treat hyperkalemia.[211] Salbutamol, a selective β_2 agonist, decreases serum potassium acutely when given by inhalation or intravenously. In 15 pediatric patients with baseline serum [K⁺] of 6.6 mEq·l⁻¹, a single infusion of salbutamol (5 μg·kg⁻¹ over 15 min) reduced serum [K⁺] to 5.7 mEq·l⁻¹ after 30 minutes and 4.9 mEq·l⁻¹ after 120 minutes.[212] In using β_2-adrenergic agents to reduce serum [K⁺], the potential for generating cardiac dysrhythmias should be recognized.[213,214]

Potassium may be removed from the body by the renal or gastrointestinal routes. Furosemide promotes kaliuresis in a dose-dependent fashion. Sodium polystyrene sulfonate resin (Kayexalate), which exchanges sodium for potassium, can be given orally (30 g) or as a retention enema (50 g in 200 ml of 20% sorbitol). However, sodium overload and hypervolemia are potential risks. Rarely, when temporizing measures are insufficient, emergency hemodialysis may remove 25–50 mEq·hr⁻¹. Peritoneal dialysis is less efficient. Mineralocorticoid deficiency can be treated with 9-α-fludrocortisone. Hyperkalemia secondary to digitalis intoxication may be resistant to therapy because attempts to shift potassium intracellularly are often ineffective. In this situation, administration of a digoxin-specific antibody may be lifesaving.

Calcium

Physiologic Role

Calcium is a divalent cation found primarily in the extracellular fluid. The free calcium concentration [Ca²⁺] in ECV is approximately 1 mM, whereas the free [Ca²⁺] in the ICV approximates 100 mM, a gradient of 10,000 to 1. Circulating calcium consists of a protein-bound fraction (40%), a chelated fraction (10%), and an ionized fraction (50%), which is the physiologically active and homeostatically regulated component.[215] Acute acidemia decreases protein-bound calcium (*i.e.,* increases ionized calcium) whereas acute alkalemia increases protein-bound calcium. Because mathematical formulae that "correct" total cal-

cium measurements for albumin concentration are inaccurate in critically ill patients,[216] ionized calcium should be directly measured.

In general, all movement that occurs in mammalian systems requires calcium. Essential for normal excitation–contraction coupling, calcium is also necessary for proper function of muscle tissue, ciliary movement, mitosis, neurotransmitter release, enzyme secretion, and hormonal secretion. Cyclic AMP (cAMP) and phosphoinositides, which are major second messengers regulating cellular metabolism, function primarily through the regulation of calcium movement. Activation of numerous intracellular enzyme systems requires calcium. Important both for generation of the cardiac pacemaker activity and for generation of the cardiac action potential, calcium is the primary ion responsible for the plateau phase of the action potential. Calcium also plays vital functions in membrane and bone structure.

Serum [Ca²⁺] is regulated by multiple factors (Fig. 9-19),[217] including a calcium receptor[218–220] and several hormones, the most important of which are parathyroid hormone (PTH) and calcitriol.[221] PTH and vitamin D (see Table 9-17), both of which mobilize calcium from bone, increase renal tubular reabsorption of calcium, and enhance intestinal absorption of calcium. Metabolites of vitamin D exert a major role in long-term control of circulating calcium. Vitamin D, after ingestion or manufacture of vitamin D in the skin under the stimulus of ultraviolet light, is 25-hydroxylated to calcidiol in the liver and then is 1-hydroxylated to calcitriol in the kidney. Calcitriol, the active metabolite, stimulates osseous calcium release, renal calcium reabsorption, and enteric calcium absorption. PTH and vitamin D can maintain a normal circulating [Ca²⁺], even in the absence of dietary calcium intake, by mobilizing calcium from bone.

Hypocalcemia

The hallmark of hypocalcemia is increased neuronal membrane irritability and tetany (Table 9-23). Early symptoms include sensations of numbness and tingling involving fingers, toes, and the circumoral region. In frank tetany, tonic contraction of respiratory muscles may lead to laryngospasm, bronchospasm, or respiratory arrest. Smooth muscle spasm can result in abdominal cramping and urinary frequency. Mental status alterations include irritability, depression, psychosis, and dementia. Hypocalcemia may impair cardiovascular function and has been associated with heart failure, hypotension, dysrhythmias, insensitivity to digitalis, and impaired β-adrenergic action.

Reduced *total* serum calcium occurs in as many as 80% of critically ill and postsurgical patients.[215] However, *ionized* hypocalcemia develops in fewer patients, including 15–20% of critically ill patients, 20% of patients after cardiopulmonary bypass, and 30–40% after multiple trauma. In these situations, ionized hypocalcemia is clinically mild ([Ca²⁺] >0.8 mM).

Initial diagnostic evaluation should concentrate on history and physical examination, laboratory evaluation of renal function, and measurement of serum phosphate concentration. Latent hypocalcemia can be diagnosed by tapping on the facial nerve to elicit Chvostek's sign or by inflating a sphygmomanometer to 20 mm Hg above systolic pressure, which produces radial and ulnar nerve ischemia, causing carpal spasm known as Trousseau's sign.[222]

The differential diagnosis of hypocalcemia can be approached by addressing four issues: age of the patient, serum phosphate concentration, general clinical status, and duration of hypocalcemia.[223] High phosphate concentrations suggest renal failure[224] or hypoparathyroidism. In renal insufficiency, reduced phosphorus excretion results in hyperphosphatemia, which downregulates the 1α-hydroxylase responsible for the renal conversion of calcidiol to calcitriol. This, in combination with decreased production of calcitriol secondary to reduced renal mass, causes reduced intestinal absorption of calcium and hypocalcemia.[221] Low or normal phosphate concentrations imply vitamin D or magnesium deficiency. An otherwise healthy

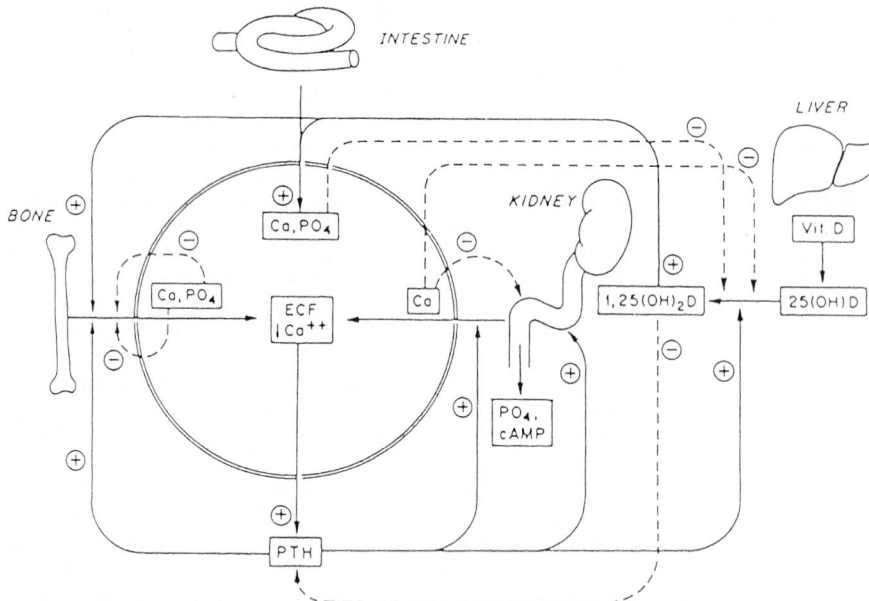

Figure 9-19. Schematic representation of the regulatory system maintaining Ca_o^{2+} homeostasis. The *solid arrows* and *lines* delineate effects of parathyroid hormone and $1,25(OH)_2D_3$ on their target tissues; *dashed arrows* and *lines* show examples of how extracellular Ca^{2+} or phosphate ions act directly on tissues regulating mineral ion metabolism. Ca = calcium; PO_4 = phosphate; ECF = extracellular fluid; PTH = parathyroid hormone; $1,25(OH)_2D_3$ = 1,25-dihydroxyvitamin D; 25(OH)D = 25-hydroxyvitamin D; minus signs indicate inhibitory actions and plus signs indicate stimulatory effects. (Reproduced with permission from Brown EM, Pollak M, Hebert SC: The extracellular calcium-sensing receptor: Its role in health and disease. Annu Rev Med 49:15, 1998.)

patient with chronic hypocalcemia probably is hypoparathyroid. Chronically ill adults with hypocalcemia often have disorders such as malabsorption, osteomalacia, or osteoblastic metastases.

Hypocalcemia (ionized $[Ca^{2+}]$ <4.0 mg · dl^{-1} or <1 mM) occurs as a result of failure of PTH or calcitriol action or because of calcium chelation or precipitation, not because of calcium deficiency alone. PTH deficiency can result from surgical damage to or removal of the parathyroid glands and from suppression of the parathyroid glands by severe hypo- or hypermagnesemia. Burns, sepsis, and pancreatitis may suppress parathyroid function and interfere with vitamin D action. Vitamin D deficiency may result from lack of dietary vitamin D or vitamin D malabsorption in patients who lack sunlight exposure. Hyperphosphatemia-induced hypocalcemia may occur as a consequence of overzealous phosphate therapy, from cell lysis secondary to chemotherapy, or as a result of cellular destruction from rhabdomyolysis. Precipitation of $CaHPO_4$ complexes occurs with hyperphosphatemia. However, ionized $[Ca^{2+}]$ only decreases approximately 0.019 mM for each 1.0 mM increase in phosphate concentration.[225] In massive transfusion, citrate may produce hypocalcemia by chelating calcium; however, decreases are usually transient and produce no cardiovascular effects. A healthy, normothermic adult who has intact hepatic and renal function can metabolize the citrate present in 20 units of blood per

hour without becoming hypocalcemic.[226] However, when citrate clearance is decreased (*e.g.*, by hepatic or renal disease or hypothermia) and when blood transfusion rates are rapid (*e.g.*, >0.5–2 ml · kg^{-1} · min^{-1}), hypocalcemia and cardiovascular compromise (usually manifested as hypotension without obvious hypovolemia) may occur. Alkalemia resulting from hyperventilation or sodium bicarbonate injection can acutely decrease $[Ca^{2+}]$.

The definitive treatment of hypocalcemia necessitates identification and treatment of the underlying cause (Table 9-24). Symptomatic hypocalcemia usually occurs when serum ionized $[Ca^{2+}]$ is <0.7 mM. The clinician should determine whether mild ionized hypocalcemia requires therapy, particularly in ischemic and septic states in which experimental evidence suggests that calcium may increase cellular damage.

Unnecessary offending drugs should be discontinued. Hypocalcemia resulting from hypomagnesemia or hyperphosphatemia is treated by repletion of magnesium or removal of phosphate. Treatment of a patient who has tetany and hyperphosphatemia requires coordination of therapy to avoid the consequences of metastatic soft tissue calcification.[227] Potassium and other electrolytes should be measured and abnormalities should be corrected. Hyperkalemia and hypomagnesemia potentiate hypocalcemia-induced cardiac and neuromuscular irritability. In contrast, hypokalemia protects against hypocalcemic tetany; therefore, correction of hypokalemia without correction of hypocalcemia may provoke tetany.

Mild, ionized hypocalcemia should not be overtreated. For instance, in most patients after cardiac surgery, administration

---

Table 9-23. HYPOCALCEMIA: CLINICAL MANIFESTATIONS

Cardiovascular	**Respiratory**
Dysrhythmias	Apnea
Digitalis insensitivity	Laryngeal spasm
ECG changes	Bronchospasm
Heart failure	
Hypotension	**Psychiatric**
	Anxiety
Neuromuscular	Dementia
Tetany	Depression
Muscle spasm	Psychosis
Papilledema	
Seizures	
Weakness	
Fatigue	

ECG = electrocardiographic.

Table 9-24. HYPOCALCEMIA: ACUTE TREATMENT

Administer calcium
 IV: 10 ml 10% calcium gluconate* over 10 min, followed by elemental calcium 0.3–2.0 mg · kg^{-1} · hr^{-1}
 Oral: 500–100 mg elemental calcium q 6 hours
Administer vitamin D
 Ergocalciferol, 1200 μg/day (T$_{1/2}$ = 30 days)
 Dihydrotachysterol, 200–400 μg/day (T$_{1/2}$ = 7 days)
 1,25-dihydroxycholecalciferol, 0.25–1.0 μg/day (T$_{1/2}$ = 1 day)
Monitor electrocardiogram

* Calcium gluconate contains 93 mg elemental calcium per 10-ml vial; T$_{1/2}$ = half-life.

of calcium only increases mean arterial blood pressure (MAP)[228] and actually attenuates the β-adrenergic effects of epinephrine.[228] In normocalcemic dogs, calcium chloride primarily acts as a peripheral vasoconstrictor, with transient reduction of myocardial contractility; in hypocalcemic dogs, calcium infusion significantly improves contractile performance and MAP (Table 9-25).[229] Therefore, calcium infusions should be of limited value during cardiac surgery unless there is demonstrable evidence of hypocalcemia.[229] Calcium salts appear to confer no benefit to patients already receiving inotropic or vasoactive agents.

The cornerstone of therapy for confirmed, symptomatic, ionized hypocalcemia ([Ca^{2+}] <0.7 mM) is calcium administration. In patients who have severe hypocalcemia or hypocalcemic symptoms, calcium should be administered intravenously. In emergency situations, in an average-sized adult, the "rule of 10s" advises infusion of 10 ml of 10% calcium gluconate (93 mg elemental calcium) over 10 minutes, followed by a continuous infusion of elemental calcium, 0.3–2 mg · kg^{-1} · hr^{-1} (i.e., 3–16 ml · hr^{-1} of 10% calcium gluconate for a 70-kg adult). Calcium salts should be diluted in 50–100 ml D5W (to limit venous irritation and thrombosis), should not be mixed with bicarbonate (to prevent precipitation), and must be given cautiously to digitalized patients because calcium increases the toxicity of digoxin. Continuous ECG monitoring during initial therapy will detect cardiotoxicity (e.g., heart block, ventricular fibrillation). During calcium replacement, the clinician should monitor serum calcium, magnesium, phosphate, potassium, and creatinine. Once the ionized [Ca^{2+}] is stable in the range of 4–5 mg · dl^{-1} (1.0–1.25 mM), oral calcium supplements can substitute for parenteral therapy. Urinary calcium should be monitored in an attempt to avoid hypercalciuria (>5 mg · kg^{-1} per 24 hours) and urinary tract stone formation.

When supplementation fails to maintain serum calcium within the normal range, or if hypercalciuria develops, vitamin D may be added. Although the principal effect of vitamin D is to increase enteric calcium absorption, osseous calcium resorption is also enhanced. When rapid changes in dosage are anticipated or an immediate effect is required (e.g., postoperative hypoparathyroidism), shorter-acting calciferols such as dihydrotachysterol may be preferable. Because the effect of vitamin D is not regulated, the dosages of calcium and vitamin D should be adjusted to raise the serum calcium into the low normal range.

Adverse reactions to calcium and vitamin D include hypercalcemia and hypercalciuria. If hypercalcemia develops, calcium and vitamin D should be discontinued and appropriate therapy given. The toxic effects of vitamin D metabolites persist in proportion to their biologic half-lives (ergocalciferol, 20–60 days;

dihydrotachysterol, 5–15 days; calcitriol, 2–10 days). Glucocorticoids antagonize the toxic effects of vitamin D metabolites.

Hypercalcemia

Although ionized [Ca^{2+}] most accurately demonstrates hypercalcemia (total serum calcium >10.5 mg · dl^{-1} or ionized [Ca^{2+}] >1.3 mM), hypercalcemia is more frequently defined in terms of total serum calcium. In hypoalbuminemic patients, total serum calcium can be estimated by assuming an increase of 0.8 mg · dl^{-1} for every 1 g · dl^{-1} of albumin concentration below 4.0 g · dl^{-1}. Patients in whom total serum calcium is less than 11.5 mg · dl^{-1} are usually asymptomatic. Patients with moderate hypercalcemia (total serum calcium 11.5–13 mg · dl^{-1}) may show symptoms of lethargy, anorexia, nausea, and polyuria. Severe hypercalcemia (total serum calcium >13 mg · dl^{-1}) is associated with more severe neuromyopathic symptoms, including muscle weakness, depression, impaired memory, emotional lability, lethargy, stupor, and coma. The cardiovascular effects of hypercalcemia include hypertension, dysrhythmias, heart block, cardiac arrest, and digitalis sensitivity.

Hypercalcemia impairs urinary concentrating ability and renal excretory capacity for calcium by irreversibly precipitating calcium salts within the renal parenchyma and by reducing RBF and GFR. In response to hypovolemia, renal tubular reabsorption of sodium enhances renal calcium reabsorption. Effective treatment of severe hypercalcemia is necessary to prevent progressive dehydration and renal failure leading to further increases in total serum calcium, because volume depletion exacerbates hypercalcemia.[230] Skeletal disease may occur secondary to direct osteolysis or humoral bone resorption.

Hypercalcemia occurs when calcium enters the ECV more rapidly than the kidneys can excrete the excess. Clinically, hypercalcemia most commonly results from an excess of bone resorption over bone formation, usually secondary to malignant disease, hyperparathyroidism, hypocalciuric hypercalcemia, thyrotoxicosis, immobilization, and granulomatous diseases. Granulomatous diseases produce hypercalciuria and hypercalcemia due to conversion by granulomatous tissue of calcidiol to calcitriol.[221]

Malignancy may produce hypercalcemia either through bone destruction or secretion by malignant tissue of hormones that promote hypercalcemia.[231] Although weakness, weight loss, and anemia associated with primary hyperparathyroidism may suggest malignancy, these may result simply from the primary disease process. Hypercalcemia associated with granulomatous diseases (e.g., sarcoidosis) results from the production of calcitriol by granulomatous tissue. To compensate for increased gut absorption or bone resorption of calcium, renal excretion can

Table 9-25. SERUM IONIZED [Ca^{2+}] CONCENTRATION AND HEMODYNAMIC VARIABLES ONE MIN AFTER CALCIUM ADMINISTRATION (5 MG/KG INTRAVENOUS BOLUS) IN NORMOCALCEMIC AND HYPOCALCEMIC (PRODUCED BY CPD ADMINISTRATION) DOGS

	Normocalcemic		Hypocalcemic		
	Baseline	*1 min*	*Baseline*	*CPD*	*1 min*
Ca^{2+} (mmol · l^{-1})	1.24 ± 0.04	1.47 ± 0.06*	1.24 ± 0.03	0.76 ± 0.03*	1.42 ± 0.22†
E$_{lves}$ (mm Hg · ml^{-1})	4.06 ± 1.00	2.16 ± 0.90*	5.03 ± 0.47	3.76 ± 0.61*	4.87 ± 0.64†
HR (beats · min^{-1})	159 ± 8	260 ± 9	154 ± 6	144 ± 7*	148 ± 6*
PAOP (mm Hg)	9 ± 2	9 ± 1	7 ± 1	10 ± 2	9 ± 2
MAP (mm Hg)	120 ± 6	137 ± 8*	157 ± 6	131 ± 6*	154 ± 6†
SVR (dyne · s · cm^{-5})	3858 ± 458	4347 ± 596*	4067 ± 550	3697 ± 479	4548 ± 904
CO (l · min^{-1})	2.7 ± 0.4	2.7 ± 0.4	3.4 ± 0.2	3.0 ± 0.3	3.1 ± 0.4

Values are mean ± sem (n = 6); E$_{lves}$, slope of the left ventricular end-systolic pressure-volume relationship; CPD, citrate-phosphate-dextrose; HR, heart rate; PAOP, pulmonary arterial occlusion pressure; MAP, mean arterial pressure; SVR, systemic vascular resistance; CO, cardiac output.
* P < 0.05 vs. baseline; † p < 0.05 vs CPD.
(Reprinted with permission from Mathru M, Rooney MW, Goldberg SA, Hirsch LJ: Separation of myocardial versus peripheral effects of calcium administration in normocalcemic and hypocalcemic states using pressure-volume (conductance) relationships. Anesth Analg 77:250, 1993.)

readily increase from 100 to more than 400 mg · day^{-1}. Factors that promote hypercalcemia may be offset by coexisting disorders, such as pancreatitis, sepsis, or hyperphosphatemia, that cause hypocalcemia.

Although definitive treatment of hypercalcemia requires correction of underlying causes, temporizing therapy may be necessary to avoid complications and to relieve symptoms. Total serum calcium exceeding 14 mg · dl^{-1} represents a medical emergency. General supportive treatment includes hydration, correction of associated electrolyte abnormalities, removal of offending drugs, dietary calcium restriction, and increased physical activity. Because anorexia and antagonism by calcium of ADH action invariably lead to sodium and water depletion, infusion of 0.9% saline will dilute serum calcium, promote renal excretion, and can reduce total serum calcium by 1.5–3 mg · dl^{-1}. Urinary output should be maintained at 200–300 ml · hr^{-1}. As GFR increases, the sodium ion increases calcium excretion by competing with the calcium ion for reabsorption in the proximal renal tubules and loop of Henle. Furosemide further enhances calcium excretion by increasing tubular sodium. Patients who have renal impairment may require higher doses of furosemide. During saline infusion and forced diuresis, careful monitoring of cardiopulmonary status and electrolytes, especially magnesium and potassium, is required. Intensive diuresis and saline administration can achieve net calcium excretion rates of 2000 to 4000 mg per 24 hours, a rate eight times greater than saline alone, but still somewhat less than the rate of removal achieved by hemodialysis (*i.e.,* 6000 mg every 8 hours). Patients treated with phosphates should be well hydrated. Slow calcium channel antagonists such as verapamil and nifedipine may also be useful in reversing hypercalcemic cardiotoxicity.[232]

Bone resorption, the primary cause of hypercalcemia, can be minimized by physical activity and drug therapy (Table 9-26).[217] Bisphosphonates, currently the first-line therapy for acute hypercalcemia, have an inhibitory effect on osteoclast function and viability. Bisphosphonates are the principal drugs for the management of hypercalcemia mediated by osteoclastic bone resorption.[233,234] Pamidronate, an aminobisphosphonate 100 times more potent than etidronate, normalized serum calcium in 70% of patients with malignancy-related hypercalcemia.[235] Pamidronate, unlike earlier bisphosphonates, does not appear to worsen renal insufficiency.[234]

Other osteoclast-inhibiting agents used to treat hypercalcemia include mithramycin and calcitonin.[236] Mithramycin, a cytotoxic agent, lowers serum calcium primarily by inhibiting bone resorption, probably because of toxicity to osteoclasts.[237] The hypocalcemia effect, usually seen within 12–24 hours following a single intravenous dose of 25 μg · kg^{-1}, peaks at 48–72 hours, and persists for 5–7 days. Major toxic effects of mithramycin, more likely to occur in renal insufficiency, include thrombocytopenia, nephrotoxicity, and hepatotoxicity. Calcitonin is useful in severe cases of hypercalcemia when added to mithramycin or bisphosphonates.[238] Usually calcitonin reduces total serum calcium by only 1–2 mg · dl^{-1}. Although calcitonin is relatively nontoxic, more than 25% of patients may not respond. Thus, calcitonin is unsuitable as a first-line drug during life-threatening hypercalcemia.

Hydrocortisone is effective in treating hypercalcemic patients with lymphatic malignancies, vitamin D or A intoxication, and diseases associated with production by tumor or granulomas of 1,25(OH)$_2$D or osteoclast-activating factor. Glucocorticoids rarely improve hypercalcemia secondary to malignancy or hyperparathyroidism. Gallium nitrate, an antineoplastic agent, reduces bone resorption by reducing the solubility of hydroxyapatite rather than by affecting osteoclasts. Nephrotoxicity is the most common side effect of gallium nitrate; therefore, the agent should not be administered to patients with SCr values greater than 2.5 mg · l^{-1} or to patients on chronic nephrotoxic drugs such as aminoglycosides or amphotericin.[239] The calcium-receptor antagonist R-568 causes a dose-dependent inhibition of parathyroid hormone secretion and decreases serum calcium,[240] but its role in management has yet to be determined.[221]

Phosphates lower serum calcium by causing deposition of calcium in bone and soft tissue. Because the risk of extraskeletal calcification of organs such as the kidneys and myocardium is less if phosphates are given orally, the intravenous route should be reserved for patients with life-threatening hypercalcemia or patients in whom other measures have failed.

Phosphate

Physiologic Role

Phosphorus, in the form of phosphate, is distributed in similar concentrations throughout intracellular and extracellular fluid. Of total body phosphorus, 90% exists in bone, 10% is intracellular, and the remainder, <1%, is found in the extracellular fluid. Phosphate circulates as the free ion (55%), complexed ion (33%), and in a protein-bound form (12%). Blood levels vary widely: the normal total serum phosphate level ranges from 2.7 to 4.5 mg · dl^{-1} in adults.

Control of phosphate concentration is achieved by altered renal excretion and redistribution within the body compartments. Absorption occurs in the duodenum and jejunum and is largely unregulated. Phosphate reabsorption in the kidney is primarily regulated by PTH, dietary intake, and insulin-like growth factor.[241] Phosphate is freely filtered at the glomerulus and its concentration in the glomerular ultrafiltrate is similar to plasma. The filtered phosphate is then reabsorbed in the proximal tubule where it is co-transported with sodium.[241] Proximal tubular reabsorption of phosphorus occurs by passive co-transport with sodium.[242] Co-transport is regulated by phosphorus intake and PTH.[243] Phosphate excretion is increased by volume expansion and decreased by respiratory alkalosis.

Table 9-26. DRUGS CURRENTLY APPROVED BY THE FOOD AND DRUG ADMINISTRATION THAT ARE EFFECTIVE IN LOWERING SERUM CALCIUM ACUTELY

Generic Name	Trade Name	Recommended Starting Dose
Synthetic human calcitonin	Cibacalcin	0.5 mg sc daily
Synthetic salmon calcitonin	Calcimar Miacalcin	4 IU · kg^{-1} body weight every 12 hours sc or intramuscularly
Etidronate	Didronel	7.5 mg · kg^{-1} body weight/day for 3 days
Pamidronate	Aredia	60–90 mg iv over 24 hours
Plicamycin	Mithracin	25 μg · kg^{-1} body weight/day iv for 3–4 days
Gallium nitrate	Ganite	200 mg · [m^2]$^{-1}$ body surface area/day for 5 days

(Reprinted with permission from Edelson GW, Kleerekoper M: Hypercalcemia crisis. Med Clin North Am 79:79, 1995.)

Table 9-27. HYPOPHOSPHATEMIA: ACUTE TREATMENT

Parenteral phosphate, 0.2 mM–0.68 mM/kg (5–16 mg·kg^{-1}) over 12 hours
  Potassium phosphate (93 mg·ml^{-1} of phosphate)
  Sodium phosphate (93 mg·ml^{-1} of phosphate)

Phosphates provide the primary energy bond in ATP and creatine phosphate. Therefore, severe phosphate depletion results in cellular energy depletion. Phosphorus is an essential element of second-messenger systems, including cAMP and phosphoinositides, and a major component of nucleic acids, phospholipids, and cell membranes. As part of 2,3-diphosphoglycerate, phosphate is important for off-loading oxygen from the hemoglobin molecule. Phosphorus also functions in protein phosphorylation and acts as a urinary buffer.

Hypophosphatemia

Hypophosphatemia is characterized by low levels of phosphate-containing cellular components, including ATP, 2,3-diphosphoglycerate, and membrane phospholipids. Serious life-threatening organ dysfunction may occur when the serum phosphate (PO_4) concentration falls below 1 mg·dl^{-1}. Neurologic manifestations of hypophosphatemia include paresthesias, myopathy, encephalopathy, delirium, seizures, and coma.[244] Hematologic abnormalities include dysfunction of erythrocytes, platelets, and leukocytes. Muscle weakness and malaise are common. Respiratory muscle failure[245] and myocardial dysfunction[246] are potential problems of particular concern to anesthesiologists. Rhabdomyolysis is a complication of severe hypophosphatemia.[247]

Common in postoperative and traumatized patients, hypophosphatemia ($PO_4 < 2.5$ mg·dl^{-1}) is caused by three primary abnormalities in PO_4 homeostasis: an intracellular shift of PO_4, an increase in renal PO_4 loss, and a decrease in gastrointestinal PO_4 absorption. Carbohydrate-induced hypophosphatemia (the "refeeding syndrome"),[248] mediated by insulin-induced cellular PO_4 uptake, is the type most commonly encountered in hospitalized patients. Hypophosphatemia may also occur as catabolic patients become anabolic, and during medical management of diabetic ketoacidosis. Acute alkalemia, which may reduce serum PO_4 to 1–2 mg·dl^{-1}, increases intracellular consumption of PO_4 by increasing the rate of glycolysis. Hyperventilation to a $Paco_2$ of 20 mm Hg may reduce the serum PO_4 level by 2–3 mg·dl^{-1}.[249] Acute correction of respiratory acidemia may also result in severe hypophosphatemia. Respiratory alkalosis probably explains the hypophosphatemia associated with gram-negative bacteremia and salicylate poisoning. Excessive renal loss of PO_4 explains the hypophosphatemia associated with hyperparathyroidism, hypomagnesemia, hypothermia, diuretic therapy, and renal tubular defects in PO_4 absorption. Excess gastrointestinal loss of PO_4 is most commonly secondary to the use of PO_4-binding antacids or to malabsorption syndromes.

Measurement of urinary PO_4 aids in differentiation of hypophosphatemia due to renal losses from that due to excessive gastrointestinal losses or redistribution of PO_4 into cells. Extrarenal causes of hypophosphatemia cause avid renal tubular PO_4 reabsorption, reducing urinary excretion to <100 mg·day^{-1}.

Patients who have severe (<1 mg·dl^{-1}) or symptomatic hypophosphatemia require intravenous phosphate administration (Table 9-27).[244] In chronically hypophosphatemic patients, 0.2–0.68 mmol·kg^{-1} (5–16 mg·kg^{-1} elemental phosphorus) should be infused over 12 hours. For moderately hypophosphatemic adult patients suffering from critical illness, the use of 15-mmol boluses (465 mg) mixed with 100 ml of 0.9% sodium chloride and given over a 2-hour period safely repletes phosphate.[250] The dosage is then adjusted as indicated by the serum PO_4 level, because the cumulative deficit cannot be predicted accurately. Oral therapy can be substituted for parenteral PO_4 once the serum PO_4 level exceeds 2.0 mg·dl^{-1}. Continued therapy with PO_4 supplements is required for 5–10 days in order to replenish body stores.

Phosphate should be administered cautiously to hypocalcemic patients because of the risk of precipitating more severe hypocalcemia. In hypercalcemic patients, PO_4 may cause soft-tissue calcification. Phosphorus must be given cautiously to patients with renal insufficiency because of impaired excretory ability. During treatment, close monitoring of serum PO_4, calcium, magnesium, and potassium is essential to avoid complications.

Hyperphosphatemia

The clinical features of hyperphosphatemia ($PO_4 > 5.0$ mg·dl^{-1}) relate primarily to the development of hypocalcemia and ectopic calcification. Hyperphosphatemia is caused by three basic mechanisms: inadequate renal excretion, increased movement of PO_4 out of cells, and increased PO_4 or vitamin D intake. Rapid cell lysis from chemotherapy, rhabdomyolysis, and sepsis can cause hyperphosphatemia, especially when renal function is impaired. Renal failure is the most common cause of hyperphosphatemia.[243] Renal excretion of PO_4 remains adequate until the GFR falls below 20–25 ml·min^{-1}.

Measurements of BUN, creatinine, GFR, and urinary PO_4 are helpful in the differential diagnosis of hyperphosphatemia. Normal renal function accompanied by high PO_4 excretion (>1500 mg·day^{-1}) indicates an oversupply of PO_4. An elevated BUN, elevated creatinine, and low GFR suggest impaired renal excretion of PO_4. Normal renal function and PO_4 excretion less than 1500 mg·day^{-1} suggest increased PO_4 reabsorption (*i.e.*, hypoparathyroidism).

Hyperphosphatemia is corrected by eliminating the cause of the PO_4 elevation and correcting the associated hypocalcemia. Calcium supplementation of hypocalcemic patients should be delayed until serum phosphate has fallen below 2.0 mmol·l^{-1} (6.0 mg·dl^{-1}).[221] The serum concentration of PO_4 is reduced by restricting intake, increasing urinary excretion with saline and acetazolamide (500 mg every 6 hours), and increasing gastrointestinal losses by enteric administration of aluminum hydroxide (30–45 ml every 6 hours). Aluminum hydroxide absorbs PO_4 secreted into the bowel lumen and increases PO_4 loss even if none is ingested. Hemodialysis and peritoneal dialysis are effective in removing PO_4 in patients who have renal failure.

Magnesium

Physiologic Role

Magnesium is an important, multifunctional, divalent cation located primarily in the intracellular space (intracellular magnesium ~2400 mg; extracellular magnesium ~280 mg). Approximately 50% of magnesium is located in bone, 25% is found in muscle, and less than 1% of total body magnesium circulates in the serum. Of the normal circulating total magnesium concentration (1.5–1.9 mEq·l^{-1} or 0.75–0.95 mmol·l^{-1} or 1.5–1.9 mg·dl^{-1}),[243] there are three components: protein-bound (30%), chelated (15%), and ionized (55%), of which only ionized magnesium is active.

Magnesium is necessary for enzymatic reactions involving DNA and protein synthesis.[251] As a primary regulator or cofactor in many enzyme systems, magnesium is important for the regulation of the sodium–potassium pump, Ca-ATPase enzymes, adenyl cyclase, proton pumps, and slow calcium channels. Magnesium has been called an endogenous calcium antagonist because regulation of slow calcium channels contributes to maintenance of normal vascular tone, prevention of vasospasm, and perhaps to prevention of calcium overload in many tissues. Because magnesium partially regulates PTH secretion and is important for the maintenance of end-organ sensitivity to both PTH and vitamin D, abnormalities in ionized magnesium concentration ($[Mg^{2+}]$) may result in abnormal calcium metabolism. Magnesium functions in potassium metabolism primarily through regulating sodium–potassium ATPase, an enzyme that controls potassium entry into cells, especially in potassium-depleted states, and controls reabsorption of potassium by the renal tubules. In addition, magnesium functions as a regulator of membrane excitability and serves as a structural component in both cell membranes and the skeleton.

Because magnesium stabilizes axonal membranes, hypomagnesemia decreases the threshold of axonal stimulation and increases nerve conduction velocity. Magnesium also influences the release of neurotransmitters at the neuromuscular junction by competitively inhibiting the entry of calcium into the presynaptic nerve terminals. The concentration of calcium required to trigger calcium release and the rate at which calcium is released from the sarcoplasmic reticulum are inversely related to the ambient magnesium concentration. Thus, the net effect of hypomagnesemia is muscle that contracts more in response to stimuli and is tetany prone.

The distal tubule of the kidney is the major site of magnesium regulation. Plasma $[Mg^{2+}]$ regulates magnesium reabsorption through the Ca^{2+}/Mg^{2+}-sensing receptor, located on the capillary side of cells in the thick ascending limb.[252] Magnesium is widely available in foods and is absorbed through the GI tract.[253] Whereas both magnesium and PO_4 are primarily regulated by intrinsic renal mechanisms,[251] PTH exerts a greater effect on renal loss of PO_4.

Magnesium has been used to help manage an impressive array of clinical problems in patients who are not hypomagnesemic.[254] Therapeutic hypermagnesemia is used to treat patients with premature labor, preeclampsia, and eclampsia. Because magnesium blocks the release of catecholamines from adrenergic nerve terminals and the adrenal glands, magnesium has been used to reduce the hypertensive response to tracheal intubation,[255] and to reduce the effects of catecholamine excess in patients with tetanus and pheochromocytoma. Magnesium administration may influence dysrhythmias by direct effects on myocardial membranes, by altering cellular potassium and sodium concentrations, by inhibiting cellular calcium entry, by improving myocardial oxygen supply and demand, by prolonging the effective refractory period, by depressing conduction, by antagonizing catecholamine action on the conducting system, and by preventing vasospasm. Administration of magnesium reduces the incidence of dysrhythmias after myocardial infarction.[256] In humans with ischemic myocardium, magnesium prevented the ischemic increase in action potential duration and membrane repolarization.[257] After acute myocardial infarction, intravenous magnesium administration decreased short-term mortality.[258] In addition, magnesium may be useful as treatment for *torsades de pointes* dysrhythmias, even in normomagnesemic patients.[259]

Hypomagnesemia

The clinical features of hypomagnesemia ($[Mg^{2+}] < 1.7$ mg·dl^{-1}), like those of hypocalcemia, are characterized by increased neuronal irritability and tetany.[260] Severe hypomagnesemia may reduce the response of adenylate cyclase to stimulation of the PTH receptor.[261] Hypomagnesemia can aggravate digoxin toxicity and congestive heart failure. Symptoms are rare when the serum $[Mg^{2+}]$ is 1.5–1.7 mg·dl^{-1}; in most symptomatic patients serum $[Mg^{2+}]$ is <1.0 mg·dl^{-1}. Patients frequently complain of weakness, lethargy, muscle spasms, paresthesias, and depression. When severe, hypomagnesemia may induce seizures, confusion, and coma. Cardiovascular abnormalities include coronary artery spasm, cardiac failure, dysrhythmias, and hypotension.

Hypomagnesemia, identified in 11% of hospitalized patients[262] and as many as 47% of blood samples collected for determination of other electrolytes,[263] is associated with hypokalemia, hyponatremia, hypophosphatemia, and hypocalcemia. Of alcoholic patients admitted to the hospital, 30% are hypomagnesemic.[264] Serum $[Mg^{2+}]$ may not reflect intracellular magnesium content. Peripheral lymphocyte magnesium concentration correlates well with skeletal and cardiac magnesium content.

Rarely resulting from inadequate dietary intake, hypomagnesemia is most commonly caused by inadequate gastrointestinal absorption, excessive magnesium losses, or failure of renal magnesium conservation. Excessive magnesium loss is associated with prolonged nasogastric suctioning, gastrointestinal or biliary fistulas, and intestinal drains. Inability of the renal tubules to conserve magnesium complicates a variety of systemic and renal diseases, although advanced renal disease with a decreased GFR may lead to magnesium retention. Polyuria, whether secondary to ECV expansion or to pharmacologic or pathologic diuresis, may result in excessive urinary magnesium excretion. Various drugs, including aminoglycosides,[265] *cis*-platinum, cardiac glycosides, and diuretics, enhance urinary magnesium excretion. Intracellular shifts of magnesium as a result of thyroid hormone or insulin administration may also decrease serum $[Mg^{2+}]$.

Measurement of 24-hour urinary magnesium excretion is useful in separating renal from nonrenal causes of hypomagnesemia. Normal kidneys can reduce magnesium excretion to less than 1–2 mEq·day^{-1} in response to magnesium depletion. Hypomagnesemia accompanied by high urinary excretion of magnesium (>3–4 mEq·day^{-1}) suggests a renal etiology. In the magnesium-loading test, urinary Mg^{2+} excretion is measured for 24 hours after an intravenous magnesium load.[226]

Magnesium deficiency is treated by the administration of magnesium supplements (Table 9-28). One gram of magnesium sulfate provides approximately 4 mmol (8 mEq, or 98 mg) of elemental magnesium. Mild deficiencies can be treated with diet alone. Replacement must be added to daily magnesium requirements (0.3–0.4 mEq·kg^{-1}·day^{-1}). Symptomatic or severe hypomagnesemia ($[Mg^{2+}] < 1.0$ mg·dl^{-1}) should be treated with parenteral magnesium: 1–2 g (8–16 mEq) of magnesium sulfate as an intravenous bolus over the first hour, followed by a continuous infusion of 2–4 mEq·hr^{-1}. Therapy should be guided subsequently by the serum magnesium level. The rate of infusion should not exceed 1 mEq·min^{-1}, even in emergency situations, and the patient should receive continuous cardiac monitoring to detect cardiotoxicity. Because magnesium antagonizes calcium, blood pressure and cardiac function should be monitored, although clinical effects on myocardial contractility and blood pressure appear to be modest. Treatment of hypomagnesemia after cardiopulmonary bypass decreased the incidence of ventricular dysrhythmias after heart surgery from 63% to 22%.[267]

Because the sodium–potassium pump is magnesium-dependent, hypomagnesemia increases myocardial sensitivity to digitalis preparations and may cause hypokalemia as a result of renal potassium wasting. Attempts to correct potassium deficits with potassium replacement therapy alone may not be successful without simultaneous magnesium therapy. Magnesium is important in the regulation of potassium channels. The interrelationships of magnesium and potassium in cardiac tissue have proba-

---

Table 9-28. HYPOMAGNESEMIA: ACUTE TREATMENT

Intravenous Mg*: 8–16 mEq bolus over 1 hour, followed by 2–4 mEq·hr^{-1} as continuous infusion
Intramuscular Mg*: 10 mEq q 4–6 hours

---

* $MgSO_4$: 1 g = 8 mEq Mg. $MgCl_2$: 1 g = 10 mEq Mg.

Table 9-29. HYPERMAGNESEMIA: CLINICAL FINDINGS

Clinical Findings	Serum [Mg^{2+}] (mg · dl^{-1})
Normal	1.7–2.4
Therapeutic range (preeclampsia)	5–8
Hypotension	3–5
Deep tendon hyporeflexia	5
Somnolence	8.5
Respiratory insufficiency, deep tendon areflexia	12
Heart block, respiratory paralysis	18
Cardiac arrest	24

bly the greatest clinical relevance in terms of dysrhythmias, digoxin toxicity, and myocardial infarction. Both severe hypomagnesemia and hypermagnesemia suppress PTH secretion and can cause hypocalcemia. Severe hypomagnesemia may also impair end-organ response to PTH.

During repletion, the patellar reflexes should be monitored frequently and magnesium withheld if they become suppressed. Patients who have renal insufficiency have a diminished ability to excrete magnesium and require careful monitoring during therapy. Repletion of systemic magnesium stores usually requires 5–7 days of therapy, after which daily maintenance doses of magnesium should be provided. Magnesium can be given orally, usually in a dose of 60–90 mEq · day^{-1} of magnesium oxide. Hypocalcemic, hypomagnesemic patients should receive magnesium as the chloride salt, because the sulfate ion can chelate calcium and further reduce the serum [Ca^{2+}].

Hypermagnesemia

Most cases of hypermagnesemia ([Mg^{2+}] >2.5 mg · dl^{-1}) are iatrogenic, resulting from the administration of magnesium in antacids, enemas, or parenteral nutrition, especially to patients with impaired renal function. Other rarer causes of mild hypermagnesemia are hypothyroidism, Addison's disease, lithium intoxication, and familial hypocalciuric hypercalcemia. Hypermagnesemia is detected in 5.7–9.3% of blood samples drawn for electrolyte determinations.[262,263] Hypermagnesemia antagonizes the release and effect of acetylcholine at the neuromuscular junction. The result is depressed skeletal muscle function and neuromuscular blockade. Magnesium potentiates the action of nondepolarizing muscle relaxants[268] and decreases potassium release in response to succinylcholine.[269] The clinical features of progressive hypermagnesemia are listed in Table 9-29.

The neuromuscular and cardiac toxicity of hypermagnesemia can be acutely, but transiently, antagonized by giving intravenous calcium (5–10 mEq) to buy time while more definitive therapy is instituted.[270] All magnesium-containing preparations must be stopped. Urinary excretion of magnesium can be increased by expanding ECV and inducing diuresis with a combination of saline and furosemide. In emergency situations and in patients with renal failure, magnesium may be removed by dialysis.

REFERENCES

1. Stewart PA: Independent and dependent variables of acid–base control. Respir Physiol 33:9, 1978
2. Eicker SW: An introduction to strong ion difference. Vet Clin North Am [Food Anim Pract] 8:45, 1990
3. Wilson RF, Gibson D, Percinel AK *et al*: Severe alkalosis in critically ill surgical patients. Arch Surg 105:197, 1972
4. Sabatini S, Arruda JAL, Kurtzman NA: Disorders of acid–base balance. Med Clin North Am 62:1223, 1978
5. Boron VF, Hediger MA, Boulpaep EL, Romero MF: The renal electrogenic Na$^+$: HCO$_3^-$ cotransporter. J Exp Biol 200(Pt 2): 263, 1997
6. Scheich A, Donnelly S, Cheema-Dhadli S *et al*: Does saline "correct" the abnormal mass balance in metabolic alkalosis associated with chloride depletion in the rat? Clin Invest Med 17:448, 1994
7. Riley LJ Jr, Elson BE, Narins RG: Acute metabolic acid–base disorders. Crit Care Clin 5:699, 1987
8. Goldring RM, Cannon PJ, Heinemann HO, Fishman AP: Respiratory adjustment to chronic metabolic alkalosis in man. J Clin Invest 47:188, 1968
9. Scheingraber S, Rehm M, Sehmisch C, Finsterer U: Rapid saline infusion produces hyperchloremic acidosis in patients undergoing gynecologic surgery. Anesthesiology 90:1265, 1999
10. Rossing TH, Maffeo N, Fencl V: Acid–base effects of altering plasma protein concentration in human blood *in vitro*. J Appl Physiol 61:2260, 1986
11. Figge J, Mydosh T, Fencl V: Serum proteins and acid–base equilibria: A follow-up. J Lab Clin Med 120:713, 1992
12. Figge J, Rossing TH, Fencl V: The role of serum proteins in acid–base equilibria. J Lab Clin Med 117:453, 1991
13. Ponce P, Santana A, Vinhas J: Treatment of severe metabolic alkalosis by "acid dialysis." Crit Care Med 19:583, 1991
14. Gluck SL: Acid–base. Lancet 352:474, 1998
15. Badrick T, Hickman PE: The anion gap: A reappraisal. Am J Clin Pathol 98:249, 1992
16. McFarlane C, Lee A: A comparison of plasmalyte 148 and 0.9% saline for intraoperative fluid replacement. Anaesthesia 49:779, 1994
17. Opie LH, Kadas T, Gevers W: Effect of pH on the function and glucose metabolism of the heart. Lancet 2:551, 1963
18. Shapiro BJ, Simmons DH, Linde LM: Pulmonary hemodynamics during acute acid–base changes in the intact dog. Am J Physiol 210:1026, 1966
19. Wildenthal K, Mierzwiak DS, Myers RW: Effects of acute lactic acidosis of left ventricular performance. Am J Physiol 241:1352, 1968
20. Stokke DB, Andersen PK, Brinklov MM *et al*: Acid–base interactions with noradrenaline-induced contractile response of the rabbit isolated aorta. Anesthesiology 60:400, 1984
21. Albert MS, Dell RB, Winters RW: Quantitative displacement of acid–base equilibrium in metabolic acidosis. Ann Intern Med 66: 312, 1967
22. Beech JS, Nolan KM, Iles RA *et al*: The effects of sodium bicarbonate and a mixture of sodium bicarbonate ("carbicarb") on skeletal muscle pH and hemodynamic status in rats with hypovolemic shock. Metabolism 43:518, 1994
23. Cooper DJ, Walley KR, Wiggs BR, Russell JA: Bicarbonate does not improve hemodynamics in critically ill patients who have lactic acidosis. A prospective, controlled clinical study. Ann Intern Med 112:492, 1990
24. Mathieu D, Neviere R, Billard V *et al*: Effects of bicarbonate therapy on hemodynamics and tissue oxygenation in patients with lactic acidosis: A prospective, controlled clinical study. Crit Care Med 19:1352, 1991
25. Mark NH, Leung JM, Arieff AI, Mangano DT: Safety of low-dose intraoperative bicarbonate therapy: A prospective, double-blind, randomized study. Crit Care Med 21:659, 1993
26. Leung JM, Landow L, Franks M *et al*: Safety and efficacy of intravenous carbicarb in patients undergoing surgery: Comparison with sodium bicarbonate in the treatment of mild metabolic acidosis. Crit Care Med 22:1540, 1994
27. Kaehny WD, Anderson RJ: Bicarbonate therapy of metabolic acidosis. Crit Care Med 22:1525, 1994
28. Stacpoole PW, Wright EC, Baumgartner TG *et al*: A controlled clinical trial of dichloroacetate for treatment of lactic acidosis in adults. N Engl J Med 327:1564, 1992
29. Nahas GG, Sutin KM, Fermon C *et al*: Guidelines for the treatment of acidaemia with THAM. Drugs 55:191, 1998
30. Severinghaus JW, Mitchell RA, Richardson BW, Singer MM: Respiratory control at high altitude suggesting active transport regulation of CSF pH. J Appl Physiol 18:1155, 1963
31. Christensen MS: Acid–base changes in cerebrospinal fluid and blood, and blood volumes changes following prolonged hyperventilation in man. Br J Anaesth 46:348, 1974
32. Elisaf MS, Tsatsoulis AA, Katopodis KP, Siamopoulos KC: Acid–base and electrolyte disturbances in patients with diabetic ketoacidosis. Diabetes Res Clin Pract 34:23, 1996
33. Jaber BL, Madias NE: Marked dilutional acidosis complicating

management of right ventricular myocardial infarction. Am J Kidney Dis 30:561, 1997

34. Prough DS, Bidani A: Hyperchloremic metabolic acidosis is a predictable consequence of intraoperative infusion of 0.9% saline. Anesthesiology 90:1247, 1999

35. Svensén C, Hahn RG: Volume kinetics of Ringer solution, dextran 70, and hypertonic saline in male volunteers. Anesthesiology 87:204, 1997

36. Stahle L, Nilsson A, Hahn RG: Modelling the volume of expandable body fluid spaces during i.v. fluid therapy. Br J Anaesth 78:138, 1997

37. Hahn RG, Svensén C: Plasma dilution and the rate of infusion of Ringer's solution. Br J Anaesth 79:64, 1997

38. Brauer KI, Prough DS, Traber LD, Traber DL: Antecedent hemorrhage increases plasma volume expansion (PVE) in response to 0.9% saline infusion in sheep. Anesth Analg 88:S135, 1999

39. Drobin D, Hahn RG: Volume kinetics of Ringer's solution in hypovolemic volunteers. Anesthesiology 90:81, 1999

40. Teitelbaum I, Kleeman CR, Berl T: The physiology of the renal concentrating and diluting mechanism. In Narins RG (ed): Clinical Disorders of Fluid and Electrolyte Metabolism. New York, McGraw-Hill, 1994

41. Fried LF, Palevsky PM: Hyponatremia and hypernatremia. In Saklayen MG (ed): The Medical Clinics of North America. Renal Disease, p 585. Philadelphia, WB Saunders, 1997

42. Abramow M, Beauwens R, Cogan E: Cellular events in vasopressin action. Kidney Int 21:S56, 1987

43. Fushimi K, Uchida S, Hara Y et al: Cloning and expression of apical membrane water channel of rat kidney collecting tubule. Nature 361:549, 1993

44. Harris HW Jr, Strange K, Zeidel ML: Current understanding of the cellular biology and molecular structure of the antidiuretic hormone-stimulated water transport pathway. J Clin Invest 88:1, 1991

45. Levin AR, Gardner DG, Samson WK: Natriuretic peptides. N Engl J Med 339:321, 1998

46. Needleman P, Greenwald JE: Atriopeptin: A cardiac hormone intimately involved in fluid, electrolyte, and blood-pressure homeostasis. N Engl J Med 314:828, 1986

47. Cernacek P, Maher E, Crawhall JC, Levy M: Renal dose response and pharmacokinetics of atrial natriuretic factor in dogs. Am J Physiol 255:R929, 1988

48. Conte G, Bellizzi V, Cianciaruso B et al: Physiologic role and diuretic efficacy of atrial natriuretic peptide in health and chronic renal disease. Kidney Int 51:S28, 1997

49. Schrier RW: Pathogenesis of sodium and water retention in high-output and low-output cardiac failure, nephrotic syndrome, cirrhosis, and pregnancy. Part 1. N Engl J Med 319:1065, 1988

50. Laragh JH: The endocrine control of blood volume, blood pressure and sodium balance: Atrial hormone and renin system interactions. J Hypertens 4(suppl 2):S143, 1986

51. Badr KF, Ichikawa I: Prerenal failure: A deleterious shift from renal compensation to decompensation. N Engl J Med 319:623, 1988

52. Henrich WL, Anderson RJ, Berns AS et al: The role of renal nerves and prostaglandins in control of renal hemodynamics and plasma renin activity during hypotensive hemorrhage in the dog. J Clin Invest 61:744, 1978

53. Henrich WL, Pettinger WA, Cronin RE: The influence of circulating catecholamines and prostaglandins on canine renal hemodynamics during hemorrhage. Circ Res 48:424, 1981

54. Murray MD, Brater DC: Adverse effect of nonsteroidal anti-inflammatory drugs on renal function. Ann Intern Med 112:559, 1990

55. Lanier WL, Stangland KJ, Scheithauer BW et al: The effects of dextrose infusion and head position on neurologic outcome after complete cerebral ischemia in primates: Examination of a model. Anesthesiology 66:39, 1987

56. Lanzino G, Kassell NF, Germanson T et al: Plasma glucose levels and outcome after aneurysmal subarachnoid hemorrhage. J Neurosurg 79:885, 1993

57. Lam AM, Winn HR, Cullen BF, Sundling N: Hyperglycemia and neurological outcome in patients with head injury. J Neurosurg 75:545, 1991

58. Longstreth WT Jr, Diehr P, Cobb LA et al: Neurologic outcome and blood glucose levels during out-of-hospital cardiopulmonary resuscitation. Neurology 36:1186, 1986

59. Roberts JP, Roberts JD Jr, Skinner C et al: Extracellular fluid deficit following operation and its correction with Ringer's lactate: A reassessment. Ann Surg 202:1, 1985

60. Böck JC, Barker BC, Clinton AG et al: Post-traumatic changes in, and effect of colloid osmotic pressure on the distribution of body water. Ann Surg 210:395, 1989

61. Peng ATC, Shamsi HH, Blancato LS et al: Euglycemic hydration with dextrose 1% in lactated Ringer's solution during epidural anesthesia for cesarean section. Reg Anesth 12:184, 1987

62. Eledjam JJ, Thomas H, Macheboef M et al: Influence of vascular loading on the secretion of the atrial natriuretic factor during epidural analgesia (EA) for labour. Anesthesiology 71:A876, 1989

63. Rout CC, Rocke DA, Levin J et al: A reevaluation of the role of crystalloid preload in the prevention of hypotension associated with spinal anesthesia for elective cesarean section. Anesthesiology 79:262, 1993

64. Mathru M, Rao TL, Kartha RK et al: Intravenous albumin administration for prevention of spinal hypotension during cesarean section. Anesth Analg 59:655, 1980

65. Demling RH: Shock and fluids. In Chernow B, Shoemaker WC (eds): Critical Care: State of the Art, p 301. Fullerton, California: Society of Critical Care Medicine, 1986

66. Uhley HN, Leeds SE, Sampson JJ, Friedman M: Role of pulmonary lymphatics in chronic pulmonary edema. Circ Res 11:966, 1962

67. Schierhout G, Roberts I: Fluid resuscitation with colloid or crystalloid solutions in critically ill patients: A systematic review of randomised trials. Br Med J 316:961, 1998

68. Cochrane Injuries Group Albumin Reviewers: Human albumin administration in critically ill patients: Systematic review of randomised controlled trials. Br Med J 317:235, 1998

69. Velanovich V: Crystalloid versus colloid fluid resuscitation: A meta-analysis of mortality. Surgery 105:65, 1989

70. Choi PTL, Yip G, Quinonez LG, Cook DJ: Crystalloids vs colloids in fluid resuscitation: A systematic review. Crit Care Med 27:200, 1999

71. Pearl RG, Halperin BD, Mihm FG, Rosenthal MH: Pulmonary effects of crystalloid and colloid resuscitation from hemorrhagic shock in the presence of oleic acid-induced pulmonary capillary injury in the dog. Anesthesiology 68:12, 1988

72. Morisaki H, Bloos F, Keys J et al: Compared with crystalloid, colloid therapy slows progression of extrapulmonary tissue in septic sheep. J Appl Physiol 77:1507, 1994

73. Rackow EC, Falk JL, Fein IA et al: Fluid resuscitation in circulatory shock: A comparison of the cardiorespiratory effects of albumin, hetastarch, and saline solutions in patients with hypovolemic and septic shock. Crit Care Med 11:839, 1983

74. Weil MH, Henning RH, Puri VK: Colloid oncotic pressure: Clinical significance. Crit Care Med 7:113, 1979

75. Virgilio RW, Rice CL, Smith DE et al: Crystalloid vs colloid resuscitation: Is one better? A randomized clinical study. Surgery 85:129, 1979

76. Stump DC, Strauss RG, Henriksen RA et al: Effects of hydroxyethyl starch on blood coagulation, particularly factor VIII. Transfusion 25:349, 1985

77. Gold MS, Russo J, Tissot M et al: Comparison of hetastarch to albumin for perioperative bleeding in patients undergoing abdominal aortic aneurysm surgery: A prospective, randomized study. Ann Surg 211:482, 1990

78. Halonen P, Linko K, Myllyla G: A study of haemostasis following the use of high doses of hydroxyethyl starch 120 and dextran in major laparotomies. Acta Anaesthesiol Scand 31:320, 1987

79. Sade RM, Crawford FA Jr, Dearing JP, Stroud M: Hydroxyethyl starch in priming fluid for cardiopulmonary bypass. J Thorac Cardiovasc Surg 84:35, 1982

80. Gan TJ, Bennett-Guerrero E, Phillips-Bute B et al: Hextend, a physiologically balanced plasma expander for large volume use in major surgery: A randomized phase III clinical trial. Anesth Analg 88:992, 1999

81. Zornow MH, Todd MM, Moore SS: The acute cerebral effects of changes in plasma osmolality and oncotic pressure. Anesthesiology 67:936, 1987

82. Kaieda R, Todd MM, Warner DS: Prolonged reduction in colloid oncotic pressure does not increase brain edema following cryogenic injury in rabbits. Anesthesiology 71:554, 1989

83. Warner DS, Boehland LA: Effects of iso-osmolal intravenous fluid therapy on post-ischemic brain water content in the rat. Anesthesiology 68:86, 1988

84. Zornow MH, Scheller MS, Todd MM, Moore SS: Acute cerebral

effects of isotonic crystalloid and colloid solutions following cryogenic brain injury in the rabbit. Anesthesiology 69:180, 1988

85. Drummond JC, Patel PM, Cole DJ, Kelly PJ: The effect of the reduction of colloid oncotic pressure, with and without reduction of osmolality, on post-traumatic cerebral edema. Anesthesiology 88:993, 1998

86. Weed LH, McKibben PS: Experimental alteration of brain bulk. Am J Physiol 48:531, 1919

87. Velasco IT, Pontieri V, Rocha e Silva M Jr, Lopes OU: Hyperosmotic NaCl and severe hemorrhagic shock. Am J Physiol 239:H664, 1980

88. Schertel ER, Valentine AK, Rademakers AM, Muir WW: Influence of 7% NaCl on the mechanical properties of the systemic circulation in the hypovolemic dog. Circ Shock 31:203, 1990

89. Vollmar B, Lang G, Menger MD, Messmer K: Hypertonic hydroxyethyl starch restores hepatic microvascular perfusion in hemorrhagic shock. Am J Physiol (Heart Circ Physiol) 266:H1927, 1994

90. Onarheim H, Missavage AE, Kramer GC, Gunther RA: Effectiveness of hypertonic saline-dextran 70 for initial fluid resuscitation of major burns. J Trauma 30:597, 1990

91. Gunn ML, Hansbrough JF, Davis JW et al: Prospective, randomized trial of hypertonic sodium lactate versus lactated Ringer's solution for burn shock resuscitation. J Trauma 29:1261, 1989

92. Prough DS, Whitley JM, Taylor CL et al: Regional cerebral blood flow following resuscitation from hemorrhagic shock with hypertonic saline: Influence of a subdural mass. Anesthesiology 75:319, 1991

93. Wisner DH, Schuster L, Quinn C: Hypertonic saline resuscitation of head injury: Effects on cerebral water content. J Trauma 30:75, 1990

94. Whitley JM, Prough DS, Brockschmidt JK et al: Cerebral hemodynamic effects of fluid resuscitation in the presence of an experimental intracranial mass. Surgery 110:514, 1991

95. Prough DS, Whitley JM, Taylor CL et al: Rebound intracranial hypertension in dogs after resuscitation with hypertonic solutions from hemorrhagic shock accompanied by an intracranial mass lesion. J Neurosurg Anesth 11:102, 1999

96. Wisner DH, Battstelia FD, Freshman SP et al: Nuclear magnetic resonance as a measure of cerebral metabolism: Effects of hypertonic saline. J Trauma 32:351, 1992

97. Vassar MJ, Fischer RP, O'Brien PE et al: A multicenter trial for resuscitation of injured patients with 7.5% sodium chloride: The effect of added dextran 70. Arch Surg 128:1003, 1993

98. Mattox KL, Maningas PA, Moore EE et al: Prehospital hypertonic saline/dextran infusion for post-traumatic hypotension. The U.S.A. Multicenter Trial. Ann Surg 213:482, 1991

99. Norenberg MD, Papendick RE: Chronicity of hyponatremia as a factor in experimental myelinolysis. Ann Neurol 15:544, 1984

100. Smith GJ, Kramer GC, Perron P et al: A comparison of several hypertonic solutions for resuscitation of bled sheep. J Surg Res 39:517, 1985

101. Gross D, Landau EH, Klin B, Krausz MM: Treatment of uncontrolled hemorrhagic shock with hypertonic saline solution. Surg Gynecol Obstet 170:106, 1990

102. Bickell WH, Wall MJ Jr, Pepe PE et al: Immediate versus delayed fluid resuscitation for hypotensive patients with penetrating torso injuries. N Engl J Med 331:1105, 1994

103. Chesnut RM: Avoidance of hypotension: *Conditio sine qua non* of successful severe head-injury management. J Trauma 42:S4, 1997

104. Zaloga GP, Hughes SS: Oliguria in patients with normal renal function. Anesthesiology 72:598, 1990

105. Lipsitz LA: Orthostatic hypotension in the elderly. N Engl J Med 321:952, 1989

106. Wong DH, O'Connor D, Tremper KK et al: Changes in cardiac output after acute blood loss and position change in man. Crit Care Med 17:979, 1989

107. Amoroso P, Greenwood RN: Posture and central venous pressure measurement in circulatory volume depletion. Lancet 2:258, 1989

108. Perel A: Assessing fluid responsiveness by the systolic pressure variation in mechanically ventilated patients. Anesthesiology 89:1309, 1998

109. Stoneham MD: Less is more. . .Using systolic pressure variation to assess hypovolaemia. Br J Anaesth 83:550, 1999

110. Tavernier B, Makhotine O, Lebuffe G et al: Systolic pressure variation as a guide to fluid therapy in patients with sepsis-induced hypotension. Anesthesiology 89:1313, 1998

111. Rooke GA, Schwid HA, Shapira Y: The effect of graded hemorrhage and intravascular volume replacement on systolic pressure variation in humans during mechanical and spontaneous ventilation. Anesth Analg 80:925, 1995

112. Shoemaker WC, Appel PL, Kram HB et al: Prospective trial of supranormal values of survivors as therapeutic goals in high-risk surgical patients. Chest 94:1176, 1988

113. Tuchschmidt J, Fried J, Astiz M, Rackow E: Elevation of cardiac output and oxygen delivery improves outcome in septic shock. Chest 102:216, 1992

114. Boyd O, Grounds RM, Bennett ED: A randomized clinical trial of the effect of deliberate perioperative increase of oxygen delivery on mortality in high-risk surgical patients. JAMA 270:2699, 1993

115. Guest JF, Boyd O, Hart WM et al: A cost analysis of a treatment policy of a deliberate perioperative increase in oxygen delivery in high risk surgical patients. Intensive Care Med 23:85, 1997

116. Wilson J, Woods I, Fawcett J et al: Reducing the risk of major elective surgery: Randomised controlled trial of preoperative optimisation of oxygen delivery. Br Med J 318:1099, 1999

117. Hayes MA, Timmins AC, Yau EHS et al: Elevation of systemic oxygen delivery in the treatment of critically ill patients. N Engl J Med 330:1717, 1994

118. Heyland DK, Cook DJ, King D et al: Maximizing oxygen delivery in critically ill patients: A methodologic appraisal of the evidence. Crit Care Med 24:517, 1996

119. Boldt J, Papsdorf M, Piper S et al: Influence of dopexamine hydrochloride on haemodynamics and regulators of circulation in patients undergoing major abdominal surgery. Acta Anaesthesiol Scand 42:941, 1998

120. Anderson RJ, Chung HM, Kluge R, Schrier RW: Hyponatremia: A prospective analysis of its epidemiology and the pathogenetic role of vasopressin. Ann Intern Med 102:164, 1985

121. Tierney WM, Martin DK, Greenlee MC et al: The prognosis of hyponatremia at hospital admission. J Gen Intern Med 1:380, 1986

122. Berl T: Treating hyponatremia: Damned if we do and damned if we don't. Kidney Int 37:1006, 1990

123. Lien YH, Shapiro JI, Chan L: Effects of hypernatremia on organic brain osmoles. J Clin Invest 85:1427, 1990

124. Moran SM, Jamison RL: The variable hyponatremic response to hyperglycemia. West J Med 142:49, 1985

125. Rothenberg DM, Berns AS, Ivankovich AD: Isotonic hyponatremia following transurethral prostate resection. J Clin Anesth 2:48, 1990

126. Campbell HT, Fincher ME, Sklar AH: Severe hyponatremia without hypoosmolality following transurethral resection of the prostate (TURP) in end stage renal disease. Am J Kidney Dis 12:152, 1988

127. Hahn RG: The transurethral resection syndrome. Acta Anaesthesiol Scand 35:557, 1991

128. Xu DL, Martin PY, Ohara M et al: Upregulation of aquaporin-2 water channel expression in chronic heart failure rat. J Clin Invest 99:1500, 1997

129. Fujita N, Ishikawa SE, Sasaki S et al: Role of water channel AQP-CD in water retention in SIADH and cirrhotic rats. Am J Physiol 269:F926, 1995

130. Ecelbarger CA, Nielsen S, Olson BR et al: Role of renal aquaporins in escape from vasopressin-induced antidiuresis in rat. J Clin Invest 99:1852, 1997

131. Kumar S, Beri T: Sodium. Lancet 352:220, 1998

132. Berendes E, Walter M, Cullen P et al: Secretion of brain natriuretic peptide in patients with aneurysmal subarachnoid haemorrhage. Lancet 349:245, 1997

133. Al-Mufti H, Arieff AI: Hyponatremia due to cerebral salt-wasting syndrome. Combined cerebral and distal tubular lesion. Am J Med 77:740, 1984

134. Kroll M, Juhler M, Lindholm J: Hyponatremia in acute brain disease. J Intern Med 232:291, 1992

135. Wijdicks EFM, Ropper AH, Hunnicutt EJ et al: Atrial natriuretic factor and salt wasting after aneurysmal subarachnoid hemorrhage. Stroke 22:1519, 1991

136. Yamaki T, Tano-oka A, Takahashi A et al: Cerebral salt wasting syndrome distinct from the syndrome of inappropriate secretion of antidiuretic hormone (SIADH). Acta Neurochir 115:156, 1992

137. Kim JK, Summer SN, Wood WM, Schrier RW: Osmotic and nonosmotic regulation of arginine vasopressin (AVP) release, mRNA, and promoter activity in small cell lung carcinoma (SCLC) cells. Mol Cell Endocrinol 123:179, 1996

138. Ayus JC, Arieff AI: Symptomatic hyponatremia: Making the diagnosis rapidly. J Crit Illn 5:846, 1990

139. Chung H, Kluge R, Schrier RW, Anderson RJ: Postoperative hyponatremia. A prospective study. Arch Intern Med 146:333, 1986

140. Gomola A, Cabrol S, Murat I: Severe hyponatraemia after plastic surgery in a girl with cleft palate, medial facial hypoplasia and growth retardation. Paediatric Anesthesia 8:69, 1998

141. Arieff AI: Postoperative hyponatraemic encephalopathy following elective surgery in children. Paediatric Anesthesia 8:1, 1998

142. Akaishi T, Sakuma Y: Estrogen-induced modulation of hypothalamic osmoregulation in female rats. Am J Physiol 258:R924, 1990

143. Stone JD, Crofton JT, Share L: Sex differences in central adrenergic control of vasopressin release. Am J Physiol 257:R1040, 1989

144. Fraser CL, Arieff AI: Fatal central diabetes mellitus and insipidus resulting from untreated hyponatremia: A new syndrome. Ann Intern Med 112:113, 1990

145. Arieff AI, Kozniewska E, Roberts TP et al: Age, gender, and vasopressin affect survival and brain adaptation in rats with metabolic encephalopathy. Am J Physiol 268:R1143, 1995

146. Steele A, Gowrishankar M, Abrahamson S et al: Postoperative hyponatremia despite near-isotonic saline infusion: A phenomenon of desalination. Ann Intern Med 126:20, 1997

147. Ayus JC, Arieff AI: Postoperative hyponatremia. Ann Intern Med 126:1005, 1997

148. Karmel KS, Bear RA: Treatment of hyponatremia: A quantitative analysis. Am J Kidney Dis 21:439, 1994

149. Sarnaik AP, Meert K, Hackbarth R, Fleischmann L: Management of hyponatremic seizures in children with hypertonic saline: A safe and effective strategy. Crit Care Med 19:758, 1991

150. Soupart A, Decaux G: Therapeutic recommendations for management of severe hyponatremia: Current concepts on pathogenesis and prevention of neurologic complications. Clin Nephrol 46:149, 1996

151. Laureno R: Central pontine myelinolysis following rapid correction of hyponatremia. Ann Neurol 13:232, 1983

152. Sterns RH, Riggs JE, Schochet SS Jr: Osmotic demyelination syndrome following correction of hyponatremia. N Engl J Med 314:1535, 1986

153. Brunner JE, Redmond JM, Haggar AM et al: Central pontine myelinolysis and pontine lesions after rapid correction of hyponatremia: A prospective magnetic resonance imaging study. Ann Neurol 27:61, 1990

154. Laureno R, Karp BI: Myelinolysis after correction of hyponatremia. Ann Intern Med 126:57, 1997

155. Verbalis JG, Drutarowsky MD: Adaptation to chronic hyposmolarity in rats. Kidney Int 34:351, 1988

156. Soupart A, Decaux G: Therapeutic recommendations for management of severe hyponatremia: Current concepts on pathogenesis and prevention of neurologic complications. Clin Nephrol 46:149, 1996

157. Adrogué HJ, Madias NE: Aiding fluid prescription for the dysnatremias. Intensive Care Med 23:309, 1997

158. Sterns RH: Vignettes in clinical pathophysiology. Neurological deterioration following treatment for hyponatremia. Am J Kidney Dis 13:434, 1989

159. Ayus JC, Arieff AI: Symptomatic hyponatremia: Correcting sodium deficits safely. Extent of replacement may be more important than infusion rate. J Crit Illn 5:905, 1990

160. Cluitmans FHM, Meinders AE: Management of severe hyponatremia: Rapid or slow correction? Am J Med 88:161, 1990

161. Narins RG: Therapy of hyponatremia: Does haste make waste? N Engl J Med 314:1573, 1986

162. Berl T: Treating hyponatremia: What is all the controversy about? Ann Intern Med 113:417, 1990

163. Marples D, Christensen S, Christensen EI et al: Lithium-induced downregulation of aquaporin-2 water channel expression in rat kidney medulla. J Clin Invest 95:1838, 1995

164. Kitiyakara C, Wilcox CS: Vasopressin V2-receptor antagonists: Panaceas for hyponatremia? Curr Opin Nephrol Hypertens 6:461, 1997

165. Hall J, Robertson G: Diabetes insipidus. Prob Crit Care 4:342, 1990

166. Ober KP: Endocrine crises: Diabetes insipidus. Crit Care Clin 7:109, 1991

167. Seckl JR, Dunger DB, Lightman SL: Neurohypophyseal peptide function during early postoperative diabetes insipidus. Brain 110:737, 1987

168. Phillips PA, Rolls BJ, Ledingham JGG et al: Reduced thirst after water deprivation in healthy elderly men. N Engl J Med 311:753, 1984

169. Rowe JW, Shock NW, DeFronzo RA: The influence of age on the renal response to water deprivation in man. Nephron 17:270, 1976

170. Strange K: Regulation of solute and water balance and cell volume in the central nervous system. J Am Soc Nephrol 3:12, 1992

171. Young RSK, Truax B: Hypernatremic hemorrhagic encephalopathy. Ann Neurol 5:588, 1979

172. Ayus JC, Armstrong DL, Arieff AI: Effects of hypernatraemia in the central nervous system and its therapy in rats and rabbits. J Physiol 492:243, 1996

173. Tannen RL, Regal EM, Dunn MJ, Schrier RW: Vasopressin-resistant hyposthenuria in advanced chronic renal disease. N Engl J Med 280:1135, 1969

174. Robertson GL: Differential diagnosis of polyuria. Annu Rev Med 39:425, 1988

175. Griffin KA, Bidani AK: How to manage disorders of sodium and water balance. Five-step approach to evaluating appropriateness of renal response. J Crit Illn 5:1054, 1990

176. Feig PU: Hypernatremia and hypertonic syndromes. Med Clin North Am 65:271, 1981

177. McManus ML, Churchwill KB, Strange K: Regulation of cell volume in health and disease. N Engl J Med 333:1260, 1995

178. Robinson AG: DDAVP in the treatment of central diabetes insipidus. N Engl J Med 294:507, 1976

179. Cobb WE, Spare S, Reichlin S: Neurogenic diabetes insipidus: Management with dDAVP (1-desamino-8-D-arginine vasopressin). Ann Intern Med 88:183, 1978

180. Shucart WA, Jackson I: Management of diabetes insipidus in neurosurgical patients. J Neurosurg 44:65, 1976

181. Chanson P, Jedynak CP, Dabrowski G et al: Ultralow doses of vasopressin in the management of diabetes insipidus. Crit Care Med 15:44, 1987

182. Halperin ML, Kamel KS: Potassium. Lancet 352:135, 1998

183. Zierler K: Insulin hyperpolarizes rat myotube primary culture without stimulating glucose uptake. Diabetes 36:1035, 1987

184. Williams ME, Gervino EV, Rosa RM et al: Catecholamine modulation of rapid potassium shifts during exercise. N Engl J Med 312:823, 1985

185. Mandal AK: Hypokalemia and hyperkalemia. In Saklayen MG (ed): The Medical Clinics of North America. Renal Disease, p 611. Philadelphia, WB Saunders, 1997

186. Rossier BC: Cum grano salis: The epithelial sodium channel and the control of blood pressure. J Am Soc Nephrol 8:980, 1997

187. Schreiber M, Schlanger LE, Chen CB et al: Antikaluretic action of trimethoprim is minimized by raising urine pH. Kidney Int 49:82, 1996

188. Greger R, Gögelein H: Role of K⁺ conductive pathways in the nephron. Kidney Int 31:1055, 1987

189. Weigand CF, Davin TD, Raij L, Kjellstrand CM: Severe hypokalemia induced by hemodialysis. Arch Intern Med 141:167, 1981

190. Jamison RL: Potassium recycling. Kidney Int 31:695, 1987

191. Sweadner KJ, Goldin SM: Active transport of sodium and potassium ions. Mechanism, function, and regulation. N Engl J Med 302:777, 1980

192. Rabinowitz L: Aldosterone and potassium homeostasis. Kidney Int 49:1738, 1996

193. Vitez TS, Soper LE, Wong KC, Soper P: Chronic hypokalemia and intraoperative dysrhythmias. Anesthesiology 63:130, 1985

194. Weiner ID, Wingo CS: Hypokalemia consequences, causes, and correction. J Am Soc Nephrol 8:1179, 1997

195. Gorden P: Glucose intolerance with hypokalemia. Failure of short-term potassium depletion in normal subjects to reproduce the glucose and insulin abnormalities of clinical hypokalemia. Diabetes 22:544, 1973

196. Schwartz WB, Relman AS: Effects of electrolyte disorders on renal structure and function. N Engl J Med 276:383, 1967

197. Adrogué HJ, Madias NE: Changes in plasma potassium concentration during acute acid–base disturbances. Am J Med 71:456, 1981

198. Kassirer JP, Harrington JT: Fending off the potassium pushers. N Engl J Med 312:785, 1985

199. Gennari FJ: Hypokalemia. N Engl J Med 339:451, 1998

200. Norgaard A, Kjeldsen K: Interrelation of hypokalaemia and potassium depletion and its implications: A re-evaluation based on studies of the skeletal muscle sodium, potassium-pump. Clin Sci 81:449, 1991

201. Tobey RE: Paraplegia, succinylcholine and cardiac arrest. Anesthesiology 32:359, 1970

202. Gronert GA, Dotin LN, Ritchey CR, Mason AD Jr: Succinylcholine-

induced hyperkalemia in burned patients—II. Anesth Analg 48:958, 1969

203. Schaner PJ, Brown RL, Kirksey TD et al: Succinylcholine-induced hyperkalemia in burned patients—I. Anesth Analg 48:764, 1969
204. Kuvin JT: Electrocardiographic changes of hyperkalemia. N Engl J Med 338:662, 1998
205. Rimmer JM, Horn JF, Gennari FJ: Hyperkalemia as a complication of drug therapy. Arch Intern Med 147:867, 1987
206. Textor SC, Bravo EL, Fouad FM, Tarazi RC: Hyperkalemia in azotemic patients during angiotensin-converting enzyme inhibition and aldosterone reduction with captopril. Am J Med 73:719, 1982
207. Maslowski AH, Nicholls MG, Ikram H, Espiner EA: Haemodynamic, hormonal, and electrolyte responses to captopril in resistant heart failure. Lancet 1:71, 1981
208. Wrenn KD, Slovis CM, Slovis BS: The ability of physicians to predict hyperkalemia from the ECG. Ann Emerg Med 20:1229, 1991
209. DeFronzo RA, Felig P, Ferrannini E, Wahren J: Effect of graded doses of insulin on splanchnic and peripheral potassium metabolism in man. Am J Physiol 238:E421, 1980
210. Vincent HH, Boomsma F, Man in't Veld AJ et al: Effects of selective and nonselective beta-agonists on plasma potassium and norepinephrine. J Cardiovasc Pharmacol 6:107, 1984
211. Allon M, Dunlay R, Copkney C: Nebulized albuterol for acute hyperkalemia in patients on hemodialysis. Ann Intern Med 110:426, 1989
212. Kemper MJ, Harps E, Müller-Wiefel DE: Hyperkalemia: Therapeutic options in acute and chronic renal failure. Clin Nephrol 46:67, 1996
213. Allon M: Treatment and prevention of hyperkalemia in end-stage renal disease. Kidney Int 43:1197, 1993
214. Salem MM, Rosa RM, Batlle DC: Extrarenal potassium tolerance in chronic renal failure: Implications for the treatment of acute hyperkalemia. Am J Kidney Dis 18:421, 1991
215. Zaloga GP, Chernow B: Hypocalcemia in critical illness. JAMA 256:1924, 1986
216. Zaloga GP, Chernow B, Cook D et al: Assessment of calcium homeostasis in the critically ill surgical patient. The diagnostic pitfalls of the McLean-Hastings nomogram. Ann Surg 202:587, 1985
217. Edelson GW, Kleerekoper M: Hypercalcemia crisis. Med Clin North Am 79:79, 1995
218. Brown EM, Pollak M, Hebert SC: The extracellular calcium-sensing receptor: Its role in health and disease. Annu Rev Med 49:15, 1998
219. Brown EM, Gamba G, Riccardi D et al: Cloning and characterization of an extracellular Ca²⁺-sensing receptor from bovine parathyroid. Nature 366:575, 1993
220. Brown EM, Pollak M, Seidman CE et al: Calcium-ion-sensing cell-surface receptors. N Engl J Med 333:234, 1995
221. Bushinsky DA, Monk RD: Calcium. Lancet 352:306, 1998
222. Lebowitz MR, Moses AM: Hypocalcemia. Semin Nephrol 12:146, 1992
223. Guise TA, Mundy GR: Evaluation of hypocalcemia in children and adults. J Clin Endocrinol Metab 80:1473, 1995
224. Bushinsky DA: The contribution of acidosis to renal osteodystrophy [clinical conference]. Kidney Int 47:1816, 1995
225. Adler AJ, Ferran N, Berlyne GM: Effect of inorganic phosphate on serum ionized calcium concentration in vitro: A reassessment of the "trade-off hypothesis." Kidney Int 28:932, 1985
226. Rutledge R, Sheldon GF, Collins ML: Massive transfusion. Crit Care Clin 2:791, 1986
227. Sutters M, Gaboury CL, Bennett WM: Severe hyperphosphatemia and hypocalcemia: A dilemma in patient management. J Am Soc Nephrol 7:2055, 1996
228. Zaloga GP, Strickland RA, Butterworth JF IV et al: Calcium attenuates epinephrine's beta-adrenergic effects in postoperative heart surgery patients. Circulation 81:196, 1990
229. Mathru M, Rooney MW, Goldberg SA, Hirsch LJ: Separation of myocardial versus peripheral effects of calcium administration in normocalcemic and hypocalcemic states using pressure-volume (conductance) relationships. Anesth Analg 77:250, 1993
230. Bilezikian JP: Clinical review 51: Management of hypercalcemia. J Clin Endocrinol Metab 77:1445, 1993
231. Mundy GR, Guise TA: Hypercalcemia of malignancy. Am J Med 103:134, 1997
232. Zaloga GP, Malcolm D, Holaday J, Chernow B: Verapamil reverses calcium cardiotoxicity. Ann Emerg Med 16:637, 1987
233. Singer FR, Minoofar PN: Bisphosphonates in the treatment of disorders of mineral metabolism. Adv Endocrinol Metab 6:259, 1995
234. Berenson JR, Lichtenstein A, Porter L et al: Efficacy of pamidronate in reducing skeletal events in patients with advanced multiple myeloma. Myeloma Aredia Study Group. N Engl J Med 334:488, 1996
235. Gucalp R, Ritch P, Wiernik PH et al: Comparative study of pamidronate disodium and etidronate disodium in the treatment of cancer-related hypercalcemia. J Clin Oncol 10:134, 1992
236. Chan FKW, Koberle LMC, Thys-Jacobs S, Bilezikian JP: Differential diagnosis, causes, and management of hypercalcemia. Curr Prob Surg 34:449, 1997
237. Kiang DT, Loken MK, Kennedy BJ: Mechanism of the hypocalcemic effect of mithramycin. J Clin Endocrinol Metab 48:341, 1979
238. Bilezikian JP: Management of acute hypercalcemia. N Engl J Med 326:1196, 1992
239. Warrell RP, Murphy WK, Schulman P: A randomized, double-blind study of gallium nitrate compared with etidronate for acute control of cancer-related hypercalcemia. J Clin Oncol 9:1467, 1991
240. Silverberg SJ, Bone HG III, Marriott TB et al: Short-term inhibition of parathyroid hormone secretion by a calcium-receptor agonist in patients with primary hyperparathyroidism. N Engl J Med 337:1506, 1997
241. Murer H, Werner A, Reshkin S et al: Cellular mechanisms in proximal tubular reabsorption of inorganic phosphate. Am J Physiol (Cell Physiol) 260:C885, 1991
242. Murer H, Markovich D, Biber J: Renal and small intestinal sodium-dependent symporters of phosphate and sulphate. J Exp Biol 196:167, 1994
243. Weisinger JR, Bellorin-Font E: Magnesium and phosphorus. Lancet 352:391, 1998
244. Peppers MP, Geheb M, Desai T: Hypophosphatemia and hyperphosphatemia. Crit Care Clin 7:201, 1991
245. Aubier M, Murciano D, Lecocguic Y et al: Effect of hypophosphatemia on diaphragmatic contractility in patients with acute respiratory failure. N Engl J Med 313:420, 1985
246. O'Connor LR, Wheeler WS, Bethune JE: Effect of hypophosphatemia on myocardial performance in man. N Engl J Med 297:901, 1977
247. Knochel JP: Hypophosphatemia and rhabdomyolysis [editorial; comment]. Am J Med 92:455, 1992
248. Brooks MJ, Melnik G: The refeeding syndrome: An approach to understanding its complications and preventing its occurrence. Pharmacology 15:713, 1995
249. Watchko J, Bifano EM, Bergstrom WH: Effect of hyperventilation on total calcium, ionized calcium, and serum phosphorus in neonates. Crit Care Med 12:1055, 1984
250. Rosen GH, Boullata JI, O'Rangers EA et al: Intravenous phosphate repletion regimen for critically ill patients with moderate hypophosphatemia. Crit Care Med 23:1204, 1995
251. Whang R, Hampton EM, Whang DD: Magnesium homeostasis and clinical disorders of magnesium deficiency. Ann Pharmacotherapy 28:220, 1997
252. Quamme GA: Renal magnesium handling: New insights in understanding old problems. Kidney Int 52:1180, 1997
253. Flink EB: Nutritional aspects of magnesium metabolism. West J Med 133:304, 1980
254. McLean RM: Magnesium and its therapeutic uses: A review. Am J Med 96:63, 1994
255. James MFM, Beer RE, Esser JD: Intravenous magnesium sulfate inhibits catecholamine release associated with tracheal intubation. Anesth Analg 68:772, 1989
256. Rasmussen HS, Suenson M, McNair P et al: Magnesium infusion reduces the incidence of arrhythmias in acute myocardial infarction. A double-blind placebo-controlled study. Clin Cardiol 10:351, 1987
257. Redwood SR, Taggart PI, Sutton PM et al: Effect of magnesium on the monophasic action potential during early ischemia in the in vivo human heart. J Am Coll Cardiol 28:1765, 1996
258. Teo KK, Yusuf S, Collins R et al: Effects of intravenous magnesium in suspected acute myocardial infarction: Overview of randomised trials. Br Med J 303:1499, 1991
259. Tzivoni D, Banai S, Schuger C et al: Treatment of torsade de pointes with magnesium sulfate. Circulation 77:392, 1988
260. Salem M, Munoz R, Chernow B: Hypomagnesemia in critical illness: A common and clinically important problem. Crit Care Clin 7:225, 1991

261. Abbott LG, Rude RK: Clinical manifestations of magnesium deficiency. Miner Electrolyte Metab 19:314, 1993
262. Wong ET, Rude RK, Singer FR, Shaw ST Jr: A high prevalence of hypomagnesemia and hypermagnesemia in hospitalized patients. Am J Clin Pathol 79:348, 1983
263. Whang R, Ryder KW: Frequency of hypomagnesemia and hypermagnesemia. Requested vs routine. JAMA 263:3063, 1990
264. Elisaf M, Merkouropoulos M, Tsianos EV, Siamopoulos KC: Pathogenetic mechanisms of hypomagnesemia in alcoholic patients. J Trace Elem Med Biol 9:210, 1995
265. Zaloga GP, Chernow B, Pock A et al: Hypomagnesemia is a common complication of aminoglycoside therapy. Surg Gynecol Obstet 158:561, 1984
266. Hebert P, Mehta N, Wang J et al: Functional magnesium deficiency in critically ill patients identified using a magnesium-loading test. Crit Care Med 25:749, 1997
267. Harris MNE, Crowther A, Jupp RA, Aps C: Magnesium and coronary revascularization. Br J Anaesth 60:779, 1988
268. Ghoneim MM, Long JP: The interaction between magnesium and other neuromuscular blocking agents. Anesthesiology 32:23, 1970
269. James MFM, Cork RC, Dennett JE: Succinylcholine pretreatment with magnesium sulfate. Anesth Analg 65:373, 1986
270. van Hook JW: Hypermagnesemia. Crit Care Clin 7:215, 1991
271. Prough DS, Johnston WE: Fluid resuscitation in septic shock: No solution yet. Anesth Analg 69:699, 1989

Clinical Anesthesia (4/e), edited by
Paul G. Barash, Bruce F. Cullen, and
Robert K. Stoelting. Lippincott Williams &
Wilkins, Philadelphia, © 2001.

CHAPTER 10

HEMOTHERAPY AND HEMOSTASIS

CHARISE T. PETROVITCH AND JOHN C. DRUMMOND

EVOLUTION OF TRANSFUSION PRACTICES

The knowledge that the acquired immune deficiency syndrome (AIDS) is transmitted by blood administration generated public fear of blood transfusion and led to dramatic changes in the way physicians approach the patient requiring blood products. For decades prior to 1985, anesthesiologists and surgeons applied, without question, the maxim that patients must have a hemoglobin (Hgb) level of $10 \text{ g} \cdot \text{dl}^{-1}$ or a hematocrit (Hct) of 30% prior to surgery. Other blood components (platelets, fresh frozen plasma) were similarly administered without reference to well-founded criteria. However, the AIDS epidemic prompted a reassessment of transfusion criteria, and contemporary practice requires that physicians take a patient-specific approach to the decision to transfuse blood components.

RBC TRANSFUSION THRESHOLDS

The Rationale

The question of what hemoglobin/hematocrit level poses greater risks to the patient than the threat of contracting a transfusion-transmitted disease has been widely discussed. However, there are no randomized controlled trials in the literature that provide a thorough risk–benefit analysis.[1] Experience with the ability of surgical patients to tolerate lower hematocrits was initially limited because the *10 &30 rule* ($10 \text{ g} \cdot \text{dl}^{-1}$ Hgb, Hct = 30%) was so widely applied. However, several patient subpopulations revealed that considerably greater degrees of anemia could be well tolerated. Chronically anemic renal failure patients tolerated many surgical procedures and anesthetics. Many surgeons had military experience that demonstrated that maintaining blood volume was more critical than correcting anemia, and these surgeons began to operate on patients with much lower hematocrits.[2] Finally, experience with Jehovah's Witnesses, who refuse blood transfusion for religious reasons, indicated that morbidity and mortality rates did not increase until hemoglobin levels fell below $7 \text{ g} \cdot \text{dl}^{-1}$.[1,3-6]

Concerns about many adverse physiologic effects of anemia have proved unfounded. There is no evidence that mild to moderate anemia impairs wound healing, increases bleeding, or increases the length of the patient's hospital stay. The cause of the anemia is thought to be more important in influencing the patient's perioperative course than the severity of the anemia.[7] In animal studies, wound healing is only impaired below a hematocrit of 15%.[6] The suspicion that anemia might increase the frequency or severity of postoperative infections has now been supplanted by evidence that transfusion, because of immunomodulatory effects (see Risks of Blood Product Administration) is actually associated with an increased incidence of postoperative infections.

The goal now is to anticipate, on a patient-by-patient basis, the minimum hemoglobin level that will avoid organ damage due to oxygen deprivation. This "transfusion trigger" requires more than a review of the patient's hemoglobin level. The physician must first consider the determinants of oxygen delivery (Do_2) and oxygen consumption (Vo_2) at the tissue level and, in addition, assess the patient's physiologic capacity for the compensatory mechanisms that enhance oxygen delivery to the tissues under conditions of anemia. Ultimately, the decision to transfuse red blood cells should be based upon the clinical judgment that the oxygen-carrying capacity of the blood must be increased to prevent oxygen consumption from outstripping oxygen delivery.

Oxygen Delivery and Oxygen Consumption

Oxygen Delivery. Oxygen delivery is a function of arterial oxygen content (Cao_2) and cardiac output. Cao_2 is, in turn, a function of hemoglobin level, hemoglobin saturation (Sao_2), and oxygen dissolved in plasma (Pao_2). Cao_2 is expressed as the number of milliliters of oxygen contained in 100 ml of blood and is calculated as follows:

$$Cao_2 = (Hgb \times 1.34 \times Sao_2) + (0.003 \times Pao_2)$$

If hemoglobin concentration is $15 \text{ g} \cdot \text{dl}^{-1}$ and the hemoglobin molecule is 100% saturated, the oxygen content of blood will be $20 \text{ ml} \cdot \text{dl}^{-1}$. The rate of oxygen delivery (Do_2) to the tissues is dependent on the product of cardiac output (CO) and the arterial oxygen content of blood. Normal average adult cardiac output is $5 \text{ l} \cdot \text{min}^{-1}$ (or $70 \text{ ml} \cdot \text{kg}^{-1}$) at rest. Oxygen delivery to the tissues is calculated as follows:

$$\text{Oxygen delivery} = CO \times Cao_2$$

$$Do_2 = 5 \text{ l} \cdot \text{min}^{-1} \times (20 \text{ ml} / 100 \text{ ml} \cdot \text{min}^{-1})$$
$$(200 \text{ ml} \cdot \text{l}^{-1} \cdot \text{min}^{-1})$$

$$= 1000 \text{ ml} \cdot \text{min}^{-1}$$

These simple calculations highlight the inadequacy of previous transfusion practices that considered hemoglobin concentration without reference to cardiac output or hemoglobin saturation.

Oxygen Consumption. Oxygen consumption can be calculated as the product of cardiac output and the difference between the arterial oxygen content and the venous ($C\bar{v}o_2$):

$$O_2 \text{ consumption} = CO \times (Cao_2 - C\bar{v}o_2)$$

The normal arteriovenous oxygen content difference is 5 vol%. Accordingly, normal oxygen consumption is $250 \text{ ml} \cdot \text{min}^{-1}$ ($5 \text{ l} \cdot \text{min}^{-1} \times 5 \text{ ml}/100 \text{ ml}$ or $50 \text{ ml} \cdot \text{l}^{-1} = 250 \text{ ml} \cdot \text{min}^{-1}$). Factors that increase oxygen extraction include sepsis, hyperthermia, and any state of increased metabolic activity, such as hyperthyroidism.

Note that these formulas provide a calculation of whole-body oxygen delivery and consumption. However, regional oxygen requirements differ substantially, and normal global oxygen delivery may occur in spite of critical levels of regional ischemia.[8]

Oxygen Extraction Ratios and the Mixed Venous Oxygen Saturation

Rather than calculating global oxygen delivery and oxygen consumption, it may be more useful to consider the extraction ratios of individual organs. The extraction ratio (ER) defines what fraction of the total oxygen delivered is consumed or extracted by the tissues as follows:

$$ER = \text{Oxygen consumption} / \text{Oxygen delivery}$$
$$ER = [CO \times (Ca_{O_2} - C\bar{v}_{O_2})] / (CO \times Ca_{O_2})$$
$$= (Ca_{O_2} - C\bar{v}_{O_2}) / Ca_{O_2}$$

Oxygen consumption for the entire body has already been calculated to be 250 ml · l^{-1} · min^{-1} and oxygen delivery to be 1000 ml · l^{-1} · min^{-1}, which produces an ER of 25%. With a normal arterial oxygen content of 20 vol% (200 ml · l^{-1}) and an extraction ratio of 25%, 5 vol% or 50 ml · l^{-1} of oxygen will be delivered to the tissues (the arteriovenous oxygen difference) and the mixed venous blood will have an oxygen content of 15 vol% (150 ml · l^{-1}) and an oxygen saturation ($S\bar{v}_{O_2}$) of 75%.

The mixed venous oxygen saturation reflects the oxygen consumption of many vascular beds, with some tissues (muscle, skin, viscera) extracting less oxygen and others (brain, heart) extracting proportionally more.[9] Under conditions of isovolemic hemodilution, increased oxygen extraction may occur in those tissue beds that normally consume a small proportion of the available oxygen (D_{O_2}). The increase in extraction ratio of these tissue beds will increase the whole-body oxygen ER and will lower the mixed venous oxygen saturation ($S\bar{v}_{O_2}$), making it a useful tool for assessing oxygen reserves in the venous blood.

In clinical practice, we cannot measure the extraction ratios of the various organs. However, it is known that the heart, under basal conditions, extracts between 55 and 70% of the oxygen delivered.[10,11] In contrast, in kidney and skin, ER is 7–10%. Organs with the greatest extraction ratios will have the least oxygen reserve. Because the heart has the highest ER, it is the organ at greatest risk under conditions of normovolemic anemia.[9] This is important to keep in mind when assessing the risks of anemia.

Compensatory Mechanisms During Anemia

When anemia develops but blood volume is maintained (isovolemic hemodilution), four compensatory mechanisms serve to maintain oxygen delivery: (1) an increase in cardiac output, (2) a redistribution of blood flow to organs with greater oxygen requirements, (3) increases in the extraction ratios of some vascular beds, and (4) alteration of oxygen–hemoglobin binding to allow the hemoglobin to deliver oxygen at lower oxygen tensions.

Increased Cardiac Output

With isovolemic hemodilution, cardiac output increases primarily because of an increase in stroke volume brought about by reductions in systemic vascular resistance (SVR). There are two principal determinants of SVR: vascular tone and the viscosity of blood.[12] As hematocrit decreases, reduction of blood viscosity decreases SVR. This decrease in SVR increases stroke volume and consequently cardiac output and blood flow to the tissues. Over a wide range of hematocrits, isovolemic hemodilution is self-correcting. Linear decreases in the oxygen-carrying capacity of the blood are matched by improvements in oxygen transport. Because oxygen transport peaks at hematocrits of 30%, oxygen delivery may remain constant between the hematocrits of 45 and 30%.[12] Transfusing red blood cells in this range of hematocrits would do little to increase oxygen delivery.[9] Further reductions in hematocrit are accompanied by increases in cardiac output, which peaks at 180% of control as the hematocrit approaches 20%.

The exact hemoglobin value at which cardiac output rises varies among individuals and is influenced by age and whether the anemia is acute or develops slowly.[3] In some patients, the cardiac output will not increase until the hemoglobin level falls to 7 or 8 g · dl^{-1}.[13] Increases in cardiac output due to changes in contractility or preload appear to play a lesser role in the maintenance of cardiac output than do increases in stroke volume.[5] Some increase in venous return is thought to occur as a result of the reduction in viscosity and a passive increase in blood flow in the postcapillary venules.[9]

Redistribution of Cardiac Output

With isovolemic hemodilution, blood flow to the tissues increases, but this increased blood flow is not distributed equally to all tissue beds. Organs with higher extraction ratios (brain and heart) receive disproportionately more of the increase in blood flow than organs with low extraction ratios (muscle, skin, viscera).

The redistribution of blood flow to the coronary circulation is the principal means by which the healthy heart compensates for anemia.[12] Coronary blood flow may increase by 400–600%. Because the heart under basal conditions already has a high extraction ratio (between 50 and 70% vs. 30% in most tissues) and the primary compensation for anemia involves cardiac work (increasing CO), the heart must rely upon redistributing blood flow to increase oxygen supply.[13] These factors make the heart the organ at greatest risk under conditions of isovolemic hemodilution. When the heart can no longer increase either cardiac output or coronary blood flow, the limits of isovolemic hemodilution are reached. Further decreases in oxygen delivery will result in myocardial injury.

Increased Oxygen Extraction

The third mechanism for adapting to isovolemic hemodilution involves increasing oxygen extraction ratios. This mechanism is thought to play an important adaptive role when the normovolemic hematocrit drops below 25%. Increased oxygen extraction in multiple tissue beds leads to an increase in the whole-body ER and consequently to a decrease in mixed venous oxygen saturation. One investigation demonstrated that as hematocrit decreases to 15%, whole-body oxygen ER increases from 38% to 60% and the $S\bar{v}_{O_2}$ decreases from 70% to 50% or less.[9] Some organs (brain and heart) already have high extraction ratios under basal conditions, and have a limited capacity to increase oxygen delivery by this mechanism.

Changes in Oxygen–Hemoglobin Affinity

The fourth mechanism of compensation for anemia involves a change in the binding of oxygen to hemoglobin. The affinity of hemoglobin for oxygen is described by the sigmoid-shaped oxygen–hemoglobin dissociation curve. This curve relates the partial pressure of oxygen in the blood to the percentage saturation of the hemoglobin molecule with oxygen.

The partial pressure of oxygen at which the hemoglobin molecule is 50% saturated with oxygen and 50% unsaturated is termed the P_{50}. P_{50} for normal adult hemoglobin at 37°C and a pH of 7.4 is 27 mm Hg. Hemoglobins differ in their P_{50} values, and changes in the acid–base status or the temperature of blood can shift the oxyhemoglobin dissociation curve to the left or right, respectively lowering or raising the P_{50} value. When the curve is shifted to the left, as with hypothermia or alkalosis, the P_{50} is lowered.[14] With a lower P_{50}, the hemoglobin molecule is more "stingy" and requires lower oxygen lower partial pressures to release oxygen to the tissues; that is, the hemoglobin molecule does not release 50% of its oxygen until an ambient P_{O_2} less than 27 mm Hg is reached. This may impair tissue oxygenation. By contrast, right-shifting of the oxygen-hemoglobin dissociation curve, as occurs with increases in temperature or acidosis, results in an increase of P_{50}, decreased hemoglobin affinity for the oxygen molecule, and release of oxygen to tissues at higher partial pressures of oxygen.

When anemia develops slowly, the affinity of hemoglobin for oxygen may be decreased (i.e., the curve is right-shifted) as a result of the accumulation in red blood cells of 2,3-phosphoglycerate (2,3-DPG).[14] Synthesis of supranormal levels of 2,3-DPG begins at a Hgb of 9 g · dl^{-1}. At Hgb levels of 6.5, the curve is shifted more prominently.[3] All stored red blood cells become depleted of 2,3-DPG. Temperature reduction and storage-related pH decreases also reduces the P$_{50}$ of stored blood. These changes, however, are quickly reversed *in vivo*, but the resynthesis of 2,3-DPG by red blood cells may require from 12 to 24 hours or longer.[13]

Isovolemic Anemia vs. Acute Blood Loss

Although the same compensatory mechanisms are operative in acute and chronic anemias, they have different degrees of importance and occur at different levels of hemoglobin. With acute blood loss, hypovolemia induces stimulation of the adrenergic nervous system, leading to vasoconstriction and tachycardia. Increased cardiac output does not contribute. In chronically anemic patients, cardiac output may not change until the hemoglobin decreases to approximately 7–8 g · dl^{-1}.[3] In these patients, the accumulation of 2,3-DPG in the red blood cells, increasing the P$_{50}$ of Hgb, is the important first mechanism for compensation.[7]

Establishing the RBC Transfusion Threshold

Guidelines

There has been extensive discussion of the red blood cell (RBC) transfusion "trigger"—the hemoglobin or hematocrit threshold that justifies RBC transfusion for individual patients. At this transfusion threshold, it is presumed that the benefits of red blood cell transfusion outweigh the risks. It was evident during the 1980s that transfusion practices varied significantly.[15] As a consequence, the National Institutes of Health convened a Consensus Conference on Perioperative Red Cell Transfusions in 1988 to review the evidence regarding the relative benefits of transfusing a patient at a given hemoglobin level versus the risk of not transfusing.[4] They concluded that no single criterion (*e.g.*, no specific Hgb level) could replace clinical judgment as the basis for decision-making. They concluded that the majority of patients with Hgb values of 10 g · dl^{-1} or greater rarely required perioperative transfusion, whereas those with hemoglobin values of less than 7 g · dl^{-1} would frequently require RBC transfusion. They recommended that clinical assessment "aided by laboratory data such as arterial oxygenation, mixed venous oxygen tension, cardiac output, the oxygen extraction ratio, and blood volume, when indicated,"[4] should guide therapy. They further concluded that there existed "no evidence that mild-to-moderate anemia contributes to perioperative morbidity."

There have been subsequent consensus statements by other bodies. These have added little to the 1988 statement other than placing greater emphasis on the development and application of perioperative blood conservation strategies[1,16,17] The focus remains on evaluation of the individual patient. Table 10-1, the contents of which follow logically from the preceding description of the mechanisms of physiologic compensation for anemia, lists conditions that may reduce patient tolerance for anemia and thereby justify transfusion of RBCs at Hgb levels greater than 7 g · dl^{-1}. The greatest emphasis in that evaluation will usually be placed on an estimation of the patient's myocardial/coronary reserve.

Myocardial/Coronary Reserve

Studies have been conducted on healthy animals with normal hearts and patent coronary arteries in an attempt to define the lowest hemoglobin or hematocrit that can be tolerated before death ensues.[5] These studies have revealed that, if normovolemia is maintained, the whole-body ER increases linearly as the Hct decreases until a critical point is reached.[18] At a hematocrit of 10% and a whole-body ER of approximately 50%, no

Table 10-1. CONDITIONS THAT MAY DECREASE TOLERANCE FOR ANEMIA AND INFLUENCE THE RBC TRANSFUSION THRESHOLD

Increased oxygen demand
  Hyperthermia
  Hyperthyroidism
  Pregnancy
Limited ability to increase cardiac output
  Coronary artery disease
  Myocardial dysfunction (infarction, cardiomyopathy)
  β-Adrenergic blockade
Inability to redistribute cardiac output
  Low SVR states (sepsis, post-cardiopulmonary bypass)
  Occlusive vascular disease (cerebral, coronary)
Left shift of O$_2$–Hgb curve
  Alkalosis
  Hypothermia
Abnormal hemoglobins
  Presence of stored Hgb (decreased 2,3-DPG)
  Hgb S (sickle cell disease)
Acute anemia (limited 2,3-DPG compensation)
Impaired oxygenation
  Pulmonary disease
  High altitude

further increases in oxygen consumption (Vo$_2$) occur; the tissues convert to anaerobic metabolism, which leads to metabolic acidosis and hemodynamic instability. Death is due to high output cardiac failure with severe tissue hypoxia. Nonetheless, survival at even lower hematocrits has occasionally been reported in humans who refuse blood for religious reasons.[2]

There is some systematically derived evidence to confirm the intuitive suspicion that patients with coronary vascular disease tolerate anemia less well than other acutely ill patients. Hebert *et al*[19] performed a prospective study of the outcome impact of a restrictive transfusion practice in a broad spectrum of critically ill patients. They observed that the restrictive approach improved outcome in some patient subsets but that the benefit was not apparent in patients with myocardial infarction or unstable angina. Although this is consistent with an adverse effect of anemia in this population, it does not allow delineation of specific transfusion thresholds. This must remain a matter of clinician judgment.

In summary, in order to establish the threshold Hgb level at which RBC transfusion is appropriate, the physician must evaluate the risks that anemia poses in the context of the patient's medical condition. The transfusion trigger for each patient will lie somewhere between a hemoglobin of 6–7 g · dl^{-1} (Hct of 18–21%) and a hemoglobin of 10 g · dl^{-1} (Hct of 30%). The lowest transfusion thresholds should be reserved for young healthy patients with acute blood loss but no other complicating factors and for those patients with well-compensated chronic anemia. The latter may be well compensated at hemoglobin values between 6 and 8 g · dl^{-1}.[6] A "middle of the road" hematocrit threshold (*e.g.*, Hct 25%) may be appropriate for the patient with well-compensated medical problems but no cardiac disease. Finally, in patients with coronary artery disease, a transfusion threshold approaching 30% may be necessary to avoid ischemia. Anticipated blood loss and the anticipated physiologic stresses of the intraoperative and postoperative course should also be factors in transfusion decisions.[20] Cardiac output, arterial and mixed venous oxygen, and the whole-body ER data should be used to provide objective criteria for these judgments when available. Mixed venous Po$_2$ of less than 25 mm Hg, a whole-body oxygen ER greater than 50%, and reduction of total oxygen consumption (Vo$_2$) to less than 50% of baseline indicate significantly impaired oxygen delivery. The final rationale for transfusion should be entered in the medical record.

COLLECTION AND PREPARATION OF BLOOD PRODUCTS FOR TRANSFUSION

Several steps are required in the preparation and selection of red blood cells for transfusion. Whole blood is first collected in bags containing citrate-phosphate-dextrose-adenine (CPDA) as a preservative and stored at 4°C. The citrate chelates the calcium present in blood and prevents coagulation. CPDA results in a longer shelf life than the once widely used acid-citrate-dextrose (ACD). Nonetheless, RBC viability at 4°C declines with time and shelf life is limited to 35–42 days. RBCs can be frozen and stored indefinitely. However, preservatives to prevent freeze/thaw-associated damage must be added and subsequently removed before administration. The process is expensive and hence not widely used.

Sequential centrifugation at various spin speeds and durations is used to separate whole blood into components including packed RBCs, platelet concentrates, cryoprecipitate, leukocyte-poor RBCs, and cell-free plasma. For preparation of platelet concentrates, centrifugation is first performed at room temperature. This separates the platelet-rich plasma fraction from the red blood cells. To separate all other blood components, centrifugation is carried out between 1° and 6°C.

The volume of the derived unit of packed RBCs is 200–220 ml with a hematocrit of 70–80% and a residual plasma volume of 50–60 ml. That plasma contains clotting factors. However, the residual concentrations of the two labile factors, V and VIII, may be too small to prevent a dilutional coagulopathy in association with very large volume transfusion. There are retained platelets but they become nonfunctional within 24 hours. Leukocytes are also present and can cause both febrile reactions and immunomodulatory effects (see White Cell–Related Transfusion Reactions). There are alternative RBC preparations that eliminate the various "passengers." Saline-washed RBCs may be used for patients who experience reactions to foreign proteins. White cells can be removed by washing, irradiation, or leukofiltration. The administration of one unit of packed RBCs will increase the Hgb and Hct of a 70-kg adult by approximately $1 \text{ g} \cdot \text{dl}^{-1}$ and 3%, respectively.

Compatibility Testing

Compatibility testing involves three separate procedures: ABO Rh blood type identification, antibody screening of donor plasma, and the donor–recipient cross-match.

ABO Rhesus Typing

Compatibility testing is carried out on both donor and recipient blood. The first step is to determine the ABO blood group type and the Rh status for both donor and recipient blood. This is a critical step because most fatal hemolytic transfusion reactions result from the transfusion of ABO-incompatible blood. Blood types are defined according to the antigens present on the surface of the red blood cell. Patients with Type A blood have type A antigens on the surface of their red cells. Type B blood has B antigens. When both antigens are present, the patient is said to have Type AB blood; and when both antigens are lacking, the patient is said to have Type O blood.

ABO typing involves determining not only which antigens are on the surface of the RBCs but also which antibodies are present in the serum. The serum constitutively contains antibodies to the AB antigens that are lacking on the RBC. Patients with Type A blood have antibodies against the B antigen and vice versa. Patients with no antigens on their cells, Type O blood, will have both anti-A and anti-B antibodies in the plasma.

Another important antigen may be present on the surface of red blood cells, the rhesus or Rho(D) antigen. Patients with this antigen are said to be Rh-positive and those who lack it are termed Rh-negative. Approximately 85% of the population is Rh-positive. In contrast to the A and B blood groups, when the

D antigen is not present on the surface of the red cells, anti-D antibodies are not constitutively present in the serum. However, Rh-negative patients exposed to donor RBCs with the D antigen (Rh-positive blood) will usually produce anti-D antibodies. There is a latency before these antibodies are synthesized. As a consequence, the reaction between the Rh-positive donor cells and the anti-D evolves slowly and may not be clinically apparent on first exposure. This process whereby a foreign antigen stimulates the synthesis of the corresponding antibody is termed *alloimmunization* and is very significant. Approximately 60–70% of Rh-negative recipients will produce anti-D antibodies after receiving Rh-positive blood.[21] Subsequent exposure of these Rh-negative individuals to Rh(D)-positive cells may result in an acute hemolytic reaction.

When determining what donor blood group types may be compatible for transfusion to a particular recipient, it is useful to focus on which antibodies will be present in the recipient serum. It is the reaction of these antibodies with donor RBC antigens that can activate complement and lead to hemolysis of the red cell. Type O+ recipients [Type O, Rh(D)-positive] will have both anti-A and anti-B antibodies, but not the anti-D antibody in their plasma. These patients must not receive Type A, Type B, or Type AB blood. They must receive Type O blood, but it may be either Rh-positive or Rh-negative. In contrast, patients with Type AB− blood (Type AB, Rh-negative) will lack both the A and B antibodies in their plasma, and may or may not have the anti-D antibody in their plasma. They can receive Type A−, Type B−, Type AB−, or Type O− blood. It should be clear that, in attempting to determine blood group and Rh compatibility between donor and recipient, patients with the fewest antigens on their cells (Type O-negative) have the most antibodies in their plasma. Patients with Type O-negative blood are called *universal donors*. In contrast patients with the most antigens on their cells (Type AB-positive) will have no antibodies to the A, B, or D antigens. These patients can receive all blood types (Types A+, A−, B+, B−, AB+, AB−, O+, and O−) and are referred to as *universal recipients* (Table 10-2).

The Antibody Screen

The second step in compatibility testing is called the antibody screen. It seeks the presence of recipient antibodies against RBC antigens. Commercially supplied RBCs, selected for the panel of antigens they possess, are mixed with both donor and recipient serum to screen for the presence of unexpected antibodies. Only about four blood donations in one thousand demonstrate unexpected antibodies. The likelihood that the antibody screen will miss a potentially dangerous antibody has been estimated to be no more than 1 in 10,000.[21] If the recipient plasma screen is positive, the antibody must be identified and the appropriate antigen-negative donor units selected. The antibody screening of recipient plasma should be repeated if the patient has been transfused since the last antibody screening test. This is because transfusions produce newly detectable antibodies in about 1% of the units used.

The Cross-match

The third phase of compatibility testing is called the cross-match. Donor RBCs are mixed with recipient serum, simulating

Table 10-2. PREVALENCE (%) OF ABO AND Rh(D) BLOOD TYPES IN THE POPULATION OF THE UNITED STATES

Antigen	O	A	B	AB	D
Caucasians	45	40	11	4	85
Blacks	49	27	20	4	92

Data from the Technical Manual (13th ed) of the American Association of Blood Banks.

the actual anticipated transfusion. This test requires about 45 minutes and is carried out in three phases: (1) the immediate phase, (2) the incubation phase, and (3) the antiglobulin phase.

The immediate phase serves primarily to ensure that there have been no errors in ABO-Rh typing. The test entails examination of a mixture of donor RBCs and patient serum for macroscopic agglutination. This immediate phase cross-match requires only 1–5 minutes and detects both ABO incompatibilities and those caused by antibodies in the MN, P, and Lewis systems. These latter antibodies are naturally occurring antibodies that are usually present in low titers and are not reactive at physiologic temperatures. For this reason, the immediate phase cross-match is carried out at room temperature.

The incubation phase requires 30–45 minutes and detects antibodies primarily in the Rh system. This phase is more time-consuming because, following the immediate cross-match, the donor RBCs and recipient serum must be incubated in albumin or low-ionic strength salt solution. This incubation phase aids in the detection of incomplete antibodies—antibodies that attach to a specific antigen but do not cause agglutination in a saline suspension of RBCs.[21]

The antiglobulin phase, or indirect antiglobulin test, involves the addition of antiglobulin sera at the end of the incubation phase. These antiglobulin sera contain antibodies that will bind to antiglobulins attached to antigens on the surface of the donor red blood cells. This phase is an attempt to identify the most incomplete antibodies (i.e., those that do not cause agglutination) from all blood group systems, including the Rh, Kell, Kidd, and Duffy blood group systems.[21] The incomplete antibodies that may be identified by the incubation and antiglobulin phases of the cross-match can cause serious hemolytic reactions.

Some have questioned the necessity for cross-matching. In patients who have been transfused previously or who may have been exposed to foreign red blood cell antigens during pregnancy, only 1 in 100 will have an antibody other than the anti-A, anti-B, and/or anti-Rh antibodies, and many of these are not reactive at physiologic temperatures. Determining the ABO blood group type and Rh status alone yields the probability that the transfusion will be compatible in 99.8% of instances. The addition of the 30–45-minute antibody screen improves the likelihood of a compatible transfusion to 99.94%; the addition of a complete cross-match increases this to 99.95%.[7] In other words, in those patients who have not previously been transfused or pregnant, the odds that an incompatible transfusion will occur when uncross-matched blood is administered is just 1 in 1000.[21] For those who have previously been exposed to foreign red blood cell antigens, the likelihood that they will have developed an antibody is about 1 in 100.[21] Nonetheless, all blood banks perform the cross-match. However, these data reveal that the administration, in emergency situations, of uncross-matched blood to patients with no history of pregnancy or transfusion entails relatively low risk.

Type and Screen Orders

When blood is ordered preoperatively for surgical cases in which transfusion is unlikely, the orders should be for a "type and screen" only. If the need arises, the blood can be cross-matched prior to transfusion. The advantage of ordering a type and screen instead of type and cross-match is twofold. First, if the blood is not needed for that particular case, the additional expense of carrying out the cross-match step is eliminated. The first two steps of compatibility testing—determining the ABO and Rh type as well as performing the antibody screen using commercially supplied RBCs—must be performed on all donor units of blood regardless of who the recipient is to be. Second, if a cross-match is performed and compatible units identified, those units are held in reserve for that specific patient and hence are at least temporarily out of the blood supply. If the blood is not used, it is returned to the general supply; however,

owing to blood's limited shelf life, this process will have contributed to wastage by outdating.

C/T Ratios

If a unit of blood that has been cross-matched and reserved for a particular patient is not needed, that unit must be cross-matched again before administration to another patient. This duplication of the cross-match procedure is costly and inefficient. Blood banks track their "cross-match-to-transfusion" (C/T) ratios and attempt to maintain ratios of 2.1–2.7.[21]

The Maximal Surgical Blood Order Schedule

The maximal surgical blood order schedule (MSBOS) is another process that seeks to decrease the number of unnecessary cross-match procedures. Blood banks accumulate data on the average number of units of red blood cells actually transfused for each type of operation performed, by each surgeon. These data are used to define the maximal number of units that the blood bank will cross-match in advance of elective surgery.

Emergency Transfusions

The exsanguinating patient may require RBCs before complete compatibility testing can be performed. If testing is to be abbreviated, there is a preferred order for selecting partially tested blood. The first choice is to transfuse type-specific, partially cross-matched blood. Only the immediate phase macroagglutination test is performed on a mixture of donor RBCs and recipient serum. This immediate phase cross-match requires 1–5 minutes. This test is useful to confirm that there are no clerical or laboratory errors in defining the blood type of the patient and of the donor. The second preference is to give type-specific uncross-matched blood. The last option is to administer O-negative (universal donor) packed RBCs. O-negative whole blood should not be used because it may contain high titers of the anti-A and anti-B hemolytic antibodies. This would be harmful unless the patient also had Type O blood. It is recommended that even if the patient's blood type becomes known and available, after 2 units of Type O-negative blood have been transfused, subsequent transfusion should continue with universal donor, Type O-negative blood. This is because even packed RBCs contain some plasma and in this plasma are antibodies. With transfusion of type O-negative blood, both anti-A and anti-B antibodies will be transfused as well. If subsequent units of donor blood are Type A, B, or AB, hemolysis may result because of a reaction between antibodies found in the plasma of the first donor units and antigens on RBCs of the new donor units. The patient should not receive his or her own type-specific blood until the transfused anti-A and anti-B antibody titers have fallen to safe levels.[21]

RISKS OF BLOOD PRODUCT ADMINISTRATION
Risks Associated with Transfusion of RBCs

The rapid transfusion of large volumes of stored blood can have several consequences. Some of these are functions of properties of the blood itself, of the agents used to preserve and anticoagulate it, and of the biochemical reactions that occur during storage.[21] There are other complications that are not unique to blood transfusions, but which may occur with the rapid transfusion of any large volume of fluid.

Citrate Intoxication

Blood is stored in a CPDA anticoagulant preservative solution. The citrate in the solution prevents coagulation of stored blood by chelating ionized calcium. When large volumes of stored blood (>1 blood volume)[22] are administered rapidly, the citrate can cause a temporary reduction in ionized calcium levels. Signs of citrate intoxication (hypocalcemia) include the following hemodynamic changes: hypotension, narrow pulse pressure, and elevated ventricular end-diastolic pressure and central venous pressure.[21] ECG changes include prolonged Q-T interval, widened QRS complexes, and flattened T waves. The hypocalcemia is directly related to the rate and volume of blood being transfused. Citrate is metabolized efficiently by the liver, and decreased ionized calcium levels should not occur unless the rate of transfusion exceeds $1 \ ml \cdot kg^{-1} \cdot min^{-1}$ or about 1 unit of blood per 5 minutes in an average-sized adult.[21] Impaired liver function or perfusion will lower the rate threshold for developing citrate intoxication. Treatment of hypocalcemia-related myocardial depression and hemodynamic instability entails iv administration of calcium, ideally after laboratory confirmation of the diagnosis.[7]

Acid–Base Changes

When citrate-phosphate-dextrose (CPD) solution is added to a unit of freshly drawn blood, pH decreases to ~7.0–7.1.[21] Further reduction of pH will occur during storage as a consequence of ongoing metabolism of glucose to lactate. At the end of 21 days, the pH may be as low as 6.9, but much of this acidity is the result of the production of CO_2, which is rapidly eliminated following the transfusion. Whether rapid infusion of this acidic bank blood leads to metabolic acidosis is debated. In the past, some clinicians administered sodium bicarbonate empirically to patients on a fixed schedule (e.g., sodium bicarbonate 44.6 mEq after each 5 units of bank blood infused). Others contend that the citrate from the CPD solution is metabolized by the patient to endogenous bicarbonate and that the acid–base disturbance is therefore self-correcting. Clinically, in the injured patient who is hypotensive, poorly perfused, and has inadequate tissue oxygenation, it is difficult to differentiate what portion of the metabolic acidosis is due to rapid transfusion and what portion is due to the production of lactic acid.[22] The appropriate course is to base bicarbonate therapy on blood gas analysis.

Decreases in 2,3-Diphosphoglycerate (2,3-DPG)

Storage of RBCs is associated with a progressive decrease in intracellular ATP and 2,3-diphosphoglycerate (2,3-DPG). The resultant left shift of the O_2–Hgb dissociation curve has been described above. Accordingly, transfusing the 2,3-DPG-depleted blood, while increasing the patient's Hgb value will result in less efficient oxygen delivery than would occur with native Hgb at the same Hct. After transfusion, 2,3-DPG levels return toward normal over 12–24 hours.[23]

Hyperkalemia

During storage, potassium moves out of the RBCs, in part to maintain electrochemical neutrality as hydrogen ions generated during storage redistribute. The potassium concentration in plasma may reach levels variously reported to be between 17 and 35 $mEq \cdot l^{-1}$ in blood stored for 21 days.[21] With normal infusion rates, the potassium is redistributed throughout the extracellular space and does not present a clinical problem. However, hazard exists if large volumes of stored blood are administered rapidly. Rates in excess of 90–120 $ml \cdot min^{-1}$ have been associated with hyperkalemia. Furthermore, while there is only 40–60 ml of plasma in a unit of packed RBCs, contemporary infusion devices allow blood to be transfused at rates of 500–1000 $ml \cdot min^{-1}$ and the replacement of four blood volumes per hour. With these infusion rates, critical hyperkalemia can occur quickly, and intraoperative arrests have been documented.[24] It is proposed that the hyperkalemia is aggravated by hypovolemia, hypothermia, and acidosis.[22] ECG changes associated with hyperkalemia include peaked T waves, a prolonged PR interval, and a widened QRS complex. If ECG changes are observed,

the transfusion should be stopped and intravenous calcium should be administered. Bicarbonate, dextrose, and insulin may also be appropriate according to the severity of the episode.[7]

Volume Overload

Circulatory volume overload occurs when blood or fluid is transfused too rapidly for compensatory fluid redistribution to take place.

Hypothermia

Packed red blood cells are stored at temperatures between 1° and 6°C, and hypothermia may result from the rapid transfusion of large volumes of cold blood. The administration of 1 unit of packed RBCs at 4°C will reduce the core temperature of a 70-kg patient by ~0.25°C. Transfusions administered rapidly or in substantial volume should be warmed to prevent hypothermia. With decreasing body temperature, cardiac output declines, tissue perfusion is impaired (as a consequence of both vasoconstriction and left-shifting of the O_2–Hgb dissociation curve), and metabolic acidosis may develop. Shivering on emergence can increase oxygen consumption by 400%. Hemostatic dysfunction (both primary hemostasis and coagulation) and ventricular irritability will become evident as body temperature declines. The latter is most likely to occur at and below 30°C and may be seen at higher core temperatures if unwarmed blood is administered, particularly through central access catheters, in a patient who is already moderately hypothermic. Hypothermia has been associated with increased postoperative morbidity and mortality including increased rates of postoperative infection.[22,25]

Microaggregate Delivery

Stored blood contains microaggregates.[22] Platelet aggregates form during the second to fifth day of storage; and after ~10 days, larger aggregates composed of fibrin, degenerated white cells, and platelets appear.[21] Macroaggregates of RBCs also develop. Standard fluid administration sets contain 170-μm filters, which will remove these larger "clots." Micropore filters, typically with a 40-μm pore size, have been advocated, but neither their efficiency at removing the microaggregates nor their contribution to patient well-being is certain. Microaggregates have been implicated in the pathogenesis of pulmonary insufficiency and the development of adult respiratory distress syndrome (ARDS), which often follows large-volume transfusions (defined as >10–12 units in 24 hours).[22,26] However, the available data do not confirm this suspicion and suggest that pulmonary injury and the occurrence of ARDS are more often related to the type of injury and the magnitude or severity of the injury than to the volume of blood transfused.[27,28] Hypotension and sepsis may play a much greater role in the development of ARDS than do microaggregates. Nonetheless, a practical consideration frequently prompts clinicians to introduce a micropore filter between the blood unit and the administration set. Unfiltered blood may clog the 170-μm filter of the standard set and it is less time-consuming to change the 40-μm filter periodically (e.g., after every fourth RBC unit) than to exchange the entire administration set.

Red blood cells are frequently diluted with crystalloid solutions to increase the rate at which the blood can be transfused. Normal saline is commonly recommended in preference to lactated Ringer's solution (LR). In fact, the amount of citrate present in stored blood is more than sufficient to bind the small amounts of calcium in the 100–300 ml of LR typically used for dilution.[29] Saline may nonetheless be preferable because, once the blood transfusion has finished, residual blood in the set may not have adequate amounts of citrate to bind the calcium in LR. It is then passed through the set, and clot formation may occur. There is no evidence that any clinically significant sequelae have resulted from the use of LR as an RBC diluent.[22]

Dilutional Coagulopathy

Administration of large volumes of fluid deficient in or devoid of platelets and clotting factors predictably leads to the development of a coagulopathy as a consequence of dilution. There has been considerable discussion of whether, in the face of massive transfusion of blood products, patients will first manifest deficiencies of platelets or clotting factors. The initial conclusion was that thrombocytopenia would develop first. In retrospect, this clinical conclusion may have been a consequence of a wider use of whole blood than prevails today. In spite of the lability of factors V and VIII, sufficient concentrations of these factors probably remain in banked whole blood to maintain coagulation function even in the face of very large transfusions. The same is probably not true when patients receive only the small residual plasma volume associated with packed RBCs. Investigations of patients receiving large-volume isovolemic transfusions suggest that clinically significant dilution of fibrinogen; factors II, V, and VIII; and platelets will occur after volume exchanges of approximately 140%, 200–230%, and 230% (i.e., 1.4, 2, and 2.3 blood volumes), respectively.[30] Resuscitation from hypovolemia will result in reaching these thresholds at smaller percentage volume exchanges. However, calculations of this nature should not be used as a guide to blood product administration but merely as a means of anticipating clinically relevant occurrences. The decision to administer fresh frozen plasma or platelets will depend on clinical and laboratory evidence of coagulopathy.

Immunologically Mediated Transfusion Reactions

Reactions to transfused blood products can occur as a result of the presence of constitutive antibodies (e.g., anti-A, anti-B); antibodies formed as a result of prior exposure to donor RBCs, white blood cells, platelets, and/or proteins[6]; or as a consequence of the effects of transfused white cells.

Reactions to RBC Antigens

Immediate Hemolytic Transfusion Reactions

The most feared of the immune reactions is the immediate hemolytic transfusion reaction against foreign red blood cells. Hemolysis of the donor RBCs often leads to acute renal failure, disseminated intravascular coagulation, and death. There are more than 300 different antigens on human red cells, but many are weak immunogens that usually do not elicit a clinically detectable antibody response. The antibodies that fix complement and commonly produce immediate intravascular hemolysis include anti-A, anti-B, anti-Kell, anti-Kidd, anti-Lewis, and anti-Duffy.[31]

The incidence of immediate hemolytic transfusion reactions is estimated to be 1 per 6000–7000 units transfused.[15] The result is commonly catastrophic, with mortality ranging from 20–60%.[21] Physician errors have been reported to be responsible for 20% of the incompatible blood transfusions that have resulted in patient death.[22]

When incompatible blood is administered, antibodies and complement in recipient plasma attack the corresponding antigens on donor RBCs. Hemolysis ensues. The hemolytic reaction may take place in the intravascular space and/or it may occur extravascularly within the endoplasmic reticulum. The antigen–antibody complexes activate Hageman factor (factor XII) which in turn acts on the kinin system to produce bradykinin. The release of bradykinin increases capillary permeability and dilates arterioles, both of which contribute to hypotension. Activation of the complement system results in the release of histamine and serotonin from mast cells, resulting in bronchospasm. Thirty to fifty percent of patients develop disseminated intravascular coagulation (DIC).[31]

Hemolysis releases hemoglobin into the blood. Initially it is bound to haptoglobin and albumin until the binding sites are saturated, then it circulates freely in the blood until it is excreted by the kidneys. Renal damage occurs for several reasons. Blood flow to the kidneys is reduced in the presence of systemic hypotension and renal vasoconstriction. Free hemoglobin and RBC stroma (not Hgb) may precipitate in the renal tubules, causing mechanical obstruction and nephrotoxicity.[21,31] Antigen–antibody complexes may be deposited in the glomeruli. If the patient develops DIC, fibrin thrombi will also be deposited in the renal vasculature, further compromising perfusion.

The signs and symptoms of a hemolytic transfusion reaction include fever, chills, nausea and vomiting, diarrhea, and rigors. The patient is hypotensive and tachycardic (bradykinin effects), and may appear flushed and dyspneic (histamine). Chest and back pains result from diffuse intravascular occlusion by agglutinated RBCs. The patient is often restless, has a headache, and feels a sense of impending doom. Hemoglobinuria will occur as well as diffuse bleeding with the development of DIC. With renal failure, oliguria develops. During general anesthesia, many signs are masked. Hypotension and hemoglobinuria and diffuse bleeding may be the only clues that a hemolytic transfusion reaction has occurred. However, hypotension and bleeding are nonspecific and fairly common in the operating room environment; thus the diagnosis may not be suspected until hemoglobinuria is observed. A reasonable index of suspicion should be maintained during administration of RBCs to anesthetized patients in order to avoid critical delay in diagnosis.

If a reaction is suspected, the transfusion should be stopped and the identity of the patient and the labeling of the blood should be rechecked. Management has three main objectives—maintenance of systemic blood pressure, preservation of renal function, and the prevention of DIC. Systemic blood pressure should be supported by administration of volume, pressors, and ionotropes as required. Urine output should be promoted by administration of fluids and the use of diuretics, either mannitol or furosemide, or both. Sodium bicarbonate can be administered to alkalinize the urine. Currently, there is no specific therapy to prevent the development of DIC. However, preventing hypotension and supporting cardiac output to prevent stasis and hypoperfusion, both of which contribute to the evolution of DIC, are important.

Blood samples should be collected in an EDTA tube. The specific tests should include (1) a repeat cross-match and (2) a direct antiglobulin (Coombs) test. The direct antiglobulin test is the definitive test for an acute hemolytic transfusion reaction. It examines recipient RBCs for the presence of surface immunoglobulins and complement. Patient serum is also examined for the presence of antibodies that react with the donor cells. Serum haptoglobin level, plasma and urine Hgb, and bilirubin assays are usually performed. However, these are evidence only of hemolysis, not specifically of an immune reaction.[31] Laboratory tests to establish baseline coagulation status—including platelet count, prothrombin time (PT), "activated" partial thromboplastin time (aPTT), thrombin time (TT), fibrinogen level, and fibrin degradation products (FDPs)—should be performed.

Examination of the patient's plasma after brief centrifugation for the pinkish discoloration caused by free hemoglobin is a simple, rapid screening test when a hemolytic transfusion reaction is suspected.[31] Hemolysis can be due to other causes including overheating prior to transfusion or inadvertent use of a hypotonic solution as a diluent. However, hemolysis should be assumed to indicate a hemolytic transfusion reaction until proven otherwise.

Delayed Hemolytic Transfusion Reactions

Numerous instances have been reported in which transfused RBCs are quickly eliminated from the circulation of the recipient after an apparently "compatible" cross-match. Many of these events are delayed hemolytic transfusion reactions. These reactions occur when the donor RBCs bear an antigen to which the recipient has previously been exposed, either by transfusion or by pregnancy. Over time, the recipient antibodies fall to levels too low to be detected by compatibility testing. When transfused again with RBCs containing the original immunizing antigen, the recipient undergoes an anamnestic response and produces more antibody, which eventually lyses the foreign RBCs. Typically, the antibody-coated RBC is sequestered extravascularly and lysis occurs in the spleen and reticuloendothelial system. Because the RBC destruction occurs extravascularly, symptoms are less severe and the reaction is less likely to be fatal. Unlike immediate hemolytic reactions, which usually involve antibodies in the ABO system, delayed hemolytic reactions commonly involve antibodies in the Rh and Kidd systems. The frequency of delayed hemolytic reactions is reported to be 1 per 800–2500 transfusions.[6,31]

Evidence of hemolysis is usually detected by the first or second week following transfusion. The reaction may be undetected or may be identified because of the combination of a low-grade fever, increased bilirubin with or without mild jaundice, and/or an unexplained reduction in hemoglobin concentration.[6] The diagnosis is confirmed by a positive direct antiglobulin test (Coombs test). The reaction is self-limiting, and the clinical manifestations resolve as the transfused cells are removed from the circulation.[31]

Transfusion Reactions to Donor Proteins

Allergic reactions to proteins in donor plasma cause urticarial reactions in 0.2–2% of all transfusions.[22] The reaction is almost always associated with the transfusion of fresh frozen plasma; but because a small volume of donor plasma is present in other blood products (RBCs, platelets), allergic reactions can occur with transfusion of these components as well. The patient may have itching, swelling, and a rash due to the release of histamine. These mild symptoms can be treated with diphenhydramine. Patients who experience severe urticarial reactions may benefit from the use of saline-washed cells.[31]

Infrequently, a more severe form of allergic reaction involving anaphylaxis will occur in which the patient experiences dyspnea, bronchospasm, hypotension, laryngeal edema, chest pain, and shock. Anaphylaxis precipitated by a transfusion is a rare, but potentially fatal, event. It occurs when patients with hereditary IgA deficiency who have been sensitized by previous transfusions or pregnancy are exposed to blood with "foreign" IgA protein. Treatment consists of discontinuation of the transfusion and administration of epinephrine and methylprednisolone. Washed RBCs, frozen deglycerolized RBCs, or RBCs from IgA-deficient donors should subsequently be used for these patients.[31]

White Cell–Related Transfusion Reactions

Febrile Reactions

Patients who receive multiple transfusions of packed RBCs or platelets often develop antibodies to the human leukocyte antigens (HLAs) on the passenger leukocytes in these products. During future RBC transfusions, febrile reactions may occur as a result of antibody attack on donor leukocytes. The leukocyte antigen–antibody reaction is thought to cause lysis of donor granulocytes with the release of chemical mediators. Phagocytosis of donor leukocyte fragments may also stimulate host macrophages to produce pyrogens.

The febrile response occurs in about 1% of all RBC transfusions. For most patients, the reaction can be characterized as troublesome and unpleasant, rather than clinically serious. Typically, the patient experiences a temperature increase of more than 1°C within 4 hours of a blood transfusion and defervesces within 48 hours.[31] Patients may experience fever only, but they may also develop chills, respiratory distress, anxiety,[26] headache, myalgias, nausea, and a nonproductive cough. Febrile reactions can be treated with acetaminophen.

A leukocyte-mediated febrile transfusion reaction should be distinguished from a hemolytic transfusion reaction (direct Coombs test), which also presents with a fever but may be life-threatening. Commercially available leukodepletion filters may be used to prevent febrile, nonhemolytic transfusion reactions.

Graft-versus-Host Disease (GVHD)

Packed RBCs and platelet concentrates both contain a significant number of viable donor lymphocytes. When transfused ("transplanted") into immunocompromised patients, the donor lymphocytes may become engrafted, proliferate, and establish an immune response against the recipient. In essence, the engrafted lymphocytes reject the host.[32]

Patients at risk for GVHD include organ transplant recipients, neonates who have undergone a blood-exchange transfusion,[31] and patients immunocompromised by many other disease processes. GVHD typically progresses rapidly to pancytopenia, and the fatality rate is very high.

Transfusion-associated GVHD has also been reported in apparently immunocompetent patients when a genetic relationship exists between the donor and the recipient. In these tragic cases, the patient shares human leukocyte antigen haplotypes with the donor lymphocytes. The patients, although immunologically competent, fail to reject the transfused cells because they do not recognize them as foreign. The transfused donor lymphocytes, however, recognize the host as foreign, and a GVHD reaction takes place.[33] Because of this phenomenon, the American Association of Blood Banks has recommended that directed donations from first-degree relatives be irradiated to inactivate donor lymphocytes.

GVHD has been reported with the transfusion of whole blood, packed RBCs, granulocytes, platelets, and fresh, not frozen, plasma. It has not occurred following transfusion of FFP, cryoprecipitate, or frozen RBCs.[33] Irradiation of cellular blood products should be done prior to transfusion in immunocompromised patients. Because of the increased probability of HLA haplotype sharing, directed donor units from relatives should always be irradiated.[26]

Transfusion-Related Acute Lung Injury (TRALI)

Transfusion-related acute lung injury is a rare reaction (~1/10,000 transfusions[34]) that occurs as a consequence of the deposition of white cell–antibody aggregates in the pulmonary vasculature. In most instances, it occurs when agents present in the plasma phase of donor blood activate leukocytes in the host.[35] Those agents are probably most often antileukocyte antibodies formed as a result of previous transfusion or pregnancy, although cytokines and biologically active lipids may also provide the trigger. In other instances, the opposite reaction, aggregation of donor leukocytes and recipient antibodies, may be the cause when the recipient has been alloimmunized to WBC antigens. The clinical picture is very similar to the adult respiratory distress syndrome (ARDS). Beginning soon after transfusion, the patient complains of dyspnea and chills and presents with a fever and noncardiogenic pulmonary edema. Chest x-ray reveals bilateral infiltrates. Severe pulmonary insufficiency develops. Treatment is largely supportive. The transfusion should be stopped if the reaction is recognized in time. The patient should be given supplemental oxygen and methylprednisolone every 6 hours. While outcome is more favorable than for ARDS, the reaction can be fatal in as many as 20% of patients. Patients who have experienced this reaction previously may benefit from the use of washed PRBCs.

Immunomodulation

Alteration of immune function has been associated with allogenic transfusion. The initial observations were of decreased rates of transplant rejection and decreased rates of spontaneous abortion in patients who had received homologous transfusions. Alteration in immune surveillance was inferred. Subsequently other, nonbeneficial effects of diminished immunocompetence were reported. These include increased incidence of postoperative infection, earlier recurrence of cancer,[36-46] and more rapid progression of HIV/AIDS.[47] Transfused white cells are thought to be the mediators of these effects, although the precise mechanisms have not been defined. These observations have led to the development and application of techniques for leukocyte depletion of donor blood products.[48]

Leukodepletion

The first widely accepted application of leukodepletion was in oncologic patients, in particular, those with leukemias who faced the prospect of multiple transfusions and were therefore at risk for the development of alloimmunization and platelet refractoriness.[49] Other benefits of leukodepletion have subsequently been demonstrated. These include: prevention of febrile reactions to RBC transfusions, reduction of postoperative infections and duration of hospitalization,[50] and prevention of transmission of cytomegalovirus (but not other viruses).[51] As noted earlier, increased rates of tumor recurrence have also been reported in cancer patients who receive transfusions. However, this association has not been consistently evident in carefully controlled trials,[48] and the relevance of leukodepletion to cancer recurrence or progression remains undefined. Blood administration has also been identified as a correlate of decreased survival in HIV infected patients, though a cause-and-effect relationship has not been established.[52] Again the relevance of leukodepletion must be viewed as unproven. Leukodepletion does not appear to prevent the occurrence of GVHD, apparently because of incomplete elimination of lymphocytes. Irradiation remains the only effective means for preventing GVHD.[48] Table 10-3 lists the benefits of leukodepletion.

Taken together, these benefits have produced substantial interest in leukodepletion. However, the issue of whether or not a clinician should request leukodepleted blood (or administer blood components through a bedside leukodepletion filter) will soon be moot. Because of the perceived benefits, many countries—including Canada, France, Portugal, and the United Kingdom—and certain states and regions within the United States have already adopted the practice of leukodepleting 100% of their blood supplies. Others will follow. Most will employ prestorage depletion to prevent the release of mediators from WBCs during storage. This is especially relevant to platelets that are stored at room temperature. In the interim, clinicians using bedside filtering should appreciate that the available filters are less efficient at higher temperatures and filtering should therefore ideally be performed before blood warms to room temperature. Clinicians should also be attentive to the possibility of severe, apparently bradykinin-mediated, hypotension in patients who receive bedside-filtered blood. The reaction appears to occur more frequently, though not exclusively, in pa-

tients receiving angiotensin-converting enzyme inhibitors (which reduce breakdown of bradykinin).[53]

Infectious Risks Associated with Blood Product Administration

The transfusion of blood products may be life-saving. However, the purpose may be in part defeated if the transfusion results in a life-threatening infectious disease. The appearance of HIV/AIDS in the early 1980s initiated a heightened consciousness of the infectious hazards of transfusion and brought new restraint to transfusion practices. The potentially transmittable diseases/agents are numerous. They include several viruses—hepatitis A, B, C, D, E, and G; the human T-cell lymphotropic viruses (HTLV-1, HTLV-2); the human immunodeficiency viruses 1 and 2; cytomegalovirus (CMV); and the Epstein-Barr virus—as well as prions (Jacob-Creutzfeldt) bacteria, parasites (malaria, Chagas' disease), and syphilis.[54,55] Bacterial and parasitic contamination of blood products is rare, and transmission of the CMV virus, though common, is usually a threat only to immunocompromised patients or neonates and infants. It is HIV and the various forms of hepatitis that pose the greatest risk to immunologically normal patients. Goodnough et al have provided a detailed review of this topic.[55]

Incidence of Viral Diseases

The rate of infectivity in the North American blood supply has decreased dramatically in the last two decades. The 1996 estimates of the risks of transmission of HIV, HTLV, hepatitis B, and hepatitis C are presented in Table 10-4. Those estimates are derived from the observed rates of seropositivity among donors and the statistical likelihood of administration of blood from donors whose infection is in the window period between contracting the virus and detectability by the available assays.

The dramatic reduction in the rate of HIV transmission after the early 1980s was the product of social screening of donors and HIV antibody testing (introduced in 1985). The 1996 transmission estimate of 1 infection per 493,000 donor exposures was made just at the time of the implementation of testing for the HIV p24 antigen. Because the HIV antigen appears prior to the antibody, the window of silent infectivity is shortened and the transmission rate should be even further decreased. A new generation of tests for HIV and HCV based on amplification of nucleic acid antigens by polymerase chain reaction has been developed recently. However, this nucleic acid antigen test (NAT) procedure will probably have only a small additional impact on absolute number of transfusion-related HIV events because the current rate is so low and because the silent window will only be reduced by an additional 6 days (from 16 to 10). The effect on HCV (hepatitis C) rates should be greater as the window is reduced from ~75 days to 30 days. Schreiber et al estimated HCV and HBV (hepatitis C) risk reductions of 72 and 42%, respectively, as a consequence of NAT testing.[56]

Post-Transfusion Viral Hepatitis (PTH)

Since the 1940s, when blood transfusions first became possible, viral hepatitis has been the foremost risk to patients who receive

Table 10-4. ESTIMATES OF THE RATE (PER DONOR EXPOSURE) OF TRANSFUSION-TRANSMITTED VIRAL DISEASE[56]

Hepatitis B (HBV)	1/63,000
Hepatitis C (HCV)	1/103,000
Human immunodeficiency virus (HIV)	1/493,000
Human T-cell lymphotrophic virus (HTLV)	1/641,000

Table 10-3. BENEFITS OF LEUKODEPLETION

CONFIRMED BENEFITS

Decreased alloimmunization/platelet refractoriness in multiply transfused leukemics
Prevention of febrile reactions to RBC transfusions
Decreased postoperative infections
Shortened hospitalization

UNCONFIRMED BENEFITS

Prevention of transfusion-related HIV acceleration
Prevention of transfusion-related increase in tumor recurrence

blood. Hepatitis B and C account for 88% of the 1/34,000 risk of a significant transfusion-related viral disease blood transfusion that prevailed in 1996 (prior to implementation of p24 and NAT testing). The hepatitis A virus, cytomegalovirus, and the Epstein-Barr virus (EBV) cause hepatitis at much lower frequencies. The diagnosis of PTH is frequently missed or delayed because fewer than 50% of patients become jaundiced during the acute phase of the disease and many are asymptomatic as well as anicteric.

Hepatitis C. HCV (the agent responsible for most of what was previously termed non-A, non-B; NANB) is more common and conveys greater patient risk than HBV. Despite HCV's commonly mild initial presentation, in 85% of patients it progresses to a chronic state with significant associated morbidity and mortality. Twenty percent of chronic carriers develop cirrhosis and 1–5% develop hepatocellular carcinoma.[57,58]

Hepatitis B. It is estimated that 35% of HBV-exposed patients will develop acute disease,[55] although ~1% will develop fulminant acute hepatitis. In ~85% of patients, the disease resolves spontaneously, 9% develop chronic persistent hepatitis, 3% develop chronic active hepatitis, 1% develop cirrhosis with or without chronic active hepatitis, and 1% develop hepatocellular carcinoma.[15] The diagnosis of HBV depends on the presence of hepatitis B surface antigen (HbsAg) or the antibody to hepatitis B core antigen (anti-HBc).

Hepatitis A

Hepatitis A does not play an important role in PTH. Blood banks do not screen for hepatitis A, and there is no carrier state for this virus. The infectious period is limited to 1–2 weeks. The diagnosis depends on hepatitis antibody seroconversion.

Human Immunodeficiency Virus (HIV)

The most feared complication of a blood transfusion is the transmission of HIV, the causative agent of the acquired immune deficiency syndrome (AIDS). It is a retrovirus, so called because its propagation requires translation of RNA to DNA. Current screening tests are directed at both HIV 1 and HIV 2, though the latter has been an extremely infrequent cause of human disease. The incidence of transfusion-related HIV infection has fallen dramatically since the implementation of serologic screening of donors. There were 714 reports to the Centers for Disease Control in 1984, but only five cases per year over the ensuing five years.[55]

Human T-Cell Lymphotropic Virus (HTLV)

HTLV-1 and HTLV-2 belong to the same retrovirus family as HIV. The incidence of clinical disease resulting from transmitted virus appears to be very low. They are associated with T-cell leukemia and lymphoma rather than the generalized immunodeficiency of AIDS. In the United States, all donor units are screened for the presence of antibody to HTLV-1 and HTLV-2.

Cytomegalovirus (CMV)

Transfusion-associated CMV infections are usually benign and self-limited. However CMV may cause serious, even fatal, infections in immunocompromised patients. Patients at risk include premature neonates, solid organ and bone marrow transplant recipients, and those patients with severely depressed immune function. CMV pneumonia is an important infectious cause of death in allogenic bone marrow transplant recipients.[51] Leukodepletion effectively prevents CMV transmission.[51]

Bacterial Contamination of Blood Components

RBCs

Bacterial contamination, estimated at 1/1,000,000 RBC units, is relatively uncommon.[59] *Yersinia enterocolitica* is the most common contaminant and is associated with substantial mortality. The patient who receives contaminated blood transfusion will rapidly experience some combination of fever, chills, tachycardia, emesis, shock, and may develop DIC and acute renal failure. The symptoms are very similar to those of immediate hemolytic transfusion reaction. The transfusion should be stopped immediately and blood cultures obtained.[31]

Platelets

Platelets, which are stored at room temperature, are more commonly contaminated. Goodnough *et al* quote the incidence as 1/12,000 and identify the organisms in order of frequency as *Staphylococcus aureus, Klebsiella Pneumoniae, Serratia marcescens,* and *Staphylococcus epidermidis.*[55] The reactions are variable in severity, and an index of suspicion should be maintained in order to distinguish these reactions from other major and minor transfusion reactions.

BLOOD CONSERVATION STRATEGIES

Autologous Donation

Preoperative donation and perioperative salvage of autologous blood have been used extensively as part of programs to reduce homologous blood administration. Autologous blood may be collected days to weeks prior to surgery (predonation); it may be donated immediately prior to surgery (isovolemic hemodilution); or it may be salvaged from the surgical field or wound drains and reinfused (blood salvage). Deciding whether any of these options is appropriate for individual patients presents another challenge in transfusion medicine.

Preoperative Autologous Donation

Preoperative donation of autologous blood (PAD) should be considered for patients undergoing elective surgical procedures in which the administration of homologous blood is expected.[60] Major orthopedic surgical procedures, such as total hip or total knee replacement, scoliosis procedures, and cardiac surgery are well suited to PAD.[61] PAD should not be recommended for patients undergoing surgery that usually does not require transfusion. The PAD procedure is more expensive than the collection of homologous blood. In addition, if autologous blood is unused, most institutions discard it and do not permit "crossover" to other patients.

Practices with respect to infectious agent testing also vary. Some institutions will store and permit return to the donor of HIV-, hepatitis-, or CMV-infected blood, while others discard it. Note also that the transfusion of autologous blood eliminates neither the chance of human error during blood collection, processing, and reinfusion nor the risk of bacterial contamination. Some institutions perform a crossmatch prior to return of blood to the donor, others do not. This underscores the caveat that no transfusion is without risk.

The medical condition of the patient must be considered prior to recommending predonation of blood.[60] Severe aortic stenosis, significant coronary disease or myocardial dysfunction, low initial hematocrit, and low blood volume (weight less than ~110 pounds) are relative contraindications to PAD.[62] If the patient's hemoglobin level, cardiac status, and general condition permit, blood can be donated at weekly intervals prior to surgery. Four units is typically the maximum donation given the shelf life of the first unit collected. The blood is stored at 4°C or, if it must be kept for longer periods of time, it can be stored as frozen RBCs.[21]

PAD has been widely, but not universally, effective in reducing exposure to homologous blood.[63] Open prostatic surgery and joint replacement have been most widely studied. Effectiveness has been limited when the patients' erythropoietic response is not vigorous, in which case the process may simply result in an anemia at the time of surgery. Patients making PAD should invariably receive supplemental iron. In addition, PAD can be supplemented with administration of recombinant erythropoietin (Epo). The effectiveness of Epo in hastening recovery of hematocrit in conjunction with PAD and in improving hematocrit in patients not submitted to PAD has been demonstrated.[64-67] However, the practice has not become widespread, in part because of the expense of the agent and in part because of the necessity for frequent (*e.g.*, thrice weekly) parenteral (sc or iv) administration of Epo. Epo is usually accepted by Jehovah's Witnesses, and its efficacy in that population has been demonstrated.[68]

Acute Normovolemic Hemodilution

Normovolemic hemodilution entails withdrawal of the patient's blood, usually *via* an intra-arterial catheter, early in the intraoperative period with concurrent administration of crystalloids or colloids to maintain normovolemia. The rationale is that during the ensuing surgery, the patient will lose blood of low hematocrit and the withdrawn blood will be available for reinfusion at the end of the operation. The end point for the initial withdrawal is an Hct of 27–33%, depending on the patient's cardiovascular[1] and respiratory reserves.[7] Selection for this technique should rely on careful evaluation of the patient for coronary or cerebral vascular disease. This procedure evolved in the anticipation that it would reduce total RBC loss and homologous blood administration. However, both mathematical modeling and empirical experience have revealed a very modest benefit with respect to reducing the necessity for homologous RBCs.[67,69-73] The technique has also been employed for the purpose of making fresh autologous blood at the end of procedures in which either a dilutional or cardiopulmonary bypass-related coagulopathy may occur. The efficacy in this context has not been confirmed by systematic study. Blood collected and reinfused for this purpose should not be passed through a 40-μm filter to avoid platelet elimination.

Perioperative Blood Salvage

Perioperative blood salvage is the recovery of shed blood from the surgical field or wound drains and readministration to the patient. In most instances, the process involves "washing" of the salvaged material with return of only the RBC component of blood. In some instances, usually those involving wound drainage, blood is returned filtered but otherwise unprocessed.

Intraoperative Blood Salvage

Intraoperative blood salvage (IBS) is employed with many surgical procedures that might otherwise necessitate homologous transfusion. Relatively simple devices that anticoagulate the suctioned blood and return it through a standard 170-μm filter without other processing are available. However, most current IBS involves more complicated apparatus ("cell savers"), entailing significant costs including that of dedicated personnel.[7] These cell saver devices anticoagulate the salvaged blood as it leaves the surgical field, separate the RBCs from other liquid and cellular elements by centrifugation, then wash the salvaged RBCs extensively with saline. The cells are typically returned to the patient in aliquots of 125 or 225 ml of saline-suspended RBCs with an Hct of 45–65%.[74] Higher hematocrits can be achieved at the expense of the time required for more prolonged centrifugation.

IBS has been used commonly during cardiovascular surgical procedures, aortic reconstruction, spinal instrumentation, joint arthroplasty, liver transplantation, resection of arteriovenous malformations,[20] and occasionally in the management of trauma patients. There have been numerous demonstrations that IBS can reduce the use of homologous RBCs.[75,76]

The presence of malignant cells has been viewed as a contraindication, as have infection and the presence of urine, bowel contents, and amniotic fluid in the operative field. However, IBS has been applied in the management of hepatic and urologic malignancies without evidence of metastasis, even though malignant cells are known to be retained with RBCs after the washing process.[77,78] At least one IBS washing device has also been shown to remove the critical procoagulant factors present in amniotic fluid,[79] and IBS has been employed successfully in cesarean section.[80]

The potential complications of IBS are largely a function of the reinfusion of materials that might remain after the washing process. These include fat, microaggregates (platelets and leukocytes), air, red cell stroma, free hemoglobin, heparin, bacteria, and debris from the surgical field. Most of these are in fact removed quite efficiently by contemporary cell saver equipment. Bacteria are the exception, and contamination of cell saver return with skin organisms is relatively common.[75] Massive air embolism has occurred as a result of user error. Direct return from the cell saver apparatus has now been largely abandoned in favor of return *via* an intermediary bag under the control of the anesthesiologist. Care should still be taken in the event that pressure infusor devices are applied to these bags.

A dilutional coagulopathy in association with large-volume IBS is to be expected because essentially all clotting factors and most platelets are removed by the washing process. Management is the same as that for a dilutional coagulopathy occurring with administration of homologous or PAD blood. However, a DIC-like coagulopathy, the "salvaged blood syndrome,"[81] has also been associated with IBS. It seems likely that this syndrome was the result of inadequate preparation of blood by older cell saver devices. Unwashed, salvaged blood has been shown to contain numerous constituents that influence the coagulation process: thromboplastic material, interleukins, complement, fibrin degradation products, and factors released from activated leukocytes and platelets.[20] The majority of these, however, are quite efficiently removed by contemporary processing devices and their presence is used as an argument against the return of unprocessed blood.[82]

An additional coagulopathy risk arises with the use of thrombin and microfibrillar collagen or cellulose products in the surgical field.[83] These agents are not reliably removed by the washing process; suction of blood to the IBS device should be discontinued during the use of these agents and resumed after the field has been irrigated.

Postoperative Blood Salvage

Post-operative recovery of blood from mediastinal chest tubes and wound drains after hip and knee replacement with immediate reinfusion of "unwashed" blood has been employed quite commonly. The many substances present in the unprocessed blood (previous section) suggest that coagulation dysfunction might result and some authorities are skeptical regarding the wisdom of this practice.[74,82] However, there have been only occasional reports of apparent adverse consequences.[84] This may reflect the fact that the recovered and reinfused volumes are usually small.

The Jehovah's Witness

In general, Jehovah's Witnesses will accept neither administration of homologous blood products nor the readministration of autologous products that have left the circulation. However, their faith allows significant personal discretion, so the wishes of each patient must be clarified. Few will permit the administration of the common whole blood components and the majority will decline PAD. But many will accept procedures that maintain extracorporeal blood in continuity with the circulation. The acceptability of cardiopulmonary bypass, acute normovolemic hemodilution, and perioperative cell salvage must be clarified with each patient individually. Most will permit administration of Epo.

THE HEMOSTATIC MECHANISM

Normal "hemostasis" involves a remarkable series of physiologic checks and balances that assure that blood remains in an invariably liquid state as it circulates throughout the body but transforms rapidly to a solid state once the vascular network is violated. The balance is delicate and complex, and it is the responsibility of the anesthesiologist to anticipate, prevent, and treat disturbances of that balance. Preoperative evaluation must identify those patients whose inherited or acquired medical conditions or whose current medications may influence these processes. With respect to medications, there are a rapidly increasing number of agents that are administered specifically for the purpose of altering the hemostatic balance, including ticlopidine, tissue plasminogen activator (t-PA), and low–molecular-weight heparin. As the patient proceeds through surgery and the postoperative period, the anesthesiologist must determine whether bleeding is surgical in nature or the result of a pre-existing or evolving hemostatic defect that will require the transfusion of hemostatic blood components—platelets, fresh frozen plasma, or cryoprecipitate—or the administration of pharmacologic agents.

Normal hemostasis involves three intertwined processes that occur almost simultaneously: primary hemostasis (formation of a friable platelet plug); coagulation or secondary hemostasis (reinforcement of the friable platelet plug by the formation of a firm fibrin clot); and fibrinolysis (clot lysis and restoration of blood flow through the recanalized vessel).

Step 1: Primary Hemostasis

Primary hemostasis begins within seconds of vascular injury and is complete within ~5 minutes. It results in the formation of a friable platelet plug that temporarily arrests bleeding until clot formation (coagulation) and vascular repair can occur. It requires the concerted actions of blood vessels and platelets.

Role of the Blood Vessels

Blood vessels are crucial to all three processes of the hemostatic mechanism. The intima of blood vessels is lined with a single layer of endothelial cells (Fig. 10-1). Deep to the endothelium is a layer of supportive collagenous tissue and smooth muscle cells. Loss of the endothelial surface is the critical event that sets the hemostatic mechanism in motion. When the endothe-

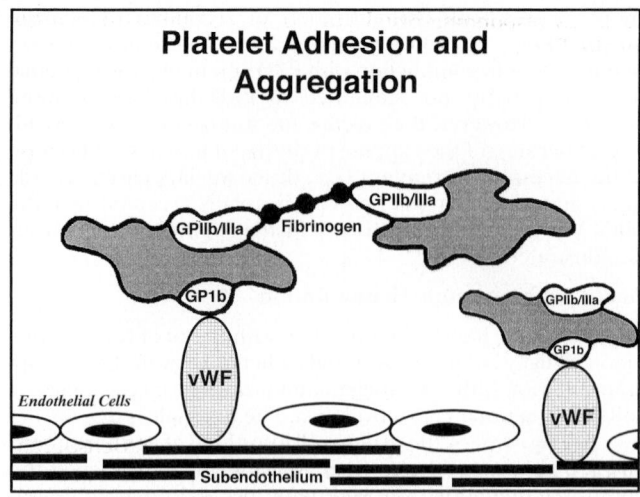

Figure 10-2. Platelet adhesion and aggregation. When the endothelium is denuded, von Willebrand factor (vWF) binds to collagen in the subendothelial layer. Platelets patrolling the blood vessel lining adhere *via* their glycoprotein (GP) 1b receptors to vWF. The binding of vWF to the GP1b receptors initiates platelet activation. Platelets change their shape from discoid to spheroid and extrude multiple pseudopods. Platelets aggregate to one another by crosslinking *via* fibrinogen (or vWF, not shown) between glycoprotein IIb/IIIa receptors expressed on the platelet surface during the process of platelet activation.

lial layer is denuded, circulating platelets are exposed to collagen and platelet activation is initiated. In addition, injured blood vessels constrict, thereby shunting blood flow away from the site of vascular injury.

Role of Platelets

Because of their small size, circulating platelets move preferentially along the walls of blood vessels where flow is slower.[85] These marginated platelets, in essence, "patrol" the vessel wall until they encounter a break in the endothelial surface. When platelets are exposed to collagen and other proteins in the subendothelial matrix, "platelet activation" occurs. Activation involves four processes: adhesion, shape change and mediator release, aggregation, and the appearance of surface phospholipid.

Platelet Adhesion. Platelet adhesion to collagen results in conformational and surface changes by the platelet. A series glycoprotein surface receptors appear. Some of these receptors facilitate platelet adhesion to collagen and other vessel wall proteins and other receptors permit platelet to platelet binding (aggregation) (Fig. 10-2). The nomenclature of platelet receptors (GPI, GPIa, GPII, GPIII, etc.) is related to their electrophoretic mobility.[85]

VON WILLEBRAND FACTOR. *In vitro* studies indicate that under conditions of stasis or low flow in the venous circulation, platelets will adhere to surfaces coated with collagen, fibronectin, or laminin. However, under the high-shear conditions that prevail in arterioles and the microcirculation, collagen, fibronectin, or laminin are insufficient to support platelet adhesion.[86] These conditions require the von Willebrand factor (vWF). vWF is a multimeric glycoprotein that circulates in plasma attached to Factor VIII. It is synthesized by endothelial cells, which both secrete it into the plasma and deposit it in the subendothelial matrix. vWF is also synthesized by megakaryocytes and stored in the alpha granules of platelets.

When the subendothelium of a vessel is damaged, circulating vWF binds to the exposed collagen. Circulating platelets adhere to the vWF *via* GPIb receptors on the platelet surface.[85,87–90] In this way, the vWF helps platelets to adhere to the collagen. Defects in vWF cause the von Willebrand syndrome, while defects

Anatomy of the Blood Vessel

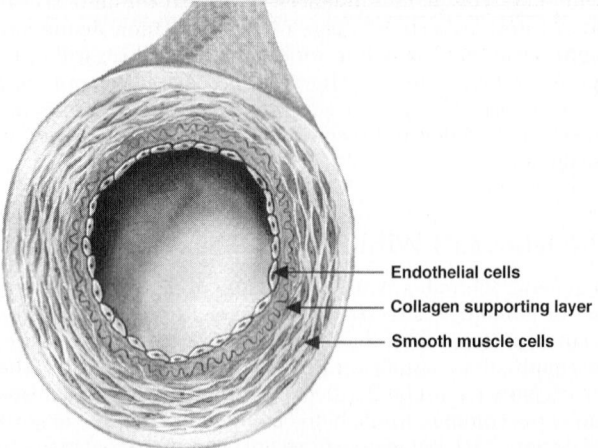

Endothelial cells
Collagen supporting layer
Smooth muscle cells

Figure 10-1. Blood vessel anatomy. The normal vascular tree resists thrombogenesis primarily because of the presence of the endothelium. By contrast, the subendothelial layer is highly thrombogenic. When exposed, proteins (collagen, fibronectin, etc.) in the subendothelium stimulate platelet adhesion and initiate the coagulation cascade.

in the corresponding platelet receptor (GPIb) are responsible for the Bernard-Soulier syndrome.[91]

Platelet Shape Change and Mediator Release. Adhesion of platelets to collagen converts the metabolically quiescent platelets to active cells which undergo rapid membrane, cytoskeletal, and metabolic changes. The activated platelets change from flattened discs to irregular spheroids which extend numerous pseudopods or "spiney" cytoplasmic processes.[85,91] This shape change is reversible in its early stages, but sustained stimuli quickly lead to irreversible shape changes and granule release.

Platelets contain both dense granules and alpha granules. In the process of platelet activation, the granule membranes are disrupted and the contents released.[92] Substances released from the alpha granules include adhesive proteins (vWF, fibrinogen, fibronectin, thrombospondin), growth modulators [*e.g.*, platelet-derived growth factor (PDGF)], and coagulation factors (V and XI, protein S, plasminogen activator inhibitor). Dense granules release calcium, ADP, ATP, serotonin, and histamine[85,93] (Fig. 10-3). The ADP released from the alpha granules is a powerful platelet activator and proaggregant which rapidly recruits other platelets to the growing platelet mass.

Platelet Aggregation. The glycoprotein receptors that appear in association with granule release and shape change allow platelets to bind to one another in a process referred to as platelet aggregation. Fibrinogen also contributes to the growth and stability of the evolving platelet plug. In the presence of Ca^+, it binds to certain of the newly exposed glycoprotein receptors on the platelet surface (glycoproteins IIb and IIIa). Fibrinogen is multi-stranded and bridges and binds many platelets simultaneously. This stage of aggregation is reversible because the fibrinogen linkage is weak. Thrombospondin (from the alpha granules) can also bind to the platelets and further strengthen the aggregation.[94]

ADP released from platelet granules promotes platelet aggregation. ADP release, in turn, is greatly increased by a potent prostaglandin, thromboxane A_2 (TxA_2), synthesized from arachidonic acid by activated platelets. Platelet activators, such as collagen and thrombin, cause mobilization of arachidonic acid from platelet membrane phospholipids. In a series of enzymatic reactions involving cyclooxygenase and thromboxane synthase, arachidonic acid is converted to TxA_2. The actions of TxA_2 are important to the control of primary hemostasis (see below).

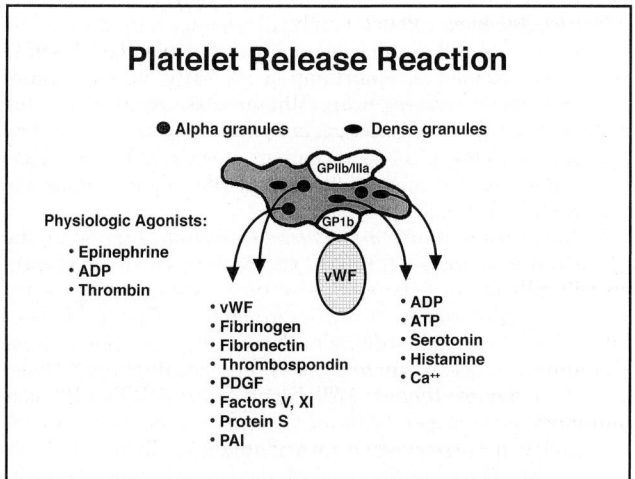

Figure 10-3. Platelet release reaction. Platelets undergo a release reaction coincident with shape change or in response to physiologic agonists including epinephrine, ADP, and thrombin. The numerous substances released from the alpha and dense granules of platelets contribute to platelet aggregation (fibrinogen, vWF), clot formation (Ca^{2+}, Factors V and XI), and adhesion and activation of additional platelets (vWF, fibronectin, and ADP).

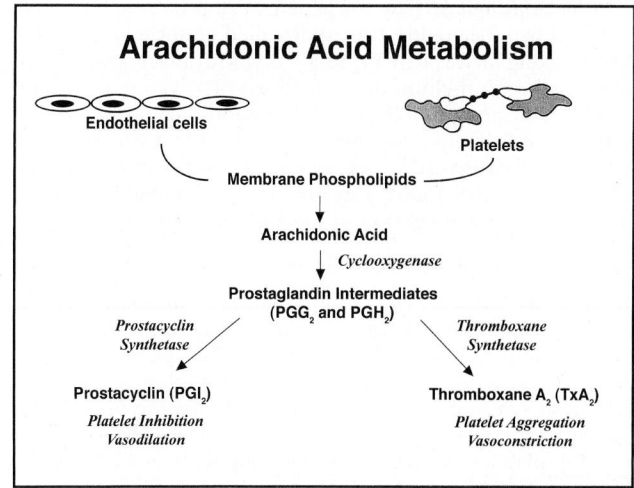

Figure 10-4. The participation of arachidonic acid metabolites in hemostasis. Prostacyclin and thromboxane A_2 are synthesized from arachidonic acid derived from phospholipids in the membranes of both endothelial cells and platelets. The balance between these two prostaglandins controls primary hemostasis and localizes clot formation to sites of vascular injury.

Appearance of New Phospholipid Procoagulant Activity. In addition to the appearance of glycoprotein receptors, platelet activation causes other surface conformation changes. Quiescent platelets possess heterogeneous phospholipids located primarily on the inner aspect of the cell membrane. With platelet activation, specific phospholipids are translocated to the outer half of the membrane. This phospholipid movement changes the surface charge of the platelet and results in procoagulant activity. This new phospholipid procoagulant property of platelets is called platelet factor-3 activity, or PF3.

The new surface phospholipids (PF3) serve as binding sites for those coagulation factors that require the formation of "reaction complexes." Those complexes involve factor pairs that must bind in a specific spatial arrangement in order to activate a third clotting factor. They depend upon the platelet phospholipid binding sites for the proper spatial interaction to occur. Factors VIIIa and IXa bind on PF3 to result in the activation of Factors X to Xa. Thereafter, Factors Va and Xa bind to the surface of the platelet and, in the presence of calcium, convert prothrombin (Factor II) to thrombin (IIa). Thrombin produced in this manner and localized to the platelet membrane surface is a potent activator of additional platelets, resulting in further release of ADP and amplification of platelet aggregation.

Control of Primary Hemostasis

The Thromboxane–Prostacyclin Balance. Primary hemostasis is, in part, controlled by the balance between the actions of two prostaglandins, thromboxane A_2 and prostacyclin. Thromboxane A_2 (TxA_2) is synthesized at the site of vascular damage by activated platelets. TxA_2 has two hemostatic effects: (1) it is a potent vasoconstrictor that causes blood vessels to constrict locally and shunt blood flow away from the site of injury; (2) it stimulates additional ADP release from platelets and thereby causes recruitment of additional platelets.[86,93]

Remote from the site of vascular damage, normal endothelial cells synthesize prostacyclin (PGI_2). PGI_2, which is also synthesized from arachidonic acid (Fig. 10-4), has actions opposite to those of TxA_2. PGI_2 inhibits platelet activation, secretion, and aggregation[95] and is a potent vasodilator. It therefore serves to prevent platelet aggregation and clot formation on the endothelial surface beyond the site of injury. An imbalance in the production of these two prostaglandins can lead to a defect in primary hemostasis.

Nitric Oxide and ADPase. The effects of prostacyclin are potentiated by nitric oxide (formerly called endothelium-dependent relaxing factor, EDRF), which is constitutively synthesized by normal endothelium and which also has vasodilatory and platelet antiaggregant effects.[88] As an additional means of preventing clot formation on the surface of normal endothelium, ADPases are expressed on the outer membrane of endothelial cells and serve to degrade "surplus" ADP which might otherwise initiate platelet aggregation on normal surfaces.

Summary of Primary Hemostasis

In summary, after vascular injury exposes collagen, platelets adhere to the injured vessel wall, largely *via* the GPIa platelet receptor and the von Willebrand factor. The platelets change shape and release the contents of their cytoplasmic granules. ADP, thus released, causes the platelets to expose the GPIIb/IIIa receptor. Fibrinogen binds *via* this GPIIb/IIIa receptor, bridging platelets together and inducing platelet aggregation. Activated platelets synthesize thromboxane A_2 which induces vasoconstriction and increases ADP release. The additional ADP further increases platelet aggregation. The aggregated platelets form the platelet plug which temporarily arrests bleeding. The aggregated platelets expose a new surface phospholipid, platelet factor 3, which serves to localize the coagulation process, which by now is underway, to the site of platelet plug formation.

Step 2: Coagulation

Coagulation is the second phase of the hemostatic process. Coagulation involves the interaction of numerous plasma proteins, referred to as clotting factors, in a cascade of reactions that generate fibrin to reinforce the friable platelet plug.

The Nomenclature of Coagulation

Understanding the coagulation process has been made more difficult by the complexity of the nomenclature. An early attempt was made to standardize it by assigning Roman numerals to each of the twelve known clotting factors. Unfortunately, especially for non-hematologists, they were numbered in the order in which they were discovered and not in the sequence in which they interact. To complicate matters, the first four of the original 12 factors are always referred to by their common names, fibrinogen, prothrombin, tissue thromboplastin (tissue factor), and calcium and not by their Roman numerals. Factor VI no longer exists; it proved to be activated Factor V. The more recently discovered clotting factors, *e.g.*, prekallikrein and high–molecular-weight kininogen have not been assigned Roman numerals. They too are identified by common names, and to further complicate matters, some have more than one name (Table 10-5).

The Broad Principles of Coagulation

Although the complexity of the coagulation mechanism appears forbidding and the nomenclature chaotic, some basic principles can help to develop a broad understanding of the process.

1. *Most clotting factors circulate in an inactive form.* Most of the clotting factors circulate in an inactive form referred to as a procoagulant or proenzyme. During the process of coagulation, a portion of this molecule is cleaved off. The remaining protein is an active cleavage enzyme, a serine protease. The "activated clotting factor" is designated by the addition of a lowercase "a" after the Roman numeral, *e.g.*, Xa. The activated clotting factor cleaves off a portion of the next procoagulant factor, thereby "activating" it in turn. Chain reaction–like, one factor "activates" another, until fibrinogen (factor I) is cleaved to yield fibrin.
2. *Most clotting factors are synthesized by the liver.* Most of the coagulation proteins are synthesized by the liver. This means that their normal structure and function are depen-

Table 10-5. CLOTTING FACTORS

Factor	Synonyms	*In Vivo* Half-life (hours)
I	Fibrinogen	100–150
II	Prothrombin	50–80
III	Tissue thromboplastin, tissue factor (TF)	
IV	Calcium ion	
V	Proaccelerin, labile factor	24
VII	Serum prothrombin conversion accelerator (SPCA), stable factor	
VIII	Antihemophiliac factor (AHF)	12
vWF	von Willebrand factor	24
IX	Christmas factor	24
X	Stuart-Prower factor	25–60
XI	Plasma thromboplastin antecedent (PTA)	40–80
XII	Hageman factor	50–70
XIII	Fibrin stabilizing factor (FSF)	150
Prekallikrein	Fletcher factor	35
HMW kininogen	Fitzgerald, Flaujeac, or Williams factor; contact activation cofactor	150

dent upon normal hepatic activity. One possible exception is Factor VIII which may have some extrahepatic synthesis.
3. *Factor VIII is a large, two-molecule complex (vWF and coagulant Factor VIII).* Factor VIII circulates as a very large complex of two distinct protein components, each under separate genetic control.[91] The high–molecular-weight portion (VIIIR:Ag) encompasses both the Factor VIII antigen (used to identify "Factor VIII" in the laboratory assay) and vWF. The vWF portion serves as a carrier protein for the second and smaller component of this macromolecular complex, VIIIC, which contains the Factor VIII coagulant activity. In addition to its role as carrier protein, the vWF has a second function. During the process of primary hemostasis when the endothelial lining has been denuded, vWF mediates adhesion of platelets to collagen. Absence of VIIIC results in hemophilia A. Absence of vWF causes two hemostatic abnormalities: (1) a defect in primary hemostasis because of a failure of platelet adhesion to the sites of vascular injury; (2) clinical hemophilia A because of an absence of circulating Factor VIIIC. Restoration of vWF levels restores normal hemostasis. Synthesis of the vWF occurs in endothelial cells and megakaryocytes. The site of synthesis of the coagulant portion of Factor VIII is unknown, but may be located in the hepatic sinusoidal endothelial cells.
4. *Four clotting factors are vitamin K–dependent.* Four of the clotting factors—II, VII, IX, and X—are said to be vitamin K–dependent factors because they require vitamin K for completion of their synthesis in the liver. Each undergoes a final enzymatic addition of a carboxyl group that requires the presence of vitamin K. The carboxyl group enables these factors to bind (with calcium as a cofactor) to phospholipid surfaces. Without vitamin K, Factors II, VII, IX, and X are produced in normal amounts but are nonfunctional. These nonfunctional factors are called PIVKAs [proteins induced by vitamin K absence/antagonist]. The anticoagulant action of vitamin K antagonists is the result of their ability to inhibit this final carboxylation step. The coumadin-like drugs compete with vitamin K for binding sites on the hepatocyte. With sufficient coumadin administration, vitamin K is displaced and the vitamin K–dependent factors are not carboxylated. Of the four vita-

min K–dependent factors, Factor VII has the shortest half-life. It is the first clotting factor to disappear from the circulation when a patient is placed on coumadin or begins to develop vitamin K deficiency.

5. *Coagulation requires the presence of a phospholipid surface.* The coagulation process involves several surface-mediated reactions that serve both to localize and control the production of fibrin. These reactions can take place on two different phospholipid surfaces. One is provided by tissue factor, which is normally extrinsic to blood[96] but which can be exposed to or released into the circulation by tissue injury. The second is provided by platelets which, when activated, expose PF3 phospholipid on their surface.

6. *Coagulation requires the formation of reaction complexes.* Many of the reactions of the coagulation cascade involve one factor activating another. However, some clotting factors are activated by the combined action of a pair of factors, bound in a particular spatial arrangement on a phospholipid surface. One factor serves as an active cleavage enzyme and the other as a "cofactor." The complex (the two factors plus phospholipid) together activate a third clotting factor, converting it into an active cleavage enzyme.

7. *Two factors, V and VIII, serve as cofactors in reaction complexes.* Factors V and VIII serve as cofactors in "reaction complexes." They do not become active cleavage enzymes. Without these cofactors in a reaction complex, the reaction may proceed, but only at a very slow rate. Thrombin modulates the activity of the cofactors (V and VIII) by a variety of feedback loops (see Protein C and Protein S).

8. *Factors V and VIII have short storage half-lives.* Factors V and VIII are also referred to as the "labile factors" because their coagulant activity is not durable in stored blood. While packed RBCs contain residual plasma with clotting factors, massive transfusion with stored blood will nonetheless lead to a dilutional coagulopathy because of diminished activity of Factors V and VII.

The Classic Model of Coagulation: Two Distinct Pathways

The cascade or waterfall description of coagulation was proposed in 1964. It proposed that coagulation could be initiated by either of two pathways: (1) an "extrinsic" pathway that required the presence of a substance "extrinsic to blood." That substance has been called tissue thromboplastin and, more recently, tissue factor (TF); (2) an "intrinsic" pathway that could proceed in a test tube containing only clotting factors intrinsic to blood. The two pathways, intrinsic and extrinsic, were thought to converge with the formation of activated Factor X. Thereafter, thrombin and subsequently fibrin were generated through a final common pathway of coagulation.

The Classic Intrinsic Pathway (coagulation initiated by contact activation). Previously, the "intrinsic pathway" was thought to be the more physiologically important of the two pathways. It was described as follows. The contact factors (Factor XII, prekallikrein, and high–molecular-weight kininogen) are activated by exposure to a negatively charged surface. They in turn activate Factor XI which then activates Factor IX. Activated Factor IX (IXa) then binds to the phospholipid surface of activated platelets (PF3) together with the cofactor, Factor VIIIC, to form a reaction complex. The IXa–VIIIC–phospholipid reaction complex then activates Factor X to produce Xa.

THE COMMON PATHWAY OF COAGULATION. With the formation of Factor Xa, the common pathway of coagulation is initiated. Factor X, once activated, binds with its cofactor, Factor V, and platelet phospholipid (PF3) and the complex activates Factor II, prothrombin, to thrombin (IIa). Thrombin, bound to PF3, cleaves fibrinogen, and "fibrin monomers" are released into the circulation (Fig. 10-5).

FROM A SOLUBLE CLOT TO A STABLE (INSOLUBLE) CLOT. Fibrin monomers aggregate end-to-end and side-by-side to form a fibrin polymer. This fibrin clot, referred to as fibrin S (soluble),

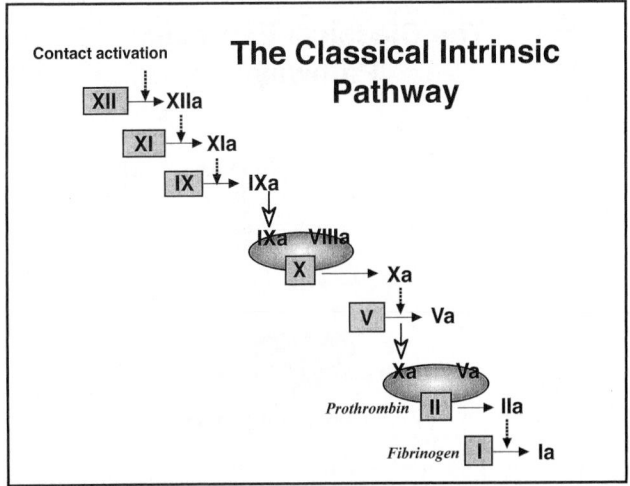

Figure 10-5. The classic intrinsic pathway of coagulation. This cascade of reactions is initiated by contact activation factors or exposure of blood to a foreign surface and leads to the formation of fibrin. The dotted arrows indicate the occurrence of an enzymatically mediated conversion of an inactive factor to its active form. The open-headed arrows indicate the translocation of an activated factor to a phospholipid surface to participate in a reaction complex. The shaded spheroids represent the phospholipid surfaces (usually provided by activated platelets).

is held together only by hydrogen bonds. Subsequently, Factor XIII (fibrin stabilizing factor), which is activated by thrombin and calcium ions, mediates the formation of covalent peptide bonds between the fibrin monomers to yield a stable (insoluble) fibrin clot (Fig. 10-6).

Although this series of reactions does occur, it probably most accurately describes clot formation in a test tube and not what occurs following tissue injury.

The Classic Extrinsic Pathway (coagulation initiated by tissue factor). Coagulation initiated by exposure to a "tissue factor" was thought to involve the activation of Factor VII and the formation of a complex of VIIa and tissue factor. This complex then activated Factor X and fibrin formation proceeded *via* the "common pathway of coagulation" just described (Fig. 10-7).

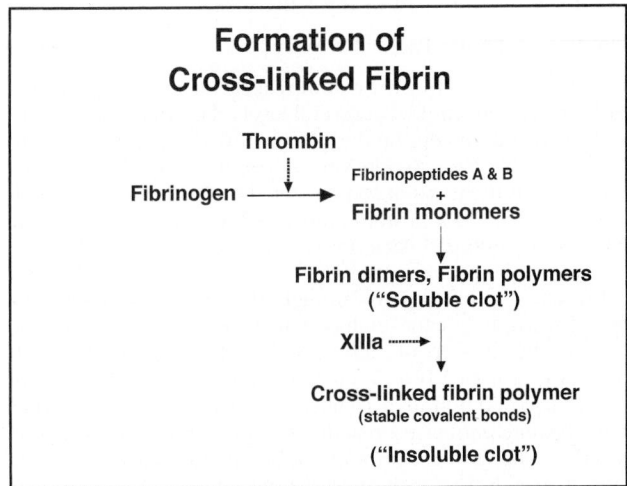

Figure 10-6. The formation of crosslinked fibrin. Several steps are required for the formation of a stable, crosslinked, insoluble fibrin clot. The dotted arrows indicate the occurrence of a reaction mediated enzymatically by an activated clotting factor.

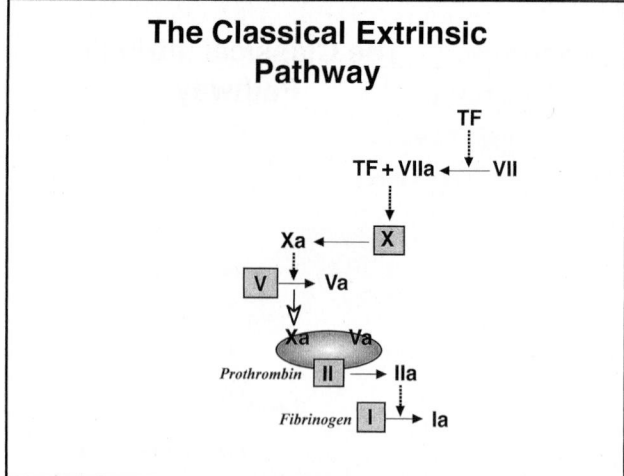

The Classical Extrinsic Pathway

Figure 10-7. The classic extrinsic pathway of coagulation. This pathway is depicted as it was originally thought to occur—*i.e.,* largely extravascularly and independent of the classic intrinsic pathway (*cf.* Fig. 10-8). The dotted arrows indicate the occurrence of an enzymatically mediated conversion of an inactive factor to its active form. The open-headed arrows indicate the translocation of an activated factor to a phospholipid surface to participate in a reaction complex. The shaded spheroid represents the phospholipid surface (usually provided by activated platelets).

Limitations of the Classic Theories.   These theories failed to explain several clinical phenomena. First, persons lacking Factor XII, prekallikrein, or high–molecular-weight kininogen do not bleed abnormally, suggesting that contact activation is not critical for normal hemostasis. Second, patients with only trace quantities of Factor XI withstand major trauma without unusual bleeding and those completely lacking Factor XI have only a mild hemorrhagic disorder. Factor XI therefore appears to have a more minor role in coagulation than that ascribed to it by classic theory. Next, deficiencies of Factor VIII and Factor IX (both in the intrinsic pathway) lead to hemophilia A and B, respectively. The classic description of two pathways of coagulation leaves it unclear why either type of hemophiliac could not simply clot *via* the unaffected pathway. Such observations suggest that the classic description represents an incomplete description of *in vivo* coagulation and have prompted some additional development of these theories.

The Single Tissue Factor Pathway

The current view is that the distinct classic intrinsic and extrinsic pathways are interlinked at several levels (Fig. 10-8). In contrast to the original conception that the intrinsic pathway was primarily responsible for coagulation *in vivo,* it is now thought that *tissue factor* is the usual *in vivo* trigger. This tissue factor has now been identified as a protein embedded in phospholipid in the surface membrane of pericytes in blood vessel walls, fibroblasts, and in a variety of other cells.[97–100]

Normal hemostasis is now thought to be initiated when endothelial disruption exposes blood to tissue factor (TF) in the subendothelial layers of blood vessels.[101] The exposed TF binds circulating Factor VII or VIIa. Although the mechanism is not clear, Factor VII bound to TF becomes an activated Factor VIIa/tissue factor complex in a reaction that probably involves Factors Xa, IXa, XIIa, and thrombin.[102] Subsequently, Factor X is activated by two distinct sequences. First, it can be activated directly by the Factor VIIa/tissue factor complex, *i.e.,* the classic extrinsic pathway. Alternatively, the Factor VIIa/tissue factor complex can activate Factor IX. Activated Factor IXa then forms the IXa/VIIIC/platelet phospholipid complex with subsequent ac-

tivation of Factor X in a reaction previously viewed as a component of the intrinsic pathway.

The Existence of Tissue Factor Pathway Inhibitor (TFPI).   The previous description appears incomplete. If Factor Xa can be formed *via* the direct action of the VIIa/TF complex, why is it that hemophiliacs bleed? Why do they appear dependent on Factors VIII and IX to produce Xa? The answer lies in the existence of a feedback inhibitor known as tissue factor pathway inhibitor (TFPI) (Fig. 10-9). TFPI, which is generated in a Factor Xa–dependent fashion, is a potent inhibitor of the formation of Factor Xa by both VIIa/TF-initiated sequences.[96] In the presence of TFPI, activation of Factor X becomes entirely dependent upon the reaction sequences of the classic intrinsic pathway. The TF pathway may initiate the first flurry of thrombin generation—enough to activate platelets and stimulate cofactors V and VIII. Thereafter, continued thrombin production appears to require the action of Factors XIa, VIIICa, and IXa.[96]

The existence of TFPI gives rise to the hope that an inhibitor of TFPI could prevent the inhibition of tissue factor–mediated coagulation by TFPI. That inhibitor might allow the TF/factor VIIa pathway to achieve hemostasis in hemophiliacs.

Tissue Factor in Disease States.   Abnormal elaboration of TF, perhaps by endothelial cells and monocytes,[103–107] or abnormal access of TF to the circulation may play a role in the initiation of hypercoagulable states or DIC in some clinical conditions, such as cancer, sepsis, amniotic fluid embolus, eclampsia, and severe cerebral injury.[96,101,108]

Control of Coagulation

Coagulation must be precisely regulated to prevent rampant, uncontrolled clotting throughout the body such as that which occurs with disseminated intravascular coagulation (DIC). Several mechanisms regulate and control coagulation. The fact that the blood remains fluid despite such intense stimuli for coagulation as massive trauma demonstrates the efficiency of these mechanisms and their effectiveness in localizing clot formation to sites of vascular injury.

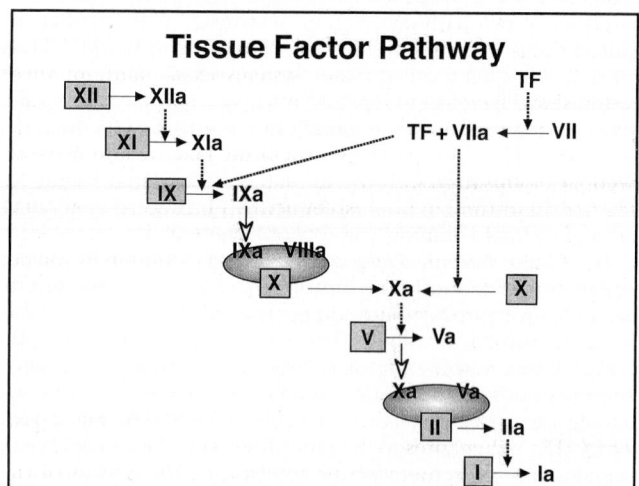

Tissue Factor Pathway

Figure 10-8. The tissue factor pathway. This figure depicts the pathway thought to be most relevant to *in vivo* coagulation. It indicates that activated Factor X (Xa) can be synthesized *via* two different pathways. The first pathway involves direct activation of Factor X by a complex formed by tissue factor (TF) and activated Factor VII (VIIa). Alternatively, activated Factor X (Xa) can be formed indirectly *via* the activation of Factor IX by this same TF and Factor VIIa complex. The dotted arrows indicate the occurrence of an enzymatically mediated conversion of an inactive factor to its active form. The open-headed arrows indicate the translocation of an activated factor to a phospholipid surface to participate in a reaction complex. The shaded spheroids represent the phospholipid surfaces (usually provided by activated platelets).

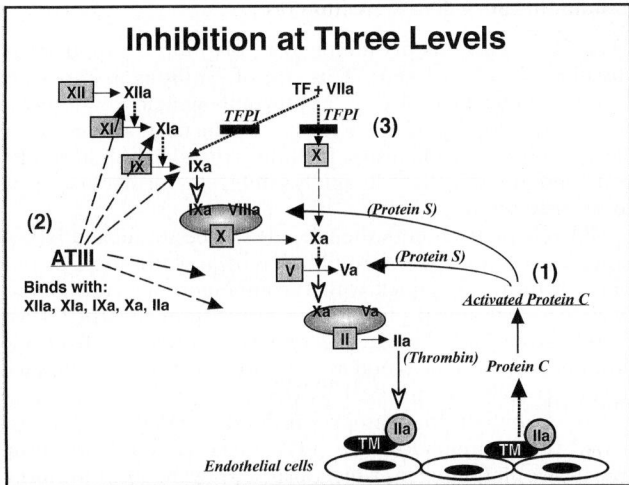

Inhibition at Three Levels

Figure 10-9. Inhibition of coagulation at three levels. Three important mechanisms that serve to control coagulation are depicted. (*1*) Thrombin, bound to thrombomodulin (TM) activates protein C which, with protein S as a cofactor, inhibits activated Factors V and VIII. (*2*) Antithrombin III (ATIII) binds, and thereby inhibits, several activated clotting factors in the classic intrinsic and common pathways (XIIa, XIa, IXa, Xa, IIa). (*3*) Tissue factor pathway inhibitor (TFPI) inhibits both of the pathways initiated by TF and VIIa that lead to the activation of Factor X (see text).

Natural Mechanisms That Modulate the Coagulation Process. Many factors serve to limit and localize clot formation. First, the clotting factors themselves circulate in an inactive form. Once they do become activated, normal blood flow dilutes their concentration and washes them away from sites of injury, limiting clot formation. Activated clotting factors are preferentially removed from the circulation by the liver and the reticuloendothelial system. And finally, the fact that some interactions of the coagulation pathway require the presence of a phospholipid surface localizes clot formation to these phospholipid surfaces.

Control of Coagulation via Anticoagulants or Inhibitors. Several specific anticoagulant inhibitor systems exist. Many of these systems work *via* thrombin which is truly the "master" coagulation enzyme (see below). It has a critical position in the coagulation cascade and orchestrates most of the positive and negative feedback loops that control coagulation. Thrombin plays a central role in primary hemostasis by activating platelets and stimulating their release of ADP, which promotes platelet aggregation and platelet plug formation. But the role of thrombin in control of the coagulation process is even more prominent because of thrombin's interaction with several naturally occurring circulating anticoagulants.

THROMBIN, THROMBOMODULIN, AND PROTEINS C AND S. Thrombin modulates the activity of the cofactors V and VIII directly, and indirectly *via* protein C and protein S (see Fig. 10-9). Thrombin, when present in low concentrations, can directly increase its own production by accelerating the activity of the two cofactors, Factors V and VIII. Thrombin can also decrease its own synthesis by inhibition of these same two cofactors. Its inhibition of V and VIII, however, occurs indirectly *via* protein C, a naturally occurring, vitamin K–dependent anticogulant protein. Protein C circulates in plasma as an inactive precursor until it is activated by thrombin.[109] The rate of thrombin-induced protein C activation can be greatly enhanced if thrombin first binds to thrombomodulin, a protein located on the vascular endothelial cell surface. The binding of thrombin to thrombomodulin alters the thrombin molecule such that it can no longer directly activate clotting factors V and VIII and cannot catalyze the conversion of fibrinogen to fibrin. Instead, the thrombin/

thrombomodulin complex rapidly converts protein C to active protein C (APC) and APC proteolytically cleaves Factors Va and VIIIa. In this way, thrombin indirectly inhibits its own synthesis.[110] The location of thrombomodulin on the endothelial surface is strategic. Where the endothelium is intact, the thrombomodulin–thrombin–protein C interaction will inhibit coagulation and maintain the "nonthrombogenic" property of the endothelial lining. Where the endothelium has been stripped away or damaged, this anticoagulant mechanism will be absent and clotting can continue unopposed.

Protein S is also an anticoagulant protein. Like protein C, it is vitamin K–dependent. Protein S acts as a cofactor in the protein C–catalyzed inactivation of Factors Va and VIIIa.[110]

The role of protein C is characteristic of that played by many participants in the hemostatic mechanism. Protein C in its native form is inactive. For its enzymatic function, it must be activated by thrombin. Protein C interacts with more than one hemostatic process. It serves as an anticoagulant (degrading cofactors Va and VIIIa) and also promotes fibrinolysis (causing the release of t-PA from endothelial cells). Its actions require the presence of a phospholipid surface to degrade factors Va and VIIIa.

THROMBIN AND ANTITHROMBIN III. Antithrombin III (ATIII) is a circulating anticoagulant that binds to thrombin to inactivate this master coagulation enzyme. Similarly, ATIII can bind and inactivate each of the activated clotting factors of the classic intrinsic coagulation cascade—Factors XIIa, XIa, IXa, and Xa[111] (see Fig. 10-9). By virtue of its broad inhibitory action, ATIII plays a central role in the regulation of hemostasis *in vivo*.

Heparin and antithrombin III. The ATIII molecule has two critical binding sites, one of which reacts with thrombin (and the other activated clotting factors), and a second to which heparin can bind. In the absence of heparin, ATIII has a relatively low affinity for thrombin. However, when heparin is bound to ATIII, the rate of binding of ATIII to thrombin is accelerated 100–1000 times. Likewise, heparin is able to accelerate dramatically the binding of ATIII to the other activated clotting factors—Factors IXa, Xa, XIa, and XIIa. The action of ATIII, which in the absence of heparin slowly inactivates thrombin, is referred to as the "progressive activity" of ATIII, while the rapid, heparin-dependent inactivation is termed the "heparin cofactor activity" of ATIII.[112] Once the ATIII/heparin complex has neutralized thrombin, heparin is released from the complex and can catalyze another ATIII inactivation.

Naturally occurring heparan sulfate and heparin. The endothelial surface is coated with a mucopolysaccharide referred to as the glycocalyx.[113] One of the constituents of this glycocalyx is a naturally occurring heparin-like component called "heparan" sulfate. Much like heparin, this naturally occurring heparan sulfate has the ability to accelerate the binding of ATIII to thrombin and the other activated clotting factors of the classic intrinsic pathway. This heparan sulfate is well positioned because it is at this blood–endothelial interface that activated factors of the coagulation cascade are being generated.[114] The presence of heparan sulfate on the endothelial surface further helps to promote the "antithrombotic" property of the endothelial lining.[114]

ATIII deficiencies. Congenital ATIII deficiency (levels 40–50% of normal) can lead to dangerous thrombotic events. Among patients with a history of deep vein thrombosis or pulmonary embolism, 2–3.5% have ATIII deficiency.[112] Arterial thromboses are reported less commonly with this deficiency.

Acquired deficiencies of ATIII may occur in a number of conditions, including liver disease, nephrotic syndrome, DIC, sepsis, pre-eclampsia, fatty liver of pregnancy, and following surgery.[115] Plasma ATIII levels are sometimes depressed by oral contraceptive use. The role of ATIII replacement therapy in acquired deficiency states remains controversial.[116]

Other antithrombins. Several other circulating proteins share the property of progressive inactivation of thrombin but are not influenced by heparin.[112] These include α_2-macroglobulin and α_1-proteinase inhibitor. These proteins are collectively called serine protease inhibitors or serpins.

TISSUE FACTOR PATHWAY INHIBITOR—AN INHIBITOR THAT DOES NOT WORK *VIA* THROMBIN. Fibrin can be generated *via* several different coagulation sequences and inhibitors exist to control each of these (see Fig. 10-9). The sequence of reactions initiated by activated Factor XII (XIIa) (the classic intrinsic pathway) can be inhibited by the thrombin–thrombomodulin–protein C interaction which inactivates Factors Va and VIIIa. The two TF-initiated sequences (the classic extrinsic pathway) which generate activated Factor X (Xa) are inhibited by TFPI. Finally, Xa and thrombin (the classic common pathway) can be inhibited by the action of ATIII.

Step 3: Fibrinolysis

The process of fibrinolysis leads to the dissolution of fibrin clots and is necessary to restore normal blood flow. Fibrinolysis can also remodel fibrin clots and "recanalize" vessels which have been occluded by thrombosis.

The Formation of Plasmin

Fibrinolysis involves primarily the production of plasmin, an active fibrinolytic enzyme capable of lysing fibrin clots. Plasmin is formed by the conversion of plasminogen to plasmin by plasminogen activator enzymes (Fig. 10-10). Plasmin does not circulate freely because it would rapidly be degraded by antiplasmins, which are present in the bloodstream in concentrations 10 times that of plasmin. Instead, plasminogen, the precursor to plasmin, circulates; and when it comes into contact with fibrin, it binds to it. In fact, when a fibrin clot is forming, plasminogen is incorporated into the growing fibrin clot together with tissue plasminogen activator (t-PA). Once bound to the fibrin surface, plasminogen is converted to plasmin by t-PA. The bound plasmin is protected from attack by circulating antiplasmins because the binding site by which the plasmin binds to the fibrin is the same site to which the antiplasmins bind.[89]

As soon as plasmin is released into the bloodstream (with its binding site exposed), α_2-antiplasmin neutralizes the plasmin in a matter of 0.1 sec. Thus, like the coagulation cascade, the fibrinolytic system relies upon surface-mediated reactions both for the production of plasmin and for the localization of fibrinolysis to the site of vascular injury.

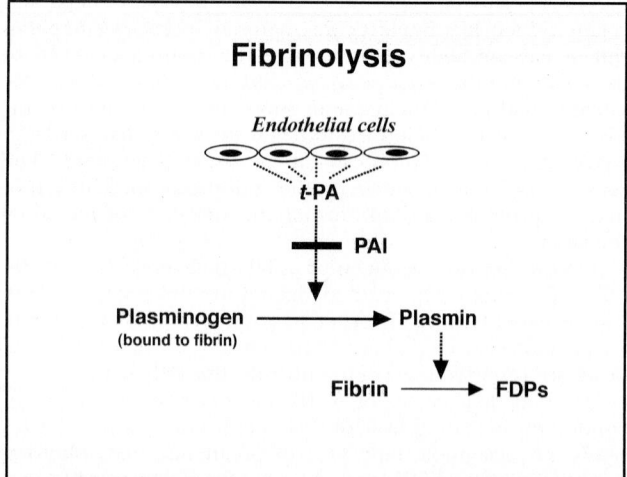

Figure 10-10. Control of fibrinolysis. Normal endothelial cells release tissue plasminogen activator (t-PA) which activates plasminogen, converting it to plasmin. This fibinolytic enzyme then degrades fibrin and fibrinogen to their various degradation products (FDPs). The action of t-PA can be inhibited by plasminogen activator inhibitor (see text).

Tissue Plasminogen Activator

t-PA, which converts plasminogen to plasmin, is produced by vascular endothelial cells. This site of synthesis is important to the maintenance of the "nonthrombogeneic" endothelial surface. If a clot should begin to form on the normal endothelial surface, several mechanisms, including the elaboration of t-PA from endothelial cells, will rapidly inhibit clot formation or lead to its dissolution.

t-PA release from endothelial cells can be stimulated by several factors. If sufficient thrombin has been synthesized, thrombin will form a complex with thrombomodulin and activate protein C. Activated protein C (APC) then stimulates the release of t-PA from endothelial cells. t-PA is also released from the endothelium into the blood in response to certain stimuli, such as venous occlusion, physical activity, stress, or vasoactive drugs (such as epinephrine, vasopressin, and DDAVP).[117] Once released from endothelial cells, t-PA selectively binds to fibrin, much like plasminogen, which also selectively binds to fibrin. Bound to fibrin, the t-PA converts plasminogen to plasmin.

t-PA does not activate circulating plasminogen. This has important implications. Because t-PA activates only plasminogen bound to fibrin, the process of fibrinolysis by plasmin is localized to the fibrin clot. Therefore, under normal circumstances, widespread, uncontrolled fibrinolysis is prevented.

Recently, a new, stable, fast-acting inhibitor of t-PA has been identified. Inhibition of t-PA reduces the amount of plasmin formed and serves to slow the fibrinolytic process (see Fig. 10-10). This t-PA inhibitor is synthesized by endothelial cells and is present in both plasma and platelets. This inhibitor plays a major role in the control and regulation of fibrinolysis. Some patients with thrombotic disorders have been found to have increased levels of this inhibitor.[117,118] A similar inhibitor is found in placental tissue. It may be that the progressive "hypercoagulable state" associated with pregnancy is related to increased levels of this t-PA inhibitor.[117]

Plasminogen Activators

There are plasminogen activators in addition to t-PA. Urokinase is present in the urine but, unlike t-PA, it has no affinity for fibrin and is not present in circulating blood.[89] Physiologic activators of the fibrinolytic system include vigorous exercise, anoxia, and stress, in addition to Factor XIIa and thrombin. Exogenous plasminogen activators include streptokinase, urokinase, and recombinant t-PA. These fibrinolytic agents all differ with respect to their action, clot specificity, systemic fibrinolytic effect, antigenic effect, and efficacy.[89] Proteins derived from streptococci and staphylococci have also been found to be activators of the fibrinolytic system. The therapeutic fibrinolytic agents, streptokinase and urokinase, differ from t-PA in that they will activate circulating plasminogen, leading to more widespread fibrinolysis. Fibrinolytic therapy has been used in the treatment of unstable angina, acute peripheral arterial occlusions, deep vein thrombosis, and pulmonary embolism and in occluded indwelling catheters and arteriovenous shunts.[89]

Fibrin Degradation Products

The primary action of plasmin is to degrade fibrin clots. The degradation products produced are called fibrin degradation products (FDPs) or fibrin split products (FSPs). Their structure varies according to whether plasmin cleaves fibrinogen and whether or not fibrin is crosslinked.[119] Under normal circumstances, FDPs are removed from the blood by the liver, kidney, and reticuloendothelial system. They normally have half-lives of ~9 hours. However, if the FDPs are produced at a rate that exceeds their normal clearance, they will accumulate. This happens when the fibrinolytic system is excessively active. In high concentrations, FDPs impair platelet function, inhibit thrombin, and prevent the crosslinking of fibrin strands.[92] The defective polymerization of the fibrin monomers results in a clot that is more readily degraded by plasmin.[117] In such high concentrations, FDPs lead to bleeding because FDPs are "inhibitors" of both primary hemostasis and coagulation.

Excess Circulating Plasmin

Under normal circumstances, once plasmin has degraded fibrin clot and escapes from the fibrin surface, it is rapidly inactivated by antiplasmins. Deficiency of α_2-antiplasmin leads to a bleeding tendency because, with reduced levels of antiplasmin in the circulation, plasmin can circulate. In addition, in pathologic conditions in which the fibrinolytic system produces large quantities of plasmin (primary fibrinolysis), the antiplasmin capacity may be exceeded and plasmin may circulate. This can also happen when fibrinolysis is stimulated in response to disseminated intravascular coagulation (secondary fibrinolysis). Excess plasmin can lead to a coagulopathy. This is primarily because plasmin degrades fibrin; but because it is a serine protease, it can also degrade other coagulation factors, such as fibrinogen, Factors V, VIII, and XIII, and also vWF.[117] Plasmin can even digest the platelet receptor GPIb. When plasmin circulates in the bloodstream (unneutralized by antiplasmins), it not only dissolves fibrin clots but also inhibits platelet function and disrupts coagulation. Widespread bleeding can occur.

Summary of the Control of Fibrinolysis

Just as the control of coagulation is multifactorial, so is the control of fibrinolysis. The mechanisms already described assure that, under normal conditions, plasmin is generated only at the site of clot formation, that it is protected from degradation while attached to fibrin, and that it is destroyed rapidly once released into the circulation.

The Complexities of the Hemostatic Mechanism

The preceding sections reveal that many mechanisms interact to maintain the liquid state of the blood under normal circumstances and to transform blood into a solid clot when injury occurs. These mechanisms include numerous feedback processes. The complexity is revealed by the occurrence of "double agents" which act, at times, as procoagulants and, at other times, as anticoagulants. Thrombin is at the heart of many of these complexities. Thrombin is primarily a procoagulant. Under normal circumstances, it promotes primary hemostasis by activating platelets, and promotes coagulation by direct activation of Factors V, VIII, and XIII. Thrombin, in the final step of the coagulation cascade, cleaves fibrinogen to fibrin. However, it also has anticoagulant effects. As described earlier, when thrombin is first synthesized, it stimulates production of tissue factor pathway inhibitor (TFPI) which slows coagulation *via* the tissue factor pathway and makes continued coagulation dependent upon the reaction complex formed by Factors VIII and IXa. Thrombin has an additional mechanism by which it can inhibit coagulation. Thrombin can bind to thrombomodulin on the surface of the endothelium, and this complex activates protein C. Activated protein C (APC) then cleaves the cofactors Va and VIIIa and inhibits coagulation. Protein C can also promote fibrinolysis. Activated protein C stimulates the release of t-PA from endothelial cells. t-PA binds to any fibrin that has formed and begins degradation of the clot. This helps to preserve the pristine "nonwettable" surface of the endothelial lining.

The Critical Role of the Vascular Endothelium

In the absence of vascular injury, the intact endothelial lining has many antithrombotic properties that serve to limit both primary hemostasis and coagulation and to induce fibrinolysis should a clot begin to form on normal endothelium.[88] These have been mentioned above and are summarized in Table 10-6.

Table 10-6. ENDOTHELIAL INVOLVEMENT IN THE THREE STAGES OF HEMOSTASIS

Endothelial control of primary hemostasis
    ADPases
    Synthesis and secretion of prostacyclin
Endothelial inhibitors of coagulation
    Thrombomodulin
    Heparan sulfate
Endothelial control of fibrinolysis
    t-PA

The Hemostatic Mechanism: Summary

Under normal circumstances, the hemostatic mechanism is quiescent with many of the potential participants in hemostasis circulating in an inactive form. Only when the endothelial lining is breached, is the hemostatic mechanism set in motion. With collagen and tissue factor exposed, the intertwined processes of platelet mediated primary hemostasis and factor mediated coagulation begin and rapidly the vascular injury is sealed by a platelet mass into which is incorporated fibrinogen, thrombin, plasminogen and t-PA. The completion of the coagulation process converts fibrinogen into fibrin and the platelet plug is transformed into a fibrin clot. Simultaneously, several properties of adjacent intact endothelium (elaboration of ADPases, prostacyclin, thrombomodulin, heparans, and t-PA) serve to prevent extension of the clot beyond the site of injury. Within the clot, plasmin, generated from the trapped plasminogen and t-PA, begins the process of fibrinolysis. Over time, the entire fibrin clot dissolves, new endothelial cells line the vessel and flow is restored.

LABORATORY EVALUATION OF THE HEMOSTATIC MECHANISM

Laboratory Evaluation of Primary Hemostasis

Platelet Count

A platelet count should be the first test ordered in the evaluation of primary hemostasis. The advantages of a platelet count include the fact that it is easy to perform, quick, accurate, and reproducible. However, it reveals only platelet numbers and gives no information regarding their function.

Normal platelet counts range between 150,000 and 440,000/mm³. Counts below 150,000/mm³ are defined as thrombocytopenia. Spontaneous bleeding is likely in patients with platelet counts of <20,000/mm³. With counts of 40,000–70,000/mm³, bleeding that is induced by surgery may be severe.

Bleeding manifestations can vary substantially from patient to patient, similar platelet counts notwithstanding. This occurs because some platelets are more effective than others. When thrombocytopenia results from peripheral destruction of platelets, the bone marrow continues to produce normal, young, large platelets that are hemostatically very effective. A patient with these platelets may have more effective primary hemostasis than a patient whose platelet count is similar but whose platelets were produced by a less active, less healthy bone marrow.

Bleeding Time

The Ivy bleeding time (BT) is the most widely accepted clinical test of platelet function. Both poor platelet function and thrombocytopenia can prolong the bleeding time. A blood pressure cuff is placed around the upper arm and inflated to 40 mm Hg. A cut is made on the volar surface of the forearm and the wound blotted at 30-sec intervals until bleeding stops. In 1977 the Simplate Bleeding Time device, which utilizes a spring-loaded lancet, was introduced to standardize the size and depth of the cut. The normal range for the Ivy BT is 2–9 m. Variations in venous pressure, blotting technique, and patient cooperation result in a lack of precision and reproducibility that make this test somewhat less reliable than other coagulation tests.

The bleeding time is purported to evaluate the time necessary for a platelet plug to form following vascular injury. This requires a normal number of circulating platelets, platelets with normal function (which can adhere and aggregate), and an appropriate platelet interaction with the blood vessel wall. A prolongation of the BT may be due to (1) thrombocytopenia, (2) platelet dysfunction (adhesion, aggregation), and (3) vascular abnormalities such as scurvy or the Ehlers-Danlos syndrome.

BTs are prolonged in patients with many conditions that cause platelet dysfunction, such as use of aspirin or uremia. However, prolonged BTs have been observed with numerous disorders that are not associated with platelet dysfunction, including vitamin K deficiency of the newborn, amyloidosis, congenital heart disease, and the presence of Factor VIII inhibitors.[120] Whether or not the BT test represents a specific measure of *in vivo* platelet function is debated. The test is unpleasant for the patient and leaves a small scar. In spite of the correlation of BT with conditions known to influence platelet function, there are no convincing data to confirm that bleeding time is a reliable predictor of the bleeding that will occur in association with surgical procedures.

Platelet Function

The ability of platelets to aggregate can be assessed quantitatively by observing the response to stimulation with ADP, epinephrine, collagen, or ristocetin. The platelet aggregometer is designed to measure platelet aggregation spectrophotometrically. Clot retraction is another function of platelets that can be assessed grossly. When maintained at 37°C, a clot should begin to retract within 2–4 hours. This test is difficult to quantify and only qualitative results (retraction vs. no retraction) are usually reported.

Laboratory Evaluation of Coagulation

Evolution of the Prothrombin Time (PT) and the Partial Thromboplastin Time (PTT)

When blood is placed in a glass test tube, clot formation occurs in response to contact with the foreign surface. No exogenous reagents are required because all of the factors necessary for contact initiated coagulation are "intrinsic" to blood. The time to formation of a clot *via* this pathway can be prolonged by deficiencies of any factors in the classic intrinsic pathway. However, the observation that, even in hemophiliacs, the addition of thromboplastin (now more commonly called tissue factor) to the test tube could shorten the time to clot formation suggested the presence of an alternative pathway of fibrin formation. That pathway required the addition of something "extrinsic to blood" and did not require the presence of Factors VIII or IX. In 1936, when Quick introduced the prothrombin time (PT) to clinical medicine, sufficient "thromboplastin" was used to yield a clotting time of ~12 sec. Under these circumstances, even patients lacking Factors VIII or IX showed normal clotting times.[121] However, when "dilute" thromboplastin (or a "partial" thromboplastin) was used in lieu of the "12-second reagent," hemophiliacs showed much longer clotting times than did healthy controls. The two different pathways could be tested individually simply by varying the amount and type of thromboplastin added to blood. If the "complete thromboplastin" were added, coagulation could proceed *via* reactions that were independent of Factors VIIIa and IXa. With a lesser thromboplastin

stimulus, coagulation would proceed *via* a sequence of reactions that required the presence of Factors VIIIa and IXa.

Basic Elements of the PT and PTT

The two common tests of coagulation, the prothrombin time (PT) and the partial thromboplastin time (PTT), differ primarily by the type of thromboplastin that is used—a standardized tissue thromboplastin (the "complete thromboplastin") or a phospholipid component that serves as a platelet substitute ("partial thromboplastin"), respectively. Calcium must also be added because of the chelating agent in the blood specimen container. The time to fibrin strand formation is then measured.

The Prothrombin Time

The PT evaluates the coagulation sequence initiated by tissue factor (TF) and leading to the formation of fibrin without the participation of Factors VIII or IX. The PT measures the time to fibrin strand formation *via* a short sequence of reactions involving only TF, Factors VII, X, V, II (prothrombin), and I (fibrinogen). Tissue factor forms a complex with VIIa and together this complex activates Factor X. From that point, coagulation proceeds *via* the common pathway of coagulation. The test evaluates neither the coagulation process initiated by the classic intrinsic pathway nor the sequence of reactions initiated by tissue factor that generate Xa *via* the reaction complex formed by factors IXa and VIIIa (see Fig. 10-8).

The normal PT is 10–12 seconds. The PT will be prolonged if deficiencies, abnormalities, or inhibitors of Factors VII, X, V, II, or I are present. The PT test has limitations. First, it is not very sensitive to deficiencies of any of these factors. In fact, the coagulant activity of these factors must drop to 30% of normal before the PT is prolonged. The PT is most sensitive to a decrease in Factor VII and least sensitive to changes in prothrombin (Factor II). When prothrombin levels are only 10% of normal, the increase in the PT may be just 2 sec. Also, PT will not be prolonged until the fibrinogen level is below $100 \text{ mg} \cdot \text{dl}^{-1}$. A prolonged PT does not define the exact hemostatic defect. However, when looking at coagulation profiles, if the aPTT ("activated" partial thromboplastin time; see below) is normal, then a prolonged PT is most likely to represent a deficiency or abnormality of Factor VII. Because it has the shortest half-life of the clotting factors synthesized in the liver, Factor VII is the clotting factor that first becomes deficient with liver disease, vitamin K deficiency, or coumadin therapy. Prolongation of the PT may also be due to deficiencies of multiple factors. However, when multiple factor deficiencies coexist, the aPTT will usually be prolonged as well.

The International Normalized Ratio. Another difficulty with the PT test is that many different thromboplastin reagents are used. This results in wide variation in normal values, rendering comparison of PT results between laboratories difficult. The International Normalized Ratio (INR) was introduced to circumvent this difficulty.[122] Each thromboplastin is compared with an internationally accepted standard thromboplastin and assigned an International Sensitivity Index (ISI). If the test thromboplastin is equivalent to the international standard, it will have an ISI index of 1. Once the ISI number has been determined, PT test times obtained with that reagent are normalized and reported as an INR.[123]

The Partial Thromboplastin Time

The PTT assesses the function of the intrinsic and final common pathways. It entails the addition of a "partial thromboplastin" (usually a chloroform extract of rabbit brain tissue phospholipid) and calcium to citrated plasma. The PTT reflects the time to fibrin strand formation *via* the classic intrinsic pathway of coagulation.

The PTT will reveal deficiencies, abnormalities, or inhibitors to one or more coagulation factors, including high–molecular-weight kininogen (HMWK), prekallikrein, and Factors XII, XI, IX, VIII, X, V, II, and I. The normal values for PTT vary widely. Times between 40 and 100 sec are usual, and the result is not considered abnormal until PTT is >120 sec.

The PTT can be made more reproducible and the range of normal values narrower by the addition of contact activator in addition to the partial thromboplastin. This test, called an "activated" partial thromboplastin time (aPTT), is the test that is most commonly used.[124] Surface activation in the laboratory parallels the contact activation phase involving Factors XII and XI, prekallikrein, and HMWK that is thought to initiate the intrinsic pathway *in vivo*. Diatomaceous earth, kaolin, celite, and ellagic acid are used as surface activators. The aPTT is much faster than the PTT because it eliminates the lengthy "natural" contact activation phase. Normal aPTT values are between 25 and 35 sec.[125] The aPTT is prolonged when there is a deficiency, abnormality, or inhibitor of Factors XII, XI, IX, VIII, X, V, II, and I (*i.e.*, all factors except VII and XIII). The aPTT is most sensitive to deficiencies of Factors VIII and IX, but, as is the case with the PT, levels of these factors must be reduced to ~30% of normal values before the test is prolonged. As with the PT, the level of fibrinogen must also be reduced to 100 mg · dl^{-1} before the aPTT is prolonged. aPTT results (like those of the PT) vary from laboratory to laboratory because of nonstandardization of the phospholipids and activators.

The Activated Clotting Time

The activated clotting time (ACT) is similar to the aPTT in that it tests the ability of blood to clot in a test tube and is dependent on factors that are all "intrinsic" to blood (the classic intrinsic pathway of coagulation). Fresh whole blood is added to a test tube that contains a particulate surface activator of Factors XII and XI. The time to clot formation is measured. Partial thromboplastin or a platelet phospholipid substitute is not added. Coagulation is therefore dependent upon the presence of adequate amounts of platelet phospholipid in the blood sample. The automated ACT is widely used to monitor heparin therapy in the operating room. Normal values are in the range of 90–120 sec.[124] The ACT is far less sensitive than the aPTT to factor deficiencies in the classic intrinsic coagulation pathway. In fact, the ACT may not be prolonged until the coagulant activity of some of the factors is reduced to 1% of normal.

The Thrombin Time

Thrombin time (TT), which is also called the "thrombin clotting time" (TCT), is a measure of the ability of thrombin to convert fibrinogen to fibrin. This test, which is performed by adding exogenous thrombin to citrated plasma, bypasses all the preceding reactions. The thrombin time may be prolonged due to conditions which affect the substrate, fibrinogen, or the action of the enzyme thrombin. The TT is prolonged when the amount of fibrinogen is inadequate (<100 mg · dl^{-1}) or when the fibrinogen molecules that are present are abnormal (dysfibrinogenemia), as in advanced liver disease. Thrombin's enzymatic function can be inhibited by inhibitors such as heparin (complexed to ATIII) or FDPs, or by inhibitors seen in patients with plasma cell myeloma and other immunoproliferative conditions.[126] The normal TT is <30 sec.

The Reptilase Time. When the thrombin time is prolonged, the reptilase time (RT) can be used to differentiate between the effects of heparin and FDPs. Reptilase, which is derived from a snake venom, converts fibrinogen to fibrin. The action of reptilase is unaffected by heparin but is inhibited by FDPs. A prolonged TT with a normal RT suggests the presence of heparin. Prolongation of both TT and RT will occur in the presence of FDPs, or when fibrinogen level is low. The normal RT is 14–21 sec.

Fibrinogen Level

Fibrinogen concentration is determined by adding large quantities of Factor IIa (thrombin) to citrated plasma and comparing the time to fibrin formation in the patient's plasma with plasma specimens of known fibrinogen levels. Normal values are between 160 and 350 mg%. Below 100 mg%, fibrinogen may be inadequate to produce a clot. Fibrinogen is rapidly depleted during DIC. Less well appreciated is the marked increase in fibrinogen that occurs following surgery and trauma. Levels in excess of 700 mg% may occur. Because of this increase, half of the fibrinogen can be consumed during a hypercoagulable state such as DIC, and the fibrinogen level may still appear to be "normal."

Laboratory Evaluation of Fibrinolysis

Fibrin Degradation Products and D-Dimer

The test to detect fibrin degradation products (FDPs) employs latex particles coated with antibodies that bind the breakdown products of fibrin (crosslinked or uncrosslinked), the breakdown products of fibrinogen, and fibrinogen itself. The particles are added to the patient's plasma and serial dilutions are made until no visible clumping is seen. The D-dimer assay is specific for a breakdown product of crosslinked fibrin. FDPs will be increased in any state of accelerated fibrinolysis, including advanced liver disease, fibrinolysis associated with cardiopulmonary bypass, administration of exogenous thrombolytics (*e.g.* streptokinase), and DIC. D-Dimer is specific to conditions in which extensive lysis of the crosslinked fibrin of mature thrombus is occurring, that is, DIC.

The Thromboelastogram

Thromboelastography provides a measure of the mechanical properties of evolving clot as a function of time. A principal advantage of this test is that the processes it measures require the integrated action of all the elements of the hemostatic process: platelet aggregation, coagulation, and fibrinolysis. The thromboelastogram (TEG) is obtained by placing a specimen of blood in a rotating cuvette into which a "piston" is lowered. As clot formation begins, the piston rotates as function of the adherence of the evolving fibrin clot to the piston. The piston is connected to a recorder and the rotation of the piston results in a to-and-fro excursion of the stylus, the amplitude of which is proportional to the speed of piston rotation. Figure 10-11 depicts a normal TEG.

Several parameters are derived from the TEG. The most commonly used ones are listed below, together with their interpretation:[127]

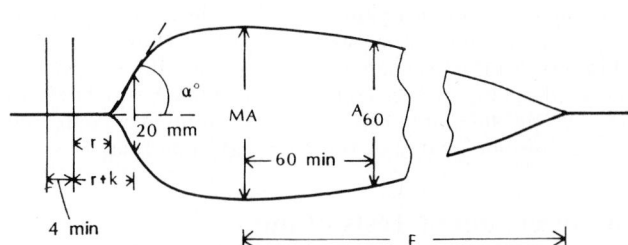

Figure 10-11. The normal thromboelastogram and the variables commonly derived from it. See text for explanation. (Reprinted with permission from Kang Y, Lewis JH, Navalgund A *et al*: ε-Aminocaproic acid for treatment of fibrinolysis during liver transplantation. Anesthesiology 66:766, 1987.)

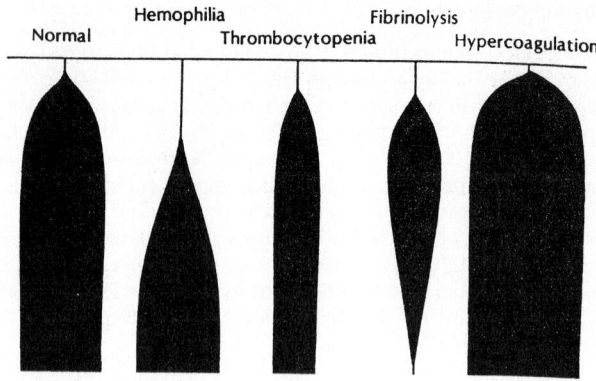

Figure 10-12. Thromboelastogram patterns seen in normal subjects and in subjects with four abnormalities of hemostasis. (Reprinted with permission from Kang YG: Monitoring and treatment of coagulation. In Winter PM, Kang YG (eds): Hepatic Transplantation: Anesthetic and Perioperative Management, p 151. New York, Praeger, 1986.)

r, the reaction time, is the interval until initial clot formation. It requires thrombin formation, and prolongation is usually indicative of an intrinsic pathway factor deficiency.

k, the clot formation time, is the interval required after *r* for the TEG to achieve a width of 20 mm. Prolongation occurs with deficiencies of thrombin formation or generation of fibrin from fibrinogen.

$\alpha°$, the alpha angle is, like *k,* a measure of the speed of clot formation. A decrease of $\alpha°$ is similar in significance to a prolongation of *k.*

MA, the maximum amplitude, is a measure of the strength of the fully formed clot. It reflects primarily platelet number and function, although it also requires proper fibrin formation to achieve normal values. MA typically occurs between 30 and 60 m.

(MA + *x*)/MA, the amplitude at a specific time interval (*x*) after MA divided by MA, is a ratio used as a measure of the rate of fibrinolysis. The (MA + 60)/MA ratio has been used most widely.[128] A ratio of <0.85 is evidence of abnormal fibrinolysis.[129] In clinical practice, particularly in liver transplantation, a nonquantitative appreciation of the typical teardrop shape (Fig. 10-12) is used more often to support a diagnosis of increased fibrinolysis than are specific numerical values.

F, the interval from MA to return to a zero amplitude, is a measure of the rate of fibrinolysis. In normal subjects *F* is sufficiently long that the test is usually terminated before this time elapses.

The TEG has been employed in cardiac surgery, major trauma, and hepatic transplantation. It is in the latter that it is used most frequently. Commonly, in that context, an increased *r* prompts the administration of FFP, a decreased MA leads to platelet administration, and the teardrop configuration of fibrinolyis leads to the administration of antifibrinolytics. The use of the TEG in liver transplantation has been shown to decrease the amount of RBCs and FFP transfused as compared with transfusion guided by routine coagulation tests.[130]

Interpretation of Tests of the Hemostatic Mechanism

The interpretation of coagulation tests requires a knowledge of the common bleeding disorders. An effective approach to the interpretation of coagulation tests is to try to appreciate in advance the constellation of test results (the coagulation "profile") that is likely to occur with each of the common

bleeding disorders (Table 10-7).[131] The most commonly ordered coagulation tests are a platelet count, aPTT, and PT and occasionally a bleeding time. When a greater disruption of the hemostatic mechanism is suspected, further tests, including fibrinogen level, TT, and assays for fibrin degradation products and the D-dimer, may be ordered.

Common Coagulation Profiles

Platelet Count Decreased (normal aPTT and PT)

Thrombocytopenia may be caused by inadequate platelet production, sequestration in the spleen, excess tissue consumption, dilution by massive transfusions, or by platelet destruction (see Bleeding Disorders, Thrombocytopenia).

Prolongation of Bleeding Time (normal platelet count, aPTT, PT)

Although the BT may be useful for evaluating primary hemostasis, it is rarely used in the intraoperative or postoperative period. As noted earlier, the BT has not been shown to be a reliable predictor of perioperative blood loss.

When the BT is prolonged and the platelet count is normal, von Willebrand's disease (vWD) should be considered. Note that when the BT is prolonged, a normal aPTT does not exclude a diagnosis of vWD. This is because although the Factor VIII:C levels may be decreased with vWD (Type 1), only 25–30% of VIII:C coagulant activity is necessary to produce a normal aPTT. Therefore, it is not uncommon for Type 1 patients with vWD to have a normal aPTT.

There are many acquired conditions that cause platelet dysfunction which can prolong the BT in the presence of a normal platelet count. These include antiplatelet drug ingestion (NSAIDS, ASA, ticlopidine, clopidogrel, etc.), uremia, liver dysfunction, the presence of FDPs (DIC or fibrinolytic therapy), and cardiopulmonary bypass. Liver disease, the presence of FDPs, and cardiopulmonary bypass, however, alter other coagulation tests as well and produce a different coagulation testing profile. Drug ingestion and uremia are the common causes of an isolated prolonged BT. The diagnosis of platelet dysfunction however, is often a diagnosis of exclusion.

Prolonged aPTT (normal platelet count and PT)

The bleeding disorders that produce this combination of test results are limited to those that affect the classic intrinsic pathway of coagulation. The clotting factors that are unique to the intrinsic pathway include prekallikrein, HMWK, and Factors XII, XI, IX, and VIII; and in the common pathway, Factors X, V, II, and I. When the coagulant activity of any of these factors falls to 30% of normal or less, the aPTT may be prolonged.

1. *Deficiency of Factor XII, HMWK, or prekallikrein:* Deficiencies of these factors are not usually associated with a significant hemostatic defect.
2. *Hemophilia A or B:* Hemophilia A (VIIIC) or B (IX) is associated with significant coagulopathies.
3. *von Willebrand's disease:* A deficiency of the von Willebrand factor, which serves as a carrier protein for the coagulant portion of Factor VIII, may prolong the aPTT. However, vWD will also affect platelet function and the patient may demonstrate problems with both primary hemostasis and coagulation.
4. *Heparin therapy:* Heparin therapy is monitored with the aPTT. Initially, only the aPTT is prolonged. At higher doses, both the aPTT and PT are prolonged.
5. *Presence of acquired Factor VIII inhibitors, circulating anticoagulants.*
6. *The lupus anticoagulant:* The lupus "anticoagulant" is an antiphospholipid antibody. It is a common cause of a prolonged aPTT. That prolongation is the result of the bind-

Table 10-7. INTERPRETATION OF COAGULATION TESTS

Platelet Count	Bleeding Time	aPTT	PT	TT	Fibrinogen	FDPs	Possible Cause	Example
↓	N or ↑	N	N	N	N	N	↓ Production, Sequestration ↑ Consumption Immune destruction	Radiation, chemotherapy Splenomagaly Extensive tissue damage HIT
N	↑	N	N	N	N	N	Platelet dysfunction	Drugs: ASA, NSAIDs, clopidogrel Uremia Mild von Willebrand's disease
N	↑	↑	N	N	N	N	Severe vWF deficiency	von Willebrand's disease
N	N	↑	N	N	N	N	Factor deficiency Factor inhibition Antiphospholid antibody	Hemophilia A or B Low-dose heparin Poor collection technique Lupus anticoagulant
N	N	N	↑	N	N	N	Factor VII deficiency	Early liver disease Early vitamin K deficiency Early coumadin therapy
N	N	↑	↑	↑	N	N	Multiple factor deficiencies	Late vitamin K deficiency Late coumadin therapy Heparin therapy*
↓	↑	↑	↑	↑	↓	N	Dilution of factors and platelets	Massive transfusion
↓	↑	↑	↑	↑	↓	↑	Hypercoagulable state ± ↓ production of factors	DIC† Advanced liver disease

↑ = increased; ↓ = decreased; N = normal; aPTT = "activated" partial thrombolastin time; PT = prothrombin time; TT = thrombin time; FDPs = fibrin degradation products; HIT = heparin-induced thrombocytopenia; vWF = von Willebrand factor; NSAIDs = nonsteroidal anti-inflammatory drugs; DIC = disseminated intravascular coagulation.
* Bleeding time may also be prolonged in association with a marked aPTT increase.
† DIC may be distinguished by the presence of D-dimers.

ing of the phospholipid used to initiate coagulation *in vitro*. The patients do not have a bleeding diathesis. In fact, they have a prothrombotic tendency that is unexplained. That tendency may occur because of activation of platelets by antibody attack directed at their surface phospholipids. This laboratory abnormality is not corrected when the patient's plasma is mixed with normal plasma because of the presence of inhibitors.

7. *Poor blood collection technique:* Poor blood collection technique can prolong just the aPTT. This is because Factors V and VIII, the labile factors, may be consumed if the blood is partially clotted prior to delivery to the laboratory.[132] The aPTT is very sensitive to Factor VIII deficiencies.

Summary. When only the PTT is prolonged, it is less likely to be due to a bleeding disorder that involves multiple factor deficiencies (such as liver disease, vitamin K deficiency, the administration of coumadin, or the coagulopathy associated with massive transfusion or DIC). Heparin therapy or congenital disorders of hemostasis are more probable.

Prolonged PT Only (normal platelet count and aPTT)

1. *Factor VII deficiency:* Deficiencies of Factor VII will prolong the extrinsic pathway.
2. *Vitamin K deficiency or coumadin administration:* Because Factor VII has the shortest half-life of the vitamin K–dependent factors, depletion of the vitamin K–dependent factors (either due to vitamin K deficiency or coumadin administration) will first prolong the PT and later prolong the aPTT as well.
3. *Liver disease:* Similarly, the development of liver disease will lead to deficiencies of Factor VII first and initially prolong only the PT. With further deterioration of liver function, both the PT and the aPTT will be prolonged. Liver disease can also lead to thrombocytopenia and platelet dysfunction.

4. *Acquired coagulation factor inhibitors:* These rare conditions can occur in patients with lymphoma or collagen vascular disease.
5. *Amyloidosis:* Patients with amyloidosis will occasionally have decreased levels of factor X with prolongation of PT.

Prolonged aPTT and PT (normal platelet count)

This coagulation profile suggests that multiple factor deficiencies exist or that there is a deficiency of one of the factors in the common pathway, such as fibrinogen. Combined prolongation of the aPTT and PT without thrombocytopenia occurs most commonly with vitamin K deficiency, coumadin therapy, or heparin therapy. With heparin therapy, the aPTT will be prolonged first, but with higher doses, both PT and aPTT will be prolonged. It is important that platelet counts be followed in patients receiving heparin because of the possibility of a heparin-induced thrombocytopenia. Although liver disease can produce multiple factor deficiencies, the platelet count is usually decreased with increasing severity of the disease, and often FDPs will also be elevated (see next page).

Prolonged PT, aPTT, and TT (normal platelet count)

The presence of "thrombin inhibitors" such as heparin or FDPs can prolong the PT, aPTT and TT simultaneously. These tests can also be prolonged by hypofibrinogenemia, *i.e.*, a fibrinogen level less than 100 mg · dl^{-1}.

Prolongation of the TT makes the diagnosis of simple vitamin K deficiency or coumadin therapy unlikely. The thrombin time is very sensitive to even minute levels of heparin and the thrombin time is also prolonged in the presence of FDPs. FDPs may be elevated with fibrinolytic therapy, DIC, or liver disease. However, DIC and liver disease usually result in a coagulation profile that includes thrombocytopenia as well. A normal platelet count makes heparin or fibrinolytic therapy more likely.

Prolonged aPTT, PT, TT; Decreased Platelet Count

The patient with a low platelet count and prolongation of all coagulation tests has a global disruption of the hemostatic mechanism. This clinical picture can be produced by DIC, the dilutional effects of massive transfusion, and by heparin. To differentiate DIC from the dilutional effects of massive transfusion and the effects of excess heparin, a fibrinogen level and an assay for FDPs and D-dimer is helpful. Both DIC and the dilutional effects of massive transfusion will reduce fibrinogen levels. DIC, however, results in the production of the D-dimer.

Fibrinogen Levels Decreased

Fibrinogen levels are decreased most commonly with hypercoagulable states such as DIC and with the coagulopathy produced by massive transfusion. Fibrinogen levels may be decreased with liver disease as well due to the decreased synthesis of this factor. Conversely, fibrinogen levels are increased with stress and pregnancy.

Fibrinogen Levels Decreased in the Presence of Circulating FDPs

An assay for FDPs is helpful in the differential diagnosis of the patient who has a low platelet count and prolonged aPTT, PT, and TT. The presence of FDPs may differentiate the coagulopathy due to massive transfusion from that produced by DIC or severe liver disease. Because FDPs are the byproduct of fibrinolysis, often their presence is used as "circumstantial evidence" that DIC is ongoing. However, elevated levels of FDPs are also seen with severe liver disease.[132] Positive tests for fibrin monomers (D-dimer) are more specific for DIC.

Summary

The interpretation of coagulation tests is best done by identifying which elements of the hemostatic mechanism have been disrupted and then attempting, in the context of the patient's medical condition, to determine the probable cause of that coagulation profile (see Table 10-7). Platelet number and platelet function disorders can be evaluated with a platelet count and bleeding time, respectively. Defects of coagulation are evaluated with the PT, aPTT, TT, and fibrinogen level. The presence of DIC is evaluated by tests for fibrin degradation products and the D-dimer. Systemic fibrinolysis is reflected by the presence of FDPs, a shortened euglobulin clot lysis time, or an abnormal TEG. Bleeding disorders which are first diagnosed in the hospitalized patient are usually acquired and often involve multiple factor deficiencies. The most common bleeding disorders include vitamin K deficiency, liver disease, DIC, systemic fibrinolysis, dilutional coagulopathy, and heparin excess. Therefore, understanding the coagulation profile produced by each of these bleeding disorders will be valuable. The interpretation of coagulation tests is made difficult by the fact that patients who develop a bleeding diathesis in the perioperative period may have more than one bleeding disorder (*e.g.*, DIC and coagulopathy due to massive transfusion) and may also have a surgical cause for bleeding.

DISORDERS OF HEMOSTASIS: DIAGNOSIS AND TREATMENT

The hemostatic mechanism involves an intricate balance that serves to limit blood loss in the event of vascular injury while maintaining the liquid character of blood at other times. Under normal circumstances, an equilibrium between clotting and bleeding is maintained with the help of multiple activators, inhibitors, cofactors, and feedback loops, both positive and negative. Under pathologic circumstances, that equilibrium may be lost, leading to either hemorrhagic or thrombotic complications. Accordingly, disorders of hemostasis can be broadly classified into those that lead to abnormal bleeding and those

that lead to abnormal clotting. The disorders may be further categorized according to whether they involve platelets, clotting factors, and/or the presence or absence of inhibitors (such as FDPs). Finally, disorders may be hereditary or acquired. These organizational frameworks will be helpful in reaching a diagnosis on the basis of the results of coagulation tests. The treatment that follows from diagnosis may require administration of hemostatic agents (platelets and/or clotting factors) or the use of pharmacologic agents. The latter may be chosen for effects on platelets (desmopressin, antiplatelet drugs), on clotting factors (vitamin K, coumadin, heparin) or on naturally occurring inhibitors (antifibrinolytic agents, protamine, fibrinolytics).

The preoperative history is invaluable in the identification of disorders of hemostasis. History will also commonly reveal whether an abnormality is one of primary hemostasis, one of coagulation, or a combined disorder. Abnormalities of primary hemostasis, usually caused by reduced platelet number or function, will be revealed by evidence of "superficial" (skin and mucosal) bleeding, including easy bruising, petechiae, prolonged bleeding from minor skin lacerations, recurrent epistaxis, and menorrhagia. Coagulation abnormalities are associated with "deep" bleeding events, including hemarthroses or hematomas after blunt trauma. Table 10-8 lists the common entities associated with these two groups of abnormalities. In the absence of a disease state or pharmacologic agent known to be associated with a bleeding disorder (discussed below), a suspicious history should lead to consideration of hereditary abnormalities of hemostasis.

Hereditary Disorders of Hemostasis

von Willebrand's Disease

von Willebrand's disease (vWD) is the most common hereditary bleeding disorder. The incidence in the general population is approximately 1%.[133] The disorder was first identified by Eric von Willebrand in 1926 among the inhabitants of the Aland Islands near the coast of Finland.[134] von Willebrand's disease is the result of abnormal synthesis of a protein, the von Willebrand factor (vWF), which is important for both primary hemostasis and coagulation. That protein is a large polymeric molecule with numerous distinct binding domains responsible for its several hemostatic functions. Those domains include sites that are specific for collagen (for adherence to the subendothelium), the platelet GPIb receptor (for platelet adhesion to collagen), the platelet GPIIb/IIIa receptor (for platelet aggregation), and Factor VIII:C (for its carrier protein function). The many different mutations of vWF lead to several quantitative and functional alterations and hence to various clinical presentations of the disease. Because of the role that vWF plays in

---

Table 10-8. ETIOLOGY OF HEMOSTATIC ABNORMALITIES IN LIVER DISEASE

Thrombocytopenia
- decreased production
- hypersplenism
- increased consumption (DIC)

Impaired platelet function
- decreased FDP clearance

Decreased factor synthesis
- decreased hepatocyte function
- vitamin K deficiency (diet, malabsorption)

Increased factor consumption
- decreased clearance of activated factors
- increased synthesis of inhibitors (protein C, protein S)

Increased fibrinolysis
- decreased synthesis of α2-antiplasmin
- decreased clearance of t-PA

primary hemostasis, the disease is often discussed in the context of platelet disorders. Without vWF, platelet function is impaired and tests of platelet function, most notably the bleeding time, are often abnormal. However, treatment of this disease does not usually involve platelet transfusion, but rather restoration of the vWF with FFP, cryoprecipitate, or the administration of desmopressin.

SYNTHESIS OF vWF.   The vWF is synthesized by endothelial cells, megakaryocytes, and platelets. Platelet vWF is stored in the platelet alpha granules. There is evidence that estrogens, corticosteroids, and thyroid hormones may influence the rate of vWF synthesis.[135,136] While the mechanisms that regulate plasma vWF are not well understood, it is known that ABO blood group status relates to vWF plasma levels. People with blood group O have 20–30% less vWF antigen than those with other blood types.[137]

ENDOTHELIAL SECRETION OF vWF.   Release of vWF from endothelial cells at sites of vascular injury can be induced by several agonists including thrombin, histamine, oxidative stress, and other mediators of thrombosis and/or inflammation.[134] These agonists, however, are thought not to influence plasma levels of vWF. Plasma levels of vWF increase in response to epinephrine and other catecholamines, vasopressin, and DDAVP (1-deamino-8-D-arginine vasopressin or desmopressin) as well as pregnancy, physical activity, and other stresses.[138] The stress-related increases in the plasma vWF level may be mediated by epinephrine.

THE ROLE OF vWF IN PRIMARY HEMOSTASIS.   vWF is essential for platelet plug formation. It mediates platelet adhesion to the subendothelial surface of blood vessels and promotes platelet-to-platelet aggregation.[139] vWF, probably principally vWF synthesized by the endothelium, is "translocated" to the subendothelium, in part in response to epinephrine and DDAVP. After binding to the subendothelium, the vWF undergoes a conformational change that allows platelets to adhere via their glycoprotein GPIb receptors. This binding can occur only after the conformational change, and in solution, platelets will not spontaneously bind to vWF. The antibiotic ristocetin can induce the platelet GPIb–vWF interaction and, accordingly, is the basis for one laboratory test of platelet function.

vWF also participates in platelet aggregation. Aggregation occurs by binding of vWF molecules to the GPIIb/IIIa receptors on the surface of several platelets. The vWF has multiple well-spaced binding sites for the platelet receptors as well as for binding to the subendothelial matrix. Fibrinogen and fibrin can also crosslink platelets by binding to the same GPIIb/IIIa sites.

CARRIER PROTEIN FOR FACTOR VIII:C.   The vWF also acts as a carrier protein for the coagulant activity of Factor VIII, referred to as VIII:C, with which it circulates in a complexed form that prolongs VIII:C's circulation time.

vWD HAS MANY PHENOTYPES.   Numerous possible mutations result in several clinical presentations. Three broad categories of the disease exist. Some patients have merely a quantitative deficiency of the factor. Others produce a vWF which is qualitatively abnormal. A third category of patients have a total vWF deficiency. The various phenotypes of the disease were classified in 1994 by a subcommittee of the International Society for Thrombosis and Hemostasis.[140]

In the most common variant of vWD (70–80% of vWD), the plasma levels of vWF are decreased, but there is no demonstrable structural or functional alteration of the protein. Patients with this form of vWD (Type 1) present with a pattern of bleeding that is characteristic of abnormalities of primary hemostasis.

Twenty to thirty percent of patients with vWD have Type 2 disease. These patients have normal or low vWF antigen levels but the vWF is structurally and functionally abnormal. There are many Type 2 subtypes. Some mutations affect the platelet interactions of vWF while others affect the Factor VIII interaction. In subtype 2B, the vWF is constitutively active and has a

high affinity for the platelet GPIb receptor without the necessity for a conformational change. The bleeding diathesis is probably the result of formation and clearance of vWF–platelet complexes and the resultant thrombocytopenia. DDAVP, which is therapeutic for other vWD variants, may aggravate this form of the disease by causing severe thrombocytopenia. In the subtype 2N (Normandy) vWD, the vWF has a markedly reduced affinity for Factor VIII. These patients demonstrate normal platelet function, but bleed because of decreased Factor VIII coagulant activity. These patients are readily misdiagnosed as having mild hemophilia A.

Type 3 vWD is characterized by a prolonged bleeding time and low to undetectable levels of vWF, resulting in a severe abnormality of both primary hemostasis and coagulation. The prevalence of this variant is very low (~1 per million).[133]

History reveals easy bruising, mucosal bleeding (epistaxis), and oozing or bleeding following prior surgery. The first line of treatment (detailed below) is DDAVP.

Diagnosis and Treatment.   History will commonly reveal abnormal bleeding from mucosal surfaces. Sixty percent of the patients will report epistaxis, 50% report menorrhagia, and 35% acknowledge gingival bleeding, easy bruising, and hematomas.[134] von Willebrand's disease should be considered in patients who give a history of unexplained postoperative bleeding, particularly following tonsillectomy or dental extraction. Although this is a hereditary disease, a clear family history is not always evident because disease severity varies substantially.

Multiple specialized laboratory tests may be required to confirm the diagnosis of vWD. What is important for the anesthesiologist to appreciate is that the results of the most commonly ordered coagulation tests—the platelet count, the aPTT, and the PT—may be normal in the patient with vWD. While the half-life of VIII:C is diminished in vWD, there is generally sufficient VIII:C to yield a normal aPTT in basal conditions. If, in fact, the aPTT is very prolonged, it is likely that the patient has a severe form of vWD. Quantitative assays of vWF are available, but interpretation can be difficult because normal values are not well established and many variables influence levels. A single normal or abnormal value for vWF cannot be viewed as definitive. The response to the infusion of plasma can be used to distinguish vWD from hemophilia A. With hemophilia A, Factor VIII level is maximal immediately after plasma or cryoprecipitate infusion. Patients with vWD demonstrate the same immediate rise in factor VIII levels, but the increase is sustained for 48 hours because the patient with vWD is able to produce factor VIII:C.[141]

DDAVP (1-deamino-8-D-arginine vasopressin), which promotes release of vWF, is effective first-line therapy for the large majority of patients with vWD, including those with Type 1 and Type 2A disease. However the recognition of subtype 2B (see above) is important because DDAVP will cause thrombocytopenia in these patients.[142] DDAVP, given intravenously in a dose of 0.3 $\mu g \cdot kg^{-1}$, increases Factor VIII:C and vWF two- to fivefold in most patients. Its effect is maximal after 30 minutes and elevated levels persist for 6–8 hours[134] (see Pharmacologic Therapy: Desmopressin below). The antifibrinolytic agents ε-aminocaproic acid and tranexamic acid are sometimes used in combination with DDAVP to manage these patients during the perioperative period. They may be given intravenously, or orally. They have also been administered topically, as mouthwashes, in patients with vWD undergoing dental extractions. Oral contraceptives (estrogens) have been used to treat patients with vWD and menorrhagia or who are undergoing elective surgery. The mechanism of action of the estrogens is not well understood, although a connection with vWF synthesis is suspected.

Cryoprecipitate contains vWF and will correct the hemostatic defect. However, its use entails exposure to multiple donors, with the associated infectious risk. Therefore, cryoprecipitate is no longer the standard form of replacement therapy. Instead virus-inactivated Factor VIII concentrates, which have significant levels of both Factor VIII and the vWF, are preferred in emergency situations if DDAVP therapy is inadequate. In situations that are less emergent, virally attenuated vWF concentrates can be used to supply vWF.[143] Over time, the infusion of vWF will increase Factor VIII levels. In those patients who do not respond to Factor VIII concentrates, platelets are sometimes administered in an attempt to correct the platelet defect caused by the deficient or abnormal vWF. Antiplatelet drugs should be avoided in patients with vWD.

The Hemophilias

The hemophilias are among the oldest disorders for which genetic counseling has been offered. Hemophilia A results from mutations that lead to either deficient or functionally defective Factor VIII:C. Hemophilia B (Christmas disease) and hemophilia C are caused by deficiency or abnormality of Factors IX and XI, respectively. The relative frequencies of the three hemophilias are: Factor VIII:C, 85%; Factor IX, 14%; and Factor XI, 1%. Both hemophilia A and B are sex-linked recessive disorders, which therefore occur almost exclusively in males. Hemophilia C is an autosomal recessive disorder that occurs almost exclusively in Ashkenazi Jews.[144] About 50% of operations in hemophiliacs are orthopedic procedures required for treatment of the arthritic consequences of hemarthroses.

Hemophilia A. Factor VIII is a very large macromolecule with two components, the coagulant Factor VIII (VIII:C) and the von Willebrand factor. The VIII:C molecule circulates bound to and protected by vWF. In hemophilia A, patients have normal levels of vWF, but exhibit reduced or defective Factor VIII:C. More than 600 abnormal Factor VIII genes have been identified.[145] Hemophilia A occurs in approximately 1 in 5000 males.[133]

Hemophiliacs experience deep tissue bleeding, hemarthroses, and hematuria most commonly. Clinically, hemophilia A can be classified as mild, moderate, and severe. Patients with mild disease have factor levels of 5–30% of normal and usually bleed abnormally only following trauma. Patients with moderate disease have factor levels of 1–5% and occasionally bleed spontaneously as well as following trauma. The great majority of hemophiliacs have the severe form of the disease. Their Factor VIII:C levels are less than 1% of normal and they frequently experience spontaneous bleeding episodes. The severity of clinical symptoms usually correlates with the level of clotting factor activity. Like the patient with von Willebrand's disease, hemophiliacs should avoid aspirin and other platelet-inhibiting agents.

DIAGNOSIS AND TREATMENT. Patients with hemophilia A will commonly report a history that reveals the X-linked recessive pattern of disease inheritance. Diagnosis of hemophilia A is made on the basis of a prolonged aPTT and specific factor assays demonstrating a deficiency of Factor VIII coagulant activity with normal levels of vWF, Factor IX, and Factor XI. The patient will have a normal prothrombin time and a normal bleeding time.

Hemophilia A is treated with plasma-derived concentrates that have been treated by viral attenuation procedures (heat-treated) or with recombinant Factor VIII. The recombinant Factor VIII is thought to provide the greatest safety from viral transmission. In the 1980s, the use of lyophilized Factor VIII concentrates made from pooled plasma from as many as 20,000 donors led to the transmission of HIV to many hemophiliacs. Recombinant factor VIII became available in 1992.

If a hemophiliac presents for elective surgery, the patient's hematologist should be consulted. Questions can also be directed to the regional hemophilia center. The National Hemophilia Foundation has listings of the regional centers. The required factor replacement will be dependent upon (1) the patient's plasma volume and (2) the desired procoagulant activity. The patient's plasma volume can be assumed to be equal to 40 ml of plasma per kilogram of body weight. A 60-kg person has a plasma volume of 2400 ml. One unit of Factor VIII procoagulant activity is defined as the amount of Factor VIII present in one milliliter of plasma in an individual with 100% of the normal level. A procoagulant level of 25% is a common target for achieving control of a bleeding episode. This would mean that a total of 600 units (25% × 2400 ml) of Factor VIII:C would be required. For elective surgery, the level of Factor VIII:C activity is usually raised to 50–100% of normal. The number of units of Factor VIII:C contained in the Factor VIII concentrates is usually noted on each bag. Cryoprecipitate contains Factor VIIIC as well, but carries a greater risk of virus transmission. Unfortunately, many hemophiliacs develop inhibitors to Factor VIII:C. The presence of the inhibitor increases the amount of Factor VIII:C that must be administered to manage a given hemostatic challenge.

DDAVP will also increase plasma Factor VIII:C and vWF concentrations. DDAVP is thought to cause the release of Factor VIII:C from liver endothelial cells. There is a large variation in patient response to DDAVP, and it is most effective in patients with Factor VIII:C levels greater than 5%.[146] It is given iv in a dose of 0.3 μg · kg^{-1} in 50 ml of saline over 15–30 min. It causes a prompt increase in Factor VIII:C.

The antifibrinolytics ε-aminocaproic acid and tranexamic acid have been used to treat hemophiliac patients prior to dental procedures. The agents are contraindicated in bleeding episodes involving joints or the urinary tract because the clots that do form may not be lysed for a long time.

Hemophilia B. Factor IX deficiency is also an X-linked recessive disorder that produces a bleeding diathesis that is clinically indistinguishable from hemophilia A. The management of this disorder is similar to that of hemophilia A. Bleeding is controlled with fresh frozen plasma or prothrombin complex, which contains Factor IX (as well as II, VII, and X). Prothrombin complex conveys a very substantial infectious risk and also entails a risk of thrombosis and DIC because of the presence of activated factors. Virus-inactivated Factor IX concentrates, which have been developed recently, should supplant the use or prothrombin complex.[144]

Protein C and Protein S Deficiency

Hereditary deficiency of proteins C and S is associated with thromboembolic events originating on the venous side of the circulation, including deep vein thromboses, pulmonary embolus, and stroke as a consequence of paradoxical embolization. The complete absence of protein C is associated with death in infancy. Patients who experience thromboembolic events and have decreased levels of protein C or S should remain on anticoagulant therapy indefinitely.

Acquired Disorders of Hemostasis

For mnemonic purposes, it is helpful to classify bleeding disorders according to which of the three hemostatic processes is involved: primary hemostasis (platelet disorders); coagulation (clotting factor disorders); fibrinolysis (production of inhibitors such as FDPs); or some combination of the three. Similarly, it is useful to use the results of coagulation tests to determine whether the clinical problem involves primary hemostasis (decreased platelet count, increased bleeding time, etc.), coagulation (prolonged PT and aPTT, decreased factor levels, etc.), fibrinolysis (increased FDPs, increased D-dimer), or some combination of the three. Ultimately, therapeutic decisions (*e.g.*, administration of platelets, FFP, or an antifibrinolytic agent) will similarly be oriented to treatment of one or more of these processes.

Acquired Disorders of Platelets

The clinical conditions that cause an isolated disorder of primary hemostasis typically involve abnormalities of either platelet number or function.

Throbocytopenia. Platelets are derived from megakaryocytes in the bone marrow in response to thrombopoietin, which is synthesized by the liver. The causes of thrombocytopenia may be categorized as follows: (1) inadequate production by the bone marrow, (2) increased peripheral consumption or destruction (non–immune-mediated), (3) increased peripheral destruction (immune-mediated), (4) dilution of circulating platelets, and (5) sequestration (Fig. 10-13).

1. Bone marrow production of platelets can be impaired in many ways. Physical and chemical agents (radiation and chemotherapy), various drugs (thiazide diuretics, sulfonamides, diphenylhydantoin, alcohol), infectious agents (hepatitis B, TB, overwhelming sepsis), and chronic disease states (uremia, liver disease) can all cause bone marrow suppression. Infiltration of the bone marrow by cancer cells or replacement by fibrosis will also result in inadequate platelet production.

2. Accelerated non–immunologically mediated consumption can occur in many conditions that cause extensive activation of coagulation with or without the occurrence of DIC. After extensive tissue damage (burns or massive crush injuries that denude vascular endothelium), the normal process of hemostasis activates platelets, leading to their consumption and to thrombocytopenia. In a similar fashion, the interaction of platelets with nonendothelialized structures such as large vascular grafts can also lead to a transient thrombocytopenia. Platelets are consumed in patients with an extensive vasculitis such as occurs with toxemia of pregnancy. The many conditions that cause DIC (see below) will also cause platelets to be consumed or destroyed faster than they can be produced.

3. Immunologicially mediated consumption can be caused by various drugs (heparin, quinidine, cephalosporins) and autoimmune disorders (systemic lupus erythematosis, rheumatoid arthritis, thrombotic thrombocytopenic purpura). Alloimmunization resulting from previous blood transfusions or pregnancy can cause refractoriness to platelet transfusions.

4. Dilution of platelets will occur in the context of massive transfusion (see below and Risks of Blood Product Adminstration above).

5. Under normal conditions approximately one third of platelets are sequestered in the spleen. When the spleen enlarges, an increasing number are sequestered and thrombocytopenia may result. This may occur in splenomegaly associated with myelodysplastic syndromes and cirrhosis of the liver, although in the latter condition decreased production also contributes to thrombocytopenia.

Disorders of Platelet Function

UREMIA. Platelet dysfunction is common in uremic patients.[147] The accumulation of compounds (guanidine, succinic acid, and hydroxyphenolic acid) is thought to contribute to this dysfunction through interference with the platelet's ability to expose the PF3 phospholipid surface. These compounds are dialyzable and, accordingly, dialysis frequently improves the hemostatic defect associated with uremia. An additional abnormality involving the interaction of von Willebrand factor with platelet receptors is also suspected. DDAVP (desmopressin), which among other effects induces immediate release of vWF from endothelial cells, rapidly improves platelet adhesiveness.[148] However, the mechanism of this effect is not understood. It is not simply a matter of restoring vWF levels, because circulating vWF is typically present in normal levels in uremia. Administration of erythropoietin and conjugated estrogens has also been observed to cause gradual improvement of the hemostatic defect associated with uremia. The mechanisms of these effects are similarly not known. Cryoprecipitate will also improve the platelet dysfunction of uremia but, given the efficacy of DDAVP, the associated risks are not justified. When life-threatening bleeding occurs in the uremic patient, platelet concentrates should be administered.

ANTIPLATELET AGENTS. Anesthesiologists will encounter patients receiving medications that are administered expressly for the purpose of platelet inhibition. These agents are given to reduce the risk of myocardial infarction, stroke,[149] and other thromboembolic complications. They induce platelet dysfunction by several mechanisms which include inhibition of cyclo-oxygenase, inhibition of phosphodiesterase, adenosine receptor antagonism, and blockade of the glycoprotein IIb/IIIa receptor. A variety of drugs given for other indications may also impair platelet function, including amitriptyline, imipramine, chlorpromazine, cocaine, diltiazem, lidocaine, various penicillins, and beta blockers.[150]

Cyclo-oxygenase inhibitors. Aspirin is the prototype. Aspirin produces irreversible inhibition of platelet cyclo-oxygenase (cox), which results in inhibition of synthesis of thromboxane A_2, a potent platelet proaggregant and vasoconstrictor. In moderate doses, there is selective sparing of the synthesis of prostacyclin (antiaggregant, vasodilator), which results in "tilting" the balance substantially in favor of platelet inhibition. Indomethacin, phenylbutazone, and all the nonsteroidal anti-inflammatory agents similarly inhibit cyclo-oxygenase. However,

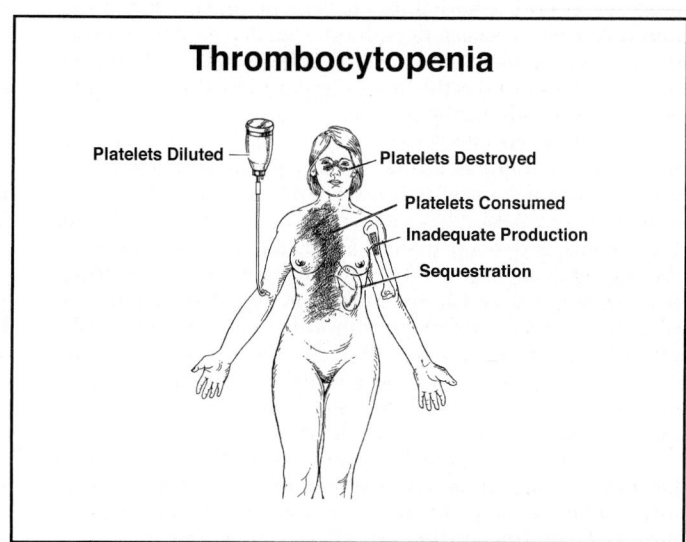

Figure 10-13. Thrombocytopenia. The figure depicts the five processes that can lead to thrombocytopenia. They include platelet destruction, as occurs immunologically in lupus erythematosis; platelet consumption, as occurs with burns or other massive tissue injury conditions; inadequate production, as can occur with marrow infiltration, chemotherapy, or radiation; sequestration as can occur in the presence of splenomegaly, and dilution occurring during massive transfusion.

their inhibition is promptly reversible with clearance of the drug. The recently introduced Cox-2 inhibitors selectively inhibit the cox isoform responsible for generating the mediators of pain and inflammation, while sparing the cox-1 isoform, whose inhibition causes gastric damage, decreased renal blood flow, and inhibition of platelet thromboxane A_2. Accordingly, platelet function should not be impaired. In fact there is concern that Cox-2 inhibitors, which should reduce prostacyclin generation by vascular endothelial cells, may actually tilt the natural balance toward platelet aggregation.[151]

Phosphodiesterase inhibitors. Cyclic AMP is an inhibitor of platelet aggregation and levels are increased by inhibition of phosphodiesterase. Dipyridamole, which is used for stroke prophylaxis alone or more commonly in combination with aspirin, appears to act primarily by this mechanism.[152] Caffeine, aminophylline, and theophylline will also similarly produce mild, reversible platelet inhibition.

Adenosine receptor antagonists. Ticlopidine and clopidogrel, which are administered for stroke prophylaxis, are antagonists of the P2 purinoceptor. They noncompetitively inhibit ADP-induced platelet aggregation and their effect is probably irreversible.[153]

Glycoprotein IIb/IIIa receptor antagonists. These newly introduced agents block platelet aggregation by blocking the GPIIb/IIIa site to which fibrinogen and vWF bind. Used principally for the management of acute coronary syndromes, these agents include abciximab (a monoclonal antibody), tirofiban, and eptifibatide. These agents all require iv administration. Their effect is reversible. Platelet function recovers rapidly (4 hours after discontinuation of tirofiban and eptifibatide) but is somewhat delayed (48 hours) after abciximab.

OTHER CONDITIONS.   Myeloproliferative and myelodysplastic syndromes produce intrinsic defects in platelets. In these disorders, the platelets may be abnormal both in morphology and function. Platelet dysfunction occurs in conjunction with conditions that also cause other hemostatic abnormalities (liver disease, fibrinolytic states including DIC, storage defects) and are discussed below.

Acquired Disorders of Clotting Factors

Vitamin K Deficiency. Hepatic synthesis of clotting Factors II, VII, IX, and X as well as protein C and protein S requires the presence of vitamin K. When synthesized in the absence of vitamin K, the factors are structurally abnormal and are called PIVKAs (proteins induced by vitamin K absence or antagonists). Vitamin K is necessary for the enzymatic carboxylation of the four vitamin K–dependent clotting factors. The carboxyl group enables these factors to bind *via* a calcium bridge to phospholipid surfaces (PF3) during the coagulation process. When vitamin K deficiency occurs, these factors are depleted in an order determined by their individual half-lives. Factor VII has the shortest half-life and is the first to be depleted, then Factors IX and X, and finally Factor II.

"Vitamin K" actually refers to a group of vitamins.[154] Vitamin K_1 (phylloquinone) is found in leafy green vegetables. The greatest quantities occur in brussels sprouts. Vitamin K_2 (menaquinone) is synthesized by the normal intestinal flora. It is rare for patients to develop vitamin K deficiency solely because of dietary deficiency, but it may occur in patients who are receiving parenteral nutrition without vitamin K supplementation and who are being treated concurrently with broad-spectrum antibiotics that destroy the gut flora. Because the body has no appreciable stores of vitamin K, deficiencies can develop in roughly one week. Newborns, who have a sterile gut at birth, have been noted to develop vitamin K deficiency.

Vitamin K is a fat-soluble vitamin, and therefore requires bile salts for absorption from the jejunum. Patients with biliary obstruction, pancreatic insufficiency, malabsorption syndromes, GI obstruction, or rapid GI transit can develop vitamin K deficiency due to inadequate absorption.

DIAGNOSIS AND TREATMENT.   Vitamin K deficiency will cause prolongation of the PT. This occurs because Factor VII is depleted first. With more prolonged deficiency, the aPTT will also be increased because of declining levels of Factors IX and X. Platelet count will be normal. Vitamin K may be administered orally, intramuscularly (im), or intravenously. Urgent treatment of vitamin K deficiency is best accomplished by im or iv administration of vitamin K (Aquamephyton) in doses of 10–20 mg. Vitamin K should be administered slowly to avoid the occurrence of hypotension. Improvement of the coagulation disturbance will be apparent within 6–8 hours.

Coumadin therapy.   Coumadin produces its anticoagulant effect by competition with vitamin K for binding sites in the liver. Administration of coumadin leads to the depletion of functional vitamin K–dependent factors (II, VII, IX, X, protein C and protein S). As with vitamin K deficiency, Factor VII is the first factor to be depleted. Subsequently, Factors IX and X are depleted, and then Factor II. Accordingly, initially only the PT will be prolonged. With higher doses of coumadin, the aPTT will be affected as well.

Coumadin is administered for the prevention of deep venous thrombosis and pulmonary embolism, and to patients with atrial fibrillation, some prosthetic heart valves, and ventricular mural thrombi in the setting of acute myocardial infarction.[155] Patients with protein S or protein C deficiency are also treated with long-term anticoagulation with coumadin. Coumadin therapy is adjusted according to the INR (see Tests of the Hemostatic Mechanism). The primary untoward effect of coumadin therapy is bleeding. Rapid reversal of coumadin effect can be accomplished by administration of vitamin K, 10–20 mg iv. INR should be rechecked at 6-hour intervals. Vitamin K administration may have to be repeated at 12-hour intervals. In situations of greater urgency FFP administration will be required.

Heparin therapy.   Heparin is used widely for anticoagulation in vascular surgery and in procedures requiring cardiopulmonary bypass (CPB). It inhibits coagulation principally through its interaction with one of the body's natural anticoagulant proteins, antithrombin III (ATIII). Heparin of higher molecular weight binds to ATIII and in so doing causes a conformational change that greatly increases ATIII's inhibitory activity. In spite of its name, anti-"thrombin" III, ATIII inhibits several activated factors, including Xa, IXa, XIa, and XIIa, in addition to IIa (thrombin). It is most active against thrombin and Xa. Heparin also increases the activity of a second native antithrombin, heparin cofactor II. Heparin cofactor II inhibits thrombin and not the other activated factors. Its contribution to the clinical effects of heparin is not clear. Resistance to heparin can occur in patients who are deficient in ATIII on either a hereditary or an acquired basis. The latter may occur in patients on sustained heparin therapy or in the presence of depletion by a consumptive coagulopathy. Heparin responsiveness can be restored by administration of ATIII (ATIII concentrates or FFP).

Heparin-induced thrombocytopenia.   Up to 5% of patients who receive heparin therapy for 5 days will develop thrombocytopenia as a result of antibodies (probably IgG) directed against platelet–heparin complexes. Onset requires several days in the heparin-naïve patient, but can occur much more quickly in those who have been previously exposed.[156]

Heparin in cardiopulmonary bypass.   A comprehensive discussion of the use and monitoring of heparin therapy in CPB is beyond the scope of this chapter. Extensive reviews are available.[157,158] In brief, the common practice is to maintain activated clotting time of >480–500 sec for the duration of bypass. There is a substantial variation in the heparin–ACT dose–response relationship, probably because of variability in heparin binding to many native surfaces including platelets, WBCs, endothelium, and plasma proteins including the vWF and ATIII.[157] While there is controversy, it appears that there is greater hazard in allowing ACT to be on the "low side" than in maintaining more complete heparinization.[159] Evidence of platelet activation is less apparent when longer ACTs are maintained. Whether this is a function of direct inhibition of platelets, which are subject to contact activation by the CPB circuit, binding of vWF, or the result of reduced formation of thrombin and inhibition of platelets by its breakdown products (FDPs) is not apparent to the authors of this review. Protamine is administered for reversal of heparin effect. Many clinicians employ a "cc for cc" technique. However, a more careful titration of protamine against ACT is ideal to avoid excessive administration of protamine, which has inherent anticoagulant effects including platelet inhibition, stimulation of t-PA release from endothelium, and inhibition of fibrinogen cleavage by thrombin.[160]

Various alternatives have been considered for the patient with heparin-induced thrombocytopenia who requires CPB.[161,162] Plasmapheresis prior to surgery with subsequent use of heparin has been employed.[156] The nonheparin alternatives for anticoagulation include specific inhibitors of thrombin (hirudin, hirulog, argatroban) and the defibrinogenating agent Ancrod (a snake venom). There are limitations. The contact activation of platelets is not inhibited and platelet inhibitors should probably be administered simultaneously. Experience is very limited and well-defined protocols are not established.

Low–molecular-weight heparins. LMW fractions of heparin have been employed principally for deep vein thrombosis prophylaxis. These agents, which also act *via* ATIII, have greater activity against Factor Xa than thrombin. Because of more consistent absorption after subcutaneous injection and less variability in binding to plasma proteins, they have more predictable dose–response characteristics than unfractionated heparin. A longer half-life allows once per day dosing. They also appear to cause less platelet inhibition and are associated with a lower incidence of heparin-induced thrombocytopenia.[163] Protamine neutralization of LMW heparins is reported to be incomplete.[164]

Acquired Combined Disorders of Platelets and Clotting Factors

Massive Transfusion. The various hazards of massive transfusion, as reviewed earlier, include two potential consequences with implications for coagulation: (1) dilutional deficiencies of factors and platelets and (2) hypothermia. Isovolemic exchange of blood with packed RBCs or other factor- and platelet-free fluids will lead to potentially significant reductions first of fibrinogen, then of Factors V and VIII, and finally platelets. These occurrences should be suspected when exchanged volumes reach 140%, 200%, and 230% of original blood volume, respectively.[30] However, as noted previously, administration of hemostasis-promoting blood products should be based on clinical and laboratory evidence of coagulopathy and not on exchange volume estimates.

Hypothermia slows coagulation (as it does all enzymatically mediated reactions) and causes sequestration of platelets. At 29°C (at which temperature the risk of cardiac dysrrythmias is critical), PT and aPTT will increase ~50% over normothermic values and platelet count will decrease by ~40%.[144] Notwithstanding a general conviction that "cold patients bleed," there have been no quantitative correlations of temperature and bleeding in the clinical setting. Temperatures of 33°C are commonly used in elective neurosurgery without clinically apparent coagulopathy. However, Ferrara *et al*[9] reviewed the clinical course of 45 patients who received massive transfusion following trauma. The duration of hypotension was similar in patients who survived and those who did not. However, the degree of acidosis and hypothermia was more extreme in the nonsurvivors, and the nonsurvivors developed coagulopathies despite adequate blood, plasma, and platelet replacement. In studies of this nature, it is difficult to separate the effects of the common clinical concomitants of hypothermia—acidosis, shock, massive transfusion, massive tissue injury—from those of hypothermia *per se*. Furthermore, the significance of hypothermia may lie in the interaction with other variables. In spite of the ambiguity,

hypothermia should be carefully avoided and aggressively corrected in the patient receiving massive transfusion.

Citrate intoxication, another potential complication of massive transfusion, can cause diminished calcium (Factor IV) availability. However, critical cardiac consequences occur before hypocalcemia has significant implications for coagulation.

Acquired Combined Disorders of Platelets and Clotting Factors with Increased Fibrinolysis

Liver Disease. Chronic liver disease is associated with abnormalities of all three phases of hemostasis: primary hemostasis, coagulation, and fibrinolysis.[147] Table 10-8 (see page 224) provides an overview of these abnormalities.

IMPAIRED PRIMARY HEMOSTASIS. Impaired primary hemostasis occurs as a result of both thrombocytopenia and impaired platelet function. The former is largely the result of decreased production which in turn is probably the result of decreased thrombopoietin secretion by the liver. Hypersplenism may also contribute but its role has been overemphasized. Platelet dysfunction can occur when liver disease is sufficiently advanced that clearance of FDPs is impaired or when DIC complicates the coagulation disturbance. The FDPs coat the surface of platelets and impair aggregation.[39] Ethanol can also directly contribute to platelet dysfunction by inhibition of the synthesis of ADP, ATP, and thromboxane A_2. Accordingly, when faced with a patient with liver disease who is bleeding, a normal platelet count cannot be assurance of intact primary hemostasis. DDAVP may be helpful, but transfusion of platelet concentrates may be necessary.[92]

DISTURBANCES OF COAGULATION. Disturbances of coagulation may occur because of both decreases in factor production and increases in factor consumption. The liver synthesizes all of the clotting factors (with the probable exception of Factor VIII). As with vitamin K deficiency, hepatic disease first leads to a deficiency of Factor VII since it has the shortest half-life. Thereafter, deficiencies will develop in Factors II, IX, and X. Dietary deficiency of vitamin K, as may occur in alcoholics, with diminished secretion of bile salts leading to malabsorption, will exaggerate these deficiencies. If impaired coagulation is the result of vitamin K deficiency and not hepatic damage, then parenteral vitamin K may be helpful in restoring factor levels of II, VII, IX, and X. Further deterioration of hepatic function will affect the remaining factors, I, V, XI, and XII. Impaired liver function can also cause a thrombotic tendency, which leads to increased consumption of clotting factors. This occurs for two reasons. First, synthesis of the natural anticoagulants—antithrombin III, protein C, and protein S—may be diminished, thereby altering the balance of pro- and anticoagulant forces; second, clearance of activated clotting factors from the circulation may be impaired, thereby allowing persistent activation of the coagulation cascade.

INCREASED FIBRINOLYSIS. Increased fibrinolysis occurs as a result of decreased clearance of t-PA from the circulation by the impaired liver and decreased hepatic synthesis of α_2-antiplasmin.[165] The combination of accelerated coagulation and increased fibrinolysis in patients with advanced liver disease can lead to a persistent, low-grade DIC. The release into the circulation of the breakdown products of necrotic hepatocytes may contribute to the development of DIC.[154] Diagnosis of DIC is often difficult because the laboratory tests used to identify DIC are already abnormal in patients with liver dysfunction. Thrombocytopenia, prolonged PT and aPTT, decreased fibrinogen level, and circulating FDPs will commonly occur in the absence of DIC. The D-dimer test is the most specific for the occurrence of DIC.

Diagnosis and Treatment.

COAGULATION ABNORMALITIES ASSOCIATED WITH LIVER DISEASE. The initial laboratory evaluation should include platelet count, PT, aPTT, fibrinogen level, and D-dimer. In the event of thrombocytopenia and clinical bleeding or pending surgery, platelet transfusions are appropriate. If the PT is prolonged (>1.5 times control), vitamin K should be administered speculatively. In the absence of a response to vitamin K (which requires a minimum of 8 hours), factor deficiencies should be treated with fresh frozen plasma (FFP) with attention to the possibility of volume overload. Cryoprecipitate is appropriate in the event of hypofibrinogenemia (fibrinogen <100–125 g · dl^{-1}). However, cryoprecipitate does not contain the vitamin K–dependent factors. While antifibrinolytics have been applied in the context of liver transplantation, they should not otherwise be used for bleeding associated with liver disease because of the catastrophic consequences of administering these agents in the face of an unrecognized DIC.[166]

Disseminated Intravascular Coagulation. Thorough and detailed reviews of DIC are available.[167,168] DIC is characterized by excessive formation of thrombin throughout the vascular tree. It is triggered by the appearance of tissue factor (TF; formerly called thromboplastin) activity in the circulation in amounts sufficient to overwhelm the mechanisms that normally restrain and localize clot formation. That appearance may be the result of either extensive endothelial injury, which exposes TF of fibroblastic origin, or the release of TF into the circulation as occurs with amniotic fluid embolus, extensive soft tissue damage, or severe head injury. Table 10-9 lists the numerous clinical conditions that can generate this TF activity. The accelerated process of clot formation causes both tissue ischemia and, ultimately, critical depletion of platelets and factors. Simultaneously, the fibrinolytic system is intensely activated and plasmin is generated to lyse the extensive fibrin clots. The mechanisms that normally serve to localize plasmin are similarly overwhelmed and plasmin circulates freely. Fibrinolysis and circulating plasmin result in extensive degradation of both fibrin and fibrinogen. The fibrin degradation products that result inhibit platelet aggregation and prevent the normal crosslinking of fibrin monomers. Depleted of platelets and clotting factors and inhibited by FDPs, the coagulation system fails and the patient bleeds.

Table 10-9 reveals that several clinical entities that are encountered frequently in anesthetic and critical care practice are associated with the development of DIC. Sepsis is the most common cause. Endotoxins or lipopolysaccharide breakdown products from bacteria incite an inflammatory response which includes the generation of cytokines (tumor necrosis factor α, various interleukins). These cytokines in turn stimulate the

Table 10-9. CLINICAL CONDITIONS ASSOCIATED WITH DISSEMINATED INTRAVASCULAR COAGULATION

Sepsis
Malignancies
Obstetric conditions
  Amniotic fluid embolus
  Fetal death *in utero*
  Abruptio placentae
  Pre-eclampsia
Extensive tissue damage
  Burns
  Trauma
  Liver failure
Extensive cerebral injury
  Head injury
  Stroke
Extensive vascular endothelial damage
  Vasculitis
  Pre-eclampsia
Hemolytic transfusion reactions
Snake venoms

release or expression of TF by endothelial cells, macrophages, and monocytes and the DIC sequence is initiated.

Several obstetric conditions can cause DIC. These include amniotic fluid embolism, placental abruption, and fetal death *in utero*. Each of these conditions can cause the direct release of TF-equivalent material into the circulation, leading to a rapid and extensive activation of the coagulation system and fulminant DIC. Pre-eclampsia is characterized by a systemic vasculitis. The associated endothelial damage causes an initially low-grade DIC which accelerates as vasculitis-related damage leads to release of TF from ischemic tissues, in particular placenta.

Large burns, extensive traumatic soft tissue injuries, severe brain injury, and hemolytic transfusion reactions can also liberate TF-equivalent material into the circulation and incite DIC. Certain malignancies, most notably promyelocytic leukemia and adenocarcinomas, are associated with DIC. However, with malignancy-associated DIC, thrombotic manifestations are more likely to appear first, whereas with the others mentioned above, the hemorrhagic diathesis is often the first clinical manifestation. A few general conditions such as acidosis, shock, and hypoxia are associated with DIC.[169] Shock which is associated with low blood flow promotes coagulation because one of the control mechanisms (rapid blood flow) is compromised. Clearance of activated clotting factors is reduced when blood flow is decreased. Acidosis and hypoxia may contribute to both tissue and endothelial damage.

The clinical manifestations of DIC are a consequence of both thrombosis and bleeding. Bleeding is a more common clinical presentation in patients with acute, fulminant DIC. Petechiae, ecchymoses, epitaxis, gingival/mucosal bleeding, hematuria, and bleeding from wounds and puncture sites may be evident. With the chronic forms of DIC, thrombotic manifestations are more likely. Organs with the greatest blood flow (*e.g.*, kidney and brain) typically sustain the greatest damage. Pulmonary function may deteriorate as a consequence of microthrombus accumulation.

DIAGNOSIS OF DIC. The typical constellation of laboratory findings includes increased PT and aPTT, thrombocytopenia, a decreased fibrinogen level, and the presence of FDPs and D-dimers. The peripheral smear may reveal schistocytes (fragmented RBCs reflecting the microangiopathy that occurs as a consequence of widespread fibrin deposition). Fibrinogen level may not be decreased initially. Fibrinogen is an "acute-phase reactant" which increases in response to stress, and the early consumption of fibrinogen may simply reduce its levels to "normal." FDPs are a sensitive measure of fibrinolytic activity although they are not specific for DIC. FDPs appear as a result of the breakdown of fibrin in any stage of clot maturation or fibrinogen itself. D-dimer (which is a breakdown product of the crosslinked fibrin in a mature clot) is much more specific for DIC and should be measured when that diagnosis is suspected.

Various other laboratory assays have been employed to support a diagnosis of DIC, but should probably not be considered part of the anesthesiologist's routine. They include levels of ATIII, α$_2$-antithrombin, and protein C (all decreased because of binding to thrombin); plasminogen (decreased); thrombin–ATIII (TAT) complexes (increased); and Factor VIII (decreased in DIC but normal with hepatic failure without DIC).

TREATMENT OF DIC. Treatment should focus on management of the underlying condition. Septicemia will require antibiotic therapy. The obstetric conditions are frequently self-limited, although evacuation of the uterus or hysterectomy may be warranted. Hypovolemia, acidosis, and hypoxemia should be corrected to prevent their contribution to the DIC process.[170]

When bleeding is or may become life-threatening, the consumptive coagulopathy must be treated. Platelets will be required for thrombocytopenia, *e.g.*, <50,000/mm^3. FFP will replace the clotting factor deficiencies. Fibrinogen level should be increased to >100 mg · dl^{-1}. When hypofibrinogenemia is severe (<50 mg · dl^{-1}), it will not be corrected by the limited amounts of fibrinogen present in FFP, and cryoprecipitate should be administered. Six units of cryoprecipitate will increase fibrinogen level by approximately 50 mg · dl^{-1} in a 70-kg patient.[168]

Heparin has been advocated. However, the contemporary practice is to restrict its use to situations in which thrombosis is clinically problematic, principally DIC associated with malignancies. There is no proven benefit in situations in which bleeding is the predominant manifestation.[167,168] Although antifibrinolytics have been considered, their administration in the face of widespread thrombosis is potentially disastrous so they should not be used. Antithrombin III concentrates have been administered. ATIII is a natural anticoagulant that binds both thrombin and the activated factors of the "intrinsic process" and is typically depleted during DIC. The hope is that its administration will serve to slow the runaway coagulation process. However, a beneficial effect on outcome from DIC has not been confirmed,[171] and its use should be viewed as experimental.

Cardiopulmonary Bypass and Coagulation. The management of anticoagulation and postcardiopulmonary bypass (CPB) bleeding are addressed in Chapter 32.

Blood Component Therapy

After observation of a clinical coagulopathy and laboratory testing, the clinician must determine which, if any, hemostatic blood products or pharmacologic agents are warranted. Brief descriptions of the preparation of and the indications for the various hemostatic blood components follow. For the collection and preparation of whole blood and packed RBCs, see the section entitled Collection and Preparation of Blood Products for Transfusion (above).

Platelets

Platelets are separated from plasma by centrifugation. They are commonly supplied as single-donor units with the platelets suspended in a small quantity of residual plasma. One unit of platelets will increase the platelet count of a 70-kg recipient by 5000–10,000/mm^3. When platelets are indicated, a common practice is to administer one unit per 10 kg of body weight. Accordingly, platelet transfusion will often entail exposure to multiple donors. Donor exposure can be minimized by the use of single-donor "platelet pheresis packs," which contain the platelet equivalent of approximately six single units. These are obtained by serial blood withdrawals from a single donor followed by centrifugation and return of the RBCs to the donor.

Platelet viability is optimal at 22°C but storage is limited to 4–5 days. The short shelf time means that platelets are usually administered before the results of the newly introduced nucleic acid amplification test (NAT) for viral agents are available. Platelets bear both ABO and human leukocyte (HLA) antigens. ABO compatibility is ideal. But even though incompatibility shortens the life span of the platelet, ABO compatibility is not absolutely necessary. Not all institutions ABO-match platelets. The HLA antigens are responsible for the platelet refractoriness exhibited in some patients who develop antibodies after multiple transfusions containing either platelets or white blood cells. Platelets do not carry the Rh antigen. However, administration of platelets from an Rh-positive donor to an Rh-negative recipient should be avoided in order to prevent sensitization as a result of passenger RBCs in the platelet preparation. This is especially important in females who may subsequently become pregnant.

Platelets should be administered to correct clinical coagulopathy associated with deficiencies in platelet number or platelet function. When platelet count falls acutely below 75,000/mm^3, bleeding is often evident in the surgical patient. However, platelets should not be given unless a clinical coagulopathy is apparent. In other patient populations, a clinical coagulopathy may not occur until much lower platelet counts are reached, *e.g.,* 10,000/mm^3 in ITP (idiopathic thrombocytopenic purpura), 20,000/mm^3 in bone marrow depression,[172] and 40,000/mm^3 during massive transfusion. Platelet dysfunction may occur and platelet administration may be warranted in situations in which platelet counts exceed 100,000/mm^3, *e.g.,* after cardiopulmonary bypass, in the presence of platelet-inhibiting drugs (ASA, ticlopidine), and uremia. Again, it is the presence of a clinical coagulopathy that justifies their administration.

Fresh Frozen Plasma (FFP)

Plasma is separated from the RBC component of whole blood by centrifugation. One unit has a volume of 200–250 ml. It will contain the preservative added at the time of collection, usually CPD-adenine. To preserve the two labile clotting factors (V and VIII), it is frozen promptly and thawed only immediately prior to administration. FFP must be ABO-compatible. Rh-positive plasma can be given to an Rh-negative recipient, but ideally this should be avoided in young females because of the possibility of alloimmunization to the Rh antigen on passenger RBCs in the FFP. Indications for FFP administration[173] include: (1) replacement of factor deficiencies indicated by a clinical coagulopathy and laboratory evidence, *e.g.,* PT >18 sec, aPTT >45 sec, fibrinogen <100 mg · dl^{-1}; (2) immediate reversal of coumadin effect; (3) deficiency of antithrombin III, protein C, protein S, or C1-esterase inhibitor; (4) treatment of thrombotic thrombocytopenic purpura and the hemolytic uremic syndrome; and (5) clinical coagulopathy associated with massive blood transfusion. FFP should not be used as a volume expander or to treat nutritional deficiency in the absence of coagulation disorders. An empirical dose of 5–10 ml of FFP per kilogram of body weight may be used.[174]

Solvent Detergent Plasma

One of the principal hazards of FFP administration has been virus transmission. Three procedures—pasteurization, photochemical treatment, and solvent detergent (SD) treatment—have been used to inactivate viruses. The SD technique is now the most widely applied, largely because it is highly effective in inactivating all of the lipid-encapsulated viruses (HIV, HCV, HGBV, HTLV). The disadvantage of the SD technique is that the process involves pooling of large numbers of single FFP units (>1000) and is not effective against nonlipid-enveloped viruses (HAV, parvovirus) or the agent of Creutzfeldt-Jacob disease. The concern with SD plasma is that the pooling process might result in wide dissemination of an infectious agent. The incidence of parvovirus viremia among donors is estimated to be between 0.03 and 0.6%.[175] Parvovirus infection has been reported as a consequence of transfusion. While the disease is usually self-limited, significant morbidity (*e.g.,* red cell aplasia, meningitis) can occur, especially in immunocompromised patients.[175] The future of SD plasma is not clear at the time of this review.

Cryoprecipitate

Cryoprecipitate can be recovered from FFP thawed at 4°C.[176,177] It is a concentrated source of Factor VIII, Factor XIII, vWF, and fibrinogen. It is stored at −20°C and thawed immediately prior to use. Indications include (1) hypofibrinogenemia (<100 mg · dl^{-1}), (2) hemophilia A (if a virus-inactivated Factor VIII concentrate is not available), (3) von Willebrand's disease, (4) Factor XIII deficiency, (5) preparation of fibrin "glue," and (6) uremia with active bleeding.

One unit of cryoprecipitate (the yield from one unit of FFP) contains sufficient fibrinogen to increase fibrinogen level 5–7 mg · dl^{-1}.[176] Accordingly, it is usually provided in bags that contain 10 or 20 units. ABO compatibility is not essential because of the limited antibody content of the associated plasma vehicle (10–20 ml). Viruses can be transmitted with cryoprecipitate.

Factor VIII and Factor IX Concentrates

Plasma concentrates of Factors VIII and IX are available. Because they are "pooled" donor products, they have an inherent risk of virus transmission. However, contemporary methods of virus inactivation have made these preparations relatively safe.[178] Factor VIII concentrate is indicated for the treatment of hemophilia A. Factor IX concentrate is indicated in hemophilia B (Christmas disease) and for deficiencies of Factors II, VII, and X, which it also contains in substantial concentrations.

Antithrombin III

Virus-treated ATIII concentrates are available. They have been employed in the treatment of congenital and acquired ATIII deficiencies.[179] The latter include DIC and fulminant hepatic failure.

Pharamacologic Therapy

Desmopressin (1-deamino-8-D-arginine vasopressin; DDAVP) is a synthetic analog of the natural hormone vasopressin. The actions of vasopressin are thought to be mediated by two general classes of receptors: those that mediate smooth muscle contraction in the peripheral vasculature (V1 receptors), and those that regulate water reabsorption in the collecting ducts of the nephron (V2 receptors). Desmopressin has no activity at the V1 receptors and accordingly has virtually no vasoconstrictor effect. It does, however, act at V2 receptors. In fact, desmopressin is a more potent antidiuretic than vasopressin and has a more prolonged activity. Desmopressin was used primarily for clinical conditions such as diabetes insipidus until its hemostatic effects were recognized.

The hemostatic effects of desmopressin are thought to be mediated by "low-affinity, extra-renal V2-like" receptors.[148] Desmopressin causes release of coagulation factor VIII:C, vWF, and tissue plasminogen activator. Desmopressin is thought to release VIII:C from the sinusoidal liver endothelial cells, and the vWF from endothelial cells. Desmopressin also increases platelet adhesiveness and shortens the bleeding time, though the mechanism of these effects is not fully understood. It appears to entail more than a simple increase in the plasma vWF level.

Desmopressin

Indications: Desmopressin has proven an effective treatment for certain types of vWD, mild hemophilia, and various conditions associated with platelet dysfunction.[148]

von Willebrand's Disease. The most common form of vWD (Type 1) involves a simple quantitative decrease in the plasma levels of vWF. Desmopressin is extremely effective in these patients. It can effectively normalize the plasma levels of vWF. However, patients with Type 2 vWD synthesize an abnormal protein, and increased release of the abnormal factor does not usually improve their bleeding defect. Patients with the 2B subtype of vWD, who produce a factor that binds spontaneously to the platelet GPIb receptor (without the need for a conformation change) may actually become thrombocytopenic following desmopressin administration. Patients with Type 3 vWD who produce virtually no vWF also do not benefit from desmopressin.[148]

Mild Hemophilia. Desmopressin is useful in patients with mild to moderate hemophilia A who synthesize enough Factor VIII:C that desmopressin can effectively liberate the needed clotting factor into the blood. In these patients, desmopressin can increase the circulating factor VIII:C concentration 2- to 6-fold.

Conditions Associated with Platelet Dysfunction. Desmopressin has been shown to reduce the bleeding time in a variety of conditions associated with platelet dysfunction. It produces rapid and temporary correction of prolonged bleeding times in uremic patients following intravenous or intranasal administration. In cirrhotics, desmopressin increases the concentrations of larger vWF multimers and shortens prolonged bleeding times. Desmopressin also decreases the prolonged bleeding times caused by many drugs including aspirin, nonsteroidal anti-inflammatory drugs (NSAIDS), dextran, ticlopidine, and heparin.[148]

Use in Cardiac Surgery. The prophylactic use of desmopressin in cardiac surgical patients has been controversial. Because one of the most common and clinically relevant hemostatic changes during CPB is the occurrence of both platelet dysfunction and thrombocytopenia, numerous studies have been performed to assess the use of desmopressin in these patients. Those that have revealed decreased blood loss or blood product administration have involved principally patients who were predisposed to blood loss, e.g., redo procedures[180–183] and patients receiving aspirin.[184] The latter observation suggests that patients at risk can safely continue aspirin up to the time of surgery.

Dosage Recommendations. Desmopressin is commonly administered iv in a dose of $0.3 \mu g \cdot kg^{-1}$. The effect of desmopressin is almost immediate. Peak levels of Factor VIII:C and vWF are achieved within 30–60 min and the effect lasts for several hours.[148] Desmopressin administration may be repeated after 8–12 hours. When used in cardiac surgery, the drug should be administered after termination of cardiopulmonary bypass. Water balance should be monitored. However, while congestive cardiac failure and hyponatremia and seizures in children have been reported, clinically significant water retention is relatively uncommon. Desmopressin may be administered as a nasal spray and is available for home use for both mild hemophiliacs and patients with vWD (Type 1). Intravenous administration causes a more rapid rise in VIII:C levels and is therefore preferable for acute hemostatic challenges.

Tachyphylaxis. There has been concern that tachyphylaxis to repeated doses might occur as a result of depletion of endogenous stores of Factor VIII:C and vWF. This has not been a problem clinically. There is a decrement in the Factor VIII:C and vWF plasma levels achieved with second and subsequent doses of desmopressin, but the response plateaus at a clinically useful level. In addition, multiple doses are rarely warranted.

Antifibrinolytics

Antifibrinolytic agents have been used frequently in situations in which exaggerated fibrinolysis is suspected of contributing to intraoperative bleeding. These situations include cardiopulmonary bypass procedures, hepatic transplantation, and prostate surgery. The use of antifibrinolytic mouthwashes in the context of dental procedures in patients with hemophilia has been mentioned elsewhere in this chapter. There are three commonly available antifibrinolytics. They are the lysine analogs ε-aminocaproic acid (EACA) and tranexamic acid (TXA) and the serine protease inhibitor aprotinin.

ε-Aminocaproic Acid and Tranexamic Acid. EACA and TXA bind to both plasminogen and plasmin molecules to produce a structural change. That structural change blocks the conversion of plasminogen to plasmin and also prevents plasmin from degrading fibrinogen and fibrin. The dual action of these agents results in two effects on the hemostatic mechanism. First, decreased synthesis of plasmin from plasminogen results in reduced fibrinolysis (clot lysis). The second effect of these drugs, the inactivation of plasmin, decreases the formation of degradation products of fibrinogen and fibrin. These FDPs have anticoagulant effects, including the inhibition of platelet aggregation and the inhibition of the crosslinking of fibrin strands, which are thereby avoided.

Aprotinin. Aprotinin produces its antifibrinolytic effect by a different mechanism. It is an inhibitor of numerous serine protease enzymes including plasmin and kallikrein. The latter participates in the process of contact activation of Factor XII.

As a consequence of its inhibition of plasmin, aprotinin, like EACA and TXA, prevents degradation of fibrinogen and fibrin. As is the case with EACA and TXA, the reduction in FDPs should improve both platelet and coagulation function. However, aprotinin is believed to have an additional beneficial effect on platelets. The mechanism of that effect is not known. Better preservation of the GP1b receptor (which is necessary for initial platelet adhesion to vascular defects) has been reported during cardiopulmonary bypass in patients who received aprotinin.[185] The relevance of any platelet specific effect remains controversial.[186]

Use of Antifibrinolytics in Cardiac Surgery. A meta-analysis of the many studies of these agents that have been performed in the context of cardiopulmonary bypass confirms that, overall, blood loss and the administration of allogeneic blood is diminished by the use of all three agents.[187] Concern has been expressed that antifibrinolysis might lead to an increased rate of graft occlusion and myocardial infarction. A recent meta-analysis did not bear out that concern.[187] There does not appear to be a clear consensus as to which of the three agents is most appropriate in the context of cardiopulmonary bypass. Various authors have argued that EACA and TXA are preferable to aprotinin because they are less expensive and have apparently similar efficacy.[188,189]

The patterns of use of antifibrinolytic agents in cardiac surgery vary substantially among institutions. Few appear to use these agents routinely for all cardiopulmonary bypass procedures. Some reserve their use for situations more likely to be associated with post-CPB bleeding (*e.g.*, redo procedures, circulatory arrest procedures). Still others appear to reserve antifibrinolytics for refractory bleeding post-CPB. The latter seems less logical because much of the activation of the hemostatic mechanism occurs during cardiopulmonary bypass.

There is a small but finite rate of allergic responses to aprotinin. Accordingly, a test dose has been recommended for patients who have had prior exposure to aprotinin. The potential for developing sensitivity has been used as a rationale for avoiding administration of aprotinin in circumstances where it is not clearly indicated (*e.g.*, first-time CABG), so that it may be used safely in the event of a redo procedure.

Use of Antifibrinolytics in Hepatic Transplantation. Accelerated fibrinolysis occurs commonly in patients undergoing hepatic transplantation. This is probably, in part, the consequence of decreased clearance of activated clotting factors by the diseased liver. More importantly, hepatic clearance ceases entirely during the anhepatic phase. In addition, with reperfusion of the donor liver, there is an "explosive" release of t-PA into the systemic circulation.[190] Aprotinin, EACA, and TXA have all been used and reported to reduce blood loss in hepatic transplantation.[190–193] However, not all studies have demonstrated a reduction in transfusion requirements.[194] In some instances, these agents have been administered prophylactically.[190] However, the more commonly used and advocated approach is to administer these agents only in response to the demonstration, typically by thromboelastography (see Fig. 10-12), of hyperfibrinolysis.[192,195]

CONCLUSION

The approach to the bleeding patient requires a knowledge of the basic hemostatic mechanism, common bleeding disorders, an ability to interpret coagulation tests, and an appreciation of the risks involved with blood component therapy.

REFERENCES

1. Consensus statement on red cell transfusion: Proceedings of a consensus conference held by the Royal College of Physicians of Edinburgh, May 9–10, 1994. Br J Anaesth 73:857, 1994
2. Simon TL: Evolution in indications for blood component transfusion. Clin Lab Med 12:655, 1992
3. Stehling L, Simon TL: The red blood cell transfusion trigger: Physiology and clinical studies. Arch Pathol Lab Med 118:429, 1994
4. Anonymous: Consensus conference: Perioperative red blood cell transfusion. JAMA 260:2700, 1988
5. Stehling L: Autologous transfusion. Int Anesthesiol Clin 28:190, 1990
6. Jain R: Use of blood transfusion in management of anemia. Med Clin North Am 76:727, 1992
7. Irving GA: Perioperative blood and blood component therapy. Can J Anaesth 39:1105, 1992
8. McClelland DLN: Therapeutic oxygen carriers: State of the art. Vox Sang 67:73, 1994
9. Crosby ET: Perioperative haemotherapy. 1. Indications for blood component transfusion. Can J Anaesth 39:695, 1992
10. Fluit C, Kunst V, Drentheschonk AM: Incidence of red cell antibodies after multiple blood transfusion. Transfusion 30:532, 1990
11. Tuman KJ: Tissue oxygen delivery: The physiology of anemia. Anesthesiol Clin North Am 8:451, 1990
12. Robertie PG, Gravlee GP: Safe Limits of isovolemic hemodilution and recommendations for erythrocyte transfusion. Int Anesthesiol Clin 28:97, 1990
13. Welch HG, Meehan KR, Goodnough LT: Prudent strategies for elective red blood cell transfusion. Ann Intern Med 116:393, 1992
14. Hamilton SM: The use of blood in resuscitation of the trauma patient. Can J Surg 36:21, 1993
15. Carson JL, Willett LR: Is a hemoglobin of 10 G/Dl required for surgery? Med Clin North Am 77:335, 1993
16. Anonymous: Consensus conference: Blood management, surgical practice guidelines. Am J Surg 170:1S, 1995
17. Stehling LC, Doherty DC, Faust RJ et al: Practice guidelines for blood component therapy: A report by the American Society of Anesthesiologists task force on blood component therapy. Anesthesiology 84:732, 1996
18. Chapler CK, Cain SM: The physiologic reserve in oxygen carrying capacity: Studies in experimental hemodilution. Can J Physiol Pharmacol 64:7, 1986
19. Hebert PC, Wells G, Blajchman MA et al: A multicenter, randomized, controlled clinical trial of transfusion requirements in critical care. N Engl J Med 340:409, 1999
20. Ereth MH, Oliver WC, Santrach PJ: Perioperative interventions to decrease transfusion of allogeneic blood products. Mayo Clin Proc 69:575, 1994
21. Miller RD, Brzica SM: Blood components, colloids and autotransfusion therapy. In: Miller RD (ed): Anesthesia, 2d ed, p 1329. New York, Churchill Livingstone, 1986
22. Crosby ET: Perioperative haemotherapy. 2. Risks and complications of blood transfusion. Can J Anaesth 39:822, 1992
23. Au Buchon JP: Minimizing donor exposure in hemotherapy. Arch Pathol Lab Med 118:380, 1994
24. Jameson LC, Popic PM, Harms BA: Hyperkalemic death during use of a high-capacity fluid warmer for massive transfusion. Anesthesiology 73:1050, 1990
25. Sessler DI: Current concepts: Mild perioperative hypothermia. N Engl J Med 336:1730, 1997
26. Klapper EB, Goldfinger D: Leukocyte-reduced blood components in transfusion medicine: Current indications and prospects for the future. Clin Lab Med 12:711, 1992
27. Snyder EL, Hezzey A, Barash PG, Palermo G: Microaggregate blood filtration in patients with compromised pulmonary function. Transfusion 22:21, 1982
28. Opelz G, Sengar DP, Mickey MR, Terasaki PI: Effect of blood transfusions on subsequent kidney transplants. Transplant Proc 5:253, 1973
29. Rock G, Tittley P, Fuller V: Effect of citrate anticoagulants on factor VIII levels in plasma. Transfusion 28:248, 1988
30. Hiippala ST, Myllyla GJ, Vahtera EM: Hemostatic factors and replacement of major blood loss with plasma-poor red cell concentrates. Anesth Analg 81:360, 1995
31. Welborn JL, Hersch J: Blood transfusion reactions—Which are life-threatening and which are not. Postgrad Med 90:125, 1991
32. Ferrara JLM, Krenger W: Graft-versus-host disease: The influence of type 1 and type 2 T cell cytokines. Transfusion Med Rev 12:1, 1998
33. Harrison CR, Sawyer PR: Special issues in transfusion medicine. Clin Lab Med 12:743, 1992
34. Walker RH: Special report: Transfusion risks. Am J Clin Pathol 88: 74, 1987

35. Silliman CC: Transfusion-related acute lung injury. Transfusion Med Rev 13:177, 1999
36. Burrows L, Tartter P, Aufses A: Increased recurrence rates in perioperatively transfused colorectal malignancy patients. Cancer Detect Prev 10:361, 1987
37. Blumberg N, Agarwal MM, Chuang C: Relation between recurrence of cancer of the colon and blood transfusion. Br Med J (Clin Res Ed) 290:1037, 1985
38. Foster RS Jr, Costanza MC, Foster JC et al: Adverse relationship between blood transfusions and survival after colectomy for colon cancer. Cancer 55:1195, 1985
39. Corman J, Arnoux R, Péloquin A et al: Blood transfusions and survival after colectomy for colorectal cancer. Can J Surg 29:325, 1986
40. Parrott NR, Lennard TW, Taylor RM et al: Effect of perioperative blood transfusion on recurrence of colorectal cancer. Br J Surg 73:970, 1986
41. Voogt PJ, van de Velde CJ, Brand A et al: Perioperative blood transfusion and cancer prognosis. Different effects of blood transfusion on prognosis of colon and breast cancer patients. Cancer 59:836, 1987
42. Stephenson KR, Steinberg SM, Hughes KS et al: Perioperative blood transfusions are associated with decreased time to recurrence and decreased survival after resection of colorectal liver metastases. Ann Surg 208:679, 1988
43. Kaneda M, Horimi T, Ninomiya M et al: Adverse affect of blood transfusions on survival of patients with gastric cancer. Transfusion 27:375, 1987
44. Tartter PI, Burrows L, Kirschner P: Perioperative blood transfusion adversely affects prognosis after resection of Stage I (subset N0) non-oat cell lung cancer. J Thorac Cardiovasc Surg 88:659, 1984
45. Hyman NH, Foster RS Jr, DeMeules JE, Costanza MC: Blood transfusions and survival after lung cancer resection. Am J Surg 149:502, 1985
46. Tartter PI, Burrows L, Papatestas AE et al: Perioperative blood transfusion has prognostic significance for breast cancer. Surgery 97:225, 1985
47. Hillyer CD, Lankford KV, Roback JD et al: Transfusion of the HIV-seropositive patient: Immunomodulation, viral reactivation, and limiting exposure to EBV (HHV-4), CMV (HHV-5), and HHV-6, 7, and 8. Transfusion Med Rev 13:1, 1999
48. Lane TA: Leukocyte reduction of cellular blood components: Effectiveness, benefits, quality control, and costs. Arch Pathol Lab Med 118:392, 1994
49. McFarland J, Menitove J, Kagen L et al: Leukocyte reduction and ultraviolet β irradiation of platelets to prevent alloimmunization and refractoriness to platelet transfusions. N Engl J Med 337:1861, 1997
50. Tartter PI, Mohandas K, Azar P et al: Randomized trial comparing packed red cell blood transfusion with and without leukocyte depletion for gastrointestinal surgery. Am J Surg 176:462, 1998
51. Bowden RA, Slichter SJ, Sayers MH et al: Use of leukocyte-depleted platelets and cytomegalovirus-seronegative red blood cells for prevention of primary cytomegalovirus infection after marrow transplant. Blood 78:246, 1991
52. Vamvakas E, Kaplan HS: Early transfusion and length of survival in acquired immune deficiency syndrome: Experience with a population receiving medical care at a public hospital. Transfusion 33:111, 1993
53. Nightingale SL: Hypotension and bedside leukocyte reduction filters. JAMA 281:1978, 1999
54. Wylie BR: Transfusion transmitted infection: Viral and exotic diseases. Anaesth Intensive Care 21:24, 1993
55. Goodnough LT, Brecher ME, Kanter MH, Au Buchon JP: Transfusion medicine. 1. Blood transfusion. N Engl J Med 340:438, 1999
56. Schreiber GB, Busch MP, Kleinman SH, Korelitz JJ: The risk of transfusion-transmitted viral infections. N Engl J Med 334:1685, 1996
57. Conry-Cantilena C, VanRaden M, Gibble J et al: Routes of infection, viremia, and liver disease in blood donors found to have hepatitis C virus infection [see comments]. N Engl J Med 334:1691, 1996
58. Tong MJ, el-Farra NS, Reikes AR, Co RL: Clinical outcomes after transfusion-associated hepatitis C [see comments]. N Engl J Med 332:1463, 1995
59. Red blood cell transfusions contaminated with *Yersinia enterocolitica*—United States, 1991–1996, and initiation of a national study to detect bacteria-associated transfusion reactions. Morbidity and Mortality Weekly Report 46:553, 1997
60. Goodnough LT, Brecher ME: Autologous blood transfusion. Intern Med 37:238, 1998
61. Leveque CM, Yawn DH: Limiting homologous blood exposure. Clin Lab Med 12:771, 1992
62. Spiess BD, Sassetti R, McCarthy RJ et al: Autologous blood donation: Hemodynamics in a high-risk patient population. Transfusion 32:17, 1992
63. Monk TG, Goodnough LT: Blood conservation strategies to minimize allogeneic blood use in urologic surgery. Am J Surg 170:S69, 1995
64. Goodnough LT: The use of erythropoietin in the enhancement of autologous transfusion therapy. Curr Opin Hematol 2:214, 1995
65. Laupacis A, Fergusson D: Erythropoietin to minimize perioperative blood transfusion: A systematic review of randomized trials. Transfusion Med 8:309, 1998
66. Milbrink J, Birgegard G, Danersund A et al: Preoperative autologous donation of 6 units of blood during rh-EPO treatment. Can J Anaesth 44:1315, 1997
67. Monk TG, Goodnough LT, Brecher ME et al: A prospective randomized comparison of three blood conservation strategies for radical prostatectomy. Anesthesiology 91:24, 1999
68. Rosengart TK, Helm RE, Klemperer J et al: Combined aprotinin and erythropoietin use for blood conservation: Results with Jehovah's Witnesses. Ann Thorac Surg 58:1397, 1994
69. Feldman JM, Roth JV, Bjoraker DG: Maximum blood savings by acute normovolemic hemodilution. Anesth Analg 80:108, 1995
70. Bryson GL, Laupacis A, Wells GA: Does acute normovolemic hemodilution reduce perioperative allogeneic transfusion? A meta-analysis. Anesth Analg 86:9, 1998
71. Boldt J, Weber A, Mailer K et al: Acute normovolaemic haemodilution vs controlled hypotension for reducing the use of allogeneic blood in patients undergoing radical prostatectomy. Br J Anaesth 82:170, 1999
72. Ness PM, Bourke DL, Walsh PC: A randomized trial of perioperative hemodilution versus transfusion of preoperatively deposited autologous blood in elective surgery. Transfusion 32:226, 1992
73. Monk TG, Goodnough LT, Birkmeyer JD et al: Acute normovolemic hemodilution is a cost-effective alternative to preoperative autologous blood donation by patients undergoing radical retropubic prostatectomy. Transfusion 35:559, 1995
74. Williamson KR, Taswell HF: Intraoperative blood salvage—A review. Transfusion 31:662, 1991
75. Desmond MJ, Thomas MJG, Gillon J, Fox MA: Perioperative red cell salvage. Transfusion 36:644, 1996
76. Huet C, Salmi LR, Fergusson D et al: A meta-analysis of the effectiveness of cell salvage to minimize perioperative allogeneic blood transfusion in cardiac and orthopedic surgery. Anesth Analg 89:861, 1999
77. Fujimoto J, Okamoto E, Yamanaka N et al: Efficacy of autotransfusion in hepatectomy for hepatocellular carcinoma. Arch Surg 128:1065, 1993
78. Hart OJ, Klimberg IW, Wajsman Z, Baker J: Intraoperative autotransfusion in radical cystectomy for carcinoma of the bladder. Surg Gynecol Obstet 168:302, 1989
79. Bernstein HH, Rosenblatt MA, Gettes M, Lockwood C: The ability of the Haemonetics® 4 cell saver system to remove tissue factor from blood contaminated with amniotic fluid. Anesth Analg 85:831, 1997
80. Potter PS, Waters JH, Burger GA, Mraovic B: Application of cell-salvage during cesarean section. Anesthesiology 90:619, 1999
81. Silvergleid AJ: Safety and effectiveness of predeposit autologous transfusions in preteen and adolescent children. JAMA 257:3403, 1987
82. Tawes RL, Sydorak GR, DuVall TB: Postoperative salvage: A technological advance in the 'washed' versus 'unwashed' blood controversy. Semin Vasc Surg 7:99, 1994
83. McKie JS, Herzenberg JE: Coagulopathy complicating intraoperative blood salvage in a patient who had idiopathic scoliosis: A case report. J Bone Joint Surg (Am) 79A:1391, 1997
84. Griffith LD, Billman GF, Daily PO, Lane TA: Apparent coagulopathy caused by infusion of shed mediastinal blood and its prevention by washing of the infusate. Ann Thorac Surg 47:400, 1989
85. Rubin BG, Santoro SA, Sicard GA: Platelet interactions with the vessel wall and prosthetic grafts. Ann Vasc Surg 7:200, 1993

86. Bennett JS: Disorders of platelet function: Evaluation and treatment. Cleveland Clin J Med 58:413, 1991

87. Shattil SJ, Bennett JS: Platelets and their membranes in hemostasis: Physiology and pathophysiology. Ann Intern Med 94:108, 1981

88. Wu KK: Endothelial cells in hemostasis, thrombosis, and inflammation. Hosp Pract 27:145, 1992

89. Diethorn ML, Weld LM: Physiologic mechanisms of hemostasis and fibrinolysis. J Cardiovasc Nursing 4:1, 1989

90. Murphy WG, Davies MJ, Eduardo A: The haemostatic response to surgery and trauma. Br J Anaesth 70:205, 1993

91. Brandt JT: Current concepts of coagulation. Clin Obstet Gynecol 28:3, 1985

92. Bick RL: Disseminated intravascular coagulation: Objective laboratory diagnostic criteria and guidelines for management. Clin Lab Med 14:729, 1994

93. Mackie IJ, Pittilo RM: Vascular integrity and platelet function. Int Anesthesiol Clin 23:3, 1985

94. Stormorken H: The hemostatic mechanism: The role of platelets in physiology and bleeding states. Scand J Gastroenterol 137(suppl):1, 1987

95. Pottmeyer E, Vassar MJ, Holcroft JW: Coagulation, inflammation, and responses to injury. Crit Care Clin 2:683, 1986

96. Broze GJ: The role of tissue factor pathway inhibitor in a revised coagulation cascade. Semin Hematol 29:159, 1992

97. Drake TA, Morrissey JH, Edgington TS: Selective cellular expression of tissue factor in human tissues. Implications for disorders of hemostasis and thrombosis. Am J Pathol 134:1087, 1989

98. Wilcox JN, Smith KM, Schwartz SM, Gordon D: Localization of tissue factor in the normal vessel wall and in the atherosclerotic plaque. Proc Natl Acad Sci USA 86:2839, 1989

99. Fleck RA, Rao LVM, Rapaport SI, Varki N: Localization of human tissue factor antigen by immunostaining with monospecific, polyclonal anti-human tissue factor antibody. Thromb Res 57:765, 1990

100. Callander NS, Varki N, Rao LVM: Immunohistochemical identification of tissue factor in solid tumors. Cancer 70:1194, 1992

101. Rapaport SI, Rao LVM: Initiation and regulation of tissue factor-dependent blood coagulation. Arterioscler Thromb 12:1111, 1992

102. Broze G, Majerus P: Human factor VII. Methods Enzymol 80(PC):228, 1982

103. Bevilacqua MP, Pober JS, Majeau GR et al: Interleukin 1 (IL-1) induces biosynthesis and cell surface expression of procoagulant activity in human vascular endothelial cells. J Exp Med 160:618, 1984

104. Bevilacqua MP, Pober JS, Majeau GR et al: Recombinant tumor necrosis factor induces procoagulant activity in cultured human vascular endothelium: Characterization and comparison with the actions of interleukin 1. Proc Natl Acad Sci USA 83:4533, 1986

105. Lerner RG, Goldstein R, Cummings G, Lange K: Stimulation of human leukocyte thromboplastic activity by endotoxin. Proc Soc Exp Biol Med 138:145, 1971

106. Muhlfelder TW, Niemetz J, Kreutzer D et al: C5 chemotactic fragment induces leukocyte production of tissue factor activity: A link between complement and coagulation. J Clin Invest 63:147, 1979

107. Rothberger H, Zimmerman TS, Spiegelberg HL, Vaughan JH: Leukocyte procoagulant activity: Enhancement of production in vitro by IgG and antigen-antibody complexes. J Clin Invest 59:549, 1977

108. Osterud B, Flaegstad T: Increased tissue thromboplastin activity in monocytes of patients with meningococcal infection: Related to an unfavourable prognosis. Thromb Haemost 49:5, 1983

109. Bauer KA: Hypercoagulability—A new cofactor in the protein C anticoagulant pathway. N Engl J Med 330:566, 1994

110. Dahlback B: Protein S and C4b-binding protein: Components involved in the regulation of the protein C anticoagulant system. Thromb Haemost 66:49, 1991

111. Mehta JL, Kitchens CS: Pharmacology of platelet-inhibitory drugs, anticoagulants, and thrombolytic agents. Cardiovasc Clin 18:163, 1987

112. High KA: Antithrombin III, protein C, and protein S. Naturally occurring anticoagulant proteins. Arch Pathol Lab Med 112:28, 1988

113. Wight TN: Vessel proteoglycans and thrombogenesis. Prog Hemost Thromb 5:1, 1980

114. Rosenberg RD: Biochemistry of heparin antithrombin interactions, and the physiologic role of this natural anticoagulant mechanism. Am J Med 87:2S, 1989

115. Büller HR, ten Cate JW: Acquired antithrombin III deficiency: Laboratory diagnosis, incidence, clinical implications, and treatment with antithrombin III concentrate. Am J Med 87:44S, 1989

116. Schwartz RS, Bauer KA, Rosenberg RD et al: Clinical experience with antithrombin III concentrate in treatment of congenital and acquired deficiency of antithrombin. The Antithrombin III Study Group. Am J Med 87:53S, 1989

117. Nilsson IM: Coagulation and fibrinolysis. Scand J Gastroenterol 137(suppl):11, 1987

118. Wessler S, Gitel SN: Pharmacology of heparin and warfarin. J Am Coll Cardiol 8:10B, 1986

119. Bone RC: Modulators of coagulation: A critical appraisal of their role in sepsis. Arch Intern Med 152:1381, 1992

120. Rodgers RPC, Levin J: A critical reappraisal of the bleeding time. Semin Thromb Hemost 16:1, 1990

121. Nemerson Y: The tissue factor pathway of blood coagulation. Semin Hematol 29:170, 1992

122. Poller L: The British system for anticoagulant control. Thromb Diath Haemorrh 33:157, 1975

123. Henriksen R: Instrumentation and quality control of hemostasis. In Lotspiech-Steininger C, Steine-Martin E, Koepke J (eds): Clinical Hematology, p 695. Philadelphia, JB Lippincott, 1992

124. Ellison N, Silberstein LE: Hemostasis in the perioperative period. In Stoelting RK, Barash PG, Gallagher TJ (eds): Advances in Anesthesia, p 67. Chicago, Year Book Medical Publishers, 1986

125. Freiberger JJ, Lumb PD: How to manage intraoperative bleeding. In Vaughn RW (ed): Perioperative Problems/Catastrophes, p 161. Philadelphia, JB Lippincott, 1987

126. Triplett DA: Overview of hemostasis. In Menitove JE, McCarthy LJ (eds): Hemostatic Disorders and the Blood Bank, p 1. Arlington, VA, American Association of Blood Banks, 1984

127. Traverso CI, Caprini JA, Arcelus JI: The normal thromboelastogram and its interpretation. Semin Thromb Hemost 21:7, 1995

128. Tuman KJ, Spiess BD, McCarthy RJ, Ivankovich AD: Effects of progressive blood loss on coagulation as measured by thromboelastography. Anesth Analg 66:856, 1987

129. Kang W: Blood coagulation during liver, kidney, and pancreas transplantation. In Lake CL, Moore RA (eds): Blood: Hemostasis, Transfusion, and Alternatives in the Perioperative Period, p 529. New York, Raven Press, 1995

130. Zuckerman L, Cohen E, Vagher JP et al: Comparison of thromboelastography with common coagulation tests. Thromb Haemost 46:752, 1981

131. Angelos MG, Hamilton GC: Coagulation studies: Prothrombin time, partial thromboplastin time, bleeding time. Emerg Med Clin North Am 4:95, 1986

132. Colonotero G, Cockerill KJ, Bowie EJW: How to diagnose bleeding disorders. Postgrad Med 90:145, 1991

133. Association of Hemophilia Clinic Directors of Canada: Hemophilia and von Willebrand's disease: 1. Diagnosis, comprehensive care and assessment. Canadian Medical Association Journal 153:19, 1995

134. Vischer UM, de Moerloose P: von Willebrand factor: From cell biology to the clinical management of von Willebrand's disease. Crit Rev Oncol Hematol 30:93, 1999

135. Harrison RL, McKee PA: Estrogen stimulates von Willebrand factor production by cultured endothelial cells. Blood 63:657, 1984

136. Dalton RG, Dewar MS, Savidge GF et al: Hypothyroidism as a cause of acquired von Willebrand's disease. Lancet 1:1007, 1987

137. Gill JC, Endres-Brooks J, Bauer PJ et al: The effect of ABO blood group on the diagnosis of von Willebrand disease. Blood 69:1691, 1987

138. Mohlke KL, Ginsburg D: von Willebrand disease and quantitative variation in von Willebrand factor. J Lab Clin Med 130:252, 1997

139. Ruggeri ZM: Structure and function of von Willebrand factor: Relationship to von Willebrand's disease. Mayo Clin Proc 66:847, 1991

140. Sadler JE, Matsushita T, Dong ZY et al: Molecular mechanism and classification of von Willebrand disease. Thromb Haemost 74:161, 1995

141. Ryden SE, Oberman HA: Compatibility of common intravenous solutions with CPD blood. Transfusion 15:250, 1975

142. Mannucci PM, Lombardi R, Bader R et al: Heterogeneity of type I von Willebrand disease: Evidence for a subgroup with an abnormal von Willebrand factor. Blood 66:796, 1985

143. Goudemand J, Mazurier C, Marey A et al: Clinical and biological evaluation in von Willebrand's disease of a von Willebrand factor

concentrate with low factor VIII activity. Br J Haematol 80:214, 1992

144. McLoughlin TM, Greilich PE: Preexisting hemostatic defects and bleeding disorders. In Lake CL, Moore RA (eds): Blood: Hemostasis, Transfusion, and Alternatives in the Perioperative Period, p 25. New York, Raven Press, 1995

145. Schrier SL: Disorders of hemostasis and coagulation. In: Care of the Surgical Patient, p 1. New York, Scientific American, 1993

146. Warrier AI, Lusher JM: DDAVP: A useful alternative to blood components in moderate hemophilia A and von Willebrand disease. J Pediatr 102:228, 1983

147. DeLoughery TG: Management of bleeding with uremia and liver disease. Curr Opin Hematol 6:329, 1999

148. Lethagen S: Desmopressin—a haemostatic drug: State-of-the-art review. Eur J Anaesthesiol 14:1, 1997

149. Bednar MM, Gross CE: Antiplatelet therapy in acute cerebral ischemia. Stroke 30:887, 1999

150. Mehta JL, Kitchens CS: Pharmacology of platelet-inhibitory drugs, anticoagulants, and thrombolytic agents. Cardiovasc Clin 18:163, 1987

151. DeWitt DL: Cox-2-selective inhibitors: The new super aspirins. Mol Pharmacol 55:625, 1999

152. Harker LA, Fuster V: Pharmacology of platelet inhibitors. J Am Coll Cardiol 8:21B, 1986

153. Schussheim AE, Fuster V: Thrombosis, antithrombotic agents, and the antithrombotic approach in cardiac disease. Prog Cardiovasc Dis 40:205, 1997

154. Staudinger T, Locker GJ, Frass M: Management of acquired coagulation disorders in emergency and intensive-care medicine. Sem Thromb Hemost 22:93, 1996

155. Raj G, Kumar R, McKinney WP: Long-term oral anticoagulant therapy: Update on indications, therapeutic ranges, and monitoring. Am J Med Sci 307:128, 1994

156. Messmore H, Upadhyay G, Farid S et al: Heparin-induced thrombocytopenia and thrombosis in cardiovascular surgery. In Pifarre R (ed): New Anticoagulants for the Cardiovascular Patient, p 83. Philadelphia, Hanley & Belfus, 1997

157. Despotis GJ, Gravlee G, Filos K, Levy J: Anticoagulation monitoring during cardiac surgery: A review of current and emerging techniques. Anesthesiology 91:1122, 1999

158. Despotis GJ, Joist JH: Anticoagulation and anticoagulation reversal with cardiac surgery involving cardiopulmonary bypass: An update. J Cardiothorac Vasc Anesth 13:18, 1999

159. Okita Y, Takamoto S, Ando M et al: Coagulation and fibrinolysis system in aortic surgery under deep hypothermic circulatory arrest with aprotinin: The importance of adequate heparinization. Circulation 96:376, 1997

160. Body SC, Morse DS: Coagulation, transfusion and cardiac surgery. In Spiess BD, Counts RB, Gould SA (eds): Perioperative Transfusion Medicine, p 419. Baltimore, Williams & Wilkins, 1998

161. Salmenpera MT, Levy JH: Pharmacologic manipulation of hemostasis. In Lake CL, Moore RA (eds): Blood: Hemostasis, Transfusion, and Alternatives in the Perioperative Period, p 105. New York, Raven Press, 1995

162. Despotis GJ, Skubas NJ, Goodnough LT: Optimal management of bleeding and transfusion in patients undergoing cardiac surgery. Semin Thorac Cardiovasc Surg 11:84, 1999

163. Schwarz RP: The preclinical and clinical pharmacology of novastan (Argatroban). In Pifarre R (ed): New Anticoagulants for the Cardiovascular Patient, p 231. Philadelphia, Hanley & Belfus, 1997

164. Ganjoo AK, Harloff MG, Johnson WD: Cardiopulmonary bypass for heparin-induced thrombocytopenia: Management with a heparin-bonded circuit and enoxaparin. J Thorac Cardiovasc Surg 112:1390, 1996

165. Mammen EF: Coagulation defects in liver disease. Med Clin North Am 78:545, 1994

166. Bakker CM, Knot EAR, Stibbe J, Wilson JHP: Disseminated intravascular coagulation in liver cirrhosis. J Hepatol 15:330, 1992

167. Rocha E, Paramo JA, Montes R, Panizo C: Acute generalized, widespread bleeding: Diagnosis and management. Haematologica 83:1024, 1998

168. Carey MJ, Rodgers GM: Disseminated intravascular coagulation: Clinical and laboratory aspects. Am J Hematol 59:65, 1998

169. Bick RL: Disseminated intravascular coagulation: Objective criteria for diagnosis and management. Med Clin North Am 78:511, 1994

170. Carr ME Jr: Disseminated intravascular coagulation: Pathogenesis, diagnosis, and therapy. J Emerg Med 5:311, 1987

171. Lechner K, Kyrle PA: Antithrombin III concentrates—Are they clinically useful? Thromb Haemost 73:340, 1995

172. Perez WE, Viets JL: Transfusion and coagulation: An overview and recent advances in practice modalities. Part I: Blood banking and transfusion practices. Nurse Anesth 1:149, 1990

173. Anonymous: Consensus conference. Fresh-frozen plasma: Indications and risks. JAMA 253:551, 1985

174. Coffin CM: Current issues in transfusion therapy. 2. Indications for use of blood components. Postgrad Med 81:343, 1987

175. Azzi A, Morfini M, Mannucci PM: The transfusion-associated transmission of parvovirus B19. Transfusion Med Rev 13:194, 1999

176. Reiner A: Massive transfusion. In Spiess B, Counts R, Gould S (eds): Perioperative Transfusion Medicine, p 351. Baltimore, Williams & Wilkins, 1998

177. Stehling L: Blood component therapy. In Lake C, Moore R (eds): Blood: Hemostasis, Transfusion, and Alternatives in the Perioperative Period, p 277. New York, Raven Press, 1995

178. Mannucci P: Clinical evaluation of viral safety of coagulation factor VIII and IX concentrates. Vox Sang 64:197, 1993

179. Vinazzer H: Clinical use of antithrombin III concentrates. Vox Sang 53:193, 1997

180. Cattaneo M, Harris AS, Stromberg U, Mannucci PM: The effect of desmopressin on reducing blood loss in cardiac surgery: A meta-analysis of double-blind, placebo-controlled trials. Thromb Haemost 74:1064, 1995

181. Salzman EW, Weinstein MJ, Weintraub RM et al: Treatment with desmopressin acetate to reduce blood loss after cardiac surgery: A double-blind randomized trial. N Engl J Med 314:1402, 1986

182. Czer LS, Bateman TM, Gray RJ: Treatment of severe platelet dysfunction and hemorrhage after cardiopulmonary bypass: Reduction in blood product usage with desmopressin. J Am Coll Cardiol 9:1139, 1987

183. Mongan PD, Hosking MP: The role of desmopressin acetate in patients undergoing coronary artery bypass surgery: A controlled clinical trial with thromboelastographic risk stratification. Anesthesiology 77:38, 1992

184. Gratz I, Koehler J, Olsen D et al: The effect of desmopressin acetate on postoperative hemorrhage in patients receiving aspirin therapy before coronary artery bypass operations. J Thorac Cardiovasc Surg 104:1417, 1992

185. Vanoeveren W, Harder MP, Roozendaal KJ et al: Aprotinin protects platelets against the initial effect of cardiopulmonary bypass. J Thorac Cardiovasc Surg 99:788, 1990

186. Lentschener C, Benhamou D: The blood sparing effect of aprotinin should be revisited. Anesthesiology 89:1598, 1998

187. Levi M, Cromheecke ME, de Jonge E et al: Pharmacological strategies to decrease excessive blood loss in cardiac surgery: A meta-analysis of clinically relevant endpoints. Lancet 354:1940, 1999

188. Munoz JJ, Birkmeyer NJO, Birkmeyer JD et al: Is ε-aminocaproic acid as effective as aprotinin in reducing bleeding with cardiac surgery? A meta-analysis. Circulation 99:81, 1999

189. Casati V, Guzzon D, Oppizzi M et al: Hemostatic effects of aprotinin, tranexamic acid and ε-aminocaproic acid in primary cardiac surgery. Ann Thorac Surg 68:2252, 1999

190. Porte RJ, Bontempo FA, Knot EA et al: Systemic effects of tissue plasminogen activator-associated fibrinolysis and its relation to thrombin generation in orthotopic liver transplantation. Transplantation 47:978, 1989

191. Grosse H, Lobbes W, Frambach M et al: The use of high dose aprotinin in liver transplantation: The influence on fibrinolysis and blood loss. Thromb Res 63:287, 1991

192. Kang Y, Lewis JH, Navalgund A et al: ε-Aminocaproic acid for treatment of fibrinolysis during liver transplantation. Anesthesiology 66:766, 1987

193. Carlier M, Veyckemans F, Scholtes JL et al: Anesthesia for pediatric hepatic transplantation: Experience of 33 cases. Transplant Proc 19:3333, 1987

194. Garcia L, Sabate A, Domenech P et al: Aprotinin in orthotopic liver transplantation. Transplant Proc 27:2290, 1995

195. Kufner RP: Antifibrinolytics and orthotopic liver transplantation. Transplant Proc 30:692, 1998

THREE

BASIC PRINCIPLES OF PHARMACOLOGY IN ANESTHESIA PRACTICE

Clinical Anesthesia (4/e), edited by Paul G. Barash, Bruce F. Cullen, and Robert K. Stoelting. Lippincott Williams & Wilkins, Philadelphia, © 2001.

CHAPTER 11

BASIC PRINCIPLES OF CLINICAL PHARMACOLOGY

ROBERT J. HUDSON

More than 30 years ago, Dr. E. M. Papper[1] emphasized the importance of understanding the pharmacology of anesthetics:

Clinical anaesthetists have administered millions of anaesthetics during more than a century with little precise information of the uptake, distribution, and elimination of inhalational and non-volatile anaesthetic agents. Considering how serious is the handi-cap of not knowing those fundamental and important facts about the drugs they have used so often, the record of success and safety in clinical anaesthesia is an extraordinary accomplishment in-deed. It can in some measure be attributed to the accumulated experience and successful teaching of a highly developed sense of intuition from generation to generation of anaesthetists. It can also be attributed in part to the ability to learn by error after ob-serving patients come uncomfortably close to injury and even to death.

In the last few years, however, sufficient fundamental informa-tion has become available to explain these clinical successes. The empirical process of giving an anaesthetic can be better understood because of the specific data provided by the studies reported in this symposium and by the work of others which has preceded them.

Understanding the principles of pharmacology and knowl-edge of the specific properties of individual drugs are even more important today. New anesthetics, opioids, and neuromuscular blockers have recently become available. We do not have the benefit of decades of experience with these new drugs, so we must depend on carefully conducted investigations for the information needed to use them optimally. As Dr. Papper wrote,

If the anaesthetist studies the pharmacology of these agents and un-derstands their pharmacokinetic properties, he can with reasonable certainty predict which of these newer anaesthetic agents will hold promise for clinical utility . . . the clinician can spare his patients much danger and his own work many hardships if he is aware of the physicochemical and pharmacological [properties] of new agents.

Our patients are also changing. Many have concomitant dis-eases that were once considered contraindications to anesthesia and surgery. Therefore, we must consider the impact of chronic diseases, and of the drugs used to treat them, on the responses to drugs administered during the perioperative period. Com-prehensive knowledge of clinical pharmacology is a prerequisite to the practice of anesthesiology.

The first sections of this chapter discuss the biologic and pharmacologic factors that influence drug absorption, distribu-tion, and elimination. Quantitative analysis of these processes is discussed in the section on pharmacokinetics. The next section presents the fundamentals of pharmacodynamics—those fac-tors that determine the relationship between drug concentra-tion and pharmacologic effects. Clinical application of pharma-cokinetics and pharmacodynamics is then reviewed. The final section briefly presents the mechanisms of drug interactions. Although specific properties of drugs are used to illustrate basic pharmacologic principles, detailed information regarding the pharmacology of drugs used in anesthesiology is presented in succeeding chapters.

TRANSFER OF DRUGS ACROSS MEMBRANES

Absorption, distribution, metabolism, and excretion of drugs require their transfer across cell membranes. Most drugs must also traverse cell membranes to reach their sites of action. Bio-logic membranes consist of a lipid bilayer with a nonpolar core and polar elements on their surfaces. Proteins are embedded in the lipid bilayer and are oriented similarly, with ionic, polar groups on the membrane surfaces and hydrophobic groups in the membrane interior. The nonpolar core hinders the passage of water-soluble molecules, so that only lipid-soluble molecules easily traverse cell membranes.

Transport Processes

Drugs can cross cell membranes either by passive processes or by active transport through the membrane. *Passive diffusion* occurs when a concentration gradient exists across a membrane. The rate of passive transfer is directly proportional to the con-centration gradient and the lipid solubility of the drug. Passage of water-soluble drugs is restricted to small aqueous channels through the membrane. These channels are so narrow that only molecules smaller than 200 D pass through them readily. Capillary endothelial cells, except those in the central nervous system (CNS), permit transfer of much larger molecules, such as albumin (molecular weight ~67,000 D). Because of these unique features, diffusion of drugs across capillary membranes outside the CNS is limited by blood flow, not by lipid solubility.[2]

Some drugs are transferred through cell membranes of hepa-tocytes, renal tubular cells, and others by *active transport*. This is an energy-requiring process that is both specific and saturable. Active transport can pump compounds against their concentra-tion gradients. *Facilitated diffusion* shares some characteristics with active transport. It is also carrier-mediated, specific, and saturable, but does not require energy and cannot overcome a concentration gradient.[2]

Effects of Molecular Properties

Most drugs are too large to pass through cellular membrane channels and must traverse the lipid component of membranes. Almost all drugs are either weak acids or weak bases, and are present in both ionized and nonionized forms at physiologic pH. The nonionized form is more lipid-soluble and able easily to traverse cell membranes. The nonionized fraction of weak acids, such as salicylates and barbiturates, is greater at low pH values, so acidic drugs become more lipid-soluble as pH de-creases. The nonionized fraction of weak bases like opioids and local anesthetics increases as the pH becomes more alkaline. The pK_a is the pH at which exactly 50% of a weak acid or base is present in each of the ionized and nonionized forms. The closer the pK_a is to the ambient pH, the greater the change in the degree of ionization for a given change in pH. If there is a pH gradient across a membrane, drug will be trapped on the side that has the higher ionized fraction, because only the nonionized drug is diffusible. This phenomenon is known as *ion trapping.* The total drug concentration is greater on the side of the membrane with the higher ionized fraction. However, at equilibrium, the concentration of nonionized drug will be the same. In most situations, the range of pH values is too small to cause major changes in the degree of ionization. However, there are major pH changes in the upper gastrointestinal (GI) tract, which can affect drug absorption.

DRUG ABSORPTION

Except after intravenous (iv) injections, drugs must be absorbed into the circulation before they can be delivered to their sites of action. Therefore, absorption is an important determinant of both the intensity and duration of drug action. Incomplete absorption limits the amount of drug reaching the site of action, reducing the peak pharmacologic effect. Rapid absorption is a prerequisite for rapid onset of action. In contrast, slow absorption permits a sustained duration of action because of the "depot" of drug at the absorptive site. The speed of absorption depends on the solubility and concentration of drug. All drugs must dissolve in water to reach the circulation. Consequently, drugs in aqueous solutions are absorbed faster than those in solid formulations, suspensions, or organic solvents, such as propylene glycol. A high concentration of drug facilitates absorption. Increased blood flow to the site of injection increases the rate of absorption. Decreased blood flow secondary to hypotension, vasoconstrictors, or other factors slows drug absorption. Vasoconstrictors added to local anesthetics delay absorption after subcutaneous injection. This prolongs the duration of action at the site of injection and lessens the chance of systemic toxicity.

Route of Administration

In general medical practice, drugs are most commonly administered orally. The advantages of oral administration are convenience, economy, and safety. Disadvantages include the requirement for a cooperative patient, incomplete absorption, and metabolism of the drug in the GI tract and liver before it reaches the systemic circulation.[2] In anesthesia, drugs are most frequently administered *via* iv and inhalational routes. Both permit rapid and reasonably predictable attainment of the desired blood concentration.

Oral Administration

Absorption from the GI tract is highly variable because of the multiple factors involved. Tablets and capsules must disintegrate before the drug can dissolve in the GI lumen. The drug must then cross the GI epithelium and pass into the portal circulation. The most important site of absorption of all drugs is the small intestine, because of its large surface area and the anatomic characteristics of its mucosa. The nonionized fraction of weak acids such as barbiturates is higher at low pH values, which favors absorption from the stomach. However, the effect of pH on ionization of acidic drugs in the stomach is offset by the small surface area and thickness of the gastric mucosa, and the rapidity of gastric emptying. Basic drugs are highly ionized at low pH, so they cannot cross the gastric mucosa. The more alkaline pH of the small intestine increases the nonionized fraction of basic drugs such as opioids, facilitating their absorption.

Once drugs enter the portal circulation, they must traverse the liver before reaching the systemic circulation. Some drugs are extensively metabolized during this initial pass through the liver, so that only a small fraction of the drug reaches the systemic circulation. This is called the *first-pass effect.* Depending on the magnitude of the first-pass effect, the oral dose must be proportionally larger than the iv dose to achieve the same

pharmacologic response. Metabolism of some drugs by the GI mucosa also contributes to the first-pass effect.[3]

Sublingual Administration

Drug absorbed from the oral mucosa passes directly into the systemic circulation, eliminating the first-pass effect. Because of the small surface area for absorption, this route is efficacious only for nonionized, highly lipid-soluble drugs, such as nitroglycerin.

Rectal Administration

The first-pass effect is less evident after rectal administration because much of the drug is absorbed into the systemic circulation. Unfortunately, absorption from the rectum is often erratic and incomplete.[2]

Transcutaneous Administration

Only lipid-soluble drugs can penetrate intact skin sufficiently to produce systemic effects. Drug "patches" applied to the skin are now widely used. These systems consist of an adhesive containing a reservoir of drug that is slowly released after the patch is applied, producing a stable pharmacologic effect. Drugs currently administered in this fashion include scopolamine (for motion sickness) and nitroglycerin. Opioid patches are used for treatment of chronic pain. Transcutaneous absorption of drugs from patches is passive, so the onset time is delayed. This disadvantage can be overcome by using an electric current to "drive" ionized drugs into the skin, a process is called *iontophoresis.* Trancutaneous iontophoretic administration of fentanyl has been described.[4]

Intramuscular and Subcutaneous Injection

Absorption of drugs from subcutaneous tissue is relatively slow, permitting a sustained effect. The rate of absorption can be altered by changes in the drug formulation. Examples of such manipulations are the various preparations of insulin and the addition of vasoconstrictors to local anesthetic solutions. Uptake of drugs after intramuscular injection is more rapid than after subcutaneous administration because of greater blood flow. Drugs in aqueous solution are very readily absorbed. The effect of drugs in nonaqueous solutions, such as diazepam in propylene glycol, is less predictable because of erratic absorption.[5]

Intrathecal, Epidural, and Perineural Injection

Intrathecal injection of local anesthetics or other drugs close to their sites of action in the spinal cord permits the use of very low doses, eliminating the risk of adverse systemic drug effects. This is not an advantage of epidural anesthesia or major perineural regional anesthesia because of the greater total dose required. The major disadvantage of these routes of injection is the expertise they require.

Inhalational Administration

Uptake of inhalational anesthetics from the pulmonary alveoli to the blood is exceedingly rapid because of their low molecular weight and high lipid solubility, the large total alveolar surface area and because alveolar blood flow is almost equal to cardiac output.

Intravenous Injection

Intravenous injection eliminates the need for absorption, so that therapeutic blood concentrations are rapidly attained. This is especially advantageous when rapid onset of action is desired. It also simplifies titration of the dose to individual patients' responses. Unfortunately, rapid onset also has its hazards;

should an adverse drug reaction or overdose occur, the effects are immediate and potentially severe.

Bioavailability

Bioavailability is defined as the fraction of the total dose that reaches the systemic circulation. Bioavailability is reduced by factors such as incomplete absorption from the site of injection or GI tract, the first-pass effect, or pulmonary uptake of drugs.

Even after iv injection, the bioavailability of drugs formulated in lipid suspensions may be less than 100%. These suspensions contain small lipid droplets. Some, but not all, of the drug diffuses from the lipid droplets into the plasma. These droplets are taken up by the liver and metabolized. Presumably, some drug is also metabolized before it is released back into the circulation. The bioavailability of the lecithin suspension of diazepam is 30% less than that of diazepam in propylene glycol, even with direct iv injection.[6]

DRUG DISTRIBUTION

After absorption or injection into the systemic circulation, drugs are distributed throughout the body. Highly perfused organs, such as the brain, heart, lungs, liver, and kidneys, receive most of the drug soon after injection. Delivery to muscle, skin, fat, and other less well perfused tissues is slower, and equilibration of distribution into these tissues may take several hours or even days.

Capillary membranes are freely permeable in most tissues, so drugs quickly pass into the extracellular space. Subsequent distribution varies according to the physicochemical properties of the drug. Distribution of highly polar, water-soluble drugs such as the neuromuscular blockers is essentially limited to extracellular fluid. Lipid-soluble drugs like propofol easily cross cell membranes and are therefore distributed much more extensively.

Distribution of drugs into the CNS is unique. Brain capillaries do not have the large aqueous channels typical of capillaries in other tissues. Consequently, diffusion of water-soluble drugs into the brain is severely restricted. In contrast, distribution of highly lipid-soluble drugs into the CNS is limited only by cerebral blood flow. For more polar compounds, the rate of entry into the brain is proportional to the lipid solubility of the nonionized drug.

Drugs accumulate in tissues because of binding to tissue components, pH gradients, or uptake of lipophilic drugs into fat. These tissue stores can act as reservoirs that prolong the duration of drug action, either in the same tissue, or by delivery to the site of action elsewhere after reabsorption into the circulation.

Binding of drugs to plasma proteins and erythrocytes influences distribution to other tissues. Only free, unbound drug can cross capillary membranes. The extent of tissue uptake of drugs depends on the affinity of drug binding to blood constituents, relative to the overall affinity of binding to tissue components.

Redistribution

The rapid entry and equally rapid egress of lipophilic drugs from richly perfused organs such as the brain and heart is referred to as *redistribution*. This phenomenon is illustrated by the events that follow an injection of thiopental. The brain concentration of thiopental peaks within 1 minute because of high blood flow to the brain and the high lipid solubility of thiopental. As the drug is taken up by other, less well perfused tissues, the plasma level rapidly decreases. This creates a concentration gradient from cerebral tissue to the blood, so that thiopental quickly diffuses back into the blood, where it is redistributed to other tissues that are still taking up drug. Ultimately, adipose tissue contains most of the drug remaining in the body

because of the high lipid solubility of thiopental. However, recovery from a single dose of thiopental depends predominantly on redistribution of thiopental from the brain to muscle, because of the larger mass and greater perfusion of muscle compared to adipose tissue.[7,8]

A single moderate dose of thiopental (<5–6 mg $\cdot$ kg^{-1}) has a very short duration of action because of redistribution. If repeated injections are given, the concentration of thiopental builds up in the peripheral tissues, and termination of drug action becomes increasingly dependent on the much slower process of drug elimination. Termination of the pharmacologic effects of other lipophilic drugs, such as fentanyl and its derivatives, and propofol, is also governed by these factors.

Placental Transfer

Most drugs cross the placenta by simple diffusion, so thiopental and other lipid-soluble drugs with low molecular weights are most readily transferred. Highly polar, water-soluble compounds such as the neuromuscular blocking drugs do not cross the placenta to a significant extent. Fetal pH is slightly lower than maternal pH. This pH gradient causes the ionized fraction of weak bases, such as opioids and local anesthetics, to be higher in the fetus. Therefore, the fetal total drug level may be higher than predicted from the maternal total drug level because of ion trapping.[9] Different total drug concentrations can also result from differences between mother and fetus in the extent of drug binding to plasma proteins. However, regardless of the effects of pH and protein binding, the concentration of free, nonionized drug is the same on both sides of the placenta once equilibrium is reached. For most drugs, this is the most important form, because it has the most pharmacologic activity.

DRUG ELIMINATION

Elimination is an inclusive term referring to all the processes that remove drugs from the body. Elimination occurs either by excretion of unchanged drug or by metabolism (biotransformation) and subsequent excretion of metabolites. The liver and kidneys are the most important organs for drug elimination. The liver eliminates drugs primarily by metabolism to less active compounds and, to a lesser extent, by hepatobiliary excretion of drugs or their metabolites. The primary role of the kidneys is the excretion of water-soluble, polar compounds. Drugs having these properties, such as most nondepolarizing neuromuscular blockers, undergo renal excretion intact.[10] The kidneys are also the primary route for excretion of water-soluble metabolites of drugs that initially undergo hepatic biotransformation. Pulmonary excretion is the major route for elimination of anesthetic gases and vapors.

The term *drug clearance*, or *elimination clearance*, describes the ability to remove drug from the blood. Drug clearance is the theoretical volume of blood from which drug is completely and irreversibly removed in a given time interval. It is analogous to creatinine clearance, which quantitatively describes the ability of the kidneys to eliminate creatinine. Like creatinine clearance, drug clearance has units of flow, milliliters per minute (mL $\cdot$ min^{-1}). Many drugs are cleared by more than one route, and multiple elimination pathways are additive. Consequently, total drug clearance is equal to the sum of the clearances of all of the elimination pathways.

Total drug clearance can be calculated with pharmacokinetic models of blood concentration *versus* time data. However, clearance by individual organs and the biologic factors influencing drug elimination cannot be estimated from blood concentration data alone. Additional data, such as the hepatic arteriovenous drug concentration difference or the rate of urinary excretion of the drug, are needed to determine the contribution of a specific organ to total drug clearance.

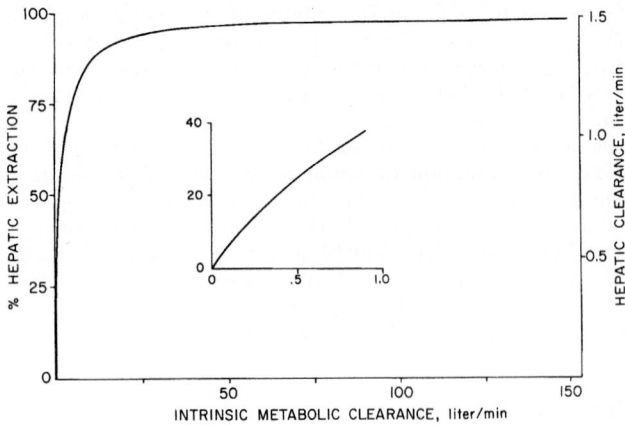

Figure 11-1. The relationship between hepatic extraction ratio, intrinsic clearance, and hepatic clearance at the normal hepatic blood flow of 1.5 L · min^{-1}. For drugs with high intrinsic clearance (>25 L · min^{-1}), increasing intrinsic clearance has little effect on hepatic extraction and total hepatic clearance. The inset demonstrates the relationship at low values of intrinsic clearance on an expanded scale. (Reprinted with permission from Wilkinson GR, Shand DG: A physiologic approach to hepatic drug clearance. Clin Pharmacol Ther 18:377, 1975.)

Hepatic Drug Clearance

Drug clearance by the liver is dependent on three biologic factors: (1) hepatic blood flow, (2) the intrinsic ability of the liver to irreversibly eliminate the drug from the blood, and (3) the extent of drug binding to plasma proteins or other blood constituents. The interrelationships between these factors have been described with the *venous equilibration model* of hepatic drug clearance.[11,12] According to this model, the unbound concentration of drug in hepatic venous blood is in equilibrium with the unbound concentration in hepatocytes. The unbound drug within the liver is the drug that can be eliminated by biotransformation or biliary excretion.

The venous equilibration model is based on two assumptions: that hepatic drug clearance is limited by delivery of drug to the liver, and that elimination is a first-order process.[11] By definition, *first-order* means that a constant fraction of the drug is eliminated per unit time. The fraction of the drug removed from the blood passing through the liver is the hepatic extraction ratio, *E*:

$$E = \frac{C_a - C_v}{C_a}, \tag{11-1}$$

where C_a is the mixed hepatic arterial–portal venous drug concentration and C_v is the mixed hepatic venous drug concentration. The total hepatic drug clearance, Cl_H, is:

$$Cl_H = Q \cdot E, \tag{11-2}$$

where Q is hepatic blood flow. Therefore, hepatic clearance is a function of hepatic blood flow and the ability of the liver to extract drug from the blood. The ability to extract drug depends on the activity of drug-metabolizing enzymes and the capacity for hepatobiliary excretion.

The concept of *intrinsic clearance* was developed to account for the effects of blood flow and drug binding in the blood on elimination.[11] Intrinsic clearance represents the ability of the liver to remove drug from the blood in the absence of any limitations imposed by blood flow or drug binding. The relationship of total hepatic drug clearance to the extraction ratio and intrinsic clearance, Cl_i, is:

$$Cl_H = Q \cdot E = Q \left(\frac{Cl_i}{Q + Cl_i} \right) \tag{11-3}$$

The right-hand side of Equation 11-3 indicates that if intrinsic clearance is very high (many times larger than hepatic blood flow), total hepatic clearance approaches hepatic blood flow. On the other hand, if intrinsic clearance is very small, hepatic clearance will be similar to intrinsic clearance. These relationships are shown in Figure 11-1.

Thus, hepatic drug clearance and extraction are determined by two independent variables, intrinsic clearance and hepatic blood flow. Changes in either will change hepatic clearance. However, the extent of the change depends on the initial intrinsic clearance. If the inherent ability of the liver to eliminate a drug (intrinsic clearance) is doubled, then the extraction ratio also increases, but not necessarily to the same extent. The extraction ratio and intrinsic clearance do not have a simple, linear relationship:

$$E = \frac{Cl_i}{Q + Cl_i} \tag{11-4}$$

If the initial intrinsic clearance is small relative to hepatic blood flow, then the extraction ratio is also small, and Equation 11-4 indicates that doubling intrinsic clearance will produce an almost proportional increment in the extraction ratio, and, consequently, clearance. However, if intrinsic clearance is much greater than hepatic blood flow, a twofold change in intrinsic clearance has a negligible effect on the extraction ratio and drug clearance. In nonmathematical terms, high intrinsic clearance indicates efficient hepatic elimination. It is hard to enhance an already efficient process, whereas it is relatively easy to improve on inefficient drug clearance due to low intrinsic clearance.

The effect of changes in hepatic blood flow also depends on the magnitude of intrinsic clearance. If extraction and intrinsic clearance are high, a decrease in hepatic blood flow causes a small increase in the extraction ratio (Fig. 11-2) that is insufficient to offset the effects of reduced hepatic flow (Eq. 11-4). Consequently, changes in hepatic blood flow produce virtually proportional changes in clearance of drugs with high extraction ratios (Fig. 11-3). For a drug with a low intrinsic clearance, a decrease in hepatic blood flow is associated with a larger, almost proportional increase in the extraction ratio (see Fig. 11-2). This largely offsets the effects of changes in blood flow, so

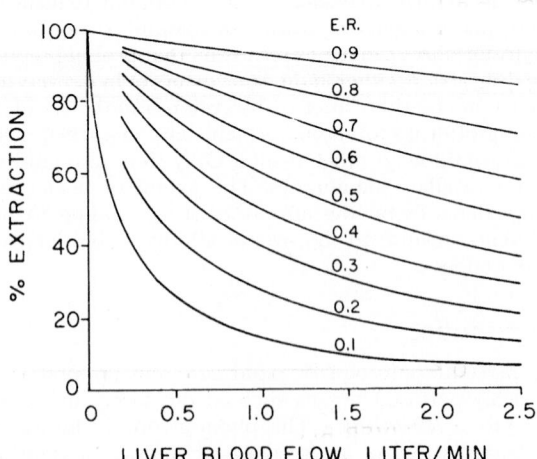

Figure 11-2. The effect of changes in hepatic blood flow on extraction of drugs with different extraction ratios. The extraction ratios at the normal hepatic blood flow of 1.5 L · min^{-1} are above the corresponding curves. (Reprinted with permission from Wood AJJ: Drug disposition and pharmacokinetics. In Wood M, Wood AJJ [eds]: Drugs and Anesthesia—Pharmacology for Anesthesiologists, p 27. Baltimore, Williams & Walkins, 1990. After Wilkinson GR, Shand DG: A physiologic approach to hepatic drug clearance. Clin Pharmacol Ther 18:377, 1975.)

that clearance of drugs with low extraction ratios is essentially independent of hepatic blood flow (see Fig. 11-3).

Hepatic clearance of drugs with extraction ratios ≤30% is independent of changes in liver blood flow, but very sensitive to the liver's ability to metabolize the drug, which can vary as a result of pathologic conditions, inhibition or induction of drug-metabolizing enzymes, or interindividual differences. In contrast, hepatic clearance of drugs with high extraction ratios (>70%) is determined primarily by liver blood flow rather than the activity of drug-metabolizing enzymes. Drugs with intermediate extraction ratios, between 30% and 70%, share characteristics with both the other groups. Drugs can be classified as having either high, intermediate, or low extraction ratios (Table 11-1). Comparing drugs with high versus low extraction ratios reveals easily discernible differences in disposition.[11]

Binding of drugs to plasma proteins and other blood constituents can also affect drug clearance. Whether drug binding influences drug clearance depends on the extraction ratio and the extent of binding. Three classes of hepatic clearance can be defined by integrating the effects of drug binding in the blood and the extraction ratio.[13] Clearance of drugs with high extraction ratios is *flow-limited* because it depends only on hepatic perfusion and is not affected by changes in drug binding or intrinsic clearance. The combination of a low extraction ratio and a high free fraction results in *capacity-limited, binding-insensitive* clearance, which is affected by changes in intrinsic clearance but is not significantly influenced by binding or hepatic perfusion. Drugs with low extraction ratios and low free fractions have capacity-limited, binding-sensitive clearance, which is not greatly affected by changes in hepatic blood flow but depends on both intrinsic clearance and the free drug concentration. Elimination of drugs with intermediate extraction ratios and binding is influenced by all three biologic factors—hepatic blood flow, intrinsic clearance, and the free drug concentration in the blood. The relative importance of these three factors cannot be predicted unless the extraction ratio and the unbound fraction in the blood are known.

Table 11-1. CLASSIFICATION OF SOME DRUGS ENCOUNTERED IN ANESTHESIOLOGY ACCORDING TO HEPATIC EXTRACTION RATIOS

Low	Intermediate	High
Diazepam	Alfentanil	Alprenolol
Lorazepam	Methohexital	Bupivacaine
Methadone	Midazolam	Diltiazem
Phenytoin	Rapacuronium	Fentanyl
Rocuronium	Vecuronium	Ketamine
Theophylline		Lidocaine
Thiopental		Meperidine
		Metoprolol
		Morphine
		Naloxone
		Nifedipine
		Propofol
		Propranolol
		Sufentanil
		Verapamil

Drugs eliminated primarily by other organs are not included in this table.

Physiologic, Pathologic, and Pharmacologic Alterations in Hepatic Drug Clearance

At rest, approximately 30% of cardiac output perfuses the liver. The hepatic artery provides roughly 25% of total hepatic flow, with the remainder supplied *via* the portal vein. Many physiologic and pathologic conditions alter hepatic blood flow, but there is little information regarding the effect of these changes in blood flow on hepatic drug clearance. The splanchnic circulation responds to a variety of stimuli, and splanchnic flow is often sacrificed to meet the demands of other tissues.

Moving from the supine to the upright position decreases cardiac output, which produces a reflex increase in systemic vascular resistance. The splanchnic circulation participates in this generalized vasoconstriction, which decreases hepatic blood flow by 30–40%.[12] Clearance of aldosterone, which has a high hepatic extraction ratio, is decreased in the upright position.[12] Postural changes probably also influence clearance of drugs with high hepatic extraction ratios, but this has not been systematically investigated.

Exercise, heat stress, and hypovolemia all decrease splanchnic blood flow in proportion to the associated increase in heart rate, which suggests that these responses are mediated by the sympathetic nervous system.[12] As expected, these conditions decrease clearance of indocyanine green, which has a high hepatic extraction ratio. In contrast, the clearance of antipyrine, a drug with a low extraction ratio, is not affected by these conditions.[14]

Decreases in cardiac output cause reflex splanchnic vasoconstriction, which reduces hepatic blood flow in proportion to the reduction in cardiac output.[15] Lidocaine clearance is reduced in patients with congestive cardiac failure.[16] Consequently, if usual doses of lidocaine are given to patients with heart failure, the risk of lidocaine toxicity is increased. Marked reduction in hepatic blood flow causes hepatocellular dysfunction; therefore, severe congestive heart failure decreases drug clearance by reducing both intrinsic clearance and hepatic blood flow.[17] Cardiovascular collapse severely compromises both liver blood flow and hepatocellular function.[12] In experimental hemorrhagic shock, clearance of lidocaine was decreased by 40%, whereas hepatic blood flow declined by 30%.[18] The reduction in clearance is too large to be caused solely by decreased hepatic perfusion, implying a concomitant reduction in intrinsic clearance secondary to hepatic ischemia.

Liver disease can decrease drug clearance because of hepatocellular dysfunction, altered hepatic blood flow, or both.[12] Cir-

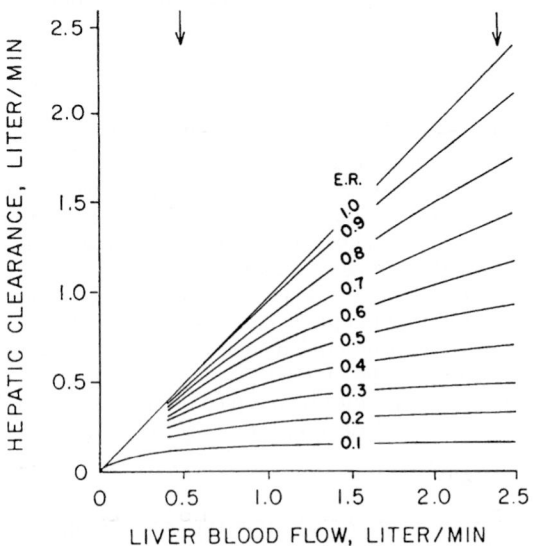

Figure 11-3. The effect of changes in hepatic blood flow on hepatic clearance of drugs with different extraction ratios. The extraction ratios for each curve at 1.5 L · min⁻¹ flow are indicated. The arrows indicate the normal physiologic range of hepatic blood flow. (Reprinted with permission from Wood AJJ: Drug disposition and pharmacokinetics. In Wood M, Wood AJJ [eds]: Drugs and Anesthesia—Pharmacology for Anesthesiologists, p 27. Baltimore, Williams & Wilkins, 1990. After Wilkinson GR, Shand DG: A physiologic approach to hepatic drug clearance. Clin Pharmacol Ther 18:377, 1975.)

rhosis reduces clearance of drugs with high extraction ratios, including lidocaine,[16] meperidine,[19,20] and propranolol.[21] This is secondary to decreased hepatic perfusion, which can be the result of reduced total liver blood flow, intrahepatic shunting, or extrahepatic shunting of portal venous blood.[12] Portosystemic shunting increases the bioavailability of orally administered drugs with high extraction ratios.[12] Cirrhosis also decreases clearance of drugs with low extraction ratios, such as diazepam,[22,23] because of impaired hepatocellular function, which decreases intrinsic clearance. Acute viral hepatitis reduces the clearance of drugs with both high (meperidine,[24] lidocaine[25]) and low (diazepam[22]) hepatic extraction ratios. These observations indicate that both acute and chronic liver diseases affect liver function and blood flow in a parallel fashion. Consequently, in chronic therapy, doses of any drug cleared by the liver should be reduced in patients with hepatic disease.

Drugs that alter splanchnic hemodynamics affect clearance of highly extracted drugs. Propranolol decreases hepatic blood flow, thus decreasing its own clearance[12] and the clearance of concomitantly administered lidocaine.[26] The volatile anesthetics all decrease hepatic blood flow, although isoflurane does so to a lesser extent than halothane or enflurane.[27,28] Intra-abdominal surgery causes a further decrease in hepatic perfusion.[27] Hypotension produced by spinal anesthesia reduces splanchnic blood flow.[29] In contrast to the volatile anesthetics, nitrous oxide, opioids, and barbiturates have little effect on hepatic blood flow.[12] Although they are potentially of great clinical importance, the effects of these hemodynamic alterations have not been thoroughly investigated. It is logical to assume that the clearance of drugs with high hepatic extraction ratios will be reduced during anesthesia and surgery.

Renal Drug Clearance

Although the kidneys do metabolize drugs, their major function in drug elimination is to excrete drugs, and metabolites produced elsewhere (primarily the liver), into the urine. Renal clearance of drugs is determined by the net effects of three processes: glomerular filtration, tubular secretion, and tubular reabsorption.[30,31]

Glomerular filtration cannot eliminate drugs efficiently. The glomerular filtration rate is approximately 20% of renal plasma flow.[32] Consequently, even if none of the drug is bound to plasma proteins, only about 20% can be removed by glomerular filtration. Drug binding to plasma proteins and erythrocytes reduces the amount filtered, because only unbound drug can pass through the glomerular membrane into the renal tubule. If a drug is neither secreted nor reabsorbed by the renal tubules, then renal drug clearance will be equal to glomerular clearance. Drugs and metabolites excreted in this fashion have low renal extraction ratios, and their renal clearance depends on the degree of binding to blood constituents. Therefore, protein binding is a major determinant of both hepatic and renal clearance of drugs with low extraction ratios.

Proximal renal tubular cells have two discrete mechanisms for secreting acidic and basic organic compounds.[30] These processes are carrier-mediated, so they are saturable. Drugs with similar physicochemical characteristics compete for available carrier molecules and interfere with each other's secretion. If a drug is very avidly secreted by tubular cells and not subsequently reabsorbed, it will have a high renal extraction ratio. Renal clearance of such drugs is largely determined by the magnitude of renal blood flow.[30] This is analogous to the importance of liver blood flow in the clearance of drugs with high hepatic extraction ratios.

Clearance of drugs filtered by the glomeruli or secreted by the proximal renal tubule may be decreased by subsequent reabsorption from the renal tubule. If this is extensive, the drug will have a very low renal extraction ratio and negligible renal clearance. Tubular reabsorption occurs by active, carrier-medi-

ated transport that is similar to active secretion. Drugs can also be reabsorbed by passive diffusion across the tubular epithelium. The progressive reabsorption of water from the renal tubule facilitates passive reabsorption of drugs by creating a tubule-to-plasma concentration gradient for the drug. Consequently, oliguria can decrease renal drug clearance.[31] Passive reabsorption is determined by the lipid solubility and degree of ionization of a drug. Highly lipophilic drugs like thiopental are almost completely reabsorbed and have virtually no renal clearance. For less lipophilic drugs, the degree of ionization is a major determinant of the extent of passive reabsorption because only the nonionized drug readily diffuses across the renal tubular epithelium. Urine pH can range from 4.5 to 8.0, which can cause large changes in the ionized fraction of weak acids and bases, particularly if the pK_a is close to or within this range. Urine pH can be manipulated to increase renal drug clearance after overdoses.

Physiologic, Pharmacologic, and Pathologic Alterations in Renal Drug Clearance

In adults, renal blood flow is approximately $1200 \text{ mL} \cdot \text{min}^{-1}$, so renal plasma flow is approximately $700 \text{ mL} \cdot \text{min}^{-1}$. About one-fifth of the plasma is filtered by the glomerulus, resulting in an average glomerular filtration rate of $125 \text{ mL} \cdot \text{min}^{-1}$. Renal blood flow and glomerular filtration rate are autoregulated, so they remain fairly constant as long as mean arterial pressure is between 70 and 160 mm Hg.[32] Consequently, renal drug clearance is more constant than hepatic clearance, because renal blood flow is more closely autoregulated than hepatic blood flow.

The capacity for excreting endogenous and exogenous compounds depends on the number of functionally intact nephrons. Decreased glomerular filtration is accompanied by a parallel loss of renal tubular function. Therefore, clearance of endogenous creatinine, which is essentially equivalent to the glomerular filtration rate, can be used to estimate overall renal function. It follows that renal drug clearance is proportional to creatinine clearance, even for drugs eliminated primarily by tubular secretion. This principle has been used to develop nomograms for reducing drug doses according to the creatinine clearance in the presence of renal dysfunction.[33] Many drugs, including lidocaine,[34] pancuronium,[35] and meperidine,[36] have pharmacologically active metabolites that are excreted by the kidneys. Therefore, both parent drugs and their metabolites can contribute to drug toxicity in patients with renal failure.

Renal function decreases progressively with age. By age 80 years, creatinine clearance is reduced by about 50%.[37] Despite the age-related decrease in glomerular filtration rate, serum creatinine is not elevated in healthy elderly patients because muscle mass, the source of creatinine, also decreases with age. Therefore, even if serum creatinine is normal, renal clearance of drugs is reduced in elderly patients.

Many drugs encountered in anesthetic practice are eliminated primarily by the kidneys (Table 11-2). In renal failure, doses of these drugs must be reduced to avoid adverse effects. In addition to renal disease, other pathologic processes can

Table 11-2. DRUGS WITH SIGNIFICANT RENAL EXCRETION ENCOUNTERED IN ANESTHESIOLOGY

Aminoglycosides	Neostigmine
Atenolol	Pancuronium
Cephalosporins	Penicillins
Digoxin	Pipecuronium
Doxacurium	Procaineamide
Edrophonium	Pyridostigmine
Nadolol	

impair kidney function. Low cardiac output states reduce renal blood flow, glomerular filtration, and, consequently, renal drug clearance.[30] Advanced hepatic cirrhosis also interferes with renal function,[30] and this combination, the *hepatorenal syndrome,* reduces elimination of almost all drugs.

DRUG METABOLISM

Unless tolerance* develops, termination of drug action depends on removal of the drug from its sites of action. Most operations are completed within a relatively short period (duration of anesthesia <2–3 hours). In such cases, drug redistribution is the primary mechanism for reducing drug concentrations in the blood. This, in turn, establishes the concentration gradient required for removal of drugs from their sites of action. Drug metabolism is more important in terminating effects of drugs that are not extensively redistributed, or when larger, or repeated, doses are administered. This could occur after prolonged anesthesia (>4–5 hours). Consideration of drug metabolism is also important in the therapeutics of critical care and pain therapy.

Drugs must usually cross biologic membranes to reach their sites of action, so most are relatively lipid-soluble. This property makes their excretion difficult, because lipophilic compounds are readily reabsorbed from the gut and the distal renal tubule. Metabolism, or *biotransformation* of drugs to more polar, water-soluble compounds, facilitates the ultimate excretion of metabolites in the bile and urine. Biotransformation is a protective mechanism for preventing the accumulation and resultant toxic effects of various lipophilic compounds acquired from the environment.

Metabolites are usually less active pharmacologically than the parent drug. However, this is not always true. Many benzodiazepines have metabolites that have similar pharmacologic effects.[5] The analgesic effects of codeine are due to its biotransformation to morphine. Metabolites can also be toxic. The major metabolite of meperidine is normeperidine, which can cause seizures.[36] If metabolites are pharmacologically active or toxic, further biotransformation or excretion is required for termination of their effects.

Metabolism of drugs and other exogenous compounds, known collectively as *xenobiotics,* occurs primarily in the liver. Other organs, including the kidneys, lungs, gut, and skin, also metabolize drugs, but extrahepatic biotransformation is quantitatively unimportant in most instances.

Biotransformation Reactions

Biotransformation reactions have classically been divided into two groups. *Phase I* reactions alter the molecular structure of xenobiotics by modifying an existing functional group of the drug, by adding a new functional chemical group to the compound, or by splitting the original molecule into two fragments. These changes in molecular structure result from oxidation, reduction, or hydrolysis of the parent compound. *Phase II* reactions consist of the coupling, or conjugation, of a variety of endogenous compounds to polar chemical groups. The polar chemical group at which conjugation occurs is frequently the result of a previous Phase I reaction, hence the "Phase I–Phase II" nomenclature. However, not all drugs are eliminated by this sequential pathway of biotransformation. Oxidation of thiopental produces its major metabolite, thiopental carboxylic

acid,[38] which undergoes renal excretion without undergoing a Phase II biotransformation. Morphine is directly conjugated to form morphine glucuronide without first undergoing a Phase I reaction.

Phase I Reactions

Phase I reactions may hydrolyze, oxidize, or reduce the parent compound. *Hydrolysis* is the insertion of a molecule of water into another molecule, which forms an unstable intermediate compound that subsequently splits apart. Thus, hydrolysis cleaves the original substance into two separate molecules. Hydrolytic reactions are the primary way amides, such as lidocaine and other amide local anesthetics, and esters, such as succinylcholine, are metabolized.

Many drugs are biotransformed by oxidative reactions. *Oxidations* are defined as reactions that remove electrons from a molecule. The common element of most, if not all, oxidations is an enzymatically mediated reaction that inserts a hydroxyl group (OH) into the drug molecule.[39] In some instances, this produces a chemically stable, more polar hydroxylated metabolite. However, hydroxylation usually creates unstable compounds that spontaneously split into separate molecules. Many different biotransformations are effected by this basic mechanism. Dealkylation (removal of a carbon-containing group), deamination (removal of nitrogen-containing groups), oxidation of nitrogen-containing groups, desulfuration, dehalogenation, and dehydrogenation all follow an initial hydroxylation.[39] Hydrolysis and hydroxylation are comparable processes. Both have an initial, enzymatically mediated step that produces an unstable compound which rapidly dissociates into separate molecules.

Some drugs are metabolized by *reductive reactions,* that is, reactions that add electrons to a molecule. In contrast to oxidations, where electrons are transferred from NADPH to an oxygen atom, the electrons are transferred to the drug molecule. Oxidation of xenobiotics requires oxygen, but reductive biotransformation is inhibited by oxygen, so it is facilitated when the intracellular oxygen tension is low.[40]

The Cytochrome P450 System. The complex of enzymes and pigmented hemoproteins that catalyzes most oxidative and some reductive biotransformations is known collectively as the *cytochrome P450 system.* These hemoproteins, when reduced by carbon monoxide, have an absorption spectrum with a peak at the 450-nm wavelength, hence their name. This system is incorporated into the smooth endoplasmic reticulum of hepatocytes. The endoplasmic reticulum is an intracellular network of tubules similar in ultrastructure to cellular membranes. Other tissues, including the kidneys, lungs, and skin, also contain cytochrome P450, but in much smaller amounts.[3] Upper intestinal enterocytes contain high concentrations of cytochrome P450, which contributes to the first-pass effect by metabolizing drugs absorbed from the GI tract before they reach the systemic circulation.[41] The cytochrome P450 complex is capable of metabolizing hundreds of compounds, including endogenous substances such as steroids and amines, as well as drugs and other exogenous compounds acquired from the environment.[42] The cytochrome P450 system oxidizes its substrates primarily by the insertion of an atom of oxygen in the form of a hydroxyl group, while another oxygen atom is reduced to water.

Cytochrome P450 is not a single entity; rather, it is a superfamily of related enzymes.[43] More than 150 cytochrome P450s have been identified.[42] More than 25 different human cytochrome P450s in 14 different families have been characterized.[44,45] There are "constitutive" forms of cytochrome P450 that are involved in the metabolism of various endogenous compounds, such as steroids, thyroxine, prostaglandins, and amines. In addition to the constitutive forms, production of cytochrome P450s can be induced by a wide variety of xenobiotics.[46] Cytochrome P450 drug-metabolizing activity increases after exposure to various

---

* Tolerance is defined as decreasing pharmacologic effect with sustained exposure to a drug. It results in higher doses (or concentrations) being required to maintain a given effect. The mechanisms responsible for tolerance are diverse. They include adaptive or reflex responses to drug effects that alter the observed effects, and alterations in the number or sensitivity of receptors.

exogenous chemicals, including many drugs.[47] The number and type of cytochrome P450s present at any time depends on exposure to different xenobiotics. The cytochrome P450 system is able to protect the organism from the deleterious effects of accumulation of exogenous compounds because of its two fundamental characteristics—broad substrate specificity and the capability to adapt to exposure to different substances by induction of different cytochrome P450 enzymes.

Biotransformations can be inhibited if different substrates compete for the drug-binding site on the same cytochrome P450. The effect of two competing substrates on each other's metabolism depends on their relative affinities for the enzyme. Biotransformation of the compound with the lower affinity is inhibited to a greater degree. This is the mechanism by which the H_2 receptor antagonist cimetidine inhibits the metabolism of many drugs, including meperidine, propranolol, and diazepam.[48–50] The newer H_2 antagonist ranitidine has a different structure and causes fewer clinically significant drug interactions.[51] Other drugs, notably calcium channel blockers and antidepressants, also inhibit oxidative drug metabolism in humans.[52,53] During the last decade, information regarding both induction and inhibition of different cytochrome P450 isoenzymes by specific drugs has become available.[53] This information allows clinicians to predict which combinations of drugs are more likely to lead to clinically significant interactions due to altered drug metabolism by the cytochrome P450 system.

Induction and inhibition of hepatic drug-metabolizing enzyme systems change the intrinsic hepatic clearance of drugs. This is most important for drugs with low hepatic extraction ratios, because intrinsic clearance is the primary determinant of their hepatic clearance. Altered drug-metabolizing enzyme activity has little effect on drugs with high hepatic extraction ratios because their clearance depends primarily on hepatic blood flow.

Phase II Reactions

Phase II reactions are also known as *conjugation* or *synthetic reactions.* Many drugs do not have a polar chemical group suitable for conjugation, so conjugation occurs only after a Phase I reaction. Other drugs, such as morphine, already have a polar group that serves as a "handle" for conjugation, and they undergo these reactions directly. Various endogenous compounds can be attached to parent drugs or their Phase I metabolites to form different conjugation products.[54] These endogenous substrates include glucuronic acid, acetate, and amino acids. Mercapturic acid conjugates result from the binding of exogenous compounds to glutathione. Other conjugation reactions produce sulfated or methylated derivatives of drugs or their metabolites. Like the cytochrome P450 system, the enzymes that catalyze Phase II reactions are inducible.[47] Phase II reactions produce conjugates that are polar, water-soluble compounds. This facilitates the ultimate excretion of the drug *via* the kidneys or hepatobiliary secretion. Like cytochrome P450, there are different families and superfamilies of the enzymes that catalyze Phase II biotransformations.[54]

Factors Affecting Biotransformation

Drug metabolism varies substantially between individuals because of variability in the genes controlling the numerous enzymes responsible for biotransformation. For most drugs, individual subjects' rates of metabolism have a unimodal distribution. However, distinct subpopulations with different rates of elimination of some drugs have been identified. The resulting multimodal distribution of individual rates of metabolism is known as *polymorphism.* For example, different genotypes result in either normal, low, or (rarely) absent plasma pseudocholinesterase activity, accounting for the well-known differences in individuals' responses to succinylcholine, which is hydrolyzed by this enzyme. Many drug-metabolizing enzymes exhibit genetic

polymorphism, including cytochrome P450 and various transferases that catalyze phase II reactions.[55]

Drug metabolism also varies with age. The fetus and neonate have less capacity for some biotransformations, especially those catalyzed by cytochrome P450.[56,57] However, cytochrome P450 activity increases dramatically in early infancy.[56,57] Neonates also have less capacity for conjugation reactions, especially glucuronidation.[56,57] Impaired conjugation of bilirubin causes "physiologic jaundice." Metabolism of some drugs may also be decreased in geriatric patients, although it is difficult to separate the effects of age *per se* from the effects of organ dysfunction, which is more prevalent in the elderly.[58,59]

Exposure to various foreign compounds can alter drug-metabolizing enzyme activity. Barbiturates, phenytoin, macrolide antibiotics, imidazole antifungal agents, and corticosteroids can cause drug interactions secondary to induction of hepatic drug-metabolizing enzymes.[47] Chronic ethanol consumption induces enzyme activity, but acute intoxication inhibits the biotransformation of some drugs.[60] Smoking increases the metabolism of many drugs secondary to enzyme induction by polycyclic hydrocarbons in tobacco smoke.[61]

Liver disease profoundly affects drug disposition. It is difficult to distinguish the impact of altered biotransformation *per se* from other effects of liver disease: altered binding of drugs to plasma proteins and decreased liver blood flow. Nonetheless, hepatic disease decreases clearance of drugs with low hepatic extraction ratios,[13,62] which implies impaired biotransformation. Congestive heart failure decreases metabolism of lidocaine and theophylline.[17] Renal failure has different effects on different biotransformation reactions. Hydrolytic and acetylation reactions are slowed, but conjugations usually are not affected, and some oxidations may actually be enhanced.[63]

Effects of Anesthesia and Surgery on Biotransformation

Drug disposition is altered in the perioperative period. Although many other factors are probably also involved, biotransformation reactions are affected by anesthesia and surgery. In dogs anesthetized with halothane, the intrinsic hepatic clearance of propranolol is decreased, which implies that hepatic drug-metabolizing ability is impaired.[64] Halothane inhibits demethylation of aminopyrine in a dose-dependent fashion. Isoflurane has less effect, and enflurane does not affect aminopyrine biotransformation.[65]

Many investigators have studied the effects of anesthesia and surgery on antipyrine clearance. Antipyrine, an antipyretic that is no longer used therapeutically, does not bind to plasma proteins, has a low hepatic extraction ratio, and is not cleared by the kidneys. Therefore, clearance of antipyrine is solely dependent on the activity of hepatic drug-metabolizing enzymes. This permits the use of antipyrine clearance as an indicator of hepatic drug-metabolizing activity.[66] Clearance of antipyrine is generally increased after surgery conducted with a wide variety of general anesthetic techniques,[67,68] although there are exceptions to this rule. General anesthesia with enflurane does not appear to increase antipyrine clearance.[69] After operations lasting more than 4 hours, antipyrine clearance is decreased.[70] Presumably, major surgical trauma interferes with drug metabolism, although the precise mechanisms are not known. Antipyrine clearance is also increased after spinal anesthesia.[68] Therefore, general anesthesia is not a prerequisite for increased rates of biotransformation in the postoperative period, and other perioperative factors also affect drug metabolism. For example, the caloric source of iv nutritional regimens influences antipyrine clearance. It is decreased when the only caloric source is 5% dextrose, and increased when amino acids are substituted for dextrose.[71]

In addition to altered rates of biotransformation, other factors, such as decreased hepatic blood flow during surgery,[27,28] can affect drug elimination in the perioperative period. In many patients the magnitude of these changes is too small to cause any clinically evident problems. However, in some patients clinically significant changes in drug elimination could occur. Decreased drug clearance can result in higher concentrations of drugs and increase the risk of adverse effects, especially after prolonged surgery. Clinicians must be aware of the potential for excessive pharmacologic effects and must tailor doses accordingly.

BINDING OF DRUGS TO PLASMA PROTEINS

After injection or ingestion, drugs are transported to their sites of action and to eliminating organs *via* the blood. Drugs are present in the blood in two fractions. Some are simply dissolved in plasma water; the rest is bound to various components of whole blood, such as plasma proteins and red blood cells. Ideally, drug concentrations should be measured in whole blood because drugs are transported in blood, not plasma, and drugs equilibrate between erythrocytes and plasma very quickly.[72] Unfortunately, measurement of total drug levels and drug binding in whole blood is technically much more difficult than in plasma or serum, so very few investigators have directly measured whole blood binding. As a compromise, the blood:plasma concentration ratio can be used to estimate whole blood binding.

Drugs bind to plasma proteins in a reversible fashion that obeys the law of mass action. The rate constants of the association and dissociation reactions are k_1 and k_2, respectively. These reactions are very rapid, having half-times of a few milliseconds. Binding of drugs to blood constituents other than proteins, such as erythrocytes, proceeds in an analogous fashion. The equilibrium dissociation constant, K_d, quantifies the affinity of drug–protein binding:

$$K_d = \frac{k_2}{k_1} = \frac{[\text{unbound drug}] \times [\text{protein}]}{[\text{drug–protein complex}]} \quad (11\text{-}5)$$

The dissociation constant has units of moles per liter $(\text{mol} \cdot \text{L}^{-1})$, and is the drug concentration at which 50% of the binding sites are occupied. The degree of binding is dependent on the affinity of the protein for the drug, the protein concentration, and the concentration of drug available for binding.

The extent of plasma–drug binding can be expressed as the *percentage of drug bound,* which is the percentage of the total drug present that is bound to plasma proteins. Alternatively, the *free fraction,* which is the percentage of drug not bound to plasma proteins, can be used. For example, approximately 83% of fentanyl is bound to plasma proteins. Therefore, the free fraction of fentanyl is about 17%.[73,74]

Protein binding is affected by many factors, including temperature and pH.[72] At high drug concentrations, binding sites become saturated and the free fraction increases. There are also qualitative differences between species in plasma proteins that affect drug binding, and binding to purified human albumin may not correlate with binding in plasma.[72] Consequently, to provide clinically useful information, *in vitro* measurement of drug binding must be conducted at physiologic temperature and pH, with human plasma, and at concentrations within the usual therapeutic range.

Drug–protein binding has important pharmacologic implications, because only unbound drug can cross cell membranes to reach its sites of action. Also, free drug is more readily available for elimination. This has led to the frequently held misconception that drug bound to plasma proteins and other blood constituents is pharmacologically inert. This is not the case. As soon as unbound drug leaves circulation, the law of mass action dictates that some drug will dissociate from binding sites, which tends to restore the free drug concentration. This occurs almost instantaneously, so that the bound fraction of drug serves as a dynamic reservoir that buffers acute changes in the free drug concentration.

As discussed earlier, clearance of some drugs depends upon the degree of protein binding. The extent of distribution of drugs throughout the body also depends on the degree of binding. At equilibrium, the portion of the total drug in the body that is in extravascular sites is determined by the relative affinity of blood binding *versus* binding to all other tissues. A drug that is highly bound to plasma proteins or erythrocytes cannot be extensively distributed unless it has even greater affinity for extravascular binding sites.

Binding Proteins

Two plasma proteins are primarily responsible for drug binding: albumin and α_1-acid glycoprotein (AAG). Drugs also bind to other plasma proteins, such as globulins or lipoproteins, and to erythrocytes. Drugs can bind to more than one protein. For example, fentanyl and sufentanil bind to albumin, AAG, globulins, and also to red blood cells.[74]

Albumin is the most important drug-binding protein. In addition to a wide range of drugs, including barbiturates, benzodiazepines, and penicillins, albumin binds endogenous compounds such as bilirubin. Many drugs bind to more than one site on the albumin molecule, and most drugs have one or two high-affinity, primary binding sites and a variable number of secondary, low-affinity sites. Studies with radioactively labeled drugs indicate that albumin has at least three discrete, high-affinity drug-binding sites. Diazepam, digitoxin, and warfarin each bind to a different site. The sites at which other drugs bind to albumin and the affinity of the drug–albumin bond can be determined by using these three markers.[75] This permits prediction of the likelihood of drug interactions due to one drug displacing another. Drugs that compete for the same binding site are more likely to displace one another than drugs that bind at different sites, and the drug with the lower affinity for the binding site will be more easily displaced.

Factors Affecting Drug Binding

The physicochemical properties of drugs influence binding to plasma proteins. Albumin is the major binding protein for organic acids, such as penicillins and barbiturates. Basic drugs also bind to albumin, but to a lesser extent. The primary binding protein for many basic drugs is AAG (Table 11-3). Basic drugs also bind to lipoproteins and globulins. AAG is an acute phase reactant, and its concentration increases in many acute and chronic illnesses.

In general, the greater the lipid solubility of a drug, the greater the binding to plasma proteins (Table 11-4). Water-soluble drugs, such as neuromuscular blocking agents, are bound to a substantially lesser extent than lipid-soluble drugs, like propofol. This is also true for drugs that belong to the same class. The degree of binding of opioids parallels their lipid solubility: morphine is the least bound, fentanyl and its derivatives are highly bound, and meperidine is intermediate. Similarly, bupivacaine is bound to a greater extent than lidocaine.

Many physiologic and pathologic states cause quantitative and qualitative changes in the primary drug-binding plasma

---

Table 11-3. DRUGS BINDING TO α_1-ACID GLYCOPROTEIN

Alfentanil	Methadone
Alprenolol	Propranolol
Bupivacaine	Quinidine
Disopyramide	Ropivacaine
Fentanyl	Sufentanil
Lidocaine	Verapamil
Meperidine	

Table 11-4. PLASMA PROTEIN BINDING OF SOME DRUGS USED IN ANESTHESIOLOGY

Class/Drug	Percent Bound	Reference
CARDIOVASCULAR DRUGS		
Digoxin	20–30	146
Diltiazem	77–80	147
Esmolol	55	148
Nifedipine	96–98	147
Propranolol	89	95
Verapamil	84–91	147
BENZODIAZEPINES		
Diazepam	97–99	149
Lorazepam	88–92	150
Midazolam	96	85
INTRAVENOUS ANESTHETICS		
Methohexital	73	151
Propofol	98	152
Thiopental	85	92
LOCAL ANESTHETICS*		
Bupivacaine	95	153
Lidocaine	70	153
Ropivacaine	94	154
NEUROMUSCULAR BLOCKERS		
Pancuronium	11–29	155, 156
Vecuronium	30	155
OPIOIDS		
Alfentanil	92	74
Fentanyl	84	74
Meperidine	53–63	84
Methadone	60–90	157
Morphine	20–35	89, 157, 158
Sufentanil	92	74

* At nontoxic concentrations. At toxic plasma concentrations, binding of local anesthetic decreases, leading to a marked increase in the free drug concentration.

proteins, albumin and AAG. Drug binding may also be affected by acid–base disturbances that alter the degree of ionization of drugs and proteins, and by accumulation of endogenous compounds that compete for drug-binding sites.

Maternal and Neonatal Drug Binding

Binding of drugs in pregnancy and in the fetus or neonate has received much attention because of its impact on placental drug transfer. Pregnant women have reduced levels of albumin, and the binding of many organic acids, such as phenytoin, is decreased at term.[76] Although thiopental is also an organic acid, unlike phenytoin, the free fraction of thiopental is not increased in patients undergoing cesarean section,[77] so that usual doses of thiopental do not result in excessive free drug levels. This is fortunate, because high free drug levels would increase the risk of side-effects and enhance placental transfer of the drug. The free fraction of diazepam, which binds primarily to albumin, is increased at term.[78] AAG levels are not changed during pregnancy.[78] However, the free fractions of lidocaine and propranolol are, nonetheless, increased at term.[78]

Neonates have decreased levels of albumin and AAG,[76–79] and neonatal albumin has less affinity for some drugs.[76,79] Consequently, the free fraction of many drugs, especially those that bind to AAG, is higher in the neonate than in the mother.[79] Although binding of many drugs is decreased in neonates, this does not affect the unbound concentration of drugs transferred across the placenta. Under near steady-state conditions, maternal and fetal free drug concentrations are the same, although the total fetal level is lower. Because the free drug is the more

pharmacologically active species, the decrease in maternal plasma protein drug binding is of greater consequence as far as placental transfer of drugs is concerned. Decreased drug binding must be considered in neonatal therapeutics.[57]

Age and Sex

The plasma concentrations of the primary drug-binding proteins change with increasing age: albumin decreases slightly, whereas AAG tends to increase.[80–82] The free fractions of lidocaine, meperidine, and propranolol, all of which bind to AAG, are not changed in the elderly.[82–84] Similarly, binding of drugs to albumin is minimally altered. The binding of midazolam does not change,[85] and diazepam binding may decrease slightly.[22,80,86] The typical magnitude of age-associated decreases in drug binding is illustrated by thiopental. The average free fraction of thiopental of 18% in young adults only increases to 22% in geriatric patients.[87] Clinically significant changes in drug binding in elderly patients are more often caused by pathologic processes than by age *per se*.

Studies comparing drug binding in men and women have not found any clinically significant differences between the sexes. This is not surprising, because the concentrations of albumin and AAG in men and women do not differ significantly.[78,81]

Hepatic Disease

The plasma albumin concentration is often decreased in patients with liver disease. Drug binding may also be affected by qualitative changes in the albumin molecule that decrease affinity for drugs, and by accumulation of endogenous substances, such as bilirubin, that compete for drug-binding sites.[13] Although hepatic diseases vary widely in pathophysiology and severity, it is possible to make some generalizations regarding their impact on drug binding. The free fractions of drugs that bind primarily to albumin are increased. This is true for organic bases such as diazepam[22,88] and morphine,[89] and for the organic acids phenytoin[89] and thiopental.[90,91] The free fractions of basic drugs, such as lidocaine[25] and meperidine,[24] are not increased in patients with acute viral hepatitis, which suggests that drug binding to AAG is minimally affected by liver disease.

Renal Disease

Albumin levels tend to decrease in all types of renal disease. However, even when albumin levels are normal, binding of thiopental[92] and phenytoin[89] is decreased. The free fraction of phenytoin is correlated with both the albumin concentration and the severity of renal dysfunction.[89] This indicates that renal failure reduces the affinity of albumin for organic acids. Dialysis does not restore the affinity of albumin for thiopental or phenytoin.[89,92] The plasma-protein binding of many other organic acids is also decreased in renal failure.[93]

The effect of renal disease on the binding of basic drugs depends on whether the drug binds primarily to albumin or to AAG, and on the type of renal disease. The free fraction of diazepam, which binds primarily to albumin, is increased in the nephrotic syndrome, renal failure, and after renal transplantation.[94] Similarly, binding of morphine is decreased in uremia.[89] Binding of other basic drugs varies according to the changes in AAG in different types of renal disease. Lidocaine binding increases in renal failure and after renal transplantation, conditions associated with increased AAG levels.[94] Likewise, propranolol binding is increased in patients with renal disease and elevated concentrations of AAG.[95] Lidocaine binding is not altered in nephrotic patients who have normal levels of AAG.[90]

Other Diseases, Surgery, and Trauma

Patients with inflammatory diseases, such as rheumatoid arthritis and Crohn's disease, have increased levels of AAG and, consequently, decreased free fractions of drugs that bind to this protein.[95,96] Malignant disease is also associated with elevated levels of AAG, and increased binding of lidocaine, propranolol, and other basic drugs has been demonstrated in patients with cancer.[97] In contrast, albumin tends to decrease in patients with malignancies, which can decrease binding of acidic drugs.[96] After acute myocardial infarction, AAG levels double and remain elevated for about 3 weeks.[98] Consequently, the binding of lidocaine and propranolol is increased.[98,99]

The catabolic state that follows surgery and trauma decreases plasma albumin levels.[100] In contrast, the concentration of AAG increases after trauma[101] and surgery[102] and remains elevated for several weeks. These changes result in alterations in drug binding. The free fraction of phenytoin increases after surgery, probably secondary to decreased levels of albumin, although the contemporaneous increase in free fatty acids may result in competition for binding sites.[100] Higher AAG levels increase binding of basic drugs, such as lidocaine and propranolol, after trauma[101] and surgery.[103,104]

PHARMACOKINETIC PRINCIPLES

The concentration of a drug at its site or sites of action is a fundamental determinant of its pharmacologic effects. Because drugs are transported to and from their sites of action in the blood, the concentration at the active site is in turn a function of the concentration in the blood. The change in drug concentration over time in the blood, at the site of action, and in other tissues is a result of complex interactions of various biologic factors with the physicochemical characteristics of the drug. Together, these factors determine the rate, extent, and pattern of drug absorption, distribution, metabolism, and excretion. The term *pharmacokinetics,* derived from the Greek words *pharmakon* (medicine) and *kinesis* (movement), refers to the quantitative analysis of the relationship between the dose of a drug and the ensuing changes in drug concentration in the blood and other tissues.

Early pharmacokinetics studies of iv and inhalational anesthetics used physiologic, or perfusion models. In these models, body tissues are classified according to similarities in perfusion and affinity for drugs.[105] Highly perfused tissues, including the brain, heart, lungs, liver, and kidneys, make up the vessel-rich group. Muscle and skin comprise the lean tissue group, and fat is considered as a separate group. The vessel-poor group, which has minimal effect on drug distribution and elimination, is composed of bone and cartilage. Physiologic pharmacokinetic models made major contributions to understanding the factors influencing recovery from thiopental. These models established that awakening after a single dose was primarily due to redistribution of thiopental from the brain to muscle and skin.[7,8] Distribution to other tissues and metabolism played minor roles. This fundamental concept, *redistribution,* also applies to all lipophilic drugs. Physiologic models have also contributed greatly to our understanding of the uptake and distribution of inhalational anesthetics.[106]

Physiologic pharmacokinetic models provide much insight into factors affecting drug action. They can predict the effects of physiologic changes, such as altered regional blood flows or reduced cardiac output, on drug distribution and elimination. The disadvantage of perfusion-based models is their complexity. Verification of these models requires measurement of drug concentrations in many different tissues, which is rarely practical.[105] Because of these disadvantages, simpler pharmacokinetic models have been developed. In these models the body is envisaged as composed of one or more *compartments.* Drug concentrations in the blood are used to define the relationship between dose and the time course of changes of the drug concentration.[107] It is critically important to understand that the different "compartments" of a compartmental pharmacokinetic model cannot be equated with the tissue groups that make up physiologic pharmacokinetic models. Compartments are theoretical entities that are used to derive pharmacokinetic parameters, such as clearance, volume of distribution, and half-times. These parameters quantify drug distribution and elimination.

Although the simplicity of compartmental models, compared to physiologic pharmacokinetic models, has its advantages, it also has some disadvantages. For example, cardiac output is not a parameter of compartmental models, and compartmental models therefore cannot be used to predict directly the effect of cardiac failure on drug disposition. However, compartmental pharmacokinetic models can still quantify the effects of reduced cardiac output on the disposition of a drug if a group of patients with cardiac failure is compared to a group of otherwise healthy subjects.

The discipline of pharmacokinetics is, to the despair of many, mathematically based. In the succeeding sections, formulas are used to illustrate the concepts needed to understand and interpret pharmacokinetic studies. Readers are encouraged to concentrate on the concepts, not the formulas.

Pharmacokinetic Concepts

Rate Constants and Half-times

The disposition of most drugs follows *first-order* kinetics. A first-order kinetic process is one in which a constant fraction of the drug is removed during a finite period of time. This fraction is equivalent to the rate constant of the process. Rate constants are usually denoted by the letter k, and have units of "inverse time," such as min^{-1} or h^{-1}. If 10% of the drug is eliminated per minute, then the rate constant is 0.1 min^{-1}. Because a constant fraction is removed per unit of time in first-order kinetics, the absolute amount of drug removed is proportional to the concentration of the drug. It follows that, in first-order kinetics, the rate of change of the concentration at any given time is proportional to the concentration present at that time. When the concentration is high, it will fall faster than when it is low. First-order kinetics apply not only to elimination, but also to absorption and distribution.[107]

Rather than using rate constants, the rapidity of pharmacokinetic processes is often described with half-times—the time required for the concentration to change by a factor of 2. Half-times are calculated directly from the corresponding rate constants with this simple equation:

$$t_{1/2} = \frac{(\ln 2)}{k} = \frac{0.693}{k} \qquad (11\text{-}6)$$

Thus, a rate constant of 0.1 min^{-1} translates into a half-time of 6.93 minutes. The half-time of any first-order kinetic process, including drug absorption, distribution, and elimination, can be calculated. First-order processes asymptotically approach completion, because a constant fraction of the drug, not an absolute amount, is removed per unit of time. However, after five half-times, the process will be almost 97% complete (Table 11-5). For practical purposes, this is close enough to 100%, and can be considered as such.

Table 11-5. HALF-TIMES AND PERCENT OF DRUG REMOVED

Number of Half-times	Percent of Drug Remaining	Percent of Drug Removed
0	100	0
1	50	50
2	25	75
3	12.5	87.5
4	6.25	93.75
5	3.125	96.875

Volumes of Distribution

The volume of distribution quantifies the extent of drug distribution. The physiologic factor that governs the extent of drug distribution is the overall capacity of tissues *versus* the capacity of blood for that drug. Overall tissue capacity for uptake of a drug is in turn a function of the total volume of the tissues into which a drug distributes and their average affinity for the drug. In compartmental pharmacokinetic models, drugs are envisaged as distributing into one or more "boxes," or compartments. These compartments cannot be equated with tissues. Rather, they are hypothetical entities that permit analysis of drug distribution and elimination, and description of the drug concentration *versus* time profile.

The volume of distribution is an "apparent" volume because it represents the size of these hypothetical boxes, or compartments, that is necessary to explain the concentration of drug in a reference compartment, usually called the *central* or *plasma compartment*. The volume of distribution, *Vd*, relates the total amount of drug present to the concentration observed in the central compartment:

$$Vd = \frac{\text{total amount of drug present}}{\text{concentration}} \quad (11\text{-}7)$$

This formula is logical. If a drug is extensively distributed, then the concentration will be lower relative to the amount of drug present, which equates to a larger volume of distribution. For example, if a total of 10 mg of drug is present and the concentration is 2 mg · L^{-1}, then the apparent volume of distribution is 5 L. On the other hand, if the concentration was 4 mg · L^{-1}, then the volume of distribution would be 2.5 L.

Simply stated, the apparent volume of distribution is a numeric index of the extent of drug distribution that does not have any relationship to the actual volume of any tissue or group of tissues. It may be as small as plasma volume, or, if overall tissue uptake is extensive, the apparent volume of distribution may greatly exceed the actual total volume of the body (Fig. 11-4). In general, lipophilic drugs have larger volumes of distribution than hydrophilic drugs (Fig. 11-4). Because the volume of distribution is a mathematical approximation, it cannot be directly correlated with the anatomic and physiologic factors that influence drug distribution. Determination of the volume of distribution from a compartmental model does not provide any information regarding the tissues into which the drug actually distributes or the concentrations in those tissues. Despite these limitations, the volume of distribution provides useful information. For example, an increase in the volume of

distribution means that a larger loading dose will be required to "fill up the box" and achieve the same concentration. Various pathologic conditions can alter the volume of distribution, necessitating therapeutic adjustments.

Total Drug Clearance

In compartmental pharmacokinetic models, the ability of the system as a whole to irreversibly eliminate a drug is quantified by the *total drug clearance* or *elimination clearance*. Elimination clearance is the portion of the volume of distribution from which drug is completely and irreversibly removed during a given time interval. It is analogous to creatinine clearance, and, like creatinine clearance, drug clearance has units of flow. Drug clearance is often corrected for weight or body surface area, in which case the units are mL · min^{-1} · kg^{-1} or mL · min^{-1} · m^{-2}, respectively.

Elimination clearance, *Cl*, can be calculated from the declining blood levels observed after an iv injection, as follows:

$$Cl = \frac{\text{dose}}{\text{area under the concentration versus time curve}} \quad (11\text{-}8)$$

Again, this formula is intuitively logical. If a drug is rapidly removed from the plasma, its concentration will fall more quickly than the concentration of a drug that is less readily eliminated. This results in a smaller area under the concentration versus time curve, which equates to greater clearance.

A significant limitation of calculating elimination clearance from compartmental pharmacokinetic models is that the relative contribution of different organs to drug elimination cannot be determined. Nonetheless, estimation of drug clearance with these models has made important contributions to clinical pharmacology. In particular, these models have provided a great deal of clinically useful information regarding altered drug elimination in various pathologic conditions.

Compartmental Pharmacokinetic Models

One-Compartment Model

Although for most drugs the one-compartment model is an oversimplification, it does serve to illustrate the basic relationships between clearance, volume of distribution, and the elimination half-time. In this model, the body is envisaged as a single homogeneous compartment. Drug distribution after injection is assumed to be instantaneous, so there are no concentration gradients within the compartment. The concentration can decrease only by elimination of drug from the system. The plasma concentration *versus* time curve for a hypothetical drug with one-compartment kinetics is shown in Figure 11-5. With the concentration plotted on a logarithmic scale, the concentration *versus* time curve becomes a straight line. The slope of the logarithm of concentration *versus* time is equal to the first-order elimination rate constant.

Immediately after injection, before any drug can be eliminated, the amount of drug present is equal to the dose. Therefore, by modifying Equation 11-7, the volume of distribution can be calculated:

$$Vd = \frac{\text{dose}}{\text{initial concentration}} \quad (11\text{-}9)$$

In the one-compartment model, drug clearance, *Cl*, is equal to the product of the elimination rate constant, k_e, and the volume of distribution:

$$Cl = k_e \cdot Vd \quad (11\text{-}10)$$

Combining Equations 11-6 and 11-10 yields:

$$Cl = \frac{0.693 \cdot Vd}{t_{1/2}}; \text{ thus: } t_{1/2} = \frac{0.693 \cdot Vd}{Cl} \quad (11\text{-}11)$$

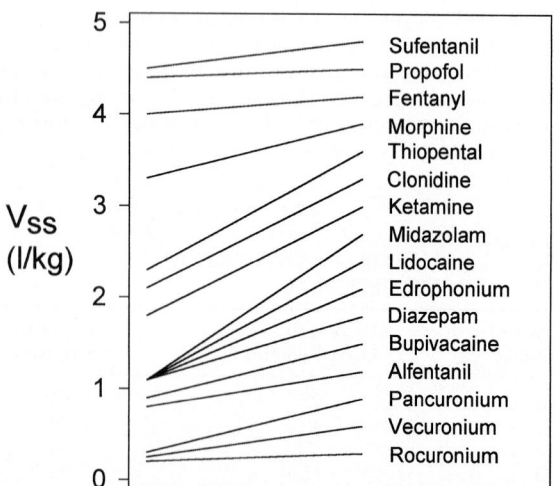

Figure 11-4. The volume of distribution of some drugs used in anesthesiology.

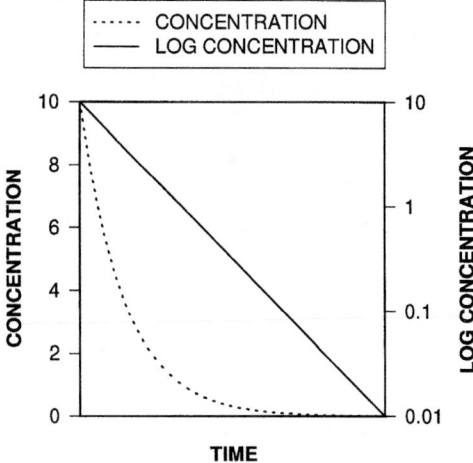

Figure 11-5. The plasma concentration, plotted on both linear (—, *left vertical axis*) and logarithmic (- - -, *right vertical axis*) scales, *versus* time for a hypothetical drug exhibiting one-compartment, first-order pharmacokinetics.

Therefore, the greater the clearance, the shorter the elimination half-time, which is easy to understand. Less obvious is the impact of the volume of distribution on the elimination half-time. It is easiest to understand if the physiologic correlate of a large volume of distribution is considered. A large volume of distribution reflects extensive tissue uptake of a drug, so that only a small fraction of the total amount of drug is in the blood and accessible to the organs of elimination. Consequently, the greater the volume of distribution, the longer the elimination half-time. For drugs that exhibit multicompartment pharmacokinetics, the relationship between clearance, volume of distribution, and the elimination half-time is not a simple linear one such as Equation 11-11. However, the same principles apply. All else being equal, the greater the clearance, the shorter the elimination half-time; the larger the volume of distribution, the longer the elimination half-time. Thus, the elimination half-time depends on two other variables, clearance and volume of distribution, that characterize, respectively, the extent of drug distribution and efficiency of drug elimination.

Two-Compartment Model

For many drugs, a graph of the logarithm of the plasma concentration *versus* time after an iv injection is similar to the schematic graph shown in Figure 11-6. There are two discrete phases in the decline of the plasma concentration. The first phase after

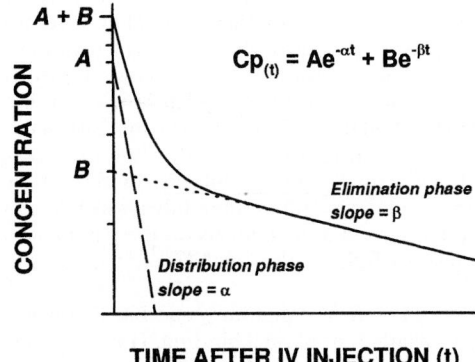

Figure 11-6. A schematic graph of the plasma concentration, on a logarithmic scale, *versus* time for a drug with a distribution phase preceding the elimination phase (two-compartment or biexponential kinetics). See text for explanation.

injection is characterized by a very rapid decrease in concentration. The rapid decrease in concentration during this "distribution phase" is largely caused by passage of drug from the plasma into tissues. The distribution phase is followed by a slower decline of the concentration owing to drug elimination. Elimination also begins immediately after injection, but its contribution to the drop in plasma concentration is initially much smaller than the fall in concentration due to drug distribution.

To account for this biphasic behavior, one must consider the body to be made up of two compartments, a central (or plasma) compartment and a peripheral compartment (Fig. 11-7). This two-compartment model assumes that it is the central compartment into which the drug is injected and from which the blood samples for measurement of concentration are obtained, and that drug is eliminated only from the central compartment. Drug distribution within the central compartment is considered to be instantaneous. In reality, this last assumption cannot be true. However, drug uptake into some of the highly perfused tissues is so rapid that it cannot be detected as a discrete phase on the plasma concentration versus time curve.

The distribution and elimination phases can be characterized by graphic analysis of the plasma concentration *versus* time curve, as shown in Figure 11-6. The elimination phase line is extrapolated back to time zero (the time of injection). At any time, the difference between the total concentration and the concentration on the extrapolated elimination phase line is equal to a corresponding point, at that time, on the distribution phase line. In Figure 11-6, the zero time intercepts of the distribution and elimination lines are points *A* and *B*, respectively. The *hybrid rate constants*, α and β, are equal to the slopes of the two lines, and are used to calculate the distribution and elimination half-times; α and β are called hybrid rate constants because they depend on both distribution and elimination processes.

At any time after an iv injection, the plasma concentration of drugs with two-compartment kinetics is equal to the sum of two exponential terms:

$$Cp_{(t)} = Ae^{-\alpha t} + Be^{-\beta t}, \qquad (11\text{-}12)$$

where t = time, $Cp_{(t)}$ = plasma concentration at time t, A = y-axis intercept of the distribution phase line, α = hybrid rate constant of the distribution phase, B = y-axis intercept of the elimination phase line, and β = hybrid rate constant of the elimination phase. The first term characterizes the distribution phase and the second term characterizes the elimination phase. Immediately after injection, the first term represents a much larger fraction of the total plasma concentration than the second term. After several distribution half-times, the value of the first term approaches zero, and the plasma concentration is essentially equal to the value of the second term (see Fig. 11-6).

In multicompartment models, the drug is initially distributed only within the central compartment. Therefore, the initial apparent volume of distribution is the volume of the central compartment. Immediately after injection, the amount of drug

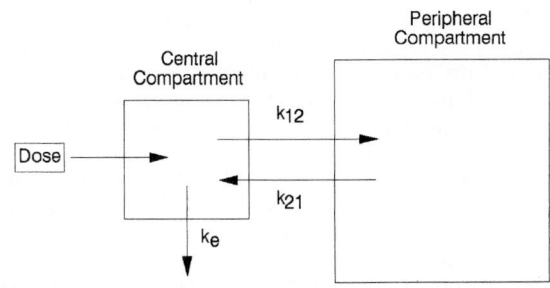

Figure 11-7. A two-compartment pharmacokinetic model. See text for explanation.

present is the dose, and the concentration is the extrapolated concentration at time $t = 0$, which is equal to the sum of the intercepts of the distribution and elimination lines. The volume of the central compartment, $V1$, is calculated by modifying Equation 11-7:

$$V1 = \frac{\text{dose}}{\text{initial plasma concentration}} = \frac{\text{dose}}{A + B} \quad (11\text{-}13)$$

The volume of the central compartment is important in clinical anesthesiology because it is the pharmacokinetic parameter that determines the peak plasma concentration after an iv bolus injection. Hypovolemia, for example, reduces the volume of the central compartment. If doses are not correspondingly reduced, the higher plasma concentrations will increase the incidence of adverse pharmacologic effects.

Immediately after iv injection, all of the drug is in the central compartment. Simultaneously, three processes begin. Drug moves from the central to the peripheral compartment, which also has a volume, $V2$. This intercompartmental transfer is a first-order process, and its magnitude is quantified by the rate constant k_{12}. As soon as drug appears in the peripheral compartment, some passes back to the central compartment, a process characterized by the rate constant k_{21}. The transfer of drug between the central and peripheral compartments is quantified by the *distributional* or *intercompartmental clearance:*

$$\text{Intercompartmental clearance} = V1 \cdot k_{12} = V2 \cdot k_{21} \quad (11\text{-}14)$$

The third process that begins immediately after administration of the drug is irreversible removal of drug from the system *via* the central compartment. As in the one-compartment model, the elimination rate constant is k_e. The rapidity of the decrease in the central compartment concentration after iv injection depends on the magnitude of the compartmental volumes, the intercompartmental clearance, and the elimination clearance.

At equilibrium, the drug is distributed among the central and the peripheral compartment, and by definition, the concentrations in the compartments are equal. Therefore, the ultimate volume of distribution, termed the volume of distribution at steady-state (V_{ss}), is the sum of $V1$ and $V2$. Extensive tissue uptake of a drug is reflected by a large volume of the peripheral compartment, which, in turn, results in a large V_{ss}. Consequently, V_{ss} can greatly exceed the actual volume of the body.

As in the single-compartment model, in multicompartment models the elimination clearance is equal to the dose divided by the area under the concentration *versus* time curve. This area, as well as the compartmental volumes, and intercompartmental clearances, can be calculated from the intercepts and hybrid rate constants, without having to reach steady-state conditions.[108]

Three-Compartment Model

After iv injection of some drugs, the initial, rapid distribution phase is followed by a second, slower distribution phase before the elimination phase becomes evident. Therefore, the plasma concentration is the sum of three exponential terms:

$$Cp_{(t)} = Ae^{-\alpha t} + Be^{-\beta t} + Ge^{-\gamma t}, \quad (11\text{-}15)$$

where t = time, $Cp_{(t)}$ = plasma concentration at time t, A = intercept of the rapid distribution phase line, α = hybrid rate constant of the rapid distribution phase, B = intercept of the slower distribution phase line, β = hybrid rate constant of the slower distribution phase, G = intercept of the elimination phase line, and γ = hybrid rate constant of the elimination phase. This triphasic behavior is explained by a three-compartment pharmacokinetic model (Fig. 11-8). As in the two-compartment model, the drug is injected into and eliminated from the central compartment. Drug is reversibly transferred between the central compartment and two peripheral compartments, which accounts for two distribution phases. Drug transfer between the central compartment and the more rapidly equilibrat-

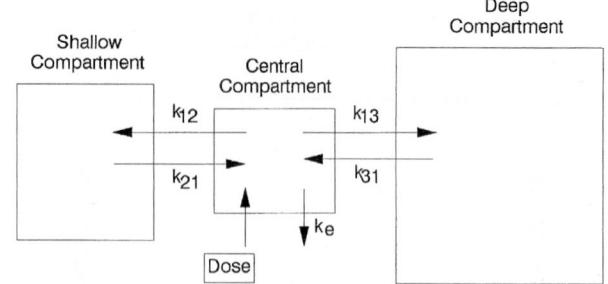

Figure 11-8. A three-compartment pharmacokinetic model. See text for explanation.

ing, or "shallow," peripheral compartment is characterized by the first-order rate constants k_{12} and k_{21}. Transfer in and out of the more slowly equilibrating, "deep" compartment is characterized by the rate constants k_{13} and k_{31}. In this model, there are three compartmental volumes: $V1$, $V2$, and $V3$, whose sum equals V_{ss}; and three clearances: the rapid intercompartmental clearance, the slow intercompartmental clearance, and elimination clearance.

The pharmacokinetic parameters of interest to clinicians, such as clearance, volumes of distribution, and distribution and elimination half-times, are determined by calculations analogous to those used in the two-compartment model. Accurate estimates of these parameters depend on accurate characterization of the measured plasma concentration versus time data. A frequently encountered problem is that the duration of sampling is not long enough to define accurately the elimination phase.[109] Similar problems arise if the assay cannot detect low concentrations of the drug. Whether a drug exhibits two- or three-compartment kinetics is of no clinical consequence. In fact, some drugs have two-compartment kinetics in some patients and three-compartment kinetics in others.[86,110] In selecting a pharmacokinetic model, the most important factor is that it accurately characterize the measured concentrations. In general, the model with the smallest number of compartments or exponents that accurately reflects the data is used.

Effects of Hepatic or Renal Disease on Pharmacokinetic Parameters

As discussed earlier, hepatic and renal disease not only affect the ability to eliminate drugs, but also change the binding of drugs to plasma proteins. Consequently, the effects of altered protein binding and the effects of impaired organ function must be considered to understand fully the impact of hepatic or renal disease on pharmacokinetic variables.

The extent of drug distribution depends on the relative affinity of blood *versus* tissues for the drug. Therefore, if the free fraction in plasma increases, the volume of distribution must also increase. The magnitude of the change depends on the initial free fraction and volume of distribution. An increase in the free fraction will produce the greatest increase in the volume of distribution for drugs that are highly bound to plasma proteins and have small volumes of distribution. In contrast, changes in plasma protein binding of drugs with large volumes of distribution have minimal effects on the volume of distribution, because so little of the total amount of drug is in the plasma.[111]

In theory, a parallel change in tissue binding would cancel the effect of changes in plasma binding. However, this appears to be uncommon. Increased volumes of distribution of propranolol[112] and diazepam[22] associated with increased free fractions have been observed in patients with hepatic disease. Decreased binding of thiopental in patients with renal failure also increases the volume of distribution.[92]

The effect of altered protein binding on total drug clearance also depends on the initial magnitude of the clearance. Increases in the free fraction of drugs with low hepatic extraction ratios and drugs eliminated primarily by glomerular filtration cause a proportional increase in clearance. In contrast, altered protein binding has little effect on drugs with high hepatic or renal clearance. The effect of an increased free fraction on elimination depends on the net effect on clearance and the volume of distribution.[111] The elimination half-time will increase if increased volume of distribution is the paramount change, or decrease if increased clearance predominates.

Diverse pathophysiologic changes preclude precise prediction of the pharmacokinetics of a given drug in individual patients with hepatic or renal disease. However, some generalizations can be made. Binding of drugs to albumin is decreased, so that doses of drugs given as an iv bolus, such as thiopental, should be reduced. In patients with hepatic disease, the elimination half-time of drugs metabolized or excreted by the liver is often increased because of decreased clearance, and, possibly, increased volume of distribution. Repeated doses of such drugs as benzodiazepines, opioids, and barbiturates may accumulate, leading to excessive and prolonged pharmacologic effects. Recovery from small doses of drugs such as thiopental and fentanyl is largely the result of redistribution, so recovery from conservative doses will be minimally affected. In patients with renal failure, similar concerns apply to the administration of drugs excreted by the kidneys. It is almost always better to underestimate a patient's dose requirement, observe the response, and give additional drug if necessary.

Nonlinear Pharmacokinetics

The physiologic and compartmental models thus far discussed are based on the assumption that drug distribution and elimination are first-order processes. Therefore, their parameters, such as clearance and elimination half-time, are independent of the dose or concentration of the drug. However, the rate of elimination of a few drugs is dose-dependent, or *nonlinear*.

Elimination of most drugs involves interactions with protein molecules, either enzymes catalyzing biotransformation reactions or carrier proteins for transmembrane transport. If sufficient drug is present, the capacity of the drug-eliminating systems can be exceeded. When this occurs, it is no longer possible to excrete a constant fraction of the drug present to the eliminating system, and a constant amount of drug is excreted per unit time. Phenytoin is a well known example of a drug that exhibits nonlinear elimination at therapeutic concentrations. In theory, all drugs are cleared in nonlinear fashion. In practice, the capacity to eliminate most drugs is so great that this is usually not evident, even with toxic concentrations.

PHARMACODYNAMIC PRINCIPLES

In its broadest sense, pharmacodynamics is the study of the effects of drugs on the body. Classically, pharmacologic effects have been quantified by dose–response studies. Advances in drug assay techniques and data analysis now allow definition of the relationship between the drug concentration and the associated pharmacologic effect *in vivo*. As a result, the term *pharmacodynamics* has acquired a more specific definition: the quantitative analysis of the relationship between the drug concentration in the blood, or at the site of action, and the resultant effects of the drug on physiologic processes.[113]

Dose–Response Curves

Dose–response studies determine the relationship between increasing doses of a drug and the ensuing changes in pharmacologic effects. Schematic dose–response curves are shown in Figure 11-9, with the dose plotted on both linear and logarithmic scales. There is a curvilinear relationship between dose and the intensity of response. Low doses produce little pharmacologic effect. Once effects become evident, a small increase in dose produces a relatively large change in effect. At near-maximal response, large increases in dose produce little change in effect. Usually the dose is plotted on a logarithmic scale (see Fig. 11-9, right panel), which demonstrates the linear relationship between the logarithm of the dose and the intensity of the response between 20% and 80% of the maximum effect.

Dose–response curves provide information regarding four aspects of the relationship of dose and pharmacologic effect. The *potency* of the drug—the dose required to produce a given effect—is determined. Potency is usually expressed as the dose required to produce a given effect in 50% of subjects, the *ED50*. The *slope* of the curve between 20% and 80% of the maximal effect indicates the rate of increase in effect as the dose is increased. The maximum effect is referred to as the *efficacy* of the drug. Finally, if curves from multiple subjects are generated, the *variability* in potency, efficacy, and the slope of the dose–response curve can be estimated.

The dose needed to produce a given pharmacologic effect varies considerably, even in "normal" patients. The patient most resistant to the drug usually requires a dose two- to three-fold greater than the patient with the lowest dose requirements. This variability is caused by differences between individuals in the relationship between drug concentration and pharmacologic effect, superimposed on differences in pharmacokinetics. Dose–response studies have the disadvantage of not being able to determine whether variations in pharmacologic response are caused by differences in pharmacokinetics, pharmacodynamics, or both.

Concentration–Response Relationships

Ideally, the concentration of drug at its site of action should be used to define the concentration–response relationship. Unfortunately, these data are rarely available, so the relationship between the concentration of drug in the blood and pharmacologic effect is studied instead. This relationship is easiest to understand if the changes in pharmacologic effect that occur during and after an iv infusion of a hypothetical drug are considered. If a drug is infused at a constant rate, the plasma concentration initially increases rapidly, and asymptotically approaches a steady-state level after approximately five elimination half-times have elapsed (Fig. 11-10). The effect of the drug initially increases very slowly, then more rapidly, and eventually also reaches a steady state. When the infusion is discontinued, indicated by point *C* in Figure 11-10, the plasma concentration immediately decreases because of drug distribution and elimination. However, the effect stays the same for a short period,

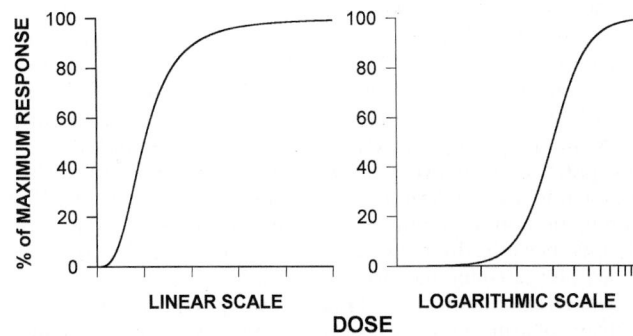

Figure 11-9. *Left panel:* A schematic curve of the effect of a drug plotted against dose. *Right panel:* The same curve, replotted with dose on a logarithmic scale. This yields the familiar sigmoid dose–response curve, which is linear between 20% and 80% of the maximal effect.

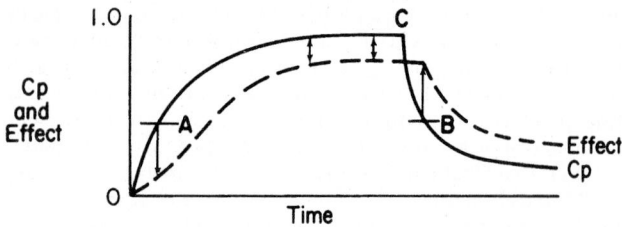

Figure 11-10. The changes in plasma drug concentration and pharmacologic effect during and after an intravenous infusion. See text for explanation. (Reprinted with permission from Stanski DR, Sheiner LB: Pharmacokinetics and pharmacodynamics of muscle relaxants. Anesthesiology 51:103, 1979.)

and then also begins to decrease—there is always a time lag between changes in plasma concentration and changes in pharmacologic response. Figure 11-10 also demonstrates that the same plasma concentration is associated with different responses if the concentration is changing. At points *A* and *B* in Figure 11-10, the plasma concentrations are the same, but the effects at each time differ. When the concentration is increasing, there is a concentration gradient from blood to the site of action. When the infusion is discontinued, the concentration gradient is reversed. Therefore, at the same plasma concentration, the concentration at the site of action is higher after, compared to during, the infusion. This is associated with a correspondingly greater effect.

In theory, there must be some degree of temporal disequilibrium between plasma concentration and drug effect for all drugs with extravascular sites of action. However, for some drugs, the time lag may be so short that it cannot be demonstrated. The magnitude of this temporal disequilibrium depends on several factors:

1. perfusion of the organ on which the drug acts
2. the tissue:blood partition coefficient of the drug
3. the rate of diffusion or transport of the drug from the blood to the cellular site of action
4. the rate and affinity of drug–receptor binding
5. the time required for processes initiated by the drug-receptor interaction to produce changes in cellular function

The consequence of this time lag between changes in concentration and changes in effects is that the plasma concentration will have an unvarying relationship with pharmacologic effect only under steady-state conditions. At steady state, the plasma concentration is in equilibrium with the concentrations throughout the body, and is thus directly proportional to the steady-state concentration at the site of action. Plotting the logarithm of the steady-state plasma concentration *versus* response generates a curve identical in appearance to the dose–response curve shown in the right panel of Figure 11-9. The $Cp_{ss}50$, the steady-state plasma concentration producing 50% of the maximal response, is determined from the concentration–response curve. Like the ED50, the $Cp_{ss}50$ is a measure of sensitivity to a drug, but the $Cp_{ss}50$ has the advantage of being unaffected by pharmacokinetic variability. Because it takes five elimination half-times to approach steady-state conditions, it is not practical to determine the $Cp_{ss}50$ directly. For drugs with long elimination half-times, the pseudoequilibrium during the elimination phase can be used to approximate steady-state conditions, because the concentrations in plasma and at the site of action are changing very slowly.

The onset and duration of pharmacologic effects depend not only on pharmacokinetic factors but also on the pharmacodynamic factors governing the degree of temporal disequilibrium between changes in concentration and changes in effect. The magnitude of the pharmacologic effect is a function of the amount of drug present at the site of action, so increasing the

dose increases the peak effect. Larger doses have a more rapid onset of action because pharmacologically active concentrations at the site of action occur sooner. Increasing the dose also increases the duration of action because pharmacologically effective concentrations are maintained for a longer time.

Integrated pharmacokinetic–pharmacodynamic models fully characterize the relationships between time, dose, plasma concentration, and pharmacologic effect.[113] This is accomplished by adding an *"effect compartment"* to a standard compartmental pharmacokinetic model. The effect compartment is also called the *biophase*. Transfer of drug between central compartment and the effect compartment, or biophase, is assumed to be a first-order process, and the pharmacologic effect is assumed to be directly related to the concentration in the biophase. By quantifying the time lag between changes in plasma concentration and changes in pharmacologic effect, these models can also define the $Cp_{ss}50$, even without steady-state conditions. These models have contributed greatly to our understanding of factors influencing the response to intravenous anesthetics,[114,115] opioids,[116,117] and nondepolarizing muscle relaxants[118,119] in humans.

Dose–response and concentration–response relationships can be altered by many factors, such as drug interactions or pathologic conditions. They are also affected by the development of tolerance, which increases the ED50 and $Cp_{ss}50$. When tolerance develops rapidly, it is referred to as *tachyphylaxis*, or *acute tolerance*.

Drug–Receptor Interactions

The biochemical and physiologic effects of drugs, neurotransmitters, and hormones result from the binding of these compounds to receptors, which initiates changes in cellular function. In addition to the well known muscarinic and nicotinic cholinergic receptors, and α- and β-adrenoceptors, there are specific receptors for histamine, serotonin, dopamine, eicosanoids, peptide hormones, steroid hormones, endorphins and exogenous opiates, benzodiazepines, and calcium channel blockers, to name a few. Subtypes of many of these receptors have been characterized. In mammals, there are dozens of distinct receptors for various endogenous and exogenous compounds.[120,121] Most receptors are protein molecules situated on the cell membrane, although some are located within the cell.

Binding of drugs to receptors, like the binding of drugs to plasma proteins, is usually reversible, and follows the law of mass action:

$$[\text{drug}] + [\text{receptor}] \rightleftharpoons [\text{drug–receptor complex}] \quad (11\text{-}16)$$

The higher the concentration of free drug or unoccupied receptor, the greater the tendency to form the drug–receptor complex. Plotting the percentage of receptors occupied by a drug against the logarithm of the concentration of the drug yields a sigmoid curve, as shown in Figure 11-11.

It is often assumed that the percentage of the maximal effect observed at any given drug concentration is equal to the percentage of receptors occupied by the drug. However, this is not always the case. At the neuromuscular junction, only 20–25% of the postjunctional nicotinic cholinoceptors need to bind acetylcholine to produce contraction of all the fibers in the muscle.[122] Thus, 75–80% of the receptors can be considered "spare receptors." The presence of spare receptors has two important consequences. Equation 11-16 indicates that the higher the concentration of unoccupied receptors, the greater the tendency to form the drug–receptor complex. Therefore, spare receptors permit near-maximal effects at very low concentrations of drugs or neurotransmitters.[123] The other corollary of the existence of spare receptors is that most of the receptors must be occupied by an antagonist before transmission is affected. This accounts for the "margin of safety" of neuromuscular transmission.[122]

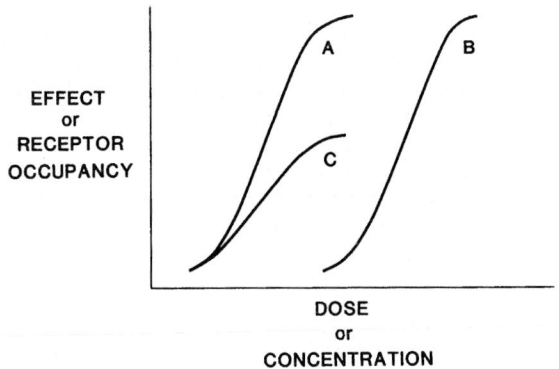

EFFECT
or
RECEPTOR
OCCUPANCY

DOSE
or
CONCENTRATION

Figure 11-11. Schematic dose–response curves representing various conditions. Either dose or concentration is plotted on the *x*-axis, and either effect or the number of receptors occupied on the *y*-axis. Curve *A* is a typical dose–response curve. Curve *B* is a parallel rightward shift of the curve, and represents a drug that is less potent than the drug depicted by curve *A*, but is a full agonist and thus capable of producing the same maximal effect. Curve *B* would also result if the drug used to generate curve *A* was studied in the presence of a competitive antagonist. Curve *C* is shifted to the right, with a reduction in slope and the maximal effect. This is the curve observed with partial agonists, and also when a full agonist (curve *A*) is studied in the presence of a noncompetitive antagonist.

The binding of drugs to receptors and the resulting changes in cellular function are the last two steps in the complex series of events between administration of the drug and production of its pharmacologic effects. There are two primary mechanisms by which the binding of an agonist to a receptor changes cellular function: receptor-linked membrane ion channels called *ionophores,* and guanine nucleotide binding proteins, referred to as *G-proteins.* The nicotinic cholinoceptor in the neuromuscular postsynaptic membrane is one example of a receptor-ionophore complex. Binding of acetylcholine opens the cation ionophore, leading to an influx of Na^+ ions, propagation of an action potential, and, ultimately, muscle contraction.[124] The γ-amino butyric acid (GABA) receptor–chloride ionophore complex is another example of this type of effector mechanism. Binding of either endogenous neurotransmitters (GABA) or exogenous agonists (benzodiazepines and iv anesthetics) increases Cl^- conductance, which hyperpolarizes the neuron and decreases its excitability.[125] β-Adrenoceptors are the prototypical receptors that alter cellular function *via* G-proteins. G-proteins change the intracellular concentrations of various so-called *second messengers,* such as Ca^{2+} and cyclic AMP.[126]

Receptors are not static entities. Rather, they are dynamic cellular components that adapt to their environment. For example, administration of β-adrenergic agonists leads to desensitization of β-adrenoceptors.[127] This occurs by several mechanisms: reduced ability to combine with G-proteins; *sequestration,* which is the removal of receptors from the cell membrane so they are no longer accessible to agonists, and by *downregulation,* a decrease in the total number of receptors. Administration of adrenoceptor antagonists increases the number of receptors.[127]

Agonists, Partial Agonists, and Antagonists

Drugs that bind to receptors and produce an effect are called *agonists.* Drugs may be capable of producing the same maximal effect, although they may differ in potency. Agonists that differ in potency but bind to the same receptors will have parallel concentration–response curves (curves *A* and *B* in Fig. 11-11). Differences in potency of agonists reflect differences in affinity for the receptor. *Partial agonists* are drugs that are not capable of producing the maximal effect, even at very high concentrations (curve *C* in Fig. 11-11).

Compounds that bind to receptors without producing any changes in cellular function are referred to as *antagonists.* Binding of agonists to receptors is inhibited by antagonists. Competitive antagonists bind reversibly to receptors, and their blocking effect can be overcome by high concentrations of an agonist. Therefore, *competitive antagonists* produce a parallel shift in the dose–response curve, but the maximum effect is not altered (see Fig. 11-11, curves *A* and *B*). *Noncompetitive antagonists* bind irreversibly to receptors. This has the same effect as reducing the number of receptors and shifts the dose–response curve downward and to the right, decreasing both the slope and the maximum effect (curves *A* and *C* in Fig. 11-11). The effect of noncompetitive antagonists is reversed only by synthesis of new receptor molecules.

Agonists produce a structural change in the receptor molecule that initiates changes in cellular function. Partial agonists may produce a qualitatively different change in the receptor, whereas antagonists bind without producing a change in the receptor that results in altered cellular function. The underlying mechanisms by which different compounds that bind to the same receptor act as agonists, partial agonists, or antagonists are not fully understood.

CLINICAL APPLICATION OF PHARMACOKINETICS AND PHARMACODYNAMICS

In anesthesia, the usual therapeutic objectives are rapidly to produce pharmacologic effects, such as unconsciousness or muscle relaxation, to maintain the optimal intensity of these effects during the anesthetic, and to have the patient recover rapidly on conclusion of surgery. Knowledge of pharmacokinetic principles and of the pharmacokinetic and pharmacodynamic properties of the drugs used in anesthesiology makes it easier to attain these objectives. If the pharmacokinetics and the therapeutic concentration of a drug are known, then the average doses required to achieve and maintain the desired pharmacologic effect can be calculated. The steady-state plasma concentration (Cp_{ss}) is a function of the rate of infusion of the drug and drug clearance:

$$Cp_{ss} = \frac{\text{Infusion rate}}{Cl}; \text{thus: Infusion rate} = Cp_{ss} \cdot Cl \quad (11\text{-}17)$$

Infusion of the drug for five elimination half-times is required to reach steady-state conditions. Therefore, for many of the iv agents used in anesthesia, it would take 24 hours or more to reach a stable plasma concentration by merely infusing the drug at a constant rate. This is obviously impractical, and does not meet the first of our therapeutic objectives.

The volume of distribution must be rapidly "filled up" with a loading dose to achieve a more rapid onset of action. The loading dose can be calculated by multiplying the volume of distribution (*Vd*) by the desired concentration:

$$\text{Loading dose} = Cp_{ss} \cdot Vd \quad (11\text{-}18)$$

Almost all drugs, including those used in anesthesia, have multicompartment pharmacokinetic properties. Therefore, their initial volume of distribution, which is equal to the volume of the central compartment (*V*1), gets progressively larger until the ultimate volume of distribution, the volume of distribution at steady state (V_{ss}), is reached. Consequently, the loading dose can vary according to specific therapeutic objectives. A minimal loading dose is the amount of drug required to "fill up" the central compartment:

$$\text{Minimal loading dose} = Cp_{ss} \cdot V1 \quad (11\text{-}19)$$

This rapidly achieves the desired concentration and effect, satisfying the first of the three therapeutic objectives. However, the concentration will decrease very quickly because of drug distribution and elimination, even if the loading dose is followed by an infusion (Figure 11-12). Consequently, the desired effect will be maintained for a very short period.

A full loading dose can be defined as the amount of drug needed to provide the desired concentration once distribution has been completed. It is calculated as follows:

$$\text{Full loading dose} = Cp_{ss} \cdot V_{ss} \qquad (11\text{-}20)$$

Figure 11-12 demonstrates the plasma concentration–time profile if a full loading dose is followed by a maintenance infusion. The concentration is initially much higher than desired, and it eventually falls to the desired concentration. The disadvantage of this combination is evident. The high initial concentration may produce adverse effects, and there may still be a high drug concentration at the conclusion of surgery, preventing rapid recovery.

As a compromise, a partial (more than the minimal, but less than the full) loading dose can be given. If this is followed by a maintenance infusion, the concentration will initially be higher than desired, and will then fall until the infusion increases the concentration, ultimately achieving the target steady-state value. Figure 11-12 demonstrates that the discrepancy between the desired and actual concentrations is less after the partial loading dose–infusion combination than with either the "full loading dose + infusion" or the "minimal loading dose + infusion" combination. The partial loading dose produces a lower initial concentration than the full loading dose, which is less likely to cause adverse effects, and there is also less likelihood of having an excessive concentration at the conclusion of the operation. The partial loading dose is less likely than the minimal loading dose to result in subtherapeutic concentrations. Therefore, the partial loading dose–maintenance infusion combination comes closest to fulfilling the three therapeutic objectives. If the nadir of the concentration results in an inadequate effect, then a supplementary bolus dose can be given. This principle can be extended by giving a minimal loading dose, followed by many progressively smaller supplementary doses, so that the concentration is close to the desired level virtually all the time.

Although the elimination half-time is often thought of as the most important pharmacokinetic parameter, it does not appear in Equations 11-17 to 11-20. The elimination half-time is not a true fundamental pharmacokinetic parameter; it is a hybrid parameter that depends on the fundamental parameters: the compartmental volumes, intercompartmental clearance (which determines the rate of equilibration between compartments),

and elimination clearance. During most anesthetics, termination of pharmacologic effects depends more on redistribution of drugs from their sites of action to other tissues than on elimination of drugs from the body, especially for lipophilic agents. The ultimate elimination half-time of propofol may be 10 hours or more.[128] However, even after infusion of propofol for 18 hours, a rapid decrease in the blood concentration occurs on termination of the infusion.[129] This is due to uptake of propofol by peripheral tissues, which permits redistribution of propofol from the brain to those tissues. Sufentanil is more lipophilic than alfentanil, and simulations suggest that the concentration of sufentanil at its sites of action actually may decrease faster than the concentration of alfentanil under conditions typical of the vast majority of anesthetics.[130] Therefore, when drugs are administered for just a few hours, the elimination half-time does not usefully predict the rapidity of recovery from lipophilic drugs because redistribution lowers the plasma, and hence brain, concentration below pharmacologically active levels. Less lipophilic agents, such as neuromuscular blockers, are less extensively taken up by tissues, and the rate of recovery from these drugs more closely parallels their elimination half-times.

The concept of the *context-sensitive half-time* has been proposed to predict the rapidity of recovery after infusions of intravenous anesthetics.[131,132] Briefly, the context-sensitive half-time is derived by plotting the time required for a 50% decrease in plasma concentration after an infusion against the duration of the infusion. The longer the infusion, the longer the context-sensitive half-time. However, for lipophilic agents with multicompartmental kinetics, the context-sensitive half-time is always shorter than the elimination half-time, even for infinitely long infusions. For example after a 3-hour infusion of fentanyl (using a pharmacokinetic model having an elimination half-time of 475 min[131]), the context-sensitive half-time is 185 min. The times for greater or lesser decreases in concentrations after infusions can also be simulated.[130,132] These simulations have provided new insights into the factors responsible for recovery from intravenous anesthetics.

Systems for Administration of Intravenous Agents

Several studies comparing the traditional intermittent bolus injection of iv anesthetics and adjuvants with continuous infusions suggest that the infusions have several advantages.[133] The pharmacologic effect is more stable, and often lower total doses are given when continuous infusions, titrated according to individual patients' requirements, are used. Administering iv infusions of iv drugs is facilitated by use of infusion pumps. In terms of operating cost, syringe pumps have a clear advantage over volumetric pumps with cassettes. The major disadvantages of syringe pumps are the relatively low volume that can be infused without interrupting the infusion to refill the syringe, and, for most pumps, a relatively low maximum infusion rate. The desirable features for iv infusion pumps are outlined in Table 11-6. Devices with the some of the programmable features listed in Table 11-6 are currently commercially available. Allowing the user to specify which drug is being delivered by the pump, and including algorithms that warn of potential overdoses is a logical extension of programmability that has yet to be fully exploited. One currently available syringe pump partly achieves this by using magnetically encoded faceplates to identify the drug to the pump, and having a microprocessor determine and control bolus and infusion doses corrected for body weight.* The pump has ranges both for bolus doses ($mg \cdot kg^{-1}$) and for maintenance infusions ($mg \cdot kg^{-1} \cdot h^{-1}$) that are specific for the drug being infused. However, the number of drugs for which faceplates

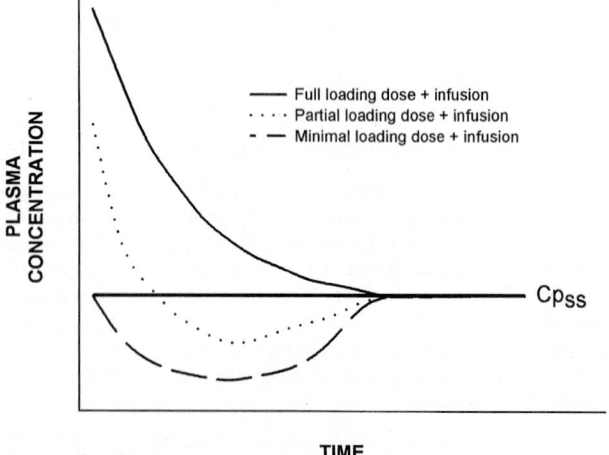

Figure 11-12. Plasma concentration *versus* time curves after administration of full, partial, and minimal loading doses, followed by a maintenance infusion at a constant rate. (See Equations 11-17 to 11-20 and accompanying text for explanation.)

* Baxter Healthcare Corporation. http://www.baxter.com/doctors/iv_therapies/index.html. October 20, 1999.

Table 11-6. DESIRABLE FEATURES FOR INTRAVENOUS INFUSION DEVICES

Low acquisition and operating costs
Accuracy over a wide range of flow rates to allow use with multiple drug formulations in adult and pediatric patients
Small size and battery backup for transporting patients
Programmability:
  Drug identification
  Ability to enter patient weight and drug concentration, allowing user to set dose in mass units rather than volumes (*i.e.,* $mg \cdot h^{-1}$ or $\mu g \cdot kg^{-1}$ instead of $ml \cdot h^{-1}$)
  Preset bolus dose in mass units or volume, with reversion to continuous infusion rate after completion of bolus
  Computer interface for data acquisition and control
  Target-controlled infusion capability
Displays:
  All programmed parameters
  Current infusion rate and cumulative dose
  Visible in low ambient light
Safety features:
  Audio and visual alarms for empty drug reservoir, air in line, occlusion, impending battery depletion, nonspecific malfunction
  Sensing and control circuits to detect discrepancies between programmed and actual flow rates
  Microprocessor-based integration of drug identification, patient weight, and set dose to alert user of potential overdoses

are available is limited. Another commercially available syringe pump allows entry of doses in either volume per time (*i.e.,* $mL \cdot h^{-1}$), mass per time (*i.e.,* $mg \cdot h^{-1}$), or mass per time corrected for weight (*i.e.,* $mg \cdot kg^{-1} \cdot h^{-1}$).*

Pharmacokinetic and pharmacodynamic principles have been used to develop computer-controlled drug infusion systems consisting of a computer linked to a volumetric pump *via* a serial interface.[134,135] Algorithms based on compartmental pharmacokinetic models determine the infusion rates necessary to achieve and maintain a target concentration in plasma or in the effect compartment. In essence, these systems give a minimal loading dose (Eq. 11-19), followed by a continuous infusion that replaces drug removed from the central compartment by both redistribution and elimination. The program continuously updates the concentration predicted by the pharmacokinetic model, then continuously adjusts the infusion rate to minimize the discrepancy between the predicted concentration and the desired target concentration. The anesthesiologist can increase or decrease the target concentration as dictated by clinical circumstances, allowing titration to the desired drug effect. This method of delivering intravenous anesthetic drugs and adjuvants is called *target-controlled infusion* (TCI).[136] In a given patient, the measured plasma concentration and the predicted concentration during TCI will differ because of individual pharmacokinetic variability. However, this bias is usually constant, at least for the duration of an anesthetic.[135,137] Compared to manually controlled devices, these systems permit more rapid, precise, proportional changes of the plasma concentration of iv agents. Preliminary investigations suggest that TCI achieved more precise control of intravenous anesthetic concentrations during cardiac surgery, compared to manually controlled continuous infusions.[138] TCI systems should facilitate attainment of the therapeutic objectives in anesthesiology—rapid onset and maintenance of the optimal effect, followed by rapid recovery at the end of surgery. A TCI system for administering propofol has recently become commercially available.†

* Sims Graseby Limited. http://www.graseby.co.uk/products/3400.htm. October 20, 1999.

† Sims Graseby Limited. http://www.graseby.co.uk/products/3500.htm. October 20, 1999.

The major disadvantage of all infusion devices is their cost. At the present time, there is no conclusive evidence that using these devices either improves patient care or reduces health care costs. Intuitively, continuous infusion of iv anesthetics seems logical—after all, we do not administer volatile agents using intermittent boluses! In the current fiscal climate, demonstration of better care or lower costs is needed to justify acquisition of sophisticated infusion systems.

DRUG INTERACTIONS

Taking into account premedication, perioperative antibiotics, iv agents used for induction or maintenance, inhalational anesthetics, opioids, muscle relaxants, the drugs used to restore neuromuscular transmission, and postoperative analgesics, 10 or more drugs may be given for a relatively "routine" anesthetic. Consequently, thorough understanding of the mechanisms of drug interactions and knowledge of specific interactions with drugs used in anesthesia are essential to the safe practice of anesthesiology. Indeed, anesthesiologists often deliberately take advantage of drug interactions. For example, when cholinesterase inhibitors are given to reverse the effects of neuromuscular blockers on nicotinic cholinoceptors, atropine or glycopyrrolate is administered concomitantly to avoid such undesirable side effects as bradycardia and bronchospasm, which would result from increased acetylcholine binding to muscarinic cholinoceptors. (See Chapter 50 for a more complete discussion.)

Drug interactions due to physicochemical properties can occur *in vitro*. Mixing acidic drugs, such as thiopental, and basic drugs, such as opioids or muscle relaxants, results in the formation of insoluble salts that precipitate.[139] Another type of *in vitro* reaction is absorption of drugs by plastics. Examples include the uptake of nitroglycerin by polyvinyl chloride infusion sets[140] and the absorption of fentanyl by the apparatus used for cardiopulmonary bypass.[141]

Drugs can alter each other's absorption, distribution, and elimination. Absorption from the GI tract is altered by drugs like ranitidine, which alters gastric pH,[51] and metoclopramide, which speeds gastric emptying.[142] Vasoconstrictors are added to local anesthetic solutions to prolong their duration of action at the site of injection and to decrease the risk of systemic toxicity from rapid absorption.

Drugs that compete for binding sites on plasma proteins have complex interactions.[72] Displacement of a drug from plasma proteins affects its distribution. The increase in the free drug concentration increases tissue uptake of the drug, increasing the volume of distribution. The extent of the effect on drug distribution depends on the fraction of the total drug in the body that is bound to plasma proteins. The change in distribution will be greatest when drugs with relatively large bound fractions and small volumes of distribution are displaced. Displacement of one drug by another may produce toxic free drug concentrations. When a steady state is re-established, the effect of decreased binding on total and free drug concentrations depends on the rate of clearance of the drug. For drugs with low extraction ratios, clearance varies with the degree of binding, and clearance increases proportionately to the increase in free fraction. Therefore, when a steady state is re-established, the total drug concentration will be lower, but the free drug level will be the same as the level before displacement. Clearance of drugs with high extraction ratios is not restricted to the free fraction and is not affected by changes in binding. Consequently, when a new steady state is reached, the total drug concentration is unchanged, and the higher free drug level will persist. Adverse interactions are thus most likely to occur if the displaced drug has high (nonrestrictive) clearance, a small volume of distribution, and relatively high binding to plasma proteins.

Drugs that inhibit or induce the enzymes that catalyze biotransformation reactions can affect clearance of other concomitantly administered drugs. Clearance can also be affected by drug-induced changes in hepatic blood flow. Drugs that are cleared by the kidneys and have similar physicochemical characteristics compete for the transport mechanisms involved in renal tubular secretion.

Pharmacodynamic interactions fall into two broad classifications. Drugs can interact, either directly or indirectly, at the same receptors. Opioid antagonists directly displace opioids from opiate receptors. Cholinesterase inhibitors indirectly antagonize the effects of neuromuscular blockers by increasing the amount of acetylcholine, which displaces the blocking drug from nicotinic receptors. Pharmacodynamic interactions can also occur if two drugs affect a physiologic system at different sites. Benzodiazepines and opioids, each acting on their own specific receptors, appear to interact synergistically.[143,144] Although receptors and mechanisms are not as well defined as for the benzodiazepine–opioid interaction, this is presumably how volatile anesthetics increase sensitivity to neuromuscular blocking drugs,[118] and also how premedication increases sensitivity to inhalational anesthetics.[145]

REFERENCES

1. Papper EM: The pharmacokinetics of inhalation anaesthetics: Clinical applications. Br J Anaesth 36:124, 1964
2. Benet LZ, Mitchell JR, Sheiner LB: Pharmacokinetics: The dynamics of drug absorption, distribution and elimination. In Gilman AG, Rall TW, Nies AS, Taylor P (eds): The Pharmacological Basis of Therapeutics, 9th ed, p 3. New York, Pergamon Press, 1996
3. Krishna DR, Klotz U: Extrahepatic metabolism of drugs in humans. Clin Pharmacokinet 26:144, 1994
4. Ashburn MA, Streisand J, Zhang J et al: The iontophoresis of fentanyl citrate in humans. Anesthesiology 82:1146, 1995
5. Greenblatt DJ, Shader RI, Abernethy DR: Current status of benzodiazepines. N Engl J Med 309:354, 410, 1983
6. Fee JPH, Collier PS, Dundee JW: Bioavailability of three formulations of intravenous diazepam. Acta Anaesthesiol Scand 30:337, 1986
7. Price HL, Kovnat PJ, Safer JN et al: The uptake of thiopental by body tissues and its relationship to the duration of narcosis. Clin Pharmacol Ther 1:16, 1960
8. Saidman LJ, Eger EI II: The effect of thiopental metabolism on duration of anesthesia. Anesthesiology 27:118, 1966
9. Brown WU Jr, Bell GC, Alper MH: Acidosis, local anesthetics and the newborn. Obstet Gynecol 48:27, 1976
10. Shanks CA: Pharmacokinetics of the nondepolarizing neuromuscular relaxants applied to calculation of bolus and infusion dosage regimens. Anesthesiology 64:72, 1986
11. Wilkinson GR, Shand DG: A physiological approach to hepatic drug clearance. Clin Pharmacol Ther 18:377, 1975
12. Nies AS, Shand DG, Wilkinson GR: Altered hepatic blood flow and drug disposition. Clin Pharmacokinet 1:135, 1976
13. Blaschke TF: Protein binding and kinetics of drugs in liver diseases. Clin Pharmacokinet 2:32, 1977
14. Swartz RD, Sidell FR, Cucinell SA: Effects of physical stress on the disposition of drugs eliminated by the liver in man. J Pharmacol Exp Ther 188:1, 1974
15. Stenson RE, Constantino RT, Harrison DC: Interrelationships of hepatic blood flow, cardiac output, and blood levels of lidocaine in man. Circulation 43:205, 1971
16. Thomson PD, Melmon KL, Richardson JA et al: Lidocaine pharmacokinetics in advanced heart failure, liver disease, and renal failure in humans. Ann Intern Med 78:499, 1973
17. Benowitz NL, Meister W: Pharmacokinetics in patients with cardiac failure. Clin Pharmacokinet 1:389, 1976
18. Benowitz NL, Forsyth RP, Melmon KL et al: Lidocaine disposition kinetics in monkey and man: II. Effects of hemorrhage and sympathomimetic drug administration. Clin Pharmacol Ther 16:99, 1974
19. Klotz U, McHorse TS, Wilkinson GR et al: The effect of cirrhosis on the disposition and elimination of meperidine in man. Clin Pharmacol Ther 16:667, 1974
20. Neal EA, Meffin PJ, Gregory PB et al: Enhanced bioavailability and decreased clearance of analgesics in patients with cirrhosis. Gastroenterology 77:96, 1979
21. Wood AJJ, Kornhauser DM, Wilkinson GR et al: The influence of cirrhosis on steady-state blood concentrations of unbound propranolol after oral administration. Clin Pharmacokinet 3:478, 1978
22. Klotz U, Avant GR, Hoyumpa A et al: The effects of age and liver disease on the disposition and elimination of diazepam in adult man. J Clin Invest 55:347, 1975
23. Klotz U, Antonin KH, Brugel H et al: Disposition of diazepam and its major metabolite desmethyldiazepam in patients with liver disease. Clin Pharmacol Ther 21:430, 1977
24. McHorse TS, Wilkinson GR, Johnson RF et al: Effect of acute viral hepatitis in man on the disposition and elimination of meperidine. Gastroenterology 68:775, 1975
25. Williams RL, Blaschke TF, Meffin PJ et al: Influence of viral hepatitis on the disposition of two compounds with high hepatic clearance: Lidocaine and indocyanine green. Clin Pharmacol Ther 20:290, 1976
26. Branch RA, Shand DG, Wilkinson GR et al: The reduction of lidocaine clearance by dl-propranolol: An example of hemodynamic drug interaction. J Pharmacol Exp Ther 184:515, 1973
27. Gelman S: Disturbances in hepatic blood flow during anesthesia and surgery. Arch Surg 111:881, 1976
28. Gelman S, Fowler KC, Smith LR: Liver circulation and function during isoflurane and halothane anesthesia. Anesthesiology 61:726, 1984
29. Cooperman LH: Effects of anaesthetics on the splanchnic circulation. Br J Anaesth 44:967, 1972
30. Duchin KL, Schrier RW: Interrelationship between renal haemodynamics, drug kinetics, and drug action. Clin Pharmacokinet 3:58, 1978
31. Garrett ER: Pharmacokinetics and clearances related to renal processes. Int J Clin Pharmacol 16:155, 1978
32. Stanton BA, Koeppen BM: Elements of renal function. In Berne RM, Levy MN (eds): Physiology, 4th ed, p 677. St. Louis, Mosby, 1998
33. Lam YW, Banerji S, Hatfield C, Talbert RL: Principles of drug administration in renal insufficiency. Clin Pharmacokinet 32:30, 1997
34. Collinsworth KA, Strong JM, Atkinson AJ et al: Pharmacokinetics and metabolism of lidocaine in patients with renal failure. Clin Pharmacol Ther 18:59, 1975
35. Miller RD, Agoston S, Booij LHDJ et al: The comparative potency and pharmacokinetics of pancuronium and its metabolites in anesthetized man. J Pharmacol Exp Ther 207:539, 1978
36. Szeto HH, Inturrisi CE, Houde R et al: Accumulation of normeperidine, an active metabolite of meperidine, in patients with renal failure or cancer. Ann Intern Med 86:738, 1977
37. Bennett WM: Geriatric pharmacokinetics and the kidney. Am J Kidney Dis 26:283, 1990
38. Stanski DR, Watkins WD: Drug Disposition in Anesthesia, p 76. New York, Grune & Stratton, 1982
39. Hollenberg PF: Mechanisms of cytochrome P450 and peroxidase-catalyzed xenobiotic metabolism. Fed Am Soc Exp Biol J 6:686, 1992
40. de Groot H, Sies H: Cytochrome P-450, reductive metabolism, and cell injury. Drug Metab Rev 20:275, 1989
41. Hall SD, Thummel KE, Watkins PB et al: Molecular and physical mechanisms of first-pass extraction. Drug Metab Dispos 27:161, 1999
42. Coon MJ, Ding X, Pernicky SJ et al: Cytochrome P450: Progress and predictions. Fed Am Soc Exp Biol J 6:669, 1992
43. Nelson DR, Kamataki T, Waxman DJ et al: The P450 superfamily: Update on new sequences, gene mapping, accession numbers, early trivial names of enzymes, and nomenclature. DNA Cell Biol 12:1, 1993
44. Guengerich FP: Catalytic selectivity of human cytochrome P450 enzymes: Relevance to drug metabolism and toxicity. Toxicol Lett 70:133, 1994
45. Chang GWM, Kam PCA: The physiological and pharmacological roles of cytochrome P450 isoenzymes. Anaesthesia 54:42, 1999
46. Gonzalez FJ, Nebert DW: Evolution of the P-450 gene superfamily: Animal–plant warfare, molecular drive and human genetic differences in drug oxidation. Trends Genet 6:182, 1990
47. Okey AB: Enzyme induction in the cytochrome P-450 system. Pharmacol Ther 45:241, 1990
48. Guay DRP, Meatherall RC, Chalmers JL et al: Cimetidine alters pethidine disposition in man. Br J Clin Pharmacol 18:907, 1984
49. Feely J, Wilkinson GR, Wood AJJ: Reduction of liver blood flow

and propranolol metabolism by cimetidine. N Engl J Med 304:692, 1981

50. Klotz U, Reimann I: Delayed clearance of diazepam due to cimetidine. N Engl J Med 302:1012, 1980

51. Smith SR, Kendall MJ: Ranitidine *versus* cimetidine: A comparison of their potential to cause clinically important drug interactions. Clin Pharmacokinet 15:44, 1988

52. Schlanz KD, Myre SA, Bottoroff MB: Pharmacokinetic interactions with calcium channel antagonists (Parts I and II). Clin Pharmacokinet 21:344, 448, 1991

53. Cupp MJ, Tracy TS: Cytochrome P450: New nomenclature and clinical implications. Am Fam Physician 57:107, 1998

54. Daly AK, Cholerton S, Gregory W *et al*: Metabolic polymorphisms. Pharmacol Ther 57:129, 1993

55. Wormhoudt LW, Commandeur JNM, Vermeulen NPE: Genetic polymorphisms of human *N*-acetyltransferase, cytochrome P450, glutathione-*S*-transferase, and epoxide hydrolase enzymes: Relevance to xenobiotic metabolism and toxicity. Crit Rev Toxicol 29:59, 1999

56. Besunder JB, Reed MD, Blumer JL: Principles of drug biodisposition in the neonate: A critical evaluation of the pharmacokinetic–pharmacodynamic interface. Clin Pharmacokinet 14:189, 261, 1988

57. Morselli PL: Clinical pharmacology of the perinatal period and early infancy. Clin Pharmacokinet 17(suppl 1):13, 1989

58. Durnas C, Loi C-M, Cusack BJ: Hepatic drug metabolism and aging. Clin Pharmacokinet 19:359, 1990

59. Woodhouse KW, James OFW: Hepatic drug metabolism and ageing. Br Med Bull 46:22, 1990

60. Lane EA, Guthrie S, Linnoila M: Effects of ethanol on drug and metabolite pharmacokinetics. Clin Pharmacokinet 10:228, 1985

61. Miller LG: Recent developments in the study of the effects of cigarette smoking on clinical pharmacokinetics and clinical pharmacodynamics. Clin Pharmacokinet 17:90, 1989

62. Williams RL, Mamelok RD: Hepatic disease and drug pharmacokinetics. Clin Pharmacokinet 5:528, 1980

63. Reidenberg MM: The biotransformation of drugs in renal failure. Am J Med 62:482, 1977

64. Reilly CS, Wood AJJ, Koshakji RP *et al*: The effect of halothane on drug disposition: Contribution of changes in intrinsic drug metabolizing capacity and hepatic blood flow. Anesthesiology 63:70, 1985

65. Wood M, Wood AJJ: Contrasting effects of halothane, isoflurane, and enflurane on in vivo drug metabolism in the rat. Anesth Analg 63:709, 1984

66. Vesell ES: The antipyrine test in clinical pharmacology: Conceptions and misconceptions. Clin Pharmacol Ther 26:275, 1979

67. Duvaldestin P, Mazze RI, Nivoche Y *et al*: Enzyme induction following surgery with halothane and neurolept anesthesia. Anesth Analg 60:319, 1981

68. Loft S, Boel J, Kyst A *et al*: Increased hepatic microsomal enzyme activity after surgery under halothane or spinal anesthesia. Anesthesiology 62:11, 1985

69. Duvaldestin P, Mauge F, Desmonts JM: Enflurane anesthesia and antipyrine metabolism. Clin Pharmacol Ther 29:61, 1981

70. Pessayre D, Allemand H, Benoist C *et al*: Effect of surgery under general anaesthesia on antipyrine clearance. Br J Clin Pharmacol 6:505, 1978

71. Pantuck EJ, Pantuck CB, Weismann C *et al*: Effects of parenteral nutrition regimens on oxidative drug metabolism. Anesthesiology 60:534, 1984

72. Wood M: Plasma drug binding—Implications for anesthesiologists. Anesth Analg 65:786, 1986

73. McLain DA, Hug CC: Intravenous fentanyl kinetics. Clin Pharmacol Ther 28:106, 1980

74. Meuldermans WEG, Hurkmans RMA, Heykants JJP: Plasma protein binding and distribution of fentanyl, sufentanil, alfentanil and lofentanil in blood. Arch Int Pharmacodynam 257:4, 1982

75. Sjoholm I, Ekman B, Kober A *et al*: Binding of drugs to serum albumin: XI. Mol Pharmacol 16:767, 1979

76. Notarianni LJ: Plasma protein binding of drugs in pregnancy and in neonates. Clin Pharmacokinet 18:20, 1990

77. Morgan DJ, Blackman GL, Paull JD *et al*: Pharmacokinetics and plasma binding of thiopental: II. Studies at cesarean section. Anesthesiology 54:474, 1981

78. Wood M, Wood AJJ: Changes in plasma drug binding and alpha$_1$-acid glycoprotein in mother and newborn infant. Clin Pharmacol Ther 29:522, 1981

79. Hill MD, Abramson FP: The significance of plasma protein binding on the fetal/maternal distribution of drugs at steady-state. Clin Pharmacokinet 14:156, 1988

80. Davis D, Grossman SH, Ketchell BB *et al*: The effects of age and smoking on the plasma protein binding of lignocaine and diazepam. Br J Clin Pharmacol 19:261, 1985

81. Verbeeck RK, Cardinal J-A, Wallace SM: Effect of age and sex on the plasma binding of acidic and basic drugs. Eur J Clin Pharmacol 27:91, 1984

82. Wallace S, Whiting B: Factors affecting drug binding in plasma of elderly patients. Br J Clin Pharmacol 3:327, 1976

83. Herman RJ, McAllister CB, Branch RA *et al*: Effect of age on meperidine disposition. Clin Pharmacol Ther 37:19, 1985

84. Holmberg L, Odar-Cederlof I, Nilsson JLG *et al*: Pethidine binding to blood cells and plasma proteins in old and young subjects. Eur J Clin Pharmacol 23:457, 1982

85. Greenblatt DJ, Abernethy DR, Locniskar A *et al*: Effect of age, gender, and obesity on midazolam kinetics. Anesthesiology 61:27, 1984

86. Greenblatt DJ, Allen MD, Harmatz JS *et al*: Diazepam disposition determinants. Clin Pharmacol Ther 27:301, 1980

87. Jung D, Mayersohn M, Perrier D *et al*: Thiopental disposition as a function of age in female patients undergoing surgery. Anesthesiology 56:263, 1982

88. Thiessen JJ, Sellers EM, Denbeigh P *et al*: Plasma protein binding of diazepam and tolbutamide in chronic alcoholics. J Clin Pharmacol 16:345, 1976

89. Olsen GD, Bennett WM, Porter GA: Morphine and phenytoin binding to plasma proteins in renal and hepatic failure. Clin Pharmacol Ther 17:677, 1975

90. Ghoneim MM, Pandya H: Plasma protein binding of thiopental in patients with impaired renal or hepatic function. Anesthesiology 42:545, 1975

91. Pandale G, Chaux F, Salvadori C *et al*: Thiopental pharmacokinetics in patients with cirrhosis. Anesthesiology 59:123, 1983

92. Burch PG, Stanski DR: Decreased protein binding and thiopental kinetics. Clin Pharmacol Ther 32:212, 1982

93. Reidenberg MM, Drayer DE: Alteration of drug–protein binding in renal disease. Clin Pharmacokinet 9(suppl 1):18, 1984

94. Grossman SH, Davis D, Kitchell BB *et al*: Diazepam and lidocaine plasma protein binding in renal disease. Clin Pharmacol Ther 31:350, 1982

95. Piafsky KM, Borga O, Odar-Cederlof I *et al*: Increased plasma protein binding of propranolol and chlorpromazine mediated by disease-induced elevations of plasma alpha$_1$-acid glycoprotein. N Engl J Med 299:1435, 1978

96. Zini R, Riant P, Barré J, Tillement J-P: Disease-induced variations in plasma protein levels. Implications for drug dosage regimens. Clin Pharmacokinet 19:147, 218, 1990

97. Jackson PR, Tucker GT, Woods HF: Altered plasma drug binding in cancer: Role of alpha$_1$-acid glycoprotein and albumin. Clin Pharmacol Ther 32:295, 1982

98. Routledge PA, Stargel WW, Wagner GS *et al*: Increased alpha$_1$-acid glycoprotein and lidocaine disposition in myocardial infarction. Ann Intern Med 93:701, 1980

99. Routledge PA, Stargel WW, Wagner GS *et al*: Increased plasma protein binding in myocardial infarction. Br J Clin Pharmacol 9:438, 1980

100. Elfstrom J: Drug pharmacokinetics in the postoperative period. Clin Pharmacokinet 4:16, 1979

101. Edwards DJ, Lalka D, Cerra F *et al*: Alpha$_1$-acid glycoprotein concentration and protein binding in trauma. Clin Pharmacol Ther 31:62, 1982

102. Fremstad D, Bergerud K, Haffner JFW *et al*: Increased plasma binding of quinidine after surgery: A preliminary report. Eur J Clin Pharmacol 10:441, 1976

103. Feely J, Forrest A, Gunn A *et al*: Influence of surgery on plasma propranolol levels and protein binding. Clin Pharmacol Ther 28:579, 1980

104. Holley FO, Ponganis KV, Stanski DR: Effects of cardiac surgery with cardiopulmonary bypass on lidocaine disposition. Clin Pharmacol Ther 35:617, 1984

105. Balant LP, Gex-Fabry M: Physiological pharmacokinetic modelling. Xenobiotica 20:1241, 1990

106. Eger EI II: Anesthetic Uptake and Action, p 79. Baltimore, Williams & Wilkins, 1974
107. Gibaldi M, Perrier D: Pharmacokinetics, 2nd ed, p 45. New York, Marcel Dekker, 1982
108. Wagner JH: Linear pharmacokinetic equations allowing direct calculation of many needed pharmacokinetic parameters from the coefficients and exponents of polyexponential equations which have been fitted to the data. J Pharmacokinet Biopharm 4:443, 1976
109. Gibaldi M, Weintraub H: Some considerations as to the determination and significance of biologic half-life. J Pharm Sci 60:624, 1971
110. Hudson RJ, Stanski DR, Burch PG: Pharmacokinetics of methohexital and thiopental in surgical patients. Anesthesiology 59:215, 1983
111. Rowland M: Protein binding and drug clearance. Clin Pharmacokinet 9(suppl 1):10, 1984
112. Branch RA, James J, Read AE: A study of factors influencing drug disposition in chronic liver disease, using the model drug (+)-propranolol. Br J Clin Pharmacol 3:243, 1976
113. Holford NHG, Sheiner LB: Understanding the dose–effect relationship: Clinical application of pharmacokinetic–pharmacodynamic models. Clin Pharmacokinet 6:429, 1981
114. Stanski DR, Hudson RJ, Homer TD et al: Pharmacodynamic modelling of thiopental anesthesia. J Pharmacokinet Biopharm 12:223, 1984
115. Stanski DR, Maitre PO: Population pharmacokinetics and pharmacodynamics of thiopental: The effect of age revisited. Anesthesiology 72:412, 1990
116. Scott JC, Ponganis KV, Stanski DR: EEG quantitation of narcotic effect: The comparative pharmacodynamics of fentanyl and alfentanil. Anesthesiology 62:234, 1985
117. Scott JC, Cooke JE, Stanski DR: Electroencephalographic quantitation of opioid effect: Comparative pharmacodynamics of fentanyl and sufentanil. Anesthesiology 74:34, 1991
118. Stanski DR, Ham J, Miller RD et al: Pharmacokinetics and pharmacodynamics of d-tubocurarine during nitrous oxide–narcotic and halothane anesthesia in man. Anesthesiology 51:235, 1979
119. Fisher DM, O'Keeffe C, Stanski DR et al: Pharmacokinetics and pharmacodynamics of d-tubocurarine in infants, children, and adults. Anesthesiology 57:203, 1982
120. Snyder SH: Drug and neurotransmitter receptors in the brain. Science 224:22, 1984
121. Birnbaumer L, Brown AM: G proteins and the mechanism of action of hormones, neurotransmitters, and autocrine and paracrine regulatory factors. Am Rev Respir Dis 141:S106, 1990
122. Waud BE, Waud DR: The margin of safety of neuromuscular transmission in the muscle of the diaphragm. Anesthesiology 37:417, 1972
123. Norman J: Drug–receptor reactions. Br J Anaesth 51:595, 1979
124. Feldman S: Neuromuscular blocking agents. In Feldman SA, Paton W, Scurr C (eds): Mechanisms of Drugs in Anaesthesia, 2nd ed, p 340. London, Hodder & Stoughton, 1993
125. Ooi R: Effects of drugs on ion channels and transmembrane signalling. In Feldman SA, Paton W, Scurr C (eds): Mechanisms of Drugs in Anaesthesia, 2nd ed, p 32. London, Hodder & Stoughton, 1993
126. Ooi R: Effects of drugs on ion channels and transmembrane signalling. In Feldman SA, Paton W, Scurr C (eds): Mechanisms of Drugs in Anaesthesia, 2nd ed, p 34. London, Hodder & Stoughton, 1993
127. Jenkinson DH: An introduction to receptors and their actions. In Feldman SA, Paton W, Scurr C (eds): Mechanisms of Drugs in Anaesthesia, 2nd ed, p 14. London, Hodder & Stoughton, 1993
128. Sebel PS, Lowdon JD: Propofol: A new intravenous anesthetic. Anesthesiology 71:260, 1989
129. McMurray TJ, Collier PS, Carson IW et al: Propofol sedation after open heart surgery: A clinical and pharmacokinetic study. Anaesthesia 45:322, 1990
130. Shafer SL, Varvel JR: Pharmacokinetics, pharmacodynamics, and rational opioid selection. Anesthesiology 74:53, 1991
131. Hughes MA, Glass PSA, Jacobs JR: Context-sensitive half-time in multicompartment pharmacokinetic models for intravenous anesthetics. Anesthesiology 76:334, 1992
132. Shafer SL, Stanski DR: Improving the clinical utility of anesthetic drug pharmacokinetics. Anesthesiology 76:327, 1992
133. White PF: Clinical uses of intravenous anesthetic and analgesic infusions. Anesth Analg 68:161, 1989
134. Alvis JM, Reves JG, Govier AV et al: Computer-assisted infusions of fentanyl during cardiac anesthesia: Comparison with a manual method. Anesthesiology 63:41, 1985
135. Shafer SL, Siegel LC, Cooke JE et al: Testing computer-controlled infusion pumps by simulation. Anesthesiology 68: 261, 1988
136. Glass PSA, Glen JB, Kenny GNC et al: Nomenclature for computer-assisted infusion devices. Anesthesiology 86:1430, 1997
137. Ausems ME, Vujk J, Hug CC Jr et al: Comparison of a computer-assisted infusion versus intermittent bolus administration of alfentanil as a supplement to nitrous oxide for lower abdominal surgery. Anesthesiology 68:851, 1988
138. Theil DR, Stanley TE, White WD et al: Midazolam and fentanyl continuous infusion anesthesia for cardiac surgery: A comparison of computer-assisted versus manual infusion systems. J Cardiothorac Vasc Anesth 7:300, 1993
139. Cullen BF, Miller MG: Drug interactions in anesthesia. Anesth Analg 58:413, 1979
140. Mutch WAC, Thomson IR: Delivery systems for intravenous nitroglycerin. Can Anaesth Soc J 30:98, 1983
141. Koren G, Goresky G, Crean P et al: Pediatric fentanyl dosing based on pharmacokinetics during cardiac surgery. Anesth Analg 63:577, 1984
142. Rawlins MD: Drug interactions and anaesthesia. Br J Anaesth 50:689, 1978
143. Vinik HR, Bradley EL Jr, Kissin I: Midazolam–alfentanil synergism for anesthetic induction in patients. Anesth Analg 69:213, 1989
144. Kissin I, Vinik HR, Castillo R, Bradley EL Jr: Alfentanil potentiates midazolam-induced unconsciousness in subanalgesic doses. Anesth Analg 71:65, 1990
145. Quasha AL, Eger EI II, Tinker JH: Determinations and applications of MAC. Anesthesiology 53:315, 1980
146. Mooradian AD: Digitalis: An update of clinical pharmacokinetics, therapeutic monitoring techniques and treatment recommendations. Clin Pharmacokinet 15:165, 1988
147. Echizen H, Eichelbaum M: Clinical pharmacokinetics of verapamil, nifedipine and diltiazem. Clin Pharmacokinet 11:425, 1986
148. Lowenthal DT, Porter RS, Saris SD et al: Clinical pharmacology, pharmacodynamics and interactions with esmolol. Am J Cardiol 56:14F, 1985
149. Mandelli M, Tognoni G, Garattini S: Clinical pharmacokinetics of diazepam. Clin Pharmacokinet 3:72, 1978
150. Greenblatt DJ: Clinical pharmacokinetics of oxazepam and lorazepam. Clin Pharmacokinet 6:89, 1981
151. Brand L, Mark LC, Snell MM et al: Physiologic disposition of methohexital in man. Anesthesiology 24:331, 1963
152. Kirkpatrick T, Cockshott ID, Douglas EJ, Nimmo WS: Pharmacokinetics of propofol (Diprivan) in elderly patients. Br J Anaesth 60:146, 1988
153. Tucker GT, Mather LM: Pharmacokinetics of local anaesthetic agents. Br J Anaesth 47:213, 1975
154. Lee A, Fagan D, Lamont M et al: Disposition kinetics of ropivacaine in humans. Anesth Analg 69:763, 1989
155. Duvaldestin P, Henzel D: Binding of tubocurarine, fazadinium, pancuronium, and Org NC45 to serum proteins in normal man and in patients with cirrhosis. Br J Anaesth 54:513, 1982
156. Wood M, Stone WJ, Wood AJJ: Plasma binding of pancuronium: Effects of age, sex, and disease. Anesth Analg 62:29, 1983
157. Säwe J: High-dose morphine and methadone in cancer patients. Clinical pharmacokinetic considerations of oral treatment. Clin Pharmacokinet 11:87, 1986
158. Patwardhan RV, Johnsson RJ, Hoyumpa A et al: Normal metabolism of morphine in cirrhosis. Gastroenterology 81:1006, 1981

Clinical Anesthesia (4/e), edited by
Paul G. Barash, Bruce F. Cullen, and
Robert K. Stoelting. Lippincott Williams &
Wilkins, Philadelphia, © 2001.

CHAPTER 12

AUTONOMIC NERVOUS SYSTEM: PHYSIOLOGY AND PHARMACOLOGY

NOEL W. LAWSON AND JOEL O. JOHNSON

AUTONOMIC PHARMACOLOGY

Anesthesiology is the practice of autonomic medicine. Drugs that produce anesthesia also produce potent autonomic side-effects. The greater part of our training and practice is spent acquiring skills in averting or utilizing the ANS (autonomic nervous system) side-effects of anesthetic drugs under a variety of pathophysiologic conditions. The success of any anesthetic depends upon how well homeostasis is maintained. The numbers that we faithfully record during the course of anesthesia reflect ANS function and not necessarily the presence of surgical anesthesia.[1,2] A knowledge of the ANS is a prerequisite to an understanding of anesthesia pharmacology.

AUTONOMIC NERVOUS SYSTEM PURPOSE

The ANS includes that part of the central and peripheral nervous system concerned with involuntary regulation of cardiac muscle, smooth muscle, glandular, and visceral functions. ANS activity refers to visceral reflexes that function essentially below the conscious level. The term *autonomic* remains the best description of this ubiquitous system, as opposed to *automatic*. Autonomic implies self-controlling, whereas automatic implies nonreflexic or intrinsic responses; however, the use of ''autonomy'' to describe this nervous system is also illusory. The ANS is also responsive to changes in somatic motor and sensory activities of the body. The physiologic evidence of visceral reflexes as a result of somatic events is abundantly clear. Psychosomatic disease is an expression of this connection. The ANS is therefore not as distinct an entity as the term suggests. Neither somatic nor ANS activity occurs in isolation.[1] The ANS organizes visceral support for somatic behavior and adjusts body states in anticipation of emotional behavior or responses to the stress of disease, *i.e.*, fight or flight.

Traditionally, the ANS has been viewed as strictly a peripheral, efferent (motor) system. This concept is no longer tenable. Afferent fibers from visceral structures are the first link in the reflex arcs of the ANS whether relaying visceral pain or changes in vessel stretch. Most ANS efferent fibers are accompanied by sensory fibers that are now commonly recognized as components of the ANS. The afferent components of the ANS cannot be as distinctively divided as can the efferent nerves.

Historically, many investigators have refused to classify any afferent fibers within the ANS because visceral sensory nerves are anatomically indistinguishable from somatic sensory nerves.[2] Visceral afferent pathways are like afferent somatic nerves in that they are unipolar. ANS efferents are bipolar (Fig. 12-1). Furthermore, afferent fibers that are anatomically aligned with ANS efferents do not differ by design, function, or drug response from somatic afferents. In addition, both somatic and visceral sensory nerves are able to initiate ANS reflexes. However, the argument is functional rather than anatomic because visceral pain can be attenuated by sympathectomy. The clinical importance of visceral afferent fibers is more closely associated with chronic pain management.

FUNCTIONAL ANATOMY

The ANS naturally falls into two divisions by anatomy, physiology, and pharmacology. Langley divided this nervous system into two parts in 1921. He retained the term *sympathetic* (sympathetic nervous system, SNS), which was introduced by Willis in 1665, for the first part and introduced the term *parasympathetic* (parasympathetic nervous system, PNS) for the second. The term *autonomic nervous system* was adopted as a comprehensive name for both. Ordinarily, activation of the SNS produces expenditure of body energy, whereas the PNS produces conservation or accumulation of energy resources. Table 12-1 lists the complementary effects of SNS (adrenergic) and PNS (cholinergic) activity of organ systems.

Central Autonomic Organization

Pure central ANS or somatic centers are not known. Extensive overlap of function occurs. And integration of ANS activity occurs at all levels of the cerebrospinal axis. Efferent ANS activity can be initiated locally and by centers located in the spinal cord, brain stem, and hypothalamus. The cerebral cortex is the highest level of ANS integration. Fainting at the sight of blood is an example of this higher level of somatic and ANS integration. ANS function has also been successfully modulated through conscious, intentional efforts, demonstrating that somatic responses are always accompanied by visceral responses and *vice versa*.

The principal site of ANS organization is the hypothalamus. SNS functions are controlled by nuclei in the posterolateral hypothalamus. Stimulation of these nuclei results in a massive discharge of the sympathoadrenal system (Table 12-2). PNS functions are governed by nuclei in the midline and some anterior nuclei of the hypothalamus. The anterior hypothalamus is involved with regulation of temperature. The supraoptic hypothalamic nuclei regulate water metabolism and are anatomically and functionally associated with the posterior lobe of the pituitary (see Interaction of Autonomic Nervous System Receptors). This hypothalamic-neurohypophyseal connection represents a central ANS mechanism that affects the kidney by means of antidiuretic hormone. Long-term blood pressure control, reactions to physical and emotional stress, sleep, and sexual reflexes are regulated through the hypothalamus.

The medulla oblongata and pons are the vital centers of acute ANS organization. Together, they integrate momentary hemodynamic adjustments and maintain the sequence and automaticity of ventilation. Integration of afferent and efferent ANS impulses at this central nervous system (CNS) level is responsible for the tonic activity exhibited by the ANS. Control of peripheral vascular resistance and blood pressure is an example of this tonic activity. Tonicity holds visceral organs in a state of intermediate activity that can either be diminished or augmented by altering the rate of nerve firing. The nucleus tractus solitarius, located within the medulla, is the primary area for relay of afferent chemoreceptor and baroreceptor information from the glossopharyngeal and vagus nerves. Increased afferent impulses from these two nerves inhibits periph-

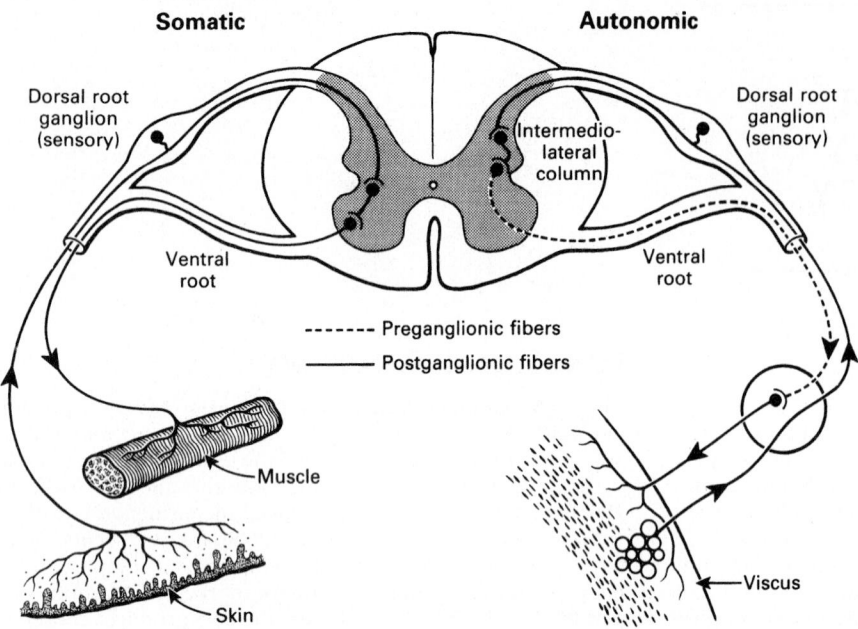

Figure 12-1. Comparison of somatic and autonomic reflex arcs. Somatic arcs are unipolar and autonomic arcs are bipolar.

Table 12-1. HOMEOSTATIC BALANCE BETWEEN ADRENERGIC AND CHOLINERGIC EFFECTS

	Response	
Organ System	*Adrenergic*	*Cholinergic*
HEART		
Sinoatrial node	Tachycardia	Bradycardia
Atrioventricular node	Increased conduction	Decreased conduction
His-purkinje	Increased automaticity and conduction velocity	Minimal
Myocardium	Increased contractility, conduction velocity, automaticity	Minimal decrease in contractility
Coronary vessels	Constriction (α_1) and dilation (β_1)	Dilation and constriction?*
BLOOD VESSELS		
Skin and mucosa	Constriction	Dilation
Skeletal muscle	Constriction (α_1) > dilation (β_2)	Dilation
Pulmonary	Constriction	?Dilation
BRONCHIAL SMOOTH MUSCLE	Relaxation	Contraction
GASTROINTESTINAL TRACT		
Gallbladder and ducts	Relaxation	Contraction
Gut motility	Decreased	Increased
Secretions	Decreased	Increased
Sphincters	Constriction	Relaxation
BLADDER		
Detrusor	Relaxes	Contracts
Trigone	Contracts	Relaxes
GLANDS		
Nasal	Vasoconstriction and reduced secretion	Stimulation of secretions
Lacrimal		
Parotid		
Submandibular		
Gastric		
Pancreatic		
SWEAT GLANDS	Diaphoresis (cholinergic)	None
APOCRINE GLANDS	Thick, odiferous secretion	None
EYE		
Pupil	Mydriasis	Miosis
Ciliary muscle	Relaxation for far vision	Contraction for near vision

* See the section on Interaction of Autonomic Nervous System Receptors.

Table 12-2. HYPOTHALAMIC NUCLEI

Anterior	Posterior
PARAVENTRICULAR NUCLEUS	**POSTERIOR HYPOTHALAMUS**
Oxytocin release	Increased blood pressure
Water conservation	Pupillary dilation
	Shivering
MEDIAL PREOPTIC AREA	Corticotropin
Bladder contraction	**DORSOMEDIAL NUCLEUS**
Decreased heart rate	Gastrointestinal stimulation
Decreased blood pressure	**PERIFORNICAL NUCLEUS**
SUPRAOPTIC NUCLEUS	Hunger
Water conservation	Increased blood pressure
	Rage
POSTERIOR PREOPTIC AND ANTERIOR HYPO-THALAMIC AREA	**VENTROMEDIAL NUCLEUS**
	Satiety
Body temperature regulation	**MAMMILLARY BODY**
Panting	Feeding reflexes
Sweating	**LATERAL HYPOTHALAMIC AREA**
Thyrotropin inhibition	Thirst and hunger

eral SNS vascular tone, producing vasodilation, and increase vagal tone, producing bradycardia. High spinal cord transection eliminates the medulla and results in hypotension. Studies of patients with high spinal cord lesions show that a number of reflex changes are mediated at the spinal or segmental level. ANS hyper-reflexia is an example of spinal cord mediation of ANS reflexes without integration of function from higher inhibitory centers.[1,3]

Peripheral Autonomic Nervous System Organization

The peripheral ANS is the efferent (motor) component of the ANS and consists of two complementary parts: the SNS and the PNS. Most organs receive fibers from both divisions (Fig. 12-2). In general, activities of the two systems produce opposite but complementary effects (see Table 12-1). Actions of the two subdivisions are supplementary in some tissues, such as the salivary glands. A few tissues, such as sweat glands and spleen, are innervated by only SNS fibers. Although the anatomy of the somatic and ANS sensory pathways is identical, the motor pathways are characteristically different. The efferent somatic motor system, like somatic afferents, is composed of a single (unipolar) neuron with its cell body in the ventral gray matter of the spinal cord. Its myelinated axon extends directly to the voluntary striated muscle unit. In contrast, the efferent (motor) ANS is a two-neuron (bipolar) chain from the CNS to the effector organ (see Fig. 12-1). The first neuron of both the SNS and PNS originates within the CNS but does not make direct contact with the effector organ. Instead, it relays the impulse to a second station known as an ANS ganglion, which contains the cell body of the second ANS (postganglionic) neuron. Its axon contacts the effector organ. Schematically, then, the motor pathways of both divisions of the ANS are a serial, two-neuron chain consisting of a preganglionic neuron and a postganglionic effector neuron (Fig. 12-3).

Preganglionic fibers of both subdivisions are myelinated, with diameters of less than 3 μm.[1] Impulses are conducted at a speed of 3–15 m · s^{-1}. The postganglionic fibers are unmyelinated and conduct impulses at slower speeds of less than 2 m · s^{-1}. They are similar to unmyelinated visceral and somatic afferent C fibers (Table 12-3). Compared with the myelinated somatic nerves, the ANS conducts impulses at speeds that preclude its participation in the immediate phase of a somatic response.

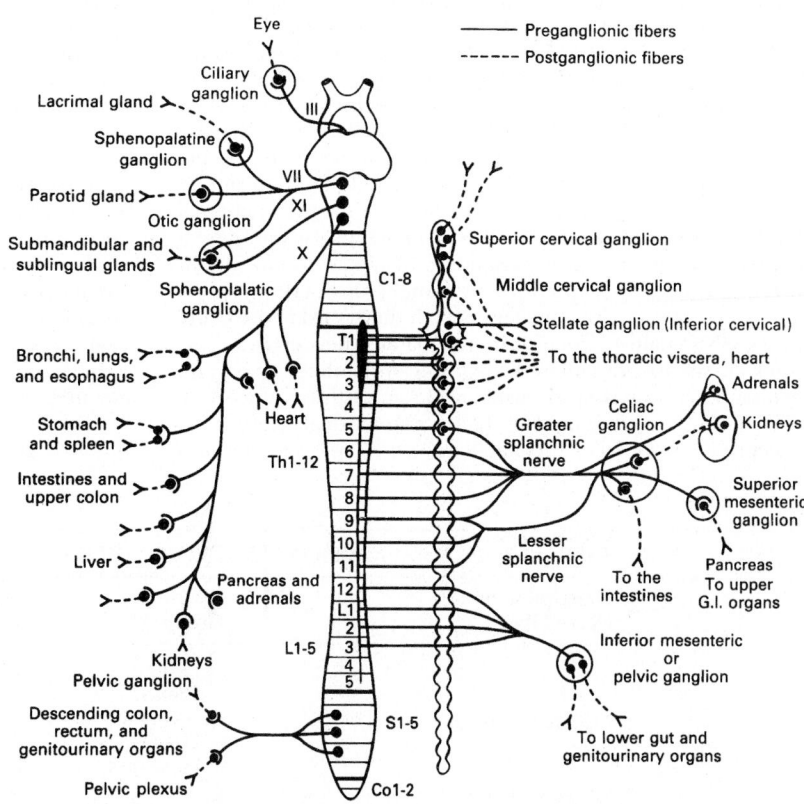

Figure 12-2. Schematic distribution of the craniosacral (parasympathetic) and thoracolumbar (sympathetic) nervous systems. Parasympathetic preganglionic fibers pass directly to the organ that is innervated. Their postganglionic cell bodies are situated near or within the innervated viscera. This limited distribution of parasympathetic postganglionic fibers is consistent with the discrete and limited effect of parasympathetic function. The postganglionic sympathetic neurons originate in either the paired sympathetic ganglia or one of the unpaired collateral plexuses. One preganglionic fiber influences many postganglionic neurons. Activation of the SNS produces a more diffuse physiologic response rather than discrete effects.

Parasympathetic nerve distribution (Craniosacral outflow)

Sympathetic nerve distribution (Thoracolumbar outflow)

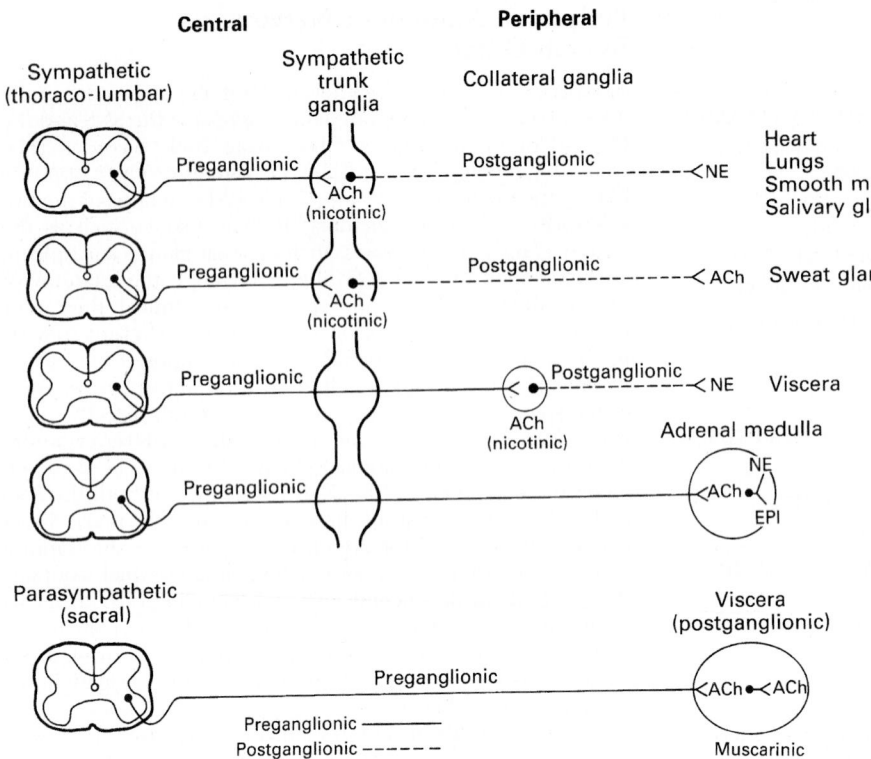

Figure 12-3. Schematic diagram of the efferent ANS. Afferent impulses are integrated centrally and sent reflexly to the adrenergic and cholinergic receptors. Sympathetic fibers ending in the adrenal medulla are preganglionic, and acetylcholine (ACh) is the neurotransmitter. Stimulation of the chromaffin cells, acting as postganglionic neurons, releases epinephrine (EPI) and norepinephrine (NE).

Sympathetic Nervous System or Thoracolumbar Division

The efferent SNS is referred to as the thoracolumbar nervous system. The origin of its preganglionic fibers provides the anatomic basis for this designation. Figure 12-2 demonstrates the distribution of the SNS and its innervation of visceral organs.

The preganglionic fibers of the SNS (thoracolumbar division) originate in the intermediolateral gray column of the 12 thoracic (T1–T12) and the first 3 lumbar segments (L1–L3) of the spinal cord. The myelinated axons of these nerve cells leave the spinal cord with the motor fibers to form the white (myelinated) communicating rami (Fig. 12-4). The rami enter one of the paired 22 sympathetic ganglia at their respective segmental levels. Upon entering the paravertebral ganglia of the lateral sympathetic chain, the preganglionic fiber may follow one of three courses: (1) synapse with postganglionic fibers in ganglia at the level of exit; (2) course upward or downward in the trunk of the SNS chain to synapse in ganglia at other levels; or (3) track for variable distances through the sympathetic chain and exit without synapsing to terminate in an outlying, unpaired, SNS collateral ganglion (Fig. 12-4). The adrenal gland is an exception to the rule. Preganglionic fibers pass directly into

the adrenal medulla without synapsing in a ganglion (see Fig. 12-3). The cells of the medulla are derived from neuronal tissue and are analogous to postganglionic neurons.[4]

The sympathetic postganglionic neuronal cell bodies are located in ganglia of the paired lateral SNS chain or unpaired collateral ganglia in more peripheral plexuses. Collateral ganglia, such as the celiac and inferior mesenteric ganglia (plexus), are formed by the convergence of preganglionic fibers with many postganglionic neuronal bodies. SNS ganglia are almost always located closer to the spinal cord than to the organs they innervate. The sympathetic postganglionic neuron can therefore originate in either the paired lateral paravertebral SNS ganglia or one of the unpaired collateral plexus. The unmyelinated postganglionic fibers then proceed from the ganglia to terminate within the organs they innervate.

Many of the postganglionic fibers pass from the lateral SNS chain back into the spinal nerves, forming the gray (unmyelinated) communicating rami at all levels of the spinal cord (Fig. 12-4). They are distributed distally to sweat glands, pilomotor muscle, and blood vessels of the skin and muscle. These nerves are unmyelinated C type fibers (Table 12-3) and are carried within the somatic nerves. Approximately 8% of the fibers in the average somatic nerve are sympathetic.[1]

Table 12-3. CLASSIFICATION OF NERVE FIBERS

Description of Nerve Fibers	Group		Diameter (μm)	Conduction Velocity (m·s⁻¹)
Myelinated somatic	A	Alpha α	20	120
		Beta β		
		Gamma γ		5–40 (pain fibers)
		Delta δ	3–4	5–40 (pain fibers)
		Epsilon ϵ	2	5
Myelinated visceral (preganglionic autonomic)	B		<3	3–15
Unmyelinated somatic	C		<2	0.5–2 (pain fibers)

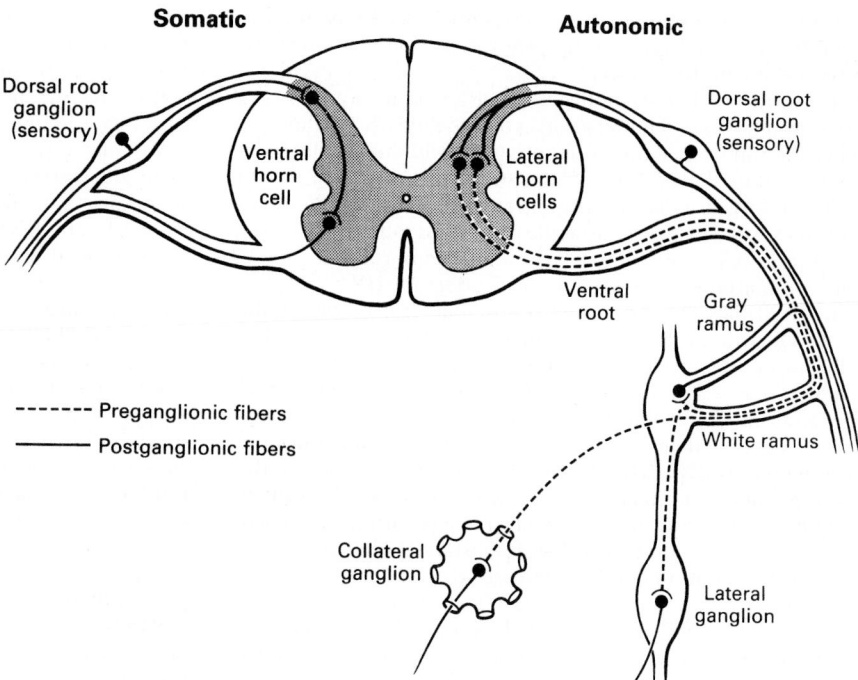

Figure 12-4. The spinal reflex arc of the somatic nerves is shown on the left. The different arrangements of neurons in the sympathetic system are shown on the right. Preganglionic fibers coming out through white rami may make synaptic connections following one of three courses: (1) synapse in ganglia at the level of exit, (2) course up or down the sympathetic chain to synapse at another level, or (3) exit the chain without synapsing to an outlying collateral ganglion.

The first four or five thoracic spinal segments generate preganglionic fibers that ascend in the neck to form three special paired ganglia. These are the superior cervical, middle cervical, and cervicothoracic ganglia. The last is known as the stellate ganglion and is actually formed by the fusion of the inferior cervical and first thoracic SNS ganglia. These ganglia provide sympathetic innervation of the head, neck, upper extremities, heart, and lungs. Afferent pain fibers also travel with these nerves, accounting for chest, neck, or upper extremity pain with myocardial ischemia.

Activation of the SNS produces a diffused physiologic response (mass reflex) rather than discrete effects. Function follows design. SNS postganglionic neurons outnumber the preganglionic neurons in an average ratio of 20:1 to 30:1.[5] One preganglionic fiber influences a larger number of postganglionic neurons, which are dispersed to many organs. In addition, the SNS response is augmented by the hormonal release of epinephrine (EPI) from the adrenal medulla.

Parasympathetic Nervous System or Craniosacral Division

The PNS, like the SNS, has both preganglionic and postganglionic neurons. This division is sometimes called the craniosacral outflow because the preganglionic cell bodies originate in the brain stem and sacral segments of the spinal cord. PNS preganglionic fibers are found in cranial nerves III (oculomotor), VII (facial), IX (glossopharyngeal), and X (vagus). The sacral outflow originates in the intermediolateral gray horns of the second, third, and fourth sacral nerves. Figure 12-2 shows the distribution of the PNS division and its innervation of visceral organs.

The vagus (cranial nerve X) nerve has the most extensive distribution of all the PNS, accounting for more than 75% of PNS activity. The paired vagus nerves supply PNS innervation to the heart, lungs, esophagus, stomach, small intestine, proximal half of the colon, liver, gallbladder, pancreas, and upper portions of the ureters. The sacral fibers form the pelvic visceral nerves, or nervi erigentes. These nerves supply the remainder of the viscera that are not innervated by the vagus. They supply the descending colon, rectum, uterus, bladder, and lower portions of the ureters and are primarily concerned with emptying. Various sexual reactions are also governed by the sacral PNS. The PNS is responsible for penile erection, but SNS stimulation governs ejaculation.

In contrast to the SNS division, PNS preganglionic fibers pass directly to the organ that is innervated. The postganglionic cell bodies are situated near or within the innervated viscera and generally are not visible. The proximity of PNS ganglia to or within the viscera provides a limited distribution of postganglionic fibers. The ratio of postganglionic to preganglionic fibers in many organs appears to be 1:1 to 3:1 compared with the 20:1 found in the SNS system. Auerbach's plexus in the distal colon is the exception, with a ratio of 8000:1. The fact that PNS preganglionic fibers synapse with only a few postganglionic neurons is consistent with the discrete and limited effect of PNS function. For example, vagal bradycardia can occur without a concomitant change in intestinal motility or salivation. Mass reflex action is not a characteristic of the PNS. The effects of organ response to PNS stimulation are outlined in Table 12-1.

Autonomic Innervation

Heart

The heart is well supplied by the SNS and PNS. These nerves affect cardiac pumping in three ways: (1) by changing the rate (chronotropism), (2) by changing the strength of contraction (inotropism), and (3) by modulating coronary blood flow. The PNS cardiac vagal fibers approach the stellate ganglia and then join the efferent cardiac SNS fibers; therefore, the vagus nerve to the heart and lungs is a mixed nerve containing both PNS and SNS efferent fibers. The PNS fibers are distributed mainly to the sinoatrial and atrioventricular (AV) nodes and to a lesser extent to the atria. There is little or no distribution to the ventricles. Therefore, the main effect of vagal cardiac stimulation to the heart is chronotropic. Vagal stimulation decreases the rate of sinoatrial node discharge and decreases excitability of the AV junctional fibers, slowing impulse conduction to the ventricles. A strong vagal discharge can completely arrest sinoatrial node firing and block impulse conduction to the ventricles. Vagal stimulation or vagotonic drugs such as methacholine reduce the vulnerability of the heart to ventricular fibrillation, decrease the frequency of premature ventricular beats, and can abolish ventricular tachycardia (see Interaction of Autonomic Nervous System Receptors).[6]

The physiologic importance of the PNS on myocardial contractility is not as well understood as that of the SNS. Cholinergic blockade can double the heart rate (HR) without altering contractility of the left ventricle. Vagal stimulation of the heart can reduce left ventricular maximum rate of tension development (dP/dT) and decrease contractile force by as much as 10–20%. However, PNS stimulation is relatively unimportant in this regard compared with its predominant effect on HR.

The SNS has the same supraventricular distribution as the PNS, but with stronger representation to the ventricles. SNS efferents to the myocardium funnel through the paired stellate ganglia. The right stellate ganglion distributes primarily to the anterior epicardial surface and the interventricular septum.[7] Right stellate stimulation decreases systolic duration and increases HR. The left stellate ganglion supplies the posterior and lateral surfaces of both ventricles. Left stellate stimulation increases mean arterial pressure and left ventricular contractility without causing a substantial change in HR. Normal SNS tone maintains contractility ~20% above that in the absence of any SNS stimulation.[8] Therefore, the dominant effect of the ANS on myocardial contractility is mediated primarily through the SNS. Intrinsic mechanisms of the myocardium, however, can maintain circulation quite well without the ANS, as evidenced by the success of cardiac transplants (see Denervated Heart).[9,10]

Early investigations, performed in anesthetized, open-chest animals, demonstrated that cardiac ANS nerves exert only slight effects on the coronary vascular bed; however, later studies on chronically instrumented, intact, conscious animals show considerable evidence for a strong SNS regulation of the small coronary resistance and larger conductance vessels (see Adrenergic Receptors).[11,12]

Different segments of the coronary arterial tree react differently to various stimuli and drugs. Large conductance vessels, the primary location for atheromatous plaques, are found on the epicardial surface, whereas the small, precapillary resistance vessels are found within the myocardium. Normally, the large conductance vessels contribute little to overall coronary vascular resistance. Fluctuations in resistance reflect changes in lumen size of the small, precapillary vessels. Blood flow through the resistance vessels is regulated primarily by the local metabolic requirements of the myocardium. The larger conductance vessels, however, can constrict markedly with neurogenic stimulation (see Adrenergic Receptor Distribution and Function). Neurogenic influence also assumes a greater role in the resistance vessels when they become hypoxic and lose autoregulation. There is a strong interaction between SNS and PNS nerves in organs with dual, antagonistic innervation. The tone of the coronary arteries is under this interacting control in a manner that is only now becoming understood (see Interaction of Autonomic Nervous System Receptors).[13]

Peripheral Circulation

The SNS nerves are by far the most important regulators of the peripheral circulation. The PNS nerves play only a minor role in this regard. The PNS dilates vessels, but only in limited areas such as the genitals. SNS stimulation produces both vasodilation and vasoconstriction, with vasoconstrictor effects predominating. The effect is determined by the type of receptors on which the SNS fiber terminates (see Receptors). SNS constrictor receptors are distributed to all segments of the circulation. This distribution is greater in some tissues than in others. Blood vessels in the skin, kidneys, spleen, and mesentery have an extensive SNS distribution, whereas those in the heart, brain, and muscle have less SNS innervation. SNS stimulation of the coronary arteries may produce vasoconstriction or vasodilation, depending upon the predomi-

nant receptor activity at the time of stimulation (see Table 12-1). Vagal stimulation may also produce coronary vasoconstriction (see β-Adrenergic Receptors). However, local autoregulatory factors usually have the predominant influence on coronary vascular tone.

Vascular tone is the sum of the muscular forces in the walls of blood vessels that oppose an increase in vessel diameter. Vasomotor tone denotes that portion of vasculature tone controlled by the ANS vasomotor nerves. Vascular tone is actively influenced also by local and circulating substances (such as hormones and metabolites), blood flow, and luminal hydrostatic pressure. An increase in blood flow increases sheer stress at the endothelial lining of the vessel wall. This triggers release of a relaxing factor from the endothelium (see Molecular Pharmacology and Effector Mechanisms). Vasodilation ensues. Conversely, an increase in intraluminal pressure directly stimulates smooth muscle contraction independent of vasomotor effects. This component of vascular tone is referred to as myogenic tone. Blood vessels have differing sensitivities to the influence of local or neurogenic control. Arterioles and venules are under strong neurogenic control and have vasomotor tone. Local autoregulation is the predominant force at the precapillary and postcapillary sphincters.[14]

Basal vasomotor tone is maintained by impulses from the lateral portion of the vasomotor center in the medulla oblongata that continually transmits impulses through the SNS, maintaining partial arteriolar and venular constriction. Circulating EPI from the adrenal medulla has additive effects. This basal ANS tone maintains arteriolar constriction at an intermediate diameter.[15] The arteriole, therefore, has the potential for either further constriction or dilation. If the basal tone were not present, the SNS could effect only vasoconstriction and not vasodilation.[1] The SNS tone in the venules produces little resistance to flow compared with the arterioles and the arteries. The importance of SNS stimulation of veins is to reduce or increase their capacity. By functioning as a reservoir for ~80% of the total blood volume, small changes in venous capacitance produce large changes in venous return and, thus, cardiac preload.

Lungs

The lungs are innervated by both the SNS and PNS.[15] Postganglionic SNS fibers from the upper thoracic ganglia (stellate) pass to the lungs to innervate the smooth muscles of the bronchi and pulmonary blood vessels. PNS innervation of these structures is from the vagus nerve.

SNS stimulation produces bronchodilation and pulmonary vasoconstriction.[16] Little else has been conclusively proved about the vasomotor control of the pulmonary vessels, other than the fact that they adjust to accommodate the output of the right ventricle. The effect of stimulation of the pulmonary SNS nerves on pulmonary vascular resistance is not great, but may be important in maintaining hemodynamic stability during stress and exercise by balancing right and left ventricular output.[17,18] Stimulation of the vagus nerve produces almost no vasodilation of the pulmonary circulation. The phenomenon of hypoxic pulmonary vasoconstriction appears to be an important force in regulation of pulmonary blood flow.[19,20] Hypoxic pulmonary vasoconstriction is a local phenomenon capable of providing a faster adjustment to needs.

Both the SNS and the vagus nerve provide active bronchomotor control. SNS stimulation causes bronchodilation, whereas vagal stimulation produces constriction. PNS stimulation may also increase secretions of the bronchial glands. Vagal receptor endings in the alveolar ducts also play an important role in the reflex regulation of the ventilation cycle.[21] The lung has important nonventilatory activity as well. It serves as a metabolic organ that removes local mediators such as norepinephrine (NE) from the circulation and converts others, such as angiotensin I, to active compounds (see Interaction with Other Regulatory Systems).[22,23]

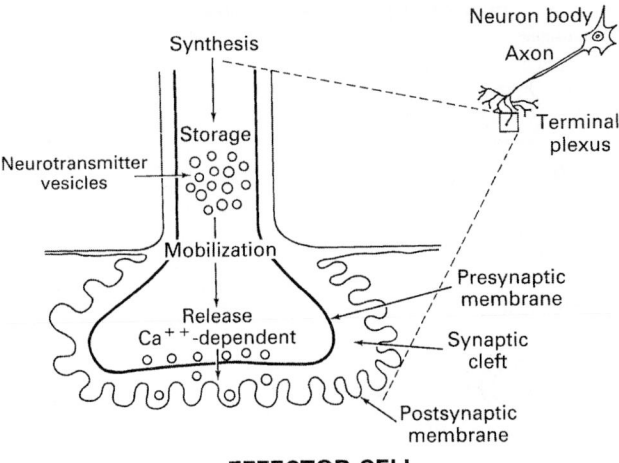

Figure 12-5. The anatomy and physiology of the terminal postganglionic fibers of sympathetic and parasympathetic fibers are similar.

AUTONOMIC NERVOUS SYSTEM: NEUROTRANSMISSION

Transmission of excitation across the terminal junctional sites (synaptic clefts) of the peripheral ANS occurs through the mediation of liberated chemicals (Fig. 12-5). Transmitters interact with a receptor on the end organ to evoke a biologic response. The ANS can be pharmacologically subdivided by the neurotransmitter secreted at the effector cell. Pharmacologic parlance designates the SNS and PNS as *adrenergic* and *cholinergic*, respectively. The terminals of the PNS postganglionic fibers release acetylcholine (ACh). With the exception of sweat glands, NE is considered the principal neurotransmitter released at the terminals of the sympathetic postganglionic fibers (see Fig. 12-3). Co-transmission of ATP, neuropeptide Y (NPY), and NE has been demonstrated at vascular sympathetic nerve terminals in a number of different tissues including muscle, intestine, kidney, and skin (see SNS Neurotransmission). The preganglionic neurons of both systems secrete ACh.

The terminations of the postganglionic fibers of both ANS subdivisions are anatomically and physiologically similar. The terminations are characterized by multiple branchings called terminal effector plexuses, or reticulae. These filaments surround the elements of the effector unit "like a mesh stocking."[14] Thus, one SNS postganglionic neuron, for example, can innervate ~25,000 effector cells, *e.g.*, vascular smooth muscle.[4,5] The terminal filaments end in presynaptic enlargements called vari-

cosities. Each varicosity contains vesicles, ~500 μm in diameter, in which the neurotransmitters are stored (Fig. 12-5). The varicosities are also heavily populated with mitochondria, which relates to the increased energy (adenosine triphosphate, ATP) requirements of ACh and NE synthesis. The rate of synthesis depends on the level of ANS activity and is regulated by local feedback. The distance between the varicosity and the effector cell (synaptic or junctional cleft) varies from 100 μm in ganglia and arterioles to as much as 20,000 μm in large arteries. This distance determines the amount of transmitter required to stimulate and the time it takes to diffuse to the effector cell. The time for diffusion is directly proportional to the width of the synaptic gap. Depolarization releases the vesicular contents into the synaptic cleft by exocytosis.

Parasympathetic Nervous System Neurotransmission

Synthesis

Classically, ACh was considered the exclusive neurotransmitter of the PNS. Current investigation suggests a role for vasoactive intestinal peptide (VIP) as an additional PNS neurotransmitter. ACh is formed in the presynaptic terminal by acetylation of choline with acetyl coenzyme A. This step is catalyzed by choline acetyl transferase (Fig. 12-6). ACh is then stored in a concentrated form in presynaptic vesicles containing ~10,000 molecules of ACh. A continual release of small amounts of ACh, called quanta, occurs during the resting state. Each quantum results in small changes in the electrical potential of the synaptic end plate without producing depolarization. These are known as miniature end-plate potentials. Arrival of an action potential causes a synchronous release of hundreds of quanta, resulting in depolarization of the end plate. Release of ACh from the vesicles is dependent on influx of calcium (Ca^{2+}) from the interstitial space.[24] Drugs that alter Ca^{2+} binding or influx may decrease ACh release and affect end-organ function. ACh is not reused like NE; therefore, it must be synthesized constantly.

Metabolism

The ability of a receptor to modulate function of an effector organ is dependent upon rapid recovery to its baseline state after stimulation. For this to occur, the neurotransmitter must be quickly removed from the vicinity of the receptor. ACh removal occurs by rapid hydrolysis by acetylcholinesterase (Fig. 12-6). This enzyme is found in neurons, at the neuromuscular junction, and in various other tissues of the body. A similar enzyme, pseudocholinesterase or plasma cholinesterase, is also found throughout the body but only to a limited extent in nervous tissue. It does not appear to be physiologically impor-

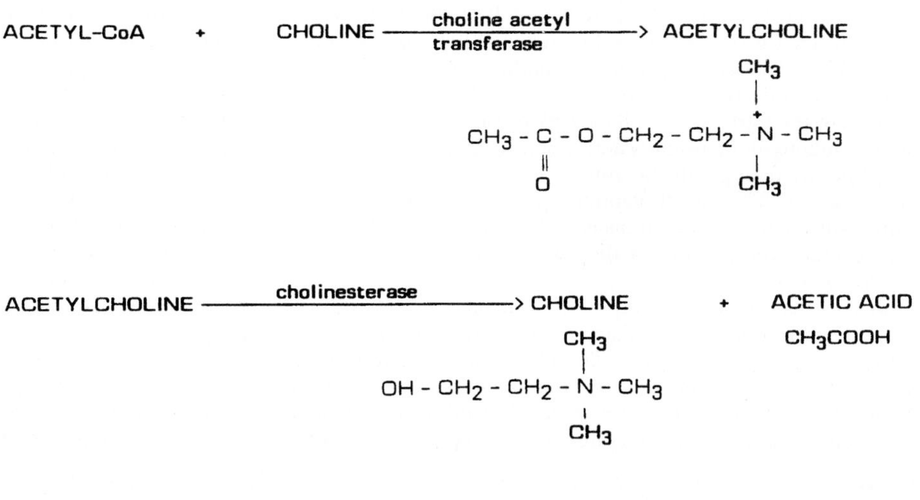

$$ACETYL-CoA \quad + \quad CHOLINE \xrightarrow{\text{choline acetyl transferase}} ACETYLCHOLINE$$

$$CH_3 - C - O - CH_2 - CH_2 - \overset{+}{\underset{CH_3}{\overset{CH_3}{N}}} - CH_3$$
$$\underset{O}{\|}$$

$$ACETYLCHOLINE \xrightarrow{\text{cholinesterase}} CHOLINE \quad + \quad ACETIC ACID$$
$$CH_3COOH$$

$$OH - CH_2 - CH_2 - \underset{CH_3}{\overset{CH_3}{N}} - CH_3$$

Figure 12-6. Synthesis and metabolism of acetylcholine.

tant in termination of the action of ACh. Both acetylcholinesterase and pseudocholinesterase hydrolyze ACh as well as other esters (such as the ester-type local anesthetics), but they may be distinguished by specific biochemical tests.[6,25]

Sympathetic Nervous System Neurotransmission

Traditionally, the catecholamines EPI and NE were considered the exclusive mediators of peripheral SNS activity. Evidence accumulated over the past two decades, though, suggests roles for ATP and NPY as additional sympathetic neurotransmitters. NE is released from localized presynaptic vesicles of nearly all postganglionic sympathetic nerves. Vascular SNS nerve terminals, though, also release ATP. Thus, ATP and NE are co-neurotransmitters. They are released directly into the site where they act. Their postjunctional effects appear to be synergistic in tissues studied to date. The function of NPY as a peripheral sympathetic neurotransmitter remains unknown.

The SNS fibers ending in the adrenal medulla are preganglionic, and ACh is the neurotransmitter (see Fig. 12-3). It interacts with the chromaffin cells in the medulla, causing release of EPI and NE. The chromaffin cells take the place of the postganglionic neurons.[4] Stimulation of the sympathetic nerves to the adrenal medulla, however, causes the release of large quantities of a mixture of EPI and NE into the circulation to become neurotransmitter hormones. The greater portion of this hormonal surge is normally EPI. EPI and NE, when released into the circulation, are classified as hormones in that they are synthesized, stored, and released from the adrenal medulla to act at distant sites.[26]

Hormonal EPI and NE have almost the same effects on effector cells as those caused by local direct sympathetic stimulation; however, the hormonal effects, although brief, last ~10 times as long as those caused by direct stimulation.[15,27] EPI has a greater metabolic effect than NE. It can increase the metabolic rate of the body as much as 100%.[1] It also increases glycogenolysis in the liver and muscle with glucose release into the blood. These functions are all necessary to prepare the body for fight or flight.

The normal resting state of secretion by the adrenal medulla is ~0.02 $\mu g \cdot kg^{-1} \cdot min^{-1}$ of EPI and ~0.02 $\mu g \cdot kg^{-1} \cdot min^{-1}$ of NE.[1,27,28] Some of the overall vascular tone results from the basal resting secretion of the adrenal medulla in addition to the tone that is maintained directly through stimulation from central vasomotor centers in the medulla.

Catecholamines: The First Messenger

The endogenous catecholamines in humans are dopamine, NE, and EPI. Dopamine is a neurotransmitter in the CNS. It is primarily involved in coordinating motor activity in the brain. It is the precursor of NE. NE is synthesized and stored in nerve endings of postganglionic SNS neurons. It is also synthesized in the adrenal medulla and is the chemical precursor of EPI. Stored EPI is located chiefly in chromaffin cells of the adrenal medulla. Eighty to eighty-five percent of the catecholamine content of the adrenal medulla is EPI and 15–20% is NE. The brain contains both noradrenergic and dopaminergic receptors, but circulating catecholamines do not cross the blood–brain barrier. The catecholamines present in the brain are synthesized there. Endogenous catecholamines are unique in that several intermediates in the synthesis function as neurotransmitters.

A catecholamine is any compound having a catechol nucleus (a benzene ring with two adjacent hydroxyl groups) and an amine-containing side chain.[29] The chemical configuration of five of the more common catecholamines in clinical use is demonstrated in Figure 12-7. A true catecholamine must possess this basic structure. Catecholamines are often referred to as

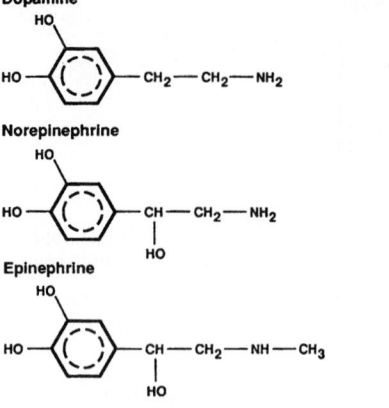

ENDOGENOUS CATECHOLAMINES

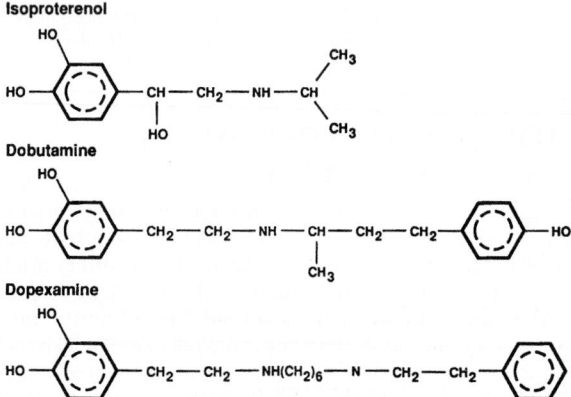

SYNTHETIC CATECHOLAMINES

Figure 12-7. The chemical configurations of three endogenous catecholamines are compared with those of three synthetic catecholamines. Sympathomimetic drugs differ in their hemodynamic effects largely because of differences in substitution of the amine group on the catechol nucleus.

adrenergic drugs because their effector actions are mediated through receptors specific for the SNS. Synthetic catecholamines can activate these same receptors because of their structural similarity. For example, clonidine is an α_2-receptor agonist that does not possess a catechol nucleus, and even has two ring systems that are aplanar to each other (Fig. 12-8). However, clonidine enjoys a remarkable spatial similarity to NE that allows it to activate the receptor.[30,31] Drugs that produce sympathetic-like effects but lack the basic catecholamine structure are defined as sympathomimetics. All clinically useful catecholamines are sympathomimetics, but not all sympathomimetics are catecholamines (Table 12-4).

The effects of endogenous or synthetic catecholamines on adrenergic receptors can be direct or indirect (Table 12-4).[32,33] Indirect-acting catecholamines have little intrinsic effect on adrenergic receptors but produce their effects by stimulating release of the stored neurotransmitter from SNS nerve terminals. Some synthetic and endogenous catecholamines stimulate adrenergic receptor sites directly, whereas others have a mixed mode of action. The actions of direct-acting catecholamines are independent of endogenous NE stores; however, the indirect-acting catecholamines are totally dependent on adequate neuronal stores of endogenous NE.

Synthesis

The main site of NE synthesis is in or near the postganglionic nerve endings. Some synthesis does occur in vesicles near the cell body that pass to the nerve endings.[34] Phenylalanine or

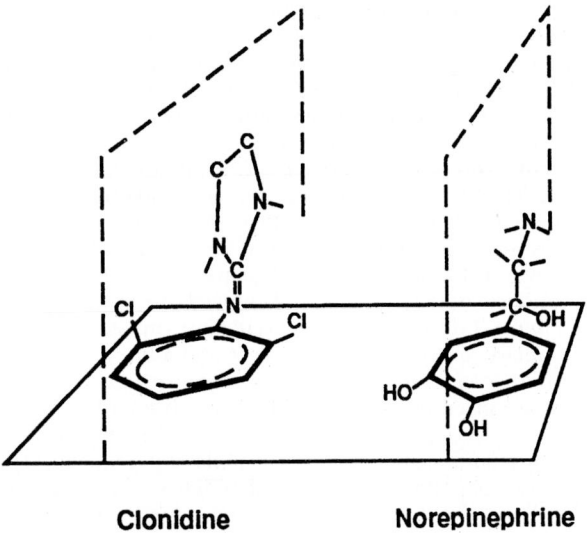

Figure 12-8. The spatial similarity of clonidine and NE allows it to activate presynaptic α_2 receptors inhibiting NE release.

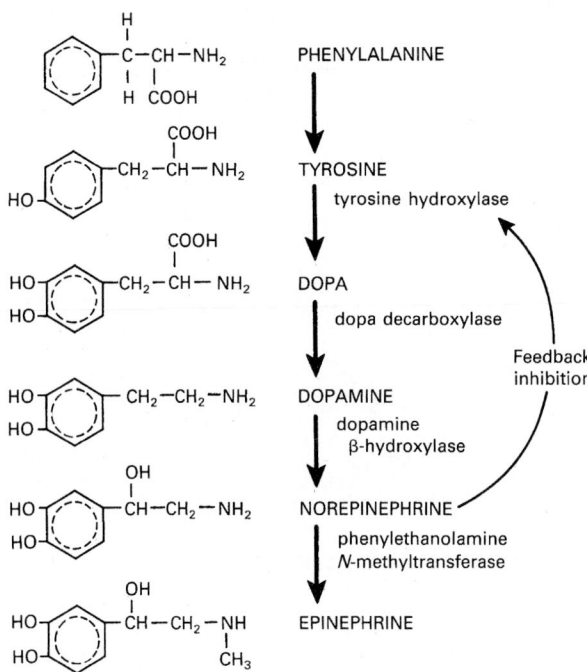

Figure 12-9. Schematic of the synthesis of catecholamines. The conversion of tyrosine to DOPA by tyrosine hydroxylase is inhibited by increased NE synthesis. Epinephrine is shown in these steps but is primarily synthesized in the adrenal medulla.

tyrosine is taken up into the axoplasm of the nerve terminal and synthesized into either NE or EPI.[4,5] Figure 12-9 demonstrates this synthesis cascade. Tyrosine hydroxylase catalyzes the conversion of tyrosine to dihydroxyphenylalanine. This is the rate-limiting step at which NE synthesis is controlled through feedback inhibition.[35] Dihydroxyphenylalanine and the subsequent compounds in this cascade are catecholamines.

Dopamine is formed from dihydroxyphenylalanine by dihydroxyphenylalanine decarboxylase. Synthesis to this point occurs in the cytoplasm of the neuron. Dopamine then enters the storage vesicles. In the brain, synthesis stops at this point

Table 12-4. SYMPATHOMIMETIC DRUGS

Drug	Trade Name
ADRENERGIC AMINES	
Catecholamines	
Epinephrine	Adrenalin
Norepinephrine	Levophed
Dopamine*	Inotropin
Dobutamine	Dobutrex
Dopexamine	
Isoproterenol	Isuprel
Noncatecholamines	
Metaraminol*†	Aramine
Mephentermine†	Wyamine
Ephedrine†	Ephedrine
Methoxamine	Vasoxyl
Phenylephrine	Neo-Synephrine
Clonidine	
NONADRENERGICS	
Xanthines	Aminophylline
Glucagon	Glucagon
Digitalis	Lanoxin
Calcium salts	
Naloxone	Narcan
Amrinone	Inocor

* Direct-acting catecholamine with some indirect action.
† Primarily indirect-acting with some direct action. Adrenergic amines produce sympathomimetic effects *via* adrenergic receptors. Nonadrenergics produce sympathomimetic effects exclusive of the adrenergic receptor.

where dopamine is the neurotransmitter. The vesicles of peripheral postganglionic neurons contain the enzyme dopamine-β-hydroxylase, which converts dopamine to NE. The adrenal medulla additionally contains phenylethanolamine-N-methyltransferase, which converts NE to EPI. This reaction takes place outside the medullary vesicles, and the newly formed EPI then enters the vesicle for storage (Fig. 12-10). All the endogenous catecholamines are stored in presynaptic vesicles and released on arrival of an action potential. Excitation-secretion coupling in sympathetic neurons is Ca^{2+}-dependent.

Regulation

Increased SNS nervous activity, as in congestive heart failure or chronic stress, stimulates the synthesis of tyrosine hydroxylase and dopamine-β-hydroxylase.[4,36] Glucocorticoids from the adrenal cortex pass through the adrenal medulla and stimulate an increase in phenylethanolamine-N-methyltransferase that methylates NE to EPI.

The release of NE is dependent upon depolarization of the nerve and an increase in calcium ion permeability. Calcium may trigger exocytosis of NE granules.[25,35,36] This release is inhibited by colchicine and prostaglandin E_2, suggesting a contractile mechanism. Blockade of prostaglandin synthesis enhances NE release. NE inhibits its own release by stimulating presynaptic (prejunctional) α_2 receptors. Phenoxybenzamine and phentolamine, α-receptor antagonists, increase the release of NE by blocking inhibitory presynaptic α_2 receptors (Fig. 12-11). Other receptors may also be important in NE regulation and are discussed later (see Other Receptors).

Inactivation

The catecholamines are removed from the synaptic cleft by three mechanisms (see Fig. 12-10).[4] These are reuptake into the presynaptic terminals, extraneuronal uptake, and diffusion. Termination of NE at the effector site is almost entirely by reuptake of NE into the terminals of the presynaptic neuron (uptake 1). Once NE is back in the nerve terminal, it is stored in the vesicles for reuse. A small amount is deaminated in

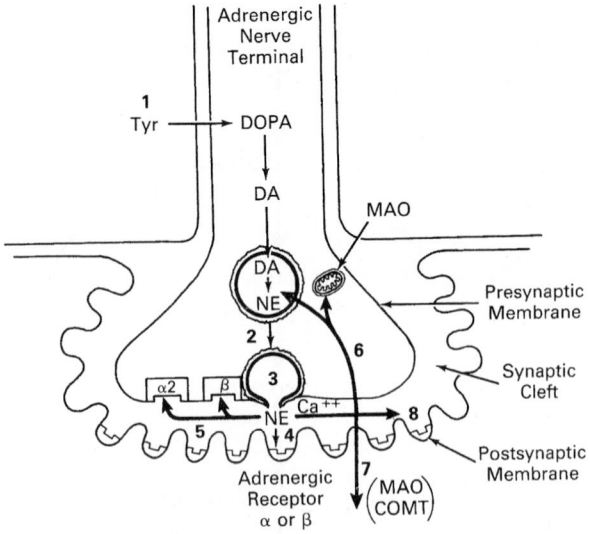

EFFECTOR CELL

Figure 12-10. Schematic of the synthesis and disposition of NE in adrenergic neurotransmission. (1) Synthesis and storage in neuronal vesicles; (2) action potential permits calcium entry with (3) exocytosis of NE into synaptic gap. (4) Released NE reacts with receptor on effector cell. NE (5) may react with presynaptic α_2 receptor to inhibit further NE release or with presynaptic β receptor to enhance reuptake of NE (6) (uptake 1). Extraneuronal uptake (uptake 2) absorbs NE into effector cell (7) with overflow occurring systemically (8). MAO = monoamine oxidase; COMT = catechol-*O*-methyltransferase; Tyr = tyrosine; DOPA = dihydroxyphenylalanine; NE = norepinephrine.

the cytoplasm of the neuron by monoamine oxidase to form dihydroxymandelic acid, which diffuses out of the nerve terminal and into the interstitial fluid. Uptake 1 is an active, energy-requiring, temperature-dependent process that can be inhibited pharmacologically.

The reuptake of NE in the presynaptic terminals is also a stereospecific process. Structurally similar compounds (guanethidine, metaraminol) may enter the vesicles and displace the neurotransmitter. Tricyclic antidepressants and cocaine inhibit the reuptake of NE, resulting in high synaptic NE concentra-

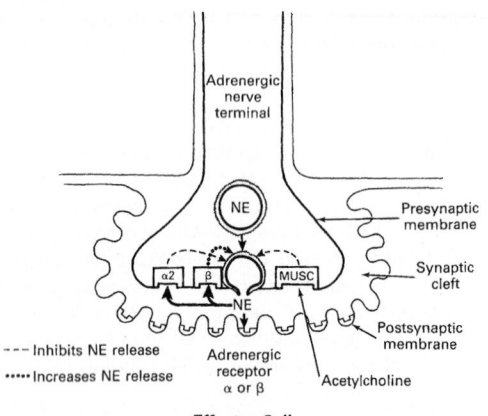

Effector Cell

Figure 12-11. This schematic demonstrates just a few of the presynaptic adrenergic receptors thought to exist. Agonist and antagonist drugs are clinically available for these receptors (see Table 12-5). The α_2 receptors serve as a negative feedback mechanism whereby NE stimulation inhibits its own release. Presynaptic β stimulation increases NE uptake, augmenting its availability. Presynaptic muscarinic (MUSC) receptors respond to ACh diffusing from nearby cholinergic terminals. They inhibit NE release and can be blocked by atropine.

tions and accentuated receptor response. In addition, recent evidence suggests that NE reuptake is mediated by a presynaptic β-adrenergic mechanism because β-blockade causes marked elevations of EPI and NE[37] (see Figs. 12-10 and 12-11), whereas α blockade does not. The clinical significance of this presynaptic β-receptor is unknown at this time.

Extraneuronal uptake (uptake 2) is a minor pathway for inactivating NE. NE is taken up by effector cells and other extraneuronal tissues. The NE that is taken up by the extraneuronal tissue is metabolized by monoamine oxidase and by catechol-*O*-methyltransferase to form vanillylmandelic acid (Fig. 12-12).[38] The minute amount of catecholamine that escapes uptake 1 and uptake 2 diffuses into the circulation (uptake 3),* where it is similarly metabolized in the liver and kidney. The importance of uptake 1 and uptake 2 is diminished when sympathomimetics are given exogenously. EPI is inactivated by the same enzymes. Whereas uptake 1 is the predominant pathway for inactivation of the endogenous catecholamines, uptake 3 is the predominant pathway for catecholamines given exogenously and is clinically important. This accounts for the longer duration of action by exogenous catecholamines than that noted at the local synapse. The former is slow (liver metabolism) and the latter is fast (uptake 1).

The final metabolic product of the catecholamines is vanillylmandelic acid. Vanillylmandelic acid constitutes the major metabolite (80–90%) of NE found in the urine. Less than 5% of released NE appears unchanged in the urine. The metabolic products excreted in the urine provide a gross estimate of SNS activity and can facilitate the clinical diagnosis of pheochromocytoma.

RECEPTORS

An *agonist* is a substance that interacts with a receptor to evoke a biologic response. ACh, NE, EPI, and ATP are the agonists of the ANS. An *antagonist* is a substance that interferes with the evocation of a response at a receptor site by an agonist. Receptors are therefore regarded as target sites on a cell that will, when activated by an agonist, lead to a response by the effector cell. Receptors are protein macromolecules and are located in the plasma membrane. Several thousand receptors have been demonstrated in a single cell. The enormity of this network is realized when it is considered that ~25,000 single cells can be innervated by a single neuron.[5,39]

Cholinergic Receptors

ACh is the neurotransmitter at three distinct classes of receptors. These receptors can be differentiated by their anatomic location and their affinity to bind various agonists and antagonists.[25] ACh mediates the "first messenger" function of transmitting impulses in the PNS, the ganglia of the SNS, and the neuroeffector junction of striated, voluntary muscle (see Fig. 12-3). The receptors are referred to as cholinoceptive or cholinergic receptors. The PNS is referred to as the cholinergic system.

Cholinergic receptors are further subdivided into muscarinic and nicotinic receptors because muscarine and nicotine stimulate them selectively.[6] However, both muscarinic and nicotinic receptors respond to ACh (see Cholinergic Drugs). Muscarine activates cholinergic receptors at the postganglionic PNS junctions of cardiac and smooth muscle throughout the body. Muscarinic stimulation is characterized by bradycardia, decreased inotropism, bronchoconstriction, miosis, salivation, gastrointestinal hypermotility, and increased gastric acid secretion (see Table 12-1). Muscarinic receptors can be blocked by atropine without effect on nicotinic receptors (see Cholinergic Drugs).

---

* Uptake 3 is used as a clinical term to describe uptake of exogenous drug administration.

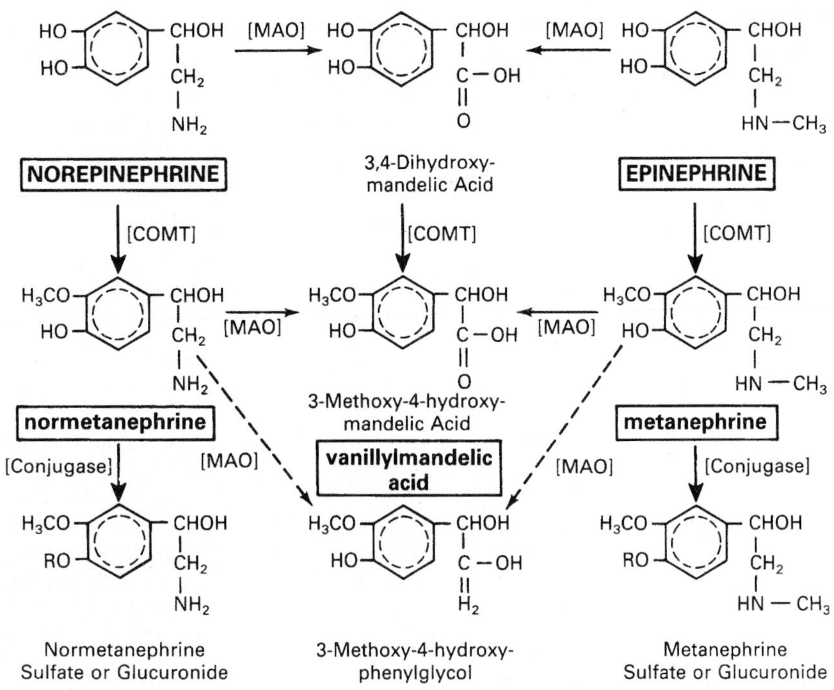

Figure 12-12. Catabolism of NE and EPI.

Muscarinic receptors are known to exist in sites other than PNS postganglionic junctions. They are found on the presynaptic membrane of sympathetic nerve terminals in the myocardium, coronary vessels, and peripheral vasculature (Fig. 12-11). These are referred to as adrenergic muscarinic receptors because of their location; however, they are stimulated by ACh. Stimulation of these receptors inhibits release of NE in a manner similar to α_2-receptor stimulation.[12,40] Muscarinic blockade removes inhibition of NE release, augmenting SNS activity. Atropine, the prototypical muscarinic blocker, may produce sympathomimetic activity in this manner as well as vagal blockade. Neuromuscular blocking drugs that cause tachycardia are thought to have a similar mechanism of action.

ACh acting on presynaptic adrenergic muscarinic receptors is a potent inhibitor of NE release.[37] The prejunctional muscarinic receptor may play an important physiologic role because several autonomically innervated tissues (*e.g.*, the heart) possess ANS plexuses in which the SNS and PNS nerve terminals are closely associated.[6] In these plexuses, ACh, released from the nearby PNS nerve terminals (vagus nerve), can inhibit NE release by activation of presynaptic adrenergic muscarinic receptors (Fig. 12-11).

Nicotinic receptors are found at the synaptic junctions of both SNS and PNS ganglia. Because both junctions are cholinergic, ACh or ACh-like substances such as nicotine will excite postganglionic fibers of both systems (see Fig. 12-3). Low doses of nicotine produce stimulation of ANS ganglia, whereas high doses produce blockade. This dualism is referred to as the nicotinic effect (see Ganglionic Drugs). Nicotinic stimulation of the SNS ganglia produces hypertension and tachycardia by causing the release of EPI and NE from the adrenal medulla. Adrenal hormone release is mediated by ACh in the chromaffin cells, which are analogous to postganglionic neurons (see Fig. 12-3). A further increase in nicotine concentration produces hypotension and neuromuscular weakness as it becomes a ganglionic blocker. The cholinergic neuroeffector junction of skeletal muscle also contains nicotinic receptors, although they are not identical to the nicotinic receptors in ANS ganglia.

Adrenergic Receptors

Von Euler differentiated the physiologic effects of EPI and NE in 1946.[31,41] The adrenergic receptors were termed adrenergic or noradrenergic, depending on their responsiveness to EPI or NE. The dissimilarities of these two drugs led Ahlquist in 1948 to propose two types of opposing adrenergic receptors, termed alpha (α) and beta (β). This postulation further implied that selective antagonism of these receptors was possible. The receptors can be classified according to the order of potency by which they are affected by SNS agonists and antagonists. Receptors that respond with an order of potency of NE $\geq$ EPI > isoproterenol are called α receptors. Those responding with an order of potency of isoproterenol > EPI $\geq$ NE are called β receptors (Table 12-5). The development of new agonists and antagonists with relatively selective activity allowed Lands to subdivide the β receptors into β_1 and β_2. α Receptors were subsequently divided into α_1 and α_2. The concept of relative selective activity arises from differential potencies among tissue groups to the same drug, such that two dose–response curves are obtained (Fig. 12-13). The sympathomimetic adrenergic drugs in current use differ from one another in their effects largely because of differences in substitution on the amine group, which influences the relative α or β effect (see Fig. 12-7).[29]

Another major peripheral adrenergic receptor specific for dopamine is termed the dopaminergic (DA) receptor. Further studies have revealed not only subsets of the α and β receptors but also the DA receptor.[41,42] These DA receptors have been identified in the CNS and in renal, mesenteric, and coronary vessels. The physiologic importance of these receptors is a matter of controversy because there are no identifiable peripheral DA neurons. Dopamine measured in the circulation is assumed to result from spillover from the brain.

The function of dopamine in the CNS has long been known, but the peripheral dopaminergic receptor (DA) has been elucidated only within the past three decades. The presence of the peripheral DA receptor was obscured because dopamine does not affect the DA receptor exclusively. It also stimulates α and β receptors in a dose-related manner.[43] However, DA receptors

Table 12-5. ADRENERGIC RECEPTORS: ORDER OF POTENCY OF AGONISTS AND ANTAGONISTS

Receptor		Agonists*	Antagonists	Location	Action
α_1	++++ +++ ++ +	Norepinephrine Epinephrine Dopamine Isoproterenol	Phenoxybenzamine† Phentolamine† Ergot alkaloids† Prazosin Tolazoline† Labetalol†	Smooth muscle (vascular, iris, radial, ureter, pilomotor, uterus, trigone, gastrointestinal, and bladder sphincters) Brain Smooth muscle (gastrointestinal) Heart Salivary glands Adipose tissue Sweat glands (localized) Kidney (proximal tubule)	Contraction Vasoconstriction Neurotransmission Relaxation Glycogenolysis Increased force,‡ glycolysis Secretion (K^+, H_2O) Glycogenesis Secretion Gluconeogenesis Na^+ reabsorption
α_2	++++ +++ ++ ++ +	Clonidine Norepinephrine Epinephrine Norepinephrine Phenylephrine	Yohimbine Piperoxan Phentolamine† Phenoxybenzamine† Tolazoline† Labetalol†	Adrenergic nerve endings Presynaptic—CNS Platelets Adipose tissue Endocrine pancrease Vascular smooth muscle—? Kidney Brain	Inhibition norepinephrine release Aggregation, granule release Inhibition lypolysis Inhibition insulin release Contraction Inhibition renin disease Neurotransmission
β_1	++++ +++ ++ +	Isoproterenol† Epinephrine Norepinephrine Dopamine	Acebutolol Practolol Propranolol† Alprenolol† Metoprolol Esmolol	Heart Adipose tissue	Increased rate, contractility, conduction velocity Coronary vasodilation Lipolysis
β_2	++++ +++ +++ +	Isoproterenol* Epinephrine Norepinephrine Dopamine	Propranolol† Butoxamine Alprenolol Esmolol Nadolol Timolol Labetalol	Liver Skeletal muscle Smooth muscle (bronchi, uterus, vascular, gastrointestinal, detrusor, spleen capsule) Endocrine pancreas Salivary glands	Glycogenolysis, gluconeogenesis Glyogenolysis, lactate release Relaxation Insulin secretion Amylase secretion
DA_1	++++ ++ + +	Fenoldopam Dopamine Epinephrine Metaclopramide	Haloperidol Droperidol Phenothiazines	Vascular smooth muscle Renal and mesentery	Vasodilation
DA_2	++ +	Dopamine Bromocriptine	Domperidone	Presynaptic—adrenergic nerve endings	Inhibits norepinephrine release

* Listed in decreasing order of potency.
† Nonselective.
‡ β_1 = adrenergic responses are greater.
Pluses indicate strength of potency.

function independently of α or β blockade and are modified by DA antagonists such as haloperidol, droperidol, and phenothiazines. Thus, there is a necessity for the addition of the DA receptor and its subsets (DA_1 and DA_2) to the Ahlquist classification.

The determination of the anatomic location and amino acid structure of receptor binding sites has been made possible through radioligand studies.[44] The distribution of adrenoreceptors in organs and tissues is not uniform, and their function differs not only by their location but also in their numbers and/or distribution.[45] Adrenoceptors are found in two loci in the sympathetic neuroeffector junction. They are found in both the presynaptic (prejunctional) and postsynaptic (postjunctional) sites as well as extrasynaptic sites (Fig. 12-14). Table 12-6 is a review of the function and synaptic location of some of the clinically important receptors that have only recently been defined.

Prejunctional receptors are considered innervated in that they are in the immediate vicinity of the neurotransmitter released by a sympathetic action potential. Postjunctional receptors are considered to be innervated or noninnervated depending upon their proximity to the synaptic cleft.[46] Receptors located directly on postjunctional membranes are considered to be innervated. However, most postsynaptic α_2 and β_2 receptors are extrasynaptic and considered noninnervated even though they are located in the vicinity of the postsynaptic membrane. These receptors are influenced more by hormonal catecholamines (EPI) than by neurotransmitter (NE). Extrasynaptic receptors also seem to be less influenced by factors causing the up- or downregulation of receptor numbers and sensitivity. This may explain the clinical observation of why EPI may work where other agonists, which work on synaptic receptors, may be ineffective. The agonist–receptor interaction of noninnervated receptors is of slower onset and longer duration as well.

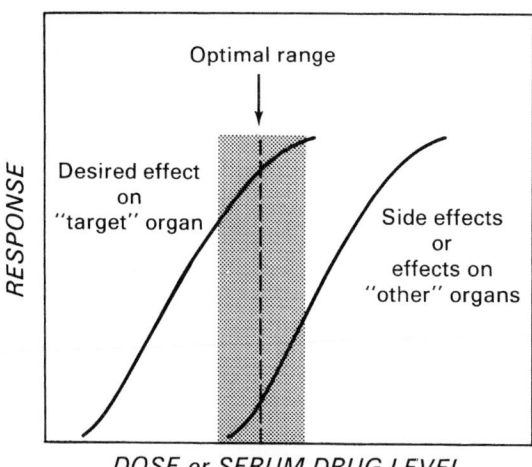

Figure 12-13. Relative dose-response relationship on target and other organs. Relative selectivity is illustrated by showing the relationship between two dose–response curves. The curve on the left represents the desired response of bronchodilation using a relatively selective β_2 agonist. The unwanted effects on other organs that occur at higher doses are represented by the curve on the right. For example, an increased HR (β_1 effect) may occur with higher doses of a relatively select β_2 agonist. The optimal range is that concentration of drug that will give the maximal desired response with minimal effects on other organs. The size of the optimal range is dependent on the therapeutic index, or the distance between the two curves. These are usually established *in vitro* where drug concentration can be precisely controlled. For many cardiovascular drugs, the optimal range is small, and wide fluctuations in serum level of the drug are common; therefore, secondary or side-effects are often seen during drug therapy.

α-Adrenergic Receptors

Two classes of α receptors have been demonstrated: α_1 and α_2. This classification is based on their response to the α-antagonists yohimbine and prazosin. Prazosin is a more potent antagonist of α_1 receptors, whereas α_2 receptors are more sensitive to yohimbine. The α_1-adrenergic receptors are also found in the smooth muscle cells of the peripheral vasculature of the coronary arteries, skin, uterus, intestinal mucosa, and splanchnic beds (see Table 12-5). The α_1 receptors serve as postsynaptic activators of vascular and intestinal smooth muscle as well as of endocrine glands. Their activation results in either decreased or increased tone, depending upon the effector organ. The response in resistance and capacitance vessels is constriction, whereas in the intestinal tract it is relaxation. There is now a large body of evidence documenting the presence of postjunctional α_1-adrenoreceptors in the mammalian heart. α_1-Adrenoreceptors have been shown to have a positive inotropic effect on cardiac tissues from most mammals studied, including humans.[33,47] Experimental work strongly supports the concept that enhanced myocardial α_1 responsiveness plays a primary role in the genesis of malignant arrhythmias induced by catecholamines during myocardial ischemia and reperfusion. Drugs possessing potent α_1-antagonist activity, such as prazosin and phentolamine, provide significant antiarrhythmic activity. Neither the clinical mechanism nor the significance of these findings is yet clear.[48,49] However, there is no doubt that α_1-adrenergic antagonists prevent catecholamine-induced ventricular arrhythmias.[50] In contrast, studies of the effects of β antagonists in experimental and clinical myocardial infarction have provided conflicting results.

The discovery of presynaptic α-adrenoreceptors and their role in the modulation of NE transmission provided the stimulus for the subclassification of receptors into α_1 and α_2 subtypes.[51,52] The successful cloning of genes for α_1 and α_2 receptors has provided unequivocal evidence for their separate identities and structures. Presynaptic α_1 receptors have not been identified and appear confined to the postsynaptic membrane. α_2 Receptors are found on both presynaptic and postsynaptic membranes

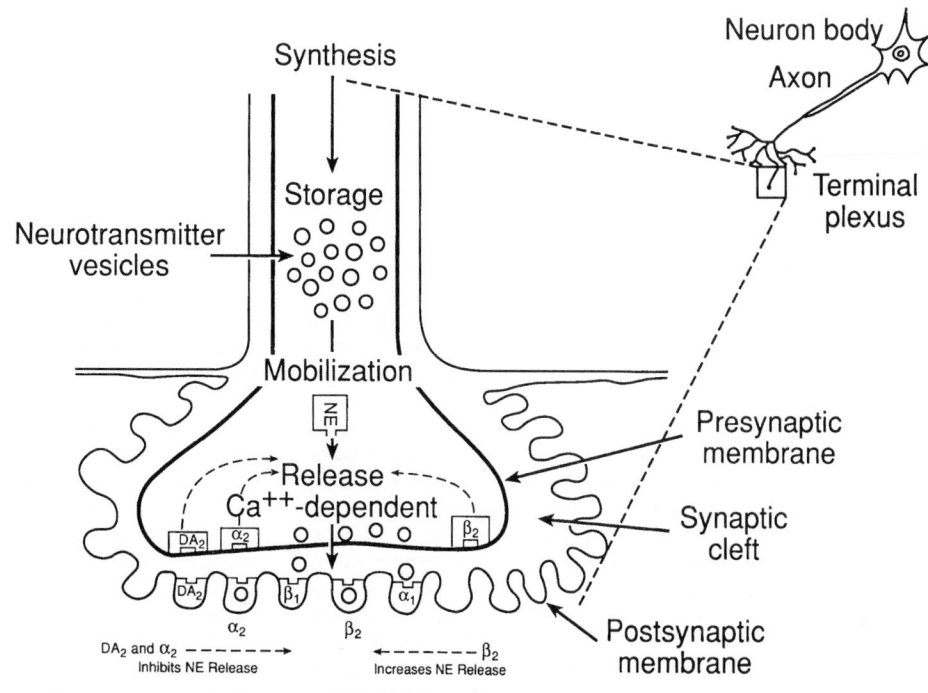

Figure 12-14. Loci of several known adrenergic receptors. The presynaptic α_2 and DA receptors serve as a negative feedback mechanism, whereby stimulation of NE inhibits its own release. Presynaptic β_2 stimulation increases NE uptake, augmenting its availability. Postsynaptic α_2 and β_2 receptors are extrasynaptic and are considered noninnervated hormonal receptors.

Table 12-6. ADRENERGIC RECEPTORS

Receptor	Synaptic Site	Anatomic Site	Action	LV Function and Stroke Volume
α_1	Postsynaptic	Peripheral vascular smooth muscle	Constriction	Decreased
		Renal vascular smooth muscle	Constriction	
		Coronary arteries, epicardial	Constriction	
		Myocardium	Positive inotropism	Improved
		30–40% of resting tone		
		Renal tubules	Antidiuresis	
α_2	Presynaptic	Peripheral vascular smooth muscle release	Inhibit NE	
			Secondary vasodilation	Improved
		Coronaries	?	
		CNS	Inhibition of CNS activity	
			Sedation	
			Decrease MAC	
	Postsynaptic	Coronaries, endocardial	Constriction	Decreased
		CNS	Inhibition of insulin release	
			Decreased bowel motility	
			Inhibition of antidiuretic hormone	
			Analgesia	
		Renal tubule	Promotes Na^{2+} and H_2O excretion	
β_1	Postsynaptic NE sensitive	Myocardium	Positive inotropism and chronotropism	Improved
		Sinoatrial (SA) node		
		Ventricular conduction		
		Kidney	Renin release	
		Coronaries	Relaxation	
β_2	Presynaptic NE sensitive	Myocardium	Accelerates NE release	Improved
		SA node ventricular conduction vessels	Opposite action to presynaptic α_2 agonism	
			Constriction	
	Postsynaptic (extrasynaptic) (EPI sensitive)	Myocardium	Positive inotropism and chronotropism	
		Vascular smooth muscle	Relaxation	Improved
		Bronchial smooth muscle	Relaxation	Improved
		Renal vessels	Relaxation	Improved
DA_1	Postsynaptic	Blood vessels (renal, mesentery, coronary)	Vasodilation	Improved
		Renal tubules	Natriuresis	
			Diuresis	
		Juxtaglomerular cells	Renin release (modulates diuresis)	
		Sympathetic ganglia	Minor inhibition	
DA_2	Presynaptic	Postganglionic sympathetic nerves	Inhibit NE release	Improved
			Secondary vasodilation	
	Postsynaptic	Renal and mesenteric vasculature	? Vasoconstriction	

of the adrenergic neuroeffector junction. Table 12-6 reviews these sites. Postsynaptic membranes contain a nearly equal mix of α_1 and α_2 receptors.[53]

The α_2-adrenoreceptors may be subdivided even further into as many as four possible subtypes. Many actions have been attributed to the postsynaptic α_2 receptor, including arterial and venous vasoconstriction, platelet aggregation, inhibition of insulin release, inhibition of bowel motility, stimulation of growth hormone release, and inhibition of antidiuretic hormone release.

α_2 Receptors can be found in cholinergic pathways as well as in adrenergic pathways. They can significantly modulate parasympathetic activity as well. Current research implies that α_2 stimulation in parasympathetic pathways plays a role in the modulation of the baroreceptor reflex (increased sensitivity), vagal mediation of heart rate (bradycardia), bronchoconstriction, and salivation (dry mouth). However, cholinergic receptors can also be found in adrenergic pathways; thus, muscarinic and nicotinic receptors have been found in presynaptic and postsynaptic locations, where they in turn modulate sympathetic activity (see Fig. 12-11). Maze speculates that although the functional role of the postsynaptic α_2 receptor in the CNS has not

been well characterized, it is probable that the features that are so desirable to the anesthesiologist, such as sedation, anxiolysis, analgesia, and hypnosis, are mediated through this site.

Stimulation of presynaptic α_2 receptors mediates inhibition of NE release into the synaptic cleft, serving as a negative feedback mechanism.[54] The central effects are primarily related to a reduction in sympathetic outflow with a concomitantly enhanced parasympathetic outflow (e.g., enhanced baroreceptor activity). This results in a decreased systemic vascular resistance, decreased cardiac output (CO), decreased inotropic state in the myocardium, and decreased HR. The peripheral presynaptic α_2 effects are similar, and NE release is inhibited in postganglionic neurons. However, stimulation of postsynaptic α_2 receptors, like the α_1 postsynaptic receptor, affects vasoconstriction.

NE acts on both α_1 and α_2 receptors. Thus, NE not only activates smooth muscle vasoconstriction (postsynaptic α_1 and α_2 receptors) but also stimulates presynaptic α_2 receptors and inhibits its own release.[55] Selective stimulation of the presynaptic α_2 receptor could produce a beneficial reduction of peripheral vascular resistance. Unfortunately, most known presynaptic α_2 agonists also stimulate the postsynaptic α_2 receptors, causing vasoconstriction. Blockade of α_2 presynaptic receptors, however, ablates normal inhibition of NE, causing vasoconstriction. Vasodilation occurs with the blockade of postsynaptic α_1 and α_2 receptors.

α Receptors in the Cardiovascular System

There is a large body of evidence documenting the presence of postsynaptic α_1 and α_2 receptors in the mammalian myocardium and coronary arteries, as well as the peripheral vasculature.[48,55]

Coronary Arteries. The presence of postsynaptic α_1 and α_2 receptors in human coronary arteries has not been established with certainty, but other mammalian models have demonstrated their presence. There is a growing consensus that sympathetic nerves cause coronary vasoconstriction, which is mediated more by postsynaptic α_2 than α_1 receptors. The larger epicardial arteries possess mainly α_1 receptors, whereas α_2 receptors and some α_1 receptors are present in the small coronary artery resistance vessels.[56] Epicardial vessels contribute only 5% to the total resistance of the coronary circulation; therefore, α_1 agonists such as phenylephrine have little influence on coronary resistance.[57]

Myocardial ischemia has been shown to increase α_2-receptor density in the coronary arteries. Ischemia has also been shown to cause a reflex increase in sympathetic activity mediated by α mechanisms. This cascade may further increase coronary constriction. Postsynaptic α_1 receptors do not rely upon extracellular Ca^{2+} to constrict the vessel, whereas the α_2-constrictor response is highly dependent upon extracellular influx and exquisitely sensitive to calcium channel inhibitors.[58]

Myocardium. The role of β receptors in mediating catecholamine-induced inotropism and arrhythmogenesis has been known for many years. Recent studies have shown the presence of postsynaptic myocardial α_1 receptors, which also exert a major, facilatory, positive inotropic effect on the myocardium of several species of mammals including humans. Their contribution to malignant reperfusion arrhythmogenesis has also been recognized.

Phenylephrine, an α_1 agonist, can increase myocardial contractility 2–3-fold compared with a 6–7-fold increase produced by isoproterenol, a pure β agonist.[59] Myocardial postsynaptic α_1 receptors mediate perhaps as much as 30–50% of the basal inotropic tone of the normal heart.[60] This contribution is reduced to about 20–30% of total inotropism when both α_1 and β_1 activation increases, as in exercise or stress. The inotropic response of the normal myocardium is more sensitive to β agonists.

Postsynaptic myocardial α_1 receptors play a more prominent inotropic role in the failing heart by serving as reserve to the normally predominant β_1 receptors. Although the response to both α_1 and β_1 agonists is reduced in the failing myocardium, the interaction between the two receptors is more apparent. Chronic heart failure is known to produce a reduced density (downregulation) of myocardial β_1 receptors as a result of high levels of circulating catecholamines. However, there is no evidence of downregulation of either α_1 or β_2 receptors with failure.[61]

The increase in density of myocardial α_1-adrenoreceptors shows a relative increase with failure and myocardial ischemia.[59,61] Thus, enhanced myocardial α_1-receptor numbers, and sensitivity, may contribute to the positive inotropism seen during ischemia as well as to the malignant arrhythmias that occur with reperfusion. Intracellular mobilization of cytosolic Ca^{2+} by the activated α_1-myocardial receptors during ischemia appears to contribute to these arrhythmias.[61] The α_1 receptor also increases the sensitivity of the contractile elements to Ca^{2+}. Drugs possessing potent α_1 antagonism such as prazosin and phentolamine have been shown to possess significant antiarrhythmic activity, although of limited usefulness because of hypotension.[62] Enhanced α_1 activity with myocardial ischemia may explain why the antiarrhythmic benefits of β antagonists in patients with acute myocardial infarction are far from certain. The contribution of β receptors to positive inotropism and arrhythmogenesis during ischemia and reperfusion may be overshadowed by the α receptors during acute failure and ischemia.

Peripheral Vessels. Activation of the presynaptic α_2-vascular receptors produces vasodilation, whereas the postsynaptic α_1- and α_2-vascular receptors subserve vasoconstriction. Presynaptic vascular α_2 receptors inhibit NE release. This represents a negative feedback mechanism by which NE inhibits its own release via the prejunctional receptor. Presynaptic α_2 agonists, such as clonidine, inhibit NE release at the neurosympathetic junction, producing vasodilatation. The effects of selective presynaptic α_2-receptor agonists to ameliorate coronary vasoconstriction in humans is unclear. Excitation of the inhibitory presynaptic α_2 receptors by endogenous or synthetic catecholamines also inhibits NE release. However, most sympathomimetics are nonselective α agonists that will excite equally presynaptic α_2 vasodilators and vasoconstrictive postsynaptic α_1 and α_2 receptors.

Postsynaptic α_1 and α_2 receptors coexist in both the arterial and venous sides of the circulation, with the relative distribution of α_2 receptors being greater on the venous side.[63,64] This may explain why pure α agonists, such as methoxamine, produce little venoconstriction, whereas many nonselective agonists produce significant venoconstriction. NE is the most potent venoconstrictor of all the catecholamines. Clinically, venoconstriction would have the effect of preloading by shifting venous capacitance centrally, whereas stimulation of arterial postsynaptic α_1 and α_2 receptors would effect afterloading by increasing arterial resistance.

α Receptors in the Central Nervous System

All subtypes of the α, β, and DA receptors have been found in various regions of the brain and spinal cord. The functional role of the cerebral α and β receptors remains under investigation, but research suggests a close association with blood pressure and HR control. Cerebral and spinal cord presynaptic α_2 receptors are also involved in inhibition of presynaptic NE release. Although the brain contains adrenergic and dopaminergic receptors, circulating catecholamines do not cross the blood–brain barrier. The catecholamines presenting in the brain are synthesized there. Many actions have been attributed to the cerebral postsynaptic α_2 receptor, including inhibition of insulin release, inhibition of bowel motility, stimulation of growth hormone release, and inhibition of antidiuretic hormone release. Postsynaptic receptors are found in specific nuclei and tracts throughout the brain and spinal cord. Central neuraxis injection of α_2 agonists, such as clonidine, act at these sites to produce analgesia, sedation, and cardiovascular depression. One might speculate that increased duration of epidural or intrathecal anesthesia by the addition of nonselective α agonists to the local anesthetic may also be producing additional analgesia through this mechanism.

α Receptors in the Kidney

The kidney has an extensive and exclusive adrenergic innervation of the afferent and efferent glomerular arterioles, proximal and distal renal tubules, ascending loop of Henle, and juxtaglomerular apparatus.[65] The greatest density of innervation is in the thick ascending loop of Henle, followed by the distal convoluted tubules and proximal tube. Both α_1 and α_2 subtypes are found in the kidney, the α_2 receptor dominating. The α_1 receptor is predominant in the renal vasculature and elicits vasoconstriction, which modulates renal blood flow. Tubular α_1 receptors enhance sodium and water reabsorption, leading to antinatriuresis, whereas tubular α_2 receptors promote sodium and water excretion.

β-Adrenergic Receptors

The β-adrenergic receptors, like the α receptor, have been divided into subtypes. They are designated as the β_1 and β_2 subtypes. The β_1 receptors predominate in the myocardium, the sinoatrial node, and the ventricular conduction system. The β_1 receptors also mediate the effects of the catecholamines on the myocardium. These receptors are equally sensitive to EPI and NE, which distinguishes them from the β_2 receptors. Effects of β_1 stimulation are outlined in Table 12-5. Table 12-6 outlines their effects specifically on the cardiovascular system.

The β_2 receptors are located in the smooth muscles of the blood vessels in the skin, muscle, mesentery, and in bronchial smooth muscle. Stimulation produces vasodilation and bronchial relaxation. The β_2 receptors are more sensitive to EPI than to NE. The β_1 receptors are suggested to be innervated receptors responding to neuronally released NE, whereas β_2 receptors are "normal" receptors responding primarily to circulating EPI.[66,67]

β Receptors are found in both presynaptic and postsynaptic membranes of the adrenergic neuroeffector junction (Table 12-6). β_1 Receptors are distributed to postsynaptic sites and have not been identified on the presynaptic membrane. Presynaptic β receptors are mostly of the β_2 subtype. The effects of activation of the presynaptic β_2 receptor are diametrically opposed to those of the presynaptic α_2 receptor. The presynaptic β_2 receptor accelerates endogenous NE release, whereas blockade of this receptor will inhibit NE release. Antagonism of the presynaptic β_2 receptors produces a physiologic result similar to activation of the presynaptic α_2 receptor.

The postsynaptic β_1 receptors are located on the synaptic membrane and are innervated receptors responding primarily to neuronal NE. The postsynaptic β_2 receptors, like the postsynaptic α_2 receptor, are considered noninnervated, extrasynaptic, normal receptors responding primarily to circulating EPI.

β Receptors in the Cardiovascular System

Myocardium. Myocardial β receptors were originally classified as β_1 receptors. Those in the vascular and bronchial smooth muscle were called the β_2 subtype. However, radioligand studies have confirmed the coexistence of β_1 and β_2 receptors in the myocardium.[67] Both β_1 and β_2 receptors are functionally coupled to adenylate cyclase, suggesting a similar involvement in the regulation of inotropism and chronotropism. Postsynaptic β_1 receptors are distributed predominantly to the myocardium, the sinoatrial node, and the ventricular conduction system. The β_2 receptors have the same distribution but are presynaptic. Activation of the presynaptic β_2 receptor accelerates the release of NE into the synaptic cleft. The β_2 receptor constitutes 20–30% of the β receptors in the ventricular myocardium and up to 40% of the β receptors in the atrium.

The increased catecholamine levels associated with heart failure lead to a proportionally greater downregulation of the β_1-receptor density with a relative sparing of the β_2 subtype and an increase in the α_1 subtype. The β_2 receptors increasingly mediate the inotropic response to catecholamines during heart failure and are facilitated by the α_1 receptor.

The effect of NE on inotropism in the normal heart is mediated entirely through the postsynaptic β_1 receptor, whereas the inotropic effects of EPI are mediated through both the β_1- and β_2-myocardial receptors. The β_2 receptors may also mediate the chronotropic responses to EPI because selective β_1 antagonists are less effective in suppressing induced tachycardia than the nonselective β_1 antagonist propranolol.

Peripheral Vessels. The postsynaptic vascular β receptors are virtually all of the β_2 subtype. The β_2 receptors are located in the smooth muscle of the blood vessels of the skin, muscle, mesentery, and bronchi. Stimulation of the postsynaptic β_2 receptor produces vasodilation and bronchial relaxation. Modest vasoconstriction occurs when subjected to blockade because the actions of the vascular postsynaptic β_2 receptors no longer oppose the actions of the α_1 and α_2 postsynaptic receptors.

β Receptor in the Kidney

The kidney contains both β_1 and β_2 receptors, the β_1 being predominant. Renin release from the juxtaglomerular apparatus is enhanced by β stimulation. β Blockers inhibit this re-

sponse. The β subtype regulating renin release is highly species-dependent. The β_1 receptor evokes renin release in humans.[68] Renal β_2 receptors also appear to regulate renal blood flow at the vascular level. They have been identified pharmacologically and mediate an expected vasodilatory response.

Dopaminergic Receptors

Dopamine, synthesized in 1910, was recognized in 1959 not only as a vasopressor and the precursor of NE and EPI, but also as an important central and peripheral neurotransmitter. Dopamine receptors (DA) have been localized in the CNS, on blood vessels and postganglionic sympathetic nerves (Table 12-6). Two major types of DA receptors have been recognized. These are the DA_1 and DA_2 receptors. The DA_1 receptors are postsynaptic, whereas the DA_2 receptors are both presynaptic and postsynaptic. The presynaptic DA_2 receptors, like the presynaptic α_2 receptor, inhibit NE release and can produce vasodilatation.[37,54,69] There is evidence that the postsynaptic DA_2 receptor may subserve vasoconstriction similar to that of the postsynaptic α_2 receptor.[70] However, postsynaptic DA_2 receptors have not been positively identified.[71] This effect is opposite to that of the postsynaptic DA_1 renal vascular receptor. Unpublished data suggest that dopamine may be the intrinsic regulator of renal function.[72] The zona glomerulose of the adrenal cortex also contains DA_2 receptors, which inhibit release of aldosterone.

Myocardium. Defining specific dopaminergic receptors has been difficult because dopamine also exerts effects on the α and β receptors.[73,74] DA receptors have not been described in the myocardium. Effects of dopamine are those related to activation of β_1 receptors, which promote positive inotropism and chronotropism. β_2 Activation would produce some systemic vasodilatation.

Peripheral Vessels. The greatest numbers of DA_1-postsynaptic receptors are found on vascular smooth muscle cells of the kidney and mesentery, but are also found in the other systemic arteries including coronary, cerebral, and cutaneous arteries. The vascular receptors are, like the β_2 receptors, linked to adenylate cyclase and mediate smooth muscle relaxation. Activation of these receptors produces vasodilatation, increasing blood flow to these organs. Concurrent activation of vascular presynaptic DA_2 receptors also inhibits NE release at presynaptic α_2 receptors, which may also contribute to peripheral vasodilatation. Higher doses of dopamine can mediate vasoconstriction via the postsynaptic α_1 and α_2 receptors. The constrictive effect is relatively weak in the cardiovascular system where the action of dopamine on adrenergic receptors is 1/35 and 1/50 as potent as that of EPI and NE, respectively.[75]

Central Nervous System. DA receptors have been identified in the hypothalamus where they are involved in prolactin release. They are also found in the basal ganglia where they coordinate motor function.[74,73] Degeneration of dopaminergic neurons of the substantia nigra is the source of Parkinson's disease. Another central action of dopamine is to stimulate the chemoreceptor trigger zone of the medulla, producing nausea and vomiting. Dopamine antagonists such as haloperidol and droperidol are clinically effective in countering this action.

Kidney and Mesentery. Apart from their effect on the vessels of the kidney and mesentery, DA receptors on the smooth muscle of the esophagus, stomach, and small intestine enhance secretion production and reduce intestinal motility.[75] Metoclopramide, a dopamine antagonist, is useful for aspiration prophylaxis by promoting gastric emptying.

The distribution of DA receptors in the renal vasculature is well known, but DA receptors have other functions within the kidney. DA_1 receptors are located on renal tubules, which inhibit sodium reabsorption with subsequent natriuresis and diuresis. The natriuresis may be the result of a combined renal vasodilatation, improved CO, and tubular action of the DA_1 receptors. Juxtaglomerular cells also contain DA_1 receptors, which increase renin release when activated. This action modulates the diuresis produced by DA_1 activation of the tubules.

Dopamine has unique autonomic effects by activating specific peripheral dopaminergic receptors, which promote natriuresis and reduce afterload *via* dilatation of the renal and mesenteric arterial beds. Peripheral dopaminergic activity serves as a natural antihypertensive mechanism.[68] Its actions are overshadowed by the opposite effect of its main biologic partner, NE.[76] Plasma NE levels are known to increase with aging, likely the result of reduced clearance. Peripheral dopaminergic activity is known to diminish. Subtle changes in the DA–NE balance with aging may account for the diminished ability of the aged kidney to excrete a salt load. This may also contribute to the uniform finding of increasing systolic blood pressure in societies with high salt consumption.

Other Receptors

Adenosine Receptors. Adenosine produces inhibition of NE release.[37,54] The effect of adenosine is blocked by caffeine and other methylxanthines. The physiologic and pharmacologic roles of adenosine-mediated inhibition of NE release are not clearly defined. The physiologic function of these receptors may be the reduction of sympathetic tone under hypoxic conditions when adenosine production is enhanced. As a consequence of reduced NE release, cardiac work would be decreased and oxygen demand reduced. Recently, adenosine has been effectively used to produce controlled hypotension.[37,76]

Serotonin. Serotonin (5-hydroxytryptamine) depresses the response of isolated blood vessels to sympathetic nervous system (SNS) stimulation and decreases release of labeled NE in these preparations. This inhibitory action of serotonin is antagonized by raising the external calcium ion concentration. Thus, serotonin may inhibit neuronal NE release by a mechanism that limits the availability of calcium ions at the nerve terminal.

Prostaglandin E_2, Histamine, and Several Opioids. Prostaglandin E_2, histamine, and several opioids have been reported to act on prejunctional receptor sites to inhibit NE release in certain sympathetically innervated tissue. However, these inhibitory receptors are unlikely to play a physiologic role in limiting NE release because inhibitors of cyclo-oxygenase, histamine antagonists, and naloxone produce no increase in NE release.

Histamine acts in a manner similar to the neurotransmitters of the SNS.[77] It has membrane receptors specific for histamine, with the individual response being determined by the type of cell being stimulated. Two receptors for histamine have been determined. These have been designated H_1 and H_2, for which it has been possible to develop specific agonists and antagonists. Stimulation of the H_1 receptors produces bronchoconstriction and intestinal contraction. The major role of the H_2 receptors is related to acid production by the parietal cells of the stomach; however, histamine is present in relatively high concentrations in the myocardium and cardiac conducting tissue, where it exerts positive inotropic and chronotropic effects while depressing dromotropism. The positive inotropic and chronotropic effects of histamine are H_2-receptor effects that are not blocked by β antagonism. These effects are blocked by H_2 antagonists, such as cimetidine, which accounts for the occasional report of cardiovascular collapse following the use of cimetidine.[78] The negative dromotropic effect and that of coronary spasm caused by histamine are H_1 receptor effects.

Adrenergic Receptor Numbers or Sensitivity

Receptors, once thought to be static entities, are now thought to be dynamically regulated by a variety of conditions and in a constant state of flux. Receptors are synthesized in the sarcoplasmic reticulum (SR) of the parent cell, where they may remain extrasynaptic or externalize to the synaptic membranes, where they may cluster. Membrane receptors may be removed or internalized to intracellular sites for either dehydration or recycling.[79] The numbers and sensitivity of adrenergic receptors can be influenced by normal, genetic, and developmental factors.[80] Changes in the number of receptors alter the response to catecholamines. Alteration in the number, or density, of receptors is referred to as either upregulation or downregulation.[81] As a rule, the number of receptors is inversely proportional to the ambient concentration of the catecholamines.[82] Extended exposure of receptors to their agonists markedly reduces, but does not ablate, the biologic response to catecholamines.[83] For example, increased adrenergic activity occurs in response to reduced perfusion as a result of acute or chronic myocardial dysfunction. Plasma catecholamines are increased. As a result, myocardial postsynaptic β_1 receptors "downregulate." This is thought to explain the diminished inotropic and chronotropic response to β_1 agonists and exercise in patients with chronic heart failure. However, calcium-induced inotropism is not impaired because β_2-receptor (extrasynaptic) numbers remain relatively intact.[84] The β_2 receptors may account for up to 40% of the inotropism of the failing heart compared with 20% in the normal heart.[85] Tachyphylaxis to infused catecholamines is also thought to be the result of acute downregulation of receptor numbers. There appears to be a reduction in numbers or sensitivity of β receptors in hypertensive patients who also have elevated plasma catecholamines. Downregulation is the presumptive explanation for the lack of correlation between plasma catecholamine levels and the blood pressure elevation in patients with pheochromocytoma. Chronic use of β agonists such as terbutaline, isoproterenol, or EPI for the treatment of asthma can result in tachyphylaxis because of downregulation. Even short-term use (1–6 hours) of β agonists may cause downregulation of receptor numbers.

Downregulation is reversible on termination of the agonist. Chronic treatment of animals with nonselective β blockade causes a 100% increase in the number of β receptors.[80,86] This accounts for the propranolol withdrawal syndrome in which the acute discontinuation of the β antagonist leaves the α receptors unopposed plus an increased number of β receptors. Clonidine withdrawal can be explained by the same mechanism.[87] Acute discontinuation of the α_2-inhibitory agonist would permit a resumption of stimulation of adrenoreceptors that upregulated during the time NE release was inhibited.

Up- or downregulation of receptor numbers may not alter sensitivity of the receptor. Likewise, sensitivity may be increased or decreased in the presence of normal numbers of receptors. The pharmacologic factors affecting up- or downregulation of the α and β receptors are similar.

MOLECULAR PHARMACOLOGY AND EFFECTOR RESPONSE

Autonomic agonists trigger a cascade of intracellular chemical reactions culminating in the cell's biologic response. The receptor is only the first link in a communication series. Understanding such ligand-triggered signaling cascades promises to be of vital importance to the anesthesiologist in management of autonomic responses to surgery and anesthesia.

A remarkable homology exists in the molecular composition of receptors and intracellular signaling cascades of the ANS. A superfamily of integral membrane proteins has been identified, which includes the adrenergic and cholinergic receptors, as well as receptors to dopamine, purines (such as adenosine and ATP), serotonin, angiotensin, vasopressin, vasoactive intestinal peptide, glucagon, histamine, leukotrienes, thrombin, γ-aminobutyric acid (GABA), opioids, and a host of others.[88–90] These receptors have two important characteristics in common: (1) each has seven hydrophobic amino acid domains, which are believed to constitute transmembrane spanning regions critical in defining ligand specificity; (2) agonist binding to the receptor is linked to the activation of one or more distinct guanine nucleotide–binding regulatory proteins (G proteins). These G proteins are a family of cytoplasmic membrane–associated proteins that act as intermediaries between the diverse array of membrane receptors and activation of a relatively smaller group of cellular effector mechanisms.[88–91] G proteins are linked to receptor binding in cells of nearly every organ system of the body.

With respect to autonomic agonists, G protein–activated mechanisms may be grouped into five principal categories: (1) activation of adenylate cyclase (AC), (2) inhibition of AC, (3) direct potassium channel activation, (4) direct calcium channel inhibition, and (5) activation of phospholipase C.

For years, the β-adrenergic receptor was considered the prototypical adrenergic receptor. This largely reflected the pioneering work of Sutherland, who revealed that the biologic activity of the β receptor is dependent upon intracellular production of cyclic adenosine monophosphate (cAMP).[92] The current understanding is that ligand binding to β_1 and β_2 receptors, as well as dopaminergic types D_1 and D_5, activates s-type (stimulatory) G protein (Gs) (Fig. 12-15). Gs, in turn, stimulates AC (also membrane-bound) to produce cAMP. cAMP acts as the cytoplasmic mediator, or second messenger, of the catecholamine-triggered cellular response. The biologic activity of cAMP is effected largely through cAMP-dependent protein kinase A (PKA). Proteins phosphorylated by PKA include ion flux channels, such as Ca^{2+}, K^+, and Cl^- channels, as well as myosin light chain kinase, troponin, and other kinases and synthases linked to cellular contraction and stimulus-secretion coupling.[88–90,93]

In the myocardium, PKA-induced protein phosphorylation results in an increase in chronotropy, inotropy, lusitropy (rate of relaxation), and dromotropy.[89,93] Phosphorylation increases depolarization-triggered Ca^{2+} influx across L-type (voltage-sensitive) channels, thereby increasing intracellular Ca^{2+} and, hence, inotropy. Ca^{2+} affinity of troponin I is decreased by PKA, and phospholamban phosphorylation by PKA increases SR Ca^{2+}–ATPase activity, allowing the more rapid Ca^{2+} cycling necessary to increase lusitropy and sustain the increase in chronotropy. Further, PKA increases sarcolemmal Cl^- and K^+ channel currents, counteracting the tendency of the increased Ca^{2+} influx to prolong depolarization. Increased pacemaker currents are

also cAMP-dependent, although the precise mechanism is unclear.

In contrast to cardiac muscle, cAMP and PKA mediate relaxation of smooth muscle. The mechanism for this may involve one or more of the following: (1) decreased cytoplasmic Ca^{2+} secondary to enhanced uptake by SR Ca^{2+}–ATPase, (2) hyperpolarization due to increased sarcolemmal K^+ conductance, and (3) phosphorylation of myosin light chain kinase, reducing its affinity for myosin light chain.[89,94,95]

In addition to β-adrenergic and D_1 and D_5 receptor systems, receptor subtypes for adenosine, serotonin, vasopressin, histamine (H_2 receptors), and glucagon, to name a few, have been identified as Gs-linked activators of AC (Table 12-7).

In contrast to Gs, i-type (inhibitory) G protein (Gi) inhibits AC, thereby reducing cytoplasmic cAMP and its subsequent effects (Fig. 12-15). Gi is linked to numerous receptor types including α_2-adrenergic, dopaminergic types D_2–D_4, and muscarinic and serotonergic subtypes (Table 12-7). Thus, opposing cellular responses to different agonists may reflect opposing activities on AC-dependent effector mechanisms.

In the case of the α_2 receptor, inhibition of AC is responsible for many but not all of its biologic effects. Coupling of the α_2 adrenoceptor with Gi or Go (other type G protein) is directly linked to membrane Ca^{2+} channel inhibition and K^+ channel activation. The subsequent hyperpolarization and decreased intracellular Ca^{2+} are believed to be responsible for α_2-mediated suppression of CNS function as well as presynaptic inhibition of NE release at sympathetic nerve terminals.[90,94] Ca^{2+} and K^+ channel conductances are similarly affected by other Gi-linked receptors. Unlike Gi, Go does not alter AC activity.

A fourth G protein, Gq, is responsible for mediating the activity of a host of other receptors including α_1-adrenoceptors, and certain muscarinic and serotonergic receptor subtypes (Table 12-7). Gq activates phospholipase C (PLC), a protein that hydrolyzes the constituent membrane phospholipid phosphatidylinositol 4,5-bisphosphate (PIP_2) to yield membrane-bound 1,2-diacylglycerol (DAG) and cytoplasmic inositol 1,4,5-

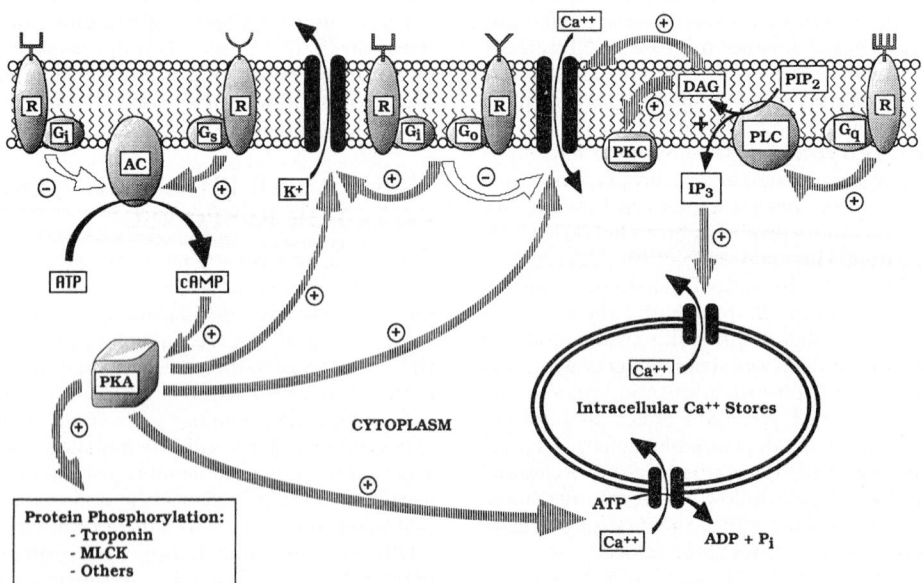

Figure 12-15. Cellular effector mechanisms of adrenergic receptors. Receptor (R) binding of the extracellular agonist activates one of five principal G protein-triggered mechanisms: (1) Activated Gs stimulates adenylate cyclase (AC) to produce free cytoplasmic cyclic AMP (cAMP), which, in turn, activates protein kinase A (PKA). PKA has a number of cellular activities including increasing K^+ and Ca^{2+} channel conductances, increasing Ca^{2+} ATPase activity, and phosphorylation of cytoplasmic proteins such as troponin and myosin light chain kinase (MLCK), which mediate cellular contractile activity. (2) Activated Gi inhibits AC. (3) Activated Gi or Go directly increases K^+ channel conductance. (4) Activated Gi or Go directly inhibits cell membrane Ca^{2+} channel conductance. (5) Activated Gq stimulates phospholipase C (PLC), which hydrolyzes phosphatidylinositol 4,5-bisphosphate (PIP_2) to yield membrane-bound 1,2-diacylglycerol (DAG) and cytoplasmic inositol 1,4,5-trisphosphate (IP_3). IP_3 interacts with its receptor on the membranes of internal Ca^{2+} stores. The IP_3 receptor is itself a Ca^{2+} channel, which, when bound to IP_3, increases its conductance, releasing Ca^{2+} into the cytoplasm. DAG increases cytoplasmic membrane Ca^{2+} conductance and activates protein kinase C (PKC).

Table 12-7. RECEPTOR-MEDIATED EFFECTOR MECHANISMS

Receptor Agonists	Principal Effector Mechanisms				
	G Protein-Linked Signal Transduction Pathways*				Endothelial Receptor Binding Releases EDRF/NO
	Gs ↑cAMP	Gi ↓cAMP	Gi/Go ↑K$^+$Efflux and ↓Ca^{2+} Influx	Gq ↑IP$_3$ and ↑DAG	↑cGMP and Other Effects of NO
β-Adrenergic agonists	✔				✔
α$_1$-Adrenergic agonists				✔	
α$_2$-Adrenergic agonists		✔	✔		
Dopaminergic agonists	✔ (D$_{1,5}$)	✔ (D$_{2,3,4}$)			
Acetylcholine (musarinic)		✔ (M$_{2,4}$)	✔ (M$_{2,4}$)	✔ (M$_{1,3,5}$)	✔
Adenosine (P$_1$-purinergic)	✔ (A$_2$)	✔ (A$_{1,3}$)	✔ (A$_1$)		
ATP and ADP (P$_2$-purinergic)				✔	✔
Serotonin	✔ (5-HT$_4$)	✔ (5-HT$_1$)	✔ (5-HT$_1$)	✔ (5-HT$_2$)	✔
Vasopressin	✔ (V$_2$)			✔ (V$_1$)	✔
Angiotensin				✔ (AT$_1$)	
Glucagon	✔				
Thrombin		✔		✔	✔
Histamine	✔ (H$_2$)			✔ (H$_1$)	✔
Bradykinin		✔		✔	✔

* Receptor subtypes are indicated in parentheses.

trisphosphate (IP$_3$) (Fig. 12-15). IP$_3$ triggers a surge in cytoplasmic free Ca^{2+} by binding to its receptor on the membranes of internal calcium stores such as the SR and the endoplasmic reticulum. The IP$_3$ receptor is itself an ion channel which, when bound to IP3, increases its conductance to Ca^{2+}. This receptor therefore acts as a gate for triggered release of Ca^{2+} into the cytoplasm of vascular smooth muscle cells, endothelial cells, and neurologic, immunologic, and endocrine tissues. The rapid rise of cytoplasmic Ca^{2+} is ultimately responsible for many of the Gq-triggered biologic responses, including cellular contraction, secretion, increased metabolism, and proliferation. Of note, the IP$_3$ receptor channel is not found in myocardium or skeletal muscle. Instead, a closely related receptor is found: the ryanodine-sensitive calcium channel, which is believed to play a principal role in the pathophysiology of malignant hyperthermia.[96]

The remainder of the effects of the Gq–PLC pathway are mediated by DAG-induced activation of protein kinase C (PKC). Activated PKC affects cellular activity by phosphorylating serine and threonine residues on numerous intracellular proteins. In vascular smooth muscle, activated PKC plays a potentiating role in agonist-induced contraction, increasing Ca^{2+} influx and sensitivity of the contractile process to Ca^{2+}.[89,90,93,95]

Gq activation has been shown to activate phospholipase A$_2$ (PLA$_2$) in addition to PKC. The physiologic role of this activation, though, remains to be determined. Hydrolysis of membrane phospholipids by PLA$_2$ produces arachidonic acid (AA). AA, in turn, inhibits myosin light chain phosphorylase. The subsequent elevation in phosphorylated (activated) myosin may increase the contractile activity of the cell.[94] On the other hand, AA is also metabolized by endothelial cells to produce prostacyclin (PGI$_2$), which is a potent vasodilator.

A new concept of endothelial control of vascular smooth muscle function has gained recognition over the past decade. An increase in endothelial cell intracellular Ca^{2+}, as triggered by compounds such as ACh, NE, histamine, bradykinin, ATP, and thrombin, has been shown to stimulate production and

release of an endothelium-dependent vasodilatory factor (EDRF).[97,98] Compounds capable of stimulating EDRF formation are termed endothelium-dependent vasodilators. With regard to adrenergic agonists, the precise physiologic and pathophysiologic roles of endothelium-dependent effects and direct smooth muscle binding effects are complex and remain to be defined.

EDRF is generally believed to be nitric oxide (NO), the synthesis of which is stimulated by Ca^{2+} bound to calmodulin in the cytoplasm (Fig. 12-16).[97,98] NO is synthesized from L-arginine by NO synthetases (NOS), which are found in neurons, vascular endothelial cells, macrophages, and several other cell types, notably excluding muscle cells. NO is a short-lived free radical that freely diffuses out of the endothelial cell to affect adjacent cells such as the smooth muscle cell. Its primary biologic effect is to stimulate production of cyclic guanosine monophosphate (cGMP) by activating cytosolic guanylate cyclase (GC).[99] cGMP stimulates cGMP-dependent protein kinase G (PKG), which reduces cytoplasmic Ca^{2+} levels and, in the case of vascular smooth muscle, inhibits contraction.[100] It is interesting to note that elevated cAMP levels are associated with activation of PKG in addition to PKA, providing, for example, an additional pathway for β adrenoceptor- and dopaminergic-induced vasorelaxation.[94,101]

In the CNS, NO is believed to function as a principal neurotransmitter. In the immune system, it is an intermediate in macrophage-induced oxidation. In addition to its role as a vasodilator, NO release by endothelium inhibits platelet aggregation and adhesion. Indeed, the ability of adrenergic agonists to affect EDRF/NO has added a new level of complexity to the scope of adrenergic activity.

Each signal must be transient in nature for these systems to be effective modulators of cell activity. This is assured by the rapid inactivation of G proteins and G protein-stimulated enzymes upon dissociation of the agonist from the receptor. cAMP and cGMP are hydrolyzed to inactive metabolites by phosphodi-

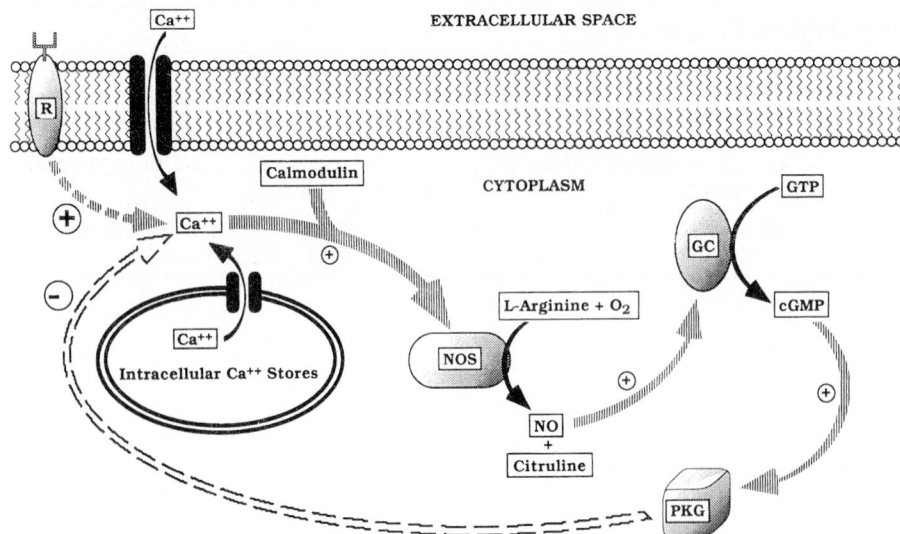

Figure 12-16. Receptor-mediated activation of nitric oxide synthase (NOS). Receptor (R) activation triggers an increase in cytoplasmic Ca^{2+} as depicted in Figure 12-15. Ca^{2+} then binds to calmodulin, and the complex of the two stimulates cytoplasmic nitric oxide synthase (NOS). NOS catalyzes the reaction of L-arginine and oxygen to form nitric oxide (NO) and citruline. The membrane-permeable free radical NO has multiple sites of activity within the cell of origin and in nearby cells. One site is cytosolic guanylate cyclase (GC), which it stimulates, converting GTP into cyclic GMP (cGMP). cGMP, in turn, activates protein kinase G (PKG), which ultimately decreases cytoplasmic Ca^{2+} levels.

esterase (PDE) enzymes. A variety of cyclic nucleotide PDEs have been identified, with variable substrate specificities for cAMP and cGMP.[102] At any moment in time, the cytoplasmic concentrations of cAMP and cGMP, and hence their activities, reflect not only their rates of production but also their rates of hydrolysis. The activities of the PDEs, like those of AC and GC, are hormonally regulated, providing an alternative mechanism for hormonal control of cyclic nucleotide second-messenger function. For instance, insulin receptor binding is linked to activation of a PDE. Furthermore, agents that increase cytoplasmic Ca^{2+} have been shown to activate a Ca^{2+}–calmodulin-dependent form of PDE. Cardiac myocyte α_1-adrenoceptors activate a cAMP-specific PDE.[48] In each case cytoplasmic levels of cAMP and/or cGMP are reduced. Lastly, cyclic nucleotides themselves are able to influence PDE function: cGMP stimulates a nonselective form of PDE and inhibits a cAMP-specific form.[100]

Therefore, the response of a receptor to a catecholamine can be regulated by (1) the concentration of the catecholamine agonists, (2) receptor numbers and binding affinity, (3) factors affecting receptor coupling to kinase or ion channel activation, (4) PDE activities, and (5) availability of ions such as calcium. All these factors can be medically manipulated, with the possible exception of receptor numbers.

AUTONOMIC NERVOUS SYSTEM REFLEXES

The ANS reflex has been compared to the computer circuit.[103] This control system, as in all reflex systems, has (1) sensors, (2) afferent pathways, (3) CNS integration, and (4) efferent pathways to the receptors and efferent organs. Fine adjustments are made at the local level according to positive and negative feedback mechanisms. The baroreceptor is an example. The variable to be controlled (blood pressure) is sensed (carotid sinus), integrated (medullary vasomotor center), and adjusted through specific effector–receptor sites. Drugs or disease can interrupt this circuit at any point. β Blockers may attenuate the effector response, whereas an α agonist such as clonidine may alter both the effector and the integrator functions of blood pressure control (see Antihypertensives).[87]

Baroreceptors

Several reflexes in the cardiovascular system help control arterial blood pressure, CO, and HR. Cardiovascular ANS reflexes are an anachronism. The business of circulation is to provide blood flow. Yet, the most important controlled variable to which

the sensors are attuned is blood pressure, a product of flow and resistance.[104]

In 1859, Etienne Marey noted that the pulse rate is inversely proportional to the blood pressure—an observation now known as Marey's law.[8] Subsequently, Hering, Koch, and others demonstrated that the alterations in HR evoked by changes in blood pressure are dependent on baroreceptors located in the aortic arch and the carotid sinuses. These pressure sensors react to alterations in stretch caused by blood pressure. Impulses from the carotid sinus and aortic arch reach the medullary vasomotor center by the glossopharyngeal and vagus nerves, respectively. Increased sensory traffic from the baroreceptors, caused by increased blood pressure, inhibits SNS effector traffic. The relative increase in vagal tone produces vasodilation, slowing of the HR, and a lowering of blood pressure.[105] Real increases in vagal tone occur when blood pressure exceeds normal limits.[103,106]

The arterial baroreceptor reflex can best be demonstrated by the Valsalva maneuver (Fig. 12-17). The Valsalva maneuver

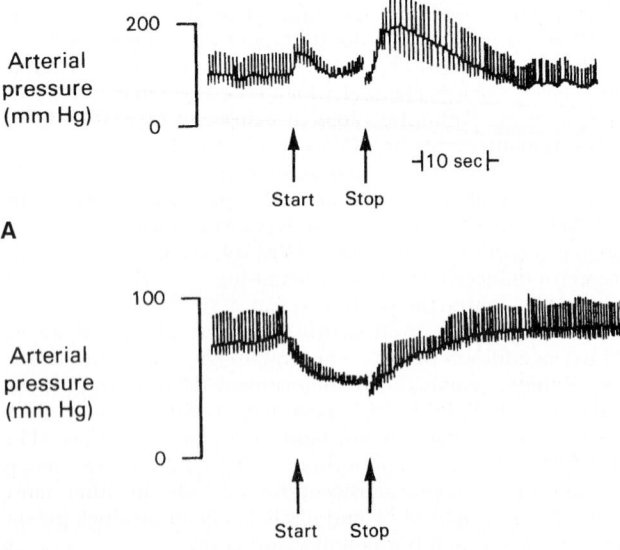

Figure 12-17. (A) The normal blood pressure response to the Valsalva maneuver is demonstrated. Pulse rate moves in a reciprocal direction according to Marey's law of the heart. (B) An abnormal Valsalva response is shown in a patient with C5 quadriplegia.

raises the intrathoracic pressure by forced expiration against a closed glottis. The arterial blood pressure rises momentarily as the intrathoracic blood is forced into the heart (preload).[5] Sustained intrathoracic pressure diminishes venous return, reduces the CO, and drops the blood pressure. Reflex vasoconstriction and tachycardia ensue. Blood pressure returns to normal with release of the forced expiration, but then briefly "overshoots" because of the vasoconstriction and increased venous return. A slowing of the HR accompanies the overshoot in pressure, according to Marey's law.

The cardiovascular responses to the Valsalva maneuver require an intact ANS circuit from peripheral sensor to peripheral adrenergic receptors. The Valsalva maneuver has been used to identify patients at risk for anesthesia due to ANS instability (Fig. 12-17). This was once a major concern in patients receiving catecholamine-depleting drugs such as reserpine. Dysfunction of the SNS is implicated if exaggerated and prolonged hypotension develops during the forced expiration phase (50% from resting mean arterial pressure).[8,103] In addition, the overshoot at the end of the Valsalva maneuver is absent. Dysfunction of the PNS can be assumed if the HR does not respond appropriately to the blood pressure changes. The Valsalva maneuver may still be a valid clinical preoperative test for detecting the autonomic dysautonomia that accompanies diabetes.

Venous baroreceptors may be more dominant in the moment-to-moment regulation of CO. Baroreceptors in the right atrium and great veins produce an increase in HR when stretched by increased right atrial pressure.[107] Reduced venous pressure decreases HR. Unlike the arterial baroreceptors, venous sensors are not thought to alter vascular tone; however, venoconstriction is postulated to occur when atrial pressures decline.[108] Stretch of the venous receptors produces changes in HR opposite to those produced when the arterial pressure sensors are stimulated. The arterial and venous pressure receptors are separately monitoring two of the four major determinants of CO: afterload and preload, respectively. Venous baroreceptors sample preload by stretch of the atrium. Arterial baroreceptors survey resistance, or afterload, as reflected in the mean arterial pressure. Afterload and preload produce opposite effects on CO; thus, one should not be surprised that the venous and arterial baroreceptors produce effects opposite those of a similar stretch stimulus, pressure.

Bainbridge described the venous baroreceptor reflex and demonstrated that it can be abolished by vagal resection. Numerous investigators have confirmed the acceleration of the HR in response to volume.[8] However, the magnitude and direction of the HR response are dependent on the prevailing HR at the time of stimulation. The exact mechanism of the Bainbridge reflex remains in doubt. The denervated, transplanted mammalian heart also accelerates in response to volume loading.[109] HR, like CO, can apparently be adjusted to the quantity of blood entering the heart.[110,111]

The Bainbridge reflex relates to the characteristic but paradoxical slowing of the heart seen with spinal anesthesia.[112] Blockade of the SNS levels of T1–T4 ablates the efferent limb of the cardiac accelerator nerves. This source of cardiac deceleration is obvious, as the vagus nerve is unopposed. However, bradycardia during spinal anesthesia is more closely related to the development of arterial hypotension than to the height of the block. The primary defect in the development of spinal hypotension is a decrease in venous return. Theoretically, the arterial hypotension should reflexly produce a tachycardia through the arterial baroreceptors. Instead, bradycardia is more common. Greene suggests that in the unmedicated person, the venous baroreceptors are dominant over the arterial. A reduced venous pressure, therefore, slows HR.[113] In contrast, humorally mediated tachycardia is the usual response to hypotension or acidosis from other causes.

Denervated Heart

Reflex modulation of the adrenergic agonists is best seen in the denervated transplant heart, which retains the recipient's innervated sinoatrial node and the donor's denervated sinoatrial node.[114] Table 12-8 is a summary of drug effects on the transplanted heart.[9,109,115] NE simultaneously activates α and β receptors of the intact heart and vessels. NE infusion in the transplanted heart produces a slowing of the recipient's atrial rate through vagal feedback as the blood pressure rises. In the unmodulated donor heart, atrial rate increases. Methoxamine-induced hypertension and nitrite-induced hypotension fail to induce deceleration and acceleration of the donor atrial rate. The baroreceptors are therefore not operant in the trans-

---

Table 12-8. DRUG EFFECTS ON THE DENERVATED HEART

Drug	Sinus Rate Recipient	Sinus Rate Donor	Atrioventricular Conduction Velocity	Intraventricular Conduction Velocity	Blood Pressure	Cardiac Output	Systemic Vascular Resistance
Resting	Normal	↑*	Normal	Normal	Normal	Normal or low	Normal
Exercise	↑	Slow ↑			↑	↑	
Atropine	↑	—	—				
Norepinephrine	↓	↑ ↑*	↑	—	↑	— or ↑	↑ ↑
Methoxamine	↓	—			↑	↓	↑ ↑
Isoproterenol	↑	↑ ↑	↑		↓	↑ ↑	↓
Glucagon	↑	↑			—	↑	
Propranolol	↓	↓	↓	—	— or ↓	↓	↑
Amyl nitrite	↑	—			↓		↓
Digoxin							
Acute	↓	—	—*	—	—	— or ↑†	
Chronic	↓	—	↓				
Quinidine	↑	↓*	↓*	↓			
Edrophonium	↓	—*	—*				
Increased preload		↑				↑ or ↓†	

↑ = increase; ↓ = decrease; — = no change.
* Opposite from normals.
† Response depends on contractile state related to rejection.
Reprinted with permission from Lawson NW, Wallfisch HK: Cardiovascular pharmacology: A new look at the "pressors." In Stoelting RK, Barash PG, Gallagher TJ (eds): Advances in Anesthesia, p 195. Chicago, Year Book Medical Publishers, 1986.

planted heart. Isoproterenol, a pure β agonist, increases the discharge rate of both the recipient and donor node by direct action, with the donor rate near doubling that of the recipient node. Atropine accelerates the recipient's atrial rate, whereas no effect is seen on the donor rate, which now controls HR.

Hypersensitivity to β cardiac stimulation in denervated dog hearts has been demonstrated. Whether or not this occurs in the human heart remains unclear. Patients who have undergone chemical sympathectomy with bretylium or guanethidine are known to be hyper-reactive to the usual doses of catecholamines.

β Blockade produces comparable slowing of the sinoatrial node of both recipient and donor. The exercise capability of the denervated heart is conspicuously reduced by β blockade, presumably because of its reliance on circulating catecholamines. Propranolol has also been demonstrated to reduce the β response to chronotropic effects of NE and isoproterenol in the transplanted heart. The CO of the transplanted heart varies appropriately with changes in preload and afterload.

INTERACTION OF AUTONOMIC NERVOUS SYSTEM RECEPTORS

Strong interactions have been noted between SNS and PNS nerves in organs that receive dual, antagonistic innervation. Release of NE at the presynaptic terminal is modified by the PNS. For example, vagal inhibition of left ventricular contractility is accentuated as the level of SNS activity is raised.[6] This interaction, termed *accentuated antagonism,* is mediated by a combination of presynaptic and postsynaptic mechanisms. The coronary arteries present an example of this phenomenon and deserve special attention.

The myocardium and coronary vessels are abundantly supplied with adrenergic and cholinergic fibers.[8,116,117] Strong activity of both α and β receptors has been demonstrated in the coronary vascular bed. Selective stimulation of both the α_1 and postsynaptic α_2 receptors increases coronary vascular resistance, whereas selective α blockade eliminates this effect. Therefore, both β_1 and α_1 adrenoreceptors are present on coronary arteries and accessible to NE from sympathetic nerves.[11,116]

The close anatomic proximity of the postganglionic vagal and SNS nerve endings in coronary arteries provides the morphologic basis for strong interaction.[6,14] SNS and PNS nerve terminals are found in such close proximity that transmitters from one can easily reach the other and affect transmitter release. In addition, the presynaptic adrenergic terminals of the myocardium and coronary vessels, like all blood vessels examined, contain muscarinic receptors.[37,118] Recent observations confirm that muscarinic agents and vagal stimulation, acting on the presynaptic, SNS muscarinic receptor, inhibit the release of NE in a manner similar to that of the presynaptic α_2 and DA_2 receptors (Fig. 12-11). Conversely, blockade of the muscarinic receptors with atropine markedly augments the positive inotropic responses to catecholamines.[6] Suppression of NE release explains, in part, vagal-induced attenuation of the inotropic response to strong SNS stimulation (accentuated antagonism) and a weak negative inotropic effect of vagal stimulation when there is low background SNS activity. This may also explain why vagal activity reduces the vulnerability of the myocardium to fibrillation during infusions of NE.

ACh may cause coronary spasm during periods of high SNS tone.[12,119] Inhibition of NE release by presynaptic adrenergic muscarinic receptors of the smooth muscle of coronary vessels would diminish the coronary relaxation normally produced by NE on the β_1 receptor (Fig. 12-11). In anesthetized dogs, the rate of NE outflow into the coronary sinus blood, evoked by cardiac SNS stimulation, is markedly diminished by simultaneous vagal efferent stimulation.[120,121] This action is known to be prevented by atropine, which also causes coronary vasodilation. Methacholine, a muscarinic parasympathomimetic agent, has

been reported to cause coronary vasoconstriction.[122] However, it simultaneously reduces ventricular irritability by reducing NE release in myocardial fibers.[6]

The concept of accentuated antagonism has yet to be clearly defined because it is unusual for high SNS and PNS activity to coexist, except during anesthesia. The importance of accentuated antagonism in the intact, conscious human has yet to be demonstrated; however, it may explain the clinical observation that angina and myocardial infarction owing to coronary spasm in humans are not often related to cardiac work, as is angina caused by sclerotic coronary disease. Attacks of angina usually occur at rest, often waking the patient from sleep. This diurnal variation also corresponds to the greatest activity of the PNS system. The mechanism by which coronary arterial spasm occurs remains unknown, but this continues to be an exciting area of investigation.

INTERACTION WITH OTHER REGULATORY SYSTEMS

The ANS is integrally related to several endocrine systems that ultimately sum to control blood pressure and regulate homeostasis. These include the renin–angiotensin system, antidiuretic hormone, glucocorticoids, and insulin.

Antidiuretic hormone, or vasopressin, is formed in the hypothalamus and released from nerve endings in the posterior pituitary gland. It causes vasoconstriction and increased reabsorption of water in the distal collecting ducts of the kidney. It therefore affects not only central blood volume but also plasma osmolality. The primary regulator of antidiuretic hormone release is plasma osmolality; however, several other stimuli may outweigh this control in stressful situations.[123] Release is also triggered by decreased central blood volume *via* low-pressure atrial receptors and hypotension *via* the carotid baroreceptors. Stress, pain, hypoxia, anesthesia, and surgery also stimulate release of antidiuretic hormone. Infusion of catecholamines may alter its release, but these effects appear to be mediated by the carotid baroreceptors. ANS drugs that induce hypotension or decreased cardiac filling may induce release of antidiuretic hormone and thus affect plasma osmolality.

Both α and β receptors have been found in the endocrine pancreas and modulate insulin release (see Table 12-5). β stimulation increases insulin release, whereas α stimulation decreases it. The overall importance of this interaction is not entirely clear, but decreased tolerance to glucose and potassium has been noted in subjects taking β-blocking drugs.[124,125]

The renin–angiotensin system is a complex endocrine system that modulates both blood pressure and water–electrolyte homeostasis (Fig. 12-18). Renin is a proteolytic enzyme contained within the cells of the juxtaglomerular apparatus of the renal cortex. When released, it acts on plasma angiotensinogen to form angiotensin I. Angiotensin I is then converted to angiotensin II by converting enzyme in the lung. Angiotensin II is a powerful direct arterial vasoconstrictor. It also acts on the adrenal cortex to release aldosterone and on the adrenal medulla to release EPI. In addition to its direct effects on vascular smooth muscle, angiotensin II augments NE release *via* presynaptic receptors, thus enhancing peripheral SNS tone. A group of drugs called angiotensin-converting enzyme inhibitors act by interfering with the formation or function of angiotensin II. These drugs have been found useful in the treatment of essential and renovascular hypertension and of congestive heart failure. Captopril, enalapril, and lisinopril inhibit the action of converting enzyme, thus preventing the conversion of angiotensin I to angiotensin II.[124–131] They have supplanted diuretics and β blockers as first-line agents in the treatment of hypertension. Saralasin is a direct angiotensin II receptor antagonist that is useful as an antihypertensive drug but is not in common use.

Renin is released in response to hyponatremia, decreased

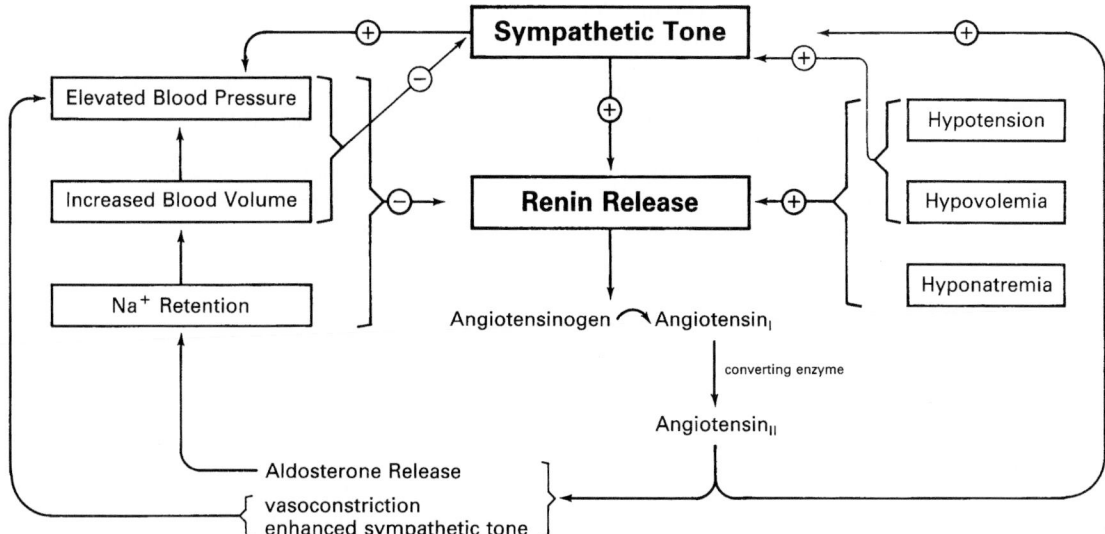

Figure 12-18. The interactions of the renin–angiotensin and SNS in regulating homeostasis are shown schematically along with the physiologic variables that modulate their function. Arrows with a plus sign (+) represent stimulation, and those with a minus sign (−) represent inhibition.

renal perfusion pressure, and ANS stimulation *via* β receptors on juxtaglomerular cells. Changes in sympathetic tone may thus alter renin release and affect homeostasis in a variety of ways. The mechanism of action of some antihypertensive agents is thought to involve alterations in activity of the renin–angiotensin system in parallel with the ANS.

The ANS is also intimately related to adrenocortical function. As outlined earlier, glucocorticoid release modulates phenylethanolamine-*N*-methyltransferase formation, and hence synthesis of EPI. Glucocorticoids are also important in regulating the response of peripheral tissues to changes in SNS tone. Thus, the ANS is intimately related to other homeostatic mechanisms.

CLINICAL AUTONOMIC NERVOUS SYSTEM PHARMACOLOGY

The clinical application of ANS pharmacology is based on knowledge of ANS anatomy, physiology, and molecular pharmacology. Drugs that modify ANS activity can be classified by their site of action, by their mechanism of action, or by the pathology for which they are most commonly used. Antihypertensive drugs are an example of the third category.

Site of Action

ANS drugs may be broadly categorized as working on the CNS or at peripheral nerve sites. This classification is a matter of degree because considerable functional overlap occurs. An example of classification by site relates to the ganglionic agonists or blocking agents. ANS drugs can be further categorized as those that act at the prejunctional membrane and those acting postjunctionally. They can then be more specifically classified by the predominant receptor or receptors on which they act.

Mode of Action

ANS drugs may be broadly classified by mode of action according to their mimetic or lytic actions. This may also be termed *agonist* or *antagonist*. Sympathomimetics, such as ephedrine, mimic SNS sympathetic activity by stimulation of adrenergic receptor sites both directly and indirectly. Sympatholytic drugs cause dissolution of SNS activity at these same receptor sites. β-Receptor blockers are examples of sympatholytic drugs.

The terms *parasympathomimetic* and *parasympatholytic* are self-explanatory and may be further divided by their site of action on the muscarinic or nicotinic receptors.

Several modes of ANS drug action become evident when one follows the cascade of neurotransmission. The mode is related to site. Drugs that act on prejunctional membranes may therefore (1) interfere with transmitter synthesis (α-methyl paratyrosine), (2) interfere with transmitter storage (reserpine), (3) interfere with transmitter release (clonidine), (4) stimulate transmitter release (ephedrine), or (5) interfere with reuptake of transmitter (cocaine). Drugs may also (6) modify metabolism of the neurotransmitter in the synaptic cleft (anticholinesterase). Drugs acting at postjunctional sites may (7) directly stimulate postjunctional receptors and (8) interfere with transmitter agonist at the postjunctional receptor.

The ultimate response of an effector organ to an agonist or antagonist depends on (1) the drug, (2) its plasma concentration, (3) the number of receptors in the effector organ, (4) binding by the receptor, (5) the concurrent activities of other drugs and hormones, (6) the cellular metabolic status, and (7) reflex adjustments by the organism. This is the source of conflicting results for drugs used in differing clinical circumstances.

Ganglionic Drugs

SNS and PNS ganglia are pharmacologically similar in that transmission through these ANS ganglia is effected by ACh (see Fig. 12-3). Most ganglionic agonists and antagonists are not selective and affect SNS and PNS ganglia equally.[132] This nonselective property creates many undesirable and unpredictable side-effects, thereby limiting the clinical usefulness of this category of drug.

Agonists

There are essentially no clinically useful ganglionic agonists. Nicotine is the prototypical ganglionic agonist. In low doses, it stimulates ANS ganglia and the neuromuscular junction of striated muscle. High doses produce ganglionic and neuromuscular blockade. Low-dose stimulation and high-dose blockade are referred to as nicotinic effects in describing any drug with similar effects. Most ganglionic agonists and antagonists produce their effects through their nicotinic effects. The protean side-effects of nicotinic stimulation render it useful only as an investigative tool.

Despite its lack of clinical usefulness, nicotine is widely used in the form of tobacco. The novice tobacco user can often describe the overlap of SNS and PNS side-effects of nicotinic stimulation, which appear as nausea and vomiting, tachycardia, bradycardia, diarrhea, and sometimes fainting as a result of high-dose ganglionic blockade.[6]

Antagonists

Drugs that interfere with neurotransmission at ANS ganglia are known as ganglionic blocking agents. Nicotine, in high doses, is the prototypical ganglionic blocking agent also; however, early stimulatory nicotinic activity can be blocked at the ganglia and muscle end plates with other ganglionic blockers and muscle relaxants, respectively, without blocking muscarinic effects.[133] Ganglionic blockers produce their nicotinic effects by competing, mimicking, or interfering with ACh metabolism. Hexamethonium, trimethaphan, and pentolinium produce a selective nondepolarizing blockade of neurotransmission at ANS ganglia without producing nicotinic neuromuscular blockade. They compete with ACh in the ganglia without stimulating the receptors. Decamethonium, a depolarizing muscle relaxant, selectively produces neuromuscular blockade in a manner similar to that of nicotine, but possesses no ganglionic effect.[6] The depolarization produced is initially associated with increased excitability, but depolarization persists. The neuron, therefore, cannot be excited, and block exists. d-Tubocurare (dTC), however, produces a competitive nondepolarizing block of both motor end plates and ANS ganglia. The action of motor paralysis predominates, but the concomitant ganglionic blockade at higher doses explains part of the hypotensive effect often seen with the use of dTC for muscle relaxation. Histamine release is the major hypotensive factor that is common to dTC and other ganglionic blockers. Anticholinesterase drugs may produce nicotinic-type ganglionic blockade by competition with ACh as well as by persistent depolarization *via* accumulated ACh.

The overall effects of ganglionic blockers on particular organ systems depend on whether the ANS activity of the system is predominantly sympathetic or parasympathetic (see Table 12-1). The overall effect on peripheral vessels is vasodilation due to release from SNS ganglionic constrictor control. The effect on the gastrointestinal tract may produce ileus. Although these drugs have a paraganglionic effect, blockade of the SNS ganglia and vascular dilation are the properties for which they were first used. They were initially used to treat chronic hypertension, but their lack of selectivity and global side-effects curtailed their popularity. The introduction of drugs that produce vasodilation directly or by action on the SNS vasomotor center has made the ganglionic blockers obsolete.

Trimethaphan is the only ganglionic blocker available in the United States. Trimethaphan produces blockade by competition with ACh for receptors, thus stabilizing the postsynaptic membrane. However, side-effects and rapid onset tachyphylaxis have markedly reduced its use in anesthesia.[134] The patient's pupils become fixed and dilated during administration, which obscures eye signs, an important consideration for neurosurgery. In this regard, it is distinctly inferior to nitroprusside. The major advantage of trimethaphan is its short duration of action, which is the result of pseudocholinesterase hydrolysis.

Pentolinium is a ganglionic blocking drug available in the United Kingdom.[135] Its mechanisms of action are similar to those of trimethaphan, but it is devoid of muscle-relaxant properties. The main disadvantage of pentolinium is its relative lack of controllability compared with trimethaphan or nitroprusside. Pupillary dilation, as with trimethaphan, occurs. Hypotension and vasomotor instability may outlast the procedure.

Cholinergic Drugs

Cholinergic drugs may be classified by the following outline, which follows physiologic response and site of action.

I. Cholinergic drugs: agonists[6]
  A. Nicotinic
    1. ANS ganglionic transmission
    2. Neuromuscular transmission
  B. Muscarinic
    1. Direct-acting
    2. Indirect-acting
II. Cholinolytic agents: antagonists
  A. Nicotinic
    1. ANS ganglionic transmission
    2. Neuromuscular transmission
  B. Muscarinic

Muscarinic Agonists

The cholinomimetic muscarinic drugs act at sites in the body where ACh is the neurotransmitter of the nerve impulse. These drugs may be divided into three groups, the first two of which are direct muscarinic agonists.[136,137] The third group acts indirectly. These groups are choline esters (ACh, methacholine, carbamylcholine, bethanechol), alkaloids (pilocarpine, muscarine, arecoline), and anticholinesterases (physostigmine, neostigmine, pyridostigmine, edrophonium, echothiophate).

Direct Cholinomimetics

ACh has virtually no therapeutic applications because of its diffuse action and rapid hydrolysis by cholinesterase (see Fig. 12-6).[136] One may encounter the use of topical ACh (1%) drops during cataract extraction when a rapid miosis is desired. Systemic effects are not usually seen because of the rapidity of ACh hydrolysis.

Other choline esters have been synthesized, mostly derivatives of ACh, which possess more selective muscarinic activity than ACh. They differ from ACh in being more resistant to inactivation by cholinesterase and thus having a more prolonged and useful action. They also differ from ACh in their relative muscarinic and nicotinic activities.[138] The best studied of these drugs are methacholine, bethanechol, and carbamylcholine.[6] The chemical structures of ACh and these choline esters are shown in Figure 12-19. Their pharmacologic actions are compared with those of ACh in Table 12-9. These are not important drugs in anesthesiology, but they deserve discussion because anesthesiologists may encounter patients who are receiving them, and they may be useful in the postoperative period to alleviate cardiac tachydysrhythmias, urinary retention, and ileus.[139]

ACh is a quaternary ammonium compound that interacts with postsynaptic receptors, causing conformational membrane changes. This results in increased permeability to small ions and, thus, depolarization. All the receptors translate the reversible binding of ACh into openings of discrete channels in excitable membranes, allowing Na^+ and K^+ ions to flow along their electrochemical gradients. Structure–activity relationships point to the presence of two important binding sites on the receptor—an esteratic site that binds the ester end of the molecule and an ionic site that binds the quaternary amine portion (see Fig. 12-6). Subtle changes in the structure of the compound can markedly alter the responses among different tissue groups. The degree of muscarinic activity falls if the acetyl group is replaced, but this confers a resistance to enzymatic hydrolysis. Carbamylcholine is synthesized by replacing the acetyl group with carbamyl (Fig. 12-19). It possesses both muscarinic and nicotinic actions but is virtually resistant to esterase hydrolysis (Table 12-9). Bethanechol is also resistant to hydrolysis but possesses mainly muscarinic activity. β-Methyl substitution produces methacholine, which is less resistant to hydrolysis but is primarily a muscarinic agonist.

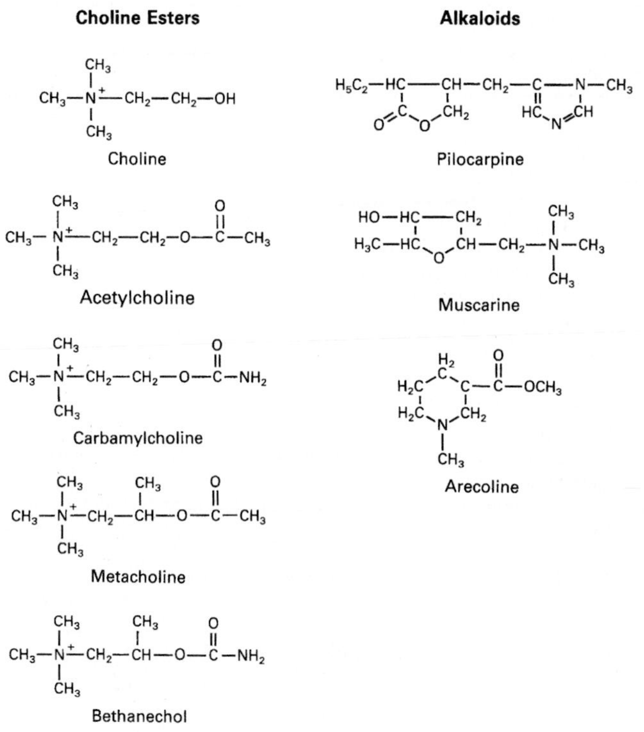

Choline Esters

CH₃
|
CH₃—N⁺—CH₂—CH₂—OH
|
CH₃
Choline

CH₃   O
| ‖
CH₃—N⁺—CH₂—CH₂—O—C—CH₃
|
CH₃
Acetylcholine

CH₃   O
| ‖
CH₃—N⁺—CH₂—CH₂—O—C—NH₂
|
CH₃
Carbamylcholine

CH₃   CH₃   O
| | ‖
CH₃—N⁺—CH₂—CH—O—C—CH₃
|
CH₃
Metacholine

CH₃   CH₃   O
| | ‖
CH₃—N⁺—CH₂—CH—O—C—NH₂
|
CH₃
Bethanechol

Alkaloids

H₅C₂—HC——CH—CH₂—C—N—CH₃
          | ‖
        O=C O—CH₂   HC   CH
                        N
Pilocarpine

HO—HC——CH₂   CH₃
   | | |
H₃C—HC O CH—CH₂—N—CH₃
                   |
                   CH₃
Muscarine

       H₂   O
H₂C——C——C—OCH₃
   | ‖
H₂C C   CH₂
     N
     |
     CH₃
Arecoline

Figure 12-19. Chemical structures of direct-acting cholinomimetic esters and alkaloids.

Methacholine is destroyed by cholinesterase less rapidly than ACh and is potentiated by anticholinesterase drugs. Its muscarinic effects are predominantly cardiovascular. Methacholine slows the heart and dilates peripheral blood vessels. It is used to terminate supraventricular tachydysrhythmias, especially paroxysmal tachycardia, when other measures have failed. It also increases intestinal tone. Methacholine should not be given to patients with asthma. Hypertensive patients may also develop marked hypotension. Side-effects are those of PNS stimulation such as nausea, vomiting, and flushed sweating. Overdose is treated with atropine.

Bethanechol has predominantly muscarinic actions that are relatively selective for the gastrointestinal and urinary tracts. In usual doses it does not slow the heart or lower the blood pressure, as does methacholine. Bethanecol is of value in treating postoperative abdominal distention (nonobstructive paralytic ileus), gastric atony following bilateral vagotomy, congenital megacolon, nonobstructive urinary retention, and some cases of neurogenic bladder. It is not a parenteral drug. Precautions are as for methacholine.

The use of carbamylcholine has largely been supplanted by better drugs because of its dual nicotinic and muscarinic effects. It is a long-acting agent because it is completely resistant to hydrolysis. Atropine will block its muscarinic actions but unmask its nicotinic effects. In this case, blood pressure will rise as sympathetic ganglia are stimulated and catecholamines released. Carbamylcholine is currently limited to use as topical ophthalmologic drops to produce miosis and for the treatment of wide-angle glaucoma.[136]

Direct-acting cholinomimetic alkaloids include muscarine, pilocarpine, and arecoline. They act at the same sites as ACh, and their effects are similar to those of ACh as described in Table 12-9. There are no uses for these drugs in anesthesiology.

Table 12-9. COMPARATIVE MUSCARINIC ACTIONS OF DIRECT CHOLINOMIMETIC AGENTS

	Systemic				
	Acetylcholine	*Methacholine*	*Carbamylcholine*	*Bethanechol*	*Pilocarpine*
Esterase Hydrolysis	+++	+	0	0	0
Eye (Topical)					
Iris	++	++	+++	+++	+++
Ciliary	++	++	+++	+++	++
Heart					
Rate	– – –	– – –	–	–	?
Contractility	–	–	–	–	
Conduction	– –	– – –	–	–	
Smooth Muscle					
Vascular	– –	– – –	–	–	– –
Bronchial	++	++	+	+	++
Gastrointestinal motility	++	++	+++	+++	++
Gastrointestinal sphincters	– –	–	– – –	– – –	++
Biliary	++	++	+++	+++	++
Bladder					
Detrusor	++	++	+++	+++	++
Sphincter	– –	–	– – –	– – –	– –
Exocrine Glands					
Respiratory	+++	++	+++	++	++++
Salivary	++	++	++	++	+++++
Pharyngeal	++	++	++	++	++++
Lacrimal	++	++	++	++	++++
Sweat	++	++	++	++	+++++
Gastrointestinal acid and secretions	++	++	++	++	++++
Nicotinic Actions	+++	+	+++	–	+++

+ = stimulation; – = inhibition.

Table 12-10. CHOLINESTERASE INHIBITORS

Drug	Trade Name	Route	Duration	Indications
Reversible				
Physostigmine	Eserine	Topical	6–12 hr	Glaucoma
Pyridostigmine	Mestinon Regonol	Oral, iv, im	4 hr	Myasthenia gravis Reversal of neuromuscular blockade
Neostigmine	Prostigmin	Oral, iv	4–6 hr	Myasthenia gravis Reversal of neuromuscular blockade
Edrophonium	Tensilon Enlon	iv	1–2 hr	Reversal of neuromuscular blockade Diagnosis of myasthenia gravis
Demecarium	Humorsol	Topical	3–5 days	Glaucoma
Ambenonium	Mytelase	Oral	4 hr	Myasthenia gravis
Nonreversible				
Echothiophate	Phospholine	Topical	3–14 days	Glaucoma
Isofluorophate		Topical	3–7 days	Glaucoma research
Malathion		Topical		Insecticide—relatively safe for mammals because of rapid hepatic metabolism
Parathion		Topical		Insecticide—highly toxic to higher animals; frequent accidental poisoning
Sarin (GB)	Nerve gas	Topical and gas		
Tabun	Nerve gas	Topical and gas		No indications for the use of nerve gas
Soman	Nerve gas	Topical and gas		

Note: Atropine should always be given prior to or with iv cholinesterase inhibitors and when only nicotinic effects are desired; muscarinic effects are dangerous when excessive.

Pilocarpine is the only drug of this group used therapeutically in the United States. Its sole use is for the treatment of glaucoma, for which it is the standard. It is used as a topical miotic drug in ophthalmologic practice to reduce intraocular pressure in glaucoma. Pilocarpine has primary muscarinic effects with minimal nicotinic effects unless given systemically, in which case hypertension and tachycardia may result. Toxicity with topical application is rare.

The benefits of muscarinic agonists must be carefully considered when one or more of their actions are likely to be dangerous (see Table 12-9). They are rarely given intravenously because of side-effects. Common side-effects are those of intense PNS stimulation, which include gastrointestinal cramping, hypotension, diaphoresis, salivation, diarrhea, and bladder pain.[6] Muscarinic agonists are particularly dangerous in patients with myasthenia gravis (who are receiving anticholinesterases), bulbar palsy, cardiac disease, asthma, peptic ulcer, progressive muscular atrophy, or mechanical intestinal obstruction or urinary retention.[140]

Indirect Cholinomimetics

The indirect-acting cholinomimetic drugs are of greater importance to the anesthesiologist than are the direct-acting drugs. These drugs produce cholinomimetic effects indirectly as a result of inhibition or inactivation of the enzyme acetylcholinesterase, which normally destroys ACh by hydrolysis. They are referred to as cholinesterase inhibitors or anticholinesterases. Table 12-10 lists therapeutic cholinesterase inhibitors and their major indications. Most of these drugs inhibit both acetylcholinesterase and pseudocholinesterase. Inhibition of acetylcholinesterase permits the accumulation of ACh transmitter in the synapse, resulting in intense PNS activity similar to that of the direct cholinomimetic agents. The action of ACh is therefore potentiated and prolonged. Their effects can be predicted from a knowledge of ANS pharmacology previously presented. Some of the acetylcholinesterase drugs (*e.g.*, edrophonium) may also stimulate cholinergic receptors by direct action.[141] The accumulation of ACh by the anticholinesterases potentially can produce all of the following: (1) stimulation of muscarinic receptors at ANS effect organs, (2) stimulation followed by depression of all ANS ganglia and skeletal muscle (nicotinic), and (3) stimulation with later depression of cholinergic receptor sites in the

CNS. All of these effects may be seen with lethal doses of anticholinesterase drugs, but therapeutic doses produce only the first two.

Of the anticholinesterase drugs, actions of therapeutic significance to the anesthesiologist concern the eye, the intestine, and the neuromuscular junction. The effects of anticholinesterases are useful in the treatment of myasthenia gravis, glaucoma, and atony of the gastrointestinal and urinary tracts. Anticholinesterase drugs are used routinely in anesthesia to reverse nondepolarizing neuromuscular block.

The most prominent pharmacologic effects of the anticholinesterase drugs are muscarinic. Their most useful actions are their nicotinic effects.[6,26] Muscarinic activity is evoked by lower concentrations of ACh than are necessary to produce the desired nicotinic effect. For example, the anticholinesterase neostigmine reverses neuromuscular blockade by increasing ACh concentration at the muscle end plate, a nicotinic receptor. Nicotinic reversal of neuromuscular blockade can usually be produced safely only when the patient has been protected by atropine or other muscarinic blockers. This prevents the untoward muscarinic effects of bradycardia, hypotension, bronchospasm, or intestinal spasm. Conversely, neuromuscular paralysis may be produced or increased if excessive anticholinesterase is used. Excess accumulation of ACh at the motor end plates produces a depolarizing block similar to that produced by succinylcholine or nicotine.

Reversal of neuromuscular blockade in patients who have had bowel anastomosis was at one time a major controversy. Some thought that the muscarinic effects of anticholinesterase drugs (hypermotility) increased the risk of anastomotic leakage,[142,143] whereas others found no association between their use and subsequent breakdown.[144,145] National experience has favored the latter opinion.

The interactions between ACh and the anticholinesterases are complex.[146] Anticholinesterase drugs inhibit hydrolysis of ACh by binding to either or both the anionic or esteratic sites of acetylcholinesterase, forming inhibitor–enzyme complexes that are more stable than ACh–enzyme complexes. These complexes prevent proper stereotactic access of ACh to the active enzyme sites; thus, hydrolysis is delayed, and ACh accumulates.

Clinically, anticholinesterase drugs may be divided into two types: the reversible and nonreversible cholinesterase inhibitors.[25,137] Reversible cholinesterase inhibitors delay the hydrolysis of ACh from 1 to 8 hours. Nonreversible drugs are so named because their inhibitory effects may last from days to weeks. The differences in duration of various anticholinesterases apparently depend on whether they inhibit the anionic or esteratic site of acetylcholinesterase.[141] Therefore, the anticholinesterase drugs have also been pharmacologically subdivided. Drugs that inhibit the anionic site are called prosthetic, competitive inhibitors. Their action is due to competition between the anticholinesterase and ACh for the anionic site. These drugs tend to be short-acting. Edrophonium is an example of this type. Drugs that inhibit the esteratic site are called acid-transferring inhibitors. These drugs include the longer-acting neostigmine, pyridostigmine, and physostigmine. Thus, the differences in the mechanism of inhibition produced by prosthetic inhibitors (edrophonium) and acid-transferring inhibitors (neostigmine) account for the longer duration of action associated with the latter agents.

Most of the reversible cholinesterase inhibitors are quaternary ammonium compounds and do not cross the blood–brain barrier. Physostigmine is a tertiary amine that readily passes into the CNS (Fig. 12-20). It produces central muscarinic stimulation, and thus is not used to reverse neuromuscular blockade but can be used to treat atropine poisoning. Conversely, atropine is used to treat physostigmine poisoning. Physostigmine has also been found to be a specific antidote in the treatment of postoperative delirium (see Central Anticholinergic Syndrome).[6,26]

The irreversible cholinesterase inhibitors are mostly organophosphate compounds. These are also considered acid-transferring inhibitors, which form a phosphorylated enzyme resistant to attack by water. The phosphorylated enzyme cannot hydrolyze ACh to any measurable degree. In addition, the organophosphate compounds are highly lipid-soluble; they readily pass into the CNS and are rapidly absorbed through the skin. They are used as the active ingredient in potent insecticides and the chemical warfare agents known as nerve gases. Table 12-10 lists some of these agents. The only therapeutic drug of this group is echothiophate, which is available in the form of topical drops for the treatment of glaucoma. Its primary advantage is its prolonged duration of action. Topical absorption is variable but considerable. Echothiophate can remain effective for 2 or 3 weeks following cessation of therapy.[147] A history of use of echothiophate is important in avoiding prolonged action of succinylcholine, which requires pseudocholinesterase for its hydrolysis.

Organophosphate poisoning manifests all the signs and symptoms of excess ACh.[148] The antidote cartridges dispensed to troops to counter the effects of anticholinesterase nerve gases contain only atropine, which would effectively counter the muscarinic effects of the gas; however, atropine does little to counter the high-dose nicotinic muscle paralysis or the central ventilation depression that contributes to death from nerve gases. Treatment requires high doses of atropine, 35–70 mg·kg⁻¹ iv every 3–10 minutes until muscarinic symptoms abate. Lower doses at less frequent intervals may be required for several days. Central ventilatory depression and nicotinic paralysis or weakness require respiratory support and specific therapy of the cholinesterase lesion. Pralidoxime has been reported to reactivate cholinesterase activity by hydrolysis of the phosphate enzyme complex. It is particularly effective with parathion poisoning and is the only cholinesterase reactivator available in the United States.[137]

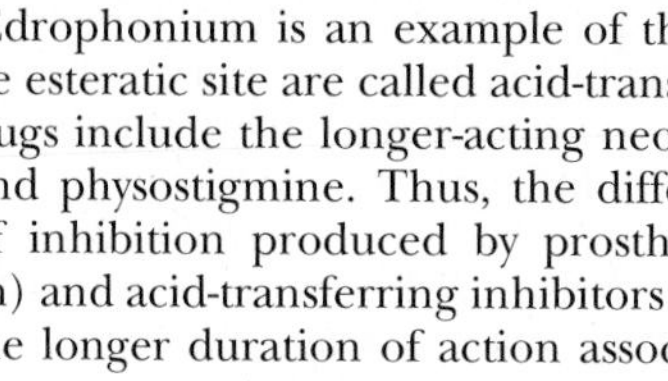

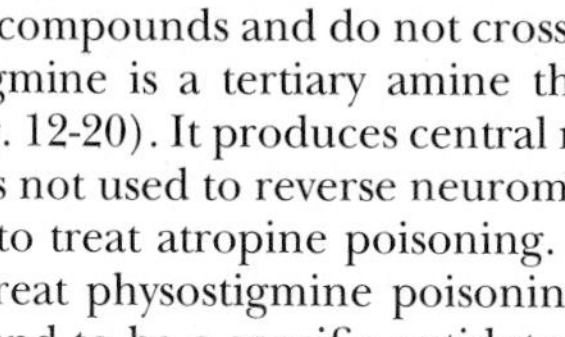

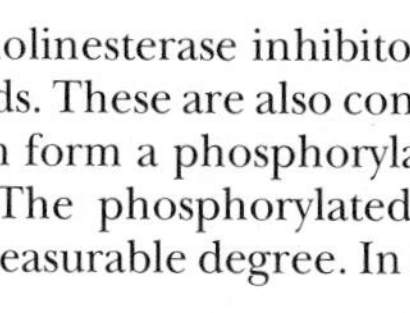

Muscarinic Antagonists

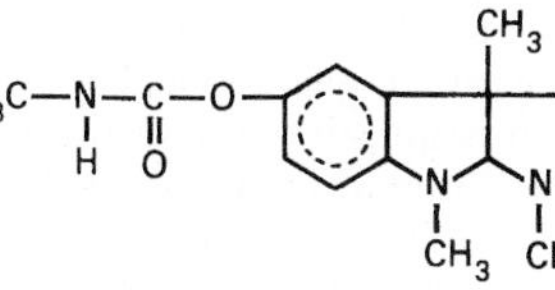

Muscarinic antagonist refers to a specific drug action for which the term anticholinergic is widely used. Any drug that interferes with the action of ACh as a transmitter can be considered an anticholinergic agent. The term anticholinergic refers to a broader classification that would include the nicotinic antagonists.

Atropinic Drugs

Atropine, scopolamine, and glycopyrrolate are the most commonly used muscarinic antagonists used in anesthesia (Fig. 12-21). The use of antimuscarinic drugs for premedication is outlined in Chapter 21.

The actions of these drugs include inhibition of salivary, bronchial, pancreatic, and gastrointestinal secretions to antagonize the muscarinic side-effects of anticholinesterases during reversal of muscle relaxants. Atropine is useful in increasing CO with sinus bradycardia due to vagal stimulation if hypoxia is ruled out. It has many uses outside of anesthesia for the treatment of renal colic, gastrointestinal spasm, gastric secretion, and asthma. Historically, atropine was introduced to anesthesia practice to prevent excessive secretions during ether anesthesia and to prevent vagal bradycardia during the administration of chloroform.[149] Atropine and scopolamine also possess antiemetic action. Atropine, however, reduces the opening pressure of the lower esophageal sphincter, which theoretically increases the risk of passive regurgitation.[150] Atropinic drugs also produce dilation of the pupil (mydriasis) and paralysis of accommodation (cycloplegia).

Antimuscarinic agents do not inhibit transmission equally, and there are marked variations in sensitivity at different muscarinic sites owing to differences in penetration and affinities of the various receptors.[151] Differences in relative potency between the different antimuscarinics are outlined in Table 12-11. For example, glycopyrrolate produces less tachycardia than atropine and is a more potent antisialogogue.

The antimuscarinic effects of the atropinic drugs are the result of competitive inhibition of ACh at the receptors of or-

Figure 12-20. Structural formulas of clinically useful reversible anticholinesterase drugs. Physostigmine is a tertiary amine and crosses the blood–brain barrier. It is useful in treating the central anticholinergic syndrome.

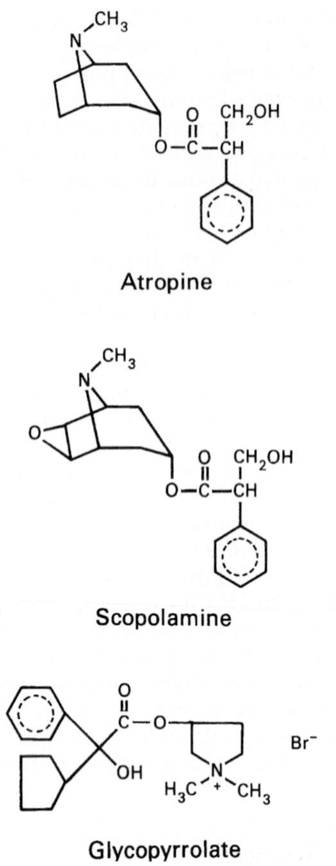

Figure 12-21. Structural formulas of the clinically useful antimuscarinic drugs.

gans innervated by cholinergic postganglionic nerves. The antagonism can be overcome by sufficient concentrations of cholinomimetic drugs or anticholinesterases that increase ACh levels at the receptor site. This explains most of the therapeutic actions of atropinic drugs; however, they are neither purely antimuscarinic nor purely antagonist.[6]

The belladonna alkaloids (atropine and scopolamine) also block ACh transmission to sweat glands, which, although they are cholinergic, are innervated by the SNS. Antimuscarinic agents produce antinicotinic actions at higher doses and result in important actions on CNS transmission that are pharmacologically similar to the postganglionic cholinergic function.[152]

Atropine and scopolamine are tertiary amines (Fig. 12-21) and easily penetrate the blood–brain barrier and placenta. Glycopyrrolate is a quaternary amine which, like the reversible anticholinesterase drugs, does not easily penetrate these barriers. Glycopyrrolate, a synthetic antimuscarinic, has gained popularity because it avoids the central effects of the other two drugs.

Atropine and scopolamine have notable CNS effects that are dissimilar. Scopolamine differs from atropine mainly in its central depressant effects, which produce sedation, amnesia, and euphoria. Such properties are widely used for premedication for cardiac patients in combination with morphine and a major tranquilizer. Atropine, as a premedicant, has slight effects on the CNS, including mild stimulation. Higher doses such as those given for reversal of muscle relaxants (1–2 mg) may produce restlessness, disorientation, hallucinations, and delirium (see Central Anticholinergic Syndrome). Excessive stimulation may be followed by depression and paralysis of respiration. Occasionally, scopolamine in low doses may cause restlessness and delirium. This syndrome is more frequently seen in the elderly and patients experiencing pain, *e.g.,* in obstetric patients.

Atropine and scopolamine are noted to produce a paradoxical bradycardia when given in low doses. Scopolamine (0.1–0.2 mg) usually causes more slowing than atropine but also produces less cardiac acceleration at higher doses. The usual intramuscular premedicant doses of scopolamine cause either a decrease or no change in HR. The paradoxical bradycardia was once thought to be caused by an early central inhibition of the medullary cardioinhibitory center. However, this phenomenon occurs in animals that have had total vagotomy. Atropine may also produce sympathomimetic effects by blocking presynaptic muscarinic receptors found on adrenergic nerve terminals.[12,37] ACh stimulation of these receptors inhibits NE release, and blockade by atropine releases this inhibition (see Cholinergic Receptors: Muscarinic).

Atropinic drugs are widely used in ophthalmology as mydriatics and cycloplegics. Atropine is contraindicated in patients with narrow-angle glaucoma. Pupillary dilation thickens the peripheral part of the iris, which narrows the iridocorneal angle. Drainage of aqueous humor is impaired, and intraocular pressure increases. Doses of atropine used for premedication have little effect in this regard, whereas equal doses of scopolamine cause mydriasis. Prudence would dictate avoidance of either agent in patients with narrow-angle glaucoma. The need for antimuscarinic premedication is questionable in this situation.[135]

Atropine is best avoided where tachycardia would be harmful, as may occur in thyrotoxicosis, pheochromocytoma, or obstructive coronary artery disease. Theoretically, antimuscarinic drugs should benefit coronary spasm, but the benefit may be offset by the oxygen cost of the ensuing tachycardia. Atropine should be avoided in hyperpyrexial patients because it inhibits sweating.

Central Anticholinergic Syndrome

The belladonna alkaloids have long been known to produce undesirable side-effects ranging from stupor (scopolamine) to delirium (atropine). This syndrome has otherwise been called postoperative delirium and atropine toxicity. The central anticholinergic syndrome appears to involve the muscarinic receptor.[6] Biochemical studies have demonstrated abundant muscarinic ACh receptors in the brain that can be affected by any drug possessing antimuscarinic activity and capable of crossing

Table 12-11. COMPARISON OF ANTIMUSCARINIC DRUGS

	Duration iv	Duration im	CNS	GI Tone	Gastric Acid	Airway Secretions*	Heart Rate
Atropine	15–30 min	2–4 hr	++	– –	–	–	+++‡
Scopolamine	30–60 min	4–6 hr	+++†	–	–	– – – –	–0‡
Glycopyrrolate	2–4 hr	6–8 hr	0	– – –	– – –	– – –	+0

* Secretions may be reduced by inspissation.
† CNS effect often manifest as sedation before stimulation.
‡ May decelerate initially.

Table 12-12. ANTIMUSCARINIC COMPOUNDS ASSOCIATED WITH CENTRAL ANTICHOLINERGIC SYNDROME

Belladonna Alkaloids
Atropine sulfate
Scopolamine hydrobromide

Synthetic and Natural Tertiary Amine Compounds
Dicyclomine (Bentyl)—antispasmodic with local anesthetic activity
Thiphenamil (Trocinate)—antispasmodic with local anesthetic activity
Procaine
Cocaine
Cyclopentolate (Cyclogyl) mydriatic

Quaternary Derivatives of Belladonna Alkaloids
Methscopolamine bromide (Pamine)—antispasmodic
Homatropine methylbromide—sedative, antispasmodic
Homatropine hydrobromide—ophthalmic solution—mydriatic

Synthetic Quaternary Compounds
Methantheline bromide (Banthine)
Propantheline bromide (Pro-Banthine)

Antihistamines
Chlorpheniramine (Ornade)
Diphenhydramine (Benadryl)

Plants
Deadly nightshade (atropine)
Bittersweet
Potato leaves and sprouts
Jimson or loco weed
Coca plant (cocaine)

Over-the-Counter
Asthma-Dor—atropine-like
Compoz—scopolamine sedation
Sleep Eze—scopolamine sedation
Sominex—scopolamine sedation

Antiparkinson Drugs
Benztropine (Cogentin)
Trihexphenidyl (Artane)
Biperiden (Akineton)
Ethopropazine (Parsidol)
Procyclidine (Kemadrin)

Antipsychotic Drugs
Chlorpromazine (Thorazine)
Thioriazine (Mellaril)
Haloperidol (Haldol)
Droperidol (Inapsine)
Promethazine (Phenegran)

Tricyclic Antidepressants
Amitriptyline (Elavil)
Imipramine (Tofranil)
Desipramine (Norpramine, Pertofrane)

Synthetic Opioids
Meperidine
Methadone

Note: Trade names are given in parentheses.

the blood–brain barrier. Hundreds of drugs meet the criteria with which this syndrome has been associated. Table 12-12 lists some of those drugs.[6,152]

High doses of atropinic alkaloids rapidly produces dryness of the mouth, blurred vision with photophobia (mydriasis), hot and dry skin (flushed), and fever.[152] Mental symptoms range from sedation, stupor, and coma to anxiety, restlessness, disorientation, hallucinations, and delirium. Convulsions and ventilatory arrest may occur if lethal poisoning has occurred. Although an alarming reaction may occur, fatalities are rare. Intoxication is usually short-lived and followed by amnesia. These reactions can be controlled by the iv injection of physostigmine.[138] Physostigmine is an anticholinesterase that, by virtue of being a tertiary amine, readily passes into the CNS to counter antimuscarinic activity. It should be given slowly in 1-mg doses, not exceeding 3 mg, to avoid producing peripheral cholinergic activity. Neostigmine, pyridostigmine, and edrophonium are not effective because they cannot pass into the CNS. Likewise, atropine is an effective antidote for physostigmine overdose.[19] The duration of physostigmine action may be shorter than that of the offending antimuscarinic agent and require repeated injection if symptoms recur. Physostigmine appears safe when used within dose recommendations and when indications are established. Central disorientation alone does not establish a diagnosis.[151] Peripheral signs of antimuscarinic activity should be present in addition to a central anticholinergic syndrome.

Physostigmine has been reported to reverse the CNS effects of many of the drugs listed in Table 12-12, including antihistamines, tricyclic antidepressants, and tranquilizers. Reversal of the sedative effects of opioids and benzodiazepines has also been reported.[153,154] However, anticholinesterase agents potentiate cholinergic synaptic transmission and increase neuronal activity, even if no receptor antagonist is present. Thus, arousal

may not be a function independent of its cholinesterase activity, and claims that physostigmine is a nonspecific CNS stimulant may be unwarranted and could, in fact, be dangerous.[6] These phenomena require more study.

Adrenergic Drugs

Adrenergic Agonists

Until recently, sympathomimetics were the most common means of treating the hypotension associated with shock.[36] A vasopressor is a drug that is used to elevate arterial blood pressure above the existing level because the pressure is too low. However, elevation of arterial blood pressure alone has repeatedly been demonstrated to be an insufficient goal in the treatment of shock.[155,156] The goal, instead, is to re-establish blood flow to vital organs. Although blood pressure has been the historical gold standard for estimating perfusion, there is no correlation between blood pressure and flow (Fig. 12-22).[157] In physiologic as well as constructed systems, flow tends to be least when pressure is highest. Flow used in this context refers to cardiac output (CO).

Oxygen transport (DO_2) is the product of the arterial oxygen content (CA_2) and CO:

$$DO_2 = CA_2 \times CO$$

Therefore, there is a close correlation between oxygen transport and CO. Unfortunately, oxygen transport is not identical to cellular oxygen supply, which can be inadequate despite normal or elevated oxygen transport. Cellular oxygen supply can be inadequate because of maldistribution of blood flow to vital organs or from the inability of the cell to use oxygen.[157,158] Improving cellular oxygen utilization remains enigmatic, but

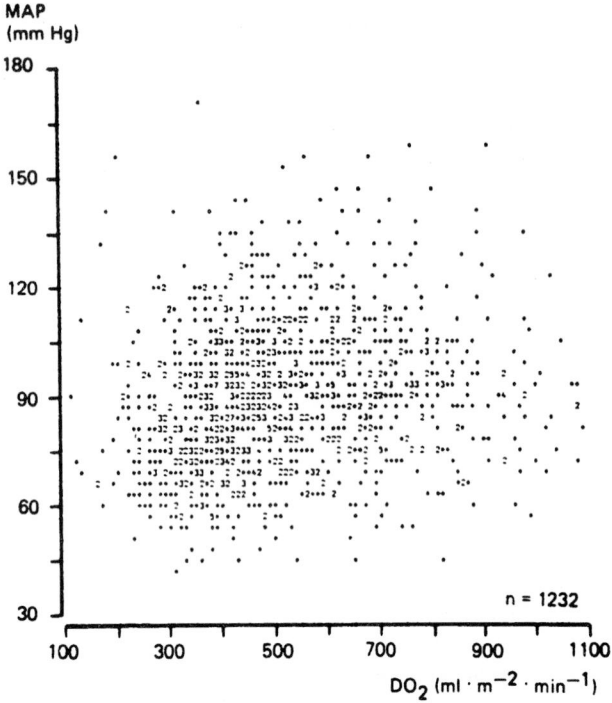

MAP
(mm Hg)

DO$_2$ (ml · m^{-2} · min^{-1})

n = 1232

Figure 12-22. Correlation between mean arterial pressure (MAP) and O$_2$ delivery (DO$_2$) during the perioperative period in patients undergoing aorta bifemoral bypass grafting. (Reprinted with permission from Reinhart K: Principles and Practice of Svo$_2$ Monitoring, pp 121–124. London, Intensive Care World, King and Worth, Publishers, vol 5, no 4, Dec 1988.)

the catecholamines can be of some assistance in the redistribution of flow.

The physiologic equation that expresses how flow (CO) is generated states that CO is the product of the HR and stroke volume (SV):

$$CO = HR \times SV$$

However, SV is determined by three factors: (1) the contractile or inotropic state of the myocardium; (2) preload, or end-diastolic myocardial fiber length; and (3) afterload, or resistance to ejection. The physiologic determinants of CO can therefore be expressed as

$$CO = HR \times (inotropism : preload : afterload)$$

Synchrony of AV contraction is an additional determinant when dysrhythmias develop. This equation is illustrated in Figure 12-23 to emphasize that the biologic mechanisms that produce and regulate flow are interdependent. Terms such as inotropism, preload, and afterload cannot be defined independently or isolated in the clinical setting. We can now measure, calculate, and manipulate each of the links in the chain of events that determine flow. Note that blood pressure is not among the determinants of flow. It is the product, not the cause. Most catecholamines affect one or more of these factors *via* the receptors and may cause changes in blood pressure by altering flow, vascular tone, or both. A measured blood pressure does not distinguish changes in flow, resistance, inotropism, or HR; therefore, blood pressure and oxygen transport do not correlate.

HEART RATE

Heart rate (HR) becomes an important support of CO when SV is decreased. A change in either HR or SV invariably causes an alteration of the other by reflex activity. Tachycardias can reduce SV by not allowing sufficient diastolic ventricular filling time. Coronary blood flow to the ventricles and especially the subendocardium, occurs primarily during diastole. The subepicardial muscle is perfused during systole as well as diastole. However, subendocardial blood flow is totally dependent upon diastolic perfusion time, diastolic pressure, and microcirculatory tone.[159]

Diastolic perfusion time becomes even more critical with ventricular hypertrophy. Increases in HR will not only shorten the percent diastolic perfusion time for the endocardium but also increase oxygen demand.[160] Increased HR, alone, has been shown to increase the severity of ischemia and the incidence of reperfusion arrhythmias. Animal studies have shown that myocardial blood flow and contractile function decrease with increased inotropic activity and tachycardia. This does not occur when increased inotropism is not accompanied by tachycardia.

Diastolic perfusion time has a curvilinear relationship with HR, increasing rapidly as rates fall below 75 beats/min (Fig. 12-24). Once HR goes above 90 beats/min in the adult, there is little further decrease in percent diastole. There is an exponential increase in percent diastole below rates of 70 beats/min.[159] Wide swings in percent diastolic time are of little consequence in the patient with normal coronary function, but can be critical in those with obstructive coronary artery disease.

Two factors actually determine the duration of systole: HR and electromechanical systole (QS$_2$). HR and QS$_2$ have an inverse relationship (Fig. 12-25).[159] Percent diastolic perfusion time is calculated as the cardiac cycle (R-R) minus QS$_2$. A decrease in HR and/or shortening in QS$_2$ will result in prolongation of the total diastolic period and *vice versa*. HR is the more important factor because small changes in the HR can produce significant changes in percent diastole as a result of the curvilinear relationship between HR and diastolic perfusion time. Changes in HR alone produce movement along that curve, whereas changes in QS$_2$ result in shifts of the curve. Dopamine

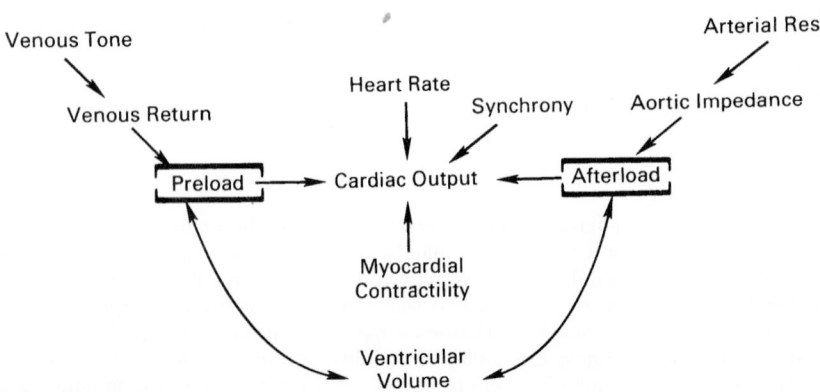

Figure 12-23. The four principal factors determining CO are demonstrated. Synchrony of AV-contraction is an additional factor becoming important with the development of cardiac dysrhythmias. (Reprinted with permission from Lawson NW, Wallfisch HK: Cardiovascular pharmacology: A new look at the "pressors." In Stoelting RK, Barash PG, Gallagher TJ (eds): Advances in Anesthesia, p 195, Chicago, Year Book Publishers, 1986.)

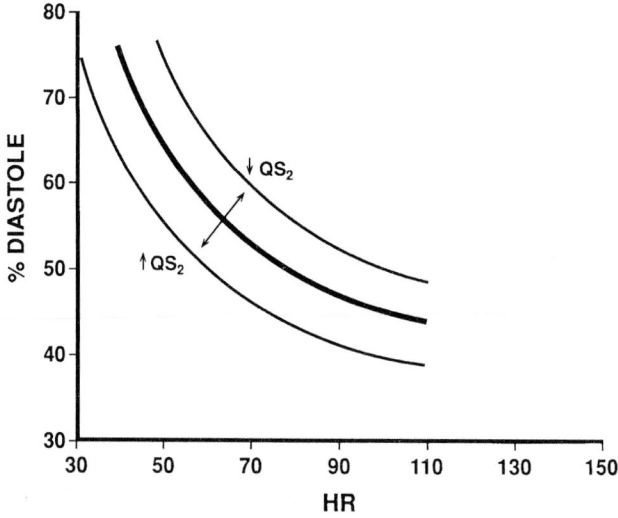

Figure 12-24. Small changes in HR produce large changes in percent diastole especially at low HRs due to the curvilinear relationship between rate and diastolic time. Shortening of electromechanical systole (QS_2) produces an upward shift of the curve. Shortening of QS_2 or a decrease in HR, or both, will increase percent diastolic perfusion time. Cardioactive drugs may affect diastolic perfusion time through either or both mechanisms.[168]

and dobutamine (DBT) affect diastolic perfusion time by altering HR and QS_2. DBT has been shown to increase percent diastole without significantly altering HR. The increase in diastolic perfusion time is due to a shortening of QS_2. Isoproterenol reduces percent diastole because it reduced QS_2 proportional to the increase in HR. Beta blockers, particularly atenolol, will significantly decrease HR and increase percent diastole because it has little effect on QS_2 in the usual clinical dose range. The beneficial effects of beta blockers on myocardial oxygen delivery and consumption can be related to a reduced HR alone, al-

though higher doses may reduce inotropism as well. Diastolic perfusion pressure may also increase with β blockade because of an unopposed relative increase in vascular tone. Lidocaine has no effect on either HR or QS_2.

PRELOAD

Preload is clinically synonymous with the volume of venous return to the heart, which establishes CO by the purported Frank–Starling mechanism. Preload has repeatedly been demonstrated to be of paramount importance in supporting cardiovascular function in the normal heart. It can be increased by adding volume to the circulation or by acute venous constriction. The catecholamines can be selected for their effect on preload by either increasing (α_1, α_2) or decreasing (β_2, DA_1, DA_2) venous tone.[64] Positive or negative preloading can be a major unrecognized benefit of some sympathomimetic agents. Although venoconstriction produces little increase in total vascular resistance (afterload), minimal venoconstriction is capable of producing large shifts of blood volume into the central circulation because the capacitance vessels contain 60–80% of the total blood volume, an effect that has largely been ignored. The central distributive effect of a catecholamine may be as important as its inotropic action in increasing the CO in the hypovolemic patient. Likewise, a central distribution of capacitance blood may be undesirable if the heart is failing, even though that agent may possess inotropic properties.

AFTERLOAD

Afterload is a measure of impedance to ventricular ejection and is the dominant factor in determining CO when inotropism is impaired. In the absence of outlet obstruction, the clinical correlate of afterload to the left ventricle is the systemic vascular resistance reflected by the mean arterial pressure. Afterload is the only factor of the four major determinants of CO that, if increased, will reduce flow. Ohm's law states that blood flow through any organ is directly related to the blood pressure gradient across that organ but is inversely proportional to the resistance (afterload).

INOTROPISM

Inotropism is defined as the force and velocity of ventricular contraction when preload and afterload are held constant. Vasoactive drugs can be described as having either a positive or negative inotropic effect. Inotropic agents, such as dopamine and DBT, represent therapeutic agents that altogether increase myocardial contractility. As yet, there are no clinically feasible means to directly measure inotropism at the bedside. We can define failure of inotropism better than we can define what it is. The myocardium permits CO to be regulated at any level below its inotropic limit.

Several direct indicators of cardiac inotropism appear useful in lieu of direct force velocity measurements. Pump function can be estimated clinically by work-pressure curves using the Frank–Starling mechanism. When inotropism is normal, CO is more dependent on extracardiac factors such as preload and afterload (Fig. 12-23).

LUSITROPISM

Lusitropism is a factor determining CO that is not depicted in Figure 12-23. Lusitropism describes abnormalities of myocardial relaxation, or diastole, as opposed to problems of inotropism. Some vasodilators such as nitroglycerin and some sympathomimetic "inodilators" are thought to improve cardiac function by promoting diastolic relaxation and hence ventricular filling (preloading) and coronary perfusion. Lusitropic dysfunction may play a larger role in chronic heart failure than hitherto

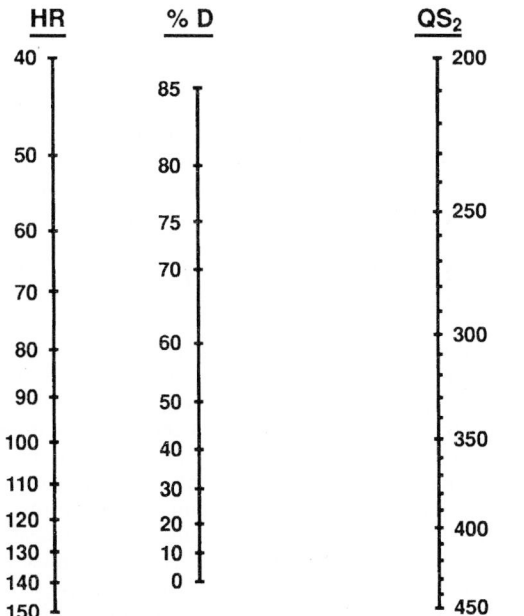

Figure 12-25. Nomogram for the relationship between electromechanical systole (QS_2), heart rate (HR), and percent diastole. The percent diastole can be obtained from QS_2 and HR.[168] (Reprinted from Boudoulas H, Rittgers SE, Lewis RP *et al:* Changes in diastolic time with various pharmacologic agents. Circulation 60:164, 1979.)

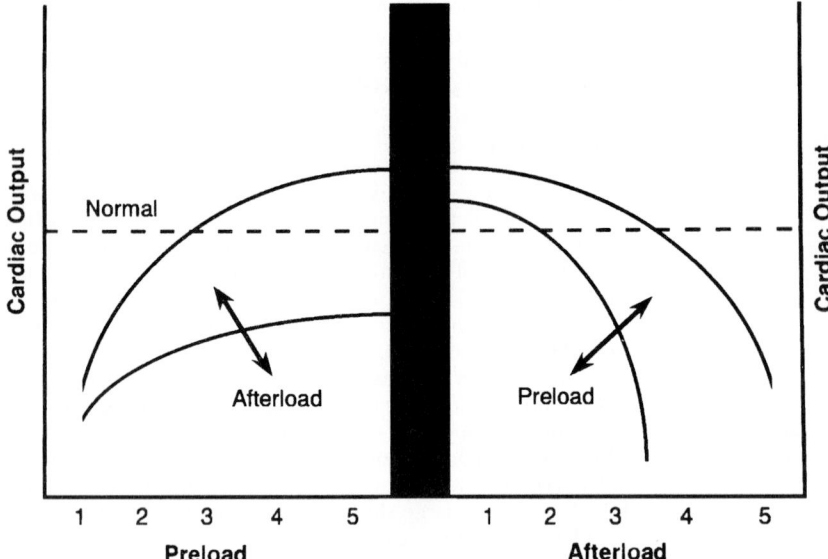

Figure 12-26. The contrasting effects of preload and afterload on CO. Increasing preload increases output in the normal myocardium, but to a lesser degree in the failing myocardium. Increased afterload is usually tolerated by the normal myocardium, but even small increases produce large reductions in output in the failing myocardium.

appreciated: it is now known to play a large role in many myocardial disease processes and may, in fact, precede inotropic dysfunction.[161] Decreased lusitropism is characteristic of the aging myocardium.

Figure 12-23 deliberately emphasizes preload and afterload as balancing forces in producing CO. They are antagonistic and assume differing degrees of dominance depending on whether the myocardium is healthy or ailing. Preload is the dominant regulator of CO in the normal cardiovascular system. Afterload dominates flow regulation when the myocardium is failing. Figure 12-26 compares the contrasting effects of preload and afterload on the CO of both the healthy and failing myocardium. Acute increases (in afterload) in the healthy patient are tolerated, up to a 4-fold increase. In contrast, even small increases in afterload produce large reductions in CO when the myocardium is depressed by disease or anesthesia.[162] The use of vasodilators for afterload reduction in the patient with a failing myocardium is based on this concept.

The problems associated with the earlier use of vasopressors are now recognized as having been caused, in large part, by an insufficient understanding of clinical cardiovascular physiology and the inability to monitor critically ill patients. We can now selectively detect and manipulate the weak links in the chain of cardiovascular events that produce blood flow and oxygen transport rather than the mindless increase in blood pressure. The term *vasopressor,* once synonymous with vasoconstriction, has now become a generic term for several species of drugs which, by whatever means, increase CO and may or may not increase blood pressure. Their uses in anesthesia include (1) maintenance or organ perfusion, (2) treatment of allergic reactions, (3) prolongation of the action of local anesthetics, and (4) for cardiopulmonary resuscitation.

Selection of Adrenergic Effect

The selection of vasoactive drugs requires a knowledge of both the hemodynamic disturbance and pharmacology of the available drugs. The catecholamines and sympathomimetic drugs continue to be the pharmacologic mainstay of cardiovascular support for the low-flow state.[32] Sustained interest in the catecholamines is related to their predictable pharmacodynamics and favorable pharmacokinetic profiles. Their effects are linearly related to plasma levels, which are directly and linearly related to the rate of infusion. There are few clinical surprises within any given dose range and the pharmacokinetics of catecholamines allow rapid titration to the effect. The half-life of most is short, ranging from 2 to 3 minutes. Undesirable side-effects dissipate within minutes of lowering or stopping the infusion. Sympathomimetics, as a group, produce a wide range of hemodynamic effects and can be used in combination to achieve a yet wider spectrum of effects. As a result, one need become familiar with but a few agents to manage most clinical situations.

The goal for managing the low-output syndrome is to establish and maintain adequate tissue perfusion. Aggressive fluid therapy will suffice in most instances. Sympathomimetics are not a substitute for volume. However, once intravascular volume is optimized, a vasoactive drug may be required to sustain CO. During the early 1990s the term *inodilator* entered our lexicon to supplant the more archaic term *vasopressor.* This neologism reflects a change in philosophy in managing low-flow states, particularly those characterized by heart failure. The new synthetic sympathomimetics have been chemically engineered to obtain inotropism and vasodilation rather than pressor effects. The potential for benefit or harm can best be understood in terms of receptor characteristics. For example, activation of the inotropic β_1 and β_2 receptors results in positive inotropism and chronotropism. Selective stimulation of the vascular β_2 receptors causes vasodilatation. Left ventricular outflow may improve as a function of increased afterload reduction and inotropism. However, chronotropism may not be a desirable feature in a patient with mitral stenosis or coronary artery disease.

CATECHOLAMINE RECEPTOR–EFFECTOR COUPLING

The net physiologic effect of a sympathomimetic is usually defined as the algebraic sum of its relative actions on the α, β, and DA receptors.[33] Most adrenergic drugs activate or block these receptors to varying degrees. Each catecholamine has a distinctive effect, qualitatively and quantitatively, on the myocardium and peripheral vasculature. Table 12-13 demonstrates the relative potency of the adrenergic amines on the various myocardial and vascular receptors. This relative potency is also dose-related, adding yet another variable. The use of pluses (+) or zeros (0) is the classical method by which the relative sensitivities of catecholamine–receptor coupling are demonstrated. The plus sign is also symbolic, suggesting the apparent summation effect of the catecholamines on the receptors. The summation effect further implies a finite number of adrenergic receptor sites to which adrenergic agonists can compete.

For many years, the focus on catecholamines was devoted,

Table 12-13. ACTIONS OF ADRENERGIC AGONISTS

Sympatho-mimetics	Receptors						Dose Dependence (α, β, or DA)	Comments
	α_1	α_2	β_1	β_2	DA$_1$	DA$_2$		
Methoxamine	+++++	?*	0	0	0		0	Vasoconstriction only
Phenylephrine	+++++	?	±	0	0		++	Primarily vasoconstriction
Norepinephrine	+++++	+++++	+++	0	0		+++	β_2 effect present but not seen clinically
Metaraminol	+++++	?	+++	0	0		+++	Releases NE
Epinephrine	+++++	+++	++++	++	0		++++	
Ephedrine	++	?	+++	++	0		++	Direct and indirect
Mephentermine	0 to ++	?	++++	+?	0		++	Cerebral stimulation
Dopamine	+ to +++++	?	++++	++	+++	?	+++++	
Dobutamine	0 to +	?	++++	++	0		++	Inotropism greater than chronotropism
Dopexamine	0	0	+	++++	+		++	
Prenalterol	+		++++	++			+	
Isoproterenol	0	0	+++++	+++++	0		0	

* The clinical significance of the effects of agonism and antagonism is not yet known.

almost entirely, to their actions on the myocardium and on arteriolar resistance vessels. Changes in venous resistance contribute little to total vascular resistance and blood pressure. However, small changes in venous capacitance result in large changes in venous return because 60–70% of the circulating blood volume is the venous circulation.[107,163] The effect of the sympathomimetic amines on the venous circulation appears to be distributive in that acute venular constriction increases the central blood volume (preload), whereas dilatation decreases venous return by the promotion of peripheral pooling.[164,165] The distributive effect of a catecholamine may be as important as its inotropic action and more important than its arteriolar effect.[23,166] Further definition should elucidate some of the complex and confusing data generated when clinical observations are limited solely to adrenergic effects on the myocardium and arteriolar vasculature.

Intravenous and intra-arterial infusions of EPI in humans have been shown to cause marked constriction of the veins. Arteriolar vasoconstriction precedes venoconstriction; however, SV does not increase until the onset of venoconstriction. The initial increase in CO seen with the infusion of EPI is more an effect of increased preload than an arteriolar or direct cardiac effect.[167] NE produces a similar effect, but the onset of venoconstriction is slower.

A differential ability of the amines to constrict veins has been noted in animals.[168] The data are expressed as the average percentage contribution of venous resistance to total change in vascular resistance (Table 12-14). Methoxamine and NE are

considered equipotent α_1 arteriolar vasoconstrictors; however, these effects differ dramatically from their effects on venoconstriction. The lack of venoconstrictor response to methoxamine has been demonstrated in humans.

A similar study in humans found similar results.[169] Table 12-15 demonstrates relative potencies of several catecholamines on resistance versus capacitance vessels. These data represent only the relative potencies of the amines within either resistance or capacitance vessels and are not a comparison of potency ratio between the two. Nevertheless, the data point out the marked differences between the agents. NE is the most potent amine with respect to arteriolar and venous constriction. Metaraminol is 1.5 times more potent than phenylephrine in constricting resistance vessels; however, phenylephrine is 1.5 times more effective in constricting capacitance vessels than metaraminol. NE proved to be 12 times more potent than metaraminol in constricting resistance vessels and 24 times more effective in constricting capacitance vessels.

Brown *et al*[170] reported the responses of resistance and capacitance vessels to catecholamines in humans on cardiopulmonary bypass. This is a unique method of examining hemodynamic drug response because flow rate (CO) is fixed, excluding the myocardial effects of the drugs. Changes in resistance or capacitance are reflected as either changes in pressure or changes in reservoir volume, respectively. The α agonist phenylephrine

Table 12-14. AVERAGE PERCENTAGES OF CONTRIBUTIONS OF INCREMENTS IN VENOUS RESISTANCE TO INCREMENTS IN TOTAL RESISTANCE (ΔVR/ΔTR × 100)

Agent	ΔVR/ΔTR × 100
Norepinephrine	13.8
Tyramine	8.0
Metaraminol	7.2
Ephedrine	3.3
Mephentermine	1.9
Phenylephrine	1.8
Methoxamine	1.4

After Zimmerman BG, Abboud FN, Eckstein JW: Comparison of the effects of sympathomimetic amines upon venous and total vascular resistance in the foreleg of the dog. J Pharmacol Exp Ther 139:290, 1963, with permission.

Table 12-15. RELATIVE POTENCIES OF SEVERAL SYMPATHOMIMETIC AMINES IN HUMANS WITH RESPECT TO CONSTRICTOR EFFECTS ON RESISTANCE VESSELS AND CAPACITANCE VESSELS

Resistance Vessels		Capacitance Vessels	
Drug	*Relative Potency*	*Drug*	*Relative Potency*
Norepinephrine	1.0000	Norepinephrine	1.0000
Metaraminol	0.0874	Phenylephrine	0.0570
Phenylephrine	0.0684	Metaraminol	0.0419
Tyramine	0.0148	Methoxamine	0.0068
Mephentermine	0.0049	Ephedrine	0.0025
Ephedrine	0.0020	Tyramine	0.0023
Methoxamine	0.0018	Mephentermine	0.0023

After Schmid PG, Eckstein JW, Abboud FM: Comparison of the effects of several sympathomimetic amines on resistance and capacitance vessels in the forearm of man. Circulation 34:III-209, 1966, with permission.

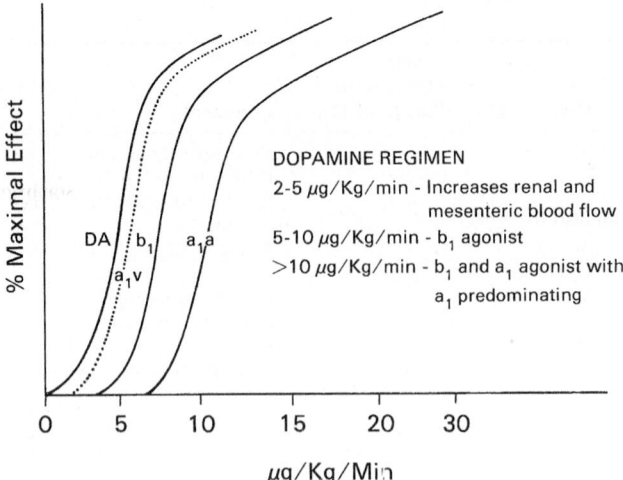

Figure 12-27. The spectrum of dose-related adrenergic activity of dopamine is demonstrated. Progressive rates of infusion produce dopaminergic (DA), β, then α activity. Infusion rates of greater than 15 $\mu g \cdot kg^{-1} \cdot min^{-1}$ produce a predominant α effect, like that of NE. Early α_1 venoconstriction may be an important redistributive feature of infused dopamine.

produced a marked decrease in venous capacitance (venoconstriction). Arteriolar resistance increased also, but to a lesser degree, confirming the study by Schmid *et al.*[169] Dopamine produces significant venoconstriction at doses that have no direct arteriolar or cardiac effect, confirming studies of dopamine in animals[166,170,171] (Fig. 12-27).

De Mey and Vanhoutte[64] compared the effects of sympathetic agonists on rings of arterial and venous vessels from dogs. Their data were similar to the information in Table 12-15. NE was the most potent arterial and venous constrictor, and relative sensitivity of the arterioles to phenylephrine and methoxamine was also similar. Their study demonstrated that the differences in response between veins and arteries lay in the uneven distribution of postjunctional α_1 and α_2 receptors. Their results indicate the presence of both receptors on venous smooth muscle, whereas arterial smooth muscle cells contain mainly postjunctional α_1 receptors.

Table 12-16 is a summary of the available data on the relative potencies of the amines on the α receptors of the resistance

and capacitance vessels. Scant data permit inaccuracies, but the table is derived from sources that demonstrate remarkable consistency. It is offered as a clinical guide to drug selection. The peripheral receptors of both resistance and capacitance vessels subserve vasoconstriction, but with divergent effects on afterload and preload; therefore, the α_1 receptors have been subdivided into α_1 arterial (α_{1a}) and α_1 venous (α_{1v}). Note that methoxamine and phenylephrine, both pure α drugs, are equipotent arterial vasoconstrictors. Phenylephrine, however, is a potent venous constrictor, and methoxamine has virtually no effect on the capacitance vessels. Dopamine has potent venoconstrictor (α_{1v}) effect at doses at which few α_{1a} or β_1 effects are noted.

Drug Dosage and Adverse Effects

The major adverse effects of the sympathomimetic amines are related to excessive α or β activity. The potential for harm can be understood in terms of receptor characteristics. Excessive β_1 activity may increase contractility but increase HR and myocardial oxygen consumption beyond supply. Severe dysrhythmias frequently accompany excess β_1 activity as a result of increased conduction velocity, automaticity, and ischemia. The β_2 activity has the potential to increase CO by reducing resistance (afterload) while reducing blood pressure. An excessive decrease in diastolic pressure, however, reduces obstructive coronary perfusion and may further aggravate myocardial ischemia. The β_1 and β_2 effects of adrenergic agonists are more useful clinically than α_1 effects and can be used for longer periods of time. Unfortunately, it is difficult to separate the inotropic, dromotropic, and chronotropic effects in the clinical setting. The characteristics of the ideal positive inotropic agent are listed in Table 12-17 for comparison with each drug as it is discussed.

Drugs with prominent α_1 agonist effects may produce a desirable increase in blood pressure but reduce total flow due to increases in arteriolar resistance (afterload). A more prominent α_1 venous constriction may improve CO by increasing preload or may precipitate failure if preload exceeds the contractile limits of the myocardium[172] (see Fig. 12-26).

In general, the α effects of the sympathomimetics are of benefit only when used for specific indications and for the briefest possible time. Other measures are usually more effective in improving flow and are indicated before a pressor should be used. The only time an adrenergic amine should be used as a pressor or in a pressor dose range without consideration of flow is when arterial perfusion pressure must be increased

Table 12-16. COMPARISON OF RELATIVE α_1 CATECHOLAMINE RESPONSES ON PERIPHERAL RESISTANCE AND CAPACITANCE VESSELS*

	Vasoconstriction		
	α_1 Arterial (α_{1a})		α_1 Venous (α_{1v})
Norepinephrine	+++++	Norepinephrine	+++++
Metaraminol	+++++	Phenylephrine	+++++
Phenylephrine	++++	Metaraminol	++++
Methoxamine	++++	Dopamine	+++
Epinephrine	0/++++†	Epinephrine	0/++++†
Dopamine	0/++++‡	Ephedrine	+++
Ephedrine	++	Mephentermine	+?
Mephentermine	++	Methoxamine	0/+?
Dobutamine	+/0	Dobutamine	?
Isoproterenol	0	Isoproterenol	0

* Drugs are listed in descending order of potency within each vascular region.
† Dose-dependent; β effects of epinephrine predominate at low doses.
‡ Dose-dependent; DA and β effects predominate at low doses.
Reprinted with permission from Lawson NW, Wallfisch HK: Cardiovascular pharmacology: A new look at the "pressors." In Stoelting RK, Barash PG, Gallagher TJ (eds): Advances in Anesthesia, p 195. Chicago, Year Book Medical Publishers, 1986.

Table 12-17. CHARACTERISTICS OF THE IDEAL POSITIVE INOTROPIC AGENT

Enhances contractile state by increasing velocity and force of myocardial fiber shortening
Lacks tolerance
Does not produce vasoconstriction
No cardiac dysrhythmias
Does not affect heart rate
Controllability—immediate onset and termination of action
Elevates perfusion pressure by raising cardiac output rather than systemic vascular resistance
Redistributes blood flow to vital organs
Direct-acting—not dependent on release of endogenous amines
Compatible with other vasoactive drugs
Effective orally or parenterally

immediately to prevent imminent death or morbidity.[173] Cardiopulmonary resuscitation is the primary example of a situation in which a pressor effect is necessary to create diastolic coronary perfusion during closed or open heart massage. Any drug with strong α agonist properties seems equally effective in this regard. EPI, with its added β properties, has been the first-line agent for this situation. Drugs that vasodilate, such as isoproterenol, have little use in this setting even if they possess inotropic properties. Another situation in which a vasoconstrictor may be justified as a temporary measure is hypotension when cerebral, coronary, or extracorporeal bypass perfusion pressure is the prime consideration.

The prolonged use of adrenergic agonists with strong α properties commonly results in tachyphylaxis. This phenomenon is probably caused by increasing plasma volume loss through ischemic capillaries and downregulation of the adrenergic receptors. Precapillary sphincters are under local myogenic control and relax when hypoxic and acidotic, despite strong α stimulation. Postcapillary sphincters are more functional in a hypoxic and acidotic milieu but are under stronger central neurogenic control. Continued postcapillary tone in the face of precapillary relaxation increases hydrostatic pressure with a net loss of intravascular volume. These events are just a few of the explanations for the once mysterious "levophed shock," in which patients could not be weaned from NE infusions.[32,38]

Dopamine is the clinically available DA agonist. This property has been put to effective clinical use in reducing resistance in the mesenteric and renal beds, mediating an improvement in perfusion of these regions in the low-flow state. Few complications have been ascribed to dopamine when used solely for this purpose.[73]

Low-Output Syndrome

Patients with the low CO syndrome have abnormalities of the heart, blood volume, or blood flow distribution.[174] Those remaining in this state for more than 1 hour usually have dysfunction of all three components. Modern hemodynamic monitoring has pinpointed hypovolemia, relative or absolute, as the most common cause of the low-output syndrome, regardless of the etiology.[174,175] Initial treatment with adrenergic amines in this setting is likely to delay volume repletion and potentiate the shock state. The proper hemodynamic management of septic shock, the most commonly seen distributive abnormality, remains controversial, but volume repletion is the primary consideration. Likewise, the initial treatment of cardiac dysfunction is optimum volume replacement because hypovolemia frequently accompanies impaired myocardial performance. Ventricular performance may be improved solely on the basis of increased preload.

The treatment of cardiogenic shock is an excellent example of the low-flow state that requires multiple autonomic interventions common to other forms of the low-output syndrome. An acute reduction of left ventricular contractility (inotropism) produces a cascade of events that worsen in cyclic fashion (Fig. 12-28).[176] One could draw this cascade beginning with any one of the five determinants of CO. Loss of contractility produces a reduction in CO, increased left ventricular end-diastolic pressure, and a host of compensatory reflexes, which are familiar. These compensatory mechanisms include the Frank–Starling law and increased sympathetic activity that augments contractility and rate. Chronic dysfunction produces a third compensatory mechanism—hypertrophy.

The attributes of the ideal inotropic drug are listed in Table 12-17. The inotropic agent needed for the patient illustrated in Figure 12-28 would be rapid-acting and short-lived and would not increase HR, preload (unless hypovolemic), afterload, or infarct size. Because the ideal inotropic drug is not available, the peripheral side-effects of any inotropic agent become critical to selection because all are multireceptor agonists.

Myocardial failure exists when the heart cannot pump enough blood to meet metabolic needs. The clinical manifestations of heart failure result from peripheral circulatory derangements that are the result of the heart's forward output lagging behind the input. Venous pressure increases and produces congestion. There are marked differences between chronic heart failure, whatever the cause, and acute failure from infarction. These differences are now fully appreciated.[177] Patients with chronic heart failure have retention of sodium and water and are typically hypervolemic, whereas patients with acute heart failure are either normovolemic or commonly hypovolemic. Cardiomegaly is a common compensatory feature of chronic heart failure but is absent with acute heart failure. Circulating catecholamines and myocardial catecholamine content are decreased in chronic failure but markedly elevated in the acute infarct. Thus, the response to inotropic drugs in chronic heart failure is influenced not only by the lack of myocardial catecholamine stores but also by downregulation of β receptors. The CO in chronic failure is borderline to decreased, whereas it is usually normal or elevated with acute failure as a result of the compensatory mechanism.

Acute failure is the most common complication of infarction, occurring in 40–50% of patients, which reflects a 20–25% involvement of the myocardium. In contrast to the patient with chronic heart failure, this dysfunction is usually transient, lasting from 48 to 72 hours. Drugs with a predominant inotropic action are used alone or in combination to acutely improve cardiac contractility. Therefore, it is a major concern that myocardial

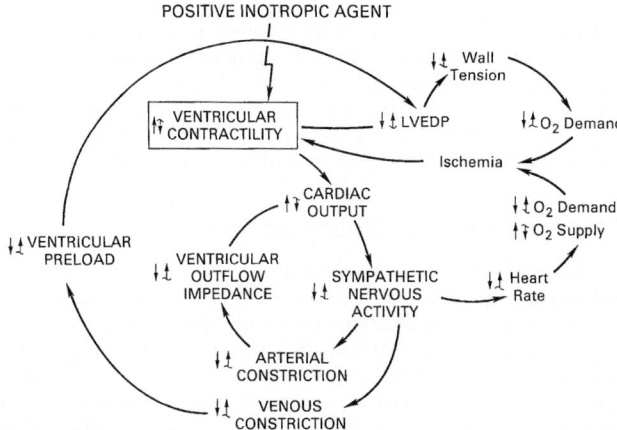

Figure 12-28. Reversal of heart failure by intervention (↑) with the ideal positive inotropic agent is depicted. (Reprinted with permission from Evans DB, Weishaar RE, Kaplan HR: Strategy for the discovery and development of a positive inotropic agent. Pharmacol Ther 16:303, 1982.)

Table 12-18. MANAGEMENT OF LOW OUTPUT SYNDROME CAUSED BY MYOCARDIAL DYSFUNCTION

1. Assure adequate ventilation and oxygenation
2. Relieve pain and symptoms of recurrent ischemia
3. Institute hemodynamic monitoring (pulmonary artery, pulmonary capillary wedge, and arterial pressures; urine output; cardiac output)
4. Optimize left ventricular filling pressure
5. Correct metabolic abnormalities
6. Control dysrhythmias (#2 priority if life-threatening)
7. Pharmacologic support
   a. Vasodilators
   b. Inotropic drugs
   c. Diuretics—chronic heart failure
8. Rule out "correctable" causes of shock (septal or left ventricle rupture, mitral regurgitation, acute aneurysm)
9. Mechanical support of circulation
10. Surgical correction if possible

Note: Hemodynamic monitoring is essential in confirming a diagnosis, optimizing filling pressures and cardiac output, selecting pharmacologic support, and avoiding complications. Adjustment of left ventricular filling pressure may require additional volume or a relative volume reduction with vasodilators. The diagnostic criteria for cardiogenic shock are not met until step 4 is accomplished.

damage not be extended during this transient period by inappropriate inotropic or chronotropic support. This is not as major a concern in the patient with hypertrophy, in whom increased inotropism may actually reduce oxygen consumption by reducing ventricular mass.

Table 12-18 presents one approach to the management of cardiogenic shock listed in order of relative importance. The use of sympathomimetic support is placed in proper perspective. It emphasizes the essential role that invasive hemodynamic monitoring and volume management play in confirming a diagnosis of cardiogenic failure. Although volume expansion and reduction of afterload may improve CO, other pharmacologic interventions may still be necessary to optimize CO and its distribution. Invasive monitoring is a prerequisite for the rational use of the vasoactive drugs to (1) establish that a sympathomimetic is necessary, (2) select drugs for the hemodynamic condition, (3) follow resultant hemodynamic changes because many of the beneficial effects of the catecholamines are hidden to the clinical eye, and (4) avoid complications of pressor therapy that are visible to all. Drug selection for the low-output state remains the most enigmatic.

Table 12-19 is a summary of the hemodynamic effects of some of the currently popular and once popular sympathomimetic drugs. Many of the hemodynamic effects are dose-related. The dose ranges are listed and a standard infusion rate cited. Standard rates of infusion are simply guidelines, and the actual dose administered should be determined by patient response.

Methoxamine and Phenylephrine

Methoxamine is the prototypical pure vasoconstrictor. Phenylephrine produces similar actions, but there are important clinical differences. Methoxamine possesses only α_1 properties and produces almost no venoconstriction. Its only pharmacologic effects are to increase arterial resistance, increase afterload, and reduce flow, even though blood pressure is elevated. Few clinical uses for methoxamine remain except for cardiopulmonary resuscitation (CPR). It has been useful for treating paroxysmal atrial tachycardias. A single iv dose of methoxamine can break a paroxysmal atrial tachycardia reflexly through baroreceptor stretch, obviating the need for digitalis or countershock. Carotid massage produces similar results by a similar mechanism.

Phenylephrine, considered a pure α drug, increases venous constriction more than arterial constriction in a dose-related manner similar to dopamine.[170,178] Venous constriction may be its most redeeming feature when compared with the purely arteriolar effect of methoxamine. One cannot discount the possibility of an inotropic effect now that α_1 receptors are known to exist in the myocardium that improve inotropism. Acutely, venoconstriction favors venous return (preload), even though arterial resistance (afterload) also increases. The net effect may result in an increase in pressure and flow. Phenylephrine, like methoxamine, does not change CO in normal individuals but can cause a decreased output in patients with ischemic heart disease.[35,162,179] It is rarely necessary to give a pure α pressor for extended periods, but phenylephrine has continued to be favored in operating rooms to sustain pressure during cardiopulmonary bypass as well as during intracranial and peripheral vascular procedures.[180] It does not produce dysrhythmia as a direct effect. Phenylephrine is also useful in reversing right-to-left shunt in tetralogy of Fallot when patients are having "spells" during anesthesia.[22] The arterial vasoconstrictors may reduce the size of an ischemic injury when used in conjunction with intra-aortic balloon pumping or nitroglycerin.[181]

Norepinephrine

NE and metaraminol produce similar hemodynamic effects. NE is the naturally occurring mediator of the SNS and the immediate precursor of EPI. It produces direct-acting hemodynamic effects on the α and β receptors in a dose-related manner when given by infusion. NE produces increased CO and blood pressure when given in low doses (see Table 12-19), primarily as a result of predominant action at this level.[182] Higher doses reduce flow because α arteriolar constriction supersedes the β effects. Reflex bradycardias may occur, as with methoxamine and phenylephrine, despite active β stimulation.

Increased plasma levels of the endogenous catecholamines NE and EPI are the sympathetic milieu in which exogenous sympathomimetics are ordinarily given. NE is the catecholamine standard against which all other catecholamines are compared. It is the endogenous neurotransmitter of the SNS. Over the years NE administered iv has gained an unseemly reputation that is perhaps unmerited.[183] Current studies indicate that NE is being used in doses that are orders of magnitude greater than that necessary to obtain its best response. Complications such as renal failure and tissue necrosis are routine and can be expected when NE is used in this manner. Personal experience and the published experience of others also indicate that if an infusion of NE is used simply to titrate to blood pressure rather than measured flow, the amount of NE infused is 5–10 times higher than necessary to obtain the best oxygen delivery and oxygen consumption.[6,184,185] Most published dose infusion rates are based on blood pressure titration, and hence are too liberal. Although NE is less commonly used in the critically ill patient than other catecholamines, a resurgence of interest in this agent is noted in the literature. It has remained clinically useful because its effects are predictable, prompt, and potent.[186,187]

Objections to the use of NE (or metaraminol) for the treatment of cardiogenic shock are based on two considerations: (1) vasoconstriction increases the pressure work of the left ventricle, with an adverse effect on the oxygen economy of the already ischemic pump; (2) these drugs cause further vasoconstriction and organ ischemia in a syndrome in which intense constriction may already have occurred.[35] The use of NE requires invasive monitoring; otherwise, complications are to be expected. It is not usually necessary to elevate the systolic blood pressure above 90–100 mm Hg. At this level of infusion, the CO will normally be increased as a β effect without excessive peripheral vasoconstriction. NE is a potent venoconstrictor, which should alter interpretation of venous filling pressures as a guide to adequate volume repletion.

Table 12-19. DOSE SCHEDULE AND HEMODYNAMIC EFFECTS OF THE ADRENERGIC AGONISTS

Drug Listed from α to β	Dosages iv Push Adults	iv infusion*	α₁ₐ	α₁ᵥ	β₁	β₂	DA	CO	Inotrop	HR	VR	TPR	RBF
Methoxamine	5–10 mg	N/R	++++	0–+?	0	0	0	−↓	−	Reflex ↓	−	↑↑	↓↓
Phenylephrine	50–100 µg	a. 10 mg/250 ml b. 40 µg·ml⁻¹ c. 0.15–0.75 µg·kg⁻¹·min⁻¹ d. 0.15 µg·kg⁻¹·min⁻¹	++++	+++++	0	0	0	−↓	−	Reflex ↓	↑↑↑	↑↑	−−↓
Norepinephrine	N/R	a. 4 mg/250 ml b. 16 µg·ml⁻¹ c. 0.01–0.1 µg·kg⁻¹·min⁻¹ d. 0.1 µg·kg⁻¹·min⁻¹	+++	+++	++++	?+	0	↑−↓	↑	Reflex ↓	↑↑↑	↑↑↑	↓↓↓
Metaraminol	N/R	a. 100 mg/250 ml b. 400 µg·ml⁻¹ c. 0.5–7 µg·kg⁻¹·min⁻¹ d. 0.5 µg·kg⁻¹·min⁻¹	++	++	+++	0	0	−↓	↑	Reflex ↓	↑	↑↑↑	↓↓↓
Epinephrine	0.3–0.5 ml 1:1000 (0.3–0.5 mg) sc—Asthma iv—Anaphylaxis 5 ml 1:10,000 (0.5 mg) cardiac arrest every 5 minutes	a. 1 mg/250 ml b. 4 µg·ml⁻¹ 0.01–0.03 µg·kg⁻¹·min⁻¹ c. 0.03–0.15 µg·kg⁻¹·min⁻¹ 0.15–0.30 µg·kg⁻¹·min⁻¹ d. 0.015 µg·kg⁻¹·min⁻¹	+ +++ +++++ +	+ +++ +++++ +	++++ ++++ ++++	++++ ++++ ++++	0 0	↑↑ ↑− ↑−↓ ↑↑	↑↑ ↑↑ ↑↑ ↑↑	↑ ↑↑ ↑↑ ↑	↑ ↑ ↑ ↑	↑ ↑↑ ↑↑↑ ↑	↑ ↓− ↓ ↑
Ephedrine	5–10 mg	N/R	++	+++	+++	++	0	↑	↑	↑	↑↑	↑	↑−↓
Mephentermine	15–30 mg	a. 500 mg/250 ml b. 2000 µg·ml⁻¹ c. 4–8 µg·kg⁻¹·min⁻¹ d. 4 µg·kg⁻¹·min⁻¹	0–++	+?	++++	+?	0	↑	↑↑	↑	↑?	↑	↓−↑
Dopamine‡	N/R	a. 200 mg/250 ml b. 800 µg·ml⁻¹ 0.05–5 µg·kg⁻¹·min⁻¹ c. 2–10 µg·kg⁻¹·min⁻¹ 10 µg·kg⁻¹·min⁻¹† d. 2 µg·kg⁻¹·min⁻¹	 + +++++ 	++++ ++++ ++++ ++++	 +++ +++++ 	 +++++ +++++ 	+++++ +++++ +++++	↑ ↑↑ ↑−↓ ↑	− ↑ ↑↑ −	− −↑ ↑↑ −	↑ ↑ ↑ ↑	−↓ −↑ ↑↑ −↓	↑ ↑ −↓ ↑
Dobutamine‡	N/R	a. 250 mg/250 ml b. 1000 µg·ml⁻¹ c. 2–30 µg·kg⁻¹·min⁻¹ d. 5 µg·kg⁻¹·min⁻¹	0–+	?	++++	++	0	↑↑	↑↑	−↑	?	−	−↑
Isoproterenol	0.004 mg (0.2 ml of 0.2 mg·ml⁻¹ solution) Third-degree heart block	a. 1 mg/250 ml b. 4 µg·ml⁻¹ c. 0.15 µg·kg⁻¹·min⁻¹ to desired effect d. 0.015 µg·kg⁻¹·min⁻¹			+++++ +++++	+++++ +++++		↑−↓	↑↑↑	↑↑↑	↓	↓↓	−↑

Site of Activity headers: α₁ₐ, α₁ᵥ, β₁, β₂, DA. Hemodynamics (↑ = increase; ↓ = decrease; − = no change): CO, Inotrop, HR, VR, TPR, RBF

* a. Mixture
  b. Concentration µg/ml⁻¹
  c. Dose range µg·kg⁻¹·min⁻¹
  d. Standard rate infusion
† "Rule of six."
‡ Dopamine and dobutamine employ the same doses. Dosage of either may quickly be calculated by multiplying patient's weight (kg) × 6 = mg added to 100 ml D5%W. The number of drops delivered through a calibrated infusor (60 drops = 1 ml) is the number of µg·kg⁻¹·min⁻¹ infused into the patient. Example: 70 kg × 6 = 420; 420 mg/100 ml = 4200 µg·kg⁻¹ or 70 µg gtt; 5 µg·kg⁻¹·min⁻¹ = 5 gtt/min.
N/R = not recommended; CO = cardiac output; Inotrop = contractility; HR = heart rate; VR = venous return (preload); TPR = peripheral resistance (afterload); RBF = renal blood flow.
Reprinted with permission from Lawson NW, Wallfisch HK: Cardiovascular pharmacology: A new look at the "pressors." In Stoelting RK, Barash PG, Gallagher TJ (eds): Advances in Anesthesia, p 195. Chicago, Year Book Medical Publishers, 1986.

NE may also not be effective initially in patients who are receiving catechol depleters. Other undesirable effects associated with the use of NE include renal arteriolar constriction and aggravation of oliguria. In addition, prolonged therapy may produce a reduction in plasma volume as a result of fluid transudation at the capillary level. Indeed, in some instances, cardiogenic shock requiring continuous NE infusions has been reversed by fluid infusions.[35] The use of the minimal effective dose NE in combination with careful invasive monitoring and attention to fluid management is the only way to avoid iatrogenic disasters. Norepinephrine should only be administered in a centrally placed iv line to avoid tissue necrosis from extravasation. It can be used for its intropic effect at low doses and titrated to effect while monitoring cardiac output. Monitoring of blood pressure alone, or titrating to a predetermined effect, is often detrimental to cardiac output. Blood pressure increases are usually due to increases in SVR and can diminish forward flow and contribute to cardiac failure. Even moderate doses of NE may have a detrimental effect on end-organ perfusion—hence the drug's ill-gotten reputation when used to tirate to pressure rather than flow. However, in clinical conditions characterized by a low perfusion pressure, high flow (vasodilatation), and maldistribution of flow, NE has been shown to improve renal and splanchnic blood flow by increasing pressure, provided the patient has been volume-resuscitated.

Epinephrine

EPI is the prototypical endogenous catecholamine. It is synthesized, stored, and released from the adrenal medulla and is the key hormonal element in the fight-or-flight response. The most widely used catecholamine in medicine, EPI is used to treat asthma, anaphylaxis, cardiac arrest, and bleeding and to prolong regional anesthesia. The cardiovascular effects of EPI, when given systemically, result from its direct stimulation of both α and β receptors. This is dose-dependent, as outlined in Table 12-19.

The effect of EPI on the peripheral vasculature is mixed.[188,200] It has predominantly α-stimulating effects in some beds (skin, mucosa, and kidney) and β-stimulating actions in others (skeletal muscle). These effects are also dose-dependent. At therapeutic doses, β-adrenergic effects predominate in the peripheral vessels, and total resistance may be reduced. Constriction, however, is maintained in the renal and cutaneous areas owing to its dominant α effect in these areas. An increase in CO with EPI may be due to a redistribution of blood to low resistance vessels in the muscle, but with further reduction in flow to vital organs. Cardiac dysrhythmias are a prominent hazard, and the strong chronotropic effects of EPI have limited its use or systematic investigation in the treatment of cardiogenic shock.

EPI is commonly used in the perioperative period in anesthesia by surgeons and anesthesiologists. It is often used to produce a bloodless field in dentistry, otolaryngology, and skin grafting, either topically or in local and field blocks. Anesthesiologists often use it to prolong regional anesthesia. The addition of EPI to arthroscopic infusions to attain a bloodless field is another area of increased EPI usage. These infusions are usually safe in maintaining a dry operative field because the solutions are very dilute at ~1:3,000,000. However, the large volumes infused and the unpredictable absorption of the epinephrine, especially in denuded cancellous bone, may expose the patient to an excessive amount of epinephrine over a short period of time despite the dilution.[189] The unexpected complications are those of epinephrine overdose: acute heart failure, pulmonary edema, or cardiac arrhythmias and arrest in the otherwise young and healthy patient. Impending problems during the infusion of intra-articular fluids will be noted by an increasing blood pressure exceeding that attributable to surgical pain or hypertension that is poorly responsive to deepening of anesthesia. Absent a pulsatile flow, oximetry may become dysfunctional. The patient will appear pale and cyanotic. Unless alert, one may unintentionally treat an unexpected acute heart failure or cardiac arrest with the very agent that caused the problem. The outcome is universally poor. Vasodilators and β blockers may save the day instead.

Some volatile anesthetics sensitize the myocardium to circulating catecholamines and induce cardiac dysrhythmias. This is especially true in the presence of hypoxia and hypercarbia. Halothane has the most pronounced cardiac-sensitizing action of the volatile anesthetics in use today. The mechanism has been thought to be related to the stimulation of α- and β-adrenergic receptors because blockade of these receptors consistently abolishes these cardiac dysrhthmias.[190] However, calcium channel blockade is equally effective.[191] This is not surprising if the shared final pathway of β and calcium-entry blockade proves to be correct.[192] The exact mechanism is further confused by studies showing that the myocardial depression produced by the volatile anesthetics is related to blockade of the slow calcium current.[193] These findings are compatible with the observations that β blockade, calcium blockade, and general anesthetics produce myocardial depression.

Intravenous and locally infiltrated adrenergic agents should be used cautiously during inhalation anesthesia, especially with halothane. The following schedule has been found to be relatively safe during halothane anesthesia:[194]

1. EPI concentrations no greater than 1:100,000–1:200,000 (1:200,000 = 5 μg $\cdot$ ml^{-1});
2. adult dose no greater than 10 ml of 1:100,000 or 20 ml of 1:200,000 within 10 min;
3. total no greater than 30 ml of 1:100,000 (60 ml of 1:200,000) within 1 hour.

The doses of submuscosally injected EPI necessary to produce ventricular cardiac dysrhythmia in 50% of patients anesthetized with a 1.25 MAC of a volatile anesthetic were 10.9, 10.9, and 6.7 μg $\cdot$ kg^{-1} during administration of halothane, enflurane, and isoflurane, respectively.[195] The incidence of cardiac dysrhythmia is eliminated when this dose is halved in patients anesthetized with halothane or isoflurane. Unlike adults, children seem to tolerate higher doses of subcutaneous EPI without developing cardiac dysrhythmia.[196]

Ephedrine

Ephedrine is one of the most commonly used noncatecholamine sympathomimetic agents. It is used extensively for treating hypotension following spinal or epidural anesthesia. Ephedrine stimulates both α and β receptors by direct and indirect actions. It is predominantly an indirect-acting pressor, producing its effects by causing NE release.[35] Tachyphylaxis develops rapidly and is probably related to the depletion of NE stores with repeated injection. The cardiovascular effects of ephedrine (see Table 12-19) are nearly identical to those of EPI but less potent.[32,33] Its effects are sustained about 10 times longer than those of EPI.

Ephedrine remains the pressor of choice in obstetrics because uterine blood flow improves linearly with blood pressure.[112,113] This effect is probably not related to its arteriolar vasoconstriction but rather to its venoconstrictive action. Ephedrine is a weak, indirect-acting sympathomimetic agent that produces venoconstriction to a greater degree than arteriolar constriction (see Table 12-16).[164,178] This may be its most important and unappreciated effect. It causes a redistribution of blood centrally, improves venous return (preload), increases CO, and restores uterine perfusion. The mild β action restores HR simultaneously with improved venous return. An increased blood pressure is noted as a result rather than a cause of these events. Mild α_1-arteriolar constriction does occur, but the net effect of improving venous return and HR is increased CO (Fig. 12-29). Uterine blood flow is spared. This response, however, depends on the patient's state of hydration.

Dopamine is an attractive alternative vasopressor for obstetrics for similar reasons. It produces strong α_1 venoconstriction and volume redistribution at infusion rates for which α_{1a} or β effects are minimal (Fig. 12-27). The primary disadvantage of dopamine is its lack of immediate availability as an iv push drug. It requires more careful titration than ephedrine. The prophylactic administration of ephedrine before spinal blockade in obstetrics can produce misleading clinical estimates of volume status because of its effects on venous return and arterial pressure.

Dopamine, Dopaminergic Agonists, and Prodrugs

Dopamine

Dopamine offers distinct advantages over many sympathomimetics in treating the low-output syndrome.[71] It is a dose-related agonist to all three types of adrenoceptors, and the desired action can be selected by changing the infusion rate. The DA receptors are most sensitive, followed by the β, and then α receptors. However, DA possesses a unique property not found with other catecholamines: it dilates renal and mesenteric vascular beds as a direct effect of its DA receptor effect. The β receptors present in the renal vasculature are not involved with DA-induced vasodilatation.

Dopamine dosage regimens have been traditionally, and arbitrarily, divided into low, medium, and high doses according to its dose–receptor sensitivity (Table 12-19). Renal and mesenteric vascular dilatation and tubular cell natriuresis are mediated through the DA receptors at low-dose infusion rates of

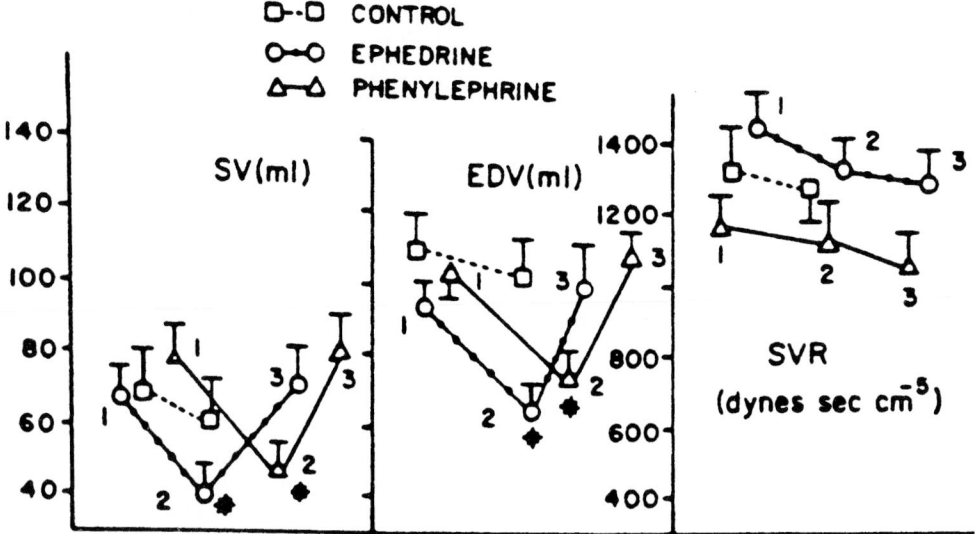

Figure 12-29. Stroke volume (SV), end-diastolic volume (EDV), and systemic vascular resistance (SVR) (1) before regional block, (2) during hypotension, and (3) after therapy with ephedrine or phenylephrine. The increase in stroke volume was related entirely to an increased venous return secondary to venoconstriction in these awake, healthy patients. The afterload effects of phenylephrine at higher doses predominate in patients with heart disease or myocardial depression and reduce CO. (Reprinted with permission from Ramanthan S, Grant G: Vasopressor therapy for hypotension due to epidural anesthesia for cesarean section. Acta Anaesthesiol Scand 32:4, 1988.)

$0.5–2.0 \ \mu g \cdot kg^{-1} \cdot min^{-1}$. This is often referred to as "renal dose dopamine" because of the enhanced renal blood flow and diuresis. The diuresis may also be attributed, in part, to inhibition of aldosterone secretion seen with low-dose DA administration.[197] A general improvement in CO from afterload reduction also contributes to improvements in renal blood flow. These effects have been well demonstrated in patients with heart failure. However, the protective effect of DA on the development of renal failure in the critically ill or injured patient, although an attractive principle, is much less certain. Prevention of renal failure by prophylactic "renal dose" DA (with or without furosemide) in the critically ill or traumatized patient has not been conclusively demonstrated, even when used early.[198] This may be related to the adrenergic milieu into which the DA is given. The vasoconstrictive effects of DA are expected to occur only at relatively high doses. However, even relatively low doses of DA can cause renal vasoconstriction when added into pre-existing high plasma levels of endogenous catecholamines[197,199] commonly seen in the acutely injured patient.

The hemodynamic effects of low-dose DA are primarily related to vasodilatation by activation of the DA_1 and DA_2 receptors. Activation of presynaptic DA_2 adrenoceptors add to the vasodilating effect of the DA_1 receptors by inhibiting presynaptic NE release in the renal and mesenteric vessels. The reduction of total systemic vascular resistance would be significant, considering that 25% of the CO goes to the kidneys alone (Fig. 12-30). A reduced diastolic blood pressure is often noted with a slight reflex increase in HR. Increasing the infusion rate of DA to $2–5 \ \mu g \cdot kg^{-1} \cdot min^{-1}$ begins to activate β receptors, increasing the CO by increasing chronotropism and contractility with early venoconstriction (preload) and systemic vasodilatation (afterload reduction). Blood pressure may not increase despite significant increases in CO. This dose range would appear optimal for managing congestive heart and lung failure because it combines inotropism and afterload reduction with diuresis. Further increases in dose activate α receptors, which will increase vascular resistance and blood pressure, but further improvements in CO may be attenuated. Infusion rates greater than $10 \ \mu g \cdot kg^{-1} \cdot min^{-1}$ produce intense α activity, which may override any beneficial DA or β vasodilation effect on total flow. High-dose dopamine behaves much like NE and, in fact, causes NE release at this dose range.[200]

Despite the apparent dose–response divisions of DA, a wide variability of individual responses has been noted. The α-adrenergic effects can be seen in some individuals in doses as low as $5 \ \mu g \cdot kg^{-1} \cdot min^{-1}$, whereas doses as high as $20 \ \mu g \cdot kg^{-1} \cdot min^{-1}$ may be required to obtain this effect in shocked patients.[200] This wide variation in dose–response has led to a re-examination of DA as a primary adrenergic for patients in cardiogenic shock or failure. Increased venous return may not be desirable in this situation, but dopamine's hemodynamic versatility continues to be useful in cardiogenic shock when combined with other complementary catecholamines such as dobutamine (Fig. 12-31) (see combinations). The venoconstriction or distributive

Systemic Vascular Resistance (SVR)

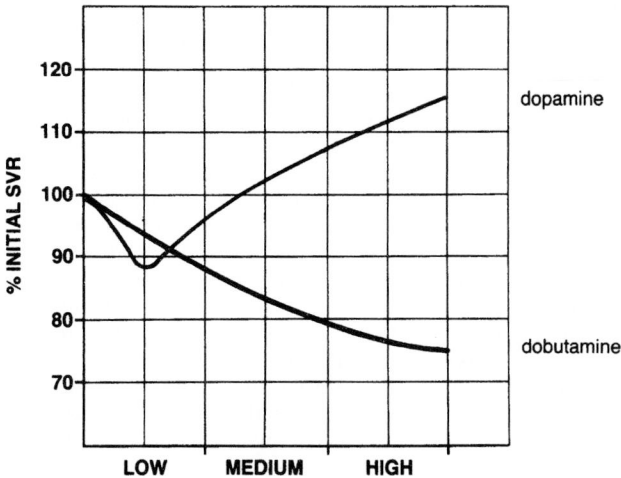

Figure 12-30. Dobutamine produces a net reduction in vascular resistance. Its weak α vasoconstrictive effects are balanced by a direct β_2 vasodilation with little change in vascular tone. However, further reflex arterial vasodilation occurs with increased CO. Low-dose dopamine dilates renal and mesentric arterial beds, which reduces afterload but increases resistance at increasing doses as a result of its predominant α effect.

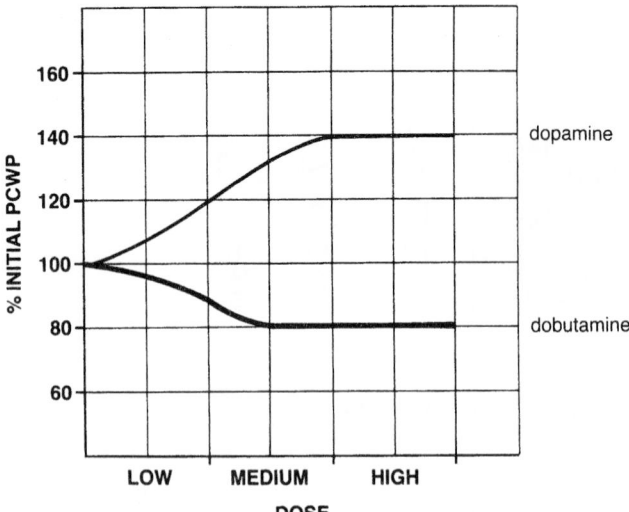

Figure 12-31. A decrease in venous capacitance has been demonstrated as an early effect of dopamine. An increase in pulmonary capillary wedge pressure may be noted. Dobutamine may decrease pulmonary capillary wedge pressure by increased inotropism as well as vasodilation with minimal effect on venous capacitance. (Redrawn with permission of Eli Lilly Co., Indianapolis, Indiana.)

effects of dopamine are useful in surgical patients in whom third-space edema and sepsis are the most common abnormalities. Dopamine increases mean pulmonary arterial pressure and is not recommended for sole support in patients with right heart failure, adult respiratory distress syndrome, or pulmonary hypertension.

Dopexamine

Dopexamine (DPX) is a "designer" catecholamine that was developed in an attempt to overcome some of the disadvantages of DA in managing cardiogenic low-flow states.[201] Afterload reduction and renal vasodilatation were desirable, but a drug was needed that did not increase myocardial oxygen consumption, or provoke arrhythmias, and whose actions could be sustained for long periods. DPX is a short-acting (t1/2b = 7 min) iv analog of DA with predominantly β_2 and DA_1 receptor agonist activity. Post-surgical patients and those with a low output show a slightly extended elimination half-life of 11 minutes. This light prolongation is not expected to cause clinical problems. It also inhibits the direct neuronal reuptake of NE. DPX provides mild positive inotropism with systemic and renal vasodilatation through its predominant receptor agonism. DPX has no direct β_1 or α_1 agonist activity like that possessed by DA.[202] It is considered an inodilator, although its inotropic actions are weak, lacking any β_1 activity except that produced by reduced NE uptake. The predominant inotropic activity is from its β_2 effect. The summed effects of DPX are due to afterload reduction *via* renal and mesenteric vasodilatation (DA_1 and β_2 receptor activation), positive inotropism (myocardial β_2 activation and reduced NE uptake), and natriuresis (DA_1 tubular receptors).[203]

The relative potency of DPX on the DA_1 and DA_2 receptors is only 0.3 and 0.17, respectively, than that of DA. It is 60 times more potent on β_2 receptors than DA. Downregulation of myocardial β_1 receptors occurs with chronic heart failure, but the β_2 subpopulation is preserved. This profile has the potential to be useful as an adjunct in increasing CO in patients with chronic heart failure because the myocardial β_2 subpopulation is preserved while the β_1 receptors are downregulated. However, adjunct inotropic agents will likely be required to realize the full benefits of its vasodilating DA_1 and β_2 properties.[61]

Doses of 2 $\mu g \cdot kg^{-1} \cdot min^{-1}$ will augment inotropism while

significantly increasing visceral blood flow.[201,204,205] DPX has been reported to improve renal function to a greater extent than could be attributed to an increased CO alone.[206] Animal studies indicate that DPX has been effective in restoring renal function to control levels following acute renal failure. However, the efficacy of DPX in preventing renal failure in humans, as in the case of dopamine, is less conclusive. DPX is a less potent direct renal vasodilator than DA. The relative contributions of dopaminergic versus β_2 receptor activation in improving renal and mesenteric blood flow has been questioned. Stephan *et al* could not demonstrate DA_1 activity of DPX in patients undergoing elective coronary artery bypass.[207] Gray found DPX at least as effective as DA for renal protection in patients undergoing liver transplantation, and Jamison *et al* were unable to demonstrate any increase in renal blood flow in patients in chronic congestive heart failure.[208,209]

The infusion rate for effective doses of DPX ranges from 0.5 to 5 $\mu g \cdot kg^{-1} \cdot min^{-1}$ depending upon the pathology. In the treatment of acute heart failure in patients following cardiac surgery DPX should be infused iv at an initial dose of 0.5 $\mu g \cdot kg^{-1} \cdot min^{-1}$.[210] It can be titrated upward in dosage increments of 1.0 $\mu g \cdot kg^{-1} \cdot min^{-1}$ according to hemodynamic response to a maximum of 6.0 $\mu g \cdot kg^{-1} \cdot min^{-1}$.[211] Infusion rates exceeding 6 $\mu g \cdot kg^{-1} \cdot min^{-1}$ can cause an intolerable tachycardia and angina in patients with pre-existing ischemic heart disease.[212] DPX inhibits hypoxic pulmonary vasoconstriction by activation of β_2 receptors. This profile has proved beneficial in both short- and long-term management of pulmonary hypertension.[213] DPX appears to be a promising catecholamine, but experience with its use in the critically ill has been limited. Its ultimate value for prolonged administration remains to be established.

Fenoldopam

Fenoldopam, a benzazepine derivative, is a selective DA_1 agonist with no α- or β-receptor activity compared to dopamine or dopexamine.[200,214,215] Oral bioavailability is poor, but it is an effective antihypertensive when given iv. The oral medication is no longer available but the iv drug is now available. Intravenous fenoldopam promotes natriuresis, diuresis, and an increase in creatinine clearance. It may offer some advantages in the acute resolution of severe hypertension, particularly if the patient has pre-existing renal impairment. Preservation or augmentation of renal blood flow during blood pressure reduction presents a potential for use during several situations in the perioperative period. Fenoldopam has an elimination half-life of 5 minutes. This property might well lend itself to producing hypotensive anesthesia while preserving renal function.[216] Aronson *et al* reported a comparative study using SNP and fenoldopam in dogs under general anesthesia. A 30% reduction in mean arterial pressure was produced by either fenoldopam or SNP. Fenoldopam maintained renal blood flow while SNP showed a reduction.[214,216,217]

Human studies have since demonstrated that fenoldopam is a potent direct renal vasodilator. It appears to improve renal function while lowering blood pressure in patients with pre-existing renal disease. Left ventricular function has been noted to improve with afterload reduction. Kien's study suggests that the improvement in renal function is a direct vasodilator effect of the drug.[216] Intravenous fenoldopam may prove to be ideal for treating conditions in which renal vasoconstriction is an expected complication. An example is cyclosporine-induced renal vasoconstriction.[218,219] Brooks *et al*, using oral fenoldopam in rats, prevented acute renal vasoconstriction in the acute phase and reversed chronic nephrotoxicity.[218] These data, also using oral medication, were reproduced in human kidney transplant recipients. Few data are available regarding the use of fenoldopam in the perioperative period. However, fenoldopam would appear to be a new option in the management of perioperative renal function.[200,220]

Bromocriptine

This compound is a selective DA_2 agonist. DA_2 agonists reduce neuronal release of NE. The magnitude of the response will be directly proportional to the background of sympathetic activity. Bromocriptine was originally found effective in humans in the treatment of Parkinson's disease and acromegaly, which can be attributed to DA_2 receptors. It also lowers blood pressure in normotensive and hypertensive individuals.

Ibopamine

This compound is an orally active prodrug that is rapidly converted into its active metabolite, epinine (*n*-methyldopamine). The pharmacologic properties of ibopamine are qualitatively similar to DA. It is a nonselective agonist of DA_1 and DA_2 receptors. Ibopamine is an effective natriuretic and diuretic in patients with congestive heart failure.

Levodopa

Levodopa has been one of the most widely used prodrugs of DA. It is the immediate precursor of DA and has been used for many years in the treatment of Parkinson's disease. It is decarboxylated (after absorption) into DA. Dose restrictions are necessary when levodopa is given alone because α-adrenergic activity can occur in higher oral doses. For this reason, it is most often combined with carbidopa, which inhibits peripheral carboxylase activity allowing therapeutic CNS levels of DA without the peripheral vascular side-effects. Oral levodopa has been used effectively in treating patients with advanced heart failure.[221] The effects noted are an increase in SV, decrease in vascular resistance, and little change in HR or blood pressure. The effects are similar to those noted in patients receiving low-dose DA. Decreased NE release may be a factor in producing vasodilatation.

Dobutamine

Dobutamine (DBT) is a synthetic catecholamine modified from the classic inodilator isoproterenol. Isoproterenol was, in turn, synthesized from dopamine. Variations and similarities in structure can be seen in Figure 12-7. Isoproterenol, the parent drug of DBT, is a potent nonselective β_1 and β_2 agonist that increases HR and contractility while reducing vascular resistance and diastolic pressure. Deleterious side-effects include serious cardiac arrhythmias, tachycardia, and reduced coronary artery perfusion. Increased myocardial oxygen demand with only a modest improvement in CO makes isoproterenol an unattractive drug for many situations, especially ischemic heart failure. It does remain useful in the temporary management of third-degree heart block, asthma, and some forms of cor pulmonale and heart transplants.

DBT has clear advantages over isoproterenol and dopamine in many clinical situations. It acts directly on β_1 receptors but exerts much weaker β_2 stimulation than isoproterenol. It does not cause NE release or stimulate DA receptors. DBT, unlike isoproterenol or DPX, possesses weak α_1 agonism, which can be unmasked by β blockade as a prompt and dramatic increase in blood pressure.[222] Ordinarily, changes in arterial blood pressure do not occur because the mild α_1 activity is countered by the β_2 activity. DBT produces strong inotropism but with weak chronotropic or vascular effects. Increases in CO are primarily through increased inotropism and secondarily by reduced afterload.

DBT increases automaticity of the SA node and increases conduction through the AV nodes and ventricles. DBT produces less increase in HR per unit gain in CO than dopamine, but it is not devoid of chronotropic activity. Troublesome tachycardias can occur in sensitive individuals and caution should be exercised in patients with established atrial fibrillation or recurrent tachycardias. Early studies found DBT preferable to dopamine,

EPI, or isoproterenol because of its lack of chronotropic effects.[223,224] DBT increases HR more than EPI for a given increase in CO.[225]

DBT may decrease diastolic coronary filling pressure because of its vasodilator properties. However, many animal and human studies show improvement of ischemia and augmentation of myocardial blood flow with DBT.[160] It appears to produce coronary vasodilation in contrast to the constriction produced by dopamine. These studies suggest that DBT produces an overall favorable metabolic climate in the ischemic myocardium despite an increase in inotropism. Improvement is rate-limited. DBT has been used effectively to improve coronary flow to differentiate, by echocardiography, responsive or unresponsive areas of dyskinesia in patients following myocardial infarction.[226]

DBT is highly controllable, with a half-life of 2 minutes. Tachyphylaxis is rare but may be noted if given over 72 hours. The net hemodynamic effects of DBT include an increase in CO, a decrease in left ventricular filling pressure, and a decrease in systemic vascular resistance without a significant increase in chronotropism at lower doses.[227,228] It has been proved to be as effective as combined dopamine and nitroprusside in treating heart failure with infarction. It is even more effective when summed with the dopaminergic properties of DA. In contrast to dopamine, DBT seems to inhibit hypoxic pulmonary vasoconstriction. Like its parent compound isoproterenol, DBT may prove to be useful in managing right ventricular failure as well.

Isoproterenol

Isoproterenol is a potent balanced β_1- and β_2-receptor agonist with no vasoconstrictor effects. It increases HR and contractility while decreasing systemic vascular resistance. Although it can increase CO, it is not useful in shock because it redistributes blood to nonessential areas by its preferential effect on the cutaneous and muscular vessels.[174] As a result, it produces variable and unpredictable results on CO and blood pressure in patients with cardiogenic shock. Isoproterenol is a potent dysrhythmogenic drug and extends myocardial ischemic areas. Deleterious effects on an evolving ischemic process include cardiac dysrhythmias, tachycardia, and reduced diastolic coronary perfusion pressure and time. Increased myocardial oxygen demand with but modest hemodynamic improvement makes it an unattractive drug for patients in shock, especially after acute myocardial infarction.

Isoproterenol is helpful in managing cardiac failure associated with bradycardia, asthma, and cor pulmonale. It is also a useful chemical pacemaker in third-degree heart block until an artificial pacemaker can be inserted or the cause can be removed. Isoproterenol might be useful in treating both idiopathic and secondary pulmonary hypertension.[34,35] It has also been reported as useful in improving the forward flow in patients with regurgitant aortic valvular disease, but it should not be used if there is an accompanying stenosis.[181,182]

COMBINATION THERAPY

Dopamine and DBT are the two most popular primary inodilators in use today. A comparison of these two drugs will underscore the importance of the extracardiac side-effects in selecting a drug either for use alone or in combination.[229] This comparison is particularly appropriate because dopamine and DBT are considered equipotent inotropic agents, and are effective in the same dose range of $2-15~\mu g \cdot kg^{-1} \cdot min^{-1}$. Their differences can be compared at low ($0.5-4~\mu g \cdot kg^{-1} \cdot min^{-1}$), medium ($5-9~\mu g \cdot kg^{-1} \cdot min^{-1}$), and high ($10-15~\mu g \cdot kg^{-1} \cdot min^{-1}$) doses. This comparison will illustrate the divergent effects of two drugs on preload and afterload while sharing the property of inotropism. Although they share several clinical indications, these drugs are pharmacologically distinct and not interchangeable. Their divergent properties, however, make them particularly valuable when used in combination.[230]

DBT is a direct-acting catecholamine that produces a positive inotropic β_1 effect but with minimal changes in β_2 HR or vascular resistance (β_2, α_1 counteraction). Thus, DBT may not alter blood pressure even though CO is markedly improved. Dopamine may do both. Low-dose dopamine can produce hemodynamic changes similar to those of DBT (inotropism and mesenteric vasodilatation) (see Fig. 12-30). Dopamine produces an increase in blood pressure at higher doses related to its direct and indirect α_1 activation. This increased afterload with dopamine may attenuate any further increase in CO comparable to that of an equal dose of DBT.

DBT does not have any clinically important venoconstrictor activity, in contrast to dopamine in which an increase in ventricular filling pressure can be noted at low doses. This contrasting effect on preload is seen in Figure 12-31. The cardiac response to all vasodilators is dependent upon the pre-existing preload status. Patients who have acute failure with normal or only slightly elevated end-diastolic volumes may not respond to afterload reduction with an increase in CO. Balanced vasodilators such as nitroprusside or venodilators such as the nitrates may actually reduce CO in these patients. Patients with dilated left ventricles and elevated filling pressures usually exhibit impressive improvement in CO with afterload reduction. This underscores the importance of monitored volume loading before proceeding apace with vasoactive drugs (Table 12-18). It is possible, indeed likely, that a portion of the reduced effectiveness of long-term vasodilator therapy results from inadequate preload, which in some circumstances can actually be a consequence of successful drug therapy.[231] Clinical studies suggest that DBT is less likely to increase HR than dopamine for a given dose, which is a major concern in the patient with coronary artery disease. DBT is a coronary artery dilator, whereas dopamine is not. A dopamine-induced tachycardia, however, may be of less concern in the septic patient who commonly has a maldistribution of volume, low vascular resistance, and a pre-existing refractory tachycardia but a previously healthy heart. The empirical preference of dopamine in surgical units and DBT in coronary units has been observed and is perhaps well founded. The surgical patient is more likely to have distributive defects and fluid shifts from major trauma and surgery. The hemodynamics of the septic patient are characterized by low vascular resistance, hypotension, high CO, and some degree of myocardial depression. The renal, distributive, inotropic, and pressor effects of dopamine would seem ideal for this condition. However, a shift of blood volume to the central circulation, tachycardia, or an unpredictable increase in afterload may not be appropriate for the patient in congestive heart failure or the patient with an acute infarct (Fig. 12-28). DBT, with its dose-related inotropism, afterload reduction, and relative lack of chronotropism would seem more appropriate for these circumstances.

Dobutamine does not cause NE release or stimulate DA receptors. Dopamine does both, but the effect is dose-related. The dopaminergic effects of increased renal perfusion is seen at low doses of DA, whereas NE is stimulated only at higher doses. Dopamine offers distinctive advantages over many sympathomimetics in managing the low-output syndrome with oliguria. This effect is ablated at higher doses. DBT does not selectively increase renal blood flow but, like DPX, does improve renal blood flow secondarily with improved CO and weak β_2 vasodilation. Much of the reduced afterload observed with the use of DBT may be related more to a reduced sympathetic tone with improved flow than to active vasodilatation. DBT belongs on the opposite end of the spectrum from amrinone. DBT is a potent inotropic agent but a weak vasodilator, whereas amrinone is a potent vasodilator but a weak inotrope.

Dopamine and DBT also have contrasting effects on the pulmonary vasculature. Dopamine has been noted to increase pulmonary artery pressure and does not inhibit the pulmonary hypoxic response. It is not recommended for patients in right heart failure. DBT does vasodilate the pulmonary vasculature and is helpful in treating right heart failure and cor pulmonale.[36] The adrenergic effects of combined sympathomimetics, like the solo drugs, also appear to be additive and competitive for receptor sites. Many combinations of adrenergic drugs have been described as having a synergistic effect. Synergism is the joint action of agents such that their combined effect is greater than the algebraic sum of their individual effects. This synergism may be a clinical interpretation of a summed receptor effect that appears synergistic. For example, infusions of the combination of dopamine and DBT have been noted to produce a greater improvement in CO, at lower doses, than can be achieved by either drug alone. Although equipotent inotropic agents, each drug dilates different vascular beds. Therefore, the summation of afterload reduction by both drugs could produce a greater improvement in CO than could be achieved by either drug alone, even at the same level of inotropism. Summation is more consistent with current receptor pharmacology and can be used to advantage in selectively avoiding unwanted side-effects of one drug while supplementing its desired attributes with another. The summation principle obviates the necessity of knowing a large number of drugs. One need become familiar with but a few agents to manage most clinical situations.

Because of summation, many combinations of vasoactive drugs have been found useful in making fine hemodynamic adjustments in the critically ill. The available sympathomimetic agents provide a wide range of hemodynamic effects, particularly when combined with vasodilators. For example, if a larger positive inotropic action and less vasoconstriction are desired, DBT could be added to dopamine. Also, nitroprusside could be added to dopamine or combined with any other appropriate inodilator.[232] Combinations are also useful in redistributing the CO to vital organs. This is why the combination of DBT and dopamine has been helpful. Dopamine could distribute the CO to the renal and mesenteric vascular bed, while DBT could provide additional afterload reduction by opening up the vascular beds of skin and muscle[233,234] (Fig. 12-32). NE has been successfully used in combination with dopamine to increase vascular resistance in septic patients while distributing a greater portion of the CO to the renal and mesenteric bed.[233]

The studied use of adrenergic combinations in patients with cardiac failure has been proposed because pathophysiology cannot be approached with the attitude that β agonism is all good and α agonism is all bad. The objective is to increase coronary perfusion and CO while decreasing afterload. This is the effect achieved by the intra-aortic balloon pump. No single vasoactive agent can achieve this, but these conditions can be approached with combination therapy. Because of receptor summation during combination therapy, standard rates of infusion (as outlined in Table 12-19) no longer apply. Invasive hemodynamic monitoring is mandatory for success; otherwise, iatrogenic disasters can be expected. Other conditions necessary for success with vasoactive drugs also require that the failing myocardium or vasculature have functional reserve, that the reserve can be stimulated, and that perfusion can be maintained.[235,236]

Tocolytics

Tocolytic simply means to stop labor. Preterm labor is defined as labor before 37 weeks gestation. It occurs in 7–10% of all births. Eighty-five percent of early neonatal deaths unrelated to lethal abnormalities are associated with premature labor.[237,238]

Contraindications to tocolysis are intrauterine infection, unexplained vaginal bleeding, and fetal distress. Tocolysis is often initiated in an attempt to prolong gestation to allow fetal maturation and reduce the complications of a premature birth. Bed

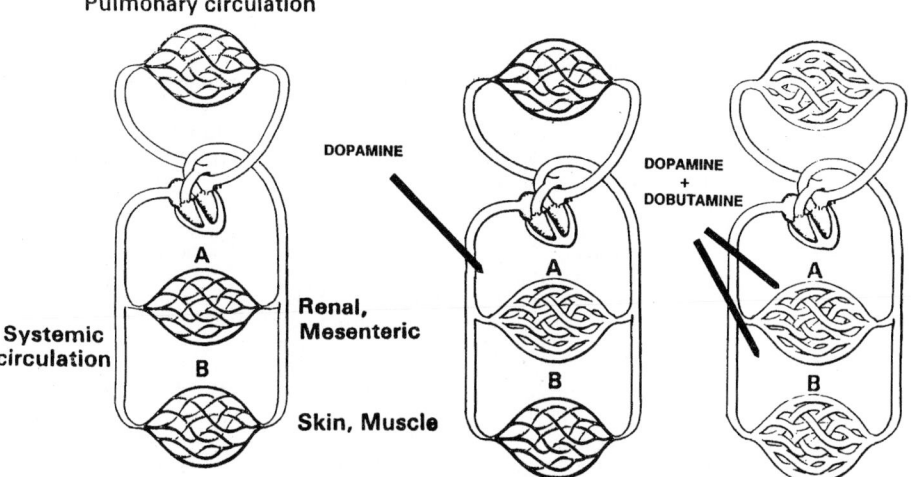

Figure 12-32. Combining low doses of dopamine and dobutamine may produce improvements in CO that are greater than can be achieved with either drug alone. This appears to be clinical synergism. However, the vasodilation of different vascular beds likely produces a summed reduction of afterload at the same level of inotropism that only appears to be synergistic. The second law of thermodynamics remains intact.

rest and hydration, often recommended, have not proved effective in halting premature labor.

Various pharmacologic agents have been used to decrease stimulus to the myometrium (alcohol) or prevent myometrial response to stimuli. Drugs belonging to the latter category include opioids, magnesium sulfate, prostaglandin inhibitors, and calcium channel inhibitors. β Agonists have now become the focus of research in this area.[239] The principal action of these drugs is to stimulate β_2 receptors of the myometrium and produce relaxation (Table 12-5).[238]

Ethanol was the earliest effective tocolytic and was used to reduce stimuli to the myometrium. It inhibits the release of oxytocin from the posterior pituitary. Intoxication of both the mother and fetus prohibited its extensive use.

Metaproterenol and isoxsuprine were the first β agonists to be used successfully. Unfortunately, these drugs are equipotent β_1 and β_2 agonists, and the side-effects of tachycardia and hypotension were unacceptable.[240,241] A second generation of β-adrenergic drugs was applied in which the predominant action is β_2. Ritodrine and terbutaline are seeing widespread use as tocolytic agents because of their predominant β_2 agonism, which minimizes the undesirable β_1 effects. Ritodrine is the only β-agonist tocolytic currently approved in the United States. It was specifically synthesized for this purpose and is structurally related to EPI.

All β-agonist tocolytic agents have both β_1 and β_2 properties but in different proportions. The circulatory effects vary from one drug to another, depending on the degree of β_1 stimulation. Table 12-18 compares the β_1 cardiovascular effects of ritodrine and terbutaline while being used as tocolytics in humans. The side-effects of these drugs may result in serious consequences. Predictable complications in pregnant women include hyperglycemia with resultant hypokalemia (see Table 12-5).[29] All manner of cardiac dysrhythmias have been described, including ischemia and chest pain. The occurrence of pulmonary edema following the use of β-agonist tocolytics with and without corticosteroids has been described, although the mechanism is not clear.[242,243] Table 12-19 outlines contraindications for the use of β agents for inhibiting labor.[244]

Table 12-20 lists the drugs that have been used as tocolytics. The majority of these prevent myometrial response to stimuli. There are no data suggesting that any of these tocolytics is effective for more than 48 hours. They may buy time for fetal lung maturation with steroids, but otherwise they are not reliable or consistent tocolystics long-term. Without a clear therapeutic advantage, the side-effects of tocolytic drugs will often determine the choice in a given patient.

Myometrial smooth muscle is endowed with both α and β receptors. β Agonists have become the focus of research in this

area. The principal action of β_2 agonists is to stimulate the β_2 receptors of the myometrium and produce relaxation. α-Adrenergic agonists increase uterine activity. However, the direct or indirect effects of the natural catecholamines on uterine activity remain unclear as both epinephrine and norepinephrine levels are markedly increased during labor. Epidural analgesia modifies this pattern, with a marked reduction in epinephrine levels but no change in norepinephrine. Epinephrine and norepinephrine are mixed α and β agonists whose effects are dose-dependent. Norepinephrine appears to stimulate uterine contraction *via* α-adrenergic receptors. The effect of epinephrine varies according to concentration.

Nonadrenergic Sympathomimetic Agents

Table 12-4 classifies the drugs that mimic the SNS into two broad categories, adrenergic or nonadrenergic. Adrenergic agonists exert their action through adrenergic receptors by direct stimulation or indirectly *via* release of NE. Adrenergic agonists may be catecholamines or noncatecholamines by chemical configuration. Nonadrenergic sympathomimetic drugs also act indirectly by influencing the cAMP–calcium cascade, exclusive of the receptors (see Fig. 12-15). The functions of the second messenger (cAMP) and the third messenger (Ca^{2+}) nearly always go together.[245] This concept reinforces the recent appreciation of the homogeneity of action of a wide variety of drugs previously thought to be unrelated. Sympathomimetics have more pharmacologic similarities than differences.

Adenosine. Adenosine, which has been around for more than 50 years, has only recently been recognized as a clinically useful drug. A by-product of ATP, it is composed of adenine and a pentose sugar. It is found in every cell in the body. Production can be increased by stimuli such as hypoxia and ischemia.[246,247] It can combine with one, two, or three phosphates to form AMP, ADP, or ATP, respectively. This ubiquitous nucleoside has potent electrophysiologic effects in addition to having a major role in regulation of vasomotor tone. Adenosine is believed to have a cardioprotective effect by regulating oxygen supply and demand. The cardiovascular effects of adenosine depend upon which of two receptor sites is activated, α_1 or α_2.[246,248] The α_1 receptors in the myocardial conduction system are the most sensitive; they mediate SA node slowing and AV nodal conduction delay. The α_1 receptor inhibits production of cAMP whose formation is stimulated by β-adrenergic activity (see Table 12-7). The α_2 smooth muscle receptors require higher concentrations of adenosine; they mediate systemic and coronary vasodilatation. The α_2 receptor directly increases the rate of formation of cAMP (Table 12-7) and functions independently of β activity. Intravenous adenosine, therefore, has significant negative chronotropic effects on the SA node as well

Table 12-20. TOCOLYTICS

Tocolytic Agent	Route of Administration and Dosage*	Efficacy†	Major Maternal Side-Effects	Major Fetal or Neonatal Side-Effects
Ethanol	No longer used	Effective	Alcoholic intoxication	May cause alcohol toxicity
Nitroglycerin	10–50 mg td every day	Unproved	Hypotension, headache	Fetal tachycardia
	100-μg bolus iv, then 1–10-μg · kg^{-1} · min^{-1} iv infusion	Unproved		
Magnesium sulfate	4–6-g iv bolus, then 2–3 g · h^{-1} iv infusion	Effective	Nausea, weakness, ileus, headache, hypotension, pulmonary edema, cardiorespiratory arrest; may cause hypocalcemia	Decreased fetal heart-rate variability, neonatal hypotonia; may cause ileus and congenital ricketic syndrome (especially with treatment 3 wk)
	Maintenance, 100–120 mg orally every 4 hr	Not effective		

β-ADRENERGIC AGONISTS

Ritodrine hydrochloride‡	50 μg · min^{-1} iv infusion (max 350 μg · min^{-1})	Effective	Jitteriness, anxiety, nausea, restlessness, vomiting, rash, cardiac arrhythmias, chest pain, myocardial ischemia, palpitations, hypostension, tachycardia (more common with isoxsuprine), pulmonary edema, paralytic ileus, hypokalemia, hyperglycemia, acidosis	Fetal tachycardia, hypotension, ileus, hyperinsulinemia, hypoglycemia (more common with isoxsuprine), hyperbilirubinemia, hypocalcemia; may cause hydrops fetalis
	5–10 mg im every 2–4 hr	Effective		
	Maintenance, 10–20 mg orally every 3–4 hr	Not effective		
Isoxsuprine hydrochloride	0.05–.5 mg · min^{-1} iv	Effective		
	10 mg orally every 8–12 hr	May be effective		
Terbutaline sulfate	2 μg · min^{-1} iv infusion (max 80 μg · min^{-1})	Effective		
	0.25 mg sc every 20 min	Effective		
	Maintenance, 2.5–5 mg orally every 4–6 hr	Not effective		
	0.05 ml · h^{-1} iv pump	Not effective		

PROSTAGLANDIN INHIBITORS

Indomethacin	25–50 mg orally every 4–6 hr	Effective / Effective	Gastrointestinal effects (nausea, heartburn), rash, headache, interstitial nephritis, increased bleeding time (more common with aspirin)	Transient oliguria and oligohydramnios, premature closure of the neonatal ductus arteriosus, pulmonary hypertension; may cause necrotizing enterocolitis and intracerebral hemorrhage
Naproxen	100 mg rectally every 12 hr	Effective		
Fenoprofen	375–500 mg orally every 6 hr	Effective		
	200–300 mg orally every 6 hr			

CALCIUM-CHANNEL BLOCKERS

Nifedipine	20–30 mg orally every 4–8 hr	Effective	Hypotension, tachycardia, headache, nausea, flushing, potentiation of the cardiac depressive effect of magnesium sulfate, hepatotoxicity	

OXYTOCIN-RECEPTOR ANTAGONIST

Atosiban	1 μM · min^{-1} iv infusion (maximum, 32 μM · min^{-1})	Effective	Nausea, headache, chest pain, arthralgias; may cause inhibition of lactation	Unknown

PHOSPHODIESTERASE INHIBITOR

Aminophylline	200 mg orally every 6–8 hr	May be effective		
	0.5–0.7 mg · kg^{-1} · h^{-1} iv	May be effective		

* iv = intravenous; sc = subcutaneous; im = intramuscular; td = transdermal.
† Efficacy is defined as the ability to delay delivery by 24–48 hours.
‡ Ritodrine hydrochloride is the only tocolytic agent approved by the Food and Drug Administration.

as negative dromotropism on the AV node. Thus, adenosine regulates atrial and ventricular rates independently of each other.

Adenosine hyperpolarizes atrial myocytes and decreases their action potential duration via an increase in outward K$^+$ current. These are the acetylcholine-regulated K$^+$ channels.[246] Adenosine mimics the effects of acetylcholine in many ways, including an extremely short plasma half-life of mere seconds. Adenosine also antagonizes the inward Ca^{2+} current produced by catecholamines. This antidysrhythmic mechanism of Ca^{2+} channel blockade is thought to be an indirect effect and important only when β stimulation is present. This trait suggests a possible role in countering catecholamine-induced dysrhythmia. Thus, adenosine exhibits some of the traits of a Class IV antidysrhythmic. However, the primary antidysrhythmic effect of adenosine is to

interrupt re-entrant AV nodal tachycardia, which most likely relates to its K$^+$ current, rather than Ca^{2+} current effects. The chief indication for adenosine is paroxysmal supraventricular tachycardia (PSVT), which it may terminate in a matter of seconds. PSVT refers to a broad category of narrow complex tachycardias with acute onset and cessation. The most common forms are AV nodal re-entry tachycardia and AV reciprocating tachycardia. PSVT accounts for about one third of all cases of perioperative dysrhythmia. Clinical studies support the use of adenosine for the treatment of W-P-W syndrome and other re-entrant tachycardias involving the AV node.[249] The same characteristics that make adenosine an effective therapeutic agent may also make it an ideal agent for diagnosing other types of dysrhythmia. The incidence of incorrect diagnosis of supraventricular dysrhythmia has been reported to be as high as 15% using conventional means.[250] This can lead to utilization of harmful medications. For example, a broad complex tachycardia can either be a VT or an SVT with aberrant conduction. Verapamil can be fatal if the dysrhythmia is VT because the drug is long-lasting.[251,252] However, the fleeting action (9–10 seconds) of adenosine assures that no harm will be done if the broad complex is of ventricular origin, providing a combined therapeutic and diagnostic test. Adenosine will stop SVT in 90% of cases in which the AV node forms one of the limbs of the re-entrant circuit, such as AV reciprocating tachycardia and AV nodal re-entry[248]; 60% will convert with the first dose. However, adenosine has no effect on ectopic atrial dysrhythmia such as ectopic foci, multifocal SVT, or flutter/fibrillation.[258] Approximately 10% of SVT do not involve AV nodal re-entry. Adenosine will nevertheless slow AV nodal conduction in these cases, decrease the ventricular rate, and allow inspection of P waves. Thus, adenosine may be useful in unmasking atrial fibrillation when fast ventricular responses are noted.

A number of side-effects have been reported with the use of adenosine, including flushing, headache, dyspnea, bronchospasm, and chest pain. The majority of these are brief (seconds) and not clinically significant. Transient new dysrhythmia (65%) will be noted at the time of cardioversion, but these disappear during the half-life of the drug. Major hemodynamic changes are rare but consist of hypotension and bradycardia. Adenosine should be given by means of a rapid iv bolus with flush because of its extremely short half-life of less than 10 seconds. The initial adult dose is 6 mg (100–150 $\mu g \cdot kg^{-1}$ pediatrics), which can be followed by 12 mg within 1–2 minutes if the initial dose is without effect.[250] The 12-mg dose may be repeated once. The antidysrhythmic effect of adenosine occurs as soon as the drug reaches the AV node.[251]

Xanthines. The clinically important xanthine is theophylline ethylenediamine (aminophylline).[181] Caffeine is a socially important xanthine. Aminophylline has been the mainstay in the treatment of asthma and bronchospasm since 1902 because of its strong β_2 mimetic effect. EPI, isoproterenol, and ephedrine are used to treat asthma for the same reason. Levels of cAMP in the cell are governed by a magnesium-dependent phosphodiesterase (PDE). This enzyme catalyzes the second messenger $3',5'$-cAMP to the less active $5'$-cAMP. Three major PDE enzymes have been discovered, designated as PDE I, PDE II, and PDE III.[102,253] The xanthines are nonspecific PDE inhibitors that interact with all three types. Inhibition of PDE results in increased levels of cAMP and β response. Increases in cAMP by this mechanism are important when reviewing the many complicated interactions of the xanthines in the clinical setting.

Catecholamines influence the accumulation of cAMP by activating adenyl cyclase. Increased catecholamine levels, combined with the xanthines, may lead to synergistic adrenergic activity by increasing production and reducing breakdown of cAMP. Cardiac dysrhythmias are common in such circumstances and are further potentiated during general anesthesia with halothane.[254] Serious cardiac dysrhythmia and arrest have been produced with this combination when it has not been carefully controlled.

Intravenous aminophylline produces an increase in CO as a result of its positive inotropic and chronotropic effects. It also reduces afterload by its β_2-vasodilating effect. The cardiac-stimulating effects are still manifest in the presence of β blockade because the xanthines are not receptor-dependent for their agonism. Thus, they may be temporarily useful in those situations in which excessive β blockade has been produced.[29] The inotropic effects are short-lived, lasting 20–30 minutes. Care must be taken during infusion because common side-effects include hypotension and dysrhythmia. Seizures have also been reported.[254]

Phosphodiesterase Inhibitors. A new group of drugs has been developed that have pharmacologic properties approaching the characteristics of the ideal inotropic agent (see Table

12-17).[176,255] They do not rely on stimulation of β and/or α receptors. They are the product of a search for a nonglycosidic, noncatecholamine inotropic agent. These drugs combine positive inotropism with vasodilator activity; like the xanthines, they are PDE inhibitors but differ in that they selectively inhibit PDE III.[102,253] PDE I and II hydrolyze all cyclic nucleotides, whereas PDE III acts specifically on cAMP. The PDE III inhibitors apparently interact with PDE III at the cell membrane and impede the breakdown of cAMP.[102,256] cAMP levels increase and protein kinases are activated to promote phosphorylation of the SR in a cascade manner similar to the effects of adrenergic drugs. In cardiac muscle, phosphorylation increases the slow inward movement of calcium current, promoting increased intracellular calcium stores. Thus, inotropism increases. In vascular smooth muscle, increased cAMP activity accounts for the vasodilation, decreased peripheral vascular resistance, and lusitropism. Amrinone, like nitroprusside and nitroglycerin, promotes diastolic relaxation, which promotes ventricular filling.[161,257]

A variety of PDE inhibitors are undergoing clinical trials.[257,258] The relative contribution of inotropism and vasodilation differs with each. Amrinone and milrinone are the only PDE inhibitors released for clinical use in the United States. Amrinone is the prototypical PDE III inhibitor. The degree of hemodynamic effect of these drugs depends on the dose, degree of inotropic reserve, and state of cAMP depletion.

AMRINONE. Amrinone is a bipyridine derivative that produces mild inotropic activity and strong vasodilatory effects. The characteristics of amrinone, compared with those of the ideal inotropic agent (Table 12-17), rank it near the ideal drug. It is the first oral inotrope available since the introduction of digitalis.[256,257] However, it is not currently prescribed in its oral form. Studies of single-dose and short-term oral and iv amrinone show dose-related improvements at rest in the cardiac index and the left ventricular stroke index (40–80% increase); left ventricular end-diastolic pressure (40% decrease); pulmonary capillary wedge pressure (16–44% decrease); pulmonary artery pressure (17–33% decrease); right atrial pressure (16–44% decrease); left ventricular ejection fraction (50% increase); and systemic vascular resistance (23–50% decrease). Significantly, HR and mean arterial pressure are not affected. Hemodynamic improvement is also noted when amrinone is used in combination with hydralazine. The improvement is greater than with either drug alone. Peak response with an iv dose occurs after 5 minutes and reveals no evidence of tolerance over short-term trials (24 hours); it is compatible with other adrenergic agonists. It is an effective inotropic agent in patients receiving β blockers. Its efficacy in the patient who has been digitalized has been demonstrated.

Intravenous amrinone therapy should be initiated with a 0.75 $mg \cdot kg^{-1}$ bolus given over 2–3 minutes. It is continued with a maintenance infusion of 5–10 $\mu g \cdot kg^{-1} \cdot min^{-1}$, adjusted by hemodynamic monitoring. An additional bolus dose of 0.75 $mg \cdot kg^{-1}$ may be given 30 minutes after initiation of therapy. Care must be taken not to give the bolus too quickly because sudden decreases in peripheral vascular resistance may occur and result in severe hypotension. Hypotension is not a major clinical problem with appropriate monitoring of ventricular filling pressures. The infusion should not exceed a total daily dose of 10 $mg \cdot kg^{-1}$, including the bolus doses. Amrinone has the same range of infusion rates as dopamine and DBT, and dose calculation follows the "rule of six" described in Table 12-19.

Amrinone has two uncommon side-effects. Dose-related thrombocytopenia occurs in some patients taking long-term oral medication. This usually responds to dose reduction. Acute iv amrinone has not produced thrombocytopenia.[258–261] Centrilobular hepatic necrosis occurs in dogs given high doses of amrinone for periods exceeding 3 months. There is no evidence of such an effect in humans, but the implications of using halothane in a patient on amrinone are obvious. If the side-effects do not prove troublesome, this will be a valuable drug.

It has a therapeutic index of approximately 100:1 compared with 1.2:1 with the digitalis glycosides.

MILRINONE. Milrinone is a bipyridine inotropic agent that is a derivative of amrinone.[262] It has nearly 20 times the inotropic potency of the parent compound. Milrinone is active both intravenously and orally and has beneficial short-term hemodynamic effects in patients with severe refractory congestive heart failure. Improvement of CO appears to result from a combination of enhanced myocardial contractility and peripheral vasodilation. Treatment with oral milrinone for up to 11 months has been effective and well tolerated without evidence of fever, thrombocytopenia, or gastrointestinal effects.[263,264] Milrinone recently has been approved for short-term iv therapy of congestive heart failure.[265] It is administered with a loading dose of 50 $\mu g \cdot kg^{-1}$ over 10 minutes. The maintenance iv infusion rate ranges from a minimum of 0.375 $\mu g \cdot kg^{-1} \cdot min^{-1}$ to a maximum of 0.75 $\mu g \cdot kg^{-1} \cdot min^{-1}$ (not to exceed 1.13 $\mu g \cdot kg^{-1} \cdot day^{-1}$). Dosage must be adjusted in renal failure patients as milrinone is excreted in the urine primarily in unconjugated form.

ENOXIMONE. Enoximone is a newer PDE III inhibitor that has proven beneficial in patients suffering from severely impaired myocardial function.[266] Enoximone is an imidazole derivative structurally unrelated to digitalis, catecholamines, or amrinone. It has not been implicated in platelet compromise. Its hemodynamic effects are similar to those produced by amrinone. It appears to be a more potent inotropic agent than amrinone, whose inotropic effect has been questioned. It produced pulmonary and systemic arteriolar vasodilation and can thus be classified as an inodilator. Any increase in myocardial oxygen consumption (MVO_2) by the increase in inotropism is countered by a decrease in afterload and reduced ventricular size. The drug has been administered by both the bolus technique and infusion. It has been used primarily in patients with cardiogenic shock and for weaning from cardiopulmonary bypass. Its use was instituted in patients who were proven refractory to catecholamine therapy. A definitive dosing therapy has not been established but several studies have given a 1–2 $mg \cdot kg^{-1}$ bolus followed by an infusion of 3–10 $\mu g \cdot kg^{-1} \cdot min^{-1}$. In all cases CI and SV increased with a decrease in ventricular filling pressure, SVR, and PVR. No increase in heart rate was noted. The bolus technique alone has been helpful in weaning patients from cardiopulmonary bypass without affecting heart rate or producing arrhythmias.

Glucagon. Glucagon is a single-chain polypeptide of 29 amino acids that is secreted by pancreas α cells in response to hypoglycemia. The liver and kidney are responsible for its degradation. Known effects of this hormone in humans include the following:[181,267]

1. Inhibition of gastric motility
2. Enhanced urinary excretion of inorganic electrolyte
3. Increased insulin secretion
4. Hepatic glycogenolysis and gluconeogenesis
5. Anorexia
6. Inotropic and chronotropic cardiac effects

Little attention was given to glucagon until 1968, when it was demonstrated to produce positive inotropic and chronotropic effects in the canine heart. Glucagon, by activation of Gs-type G protein (Table 12-7), enhances the activation of adenyl cyclase in a manner similar to that of NE, EPI, and isoproterenol. These cardiac actions of glucagon are not blocked by β blockade or catecholamine depletion. Glucagon, in contrast to the xanthines, rarely causes dysrhythmia, even in the face of ischemic heart disease, hypokalemia, and digitalis toxicity. Glucagon may possess antidysrhythmic activity in digitalis toxicity because it has been shown to enhance AV nodal conduction in patients with varying degrees of AV block. It should be used carefully in patients with atrial fibrillation. In humans, an iv dose of 1–5 mg of glucagon increases cardiac index, mean arterial pressure, and ventricular contractility, even in the presence of digitalis therapy. Glucagon can be mixed in 5% dextrose in water and is stable for long periods. After a bolus dose, its action dissipates in approximately 30 minutes. A continuous infusion of 5 $\mu g \cdot kg^{-1} \cdot min^{-1}$ is augmented by an initial bolus of 50 $\mu g \cdot kg^{-1}$. Onset of action occurs in 1–3 minutes and peaks at 10–15 minutes.

Nausea and vomiting are common side-effects in the awake patient, especially following a bolus dose. Hypokalemia, hypoglycemia, and hyperglycemia are also seen. Despite the obvious benefits of glucagon in cardiac patients, its use has not become popular. This may be related to its high cost and the multiple metabolic and physiologic effects that are common after its administration.

This pancreatic hormone may be of benefit when more conventional approaches have proved refractory in the following settings: (1) low CO syndrome following cardiopulmonary bypass, (2) low CO syndrome with myocardial infarction, (3) chronic congestive heart failure, and (4) excessive β-adrenergic blockade.

Digitalis Glycosides. The most important actions of the digitalis glycosides are those affecting myocardial contractility, conduction, and rhythm. The glycoside most likely to be used by the anesthesiologist is digoxin. The principal uses of digoxin are for the treatment of congestive heart failure and to control supraventricular cardiac dysrhythmia such as atrial fibrillation. Digoxin is one of the few positive inotropes that does not increase HR. Digoxin enhances myocardial inotropism and automaticity but slows impulse propagation through the conduction tissues.[268] Despite nearly two centuries of use, its mechanism of action is only modestly certain. Digitalis reciprocally facilitates calcium entry into the myocardial cell by blocking the Na^+, K^+-adenosine triphosphatase pump.[269] This calcium influx may account for its positive inotropic action because this inotropic response is not catecholamine- or β-receptor–dependent and is therefore effective in patients taking β-blocking drugs. The inhibition of this enzyme transport mechanism also results in a net K^+ loss from the myocardial cell. This contributes to digitalis toxicity with hypokalemia. Calcium potentiates the toxic effects of digitalis. Extreme caution should be observed when calcium is given to a patient taking digitalis or when digitalis administration is contemplated in the patient with hypercalcemia.

A common indication for the glycosides is in the chronic management of cardiac tachydysrhythmias. Cardiac dysrhythmias are, paradoxically, their most common side-effect. Synchrony of the cardiac beat is an important determinant of CO, and digoxin can be beneficial when heart failure is caused by a tachydysrhythmia, even in ischemic myocardial disease. However, the use of β or calcium channel blockers is increasing in this regard because they both reduce overall myocardial oxygen consumption. The positive inotropic effects of digoxin are potentially beneficial in selected cases of the low CO syndrome. Digoxin produces a dose-related increase in contractility in both normal and failing hearts. Limits are imposed on the upper reaches of inotropism by the development of serious dysrhythmia.

Confusion has arisen in the past about whether digitalis increases or decreases myocardial oxygen consumption. This was based on the observation that the increased inotropism of digoxin increases MVO_2 in patients with normal hearts but decreases it in patients with heart failure. The tension developed within the ventricular wall is a prime determinant of oxygen consumption. By augmenting contractility, wall tension and MVO_2 at any given afterload will be decreased, with a reduction in ventricular radius and HR.[235] This may underlie the clinical observation that angina is often decreased by digoxin in patients with cardiomegaly, whereas angina may be markedly increased by digitalis in patients with ischemic disease without cardiomegaly.

Digitalis tends to increase the tone of the peripheral resistance vessels in normal subjects by a direct vasoconstrictor effect. Untreated congestive heart failure is accompanied by high peripheral vascular resistance owing to compensatory SNS activation. Successful treatment with digitalis usually reduces resistance as increased contractility improves CO. This is the result of SNS release associated with improved cardiac function. Caution must be exercised, however, in giving iv digoxin or ouabain in a setting in which an increase in afterload would be deleterious. An immediate peripheral vasoconstrictor effect can occur, producing a transient worsening of congestive heart failure. Inconsistent hemodynamic benefit has occurred with digitalis in congestive heart failure following myocardial infarction. It has been of no benefit in cardiogenic shock and has proved potentially injurious in patients with uncomplicated myocardial infarction because of its vasoconstrictive properties and effects on myocardial oxygen consumption in the absence of cardiomegaly.

Digoxin is of potential value in patients with signs and symptoms of congestive heart failure caused by ischemic, valvular, hypertensive, and congenital heart disease. Patients with cardiomyopathies and cor pulmonale may also benefit. Care must be taken to rule out conditions in which the use of digitalis is of no benefit and is potentially harmful. These include mitral stenosis with normal sinus rhythm and constrictive pericarditis with tamponade. Signs and symptoms of idiopathic hypertrophic subaortic stenosis are often exacerbated by digitalis. With increased strength of contraction, the muscular obstruction can be markedly increased. The same is true for the use of digitalis in patients with infundibular pulmonic stenosis, as occurs with tetralogy of Fallot. Any augmentation of contractility may further reduce an already diminished pulmonary blood flow. Beware of digitalis toxic reactions in the older age group and in patients suffering from arterial hypoxemia, acidosis, renal compromise, hypothyroidism, hypokalemia, or hypomagnesemia as well as in patients receiving quinidine or calcium channel blockers. In patients with diminished cardiac reserve who are about to undergo major surgical procedures the issue of prophylactic digitalization remains controversial.[268,269] Indications for preoperative digitalis in which the prophylactic administration of digoxin should be considered include the following: (1) previous heart failure, (2) increased heart size, (3) coronary flow disturbances according to electrocardiogram, (4) age over 60 years, (5) age over 50 years before lung surgery, (6) anticipated massive blood loss, (7) atrial flutter or fibrillation, (8) cardiovascular surgery, and (9) rheumatic valvular lesions.

When entertaining the possibility of perioperative digitalis administration, the following points must be considered:

1. Myocardial oxygen balance is threatened in the nonfailing, nondilated heart.
2. The therapeutic-to-toxic ratio of digitalis is narrow.
3. Inotropic drugs that are less toxic and may be stopped immediately are readily available.
4. Verapamil or β blockers are more efficacious for supraventricular tachydysrhythmias not initiated by heart failure.
5. Digitalis may cause serious dysrhythmia in the unstable patient.
6. Serum potassium concentrations may fluctuate in the surgical patient who is critically ill.
7. Any cardiac dysrhythmia that occurs in the presence of digitalis must be considered a toxic phenomenon.

8. Digitalis-induced cardiac dysrhythmias are difficult to treat.
9. Renal compromise will result in toxic effects with standard maintenance doses.
10. Cardioversion may be dangerous after digitalis administration.
11. After initiation of digitalis therapy, the administration of alternative drugs becomes more complicated.

Calcium Salts.   Ringer established the importance of calcium in cardiac contraction more than 150 years ago. It is of great importance in the genesis of the cardiac action potential and is the key to controlling intracellular energy storage and utilization.[270] Movement of extracellular calcium across membranes also governs the function of uterine smooth muscle as well as the smooth muscle of the blood vessels. Only recently have we begun to appreciate the critical role that calcium plays in a wide spectrum of biologic processes, from coagulation to neuromuscular transmission. The sympathomimetic drugs promote the transmembrane influx of calcium, whereas the β blockers and calcium channel blockers inhibit such movement.

Despite its molecular simplicity, calcium is one of the least understood drugs.[271] Calcium chloride is often part of the treatment of ventricular fibrillation, even though the published data to support this indication are scanty. There are data confirming its capability to initiate ventricular fibrillation in a manner similar to that of EPI. Although many of the effects of EPI are mediated by calcium, the two drugs are clearly not identical. The fact that EPI can improve defibrillation success by strengthening the fibrillatory pattern is the apparent basis for the use of calcium salts in this setting. This assumption has not been experimentally or clinically documented.[272] The American Heart Association has recently recommended against the use of calcium during cardiac arrest except when hyperkalemia, hypocalcemia, or calcium-entry inhibitor toxicity is present.[273]

Traditionally, calcium gluconate has been preferred in pediatric patients and calcium chloride in adult patients. Previous data suggested that calcium chloride produced consistently higher and more predictable levels of ionized calcium than an equivalent dose of the other preparations.[274] Recent studies have shown, however, that ionization of any of the preparations is immediate and equally effective.[275,276] Intravenous calcium appears effective for the transient reversal of hypotension thought to be the result of myocardial depression from the potent volatile anesthetic drugs.[277] Some clinicians feel that recurrent intraoperative hypotension response to calcium chloride may be an indication for the administration of digoxin. Calcium chloride is also given at the termination of cardiopulmonary bypass to offset the myocardial depression associated with hypothermic potassium cardioplegia. The use of calcium salts is clearly indicated during rapid or massive transfusions of citrated blood.[278] Citrate binds calcium, and rapid infusion rates of citrated blood result in myocardial depression which is reversible by calcium.

Three forms of calcium salts are available: calcium chloride, calcium gluconate, and calcium gluceptate. Calcium chloride produces only transient (10–20 minutes) increases in CO.[268] If inotropic effects are needed for a longer period of time, other inotropic agents should be selected. Bolus doses of 2–10 $\mu g \cdot kg^{-1}$ ($1.5 \ \mu g \cdot kg^{-1} \cdot min^{-1}$) of calcium chloride can produce moderate improvement in contractility. The rapid administration of calcium salts, if the heart is beating, can produce bradycardia and must be used cautiously in the patient who is digitalized because of the hazard of producing toxic effects. Calcium gluceptate can be given in a dose of 5–7 ml (4.5–6.3 mEq) and calcium gluconate in a dose of 10–15 ml (4.8–7.2 mEq). These doses are approximately equivalent to that suggested for calcium chloride. Calcium gluconate is unstable and is no longer in frequent use. All of the calcium salts will precipitate as calcium carbonate if mixed with sodium bicarbonate.

Antidepressant Drugs

Monoamine Oxidase Inhibitors

Monoamine oxidase inhibitors (MAOIs) and the tricyclic antidepressants are used to treat psychotic depression. These drugs are not used in the practice of anesthesia but are a source of potentially serious interactions in patients who are taking them chronically. Their use is rapidly declining as the nontricyclic antidepressants such as Prozac are more efficacious and produce fewer side-effects. These drugs were a source of potentially serious interactions in the practice of anesthesia. Table 12-21 lists the antidepressants that have been in use and is offered to be historically complete. Few of the MAO inhibitors or tricyclic antidepressants will be encountered in an anesthesia practice today, with the exceptions of phenelzine (Nardil) and amitriptyline (Amitril, Elavil). Their pharmacologic actions and side-effects are a direct result of their effect on the cascade of catecholamine metabolism. The nontricyclics also produce their antidepressant effects *via* this cascade but linked to their inhibition of CNS neuronal uptake of serotonin.

MAOIs (Table 12-21) block the oxidative deamination of endogenous catecholamines into inactive vanillylmandelic acid (see Fig. 12-12). They do not inhibit synthesis.[279] Thus, blockade of monoamine oxidase would produce an accumulation of NE, EPI, dopamine, and 5-hydroxytryptamine in adrenergically active tissues, including the brain. Alleviation of depression may be related to elevations of the endogenous catecholamines. Overdose with MAOIs is expressed as SNS hyperactivity. They may produce agitation, hallucinations, hyperpyrexia, convulsions, hypertension, and hypotension. Orthostatic hypotension is a common complaint in patients taking MAOIs.[280]

The action of sympathomimetic amines is potentiated in patients taking MAOIs. Indirect-acting sympathomimetics (ephedrine, tyramine) produce an exaggerated response as they trigger the release of accumulated catecholamines. Foods with a high tyramine content (cheese, red Italian wine, pickled herring) can also precipitate hypertensive crises.[280] SNS reflex stimulation is also intensified by tyramine. Meperidine has been reported to produce hypertensive crisis, convulsions, and coma with MAO inhibitors. Hepatotoxicity has been reported that does not seem to be related to dosage or duration of treatment. Its incidence is low but remains a factor in selecting anesthesia.

The MAOIs produce long-lasting, irreversible enzyme inhibition that is unrelated to duration of treatment. Regeneration of monoamine oxidase may therefore take weeks and has much the same effect on adrenergic metabolism as organophosphates on the cholinesterase system. MAOIs are known to intensify CNS depression caused by ethanol, analgesics, and general anesthesia. The depressive mechanism is not known.

The anesthetic management of patients taking MAOIs remains controversial, although recent data question the need to discontinue them preoperatively. Currently, recommendations for management include discontinuation of the drugs for at least 2 weeks before surgery. However, this recommendation is not based on controlled studies but rather is the result of limited case reports that suggest potent drug interactions.[279,281,282] A small number of studies found few adverse effects in humans taking MAOIs given analgesics, opioid anesthesia, or regional blocks. However, opioids that cause release of catecholamines (meperidine) should be avoided in these patients.

Symptoms of SNS overdose or interactions due to MAOIs can be treated effectively with α blockers, ganglionic blockers, or direct-acting vasodilators. Tricyclic antidepressants should not be substituted for the MAOIs in the perioperative period. Adverse CNS interactions similar to those encountered with the indirect sympathomimetic amines have been reported. A 2-week washout period is recommended before introducing tricyclic antidepressants to a patient taking an MAOI.

Tricyclic Antidepressants

This group of antidepressant drugs is referred to as tricyclic antidepressants because of their structure. The important tricyclic antidepressants are listed in Table 12-21. These drugs have almost replaced the MAOIs because they cause fewer side-effects.[279] The manner in which the tricyclic antidepressants relieve depression is not clear, but all of these agents block uptake of NE into adrenergic nerve endings. Just as with the MAOIs, high doses of the tricyclic antidepressants can induce seizure activity that is responsive to diazepam.

Neuroleptic drugs may potentiate the effects of tricyclic antidepressants by competition with metabolism in the liver. Chronic barbiturate use increases metabolism of the tricyclic antidepressants by microsomal enzyme induction. Other sedatives, however, potentiate the tricyclic antidepressants in a manner similar to that occurring with the MAOIs. Atropine also has an exaggerated effect because of the anticholinergic effect of tricyclic antidepressants. Prolonged sedation from thiopental has been reported. Ketamine may also be dangerous in patients taking tricyclic antidepressants by producing acute hypertension and cardiac dysrhythmia. Likewise, muscle relaxants that produce tachycardia (pancuronium, gallamine) have been observed to produce serious ventricular cardiac dysrhythmia in humans and dogs pretreated with imipramine.

Despite these serious interactions, discontinuation of these drugs before surgery is probably unnecessary. The latency of onset of these drugs is from 2 to 5 weeks; however, the excretion of tricyclic antidepressants is rapid, with approximately 70% of a dose appearing in the urine during the first 72 hours. One might consider a discontinuation of the drug for 72 hours, but the risk of recurrent depression may be greater than that of any untoward drug reaction. The long latency period for resumption of treatment militates against interrupted treatment. A thorough knowledge of the possible drug interactions and autonomic countermeasures obviates postponement.

Nontricyclic Antidepressants

The nontricyclic antidepressants are listed in Table 12-21. Their mechanism of action is not fully known, but all have in common selective inhibition of neuronal uptake of serotonin. This potentiates the behavioral changes induced by the serotonin precursor, 5-hydroxytryptophan.[283,284]

Desyrel has been associated with the occurrence of priapism and should not be used in those patients with a propensity for cardiac arrhythmias. Little is known about the interaction

---

Table 12-21. ANTIDEPRESSANT DRUGS

Nonproprietary Name	Trade Name
Monamine Oxidase Inhibitors	
Isocarboxazid	Marplan
Pargyline	Eutonyl
Phenelzine	Nardil
Tranylcypromine	Parnate
Tricyclic Antidepressants	
Imipramine	Imavate, Janimine, Presamine, SK-Pramine, Tofranil
Desipramine	Norpramin, Pertofrane
Amitriptyline	Amitril, Elavil, Endep
Nortriptyline	Aventyl, Pamelor
Doxepin	Adapin, Sinequan
Protriptyline	Vivactil
Amoxapine	Asendin
Maprotiline	Ludiomil
Nontricyclics	
Trazodone	Desyrel
Fluoxetine	Prozac
Buproprion	Wellbutrin

between Desyrel and general anesthesia. It has an elimination half-life of 6 hours, posing the question of whether to discontinue its use before elective surgery. Currently there is no information about potential risk factors of discontinuance versus the benefits of therapy. The availability of sympathetic antagonists for possible side-effects during anesthesia weighs in favor of continuation of therapy versus the risk of exacerbation of a severe depression.[285]

Prozac (fluoxetine) is a popular oral nontricyclic antidepressant. Unlike Desyrel, Prozac has an elimination half-life of 1–3 days, which can lead to significant accumulation of the drug. Prozac's metabolism, like that of other compounds including tricyclic antidepressants, phenobarbital, ethanol, and pentothal, involves the $P_{450}IID_6$ system; thus, concomitant therapy with drugs also metabolized by this enzyme system may lead to drug interactions and prolongation of effect of the benzodiazepines.

Wellbutrin and Zyban are the same drug—buproprion hydrochloride. Zyban, however, is a sustained-release drug. Wellbutrin is used as an antidepressant whereas Zyban is marketed as a non-nicotine aid to smoking cessation. These drugs should not be used concomitantly. Overdose is possible, with resultant seizures. Seizure activity is dose-related. The neurochemical mechanism of the antidepressant effect of buproprion is not known. It does not inhibit monoamine oxidase and is a weak blocker of the neuronal uptake of serotonin and norepinephrine. It does, however, inhibit the neuronal uptake of dopamine to some extent. No systematic data have been collected on the interactions of buproprion with other drugs. The mechanism by which Zyban enhances the ability to abstain from smoking is unknown but perhaps it assists the patient through the mental vicissitudes of nicotine withdrawal. The primary untoward side-effects of therapeutic levels of Zyban are insomnia and a dry mouth. Doses higher than 300 mg can result in seizures.[286]

Adrenergic Antagonists

α Antagonists

Drugs that bind selectively to α-adrenergic receptors block the action of endogenous catecholamines at effector sites and alter the autonomic response. The resultant effects may be ascribed to unopposed β-adrenergic receptors and are dependent upon the prevailing adrenergic tone. In the vasculature, for example, the response to the α blocker phenoxybenzamine may vary over a wide range in a single vascular bed, depending on its intrinsic state of constriction. Vessels with higher initial tone have a greater response to a blockade. Classically, α blockers are defined as drugs that convert the vascular response to EPI from constriction to vasodilation.[287] Prominent clinical effects of α blockers include hypotension, tachycardia, and miosis. Nasal stuffiness, diarrhea, and inhibition of ejaculation are common side-effects.

The α blockers may be classified according to binding characteristics (Table 12-22). Phenoxybenzamine is a drug that binds covalently to the receptors and produces an irreversible blockade. It is relatively nonspecific and has antagonistic activity at several other receptor types as well.[288] Phentolamine, tolazoline, and prazosin are characterized by reversible binding and antagonism.

Table 12-22. α-ADRENERGIC BLOCKING DRUGS

	Type of Antagonism	Selectivity
Phenoxybenzamine	Noncompetitive	$\alpha_1 > \alpha_2$
Phentolamine	Competitive	$\alpha_1 = \alpha_2$
Tolazoline	Competitive	$\alpha_1 = \alpha_2$
Prazosin	Competitive	$\alpha_1 \gg \alpha_2$
Yohimbine	Competitive	$\alpha_2 \gg \alpha_1$

There are also important differences between the individual drugs with regard to relative receptor specificity. As with the β blockers, some show greater affinity for one subset of α receptors than another. Phenoxybenzamine, for example, is 100 times more potent on α_1 than on α_2 receptors. Prazosin is also markedly specific for α_1 receptors, whereas phentolamine has nearly equal blocking activity on both subsets. Phentolamine, therefore, by blocking presynaptic inhibitory α_2 receptors, causes greater NE release from the presynaptic terminal. The tachycardia and the reflex response to hypotension seen commonly with phentolamine are thought to be secondary to this enhanced NE release.

The α blockers in use today include prazosin and phentolamine (see Table 12-22). Phentolamine is used almost exclusively in the diagnosis and treatment of pheochromocytoma. Prazosin is now commonly used to treat essential hypertension. When patients taking these drugs are to undergo anesthesia, one should keep in mind that the normal ANS response to stress and inhalation anesthetic drugs may be completely blocked at the vascular effector site; therefore, elevations of catecholamines will not reflexly increase peripheral vascular resistance and may actually decrease it if vascular β receptors are left unopposed. In the presence of a blockade, we suggest preloading with iv fluids to ensure adequate central volume and careful titration of halogenated anesthetic drugs.

Phenoxybenzamine.   Phenoxybenzamine is a haloalkylamine with predominantly α_1 antagonist activity. Because of the non-competitive nature of the block, as discussed above, it has a relatively long duration of 24 hours. In the past it was the drug of choice for treating patients with pheochromocytoma in preparation for surgery. It has now been replaced with shorter-acting, more specific drugs such as phentolamine.

Phentolamine.   Phentolamine is an imidazoline, which is a competitive antagonist at α_1 and α_2 receptors. The imidazolines also have some antihistaminic and cholinomimetic activity. The cholinomimetic activity may result in abdominal cramping and diarrhea, both of which are blocked by atropine. Tachycardia and hypotension are also common side-effects.[287] It also is commonly used in the diagnosis and treatment of pheochromocytoma. It is usually given in 2–5-mg iv boluses until adequate control of blood pressure is obtained.

Tolazoline.   Tolazoline is also an imidazoline derivative and acts like phentolamine. It is less potent on peripheral α receptors, however, and some of its vasodilatory action has been ascribed to histamine-like activity. It effectively decreases pulmonary vascular resistance and has been used in neonates with respiratory distress syndrome to improve pulmonary blood flow. The effects, however, were detrimental and inconsistent.[289,290]

Prazosin.   Prazosin is a piperazine derivative that has relative selectivity for α_1 receptors and, as a result, does not cause the tachycardia seen with phentolamine. Cardiovascular effects include decreased peripheral vascular resistance and venous return with little change in HR or CO. When used alone, it is not remarkably effective in treatment of essential hypertension resulting from fluid retention. When combined with a diuretic, however, it is an effective antihypertensive drug. It should not be used with clonidine or α-methyldopa (discussed below), as it appears to decrease their effectiveness. Prazosin also may cause bronchodilation, and it decreases serum cholesterol and triglyceride levels.[291]

Yohimbine.   Yohimbine is an α_2 antagonist (see Table 12-5). It blocks the action of clonidine on presynaptic receptors and increases NE release. It is mostly used as a research tool but has been used in the treatment of impotence and orthostatic hypotension.[292]

β Antagonists

The use of β-blocking drugs has markedly escalated in the last 10 years as more indications for their use have been found and more compounds have been developed.[293] They are among the

Table 12-23. *β*-ADRENERGIC BLOCKING DRUGS

Drug	Trade Name	Relative β_1 Selectivity	Membrane-Stabilizing Activity	Intrinsic Sympathomimetic Activity	Plasma Half-Life (hr)	Oral Availability (%)	Lipid Solubility	Elimination	Preparations
Propranolol	Inderal	0	+	0	3–4	36	+++	Hepatic	Oral, iv
Nadolol	Cogard	0	0	0	14–24	34	0	Renal	Oral
Timolol	Blocadren	0	0	0	4–5	50	+	Hepatic and renal	Oral, eye drops
Pindolol	Visken	0	+	++	3–4	86	+	Hepatic and renal	Oral
Esmolol	Brevibloc	++	0	0	0–16	—	?	RBC esterase	iv
Acebutolol	Sectral	+	+	+	3–4	37*	0	Hepatic*	Oral
Atenolol	Tenormin	++	0	0	6–9	57	0	Renal	Oral
Metoprolol	Lopressor	++	0	0	3–4	38	+	Hepatic	Oral
Betaxolol	Kerlone	+++	+	0	14–22	89	0	Hepatic*	Oral
Penbutolol	Levatol	0	0	+	5	85	0	Hepatic*	Oral
Carteolol	Cartrol	0	0	+	6	85	0	Renal	Oral

* Primarily hepatic, but active metabolites are formed that must be renally excreted.

most common drugs used in the treatment of cardiovascular disease, and frequently the anesthesiologist must deal with their effects and side-effects during anesthesia. There are now a variety of drugs available with β-blocking activity that may be distinguished by differing pharmacokinetic and pharmacodynamic characteristics.[294,295] Examples of drugs available for clinical use

in the United States and their characteristics are listed in Table 12-23. Their structures are shown in Figure 12-33.

Several of these drugs are marketed on the basis of cardioselectivity, *i.e.*, antagonist activity is greater at β_1 than β_2 receptors in an isolated muscle preparation. Theoretically, this implies that these agents would be of greater benefit in treatment of

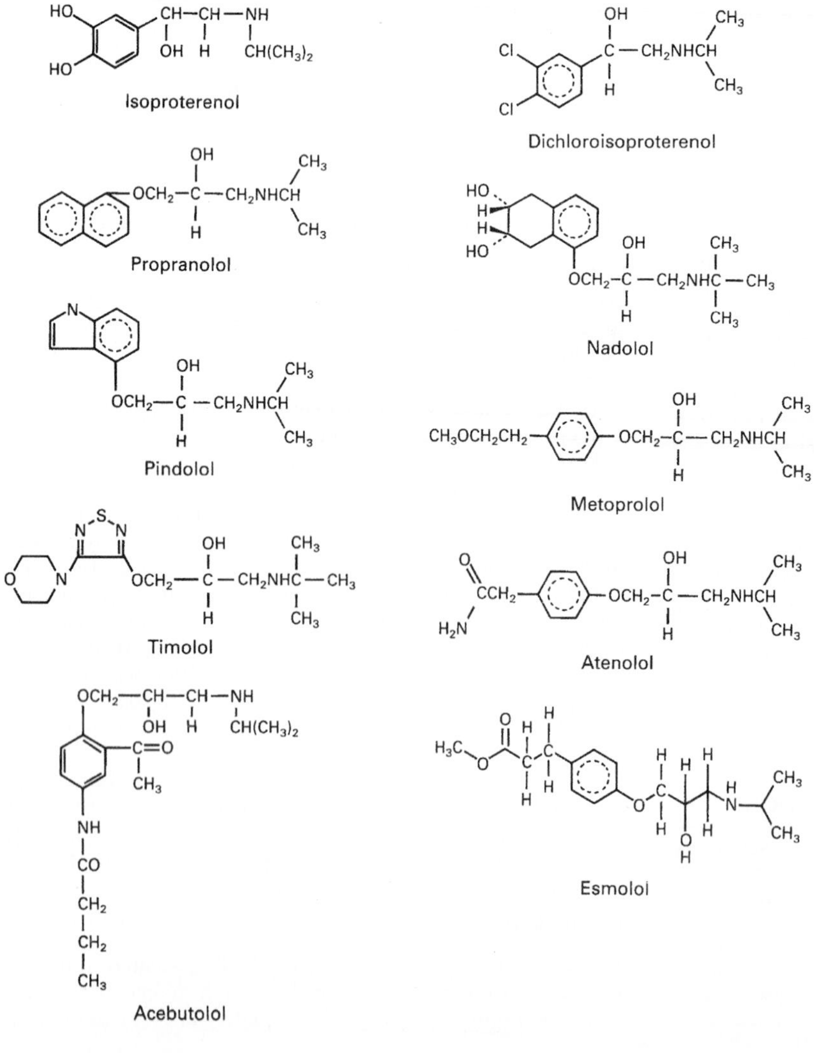

Figure 12-33. The structures of the commonly used β blockers are compared with the pure β agonist isoproterenol, and the partial agonist dichloroisoproterenol.

patients with obstructive airway disease, diabetes mellitus, or peripheral vascular disease.[296] The practitioner must keep in mind, however, that this means relative selectivity, not specificity, and that β-blocking effects may be seen in all tissues if higher blood levels are reached (see Fig. 12-13). Clinical studies have not shown greater effectiveness of cardioselective β blockers in treatment of hypertension[297] or diabetes mellitus,[298] and their relative effectiveness in the case of peripheral vascular disease is still controversial.[296]

The use of β_1-selective blockers in patients with obstructive airway disease is also controversial. The degree of bronchoreactivity is an important consideration in their use. Patients with reactive airway disease may develop serious reductions in ventilatory function even with β-selective drugs.[299] No β blocker can be considered safe in patients with obstructive airway disease, and other types of drugs are available for treatment of supraventricular arrhythmias and hypertension.

SNS activation generally results in increased circulating glucose levels secondary to enhanced glycogenolysis, lipolysis, and gluconeogenesis. Administration of β blockers to insulin-dependent diabetics reduces their ability to recover from hypoglycemic episodes, primarily due to β_2-adrenoceptor antagonism. Thus, β blockers must be used with caution in diabetic patients on insulin therapy, to avoid potentially life-threatening hypoglycemic episodes. When necessitated, β_1-selective antagonists are preferable.

β-Adrenergic receptor blockers are also commonly used now in the treatment of hypertension. They have been discussed in detail above, but certain comments about their perioperative use are pertinent here (see Table 12-23). Following the introduction of propranolol, several deleterious interactions (in particular, the enhanced negative inotropic and chronotropic effects of halothane) were noted with anesthetics. This resulted in a debate over whether or not the blocker should be discontinued preoperatively. β-Blocker therapy should be continued up until the time of operation. A withdrawal syndrome has been noted after acute discontinuation of chronic β-blocker therapy.[300,301] Also, the control of HR and blood pressure perioperatively is easier if chronic medications are continued and the anesthetic plan is altered rather than acutely stopping the chronic medications and administering a routine anesthetic plan.[302] HR is a major determinant of myocardial oxygen demand. Tachycardia has recently been shown to increase the risk of poor outcome in patients with ischemic heart disease.[303] Therefore, the control of HR and blood pressure is important perioperatively, and β-blocker therapy should be continued to maximize this control.

Some β antagonists have partial agonist activity at low doses. This is referred to as intrinsic sympathomimetic activity. Drugs with intrinsic sympathomimetic activity decrease resting HR less than those without it.[304] In the presence of similar degrees of β blockade, however, all β blockers blunt exercise-induced increases in HR to a similar extent.[298] The clinical relevance of this is unclear, but it has been implied that intrinsic sympathomimetic activity would be advantageous in patients treated with nonselective β blockers who are troubled by bradycardia or worsening ventricular failure.[305] A distinct advantage to intrinsic sympathomimetic activity in β blockers has not been clearly shown in clinical studies.

Several of the β blockers listed in Table 12-23 also have a local anesthetic–like effect on myocellular membranes at high doses. This effect is similar to that of quinidine in that Phase 0 of the cardiac action potential is depressed, slowing conduction. This membrane-stabilizing activity is caused by the D-isomer, whereas the L-isomer is responsible for β-blocking activity. The clinical significance of membrane-stabilizing activity is also unclear.[295]

Propranolol. Propranolol is the prototypical β-blocking drug against which all others are compared. It is nonselective and has no intrinsic sympathomimetic activity but does have membrane-stabilizing activity at higher doses. It is available in both iv and oral forms. It is highly lipophilic and is metabolized by the liver to more water-soluble metabolites, one of which, 17-OH propranolol, has weak β-blocking activity. There is a significant first-pass effect by the liver after oral administration of the drug. It is highly protein-bound, and the free drug level may be altered by other highly bound drugs. The elimination half-life is approximately 4 hours, but the pharmacologic half-life is around 10 hours.

Hemodynamic effects include decreased HR and contractility. The major factors contributing to the decrease in blood pressure by propranolol are decreased CO and renin release. Systemic vascular resistance may increase upon acute administration owing to blockade of β_2 receptors in the peripheral vasculature. With chronic administration, however, peripheral vascular resistance decreases. This is thought to be secondary to decreased renin release and, possibly, decreased central SNS outflow.[292,306] Complications with the use of propranolol include bradycardia, heart block, worsening of congestive heart failure, bronchospasm, and sedation. During anesthesia with halothane, it may cause severe bradydysrhythmias.

Nadolol. Nadolol is a noncardioselective β blocker with no membrane-stabilizing activity or intrinsic sympathomimetic activity. It is approximately equipotent to propranolol, but its effects are prolonged owing to slower elimination. It is relatively lipid-insoluble and is excreted 70% unchanged in urine and 20% in the feces. The elimination half-life is 24 hours. Because it is lipid-insoluble, it does not cross the blood–brain barrier, and sedation is less of a problem than with propranolol. Hemodynamic effects are the same as for propranolol. The main advantage of the drug is the capability for once per day dosing.

Timolol. Timolol is also noncardioselective with little intrinsic sympathomimetic activity and no membrane-stabilizing activity. It is the only β blocker used as the L-isomer rather than the racemic mixture. It is 5–10 times as potent as propranolol. Hepatic metabolism accounts for approximately 66% of its elimination, and another 20% is found unchanged in the urine. The elimination half-life is 5.6 hours, and the pharmacologic half-life is approximately 15 hours. It was first used topically for treatment of glaucoma but is now used in hypertension and has been shown to decrease the risk of reinfarction and death following myocardial infarction.[307] Its hemodynamic effects and side-effects are similar to those of other β blockers. The anesthesiologist should also be aware that timolol eye drops may be absorbed systemically and cause bradycardia and hypotension that are refractory to treatment with atropine.[308]

Pindolol. Pindolol is a nonselective β blocker with membrane-stabilizing activity and intrinsic sympathomimetic activity. It is 10–40 times as potent as propranolol. It is lipid-soluble and metabolized by the liver but not as avidly extracted; therefore, its biologic availability after oral administration is more predictable. It is excreted 40% unchanged in the urine. The elimination half-life is 3.5 hours. It is useful in the treatment of angina pectoris, cardiac dysrhythmia, and hypertension. As discussed above, the clinical usefulness of the intrinsic sympathomimetic activity property is unclear.

Oxprenolol. Oxprenolol is similar to pindolol except for less intrinsic sympathomimetic activity and lower potency.

Metoprolol. Metoprolol is a relatively selective β-blocking drug with β-blocking effects at moderate and high doses. It has neither intrinsic sympathomimetic activity nor membrane-stabilizing activity. It has a possible advantage in patients with reactive airway disease at oral doses up to 100 mg · day^{-1}.[309] In this case, it should probably be used with a β_2-mimetic drug. It is mostly metabolized in the liver, with only about 5% excreted unchanged in the urine. The elimination half-life is 3.5 hours. It has recently become available in iv as well as oral form; therefore, it may be useful during anesthesia.

Atenolol. Atenolol is similar to metoprolol in that it is relatively cardioselective and has no intrinsic sympathomimetic activity or membrane-stabilizing activity. It is less lipophilic, however, and is eliminated primarily by renal excretion. The elimination half-life is 6–7 hours. The lack of first-pass metabolism results in more predictable blood levels after oral dosing.

Acebutolol. Acebutolol is a cardioselective β blocker with intrinsic sympathomimetic activity and membrane-stabilizing activity.[310] It is metabolized in the liver and is subject to extensive first-pass metabolism. The primary metabolite is diacetolol, which has a pharmacologic profile similar to that of the parent drug and is excreted renally.[311] The pharmacologic effects of the drug, therefore, are dependent on both hepatic transformation and renal excretion. The elimination half-life of acebutolol is 3–4 hours and of diacetolol 8–13 hours. Elimination is prolonged in the elderly and patients with renal disease. Acebutolol, like pindolol, has intrinsic sympathetic activity that makes it more advantageous than the other β blockers in patients with bradydysrhythmias or myocardial failure.

Esmolol. Esmolol has several uses in the perioperative period.[312,313] The most distinctive feature of the drug is the ester function that is incorporated into the phenoxypropanolamine structure. This allows for rapid degradation by esterases in the red blood cells and a resultant pharmacologic half-life of 10–20 minutes.[313] Esmolol is cardioselective and appears to have little effect on bronchial or vascular tone at doses that decrease HR in humans. It has been used successfully in low doses in patients with asthma,[314] but caution is again advised when using β blockers in these patients.[296] Esmolol is metabolized rapidly in the blood by an esterase located in the red blood cell cytoplasm. It is different from the plasma cholinesterase and is not inhibited to a significant degree by physostigmine or echothiophate but is markedly inhibited by sodium fluoride. There are no apparent important clinical interactions between esmolol and other ester-containing drugs. At the highest infusion rates (500 $\mu g \cdot kg^{-1} \cdot min^{-1}$), esmolol does not prolong neuromuscular blockade by succinylcholine.[315]

Esmolol has proved useful in the perioperative period because of its capability to be administered intravenously and its short half-life.[316] This feature permits a trial of β blockade in doubtful situations. Esmolol has been shown to blunt the response to intubation of the trachea[313,317] and is moderately effective in treating postoperative hypertension.[317,318] Most reported studies in humans have used doses of 50–500 $\mu g \cdot kg^{-1} \cdot min^{-1}$. The most beneficial approach seems to be a loading dose of 500 $\mu g \cdot kg^{-1}$ over 30 seconds, followed by continuous infusion of 50–300 $\mu g \cdot kg^{-1} \cdot min^{-1}$. Peak blockade appears to occur within 5 minutes. On discontinuation of the infusion, serum levels decline with an elimination half-life of 9 minutes. The HR response to isoproterenol returns to control in 20 minutes.

Betaxolol. Betaxolol hydrochloride is a β_1-selective (cardioselective) adrenergic receptor antagonist and is freely soluble in water. It has weak membrane-stabilizing activity and no intrinsic sympathomimetic (partial agonist) activity. The preferential effect on β_1 receptors is not absolute. Some β_2-inhibitory activity can be expected in the bronchial and vascular musculature at higher doses. Absorption of an oral dose is complete, with an absolute bioavailability of 90% that is unaffected by ingestion of food or alcohol. The mean elimination half-life is from 11 to 22 hours. It is eliminated primarily by the liver but secondarily through the kidneys. Betaxolol is indicated in the management of hypertension. It may be used alone or concomitantly with other antihypertensive agents.

Penbutolol. Penbutolol is a synthetic β-receptor antagonist for oral administration. It is a nonselective β-receptor antagonist with some intrinsic sympathomimetic activity. Penbutolol does not appear to have any membrane-stabilizing properties, as does propranolol. Plasma elimination half-life is 5 hours in normal subjects. Ninety percent of radioactive penbutolol was found to be excreted in the urine. There is no change in the effective half-life of penbutolol in healthy patients versus those on renal

dialysis. It is indicated primarily for the treatment of hypertension and may be used in combination with other antihypertensives.

Carteolol. Carteolol is a synthetic, nonselective, β-adrenergic receptor-blocking agent with intrinsic sympathetic activity. It possesses no significant membrane-stabilizing (local anesthetic) activity and is without value in treating intrinsic arrhythmias. Carteolol has equivocal effects on renin secretion because of its intrinsic sympathomimetic activity, in contrast to β blockers without such activity, which inhibit renin. Carteolol is well absorbed with a half-life of approximately 6 hours. About 50–75% of the drug is eliminated by the kidneys; thus, renal impairment increases its half-life in proportion to the reduction in creatinine clearance. Carteolol is primarily indicated for the management of hypertension but may be used in combination with other potent drugs.

Mixed Antagonists

Labetalol. Labetalol is an antihypertensive drug with blocking activity at both α and β receptors. The relative α/β-blocking effects are dependent upon the route of administration. After oral administration, the ratio of α/β effectiveness is 1 : 3; however, when given intravenously, it is 1 : 7 (i.e., it is 3 and 7 times more potent on β than on α receptors, respectively). The α effects are primarily on α_1 receptors, whereas the β effects are nonselective.

Hemodynamic effects consist primarily of decreased peripheral resistance and decreased or unchanged HR with little change in CO.[316] Serum renin activity is decreased. Maintenance of lower HRs in the presence of decreased systemic blood pressure is beneficial in controlling the myocardial oxygen supply/demand ratio and is a major benefit of labetalol in patients with coronary artery disease.[319]

Labetalol is eliminated by hepatic glucuronide conjugation. The elimination half-life after iv administration is 5.5 hours and 6–8 hours after oral use. Elimination is not markedly prolonged in patients with hepatic or renal failure. Another advantage of the drug is the ability to convert from iv to oral forms of the same drug after the patient is stable.[320,321] For treatment of hypertension when used as a bolus, the initial dose is 0.25 mg $\cdot$ kg^{-1} iv over 2 minutes, then repeat every 10 minutes to a total of 300 mg. When used as a continuous infusion, it is usually started at 2 mg $\cdot$ min^{-1} and titrated to effect. Because there is an enhanced effect by inhalation anesthetics, these doses should be decreased when used intraoperatively.

Complications and contraindications are similar to those for the β blockers. Labetalol should be used with caution in patients with compromised myocardial function because it may worsen heart failure. Also, owing to β-blocking activity, the drug may induce bronchospasm in asthmatics. As with other β blockers, abrupt withdrawal is not recommended.

Calcium Entry Blockers

Calcium is regarded as the universal messenger in cells and plays a critical role in a number of biologic processes.[245] It is involved in blood coagulation, a broad array of enzymatic reactions, the metabolism of bone, neuromuscular transmission, the electrical activation of various excitable membranes and endocrine secretion, and muscle contraction. Calcium initiates several physiologic events in the specialized automatic and conducting cells in the heart.[322] It is involved in the genesis of the cardiac action potential, and it links excitation to contraction and controls energy stores and utilization. Movement of extracellular calcium across membranes also governs the function of smooth muscle in bronchi and in coronary, pulmonary, and systemic arterioles. Its role in adrenergic effector response has been outlined in detail (see Molecular Pharmacology and Effector Response).

There are membrane calcium channels that provide a pathway for calcium influx across cell membranes that differs from

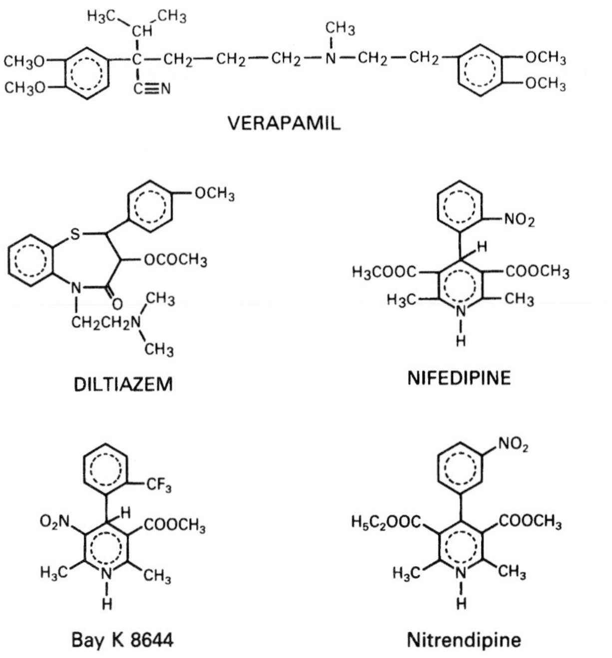

Figure 12-34. Structural formulas of the calcium entry blockers demonstrate dissimilar structures consistent with their dissimilar electrophysiologic and pharmacologic properties. They also share some similarities but cannot be considered therapeutically interchangeable. Nifedipine and nitrendipine are structurally similar and are both potent vasodilators; BAY K 8644 is also similar but is a calcium channel agonist.

Table 12-25. USES OF CALCIUM CHANNEL BLOCKERS

Vascular Disorders	Nonvascular Disorders
Systemic hypertension	Bronchial asthma
Pulmonary hypertension	Esophageal spasm
Cerebral arterial spasm	Dysmenorrhea
Raynaud's phenomenon	Premature labor
Migraine	

The molecular structures of three clinically useful calcium entry blockers are shown in Figure 12-34. Calcium entry blockers are a heterogeneous group of drugs with dissimilar structures and electrophysiologic and pharmacologic properties.[192] Despite structural dissimilarities, this group shares some important actions that are consistent with the known importance of extracellular calcium and adrenergic function. Any drug that alters slow-channel kinetics could be expected to produce vasodilatation, to depress cardiac conduction velocity (dromotropism), to depress contractility (inotropism), and to decrease HR (chronotropism). All calcium entry blockers do this, but with varying degrees of potency in the intact human and *in vitro* (Table 12-24).[327,328] Thus, despite their similarities, these drugs cannot be considered therapeutically interchangeable. Clinically, nifedipine is a potent coronary artery vasodilator with little direct effect on cardiac conduction. It may reduce dysrhythmia secondarily when increased coronary blood flow is of benefit. Verapamil is valued for its specific antidysrhythmic activity, but it is a myocardial depressant with little vasodilator activity. Verapamil also has slightly greater local anesthetic activity (fast-channel inhibition) than procaine on an equimolar basis.[329] The significance of this observation in humans has not been established. The structural heterogeneity of this group of drugs also suggests more than one site and mechanism of action. Although the molecular basis of the action of these compounds is unknown, they are lipophilic, and it appears likely that they work by producing conformational changes in the cell membranes (see Molecular Pharmacology and Effector Response).

The useful pharmacologic effects of the calcium entry blockers have been confined almost solely to the cardiovascular system, although the list of uses will likely grow.[193] Table 12-25 lists some of the areas of investigation in which they appear to be of clinical benefit.[123,330] Calcium entry blockers have been described, perhaps erroneously, as selective slow-channel blockers. A review of the literature, however, suggests that these agents are not selective, but rather that the slow-channel effects on the cardiovascular system are just more apparent. Their lack of selectivity should not be surprising considering the critical role calcium plays in a wide variety of biologic processes. The sensitivity of a given tissue to the calcium entry blockers is related to that tissue's dependence on extracellular calcium for its function. This would explain the sensitivity of the calcium-dependent myocardium and smooth muscle to these blockers on the one hand and the apparent insensitivity of striated muscle on the other.[331] Extracellular calcium is relatively insignifi-

that of calcium efflux movements associated with active pumps or exchange.[323] The inward calcium channel exhibits two distinguishing properties: (1) selectivity, in that they have the ability to distinguish between ion species; (2) excitability, in that they have the property of responding to changes in membrane potential.[324] Separate, ion-specific channels for sodium and calcium influx are thought to exist. The status of these channels can vary to produce three kinetic states: resting, activated, and inactivated. Sodium channels are referred to as fast channels because the transition among resting, activated, and inactivated states is more rapid than among the calcium channels. Thus, calcium channels are often referred to as membrane "slow channels."[193]

Classification of calcium entry blockers has been difficult since their discovery. They were initially thought to be β-adrenergic blocking drugs because of their sympatholytic action. Later they were called calcium antagonists.[325] It is clear, however, that these drugs are not true pharmacologic antagonists of calcium. Instead, they interact with the cell membrane to control the intracellular concentration of calcium. The correct terminology for this group of drugs appears to be calcium entry blockers.[326] Slow channel inhibitors or calcium channel blockers are alternative terms.

Table 12-24. AUTONOMIC EFFECTS OF CALCIUM ENTRY BLOCKERS IN INTACT HUMANS

	Verapamil	Diltiazem	Nifedipine	Lidoflazine
Negative inotropic	+	0/+	0	0
Negative chronotropic	+	0/+	0	0
Negative dromotropic	++++	+++	0	0
Coronary vasodilation	++	+++	++++	++++
Systemic vasodilation	++	++	++++	+++
Bronchodilation	0/+		0/+	

Table 12-26. COMPARATIVE PHARMACOLOGY OF CALCIUM ENTRY BLOCKERS

	Verapamil	Diltiazem	Nifedipine
Dose			
Oral	80–160 mg tid	60–90 mg tid	10–20 mg tid
iv	75–150 $\mu g \cdot kg^{-1}$	75–150 $\mu g \cdot kg^{-1}$	5–15 $\mu g \cdot kg^{-1}$
Absorption			
Oral (%)	>90%	>90%	>90%
Bioavailability			
Oral (%)	<20%	?<20%	60–70%*
Onset			
Oral	15–20 min	20–30 min	15–20 min
iv	1 min	?	1 min
Sublingual	—	—	3 min
Peak Effect			
Oral	5 hr	30 min	1–2 hr
iv	5–30 min	?	1–3 hr
Elimination half-life	2–7 hr	4 hr	4–5 hr
Plasma protein binding	90%	80%	90%
Metabolism	70% First-pass hepatic	Deacetylated	80% to lactone
Elimination			
Renal	75%	35%	70%
Gastrointestinal (liver)	15%	75%	<15%
Side-effects	Constipation, headache, vertigo, hypotension, atrioventricular conduction disturbances	Headache, dizziness, flushing, atrioventricular conduction disturbances, constipation	Headache, hypotension, flushing, digital dysesthesias, leg edema

* Light-sensitive.

cant in the function of striated muscle, where the SR is the major storage organelle of calcium. Striated muscle can recycle intracellular calcium for prolonged periods, which is in keeping with its function of sustained contraction as opposed to the rhythmic or cyclic contraction of the myocardium and smooth muscle.

The drugs are all absorbed *via* the gastrointestinal tract, but the extensive first-pass hepatic extraction of verapamil limits its bioavailability orally (Table 12-26). Onset of action is equivalent for all three drugs and is consistent with rapid membrane transport. All three drugs are extensively protein-bound and subject to the effect of changes in plasma protein concentration and competition from other protein-bound drugs and metabolites, but final elimination of verapamil and nifedipine is primarily renal.

Verapamil. Verapamil is a calcium entry blocker that is administered intravenously for terminating supraventricular tachydysrhythmias.[332,333] Nearly all forms of supraventricular tachydysrhythmias are caused by re-entry using either the sinoatrial or the AV node as part of the circuit. Verapamil terminates these cardiac dysrhythmias by decreasing nodal conductivity, converting the unidirectional block of re-entry to a bidirectional block. In this regard, its action on supraventricular dysrhythmia is similar to that of quinidine on ventricular re-entry cardiac dysrhythmia.

Verapamil does not alter the action potential upstroke in fibers whose resting membrane potential is more negative than −60 mV, *i.e.*, fast action potentials.[334] It does slow or prevent depolarization in cardiac tissue with a resting membrane potential that is less negative than −50 mV, *i.e.*, calcium-dependent upstroke. Verapamil, therefore, has profound effects on pacemaker cells, which depend on the calcium current for depolarization.[335] It depresses the rate of sinus discharge, reduces conduction velocity, and increases refractoriness of the AV node.

A dose-dependent increase in the PR interval and AV interval is produced on the electrocardiogram. This has been described as a quinidine-like effect similar to that produced by Class IA antidysrhythmic drugs (*e.g.*, procainamide), which are also effective for supraventricular dysrhythmia. In contrast to the procainamide, verapamil does not increase the QRS or Q-T interval because it lacks activity on the sodium-dependent action potentials.

Verapamil is a first-line drug for treatment of supraventricular tachydysrhythmias (Table 12-27). The incidence of successful termination of paroxysmal atrial tachycardia with verapamil in adults has approached 90%.[336] It is also effective in treating atrial fibrillation and atrial flutter by either converting to a sinus rhythm or slowing the ventricular response. The ventricular rate will slow as a result of decreased conduction velocity through the AV node even when conversion is not produced. Caution must be exercised in treating patients when the underlying cause of the atrial tachycardia, atrial fibrillation, or atrial flutter is the Wolff-Parkinson-White syndrome.[337] An accessory bypass tract lies near the AV node that participates in the re-entry of these tachydysrhythmias. Verapamil may terminate the tachydysrhythmia by its specific depressant effects on the AV node, which is one limb of the re-entrant pathway. It may also increase conduction velocity in the accessory tract, in which case the HR may actually increase.

Verapamil has no adverse effects on bronchial asthma or obstructive lung disease and may be selected over propranolol in patients with these conditions.[123] It should be avoided in patients with sick sinus syndrome, AV block, and the presence of heart failure, unless the heart failure is the result of a supraventricular tachycardia.

Studies further support the hypothesis that Ca^{2+} participates directly in the genesis of ventricular dysrhythmia.[337,338] When sodium channels are inactivated by hypoxia, stretch, or hyperka-

Table 12-27. ACTIONS OF CALCIUM ENTRY BLOCKERS

Verapamil

Vasodilator
  ↓ systemic vascular resistance → ↑ heart rate
  → ↑ ejection fraction and cardiac output
Small decrease in left ventricular dP/dt
Little or no change in coronary resistance
↓ conduction through atrioventricular node (↑ P-R interval)
Should not be given with digitalis or β blockers

Diltiazem

More like verapamil than nifedipine
Dilates coronary more than systemic vessels and has less marked
  hemodynamic effects than nifedipine or verapamil
Little effect on cardiac output
Does not cause tachycardia
Effects on conduction system similar to those of verapamil
Less inotropic effect than verapamil

Nifedipine

Rapid onset of action, may be used sublingually
Potent peripheral vasodilator, may be useful in treatment of hyper-
  tension
Has little clinically important negative inotropic activity
Less tendency to produce cardiac decompensation than verapamil
Little effect on nodal activity and no antiarrhythmic activity; there-
  fore causes no electrocardiographic changes
Increased coronary blood flow in normal and ischemic myo-
  cardium

---

lemia, the remaining Ca^{2+} can produce a depolarizing current in these abnormal cells, especially in the presence of catechol-amines. The conversion of a fast response cell to a cell with slow response characteristics presents all the necessary ingredients for the re-entry phenomenon: slow depolarization and delayed conduction. The resulting ventricular dysrhythmia can usually be terminated with one of the Class I drugs as long as the resting membrane potential of the slow response is between −80 and −60 mV. Verapamil has been effective in terminating ventricular tachycardias and premature depolarizations in about two thirds of the treatment trials when other drugs have failed. The resting membrane potential of these abnormal "slow response" foci has been postulated to be less negative than −60 mV, a range in which lidocaine would be ineffective on the calcium current conduction and depolarization. More information is needed before recommendations can be made for verapamil in treating dysrhythmia other than supraventricular tachydysrhythmias. Other drugs are significantly more effective for the initial treatment of ventricular dysrhythmia.

The important side-effects of verapamil are directly related to its predominant pharmacologic action (see Table 12-27). It may produce unwanted AV conduction delays and bradycardia, resulting in cardiovascular collapse. Verapamil must be used carefully, if at all, in the presence of propranolol. The combined effect has produced complete heart block in animals and humans. It must be used carefully in digitalized patients for the same reason. No such interactions exist with nifedipine. The combination of β blockade and nifedipine may be beneficial in patients with ischemic heart disease because the reflex tachycardia seen with nifedipine can be countered with β blockade.

Nifedipine. Nifedipine is the most potent calcium entry blocker when tested in isolated tissue preparations. It is an equipotent cardiac depressant and vasodilator. Depression of inotropism and cardiac conduction, however, is not evident in the intact human. It does not effect baroreflex mechanisms and, as a result, the marked vasodilation is accompanied by increased SNS tone and afterload reduction (see Table 12-27).[193]

A compensatory tachycardia may result, and CO may actually increase as a result of the afterload reduction.

The most specific therapeutic application for nifedipine is coronary vasospasm (variant of Prinzmetal's angina).[192,328] It has been more successful than nitroglycerin for this purpose because it produces a more profound and predictable coronary vasodilation. It has also been extremely useful in other types of ischemic heart disease ranging from unstable angina to myocardial infarction. The decrease in myocardial oxygen demand that results from the reduced afterload and reduced left ventricular volume appears to be the mechanism for the relief of angina. Coronary vasodilation is another factor, but it is not known if this is the antianginal effect in patients with coronary artery disease. The dilating effect may last only 5 minutes, but the antianginal effect may last more than 1 hour.

Nifedipine is not available for iv use, but clinical practice has demonstrated that sublingual nifedipine is an effective therapeutic application with a nearly immediate onset of action.[192] One need only puncture the end of a nifedipine capsule and squirt it under the patient's tongue. Use of this technique is particularly applicable for the anesthesiologist in situations in which oral medication cannot be given. We have also used sublingual nifedipine effectively in situations in which perioperative hypertension and evidence of acute coronary ischemia coexist. In these circumstances, a reduction in afterload, coronary vasodilation, and reduced blood pressure are all achieved with the same drug.[339] Reflex tachycardia, if it occurs, can be managed with β blockade without significant interaction with nifedipine.

Diltiazem. The hemodynamic effects of diltiazem lie somewhere between those of verapamil and nifedipine.[193] It is less potent than either of these two agents.[340] Diltiazem is a good coronary artery dilator but a poor peripheral vasodilator. It often produces bradycardia and delayed conduction, and reflex tachycardia is not a problem.[337] It appears to be an effective oral drug for the treatment of coronary disease in which cardiac dysrhythmias are troublesome. Cardiac dysrhythmias are noticeably a part of the clinical picture in patients suffering from coronary spasm. Intravenous administration of diltiazem is effective therapy for supraventricular tachycardias including PSVT, atrial fibrillation, atrial flutter, and re-entrant tachycardias such as Wolff-Parkinson-White syndrome.[341] Like verapamil, diltiazem acts by prolonging AV nodal conduction. The peripheral vascular effects of diltiazem, though, are less severe, making it a more desirable therapeutic choice in most cases. A bolus dose of $0.25 \text{ mg} \cdot \text{kg}^{-1}$ is administered over 2 minutes and may be repeated at $0.35 \text{ mg} \cdot \text{kg}^{-1}$ if necessary after 15 minutes. An infusion of $5\text{–}15 \text{ mg} \cdot \text{hr}^{-1}$ may be necessary to maintain the reduction of HR.

Nicardipine. Nicardipine hydrochloride is a calcium channel blocker that can be administered orally and intravenously. It is the only calcium channel blocker that can be titrated intravenously to achieve blood pressure response. Nicardipine is a smooth muscle relaxant producing vasodilation of peripheral and coronary arteries. It has a rapid onset of action, and the major effects last 10–15 minutes. Toxic metabolic products are not produced.[342] It has minimal cardiodepressant effects and does not decrease the rate of the sinus node pacemaker or slow conduction through the AV node. Renal failure does not affect the dosage, but the dosage should be reduced in the elderly and those with hepatic dysfunction. It is compatible with most crystalloid solutions. Side-effects of nicardipine include headache, lightheadedness, flushing, and hypotension. Reflex tachycardia is not a frequent finding with nicardipine, as is the case with nitroprusside, hydralazine, or nifedipine.

Nimodipine. Nimodipine is highly lipophilic. It has a greater vasodilating effect on cerebral arteries than on vessels elsewhere because of its lipophilism, which promotes crossing the blood–brain barrier. Clinical studies demonstrate a favorable effect on the severity of neurologic deficits caused by cerebral vasospasm following subarachnoid hemorrhage. However, no radiographic evidence has been presented that nimodipine either prevents or relieves spasm of these arteries. The mechanism for clinical improvement is not known. It is primarily an oral drug that is rapidly absorbed, with a T-terminal half-life of approximately 8–9 hours. Earlier elimination rates are much more rapid, which results in a need to redose every 4 hours. The bioavailability of an oral dose is only 13%. Dosage should be reduced in patients with hepatic dysfunction. The primary indication for nimodipine is for the improvement of neurologic deficits caused by spasm following subarachnoid hemorrhage from a ruptured congenital aneurysm.

Felodipine. Felodipine is a second-generation calcium channel inhibitor that is currently under investigation by the Federal Drug Administration. Nimodipine and felodipine have demonstrated selectivity for vascular tissue beds. Whereas nimodipine preferentially dilates cerebral vessels, felodipine preferentially dilates peripheral resistance vessels. Neither has significant effects on cardiac muscle. This has important clinical implications in the treatment of hypertension. Early studies indicate that 10–20 mg of felodipine daily will reduce blood pressure without reducing CO or HR. Coronary blood flow increases, but no effect on ventricular contraction or relaxation has been reported. This would make the drug appropriate for the active hypertensive patient.

Calcium Entry Blockers and Anesthesia

Evidence indicates that halothane depresses slow-channel kinetics. All of the potent inhalation anesthetics behave in a similar fashion in that they depress myocardial contractility and vascular tone in a dose-related manner.[343,344] Most studies indicate that the calcium entry blockers and inhalation anesthetics exert additive effects on the inward calcium current.[192,328] Opioid anesthetics do not appear to add anything to the effects of the calcium entry blockers. Several recent studies indicate an interaction between the calcium entry blockers and the neuromuscular blocking drugs similar to that seen with the mycin antibiotics.[193] This interaction is not well defined, but *in vitro* and *in vivo* studies indicate a reduced margin of safety with these drug combinations. Calcium entry blockers appear to augment the effects of both depolarizing and nondepolarizing muscle relaxants.[345] These observations serve as a word of caution because their clinical significance has not been defined. Prolonged apnea and relaxation have been reported when verapamil was used to treat a supraventricular tachycardia in a patient with Duchenne's muscular dystrophy.[346]

Calcium entry blockers should be continued until the time of surgery to maintain control of angina pectoris, hypertension, or cardiac dysrhythmia.[193] It could be anticipated that sudden discontinuation of these drugs theoretically could produce a rebound of symptoms, although this phenomenon has not been reported. Upregulation of calcium receptors would probably occur during periods of entry blockade.[347]

Verapamil may increase the toxicity of digoxin, the benzodiazepines, carbamazepine, oral hypoglycemics, and possibly quinidine and theophylline.[348] Cardiac failure, AV conduction disturbances, and sinus bradycardia may be more frequent with concurrent use of β blockers, and severe hypotension and bradycardia may occur with bupivacaine. Decreased lithium effect and lithium neurotoxicity have both been reported with the concurrent use of verapamil.[349] The effects of verapamil may also be increased by cimetidine.[350]

Antihypertensives

Increased awareness and treatment of hypertension over the last 20 years has resulted in increasing numbers of patients presenting for anesthesia and surgery who are taking one or more antihypertensive medications. These drugs are numerous, affect multiple organ systems, and have the potential for many deleterious interactions in the perioperative period. Most antihypertensive drugs blunt the ANS or its effector organs or cause reflex increases in ANS outflow. Most anesthetic agents also inhibit ANS tone to some degree[348] and may therefore have additive effects with antihypertensive drugs. In addition, patients with hypertension may exhibit greater liability in blood pressure intraoperatively and rebound hypertension in the postoperative period.[351,352] The anesthesiologist should therefore maintain a thorough understanding of the commonly used antihypertensive drugs. A rational approach to their perioperative use includes decisions as to holding or continuing them preoperatively, possible interactions with anesthetic drugs, and resumption of treatment postoperatively. The commonly used antihypertensive drugs are grouped below according to their primary mechanism of action and discussed briefly with emphasis on consideration for the anesthesiologist.

Diuretics

Diuretics are the most common prescribed drugs for hypertension. Their basic mechanisms of action are decreased plasma and extracellular volumes. Although the thiazides and furosemide have been shown to have vasodilating properties, the clinical significance of this effect is unclear. Chronic diuretic therapy results in decreased intravascular volume. The cardiovascular response to induction of anesthesia may therefore be accentuated, resulting in hypotension and tachycardia. Other problems associated with diuretic use include hypokalemia, hyponatremia, hypocalcemia, and hyperglycemia. Chronic hypokalemia is common with diuretic therapy and may predispose the patient to cardiac arrhythmias.[353] The clinical relevance of perioperative hypokalemia is unclear and has stirred considerable debate among anesthesiologists as to whether surgery should be postponed until plasma potassium levels are treated.[354,355]

Sympatholytics

Sympatholytic drugs include those that block central SNS outflow or NE release from the presynaptic neuron at the effector site. Currently included in this group are α-methyldopa and clonidine.

α-Methyldopa. α-Methyldopa is a catechol derivative that is enzymatically converted to active compounds by enzymes in the catecholamine synthesis chain (see Fig. 12-9). α-Methyldopamine and α-methylnorepinephrine are the primary metabolites. The precise mechanism responsible for decreased SNS tone is unclear, but it is thought that α-methylnorepinephrine, which is stored in presynaptic vesicles, is released and stimulates presynaptic α_2 receptors, thereby inhibiting NE release.[292] Because of the unique metabolism of α-methyldopa to the active compound and the storage of the metabolite in presynaptic vesicles, both the time to onset and duration of action are long. Even after iv administration, the peak effect may not be seen for several hours. Although the elimination half-life is 2 hours, the effect of an oral dose may last up to 24 hours.

Clonidine. Clonidine stimulates presynaptic α_2 receptors and inhibits NE release from both central and peripheral adrenergic terminals. It also has some α_1-agonist activity and in high oral doses may cause paradoxical hypertension by stimulating vascular α_1 receptors. Under normal circumstances, the α_2 effects predominate. The prominent antihypertensive effect is thought to be secondary to stimulation of α_2 receptors in the vasomotor centers of the medulla oblongata.[292] Whether these are presynaptic or postsynaptic receptors remains controversial[287]; however, the end result is decreased SNS and enhanced vagal tone. Peripherally, there is decreased plasma renin activity as well as decreased EPI and NE levels.[356]

Cardiovascular effects of clonidine include decreased peripheral vascular resistance and HR.[357] The cardiovascular response to exercise is usually maintained. Prominent side-effects include hypotension, sedation, and dry mouth.[358,359] One of the more worrisome complications of clonidine use is the occurrence of a withdrawal syndrome on acute discontinuation of the drug. This usually occurs about 18 hours after discontinuation and consists of hypertension, tachycardia, insomnia, flushing, headache, apprehension, sweating, and tremulousness. It lasts for 24–72 hours and is most likely to occur in patients taking more than 1.2 mg · day^{-1} of clonidine. The withdrawal syndrome has been noted postoperatively in patients who were taken off clonidine for surgery.[360] It can be confused with anesthesia emergence symptoms, particularly in a patient with uncontrolled hypertension. Clonidine is not available for iv use, but symptoms of the withdrawal syndrome as well as routine postoperative hypertension can be treated with clonidine administered transdermally or rectally.[361] Withholding clonidine prior to surgery is not recommended.

Dexmedetomidine. Dexmedetomidine is a more selective α_2 agonist than clonidine.[362] It has a much shorter half-life (about 1.5 hours) and a more rapid onset of action (<5 minutes). The time to peak effect is 15 minutes. Intravenous dexmedetomidine provides excellent sedation, lowering of blood pressure and HR, and profound decreases in plasma catecholamines. Little respiratory depression is evident. Other studies have shown it to be an effective anxiolytic and sedative when used as premedication for anesthesia for minor gynecologic surgery. In an animal model, dexmedetomidine produces stereospecific and dose-dependent decreases in MAC.[363]

Flacke listed the potential uses of sympatholytic drugs in the future. In addition to the reducing effect of MAC and the absent respiratory depression, the following properties seem particularly valuable to the anesthesiologist[363]:

1. They are potent analgesics.
2. They are sedatives and anxiolytics.
3. They are antisialogogues.
4. They may promote hemodynamic stability.
5. Homeostatic reflexes remain intact.
6. They attenuate opioid rigidity (in animals).
7. Their circulatory actions can be reversed.

Clonidine has also been used successfully as a substitute for opiates and nicotine during withdrawal. It reduces sympathetic hyperactivity with head injury and can be used as an analgesic in the subarachnoid and epidural spaces for the treatment of pain.

Converting Enzyme Inhibitors

The renin-angiotensin system is integrally related to the ANS in controlling blood pressure (see Fig. 12-18). The central role of the renin-angiotensin-aldosterone system in the regulation of fluid balance and hemodynamics was not fully appreciated

until the discovery and clinical application of inhibitors of the angiotensin-converting enzyme (ACE).[126,127] Captopril, enalapril, and lisinopril inhibit converting enzyme and thereby prevent the conversion of angiotensin I to the active angiotensin II. These drugs have been highly effective in the treatment of all levels of essential hypertension as well as renovascular and malignant hypertension.[128,129] The cardiovascular effects normally involve only decreased peripheral vascular resistance. CO may remain normal or increase while the filling pressure remains unchanged. Thus, these drugs have been effective in the management of congestive heart failure as well.[364–366,367] There is usually no increase in SNS tone in response to the lowered blood pressure. ACE inhibition generally results in reductions in angiotensin-aldosterone, NE, and plasma antidiuretic hormone. This suppression is accompanied by a decrease in aldosterone and an improvement in cumulative plasma potassium levels, which are beneficial in both congestive heart failure and hypertension. It can be concluded that the major humoral responses to chronic congestive heart failure, even overlooking the effects of the diuretics, are affected by the release of angiotensin, aldosterone, and increased SNS tone.

Captopril, the first orally active compound, has proved highly effective in the treatment of all levels of hypertension and congestive heart failure (Table 12-28). Enalapril is a second-generation (nonsulfhydryl) ACE inhibitor. The omission of the sulfhydryl group possibly diminishes side-effects. Both captopril and enalapril combine a high degree of clinical efficacy with a low rate of side-effects. Both are eliminated *via* renal excretion and should be given in reduced doses in patients with renal dysfunction. Captopril has a shorter half-life and requires more frequent dosing than enalapril. Enalapril has to be converted by esterase in the liver and other tissues into the active compound enalaprilat. Many new ACE inhibitors are being developed that are eliminated *via* hepatic routes and may prove advantageous in renal failure. Lisinopril is one of these ACE inhibitors that is absorbed as the active form and is very long-acting.

The ACE inhibitors are associated with few side-effects and are increasingly popular in treating hypertension. Captopril may produce reversible neutropenia, dermatitis, and angioedema. Enalapril produces syncope, headache, and dizziness in about 1% of elderly patients. All ACE inhibitors may cause hypotension in patients who are hypovolemic and taking diuretic therapy. Diuretic therapy should be discontinued 1 week before starting ACE inhibitor therapy. The hypotensive effects are also enhanced by the concomitant use of calcium channel blockers. The ACE inhibitors blunt the hypokalemic effects of thiazide diuretics and may magnify the potassium-sparing effects of spironolactone, triamterene, and amiloride. In addition, non-

Tabe 12-28. THE ANGIOTENSIN-CONVERTING ENZYME (ACE)

Agent	Major Studies	Characteristics
Captopril	Quality of life; SAVE; diabetic nephropathy; ISIS-IV (early Stage AMI, trial negative)	The first ACE inhibitor; overall the best studied
Enalapril	CONSENSUS; SOLVD (prevention and treatment arms); V-HeFT I and II	Longer-acting; the best-studied in heart failure
Benazepril	None	Long plasma half-life (22 hr)
Cilazepril	None	Long tissue half-life
Fosinopril	None	Renal and hepatic elimination may allow safer use in renal or hepatic failure
Perindopril	None	Long plasma half-life (35 hr), less initial hypotension
Quinapril	QUIET (Quinapril Ischemic Event Trial: post-angioplasty, end points AMI, sudden death; ready 1995)	Potent binding to tissue ACE prolongs effective half-life
Ramipril	AIRE (acute infarction ramipril efficacy)	Long plasma half-life (>33 hr), proven use in postinfarct CHF
Trandolapril	TRACE (Trandolapril Cardiac Evaluation Study) on high-risk AMI patients; ready 1995	Long plasma half-life (20 hr); highly lipid-soluble with potential for tissue binding
Lisinopril	GISSI-III: early-stage AMI, mortality reduced by 11%	Active as is; water-soluble; long-acting

CHF = congestive heart failure.

steroidal anti-inflammatory drugs, including aspirin, may magnify the potassium-retaining effects of ACE inhibitors.

Vasodilators

The drugs that directly relax smooth muscle to cause vasodilation reflexively increase ANS tone and are included here for the sake of a complete discussion of antihypertensive drugs.[134] These are discussed with emphasis on perioperative use.

Hydralazine. Hydralazine is the most commonly used vasodilator and can be given by the im, iv, and oral routes. It relaxes smooth muscle tone directly, without interacting with adrenergic or cholinergic receptors. The mechanism of action is unknown. It is most potent in coronary, splanchnic, renal, and cerebral vessels, causing increased blood flow in each of these organs. The decrease in cardiac afterload is beneficial, but, unfortunately, there is usually a concomitant reflex tachycardia that may be severe. It is commonly combined with a β blocker such as propranolol. It may also cause fluid retention and is usually given chronically with a diuretic.[292] Hydralazine is metabolized by hepatic acetylation, and oral bioavailability may be low owing to first-pass metabolism. The elimination half-life is about 4 hours, but the pharmacologic half-life is much longer as a result of avid binding of the drug to smooth muscle. The effective half-life is approximately 100 hours.[368] Side-effects include a lupus-like syndrome, drug fever, skin rash, pancytopenia, and peripheral neuropathy. The iv dose we recommend for perioperative use is 5–10 mg in an iv bolus every 15–20 minutes until blood pressure control is achieved. It may also be given 10–40 mg im, but the response is slower.

Sodium Nitroprusside. Sodium nitroprusside is an extremely potent vasodilator that is available only for iv administration. It acts directly on smooth muscle, causing both arterial and venous dilation.[134,369] The mechanism of action is not entirely clear but appears to involve binding to α receptor on the surface of the myocyte, followed by activation of an intracellular vasodilator intermediate. The action of sodium nitroprusside on both venous and arterial sides of the circulation causes decreases in cardiac preload as well as afterload. This results in decreased cardiac work; however, it has been suggested that sodium nitroprusside may further compromise ischemic myocardium in the presence of occlusive coronary artery disease by shunting blood away from the ischemic zone.[370]

Sodium nitroprusside is useful during the perioperative period. It lowers blood pressure within 1–2 minutes, with the effect dissipating within 2 minutes after infusion is stopped. It is extremely potent and should be administered through a central venous line by infusion pump while continuously monitoring arterial pressure. The starting dose is $0.25–0.5\ \mu g \cdot kg^{-1} \cdot min^{-1}$. It can be increased slowly as needed to control blood pressure, but chances for toxicity are greater if the dose of 10 $\mu g \cdot kg^{-1} \cdot min^{-1}$ is exceeded. The dose required for steady-state-induced hypotension is variable.

Chemically, sodium nitroprusside consists of a ferrous iron atom bound with five cyanide molecules and one nitric group. The ferrous iron reacts with sulfhydryl groups in red blood cells and releases cyanide.[371] Cyanide is reduced to thiocyanate in the liver and excreted in the urine. The half-life of thiocyanate is 4 days, and it accumulates in the presence of renal failure.[372] There is no evidence, however, that pre-existing hepatic or renal failure increases the likelihood of cyanide toxicity. Administration of high doses of sodium nitroprusside can result in cyanide toxicity. The cyanide molecule binds to cytochrome oxidase, interfering with electron transport and causing cellular hypoxia. This can be recognized by increasing tolerance to the drug, elevated mixed venous Pa_{O_2}, and metabolic acidosis. The treatment of cyanide toxicity consists of (1) administration of amyl nitrate (by inhalation or directly into the anesthesia circuit), (2) infusion of sodium nitrite 5 $mg \cdot kg^{-1}$ over 4–5 minutes, and (3) administration of sodium thiosulfate 150 $mg \cdot kg^{-1}$ in 50 ml water over 15 minutes.

The hypotensive effects of sodium nitroprusside may be potentiated by inhalation anesthetics and blood loss; therefore, close perioperative monitoring is essential. It is commonly used to induce hypotension for decreasing blood loss in patients predisposed to major hemorrhage. Administration of sodium nitroprusside causes a reflex increase in sympathetic tone and renin release.[373] Drugs that blunt these reflexes markedly enhance its effects. Preoperative treatment with propranolol or captopril decreases the amount of sodium nitroprusside required for producing hypotension and thus decreases the potential for toxicity.[374,375]

Glyceril Trinitrate. Glyceril trinitrate, or nitroglycerin, is a venodilator used to treat myocardial ischemia. Its predominant action is on venules, causing increased venous capacitance and decreased cardiac preload. Effects on the arterial side are minimal except at very high doses. Upon iv administration, effects can be seen within 2 minutes, and they usually resolve within 5 minutes of discontinuing the drug. Side-effects are minimal, and there is no potential for cyanide toxicity as with nitroprusside. Use of nitroglycerin for control of perioperative hypertension has been reported,[376] but because of its relatively weak arteriolar action it is not as useful as other drugs as an antihypertensive agent. In obstetric patients with pre-eclampsia, however, it may be chosen over nitroprusside to circumvent potential cyanide toxicity to the fetus.[377]

Diazoxide. Diazoxide is a direct-acting vasodilator that may be given iv and is useful in hypertensive emergencies. It has a greater effect on resistance than capacitance vessels, thus decreasing cardiac afterload with little effect on preload. It also causes fluid retention and induces a reflex sympathetic response.[292] The hypotensive effect is potentiated by diuretics, sympatholytics, and hypovolemia. Diazoxide is usually administered as an iv bolus of 300 mg for a 70-kg adult. It is 90% bound to serum albumin; therefore, a substantial portion of the initial bolus may not reach the site of action. Rapid boluses (30 seconds) of 100 mg every 5 minutes are often recommended as an alternative to allow more free drug to reach the arterioles.[292] The hypotensive effect is usually obtained in 5–10 minutes and lasts 5–12 hours.

Calcium Entry Inhibitors

The calcium entry blockers verapamil, nifedipine, and nitrendipine may also be useful for treating hypertension in the perioperative period[378,379] (see Adrenergic Antagonists: Calcium Channel Blockers).

Treatment of Postoperative Hypertension

The wide variety of antihypertensive agents discussed previously makes the treatment of hypertension in the recovery room easier because we can now choose from among multiple routes of administration and variable onsets and durations of action of the different agents.[380,381] However, treatment may become confusing unless the basic pharmacology of each drug is understood. Those drugs available for only oral administration are not routinely used because of unreliable gastrointestinal function during this period. The etiology of postoperative hypertension in each case should be considered. A determination should be made as to whether this requires emergency therapy or is just urgent. Pain should be eliminated by assurance of adequate analgesia prior to therapy with antihypertensive agents. Also, because of the complex pathophysiology of hypertension, a thorough knowledge of each patient and his or her condition is mandatory in choosing a treatment regimen. The medications required for preoperative control may provide the most information in determining what will be necessary postoperatively. In particular, the use of drugs that may have an associated withdrawal syndrome, such as clonidine or β blockers, should be noted as well as if they were withheld prior to surgery. The volume status of the patient is also important. Fluid overload may require diuretic therapy. Volume depletion or hemorrhage may predispose to severe hypotension in response to routine doses of sympatholytics or vasodilators.

For severe elevations of blood pressure that require immediate treatment, sodium nitroprusside is the drug of choice. Diazoxide and nifedipine (sublingual) are also useful but may take 5–10 minutes to work. Intravenous nicardipine can be given and effective before a sodium nitroprusside infusion can be prepared. Labetalol, metoprolol, and esmolol may also be used intravenously. Esmolol has the advantage of being rapidly titratable.[382] α-Methyldopa may be used intravenously but takes much longer to work than clonidine. Clonidine can be given per rectum and begins to act in 10–20 minutes.[361] If conditions permit, it is helpful to use the drugs the patient was taking preoperatively to ease the transition in the postoperative period. Caution must be exercised if the hypertension is the result of excessive exogenous catecholamines, pheochromocytoma, or thyrotoxicosis. α Blockade should be started before β blockade. The hypertension may, in fact, worsen if β receptors are blocked first, leaving the α receptors unopposed.

REFERENCES

1. Guyton AC: The autonomic nervous system: The adrenal medulla. In Guyton AC (ed): Textbook of Medical Physiology, p. 686. Philadelphia, WB Saunders, 1986
2. Willis WD: The pain system: The neural basis of nociceptive transmission in the mammalian nervous system. In Gildenberg PL (ed): Pain and Headache, New York, Karger, 1985
3. Kewalramani LS: Autonomic dysreflexia in traumatic myelopathy. Am J Phys Med 59:1, 1980
4. Lake CR, Chernow B, Feuerstein G: The sympathetic nervous system in man: Its evaluation and the measurement of plasma NE. In Ziegler MG, Lake CR (eds): Norepinephrine, p 1. Baltimore, Williams & Wilkins, 1984
5. Axelrod J, Weinshilboum R: Catecholamines. N Engl J Med 287:237, 1972
6. Flacke WE, Flacke JW: Cholinergic and anticholinergic agents. In Smith NT, Corbascio AN (eds): Drug Interaction in Anesthesia, p 160. Philadelphia, Lea & Febiger, 1986
7. Yanowitz F, Preston JB, Abildskov JA: Functional distribution of right and left stellate innervation to the ventricles. Production of neurogenic electrocardiographic changes by unilateral alteration of sympathetic tone. Circ Res 18:416, 1966
8. Berne RM, Levy MN: Control of the heart. In Berne RM, Levy MN (eds): Cardiovascular Physiology, p 221. St. Louis, Mosby, 1977
9. Bexton RS, Milne JR, Cory-Pearce R et al: Effect of beta blockade on exercise response after cardiac transplantation. Br Heart J 49:584, 1983
10. Manger WM: Catecholamines in normal and abnormal cardiac function. In Kellerman JJ (ed): Advances in Cardiology, p 30. New York, Karger, 1982
11. Vatner SF: Regulation of coronary resistance vessels and large coronary arteries. Am J Cardiol 56:16E, 1985
12. Shepherd JT, Vanhoutte PM: Spasm of the coronary arteries: Causes and consequences (the scientist's viewpoint). Mayo Clin Proc 60:33, 1985
13. Anonymous: A symposium: Experimental and clinical aspects of coronary vasoconstriction. November 10, 1984, Miami, Florida. Am J Cardiol 56:1E, 1985
14. Bevan JA: Some bases of differences in vascular response to sympathetic activity. Circ Res 45:161, 1979
15. Koizumi K, Brooks CC: The autonomic nervous system and its role in controlling visceral activities. In Mountcastle VB (ed): Medical Physiology, p 783. St. Louis, CV Mosby, 1974
16. O'Rourke ST, Vanhoutte PM: Adrenergic and cholinergic regulation of bronchial vascular tone. Am Rev Respir Dis 146:S11, 1992
17. Benumof JL: The pulmonary circulation. In Kaplan JA (ed): Thoracic Anesthesia, p 249. New York, Churchill-Livingstone, 1983
18. Guyton AC: The pulmonary circulation. In Guyton AC (ed): Textbook of Medical Physiology, p 287. Philadelphia, WB Saunders, 1986
19. Benumof JL: One-lung ventilation and hypoxic pulmonary vasoconstriction: Implications for anesthetic management. Anesth Analg 64:821, 1985
20. Carlsson AJ, Bindslev L, Hedenstierna G: Hypoxia-induced pulmonary vasoconstriction in the human lung. The effect of isoflurane anesthesia. Anesthesiology 66:312, 1987
21. Comroe JH: Reflexes from the lungs. In Comroe JH (ed): Physiology of Respiration, p 72. Chicago, Year Book, 1979
22. Junod AF: Metabolism of vasoactive agents in lung. Am Rev Respir Dis 115:51, 1977
23. Pearl RG, Maze M, Rosenthal MH: Pulmonary and systemic hemodynamic effects of central venous and left atrial sympathomimetic drug administration in the dog. J Cardiothorac Anesth 1:29, 1987
24. Miller RJ: Multiple calcium channels and neuronal function. Science 235:46, 1987
25. Wood M: Cholinergic and parasympathomimetic drugs: Cholinesterases and anticholinesterases. In Wood M, Wood AJJ (eds): Drugs and Anesthesia, p 111. Baltimore, Williams & Wilkins, 1982
26. Oparil S, Katholi R: Humoral control of the circulation. In Garfein OB (ed): Current Concepts in Cardiovascular Physiology, p 208. San Diego, Academic Press, 1990
27. Thomas J, Fouad FM, Tarazi RC, Bravo EL: Evaluation of plasma catecholamines in humans. Correlation of resting levels with cardiac responses to beta-blocking and sympatholytic drugs. Hypertension 5:858, 1983
28. Lake CR, Ziegler MG, Kopin IJ: Use of plasma norepinephrine for evaluation of sympathetic neuronal function in man. Life Sci 18:1315, 1976
29. Stoelting RK: Sympathomimetics. In Stoelting RK (ed): Pharmacology and Physiology in Anesthetic Practice, p 251. Philadelphia, JB Lippincott, 1987
30. Hoefke W: Clonidine Pharmacology of Antihypertensive Drugs. New York, Raven Press, 1980
31. Lawson N: Catecholamines: The first messengers. In Skarvan K (ed): Bailliere's Clinical Anesthesiology, p 27. London, Bailliere Tindall, 1994
32. Zaimis E: Vasopressor drugs and catecholamines. Anesthesiology 29:732, 1968
33. Smith NT, Corbascio AN: The use and misuse of pressor agents. Anesthesiology 33:58, 1970
34. Shepherd JT, Vanhoutte PM: Neurohumoral regulation. In The Human Cardiovascular System, p 368. New York, Raven Press, 1984
35. Zaritsky AL, Chernow B: Catecholamines, sympathomimetics. In Ziegler MG, Lake CR (eds): Frontiers of Clinical Neuroscience, p 481. Baltimore, Williams & Wilkins, 1984
36. Chernow B, Rainey TG, Lake CR: Catecholamines in critical care medicine. In Ziegler MG, Lake CR (eds): Frontiers of Clinical Neuroscience, p 368. Baltimore, Williams & Wilkins, 1984
37. Fuder H: Selected aspects of presynaptic modulation of noradrenaline release from the heart. J Cardiovasc Pharmacol 7(suppl 5):S2, 1985
38. Kopin IJ: Metabolic degradation of catecholamines and relative importance of different pathways under physiological conditions and after the administration of drugs. In Blaschko H, Muscholl E (eds): Catecholamines: Handbook of Experimental Pharmacology, p 270. New York, Springer Verlag, 1972
39. Maze M: Clinical implications of membrane receptor function in anesthesia. Anesthesiology 55:160, 1981
40. Rardon DP, Bailey JC: Direct effects of cholinergic stimulation on ventricular automaticity in guinea pig myocardium. Circ Res 52:105, 1983
41. Prys-Roberts C: Structure and function of adrenoreceptors. In Skarvan K (ed): Bailliere's Clinical Anesthesiology, p 1. London, Bailliere Tindall, 1994
42. Kebabian JW, Calne DB: Multiple receptors for dopamine. Nature 277:93, 1979
43. Goldberg LI: The role of dopamine receptors in the treatment of congestive heart failure. J Cardiovasc Pharmacol 14(suppl 5):S19, 1989
44. Motulsky HJ, Insel PA: Radioligand binding to adrenergic receptors in humans. In Ziegler MG, Lake CR (eds): Norepinephrine, p 71. Baltimore, Williams & Wilkins, 1984
45. Vanhoutte PM, Flavahan NA: The heterogenicity of adrenergic receptors. In Szabadi E, Bradshaw CM, Nohovski SR (eds): Pharmacology of Adrenoreceptors, p 43. VCH, VCH Verlagsgesellschaft, Germany, 1985
46. Van Zwieten PA: The role of adrenoceptors in circulatory and metabolic regulation. Am Heart J 116:1384, 1988
47. Davey MJ: Alpha adrenoceptors—An overview. J Mol Cell Cardiol 18(suppl 5):1, 1986

48. Terzic A, Puceat M, Vassort G, Vogel SM: Cardiac α_1-adrenoceptors: An overview. Pharmacol Rev 45:147, 1993

49. Maze M, Hayward EJ, Gaba DM: α_1-Adrenergic blockade raises epinephrine-arrhythmia threshold in halothane-anesthetized dogs in a dose-dependent fashion. Anesthesiology 63:611, 1985

50. Aubry ML, Davey MJ, Petch B: Cardioprotective and antidysrhythmic effects of α_1-adrenoceptor blockade during myocardial ischaemia and reperfusion in the dog. J Cardiovasc Pharmacol 7(suppl 6):S93, 1985

51. Berthelsen S, Pettinger WA: A functional basis for classification of alpha-adrenergic receptors. Life Sci 21:595, 1977

52. Hoffman BB, Lefkowitz RJ: Alpha-adrenergic receptor subtypes. N Engl J Med 302:1390, 1980

53. Langer SZ, Hicks PE: Alpha-adrenoreceptor subtypes in blood vessels: Physiology and pharmacology. J Cardiovasc Pharmacol 6(suppl 4):S547, 1984

54. Langer SZ: Presynaptic regulation of catecholamine release. Biochem Pharmacol 23:1793, 1974

55. Hoffman JIE: Coronary physiology. In Garfein OB (ed): Current Concepts in Cardiovascular Physiology, p 289. San Diego, Academic Press, 1990

56. Cohen RA, Shepherd JT, Vanhoutte PM: Effects of the adrenergic transmitter on epicardial coronary arteries. Fed Proc 43:2862, 1984

57. Griggs DMJ, Chilian WM, Boatwright RB et al: Evidence against significant resting alpha-adrenergic coronary vasoconstrictor tone. Fed Proc 43:2873, 1984

58. Timmermans PB, Van Zwieten PA: α_2-Adrenoceptors: Classification, localization, mechanisms, and targets for drugs. J Med Chem 25:1389, 1982

59. Schmitz W, Kohl C, Neumann J et al: On the mechanism of positive inotropic effects of alpha-adrenoceptor agonists. Basic Res Cardiol 84(suppl 1):23, 1989

60. Osnes JB, Aass H, Skomedal T: Adrenoceptors in myocardial regulation: Concomitant contribution from both α- and β-adrenoceptor stimulation to the inotropic response. Basic Res Cardiol 84(suppl 1):9, 1989

61. Bohm M, Diet F, Feiler G et al: α-Adrenoceptors and α-adrenoceptor-mediated positive inotropic effects in failing human myocardium. J Cardiovasc Pharmacol 12:357, 1988

62. Murdock CJ, Hickey GM, Hockings BE et al: Effect of α_1-adrenoceptor blockade on ventricular ectopic beats in acute myocardial infarction. Int J Cardiol 26:45, 1990

63. Maze M, Tranquilli W: α_2-Adrenoceptor agonists: Defining the role in clinical anesthesia. Anesthesiology 74:581, 1991

64. De Mey J, Vanhoutte PM: Uneven distribution of postjunctional α_1- and α_2-like adrenoceptors in canine arterial and venous smooth muscle. Circ Res 48:875, 1981

65. DiBona GF: Update on renal neurology: Role of the renal nerves in formation of edema. Mayo Clin Proc 64:469, 1989

66. Bryan LJ, Cole JJ, O'Donnell SR, Wanstall JC: A study designed to explore the hypothesis that β_1-adrenoceptors are "innervated" receptors and β_2-adrenoceptors are "hormonal" receptors. J Pharmacol Exp Ther 216:395, 1981

67. Summers RJ, Molnaar P, Russell F et al: Coexistence and localization of β_1- and β_2-adrenoceptors in the human heart. Eur Heart J 10(suppl B):11, 1989

68. Keeton TK, Campbell WB: The pharmacologic alteration of renin release. Pharmacol Rev 32:81, 1980

69. Goldberg LI: Dopamine receptors and hypertension. Physiologic and pharmacologic implications. Am J Med 77:37, 1984

70. Kuchel OG, Kuchel GA: Peripheral dopamine in pathophysiology of hypertension. Interaction with aging and lifestyle. Hypertension 18:709, 1991

71. Goldberg LI: Pharmacological bases for the use of dopamine and related drugs in the treatment of congestive heart failure. J Cardiovasc Pharmacol 14(suppl 8):S21, 1989

72. Burns AM: Dopamine: Past, present and future (editorial). Clin Intensive Care 1:148, 1990

73. Yahr MD: Levodopa. Ann Intern Med 83:677, 1975

74. Miller R: Metoclopramide and dopamine receptor blockade. Neuropharmacology 15:463, 1976

75. Hilberman M, Maseda J, Stinson EB et al: The diuretic properties of dopamine in patients after open-heart operation. Anesthesiology 61:489, 1984

76. Owall A, Gordon E, Lagerkranser M et al: Clinical experience with adenosine for controlled hypotension during cerebral aneurysm surgery. Anesth Analg 66:229, 1987

77. Manchikanti L, Kraus JW, Edds SP: Cimetidine and related drugs in anesthesia. Anesth Analg 61:595, 1982

78. Lineberger AS, Sprague DH, Battaglini JW: Sinus arrest associated with cimetidine. Anesth Analg 64:554, 1985

79. Insel PA: Structure and function of α-adrenergic receptors. Am J Med 87:12S, 1989

80. Williams LT, Lefkowitz RJ: Receptor Binding Studies in Adrenergic Pharmacology. New York, Raven Press, 1979

81. Motulsky HJ, Insel PA: Adrenergic receptors in man: Direct identification, physiologic regulation, and clinical alterations. N Engl J Med 307:18, 1982

82. Tell GP, Haour F, Saez JM: Hormonal regulation of membrane receptors and cell responsiveness: A review. Metabolism 27:1566, 1978

83. Prichard BN, Owens CW, Smith CC, Walden RJ: Heart and catecholamines. Acta Cardiol 46:309, 1991

84. Prys-Roberts C: The changing face of adrenergic pharmacology. Curr Opin Anesth 5:113, 1992

85. Brodde OE: β-Adrenoceptors in cardiac disease. Pharmacol Ther 60:405, 1993

86. Glaubiger G, Lefkowitz RJ: Elevated β-adrenergic receptor number after chronic propranolol treatment. Biochem Biophys Res Commun 78:720, 1977

87. Hoefke W: Clonidine. In Scriabine A (ed): Pharmacology of Antihypertensive Drugs, p 55. New York, Raven Press, 1980

88. Watson S, Arkinstall S: Seven transmembrane proteins. In The G-Protein Linked Receptor Facts Book, p 2. London, Academic Press, 1994

89. Lynch CL III, Jaeger JM: The G protein cell signaling system. In Lake CL, Barash PG, Sperry RJ (eds): Advances in Anesthesia, p 65. St. Louis, Mosby–Year Book, 1994

90. Yost CS: G proteins: Basic characteristics and clinical potential for the practice of anesthesia. Anesth Analg 77:822, 1993

91. Gilman AG: G proteins: Transducers of receptor-generated signals. Annu Rev Biochem 56:615, 1987

92. Sutherland EW, Robison GA: The role of cyclic-3',5'-AMP in responses to catecholamines and other hormones. Pharmacol Rev 18:145, 1966

93. Fleming JW, Wisler PL, Watanabe AM: Signal transduction by G proteins in cardiac tissues. Circulation 85:420, 1992

94. Bosnjak ZJ: Ion channels in vascular smooth muscle: Physiology and pharmacology. Anesthesiology 79:1392, 1993

95. Stull JT, Gallagher PJ, Herring BP, Kamm KE: Vascular smooth muscle contractile elements: Cellular regulation. Hypertension 17:723, 1991

96. Lenzen C, Roewer N, Wappler F et al: Accelerated contractures after administration of ryanodine to skeletal muscle of malignant hyperthermia susceptible patients. Br J Anaesth 71:242, 1993

97. Johns RA: Endothelium, anesthetics, and vascular control. Anesthesiology 79:1381, 1993

98. Moncada S, Palmer RM, Higgs EA: Nitric oxide: Physiology, pathophysiology, and pharmacology. Pharmacol Rev 43:109, 1991

99. Murad F, Forstermann U, Nakanme M et al: The nitric oxide–cyclic GMP signal transduction system for intracellular and intercellular communication. In Brown BL, Dobson PRM (eds): Phosphoprotein Research, p 101. New York, Raven Press, 1993

100. Lincoln TM, Cornwell TL: Intracellular cyclic GMP receptor proteins. FASEB J 7:328, 1993

101. Torphy TJ: β-Adrenoceptors, cAMP and airway smooth muscle relaxation: Challenges to the dogma. Trends Pharmacol Sci 15:370, 1994

102. Conti M, Jin SL, Monaco L et al: Hormonal regulation of cyclic nucleotide phosphodiesterases. Endocr Rev 12:218, 1991

103. Krieger EM: Time course of baroreceptor resetting in acute hypertension. Am J Physiol 218:486, 1970

104. Flacke WE, Flacke JW: Cardiovascular physiology and circulatory control. Semin Anesth 1:185, 1982

105. Takeshima R, Dohi S: Circulatory responses to baroreflexes, Valsalva maneuver, coughing, swallowing, and nasal stimulation during acute cardiac sympathectomy by epidural blockade in awake humans. Anesthesiology 63:500, 1985

106. Berne RM, Levy MN: Coronary circulation and cardiac metabolism. In Berne RM, Levy MN (eds): Cardiovascular Physiology, p 221. St. Louis, CV Mosby, 1977

107. Guyton AC: Cardiac output, venous return, and their regulation. In Guyton AC (ed): Textbook of Medical Physiology, p 272. Philadelphia, WB Saunders, 1986

108. Sharpey-Schafer EP: Venous tone: Effects of reflex changes, humoral agents and exercise. Br Med Bull 19:115, 1963

109. Blinks JR: Positive chronotropic effect of increasing right atrial pressure in the isolated mammalian heart. Am J Physiol 196:299, 1956

110. Baron JF, Decaux-Jacolot A, Edouard A et al: Influence of venous return on baroreflex control of heart rate during lumbar epidural anesthesia in humans. Anesthesiology 64:188, 1986

111. Kotrly KJ, Ebert TJ, Vucins EJ et al: Baroreceptor reflex control of heart rate during morphine sulfate, diazepam, N₂O/O₂ anesthesia in humans. Anesthesiology 61:558, 1984

112. Greene NM: The cardiovascular system. In Greene NM (ed): Physiology of Spinal Anesthesia, p 43. New York, 1976

113. Greene NM: Perspectives in spinal anesthesia. Reg Anesth 7:55, 1982

114. Bailey PL, Stanley TH: Anesthesia for patients with a prior cardiac transplant. J Cardiothorac Anesth 4:38, 1990

115. Orlick AE, Ricci DR, Alderman EL et al: Effects of α adrenergic blockade upon coronary hemodynamics. J Clin Invest 62:459, 1978

116. Shepherd JT, Vanhoutte PM: Why nerves to coronary vessels? Fed Proc 43:2855, 1984

117. Moreland RS, Bohr DF: Adrenergic control of coronary arteries. Fed Proc 43:2857, 1984

118. Vanhoutte PM, Cohen RA: Effects of acetylcholine on the coronary artery. Fed Proc 43:2878, 1984

119. Feigl EO: Parasympathetic control of coronary blood flow. Fed Proc 43:2881, 1984

120. Loffelholz K, Muscholl E: A muscarinic inhibition of the noradrenaline release evoked by postganglionic sympathetic nerve stimulation. Naunyn-Schmiedebergs Arch Pharmakol 265:1, 1969

121. Levy MN, Blattberg B: Effect of vagal stimulation on the overflow of norepinephrine into the coronary sinus during cardiac sympathetic nerve stimulation in the dog. Circ Res 38:81, 1976

122. Yasue H, Touyama M, Shimamoto M et al: Role of autonomic nervous system in the pathogenesis of Prinzmetal's variant form of angina. Circulation 50:534, 1974

123. Schrier RW, Berl T, Anderson RJ: Osmotic and nonosmotic control of vasopressin release. Am J Physiol 236:F321, 1979

124. Coore HG, Randle PJ: Regulation of insulin secretion studied with pieces of rabbit pancreas incubated in vitro. Biochem J 93:66, 1964

125. Torretti J, Gerson JI, Oates RP, Lange JS: β-Adrenoceptor blockade and tolerance to potassium. Anesthesiology 64:846, 1986

126. Todd PA, Heel RC: Enalapril: A review of its pharmacodynamic and pharmacokinetic properties, and therapeutic use in hypertension and congestive heart failure. Drugs 31:198, 1986

127. Frohlich ED: Angiotensin converting enzyme inhibitors: Present and future. Hypertension 13:I125, 1989

128. Dzau VJ: Mechanism of action of angiotensin-converting enzyme (ACE) inhibitors in hypertension and heart failure. Role of plasma versus tissue ACE. Drugs 39(suppl 2):11, 1990

129. Weinberger MH: Angiotensin-converting enzyme inhibitors. Med Clin North Am 71:979, 1987

130. Stoelting RK: Antihypertensive drugs. In Stoelting RK (ed): Pharmacology and Physiology in Anesthetic Practice, p 294. Philadelphia, JB Lippincott, 1987

131. MacGregor GA, Dawes PM: Agonist and antagonist effects of Sar¹-Ala⁸–angiotensin II in salt-loaded and salt-depleted normal man. Br J Clin Pharmacol 3:483, 1976

132. Taylor P: Ganglionic stimulating and blocking agents. In Gilman AG, Goodman LS, Rall TW, Murad F (eds): The Pharmacological Basis of Therapeutics, p 315. New York, Macmillan, 1985

133. Vickers MD, Wood-Smith FG, Stewart HC: Cardiovascular drugs. In Vickers MD, Wood-Smith FG, Stewart HC (eds): Drugs in Anesthetic Practice, p 337. Boston, Butterworth, 1979

134. Stoelting RK: Peripheral vasodilators. In Stoelting RK (ed): Pharmacology and Physiology in Anesthetic Practice, p 307. Philadelphia, JB Lippincott, 1987

135. Wood M: Anticholinergic drugs: Anesthetic premedication. In Wood M, Wood AJJ (eds): Drugs and Anesthesia: Pharmacology for Anesthesiologists, p 141. Baltimore, Williams & Wilkins, 1982

136. Taylor P: Cholinergic agonists. In Gilman AG, Goodman LS, Rall TW, Murad F (eds): The Pharmacologic Basis of Therapeutics, p 100. New York, Macmillan, 1985

137. Stoelting RK: Anticholinesterase drugs and cholinergic agonists. In Stoelting RK (ed): Pharmacology and Physiology in Anesthetic Practice, p 217. Philadelphia, JB Lippincott, 1987

138. Duvoisin RC, Katz R: Reversal of central anticholinergic syndrome in man by physostigmine. JAMA 206:1963, 1968

139. Vickers MD, Wood-Smith FG, Stewart HC: Parasympathomimetic and cholinergic agents: Anticholinesterases. In Vickers MD, Wood-Smith FG, Stewart HC (eds): Drugs in Anesthetic Practice, p 306. Boston, Butterworth, 1979

140. Westfall TC: Muscarinic agents. In Bevan JA (ed): Essentials of Pharmacology, p 116. New York, Harper & Row, 1976

141. Westfall TC: Cholinesterase inhibitors. In Bevan JA (ed): Essentials of Pharmacology, p 120. New York, Harper & Row, 1976

142. Bell CM, Lewis CB: Effect of neostigmine on integrity of ileorectal anastomoses. Br Med J 3:587, 1968

143. Wilkins JL, Hardcastle JD, Mann CV, Kaufman L: Effects of neostigmine and atropine on motor activity of ileum, colon, and rectum of anaesthetized subjects. Br Med J 1:793, 1970

144. Brown EN, Daugherty MJ, Petty WC: Integrity of intestinal anastomoses following muscle relaxant reversal with neostigmine. Anesth Analg 52:117, 1973

145. Child CS: Prevention of neostigmine-induced colonic activity: A comparison of atropine and glycopyrronium. Anaesthesia 39:1083, 1984

146. Taylor P: Anticholinesterase agents. In Gilman AG, Goodman LS, Rall TW, Murad F (eds): The Pharmacological Basis of Therapeutics, p 110. New York, Macmillan, 1985

147. De Roeth AJ, Wong A, Dettbarn W et al: Blood cholinesterase activity of glaucoma patients treated with phospholine iodide. Am J Ophthalmol 62:834, 1966

148. Milby TH: Prevention and management of organophosphate poisoning. JAMA 216:2131, 1971

149. Stoelting RK: Anticholinergic drugs. In Stoelting RK (eds): Pharmacology and Physiology in Anesthetic Practice, p 232. Philadelphia, JB Lippincott, 1987

150. Price NM, Schmitt LG, McGuire J et al: Transdermal scopolamine in the prevention of motion sickness at sea. Clinical Pharmacol Ther 29:414, 1981

151. Brown JH: Atropine, scopolamine, and related antimuscarinic drugs. In Gilman AG, Rall TW, Nies AS, Taylor P (eds): The Pharmacological Basis of Therapeutics, 8th ed, p 150. New York, Macmillan, 1990

152. Westfall TC: Antimuscarinic agents. In Bevan JA (ed): Essentials of Pharmacology, p 128. New York, Harper & Row, 1976

153. Spaulding BC, Choi SD, Gross JB et al: The effect of physostigmine on diazepam-induced ventilatory depression: A double-blind study. Anesthesiology 61:551, 1984

154. Snir-Mor I, Weinstock M, Davidson JT, Bahar M: Physostigmine antagonizes morphine-induced respiratory depression in human subjects. Anesthesiology 59:6, 1983

155. Shoemaker WC, Kram HB, Appel PL: Therapy of shock based on pathophysiology, monitoring, and outcome prediction. Crit Care Med 18:S19, 1990

156. Shoemaker WC, Patil R, Appel PL, Kram HB: Hemodynamic and oxygen transport patterns for outcome prediction, therapeutic goals, and clinical algorithms to improve outcome. Feasibility of artificial intelligence to customize algorithms. Chest 102:617S, 1992

157. Reinart K: Principles and practice of SvO₂ monitoring. In King, Worth (eds): Intensive Care World, p 121. London, vol 5, 1988

158. Astiz ME, Rackow EC, Falk JL et al: Oxygen delivery and consumption in patients with hyperdynamic septic shock. Crit Care Med 15:26, 1987

159. Boudoulas H, Rittgers SE, Lewis RP et al: Changes in diastolic time with various pharmacologic agents: Implication for myocardial perfusion. Circulation 60:164, 1979

160. Royster RL: Intraoperative administration of inotropes in cardiac surgery patients. J Cardiothorac Anesth 4(suppl 5):17, 1990

161. Pagel PS, Grossman W, Haering JM, Warltier DC: Left ventricular diastolic function in the normal and diseased heart: Perspectives for the anesthesiologist (2). Anesthesiology 79:1104, 1993

162. Schwinn DA, Reves JG: Time course and hemodynamic effects of α₁-adrenergic bolus administration in anesthetized patients with myocardial disease. Anesth Analg 68:571, 1989

163. Rothe CF: Physiology of venous return: An unappreciated boost to the heart. Arch Intern Med 146:977, 1986

164. Stanton-Hicks M, Hock A, Stuhmeier KD, Arndt JO: Venoconstrictor agents mobilize blood from different sources and increase

intrathoracic filling during epidural anesthesia in supine humans. Anesthesiology 66:317, 1987

165. Lundberg J, Norgren L, Thomson D, Werner O: Hemodynamic effects of dopamine during thoracic epidural analgesia in man. Anesthesiology 66:641, 1987

166. Butterworth JF, Austin JC, Johnson MD et al: Effect of total spinal anesthesia on arterial and venous responses to dopamine and dobutamine. Anesth Analg 66:209, 1987

167. Sharpey-Schafer EP, Ginsburg J: Humoral agents and venous tone: Effects of catecholamines, 5-hydroxytryptamine, histamine and nitrates. Lancet 2:1337, 1962

168. Zimmerman BG, Abboud FM, Eckstein JW: Comparison of the effects of sympathomimetic amines upon venous and total vascular resistance in the foreleg of the dog. J Pharmacol Exp Ther 139:290, 1966

169. Schmid PG, Eckstein JW, Abboud FM: Comparison of the effects of several sympathomimetic amines on resistance and capacitance vessels in the forearm of man. Circulation 34:209, 1966

170. Brown BR Jr.: Selective venoconstriction by dopamine in comparision with isoproterenol and phenylephrine. Anesthesiology 43:570, 1975

171. McNay JL, McDonald RA, Goldberg LI: Direct renal vasodilatation produced by dopamine in the dog. Circ Res 16:510, 1965

172. Rude RE: Pharmacologic support in cardiogenic shock. Adv Shock Res 10:35, 1983

173. Rajfer SI, Goldberg LI: Sympathetic amines in the treatment of shock. In Shoemaker WC, Thompson WL, Holbrook PR (eds): Textbook of Critical Care, p 490. Philadelphia, WB Saunders, 1984

174. Houston MC, Thompson WL, Robertson D: Shock. Diagnosis and management. Arch Intern Med 144:1433, 1984

175. Shoemaker WC: Fluid management. Semin Anesth 2:251, 1983

176. Makabali C, Weil MH, Henning RJ: Dobutamine and other sympathomimetic drugs for the treatment of low cardiac output failure. Semin Anesth 1:63, 1982

177. Roberts R: The role of diuretics and inotropic therapy in failure associated with myocardial infarction. Arch Physiol Biochem 92:S33, 1984

178. Ramanathan S, Grant GJ: Vasopressor therapy for hypotension due to epidural anesthesia for cesarean section. Acta Anaesthesiol Scand 32:559, 1988

179. Rooke GA, Freund PR, Jacobson AF: Hemodynamic response and change in organ blood volume during spinal anesthesia in elderly men with cardiac disease. Anesth Analg 85:99, 1997

180. Evans DB, Weishaar RE, Kaplan HR: Strategy for the discovery and development of a positive inotropic agent. Pharmacol Ther 16:303, 1982

181. Hug CC, Kaplan JA: Pharmacology-cardiac drugs. In Kaplan JA (ed): Cardiac Anesthesia, p 39. New York, Grune & Stratton, 1979

182. Bourdarias JP, Dubourg O, Gueret P et al: Inotropic agents in the treatment of cardiogenic shock. Pharmacol Ther 22:53, 1983

183. Mueller HS: Catecholamine support of the critically ill cardiac patient: Inotropic agents versus vasopressors α- or β-adrenergic agonists or both? Intensive Crit Care Dig 5:36, 1986

184. Desjars P, Pinaud M, Bugnon D, Tasseau F: Norepinephrine therapy has no deleterious renal effects in human septic shock. Crit Care Med 17:426, 1989

185. Meadows D, Edwards JD, Wilkins RG, Nightingale P: Reversal of intractable septic shock with norepinephrine therapy. Crit Care Med 16:663, 1988

186. Desjars P, Pinaud M, Potel G et al: A reappraisal of norepinephrine therapy in human septic shock. Crit Care Med 15:134, 1987

187. Stuart-Taylor ME, Crosse MM: A plea for noradrenaline. Anaesthesia 44:916, 1989

188. Tarnow J, Muller RK: Cardiovascular effect of low-dose epinephrine infusions in relation to the extent of preoperative β-adrenoceptor blockade. Anesthesiology 74:1035, 1991

189. Karns JL: Epinephrine-induced potentially lethal arrhythmia during arthroscoic shoulder surgery: A case report. Am Assoc Nurse Anes J 67:419, 1999

190. Maze M, Smith CM: Identification of receptor mechanism mediating epinephrine-induced arrhythmias during halothane anesthesia in the dog. Anesthesiology 59:322, 1983

191. Kapur PA, Flacke WE: Epinephrine-induced arrhythmias and cardiovascular function after verapamil during halothane anesthesia in the dog. Anesthesiology 55:218, 1981

192. Reves JG, Kissin I, Lell WA, Tosone S: Calcium entry blockers:

Uses and implications for anesthesiologists. Anesthesiology 57:504, 1982

193. Stoelting RK: Calcium entry blockers. In Stoelting RK (ed): Pharmacology and Physiology in Anesthetic Practice, p 355. Philadelphia, JB Lippincott, 1987

194. Wood M: Drugs and the sympathetic nervous system. In Wood M, Alistair JJ (eds): Drugs and Anesthesia, p 407. Baltimore, Williams & Wilkins, 1982

195. Johnston RR, Eger EI II, Wilson C: A comparative interaction of epinephrine with enflurane, isoflurane, and halothane in man. Anesth Analg 55:709, 1976

196. Karl HW, Swedlow DB, Lee KW, Downes JJ: Epinephrine-halothane interactions in children. Anesthesiology 58:142, 1983

197. Olsen NV, Lund J, Jensen PF et al: Dopamine, dobutamine, and dopexamine: A comparison of renal effects in unanesthetized human volunteers. Anesthesiology 79:685, 1993

198. Vincent J: Do we need a dopaminergic agent in the management of the critically ill? Auton Pharmacol 10:123, 1990

199. Garwood S, Hines R: Perioperative renal preservation: Dopexamine and fenoldopam—New agents to augment renal performance. Semin Anesth 17:308, 1998

200. Murphy MB, Elliott WJ: Dopamine and dopamine receptor agonists in cardiovascular therapy. Crit Care Med 18:S14, 1990

201. Leier CV, Binkley PF, Carpenter J et al: Cardiovascular pharmacology of dopexamine in low output congestive heart failure. Am J Cardiol 62:94, 1988

202. Lokhandwala MF, Hegde SS: Cardiovascular pharmacology of adrenergic and dopaminergic receptors: Therapeutic significance in congestive heart failure. Am J Med 90:2S, 1991

203. Jaski BE, Peters C: Inotropic, vascular and neuroendocrine effects of dopexamine hydrochloride and comparison with dobutamine. Am J Cardiol 62:63C, 1988

204. Gollub SB, Elkayam U, Young JB et al: Efficacy and safety of a short-term (6-h) intravenous infusion of dopexamine in patients with severe congestive heart failure: A randomized, double-blind, parallel, placebo-controlled multicenter study. J Am Coll Cardiol 18:383, 1991

205. Poelaert JI, Mungroop HE, Koolen JJ, Van den Berg PC: Hemodynamic effects of dopexamine in patients following coronary artery bypass surgery. J Cardiothorac Anesth 3:441, 1989

206. Lokhandwala MF: Renal actions of dopexamine hydrochloride. Clin Intensive Care 1:163, 1990

207. Stephan H, Sonntag H, Henning H, Yoshimine K: Cardiovascular and renal haemodynamic effects of dopexamine: Comparison with dopamine. Br J Anaesth 65:380, 1990

208. Gray PA, Bodenham AR, Park GR: A comparison of dopexamine and dopamine to prevent renal impairment in patients undergoing orthotopic liver transplantation. Anaesthesia 46:638, 1991

209. Jamison M, Widerhorn J, Weber L et al: Central and renal hemodynamic effects of a new agonist at peripheral dopamine- and β_2-adrenoreceptors (dopexamine) in patients with heart failure. Am Heart J 117:607, 1989

210. Ghosh S, Gray B, Oduro A, Latimer RD: Dopexamine hydrochloride: pharmacology and use in low cardiac output states. J Cardiothorac Anesth 5:382, 1991

211. Fitton A, Benfield P: Dopexamine hydrochloride: A review of its pharmacodynamic and pharmacokinetic properties and therapeutic potential in acute cardiac insufficiency. Drugs 39:308, 1990

212. Meinertz T, Drexler H, Just H: Dopexamine in congestive heart failure: How do the pharmacological activities translate into the clinical situation? Basic Res Cardiol 84(suppl 1):177, 1989

213. Hunter DN, Gray H, Mudaliar Y et al: The effects of dopexamine hydrochloride on cardiopulmonary haemodynamics following cardiopulmonary bypass surgery. Int J Cardiol 23:365, 1989

214. Aronson S, Goldberg LI, Roth S et al: Preservation of renal blood flow during hypotension induced with fenoldopam in dogs. Can J Anaesth 37:380, 1990

215. Aronson S, Goldberg LI, Glock D et al: Effects of fenoldopam on renal blood flow and systemic hemodynamics during isoflurane anesthesia. J Cardiothorac Anesth 5:29, 1991

216. Kien ND, Moore PG, Jaffe RS: Cardiovascular function during induced hypotension by fenoldopam or sodium nitroprusside in anesthetized dogs. Anesth Analg 74:72, 1992

217. Shusterman NH, Elliott WJ, White WB: Fenoldopam, but not nitroprusside, improves renal function in severely hypertensive patients with impaired renal function. Am J Med 95:161, 1993

218. Brooks DP, Drutz DJ, Ruffolo RR Jr.: Prevention and complete

reversal of cyclosporine A-induced renal vasoconstriction and nephrotoxicity in the rat by fenoldopam. J Pharmacol Exp Ther 254:375, 1990

219. White WB, Radford MJ, Gonzalez FE *et al:* Selective dopamine-1 agonist therapy in severe hypertension: Effects of intravenous fenoldopam. Am J Med 95:161, 1988

220. Oparil S, Aronson S, Deeb GM *et al:* Fenoldopam: A new parenteral antihypertensive. Consensus roundtable on the management of perioperative hypertension and hypertensive crises. Am J Hypertension 12:653, 1999

221. Rajfer SI, Rossen JD, Nemanich JW *et al:* Sustained hemodynamic improvement during long-term therapy with levodopa in heart failure: Role of plasma catecholamines. J Am Coll Cardiol 10:1286, 1987

222. Tarnow J, Komar K: Altered hemodynamic response to dobutamine in relation to the degree of preoperative β-adrenoceptor blockade. Anesthesiology 68:912, 1988

223. Steen PA, Tinker JH, Pluth JR *et al:* Efficacy of dopamine, dobutamine, and epinephrine during emergence from cardiopulmonary bypass in man. Circulation 57:378, 1978

224. Maekawa K, Liang CS, Hood WB Jr.: Comparison of dobutamine and dopamine in acute myocardial infarction: Effects of systemic hemodynamics, plasma catecholamines, blood flows and infarct size. Circulation 67:750, 1983

225. Butterworth JF, Prielipp RC, Royster RL *et al:* Dobutamine increases heart rate more than epinephrine in patients recovering from aortocoronary bypass surgery. J Cardiothorac Anesth 6:535, 1992

226. Pierard LA, De Landsheere CM, Berthe C *et al:* Identification of viable myocardium by echocardiography during dobutamine infusion in patients with myocardial infarction after thrombolytic therapy: Comparison with positron emission tomography. J Am Coll Cardiol 15:1021, 1990

227. McGhie AI, Golstein RA: Pathogenesis and management of acute heart failure and cardiogenic shock: Role of inotropic therapy. Chest 102:626S, 1992

228. Teich S, Chernow B: Specific cardiovascular drugs utilized in the critically ill. Crit Care Clin 1:491, 1985

229. Harkin CP, Farber NE: New cardiac inotropic drugs. In Advances in Anesthesiology, p 461. St. Louis, Mosby, 1996

230. Lawson N: Therapeutic combinations of vasopressors and inotropic agents. Semin Anesthesiol 9:270, 1990

231. Braunwald E, Colucci WS: Vasodilator therapy of heart failure. Has the promissory note been paid? N Engl J Med 310:459, 1984

232. Banic A, Krejci V, Erni D *et al:* Effects of sodium nitroprusside and phenylephrine on blood flow in free musculocutaneous flaps during general anesthesia. Anesthesiology 90:147, 1999

233. el Allaf D, Cremers S, D'Orio V, Carlier J: Combined haemodynamic effects of low doses of dopamine and dobutamine in patients with acute infarction and cardiac failure. Arch Int Physiol Biochem 92:S49, 1984

234. Royster RL, Butterworth JF, Prielipp RC *et al:* Combined inotropic effects of amrinone and epinephrine after cardiopulmonary bypass in humans. Anesth Analg 77:662, 1993

235. Richard C, Ricome JL, Rimailho A *et al:* Combined hemodynamic effects of dopamine and dobutamine in cardiogenic shock. Circulation 67:620, 1983

236. Tinker JH: Perioperative myocardial infarction. Semin Anesthesiol 253, 1982

237. Ferguson JE, Hensleigh PA, Kredenster D: Adjunctive use of magnesium sulfate with ritodrine for preterm labor tocolysis. Am J Obstet Gynecol 148:166, 1984

238. Schwarz R, Retzke U: Cardiovascular effects of terbutalin in pregnant women. Acta Obstet Gynecol Scand 62:419, 1983

239. Segal S, Csavoy AN, Datta S: The tocolytic effect of catecholamines in the gravid rat uterus. Anesth Analg 87:864, 1998

240. Beneditti TJ: Maternal complications of parenteral β-sympathetic therapy for premature labor. Am J Obstet Gynecol 145:1, 1983

241. Norwitz ER, Robinson JN, Challis JRG: The control of labor. N Engl J Med 341:660, 1999

242. Pou-Martinez A, Kelly SH, Newell FD, Culbert CM: Postpartum pulmonary edema after ritodrine and betamethasone use. J Reprod Med 27:428, 1982

243. Semchyshyn S, Zuspan FP, O'Shaughnessy R: Pulmonary edema associated with the use of hydrocortisone and a tocolytic agent for the management of premature labor. J Reprod Med 28:47, 1983

244. Spielman RJ: Maternal effects and complications of β-adrenergic therapy for premature labor. Res Staff Phys 32:102, 1986

245. Rasmussen H: Cell communication, calcium ion, and cyclic adenosine monophosphate. Science 170:404, 1970

246. Belardinelli L, Isenberg G: Isolated atrial myocytes: Adenosine and acetylcholine increase potassium conductance. Am J Physiol 244:H734, 1983

247. Marsch SCU: Adenosine. In Clinical Pharmacology, p 201. London, Bailliere Tindall, 1994

248. DiMarco JP, Miles W, Akhtar M *et al:* Adenosine for paroxysmal supraventricular tachycardia: Dose ranging and comparison with verapamil. Assessment in placebo-controlled, multicenter trials. Ann Intern Med 113:104, 1990

249. Dreifus LS, Hessen SE: Supraventricular tachycardia: Diagnosis and treatment. Cardiology 77:259, 1990

250. Rossi AF, Steinberg LG, Kipel G *et al:* Use of adenosine in the management of perioperative arrhythmias in the pediatric cardiac intensive care unit. Crit Care Med 20:1107, 1992

251. Opie LH: Antiarrhythmic agents. In Opie LH (ed): Drugs for the Heart, p 180. Philadelphia, WB Saunders, 1991

252. Freilich A, Tepper D: Adenosine and its cardiovascular effects. Am Heart J 123:1324, 1992

253. Rutman HI, LeJemtel TH, Sonnenblick EH: Newer cardiotonic agents: implications for patients with heart failure and ischemic heart disease. J Cardiothorac Anesth 1:59, 1987

254. Stirt JA, Sullivan SF: Aminophylline. Anesth Analg 60:587, 1981

255. Boldt J, Hempelmann G: Phosphodiesterase inhibitors. In Clinical Pharmacology, p 59. London, Bailliere Tindall, 1994

256. Levy JH, Bailey JM: Amrinone: Pharmacokinetics and pharmacodynamics. J Cardiothorac Anesth 3:10, 1989

257. Hines R: Clinical applications of amrinone. J Cardiothorac Anesth 3:24, 1989

258. Pagel PS, Hettrick DA, Warltier DC: Amrinone enhances myocardial contractility and improves left ventricular diastolic function in conscious and anesthetized chronically instrumented dogs. Anesthesiology 79:753, 1993

259. Baunwald E: Newer positive inotropic agents. Circulation 73:III1, 1986

260. Benotti JR, Grossman W, Braunwald E, Carabello BA: Effects of amrinone on myocardial energy metabolism and hemodynamics in patients with severe congestive heart failure due to coronary artery disease. Circulation 62:28, 1980

261. Ward A, Brogden RN, Heel RC *et al:* Amrinone: A preliminary review of its pharmacological properties and therapeutic use. Drugs 26:468, 1983

262. Baim DS, McDowell AV, Cherniles J *et al:* Evaluation of a new bipyridine inotropic agent—milrinone—in patients with severe congestive heart failure. N Engl J Med 309:748, 1983

263. Mollhoff T, Loick HM, Van Aken H *et al:* Milrinone modulates endotoxemia, systemic inflammation, and subsequent acute phase response after cardiopulmonary bypass (CPB). Anesthesiology 90:72, 1999

264. Yndgaard S, Lippert FK, Berthelsen PG: Are patients chronically treated with β₁-adrenoceptor antagonists in fact beta-blocked? J Cardiothorac Anesth 11:32, 1997

265. Doolan LA, Jones EF, Kalman J *et al:* A placebo-controlled trial verifying the efficacy of milrinone in weaning high-risk patients from cardiopulmonary bypass. J Cardiothorac Anesth 11:37, 1997

266. Boldt J, Kling D, Moosdorf R, Hempelmann G: Enoximone treatment of impaired myocardial function during cardiac surgery: Combined effects with epinephrine. J Cardiothorac Anesth 4:462, 1990

267. Zaloga GP, Chernow B: Insulin, glucagon and growth hormone. In Chernow B, Lake CR (eds): The Pharmacologic Approach to the Critically Ill Patient, p 562. Baltimore, Williams & Wilkins, 1983

268. Stoelting RK: Digitalis and related drugs. In Stoelting RK (ed): Pharmacology and Physiology in Anesthetic Practice, p 269. Philadelphia, JB Lippincott, 1987

269. Haustein KO: Digitalis. Pharmacol Ther 18:1, 1982

270. Butterworth JF, Zaloga GP: Calcium and magnesium as vasoactive drugs. In Clinical Pharmacology, p 109. London, Bailliere Tindall, 1994

271. Silverberg RA, Weil MH: Cardiopulmonary resuscitation. In Chernow B, Lake CR (eds): The Pharmacologic Approach to the Critically Ill Patient, p 140. Baltimore, Williams & Wilkins, 1983

272. Blecic S, De Backer D, Huynh CH *et al:* Calcium chloride in

experimental electromechanical dissociation: A placebo-controlled trial in dogs. Crit Care Med 15:324, 1987

273. Montgomery WH, Donegan J, McIntyre K: Standards and guidelines for cardiopulmonary resuscitation and emergency cardiac care. Circulation 74:IV1, 1986

274. White RD, Goldsmith RS, Rodriguez R et al: Plasma ionic calcium levels following injection of chloride, gluconate, and gluceptate salts of calcium. J Thorac Cardiovasc Surg 71:609, 1976

275. Oshida J, Goto H, Benson KT, Arakawa K: Effects of calcium chloride on verapamil- and diltiazem-pretreated isolated rat hearts. J Cardiothorac Anesth 7:717, 1993

276. Cote CJ, Drop LJ, Daniels AL, Hoaglin DC: Calcium chloride versus calcium gluconate: Comparison of ionization and cardiovascular effects in children and dogs. Anesthesiology 66:465, 1987

277. Desai TK, Carlson RW, Thill-Baharozian M, Geheb MA: A direct relationship between ionized calcium and arterial pressure among patients in an intensive care unit. Crit Care Med 16:578, 1988

278. Marquez J, Martin D, Virji MA et al: Cardiovascular depression secondary to ionic hypocalcemia during hepatic transplantation in humans. Anesthesiology 65:457, 1986

279. Wong KC, Everett JD: Sympathomimetic drugs. In Smith NT, Corbascio AN (eds): Drug Interactions in Anesthesia, p 71. Philadelphia, Lea & Febiger, 1986

280. Stoelting RK: Drugs used in treatment of psychiatric disease. In Stoelting RK (ed): Pharmacology and Physiology in Anesthetic Practice, p 347. Philadelphia, JB Lippincott, 1987

281. Wong KC, Ashburn MA: Monoamine oxidase inhibitors and anesthesia. In Literature Scan: Anesthesiology Current Insights. Cedar Knoll, New Jersey, Word Medical Communication, 1990

282. Wells DG, Bjorksten AR: Monoamine oxidase inhibitors revisited. Can J Anaesth 36:64, 1989

283. Bhatara VS, Magnus RD, Paul KL, Preskorn SH: Serotonin syndrome induced by venlafaxine and fluoxetine: A case study in polypharmacy and potential pharmacodynamic and pharmacokinetic mechanisms. Ann Pharmacother 32:432, 1998

284. Harvey AT, Preskorn SH: Cytochrome P450 enzymes: Interpretation of their interactions with selective serotonin reuptake inhibitors. J Clin Psychopharm 16:273, 1997

285. Catterson ML, Preskorn SH, Martin RL: Pharmacodynamic and pharmacokinetic considerations in geriatric psychopharmacology. Psychiatr Clin North Am 20:205, 1997

286. Zacny JP, Galinkin JL: Psychotropic drugs used in anesthesia practice. Anesthesiology 90:269, 1999

287. Weiner N: Drugs that inhibit adrenergic nerves and block adrenergic receptors. In Gilman AG, Goodman LS, Rall TW, Murad F (eds): The Pharmacological Basis of Therapeutics, p 181. New York, Macmillan, 1985

288. Nickerson M, Goodman LS: Pharmacological properties of a new adrenergic blocking agent: N,N-Dibenzyl-b-chlorethylamine (dibenamine). J Pharmacol Exp Ther 89:167, 1947

289. Hickey PR, Hansen DD: Anesthesia and cardiac shunting in the neonate: Ductus arteriosus, transitional circulation, and congenital heart disease. Semin Anesthesiol 3:106, 1984

290. Grover RF, Reeves JT, Blount SG: Tolazoline hydrochloride (priscoline) and effective pulmonary vasodilator. Am Heart J 61:5, 1961

291. Koch-Weser J, Graham RM, Pettinger WA: Drug therapy: Prazosin. N Engl J Med 300:232, 1979

292. Ziegler MG: Antihypertensives. In Chernow B, Lake CR (eds): The Pharmacologic Approach to the Critically Ill Patient, p 303. Baltimore, Williams & Wilkins, 1983

293. Lowenthal DT, Saris SD, Packer J et al: Mechanisms of action and the clinical pharmacology of β-adrenergic blocking drugs. Am J Med 77:119, 1984

294. Wood AJ: Pharmacologic differences between beta blockers. Am Heart J 108:1070, 1984

295. Shand DG: Comparative pharmacology of the β-adrenoreceptor blocking drugs. Drugs 25:92, 1983

296. McDevitt DG: Clinical significance of cardioselectivity. Prim Cardiol (supp 1):165, 1983

297. Clausen N, Damsgaard T, Mellemgaard K: Antihypertensive effect of a nonselective (propranolol) and a cardioselective (metoprolol) β-adrenoceptor blocking agent at rest and during exercise. Br J Clin Pharmacol 7:379, 1979

298. Woods KL, Wright AD, Kendall MJ, Black E: Lack of effect of propranolol and metoprolol on glucose tolerance in maturity-onset diabetics. Br Med J 281:1321, 1980

299. Chang LC: Use of practolol in asthmatics: A plea for caution. Lancet 2:321, 1971

300. Boudoulas H, Lewis RP, Kates RE, Dalamangas G: Hypersensitivity to adrenergic stimulation after propranolol withdrawal in normal subjects. Ann Intern Med 87:433, 1977

301. Stoelting RK: Alpha- and beta-adrenergic receptor antagonists. In Stoelting RK (ed): Pharmacology and Physiology in Anesthetic Practice, p 280. Philadelphia, JB Lippincott, 1987

302. Avorn J, Everitt DE, Weiss S: Increased antidepressant use in patients prescribed beta-blockers. JAMA 255:357, 1986

303. Slogoff S, Keats AS: Does perioperative myocardial ischemia lead to postoperative myocardial infarction? Anesthesiology 62:107, 1985

304. Silke B, Verma SP, Ahuja RC et al: Is the intrinsic sympathomimetic activity (ISA) of beta-blocking compounds relevant in acute myocardial infarction? Eur J Clin Pharmacol 27:509, 1984

305. Taylor SH, Silke B, Lee PS: Intravenous beta-blockade in coronary heart disease: Is cardioselectivity or intrinsic sympathomimetic activity hemodynamically useful? N Engl J Med 306:631, 1982

306. Reid JL, Dean CR, Jones DH: Central actions of anti-hypertensive drugs. Cardiovasc Med 2:1185, 1977

307. Pratt CM, Young JB, Roberts R: The role of beta-blockers in the treatment of patients after infarction. Cardiol Clin 2:13, 1984

308. Frishman WH: Drug therapy: Atenolol and timolol, two new systemic β-adrenoceptor antagonists. N Engl J Med 306:1456, 1982

309. Formgren H: Broncho- and cardioselective β-receptor active drugs in the treatment of asthmatic patients. Clinical studies of effects and side-effects of terbutaline, practolol and metoprolol. Scand J Respir Dis 97(suppl):1, 1977

310. Wollam GL, Cody RJJ, Tarazi RC, Bravo EL: Acute hemodynamic effects and cardioselectivity of acebutolol, practolol, and propranolol. Clinical Pharmacol Ther 25:813, 1979

311. Basil B, Jordan R: Pharmacological properties of diacetolol, a major metabolite of acebutolol. Eur J Pharmacol 80:47, 1982

312. Girard D, Shulman BJ, Thys DM et al: The safety and efficacy of esmolol during myocardial revascularization. Anesthesiology 65:157, 1986

313. Menkhaus PG, Reves JG, Kissin I et al: Cardiovascular effects of esmolol in anesthetized humans. Anesth Analg 64:327, 1985

314. Steck J, Sheppard D, Byrd R et al: Pulmonary effects of esmolol. Clin Res 33:472A, 1985

315. Gorczynski RJ: Basic pharmacology of esmolol. Am J Cardiol 56:3F, 1985

316. de Bruijn NP, Reves JG, Croughwell N et al: Pharmacokinetics of esmolol in anesthetized patients receiving chronic beta blocker therapy. Anesthesiology 66:323, 1987

317. Gold MI, Sacks DJ, Grosnoff DB et al: Use of esmolol during anesthesia to treat tachycardia and hypertension. Anesth Analg 68:101, 1989

318. Jordan D, Shulman SM, Miller ED Jr: Esmolol hydrochloride, sodium nitroprusside, and isoflurane differ in their ability to alter peripheral sympathetic responses. Anesth Analg 77:281, 1993

319. Wilson DJ, Wallin JD, Vlachakis ND et al: Intravenous labetalol in the treatment of severe hypertension and hypertensive emergencies. Am J Med 75:95, 1983

320. Gagnon RM, Morissette M, Presant S et al: Hemodynamic and coronary effects of intravenous labetalol in coronary artery disease. Am J Cardiol 49:1267, 1982

321. Lebel M, Langlois S, Belleau LJ, Grose JH: Labetalol infusion in hypertensive emergencies. Clin Pharmacol Ther 37:615, 1985

322. Atlee JA: Normal electrical activity of the heart. In Atlee JA (ed): Perioperative Cardiac Dysrhythmias, p 16. Chicago, Year Book, 1985

323. Nayler WG, Poole-Wilson P: Calcium antagonists: Definition and mode of action. Basic Res Cardiol 76:1, 1981

324. Triggle DJ: Calcium antagonists: Basic chemical and pharmacological aspects. In Weiss GB (ed): New Perspectives on Calcium Antagonists, p 1. Baltimore, Williams & Wilkins, 1981

325. Marty J: Calcium antagonists and urapidil. In Clinical Pharmacology, p 137. London, Bailliere Tindall, 1994

326. Henry PD: Comparative pharmacology of calcium antagonists: Nifedipine, verapamil and diltiazem. Am J Cardiol 46:1047, 1980

327. Millard RW, Lathrop DA, Grupp G et al: Differential cardiovascular effects of calcium channel blocking agents: Potential mechanisms. Am J Cardiol 49:499, 1982

328. Reves JG: The relative hemodynamic effects of Ca²⁺ entry blockers. Anesthesiology 61:3, 1984

329. Kraynack BJ, Lawson NW, Gintautas J: Local anesthetic effect of verapamil in vitro. Reg Anaesth 7:114, 1982

330. McLeod AA, Jewitt DE: Drug treatment of primary pulmonary hypertension. Drugs 31:177, 1986

331. Fleckenstein A: Specific pharmacology of calcium in myocardium, cardiac pacemakers, and vascular smooth muscle. Ann Rev Pharmacol Toxicol 17:149, 1977

332. Atlee JA: Drugs used for treatment of cardiac dysrhythmias. In Atlee JA (ed): Perioperative Cardiac Dysrhythmias, p. 272. Chicago, Year Book, 1985

333. Haft JI, Habbab MA: Treatment of atrial arrhythmias: Effectiveness of verapamil when preceded by calcium infusion. Arch Intern Med 146:1085, 1986

334. Stone PH, Antman EM, Muller JE, Braunwald E: Calcium channel blocking agents in the treatment of cardiovascular disorders. Part II: Hemodynamic effects and clinical applications. Ann Intern Med 93:886, 1980

335. Morad M, Tung L: Ionic events responsible for the cardiac resting and action potential. Am J Cardiol 49:584, 1982

336. Klein HO, Kaplinsky E: Digitalis and verapamil in atrial fibrillation and flutter. Is verapamil now the preferred agent? Drugs 31:185, 1986

337. Atlee JA: Management of specific cardiac dysrhythmias. In Atlee JA (ed): Perioperative Cardiac Dysrhythmias, p 380. Chicago, Year Book, 1985

338. Clusin WT, Bristow MR, Karagueuzian HS et al: Do calcium-dependent ionic currents mediate ischemic ventricular fibrillation? Am J Cardiol 49:606, 1982

339. Given BD, Lee TH, Stone PH, Dzau VJ: Nifedipine in severely hypertensive patients with congestive heart failure and preserved ventricular systolic function. Arch Intern Med 145:281, 1985

340. Kraynack BJ: Calcium channel blocking agents: Side effects and drug interactions. In Annual Refresher Course Lecture 238. Chicago, American Society of Anesthesiology, 1983

341. Merin RG: Calcium (slow) channel blocking drugs. In Annual Refresher Course Lecture 101. Chicago, American Society of Anesthesiology, 1982

342. Halpern NA, Sladen RN, Goldberg JS et al: Nicardipine infusion for postoperative hypertension after surgery of the head and neck. Crit Care Med 18:950, 1990

343. Merin RG: Are the myocardial functional and metabolic effects of isoflurane really different from those of halothane and enflurane? Anesthesiology 55:398, 1981

344. Merin RG, Chelly JE, Hysing ES et al: Cardiovascular effects of and interaction between calcium blocking drugs and anesthetics in chronically instrumented dogs. IV. Chronically administered oral verapamil and halothane, enflurane, and isoflurane. Anesthesiology 66:140, 1987

345. Carpenter RL, Mulroy MF: Edrophonium antagonizes combined lidocaine-pancuronium and verapamil-pancuronium neuromuscular blockade in cats. Anesthesiology 65:506, 1986

346. Zalman F, Perloff JK, Durant NN, Campion DS: Acute respiratory failure following intravenous verapamil in Duchenne's muscular dystrophy. Am Heart J 105:510, 1983

347. Snyder SH, Reynolds IJ: Calcium-antagonist drugs: Receptor interactions that clarify therapeutic effects. N Engl J Med 313:995, 1985

348. Roizen MF, Moss J, Muldoon SM: The effects of anesthesia, anesthetic adjuvant drugs, and surgery on plasma norepinephrine. In Ziegler MG, Lake CR (eds): Frontiers of Clinical Neuroscience, p 227. Baltimore, Williams & Wilkins, 1984

349. Price WA, Giannini AJ: Neurotoxicity caused by lithium-verapamil synergism. J Clin Pharmacol 26:717, 1986

350. Anonymous: Verapamil for hypertension. Med Lett Drugs Ther 29:37, 1987

351. Goldman L, Caldera DL: Risks of general anesthesia and elective operation in the hypertensive patient. Anesthesiology 50:285, 1979

352. James TN: A cardiogenic hypertensive chemoreflex. Anesth Analg 69:633, 1989

353. Holland OB: Diuretic-induced hypokalaemia and ventricular arrhythmias. Drugs 28(suppl 1):86, 1984

354. Vitez TS, Soper LE, Wong KC, Soper P: Chronic hypokalemia and intraoperative dysrhythmias. Anesthesiology 63:130, 1985

355. McGovern B: Hypokalemia and cardiac arrhythmias. Anesthesiology 63:127, 1985

356. Maze M, Segal IS, Bloor BC: Clonidine and other α_2 adrenergic agonists: Strategies for the rational use of these novel anesthetic agents. J Clin Anesth 1:146, 1988

357. Flacke JW, Bloor BC, Flacke WE et al: Reduced narcotic requirement by clonidine with improved hemodynamic and adrenergic stability in patients undergoing coronary bypass surgery. Anesthesiology 67:11, 1987

358. Heidemann SM, Sarnaik AP: Clonidine poisoning in children. Crit Care Med 18:618, 1990

359. Payen D, Quintin L, Plaisance P et al: Head injury: Clonidine decreases plasma catecholamines. Crit Care Med 18:392, 1990

360. Brodsky JB, Bravo JJ: Acute postoperative clonidine withdrawal syndrome. Anesthesiology 44:519, 1976

361. Johnston RV, Nicholas DA, Lawson NW et al: The use of rectal clonidine in the perioperative period. Anesthesiology 64:288, 1986

362. Aantaa R, Kanto J, Scheinin M et al: Dexmedetomidine, an α_2-adrenoceptor agonist, reduces anesthetic requirements for patients undergoing minor gynecologic surgery. Anesthesiology 73:230, 1990

363. Muzi M, Goff DR, Kampine JP et al: Clonidine reduces sympathetic activity but maintains baroreflex responses in normotensive humans. Anesthesiology 77:864, 1992

364. Fyhrquist F: Clinical pharmacology of the ACE inhibitors. Drugs 32(suppl 5):33, 1986

365. Brunner HR, Nussberger J, Waeber B: Effects of angiotensin converting enzyme inhibition: A clinical point of view. J Cardiovasc Pharmacol 7(suppl 4):S73, 1985

366. Colson P: Angiotensin-converting enzyme inhibitors in cardiovascular anesthesia. J Cardiothorac Anesth 7:734, 1993

367. Mets B, Miller ED: Angiotensin and angiotensin-converting enzyme inhibitors. In Clinical Pharmacology, p 151. London, Baillere Tindall, 1994

368. O'Malley K, Segal JL, Israili ZH et al: Duration of hydralazine action in hypertension. Clin Pharmacol Ther 18:581, 1975

369. Cohn JN, Burke LP: Nitroprusside. Ann Intern Med 91:752, 1979

370. Chiariello M, Gold HK, Leinbach RC et al: Comparison between the effects of nitroprusside and nitroglycerin on ischemic injury during acute myocardial infarction. Circulation 54:766, 1976

371. Tinker JH, Michenfelder JD: Sodium nitroprusside: Pharmacology, toxicology and therapeutics. Anesthesiology 45:340, 1976

372. Tinker JH, Michenfelder JD: Increased resistance to nitroprusside-induced cyanide toxicity in anuric dogs. Anesthesiology 52:40, 1980

373. Miller EDJ, Ackerly JA, Vaughan EDJ et al: The renin-angiotensin system during controlled hypotension with sodium nitroprusside. Anesthesiology 47:257, 1977

374. Khambatta HJ, Stone JG, Khan E: Propranolol alters renin release during nitroprusside-induced hypotension and prevents hypertension on discontinuation of nitroprusside. Anesth Analg 60:569, 1981

375. Woodside JJ, Garner L, Bedford RF et al: Captopril reduces the dose requirement for sodium nitroprusside induced hypotension. Anesthesiology 60:413, 1984

376. Fremes SE, Weisel RD, Mickle DA et al: A comparison of nitroglycerin and nitroprusside: II. The effects of volume loading. Ann Thorac Surg 39:61, 1985

377. Hood DD, Dewan DM, James FM et al: The use of nitroglycerin in preventing the hypertensive response to tracheal intubation in severe preeclampsia. Anesthesiology 63:329, 1985

378. Goa KL, Sorkin EM: Nitrendipine: A review of its pharmacodynamic and pharmacokinetic properties, and therapeutic efficacy in the treatment of hypertension. Drugs 33:123, 1986

379. Guazzi M, Olivari MT, Polese A et al: Nifedipine, a new antihypertensive with rapid action. Clin Pharmacol Ther 22:528, 1977

380. Ferguson RK, Vlasses PH: Hypertensive emergencies and urgencies. JAMA 255:1607, 1986

381. Abramowicz M: Drugs for hypertension. Med Lett Drugs Ther 29:1, 1987

382. Reves JG, Flezzani P: Perioperative use of esmolol. Am J Cardiol 56:57F, 1985

Clinical Anesthesia (4/e), edited by
Paul G. Barash, Bruce F. Cullen, and
Robert K. Stoelting. Lippincott Williams &
Wilkins, Philadelphia, © 2001.

CHAPTER 13

NONOPIOID INTRAVENOUS ANESTHESIA

JEN W. CHIU AND PAUL F. WHITE

The concept of intravenous (iv) anesthesia has evolved from primarily induction of anesthesia to that of total iv anesthesia (TIVA). This change has been spurred by the development of rapid, short-acting iv hypnotic, analgesic, and muscle relaxant drugs; by pharmacokinetic and pharmacodynamic-based "closed-loop" infusion delivery systems; and by the development of the electroencephalogram (EEG) bispectral index (BIS) monitor, which measures the hypnotic component of the anesthetic state. This chapter focuses on the pharmacologic properties and clinical uses of the currently available nonopioid iv anesthetics.

Since its introduction into clinical practice in 1934, thiopental has become the "gold standard" of iv anesthetics against which all newer drugs must be compared. Many different hypnotic drugs are currently available for use during iv anesthesia (Fig. 13-1). However, the "ideal" iv anesthetic has not yet been developed. The most important physical and pharmacologic properties that an iv anesthetic should possess include the following:

1. Drug compatibility and stability in solution
2. Lack of pain on injection, venoirritation, or tissue damage from extravasation
3. Low potential to release histamine or precipitate hypersensitivity reactions
4. Rapid and smooth onset of action without excitatory activity
5. Rapid metabolism to pharmacologically inactive metabolites
6. A steep dose–response relationship that enhances titratability and minimizes accumulation
7. Lack of acute cardiovascular and respiratory depression
8. Decreases in cerebral metabolism and intracranial pressure
9. Rapid and smooth return of consciousness and cognitive skills
10. Absence of postoperative nausea and vomiting, amnesia, psychomimetic reactions, dizziness, headache, or prolonged sedation ("hangover")

Despite thiopental's proven clinical usefulness, safety, and widespread acceptance, it is far from the "ideal" iv anesthetic. Many of the sedative-hypnotic drugs that have been introduced into clinical practice over the last few decades have proved extremely valuable in specific clinical situations. These newer compounds combine many of the characteristics of the ideal iv anesthetic but fail in aspects where other drugs succeed. For some of these sedative-hypnotics, disadvantages have led to restricted indications (*e.g.*, ketamine, etomidate) or withdrawal from clinical use (*e.g.*, althesin, propanidid, eltanolone). Because the desired pharmacologic properties are not equally important in every clinical situation, the anesthesiologist must make the choice that best fits the needs of the individual patient and the operative procedure. Not surprisingly, the search for better iv sedative-hypnotics continues.

GENERAL PHARMACOLOGY OF INTRAVENOUS HYPNOTICS

Mechanism of Action

A widely accepted theory of anesthetic action is that both iv and inhalational anesthetics exert their primary sedative and hypnotic effects through an interaction with the inhibitory γ-aminobutyric acid (GABA) neurotransmitter system.[1] GABA is the principal inhibitory neurotransmitter within the central nervous system (CNS). The GABA and adrenergic neurotransmitter systems counterbalance the action of excitatory neurotransmitters. The GABA type A (GABA_A) receptor is a receptor complex consisting of up to five glycoprotein subunits. When the GABA_A receptor is activated, transmembrane chloride conductance increases, resulting in hyperpolarization of the postsynaptic cell membrane and functional inhibition of the postsynaptic neuron. Sedative-hypnotic drugs interact with different components of the GABA receptor complex (Fig. 13-2). However, the allosteric (structural) requirements for activation of the receptor are different for iv and volatile anesthetics.[2]

Benzodiazepines bind to specific receptor sites that are part of the GABA_A receptor complex. The binding of benzodiazepines to their receptor site increases the efficiency of the coupling between the GABA receptor and the chloride ion channel. The degree of modulation of the GABA-receptor function is limited, which explains the "ceiling effect" produced by benzodiazepines with respect to CNS depression. The CNS properties of benzodiazepines (*e.g.*, hypnosis, sedation, anxiolysis, anticonvulsant effects) are presumed to be associated with the stimulation of different receptor subtypes and/or concentration-dependent receptor occupancy. It has been suggested that a benzodiazepine receptor occupancy of 20% provides anxiolysis, while 30–50% receptor occupancy is associated with sedation and >60% receptor occupancy is required for hypnosis (unconsciousness).

The interaction of barbiturates (and propofol) with specific membrane structures appears to decrease the rate of dissociation of GABA from its receptor, thereby increasing the duration of the GABA-activated opening of the chloride ion channel (Fig. 13-2). Barbiturates can also mimic the action of GABA by directly activating the chloride channels. Etomidate augments GABA-gated chloride currents (*i.e.*, indirect modulation) and, at higher concentrations, evokes chloride currents in the absence of GABA (*i.e.*, direct activation). Although the mechanism of action of propofol is similar to that of the barbiturates (*i.e.*, enhancing the activity of the GABA-activated chloride channel), it also possesses ion channel blocking effects in cerebral cortex tissue and nicotinic acetylcholine receptors, as well as an inhibitory effect on lysophosphatidate signaling in lipid mediator receptors.[3]

Ketamine produces a functional dissociation between the thalamocortical and limbic systems, a state that has been termed "dissociative" anesthesia. Ketamine depresses neuronal function in the cerebral cortex and thalamus, while simultaneously activating the limbic system. Ketamine's effect on the medial medullary reticular formation may be involved in the affective

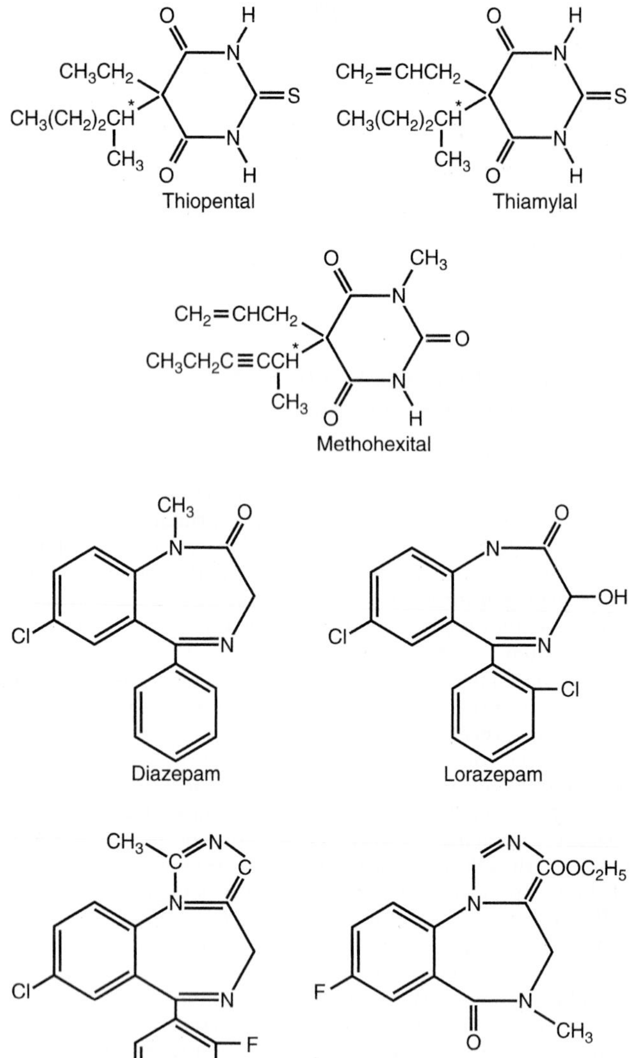

Figure 13-1. Chemical structures of currently available nonopioid iv anesthetics.

component of its nociceptive activity. The CNS effects of ketamine appear to be primarily related to its antagonistic activity at the N-methyl-D-aspartate (NMDA) receptor (Fig. 13-2). Unlike the other iv anesthetics, ketamine does not interact with GABA receptors; however, it binds to non-NMDA glutamate receptors and to nicotinic, muscarinic, monoaminergic, and opioid receptors. In addition, it also inhibits neuronal sodium channels (accounting for a modest local anesthetic action) and calcium channels (causing cerebral vasodilatation).

Pharmacokinetics and Metabolism

An understanding of basic pharmacokinetic principles is integral to the understanding the pharmacologic actions and interactions of iv anesthetic and adjunctive drugs, and will allow the anesthesiologist to develop more optimal dosing strategies when using iv techniques. Although lipid solubility facilitates diffusion of iv anesthetics across cellular membranes including the blood–brain barrier, only the nonionized form is able to readily cross neuronal membranes. The ratio of the nonionized-to-ionized fraction depends on the pK_a of the drug and the pH of the body fluids.

The rapid onset of the CNS effect of most iv anesthetics can be explained by their high lipid solubility and the relatively high proportion of the cardiac output (20%) perfusing the brain. However, a substantial degree of hysteresis may exist between the blood concentration of the hypnotic drug and its onset of action on the CNS. The hysteresis is related in part to diffusion of these drugs into brain tissue and nonspecific CNS receptor binding. However, the number of CNS binding sites is usually saturable, and only a small fraction of the available binding sites needs to be occupied to produce clinical effects. Although the total amount of drug in the blood is available for diffusion, the diffusion rate will be more limited for iv anesthetics with a high degree of plasma protein binding (>90%) because only the "free" unbound drug can diffuse across membranes and exert central effects. When several drugs compete for the same binding sites, or when the protein concentration in the blood is decreased by pre-existing disease (*e.g.*, hepatic failure), a higher fraction of the unbound drug will be available to exert effects on the CNS. Since only unbound drug is available for uptake and metabolism in the liver, highly protein-bound drugs may have a lower rate of hepatic metabolism as a result of their decreased hepatic extraction ratio (*i.e.*, the fraction of the hepatic blood flow that is cleared of the drug).

The pharmacokinetics of iv hypnotics are characterized by rapid distribution and subsequent redistribution into several hypothetical compartments, followed by elimination (Table 13-1). The initial pharmacologic effects are related to the activity of the drug in the central compartment. The primary mechanism for terminating the central effects of iv anesthetics administered for induction of anesthesia is redistribution from the central highly perfused compartment (brain) to the larger but less well perfused "peripheral" compartments (muscle, fat). Even for drugs with a high hepatic extraction ratio, elimination does not usually play a major role in terminating the drug's CNS effects because elimination of the drug can only occur from the central compartment. The rate of elimination from the central compartment, the amount of drug present in the peripheral compartments, and the rate of redistribution from the peripheral compartments "back" into the central compartment determine the time necessary to eliminate the drug from the body.

Most iv anesthetic agents are eliminated *via* hepatic metabolism followed by renal excretion of more water-soluble metabolites. Some metabolites have pharmacologic activity and can produce prolonged drug effects (*e.g.*, oxazepam, desmethyldiazepam, norketamine). Moreover, there is considerable interpatient variability in the clearance rates for commonly used iv

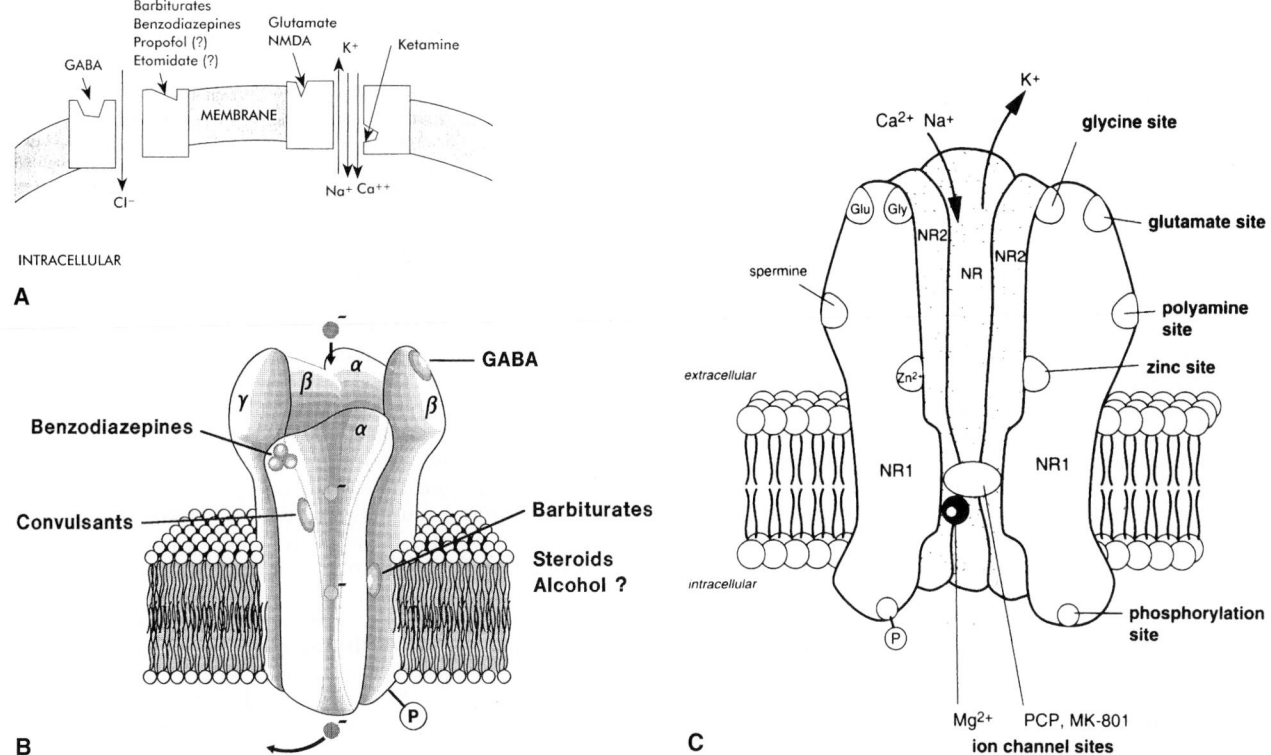

Figure 13-2. (*A*) A model depicting the postsynaptic site of GABA and glutamate within the CNS. GABA decreases the excitability of neurons by its action at the GABA$_A$ receptor complex. When GABA occupies the binding site of this complex, it allows inward flux of chloride ion, resulting in hyperpolarization of the cell and subsequent resistance of the neuron to stimulation by excitatory transmitters. Barbiturates, benzodiazepines, propofol, and etomidate decrease neuronal excitability by enhancing the effect of GABA at this complex, facilitating this inhibitory effect on the postsynaptic cell. Glutamate and its analog *N*-methyl-D-aspartate (NMDA) are excitatory amino acids. When glutamate occupies the binding site on the NMDA subtype of the glutamate receptor, the channel opens and allows Na$^+$, K$^+$, and Ca^{2+} to enter or leave the cell. Flux of these ions leads to depolarization of the postsynaptic neuron and initiation of an action potential and activation of other pathways. Ketamine blocks this open channel and prevents further ion flux, thus inhibiting the excitatory response to glutamate. (Reprinted with permission from Van Hemelrijck J, Gonzales JM, White PF: Use of intravenous sedative agents. In Rogers MC, Tinker JH, Covino BG, Longnecker DE (eds): Principles and Practice of Anesthesiology, p 1131. St. Louis, Mosby, 1992.) (*B*) Schematic model of the GABA$_A$ receptor complex illustrating recognition sites for many of the substances that bind to the receptor. (Reprinted with permission from Rochelle D. Schwartz.) (*C*) Model of the NMDA receptor showing sites for antagonist action. Ketamine binds to the site labeled PCP (phencyclidine). The pentameric structure of the receptor, composed of a combination of the subunits NR 1 and NR 2, is illustrated. (Altered with permission from Leeson TD, Iversen LL: The glycine site on the NMDA receptor: Structure–activity relationships and therapeutic potential. J Med Chem 37:4054, 1994.)

anesthetic drugs. The elimination clearance is the distribution volume cleared of drug over time and is a measure of the efficacy of the elimination process. The slow elimination of some anesthetics is due in part to their high degree of protein binding, which reduces their hepatic extraction ratio. Other drugs may have a high hepatic extraction ratio and elimination clearance despite extensive plasma protein binding (*e.g.*, propofol), indicating that protein binding is not always a rate-limiting factor.

For most drugs, the hepatic enzyme systems are not saturated at clinically relevant drug concentrations, and the rate of drug elimination will decrease as an exponential function of the drug's plasma concentration (first-order kinetics). However, when high steady-state plasma concentrations are achieved with prolonged infusions, hepatic enzyme systems can become saturated and the elimination rate becomes independent of the drug concentration (zero-order kinetics). The elimination half-life (t$_{1/2}\beta$) is the time required for the anesthetic concentration to decrease by 50% during the terminal phase of the plasma

Table 13-1. PHARMACOKINETIC VALUES FOR THE CURRENTLY AVAILABLE INTRAVENOUS SEDATIVE-HYPNOTIC DRUGS

Drug Name	Distribution Half-life (min)	Protein Binding (%)	Distribution Volume at Steady State (L·kg^{-1})	Clearance (ml·kg^{-1}·min^{-1})	Elimination Half-life (h)
Thiopental	2–4	85	2.5	3.4	11
Methohexital	5–6	85	2.2	11	4
Propofol	2–4	98	2–10	20–30	4–23
Midazolam	7–15	94	1.1–1.7	6.4–11	1.7–2.6
Diazepam	10–15	98	0.7–1.7	0.2–0.5	20–50
Lorazepam	3–10	98	0.8–1.3	0.8–1.8	11–22
Etomidate	2–4	75	2.5–4.5	18–25	2.9–5.3
Ketamine	11–16	12	2.5–3.5	12–17	2–4

decay curve. The $t_{1/2}\beta$ is dependent on the volume to be cleared (the distribution volume) and the efficiency of the metabolic clearance system. Because their volumes of distribution are similar, the wide variation in elimination half-life values for the iv anesthetics is a reflection of differences in their clearance values.

When a drug infusion is administered without a loading dose, 3–5 times the $t_{1/2}\beta$ value may be required to reach a "steady-state" plasma concentration. The steady-state concentration obtained during an anesthetic infusion depends on the rate of drug administration and its clearance rate. When an infusion is discontinued, the rate at which the plasma concentration decreases is largely dependent on the clearance rate (as reflected by the terminal elimination half-life value). For drugs with shorter elimination half-lives, plasma concentration will decrease at a rate that allows for a more rapid recovery (*e.g.*, propofol). Drugs with long elimination half-life values (*e.g.*, thiopental and diazepam) are usually only administered by continuous iv infusion when the medical condition requires long-term treatment [elevated intracranial pressure (ICP), prolonged sedation in the ICU, or anticonvulsive treatment].

Careful titration of an anesthetic drug to achieve the desired clinical effect is necessary to avoid drug accumulation and the resultant prolonged CNS effects after the infusion has been discontinued. Although the value of the terminal half-life indicates how fast a drug is eliminated from the body, a more useful indicator of the acceptability of an hypnotic infusion for maintenance of anesthesia or sedation is the context-sensitive half-time, a value derived from computer simulations of drug infusions.[4] The context-sensitive half-time is defined as the time necessary for the effect-compartment concentration to decrease by 50% in relation to the duration of the infusion. The context-sensitive half-time becomes particularly important in determining recovery after variable-length infusions of sedative-hypnotic drugs. Drugs (*e.g.*, propofol) may have a relatively short context-sensitive half-time despite the fact that a large amount of drug remains present in the "deep" (less well perfused) compartment. The slow return of the anesthetic from the deep compartment contributes little to the concentration of drug in the central compartment from which it is rapidly cleared. Therefore, the concentration in the central compartment rapidly declines below the hypnotic threshold after discontinuation of the infusion, contributing to short emergence times despite the fact that a substantial quantity of anesthetic drug may remain in the body.

Marked interpatient variability exists in the pharmacokinetics of iv sedative-hypnotic drugs. Factors that can influence anesthetic drug disposition include the degree of protein binding, the efficiency of hepatic and renal elimination processes, physiologic changes with aging, pre-existing disease states, the operative site, body temperature, and drug interactions (*e.g.*, co-administration of volatile anesthetics). For example, with increasing age, lean body mass, and total body water decrease, resulting in an increase in the steady-state volume of distribution of most iv anesthetics. The increased distribution volume and decreased hepatic clearance lead to a prolongation of their $t_{1/2}\beta$ values. Moreover, a decrease of the volume of the central compartment may result in higher initial drug concentrations, and can at least partially explain the decreased induction requirement in the elderly. Additionally, the slower redistribution from the vessel-rich tissues to intermediate compartments (muscles) also contributes to the age-related decrease in the induction dose requirements.[5] Although prolongation of the elimination half-time does not provide an explanation for the decreased induction dose requirement, it is responsible for producing higher steady-state plasma concentrations at any given infusion rate.

The hepatic clearance of iv anesthetics with a high (etomidate, propofol, ketamine) or intermediate (methohexital, midazolam) extraction ratio is largely dependent on hepatic blood flow, with most of the drug being removed from the blood as it flows through the liver (so-called perfusion-limited clearance). The elimination rate of drugs with low hepatic extraction ratios (thiopental, diazepam, lorazepam) is dependent upon the enzymatic activity of the liver and is less dependent of hepatic blood flow (so-called capacity-limited clearance). Hepatic blood flow decreases during upper abdominal surgery, and as a result, higher blood levels of drugs with perfusion-limited clearance are achieved at any given infusion rate. With aging, a decreased cardiac output and a redistribution of blood flow can partly explain the lower clearance rate for drugs with perfusion-limited clearance. While concomitant administration of volatile anesthetics (which are known to decrease liver blood flow) has little influence on the elimination of thiopental, they can decrease the clearance of etomidate, ketamine, methohexital, and propofol. Other factors that decrease hepatic blood flow include hypocapnia, congestive heart failure, intravascular volume depletion, circulatory collapse, β-adrenergic blockade, and norepinephrine administration.

Hepatic disease can influence the pharmacokinetics of drugs by the following: (1) altering the plasma-protein content and changing the degree of protein binding, (2) decreasing hepatic blood flow and producing intra-hepatic shunting, and (3) depressing the metabolic enzymatic activity of the liver. Therefore, the influence of hepatic disease on the pharmacokinetics and dynamics of iv anesthetics is difficult to predict. Renal disease can also alter the concentration of plasma and tissue proteins, as well as the degree of protein binding, thereby producing changes in free drug concentrations. Because iv anesthetic agents are primarily metabolized by the liver, renal insufficiency has little influence on their rate of metabolic inactivation or elimination of the primary compound.

Pharmacodynamics

The principal pharmacologic effect of iv anesthetics is to produce sedation and hypnosis as a result of dose-dependent CNS depression. However, all sedative-hypnotics also directly or indirectly affect other major organ systems. The relationship between the dose of a sedative-hypnotic and its CNS effects can be defined by dose–response curves. Although most iv anesthetics are characterized by steep dose–response curves, they are not always parallel (Fig. 13-3). The characteristics of a dose–response curve can only be interpreted in relation to the specific response for which it was constructed.

When steady-state plasma concentrations are achieved, it can be presumed that the plasma concentration is in equilibrium with the effect-site concentration. Under these circumstances, it is possible to describe the relationship between drug and effect using a concentration–effect curve (Fig. 13-4). Because of the pharmacodynamic variability that exists among individuals, the plasma drug concentration necessary to obtain a particular effect is often described in terms of an effective concentration range, the so-called therapeutic window. Efficacy of an iv anesthetic relates to the maximum effect that can be achieved with respect to some measure of CNS function. Depending on the drug effect under consideration, the efficacy of sedative-hypnotics may appear to be less than 100%. For example, it is virtually impossible to produce a burst-suppressive EEG pattern with a benzodiazepine. Potency, on the other hand, relates to the quantity of drug necessary to obtain the maximum CNS effect. The relative potency of sedative-hypnotics also varies depending on the end point chosen. In the presence of an antagonist drug (*e.g.*, flumazenil), the maximal response that can be obtained with a benzodiazepine agonist is reduced due to competition for the same CNS receptor binding sites.

The influence of sedative-hypnotics on cerebral metabolism, cerebral hemodynamics, and ICP is of particular importance during neuroanesthesia. In patients with reduced cerebral compliance, a small increase in cerebral blood volume can cause a

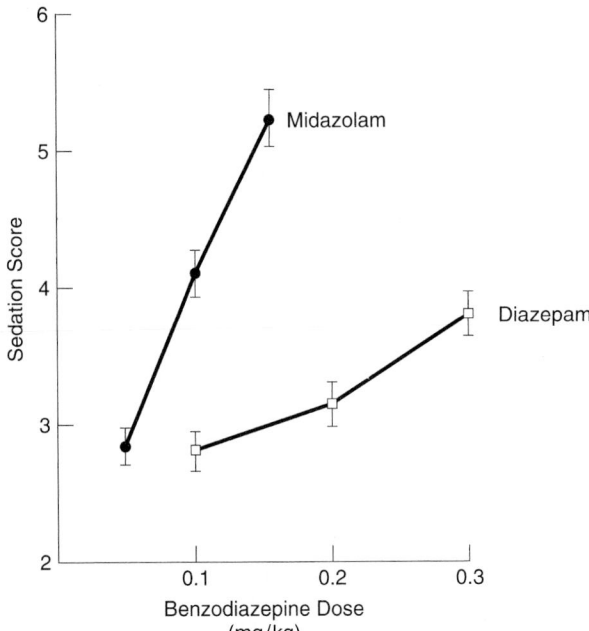

Figure 13-3. Dose–response relationships for sedation with midazolam (●) and diazepam (□). The level of sedation (2 = awake and alert to 6 = asleep and unarousable) was assessed 5 min after bolus doses of midazolam (0.05, 0.1, or 0.15 mg·kg^{-1}) or diazepam (0.1, 0.2, or 0.3 mg·kg^{-1}). Values represent mean values ± SEM. (Reprinted with permission from White PF, Vascones LO, Mathes SA, Way WL, Wender LA: Comparison of midazolam and diazepam for sedation during plastic surgery. J Plast Reconstruct Surg 81:703, 1988.)

and inhibitory subcortical centers, produced by an unequal degree of suppression of these brain centers by low concentrations of hypnotic drugs.

Although some induction drugs can increase airway sensitivity, coughing and airway irritation (bronchospasm) are usually due to manipulation of the airway during "light" levels of anesthesia rather than to a direct drug effect. With the exception of ketamine (and to a lesser extent etomidate), iv anesthetics produce dose-dependent respiratory depression which is enhanced in patients with chronic obstructive pulmonary disease. The respiratory depression is characterized by a decrease in tidal volume and minute ventilation, as well as a transient rightward shift in the CO_2 response curve. Following the rapid injection of a large bolus dose of an iv anesthetic, transient apnea lasting 30–90 sec is usually produced. Ketamine causes minimal respiratory depression when administered in the usual induction doses, while etomidate is associated with less respiratory depressant effects than the barbiturate compounds or propofol.

Many different factors contribute to the hemodynamic changes associated with iv induction of anesthesia, including the patient's pre-existing cardiovascular and fluid status, resting sympathetic nervous system tone, chronic cardiovascular drugs, preanesthetic medication, the speed of drug injection, and the onset of unconsciousness. In addition, cardiovascular changes can be attributed to the direct pharmacologic actions of anesthetic and analgesic drugs on the heart and peripheral vasculature. Intravenous anesthetics can depress the CNS and peripheral nervous system responses, blunt the compensatory baroreceptor reflex mechanisms, produce direct myocardial

life-threatening increase in ICP. Most sedative-hypnotic drugs cause a proportional reduction in cerebral metabolism ($CMRO_2$) and cerebral blood flow (CBF), resulting in a decrease in ICP. Although a decrease in $CMRO_2$ probably provides only a modest degree of protection against CNS ischemia or hypoxia, some hypnotics appear to possess cerebroprotective potential. Explanations for the alleged neuroprotective effects of these compounds include a biochemical role as free-radical scavengers and membrane stabilizers (barbiturates and propofol), or NMDA-receptor antagonists (ketamine). With the exception of ketamine, all sedative-hypnotics also lower intraocular pressure (IOP). The changes in IOP generally reflect the effects of the iv agent on systemic arterial pressure and intracranial hemodynamics. However, none of the available sedative-hypnotic drugs protects against the transient increase in IOP that occurs with laryngoscopy and intubation.

Most iv hypnotics have similar electroencephalographic (EEG) effects. Activation of high-frequency EEG activity (15–30 Hz) is characteristic of low concentrations (so-called sedative doses) of iv anesthetics. At higher concentrations, an increase in the relative contribution of the lower-frequency higher-amplitude waves is observed. At high concentrations, a burst-suppressive pattern develops with an increase in the isoelectric periods. Most sedative-hypnotic drugs have been reported to cause occasional EEG seizure-like activity. Interestingly, the same drugs also possess anticonvulsant properties.[6] When considering possible epileptogenic properties of CNS depressant drugs, it is important to differentiate between true epileptogenic activity and myoclonic-like phenomena. Epileptic activity refers to a sudden alteration in CNS activity resulting from a high-voltage electrical discharge at either cortical or subcortical sites, with subsequent spreading to the thalamic and brainstem centers. Myoclonus can have an epileptic or nonepileptic origin, depending on the EEG findings. Myoclonic activity is generally considered to be the result of an imbalance between excitatory

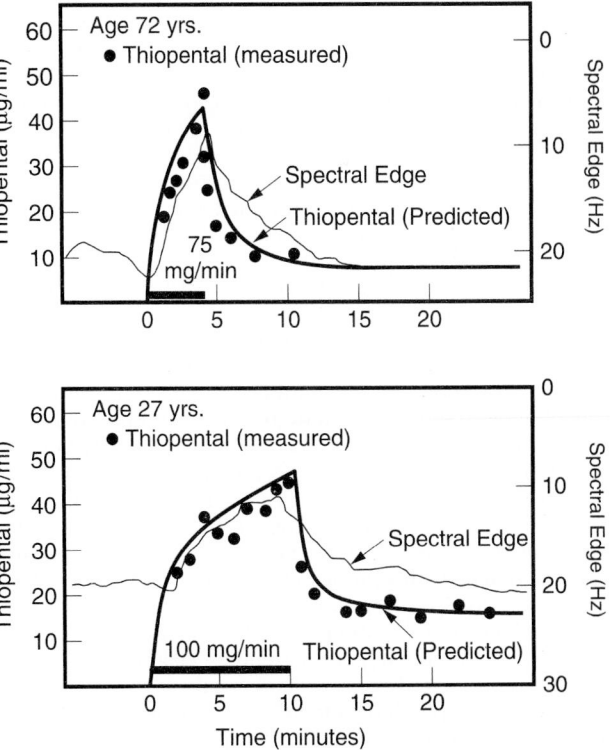

Figure 13-4. The concentration of thiopental *versus* time and spectral edge in an elderly patient (*top*) and in a younger patient (*bottom*). Solid horizontal bars represent the length of thiopental infusion. Filled circles represent the measured thiopental concentration (linear scale), and the solid line next to them represents the fitted data from the pharmacokinetic model. The axis for spectral edge has been inverted for visual clarity. (Reprinted with permission from Homer TD, Stanski DR: The effect of increasing age on thiopental disposition and anesthetic requirement. Anesthesiology 62:714, 1985.)

depression, and lower peripheral vascular resistance (and/or dilate venous capacitance vessels), thereby decreasing venous return. Profound hemodynamic effects occur at induction in the presence of hypovolemia because a higher than expected drug concentration is achieved in the central compartment. Not surprisingly, the acute cardiocirculatory depressant effects of all iv anesthetics are accentuated in the elderly, as well as in the presence of pre-existing cardiovascular disease.

The effects of intravenous anesthetics on neuroendocrine function are influenced by the surgical stimuli. For example, although iv anesthetics are alleged to increase antidiuretic hormone (vasopressin) secretion, it is probably secondary to the surgical stress. Increases in this stress hormone can result in increased peripheral vascular resistance and a reduction of urine output. Similarly, glucose tolerance appears to be decreased by surgical stress, resulting in hyperglycemia. Most iv sedative-hypnotic drugs lack intrinsic analgesic activity. In fact, thiopental has been alleged to possess so-called antianalgesic activity (*i.e.*, it appears to lower the pain threshold, but this is unproven). On the other hand, ketamine has analgesic-like activity.

Hypersensitivity (Allergic) Reactions

Allergic reactions to iv anesthetics and/or their solubilizing agents can be severe and even life-threatening. Intravenous drug administration bypasses the normal "protective barriers" against entrance of foreign molecules into the body. With the exception of etomidate, all iv induction agents have been alleged to cause some histamine release. However, the incidence of severe anaphylactic reactions is low with the currently available induction agents. The high frequency of allergic reactions to the cremophor EL-containing formulations led to the early withdrawal of several iv anesthetics containing this solubilizing agent (*e.g.*, propofol EL, propanidid, Althesin). The possible mechanisms for immunologic reactions include the following: (1) direct action on mast cells, (2) classic complement activation after previous exposure and antibody formation, (3) complement activation through the alternative pathway without previous antigen exposure, (4) antigen–antibody reactions, and (5) the "mixed type" of anaphylactoid reactions.

Following thiopental administration, the plasma level of histamine increases to ~350% of normal and decreases to the normal range after ~10 min. A transient urticarial skin rash can be associated with the use of barbiturates. Although severe anaphylactic reactions are extremely uncommon, profound hypotension attributed to non-immunologically mediated histamine release has been reported with thiopental use. The incidence of allergic reactions to the emulsion formulation of propofol, ketamine, and benzodiazepines also appears to be extremely low. Although anaphylactic reactions to etomidate have been reported, it does not appear to release histamine and is considered to be the most "immunologically safe" iv anesthetic. While propofol does not normally trigger histamine release, life-threatening anaphylactoid reactions have been reported most often in patients with a previous history of drug allergies. Barbiturates may precipitate episodes of acute intermittent porphyria (AIP) and their use is contraindicated in patients who are predisposed to AIP. Although benzodiazepines, ketamine, and etomidate are reported to be safe in humans, these drugs have been shown to be porphyrinogenic in animal models. Propofol has been used with no evidence of porphyrinogenicity in AIP-susceptible patients.

PHARMACOLOGY OF INTRAVENOUS SEDATIVE-HYPNOTICS

Barbiturates

The most commonly used barbiturates are thiopental [5-ethyl-5-(1-methylbutyl)-2-thiobarbituric acid], methohexital [1-methyl-

5-allyl-5-(1-methyl-2-pentynyl)barbituric acid], and thiamylal [5-allyl-5-(1-methylbutyl)-2-thiobarbituric acid]. Thiopental (Pentothal) and thiamylal (Surital) are thiobarbiturates, while methohexital (Brevital) is an oxybarbiturate. Thiamylal is slightly more potent than thiopental but has a similar pharmacologic profile. Although the L-isomers of thiopental and thyamylal are twice as potent as the D-isomers, both hypnotics are commercially available as racemic mixtures. Because methohexital has two asymmetric centers, it has four stereoisomers. The β-L-isomer is 4–5 times more potent than the α-L-isomer, but it produces excessive motor responses. Therefore, methohexital is marketed as the racemic mixture of the two α-isomers.

All three barbiturates are available as sodium salts and must be dissolved in isotonic sodium chloride (0.9%) or water to prepare solutions of 2.5% thiopental, 1–2% methohexital, and 2% thiamylal. If refrigerated, solutions of the thiobarbiturates are stable for up to 2 weeks. Solutions of methohexital are stable for up to 6 weeks. When barbiturates are added to Ringer's lactate or an acidic solution containing other water-soluble drugs, precipitation will occur and can occlude the iv catheter. Although the typical solution of thiopental (2.5%) is highly alkaline (*p*H >9) and can be irritating to the tissues if injected extraneously, it does not cause pain on injection and venoirritation is rare. In contrast, a 1% methohexital solution frequently causes discomfort when injected into small veins. Intra-arterial injection of thiobarbiturates is a serious complication as crystals can form in the arterioles and capillaries, causing intense vasoconstriction, thrombosis, and even tissue necrosis. Accidental intra-arterial injections should be treated promptly with intra-arterial administration of papaverine and lidocaine (or procaine), as well as a regional anesthesia-induced sympathectomy (stellate ganglion block, brachial plexus block) and heparinization.

Thiopental is metabolized in the liver to hydroxythiopental and the carboxylic acid derivative, which are more water-soluble and have little CNS activity. When high doses of thiopental are administered, a desulfuration reaction can occur with the production of pentobarbital, which has long-lasting CNS-depressant activity. The low elimination clearance of thiopental ($3.4 \ ml \cdot kg^{-1} \cdot min^{-1}$) contributes to a long elimination half-life ($t_{1/2}\beta$ of 12 h). Pre-existing hepatic and renal disease results in decreased plasma protein binding, thereby increasing the free fraction of thiopental and enhancing its CNS and cardiovascular-depressant properties. During prolonged continuous administration of thiopental, the concentration in the tissues approaches the concentration in the central compartment, with termination of its CNS effects becoming solely dependent on elimination by nonlinear hepatic metabolism. Methohexital is metabolized in the liver to inactive hydroxy derivatives. The clearance of methohexital ($11 \ ml \cdot kg^{-1} \cdot min^{-1}$) is higher and more dependent on hepatic blood flow than thiopental, resulting in a shorter elimination half-life ($t_{1/2}\beta$ 3–6 h).

The usual induction dose of thiopental is $3–5 \ mg \cdot kg^{-1}$ in adults, $5–6 \ mg \cdot kg^{-1}$ in children, and $6–8 \ mg \cdot kg^{-1}$ in infants. Because methohexital is approximately 2.7 times more potent than thiopental, a dose of $1.5 \ mg \cdot kg^{-1}$ is equivalent to $4 \ mg \cdot kg^{-1}$ of thiopental in adults. The dose of barbiturates necessary to induce anesthesia is reduced in premedicated patients, patients in early pregnancy (7–13 weeks' gestation) and those of more advanced ASA physical status (III or IV). Geriatric patients require a 30–40% reduction in the usual adult dose because of a decrease of the volume of the central compartment and slowed redistribution of thiopental from the vessel-rich tissues to lean muscle.[5] When the calculation of the induction dose is based on the lean body mass rather than total body weight, dosage adjustments for age, sex, or obesity are not necessary. Thiopental infusion is seldom used to maintain anesthesia because of the long context-sensitive half-time and prolonged recovery period. Plasma thiopental levels necessary to maintain a hypnotic state range between 10 and 20 $\mu g \cdot ml^{-1}$.

A typical infusion rate necessary to treat intracranial hypertension or intractable convulsions is $2-4$ mg $\cdot$ kg^{-1} $\cdot$ h^{-1}. The plasma concentration of methohexital needed to maintain hypnosis during anesthesia ranges between 3 and 5 μg $\cdot$ ml^{-1} and can be achieved with an infusion rate of $50-120$ μg $\cdot$ kg^{-1} $\cdot$ min^{-1}.

Barbiturates produce a proportional decrease in CMRO$_2$ and CBF, thereby lowering ICP. The maximal decrease in CMRO$_2$ (55%) occurs when the EEG becomes isoelectric (burst-suppressive pattern). An isoelectric EEG can be maintained with a thiopental infusion rate of $4-6$ mg $\cdot$ kg^{-1} $\cdot$ h^{-1} (resulting in plasma concentrations of $30-50$ μg $\cdot$ ml^{-1}). Because the decrease in systemic arterial pressure is usually less than the reduction in ICP, thiopental should improve cerebral perfusion and compliance. Therefore, thiopental is widely used to improve brain relaxation during neurosurgery and to improve cerebral perfusion pressure (CPP) after acute brain injury. Although barbiturate therapy is widely used to control ICP after brain injury, the results of outcome studies are no better than with other aggressive forms of cerebral antihypertensive therapy.

It has been suggested that barbiturates also possess "neuroprotective" properties secondary to their ability to decrease oxygen demand. Alternative explanations that have been suggested, including a reverse steal ("Robin Hood effect") on CBF, free-radical scavenging, stabilization of liposomal membranes, as well as excitatory amino acid (EAA) receptor blockade. Based on evidence from experimental studies and a large randomized prospective multi-institutional study,[7] it has been concluded that barbiturates have no place in the therapy following resuscitation of a cardiac arrest patient. In contrast, barbiturates are frequently used for cerebroprotection during incomplete brain ischemia (e.g., carotid endarterectomy, temporary occlusion of cerebral arteries, profound hypotension, cardiopulmonary bypass). By improving the brain's tolerance of incomplete ischemia in patients undergoing open heart surgery with cardiopulmonary bypass, barbiturates are alleged to decrease the incidence of post-bypass neuropsychiatric disorders.[8] However, during valvular open heart cardiac surgery, a protective effect of barbiturate loading could not be demonstrated.[9] The routine use of barbiturates during cardiac surgery is not recommended because recent evidence would suggest that the use of moderate degrees of hypothermia ($33-34°C$) may provide superior neuroprotection without prolonging the recovery phase.

Barbiturates cause predictable, dose-dependent EEG changes and possess potent anticonvulsant activity. Continuous infusions of thiopental have been used to control refractory status epilepticus. However, low doses of thiopental may induce spike wave activity in epileptic patients. Methohexital has well-established epileptogenic effects in patients with psychomotor epilepsy. Low-dose methohexital infusions are frequently used to activate cortical EEG seizure discharges in patients with temporal lobe epilepsy. Yet, the frequency of epileptiform EEG activity during induction of anesthesia with methohexital is significantly less than that which occurs during normal periods of sleep in epileptic patients, suggesting that even methohexital has some anticonvulsant activity.[6] Methohexital frequently causes myoclonic-like muscle tremors and other signs of excitatory activity (hiccoughing).

Barbiturates cause dose-dependent respiratory depression.[10] However, bronchospasm or laryngospasm following induction with thiopental is usually the result of airway manipulation in "lightly" anesthetized patients. Laryngeal reflexes appear to be more active after induction with thiopental than with propofol. The cardiovascular effects of thiopental and methohexital include decreases in cardiac output, systemic arterial pressure, and peripheral vascular resistance. The depressant effects of thiopental on cardiac output are primarily due to a decrease in venous return caused by peripheral pooling, as well as to a direct myocardial depressant effect, which assumes increasing importance in the presence of hypovolemia and myocardial

disease.[11] An equipotent dose of methohexital produces somewhat less hypotension than thiopental due to a greater tachycardic response to the blood pressure–lowering effects of the drug. If the blood pressure remains stable, the myocardial oxygen demand–supply ratio remains normal despite the increase in heart rate because of a concurrent decrease in coronary vascular resistance.

Propofol

Propofol [2,6-diisopropylphenol], an alkylphenol compound, is virtually insoluble in aqueous solution. The initial cremophor EL formulation of propofol was withdrawn from clinical testing because of the high incidence of anaphylactic reactions. Subsequently, propofol (10 mg $\cdot$ ml^{-1}) has been reintroduced as an egg lecithin emulsion formulation (Diprivan), consisting of 10% soybean oil, 2.25% glycerol, and 1.2% egg phosphatide. Pain on injection occurs in $32-67\%$ of patients when injected into small hand veins, but can be minimized by injection into larger veins and by prior administration of either 1% lidocaine or a potent opioid analgesic. Diluting the formulation with additional solvent (Intralipid) or changing the lipid carrier (Lipofundin) also reduced injection pain, probably due to a decrease in the concentration of free propofol in the aqueous phase of the emulsion. A new propofol formulation with sodium metabisulfite (instead of disodium edetate) as an antimicrobial, has recently been shown to be associated with less pain on injection. However, the presence of the metabisulfite has raised concerns regarding its use in sulfite-allergic patients. Of interest, a 2% formulation is available for long-term sedation to decrease the volume infused as well as the lipid load.

Propofol's pharmacokinetics have been studied using single-bolus dosing and continuous infusions.[12] In studies using a two-compartment kinetic model, the initial distribution half-life is $2-8$ min and the elimination half-life is $1-3$ h. Using a three-compartment model the initial and slow distribution half-life values are $1-8$ min and $30-70$ min, respectively. The elimination half-life depends largely on the sampling time after discontinuing the administration of propofol and ranges from 2 to 24 h. This long elimination half-life is indicative of the existence of a poorly perfused compartment from which propofol slowly diffuses back into the central compartment. Propofol is rapidly cleared from the central compartment by hepatic metabolism and the context-sensitive half-life for propofol infusions up to 8 h is less than 40 min.[4] Propofol is rapidly and extensively metabolized to inactive, water-soluble sulfate and glucuronic acid metabolites, which are eliminated by the kidneys. Propofol's clearance rate ($1.5-2.2$ l $\cdot$ min^{-1}) exceeds hepatic blood flow, suggesting that an extrahepatic route of elimination (lungs) also contributes to its clearance. Nevertheless, changes in liver blood flow would be expected to produce marked alterations in propofol's clearance rate. Surprisingly, few changes in propofol's pharmacokinetics have been reported in the presence of hepatic or renal disease.

The induction dose of propofol in healthy adults is $1.5-2.5$ mg $\cdot$ kg^{-1}, with blood levels of $2-6$ μg $\cdot$ ml^{-1}, producing unconsciousness depending on the associated medication, the patient's age and physical status, and the extent of the surgical stimulation.[13] The recommended maintenance infusion rate of propofol varies between 100 and 200 μg $\cdot$ kg^{-1} $\cdot$ min^{-1} for hypnosis and $25-75$ μg $\cdot$ kg^{-1} $\cdot$ min^{-1} for sedation. Awakening typically occurs at plasma propofol concentrations of $1-1.5$ μg $\cdot$ ml^{-1}.[14] Because a 50% decrease in the plasma propofol concentration is usually required for awakening, emergence following anesthesia is rapid, even following prolonged infusions. Analogous to the barbiturates, children require higher induction and maintenance doses of propofol on a milligram-per-kilogram basis as a result of their larger central distribution volume and higher clearance rate. Elderly and patients in poor health require lower induction and maintenance doses of propofol as a result of their smaller central distribution volume and decreased clearance rate. Although subhypnotic doses of propofol produce sedation and amnesia,[14] awareness has been reported even at higher infusion rates when propofol is used as the sole anesthetic.[15] Propofol often produces a subjective feeling of well-being and even euphoria,[16] and may have abuse potential as a result of these effects.

Propofol decreases $CMRO_2$ and CBF, as well as ICP.[17] However, when larger doses are administered, the marked depressant effect on systemic arterial pressure can significantly decrease CPP. Cerebrovascular autoregulation in response to changes in systemic arterial pressure and reactivity of the cerebral blood flow to changes in carbon dioxide tension are not affected by propofol. Evidence for a possible neuroprotective effect has been reported in *in vitro* preparations, and the use of propofol to produce EEG burst suppression has been proposed as a method for providing neuroprotection during aneurysm surgery. Its neuroprotective effect may at least partially be related to the antioxidant potential of propofol's phenol ring structure, which may act as a free-radical scavenger, decreasing free-radical–induced lipid peroxidation. Although total iv anesthesia with propofol and an opioid analgesic is a safe and effective alternative to standard "balanced" techniques for maintenance of neuroanesthesia, concerns have been raised regarding the cost-effectiveness of this technique.

Propofol produces cortical EEG changes that are similar to those of thiopental. However, sedative doses of propofol increase β-wave activity analogous to the benzodiazepines. Induction of anesthesia with propofol is occasionally accompanied by excitatory motor activity (so-called nonepileptic myoclonia). In a study involving patients without a history of seizure disorders, excitatory movements following propofol were not associated with EEG seizure activity.[18] Propofol appears to possess profound anticonvulsant properties.[19] Propofol has been reported to decrease spike activity in patients with cortical electrodes implanted for resection of epileptogenic foci and has been used successfully to terminate status epilepticus. The duration of motor and EEG seizure activity following electroconvulsive therapy is shorter with propofol than with methohexital anesthesia. Propofol produces a decrease in the early components of somatosensory and motor-evoked potentials but does not influence the early components of the auditory-evoked potentials.

Propofol produces dose-dependent respiratory depression, with apnea occurring in 25–35% of patients after a typical induction dose. A maintenance infusion of propofol decreases tidal volume and increases respiratory rate. The ventilatory response to carbon dioxide and hypoxia is also significantly decreased by propofol.[10] Propofol can produce bronchodilation in patients with chronic obstructive pulmonary disease and does not inhibit hypoxic pulmonary vasoconstriction.

Propofol's cardiovascular depressant effects are generally considered to be more profound than those of thiopental.[11] Both direct myocardial depressant effects and decreased systemic vascular resistance have been implicated as important factors in producing cardiovascular depression. Direct myocardial depression and peripheral vasodilation are dose- and concentration-dependent. In addition to arterial vasodilation, propofol produces venodilation (due both to a reduction in sympathetic activity and to a direct effect on the vascular smooth muscle), which further contributes to its hypotensive effect. The relaxation of the vascular smooth muscle may be due to an effect on intracellular calcium mobilization or to an increase in the production of nitric oxide. Experiments in isolated myocardium suggest that the negative inotropic effect of propofol results from a decrease in intracellular calcium availability secondary to inhibition of trans-sarcolemmal calcium influx. Propofol alters the baroreflex mechanism, resulting in a smaller increase in heart rate for a given decrease in arterial pressure.[20] The smaller increase in heart rate with propofol may account for the larger decrease in arterial pressure than with an equipo-

tent dose of thiopental. Recent research suggests that induction of anesthesia with propofol attenuates desflurane-mediated sympathetic activation.[21] Age enhances the cardiodepressant response to propofol and dosage adjustments are required in the elderly. Patients with limited cardiac reserve seem to tolerate the cardiac depression and systemic vasodilation produced by carefully titrated doses of propofol, and maintenance infusions are increasingly used during coronary artery surgery when early extubation is desired.

Propofol appears to possess antiemetic properties that contribute to a low incidence of emetic sequelae after propofol anesthesia. In fact, subanesthetic doses of propofol (10–20 mg) have also been successfully used to treat nausea and emesis in the early postoperative period.[22] The postulated mechanisms include antidopaminergic activity, depressant effect on the chemoreceptor trigger zone and vagal nuclei, decreased release of glutamate and aspartate in the olfactory cortex, and reduction of serotonin concentrations in the area postrema. Interestingly, propofol also decreases the pruritus associated with spinal opioids, as well as with cholestatic liver disease.

Propofol does not trigger malignant hyperthermia (MH) and may be considered the induction agent of choice in MH-susceptible patients. The use of propofol infusions for sedation in the pediatric intensive care unit has been linked to several deaths following prolonged administration. Although clinical doses of propofol do not affect cortisol synthesis or the response to adrenocorticotropic hormone (ACTH) stimulation, propofol has been reported to inhibit phagocytosis and killing of bacteria *in vitro* and to reduce proliferative responses when added to lymphocytes from critically ill patients.[23] Because fat emulsions are known to support the growth of microorganisms, contamination can occur as a result of dilution or fractionated use.[24]

Benzodiazepines

The benzodiazepines of primary interest to anesthesiologists are diazepam (Valium), lorazepam (Ativan), and midazolam (Versed), as well as the antagonist flumazenil (Romazicon). Diazepam and lorazepam are insoluble in water and their formulation contains propylene glycol, a tissue irritant that causes pain on injection and venous irritation. Diazepam is available in a lipid emulsion formulation (Diazemuls or Dizac), which does not cause pain or thrombophlebitis but is associated with a slightly lower bioavailability. Midazolam is a water-soluble benzodiazepine that is available in an acidified (pH 3.5) aqueous formulation that produces minimal local irritation after iv or im injection.[25] At physiologic pH, an intramolecular rearrangement changes the physicochemical properties of midazolam such that it becomes more lipid-soluble.

Benzodiazepines undergo hepatic metabolism *via* oxidation and glucuronide conjugation. Oxidation reactions are susceptible to hepatic dysfunction and co-administration of other anesthetic drugs. Diazepam is metabolized to active metabolites (desmethyldiazepam, 3-hydroxydiazepam), which can prolong its residual sedative effects. These metabolites undergo secondary conjugation to form inactive water-soluble glucuronide conjugates. Drugs that inhibit the oxidative metabolism of diazepam include the H_2-receptor blocking drug cimetidine. Severe liver disease reduces diazepam's protein-binding and hepatic clearance rate, increases volume of distribution, and thereby prolongs the $t_{1/2}\beta$ value. Chronic renal disease decreases protein binding and increases the free drug fraction, resulting in enhanced hepatic metabolism and a shorter $t_{1/2}\beta$ value. In elderly patients, the clearance rate of diazepam is significantly decreased, prolonging its $t_{1/2}\beta$ to 75–150 h.

Lorazepam is directly conjugated to glucuronic acid to form pharmacologically inactive metabolites. Age and renal disease have little influence on the kinetics of lorazepam; however, severe hepatic disease decreases its clearance rate.

Midazolam undergoes extensive oxidation by hepatic enzymes to form water-soluble hydroxylated metabolites, which are excreted in the urine. However, the primary metabolite, 1-hydroxymethylmidazolam, has some CNS-depressant activity. The hepatic clearance rate of midazolam is 5 times greater than that of lorazepam and 10 times greater than that of diazepam. Although changes in liver blood flow can affect the clearance of midazolam, age has relatively little influence on midazolam's elimination half-life.

The benzodiazepines used in anesthesia are classified as either short- (midazolam, flumazenil), intermediate- (diazepam), or long-acting (lorazepam). Because the distribution volumes are similar, the large difference in the elimination half-times is due to differences in their clearance rates (see Table 13-1). The context-sensitive half-times for diazepam and lorazepam are very long; therefore, only midazolam should be used for continuous infusion.

All benzodiazepines have anxiolytic, amnestic, sedative, hypnotic, anticonvulsant, and spinally mediated muscle relaxant properties. Benzodiazepines differ in potency and efficacy with regard to their distinctive pharmacologic properties.[25] The dose-dependent pharmacologic activity implies that the CNS effects of various benzodiazepine compounds depend on the affinity for receptor subtypes and their degree of receptor binding. Although benzodiazepines can be used as hypnotics, they are primarily used as premedicants and adjuvant drugs because of their anxiolytic, sedative, and amnestic properties. For example, midazolam ($0.04-0.08$ mg·kg^{-1} iv/im) is a commonly used premedicant. In addition, midazolam, $0.4-0.8$ mg·kg^{-1} administered orally 10–15 min before parental separation is an excellent premedicant in children. In contrast to lorazepam, both diazepam and midazolam can be used to induce anesthesia because they have a relatively short onset time after iv administration. The half-life of equilibration between the plasma concentration of midazolam and its maximal EEG effect is only 2–3 min. The therapeutic window to maintain unconsciousness with midazolam is reported to be $100-200$ ng·ml^{-1}, with awakening occurring at plasma concentrations below 50 ng·ml^{-1}. However, significant hypnotic synergism occurs when midazolam and opioid analgesics are administered in combination.

The usual induction dose of midazolam in premedicated patients is $0.1-0.2$ mg·kg^{-1} iv, with infusion rates of $0.25-1$ μg·kg^{-1}·min^{-1} required to maintain hypnosis and amnesia in combination with inhalational agents and/or opioid analgesics. Higher maintenance infusion rates and prolonged administration will result in accumulation and prolonged recovery times. Lower infusion rates are sufficient to provide sedation and amnesia during local and regional anesthesia.[26] Patient-controlled administration of midazolam during procedures under local anesthesia is well accepted by patients and associated with few perioperative complications.[27]

Benzodiazepines decrease both CMRO$_2$ and CBF analogous to the barbiturates and propofol. However, in contrast to these compounds, midazolam is unable to produce a burst-suppressive (isoelectric) pattern on the EEG. Accordingly, there is a "ceiling" effect with respect to the decrease in CMRO$_2$ produced by increasing doses of midazolam. Midazolam induces dose-dependent changes in regional cerebral perfusion in the parts of the brain that subserve arousal, attention, and memory. Cerebral vasomotor responsiveness to carbon dioxide is preserved during midazolam anesthesia. In patients with severe head injury, a bolus dose of midazolam may decrease CPP with little effect on ICP. Although midazolam may improve neurologic outcome after incomplete ischemia in animal experiments, benzodiazepines have not been shown to possess neuroprotective activity in humans. Like the other sedative-hypnotic drugs, the benzodiazepines are potent anticonvulsants that are commonly used to treat status epilepticus.

Benzodiazepines produce dose-dependent respiratory depression. In healthy patients, the respiratory depression associated with benzodiazepine premedication is insignificant. How-ever, the depressant effect is enhanced in patients with chronic respiratory disease, and synergistic depressant effects occur when benzodiazepines are co-administered with opioid analgesics. Benzodiazepines also depress the swallowing reflex and decrease upper airway reflex activity.

Both midazolam and diazepam produce decreases in systemic vascular resistance and blood pressure when large doses are administered for induction of anesthesia. However, the cardiovascular depressant effects of benzodiazepines are frequently "masked" by the stimulus of laryngoscopy and intubation. The cardiovascular depressant effects are directly related to the plasma concentration; however, a plateau plasma concentration appears to exist above which little further change in arterial blood pressure occurs. In the presence of heart failure, the decrease in preload and afterload produced by benzodiazepines may be beneficial in improving cardiac output. However, the cardiodepressant effect of benzodiazepines may be more marked in hypovolemic patients.

Ro 48-6791, 3-(5-dipropylaminomethyl-1,2,4-oxadiazol-3-yl)-8-fluoro-5-methyl-5,6-dihydro-4H-imidazol[1,5-a][1,4]benzodiazepin-6-one) is a new water-soluble benzodiazepine that has full agonistic activity at CNS benzodiazepine receptors. Compared with midazolam, it is 2 to 2.5-fold more potent, has a higher plasma clearance rate, and a similar onset and duration of action.[28] In a recent study involving outpatients undergoing endoscopy procedures, the times to ambulation and to recovery from psychomotor impairment were decreased compared to midazolam, although the later recovery end points (*e.g.*, "fitness-for-discharge") were similar.[29]

In contrast to all other sedative-hypnotic drugs, there is a specific antagonist for benzodiazepines. Flumazenil, a 1,4-imidazobenzodiazepine derivative, has a high affinity for the benzodiazepine receptor but minimal intrinsic activity.[30] Flumazenil's molecular structure is similar to that of other benzodiazepines except for the absence of a phenyl group, which is replaced by a carbonyl group. It is water-soluble and possesses moderate lipid solubility at physiologic pH. Flumazenil is rapidly metabolized in the liver, and its metabolites are excreted in the urine as glucuronide conjugates. Flumazenil acts as a competitive antagonist in the presence of benzodiazepine agonist compounds. The residual activity of the benzodiazepines in the presence of flumazenil depends on the relative concentrations of the agonist and antagonist drugs. As a result, it is possible to reverse benzodiazepine-induced anesthesia (or deep sedation) either completely or partially depending on the dose of flumazenil. Flumazenil is short-acting, with an elimination half-life of ~1 h.

Recurrence of the central effects of benzodiazepines (resedation) may occur after a single dose of flumazenil due to residual effects of the more slowly eliminated agonist drug.[31] If sustained antagonism is desired, it may be necessary to administer flumazenil as repeated bolus doses or a continuous infusion. In general, 45–90 min of antagonism can be expected following flumazenil 1–3 mg iv. However, the respiratory depression produced by benzodiazepines is not completely reversed by flumazenil.[32] Reversal of benzodiazepine sedation with flumazenil is not associated with adverse cardiovascular effects or evidence of an acute stress response.[33] Although flumazenil does not appear to change CBF or CMRO$_2$ following midazolam anesthesia for craniotomy, acute increases in ICP have been reported in head-injured patients receiving flumazenil.

Etomidate

Etomidate is a carboxylated imidazole-containing anesthetic compound [R-1-ethyl-1-(a-methylbenzyl) imidazole-5-carboxylate] which is structurally unrelated to any other iv anesthetic. Only the D-isomer of etomidate possesses anesthetic activity. Analogous to midazolam (which also contains an imidazole nucleus), etomidate undergoes an intramolecular rearrangement at physiologic pH, resulting in a closed-ring structure with enhanced lipid solubility. The aqueous solution of etomidate (Amidate) is unstable at physiologic pH and is formulated in a 0.2% solution with 35% propylene glycol (pH 6.9), contributing to a high incidence of pain on injection, venoirritation, and hemolysis. A new lipid emulsion formulation (Etomidate-Lipuro) has recently been introduced in Europe and appears to be associated with a lower incidence of side effects compared to the original propylene glycol formulation.

The standard induction dose of etomidate ($0.2-0.4$ mg · kg^{-1} iv) produces a rapid onset of anesthesia. Involuntary myoclonic movements are common during the induction period as a result of subcortical disinhibition, and are unrelated to cortical seizure activity. The frequency of this myoclonic-like activity can be attenuated by prior administration of opioid analgesics, benzodiazepines, or small sedative doses of etomidate ($0.03-0.05$ mg · kg^{-1}) prior to induction of anesthesia.[34] Emergence time after etomidate anesthesia is dose-dependent but remains short even after administration of repeated bolus doses or continuous infusions. For maintenance of hypnosis, the target concentration is $300-500$ ng · ml^{-1} and can be rapidly achieved by administering a two- or three-stage infusion (e.g., 100 μg · kg^{-1} · min^{-1} for 10 min followed by 10 μg · kg^{-1} · min^{-1} or 100 μg · kg^{-1} · min^{-1} for $3-5$ min, followed by 20 μg · kg^{-1} · min^{-1} for $20-30$ min, and then 10 μg · kg^{-1} · min^{-1}). The pharmacokinetics of etomidate are optimally described by a three-compartment open model.[35] The high clearance rate of etomidate ($18-25$ ml · kg^{-1} · min^{-1}) is a result of extensive ester hydrolysis in the liver (forming inactive water-soluble metabolites). A significant decrease in plasma protein binding has been reported in the presence of uremia and hepatic cirrhosis. Severe hepatic disease causes a prolongation of the elimination half-life secondary to an increased volume of distribution and a decreased plasma clearance rate.

Analogous to the barbiturates, etomidate decreases CMRO$_2$, CBF, and ICP. However, the hemodynamic stability associated with etomidate will maintain adequate CPP. Etomidate has been used successfully for both induction and maintenance of anesthesia for neurosurgery. Etomidate's well-known inhibitory effect on adrenocortical synthetic function[36] limits its clinical usefulness for long-term treatment of elevated ICP. Although clear evidence for a neuroprotective effect in humans is lacking, etomidate is frequently used during temporary arterial occlusion and intraoperative angiography (for the treatment of cerebral aneurysms). Etomidate produces an EEG pattern that is similar to thiopental except for the absence of increased β activity at lower doses. Etomidate can induce convulsion-like EEG potentials in epileptic patients without the appearance of myoclonic or convulsant-like motor activity, a property that has been proven useful for intraoperative mapping of seizure foci. Etomidate also possesses anticonvulsant properties, and it has been used to terminate status epilepticus.[6] Etomidate produces a significant increase of the amplitude of somatosensory evoked potentials while only minimally increasing their latency. Consequently, etomidate can be used to facilitate the interpretation of somatosensory evoked potentials when the signal quality is poor.

Etomidate causes minimal cardiorespiratory depression even in the presence of cardiovascular and pulmonary disease.[37] The drug does not induce histamine release and can be safely used in patients with reactive airway disease. Consequently, etomidate is considered to be the induction agent of choice for poor-risk patients with cardiorespiratory disease, as well as in those situations in which preservation of a normal blood pressure is crucial (e.g., cerebrovascular disease). However, etomidate does not effectively blunt the sympathetic response to laryngoscopy and intubation unless combined with a potent opioid analgesic.

Etomidate is associated with a high incidence of postoperative nausea and emesis when used in combination with opioids for short outpatient procedures. In addition, the increased mortality in critically ill patients sedated with an etomidate infusion

has been attributed to its inhibitory effect on cortisol synthesis.[36] Etomidate inhibits the activity of 11-β-hydroxylase, an enzyme necessary for the synthesis of cortisol, aldosterone, 17-hydroxy-progesterone, and corticosterone. Even after a single induction dose of etomidate,[38] adrenal suppression persists for $5-8$ h. Although the clinical significance of short-term blockade of cortisol synthesis is not known, the use of etomidate for maintenance of anesthesia has been questioned. In spite of its side-effect profile, etomidate remains a valuable induction drug for specific indications (in patients with severe cardiovascular and cerebrovascular disease).

Ketamine

Ketamine (Ketalar or Ketaject) is an arylcyclohexylamine that is structurally related to phencyclidine.[39] Ketamine is a water-soluble compound with a pK_a of 7.5, and is available in 1%, 5%, and 10% aqueous solutions. The ketamine molecule contains a chiral center producing two optical isomers. The $S(+)$ isomer of ketamine possesses more potent anesthetic and analgesic properties despite having a similar pharmacokinetic and pharmacodynamic profile to that of the racemic mixture [or the $R(-)$ isomer].[40] However, apart from some European countries where $S(+)$-ketamine is approved for clinical use, the commercially available solution is a racemic mixture of the two isomers and the preservative is benzethonium chloride. Ketamine is extensively metabolized by hepatic microsomal cytochrome P-450 enzymes, and its primary metabolite, norketamine, is one-third to one-fifth as potent as the parent compound. The metabolites of norketamine are excreted by the kidney as water-soluble hydroxylated and glucuronidated conjugates. Analogous to the barbiturates and propofol, ketamine has relatively short distribution and redistribution half-life values. Ketamine also has a high hepatic clearance rate (1 l · min^{-1}) and a large distribution volume (3 l · kg^{-1}), resulting in an elimination half-life of $2-3$ h. The high hepatic extraction ratio suggests that alterations in hepatic blood flow can significantly influence ketamine's clearance rate.

Ketamine produces dose-dependent CNS depression leading to a so-called dissociative anesthetic state characterized by profound analgesia and amnesia, even though patients may be conscious and maintain protective reflexes. The proposed mechanism for this cataleptic state includes electrophysiologic inhibition of thalamocortical pathways and stimulation of the limbic system. Although it is most commonly administered parenterally, oral and intranasal administration of ketamine (6 mg · kg^{-1}) has been used for premedication of pediatric patients. Following benzodiazepine premedication, ketamine $1-2$ mg · kg^{-1} iv (or $4-8$ mg · kg^{-1} im) can be used for induction of anesthesia. The duration of ketamine-induced anesthesia is in the range of $10-20$ min after a single induction dose; however, recovery to full orientation may require an additional $60-90$ min. Emergence times are even longer following repeated bolus injections or a continuous infusion. $S(+)$-Ketamine has a shorter recovery time compared with the racemic mixture. The therapeutic window for maintenance of unconsciousness with ketamine is between 0.6 and 2 mg · ml^{-1} in adults and between 0.8 and 4 mg · ml^{-1} in children. Analgesic effects are evident at subanesthetic doses of $0.1-0.5$ mg · kg^{-1} iv and plasma concentrations of between 85 and 160 ng · ml^{-1}. A low-dose infusion of 4 μg · kg^{-1} · min^{-1} iv was reported to result in equivalent postoperative analgesia as an iv morphine infusion of 2 mg · h^{-1}.

As a result of its NMDA receptor blocking activity, it has been suggested that ketamine should be highly effective for pre-emptive analgesia and opioid-resistant chronic pain states.[41] Unfortunately, a recent well-controlled study failed to demonstrate a pre-emptive effect when ketamine was administered prior to the surgical incision.[42]

An important consideration in the use of ketamine anesthesia relates to the high incidence of psychomimetic reactions (namely, hallucinations, nightmares, altered short-term memory and cognition) during the early recovery period. The incidence of these reactions is dose-dependent and can be reduced by co-administration of benzodiazepines, barbiturates, or propofol. Ketamine has been traditionally contraindicated for patients with increased ICP or reduced cerebral compliance because it increases $CRMO_2$, CBF, and ICP. However, there is recent evidence that iv induction doses of ketamine actually decreases ICP in traumatic brain injury patients during controlled ventilation with propofol sedation.[43] Prior administration of thiopental or benzodiazepines can blunt ketamine-induced increases in CBF. Since ketamine has antagonistic activity at the NMDA receptor, it has been suggested that it possesses some inherent protective effects against brain ischemia. Nevertheless, ketamine can adversely affect neurologic outcome in the presence of brain ischemia despite its NMDA-receptor blocking activity. Cortical EEG recordings following ketamine induction are characterized by the appearance of fast β activity (30–40 Hz) followed by moderate-voltage θ activity, mixed with high-voltage δ waves recurring at 3–4 sec intervals. At higher dosages, ketamine produces a unique EEG burst suppression pattern (Fig. 13-5). Although ketamine-induced myoclonic and seizure-like activity has been observed in normal (nonepileptic) patients, ketamine appears to possess anticonvulsant activity.[6]

Ketamine has well-characterized bronchodilatory activity. In the presence of active bronchospasm, ketamine is considered to be the iv induction agent of choice. Ketamine has been used in subanesthetic dosages to treat persistent bronchospasm in the operating room and ICU. It is also used in combination with midazolam to provide sedation and analgesia for asthmatic patients. In contrast to the other iv anesthetics, protective airway reflexes are more likely to be preserved with ketamine. However, it must be emphasized that the use of ketamine does not obviate the need for tracheal intubation in the patient with a full stomach (because tracheal soiling has been reported in this situation). Ketamine causes minimal respiratory depression in clinically relevant doses and can facilitate the transition from mechanical to spontaneous ventilation after anesthesia. How-

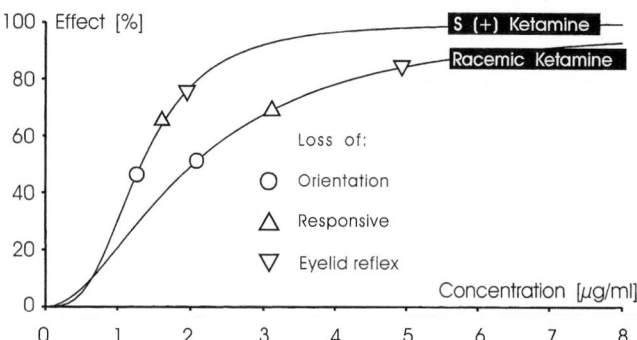

Figure 13-6. Concentration–response relationship for racemic ketamine and $S(+)$-ketamine in relation to specific clinical end points. The slowing of the median EEG frequency was used as the effect (end point) and was related to the arterial blood concentrations of ketamine. (Reprinted with permission from Schüttler J, Kloos S, Ihmsen H, Pelzer E: Pharmacokinetic–pharmacodynamic properties of $S(+)$-ketamine *versus* racemic ketamine: A randomized double-blind study in volunteers. Anesthesiology 77:A330, 1992.)

ever, its ability to increase oral secretions can lead to laryngospasm during ''light'' anesthesia.

Ketamine has prominent cardiovascular stimulating effects secondary to direct stimulation of the sympathetic nervous system. Induction of anesthesia with ketamine often produces significant increases in arterial blood pressure and heart rate. Although the mechanism of the cardiovascular stimulation is not entirely clear, it appears to be centrally mediated. There is evidence to suggest that ketamine attenuates baroreceptor activity *via* an effect on NMDA receptors in the nucleus tractus solitarius. Owing to the increased cardiac work and myocardial oxygen consumption, ketamine negatively affects the balance between myocardial oxygen supply and demand. Consequently, its use is not recommended in patients with severe coronary artery disease. In contrast to the secondary cardiovascular stimulation, ketamine has intrinsic myocardial depressant properties that become apparent only in the seriously ill patient with depleted catecholamine reserves. Because ketamine can also increase pulmonary artery pressure, its use is contraindicated in adult patients with poor right ventricular reserve. Interestingly, the effect on the pulmonary vasculature seems to be attenuated in children.

The anesthetic and analgesic potency of $S(+)$-ketamine is 3 times greater than that of $R(-)$-ketamine and twice that of the racemic mixture (Fig. 13-6), reflecting its 4-fold greater affinity at the phencyclidine binding site on the NMDA receptor compared with the $R(-)$ isomer.[40] The therapeutic index of $S(+)$-ketamine is 2.5 times greater than both the $R(-)$ and the racemic forms. In addition, hepatic biotransformation of $S(+)$-ketamine occurs 20% faster than that of the $R(-)$ enantiomer, contributing to shorter emergence times and a faster return of cognitive function. Both isomers produce similar cardiovascular stimulating effects and hormonal responses during surgery. Although the incidence of dreaming is similar with $S(+)$-ketamine and the racemic mixture, subjective mood and patient acceptance are higher with the $S(+)$ isomer. Of interest is the fact that $S(+)$-ketamine has been reported to have possible neuroregenerative properties.[44]

CLINICAL USES OF INTRAVENOUS ANESTHETICS
Use of Intravenous Anesthetics as Induction Agents

The induction characteristics and recommended dosages of the available iv anesthetic agents are summarized in Table 13-2. As a

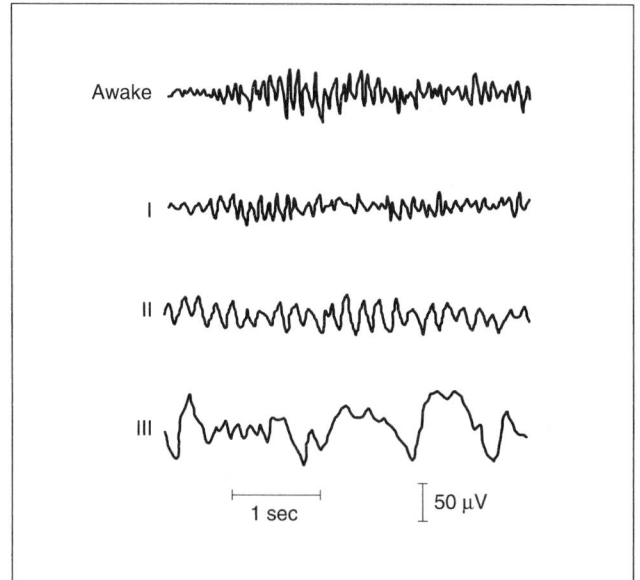

Figure 13-5. Progressive changes in the EEG produced by ketamine. Stages I–III are achieved with racemic ketamine and its $S(+)$ isomer. With $R(-)$ketamine, Stage II was the maximal EEG depression produced. (Reprinted with permission from Schüttler J, Stanski DR, White PF *et al:* Pharmacodynamic modeling of the EEG effect of ketamine and its enantiomers in man. J Pharmacokinet Biopharm 15:241, 1987.)

Table 13-2. INDUCTION CHARACTERISTICS AND DOSAGE REQUIREMENTS FOR THE CURRENTLY AVAILABLE SEDATIVE-HYPNOTIC DRUGS

Drug Name	Induction Dose (mg·kg^{-1})	Onset (sec)	Duration (min)	Excitatory Activity*	Pain on Injection*	Heart Rate†	Blood Pressure†
Thiopental	3–6	<30	5–10	+	0–+	↑	↓
Methohexital	1–3	<30	5–10	++	+	↑↑	↓
Propofol	1.5–2.5	15–45	5–10	+	++	0–↓	↓↓
Midazolam	0.2–0.4	30–90	10–30	0	0	0	0/↓
Diazepam	0.3–0.6	45–90	15–30	0	+/+++	0	0/↓
Lorazepam	0.03–0.06	60–120	60–120	0	++	0	0/↓
Etomidate	0.2–0.3	15–45	3–12	+++	+++	0	0
Ketamine	1–2	45–60	10–20	+	0	↑↑	↑↑

* 0 = none; + = minimal; ++ = moderate; +++ = severe.
† ↓ = decrease; ↑ = increase.

result of differences in pharmacokinetic (*e.g.,* altered clearance and distribution volumes) and pharmacodynamic (altered brain sensitivity) variables, the induction dosages of all iv anesthetics need to be adjusted to meet the needs of individual patients. For example, advanced age, pre-existing diseases (*e.g.,* hypothyroidism, hypovolemia), premedication (*e.g.,* benzodiazepines), and co-administration of adjuvant drugs (*e.g.,* opioids, α_2-agonists) decrease the induction dose requirements. When there is concern regarding a possible abnormal response, assessing the effect of a small "test dose" (equal to 10–20% of the usual induction dose) will often identify those patients for whom a dosage adjustment is required. Before administering additional medication, adequate time should be allowed for the anesthetic to exert its effect, especially when using drugs with a slow onset of action (midazolam) or in the presence of a "slow" circulation time in elderly patients and those with congestive heart failure.

The clinical uses of propofol have expanded greatly since its introduction into clinical practice in 1989.[45] Intravenous administration of propofol results in a rapid loss of consciousness (usually within one arm-to-brain circulation) comparable to that of barbiturates. Although an induction dose of 2.5 mg · kg^{-1} was initially recommended, the use of smaller induction doses of propofol (1–2 mg · kg^{-1}) has minimized its acute cardiovascular and respiratory depressant effects. Recovery from propofol's sedative-hypnotic effects is rapid, with less residual sedation, fatigue ("hangover"), and cognitive impairment than with other available sedative-hypnotic drugs after short surgical procedures. Consequently, propofol has become the iv drug of choice for outpatients undergoing ambulatory surgery.

With benzodiazepines, there is wide variation in the dose–response relationships in unpremedicated elective surgery patients. Compared to midazolam, diazepam and lorazepam have slower onset times to achieve a peak effect and their dose–effect relationship is less predictable. As a result, diazepam and lorazepam are rarely used for induction of general anesthesia. In addition, the slow hepatic clearance of diazepam and lorazepam may contribute to prolonged residual effects (sedation, amnesia, fatigue) when they are used for premedication. Midazolam has a slightly more rapid onset and may be a useful induction agent for special indications (when nitrous oxide is contraindicated, or as part of a total iv anesthetic technique). However, when midazolam is used for induction and/or maintenance of anesthesia, return of consciousness takes substantially longer than with other sedative-hypnotic drugs. In spite of its extensive hepatic metabolism, recovery of cognitive function is still slower after midazolam compared with thiopental, methohexital, etomidate, or propofol.

In an effort to optimize the clinical use of midazolam during the induction period, it is utilized increasingly as a co-induction agent with other sedative-hypnotic drugs (propofol, ketamine). Midazolam 2–5 mg iv can provide for increased sedation, amne-

sia, and anxiolysis during the preinduction period. When midazolam is used in combination with propofol, 1.5–2 mg · kg^{-1} iv, or ketamine, 0.75–1 mg · kg^{-1} iv, it facilitates the onset of anesthesia without delaying emergence times.[46] Midazolam attenuates the cardiostimulatory response to ketamine, as well as its psychomimetic emergence reactions. Use of midazolam, 2–3 mg iv, with propofol reduces recall during the induction period; however, larger doses of midazolam (>5 mg iv) will delay emergence after brief surgical procedures.

Owing to their side-effect profiles, the clinical use of etomidate and ketamine for induction of anesthesia is restricted to specific situations where their unique pharmacologic profiles offer advantages over other available iv anesthetics. For example, etomidate can facilitate maintenance of a stable blood pressure in high-risk patients with critical stenosis of the cerebral vasculature and in patients with severe cardiac impairment or unstable angina. Ketamine is a useful induction agent for hypovolemic patients, as well as in patients with reactive airway disease or a compromised upper airway.

Use of Intravenous Drugs for Maintenance of Anesthesia

The continued popularity of volatile anesthetics for maintenance of anesthesia is due primarily to their rapid reversibility and ease of administration when using conventional vaporizer delivery system for titrating to the desired end point. The availability of iv drugs with more rapid onset and shorter recovery profiles, as well as user-friendly infusion delivery systems, has facilitated the maintenance of anesthesia with continuous infusions of iv drugs, producing an anesthetic state (namely, TIVA) that compares favorably with that of the volatile anesthetics.

The traditional intermittent bolus administration of iv drugs results in a "depth" of anesthesia (and analgesia) that oscillates above and below the desired level.[47] Owing to rapid distribution and redistribution of the iv anesthetics, the high peak blood concentration after each bolus is followed by a rapid decrease, producing fluctuating drug levels in the blood, and hence the brain. The magnitude of the drug level fluctuation is dependent on the size of the bolus dose and the frequency of its administration. Wide variation in the plasma drug concentrations can result in hemodynamic and respiratory instability due to changes in the depth of anesthesia or sedation. By providing more stable blood (and brain) concentrations with a continuous iv infusion, it might be possible to improve anesthetic conditions and hemodynamic stability, as well as decreasing side effects and recovery times with iv anesthetics.[48] Administration of iv anesthetics by a variable-rate infusion is a logical extension of the incremental bolus method of drug titration, as a continuous infusion is equivalent to the sequential administration of infinitely small bolus doses.

Although an iv anesthetic can be titrated to achieve and maintain the desired clinical effect, a knowledge of basic pharmacokinetic principles is helpful in more accurately predicting the optimal dosage requirements. The required plasma concentration depends on the desired pharmacologic effect (hypnosis, sedation), the concomitant use of other adjunctive drugs (opioid analgesics, muscle relaxants, cardiovascular drugs), the type of operation (superficial, intra-abdominal, intracranial), and the patient's sensitivity to the drug (age, drug history, pre-existing diseases). Pre-existing diseases (cirrhosis, congestive heart failure, renal failure) can markedly alter the pharmacokinetic variables of the highly protein-bound, lipophilic iv anesthetic drugs. In general, children have higher clearance rates, while the elderly have reduced clearance values. Various intraoperative interventions (laryngoscopy, tracheal intubation, skin incision, entry into body cavities) transiently increase the anesthetic and analgesic requirements. Therefore, the infusion scheme should be tailored to provide peak concentrations during the periods of most intense stimulation. For specific surgical interventions, the so-called therapeutic window of an iv anesthetic is defined as the blood concentration range required to produce a given effect (Table 13-3). It must be emphasized that the therapeutic window for sedative-hypnotics is markedly influenced by the presence of adjunctive drugs (opioids, α_2-agonists, nitrous oxide).

The use of iv anesthetic techniques requires continuous titration of the drug infusion rate to the desired pharmacodynamic end point. Most anesthesiologists rely on somatic and autonomic signs for assessing depth of iv anesthesia, analogous to the manner in which they titrate the volatile anesthetics. The most sensitive clinical signs of depth of anesthesia appear to be changes in muscle tone and ventilatory pattern.[49] However, if the patient has been given muscle relaxants, the anesthesiologist must rely on signs of autonomic hyperactivity (tachycardia, hypertension, lacrimation, diaphoresis). Unfortunately, the anesthetic drugs (ketamine), as well as adjunctive agents (α_2-agonists, β-blockers, adenosine, calcium-channel blockers), can influence the cardiovascular response to surgical stimulation. Although the cardiovascular signs of autonomic nervous system hyperactivity may be masked, other autonomic signs (*e.g.*, diaphoresis) and purposeful movements are more reliable indicators of depth of anesthesia than blood pressure because the latter depends upon the ability of the heart to maintain the cardiac output in the face of acute changes in afterload. The heart rate response to surgical stimulation appears to be more useful than the blood pressure response in determining the need for additional analgesic medication. Moreover, it would appear that blood pressure and heart rate responses to surgical stimulation are a less useful guide with iv techniques than with volatile anesthetics.

An important problem with the clinical assessment of anesthetic depth is that modern iv anesthesia uses a combination of hypnotics, opioids, muscle relaxants, and adjuvant drugs. The interactions between these drugs can result in additive, supra-additive, infra-additive, or even antagonistic effects. An ideal "depth of anesthesia" indicator would integrate the physiologic information from all aspects of the anesthetic state. In the absence of a global cerebral function monitor, the "depth of anesthesia" device should provide an indication of one or more of the key components of general anesthesia (*e.g.*, hypnosis, analgesia, amnesia, suppression of the stress response, or muscle relaxation). A simple, noninvasive monitor of the depth of anesthesia, which would reliably predict a patient's response to surgical stimulation, would be extremely valuable when utilizing iv anesthetic techniques.

Electromyographic (EMG) activity of the frontalis muscles increases significantly in patients who move in response to a specific surgical stimuli[49]; however, EMG changes occur late and their interpretation can be obscured by muscle relaxant drugs. The EEG changes depend largely on the type of anesthetic drugs used. Although a common EEG pattern can be recognized with increasing depression of CNS function by sedative-hypnotics and opioid analgesics, there is no characteristic EEG pattern associated with unconscious and amnestic states.[50] Univariate descriptors of EEG activity appear to be of limited clinical utility, and no meaningful correlation could be found between EEG spectral edge frequency and hemodynamic response to surgical stimuli during propofol anesthesia.[51] Although EEG variables (spectral edge frequency, median frequency) appear to be useful indicators of the CNS effects of anesthetic and analgesic drugs in the experimental setting, their usefulness in clinical practice is limited owing to the many confounding factors during the operation (changing drug levels and surgical stimulation). The bispectral index (BIS), a novel approach to the analysis of the spontaneous EEG, may prove to be a useful indicator of anesthetic (hypnotic) depth.[52] A study showed that the BIS index reliably predicted fast-track eligibility after ambulatory surgery.[53]

An attractive alternative to the spontaneous EEG is the evoked responses of the EEG to sensory stimuli. The ability to quantitatively assess the response of the body to varying levels of stimulation (sensory or auditory evoked responses) may be the key to assessing depth of anesthesia.[54] Although all sedative-hypnotic drugs affect the brainstem-evoked potentials, uncertainty still exists regarding the most useful evoked response(s) to measure. In addition, the technical and practical complexity associated with recording evoked responses is much greater than recording the spontaneous EEG. The evoked response is also critically dependent on technical factors (stimulus intensity, stimulus rate, electrode position), body temperature, and the anesthetic drugs. Although most iv anesthetics produce dose-dependent changes in the somatosensory evoked potentials, the correlation between the acute hemodynamic changes to surgical stimuli and the early auditory evoked responses is poor. However, the early cortical (mid-latency) auditory evoked response might be useful in detecting awareness under anesthesia. Furthermore, the auditory evoked potential index (AEPi), a mathematical derivative of the morphology of the auditory

Table 13-3. THERAPEUTIC BLOOD CONCENTRATIONS WHEN INTRAVENOUS ANESTHETICS ARE INFUSED FOR HYPNOSIS OR SEDATION

Drug Name	Major Surgery Procedures	Minor Surgery Procedures	Sedative Concentration	Awakening Concentration
Thiopental	10–20 μg · ml^{-1}	10–20 μg · ml^{-1}	4–8 μg · ml^{-1}	4–8 μg · ml^{-1}
Methohexital	6–15 μg · ml^{-1}	5–10 μg · ml^{-1}	1–3 μg · ml^{-1}	1–3 μg · ml^{-1}
Propofol	4–6 μg · ml^{-1}	2–4 μg · ml^{-1}	1–2 μg · ml^{-1}	1–1.5 μg · ml^{-1}
Midazolam	100–200 ng · ml^{-1}	50–200 ng · ml^{-1}	40–100 ng · ml^{-1}	50–150 ng · ml^{-1}
Etomidate	500–1000 ng · ml^{-1}	300–600 ng · ml^{-1}	100–300 ng · ml^{-1}	200–350 ng · ml^{-1}
Ketamine	1–4 μg · ml^{-1}	0.6–2 μg · ml^{-1}	0.1–1 μg · ml^{-1}	NA

NA = not available.

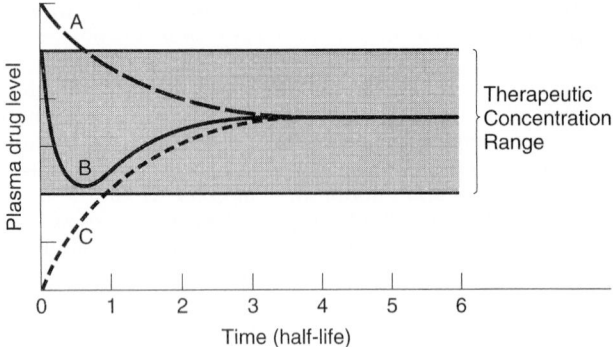

Figure 13-7. Simulated drug level curves when a constant infusion is administered following a "full" loading dose equal to $Cp \cdot Vd_{ss}$ (curve A), a smaller loading dose equal to $Cp \cdot Vc$ (curve B), or in the absence of a loading (curve C). (Reprinted with permission from White PF: Clinical uses of intravenous anesthetic and analgesic infusions. Anesth Analg 68:161, 1989.)

evoked potential waveform, may be more discriminatory than BIS in characterizing the transition from wakefulness to unresponsiveness.[55]

As a result of the availability of more rapid and shorter-acting sedative-hypnotics, sophisticated computer technology, and new insights into pharmacokinetic-dynamic interactions, use of TIVA techniques has been increasing. When utilizing constant-rate iv infusions, 4–5 half-lives may be required to achieve a steady-state anesthetic concentration (Fig. 13-7). To more rapidly achieve a therapeutic blood concentration, it is necessary to administer a loading (priming) dose and to maintain the desired drug concentration using a maintenance infusion. The loading dose (LD) and initial maintenance infusion rate (MIR) can be calculated from previously determined population kinetic values using the following equations:

$$LD = Cp(mg \cdot ml^{-1}) \cdot Vd(ml \cdot kg^{-1})$$

$$MIR = Cp(ml \cdot kg^{-1}) \cdot Cl(ml \cdot kg^{-1} \cdot min^{-1})$$

where Cp = plasma drug concentration; Vd = distribution volume; Cl = drug clearance.

The use of the smaller central volume of distribution (Vc) for the Vd component of the LD equation will underestimate the LD, whereas use of the larger steady-state volume of distribution (Vd_{ss}) will result in drug levels that transiently exceed those that are desired. If a smaller LD is administered, a higher initial MIR will be required to compensate for the drug that is removed from the brain by both redistribution and elimination processes. As the redistribution phase assumes less importance, the MIR will decrease because it becomes solely dependent on the drug's elimination and the desired plasma concentration.

An alternative approach is to begin with a rapid loading infusion with a bolus-elimination transfer (BET) scheme that combines three functions as shown in the following equation:

$$Input = V1 \cdot C_{ss} + Cl \cdot C_{ss} + V1 \cdot C_{ss}(k_{12} \cdot e^{-k_{21}t})$$

where $V1$ = distribution volume of the central compartment; C_{ss} = steady-state plasma concentration; Cl = drug clearance; k_{12} = redistribution constant from the central to the peripheral compartment; k_{21} = redistribution constant from the peripheral to the central compartment. Implementation of the BET infusion scheme requires the use of a microprocessor-controlled pump. If a continuous infusion is to be used in an optimal manner to suppress responses to surgical stimuli, the MIR should be varied according to the individual patient responses (Fig. 13-8). Using an MIR large enough to suppress responses to the most intense surgical stimuli will lead to excessive drug accumulation, postoperative side effects, and delayed recovery.

More gradual signs of inadequate or excessive anesthesia can be treated by making 50–100% changes in the MIR. Abrupt increases in autonomic activity can be treated by giving a small bolus dose equal to 10–25% of the initial loading dose and increasing the MIR.

Automated iv infusion devices are becoming more readily available for clinical practice. Despite the marked pharmacokinetic and pharmacodynamic variability that exists among surgical patients, computer programs have been developed that allow reasonable predictions of concentration–time profiles for iv anesthetics and analgesics. This new technology has led to the concept of target-controlled infusions (TCI), whereby the anesthesiologist chooses a "target" drug concentration and the microprocessor-controlled infusion pump infuses the drug at the rate needed to rapidly achieve and maintain the desired concentration based on population pharmacokinetic data.[56] It is obvious that the target concentration must be altered depending on the observed pharmacodynamic effect and the anticipated changes in surgical stimulation. Closed-loop control based on plasma drug concentrations is not possible because there is no available methodology to obtain frequent measurements of drug concentrations in real time. A more advanced form of TCI uses a feedback signal generated by simulating a mathematical model of the control process. Clearly, the precision of control achievable with a model-based system is only as accurate as the model. The performance of automated drug delivery devices is defined by the percent performance error (the difference between the measured and predicted drug values divided by the predicted value and multiplied by 100). An example of a model-based drug delivery system is the computer-assisted continuous infusion (CACI) system. An ideal automatic anesthesia delivery device would titrate anesthetic to meet the needs of the individual patient using an acquired feedback signal consisting of a measured value (*e.g.*, evoked responses, EEG parameters) that reflects the adequacy of the anesthetic state. The most successful efforts at feedback control of anesthesia have utilized the BIS and cortical auditory evoked responses to assess the pharmacodynamic end point.[52, 55]

The rapid, short-acting, sedative-hypnotics and opioids are better suited for continuous administration techniques than the more traditional anesthetic and analgesic agents because they can be more precisely titrated to meet the unique and changing needs of the individual patient. Traditionally, the

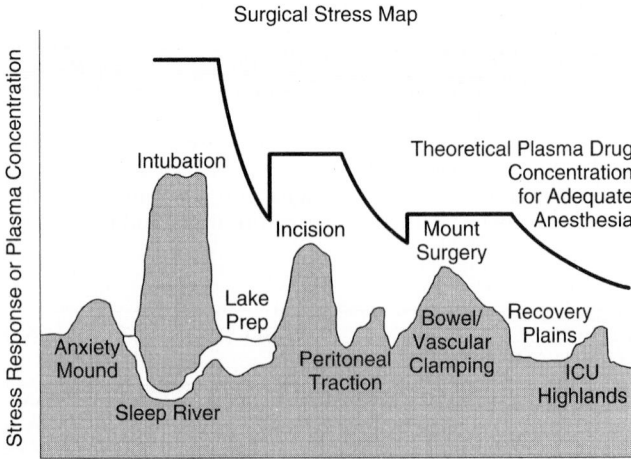

Figure 13-8. The "landscape" of surgical anesthesia. The surgical stimuli are not constant during an operation; therefore, the plasma concentration of an iv anesthetic should be titrated to match the needs of the individual patient. (Reprinted with permission from Glass PSA, Shafer SL, Jacobs JR, Reves JG: Intravenous drug delivery systems. In Miller's Anesthesia, 4th ed, p 391. New York, Churchill Livingstone, 1994.)

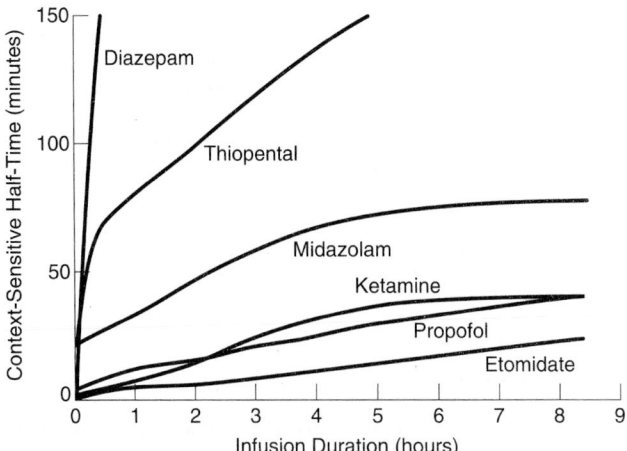

Figure 13-9. Context-sensitive half-time values as a function of infusion duration for iv anesthetics, including thiopental, midazolam, diazepam, ketamine, etomidate, and propofol. The context-sensitive half-time for thiopental and diazepam is significantly longer compared with etomidate, propofol, and midazolam with an increasing infusion duration increase. (Reprinted with permission from Hughes MA, Jacobs JR, Glass PSA: Context-sensitive half-time in multicompartment pharmacokinetic models for intravenous anesthesia. Anesthesiology 76:334, 1992.)

elimination half-life of a particular drug has been used in attempting to predict the duration of drug action and the time to awakening after discontinuation of the anesthetic infusion. Using conceptual modeling techniques, it has been shown that the concept of context-sensitive half-time is more appropriate in choosing drugs for continuous iv administration (Fig. 13-9).[4] Because none of the currently available iv drugs can provide for a complete anesthetic state without producing prolonged recovery times and undesirable side effects, it is necessary to administer a combination of iv drugs that provide for hypnosis, amnesia, hemodynamic stability, analgesia, and muscle relaxation. Selecting a combination of drugs with similar pharmacokinetics and compatible pharmacodynamic profiles should improve the anesthetic and surgical conditions. Sedative-hypnotics (methohexital, midazolam, propofol, etomidate, ketamine), opioids (fentanyl, alfentanil, sufentanil, remifentanil), and muscle relaxants (*cis*-atracurium, mivacurium, rocuronium, rapacuronium) can be successfully administered using continuous infusion TIVA techniques as alternatives to the volatile anesthetics and nitrous oxide.

Use of Intravenous Anesthetics for Sedation

The use of sedative-hypnotic drugs as part of a monitored anesthesia care (MAC) technique in combination with local anesthetics is becoming increasingly popular. During local or regional anesthesia, subhypnotic dosages of iv anesthetics can be infused to produce sedation, anxiolysis, and amnesia and enhance patient comfort. The optimum sedation technique achieves the desired clinical end points without producing perioperative side effects (respiratory depression, nausea, and vomiting). In addition, it should provide for ease of titration to the desired level of sedation while providing for a rapid return to a "clearheaded" state upon completion of the surgical procedure. Sedation also constitutes an essential element in the management of patients in the ICU. The ideal sedative agent for critically ill patients would have minimal depressant effects on the respiratory and cardiovascular systems, would not influence biodegradation of other drugs, and would be independent of renal and hepatic function for its elimination. The BIS monitor has been used to monitor the depth of sedation in the ICU. For patients undergoing cardiac surgery, rapid reversibility of the sedative

state may result in earlier extubation and lead to a shorter stay in the ICU. Although intermittent bolus injections of sedative-hypnotic drugs (*e.g.*, diazepam 2.5–5 mg, lorazepam 0.5–1 mg, midazolam 1.25–2.5 mg) are often administered, continuous infusion techniques with propofol are becoming increasingly popular for maintaining a stable level of sedation in the OR and ICU settings.

Benzodiazepines, particularly midazolam, are still the most widely used for sedation in the ICU and for relief of acute situational anxiety during local and regional anesthesia. Midazolam has a steeper dose–response curve than diazepam (Fig. 13-3)[57]; therefore, careful titration is necessary to avoid oversedation and respiratory depression. Midazolam infusion, 0.05–5 $mg \cdot kg^{-1} \cdot min^{-1}$, can be highly effective in providing sedation for hemodynamically unstable patients in the ICU.[58] Use of a midazolam infusion has been shown to control agitation and decrease analgesic requirements without producing cardiovascular or respiratory instability. However, marked variability exists for midazolam in the individual patient dose–effect relationships.[59] In addition, marked tolerance may develop to the CNS effects of midazolam with prolonged administration.

Propofol sedation offers advantages over the other sedative-hypnotics (including midazolam) because of its rapid recovery and favorable side-effect profile.[31, 60] In addition, the degree of sedation is readily changeable from "light" to "deep" levels by varying the MIR. Following a propofol LD of 0.25–0.5 $mg \cdot kg^{-1}$, a carefully titrated subhypnotic infusion of 25–75 $\mu g \cdot kg^{-1} \cdot min^{-1}$ produces a stable level of sedation with minimal cardiorespiratory depression and a short recovery period. Because even low concentrations of propofol can depress the ventilatory response to hypoxia, supplemental oxygen should always be provided. Sedative infusions of propofol produce less perioperative amnesia than midazolam,[60] and propofol-induced amnesia appears to be directly related to the infusion rate.

A small dose of midazolam (2 mg iv) administered immediately before a variable-rate infusion of propofol has also been shown to significantly decrease intraoperative anxiety and recall of uncomfortable events without compromising the rapid recovery from propofol sedation.[61] Propofol sedation can also be supplemented with potent opioid and nonopioid analgesics to provide sedation-analgesia.[62] In comparing propofol and midazolam for patient-controlled sedation,[27] midazolam was associated with less intraoperative recall and pain on injection than propofol, while propofol was associated with less residual impairment of cognitive function. Compared with midazolam in the ICU setting, use of propofol sedation allowed for more rapid weaning of critically ill patients from artificial ventilation.[63] It has been suggested that the more rapid weaning after propofol sedation may be cost-saving compared with midazolam when only a limited period of sedation (<48 h) is required.[64] Although a pharmacokinetic study yielded no evidence of a change in receptor sensitivity or drug accumulation over a 4-day study period, preliminary data suggest that tolerance to the CNS effects of propofol may develop with more prolonged administration (>1 week).

Concerns have been raised about elevated lipid plasma levels in patients sedated with propofol for several days, especially when high infusion rates (>6 $mg \cdot kg^{-1} \cdot h^{-1}$) are utilized. However, the availability of a 2% concentration of propofol should decrease the risk of this problem. Due to conflicting evidence regarding increased mortality as a result of myocardial failure when propofol was used for sedation in the neonatal ICU,[65, 66] more safety data are needed to define the indications for the use of prolonged propofol infusions, especially in the pediatric population.[67] Low-dose ketamine infusions (5–25 $\mu g \cdot kg^{-1} \cdot min^{-1}$) can also be used for sedation and analgesia during local or regional anesthetic procedures, as well as in the ICU setting.[39] Midazolam, 0.07–0.15 $mg \cdot kg^{-1}$ infused over 3–5 min, followed by ketamine, 0.25–0.5 $mg \cdot kg^{-1}$ iv over

1–3 min, produced excellent sedation, amnesia, and analgesia without significant cardiorespiratory depression.

SUMMARY

It is obvious that many of the goals desirable in an ideal iv anesthetic have not been achieved with the currently available drugs. Nevertheless, each of these sedative-hypnotic drugs possesses characteristics that may be useful in specific clinical situations. For example, thiopental remains a widely used iv anesthetic even though it is unstable in solution, produces significant cardiovascular and respiratory depression, and is associated with a high incidence of postoperative drowsiness and sedation. Although recovery from anesthesia with methohexital appears to be more rapid than with thiopental (and thiamylal), it produces more pain on injection and excitatory side effects (*e.g.*, myoclonus, hiccoughing) than the other barbiturates.

Propofol is the iv drug of choice when a rapid and smooth recovery is required (*e.g.*, outpatient anesthesia). Recovery from propofol anesthesia is characterized by the absence of a "hangover effect" and less postoperative nausea and vomiting when used for maintenance anesthesia. The cardiovascular depressant effects produced by propofol appear to be more pronounced than those of thiopental, but can be minimized by careful titration and the use of a variable-rate infusion. Propofol, with its favorable pharmacokinetic-dynamic profile, has greatly facilitated the use of TIVA techniques, especially when combined with remifentanil (a potent opioid analgesic that has a very short context-sensitive half-life and propofol-sparing activity), because this will provide for an even more rapid emergence from propofol-based anesthesia.

When administered alone for induction of anesthesia, benzodiazepines are associated with a prolonged recovery profile. In the usual induction doses, benzodiazepines are associated with minimal cardiorespiratory depression and the reliable amnestic effects are particularly valuable during iv anesthesia (*e.g.*, for acute sedation prior to induction of anesthesia, in the absence of nitrous oxide as part of a TIVA technique). Recently, midazolam has become an important adjunct during the induction period as part of a co-induction (or co-sedation) technique.

A new benzodiazepine with a favorable pharmacokinetic profile, Ro 48-6791, may find a niche in the future.

Etomidate has minimal cardiovascular and respiratory depressant effects and is therefore an extremely useful induction agent in "high-risk" patients. Unfortunately, pain on injection, excitatory phenomena, adrenocortical suppression, and a high incidence of postoperative nausea and vomiting have limited the use of etomidate to special situations in which it offers significant advantages over other available iv anesthetics. The new lipid formulation, with its fewer side effects, may allow this iv anesthetic to gain wider clinical acceptance.

Ketamine produces a wide spectrum of pharmacologic effects, including sedation, hypnosis, somatic analgesia, bronchodilation, and sympathetic nervous system stimulation. Induction of anesthesia can be rapidly achieved following im injection, making it the drug of choice when iv access is difficult to establish in an emergency situation. Ketamine is also indicated for induction of anesthesia in the presence of hypovolemic shock, acute bronchospastic states, right-to-left intracardiac shunts, and cardiac tamponade. The adverse cardiovascular, cerebrodynamic, and psychomimetic effects of ketamine can be minimized by prior administration of benzodiazepines (*e.g.*, midazolam) and sedative-hypnotic drugs (*e.g.*, thiopental, propofol), making it useful as part of a co-induction technique. The recent introduction of $S(+)$-ketamine may increase its use in low-doses ($100-250\ \mu g \cdot kg^{-1}$) as an adjuvant with anesthetic and analgesic-sparing activity.

In conclusion, iv anesthesia has evolved from being used mainly for induction of anesthesia to providing unconsciousness and amnesia for surgical procedures performed under local, regional, and general anesthesia. New insights into the pharmacokinetics and dynamics of iv anesthetics, as well as the development of computer technology to facilitate iv drug delivery, have greatly enhanced the use of total iv anesthetic techniques. The shorter context-sensitive half-life values of the newer sedative-hypnotic drugs make these compounds more useful as continuous infusions for maintenance of anesthesia or sedation. While the search for the ideal iv anesthetic continues, the challenge for the anesthesiologist is to choose the sedative-hypnotic that most closely matches the needs of the specific clinical situation in the most cost-effective manner.

REFERENCES

1. Franks NP, Lieb WR: Molecular and cellular mechanisms of general anaesthesia. Nature 367:607, 1994
2. Krasowski MD, Koltchine VV, Rick CE *et al:* Propofol and other intravenous anesthetics have sites of action on the gamma-aminobutyric acid type A receptor distinct from that for isoflurane. Mol Pharmacol 53:530, 1998
3. Rossi MA, Chan CK, Christensen JD *et al:* Interactions between propofol and lipid mediator receptors: Inhibition of lysophosphatidate signaling. Anesth Analg 83:1090, 1996
4. Hughes MA, Jacobs JR, Glass PSA: Context-sensitive half-time in multicompartment pharmacokinetic models for intravenous anesthesia. Anesthesiology 76:334, 1992
5. Avram J, Krejcie TC, Henthorn TK: The relationship of age to pharmacokinetics of early drug distribution: The concurrent disposition of thiopental and indocyanine green. Anesthesiology 72:403, 1990
6. Modica PA, Tempelhoff R, White PF: Pro- and anticonvulsant effects of anesthetics (Part II). Anesth Analg 70:433, 1990
7. Abramson N: Randomized clinical study of thiopental loading in comatose survivors of cardiac arrest. N Engl J Med 314:397, 1986
8. Gunaydin B, Babacan A: Cerebral hypoperfusion after cardiac surgery and anesthetic strategies: A comparative study with high-dose fentenyl and barbiturate anesthesia. Ann Thorac Cardiovasc Surg 4:12, 1998
9. Newman MF, Croughwell ND, White WD *et al:* Pharmacologic electroencephalographic suppression during cardiopulmonary bypass: A comparison of thiopental and isoflurane. Anesth Analg 86:246, 1998
10. Blouin RT, Conard PF, Gross JB: Time course of ventilatory depression following induction doses of propofol and thiopental. Anesthesiology 75:940, 1991
11. Vohra A, Thomas AN, Harper NJN, Pollard BJ: Non-invasive measurement of cardiac output during induction of anaesthesia and tracheal intubation: Thiopentone and propofol compared. Br J Anaesth 67:64, 1991
12. Shafer A, Doze VA, Shafer SL, White PF: Pharmacokinetics and pharmacodynamics of propofol infusions during general anesthesia. Anesthesiology 69:348, 1988
13. Sebel PS, Lowdon JD: Propofol: A new intravenous anesthetic. Anesthesiology 71:260, 1989
14. Smith I, White PF, Nathanson M, Gouldson R: Propofol: An update on its clinical use. Anesthesiology 81:1005, 1994
15. Glass PSA: Prevention of awareness during total intravenous anesthesia. Anesthesiology 78:399, 1993
16. Oxorn D, Orser B, Ferris LE, Harrington E: Propofol and thiopental anesthesia: A comparison of the incidence of dreams and perioperative mood alterations. Anesth Analg 79:553, 1994
17. Pinaud M, Lelausque JN, Chetanneau A *et al:* Effects of propofol on cerebral hemodynamics and metabolism in patients with brain trauma. Anesthesiology 73:404, 1990
18. Reddy RV, Moorthy SS, Dierdorf SF *et al:* Excitatory effects and electroencephalographic correlation of etomidate, thiopental, methohexital, and propofol. Anesth Analg 77:1008, 1993
19. Ebrahim ZY, Schubert A, Van Ness P *et al:* The effect of propofol on the electroencephalogram of patients with epilepsy. Anesth Analg 78:275, 1994
20. Sellgren J, Ejnell H, Elam M *et al:* Sympathetic muscle nerve activity, peripheral blood flows, and baroreceptor reflexes in humans during propofol anesthesia and surgery. Anesthesiology 80:534, 1994
21. Lopatka CW, Muzi M, Ebert TJ: Propofol, but not etomidate, reduces desflurane-mediated sympathetic activation in humans. Can J Anaesth 46:342, 1999

22. Gan TJ, Glass PSA, Howell ST *et al:* Determination of plasma concentrations associated with 50% reduction in postoperative nausea. Anesthesiology 87:779, 1997

23. Krumholz W, Endrass J, Hempelmann G: Propofol inhibits phagocytosis and killing of *Staphylococcus aureus* and *Escherichia coli* by polymorphonuclear leukocytes *in vitro.* Can J Anaesth 41:446, 1994

24. Crowther J, Hrazdil J, Jolly DT *et al:* Growth of microorganisms in propofol, thiopental, and a 1:1 mixture of propofol and thiopental. Anesth Analg 82:475, 1996

25. Reves JG, Fragen RJ, Vinik HR, Greenblatt DJ: Midazolam—Pharmacology and uses. Anesthesiology 62:310, 1985

26. Urquhart ML, White PF: Comparison of sedative infusions during regional anesthesia: Methohexital, etomidate, and midazolam. Anesth Analg 68:249, 1988

27. Ghouri A, Taylor E, White PF: Patient-controlled drug administration during local anesthesia: A comparison of midazolam, propofol, and alfentanil. J Clin Anesth 4:476, 1992

28. Dingemanse J, van Gerven JMA, Schoemaker RC *et al:* Integrated pharmacokinetics and pharmacodynamics of Ro 48-6791, a new benzodiazepine, in comparison with midazolam during first administration to healthy male subjects. Br J Clin Pharmacol 44:477, 1997

29. Tang J, Wang B, White PF *et al:* Comparison of the sedation and recovery profiles of Ro 48-6791, a new benzodiazepine, and midazolam in combination with meperidine for outpatient endoscopic procedures. Anesth Analg 89:893, 1999

30. Brodgen RN, Goa KL: Flumazenil. Drugs 42:1061, 1991

31. Ghouri AF, Ramirez Ruiz MA, White PF: Effect of flumazenil on recovery after midazolam and propofol sedation. Anesthesiology 81:333, 1994

32. Flogel CM, Ward DS, Wada DR, Ritter JW: The effects of large-dose flumazenil on midazolam-induced ventilatory depression. Anesth Analg 77:1207, 1993

33. White PF, Shafer A, Boyle WA *et al:* Benzodiazepine antagonism does not provoke a stress response. Anesthesiology 70:636, 1989

34. Doenicke AW, Roizen MF, Kugler J *et al:* Reducing myoclonus after etomidate. Anesthesiology 90:113, 1999

35. Van Hamme MJ, Ghoneim MM, Amber JJ: Pharmacokinetics of etomidate, a new intravenous anesthetic. Anesthesiology 49:274, 1978

36. Wagner RL, White PF, Kan PB *et al:* Inhibition of adrenal steroidogenesis by the anesthetic etomidate. N Engl J Med 310:1415, 1984

37. Gooding JM, Weng JT, Smith RA *et al:* Cardiovascular and pulmonary response following etomidate induction of anesthesia in patients with demonstrated cardiac disease. Anesth Analg 50:40, 1979

38. Wagner RL, White PF: Etomidate inhibits adrenocortical function in surgical patients. Anesthesiology 61:647, 1984

39. Schüttler J, Zsigmond EK, White PF: Ketamine and its isomers. In White PF (ed): Textbook of Intravenous Anesthesia. Baltimore, Williams & Wilkins, 1997

40. Kohrs R, Durieux ME: Ketamine: Teaching an old drug new tricks. Anesth Analg 87:1186, 1998

41. Rabben T, Skjelbred P, Oye I: Prolonged analgesia effect of ketamine, an *N*-methyl-D-aspartate receptor inhibitor, in patients with chronic pain. J Pharmacol Ther 289:1060, 1999

42. Adam F, Libier M, Oszustowicz T *et al:* Preoperative small-dose ketamine has no preemptive analgesic effect in patients undergoing total mastectomy. Anesth Analg 89:444, 1999

43. Albanese J, Arnaud S, Rey M *et al:* Ketamine decreases intracranial pressure and electroencephalographic activity in traumatic brain injury patients during propofol sedation. Anesthesiology 87:1328, 1997

44. Himmelseher S, Pfenninger E, Georgieff M: The effects of ketamine-isomers on neuronal injury and regeneration in rat hippocampal neurons. Anesth Analg 83:505, 1996

45. Smith I, White PF, Nathanson M, Gouldson R: Propofol: An update on its clinical use. Anesthesiology 81:1005, 1994

46. White PF: Comparative evaluation of intravenous agents for rapid sequence induction: Thiopental, ketamine, and midazolam. Anesthesiology 57:279, 1982

47. White PF: Use of continuous infusion versus intermittent bolus administration of fentanyl or ketamine during outpatient anesthesia. Anesthesiology 59:294, 1983

48. White PF: Clinical uses of intravenous anesthetic and analgesic infusions. Anesth Analg 68:161, 1989

49. Chang T, Dworsky WA, White PF: Continuous electromyography for monitoring depth of anesthesia. Anesth Analg 53:315, 1980

50. Plourde G: Depth of anaesthesia. Can J Anaesth 31:270, 1991

51. White PF, Boyle WA: Relationship between hemodynamic and electroencephalographic changes during general anesthesia. Anesth Analg 68:177, 1989

52. Struys M, Versichelen L, Mortier E *et al:* Comparison of spontaneous frontal EMG, EEG power spectrum and bispectral index to monitor propofol drug effect and emergence. Acta Anaesthesiol Scand 42:628, 1998

53. Song D, van Vlymen J, White PF: Is the bispectral index useful in predicting fast-track eligibility after ambulatory anesthesia with propofol and desflurane? Anesth Analg 87:1245, 1998

54. Sebel PS, Glass P, Neville WK: Do evoked potentials measure depth of anesthesia? Int J Clin Monit Comp 5:163, 1988

55. Schraag S, Bothner U, Gajraj R *et al:* The performance of electroencephalogram bispectral index and auditory evoked potential index to predict loss of consciousness during propofol infusion. Anesth Analg 89:1311, 1999

56. Milne SE, Kenny GN: Future applications for TCI systems. Anaesthesia 53(suppl 1):56, 1998

57. White PF, Vascones LO, Mathes SA *et al:* Comparison of midazolam and diazepam for sedation during plastic surgery. J Plast Reconstruct Surg 81:703, 1988

58. Shapiro HM, Westphal LM, White PF *et al:* Midazolam infusion for sedation in the intensive care unit: Effect on adrenal function. Anesthesiology 66:396, 1986

59. Shafer A, Doze VA, White PF: Pharmacokinetic variability of midazolam infusions in critically ill patients. Crit Care Med 18:1039, 1990

60. White PF, Negus JB: Sedative infusions during local or regional anesthesia: A comparison of midazolam and propofol. J Clin Anesth 3:32, 1991

61. Taylor E, Ghouri AF, White PF: Midazolam in combination with propofol for sedation during local anesthesia. J Clin Anesth 4:213, 1992

62. Sá Rêgo MM, Watcha MF, White PF: The changing role of monitored anesthesia care in the ambulatory setting. Anesth Analg 85:1020, 1997

63. Aitkenhead AR, Pepperman ML, Willatts SM *et al:* Comparison of propofol and midazolam for long-term sedation in critically ill patients. Lancet 2:704, 1989

64. Carrasco G, Molina R, Costa J *et al:* Propofol vs. midazolam in short-, medium-, and long-term sedation of critically ill patients: A cost–benefit analysis. Chest 103:557, 1993

65. Parke TJ, Steven JE, Rice ASC *et al:* Metabolic acidosis and fatal myocardial failure after propofol infusion in children: Five case reports. Br Med J 305:613, 1992

66. Martin PH, Murphy BVS, Petros AJ: Metabolic, biochemical and haemodynamic effects of infusion of propofol for long-term sedation of children undergoing intensive care. Br J Anaesth 79:276, 1997

67. McFarlan CS, Anderson BJ, Short TG: The use of propofol infusions in paediatric anaesthesia: a practical guide. Paediatr Anaesth 9:209, 1999

Clinical Anesthesia (4/e), edited by
Paul G. Barash, Bruce F. Cullen, and
Robert K. Stoelting. Lippincott Williams &
Wilkins, Philadelphia, © 2001.

CHAPTER 14

OPIOIDS

BARBARA A. CODA

HISTORY

Opioids have been used in the treatment of pain for thousands of years. The drug opium is obtained from the exudate of seed pods of the poppy *Papaver somniferum,* and the word "opium" is derived from *opos,* the Greek word for juice. The first undisputed reference to poppy juice is found in the third-century (B.C.E.) writings of Theophrastus.[1] Opium contains more than 20 alkaloids. The German pharmacist Sertuener isolated what he called the "soporific principle" in opium in 1806, and in 1817 named it morphine, after the Greek god of dreams, Morpheus.[2] Isolation of other opium alkaloids followed, and by the mid-1800s, the medical use of pure alkaloids rather than crude opium preparations began to spread.[1] In 1828, Bally published a memoir dealing with the use of morphine in nearly 800 patients. His observations described oral morphine's therapeutic indications, side effects, and dosage, as well as the development of tolerance and potential abuse.[2] Morphine was used widely to treat wounded soldiers during the American Civil War, and in 1869, its use as a premedication was described by Claude Bernard. However, in the absence of muscle relaxants and controlled ventilation, opioids were associated with a significant risk of severe respiratory depression and death. Thus its use in anesthesia was limited at that time.

With the advent of cardiac surgery in the late 1950s came the development of "opioid anesthesia." A decade later, Lowenstein reported the use of progressively higher doses of morphine (0.5–3 mg · kg^{-1}) without adverse circulatory effects, but two years later described limitations of the technique, including incomplete suppression of the stress response, hypotension, and awareness during anesthesia. Stanley found that much higher doses of morphine were associated with increased fluid and blood requirements.[3]

Phenoperidine, a derivative of normeperidine, was synthesized in 1957, and fentanyl, a 4-anilinopiperidine derivative, was synthesized in 1960.[4] These completely synthetic opioids were more potent and had a better safety margin (ratio of median lethal dose to lowest effective dose for surgery) than meperidine. Advances in surgical techniques have created the need for potent opioids with a rapid onset and a brief, predictable duration of action as well as a maximal safety margin for use in clinical anesthesia. Development of sufentanil, alfentanil, and other fentanyl derivatives between 1974 and 1976 was guided by these needs. The newest potent opioid, remifentanil, has an ultrashort duration of action owing to its rapid metabolism by ester hydrolysis. It remains to be seen whether these characteristics provide more safety and flexibility in the clinical setting.

The search for opioid analgesics having no potential for dependence was stimulated by concerns about opioid addiction, and led eventually to the identification of multiple opioid receptor types. In the mid 1960s, nalorphine, a drug known to antagonize the effects of morphine, was also found to have analgesic properties. Two other compounds, pentazocine and cyclazocine, antagonized some of morphine's effects. Pentazocine also produced analgesia, and both produced some psychotropic effects that morphine did not. These and other observations led Martin to propose the theory of receptor dualism. Intrinsic to this theory were two key concepts: (1) the existence of multiple opioid receptors (originally only two were proposed); (2) the idea of pharmacologic redundancy (*i.e.,* more than one receptor could mediate a physiologic function, such as analgesia).[5] Thus, a drug could be a strong agonist, a partial agonist, or a competitive antagonist at one or more of the different receptor types. Subsequent research has revealed three distinct families of opioid peptides and multiple categories of opioid receptors. Future research may identify compounds that provide potent analgesia but fewer side effects or propensity for abuse based on receptor selectivity.

TERMINOLOGY

The term *opiate* was originally used to refer to drugs derived from opium, including morphine, its semisynthetic derivatives, and codeine. The more general term *opioid* was introduced to designate all drugs, both natural and synthetic, with morphine-like properties, including endogenous peptides. However, the use of the term "opioid" has expanded to include reference to antagonists and receptors as well. The nonspecific term *narcotic,* which is derived from the Greek *narkotikos* (benumbing or deadening), has been used to refer to morphine and potent morphine-like analgesics. However, because of its use in a legal context, referring to any drug (including nonopioids, such as cocaine) that can produce dependence, the term "narcotic" is not useful in a pharmacologic or clinical context.[1]

In its broadest sense, the term "opioid" can refer to agonists, partial agonists, mixed agonist–antagonists, and competitive antagonists. Differentiation of these terms requires understanding of receptor–ligand interactions. Receptor theory states that drugs have two independent characteristics at receptor sites: affinity, the ability to bind a receptor to produce a stable complex; and intrinsic activity or efficacy, which is described by the dose–effect curve resulting from the drug–receptor combination. Efficacy can range from zero (*i.e.,* no effect) to the maximum possible effect, depicted graphically as the plateau of the dose–effect curve (Fig. 14-1). Given a high enough dose, an agonist will produce the maximum possible effect of binding with the receptor, whereas an antagonist produces no direct effect when it binds the receptor. A partial agonist has a dose–effect ceiling that is lower than the maximum possible effect produced by a full agonist, as well as a dose–effect curve that is less steep than that of a full agonist. A mixed agonist–antagonist acts as an agonist (or partial agonist) at one receptor and an antagonist at another. It is important to differentiate the term "potency" from "efficacy." Whereas efficacy defines the range in magnitude of an effect produced by a drug–receptor combination relative to the maximum possible effect, potency refers to the relative dose required to achieve an effect, and is related to receptor affinity. Thus, at the lower end of the effect range, a partial agonist may be more potent than a full agonist (Fig. 14-1). However, even at very large doses the efficacy, or maximum effect achieved by the partial agonist, will be less than the maximum possible effect of a full agonist.

ENDOGENOUS OPIOIDS AND OPIOID RECEPTORS

Opioid receptors were discovered in brain tissue before endogenous opioids were isolated. In 1975, Hughes *et al*[6] identified two pentapeptides with potent opioid activity, and within 10 years, more than 20 opioid peptides had been identified. All of the endogenous opioids are derived from three prohormones—proenkephalin, prodynorphin, and pro-opiomelanocortin (POMC)—and each of these precursors is encoded by

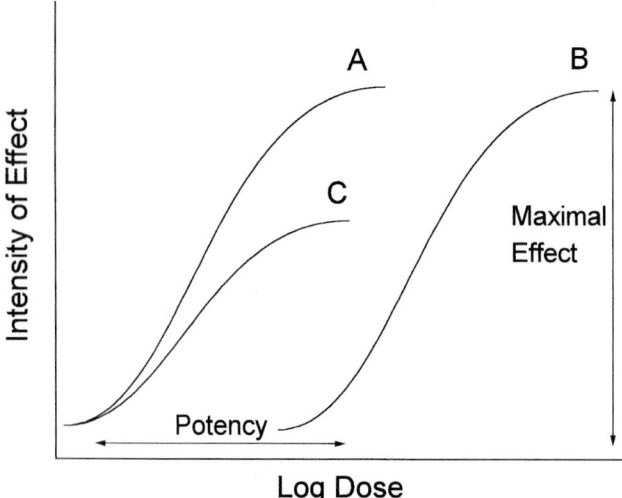

Figure 14-1. Log dose–effect curves for two agonists (A and B) with equal efficacy but different potency, and a partial agonist (C). Note that the potencies of A and C are similar, but the efficacy is less and the slope of the dose–response curve is shallower for the partial agonist. Note also that at lower doses, the partial agonist C is more potent than the full agonist B.

a separate gene. The three families of peptides differ in their distribution, receptor selectivity, and neurochemical role,[7] but they also share some features. For example, endogenous opioids from all three families begin with the pentapeptide sequences of [Leu]- or [Met]-enkephalin. Proenkephalin includes the pentapeptide sequences for [Met]- and [Leu]-enkephalin, and cells that synthesize proenkephalin are widely distributed throughout the brain and spinal cord as well as peripheral sites, particu-

larly the adrenal medulla.[8] Pro-opiomelanocortin is the common precursor of several peptides, including β-endorphin, adrenocorticotropic hormone (ACTH), and melanocyte-stimulating hormone (MSH). The term *endorphin* is reserved for peptides of the POMC family. The major site of POMC synthesis is the pituitary, but it is also found in the pancreas and placenta. Prodynorphin was formerly known as proenkephalin B. The dynorphin peptides all begin with the [Leu]-enkephalin sequence. Like the enkephalins, the dynorphins are widely distributed throughout the brain and spinal cord as well as peripheral sites.

Endogenous opioid peptides bind to a number of opioid receptors to produce their effects. Opioid receptor classification is continually being expanded and revised. Martin's initial classification of opioid receptors into the three types was based on binding activity of the exogenous ligands morphine, ketocyclazocine, and SKF10,047 at mu (μ), kappa (κ), and sigma (σ) receptors, respectively. Other opioid receptors identified since that time are delta (δ) receptors, bound by enkephalins, and epsilon (ε) receptors, bound by endorphin.[7,8] Of the above receptors, only the μ, κ, and δ receptor classes are firmly established as opioid receptors at this time.[7] There is also evidence supporting the existence of two μ, two δ, and three κ receptor subtypes.[8] While it appears that specific opioid receptors are responsible for different opioid effects and that synthetic opioids may be highly selective for a receptor type or subtype, it is important to note that very few endogenous opioids exhibit great selectivity for a single receptor type.[7] Remember also, that the theory of receptor dualism includes the concept of pharmacologic redundancy of receptor function. Thus, observed opioid effects typically involve complex interactions among the different receptor systems at supraspinal, spinal, and peripheral sites. Table 14-1 summarizes our current understanding of which opioid receptors are responsible for mediating opioid analgesic and side effects. One caveat in interpreting this summary is that species differences in opioid receptor sys-

Table 14-1. TENTATIVE CLASSIFICATION OF OPIOID RECEPTOR SUBTYPES AND THEIR ACTIONS

Receptor	Analgesia	Respiratory	Gastrointestinal	Endocrine	Other
μ	Peripheral		↓ Gastric secretion ↓ GI transit—supraspinal and peripheral Antidiarrheal	Skeletal muscle rigidity	Pruritus ?Urinary retention (and/or δ) Biliary spasm (probably >1 receptor type)
μ₁	Supraspinal			Prolactin release	Acetylcholine turnover Catalepsy
μ₂	Spinal Supraspinal (synergism with spinal)	Respiratory depression	↓ GI transit—spinal and supraspinal		Most cardiovascular effects
κ	Peripheral			↓ ADH release	Sedation
κ₁	Spinal				
κ₂	?				(Pharmacology unknown)
κ₃	Supraspinal				
δ	Peripheral	?Respiratory depression	↓ GI transit—spinal Antidiarrheal—spinal and supraspinal	?Growth hormone release	?Urinary retention (and/or μ)
δ₁	Spinal				Dopamine turnover
δ₂	Supraspinal				
Unknown (receptor type not identified)	Supraspinal				Pupillary constriction Nausea and vomiting

Adapted from Pasternak GW: Pharmacological mechanisms of opioid analgesics. Clin Neuropharmacol 16:1, 1993.

tems exist, so the results of animal studies, from which most of this information is derived, may not always be directly applicable to humans. Most opioids used in clinical anesthesia today (*e.g.,* fentanyl and morphine and their derivatives) are highly selective for μ opioid receptors. Naloxone, the most commonly used opioid antagonist, is not selective for opioid receptor type. In fact, current identification of an opioid-receptor–mediated drug effect requires demonstration of naloxone reversibility. Development of selective opioid receptor subtype antagonists is in progress. Such antagonists will be helpful tools in improving our understanding of which receptor subtypes mediate specific opioid effects.

At the cellular level, endogenous opioid peptides and exogenous opioids produce their effects by altering patterns of interneuronal communication. Receptor binding initiates a series of physiologic functions resulting in cellular hyperpolarization and inhibition of neurotransmitter release, effects that are mediated by second messengers. All opioid receptors appear to be coupled to G-proteins,[7] which regulate the activity of adenylate cyclase as well as performing other functions. G-protein interactions, in turn, affect ion channels. There may be different ion conductances involved at different opioid receptor types.[9] μ Opioid receptors are coupled to a potassium conductance; receptor activation increases potassium conductance, which inhibits neurotransmitter release and hyperpolarizes the cell membrane. δ Receptor activation increases potassium conductance in a similar manner, but may also affect a voltage-dependent calcium current. κ Opioids appear to inhibit calcium entry via voltage-dependent calcium channels.

STRUCTURE–ACTIVITY RELATIONSHIPS

The wide array of different molecules that produce morphine-like analgesia and side effects, including endogenous opioid peptides, all share some common structural characteristics. Horn and Rodgers[10] suggested that the tyrosine moiety at the amino terminal of the enkephalins formed the basis of a significant conformational relationship between the enkephalins and opiates. The structure of the phenanthrene class of opium alkaloids is complex, and consists of five or six fused rings. Morphine, one of three phenanthrenes, has a rigid five-ring structure that conforms to a "T" shape, with a phenylpiperidine ring forming the crossbar and a hydroxylated aromatic ring in the vertical axis (Fig. 14-2).[11] The other phenanthrenes are codeine, a derivative of morphine, and thebaine, a precursor of oxycodone and naloxone. Progressively reducing the number of fused rings from the phenanthrenes yields the morphinans, with four rings; the benzomorphans, with three rings; the phenylpiperidines, with two rings; and finally, the tyramine moiety of the endogenous opioid peptides, with a single hydroxylated ring. All of these distinct classes of drugs possess morphine-like activity. Thorpe[11] has proposed an opiate receptor model based on these structural similarities with two aromatic binding sites and one anionic site responsible for binding the positively charged nitrogen. In this model, differences in binding at the aromatic or anionic sites could potentially account for receptor specificity or for agonist *versus* antagonist activity. Structural modifications alter such important properties as opioid receptor affinity, agonist *versus* antagonist activity, resistance to metabolic breakdown, lipid solubility, and pharmacokinetics.[1]

PHARMACOKINETICS AND PHARMACODYNAMICS

Basic Considerations

Opioid effects are initiated by the combination of an opioid with one or more receptors at specific tissue sites. The relationship between opioid dose and effects depends on both pharmacokinetic and pharmacodynamic variables. Pharmacokinetics deter-

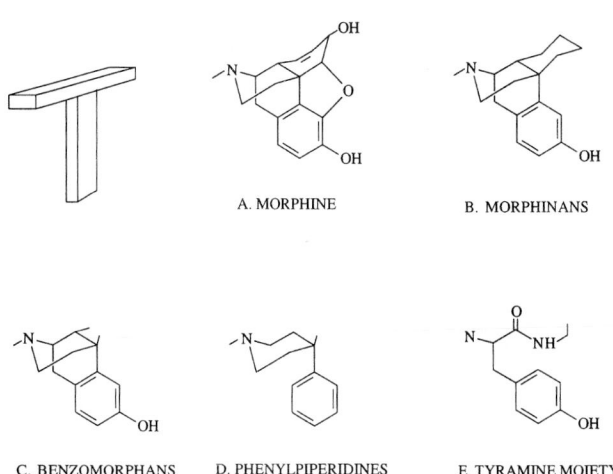

Figure 14-2. "T"-shape conformation of opioid molecules. (*A*) Morphine, one of the phenanthrene alkaloids, has a rigid five-ring structure, with a phenylpiperidine ring forming a crossbar and a hydroxylated aromatic ring in the vertical axis. (*B*) Reducing the number of fused rings to four yields the morphinan class of opium alkaloids. (*C*) Benzomorphans have three fused rings. (*D*) Phenylpiperidines and the 4-anilinopiperidines such as fentanyl have a flexible two-ring structure. (*E*) Finally, the tyramine moiety, which is the amino terminal peptide of both [Leu]- and [Met]-enkephalin, is shown, with a single aromatic ring. Another key feature is the positively charged basic nitrogen equidistant (4.55 Å) from the aromatic ring. (Adapted with permission from Thorpe DH: Opiate structures and activity: A guide to understanding the receptor. Anesth Analg 63:143, 1984.)

mines the relationship between drug dose and its concentration at the effect site(s). Pharmacodynamic variables relate the concentration of a drug at its site of action, in this case opioid receptors in the brain and other tissues, and the intensity of its effects. It is not generally possible to measure tissue drug concentrations directly, but tissue concentration bears a definable relationship to drug concentration in blood or plasma. Therefore, *pharmacokinetics* generally refers to the study of plasma drug concentration *versus* time because blood is easy to sample and because the blood is the medium by which drugs are distributed throughout the body. Changes in drug concentration over time in the blood, at the effect site and at other sites, are determined by physicochemical properties of the drug as well as a multitude of biologic functions involved in the processes of absorption, redistribution, biotransformation, and elimination.

In clinical anesthesia practice, opioids are typically administered intravenously. After an intravenous bolus dose or brief infusion, with no delay in absorption, peak plasma opioid concentrations occur within minutes. Plasma drug concentrations then fall rapidly as the drug is distributed to extravascular sites, including sites of action, noneliminating tissues, and eliminating organs. Compartmental models describe the time course of change in plasma concentration; typically, opioids used in anesthesia are characterized by two- or three-compartment models (see Chapter 11). The early rapid decline in plasma concentration after the peak is called the *distribution phase,* and the subsequent slower decline is the *elimination phase.* From a mathematical curve fitted to measured plasma concentration *versus* time data, distribution and elimination half-lives, systemic clearance, compartment volumes, and intercompartmental transfer rate constants can be calculated. Table 14-2 summarizes the estimates of key pharmacokinetic parameters as well as physicochemical characteristics for some of the most commonly used opioids in clinical anesthesia.

It is important to note that there is tremendous variability in the values published for opioid pharmacokinetic parameters. This is due, in part, to real population differences (*e.g.,* age,

Table 14-2. PHYSICOCHEMICAL CHARACTERISTICS AND PHARMACOKINETICS OF COMMONLY USED OPIOID AGONISTS IN ADULTS

Parameter	Morphine	Meperidine	Fentanyl	Sufentanil	Alfentanil	Remifentanil
pK_a	7.9	8.5	8.4	8.0	6.5	7.26*
% nonionized (pH 7.4)	23	7	8.5	20	89	58*
λ_{OW}	1.4	39	816	1757	128	17.9†
Protein binding (%)	35	70	84	93	92	66–93*
Clearance (ml · min^{-1})	1050	1020	1530	900	238	4000
Vd$_{ss}$ (L)	224	305	335	123	27	30
Rapid distribution half-life ($T_{1/2}\pi$, min)			1.2–1.9	1.4	1.0–3.5	0.4–0.5
Slow redistribution half-life ($T_{1/2\alpha}$, min)	1.5–4.4	4–16	9.2–19	17.7	9.5–17	2.0–3.7
Elimination half-life ($T_{1/2}\beta$, h)	1.7–3.3	3–5	3.1–6.6	2.2–4.6	1.4–1.5	0.17–0.33

λ_{OW} = octanol:water partition coefficient, Vd$_{ss}$ = steady-state volume of distribution.
Adapted from Bovill JG: Pharmacokinetics and pharmacodynamics of opioid agonists. Anaesth Pharmacol Rev 1:122, 1993.
* Unpublished information from Glaxo. JG Bovill, personal communication.
† Glass PSA *et al*: Anesth Analg 89:S7, 1999.

diseases), and in part to differences in study design (*e.g.*, sampling site, duration, concomitant events such as surgery, or other drugs that may affect differential flow to sites of action, metabolism, or elimination). In addition, the distributional and elimination half-lives are of limited use in predicting the onset and duration of opioid action in clinical anesthesia. For drugs with multicompartment characteristics, contributions of distribution processes between compartments vary with time. In an effort to relate pharmacokinetics to the time of onset and duration of action, concepts such as *effect compartment* in pharmacodynamic modeling,[12] and *context-sensitive half-times*[13] have been developed. The application of these concepts will be considered later in this chapter.

Physicochemical properties of opioids influence both pharmacokinetics and pharmacodynamics. In order to reach its effector sites in the central nervous system (CNS), an opioid must cross biologic membranes from the blood to receptors on neuronal cell membranes. The ability of opioids to cross this blood–brain barrier depends on such properties as molecular size, ionization, lipid solubility, and protein binding (see Table 14-2). Of these characteristics, lipid solubility and ionization assume major importance in determining the rate of penetration to the CNS. In the laboratory, lipid solubility is measured as an octanol:water or octanol:buffer partition coefficient. Drug ionization is also an important determinant of lipid solubility; nonionized drugs are 1000 to 10,000 times more lipid-soluble than the ionized form.[14] The degree of ionization depends on the pK_a of the opioid and the pH of the environment. An opioid with a pK_a much lower than 7.4 will have a much greater nonionized fraction in plasma than one with a pK_a close to or greater than physiologic pH. While greater lipid solubility correlates with membrane permeability, the relationship is not simply a linear one. Hansch[15] has shown that there is an optimal hydrophobicity for blood–brain barrier penetration, and Bernards[16] has demonstrated a similar biphasic relationship between the octanol:buffer distribution coefficient and spinal meningeal permeability. Plasma protein binding also affects opioid redistribution because only the unbound fraction is free to diffuse across cell membranes. The major plasma proteins to which opioids bind are albumin and α_1-acid glycoprotein (AAG). Alterations in AAG concentration occur in a variety of conditions and disease states, and result in acute or chronic changes in opioid requirements.

Two main mechanisms are responsible for drug elimination: *biotransformation* and *excretion*. Opioids are biotransformed in the liver by two types of metabolic processes. Phase I reactions include oxidative and reductive reactions, such as those cata-lyzed by cytochrome P-450 system, and hydrolytic reactions. Phase II reactions involve conjugation of a drug or its metabolite to an endogenous substrate, such as D-glucuronic acid.[14] A new phenylpiperidine, remifentanil, is metabolized via ester hydrolysis, which is unique for an opioid. With the exceptions of the N-deallylated metabolite of meperidine and the 6- and possibly 3-glucuronides of morphine, opioid metabolites are generally inactive. Opioid metabolites and, to a lesser extent, their parent compounds are excreted primarily by the kidneys. The biliary system and gut are other routes of opioid excretion.

Morphine

Morphine produces its major therapeutic as well as adverse effects in the central nervous system (brain and spinal cord) and the gastrointestinal system, but other systems are also affected. CNS effects include analgesia, sedation, changes in affect, respiratory depression, nausea and vomiting, pruritus, and changes in pupil size. Morphine also affects gastric secretions and gut motility, and has endocrine, urinary, and autonomic nervous system effects. Morphine mimics the effects of endogenous opioids by acting as an agonist at μ_1 and μ_2 opioid receptors throughout the body, and is considered the standard agonist to which other μ agonists are compared.

Analgesia

Opioids are administered primarily for their analgesic effect. Morphine analgesia results from complex interactions at a number of discrete sites in the brain, spinal cord, and under certain conditions, peripheral tissues, and involves both μ_1 and μ_2 opioid effects. Morphine and related opioids act selectively on neurons that transmit and modulate nociception, leaving other sensory modalities as well as motor function intact. At the spinal cord level, morphine acts presynaptically on primary afferent nociceptors to decrease the release of substance P, and also hyperpolarizes post-synaptic neurons in the substantia gelatinosa of the dorsal spinal cord to decrease afferent transmission of nociceptive impulses.[17] Spinal morphine analgesia is mediated by μ_2 opioid receptors. Supraspinal opioid analgesia originates in the periaqueductal gray matter (PAG), the locus ceruleus (LC), and nuclei within the medulla, notably the nucleus raphe magnus (NRM), and primarily involves μ_1 opioid receptors. Microinjections of morphine into any of these regions activates the respective descending modulatory systems to produce profound analgesia.[8,17] A more detailed description of the endogenous pain transmission and modulation pathways is given in Chapter 55. Morphine can act at a number of these discrete regions in the CNS to produce synergistic analgesic effects. For example, coadministration at the level of the brain and spinal cord increases morphine's analgesic potency nearly 10-fold,[18] an effect mediated by μ_2 opioid receptors.[8,19] There are also synergistic interactions between supraspinal sites of opioid action (*e.g.*, between the PAG and the NRM).[8] Recent animal studies as well as preliminary clinical studies in humans[20] suggest that morphine can also produce analgesia by peripheral mechanisms, most likely by activating opioid receptors on primary afferent neurons. However, it appears that peripheral opioid analgesia occurs only when inflammation is present.[20,21]

Although rapidly changing plasma morphine concentrations, such as those that follow bolus dosing, do not correlate well with analgesic effects, constant or very slowly changing (*i.e.*, steady-state) plasma concentrations do correlate with effect intensities. This observation has practical implications for postoperative analgesia. For example, patients using patient-controlled analgesia systems achieve more constant plasma opioid concentrations than those receiving intramuscular injections, and are able to maintain plasma morphine concentrations within an effective range for analgesia. In these patients, Dahlström measured the minimum effective analgesic concentration (MEAC) of morphine for postoperative pain relief at 10–15 $ng \cdot ml^{-1}$.[22] Cancer patients with severe oropharyngeal mucositis maintained their plasma morphine concentrations at a slightly higher level, 30–50 $ng \cdot ml^{-1}$, to achieve adequate analgesia.[23]

Effect on MAC of Volatile Anesthetics

In awake patients, therapeutic doses of morphine are effective in relieving clinical pain as well as increasing the ability of subjects to tolerate experimentally induced pain. μ Agonists are used extensively in conjunction with nitrous oxide (N_2O) with or without volatile anesthetics to provide "balanced anesthesia." Roizen *et al*[24] demonstrated that electrical stimulation of the periaqueductal gray (PAG) matter 1 hour prior to surgery reduced the MAC [minimum alveolar concentration] of halothane in 60% N_2O by 70%. One possible mechanism for this effect is the release of endogenous opioids following PAG stimulation. In animals morphine decreases the MAC of volatile anesthetics in a dose-dependent manner,[25–27] but there appears to be a ceiling effect to the anesthetic-sparing ability of morphine, with a plateau at 65% MAC.[25] Measurement of the maximum effect of very high morphine doses on MAC is limited by undesirable side effects such as hypotension and abdominal wall rigidity. Morphine 1 $mg \cdot kg^{-1}$ administered with 60% N_2O blocked the adrenergic response to skin incision in 50% of patients.[28] Neuraxial morphine may also reduce MAC. Epidural morphine 4 mg given 90 minutes prior to incision reduced halothane MAC by nearly 30%.[29] The effect of intrathecal morphine on MAC is unclear. In one study, a relatively large dose of intrathecal morphine (0.750 μg) reduced halothane MAC approximately 40%,[30] but an equally large dose (15 $\mu g \cdot kg^{-1}$) failed to reduce halothane MAC in another.[31] The reason for this discrepancy is unclear.

Other CNS Effects

Morphine can produce sedation, as well as cognitive and fine motor impairment, even at plasma concentrations commonly achieved during management of moderate to severe pain.[32] Other subjective side effects include euphoria, dysphoria, and sleep disturbances. High doses of morphine and similar opioids produce a slowing of electroencephalogram (EEG) activity associated with a marked shift toward increased voltage and decreased frequency.[1,33] Morphine can also produce sleep disturbances, including reduction in REM and slow wave sleep,[1] as well as vivid dreams with routine doses used for pain management. In extremely high doses, morphine can produce seizure activity in animals, but this toxic effect is not seen with doses used clinically in humans.

While there are significant species differences in opioid effects on pupil size, morphine produces dose-dependent pupillary constriction (miosis) in humans. This effect is thought to be mediated via the Edinger-Westphal nucleus of the oculomotor nerve.[1] A near maximal degree of miosis is seen with 0.5 $mg \cdot kg^{-1}$ of morphine.[34] In the absence of other drugs, miosis appears to correlate with opioid-induced ventilatory depression. However, hypoxemia from severe opioid-induced respiratory depression will cause pupillary dilation.

Systemic and neuraxial administration of morphine can produce pruritus, although this symptom is more common with spinal administration.[1] Pruritus appears to be a μ receptor–mediated effect which is produced at the level of the medullary dorsal horn (MDH).[35] Clinically, antihistamines are often used to treat this side effect, but pruritus induced by morphine microinjection into the MDH is not histamine-mediated.[36] Thus, their effectiveness is probably related to nonspecific sedative effects.

Morphine can also affect the release of several pituitary hormones, both directly and indirectly. Inhibition of corticotropin-releasing factor and gonadotropin-releasing hormone decreases circulating concentrations of ACTH, β-endorphin, follicle-stimulating hormone, and luteinizing hormone. Prolactin and growth hormone concentrations may be increased by opioids, and antidiuretic hormone (ADH) release is inhibited by opioids (see Table 14-1).[1]

Respiratory Depression

Morphine and other μ agonists produce dose-dependent ventilatory depression primarily by decreasing the responsivity of the medullary respiratory center to CO_2.[34] Standard therapeutic doses of morphine can produce a shift to the right and a decrease in slope of the ventilatory response to CO_2 curve, as well as abnormal breathing patterns.[37,38] Figure 14-3 illustrates the prolonged duration of an individual ventilatory response to CO_2 after high dose morphine (2 $mg \cdot kg^{-1}$). Ventilatory depression, seen as a shift to the right and decrease in slope, was partially reversed by 1 hour after a naloxone loading dose (3.66 $\mu g \cdot kg^{-1}$) plus continuous infusion (3.66 $\mu g \cdot kg^{-1} \cdot h^{-1}$). During and after the 10-hour naloxone infusion, end-tidal CO_2 and ventilatory drive gradually returned to control values by 21 hours after the morphine dose.[39] The respiratory depressant effects of morphine are similar for young and elderly patients,[37,38] but normal sleep markedly potentiates the effect of morphine on the venti-

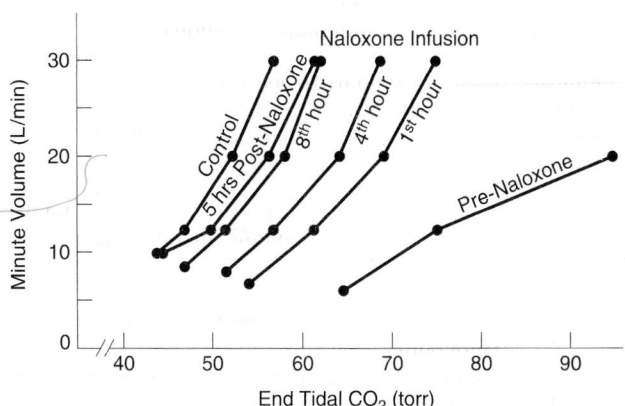

Figure 14-3. Ventilatory response to CO_2 after morphine 2 $mg \cdot kg^{-1}$, and antagonism by naloxone in a single subject. The control curve was obtained before morphine, and the prenaloxone curve 6 hours after morphine administration. The naloxone infusion was initiated 6 hours after morphine administration, and was continued at 4 $\mu g \cdot kg^{-1} \cdot h^{-1}$ for 10 hours. The 5-hour postnaloxone curve was obtained 31 hours after the initial morphine dose. (Reprinted with permission from Johnstone RE, Jobes DR, Kennell *et al:* Reversal of morphine anesthesia with naloxone. Anesthesiology 41:361, 1974.)

latory response to CO_2.[40] Frequent periods of oxygen desaturation associated with obstructive apnea, paradoxic breathing, and slow respiratory rate have been reported in patients who were receiving morphine infusions for postoperative analgesia. These episodes occurred only when the patients were asleep.[41] Such reports emphasize the need to consider both the expected severity of postoperative pain as well as diurnal variations in pain and opioid sensitivity when including long-acting opioids such as morphine in the anesthetic. With increasing doses, periodic breathing resembling Cheyne-Stokes breathing, decreased hypoxic ventilatory drive, and apnea can occur.[42] However, even with severe ventilatory depression, patients are usually arousable and will breathe on command.

Cough Reflex

Morphine and related opioids depress the cough reflex, at least in part by a direct effect on the medullary cough center. Doses required to attenuate the cough reflex are smaller than the usual analgesic dosage, and receptors mediating this effect appear to be less stereospecific and less sensitive to naloxone than those responsible for analgesia.[1] Dextroisomers of opioids, which do not produce analgesia, are also effective cough suppressants.[1]

Muscle Rigidity

Large doses of iv morphine ($2 \text{ mg} \cdot \text{kg}^{-1}$ infused at $10 \text{ mg} \cdot \text{min}^{-1}$) can produce abdominal muscle rigidity and decrease thoracic compliance; this effect reaches a plateau 10 minutes after morphine administration is complete.[43] Subjects receiving smaller doses of iv morphine (10–15 mg) also report feelings of muscle tension, most frequently in the neck or legs, but occasionally around the chest (unpublished observations). Muscle rigidity is drastically increased by the addition of 70% N_2O.[43] Myoclonus, sometimes resembling seizures, but without EEG evidence of seizure activity, has also been observed with high-dose opioids.[44] Opioid-induced muscle rigidity appears to be mediated by μ receptors[45] at supraspinal sites, including the nucleus raphe pontis and sites immediately lateral to it in the hindbrain.[46] In clinical practice, opioid-induced muscle rigidity and myoclonus are most often observed on induction, but have been observed postoperatively,[47] and can be severe enough to interfere with manual or mechanical ventilation. These effects are reduced or eliminated by naloxone,[47] drugs that facilitate GABA agonist activity (such as thiopental[43] and diazepam), and muscle relaxants.[47]

Nausea and Vomiting

Nausea and vomiting are among the most distressing side effects of morphine and its derivatives. Increased postoperative vomiting is seen with morphine premedication as well as with the use of intraoperative opioids as part of a balanced anesthesia technique.[48] The incidence of opioid-induced nausea appears to be similar irrespective of the route of administration, including oral, intravenous, intramuscular, subcutaneous, transmucosal, transdermal, intrathecal, and epidural.[48] Furthermore, laboratory investigations and clinical postoperative studies comparing the incidence or severity of nausea and vomiting have found no differences among opioids, including morphine, meperidine, fentanyl, sufentanil, and alfentanil.[32,48,49] Morphine causes dose-dependent nausea and vomiting, but the physiology and neuropharmacology of opioid-induced nausea and vomiting are complex (Fig. 14-4). The vomiting center receives input from the chemotactic trigger zone (CTZ) in the area postrema of the medulla, as well as from the pharynx, gastrointestinal tract, mediastinum, and visual center.[48,50] The CTZ is rich in opioid, dopamine (D_2), serotonin ($5\text{-}HT_3$), histamine, and (muscarinic) acetylcholine receptors, and also receives input from the vestibular portion of the eighth cranial nerve. Morphine and related opioids induce nausea by direct stimulation of the CTZ, and can also produce increased vestibular sensitivity.[1] Therefore, vestibular stimulation such as ambulation markedly increases the nauseant and emetic effects of morphine. High doses of morphine and other opioids also have naloxone-reversible antiemetic effects at the level of the vomiting center.[51] In volunteer studies, morphine-induced nausea and vomiting increase after a morphine infusion is stopped,[52] which suggests that antiemetic effects are more short-lived than emetic effects. Another possible explanation for this observation is that the active metabolite morphine-6-glucuronide continues to accumulate and worsens nausea. Prophylaxis and treatment of opioid-induced nausea and vomiting includes the use of drugs that act as antagonists at the various receptor sites (above) in the CTZ as well as others, such as propofol and benzodiazepines, whose antiemetic mechanisms are unknown.[48]

Gastrointestinal Motility and Secretion

Morphine and other opioids also affect gastrointestinal motility and propulsion, as well as gastric and pancreatic secretions via stimulation of opioid receptors in the brain, spinal cord, enteric muscle, and smooth muscle.[42,53] Selective activation of μ, κ, and

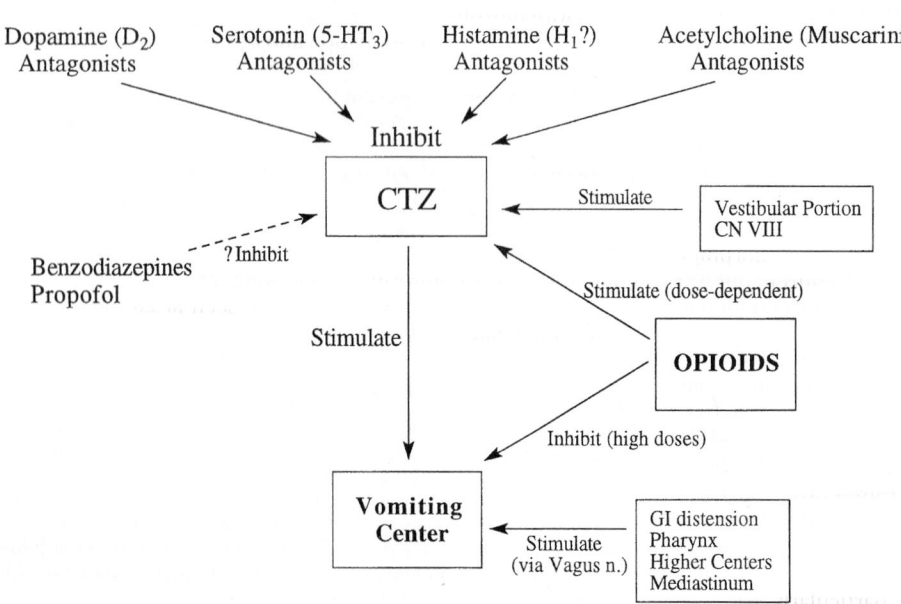

Figure 14-4. Pharmacology of nausea and vomiting. The chemotactic trigger zone (CTZ), located in the area postrema of the brain stem, contains dopamine, serotonin, histamine, and muscarinic acetylcholine as well as opioid receptors. The vomiting center receives input from the CTZ as well as peripheral sites via the vagus nerve. As illustrated, the role of opioids is complex, and they appear to have both emetic and antiemetic effects.

δ opioid receptors at different anatomic sites affects each of these gastrointestinal functions differently.[53,54] In rodents, μ agonists inhibit gastric secretion, decrease gastrointestinal motility and propulsion, and suppress diarrhea when administered by intracerebroventricular, intrathecal, and peripheral injection.[53] A study in human volunteers demonstrated that methylnaltrexone, an opioid antagonist that does not cross the blood–brain barrier, attenuated morphine-induced delay in gastric emptying,[55] suggesting that this effect is mediated primarily by a peripheral opioid mechanism. Morphine decreases lower esophageal sphincter tone and produces symptoms of gastroesophageal reflux in patients as well as normal volunteers,[42] and diamorphine, a morphine derivative, significantly slows gastric emptying in postoperative patients. This may increase the risk of regurgitation and aspiration of gastric contents in anesthetized or sedated patients. Like other opioid effects, gastrointestinal effects are probably dose-related. In both the small and large bowel tone is increased, but propulsive activity is decreased, leading to constipation. Epidural morphine can also delay gastric emptying. A single epidural dose (4 mg) of morphine slowed gastric emptying, while an intramuscular dose did not.[56] How the effects of equianalgesic or repeated doses would compare is unknown.

Biliary Tract

Morphine and other opioids increase the tone of the common bile duct and sphincter of Oddi. Symptoms accompanying increases in biliary pressure can vary from epigastric distress to typical biliary colic, and may even mimic angina. While not consistently produced by therapeutic doses of morphine, biliary spasm can produce elevations in plasma amylase and lipase that may persist for up to 24 hours.[1] Morphine and other μ agonists such as fentanyl have been used in provocative tests to evaluate sphincter of Oddi dysfunction and biliary-type pain.[57] In volunteers, morphine caused a greater delay in gallbladder emptying[58] and an increase in contractions of the sphincter of Oddi[59] than meperidine. Nitroglycerine, atropine, and naloxone can reverse opioid-induced increases in biliary pressure.[1] It has been suggested that morphine causes biliary tract contraction via histamine release. Antagonism of morphine's biliary effects by diphenhydramine supports this hypothesis.[60]

Genitourinary Effects

Urinary retention, seen after both systemic and spinal morphine administration, is due to complex effects on central and peripheral neurogenic mechanisms. It results in dyssynergia between the bladder detrusor muscle and the urethral sphincter, due to a failure of sphincter relaxation.[1,61] Estimates of the incidence of this bothersome side effect vary widely, and are confounded by the effects of anesthesia and surgery on urinary retention, but it is probably more common after spinal administration. Spinal morphine appears to cause naloxone-reversible urinary retention via μ and/or δ, but not κ opioid receptors.[61] The dopamine agonist apomorphine was also effective in treatment of spinal morphine-induced urinary retention in an animal model,[62] but this treatment is not recommended for clinical practice because of the potent emetic effects of apomorphine. In the same study cholinomimetic agents and α-adrenergic agonists aggravated high intravesical pressures, and therefore may be harmful agents to use for treatment of morphine-induced urinary retention.

Histamine Release

Opioids stimulate the release of histamine from circulating basophils as well as from tissue mast cells in skin and lung in a heterogeneous manner.[63,64] Morphine causes dose-dependent histamine release; intradermal injection of morphine in a concentration of $1 \text{ mg} \cdot \text{ml}^{-1}$ induces an urticarial wheal and flare.[64] In human basophil and mast cell preparations, this effect appears to be selective for mast cells,[63,64] particularly skin mast

cells.[63] However, in an isolated perfused lung model, morphine increased pulmonary vascular resistance, which was reversed by histamine H_1-receptor antagonism.[65] Morphine-induced histamine release is not prevented by pretreatment with naloxone,[64] suggesting that histamine release is not mediated by opioid receptors. Morphine-induced histamine release has clinical relevance. The decrease in peripheral vascular resistance seen with high-dose morphine ($1 \text{ mg} \cdot \text{kg}^{-1}$) correlates well with elevated plasma histamine concentration.[66] Furthermore, differences in the release of histamine could account for most of the hemodynamic differences between morphine and fentanyl (Fig. 14-5).[66] Histamine release may also be responsible for increased pulmonary vascular resistance and acute pulmonary edema associated with intravenous opioid abuse.[65]

Cardiovascular Effects

Opioids are popular in clinical anesthesia because they reliably produce analgesia and stable hemodynamics. In doses typically used for pain management or as part of balanced anesthesia, morphine has little effect on blood pressure or heart rate and rhythm in the supine, normovolemic patient. However, therapeutic doses of morphine can produce arteriolar and venous dilation, decreased peripheral resistance, and inhibition of baroreceptor reflexes,[1] which can lead to postural hypotension. Peripheral vasodilation is thought to be mediated by central sympatholytic activity. Thus, morphine's effect on vascular resistance is greater under conditions of high sympathetic tone.[67] The clinical implications of this finding are important. Patients who are critically ill (e.g., patients with severe trauma or cardiac disease) can be expected to have high sympathetic tone, and thus may experience hypotension in response to doses of morphine which would not normally produce hemodynamic instability. Morphine may also have some direct action on vascular smooth muscle,[67] but the primary mechanism for morphine-mediated vasodilation appears to be histamine release, as discussed earlier. At clinically relevant doses, morphine does not suppress myocardial contractility.[1,68] However, opioids do produce dose-dependent bradycardia, probably by both sympatholytic and parasympathomimetic mechanisms.[69] In clinical anesthesia practice, opioids are often used to prevent tachycardia and reduce myocardial oxygen demand. Patients undergoing cardiovascular surgery who received morphine $1–2 \text{ mg} \cdot \text{kg}^{-1}$ experienced minimal changes in heart rate, mean arterial pressure, cardiac index, and systemic vascular resistance. However, outcome was no different from that achieved with carefully administered inhalation-based anesthesia.[69]

Morphine does not directly affect cerebral circulation. However, with morphine-induced respiratory depression, CO_2 retention causes cerebral vasodilation and an elevation in cerebrospinal fluid pressure. This effect is not seen when mechanical ventilation is used to prevent hypercarbia.[1] Thus, morphine and other potent opioids must be used with caution in spontaneously breathing patients with head injury or other conditions associated with elevated intracranial pressure.

Disposition Kinetics

Morphine is rapidly absorbed after intramuscular, subcutaneous, and oral administration. Following intramuscular administration, peak plasma concentration is seen at 20 minutes and absorption half-life is estimated at 7.7 minutes (range 2–15 min).[70] After intravenous administration morphine undergoes rapid redistribution, with a mean redistribution half-time between 1.5 and 4.4 minutes in awake and anesthetized adults.[70-72] Morphine has a terminal elimination half-life between 1.7 and 3.3 hours.[71-73] Age affects morphine pharmacokinetics. The average elimination half-life of morphine is 7–8 hours in neonates less than 1 week of age, and 3–5 hours in older infants.[74] Patients between 61 and 80 years were found to have a terminal elimination half-life of 4.5 hours compared to 2.9 hours in younger patients.[70]

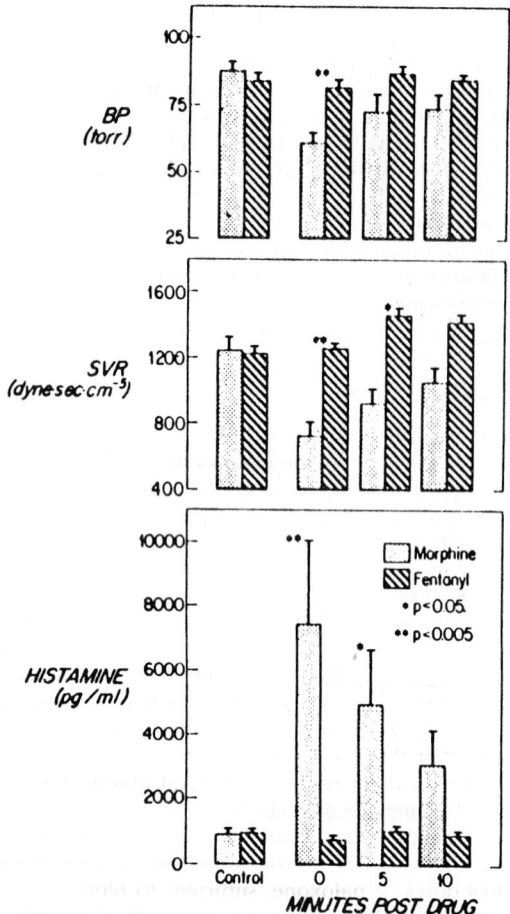

Figure 14-5. Mean arterial pressure (BP), systemic vascular resistance (SVR), and plasma histamine concentration (mean ± SE) before and after morphine 1 mg · kg^{-1} and fentanyl 50 μg · kg^{-1} (both infused over 10 minutes). Morphine, but not fentanyl, causes significant decrements in BP and SVR, which parallel the increase in plasma histamine concentration. (Reprinted with permission from Rosow CE, Moss J, Philbin DM *et al*: Histamine release during morphine and fentanyl anesthesia. Anesthesiology 56:93, 1982.)

Morphine is about 35% protein-bound, mostly to albumin.[14] Its steady-state volume of distribution is large, with estimates in the range of 3–41 · kg^{-1} in normal adults.[70–72] Morphine's major metabolic pathway is phase II conjugation. In the liver, morphine undergoes extensive conjugation to form morphine-3-glucuronide (M3G) and morphine-6β-glucuronide (M6G). 3-Glucuronidation is the predominant pathway, and following a single intravenous morphine dose, 40% and 10% of the dose are excreted in the urine as M3G and M6G, respectively.[75] Unchanged morphine in the urine accounts for only about 10% of the dose. Other minor metabolites in urine are morphine-3, 6-digluguronide, morphine-3-ethereal sulfate, normorphine, and its 3- and 6-glucuronides. The rate of hepatic clearance of morphine is high, with a hepatic extraction ratio of 0.7.[70] Thus, morphine elimination may be slowed by processes that decrease hepatic blood flow.[72] Extrahepatic sites, such as kidney, intestine, and lung, have been suggested for morphine glucuronidation, but their importance in humans is unknown.

Active Metabolites

M6G possesses significant μ receptor affinity and potent antinociceptive activity.[76] Appreciable plasma concentrations of M6G and M3G have been measured in cancer patients receiving high doses of oral morphine. During chronic oral morphine therapy, plasma M6G concentrations can be higher than those of the parent morphine compound.[77] Because morphine glucuronides are eliminated by the kidney, it is not surprising that very high M6G:morphine ratios have been reported in patients with renal dysfunction. This accumulation of the active metabolite is thought to be responsible for the unusual sensitivity of renal failure patients to morphine. While common wisdom suggests that glucuronide conjugates do not penetrate the blood–brain barrier, M6G concentration in cerebrospinal fluid (CSF) is 20–80% that of morphine.[78] Despite a mounting volume of animal literature demonstrating the analgesic potency of M6G, there is little information in humans concerning the magnitude of analgesia and side effects of M6G relative to morphine. Portenoy *et al*[78] demonstrated that in cancer patients on chronic morphine therapy, pain relief correlated positively with the M6G:morphine ratio, suggesting a contributing role of M6G to overall morphine analgesia. In a study of cancer patients with severe pain who received synthetic M6G (up to 60 μg · kg^{-1}), 17 of 19 patients experienced effective analgesia, with no changes in blood pressure or minute ventilation, and no nausea.[79] However, side effects such as dizziness, nausea, sedation, muscle aches, and respiratory depression have been reported in volunteers who received M6G.[77] While the contribution of M6G to morphine-induced analgesia and side effects remains to be determined, morphine should probably be administered cautiously to patients with renal failure.

Dosage and Administration of Morphine

In clinical practice morphine is used as a premedicant, a component of balanced anesthesia, in high-dose opioid anesthesia, and for postoperative analgesia. Intravenous analgesic doses of morphine for adults typically range from 0.01 to 0.20 mg · kg^{-1}. When used in a balanced anesthetic technique with N_2O, morphine can be given in total doses of up to 3 mg · kg^{-1} with remarkable hemodynamic stability. However, with the use of morphine 3 mg · kg^{-1} as the sole "anesthetic" agent, awareness (but not pain) has been reported.[3] When used in conjunction with other inhalation agents, it is unlikely that more than 1-2 mg · kg^{-1} of morphine is necessary. Because of its hydrophilicity, morphine crosses the blood–brain barrier relatively slowly; and while its onset can be observed within 5 minutes, peak effects may be delayed for 10 minutes or longer. Because of its delay in action, morphine can be more difficult to titrate as an anesthetic supplement than the more rapidly acting opioids. Patients may experience prolonged analgesia and adverse side effects such as respiratory depression even when plasma morphine concentration is low. However, Gross and Alexander[80] reported that a single dose of morphine 0.1 mg · kg^{-1} given 80 minutes prior to the end of surgery did not affect the time to awakening or the awakening concentration of isoflurane.

Meperidine

Meperidine, a phenylpiperidine derivative (Fig. 14-6), was the first totally synthetic opioid, described in 1939 by Eisleb and Schaumann. It was initially studied as an anticholinergic agent, but was found to have significant analgesic activity.[1]

Analgesia and Effect on MAC of Volatile Anesthetics

Meperidine's analgesic potency is about one tenth that of morphine's and is most likely mediated by μ opioid receptor activation. However, meperidine also has moderate affinity for κ and δ opioid receptors.[1,81] Unlike morphine, meperidine plasma concentrations correlate reasonably well with analgesic effects.[82,83] While there is considerable interpatient variability, the minimum effective analgesia concentration of meperidine is approximately 200 ng · ml^{-1}. There is very little information available on the effect of meperidine on MAC of inhaled anesthetics, but a study in dogs demonstrated a dose-dependent reduction in the MAC of halothane.[84]

Meperidine also has well recognized weak local anesthetic

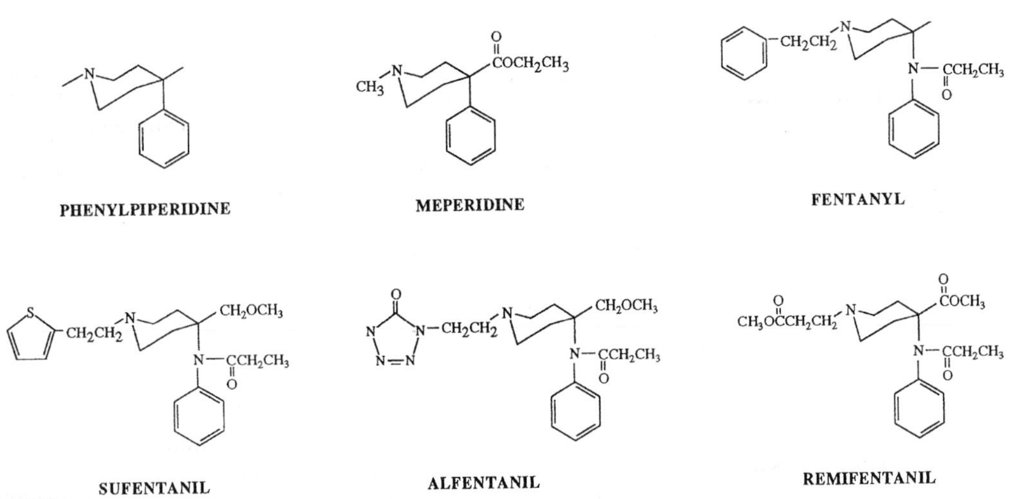

Figure 14-6. Chemical structures of phenylpiperidine, meperidine, and the 4-anilinopiperidine derivatives fentanyl, sufentanil, alfentanil, and remifentanil.

properties. Compared to morphine, fentanyl, and buprenorphine injected perineurally, only meperidine alters nerve conduction and produces analgesia.[85,86] This has led to its increasing popularity for epidural and subarachnoid administration, particularly in obstetric anesthesia. But because of its local anesthetic effects, spinal meperidine may also produce sensory and motor blockade as well as sympatholytic effects that are not seen with other opioids.

Side Effects

Like morphine, therapeutic doses of meperidine can produce sedation, pupillary constriction, and euphoria. Very high doses of meperidine are associated with CNS excitement and seizures (see below). In equianalgesic doses, meperidine produces respiratory depression equal to that of morphine, as well as nausea, vomiting, and dizziness, particularly in ambulatory patients.[1]

Like other opioids, meperidine causes significant delay in gastric emptying. While meperidine does increase common bile duct pressure and delay gall bladder emptying, this occurs to a lesser extent than with equianalgesic doses of morphine and fentanyl (Fig. 14-7).[58,89]

Analgesic doses of meperidine in awake patients are not associated with hemodynamic instability. However, patients with cardiac disease who received 1 mg · kg^{-1} of meperidine experienced decreases in heart rate, cardiac index, and rate–pressure product.[90] In an isolated papillary muscle preparation, high concentrations of meperidine depressed contractility. This effect was not naloxone-reversible and is consistent with a nonspecific, local anesthetic effect.[91] In higher doses, meperidine causes significantly more hemodynamic instability than morphine or fentanyl and its derivatives.[92] This may be at least partially related to histamine release. In a comparison of opioids administered as part of balanced anesthesia, Flacke *et al*[92] found that 4 of 16 patients in the meperidine group did not receive the total planned induction dose (5 mg · kg^{-1}) because of hypotension. Five patients developed tachycardia, three of these with marked flushing. These five patients were found to have abnormally elevated plasma histamine concentrations. Interestingly, only one patient in the morphine group (0.6 mg · kg^{-1} morphine given) had a similar histamine plasma concentration. Thus, meperidine is not recommended in high doses for clinical anesthesia.

Shivering

Meperidine is effective in reducing shivering from diverse causes, including general and epidural anesthesia, fever, experimentally induced cold, transfusion reactions, and administra-

tion of amphotericin B. Intravenous doses of 25–50 mg reduce or eliminate visible shivering as well as the accompanying increase in oxygen consumption[93,94] following general and epidural anesthesia. Equianalgesic doses of fentanyl (25 μg) and morphine (2.5 mg) did not reduce postoperative shivering,[95] suggesting that the antishivering effect of meperidine is not mediated by μ-opioid receptors. Several observations suggest that this effect may be mediated by κ-opioid receptors. Butorphanol, a drug with significant κ agonist activity, effectively reduces postoperative shivering in a dose of 1 mg.[96] Furthermore, low doses of naloxone, sufficient to block μ receptor-mediated miosis, did not reverse meperidine's antishivering effect, but high-dose naloxone, designed to block both μ and κ receptors, did reverse the antishivering effect.[81] However, infusion of alfentanil, a pure μ agonist, has been shown to impair thermoregulation, including reducing the shivering threshold and raising the sweating threshold.[97] The plasma alfentanil concentrations measured in this study were typical of those used during alfentanil anesthesia. Whether a smaller dose of alfentanil can eliminate postoperative shivering has not been evaluated. The observation that other types of drugs, such as α$_1$-adrenergic agonists and serotonin (5-HT$_2$) antagonists[98] as well as propofol,[99] can also reduce postoperative shivering suggests that a nonopioid mechanism may be involved. Physostigmine can also prevent postoperative shivering, suggesting a role for the cholinergic system. Horn[100] and others[97] suggest that a central inhibition of thermoregulatory control is the mechanism by which many classes of drugs reduce or prevent shivering. Perhaps meperidine's greater antishivering effect, relative to other opioids, is due to additive thermoregulatory impairment by more than one mechanism.

Disposition Kinetics

Following intravenous administration, meperidine plasma concentration falls rapidly, and has been described by both two- and three-compartment models. Meperidine's redistribution phase is rapid, with a half-life of 4–16 minutes,[101,102] and its terminal elimination half-life is between 3 and 5 hours.[101-103] The elimination half-life is not prolonged in patients 60–80 years old. However, in neonates and infants, a median elimination half-life, 8–10 hours, with greater individual variability (3–5-fold) compared to adults, has been reported. Absorption after intramuscular administration was complete in normal volunteers, with peak plasma concentration at 5–15 minutes after injection; but in postoperative patients, intramuscular meperidine absorption can be more variable, with time to reach peak concentration between 5 and 110 minutes.[82]

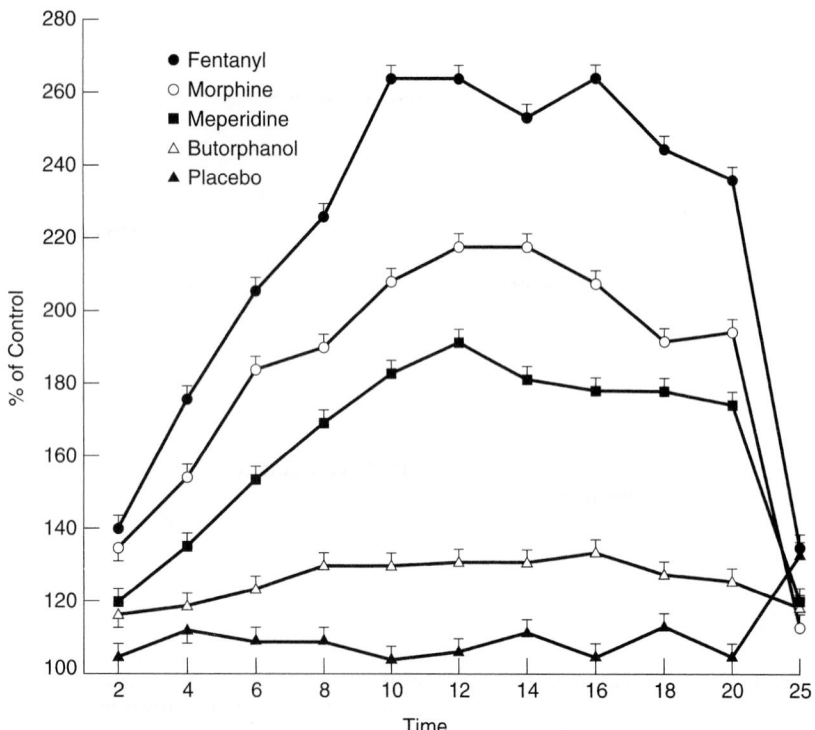

Figure 14-7. The effect of several opioids on common bile duct pressures in patients anesthetized with enflurane and N_2O–O_2. Patients received either fentanyl 100 $\mu g \cdot 70$ kg^{-1}, morphine 10 mg $\cdot$ 70 kg^{-1}, meperidine 75 mg $\cdot$ 70 kg^{-1}, or butorphanol 2 mg $\cdot$ 70 kg^{-1}. After 20 minutes, the effects were reversed with naloxone. (Reprinted with permission from Radnay PA, Duncalf D, Novakovik M, Lesser ML: Common bile duct pressure changes after fentanyl, morphine, meperidine, butorphanol, and naloxone. Anesth Analg 63:441, 1984.)

Meperidine is moderately lipid-soluble, and is about 40–70% protein-bound, mostly to albumin and α_1-acid glycoprotein (Table 14-2).[104] Meperidine has a large steady-state volume of distribution, with estimates in the range of 3.5–5 l $\cdot$ kg^{-1} in adults.[101,102] The high clearance rate (10 ml $\cdot$ kg^{-1} $\cdot$ min^{-1}) reflects a high hepatic extraction ratio. Meperidine is metabolized mainly in the liver by N-demethylation to form normeperidine, the principal metabolite, and by hydrolysis to form meperidinic acid. Both of these metabolites may then be conjugated[1] and excreted renally. Normeperidine is pharmacologically active and potentially toxic (see below).

Active Metabolites

Normeperidine has appreciable pharmacologic activity, and can produce signs of central nervous system excitation. In humans, mood alterations such as apprehension and restlessness, as well as neurotoxic effects such as tremors, myoclonus, and seizures, have been reported.[105] The elimination half-life of the metabolite normeperidine (14–21 hours) is considerably longer than the parent compound, and therefore is likely to accumulate with repeated or prolonged administration, particularly in patients with renal dysfunction.[105] Myoclonus and seizures have been reported in patients receiving meperidine for postoperative or chronic pain. Patients who developed seizures had a mean plasma normeperidine concentration of 0.81 $\mu g \cdot ml^{-1}$,[105] and it appears that a total daily dosage of 1000 mg is associated with an increased risk of seizures.

Dosage and Administration of Meperidine

A single dose of meperidine is approximately one tenth as potent as morphine when given parenterally, but has a shorter duration of action. Intravenous analgesic doses of meperidine for adults typically range from 0.1 to 1 mg $\cdot$ kg^{-1}. Doses of 25–50 mg are generally effective in reducing postoperative shivering, but doses as low as 12.5 mg may be effective in some individuals. As discussed above, high doses of meperidine for intraoperative use are not recommended due to hemodynamic instability. In addition very high single doses or prolonged administration may produce seizures due to the metabolite normeperidine; thus the total daily dose should not exceed 1000 mg/24 hours.

Methadone

Methadone, a synthetic opioid introduced in the 1940s, is primarily a μ agonist with pharmacologic properties that are similar to morphine. While its chemical structure is very different from that of morphine, steric factors force the molecule to simulate the pseudopiperidine ring conformation that appears to be required for opioid activity.[1] Because of its long elimination half-life, methadone is most often used for long-term pain management and in treatment of opioid abstinence syndromes.

Analgesia and Use in Anesthesia

Following parenteral administration, the onset of analgesia is rapid, within 10–20 minutes. After single doses of up to 10 mg, the duration of analgesia is similar to morphine,[1] but with large or repeated parenteral doses, prolonged analgesia can be obtained. Several investigators have administered methadone intra- and postoperatively with the aim of providing prolonged postoperative analgesia.[106–108] Patients who received 20 mg methadone intraoperatively and up to 20 mg additional methadone in the immediate postoperative period had a median duration of postoperative analgesia of over 20 hours.[106,107] Gourlay *et al*[107] found that for relief of postoperative pain, the minimum effective concentration of methadone in blood is 58 ng $\cdot$ ml^{-1} (range 34–80 ng $\cdot$ ml^{-1}). The effect of methadone on the MAC of volatile anesthetics has not been reported.

Side Effects

Side effects of methadone are similar in magnitude and frequency to those of morphine.[1,106] Patients who received 20 mg methadone at the beginning of surgery were sedated in the immediate postoperative period, but did not appear to have clinically significant respiratory depression. About 50% experienced nausea or vomiting, which was easily treated with standard antiemetic therapy.[106] Methadone produces typical opioid effects on smooth muscle. Like morphine, it markedly decreases intestinal propulsive activity, and can cause constipation as well as biliary spasm.[1]

Disposition Kinetics

Following an intravenous dose, the plasma concentration-time data for methadone are described by a biexponential equation. The mean redistribution half-time is 6 minutes (range 1–24 min), and the mean terminal elimination half-time is 34 hours (range 9–87 h).[107] Methadone is well absorbed after an oral dose, with bioavailability approximately 90%, and reaches peak plasma concentration at 4 hours after oral administration.[1] It is nearly 90% plasma protein–bound, and undergoes extensive metabolism in the liver, mostly N-demethylation and cyclization to form pyrrolidines and pyrroline.[1]

Dosage and Administration of Methadone

The use of methadone in clinical anesthesia has focused on attempts to achieve prolonged postoperative analgesia, providing that an adequate initial dose is administered. Because adverse effects can also be prolonged, careful titration of the dose is necessary. In general, an initial single dose of 20 mg can provide analgesia without significant postoperative respiratory depression.[106] Wangler[108] described a technique to avoid respiratory depression in which 8–12 mg methadone is administered to the awake patient until the threshold of respiratory depression (respiratory rate of 6–8 min^{-1}) is reached. Immediately prior to incision, an additional dose equal to half the initial dose is given. For patients who need supplemental analgesic doses in the immediate postoperative period, Gourlay et al[109] have suggested that to avoid respiratory depression, the patients must meet the following criteria prior to each supplementary dose of methadone 5 mg:

1. The patient complains of significant postoperative pain
2. The respiratory rate is >10 breaths per minute
3. No marked depression of the level of consciousness is observed

They also recommend that 30–40 minutes (5–6 times the mean distribution half-life) should elapse between supplementary doses to allow full assessment of the effects of the previous dose.

Fentanyl

Fentanyl and its analogs sufentanil and alfentanil are the most frequently used opioids in clinical anesthesia today. Fentanyl, first synthesized in 1960, is structurally related to the phenylpiperidines (see Fig. 14-6), and has a clinical potency ratio 50–100 times that of morphine. Clear plasma concentration–effect relationships have been demonstrated for fentanyl (Table 14-3). Scott et al[110] demonstrated progressive EEG changes with in-creasing serum fentanyl concentration (Fig. 14-8). During a 5-minute fentanyl infusion, the time lag between increasing serum fentanyl concentration and EEG slowing was 3–5 minutes. After the infusion was stopped, the resolution of EEG changes lagged behind decreasing serum fentanyl concentration by 10–20 minutes.

Analgesia

Fentanyl is a μ-opioid receptor agonist that produces profound dose-dependent analgesia, ventilatory depression, sedation, and at high doses can produce unconsciousness. In postoperative patients receiving fentanyl by a patient-controlled analgesia system, the mean fentanyl dose requirement was 55.8 $\mu g \cdot h^{-1}$, and mean minimum effective analgesic concentration (MEAC) in blood was 0.63 $ng \cdot ml^{-1}$.[111] A large interpatient variability in MEAC (0.23–1.18 $ng \cdot ml^{-1}$) typical of opioids was observed, but over the 2-day study period, the MEAC for any individual patient remained relatively constant. In a volunteer study, a mean plasma fentanyl concentration of 1.3 $ng \cdot ml^{-1}$ reduced experimental pain intensity ratings by 50%.[49] This is consistent with other estimates of plasma fentanyl concentrations associated with mild to moderate analgesia.[112]

Effect on MAC of Volatile Anesthetics and Use in Anesthesia

Fentanyl reduces the MAC of volatile anesthetics in a concentration- or dose-dependent fashion. A single intravenous bolus dose of fentanyl 3 $\mu g \cdot kg^{-1}$, given 25–30 minutes prior to incision, reduced both isoflurane and desflurane MAC by approximately 50%.[113] Fentanyl 1.5 $\mu g \cdot kg^{-1}$ administered 5 minutes prior to skin incision reduces the minimum alveolar concentration which blocks adrenergic responses to stimuli (MAC-BAR) of isoflurane or desflurane in 60% N_2O by 60–70%.[114] No further drop is seen with an increase in fentanyl dose to 3 $\mu g \cdot kg^{-1}$. Utilizing a computer-assisted continuous infusion (CACI) designed to provide constant fentanyl concentrations, a 50% reduction of isoflurane MAC was associated with plasma fentanyl concentrations of 0.5–1.7 $ng \cdot ml^{-1}$.[115,116] Fentanyl produces a steep concentration-related reduction in sevoflurane MAC.[117] Fentanyl 3 $ng \cdot ml^{-1}$ provides a 59% reduction. Further increases in fentanyl concentration produce a ceiling effect, such that a 3-fold increase to 10 $ng \cdot ml^{-1}$ reduced MAC by only an additional 17%.

Epidural fentanyl reduces halothane MAC in patients undergoing hysterectomy.[118] Epidural fentanyl 1, 2, and 4 $\mu g \cdot kg^{-1}$ reduced halothane MAC by 45, 58, and 71%, respectively, while the same doses of fentanyl given iv reduced halothane MAC by 8, 40, and 49%, respectively.

Combining opioids with propofol rather than an inhalation

Table 14-3. PLASMA CONCENTRATION RANGES (ng · ml⁻¹) FOR VARIOUS THERAPEUTIC AND NONTHERAPEUTIC OPIOID EFFECTS

Effect	Morphine	Meperidine	Fentanyl	Sufentanil	Alfentanil	Remifentanil
MEAC	10–15	200	0.6	0.03	15	
Moderate to strong analgesia	20–50	400–600	1.5–5	0.05–0.10	40–80	
50% MAC reduction	NA	>500	0.5–2	0.145	200	1.3
Surgical analgesia with ~70% N₂O	NA	NA	15–25	NA	300–500	
Respiratory depression threshold	25	200	1	0.02–0.04	50–100	
50% ↓ ventilatory response to CO₂	50	NA	1.5–3	0.04	120–350	2.07–2.97
Apnea	NA	NA	7–22	NA	300–600	
Unconsciousness (not reliably achieved with opioids alone)		(Seizures)	15–20	NA	500–1500	

Effects were generally achieved during continuous infusions or patient-controlled analgesia systems. Note that plasma concentrations associated with measurable depression of ventilatory drive are similar to those associated with analgesia for all opioids.
MEAC = minimum effective analgesic concentration, defined in most studies as the plasma opioid concentration associated with just perceptible analgesia; NA = information not available.

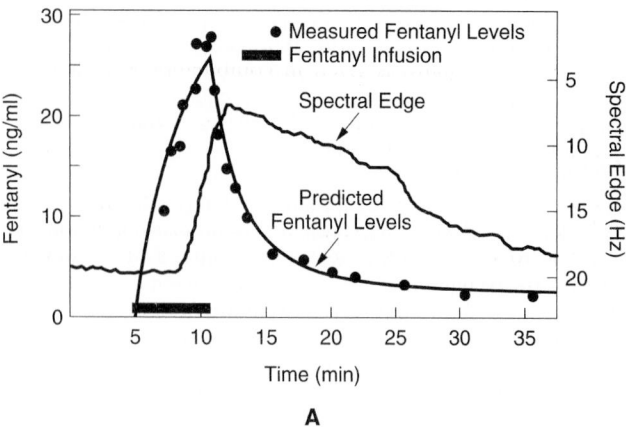
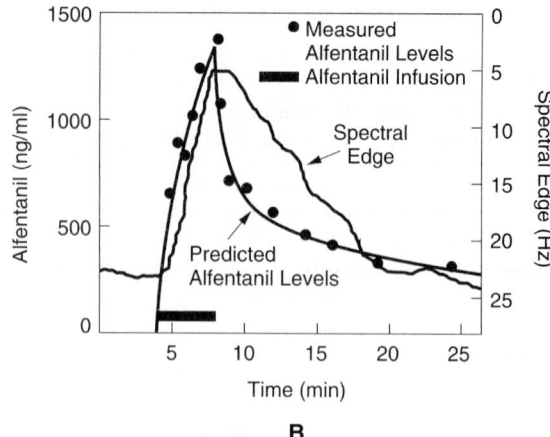

A   **B**

Figure 14-8. The time course of EEG spectral edge and serum concentrations of fentanyl (*A*) and alfentanil (*B*). Infusion rates were 150 μg · min^{-1} fentanyl and 1500 μg · min^{-1} alfentanil. Increasing opioid effect is seen as a decrease in spectral edge. Changes in spectral edge follow serum concentrations more closely with alfentanil than with fentanyl. (Reprinted with permission from Scott JC, Ponganis KV, Stanski DR: EEG quantitation of narcotic effect: The comparative pharmacodynamics of fentanyl and alfentanil. Anesthesiology 62:234, 1985.)

agent is another common technique for providing general anesthesia, and is often referred to as "total intravenous anesthesia" or TIVA. For an intravenous anesthetic, the potency index is described as the plasma concentration required to prevent a response in 50% (CP$_{50}$) or 95% (CP$_{95}$) of patients to various surgical stimuli. Plasma concentrations of fentanyl and propofol that reduce hemodynamic or somatic responses to various surgical stimuli in 50% of patients have been determined using computer-assisted continuous infusion.[119] Fentanyl plasma concentrations of 1.2, 1.8, and 2.8 ng · ml^{-1} were required for 50% reductions in propofol's CP$_{50}$s for skin incision, peritoneal incision, and abdominal retraction, respectively. Greater fentanyl concentrations were required to suppress hemodynamic responses to these same stimuli. Thus, fentanyl reduces requirements for both volatile agents and propofol by a similar proportion.

Several other investigators have also used computer-assisted continuous infusion to administer fentanyl as a component of a balanced anesthetic technique.[120-122] In combination with 50% N$_2$O in oxygen, loss of consciousness is achieved at a plasma fentanyl concentration between 15 and 25 ng · ml^{-1}. Patients whose plasma fentanyl concentrations are maintained greater than 3.7 ng · ml^{-1} did not respond to skin incision, and concentration requirements during the course of surgery varied between 1 and 9 ng · ml^{-1}. Finally, spontaneous ventilation upon emergence from anesthesia was seen when the fentanyl concentration dropped to 1.5–2 ng · ml^{-1}.[120,121] Given with 70% N$_2$O, similar plasma fentanyl concentrations were required to prevent movement and hemodynamic response to skin incision in 50% of patients.[122]

Fentanyl has also been used as the sole agent for anesthesia, a technique that requires a large initial dose of 50–150 μg · kg^{-1} or stable plasma fentanyl concentrations in the range of 20–30 ng · ml^{-1}.[112] The major advantage of this technique, particularly in patients with coronary disease, is in the reliable hemodynamic stability that is achieved. High doses of fentanyl significantly blunt the "stress response"—*i.e.*, hemodynamic and hormonal responses to surgical stimuli—while producing only minimal cardiovascular depression. Thus, the technique is sometimes referred to as "stress-free anesthesia." There are also disadvantages to using high-dose fentanyl as the sole anesthetic agent. It appears that no dose of fentanyl will completely block hemodynamic or hormonal responses in all patients.[123] Furthermore, although high doses generally result in unconsciousness, there have been reports of intraoperative awareness and recall in patients who received 5000 μg of fentanyl.[124] Because opioids do not produce muscle relaxation, and high-dose fentanyl can

produce muscle rigidity, a muscle relaxant is generally required to achieve adequate surgical conditions. This can potentially increase the difficulty in detecting signs of intraoperative awareness. EEG monitoring has been used to assess the depth of anesthesia achieved with high-dose opioids, and high-dose fentanyl produces typical opioid effects on the EEG. That is, a marked shift to the left in frequency and amplitude, including an increased low-frequency amplitude (δ waves) and a decrease in higher frequency amplitudes (α and β).[33]

Other CNS Effects

The effects of fentanyl on cerebral blood flow (CBF) and intracranial pressure (ICP) have been studied in normal patients as well as in those with neurologic disease. An induction dose of 16 μg · kg^{-1} increased middle cerebral artery flow by 25% in normal patients having noncranial neurosurgery.[125] A smaller dose (3 μg · kg^{-1}) resulted in an elevation in ICP in ventilated patients with head trauma.[126] However, in brain tumor patients anesthetized with N$_2$O–O$_2$, a dose of 5 μg · kg^{-1} of fentanyl did not result in elevated ICP.[127] In all cases of elevation in ICP and CBF, there were decreases in mean arterial pressure, which may have contributed to these changes.

Muscle rigidity is often seen on induction with high-dose fentanyl and its derivatives. When rigidity is intense, it may be difficult or impossible to ventilate the patient. In a study in normal volunteers, 1500 μg fentanyl infused over 10 minutes produced rigidity in 50% of subjects.[128] A similar incidence, 35%, was seen in patients receiving 750–1000 μg fentanyl during induction of general anesthesia,[45] and up to 80% of patients receiving 30 μg · kg^{-1} developed moderate to severe rigidity.[129] Muscle rigidity seen with high doses of fentanyl increases with age,[129] and is accompanied by unconsciousness and apnea[128,129]; but lower doses, 7–8 μg · kg^{-1}, have produced chest wall rigidity without unconsciousness or apnea. Streisand *et al*[128] hypothesized that hypercarbia from fentanyl-induced respiratory depression may have influenced fentanyl ionization and cerebral blood flow, and hence the delivery of fentanyl to brain tissue. It would follow that patients instructed to deep-breathe during fentanyl induction may experience less rigidity during induction of anesthesia. This is consistent with observations by Lunn *et al*.[130] During high-dose fentanyl induction (75 μg · kg^{-1}), PaCO$_2$ was maintained at 35–40 torr by assisting and then controlling respirations at 10–15 breaths/minute. Chest wall compliance was reduced in 4 of 18 patients, but no patient developed rigidity sufficient to impair ventilation.

Fentanyl has also been associated with seizure-like movements during anesthetic induction. However, this activity is not associated with seizure activity on the EEG.[131] Whereas fentanyl can induce seizures in other animals, the doses required to produce EEG-documented seizures is generally higher than that used in humans. Such activity may represent myoclonus, due to opioid-mediated blockade of inhibitory motor pathways of cortical origin, or may represent exaggerations of opioid-induced muscle rigidity.[131] Manninen demonstrated that both fentanyl and alfentanil activate epileptiform EEG activity in patients having surgery under general anesthesia for intractable temporal lobe epilepsy.[132]

Fentanyl-induced pruritus often presents as facial itching, but can be generalized. A comparison of iv fentanyl with morphine and alfentanil demonstrated that the intensity of pruritus was equivalent among all three opioids at equianalgesic plasma concentrations.[49] Fentanyl has also been reported to have a tussive effect. Twenty-eight percent of patients coughed within 1 minute after receiving a bolus dose of fentanyl (1.5 $\mu g \cdot kg^{-1}$). While the mechanism of this tussive effect is unclear, it was attenuated by pretreatment with morphine but not by atropine or midazolam.[133]

Respiratory Depression

Fentanyl produces approximately the same degree of ventilatory depression as equianalgesic doses of morphine.[49] Respiratory depression—expressed as an elevation in end-tidal CO_2, a decrease in the slope of the CO_2 response curve, or the minute ventilation at an end-tidal CO_2 of 50 mm Hg (V_E50)—develops rapidly, reaching a peak in ~5 minutes,[110,134,135] and the time course closely follows plasma fentanyl concentration,[134,136] as illustrated in Figure 14-9. Even at plasma concentrations associated with mild analgesia, ventilatory depression can be detected, and the magnitude of respiratory depression is linearly related to intensity of analgesia (Table 14-3).[49,137] In postoperative pa-

tients, plasma fentanyl concentrations of 1.5–3.0 $ng \cdot ml^{-1}$ were associated with a 50% reduction in CO_2 responsiveness.[138]

The magnitude of respiratory depression can be greatly increased when fentanyl is given in combination with another respiratory depressant such as midazolam. Bailey et al[135] determined that midazolam alone (0.05 $mg \cdot kg^{-1}$) did not depress ventilation or cause hypoxemia. Fentanyl alone (2 $\mu g \cdot kg^{-1}$) reduced the slope of the CO_2 response curve and the V_E50 by 50%, and 6 of 12 subjects became hypoxemic. Fentanyl and midazolam produced no greater depression of the ventilatory response to CO_2 than fentanyl alone, but 11 of 12 subjects became hypoxemic and 6 of 12 became apneic within 5 minutes. These observations suggest that this frequently used combination blunts the hypoxic ventilatory drive to a greater extent than the hypercarbic ventilatory drive. Precautions such as supplemental oxygen and pulse oximetry monitoring are recommended when such drug combinations are used.

Airway Reflexes

Although obtundation of airway reflexes by general inhalation anesthetics is well described, little is known about the direct effects of opioids on these protective reflexes. Tagaito et al examined the dose-related effects of fentanyl on airway responses to laryngeal irritation during propofol anesthesia in humans.[139] All patients had laryngeal mask airways; half breathed spontaneously, and half had ventilation controlled to maintain an end-tidal CO_2 of 38 mm Hg. In both groups, stimulation of the larynx (application of water to mucosa) elicited a forced expiration, followed by spasmodic panting mingled with cough reflexes and brief laryngospasm. With three cumulative fentanyl doses (50, 50, and 100 μg), expiration, panting, and coughing decreased in a dose-dependent fashion. After the first dose of fentanyl, apnea with laryngospasm replaced the other reflexes, and with cumulative fentanyl dosing, the duration of laryngospasm shortened. These investigators also described specific characteristic laryngeal behaviors, which were observed endoscopically during laryngeal stimulation. Cough was the airway reflex most vulnerable to depression by fentanyl. While attenuation of airway reflexes is desirable during general anesthesia, it is equally desirable that these protective reflexes should return to baseline rapidly after emergence. Doses required to suppress cough and other reflexes in awake or sedated individuals have not been characterized.

Cardiovascular and Endocrine Effects

Isolated heart muscle models have shown concentration-dependent negative inotropic effects of opioids, including morphine, meperidine, and fentanyl.[69] Fentanyl concentrations up to 1 $\mu g \cdot ml^{-1}$ had no significant effects on papillary muscle mechanics, while 10 $\mu g \cdot ml^{-1}$ reduced contractility by 50%. In clinical practice, high-dose fentanyl administration (up to 75 $\mu g \cdot kg^{-1}$) produces much lower plasma concentrations, i.e., in the range of 50 $ng \cdot ml^{-1}$,[130] and is associated with remarkable hemodynamic stability. Patients who received 7 $\mu g \cdot kg^{-1}$ fentanyl at induction of anesthesia had a slight decrease in heart rate, but no change in mean arterial pressure compared to control.[92] Fentanyl-induced bradycardia is more marked in anesthetized than conscious subjects, but atropine is usually effective in treating opioid-induced bradycardia. Fentanyl doses in the range of 20–25 $\mu g \cdot kg^{-1}$ can decrease heart rate, mean arterial pressure, systemic and pulmonary vascular resistance, and pulmonary capillary wedge pressure by approximately 15% in patients with coronary artery disease.[130,140] Higher doses, up to 75 $\mu g \cdot kg^{-1}$ produced no further hemodynamic changes. All of these patients had been premedicated with a valium or pentobarbital and scopolamine or atropine. In unpremedicated patients undergoing noncardiac surgery, induction with fentanyl 30 $\mu g \cdot kg^{-1}$ produced no changes in heart rate or systolic blood pressure.[129] Hypertension in response to sternotomy is the most common hemodynamic disturbance during high-dose fentanyl

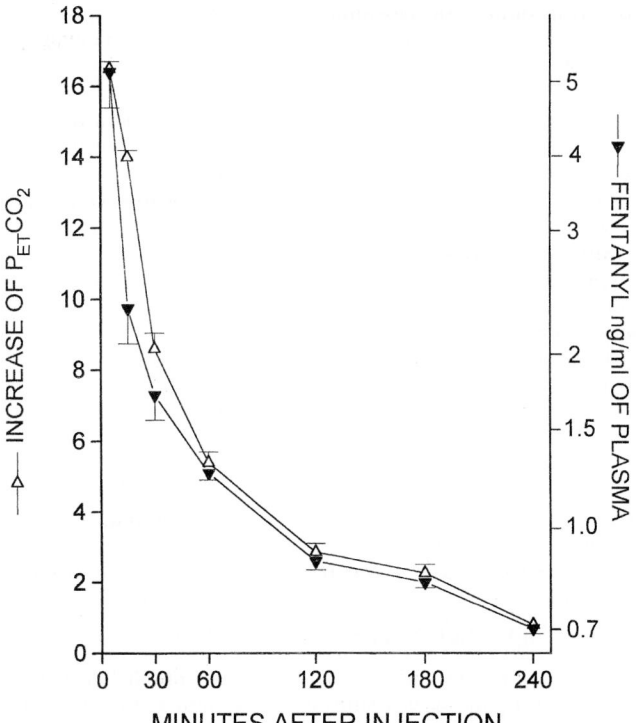

Figure 14-9. Comparison of the decline in plasma fentanyl concentration in 5 subjects given fentanyl 6.4 $\mu g \cdot kg^{-1}$ with 10 different subjects who received fentanyl 6 $\mu g \cdot kg^{-1}$ intravenously. A close correlation is seen between changes in plasma fentanyl concentration and ventilatory depression. (Reprinted with permission from McClain DA, Hug CC Jr: Intravenous fentanyl kinetics. Clin Pharmacol Ther 28:106, 1980.)

anesthesia. The incidence varies widely, and is reported to be between 40 and 100% in patients receiving 50–100 $\mu g \cdot kg^{-1}$.[141] Unlike morphine and meperidine, which induce hypotension, at least in part due to histamine release,[67,142] high-dose fentanyl ($50 \mu g \cdot kg^{-1}$) is not associated with significant histamine release (see Fig. 14-5).

While high doses of fentanyl are associated with minimal cardiovascular changes, combining fentanyl with other drugs can compromise hemodynamic stability. The combination of fentanyl and diazepam produces significant cardiovascular depression.[129,140] Diazepam 10 mg given after 20–50 $\mu g \cdot kg^{-1}$ of fentanyl decreased stroke volume, cardiac output, systemic vascular resistance, and mean arterial pressure, and increased central venous pressure significantly.[140] In an animal model, these negative inotropic effects were shown to be simply additive.[143] The addition of 60% N_2O to high-dose fentanyl produced a significant decrease in cardiac output as well as increases in systemic and pulmonary vascular resistance.[130]

High-dose fentanyl ($100 \mu g \cdot kg^{-1}$) prevented increases in plasma epinephrine, cortisol, glucose, free fatty acids, and growth hormone (the "stress response") during surgery. Lower dose fentanyl ($5 \mu g \cdot kg^{-1}$ followed by an infusion of 3 $\mu g \cdot kg^{-1} \cdot h^{-1}$) failed to block increases in plasma epinephrine and cortisol.[144]

Smooth Muscle and Gastrointestinal Effects

Fentanyl, like morphine and meperidine, significantly increases common bile duct pressure (see Fig. 14-7).[89] Like other opioids, fentanyl can cause nausea and vomiting, particularly in ambulatory patients, and can delay gastric emptying and intestinal transit.

Disposition Kinetics

Fentanyl's extreme lipid solubility (see Table 14-2) allows it to cross biologic membranes quickly and to be taken up rapidly by the highly perfused tissue groups, including the brain, heart, and lung. Thus, after a single bolus dose, the onset of effects is rapid and the duration brief. Hug and Murphy[145] determined the relationships between fentanyl effects and its concentration over time in plasma and various tissues in rats given fentanyl 50 $\mu g \cdot kg^{-1}$ (Fig. 14-10). The onset of opioid effects occurred

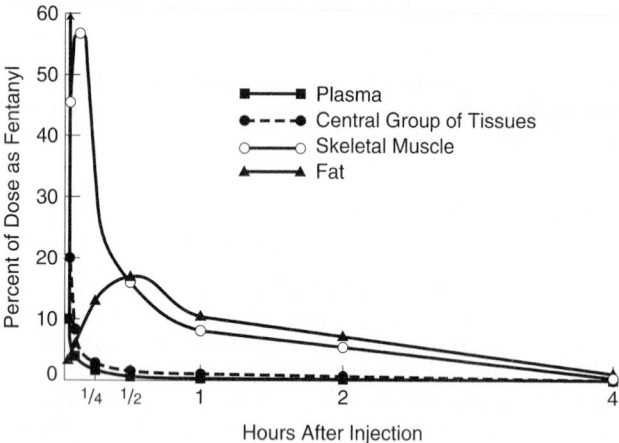

Figure 14-10. Fentanyl uptake and elimination in various tissues of the rat following intravenous injection. Unchanged fentanyl tissue concentrations (means for 6 fats) are expressed as percentage of dose. "Central" represents the combined content of brain, heart, and lung tissues. The large mass of muscle (50% body weight of the rat) and high affinity of fat for fentanyl (despite slow equilibration) serve as a drain on the central compartment. (Reprinted with permission from Hug CC, Murphy MR: Tissue redistribution of fentanyl in terms of its effects in rats. Anesthesiology 55:369, 1981.)

within 10 seconds, and correlated with a rapid increase in brain tissue fentanyl concentration, which equilibrated with plasma by 1.5 minutes. Recovery from fentanyl effects started within 5 minutes and was complete by 60 minutes. Elimination from the "central tissues" (brain, heart, and lung) was also rapid, as fentanyl was redistributed to other tissues, particularly muscle and fat. Peak muscle concentration was seen at 5 minutes, while fat concentration reached a maximum approximately 30 minutes after the dose. The delay in fat uptake despite fentanyl's high lipid solubility is due to the limited blood supply to that tissue. Thus, redistribution to muscle and fat limits the duration of a bolus dose of fentanyl, and accumulation in peripheral tissue compartments can be extensive because of the large mass of muscle and high affinity of fentanyl for fat. With prolonged administration of fentanyl, fat can act as a reservoir of drug.

Fentanyl pharmacokinetics have been studied in normal volunteers as well as patients under general anesthesia. After an iv dose, plasma fentanyl concentration falls rapidly, and the concentration–time curve has been described by both two- and three-compartment models.[146] McClain and Hug[134] administered a 3.2 or 6.4 $\mu g \cdot kg^{-1}$ dose of fentanyl to healthy male volunteers and found that nearly 99% of the dose was eliminated from plasma by 60 minutes. These investigators found both rapid and slower distribution phases, with half-times of 1.2–1.9 minutes and 9.2–19 minutes, respectively. The terminal elimination half-time ranged from 3.1 to 6.6 hours, which is somewhat longer than that for morphine. Similar values were noted in surgical patients less than 50 years old,[146,147] including morbidly obese patients.[146] Reports of age effects on fentanyl kinetics are conflicting. Scott and Stanski[148] found a decrease in fentanyl requirement with increasing age (20–89 years), but they did not observe differences in pharmacokinetic parameters. In contrast, Bentley *et al*[147] observed a marked decrease in clearance and an increase in terminal elimination half-time to approximately 15 hours in patients over 60 years old compared to 4.4 hours in patients less than 50 years old. However, another comparison between older (>70 years old) and younger (<42 years old) patients anesthetized in a manner similar to that used in Bailey's study failed to show any differences in plasma clearance and elimination half-times between the two groups.[149]

Unlike its derivatives, fentanyl is significantly bound to red blood cells, approximately 40%, and has a blood:plasma partition coefficient of approximately 1.[146] Plasma fentanyl is highly protein-bound, with estimates in the range of 79–87%. It binds avidly to α_1-acid glycoprotein, but also binds to albumin.[146,150] Fentanyl protein binding is pH-dependent, such that a decrease in pH will increase the proportion of fentanyl that is unbound.[146] Mean values for unbound fractions of fentanyl in plasma have been estimated between 13 and 21%.[146]

Clearance of fentanyl is primarily by metabolism, which occurs rapidly and extensively in the liver. Clearance estimates[134,148] of 8–21 $ml \cdot kg^{-1} \cdot min^{-1}$ approach liver blood flow, and indicate a high hepatic extraction ratio. Thus, hepatic metabolism of fentanyl is expected to be dependent on liver blood flow. Metabolism is primarily by N-dealkylation to norfentanyl, and by hydroxylation of both the parent and norfentanyl to hydroxyproprionylfentanyl and hydroxyproprionylnorfentanyl.[146] Only about 6% of the dose of fentanyl is excreted unchanged in the urine.[134]

Dosage and Administration of Fentanyl

From administration as a single bolus dose, fentanyl developed an early reputation as a short-acting opioid. Experience with very large doses and multiple doses revealed that prolonged respiratory depression and delayed recovery could occur. These observations demonstrate that fentanyl's clinical duration is limited by redistribution, and that with prolonged administration, accumulation can occur.

Fentanyl can be useful as a sedative/analgesic premedication when given a short time prior to induction. For this use incremental doses of 25–50 μg can be used and titrated until the desired effect is achieved. It is important to note that although the onset of fentanyl's effects is rapid, peak effect lags behind peak plasma concentration by up to 5 minutes.[110] A transmucosal delivery system for fentanyl is also available, and has been shown to be an effective premedicant for pediatric as well as adult patients. In children, doses of 10–20 μg · kg^{-1}, and in adults, 400–800 μg, administered 30 minutes prior to induction or a painful procedure are safe and effective.[151,152] However, dose-dependent side effects typical of opioids are reported, including sedation, respiratory depression, nausea, and pruritus.[151-153] Because respiratory depression and hypoxemia can occur, transmucosal fentanyl should be administered in a monitored environment.

Fentanyl is also used frequently as an adjunct to induction agents such as thiopental to blunt the hemodynamic response to laryngoscopy and tracheal intubation, which can be particularly severe in patients with hypertension or cardiovascular disease. In patients undergoing major vascular surgery, induction with 3 mg · kg^{-1} thiopental and pancuronium was followed by fentanyl 8 μg · kg^{-1}, administered over 2 minutes. Patients who received this combination experienced no significant increase in heart rate or blood pressure compared to baseline, preinduction values compared to those who received 6 mg · kg^{-1} thiopental.[154] Patients in both groups experienced a 20% drop in mean arterial pressure after induction but prior to laryngoscopy. Common clinical practice involves titration of fentanyl in doses of 1.5–5 μg · kg^{-1} prior to administration of a barbiturate or other induction agent. Because fentanyl's peak effect lags behind peak plasma concentration by 3–5 minutes, fentanyl titration should be complete approximately 3 minutes prior to laryngoscopy in order to maximally blunt hemodynamic responses to tracheal intubation. When fentanyl was administered with 50% N$_2$O in oxygen for induction, the effective dose for loss of consciousness was 8–23 μg · kg^{-1}.[121] Recall, however, that the combination of N$_2$O and a moderate to high dose of opioid may cause significant muscle rigidity, which can be attenuated by a variety of adjuvants, including benzodiazepines, barbiturates, and muscle relaxants.

Perhaps the most common clinical use of fentanyl and its derivatives is as an analgesic component of balanced general anesthesia. With this technique, incremental doses of fentanyl 0.5–2.5 μg · kg^{-1} are administered intermittently as dictated by the intensity of the surgical stimulus, and may be repeated approximately every 30 minutes. Generally, administration of up to 3–5 μg · kg^{-1} · h^{-1} will allow recovery of spontaneous ventilation at the end of surgery. As an alternative to intermittent dosing, a loading dose of 5–10 μg · kg^{-1} and continuous fentanyl infusion at a rate between 2 and 10 μg · kg^{-1} · h^{-1} are recommended.[121] It is important to remember, however, that anesthetic requirements vary with age, concurrent diseases, and the surgical procedure. For example, fentanyl requirements decrease by 50% as age increases from 20 to 89 years.[148] Fentanyl requirements can also be expected to decrease with the duration of infusion (see discussion of context-specific half-times at the end of this chapter).

Fentanyl can also be used in combination with droperidol, a butyrophenone, and nitrous oxide, in a technique called neuroleptanesthesia.[155] This technique entails premedication with intramuscular (im) diphenhydramine (50–100 mg), scopolamine (0.3–0.4 mg), and an opioid such as meperidine (25–75 mg) in order to minimize the side effects of high-dose droperidol, which include dysphoria and extrapyramidal motor effects. Induction consists of infusion of 0.15 mg · kg^{-1} droperidol followed by a small dose (20–60 μg) of fentanyl. Nitrous oxide 60–70% is added to induce sleep, and then fentanyl is further titrated in small increments. The total loading dose of fentanyl is in the range of 2–2.5 μg · kg^{-1}, and the average total fentanyl

dose is approximately 2 μg · kg^{-1} · h^{-1}. Because this technique does not provide muscle relaxation, neuromuscular blockers are generally required.

High dose (e.g., 50–150 μg · kg^{-1}) fentanyl "anesthesia" has been used extensively for cardiac surgery. With this technique, a mean plasma fentanyl concentration of 15 ng · ml^{-1}, which prevents hemodynamic changes in response to noxious stimuli,[156] can be achieved with a loading dose of 50 μg · kg^{-1}, followed by a continuous infusion of 30 μg · kg^{-1} · h^{-1}. With high-dose fentanyl, muscle relaxants and mechanical ventilation are required. Whether opioids alone are suitable as the sole "anesthetic" agent continues to be debated.

Finally, fentanyl has been used as an analgesic in management of postoperative as well as cancer pain. For acute pain, fentanyl is administered as a continuous iv infusion, or via an on-demand system, such as a patient-controlled analgesia (PCA) pump. Effective continuous infusion rates for nontolerant individuals are generally in the range of 50–100 μg · h^{-1}. A reasonable starting dose regimen for PCA includes a background continuous infusion of 20–50 μg · h^{-1} plus a bolus "demand" dose of 10–25 μg, and a lockout period of 5 minutes. Transdermal fentanyl has also been used for postoperative analgesia; a nominal delivery rate of 100 μg · h^{-1} produces a serum fentanyl concentration of 2 ng · ml^{-1}. However, the slow increase to a stable serum concentration (approximately 15 hours) and the long apparent elimination half-life (21 hours) make this a reasonable choice for long-term pain relief. Thus transdermal delivery is an impractical method to use when drug titration is necessary and fairly rapid (e.g., over hours to days) changes in opioid dose and plasma concentrations are required. Both transdermal and transmucosal fentanyl delivery systems have proved effective for cancer pain relief. The transmucosal system is particularly useful for therapy of acute pain exacerbation episodes, or "breakthrough" pain.

Sufentanil

Sufentanil, a thienyl derivative of fentanyl (see Fig. 14-6) first described in the mid 1970s, has a clinical potency ratio 2000–4000 times that of morphine and 10–15 times that of fentanyl.[157,158] Like fentanyl, sufentanil equilibrates rapidly between blood and brain, and demonstrates clear plasma concentration-effect relationships. In a study comparing sufentanil and fentanyl pharmacodynamics, using EEG changes as a measure of opioid effects, Scott et al[158] noted similar profiles. During a 4-minute sufentanil infusion, the change in spectral edge lagged behind rising sufentanil concentration by approximately 2–3 minutes, while resolution of the EEG changes lagged behind plasma concentration changes by 20–30 minutes.

Analgesia

Sufentanil is a highly selective μ opioid receptor agonist, and exerts potent analgesic effects in animals when given by either systemic or spinal routes.[159] While the literature describing clinical experience with sufentanil as a component of general anesthesia is extensive, available information regarding the analgesic potency of systemically administered sufentanil in humans is limited. Geller et al[160] titrated an iv infusion rate to adequate postoperative analgesia, and noted that a mean rate of 8–17 μg · h^{-1} was required during the first 48 hours. This was associated with a 5-fold range in plasma sufentanil concentrations, between 0.02 and 0.1 ng · ml^{-1}. Lehmann et al[161] found similar sufentanil requirements (including a wide interpatient variability) in postoperative patients, and estimated that the minimum effective analgesic concentration of sufentanil is near 0.03 ng · ml^{-1}. A laboratory study using normal volunteers found that a steady-state plasma sufentanil concentration of 0.05 ng · ml^{-1} was associated with a 50% pain reduction.[162]

Effect on MAC of Volatile Anesthetics and Use in Anesthesia

Animal studies have shown that sufentanil decreases the MAC of volatile anesthetics in a dose-dependent manner.[163,164] The maximum reduction of enflurane or halothane MAC by sufentanil in animals is between 70 and 90%. A study in humans found that a plasma sufentanil concentration of 0.145 ng $\cdot$ ml^{-1} was associated with a 50% reduction in isoflurane MAC[165]. Increasing the plasma sufentanil concentration to 0.5 ng $\cdot$ ml^{-1} reduced isoflurane MAC by 78%, and a ceiling effect was approached with greater plasma sufentanil concentrations. The maximum MAC reduction seen in humans was 89%, at a sufentanil concentration of 1.4 ng $\cdot$ ml^{-1}.

In clinical anesthesia practice, sufentanil is used as a component of balanced anesthesia, and has been employed extensively in high doses (10–30 μg $\cdot$ kg^{-1}) with oxygen and muscle relaxants for cardiac surgery. In this dose range, sufentanil is at least as effective as fentanyl in its ability to produce and maintain hypnosis. In addition, hemodynamic stability appears to be as good as or better than that achieved with fentanyl.[92,157] Bailey et al[166] used a computer-assisted continuous infusion system to determine sufentanil plasma concentration–response to various noxious stimuli during high-dose sufentanil anesthesia for cardiac surgery. They estimated the plasma concentration associated with a 50% probability of no response (movement, hemodynamic, or sympathetic) to intubation, incision, sternotomy, and mediastinal dissection (CP_{50}). The CP_{50} for intubation, incision, and sternotomy (pooled data) was 7.06 ng $\cdot$ ml^{-1}, and for mediastinal dissection CP^{50} was 12.1 ng $\cdot$ ml^{-1}. As is typical of opioids, a wide intersubject variability was noted in sufentanil concentration requirements (3–10-fold) to suppress responses to these stimuli. However, even at high doses, when used as the sole anesthetic agent, sufentanil may not completely block the hemodyamic responses to noxious stimuli.[123]

Other CNS Effects

Equianalgesic doses of sufentanil and fentanyl produce similar changes in the EEG.[157,158] In cardiac patients who received sufentanil 15 μg $\cdot$ kg^{-1}, α activity became prominent within a few seconds, and within 3 minutes, the EEG consisted almost entirely of slow δ activity.[157] Rigidity and myoclonic activity have been reported during induction of, and on emergence from, anesthesia with sufentanil in doses of approximately 1–2 μg $\cdot$ kg^{-1}.[44,47,167] While the observed myoclonic activity resembles seizures, it has not been associated with EEG evidence of seizures.[44,167]

There has been considerable investigation of the effects of sufentanil on cerebral hemodynamics and intracranial pressure. In patients with intracranial tumors, sufentanil 1 μg $\cdot$ kg^{-1} was associated with an elevation in spinal cerebrospinal pressure, and a decrease in cerebral perfusion pressure.[168] As in patients with elevated intracranial pressure and cerebral blood flow after fentanyl, mean arterial pressure had dropped significantly in these patients. In normal volunteers, a smaller dose of sufentanil (0.5 μg $\cdot$ kg^{-1}) was not associated with changes in cerebral blood flow.[169] In dogs that received very large doses of sufentanil (20 μg $\cdot$ kg^{-1}) cerebral blood flow decreased in proportion to a decrease in cerebral metabolism, and intracranial pressure did not change.[170]

Respiratory Depression

Like other μ opioid agonists, sufentanil causes respiratory depression in doses associated with clinical analgesia.[136,137] Respiratory depression can be especially marked in the presence of inhalation anesthetics. In spontaneously breathing patients anesthetized with 1.5% halothane in N_2O and 33% oxygen, a small dose of sufentanil (approximately 2.5 μg) reduced mean minute ventilation by 50%, and 4 μg reduced mean respiratory rate by 50%.[171] Postoperative respiratory depression after apparent recovery from anesthesia has been reported for both sufentanil and fentanyl.[172] The occurrence of secondary peaks in plasma drug concentration has been suggested as a mechanism, but a lack of exogenous stimulation in the early postoperative period may be just as important a factor.

Results of one study in normal volunteers who received bolus doses of fentanyl and sufentanil suggest that sufentanil may cause less respiratory depression than fentanyl.[136] The magnitude and time course of change in end-tidal CO_2 were the same for fentanyl and sufentanil, but the slope of the ventilatory response to CO_2 was depressed to a greater extent by fentanyl. In another study with normal volunteers, equianalgesic steady plasma concentrations of morphine (25, 50, and 100 ng $\cdot$ ml^{-1}) and sufentanil (0.02, 0.04, and 0.08 ng $\cdot$ ml^{-1}) produced equivalent respiratory depression, measured as increased end tidal CO_2 and a decreased ventilatory response to CO_2.[162]

Cardiovascular and Endocrine Effects

In animal studies, sufentanil has been shown to cause vasodilation by a sympatholytic mechanism, but may also have a direct smooth muscle effect.[163] Clinically, a prominent feature of many clinical trials involving sufentanil is the remarkable hemodynamic stability achieved during balanced and high dose (up to 30 μg $\cdot$ kg^{-1}) opioid anesthesia. In general, only a modest decrease in mean arterial pressure is observed when sufentanil (approximately 15 μg $\cdot$ kg^{-1}) is used for induction of anesthesia.[92,173] Intraoperatively, sufentanil in moderate or high doses does not completely abolish the hypertensive response to sternotomy or other noxious stimuli.[123,173–175] In general, sufentanil and fentanyl have been found to be equivalent for use in balanced and high-dose opioid anesthesia,[123,173,175] but two clinical comparisons between fentanyl and sufentanil suggest that sufentanil may be associated with less respiratory depression[176] and better analgesia[176,177] in the immediate postoperative period.

The choice of premedication and muscle relaxant may significantly affect hemodynamics during induction and maintenance of anesthesia with sufentanil. Combining vecuronium and sufentanil can cause a decrease of 10–15 torr in mean arterial pressure during induction,[178] and significant bradycardia and sinus arrest[179] have been reported. Bradycardia is not seen when pancuronium is used during anesthesia with sufentanil.[180]

Sufentanil, like fentanyl, reduces the endocrine and metabolic responses to surgery.[157] However, even a large induction dose (20 μg $\cdot$ kg^{-1}) did not prevent increases in cortisol, catecholamines, glucose, and free fatty acids during and after cardiopulmonary bypass.[181]

Disposition Kinetics

Sufentanil is an extremely lipophilic opioid, and has pharmacokinetic properties similar to that of fentanyl. Because of a higher degree of ionization at physiologic pH and higher degree of plasma protein binding, its volume of distribution is somewhat smaller and its elimination half-life shorter than that of fentanyl (see Table 14-2). Sufentanil pharmacokinetics have been studied in patients under general anesthesia who had received methohexital for anesthetic induction, followed by the sufentanil dose of 5 μg $\cdot$ kg^{-1}, and N_2O in oxygen 33%.[182] After an iv bolus dose, plasma sufentanil concentration drops very rapidly, and 98% of the drug is cleared from plasma within 30 minutes. Plasma concentration–time data in this study were best fitted to a three-compartment model. The rapid and slower distribution half-times were 1.4 and 17.7 minutes, respectively, and the elimination half-life was 2.7 hours. In other pharmacokinetic studies involving anesthetized patients, mean elimination half-lives were in the range of 2.2–4.6 hours.[183–185] In contrast, Hudson[186] reported a much longer elimination half-life (12.2 hours). In this study, patients undergoing aortic surgery received larger sufentanil doses (12.5 μg $\cdot$ kg^{-1}) during abdominal aortic surgery, and a significant correlation between increasing age and elimination half-life was noted. Obese patients were found to have a larger total volume of distribution and a longer elimination half-life (3.5 vs. 2.2 hours) compared to nonobese patients.[183]

Sufentanil is less red cell–bound than fentanyl (22% compared to 40%), and has a whole blood:plasma concentration ratio of 0.741.[146] Plasma sufentanil is approximately 92% protein-bound at pH 7.4, mostly to α_1-acid glycoprotein. Clearance of sufentanil is rapid, and like fentanyl, sufentanil has a high hepatic extraction ratio.[146] Metabolism in the liver is by N-dealkylation and O-demethylation. However, sufentanil clearance in patients with cirrhosis was similar to controls, as was the elimination half-life.[184]

Dosage and Administration of Sufentanil

Like fentanyl, sufentanil is most often used as a component of balanced anesthesia, or as a single agent in high doses, particularly for cardiac surgery. Several investigations have found similar sufentanil dose requirements for induction of anesthesia.[92,166,187] When sufentanil is titrated during induction, loss of consciousness is seen with total doses between 1.3–2.8 $\mu g \cdot kg^{-1}$. Doses in the range of 0.3–1.0 $\mu g \cdot kg^{-1}$ given 1–3 minutes prior to laryngoscopy can be expected to blunt hemodynamic responses to intubation. Muscle rigidity can occur, particularly in the elderly, even at these lower doses.

For maintenance of balanced anesthesia, intermittent bolus doses or a continuous infusion can be used. With bolus doses in the range of 0.1–0.5 $\mu g \cdot kg^{-1}$, mean maintenance requirements of 0.35 $\mu g \cdot kg^{-1} \cdot h^{-1}$ have been reported.[92] Cork et al[185] administered an initial bolus of 0.5 $\mu g \cdot kg^{-1}$ followed by an infusion of 0.5 $\mu g \cdot kg^{-1} \cdot h^{-1}$, which was varied according to patient need. This regimen of sufentanil in combination with N_2O 70% in oxygen provided satisfactory anesthesia with good hemodynamic stability, and stable plasma sufentanil concentrations of approximately 0.15–0.25 $ng \cdot ml^{-1}$. Thus, for balanced anesthesia, sufentanil can be administered as repeated bolus doses or continuous infusion, with an expected dose requirement in the range of 0.3–1 $\mu g \cdot kg^{-1} \cdot h^{-1}$. Much higher bolus doses and/or infusion rates are required to achieve the plasma sufentanil concentration range of 6–60 $ng \cdot ml^{-1}$ required during cardiac anesthesia using sufentanil as the sole agent. For "complete anesthesia" total sufentanil doses in the range of 8–50 $\mu g \cdot kg^{-1}$ are required.[166]

Alfentanil

Alfentanil, a tetrazole derivative of fentanyl (see Fig. 14-6), was synthesized two years after sufentanil and introduced into clinical practice in the early 1980s. On a milligram basis, its clinical potency is approximately ten times that of morphine and one fourth to one tenth that of fentanyl when given in single doses. Alfentanil differs from fentanyl in its pharmacokinetics as well as in its speed of equilibration between plasma and effect site in the brain. In a comparison using EEG spectral edge effects to quantify fentanyl and alfentanil pharmacodynamics, Scott et al[110] demonstrated that alfentanil's effect followed serum drug concentration more closely than fentanyl (see Fig. 14-8). Peak effect lagged behind peak plasma concentration by less than 1 minute, and resolution of effect followed decreasing serum alfentanil concentration by no more than 10 minutes. Alfentanil is a μ-opioid receptor agonist, and produces typical naloxone-reversible analgesia and side effects such as sedation, nausea, and respiratory depression.

Analgesia

Alfentanil has been administered intravenously for treatment of postoperative and cancer-related pain, as well as in laboratory pain models with normal volunteers. Clear concentration and dose-related analgesic effects have been demonstrated for alfen-

tanil, but individual requirements in terms of dosage or plasma concentrations vary widely. For postoperative analgesia, the MEAC is approximately 10 $ng \cdot ml^{-1}$, with a range of 2 to >40 $ng \cdot ml^{-1}$.[188] In a laboratory investigation, pain intensity ratings decreased in a plasma concentration-dependent fashion, and 80 $ng \cdot ml^{-1}$ was associated with a 50% reduction in pain intensity.[49] Clinical studies have shown that in patients receiving continuous iv infusion of alfentanil, mean plasma concentrations required for relief of moderate to severe pain are approximately 40–80 $ng \cdot ml^{-1}$ (see Table 14-3).[189,190] Following an adequate loading dose, average alfentanil requirements for postoperative analgesia are approximately 10–20 $\mu g \cdot kg^{-1} \cdot h^{-1}$.[189,191,192]

Effect on MAC of Volatile Anesthetics and Use in Anesthesia

Like other opioids, alfentanil decreases the MAC of enflurane in a curvilinear fashion up to a plateau in dogs.[26,193] An infusion rate of 8 $\mu g \cdot kg^{-1} \cdot min^{-1}$ achieved a plasma concentration of 223 $ng \cdot ml^{-1}$ and reduced enflurane MAC by 69%. Increasing the infusion rate 4-fold did not reduce enflurane MAC further.[193] In rats, an infusion of 15 $\mu g \cdot kg^{-1} \cdot min^{-1}$ reduced the MAC of halothane by 48%, but evaluation of higher doses was precluded by the development of muscle rigidity.[26]

In humans, alfentanil plasma concentrations required to supplement nitrous oxide anesthesia for various noxious stimuli have been determined.[194] Patients received a loading dose of 150 $\mu g \cdot kg^{-1}$, followed by an infusion that was titrated between 25 and 150 $\mu g \cdot kg^{-1} \cdot h^{-1}$ according to the patients' responses to surgical stimuli, and steep concentration–effect curves were demonstrated. Plasma concentrations required along with 66% N_2O to obtund somatic, autonomic, and hemodynamic responses to stimuli in 50% of patients were 475, 279, and 150 $ng \cdot ml^{-1}$ for tracheal intubation, skin incision, and skin closure, respectively. The plasma alfentanil concentration associated with spontaneous ventilation after discontinuation of N_2O was 223 $ng \cdot ml^{-1}$. Nearly identical results were obtained in a similar study using computer-controlled infusions to deliver alfentanil (Fig. 14-11).[195] Plasma alfentanil concentrations required in combination with propofol to obtund responses to intubation and surgical stimuli have also been determined. Vuyk et al[196] found alfentanil requirements with 66% N_2O that were nearly identical to those of Ausems.[194,195] In contrast, much lower alfen-

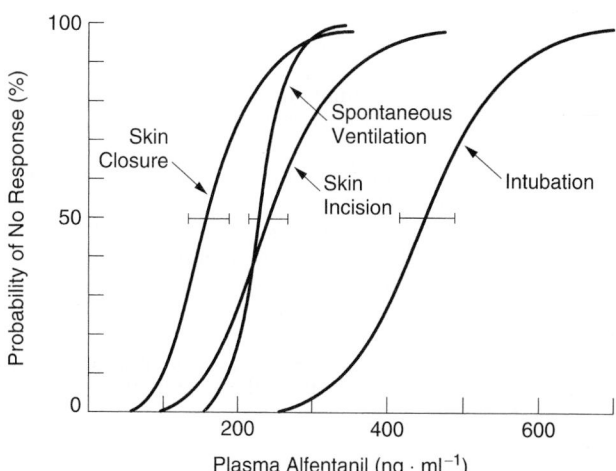

Figure 14-11. The relationship between alfentanil plasma concentration (with 66% N_2O) and the probability of no response for intubation, skin incision, and skin closure; and the relationship of plasma alfentanil concentration (without N_2O) and the recovery of adequate spontaneous ventilation. (Reprinted with permission from Ausems ME, Vuyk J, Hug CC et al: Comparison of a computer-assisted infusion *versus* intermittent bolus administration of alfentanil as a supplement to nitrous oxide for lower abdominal surgery. Anesthesiology 68:851, 1988.)

tanil plasma concentrations, 55–92 ng · ml^{-1}, were required to prevent responses in 50% of patients when alfentanil was combined with propofol at a plasma concentration of 3 μg · ml^{-1} (Fig. 14-12).

High-dose alfentanil has been used as an induction agent for patients with and without cardiac disease,[197] and for induction and maintenance of cardiac anesthesia.[141,198,199] Patients with cardiac (valvular or coronary artery) disease required half as much alfentanil to induce unconsciousness.[197] When used as the sole anesthetic agent, mean plasma alfentanil concentrations required to significantly blunt hemodynamic responses to intubation and sternotomy were 700–830 ng · ml^{-1} and 1200–1800 ng · ml^{-1}, respectively.[198,200] These values are approximately twice those reported for alfentanil in combination with 66% nitrous oxide.[194,195] However, even doses that produced very high plasma alfentanil concentrations (1200 to >2000 ng · ml^{-1}) did not eliminate responses to intubation and intraoperative stimuli in all patients.[199] In contrast to fentanyl and sufentanil, the duration of even very large doses of alfentanil is short. Thus, for cardiac anesthesia, repeated doses or a continuous infusion of alfentanil is required.

Other CNS Effects

Alfentanil produces the typical generalized slowing of the EEG[110,201]; a plasma concentration of approximately 1400 ng · ml^{-1} is associated with the onset of δ-wave activity. Unlike fentanyl and sufentanil, alfentanil produced less synchronization of the EEG as well as spindle activity in most patients.[201] Like fentanyl, alfentanil can increase epileptiform EEG activity in patients with intractable temporal lope epilepsy having surgery under general anesthesia.[132] Like fentanyl and sufentanil, alfentanil can produce intense muscle rigidity accompanied by loss of consciousness. In 90–100% of patients, induction doses of 150–175 μg · kg^{-1} were associated with muscle rigidity, which was not limited to the chest wall or trunk. Rather, electromyogra-

phy has shown increased activity of comparable magnitude in muscles of the neck, extremities, chest wall, and abdomen.[44,202] Studies in rats suggest that specific nuclei of the reticular formation, including the periaqueductal gray, are important in alfentanil-mediated rigidity.[46]

Alfentanil has been reported to increase cerebrospinal fluid pressure in patients with brain tumors, whereas fentanyl does not.[127] This effect is thought to be due to cerebrovasodilation, but a study in dogs failed to confirm this hypothesis. Mayberg et al[203] examined the effect of 25 and 50 μg · kg^{-1} of alfentanil on cerebral blood flow velocity and intracranial pressure in neurosurgical and orthopedic patients under general anesthesia with isoflurane and 50% N$_2$O. Ventilation was controlled to maintain normocapnea, and blood pressure was maintained at baseline for neurosurgical patients. No clinically significant changes in ICP and no evidence of cerebral vasodilation or vasoconstriction were seen.

Respiratory Depression

The relationships among plasma alfentanil concentration, analgesia, and respiratory depression have been examined in animals and human subjects.[49,204] In dogs, 50% maximal nociceptive and ventilatory responses were seen at plasma alfentanil concentrations between 20 and 80 ng · ml^{-1}, and maximal responses at 200 ng · ml^{-1}.[204] Importantly, antinociceptive effects could not be separated from respiratory depression. A human study involving normal volunteers reported similar findings. Mild ventilatory depression (increased end-tidal CO$_2$; decreased slope of the CO$_2$ response curve) was seen at plasma concentrations as low as 20 ng · ml^{-1}. At plasma concentrations associated with 50% reduction in pain intensity, respiratory depression was equivalent for alfentanil, fentanyl, and morphine.[49] A clinical study examined analgesia and respiratory effects of alfentanil administered by a patient-controlled analgesia system for postoperative pain control.[205] In patients who received a continuous

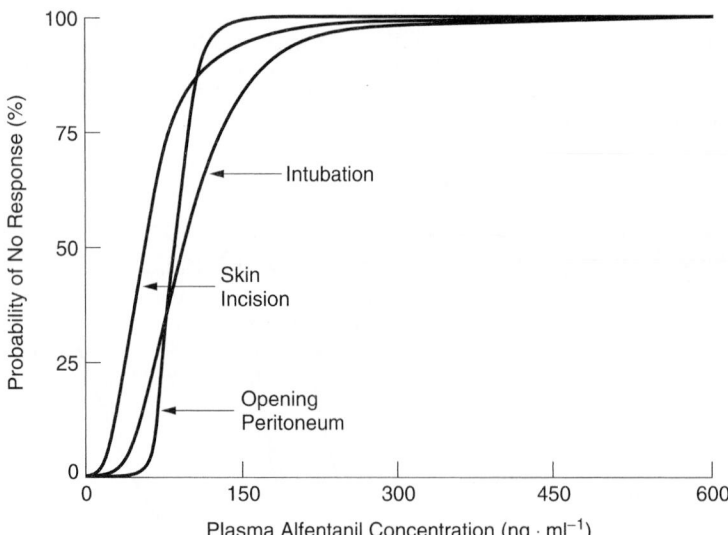

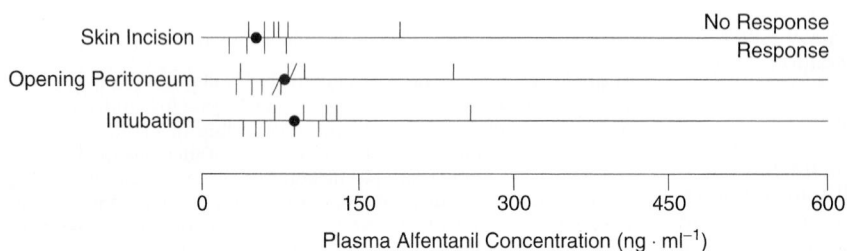

Figure 14-12. The alfentanil plasma concentration–effect relationships for intubation, skin incision, and the opening of the peritoneum when given as a supplement to propofol. (Reprinted with permission from Vuyk J, Lim T, Engbers FHM, *et al:* Pharmacodynamics of alfentanil as a supplement to propofol or nitrous oxide for lower abdominal surgery in female patients. Anesthesiology 78:1036, 1993.)

alfentanil infusion at 900 $\mu g \cdot h^{-1}$ plus 100–200-μg doses as needed, 3 of 10 patients developed respiratory depression (respiratory rate < 8/min). Mean alfentanil blood concentration in this group of patients was 80 ng $\cdot$ ml^{-1}.

Two clinical studies have examined the intensity and duration of respiratory depressant effects of alfentanil in the immediate postoperative period.[206,207] Intraoperative anesthesia was maintained with alfentanil 20–100 $\mu g \cdot kg^{-1} \cdot h^{-1}$ and 67% N_2O with or without 0.5% halothane. At the end of surgery the infusion was decreased to 20 $\mu g \cdot kg^{-1} \cdot h^{-1}$, which produced plasma alfentanil concentrations between 106 and 120 ng $\cdot$ ml^{-1}, and good analgesia. With this regimen, ventilatory response to CO_2 was decreased to 50% of the baseline value, but $PaCO_2$ was only moderately elevated (42–48 torr). By 2 hours after alfentanil was discontinued, respiratory function was near baseline. When compared to fentanyl, the recovery of ventilatory function was faster with alfentanil.[207] Another comparison found that for anesthetics of 1.5–2 hours duration, recovery of respiratory function was similar with alfentanil and fentanyl.[208] Like its congeners, alfentanil has been associated with apnea and unconsciousness after apparent recovery from anesthesia.[209]

Cardiovascular Effects

The cardiovascular effects of alfentanil are influenced by preoperative medication, the muscle relaxant used, the method of administration, and the degree of surgical stimulation.[210] In general, heart rate and mean arterial pressure are unchanged or slightly decreased during induction with alfentanil 40–120 $\mu g \cdot kg^{-1}$,[197,210] but rapid induction with 150–175 $\mu g \cdot kg^{-1}$ alfentanil can decrease mean arterial pressure by 15–20 torr.[202] After induction with etomidate, alfentanil 120 $\mu g \cdot kg^{-1}$ decreased mean arterial pressure by approximately 30 torr,[211] and following thiopental (3–5 mg $\cdot$ kg^{-1}) induction, a smaller dose of alfentanil (40 $\mu g \cdot kg^{-1}$) decreased mean arterial pressure by approximately 40 torr.[212] In combination with lorazepam premedication or thiopental induction, moderate doses (10–50 $\mu g \cdot kg^{-1}$) of alfentanil blunt the cardiovascular and catecholamine responses to laryngoscopy and intubation,[200,212] but for patients over 70 years old, doses greater than 10 $\mu g \cdot kg^{-1}$ given with thiopental can produce significant hypotension after induction.[213] Alfentanil can also cause bradycardia, but this effect is minimized by premedication with atropine, and by the vagolytic effect of pancuronium.[210] Alfentanil is commonly administered with propofol for induction and maintenance of anesthesia, but both of these agents act centrally to produce bradycardia. Skues et al[214] found that patients who received alfentanil 50 $\mu g \cdot kg^{-1}$ plus propofol 1 mg $\cdot$ kg^{-1} for induction of anesthesia experienced significant bradycardia, accompanied by hypotension, after intubation. Premedication with both atropine and glycopyrrolate prevented the bradycardia, but only glycopyrrolate prevented hypotension. Like fentanyl, alfentanil does not appear to have negative inotropic effects,[211] but severe hypotension has been observed when alfentanil is given after 0.125 mg $\cdot$ kg^{-1} diazepam.[215]

Nausea and Vomiting

Early clinical reports noted frequent nausea during recovery from balanced anesthesia using alfentanil, and suggested that perhaps this side effect was worse with alfentanil compared to fentanyl.[216] However, a clinical comparison between alfentanil and sufentanil in combination with N_2O revealed the same incidence of nausea and vomiting with both drugs.[217] Similarly, fentanyl and alfentanil with N_2O both produced a similar degree of nausea in pediatric patients undergoing appendectomy.[218] In normal volunteers receiving computer-controlled opioid infusions, the severity of nausea at equianalgesic plasma concentrations was equivalent for alfentanil, fentanyl, and morphine.[49] Furthermore, alfentanil-induced nausea and vomiting in volunteers resolves more quickly than morphine- or fentanyl-induced vomiting (Coda BA, unpublished observations).

Disposition Kinetics

Alfentanil pharmacokinetics differ from those of fentanyl and sufentanil in several respects (see Table 14-3). A unique characteristic is that alfentanil is a weaker base than other opioids. Whereas other opioids have pK_a above 7.4, the pK_a of alfentanil is 6.8; consequently, nearly 90% of unbound plasma alfentanil is nonionized at pH 7.4.[146] This property, together with its moderate lipid solubility, enables alfentanil to cross the blood–brain barrier rapidly and accounts for its rapid onset of action. Compared to fentanyl and sufentanil, which have mean plasma–brain equilibration half-times of 6.4 and 6.2 minutes, respectively,[110,158] alfentanil has a blood–brain equilibration half-time of 1.1 minutes.[110] Alfentanil also has a smaller volume of distribution than fentanyl, which is a result of lower lipid solubility and high protein binding.[219] Approximately 92% of alfentanil is protein-bound, mostly to α_1-acid glycoprotein.[146,150]

After a bolus dose or rapid iv infusion, plasma alfentanil concentration falls rapidly; 90% of the administered dose has left the plasma by 30 minutes.[220] This initial rapid decline is mostly due to alfentanil's distribution to highly perfused tissues. Plasma concentration decay curves in patients most often fit a three-compartment model.[23,220] Like fentanyl, alfentanil is quickly distributed, with rapid and slow distribution half-times of 1.0–3.5 minutes and 9.5–17 minutes, respectively. However, alfentanil has a terminal elimination half-life of 84–90 minutes, which is considerably shorter than those of fentanyl and sufentanil. Clearance of alfentanil, 6.4 ml $\cdot$ kg$^{-1} \cdot$ min^{-1}, is just half that of fentanyl, but because alfentanil's volume of distribution is 4 times smaller than fentanyl's, relatively more of the body burden is available to the liver for metabolism.[221] Chauvin et al[222] found that alfentanil has an intermediate hepatic extraction coefficient (32–53%) in humans, and that its elimination is dependent on hepatic plasma flow.

In animals, alfentanil undergoes N-dealkylation and O-demethylation in the liver to form inactive metabolites.[146] Liver disease can significantly prolong the elimination half-life of alfentanil. Patients with moderate hepatic insufficiency due to cirrhosis have reduced binding to α_1-acid glycoprotein, and a plasma clearance one half that of control patients. These changes result in a marked increase in the elimination half-life, 219 minutes versus 90 minutes in controls.[223] Renal disease also decreases alfentanil protein binding, but does not result in decreased plasma clearance or a prolonged terminal elimination half-life.[224] Alfentanil's elimination half-life is prolonged by about 30% in the elderly, and appears to be much shorter (about 40 minutes) in children 5–8 years old.[225] Obesity is also associated with a 50% decrease in alfentanil clearance and a prolonged (172 minutes) elimination half-life.[225]

The combination of moderate lipid solubility and short elimination half-life suggests that both redistribution and elimination are important in the termination of alfentanil's effects.[221] After a single bolus dose, redistribution will be the most important mechanism, but after a very large dose, repeated small doses, or a continuous infusion, elimination will be a more important determinant of the duration of alfentanil's effects.

Dosage and Administration of Alfentanil

Because of its rapid onset, alfentanil has been used as an induction agent alone or in combination with other drugs. In healthy patients, doses of about 120 $\mu g \cdot kg^{-1}$ produce unconsciousness in 2–2.5 minutes. Premedication with a benzodiazepine (e.g., lorazepam 0.08 mg $\cdot$ kg^{-1}) is associated with a lower dose requirement, 40–50 $\mu g \cdot kg^{-1}$, and a faster onset of unconsciousness, within 1.5 minutes,[197] but may also produce hypotension.

Alfentanil is used as a supplement to maintain general anesthesia and, owing to its brief duration of action, can be useful in short surgical procedures, particularly in outpatient surgery. In this setting, loading doses of 5–10 $\mu g \cdot kg^{-1}$ provide good analgesia with rapid recovery.[219] For longer procedures, alfentanil can be administered as needed in repeated small bolus doses, but its pharmacokinetic properties make it ideal for administration as a continuous infusion. After induction of anesthesia, a loading dose of alfentanil $10-50$ $\mu g \cdot kg^{-1}$ is followed with supplemental bolus doses of $3-5$ $\mu g \cdot kg^{-1}$ as needed or a continuous infusion starting at $25-100$ $\mu g \cdot kg^{-1} \cdot h^{-1}$ with $60-70\%$ N_2O[194,195,219] or a propofol infusion.

When high-dose alfentanil is used as the sole anesthetic agent for cardiac surgery, a continuous infusion of up $150-600$ $\mu g \cdot kg^{-1} \cdot h^{-1}$ is adjusted according to the patient's responses to stimuli.[198] Others have reported that much lower doses can be effective for cardiac surgery if adequate premedication is given.[199]

Remifentanil

Remifentanil (initially known as GI 87084B), a 4-anilidopiperidine with a methyl ester side chain (see Fig. 14-6) first described in 1990 and approved for clinical use in 1996, was developed to meet the need for an ultrashort-acting opioid. Because its ester side chain is susceptible to metabolism by blood and tissue esterases, remifentanil is rapidly metabolized to a substantially less active compound. Thus, because its ultrashort action is due to metabolism rather than to redistribution, it does not accumulate with repeated dosing or prolonged infusion. Remifentanil demonstrates potent, naloxone-reversible μ-opioid agonist activity in guinea pig ileum and mouse vas deferens assays.[226] Testing with κ- and δ-selective antagonists yielded no evidence that remifentanil is active at either of these opioid receptor subtypes.

Analgesia

In animals and humans, remifentanil produces dose-dependent analgesic effects. In a volunteer study, Glass et al[227] quantified analgesic and side effects of increasing doses of remifentanil and compared them to the effects of alfentanil. Across a range of $0.0625-2.0$ $\mu g \cdot kg^{-1}$, remifentanil produced dose-dependent analgesia, measured as an increase in tolerance to tibial pressure, with a peak analgesic effect between 1 and 3 minutes. On a milligram basis, the relative analgesic potency of single doses of remifentanil was $22-47$ times as potent as alfentanil. Remifentanil 1.5 $\mu g \cdot kg^{-1}$ and alfentanil 32 $\mu g \cdot kg^{-1}$ produced a similar magnitude and duration (approximately 10 minutes) of analgesia.

Effect on MAC of Volatile Anesthetics and Use in Anesthesia

The effect of remifentanil on MAC of volatile anesthetics is characterized by steep dose–effect or concentration–effect curves typical of other μ-opioid agonists. In a canine study, continuous infusion of remifentanil decreased enflurane MAC in a dose-dependent fashion up to a maximum near 65%, similar to the maximum reduction of MAC seen with fentanyl.[228] In humans who received computer-assisted continuous infusions (CACI) of remifentanil to achieve target blood concentrations of $0-32$ $ng \cdot ml^{-1}$, isoflurane MAC was reduced logarithmically in a concentration-dependent fashion,[229] and was influenced by age. Isoflurane MAC was reduced by 50% at a whole blood remifentanil concentration of approximately 1.3 $ng \cdot ml^{-1}$, and a ceiling effect on MAC reduction was seen at 85% with a remifentanil concentration of $8-12$ $ng \cdot ml^{-1}$. In 1999, Peacock and Philip[230] summarized results from an early clinical study[231] that evaluated various combinations of remifentanil and propofol. Remifentanil concentration (EC_{50}) and dosage (ED_{50}) to prevent patient responses to intubation and skin incision in 50% of patients were determined at different target propofol concentrations achieved with CACI. At a propofol target plasma concentration of 1 $\mu g \cdot ml^{-1}$ (mean infusion rate 44 $\mu g \cdot kg^{-1} \cdot min^{-1}$), remifentanil EC_{50} was 14.3 $ng \cdot ml^{-1}$ (infusion rate 0.44 $\mu g \cdot kg^{-1} \cdot min^{-1}$) for intubation, while at a propofol target concentration of 4 $\mu g \cdot ml^{-1}$ (mean infusion rate 200 $\mu g \cdot kg^{-1} \cdot$

min^{-1}), remifentanil EC_{50} was 1.4 $ng \cdot ml^{-1}$ (infusion rate 0.07 $\mu g \cdot kg^{-1} \cdot min^{-1}$) for intubation. Response to intubation was prevented in 80% of patients by approximately doubling the remifentanil doses or concentrations.

The rapid onset and brief duration of remifentanil suggest that it is suitable for induction of anesthesia. A clinical study comparing a range of remifentanil doses ($2-20$ $\mu g \cdot kg^{-1}$) to alfentanil ($40-200$ $\mu g \cdot kg^{-1}$) for induction of anesthesia[232] showed that loss of consciousness was not reliably achieved with opioids alone. The median dose of remifentanil required for loss of consciousness in 50% of patients was 12 $\mu g \cdot kg^{-1}$,[232] while doses less than 5 $\mu g \cdot kg^{-1}$ did not produce loss of consciousness in any patients. Furthermore, as is common with other opioids, a high incidence of muscle rigidity and purposeless movement was seen. Even at the lowest remifentanil dose, moderate muscle rigidity was seen in 40% of patients, and at the highest dose, 60% of patients had severe muscle rigidity. This effect limits the utility of opioids as sole agents for induction of anesthesia.

Early clinical experience suggested that for maintenance of anesthesia with 66% N_2O, an infusion rate of 0.05 $\mu g \cdot kg^{-1} \cdot min^{-1}$ prevents motor and hemodynamic responses to tracheal intubation and skin incision in 50% of patients.[233] Higher infusion rates (0.6 $\mu g \cdot kg^{-1} \cdot min^{-1}$) are necessary to prevent responses to subsequent surgical stimuli. Randel et al[234] similarly found that a remifentanil infusion rate of 0.4 $\mu g \cdot kg^{-1} \cdot min^{-1}$ was reliably associated with prevention of response to surgical stimuli in the presence of 66% N_2O. In this study, remifentanil EC_{50} for no responses to intubation and incision were approximately 2.0 and 1.5 $ng \cdot ml^{-1}$, respectively. It is important to note that these studies included induction with propofol $2-2.5$ $mg \cdot kg^{-1}$, and supplementation with low-dose isoflurane if titration of remifentanil alone could not control hemodynamics. Drover and Lemmens[235] used computer-assisted infusions to determine the blood concentrations of remifentanil required to supplement 66% N_2O in patients having abdominal surgery. A range of $0.5-7.8$ $ng \cdot ml^{-1}$ target concentrations was used, and other than premedication with $1-2$ mg midazolam, no sedatives or hypnotics were given. These investigators were unable to determine an EC_{50} for either intubation or incision because they could not identify a concentration low enough to result in a consistent response to stimuli, or a concentration high enough to consistently prevent a response. During surgery, however, the remifentanil blood concentration associated with a 50% probability of adequate anesthesia (EC_{50}) was 4.1 $ng \cdot ml^{-1}$ for men and 7.5 $ng \cdot ml^{-1}$ for women. The reason for gender differences in these results was not clear, but could have been related to different types of surgeries. Thus propofol, and perhaps other agents, used for induction appear to reduce subsequent remifentanil requirements by as much as $2-4$-fold.

Another increasingly common clinical use of remifentanil is in conjunction with propofol infusion for maintenance of total intravenous anesthesia (TIVA). This combination has been used successfully for a variety of inpatient procedures, including CABG, other major thoracic, abdominal, and orthopedic procedures[236,237] as well as for ambulatory surgery procedures.[230,238,239] Optimum regimens are still being evaluated.

Recovery from remifentanil is rapid, with return of spontaneous ventilation in $2-5$ minutes, even when it is continued until after skin closure is complete.[233] The drawback of this characteristic is that patients require analgesics very soon after remifentanil is discontinued. This problem can be overcome by continuing a low dose of remifentanil until the patient arrives in the recovery room.

Other CNS Effects

Remifentanil produces classic μ-opioid agonist effects on the EEG, i.e., a concentration-dependent slowing. The plasma concentration associated with 50% maximal EEG changes (EC_{50}) is $15-20$ $ng \cdot ml^{-1}$.[240,241] Remifentanil has an onset of action similar to that of alfentanil, but the duration is much shorter.

This is seen as an extremely close tracking of changes in EEG spectral edge with plasma remifentanil concentration.[240,241] In dogs anesthetized with 1% isoflurane and 50% nitrous oxide in oxygen, low- and high-dose remifentanil and alfentanil infusions produced a similar magnitude of EEG slowing, and similar decreases in cerebral blood flow and intracranial pressure.[242] Mean arterial pressure also decreased in response to both opioids, but when blood pressure was maintained with phenylephrine, remifentanil produced similar decreases in cerebral blood flow and intracranial pressure.[242]

Several clinical reports have described cerebral hemodynamics in humans. In the first clinical report,[243] bolus doses of remifentanil (0.5 or 1.0 $\mu g \cdot kg^{-1}$) or alfentanil (10 or 20 $\mu g \cdot kg^{-1}$) were given after the first burr hole was drilled. Under conditions of background isoflurane/N_2O anesthesia and controlled ventilation, neither opioid affected intracranial pressure and both produced modest, dose-dependent decreases in mean arterial pressure. A multicenter clinical trial followed, in which remifentanil/N_2O anesthesia was compared to fentanyl/N_2O anesthesia.[244] Opioid infusions were started prior to induction; then the rates were decreased after intubation and titrated to maintain stable hemodynamics. Intracranial pressure (remifentanil 13 ± 10; fentanyl 14 ± 13 mm Hg) and cerebral perfusion pressure (remifentanil 78 ± 14; fentanyl 76 ± 19 mm Hg) were similar with the two regimens. Under conditions of controlled ventilation and maintenance of blood pressure with vasoactive adjuvants as necessary, cerebral blood flow was similar, and cerebral vascular reactivity to CO_2 was found to be intact during both remifentanil/N_2O and fentanyl/N_2O anesthesia[245] for craniotomy. Another report described the effect of two infusion rates of remifentanil on cerebral blood flow velocity in patients scheduled for coronary artery bypass graft surgery.[246] No inhalation agents were used, ventilation was controlled to maintain isocapnea, and mean arterial pressure was maintained with phenylephrine. Cerebral blood flow velocity decreased significantly in patients who received high dose (5 $\mu g \cdot kg^{-1}$, followed by 3 $\mu g \cdot kg^{-1} \cdot min^{-1}$) but not in those with modest dose (2 $\mu g \cdot kg^{-1}$, followed by 1 $\mu g \cdot kg^{-1} \cdot min^{-1}$) remifentanil.

Respiratory Depression

Remifentanil produces dose-dependent respiratory depression as measured by increases in end-tidal CO_2 and decreased oxygen saturation. In a dose-escalation study in normal volunteers, the respiratory depressant effects of remifentanil and alfentanil were compared.[227] Peak respiratory depression occurred at 5 minutes after each dose of remifentanil and alfentanil, and the maximal respiratory depressant effect seen after 2 $\mu g \cdot kg^{-1}$ remifentanil was similar to that caused by 32 $\mu g \cdot kg^{-1}$ alfentanil. The duration of respiratory depression, measured as time to return of blood gases to within 10% of baseline values, was 10 minutes after 1.5 $\mu g \cdot kg^{-1}$ and 20 minutes after 2 $\mu g \cdot kg^{-1}$ remifentanil compared to 30 minutes after 32 $\mu g \cdot kg^{-1}$ alfentanil. During continuous opioid infusion, minute ventilation, in the presence of 8% inspired CO_2, decreased by approximately 30, 45, and 60% in response to 4-hour remifentanil infusions of 0.025, 0.050, and 0.075 $\mu g \cdot kg^{-1} \cdot min^{-1}$, respectively.[247] Recovery from remifentanil-induced respiratory depression was rapid, and minute ventilation returned to baseline by 8 (range 5–15) minutes after the infusion was stopped for all infusion rates. In contrast, a 50% decrease in minute ventilation produced by a 4-hour continuous infusion of alfentanil at 0.5 $\mu g \cdot kg^{-1} \cdot min^{-1}$ required 61 (range 5–90) minutes to return to baseline.[228] In a volunteer study, Glass et al reported that the blood remifentanil concentration needed to depress minute ventilation in the presence of 8% inspired CO_2 by 50% (EC_{50}) was 1.17 $ng \cdot ml^{-1}$.[248]

While the time course for recovery of normal ventilatory drive is rapid in patients as well as volunteers, maintenance of spontaneous respiration during general anesthesia with remifentanil and volatile agents or propofol may not be feasible unless low doses of remifentanil are used.[249] Clinical experience

in spontaneously breathing humans receiving remifentanil combined with either isoflurane or propofol has demonstrated dose-dependent respiratory depression.[230] Respiratory depression is seen in 10–35% of patients receiving remifentanil at 0.025 $\mu g \cdot kg^{-1} \cdot min^{-1}$. It increases to nearly 50% in patients receiving 0.05 $\mu g \cdot kg^{-1} \cdot min^{-1}$ and to >90% in patients receiving remifentanil at 0.075 $\mu g \cdot kg^{-1} \cdot min^{-1}$.

Hemodynamic Effects

In healthy volunteers, remifentanil in bolus doses greater than 1.0 $\mu g \cdot kg^{-1}$ produces brief increases in systolic blood pressure (5–20 torr) and heart rate (10–25 beats/min), which return to baseline by 10 minutes.[227] In patients anesthetized with isoflurane and 66% N_2O in oxygen, remifentanil (up to 5 $\mu g \cdot kg^{-1}$) produces dose-dependent decreases in systolic blood pressure and heart rate. These effects are attenuated by premedication with glycopyrrolate 0.3–0.4 mg, and are readily reversed with ephedrine or phenylephrine.[250] Sebel et al[251] evaluated hemodynamic responses in patients receiving 2–30 $\mu g \cdot kg^{-1}$ (escalating doses) given during general anesthesia. Remifentanil was associated with systolic heart rate decreases in excess of 20% for doses greater than 2 $\mu g \cdot kg^{-1}$. There were no alterations in histamine concentrations, indicating that hemodynamic effects are not mediated by histamine release. Another series of case reports[252] described severe bradycardia (HR < 30 beats/min) and hypotension (systolic BP < 80 mm Hg) in six patients scheduled for coronary artery bypass grafting, who received remifentanil 1 $\mu g \cdot kg^{-1}$ followed by a continuous infusion at 0.1–0.2 $\mu g \cdot kg^{-1} \cdot min^{-1}$. Of particular note, the bolus dose was given more rapidly than is recommended, i.e., over less than 30 seconds versus 30–60 seconds. Hypotension in all cases was effectively treated by ephedrine and temporary discontinuation of remifentanil. Preoperative use of beta blockers or calcium channel blockers did not predispose patients to bradycardia. Smaller bolus doses of remifentanil (0.3–0.5 $\mu g \cdot kg^{-1}$) are apparently not associated with severe bradycardia and hypotension. The most likely mechanisms for these hemodynamic effects include centrally mediated decrease in sympathetic tone and vagally induced bradycardia.

Other Side Effects

Like other μ agonists, remifentanil can cause nausea and vomiting. Preliminary results suggested that the incidence of nausea and vomiting with remifentanil might be lower than with alfentanil after single bolus doses in volunteers[227] as well as in patients sedated with low-dose opioid infusions (0.05 $\mu g \cdot kg^{-1} \cdot min^{-1}$ remifentanil) during regional anesthesia.[253] With high infusion rates (1–8 $\mu g \cdot kg^{-1} \cdot min^{-1}$) nausea occurred in 70% of subjects, and muscle rigidity was noted in all subjects.[240] In pediatric patients who received desflurane with and without remifentanil 0.2 $\mu g \cdot kg^{-1} \cdot min^{-1}$,[254] nausea and vomiting on emergence from general anesthesia was evaluated. In this study, the addition of remifentanil produced no increase in the incidence of postoperative nausea or vomiting after dental surgery; nausea and vomiting occurred in <5% of patients who received remifentanil. Philip et al[238] compared nausea and vomiting at multiple time points in outpatient adults for laparoscopic surgery who received remifentanil or alfentanil combined with propofol. In this study remifentanil was infused at 0.25–0.5 $\mu g \cdot kg^{-1} \cdot min^{-1}$ and alfentanil was infused at 1–2 $\mu g \cdot kg^{-1} \cdot min^{-1}$ after induction. Overall, the incidence of nausea was 44% and 53% for remifentanil and alfentanil, respectively; the incidence of vomiting was 21% and 29% for remifentanil and alfentanil, respectively. Thus, remifentanil appears to produce dose-dependent nausea and vomiting similar to other short-acting μ-agonist opioids.

Disposition Kinetics

The key structural feature of remifentanil is an ester functional group that is susceptible to hydrolysis by blood and tissue nonspecific esterases, which results in very rapid metabolism. Because butyrocholinesterase (pseudocholinesterase) does not appear to metabolize remifentanil, plasma cholinesterase deficiency and anticholinergic administration were not expected to affect remifentanil clearance. This expectation has been confirmed.[255] Unlike other opioids, remifentanil clearance is mainly due to enzymatic hydrolysis, with redistribution playing only a minor role. This property reduces its pharmacokinetic variability compared to other opioids. Several investigators have evaluated the pharmacokinetics of remifentanil in humans.[227,240,241,256,257] Both two- and three-compartment models have been used to describe the plasma concentration decay curve of remifentanil. Glass et al[227] administered bolus doses of up to 2 μg $\cdot$ kg^{-1} to normal volunteers. They reported a small volume of distribution, 0.39 l $\cdot$ kg^{-1}, and a high clearance, 41 ml $\cdot$ kg^{-1} $\cdot$ min^{-1}. A rapid distribution phase of 0.9 minutes and a very short terminal elimination half-life of 9.5 minutes characterized a two-compartment model. Westmoreland et al[257] found similar pharmacokinetic parameters in anesthetized patients given 2–30 μg $\cdot$ kg^{-1}, but observed that a three-compartment model best described the pharmacokinetics of remifentanil. The rapid and slow distribution half-times were 0.4–0.5 and 2–3.7 minutes, respectively, and the elimination half-time was 10–20 minutes. The investigators reported a similar volume of distribution (approximately 0.3–0.5 l $\cdot$ kg^{-1}) and high total clearance (250–300 l $\cdot$ h^{-1}), approximately 3–4 times normal hepatic blood flow.

Although pharmacokinetic parameters of remifentanil are unchanged in patients with severe liver disease[258] or renal failure,[259] patients with hepatic disease appear to be more sensitive to remifentanil-induced respiratory depression (measured by hypercarbic challenge). As for other fentanyl congeners, gender does not affect remifentanil pharmacokinetics, but advanced age is associated with a decrease in clearance and volume of distribution, as well as an increase in potency.[260] Egan et al demonstrated that remifentanil pharmacokinetics are similar in lean (within 20% ideal body weight) and obese (at least 80% over ideal body weight) patients, and recommended that remifentanil dosing should be based on lean body mass.[261]

Dosage and Administration of Remifentanil

Clinical trials to develop ideal dosage combinations and regimens for a variety of inpatient and ambulatory procedures are ongoing. However, since its approval for clinical use, numerous reports have described dosing regimens for remifentanil alone or in combination with other agents for induction and maintenance of general anesthesia, and as a component of sedation and monitored anesthesia care. Because of its extremely short duration of action, remifentanil is best administered as a continuous infusion, although administration as repeated bolus doses has also been reported to be effective.

As described earlier, remifentanil alone has not been found to be a satisfactory single agent for induction of anesthesia because of unreliability in loss of consciousness as well as significant muscle rigidity. Several clinical trials have described dosing regimens of remifentanil and propofol for induction of anesthesia. Hogue et al[237] described a dose of remifentanil 1 μg $\cdot$ kg^{-1} followed by an infusion of 1 μg $\cdot$ kg^{-1} $\cdot$ min^{-1}; 3 minutes later, propofol 0.5–1 mg $\cdot$ kg^{-1} was given. This regimen resulted in minimal hemodynamic response to tracheal intubation, but 15% of patients experienced hypotension (systolic BP < 80 mm Hg or MAP < 60 mm Hg). Song et al[262] compared bolus doses of fentanyl 1 μg $\cdot$ kg^{-1}, remifentanil 0.5 μg $\cdot$ kg^{-1}, and remifentanil 1 μg $\cdot$ kg^{-1} followed 1 minute later by propofol 2 mg $\cdot$ kg^{-1}. Both remifentanil doses compared favorably to the fentanyl dose; remifentanil 1 μg $\cdot$ kg^{-1} provided the best hemodynamic control without hypotension.

Early experience with remifentanil suggests that when administered as part of a balanced anesthetic with 66% N$_2$O, remifentanil infusion rates of 0.3–1 μg $\cdot$ kg^{-1} $\cdot$ min^{-1} are optimal to prevent hemodynamic responses to surgical stimuli.[233,234] When infusion rates as high as 2 μg $\cdot$ kg^{-1} $\cdot$ min^{-1} are continued until placement of the last suture, spontaneous ventilation returns within 7 minutes. Peacock and Philip[230] have suggested that an infusion of remifentanil at 0.02–0.05 μg $\cdot$ kg^{-1} $\cdot$ min^{-1} administered with isoflurane at an end-tidal concentration of 0.8–1.3% will provide adequate maintenance of anesthesia. Combined with a propofol infusion of 75 μg $\cdot$ kg^{-1} $\cdot$ min^{-1}, mean remifentanil infusion rates of approximately 0.25–0.4 μg $\cdot$ kg^{-1} $\cdot$ min^{-1} appear to provide good hemodynamic control and allow for rapid emergence from anesthesia.[237,238] With higher propofol infusion rates, 120–140 g $\cdot$ kg^{-1} $\cdot$ min^{-1}, the remifentanil infusion can be reduced to 0.02–0.05 μg $\cdot$ kg^{-1} $\cdot$ min^{-1}.[230] For cardiac surgery, remifentanil infusion rates from 1 to 3 μg $\cdot$ kg^{-1} $\cdot$ min^{-1} combined with a low-dose propofol infusion of 50 μg $\cdot$ kg^{-1} $\cdot$ min^{-1} effectively suppressed responses to skin incision, sternotomy, and aortic cannulation.[236]

A potential disadvantage of remifentanil is also related to its short duration of action. Upon emergence from anesthesia, patients may experience substantial pain. Thus, if moderate to severe postoperative pain is anticipated, continuing the remifentanil infusion at a lower rate may prevent this problem. Bowdle et al used this approach in patients undergoing a variety of orthopedic, abdominal, and thoracic procedures.[263] At the time of the completion of skin sutures, the infusion rate was decreased to 0.05 μg $\cdot$ kg^{-1} $\cdot$ min^{-1}, and subsequently titrated to patient comfort (pain rated as "none" to "mild"). Nearly half of these patients required no further adjustment of the remifentanil rate for immediate postoperative analgesia; 78% had adequate analgesia with remifentanil infusion rates from 0.05 to 0.15 μg $\cdot$ kg^{-1} $\cdot$ min^{-1}. When only mild postoperative pain is anticipated, intraoperative administration of a nonsteroidal anti-inflammatory drug 30–60 minutes before the end of surgery may provide effective analgesia without additional opioids.

Remifentanil can also be used as an adjunct for sedation or analgesia during regional anesthesia, for block placement, or as part of monitored anesthesia care (MAC). A dose of 1 μg $\cdot$ kg^{-1} with or without a subsequent infusion of 0.2 μg $\cdot$ kg^{-1} $\cdot$ min^{-1} administered 90 seconds prior to placement of ophthalmologic block resulted in up to 80% of patients reporting no pain at the time of the block.[264] However, 14% of patients who received an infusion experienced respiratory depression. During regional anesthesia, a maintenance infusion rate in the range of 0.05–0.1 μg $\cdot$ kg^{-1} $\cdot$ min^{-1} can provide adequate sedation and analgesia during surgery performed under local or regional nerve block.[265] In general, bolus doses of remifentanil during MAC have been discouraged because of the increased risk of respiratory depression and muscle rigidity, but this may be reduced somewhat by administering single doses slowly, i.e., over >30 seconds. Finally, the dose requirement of remifentanil for sedation/analgesia is reduced substantially when combined with midazolam or propofol. Gold et al[266] found that remifentanil requirement was reduced by approximately 50% (0.06 vs. 0.12 μg $\cdot$ kg^{-1} $\cdot$ min^{-1}) when 1–2 mg of midazolam was given at the beginning of procedures performed under local anesthesia. A clinical study evaluated several regimens of remifentanil plus propofol for extracorporeal shock wave lithotripsy. Combined with propofol 50 μg $\cdot$ kg^{-1} $\cdot$ min^{-1}, small intermittent remifentanil doses (25 μg $\cdot$ kg^{-1}), administered over 15–30 seconds, or a low-dose continuous infusion (0.05 μg $\cdot$ kg^{-1} $\cdot$ min^{-1}) supplemented by 12.5 μg $\cdot$ kg^{-1} bolus doses provided good analgesia, without an undue risk of respiratory depression.[267]

Partial Agonists and Mixed Agonist–Antagonists

The partial agonist and mixed agonist–antagonist opioids are synthetic or semisynthetic compounds that are structurally related to morphine. They are characterized by binding activity at

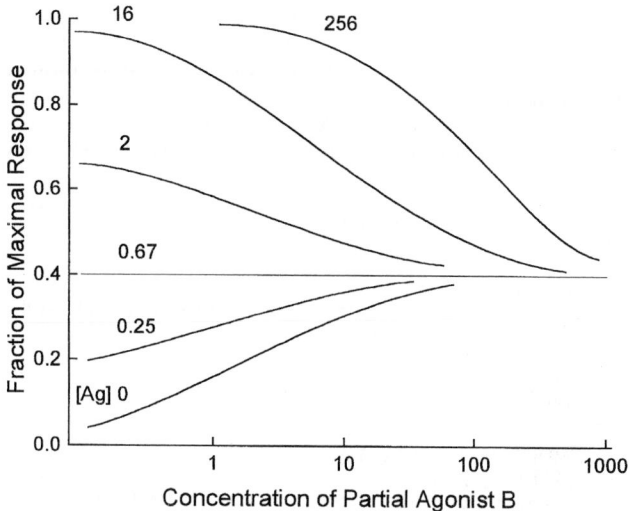

Figure 14-13. Hypothetical log dose–effect curves for the combination of a partial agonist, B (intrinsic efficacy of 0.4), with a range of concentrations of a full agonist, A. The observed effect of the combination of A and B is expressed as a fraction of the maximal effect of the full agonist. As the concentration of the partial agonist increases, the effect of the combination converges on the maximum effect of the partial agonist. When added to a low concentration (*e.g.,* [A] = 0.25) of agonist, the partial agonist increases the response; but when added to a large concentration of the agonist, the response decreases—that is, B acts like an antagonist. (Modified with permission from Bowdle TA: Partial agonist and agonist–antagonist opioids: Basic pharmacology and clinical applications. Anaesth Pharmacol Rev 1:135, 1993.)

multiple opioid receptors and their differential effects (agonist, partial agonist, or antagonist) at each receptor type. The clinical effect of a partial agonist at the μ-opioid receptor is complex (Fig. 14-13). Administered alone, a partial agonist has a more shallow dose–response curve and a lower maximal effect than a full agonist (see Fig. 14-1 and the lowermost curve in Fig. 14-13). Combined with a low concentration (*cf.* curve indicated by [Ag] = 0.25 in Fig. 14-13) of a full agonist, the effects of the partial agonist are additive up to the maximum effect of the partial agonist. Combined with increasing concentrations ([Ag] = 0.67–256) of full agonist, the partial agonist will act as an antagonist. These drugs mediate their clinical effects via μ- and κ-opioid receptors, as summarized in Table 14-4. The classification scheme presented may change as our understanding of these drugs and of opioid receptors continues to grow. Bowdle extensively reviewed the pharmacology and clinical uses of these and other drugs in this class.[268] Only nalbuphine, butorphanol, and buprenorphine are considered in this chapter.

The major role of the opioid agonist–antagonist and partial agonist drugs continues to be in the provision of postoperative analgesia, but they have also been used for intraoperative sedation, as adjuncts during general anesthesia, and to antagonize some of the effects of full μ-opioid agonists.

Nalbuphine

Nalbuphine is a phenanthrene opioid derivative. Although it is often classified as a κ agonist and μ antagonist, it is more accurately described as a partial agonist at both κ and μ receptors.[268] While MAC [minimum alveolar concentration] reduction studies have not been done in humans, Murphy and Hug[25] reported that a 0.5 mg · kg^{-1} dose reduced enflurane MAC by 8% in dogs. However, increasing the dose 8-fold produced no further reduction in enflurane MAC. This modest MAC reduction, compared to 65% for morphine, suggests that nalbuphine may not be a useful adjunct for general anesthesia. However,

several investigators have examined its effectiveness as a component of balanced anesthesia for cardiac[269] and lower abdominal surgery.[25,270] Combined with diazepam 0.4 mg · kg^{-1} and 50% N$_2$O in oxygen, a loading dose of 3 mg · kg^{-1} was followed by additional doses of 0.25 mg · kg^{-1} as needed throughout surgery. No significant increases in blood pressure, stress hormones, or histamine were seen, and emergence from anesthesia was uncomplicated.[269] Nalbuphine 0.2 mg · kg^{-1} was compared to meperidine 0.5 mg · kg^{-1} as an adjuvant to general anesthesia with 1% halothane and 70% N$_2$O in oxygen in spontaneously breathing patients undergoing inguinal hernia repair.[271] Both drugs produced a similar degree of respiratory depression as well as postoperative analgesia and side effects. The most common side effect was drowsiness. In a double-blind comparison with fentanyl for gynecologic surgery, fentanyl was found to better attenuate hypertensive responses to intubation and surgical stimulation.[270] However, significant respiratory depression was seen in 8 of 30 patients who received fentanyl, and 4 required naloxone, compared to no respiratory depression in the nalbuphine group. Analgesia was similar, and as in other studies, postoperative sedation was common in the nalbuphine group.

The respiratory depression produced by nalbuphine, an effect most likely mediated by μ-opioid receptors, has a ceiling effect equivalent to that produced by 30 mg / 70 kg morphine.[268] Analgesia is mediated by both κ and μ receptors. Because of these effects, nalbuphine has been used to antagonize the respiratory depressant effects of full agonists while still providing analgesic effects. In a double-blind comparison, nalbuphine and naloxone both effectively antagonized fentanyl-induced postoperative respiratory depression.[272] However, patients who received naloxone subsequently required analgesics more often than did those who received nalbuphine. Nalbuphine has also been effective in antagonizing respiratory depression due to residual fentanyl effect following high-dose (100–120 μg · kg^{-1}) fentanyl anesthesia for cardiac surgery.[273] Only 3 of 21 patients experienced pain after nalbuphine administration, and this was adequately treated with additional nalbuphine. However, in a volunteer study, nalbuphine 0.21 mg · kg^{-1} did not antagonize the respiratory depressant effects of 0.21 mg · kg^{-1} morphine.[274]

While nalbuphine and other agonist–antagonists have ceiling analgesic effects as well as respiratory depressant effects, they can be as effective as full μ agonists in providing postoperative analgesia. Nalbuphine 5–10 mg has also been used to antagonize pruritus induced by epidural and intrathecal morphine. The usual adult dose of nalbuphine is 10 mg as often as every 3 hours. It is important to be aware that nalbuphine can precipitate withdrawal symptoms in patients who are physically dependent on opioids.

Table 14-4. ACTIONS OF THE NALBUPHINE, BUTORPHANOL, AND BUPRENORPHINE AT OPIOID RECEPTORS

Drug	μ Receptor	κ Receptor
Nalbuphine	Partial agonist	Partial agonist
Butorphanol	Partial agonist	Partial agonist
Buprenorphine	Partial agonist	?Antagonist

Although nalbuphine and butorphanol have been reported to be antagonists at the μ-opioid receptor, they do cause respiratory depression, which is not a function of κ agonists. Thus, they appear to have at least partial agonist activity at the μ-opioid receptor.
Adapted from Bowdle TA: Partial agonist and agonist–antagonist opioids: Basic pharmacology and clinical applications. Anesth Pharmacol Rev 1:135, 1993.

Butorphanol

Butorphanol, a morphinan congener, has partial agonist activity at κ and μ opioid receptors, similar to those of nalbuphine. Compared to nalbuphine and similar drugs, however, butorphanol has a pronounced sedative effect, which is probably mediated by κ receptors. In a laboratory study as well as in clinical use as a premedicant, butorphanol produced dose-dependent sedation comparable to that of midazolam.[275] Like nalbuphine, butorphanol decreases enflurane MAC, in dogs, by a modest amount: 11%, at the lowest dose evaluated $(0.1 \text{ mg} \cdot \text{kg}^{-1})$.[25] Increasing the butorphanol dose 40-fold does not produce a further reduction. However, like nalbuphine, butorphanol has also been reported to be an effective component of balanced general anesthesia in cardiac surgery patients. Combined with diazepam and nitrous oxide, butorphanol and morphine provided equally satisfactory anesthesia.[268]

Given alone, butorphanol produces respiratory depression; but like nalbuphine, it has a ceiling effect below that of full μ agonists. In postoperative patients a parenteral dose of 3 mg produces respiratory depression approximately equal to that of 10 mg morphine.[1] It has been used to antagonize the respiratory depressant effects of fentanyl.[276] Patients who had been anesthetized with isoflurane, nitrous oxide, and fentanyl $5 \ \mu\text{g} \cdot \text{kg}^{-1}$ followed by an infusion of $3 \ \mu\text{g} \cdot \text{kg}^{-1} \cdot \text{h}^{-1}$ received three sequential doses of butorphanol 1 mg at 10–15-minute intervals. After the first 1-mg dose, respiratory rate and ventilatory response to CO_2 increased, while end-tidal CO_2 decreased significantly. Further progressive changes in all parameters were not significantly different from the initial response to butorphanol. Analgesia was not significantly affected in 21 of 22 patients.

In contrast to morphine, fentanyl, and even meperidine, butorphanol does not produce significant elevation in intrabiliary pressure[89] (see Fig. 14-7). Butorphanol has also been shown to be effective in the treatment of postoperative shivering,[96] but the mechanism for this effect is unknown.

Butorphanol is indicated for sedation as well as treatment of moderate to severe postoperative pain. Preliminary clinical experience suggests that butorphanol administered as patient-controlled analgesia is associated with a lower incidence of opioid-induced ileus compared to μ-selective opioids (Dunbar PJ, personal communication). A dose as low as 0.5 mg can provide clinically useful sedation, while single analgesic doses range from 0.5 to 2 mg. Butorphanol has also been administered epidurally and transnasally.

Buprenorphine

Buprenorphine is a highly lipophilic thebaine derivative, which at small to moderate doses is 25–50 times more potent than morphine.[1] Unlike nalbuphine and butorphanol, buprenorphine does not appear to have agonist, and may have antagonist, activity at the κ-opioid receptor (see Table 14-4).[268] Another unique characteristic of buprenorphine is its slow dissociation from μ receptors, which can lead to prolonged effects not easily antagonized by naloxone. Buprenorphine also appears to have an unusual bell-shaped dose–response curve such that, at very high doses, buprenorphine produces progressively less analgesia.[268] In a clinical study, Pedersen[277] found that patients who received 10 or 20 $\mu\text{g} \cdot \text{kg}^{-1}$ buprenorphine during surgery were pain-free postoperatively, but half of the patients who received 30 or 40 $\mu\text{g} \cdot \text{kg}^{-1}$ had significant postoperative pain. This observation is consistent with buprenorphine's bell-shaped dose–effect curve. Patients who received very high buprenorphine doses probably had plasma drug concentrations in the range at which declining analgesia is seen.

Buprenorphine also appears to have a ceiling effect to its respiratory depressant dose–response curve. However, although buprenorphine-induced respiratory depression can be prevented by prior naloxone administration, it is not easily reversed by naloxone once the effects have been produced.[1] A dose of 0.3 mg buprenorphine reduces CO_2 responsiveness to about 50% of control values.[278] Large doses of naloxone (5–10 mg) were required to antagonize buprenorphine respiratory depression in volunteers, while 1-mg doses were not effective. In addition, the maximum antagonist effect did not occur until 3 hours after naloxone administration, an observation consistent with buprenorphine's slow dissociation from μ receptors. Buprenorphine has been compared to naloxone in its ability to antagonize fentanyl-induced respiratory depression, and appears to increase respiratory rate without antagonizing analgesic effects in slowly administered doses up to 0.5 mg.[279]

Buprenorphine can be effective in treatment of moderate to severe pain. Its onset can be slow, but analgesic duration can be more than 6 hours. A single dose of 0.3–0.4 mg appears to produce analgesia equivalent to 10 mg morphine.[1]

Antagonists (Naloxone and Naltrexone)

Under normal conditions, opioid antagonists produce few effects. They are competitive inhibitors of the opioid agonists, so the effect profile depends on the type and dose of agonist administered as well as the degree to which physical dependence on the opioid agonist has developed. The most widely used opioid antagonist is naloxone, which is structurally related to morphine and oxymorphone, and is a pure antagonist at μ-, κ-, and δ-opioid receptors.[1] Naltrexone is a long-acting oral agent, which also has relatively pure antagonist activity. In some circumstances, naloxone can antagonize effects that appear to be mediated by endogenous opioids. For example, naloxone can reverse "stress analgesia" in animals and man; it can antagonize analgesia produced by low-frequency stimulation with acupuncture needles, and it can also reverse analgesia produced by placebo medications.[1]

In clinical anesthesia practice, naloxone is administered to antagonize opioid-induced respiratory depression and sedation. Because opioid antagonists will reverse all opioid effects, including analgesia, naloxone should be carefully titrated to avoid producing sudden, severe pain in postoperative patients. Sudden, complete antagonism of opioid effects with naloxone has been reported to cause severe hypertension, tachycardia, ventricular dysrhythmias, and acute, sometimes fatal, pulmonary edema.[280] Naloxone-induced pulmonary edema can occur even in healthy young patients who have received relatively small doses (80–500 μg) of naloxone.[281, 282] The mechanism for this phenomenon is thought to be centrally mediated catecholamine release, which causes acute pulmonary hypertension. Because most patients with opioid-induced respiratory depression will often breathe on command, it is important to stimulate them in addition to administering carefully titrated naloxone doses in the immediate postoperative period. It is also essential to monitor vital signs and oxygenation closely after naloxone is administered in order to detect occurrence of any of these potentially serious complications.

Naloxone will precipitate opioid withdrawal symptoms in opioid-dependent individuals. Clinicians tend to be aware of this risk when treating patients with known opioid addiction, but it is important to consider the potential for opioid withdrawal syndrome when treating nonaddicts who use opioids chronically, such as cancer patients and severe burn and trauma patients with protracted recovery courses.

Naloxone has a very fast onset of action, and thus is easily titrated. Peak effects occur within 1–2 minutes, and duration is dose-dependent, but total doses of 0.4–0.8 mg generally last 1–4 hours.[1] Suggested incremental doses for intravenous titration are 20–40 μg given every few minutes until the patient's ventilation improves, but analgesia is not completely reversed. Because naloxone has a short duration of action, respiratory depression may recur if large doses and/or long-acting opioid agonists have been administered. When prolonged ventilatory depression is anticipated, an initial loading dose followed by a naloxone infusion can be used. Infusion rates between 3 and 10 $\mu g \cdot h^{-1}$ have been effective in antagonizing respiratory depression from systemic as well as epidural opioids.[39,283]

USE OF OPIOID AGONISTS IN CLINICAL ANESTHESIA

Opioids are used alone or in combination with other agents, such as sedatives or anticholinergic agents, as "premedications." For this purpose, longer acting opioids such as morphine are administered as single doses that are generally within the "analgesic" range. The goal of opioid premedication is to provide moderate sedation, anxiolysis, and analgesia while maintaining hemodynamic stability. Potential risks of opioid premedication include oversedation, respiratory depression, and nausea and vomiting. For induction of anesthesia, opioids are often used to blunt or prevent the hemodynamic responses to tracheal intubation. Opioids with rapid onset of action, such as fentanyl and its derivatives, are appropriate for this use.

Intraoperatively, opioids are administered as components of balanced anesthesia and neuroleptanesthesia, or alone in high-dose opioid anesthesia. During maintenance of general anesthesia, opioid dosage is titrated to the desired effect based on the surgical stimulus as well as individual patient characteristics, such as age, volume status, neurologic status, liver dysfunction, or other systemic disease states. Plasma opioid concentrations required to blunt hemodynamic responses to laryngoscopy, tracheal intubation, and various surgical stimuli, as well as plasma opioid concentration associated with awakening from anesthesia, have been determined for several opioids. Titration to achieve these plasma concentrations (see Table 14-3), which reflect brain (effect site) concentrations, can be accomplished by administering repeated small bolus doses or by infusing the opioid at variable rates.

Fentanyl and its derivatives sufentanil and alfentanil are the opioids most widely used as supplements to general anesthesia. All of these opioids are more easily titrated than morphine because of their rapid onset of action. However, Shafer and Varvel[12] have emphasized that making a rational choice among these opioids requires an understanding of the relationships between their pharmacokinetics and pharmacodynamics. They have used elegant computer models to simulate the rate of decrease in plasma and effect site (brain) concentrations after various administration methods, including bolus doses, brief infusion, and prolonged infusion. Decreases in effect site concentration will determine time to recovery from various opioid effects. Comparable simulations have also been done for the newer opioid remifentanil.[240] Important pharmacokinetic differences among these opioids include volumes of distribution and intercompartmental (distributional) and central (elimination) clearances. A smaller distribution volume tends to shorten recovery time, and a reduction in clearance tends to increase recovery time.[12] The major pharmacodynamic differences among these opioids are potency and the equilibration times between the plasma and the site of drug effect. Equilibration half-times between plasma and effect site are 5–6 minutes for fentanyl and sufentanil and 1.3–1.5 minutes for alfentanil and remifentanil.[12,227] Computer simulations demonstrate that simply comparing elimination half-lives will not predict the relative rate of decline in drug concentration at the effect site after either bolus doses or continuous infusion of fentanyl, sufentanil, and alfentanil. The rate of recovery after a continuous infusion will depend on the duration of the infusion as well as the magnitude of decline that is required. Figure 14-14 demonstrates how the times required for 20, 50, and 80% decrements in effect site (i.e., brain) concentrations vary with each opioid depending on infusion duration. If only a 20% drop in effect site concentration is required (upper panel), recovery from all three opioids will be rapid, although recovery time increases for fentanyl after 3 hours of drug infusion. However, if a 50%

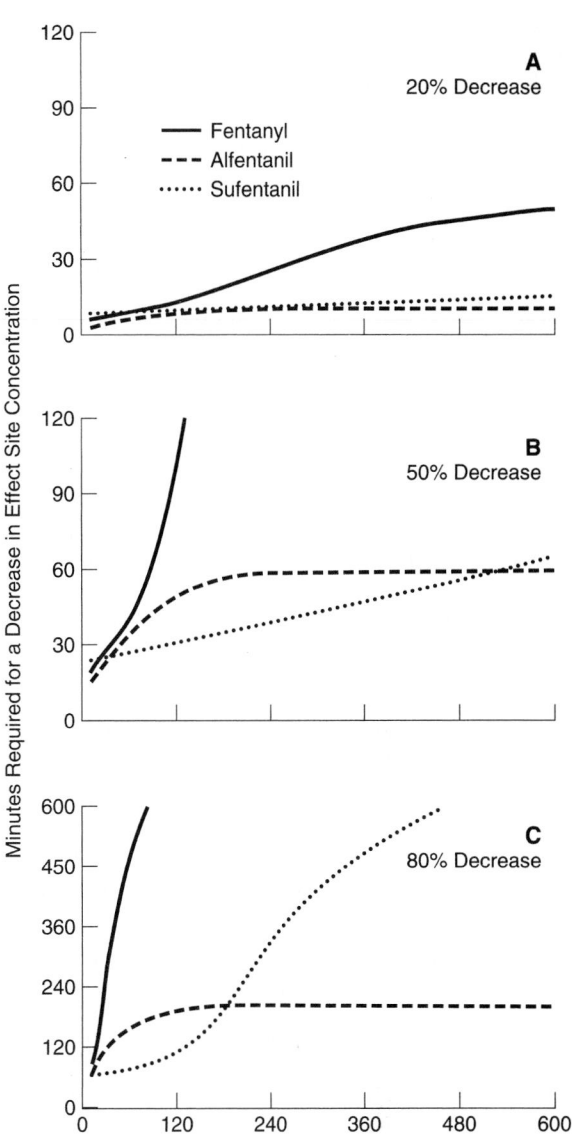

Figure 14-14. Recovery curves for fentanyl, sufentanil, and alfentanil showing the time required for decreases of 20% (*A*), 50% (*B*), and 80% (*C*) from maintained intraoperative effect site (brain) concentrations after termination of the infusion. (Reprinted with permission from Shafer SL, Varvel JR: Pharmacokinetics, pharmacodynamics, and rational opioid selection. Anesthesiology 74:53, 1991.)

decrease is required, recovery from sufentanil will be fastest for infusions less than 6–8 hours in duration, but more rapid for alfentanil if infusions are continued for more than 8 hours.

Context-Sensitive Half-time

Hughes *et al*[13] expanded the concepts of Shafer and Varvel to define the relative contributions of distribution compartments to central compartment (plasma) drug distribution. These relative contributions vary according to infusion duration. Hughes devised the concept of "context-sensitive half-time," which is defined as the time required for the drug concentration in the central compartment to decrease by 50%, and demonstrated how this half-time changes as drug infusion duration increases. During an infusion, the peripheral (fast and slow) compartments begin to fill up. After the infusion is stopped, drug will be eliminated, but will also continue to be redistributed as long as the concentration in a peripheral compartment is lower than that in the central compartment. This leads to a rapid drop in central compartment drug concentration. When central compartment (plasma) concentration drops below that of the peripheral compartment(s), the direction of drug redistribution will reverse, and will slow the decline in plasma concentration. The degree to which redistribution will affect the rate of drug elimination depends on the ratio of the distributional to elimination time constants. Thus, a drug that can rapidly redistribute will have a correspondingly larger contribution from the peripheral compartment(s), and plasma concentration will drop progressively more slowly as infusion duration continues. Figure 14-15 illustrates the context-sensitive half-times for fentanyl, alfentanil, sufentanil, and remifentanil. This model predicts the time to a 50% concentration decrease in the plasma, which will reflect but not be equal to, effect site concentrations depicted in Figure 14-14.

It is important to point out that these are theoretical predictions based on computer models, which require testing in humans for validation. Kapila et al[284] compared modeled context-sensitive half-times with measured decreases in drug concentration and drug effect (respiratory depression) in volunteers receiving remifentanil and alfentanil. After 3-hour opioid infusions, measured whole blood opioid concentrations and recovery of ventilatory drive corresponded closely to modeled values for both drugs. To date, these predictions have not been validated during anesthesia for surgical procedures. Although the concept of a context-sensitive half-time appears to be useful, Hughes et al[13] noted that it is unknown whether a decrement of 50% provides the most clinically useful description of the rate of offset of opioid effects. If one closely titrates infusions so that minimum effective concentrations are achieved, perhaps much smaller decrements will be necessary. In practice, it is relatively easy to administer higher than necessary doses of opioids, particularly to mechanically ventilated patients, because hemodynamic consequences are minimal. Titrating against a quantifiable parameter, such as minute ventilation in a spontaneously breathing patient, may allow a tighter dose titration. It does seem clear, however, that some context-sensitive index is more useful than the elimination half-life. Understanding these concepts can be useful when deciding which opioid to use, as well as in adapting guidelines for opioid dosage and infusion rates depending on the duration of anesthesia.

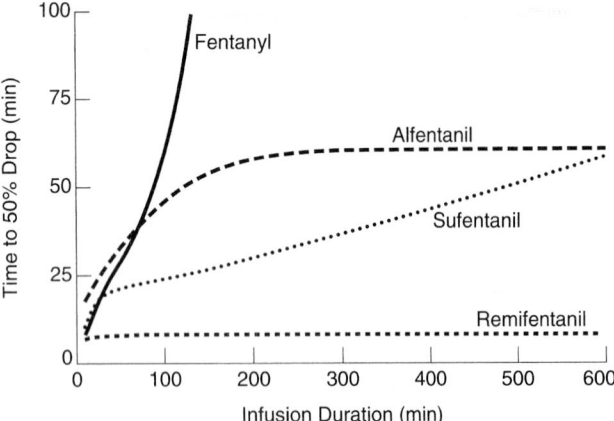

Figure 14-15. Contex-sensitive half-times for fentanyl, sufentanil, alfentanil, and remifentanil. This computer simulation depicts the time necessary to achieve a 50% reduction in plasma opioid concentration as a function of infusion duration. (Reprinted with permission from Egan TD, Lemmens HJM, Fiset P *et al:* The pharmacokinetics of the new short-acting opioid remifentanil (GI87084B) in healthy adult male volunteers. Anesthesiology 79:881, 1993.)

REFERENCES

1. Jaffe JH, Martin WR: Opioid analgesics and antagonists. In Gilman AG, Goodman LS, Rall TW, Murad F (eds): The Pharmacological Basis of Therapeutics, p 491. New York, Macmillan, 1985
2. Rey A: L'Examen Clinique en Psychologie. Paris, Presses Universitaires de France, 1964
3. Lowenstein E: "Morphine anesthesia": A perspective. Anesthesiology 35:563, 1971
4. Janssen PA: The development of new synthetic narcotics. In Estafanous FG (ed): Opioids in Anesthesia, p 37. Boston, Butterworth, 1984
5. Martin WR: Multiple opioid receptors. Life Sci 128:1547, 1981
6. Hughes J, Smith TW, Kosterlitz HW et al: Identification of two related pentapeptides from the brain with potent opioid agonist activity. Nature 258:577, 1975
7. Pleuvry BJ: The endogenous opioid system. Anaesth Pharmacol Rev 1:114, 1993
8. Pasternak GW: Pharmacologic mechanisms of opioid analgesics. Clin Neuropharmacol 16:1, 1993
9. McFadzean I: The ionic mechanisms underlying opioid mechanisms. Neuropeptides 11:173, 1988
10. Horn AS, Rodgers JR: Structural and conformational relationships between the enkephalins and the opiates. Nature 260:795, 1976
11. Thorpe DH: Opiate structures and activity: A guide to underlying opioid actions. Anesth Analg 63:143, 1984
12. Shafer SL, Varvel JR: Pharmacokinetics, pharmacodynamics, and rational opioid selection. Anesthesiology 74:53, 1991
13. Hughes MA, Glass PSA, Jacobs JR: Context-sensitive half-time in multicompartment pharmacokinetic models for intravenous anesthetic drugs. Anesthesiology 76:334, 1992
14. Bovill JG: Pharmacokinetics and pharmacodynamics of opioid agonists. Anaesth Pharmacol Rev 1:122, 1993
15. Hansch C, Dunn WJ: Linear relationships between lipophilic character and biological activity of drugs. J Pharm Sci 61:1, 1972
16. Bernards CM, Hill HF: Physical and chemical properties of drug molecules governing their diffusion through the spinal meninges. Anesthesiology 77:750, 1992
17. Lipp J: Possible mechanisms of morphine analgesia. Clin Neuropharmacol 14:31, 1991
18. Yeung JC, Rudy TA: Multiplicative interaction between narcotic agonisms expressed at spinal and supraspinal sites of antinociceptive action as revealed by concurrent intrathecal and intracerebroventricular injections of morphine. J Pharmacol Exp Ther 215:633, 1980
19. Pick CG, Roques B, Gacel G, Pasternak GW: Supraspinal μ_2-opioid receptors mediate spinal/supraspinal morphine synergy. Eur J Pharmacol 220:275, 1992
20. Stein C: Peripheral mechanisms of opioid analgesia. Anesth Analg 76:182, 1993
21. Stein C, Millan MJ, Shippenberg TS et al: Peripheral opioid receptors mediating antinociception in inflammation: Evidence for involvement of μ, δ and κ receptors. J Pharmacol Exp Ther 248:1269, 1989
22. Dahlstrom B, Tamsen A, Psalzow I, Hartvig P: Patient-controlled analgesia therapy. Part IV: Pharmacokinetics and analgesic plasma concentrations of morphine. Clin Pharmacokinetics 7:266, 1982
23. Hill HF, Coda BA, Mackie AM, Iverson K: Patient-controlled analgesic infusions: alfentanil versus morphine. Pain 49:301, 1992
24. Roizen MF, Newfield P, Eger E et al: Reduced anesthetic requirement after electrical stimulation of periaqueductal gray matter. Anesthesiology 62:120, 1985
25. Murphy MR, Hug CC: The enflurane-sparing effect of morphine, butorphanol, and nalbuphine. Anesthesiology 57:489, 1982
26. Lake CL, DiFazio CA, Moscicki JC et al: Reduction in halothane MAC: Comparison of morphine and alfentanil. Anesth Analg 64:807, 1985
27. Steffey EP, Eisele JH, Baggot JD et al: Influence of inhaled anesthetics on the pharmacokinetics and pharmacodynamics of morphine. Anesth Analg 77:346, 1993
28. Roizen MF, Horrigan RW, Frazer BM: Anesthetic doses blocking adrenergic (stress) and cardiovascular responses to incision-MAC BAR. Anesthesiology 54:390, 1981
29. Schweiger IM, Klopfenstein CE, Forster A: Epidural morphine reduces halothane MAC in humans. Can J Anaesth 39:911, 1992
30. Drasner K, Bernards CM, Ozanne GM: Intrathecal morphine reduces the minimum alveolar concentration of halothane in humans. Anesthesiology 69:310, 1988

31. Licina MG, Schubert A, Tobin JE *et al:* Intrathecal morphine dose not reduce minimum alveolar concentration of halothane in humans: Results of a double-blind study. Anesthesiology 74:660, 1991

32. Coda BA, Hill HF, Hunt EB *et al:* Cognitive and motor function impairments during continuous opioid analgesic infusions. Hum Psychopharmacol 8:383, 1993

33. Smith NT, Dee-Silver H, Sanford TJ *et al:* EEGs during high-dose fentanyl–, sufentanil–, or morphine–oxygen anesthesia. Anesth Analg 63:386, 1984

34. Martin WR: Pharmacology of opioids. Pharmacol Rev 35:283, 1984

35. Thomas DA, Williams GM, Iwata K *et al:* Multiple effects of morphine on facial scratching in monkeys. Anesth Analg 77:933, 1993

36. Thomas DA, Williams GM, Iwata K *et al:* The medullary dorsal horn: A site of action of morphine in producing facial scratching in monkeys. Anesthesiology 79:548, 1993

37. Arunasalam K, Davenport HT, Painter S *et al:* Ventilatory response to morphine in young and old subjects. Anaesthesia 38:529, 1983

38. Daykin AP, Bowen DJ, Saunders DA, Norman J: Respiratory depression after morphine in the elderly. Anaesthesia 41:910, 1986

39. Johnstone RE, Jobes DR, Kennell EM *et al:* Reversal of morphine anesthesia with naloxone. Anesthesiology 41:361, 1974

40. Forrest WH, Bellville JW: The effect of sleep plus morphine on the respiratory response to carbon dioxide. Anesthesiology 25:137, 1964

41. Catley DM, Thornton C, Jordan C *et al:* Pronounced episodes of oxygen desaturation on the postoperative period: Its association with ventilatory pattern and analgesic regimen. Anesthesiology 63:20, 1985

42. Duthie DJR, Nimmo WS: Adverse effects of opioid analgesic drugs. Br J Anaesth 59:61, 1987

43. Freund FG, Martin WE, Wong KC *et al:* Abdominal-muscle rigidity induced by morphine and nitrous oxide. Anesthesiology 38:358, 1973

44. Smith NT, Benthuysen JL, Bickford RG *et al:* Seizures during opioid anesthetic induction: Are they opioid-induced rigidity? Anesthesiology 71:852, 1989

45. Havemann U, Kuschinsky K: Further characterization of opioid receptors in the striatum mediating muscular rigidity in rats. Naunyn Schmiedebergs Arch Pharmakol 317:321, 1981

46. Weinger MB, Cline EJ, Smith NT *et al:* Localization of brainstem sites which mediate alfentanil-induced muscle rigidity in the rat. Pharmacol Biochem Behav 29:573, 1988

47. Bowdle TA, Rooke GA: Postoperative myoclonus and rigidity after anesthesia with opioids. Anesth Analg 78:783, 1994

48. Watcha MF, White PF: Postoperative nausea and vomiting. Anesthesiology 77:162, 1992

49. Hill HF, Chapman CR, Saeger LS *et al:* Steady-state infusions of opioids in human. II. Concentration–effect relationships and therapeutic margins. Pain 43:69, 1990

50. Peroutka SJ, Snyder SH: Antiemetics: Neurotransmitter receptor binding predicts therapeutic actions. Lancet 20:659, 1982

51. Costello DJ, Borison HL: Naloxone antagonizes narcotic self blockade of emesis in the cat (abs). J Pharmacol Exp Ther 203:222, 1977

52. Coda BA, Mackie A, Hill HF: Influence of alprazolam on opioid analgesia and side effects during steady-state morphine infusions. Pain 50:309, 1992

53. Burks TF, Fox DA, Hirning LD *et al:* Regulation of gastrointestinal function by multiple opioid receptors. Life Sci 43:2177, 1988

54. Porreca F, Mosberg HI, Hurst R *et al:* Roles of mu, delta and kappa opioid receptors in spinal and supraspinal mediation of gastrointestinal transit effects and hot-plate analgesia in the mouse. J Pharmacol Exp Ther 230:341, 1984

55. Murphy DB, Sutton JA, Prescott LF, Murphy MB: Opioid-induced delay in gastric emptying: A peripheral mechanism in humans. Anesthesiology 87(4):765, 1997

56. Thorén T, Wattwil M: Effects on gastric emptying of thoracic epidural analgesia with morphine or bupivicaine. Anesth Analg 67:687, 1988

57. Steinberg WM: Sphincter of Oddi dysfunction: A clinical controversy. Gastroenterology 95:1409, 1988

58. Hahn M, Baker R, Sullivan S: The effect of four narcotics on cholecystokinin octapepetide stimulated gallbladder contraction. Aliment Pharmacol Ther 2:129, 1988

59. Thune A, Baker RA, Saccone GT *et al:* Differing effects of pethidine and morphine on human sphincter of Oddi motility. Br J Surg 77:992, 1990

60. Ehrenpreis S, Kimura I, Kobayashi T *et al:* Histamine release as the basis for morphine action on bile duct and sphincter of Oddi. Life Sci 40:1695, 1987

61. Dray A: Epidural opiates and urinary retention: New models provide new insights. Anesthesiology 68:323, 1988

62. Durant PAC, Yaksh TL: Drug effects on urinary bladder tone during spinal morphine-induced inhibition of the micturition reflex in unanesthetized rats. Anesthesiology 68:325, 1988

63. Stellato C, Cirillo R, de Paulis A *et al:* Human basophil/mast cell releasability: IX. Heterogeneity of the effects of opioids on mediator release. Anesthesiology 77:32, 1992

64. Hermens JM, Ebertz JM, Hanifin JM, Hirshman CA: Comparison of histamine release in human skin mast cells induced by morphine, fentanyl, and oxymorphone. Anesthesiology 62:124, 1985

65. Hakim TS, Grunstein MM, Michel RP: Opiate action in the pulmonary circulation. Pulm Pharmacol 5:159, 1992

66. Rosow CE, Moss J, Philbin DM *et al:* Histamine release during morphine and fentanyl anesthesia. Anesthesiology 56:93, 1982

67. Lowenstein E, Whiting RB, Bittar DA *et al:* Local and neurally mediated effects of morphine on skeletal muscle vascular resistance. J Pharmacol Exp Ther 180:359, 1972

68. Strauer BE: Contractile responses to morphine, piritramide, meperidine, and fentanyl: A comparative study of the effects on the isolated ventricular myocardium. Anesthesiology 37:304, 1972

69. Roizen MF: Does the chioce of anesthetic (narcotic *versus* inhalational) significantly affect cardiovascular outcome after cardiovascular surgery? In Estafanous FG (ed): Opioids in Anesthesia, p 180. Boston, Butterworth, 1984

70. Stanski DR, Greenblatt DJ, Lowenstein E: Kinetics of intravenous and intramuscular morphine. Clin Pharmacol Ther 24:52, 1978

71. Murphy MR, Hug CC: Pharmacokinetics of intravenous morphine in patients anesthetized with enflurane–nitrous oxide. Anesthesiology 54:187, 1981

72. Mazoit JX, Sandouk P, Zetlaoui P: Pharmacokinetics of unchanged morphine in normal volunteers. Anesth Analg 66:293, 1987

73. Sear JW, Hand CW, Moore RA, McQuay HJ: Studies on morphine disposition: influence of general anesthesia on plasma concentrations of morphine and its metabolites. Br J Aneasth 662:22, 1989

74. Lynn AM, Slattery JT: Morphine pharmacokinetics in early infancy. Anesthesiology 66:136, 1987

75. Osborne R, Joel S, Trew D *et al:* Morphine and metabolite behavior after different routes of morphine administration: Demonstration of the importance of the active metabolite morphine-6-glucuronide. Clin Pharmacol Ther 47:12, 1990

76. Pasternak GW, Bodnar RJ, Clark JA, Inturrisi CE: Morphine-6-glucuronide: A potent mu agonist. Life Sci 41:2845, 1987

77. Lehmann KA, Zech D: Morphine-6-glucuronide, a pharmacologically active morphine metabolite: A review of the literature. Eur J Pain 14:28, 1993

78. Portenoy RK, Thaler HT, Inturrisi CE *et al:* The metabolite morphine-6-glucuronide contributes to the analgesia produced by morphine infusion in patients with pain and normal renal function. Clin Pharmacol Ther 51:422, 1992

79. Osborne R, Thompson P, Joel S *et al:* The analgesic activity of morphine-6-glucuronide. Br J Clin Pharmacol 34:130, 1992

80. Gross JB, Alexander CM: Awakening concentrations of isoflurane are not affected by analgesic doses of morphine. Anesth Analg 67:27, 1988

81. Kurz M, Belani KG, Sessler DI *et al:* Naloxone, meperidine, and shivering. Anesthesiology 79:1193, 1993

82. Austin KL, Stapleton JV, Mather LE: Relationship between blood meperidine concentrations and analgesic response: A preliminary report. Anesthesiology 53:460, 1980

83. Tamsen A, Hartvig P, Fagerlund C *et al:* Patient-controlled analgesic therapy, part II: Individual analgesic demand and analgesic plasma concentrations of pethidine in postoperative pain. Clin Pharmacokinet 7:164, 1982

84. Steffey EP, Martucci R, Howland D *et al:* Meperidine–halothane interaction in dogs. Can Anaesth Soc J 24:459, 1977

85. Kaya K, Babacan A, Beyazova M *et al:* Effects of perineural opioids on nerve conduction of N. suralis in man. Acta Neurol Scand 85:337, 1992

86. Hassan HG, Pilcher CW, Akerman B *et al:* Antinociceptive effects of localized administration of opioids compared with lidocaine. Reg Anesth 14:138, 1989

87. Kaza R, Lawlor M, Allen W *et al:* Epidural meperidine provides

surgical anesthesia for critically ill patients undergoing major surgery. Anesth Analg 77:1077, 1993

88. Kafle SK: Intrathecal meperidine for elective caesarean section: A comparison with lidocaine. Can J Anaesth 40:718, 1993

89. Radnay PA, Duncalf D, Novakovic M et al: Common bile duct pressure changes after fentanyl, morphine, meperidine, butorphanol, and naloxone. Anesth Analg 63:441, 1984

90. Yrjola H, Heinonen J, Tuominen M et al: Comparison of haemodynamic effects of pethidine and anileridine in anaesthetised patients. Acta Anaesthesiol Scand 25:412, 1981

91. Rendig SV, Amsterdam EA, Henderson GL, Mason DT: Comparative cardiac contractile actions of six narcotic analgesics: Morphine, meperidine, pentazocine, fentanyl, methadone and L-α-acetylmethadol (LAAM). J Pharmacol Exp Ther 215:259, 1980

92. Flacke JW, Bloor BC, Kripke BJ et al: Comparison of morphine, meperidine, fentanyl, and sufentanil in balanced anesthesia: A double-blind study. Anesth Analg 64:897, 1985

93. Macintyre PE, Pavlin EG, Dwersteg JF: Effect of meperidine on oxygen consumption, carbon dioxide production, and respiratory gas exchange in postanesthesia shivering. Anesth Analg 66:751, 1987

94. Casey WF, Smith CE, Katz JM et al: Intravenous meperidine for control of shivering during caesarean section under epidural anaesthesia. Can J Anaesth 35:128, 1988

95. Pauca AL, Savage RT, Simpson S et al: Effect of pethidine, fentanyl and morphine on post-operative shivering in children. Acta Anaesthesiol Scand 28:138, 1984

96. Vogelsang J, Hayes SR: Butorphanol tartrate (Stadol) relieves postanesthesia shaking more effectively than meperidine (Demerol) or morphine. J Post Anesth Nurs 7:94, 1992

97. Kurz A, Go JC, Sessler DI, Kaer K et al: Alfentanil slightly increases the sweating threshold and markedly reduces the vasoconstriction and shivering thresholds. Anesthesiology 83:293, 1995

98. Joris J, Banache M, Bonnet F et al: Clonidine and ketanserin both are effective treatment for postanesthetic shivering. Anesthesiology 79:532, 1993

99. Matsukawa T, Kurz A, Sessler DI et al: Propofol linearly reduces the vasoconstriction and shivering thresholds. Anesthesiology 82:1169, 1995

100. Horn E-P, Standl T, Sessler DI et al: Physostigmine prevents postanesthetic shivering as does meperidine or clonidine. Anesthesiology 88:108, 1998

101. Mather LE, Tucker GT, Pflug AE et al: Meperidine kinetics in man: Intravenous injection in surgical patients and volunteers. Clin Pharmacol Ther 17:27, 1975

102. Koska AJ, Kramer WG, Romagnoli A et al: Pharmacokinetics of high-dose meperidine in surgical patients. Anesth Analg 60:8, 1981

103. Verbeeck RK, Branch RA, Wilkinson GR: Meperidine disposition in man: Influence of urinary pH and route of administration. Clin Pharmacol Ther 30:619, 1981

104. Wong YC, Chan K, Lau OW et al: Protein binding characterization of pethidine and norpethidine and lack of interethnic variability. Methods Find Exp Clin Pharmacol 13:273, 1991

105. Kaiko RF, Foley KM, Grabinski PY et al: Central nervous system excitatory effects of meperidine in cancer patients. Ann Neurol 13:180, 1983

106. Gourlay GK, Wilson PR, Glynn CJ: Pharmacodynamics and pharmacokinetics of methadone during the perioperative period. Anesthesiology 57:458, 1982

107. Gourlay GK, Willis RJ, Wilson PR: Postoperative pain control with methadone: Influence of supplementary methadone doses and blood concentration–response relationships. Anesthesiology 61:19, 1984

108. Wangler MA, Rosenblatt RM: Methadone titration to avoid excessive respiratory depression. Anesthesiology 59:363, 1983

109. Gourlay GK, Willis RJ, Wilson PR: Methadone titration to avoid excessive respiratory depression. Anesthesiology 59:364, 1983

110. Scott JC, Ponganis KV, Stanski DR: EEG quantitation of of narcotic effect: The comparative pharmacodynamics of fentanyl and alfentanil. Anesthesiology 62:234, 1985

111. Gourlay GK, Kowalski SR, Plummer JL et al: Fentanyl blood concentration–analgesic response relationship in the treatment of postoperative pain. Anesth Analg 67:329, 1988

112. Hug CC: Pharmacokinetics of new synthetic narcotic analgesics. In Estafanous FG (ed): Opioids in Anesthesia, p 50. Boston, Butterworth, 1984

113. Sebel PS, Glass PSA, Fletcher JE et al: Reduction of the MAC of desflurane with fentanyl. Anesthesiology 76:52, 1992

114. Daniel M, Weiskopf RB, Noorani M, Eger EI: Fentanyl augments the blockade of the sympathetic response to incision (MAC-BAR) produced by desflurane and isoflurane. Anesthesiology 88:43, 1998

115. Westmoreland CL, Sebel PS, Gropper A: Fentanyl or alfentanil decreases the minimum alveolar anesthetic concentration of isoflurane in surgical patients. Anesth Analg 78:23, 1994

116. McEwan AI, Smith C, Dyar O et al: Isoflurane minimum alveolar concentration reduction by fentanyl. Anesthesiology 78:864, 1993

117. Katoh T, Ikeda K: The effects of fentanyl on sevoflurane requirements for loss of consciousness and skin incision. Anesthesiology 88:18, 1998

118. Inagaki Y, Mashimo T, Yoshiya I: Segmental analgesic effect and reduction of halothane MAC from epidural fentanyl in humans. Anesth Analg 74:856, 1992

119. Kazama T, Ikeda K, Morita K: The pharmacodynamic interaction between propofol and fentanyl with respect to the suppression of somatic or hemodynamic responses to skin incision, peritoneum incision, and abdominal wall retraction. Anesthesiology 89:894, 1998

120. Shafer SL, Varvel JR, Aziz N et al: Pharmacokinetics of fentanyl administered by computer-controlled infusion pump. Anesthesiology 73:1091, 1990

121. Glass PSA, Jacobs JR, Smith LR et al: Pharmacokinetic model-driven infusion of fentanyl: Assessment of accuracy. Anesthesiology 73:1082, 1990

122. Glass PSA, Doherty M, Jacobs JR et al: Plasma concentration of fentanyl with 70% nitrous oxide, to prevent movement at skin incision. Anesthesiology 78:842, 1993

123. Philbin DM, Rosow CE, Schneider RC et al: Fentanyl and sufentanil anesthesia revisited: How much is enough? Anesthesiology 73:5, 1990

124. Mummaneni N, Rao TLK, Montoya A: Awareness and recall with high-dose fentanyl–oxygen anesthesia. Anesth Analg 59:948, 1980

125. Trindle MR, Dodson BA, Rampil IJ: Effects of fentanyl versus sufentanil in equianesthetic doses on middle cerebral artery blood flow volume. Anesthesiology 78:454, 1993

126. Sperry RJ, Bailey PL, Reichman MV et al: Fentanyl and sufentanil increase intracranial pressure in head trauma patients. Anesthesiology 77:416, 1992

127. Jung R, Shah N, Reinsel R et al: Cerebrospinal fluid pressure in patients with brain tumors: Impact of fentanyl versus alfentanil during nitrous oxide–oxygen anesthesia. Anesth Analg 71:419, 1990

128. Streisand JB, Bailey PL, LeMaire L et al: Fentanyl-induced rigidity and unconsciousness in human volunteers. Anesthesiology 78:629, 1993

129. Bailey PL, Wilbrink J, Zwanikken P et al: Anesthetic induction with fentanyl. Anesth Analg 64:48, 1985

130. Lunn JK, Stanley TH, Eisele J et al: High dose fentanyl anesthesia for coronary artery surgery: Plasma fentanyl concentrations and influence of nitrous oxide on cardiovascular responses. Anesth Analg 58:390, 1979

131. Scott JC, Sarnquist FH: Seizure-like movements during a fentanyl infusion with absence of seizure activity in a simultaneous EEG recording. Anesthesiology 62:812, 1985

132. Manninen PH, Burke SJ, Wennberg R et al: Intraoperative localization of epileptogenic focus with alfentanil and fentanyl. Anesth Analg 88:1101, 1999

133. Phua WT, Teh BT, Jong W et al: Tussive effect of a fentanyl bolus. Can J Anaesth 38:330, 1991

134. McClain DA, Hug CC: Intravenous fentanyl kinetics. Clin Pharmacol Ther 28:106, 1980

135. Bailey PL, Pace NL, Ashburn MA et al: Frequent hypoxemia and apnea after sedation with midazolam and fentanyl. Anesthesiology 73:826, 1990

136. Bailey PL, Streisand JB, East KA et al: Differences in magnitude and duration of opioid-induced respiratory depression and analgesia with fentanyl and sufentanil. Anesth Analg 70:8, 1990

137. Knill RL: Does sufentanil produce less ventilatory depression than fentanyl? Anesth Analg 71:564, 1990

138. Cartwright P, Prys-Roberts C, Gill K et al: Ventilatory depression related to plasma fentanyl concentrations during and after anesthesia in humans. Anesth Analg 62:966, 1983

139. Tagaito Y, Isono S, Nishino T: Upper airway reflexes during a

combination of propofol and fentanyl anesthesia. Anesthesiology 88:1459, 1998

140. Stanley TH, Webster LR: Anesthetic requirements and cardiovascular effects of fentanyl–oxygen and fentanyl–diazepam–oxygen anesthesia in man. Anesth Analg 57:411, 1978

141. Bovill JG, Sebel PS, Stanley TH: Opioid analgesics in anesthesia: With special reference to their use in cardiovascular anesthesia. Anesthesiology 61:731, 1984

142. Flacke JW, Flacke WE, Bloor BC et al: Histamine release by four narcotics: A double-blind study in humans. Anesth Analg 66:723, 1987

143. Reves JG, Kissin I, Fournier SE et al: Additive negative inotropic effet of a combination of diazepam and fentanyl. Anesth Analg 63:97, 1984

144. Giesecke K, Hamberger B, Järnberg PO et al: High- and low-dose fentanyl anaesthesia: Hormonal and metabolic responses during cholecystectomy. Br J Anaesth 61:575, 1988

145. Hug CC, Murphy MR: Tissue redistribution of fentanyl and termination of its effects in rats. Anesthesiology 55:369, 1981

146. Mather LE: Clinical pharmacokinetics of fentanyl and its newer derivatives. Clin Pharmacokinetics 8:422, 1983

147. Bentley JB, Borel JD, Nenad RE et al: Age and fentanyl pharmacokinetics. Anesth Analg 61:968, 1982

148. Scott JC, Stanski DR: Decreased fentanyl and alfentanil dose requirements with age: A simultaneous pharmacokinetic and pharmacodynamic evaluation. J Pharmacol Exp Ther 240:159, 1987

149. Singleton MA, Rosen JI, Fisher DM: Pharmacokinetics of fentanyl in the elderly. Br J Anaesth 60:619, 1986

150. Meuldermans WEG, Hurkmans RMA, Heykants JJP: Plasma protein binding and distribution of fentanyl, sufentanil, alfentanil and lofentanil in blood. Arch Int Pharmacodyn 257:4, 1982

151. Streisand JB, Stanski DR, Hague B et al: Oral transmucosal fentanyl citrate premedication in children. Anesth Analg 69:28, 1989

152. Gerwels JW, Bezzant JL, Le Maire L et al: Oral transmucosal fentanyl citrate for painful procedures in patients undergoing outpatient dermatologic procedures. J Dermatol Surg Oncol 20:823, 1994

153. Stanley TH, Hague B, Mock DL et al: Oral transmucosal fentanyl citrate (lollipop) premedication in volunteers. Anesth Analg 69:21, 1989

154. Martin DE, Rosenberg H, Aukberg SJ et al: Low-dose fentanyl blunts circulatory responses to tracheal intubation. Anesth Analg 61:680, 1982

155. Foldes FF: Neuroleptanesthesia for general surgery. In Oyama T (ed): International Anesthesiology Clinics, p 1. Boston, Little, Brown, 1973

156. Sprigge JS, Wynands JE, Whalley DG et al: Fentanyl infusion anesthesia for aortocoronary bypass surgery: Plasma levels and hemodynamic response. Anesth Analg 61:972, 1982

157. Monk JP, Beresford R, Ward A: Sufentanil: A review of its pharmacological properties and therapeutic use. Drugs 36:286, 1988

158. Scott JC, Cooke JE, Stanski DR: Electroencephalographic quantitation of opioid effect: Comparitive pharmacodynamics of fentanyl and sufentanil. Anesthesiology 74:34, 1991

159. Colpaert FC, Leysen JE, Michiels M et al: Epidural and intravenous sufentanil in the rat: Analgesia, opiate receptor binding, and drug concentrations in plasma and brain. Anesthesiology 65:41, 1986

160. Geller E, Chrubasik J, Graf R et al: A randomized double-blind comparison of epidural sufentanil versus intravenous sufentanil or epidural fentanyl analgesia after major abdominal surgery. Anesth Analg 76:1243, 1993

161. Lehmann KA, Gerhard A, Horrichs-Haermeyer G et al: Postoperative patient-controlled analgesia with sufentanil: Analgesic efficacy and minimum effective concentrations. Acta Anaesthesiol Scand 35:221, 1991

162. Coda BA, Hill HF, Bernards C et al: Comparison of therapeutic margins of sufentanil and morphine during steady-state infusions in volunteers. Anesthesiology 75:A673, 1991

163. Hecker BR, Lake CL, DiFazio CA et al: The decrease of the minimum alveolar anesthetic concentration produced by sufentanil in rats. Anesth Analg 62:987, 1983

164. Hall RI, Murphy MR, Hug CC: The enflurane sparing effect of sufentanil in dogs. Anesthesiology 67:518, 1987

165. Brunner MD, Braithwaite P, Jhaveri R et al: MAC reduction of isoflurane by sufentanil. Br J Anaesth 72:42, 1994

166. Bailey JM, Schweiger IM, Hug CC: Evaluation of sufentanil anesthesia obtained by a computer-controlled infusion for cardiac surgery. Anesth Analg 76:247, 1993

167. Bowdle TA: Myoclonus following sufentanil without EEG seizure activity. Anesthesiology 67:593, 1987

168. Marx W, Shah N, Long C et al: Sufentanil, alfentanil, and fentanyl: Impact on cerebrospinal fluid pressure in patients with brain tumors. J Neurosurg Anesth 1:3, 1989

169. Mayer N, Weinstabl C, Podreka I et al: Sufentanil does not increase cerebral blood flow in healthy human volunteers. Anesthesiology 73:240, 1990

170. Werner C, Hoffman WE, Baughman VL et al: Effects of sufentanil on cerebral blood flow, cerebral blood flow velocity, and metabolism in dogs. Anesth Analg 72:177, 1991

171. Welchew EA, Herbert P: Effects of sufentanil on respiration and heart rate during nitrous oxide and halothane anaesthesia. Br J Anaesth 58:120P, 1986

172. Robinson D: Respiratory arrest after recovery from anaesthesia supplemented with sufentanil. Can J Anaesth 35:101, 1988

173. Karasawa F, Iwanov V, Moulds RF: Sufentanil and alfentanil cause vasorelaxation by mechanisms independent of the endothelium. Clin Exp Pharmacol Physiol 20:705, 1993

174. Sebel PS, Bovil JG: Cardiovascular effects of sufentanil. Anesth Analg 61:115, 1982

175. Rosow CE: Cardiovascular effects of opioid analgesia. Mt Sinai J Med 54:273, 1987

176. Clark NJ, Meuleman T, Liu W et al: Comparison of sufentanil–N_2O and fentanyl–N_2O in patients without cardiac disease undergoing general surgery. Anesthesiology 66:130, 1987

177. Gauzit R, Marty J, Couderc E et al: Comparison of sufentanil and fentanyl to supplement N_2O–halothane anesthesia for total hip arthroplasty in elderly patients. Anesth Analg 72:756, 1991

178. Thomson IR, MacAdams CL, Hudson RJ et al: Drug interactions with sufentanil. Anesthesiology 76:922, 1992

179. Schmeling WT, Bernstein JS, Vucins EJ et al: Persistent bradycardia with episodic sinus arrest after sufentanil and vecuronium administration: Successful treatment with isoproterenol. J Cardiothorac Anesth 4:89, 1990

180. Sonntag H, Stephan H, Lange H et al: Sufentanil does not block sympathetic responses to surgical stimuli in patients having coronary artery revascularization surgery. Anesth Analg 68:584, 1989

181. Bovill JG, Sebel PS, Fiolet JWT et al: The influence of sufentanil on endocrine and metabolic responses to cardiac surgery. Anesth Analg 62:391, 1983

182. Bovill JG, Sebel PS, Blackburn CL et al: The pharmacokinetics of sufentanil in surgical patients. Anesthesiology 61:502, 1984

183. Schwartz AE, Matteo RS, Ornstein E et al: Pharmacokinetics of sufentanil in obese patients. Anesth Analg 73:790, 1991

184. Chauvin M, Ferrier C, Haberer JP et al: Sufentanil pharmacokinetics in patients with cirrhosis. Anesth Analg 68:1, 1989

185. Cork RC, Gallo JA, Weiss LB et al: Sufentanil infusion: Pharmacokinetics compared to bolus. Anesth Analg 67:S1, 1988

186. Hudson RJ, Bergstrom RG, Thomson IR et al: Pharmacokinetics of sufentanil in patients undergoing abdominal aortic surgery. Anesthesiology 70:426, 1989

187. Bowdle TA, Ward RJ: Induction of anesthesia with small doses of sufentanil or fentanyl: Dose versus EEG response, speed of onset, and thiopental requirement. Anesthesiology 70:26, 1989

188. Lehmann KA: The pharmacokinetics of opioid analgesics with special reference to patient-controlled administration. In Harmer M, Rosen M, Vickers MD (eds): Patient-Controlled Analgesia, p 18. Oxford, Blackwell Scientific, 1985

189. Camu F, Debucquoy F: Alfentanil infusions for postoperative pain: A comparison of epidural and intravenous routes. Anesthesiology 75:171, 1991

190. van den Nieuwenhuyzen MCO, Engbers FHM, Burm AGL et al: Computer-controlled infusion of alfentanil for postoperative analgesia: A pharmacokinetic and pharmacodynamic evaluation. Anesthesiology 79:481, 1993

191. Welchew EA, Hosking J: Patient-controlled postoperative analgesia with alfentanil. Anaesthesia 40:1172, 1985

192. Chauvin M, Hongnat JM, Mourgeon E et al: Equivalence of postoperative analgesia with patient-controlled intravenous or epidural alfentanil. Anesth Analg 76:1251, 1993

193. Hall RI, Szlam F, Hug CC: The enflurane-sparing effect of alfentanil in dogs. Anesth Analg 66:1287, 1987

194. Ausems ME, Hug CC, Stanski DR et al: Plasma concentrations of

alfentanil required to supplement nitrous oxide anesthesia for general surgery. Anesthesiology 65:362, 1986

195. Ausems ME, Vuyk J, Hug CC *et al:* Comparison of a computer-assisted infusion *versus* intermittent bolus administration of alfentanil as a supplement to nitrous oxide for lower abdominal surgery. Anesthesiology 68:851, 1988

196. Vuyk J, Lim T, Engbers FHM *et al:* Pharmacodynamics of alfentanil as a supplement to propofol or nitrous oxide for lower abdominal surgery in female patients. Anesthesiology 78:1036, 1993

197. Nauta J, de Lange S, Koopman D *et al:* Anesthetic induction with alfentanil: A new short-acting narcotic analgesic. Anesth Analg 61:267, 1982

198. de Lange S, de Bruijn NP: Alfentanil–oxygen anaesthesia: Plasma concentrations and clinical effects during variable-rate continuous infusion for coronary artery surgery. Br J Anaesth 55:183S, 1983

199. Hug CC, Hall RI, Angert KC *et al:* Alfentanil plasma concentration *vs.* effect relationships in cardiac surgical patients. Br J Anaesth 61:435, 1988

200. Hynynen M, Takkunen O, Salmenperä M *et al:* Continuous infusion of fentanyl or alfentanil for coronary artery surgery. Br J Anaesth 58:1252, 1986

201. Bovill JG, Sebel PS, Wauquier A *et al:* Influence of high-dose alfentanil anaesthesia on the electroencephalogram: Correlation with plasma concentrations. Br J Anaesth 55:199, 1983

202. Benthuysen JL, Smith NT, Sanford TJ *et al:* Physiology of alfentanil-induced rigidity. Anesthesiology 64:440, 1986

203. Mayberg TS, Lam AM, Eng CC *et al:* The effect of alfentanil on cerebral blood flow velocity and intracranial pressure during isoflurane–nitrous oxide anesthesia in humans. Anesthesiology 78:288, 1993

204. Arndt JO, Bednarski B, Parasher C: Alfentanil's analgesic, respiratory, and cardiovascular actions in relation to dose and plasma concentration in unanesthetized dogs. Anesthesiology 64:345, 1986

205. Owen H, Currie JC, Plummer JL: Variation in the blood concentration/analgesic response relationship during patient-controlled analgesia with alfentanil. Anaesth Intens Care 19:555, 1991

206. O'Connor M, Escarpa A, Prys-Roberts C: Ventilatory depression during and after infusion of alfentanil in man. Br J Anaesth 55:217S, 1983

207. Andrews CJH, Sinclair M, Prys-Roberts C *et al:* Ventilatory effects during and after continuous infusion of fentanyl or alfentanil. Br J Anaesth 55:211S, 1983

208. Stanley TH, Pace NL, Liu WS *et al:* Alfentanil–N₂O vs fentanyl–N₂O balanced anesthesia: Comparison of plasma hormonal changes, early postoperative respiratory function, and speed of postoperative recovery. Anesth Analg 62:245, 1983

209. Hudson RJ: Apnoea and unconsciousness after apparent recovery from alfentanil-supplemented anaesthesia. Can J Anaesth 37:255, 1990

210. Reitz JA: Alfentanil in anesthesia and analgesia. Drug Intell Clin Pharm 20:355, 1986

211. Rucquoi M, Camu F: Cardiovascular responses to large doses of alfentanil and fentanyl. Br J Anaesth 55:223S, 1983

212. Crawford DC, Fell D, Achola KJ *et al:* Effects of alfentanil on the pressor and catecholamine responses to tracheal intubation. Br J Anaesth 59:707, 1987

213. Kirby IJ, Northwood D, Dodson ME: Modification by alfentanil of the haemodynamic response to tracheal intubation in elderly patients. Br J Anaesth 60:384, 1988

214. Skues MA, Richards MJ, Jarvis A, Prys-Roberts C: Preinduction atropine or glycopyrrolate and hemodynamic changes associated with induction and maintenance of anesthesia with propofol and alfentanil. Anesth Analg 69:386, 1989

215. Silbert BS, Rosow CE, Keegan CR *et al:* The effect of diazepam on induction of anesthesia with alfentanil. Anesth Analg 65: 71, 1986

216. Kay B, Stephenson DK: Alfentanil (R39209): Initial clinical experience with a new narcotic analgesic. Anaesthesia 35:1197, 1980

217. Bloomfield EL: The incidence of postoperative nausea and vomiting: A retrospective comparison of alfentanil *versus* sufentanil. Mil Med 157:59, 1992

218. Sfez M, Mapihan YL, Gaillard JL *et al:* Analgesia for appendectomy: A comparison of fentanyl and alfentanil in children. Acta Anaesthesiol Scand 34:30, 1990

219. Bovill JG: Which potent opioid? Important criteria for selection. Drugs 33:520, 1987

220. Bovill JG, Sebel PS, Blackburn CL *et al:* The pharmacokinetics of alfentanil (R39209): A new opioid analgesic. Anesthesiology 57:439, 1982

221. Stanski DR, Hug CC: Alfentanil: A kinetically predictable narcotic analgesic. Anesthesiology 57:435, 1982

222. Chauvin M, Bonnet F, Montembault C *et al:* The influence of hepatic plasma flow on alfentanil plasma concentration plateaus achieved with an infusion model in humans: Measurement of alfentanil hepatic extraction coefficient. Anesth Analg 65:999, 1986

223. Ferrier C, Marty J, Bouffard Y *et al:* Alfentanil pharmacokinetics in patients with cirrhosis. Anesthesiology 62:480, 1985

224. Chauvin M, Lebrault C, Levron JC *et al:* Pharmacokinetics of alfentanil in chronic renal failure. Anesth Analg 66:53, 1987

225. Larijani GE, Goldberg ME: Alfentanil hydrochloride: A new short-acting narcotic analgesic for surgical procedures. Clin Pharm 6:275, 1987

226. James MK, Feldman PL, Schuster SV *et al:* Opioid receptor activity of GI87084B, a novel ultra-short acting analgesic, in isolated tissues. J Pharmacol Exp Ther 259:712, 1991

227. Glass PSA, Hardman D, Kamiyama Y *et al:* Preliminary pharmacokinetics and pharmacodynamics of an ultra-short-acting opioid: Remifentanil (GI87084B). Anesth Analg 77:1031, 1993

228. Michlesen LG, Salmenpera M, Hug CC *et al:* Anesthetic potency of remifentanil in dogs. Anesthesiology 84:865, 1996

229. Lang E, Kapila A, Shlugman D *et al:* Reduction of isoflurane minimal alveolar concentration by remifentanil. Anesthesiology 85:721, 1996

230. Peacock JE, Philip BK: Ambulatory anesthesia experience with remifentanil. Anesth Analg 89(suppl 4):S22, 1999

231. Fragen RJ, Randel GI, Librojo ES *et al:* The interaction of remifentanil and propofol to prevent response to tracheal intubation and the start of surgery for outpatient knee arthroscopy. Anesthesiology 81:A376, 1994

232. Jhaveri R, Joshi P, Batenhorst R *et al:* Dose comparison of remifentanil and alfentanil for loss of consciousness. Anesthesiology 87:253, 1997

233. Dershwitz M, Randel GI, Rosow CE *et al:* Initial clinical experience with remifentanil, a new opioid metabolized by estersases. Anesth Analg 81:619, 1995

234. Randel GI, Fragen RJ, Librojo ES *et al:* Remifentanil blood concentration effect relationship at intubation and skin incision in surgical patients compared to alfentanil. Anesthesiology 81:A375, 1994

235. Drover DR, Lemmens HJ: Population pharmacodynamics and pharmacokinetics of remifentanil as a supplement to nitrous oxide anesthesia for elective abdominal surgery. Anesthesiology 89(4): 869, 1998

236. Camu F, Royston D: Inpatient experience with remifentanil. Anesth Analg 89(suppl 4):S15, 1999

237. Hogue CW Jr, Bowdle TA, O'Leary C *et al:* A multicenter evaluation of total intravenous anesthesia with remifentanil and propofol for elective inpatient surgery. Anesth Analg 83(2):279, 1996

238. Philip BK, Scuderi PE, Chung F *et al:* Remifentanil compared with alfentanil for ambulatory surgery using total intravenous anesthesia. The Remifentanil/Alfentanil Outpatient TIVA Group. Anesth Analg 84(3):515, 1997

239. Cartwright DP, Kvalsvik O, Cassuto J *et al:* A randomized, blind comparison of remifentanil and alfentanil during anesthesia for outpatient surgery. Anesth Analg 85(5):1014, 1997

240. Egan TD, Lemmens HJM, Fiset P *et al:* The pharmacokinetics and pharmacodynamics of the new short-acting opioid remifentanil (GI87084B) in healthy adult male volunteers. Anesthesiology 79:881, 1993

241. Egan TD, Minto CF, Hermann DJ *et al:* Remifentanil *versus* alfentanil: Comparative pharmacokinetics and pharmacodynamics in healthy adult male volunteers [published erratum appears in Anesthesiology 85(3):695, 1996]. Anesthesiology 84(4):821, 1996

242. Hoffman WE, Cunnungham F, James MK *et al:* Effects of remifentanil, a new short-acting opioid, on cerebral blood flow, brain electrical activity, and intracranial pressure in dogs anesthetized with isoflurane and nitrous oxide. Anesthesiology 79:107, 1993

243. Warner DS, Hindman BJ, Todd MM *et al:* Intracranial pressure and hemodynamic effects of remifentanil *versus* alfentanil in patients undergoing supratentorial craniotomy. Anesth Analg 83(2):348, 1996

244. Guy J, Hindman BJ, Baker KZ *et al:* Comparison of remifentanil and fentanyl in patients undergoing craniotomy for supratentorial

space-occupying lesions [see comments]. Anesthesiology 86(3): 514, 1997

245. Ostapkovich ND, Baker KZ, Fogarty-Mack P *et al:* Cerebral blood flow and CO₂ reactivity is similar during remifentanil/N₂O and fentanyl/N₂O anesthesia. Anesthesiology 89(2):358, 1998

246. Paris A, Scholz J, von Knobelsdorff G *et al:* The effect of remifentanil on cerebral blood flow velocity. Anesth Analg 87(3):569, 1998

247. Glass PSA, Hardman HD, Kamiyama Y *et al:* Pharmacodynamic comparison of GI87084B (GI), a novel ultra-short acting opioid, and alfentanil. Anesth Analg 74:S113, 1992

248. Glass PS, Gan TJ, Howell S: A review of the pharmacokinetics and pharmacodynamics of remifentanil. Anesth Analg 89(suppl 4):S7, 1999

249. Daqing M, Chakrabarti MK, Whitwam JG: The combined effects of sevoflurane and remifentanil on central respiratory activity and nociceptive cardiovascular responses in anesthetized rabbits. Anesth Analg 89:453, 1999

250. Pitts MC, Palmore MM, Salmenpera MT *et al:* Pilot study: Hemodynamic effects of intravenous GI87084B (GI) in patients undergoing elective surgery. Anesthesiology 77:A101, 1992

251. Sebel PS, Hoke JF, Westmoreland C *et al:* Histamine concentrations and hemodynamic responses after remifentanil. Anesth Analg 80:990, 1995

252. DeSouza G, Lewis MC, TerRiet MF: Severe bradycardia after remifentanil [letter]. Anesthesiology 87(4):1019, 1997

253. Sung YF, Stulting RD, Beatie CD *et al:* Intraocular pressure (IOP) effects of remifentanil (R) (GI87084B) and alfentanil. Anesthesiology 81:A35, 1994

254. Pinsker MC, Carroll NV: Quality of emergence from anesthesia and incidence of vomiting with remifentanil in a pediatric population. Anesth Analg 89(1):71, 1999

255. Manullang J, Egan TD: Remifentanil's effect is not prolonged in a patient with pseudocholinesterase deficiency. Anesth Analg 89(2):529, 1999

256. Glass PSA, Gan TJ, Howell S: A review of the pharmacokinetics and pharmacodynamics of remifentanil. Anesth Analg 89:S7, 1999

257. Westmoreland CL, Hoke JF, Sebel PS *et al:* Pharmacokinetics of remifentanil (GI87084B) and its major metabolite (GI90291) in patients undergoing elective inpatient surgery. Anesthesiology 79:893, 1993

258. Dershwitz M, Hoke JF, Rosow CE *et al:* Pharmacokinetics and pharmacodynamics of remifentanil in volunteer subjects with severe liver disease. Anesthesiology 84(4):812, 1996

259. Hoke JF, Shlugman D, Dershwitz M *et al:* Pharmacokinetics and pharmacodynamics of remifentanil in persons with renal failure compared with healthy volunteers. Anesthesiology 87(3):533, 1997

260. Minto CF, Schnider TW, Egan TD *et al:* Influence of age and gender on the pharmacokinetics and pharmacodynamics of remifentanil. I. Model development. Anesthesiology 86(1):10, 1997

261. Egan TD, Huizinga B, Gupta SK *et al:* Remifentanil pharmacokinetics in obese *versus* lean patients [see comments]. Anesthesiology 89(3):562, 1998

262. Song D, Whitten CW, White PF: Use of remifentanil during anesthetic induction: A comparison with fentanyl in the ambulatory setting. Anesth Analg 88(4):734, 1999

263. Bowdle TA, Camporesi EM, Maysick L *et al:* A multicenter evaluation of remifentanil for early postoperative analgesia. Anesth Analg 83(6):1292, 1996

264. Ahmad S, Leavell ME, Fragen RJ *et al:* Remifentanil *versus* alfentanil as analgesic adjuncts during placement of ophthalmologic nerve blocks. Reg Anesth Pain Med 24(4):331, 1999

265. Servin F, Desmonts JM, Watkins WD: Remifentanil as an analgesic adjunct in local/regional anesthesia and in monitored anesthesia care. Anesth Analg 89(suppl 4):S28, 1999

266. Gold MI, Watkins WD, Sung YF *et al:* Remifentanil *versus* remifentanil/midazolam for ambulatory surgery during monitored anesthesia care. Anesthesiology 87(1):51, 1997

267. Sá Rêgo MM, Inagaki Y, White PF: Remifentanil administration during monitored anesthesia care: Are intermittent boluses an effective alternative to a continuous infusion? Anesth Analg 88:518, 1999

268. Bowdle TA: Partial agonist and agonist–antagonist opioids: Basic pharmacology and clinical applications. Anaesth Pharmacol Rev 1:135, 1993

269. Zsigmond EK, Winnie AP, Raza SMA *et al:* Nalbuphine as an analgesic component in balanced anesthesia for cardiac surgery. Anesth Analg 66:1155, 1987

270. Rawal N, Wennhager M: Influence of perioperative nalbuphine and fentanyl on postoperative respiration and analgesia. Acta Anaesthesiol Scand 34:197, 1990

271. O'Connor SA, Wilkinson DJ: A double-blind study of the respiratory effects of nalbuphine hydrochloride in spontaneously breathing anesthetized patients. Anesth Analg 67:324, 1988

272. Bailey PL, Clark NJ, Pace NL *et al:* Antagonism of postoperative opioid-induced respiratory depression: Nalbuphine *versus* naloxone. Anesth Analg 66:1109, 1987

273. Moldenhauer CC, Roach GW, Finlayson DC *et al:* Nalbuphine antagonism of ventilatory depression following high-dose fentanyl anesthesia. Anesthesiology 62:647, 1985

274. Bailey PL, Clark NJ, Pace NL *et al:* Failure of nalbuphine to antagonize morphine: A double-blind comparison with naloxone. Anesth Analg 65:605, 1986

275. Dershwitz M, Rosow CE, DiBiase PM *et al:* Comparison of the sedative effects of butorphanol and midazolam. Anesthesiology 74:717, 1991

276. Bowdle TA, Greichen SL, Bjurstrom RI *et al:* Butorphanol improves CO₂ response and ventilation after fentanyl anesthesia. Anesthesiol Analg 66:517, 1987

277. Pedersen JE: Perioperative buprenorphine: Do high doses shorten analgesia postoperatively? Acta Anaesthesiol Scand 30:660, 1986

278. Gal TL: Naloxone reversal of buprenorphine-induced respiratory depression. Clin Pharmacol Ther 45:66, 1989

279. Boysen K, Hertel S, Chraemmer-Jorgansen B *et al:* Buprenorphine antagonism of ventilatory depression following fentanyl anaesthesia. Acta Anaesthesiol Scand 32:490, 1988

280. Pallasch TJ, Gill CJ: Naloxone-associated morbidity and mortality. Oral Surg Oral Med Oral Pathol 52:602, 1981

281. Partridge BL, Ward CF: Pulmonary edema following low-dose naloxone administration. Anesthesiology 65:709, 1986

282. Prough DS, Roy R, Bumgarner J *et al:* Acute pulmonary edema in healthy teenagers following conservative doses of intravenous naloxone. Anesthesiology 60:485, 1984

283. Rawal N, Schött U, Dahlström B *et al:* Influence of naloxone infusion on analgesia and respiratory depression following epidural morphine. Anesthesiology 64:194, 1986

284. Kapila A, Glass PSA, Jacobs JR *et al:* Measured context-sensitive half-times of remifentanil and alfentanil. Anesthesiology 83:968, 1995

Clinical Anesthesia (4/e), edited by
Paul G. Barash, Bruce F. Cullen, and
Robert K. Stoelting. Lippincott Williams &
Wilkins, Philadelphia, © 2001.

CHAPTER 15

INHALATION ANESTHESIA

THOMAS J. EBERT AND PHILLIP G. SCHMID III

Inhalation anesthetics are the most common drugs used for the provision of general anesthesia. Adding as little as 1% of a volatile anesthetic to the inspired oxygen results in a state of unconsciousness and amnesia, which are essential components of general anesthesia. When combined with intravenous adjuvants, such as opioids or benzodiazepines, a balanced technique is achieved that results in further sedation/hypnosis and analgesia. The popularity of the inhaled anesthetics for establishing general anesthesia is based upon their ease of administration (*i.e., via* inhalation) and the ability to predictably monitor their effects (*i.e.,* clinical signs and end-tidal concentrations). In contrast to intravenous anesthetics, the tissue concentrations of the inhaled anesthetics can be closely estimated from the end-tidal concentrations of these agents. In addition, the volatile anesthetic gases are relatively inexpensive in terms of the overall cost of the anesthesia care of the patient. The most significant nonideal characteristic of the inhaled anesthetics is the narrow range between therapeutic and lethal doses. This is easily dealt with, however, by monitoring tissue concentrations and by titrating to common clinical endpoints.

The most popular potent inhaled anesthetics used in adult surgical procedures are isoflurane and the two new volatile anesthetics, sevoflurane and desflurane (Fig. 15-1). In pediatrics, halothane and sevoflurane are most commonly employed. Although there are many similarities in terms of the overall effects of the volatile anesthetics (*e.g.,* they all have a dose-dependent effect to decrease blood pressure), there are some unique differences that affect the clinician's selection for use. These differences are balanced with the patient's health and with the particular effects of the planned surgical procedure. Discussion of the four most popular inhaled anesthetics provides the major emphasis of this chapter. For the sake of completeness and for historical purposes related to metabolism and renal toxicity, reasonably detailed comments on both enflurane and methoxyflurane are included.

HISTORY

The volatile anesthetics in early clinical use consisted of flammable gases, including diethyl ether, cyclopropane, and divinyl ether. Several nonflammable compounds were available, including chloroform and trichloroethylene, but these were associated with hepatic toxicity and neurotoxicity and enjoyed but a brief period of clinical use. In the early 1930s studies on derivatives of the halogenated compound chloroform indicated that noncombustible anesthetic gases might be derived using organic fluoride compounds. Advances in fluorine chemistry in the 1940s allowed safe incorporation of fluorine into molecules at a reasonable expense. The advances in fluorine chemistry were driven by an appreciation of the role of fluorine in the production of high-octane aviation fuel and in the enrichment of uranium-235, both important issues in the war time effort. These advances proved to be pivotal to the development of modern-day anesthetics. There were approximately 46 fluorine-containing compounds synthesized by Dr. Earl McBee in research supported from the secret Manhattan project and from the Mallinkrodt Company. Although none of these ultimately proved to be useful as anesthetics in humans, several were very close in structure to what we now know as halothane. Fluorine is the halogen with the lowest atomic weight (18.998; chlorine = 35.45; bromine = 79.90; iodine = 126.9). Fluorine substitu-

tions for other halogens on the ether molecule lowered the boiling point, increased stability, and generally decreased toxicity. The fluoride ion also damped the flammable hydrocarbon of the ether anesthetic framework.

In 1951, halothane was synthesized and extensively tested in animals by Suckling, working at ICI Laboratory in England.[1] Halothane was introduced into clinical practice in 1956 and was rapidly embraced, owing in part to its nonflammability and in part to its lower tissue solubility. Halothane also had a relatively low pungency and a high potency; thus, it could be administered in high inspired concentrations (relative to its potency) to induce anesthesia. It proved to be well accepted *via* inhalation in both adults and children. Another advantage of halothane over the older volatile anesthetics was the lower incidence of nausea and vomiting associated with its use.

Despite these desirable properties of halothane, some concerns and drawbacks remained. Most notable were the effects of halothane on sensitizing the myocardium to catecholamines and the later described role of its intermediate metabolite in hepatic necrosis. Thus, the search for better agents continued. Between 1959 and 1966, Terrell and colleagues at Ohio Medical Products (subsequently called Anaquest, Ohmeda, and most currently, Baxter) synthesized more than 700 compounds.[2-4] The 347th and 469th compounds in the series were the methyl ethyl ethers enflurane and isoflurane, which were halogenated with fluorine and chlorine. Clinical trials of enflurane and isoflurane proceeded nearly in parallel, involving both human volunteer and patient studies. Years later, several compounds in Terrell's series were reexamined. One of these (the 653rd) was difficult to synthesize because of a potentially explosive step using elemental fluorine, and because the compound had a vapor pressure close to 1 atm, making it impossible to deliver with a standard wicked vaporizer. However, this particular compound was completely halogenated with fluorine and hence was predicted to have a very low solubility in blood. As synthesis and delivery problems were resolved, this compound, now known as desflurane, was introduced into clinical practice in 1993.

Other new compounds were described in the early 1970s by Wallin and colleagues at Travenol Laboratories during the course of evaluating fluorinated isopropyl ethers. One of these proved to be a potent anesthetic agent and became known as sevoflurane.[5] Like desflurane, it had a low solubility owing to fluorination of the ether molecule. It was noted that sevoflurane released organic and inorganic fluorides in both animals and humans; thus, the drug was not aggressively developed and marketed. When the patent rights were transferred to Ohio Medical Products, further testing revealed significant breakdown of sevoflurane in the presence of soda lime, raising safety concerns that limited further evaluation. As the patent rights expired, Maruishi Pharmaceutical in Japan undertook testing and development of sevoflurane, releasing the drug for general use in Japan in July, 1990. Because of the rapid acceptance and safety record of sevoflurane in Japan, Abbott Laboratories began pursuing laboratory and clinical trials with sevoflurane in the United States. After its safety was established, sevoflurane was introduced in U.S. clinical practice in 1995.

The new inhaled anesthetics sevoflurane and desflurane differ from isoflurane most importantly in their kinetic behavior. They both have significantly lower solubility in blood, which increases their speed for wash-in/wash-out and their speed in adjustment of anesthetic depth (Table 15-1). These characteris-

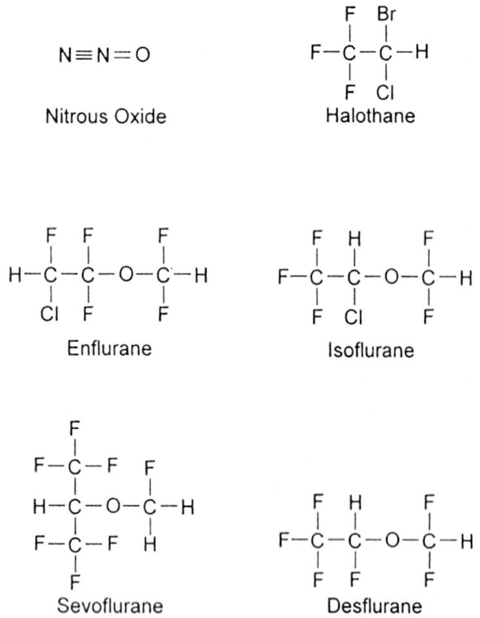

Figure 15-1. Chemical structure of inhaled anesthetics. Halothane is an alkane, a halogen-substituted ethane derivative. Isoflurane and enflurane are isomers that are methyl ethyl ethers. Desflurane differs from isoflurane in the substitution of a fluorine for a chlorine atom and sevoflurane is a methyl isopropyl ether.

tics mesh well with the ambulatory anesthesia environment of modern-day practice.

PHARMACOKINETIC PRINCIPLES

Pharmacokinetics as a discipline began with the study of noninhaled drugs before the concepts were applied to the inhaled anesthetics. Kety in 1950 was the first to examine the pharmacokinetics of inhaled agents in a systematic fashion.[6] Eger and colleagues accomplished much of the early research in the field, leading to his landmark text on the subject in 1974.[7] The inhaled anesthetics differ substantially from nearly all other drugs because they are gases given *via* inhalation. This makes their pharmacokinetics unique as well, and most major textbooks of anesthesia continue to devote considerable space to pharmacokinetic principles of currently used agents. Before delving into the particulars of inhaled anesthetic pharmacokinetics, however, a review of basic pharmacokinetic concepts is useful.

Drug pharmacology is classically divided into two disciplines, pharmacodynamics and pharmacokinetics. *Pharmacodynamics* can be defined as what drugs do to the body. It describes the desired and undesired effects of drugs, as well as the cellular and molecular changes leading to these effects. *Pharmacokinetics* can be defined as what the body does to drugs. It describes where drugs go, how they are transformed, and the cellular and molecular mechanisms underlying these processes.

Systemic drug pharmacokinetics has four phases: absorption, distribution, metabolism, and excretion. *Absorption* is the phase in which drug is transferred from the administration site (*e.g.*, digestive tract, lung, muscle) into the bloodstream. Intravenous drugs have no absorption phase because they are delivered directly into the bloodstream. *Distribution* is the phase in which drug is transferred to tissue sites throughout the body. *Metabolism* refers to the physiochemical processes by which substances in a living organism are synthesized (anabolism) or altered (catabolism); but in the context of anesthetic drugs, only drug alteration is pertinent. Finally, *excretion* is the phase in which changed or unchanged drug is transferred from tissues or blood into some vehicle (*e.g.*, bile, exhaled air, urine) for removal from the body.

Tissues are often grouped into hypothetical *compartments* based on perfusion. An important implication of different compartments and perfusion rates is the concept of *redistribution*. After a given amount of drug is administered, it reaches highly perfused tissue compartments first where it can equilibrate rapidly and exert its effects. With time, however, compartments with lower perfusion rates receive the drug and additional equilibria are established between blood and these tissues. As the tissues with lower perfusion absorb drug, maintenance of equilibria throughout the body requires drug transfer from highly perfused compartments back into the bloodstream. This lowering of drug concentration in one compartment by delivery into another compartment is called redistribution.

In discussions of the inhaled anesthetics, the terminology just described is subject to some minor differences. The absorption phase is usually called *uptake*, the metabolic phase is usually called *biotransformation*, and the excretion phase is usually called *elimination*. The terms are completely interchangeable.

Unique Features of Inhaled Anesthetics

Speed, Gas State, and Route of Administration

The inhaled anesthetics are among the most rapidly acting drugs in existence, and when administering a general anesthetic this speed provides a margin of safety. The ability to quickly increase or decrease anesthetic levels as necessary can mean

Table 15-1. PHYSIOCHEMICAL PROPERTIES OF VOLATILE ANESTHETICS

	Sevoflurane	Desflurane	Isoflurane	Enflurane	Halothane	N_2O
Boiling point (°C)	59	24	49	57	50	−88
Vapor pressure at 20°C (mm Hg)	157	669	238	172	243	38,770
Molecular weight (g)	200	168	184	184	197	44
Oil:gas partition coefficient	47	19	91	97	224	1.4
Blood:gas partition coefficient	0.65	0.42	1.46	1.9	2.50	0.46
Brain:blood solubility	1.7	1.3	1.6	1.4	1.9	1.1
Fat:blood solubility	47.5	27.2	44.9	36	51.1	2.3
Muscle:blood solubility	3.1	2.0	2.9	1.7	3.4	1.2
MAC in O_2, 30–60 yr, at 37°C P_B760 (%)	1.8	6.6	1.17	1.63	0.75	104
MAC in 60–70% N_2O (%)	0.66	2.38	0.56	0.57	0.29	
MAC, >65 yr (%)	1.45	5.17	1.0	1.55	0.64	—
Preservative	No	No	No	No	Thymol	No
Stable in moist CO_2 absorber	No	Yes	Yes	Yes	No	Yes
Flammability (%) (in 70% N_2O/30% O_2)	10	17	7	5.8	4.8	
Recovered as metabolites (%)	2–5	0.02	0.2	2.4	20	

the difference between an anesthetic state and an anesthetic misadventure. Speed also means efficiency. Rapid induction and recovery may lead to faster operating room turnover times, shorter recovery room stays, and earlier discharges to home.

Technically, nitrous oxide is the only true gas, while the potent anesthetics are the vapors of volatile liquids. But for simplicity, all of them are called gases because they are all in the gas phase when administered *via* the lungs. As gases, none deviates significantly from ideal-gas behavior. These agents are all nonionized and have low molecular weights. This allows them to diffuse rapidly without the need for facilitated diffusion or active transport from bloodstream to tissues. The other advantage of gases is that they can be delivered to the bloodstream *via* a unique route available in all patients: the lungs.

The lung route of administration is unique to the inhaled anesthetics, except for bronchodilators or endotracheal administration of cardiac resuscitation drugs. These exceptions are, however, a "one-way street" because their route of delivery is different from their elimination route. Inhaled anesthetics have a "two-way street" in the lungs; they are delivered and primarily eliminated *via* this route.

Speed, gaseous state, and the lung route of administration combine to form the major beneficial feature of the inhaled anesthetics—the ability to decrease plasma concentrations as easily and as rapidly as they are increased.

Physical Characteristics of Inhaled Anesthetics

The goal of delivering inhaled anesthetics is to produce the anesthetic state by establishing a specific concentration of anesthetic molecules in the central nervous system (CNS). This is done by establishing the specific partial pressure of the agent in the lungs, which ultimately equilibrates with the brain and spinal cord. Equilibration is due to three factors:

1. Inhaled anesthetics are gases rapidly transferred bidirectionally *via* the lungs to and from the bloodstream, and subsequently to and from CNS tissues as partial pressures equilibrate.
2. Plasma and tissues have a low capacity to absorb the inhaled anesthetics relative to the amount we can deliver to the lungs, allowing us to quickly establish or abolish anesthetizing concentrations of anesthetic in the bloodstream and, ultimately, the CNS.
3. Metabolism, excretion, and redistribution of the inhaled anesthetics are minimal relative to the rate at which they are delivered or removed from the lungs. This permits easy maintenance of blood and CNS concentrations.

At equilibrium, CNS partial pressure equals blood partial pressure, which in turn equals alveolar partial pressure:

$$P_{CNS} = P_{blood} = P_{alveoli} \qquad (15\text{-}1)$$

where P is partial pressure. The physical characteristics of inhaled anesthetics are shown in Table 15-1.

Inhaled anesthetics are delivered to the lung as gases and follow the ideal gas law, $PV = nRT$, where P is pressure, $\dot{V}$ is volume, n is number of moles of gas, R is the gas constant, and T is absolute temperature. If a gas is heated in a fixed volume, pressure will increase. If a gas is heated or if molecules of gas are added while keeping its pressure constant, its volume must increase. If the number of molecules of gas is increased into a fixed volume, pressure will increase.

Just about any substance at a high enough temperature (if the substance is not destroyed by that temperature) can exist as a gas. The so-called *permanent gases,* such as oxygen and nitrogen, exist only as gases at ambient temperatures. Gases such as nitrous oxide can be compressed into liquids under high pressure at ambient temperature. Most *potent volatile anesthetics* are liquids at ambient temperature and pressure. Some molecules with sufficient energy escape the liquid and enter a

gas phase above the surface of the liquid as a vapor. If left open to air, gas molecules rapidly diffuse, seeking to equalize with atmospheric pressure until all of the liquid is gone. Pure gases always diffuse from an area of high pressure to an area of low pressure because of their *chemical potential,* μ. Chemical potential, also called the escaping tendency, is a thermodynamic concept. It is similar to an electrical potential. In this case, however, it is gases that continue to seek equilibrium until μ is equal throughout the system. Chemical potential depends on the substance and characteristics of the system in which it exists, such as temperature, pressure, and presence of other substances.

If the system in which the volatile liquid resides is a closed container, molecules of the substance will equilibrate between the liquid and gas phases (to equalize μ). At equilibrium the pressure exerted by molecular collisions of the gas against the container walls is the *vapor pressure.* One important property of vapor pressure is that as long as *any* liquid remains in the container, the vapor pressure is independent of the volume of that liquid. As with any gas, however, vapor pressure is proportional to temperature.

For all of the potent agents at 20°C the vapor pressure is below atmospheric pressure. Thus, transfer of molecules between liquid and gas phases occurs only at the liquid:gas interface at the surface of the liquid. If the temperature is raised, however, the vapor pressure increases. The *boiling point* of a liquid is the temperature at which its vapor pressure exceeds atmospheric pressure in an open container. Above this temperature molecules convert into the gas phase within the liquid, rising through the liquid because of their lower density; that is, the substance boils. Desflurane is bottled in a special container because its boiling point of 23.5°C makes it boil at typical room temperatures. Boiling does not occur within the bottle because it is countered by build-up of vapor pressure within the bottle; but once opened to air, the desflurane would quickly boil away. The bottle is designed to allow transfer of desflurane from bottle to vaporizer without exposure to the atmosphere.

Gases in Mixtures

For any mixture of gases in a closed container, each gas exerts a pressure proportional to its *fractional mass* (or fractional *volume* according to $PV = nRT$, since "volume" is a more familiar term when dealing with gases). This is its *partial pressure.* The sum of the partial pressures of each gas in a mixture of gases equals the total pressure of the entire mixture (Dalton's law):

$$P_{total} = P_{gas1} + P_{gas2} + \ldots + P_{gasN} \qquad (15\text{-}2)$$

The entire mixture behaves just as if it were a single gas according to the ideal gas law.

Gases in Solution

Partial pressures of gases in solution are more complicated. Any gas/vapor dissolved in a liquid exerts a force to drive molecules out of solution and into the gas phase. Molecules in the gas phase counter this by exerting a force that drives them into the liquid phase. Only at a given concentration of molecules in the gas phase will the forces (hence chemical potentials) be equal and the system in equilibrium. This force is called the *tension,* and the concentration of molecules in the gas phase at equilibrium will determine the pressure of that phase according to the ideal gas law. Tension is conveniently described by the partial pressure of the gas in equilibrium with the liquid phase. The terms "tension" and "partial pressure" are used synonymously in this chapter.

The *concentration* of gas molecules in solution is more complicated still, owing to intermolecular interaction. Gas molecules within a liquid interact with solvent molecules to a much larger extent than do molecules in the gas phase, in which there are almost no intermolecular interactions. The gas molecules will be present in the liquid only to the extent that this equalizes the chemical potential between the liquid and gas phases. The chemical potential of the gas in a liquid depends dramatically on the liquid itself and the energy state of that liquid. *Solubility* is the term used to describe the tendency of a gas to equilibrate with a solution, hence determining its concentration in solution. The solubility coefficient, λ, is an expression of this tendency:

$$\lambda = V_{\text{dissolved gas}} / V_{\text{liquid}} \quad \text{(at 37°C)} \qquad (15\text{-}3)$$

where V = volume.

The principles of partial pressures and solubility apply in mixtures of gases in solution. That is, the concentration of any one gas in a mixture of gases in solution depends upon two factors: (1) its partial pressure in the gas phase in equilibrium with the solution, and (2) its solubility within that solution. Thus, the partial pressure of a particular gas is proportional to its fractional volume in the gas phase, but is *not* proportional to its fractional volume in solution.

The implications of these properties are profound. Anesthetic gases administered *via* the lungs diffuse into blood until the partial pressures in alveoli and blood are equal. The concentration of anesthetic in the blood depends upon the partial pressure at equilibrium and the blood solubility. Likewise, transfer of anesthetic from blood to target tissues also proceeds toward equalizing partial pressures. The concentration of anesthetic in target tissue depends on the partial pressure at equilibrium and the target tissue solubility. Because inhaled anesthetics are gases, and because partial pressures of gases equilibrate throughout a system, monitoring the alveolar concentration of inhaled anesthetics provides an index of their effects in the brain.

In summary:

1. Inhaled anesthetics equilibrate based on their partial pressures in each tissue (or tissue compartment), *not* based on their concentrations.
2. The partial pressure of a gas in solution is always defined by the partial pressure in the gas phase with which it is in equilibrium.
3. The concentration of anesthetic in a tissue depends on its partial pressure and tissue solubility.

Finally, the particular terminology used when referring to gases in the gas phase or absorbed in plasma or tissues is important. Inspired concentrations or fractional volumes of inhaled anesthetic are typically used rather than partial pressure. For most drugs, concentration is expressed as mass (mg) per volume (ml), but it can also be expressed in percent by weight or volume. Since volume of a gas in the gas phase is directly proportional to mass according to the ideal gas law, it is easier to express this fractional concentration as a percent by volume. Tension and partial pressure, on the other hand, are expressed in mm Hg, or torr (1 torr = 1 mm Hg), or kPa (kilopascals). In the gas phase, fractional concentration is equal to the partial pressure (or tension) divided by ambient pressure, usually atmospheric, or:

$$\text{Fractional volume} = P_{\text{anesthetic}} / P_{\text{barometric}} \qquad (15\text{-}4)$$

Anesthetic Transfer: Machine to CNS

Anesthetics follow a multistep route from anesthesia machine to patient (and back). Each of these steps represents a transfer point or interface between hypothetical compartments. The compartments are organized by location or pharmacokinetic properties in an effort to simplify the concept of anesthetic flow. For example, one-way flow occurs from the fresh gas outlet to the anesthesia circuit and to the waste gas scavenging system. Equilibrium flow occurs between the anesthesia circuit and the airways (and alveoli) and between the alveoli and pulmonary blood. Bulk flow of blood accounts for anesthetic transfer to systemic blood, and equilibrium flow occurs between systemic blood and tissues. The flow of anesthetic from compartment to compartment can be characterized by pharmacokinetics. Technically, the flow from fresh gas outlet (FGO) to circuit is not a pharmacokinetic concern because it does not characterize what the body does to the drug. But it is typically discussed as a pharmacokinetic parameter because it has important clinical implications.

When the fresh gas flow and the vaporizer are turned on, fresh gas with a fixed fractional concentration of anesthetic leaves the FGO and mixes with the gas in the circuit—the bag, tubing, absorbent canister, and piping. It is immediately diluted to a lower fractional concentration, then slowly rises as this compartment equilibrates with the fresh gas flow. With spontaneous patient ventilation by mask, the anesthetic gas passes from circuit to airways. The fractional concentration of anesthetic leaving the circuit is designated as F_I (fraction inspired). In the lungs the gas comprising the dead space in the airways (trachea, bronchi) and the alveoli further dilutes the circuit gas. The fractional concentration of anesthetic present in the alveoli is designated as F_A (fraction alveolar). The anesthetic then passes across the alveolar–capillary membrane and dissolves in pulmonary blood according to the partial pressure of the gas and its solubility. It is further diluted and travels *via* bulk blood flow throughout the vascular tree. The anesthetic then passes *via* simple diffusion from blood to tissues as well as between tissues.

The general direction of *diffusion* of gas at all times depends on partial pressure gradients. *Bulk gas flow,* on the other hand, is generally one-way, depending on the phase of the respiratory cycle. Various equilibria are being established between the compartments *via* diffusion during and between periods of bulk flow.

The vascular system delivers blood to three physiologic tissue groups: the vessel-rich group (VRG), the muscle group, and the fat group. The VRG includes the brain, heart, kidney, liver, digestive tract, and glandular tissues. The percent body mass and perfusion of each are shown in Table 15-2. The CNS tissues of the VRG are referred to as *tissues of desired effect*. The other tissues of the VRG comprise the compartment frequently referred to as *tissues of undesired effects*. The tissues of the muscle and fat groups comprise the *tissues of accumulation*.

Anesthetic is delivered most rapidly to the VRG, where it diffuses according to partial pressure gradients. CNS tissue takes in the anesthetic according to the tissue solubility, and at a high enough tissue concentration unconsciousness is achieved. Increasing CNS tissue concentrations cause progressively

Table 15-2. CHARACTERISTICS OF PHYSIOLOGIC TISSUE COMPARTMENTS

Group	% Body Mass	% Cardiac Output	Perfusion (ml · min^{-1} · 100 g^{-1})
Vessel-rich	10	75	75
Muscle	50	19	3
Fat	20	6	3

deeper stages of anesthesia. As this is occurring, anesthetic is also distributing to other VRG tissues, mostly causing undesired effects, which must be monitored closely and sometimes treated. Also coincident with delivery to the CNS, anesthetic is being delivered—albeit more slowly owing to lower perfusion—to muscle and fat where it accumulates and can affect the speed of emergence from the anesthetic. The concentration of inhaled anesthetic in a given tissue at a particular time during the administration depends not only on tissue blood flow, but also on tissue solubility, which governs how the inhaled anesthetics partition themselves between blood and tissue. Partitioning depends on the relative solubilities of the anesthetic for each compartment. These relative solubilities are expressed by a partition coefficient, δ, which is the ratio of dissolved gas (by volume) in two tissue compartments at equilibrium. Alternatively, it is the ratio of tissue:gas solubilities in the two compartments. For a pure gas in the gas phase, $\lambda = 1$; that is, $V_{\text{dissolved gas}}/V_{\text{gas}} = 1$. Thus, the blood:gas partition coefficient is the same as blood solubility:

$$\delta_{\text{b/g}} = \lambda_{\text{blood}}/\lambda_{\text{gas}} = \lambda_{\text{blood}}/1 = \lambda_{\text{blood}} \quad (15\text{-}5)$$

where $\delta_{\text{b/g}}$ is the blood:gas partition coefficient. For other partition coefficients such as brain:blood ($\delta_{\text{br/bl}}$), the volume of anesthetic dissolved in brain is divided by the volume of anesthetic dissolved in blood:

$$\delta_{\text{br/bl}} = \lambda_{\text{brain}}/\lambda_{\text{blood}} \quad (15\text{-}6)$$

Some of the partition coefficients for the inhaled anesthetics are shown in Table 15-1.

As explained earlier, one of the reasons why inhaled anesthetics are rapidly titratable is that their tissue solubilities are low relative to delivery rate; thus delivery of a desired partial pressure to the CNS is possible despite redistribution and accumulation of anesthetic in other tissues. Over a longer delivery period, however, accumulation in the non-VRGs becomes significant for some anesthetics and can delay emergence.

Uptake and Distribution

F_A/F_I

A simple, common way to assess anesthetic uptake is to follow the ratio of fractional concentration of alveolar anesthetic to inspired anesthetic (F_A/F_I) over time. Experimentally derived data for F_A/F_I versus time during induction are shown in Figure 15-2.

The inhaled anesthetics with the lowest solubilities in blood show the fastest rise in F_A/F_I. The shape of these curves has several regions with different origins. As fresh gas carrying anesthetic begins to flow into the air-filled circuit (assuming complete mixing), the concentration in the circuit (F_I) will rise according to first-order kinetics:

$$F_I = F_{\text{FGO}}(1 - e^{-T/\tau}) \quad (15\text{-}7)$$

F_{FGO} is the fraction of inspired anesthetic in the gas leaving the fresh gas outlet (*i.e.*, the vaporizer setting), T is time, and τ is a time constant. Because all anesthetics in the circuit are in the gas phase, F (fractional volume or concentration) is also P (partial pressure) divided by P_B (barometric pressure), and inspired anesthetic can be expressed as either F_I or P_I. The time constant is simply the volume or "capacity" of the circuit (V_C) divided by the fresh gas flow (FGF) or $\tau = V_C/\text{FGF}$. For example, if the bag, tubing, absorbent canister, and piping comprise 8 l, and the fresh gas flow is 2 l, the time constant $\tau = 8/2 = 4$. One of the characteristics of first-order kinetics is that 95% of maximum is reached after three time constants—in this case, $3 \times 4 = 12$ minutes.

Because 12 minutes is relatively long, the rate of rise of F_I can be increased by starting with a higher F_{FGO}. Using the example above with $\tau = 4$, by first-order kinetics 63% of maximum

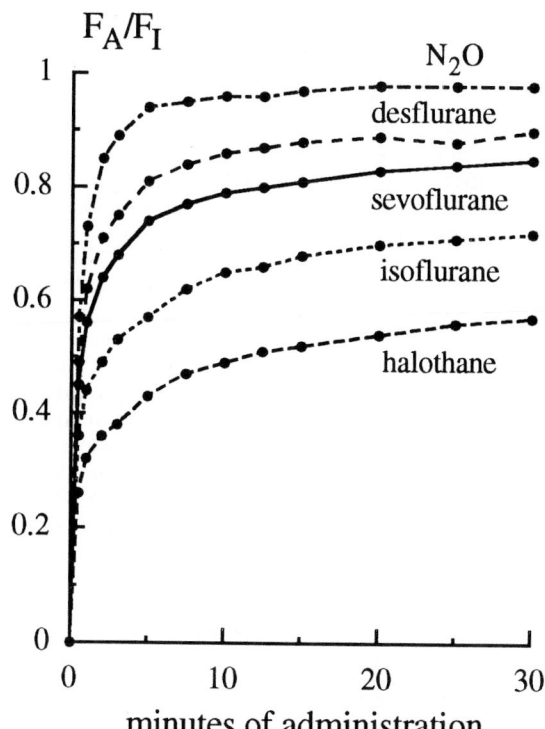

Figure 15-2. The rise in alveolar (F_A) anesthetic concentration toward the inspired (F_I) concentration is most rapid with the least soluble anesthetics nitrous oxide, desflurane, and sevoflurane. It rises most slowly with the more soluble anesthetics, *e.g.*, halothane. All data are from human studies. (Adapted from Yasuda N, Lockhart SH, Eger EI II *et al:* Kinetics of desflurane, isoflurane, and halothane in humans. Anesthesiology 74:489, 1991; and Yasuda N, Lockhart SH, Eger EI II *et al:* Comparison of kinetics of sevoflurane and isoflurane in humans. Anesth Analg 72:316, 1991.)

is reached after one time constant, or 4 minutes. To attain an F_I of 2% at 4 instead of 12 minutes, the F_{FGO} can be set to 3.2% (2% divided by 0.63) and then lowered to 2% at the 4-minute mark.

Other ways to speed the increase in F_I include increasing the fresh gas flow (FGF), thus decreasing τ. Furthermore, the rebreathing bag can be collapsed prior to starting the FGF, such that the capacity in the circuit (V_C) is less, which also decreases τ. Finally, at high flows ($>4\,l \cdot \text{min}^{-1}$) there is far less mixing because fresh gas pushes "old" gas out of the circuit *via* the pop-off valve before complete mixing occurs, causing F_I to increase at a greater rate.

One factor that delays the rate of rise of F_I arises from the fact that CO_2 absorbent can adsorb and decompose the inhaled anesthetics. From a practical standpoint, this does not affect the rate of rise in F_I to a significant extent compared to other factors. Another factor that delays the rate of rise of F_I is solubility of the inhaled anesthetics in some of the plastic and rubber parts of the anesthesia circuit. This absorption has been quantified,[8,9] but plays only a small role in decreasing the rate of rise of F_I. More significant is its tendency to delay emergence at the end of an anesthetic.

Rise in F_A in the Absence of Uptake

The rate of rise in F_I discussed above assumes that no anesthetic is mixing with gas in the patient's lungs. In reality, circuit gas mixes with exhaled gases from the lung with each breath. If extremely high fresh gas flows (producing a high volume of gas at the desired concentration) are used, little mixing with exhaled air occurs and F_I is relatively fixed. In this situation, circuit gas enters the lungs where it mixes with alveolar gas. If there were no blood flow to the lungs, F_A would rise in a fashion analogous to F_I; that is:

$$F_A = F_I(1 - e^{-T/\tau}) \tag{15-8}$$

In this equation, τ is the time constant for alveolar rise in anesthetic concentration and equals the functional residual capacity (FRC) of the patient's lungs divided by minute ventilation, $\dot{V}_A$. There are two ways to speed the equilibration of F_A with F_I, that is, to decrease τ. One way is to increase minute ventilation, and the other is to decrease FRC. Both of these methods can be used to speed induction by mask: the patient can exhale deeply before applying the mask (to decrease the initial FRC), and the patient can breathe deeply and rapidly (to increase $\dot{V}_A$) after the mask is applied. One of the reasons that pediatric inductions by spontaneous breathing of inhaled anesthetics are so much quicker than adult inductions is that the low FRC relative to $\dot{V}_A$ of children makes for a low time constant, and hence a rapid increase in F_A/F_I. One important caveat about the relationship of F_A to FRC is that FRC includes airway dead space; thus, in reality, F_A by Eq. (15-8) is not just the concentration of inhaled anesthetic in the alveoli but the concentration in the entire lung. However, it is simply called the alveolar concentration because the dead space in the airways is relatively insignificant and only the alveolar gas is exchanging anesthetic with the blood.

Rise in F_A in the Presence of Uptake

Because in reality there *is* pulmonary blood flow, the most important factor in the rate of rise of F_A/F_I is uptake of anesthetic from the alveoli into the bloodstream. The rate of rise of F_A/F_I (the slope of the curves seen in Fig. 15-2) reflects the speed at which alveolar anesthetic (F_A) equilibrates with that being delivered to the lungs (F_I). F_A is not solely a function of F_I and time. Inhaled anesthetics so avidly transfer into and are diluted by the bloodstream that uptake into blood is a primary determinant of F_A. The greater the uptake, the slower the rate of rise of F_A/F_I. Uptake is proportional to tissue solubility. The more soluble the anesthetic (such as halothane), the greater its uptake and the slower it is to reach equilibrium. For any fixed volume of halothane delivered to the lungs, a greater number of molecules of halothane are transferred from alveoli to bloodstream as partial pressures equilibrate when compared to the less soluble anesthetics, desflurane and sevoflurane.

Consider a hypothethical example. Suppose that halothane and desflurane are soluble in blood, but insoluble in all other tissues. Suppose further that total lung capacity and blood volume are both 5 l. If a fixed volume of anesthetic is delivered to the lungs (by asking the patient to take one deep breath and hold it), according to partition coefficients, 70.6% of the delivered halothane will be transferred to the blood while 29.4% remains in the alveoli (70.6/29.4 = 2.4). In contrast, 29.6% of the desflurane will be transferred to the blood while 70.4% remains in the alveoli (29.6/70.4 = 0.42). Therefore, 2.4 times (70.6/29.6) more halothane than desflurane (by volume or number of molecules) will be transferred from alveoli to bloodstream before partial pressures equilibrate. At equilibrium, the partial pressures of halothane and desflurane are 29.4% and 70.4% of their inhaled values, respectively.

But anesthetics *are* soluble in tissues, and they are delivered *continuously* rather than in a "one-shot" fashion; thus they are again characterized by first-order kinetics:

$$P_{bl} = P_A \times (1 - e^{-T/\tau}), \quad \text{where } P_A = F_A \times P_B \tag{15-9}$$

Here, P_B is the barometric pressure, and the time constant, τ, equals "capacity" (volume of anesthetic dissolved in blood at the desired alveolar partial pressure) divided by flow (volume of anesthetic delivered per unit time). For any given flow of anesthetic into the system, this capacity for the more soluble halothane is greater than the capacity for the less soluble desflurane; thus, τ for halothane is greater than that for desflurane.

The more soluble an inhaled anesthetic, the larger the capacity of the blood and tissues for that anesthetic, and the longer it takes to saturate at any given delivery rate.

Anesthetic flow can be described by a series of first-order rate equations: F_I as a function of F_{FGO}, F_A as a function of F_I, blood uptake as a function of F_A, and so on. These differential equations can then be solved to determine any value as a function of time. Relatively straightforward equations help describe which parameters determine the rate of rise of F_A/F_I.

Let $\dot{V}_{inspired}$ be the rate of anesthetic delivery to the alveoli. Assuming an ideal situation in which inspired gas is not diluted in the circuit by expired gas, $\dot{V}_{inspired}$ equals the inspired fraction of anesthetic, F_I, multiplied by the alveolar ventilation, $\dot{V}_A$:

$$\dot{V}_{inspired} = F_I \times \dot{V}_A \tag{15-10}$$

Let $\dot{V}_{expired}$ be the flow of anesthetic not participating in gas exchange with the bloodstream and let $\dot{V}_B$ be the rate of anesthetic uptake into the bloodstream. Then

$$\dot{V}_{expired} = \dot{V}_{inspired} - \dot{V}_B \tag{15-11}$$

During any given period of time, the alveolar anesthetic fraction, F_A, as a proportion of the inspired anesthetic fraction, F_I, will equal the ratio of $\dot{V}_{expired}$ to $\dot{V}_{inspired}$; that is:

$$F_A/F_I = \dot{V}_{expired}/\dot{V}_{inspired} \tag{15-12}$$

For example, at steady state, if 10 ml of an inhaled anesthetic were inspired and 5 ml were expired (5 ml transferred to the blood), then the alveolar fraction (F_A) would be only half of the inspired fraction (F_I) since 50% of the anesthetic is taken up. Substituting for $\dot{V}_{expired}$ according to Eq. (15-11), we have

$$F_A/F_I = (\dot{V}_{inspired} - \dot{V}_B)/\dot{V}_{inspired} = 1 - \dot{V}_B/\dot{V}_{inspired} \tag{15-13}$$

Substituting for $\dot{V}_{inspired}$ according to Eq. (15-10),

$$F_A/F_I = 1 - \dot{V}_B/F_I \times \dot{V}_A \tag{15-14}$$

If F_A/F_I is zero and starts to increase as inhaled anesthetic reaches the alveoli from the circuit but uptake of anesthetic in the pulmonary blood ($\dot{V}_B$) nearly equals its delivery to the alveoli ($F_I \times \dot{V}_A$), then F_A/F_I will not rise. All of the anesthetic arriving at alveoli is transferred immediately to the blood. Since blood capacity to absorb anesthetic is finite, F_A will eventually begin to rise relative to F_I. $\dot{V}_B$ can never exceed $F_I \times \dot{V}_A$ by definition. If, on the other hand, blood uptake is very small, F_A and F_I quickly become nearly equal.

Blood uptake of anesthetic is expressed by the equation

$$\dot{V}_B = \delta_{b/g} \times Q \times ((P_A - P_v)/P_B) \tag{15-15}$$

where $\dot{V}_B$ is blood uptake, $\delta_{b/g}$ is the blood:gas partition coefficient, Q is cardiac output, P_A is alveolar partial pressure of anesthetic, P_v is mixed venous partial pressure of anesthetic, and P_B is barometric pressure. This is the Fick equation applied to blood uptake of inhaled anesthetics. Combining Eqs. (15-14) and (15-15) gives

$$F_A/F_I = 1 - (\lambda_B/F_I)(Q/\dot{V}_A)((P_A - P_v)/P_B) \tag{15-16}$$

Based on Eq. (15-16), the parameters that increase or decrease the rate of rise in F_A/F_I during induction can be clearly defined and these important factors have been substantiated in experimental models (Table 15-3).

Before induction, P_V is zero because no anesthetic is present in the bloodstream. P_A is established with the first inspiration of anesthetic, and the alveolar to pulmonary blood partial pressure gradient, $P_A - P_v$, determines the rate of increase in F_A/F_I. Initially, P_A climbs at a much greater rate than P_V because circulation and dilution as well as tissue uptake together keep P_V low. As significant tissue concentrations of anesthetic start to accumulate, P_V rapidly climbs as the pulmonary blood, originally carrying no anesthetic, becomes saturated with anesthetic. This early rapid rise in F_A/F_I followed by slowing is seen in Figure 15-2.

Table 15-3. FACTORS THAT INCREASE OR DECREASE THE RATE OF RISE OF F_A/F_I

Increase	Decrease	
Low λ_B	High λ_B	The lower the blood:gas solubility, the faster the rise in F_A/F_I[15,29,30,409]
Low Q	High Q	The lower the cardiac output, the faster the rise in F_A/F_I[15,17]
High $\dot{V}_A$	Low $\dot{V}_A$	The higher the minute ventilation, the faster the rise in F_A/F_I[17,21,409–411]
High (P_A-P_v)	Low (P_A-P_v)	At the beginning of induction, P_v is zero but rises rapidly (thus $[P_A - P_v]$ falls rapidly) and F_A/F_I increases rapidly. Later during induction and maintenance, P_v rises more slowly so F_A/F_I rises more slowly.

Parameters as described in Eq. (15-16): λ_B = blood solubility; Q = cardiac output; $\dot{V}$ = minute ventilation; P_A, P_V= pulmonary arterial and venous blood partial pressure

Distribution (Tissue Uptake)

Until P_V starts to increase, the maximum F_A/F_I at a given inspired concentration of anesthetic, cardiac output, and minute ventilation is entirely dependent on the solubility of that drug in the blood as characterized by the blood:gas partition coefficient $\delta_{b/g}$. This can be seen in the time curves for the rise in F_A/F_I during induction for the various inhalation anesthetics shown in Figure 15-2. The first "knee" in each curve in Figure 15-2 represents the point at which the rapid rise in P_V begins to taper off, that is, when significant inhaled anesthetic concentrations begin to build up in the bloodstream because of distribution to and equilibration with the various tissue compartments.

Each of the three perfusion compartments—VRG, muscle, and fat—takes up anesthetic based on the Fick equation:

$$\dot{V}_{Compart} = \lambda_{Compart} \times Q_{Compart} \times ((P_{aCompart} - P_{vCompart})/P_B) \quad (15\text{-}17)$$

where $P_{aCompart}$ and $P_{vCompart}$ are arterial and venous partial pressures in the tissue compartment. Mixed venous partial pressure of anesthetic in the pulmonary outflow, P_v, depends on the relative uptake in each of these perfusion compartments. To the extent that the mass and blood flow to each of these compartments differ, anesthetic uptake will differ.

As blood is equilibrating with alveolar gas, it also begins to equilibrate with the VRG, muscle, and, more gradually, the fat compartments based on perfusion. Muscle is not that different from the VRG, having partition coefficients that range from 1.2 (nitrous oxide) to 3.4 (halothane), just under a threefold difference; and for each anesthetic except nitrous oxide, the muscle partition coefficient is approximately double that for the VRG. Although both VRG and muscle are lean tissues, the muscle compartment equilibrates far more slowly than the VRG. The explanation comes from Eq. (15-17) and the mass of the compartments relative to perfusion. The perfusion of the VRG is about 75 ml·min^{-1}·100 g^{-1} of tissue, whereas it is only 3 ml·min^{-1}·100 g^{-1} of tissue in the muscle (see Table 15-2). This 25-fold difference in perfusion between VRG (especially brain) and muscle means that even if the partition coefficients were equal, the muscle would still take 25 times longer to equilibrate with blood.

Fat is perfused to an extent similar to muscle but its time for equilibration with blood is considerably slower because the partition coefficients are so much greater. All of the potent agents are highly lipid-soluble. Partition coefficients range from 27 (desflurane) to 51 (halothane). On average, the solubility for these agents is about 25 times greater in fat than in the VRG group. Thus fat equilibrates far more slowly with the blood and does not play a significant role in determining speed of induction. However, after long anesthetic exposures, the high saturation of fat tissue can play a significant role in delaying emergence.

Nitrous oxide represents an exception. Its partition coefficients are fairly similar in each tissue, it does not accumulate to any great extent, and it is not a very potent anesthetic. Its utility lies as an adjunct to the potent agents, and as a vehicle to speed induction.

Metabolism

Data suggest that the enzymes responsible for biotransformation of inhaled anesthetics become saturated at less than anesthetizing doses of these drugs, such that metabolism plays little role in opposing induction.[10] It may, however, have some significance to recovery from anesthesia, as discussed later.

Overpressurization and the Concentration Effect

There are several ways to speed uptake and induction of anesthesia with the inhaled anesthetics. The first is *overpressurization*, which is analogous to an iv bolus. This is the administration of a higher partial pressure of anesthetic (F_I) than the alveolar concentration (F_A) actually desired for the patient.

Inspired anesthetic concentration (F_I) can influence both F_A and the *rate of rise* of F_A/F_I.[11,12] The greater the inspired concentration of an inhaled anesthetic, the greater the rate of rise. This *concentration effect* has two components. The first is a concentrating effect, and the second is an augmented gas inflow effect.

For example, consider the administration of 10% anesthetic (10 parts anesthetic and 90 parts other gas) to a patient in which 50% of the anesthetic in the alveoli is absorbed by the blood. In this case, 5 parts (0.5×10) anesthetic remain in the alveoli, 5 parts enter the blood, and 90 parts remain as other alveolar gas. The alveolar concentration is now $5/(90 + 5) = 5.3\%$. Consider next administering 50% anesthetic with the same 50% uptake. Now 25 parts anesthetic remain in alveoli, 25 parts pass into blood, and 50 parts remain as other alveolar gas. The alveolar concentration becomes $25/(50 + 25) = 33\%$. Giving 5 times as much anesthetic leads to an alveolar concentration that is $33\%/5.3\% = 6.2$ times greater. The higher the F_I, the greater the effect. Thus, nitrous oxide, typically given in concentrations of 50–70%, has the greatest concentrating effect. This is why the F_A/F_I versus time curve in Figure 15-2 rises most quickly with nitrous oxide, even though desflurane has a lower blood:gas solubility. However, this concentrating effect becomes most prominent with the most soluble anesthetic. Therefore, halothane and isoflurane *should* benefit most at any particular concentration of anesthetic, F_I. But because equipotent concentrations for halothane and isoflurane are lower than those of the less soluble anesthetics, sevoflurane and desflurane, these agents benefit from the concentration effect less than expected—that is, *concentration outweighs solubility*. The typical inspired concentrations of N_2O are so much greater than the

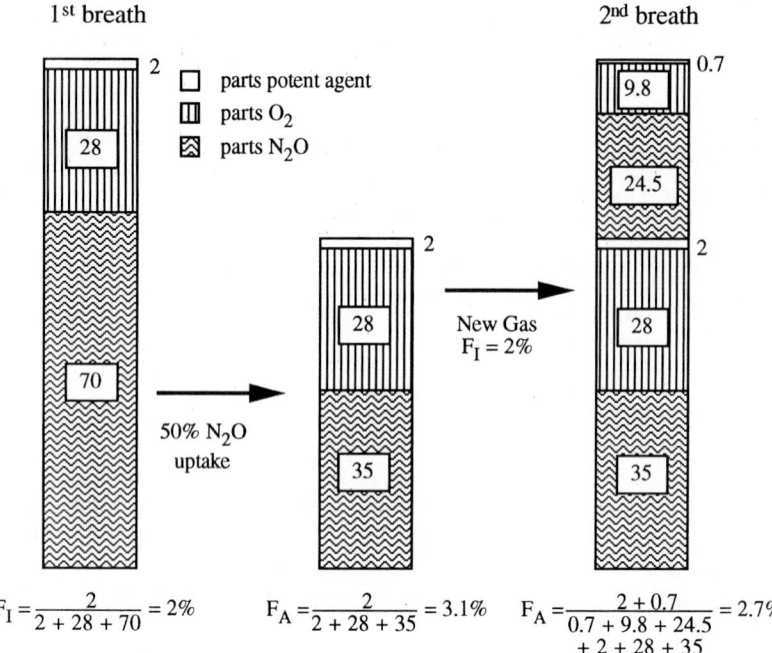

1st breath

□ parts potent agent
▥ parts O_2
▨ parts N_2O

2nd breath

$$F_I = \frac{2}{2 + 28 + 70} = 2\%$$

$$F_A = \frac{2}{2 + 28 + 35} = 3.1\%$$

50% N_2O uptake

New Gas $F_I = 2\%$

$$F_A = \frac{2 + 0.7}{0.7 + 9.8 + 24.5 + 2 + 28 + 35} = 2.7\%$$

Figure 15-3. The second-gas effect. In this hypothetical example, the second gas is set at 2% of a potent anesthetic and the model is set for 50% uptake of the first gas (N_2O) in the first inspired breath. The second gas is concentrated because of the uptake of N_2O (middle panel). On replenishing the inspired second gas (F_I = 2%) in the next breath, the second gas has been concentrated to be 2.7% because of the uptake of N_2O in the previous breath.

potent anesthetics that its low tissue solubility is of no consequence.

This isn't the complete picture; there is yet another factor to consider. As gas is leaving the alveoli for the blood, new gas at the original F_I is entering to replace that which is lost. This other aspect of the concentration effect has been called *augmented gas inflow*. Again, take the example of 10% anesthetic delivered with 50% uptake into the bloodstream. The 5 parts anesthetic absorbed by the bloodstream are replaced by gas in the circuit that is still 10% anesthetic. The 5 parts anesthetic and 90 parts other gas left in the lungs mix with 5 parts replacement gas, or $5 \times 0.10 = 0.5$ parts anesthetic. Now the alveolar concentration is $(5 + 0.5)/(100\%) = 5.5\%$ (as compared to 5.6% without augmented inflow). For 50% anesthetic and 50% uptake, 25 parts of anesthetic removed from the alveoli are replaced with 25 parts of 50% anesthetic, giving a new alveolar concentration of $(25 + 12.5)/(100\%) = 37.5\%$ (as compared to 50% without augmented inflow). Thus 5 times the F_I leads to $37.5/5.5 = 6.8$ times greater F_A (compared to 6.2 times without augmented gas inflow). Of course, this cycle of absorbed gas being replaced by fresh gas inflow is continuous and has a finite rate, so our example is a simplification.

Second-Gas Effect

A special case of concentration effect applies to administration of a potent anesthetic with nitrous oxide—that is, two gases simultaneously. Along with the concentration of potent agent in the alveoli *via* its uptake, there is further concentration *via* the uptake of nitrous oxide. This process, called the *second-gas effect,* has been confirmed in dogs.[13] Some confusion attends the question of which is the second gas, the nitrous oxide or the potent anesthetic. As originally proposed[14] the second gas is the potent agent. Terminology aside, the principle is simple (Figs. 15-3 and 15-4). Consider, for example, administering 2% of a potent anesthetic in 70% nitrous oxide and 28% oxygen. In this case, nitrous oxide, with its extremely high vapor pressure (despite low solubility), partitions into the blood more rapidly than the potent anesthetic, decreasing the alveolar N_2O concentration by some amount (*e.g.,* by 50%). Ignoring uptake of the potent anesthetic, the uptake of N_2O is 35 parts, leaving 35 parts N_2O, 28 parts O_2, and 2 parts potent agent in the alveoli.

The second gas is now present in the alveoli at a concentration of $2/(2 + 35 + 28) = 3.1\%$. The second gas has been concentrated.

Ventilation Effects

As indicated by Figure 15-2 and Eq. (15-16), inhaled anesthetics with very low tissue solubility have an extremely rapid rise in

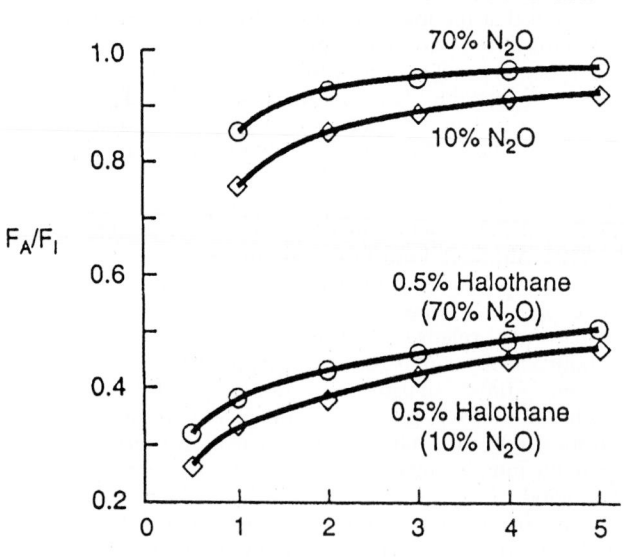

Concentration & Second-Gas Effects

70% N_2O
10% N_2O
F_A/F_I
0.5% Halothane (70% N_2O)
0.5% Halothane (10% N_2O)

minutes

Figure 15-4. The concentration and second-gas effects in dogs receiving nitrous oxide. (*Upper curves*) The concentration effect: Administration of 70% N_2O produces a more rapid rise in the F_A/F_I ratio of nitrous oxide than does administration of 10% N_2O. (*Lower curves*) The second-gas effect: The F_A/F_I ratio for 0.5% halothane rises more rapidly when given with 70% N_2O than when given with 10% N_2O. (Adapted from Epstein R, Rackow H, Salanitre E *et al:* Influence of the concentration effect on the uptake of anesthetic mixtures: The second-gas effect. Anesthesiology 25:364, 1964.)

F_A/F_I with induction. This suggests that there is very little room to improve this rate by increasing or decreasing ventilation. This is consistent with the experimental evidence shown in Figure 15-5.[15] The greater the solubility of an inhaled anesthetic, the more rapidly it is absorbed by the bloodstream, such that anesthetic delivery to the lungs may be rate-limiting. Therefore, for more soluble anesthetics, augmentation of anesthetic delivery by increasing minute ventilation also increases the rate of rise in F_A/F_I.

Spontaneous minute ventilation is not static, however, and to the extent that the inhaled anesthetics depress spontaneous ventilation with increasing inspired concentration, $\dot{V}_A$ will decrease and so will the rate of rise of F_A/F_I.[16–19] This negative feedback should not be considered a drawback of the inhaled anesthetics, because the respiratory depression produced at high anesthetic concentrations essentially slows the rise in F_A/F_I. This might arguably add a margin of safety in preventing an overdose.

Perfusion Effects

As with ventilation, cardiac output is not static during the course of induction. For the insoluble agents, changes in cardiac output do not affect the rate of rise of F_A/F_I to a great extent, but for the more soluble agents the effect is noticeable, as seen in Figure 15-6.[20] However, as inspired concentration increases, greater cardiovascular depression reduces anesthetic uptake and actually increases the rate of rise of F_A/F_I. This positive feedback can rapidly lead to profound cardiovascular depression. Figure 15-6 presents experimental data in which lower cardiac outputs lead to a much more rapid rise in F_A/F_I when $\dot{V}_A$ is held constant.[21] This more rapid rise is greater than can be accounted for just by concentration effect.

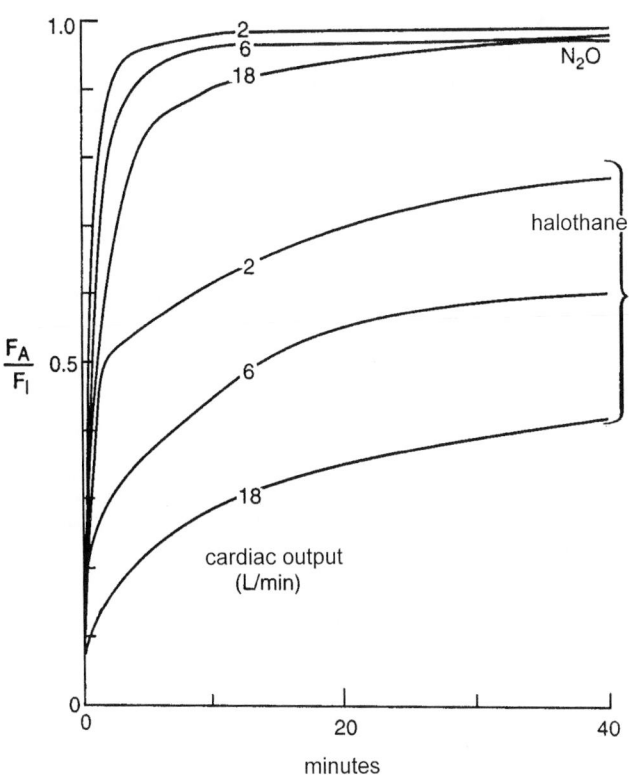

Figure 15-6. If ventilation is fixed, an increase in cardiac output from 2 to 18 L · min⁻¹ will decrease the alveolar anesthetic concentration by augmenting uptake, thereby slowing the rise of the F_A/F_I ratio. This effect is most prominent with the more soluble anesthetics (halothane) than with the less soluble anesthetics (nitrous oxide). (Adapted from Eger EI II: Ventilation, circulation and uptake. In Anesthetic Uptake and Action, p 131. Baltimore, Williams & Wilkins, 1974.)

Ventilation–Perfusion Mismatching

Ventilation and perfusion are normally fairly well matched in healthy patients such that P_A (alveolar partial pressure) $/P_I$ and P_a (arterial partial pressure) $/P_I$ are the same curve. If significant intrapulmonary shunt occurs, however, as in the case of inadvertent bronchial intubation, the rate of rise of alveolar and arterial anesthetic partial pressures can be affected. The effects, however, depend on the solubility of the anesthetic, as seen in Figure 15-7. Ventilation of the intubated lung is dramatically increased while perfusion increases slightly. The nonintubated lung receives no ventilation, while perfusion decreases slightly. For the less soluble anesthetics, increased ventilation of the intubated lung cannot appreciably increase alveolar partial pressure relative to inspired concentration on that side, but alveolar partial pressure on the nonintubated side is essentially zero. Pulmonary mixed venous blood therefore comprises nearly equal parts blood containing normal amounts of anesthetic and blood containing no anesthetic, that is, diluted relative to normal. Thus the rate of rise in P_a relative to P_I is significantly reduced. There is less total anesthetic uptake, so the rate of rise of P_A relative to P_I increases even though induction of anesthesia is slowed because CNS partial pressure equilibrates with P_a. For the more soluble anesthetics, increased ventilation of the intubated lung *does* increase the alveolar partial pressure relative to inspired concentration on that side. Pulmonary venous blood from the intubated side contains a higher concentration of anesthetic that lessens the dilution by blood from the nonintubated side. Thus the rate of rise of P_a/P_I is not as depressed as that for the less soluble anesthetics, and induction of anesthesia is less delayed.

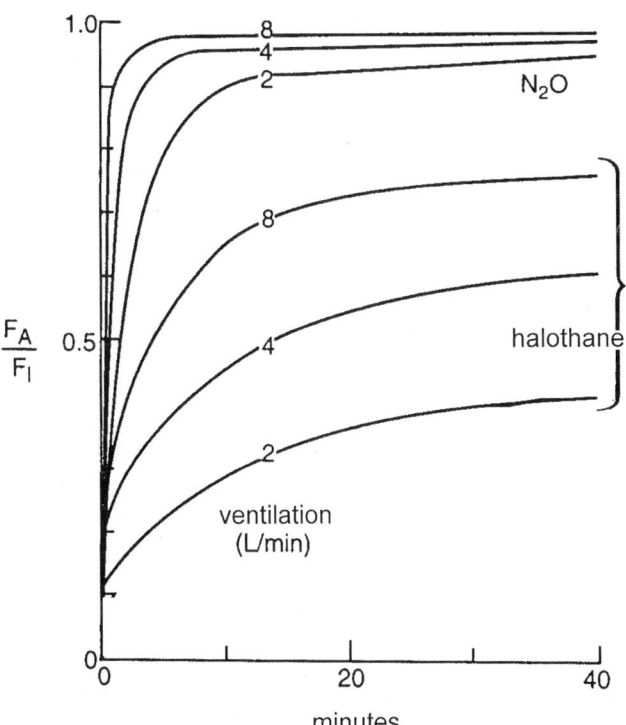

Figure 15-5. The F_A/F_I ratio rises more rapidly if ventilation is increased from 2 to 8 L · min⁻¹. Solubility modifies this impact of ventilation; *e.g.*, the effect is least with the least soluble anesthetic, nitrous oxide, and greatest with the more soluble anesthetic, halothane. (Adapted from Eger EI II: Ventilation, circulation and uptake. In Anesthetic Uptake and Action, p 123. Baltimore, Williams & Wilkins, 1974.)

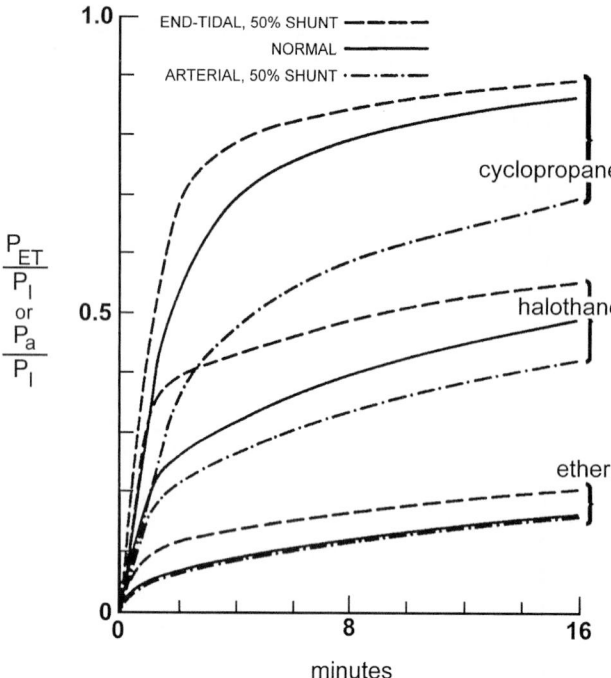

Figure 15-7. When no ventilation/perfusion abnormalities exist, the alveolar (P_A) or end-tidal (P_{ET}) and arterial (P_a) anesthetic partial pressures rise together (continuous lines) toward the inspired partial pressure (P_I). When 50% of the cardiac output is shunted through the lungs, the rate of rise of the end-tidal partial pressure (dashed lines) is accelerated while the rate of rise of the arterial partial pressure (dot-dashed lines) is retarded. The greatest effect of shunting is found with the least soluble anesthetic, cyclopropane. (Adapted from Eger EI II, Severinghaus JW: Effect of uneven pulmonary distribution of blood and gas on induction with inhalation anesthetics. Anesthesiology 25:620, 1964.)

Elimination

Percutaneous and Visceral Loss

Although the loss of inhaled anesthetics *via* the skin is very small, it does occur[22-25] and is the greatest for nitrous oxide. These anesthetics also pass across gastrointestinal viscera and the pleura. During open abdominal or thoracic surgery there is some anesthetic loss *via* these routes.[26] Relative to losses by all other routes, losses *via* percutaneous and visceral routes are insignificant.

Diffusion between Tissues

Using more elaborate mathematical modeling of inhaled anesthetic pharmacokinetics than presented here, several laboratories have derived a five-compartment model that best describes tissue compartments.[27-30] These compartments are the alveoli, the VRG, the muscle, the fat, and one additional compartment. Current opinion is that this fifth compartment represents adipose tissue adjacent to lean tissue that receives anesthetic *via* intertissue diffusion. This transfer of anesthetic is not insignificant and may account for up to one-third of uptake during long administration.

Metabolism

Inhaled anesthetic biotransformation is discussed in more depth elsewhere in this chapter. Metabolism is greatest for halothane, up to 50% of loss.[31] In fact, there is evidence that decreases in the alveolar concentrations of halothane during emergence outpace those for isoflurane, presumably because of this significant metabolism.[27,28] Experimentally, it has been determined that metabolism does not significantly affect recov-

ery from isoflurane and desflurane,[29,30] but may have a slight influence for sevoflurane.[32]

Exhalation and Recovery

Recovery from anesthesia, like induction, depends on anesthetic solubility, cardiac output, and minute ventilation. Solubility is the primary determinant of the rate of fall of F_A (Fig. 15-8).[33] The greater the solubility of inhaled anesthetic, the larger the capacity for absorption in the bloodstream and tissues. The "reservoir" of anesthetic in the body at the end of administration depends on tissue solubility (which determines the capacity) and the dose and duration of anesthetic (which determine how much of that capacity is filled). Recovery from anesthesia, or "washout," is usually expressed as the ratio of expired fractional concentration of anesthetic (F_E) to the expired concentration at time zero (F_{E0}) when the anesthetic was discontinued (or F_A/F_{A0}). Elimination curves of nitrous oxide and halothane are shown in Figure 15-9. The longer the duration of anesthetic, the greater the reservoir of anesthetic in the body, and the higher the curve seen in Figure 15-9.

There are two major pharmacokinetic differences between recovery and induction. First, whereas overpressurization can increase the speed of induction, there is no "underpressurization." Both induction and recovery rates depend on the P_A to P_V gradient, and P_A can never fall below zero. Second, whereas all tissues begin induction with zero anesthetic, each begins recovery with quite different anesthetic concentrations. The VRG tissues begin recovery with the same anesthetic partial pressure as that in alveoli, since $P_{CNS} = P_{blood} = P_{alveoli}$. The partial pressures in muscle and fat depend on the inspired concentration during anesthesia, the duration of administration, and the anesthetic tissue solubilities. As long as an arterial-to-tissue partial pressure gradient exists, these tissues will absorb anesthetic—especially fat, since it is a huge potential reservoir whose anesthetic partial pressures are typically low after hours of anesthesia. After discontinuation of anesthesia, muscle and fat may continue to absorb anesthetic, even hours later. This is essen-

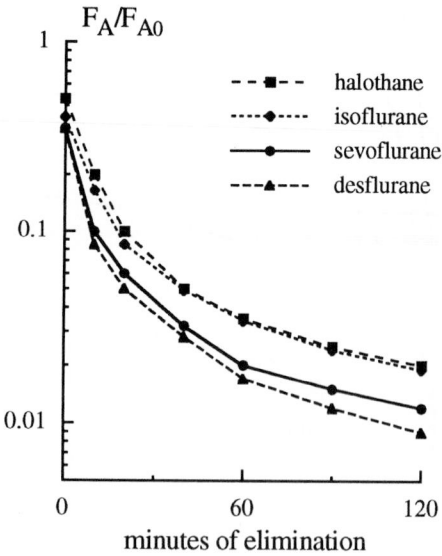

Figure 15-8. Elimination of anesthetic gases is defined as the ratio of end-tidal anesthetic concentration (F_A) to the last F_A during administration and immediately before the beginning of elimination (F_{A0}). During the 120-min period after ending the anesthetic delivery, the elimination of sevoflurane and desflurane is 2–2.5 times faster than that of isoflurane or halothane (note logarithmic scale for the ordinate). (Adapted from Yasuda N, Lockhart SH, Eger EI II *et al:* Kinetics of desflurane, isoflurane, and halothane in humans. Anesthesiology 74:489, 1991; and Yasuda N, Lockhart SH, Eger EI II *et al:* Comparison of kinetics of sevoflurane and isoflurane in humans. Anesth Analg 72:316, 1991.)

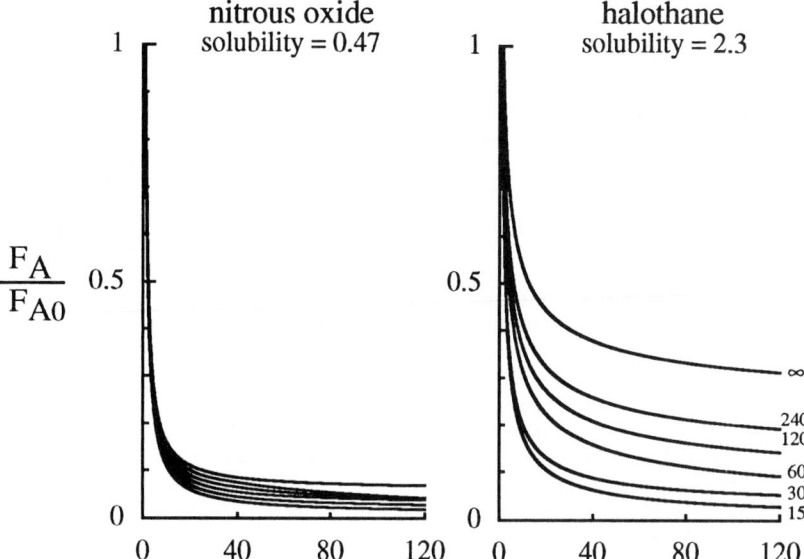

Figure 15-9. Both solubility and duration of anesthesia affect the decrease of the alveolar concentration (F_A) from its value immediately preceding the cessation of anesthetic administration (F_{A0}). A longer anesthetic time (from 15 min to 240 min) slows the decrease, as does a greater solubility of the agent (halothane). (Adapted from Stoelting RK, Eger EI II: The effects of ventilation and anesthetic solubility on recovery from anesthesia: An *in vivo* and analog analysis before and after equilibrium. Anesthesiology 30:290, 1969.)

tially redistribution, which continues until blood/alveolar anesthetic partial pressure falls below tissue partial pressure. This redistribution causes the early rate of decline in alveolar anesthetic concentration during recovery to exceed its increase during induction.[34,35]

Because VRG tissues are highly perfused and washout of anesthetic is mostly *via* elimination from these tissues early in recovery, all anesthetics, regardless of duration of administration, have approximately the same rate of elimination to 50% of F_{E0}.[36] Unfortunately, halving the CNS concentration of anesthetic is rarely sufficient for waking the patient. More commonly, 80–90% of inhaled anesthetic must be eliminated before emergence. At these amounts of washout, the more soluble anesthetics are eliminated much more slowly than less soluble agents.[36]

Diffusion Hypoxia

During recovery from anesthesia, washout of high concentrations of nitrous oxide can lower alveolar concentrations of oxygen[37-39] and carbon dioxide,[39] a phenomenon called *diffusion hypoxia*. The resulting alveolar hypoxia can cause hypoxemia, and alveolar hypocarbia can depress respiratory drive, which may exacerbate hypoxemia. It is therefore appropriate to initiate recovery from nitrous oxide anesthesia with 100% oxygen rather than less concentrated O_2/air mixtures.

CLINICAL OVERVIEW OF CURRENT INHALED ANESTHETICS

Halothane

Halothane, a relatively nonflammable liquid, is the most potent of the currently used volatile anesthetics. It is an alkane—a halogen-substituted ethane derivative (see Fig. 15-1)—that was placed into clinical use in 1956. The halogenated structure provided nonflammability. It has an intermediate blood solubility and is relatively nonpungent; hence it can be inhaled *via* the facemask. The carbon–fluorine bond is important in providing nonflammability of halothane at room temperature and the trifluorocarbon group contributes to its molecular stability. Despite its chemical stability, halothane oxidizes spontaneously and is broken down by ultraviolet light. It decomposes to hydrochloric acid (HCl), hydrobromic acid (HBr), chloride (Cl^-), bromide (Br^-), and phosgene ($COCl_2$). To prevent this decomposition, halothane is stored in amber-colored bottles and 0.01% thymol is added as a preservative to prevent spontaneous oxidative decomposition. The thymol preservative can "gum

up" vaporizers, mandating a more difficult and more frequent cleaning schedule than that for vaporizers specific to other volatile anesthetics. Halothane also is adsorbed by contact with dry soda lime and broken down to BCDFE (2-bromo-2-chloro-1,1-difluoroethene), which has organ toxicity in animal models. In humans, halothane has been associated with an immune-mediated hepatitis and a sensitization to epinephrine resulting in arrhythmias. It also has been associated with bradycardia when used in the pediatric population.

Enflurane

Enflurane, a halogenated methyl ethyl ether, is an isomer of isoflurane (see Fig. 15-1). It is a nonflammable liquid at room temperature and is pungent. Its use in high concentrations has been associated with seizure-like activity on the EEG. Its metabolism has resulted in an increase in blood fluoride concentration and, rarely, with a renal concentrating deficiency. Its popularity has generally been reserved owing to competition from isoflurane—the near-simultaneously introduced volatile anesthetic, which has proven to be associated with very few side effects. In recent years, the use of enflurane has been further diminished with the introduction of new anesthetics with lower solubilities.

Isoflurane

Isoflurane, a halogenated methyl ethyl ether, is a clear, nonflammable liquid at room temperature and has a high degree of pungency (see Fig. 15-1). The second most potent of the volatile anesthetics in clinical use, isoflurane has great physical stability and undergoes essentially no deterioration during storage for up to five years or on exposure to sunlight. It has become the "gold standard" anesthetic since its introduction in the 1970s. There has been a brief period of controversy concerning the use of isoflurane in patients with coronary disease because of the possibility for coronary "steal," arising from isoflurane's potent effects on coronary vasodilation. In clinical use, however, this has been, at most, a rare occurrence.

Desflurane

Desflurane is a fluorinated methyl ethyl ether that differs from isoflurane by just one atom: a fluorine atom is substituted for a chlorine atom on the α-ethyl component of isoflurane (see Fig. 15-1). The process of completely fluorinating the ether molecule has several effects. It decreases blood and tissue solubility (the blood:gas solubility of desflurane equals that of nitrous oxide), and it results in a loss of potency (the MAC of desflurane is 5 times higher than that of isoflurane). Moreover, the complete fluorination of the methyl ether molecule results in a high vapor pressure (owing to decreased intermolecular attraction). Thus, a new vaporizer technology has been developed to deliver a regulated concentration of desflurane as a gas. A heated, pressurized vaporizer requiring electrical power is required. One of the advantages of desflurane is the near-absent metabolism to serum trifluoroacetate. This makes immune-mediated hepatitis extremely unlikely. The most pungent of the volatile anesthetics, desflurane cannot be administered *via* the facemask as it results in coughing, salivation, breath holding, and laryngospasm. In extremely dry CO_2 absorbers, desflurane (and, to a lesser extent, isoflurane and enflurane) degrades to form carbon monoxide. Desflurane has the lowest blood:gas solubility of the potent volatile anesthetics; moreover, its fat solubility is roughly half that of the other volatile anesthetics. Thus, desflurane offers a theoretical advantage in long surgical procedures by virtue of decreased tissue saturation. Desflurane also has been associated with transient periods of sympathetic activation, hypertension, and tachycardia when used in high concentrations or when rapidly increasing the inspired concentration.

Sevoflurane

Sevoflurane is a sweet-smelling, completely fluorinated methyl isopropyl ether (see Fig. 15-1). Its vapor pressure is most similar to that of enflurane and it can be used in a conventional vaporizer. The blood:gas solubility of sevoflurane is second only to desflurane in terms of potent volatile anesthetics. Sevoflurane is approximately half as potent as isoflurane, and some of the preservation of potency, despite fluorination, is due to the bulky propyl side chain on the ether molecule. Sevoflurane has minimal odor, no pungency, and is a potent bronchodilator. These attributes make sevoflurane an excellent candidate for administration *via* the facemask on induction of anesthesia in both children and adults. As a coronary vasodilator, sevoflurane is half as potent as isoflurane, but it is 10–20 times more vulnerable to metabolism than isoflurane. Like that of enflurane and methoxyflurane, the metabolism of sevoflurane results in inorganic fluoride; but the increase in plasma fluoride after sevoflurane administration has not been associated with renal concentrating defects, as is the case with methoxyflurane. Unlike other potent volatile anesthetics, sevoflurane is not metabolized to trifluoroacetate; rather, it is metabolized to an acyl halide (hexafluoroisopropanol). This does not stimulate formation of antibodies, and immune-mediated hepatitis has not been reported with sevoflurane. Sevoflurane does not form carbon monoxide during exposure to dry CO_2 absorbents. Rather, sevoflurane breaks down in the presence of the carbon dioxide absorber to form a vinyl halide called compound A. Compound A has been shown to be a dose-dependent nephrotoxin in rats, but has not been associated with renal injury in human volunteers and patients, even when fresh gas flows are $1 \, l \cdot min^{-1}$ or less.

Xenon

Xenon is an inert gas. Difficult to obtain, and hence extremely expensive, it has received considerable interest in the last few years because it has many characteristics approaching those of an "ideal" inhaled anesthetic.[40,41] Its blood:gas partition coefficient is 0.14; and unlike the other potent volatile anesthetics (except methoxyflurane), xenon provides some degree of analgesia. Unfortunately, the MAC in humans is 71%, which might prove to be a limitation. It is nonexplosive, nonpungent, and odorless, and thus can be inhaled with ease. In addition, it does not produce significant myocardial depression.[41] Because of

its scarcity and high cost, new anesthetic systems need to be developed to provide for recycling of xenon. If this proves to be too difficult from either a technical or patient safety standpoint, it may be necessary to use it in a very low, or closed, fresh gas flow system to reduce wastage.

Nitrous Oxide

Nitrous oxide is a sweet-smelling, nonflammable gas of low potency (MAC = 104%) and is relatively insoluble in blood. It is most commonly administered as an anesthetic adjuvant in combination with opioids or volatile anesthetics during the conduct of general anesthesia. Although not flammable, nitrous oxide will support combustion. Unlike the potent volatile anesthetics in clinical use, nitrous oxide does not produce significant skeletal muscle relaxation, but it does have documented analgesic effects. Despite a long track record of use, controversy has surrounded nitrous oxide in four areas: its role in postoperative nausea and vomiting, its potential toxic effects on cell function *via* inactivation of vitamin B_{12}, its adverse effects related to absorption and expansion into air-filled structures and bubbles, and its effect on embryonic development. The one concern that seems most valid and most clinically relevant is the ability of nitrous oxide to expand air-filled spaces because of its greater solubility in blood compared to nitrogen. Several closed gas spaces, such as the bowel and middle ear, exist in the body and other spaces, such as a pneumothorax, may occur as a result of disease or surgery. Nitrogen cannot be removed readily *via* the bloodstream. Unfortunately, nitrous oxide delivered to a patient diffuses from the blood into these closed gas spaces quite easily, in which case the spaces must increase pressure and may expand.[42] Movement of nitrous oxide into these spaces continues until the partial pressure equals that of the blood and alveoli. Compliant spaces will continue to expand until sufficient pressure is generated to oppose further N_2O flow into the space. The higher the inspired concentration of nitrous oxide, the higher the partial pressure required for equilibration.

Seventy-five percent N_2O can expand a pneumothorax to double or triple its size in 10 and 30 minutes, respectively.[42] Air-filled cuffs of pulmonary artery catheters and endotracheal tubes also expand with the use of N_2O, possibly causing tissue damage *via* increased pressure in the pulmonary artery or trachea, respectively.[43–45] In a rabbit model, the volume of air required to create an air embolus that results in cardiovascular compromise is less during coadministration of nitrous oxide.[46] Accumulation of nitrous oxide in the middle ear can diminish hearing postoperatively,[47] and is relatively contraindicated for tympanoplasty because the increased pressure can dislodge a tympanic graft.[48]

NEUROPHARMACOLOGY OF INHALED ANESTHETICS

The inhaled anesthetics establish the anesthetic state by effects on spontaneous neuronal activity and metabolism. The exact anesthetic mechanisms of inhaled agents remain poorly understood, and the associated nervous system effects may be mediated in part by undetermined mechanisms. Therefore, as a whole, the current understanding of inhaled anesthetic neuropharmacology tends to be more descriptive than mechanistic in nature.

The mechanisms of anesthesia are elusive partly because no uniform definition exists as to when the brain is anesthetized; however, the anesthetized brain may be usefully defined as one that is incapable of self-awareness or subsequent recall.[49] This definition is helpful conceptually, but practical questions remain: How do we know when the brain is no longer self-aware or will have no recall? And what is the dose of inhaled anesthetic at this point? The ability to determine, establish, and maintain this level of anesthesia is part of the art of anesthesia. It depends on the integration of knowledge of inhaled anesthetic pharmacokinetics and pharmacodynamics and direct observation of the patient and interpretation of data from a complex array of monitors. The BIS monitor, the first, albeit crude, index of anesthetic "depth" *via* continuous real-time analysis of the patient's electroencephalogram (EEG) might provide relevant information. The utility of this device remains controversial, however.

Minimum Alveolar Concentration (MAC)

The pharmacodynamic effects of inhaled anesthetics must be based on a dose, and this dose is the *minimum alveolar concentration* (MAC). MAC is the alveolar concentration of an anesthetic at 1 atm (1 atm = 760 mm Hg) that prevents movement in response to a surgical stimulus in 50% of patients.[50,51] It is analogous to the ED_{50} expressed for intravenous drugs. A variety of surgical stimuli have been used to establish the MAC for each inhaled anesthetic, but the classic defining noxious stimulus is incision of the abdomen. Likewise, skeletal muscle movement is the defining patient response, but other responses have been used to establish MAC as well. Experimentally determined MAC values for humans for the inhaled anesthetics are shown in Table 15-1.

The 95% confidence ranges for MAC are approximately ±25% of the listed MAC values. Manufacturers' recommendations and clinical experience establish 1.2–1.3 times MAC as a dose that consistently prevents patient movement during surgical stimuli. Presumably, loss of consciousness precedes the absence of stimulus-induced movement by a wide margin. While these 1.2–1.3 MAC values do not *absolutely* ensure the defining criteria for brain anesthesia (the absence of self-awareness and recall), vast clinical experience suggests it is extremely unlikely for a patient to be aware of, or to recall, the surgical incision at these anesthetic concentrations.

Concentrations of inhaled anesthetics that provide loss of self-awareness and recall are about 0.4–0.5 MAC. Several lines of reasoning lead to this conclusion. First, most patients receiving only 50% nitrous oxide (approximately 0.4–0.5 MAC), as in a typical dentist's office, will have no recall of their procedure during N_2O administration. Second, various studies have shown that a shift in EEG dominance to the anterior leads (*i.e.*, the shift from self-aware to non-self-aware) accompanies loss of consciousness; and in primates, the EEG shift and loss of consciousness occur at 0.5 MAC.[52] Third, in dogs, loss of consciousness accompanies a sudden nonlinear fall in cerebral metabolic rate at approximately 0.5 MAC (Fig. 15-10).

MAC values can be established for any measurable response. MAC-awake, the alveolar concentration of anesthetic at which a patient opens his or her eyes to command, varies from 0.15 to 0.5 MAC.[53,54] Interestingly, transition from awake to unconscious and back typically shows some hysteresis, in that it quite consistently takes 0.4–0.5 MAC to lose consciousness, but less than that (as low as 0.15 MAC) to regain consciousness. MAC-BAR, the alveolar concentration of anesthetic that blunts adrenergic responses to noxious stimuli, has likewise been established and is approximately 50% higher than standard MAC.[55] MAC also has been established for discrete levels of EEG activity, such as onset of burst suppression or isoelectricity. Attempts to establish MAC values for particular EEG bispectral index (BIS) values are underway.

Standard MAC values are roughly additive.[56,57] Administering 0.5 MAC of a potent agent and 0.5 MAC of nitrous oxide is equivalent to 1 MAC of potent agent in terms of preventing patient movement, although this does not hold over the entire range of N_2O doses.[58] MAC effects for other response parameters are not necessarily additive. Because MAC-movement probably differs from MAC for various secondary side effects (such hypothetical situations as "MAC-dysrhythmia," "MAC-hypotension," or "MAC-tachycardia"), combinations of a potent agent and nitrous oxide may decrease or increase these secondary

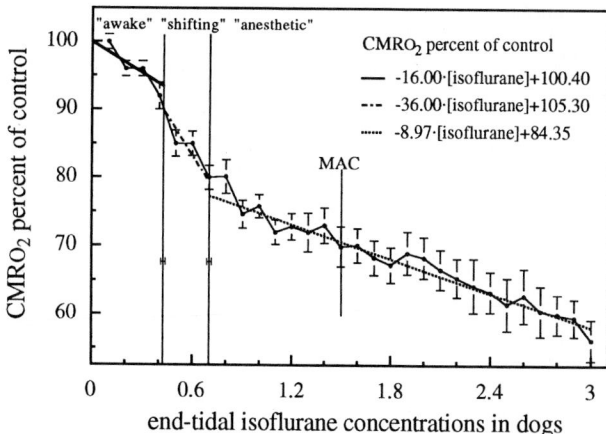

Figure 15-10. The effects of halothane on $CMRO_2$ (cerebral metabolic rate) as a percentage of control ("awake"). $CMRO_2$ is plotted versus end-tidal isoflurane concentration. Regression lines for changes in $CMRO_2$ are drawn for each EEG-determined area. The pattern depicted here is characteristic of all of the anesthetics examined (enflurane, halothane, and isoflurane). (Adapted from Stullken EH Jr, Milde JH, Michenfelder JD *et al*: The non-linear responses of cerebral metabolism to low concentrations of halothane, enflurane, isoflurane and thiopental. Anesthesiology 46:28, 1977.)

effects relative to potent agent alone. For example, combining 0.6 MAC of nitrous oxide with 0.6 MAC of halothane produces less hypotension than 1.2 MAC of halothane alone because halothane is a more potent vasodilator and myocardial depressant than N_2O at equivalent MAC.

Various factors increase (Table 15-4) or decrease (Table 15-5) MAC. Unfortunately, no single mechanism explains these alterations in MAC, supporting the view that anesthesia is the net result of numerous and widely varying physiologic alterations. In general, factors that increase CNS metabolic activity and neurotransmission,[59,60] increase CNS neurotransmitter levels,[61] and up regulate CNS responses to chronically depressed neurotransmitter levels (as in chronic alcoholism) seem to increase MAC. And factors that decrease CNS metabolic activity and neurotransmission,[62–64] decrease CNS neurotransmitter levels, and down regulate CNS responses to chronically elevated neurotransmitter levels[65] seem to decrease MAC. But many notable factors do *not* alter MAC, including duration of inhaled anesthetic administration, gender, type of surgical stimulation, thyroid function, hypo- or hypercarbia, metabolic alkalosis, hyperkalemia, and magnesium levels.

Effect of Age on MAC

The MAC for each of the potent anesthetic gases shows a clear, age-related change (Fig. 15-11).[64,66,67] MAC decreases with age and there are similarities between agents in the decline in MAC and age. Excluding data in patients less than 1 year of age (where MAC can be lower[60]), there is a linear model that describes the decrease in MAC with increasing age.[67] The slope of this model is MAC = $a(10^{bx})$, where *a* is the MAC at age 40, *x* is the

---

Table 15-4. FACTORS THAT INCREASE MAC

- Increased central neurotransmitter levels (monoamine oxidase inhibitors, acute dextroamphetamine administration, cocaine, ephedrine, levodopa)
- Hyperthermia
- Chronic ethanol abuse (determined in humans)
- Hypernatremia

Table 15-5. FACTORS THAT DECREASE MAC

- Increasing age
- Metabolic acidosis
- Hypoxia (Pao_2, 38 mm Hg)
- Induced hypotension (MAP < 50 mm Hg)
- Decreased central neurotransmitter levels (α-methyldopa, reserpine, chronic dextroamphetamine administration, levodopa)
- Alpha-2 agonists
- Hypothermia
- Hyponatremia
- Lithium
- Hypo-osmolality
- Pregnancy
- Acute ethanol administration*
- Ketamine
- Pancuronium*
- Physostigmine (10 times clinical doses)
- Neostigmine (10 times clinical doses)
- Lidocaine
- Opioids
- Opioid agonist–antagonist analgesics
- Barbiturates*
- Chlorpromazine*
- Diazepam*
- Hydroxyzine*
- Δ-9-Tetrahydrocannabinol
- Verapamil
- Anemia (<4.3 ml/$O_2 \cdot dl^{-1}$ blood)

* Determined in humans.

difference in age in years from 40, and $b = -0.00269$. This equation defines a change in MAC of ~6% per decade, a 22% decrease in MAC from age 40 to age 80, and a 27% decrease in MAC from age 1 to 40 years. MAC is typically expressed for an intermediate age (40 years), and these are:

Halothane	0.75%
Isoflurane	1.17%
Enflurane	1.63%
Sevoflurane	1.8%
Desflurane	6.6%
Nitrous oxide	104%

Other Alterations in Neurophysiology

The four potent agents currently in widespread use—halothane, isoflurane, desflurane, and sevoflurane—all have qualitatively similar effects on a wide range of parameters, including cerebral metabolic rate (CMR), the electroencephalogram (EEG), cerebral blood flow (CBF), CBF autoregulation, and flow–metabolism coupling. There are notable differences in effects on intracerebral pressure (ICP), cerebrospinal fluid (CSF) production and reabsorption, CO_2 vasoreactivity, and cerebral protection. Nitrous oxide departs from the potent agents in several important respects, and is therefore discussed separately.

Cerebral Metabolic Rate (CMR) and EEG

All of the potent agents depress CMR to varying degrees in a nonlinear fashion. In isoflurane-anesthetized dogs, there is a sudden decrease in $CMRo_2$ paralleling a change in the EEG from an awake to anesthetized pattern at about 0.4–0.6 MAC as seen in Figure 15-10.[68] For most of the potent agents, CMR is decreased only to the extent that spontaneous cortical neuronal activity (as reflected in the EEG) is decreased.[69] With gradually increasing inspired concentrations of anesthetic, after spontaneous cortical neuronal activity vanishes (an isoelectric EEG), no further decreases in CMR are generated. Halothane is the

exception. Halothane causes a 20–30% decrease in CMR at normal clinical concentrations.[70] However, halothane at 4.5% produces an isoelectric EEG, and further increases in inspired concentration cause further decreases in $CMRo_2$. This further depression of $CMRo_2$ is due to toxic effects on oxidative phosphorylation. Toxic effects begin at concentrations as low as 2.3%, at which point brain lactate concentrations increase,[71] but this dose is typically well above those used clinically for halothane.

Isoflurane causes a larger MAC-dependent depression of CMR than halothane does, and does not depress $CMRo_2$ once an isoelectric EEG is produced.[72] Because of this greater depression in neuronal activity on a per-MAC basis, isoflurane abolishes EEG activity at doses used clinically and can usually be tolerated from a hemodynamic standpoint.[69] Desflurane and sevoflurane both cause decreases in CMR similar to that of isoflurane.[73–75] Interestingly, while both desflurane and sevoflurane depress the EEG and abolish activity at clinically tolerated doses of approximately 2 MAC,[75,76] in *dogs* desflurane-induced isoelectric EEG reverts to continuous activity with time despite an unchanging MAC—a property unique to desflurane.[76] In *cats,* sevoflurane at isoelectric EEG concentrations is not associated with a reversion to continuous EEG activity, although species differences could account for the differing results.[77] The reversion of an isoelectric to continuous EEG does not occur in desflurane-anesthetized swine,[78] and there are no case reports of this phenomenon in humans.

Potential for cerebral toxicity has been studied for sevoflurane as compared to halothane. At normal CO_2 and blood pressure no evidence of sevoflurane toxicity exists.[79] With extreme hyperventilation to decrease cerebral blood flow by half, brain lactate levels increase, but significantly less so than with halothane. There are conflicting data as to whether sevoflurane has a proconvulsant effect.[75,77,80] Many neuroanesthesiologists use sevoflurane routinely since any proconvulsant effects do not appear to be clinically relevant.

Cerebral Blood Flow (CBF), Flow–Metabolism Coupling, and Autoregulation

All of the potent agents increase CBF in a dose-dependent manner. Halothane is a very potent cerebral vasodilator[70,81,82] and causes the greatest increase in CBF per MAC multiple.

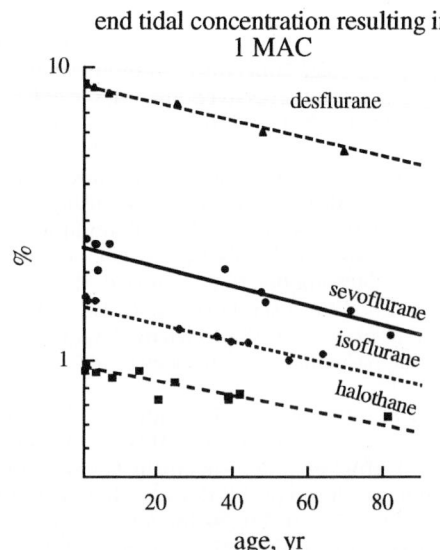

Figure 15-11. Effect of age on MAC. Regression lines are fitted to published values from separate studies. Data are from patients aged 1 to 80 years. (Adapted from Mapleson WW: Effect of age on MAC in humans: A meta-analysis. Br J Anaesth 76:179, 1996.)

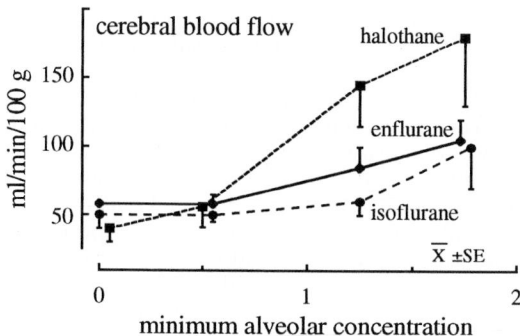

Figure 15-12. Cerebral blood flow measured in the presence of normocapnia and in the absence of surgical stimulation in volunteers. At light levels of anesthesia, enflurane or halothane (but not isoflurane) increased cerebral blood flow. All three agents increased cerebral blood flow at 1.6 MAC. (Adapted from Eger EI II: Isoflurane (Forane): A compendium and reference. Madison, Ohio Medical Products, 1985.)

Because of this, halothane is rarely used in neurosurgery today, even though it was the dominant anesthetic for these cases until the early 1970s. Despite causing the greatest increase in CBF, the vasodilating effects of halothane are blunted by hyperventilating subjects to a $Paco_2$ of 25 mm Hg prior to or simultaneous with the administration of halothane.[83]

Isoflurane causes far less cerebral vasodilation per MAC multiple than does halothane,[82,84,85] and is the predominant volatile anesthetic used in neurosurgical cases today (Fig. 15-12). In human studies, isoflurane produces insignificant[86] or no changes in CBF.[87] Desflurane and sevoflurane both influence CBF in a fashion similar to isoflurane.[73–75,88] All of these inhaled anesthetic agents affect CBF in a time-dependent as well as a dose-dependent manner. In both goats and dogs, an initial dose-dependent increase in CBF with halothane and isoflurane administration recovers to preinduction levels approximately 2–5 hours after induction.[89–91] The mechanism of this recovery is unclear.

The increase in CBF with increasing dose caused by the potent agents occurs despite decreases in CMR. This phenomenon has been called "uncoupling," but from a mechanistic standpoint, true uncoupling of flow from metabolism may not occur. That is, as CMR is depressed by the volatile anesthetics, there is still a coupled decline in tonic vasodilating influences on the cerebral vasculature, but a coincident direct vasodilatory effect on the cerebral blood vessels. The net effect on the cerebral vessels depends on the sum of indirect "vasoconstricting" and direct vasodilating influences.

This view is supported by several facts. First, at low doses, both halothane ($< 0.375\%$) and isoflurane (0.5%) can actually decrease CBF.[92,93] This probably reflects intact coupling of CBF to CMR, with the depression in neuronal activity and metabolism causing a coupled decline in perfusion. At higher doses, increases in CBF occur presumably because direct vasodilation at these doses outweighs indirect vasoconstriction. Second, if CMR is maximally or near-maximally depressed with a barbiturate, halothane and isoflurane produce similar increases in CBF.[94] This is consistent with the greater depression of CMR seen with isoflurane. From a starting point of normal CMR, isoflurane causes a greater dose-dependent decrease in CMR, resulting in greater indirect vasoconstriction and less vasodilation. When CMR is maximally depressed prior to isoflurane or halothane administration, no further indirect vasoconstriction is possible, and the two agents dilate cerebral vessels to a similar extent. Third, CBF:$CMRo_2$ ratios are the same for many volatile anesthetics at equivalent MAC, and increase with increasing dose in a similar fashion.[95] Finally, regional CBF–CMR relationships are arguably better indicators of coupling than the global CBF:CMR ratio, and both isoflurane and halothane show strong

coupling between decreases in CMR and CBF in individual brain regions.[96]

Autoregulation is the intrinsic myogenic regulation of vascular tone. In normal brain, the mechanisms of autoregulation of CBF over a range of mean arterial pressures from 50 to 150 mm Hg are incompletely understood. Because the volatile anesthetics are direct vasodilators, all are considered to diminish autoregulation in a dose-dependent fashion such that CBF is essentially pressure-passive at high anesthetic doses. There are data documenting impaired autoregulation with halothane and relatively preserved autoregulation with isoflurane in studies specifically aimed at investigating the relationship between the two (Fig. 15-13).[97,98] Sevoflurane preserves autoregulation up to approximately 1 MAC.[75]

Intracerebral Pressure (ICP)

Probably the area of greatest clinical interest to the anesthesiologist is the effect of volatile anesthesia on ICP. In general, ICP will increase or decrease in proportion to changes in cerebral blood flow.[99,100] Halothane increases ICP to the greatest extent, reflecting its effects on CBF which are the largest of the potent agents'.[82,83] In fact, brain protrusion during craniotomy is greater with halothane than with isoflurane, consistent with the greater increase in ICP by halothane.[101] At concentrations of 0.5 MAC or less, halothane alone insignificantly increases ICP; above this, however, halothane has the propensity to increase CBF and ICP. This, in association with a tendency to lower mean arterial blood pressure, may cause profound decreases in cerebral perfusion pressure. Preinduction hyperventilation prevents—and simultaneous hyperventilation with induction blunts—the increases in ICP seen with halothane administration.[83] Barbiturate coadministration likewise blunts or prevents halothane-induced increases in ICP.

In contrast to halothane, isoflurane increases ICP minimally in animals both with and without brain pathology, including those with an already elevated ICP.[82] In human studies there usually are mild increases in ICP with isoflurane administration that, as with halothane, are blocked or blunted by hyperventilation or barbiturate coadministration.[102,103] There are some contradictory data, however. In an animal model, edema caused by cryogenic brain lesions was greater with isoflurane anesthesia than with halothane anesthesia[104]; and in another, hypocapnia prior to the lesions did not prevent increases in ICP under isoflurane anesthesia. In one human study, hypocapnia did not prevent elevations in ICP with isoflurane administration in patients with space-occupying brain lesions.[105] In any case, the increase in ICP with or without brain pathology is far less for isoflurane than for halothane. Furthermore, any isoflurane-induced increases in ICP tend to be of short duration—in one

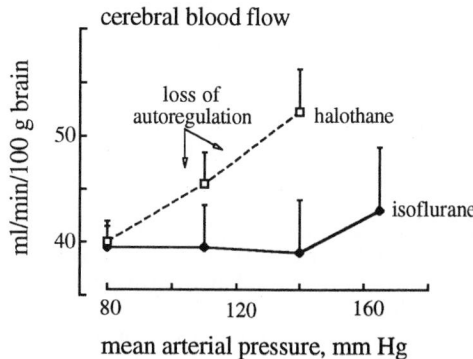

Figure 15-13. Autoregulation of cerebral blood flow (mean ± SE) is preserved in animals receiving isoflurane, but impaired during halothane anesthesia. (Adapted from Eger EI II: Pharmacology of isoflurane. Br J Anaesth 56:71S, 1984.)

study, just 30 minutes[106] —as opposed to halothane, in which case the ICP increase may last for hours.

Like isoflurane, both sevoflurane and desflurane produce mild increases in ICP, paralleling their mild increases in CBF.[74-76] One potential advantage of sevoflurane is that its lower pungency and airway irritation may diminish the risk of coughing and bucking and the associated rise in ICP as compared to desflurane or isoflurane. Ultimately, all four potent agents may be used at appropriate doses, especially with compensatory therapies, in virtually any neurosurgical procedure. For example, many neuroanesthesiologists maintain that halothane can be safely used in neurosurgery at doses of 1 MAC or less, and perhaps slightly more with hyperventilation or barbiturate administration. However, patients with traumatic head injuries, elevated ICP, or space-occupying brain lesions are probably better served with isoflurane or the newer volatile anesthetics.

Cerebrospinal Fluid (CSF) Production and Reabsorption

Studies indicate that 1 MAC halothane decreases CSF production but increases resistance to reabsorption,[107,108] the net effect being an increase in CSF volume.[100] Isoflurane does not appear to alter CSF production,[106,107] but may increase, decrease, or leave unchanged the resistance to reabsorption depending on dose.[109] Sevoflurane at 1 MAC depresses CSF production up to 40%.[110] Desflurane at 1 MAC leaves CSF production unchanged or increased.[111,112] CSF dynamics may play a clinically relevant role in raising or lowering ICP, depending on the relationship of CSF production to CSF reabsorption and the associated changes in cerebral blood volume. At this time, however, no clear recommendations can be made as to which volatile anesthetics are better or worse for a given clinical situation. In general, anesthetic effects on ICP *via* changes in CSF dynamics are clinically much less important than anesthetic effects on CBF.

CBF Response to Hyper- and Hypocapnia

Significant hypercapnia is associated with dramatic increases in CBF, whether or not volatile anesthetics are administered. As discussed earlier, hypocapnia can blunt or abolish anesthetic-induced increases in CBF, depending on when the hypocapnia is produced. This vasoreactivity to CO_2 may be somewhat altered by the volatile anesthetics as compared to normal. Neither isoflurane nor halothane abolishes hypocapnic vasoconstriction, and at least two studies suggest that halothane actually enhances CO_2 reactivity.[84,113] CO_2 vasoreactivity under desflurane anesthesia is normal up to 1.5 MAC,[114] but CO_2 vasoreactivity for sevoflurane may be slightly less, relative to other potent agents.[75,115]

Cerebral Protection

Because all of the potent agents significantly depress CMR, one might reason that each could offer some degree of neuroprotection. Unfortunately, this is not the case. In halothane-anesthetized dogs, focal ischemia caused by middle cerebral artery occlusion led to larger infarct size and worse neurologic outcome than for awake animals.[116] Fortunately, it was shown that the well known neuroprotective effects of pentobarbital are preserved with halothane, since pentobarbital coadministration minimized the pathologic and functional damage.[117]

In comparison, isoflurane may provide some neuroprotective effects in both mice and dogs during hypoxemia or ischemia.[118,119] In one study, cerebral hypoperfusion due to induced hypotension with isoflurane was associated with better tissue oxygen content than during hypotension by other means, consistent with the profound decrease in $CMRo_2$ seen with isoflurane.[120] The most compelling evidence for isoflurane's superiority to halothane for neuroprotection was shown in two studies of human carotid endarterectomy surgery. In these patients, the incidence of ischemic EEG changes was lower with isoflur-

ane than with halothane,[121] and ischemic EEG changes occurred at a lower CBF with isoflurane than with halothane.[122]

Both sevoflurane and desflurane have been shown to improve neurologic outcome in comparison to N_2O–fentanyl after incomplete cerebral ischemia in a rat model.[123,124] Desflurane has been shown to increase brain tissue Po_2 during administration and to maintain Po_2 to a greater extent than thiopental during temporary cerebral artery occlusion in humans undergoing cerebrovascular surgery.[125] No human neuroprotection outcome studies for sevoflurane and desflurane have been published. Interpretation of the published data suggests that surgical cases in which temporary cerebral arterial occlusion is planned or probable would benefit more from isoflurane (or sevoflurane or desflurane?) than halothane anesthesia, but further studies are necessary.

Nitrous Oxide

The effects of nitrous oxide on cerebral physiology are not clear. Both the MAC for N_2O and its effects on CMR vary widely depending on species.[126-130] The difference in CMR effects may in part be accounted for by differences in MAC, but MAC-equivalent effects on CMR also differ. According to several studies in dogs, goats, and swine, N_2O causes an increase in $CMRo_2$ and CBF,[129-131] while in rodents no such increases[127,132,133] or only slight increases occur.[126,132] In human studies, N_2O administration preserved CBF but decreased $CMRo_2$.[95]

Another problem is the fact that N_2O is a co-anesthetic used to supplement potent agents, not a complete anesthetic in itself, so that CMR effects may differ depending on presence or absence of potent agent as well as the particular agent and dose. N_2O causes a greater increase in CBF and CMR in dogs at 0.2% halothane than at 0.8% halothane. In contrast, addition of N_2O to 1 or 2.2 MAC isoflurane does not alter $CMRo_2$,[134] but does increase CBF at 1 MAC and not at 2.2 MAC.

Barbiturates,[130] narcotics,[135] or combinations of the two[136] appear to decrease or eliminate the increases in CMR and CBF produced by N_2O. The effect of pentobarbital/N_2O is dose-dependent, with preserved increases in CMR by N_2O at low-dose pentobarbital, and no changes in CMR at high-dose pentobarbital.[137] N_2O and benzodiazepine coadministration is particularly confusing. Midazolam/N_2O in dogs increased CBF but did not alter $CMRo_2$[138] while the opposite was true in rats,[139] and both CBF and $CMRo_2$ declined in rats given diazepam/N_2O. N_2O administration increases ICP,[130] but as is the case for CMR and CBF, changes in ICP are decreased or eliminated by a variety of co-anesthetics and, more importantly, by hypocapnia.[130,140]

N_2O appears to have an anti-neuroprotective effect, as addition of N_2O to isoflurane during temporary ischemia is associated with greater tissue damage and worsened neurologic outcome.[141] In a study in mice, survival time after a hypoxic event was decreased by addition of N_2O.[142] Given the conflicting data on the effects of N_2O on CMR, CBF, and ICP, and its apparent anti-neuroprotective effect, avoidance or discontinuation of its use should be considered in surgical cases with a high likelihood of elevated ICP or significant cerebral ischemia.

THE CIRCULATORY SYSTEM

Hemodynamics

The cardiac vascular and autonomic effects of the volatile anesthetics have been carefully defined by a number of studies carried out in human volunteers not undergoing surgery.[143-152] In general, the information from these volunteer studies has translated well to the patient population commonly exposed to these anesthetics during elective and emergent surgeries. There are clearly modifying factors in describing the volatile anesthetic effects on the circulation, such as interactions with anesthetic adjuvants and modifications in response due to underlying disease.

A very clear and common effect of the potent volatile anesthetics halothane, enflurane, isoflurane, desflurane, and sevoflurane has been a dose-related decrease in arterial blood pressure.[153,154] No essential differences are seen among the volatile anesthetics when examining their effect on blood pressure at steady-state equi-anesthetic concentrations (Fig. 15-14). However, the mechanism by which they decrease arterial blood pressure is somewhat more specific for each anesthetic. Halothane is notable for its decrease in cardiac output—an effect that contributes importantly to its blood pressure lowering effect (Fig. 15-15).[143,155,156] The mechanism by which halothane decreases cardiac output primarily involves a profound depression of myocardial contractility and has been associated with an increase in right atrial pressure (Fig. 15-15).[143,157] In contrast, desflurane, sevoflurane, and isoflurane are known to maintain cardiac output.[149,153,154,158] Their primary mechanism to decrease blood pressure with increasing dose is related to their potent effects on regional and systemic vascular resistance (Fig. 15-15).[145,150,159] Enflurane falls somewhere between halothane and the newer volatile anesthetics in terms of its effects on cardiac output and peripheral resistance. Enflurane is associated with some myocardial depression, a decrease in cardiac output, and a measurable increase in right atrial pressure.[144,160-162]

In terms of the effects of the volatile anesthetics on heart rate, data from animal studies indicate that desflurane consistently increases heart rate,[161,163-165] whereas sevoflurane provides a relatively stable heart rate.[88,166-168] In volunteers, sevoflurane and halothane up to about 1 MAC result in minimal, if any, changes

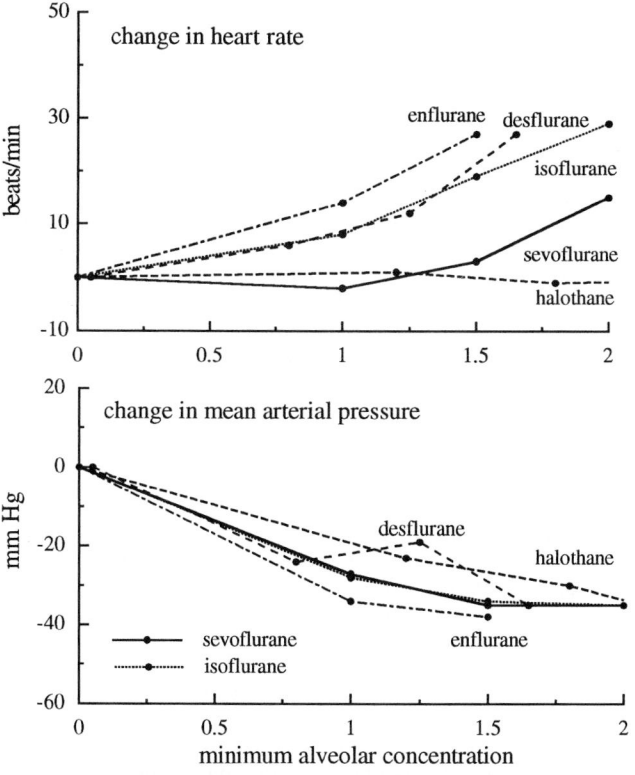

Figure 15-14. Heart rate and blood pressure changes (from awake baseline) in volunteers receiving general anesthesia with a potent anesthetic. Halothane and sevoflurane produced little change in heart rate at less than 1.5 MAC. All anesthetics caused similar decreases in blood pressure. (Adapted from Calverley RK, Smith NT, Prys-Roberts C *et al:* Cardiovascular effects of enflurane anesthesia during controlled ventilation in man. Anesth Analg 57:619, 1978; Weiskopf RB, Cahalan MK, Eger EI II *et al:* Cardiovascular actions of desflurane in normocarbic volunteers. Anesth Analg 73:143, 1991; and Malan TP, DiNardo JA, Isner RJ *et al:* Cardiovascular effects of sevoflurane compared with those of isoflurane in volunteers. Anesthesiology 83:918, 1995.)

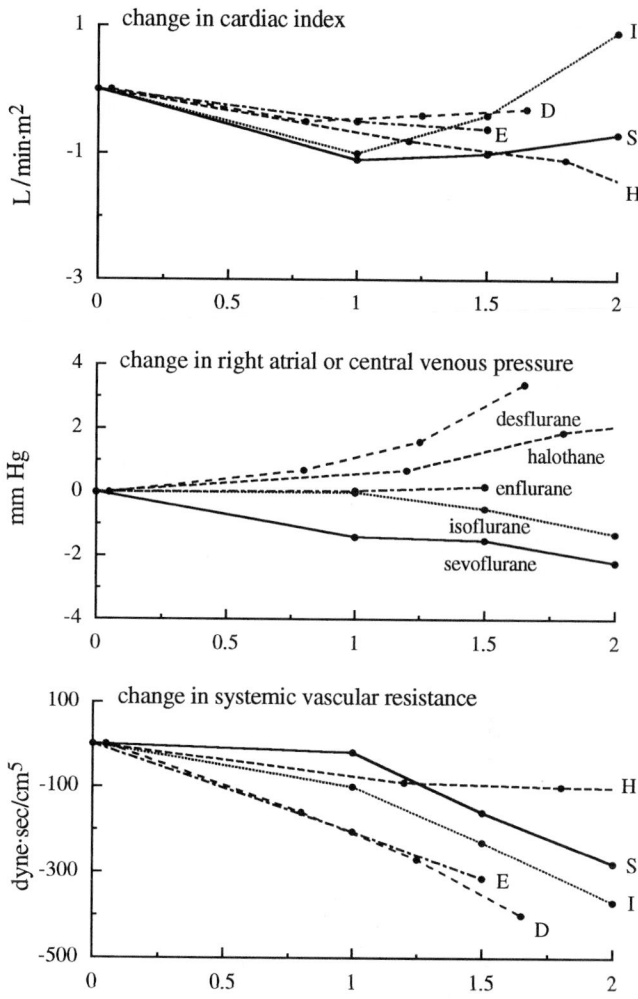

Figure 15-15. Cardiac index, systemic vascular resistance, and central venous pressure (or right atrial pressure) changes (from awake baseline) in volunteers receiving general anesthesia with a potent anesthetic. Increases in central venous pressure from halothane and desflurane might be due to different mechanisms. With halothane, the increase might be due to myocardial depression, whereas with desflurane, the increase is more likely due to venoconstriction. (Adapted from Calverley RK, Smith NT, Prys-Roberts C *et al:* Cardiovascular effects of enflurane anesthesia during controlled ventilation in man. Anesth Analg 57:619, 1978; Weiskopf RB, Cahalan MK, Eger EI II *et al:* Cardiovascular actions of desflurane in normocarbic volunteers. Anesth Analg 73:143, 1991; and Malan TP, DiNardo JA, Isner RJ *et al:* Cardiovascular effects of sevoflurane compared with those of isoflurane in volunteers. Anesthesiology 83:918, 1995.)

in steady-state heart rate (Fig. 15-14).[149,153,154] In contrast, both enflurane and isoflurane have been associated with an increase in heart rate of 10–20% at 1 MAC.[154] At anesthetic levels >1 MAC, desflurane has been associated with an increase in heart rate equal to that of isoflurane.[159] This is generally reflected as a 10–15 beats/min increase in heart rate. Both desflurane and, to a lesser extent, isoflurane have been associated with transient and significant increases in heart rate during rapid increases in the inspired concentration of either anesthetic.[159,169] Although the mechanism(s) underlying these transient heart rate surges are not known, it is conjectured that the relative pungency of these anesthetics activates airway receptors, leading to a reflex tachycardia.[170,171] This tachycardia can be lessened with fentanyl or alfentanil pretreatment.[172-174]

Myocardial Contractility

Myocardial contractility indices have been directly evaluated in animals and indirectly evaluated in humans during the administration of each of the volatile anesthetics. The older anesthetics, halothane and enflurane, have been studied in humans using a relatively imprecise technique called ballistocardiography which permits an indirect measure of contractility (IJ amplitude). At 1 MAC, enflurane caused a 40% decrease in IJ amplitude, whereas halothane caused a 30% decrease in IJ amplitude.[143,144] At 1.5 MAC, greater depression of myocardial contractility was noted for both volatile anesthetics. These changes were noted in conjunction with approximately 20% decreases in cardiac output at 1 MAC halothane and enflurane. Animal and human studies indicate that the myocardial depression from halothane is greater than for isoflurane and enflurane.[175-180] In contrast, human studies with the newer volatile anesthetics, isoflurane, sevoflurane, and desflurane, have not demonstrated significant changes in echocardiographic-determined indices of myocardial function, including the more noteworthy measurement of the velocity of circumferential fiber shortening (Fig. 15-16).[147,149] More precise indices of myocardial contractility have been obtained for sevoflurane, isoflurane, and desflurane in chronically instrumented dogs after autonomic innervation of the heart was blocked by pharmacologic means. This allowed the evaluation of the direct effects of the anesthetics on the heart. The data indicate that isoflurane, desflurane, and sevoflurane cause dose-dependent depression of myocardial function with no differences among the three anesthetics (Fig. 15-17).[153,181,182] Thus, the direct effect of volatile anesthetics is a dose-dependent myocardial depression; however, halothane and enflurane have greater effects on myocardial contractility than do isoflurane, sevoflurane, and desflurane. Not unexpectedly, when the circulatory effects of isoflurane have been compared to halothane in patients with ischemic heart disease, similar effects on lowering blood pressure have been noted; however, cardiac output was decreased to a greater degree with halothane. Halothane also was associated with increases in systemic vascular resistance, whereas isoflurane caused no clinically relevant change in systemic vascular resistance.[155]

Other Circulatory Effects

The majority of the volatile anesthetics have been studied during both controlled and spontaneous ventilation.[18,149,183-185] The

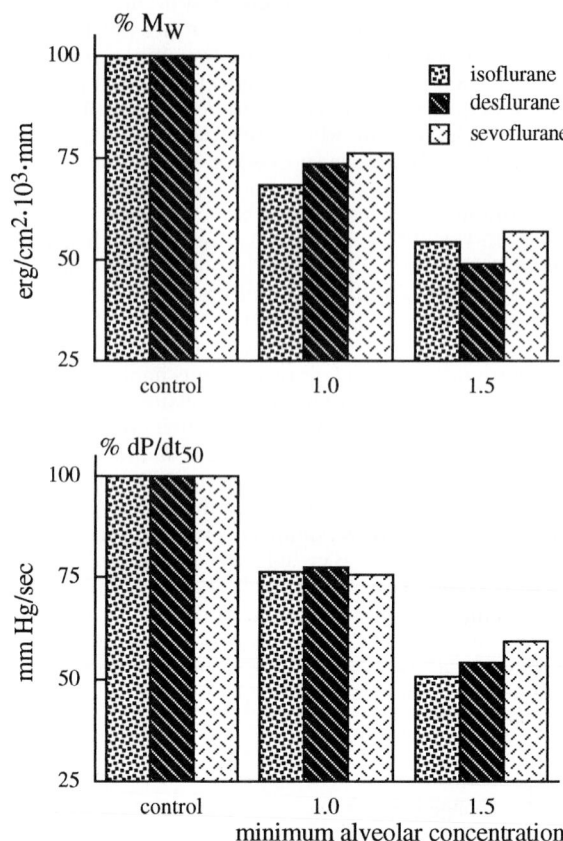

myocardial contractility indices

Figure 15-17. Myocardial contractility indices from chronically instrumented dogs. For these measurements, pharmacologic blockade of the autonomic nervous system was established to eliminate neural or circulating humoral influences on the inotropic state of the heart. The conscious control data were assigned 100%, and subsequent reductions in the inotropic state are depicted for both 1 and 1.5 minimum alveolar anesthetic concentrations of sevoflurane, desflurane, and isoflurane. There were no differences between these three volatile anesthetics. M_w = slope of the regional preload recruitable stroke work relationship; dP/dt_{50} = change in pressure per unit of time. (Adapted from Harkin CP, Pagel PS, Kersten JR et al: Direct negative inotropic and lusitropic effects of sevoflurane. Anesthesiology 81:156, 1994; and Pagel PS, Kampine JP, Schmeling WT et al: Influence of volatile anesthetics on myocardial contractility in vivo: Desflurane versus isoflurane. Anesthesiology 74:900, 1991.)

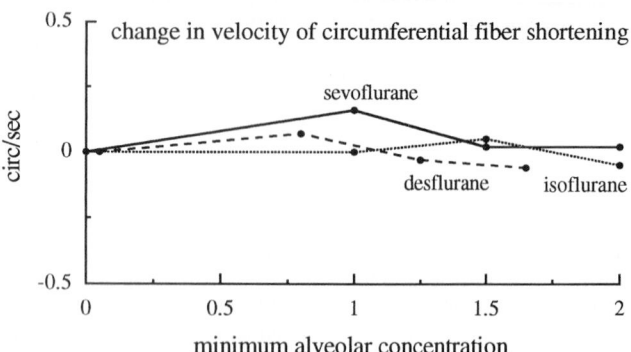

Figure 15-16. Noninvasive assessment of myocardial contractility with echocardiography during anesthesia in volunteers. Sevoflurane, desflurane, and isoflurane did not cause changes suggestive of myocardial depression. (Adapted from Calverley RK, Smith NT, Prys-Roberts C et al: Cardiovascular effects of enflurane anesthesia during controlled ventilation in man. Anesth Analg 57:619, 1978; Weiskopf RB, Cahalan MK, Eger EI II et al: Cardiovascular actions of desflurane in normocarbic volunteers. Anesth Analg 73:143, 1991; and Malan TP, DiNardo JA, Isner RJ et al: Cardiovascular effects of sevoflurane compared with those of isoflurane in volunteers. Anesthesiology 83:918, 1995.)

process of spontaneous ventilation results in a reduction of the high intrathoracic pressures associated with positive pressure ventilation. The negative intrathoracic pressure during the inspiratory phase of spontaneous ventilation augments venous return and cardiac filling and improves cardiac output and, hence, blood pressure. A second result of spontaneous ventilation is higher $Paco_2$, and this change causes cerebral and systemic vascular relaxation and further contributes to an improved cardiac output via afterload reduction. Thus, there is a decrease in systemic vascular resistance and an increase in heart rate, cardiac output, and stroke volume when spontaneous ventilation is contrasted to positive pressure ventilation. It has been suggested that spontaneous ventilation might improve the safety of inhaled anesthetic administration because the concentration of the volatile anesthetics that produces cardiovascular collapse exceeds the concentration resulting in apnea.[186]

A curious observation with the volatile anesthetics has been an alteration in the cardiovascular effects during prolonged anesthetic exposures. Prolonged exposures to halothane, enflurane, sevoflurane, isoflurane, and desflurane have been associated with small increases in heart rate, an improvement in cardiac index, and gradual decreases in systemic vascular resistance.[144,147,149,154,185] There has been no evidence of worsening (or improvement) of myocardial contractility indices during prolonged anesthesia.[147,149] Activation of β-sympathetic receptors has been suggested as a mechanism contributing to the increased heart rate and cardiac output from prolonged anesthesia with halothane[187]; however, this possibility has been questioned based on recent studies with prolonged exposure to enflurane[144] and desflurane anesthesia.[147]

Nitrous oxide is commonly combined with potent volatile anesthetics to maintain general anesthesia. Nitrous oxide has unique cardiovascular actions.[151,152,188] It increases sympathetic nervous system activity when given in a 40% concentration.[188] At the same time, increases in forearm vascular resistance and circulating catecholamines can be observed.[151,152] When nitrous oxide is combined with volatile anesthetics and compared to equipotent concentrations of the volatile anesthetic without nitrous oxide, there still is evidence of sympathetic nervous system activation, with an increased systemic vascular resistance and an improved arterial pressure with little effect on cardiac output.[149,189–192] Some of these effects might not be due to the nitrous oxide *per se*, but may simply be attributed to a decrease in the concentration of the coadministered potent volatile anesthetic to achieve a MAC equivalent when using nitrous oxide.

Oxygen consumption is decreased approximately 10–15% during general anesthesia.[193] The distribution of cardiac output also is altered by anesthesia. Blood flow to liver, kidneys, and gut is decreased, particularly at deep levels of anesthesia. In contrast, blood flow to the brain, muscle, and skin is increased or unchanged during general anesthesia.[163,194,195] With respect to changes in muscle blood flow, data from human volunteer studies comparing isoflurane to desflurane and sevoflurane indicate increases in blood flow with very little difference between anesthetics at equipotent concentrations.[145,153]

In contrast to halothane, the ether-based anesthetics (isoflurane, enflurane, sevoflurane, and desflurane) have neither predisposed patients to ventricular arrhythmias nor sensitized the heart to the dysrhythmogenic effects of epinephrine (Fig. 15-18).[196–198] The use of iv lidocaine can lessen the epinephrine effect during halothane anesthesia.[197] Some of the differences between volatile anesthetics in their ability to promote dysrhythmias during epinephrine administration can be attributed to their direct effects on cardiac pacemaker cells and conduction pathways.[199] The volatile anesthetics slow the SA node discharge rate[200]; in addition, they prolong conduction in the His–Purkinje system and conduction pathways in the ventricle.[199,201] A greater slowing by halothane over isoflurane in the His–Purkinje system might promote dysrhythmias *via* a re-entry phenomenon.[201]

Coronary Steal

The fact that potent volatile anesthetics relax vascular smooth muscle and lead to vasodilation has raised concerns related to abnormal distribution of blood flow in coronary blood vessels of patients with ischemic heart disease. This effect, called *coronary steal,* became a concern with the introduction of isoflurane to clinical practice. Isoflurane (and most other potent volatile anesthetics) increases coronary blood flow many times beyond that of the myocardial oxygen demand, thereby creating potential for "steal." "Steal" is the diversion of blood from a myocardial bed with limited or inadequate perfusion to a bed with more adequate perfusion—especially one that has a remaining element of autoregulation. In instrumented animal models, the pronounced coronary vasodilation produced by isoflurane was shown to cause steal,[202] and early patient studies provided additional support.[203,204] However, more recent work in a chronically instrumented canine model of multivessel coronary artery obstruction has shown that isoflurane, sevoflurane, and desflurane at concentrations up to 1.5 MAC do not result in abnormal collateral coronary blood flow redistribution (steal), whereas adenosine, a potent coronary vasodilator, clearly resulted in abnormal flow distribution.[181,205–207] Interestingly, sevoflurane preferentially increased collateral coronary blood flow in this instrumented animal model when aortic pressure was held constant (as might be seen with systemic blood pressure support).[205] Isoflurane has been shown to increase the tolerance to pacing-induced myocardial ischemia in patients with coronary disease.[208]

Myocardial Ischemia and Cardiac Outcome

Not surprisingly, the clinical relevance of coronary steal with isoflurane has been debated and is generally thought to be minimal.[209,210] Outcome studies have failed to associate the use of isoflurane in patients undergoing coronary artery bypass operations with an increased incidence of myocardial infarction or perioperative death.[210–212] Most studies suggest that determinants of myocardial oxygen supply and demand, rather than the anesthetic, are of far greater importance to patient outcomes.

Several studies have evaluated the two new anesthetics, sevoflurane and desflurane, to comparator anesthetics, in terms of myocardial ischemia and outcome in patients with coronary artery disease undergoing either noncardiac or coronary artery bypass graft (CABG) surgery.[213,214] In both populations, sevoflurane appears to be essentially equivalent to isoflurane in terms of the incidence of myocardial ischemia and adverse cardiac outcomes. In cardiac patients having CABG, desflurane and isoflurane appear to result in similar outcome effects,[215] with one exception. When desflurane was given without opioids

Figure 15-18. The dose of epinephrine associated with cardiac arrhythmias in animal and human models was least with halothane. The ether anesthetics, isoflurane, desflurane, and sevoflurane, required 3–6-fold greater doses of epinephrine to cause dysrhythmias. (Adapted from Hayashi Y, Sumikawa K, Tashiro C *et al:* Arrhythmogenic threshold of epinephrine during sevoflurane, enflurane, and isoflurane anesthesia in dogs. Anesthesiology 69:145, 1988; Weiskopf RB, Eger EI II, Holmes MA *et al:* Epinephrine-induced premature ventricular contractions and changes in arterial blood pressure and heart rate during I-653, isoflurane, and halothane anesthesia in swine. Anesthesiology 70:293, 1989; Navarro R, Weiskopf RB, Moore MA *et al:* Humans anesthetized with sevoflurane or isoflurane have similar arrhythmic response to epinephrine. Anesthesiology 80:545, 1994; and Moore MA, Weiskopf RB, Eger EI II *et al:* Arrhythmogenic doses of epinephrine are similar during desflurane or isoflurane anesthesia in humans. Anesthesiology 79:943, 1993.)

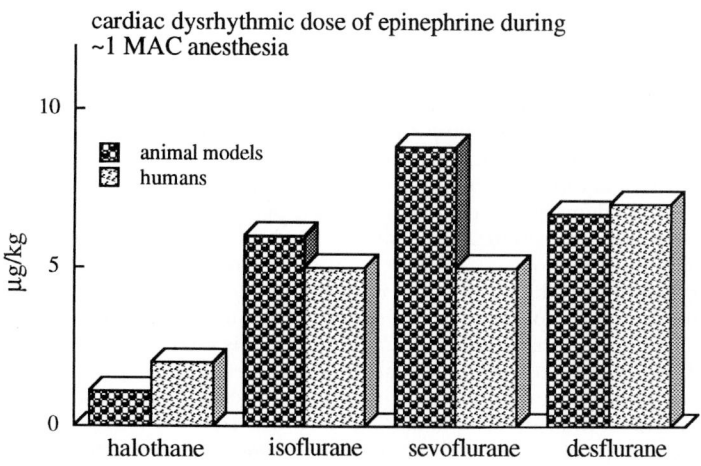

cardiac dysrhythmic dose of epinephrine during ~1 MAC anesthesia

animal models
humans

halothane   isoflurane   sevoflurane   desflurane

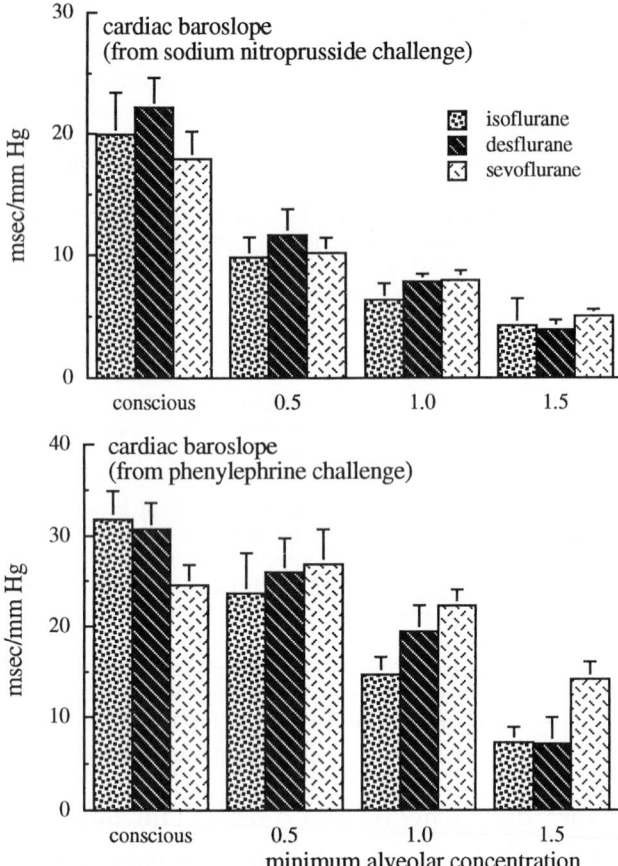

Figure 15-19. Summary data of the baroreflex regulation of heart rate (R–R interval) in response to a decreasing pressure stimulus (sodium nitroprusside) or in response to an increasing pressure stimulus (phenylephrine). These data were acquired in healthy volunteers who were randomized to receive isoflurane, desflurane, or sevoflurane. With increasing MAC, each of the volatile anesthetics led to a progressive reduction in the cardiac baroslope (an index of baroreflex sensitivity derived by relating changes in mean pressure to changes in R–R interval). There were no statistical differences between anesthetics. (Adapted from Ebert TJ, Harkin CP, Muzi M: Cardiovascular responses to sevoflurane: A review. Anesth Analg 81:S11, 1995.)

to patients with coronary artery disease requiring CABG, significant ischemia was noted, mandating the use of beta blockers.[216] Desflurane has not been evaluated in terms of ischemia and outcome in a patient population with coronary disease undergoing noncardiac surgery.

Autonomic Nervous System

Studies that have focused on the efferent activity of the parasympathetic and sympathetic nervous systems indicate that the volatile anesthetics depress their activity in a dose-dependent fashion.[217-219] However, because the autonomic nervous system is importantly modulated by baroreceptor reflex mechanisms, the effects of anesthetics on the efferent system cannot be reported without taking into account their effects on different components of the baroreflex arc. Thus, although both limbs of the autonomic nervous system have been shown to be attenuated by anesthetics, the afferent activity from the arterial baroreceptors has been found to be increased with some anesthetics, including halothane and isoflurane.[218,220,221] This increased discharge of the baroreceptors actually contributes to the depression of the entire baroreflex arc by tonically lowering the overall level of outflow of the sympathetic nervous system. From the perspective of clinical relevance, studies have examined the

behavior of the arterial baroreflex system during a hypotensive or hypertensive stimulus by evaluating changes in heart rate and sympathetic nerve activity. The arterial baroreflex is the most rapid system responding to blood pressure pertubations. Early investigations focused primarily on the regulation of heart rate (which reflects primarily a vagally mediated endpoint). Halothane,[222,223] enflurane,[223,224] and isoflurane[223,225] all depress the arterial baroreflex control of heart rate in a dose-dependent fashion, although there was a suggestion that isoflurane had a less prominent effect than halothane or enflurane.[225] Similar effects on the reflex control of heart rate have been demonstrated with sevoflurane and desflurane (Fig. 15-19).[153,226-228]

There is greater difficulty in evaluating the sympathetic component of the baroreflex arc in humans. Recently, a technique called sympathetic microneurography has been utilized to directly record vasoconstrictor impulses directed to blood vessels in humans.[150,159,229] There is a dose-dependent depression of the reflex control of sympathetic outflow that appears to be relatively equivalent for isoflurane, sevoflurane, and desflurane (Fig. 15-20).[153,228] Importantly, at low levels of anesthesia (e.g., 0.5 MAC), there is little if any depression of reflex function, and this might have important implications in the compromised patient population. Opioid and benzodiazepine adjuvants have only minimal effects on reflex function, and combining these with low levels of potent anesthetics might preserve reflex function.[230-232] Another important observation has been the more rapid return of baroreflex function with the less soluble anesthetic sevoflurane relative to isoflurane.[233] This might add to hemodynamic stability in the postoperative period when tissue concentrations of the volatile anesthetics are declining.

Desflurane has a unique and prominent effect on sympathetic outflow in humans—an effect that is not apparent in animal models. With increasing steady-state concentrations of desflurane, there is a progressive increase in resting sympathetic nervous system activity and plasma norepinephrine levels.[150,159,234] Despite this increase in tonic sympathetic outflow, blood pressure decreases similarly to sevoflurane and isoflurane. This raises the question as to whether desflurane has the ability to uncouple neuroeffector responses. In addition, desflurane can cause marked activation of the sympathetic nervous system when the inspired concentration is increased, especially to concentrations above 5–6% (Fig. 15-21).[150,159,169,234,235] There is a transient

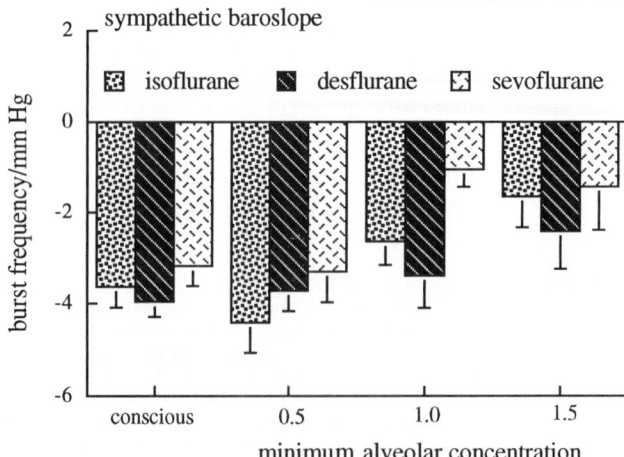

Figure 15-20. The sympathetic baroreflex function of healthy volunteers randomized to receive isoflurane, desflurane, or sevoflurane. The slope (sensitivity) is the relationship between decreasing diastolic pressure and increasing efferent sympathetic nerve activity. The reflex regulation of sympathetic outflow was fairly well preserved at 0.5 and 1.0 MAC of anesthetic. At 1.5 MAC, there was a 50% decrease in the slope with all anesthetics. (Adapted from Ebert TJ, Harkin CP, Muzi M: Cardiovascular responses to sevoflurane: A review. Anesth Analg 81:S11, 1995.)

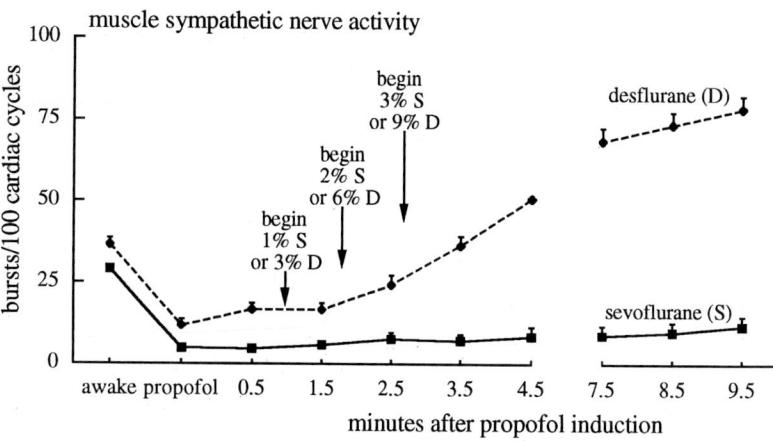

Figure 15-21. Consecutive measurements of sympathetic nerve activity (SNA; mean ± SEM) from human volunteers during induction of anesthesia with propofol and the subsequent mask administration of sevoflurane or desflurane for a 10-min period. The inspired concentration of these anesthetics was increased at 1-min intervals beginning precisely 2 min after propofol administration (0.41 MAC of sevoflurane 1% and of desflurane 3%). In both groups, propofol reduced SNA and MAP. Desflurane resulted in significant increases in neurocirculatory variability that persisted throughout the 10-min mask administration period. (Adapted from Ebert TJ, Muzi M, Lopatka CW: Neurocirculatory responses to sevoflurane in humans. A comparison to desflurane. Anesthesiology 83:88, 1995.)

surge in sympathetic outflow, leading to hypertension and tachycardia. In addition, the endocrine axis is activated, as evidenced by 15–20-fold increases in plasma antidiuretic hormone and epinephrine (Fig. 15-22).[169] The hemodynamic response persists for 4–5 minutes and the endocrine response persists for 15–25 minutes. Administration of adequate concentrations of fentanyl prior to increasing the concentration of desflurane has been shown to attenuate these responses.[172,173] The source of the neuroendocrine activation has been actively sought. It would appear that there are receptors in the upper and the lower airways—and/or perhaps in highly perfused tissue near the airways—that initiate the sympathetic activation.[170,171] The possibility that desflurane activates airway irritant receptors is quite strong, since desflurane is the most pungent of the anesthetics available for clinical use.[237-239]

Cardioprotection from Volatile Anesthetics

There is a new body of literature describing the potential for organ-protective effects (particularly cardioprotective effects) of the potent inhaled agents.[240-244] Organ protection may be defined as "reducing tissue damage after hypoxic ischemia or toxic insult." A standard model to reduce tissue damage after ischemia has been termed "ischemic preconditioning." Preconditioning is a process that protects the myocardium by providing a brief episode of ischemia, which exerts a protective effect against subsequent, more prolonged ischemia. Numerous factors may be involved in preconditioning, including the sodium:hydrogen exchanger, the adenosine receptor (particularly α_1 and α_2 subtypes), inhibitory G proteins, protein kinase C, tyrosine kinase, map kinases, dag, and pkg. Blocking any of these compounds (e.g., with adenosine blockers, δ_1 opioids, pertussis toxin, glibenclamide) reduces the cardioprotective effect of ischemic preconditioning and of the volatile anesthetics. Alternatively, administration of certain drugs can mimic ischemic preconditioning. These include adenosine, opioid agonists, and potassium (K^+–ATP) channel openers. Unlike volatile anesthetics, which can be safely administered via inhalation, these cardioprotective drugs must be given in a coronary artery because systemic administration has serious side effects. Among other cardioprotective effects, inhalation anesthetics are known to:

- Reduce vascular reperfusion damage
- Reduce infarct size
- Reduce ST segment depression
- Improve metabolism
- Reduce dysrhythmias
- Improve vasodilation
- Activate adenosine α_1 receptors
- Produce acidosis by inhibiting sodium:hydrogen exchange
- Spare ATP levels, allowing K^+–ATP channels to open
- Depress calcium currents
- Reduce oxygen free radicals
- Reduce troponin I production

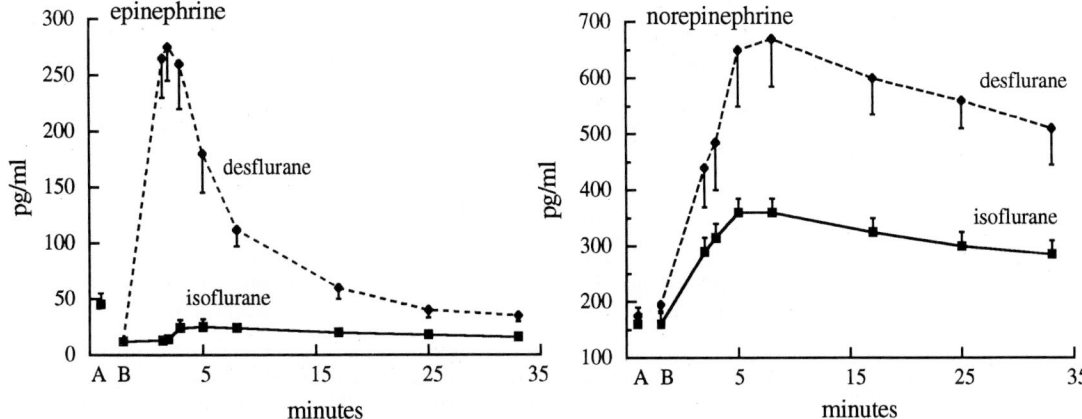

Figure 15-22. Stress hormone responses to a rapid increase in anesthetic concentration, from 4 to 12% inspired. Volunteers given desflurane (diamonds) showed a larger increase in plasma epinephrine and norepinephrine concentrations than when given isoflurane (squares). Data are mean ± SE. (A) Awake value; (B) value after 32 min of 0.55 MAC. Time represents minutes after the first breath of increased anesthetic concentration. (Adapted from Weiskopf RB, Moore MA, Eger EI II et al: Rapid increase in desflurane concentration is associated with greater transient cardiovascular stimulation than with rapid increase in isoflurane concentration in humans. Anesthesiology 80:1035, 1994.)

Approximately 30–40% of the cardioprotection from the volatile anesthetics appears to be related to a reduced loading of calcium into the myocardial cells during ischemia.[243] As nearly all of these evolving data derive from animal models, a number of important questions remain for clinical studies in humans. What quantity of volatile anesthetic and what duration is needed to offer cardioprotective effects? How long is the "memory" of preconditioning after exposure to a volatile anesthetic? Are there dose-related effects? When is the best time to administer the anesthetic prior to the ischemic insult? These and other questions will undoubtedly be addressed and answered in the upcoming years, keeping in mind that good surgical technique might far outweigh any potential for cardiac protection from the volatile anesthetics.

THE PULMONARY SYSTEM

The volatile anesthetics have multiple and important effects on many aspects of pulmonary physiology, including respiratory rate and tidal volume, responses to CO_2 and hypoxia, and effects on bronchiolar smooth muscle tone and mucociliary function. Less pronounced, but still important effects have been ob-

served on pulmonary vascular resistance and pulmonary blood flow.

General Ventilatory Effects

All volatile anesthetics decrease tidal volume but have lesser effects on decreasing minute ventilation because of an offsetting response to increasing respiratory rate (Fig. 15-23).[154,245–250] These effects are dose-dependent, with higher concentrations of volatile anesthetics resulting in greater decreases in tidal volume[248–250] and greater increases in respiratory rate.[245–249] The net effect of a gradual decrease in minute ventilation has been associated with increasing resting $Paco_2$. The relative increases in $Paco_2$ as an index of respiratory depression with volatile anesthetics evaluated at <1.24 MAC are as follows: enflurane > desflurane = isoflurane > sevoflurane = halothane. The respiratory depression can be partially antagonized during surgical stimulation where respiratory rate has been shown to increase, resulting in a decrease in the $Paco_2$ (Fig. 15-24).[251] In addition, resting $Paco_2$ during desflurane or sevoflurane anesthesia is significantly decreased (returned toward normal) with the addition of nitrous oxide.[248,251] This comparison (with and without

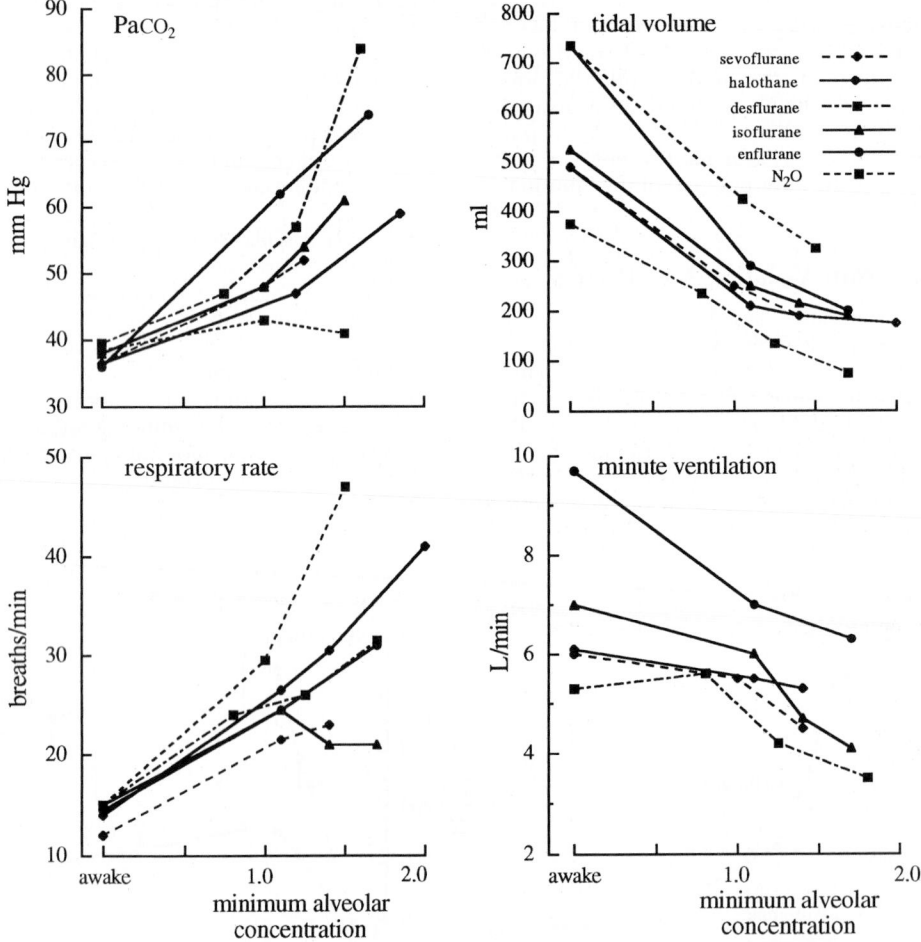

Figure 15-23. Comparison of mean changes in resting $Paco_2$, tidal volume, respiratory rate, and minute ventilation in patients anesthetized with either halothane, isoflurane, enflurane, sevoflurane, desflurane, or nitrous oxide. Anesthetic-induced tachypnea compensates in part for the ventilatory depression caused by all volatile anesthetics (decrease in minute ventilation and tidal volume and concomitant increase in $Paco_2$). Desflurane results in the greatest increase in $Paco_2$ with corresponding reductions in tidal volume and minute ventilation. Isoflurane, like all other inhaled agents, increases respiratory rate; however, isoflurane does not result in dose-dependent tachypnea. (Adapted from Calverley RK, Smith NT, Jones CW *et al:* Ventilatory and cardiovascular effects of enflurane anesthesia during spontaneous ventilation in man. Anesth Analg 57:610, 1978; Lockhart SH, Rampil IJ, Yasuda N *et al:* Depression of ventilation by desflurane in humans. Anesthesiology 74:484, 1991; Fourcade HE, Stevens WC, Larson CPJ *et al:* The ventilatory effects of Forane, a new inhaled anesthetic. Anesthesiology 35:26, 1971; and Doi M, Ikeda K: Respiratory effects of sevoflurane. Anesth Analg 66:241, 1987.)

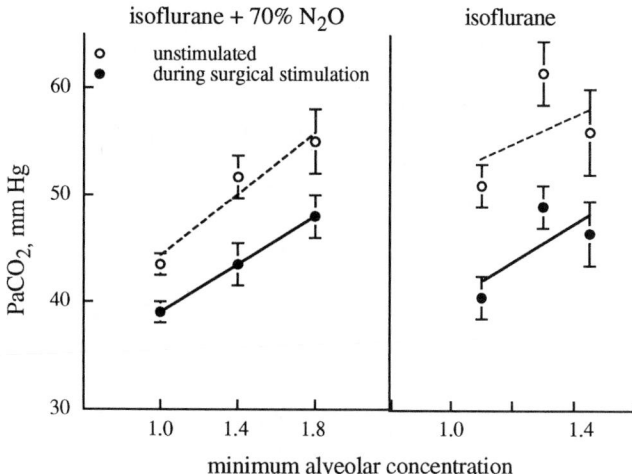

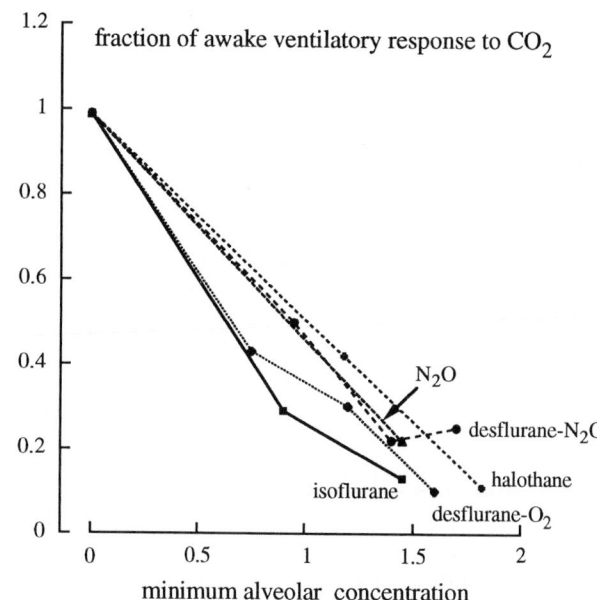

Figure 15-24. The effect of surgical stimulation on the ventilatory depression of inhaled anesthesia with isoflurane in the presence and absence of nitrous oxide. Surgical stimulation increased alveolar ventilation and decreased $PaCO_2$ at all depths of anesthesia examined. (Adapted from Eger EI II, Dolan WM, Stevens WC *et al*: Surgical stimulation antagonizes the respiratory depression produced by forane. Anesthesiology 36:544, 1972.)

Figure 15-25. All inhaled anesthetics produce similar dose-dependent decreases in the ventilatory response to carbon dioxide. (Adapted from Eger EI II: Desflurane. Anesth Rev 20:87, 1993.)

nitrous oxide) requires a lessening of the potent volatile anesthetic to maintain an equi-MAC concentration when adding nitrous oxide to the inspired gas, and this probably contributes to the return of $PaCO_2$ toward normal. The degree of respiratory depression from inhaled anesthetics appears to be lessened during prolonged administration of the anesthetic.[247,252]

Ventilatory Mechanics

The decrease in functional residual capacity during general anesthesia has been explained by a number of mechanisms, including a decrease in the intercostal muscle tone, alteration in diaphragm position, changes in thoracic blood volume, and the onset of phasic expiratory activity of respiratory muscles.[253-256] About 40% of the muscular work of breathing is *via* intercostal muscles and about 60% is from the diaphragm. The diaphragmatic muscle function is relatively spared when contrasted to the parasternal intercostal muscles.[253,254] However, inspiratory rib cage expansion is reasonably well maintained during anesthesia because of preserved activity of the scalene muscles.[254] Expiration is generally considered a passive function mediated by the elastic recoil of the lung. The process of applying a resistance or load to expiration typically results in a slowing of respiration; but under anesthesia, additional responses have been noted, including a substantial asynchrony of the thoracic movements with respiration.[257] This suggests that in patients with pulmonary disease associated with increased expiratory resistance, the act of spontaneous ventilation during general anesthesia might be associated with increased risk.[258]

Response to Carbon Dioxide and Hypoxemia

In normal subjects not under anesthesia, increases in minute ventilation of approximately $3\ l \cdot min^{-1}$ for each 1 mm Hg increase in $PaCO_2$ have been demonstrated. This relatively high sensitivity to CO_2 is mediated by central chemoreceptors and has been used as an index of ventilatory drive. All of the inhaled anesthetics produce a dose-dependent depression of the ventilatory response to hypercarbia (Fig. 15-25).[154,245,246,248,249] Early studies suggested that the addition of nitrous oxide to halothane depressed ventilation less than an equi-MAC dose of halothane alone[259]; however, this does not appear to be the case for desflurane (Fig. 15-25).[248] During anesthesia with spontaneous ven-

tilation, an apneic threshold can be determined which is generally 4–5 mm Hg below the prevailing resting $PaCO_2$, and this threshold is not related to the slope of the CO_2 response curves or to the level of the resting $PaCO_2$. The clinical relevance of this threshold may be important when assisting ventilation in an anesthetized patient who is breathing spontaneously. This only serves to lower the $PaCO_2$ to approach that of the apneic threshold, thus mandating more control of ventilation.

Inhaled anesthetics, including nitrous oxide, also produce dose-dependent attenuation of the ventilatory response to hypoxia.[260-264] This action appears to be dependent on the peripheral chemoreceptors. In fact, even subanesthetic concentrations of volatile anesthetics (0.1 MAC) have profound effects on the ventilatory drive to hypoxia (Fig. 15-26).[265,266] Studies indicate

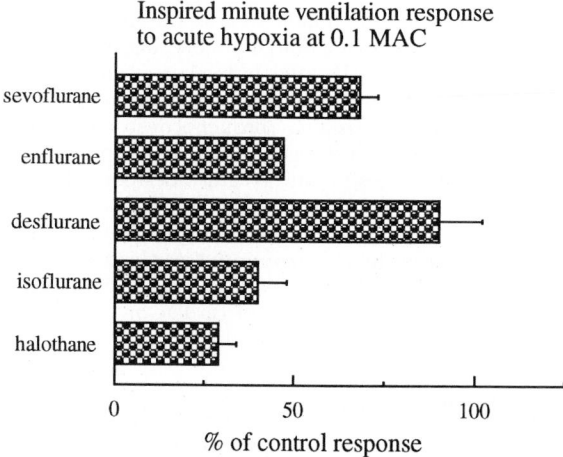

Figure 15-26. Influence of 0.1 MAC of five volatile anesthetic agents on the ventilatory response to a step decrease in end-tidal oxygen concentration. Values are mean ± SD. Subanesthetic concentrations of the volatile anesthetics, except desflurane and sevoflurane, profoundly depress the response to hypoxia. (Adapted from Sarton E, Dahan A, Teppema L *et al*: Acute pain and central nervous system arousal do not restore impaired hypoxic ventilatory responses during sevoflurane sedation. Anesthesiology 85:295, 1996.)

anywhere from 15–75% depression of the response to hypoxia with 0.1 MAC of a volatile anesthetic. This has important clinical implications. The extreme sensitivity of the volatile anesthetics in terms of inhibiting hypoxic responsiveness may persist in patients during their stay in the recovery room because of residual effects. In this regard, the short-acting anesthetics (sevoflurane and desflurane) may prove advantageous because of their more rapid washout. In addition, they appear to have the least effect on hypoxic sensitivity at subanesthetic concentrations (Fig. 15-26). The effects of the volatile anesthetics on hypoxic drive may play an even more important role in patients who rely on hypoxic drive to set their level of ventilation, such as those with chronic respiratory failure. In these situations, consideration should be given to the need for more prolonged mechanical ventilation in the postoperative period until the residual effects of the volatile anesthetics have resolved.

Bronchiolar Smooth Muscle Tone

Bronchoconstriction under anesthesia occurs because of direct stimulation of the laryngeal and tracheal areas, the administration of adjuvant drugs that cause histamine release, and from noxious stimuli, especially in lightly anesthetized patients.[267] These responses are enhanced in patients with known reactive airway disease (including those requiring bronchodilator therapy or those with chronic smoking histories). Airway smooth muscle, which extends as far distally as the terminal bronchioles, is under the influence of both parasympathetic and sympathetic nerves. The parasympathetic nerves mediate baseline airway tone and reflex bronchoconstriction, and this has been attributed to M_3 muscarinic receptors on the airway smooth muscle that promote increases in intracellular cGMP. Adrenergic receptors also are located on bronchial smooth muscle, with the β_2 receptor subtype playing an important role in promoting bronchiolar muscle relaxation through an increase in intracellular cAMP. The volatile anesthetics relax airway smooth muscle by directly depressing smooth muscle contractility, and indirectly by inhibiting the reflex neural pathways.[268] They also may have protective effects by acting on the bronchial epithelium *via* a nonadrenergic, noncholinergic mechanism, possibly involving the nitric oxide pathway.[269] Based upon computerized tomography (CT) scans in dogs, halothane has been shown to be a better bronchodilator than isoflurane.[270,271] A study in patients comparing isoflurane, halothane, and sevoflurane to a control group receiving thiopental indicated that sevoflurane may be a better bronchodilator than isoflurane or halothane (Fig. 15-27).[272] Studies from our laboratory suggest that desflurane administration shortly after induction of anesthesia with thiopental and tracheal intubation results in a transient increase in respiratory system resistance (bronchoconstriction), and we have attributed this to a direct effect from the pungency and airway irritability of desflurane. Volatile anesthetics have been used effectively to treat status asthmaticus when other conventional treatments have failed.[273–276] Although halothane has been successfully used in these situations, newer volatile anesthetics may be a better choice because of their absence of cardiovascular depression and reduced risk of cardiac arrhythmias compared to halothane.

Mucociliary Function

Adequate mucociliary function may be important in preventing postoperative atelectasis and hypoxemia. There are a number of factors involved in diminished mucociliary function, particularly in the mechanically ventilated patient, and anesthesia plays an as yet poorly defined role. Halothane, enflurane, and nitrous oxide with halothane have been shown to decrease, in a dose-dependent fashion, mucociliary movement.[277,278] It also is known that smokers have impaired mucociliary function compared to nonsmokers, and the combination of a volatile anesthetic in a

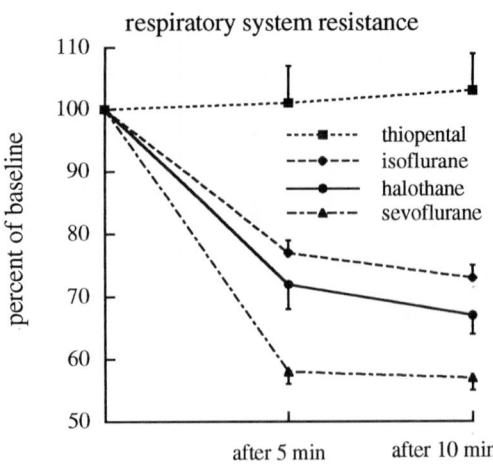

Figure 15-27. Respiratory system resistance decreased (bronchodilation) in the presence of 1.1 MAC isoflurane, halothane, and sevoflurane, whereas no change occurred in patients receiving thiopental 1.25 $mg \cdot kg^{-1} \cdot min^{-1}$ plus 50% nitrous oxide. The greatest decrease in resistance occurred with sevoflurane. (Adapted from Rooke GA, Choi J-H, Bishop MJ: The effect of isoflurane, halothane, sevoflurane, and thiopental/nitrous oxide on respiratory system resistance after tracheal intubation. Anesthesiology 86:1294, 1997.)

smoker who is mechanically ventilated sets up a scenario for inadequate clearing of secretions, mucous plugging, atelectasis, and hypoxemia.

Pulmonary Vascular Resistance

Although vascular smooth muscle is clearly affected by the volatile anesthetics, the pulmonary vasodilator action of the inhaled anesthetics, including halothane, isoflurane, enflurane, sevoflurane, and desflurane, in normal lungs is minimal.[279–281] In addition, any decrease in cardiac output that might occur from a volatile anesthetic tends to offset the direct vasodilator action of the anesthetic, resulting in little or no change in pulmonary artery pressures and pulmonary blood flow. Even nitrous oxide, which has little effect on cardiac output and pulmonary blood flow, has at best a small effect to increase pulmonary vascular resistance. However, the effect of nitrous oxide may be magnified in patients with resting pulmonary hypertension.[282,283] Perhaps more important in terms of volatile anesthetics and pulmonary blood flow is their ability to modulate hypoxic pulmonary vasoconstriction (HPV). During periods of hypoxemia, HPV reduces blood flow to underventilated areas of the lung, thereby shunting blood flow to areas of the lung with greater oxygen concentrations. The net effect is to improve the $\dot{V}/\dot{Q}$ matching. Although all of the inhaled anesthetics have been shown to attenuate HPV in animal models,[279–281] the situation is less clear in patient studies. This may reflect the multiple effects of the volatile anesthetics on factors involved in pulmonary blood flow, including their cardiovascular, autonomic, and humoral actions. In patients undergoing one-lung ventilation during thoracic surgery, minimal effects on PaO_2 and intrapulmonary shunt fraction (Q_s/Q_t) have been noted when changing from two-lung to one-lung ventilation during halothane, isoflurane, enflurane, and desflurane anesthesia (Fig. 15-28).[284–286] Isoflurane appears to be less inhibitory on HPV than halothane and, although this effect is subtle,[286] it might be attributed to the greater maintenance of cardiac output known to occur with isoflurane.

HEPATIC EFFECTS

Although postoperative liver dysfunction has been associated with most of the volatile anesthetics in current use, the most

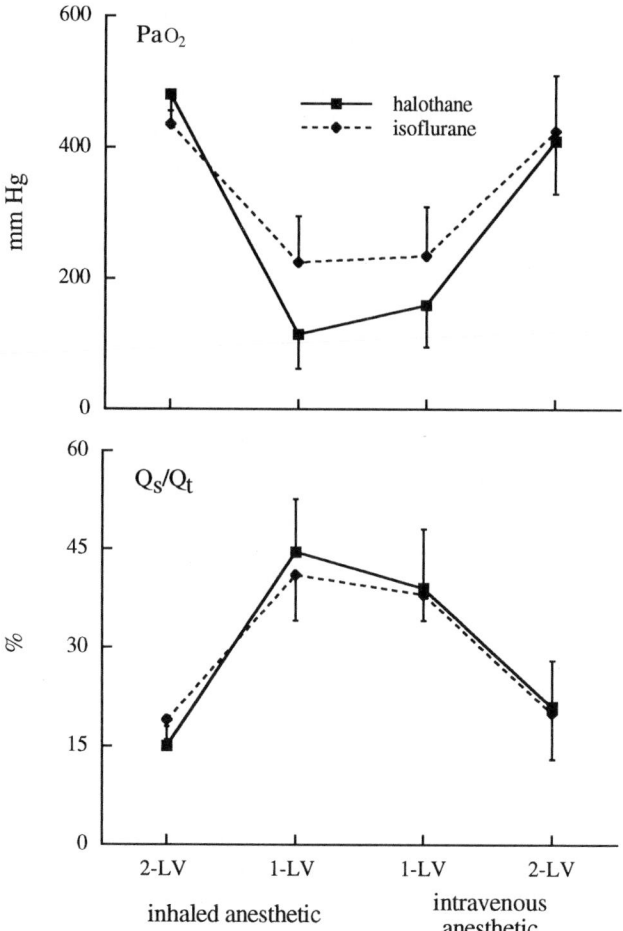

Figure 15-28. Arterial oxygenation (PaO_2) and intrapulmonary shunt ($\dot{Q}_s/\dot{Q}_t$) in patients ventilated with both lungs (2-LV) or with one lung (1-LV). Patients received either an inhalational agent, halothane or isoflurane, or a continuous intravenous anesthetic, thiopental. Note the minimal effect on PaO_2 and shunt that occurs on changing from a volatile anesthetic to an iv agent. (Adapted from Benumof JL, Augustine SD, Gibbons JA: Halothane and isoflurane only slightly impair arterial oxygenation during one-lung ventilation in patients undergoing thoracotomy. Anesthesiology 67:910, 1987.)

focused attention has been directed to halothane. There appear to be two distinct mechanisms by which halothane can cause hepatitis. One is more common but relatively mild, does not require a previous exposure, and has a low morbidity. The other, which is associated with repeat exposure and probably represents an immune reaction to oxidatively derived metabolites of halothane, has been implicated in severe liver damage and fulminant hepatic failure.

The liver has two blood supplies. One is the well-oxygenated blood from the hepatic artery and the other is the poorly oxygenated blood supply from the portal vein. Hepatocyte hypoxia is a significant contributor to postoperative hepatic injury. A pleasant attribute of the ether-based anesthetics (isoflurane, sevoflurane, and desflurane) is their ability to maintain or increase hepatic artery blood flow while decreasing (or not changing) portal vein blood flow.[163,287] This contrasts with halothane where decreases in portal vein blood flow are not compensated by increases in hepatic artery blood flow (Fig. 15-29).[288] Rather, halothane causes selective hepatic artery vasoconstriction.[289] According to animal model estimates, there is a 65% reduction in oxygen availability during halothane anesthesia while the reduction in availability is just 35% during isoflurane anesthesia.[290]

Situations that decrease hepatic blood flow or increase hepatic oxygen demand make patients vulnerable to the unwanted effects of halothane on hepatic blood flow. For example, surgery in the area of the liver (or elsewhere in the abdominal cavity) that might compromise hepatic blood flow puts patients at risk for hepatic cell injury. In addition, enzyme induction, which increases oxygen demand, enhances the vulnerability of patients to the effects of halothane. Furthermore, patients who are critically dependent upon oxygen supply for survival of remaining liver tissue, such as the cirrhotic patient, are at higher risk for further hepatic injury than noncirrhotic individuals.[291] Whether this injury is attributable to a direct effect of halothane during hypoxic conditions or to reductive metabolism of halothane that is enhanced under hypoxic conditions is not entirely clear.[292]

Changes in liver function tests have been used as an index of hepatic injury during anesthesia. Transient increases in plasma alanine aminotransferase (ALT) activity followed the administration of enflurane, but not desflurane, isoflurane, or sevoflurane in human volunteers (Fig. 15-30).[287,293,294] Although changes in the ALT or aspartate aminotransferase (AST) are accepted indices of liver cell damage, these measures may not accurately reflect the extent of hepatic injury and are not uniquely specific to the liver. Most cases of halothane hepatitis demonstrate lesions in the centrilobular area of the liver, and, not coincidentally, this area is most susceptible to hypoxia. Therefore, a more sensitive measure of injury may be glutathione-*S*-transferase (GST), which is distributed primarily in the centrilobular hepatocytes.[295] In patient studies comparing halothane anesthesia to isoflurane and enflurane,[296,297] significant increases in GST occurred after halothane (24–50%) and enflurane (20%), but not after isoflurane. There were two peaks in the GST responses; the first was 3–6 hours after halothane and the second was approximately 24 hours after halothane. It has been suggested that the early peak reflects direct damage or impaired liver blood flow and the second peak may be caused by metabolites or an immune response. (The immune mechanism of hepatitis is considered later in this chapter; see Anesthetic Metabolism.)

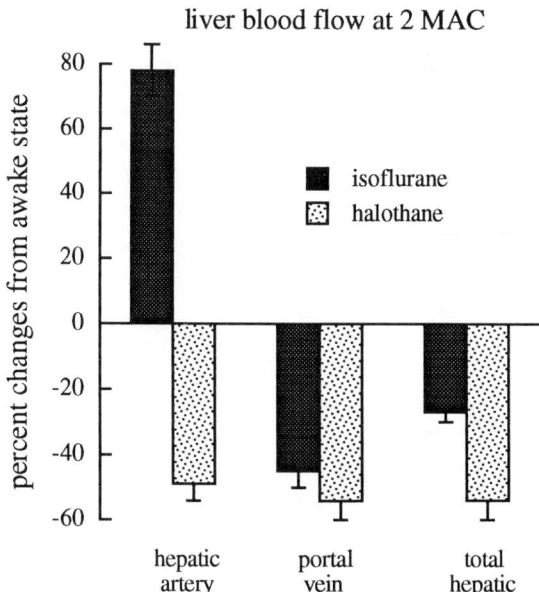

Figure 15-29. Changes (%, mean ± SE) in hepatic blood flow during administration of isoflurane or halothane. Decreases in portal vein blood flow produced by 2 MAC isoflurane are offset by increases in hepatic artery blood flow (autoregulation). Halothane resulted in decreases in both portal vein and hepatic artery blood flow, thereby significantly compromising total hepatic artery blood flow. (Adapted from Gelman S, Fowler KC, Smith LR: Liver circulation and function during isoflurane and halothane anesthesia. Anesthesiology 61:726, 1984.)

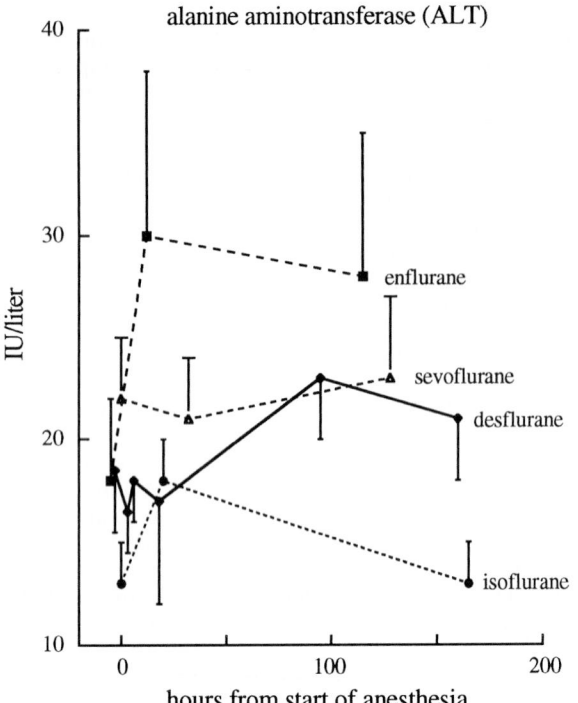

Figure 15-30. Plasma alanine aminotransferase (ALT) levels do not change significantly when sevoflurane, enflurane, desflurane, or isoflurane are administered to healthy volunteers (mean ± SEM). (Adapted from Weiskopf RB, Eger EI II, Ionescu P *et al:* Desflurane does not produce hepatic or renal injury in human volunteers. Anesth Analg 74:570, 1992; Frink EJ Jr, Malan TP Jr, Isner RJ *et al:* Renal concentrating function with prolonged sevoflurane or enflurane anesthesia in volunteers. Anesthesiology 80:1019, 1994; Eger EI II, Calverley RK, Smith NT: Changes in blood chemistries following prolonged enflurane anesthesia. Anesth Analg 55:547, 1976; and Stevens WC, Eger EI II, Joas TA *et al:* Comparative toxicity of isoflurane, halothane, fluroxene and diethyl ether in human volunteers. Can J Anaesth 20:357, 1973.)

NEUROMUSCULAR SYSTEM AND MALIGNANT HYPERTHERMIA

Compared to the alkane halothane, the ether-derived fluorinated volatile anesthetics produce about twofold greater skeletal muscle relaxation. Nitrous oxide does not relax skeletal muscles; in fact, in doses greater than 1 MAC, it may produce skeletal muscle rigidity.[298] Interestingly, the inhaled anesthetics, in addition to the direct effects of relaxing skeletal muscle, also potentiate the action of neuromuscular blocking drugs. Although the mechanism of this potentiation is not entirely clear, it appears that it is largely due to a postsynaptic effect at the neuromuscular junction (see Chapter 17).

All of the potent volatile anesthetics serve as triggers for malignant hyperthermia in genetically susceptible patients.[299–302] In contrast, nitrous oxide is a weak trigger for malignant hyperthermia.[302] Studies evaluating caffeine-induced contractures indicate that augmentation of the contractures by nitrous oxide is 1.3, whereas for isoflurane it is 3-fold, for enflurane 4-fold, and for halothane 11-fold.[302] Thus, halothane is the most potent trigger of the volatile anesthetics for malignant hyperthermia.

GENETIC EFFECTS

In tests employed to identify chemicals that cause a mutagenic or carcinogenic response, all of the volatile anesthetics, including nitrous oxide, have proven to be negative. The Ames test, which identifies chemicals that act as mutagens and carcinogens, has been shown to be negative for enflurane, isoflurane, desflurane, sevoflurane, and nitrous oxide.[236,291,303] Although halothane results in a negative Ames test, metabolites may be positive.[304]

Virtually every volatile anesthetic agent has been shown to be teratogenic in animal studies, but none has been shown to be teratogenic in humans. Animal studies have indicated that nitrous oxide exposure in the early periods of gestation may result in adverse effects, including an increased incidence of fetal resorption.[305,306] The same vulnerability does not exist during the administration of the potent volatile anesthetics.[307] However, learning function may be impaired in newborn animals exposed *in utero* to inhaled anesthetics.[308,309]

There has been an ongoing concern about the incidence of spontaneous abortions in operating room personnel chronically exposed to trace concentrations of inhaled anesthetics, especially nitrous oxide.[306] Animal studies using intermittent exposure to trace concentrations of nitrous oxide, halothane, enflurane, and isoflurane have not revealed harmful reproductive effects.[310] Methionine synthetase and thymidylate synthetase are vitamin B_{12}-dependent enzymes that have been shown to decrease in activity during nitrous oxide exposure. The mechanism appears to be an irreversible oxidation of the cobalt atom

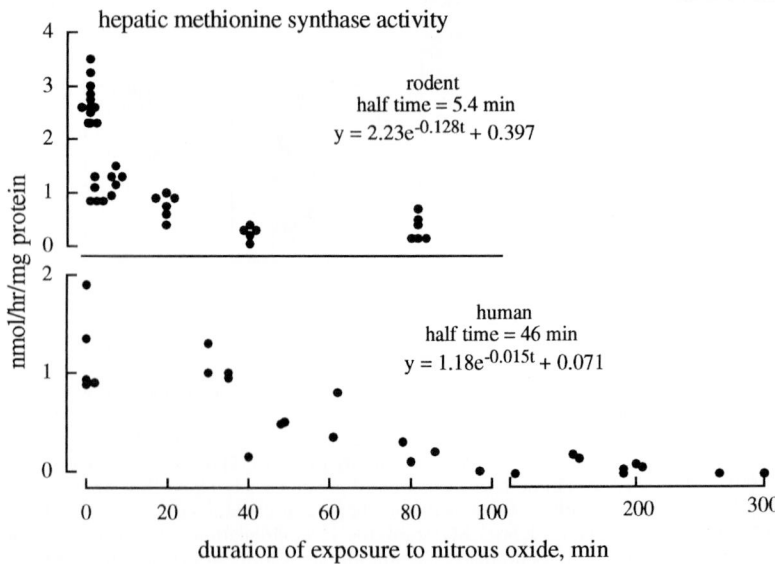

Figure 15-31. Time course of inactivation of hepatic methionine synthase (synthetase) activity during administration of 50% nitrous oxide to rats or 70% nitrous oxide to humans. The half-life was substantially less in rats. (Adapted from Royston BD, Nunn JF, Weinbren HK *et al:* Rate of inactivation of human and rodent hepatic methionine synthase by nitrous oxide. Anesthesiology 68:213, 1988.)

of vitamin B_{12} by nitrous oxide. The half-time for inactivation of methionine synthetase is 46 min when 70% nitrous oxide is administered to patients (Fig. 15-31).[311] Methionine synthetase and thymidylate synthetase are involved in the formation of myelin and the formation of DNA, respectively. Thus, the concern that these changes might have an effect on a rapidly developing embryo/fetus seems appropriate. Inhibition of these enzymes could also manifest as depression of bone marrow function and neurologic disturbances. Animals exposed to 15% nitrous oxide for up to 15 days developed a neuropathy presented as ataxia and spinal cord and peripheral nerve degeneration. A sensory motor polyneuropathy that is often combined with signs of posterior lateral spinal cord degeneration resembling pernicious anemia has been described in humans who chronically inhale nitrous oxide for recreational use.[312] These effects have been attributed to reduced activity of the vitamin B_{12}-dependent enzymes.

Despite the unproved influence of trace concentrations of the volatile anesthetics on congenital development and spontaneous abortions, these concerns have resulted in the use of scavenging systems to remove anesthetic gases from the operating room and the establishment of OSHA standards for waste gas exposure. The NIOSH (National Institute for Occupational Safety and Health) recommended exposure level for nitrous oxide is 25 parts per million (ppm) as a time-weighted average over the time of exposure. The exposure limit for halogenated anesthetics (without nitrous oxide exposure) is 2 ppm.[313]

BONE MARROW FUNCTION

Long administration of nitrous oxide has been associated with megaloblastic changes and agranulocytosis in bone marrow, presumably due to interference with DNA synthesis. Much of the concern about the volatile anesthetics in terms of bone marrow (and fetal development) is in relation to the effects on DNA synthesis and myelin formation in rapidly dividing cells. Nunn reported megaloblastic bone marrow changes in a seriously ill patient after 105 min of nitrous oxide anesthesia. These changes appeared to be prevented by administering 30 mg of folinic acid before the nitrous oxide. Megaloblastic changes in bone marrow are consistently observed in patients exposed to nitrous oxide for 24 hours,[311] and four days of exposure to nitrous oxide has resulted in agranulocytosis. Two considerations related to these effects have proved irrelevant. First, in patients undergoing bone marrow transplantation, exposure to nitrous oxide has not altered *via*bility of the bone marrow. Second, the use of nitrous oxide to treat leukemia has proved only that the potentially beneficial suppressive effects of nitrous oxide on cell synthesis are transient.[314]

OBSTETRIC EFFECTS

As with vascular smooth muscle, the volatile anesthetics produce a dose-dependent decrease in uterine smooth muscle contractility and blood flow, and the effects appear to be similar with most of the volatile anesthetics.[294,315,316] Because of the dose dependency, a common technique to provide general anesthesia for urgent cesarean sections is to use them in low concentrations, such as 0.5 MAC, combined with nitrous oxide. This decreases the likelihood of uterine atony and blood loss, especially after delivery when uterine contraction is essential. Uterine relaxation becomes substantial at concentrations of volatile anesthesia greater than 1 MAC, and this is not altered by the use of nitrous oxide. In some situations, uterine relaxation may be desirable, as in removal of a retained placenta. In this case, a brief high concentration of a volatile anesthetic may prove advantageous. In terms of neonatal effects, APGAR scores and acid–base balance are not affected by anesthetic technique (*e.g.*, spinal vs. general). More sensitive measures of neurologic and

behavioral function, such as the Scanlon early neonatal neurobehavioral scale (ENNS) and the neurologic and adaptive capacities score (NACS), indicate some transient depression of scores following general anesthesia that did not persist at 24-hour post-delivery measurements.[317,318] Fetal loss seems to increase following surgery in the first or second trimester, but the majority of these findings have been in patients following acute abdomen or trauma in emergency settings. Generally, elective surgeries are delayed until at least six weeks post-partum, or until the late second or early third trimester. Perhaps the most important factor in promoting good fetal outcome is maintaining good uterine blood flow during anesthesia and surgery.

ANESTHETIC DEGRADATION BY CARBON DIOXIDE ABSORBERS

Most adult general anesthesia is given through closed or semiclosed breathing circuits. This mandates the use of a carbon dioxide absorbent in the circuit. One of the problems with the CO_2 absorbents in use today is their content, which consists of monovalent hydroxide bases. These strong bases result in breakdown or degradation of all potent anesthetics (halothane, sevoflurane, enflurane, desflurane, and isoflurane).[319] The initial step in this degradation is removal of a labile proton. Currently, CO_2 absorbers contain the alkali bases—potassium and sodium hydroxide. Degradation of the anesthetics is slightly greater with potassium hydroxide.[320] Barium hydroxide lime, which contains potassium but not sodium hydroxide, degrades the anesthetics more so than soda lime (which contains less potassium hydroxide and some sodium hydroxide).[321] In the case of halothane and sevoflurane, the reaction with carbon dioxide absorbents results in degradation of these anesthetics to haloalkenes.[5,322,323] Halothane degrades to form trace amounts of BCDFE (2-bromo-2-chloro-1,1-difluoroethene) and sevoflurane degrades to form trace amounts of compound A [2,2-difluoro-1-(trifluoromethyl)vinyl ether]. These haloalkenes have been shown to be nephrotoxic in rats,[324,325] although clinically significant renal effects of haloalkene formation in surgical patients have not been reported. In the case of desflurane, enflurane, and isoflurane, degradation occurs only in dehydrated carbon dioxide absorbents and results in carbon monoxide formation.[320,326]

Special mention of a novel carbon dioxide absorbent that does not contain sodium or potassium hydroxide is warranted prior to delving into the controversial discussion of compound A and carbon monoxide. This new absorbent, called Amsorb, consists of calcium hydroxide with a compatible humectant, calcium chloride. Hardness and porosity have been established with two setting agents, calcium sulfate and polyvinyl pyrrolidine. This new material is chemically unreactive with sevoflurane, enflurane, isoflurane, and desflurane, and thus prevents the degradation of these compounds to carbon monoxide and compound A.[327]

Compound A

Sevoflurane undergoes base-catalyzed degradation in carbon dioxide absorbents to form a vinyl ether called compound A. The production of compound A is enhanced in low-flow or closed-circuit breathing systems (Fig. 15-32) and by warm or very dry CO_2 absorbents.[328–330] Barium hydroxide lime produces more compound A than does soda lime, and this can be attributed to slightly higher absorbent temperature during CO_2 extraction.[321]

Studies in rats where compound A has been administered in the inspired gas have identified a threshold for renal tubular necrosis between 290 and 340 ppm · h (50 ppm × 6 hr = 300 ppm · hr) (Fig. 15-33).[331–334] The histology of the nephrotoxicity is characterized by cell necrosis of the cortical medullary tubules located in the proximal tubules.[325,331,332] The biochemical mark-

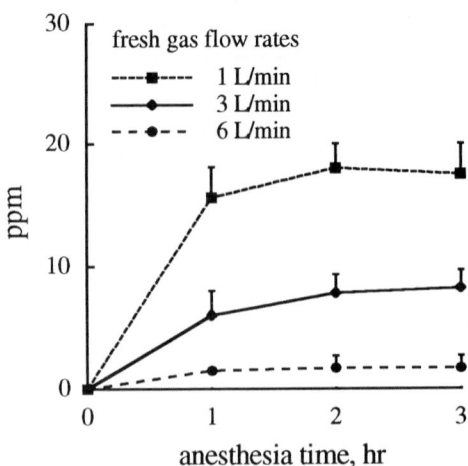

Figure 15-32. Inhaled compound A concentrations during administration of sevoflurane at fresh gas flow rates of 1, 3, or 6 L·min⁻¹ in humans (*$P < 0.05$ versus 3 L·min⁻¹; **$P < 0.05$ versus 6 L·min⁻¹). (Adapted from Bito H, Ikeda K: Effect of total flow rate on the concentration of degradation products generated by reaction between sevoflurane and soda lime. Br J Anaesth 74:667, 1995.)

ers of this necrosis include elevations of serum BUN and creatinine, glucosuria, and proteinuria.[325,333] In addition, several enzymes from the tubule cells have been used as markers of cell injury including increases in urinary excretion of n-acetyl-β-D-glucosaminidase (NAG) and α-glutathione-S-transferase (αGST).[325,333]

There are species differences in the threshold for compound A-induced nephrotoxicity. The threshold is approximately 300 ppm·hr in 250-g rats,[331-333] greater than 612 ppm·hr in pigs,[335] and 600–800 ppm·hr in monkeys.[336] In patients and volunteers receiving sevoflurane in low-flow delivery systems, inspired compound A concentrations averaged 8–24 and 20–32 ppm with soda lime and barium hydroxide lime, respectively.[337-342] Total exposures as high as 320–400 ppm·hr have had no clear effect on clinical markers of renal function.[343-345] In randomized and prospective studies, the effects of low-flow (1 l·min⁻¹) or closed-circuit sevoflurane anesthesia on renal function in humans have been examined using both standard clinical markers of renal function (serum creatinine and BUN concentrations) and experimental markers of renal function and structural integrity (proteinuria, glucosuria, and enzymuria).[337,339-341,344,346] In only one study to date has the administration of sevoflurane (to volunteers at a fresh gas flow of 2 l·min⁻¹ for 8 hr) been associated with significant increases in urinary excretion rates of glucose, protein, and enzyme markers.[345] These increases

were transient, resolving after several days, were not associated with significant changes in BUN and creatinine, and have not been reproduced by independent investigations employing volunteers in identical protocols.[344,346] In addition, recent evidence from patients undergoing elective surgery indicates that transient proteinuria, glucosuria, and enzymuria also occur after desflurane and isoflurane anesthesia, without changes in serum BUN and creatinine.[341,342] Proteinuria also has been documented to occur after surgery employing only epidural anesthesia.[347] Thus, it is unclear if renal injury can be inferred from transient changes in urinary glucose or protein. This has fueled the argument that the only clinically accepted and relevant outcome markers of renal injury or renal functional impairment are serum BUN and creatinine.[348]

Aside from the high probability that the absence of renal injury in patients is due to low compound A levels during the clinical use of sevoflurane in a low-flow system, another probable explanation must be considered. Compound A is not itself toxic to organs. Rather, it is the biodegradation of compound A to cysteine conjugates and the further action of a renal enzyme called β-lyase on the conjugates that can result in formation of a potentially toxic thiol (Fig. 15-34).[334,349,350] There is clear evidence for species differences in the biotransformation of compound A to cysteine-s conjugates.[351] Recent evidence suggests that the cysteine conjugates can be handled in one (or both) of two ways.[352] They can be acetylated to mercapturic acid through a detoxification pathway, which results in no organ toxicity; or they can be acted upon by an enzyme in the kidneys, renal β-lyase, to form reactive intermediates (toxification pathway). These reactive intermediates are responsible for the renal cell necrosis seen in rats. The β-lyase-dependent metabolism pathway in humans is far less extensive than the β-lyase pathway in rats (8–30 times less active).[351] Thus, compared with rats, humans receive markedly lower doses of compound A and metabolize a lower fraction via the renal β-lyase pathway. This may account for the safety of sevoflurane in both human volunteers and patients when compared to rat models. Because there has been limited experience with the use of sevoflurane in patients with renal impairment, caution is still advised when sevoflurane is applied to this patient population. An ongoing, multicenter phase IV study of sevoflurane versus isoflurane in patients with renal insufficiency is underway and new information should soon be available to the clinician.

Carbon Monoxide

CO_2 absorbents degrade desflurane, enflurane, and isoflurane to carbon monoxide when the normal water content of the absorbent (13–15%) is markedly decreased.[320,326,353] The degradation has resulted in occasional patient exposure to toxic CO concentrations.[354-358] The instances of CO poisoning have been reported in situations where the CO_2 absorbent has presumably been dried (desiccated) because an anesthetic machine has

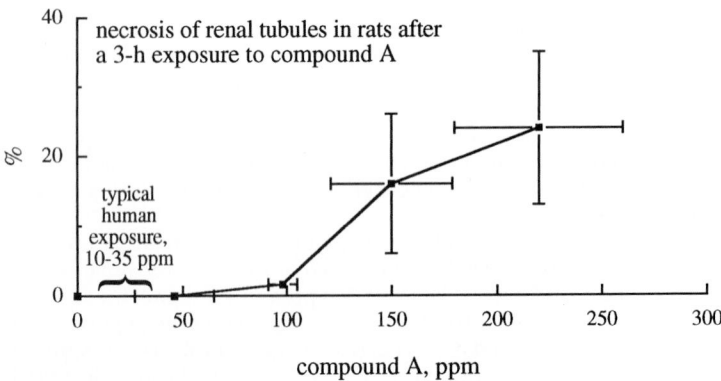

Figure 15-33. Renal biopsy results from rats inhaling different concentrations of compound A for 3 hours. The derived threshold to cause renal necrosis is about 100 ppm (300 ppm·h). The typical human exposure during the administration of sevoflurane in a semi-closed circuit is between 10 and 35 ppm of compound A, which falls well below the threshold to cause renal injury in rats. (Adapted from Kharasch ED, Hoffman GM, Thorning D et al: Role of the renal cysteine conjugate β-lyase pathway in inhaled compound A nephrotoxicity in rats. Anesthesiology 88:1624, 1998.)

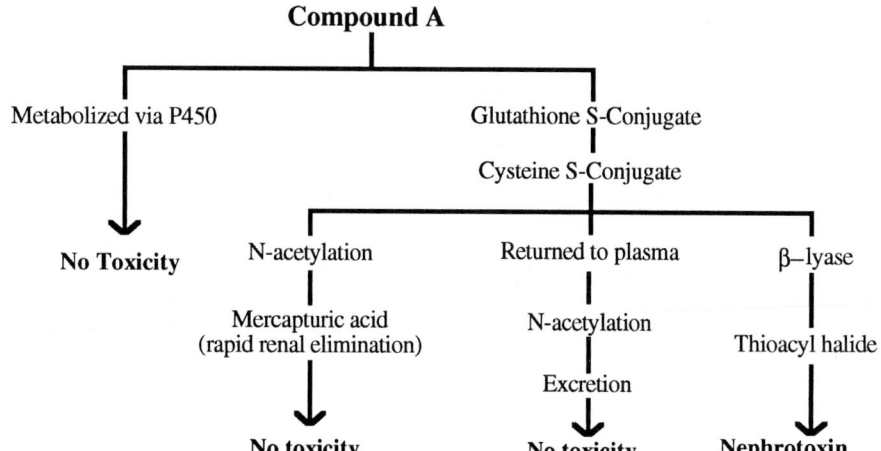

Figure 15-34. Known pathways for metabolism and elimination of compound A in humans. A potential toxin only results from the action of renal β-lyase on cysteine S-conjugates. The activity of this enzyme in humans is 8–30-fold less than in rats. Considerable handling of the cysteine S-conjugates in humans is *via N*-acetylation to mercapturic acid. (Adapted from Kharasch ED, Jubert C: Compound A uptake and metabolism to mercapturic acids and 3,3,3-trifluoro-2-fluoromethoxy-propanoic acid during low-flow sevoflurane anesthesia. Anesthesiology 91:1267, 1999.)

been left on with a high fresh gas flow passing through the CO_2 absorbent over an extended period of time. The anesthetic molecular structure and the presence of a strong base in the carbon dioxide absorbent are involved in the formation of CO.[320] Desflurane, enflurane, and isoflurane contain an essential difluoromethoxy moiety, not found in the sevoflurane or halothane molecules, which is essential for the formation of CO. In addition, high absorbent temperatures increase CO formation.

As discussed in a recent editorial, the availability of a new CO_2 absorbent that does not degrade anesthetics (to either compound A or carbon monoxide) should change the way the clinicians deliver inhaled anesthetic, both domestically and worldwide: "From a patient safety perspective, widespread adoption of a nondestructive CO_2 absorbent should be axiomatic."[319] Although the cost of this new CO_2 absorbent has not been established, it is likely to be somewhat greater than the cost of the currently employed CO_2 absorbents; however, the benefit may be substantial. The use of a nondestructive absorbent eliminates all the potential complications related to anesthetic breakdown and therefore minimizes the possibility of additional costs from complications including additional lab tests, hospital days, and medical/legal expenses from any serious outcome.

ANESTHETIC METABOLISM
Fluoride-Induced Nephrotoxicity

Nephrotoxicity due to metabolism (biotransformation) of halogenated anesthetics to free inorganic fluoride is now an accepted fact for methoxyflurane.[359] The metabolism of methoxyflurane and, to a lesser extent, enflurane has resulted in a well described injury to renal collecting tubules.[360-362] The nephrotoxicity associated with these anesthetics is a high output renal insufficiency, characterized by dilute polyuria, dehydration, serum hypernatremia, hyperosmolality, and elevated BUN and creatinine, that is unresponsive to vasopressin. An association between increased plasma fluoride concentrations that occur as a result of metabolism of these anesthetics was noted early on and detailed by Mazze and colleagues.[360,363] This work led to a "fluoride hypothesis." Nephrotoxicity is caused by metabolism of the volatile anesthetics to fluoride, and the inorganic fluoride is the ultimate substance producing the renal injury. This traditional hypothesis has been reexamined recently, in part because sevoflurane, a newer potent volatile anesthetic, also undergoes metabolism, resulting in transient increases in serum fluoride concentrations, but has not been associated with a renal concentrating defect.[345,362] The traditional hypothesis stated that both the duration of the high systemic fluoride concentrations (area under the fluoride–time curve) and the

peak fluoride concentration (peaks above $50\mu M$ appear to represent the toxic threshold) were important in determining nephrotoxicity (Fig. 15-35).[360,361,363] One theory for the safety of sevoflurane and relative safety of enflurane with regard to fluoride concentrations has been the more rapid elimination of these less soluble anesthetics compared to methoxyflurane. This provides a rapid decline in the plasma fluoride concentrations and less availability of the anesthetic for metabolism.[364]

Another report further clarifies this issue and has led to a modification of the traditional fluoride hypothesis for renal toxicity.[365] This modification is based upon the likely contribution of intrarenal metabolism of anesthetics to fluoride to the

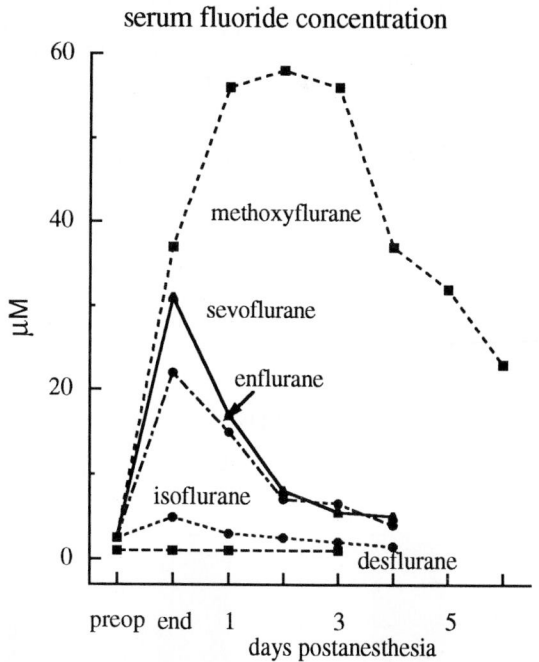

Figure 15-35. Plasma inorganic fluoride concentrations (mean ± SE) before and after 2–4 hours of methoxyflurane, enflurane, sevoflurane, isoflurane, and desflurane anesthesia. (Adapted from Kharasch ED, Armstrong AS, Gunn K *et al:* Clinical sevoflurane metabolism and disposition. II. The role of cytochrome P450 2E1 in fluoride and hexafluoroisopropanol formation. Anesthesiology 82:1379, 1995; Mazze RI: Metabolism of the inhaled anaesthetics: Implications of enzyme induction. Br J Anaesth 56(suppl):27S, 1984; and Sutton TS, Koblin DD, Gruenke LD *et al:* Fluoride metabolites after prolonged exposure of volunteers and patients to desflurane. Anesth Analg 73:180, 1991.)

resulting toxicity. It is well known that the human kidneys can metabolize volatile anesthetics, and recent work indicates that metabolism of methoxyflurane to fluoride in the kidney is significantly greater than that of sevoflurane and enflurane. This may be related to the multiple cytochrome P450 enzymes in the kidney responsible for metabolism of methoxyflurane (P450-2A6, P450-3A, P450-2E1).[365] In contrast, sevoflurane and enflurane are primarily metabolized by the cytochrome P450-2E1. The theory now holds that the intrarenal fluoride generated from methoxyflurane metabolism and/or the multiple P450 isoenzymes involved in methoxyflurane metabolism account for the nephrotoxicity from this anesthetic. Despite the potential for relatively high plasma levels of fluoride following long exposure to newer anesthetics, the minimal amount of sevoflurane and enflurane renal defluorination may explain the relative absence of renal concentrating defects with these anesthetics (Fig. 15-36).[345,362,365]

Factors such as total dose of anesthetic, enzyme induction, and obesity have been proved to enhance biotransformation. The activity of hepatic cytochrome P450 enzymes is increased by a variety of drugs, including phenobarbital, phenytoin, and isoniazid.[236,366] Obesity causes increased metabolism (defluorination) in halothane, enflurane, and isoflurane.[367–369] However, the effects of obesity on the defluorination of sevoflurane are less clear.[370,371]

Hepatic Injury from Metabolism: Halothane Hepatitis

Although postoperative liver dysfunction has been associated with most of the volatile anesthetics in current use, the most focused attention has been directed to halothane. This is due, in part, to the relatively recent demonstration of binding of an oxidatively derived metabolite of halothane to liver cytochromes that could then act as a hapten and induce an immune reaction. This hypersensitivity reaction has been associated with severe liver damage and fulminant hepatic failure. There are many causes of postoperative jaundice and abnormal liver function tests, including viral hepatitis, coexisting liver disease (such as Gilbert's disease), blood transfusions, septicemia, drug reactions, intra- and postoperative hypoxia and hypotension, and direct tissue trauma as a result of the surgical procedure.[292] The diagnosis of halothane hepatitis is generally made based on "incomplete exclusion," defined as the appearance of liver damage within 28 days of halothane exposure in a person in whom other known causes of liver disease have been excluded.

Halothane was introduced into clinical practice in 1956, and case reports of unexplained jaundice following anesthesia with halothane began to appear in 1958. By 1963, at least 350 putative cases of "halothane hepatitis" had been reported. The common thinking in the early 1950s was that inhaled anesthetics (except trichloroethylene) were metabolically unaltered by the body's biochemical machinery. However, in 1967, it was determined that approximately 18% of halothane was metabolized in humans.[372] The metabolites were oxidatively derived. It is now known that oxidative metabolism of halothane produces an intermediate that binds to liver tissue and can produce an immune response in certain individuals. However, halothane-associated hepatitis can present as one of two clinical syndromes, and it is likely that only one syndrome can be explained by an immune mechanism.[292,373,374] Each may develop after an uneventful anesthesia and surgery with no apparent time-to-dose relationship. The most common syndrome, which occurs in close to 20% of the adult patients receiving halothane, is a mild, self-limited postoperative toxicity that has been ascribed to reductive metabolism of halothane; this route of metabolism is enhanced under low-oxygen or hypoxic conditions. Reductive metabolism of isoflurane, desflurane, sevoflurane, and enflurane does not occur. The typical presentation of hepatitis from reductive metabolism is a rapid (1–3 days) but mild, unprogressing pattern of liver injury characterized by nausea, lethargy, fever, moderately increased concentrations of liver transaminases, and, rarely, transient jaundice. It does not require a repeat exposure, as does the immune mechanism of hepatitis; it can occur on the first exposure to halothane.

Historically, an immune-mediated mechanism for halothane hepatitis seemed unlikely. Halothane is a small molecule, and thus seemed unlikely to be immunoreactive, although reductive metabolites have been shown to bind to rat liver microsomes, which contain the cytochrome P450 system. Several more recent observations suggest that reductive metabolism is not an important mechanism in the evolution of the immune-mediated halothane hepatitis.[292] The possibility still existed that binding of a metabolite of halothane to the liver cytochromes could act as a hapten and induce a hypersensitivity response.[375] Supporting this possibility were the clinical manifestations of hepatitis, including eosinophilia, fever, rash, and arthralgia, and prior exposure to halothane. The possibility of a genetic susceptibility factor is suggested by case reports of halothane hepatitis in closely related patients.[373] The most compelling evidence for an immune-mediated mechanism is the presence of circulating immunoglobulin g antibodies in up to 70% of patients with diagnosis of halothane hepatitis.[292,375] This antibody is not directed against the reductive metabolite of halothane, but against an oxidative compound, trifluoroacetyl halide, which is incorporated onto the surface of the hepatocyte (Fig. 15-37).[376,377]

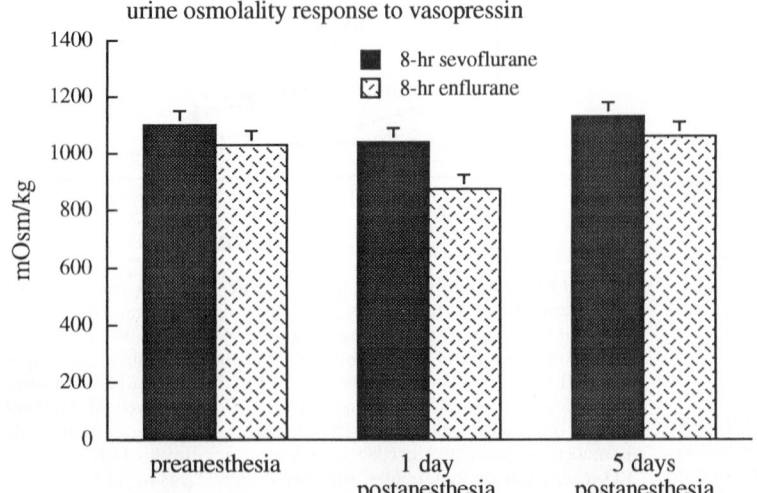

urine osmolality response to vasopressin

■ 8-hr sevoflurane
▨ 8-hr enflurane

Figure 15-36. Maximal urinary osmolalities (mean ± SE) in adult male volunteers after administration of desmopressin before and after prolonged administration (>9 MAC hours) of enflurane or sevoflurane. (Adapted from Frink EJ Jr, Malan TP Jr, Isner RJ *et al:* Renal concentrating function with prolonged sevoflurane or enflurane anesthesia in volunteers. Anesthesiology 80:1019, 1994.)

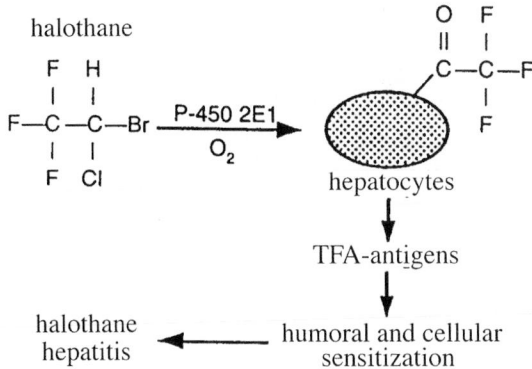

Figure 15-37. Halothane is metabolized to a trifluoroacetylated (TFA) adduct that binds to liver proteins. In susceptible patients, this adduct (altered protein) is seen as non-self (neoantigen), generating an immune response (production of antibodies). Subsequent exposure to halothane may result in hepatotoxicity. A similar process may occur in genetically susceptible individuals after anesthetic exposure to other fluorinated volatile anesthetics (enflurane, isoflurane, desflurane) that also generate a TFA adduct. (Adapted from Njoku D, Laster MJ, Gong DH *et al:* Biotransformation of halothane, enflurane, isoflurane, and desflurane to trifluoroacetylated liver proteins: Association between protein acylation and hepatic injury. Anesth Analg 84:173, 1997.)

Trifluoroacetyl proteins (TFA) have been identified from the liver of rats after halothane exposure with enzyme-linked immunosorbent assays and immunoblotting techniques. These altered proteins can be seen by the immune system as non-self (*i.e.*, neoantigen), resulting in production of antibodies. These can now be identified from serum samples of humans by identifying anti-TFA albumin activity on an ELISA screening evaluation and by using a competitive, direct ELISA to test the ability of trifluoroacetylated lysine to block antibody binding to TFI-albumin.[378,379]

This metabolic pathway involving the cytochrome P450 system during halothane exposure is identical to the metabolic pathway noted with enflurane, isoflurane, and desflurane (Fig. 15-38). However, the expression of the neoantigens should be related to the amount of metabolism of each agent. This would suggest that, in terms of antigenic load, halothane > enflurane > isoflurane > desflurane. Indeed, case reports have appeared in the literature linking each of these anesthetics with immune-mediated hepatitis.[374,379–383] If the incidence of fulminant hepatic failure after halothane is 1 in 35,000,[384] hepatic failure caused by isoflurane may occur in only 1 per 3,500,000 isoflurane anesthetics, and a lower incidence would be expected with desflurane. Desflurane is the least metabolized of the volatile anesthetics, resulting in very small amounts of adduct, and only one case report of hepatotoxicity from desflurane has been described.[379] Sensitization of this patient by two exposures to halothane (18 years and 12 years previously), precipitated massive hepatotoxicity. Anti-TFA antibodies were identified in the serum.

Immunologic memory resulting in hepatitis has been reported 28 years after an initial halothane exposure.[385] In addition, cross-sensitivity has been reported in which exposure to one anesthetic can sensitize patients to a second, but different anesthetic.[379,386] There are no reports of fulminant hepatic necrosis associated with sevoflurane in humans. Sevoflurane is not metabolized to a trifluoroacetyl halide; rather, it is metabolized to hexafluoroisopropanol that does not serve as a neoantigen (Fig. 15-39).[287]

It is worth recalling that, despite case reports of hepatic damage associated with halothane that appeared in the literature within two years of its introduction, it has taken some 35 years of research and debate to reach the current consensus on the mechanism of halothane-associated hepatitis and fulmi-

nant hepatic failure. It is the opinion of these authors that halothane should not be used in adult surgical cases and should be strongly discouraged in the pediatric population. Although the incidence of hepatitis appears to be much lower in the pediatric population, our concern is related to immunologic memory resulting in hepatitis later in life during a repeat exposure to anesthesia. The new volatile anesthetics have an extremely low potential for hepatotoxicity, and the possibility of avoiding even one case of fulminant hepatic failure from a volatile anesthetic is sufficiently compelling to discourage use of the older, more metabolized anesthetics including halothane and enflurane.

CLINICAL UTILITY OF VOLATILE ANESTHETICS
For Induction of Anesthesia

Although current practices for establishing the anesthetic state consist of initial administration of an iv sedative/hypnotic, there is increasing interest in the use of volatile anesthetics *via* the facemask. Facemask use is commonplace in pediatric anesthesia but relatively rare in adult anesthesia. Historically, in the days of ether and cyclopropane, the standard induction technique was a mask induction. The renewed interest in this technique is primarily attributable to the advent of the newer potent and poorly soluble anesthetic sevoflurane, which is nonpungent and hence easily inhaled.[387] An important attribute of the gaseous induction technique is the ability to take the patient "deep" in a rapid fashion, thereby avoiding some of the unwanted side effects of stage 2 anesthesia (excitation, salivation, coughing, movement). The classic stages of anesthesia (stages 1–4) were described with the use of ether anesthesia. This volatile agent was far more soluble than sevoflurane, and therefore resulted in a slow and sometimes stormy induction of anesthesia. These older anesthetic agents were replaced by halothane in the 1950s, and the success of halothane was based primarily on its nonflammability and potency. Induction of anesthesia with halothane in the pediatric population is quite common. Interestingly, induction of anesthesia with halothane in adults was also practiced, but was not exceptionally popular. Ruffle and colleagues[388,389] described a single-breath induction with 4% halothane in adults that achieved loss of consciousness in most patients within two minutes. However, the development of the barbiturates (described in the 1930s) and iv technology and the importance of iv fluid administration were advanced through the middle of the 20th century. These factors, along with the speed of iv induction with thiopental, promoted the popularity of iv over inhaled inductions in adults. The resurgence of interest in mask induction in the adult population centers on the potential safety and utility of this technique when using sevoflurane.[390–393] The safety issues center primarily on the fact that spontaneous ventilation is preserved with a gas induction, and patients essentially regulate their own depth of anesthesia, as excessive sevoflurane would, in fact, suppress ventilation. Safety would be compromised if stage 2 excitation were a problem; however, clinical studies indicate that this is not the case. It is likely that the low blood:gas solubility of sevoflurane makes for a rapid induction, and typical times to loss of consciousness average ~1 minute when delivering sevoflurane *via* the facemask. Sevoflurane also has been used in the approach to the difficult adult airway because of the preservation of spontaneous ventilation, the lack of excitation, and absence of salivation with this technique.[394] The traditional "awake look" in the suspected difficult airway (where iv drugs are titrated to a level that allows direct laryngoscopy in the awake patient) has been modified to consist of spontaneous ventilation of high concentrations of sevoflurane until laryngoscopic evaluation is tolerated. Laryngeal mask placement can be successfully achieved two minutes after administering 7% sev-

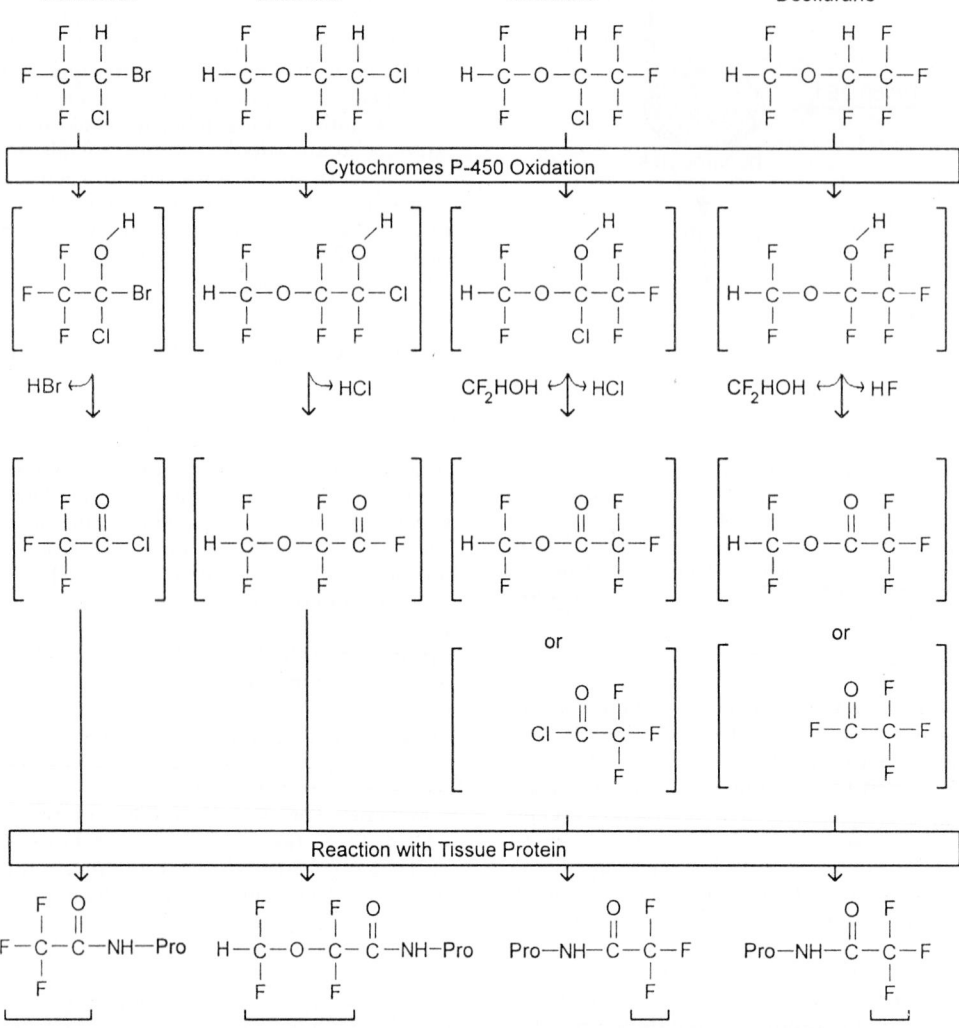

Figure 15-38. Pathways for the oxidative metabolism of fluorinated volatile anesthetics by cytochrome P450 enzymes to form acetylated protein adducts. In genetically susceptible individuals, the resulting trifluoroacetylates are thought to produce an immune response manifesting clinically as drug-induced hepatitis. (Adapted from Martin JL, Plevak DJ, Flannery KD *et al:* Hepatotoxicity after desflurane anesthesia. Anesthesiology 83:1125, 1995.)

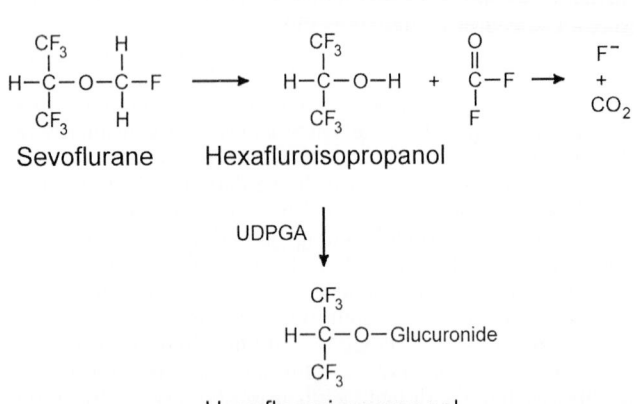

Figure 15-39. Pathway for oxidative metabolism of sevoflurane (UDPGA, uridine diphosphate glucuronic acid). Trifluoroacetylated (TFA) adducts are not formed from the metabolism of sevoflurane. (Adapted from Frink EJ Jr, Ghantous H, Malan TP *et al:* Plasma inorganic fluoride with sevoflurane anesthesia: Correlation with indices of hepatic and renal function. Anesth Analg 74:231, 1992.)

oflurane *via* the facemask. Although the addition of nitrous oxide to the inspired gas mixture does not add significantly to the induction sequence, most practitioners favor high concentrations of sevoflurane with oxygen. The gas induction technique is promoted by pretreatment with benzodiazepines but complicated by apnea with opioid pretreatment.[392] Of course, the utility of this technique is that clinicians simply need to pay attention to the airway during the induction sequence, rather than reaching for drugs and injecting them through an iv port. End-tidal gas concentrations can be reasonably obtained (although not precisely obtained because of mixing in the facemask during the induction sequence) and pupil responses and ventilation can be evaluated. Importantly, patient acceptance of this technique has been relatively high, exceeding 90% of the cases.[393] There have been a number of techniques described to use sevoflurane for induction of anesthesia *via* facemask. These include: priming the circuit (emptying the rebreathing bag, opening the "pop-off" valve, dialing the vaporizer to 8% while using a fresh gas flow of 8 l · min⁻¹, and maintaining this for 60 seconds prior to applying the facemask to the patient); a single-breath induction from end-expiratory volume to maximum inspired volume; and simply deep breathing. All seem to have the successful end result of loss of consciousness, generally within one minute.

For Maintenance of Anesthesia

The volatile anesthetics are clearly the most popular drugs used to maintain anesthesia. They are easily administered *via* inhalation, they are readily titrated, they have a high safety ratio in terms of preventing recall, and the depth of anesthesia can be quickly adjusted in a predictable way while monitoring tissue levels *via* end-tidal concentrations. They are effective regardless of age or body habitus, and are associated with clinical signs that give an indication of anesthetic depth, irrespective of end-tidal gas monitoring. Moreover, they have some properties that prove beneficial in the operating room, including relaxation of skeletal muscle, in most cases preservation of cardiac output and cerebral blood flow, and relatively predictable recovery profiles. Some of the drawbacks to the use of the current volatile anesthetics are the absence of analgesic effects and their association with postoperative nausea and vomiting. In addition, as mentioned earlier, various inhaled anesthetics have been associated with cellular toxicity in animal models, although in patients in a clinical setting these issues have not resulted in any discernible effect on outcome. The exceptions are halothane and desflurane. Halothane has a well-described immunologic effect in producing hepatitis, it sensitizes the myocardium to epinephrine-induced arrhythmias, and it has been associated with bradycardia and bradyarrhythmias (coronary steal). Desflurane has been associated with tachycardia, hypertension, and, in select cases, myocardial ischemia when used in high concentrations or rapidly increasing the inspired concentrations (without using opioid adjuvants to prevent such a response).

PHARMACOECONOMICS AND VALUE-BASED DECISIONS

In the current environment of cost containment, clinicians are constantly being pressured to use less expensive anesthetic agents, including neuromuscular blocking drugs and volatile anesthetics. In succumbing to these pressures, the clinician must focus on providing value-based anesthesia—that is, obtaining the best results at the most practical cost. Factors involved in the value-based decision include the efficacy of the drug, its side effects, its direct costs, and its indirect effects. In terms of efficacy, all of the volatile anesthetics are reasonably similar: each can be used to establish state of anesthesia for surgical interventions and can be reversed easily.

In terms of side effects, the things to consider are serious side effects or toxicities versus manageable side effects, and to what extent these manageable side effects increase the cost. With respect to serious side effects, halothane is the least expensive of the volatile anesthetics, but it has definite life-threatening potential in terms of sensitization of the heart to arrhythmias and the development of an immune response that can cause fulminant hepatic necrosis. One can make a strong argument that halothane does not belong in the operating room. Other side effects of the volatile anesthetics are nausea and vomiting. The need for rescue medications to treat nausea and vomiting after volatile anesthesia must be weighed into any legitimate cost analysis.

Direct costs are not simply the cents per milliliter of liquid or dollars per bottle of anesthetic. Rather, they reflect the combination of the potency of the drug to establish a MAC level, the fresh gas flow, and the cost of the anesthetic. At $2 \, l \cdot min^{-1}$ fresh gas flow, delivering 1 MAC, both desflurane and sevoflurane cost about $10.00 per hour. This contrasts to isoflurane, which costs $2.00–$3.00 per MAC-hour when delivered at 2 $l \cdot min^{-1}$ because of generic price pressures.[395]

The indirect costs are probably the most difficult to pinpoint, but may be the most important to evaluating the cost of using the new volatile anesthetics. Examples of indirect costs include costs associated with OR time, time in the PACU versus bypassing the PACU to a step-down unit, labor costs, and outcome-

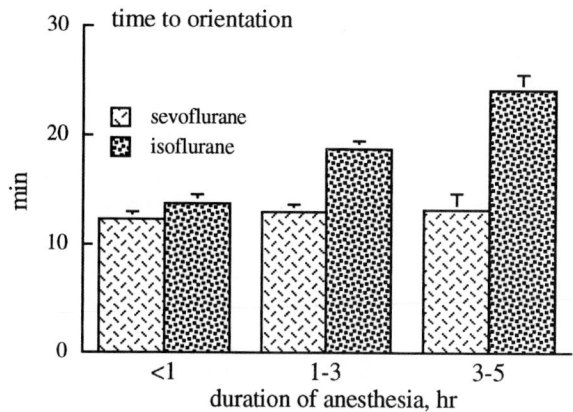

Figure 15-40. The recovery times to orientation after anesthesia of varying durations. With the less soluble anesthetic sevoflurane, the time to orientation was independent of the anesthetic duration. In contrast, long anesthetics with isoflurane were associated with delayed times to orientation. (Adapted from Ebert TJ, Robinson BJ, Uhrich TD *et al:* Recovery from sevoflurane anesthesia. Anesthesiology 89:1524, 1998.)

related costs, such as litigation to defend a bad outcome from an anesthetic drug.

One of the arguments for using the newer, more expensive volatile anesthetics, sevoflurane and desflurane, has been their relative speed in terms of emergence from anesthesia. It seems that this speed matches the ambulatory anesthesia environment in which we practice and the "move 'em in/move 'em out" approach to surgical patients. This argument has been tempered somewhat by the basic knowledge that one of the skills of the clinician is the titration of the volatile anesthetics. Even the more soluble drugs can be titrated based on clinical experience or with the aid of processed EEG monitors (such as the bispectral index system), permitting fast wakeups regardless of the choice of anesthetic agent. However, there is solid evidence to support the use of the less soluble drugs in the longest surgical cases, even though these agents have the highest direct costs (Fig. 15-40).[33,396] In these cases the improved recovery profile of the less soluble drugs over the more soluble drugs includes a more rapid time to emergence and a more rapid discharge from the recovery room. This discharge advantage with new agents has been difficult to show after shorter surgical procedures. Clearly, the use of the most expensive drugs in the longest procedures adds to the direct cost of managing that case, but may provide substantial cost savings in terms of side effects and indirect costs.

REFERENCES

1. Jones RM: Desflurane and sevoflurane: Inhalation anaesthetics for this decade? Br J Anaesth 65:527, 1990
2. Vitcha JF: A history of forane. Anesthesiology 35:4, 1971
3. Terrell RC: Physical and chemical properties of anaesthetic agents. Br J Anaesth 56:3S, 1984
4. Terrell RC, Speers L, Szur AJ *et al:* General anesthetics. 1. Halogenated methyl ethyl ethers as anesthetic agents. J Med Chem 14:517, 1971
5. Wallin RF, Regan BM, Napoli MD *et al:* Sevoflurane: A new inhalational anesthetic agent. Anesth Analg 54:758, 1975
6. Kety SS: The physiological and physical factors governing the uptake of anesthetic gases by the body. Anesthesiology 11:517, 1950
7. Eger EI II: Anesthetic Uptake and Action. Baltimore, Williams & Wilkins, 1974
8. Targ AG, Yasuda N, Eger EI II: Solubility of I-653, sevoflurane, isoflurane, and halothane in plastics and rubber composing a conventional anesthetic circuit. Anesth Analg 68:218, 1989
9. Eger E, Larson P, Severinghaus J: The solubility of halothane in rubber, soda lime and various plastics. Anesthesiology 23:356, 1962
10. Munson ES, Eger EI II, Tham MK *et al:* Increase in anesthetic

uptake, excretion, and blood solubility in man after eating. Anesth Analg 57:224, 1978

11. Eger EI II: The effect of inspired concentration on the rate of rise of alveolar concentration. Anesthesiology 24:153, 1963

12. Eger EI II: Application of a mathematical model of gas uptake. In Uptake and Distribution of Anesthetic Agents, p 88. New York, McGraw-Hill, 1963

13. Epstein R, Rackow H, Salanitre E et al: Influence of the concentration effect on the uptake of anesthetic mixtures: The second gas effect. Anesthesiology 25:364, 1964

14. Stoelting RK, Eger EI II: An additional explanation for the second gas effect: A concentrating effect. Anesthesiology 30:273, 1969

15. Eger EI II: Ventilation, circulation and uptake. In Anesthetic Uptake and Action, p 123. Baltimore, Williams & Wilkins, 1974

16. Munson ES, Eger EI II, Bowers DL: Effects of anesthetic-depressed ventilation and cardiac output on anesthetic uptake. Anesthesiology 38:251, 1973

17. Fukui Y, Smith NT: Interactions among ventilation, the circulation, and the uptake and distribution of halothane—Use of a hybrid computer multiple model: I. The basic model. Anesthesiology 54:107, 1981

18. Calverley RK, Smith NT, Jones CW et al: Ventilatory and cardiovascular effects of enflurane anesthesia during spontaneous ventilation in man. Anesth Analg 57:610, 1978

19. Lockhart SH, Rampil IJ, Yasuda N et al: Depression of ventilation by desflurane in humans. Anesthesiology 74:484, 1991

20. Eger EI II: Ventilation, circulation, and uptake. In Anesthetic Uptake and Action, p. 131. Baltimore, Williams & Wilkins, 1974

21. Gibbons RT, Steffey EP, Eger EI II: The effect of spontaneous versus controlled ventilation on the rate of rise of alveolar halothane concentration in dogs. Anesth Analg 56:32, 1977

22. Fassoulaki A, Lockhart S, Freire BA et al: Percutaneous loss of desflurane, isoflurane and halothane in humans. Anesthesiology 74:479, 1991

23. Lockhart SH, Yasuda Y, Peterson N et al: Comparison of percutaneous losses of sevoflurane and isoflurane in humans. Anesth Analg 72:212, 1991

24. Cullen BF, Eger EI II: Diffusion of nitrous oxide, cyclopropane, and halothane through human skin and amniotic membrane. Anesthesiology 36:168, 1972

25. Stoelting RK, Eger EI II: Percutaneous loss of nitrous oxide, cyclopropane, ether and halothane in man. Anesthesiology 30:278, 1969

26. Laster MJ, Tahari S, Eger EI II et al: Visceral losses of desflurane, isoflurane, and halothane in swine. Anesth Analg 73:209, 1991

27. Carpenter RL, Eger EI II, Johnson BH et al: Does the duration of anesthetic administration affect the pharmacokinetics or metabolism of inhaled anesthetics in humans? Anesth Analg 66:1, 1987

28. Carpenter RL, Eger EI II, Johnson BH et al: Pharmacokinetics of inhaled anesthetics in humans: Measurements during and after the simultaneous administration of enflurane, halothane, isoflurane, methoxyflurane, and nitrous oxide. Anesth Analg 65:575, 1986

29. Yasuda N, Lockhart SH, Eger EI II et al: Kinetics of desflurane, isoflurane, and halothane in humans. Anesthesiology 74:489, 1991

30. Yasuda N, Lockhart SH, Eger EI II et al: Comparison of kinetics of sevoflurane and isoflurane in humans. Anesth Analg 72:316, 1991

31. Carpenter RL, Eger EI II, Johnson BH et al: The extent of metabolism of inhaled anesthetics in humans. Anesthesiology 65:201, 1986

32. Eger EI II, Gong D, Koblin DD et al: The effect of anesthetic duration on kinetic and recovery characteristics of desflurane versus sevoflurane, and on the kinetic characteristics of compound A, in volunteers. Anesth Analg 86:414, 1998

33. Eger EI II, Johnson BH: Rates of awakening from anesthesia with I-653, halothane, isoflurane, and sevoflurane: A test of the effect of anesthetic concentration and duration in rats. Anesth Analg 66:977, 1987

34. Stoelting RK, Eger EI II: The effects of ventilation and anesthetic solubility on recovery from anesthesia: An in vivo and analog analysis before and after equilibrium. Anesthesiology 30:290, 1969

35. Mapleson WW: Quantitative prediction of anesthetic concentrations. In Uptake and Distribution of Anesthetic Agents, p 104. New York, McGraw-Hill, 1963

36. Bailey JM: Context-sensitive half-times and other decrement times of inhaled anesthetics. Anesth Analg 85:681, 1997

37. Fink BR: Diffusion anoxia. Anesthesiology 16:511, 1955

38. Sheffer L, Steffenson JL, Birch AA: Nitrous oxide-induced diffusion hypoxia in patients breathing spontaneously. Anesthesiology 37:436, 1972

39. Rackow H, Salanitre E, Frumin MH: Dilution of alveolar gases during nitrous oxide excretion in man. J Appl Physiol 16:723, 1961

40. Nakata Y, Goto T, Morita S: Comparison of inhalation inductions with xenon and sevoflurane. Acta Anaesthesiol Scand 41:1157, 1997

41. Hettrick DA, Pagel PS, Kersten JR et al: Cardiovascular effects of xenon in isoflurane-anesthetized dogs with dilated cardiomyopathy. Anesthesiology 89:1166, 1998

42. Eger EI II, Saidman LJ: Hazards of nitrous oxide anesthesia in bowel obstruction and pneumothorax. Anesthesiology 26:61, 1965

43. Stanley TH, Kawamura R, Graves C: Effects of nitrous oxide on volume and pressure of endotracheal tube cuffs. Anesthesiology 41:256, 1974

44. Eisenkraft JB, Eger EI II: Nitrous oxide anesthesia may double the balloon gas volume of Swan-Ganz catheters. Mt Sinai J Med 49:430, 1982

45. Kaplan R, Abramowitz MD, Epstein BS: Nitrous oxide and air-filled balloon-tipped catheters. Anesthesiology 55:71, 1981

46. Munson ES, Merrick HC: Effect of nitrous oxide on venous air embolism. Anesthesiology 27:783, 1966

47. Waun JE, Sweitzer RS, Hamilton WK: Effect of nitrous oxide on middle ear mechanics and hearing acuity. Anesthesiology 28:846, 1987

48. Graham MD, Knight PR: Atelectative tympanic membrane reversal by nitrous oxide supplemented general anesthesia and polyethylene ventilation tube insertions: A preliminary report. Laryngoscope 41:1469, 1981

49. Black S, Michenfelder JD: Cerebral blood flow and metabolism. In Clinical Neuroanesthesia, 2nd ed, p 11. New York, Churchill Livingstone, 1998

50. Saidman LJ, Eger EI II, Munson ES et al: Minimum alveolar concentrations of methoxyflurane, halothane, ether and cyclopropane in man: Correlation with theories of anesthesia. Anesthesiology 28:994, 1967

51. Quasha AL, Eger EI II, Tinker JH: Determination and applications of MAC. Anesthesiology 53:315, 1980

52. Tinker JH, Sharbrough FW, Michenfelder JD: Anterior shift of the dominant EEG rhythm during anesthesia in the Java monkey: Correlation with anesthetic potency. Anesthesiology 46:252, 1977

53. Stoelting RK, Longnecker DE, Eger EI II: Minimum alveolar concentrations in man on awakening from methoxyflurane, halothane, ether and fluroxene anesthesia: MAC awake. Anesthesiology 33:5, 1970

54. Gross JB, Alexander CM: Awakening concentrations of isoflurane are not affected by analgesic doses of morphine. Anesth Analg 67:27, 1988

55. Roizen MF, Horrigan RW, Frazer BM: Anesthetic doses blocking adrenergic (stress) and cardiovascular responses to incision—MAC BAR. Anesthesiology 54:390, 1981

56. Cullen SC, Eger EI II, Cullen BF et al: Observations on the anesthetic effect of the combination of xenon and halothane. Anesthesiology 31:305, 1969

57. Miller RD, Wahrenbrock EA, Schroeder CF et al: Ethylene–halothane anesthesia: Addition or synergism? Anesthesiology 31:301, 1969

58. Cole DJ, Kalichman MW, Shapiro HM et al: The nonlinear potency of sub-MAC concentrations of nitrous oxide in decreasing the anesthetic requirement of enflurane, halothane, and isoflurane in rats. Anesthesiology 73:93, 1990

59. Johnston RR, Way WL, Miller RD: Alteration of anesthetic requirement by amphetamine. Anesthesiology 36:357, 1972

60. LeDez KM, Lerman J: The minimum alveolar concentration (MAC) of isoflurane in preterm neonates. Anesthesiology 67:301, 1987

61. Miller RD, Way WL, Eger EI II: The effects of alpha-methyldopa, reserpine, guanethidine, and iproniazid on minimum alveolar anesthetic requirement (MAC). Anesthesiology 29:1153, 1968

62. Sebel PS, Glass PSA, Fletcher JE et al: Reduction of the MAC of desflurane with fentanyl. Anesthesiology 76:52, 1992

63. Cullen DJ, Cotev S, Severinghaus JW et al: The effects of hypoxia and isovolemic anemia on the halothane requirement (MAC) of dogs. II. The effects of acute hypoxia on halothane requirement and cerebral-surface PO_2, PCO_2, pH and HCO_3. Anesthesiology 32:35, 1970

64. Gregory GA, Eger EI II, Munson ES: The relationship between age and halothane requirement in man. Anesthesiology 30:488, 1969

65. Johnston RR, White PF, Way WL et al: The effect of levodopa on halothane anesthetic requirements. Anesth Analg 54:178, 1975

66. Stevens WC, Dolan WM, Gibbons RT et al: Minimum alveolar concentrations (MAC) of isoflurane with and without nitrous oxide in patients of various ages. Anesthesiology 42:197, 1975

67. Mapleson WW: Effect of age on MAC in humans: A meta-analysis. Br J Anaesth 76:179, 1996

68. Stullken EH Jr, Milde JH, Michenfelder JD et al: The non-linear responses of cerebral metabolism to low concentrations of halothane, enflurane, isoflurane and thiopental. Anesthesiology 46:28, 1977

69. Newberg LA, Milde JH, Michenfelder JD: The cerebral metabolic effects of isoflurane at and above concentrations that suppress cortical electrical activity. Anesthesiology 59:23, 1983

70. Theye RA, Michenfelder JD: The effect of halothane on canine cerebral metabolism. Anesthesiology 29:1113, 1968

71. Michenfelder JD, Theye RA: *In vivo* toxic effects of halothane on canine cerebral metabolic pathways. Am J Physiol 229:1050, 1975

72. Michenfelder JD: The *in vivo* effects of massive concentrations of anesthetics on canine cerebral metabolism. In Molecular Mechanisms of Anesthesia, p 537. New York, Raven Press, 1975

73. Young WL: Effects of desflurane on the central nervous system. Anesth Analg 75:S32, 1992

74. Scheller MS, Tateishi A, Drummond JC et al: The effects of sevoflurane on cerebral blood flow, cerebral metabolic rate for oxygen, intracranial pressure, and the electroencephalogram are similar to those of isoflurane in the rabbit. Anesthesiology 68:548, 1988

75. Scheller MS, Nakakimura K, Fleischer JE et al: Cerebral effects of sevoflurane in the dog: Comparison with isoflurane and enflurane. Br J Anaesth 65:388, 1990

76. Lutz LJ, Milde JH, Milde LN: The cerebral functional, metabolic, and hemodynamic effects of desflurane in dogs. Anesthesiology 73:125, 1990

77. Osawa M, Shingu K, Murakawa M et al: Effects of sevoflurane on central nervous system electrical activity in cats. Anesth Analg 79:52, 1994

78. Rampil IJ, Laster M, Dwyer RC et al: No EEG evidence of acute tolerance to desflurane in swine. Anesthesiology 74:889, 1991

79. Fujibayashi T, Sugiura Y, Yanagimoto M et al: Brain energy metabolism and blood flow during sevoflurane and halothane anesthesia: Effects of hypocapnia and blood pressure fluctuations. Acta Anaesthesiol Scand 38:413, 1994

80. Yli-Hankala A, Vakkuri A, Särkelä M et al: Epileptiform electroencephalogram during mask induction of anesthesia with sevoflurane. Anesthesiology 91:1596, 1999

81. McDowall DG: The effects of clinical concentrations of halothane on the blood flow and oxygen uptake of the cerebral cortex. Br J Anaesth 39:186, 1967

82. Todd MM, Drummond JC: A comparison of the cerebrovascular and metabolic effects of halothane and isoflurane in the cat. Anesthesiology 60:276, 1984

83. Adams RW, Gronert GA, Sundt TMJ et al: Halothane, hypocapnia, and cerebrospinal fluid pressure in neurosurgery. Anesthesiology 37:510, 1972

84. Drummond JC, Todd MM: The response of the feline cerebral circulation to Pa_{CO_2} during anesthesia with isoflurane and halothane and during sedation with nitrous oxide. Anesthesiology 62:268, 1985

85. Scheller MS, Todd MM, Drummond JC: Isoflurane, halothane, and regional cerebral blood flow at various levels of Pa_{CO_2} in rabbits. Anesthesiology 64:598, 1986

86. Eintrei C, Leszniewski W, Carlsson C: Local application of ^{133}Xe for measurement of regional cerebral blood flow (rCBF) during halothane, enflurane, and isoflurane anesthesia in humans. Anesthesiology 63:391, 1985

87. Algotsson L, Messeter K, Nordström CH et al: Cerebral blood flow and oxygen consumption during isoflurane and halothane anesthesia in man. Acta Anaesthesiol Scand 32:15, 1988

88. Conzen PF, Vollmar B, Habazettl H et al: Systemic and regional hemodynamics of isoflurane and sevoflurane in rats. Anesth Analg 74:79, 1992

89. Albrecht RF, Miletich DJ, Madala LR: Normalization of cerebral blood flow during prolonged halothane anesthesia. Anesthesiology 58:26, 1983

90. Boarini DJ, Kassell NF, Coester HC et al: Comparison of systemic and cerebrovascular effects of isoflurane and halothane. Neurosurgery 15:400, 1984

91. Warner DS, Boarini DJ, Kassell NF: Cerebrovascular adaptation to prolonged halothane anesthesia is not related to cerebrospinal fluid pH. Anesthesiology 63:1985

92. Brüssel T, Fitch W, Brodner G et al: Effects of halothane in low concentrations on cerebral blood flow, cerebral metabolism, and cerebrovascular autoregulation in the baboon. Anesth Analg 73:758, 1991

93. Van Aken H, Fitch W, Graham DI et al: Cardiovascular and cerebrovascular effects of isoflurane-induced hypotension in the baboon. Anesth Analg 65:565, 1986

94. Drummond JC, Todd MM, Scheller MS et al: A comparison of the direct cerebral vasodilating potencies of halothane and isoflurane in the New Zealand white rabbit. Anesthesiology 65:462, 1986

95. Smith AL, Wollman H: Cerebral blood flow and metabolism: Effects of anesthetic drugs and techniques. Anesthesiology 36:378, 1972

96. Hansen TD, Warner DS, Todd MM et al: The role of cerebral metabolism in determining the local cerebral blood flow effects of volatile anesthetics: Evidence for persistent flow-metabolism coupling. J Cereb Blood Flow Metab 9:323, 1989

97. Miletich DJ, Ivankovich AD, Albrecht RF et al: Absence of autoregulation of cerebral blood flow during halothane and enflurane anesthesia. Anesth Analg 55:100, 1976

98. Eger EI II: Pharmacology of isoflurane. Br J Anaesth 56:71S, 1984

99. Archer DP, Labrecque P, Tyler JL et al: Cerebral blood volume is increased in dogs during administration of nitrous oxide or isoflurane. Anesthesiology 67:642, 1987

100. Artru AA: Relationship between cerebral blood volume and CSF pressure during anesthesia with halothane or enflurane in dogs. Anesthesiology 58:533, 1983

101. Drummond JC, Todd MM, Toutant SM et al: Brain surface protrusion during enflurane, halothane, and isoflurane anesthesia in cats. Anesthesiology 59:288, 1983

102. Adams RW, Cucchiara RF, Gronert GA et al: Isoflurane and cerebrospinal fluid pressure in neurosurgical patients. Anesthesiology 54:97, 1981

103. Campkin TV: Isoflurane and cranial extradural pressure. A study in neurosurgical patients. Br J Anaesth 56:1083, 1984

104. Kaieda R, Todd MM, Weeks JB et al: A comparison of the effects of halothane, isoflurane, and pentobarbital anesthesia on intracranial pressure and cerebral edema formation following brain injury in rabbits. Anesthesiology 71:571, 1989

105. Grosslight K, Foster R, Colohan AR et al: Isoflurane for neuroanesthesia: Risk factors for increases in intracranial pressure. Anesthesiology 63:533, 1985

106. Artru AA: Isoflurane does not increase the rate of CSF production in the dog. Anesthesiology 60:193, 1984

107. Artru AA: Effects of enflurane and isoflurane on resistance to reabsorption of cerebrospinal fluid in dogs. Anesthesiology 61:529, 1984

108. Artru AA: Effects of halothane and fentanyl anesthesia on resistance to reabsorption of CSF. J Neurosurg 60:252, 1984

109. Artru AA: Concentration-related changes in the rate of CSF formation and resistance to reabsorption of CSF during enflurane and isoflurane anesthesia in dogs receiving nitrous oxide. J Neurosurg Anesthesiol 1:256, 1989

110. Sugioka S: Effects of sevoflurane on intracranial pressure and formation and absorption of cerebrospinal fluid in cats. Masui—Japanese Journal of Anesthesiology 41:1434, 1992

111. Artru AA: Rate of cerebrospinal fluid formation, resistance to reabsorption of cerebrospinal fluid, brain tissue water content, and electroencephalogram during desflurane anesthesia in dogs. J Neurosurg Anesthesiol 5:178, 1993

112. Muzzi DA, Losasso TJ, Dietz NM et al: The effect of desflurane and isoflurane on cerebrospinal fluid pressure in humans with supratentorial mass lesions. Anesthesiology 76:720, 1992

113. Wollman H, Alexander C, Cohen PJ et al: Cerebral circulation during general anesthesia and hyperventilation in man. Thiopental induction to nitrous oxide and D-tubocurarine. Anesthesiology 26:329, 1965

114. Lutz LJ, Milde JH, Milde LN: The response of the canine cerebral circulation to hyperventilation during anesthesia with desflurane. Anesthesiology 74:504, 1991

115. Nishiyama T, Matsukawa T, Yokoyama T et al: Cerebrovascular

carbon dioxide reactivity during general anesthesia: A comparison between sevoflurane and isoflurane. Anesth Analg 89:1437, 1999

116. Hoff J, Schmith A, Nielsen S et al: Effects of barbiturate and halothane anaesthesia on focal cerebral infarction in the dog. Surg Forum 24:449, 1973

117. Michenfelder JD, Milde JH, Sundt JM Jr: Cerebral protection by barbiturate anesthesia. Use after middle cerebral artery occlusion in Java monkeys. Arch Neurol 33:1976

118. Newberg LA, Michenfelder JD: Cerebral protection by isoflurane during hypoxemia or ischemia. Anesthesiology 59:29, 1983

119. Newberg LA, Milde JH, Michenfelder JD: Systemic and cerebral effects of isoflurane-induced hypotension in dogs. Anesthesiology 60:541, 1984

120. Seyde WC, Longnecker DE: Cerebral oxygen tension in rats during deliberate hypotension with sodium nitroprusside, 2-chloroadenosine, or deep isoflurane anesthesia. Anesthesiology 64:480, 1986

121. Michenfelder JD, Sundt TM, Fode N et al: Isoflurane when compared to enflurane and halothane decreases the frequency of cerebral ischemia during carotid endarterectomy. Anesthesiology 67:336, 1987

122. Messick JM Jr, Casement B, Sharbrough FW et al: Correlation of regional cerebral blood flow (rCBF) with EEG changes during isoflurane anesthesia for carotid endarterectomy: Critical rCBF. Anesthesiology 66:344, 1987

123. Werner C, Möllenberg O, Kochs E et al: Sevoflurane improves neurological outcome after incomplete cerebral ischaemia in rats. Br J Anaesth 75:756, 1995

124. Engelhard K, Werner C, Reeker W et al: Desflurane and isoflurane improve neurological outcome after incomplete cerebral ischaemia in rats. Br J Anaesth 83:415, 1999

125. Hoffman WE, Charbel FT, Edelman G et al: Thiopental and desflurane treatment for brain protection. Neurosurgery 43:1050, 1998

126. Crosby G, Crane AM, Sokoloff L: A comparison of local rates of glucose utilization in spinal cord and brain in conscious and nitrous oxide or pentobarbital treated rats. Anesthesiology 61:1984

127. Dahlgren N, Ingvar M, Yokoyama H et al: Influence of nitrous oxide on local cerebral blood flow in awake minimally restrained rats. J Cereb Blood Flow Metab 1:211, 1981

128. Seyde WC, Ellis JE, Longnecker DE: The addition of nitrous oxide to halothane decreases renal and splanchnic flow and increases cerebral blood flow in rats. Br J Anaesth 58:63, 1986

129. Theye RA, Michenfelder JD: The effect of nitrous oxide on canine cerebral metabolism. Anesthesiology 29:1119, 1968

130. Sakabe T, Kuramoto T, Inoue S et al: Cerebral effects of nitrous oxide in the dog. Anesthesiology 48:195, 1978

131. Manohar M, Parks CM: Regional distribution of brain and myocardial perfusion in swine while awake and during 1.0 and 1.5 MAC isoflurane anaesthesia produced without or with 50% nitrous oxide. Cardiovasc Res 18:344, 1984

132. Baughman VL, Hoffman WE, Miletich DJ et al: Cerebrovascular and cerebral metabolic effects of N_2O in unrestrained rats. Anesthesiology 73:269, 1990

133. Carlsson C, Smith DS, Keykhah MN et al: The effects of high dose fentanyl on cerebral circulation and metabolism in rats. Anesthesiology 57:375, 1982

134. Roald OK, Forsman M, Heier MS et al: Cerebral effects of nitrous oxide when added to low and high concentrations of isoflurane in the dog. Anesth Analg 72:75, 1991

135. Drummond JC, Scheller MS, Todd MM: The effect of nitrous oxide on cortical cerebral blood flow during anesthesia with halothane and isoflurane, with and without morphine, in the rabbit. Anesth Analg 66:1083, 1987

136. Kaieda R, Todd MM, Warner DS: The effects of anesthetics and $Paco_2$ on the cerebrovascular, metabolic, and electroencephalographic responses to nitrous oxide in the rabbit. Anesth Analg 68:135, 1989

137. Sakabe T, Tsutsui T, Maekawa T et al: Local cerebral glucose utilization during nitrous oxide and pentobarbital anesthesia in rats. Anesthesiology 63:262, 1985

138. Fleischer JE, Milde JH, Moyer TP et al: Cerebral effects of high-dose midazolam and subsequent reversal with Ro 15-1788 in dogs. Anesthesiology 68:234, 1988

139. Hoffman WE, Miletich DJ, Albrecht RF: The effects of midazolam on cerebral blood flow and oxygen consumption and its interaction with nitrous oxide. Anesth Analg 65:729, 1986

140. Phirman JR, Shapiro HM: Modification of nitrous oxide-induced intracranial hypertension by prior induction of anesthesia. Anesthesiology 46:150, 1977

141. Baughman VL, Hoffman WE, Thomas C et al: The interaction of nitrous oxide and isoflurane with incomplete cerebral ischemia in the rat. Anesthesiology 70:767, 1989

142. Hartung J, Cottrell JE: Nitrous oxide reduces thiopental-induced prolongation of survival in hypoxic and anoxic mice. Anesth Analg 66:1987

143. Eger EI II, Smith NT, Stoelting RK et al: Cardiovascular effects of halothane in man. Anesthesiology 32:396, 1970

144. Calverley RK, Smith NT, Prys-Roberts C et al: Cardiovascular effects of enflurane anesthesia during controlled ventilation in man. Anesth Analg 57:619, 1978

145. Stevens WC, Cromwell TH, Halsey MJ et al: The cardiovascular effects of a new inhalation anesthetic, Forane, in human volunteers at a constant arterial carbon dioxide tension. Anesthesiology 35:8, 1971

146. Jones RM, Cashman JN, Mant TGK: Clinical impressions and cardiorespiratory effects of a new fluorinated inhalation anaesthetic, desflurane (I-653), in volunteers. Br J Anaesth 64:11, 1990

147. Weiskopf RB, Cahalan MK, Eger EI II et al: Cardiovascular actions of desflurane in normocarbic volunteers. Anesth Analg 73:143, 1991

148. Holaday DA, Smith FR: Clinical characteristics and biotransformation of sevoflurane in healthy human volunteers. Anesthesiology 54:100, 1981

149. Malan TP, DiNardo JA, Isner RJ et al: Cardiovascular effects of sevoflurane compared with those of isoflurane in volunteers. Anesthesiology 83:918, 1995

150. Ebert TJ, Muzi M, Lopatka CW: Neurocirculatory responses to sevoflurane in humans. A comparison to desflurane. Anesthesiology 83:88, 1995

151. Eisele JH, Smith NT: Cardiovascular effects of 40 percent nitrous oxide in man. Anesth Analg 51:956, 1972

152. Ebert TJ, Kampine JP: Nitrous oxide augments sympathetic outflow: Direct evidence from human peroneal nerve recordings. Anesth Analg 69:444, 1989

153. Ebert TJ, Harkin CP, Muzi M: Cardiovascular responses to sevoflurane: A review. Anesth Analg 81:S11, 1995

154. Eger EI II: Isoflurane: A review. Anesthesiology 55:559, 1981

155. Bastard OG, Carter JG, Moyers JR et al: Circulatory effects of isoflurane in patients with ischemic heart disease: A comparison with halothane. Anesth Analg 63:635, 1984

156. Holzman RS, van der Velde ME, Kaus SJ et al: Sevoflurane depresses myocardial contractility less than halothane during induction of anesthesia in children. Anesthesiology 85:1260, 1996

157. Pagel PS, Kampine JP, Schmeling WT et al: Alteration of left ventricular diastolic function by desflurane, isoflurane, and halothane in the chronically instrumented dog with autonomic nervous system blockade. Anesthesiology 74:1103, 1991

158. Eger EI II: New inhaled anesthetics. Anesthesiology 80:906, 1994

159. Ebert TJ, Muzi M: Sympathetic hyperactivity during desflurane anesthesia in healthy volunteers. A comparison with isoflurane. Anesthesiology 79:444, 1993

160. Moffitt EA, Imrie DD, Scovil JE et al: Myocardial metabolism and haemodynamic responses with enflurane anaesthesia for coronary artery surgery. Can Anaesth Soc J 31:604, 1984

161. Pagel PS, Kampine JP, Schmeling WT et al: Comparison of the systemic and coronary hemodynamic actions of desflurane, isoflurane, halothane and enflurane in the chronically instrumented dog. Anesthesiology 74:539, 1991

162. Shimosato S, Iwatsuki N, Carter JG: Cardio-circulatory effects of enflurane anaesthesia in health and disease. Acta Anaesthesiol Scand 71:69, 1979

163. Merin RG, Bernard J, Doursout M et al: Comparison of the effects of isoflurane and desflurane on cardiovascular dynamics and regional blood flow in the chronically instrumented dog. Anesthesiology 74:568, 1991

164. Pagel PS, Kampine JP, Schmeling WT et al: Evaluation of myocardial contractility in the chronically instrumented dog with intact autonomic nervous system function: Effects of desflurane and isoflurane. Acta Anaesthesiol Scand 37:203, 1993

165. Weiskopf RB, Holmes MA, Eger EI II et al: Cardiovascular effects of I653 in swine. Anesthesiology 69:303, 1988

166. Bernard J-M, Wouters PF, Doursout M-F et al: Effects of sevoflurane and isoflurane on cardiac and coronary dynamics in chronically instrumented dogs. Anesthesiology 72:659, 1990

167. Manabe M, Ookawa I, Nonaka A et al: Effects of sevoflurane with or without nitrous oxide on cardiac contractility and sinoatrial node rate. J Anesth 3:145, 1989

168. Frink EJ Jr, Morgan SE, Coetzee A et al: The effects of sevoflurane, halothane, enflurane, and isoflurane on hepatic blood flow and oxygenation in chronically instrumented greyhound dogs. Anesthesiology 76:85, 1992

169. Weiskopf RB, Moore MA, Eger EI II et al: Rapid increase in desflurane concentration is associated with greater transient cardiovascular stimulation than with rapid increase in isoflurane concentration in humans. Anesthesiology 80:1035, 1994

170. Weiskopf RB, Eger EI II, Daniel M et al: Cardiovascular stimulation induced by rapid increases in desflurane concentration in humans results from activation of tracheopulmonary and systemic receptors. Anesthesiology 83:1173, 1995

171. Muzi M, Ebert TJ, Hope WG et al: Site(s) mediating sympathetic activation with desflurane. Anesthesiology 85:737, 1996

172. Pacentine GG, Muzi M, Ebert TJ: Effects of fentanyl on sympathetic activation associated with the administration of desflurane. Anesthesiology 82:823, 1995

173. Weiskopf RB, Eger EI II, Noorani M et al: Fentanyl, esmolol, and clonidine blunt the transient cardiovascular stimulation induced by desflurane in humans. Anesthesiology 81:1350, 1994

174. Yonker-Sell AE, Muzi M, Hope WG et al: Alfentanil modifies the neurocirculatory responses to desflurane. Anesth Analg 82:162, 1996

175. Khambatta HJ, Sonntag H, Larsen R et al: Global and regional myocardial blood flow and metabolism during equipotent halothane and isoflurane anesthesia in patients with coronary artery disease. Anesth Analg 67:936, 1988

176. Sonntag H, Donath U, Hillebrand W et al: Left ventricular function in conscious man and during halothane anesthesia. Anesthesiology 48:320, 1978

177. Merin RG, Kumazawa T, Luka NL: Myocardial function and metabolism in the conscious dog and during halothane anesthesia. Anesthesiology 44:402, 1976

178. Morrow DH, Morrow AG: The effects of halothane on myocardial contractile force and vascular resistance. Anesthesiology 22:537, 1961

179. Delaney TJ, Kistner JR, Lake CL et al: Myocardial function during halothane and enflurane anesthesia in patients with coronary artery disease. Anesth Analg 59:240, 1980

180. Housmans PR, Murat I: Comparative effects of halothane, enflurane, and isoflurane at equipotent anesthetic concentrations on isolated ventricular myocardium of the ferret. II. Relaxation. Anesthesiology 69:464, 1988

181. Harkin CP, Pagel PS, Kersten JR et al: Direct negative inotropic and lusitropic effects of sevoflurane. Anesthesiology 81:156, 1994

182. Pagel PS, Kampine JP, Schmeling WT et al: Influence of volatile anesthetics on myocardial contractility in vivo: Desflurane versus isoflurane. Anesthesiology 74:900, 1991

183. Cromwell TH, Stevens WC, Eger EI II et al: The cardiovascular effects of compound 469 (Forane®) during spontaneous ventilation and CO₂ challenge in man. Anesthesiology 35:17, 1971

184. Weiskopf RB, Cahalan MK, Ionescu P et al: Cardiovascular actions of desflurane with and without nitrous oxide during spontaneous ventilation in humans. Anesth Analg 73:165, 1991

185. Bahlman SH, Eger EI II, Halsey MJ et al: The cardiovascular effects of halothane in man during spontaneous ventilation. Anesthesiology 36:494, 1972

186. Weiskopf RB, Holmes MA, Rampil IJ et al: Cardiovascular safety and actions of high concentrations of I-653 and isoflurane in swine. Anesthesiology 70:793, 1989

187. Price HL, Skovsted P, Pauca AL et al: Evidence for beta-receptor activation produced by halothane in normal man. Anesthesiology 32:389, 1970

188. Ebert TJ: Differential effects of nitrous oxide on baroreflex control of heart rate and peripheral sympathetic nerve activity in humans. Anesthesiology 72:16, 1990

189. Smith NT, Eger EI II, Stoelting RK et al: The cardiovascular and sympathomimetic responses to the addition of nitrous oxide to halothane in man. Anesthesiology 32:410, 1970

190. Smith NT, Calverley RK, Prys-Roberts C et al: Impact of nitrous oxide on the circulation during enflurane anesthesia in man. Anesthesiology 48:345, 1978

191. Dolan WM, Stevens WC, Eger EI II et al: The cardiovascular and respiratory effects of isoflurane–nitrous oxide anaesthesia. Can Anaesth Soc J 21:557, 1974

192. Cahalan MK, Weiskopf RB, Eger EI II et al: Hemodynamic effects of desflurane/nitrous oxide anesthesia in volunteers. Anesth Analg 73:157, 1991

193. Theye RA, Michenfelder JD: Whole-body and organ Vo₂ changes with enflurane, isoflurane, and halothane. Br J Anaesth 47:813, 1975

194. Crawford MW, Lerman J, Saldivia V et al: Hemodynamic and organ blood flow responses to halothane and sevoflurane anesthesia during spontaneous ventilation. Anesth Analg 75:1000, 1992

195. Gelman S, Fowler KC, Smith LR: Regional blood flow during isoflurane and halothane anesthesia. Anesth Analg 63:557, 1984

196. Hayashi Y, Sumikawa K, Tashiro C et al: Arrhythmogenic threshold of epinephrine during sevoflurane, enflurane, and isoflurane anesthesia in dogs. Anesthesiology 69:145, 1988

197. Johnston RR, Eger EI II, Wilson C: A comparative interaction of epinephrine with enflurane, isoflurane, and halothane in man. Anesth Analg 55:709, 1976

198. Weiskopf RB, Eger EI II, Holmes MA et al: Epinephrine-induced premature ventricular contractions and changes in arterial blood pressure and heart rate during I-653, isoflurane, and halothane anesthesia in swine. Anesthesiology 70:293, 1989

199. Atlee JLI, Bosnjak ZJ: Mechanisms for cardiac dysrhythmias during anesthesia. Anesthesiology 72:347, 1990

200. Bosnjak ZJ, Kampine JP: Effects of halothane, enflurane, and isoflurane on the SA node. Anesthesiology 58:314, 1983

201. Atlee JLI, Brownlee SW, Burstrom RE: Conscious-state comparisons of the effects of inhalation anesthetics on specialized atrioventricular conduction times in dogs. Anesthesiology 64:703, 1986

202. Buffington CW, Romson JL, Levine A et al: Isoflurane induces coronary steal in a canine model of chronic coronary occlusion. Anesthesiology 66:280, 1987

203. Reiz S, Balfors E, Sorensen MB et al: Isoflurane—a powerful coronary vasodilator in patients with coronary artery disease. Anesthesiology 59:91, 1983

204. Inoue K, Reichelt W, El-Banayosy A et al: Does isoflurane lead to a higher incidence of myocardial infarction and perioperative death than enflurane in coronary artery surgery? Anesth Analg 71:469, 1990

205. Kersten JR, Brayer AP, Pagel PS et al: Perfusion of ischemic myocardium during anesthesia with sevoflurane. Anesthesiology 81:995, 1994

206. Hartman JC, Kampine JP, Schmeling WT et al: Steal-prone coronary circulation in chronically instrumented dogs: Isoflurane versus adenosine. Anesthesiology 74:744, 1991

207. Hartman JC, Pagel PS, Kampine JP et al: Influence of desflurane on regional distribution of coronary blood flow in a chronically instrumented canine model of multivessel coronary artery obstruction. Anesth Analg 72:289, 1991

208. Tarnow J, Markschies-Hornung A, Schulte-Sasse U: Isoflurane improves the tolerance to pacing-induced myocardial ischemia. Anesthesiology 64:147, 1986

209. Slogoff S, Keats AS: Randomized trial of primary anesthetic agents on outcome of coronary artery bypass operations. Anesthesiology 70:179, 1989

210. Slogoff S, Keats AS, Dear WE et al: Steal-prone coronary anatomy and myocardial ischemia associated with four primary anesthetic agents in humans. Anesth Analg 72:22, 1991

211. Tuman KJ, McCarthy RJ, Spiess BD et al: Does choice of anesthetic agent significantly affect outcome after coronary artery surgery? Anesthesiology 70:189, 1989

212. O'Young J, Mastrocostopoulos G, Hilgenberg A et al: Myocardial circulatory and metabolic effects of isoflurane and sufentanil during coronary artery surgery. Anesthesiology 66:653, 1987

213. Searle NR, Martineau RJ, Conzen P et al: Comparison of sevoflurane/fentanyl and isoflurane/fentanyl during elective coronary artery bypass surgery. Can J Anaesth 43:890, 1996

214. Ebert TJ, Kharasch ED, Rooke GA et al: Myocardial ischemia and adverse cardiac outcomes in cardiac patients undergoing noncardiac surgery with sevoflurane and isoflurane. Anesth Analg 85:993, 1997

215. Thomson IR, Bowering JB, Hudson RJ et al: A comparison of desflurane and isoflurane in patients undergoing coronary artery surgery. Anesthesiology 75:776, 1991

216. Helman JD, Leung JM, Bellows WH et al: The risk of myocardial ischemia in patients receiving desflurane versus sufentanil anesthe-

sia for coronary artery bypass graft surgery. Anesthesiology 77:47, 1992

217. Skovsted P, Sapthavichaikul S: The effects of isoflurane on arterial pressure, pulse rate, autonomic nervous activity, and barostatic reflexes. Can Anaesth Soc J 24:304, 1977

218. Seagard JL, Hopp FA, Donegan JH et al: Halothane and the carotid sinus reflex: Evidence for multiple sites of action. Anesthesiology 57:191, 1982

219. Seagard JL, Hopp FA, Bosnjak ZJ et al: Sympathetic efferent nerve activity in conscious and isoflurane-anesthetized dogs. Anesthesiology 61:266, 1984

220. Seagard JL, Hopp FA, Bosnjak ZJ et al: Extent and mechanism of halothane sensitization of the carotid sinus baroreceptors. Anesthesiology 58:432, 1983

221. Seagard JL, Elegbe EO, Hopp FA et al: Effects of isoflurane on the baroreceptor reflex. Anesthesiology 59:511, 1983

222. Duke PC, Fownes D, Wade JG: Halothane depresses baroreflex control of heart rate in man. Anesthesiology 46:184, 1977

223. Muzi M, Ebert TJ: A randomized, prospective comparison of halothane, isoflurane and enflurane on baroreflex control of heart rate in humans. In Advances in Pharmacology, Vol. 31: Anesthesia and Cardiovascular Disease, p 379. San Diego, Academic Press, 1994

224. Morton M, Duke PC, Ong B: Baroreflex control of heart rate in man awake and during enflurane and enflurane–nitrous oxide anesthesia. Anesthesiology 52:221, 1980

225. Kotrly KJ, Ebert TJ, Vucins EJ et al: Human baroreceptor control of heart rate under isoflurane anesthesia. Anesthesiology 60:173, 1984

226. Tanaka M, Nishikawa T: Arterial baroreflex function in humans anaesthetized with sevoflurane. Br J Anaesth 82:350, 1999

227. Muzi M, Ebert TJ: A comparison of baroreflex sensitivity during isoflurane and desflurane anesthesia in humans. Anesthesiology 82:919, 1995

228. Ebert TJ, Perez F, Uhrich TD et al: Desflurane-mediated sympathetic activation occurs in humans despite preventing hypotension and baroreceptor unloading. Anesthesiology 88:1227, 1998

229. Wallin BG: Recordings of impulses in unmyelinated nerve fibres in man: Sympathetic activity. Acta Anaesthesiol Scand 70:130, 1978

230. Kotrly KJ, Ebert TJ, Vucins EJ et al: Effects of fentanyl–diazepam–nitrous oxide anaesthesia on arterial baroreflex control of heart rate in man. Br J Anaesth 58:406, 1986

231. Ebert TJ, Kotrly KJ, Madsen KS et al: Fentanyl–diazepam anesthesia with or without N₂O does not attenuate cardiopulmonary baroreflex-mediated vasoconstrictor responses to controlled hypovolemia in humans. Anesth Analg 67:548, 1988

232. Kotrly KJ, Ebert TJ, Vucins EJ et al: Baroreceptor reflex control of heart rate during morphine sulfate, diazepam, N₂O/O₂ anesthesia in humans. Anesthesiology 61:558, 1984

233. Tanaka M, Nishikawa T: Sevoflurane speeds recovery of baroreflex control of heart rate after minor surgical procedures compared with isoflurane. Anesth Analg 89:284, 1999

234. Muzi M, Lopatka CW, Ebert TJ: Desflurane-mediated neurocirculatory activation in humans: Effects of concentration and rate of change on responses. Anesthesiology 84:1035, 1996

235. Moore MA, Weiskopf RB, Eger EI II et al: Rapid 1% increases of end-tidal desflurane concentration to greater than 5% transiently increase heart rate and blood pressure in humans. Anesthesiology 81:94, 1994

236. Kharasch ED: Biotransformation of sevoflurane. Anesth Analg 81:S27, 1995

237. Bunting HE, Kelly MC, Milligan KR: Effect of nebulized lignocaine on airway irritation and haemodynamic changes during induction of anaesthesia with desflurane. Br J Anaesth 75:631, 1995

238. Smiley RM: An overview of induction and emergence characteristics of desflurane in pediatric, adult, and geriatric patients. Anesth Analg 75:S38, 1992

239. Zwass MS, Fisher DM, Welborn LG et al: Induction and maintenance characteristics of anesthesia with desflurane and nitrous oxide in infants and children. Anesthesiology 76:373, 1992

240. Mathur S, Farhangkhgoee P, Karmazyn M: Cardioprotective effects of propofol and sevoflurane in ischemic and reperfused rat hearts: Role of K(ATP) channels and interaction with the sodium–hydrogen inhibitor HOE 642 (cariporide). Anesthesiology 91:1349, 1999

241. Toller WG, Kersten JR, Pagel PS et al: Sevoflurane reduces myocar-

dial infarct size and decreases the time threshold for ischemic preconditioning in dogs. Anesthesiology 91:1437, 1999

242. Kersten JR, Schmeling TJ, Pagel PS et al: Isoflurane mimics ischemic preconditioning via activation of K–ATP channels. Anesthesiology 87:361, 1997

243. Novalija E, Fujita S, Kampine JP et al: Sevoflurane mimics ischemic preconditioning effects on coronary flow and nitric oxide release in isolated hearts. Anesthesiology 91:701, 1999

244. Novalija E, Stowe DF: Prior preconditioning by ischemia or sevoflurane improves cardiac work per oxygen use in isolated guinea pig hearts after global ischemia. Adv Exp Med Biol 454:533, 1998

245. Hickey RF, Severinghaus JW: Regulation of breathing: Drug effects. In Regulation of Breathing, p 1251. New York, Marcel Dekker, 1981

246. Fourcade HE, Stevens WC, Larson CPJ et al: The ventilatory effects of Forane, a new inhaled anesthetic. Anesthesiology 35:26, 1971

247. Calverley RK, Smith NT, Jones CW et al: Ventilatory and cardiovascular effects of enflurane anesthesia during spontaneous ventilation in man. Anesth Analg 57:610, 1978

248. Lockhart SH, Rampil IJ, Yasuda N et al: Depression of ventilation by desflurane in humans. Anesthesiology 74:484, 1991

249. Doi M, Ikeda K: Respiratory effects of sevoflurane. Anesth Analg 66:241, 1987

250. Green WB Jr: The ventilatory effects of sevoflurane. Anesth Analg 81:S23, 1995

251. Eger EI II, Dolan WM, Stevens WC et al: Surgical stimulation antagonizes the respiratory depression produced by forane. Anesthesiology 36:544, 1972

252. Fourcade HE, Larson CP Jr, Hickey RF et al: Effects of time on ventilation during halothane and cyclopropane anesthesia. Anesthesiology 36:83, 1972

253. Tusiewicz K, Bryan AC, Froese AB: Contributions of changing rib cage–diaphragm interactions to the ventilatory depression of halothane anesthesia. Anesthesiology 47:327, 1977

254. Warner DO, Warner MA, Ritman EL: Mechanical significance of changing rib cage–diaphragm interactions to the ventilatory depression of halothane anesthesia. Anesthesiology 84:309, 1996

255. Warner DO, Warner MA, Ritman EL: Human chest wall function while awake and during halothane anesthesia. I: Quiet breathing. Anesthesiology 82:6, 1995

256. Warner DO, Warner MA, Ritman EL: Atelectasis and chest wall shape during halothane anesthesia. Anesthesiology 85:49, 1996

257. Kochi T, Ide T, Isono S et al: Different effects of halothane and enflurane on diaphragmatic contractility in vivo. Anesth Analg 70:362, 1990

258. Pietak S, Weenig CS, Hickey R et al: Anesthetic effects on ventilation in patients with chronic obstructive pulmonary disease. Anesthesiology 42:160, 1975

259. Hornbein TF, Martin WE, Bonica JJ et al: Nitrous oxide effects on the circulatory and ventilatory responses to halothane. Anesthesiology 31:250, 1969

260. Knill RL, Manninen PH, Clement JL: Ventilation and chemoreflexes during enflurane sedation and anaesthesia in man. Can Anaesth Soc J 26:353, 1979

261. Knill RL, Gelb AW: Ventilatory responses to hypoxia and hypercapnia during halothane sedation and anesthesia in man. Anesthesiology 49:244, 1978

262. Weiskopf RB, Raymond LW, Severinghaus JW: Effects of halothane on canine respiratory responses to hypoxia with and without hypercarbia. Anesthesiology 41:350, 1974

263. Hirshman CA, McCullough RE, Cohen PJ et al: Depression of hypoxic ventilatory response by halothane, enflurane and isoflurane in dogs. Br J Anaesth 49:957, 1977

264. Yacoub O, Doell D, Kryger MH et al: Depression of hypoxic ventilatory response by nitrous oxide. Anesthesiology 45:385, 1976

265. Sarton E, Dahan A, Teppema L et al: Acute pain and central nervous system arousal do not restore impaired hypoxic ventilatory responses during sevoflurane sedation. Anesthesiology 85:295, 1996

266. van den Elsen M, Sarton E, Teppema L et al: Influence of 0.1 minimum alveolar concentration of sevoflurane, desflurane and isoflurane on dynamic ventilatory response to hypercapnia in humans. Br J Anaesth 80:174, 1998

267. Hirshman CA, Bergman NA: Factors influencing intrapulmonary airway calibre during anaesthesia. Br J Anaesth 65:30, 1990

268. Hirshman CA, Edelstein G, Peetz S et al: Mechanism of action of inhalational anesthesia on airways. Anesthesiology 56:107, 1982

269. Lindeman KS, Baker SG, Hirshman CA: Interaction between halothane and the nonadrenergic, noncholinergic inhibitory system in porcine trachealis muscle. Anesthesiology 81:641, 1994

270. Brown RH, Zerhouni EA, Hirshman CA: Comparison of low concentrations of halothane and isoflurane as bronchodilators. Anesthesiology 65:1097, 1986

271. Yamamoto K, Morimoto N, Warner DO et al: Factors influencing the direct actions of volatile anesthetics on airway smooth muscle. Anesthesiology 78:1102, 1993

272. Rooke GA, Choi J-H, Bishop MJ: The effect of isoflurane, halothane, sevoflurane, and thiopental/nitrous oxide on respiratory system resistance after tracheal intubation. Anesthesiology 86:1294, 1997

273. Schwartz SH: Treatment of status asthmaticus with halothane. JAMA 251:2688, 1984

274. Johnston RG, Noseworthy TW, Friesen EG et al: Isoflurane therapy for status asthmaticus in children and adults. Chest 97:698, 1990

275. Parnass SM, Feld JM, Chamberlin WH et al: Status asthmaticus treated with isoflurane and enflurane. Anesth Analg 66:193, 1987

276. Mori N, Nagata H, Ohta S et al: Prolonged sevoflurane inhalation was not nephrotoxic in two patients with refractory status asthmaticus. Anesth Analg 83:189, 1996

277. Forbes AR: Halothane depresses mucociliary flow in the trachea. Anesthesiology 45:59, 1976

278. Forbes AR, Horrigan RW: Mucociliary flow in the trachea during anesthesia with enflurane, ether, nitrous oxide, and morphine. Anesthesiology 46:319, 1977

279. Marshall C, Lindgren L, Marshall BE: Effects of halothane, enflurane, and isoflurane on hypoxic pulmonary vasoconstriction in rat lungs in vitro. Anesthesiology 60:304, 1984

280. Ishibe Y, Gui X, Uno H et al: Effect of sevoflurane on hypoxic pulmonary vasoconstriction in the perfused rabbit lung. Anesthesiology 79:1348, 1993

281. Loer SA, Scheeren TW, Tarnow J: Desflurane inhibits hypoxic pulmonary vasoconstriction in isolated rabbit lungs. Anesthesiology 83:552, 1995

282. Lilleaasen P, Semb B, Lindberg H et al: Haemodynamic changes with the administration of nitrous oxide during coronary artery surgery. Acta Anaesthesiol Scand 25:533, 1981

283. Reiz S: Nitrous oxide augments the systemic and coronary haemodynamic effects of isoflurane in patients with ischaemic heart disease. Acta Anaesthesiol Scand 27:464, 1983

284. Benumof JL: One-lung ventilation and hypoxic pulmonary vasoconstriction: Implications for anesthetic management. Anesth Analg 64:821, 1985

285. Pagel PS, Fu JL, Damask MC et al: Desflurane and isoflurane produce similar alterations in systemic and pulmonary hemodynamics and arterial oxygenation in patients undergoing one-lung ventilation during thoracotomy. Anesth Analg 87:800, 1998

286. Benumof JL, Augustine SD, Gibbons JA: Halothane and isoflurane only slightly impair arterial oxygenation during one-lung ventilation in patients undergoing thoracotomy. Anesthesiology 67:910, 1987

287. Frink EJ Jr, Ghantous H, Malan TP et al: Plasma inorganic fluoride with sevoflurane anesthesia: Correlation with indices of hepatic and renal function. Anesth Analg 74:231, 1992

288. Gelman S, Fowler KC, Smith LR: Liver circulation and function during isoflurane and halothane anesthesia. Anesthesiology 61:726, 1984

289. Benumof NL, Bookstein JJ, Saidman LJ et al: Diminished hepatic arterial flow during halothane administration. Anesthesiology 45:545, 1976

290. Hursh D, Gelman S, Bradley EL: Hepatic oxygen supply during halothane or isoflurane anesthesia in guinea pigs. Anesthesiology 67:701, 1987

291. Baden JM, Serra M, Fujinaga M et al: Halothane metabolism in cirrhotic rats. Anesthesiology 67:660, 1987

292. Elliott RH, Strunin L: Hepatotoxicity of volatile anaesthetics. Br J Anaesth 70:339, 1993

293. Weiskopf RB, Eger EI II, Ionescu P et al: Desflurane does not produce hepatic or renal injury in human volunteers. Anesth Analg 74:570, 1992

294. Eger EI II. Isoflurane (Forane): A compendium and reference. Madison, Ohio Medical Products, 1985

295. Van Dyke RA: Hepatic centrilobular necrosis in rats after exposure to halothane, enflurane or isoflurane. Anesth Analg 61:812, 1982

296. Allan LG, Howie J, Smith AF et al: Hepatic glutathione-S-transferase release after halothane anaesthesia: Open randomised comparison with isoflurane. Lancet 1:771, 1987

297. Hussey AJ, Aldridge LM, Paul D et al: Plasma glutathione-S-transferase concentration as a measure of hepatocellular integrity following a single general anaesthetic with halothane, enflurane or isoflurane. Br J Anaesth 60:130, 1988

298. Hornbein TF, Eger EI II, Winter PM et al: The minimum alveolar concentration of nitrous oxide in man. Anesth Analg 61:553, 1982

299. Allen GC, Brubaker CL: Human malignant hyperthermia associated with desflurane anesthesia. Anesth Analg 86:1328, 1998

300. Ducart A, Adnet P, Renaud B et al: Malignant hyperthermia during sevoflurane administration. Anesth Analg 80:609, 1995

301. Fu ES, Scharf JE, Mangar D et al: Malignant hyperthermia involving the administration of desflurane. Can J Anaesth 43:687, 1996

302. Reed SB, Strobel GE: An in vitro model of malignant hyperthermia: Differential effects of inhalation anesthetics on caffeine-induced muscle contractures. Anesthesiology 48:254, 1978

303. Baden J, Kelley M, Mazze R: Mutagenicity of experimental inhalational anesthetic agents: Sevoflurane, synthane, dioxychlorane, and dioxyflurane. Anesthesiology 56:462, 1982

304. Sachder K, Cohen EN, Simmou VF: Genotoxic and mutagenic assays of halothane metabolites in Bacillus subtilis and Salmonella typhimurium. Anesthesiology 53:31, 1980

305. Bussard DA, Stoelting RK, Peterson C et al: Fetal changes in hamsters anesthetized with nitrous oxide and halothane. Anesthesiology 41:275, 1974

306. Lane GA, Nahrwold ML, Tait AR: Anesthetics as teratogens: Nitrous oxide is fetotoxic, xenon is not. Science 210:899, 1980

307. Mazze RI, Fujinaga M, Rice SA et al: Reproductive and teratogenic effects of nitrous oxide, halothane, isoflurane, and enflurane in Sprague-Dawley rats. Anesthesiology 64:339, 1986

308. Mazze RI, Wilson AI, Rice SA et al: Effects of isoflurane on reproduction and fetal development in mice. Anesth Analg 63:249, 1984

309. Chalon J, Ramanathan S, Turndorf H: Exposure to isoflurane affects learning function of murine progeny. Anesthesiology 57:A360, 1982

310. Mazze RI: Fertility, reproduction, and postnatal survival in mice chronically exposed to isoflurane. Anesthesiology 63:663, 1985

311. Royston BD, Nunn JF, Weinbren HK et al: Rate of inactivation of human and rodent hepatic methionine synthase by nitrous oxide. Anesthesiology 68:213, 1988

312. Layzer RB, Fishman RA, Schafer JA: Neuropathy following use of nitrous oxide. Neurology 28:504, 1978

313. Hoerauf KH, Wallner T, Akça O et al: Exposure to sevoflurane and nitrous oxide during four different methods of anesthetic induction. Anesth Analg 88:925, 1999

314. Koblin DD: Nitrous oxide: A cause of cancer or chemotherapeutic adjuvant? Semin Surg Oncol 6:141, 1990

315. Munson ES, Embro WJ: Enflurane, isoflurane and halothane and isolated human uterine muscle. Anesthesiology 46:11, 1977

316. Palahniuk RJ, Shnider SM: Maternal and fetal cardiovascular and acid-base changes during halothane and isoflurane anesthesia in the pregnant ewe. Anesthesiology 41:462, 1974

317. Warren TM, Datta S, Ostheimer GW et al: Comparisons of the maternal and neonatal effects of halothane, enflurane and isoflurane for cesarean delivery. Anesth Analg 62:516, 1983

318. Abboud TK, Nagappala S, Murakawa K et al: Comparison of the effects of general and regional anesthesia for cesarean section on neonatal neurologic and adaptive capacity scores. Anesth Analg 64:996, 1985

319. Kharasch ED: Putting the brakes on anesthetic breakdown. Anesthesiology 91:1192, 1999

320. Baxter PJ, Garton K, Kharasch ED: Mechanistic aspects of carbon monoxide formation from volatile anesthetics. Anesthesiology 89:929, 1998

321. Frink EJ, Malan TP, Morgan SE et al: Quantification of the degradation products of sevoflurane in two CO_2 absorbents during low-flow anesthesia in surgical patients. Anesthesiology 77:1064, 1992

322. Raventos J, Lemon PG: The impurities in fluothane: Their biological significance. Br J Anaesth 37:716, 1965

323. Sharp JH, Trudell JR, Cohen EN: Volatile metabolites and decomposition products of halothane in man. Anesthesiology 50:2, 1979

324. Finkelstein MB, Baggs RB, Anders MW: Nephrotoxicity of the glutathione and cysteine conjugates of 2-bromo-2-chloro-1,1-difluoroethene. J Pharmacol Exp Ther 261:1248, 1992

325. Jin L, Baillie TA, Davis MR et al: Nephrotoxicity of sevoflurane compound A [fluoromethyl-2,2-difluoro-1-(trifluoromethyl)vinyl

ether] in rats: Evidence for glutathione and cysteine conjugate formation and the role of renal cysteine conjugate beta-lyase. Biochem Biophys Res Commun 210:498, 1995

326. Fang ZX, Eger EI II, Laster MJ *et al:* Carbon monoxide production from degradation of desflurane, enflurane, isoflurane, halothane, and sevoflurane by soda lime and baralyme. Anesth Analg 80:1187, 1995

327. Murray JM, Renfrew CW, Bedi A *et al:* Amsorb. A new carbon dioxide absorbent for use in anesthetic breathing systems. Anesthesiology 91:1342, 1999

328. Funk W, Gruber M, Wild K *et al:* Dry soda lime markedly degrades sevoflurane during simulated inhalation induction. Br J Anaesth 82:193, 1999

329. Fang ZX, Kandel L, Laster MJ *et al:* Factors affecting production of compound A from the interaction of sevoflurane with Baralyme and soda lime. Anesth Analg 82:775, 1996

330. Ruzicka JA, Hidalgo JC, Tinker JH *et al:* Inhibition of volatile sevoflurane degradation product formation in an anesthesia circuit by a reduction in soda lime temperature. Anesthesiology 81:238, 1994

331. Gonsowski CT, Laster MJ, Eger EI II *et al:* Toxicity of compound A in rats. Effect of increasing duration of administration. Anesthesiology 80:566, 1994

332. Gonsowski CT, Laster MJ, Eger EI II *et al:* Toxicity of compound A in rats. Effect of a 3-hour administration. Anesthesiology 80:556, 1994

333. Kharasch ED, Hoffman GM, Thorning D *et al:* Role of the renal cysteine conjugate β-lyase pathway in inhaled compound A nephrotoxicity in rats. Anesthesiology 88:1624, 1998

334. Kharasch ED, Thorning DT, Garton K *et al:* Role of renal cysteine conjugate β-lyase in the mechanism of compound A nephrotoxicity in rats. Anesthesiology 86:160, 1997

335. Steffey EP, Laster MJ, Ionescu P *et al:* Dehydration of Baralyme increases compound A resulting from sevoflurane degradation in a standard anesthetic circuit used to anesthetize swine. Anesth Analg 85:1382, 1997

336. Mazze RI, Friedman M, Delgado-Herrara L *et al:* Renal toxicity of compound A plus sevoflurane compared with isoflurane in nonhuman primates. Anesthesiology 89:A490, 1998

337. Bito H, Ikeda K: Closed-circuit anesthesia with sevoflurane in humans. Effects on renal and hepatic function and concentrations of breakdown products with soda lime in the circuit. Anesthesiology 80:71, 1994

338. Bito H, Ikeda K: Plasma inorganic fluoride and intracircuit degradation product concentrations in long-duration, low-flow sevoflurane anesthesia. Anesth Analg 79:946, 1994

339. Bito H, Ikeda K: Renal and hepatic function in surgical patients after low-flow sevoflurane or isoflurane anesthesia. Anesth Analg 82:173, 1996

340. Bito H, Ikeuchi Y, Ikeda K: Effects of low-flow sevoflurane anesthesia on renal function. Comparison with high-flow sevoflurane anesthesia and low-flow isoflurane anesthesia. Anesthesiology 86:1231, 1997

341. Kharasch ED, Frink EJ Jr, Zager R *et al:* Assessment of low-flow sevoflurane and isoflurane effects on renal function using sensitive markers of tubular toxicity. Anesthesiology 86:1238, 1997

342. Ebert TJ, Arain SR: Renal effects of low-flow anesthesia with desflurane and sevoflurane in patients. Anesthesiology 91:A404, 1999

343. Eger EI II, Gong D, Koblin DD *et al:* Dose-related biochemical markers of renal injury after sevoflurane versus desflurane anesthesia in volunteers. Anesth Analg 85:1154, 1997

344. Ebert TJ, Frink EJ, Kharasch ED: Absence of biochemical evidence for renal and hepatic dysfunction after 8 hours of 1.25 minimum alveolar concentration sevoflurane anesthesia in volunteers. Anesthesiology 88:601, 1998

345. Eger EI II, Koblin DD, Bowland T *et al:* Nephrotoxicity of sevoflurane versus desflurane anesthesia in volunteers. Anesth Analg 84:160, 1997

346. Ebert TJ, Messana LD, Uhrich TD *et al:* Absence of renal and hepatic toxicity after four hours of 1.25 MAC sevoflurane anesthesia in volunteers. Anesth Analg 86:662, 1998

347. Ali A, Panagopoulos G, Salimi, B *et al:* Micro-albuminuria following epidural anesthesia. Unpublished, 1997

348. Mazze RI, Jamison RL: Low-flow (1 l/min) sevoflurane: Is it safe? Anesthesiology 86:1225, 1997

349. Kharasch ED, Karol MD, Lanni C *et al:* Clinical sevoflurane metabo-

lism and disposition. I. Sevoflurane and metabolite pharmacokinetics. Anesthesiology 82:1369, 1995

350. Spracklin D, Kharasch ED: Evidence for the metabolism of fluoromethyl-1,1-difluoro-1-(trifluoromethyl)vinyl ether (compound A), a sevoflurane degradation product, by cysteine conjugate β-lyase. Chem Res Toxicol 9:696, 1996

351. Iyer RA, Anders MW: Cysteine conjugate β-lyase-dependent biotransformation of the cysteine S-conjugates of the sevoflurane degradation product compound A in human, nonhuman, nonhuman primate, and rat kidney cytosol and mitochondria. Anesthesiology 85:1454, 1996

352. Kharasch ED, Jubert C: Compound A uptake and metabolism to mercapturic acids and 3,3,3-trifluoro-2-fluoromethoxypropanoic acid during low-flow sevoflurane anesthesia. Anesthesiology 91:1267, 1999

353. Fang ZX, Eger EI II: Source of toxic CO explained: −CHF₂ anesthetic + dry absorbent. UCSF research shows CO comes from CO₂ absorbent. APSF Newsletter 9:25, 1994

354. Woehlck HJ, Dunning M, Connolly LA: Reduction in the incidence of carbon monoxide exposures in humans undergoing general anesthesia. Anesthesiology 87:228, 1997

355. Woehlck HJ, Dunning MI, Gandhi S *et al:* Indirect detection of intraoperative carbon monoxide exposure by mass spectrometry during isoflurane anesthesia. Anesthesiology 83:213, 1995

356. Lentz RE: CO poisoning during anesthesia poses puzzle. APSF Newsletter 9:13, 1994

357. Woehlck HJ: Severe intraoperative CO poisoning. Anesthesiology 90:353, 1999

358. Berry PD, Sessler DI, Larson MD: Severe carbon monoxide poisoning during desflurane anesthesia. Anesthesiology 90:613, 1999

359. Mazze RI, Shue GL, Jackson SH: Renal dysfunction associated with methoxyflurane anaesthesia: A randomized, prospective clinical evaluation. JAMA 216:278, 1971

360. Cousins MJ, Mazze RI: Methoxyflurane nephrotoxicity: A study of dose–response in man. JAMA 225:1611, 1973

361. Mazze RI, Calverley RK, Smith NT: Inorganic fluoride nephrotoxicity: Prolonged enflurane and halothane anesthesia in volunteers. Anesthesiology 46:265, 1977

362. Frink EJ Jr, Malan TP Jr, Isner RJ *et al:* Renal concentrating function with prolonged sevoflurane or enflurane anesthesia in volunteers. Anesthesiology 80:1019, 1994

363. Mazze RI, Trudell JR, Cousins MJ: Methoxyflurane metabolism and renal dysfunction: Clinical correlation in man. Anesthesiology 35:247, 1971

364. Mazze RI: The safety of sevoflurane in humans. Anesthesiology 77:1062, 1992

365. Kharasch ED, Hankins DC, Thummel KE: Human kidney methoxyflurane and sevoflurane metabolism. Intrarenal fluoride production as a possible mechanism of methoxyflurane nephrotoxicity. Anesthesiology 82:689, 1995

366. Malan TP Jr, Kadota Y, Mata H *et al:* Renal function after sevoflurane or enflurane anesthesia in the Fischer 344 rat. Anesth Analg 77:817, 1993

367. Miller MS, Gandolfi AJ, Vaughan RW *et al:* Disposition of enflurane in obese patients. J Pharmacol Exp Ther 215:292, 1980

368. Strube PJ, Hulands GH, Halsey MJ: Serum fluoride levels in morbidly obese patients: Enflurane compared with isoflurane anaesthesia. Anaesthesia 42:685, 1987

369. Young SR, Stoelting RK, Peterson C *et al:* Anesthetic biotransformation and renal function in obese patients during and after methoxyflurane or halothane anesthesia. Anesthesiology 42:451, 1975

370. Higuchi H, Sumikura H, Sumita S *et al:* Renal function in patients with high serum fluoride concentrations after prolonged sevoflurane anesthesia. Anesthesiology 83:449, 1995

371. Frink EJ Jr, Malan TP Jr, Brown EA *et al:* Plasma inorganic fluoride levels with sevoflurane anesthesia in morbidly obese and nonobese patients. Anesth Analg 76:1333, 1993

372. Rehder K, Forbes J, Alter H *et al:* Halothane biotransformation in man: A quantitative study. Anesthesiology 28:711, 1967

373. Brown BR Jr, Gandolfi AJ: Adverse effects of volatile anaesthetics. Br J Anaesth 59:14, 1987

374. National Halothane Study: A study of the possible association between halothane anaesthesia and post operative hepatic necrosis. Washington D.C., US Government Printing Office 1969

375. Kenna G, Satoh H, Christ DD *et al:* Metabolic basis for drug hypersensitivity; antibodies in sera from patients with halothane

hepatitis is recognise liver neo-antigens that contain the tri-fluoro-acetyl group derived from halothane. J Pharmacol Exp Ther 245:1103, 1988

376. Kenna JG, Martin JL, Satoh H *et al:* Factors affecting the expression of trifluoroacetylated liver microsomal protein neoantigens in rats treated with halothane. Drug Metabolism and Disposition 18:188, 1990

377. Kenna JG, Neuberger J, Williams R: Specific antibodies to halothane induced liver antigens in halothane associated hepatitis. Br J Anaesth 59:1286, 1987

378. Martin JL, Kenna JG, Pohl LR: Antibody assays for the detection of patients sensitised to halothane. Anesth Analg 2:154, 1990

379. Martin JL, Plevak DJ, Flannery KD *et al:* Hepatotoxicity after desflurane anesthesia. Anesthesiology 83:1125, 1995

380. Carrigan TW, Staughen WJ: A report of hepatic necrosis and death following isoflurane anesthesia. Anesthesiology 67:581, 1987

381. Lewis JH, Zimmerman HJ, Ishak KG *et al:* Enflurane hepatotoxicity. A clinicopathologic study of 24 cases. Ann Intern Med 98:984, 1983

382. Stoelting RK, Blitt CD, Cohen PF *et al:* Hepatic dysfunction after isoflurane anesthesia. Anesth Analg 66:147, 1987

383. Eger EI II, Smuckler EA, Ferrel LD *et al:* Is enflurane hepatotoxic? Anesth Analg 65:21, 1986

384. Ray DC, Drummond GB: Halothane hepatitis. Br J Anaesth 67:84, 1991

385. Martin JL, Dubbink DA, Plevak DJ *et al:* Halothane hepatitis 28 years after primary exposure. Anesth Analg 74:605, 1992

386. Sigurdsen J, Hreidarsson AB, Thiodleifsson B: Enflurane hepatitis. A report of a case with a previous history of halothane hepatitis. Acta Anaesthesiol Scand 29:495, 1985

387. Doi M, Ikeda K: Airway irritation produced by volatile anaesthetics during brief inhalation: Comparison of halothane, enflurane, isoflurane and sevoflurane. Can J Anaesth 40:122, 1993

388. Ruffle JM, Snider MT, Rosenberger JL *et al:* Rapid induction of halothane anaesthesia in man. Br J Anaesth 57:607, 1985

389. Ruffle JM, Snider MT: Comparison of rapid and conventional inhalation inductions of halothane oxygen anesthesia in healthy men and women. Anesthesiology 67:584, 1987

390. Tanaka S, Tsuchida H, Nakabayashi K *et al:* The effects of sevoflurane, isoflurane, halothane, and enflurane on hemodynamic responses during an inhaled induction of anesthesia via a mask in humans. Anesth Analg 82:821, 1996

391. Muzi M, Robinson BJ, Ebert TJ *et al:* Induction of anesthesia and tracheal intubation with sevoflurane in adults. Anesthesiology 85:536, 1996

392. Muzi M, Colinco MD, Robinson BJ *et al:* The effects of premedication on inhaled induction of anesthesia with sevoflurane. Anesth Analg 85:1143, 1997

393. Thwaites A, Edmends S, Smith I: Inhalation induction with sevoflurane: A double-blind comparison with propofol. Br J Anaesth 78:356, 1997

394. Mostafa SM, Atherton AMJ: Sevoflurane for difficult tracheal intubation. Br J Anaesth 79:392, 1997

395. Dion P: The cost of anesthetic vapors. Can J Anaesth 39:633, 1992

396. Ebert TJ, Robinson BJ, Uhrich TD *et al:* Recovery from sevoflurane anesthesia. Anesthesiology 89:1524, 1998

397. Eger EI II, Severinghaus JW: Effect of uneven pulmonary distribution of blood and gas on induction with inhalation anesthetics. Anesthesiology 25:620, 1964

398. Navarro R, Weiskopf RB, Moore MA *et al:* Humans anesthetized with sevoflurane or isoflurane have similar arrhythmic response to epinephrine. Anesthesiology 80:545, 1994

399. Moore MA, Weiskopf RB, Eger EI II *et al:* Arrhythmogenic doses of epinephrine are similar during desflurane or isoflurane anesthesia in humans. Anesthesiology 79:943, 1993

400. Doi M, Ikeda K: Respiratory effects of sevoflurane. Anesth Analg 66:241, 1987

401. Eger EI II: Desflurane. Anesth Rev 20:87, 1993

402. Eger EI II, Calverley RK, Smith NT: Changes in blood chemistries following prolonged enflurane anesthesia. Anesth Analg 55:547, 1976

403. Stevens WC, Eger EI II, Joas TA *et al:* Comparative toxicity of isoflurane, halothane, fluroxene and diethyl ether in human volunteers. Can J Anaesth 20:357, 1973

404. Bito H, Ikeda K: Effect of total flow rate on the concentration of degradation products generated by reaction between sevoflurane and soda lime. Br J Anaesth 74:667, 1995

405. Kharasch ED, Armstrong AS, Gunn K *et al:* Clinical sevoflurane metabolism and disposition. II. The role of cytochrome P450 2E1 in fluoride and hexafluoroisopropanol formation. Anesthesiology 82:1379, 1995

406. Mazze RI: Metabolism of the inhaled anaesthetics: Implications of enzyme induction. Br J Anaesth 56(suppl):27S, 1984

407. Sutton TS, Koblin DD, Gruenke LD *et al:* Fluoride metabolites after prolonged exposure of volunteers and patients to desflurane. Anesth Analg 73:180, 1991

408. Njoku D, Laster MJ, Gong DH *et al:* Biotransformation of halothane, enflurane, isoflurane, and desflurane to trifluoroacetylated liver proteins: Association between protein acylation and hepatic injury. Anesth Analg 84:173, 1997

409. Eger EI II: Uptake of inhaled anesthetics: The alveolar to inspired anesthetic difference. In Anesthetic Uptake and Action, p 77. Baltimore, Williams & Wilkins, 1974

410. Yamamura H, Wakasugi B, Okuma Y *et al:* The effects of ventilation on the absorption and elimination of inhalation anaesthetics. Anaesthesia 18:427, 1963

411. Yamamura, H: The effect of ventilation and blood volume on the uptake and elimination of inhalation anesthetic agents. Progress in Anaesthesiology. Proceedings of the Fourth World Congress of Anesthesiologists. International Congress Series 200, 394–399. 68, Excerpta Medica.

Clinical Anesthesia (4/e), edited by
Paul G. Barash, Bruce F. Cullen, and
Robert K. Stoelting. Lippincott Williams &
Wilkins, Philadelphia, © 2001.

CHAPTER 16

MUSCLE RELAXANTS

DAVID R. BEVAN AND FRANÇOIS DONATI

PHYSIOLOGY AND PHARMACOLOGY

Structure

The cell bodies of motor neurons supplying skeletal muscle lie in the spinal cord. They receive and integrate information from the central nervous system. This information is carried *via* an elongated structure, the axon, to distant parts of the body. Each nerve cell supplies many muscle cells (or fibers) a short distance after branching into nerve terminals. The terminal portion of the axon is a specialized structure, the synapse, designed for the production and release of acetylcholine (ACh). The synapse is separated from the endplate of the muscle fiber by a narrow gap, called the synaptic cleft, which is approximately 50 nm in width (0.05 μm).[1] The nerve terminal is surrounded by a Schwann cell, and the synaptic cleft has a basement membrane and contains filaments that anchor the nerve terminal to the muscle.

The endplate is a specialized portion of the membrane of the muscle fiber where nicotinic ACh receptors are concentrated. During development, multiple connections are made between nerve terminals and a single muscle fiber. The presence of these connections promotes clustering of receptors. As maturation continues, most of these connections atrophy and disappear, usually leaving only one connection per muscle fiber. This endplate continues to differentiate from the rest of the muscle fiber. As the nerve terminal enlarges and folds appear, the density of ACh receptors increases at the endplate and decreases to almost zero in extrajunctional areas.[2] Mammalian endplates usually have an oval shape with the short axis perpendicular to the fiber. The width of the endplate is sometimes as large as the diameter of the fiber, but is usually smaller. However, its length is only a small fraction of that of the fiber.[3]

Nerve Stimulation

Under resting conditions, the electrical potential of the inside of a nerve cell is negative with respect to the outside (typically −90 mV). If this potential is made less negative (depolarization), sodium channels open and allow sodium to enter the cell. This influx of positive ions makes the potential inside the membrane positive with respect to the outside. This potential change in turn causes depolarization of the next segment of membrane, causing more sodium channels to open, and an electrical impulse, or action potential, propagates. The duration of the action potential is brief (<1 msec), because inactivation of sodium channels occurs within a short period of time and because potassium channels, which produce outward movement of potassium ions, open and make the inside potential more negative. An action potential also triggers the opening of calcium channels, allowing calcium to penetrate the cell, and this entry of calcium has special importance at the nerve terminal.

Sodium channels are made up of three protein subunits. The ion channel *per se* is surrounded by the α subunit, a funnel-shaped protein that crosses the membrane completely. The wider end of the protein lies inside the membrane. The two smaller subunits (β_1 and β_2) lie on opposite sides of the α subunit. They do not cross the membrane entirely and face outward.[4] When a nerve stimulator is used, an action potential may be generated if enough current is applied to depolarize the axon above a certain threshold. The magnitude of the depolarization depends both on the current applied and the duration of the stimulus.

A peripheral nerve is made up of a large number of axons of different thresholds, different sizes, and different distances from the stimulating electrode. Although each axon responds in an all-or-none fashion to the stimulus applied, not all axons may respond to a given stimulus. Thus, in the absence of neuromuscular blockers, the relationship between the amplitude of the muscle contraction and current applied is sigmoid.[5] At low currents, the depolarization is insufficient in all axons. As current increases, more and more axons are depolarized to threshold and the strength of the muscle contraction increases. When the stimulating current reaches a certain level, all axons are depolarized to threshold and propagate an action potential. Increasing current beyond this point does not increase the amplitude of muscle contraction: the stimulation is supramaximal (Fig. 16-1).

After firing once, a nerve axon cannot respond to further stimulation for a short time (usually 0.5−1 msec) known as the refractory period. If the duration of stimulation is longer than the refractory period, repetitive stimulation of the axon may result.[1] For this reason, the current pulse applied must be brief, <0.5 msec. Most commercially available stimulators deliver impulses lasting 0.1−0.2 msec.

Release of Acetylcholine

Acetylcholine is synthesized from choline and acetate. It is then packaged into 45-nm vesicles, which tend to concentrate in the area of the nerve terminal closest to the endplate. Some of these vesicles cluster near the cell membrane opposite the crests of the junctional folds of the endplate, in areas called active zones (Fig. 16-2).[6] Each vesicle contains about 5000−10,000 ACh molecules.

Although there have been doubts regarding the vesicular hypothesis, it is now widely accepted that ACh is released in packets, or quanta, and that a quantum represents the contents of one vesicle, which amounts to 5000−10,000 molecules.[7] In the absence of nerve stimulation, quanta are released spontaneously, at random, and this is seen as small depolarizations of the endplate (miniature endplate potential; MEPP). When an action potential invades the nerve terminal, ~200−400 quanta are released simultaneously, unloading ~1−4 million ACh molecules into the synaptic cleft.[1,7] Calcium, which enters the nerve terminal through channels that open in response to depolarization, is required for vesicle fusion and release. Calcium channels are located near docking proteins, and this special geometric arrangement provides high intracellular concentrations of calcium to allow binding of specialized proteins on the ACh vesicular membrane with docking proteins. Binding produces fusion of the membranes and release of ACh ensues.[8] After release, vesicles are most likely recycled, and there is evidence that these newly re-formed vesicles are released preferentially.[7] When the calcium concentration is decreased, or if the action of calcium is antagonized by magnesium, the release process is inhibited and transmission failure may occur. Other proteins regulate storage and mobilization of ACh vesicles. Recent research on the identification of the numerous proteins regulating movement of vesicles at the nerve terminal and the study of their function has corroborated the concepts of a small, immediately releasable pool and a much larger reserve pool. Each impulse

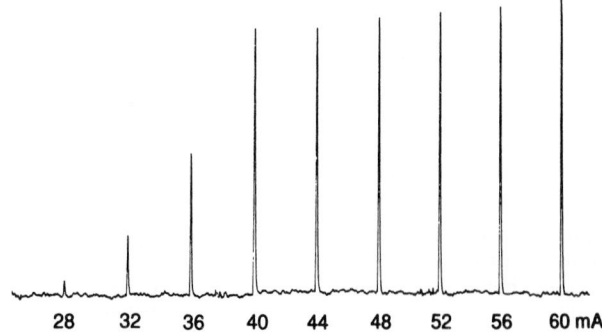

Figure 16-1. Example of increasing stimulating current in one patient. Current pulses, 0.2-msec duration, were delivered to the ulnar nerve at the wrist every 10 sec. The force of contraction of the adductor pollicis was measured and appears as spikes. No twitch was seen if the current was <28 mA. At current strengths of ≥40 mA, the current became supramaximal; increasing the current produced little change in force.

releases 0.2–0.5% of the 75,000–100,000 vesicles in the nerve terminal.[7] With repetitive stimulation, the amount of ACh released decreases rapidly because only a small fraction of the vesicles is in a position to be released immediately. To sustain release during high-frequency stimulation, vesicles must be released from the reserve pool, and this process requires calcium.[7]

Postsynaptic Events

The 1–10 million receptors located at the endplate are made up of five glycoprotein subunits arranged in the form of a rosette and lying across the whole cell membrane (Fig. 16-3). Two of these noncontiguous subunits, designated α, are similar and each must bind simultaneously to an ACh molecule to induce a conformational change in the receptor structure such that an opening is made in the center of the rosette, allowing small ions to pass through the channel.[1,9] Sodium ions move inside along their concentration and electrical gradients, making the inside less negative, thus depolarizing the cell membrane. There is a high density of sodium channels in the folds of synaptic clefts and in the perijunctional area.[10] These channels open when the membrane is depolarized beyond a critical point, allowing more sodium to enter the cell, and producing further

depolarization. The high density of sodium channels in the junctional and perijunctional areas contributes to the generation of an action potential, which propagates by activation of sodium channels along the whole length of the muscle fiber.

There are two categories of nicotinic ACh receptors. The type normally present at the endplate has an ε subunit. Fetal receptors and those present on the muscle outside the endplate, also called extrajunctional receptors, have a γ subunit instead of an ε subunit. Both types of receptor differ by their sensitivity to agonist and antagonist drugs. However, in both types, each subunit has four transmembrane domains; that is, each is a string of amino acids that crosses the membrane four times. The binding site for acetylcholine is before the first membrane domain of the α subunit on the outside of the membrane.[9,11]

Depolarization above threshold in a muscle fiber is followed by two distinct but related phenomena: an electrical event, the action potential; and a mechanical event, muscle contraction. The activity of a whole muscle is the sum of the responses of the individual fibers and can be measured either in terms of its electrical activity (by electromyography, EMG) or its contractile force (by mechanomyography, MMG). The EMG response of the muscles of the hand is 5–10 msec in duration, but the MMG lasts ~150 msec (Fig 16-4). Thus, for frequencies up to 100 Hz, the EMG response can be distinguished for each stimulus. However, summation of individual twitch responses occurs for frequencies >7–10 Hz, and a tetanic response, greater in intensity than a muscle twitch, can be observed.

The main action of nondepolarizing neuromuscular blocking drugs is to block the postsynaptic ACh receptor by binding to at least one of the two α subunits, thus preventing access by ACh. Under normal circumstances, only a small fraction of available receptors must bind to ACh to produce sufficient depolarization to trigger a muscle contraction. In other words, there is a wide "margin of safety." This implies that neuromuscular blocking drugs must be bound to a large number of receptors before any blockade is detectable. Animal studies suggest that 75% of receptors must be occupied before twitch height decreases in the presence of *d*-tubocurarine, and blockade is complete when 92% of receptors are occupied.[12] The actual number depends on species and type of muscle, and humans might have a reduced margin of safety.[13] However, the general concept is applicable to clinical practice; that is, detectable blockade occurs over a narrow range of receptor occupancy.

ACh is hydrolyzed rapidly by the enzyme acetylcholinesterase, which is present in the folds of the endplate as well as embedded

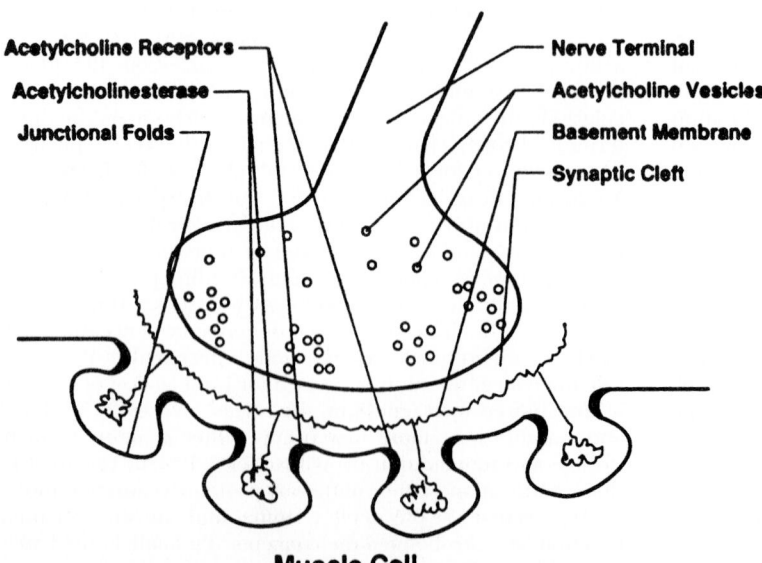

Muscle Cell

Figure 16-2. Diagram of neuromuscular junction.

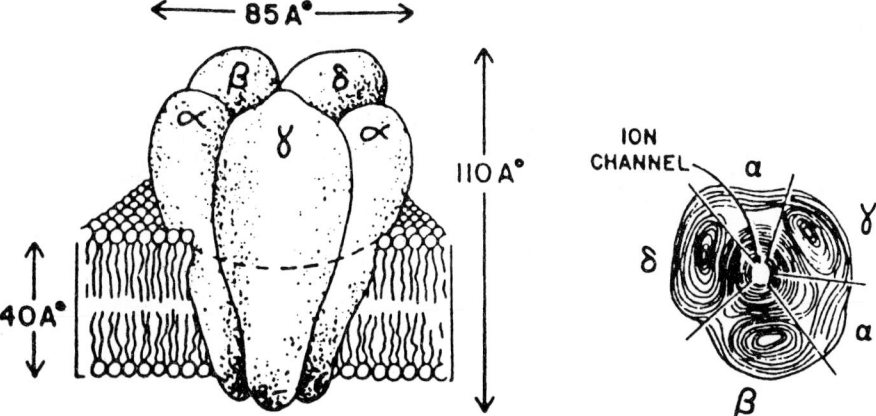

Figure 16-3. The nicotinic acetylcholine receptor consists of five glycoprotein subunits arranged to form an ion channel. The α subunits carry a recognition site for agonists and antagonists. (Reprinted with permission from Taylor P: Are neuromuscular blocking agents more efficacious in pairs? Anesthesiology 63:1, 1985.)

in the basement membrane of the synaptic cleft. The presence of the enzyme in the synaptic cleft suggests that not all the ACh released reaches the endplate; some is hydrolyzed en route.[7]

Presynaptic Events

The release of ACh normally decreases during high-frequency stimulation because the pool of readily releasable ACh becomes depleted faster than it can be replenished. However, the reduced amount released is well above what is required to produce muscle contraction because of the high margin of safety at the neuromuscular junction. However, during partial nondepolarizing blockade this decrease in transmitter output produces fade—a progressive decrease in muscle response with each stimulus. Nondepolarizing neuromuscular blocking drugs probably accentuate the fade by blocking presynaptic nicotinic receptors, which differ structurally from postsynaptic receptors.[14] The function of the presynaptic receptors is to sustain ACh mobilization in the face of continuing stimulation. One possible mechanism of action could be to break the link between a vesicular protein and a cytoplasmic filament, which prevents mobilization of the vesicle.[15] The affinity of agonists and antagonists is not the same for presynaptic receptors. Only small doses of nondepolarizing relaxants are needed to block presynaptic receptors.[16] Whatever the exact mechanism of fade, it remains a key property of nondepolarizing neuromuscular blocking drugs and is useful for monitoring purposes.

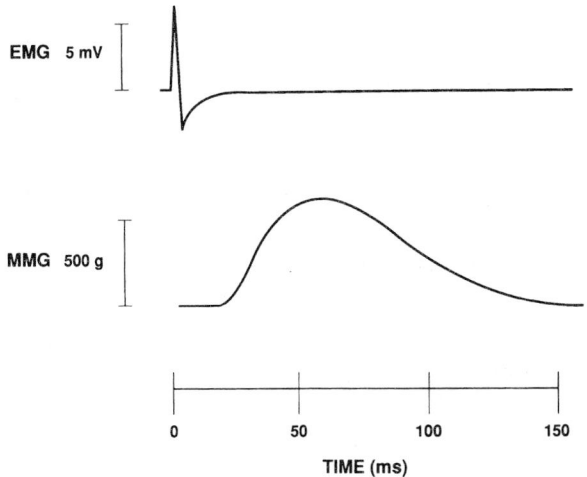

Figure 16-4. Typical electromyographic (EMG) and mechanomyographic (MMG) tracings of the adductor pollicis after single stimulation of the ulnar nerve. Note the longer duration and latency of the MMG response.

NEUROMUSCULAR PHARMACOLOGY

Neuromuscular blocking drugs interact with the ACh receptor either by depolarizing the endplate or by competing with ACh for binding sites. The former mechanism is characteristic of depolarizing drugs and the latter of nondepolarizing agents. The only depolarizing agent still in use is succinylcholine. All others are of the nondepolarizing type.

The effect of all neuromuscular blocking drugs is measured as the depression of adductor muscle contraction (twitch) following electrical stimulation of the ulnar nerve. Potency of each drug is determined by constructing dose–response curves, which describe the relationship between twitch depression and dose. Then, the effective dose 95, or ED_{95}, which is the median dose corresponding to 95% twitch depression, is obtained. In addition to potency data, it is necessary to describe the time course of blockade by specifying onset (time to maximum blockade) and duration of action (time from injection to 25% recovery of twitch height). Both onset and duration depend on dose, so $2 \times ED_{95}$ has been retained for comparison purposes. Recently, categories were proposed for neuromuscular blocking drugs, which may be defined according to their onset and duration of action at the adductor pollicis to $2 \times ED_{95}$ doses (Table 16-1).[17] Muscles other than the adductor pollicis may have very different onset, ED_{95}, and duration of action.

Depolarizing Blocking Drugs: Succinylcholine

Among drugs that depolarize the endplate, only succinylcholine and decamethonium were introduced into clinical practice in North America. Decamethonium, a drug with a slow onset and intermediate duration, has been replaced by nondepolarizing alternatives. However, succinylcholine still enjoys some popularity, despite a long list of undesired effects, because it is the only ultra-rapid onset, ultra-short duration neuromuscular blocking drug (NMBD) available. Although successful tracheal intubation can be achieved by a combination of propofol and remifentanil[18] or alfentanil,[19] intubation conditions are improved by the addition of NMBDs.

Neuromuscular Effects

The effects of succinylcholine at the neuromuscular junction are not completely understood. The drug binds to presynaptic, postsynaptic, and extrajunctional receptors. When it first reaches any of these receptors, succinylcholine exhibits ACh-like activity; that is, depolarization is produced.[20] However, when the receptor is in contact with any agonist, including ACh, for a prolonged time, it ceases to respond to the agonist. Normally, the rapid breakdown of ACh (<1 msec) does not allow this desensitization process to take place. However, succinylcholine remains at the endplate for much longer, and desensitization

Table 16-1. DEFINITION OF NEUROMUSCULAR BLOCKING DRUGS ACCORDING TO ONSET AND DURATION OF BLOCK AT ADDUCTOR POLLICIS

Onset to Maximum Block (min)			
Ultra-rapid (<1)	*Rapid (1–2)*	*Intermediate (2–4)*	*Long (>4)*
Succinylcholine	Rapacuronium Rocuronium	Atracurium Mivacurium Vecuronium d-Tubocurarine Gallamine Metocurine Pancuronium Pipecuronium	Cisatracurium Doxacurium

Duration to 25% Recovery T$_1$ (min)			
Ultra-short (<8)	*Short (8–20)*	*Intermediate (20–50)*	*Long (>50)*
Succinylcholine	Mivacurium Rapacuronium	Atracurium Cisatracurium Rocuronium Vercuronium	Doxacurium d-Tubocurarine Gallamine Metocurine Pancuronium Pipecuronium

The definition of categories according to: Bedford RE: From the FDA. Anesthesiology 82:33A, 1995. Drugs are listed that best fit the categories under optimal circumstances. It must be noted that onset and duration depend on patient, dose, and method of measurement. Also, appreciable differences may exist within categories. For example, onset of rapacuronium and rocuronium are in the 1–2-min category, but rapacuronium is close to 1 min and rocuronium is close to 2 min.

can develop. Another possible mechanism is the inactivation of sodium channels in the junctional and perijunctional area, which occurs when the membrane remains depolarized. This inactivation prevents the propagation of the action potential. These two possible mechanisms are probably not mutually exclusive.

Succinylcholine-induced fasciculations are probably due to depolarization of the nerve terminal produced by activation of presynaptic receptors. This is observed clinically as disorganized muscular activity following the injection of succinylcholine. The effectiveness of small doses of nondepolarizing drugs in reducing the incidence of fasciculations suggests that the presynaptic receptors are relatively sensitive to these drugs.[21]

Succinylcholine has yet another neuromuscular effect. In some muscles, like the masseter and to a lesser extent the adductor pollicis, a sustained increase in tension that may last for several minutes can be observed.[22,23] The mechanism of action of this tension change is uncertain but is most likely mediated by ACh receptors because it is blocked by large amounts of nondepolarizing drugs.[24] The increase in masseteric tone, which is probably always present to some degree, may lead to imperfect intubating conditions and is the probable reason for the poor conditions seen in 5% of pediatric patients as described by Hanallah and Kaplan.[25] More subtle measurements of the force on the laryngoscope blade necessary to achieve the best view of the vocal cords suggest that experienced anesthetists use more force after succinylcholine than after vecuronium.[26] Masseter spasm, which has been associated with malignant hyperthermia (MH), may be an exaggerated form of this response.

Characteristics of Depolarizing Blockade

After injection of succinylcholine, single-twitch height is decreased. However, the response to high-frequency stimulation is sustained: train-of-four fade and tetanic fade are not observed. The block is antagonized by nondepolarizing agents so that the intubating dose of succinylcholine must be increased from 1.0 to 1.5 or 2 mg · kg⁻¹ after precurarization with a nondepolarizing

NMB. Isobolographic analysis has shown that mixture of succinylcholine with either mivacurium or atracurium is antagonistic.[27] Succinylcholine is potentiated by inhibitors of acetylcholinesterase, such as neostigmine and edrophonium.[28]

Phase II Block

After prolonged exposure to succinylcholine, the characteristics of the block change, and features of nondepolarizing blockade appear. Train-of-four and tetanic fade become apparent after the administration of 7–10 mg · kg⁻¹, which corresponds to 30–60 min of paralysis. Neostigmine or edrophonium can antagonize this block, which has been termed "nondepolarizing," "dual," or "Phase II block." The last term is preferable because it does not imply any specific mechanism of action. The onset of Phase II block coincides with tachyphylaxis, as more succinylcholine is required for the same effect.[29]

Pharmacology of Succinylcholine

Succinylcholine is rapidly hydrolyzed by plasma cholinesterase to choline and succinylmonocholine,[30] with an elimination half-life of <1 min in patients. Because of the rapid disappearance of succinylcholine from plasma, the maximum effect is reached quickly. Subparalyzing doses (up to 0.3–0.5 mg · kg⁻¹) reach their maximal effect within ~1.5–2 min at the adductor pollicis,[31] and within 1 min at more central muscles, such as the masseter and the larynx (Fig. 16-5).[32] With larger doses (1–2 mg · kg⁻¹), abolition of twitch response can be reached even more rapidly.

The mean dose producing 50% blockade (ED$_{50}$) at the adductor pollicis is 0.15–0.2 mg · kg⁻¹ with opioid–nitrous oxide anesthesia,[33] and the ED$_{95}$ is in the range of 0.30–0.35 mg · kg⁻¹. In the absence of nitrous oxide, the ED$_{50}$ and ED$_{95}$ are increased to 0.3 and 0.5 mg · kg⁻¹, respectively.[31] These values are doubled if d-tubocurarine, 0.05 mg · kg⁻¹, is given as a defasciculating agent.[31] The time until full recovery of MMG is 10–12 min after a dose of 1 mg · kg⁻¹ (Fig. 16-6).[34]

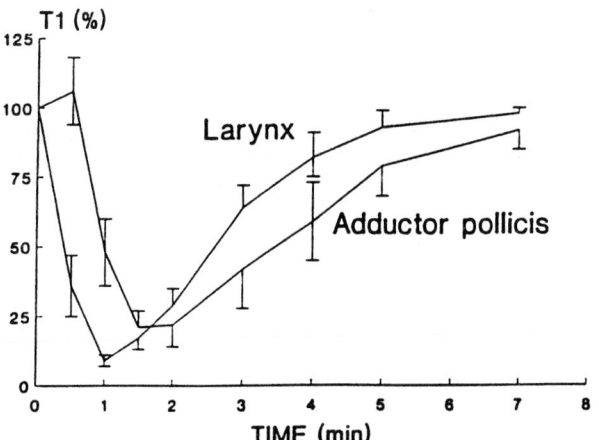

Figure 16-5. Onset and intensity of succinylcholine neuromuscular block at the adductor pollicis and laryngeal adductor muscles. (Reproduced with permission from Meistelman C, Plaud B, Donati, F: Neuromuscular effects of succinylcholine on the vocal cords and adductor pollicis muscles. Anesth Analg 73:278, 1991.)

Side Effects

Cardiovascular. Because of its structural similarity to ACh, succinylcholine is expected to have some parasympathetic activity. Sinus bradycardia with nodal or ventricular escape beats (or both) may occur, especially in children, and asystole has been described after a second dose of succinylcholine in adults. However, parasympathetic effects are infrequent and can be attenuated with atropine or glycopyrrolate.[35] Succinylcholine increases catecholamine release, and this effect may explain, in part, the low incidence of bradycardia. The exact nature of the interaction of succinylcholine with muscarinic receptors is, however, poorly understood, and the mechanism for the enhanced bradycardic effect of a second dose is not known.

Anaphylaxis. Succinylcholine has been incriminated as the trigger of allergic reactions more often than any other intravenous (iv) drug used in anesthesia. However, the prevalence is uncertain and the number of reported cases is low, given the widespread use of the drug. Anaphylactic reactions to succinylcholine and rocuronium have been described in two members of the same family with intradermal testing, as has sensitivity to pancuronium, atracurium, and mivacurium.[36] However, the sensitivity and specificity of skin testing are not known.

Fasciculations. The prevalence of fasciculations is high after the rapid injection of succinylcholine, especially in muscular adults. Although this is a benign side effect of the drug, most clinicians prefer to prevent fasciculations. In this respect, a small dose of a nondepolarizing neuromuscular blocking drug given 3–5 min before succinylcholine is effective. *d*-Tubocurarine 0.05 mg · kg^{-1}, gallamine 0.2 mg · kg^{-1}, atracurium 0.03 mg · kg^{-1}, or rocuronium 0.06 mg · kg^{-1} may be given for this purpose, of which *d*-tubocurarine and rocuronium are the most effective[37,38] if an interval of 3–5 min is allowed before administration of succinylcholine.[39] Pancuronium, 0.01 mg · kg^{-1}, and vecuronium, 0.007 mg · kg^{-1}, are probably less effective as defasciculants. After these nondepolarizing drugs, the dose of succinylcholine must be increased from 1 mg · kg^{-1} to 1.5–2 mg · kg^{-1} because of the antagonism between depolarizing and nondepolarizing drugs.[31] Care must be taken not to exceed these doses of nondepolarizing agents to avoid partial neuromuscular blockade in awake patients. The most common symptoms are blurred vision, heavy eyelids, and, occasionally, difficulty in swallowing or breathing. Other drugs, such as diazepam, lidocaine, fentanyl, calcium, vitamin C, magnesium, and dantrolene have all been used to prevent fasciculations. The results are no better than with nondepolarizing relaxants, and they may have undesirable effects of their own. "Self-taming," the administration of small (10-mg) doses of succinylcholine 1 min before the intubating dose, is an effective tactic but has largely been abandoned owing to the considerable blockade that may be produced by the "taming" dose.[1]

Muscle Pains. Generalized aches and pains, similar to the myalgias that follow violent exercise, are common 24–48 hr after succinylcholine administration. The relationship between muscle pains and fasciculations is not firmly established. Although many studies have failed to confirm that precurarization with a nondepolarizing neuromuscular blocking drug is of any value in the prevention of myalgias, the available evidence suggests that there is a protective effect.[40]

Intragastric Pressure. Succinylcholine increases intragastric pressure, and this effect is blocked by precurarization. However, succinylcholine causes even greater increases in lower esophageal sphincter pressure.[41] Thus, succinylcholine does not appear to increase the risk of aspiration of gastric contents unless the esophageal sphincter is incompetent.

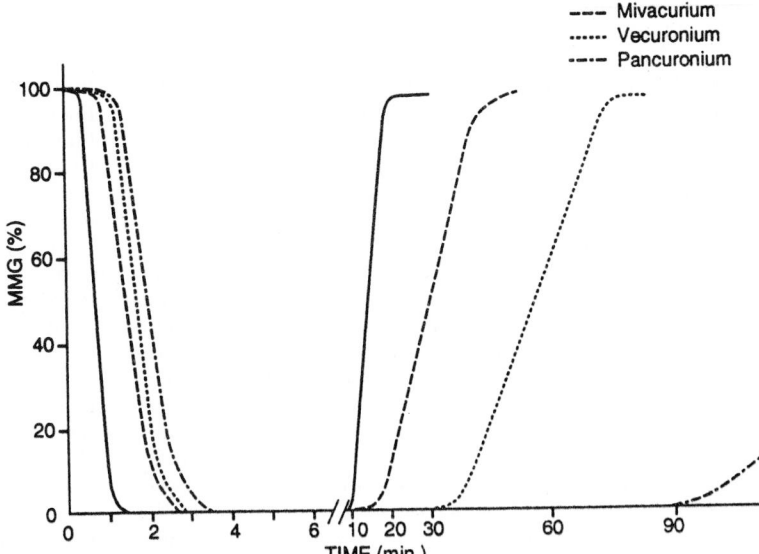

Figure 16-6. Approximate onset and recovery profiles for an ultra-short-acting drug, succinylcholine 1.0 mg · kg^{-1}; a short-acting drug, mivacurium 0.2 mg · kg^{-1}; an intermediate-acting drug, vecuronium 0.1 mg · kg^{-1}; and a long-acting drug, pancuronium 0.15 mg · kg^{-1}. Doses given are 2–2.5 × ED$_{95}$ for all four drugs.

Intraocular Pressure. Intraocular pressure increases by 5–15 mm Hg after injection of succinylcholine. The mechanism is unknown but occurs after detachment of extraocular muscle, suggesting an intraocular etiology.[42] Precurarization with a nondepolarizing blocker has little or no effect on this increase, so that large doses of nondepolarizing neuromuscular blocking drugs are recommended in the presence of open eye injuries. However, it must be appreciated that other factors, such as inadequate anesthesia, elevated systemic blood pressure, and insufficient neuromuscular blockade during laryngoscopy and tracheal intubation, might increase intraocular pressure more than succinylcholine.[43]

Intracranial Pressure. Succinylcholine may increase intracranial pressure (ICP), and this response is probably diminished by precurarization.[44] Most of this change may be due to an increase in PCO_2 produced by fasciculations.[45] Again, laryngoscopy and tracheal intubation with inadequate anesthesia or muscle relaxation are likely to increase ICP even more than succinylcholine. Any direct effect of succinylcholine on ICP is small; no changes in ICP, cerebral blood flow velocity, or EEG were observed when succinylcholine was given to patients with neurologic injury receiving mechanical ventilation.[46]

Hyperkalemia. Serum potassium increases by 0.5–1.0 $mEq \cdot l^{-1}$ after injection of succinylcholine. This increase is not prevented completely by precurarization. In fact, only large doses of nondepolarizing blockers abolish this effect.[47] Subjects with pre-existing hyperkalemia, such as patients in renal failure, do not have a greater increase in potassium levels, but the absolute level might reach the toxic range. However, severe hyperkalemia, occasionally leading to cardiac arrest, has been described in patients after major denervation injuries, spinal cord transection, peripheral denervation, stroke, trauma, extensive burns, and prolonged immobility with disease,[1,48] and may be related to potassium loss *via* a proliferation of extrajunctional receptors. Severe hyperkalemia after succinylcholine resulting in cardiac arrest has also been observed in acidotic hypovolemic patients.[49] It is likely that acidosis encourages the intracellular to extracellular shift of potassium that is exacerbated by succinylcholine. The source of potassium in this situation is likely to be liver and not the muscles.[50]

Abnormal Plasma Cholinesterase. Plasma cholinesterase activity can be reduced by a number of endogenous and exogenous causes, such as pregnancy, liver disease, uremia, malnutrition, burns, plasmapheresis, and oral contraceptives. These conditions usually lead to a slight, clinically unimportant increase in the duration of action of succinylcholine.[51] Plasma cholinesterase activity is reduced by some anticholinesterases (*e.g.,* neostigmine) so that the duration of succinylcholine given after neostigmine, but not after edrophonium, is increased from 10 to 24 min.[52] In the absence of plasma cholinesterase, the onset of action of succinylcholine is prolonged.[53]

A small proportion of patients (1:1500 to 1:2000 in the general population) have a genetically determined inability to metabolize succinylcholine. Either plasma cholinesterase is absent or an abnormal form of the enzyme is present. Only patients homozygous for the condition have prolonged paralysis (3–6 hr) after usual doses of succinylcholine (1–1.5 $mg \cdot kg^{-1}$). In heterozygous patients, the duration of action is only slightly prolonged. Traditional methods for identifying plasma cholinesterase phenotype by measurement of enzyme activity with a variety of substrates, such as benzoyl choline and ACh, and their inhibition with dibucaine, fluoride, and so forth are only capable of identifying some enzyme variants. The complete amino acid sequence of plasma cholinesterase has now been determined using molecular genetics techniques.[54] The cholinesterase gene is located on chromosome 3 at q26,[55] and 20 mutations in the coding region of the plasma cholinergic gene have been identified. It now seems likely that the failure to identify abnormal phenotypes using conventional techniques (prolonged reaction to succinylcholine but homozygous for normal plasma cholinesterase) will be corrected as more mutations are discovered.[56] Although whole blood or fresh frozen plasma can be given to accelerate succinylcholine metabolism in patients with low or absent plasma cholinesterase, the best course of action is probably mechanical ventilation of the lungs until full recovery of neuromuscular function can be demonstrated. Neostigmine and edrophonium are unpredictable in the reversal of abnormally prolonged succinylcholine blockade[57] and are best avoided.

Clinical Uses

The main indication for succinylcholine is to facilitate tracheal intubation. The dose required is ~1.0 $mg \cdot kg^{-1}$, and must be increased to 1.5–2.0 $mg \cdot kg^{-1}$ if a precurarizing dose of nondepolarizing blocker has been used. Intubating conditions are optimal within 1–1.5 min.

Succinylcholine has also been used for maintenance of relaxation for up to 3 h. However, because of the availability of short and intermediate nondepolarizing drugs for this purpose, succinylcholine infusions are seldom used to maintain relaxation. Infusion rates for 90–95% blockade are ~50–100 $mg \cdot kg^{-1} \cdot min^{-1}$ and need to be adjusted upward after 30–60 min, because of tachyphylaxis.[29]

Children are slightly more resistant to succinylcholine than adults[23] and doses of 1–2 $mg \cdot kg^{-1}$ are required to facilitate intubation. In infants, 2–3 $mg \cdot kg^{-1}$ may be required. Precurarization is not necessary in patients younger than 10 years because fasciculations are uncommon in this age group. Bradycardia is common in children unless atropine or glycopyrrolate is given.[35] Succinylcholine may also be given intramuscularly in a dose of 4 $mg \cdot kg^{-1}$ in children with difficult intravenous access, and provides adequate conditions for tracheal intubation in about 4 min.[58]

Nondepolarizing Drugs

Effects at the Neuromuscular Junction

Nondepolarizing neuromuscular blocking drugs bind to the postsynaptic receptor in a competitive fashion. An excess of ACh can tilt the balance in favor of neuromuscular transmission. To exert their effect, the nondepolarizing neuromuscular blocking drugs must bind to only one of the α subunits of the receptor, because two ACh molecules must be present on the same receptor to activate it.[2]

Neuromuscular blockade in a given muscle is not apparent until a large proportion of receptors are occupied.[12] To reach 100% blockade, a greater fraction of receptors must be occupied. For example, in the cat tibialis anterior, it has been estimated that blockade takes place in the range of 75–92% receptor occupancy. This means that neurotransmission fails in some fibers when receptors are 75% occupied, but the most resistant fibers in the same muscle require as much as 92% occupancy to block. In other words, partial neuromuscular blockade (between 0% and 100%) is not due to reduced contraction in all fibers, but to total blockade at some endplates.

The margin of safety is reduced when high-frequency stimulation is used owing to a decrease in ACh release. Thus, fade following either train-of-four or tetanic stimulation will be detected at lower levels of receptor occupancy than that with depression of single-twitch response. For example, in the cat tibialis anterior, train-of-four fade occurs at 70% receptor occupancy.[59] The actual number, however, depends on species and varies from muscle to muscle within the same individual. So, although the principle of decreased margin of safety for high-frequency stimulation should be retained, it is futile to correlate receptor occupancy data obtained in cats with certain clinical tests in humans, such as hand grip and head lift, which involve different muscle groups.

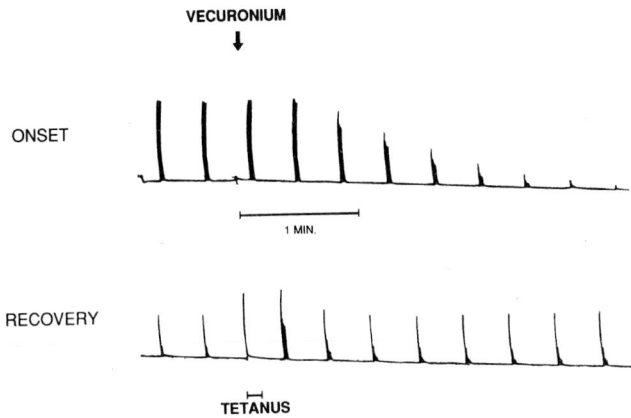

Figure 16-7. Characteristics of nondepolarizing blockade. Train-of-four responses are equal before the administration of vecuronium (arrow). For a given first-twitch depression, fade is less during onset (*top*) than during recovery (*bottom*). Fade also occurs with a 5-sec, 50-Hz tetanus (*bar*). Facilitation is apparent after the tetanus; *i.e.*, first-twitch height and train-of-four ratio are increased, but only for the first two trains.

Characteristics of Nondepolarizing Blockade

The fade observed in response to high-frequency stimulation (>0.1–0.15 Hz) is characteristic of nondepolarizing blockade. When EMG recordings are made in humans, fade reaches a maximum at 2 Hz and stays constant for frequencies up to 50 Hz.[60] With mechanical recordings, fusion of several individual responses occurs when the stimulation frequency exceeds the duration of the twitch. Thus, the initial peak is made up of the first few responses, the first being the strongest, and fade follows.

Tetanic stimulation is followed by post-tetanic facilitation, which is due to an increase in ACh release when the stimulation occurs soon after the tetanus. Thus, the response to nerve stimulation is increased. The intensity and duration of this effect depend on the frequency and duration of the tetanic stimulation. With a 50-Hz tetanus of 5-sec duration, twitch responses have been found to fall within 10% of their pretetanic values in 1–2 min, and in most cases in 1 min (Fig. 16-7).[61]

Finally, nondepolarizing blockade can be antagonized with anticholinesterase agents such as edrophonium, neostigmine, or pyridostigmine. It is also antagonized by depolarizing agents, such as succinylcholine, provided that the nondepolarizing

blockade is intense and that the succinylcholine dose is too small to produce a block of its own.

Pharmacokinetics

Plasma concentrations have been measured for all the nondepolarizing agents used clinically. The pharmacokinetic variables derived from these experiments depend on the dose given, the sampling schedule used, the accuracy of the assay, and the model chosen. As is the case for other drugs used in anesthesia, the elimination half-life of neuromuscular blocking agents does not always correlate with duration of action because termination of action sometimes depends on redistribution instead of elimination. However, knowledge of the kinetics of the drug helps us understand the behavior of the drug in special situations (prolonged administration, disease of the organs of elimination, and so on).

Several mechanisms can explain the various categories of durations of action listed in Table 16-1:

1. Long-acting drugs all have a long (1–2 hr) elimination half-life and depend on liver and/or kidney function for termination of action.
2. Intermediate-duration drugs either have an intermediate elimination half-life (atracurium and cisatracurium); or they have long elimination half-lives (1–2 hr) but depend on redistribution rather than elimination for termination of effect (vecuronium and rocuronium) (Fig. 16-8).
3. Short-duration drugs have either short elimination half-lives (the active isomers of mivacurium)[62] or long elimination half-life but extensive redistribution (rapacuronium).[63]
4. Ultra-short-duration drugs have a very short elimination half-life (succinylcholine).

Nevertheless, pharmacokinetic analysis illustrates some of the common properties of these drugs (Table 16-2). Each has a volume of distribution that is approximately equal to extracellular fluid (ECF) volume (0.2–$0.4\ 1\cdot kg^{-1}$). In infants, in whom the ECF volume, as a proportion of body weight, is increased, the volume of distribution of *d*-tubocurarine parallels ECF volume closely.[64]

Onset and Duration of Action

The duration of action of nondepolarizing drugs is determined by the time required for plasma concentrations to decrease below a critical level. However, onset is not determined by

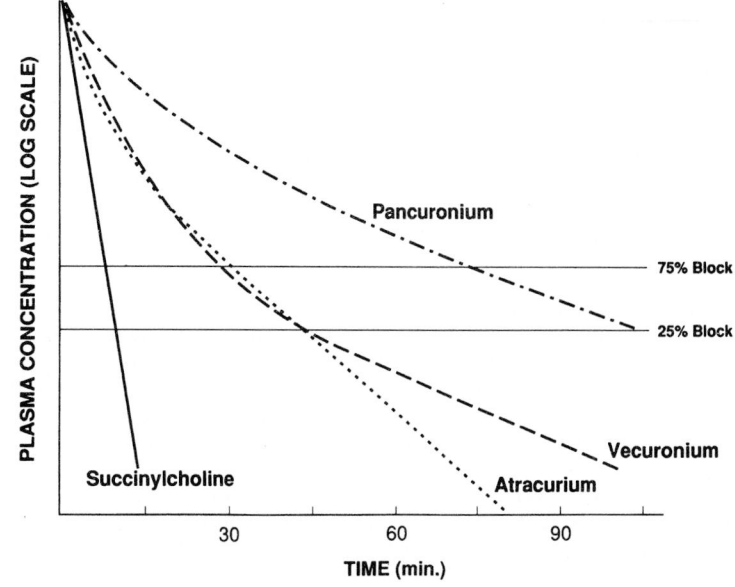

Figure 16-8. Plasma concentrations versus time for four representative muscle relaxants. Concentrations are expressed as a function of each drug's concentration corresponding to 25% and 75% block. Succinylcholine is broken down rapidly in the plasma: it is a short-acting drug. Pancuronium is a long-acting drug because of its long elimination time. Atracurium is an intermediate-duration drug and has an intermediate half-life. Vecuronium has an elimination half-life comparable to that of pancuronium. However, redistribution of the drug is important and the duration of action is comparable to that of atracurium.

Table 16-2. TYPICAL PHARMACOKINETIC DATA FOR NONDEPOLARIZING BLOCKERS IN ADULTS, EXCEPT WHERE STATED

Relaxant	V_D (L·kg^{-1})	Cp (ml·kg^{-1}·min^{-1})	$T_{1/2}\beta$ (min)
d-Tubocurarine			
adults 30–60 yr	0.3–0.6	1–3	90–350
elderly 70–87 yr	0.3	0.8	270
neonates	0.5	1.1	310
infants 1–12 mo	0.5	1.0	305
children 1–12 yr	0.3	1.5	170
Atracurium	0.2	5.5	20
Doxacurium	0.2	2.5	95
Metocurine	0.4	1.3	220
Mivacurium			
cis–trans	0.3	105	1.8
trans–trans	0.2	60	1.9
cis–cis	0.3	4.6	53
Pancuronium	0.3	1–2	100–130
Rapacuronium	0.2	73	99
Rocuronium	0.3	4.0	130
Vecuronium	0.4	4.5	110

plasma concentrations. Peak plasma concentrations are obtained less than 1 min after injection of the drug, but maximum blockade is reached after only 2–7 min if subparalyzing doses are given. This discrepancy between concentration and block has been modeled mathematically by introducing the concept of a compartment, in which the drug concentration is directly related to its effect. The access to this "effect compartment" is controlled by a rate constant (k_{eo}).[65] This rate constant corresponds to half-times of 5–10 min for most nondepolarizing drugs.[66]

The delay between peak plasma concentrations and blockade, represented by k_{eo}, is determined by all the factors that modify access of the drug to, and its removal from, the neuromuscular junction. These include cardiac output, distance of the muscle from the heart, and muscle blood flow.[66] Thus, onset times are not the same in all muscles because of different blood flows. If metabolism or redistribution is very rapid, the onset time is accelerated. This probably plays a role only for succinylcholine and mivacurium. Finally, there is growing evidence that potent drugs have a slower onset of action than less potent agents (Fig. 16-9).[67–69] This is because spare receptors must be occupied before blockade can be observed. Blockade of these spare receptors will occur faster, and onset will be more rapid, if more drug molecules are available, i.e., if potency is low.[66]

Time to maximal blockade is independent of dose if maximum block attained is less than 100%. For most drugs, this value is 5–7 min.[66] For doxacurium, the most potent drug tested in humans, 10–15 min is required.[70] For rapacuronium, the least potent drug available, this delay is 2–3 min. Once 100% block has been achieved, the time to disappearance of the twitch decreases with increasing dose. Onset and recovery times for nondepolarizing relaxants are shown in Table 16-3.

Individual Nondepolarizing Relaxants

Since 1942, nearly 50 nondepolarizing relaxants have been introduced into clinical anesthesia. This section covers only those drugs currently available in North America and Europe. The first relaxant to undergo clinical investigation was Intocostrin, the purified and standardized product of curare obtained from the plant *Chondodendrum tomentosum*. The pharmacologic action of d-tubocurarine is discussed first as the prototypical muscle relaxant.

d-Tubocurarine. d-Tubocurarine is a monoquaternary ammonium compound. However, at body pH, the second nitrogen atom becomes protonated so that it possesses two positively charged centers. The molecule undergoes minimal metabolism

so that 24 hr after its administration about 10% of the compound is found in the urine and 45% in the bile. It is 30–50% protein-bound, but altered plasma protein concentration does not appear to modify the pharmacokinetic or pharmacodynamic behavior.[71]

The development of a sensitive radioimmunoassay allowed the relationship between plasma concentration of d-tubocurarine and recovery from neuromuscular block to be demonstrated (Fig. 16-10).[72] As for most nondepolarizing relaxants, excretion is impaired in renal failure with an increase in elimination half-life ($T_{1/2}\beta$).[73]

CARDIOVASCULAR EFFECTS. Hypotension frequently accompanies the administration of d-tubocurarine. In cats, autonomic

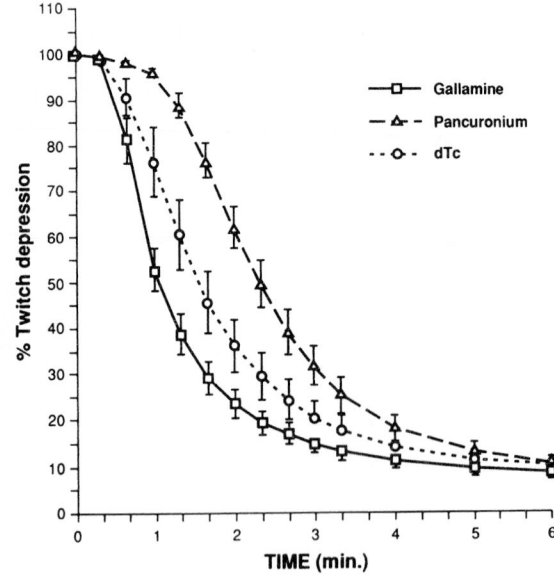

Figure 16-9. Onset times of single-twitch depression of adductor pollicis after pancuronium (0.07 mg·kg^{-1}), d-tubocurarine (0.45 mg·kg^{-1}), and gallamine (2.4 mg·kg^{-1}). Although the maximum effect was identical in all three groups, the onset of blockade was fastest after gallamine. The mean time to 50% depression was 141 sec for pancuronium, 99 sec for d-tubocurarine, and 66 sec for gallamine. (Reprinted with permission from Kopman AF: Pancuronium, gallamine, and d-tubocurarine compared: Is speed of onset inversely related to drug potency? Anesthesiology 70:915, 1989.)

Table 16-3. TYPICAL NEUROMUSCULAR ACTIVITY OF NONDEPOLARIZING BLOCKING DRUGS: POTENCY (ED$_{95}$), ONSET TO MAXIMUM EFFECT, 25–75% RECOVERY INDEX (RI), AND TIME TO 90% T$_1$ RECOVERY (T$_{90}$) AFTER AN ED$_{95}$ DOSE IN ADULTS

Relaxant	ED$_{95}$ ($\mu g \cdot kg^{-1}$)	Onset (min)	RI (min)	T$_{90}$ (min)
d-Tubocurarine	500	6	25–35	70–90
Atracurium	200	5–6	10–15	20–25
Cisatracurium	50	5–6	10–15	20–25
Doxacurium	25	10–14	30–50	80–100
Metocurine	280	5	30–40	80–90
Mivacurium	80–150	2–3	10–15	20
Pancuronium	60	4–5	25	60
Rapacuronium	1000	1.5–2.5	8–10	20
Rocuronium	300	2–3	10–15	20
Vecuronium	80	5–6	10–15	20

ganglionic blockade occurs at doses similar to those that produce neuromuscular blockade.[74] In addition, *d*-tubocurarine causes vagal and sympathetic blockade, although, clinically, bradycardia is more common than tachycardia.

In humans, *d*-tubocurarine causes dose-related histamine release,[75] and skin flushing is frequently observed. The hypotension can be reduced by pretreatment with the antihistamine promethazine or by administering *d*-tubocurarine slowly over 3 min. Thus, in humans, histamine release is probably more important than ganglionic blockade in the production of hypotension. Alternatively, a bolus injection of *d*-tubocurarine may induce the release of prostacyclin, which acts *via* H$_1$ receptors to produce hypotension.[76]

AGE. The potency of *d*-tubocurarine on a mg · kg^{-1} basis is similar at all ages. However, the increased sensitivity of the neuromuscular junction in infants is concealed by the increased volume of distribution (see Table 16-2).[64,77] The onset of action is more rapid in the young as a result of a more rapid circulation time. However, the decreased glomerular filtration rate (GFR) in the very young and the very old results in an increase in T$_{1/2}\beta$ and prolonged duration of action.[78]

BURNS. Patients with massive burns demonstrate resistance to *d*-tubocurarine and other nondepolarizing drugs that is dependent upon the size of the burn and the time since injury.[79] The pharmacokinetic behavior of atracurium is unaffected in

burn patients. Resistance is associated with higher concentrations of the free drug to produce a given degree of twitch depression compared with nonthermally injured patients. As in denervation injury, there is an increase in the number of acetylcholine receptors in the diaphragm of the rat after burn injury to 45% of the body surface area.[80] Circulatory mediators such as catecholamines and prostaglandins may play a role in producing these effects, which are at a distance from the burn areas.[81]

CLINICAL USE. The slow onset and long duration of *d*-tubocurarine have restricted its use, in doses of 15–30 mg · 70 kg^{-1}, to the maintenance of relaxation during surgery. However, the dose-related cardiovascular effects were a stimulus for the production of alternative agents. Initially, this led to the introduction of pancuronium, which replaced the hypotension of *d*-tubocurarine with hypertension and tachycardia. More recently, drugs of intermediate duration (atracurium, vecuronium, and rocuronium) have almost eliminated the use of *d*-tubocurarine because they have minimal cardiovascular activity. Its use is mainly confined to small doses of *d*-tubocurarine (3 mg · 70 kg^{-1}) before succinylcholine ("precurarization") to reduce the incidence of fasciculations and muscle pains.

Atracurium. Atracurium is a bisquaternary ammonium benzylisoquinoline compound that was developed in an attempt to produce a short-acting muscle relaxant that was independent of the liver and the kidney for termination of its action.[82] Its ED$_{95}$ is 0.2–0.25 mg · kg^{-1}. In humans, atracurium is metabolized both by the Hofmann reaction (nonenzymatic degradation at body temperature and pH) and ester hydrolysis to several compounds (Fig. 16-11). It has been estimated that two thirds of atracurium is degraded by ester hydrolysis and one third by Hofmann reaction.[83]

The metabolites of atracurium may be toxic. The quaternary monoacrylate, quaternary alcohol, and monoquaternary analogs produce neuromuscular blockade in high doses. Also, the quaternary monoacrylate, laudanosine, the quaternary alcohol, metholaudanosine, and the monoquaternary analog decrease blood pressure but at concentrations higher than those found in clinical practice.[84]

Laudanosine has been suspected of causing cerebral excitation. It has been shown to increase the MAC of halothane in rabbits.[85] At doses of 2–8 mg · kg^{-1} it produced wakening from halothane anesthesia, and at 14–22 mg · kg^{-1} seizure activity was observed in dogs.[86] However, such doses are not used in humans. The clinical effects of laudanosine have been sought extensively but unsuccessfully. There is also interest in the potential toxic effects of the highly reactive acrylates.[87]

PHARMACOKINETICS. The plasma concentration of atracurium decreases rapidly following iv administration (see Fig. 16-8). The conventional pharmacokinetic model that is used

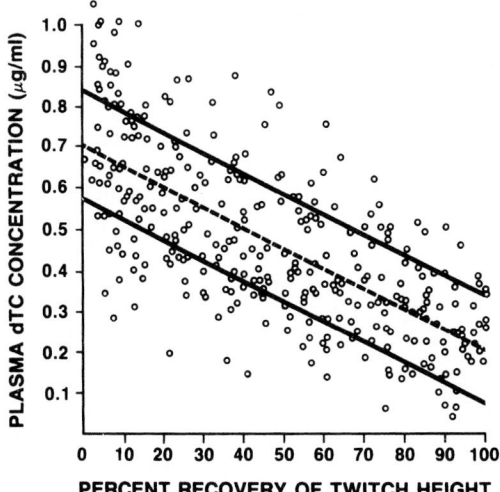

Figure 16-10. Relationship between twitch height and plasma *d*-tubocurarine concentration. (Reprinted with permission from Matteo RS, Spector S, Horowitz PE: Relation of serum *d*-tubocurarine concentration to neuromuscular blockade. Anesthesiology 41:441, 1974.)

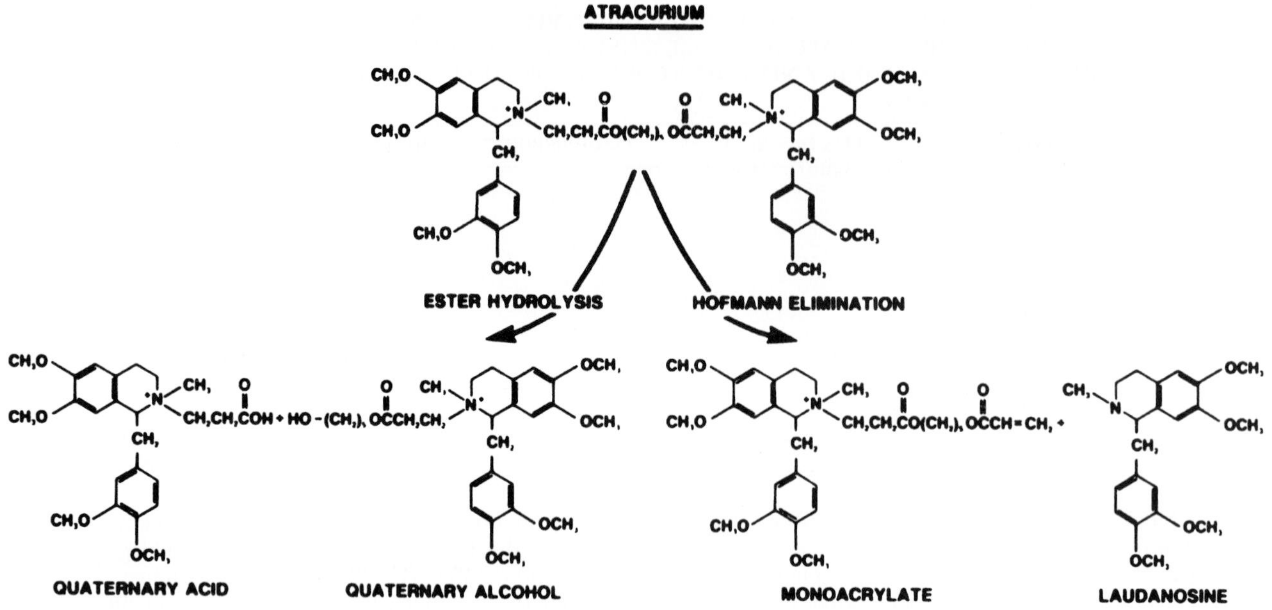

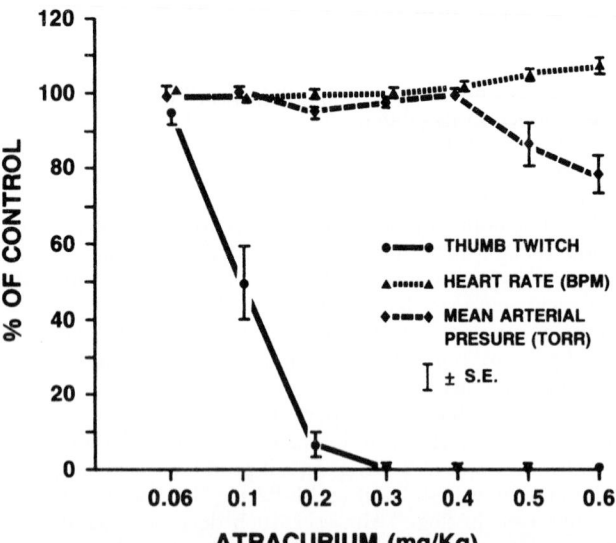

Figure 16-11. Atracurium and its major metabolites.

for other nondepolarizing relaxants may not be suitable for atracurium because it undergoes nonenzymatic degradation in the tissues as well as in plasma.

The *onset of action* of equipotent doses is similar for atracurium, pancuronium, *d*-tubocurarine, and vecuronium. It is slower than succinylcholine but can be reduced if the dose is increased.[89] However, such acceleration is limited by hypotension and histamine release after large doses. The duration of action is also dose-related. The time to 25% recovery of T_1 after 0.4 mg $\cdot$ kg^{-1} is rapid: $\approx$30 min (see Table 16-3).

CARDIOVASCULAR EFFECTS. Atracurium is associated with few cardiovascular effects unless large doses (2 × ED$_{95}$) are administered. The most common cardiovascular abnormality following smaller doses is the bradycardia that is most likely due to con-

comitant administration of opioids[90] or to vagal traction. Hypotension and tachycardia may accompany doses exceeding 0.4 mg $\cdot$ kg^{-1} (Fig. 16-12); these effects occur as a result of dose-related histamine release.[91] Similar changes occur after the use of *d*-tubocurarine or metocurine but at much lower doses (Table 16-4). The most obvious clinical manifestation of histamine release is skin flushing, but this is seldom associated with hypotension or bronchospasm. These responses can be avoided by slow injection over 1–3 min or by pretreatment with H$_1$ and H$_2$ receptor blockade.[92] Profound bronchospasm has been described following administration of even small doses of atracurium to patients with a history of bronchial asthma.[93] Anaphylactoid reactions to atracurium have been described, but no more frequently than after other neuromuscular blocking drugs.[94]

AGE. The potency of atracurium is similar in adults and children. When atracurium is given by infusion to the elderly, the reduction in dose requirement and the slower recovery time observed with vecuronium are not seen,[95] presumably reflecting the organ independence of atracurium's elimination.

OBESITY. The dose of atracurium, as for all NMDs, should be reduced on a mg $\cdot$ kg^{-1} basis to reflect lean body mass,[96] although reversal from similar degrees of block is similar to that in nonobese subjects[97]

CLINICAL USES. The short duration of action, rapid recovery, and absence of severe cardiovascular and cumulative drug effects have encouraged the use of atracurium as a continuous infusion (5–10 μg $\cdot$ kg^{-1} $\cdot$ min^{-1}) or as intermittent injections in several situations including ambulatory surgery, cardiopulmonary bypass surgery, pheochromocytoma resection, and renal and hepatic disease. Large doses (0.5–0.6 mg $\cdot$ kg^{-1}) must be given if atracurium is used to produce rapid paralysis to facilitate tracheal intubation when conditions will also be influenced by the depth of anesthesia, airway reactivity, and strength of the patient.

Cisatracurium. Cisatracurium is a potent (ED$_{95}$ 0.05 mg $\cdot$ kg^{-1}), long-onset, intermediate-duration benzylisoquinolinium neuromuscular blocking drug.[98] It is one of the ten isomers of atracurium that is devoid of cardiovascular effects. It is more potent than atracurium, and thus has a slower onset of maximum block. Otherwise this drug resembles atracurium in duration of action and rate of recovery. After 0.1 mg $\cdot$ kg^{-1}, the mean onset is 3.1 min (versus 2.3 min after 0.5 mg $\cdot$ kg^{-1} for

Figure 16-12. Neuromuscular, heart rate, and blood pressure responses to atracurium at various doses. (Reprinted with permission from Savarese JJ, Basta SJ, Ali HH *et al:* Neuromuscular and cardiovascular effects of BW33A [atracurium] in patients under halothane anesthesia. Anesthesiology 57:A262, 1982.)

atracurium)[99] with spontaneous recovery to TOF 0.8 of 74 min, which is reduced to 48 and 50 min after reversal with neostigmine at 10% and 25% spontaneous recovery, respectively.[100] The potency is increased and the duration prolonged in the presence of volatile anesthetics.[101] In children it is slightly more potent (ED$_{95}$ 0.04 mg·kg^{-1}), has a slightly quicker onset (2.5 min), and shorter recovery (TOF > 0.7 at 53 min).[102] Clearance, by Hofmann elimination, is greater than that of atracurium (77% versus 39%)[103] (see Table 16-2). Mixtures of cisatracurium and rocuronium are highly synergistic.[104] Unlike atracurium, cisatracurium does not undergo significant hydrolysis by non-specific plasma esterases. The metabolites of cisatracurium include laudanosine and a monoquaternary acrylate. The peak plasma concentration of laudanosine following the administration of 2 × ED$_{95}$ of cisatracurium is about 5-fold less than was present following a similar dose of atracurium. Presumably, the greater potency of cisatracurium compared with atracurium results in fewer molecules being administered, and hence in lower plasma concentrations of metabolites.

In contrast to atracurium, cisatracurium is devoid of histamine-releasing properties even at high doses (8 × ED$_{95}$), although anaphylactic reactions have been described.[105] Also, it lacks cardiovascular effects.[106] Neuromuscular blockade is easily maintained at a stable level by continuous intravenous infusion of cisatracurium at a constant rate and does not change with time, suggesting the lack of a significant cumulative drug effect and lack of dependence on renal and/or hepatic clearance mechanisms. The rate of recovery is independent of the dose of cisatracurium and the duration of the administration. Recovery from drug-induced neuromuscular blockade can be facilitated by administration of an anticholinesterase drug.

Doxacurium. Doxacurium is a long-acting bisquaternary ammonium compound that is devoid of histamine-releasing or cardiovascular side effects. The pharmacokinetic behavior of doxacurium resembles that of pancuronium with respect to T$_{1/2}\beta$ and dependence on renal clearance for elimination from the circulation (see Table 16-2).[107] In the elderly, elimination half-life is prolonged and plasma clearance reduced without any change in volume of distribution.[108] Doxacurium is also a weak substrate for plasma cholinesterase. The ED$_{95}$ for doxacurium is 25 µg·kg^{-1} (see Table 16-3).[109] Volatile anesthetics decrease doxacurium dose requirements by 20–40% compared with doses needed during N$_2$O–fentanyl anesthesia.[110] Doxacurium has a limited place in clinical practice because of its very slow onset and long duration of action. Nevertheless, it may be useful in patients with ischemic heart disease who are undergoing prolonged anesthesia or long-term mechanical ventilation of the lungs. The slow onset time, prolonged duration of action, and slow recovery make doxacurium unsuitable for facilitating tracheal intubation or for providing skeletal muscle relaxation during brief surgical procedures. When infused for more than 4 days to patients in the ICU, recovery after stopping the infusion exceeded 10 h.[111]

Metocurine. Metocurine, produced by methylation of two hydroxy groups of d-tubocurarine, is twice as potent as the parent compound and produces less histamine release. Like d-tubocurarine, it undergoes minimal metabolism. Within 48 hr of administration, approximately half appears in the urine and another 2% appears in the bile.[112] Because metocurine is more dependent on renal function for excretion than is d-tubocurarine, clearance is disturbed to a greater degree in renal failure and in the elderly.

CARDIOVASCULAR EFFECTS. In animals the separation between autonomic and neuromuscular effects of metocurine is greater than for d-tubocurarine[74] and metocurine causes less histamine release than does d-tubocurarine.[113] Consequently, changes in blood pressure and heart rate are not seen until doses greater than the ED$_{95}$ are administered.

BURNS. Patients with burn injuries are resistant to all nondepolarizing relaxants, and the resistance to metocurine may be extensive. For example, an 8-year-old boy with a 35% surface burn required 12 times the normal dose of metocurine and 8 times the plasma concentration during the acute phase of the burn to produce complete neuromuscular block.[114]

CLINICAL USE. Because of its lack of cardiovascular effects, metocurine enjoyed a brief period of popularity before the introduction of atracurium and vecuronium. The combination of metocurine and pancuronium augmented neuromuscular block with opposing cardiovascular effects and was recommended for use in patients with severe cardiovascular disease.[115] However, the introduction of intermediate- and long-acting relaxants without cardiovascular effects has made metocurine obsolete.

Mivacurium. Mivacurium is an intermediate-onset, short-duration, nondepolarizing neuromuscular blocking drug that is hydrolyzed by plasma cholinesterase.[116] The drug is presented as a mixture of three isomers. Two, the cis–trans and trans–trans, have short half-lives, but the cis–cis isomer has a much longer half-life (2 versus 53 min, respectively). The cis–cis isomer accounts for 10% of the mixture, has less than one tenth the potency of the other isomers, and thus contributes little if anything to neuromuscular block during anesthesia.[62] Under steady-state conditions, the ED$_{95}$ of mivacurium is 0.08 mg·kg^{-1}, the time to onset of action is 3.3 min, and spontaneous recovery to 95% twitch height occurs in about 25 min (see Table 16-3). At 2 × ED$_{95}$ the onset time is 2.5 min and recovery to 95% twitch height occurs in about 31 min. In infants and children the ED$_{95}$ is greater than in adults, 120–150 µg·kg^{-1}, and the onset of block is more rapid.[117,118] The recovery time after discontinuing an infusion of mivacurium is about half that for atracurium or vecuronium infusions and is similar to that for succinylcholine.[119,120] The effect of anticholinesterase drugs is additive to the rapid rate of spontaneous recovery from mivacurium-induced neuromuscular blockade. Therefore, mivacurium is more rapidly reversed than are the longer-acting nondepolarizing neuromuscular blocking drugs.[121] However, reversal of intense neuromuscular block with neostigmine has been shown to delay recovery,[122] presumably as a result of plasma cholinesterase inhibition by neostigmine.[123] Spontaneous recovery is so rapid that it has been suggested that reversal is unnecessary and that

Table 16-4. DOSES OF DRUGS ASSOCIATED WITH CARDIOVASCULAR CHANGES

	Dose (mg·kg^{-1})	ED$_{95}$ (multiple)	% Control		
			HR	BP	Hist conc
d-Tubocurarine	0.5	1	78	116	410
Metocurine	0.5	2	79	119	212
Atracurium	0.6	3	80	108	192

Adapted with permission from Basta SJ, Savarese JJ, Ali HH *et al:* Histamine releasing potencies of atracurium, dimethyl tubocurarine, and tubocurarine. Br J Anaesth 55:105S, 1983.

its avoidance may reduce the incidence of postoperative nausea and vomiting.[124] However, this may result in residual block on arrival in the PACU, particularly if large doses of mivacurium are used up to the end of anesthesia.[125] In addition, careful meta-analysis has shown that avoidance of reversal of mivacurium has only a marginal effect in reducing PONV at the risk of residual weakness.[126]

PLASMA CHOLINESTERASE. Mivacurium is metabolized by plasma cholinesterase more slowly than succinylcholine. Duration of action is correlated with plasma cholinesterase activity, and hence is prolonged when plasma cholinesterase concentrations are decreased (*e.g.*, in pediatric[127] and obstetric patients[128]). Reversal can be accelerated with human plasma cholinesterase.[129] Patients homozygous for atypical plasma cholinesterase may show very prolonged block. After a "test-dose" of 0.14 $mg \cdot kg^{-1}$, full recovery took 7 hours.[130] Inhibition of enzymatic degradation of mivacurium by plasma cholinesterase also results in slower onset.[53]

The cardiovascular response to mivacurium is minimal at doses of $2-3 \times ED_{95}$, whereas administration of $3 \times ED_{95}$ over 10–15 sec evokes sufficient histamine release to decrease mean arterial blood pressure transiently by about 15%.[116,131] Therefore, the cardiovascular effects are similar to those of atracurium.

CLINICAL USE. Mivacurium is well suited to surgical procedures requiring brief muscle relaxation, particularly those in which rapid recovery is required, such as ambulatory and laparoscopic surgery. Because of its slow onset, conditions for tracheal intubation are unsatisfactory unless large bolus doses, at least $0.2 \ mg \cdot kg^{-1}$, are given and a delay of at least 2 min is allowed before intubation is attempted.[132] However, by using two doses of 0.15 and $0.1 \ mg \cdot kg^{-1}$ separated by 30 sec, good to excellent intubation conditions have been achieved in almost 90% of patients, an onset similar to that of succinylcholine.[133] Small doses of mivacurium ($0.04-0.08 \ mg \cdot kg^{-1}$) have been suggested to facilitate insertion of a Laryngeal Mask Airway,[134] although this is seldom necessary. The rapid recovery makes it necessary to monitor neuromuscular activity continuously during its administration, which is accomplished more easily by constant infusion ($5-10 \ \mu g \cdot kg^{-1} \cdot min^{-1}$) than by intermittent bolus injection.

Pancuronium. Pancuronium is a long-acting, synthetic, nondepolarizing neuromuscular blocking drug developed from a series of bisquaternary aminosteroid compounds.[135] The two quaternary groups were attached to a rigid steroid structure to maintain a constant interonium distance. It is metabolized to a 3-OH compound, which has one half the neuromuscular blocking activity of the parent compound. Although values for protein binding varying from 20% to 87% have been described for pancuronium, the extent of binding does not appear to be important for its clinical activity. Clearance is decreased in renal and hepatic failure, demonstrating that excretion is dependent upon both organs. The onset of action is more rapid in infants and children than in adults and recovery is slower in the elderly.

CARDIOVASCULAR EFFECTS. Pancuronium is associated with increases in heart rate, blood pressure, and cardiac output, particularly after large doses ($2 \times ED_{95}$). The cause is uncertain but includes a vagolytic effect at the postganglionic nerve terminal, a sympathomimetic effect as a result of blocking of muscarinic receptors that normally exert some braking on ganglionic transmission, and an increase in catecholamine release.[2] Pancuronium does not release histamine.

CLINICAL USE. The slow onset of action of pancuronium limits its usefulness in facilitating tracheal intubation. Administration in divided doses (priming principle) produces a small but measurable acceleration,[136] but the intermediate- and short-acting compounds are more suitable when succinylcholine is contraindicated prior to tracheal intubation. In patients with myocardial ischemia, tachycardia should be avoided. Because these patients are often anesthetized with high doses of opioids, the use of pancuronium to provide muscle relaxation may offer some advantage over the use of cardiovascularly neutral relaxants. The continued popularity of pancuronium is dependent upon cost: generic pancuronium is cheaper than other nondepolarizing relaxants. Its use is associated with a high incidence of residual block in the PACU, at least in adults. Pancuronium neuromuscular block is more difficult to reverse than that of the intermediate NMBDs.[137]

Rapacuronium. Rapacuronium is the most recently introduced aminosteroid NMBD.[138] It is less potent than rocuronium, and thus has a more rapid onset of action and faster recovery. Following $1.5 \ mg \cdot kg^{-1}$, good to excellent intubation conditions are produced at 60 sec,[139] clinical duration (25% T_1 recovery) occurs in 17 min and spontaneous recovery to TOF 0.7 occurs in 35 min.[140] Rapacuronium is metabolized to a 17-OH derivative (ORG 9488) that has ½ times the neuromuscular blocking activity of the parent compound and is excreted slowly *via* the kidneys.[63,141] Thus it has been recommended that rapacuronium be used only for short procedures requiring neuromuscular blockade for 30 min or less. Repeated boluses produce increasing duration of block.[142] When 0.05 or $0.07 \ mg \cdot kg^{-1}$ neostigmine was given 2 or 5 min after $1.5 \ mg \cdot kg^{-1}$ rapacuronium, recovery was accelerated so that TOF 0.7 was achieved in 17 min,[143] which was very much more rapid than after rocuronium ($0.45 \ mg \cdot kg^{-1}$).[144] Although this duration is longer than that of succinylcholine, rapacuronium has the most rapid onset and recovery of any nondepolarizing NMBD. Rapacuronium produces mild dose-related tachycardia and hypotension, and these cardiovascular changes do not appear to be due to histamine release.[145] Increased airway pressure and bronchospasm have been reported in some patients.[139,145]

Rocuronium. Rocuronium is an aminosteroid neuromuscular relaxant. It has one sixth the potency of vecuronium, a more rapid onset, but a similar duration of action[146] and similar pharmacokinetic behavior.[147] Bartkowski *et al* showed that, with equipotent doses, rocuronium onset at the adductor pollicis was much faster than that of atracurium and vecuronium[148] (Fig. 16-13). After doses of $600 \ \mu g \cdot kg^{-1}$ ($2 \times ED_{95}$, $4 \times ED_{50}$) maximal block occurs in ~60–90 s. In a multicenter study of 349 patients, intubating conditions at 60 s after $1.0 \ mg \cdot kg^{-1}$ rocuronium were similar to those after $1 \ mg \cdot kg^{-1}$ succinylcholine and superior to those after $0.6 \ mg \cdot kg^{-1}$ rocuronium (92 versus 77% good–excellent).[149] As for other nondepolarizing

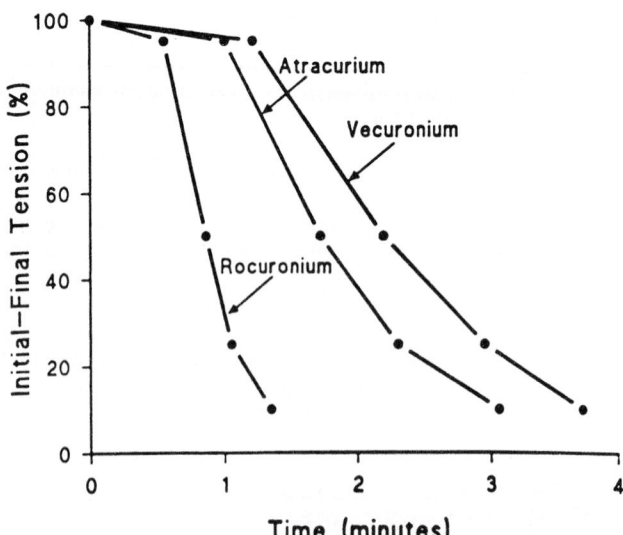

Figure 16-13. Onset of block of adductor after rocuronium, vecuronium, or atracurium. (Reproduced with permission from Bartkowski RR, Witkowski TA, Azad S *et al*: Rocuronium onset of action: A comparsion with atracurium and vercuronium. Anesth Analg 77:574, 1993.)

relaxants the onset of action of rocuronium is more rapid at the diaphragm[150] and laryngeal muscle[151] than at the adductor pollicis, and approximately twice as much is required to produce the same degree of paralysis at the diaphragm.[150] The potency, onset time, recovery index, and duration of action are similar in infants, children, and adults during nitrous oxide-alfentanil anesthesia[152] in contrast to vecuronium, which is a long-acting relaxant in infants.[153]

CARDIOVASCULAR EFFECTS.   No hemodynamic changes (blood pressure, heart rate, or ECG) were seen in humans, and there were no increases in plasma histamine concentrations after doses of up to $4 \times ED_{95}$,[154] although anaphylactic reactions have been described.[36] Similarly, when rocuronium $0.6 \; mg \cdot kg^{-1}$ was given to patients before coronary artery bypass grafting, the slight hemodynamic changes observed were no different from those following equivalent doses of vecuronium.[155]

CLINICAL USE.   The rapid onset and intermediate duration of action makes this agent a potential replacement for succinylcholine in conditions where rapid tracheal intubation is indicated. However, large doses are required with a prolonged duration of action. A "timing principle" has been described in which $0.6 \; mg \cdot kg^{-1}$ rocuronium is given *before* the induction agent, which is administered at the onset of ptosis. Used in this fashion, intubation conditions are similar to those after succinylcholine.[156] Rocuronium has replaced vecuronium as an intermediate-duration relaxant because of its more rapid onset and lack of active metabolites, and because it is unnecessary to reconstitute the drug from a lyophilized base. Initial doses of $0.6 \; mg \cdot kg^{-1}$ iv will usually produce good intubating conditions within 90 sec. Subsequent doses of $0.075-0.225 \; mg \cdot kg^{-1}$ will provide clinical relaxation for 10–20 min.[157] Alternatively, rocuronium might be given by continued infusion, titrated with the help of a nerve stimulator.

Vecuronium.   Vecuronium is an intermediate-acting aminosteroid neuromuscular relaxant without cardiovascular effects. Its ED_{95} is $0.04-0.05 \; mg \cdot kg^{-1}$. It is a monoquaternary ammonium compound produced by demethylation of the pancuronium molecule at the 2-piperidino position.[158] The demethylation reduces the ACh-like characteristics of the molecule and increases its lipophilicity, which encourages hepatic uptake. Vecuronium undergoes spontaneous deacetylation to produce 3-OH, 17-OH, and $3,17-(OH)_2$ metabolites. The most potent, 3-OH vecuronium, has about 60% of the activity of vecuronium, is excreted by the kidney, and has been found to be responsible for prolonged paralysis in patients in the intensive care unit.[159] Vecuronium is less potent and has a shorter duration of action in men than in women,[160] probably as a result of a decrease in the volume of distribution which results in increased plasma concentrations in women.[161]

The pharmacokinetic variables of vecuronium are similar to those of pancuronium, and the reason for vecuronium's shorter duration of action is that the plasma concentration decreases through the effective range far more rapidly so that duration and recovery depend more on distribution than on elimination[162] (Fig. 16-8). Recovery after long-term infusions of vecuronium (in excess of 6 h) is slower than after a bolus dose[163] because the peripheral storage sites have become saturated and a decrease in plasma concentration is then dependent upon metabolism and excretion and not upon redistribution.

Attempts have been made to reduce the time of onset of action of vecuronium, and other nondepolarizing blocking drugs, by using the priming principle.[164] This refers to the administration of a small, subparalyzing dose several minutes before the principal dose is given. For vecuronium, the best results have been obtained with a priming dose of $0.01 \; mg \cdot kg^{-1}$ followed 3–4 min later by $0.1 \; mg \cdot kg^{-1}$. The time to onset of maximal block is reduced by about 25%, but intubating conditions 2 min later are not as good as after succinylcholine.[165] However, the introduction of rocuronium is likely to make this practice obsolete.

CARDIOVASCULAR EFFECTS.   Vecuronium usually produces no cardiovascular effects with clinical doses. It does not induce histamine release, although it may interfere with histamine metabolism.[166] Allergic reactions have been described, but no more frequently than after the use of other neuromuscular blocking drugs.

CLINICAL USE.   The cardiovascular neutrality and intermediate duration of action make vecuronium a suitable agent for use in patients with ischemic heart disease or those undergoing short, ambulatory surgery. Care should be taken when vecuronium is administered immediately after thiopental because a precipitate of barbituric acid may be formed that may obstruct the intravenous cannula.[167]

Large doses, $0.1-0.2 \; mg \cdot kg^{-1}$, with or without priming, are frequently used to facilitate tracheal intubation in place of succinylcholine. For maintenance of relaxation, vecuronium may be given using intermittent boluses, $0.01-0.02 \; mg \cdot kg^{-1}$, or by continuous infusion. Infusion rates to maintain constant neuromuscular block vary considerably, and doses of $1-2 \; \mu g \cdot kg^{-1} \cdot min^{-1}$ have been necessary to maintain 90% block. However, the rate of spontaneous recovery of neuromuscular function is slower after administration by infusion than by intermittent boluses.[168] The wide individual variation suggests that dosing should be titrated with the help of neuromuscular monitoring. Vecuronium has now largely been replaced by the more rapid rocuronium.

DRUG INTERACTIONS

Interactions between neuromuscular blocking drugs and several anesthetic and nonanesthetic drugs have been suggested. Although some interactions have been confirmed, many remain as isolated case reports or theoretical possibilities.

Interactions with Anesthetic Agents

Inhalational Agents

The anesthetic vapors potentiate neuromuscular blockade when administered in high concentration. At clinical doses, shifts in the dose–response curves of *d*-tubocurarine, gallamine, pancuronium, metocurine–pancuronium combinations, atracurium, and vecuronium have been demonstrated.[169–173] Enflurane and isoflurane are more potent than halothane in potentiating the effect of *d*-tubocurarine and pancuronium, but enflurane produces greater potentiation of vecuronium than do halothane or isoflurane.[172] When atracurium was given by continuous infusion to children, the dose required to maintain constant blockade was reduced by about 30% during halothane (0.8%) or isoflurane (1.0%) administration.[174] Also, isoflurane[169] and nitrous oxide[175] have been shown to potentiate the effect of succinylcholine.

The influence of anesthetic vapors on the effect of initial doses of NMBDs is minimal unless equilibration of the anesthetic agent is allowed to occur before administration of the NMBD.[176] More pronounced effects may be seen in the presence of sevoflurane and desflurane[177] that equilibrate more rapidly. Nevertheless, the mivacurium infusion rate required to maintain 90% neuromuscular block continues to decrease for 45 min after the start of sevoflurane inhalation.[127]

The cause of the potentiation is unknown, but the greater effect on tetanic and train-of-four responses than on single-twitch responses suggests that prejunctional mechanisms are involved.[178]

Intravenous Anesthetics

Some slight potentiation of nondepolarizing neuromuscular blocking drugs has been demonstrated with most iv induction agents in animals,[179] but this is of limited clinical importance.

Local Anesthetics

Lidocaine, procaine, and other local anesthetic agents produce neuromuscular blockade in their own right as well as potentiating the effects of depolarizing and nondepolarizing neuromuscular blocking drugs.[180] Gentamicin and lidocaine have additive effects, and profound neuromuscular block has been observed after their combined use in a patient given *d*-tubocurarine.[181]

Neuromuscular Blocking Drugs

Nondepolarizing–Nondepolarizing Interactions

Combinations of similar drugs—*e.g.,* pancuronium–vecuronium, *d*-tubocurarine–metocurine, and atracurium–mivacurium[182]—have additive effects. Other combinations tend to show potentiation. The first such synergism was demonstrated for pancuronium–metocurine combinations, and it was suggested that the combination may be used to reduce unwanted hemodynamic effects without prejudicing neuromuscular block.[115] Other combinations have also been shown to be synergistic (atracurium with *d*-tubocurarine, metocurine, mivacurium,[183] or pancuronium; vecuronium with atracurium or *d*-tubocurarine; *d*-tubocurarine with gallamine or vecuronium). Combinations of rocuronium and cisatracurium are also synergistic. The rapid onset of rocuronium was preserved,[184] while with mivacurium and pancuronium combinations the combination produced rapid recovery,[185] suggesting that the better features of each of the drugs might be conserved in the mixtures.

Administration of a combination of relaxants does not affect the degree of protein binding of either drug, so the potentiation is not the result of an increase in unbound drug. An alternative is that one drug of the pair has predominantly presynaptic activity and the other acts postsynaptically.[186] Finally, the potentiation may be entirely of postsynaptic origin as a result of asymmetric binding of different relaxants to the α subunits of the ACh receptor.[187]

Nondepolarizing–Depolarizing Interactions

Depolarizing and nondepolarizing relaxants are mutually antagonistic. When *d*-tubocurarine or other nondepolarizing agents are given before succinylcholine to prevent fasciculations and muscle pain, the succinylcholine is less potent and has a shorter duration of action[188] except after pancuronium administration when the duration of action is prolonged, presumably because pancuronium inhibits plasma cholinesterase.[189] Conversely, the potency of the nondepolarizing drugs is enhanced when they are administered after succinylcholine.[190] Isobolographic evaluation of mixtures of succinylcholine with mivacurium or atracurium demonstrate antagonism.[191] Finally, the response to a small dose of succinylcholine at the end of an anesthetic in which a nondepolarizing agent has been used is difficult to predict. It may either antagonize or potentiate the blockade, depending on the degree of nondepolarizing block.[192] In part, the ability of succinylcholine to reverse nondepolarizing block is a result of enhanced ACh release.[193] If anticholinesterase has been given, the effect of the succinylcholine is potentiated because of inhibition of plasma cholinesterase.

Antibiotics

Neomycin and streptomycin are the most potent of the aminoglycosides in depressing neuromuscular function.[194] They augment both depolarizing and nondepolarizing block and their effects are potentiated by magnesium and antagonized by calcium but only partly by anticholinesterases. Other aminoglycosides (*e.g.,* gentamicin, netilmicin) also potentiate nondepolarizing neuromuscular blockade.

The polymixins are the most potent of all antibiotics in their action at the neuromuscular junction. Their effect appears to be predominantly postjunctional. Reversal of the block is difficult: calcium and anticholinesterases are both inconsistent.

The lincosamines clindamycin and lincomycin have prejunctional and postjunctional effects, and the block cannot be reversed with calcium or anticholinesterases.

Management of a prolonged block that is suspected to have arisen from a combination of antibiotics and neuromuscular blocking drugs is difficult. Only that portion of the block due to the neuromuscular blocking drug can be reversed with anticholinesterases. Management includes mechanical support of ventilation until spontaneous breathing resumes. It is better to avoid the syndrome by administering small doses of the most potent antibiotics, particularly when they are given by the iv, intraperitoneal, or intrapleural routes.

Anticonvulsants

Resistance to pancuronium, metocurine, vecuronium, and rocuronium, but not to atracurium or mivacurium, has been demonstrated in patients receiving chronic anticonvulsant therapy with carbamazepine or phenytoin, probably as a result of up-regulation of the receptor.[195–198] Acute administration of phenytoin produces augmentation of neuromuscular block.[199]

Miscellaneous

Altered reactions to several other agents have been described.[78] These include potentiation of depolarizing and nondepolarizing blockade with β-agonist and calcium channel blockers as well as abnormal reactions in the presence of diuretics, corticosteroids, immunosuppressants, hypotensive agents, and several psychotropic drugs. Management of neuromuscular blockade in patients receiving other drugs is by titration of the dose with the help of a nerve stimulator.

ALTERED RESPONSES TO MUSCLE RELAXANTS

Muscle Relaxants in the Intensive Care Unit

There are several reports of critically ill patients who demonstrated residual weakness for unexpectedly long periods after discontinuation of a neuromuscular relaxant, which had been used to facilitate mechanical ventilation. In some, recovery took several months. A majority have occurred in asthmatics receiving high doses of methylprednisolone.[200] Pancuronium or vecuronium has been the relaxant used most frequently, but recent descriptions of similar syndromes after atracurium[201] suggest that this reflects their popularity rather than a particular association with steroid-based relaxants.[200] Some cases are the result of impaired organ excretion of the drug or an active metabolite, such as high concentrations of 3-hydroxyvecuronium in patients with renal failure.[159] Electromyographic studies have shown variable lesions from myopathy to axonal degeneration of motor and sensory fibers. The picture is complicated by the syndrome of "critical illness neuropathy," which occurs in patients with sepsis and multiorgan failure. Symptoms include failure to wean from mechanical ventilation, limb weakness, and impaired deep tendon reflexes, but sensory function is usually not affected.[202] Other predisposing conditions include electrolyte abnormality,[203] acid–base disturbance,[204] aminoglycoside antibiotics,[194] and cyclosporine.[78] There are no controlled clinical studies to allow the several initiating factors to be identified and matched with particular syndromes.

Studies in ICU patients in whom the administration of relaxant was adjusted according to strict neuromuscular monitoring criteria have shown considerable variation in the requirement for NMBD to maintain the same effect among patients[205] and a wide within-patient pharmacokinetic variability[206] but failed to demonstrate prolonged block,[207,208] suggesting that the prolonged effects were due to overdose, but this has not been confirmed. Although the most likely site of the lesion is in the motor nerve or muscle, prolonged administration of muscle relaxants may result in transmission failure from prejunctional or postjunctional mechanisms. These may include failure of synthesis and release of ACh, interference with calcium ion currents, disorganization of the postjunctional membrane, channel block, or down-regulation of the receptor.[209] These reports suggest the need for more careful monitoring of neuromuscular block in ICU patients, although the optimal method and level of block to be achieved are uncertain.[210]

Myasthenia Gravis

Myasthenia gravis is an autoimmune disease in which circulating antibodies produce a functional reduction in the number of ACh receptors.[1,211,212] The lesion is postsynaptic: the number of ACh quanta is normal and their content is either normal or increased.[213]

Diagnosis

The characteristic EMG finding in myasthenia gravis is a voltage decrement to repeated stimulation. Stimuli at 3 Hz show a fade in response to the second stimulus, and myasthenia gravis is diagnosed if the response to the fifth is reduced by 10%.[214] Latent myasthenia gravis may be revealed by testing after exercise. The diagnosis can be confirmed with the regional curare test.[215] A forearm tourniquet is applied, 0.5 mg d-tubocurarine is given iv, and the tourniquet is released after 4–5 min. Myasthenia is characterized by pronounced fade in response to train-of-nine stimulation. Edrophonium, 2–8 mg, produces brief recovery from myasthenia gravis. Finally, the diagnosis can be made by recognizing circulating ACh antibody.[216]

Response to Muscle Relaxants

Patients with myasthenia gravis are usually slightly resistant to succinylcholine,[217] but, during recovery, Phase II block develops rapidly and recovery is slow.[218] Sensitivity to nondepolarizing neuromuscular blocking drugs led to the avoidance of d-tubocurarine or pancuronium except for diagnosis. The dose required to produce neuromuscular block is reduced by about 75%. Dose–response curves for atracurium and vecuronium have characterized the response more clearly.[219,220]

Anesthesia in Myasthenia Gravis

Traditionally, neuromuscular blocking drugs have been avoided in the patient with myasthenia gravis by the use of inhalational vapors with or without local anesthesia. More recently, there have been several reports of the successful use of atracurium,[221] mivacurium,[222] or vecuronium[223] when these drugs are administered under neuromuscular monitoring. The use of atracurium or mivacurium and the avoidance of anticholinesterases seem to be particularly appropriate.

Two problems remain after thymectomy: postoperative anticholinesterase therapy and predicting the need for mechanical support of ventilation. In most patients, the dose of anticholinesterases is reduced for 1–2 days after surgery. The need for mechanical ventilation of the lungs can be predicted by preoperative lung function tests.[224] Previous suggestions that the need correlated with long-standing disease or patients taking high doses of pyridostigmine have not been confirmed.

Myotonia

Myotonia is characterized by an abnormal delay in muscle relaxation after contraction. It exists in three forms: myotonic dystrophy (dystrophia myotonica, myotonia atrophica, Steinert's disease), myotonia congenita (Thomsen's disease), and paramyotonia congenita.

Diagnosis

Repeated nerve stimulation leads to a gradual but persistent increase in muscle tension. The EMG is pathognomonic; myotonic after-discharges are seen in peripheral muscle, consisting of rapid bursts of potential produced by tapping the muscle or moving the needle. They produce typical "dive-bomber" sounds on the loudspeaker.

Response to Muscle Relaxants

The characteristic abnormality is a sustained, dose-related contracture after succinylcholine that makes ventilation difficult for 2–5 min.[225] The response to nondepolarizing drugs is normal, although myotonic responses have been observed after reversal with neostigmine.[226]

Anesthesia

Succinylcholine should be avoided and respiratory depressants used with care. Atracurium or mivacurium, without reversal, is an appropriate choice for relaxation.

Muscular Dystrophy

An increased incidence of morbidity and mortality has been described after anesthesia in the patient with Duchenne-type muscular dystrophy (DMD). In particular, there are several reports of cardiac arrest after administration of succinylcholine.[227,228] In 1993, the number of such reports[229,230] encouraged Burroughs Wellcome, the manufacturer of Anectine (succinylcholine), to state that "succinylcholine [is] contraindicated in children and adolescents except when used for emergency tracheal intubation." After further discussion the recommendation was modified to a warning. Nevertheless, it is recognized that in these patients succinylcholine-induced hyperkalemic cardiac arrest is difficult to treat[231] and carries a high mortality.

Response to Muscle Relaxants

The response to depolarizing and nondepolarizing relaxants seems to be normal, although the regional curare test demonstrates a normal blockade that lasts for longer than normal[232] and increased sensitivity to, and delayed recovery from, vecuronium has been reported.[233] Patients with the rare syndrome, ocular muscular dystrophy, exhibited extreme sensitivity to d-tubocurarine, but showed little response to anticholinesterases.[234] There is considerable controversy over whether DMD patients are susceptible to MH.[235,236]

Anesthesia

Succinylcholine should be avoided in patients with DMD. The possibility of latent or unrecognized DMD in young males (less than 10 years old) may be a reason to avoid succinylcholine in this patient population.

Upper Motor Neuron Lesions

Response to Muscle Relaxants

Patients with hemiplegia or quadriplegia as a result of central nervous system lesions show an abnormal response to depolarizing and nondepolarizing relaxants. Hyperkalemia and cardiac arrest have been described after succinylcholine, probably as a result of extrajunctional receptor spread. Hyperkalemia is usually seen from 1 week to 6 months after the lesion, so that recommendations for the avoidance of succinylcholine[237] may not be indicated in the patient with chronic weakness.[238]

Hemiplegic patients are resistant to nondepolarizing neuromuscular blocking drugs. Monitoring of the affected side shows that the block is less intense and recovery is more rapid than on the unaffected side. However, the apparently normal side also demonstrates some weakness.[239]

Miscellaneous

Denervated muscle demonstrates potassium release after succinylcholine and resistance to nondepolarizing relaxants. Contractures in response to succinylcholine have also been observed in amyotrophic lateral sclerosis, myotonia, and multiple sclerosis.[218] Succinylcholine is usually avoided in several neurologic diseases, including Friedrich's ataxia, polyneuritis, and Parkinson's disease, because of isolated reports of hyperkalemia. Hyperkalemia and cardiac arrest have also been reported in burn patients starting 24–48 hr after injury. Resistance to nondepolarizing drugs may also develop.[79]

MONITORING NEUROMUSCULAR BLOCKADE
Why Monitor?

Deep levels of paralysis are usually desired during anesthesia to facilitate tracheal intubation and to obtain an immobile surgical field. However, complete return of respiratory function must be attained before the trachea is extubated. Ventilatory depression is an important cause of anesthesia-related mortality and morbidity, and the presence of residual neuromuscular block in this setting is undoubtedly an important factor.[240,241] Administration of neuromuscular blocking drug must be individualized because blockade occurs over a narrow range of receptor occupancy,[12,59] and because there is considerable interindividual variability in response.[242] Thus, it is important for the clinician to assess the effect of neuromuscular blocking drugs without the confounding influence of volatile agents, iv anesthetics, and opioids. To test the function of the neuromuscular junction, a peripheral nerve is stimulated electrically, and the response of the muscle is assessed.

Stimulator Characteristics

The response of the nerve to electrical stimulation depends on three factors: the current applied, the duration of the current, and the position of the electrodes. Stimulators should deliver a maximum current in the range of 60–80 mA.[5] Most stimulators available for clinical use are designed to provide constant current, irrespective of impedance changes due to drying of the electrode gel, cooling, decreased sweat gland function, and so forth. However, this constant current feature does not hold for high impedances (>5 kΩ). Thus, electrodes should be firmly applied to the skin. A current display monitor on the stimulator is an asset, because accidental disconnection can be identified easily by a current approaching 0 mA. The duration of the current pulse should be long enough for all axons in the nerve to depolarize but short enough to avoid the possibility of exceeding the refractory period of the nerve. In practice, pulse durations of 0.1–0.2 msec are acceptable. At least one electrode should be on the skin overlying the nerve to be stimulated. If the negative electrode is used for this purpose, the threshold to supramaximal stimulation is less than for the positive electrode.[243,244] However, the difference is not large in practice. The position of the other electrode is not critical, but it should not be placed in the vicinity of other nerves. There is no need to use needle electrodes. Silver–silver chloride surface electrodes, used to monitor the electrocardiogram, are adequate for peripheral nerve stimulation, without the risk of bleeding, infection, and burns. In practice, applying these electrodes along the course of a nerve gives the best results.

Monitoring Modalities

Different stimulation modalities were introduced into clinical practice to take advantage of the characteristic features of nondepolarizing neuromuscular blockade: fade and post-tetanic facilitation with high-frequency stimulation. Thus, the following discussion refers mostly to nondepolarizing block.

Single Twitch

The simplest way to stimulate a nerve is to apply a single stimulus, at intervals of >10 sec. The amplitude of response is compared with a control, prerelaxant twitch height. However, because a control is required, the clinical usefulness of this mode of stimulation is limited.

Tetanus

When stimulation is applied at a frequency of ≥30 Hz, individual EMG responses can be discerned while the mechanical response of the muscle is fusion of individual twitch responses. During nondepolarizing blockade, the mechanical response appears as a peak, followed by a fade (see Fig. 16-7). In the absence of neuromuscular blocking drugs, no fade is present and the response is sustained. The sensitivity of tetanic stimulation in the detection of residual neuromuscular blockade is greater than that of single twitch, and this sensitivity increases with frequency.[59] However, at frequencies >100 Hz, some fade may be seen even in the absence of neuromuscular blocking drugs.[170] To avoid this problem, a 50-Hz, 5-sec train is used most commonly in practice. However, 100-Hz frequencies are most useful in the detection of residual block. No control prerelaxant response is required, as the degree of muscle paralysis can be assessed by the degree of fade following tetanic stimulation. However, the main disadvantage of this mode of stimulation is post-tetanic facilitation (Fig. 16-7), the extent of which depends on the frequency and duration of the tetanic stimulation. For a 50-Hz tetanus applied for 5 sec, the duration of this interval appears to be at least 1–2 min.[61] If a single-twitch stimulation is performed during that time, the response is spuriously exaggerated.

Train-of-Four

With 2-Hz stimulation, the mechanical or electrical response decreases little after the fourth stimulus, and the degree of fade is similar to that found at 50 Hz.[60] Thus, applying train-of-four stimulation at 2 Hz provides approximately the same sensitivity as tetanic stimulation at 50 Hz. In addition, this relatively low frequency allows the response to be evaluated manually or visually. Moreover, the presence of a small number of impulses eliminates the problem of post-tetanic facilitation. Train-of-four stimulation can be repeated after a pause of 10 sec. There is a fairly close relationship between single-twitch depression and train-of-four response, and no control is required for the latter.[245] With single-twitch blockade of >70–75%, four responses are not all visible. With blockade of >85–90%, only the first twitch is visible. In the range of 70–85% block, two to four twitches are visible. The train-of-four ratio, the height of the fourth twitch to that of the first twitch, is linearly related to first twitch height when blockade is <70%. When single-twitch height has recovered to 100%, the train-of-four ratio is ~70%. Thus, train-of-four stimulation is a more sensitive indicator of neuromuscular blockade than single-twitch stimulation.

Post-Tetanic Count

During profound neuromuscular blockade, there is no response to single-twitch, tetanic, or train-of-four stimulation. To estimate the time required before the return of a response, one may use a technique that depends upon the principle of post-tetanic facilitation. A 50-Hz tetanus is applied for 5 sec, followed by a 3-sec pause and by stimulation at 1 Hz. The train-of-four and tetanic responses are undetectable, but facilitation produces a certain number of visible post-tetanic twitches (Fig. 16-14). For a given drug, the number of visible twitches correlates inversely with the time required for a return of single-twitch or train-of-four responses.[246]

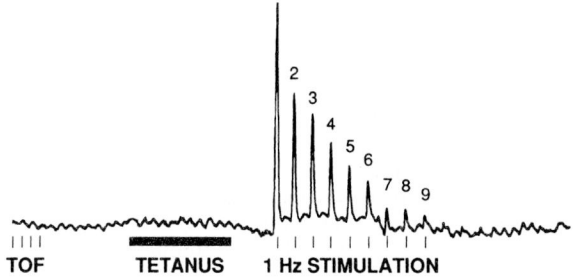

Figure 16-14. Post-tetanic count. During profound blockade, no response can be seen after train-of-four or tetanic stimulation. However, if 1-Hz stimulation is applied after the tetanus, some twitches can be seen.

Double-Burst Stimulation

Train-of-four fade may be difficult to evaluate by visual or tactile means during recovery from neuromuscular blockade.[247] This can be overcome, to a certain extent, by applying two short tetanic stimulations and evaluating the ratio of the second to the first response. Many patterns have been suggested, but the most promising consists of two trains of three impulses at 50 Hz, separated by 750 msec.[248] The double-burst stimulation ratio correlates closely with the train-of-four ratio (Fig. 16-15)[248,249] but is easier to detect manually.[249,250] At least 12–15 sec must elapse between two consecutive double-burst stimulations.[248,249]

Recording the Response

Visual and Tactile Evaluation

When electrical stimulation is applied to a nerve, the easiest and least expensive way to assess the response is to observe or feel the response of the muscle. This method is easily adaptable to any superficial muscle. However, serious errors in assessment can be made. In the case of evaluating the response of the adductor pollicis to ulnar nerve stimulation, the train-of-four count can be made reliably during a surgical procedure,[251] but the quantitative assessment of train-of-four ratio is difficult to make during recovery. Several investigations suggest that train-of-four ratios as low as 0.3[249,250] can remain undetected. The detection rate for tetanic fade (50 Hz) is no better.[252] With

double-burst stimulation, fade can be detected reliably up to train-of-four ratios in the range of 0.5–0.6.[249,250]

Measurement of Force

A force transducer can overcome the shortcomings of one's senses. If applied correctly, the device provides accurate and reliable responses, displayed as either a digital or an analog signal on a monitor, such as an electrocardiogram screen. Unfortunately, transducers are applicable to only one muscle, usually the adductor pollicis. Force measurement can be used with single-twitch, tetanus, train-of-four, double-burst, or post-tetanic stimulation. However, the availability of tetanus and double-burst stimulation is superfluous if accurate recording of the train-of-four response can be made.

Electromyography

It is possible to measure the electrical instead of the mechanical response of the muscle (see Fig. 16-4). One electrode should be positioned over the neuromuscular junction, which is usually close to the midportion of the muscle, and the other near the insertion of the muscle. A third, neutral electrode can be located anywhere else. Theoretically, any superficial muscle can be used for EMG recordings. In practice, such recordings are limited to the hypothenar eminence, the first dorsal interosseous, and the adductor pollicis muscles, which are supplied by the ulnar nerve. Most EMG recording devices compute the area under the EMG curve during a specified time window (usually 3–18 msec) after the stimulus is applied.[253] This integrated EMG response is considered a better representation of the overall muscular activity than the measurement of peak response. There is usually good correlation between EMG and force of the adductor pollicis if the EMG signal is taken from the thenar eminence.[254] The signal obtained from the hypothenar eminence is larger and less subject to movement artifacts, but it can underestimate the degree of paralysis when compared with the adductor pollicis.[255]

Accelerometry

Accelerometers respond to acceleration, which, according to Newton's law, is proportional to force if mass remains unchanged. The device is usually attached to the tip of the thumb and a digital read-out is obtained. The setup is sensitive to inadvertent displacement of the thumb and, in the absence of neuromuscular blocking drugs, train-of-four ratios > 100% can be obtained.[256]

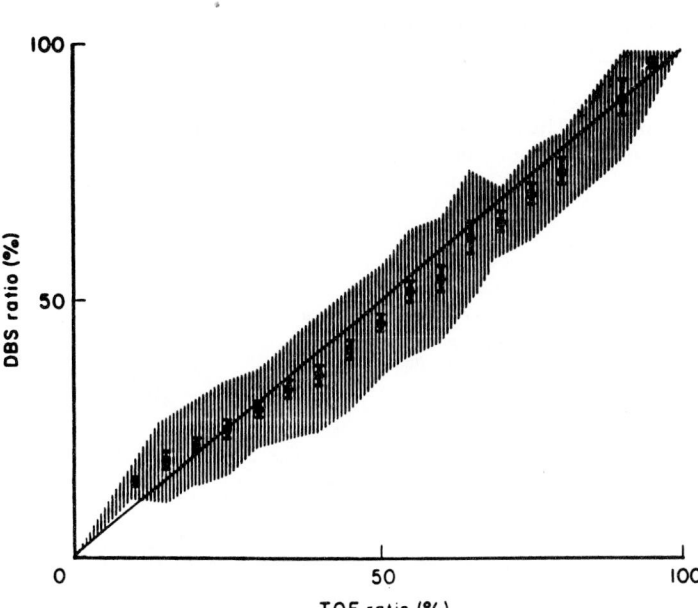

Figure 16-15. Relationship between double-burst stimulation (DBS) and train-of-four stimulation (TOF). The shaded zone shows 95% confidence limits and the line is the line of identity. (Reprinted with permission from Gill S, Donati F, Bevan DR: Clinical evaluation of double burst stimulation: Its relationship to train-of-four stimulation. Anaesthesia 45:543, 1989.)

Choice of Muscle

Muscles do not respond in a uniform fashion to neuromuscular blocking drugs. After administration of a neuromuscular blocking agent, differences can be measured with respect to onset time, maximum blockade, and duration of action. Ideally, it would be best to monitor the muscles of practical importance, such as those that must be relaxed during surgery (*e.g.,* the abdominal muscles), or the respiratory and airway that must recover postoperatively. One approach is to choose a monitoring site that has a response similar to the muscle of interest. For example, monitoring the response of the facial nerve around the eye is a good indicator of intubating conditions, and the use of the adductor pollicis during recovery reflects upper airway muscle function. If one prefers not to change sites depending on circumstances, one has to interpret the information provided by monitoring, usually at the adductor pollicis, from knowledge of the possible differences among muscles (Fig. 16-16).

Adductor Pollicis

The adductor pollicis, supplied by the ulnar nerve, is accessible during most surgical procedures. Its force of contraction can be measured easily, and it has become a standard in research. After injection of a dose of muscle relaxant, the time to maximal blockade is longer than in centrally located muscles.[257,258] The adductor pollicis is relatively sensitive to nondepolarizing neuromuscular blocking drugs, and during recovery it is blocked more than some respiratory muscles such as the diaphragm,[257,258] laryngeal adductors,[259] and rectus abdominis.[260]

Other Muscles of the Hand

Ulnar nerve stimulation also produces flexion and abduction of the fifth finger, which usually recovers before the adductor pollicis, the discrepancy in first twitch or train-of-four ratio being of the order of 15–20%.[255] Relying on the response of the fifth finger might overestimate recovery from blockade. Abduction of the index finger also results from stimulation of the ulnar nerve because of contraction of the first dorsal interosseous, the sensitivity of which is comparable to that of the adductor pollicis.[254] The hypothenar eminence (near the fifth finger) and the first dorsal interosseous are particularly well suited for EMG recordings.[253]

Muscles Surrounding the Eye

There seem to be major differences in the response of muscles innervated by the facial nerve and located around the eye. The response of the orbicularis oculi over the eyelid is similar to that of the adductor pollicis,[261] but recordings over the eyebrow are similar to that of the laryngeal adductors.[262] Onset of blockade is more rapid and recovery occurs sooner than at the adductor pollicis.[257] Thus, facial nerve stimulation with inspection of the response of the eyebrow (which most likely represents the effect of the corrugator supercilii, not the orbicularis oculi) is indicated to predict intubating conditions and to monitor profound blockade. The facial nerve can be stimulated 2–3 cm posterior to the lateral border of the orbit.

Muscles of the Foot

The posterior tibial nerve, which can be stimulated behind the internal malleolus, produces flexion of the big toe by contraction of the flexor hallucis. The response of this muscle is comparable to that of the adductor pollicis.[263] Stimulation of the external peroneal nerve produces dorsiflexion, but the sensitivity of the muscles involved has not been measured.

Clinical Applications

Monitoring Onset

The quality of intubating conditions depends chiefly on the state of relaxation of muscles of the jaw, pharynx, larynx, and respiratory system. Onset of action is faster in all these muscles than in the hand or foot because they are closer to the central circulation and they receive a greater blood flow. Among these central muscles, the diaphragm and especially the laryngeal adductors are the most resistant to nondepolarizing agents. Data on laryngeal muscles are important not only because easy passage of the tracheal tube can be performed if vocal cords are relaxed, but also because all other muscles can be presumed to be blocked if the resistant laryngeal muscles are blocked. The relationship between onset time in laryngeal and hand muscles depends on dose. At relatively low doses (*e.g.,* rocuronium, 0.4–0.6 mg · kg^{-1}), onset time is slower at the adductor pollicis than at the laryngeal muscles. If the dose is increased (*e.g.,* rocuronium, 0.8–1.0 mg · kg^{-1}), onset is faster at the adductor pollicis because these doses produce 100% blockade at the adductor pollicis without blocking laryngeal muscles completely.[264] Onset time decreases considerably in any muscle if the dose given is sufficient to reach 100%. Finally, if the dose is large enough to block the laryngeal muscles completely, onset time again becomes shorter at the larynx. It is not surprising that monitoring the adductor pollicis muscle predicts intubating conditions poorly. Facial nerve stimulation with visual observation of the response over the eyebrow gives better results because the response of the corrugator supercilii is close to that of the vocal cords. Train-of-four fade takes longer to develop than single-twitch depression (see Fig. 16-7), and train-of-four stimulation does not have any advantages over single-twitch stimulation at 0.1 Hz.

Surgical Relaxation

Adequate surgical relaxation is usually obtained when fewer than two or three visible twitches are observed at the adductor pollicis. However, this criterion might prove inadequate in certain circumstances when profound relaxation is required owing

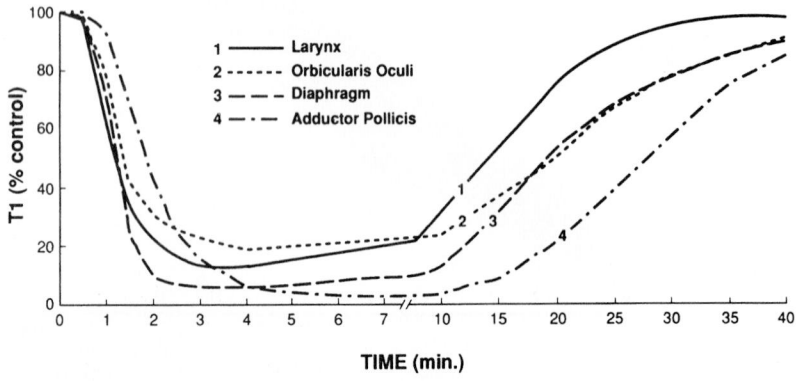

Figure 16-16. Onset and recovery after vecuronium, 0.07 mg · kg^{-1}, at various muscles, versus time. Onset of action is more rapid at the larynx, orbicularis oculi, and diaphragm than at the adductor pollicis. Recovery occurs first at the larynx and last at the adductor pollicis. (Reprinted with permission from Donati F, Meistelman C, Plaud B: Vecuronium neuromuscular blockade at the diaphragm, the orbicularis oculi, and adductor pollicis muscles. Anesthesiology 73:870, 1990.)

to the discrepancy between the adductor pollicis and other muscles. In this case, the post-tetanic count can be used at the adductor pollicis,[246] provided that this type of stimulation is not repeated more often than every 2–3 min. A suitable alternative is stimulation of the facial nerve with observation of the response over the eyebrow, which recovers at the same rate as such resistant muscles as the diaphragm.[257]

Monitoring Recovery

Complete return of neuromuscular function should be achieved at the conclusion of surgery unless mechanical ventilation is planned. Thus, monitoring is useful in determining whether spontaneous recovery has progressed to a degree that allows reversal agents to be given and to assess the effect of these agents.

The effectiveness of anticholinesterases depends directly on the degree of recovery present when they are administered. Preferably, reversal agents should be given only when four twitches are visible, which corresponds to a first-twitch recovery of >25%. The dose of anticholinesterase can also be adjusted according to the extent of recovery. For this assessment, using the adductor pollicis is preferable. The presence of spontaneous respiration is not a sign of adequate neuromuscular recovery. The diaphragm recovers earlier than the much more sensitive upper airway muscles. For example, the geniohyoid recovers, on average, at the same time as the adductor pollicis.[265] To prevent upper airway obstruction after extubation, it is preferable to use the adductor pollicis to monitor recovery, instead of the more resistant muscles of the hypothenar eminence[255] or those around the eye.[257]

Finally, the adequacy of recovery should be assessed. Traditionally, a train-of-four ratio of 0.7 was considered to be the threshold below which residual weakness of the respiratory muscles could be present.[266] There is abundant evidence that significant weakness may occur up to train-of-four values of 0.9. Awake volunteers given mivacurium failed to perform the head-lift test when the train-of-four ratio at the adductor pollicis decreased below 0.62, but needed a train-of-four ratio of at least 0.86 to hold a tongue depressor between their teeth.[267] This suggests that the head-lift test does not guarantee full recovery, and that the upper airway muscles used to retain a tongue depressor are very sensitive to the residual effects of neuromuscular blocking drugs. Furthermore, impairment in swallowing and laryngeal aspiration of a pharyngeal fluid was observed at train-of-four ratios as high as 0.9 in volunteers given vecuronium.[268]

Anesthetized patients appear considerably more sensitive to the ventilatory effects of neuromuscular blocking drugs than are awake patients.[269] Whereas tidal volume is preserved in awake patients receiving relatively high doses of neuromuscular blocking drugs, anesthetized adults have a decreased tidal volume and increased PCO_2 with doses of pancuronium as low as 0.5 mg (Fig. 16-17). In conscious volunteers, administration of small doses of vecuronium to maintain train-of-four at less than 0.9 leads to severe impairment of the ventilatory response to hypoxia. The response to hypercapnia is maintained, and this indicates that the response to hypoxia is not due to respiratory muscle weakness.[270]

Taken together, the results of these investigations indicate that normal respiratory and upper airway function does not return to normal unless the train-of-four ratio at the adductor pollicis is 0.9 or more. However, it has become apparent that human senses fail to detect either a train-of-four or tetanic fade when the train-of-four ratio is as low as 0.3.[247,250] With double-burst stimulation, detection failures may occur at train-of-four ratios of 0.5–0.6.[249,250] The detection rate may be improved somewhat with train-of-four or double burst if submaximal (less than supramaximal) currents are used,[271] and/or if the movement of the first dorsal interosseous is assessed at the index finger.[272] Compared with the train-of-four, the ability to detect fade is

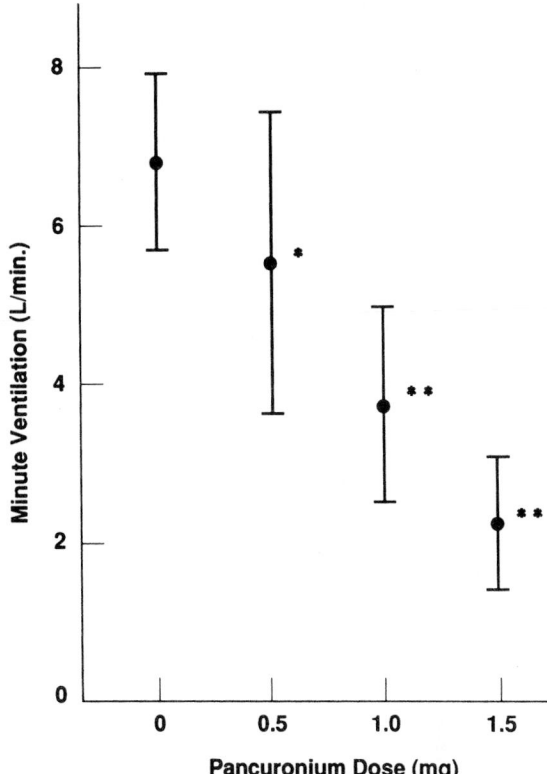

Figure 16-17. Minute ventilation in adults anesthetized with enflurane given the cumulative dose of pancuronium indicated. (Reprinted with permission from Nishino T, Yokokawa N, Hiraga K *et al:* Breathing pattern of anesthetized humans during pancuronium-induced partial paralysis. J Appl Physiol 64:78, 1988.)

not improved by using tetanic stimulation at 50 Hz for 5 sec.[252] However, tetanic fade can be felt manually at train-of-four ratios of 0.8–0.9 by using 100-Hz tetanic stimulation.[273] Because of the presence of post-tetanic facilitation, this test should not be used more often than every 2 min. Mechanographic and EMG equipment give reliable values of train-of-four ratio, but the use of this equipment is limited by size, cost, and convenience. Accelerometers are less bulky and cheaper, but they can overestimate the value of train-of-four ratio during recovery. In any event, clinicians must be aware of the limitations of the tests they are using and complete their evaluations with clinical tests.

Factors Affecting the Monitoring of Neuromuscular Blockade

Many drugs interfere with neuromuscular function and these are dealt with elsewhere. However, certain situations make the interpretation of data on neuromuscular function difficult. For example, hypothermia decreases the response when neuromuscular blocking drugs are given. Thus, if the monitored hand is cold, the degree of paralysis will appear to be increased.[274] Resistance to nondepolarizing neuromuscular blocking drugs occurs with nerve damage, including peripheral nerve trauma, cord transection, and stroke. In this case, monitoring of the involved limb would tend to underestimate the degree of muscle paralysis.[275,276] A noninvolved extremity should be used. The level of paralysis should also be adjusted for the type of patient, as well as the type of surgery. For example, it is not necessary to paralyze frail individuals or patients at the extremes of age to the same extent as young muscular adults. The same applies to patients with debilitating muscular diseases.

It may be argued that neuromuscular monitoring has limited usefulness because the response of one skeletal muscle cannot be taken as representative of the whole body, and because major errors in assessment can be made. In two studies, monitoring did not influence the amount of relaxant given or the incidence of postoperative residual block.[277,278] In at least two other investigations, monitoring and administration of neuromuscular blocking reversal drugs according to rigid criteria decreased the incidence of residual paralysis.[279,280] It must be recognized that the effect of the neuromuscular blocking drug is the same whether or not monitoring is used. Neuromuscular monitoring can help in the diagnosis of inadequate skeletal muscle relaxation during surgery or insufficient recovery after surgery, but does not, in itself, treat these conditions.

ANTAGONISM OF NEUROMUSCULAR BLOCK

The aim in the reversal of neuromuscular blockade is to ensure that the patient leaves the operating room with unimpaired muscle strength. In some circumstances, however, this is not desirable—for example, when it has been decided to continue mechanical support of ventilation into the postoperative period. And occasionally, complete recovery is unattainable.

Assessment of Neuromuscular Blockade

The principal goal of reversal is the re-establishment of spontaneous respiration and the ability to protect the airway from aspiration. Sensitive tests of pulmonary function, such as vital capacity, maximum voluntary ventilation, and forced expiratory flow rate, are difficult to perform in everyday practice, particularly when the patient is recovering from general anesthesia. Consequently, several indirect indices, which are easier to measure, have been correlated with the more specific tests of ventilatory function. Spontaneous ventilation, adequate to prevent hypercapnia, can be maintained despite considerable measurable skeletal muscle weakness if a patent airway is ensured.

Clinical Evaluation

Several crude tests have been suggested, including head lift for 5 sec, tongue protrusion, and the ability to lift the legs off the bed. The maximum inspiratory pressure (MIP) has been correlated with tests of skeletal muscle strength (vital capacity, head lift, hand grip, leg raising) and of airway musculature (ability to swallow, approximate the vocal cords, maintain a patent airway, and to elevate the mandible) in conscious volunteers receiving subparalyzing doses of d-tubocurarine.[281] The MIP was reduced successively. Head lift and leg raising were affected first, typically at an MIP of −53 and −50 cm H_2O, respectively. At an MIP of −20 to −25 cm H_2O, none of the subjects could swallow or maintain a patent airway, and hand grip was abolished. Nevertheless, as long as the mandible was elevated by an observer, the vital capacity was 40% of control and PET_{CO_2} was normal. Thus, the ability to maintain head lift for 5 sec usually indicates sufficient strength to protect the airway and support ventilation.[281] Grip strength is more sensitive, but its assessment requires a dynamometer and preoperative control values so that it is a less useful clinical tool. In infants and neonates the ability to lift both legs off the table as a reflex response[282] appears to be as sensitive as the head lift in adults. Kopman has shown, in volunteers, that the most sensitive test is the ability to clamp the jaws shut and prevent removal of a wooden spatula. This correlated with a TOF of >0.86, whereas 5-sec leg lift correlated with a TOF of 0.6. All subjects complained of visual symptoms until TOF > 0.9.[267]

Evoked Responses to Nerve Stimulation

Clinical tests may be unobtainable in the patient recovering from anesthesia. Also, head lift may be impaired as a result of pain. Evoked responses to nerve stimulation are then appropriate. When the mechanical train-of-four ratio at the adductor pollicis is 0.7, most clinical tests of neuromuscular function

have returned to normal,[266,283] although, in some patients, head lift may be impaired unless train-of-four is 0.9.[284] This assumes that such a level of train-of-four recovery can be recognized, but subjective assessment of train-of-four fade is unreliable and is usually undetected until values are less than 0.4–0.5.[249,250] Double-burst stimulation is more sensitive, but 28–58% of cases of TOF 0.4–0.7 may be missed.[249,250] The most sensitive test is the ability to maintain sustained contraction to 100-Hz tetanus for 5 sec.[273]

Detection of residual neuromuscular block is difficult unless the patient is awake and cooperative. Small degrees of paralysis will not be detected by train-of-four monitoring. However, this should not be an excuse to avoid neuromuscular monitoring. Rather, train-of-four monitoring should be done to ensure that there is no detectable fade when the patient leaves the operating room. This will not guarantee full recovery, which awaits confirmation in the PACU when the patient is awake.

Residual Paralysis

Several studies have demonstrated that residual neuromuscular blockade is frequent in patients in the recovery room after surgery. Viby-Mogensen et al found in 72 adult patients given d-tubocurarine, gallamine, or pancuronium that the train-of-four ratio was 0.7 in 30 (42%) patients, and 16 of the 68 patients who were awake were unable to sustain head lift for 5 sec.[285] Similar results have been obtained in Sweden,[286] Australia,[287] Canada,[284] and the United States.[288] The incidence of train-of-four ratio 0.7 is about 30% following the use of the longer acting agents d-tubocurarine, pancuronium, alcuronium, and gallamine, but is reduced to 10% after using atracurium or vecuronium for operations lasting 2 h.[284,289] Recovery from mivacurium is more rapid. However, if neuromuscular blockade is maintained up to the end of surgery and patients are moved rapidly to the PACU, residual block may be detected.[290]

Clinical Importance

Until recently, it was difficult to determine the importance of residual neuromuscular blockade. In a report on deaths occurring within 6 days of surgery, 11 of the 32 deaths due entirely to anesthesia were caused by postoperative ventilatory failure. The presence of neuromuscular block was considered to be contributory in 6 of those deaths.[291] Although intense residual block has been demonstrated in patients arriving in the PACU after cardiac surgery,[292,293] the choice of intermediate or long-acting NMBD has not affected ICU or hospital length of stay.[294] However, in 1997 Berg et al studied nearly 700 patients who randomly received pancuronium, vecuronium, or atracurium to produce surgical relaxation. In patients whose TOF ratio was <0.7 on arrival in the PACU and who had received pancuronium, the incidence of postoperative partial paralysis was three times greater than in patients receiving either of the two intermediate-acting drugs.[289] Residual block is important.

Although TOF 0.7 has been taken as the gold standard for recovery of neuromuscular block, less intense blockade is associated with physiologic disturbances. Eriksson et al showed that, in volunteers, TOF 0.7 was associated with impaired ventilatory responses to hypoxia and disturbed esophageal motility,[270] both of which may predispose to respiratory sequelae.

Anticholinesterase Pharmacology

The pharmacologic principle involved in the reversal of muscle relaxants is the reduction of the effect of competitive blocking drugs by increasing the concentration of ACh at the neuromuscular junction.

Mechanism of Action

Neostigmine, edrophonium, and pyridostigmine inhibit acetylcholinesterase, but this may not be the only mechanism by which blockade is antagonized.

Neostigmine and pyridostigmine are attached to the anionic and esteratic sites of the acetylcholinesterase molecule and produce longer-lasting inhibition than edrophonium. Neostigmine and pyridostigmine are inactivated by the interaction with the enzyme, whereas edrophonium is unaffected.[295]

Inhibition of acetylcholinesterase results in an increase in the amount of ACh that reaches the receptor and in the time that ACh remains in the synaptic cleft. This causes an increase in the size and duration of the endplate potentials.[296,297] Anticholinesterases also have presynaptic effects. In the absence of neuromuscular blocking drugs, they potentiate the normal twitch response in a way similar to succinylcholine, probably as a result of the generation of action potentials that spread antidromically.[16]

Anticholinesterases have other effects at the junction than inhibition of acetylcholinesterase. For example, the relationship between the train-of-four ratio and T1 depression is not the same for all agents.[298] Also, anticholinesterases react with single ACh receptors *in vitro* to decrease channel open time.[299]

The three anticholinesterases have a ceiling effect, at least *in vitro*.[300] Also, the effect of neostigmine may be modified by atropine[301] and by epinephrine, both of which augment the ability of neostigmine to reverse the blockade.

Neostigmine Block

Large doses of anticholinesterases, greater than those used clinically, may produce neuromuscular blockade. Fade of both EMG and MMG responses has been observed during tetanic stimulation after clinical doses of neostigmine[302] but not edrophonium[303] were given to reverse neuromuscular blockade. Paradoxically, this neostigmine effect is antagonized with small doses of nondepolarizing relaxants. The mechanism involved is uncertain, but it appears to be of little clinical importance.

Potency

Dose–response curves have been constructed for edrophonium, neostigmine, and pyridostigmine. During a constant infusion of neuromuscular blocking drugs, the curves are obtained by plotting the peak effect versus the dose of reversal agent. In this situation, neostigmine was found to be ~12 times as potent as edrophonium.[304] A similar relationship has been found during spontaneous recovery when the reversal agent was given at 10% T_1 recovery, and the values obtained at 10 min were used to construct the curves.[305] Potency ratios are difficult to determine because the slopes of the edrophonium and neostigmine curves are not parallel. In addition, the slope for edrophonium is flatter for train-of-four recovery than for T_1 recovery,[306] and the curves were shifted to the right when reversal of a more intense (99%) block was attempted[307] (Fig. 16-18). There is no difference in the dose–response relationship of anticholinesterases if vecuronium is infused instead of pancuronium.[308] However, there is a marked shift to the left for the curves obtained during vecuronium block if the reversal agent is given during spontaneous recovery.[309]

Pharmacokinetics

Following bolus iv injection, the plasma concentration of the anticholinesterases decreases rapidly during the first 5–10 min and then more slowly. Two-compartment analysis has demonstrated similar values for the three drugs.[310,311] Volumes of distribution are in the range of 0.7–1.4 $1 \cdot kg^{-1}$ and the $T_{1/2}\beta$ is 60–120 min. The drugs are water-soluble, ionized compounds so that their principal route of excretion is the kidney. Their clearances are in the range of 8–16 $ml \cdot kg^{-1} \cdot min^{-1}$, which is much greater than the GFR because they are actively secreted into the tubular lumen.[312] Their clearance is reduced markedly in patients in renal failure.

Pharmacodynamics

The onset of action of edrophonium (1–2 min) to peak effect is much more rapid than that of neostigmine (7–11 min) or

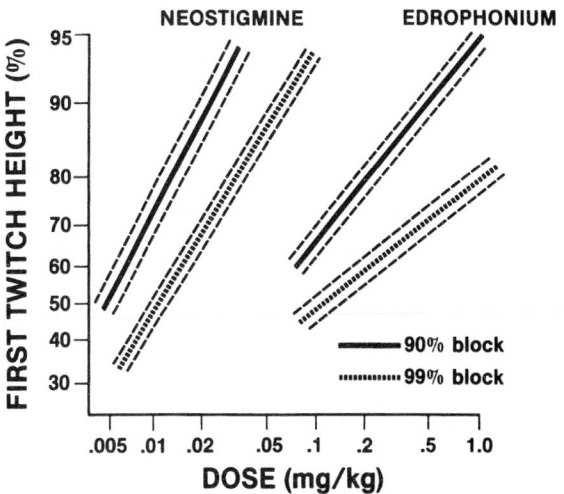

Figure 16-18. Dose–response curves for edrophonium and neostigmine in reversing 90% and 99% atracurium block. (Reprinted with permission from Donati F, Smith CE, Bevan DR: Dose–response relationships for edrophonium and neostigmine as antagonists of moderate and profound aztracurium blockade. Anesth Analg 68:13, 1989.)

pyridostigmine (15–20 min) (Fig. 16-19).[304,313–315] The reason for the differences is uncertain, but may be related to the different rates of binding to the enzyme.

The duration of action corresponds to their pharmacokinetic behavior. In practice, the recovery of neuromuscular activity after reversal has two components: slow recovery from the relaxant and rapid, augmented recovery induced by the reversal agent. No recurarization should be expected after reversal unless the duration of action of the relaxants exceeds that of the reversal agents.

Factors Affecting Reversal

Several factors modify the rate of recovery of neuromuscular activity after reversal.

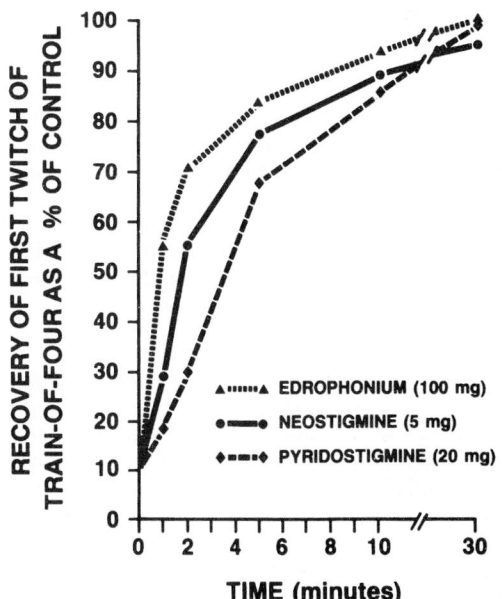

Figure 16-19. Onset of action of edrophonium, neostigmine, and pyridostigmine in the reversal of 90% pancuronium block. (Data from Ferguson A, Egerszegi P, Bevan DR: Neostigmine, pyridostigmine, and edrophonium as antagonists of pancuronium. Anesthesiology 53:300, 1980.)

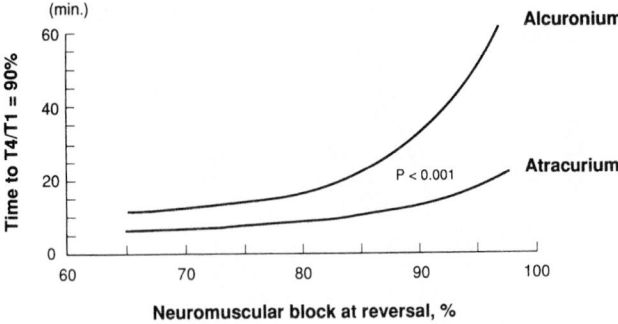

Figure 16-20. Relationship between time to recovery and prereversal twitch height after reversal of alcuronium, a long-acting relaxant, or atracurium with edrophonium in children. (Reprinted with permission from Meretoja OA, Gebert R: Postoperative neuromuscular block following atracurium in children. Can J Anaesth 37:743, 1990.)

Block Intensity

The more intense the block at the time of reversal, the longer the recovery of neuromuscular activity[316,317] (Fig. 16-20). In addition, neostigmine is more effective than edrophonium or pyridostigmine in antagonizing intense (90%) blockade.[307] When reversal is administered after spontaneous recovery to $\geq 25\%$ T_1 has occurred, recovery is rapid and the time from reversal to TOF 0.7 is usually only a few minutes, although recovery after pancuronium may not be complete.[318] Thus, it has been recommended that reversal should not be attempted until $T_1 \geq 25\%$[319] when four twitches to TOF stimulation are visible. The duration of action of atracurium (time from administration to TOF 0.7) is least when reversal is performed at TOF 0.04.[320] Reversal can be attempted earlier, at least after small doses of rocuronium, vecuronium, and rapacuronium, even as early as 2–5 min after administration of relaxant. However, the earlier that reversal is attempted, the longer is the time from reversal administration to TOF 0.7. In fact, the relaxant recovery time is similar when reversal is attempted at $T_1 \leq 25\%$: shorter for rapacuronium (17 min[143]) than for rocuronium and vecuronium (27 min[144]). Thus, there is little advantage in attempting early reversal except in situations where tracheal intubation and pulmonary ventilation are compromised.

Anticholinesterase Dose

With more intense block a certain degree of recovery (TOF 0.7) can be obtained within a reasonable time (10 min) by increasing the dose of reversal agent. However, because of the ceiling effect, there is little benefit in administering >0.07 $mg \cdot kg^{-1}$ neostigmine.

Attempts have been made to accelerate reversal by administering the anticholinesterase in divided doses, the priming principle. Although some acceleration can be demonstrated, the effect is small and of limited clinical importance.[321]

Choice of Relaxant

Recovery of neuromuscular activity after reversal is dependent on the rate of spontaneous recovery as well as the acceleration induced by the reversal agent. Consequently, the overall recovery of short-acting agents (atracurium, vecuronium, mivacurium, rocuronium) following the same dose of anticholinesterase is more rapid than after pancuronium, *d*-tubocurarine, or gallamine.[306–309] Conversely, the doses of reversal agent required to achieve the same degree of recovery are greater after the long-acting than the short-acting relaxants. For example, the dose of neostigmine required to achieve 80% twitch activity 10 min after reversal of 90% block is ~40–50 $\mu g \cdot kg^{-1}$ with pancuronium and *d*-tubocurarine; 20–30 $\mu g \cdot kg^{-1}$ with atracurium, vecuronium,[309] and rocuronium[322]; and 5 $\mu g \cdot kg^{-1}$ with mivacurium.[323] However, after prolonged infusions of vecuro-

nium, spontaneous recovery becomes dependent upon elimination and metabolism rather than redistribution. Thus, the difference between vecuronium and pancuronium will be diminished because of their similar $T_{1/2}\beta$.[162]

Age

Recovery of neuromuscular activity occurs more rapidly[324] with smaller doses[325] of anticholinesterases in infants and children than in adults (Fig. 16-21). Thus, residual weakness in the PACU is found less frequently in children than in adults.[326] Although the clearance of nondepolarizing relaxants is decreased in the elderly, the speed and extent of recovery after reversal are not affected, probably because the elimination of anticholinesterases is also reduced.

Drug Interaction

Several drugs potentiate the action of neuromuscular blocking drugs, but there are few reports of impaired reversal. In the presence of enflurane and isoflurane, the reversal of pancuronium and vecuronium blockade is impaired, but only if the administration of the vapor is continued during reversal.[327]

Renal Failure

Anticholinesterases are actively secreted into the tubular lumen[312] so that their clearance is reduced in renal failure.[310–311] The rate and extent of recovery of pancuronium in renal failure after neostigmine are not impaired in renal failure, and "recurarization" does not occur.[328]

Acid–Base Balance, Electrolytes

The influence of acid–base disturbances on the reversal of neuromuscular blockade is poorly understood. Although it has been suggested that reversal is impaired in the ill, cachectic patient (neostigmine-resistant curarization) as a result of acidosis, this has been difficult to confirm in the laboratory.[329]

In addition to the prolonged block induced by magnesium sulfate, the recovery of vecuronium-induced block was prolonged in patients who had received 60 $\mu g \cdot kg^{-1}$ MgSO$_4$.[330]

Other Effects

Cardiovascular

Anticholinesterases provoke profound vagal stimulation. The time course of the vagal effects parallels the reversal of block:

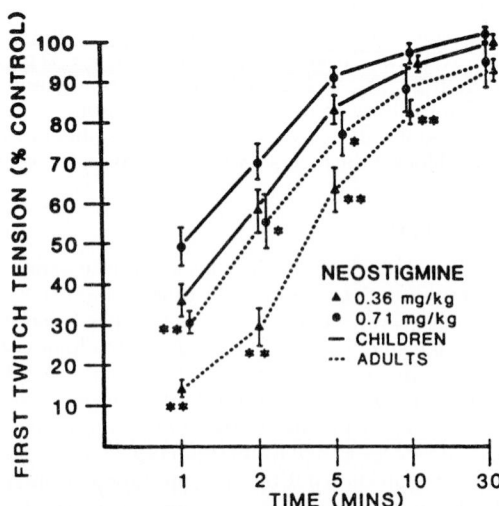

Figure 16-21. Comparison of recovery after reversal of 90% pancuronium blockade with neostigmine in adults and children. (Reprinted with permission from Meakin G, Sweet PT, Bevan JC *et al:* Neostigmine and edrophonium as antagonists of pancuronium in infants and children. Anesthesiology 59:316, 1983.)

rapid for edrophonium and slower for neostigmine. However, the bradycardia and bradyarrhythmias can be prevented with anticholinergic agents. Atropine has a rapid onset of action (1 min), duration of 30–60 min, and crosses the blood–brain barrier. Its time course makes it appropriate for use in combination with edrophonium,[304] whereas glycopyrrolate (onset 2–3 min) is more suitable with neostigmine or pyridostigmine. Because glycopyrrolate does not cross the blood–brain barrier, the incidence of memory deficits after anesthesia is less than that after atropine.[314] If atropine is given with neostigmine, the dose is approximately half that of neostigmine (atropine 20 $\mu g \cdot kg^{-1}$ versus neostigmine 40 $\mu g \cdot kg^{-1}$). Such a combination leads to an initial tachycardia followed by a slight bradycardia. Atropine requirements are less with edrophonium (atropine 7–10 $\mu g \cdot kg^{-1}$ versus edrophonium 0.5 mg $\cdot kg^{-1}$).

Other Cholinergic Effects

Anticholinesterases produce increased salivation and bowel motility. Although atropine blocks the former, it appears to have little effect on peristalsis. Some reports claim an increase in bowel anastomotic leakage after the reversal of neuromuscular blockade.[331] Others have held the use of anticholinesterases to be responsible for an increased incidence of vomiting after ambulatory surgery.[332]

Respiratory Effects

Anticholinesterases may cause an increase in airway resistance, but anticholinergics reduce this effect. Several other factors, such as pain, the presence of an endotracheal tube, or light anesthesia, may predispose to bronchoconstriction at the end of surgery so that it is difficult to incriminate the reversal agents.

Clinical Use

Several reversal regimens have been proposed and are effective. In general, the more intense the block, the greater the dose of anticholinesterase that is required. However, there does not seem to be any advantage in giving more than the equivalent of neostigmine 0.07 mg $\cdot kg^{-1}$. Neostigmine is preferred to edrophonium for intense block, but the rapid action of edrophonium has the advantage of allowing the extent of reversal to be assessed in the operating room.

REFERENCES

1. Boonyapisit K, Kaminski HJ, Ruff RL: Disorders of neuromuscular junction ion channels. Am J Med 106:97,1999
2. Sanes JR, Lichtman JW: Development of the vertebrate neuromuscular junction. Annu Rev Neurosci 22:389,1999
3. Ibebunjo C, Srikant CB, Donati F: Properties of fibres, endplates and acetylcholine receptors in the diaphragm, masseter, laryngeal, abdominal and limb muscles in the goat. Can J Anaesth 43:475, 1996
4. Catterall WA: Cellular and molecular biology of voltage-gated sodium channels. Physiol Rev 72:S15, 1992
5. Kopman AF, Lawson D: Milliamperage requirements for supramaximal stimulation of the ulnar nerve with surface electrodes. Anesthesiology 61:83, 1984
6. Ellisman MH, Rash JE, Staehelin A, Porter KR: Studies of excitable membranes: II. A comparison of specialization at neuromuscular junctions and nonjunctional sarcolemmas of mammalian fast and slow twitch muscle fibers. J Cell Biol 68:752, 1976
7. Van der Kloot W, Molgo J: Quantal acetylcholine release at the vertebrate neuromuscular junction. Physiol Rev 74:899, 1994
8. Calakos N, Scheller RH: Synaptic vesicle biogenesis, docking, and fusion: A molecular description. Physiol Rev 76:1, 1996
9. Sastry BVR: Nicotinic receptor. Anaesth Pharmacol Rev 1:6, 1993
10. Wood SJ, Slater CR: The contribution of postsynaptic folds to the safety factor for neuromuscular transmission in rat fast- and slow-twitch muscles. J Physiol (Lond) 500 (Pt 1):165, 1997
11. Anderson OS, Koeppe RE: Molecular determinants of channel function. Physiol Rev 72:S89, 1992
12. Paton WDM, Waud DR: The margin of safety of neuromuscular transmission. J Physiol 191:59, 1967
13. Vincent A, Newland C, Croxen R, Beeson D: Genes at the junction—candidates for congenital myasthenic syndromes. Trends Neurosci 20:15, 1997
14. Gibb AJ, Marshall IG: Pre- and post-junctional effects of tubocurarine and other nicotinic antagonists during repetitive stimulation in the rat. J Physiol 351:275, 1984
15. MacDermott AB, Role LW, Siegelbaum SA: Presynaptic ionotropic receptors and the control of transmitter release. Annu Rev Neurosci 22:443, 1999
16. Baker T, Stanec A: Drug actions at mammalian motor endings: The suppression of neostigmine-induced fasciculations by vecuronium and isoflurane. Anesthesiology 67:942, 1987
17. Bedford RE: From the FDA. Anesthesiology 82:33A, 1995
18. Stevens JB, Wheatley L: Tracheal intubation in ambulatory surgery patients: Using remifentanil and propofol without relaxants. Anesth Analg 86:45, 1998
19. Barclay K, Eggers K, Asai T: Low-dose rocuronium improves conditions for tracheal intubation after induction of anaesthesia with propofol and alfentanil. Br J Anaesth 78:92, 1997
20. Waud DR: The nature of "depolarization block." Anesthesiology 29:1014, 1968
21. Hartman GS, Flamengo SA, Riker WF: Succinylcholine: Mechanism of fasciculations and their prevention by d-tubocurarine or diphenylhydantoin. Anesthesiology 65:405, 1986
22. Van der Spek AFL, Fang WB, Ashton-Miller JA et al: The effects of succinylcholine on mouth opening. Anesthesiology 67:459, 1987
23. Plumley MH, Bevan JC, Saddler JM et al: Dose–related effects of succinylcholine on the adductor pollicis and masseter muscles in children. Can J Anaesth 37:15, 1990
24. Smith CE, Saddler JM, Bevan JC et al: Pretreatment with nondepolarizing neuromuscular blocking agents and suxamethonium-induced increases in resting jaw tension in children. Br J Anaesth 64:577, 1990
25. Hanallah RS, Kaplan RF: Jaw relaxation after a halothane/succinylcholine sequence in children. Anesthesiology 81:99, 1994
26. Bucx MJL, Van Geel RTM, Meursing AEE et al: Forces applied during laryngoscopy in children: Are volatile anaesthetics essential for suxamethonium induced muscle rigidity? Acta Anaesthesiol Scand 38:448, 1994
27. Kim KS, Na DJ, Chon SU: Interactions between suxamethonium and mivacurium or atracurium. Br J Anaesth 77:612, 1996
28. Lee C: Train-of-four fade and edrophonium antagonism of neuromuscular block by succinylcholine in man. Anesth Analg 55:663, 1976
29. Donati F, Bevan DR: Long-term succinylcholine infusion during isoflurane anesthesia. Anesthesiology 58:6, 1983
30. Gao H, Roy S, Donati F, Varin F: Determination of succinylcholine in human plasma by high-performance liquid chromatography with electrochemical detection. J Chromatogr B Biomed Sci Appl 718:129,1998.
31. Szalados JE, Donati F, Bevan DR: Effect of d-tubocurarine pretreatment on succinylcholine twitch augmentation and neuromuscular blockade. Anesth Analg 71:55, 1990
32. Meistelman C, Plaud B, Donati F: Neuromuscular effects of succinylcholine on the vocal cords and adductor pollicis muscles. Anesth Analg 73:278, 1991
33. Smith CE, Donati F, Bevan DR: Dose–response curves for succinylcholine: Single versus cumulative techniques. Anesthesiology 69:338, 1988
34. Vanlinthout LE, van Egmond J, de Boo T et al: Factors affecting magnitude and time course of neuromuscular block produced by suxamethonium. Br J Anaesth 69:29,1992.
35. Lerman J, Chinyanga HM: The heart rate response to succinylcholine in children: A comparison of atropine and glycopyrrolate. Can Anaesth Soc J 30:377, 1983
36. Duvaldestin P, Wigdorowicz C, Gabriel I: Anaphylactic shock to neuromuscular blocking agent: A familial history. Anesthesiology 90:1211, 1990
37. Erkola O, Salmenpera A, Kuoppamaki R: Five nondepolarizing muscle relaxants in precurarization. Acta Anesthesiol Scand 27:427, 1983
38. Martin R, Carrier J, Pirlet M et al: Rocuronium is the best nondepolarizing relaxant to prevent succinylcholine fasciculations and myalgia. Can J Anaesth 45:521, 1998
39. Pinchak AC, Smith CE, Shepard LS, Patterson L: Waiting time

after nondepolarizing relaxants and muscle fasciculation response to succinylcholine. Can J Anaesth 41:206, 1994

40. Pace NL: Prevention of succinylcholine myalgias: A meta-analysis. Anesth Analg 70:77, 1990

41. Smith G, Dalling R, Williams TIR: Gastro-oesophageal pressure gradient changes produced by induction of anaesthesia and suxamethonium. Br J Anaesth 50:1137, 1978

42. Kelly RE, Dimer M, Turneer LS et al: Succinylcholine increases intraocular pressure in the human eye with the extraocular muscles detached. Anesthesiology 79:948, 1993

43. Wynands JE, Crowell DE: Intraocular tension in association with succinylcholine and endotracheal intubation: A preliminary report. Can Anaesth Soc J 7:39, 1960

44. Stirt JA, Grosslight KR, Bedford RF, Vollmer D: "Defasciculation" with metocurine prevents succinylcholine-induced increases in intracranial pressure. Anesthesiology 67:50, 1987

45. Lanier WL, Milde JH, Michenfelder JD: Cerebral stimulation following succinylcholine in dogs. Anesthesiology 64:551, 1986

46. Kovarik WD, Mayberg TS, Lam AM et al: Succinylcholine does not change intracranial pressure, cerebral blood flow velocity, or the encephalogram in patients with neurological injury. Anesthesiology 78:469, 1994

47. Bali IM, Coppel DL, Dundee JW: The effect of non-depolarizing muscle relaxants on plasma potassium. Br J Anaesth 47:505, 1975

48. Gronert GA, Theye RA: Pathophysiology of hyperkalemia induced by succinylcholine. Anesthesiology 43:89, 1975

49. Schwartz DE, Kelly B, Caldwell JE et al: Succinylcholine-induced hyperkalemic arrest in a patient with severe metabolic acidosis and exsanguinating hemorrhage. Anesth Analg 75: 291, 1992

50. Antognini JF: Splanchnic release of potassium after hemorrhage and succinylcholine in rabbits. Anesth Analg 78:687, 1994

51. Whittaker M: Plasma cholinesterase variants and the anaesthetist. Anaesthesia 35:174, 1980

52. Fleming NW, Macres S, Antognini JF, Vengco J: Neuromuscular blocking action of suxamethonium after antagonism of vecuronium by edrophonium, pyridostigmine or neostigmine. Br J Anaesth 77:492, 1996

53. Beaufort TM, Nigrovic V, Proost JH et al: Inhibition of the enzymatic degradation of suxamethonium and mivacurium increases the onset time of submaximal neuromuscular block. Anesthesiology 89:707, 1998

54. Lockridge O, Bartels CF, Vaughan TA et al: Complete amino acid sequence of human plasma cholinesterase. J Biol Chem 262:549, 1987

55. Allerdice PW, Gardner HAR, Galutira D et al: The cloned butyrylcholinesterase (BCHE) gene maps to a single chromosome site q26.2. Genomics 11:452, 1991

56. Pantuck EJ: Plasma cholinesterase: Gene and variations. Anesth Analg 77:380, 1993

57. Viby-Mogensen J: Succinylcholine neuromuscular blockade in subjects homozygous for atypical plasma cholinesterase. Anesthesiology 55:429, 1981

58. Liu LMP, DeCook TH, Goudsouzian NG et al: Dose response to intramuscular succinylcholine in children. Anesthesiology 55: 599, 1981

59. Waud BE, Waud DR: The relation between the response to "train-of-four" stimulation and receptor occlusion during competitive neuromuscular block. Anesthesiology 37:413, 1972

60. Lee C, Katz RL: Fade of neurally evoked compound electromyogram during neuromuscular block by d-tubocurarine. Anesth Analg 56:271, 1977

61. Brull SJ, Connelly NR, O'Connor TZ, Silverman DG: Effect of tetanus on subsequent neuromuscular monitoring in patients receiving vecuronium. Anesthesiology 74:64, 1991

62. Lien CA, Schmith VD, Embree PB et al: The pharmacokinetics and pharmacodynamics of the stereoisomers of mivacurium in patients receiving nitrous oxide/opioid/barbiturate anesthesia. Anesthesiology 80:1296, 1994

63. Schiere S, Proost JH, Schuringa M, Wierda JM: Pharmacokinetics and pharmacokinetic–dynamic relationship between rapacuronium (Org 9487) and its 3-desacetyl metabolite (Org 9488). Anesth Analg 88:640, 1999

64. Fisher DM, O'Keefe C, Stanski DR et al: Pharmacokinetics and pharmacodynamics of d-tubocurarine in infants, children, and adults. Anesthesiology 57:203, 1982

65. Sheiner LB, Stanski DR, Vozeh S et al: Simultaneous modeling

66. of pharmacokinetics and pharmacodynamics: Application to d-tubocurarine. Clin Pharmacol Ther 25:358, 1979

66. Donati F: Onset of action of relaxants. Can J Anaesth 35:S52, 1988

67. Bowman WC, Rodger IW, Houston J et al: Structure : action relationships among some desacetoxy analogues of pancuronium and vecuronium in the anesthetized cat. Anesthesiology 69:57, 1988

68. Law Min JC, Bekavac I, Glavinovic MI et al: Iontophoretic study of speed of action of various muscle relaxants. Anesthesiology 77:351, 1992

69. Kopman AF: Pancuronium, gallamine, and d-tubocurarine compared: Is speed of onset inversely related to drug potency? Anesthesiology 70:915, 1989

70. Basta SJ, Savarese JJ, Ali HH et al: Clinical pharmacology of doxacurium chloride: A new long-acting nondepolarizing relaxant. Anesthesiology 69:478, 1988

71. Ghoneim MM, Kramer E, Barrow R et al: Binding of d-tubocurarine to plasma protein in health and disease. Anesth Analg 62:870, 1983

72. Matteo RS, Spector S, Horowitz PE: Relation of serum d-tubocurarine concentration to neuromuscular blockade. Anesthesiology 41:441, 1974

73. Miller RD, Matteo RS, Benet LZ et al: The pharmacokinetics of d-tubocurarine in man with and without renal failure. J Pharmacol Exp Ther 202:1, 1977

74. Hughes R, Chapple DJ: Effect of non-depolarizing neuromuscular blocking agents on peripheral autonomic mechanisms in cats. Br J Anaesth 48:59, 1976

75. Moss J, Roscow CE, Savarese JJ et al: Role of histamine in the hypotensive action of d-tubocurarine in humans. Anesthesiology 55:19, 1981

76. Hatano Y, Arai T, Noda J et al: Contribution of prostacyclin to d-tubocurarine-induced hypotension in humans. Anesthesiology 72:28, 1984

77. Matteo RS, Backus WW, McDaniel DD et al: Pharmacokinetics and pharmacodynamics of d-tubocurarine and metocurine in the elderly. Anesth Analg 64:23, 1985

78. Bevan DR, Bevan JC, Donati F: Muscle Relaxants in Clinical Anesthesia. Chicago, Year Book Medical Publishers, 1988

79. Martyn JAJ, Szyfelbein SK, Ali HH et al: Increased d-tubocurarine requirement following major thermal injury. Anesthesiology 52:352, 1980

80. Kim C, Fuke N, Martyn JAJ: Burn injury to rat increases nicotinic acetylcholine receptors in the diaphragm. Anesthesiology 68: 401, 1988

81. Martyn JAJ, White DA, Groneret GA et al: Up- and down-regulation of skeletal muscle acetylcholine receptors. Anesthesiology 76: 822, 1992

82. Stenlake JB, Waigh RB, Urwin J et al: Atracurium: Conception and inception. Br J Anaesth 55:3S, 1983

83. Stiller RL, Cook DR, Chakravorti S: In vitro degradation of atracurium in human plasma. Br J Anaesth 57:1085, 1985

84. Chapple DJ, Clark JS: Pharmacological action of breakdown products of atracurium and related substances. Br J Anaesth 55:11S, 1983

85. Shi WZ, Fahey MR, Fisher DM et al: Laudanosine (a metabolite of atracurium) increases the minimal alveolar concentration of halothane in rabbits. Anesthesiology 63:584, 1985

86. Hennis PJ, Fahey MR, Canfell PC et al: Pharmacology of atracurium during isoflurane anesthesia in normal and anephric patients. Anesth Analg 65:743, 1986

87. Nigrovic V, Pandya JB, Klaunig JE, Fry K: Reactivity and toxicity of atracurium and its metabolites in vitro. Can J Anaesth 36:262, 1989

88. Miller RD, Rupp SM, Fisher DM et al: Clinical pharmacology of vecuronium and atracurium. Anesthesiology 61:444, 1984

89. Mirakhur RK, Lavery GG, Clarke RSJ et al: Atracurium in clinical anaesthesia: Effect of dosage on onset, duration and conditions for tracheal intubation. Anaesthesia 40:801, 1985

90. Hunter JM: Bradycardia after the use of atracurium. Br Med J 287:759, 1983

91. Savarese JJ, Basta SJ, Ali HH et al: Neuromuscular and cardiovascular effects of BW 33A (atracurium) in patients under halothane anesthesia. Anesthesiology 57:A262, 1982

92. Scott RPF, Savarese JJ, Basta SJ et al: Atracurium: Clinical strategies for preventing histamine release and attenuating the haemodynamic response. Br J Anaesth 57:550, 1985

93. Oh TE, Horton JM: Adverse reactions to atracurium. Br J Anaesth 62:467, 1989

94. Jick H, Andrews EB, Tilson HH et al: Atracurium—a post-market-

ing surveillance study: Methods and US experience. Br J Anaesth 62:590, 1989

95. d'Hollander AA, Luyckx C, Barvais L et al: Clinical evaluation of atracurium besylate requirement for stable muscle relaxation during surgery: Lack of age-related effects. Anesthesiology 59:237, 1983

96. Kirkegaard-Nielsen H, Helbo-Hansen HS, Lindholm P et al: Anthropometric variables as predictors for the duration of action of atracurium-induced neuromuscular blockade. Anesth Analg 83:1076, 1996

97. Kirkegaard-Nielsen H, Lindholm P, Petersen HS, Severinsen IK: Antagonism of atracurium-induced block in obese patients. Can J Anaesth 45:39, 1998

98. Lien CA, Schmith VD, Belmont MR et al: Pharmacokinetics of cisatracurium in patients receiving nitrous oxide/opioid/barbiturate anesthesia. Anesthesiology 84:300, 1996

99. Mellinghof H, Radbruch L, Diefenbach C, Buzello W: A comparison of cisatracurium and atracurium: Onset of neuromuscular block after bolus injection and recovery after subsequent infusion. Anesth Analg 83:1072, 1996

100. Carroll MT, Mirakhur RK, Lowry D et al: A comparison of the neuromuscular blocking effects and reversibility of cisatracurium and atracurium. Anaesthesia 53:744, 1998

101. Wulf H, Kahl M, Ledowski T: Augmentation of the neuromuscular blocking effects of cisatracurium during desflurane, sevoflurane, isoflurane or total i.v. anaesthesia. Br J Anaesth 80:308, 1998

102. Meretoja OA, Taivainen T, Wirtavuori K: Pharmacodyamic effects of 51W89, an isomer of atracurium, in children during halothane anaesthesia. Br J Anaesth 74:6, 1995

103. Kisor DF, Schmith VD, Wargin WA et al: Importance of organ-independent elimination of cisatracurium. Anesth Analg 83:1065, 1996

104. Naguib M, Samarkandi AH, Ammar A et al: Comparative clinical pharmacology of rocuronium, cisatracurium, and their combination. Anesthesiology 89:1116, 1998

105. Toh KW, Deacock SJ, Fawcett WJ: Severe anaphylactic reaction to cisatracurium. Anesth Analg 88:462, 1999

106. Lien CA, Belmont MR, Abalos A et al: The cardiovascular effects and histamine-releasing properties of 51W89 in patients receiving nitrous oxide/opioid/barbiturate anesthesia. Anesthesiology 82:1131, 1995

107. Dressner DL, Basta SJ, Ali HH et al: Pharmacokinetics and pharmacodynamics of doxacurium in young and elderly patients during isoflurane anesthesia. Anesth Analg 71:498, 1990

108. Gariepy LP, Varin F, Donati F et al: Influence of aging on the pharmacokinetics and pharmacodynamics of doxacurium. Clin Pharmacol Ther 53:340, 1993

109. Lennon RL, Hosking MP, Houck PC et al: Doxacurium chloride for neuromuscular blockade before tracheal intubation and surgery during nitrous oxide–oxygen–narcotic–enflurane anesthesia. Anesth Analg 68:255, 1989

110. Katz JA, Fragen RJ, Shanks CA et al: Dose–response relationship of doxacurium chloride in humans during anesthesia with nitrous oxide and fentanyl, enflurane, isoflurane, or halothane. Anesthesiology 70:432, 1989

111. Brandom BW, Yellon RF, Lloyd ME et al: Recovery from doxacurium infusion administered to produce immobility for more than four days in pediatric patients in the intensive care unit. Anesth Analg 84:307, 1997

112. Meijer DKF, Weitering JG, Vermeer GA et al: Comparative pharmacokinetics of d-tubocurarine and metocurine in man. Anesthesiology 51:402, 1979

113. McCullogh LS, Stone WA, Delaunis AL et al: The effects of dimethyltubocurarine iodide on cardiovascular parameters, postganglionic sympathetic activity and histamine release. Anesth Analg 51:554, 1972

114. Martyn JAJ, Matteo RS, Szyfellelbein SK et al: Unprecedented resistance to neuromuscular blocking effects of metocurine with persistence after complete recovery in a burned patient. Anesth Analg 61:614, 1982

115. Lebowitz PW, Ramsey FM, Savarese JJ et al: Combination of pancuronium and metocurine: Neuromuscular and hemodynamic advantages over pancuronium alone. Anesth Analg 60:12, 1981

116. Savarese JJ, Ali HH, Basta SJ et al: The clinical neuromuscular pharmacology of mivacurium chloride (BW 1090U): A short acting nondepolarizing ester neuromuscular blocking drug. Anesthesiology 68:723, 1988

117. Meretoja OA, Taivainen T, Wirtavuori K: Pharmacodynamics of mivacurium in infants. Br J Anaesth 73:490, 1994

118. Meretoja OA, Olkkola KT: Pharmacodynamics of mivacurium in children, using a computer-controlled infusion. Br J Anaesth 71:232, 1993

119. Ali HH, Savarese JJ, Embree PT et al: Clinical pharmacology of mivacurium chloride (BW 1090U) infusion: Comparison with vecuronium and atracurium. Br J Anaesth 61:541, 1988

120. Brandom BW, Woelfel SK, Cook DR et al: Comparison of mivacurium and suxamethonium administered by bolus and infusion. Br J Anaesth 62:488, 1989

121. Naguib M, Abdulatif M, Al-Ghamdi A et al: Dose–response relationships for edrophonium and neostigmine antagonism of mivacurium-induced neuromuscular block. Br J Anaesth 71:709, 1993

122. Kao YJ, Le ND: The reversal of profound mivacurium-induced neuromuscular blockade. Can J Anaesth 43:1128, 1996

123. Symington MJJ, Mirakhur RK, Kumar N: Neostigmine but not edrophonium prolongs the action of mivacurium. Can J Anaesth 43:1220, 1996

124. Ding Y, Fredman B, White PF: Use of mivacurium during laparoscopic surgery: Effect of reversal drugs on postoperative recovery. Anesth Analg 78:440, 1994

125. Bevan DR, Kahwaji R, Ansermino JM et al: Residual block after mivacurium with or without edrophonium reversal in adults and children. Anesthesiology 84:362, 1996

126. Tramèr MR, Fuchs-Buder T: Omitting antagonism of neuromuscular block: Effect on postoperative nausea and vomiting and risk of residual paralysis: a systematic review. Br J Anaesth 82:379, 1999

127. Bevan JC, Reimer EJ, Smith MF et al: Decreased mivacurium requirements and delayed neuromuscular recovery during sevoflurane anesthesia in children and adults. Anesth Analg 87:772, 1998

128. Gin T, Derrick JL, Chan MTV et al: Postpartum patients have slightly prolonged neuromuscular block after mivacurium. Anesth Analg 86:82, 1998

129. Naguib M, Samarkandi AH, Bakhamees HS et al: Edrophonium and human plasma cholinesterase combination for antagonism of mivacurium-induced neuromuscular blockade. Br J Anaesth 77:424, 1997

130. Vanlinthout LE, Bartels CF, Lockridge O et al: Prolonged paralysis after a test dose of mivacurium in a patient with atypical serum cholinesterase. Anesth Analg 87:1199, 1998

131. Stoops CM, Curtis CA, Kovach DA et al: Hemodynamic effects of mivacurium chloride administered to patients during oxygen–sufentanil anesthesia for coronary artery bypass grafting or valve replacement. Anesth Analg 68:333, 1989

132. Maddineni VR, Mirakhur RK, McCoy EP et al: Neuromuscular effects and intubating conditions following mivacurium: A comparison with suxamethonium. Anaesthesia 48:940, 1993

133. Ali HH, Lien CA, Witkowski T et al: Efficacy and safety of divided dose administration of mivacurium for a 90 second tracheal intubation. J Clin Anesth 8:276, 1996

134. Chui PT, Cheam EWS: The use of low-dose mivacurium to facilitate insertion of the laryngeal mask airway. Anaesthesia 53:491, 1998

135. Buckett WR, Hewitt CL, Savage DS: Pancuronium bromide and other steroidal neuromuscular blocking agents containing acetylcholine fragments. J Med Chem 16:1116, 1973

136. Doherty WG, Breen PJ, Donati F et al: Accelerated onset of pancuronium with divided doses. Can Anaesth Soc J 32:1, 1985

137. Baurain MJ, Hoton F, D'Hollander AA, Cantraine FR: Is recovery of neuromuscular transmission complete after the use of neostigmine to antagonise block produced by rocuronium, vecuronium, atracurium and pancuronium? Br J Anaesth 77:496, 1996

138. Wierda JMKH, van den Broek L, Proost JH et al: Time course of action and endotracheal intubating conditions of Org 9487, a new short-acting steroidal muscle relaxant: A comparison with succinylcholine. Anesth Analg 77:579, 1993

139. Sparr HJ, Mellinghoff H, Blobner M, Nüldge-Schomberg G: Comparison of intubating conditions after rapacuronium (Org 9487) and succinylcholine following rapid sequence induction in adult patients. Br J Anaesth 82:537, 1999

140. Kahwaji R, Bevan DR, Bikhazi G et al: Dose-ranging study in younger adult and elderly patients of ORG 9487, a new, rapid-onset, short duration muscle relaxant. Anesth Analg 84:1011, 1997

141. Szenohradszky J, Caldwell JE, Wright PMC et al: Influence of renal failure on the pharmacokinetics and neuromuscular blocking effects of a single dose of rapacuronium bromide. Anesthesiology 90:24, 1999

142. Van den Broek L, Wierda JMKH, Smeulers NJ, Proost JH: Pharmacodynamics and pharmacokinetics of an infusion of Org 9487, a new short-acting steroidal neuromuscular blocking agent. Br J Anaesth 73:331, 1994

143. Purdy R, Bevan DR, Donati F, Lichtor JL: Early reversal of rapacuronium with neostigmine. Anesthesiology 91:51, 1999

144. Bevan JC, Collins L, Fowler C et al: Early and late reversal of rocuronium and vecuronium with neostigmine in adults and children. Anesth Analg 89:333, 1999

145. Levy JH, Thanopoulos A, Szlam F et al: The effects of rapacuronium on histamine release and hemodynamics in adult patients undergoing general anesthesia. Anesth Analg 89:290, 1999

146. Wierda JMKH, de Wit APM, Kuizenga K, Agoston S: Clinical observations on the neuromuscular blocking action of ORG 9426, a new steroidal non-depolarizing agent. Br J Anaesth 64:521, 1990

147. Wierda JMKH, Kleef UW, Lambalk LM et al: The pharmacodynamics and pharmacokinetics of ORG 9426. A new non-depolarizing neuromuscular blocking agent in patients anaesthetized with nitrous oxide, halothane and fentanyl. Can J Anaesth 38:430, 1991

148. Bartkowski RR, Witkowski TA, Azad S et al: Rocuronium onset of action: A comparison with atracurium and vecuronium. Anesth Analg 77:574, 1993

149. Andrews JL, Kumar N, Van den Brom RHG et al: A large sample randomized trial of rocuronium versus succinylcholine in rapid-sequence induction of anaesthesia along with propofol. Acta Anaesthesiol Scand 43:4, 1999

150. Cantineau JP, Porte F, d'Honneur G, Duvaldestin P: Neuromuscular effects of rocuronium on the diaphragm and adductor pollicis muscles in anesthetized patients. Anesthesiology 81:585, 1994

151. Girling KJ, Bedforth NM, Spendlove JL, Mahajan RP: Assessing neuromuscular block at the larynx: The effect of change in resting cuff pressure and a comparison with video imaging in anesthetized humans. Anesth Analg 88:426, 1999

152. Taivainen T, Meretoja OA, Erkola O et al: Rocuronium in infants, children and adults. Anesthesiology 81:A1074, 1994

153. Meretoja OA: Is vecuronium a long-acting neuromuscular blocking drug in neonates and infants? Br J Anaesth 69:184, 1989

154. Levy JH, Davis GK, Duggan J, Szalm F: Determination of the hemodynamics and histamine release of rocuronium (Org 9426) when administered in increased doses under N_2O/O_2-sufentanil anesthesia. Anesth Analg 78:318, 1994

155. McCoy EP, Maddineni VR, Elliott P et al: Haemodynamic effects of rocuronium during fentanyl anaesthesia: Comparison with vecuronium. Can J Anaesth 40:703, 1993

156. Sieber TJ, Zbinden AM, Curatolo M, Shorten GD: Tracheal intubation with rocuronium using the "timing principle." Anesth Analg 86:1137, 1996

157. Khuenl-Brady KS, Pühringer F, Koller J, Mitterschiffthaler G: Evaluation of the time course of action of maintenance doses of rocuronium (ORG 9426) under halothane anaesthesia. Acta Anaesthesiol Scand 37:137, 1993

158. Savage DS, Sleigh T, Carlyle I: The emergence of ORG NC 45, 1-[(2-β, 3-α, 5,16-β, 17β)-3,17-bis(acetoxy)-2-(piperidinyl)androstan-16-yl]-1-methylpiperidinium bromide, from the pancuronium series. Br J Anaesth 52:3S, 1980

159. Segredo V, Malthay MA, Sharma ML et al: Prolonged neuromuscular blockade after long-term administration of vecuronium in two critically ill patients. Anesthesiology 72:566, 1990

160. Xue FS, Liao X, Liu JH et al: Dose–response curves and time-course of effect of vecuronium in male and female patients. Br J Anaesth 80:720, 1998

161. Xue FS, An G, Liao X et al: The pharmacokinetics of vecuronium in male and female patients. Anesth Analg 86:1322, 1998

162. Sohn YJ, Bencini AF, Scaf AHJ et al: Comparative pharmacokinetics and dynamics of vecuronium and pancuronium in anesthetized patients. Anesth Analg 65:233, 1986

163. Noeldge G, Hinsken H, Buzello W: Comparison between the continuous infusion of vecuronium and the intermittent administration of pancuronium and vecuronium. Br J Anaesth 56:473, 1984

164. Schwartz S, Ilias W, Lackner F et al: Rapid tracheal intubation with vecuronium: The priming principle. Anesthesiology 62:388, 1985

165. Mirakhur RK, Ferres CJ, Clarke RSJ et al: Clinical evaluation of ORG NC45. Br J Anaesth 55:119, 1983

166. Futo J, Kupferberg JP, Moss J et al: Vecuronium inhibits histamine N-methyltransferase. Anesthesiology 69:92, 1988

167. Taniguchi T, Yamamoto K, Kobayashi T: Precipitate formed by thiopentone and vecuronium causes pulmonary embolism. Can J Anaesth 45:347, 1998

168. Diefenbach C, Mellinghoff H, Grond S, Buzello W: Atracurium and vecuronium: Repeated bolus injection versus infusion. Anesth Analg 74:519, 1992

169. Miller RD, Way WL, Dolan WM et al: Comparative neuromuscular effects of pancuronium, gallamine, and succinylcholine during Forane and halothane anesthesia in man. Anesthesiology 35:509, 1971

170. Fogdall RP, Miller RD: Neuromuscular blocking effects of enflurane, alone and combined with d-tubocurarine, pancuronium, and succinylcholine in man. Anesthesiology 42:173, 1975

171. Bennett MJ, Hahn JF: Potentiation of the combination of pancuronium and metocurine by halothane and isoflurane in humans with and without renal failure. Anesthesiology 62:759, 1985

172. Rupp SM, Miller RD, Gencarelli PJ: Vecuronium-induced neuromuscular blockade during enflurane, isoflurane, and halothane anesthesia in humans. Anesthesiology 60:102, 1984

173. Chapple DJ, Clark JS, Hughes R: Interaction between atracurium and drugs used in anaesthesia. Br J Anaesth 55:17S, 1983

174. Brandom BW, Rudd GD, Cook DR: Clinical pharmacology of atracurium in paediatric patients. Br J Anaesth 55:117S, 1983

175. Szalados JE, Donati F, Bevan DR: Nitrous oxide potentiates succinylcholine neuromuscular blockade in humans. Anesth Analg 72:18, 1991

176. Wulf H, Kahl M, Ledowski T: Augmentation of the neuromuscular blocking effects of cisatracurium during desflurane, sevoflurane, isoflurane or total i.v. anaesthesia. Br J Anaesth 80:308, 1998

177. Wulf H, Ledowski T, Linstedt U et al: Neuromuscular blocking effects of rocuronium during desflurane, isoflurane, and sevoflurane anesthesia. Can J Anaesth 45:526, 1998

178. Waud BE, Waud DR: Effects of volatile anesthetics on directly and indirectly stimulated skeletal muscle. Anesthesiology 50:103, 1979

179. McIndewar IC, Marshall RJ: Interaction between the neuromuscular block of ORG NC45 and some anaesthetic, analgesic and antimicrobial agents. Br J Anaesth 53:785, 1981

180. Matsuo S, Rao DBS, Chaudry I et al: Interaction of muscle relaxants and local anesthetics at the neuromuscular junction. Anesth Analg 57:580, 1978

181. Usubiaga JF, Wikinski JA, Morales RL: Interaction of intravenously administered procaine, lidocaine and succinylcholine in anesthetized subjects. Anesth Analg 46:39, 1967

182. Naguib M, Abdulatif M, Al-Ghamdi A et al: Interactions between mivacurium and atracurium. Br J Anaesth 73:484, 1994

183. Naguib M: Neuromuscular effects of rocuronium bromide and mivacurium chloride administered alone and in combination. Anesthesiology 81:388, 1994

184. Naguib M, Samarkandi AH, Ammar A et al: Comparative clinical pharmacology of rocuronium, cisatracurium, and their combination. Anesthesiology 89:1116, 1998

185. Rautoma P, Erkola O, Meretoja O: Potency and maintenance requirement of combinations of mivacurium and pancuronium in adults. Can J Anaesth 45:212,1998

186. Su PC, Su WL, Rosen AD: Pre- and post-synaptic effects of pancuronium at the neuromuscular junction of the mouse. Anesthesiology 50:199, 1979

187. Waud BE, Waud DR: Interaction among agents that block end-plate depolarization competitively. Anesthesiology 61:420, 1984

188. Ferguson A, Bevan DR: Mixed neuromuscular block: The effect of precurarization. Anaesthesia 36:661, 1981

189. Stovner J, Oftedal N, Holmboe J: The inhibition of cholinesterase by pancuronium. Br J Anaesth 47:949, 1975

190. Krieg N, Hendrickx HHL, Crul JF: Influence of suxamethonium on the potency of ORG NC45 in anaesthetized patients. Br J Anaesth 53:259, 1981

191. Kim NS, Na DJ, Chon SU: Interactions with suxamethonium and mivacurium or atracurium. Br J Anaesth 77:612, 1996

192. Rouse JM, Bevan DR: Mixed neuromuscular block. Anaesthesia 34:608, 1979

193. Braga MFM, Rowan EG, Harvey AL, Bowman WC: Interactions between suxamethonium and non-depolarizing neuromuscular blocking drugs. Br J Anaesth 74:198, 1994

194. Argov Z, Mastaglia FL: Disorders of neuromuscular transmission caused by drugs. N Engl J Med 301:409, 1979

195. Ornstein E, Matteo RS, Silverberg PA et al: Dose–response relationships for vecuronium in the presence of chronic phenytoin therapy. Anesth Analg 65:S116, 1986

196. Ornstein E, Schwartz AE, Matteo RS *et al:* Predictability of atracurium effect in phenytoin exposed patients. Anesthesiology 65:A112, 1986
197. Spacek A, Neiger FX, Krenn CG *et al:* Rocuronium-induced neuromuscular block is affected by chronic carbamazepine therapy. Anesthesiology 90:109, 1999
198. Spacek A, Nager FX, Spiss CK, Kress HG: Chronic carbamazepine therapy does not influence mivacurium-induced neuromuscular block. Br J Anaesth 77:500, 1996
199. Spacek A, Nicki S, Neiger FX *et al:* Augmentation of the rocuronium-induced neuromuscular block by the acutely administered phenytoin. Anesthesiology 90:1551, 1999
200. Griffin D, Fairman N, Coursin D *et al:* Acute myopathy during treatment of status asthmaticus with corticosteroids and steroidal muscle relaxants. Chest 102:510, 1992
201. Branney SW, Haenel JB, Moore FA *et al:* Prolonged paralysis with atracurium infusion: A case report. Crit Care Med 22:1699, 1994
202. Zochodne DW, Bolton CF, Wells GA *et al:* Critical illness neuropathy: A complication of sepsis and multiple organ failure. Brain 110:819, 1987
203. Buck ML, Reed MD: Use of non-depolarizing neuromuscular blocking agents in mechanically ventilated patients. Clin Pharm 10:32, 1991
204. Cody M, Dormon F: Recurarization after vecuronium in a patient with renal failure. Anesthesiology 42:993, 1987
205. Tobias JD: Continuous infusion of rocuronium in a paediatric intensive care unit. Can J Anaesth 43:353, 1996
206. Segredo V, Caldwell JE, Wright PMC *et al:* Do the pharmacokinetics of vecuronium change during prolonged administration in critically ill patients? Br J Anaesth 80:715, 1998
207. Darrah W, Johnston J, Mirakhur R: Vecuronium infusions for prolonged muscle relaxation in the intensive care unit. Crit Care Med 17:1297, 1989
208. Khuenl-Brady KS, Reitstätter B, Schlager A *et al:* Long-term administration of pancuronium and pipecuronium in the intensive care unit. Anesth Analg 78:1082, 1994
209. Bowman WC: Physiology and pharmacology of neuromuscular transmission, with special reference to the possible consequences of prolonged blockade. Intensive Care Med 19:S45, 1993
210. Greer R, Harper NJN, Pearson AJ: Neuromuscular monitoring by intensive care nurses: Comparison of acceleromyography and tactile assessment. Br J Anaesth 80:384, 1998
211. Bender AN, Engel WK, Reingel SP *et al:* Myasthenia gravis: A serum factor blocking acetylcholine receptors of the human neuromuscular junction. Lancet 1:607, 1975
212. Drachman DB, Kao I, Pestronk A *et al:* Myasthenia gravis as a receptor disorder. Ann NY Acad Sci 274:226, 1976
213. Cull-Candy SG, Miledi R, Trautmann A *et al:* On the release of transmitter at normal, myasthenia gravis, and myasthenic syndrome affected human end-plates. J Physiol (Lond) 299:621, 1980
214. Ozdemiv C, Young RR: The results to be expected from electrical testing in the diagnosis of myasthenia gravis. Ann NY Acad Sci 274:203, 1976
215. Brown JC, Charlton JE: A study of sensitivity to curare in myasthenic disorders using a regional technique. J Neurol Neurosurg Psychiatry 38:27, 1975
216. Wojciechowski ARJ, Hanning CD, Pohl JEF: Postoperative apnoea and latent myasthenia gravis. Anaesthesia 40:882, 1985
217. Eisencraft JB, Book WJ, Mann SM *et al:* Resistance to succinylcholine in myasthenia gravis: A dose–response study. Anesthesiology 69:760, 1988
218. Azar I: The response of patients with neuromuscular disorders to muscle relaxants: A review. Anesthesiology 61:173, 1984
219. Smith CE, Donati F, Bevan DR: Cumulative dose–response curves for atracurium in patients with myasthenia gravis. Can J Anaesth 36:402, 1989
220. Nilsson E, Meretoja OA: Vecuronium dose–response and maintenance requirements in patients with myasthenia gravis. Anesthesiology 73:28, 1990
221. Green SJ, Shanks CA, Ronai AK *et al:* Atracurium-induced neuromuscular blockade in five myasthenic patients. Anesth Analg 64:221, 1985
222. Paterson IG, Hood JR, Russell SH *et al:* Mivacurium in the myasthenic patient. Br J Anaesth 73:494, 1994
223. Buzello W, Noeldge G, Krieg N *et al:* Vecuronium for muscle relaxation in patients with myasthenia gravis. Anesthesiology 64:507, 1986
224. Naguib M, Dawlatly AA, Ashour M, Bamgboye EA: Multivariate determinants of the need for postoperative ventilation in myasthenia gravis. Can J Anaesth 43:1014, 1996
225. Paterson IS: Generalized myotonia following suxamethonium. Br J Anaesth 34:340, 1962
226. Buzello W, Krieg N, Schlickewei A: Hazards of neostigmine in patients with neuromuscular disorders. Br J Anaesth 54:529, 1982
227. Smith CL, Bush GH: Anaesthesia and progressive muscular dystrophy. Br J Anaesth 57:1113, 1985
228. Larsen UT, Juhl B, Hein-Sørensen O, Olivarius B de F: Complications during anaesthesia in patients with Duchenne's muscular dystrophy. Can J Anaesth 36:418, 1989
229. Rosenberg H, Gronert GA: Intractable cardiac arrest in children given succinylcholine (letter). Anesthesiology 77:1054, 1992
230. Sullivan M, Thompson WK, Hill GD: Succinylcholine-induced cardiac arrest in children with undiagnosed myopathy. Can J Anaesth 41:497, 1994
231. Schulte-Sasse Von U, Eberlein HJ, Schmücker I *et al:* Solte die verwendung von succinylcholin in der Kinderanästhesie neu überdacht werden. Anaesthesiol Reanimat 18:13, 1993
232. Brown JC, Charlton JE: Study of sensitivity to curare in certain neurological disorders using a regional technique. J Neurol Neurosurg Psychiatry 38:34, 1975
233. Ririe DG, Shapiro F, Sethna NF: The response of patients with Duchenne's muscular dystrophy to neuromuscular blockade with vecuronium. Anesthesiology 88:351, 1998
234. Robertson JA: Ocular muscular dystrophy: A cause of curare sensitivity. Anaesthesia 39:251, 1984
235. Gronert GA: Controversies in malignant hyperthermia. Anesthesiology 59:273, 1983
236. Rosenberg H, Heiman-Patterson T: Duchenne's muscular dystrophy and malignant hyperthermia: Another warning. Anesthesiology 59:362, 1983
237. Stone WA, Beach TP, Hamelberg W: Succinylcholine-danger in the spinal-cord–injured patient. Anesthesiology 32:168, 1970
238. Kardash K, Abou-Madi M, Trop D, Delorme M: Succinylcholine, motor dysfunction and potassium in brain tumor patients. Anesthesiology 71:A1139, 1989
239. Graham DH: Monitoring neuromuscular block may be unreliable in patients with upper motor-neuron lesions. Anesthesiology 52:74, 1980
240. Cooper AL, Leigh JM, Tring IC: Admissions to the intensive care unit after complication of anaesthetic techniques over 10 years: I. The first 5 years. Anaesthesia 44:953, 1989
241. Tiret L, Desmonts JM, Hatton F, Vourc'h G: Complications associated with anaesthesia: A prospective study in France. Can Anaesth Soc J 33:336, 1986
242. Katz RL: Neuromuscular effects of *d*-tubocurarine, edrophonium and neostigmine in man. Anesthesiology 28:327, 1967
243. Rosenberg H, Greenhow DE: Peripheral nerve stimulator performance: The influence of output polarity and electrode placement. Can Anaesth Soc J 25:424, 1978
244. Hudes E, Lee KC: Clinical use of nerve stimulators in anaesthesia. Can J Anaesth 34:525, 1987
245. Ali HH, Utting JE, Gray TC: Quantitative assessment of residual antidepolarizing block. I. Br J Anaesth 43:473, 1971
246. Viby-Mogensen J, Howardy-Hansen P, Chraemmer-Jorgensen B *et al:* Posttetanic count (PTC): A new method of evaluating an intense nondepolarizing neuromuscular blockade. Anesthesiology 55:458, 1981
247. Viby-Mogensen J, Jensen NH, Engbaek J *et al:* Tactile and visual evaluation of the response to train-of-four nerve stimulation. Anesthesiology 63:440, 1985
248. Engbaek J, Ostergaard D, Viby-Mogensen J: Double burst stimulation (DBS): A new pattern of nerve stimulation to identify residual neuromuscular block. Br J Anaesth 62:274, 1989
249. Gill S, Donati F, Bevan DR: Clinical evaluation of double burst stimulation: Its relationship to train-of-four stimulation. Anaesthesia 45:543, 1989
250. Drenck DE, Ueda N, Olsen NV *et al:* Manual evaluation of residual curarization using double burst stimulation: A comparison with train-of-four. Anesthesiology 70:578, 1989
251. O'Hara DA, Fragen RJ, Shanks CA: Comparison of visual and measured train-of-four recovery after vecuronium-induced neuromuscular blockade using two anaesthetic techniques. Br J Anaesth 58:1300, 1986
252. Dupuis JY, Martin R, Tessonier JM, Tétrault JP: Clinical assessment

of the muscular response to tetanic nerve stimulation. Can J Anaesth 37:397, 1990

253. Kalli I: Effect of surface electrode position on the compound action potential evoked by ulnar nerve stimulation during isoflurane anaesthesia. Br J Anaesth 66:734, 1991

254. Kopman AF: The dose–effect relationship of metocurine: The integrated electromyogram of the first dorsal interosseous muscle and the mechanomyogram of the adductor pollicis compared. Anesthesiology 68:604, 1988

255. Kopman AF: The relationship of evoked electromyographic and mechanical responses following atracurium in humans. Anesthesiology 63:208, 1985

256. Viby-Mogensen J, Jensen E, Werner M, Kirkegaard Nielsen H: Measurement of acceleration: A new method of monitoring neuromuscular function. Acta Anaesthesiol Scand 32:45, 1988

257. Donati F, Meistelman C, Plaud B: Vecuronium neuromuscular blockade at the diphragm, the orbicularis oculi, and adductor pollicis muscles. Anesthesiology 73:870, 1990

258. Chauvin M, Lebrault C, Duvaldestin P: The neuromuscular blocking effect of vecuronium on the human diaphragm. Anesth Analg 66:117, 1987

259. Donati F, Meistelman C, Plaud B: Vecuronium neuromuscular blockade at the adductor muscles of the larynx and adductor pollicis. Anesthesiology 74:833, 1991

260. Saddler JM, Norman J: Comparison of atracurium-induced neuromuscular blockade in rectus abdominis and hand muscles in man. Br J Anaesth 69:26, 1992

261. Rimaniol JM, Dhonneur G, Sperry L, Duvaldestin P: A comparison of the neuromuscular blocking effects of atracurium, mivacurium, and vecuronium on the adductor pollicis and the orbicularis oculi muscle in humans. Anesth Analg 83:808, 1996

262. Plaud B, Donati F: The corrugator supercilii, not the orbicularis oculi, reflects rocuronium neuromuscular blockade of the adductro laryngeal muscles. Anesthesiology 91:A1032, 1999

263. Sopher MJ, Sears DH, Walts LF: Neuromuscular monitoring comparing the flexor hallucis brevis and adductor pollicis muscles. Anesthesiology 69:129, 1988

264. Wright PM, Caldwell JE, Miller RD: Onset and duration of rocuronium and succinylcholine at the adductor pollicis and laryngeal adductor muscles in anesthetized humans. Anesthesiology 81:1110, 1994

265. D'Honneur G, Guignard B, Slavov V et al: Comparison of the neuromuscular blocking effect of atracurium and vecuronium on the adductor pollicis and the geniohyoid muscle in humans. Anesthesiology 82:649, 1995

266. Ali HH, Wilson RS, Savarese JJ, Kitz RJ: The effect of tubocurarine on indirectly elicited train-of-four muscle response and respiratory measurements in humans. Br J Anaesth 47:570, 1975

267. Kopman AF, Yee PS, Neuman GG: Relationship of the train-of-four fade ratio to clinical signs and symptoms of residual paralysis in awake volunteers. Anesthesiology 86:765, 1997

268. Eriksson LI, Sundman E, Olsson R et al: Functional assessment of the pharynx at rest and during swallowing in partially paralyzed humans. Anesthesiology 87:1045, 1997

269. Nishino T, Yokokawa N, Hiraga K et al: Breathing pattern of anesthetized humans during pancuronium-induced partial paralysis. J Appl Physiol 64:78, 1988

270. Eriksson LI, Sato M, Severinghaus JW: Effect of vecuronium-induced partial neuromuscular block on hypoxic ventilatory response. Anesthesiology 78:693, 1993

271. Brull SJ, Silverman DG: Visual assessment of train-of-four and double-burst induced fade at submaximal stimulating currents. Anesth Analg 73:627, 1991

272. Saitoh Y, Nakazawa K, Makita K et al: Evaluation of residual neuromuscular block using train-of-four and double burst stimulation at the index finger. Anesth Analg 84:1354, 1997

273. Baurain MJ, Hennart DA, Godschalx A et al: Visual evaluation of residual curarization in anesthetized patients using one hundred-Hertz, five-second tetanic stimulation at the adductor pollicis muscle. Anesth Analg 87:185, 1998

274. Thornberry EA, Mazumdar D: The effect of changes in temperature on neuromuscular monitoring in the presence of atracurium blockade. Anaesthesia 43:447, 1988

275. Moorthy SS, Hildenberg JC: Resistance to non-depolarizing muscle relaxants in paretic upper extremities of patients with residual hemiplegia. Anesth Analg 59:624, 1980

276. Laycock JRD, Smith CE, Donati F, Bevan DR: Sensitivity of the

277. Pedersen T, Viby-Mogensen J, Bang U et al: Does perioperative tactile evaluation of the train-of-four response influence the frequency of postoperative residual neuromuscular blockade. Anesthesiology 73:835, 1990

278. Martin R, Bourdua I, Theriault S et al: Neuromuscular monitoring: Does it make a difference? Can J Anaesth 43:585, 1996

279. Mortensen CR, Berg H, el-Mahdy A, Viby-Mogensen J: Perioperative monitoring of neuromuscular transmission using acceleromyography prevents residual neuromuscular block following pancuronium. Acta Anaesthesiol Scand 39:797, 1995

280. Ansermino JM, Sanderson PM, Bevan JC, Bevan DR: Acceleromyography improves detection of residual neuromuscular blockade in children. Can J Anaesth 43:589, 1996

281. Pavlin EG, Holle RH, Schoene RB: Recovery of airway protection compared with ventilation in humans after paralysis with curare. Anesthesiology 70:381, 1989

282. Mason LJ, Betts EK: Leg lift and maximum inspiratory force, clinical signs of neuromuscular blockade reversal in infants and children. Anesthesiology 52:441, 1980

283. Brand JB, Cullen DJ, Wilson NE, Ali HH: Spontaneous recovery from nondepolarizing neuromuscular blockade: Correlation between clinical and evoked responses. Anesth Analg 56:55, 1977

284. Bevan DR, Smith CE, Donati F: Postoperative neuromuscular blockade: A comparison between atracurium, vecuronium, and pancuronium. Anesthesiology 69:272, 1988

285. Viby-Mogensen J, Jorgensen BC, Ording H: Residual curarization in the recovery room. Anesthesiology 50:539, 1979

286. Lennmarken C, Löfström JB: Partial curarization in the postoperative period. Acta Anaesthesiol Scand 28:260, 1984

287. Beemer GH, Rozental P: Postoperative neuromuscular function. Anaesth Intensive Care 14:41, 1986

288. Brull SJ, Silverman DG, Ehrenwerth J: Problems of recovery and residual neuromuscular blockade: Pancuronium vs. vecuronium. Anesthesiology 69:A473, 1988

289. Berg H, Viby-Mogensen J, Roed J et al: Residual neuromuscular block is a risk factor for postoperative pulmonary complications. Acta Anaesthesiol Scand 41:1095, 1997

290. Bevan DR, Kahwaji R, Ansermino JM et al: Residual block after mivacurium with or without edrophonium reversal in adults and children. Anesthesiology 84:362, 1996

291. Lunn JN, Hunter AR, Scott DB: Anaesthesia-related surgical mortality. Anaesthesia 38:1090, 1983

292. McEwin L, Merrick PM, Bevan DR: Residual neuromuscular block after cardiac surgery: Pancuronium vs. rocuronium. Can J Anaesth 44:891, 1997

293. Van Oldenbeek C, Knowles P, Harper NJN: Residual neuromuscular block caused by pancuronium after cardiac surgery. Br J Anaesth 83:338, 1999

294. Butterworth J, James R, Prielipp RC et al: Do shorter neuromuscular blocking drugs or opioids associate with reduced intensive care unit or hospital lengths of stay after coronary artery bypass grafting? Anesthesiology 88:1437, 1998

295. Kitz RJ: The chemistry of anticholinesterase activity. Acta Anaesthesiol Scand 8:197, 1964

296. Fiekers JF: Interactions of edrophonium, physostigmine and methanesulfonyl fluoride with the snake end-plate acetylcholine receptor-channel complex. J Pharmacol Exp Ther 234:539, 1985

297. Kordas M, Brzin M, Majcen Z: A comparison of the effect of cholinesterase inhibitors on end-plate current and on cholinesterase activity in frog muscle. Neuropharmacology 14:791, 1975

298. Donati F, Ferguson A, Bevan DR: Twitch depression and train-of-four ratio after antagonism of pancuronium with edrophonium, neostigmine, or pyridostigmine. Anesth Analg 62:314, 1983

299. Wachtel RE: Comparison of anticholinesterases and their effects on acetylcholine-activated ion channels. Anesthesiology 72:496, 1990

300. Bartkowski RR: Incomplete reversal of pancuronium neuromuscular blockade by neostigmine, pyridostigmine, and edrophonium. Anesth Analg 66:594, 1987

301. Alves-do-Prado W, Corrado AP, Prado WA: Reversal by atropine of tetanic fade induced in cats by antinicotinic and anticholinesterase agents. Anesth Analg 66:492, 1987

302. Goldhill DR, Wainwright AP, Stuart CS, Flynn PJ: Neostigmine after spontaneous recovery from neuromuscular blockade: Effect

on depth of blockade monitored with train-of-four and tetanic stimuli. Anaesthesia 44:293, 1989

303. Astley BA, Katz RL, Payne JP: Electrical and mechanical responses after neuromuscular blockade with vecuronium, and subsequent antagonism with neostigmine or edrophonium. Br J Anaesth 59:983, 1987

304. Cronnelly R, Morris RB, Miller RD: Edrophonium: Duration of action and atropine requirement in humans during halothane anesthesia. Anesthesiology 57:261, 1982

305. Breen PJ, Doherty WG, Donati F et al: The potencies of edrophonium and neostigmine as antagonists of pancuronium. Anaesthesia 40:844, 1985

306. Donati F, McCarroll SM, Antzaca C et al: Dose–response curves for edrophonium, neostigmine, and pyridostigmine after pancuronium and d-tubocurarine. Anesthesiology 66:471, 1987

307. Donati F, Smith CE, Bevan DR: Dose–response relationships for edrophonium and neostigmine as antagonists of moderate and profound atracurium blockade. Anesth Analg 68:13, 1989

308. Gencarelli PJ, Miller RD: Antagonism of ORG NC45 (vecuronium) and pancuronium neuromuscular blockade by neostigmine. Br J Anaesth 54:53, 1982

309. Smith CE, Donati F, Bevan DR: Dose–response relationships for edrophonium and neostigmine as antagonists of atracurium and vecuronium neuromuscular blockade. Anesthesiology 71:37, 1989

310. Cronnelly R, Stanski DR, Miller RD et al: Renal function and the pharmacokinetics of neostigmine in anesthetized man. Anesthesiology 51:222, 1979

311. Morris RB, Cronnelly R, Miller RD et al: Pharmacokinetics of edrophonium in anephric and renal transplant patients. Br J Anaesth 53:1311, 1981

312. Rennick BR: Renal tubule transport of organic cations. Am J Physiol 9:F83, 1981

313. Miller RD, Van Nyhuis LS, Eger EI et al: Comparative times to peak effect and durations of action of neostigmine and pyridostigmine. Anesthesiology 41:27, 1974

314. Mirakhur RK: Antagonism of neuromuscular block in the elderly: A comparison of atropine and glycopyrrolate in a mixture with neostigmine. Anaesthesia 40:254, 1985

315. Ferguson A, Egerszegi P, Bevan DR: Neostigmine, pyridostigmine, and edrophonium as antagonists of pancuronium. Anesthesiology 53:390, 1980

316. Rupp SM, McChristian JW, Miller RD et al: Neostigmine and edrophonium antagonism of varying intensity neuromuscular blockade induced by atracurium, pancuronium, or vecuronium. Anesthesiology 64:711, 1986

317. Meretoja OA, Gebert R: Postoperative neuromuscular block following atracurium in children. Can J Anaesth 37:743, 1990

318. Baurain MJ, Hoton F, d'Hollander AA, Cantraine FR: Is recovery of neuromuscular transmission complete after the use of neostigmine to antagonise block produced by rocuronium, vecuronium, atracurium and pancuronium? Br J Anaesth 77:496, 1996

319. Baurain MJ, Dernovoi BS, d'Hollander AA et al: Conditions to optimise the reversal action of neostigmine upon a vecuronium-induced neuromuscular block. Acta Anaesthesiol Scand 40:574, 1996

320. Kirkegaard-Nielsen H, Hjelbo-Hansen HS, Lindholm P et al: Optimum time for neostigmine reversal of atracurium-induced neuromuscular blockade. Can J Anaesth 43:932, 1996

321. Szalados JE, Donati F, Bevan DR: Edrophonium priming for antagonism of atracurium neuromuscular blockade. Can J Anaesth 37:197, 1990

322. Naguib M, Abdulatif M, Al-Ghamdi A: Dose–response relationships for edrophonium and neostigmine antagonism of rocuronium bromide (Org 9426)-induced neuromuscular blockade. Anesthesiology 79:739, 1993

323. Naguib M, Abdulatif M, Al-Ghamdi A et al: Dose–response relationships for edrophonium and neostigmine antagonism of mivacurium-induced neuromuscular blockade. Br J Anaesth 71:709, 1993

324. Meakin G, Sweet PT, Bevan JC, Bevan DR: Neostigmine and edrophonium as antagonists of pancuronium in infants and children. Anesthesiology 59:316, 1983

325. Fisher DM, Cronnelly R, Miller RD, Sharma M: The neuromuscular pharmacology of neostigmine in infants and children. Anesthesiology 59:220, 1983

326. Baxter MM, Bevan JC, Samuel J et al: Postoperative neuromuscular function in pediatric day-care patients. Anesth Analg 72:504, 1991

327. Gill SS, Bevan DR, Donati F: Edrophonium antagonism of atracurium during enflurane anaesthesia. Br J Anaesth 64:300, 1990

328. Bevan DR, Archer DP, Donati F et al: Antagonism of pancuronium in renal failure: No recurarization. Br J Anaesth 54:63, 1982

329. Wirtavouri K, Salmenperä M, Tammisto T: Effect of hypocarbia and hypercarbia on the antagonism of pancuronium-induced neuromuscular blockade with neostigmine in man. Br J Anaesth 54:57, 1982

330. Fuchs-Buder T, Ziegenfuß T, Lysakowski K, Tassonyi E: Antagonism of vecuronium-induced neuromuscular block in patients pretreated with magnesium sulphate: Dose–effect relationship of neostigmine. Br J Anaesth 82:61,1999

331. Aitkenhead AR: Anaesthesia and bowel surgery. Br J Anaesth 56:95, 1984

332. King MJ, Milazkiewicz R, Carli F, Deacock AR: Influence of neostigmine on postoperative vomiting. Br J Anaesth 61:403, 1988

Clinical Anesthesia (4/e), edited by Paul G. Barash, Bruce F. Cullen, and Robert K. Stoelting. Lippincott Williams & Wilkins, Philadelphia, © 2001.

CHAPTER 17

LOCAL ANESTHETICS

SPENCER S. LIU AND PETER S. HODGSON

INTRODUCTION

Local anesthetics block the generation, propagation, and oscillations of electrical impulses in electrically excitable tissue. Use of local anesthetics in clinical anesthesia is varied and includes direct injection into tissues, topical application, and intravenous administration to produce clinical effects at varied locations including the central neuraxis, peripheral nerves, mucosa, skin, heart, and airway. Detailed knowledge of pertinent anatomy and pharmacology will aid in optimal therapeutic use of local anesthetics. Care should be taken to avoid potential central nervous system and cardiovascular toxicity from local anesthetics.

Cocaine was the first local anesthetic used (1884) but eventually fell into disfavor owing to its toxicity and addiction potential. The first aminoester local anesthetic, procaine, was introduced in 1905, and the first aminoamide local anesthetic, lidocaine, was introduced in 1944. Commercial release of these agents, which possessed high efficacy and low toxicity, revitalized the use of local anesthetics for regional anesthesia and other clinical applications. Many local anesthetics have been introduced since then, with ropivacaine (1996) and *levo*-bupivacaine (2000) representing the latest offerings. This chapter reviews: (1) mechanisms of action of local anesthetics for neural blockade; (2) pharmacology and pharmacodynamics of local anesthetics; (3) pharmacokinetics of local anesthetics; (4) clinical use of local anesthetics; (5) toxicity of local anesthetics; and (6) new local anesthetics and local anesthetic preparations.

MECHANISMS OF ACTION OF LOCAL ANESTHETICS

Anatomy of Nerves

Local anesthetics are often used to block nerves either peripherally or centrally. Knowledge of the anatomy of nerves will aid in understanding mechanism of action of local anesthetics. Peripheral nerves are mixed nerves containing afferent and efferent fibers that may be myelinated or unmyelinated. Each axon within the nerve fiber is surrounded by endoneurium composed of nonneural glial cells. Individual nerve fibers are gathered into fascicles and surrounded by perineurium composed of connective tissue. Finally, the entire peripheral nerve is encased by epineurium composed of dense connective tissue (Fig. 17-1). Thus, several layers of protective tissue surround individual axons, and these layers act as barriers to the penetration of local anesthetics.[1] In addition to the enveloping connective tissue, all mammalian nerves with a diameter greater than 1 μm are myelinated. Myelinated nerve fibers are segmentally enclosed by Schwann cells forming a bilayer lipid membrane that is wrapped several hundred times around each axon.[2] Thus, myelin accounts for over half the thickness of nerve fibers >1 μm (Fig. 17-2). Separating the myelinated regions are the nodes of Ranvier where structural elements for neuronal excitation are concentrated (Fig. 17-3).[3] The nodes are covered by interdigitations from nonmyelinating Schwann cells[4] and by negatively charged glycoproteins. Although axonal membranes are not freely in contact with their environment at the nodes, these areas do allow passage of drugs and ions.[5] Furthermore, the negatively charged proteins may bind basic local anesthetics and thus act as a depot. Unmyelinated nerve fibers (diameter

<1 μm) are encased by a Schwann cell that covers several (5–10) fibers at once (Fig. 17-2). These fibers are continuously encased by Schwann cells and do not possess interruptions (nodes of Ranvier). The existence of multiple protective layers around both myelinated and unmyelinated nerve fibers presents a substantial barrier to the entry of clinically used local anesthetics. For example, animal models suggest that only 1.6% of an injected dose of local anesthetic penetrates into the nerve following performance of peripheral nerve blocks.[6]

Nerve fibers are commonly classified by size, conduction velocity, and function (Table 17-1). In general, increasing myelination and nerve diameter lead to increased conduction velocity. The presence of myelin accelerates conduction velocity due to increased electrical insulation of nerve fibers and saltatory conduction. Increased nerve diameter accelerates conduction velocity both by increased myelination and by improved electrical cable conduction properties of the nerve. Myelinated and unmyelinated nerves carry out both afferent and efferent functions.

Electrophysiology of Neural Conduction

Ionic disequilibria across semipermeable membranes form the basis for neuronal resting potentials and for the potential energy needed to initiate and maintain electrical impulses. The resting potential of neural membranes averages −60 to −70 mV, with the interior being negative to the exterior. This resting potential is predominantly maintained by a potassium gradient with 10 times greater concentration of potassium within the cell. This gradient is maintained by an active protein pump that transports potassium into the cell and sodium out of the cell through voltage-gated potassium channels that are open at resting potentials.[7] Potassium equilibrium is not the only factor in resting potential, as a resting potential of approximately −90 mV is predicted by the Nernst equation if only potassium is considered. In addition to potassium channels, voltage-independent channels that allow "leak" currents of sodium, chloride, and other ions affect the resting potential.

In contrast to the dependence of resting membrane potential on potassium disequilibria, generation of action potentials is primarily due to activation of voltage-gated sodium channels.[7] These channels are protein structures spanning the bilayer lipid membrane composed of structural elements, an aqueous pore, and voltage-sensing elements that control passage of ions through the pore (Fig. 17-4).[8] Sodium channels exist in several conformations depending on membrane potential and time. At resting membrane potential, sodium channels predominantly exist in a resting (closed) conformation.[7,9] During membrane depolarization, channels open within a few hundred microseconds and allow passage of 10^7 ions · sec^{-1}. Sodium channels are relatively selective, but other monovalent ions can also gain passage through the channel. For example, lithium traverses about as well as sodium, whereas potassium only about one tenth as well. Following activation (opening) of the sodium channel and depolarization, the channel will spontaneously close into an inactivated state in a time-dependent fashion to allow repolarization, then revert to a resting conformation.[10] Thus, a three-state kinetic scheme (Fig. 17-5) conceptualizes the changes in sodium channel conformation that account for changes in sodium conductance during depolarization and repolarization.

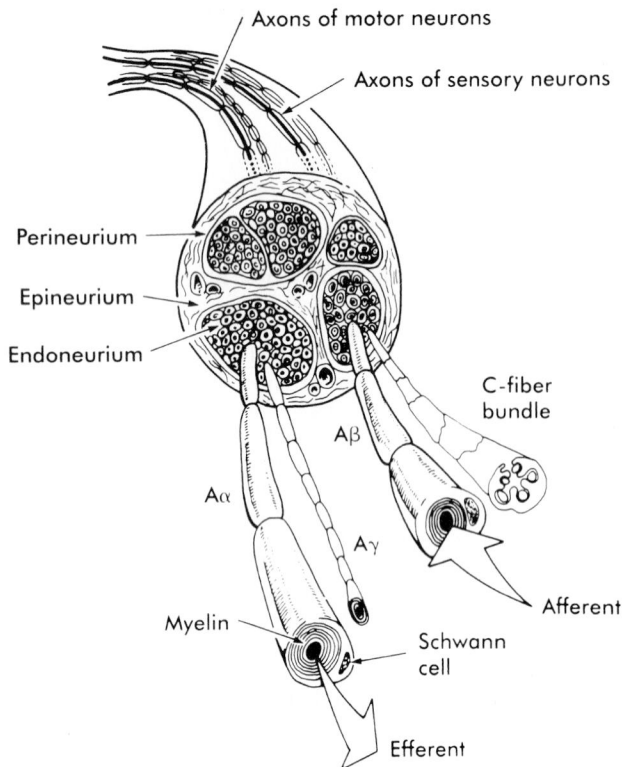

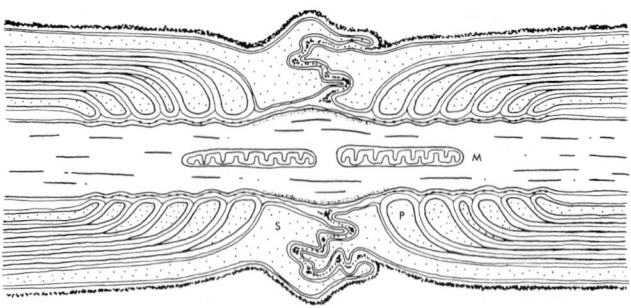

Figure 17-3. Diagram of node of Ranvier displaying mitochondria (M), tight junctions in paranodal area (P), and Schwann cell (S) surrounding node. (Adapted with permission from Strichartz GR: Mechanisms of Action of Local Anesthetic Agents. In Rogers MC, Tinker JH, Covino BG, Longnecker DE (eds): Principles and Practice of Anesthesiology, p 1197. St. Louis, Mosby–Year Book, 1993.)

Figure 17-1. Schematic cross section of typical peripheral nerve. The epineurium, consisting of collagen fibers, is oriented along the long axis of the nerve. The peineurium is a discrete cell layer, whereas the endoneurium is a matrix of connective tissue. Both afferent and efferent axons are shown. Sympathetic axons (not shown) are also present in mixed peripheral nerves. (Adapted with permission from Strichartz GR: Neural physiology and local anesthetic action. In Cousins MJ, Bridenbaugh PO (eds): Neural Blockade in Clinical Anesthesia and Management of Pain, p 35. Philadelphia, Lippincott–Raven, 1998.)

slowly create an action potential. As the stimulus slowly increases, initially activated sodium channels will spontaneously inactivate, so there will never be enough open channels at one time to generate an action potential. Furthermore, voltage-sensitive potassium channels would begin to increase potassium conductance that would further inhibit generation of an action potential. Thus, successful generation of an action potential requires a depolarizing stimulus of correct intensity and duration.

Once an action potential is generated, propagation of the potential along the nerve fiber is required for information to be transmitted. Both impulse generation and propagation are "all or nothing" phenomena. In the case of impulse propagation, either the locally generated action potential reaches the threshold potential of adjacent segments and causes propagation along the nerve, or the local depolarization ends. Nonmyelinated fibers require achievement of threshold potential at the immediately adjacent membrane, whereas myelinated fibers require generation of threshold potential at a subsequent node of Ranvier.

Repolarization after action potential generation and propagation rapidly follows owing to increasing equilibria of internal and external sodium ions, a time-controlled decrease in sodium conductance, and a voltage-controlled increase in potassium conductance.[11] In addition, active internal concentration of potassium occurs *via* the membrane-bound enzyme Na^+/K^+-ATPase which extrudes three sodium ions for every two potassium ions that are absorbed. Although many mammalian nonmyelinated nerve fibers develop a period of hyperpolarization after the action potential, myelinated nerve fibers return directly to resting membrane potential.[11]

An action potential will be generated by depolarization when the impulse firing threshold of the axon is reached. That is the point at which no further depolarization is required for local processes to generate a complete action potential. This threshold is not an absolute voltage, but rather depends on the dynamics of the sodium and potassium channels. For example, a brief maximally depolarizing stimulus will not generate an action potential because there is insufficient time for sodium channels to open. Nor will a depolarizing stimulus that increases too

Molecular Mechanisms of Action of Local Anesthetics

Most evidence indicates that the sodium channel is the key target of local anesthetic activity. The wide variety of compounds that exhibit local anesthetic activity combined with the different effects of neutral and charged local anesthetics suggests that local anesthetics may act on the sodium channel either by modification of the lipid membrane surrounding it or by direct interaction with its protein structure.

Previous studies have demonstrated that anesthetics can reduce sodium conductance through sodium channels by interacting with the surrounding lipid membrane.[12] Alterations in neuronal membranes by local anesthetics can occur by altering the fluidity of the membrane that causes membrane expansion and subsequent closure of the sodium channel. Furthermore, alterations in membrane composition may lower the probability of occurrence of the open sodium channel state. Such observa-

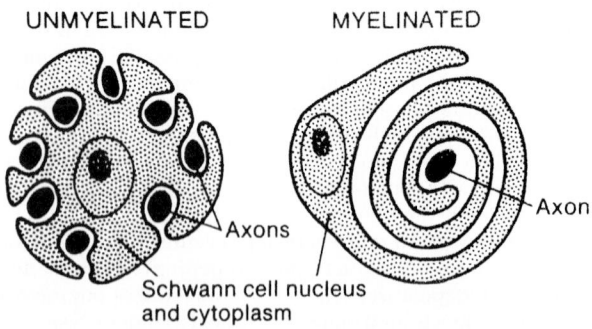

Figure 17-2. Schwann cells form myelin around one myelinated axon or encompass several unmyelinated axons. (Adapted with permission from Carpenter RL, Mackey DC: Local anesthetics. In Barash PG, Cullen BF, Stoelting RF (eds): Clinical Anesthesia, p 413. Philadelphia, Lippincott–Raven, 1996.)

Table 17-1. CLASSIFICATION OF NERVE FIBERS

Classification	Diameter (μm)	Myelin	Conduction (m · sec^{-1})	Location	Function
A alpha A beta	6–22	+	30–120	Afferents to and efferents from muscles and joints	Motor and proprioception
A gamma	3–6	+	15–35	Efferent to muscle spindle	Muscle tone
A delta	1–4	+	5–25	Afferent sensory nerve	Pain Touch Temperature
B	<3	+	3–15	Preganglionic sympathetic	Autonomic function
C	0.3–1.3	−	0.7–1.3	Postganglionic sympathetic Afferent sensory nerve	Autonomic function Pain Temperature

tions can account for local anesthetic actions of neutral and lipophilic local anesthetics, but do not explain the different activity of clinically used, tertiary amine local anesthetics (*e.g.*, lidocaine).

Instead, the mechanisms of action of these local anesthetics are best explained by direct interaction with the sodium channel (modulated receptor theory).[13,14] The commonly used tertiary amine local anesthetics exist in free equilibrium as both a lipid-soluble neutral form and a hydrophilic, charged form depending on pK_a and environmental pH. Although the neutral form may exert anesthetic actions as described above, the cationic species is clearly the more potent form (see Fig. 17-4).[14] These tertiary amine local anesthetics also demonstrate greater sodium channel blockade when the neural membrane is repetitively depolarized (1-100 Hz),[15,16] whereas neutral local anesthetics exhibit little change in activity with increased frequency of stimulation (use-dependent block). Increasing frequency of stimulation increases the probability that sodium channels will exist in the open and inactive forms as compared to the unstimulated state. Thus, differences in activity of tertiary amine local anesthetics between use-dependent (repetitive stimulation) and

tonic (unstimulated) block are well explained by the existence of a single local anesthetic receptor within the sodium channel that possesses different affinities during different channel conformations (resting, open, inactive). Specifically, higher affinities occur during the open and inactive phases. In support of this theory, when the affinity of inactive channels for local anesthetics is decreased through genetic manipulation, use-dependent block is abolished.[17]

Molecular manipulation of the sodium channel is beginning to reveal specifics of the local anesthetic receptor. Binding sites to local anesthetics are located on the intracellular side of the sodium channel, may have different binding areas during the open and inactivated conformations of the sodium channel, and possess stereoselectivity with preference for the *R* isomers.[9,18,19] The use of molecular techniques to determine exact binding sites for different actions of local anesthetics and the development of tailored agonists to these binding sites may, in future, create more effective local anesthetics that are specific for tonic or use-dependent block.

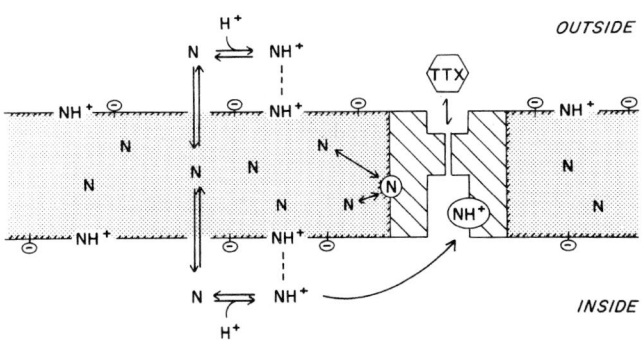

Figure 17-4. Diagram of bilayer lipid membrane of conductive tissue with sodium channel (cross-hatching) spanning the membrane. Tertiary amine local anesthetics exist as neutral base (N) and protonated, charged form (NH$^+$) in equilibrium. The neutral base (N) is more lipid-soluble, preferentially partitions into the lipophilic membrane interior, and easily passes through the membrane. The charged form (NH$^+$) is more water-soluble and binds to the sodium channel at the negatively charged membrane surface. Both forms can affect function of the sodium channel. The N form can cause membrane expansion and closure of the sodium channel. The NH$^+$ form will directly inhibit the sodium channel by binding with a local anesthetic receptor. The natural "local anesthetic" tetrodotoxin (TTX) binds at the external surface of the sodium channel and has no interaction with clinically used local anesthetics. (Adapted with permission from Strichartz GR: Neural physiology and local anesthetic action. In Cousins MJ, Bridenbaugh PO (eds): Neural Blockade in Clinical Anesthesia and Management of Pain, p 35. Philadelphia, Lippincott–Raven, 1998.)

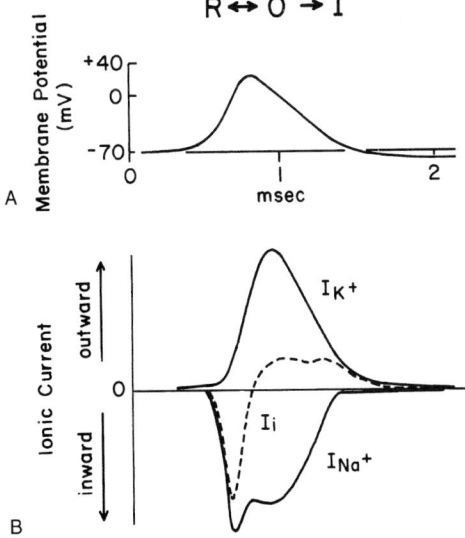

Figure 17-5. Illustration of dominant form of sodium channel during generation of an action potential. R = resting form; O = open form; I = inactive form. (*A*) The concurrent generation of an action potential as the membrane depolarizes from resting potential. (*B*) Concurrent changes in ion flux, as inward sodium current (I_{Na+}) and outward potassium current (I_{K+}) together yield the net ionic current across the membrane (I_i). (Adapted with permission from Strichartz GR: Neural physiology and local anesthetic action. In Cousins MJ, Bridenbaugh PO (eds): Neural Blockade in Clinical Anesthesia and Management of Pain, p 35. Philadelphia, Lippincott–Raven, 1998.)

Mechanism of Blockade of Peripheral Nerves

Local anesthetics may block function of peripheral nerves through several mechanisms. As discussed above, sodium channel blockade leads to attenuation of neural action potential formation and propagation. Although it remains unknown in humans by what percent the neural action potential must be decreased before functional block occurs, recent animal studies suggest that the action potential must be decreased by at least 50% before measurable loss of function is observed.[6] Previous studies have examined the differences in susceptibility of nerve fiber to local anesthetic blockade based on size, myelination, and length of fiber exposed to local anesthetic. Clinically, one can often discern a differential pattern of sensory block after application of local anesthetic to a peripheral nerve.[20] Classically, the sensation of temperature is lost, followed by sharp pain, then light touch. Thus, an initial assumption was that small, unmyelinated (C) fibers conducting temperature sensation were inherently more susceptible to local anesthetic blockade than large, myelinated (A) fibers conducting touch. However, experimental studies reveal a more complex picture. When local anesthetic block is restricted to ≤1 cm of the length of a nerve, A fibers exhibit a greater susceptibility to tonic block than do C fibers. In contrast, C fibers are more susceptible to use-dependent block.[16] Differential block of large and small nerve fibers is also affected by choice of local anesthetic. Those with an amide group, high pK_a, and lower lipid solubility are more potent blockers of C fibers. Thus, experimental studies indicate that local anesthetic block of nerve fibers will intrinsically depend on type (size) of fiber, frequency of membrane stimulation, and choice of local anesthetic.[15,21]

During clinical applications, it is likely that >1 cm of the peripheral nerve is exposed to local anesthetic. For example, sciatic nerve blocks in humans probably result in 5–10 cm of affected nerve length.[6] In such a situation, the exposure length of the nerve fiber becomes an important determinant of blocking susceptibility.[22,23] Small nerve fibers require a shorter length of fiber exposed to local anesthetic for block to occur than do large fibers. It is theorized that this observation is due to *decremental conduction.*[23] This phenomenon describes the decreased ability of successive nodes of Ranvier to propagate an impulse in the presence of local anesthetic (Fig. 17-6). As

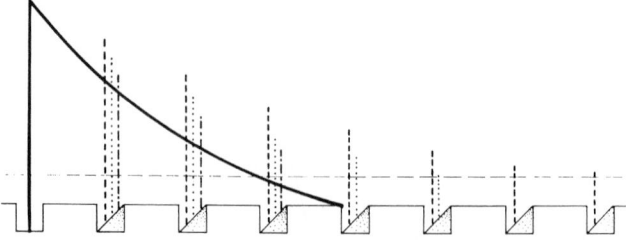

Figure 17-6. Diagram illustrating the principle of decremental conduction block by local anesthetic at a myelinated axon. The first node of Ranvier at left contains no local anesthetic and gives rise to a normal action potential (*solid curve*). If the nodes succeeding the first are occupied by a concentration of local anesthetic high enough to block 74–84% of the sodium conductance, the action potential amplitudes decrease at successive nodes (amplitudes are indicated by interrupted bars representing three increasing concentrations of local anesthetic). Eventually, the impulse decays to below-threshold amplitude if the series of local anesthetic containing nodes is long enough. Propagation of the impulse has then been blocked by decremental conduction, even though none of the nodes is completely blocked. Concentrations of local anesthetic that block more than 84% of the sodium conductance at three successive nodes prevent any impulse propagation at all. (Adapted with permission from Fink BR: Mechanisms of differential axial blockade in epidural and spinal anesthesia. Anesthesiology 70:851, 1989.)

internodal distances become greater with increasing nerve fiber size,[24] larger nerve fibers will demonstrate increasing resistance to local anesthetic block. Thus, this theory provides an explanation for the clinical occurrence of differential sensory block.

A final mechanism whereby local anesthetics may block peripheral nerve function is *via* degradation of transmitted electrical patterns. It is theorized that a large part of the sensory information transmitted *via* peripheral nerves is carried *via* coding of electrical signals in after-potentials and after-oscillations.[25] Evidence for this theory is found in studies demonstrating loss of sensory nerve function after incomplete local anesthetic blockade. For example, sensation of temperature of the skin can be lost despite unimpeded conduction of small fibers.[26] Furthermore, a surgical depth of epidural and peripheral nerve block anesthesia can be obtained with only minor changes in somatosensory-evoked potentials from the anesthetized area.[27,28] Previous studies have demonstrated that application of subblocking concentrations of local anesthetic will suppress normally occurring after-potentials and after-oscillations without significantly affecting action potential conduction.[29] Thus, disruption of coding of electrical information by local anesthetics may be another mechanism for block of peripheral nerves.

Mechanism of Blockade of Central Neuraxis

Central neuraxial block *via* spinal or epidural administration of local anesthetics involves the same mechanisms at the level of spinal nerve roots, either intra- or extradural, as discussed above. In addition, central neuraxial administration of local anesthetics allows multiple potential actions of local anesthetics within the spinal cord at different sites. For example, within the dorsal horn, local anesthetics can exert familiar ion channel block of sodium and potassium channels in dorsal horn neurons and inhibit generation and propagation of nociceptive electrical activity.[30] Similar actions in the ventral horn may contribute to block of motor activity from central neuraxial administration of local anesthetics. Other spinal cord neuronal ion channels, such as calcium channels, are also important for afferent and efferent electrical activity. Administration of calcium channel blockers to spinal cord N (neuronal) calcium channels results in hyperpolarization of cell membranes, resistance to electrical stimulation from nociceptive afferents, and intense analgesia.[31] Local anesthetics appear to have similar actions on calcium channels, which may contribute to analgesic actions of central neuraxially administered local anesthetics.[32]

In addition to ion channels, multiple neurotransmitters are involved in nociceptive transmission in the dorsal horn of the spinal cord.[33] For example, substance P, the archetypal tachykinin, is an important neurotransmitter that modulates nociception from C fibers and is released from presynaptic terminals of dorsal root ganglion cells.[34] Administration of local anesthetics in concentrations that occur after spinal and epidural anesthesia inhibits release of substance P and may exert analgesic actions by presynaptic actions.[35] Other neurotransmitters that are important for nociceptive processing in the spinal cord, such as acetylcholine and γ-aminobutyric acid (GABA), are also affected by local anesthetics in the presynaptic area. Local anesthetics can affect these analgesic pathways by either directly binding to receptors or by altering local pharmacokinetics of endogenous agonists.[36–38] Finally, local anesthetics can also affect the postsynaptic effects of nociceptive neurotransmitters. Administration of clinically relevant concentrations of local anesthetics inhibits binding of substance P to its receptor in the central neuraxis in a noncompetitive fashion.[39] These studies suggest that antinociceptive effects of central neuraxial local anesthetic block may be mediated *via* complex interactions at neural synapses in addition to ion channel blockade.

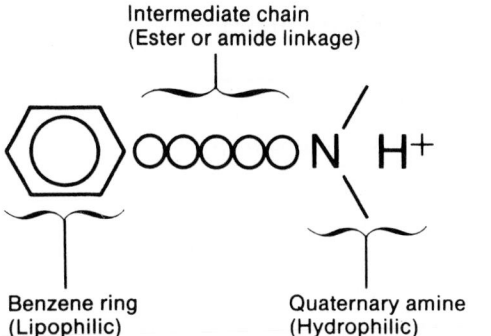

Figure 17-7. General structure of clinically used local anesthetics. (Adapted with permission from Carpenter RL, Mackey DC: Local anesthetics. In Barash PG, Cullen BF, Stoelting RF (eds): Clinical Anesthesia, p 413. Philadelphia, Lippincott–Raven, 1996.)

PHARMACOLOGY AND PHARMACODYNAMICS

Chemical Properties and Relationship to Activity and Potency

The clinically used local anesthetics consist of a lipid-soluble, substituted benzene ring linked to an amine group (tertiary or quaternary depending on pK_a and pH) *via* an alkyl chain containing either an amide or ester linkage (Fig. 17-7). The type of linkage separates the local anesthetics into either *aminoamides*, metabolized in the liver, or *aminoesters*, metabolized by plasma cholinesterases. Several chemical properties of local anesthetics will affect their efficacy and potency.

All clinically used local anesthetics are weak bases that can exist as either the lipid-soluble, neutral form or as the charged, hydrophilic form. The combination of pH of the environment and pK_a, or dissociation constant, of a local anesthetic determines how much of the compound exists in each form (Table 17-2). As previously discussed, the primary site of action of local anesthetics appears to exist on the intracellular side of the sodium channel, and the charged form appears to be the predominantly active form.[14] Penetration of the lipid-soluble form through the lipid neural membrane appears to be the primary form of access of local anesthetic molecules, although some access by the charged form can be gained *via* the aqueous

sodium channel pore (see Fig. 17-4).[40] Thus, decreasing pK_a for a given environmental pH will increase the percentage of lipid-soluble forms in existence, hastening penetration of neural membranes and onset of action.

Lipid solubility is another important determinant of activity. Although increasing lipid solubility may hasten penetration of neural membranes, increasing solubility may also result in increased sequestration of local anesthetic in myelin and other lipid-soluble compartments. Thus, increasing lipid solubility usually slows the rate of onset of action.[41] Similarly, duration of action is increased as absorption of local anesthetic molecules into myelin and surrounding neural compartments creates a depot for slow release of local anesthetics.[41] Finally, increased lipid solubility increases potency of the local anesthetic.[12,13] This observation may be explained by a correlation between lipid solubility and both sodium channel receptor affinity and ability to alter sodium channel conformation by direct effects on lipid cell membranes.

Degree of protein binding also affects activity of local anesthetics, as only the unbound form is free for pharmacologic activity. In general, increasing protein binding is associated with increased duration of action. Although the sodium channel is a protein structure, it does not appear that degree of local anesthetic protein binding correlates with binding to the local anesthetic receptor. Studies suggest that dissociation of local anesthetic molecules from the sodium channel occurs in a matter of seconds regardless of degree of protein binding of the local anesthetic.[42] Thus, prolongation in duration of action associated with an increased degree of protein binding must involve other extracellular or membranous proteins.

A final physical property of current interest is stereoisomeric mixture of the commercially available local anesthetics. All currently available local anesthetics are racemic mixtures with the exception of lidocaine (achiral), ropivacaine (*S*), and *levo*-bupivacaine (*l = S*).[43,44] Stereoisomers of local anesthetics appear to have potentially different effects on anesthetic potency, pharmacokinetics, and systemic toxicity.[43,45] For example, *R* isomers appear to have greater *in vitro* potency for block of both neural and cardiac sodium channels and may thus have greater therapeutic efficacy and potential systemic toxicity.[19,46] A complete analysis of clinical effects resulting from the potential differences in pharmacology between optical isomers has not been undertaken, nor have optimal mixtures of optical isomers been determined. Future production and commercial release of specific local anesthetic isomers may allow for precise selection of

Table 17-2. PHYSICOCHEMICAL PROPERTIES OF CLINICALLY USED LOCAL ANESTHETICS

Local Anesthetic	pK_a	% Ionized (at pH 7.4)	Partition Coefficient (lipid solubility)	% Protein Binding
AMIDES				
Bupivacaine*	8.1	83	3420	95
Etidocaine	7.7	66	7317	94
Lidocaine	7.9	76	366	64
Mepivacaine	7.6	61	130	77
Prilocaine	7.9	76	129	55
Ropivacaine	8.1	83	775	94
ESTERS				
Chloroprocaine	8.7	95	810	N/A
Procaine	8.9	97	100	6
Tetracaine	8.5	93	5822	94

N/A = not available.
Data from Liu SS: Local anesthetics and analgesia. In Ashburn MA, Rice LJ (eds): The Management of Pain, p 141. New York, Churchill Livingstone, 1997.
* *levo*-Bupivacaine has the same physicochemical properties as the racemate.

Table 17-3. RELATIVE POTENCY OF LOCAL ANESTHETICS FOR BLOCK OF DIFFERENT NERVE FIBERS

| | Nerve Fiber | | | | | |
| | Tonic Block | | | Use-Dependent Block | | |
Local Anesthetic	A	B	C	A	B	C
Bupivacaine	12.3	8.4	5.9	16	21.3	24.7
levo-Bupivacaine	16.4	11.2	7.8	24	32	37
Etidocaine	22.9	20	14.5	35.5	26.7	21.3
Lidocaine	3	2.3	0.8	3.4	4.8	3.4
Mepivacaine	1.7	1.3	0.7	2	2.9	2
Procaine	1	0.7	0.3	1.1	1.1	0.5
Ropivacaine	9.4	6.4	3.5	10.7	15.2	9.7

Data from Wildsmith JA: Br J Anaesth 63:444, 1989 and Lee-Son MB, Wang GK, Concus *et al*: Stereoselective inhibition of neuronal sodium channels by local anesthetics. Anesthesiology 77:324, 1992.

not only type of local anesthetic but also exact racemic mixtures for specific applications. (Ropivacaine and *levo*-bupivacaine are discussed in the section on New and Future Local Anesthetics.)

Relative *in vitro* potencies of the clinically used local anesthetics have been identified and vary depending on individual nerve fibers and frequency of stimulation (Table 17-3). As previously mentioned, increasing nerve size and increasing rate of electrical stimulation increase susceptibility to local anesthetic blockade for affected nerve length <1 cm. In general, increasing lipid solubility of local anesthetic correlates with increasing anesthetic potency (see Table 17-2).[47] However, clinical use of local anesthetics is more complex than the bathing of nerve fibers in solutions, and *in vivo* potencies often do not correlate with *in vitro* determinants.[48] Local factors affecting diffusion and spread of anesthetic will have great impact on clinical effects and will vary with different applications (*e.g.*, peripheral nerve block vs. spinal injection). Furthermore, clinical use may not require absolute suppression of the compound action potential, but rather a disruption of information coding in the pattern of discharges. Few rigorous studies have been performed to evaluate relative clinical potencies of local anesthetics, and commonly accepted values are listed in Table 17-4.

Mixtures of Local Anesthetics

Combining a quick-acting local anesthetic (chloroprocaine, lidocaine, prilocaine) with one having a long duration of action (bupivacaine, etidocaine) is practiced by some clinicians. The value of such combinations is unclear, as previous studies have reported inconsistent effects on onset and duration of action that may vary with type of local anesthetic, ratio of local anesthetic mixtures, and type of neural block.[49,50] These disparate findings may reflect the complexity of potential interactions of mixtures of local anesthetics. Actions of local anesthetic combi-

nations could be due to additive, antagonistic, or synergistic actions at the local anesthetic receptor; to effects on permeability of component local anesthetics through tissue barriers; or to changes in uptake of component local anesthetics.[50] Thus, current evidence does not allow conclusions regarding effectiveness of mixing local anesthetics. However, systemic toxicity appears to be additive, and caution should be used to limit total doses of local anesthetic mixtures.[51,52]

Tachyphylaxis to Local Anesthetics

Tachyphylaxis to local anesthetics is a clinical phenomenon whereby repeated injection of the same dose of local anesthetic leads to decreasing efficacy. Tachyphylaxis has been described after central neuraxial blocks, peripheral nerve blocks, and for different local anesthetics.[53,54] An interesting clinical feature of tachyphylaxis to local anesthetics is its dependence on dosing interval. If dosing intervals are short enough such that pain does not occur, tachyphylaxis does not develop. Conversely, longer periods of patient discomfort before redosing hastens development of tachyphylaxis.[53] Previous studies investigating the etiology of tachyphylaxis have found little pharmacokinetic or -dynamic change after repeated doses of local anesthetics. For example, with the development of clinical tachyphylaxis, there is no difference in local anesthetic spread within or clearance from the epidural space.[55] Changes in pH of the surrounding tissues do not affect the development of tachyphylaxis.[54] Prolonged exposure of peripheral nerve and neural cells to local anesthetic does not affect either flux through sodium channels[56] or propagation of the action potential over time.[57] The lack of an etiology, coupled with the observation that pain is important for the development of tachyphylaxis, led to speculation that there is a central, spinal mechanism for tachyphylaxis *via* spinal cord sensitization. A series of studies in 1994 lend

Table 17-4. RELATIVE POTENCY OF LOCAL ANESTHETICS FOR DIFFERENT CLINICAL APPLICATIONS

	Bupivacaine	Chloroprocaine	Etidocaine	Lidocaine	Mepivacaine	Prilocaine
Peripheral nerve	3.6	N/A	0.7	1	2.6	0.8
Spinal	9.6	N/A	6.7	1	1	N/A
Epidural	4	0.5	2	1	1	1

N/A = not available.
Data from Hassan HG: Acta Anaesth Scand 38:505, 1994; Langerman L: Br J Anaesth 72:456, 1994; Langerman L: Anesth Analg 79:490, 1994; Smith C: Br J Hosp Med 52:455, 1994; Morrison LM: Br J Anaesth 72:164, 1994; Wahedi W: Reg Anaesth 13:66, 1990; Nolte H: Reg Anesth 15:118, 1990; Pateromichelakis S: Acta Anaesth Scand 32:672, 1988; and Vainionpaa VA: Anesth Analg 81:534, 1995.

support to this theory.[58] Rats receiving repeated sciatic nerve blocks with 2-chloroprocaine and lidocaine failed to develop tachyphylaxis in the absence of noxious stimulation. Exposure of the rats to increasingly noxious degrees of thermal stimulation increasingly hastened development of tachyphylaxis, whereas pretreatment with a NMDA antagonist (MK-801) that prevents spinal cord sensitization also prevented development of tachyphylaxis. Second-messenger effects of nitric oxide for NMDA pathways may be especially important, as administration of nitric oxide synthase inhibitors prevented development of tachyphylaxis in a dose-dependent manner in the same model.[59] The clinical relevance of these findings needs to be explored, but the development of a plausible etiology for local anesthetic tachyphylaxis may lead to useful clinical means for its prevention.

Additives to Increase Local Anesthetic Activity

Epinephrine

Epinephrine has been added to local anesthetics since the early 1890s.[60] Reported benefits of epinephrine include prolongation of local anesthetic block,[61] increased intensity of block,[62] and decreased systemic absorption of local anesthetic.[63] The mechanism whereby epinephrine augments local anesthetic actions remains uncertain. It is commonly theorized that vasoconstriction plays an important role,[64] as most local anesthetics, with the exception of ropivacaine,[65] produce local vasodilation.[66] Local vasoconstriction would theoretically inhibit systemic absorption of local anesthetic, thus allowing a greater amount available for blocking activity. Further analgesic effects from epinephrine may also occur *via* interaction with α_2-adrenergic receptors in the brain and spinal cord,[67] especially since local anesthetics increase the vascular uptake of epinephrine.[68] Although most reports support the practice of adding epinephrine, reported effectiveness depends on amount of epinephrine added, local anesthetic used, and type of regional block (Table 17-5). It is unfortunate that few data are available concerning the optimal amount of epinephrine as an additive. The smallest dose should be used, as epinephrine combined with local anesthetics may have toxic effects on tissue,[69] the cardiovascular system,[70] peripheral nerves, and the spinal cord.[33,60]

Alkalinization of Local Anesthetic Solution

Since the late 1800s, local anesthetic solutions have been alkalinized in order to hasten onset of neural block.[71] The pH of commercial preparations of local anesthetics ranges from 3.9 to 6.47 and is especially acidic if prepackaged with epinephrine.[72] As the pK_a of commonly used local anesthetics ranges from 7.6 to 8.9 (see Table 17-2), less than 3% of the commercially prepared local anesthetic exists as the lipid-soluble neutral form. As previously discussed, the neutral form is believed to be the most important for penetration into the neural cytoplasm, whereas the charged form primarily interacts with the local anesthetic receptor within the sodium channel. Therefore, the initial rationale for alkalinization was to increase the percentage of local anesthetic existing as the lipid-soluble neutral form. However, clinically used local anesthetics cannot be alkalinized beyond a pH of 6.05–8 before precipitation occurs,[72] and such pHs will only increase the neutral form to about 10%. Although a tripling of available local anesthetic (from 3% to 10%) will improve efficacy, recent studies have proposed several other mechanisms for the effects of alkalinization.

In general, clinical studies demonstrate increased activity of alkalinized local anesthetic only when epinephrine is present, either prepackaged or freshly added.[73] Although prepackaged epinephrine-containing solutions are quite acidic, fresh addition of epinephrine does not alter the pH of the more alkaline, plain local anesthetic solutions.[72] Thus, the association between increased local anesthetic activity with alkalinization and epinephrine does not appear to be due solely to increased acidity with epinephrine. On the other hand, the vasoconstrictive effects of epinephrine are also pH-dependent. At a pH less than 5.6, little vasoconstriction is seen, and maximal vasoconstriction occurs around a pH of 7.8. Therefore, alkalinization may affect activity of local anesthetic by activation of vasoconstrictive effects of epinephrine.

A series of studies examining desheathed nerve fibers suggested multiple mechanisms of interaction between bicarbonate and local anesthetic independent of neural penetration.[74] Alkalinization of the local environment by itself inhibited neural impulse conduction. Furthermore, addition of bicarbonate potentiates local anesthetic block of impulse conduction specific to type of local anesthetic. This finding suggests a specific inter-

Table 17-5. EFFECTS OF ADDITION OF EPINEPHRINE TO LOCAL ANESTHETICS

	Increase Duration	Decrease Blood Levels (%)	Dose/Concentration of Epinephrine
NERVE BLOCK			
Bupivacaine*	++	10–20	1:200,000
Lidocaine	++	20–30	1:200,000
Mepivacaine	++	20–30	1:200,000
Ropivacaine	−	0	1:200,000
EPIDURAL			
Bupivacaine*	++	10–20	1:300,000–1:200,000
Chloroprocaine	++		1:200,000
Lidocaine	++	20–30	1:600,000–1:200,000
Mepivacaine	++	20–30	1:200,000
Ropivacaine	−	0	1:200,000
SPINAL			
Bupivacaine*	++		0.2 mg
Lidocaine	++		0.2 mg
Tetracaine	++		0.2 mg

++ overall supported; − overall not supported.
Data from Liu SS: Local anesthetics and analgesia. In Ashburn MA, Rice LJ (eds): The Management of Pain, p 141. New York, Churchill Livingstone, 1997.
* Effects of epinephrine on *levo*-bupivacaine are unknown.

action at the local anesthetic receptor within the sodium channel. Thus, it is likely that alkalinization of local anesthetics works through multiple mechanisms to affect local anesthetic activity. Alkalinization of local anesthetics presents an easy, attractive means to alter activity of local anesthetics,[73] especially as toxicity is not increased.[60]

Opioids

Addition of opioids to local anesthetics has gained popularity. Opioids have multiple central neuraxial and peripheral mechanisms of analgesic action (see Chapter 14). Supraspinal administration of opioids results in analgesia *via* opiate receptors in multiple sites,[75] *via* activation of descending spinal pathways,[76] and *via* activation of nonopioid analgesic pathways.[77] Spinal administration of opioids provides analgesia primarily by attenuating C fiber nociception,[78] and is independent of supraspinal mechanisms.[79] Co-administration of opioids with most local anesthetics epidurally[80] and intrathecally[81] results in synergistic analgesia.[82] An exception to this analgesic synergy is 2-chloroprocaine, which appears to decrease the effectiveness of epidural opioids when used for epidural anesthesia.[83] The mechanism for this action is unclear but does not appear to involve direct antagonism of opioid receptors.[84] Overall, clinical studies support the practice of central neuraxial co-administration of local anesthetics and opioids in humans for prolongation and intensification of analgesia and anesthesia[85]; however, the optimal mixtures have yet to be determined.[86]

The discovery of peripheral opioid receptors offers yet another circumstance in which the co-administration of local anesthetics and opioids may be useful.[87] The most promising clinical results have been from intra-articular and peri-incisional administration of local anesthetic and opioid for postoperative analgesia,[88,89] whereas combining local anesthetics and opioids for nerve blocks appears to be ineffective.[90] There are several reasons for a predicted lack of effect of co-administration of local anesthetic and opioid for peripheral nerve blocks. Anatomically, peripheral opioid receptors are found primarily at the end terminals of afferent fibers.[91] However, peripheral nerves are commonly blocked by deposition of anesthetic proximal to the end terminals of nerve fibers. In addition, common sites for peripheral nerve blocks are encased in multiple layers of connective tissue which the anesthetics must traverse before gaining access to peripheral opioid receptors. Finally, previous studies have demonstrated the importance of concomitant local tissue inflammation for analgesic effectiveness of peripheral opioid receptors.[92] The mechanism for the underlying dependence on local inflammation is speculative and may involve up-regulation or activation of peripheral opioid receptors or ''loosening'' of intercellular junctions to allow passage of opioids to receptors. Nonetheless, lack of inflammation at the site of a peripheral nerve block may also reduce the effects of co-administration of local anesthetic and opioid. All of these factors combine to decrease the theoretical effectiveness of combinations of local anesthetics and opioids for peripheral nerve blocks. In summary, co-administration of opioids and local anesthetic in the central neuraxis appears to be an effective, nontoxic[33] means to improve activity of local anesthetic, whereas there is little theoretical reason to expect the mixture to enhance peripheral nerve block.

α_2-Adrenergic Agonists

α_2-Adrenergic agonists can be a useful adjuvant to local anesthetics. α_2 Agonists, such as clonidine, produce analgesia *via* supraspinal and spinal adrenergic receptors.[93] Clonidine also has direct inhibitory effects on peripheral nerve conduction (A and C nerve fibers).[94] Thus, addition of clonidine may have multiple routes of action depending on type of application. Preliminary evidence suggests that co-administration of α_2 agonist and local anesthetic results in central neuraxial and peripheral nerve analgesic synergy,[95] whereas systemic (supraspinal)

effects are additive.[96] Overall, clinical trials indicate that clonidine enhances intrathecal and epidural anesthesia,[93,97] peripheral nerve blocks,[98] and intravenous regional anesthesia[99] without evidence for neurotoxicity.[33]

PHARMACOKINETICS OF LOCAL ANESTHETICS

Clearance of local anesthetic from neural tissue and from the body governs both duration of effect and potential toxicity. Clinical effects of neural block from local anesthetics are primarily dependent on local factors as discussed in the Pharmacology section. However, systemic toxicity is primarily dependent on blood levels of local anesthetics. Resultant blood levels after administration of local anesthetics for neural blockade depend on absorption, distribution, and elimination of local anesthetics.

Systemic Absorption

In general, local anesthetics with decreased systemic absorption will have a greater margin of safety in clinical use. The rate and extent of absorption will depend on numerous factors, of which the most important are the site of injection, the dose of local anesthetic, the physicochemical properties of the local anesthetic, and the addition of epinephrine.

The relative amounts of fat and vasculature surrounding the site of local anesthetic injection will interact with the physicochemical properties of the local anesthetic to affect rate of systemic uptake. In general, areas with greater vascularity will have more rapid and complete uptake as compared to those with more fat, regardless of type of local anesthetic. Thus, rates of absorption from injection of local anesthetic into various sites generally decrease in the following order: intercostal > caudal > epidural > brachial plexus > sciatic/femoral (Table 17-6).[100,101]

The greater the total dose of local anesthetic injected, the greater the systemic absorption and peak blood levels (C_{max}). This relationship is nearly linear (Fig. 17-8) and is relatively unaffected by anesthetic concentration[102] and speed of injection.[100,101]

Physicochemical properties of local anesthetics will affect systemic absorption. In general, the more potent agents with greater lipid solubility and protein binding will result in lower systemic absorption and C_{max} (Fig. 17-9).[101] Increased binding to neural and nonneural tissue probably explains this observation.

Effects of epinephrine have been previously discussed. In brief, epinephrine can counteract the inherent vasodilating characteristics of most local anesthetics. The reduction in C_{max} with epinephrine is most effective for the less lipid-soluble, less potent, shorter-acting agents (see Table 17-5), as increased tissue binding rather than local blood flow may be a greater determinant of absorption for the long-acting agents.

Distribution

After systemic absorption, local anesthetics are rapidly distributed to the body. Regional distribution of local anesthetic will depend on organ blood flow, partition coefficient of local anesthetic between compartments, and plasma protein binding. The end organs of main concern for toxicity are within the cardiovascular and the central nervous systems. Both are considered members of the ''vessel-rich group'' and will have local anesthetic rapidly distributed to them. Despite the high blood perfusion, regional blood and tissue levels of local anesthetics within these organs will not initially correlate with systemic blood levels due to hysteresis.[103] As regional, rather than systemic, pharmacokinetics govern subsequent pharmacodynamic effects, systemic blood levels may not correlate with effects of local anesthetics on end organs.[104] Regional pharmacokinetics of local anesthetics for the heart and brain have not been fully delineated; thus the volume of distribution at steady state (VDss) is often

Table 17-6. TYPICAL C_{max} AFTER REGIONAL ANESTHETICS WITH COMMONLY USED LOCAL ANESTHETICS

Local Anesthetic	Technique	Dose (mg)	C_{max} ($\mu g \cdot ml^{-1}$)	T_{max} (min)	Toxic Plasma Concentration ($\mu g \cdot ml^{-1}$)
Bupivacaine*	Brachial plexus	150	1.00	20	3
	Celiac plexus	100	1.50	17	
	Epidural	150	1.26	20	
	Intercostal	140	0.90	30	
	Lumbar sympathetic	52.5	0.49	24	
	Sciatic/femoral	400	1.89	15	
Lidocaine	Brachial plexus	400	4.00	25	5
	Epidural	400	4.27	20	
	Intercostal	400	6.80	15	
Mepivacaine	Brachial plexus	500	3.68	24	5
	Epidural	500	4.95	16	
	Intercostal	500	8.06	9	
	Sciatic/femoral	500	3.59	31	
Ropivacaine	Brachial plexus	190	1.30	53	4
	Epidural	150	1.07	40	
	Intercostal	140	1.10	21	

C_{max} = peak plasma levels; T_{max} = time until C_{max}.
Data from Liu SS: Local anesthetics and analgesia. In Ashburn MA, Rice LJ (eds): The Management of Pain, p 141. New York, Churchill Livingstone, 1997; and Berrisford RG, Sabanathan S, Mearns AJ et al: Plasma concentrations of bupivacaine and its enantiomers during continuous extrapleural intercostal nerve block. Br J Anaesth 70:201, 1993.
* C_{max} and T_{max} after *levo*-bupivacaine are expected to be similar to those of the racemate.[1]

used to describe local anesthetic distribution (Table 17-7). However, VDss describes the extent of total body distribution and may be inaccurate for specific organ systems.

Elimination

Clearance (CL) of aminoester local anesthetics is primarily dependent on plasma clearance by cholinesterases,[105] whereas aminoamide local anesthetic clearance is dependent on clearance by the liver.[106] Thus, hepatic extraction, hepatic perfusion, hepatic metabolism, and protein binding (Table 17-7) will primarily determine the rate of clearance of aminoamide local anesthetics. In general, local anesthetics with higher rates of clearance will have a greater margin of safety.[101]

Clinical Pharmacokinetics

The primary benefit of a knowledge of the systemic pharmacokinetics of local anesthetics is the ability to predict C_{max} after the agents are administered, thereby avoiding the administration

of toxic doses (Tables 17-6, 17-8, and 17-9). However, pharmacokinetics are difficult to predict in any given circumstance as both physical and pathophysiologic characteristics will affect the individual pharmacokinetics. There is some evidence for increased systemic levels of local anesthetics in the very young and in the elderly owing to decreased clearance and increased absorption,[101] whereas correlation of resultant systemic blood levels between dose of local anesthetic and patient weight is often inconsistent (Fig. 17-10).[107] Effects of gender on clinical pharmacokinetics of local anesthetics have not been well defined, although pregnancy may decrease clearance.[101] Patho-

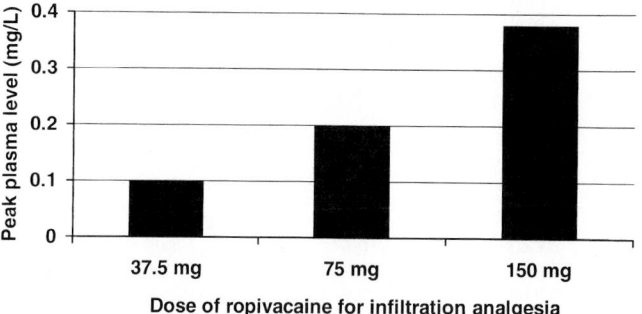

Figure 17-8. Increasing doses of ropivacaine used for wound infiltration result in linearly increasing maximal plasma concentrations (C_{max}). (Data from Mulroy MF, Burgess FW, Emanuelsson B-M: Ropivacaine 0.25% and 0.5%, but not 0.125%, provide effective wound infiltration analgesia after outpatient hernia repair, but with sustained plasma drug levels. Reg Anesth Pain Med 24:136, 1999.)

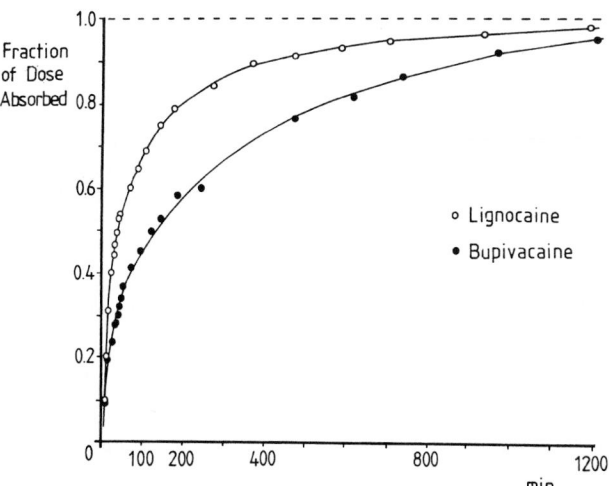

Figure 17-9. Fraction of dose absorbed into the systemic circulation over time from epidural injection of lidocaine or bupivacaine. Bupivacaine is a more lipid-soluble, more potent agent with less systemic absorption over time. (Adapted with permission from Tucker GT, Mather LE: Properties, absorption, and disposition of local anesthetic agents. In Cousins MJ, Bridenbaugh PO (eds): Neural Blockade in Clinical Anesthesia and Management of Pain, p 55. Philadelphia, Lippincott–Raven, 1998.)

Table 17-7. PHARMACOKINETIC PARAMETERS OF CLINICALLY USED LOCAL ANESTHETICS

Local Anesthetic	VD_{SS} (l·kg^{-1})	CL (l·kg^{-1}·hr^{-1})	$T_{1/2}$ (hr)
Bupivacaine	1.02	0.41	3.5
levo-Bupivacaine	0.78	0.32	2.6
Chloroprocaine	0.50	2.96	0.11
Etidocaine	1.9	1.05	2.6
Lidocaine	1.3	0.85	1.6
Mepivacaine	1.2	0.67	1.9
Prilocaine	2.73	2.03	1.6
Procaine	0.93	5.62	0.14
Ropivacaine	0.84	0.63	1.9

Data from Denson DD: Physiology and pharmacology of local anesthetics. In Sinatra RS, Hord AH, Ginsberg B, Preble LM (eds): Acute Pain: Mechanisms and Management, p 124. St. Louis, Mosby–Year Book, 1992; and Burm AG, van der Meer, van Kleef JW *et al*: Pharmacokinetics of the enantiomers of bupivacaine following intravenous administration of the racemate. Br J Clin Pharm 38:125, 1994.

Table 17-8. RELATIVE POTENCY FOR SYSTEMIC CENTRAL NERVOUS SYSTEM TOXICITY BY LOCAL ANESTHETICS AND RATIO OF DOSAGE NEEDED FOR CARDIOVASCULAR SYSTEM:CENTRAL NERVOUS SYSTEM (CVS:CNS) TOXICITY

Agent	Relative Potency for CNS Toxicity	CVS:CNS
Bupivacaine	4.0	2.0
levo-Bupivacaine	2.9	2.0
Chloroprocaine	0.3	3.7
Etidocaine	2.0	4.4
Lidocaine	1.0	7.1
Mepivacaine	1.4	7.1
Prilocaine	1.2	3.1
Procaine	0.3	3.7
Ropivacaine	2.9	2.2
Tetracaine	2.0	

Data from Liu SS: Local anesthetics and analgesia. In Ashburn MA, Rice LJ (eds): The Management of Pain, p 141. New York, Churchill Livingstone, 1997.

Table 17-9. CLINICAL PROFILE OF LOCAL ANESTHETICS

Local Anesthetic	Concentration (%)	Clinical Use	Onset	Duration (hr)	Recommended Maximal Single Dose (mg)
AMIDES					
Bupivacaine	0.25	Infiltration	Fast	2–8	175/225 + epinephrine
	0.25–0.5	Peripheral nerve block	Slow	4–12	175/225 + epinephrine
	0.5–0.75	Epidural anesthesia	Moderate	2–5	175/225 + epinephrine
	0.03–0.25	Epidural anesthesia	NA	NA	NA
	0.5–0.75	Spinal anesthesia	Fast	1–4	20
Etidocaine	0.5	Infiltration	Fast	2–8	300/400 + epinephrine
	0.5–1	Peripheral nerve block	Fast	3–12	300/400 + epinephrine
	1–1.5	Epidural anesthesia	Fast	2–4	300/400 + epinephrine
Lidocaine	0.5–1	Infiltration	Fast	1–4	300/500 + epinephrine
	0.25–0.5	iv regional anesthesia	Fast	0.5–1	300
	1–1.5	Peripheral nerve block	Fast	1–3	300/500 + epinephrine
	1.5–2	Epidural anesthesia	Fast	1–2	300/500 + epinephrine
	1.5–5	Spinal anesthesia	Fast	0.5–1	100
	4	Topical	Fast	0.5–1	300
Mepivacaine	0.5–1	Infiltration	Fast	1–4	400/500 + epinephrine
	1–1.5	Peripheral nerve block	Fast	2–4	400/500 + epinephrine
	1.5–2	Epidural anesthesia	Fast	1–3	400/500 + epinephrine
	2–4	Spinal anesthesia	Fast	1–2	100
Prilocaine	0.5–1	Infiltration	Fast	1–2	600
	0.25–0.5	iv regional anesthesia	Fast	0.5–1	600
	1.5–2	Peripheral nerve block	Fast	1.5–3	600
	2–3	Epidural anesthesia	Fast	1–3	600
Ropivacaine	0.2–0.5	Infiltration	Fast	2–6	200
	0.5–1	Peripheral nerve block	Slow	5–8	250
	0.5–1	Epidural anesthesia	Moderate	2–6	200
	0.05–0.2	Epidural anesthesia	NA	NA	NA
MIXTURE					
Lidocaine + prilocaine	2.5/2.5	Skin topical	Slow	3–5	20 g
ESTERS					
Benzocaine	Up to 20%	Topical	Fast	0.5–1	200
Chloroprocaine	1	Infiltration	Fast	0.5–1	800/1000 + epinephrine
	2	Peripheral nerve block	Fast	0.5–1	800/1000 + epinephrine
	2–3	Epidural anesthesia	Fast	0.5–1	800/1000 + epinephrine
Cocaine	4–10	Topical	Fast	0.5–1	150
Procaine	10	Spinal anesthesia	Fast	0.5–1	1000
Tetracaine	2	Topical	Fast	0.5–1	20
	0.5	Spinal anesthesia	Fast	2–6	20

Adapted with permission from Covino BG, Wildsmith JAW: Clinical pharmacology of local anesthetic agents. In Cousins MJ, Bridenbaugh PO (eds): Neural Blockade in Clinical Anesthesia and Management of Pain, p 97. Philadelphia, Lippincott–Raven, 1998.

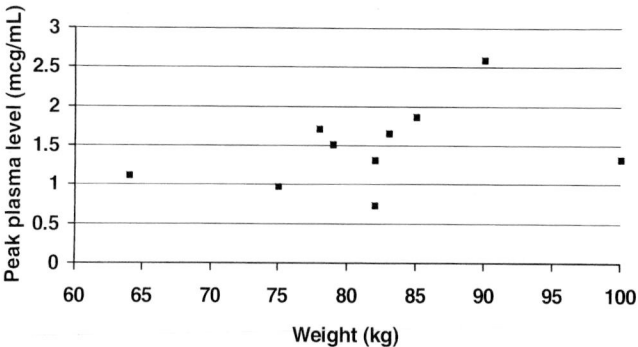

Figure 17-10. Lack of correlation between patient weight and peak plasma concentration after epidural administration of 150 mg of bupivacaine. (Data from Sharrock NE, Mather LE, Go G *et al:* Arterial and pulmonary concentrations of the enantiomers of bupivacaine after epidural injection in elderly patients. Anesth Analg 86:812, 1998.)

physiologic states such as cardiac and hepatic disease will alter expected pharmacokinetic parameters (Table 17-10), and lower doses of local anesthetics should be used for these patients. As expected, renal disease has little effect on pharmacokinetic parameters of local anesthetics (Table 17-10). Finally, the skill of the anesthesiologist should be considered, as a large dose of local anesthetic placed in the correct location may have much less potential for systemic toxicity than a small dose incorrectly injected intravascularly. All of these factors should be considered when utilizing local anesthetics and minimizing systemic toxicity, the commonly accepted maximal dosages (Table 17-9) notwithstanding.

CLINICAL USE OF LOCAL ANESTHETICS

Local anesthetics are used in a variety of ways in clinical anesthesia practice. Probably, the most common clinical use of local anesthetics for anesthesiologists is for regional anesthesia and analgesia. Central neuraxial anesthesia and analgesia can be accomplished by epidural or spinal injections of local anesthetics. Placement of epidural and spinal catheters can allow continuous infusion of local anesthetics and other analgesics for extended durations. Intravenous regional anesthesia and peripheral nerve blocks allow for anesthesia of the head and neck including the airway, upper extremities, trunk, and lower extremities. Newly developed catheters for continuous peripheral nerve blocks can also be placed to allow continuous infusions of local anesthetics and other analgesics for prolonged analgesia in a fashion similar to continuous epidural analgesia. Topical application of local anesthetics to the airway, eye, and skin provides sufficient anesthesia for painless performance of minor anesthetic and surgical procedures such as tracheal intubation, intravenous catheter placement, or spinal puncture.[108] Typical applications for each local anesthetic are listed in Table 17-9.[49]

Other common clinical uses for local anesthetics include administration of lidocaine to blunt responses to tracheal instrumentation and to suppress cardiac dysrhythmias. Intravenous or topical administration of lidocaine have been used with variable success to blunt hemodynamic response to tracheal intubation and extubation.[109,110] In addition to hemodynamic responses, instrumentation of the airway can result in coughing, brochoconstriction, and other airway responses. Intravenous lidocaine can be effective for decreasing airway sensitivity to instrumentation by depressing airway reflexes and decreasing calcium flux in airway smooth muscle.[111,112] Doses of intravenous lidocaine from 2 to 2.5 mg · kg^{-1} are needed to consistently blunt hemodynamic and airway responses to tracheal instrumentation.[111–113] Intravenous lidocaine is also effective for attenuating increases in intraocular pressure, intracranial pressure, and intraabdominal pressure during airway instrumentation.[114] Attenuation of all these responses may be beneficial in selected clinical situations (*e.g.,* corneal laceration or increased intracranial pressure). Intravenous lidocaine has well recognized antidysrhythmic effects and is easy to administer as an intravenous bolus followed by infusion for treatment of ventricular dysrhythmias.[115]

Finally, intravenous lidocaine (1–5 mg · kg^{-1}) is an effective analgesic and has been used to treat postoperative[116] and chronic neuropathic pain.[117] The mechanism of analgesia remains unclear,[118] but does not involve typical block of impulse conduction in peripheral nerves.[119,120] Both peripheral inhibition of spontaneous electrical activity in injured C nerve fibers, Aδ nerve fibers,[120] and dorsal root ganglia[119] and central inhibition of activity of hippocampal and thalamic neurons[121,122] probably contribute to systemic analgesic effects of local anesthetics. The ability of local anesthetics to provide systemic analgesic effects at central and peripheral sites may in part explain the ability of a single neural block to provide long-lasting analgesia from neuropathic pain.[118,123] In addition, orally administered tocainide and mexiletine (Class I anti-arrhythmic agents that are similar to lidocaine) have been successfully used to treat chronic pain conditions such as peripheral neuropathies[124,125] and central spinal cord pain.[126]

TOXICITY OF LOCAL ANESTHETICS
Systemic Toxicity of Local Anesthetics
Central Nervous System (CNS) Toxicity

Local anesthetics readily cross the blood–brain barrier, and generalized central nervous system toxicity may occur from systemic absorption or direct vascular injection. Signs of generalized CNS toxicity due to local anesthetics are dose–dependent (Table 17-11). Low doses produce CNS depression, and higher doses result in CNS excitation and seizures.[127] The rate of intravenous administration of local anesthetic will also affect signs of CNS toxicity, as higher rates of infusion of the same dose will lessen the appearance of CNS depression while leaving excitation intact.[128] This dichotomous reaction to local anes-

Table 17-10. EFFECTS OF CARDIAC, HEPATIC, AND RENAL DISEASE ON LIDOCAINE PHARMACOKINETICS

	VD$_{SS}$ (l · kg^{-1})	CL (ml · kg^{-1} · min^{-1})	T$_{1/2}$ (hr)
Normal	1.32	10.0	1.8
Cardiac failure	0.88	6.3	1.9
Hepatic disease	2.31	6.0	4.9
Renal disease	1.2	13.7	1.3

VD$_{SS}$ = volume of distribution at steady state; CL = total body clearance; T$_{1/2}$ = terminal elimination half-life.
Data from Thomson PD: Ann Intern Med 78:499, 1973.

Table 17-11. DOSE-DEPENDENT SYSTEMIC EFFECTS OF LIDOCAINE

Plasma Concentration ($\mu g \cdot ml^{-1}$)	Effect
1–5	Analgesia
5–10	Lightheadedness
	Tinnitus
	Numbness of tongue
10–15	Seizures
	Unconsciousness
15–25	Coma
	Respiratory arrest
>25	Cardiovascular depression

thetics may be due to a greater sensitivity of cortical inhibitory neurons to the impulse blocking effects of local anesthetics.[129] As expected, incidences of seizures vary after regional anesthetic techniques owing to differences in systemic absorption and the likelihood of unintentional vascular injection (Table 17-12).[130,131]

Local anesthetic potency for generalized CNS toxicity approximately parallels action potential blocking potency (Tables 17-4 and 17-8). In general, decreased local anesthetic protein binding and clearance will increase potential CNS toxicity.[63] External factors can increase potency for CNS toxicity, such as acidosis and increased Pco_2, perhaps *via* increased cerebral perfusion or decreased protein binding of local anesthetic.[127] There are also external factors that can decrease local anesthetic potency for generalized CNS toxicity. For example, seizure thresholds of local anesthetics are increased by administration of barbiturates and benzodiazepines.[132]

Addition of vasoconstrictors such as epinephrine may reduce or promote the potential for generalized local anesthetic CNS toxicity. Addition of epinephrine to local anesthetics will decrease systemic absorption and peak blood levels and increase the safety margin. On the other hand, the convulsive threshold for intravenous administration of lidocaine in the rat is decreased by about 42% when epinephrine (1:100,000), norepinephrine, or phenylephrine is added to the plain solution.[133] The mechanisms of increased toxicity with addition of epinephrine are unclear, but appear to depend on the development of hypertension from vasoconstriction. A hyperdynamic circulatory system may enhance the toxic effects of local anesthetics by causing increased cerebral blood flow and delivery of lidocaine to the brain[134,135] or through disruption of the blood–brain barrier.[136] In addition to enhancing distribution of local anesthetic to the brain, hyperdynamic circulatory changes can also decrease clearance of local anesthetic from the body due to changes in distribution of blood flow away from the liver. Changes in total body clearance from hyperdynamic circulatory

changes induced by local anesthetic seizures have been studied in dogs.[137] Seizures significantly increased heart rate, blood pressure, and cardiac output while significantly decreasing total body clearance (29–68%) of lidocaine, mepivacaine, bupivacaine, and etidocaine.

Cardiovascular (CV) Toxicity of Local Anesthetics

In general, much greater doses of local anesthetics are required to produce CV toxicity then CNS toxicity. Similar to CNS toxicity, potency for CV toxicity reflects the anesthetic potency of the agent (Tables 17-4 and 17-8). Recent attention has focused on the apparently exceptional cardiotoxicity of the more potent, more lipid-soluble agents (bupivacaine, *levo*-bupivacaine, etidocaine, ropivacaine).[43,138] These agents appear to have a different sequence of CV toxicity than less potent agents. For example, increasing doses of lidocaine lead to hypotension, bradycardia, and hypoxia, whereas bupivacaine often results in sudden cardiovascular collapse due to ventricular dysrhythmias that are resistant to resuscitation.[139] Subsequent studies have identified multiple mechanisms in the CNS and CV system for increased cardiotoxicity from potent local anesthetics.

Cardiovascular Toxicity Mediated at the CNS. It has been demonstrated that the central and peripheral nervous systems may be involved in the increased cardiotoxicity with bupivacaine. The nucleus tractus solitarii in the medulla is an important region for autonomic control of the cardiovascular system.[140] Neural activity in the nucleus tractus solitarii of rats is markedly diminished by intravenous doses of bupivacaine immediately prior to development of hypotension.[140] Furthermore, direct intracerebral injection of bupivacaine can elicit sudden dysrhythmias and cardiovascular collapse.[141]

Peripheral effects of bupivacaine on the autonomic and vasomotor systems may also augment its CV toxicity. Bupivacaine possesses a potent peripheral inhibitory effect on sympathetic reflexes[142] that have been observed even at blood concentrations similar to those measured after uncomplicated regional anesthesia.[143] Finally, bupivacaine also has potent direct vasodilating properties which may exacerbate cardiovascular collapse.[66,144]

Cardiovascular Toxicity Mediated at the Heart. The more potent local anesthetics appear to possess greater potential for direct cardiac electrophysiologic toxicity. A previous study examining lidocaine, bupivacaine, and ropivacaine in rats has demonstrated equivalent peak effects on myocardial contractility but much greater effects on electrophysiology (prolongation of QRS) from bupivacaine and ropivacaine than lidocaine (Fig. 17-11).[145] Although all local anesthetics block the cardiac conduction system *via* a dose-dependent block of sodium channels, two features of bupivacaine's sodium channel blocking abilities may enhance its cardiotoxicity. First, bupivacaine exhibits a much stronger binding affinity to resting and inactivated sodium channels than lidocaine.[146] Second, local anesthetics bind to sodium channels during systole and dissociate during diastole (Fig. 17-12). Bupivacaine dissociates from sodium channels dur-

Table 17-12. INCIDENCE OF SEIZURES AFTER REGIONAL ANESTHESIA IN THE UNITED STATES AND EUROPE

Anesthesia	Total Number of Procedures	Total Number of Seizures	Incidence of Seizures
Peripheral nerve blocks*	28,810	31	11/10,000
Epidural*	45,578	15	3/10,000
Intravenous regional	11,220	3	3/10,000

* Increased incidence of seizures with bupivacaine vs. lidocaine.
Data from Auroy Y, Narchi P, Messiah A *et al*: Serious complications related to regional anesthesia: Results of a prospective survey in France. Anesthesiology 87:479, 1997; and Brown DL, Ransom DM, Hall JA *et al*: Regional anesthesia and local anesthetic-induced systemic toxicity: Seizure frequency and accompanying cardiovascular changes. Anesth Analg 81:321, 1995.

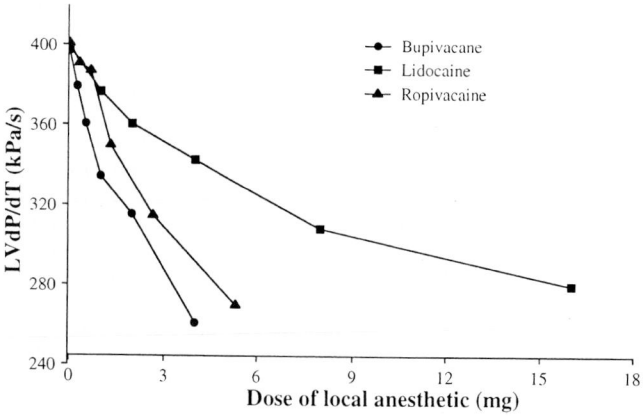

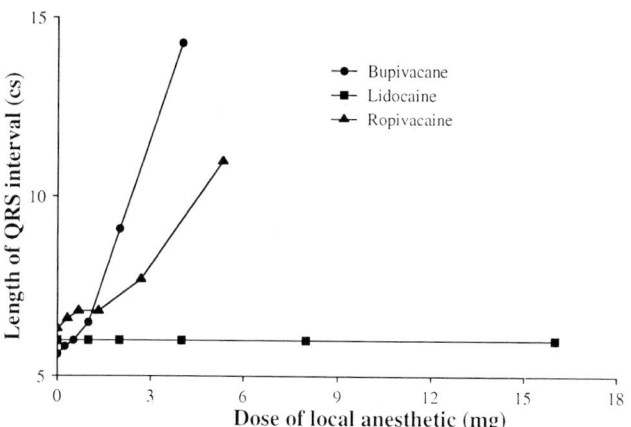

Figure 17-11. Dose-related effects of bupivacaine, lidocaine, and ropivacaine on myocardial contractility (LV *dp/dt*) and on QRS prolongation in rats. Relative potencies of bupivacaine:ropivacaine:lidocaine for myocardial depression are 4:1:3 and for QRS prolongation are 15:1:7. (Data from Reiz S, Haggmark S, Johansson G *et al:* Cardiotoxicity of ropivacaine—a new amide local anaesthetic agent. Acta Anaesthesiol Scand 33:93, 1989.)

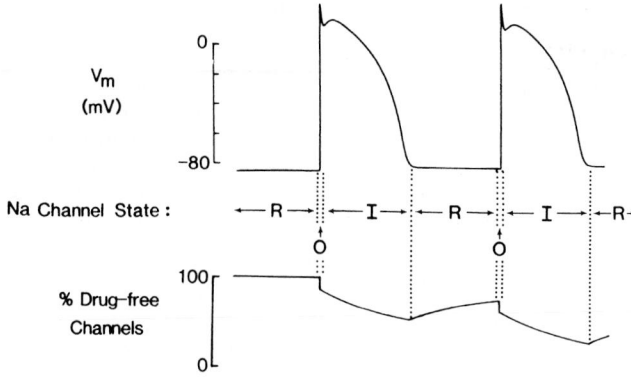

Figure 17-12. Diagram illustrating relationship between cardiac action potential (*top*), sodium channel state (*middle*), and block of sodium channels by bupivacaine (*bottom*). R = resting, O = open, and I = inactive forms of the sodium channel. Sodium channels are predominantly in the resting form during diastole, open transiently during the action potential upstroke, and are in the inactive form during the action potential plateau. Block of sodium channels by bupivacaine accumulates during the action potential (systole) with recovery occurring during diastole. Recovery of sodium channels is from dissociation of bupivacaine and is time-dependent. Recovery during each diastolic interval is incomplete and results in accumulation of sodium channel block with successive heart beats. (Adapted with permission from Clarkson CW, Hondeghem LM: Mechanisms for bupivacaine depression of cardiac conduction: Fast block of sodium channels during the action potential with slow recovery from block during diastole. Anesthesiology 62:396, 1985.)

nels,[151] release of calcium from sarcoplasmic reticulum,[152] and mitochondrial energy metabolism.[153] Thus, multiple direct effects of bupivacaine on activity of the cardiac myocyte may enhance the cardiotoxicity of bupivacaine.

The multitude of different cardiac and neural mechanisms of cardiotoxicity may in part explain the reported difficulties of resuscitation after cardiovascular collapse from bupivacaine.[138] An additional contributing factor may be bupivacaine's ability to inhibit cyclic AMP production.[154] Cyclic AMP is an

ing cardiac diastole much more slowly than lidocaine. Indeed, bupivacaine dissociates so slowly that the duration of diastole at physiologic heart rates (60–180 bpm) does not allow enough time for complete recovery of sodium channels and bupivacaine conduction block accumulates. In contrast, lidocaine fully dissociates from sodium channels during diastole and little accumulation of conduction block occurs (Fig. 17-13).[146,147] Thus, enhanced electrophysiologic effects of more potent local anesthetics on the cardiac conduction system may explain their increased potential to produce sudden cardiovascular collapse *via* cardiac dysrhythmias.

Increased potency for direct myocardial depression from the more potent local anesthetics is another contributing factor to increased cardiotoxicity. However, potency of myocardial depression roughly parallels anesthetic potency (Fig. 17-11);[145] thus, appropriate use of bupivacaine, *levo*-bupivacaine, etidocaine, and ropivacaine will not lead to excessive myocardial depression. Indeed, blood concentrations of bupivacaine and ropivacaine that typically occur from systemic absorption after regional blocks do not result in significant myocardial depression in animals or humans.[43,148,149] Again, multiple mechanisms may account for the increased potency for myocardial depression from more potent local anesthetics. Bupivacaine, the most completely studied potent local anesthetic, possesses a high affinity for sodium and potassium channels in the cardiac myocyte.[150,151] Furthermore, bupivacaine inhibits calcium chan-

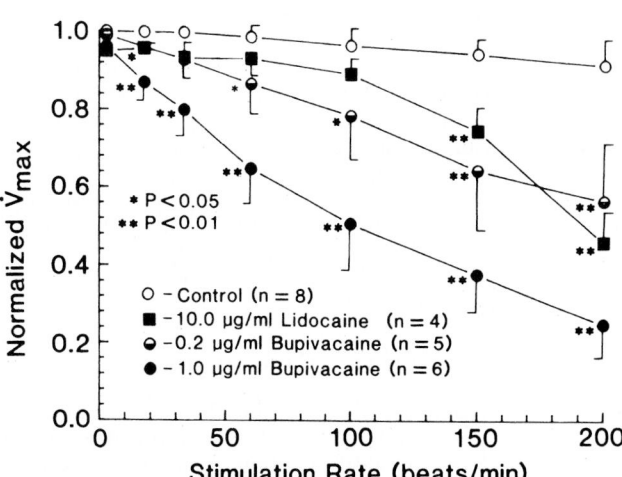

Figure 17-13. Heart rate–dependent effects of lidocaine and bupivacaine on velocity of the cardiac action potential (V_{max}). Bupivacaine progressively decreases V_{max} at heart rates above 3 bpm due to accumulation of sodium channel block, whereas lidocaine does not decrease V_{max} until heart rate exceeds 150 bpm. (Adapted with permission from Clarkson CW, Hondeghem LM: Mechanisms for bupivacaine depression of cardiac conduction: Fast block of sodium channels during the action potential with slow recovery from block during diastole. Anesthesiology 62:396, 1985.)

important second messenger for the adrenergic receptor system, and thus modulates the resuscitative effects of epinephrine. Bupivacaine inhibition of cyclic AMP suggests that large doses of epinephrine may be necessary during resuscitation from overdose, as has been previously reported.[155] Once cardiovascular collapse occurs, maintenance of respiration and myocardial perfusion are vital, as hypercapnia, hypoxia, acidosis, hypothermia, hyperkalemia, hyponatremia, and myocardial ischemia will all sensitize the heart to bupivacaine cardiotoxicity.[156,157]

Treatment of Systemic Toxicity from Local Anesthetics

The best method for avoiding systemic toxicity from local anesthetics is through prevention. Toxic systemic levels can occur by unintentional intravenous or intra-arterial injection or by systemic absorption of excessive doses placed in the correct area. Unintentional intravascular and intra-arterial injections can be minimized by frequent syringe aspiration for blood, use of a small test dose of local anesthetic (~3 ml) to test for subjective systemic effects from the patient (e.g., tinnitus, circumoral numbness), and either slow injection or fractionation of the rest of the dose of local anesthetic.[138] Detailed knowledge of local anesthetic pharmacokinetics will also aid in reducing the administration of excessive doses of local anesthetics. Ideally, heart rate, blood pressure, and the electrocardiogram should be monitored during administration of local anesthetics.

Treatment of systemic toxicity is primarily supportive. Injection of local anesthetic should be stopped. Oxygenation and ventilation should be maintained, as systemic toxicity of local anesthetics is enhanced by hypoxemia, hypercarbia, and acidosis.[156,157] If needed, the patient's trachea should be intubated and positive pressure ventilation instituted. As previously discussed, signs CNS of toxicity will typically occur prior to CV events. Seizures can increase body metabolism and cause hypoxemia, hypercarbia, and acidosis. Pharmacologic treatment to terminate seizures may be needed if oxygenation and ventilation cannot be maintained. Intravenous administration of thiopental (50–100 mg), midazolam (2–5 mg), and propofol (1 mg · kg^{-1}) can terminate seizures from systemic local anesthetic toxicity.[49,158] Succinylcholine (50 mg) can terminate muscular activity from seizures and facilitate ventilation and oxygenation. However, succinylcholine will not terminate seizure activity in the CNS, and increased cerebral metabolic demands will continue unabated.[49]

Cardiovascular depression from less potent local anesthetics (e.g., lidocaine) is usually mild and caused by mild myocardial depression and vasodilation. Hypotension and bradycardia can usually be treated with ephedrine (10–30 mg) and atropine (0.4 mg). As previously discussed, potent local anesthetics (e.g., bupivacaine) can produce profound cardiovascular depression and malignant dysrhythmias that should be promptly treated. Oxygenation and ventilation must be immediately instituted, with cardiopulmonary resuscitation if needed. Ventricular dysrhythmias may be difficult to treat and may need large and multiple doses of electrical cardioversion, epinephrine, bretylium, and magnesium.[49,115]

Neural Toxicity of Local Anesthetics

In addition to systemic toxicity, local anesthetics can cause injury to the central and peripheral nervous system from direct exposure. Mechanisms for local anesthetic neurotoxicity remain speculative, but previous studies have demonstrated local anesthetic–induced injury to Schwann cells, inhibition of fast axonal transport, disruption of the blood–nerve barrier, and decreased neural blood flow with associated ischemia.[159] Although all clinically used local anesthetics can cause concentration-dependent nerve fiber damage in peripheral nerves when used in high enough concentrations, previous studies have demonstrated that local anesthetics in clinically used concentrations are generally safe for peripheral nerves.[160] The spinal cord and

the nerve roots, on the other hand, are more prone to injury. Spinal cord or nerve root toxicity may manifest itself as neurohistopathologic, physiologic, or behavioral/clinical changes such as pain, motor and sensory deficits, and bowel and bladder dysfunction.

In 1985 Ready et al evaluated the neurotoxic effects of single intrathecal injections of clinically relevant concentrations of tetracaine, lidocaine, bupivacaine, or chloroprocaine in rabbits, after which spinal cord histopathology remained normal and persistent behavioral deficits were not seen.[161] However, histopathologic changes and neurologic deficits did occur with higher concentrations of tetracaine (1%) and lidocaine (8%). Desheathed peripheral nerve models, designed to mimic unprotected nerve roots in the cauda equina, have been used to further assess electrophysiologic neurotoxicity of local anesthetics.[162–164] Lidocaine 5% and tetracaine 0.5% caused irreversible conduction block in these models, whereas lidocaine 1.5%, bupivacaine 0.75%, and tetracaine 0.06% did not. Electrophysiologic toxicity of lidocaine in isolated nerve preparations represented by incomplete recovery of neuromuscular function occurs at 40 mM (~1%) (Fig. 17-14) with irreversible ablation of the compound action potential seen at 80 mM (~2%). Although such studies do not reflect in vivo conditions, they suggest that lidocaine and tetracaine may be especially neurotoxic in a concentration-dependent fashion, and that neurotoxicity could theoretically occur with clinically used solutions. Local anesthetic effects on spinal cord blood flow, another possible etiology of neurotoxicity from direct drug exposure, appear benign. Spinal administration of bupivacaine, lidocaine, mepivacaine, and tetracaine cause vasodilation and increase spinal cord blood flow, whereas ropivacaine causes vasoconstriction and reduction in spinal cord blood flow in a concentration-dependent fashion.[165]

Neurohistopathologic data in humans after intrathecal exposure to local anesthetics is not available. Electrophysiologic parameters such as somatosensory-evoked potentials, monosynaptic H-reflex,[166] and cutaneous current perception thresholds[167] have been used to evaluate recovery after spinal anesthesia. These measurements have shown complete return to baseline activity after 5% lidocaine spinal anesthesia in very small study populations. Epidemiologic studies in 1999 report an incidence of 0–0.7% postoperative neurologic injury in patients undergoing spinal anesthesia.[33] Thus, despite findings that all local anesthetics have the potential for neurotoxicity in laboratory and

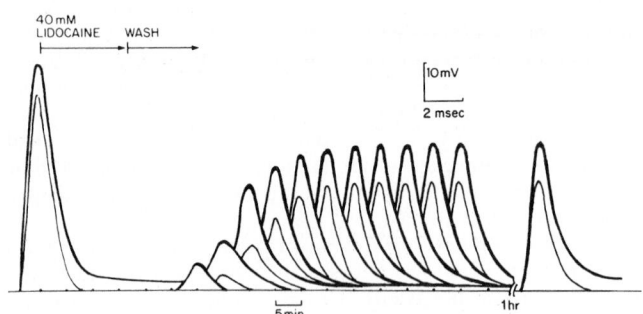

Figure 17-14. The nonreversible effect of 40 mM lidocaine on the compound action potential (CAP) of frog sciatic nerve. Lidocaine was applied to a stable nerve preparation for 15 min and then washed with frog Ringer's solution for 2 hr. Tracings represent CAPs in response to stimulus (1-Hz stimulus = heavy line; 40-Hz stimulus = thin line). 40 mM lidocaine completely ablated the CAP when applied to the nerve. The 1-Hz CAP response began to return after 10–15 min of washing and reached a new level in 45 min, where it was stable for the subsequent 2 hr of observation. The recovered 1-Hz CAP is only 65% of the original. (Adapted with permission from Bainton C: Concentration dependence of lidocaine-induced irreversible conduction loss frog nerve. Anesthesiology 81:657, 1994.)

Table 17-13. INCIDENCE OF TRANSIENT NEUROLOGIC SYMPTOMS (TNS) AFTER SPINAL ANESTHESIA

Agent	Preparation	Position	Approximate TNS Incidence
Lidocaine	Hyperbaric 2–5%	Lithotomy	30–40%
	Hyperbaric 0.5–5%	Knee arthroscopy	20–30%
	Hyperbaric 5%	Supine/unspecified	5–10%
Bupivacaine	Isobaric/hyperbaric	Lithotomy/other	Rare
Tetracaine	Hyperbaric	General use	Rare
	Hyperbaric + phenylephrine	Lower extremity/perineal	12%
Procaine	Hyperbaric 5%	Knee arthroscopy	6%
	Isobaric 5%	Supine/other	1%
Mepivacaine	Hyperbaric 4%	Lithotomy/other	30–40%
	Isobaric 1.5%	Knee arthroscopy	Rare
Ropivacaine	Hyperbaric 0.25%	Supine volunteers	Rare

Data from Hodgson PS, Neal JM, Pollock JE *et al*: The neurotoxicity of drugs given intrathecally (spinal). Anesth Analg 88:797, 1999.

animal models, spinally administered local anesthetics have not notably manifested their neurotoxic potential in human studies to date.

Transient Neurologic Symptoms (TNS) after Spinal Anesthesia

Prospective, randomized studies reveal a 4–40% incidence of transient neurologic symptoms (TNS), including pain or sensory abnormalities in the lower back, buttocks, or lower extremities, after lidocaine spinal anesthesia.[33,168,169] These symptoms have been reported with other local anesthetics as well (Table 17-13). The incidence of TNS varies with the type of surgical procedure and positioning and is apparently unaffected by baricity or dose. Contemporary reports of cauda equina syndrome after single-bolus administration, as well as continuous, lidocaine spinal anesthesia, and the potential concentration-dependent neurotoxicity of lidocaine, have led several authors to label TNS as a manifestation of subclinical neurotoxicity.[170]

As previously discussed, laboratory work in both intrathecal and desheathed peripheral nerve models has proved that the concentration of lidocaine is a critical factor in neurotoxicity. As concentrations of lidocaine below 40 mM (~1.0%) are not neurotoxic to desheathed peripheral nerve, such dilute concentrations of spinal lidocaine should not cause TNS if the syndrome is due to subclinical concentration-dependent neurotoxicity. However, the dilution of lidocaine to as low as 0.5% does not decrease the incidence of TNS.[168] The high incidence of TNS observed with lidocaine concentrations <1% despite further dilution in cerebrospinal fluid would appear to lessen the plausibility of a concentration-dependent neurotoxic etiology. Other potential etiologies for TNS include patient positioning, early mobilization, needle trauma, neural ischemia, pooling of local anesthetics secondary to maldistribution by pencil-point needles or the addition of glucose, muscle spasm, myofascial trigger points, and irritation of dorsal ganglia.[168] Clearly, the etiology of TNS remains undetermined, and further studies are needed to elucidate the underlying mechanism.

In summary, local anesthetics all have the potential to be neurotoxic, particularly in concentrations and doses greater than those used clinically. In neurohistopathologic, electrophysiologic, behavioral, and *in vitro* models, lidocaine and tetracaine appear to have greater potential for neurotoxicity than bupivacaine at clinically relevant concentrations. Nonetheless, large-scale surveys of the complications of spinal anesthesia attest to the relative safety of spinally administered local anesthetics.

Allergic Reactions to Local Anesthetics

True allergic reactions to local anesthetics are rare and usually involve Type I (IgE) or Type IV (cellular immunity) reactions.[171,172] Type I reactions are worrisome, as anaphylaxis may occur, and are more common with ester than amide local anesthetics.[127] True Type I allergy to aminoamide agents is extremely rare.[172] Increased allergenic potential with esters may be due to hydrolytic metabolism to *para*-aminobenzoic acid which is a documented allergen.[173] Added preservatives such as methylparaben and metabisulfite can also provoke an allergic response.[174] Skin testing with intradermal injections of preservative-free local anesthetics has been advocated as a means to determine tolerance to local anesthetic.[174] These tests should be undertaken with caution, as potentially severe and even fatal reactions can occur in truly allergic patients.[172]

NEW AND FUTURE LOCAL ANESTHETICS

Local Anesthetics with Decreased Systemic Toxicity

In 1979, an editorial drew attention to the potential for sudden cardiovascular collapse with unintentional intravascular injection of potent local anesthetics such as bupivacaine.[44] Enhanced awareness of potential cardiovascular toxicity with long-acting local anesthetics led to withdrawal of FDA approval of high concentrations of bupivacaine (0.75%) for obstetric use in the

Table 17-14. ANIMAL STUDIES EVALUATING RELATIVE CARDIOTOXICITY OF LIDOCAINE, ROPIVACAINE, AND BUPIVACAINE

Species	Measurement	Lidocaine	Ropivacaine	Bupivacaine
Dog	Ventricular fibrillation (%)	0	33	83
	Resuscitate (%)	75	100	66
Sheep	Ventricular fibrillation (%)	—	40	75
Pig	Myocardial depression (%)	13	38	50
	Death (%)	0	0	25

Data from Carpenter RL: Am J Anesth 24:4, 1997.

Table 17-15. COMPARISON OF SYSTEMIC TOXICITY OF INTRAVENOUS *levo*-**BUPIVACAINE TO RACEMIC BUPIVACAINE IN SHEEP**

Dose (mg)	Seizures (%)	QT_c (msec)	Ventricular Dysrhythmias (#)
levo-**BUPIVACAINE**			
75	43	430	0
100	83	403	0*
150	100	413	44*
200	100	315	100*
RACEMIC BUPIVACAINE			
75	83	445	0
100	100	473	92
150	100	523	183
200	100	505	231

* Different from the same dose of bupivacaine ($p < 0.05$).
Data from Huang YF, Pryor ME, Mather LE *et al:* Cardiovascular and central nervous system effects of intravenous *levo*-bupivacaine and bupivacaine in sheep. Anesth Analg 86:797, 1998.

United States and to changes in clinical practice, such as the use of test doses, intermittent aspiration, and incremental injection of local anesthetic.[138] Indeed, reports suggest that current clinical use of potent local anesthetics is very safe, with an incidence of CNS toxicity with epidural injection approximating 3/10,000 and an incidence of 11/10,000 with peripheral nerve blocks (Table 17-12).[130,131] There appears to be a higher incidence of continued unintentional intravascular injection of local anesthetic during peripheral nerve blocks, perhaps due to differences in practice or less clinical awareness. This observation is consistent with Albright's original editorial, as four out of six of the initial reports were observed during performance of peripheral nerve blocks. Thus, current concerns for systemic toxicity for local anesthetics should be focused on clinical practice involving placement of peripheral nerve blocks rather than that associated with epidural anesthesia.

The recent release of single–optical isomer (S/L) preparations of ropivacaine and impending release of *levo*-bupivacaine appear well suited to fill this niche. Both ropivacaine and *levo*-bupivacaine appear to be approximately equipotent to racemic bupivacaine for epidural and plexus anesthesia (see Table 17-4).[175–178] Both ropivacaine and *levo*-bupivacaine appear to have approximately 30–40% less systemic toxicity on a mg:mg basis in both animal[44,179] (Tables 17-14 and 17-15) and human[180,181] volunteer studies (Figs. 17-15 and 17-16), which is likely due to reduced affinity for brain and myocardial tissue from their single isomer preparation.[46,182] It is hoped that, with

the introduction of these new agents, the incidence of systemic local anesthetic toxicity will be reduced.

Extended-Duration Local Anesthetics

There are potential clinical applications for extended-duration local anesthetics that act for 2–7 days. Central neuraxial use of such extended-duration local anesthetics would probably be limited to treatment of chronic and cancer pain because of the associated extended duration of motor block. Use of extended-duration local anesthetics for infiltration anesthesia/analgesia and for peripheral nerve blocks could result in an increased use for both forms of anesthesia for treatment of acute and chronic pain. Current technology for extending the duration of action typically involves modification of the method of delivery rather than development of new local anesthetics. Such delivery systems include encapsulation of local anesthetic in liposomes, microspheres, or polymers with slow degradation and release (Fig. 17-17).[183] Animal studies with these extended-duration preparations demonstrate the ability to provide peripheral nerve block analgesia from 2 days to >2 weeks (Fig. 17-18).[184] In addition to extended clinical duration, these delivery systems also appear to decrease potential for both CNS and cardiovascular toxicity due to slow release of local anesthetic and altered tissue uptake (Fig. 17-19).[185] Commercial release of these products has the potential to markedly change the practice of anesthesia and analgesia. For example, anesthesia could be initiated

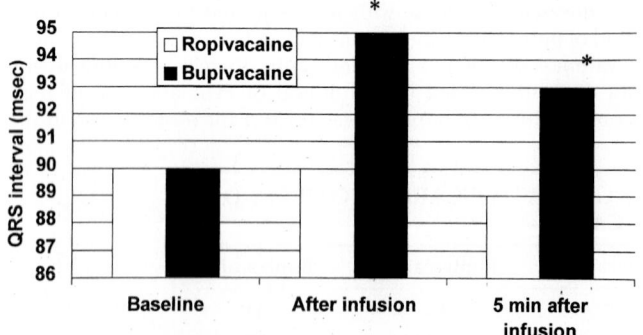

Figure 17-15. Effects of intravenous infusion of ropivacaine (150 mg) and bupivacaine (150 mg) on QRS interval in human volunteers. * = different from ropivacaine ($p < 0.05$). (Data from Scott B, Lee AL, Fagen D: Acute toxicity of ropivacaine compared with that of bupivacaine. Anesth Analg 69:563, 1989.)

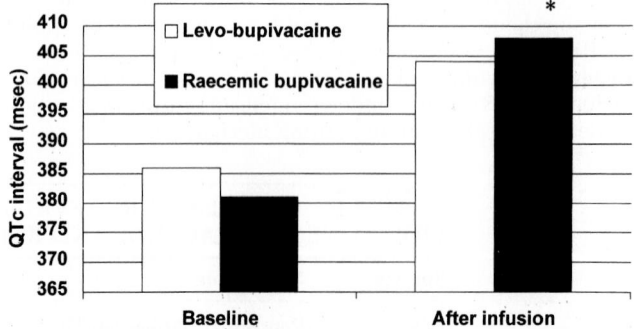

Figure 17-16. Effects of intravenous infusion of *levo*-bupivacaine (56 mg) and racemic bupivacaine (48 mg) on QT_c interval in human volunteers. * = different from baseline ($p < 0.05$). (Data from Bardsley H, Gristwood R, Baker H *et al:* A comparison of the cardiovascular effects of *levo*-bupivacaine and rac-bupivacaine following intravenous administration to healthy volunteers. Br J Clin Pharmacol 46:245, 1998.)

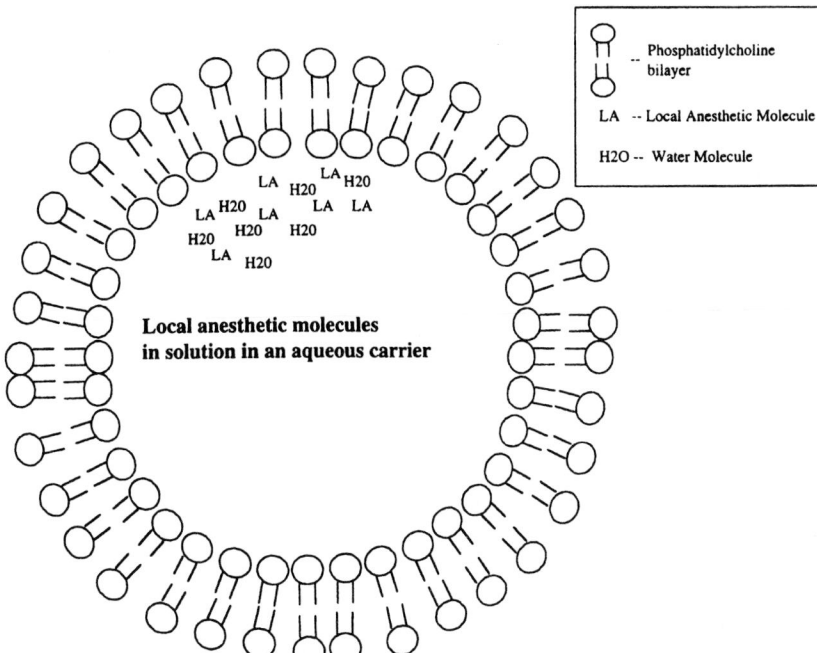

Figure 17-17. Schematic structure of a liposome. (Adapted with permission from Kuzma PJ, Kline MD, Calkins MD *et al:* Progress in the development of ultra-long-acting local anesthetics. Reg Anesth 22:543, 1997.)

in the pre-op clinic while peripheral nerve blocks and infiltration analgesia may be increasingly utilized for treatment of acute and chronic pain.

Local Anesthetics with Combined Mechanisms of Action

An increased understanding of the mechanisms of pain has led to the realization that numerous neurotransmitters are involved in the spinal cord and peripheral nervous system, and these may result in central sensitization of the CNS responses to pain.[33,186] Local anesthetics are somewhat effective for prevention of pain and central sensitization when delivered either centrally or peripherally.[187,188] However, targeted modulation of the multiple receptors involved in the mechanisms of pain and central sensitization could produce multimodal analgesia, with added efficacy and decreased side effects, in contrast to local anesthetics alone. Molecules that have local anesthetic activity

in combination with analgesic activities *via* other mechanisms (opioid receptors, α-adrenergic receptors, etc.) could potentially provide this multimodal analgesia by either central neuraxial or peripheral delivery. Sameridine is a mixed local anesthetic and opioid agonist compound that is undergoing clinical trials as a spinal agent,[189] and other mixed function compounds may soon undergo testing.

Very Short-Duration Local Anesthetics

The popularity of ambulatory surgery continues to grow, with 60–70% of surgery in the United States being performed on an outpatient basis. Current popular general anesthetic agents such as propofol or desflurane have a very brief duration of action, allowing for rapid recovery and patient discharge. Regional anesthetic techniques with local anesthetics for ambulatory surgery are somewhat hampered by the lack of a similar agent with 5–10 min offset time after cessation of infusion. Unfortunately, no such rapid-acting local anesthetic is near commercial release.

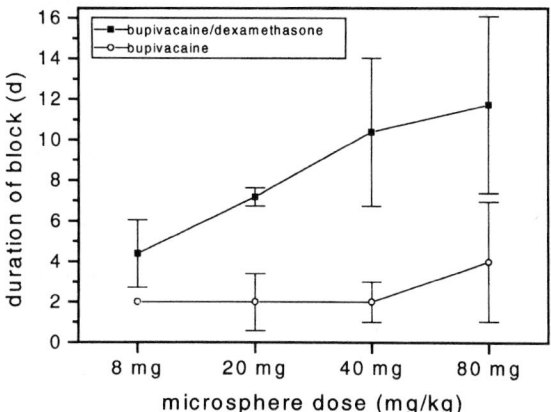

Figure 17-18. Duration of intercostal block in sheep for doses from 8 to 80 mg · kg⁻¹ of bupivacaine microspheres and bupivacaine/dexamethasone microspheres. (Adapted with permission from Drager C, Benzinger D, Gao F *et al:* Prolonged intercostal nerve blockade in sheep using controlled release of bupivacaine and dexamethasone from polymer microspheres. Anesthesiology 89:969, 1998.)

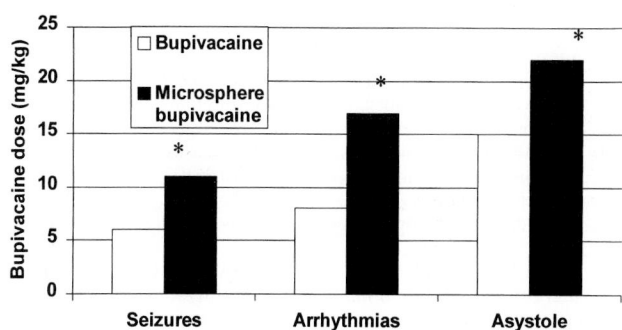

Figure 17-19. Dose of bupivacaine required to produce seizures, ventricular arrhythmias, and asystole in rabbits. * = different from plain bupivacaine ($p < 0.05$). (Adapted with permission from Boogaerts J, Declercq A, Lafont N *et al:* Toxicity of bupivacaine encapsulated into liposomes and injected intravenously: Comparison with plain solutions. Anesth Analg 76:553, 1993.)

REFERENCES

1. Ritchie JM, Ritchie B, Greengard P: The effect of the nerve sheath on the action of local anesthetics. J Pharmacol Exp Ther 150:160, 1965
2. Coggeshall RE: A fine structured analysis of the myelin sheath in rat spinal roots. Anat Rec 194:201, 1979
3. Waxman SG, Ritchie JM: Molecular dissection of the myelinated axon. Ann Neurol 33:121, 1993
4. Landon N, Williams PL: Ultrastructure of the node of Ranvier. Nature 199:575, 1963
5. London DN, Langely OK: The local chemical environment of nodes of Ranvier: A study of cation binding. J Anat 108:419, 1971
6. Popitz-Berger FA, Leeson S, Strichartz GR et al: Relation between functional deficit and intraneural local anesthetic during peripheral nerve block. Anesthesiology 83:583, 1995
7. Wann KT: Neuronal sodium and potassium channels: Structure and function. Br J Anaesth 71:2, 1993
8. Stuhmer W, Conti F, Suzuki H et al: Structural parts involved in activation and inactivation of the sodium channel. Nature (Lond) 339:597, 1989
9. French RJ, Zamponi GW, Sierralta IE: Molecular and kinetic determinants of local anaesthetic action on sodium channels. Toxicol Lett 100:247, 1998
10. Caterall WA: The molecular basis of neuronal excitability. Science 223:653, 1984
11. Chiu SY, Ritchie JM, Rogart RB: A quantitative description of membrane current in rabbit myelinated nerve. J Physiol (Lond) 292:149, 1979
12. Mateu L, Moran O, Padron R et al: The action of local anesthetics on myelin structure and nerve conduction in toad sciatic nerve. Biophys J 72:2581, 1997
13. Brau ME, Vogel W, Hempelmann G: Fundamental properties of local anesthetics: Half-maximal blocking concentrations for tonic block of Na^+ and K^+ channels in peripheral nerve. Anesth Analg 87:885, 1998
14. Butterworth JF, Strichartz GR: Molecular mechanisms of local anesthesia: A review. Anesthesiology 72:711, 1990
15. Huang JH, Thalhammer JG, Raymond SA et al: Susceptibility to lidocaine of impulses in different somatosensory afferent fibers of rat sciatic nerve. J Pharmacol Exp Ther 282:802, 1997
16. Wildsmith JA, Brown DT, Paul D et al: Structure–activity relationships in differential nerve block at high and low frequency stimulation. Br J Anaesth 63:444, 1989
17. Ragsdale DS, McPhee JC, Scheuer T et al: Molecular determinants of state-dependent block of Na^+ channels by local anesthetics. Science 265:1724, 1994
18. Li HL, Galue A, Meadows L et al: A molecular basis for the different local anesthetic affinities of resting versus open and inactivated states of the sodium channel. Mol Pharmacol 55:134, 1999
19. Lee-Son MB, Wang GK, Concus A et al: Stereoselective inhibition of neuronal sodium channels by local anesthetics. Anesthesiology 77:324, 1992
20. Butterworth J, Ririe DG, Thompson RB et al: Differential onset of median nerve block: Randomized, double-blind comparison of mepivacaine and bupivacaine in healthy volunteers. Br J Anaesth 81:515, 1998
21. Jaffe RA, Rowe MA: Differential nerve block: Direct measurements on individual myelinated and unmyelinated dorsal root axons. Anesthesiology 84:1455, 1996
22. Raymond SA, Steffensen SC, Gugino LD et al: The role of length of nerve exposed to local anesthetics in impulse blocking action. Anesth Analg 68:563, 1989
23. Fink BR: Mechanisms of differential axial blockade in epidural and spinal anesthesia. Anesthesiology 70:851, 1989
24. Ritchie JM: On the relation between fiber diameter and conduction velocity in myelinated nerve fibers. Proc R Soc Lond 29:B217, 1982
25. Waikar SS, Thalhammer JG, Raymond SA et al: Mechanoreceptive afferents exhibit functionally-specific activity dependent changes in conduction velocity. Brain Res 721:91, 1996
26. Mackenzie RA, Burke D, Skuse NF: Fibre function and perception during cutaneous nerve block. J Neurol Neurosurg Psychiatry 38:865, 1975
27. Narita Y, Nagai M, Kuzuhara S: Trigeminal somatosensory evoked potentials before, during and after an inferior alveolar nerve block in normal subjects. Psych Clin Neurosci 51:241, 1997
28. Zaric D, Hallgren S, Leissner L et al: Evaluation of epidural sensory block by thermal stimulation, laser stimulation, and recording of somatosensory evoked potentials. Reg Anesth 21:124, 1996
29. Raymond SA: Subblocking concentrations of local anesthetics: Effects on impulse generation and conduction in single myelinated sciatic nerve axons in frog. Anesth Analg 75:906, 1992
30. Olschewski A, Hempelmann G, Vogel W et al: Blockade of Na^+ and K^+ currents by local anesthetics in the dorsal horn neurons of the spinal cord. Anesthesiology 88:172, 1998
31. Bowersox SS, Luther R: Pharmacotherapeutic potential of omega-conotoxin MVIIA (SNX-111), an N-type neuronal calcium channel blocker found in the venom of Conus magus. Toxicon 36:1651, 1998
32. Xiong Z, Strichartz GR: Inhibition by local anesthetics of Ca^{2+} channels in rat anterior pituitary cells. Eur J Pharmacol 363:81, 1998
33. Hodgson PS, Neal JM, Pollock JE et al: The neurotoxicity of drugs given intrathecally (spinal). Anesth Analg 88:797, 1999
34. Too HP, Maggio JE: Immunocytochemical localization of neuromedin K (neurokinin B) in rat spinal ganglia and cord. Peptides 12:431, 1991
35. Sugiyama K, Muteki T: Local anesthetics depress the calcium current of rat sensory neurons in culture. Anesthesiology 80:1369, 1994
36. Ryan SE, Baenziger JE: A structure-based approach to nicotinic receptor pharmacology. Mol Pharmacol 55:348, 1999
37. Pascual JM, Karlin A: Delimiting the binding site for quaternary ammonium lidocaine derivatives in the acetylcholine receptor channel. J Gen Physiol 112:611, 1998
38. Nordmark J, Rydqvist B: Local anaesthetics potentiate GABA-mediated Cl^- currents by inhibiting GABA uptake. Neuroreport 8:465, 1997
39. Li Y-M, Wingrove DE, Too HP et al: Local anesthetics inhibit substance P binding and evoked increases in intracellular Ca^{++}. Anesthesiology 82:166, 1995
40. Frazier DY, Narahashi T, Yamada M: The site of action and active form of local anesthetic. II. Experiments with quaternary compounds. J Pharmacol Exp Ther 171:45, 1970
41. Gissen AJ, Covino BG, Gregus J: Differential sensitivity of fast and slow fibers in mammalian nerve. II. Margin of safety for nerve transmission. Anesth Analg 61:561, 1982
42. Ulbricht W: Kinetics of drug action and equilibrium results at the node of Ranvier. Physiol Rev 61:785, 1981
43. McClellan KJ, Spencer CM: Levobupivacaine. Drugs 56:355; discussion 363, 1998
44. McClure JH: Ropivacaine. Br J Anaesth 76:300, 1996
45. Burm AG, van der Meer AD, van Kleef JW et al: Pharmacokinetics of the enantiomers of bupivacaine following intravenous administration of the racemate. Br J Clin Pharmacol 38:125, 1994
46. Valenzuela C, Snyders DJ, Bennett PB et al: Stereoselective block of cardiac sodium channels by bupivacaine in guinea pig ventricular myocytes. Circulation 92:3014, 1995
47. Strichartz GR, Sanchez V, Arthur GR: Fundamental properties of local anesthetics. II. Measured octanol:buffer partition coefficients and pK_a values of clinically used drugs. Anesth Analg 71:158, 1990
48. Pateromichelakis S, Prokopiou AA: Local anaesthesia efficacy: Discrepancies between in vitro and in vivo studies. Acta Anaesthesiol Scand 32:672, 1988
49. Covino BG, Wildsmith JAW: Clinical pharmacology of local anesthetic agents. In Cousins MJ, Bridenbaugh PO (eds): Neural Blockade in Clinical Anesthesia and Management of Pain, 3d ed, p 97. Philadelphia, Lippincott–Raven Publishers, 1998
50. Hassan HG, Youssef H, Renck H: Duration of experimental nerve block by combinations of local anesthetic agents. Acta Anaesthesiol Scand 37:70, 1993
51. Mets B, Janicki PK, James MF et al: Lidocaine and bupivacaine cardiorespiratory toxicity is additive: A study in rats. Anesth Analg 75:611, 1992
52. Spiegel DA, Dexter F, Warner DS: Central nervous system toxicity of local anesthetic mixtures in the rat. Anesth Analg 75:922, 1992
53. Bromage PR, Pettigrew RT, Crowell DE: Tachyphylaxis in epidural analgesia: I. Augmentation and decay of local anesthetic. J Clin Pharmacol 9:30, 1969
54. Baker CE, Berry RL, Elston RC: Effects of pH of bupivacaine on duration of repeated sciatic nerve blocks in the albino rat: Local anesthetics for neuralgia study group. Anesth Analg 72:773, 1991
55. Mogensen T, Simonsen L, Scott NB: Tachyphylaxis associated with repeated epidural injections of lidocaine is not related to changes

in distribution or the rate of elimination from the epidural space. Anesth Analg 69:71, 1989

56. Wilder RT, Chickalingaiah R, Berde CB et al: Chronic exposure to lidocaine does not alter flux through sodium channels in cultured neuronal cells. Reg Anesth 18:283, 1993

57. Lipfert P, Holthusen H, Arndt JO: Tachyphylaxis to local anesthetics does not result from reduced drug effectiveness itself. Anesthesiology 70:71, 1989

58. Lee K-C, Wilder RT, Smith RL et al: Thermal hyperalgesia accelerates and MK-801 prevents the development of tachyphylaxis to rat sciatic nerve blockade. Anesthesiology 81:1284, 1994

59. Wilder RT, Sholas MG, Berde CB: NG-nitro-L-arginine methyl ester (L-NAME) prevents tachyphylaxis to local anesthetics in a dose-dependent manner. Anesth Analg 83:1251, 1996

60. Rowlingson JC: Toxicity of local anesthetic additives. Reg Anesth 18:453, 1993

61. Kito K, Kato H, Shibata M et al: The effect of varied doses of epinephrine on duration of lidocaine spinal anesthesia in the thoracic and lumbosacral dermatomes. Anesth Analg 86:1018, 1998

62. Chiu AA, Liu S, Carpenter RL: Effects of epinephrine on lidocaine spinal anesthesia: A crossover study. Anesth Analg 80:735, 1995

63. Tucker GT: Safety in numbers. The role of pharmacokinetics in local anesthetic toxicity: The 1993 ASRA Lecture. Reg Anesth 19:155, 1994

64. Liu S, Carpenter RL, Chiu AA: Epinephrine prolongs duration of subcutaneous infiltration of local anesthetics in a dose related manner: Correlation with magnitude of vasoconstriction. Reg Anesth 20:378, 1995

65. Cederholm I, Evers H, Lofstrom JB: Skin blood flow after intradermal injection of ropivacaine in various concentrations with and without epinephrine evaluated by laser Doppler flowmetry. Reg Anesth 17:322, 1992

66. Lofstrom JB: 1991 Labat Lecture. The effect of local anesthetics on the peripheral vasculature. Reg Anesth 17:1, 1992

67. Curatolo M, Petersen-Felix S, Arendt-Nielsen L et al: Epidural epinephrine and clonidine: Segmental analgesia and effects on different pain modalities. Anesthesiology 87:785, 1997

68. Ueda W, Hirakawa M, Mori K: Acceleration of epinephrine absorption by lidocaine. Anesthesiology 63:717, 1985

69. Magee C, Rodeheaver GT, Edgerton MT et al: Studies of the mechanisms by which epinephrine damages tissue defenses. J Surg Res 23:126, 1977

70. Hall JA, Ferro A: Myocardial ischaemia and ventricular arrhythmias precipitated by physiological concentrations of adrenaline in patients with coronary artery disease. Br Heart J 67:419, 1992

71. Curatolo M, Petersen-Felix S, Arendt-Nielsen L et al: Adding sodium bicarbonate to lidocaine enhances the depth of epidural blockade. Anesth Analg 86:341, 1998

72. Ikuta PT, Raza SM, Durrani Z: pH adjustment schedule for the amide local anesthetics. Reg Anesth 14:229, 1989

73. Capogna G, Celleno D, Laudano D: Alkalinization of local anesthetics: Which block, which local anesthetic? Reg Anesth 20:369, 1995

74. Wong K, Strichartz GR, Raymond SA: On the mechanisms of potentiation of local anesthetics by bicarbonate buffer: Drug structure–activity studies on isolated peripheral nerve. Anesth Analg 76:131, 1993

75. Rossi GC, Pasternak GW, Bodnar RJ: Synergistic brainstem interactions for morphine analgesia. Brain Res 624:171, 1993

76. Matos FF, Rollema H, Brown JL et al: Do opioids evoke the release of serotonin in the spinal cord? An in vivo microdialysis study of the regulation of extracellular serotonin in the rat. Pain 48:439, 1992

77. Barke KE, Hough LB: Simultaneous measurement of opiate-induced histamine release in the periaqueductal gray and opiate antinociception: An in vivo microdialysis study. J Pharmacol Exp Ther 266:934, 1993

78. Wang C, Chakrabarti MK, Galletly DC et al: Relative effects of intrathecal administration of fentanyl and midazolam on A delta and C fibre reflexes. Neuropharmacology 31:439, 1992

79. Niv D, Nemirovsky A, Rudick V: Antinociception induced by simultaneous intrathecal and intraperitoneal administration of low doses of morphine. Anesth Analg 80:886, 1995

80. Kaneko M, Saito Y, Kirihara Y et al: Synergistic antinociception after epidural coadministration of morphine and lidocaine in rats. Anesthesiology 80:137, 1994

81. Saito Y, Kaneko M, Kirihara Y et al: Interaction of intrathecally infused morphine and lidocaine in rats (part I): Synergistic antinociceptive effects. Anesthesiology 89:1455, 1998

82. Solomon RE, Gebhart GF: Synergistic antinociceptive interactions among drugs administered to the spinal cord. Anesth Analg 78:1164, 1994

83. Karambelkar DJ, Ramanathan S: 2-Chloroprocaine antagonism of epidural morphine analgesia. Acta Anaesth Scand 41:774, 1997

84. Coda B, Bausch S, Haas M et al: The hypothesis that antagonism of fentanyl analgesia by 2-chloroprocaine is mediated by direct action on opioid receptors. Reg Anesth 22:43, 1997

85. Curatolo M, Petersen-Felix S, Scaramozzino P et al: Epidural fentanyl, adrenaline and clonidine as adjuvants to local anaesthetics for surgical analgesia: Meta-analyses of analgesia and side-effects. Acta Anaesthesiol Scand 42:910, 1998

86. Curatolo M: Optimization of epidural analgesia. Anesthesiology. In Press

87. Stein C, Yassouridis A: Peripheral morphine analgesia. Pain 71:119, 1997

88. Likar R, Sittl R, Gragger K et al: Peripheral morphine analgesia in dental surgery. Pain 76:145, 1998

89. Allen GC, St Amand MA, A.C.P.L et al: Postarthroscopy analgesia with intraarticular bupivacaine/morphine. Anesthesiology 79:475, 1993

90. Kardash K, Schools A, Concepcion M: Effects of brachial plexus fentanyl on supraclavicular block. Reg Anesth 20:311, 1995

91. Fields HL, Emson PC, Leigh BK: Multiple opiate receptor sites on primary afferent fibres. Nature 284:351, 1980

92. Zhou L, Zhang Q, Stein C et al: Contribution of opioid receptors on primary afferent versus sympathetic neurons to peripheral opioid analgesia. J Pharm Exp Ther 286:1000, 1998

93. Eisenach JC, De Kock M, Klimscha W: Alpha(2)-adrenergic agonists for regional anesthesia: A clinical review of clonidine (1984–1995). Anesthesiology 85:655, 1996

94. Butterworth JF, Strichartz GR: The α_2-adrenergic agonists clonidine and guanfacine produce tonic and phasic block of conduction in rat sciatic nerve fibers. Anesth Analg 76:295, 1993

95. Gaumann DM, Brunet PC, Jirounek P: Clonidine enhances the effects of lidocaine on C fiber action potential. Anesth Analg 74:719, 1992

96. Pertovaara A, Hamalainen MM: Spinal potentiation and supraspinal additivity in the antinociceptive interaction between systemically administered α_2-adrenoreceptor agonist and cocaine in the rat. Anesth Analg 79:261, 1994

97. Klimscha W, Chiari A, Lorber C et al: Additives in neuraxial anesthesia: Opioids, alpha-2 adrenergic agonists, and neostigmine as a possible future drug for perioperative pain management. Acta Anaesth Scand 109(suppl):176, 1996

98. Bernard JM, Macaire P: Dose–range effects of clonidine added to lidocaine for brachial plexus block. Anesthesiology 87:277, 1997

99. Reuben SS, Steinberg RB, Klatt JL et al: Intravenous regional anesthesia using lidocaine and clonidine. Anesthesiology 91:654, 1999

100. Tucker GT, Moore DC, Bridenbaugh PO: Systemic absorption of mepivacaine in commonly used regional block procedures. Anesthesiology 37:277, 1972

101. Tucker GT, Mather LE: Properties, absorption, and disposition of local anesthetic agents. In Cousins MJ, Bridenbaugh PO (eds): Neural Blockade in Clinical Anesthesia and Management of Pain, 3d ed, p 55. Philadelphia, Lippincott–Raven, 1998

102. Morrison LM, Emanuelsson BM, McClure JH: Efficacy and kinetics of extradural ropivacaine: Comparison with bupivacaine. Br J Anaesth 72:164, 1994

103. Huang YF, Upton RN, Runciman WB: I.V. bolus administration of subconvulsive doses of lignocaine to conscious sheep: Myocardial pharmacokinetics. Br J Anaesth 70:326, 1993

104. Huang YF, Upton RN, Runciman WB: I.V. bolus administration of subconvulsive doses of lidocaine to conscious sheep: Relationships between myocardial pharmacokinetics and pharmacodynamics. Br J Anaesth 70:556, 1993

105. Kuhnert BR, Kuhnert PM, Philipson EH: The half-life of 2-chloroprocaine. Anesth Analg 65:273, 1986

106. Rutten AJ, Mather LE, Nancarrow C: Cardiovascular effects and regional clearances of intravenous ropivacaine in sheep. Anesth Analg 70:577, 1990

107. Braid DP, Scott DB: Dosage of lignocaine in epidural block in relation to toxicity. Br J Anaesth 38:596, 1966

108. Koscielniak-Nielsen Z, Hesselbjerg L, Brushoj J et al: EMLA patch

for spinal puncture: A comparison of EMLA patch with lignocaine infiltration and placebo patch. Anaesthesia 53:1218, 1998

109. Paulissian R, Salem MR, Joseph NJ et al: Hemodynamic responses to endotracheal extubation after coronary artery bypass grafting. Anesth Analg 73:10, 1991

110. Kindler CH, Schumacher PG, Schneider MC et al: Effects of intravenous lidocaine and/or esmolol on hemodynamic responses to laryngoscopy and intubation: A double-blind, controlled clinical trial. J Clin Anesth 8:491, 1996

111. Gonzalez RM, Bjerke RJ, Drobycki T et al: Prevention of endotracheal tube-induced coughing during emergence from general anesthesia. Anesth Analg 79:792, 1994

112. Yukioka H, Hayashi M, Terai T et al: Intravenous lidocaine as a suppressant of coughing during tracheal intubation in elderly patients. Anesth Analg 77:309, 1993

113. Helfman SM, Gold MI, DeLisser EA et al: Which drug prevents tachycardia and hypertension associated with tracheal intubation: Lidocaine, fentanyl, or esmolol? [see comments]. Anesth Analg 72:482, 1991

114. Nakayama M, Fujita S, Kanaya N et al: Effect of intravenous lidocaine on intraabdominal pressure response to airway stimulation. Anesth Analg 78:1149, 1994

115. Chamberlain DA: Antiarrhythmic drugs in resuscitation. Heart 80:408, 1998

116. Cassuto J, Wallin G, Hogstrom S et al: Inhibition of postoperative pain by continuous low-dose intravenous infusion of lidocaine. Anesth Analg 64:971, 1985

117. Marchettini P, Lacerenza M, Marangoni C: Lidocaine test in neuralgia. Pain 48:377, 1992

118. Chaplan SR, Bach FW, Shafer SL et al: Prolonged alleviation of tactile allodynia by intravenous lidocaine in neuropathic rats. Anesthesiology 83:775, 1995

119. Devor M, Wall PD, Catalan N: Systemic lidocaine silences neuroma and DRG discharge without blocking nerve conduction. Pain 48:261, 1992

120. Tanelian DL, MacIver MB: Analgesic concentrations of lidocaine suppress tonic A-delta and C fiber discharges produced by acute injury. Anesthesiology 74:934, 1991

121. Schwarz SK, Puil E: Analgesic and sedative concentrations of lignocaine shunt tonic and burst firing in thalamocortical neurones. Br J Pharmacol 124:1633, 1998

122. Butterworth J, Marlow G: Inhibition of brain cell excitability by lidocaine, QX314, and tetrodotoxin: A mechanism for analgesia from infused local anesthetics? Acta Anaesth Scand 37:516, 1993

123. Arner S, Lindblom Y, Meyerson BA: Prolonged relief of neuralgia after regional anesthetic blocks: A call for further experimental and systematic clinical studies. Pain 43:28, 1990

124. Jarvis B, Coukell AJ: Mexiletine. A review of its therapeutic use in painful diabetic neuropathy. Drugs 56:691, 1998

125. Kemper CA, Kent G, Burton S et al: Mexiletine for HIV-infected patients with painful peripheral neuropathy: A double-blind, placebo-controlled, crossover treatment trial. J Acquired Immune Deficiency Syndromes Hum Retrovirol 19:367, 1998

126. Chiou-Tan FY, Tuel SM, Johnson JC et al: Effect of mexiletine on spinal cord injury dysesthetic pain. Am J Phys Med Rehab 75:84, 1996

127. McCaughey W: Adverse effects of local anaesthetics. Drug Safety 7:178, 1992

128. Shibata M, Shingu K, Murakawa M: Tetraphasic actions of local anesthetics on central nervous system electrical activity in cats. Reg Anesth 19:255, 1994

129. Tanaka K, Yamasaki M: Blocking of cortical inhibitory synapses by intravenous lidocaine. Nature 209:207, 1966

130. Brown DL, Ransom DM, Hall JA et al: Regional anesthesia and local anesthetic-induced systemic toxicity: Seizure frequency and accompanying cardiovascular changes [see comments]. Anesth Analg 81:321, 1995

131. Auroy Y, Narchi P, Messiah A et al: Serious complications related to regional anesthesia: Results of a prospective survey in France [see comments]. Anesthesiology 87:479, 1997

132. Bernards CM, Carpenter RL, Rupp SM: Effects of midazolam and diazepam premedication on central nervous system and cardiovascular toxicity of bupivacaine. Anesthesiology 70:318, 1989

133. Yokoyama M, Hirakawa M, Goto H: Effect of vasoconstrictive agents added to lidocaine on intravenous lidocaine-induced convulsions in rats. Anesthesiology 82:574, 1995

134. Yamauchi Y, Kotani J, Ueda Y: The effects of exogenous epineph-

rine on a convulsive dose of lidocaine: Relationship with cerebral circulation. J Neurosurg Anesth 10:178, 1998

135. Sokrab TEO, Johansson BB: Regional cerebral bloodflow in acute hypertension induced by adrenaline, noradrenaline, and phenylephrine in the conscious rat. Acta Physiol Scand 137:101, 1989

136. Mayhan WG, Faraci FM, Siems JL: Role of molecular charge in disruption of the blood–brain barrier during acute hypertension. Circ Res 64:658, 1989

137. Arthur GR, Feldman HS, Covino BG: Alterations in the pharmacokinetic properties of amide local anaesthetics following local anaesthetic induced convulsions. Acta Anaesthesiol Scand 32:522, 1988

138. Mulroy MF, Norris MC, Liu SS: Safety steps for epidural injection of local anesthetics: Review of the literature and recommendations. Anesth Analg 85:1346, 1997

139. Nancarrow C, Rutten A, Runciman W: Myocardial and cerebral drug concentrations and the mechanisms of death after fatal intravenous doses of lidocaine, bupivacaine, and ropivacaine in sheep. Anesth Analg 69:276, 1989

140. Denson DD, Behbehani MM, Gregg RV: Effects of an intravenously administered arrhythmogenic dose of bupivacaine at the nucleus tractus solitarius in the conscious rat. Reg Anesth 15:76, 1990

141. Bernards CM, Artruu AA: Hexamethonium and midazolam terminate dysrhythmias and hypertension caused by intracerebroventricular bupivacaine in rabbits. Anesthesiology 74:89, 1991

142. Szocik JF, Gardner CA, Webb RC: Inhibitory effects of bupivacaine and lidocaine on adrenergic neuroeffector junctions in rat tail artery. Anesthesiology 78:911, 1993

143. Chang KSK, Yang M, Andresen MC: Clinically relevant concentrations of bupivacaine inhibit rat aortic baroreceptors. Anesth Analg 78:501, 1994

144. Hogan QH, Stadnicka A, Bosnjak ZJ et al: Effects of lidocaine and bupivacaine on isolated rabbit mesenteric capacitance veins. Reg Anesth Pain Med 23:409, 1998

145. Reiz S, Haggmark S, Johansson G et al: Cardiotoxicity of ropivacaine—a new amide local anaesthetic agent. Acta Anaesthesiol Scand 33:93, 1989

146. Guo XT, Castle NA, Chernoff DM et al: Comparative inhibition of voltage-gated cation channels by local anesthetics. Ann N Y Acad Sci 625:181, 1991

147. Clarkson CW, Hondeghem LM: Mechanisms for bupivacaine depression of cardiac conduction: Fast block of sodium channels during the action potential with slow recovery from block during diastole. Anesthesiology 62:396, 1985

148. Scott B, Lee AL, Fagen D: Acute toxicity of ropivacaine compared with that of bupivacaine. Anesth Analg 69:563, 1989

149. Coyle DE, Porembka DT, Selhorst CS: Echocardiographic evaluation of bupivacaine cardiotoxicity. Anesth Analg 79:335, 1994

150. Berman MF, Lipka LJ: Relative sodium current block by bupivacaine and lidocaine in neonatal rat myocytes. Anesth Analg 79:350, 1994

151. Sanchez-Chapula J: Effects of bupivacaine on membrane current of guinea pig ventricular myocytes. Eur J Pharmacol 156:303, 1988

152. Lynch C: Depression of myocardial contractility in vitro by bupivacaine, etidocaine, and lidocaine. Anesth Analg 65:551, 1986

153. Sztark F, Malgat M, Dabadie P et al: Comparison of the effects of bupivacaine and ropivacaine on heart cell mitochondrial bioenergetics. Anesthesiology 88:1340, 1998

154. Butterworth JF, Brownlow RC, Leith JP: Bupivacaine inhibits cyclic-3′,5′-adenosine monophosphate production: A possible contributing factor to cardiovascular toxicity. Anesthesiology 79:88, 1993

155. Davis NL, de Jong RH: Successful resuscitation following massive bupivacaine overdose. Anesth Analg 61:62, 1982

156. Freysz M, Timour Q, Bertrix L et al: Bupivacaine hastens the ischemia-induced decrease of the electrical ventricular fibrillation threshold. Anesth Analg 80:657, 1995

157. Heavner JE, Badgwell JM, Dryden CF: Bupivacaine toxicity in lightly anesthetized pigs with respiratory imbalance plus or minus halothane. Reg Anesth 20:20, 1995

158. Heavner JE, Rosenberg P: Propofol for lidocaine-induced seizures [letter]. Anesth Analg 88:1193, 1999

159. Kalichman MW: Physiologic mechanisms by which local anesthetics may cause injury to nerve and spinal cord. Reg Anesth 18:448, 1993

160. Selander D: Neurotoxicity of local anesthetics: Animal data. Reg Anesth 18:461, 1993

161. Ready LB, Plumer MH, Haschke RH et al: Neurotoxicity of intrathecal local anesthetics in rabbits. Anesthesiology 63:364, 1985

162. Bainton C, Strichartz G: Concentration dependence of lidocaine-induced irreversible conduction loss in frog nerve. Anesthesiology 81:657, 1994

163. Kanai T, Katsuki H, Takasake M: Graded, irreversible changes in crayfish giant axon as manifestations of lidocaine neurotoxicity in vitro. Anesth Analg 86:569, 1998

164. Lambert L, Lambert D, Strichartz G: Irreversible conduction block in isolated nerve by high concentrations of local anesthetics. Anesthesiology 80:1082, 1994

165. Iida H, Watanabe Y, Dohi S et al: Direct effects of ropivacaine and bupivacaine on spinal pial vessels in canine. Anesthesiology 87:75, 1997

166. Chabal C, Jacobson L, Little J: Effects of intrathecal fentanyl and lidocaine on somatosensory-evoked potentials, the H-reflex, and clinical responses. Anesth Analg 67:509, 1988

167. Liu S, Kopacz D, Carpenter R: Quantitative assessment of differential sensory nerve block after lidocaine spinal anesthesia. Anesthesiology 82:60, 1995

168. Pollock JE, Liu SS, Neal JM et al: Dilution of lidocaine does not decrease the incidence of transient neurologic symptoms. Anesthesiology 90:445, 1999

169. Hampl KF, Heinzmann-Wiedmer S, Luginbuehl I et al: Transient neurologic symptoms after spinal anesthesia. Anesthesiology 88:629, 1998

170. Drasner K: Lidocaine spinal anesthesia: A vanishing therapeutic index? Anesthesiology 87:469, 1997

171. Bircher AJ, Messmer SL, Surber C et al: Delayed-type hypersensitivity to subcutaneous lidocaine with tolerance to articaine: Confirmation by in vivo and in vitro tests. Contact Dermatitis 34:387, 1996

172. Ogunsalu CO: Anaphylactic reaction following administration of lignocaine hydrochloride infiltration. Case report. Australian Dent J 43:170, 1998

173. Chen AH: Toxicity and allergy to local anesthesia. J California Dent Assoc 26:683, 1998

174. Glinert RJ, Zachary CB: Local anesthetic allergy: Its recognition and avoidance. J Dermatol Surg Oncol 17:491, 1991

175. Cox CR, Checketts MR, Mackenzie N et al: Comparison of S(−)-bupivacaine with racemic (R,S)-bupivacaine in supraclavicular brachial plexus block. Br J Anaesth 80:594, 1998

176. Cox CR, Faccenda KA, Gilhooly C et al: Extradural S(−)-bupivacaine: Comparison with racemic R,S-bupivacaine. Br J Anaesth 80:289, 1998

177. McGlade DP, Kalpokas MV, Mooney PH et al: A comparison of 0.5% ropivacaine and 0.5% bupivacaine for axillary brachial plexus anaesthesia. Anaesth Intens Care 26:515, 1998

178. McGlade DP, Kalpokas MV, Mooney PH et al: Comparison of 0.5% ropivacaine and 0.5% bupivacaine in lumbar epidural anaesthesia for lower limb orthopaedic surgery. Anaesth Intens Care 25:262, 1997

179. Huang YF, Pryor ME, Mather LE et al: Cardiovascular and central nervous system effects of intravenous levobupivacaine and bupivacaine in sheep. Anesth Analg 86:797, 1998

180. Knudsen K, Beckman Suurkula M, Blomberg S et al: Central nervous and cardiovascular effects of i.v. infusions of ropivacaine, bupivacaine and placebo in volunteers. Br J Anaesth 78:507, 1997

181. Bardsley H, Gristwood R, Baker H et al: A comparison of the cardiovascular effects of levobupivacaine and rac-bupivacaine following intravenous administration to healthy volunteers. Br J Clin Pharmacol 46:245, 1998

182. Thomas JM, Schug SA: Recent advances in the pharmacokinetics of local anaesthetics. Long-acting amide enantiomers and continuous infusions. Clin Pharmacokin 36:67, 1999

183. Kuzma PJ, Kline MD, Calkins MD et al: Progress in the development of ultra-long-acting local anesthetics. Reg Anesth 22:543, 1997

184. Drager C, Benzinger D, Gao F et al: Prolonged intercostal nerve blockade in sheep using controlled release of bupivacaine and dexamethasone from polymer microspheres. Anesthesiology 89:969, 1998

185. Boogaerts J, Declercq A, Lafont N et al: Toxicity of bupivacaine encapsulated into liposomes and injected intravenously: Comparison with plain solutions. Anesth Analg 76:553, 1993

186. Cousins MJ: Pain: The past, present, and future of anesthesiology. The E.A. Rovenstine Memorial Lecture. Anesthesiology 91:538, 1999

187. Curatolo M, Petersen-Felix S, Arendt-Nielsen L et al: Spinal anaesthesia inhibits central temporal summation. Br J Anaesth 78:88, 1997

188. Abram SE, Yaksh TL: Systemic lidocaine blocks nerve injury-induced hyperalgesia and nociceptor driven spinal sensitization in rats. Anesthesiology 80:383, 1994

189. Mulroy MF, Greengrass R, Ganapathy S et al: Sameridine is safe and effective for spinal anesthesia: A comparative dose-ranging study with lidocaine for inguinal hernia repair. Anesth Analg 88:815, 1999

FOUR

PREPARING FOR ANESTHESIA

Clinical Anesthesia (4/e), edited by
Paul G. Barash, Bruce F. Cullen, and
Robert K. Stoelting. Lippincott Williams &
Wilkins, Philadelphia, © 2001.

CHAPTER 18

PREOPERATIVE EVALUATION

LEE A. FLEISHER

INTRODUCTION

The past decade has been marked by an intense interest in better refining the optimal perioperative evaluation before surgery. The impetus for this focus is a desire to save costs and make the perioperative process more efficient. Within the general context of using the best evidence to define medical practice, preoperative testing represents a unique and complex problem of relating a diagnostic test to an intervention whose outcome would be different if the test were not performed. Except for high-risk populations, such as patients undergoing major vascular surgery or with known cardiovascular disease, extremely large sample sizes are needed to identify differences in final outcomes such as stroke, myocardial infarction, or death. In lower-risk groups, the difficulty is in linking the value of preoperative testing to the rare morbid events; therefore, the trend in the literature is toward assessing surrogate outcomes such as costs, resource utilization, and cancellation of cases. In many cases, studies are undertaken to prove that a test does not affect outcome in lower-risk populations. Most importantly, all of these studies emphasize an initial history and physical examination to define those patients who might benefit from further evaluation and diagnostic testing.

In defining the components and extent of the anesthesia evaluation of the patient prior to surgery, it is important to acknowledge that it serves multiple purposes. The Joint Commission for the Accreditation of Health Care Organizations (JCAHO) requires that all patients receive a preoperative anesthetic evaluation. The American Society of Anesthesiologists approved Basic Standards for Preanesthetic Care, which outline minimum requirements for the preoperative evaluation.[1] A preoperative evaluation is also an important component of perioperative management. In a study evaluating methods of reducing preoperative anxiety, a thorough preoperative evaluation can be as effective as an anxiolytic premedication.[2] Finally, the preoperative evaluation serves to establish a database upon which a risk assessment and perioperative management decisions can be made.

The concept of establishing a data base is predicated upon the assumption that information regarding the patient's medical condition can be used to modify care, and that this will result in improved outcome. Although there are no hard data in the form of randomized controlled trials to support such an assumption, there are several decision analyses regarding preoperative cardiac evaluation that highlight the potential benefits of testing and coronary revascularization.[3-5]

In an ideal world, the preoperative database would be complete and contain confirmatory evidence of the pertinent disease processes. It is important for anesthesiologists to determine the presence or absence of certain pathophysiologic processes in all patients, but frequently the evaluation is abbreviated and focuses on the systems of interest. For example, the patient undergoing a carotid endarterectomy may have a more extensive neurologic evaluation than a patient undergoing an elective cholecystectomy. Bleeding history may require more extensive evaluation in the patient for whom an epidural anesthetic is planned than if general anesthesia is planned. Therefore, the anesthesiologist frequently applies clinical judgment in the decision to further assess the probability of disease.

In this chapter, the clinical risk factors that raise the probability of disease and the use of tests to confirm the diagnosis are outlined. In addition, the cost–benefit issues of a more detailed database are discussed. This chapter provides an overview of the preoperative evaluation process; for more specific details, the reader is referred to chapters focusing on given organ systems.

THE EVOLVING CONCEPTS OF PREOPERATIVE SCREENING

It is now the exception rather than the rule for patients to be admitted to the hospital the day prior to surgery. Even patients undergoing coronary artery bypass grafting are being admitted the morning of surgery. In order to obtain a thorough history in these patients, preoperative screening clinics have been created. There are multiple approaches to obtaining a preoperative evaluation in such settings. In some practice settings, these centers are staffed entirely by attending anesthesiologists. This poses a significant financial burden, since it represents time away from the operating rooms. If this activity is combined with other responsibilities, the preoperative evaluations performed may be cursory. In order to balance the financial burden of utilizing attending staff with issues of appropriate medical supervision, many centers employ nurse specialists, with questions referred to anesthesiologists. Since the system to evaluate all patients would require extensive resources at high expense, alternative means of obtaining an adequate evaluation are necessary. In many practice settings, the internist or primary caregiver provides a preoperative evaluation, with the anesthesiologist performing a brief history at the time of surgery. Alternatively, the surgeon may identify healthy patients for whom a telephone interview may suffice or whose evaluation may occur the day of surgery. Managed care organizations may also restrict the number and nature of preoperative tests performed, and the anesthesiologist may not be able to evaluate the patient prior to surgery. It is important for the anesthesiologist to take an active role in the design and implementation of the preoperative screening clinic, since it is area in which they can reduce total health care expenditures by reducing unnecessary testing.

Several systems have been developed to ensure accuracy and completeness of the information from the preoperative evaluation. Multiple preoperative questionnaires have been developed and tested against traditional physician interviewing. These questionnaires are at least as accurate as, if not more accurate than, physician interviews.[6] Computer-driven programs have also been developed, which demonstrate good success.[7] In both cases, repetition of critical questions is essential. The precise method of obtaining the history is not as important as its completeness and its accurate ability to dictate appropriate care.

Increasingly, the systems by which a preoperative evaluation is obtained are being evaluated for their value in improving the efficiency of the perioperative process. By assuming responsibility for ordering tests, the anesthesiologist can obtain a more appropriate laboratory panel and potentially reduce cancellations the day of surgery arising from an inadequate evaluation. Additionally, laboratories can be centralized and patient and family perioperative education can occur within the confines of these centers. Fisher et al demonstrated the cost-effectiveness of establishing a preoperative evaluation clinic at Stanford by reducing both testing and cancellations.[8,9] Starsnic and colleagues at Thomas Jefferson University compared a group whose testing was primarily ordered by surgeons augmented by anesthesiologists in the preoperative evaluation clinic versus a group whose testing was ordered primarily by anesthesiologists augmented by the surgeons as deemed necessary during two consecutive time periods in 1992.[10] They demonstrated an average cost savings of $20.89 per patient when the anesthesiologist was the primary physician determining testing. Importantly, there were no recorded cancellations or alterations in intraoperative management attributable to inadequate testing. Similarly, Allison and Bromley performed an analysis of the cost savings of unnecessary testing at the Department of Veterans Affairs Medical Center in South Carolina and demonstrated a potential savings of $11,757.50 per year.[11] Vogt and Henson performed a retrospective chart review and estimated a potential hospital savings of approximately $80,000 by eliminating unindicated tests for the 5100 patients seen in the preoperative clinic annually.[12]

An alternative approach to the construction of a preoperative evaluation clinic is through the simple dissemination of guidelines. Mancuso studied the impact of new guidelines on physicians' ordering of preoperative tests at an orthopedic hospital.[13] A simple memo was distributed to the participating surgeons after the establishment of ordering patterns by a multidisciplinary group. They demonstrated a marked reduction in the number of tests without an increase in cancellations or untoward events. A savings in charges of $34,000 was realized. Although the compliance of the physicians was variable, this simple approach did demonstrate efficacy in reducing costs. These studies suggest that the anesthesiologist's involvement in the design of the system to determine the preoperative testing algorithm is essential for economic success.

APPROACH TO THE PATIENT: HISTORY

The approach to the patient should always begin with a thorough history. A thorough history may frequently be sufficient (without additional routine laboratory tests) prior to certain procedures. In fact, Schein *et al* studied approximately 20,000 patients undergoing cataract procedures, randomizing half of the patients to no routine testing prior to surgery.[14] They found no difference in outcome between those who received testing and those who did not if the primary physician evaluated the patient within 30 days and determined that the patient's medical condition was stable.

The indication for the surgical procedure is part of the preoperative history, since it will help determine the urgency of the surgery. True emergent procedures, which are associated with an accepted higher morbidity and mortality, require a more abbreviated evaluation.[15] The difficult area is with regard to urgent procedures. For example, ischemic limbs or malignant tumors require surgery soon after presentation, but can usually be delayed for 24 hours for further evaluation. The indication for the surgical procedure may also have implications on other aspects of perioperative management. For example, the presence of a small bowel obstruction has implications regarding the risk of aspiration and the need for a rapid sequence induction. The extent of a lung resection will dictate the need for further pulmonary testing and perioperative monitoring. Patients undergoing carotid endarterectomy may require a more extensive neurologic examination. Frequently, further information will be required that necessitates contacting the surgeon.

Information regarding previous anesthetics is important in order to evaluate for the presence of a difficult airway, a history of malignant hyperthermia, and the individual's response to surgical stress and specific anesthetics. A history of a previous surgical procedure performed without complications under general anesthesia reduces the probability of a major airway problem, although it does not eliminate it. The ability to review previous anesthetic records is required to confirm a previous easy intubation, assuming the patient's body habitus has not changed in the interim. The patient should be questioned regarding any previous difficulty with anesthesia or other family members' having a history of difficulty with anesthesia. Frequently, the patient will relate an "allergy" to anesthesia, which may indicate a history of malignant hyperthermia.

The history should include a complete list of medications in order to adequately define a preoperative medication regimen, anticipate potential drug interactions, and provide clues to underlying disease. A complete list of drug allergies, including previous reactions, should also be obtained. Once the general issues are completed, the preoperative history can focus on specific organ systems.

Specific Organ Systems

Cardiac Disease

Cardiovascular disease has traditionally been approached from two perspectives: multifactorial risk indices and evaluation of new preoperative testing modalities in specific patient groups. The first area was popularized by the pioneering work of Drs. Saklad and Dripps and the American Society of Anesthesiologists (Physical Status Index) (Table 18-1) and that of Dr. Lee Goldman and colleagues (Cardiac Risk Index).[1,15] The second area involves the assessment of new, noninvasive testing modalities and has received extensive attention during the previous two decades. Specific testing modalities will be addressed later in the chapter.

In interpreting studies that develop a multifactorial index of risk, three basic assumptions are made. The first is that data on all of the potentially important variables are available. For example, if angina was not included in the data base, it could not be included in the final index. Second, eliminating variables from the model must be based upon biological significance, not just on statistical significance. In the original Goldman Cardiac Risk Index, New York Heart Association (NYHA) Class IV angina was not found to be a risk factor; however, the number of patients who fit this criteria was too small to achieve statistical significance.[15] Therefore, it was eliminated, probably erroneously, from the model. Third, if a factor is identified as placing the patient at significant risk, and if the anesthesiologist can use the information to modify and reduce that risk, then the factor may no longer appear to be significant. In other words, the perioperative period cannot be used as a black box. Should perioperative hemodynamic management decisions not include the hypertensive status of a patient, then lack of hypertensive management in subsequent patients may lead to increased morbidity.

Table 18-1. AMERICAN SOCIETY OF ANESTHESIOLOGISTS PHYSICAL STATUS CLASSIFICATION

Status	Disease State
ASA Class 1	No organic, physiologic, biochemical, or psychiatric disturbance
ASA Class 2	Mild to moderate systemic disturbance that may not be related to the reason for surgery
ASA Class 3	Severe systemic disturbance that may or may not be related to the reason for surgery
ASA Class 4	Severe systemic disturbance that is life-threatening with or without surgery
ASA Class 5	Moribund patient who has little chance of survival but is submitted to surgery as a last resort (resuscitative effort)
Emergency operation (E)	Any patient in whom an emergency operation is required

From information in American Society of Anesthesiologists: New classification of physical status. Anesthesiology 24:111, 1963.

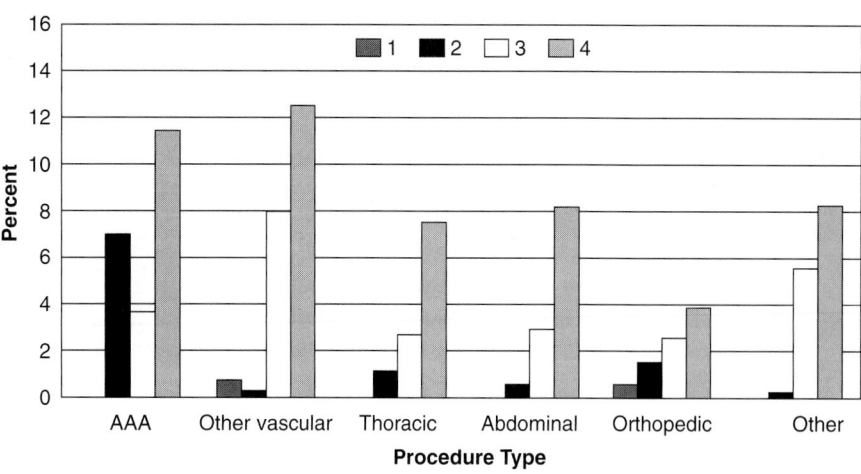

Figure 18-1. CRI cardiac risk index. Bars represent rate of major cardiac complications in entire patient population (both derivation and validation cohorts combined) for patients in revised CRI classes according to type of procedure performed. AAA = abdominal aortic aneurysm. Note that, by definition, patients undergoing AAA, thoracic, and abdominal procedures were excluded from Class I. In all subsets except patients undergoing AAA, there was a statistically significant trend toward greater risk with higher-risk class. See text for details. (Reproduced with permission from Lee TH, Marcantonio ER, Mangione CM *et al:* Derivation and prospective validation of a simple index for prediction of cardiac risk of major noncardiac surgery. Circulation 100:1043, 1999.)

Noncardiac Risk Indices

In 1977, Goldman and colleagues published their landmark article studying 1001 patients undergoing noncardiac surgical procedures, excluding transurethral resection of the prostate (TURP).[15] The authors excluded this surgery because of their impression of a low morbidity rate when performed under spinal anesthesia. They identified nine risk factors and gave each factor a certain number of points (Goldman Cardiac Risk Index, or CRI). A myocardial infarction and S3 gallop were identified as the most significant risk factors. By adding up the total number of points, patients were placed in one of four classes. The patient's class could then be compared to the rates of morbidity and mortality from the original cohort.

The CRI was subsequently validated in another cohort of patients; however, it has not been found to be predictive in patients undergoing major vascular surgery.[16,17] Multiple studies have demonstrated that major vascular surgery is associated with a higher rate of morbidity and mortality compared to nonvascular surgery.[15,18–20] In order to rectify this problem, Detsky and colleagues proposed a modification of the CRI for vascular patients.[21]

Although both of these indices were extremely useful when initially proposed, perioperative care has changed significantly in the intervening years. Goldman Class III and IV continues to represent a high-risk cohort; however, recent mortality has been lower than originally reported.[22] In addition, many vascular surgery patients would be classified as low-risk, but would benefit from further risk stratification.[17] Significant changes in the medical care of the patient with coronary artery disease has had profound impact on the perioperative period.

In an attempt to update the original CRI, Goldman and colleagues studied 4315 patients aged 50 years who were undergoing elective major noncardiac procedures in a tertiary-care teaching hospital.[23] Six independent predictors of complications were identified and included in a revised CRI: high-risk type of surgery, history of ischemic heart disease, history of congestive heart failure, history of cerebrovascular disease, preoperative treatment with insulin, and preoperative serum creatinine >2.0 mg · dl^{-1}. Rates of major cardiac complication with 0, 1, 2, or 3 of these factors were 0.5%, 1.3%, 4%, and 9%, respectively, in the derivation cohort and 0.4%, 0.9%, 7%, and 11%, respectively, among 1422 patients in the validation cohort (Fig. 18-1).

A primary issue with all of these indices from the anesthesiologist's perspective is that a simple estimate of risk does not help in refining perioperative management, but may provide information to assess the probability of risk. In contrast, the anesthesiologist is most concerned with defining the cardiovascular risk factors and symptoms or signs of unstable cardiac disease states, such as myocardial ischemia, congestive heart failure, valvular heart disease, and significant cardiac arrhythmias.

In patients with symptomatic coronary disease, the preoperative evaluation may lead to the recognition of a change in the frequency or pattern of anginal symptoms. Symptoms of cardiovascular disease should be carefully determined, especially the characteristics of chest pain, if present. Certain populations of patients—the elderly, for example, or women or diabetics—may present with more atypical features. The presence of unstable angina has been associated with a high perioperative risk of myocardial infarction (MI).[24] The perioperative period is associated with a hypercoagulable state and surges in endogenous catecholamines, both of which may exacerbate the underlying process in unstable angina, increasing the risk of acute infarction.[25] The preoperative evaluation can affect both a patient's short- and long-term health by instituting treatment of unstable angina.

The patient with stable angina represents a continuum from mild angina with extreme exertion to dyspnea with angina after walking up a few stairs. The patient who manifests angina only after strenuous exercise does not demonstrate signs of left ventricular dysfunction and would not be a candidate for changes in management. In contrast, a patient with dyspnea on mild exertion would be at high risk for developing perioperative ventricular dysfunction, myocardial ischemia, and possible MI. These patients have an extremely high probability of having extensive coronary artery disease, and additional monitoring or cardiovascular testing should be contemplated, depending upon the surgical procedure and institutional factors.

In virtually all studies, the presence of active congestive heart failure preoperatively has been associated with an increased incidence of perioperative cardiac morbidity.[15,21] Stabilization of ventricular function and treatment for pulmonary congestion are prudent prior to elective surgery. Also, it is important to determine the etiology of the left heart failure. Congestive symptoms may be due to nonischemic cardiomyopathy or mitral or aortic valvular insufficiency and/or stenosis. Since the type of perioperative monitoring and treatments would be different, clarifying the cause of cardiac congestion is important.

Patients with a prior MI have coronary artery disease, although a small group of patients may sustain a MI from a nonatherosclerotic mechanism. Traditionally, risk assessment for noncardiac surgery was based upon the time interval between the MI and surgery. Multiple studies have demonstrated an increased incidence of reinfarction if the MI was within 6 months of surgery.[26–28] With improvements in perioperative care, this difference has decreased. Therefore, the importance of the intervening time interval may no longer be valid in the current era of thrombolytics, angioplasty, and risk stratification after an acute MI. Although many patients with an MI may continue to have myocardium at risk for subsequent ischemia and infarction, other patients may have their critical coronary stenosis either totally occluded or widely patent. For example, the use of percutaneous transluminal coronary angioplasty, thrombolysis, and early coronary artery bypass grafting has changed the natural history of the disease.[29,30] Therefore, patients should be evaluated from the perspective of their risk for ongoing ischemia. The American Heart Association/American College of Cardiology Task Force on Perioperative Evaluation of the Cardiac Patient Undergoing Noncardiac Surgery has defined three risk groups—major, intermediate, and minor[31] (Table 18-2). They indicate that recent MI (MI < 30 days) places patients in the group at highest risk; after that period, a prior MI places the patient at intermediate risk.[31]

Patients at Risk for Coronary Artery Disease (CAD)

For those patients without overt symptoms or history, the probability of CAD varies with the type and number of atherosclerotic risk factors present. Peripheral arterial disease has been shown to be associated with CAD in multiple studies. Hertzer and colleagues studied 1000 consecutive patients scheduled for major vascular surgery and found that approximately 60% of patients had at least one coronary artery with a critical stenosis.[32]

Diabetes mellitus is common in the elderly and represents a

Table 18-2. CLINICAL PREDICTORS OF INCREASED PERIOPERATIVE CARDIOVASCULAR RISK (MYOCARDIAL INFARCTION, CONGESTIVE HEART FAILURE, DEATH)

Major

Unstable coronary syndromes
• Recent myocardial infarction* with evidence of important ischemic risk by clinical symptoms or noninvasive study
• Unstable or severe† angina (Canadian Class III or IV)‡
Decompensated congestive heart failure
Significant arrhythmias
• High-grade atrioventricular block
• Symptomatic ventricular arrhythmias in the presence of underlying heart disease
• Supraventricular arrhythmias with uncontrolled ventricular rate
Severe valvular disease

Intermediate

Mild angina pectoris (Canadian Class I or II)
Prior myocardial infarction by history or pathological Q waves
Compensated or prior congestive heart failure
Diabetes mellitus

Minor

Advanced age
Abnormal ECG (left ventricular hypertrophy, left bundle branch block, ST-T abnormalities)
Rhythm other than sinus (e.g., atrial fibrillation)
Low functional capacity (e.g., inability to climb one flight of stairs with a bag of groceries)
History of stroke
Uncontrolled systemic hypertension

---

* The American College of Cardiology National Database Library defines recent MI as greater than 7 days but less than or equal to 1 month (30 days).
† May include "stable" angina in patients who are unusually sedentary.
‡ Campeau L: Grading of angina pectoris. Circulation 54:522, 1976.
Reproduced with permission from Eagle K, Brundage B, Chaitman B et al: Guidelines for perioperative cardiovascular evaluation of the noncardiac surgery. A report of the American Heart Association/American College of Cardiology Task Force on Assessment of Diagnostic and Therapeutic Cardiovascular Procedures. Circulation 93:1278, 1996.

Table 18-3. BLOOD PRESSURE (mm Hg)

Category	Systolic		Diastolic
Optimal	<120	and	<80
Normal	<130	and	<85
High-normal	130–139	or	85–89
Hypertension			
Stage 1	140–159	or	90–99
Stage 2	160–179	or	100–109
Stage 3	≥180	or	≥110

Reproduced with permission from Sixth report of the Joint National Committee on Prevention, Detection, Evaluation, and Treatment of High Blood Pressure. Arch Intern Med 157:2413, 1997.

---

disease that affects multiple organ systems. Complications of diabetes mellitus are frequently the cause of urgent or emergent surgery, especially in the elderly. Diabetes accelerates the progression of atherosclerosis, which can frequently be silent. Diabetics have a higher probability of CAD than nondiabetics do. There is a high incidence of both silent myocardial infarction and myocardial ischemia.[33] Eagle et al demonstrated that diabetes is an independent risk factor for perioperative cardiac morbidity.[34] In attempting to determine the degree of this increased probability, the length of the disease and other associated end-organ dysfunction should be taken into account. Autonomic neuropathy has been found to be the best predictor of silent coronary artery disease.[35] Since these patients are at very high risk for silent MI, the electrocardiogram should be obtained to examine for the presence of Q waves.

Hypertension has also been associated with an increased incidence of silent myocardial ischemia and infarction.[33] Hypertensive patients who have left ventricular hypertrophy and are undergoing noncardiac surgery are at a higher perioperative risk than nonhypertensive patients.[36] Investigators have suggested that the presence of a strain pattern on ECG suggests a chronic ischemic state.[37] Therefore, these patients should also be considered to have an increased probability of CAD and developing cardiovascular morbidity.

There is a great deal of debate regarding a trigger to delay or cancel a surgical procedure in a patient with poorly or untreated hypertension. Hypertension has been divided into three stages, with Stage 3 denoting that which might be used as a cut-off (Table 18-3).[38] Aggressive treatment of blood pressure is associated with increasing reduction in long-term risk, although the effect diminishes in all but diabetic patients as diastolic blood pressure is reduced below 90 mm Hg.[39] Although there has been a suggestion in the literature that a case should be delayed if the diastolic pressure is greater than 110 mm Hg, the study often quoted as the basis for this determination demonstrated no major morbidity in this small cohort of individuals in their study.[40] In fact, the authors actually suggested that proceeding with elective surgery is safe with a diastolic blood pressure up to 110 mm Hg, and that the sample size was too small to make comments above this level. In the absence of end-organ changes, such as renal insufficiency or left ventricular hypertrophy with strain, it would seem appropriate to proceed with surgery. In contrast, a patient with a markedly elevated blood pressure and new onset of a headache should have surgery delayed for further treatment.

Several other risk factors have been used to suggest an increased probability of CAD. These include the atherosclerotic processes associated with tobacco use and hypercholesterolemia. Although these risk factors increase the probability of developing coronary artery disease, they have not been shown to increase perioperative risk. When attempting to determine the overall probability of disease, the number and severity of the risk factors are important.

Table 18-4. CARDIAC RISK* STRATIFICATION FOR NONCARDIAC SURGICAL PROCEDURES

HIGH	(Reported cardiac risk often >5%) • Emergent major operations, particularly in the elderly • Aortic and other major vascular • Peripheral vascular • Anticipated prolonged surgical procedures associated with large fluid shifts and/or blood loss
INTERMEDIATE	(Reported cardiac risk generally <5%) • Carotid endarterectomy • Head and neck • Intraperitoneal and intrathoracic • Orthopedic • Prostate
LOW†	(Reported cardiac risk generally <1%) • Endoscopic procedures • Superficial procedure • Cataract • Breast

* Combined incidence of cardiac death and nonfatal myocardial infarction.
† Do not generally require further preoperative cardiac testing.
Reproduced with permission from Eagle K, Brundage B, Chaitman B et al: Guidelines for perioperative cardiovascular evaluation of the noncardiac surgery. A report of the American Heart Association/American College of Cardiology Task Force on Assessment of Diagnostic and Therapeutic Cardiovascular Procedures. Circulation 93:1278, 1996.

Importance of Surgical Procedure

The surgical procedure influences the extent of the preoperative evaluation required by determining the potential range of changes in perioperative management. For example, a pulmonary artery catheter or transesophageal echocardiography may be appropriate for a patient undergoing major abdominal or vascular surgery, but would not be considered appropriate for ambulatory surgery. Similarly, coronary revascularization may be beneficial for procedures associated with a high incidence of morbidity and mortality, but not those associated with a low incidence, as described below. There are few hard data to define the surgery-specific incidence of complications. It is known that peripheral procedures, such as those included in a study of

ambulatory surgery completed at the Mayo Clinic, are associated with an extremely low incidence of morbidity and mortality.[41] Similarly, major vascular procedures are associated with the highest incidence of complications, with a similar incidence documented for infra-inguinal and aortic surgery.[42] Eagle et al published data on the incidence of perioperative myocardial infarction and mortality by procedure for patients enrolled in the Coronary Artery Surgery Study (CASS).[43] They determined the overall risk of perioperative morbidity in patients with known coronary artery disease on medical treatment and the potential reduced rate of perioperative morbidity in those patients who had a prior coronary artery bypass grafting. High-risk procedures include major vascular, abdominal, thoracic, and orthopedic surgery. The American Heart Association/American College of Cardiology Guidelines defined three tiers of surgical stress, which are shown in Table 18-4.[31]

Importance of Exercise Tolerance

Exercise tolerance is one of the most important determinants of perioperative risk and the need for invasive monitoring.[44] An excellent exercise tolerance, even in patients with stable angina, suggests that the myocardium can be stressed without becoming dysfunctional. If a patient can walk a mile without becoming short of breath, the probability of extensive coronary artery disease is small. Alternatively, if patients experience dyspnea associated with chest pain during minimal exertion, the probability of extensive coronary artery disease is high. A greater degree of coronary artery disease has been associated with a higher perioperative risk.[45] Additionally, these patients are at risk for developing hypotension with ischemia, and therefore may benefit from more extensive monitoring or coronary revascularization. Exercise tolerance can be assessed with formal treadmill testing or with a questionnaire that assesses activities of daily living (Table 18-5).[31]

Reilly et al have evaluated the predictive value of self-reported exercise tolerance for serious perioperative complications, and demonstrated that a poor exercise tolerance (could not walk 4 blocks and climb 2 flights of stairs) independently predicted a complication with an odds ratio of 1.94.[46] The likelihood of a serious adverse event was inversely related to the number of blocks that could be walked. Therefore, there is good evidence to suggest that minimal additional testing is necessary if the patient is able to relate a good exercise tolerance.

Table 18-5. ESTIMATED ENERGY REQUIREMENT FOR VARIOUS ACTIVITIES*

1 MET	Can you take care of yourself? Eat, dress, or use the toilet? Walk indoors around the house? Walk a block or two on level ground at 2–3 mph or 3.2–4.8 km/hr? Do light work around the house like dusting or washing dishes?	4 METs	Walk on level ground at 4 mph or 6.4 km/hr? Run a short distance Do heavy work around the house like scrubbing floors or lifting or moving heavy furniture? Participate in moderate recreational activities like golf, bowling, dancing, doubles tennis, or throwing a baseball or football?
4 METs	Climb a flight of stairs or walk up a hill?	>10 METs	Participate in strenuous sports like swimming, singles tennis, football, basketball, or skiing?

MET = metabolic equivalent.
* Adapted from the Duke Activity Status Index and AHA Exercise Standards.
Reproduced with permission from Eagle K, Brundage B, Chaitman B et al: Guidelines for perioperative cardiovascular evaluation of the noncardiac surgery. A report of the American Heart Association/American College of Cardiology Task Force on Assessment of Diagnostic and Therapeutic Cardiovascular Procedures. Circulation 93:1278, 1996.

APPROACH TO THE PATIENT: FURTHER TESTING

Multiple algorithms have been proposed to determine who requires further testing. As described previously, the risk associated with the proposed surgical procedure influences the decision to perform further diagnostic testing and interventions. These Guidelines must be tempered by recent studies in which perioperative cardiac morbidity was greatly reduced by perioperative β-adrenergic blockade administration.[47,48] With the reduction in perioperative morbidity, it has been suggested that extensive cardiovascular testing is not necessary.[49] However, until these findings can be translated into routine use with similar outcomes, further testing may be warranted.

The algorithm to determine the need for testing proposed by the American College of Cardiology/American Heart Association Task Force is based upon the available evidence and expert opinion and integrates clinical history, surgery-specific risk, and exercise tolerance (Fig. 18-2).[31] First, the clinician must evaluate the urgency of the surgery and the appropriateness of a formal preoperative assessment. Next, determine if the patient has undergone a previous revascularization procedure or coronary evaluation. Those patients with unstable coronary syndromes should be identified, and appropriate treatment instituted. Finally, the decision to undergo further testing depends upon the interaction of the clinical risk factors, surgery-specific risk,

and functional capacity. For patients at intermediate clinical risk, both the exercise tolerance and the extent of the surgery are taken into account with regard to the need for further testing. Importantly, no preoperative cardiovascular testing should be performed if the results will not change perioperative management.

The American College of Physician Guidelines attempt to apply the evidence-based approach.[50] The initial decision point is the assessment of risk using the Detsky modification of the CRI.[21] If patients are Class II or III, they are considered high-risk. If they are Class I, the presence of other clinical factors (according to work by Eagle et al[31] or Vanzetto et al[51]) is used to further stratify risk. Those who exhibit multiple markers for cardiovascular disease according to these risk indices and who are undergoing major vascular surgery are considered appropriate for further diagnostic testing, either by dipyridamole imaging or by dobutamine stress echocardiography. The Guidelines suggest that there is insufficient evidence to recommend diagnostic testing for nonvascular surgery patients.

Pulmonary Disease

Although a great deal of attention has been focused on the cardiovascular system, perioperative pulmonary complications occur frequently and lead to significant morbidity. The presence

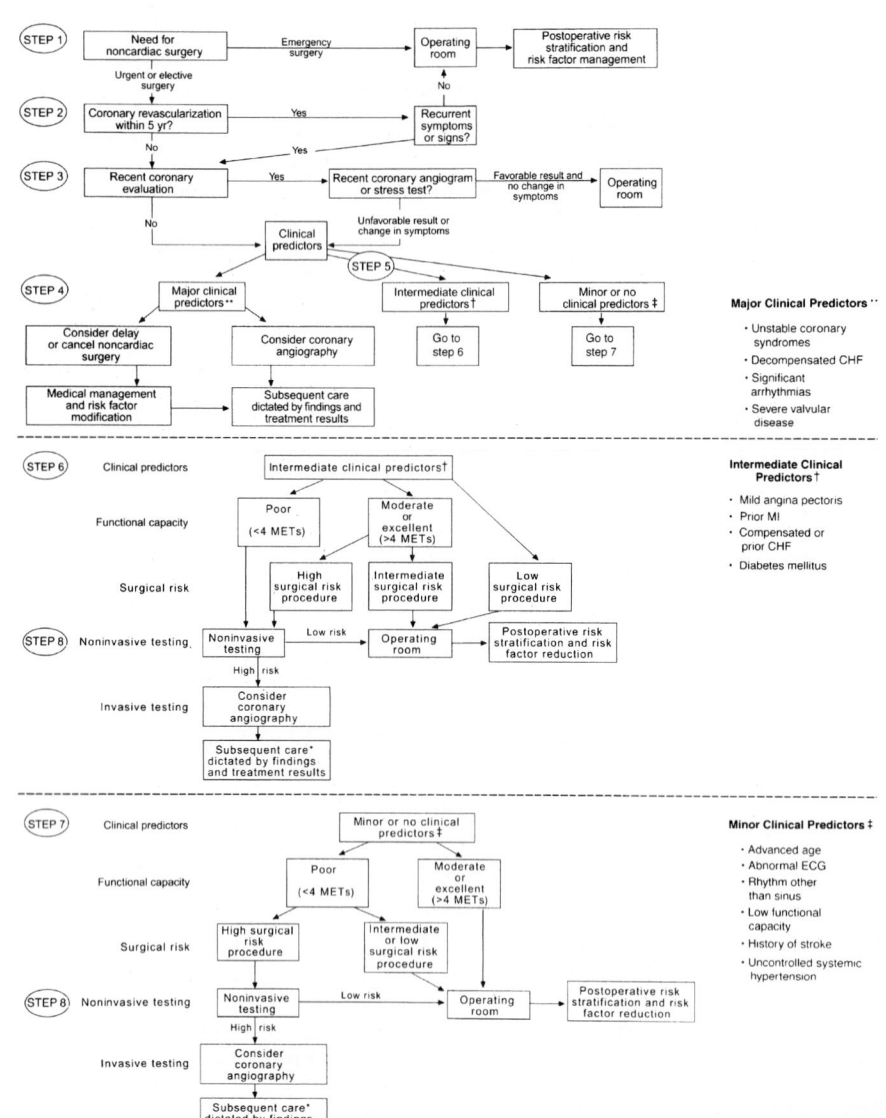

Major Clinical Predictors
- Unstable coronary syndromes
- Decompensated CHF
- Significant arrhythmias
- Severe valvular disease

Intermediate Clinical Predictors†
- Mild angina pectoris
- Prior MI
- Compensated or prior CHF
- Diabetes mellitus

Minor Clinical Predictors‡
- Advanced age
- Abnormal ECG
- Rhythm other than sinus
- Low functional capacity
- History of stroke
- Uncontrolled systemic hypertension

Figure 18-2. The American Heart Association/American College of Cardiology Task Force on Perioperative Evaluation of Cardiac Patients Undergoing Noncardiac Surgery has proposed an algorithm for decisions regarding the need for further evaluation. This represents one of multiple algorithms proposed in the literature. It is based upon expert opinion, and incorporates six steps. First, the clinician must evaluate the urgency of the surgery and the appropriateness of a formal preoperative assessment. Next, he or she must determine whether the patient has had a previous revascularization procedure or coronary evaluation. Those patients with unstable coronary syndromes should be identified, and appropriate treatment should be instituted. The decision to have further testing depends on the interaction of the clinical risk factors, surgery-specific risk, and functional capacity. (Adapted with permission from Eagle K, Brundage B, Chaitman B et al: Guidelines for perioperative cardiovascular evaluation of noncardiac surgery. A report of the American Heart Association/American College of Cardiology Task Force on Assessment of Diagnostic and Therapeutic Cardiovascular Procedures. Circulation 93:1278, 1996.)

Table 18-6. POTENTIAL PATIENT-RELATED RISK FACTORS FOR POSTOPERATIVE PULMONARY COMPLICATIONS

Potential Risk Factor*	Type of Surgery	Unadjusted Relative Risk Associated with Factor
Smoking	Coronary bypass	3.4
	Abdominal	1.4–4.3
ASA class > II	Unselected	1.7
	Thoracic or abdominal	1.5–3.2
Age > 70 yr	Unselected	1.9–2.4
	Thoracic or abdominal	0.9–1.9
Obesity	Unselected	1.3
	Thoracic or abdominal	0.8–1.7
COPD	Unselected	2.7–3.6
	Thoracic or abdominal	4.7

* ASA = American Society of Anesthesiologists; COPD = chronic obstructive pulmonary disease.
Adapted from Smetana GW: Preoperative pulmonary evaluation. N Engl J Med 340(12):942, 1999.

of pulmonary disease places the patient at markedly increased risk of perioperative complications, including such problems as an intraoperative bronchospasm, the need for postoperative ventilation, and the development of atelectasis and pneumonia (Table 18-6). Several strategies have been proposed to reduce this risk and its associated perioperative morbidity (Table 18-7), but all are associated with utilization of both time and resources.

The evaluation of the patients should include a determination of the type of pulmonary disease, severity, and reversibility. A history of reactive airway disease places the patient at risk for developing bronchospasm perioperatively. In patients with asthma, it is important to determine the reversibility of symptoms, i.e., if the disease is currently active or if the patient is in "optimal" medical condition. Frequently, severe asthmatics may wheeze despite intensive medical therapy. Current medications, as well as the recent use of steroids, can be used to determine the optimal preoperative medical regimen. A steroid

Table 18-7. RISK-REDUCTION STRATEGIES

Preoperative

Encourage cessation of cigarette smoking for at least 8 wks
Treat airflow obstruction in patients with chronic obstructive pulmonary disease or asthma
Administer antibiotics and delay surgery if respiratory infection is recent
Begin patient education regarding lung-expansion maneuvers

Intraoperative

Limit duration of surgery to less than 3 hr
Use spinal or epidural anesthesia*
Avoid use of pancuronium
Use laparoscopic procedures when possible
Substitute less ambitious procedure for upper abdominal or thoracic surgery when possible

Postoperative

Use deep-breathing exercises or incentive spirometry
Use continuous positive airway pressure
Use epidural analgesia*
Use intercostal nerve blocks*

* This strategy is recommended, although variable efficacy has been reported in the literature.
Adapted from Smetana GW: Preoperative pulmonary evaluation. N Engl J Med 340(12):942, 1999.

pulse is warranted in many patients with significant asthma undergoing a major surgical procedure.

The evaluation of the patient with chronic obstructive pulmonary disease (COPD) is complex and depends upon the extent of the surgical procedure. In severe COPD, the patient develops a barrel chest, distant breath sounds, and use of accessory muscles of respiration. Determination of any symptoms of wheezing is as important as in the asthmatic. The onset or exacerbation of wheezing symptoms may indicate a new pulmonary process, such as bronchitis or pulmonary infection. Such patients will frequently benefit from delay of surgery and institution of antibiotic therapy. Symptoms of dyspnea and reduced exercise tolerance identify those at increased risk, while the absence of such symptoms with moderate exercise is rarely associated with advanced disease. Dales et al, using a modified pneumoconiosis research unit questionnaire concerning dyspnea, demonstrated an incidence of complications after thoracotomy that was approximately double (53%) in the group who were "unable to walk more than 100 yards on the level without a rest" or "breathless on talking, dressing, or unable to leave the house because of breathlessness" compared with those having no abnormal dyspnea.[52] The use of further noninvasive tests prior to thoracotomy has been reviewed extensively elsewhere[53-55] (see also Chapter 30). Although preoperative testing can identify patients at high risk for complications, implementation of perioperative interventions to reduce morbidity may be the most effective approach.[56]

Patients should also be evaluated for a history of sleep apnea. Sleep apnea suggests intermittent airway obstruction, which is associated with difficulty in controlled ventilation. Additionally, these patients frequently have a difficult airway. Although central sleep apnea may not be as difficult as sleep apnea caused by airway issues, a thorough evaluation is frequently required to identify those patients in whom a fiberoptic intubation is prudent.

Smoking is an important risk factor for both cardiac and pulmonary disease. The value of smoking cessation has been reviewed.[57] Acute cessation of smoking for 24 hours does reduce the quantity of methemoglobin and can improve oxygenation. However, cessation between 24 hours and 6 weeks is associated with an increased incidence of morbidity, presumably secondary to decreased mucociliary clearance.[58] Cessation greater than 6 weeks returns oxygenation and mucociliary clearance to baseline, although not necessarily to normal.

The management of the patient with a recent cough or cold represents a difficult dilemma. The evidence regarding the increased risk of respiratory complications in such patients is controversial. One large retrospective series did not demonstrate an increased risk of complications in patients with uncomplicated upper respiratory infections, whereas several other studies did demonstrate a difference, especially if endotracheal intubation was performed.[59-63] If the procedure is urgent or emergent, surgery should proceed. However, if surgery is elective, the risk of delay for several weeks must be balanced against proceeding with surgery at a potentially increased risk.

Endocrinopathies

There are several endocrine diseases that have implications to the anesthesiologist, many of which are covered in greater detail in Chapter 41. Diabetes is an example of a disease that affects multiple organ systems. Diabetes accelerates the progression of atherosclerosis, which is frequently silent. Although the duration of diabetes affects the development of end-organ damage, the presence of autonomic dysfunction identifies the group at highest risk for silent myocardial ischemia.[35] Autonomic dysfunction is also associated with a greater hemodynamic lability during induction of anesthesia.[64] It is important to determine the current medication regimen and recent changes. One method of determining current control is a history of recent episodes of hypo- or hyperglycemia and the need for acute medical interventions. This information is critical in determining an appropriate glucose management plan perioperatively. Several options for appropriate management are outlined in Table 18-8.

Both thyroid and parathyroid disease have systemic manifestations that can affect the perioperative plan (Table 18-9). Although thyroid function tests are the best method of determining a euthyroid state, clinical history is frequently sufficient. Part of the preoperative evaluation should focus on identifying the presence or absence of signs and symptoms of hyperthyroidism or hypothyroidism. The presence of hypothyroidism is marked by a susceptibility to depressant drugs and the tendency to develop hypothermia, hypoventilation, hyponatremia, and hypoglycemia. In the case of hyperthyroidism, the anesthesiologist should be most concerned with the development of thyroid storm, with its manifestation of a hypermetabolic state. In addition to the systemic manifestations of the disease, a large thyroid mass may distort the airway. If the thyroid causes significant airway obstruction, the patient may have symptoms of wheezing, especially on lying flat. In such patients, a chest x-ray is indicated to evaluate for tracheal narrowing or deviation. If the symptoms are severe, a CT scan of the trachea may provide additional details of the area of narrowing and minimal diameter. Patients with hyperparathyroidism have hypercalcemia, and a preopera-

tive serum calcium level should be obtained. Preoperative preparation of the patient with hypercalcemia includes correction of hypovolemia and dilution of the hypercalcemia.

Mortality for surgical resection of a pheochromocytoma has decreased during the last several decades, presumably due to improved perioperative care.[65] The critical issue is to identify patients with a pheochromocytoma prior to other types of surgical procedure, since surgery in a patient with an undiagnosed pheochromocytoma can still lead to significant morbidity and mortality. The classic findings include intermittent hypertension, headache, sweating, and tachycardia. In patients with other endocrine tumors, a pheochromocytoma should be excluded as a cause of unexplained hypertension as part of a multiple endocrine neoplasia syndrome. The preoperative preparation of the patient with a pheochromocytoma is complex, and a full discussion can be found in Chapter 41.

Adrenal cortical suppression can be seen perioperatively in a significant percentage of surgical patients. There are multiple etiologies including primary tumors of the adrenal cortex, tumors of the pituitary gland, and, most commonly, recent or prolonged steroid use. In patients with prolonged use of glucocorticoids, Cushing's syndrome can develop. The hallmark of this syndrome includes truncal obesity, moon facies, skin striations, easy bruisability, hypertension, and hypovolemia. Preoperative preparation includes correction of fluid and electrolyte

---

Table 18-8. PROTOCOL FOR TIGHT METABOLIC DIABETES MELLITUS CONTROL

Indications

Labor and delivery
Neurosurgical procedures
Brittle diabetes

Rationale

The amounts of insulin and glucose given should be related. Investigators have shown that an infusion of 0.25–0.33 $U \cdot g^{-1}$ of glucose provides good glycemic control.

Regimen

Preoperatively:
  Discontinue subcutaneous insulin
  Obtain baseline blood glucose
  NPO after midnight
  Add 5 U regular insulin to 500 ml of 5% dextrose solution and run at 100 $ml \cdot hr^{-1}$
Intraoperatively and postoperatively:
  The infusion is continued until the patient is taking well PO and preoperative insulin therapy can be reinstituted. Glucose determinations are made every 2–4 hr.

Adjustments

If blood glucose is <100 mg, decrease the infusion to 3 U insulin per 500 ml.
A blood glucose >200 $mg \cdot dl^{-1}$ is treated with an increase in insulin of 8–10 U per 500 ml 5% dextrose solution.
Conditions that increase insulin requirements include patients receiving insulin >1.5 $U \cdot kg^{-1} \cdot day^{-1}$, obesity, steroids, infection, liver disease, and cardiopulmonary bypass.

Indications

Most surgical cases involving diabetic patients, especially when lack of personnel or outpatient surgery is a concern.

Rationale

Principle 5 (see text)

Regimen

Preoperative:
  NPO after midnight
Intraoperatively and postoperatively:
  On the morning of surgery, start iv solution containing 5% dextrose at a maintenance rate; give one half to two thirds of AM dose of insulin as subcutaneous NPH early in the morning and continue glucose infusion intraoperatively and postoperatively; continue blood glucose monitoring every 2–4 hr intraoperatively and postoperatively using sliding scale coverage with regular insulin; reinstitute preoperative insulin regimen when patient is taking PO adequately.

Data from Sieber FE: Diabetes mellitus. In Rogers MC (ed): Current Practice in Anesthesiology. St. Louis, Mosby–Year Book, 1990.

Table 18-9. CLINICAL MANIFESTATIONS OF THYROID AND PARATHYROID DISEASES

	Hyperthyroidism	Hypothyroidism	Hyperparathyroidism
General	Weight loss; heat intolerance; warm, moist skin	Cold intolerance	Weight loss, polydipsia
Cardiovascular	Tachycardia, atrial fibrillation, congestive heart failure	Bradycardia, congestive heart failure, cardiomegaly, pericardial or pleural effusion	Hypertension, heart block
Neurologic	Nervousness, tremor, hyperactive reflexes	Slow mental function, minimal reflexes	Weakness, lethargy, headache, insomnia, apathy, depression
Musculoskeletal	Muscle weakness, bone resorption	Large tongue, amyloidosis	Bone pains, arthritis, pathologic fractures
Gastrointestinal	Diarrhea	Delayed gastric emptying	Anorexia, nausea, vomiting, constipation, epigastric pain
Hematologic	Anemia, thrombocytopenia		
Renal		Impaired free water clearance	Polyuria, hematuria

Adapted from Roizen MF: Anesthesia for the patient with endocrine disease, Part 1. Curr Rev Clin Anesth 6:43, 1987.

abnormalities. In patients on long-term corticosteroids, perioperative steroid supplementation is indicated to cover the stress of anesthesia and surgery. In patients who have had a short course of steroids within the 12 months prior to surgery, the use of supplemental steroids is somewhat controversial, although most clinicians favor their use (Table 18-10).[66]

Other Organ Systems

The anesthesiologist should evaluate for the presence of hepatic or renal disease. For patients with liver disease, the synthetic function may be decreased and the volume of distribution is increased. Both of these factors may influence the effects of anesthetic drugs. Most of the coagulation factors are produced in the liver, and hepatic dysfunction is associated with coagulopathies perioperatively. For patients in whom poor synthetic function is suspected, prothrombin time is the best screening test.

The presence of renal disease has important implications for both the metabolism of drugs and fluid management. As part of the preoperative evaluation, it is important to determine the type of dialysis, the last dialysis, the serum potassium, and hematocrit level. Patients with chronic renal failure, especially those on dialysis, are prone to congestive heart failure, hyperkalemia, and platelet dysfunction. After hemodialysis, patients may actually be hypovolemic, and require administration of fluid prior to induction of general anesthesia. Patients frequently exhibit chronic anemia, which is responsive to erythropoietin treatment.[67] These patients exhibit multiple mechanisms to compensate for the low hematocrit level, which allow them to tolerate a lower hematocrit perioperatively than other patients. However, these compensatory mechanisms must be balanced against the high incidence of coronary artery disease in selected renal patients.

The anesthesiologist must be concerned with the presence of infectious diseases. Part of the questioning should be directed at determining the presence of hepatitis and human immunodeficiency virus (HIV) infection. Although universal precautions should be used in all patients, knowledge of disease state should increase safety.

Multiple hematologic problems can have an impact on the anesthesiologist. Patients who demonstrate anemia (hematocrit $< 10 \mathrm{g} \cdot \mathrm{dl}^{-1}$) preoperatively should be evaluated for the cause, although anemia of chronic disease is frequently the etiology. In patients with gastrointestinal bleeds or systemic diseases such as chronic renal failure, further evaluation is unnecessary. However, a low hematocrit level may signify sickle cell disease or thalassemia. The perioperative management of hemoglobinopathies is reviewed in Chapter 19.

An area of major concern and continued debate is the evaluation for coagulation disorders. A coagulation disorder can affect the anesthesiologist's decision to perform regional anesthesia and direct perioperative utilization of blood products. The patient should be questioned regarding a history of a bleeding diathesis, such as easy bruising, bloody noses, or bleeding from the gums. The use of any medications that can affect platelet function (aspirin, other NSAIDs, anticoagulants) should be determined. Platelet dysfunction is associated with bleeding of the mucocutaneous surfaces, such as petechiae, epistaxis, hematuria. The anesthesiologist should also review any in-hospital medications to determine whether low-molecular-weight heparins have been given.

Table 18-10. PERIOPERATIVE CORTICOSTEROID COVERAGE

For minor surgery	The patient should take 1.5–2 times his or her usual prednisone dosage on the morning of surgery. The following day the patient should take his or her normal prednisone dose (or parenteral equivalent if gut cannot be used). The surgeon and anesthesiologist should be aware that the patient is glucocorticoid-dependent and should be prepared to administer more "steroids" if the surgery becomes prolonged or more extensive.
For moderate surgery	The patient should be given 2 times his or her usual glucocorticoid dosage orally (if possible) on the morning of surgery and/or 25 mg hydrocortisone iv before the operation, then 75 mg hydrocortisone iv during the operation, and 50 mg hydrocortisone iv after the operation; then the dose should be rapidly tapered over 48 hr to the usual dose—if the postoperative course is uncomplicated.
For major surgery	The patient should be given 2 times his or her usual glucocorticoid dosage orally (if possible) on the morning of surgery and/or 50 mg hydrocortisone iv before the operation, then 100 mg hydrocortisone iv during the operation. After the operation, 100 mg iv q 8 hr × 24 hr should be administered and then rapidly tapered (over 48–72 hr) to the patient's usual glucocorticoid dosage—if the postoperative course is uncomplicated.

Adapted from Brussel T, Chernow B: Perioperative management of endocrine problems: Thyroid, adrenal cortex, pituitary. Am Soc Anesthesiol 3:48, 1990.

Musculoskeletal disorders can present physical obstacles to the anesthesiologist, as well as having systemic manifestations. The presence of muscular disorders has been associated with an increased risk for malignant hyperthermia, and should be included in the preoperative history.[68] Osteoarthritis is common in the population, and may lead to a more difficult intubation or difficulty in positioning for regional anesthesia. Rheumatoid arthritis is less common, but may lead to greater problems perioperatively. These patients may have atlanto-occipital instability and are at risk for myocarditis, pleuritis, and restrictive lung disease. It is important in such patients to perform a thorough review of systems.

The extent of the neurologic history frequently depends upon the surgical procedure. Neurologic deficits can be divided into those primarily affecting the central versus peripheral system. A history of stroke identifies patients with increased risk of perioperative stroke. Evaluation of any residual neurologic defects as a baseline status should be performed in order to compare any changes postoperatively. In patients with a recent trauma, signs of increased intracranial pressure should be elicited. The presence of a change in mental status, lethargy, headache, or change in vision should alert the anesthesiologist to increased intracranial pressure and a risk for herniation. The *Glasgow Coma Scale* is frequently used to assess the level of consciousness (Table 18-11). Physical signs may include hypertension, bradycardia, arrhythmias, focal sensory or motor deficits, and slurred speech.

PHYSICAL EXAMINATION

The physical examination can be divided into two parts: a general examination and a specific examination guided by the preoperative history. As anesthesiologists, we are acutely concerned with the airway. Evaluation of the airway involves determining the thyromental distance, the ability to flex and extend the neck, and aperture opening. Recently, the Mallampati classification has been used as a method of assessing the airway (Table 18-12).[69] The Mallampati class has met with only moderate success (low positive predictive value) in identifying patients with a difficult intubation.[70,71] In patients who have sustained a recent trauma, assessment of the stability of the cervical spine is critical. In appropriate patients, the presence of pain on movement should be assessed. Otherwise, radiographic examination may be required.

The cardiovascular examination includes determination of blood pressure and auscultation of the heart. Determination

Table 18-11. GLASGOW COMA SCALE

Response	Score
Eye Opening	
Spontaneous	4
To speech	3
To pain	2
Nil	1
Best Motor Response	
Obeys	6
Localizes	5
Withdraws (flexion)	4
Abnormal flexion	3
Extensor response	2
Nil	1
Verbal Response	
Oriented	5
Confused conversation	4
Inappropriate words	3
Incomprehensible sounds	2
Nil	1

Table 18-12. AIRWAY CLASSIFICATION SYSTEM

Class	Direct Visualization, Patient Seated	Laryngoscopic View
I	Soft palate, fauces, uvula, pillars	Entire glottic
II	Soft palate, fauces, uvula	Posterior commissure
III	Soft palate, uvular base	Tip of epiglottis
IV	Hard palate only	No glottal structures

Modified with permission from Mallampati RS, Gatt SP, Gugino LD et al: A clinical sign to predict difficult tracheal intubation: A prospective study. Can Anaesth Soc J 32:429, 1985.

of blood pressure can vary between examinations and between extremities. Frank *et al* demonstrated a marked difference between left- and right-arm blood pressures in patients with vascular disease.[72] This may have important implications in patients with altered cerebrovascular autoregulation and in determining appropriate blood pressure limits. In addition, blood pressure measurements exhibit a circadian variation in normal individuals. Many demonstrate "white coat hypertension"—that is, their blood pressure is elevated only in an examination setting.[73] The preoperative setting may also be a circumstance that occasions abnormally elevated measurements owing to anxiety. However, Bedford *et al* reported that the admission blood pressure was the best predictor of response to laryngoscopy.[74] Therefore, the initial blood pressure may also provide prognostic information.

The cardiac examination should include determination of the rhythm, the presence of murmurs and the presence of third or fourth heart sounds. If a murmur is present, it is important to determine its relation to the phase of the cardiac cycle and radiation pattern. Frequently, soft murmurs are more significant than loud murmurs. Since a diagnosis of aortic stenosis carries a high risk of perioperative morbidity and mortality, a systolic murmur radiating to the carotids frequently deserves further evaluation, particularly if symptoms are present (angina, congestive heart failure, syncope).[15]

Further examination of the cardiovascular system should be directed by the history. For example, more extensive examination of peripheral pulses for both strength and murmurs may be indicated in patients with vascular disease.

Examination of the lungs should focus on auscultation for sounds of rales suggestive of congestive heart failure and the presence of wheezing indicative of reactive airway disease. In patients who wheeze, the relationship of the wheezing to the phase of the respiratory cycle and position can help differentiate the etiology.

The neurologic examination may be cursory in healthy patients, or extensive in patients with co-existing disease. Testing of strength, reflexes, and sensation may be important in patients if the anesthetic plan or surgical procedure may result in a change in the condition. For example, the presence of a peripheral neuropathy is important information in a patient scheduled for a toe amputation since these patients frequently require minimal anesthesia if the neuropathy is severe. Similarly, patients undergoing carotid endarterectomy may have a baseline neurologic deficit, which affects the postoperative examination.

ROUTINE LABORATORY DATA (Table 18-13)

The Value of Preoperative Testing: Normal Values

In attempting to determine the optimal choice of preoperative tests, it is important to understand the interpretation of the results. Ideally, tests would either confirm or exclude the presence of a disease; however, the vast majority of tests only increase or decrease the probability of disease. In determining reference ranges for diagnostic tests, values that fall outside of the 95% confidence intervals for normal individuals are considered abnormal. Therefore, up to 5% of normal individuals can have "abnormal" test results. In order to determine its clinical relevance, a test must be interpreted within the context of the clinical situation. Performing tests in patients with no risk for having the pathophysiologic process of interest can yield a high number of false-positive results. For example, a low potassium (3.0 mg · dl^{-1}) in an otherwise healthy individual is most likely a normal result. Interpreting this test as abnormal, and initiating treatment, could lead to harm without any benefit.

Table 18-13. RECOMMENDED LABORATORY TESTING SYSTEM UTILIZED AT THE JOHNS HOPKINS HOSPITAL

ELECTROCARDIOGRAM

Age 50 or older
Significant cardiocirculatory disease
Diabetes mellitus (age 40 or older)
Renal disease
Other major metabolic disease
Procedure level 5*

CHEST X-RAY

Asthma or COPD that is debilitating or with change of symptoms or acute episode within past 6 months
Cardiothoracic procedure
Procedure level 4

SERUM CHEMISTRIES

Renal disease
Adrenal or thyroid disorders
Diuretic therapy
Chemotherapy
Procedure level 5

URINALYSIS

Diabetes mellitus
Renal disease
Genitourologic procedure
Recent genitourinary infection
Metabolic disorder involving renal function
Procedure level 5

COMPLETE BLOOD COUNT

Hematologic disorder
Vascular procedure
Chemotherapy
Procedure level 4

COAGULATION STUDIES

Anticoagulation therapy
Vascular procedure
Procedure level 5

PREGNANCY TESTING

Patients for whom pregnancy might complicate the surgery
Patients of uncertain status by history

---

* Five surgical categories are defined, with a higher category denoting increasing invasiveness. Blood loss and estimated risk are also taken into account in this system. Procedure level 4, defined as highly invasive procedures with blood loss >1500 ml and major risk to patients independent of anesthesia, includes major orthopedic surgery, reconstruction of the GI tract, and vascular repair without an ICU stay. Procedure level 5 is similar to level 4, but includes a usual postoperative ICU stay with invasive monitoring.
Reproduced with permission from Pasternak LR: Screening patients: Strategies and studies. In McGoldrick K (ed): Ambulatory Anesthesiology: A Problem-Oriented Approach, p 15. Baltimore, Williams & Wilkins, 1995.

The Value of Preoperative Testing: Bayesian Analysis

The use of noninvasive testing is another area in which the clinical situation significantly affects the interpretation. It is rare for a test result to be pathognomonic for a disease state; that is, no test is 100% sensitivity and specific. For example, exercise or pharmacologic stress testing has sensitivities ranging from 60–90% and specificities ranging from 60–80% for a significant coronary artery stenosis. In order to interpret the results of a noninvasive test, it is important to know the prevalence of disease in the population as well as the sensitivity and specificity of the test. If a test is used in a population with a very low prevalence of disease, a positive result is frequently a false positive. Similarly, a negative result in a population with a very high prevalence of disease may be a false negative. Bayes' theorem suggests a test is most useful in a population with a moderate probability of disease.[75]

Risks and Costs Versus Benefits

The use of medical testing is associated with significant cost, both in real dollars and in lost opportunity and potential harm. Cardiovascular testing in vascular surgery patients alone has been estimated to cost more than $1 billion annually.[76] Routine preoperative testing has been estimated to cost $3 billion annually. In an era of limited resources and capitated care, resources spent on inappropriate testing may lead to a lack of resources for other areas of medical care or potentially a decrease in reimbursement of physicians. From the patient's perspective, each test is associated with time away from other areas, i.e., lost opportunity. Finally, an "abnormal" test that is later determined to be a false result can lead to significant cost and real harm. For example, a positive exercise electrocardiographic stress test in a healthy 40-year-old female may lead to coronary angiography. Coronary angiography is not a benign procedure, and can lead to vascular injuries. Based upon Bayesian analysis, a positive test result in this patient is most likely a false positive, and the test was inappropriately used. Therefore, the woman and her physician would gain no additional information, thousands of dollars in medical costs would accrue, and she would sustain morbidity.

Several studies have evaluated the implications of reduced testing. Kaplan et al studied the preoperative laboratory screening pattern from 2000 patients undergoing elective surgery over a 4-month period.[77] Of the routinely ordered tests, 60% would not have been performed if testing had been done only for defined indications, and only 0.22% of these demonstrated abnormalities that might influence perioperative management. The authors concluded that routine testing contributed little to patient care.

Golub et al retrospectively reviewed the records of 325 patients who had undergone preadmission testing prior to ambulatory surgery.[78] Of these, 272 (84%) had at least one abnormal screening test result, while only 28 surgeries were delayed or canceled. The authors estimated that only three patients potentially benefited from preadmission testing, including a new diagnosis of diabetes in one and nonspecific ECG changes in two, one of which had known ischemic heart disease.

In a study published in 1991, Narr and colleagues at the Mayo Clinic demonstrated minimal benefits from routine testing and proposed that routine laboratory screening tests were not required in healthy patients.[79] In a follow-up study published in 1997, a cohort of patients who had no preoperative testing during 1994 was reviewed and found to include no deaths or major perioperative morbidity.[80] They concluded that current anesthetic and medical practices rapidly identify indications for laboratory evaluation when necessary and therefore routine testing was not indicated in this healthy cohort.

Even if testing better defines a disease state, the risks of any

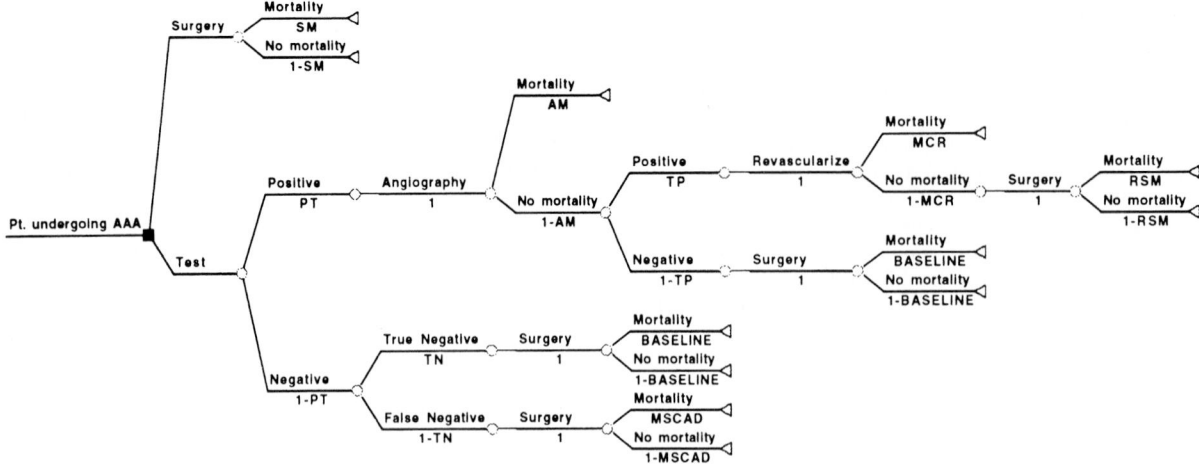

Figure 18-3. A decision algorithm evaluating the decision between vascular surgery alone or coronary artery revascularization before vascular surgery. There are currently no randomized trials to address the optimal strategy. By outlining the multiple decision points at which a patient can sustain mortality by choosing to undergo coronary revascularization first, the optimal strategy for preoperative evaluation can be demonstrated. Specifically, variation in mortalities at each decision point can change the optimal strategy. (Reproduced with permission from Fleisher LA, Skolnick ED, Holroyd KJ, Lehmann HP: Coronary artery revascularization before abdominal aortic aneurysm surgery: A decision analytic approach. Anesth Analg 79:661, 1994.)

intervention based upon the results may outweigh the benefit. Cardiovascular testing is a classic example (Fig. 18-3). If a noninvasive test is positive, coronary angiography may be performed. A positive angiogram may then result in coronary artery bypass grafting prior to the planned noncardiac surgery. Although cardiovascular morbidity and mortality may be reduced in patients with significant coronary artery disease who have undergone coronary revascularization, the morbidity associated with both the testing and revascularization procedure may be greater than any potential benefit. Fleisher *et al* has suggested the use of decision analysis as a method of quantifying these risks and benefits.[4]

Complete Blood Count and Hemoglobin Concentration

The use of a preoperative hemoglobin has been suggested as the only test necessary in many patients prior to elective surgery; however, even this minimal standard has been questioned. Baron *et al* reviewed the records of 1863 pediatric patients scheduled for elective outpatient procedures.[81] In only 1.1% of patients was the hematocrit abnormal, and in none of these patients was the procedure canceled or anesthetic plan modified. However, a baseline hematocrit is still indicated in any procedure with a risk of blood loss.

The standard regarding the lowest acceptable perioperative hematocrit and indication for a preoperative transfusion has changed during the past decade. Traditionally, the minimum hematocrit was considered to be 10 g · dl^{-1}. However, concern over blood-borne infections has resulted in a general acceptance of lower levels. The current recommendations of the National Blood Resource Education Committee is that a hemoglobin of 7 g · dl^{-1} is acceptable in patients without systemic disease.[82] In patients with systemic disease, signs of inadequate systemic oxygen delivery (tachycardia, tachypnea) are an indication for transfusion. In a retrospective study, a hematocrit of <29% postoperatively in vascular surgery patients was associated with a significantly increased incidence of myocardial ischemia and infarction.[83] Therefore, in patients with active coronary artery disease, a higher hematocrit may be indicated.

Electrolytes

In the past, patients routinely received a chemistry panel prior to surgery. These panels can include as few as 7 tests and may include more than 36 tests. Because of technology issues, it may be cheaper to obtain a standard battery than to determine one particular test. However, testing rarely leads to any change in perioperative management.

There are numerous guidelines regarding the need for preoperative electrolytes. The only consensus is the lack of routine testing in asymptomatic adults, although a creatinine and glucose has been recommended in older patients. In patients with systemic diseases or on medications that affect the kidneys, a BUN and creatinine are indicated.

Coagulation Studies

Coagulation disorders can have significant impact on the surgical procedure and perioperative management. However, abnormal laboratory studies in the absence of clinical abnormalities will rarely lead to perioperative problems. Patients with known inherited coagulopathies, such as hemophilia or von Willebrand's disease, require preoperative preparation of the patient. It is important to identify such disorders from prior history or bleeding problems. A prothrombin, partial thromboplastin time analysis is indicated in the presence of previous bleeding disorders such as following injuries, after tooth extraction or surgical procedures, and in patients with known or suspected liver disease, malabsorption or malnutrition, and on certain medications such as antibiotics and chemotherapeutic agents.

Bleeding time has been advocated as a means of determining the presence of a qualitative platelet defect. It can be performed in patients with low platelets (<100,000/mm^3), patients with medical conditions that affect platelets (*e.g.,* uremia), or patients on anti-platelet agents. Although this information may be important from the surgeon's perspective, it rarely affects anesthetic care unless a regional technique is planned. However, several recent reviews have questioned the value of this test in clinical practice.[84,85] The test is extremely operator-dependent, and may be invalid in inexperienced hands. It would therefore be best to determine the limits for the individual performing the test. Since this is rare in clinical practice, some authors have suggested that the test should be abandoned in favor of clinical history. In the absence of a clinical bleeding diathesis, complications are extremely rare. If such a history exists, it may be prudent to avoid regional anesthesia.

Urinary Analysis

A routine preoperative urinary analysis (UA) is rarely indicated. O'Connor and Drasner reviewed the records of 486 elective surgeries in children, of which only two demonstrated an abnormal UA result.[86] One of these results was contaminated, and the cancellation of surgery resulted in a complication (incarcerated inguinal hernia) requiring emergency surgery. The other abnormal test was a probable asymptomatic bacteriuria. The authors suggest that a routine UA adds little to the preoperative evaluation of a healthy child, and should be omitted. Lawrence *et al* determined the cost-effectiveness of preoperative urinalysis in non-prosthetic knee procedures and estimated the costs at $1,500,000 per wound infection prevented.[87] Therefore, preoperative UA is rarely performed currently.

Pregnancy Testing

Routine pregnancy testing in women of child-bearing potential is a subject of considerable debate. The rationale is that specific agents may be avoided, or surgery may be delayed. Information regarding the last menstrual period can help define the potential, but does not eliminate the possibility. Roizen and Cohn suggest that pregnancy testing should be limited to females who believe they are pregnant or cannot tell if they are pregnant.[88] However, a number of studies have evaluated the validity of history as a means of assessing pregnancy status in adolescents with conflicting results.[89–91] Current practice varies dramatically among centers and anesthesiologists, and may be a function of the population served with regard to the need to routinely test those women with a negative pregnancy history.[92]

Chest Radiographs

A preoperative chest x-ray can identify abnormalities that may lead to either delay or cancellation of the planned surgical procedure or modification of perioperative care. For example, identification of pneumonia, pulmonary edema, pulmonary nodules, or a mediastinal mass could all lead to modification of care. However, routine testing in the population without risk factors can lead to more harm than benefit. Roizen has demonstrated substantial harm from additional procedures based upon shadows performed solely as a routine preoperative chest x-ray.[88]

The American College of Physicians suggests that a chest x-ray is indicated in the presence of active chest disease or an intrathoracic procedure, but not solely on the basis of advanced age alone.[93] Other guidelines suggest that a preoperative chest x-ray is reasonable in patients over the age of 60 years. In a meta-analysis, Archer *et al* reviewed the published reports from 1966 to 1992 in the English, French, and Spanish literature.[94] Twenty-one reports were identified with sufficient data to evaluate the use of testing. On average, abnormalities were reported in 10% of routine preoperative chest x-rays, of which only 1.3% were unexpected. These findings result in modification in management in only 0.1% of patients, with unknown influence on outcome. The authors estimated that each finding that influenced management would cost $23,000, concluding that routine chest x-rays without a clinical indication were not justified. Therefore, a preoperative chest x-ray is indicated in patients with a history or clinical evidence of active pulmonary disease, and *may* be indicated routinely only in patients with advanced age.

Cardiovascular Tests

Electrocardiogram

The preoperative 12-lead electrocardiogram can provide important information on the status of the patient's myocardium and coronary circulation. Evidence of active ischemia can be detected and usually requires changes in at least two leads. The sensitivity of abnormalities on the 12-lead ECG as a marker for specific types of heart disease depends on the prevalence of the disease in that patient population. Abnormal Q waves in high-risk patients are highly suggestive of a past myocardial infarction. Patients with Q-wave infarctions are known to be at increased risk of a perioperative cardiac event, and have a worse long-term prognosis.

It has been estimated that approximately 30% of infarctions are silent and only detected on routine ECG, with the highest incidence in patients with diabetes or hypertension. According to the Framingham study, long-term prognosis is not altered by the lack of symptoms.[33] The absence of Q waves on the 12-lead ECG does not exclude the occurrence of a Q-wave myocardial infarction in the past. It has been shown that 5–27.1% of Q waves disappear over a 10-year period.[95] Those patients in whom the electrocardiogram reverts to normal have improved survival compared with those with persistent abnormalities, with or without Q waves. The presence of Q waves on a preoperative ECG in a high-risk patient, regardless of symptoms, should alert the anesthesiologist to the increased perioperative risk and the possibility of active ischemia in that patient.

It has not been established that the information obtained from the preoperative 12-lead electrocardiogram affects clinical care. In a retrospective study conducted in the early 1970s to determine how the preoperative ECG was used, no operations were delayed based upon preoperative ECG, even in the presence of new Q-waves.[96] Carliner *et al* found that preoperative 12-lead ST-T wave abnormalities occurred more frequently in patients who subsequently had more complicated postoperative courses.[97] Although changes on the preoperative electrocardiogram may not result in delay of surgical procedures, the increased vigilance by the anesthesiologist may influence intraoperative monitoring and treatment. However, in a retrospective review of adults undergoing ambulatory surgery, 42.7% had electrocardiographic abnormalities.[98] The preoperative electrocardiogram was not predictive of perioperative complications, which occurred in only 1.6% of the patients. The authors concluded that a preoperative electrocardiogram rarely helps perioperative management in this group. In contrast, Landesberg *et al* reported a significantly increased risk of a perioperative cardiac event in patients with left ventricular hypertrophy or ST segment changes on the preoperative ECG.[99] Current recommendations vary, but include the need for a preoperative electrocardiogram in the presence of systemic cardiovascular disease (*e.g.*, hypertension, peripheral vascular disease), age over 40 in males and over 50 in females.

Noninvasive Cardiovascular Testing

The exercise electrocardiogram has been the traditional method of evaluating individuals for the presence of coronary artery disease. It represents the least invasive and most cost-effective method of detecting ischemia, with a reasonable sensitivity (68–81%) and specificity (66–77%) for identifying coronary artery disease.[100] The goal of the test is to provoke ischemia by exercise, thus causing an increase in myocardial oxygen demand relative to myocardial oxygen supply. Electrocardiographic signs of myocardial ischemia and clinical signs of left ventricular dysfunction are considered positive. A decrease in blood pressure in response to exercise has been associated with global ventricular dysfunction in humans. Syncope during the test also signifies decreased cardiac output. Either sign signifies poor dynamic function, and is much more ominous than ST segment depression alone. A positive exercise electrocardiographic stress test can alert the anesthesiologist that the patient is at risk for ischemia at a wide range of heart rates, with the greatest risk in those who develop ischemia at low workloads during the test. However, as outlined above, the ability to exercise suggests that no further testing is necessary, and therefore exercise electrocardiography is rarely indicated.

A significant number of high risk patients are either unable to exercise or have contraindications to exercise. In surgical patients, this phenomenon is most evident in those patients with claudication or an abdominal aortic aneurysm undergoing vascular surgery, both of which have a high rate of perioperative cardiac morbidity. Therefore, pharmacologic stress testing and ambulatory electrocardiography have become popular, particularly as preoperative tests in vascular surgery patients.

Pharmacologic stress for the detection of CAD can be divided into two categories: (1) those that result in coronary artery vasodilation, such as dipyridamole, and (2) those that increase myocardial oxygen demand, such as dobutamine. The coronary artery vasodilators work by producing differential flows in normal coronary arteries when compared to those with a stenosis. Several authors have shown that the presence of a redistribution defect on dipyridamole thallium imaging in patients undergoing peripheral vascular surgery is predictive of postoperative cardiac events (Fig. 18-4).[101–104] This work has been extended to include patients undergoing nonvascular surgery.[45] In order to increase the predictive value of the test, several strategies have been suggested. Lung uptake, left ventricular cavity dilation, and redistribution defect size have all been shown to be predictive of subsequent morbidity. Fleisher et al demonstrated that the delineation of "low" and "high" risk thallium scans markedly improved the tests predictive value.[45] They demonstrated that only patients with "high" risk thallium scans were

at increased risk for perioperative morbidity and long-term mortality.

The ambulatory ECG (AECG or Holter) provides a means of continuously monitoring the electrocardiogram for significant ST segment changes during the preoperative period. Raby demonstrated that the presence of silent ischemia is a strong predictor of outcome, while its absence was associated with a good outcome in 99% of patients.[105] Other investigators have demonstrated the value of silent AECG monitoring, although the negative predictive values have not been as high as originally reported.[45] Fleisher et al demonstrated a similar predictive value of dipyridamole thallium imaging and AECG monitoring; however, the quantity of silent ischemia could not be used to identify those patients at greatest risk who might benefit from further testing and coronary revascularization.[45]

Stress echocardiography has received attention as a preoperative test. The appearance of new or worsened regional wall motion abnormalities is considered a positive test. These represent areas at risk for myocardial ischemia. The advantage of this test is that it is a dynamic assessment of ventricular function. Dobutamine echocardiography has also been studied and found to have among the best positive and negative predictive.[106] Poldermans et al demonstrated that the group at greatest risk comprised those who demonstrated regional wall motion abnormalities at low heart rates.[107,108]

Several groups have published meta-analyses of preoperative diagnostic tests. Mantha et al demonstrated good predictive values of AECG monitoring, radionuclide angiography, dipyridamole thallium imaging, and dobutamine stress echocardiography.[109] Shaw et al also demonstrated good predictive values of dipyridamole thallium imaging and dobutamine stress echocardiography.[110] Both studies demonstrated the superior predictive value of dobutamine stress echocardiography; however, there was significant overlap of the confidence intervals with other tests. However, the most important determinant with respect to the choice of preoperative testing is the expertise at the local institution. The decision to perform further invasive testing and management should be based on the principles outlined above, *i.e.*, the ability of the intervention to affect both short- and long-term health.

Assessment of Ventricular and Valvular Function

There are multiple methods to assess ejection fraction and valvular function. The least invasive method is echocardiography. Echocardiography can be used to assess static function or can be combined with exercise or pharmacologic stress to assess dynamic function. It is also very effective in evaluating valvular function and diagnosing valve area. Radionuclide angiography has also been used as a both a static and dynamic measure of ejection fraction.

A preoperative resting echocardiography can determine the presence of ventricular dysfunction, regional wall motion abnormalities, ventricular wall thickness, and valvular function. Pulse wave Doppler can be used to obtain the velocity time integral. Ejection fraction can then be calculated by determining the cross-sectional area of the ventricle. Several investigators have examined the predictive value of ejection fraction using either echocardiographic or radionuclide measurements. Kazmers and colleagues found that a poor ejection fraction (<35%) was the best predictor of perioperative outcome after vascular surgery.[111] In contrast, Franco and colleagues found no difference in perioperative morbidity based upon ejection fraction.[112] Similarly, McEnroe and colleagues were unable to demonstrate a difference.[17] Importantly, Halm et al demonstrated that the ejection fraction did not add additional prognostic information over standard clinical history.[113]

Echocardiography can provide important information regarding valvular function. This information may have important implications for both cardiac and noncardiac surgery, and is discussed more fully later in the book. In particular, aortic

Figure 18-4. A dipyridamole-thallium SPECT image demonstrating a reversible defect. The top image demonstrates defects consistent with areas of low perfusion or ischemia, which fills in on subsequent imaging (*bottom*). (See upper left portion of image.)

stenosis has been associated with a worse prognosis in noncardiac surgical procedures, and knowledge of valve lesions can modify management chances and treatment of hemodynamic dysfunction.[15]

Coronary Angiography

Coronary angiography represents the gold standard for defining coronary anatomy. Information regarding ventricular and valvular function can also be assessed. Finally, hemodynamic indices can be determined. For example, ventricular pressure and gradients across valves can be calculated.

In patients undergoing coronary artery bypass grafting, the information is routinely available. As described above, certain lesions, *i.e.,* left main disease, may be associated with greater perioperative risk. Certain disease types may also increase risk. Diffuse atherosclerosis in small vessels, as seen in diabetics, may lead to incomplete revascularization, and a risk for developing post-bypass ischemia.

In patients undergoing noncardiac surgery, the decision to perform coronary angiography may be the result of a positive preoperative test or may be the first test in a patient with a very high probability of significant disease. The test is then used by the cardiologist to determine whether coronary artery revascularization is an option.

Unlike the exercise or pharmacologic stress tests described above, coronary angiography provides the clinician with anatomic, not functional, information. Although a critical stenosis delineates an area at risk for developing myocardial ischemia, the functional response to that ischemia cannot be determined by angiography alone. Although coronary artery disease is undoubtedly the substrate for a perioperative MI, the critical stenosis may not be the underlying pathophysiology. In the ambulatory population, many infarctions are the result of acute thrombosis of a noncritical stenosis. Therefore, the value of routine angiography prior to noncardiac surgery depends on the ability to correct the lesions that cause morbidity.

Pulmonary Function Tests

Pulmonary function tests can be generally divided into two categories, spirometry and an arterial blood gas. Spirometry can provide information on forced vital capacity (FVC), forced expiratory volume in 1 sec (FEV_1), ratio of FEV_1/FVC, and average forced expiratory flow from 25 to 75%. Although each of these measures has a sound physiologic basis, their practical assessment can vary greatly among healthy persons. Objective measures defining high risk for pulmonary resection have been proposed.[53] For nonpulmonary surgery, they rarely provide additional information beyond that obtained from history. The one possible indication is the use of pulmonary function testing with bronchodilator therapy to assess responsiveness in a patient who is wheezing.

With the advent of the pulse oximeter, the use of preoperative arterial blood gas sampling has become less important. It may still be indicated, since determining the baseline CO_2 is useful in managing postoperative ventilation settings and resting hypercapnia is associated with increased perioperative risk. However, the physical act of obtaining an arterial blood gas can lead to hyperventilation and change the Pa_{CO_2}. One method of assessing the probability of CO_2 retention is evaluation of the serum bicarbonate. A normal serum bicarbonate will virtually exclude the diagnosis of CO_2 retention. If the serum bicarbonate is elevated, then an arterial blood gas either preoperatively on immediately prior to induction may be indicated.

Another indication for an arterial blood gas has been determination of oxygen concentration. With the advent and availability of pulse oximetry in the preoperative screening clinic, this is rarely an indication.

SUMMARY

The preoperative evaluation of the surgical patient continues to be an important component of the anesthesiologist's role. A thorough history and physical examination can be used to identify those medical conditions that might affect perioperative management and direct further laboratory testing. In the current era of capitated care and the desire to reduce inappropriate utilization of medical technology, the anesthesiologist can have a significant impact on health resource utilization by performing appropriate laboratory tests. By combining data from the history, physical examination, exercise tolerance, and the stress of the surgical procedure, inappropriate testing can be reduced; but more importantly, appropriate screening tests will be performed.

REFERENCES

1. Keats AS: The ASA classification of physical status: A recapitulation. Anesthesiology 49:233, 1978
2. Egbert LD, Battit GE, Turndorf H, Beecher HK: The value of the preoperative visit by an anesthetist: A study of doctor–patient rapport. JAMA 185:553, 1963
3. Mason JJ, Owens DK, Harris RA *et al:* The role of coronary angiography and coronary revascularization before noncardiac surgery. JAMA 273:1919, 1995
4. Fleisher LA, Skolnick ED, Holroyd KJ, Lehmann HP: Coronary artery revascularization before abdominal aortic aneurysm surgery: A decision analytic approach. Anesth Analg 79:661, 1994
5. Glance LG: Selective preoperative cardiac screening improves five-year survival in patients undergoing major vascular surgery: A cost-effectiveness analysis. J Cardiothorac Vasc Anesth 13:265, 1999
6. Lutner RE, Roizen MF, Stocking CB *et al:* The automated interview versus the personal interview. Do patient responses to preoperative health questions differ? Anesthesiology 75:394, 1991
7. Roizen MF, Coalson D, Hayward RS *et al:* Can patients use an automated questionnaire to define their current health status? Med Care 30:MS74, 1992
8. Fischer SP: Development and effectiveness of an anesthesia preoperative evaluation clinic in a teaching hospital. Anesthesiology 85:196, 1996
9. Fischer SP: Cost-effective preoperative evaluation and testing. Chest 115:96S, 1999
10. Starsnic MA, Guarnieri DM, Norris MC: Efficacy and financial benefit of an anesthesiologist-directed university preadmission evaluation center. J Clin Anesth 9:299, 1997
11. Allison JG, Bromley HR: Unnecessary preoperative investigations: Evaluation and cost analysis. Am Surg 62:686, 1996
12. Vogt AW, Henson LC: Unindicated preoperative testing: ASA physical status and financial implications. J Clin Anesth 9:437, 1997
13. Mancuso CA: Impact of new guidelines on physicians' ordering of preoperative tests. J Gen Intern Med 14:166, 1999
14. Schein OD, Katz J, Bass EB *et al:* Preoperative medical testing for routine cataract surgery: Time to abandon the routine. N Engl J Med 342:168, 2000
15. Goldman L, Caldera DL, Nussbaum SR *et al:* Multifactorial index of cardiac risk in noncardiac surgical procedures. N Engl J Med 297:845, 1977
16. Zeldin RA: Assessing cardiac risk in patients who undergo noncardiac surgical procedures. Can J Surg 27:402, 1984
17. McEnroe CS, O'Donnell TF, Yeager A *et al:* Comparison of ejection fraction and Goldman risk factor analysis to dipyridamole thallium-201 imaging studies in the evaluation of cardiac morbidity after aortic aneurysm surgery. J Vasc Surg 11:497, 1990
18. Fleisher L, Rosenbaum S, Nelson A, Barash P: The predictive value of preoperative silent ischemia for postoperative ischemic cardiac events in vascular and nonvascular surgical patients. Am Heart J 122:980, 1991
19. Calvin JE, Kieser TM, Walley VM *et al:* Cardiac mortality and morbidity after vascular surgery. Can J Surg 29:93, 1986
20. Mangano DT, Browner WS, Hollenberg M *et al:* Association of perioperative myocardial ischemia with cardiac morbidity and mortality in men undergoing noncardiac surgery. N Engl J Med 323:1781, 1990
21. Detsky A, Abrams H, McLaughlin J *et al:* Predicting cardiac compli-

cations in patients undergoing non-cardiac surgery. J Gen Intern Med 1:211, 1986

22. Shah K, Kleinman B, Rao T et al: Reduction in mortality from cardiac causes in Goldman class IV patients. J Cardiothorac Anesth 2:789, 1988

23. Lee TH, Marcantonio ER, Mangione CM et al: Derivation and prospective validation of a simple index for prediction of cardiac risk of major noncardiac surgery. Circulation 100:1043, 1999

24. Shah KB, Kleinman BS, Rao T et al: Angina and other risk factors in patients with cardiac diseases undergoing noncardiac operations. Anesth Analg 70:240, 1990

25. Tuman KJ, McCarthy RJ, March RJ et al: Effects of epidural anesthesia and analgesia on coagulation and outcome after major vascular surgery. Anesth Analg 73:696, 1991

26. Tarhan S, Moffitt EA, Taylor WF, Giuliani ER: Myocardial infarction after general anesthesia. JAMA 220:1451, 1972

27. Rao TL, Jacobs KH, El-Etr AA: Reinfarction following anesthesia in patients with myocardial infarction. Anesthesiology 59:499, 1983

28. Shah KB, Kleinman BS, Sami H et al: Reevaluation of perioperative myocardial infarction in patients with prior myocardial infarction undergoing noncardiac operations. Anesth Analg 71:231, 1990

29. Califf RM, Topol EJ, George BS et al: One-year outcome after therapy with tissue plasminogen activator: Report from the Thrombolysis and Angioplasty in Myocardial Infarction trial. Am Heart J 119:777, 1990

30. Rouleau JL, Talajic M, Sussex B et al: Myocardial infarction patients in the 1990s—their risk factors, stratification and survival in Canada: The Canadian Assessment of Myocardial Infarction (CAMI) study. J Am Coll Cardiol 27:1119, 1996

31. Eagle K, Brundage B, Chaitman B et al: Guidelines for perioperative cardiovascular evaluation of the noncardiac surgery. A report of the American Heart Association/American College of Cardiology Task Force on Assessment of Diagnostic and Therapeutic Cardiovascular Procedures. Circulation 93:1278, 1996

32. Hertzer NR, Bevan EG, Young JR et al: Coronary artery disease in peripheral vascular patients: A classification of 1000 coronary angiograms and results of surgical management. Ann Surg 199:223, 1984

33. Kannel W, Abbott R: Incidence and prognosis of unrecognized myocardial infarction: An update on the Framingham study. N Engl J Med 311:1144, 1984

34. Eagle KA, Coley CM, Newell JB et al: Combining clinical and thallium data optimizes preoperative assessment of cardiac risk before major vascular surgery. Ann Int Med 110:859, 1989

35. Acharya DU, Shekhar YC, Aggarwal A, Anand IS: Lack of pain during myocardial infarction in diabetics: Is autonomic dysfunction responsible? Am J Cardiol 68:793, 1991

36. Hollenberg M, Mangano DT, Browner WS et al: Predictors of postoperative myocardial ischemia in patients undergoing noncardiac surgery. The Study of Perioperative Ischemia Research. JAMA 268:205, 1992

37. Pringle SD, MacFarlane PW, McKillop JH et al: Pathophysiologic assessment of left ventricular hypertrophy and strain in asymptomatic patients with essential hypertension. J Am Coll Cardiol 13:1377, 1989

38. Sixth report of the Joint National Committee on Prevention, Detection, Evaluation, and Treatment of High Blood Pressure. Arch Intern Med 157:2413, 1997

39. Hansson L, Zanchetti A, Carruthers SG et al: Effects of intensive blood-pressure lowering and low-dose aspirin in patients with hypertension: Principal results of the Hypertension Optimal Treatment (HOT) randomised trial. Lancet 351:1755, 1998

40. Goldman L, Caldera DL: Risks of general anesthesia and elective operation in the hypertensive patient. Anesthesiology 50:285, 1979

41. Warner MA, Shields SE, Chute CG: Major morbidity and mortality within 1 month of ambulatory surgery and anesthesia. JAMA 270:1437, 1993

42. Krupski WC, Layug EL, Reilly LM et al: Comparison of cardiac morbidity between aortic and infrainguinal operations. Study of Perioperative Ischemia (SPI) Research Group. J Vasc Surg 15:354, 1992

43. Eagle KA, Rihal CS, Mickel MC et al: Cardiac risk of noncardiac surgery: Influence of coronary disease and type of surgery in 3368 operations. CASS Investigators and University of Michigan Heart Care Program. Circulation 96:1882, 1997

44. McPhail N, Calvin JE, Shariatmadar A et al: The use of preoperative exercise testing to predict cardiac complications after arterial reconstruction. J Vasc Surg 7:60, 1988

45. Fleisher LA, Rosenbaum SH, Nelson AH et al: Preoperative dipyridamole thallium imaging and Holter monitoring as a predictor of perioperative cardiac events and long tem outcome. Anesthesiology 83:906, 1995

46. Reilly DF, McNeely MJ, Doerner D et al: Self-reported exercise tolerance and the risk of serious perioperative complications. Arch Intern Med 159:2185, 1999

47. Poldermans D, Boersma E, Bax JJ et al: The effect of bisoprolol on perioperative mortality and myocardial infarction in high-risk patients undergoing vascular surgery. N Engl J Med 341:1789, 1999

48. Mangano DT, Layug EL, Wallace A, Tateo I: Effect of atenolol on mortality and cardiovascular morbidity after noncardiac surgery. Multicenter Study of Perioperative Ischemia Research Group. N Engl J Med 335:1713, 1996

49. Lee TH: Reducing cardiac risk in noncardiac surgery. N Engl J Med 341:1838, 1999

50. Physicians ACo: Guidelines for assessing and managing the perioperative risk from coronary artery disease associated with major noncardiac surgery. Ann Intern Med 127:313, 1997

51. Vanzetto G, Machecourt J, Blendea D et al: Additive value of thallium single-photon emission computed tomography myocardial imaging for prediction of perioperative events in clinically selected high cardiac risk patients having abdominal aortic surgery. Am J Cardiol 77:143, 1996

52. Dales RE, Dionne G, Leech JA et al: Preoperative prediction of pulmonary complications following thoracic surgery. Chest 104:155, 1993

53. Zibrak JD, O'Donnell CR: Indications for preoperative pulmonary function testing. Clin Chest Med 14:227, 1993

54. Reilly JJ Jr, Mentzer SJ, Sugarbaker DJ: Preoperative assessment of patients undergoing pulmonary resection. Chest 103:342S, 1993

55. Smetana GW: Preoperative pulmonary evaluation. N Engl J Med 340:937, 1999

56. Dunn WF, Scanlon PD: Preoperative pulmonary function testing for patients with lung cancer. Mayo Clin Proc 68:371, 1993

57. Egan TD, Wong KC: Perioperative smoking cessation and anesthesia: A review. J Clin Anesth 4:63, 1992

58. Warner MA, Offord KP, Warner ME et al: Role of preoperative cessation of smoking and other factors in postoperative pulmonary complications: A blinded prospective study of coronary artery bypass patients. Mayo Clin Proc 64:609, 1989

59. Rolf N, Cote CJ: Frequency and severity of desaturation events during general anesthesia in children with and without upper respiratory infections. J Clin Anesth 4:200, 1992

60. Cohen MM, Cameron CB: Should you cancel the operation when a child has an upper respiratory tract infection? Anesth Analg 72:282, 1991

61. Tait AR, Knight PR: Intraoperative respiratory complications in patients with upper respiratory tract infections. Can J Anaesth 34:300, 1987

62. Martin LD: Anesthetic implications of an upper respiratory infection in children. Pediatr Clin North Am 41:121, 1994

63. Levy L, Pandit UA, Randel GI et al: Upper respiratory tract infections and general anaesthesia in children. Peri-operative complications and oxygen saturation. Anaesthesia 47:678, 1992

64. Burgos L, Ebert T, Asiddao C, Turner L: Increased intraoperative cardiovascular morbidity in diabetics with autonomic neuropathy. Anesthesiology 70:591, 1989

65. Roizen MF, Hunt TK, Beaupre PN et al: The effect of alpha-adrenergic blockade on cardiac performance and tissue oxygen delivery during excision of pheochromocytoma. Surgery 94:941, 1983

66. Salem M, Tainsh RE Jr, Bromberg J et al: Perioperative glucocorticoid coverage. A reassessment 42 years after emergence of a problem. Ann Surg 219:416, 1994

67. Paganini EP, Miller T: Erythropoietin therapy in renal failure. Adv Intern Med 38:223, 1993

68. Wedel DJ: Malignant hyperthermia and neuromuscular disease. Neuromusc Disord 2:157, 1992

69. Mallampati RS, Gatt SP, Gugino LD et al: A clinical sign to predict difficult tracheal intubation: A prospective study. Can Anaesth Soc 32:429, 1985

70. Frerk CM: Predicting difficult intubation. Anaesthesia 46:1005, 1991

71. Savva D: Prediction of difficult tracheal intubation. Br J Anaesth 73:149, 1994

72. Frank SM, Norris EJ, Christopherson R, Beattie C: Right- and left-arm blood pressure discrepancies in vascular surgery patients. Anesthesiology 75:457, 1991

73. Lavie CJ, Schmieder RE, Messerli FH: Ambulatory blood pressure monitoring: Practical considerations. Am Heart J 116:1146, 1988

74. Bedford R, Feinstein B: Hospital admission blood pressure, a predictor for hypertension following endotracheal intubation. Anesth Analg 59:367, 1980

75. Shuman P: Bayes' theorem: A review. Cardiol Clin 2:319, 1984

76. Fleisher LA, Beattie C: Current practice in the preoperative evaluation of patients undergoing major vascular surgery: A survey of cardiovascular anesthesiologists. J Cardiothorac Vasc Anesth 7:650, 1993

77. Kaplan EB, Sheiner LB, Boeckmann AJ, et al: The usefulness of preoperative laboratory screening. JAMA 253:3576, 1985

78. Golub R, Cantu R, Sorrento JJ, Stein HD: Efficacy of preadmission testing in ambulatory surgical patients. Am J Surg 163:565(discussion 571), 1992

79. Narr BJ, Hansen TR, Warner MA: Preoperative laboratory screening in healthy Mayo patients: Cost-effective elimination of tests and unchanged outcomes. Mayo Clin Proc 66:155, 1991

80. Narr BJ, Warner ME, Schroeder DR, Warner MA: Outcomes of patients with no laboratory assessment before anesthesia and a surgical procedure. Mayo Clin Proc 72:505, 1997

81. Baron MJ, Gunter J, White P: Is the pediatric preoperative hematocrit determination necessary? South Med J 85:1187, 1992

82. Perioperative red cell transfusion. Consensus Conference. JAMA 260:2700, 1988

83. Nelson AH, Fleisher LA, Rosenbaum SH: Relationship between postoperative anemia and cardiac morbidity in high-risk vascular patients in the intensive care unit. Crit Care Med 21:860, 1993

84. Bick RL: Platelet function defects: A clinical review. Semin Thromb Hemost 18:167, 1992

85. Lind SE: The bleeding time does not predict surgical bleeding [see comments]. Blood 77:2547, 1991

86. O'Connor ME, Drasner K: Preoperative laboratory testing of children undergoing elective surgery. Anesth Analg 70:176, 1990

87. Lawrence VA, Gafni A, Gross M: The unproven utility of the preoperative urinalysis: Economic evaluation. J Clin Epidemiol 42:1185, 1989

88. Roizen MF, Cohn S: Preoperative evaluation for elective surgery: What laboratory tests are needed? In Advances in Anesthesia, p 25. St Louis, Mosby–Year Book, 1993

89. Wheeler M, Cote CJ: Preoperative pregnancy testing in a tertiary care children's hospital: A medico-legal conundrum. J Clin Anesth 11:56, 1999

90. Malviya S, D'Errico C, Reynolds P et al: Should pregnancy testing be routine in adolescent patients prior to surgery? Anesth Analg 83:854, 1996

91. Azzam FJ, Padda GS, DeBoard JW et al: Preoperative pregnancy testing in adolescents. Anesth Analg 82:4, 1996

92. Kempen PM: Preoperative pregnancy testing: A survey of current practice. J Clin Anesth 9:546, 1997

93. Sox HCJ: Common Diagnostic Tests: Use and Interpretation. Philadelphia, American College of Physicians, 1990

94. Archer C, Levy AR, McGregor M: Value of routine preoperative chest x-rays: A meta-analysis. Can J Anaesth 40:1022, 1993

95. Kalbfleisch JM, Shudaksharappa KS, Conrad LL, Sarkar NK: Disappearance of the Q deflection following myocardial infarction. Am Heart J 76:193, 1968

96. Rabkin SW, Horne JM: Preoperative electrocardiography: Effect of new abnormalities on clinical decisions. Can Med Assoc J 128:146, 1983

97. Carliner NH, Fischer ML, Plotnick GD et al: The preoperative electrocardiogram as an indicator of risk in major noncardiac surgery. Can J Cardiol 2:134, 1986

98. Gold BS, Young ML, Kinman JL et al: The utility of preoperative electrocardiograms in the ambulatory surgical patient. Arch Intern Med 152:301, 1992

99. Landesberg G, Einav S, Christopherson R et al: Perioperative ischemia and cardiac complications in major vascular surgery: Importance of the preoperative twelve-lead electrocardiogram. J Vasc Surg 26:570, 1997

100. Detrano R, Gianrossi R, Mulvihill D et al: Exercise-induced ST segment depression in the diagnosis of multivessel coronary disease: A meta analysis. J Am Coll Cardiol 14:1501, 1989

101. Boucher CA, Brewster DC, Darling RC et al: Determination of cardiac risk by dipyridamole-thallium imaging before peripheral vascular surgery. N Engl J Med 312:389, 1985

102. Eagle KA, Singer DE, Brewster DC et al: Dipyridamole-thallium scanning in patients undergoing vascular surgery. Optimizing preoperative evaluation of cardiac risk. JAMA 257:2185, 1987

103. Cutler BS, Leppo JA: Dipyridamole–thallium-201 scintigraphy to detect coronary artery disease before abdominal aortic surgery. J Vasc Surg 5:91, 1987

104. Lette J, Waters D, Cerino M et al: Preoperative coronary artery disease risk stratification based on dipyridamole imaging and a simple three-step, three-segment model for patients undergoing noncardiac vascular surgery or major general surgery. Am J Cardiol 69:1553, 1992

105. Raby KE, Goldman L, Creager MA et al: Correlation between perioperative ischemia and major cardiac events after peripheral vascular surgery. N Engl J Med 321:1296, 1989

106. Poldermans D, Fioretti PM, Forster T et al: Dobutamine stress echocardiography for assessment of perioperative cardiac risk in patients undergoing major vascular surgery. Circulation 87:1506, 1993

107. Poldermans D, Arnese M, Fioretti PM et al: Improved cardiac risk stratification in major vascular surgery with dobutamine-atropine stress echocardiography. J Am Coll Cardiol 26:648, 1995

108. Poldermans D, Arnese M, Fioretti PM et al: Sustained prognostic value of dobutamine stress echocardiography for late cardiac events after major noncardiac vascular surgery. Circulation 95:53, 1997

109. Mantha S, Roizen MF, Barnard J et al: Relative effectiveness of four preoperative tests for predicting adverse cardiac outcomes after vascular surgery: A meta-analysis. Anesth Analg 79:422, 1994

110. Shaw LJ, Eagle KA, Gersh BJ, Miller DD: Meta-analysis of intravenous dipyridamole–thallium-201 imaging (1985 to 1994) and dobutamine echocardiography (1991 to 1994) for risk stratification before vascular surgery. J Am Coll Cardiol 27:787, 1996

111. Kazmers A, Moneta GL, Cerqueira MD et al: The role of preoperative radionuclide ventriculography in defining outcome after revascularization of the extremity. Surg Gynecol Obstet 171:481, 1990

112. Franco CD, Goldsmith J, Veith FJ et al: Resting gated pool ejection fraction: A poor predictor of perioperative myocardial infarction in patients undergoing vascular surgery for infrainguinal bypass grafting. J Vasc Surg 10:656, 1989

113. Halm EA, Browner WS, Tubau JF et al: Echocardiography for assessing cardiac risk in patients having noncardiac surgery. Study of Perioperative Ischemia Research Group. Ann Intern Med 125:433, 1996

Clinical Anesthesia (4/e), edited by
Paul G. Barash, Bruce F. Cullen, and
Robert K. Stoelting. Lippincott Williams &
Wilkins, Philadelphia, © 2001.

CHAPTER 19

ANESTHESIA FOR PATIENTS WITH RARE AND COEXISTING DISEASES

STEPHEN F. DIERDORF

Knowledge of the pathophysiologic characteristics of coexisting diseases and an understanding of the implications of concomitant drug therapy are essential for the optimal management of anesthesia for an individual patient. In many instances, the nature of the coexisting disease has more impact on the management of anesthesia than does the actual surgical procedure. A variety of rare disorders may influence the selection and conduct of anesthesia (Table 19-1). Economic constraints have increased the likelihood that patients with these diseases will present for outpatient surgery with little time for complete preoperative evaluation. Recent advances in molecular genetics and cellular biology have clarified the understanding of the pathophysiology of many uncommon diseases. Consequently, anesthesiologists must periodically update their diagnostic skills and clinical knowledge to recognize when additional evaluation or treatment may be required.

MUSCULOSKELETAL DISEASES

Muscular Dystrophy

Research in the past ten years has dramatically increased the understanding of the defects in the cellular architecture of muscle in patients with muscular dystrophy. The key discovery was that patients with Duchenne's muscular dystrophy lack the muscle protein dystrophin, an important component of the cytoskeleton of muscle cells.[1] Since the discovery of dystrophin, a number of other proteins have been identified that also contribute to the stability of muscle cell membranes. These proteins include merosin, dystroglycans, sarcoglycans, utrophin, syntrophin, and dystrobrevin.[2,3] It is now known that dystrophin and the dystrophin-associated proteins form a complex structural network extending from the extracellular matrix to the submembrane complex that maintains the integrity of the muscle cell membrane (Fig. 19-1). The absence or deficiency of one of these proteins will result in a weakened muscle membrane that is susceptible to damage (Table 19-2).

The muscular dystrophies are characterized by a progressive but variable rate of loss of skeletal muscle function. Although many of the initial signs and symptoms of muscular dystrophy are a result of skeletal muscle dysfunction, many studies have demonstrated that cardiac and smooth muscle are also affected. Consequently, the evaluation of cardiac function is important in patients with muscular dystrophy. In some types of muscular dystrophy, cardiac muscle dysfunction may be more significant than skeletal muscle dysfunction.

Duchenne's Muscular Dystrophy

Duchenne's muscular dystrophy, the most severe of the muscular dystrophies, is produced by a genetic abnormality resulting in a lack of production of dystrophin. Duchenne's dystrophy is characterized by painless degeneration and atrophy of skeletal muscle. This disorder is a sex-linked recessive trait that is clinically evident in boys. Progressive skeletal muscle weakness produces symptoms between the ages of 2 and 5 years. Progressive limitation of movement usually confines the patient to a wheelchair by 12 years of age. Axial skeletal muscle imbalance produces kyphoscoliosis, which often requires operative instrumen-

tation for stabilization. Death occurs when patients are between 15 and 25 years old and is usually secondary to congestive heart failure or pneumonia. Serum creatine kinase levels reflect the progression of the disease. Early in the patient's life, the creatine kinase level is elevated. Later, as significant amounts of skeletal muscle have degenerated, the creatine kinase level decreases.

It is very evident that smooth muscle and cardiac muscle are also affected in patients with muscular dystrophy. Smooth muscle involvement results in intestinal tract hypomotility, delayed gastric emptying, and acute gastroparesis.[4,5] Most patients with Duchenne's muscular dystrophy have evidence of myocardial degeneration. The degeneration of myocardial tissue is reflected in the progressive loss of R-wave amplitude in the lateral precordial electrocardiogram (ECG) leads with aging.[6,7] Progressive loss of myocardial tissue can result in reduced myocardial contractility, dilated cardiomyopathy, ventricular dysrhythmias, mitral regurgitation (papillary muscle dysfunction), and right ventricular outflow obstruction.[8,9]

Degeneration of respiratory muscles can be measured by pulmonary function testing, which reveals a restrictive disease pattern. Diminished muscle strength produces an ineffective cough, resulting in retention of pulmonary secretions, pneumonia, and death.

Although the genetic defect for Duchenne's muscular dystrophy is known, successful genetic therapy remains elusive. Other therapeutic modalities include myoblast transplantation and administration of muscle protein precursors. Most therapy is directed at prevention of musculoskeletal deformities. Treatment of selected patients with ACE inhibitors and/or β-adrenergic blockers may retard the development of congestive heart failure.[9]

Becker's Muscular Dystrophy

Becker's muscular dystrophy is similar to Duchenne's muscular dystrophy, but the onset is later in life and slower in progression. Patients afflicted with Becker's muscular dystrophy often remain ambulatory until 60 years of age. Patients with Becker's muscular dystrophy have abnormal dystrophin or reduced levels of normal dystrophin, which explains the milder clinical course when compared to Duchenne's muscular dystrophy. Recent research has established that cardiac abnormalities such as cardiomyopathy and ventricular dysrhythmias are common in patients with Becker's muscular dystrophy.[10-12]

Emery-Dreifuss Muscular Dystrophy

Emery-Dreifuss muscular dystrophy is an X-linked recessive disease that is characterized by contractures of the elbows, ankles, and spine as well as humeropectoral weakness. The skeletal muscle manifestations are usually mild, whereas cardiac conduction defects can be fatal.[13,14] Emery-Dreifuss muscular dystrophy is caused by a deficiency of emerin, a protein found in the nucleus of skeletal muscle cells and near the intercalated disks of cardiac muscle.[15] This distribution of emerin may explain why cardiac muscle is more severely affected than skeletal muscle.

Limb Girdle Muscular Dystrophy

Patients with limb girdle dystrophy exhibit weakness of the muscles of the shoulder and pelvic girdles. Although most cases

Table 19-1. COEXISTING DISEASES THAT INFLUENCE ANESTHESIA MANAGEMENT

MUSCULOSKELETAL

Muscular dystrophy
Myotonic dystrophy
Familial periodic paralysis
Myasthenia gravis
Lambert-Eaton (myasthenic) syndrome
Guillain-Barré syndrome

CENTRAL NERVOUS SYSTEM

Multiple sclerosis
Epilepsy
Parkinson's disease
Huntington's disease
Alzheimer's disease
Amyotrophic lateral sclerosis
Creutzfeldt-Jakob disease

ANEMIAS

Nutritional deficiency
Hemolytic
Hemoglobinopathies
Thalassemias

COLLAGEN VASCULAR

Rheumatoid arthritis
Systemic lupus erythematosus
Scleroderma
Polymyositis

SKIN

Epidermolysis bullosa
Pemphigus

of limb girdle dystrophy are inherited as an autosomal recessive trait, some forms are inherited as autosomal dominant traits. Limb girdle dystrophy is caused by an abnormality in the sarcoglycan proteins.[16] Cardiac abnormalities such as dilated cardiomyopathy and atrioventricular conduction disturbances have been reported in patients with limb girdle muscular dystrophy.[17,18]

Facioscapulohumeral Muscular Dystrophy

Facioscapulohumeral muscular dystrophy is inherited as an autosomal dominant trait. Patients with this abnormality have diverse clinical manifestations. In addition to weakness of the facial, scapulohumeral, anterior tibial, and pelvic girdle muscles, retinal vascular disease, deafness, and neurologic abnor-

malities have also been described.[13] Of patients with facioscapulohumeral muscular dystrophy, 5% have cardiac conduction defects and cardiac dysrhythmias.[19]

Oculopharyngeal Muscular Dystrophy

Oculopharyngeal muscular dystrophy typically presents in late adulthood. The primary clinical manifestations are ptosis and dysphagia. Weakness of the muscles of the head, neck, and arms may also develop. Although dysphagia has been attributed to weakness of pharyngeal skeletal muscle, esophageal smooth muscle dysfunction occurs in most patients.[20]

Congenital Muscular Dystrophy

Congenital muscular dystrophy is characterized by early onset (*in utero* or infancy), muscle weakness, and mental retardation. These types of muscular dystrophy are caused by genetic defects that affect production of muscle proteins of the surface of the sarcolemma. Included in this group of muscular dystrophy are merosin-deficient muscular dystrophy, Fukuyama muscular dystrophy, Walker-Warburg syndrome, Ullrich's disease, and muscle-eye-brain (MEB) disease.[21]

Management of Anesthesia

Most of the significant complications from anesthesia in patients with muscular dystrophy are secondary to the effects of anesthetic drugs on myocardial and skeletal muscle. Myocardial dysfunction makes these patients more sensitive to the myocardial depressant effects of potent inhaled anesthetics. There are numerous reports of cardiac arrest having occurred during induction of anesthesia.[22] These arrests are associated with rhabdomyolysis and hyperkalemia and have occurred with volatile anesthetics alone or in combination with succinylcholine. In view of the weakened muscle structure of patients with muscular dystrophy, succinylcholine may produce muscle membrane damage and release of intracellular contents. Consequently, succinylcholine is best avoided in patients with muscular dystrophy. The effect of volatile anesthetics on abnormal skeletal muscle is not known. However, it could be speculated that volatile anesthetics, by releasing calcium from the sarcoplasmic reticulum, could produce muscle membrane damage and rhabdomyolysis. Sevoflurane is a less potent stimulus for release of calcium from the sarcoplasmic reticulum and may be the preferred volatile agent for patients with Duchenne's muscular dystrophy.[23] Some patients with muscular dystrophy may be susceptible to malignant hyperthermia, but this is unpredictable.[24–26]

Nondepolarizing muscle relaxants can be used, although patients with Duchenne's muscular dystrophy may require a

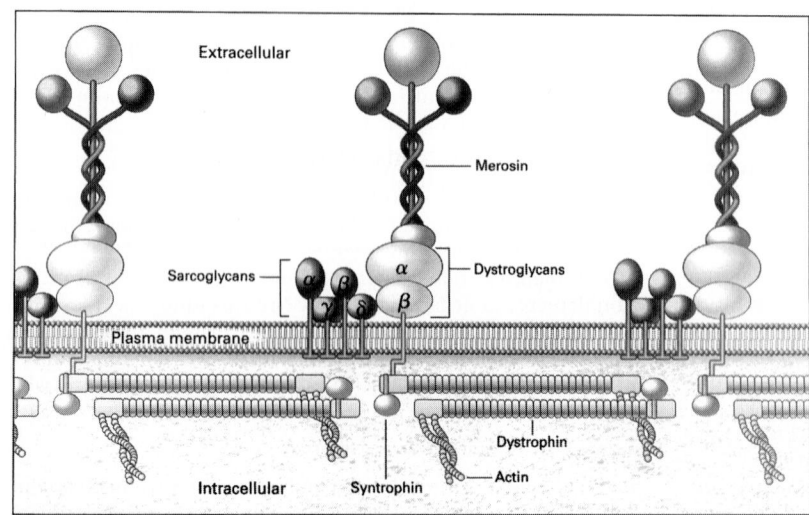

Figure 19-1. Muscle cell cytoskeleton. (Reprinted with permission from Duggan DJ, Gorospe JR, Fanin M *et al:* Mutations in the sarcoglycan genes in patients with myopathy. N Engl J Med 336:618, 1997.)

Table 19-2. TYPES OF MUSCULAR DYSTROPHY

Duchenne
Becker
Emery-Dreifuss
Limb-girdle
Oculopharyngeal
Facioscapulohumeral
Congenital muscular dystrophy

longer recovery time.[27] The response to mivacurium, however, is normal.[28] The response of patients with other forms of muscular dystrophy is variable.[29] Consequently, close monitoring of neuromuscular function is indicated. Degeneration of gastrointestinal smooth muscle with hypomotility of the intestinal tract and delayed gastric emptying in conjunction with impaired swallowing mechanisms may increase the risk of perioperative aspiration of gastric contents.

After surgery, the patient with Duchenne's muscular dystrophy must be closely monitored for evidence of pulmonary dysfunction and retention of pulmonary secretions. Vigorous respiratory therapy and ventilatory support may be required.

The Myotonias

The myotonias comprise a group of diseases having very different genetic and molecular origins but exhibiting a common clinical feature. Myotonia, the delayed relaxation of skeletal muscle after voluntary contraction, is the basic clinical feature of these diseases.[30] Typically, a myotonic contracture is not relieved by regional anesthesia, nondepolarizing muscle relaxants, or deep anesthesia. Relaxation may be induced by infiltration of the muscle with local anesthetic.

Recent advances in molecular biology and genetics have clarified much of the confusion about the myotonic disorders. Myotonic diseases are caused by genetic abnormalities that produce defects in sodium or chloride channels or proteins which alter ion channel function in muscle cells (Table 19-3).[31] Since myotonia is caused by abnormal ion channel activity, administration of drugs that depress sodium influx into the cell and delay return of membrane excitability, such as quinine, tocainide, or mexilitene, may relax myotonic contracture.[32] Examples of myotonic disorders are myotonic dystrophy, hyperkalemic periodic paralysis, paramyotonia congenita, congenital myotonia, and proximal myotonic myopathy.

Myotonic Dystrophy (Steinert's Disease)

Myotonic dystrophy is the most common form of the myotonias. Myotonic dystrophy is an autosomally dominant inherited disorder (incidence 1 in 8000) with symptoms occurring during the second and third decades of life. In addition to myotonia, other clinical features associated with myotonic dystrophy include muscle degeneration, cataracts, premature balding, diabetes mellitus, thyroid dysfunction, adrenal insufficiency, gonadal atrophy, and cardiac conduction abnormalities. Myotonic dystrophy is the result of an enlarged trinucleotide repeat of cytosine, thymine, and guanine (CTG) on chromosome 19. This defect produces a decrease in protein kinase which results in degeneration of the sarcoplasmic reticulum.[33]

Cardiac abnormalities have been well described in patients with myotonic dystrophy. Although myocardial contractile tissue degenerates and may reduce ventricular function, as evidenced by left ventricular diastolic dysfunction, cardiac failure is rare.[34] Prominent cardiac features of myotonic dystrophy include conduction delays (atrioventricular block), atrial flutter and fibrillation, and ventricular dysrhythmias.[35,36] First-degree atrioventricular block may actually precede the onset of clinical symptoms of myotonic dystrophy. Sudden death may be a result of the abrupt onset of third-degree atrioventricular block. Although mitral valve prolapse occurs in 20% of patients with myotonic dystrophy, the prolapse is secondary to geometric changes of the heart caused by thoracic deformation. Systemic complications from mitral valve prolapse usually do not occur in patients with myotonic dystrophy.[37]

Pulmonary function studies demonstrate restrictive lung disease, mild arterial hypoxemia, and diminished ventilatory responses to hypoxia and hypercapnia.[38] Brain stem respiratory control mechanisms may also be defective.[39] Weakness of respiratory muscles diminishes the effectiveness of cough and may lead to pneumonia. Myotonia of respiratory muscles can produce intense dyspnea, requiring therapy with procainamide.[40] Alteration of smooth muscle function produces gastric atony and intestinal hypomotility. Pharyngeal muscle weakness in conjunction with delayed gastric emptying increases the risk for aspiration of gastric contents.[41]

Pregnancy often produces an exacerbation of myotonic dystrophy. It has been suggested that increased progesterone levels of pregnancy contribute to increased symptoms. Congestive heart failure is also more likely to occur during pregnancy.[42] Cesarean section must often be performed because of uterine smooth muscle dysfunction.[43]

Therapy for patients with myotonic dystrophy has been mostly palliative and includes respiratory muscle training and the administration of androgenic steroids.[44,45] Patients with cardiac dysrhythmias may require pacemaker implantation, cardioversion, or catheter ablation of ventricular reentry pathways. Embryo preimplantation diagnosis of myotonic dystrophy may also be effective in reducing the number of infants born with myotonic dystrophy.[46]

Other Myotonias

Congenital myotonic dystrophy is an early-onset form of myotonic dystrophy. Some patients have very mild symptoms such as a swallowing dysfunction as a result of the inability to relax the oropharyngeal muscles. This condition often improves with age and does not affect a patient's life expectancy. Some infants, however, have an early-onset form characterized by hypotonia, respiratory distress, and aspiration pneumonia. Mechanical ventilation is often required and mortality during infancy is high.[47]

Paramyotonia is the rarest of the myotonic diseases. Myotonic contracture develops when the patient is exposed to cold, and warming relaxes the contracted muscle. Hypokalemia has also been reported to produce skeletal muscle weakness in patients with paramyotonia.[48]

Proximal myotonic myopathy was described in 1994. Patients with proximal myotonic myopathy have many of the clinical features that patients with myotonic dystrophy have. Patients with proximal myotonic myopathy, however, do not have the same chromosomal abnormalities as patients with myotonic dystrophy. Muscle pain is a prominent feature of proximal myotonic dystrophy.[49]

Table 19-3. CLASSIFICATION OF MYOTONIC DYSTROPHY

Protein kinase deficiency
    Myotonic dystrophy
Sodium channel diseases
    Hyperkalemic periodic paralysis
    Paramyotonia congenita
Chloride channel diseases
    Myotonia congenita (Thomsen)
    Recessive myotonia
Unknown defect
    Proximal myotonic dystrophy

Management of Anesthesia

Considerations for anesthesia in patients with myotonic dystrophy include the presence of cardiac and respiratory muscle disease and the abnormal responses to drugs used during anesthesia.[50] Succinylcholine produces an exaggerated contracture and its use should be avoided (Fig. 19-2). Succinylcholine-induced myotonia can make ventilation of the lungs and tracheal intubation difficult or impossible.[51] Most patients with myotonic dystrophy develop a chronic myopathy. Consequently, the response to nondepolarizing muscle relaxants may be unpredictable. It would be prudent to use shorter-acting muscle relaxants such as mivacurium or atracurium and monitor the response to the muscle relaxant.[52,53]

Mivacurium is an especially attractive choice, as reversal of neuromuscular blockade is usually not necessary. Neostigmine has been reported to induce myotonia.[54] The response to a peripheral nerve stimulator must be carefully interpreted because muscle stimulation may produce myotonia, which can be misinterpreted as sustained tetanus when significant neuromuscular blockade still exists (personal observation). Patients with myotonic dystrophy are quite sensitive to the respiratory depressant effects of opioids, barbiturates, benzodiazepines, and inhaled anesthetics. Severe respiratory depression has also been reported after the administration of epidural morphine for postoperative analgesia.[55] Increasing respiratory depression parallels the progression of the disease and may develop as a result of depression of central respiratory centers as well as a peripheral muscle effect.[56] In a study of more than 200 patients with myotonic dystrophy undergoing surgery, respiratory complications were more likely to occur in the early postoperative period after upper abdominal surgery or in those patients in whom preoperative upper extremity weakness was clinically evident.[57] Although no specific anesthetic technique has been shown to be preferable, reported responses to propofol have been varied. One report described an uneventful intraoperative course and rapid emergence, while other reports described exaggerated respiratory depression, hypotension, and generalized myotonia.[58–60] Since smooth muscle function is affected by myotonia, gastrointestinal motility is decreased and gastric emptying is delayed. Consequently, precautions should be used to prevent pulmonary aspiration.[61]

Because patients with myotonic dystrophy have cardiac conduction abnormalities and mitral valve prolapse, cardiac dysrhythmias may occur. The preoperative ECG should be carefully examined for signs of atrioventricular conduction delay. Use

Table 19-4. CLINICAL FEATURES OF FAMILIAL PERIODIC PARALYSIS

HYPOKALEMIC
Calcium channel defect
Potassium level <3 mEq $\cdot$ l^{-1} during symptoms
Precipitating factors
    High-glucose meals
    Strenuous exercise
    Glucose–insulin infusions
    Stress
    Hypothermia
Other Features
    Cardiac dysrhythmias
    Signs of hypokalemia on ECG

HYPERKALEMIC
Sodium channel defect
Potassium level normal or >5.5 mEq $\cdot$ l^{-1} during symptoms
Precipitating factors
    Rest after exercise
    Potassium infusions
    Metabolic acidosis
    Hypothermia
Other Features
    Skeletal muscle weakness may be localized to tongue and eyelids

of anesthetics known to delay conduction in the His-Purkinje system, specifically halothane, should be avoided.

Skeletal muscle weakness and myotonia are exacerbated during pregnancy. Labor is typically prolonged, and there is an increased incidence of postpartum hemorrhage from placenta accreta.[62] Although regional anesthesia may not prevent myotonia, spinal and epidural anesthesia have been successfully used for both pregnant and nonpregnant patients with myotonic dystrophy.[63,64] If general anesthesia is administered, it should be anticipated that these patients will be sensitive to respiratory depressant drugs and will have a decreased ability to clear pulmonary secretions.[65]

Familial Periodic Paralysis

Traditionally, there were three recognized forms of familial periodic paralysis: hyperkalemic, normokalemic, and hypokalemic. In recent years, however, the normokalemic form was found to be a variant of the hyperkalemic type and is no longer recognized as a separate disease. Although the hyperkalemic and hypokalemic forms of familial periodic paralysis are both autosomally dominant inherited diseases that share the common clinical feature of intermittent, acute episodes of skeletal muscle weakness, these disorders have very different cellular mechanisms (Table 19-4).

Hyperkalemic Periodic Paralysis. Patients with hyperkalemic periodic paralysis have evidence of myotonia as well as episodes of muscle weakness. Hyperkalemic periodic paralysis is caused by a sodium channel mutation.[66] Episodes of weakness lasting several hours can occur during rest after exercise, infusions of potassium, metabolic acidosis, or hypothermia. The weakness may be so severe as to produce respiratory distress. The hyperkalemia is often transient, occurring only at the onset of weakness. Consequently, potassium levels measured during the episode of weakness may be normal or even decreased. Treatment consists of a low-potassium diet and the administration of thiazide diuretics.

Hypokalemic Periodic Paralysis. Hypokalemic periodic paralysis is caused by a calcium channel mutation.[67] Paralysis may be produced by ingestion of carbohydrate loads, strenuous exercise, and infusion of glucose and insulin. Paralysis is usually incomplete, affecting the limbs and trunk, but sparing the dia-

Succinylcholine (mg/kg)

0.1   0.2

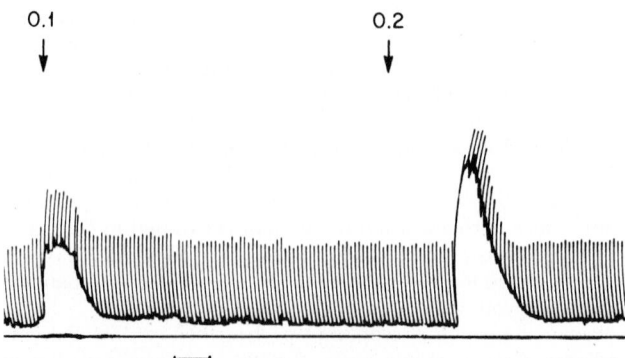

Figure 19-2. Administration of low doses of succinylcholine to a patient with myotonic dystrophy produces an exaggerated contraction of skeletal muscle. (Reprinted with permission from Mitchell MM, Ali HH, Savarese JJ: Myotonia and neuromuscular blocking drugs. Anesthesiology 49:44, 1978.)

phragm. Respiratory distress may, however, be caused by vocal cord paralysis.[68] The low potassium levels present during acute episodes often produce cardiac dysrhythmias and may require treatment with calcium channel blockers.[69] Treatment consists of potassium infusion and the administration of acetazolamide, a carbonic anhydrase inhibitor.[70] Permanent skeletal muscle weakness occurs in most patients with hypokalemic periodic paralysis as they age.[71]

Management of Anesthesia

The primary goal of perioperative management of patients with both forms of periodic paralysis is maintenance of normal potassium levels and avoidance of events that may precipitate weakness.[72,73] If possible, any electrolyte abnormality should be corrected before surgery. During periods of weakness these patients may be sensitive to nondepolarizing muscle relaxants. Doses of these drugs should be reduced and the response monitored with a peripheral nerve stimulator.[74] Short-acting muscle relaxants are preferred to longer-acting neuromuscular blockers. Succinylcholine is best avoided as its administration may alter serum potassium levels. Metabolic changes (acidosis or alkalosis) or medications (glucose and insulin, diuretics, β-adrenergic agonists) that reduce potassium levels may initiate an episode of paralysis. Since changes in potassium levels may actually precede the onset of clinical muscle weakness, serial measurement of potassium levels during prolonged surgical procedures and in the early postoperative period should be considered.[75,76] The ECG should be continuously monitored for evidence of potassium-related dysrhythmias. Other recommendations include the avoidance of large carbohydrate loads and hypothermia. It should be remembered that any cause of severe potassium depletion, such as renal tubular acidosis or chronic diarrhea, can produce muscle weakness in patients with the hypokalemic form of periodic paralysis.[77,78]

After surgery, adequate skeletal muscle strength must be ascertained before mechanical ventilation of the lungs is discontinued. Regional anesthesia may also be considered.[79,80] Malignant hyperthermia has been associated with both forms of familial periodic paralysis.[81,82]

Myasthenia Gravis

Myasthenia gravis is a disease of the neuromuscular junction caused by a decrease in the population of acetylcholine receptors. The incidence is 1 in 20,000, and women are affected twice as frequently as men. Myasthenia gravis is an autoimmune disease because 70–90% of myasthenic patients have circulating anti-acetylcholine receptor antibodies.[83] Anti-acetylcholine receptor antibodies damage the postsynaptic membrane *via* a complement-mediated reaction. This results in increased degradation and decreased formation of acetylcholine receptors.[84] There is an apparent breakdown in tolerance of T and B cells to the acetylcholine receptor. This lack of tolerance activates T-helper cells, which produce antibodies specific for acetylcholine receptors. This process most likely originates in the thymus, as 90% of patients have histologic abnormalities of the thymus gland, including thymoma, hyperplasia, or atrophy.[85] Thymomas are more likely to occur in patients older than 30 years, whereas thymic hyperplasia occurs in younger patients. Although the evidence implicating anti-acetylcholine receptor antibodies is compelling, there is a poor correlation between levels of circulating antibodies and the clinical severity of the disease. Many myasthenic patients also have detectable anti-nuclear, anti-thyroid, and anti-muscle antibodies. Consequently, other autoimmune diseases such as systemic lupus erythematosus, rheumatoid arthritis, pernicious anemia, and thyroiditis are associated with myasthenia gravis.

The clinical hallmark of myasthenia gravis is skeletal muscle weakness. Typically, the weakness is exacerbated by repetitive muscle use and there are periods of exacerbation alternating with remission. Any skeletal muscle may be affected, although there is a predilection for muscles innervated by cranial nerves, which leads to dysphagia, dysarthria, and pulmonary aspiration. Initial symptoms include diplopia, difficulty speaking and swallowing, or limb muscle weakness.[86] Although respiratory insufficiency is not a common presenting symptom, its presentation can be quite dramatic.[87] Consequently, undiagnosed myasthenia gravis should be included in the differential diagnosis of respiratory failure.

There are several types of myasthenia gravis. The classification is based on skeletal muscle groups affected as well as the age of onset (Table 19-5). Types of myasthenia include generalized, ocular, bulbar, and shoulder-girdle. A staging system (Osserman) based on the severity of the disease is commonly used.[88] Type I presents with ocular signs and symptoms only; Type IIA comprises generalized mild muscle weakness; Type IIB is characterized by generalized moderate weakness or bulbar dysfunction or both; Type III includes acute fulminant presentation or respiratory dysfunction or both; and Type IV is late, severe generalized myasthenia.

Many conditions such as viral infections, pregnancy, extreme heat, stress, and surgery may initiate or exacerbate the symptoms of myasthenia gravis, but the responses are very unpredictable. Although some pregnant myasthenics undergo a remission of symptoms during pregnancy, 20–40% report an increased severity of symptoms during gestation.[89] Postpartum respiratory failure and death can occur. Of neonates born to myasthenic women, 15–20% have transient myasthenia resulting from the

---

Table 19-5. DIFFERENT PRESENTATIONS OF MYASTHENIA GRAVIS

	Etiology	Onset	Sex	Thymus	Course
Neonatal myasthenia	Passage of antibodies from myasthenic mothers across the placenta	Neonatal	Both sexes	Normal	Transient
Congenital myasthenia	Congenital end-plate pathology, genetic, autosomal recessive pattern of inheritance	0–2 yr	Male > female	Normal	Nonfluctuating, compatible with long survival
Juvenile myasthenia	Autoimmune disorder	2–20 yr	Female > male (4:1)	Hyperplasia	Slowly progressive, tendency to relapse and remission
Adult myasthenia	Autoimmune disorder	20–40 yr	Female > male	Hyperplasia > thymoma	Maximum severity within 3–5 yr
Elderly myasthenia	Autoimmune disorder	>40 yr	Male > female	Thymoma (benign or locally invasive)	Rapid progress, higher mortality

Reproduced with permission from Baraka A: Anesthesia and myasthenia gravis. Can J Anaesth 39:476, 1992.

passive placental transfer of anti-acetylcholine receptor antibodies. Neonatal myasthenia begins 12–48 hours after birth and may persist for several weeks. Neonatal skeletal muscle strength must be carefully monitored during the early neonatal period.[90]

Patients with a thymoma and myasthenia gravis frequently have related heart disease that manifests as focal myocarditis and atrial fibrillation or atrioventricular block.[91] Although left ventricular systolic function is usually normal, left ventricular diastolic filling may be impaired, heralding the early stages of a decrease in cardiac performance.[92]

A myasthenic crisis will occur in 15–20% of patients during the course of their disease. Myasthenic crises are often precipitated by pneumonia or upper respiratory infections and result in respiratory failure requiring mechanical ventilation.[93]

The diagnosis of myasthenia gravis is based on the clinical history, the edrophonium test, electromyography, and the detection of circulating anti-acetylcholine receptor antibodies.[94] No single test is, however, definitive. For example, the administration of edrophonium can improve strength both in myasthenics and in patients with other neuromuscular disorders.

Treatment modalities for myasthenia gravis include cholinesterase inhibitors, thymectomy, corticosteroids, plasmapheresis, and immunosuppressants. The primary treatment for myasthenia gravis since the 1940s has been the administration of cholinesterase inhibitors such as physostigmine and neostigmine.[86] These drugs function by effectively increasing the concentration of acetylcholine at the nicotinic postsynaptic membrane. Consistent control of myasthenia with cholinesterase inhibitors can be quite challenging. For example, underdosage will result in increased skeletal muscle weakness, whereas overdosage will produce a "cholinergic crisis." Excessive doses of cholinesterase inhibitors produce abdominal cramping, vomiting, diarrhea, salivation, bradycardia, and skeletal muscle weakness that mimics the weakness of myasthenia. Corticosteroids produce remission in 80% of patients with myasthenia but also produce significant drug side effects during long-term therapy. Immunosuppressive therapy with azathioprine, cyclophosphamide, or cyclosporine has been shown to reduce anti-acetylcholine receptor antibody levels and produce clinical improvement. Hazards of immunosuppressive therapy include infection and malignancy. Plasmapheresis, by reducing anti-acetylcholine receptor antibody levels, produces improved muscle strength and is a very effective treatment for patients in myasthenic crisis.[95] The effects of plasmapheresis are short-lived, and long-term therapy with plasmapheresis is impractical. The administration of intravenous immunoglobulin may also improve strength in some patients with myasthenia.[96]

Thymectomy is highly effective for the treatment of myasthenia gravis and is usually recommended for adults with myasthenia. There is, however, considerable controversy among surgeons with regard to the timing of thymectomy and the surgical approach (transsternal versus transcervical).[97,98] There is no universally reliable single therapy for myasthenia gravis. Successful management depends on an experienced neurologist or internist who can orchestrate the different therapeutic modalities at the proper time.[99]

Management of Anesthesia

The primary concern in anesthesia for the patient with myasthenia gravis is the potential interaction between the disease, treatment of the disease, and neuromuscular blocking drugs. The uncontrolled or poorly controlled myasthenic patient is exquisitely sensitive to nondepolarizing muscle relaxants. Even small, defasciculating doses of nondepolarizers can produce significant respiratory muscle paralysis and respiratory distress.[100] It should be anticipated that any patient with myasthenia, no matter how localized, will have increased sensitivity to nondepolarizing muscle relaxants (Fig. 19-3). Numerous studies have demonstrated this increased sensitivity.[101,102] Because of rapid elimination, however, mivacurium, atracurium, rocuronium,

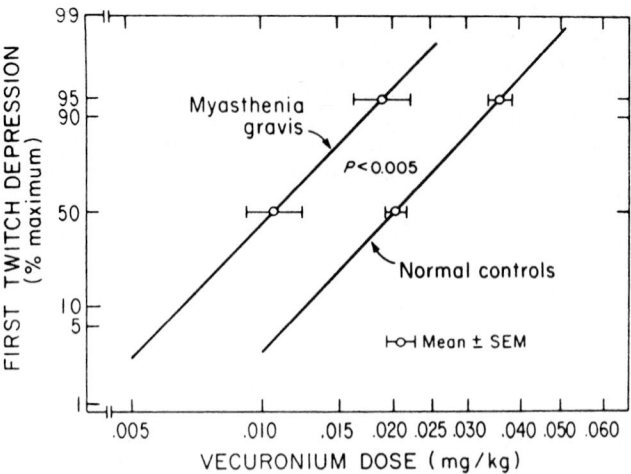

Figure 19-3. Dose–response for vecuronium in normal patients and patients with myasthenia gravis. (Reprinted with permission from Eisenkraft JB, Book WJ, Papatestas AE: Sensitivity to vecuronium in myasthenia gravis: A dose–response study. Can J Anaesth 37:301, 1990.)

and rapacuronium can be effectively titrated to produce satisfactory muscle relaxation with minimal risk of prolonged postoperative paralysis.[103–107] Treatment of myasthenia with cholinesterase inhibitors can influence the response to both depolarizing and nondepolarizing neuromuscular blocking drugs.[108] The response to succinylcholine is unpredictable. The untreated myasthenic is usually resistant to the effects of succinylcholine; however, the myasthenic patient treated with cholinesterase inhibitors may exhibit resistant, prolonged, or normal responses to succinylcholine.[109,110] As would be anticipated, the duration of neuromuscular blockade produced by succinylcholine is inversely related to the plasma cholinesterase level.[111] Successive doses of succinylcholine can produce a progressive prolongation of neuromuscular blockade in patients with myasthenia.[112] Because of the myasthenic patient's unpredictable response to succinylcholine, a short-acting nondepolarizing muscle relaxant is preferred.

The tremendous variability in the response of myasthenic patients to the different types of neuromuscular blocking drugs warrants careful monitoring with a peripheral nerve stimulator and correlation with clinical signs of recovery from neuromuscular blockade. Since halogenated inhaled anesthetics depress neuromuscular transmission in myasthenic patients, neuromuscular blocking drugs may not be required.[113,114] There is no specific anesthetic technique that is superior to others for patients with myasthenia. Inhaled and intravenous anesthetics have been successfully employed.[115] Analgesic techniques such as regional anesthesia and/or neuraxial narcotic administration may decrease the likelihood of postoperative respiratory depression from the systemic administration of opioids.[116,117] At the conclusion of surgery, complete recovery from neuromuscular blockade must be established before tracheal extubation and withdrawal of ventilatory support. Risk factors that increase the likelihood of postoperative ventilatory insufficiency include: (1) duration of myasthenia of > 6 years; (2) history of chronic respiratory disease; (3) treatment doses of pyridostigmine > 750 mg · day^{-1}; and (4) preoperative vital capacity < 2.9 l.[118] The need for postoperative ventilatory support after thymectomy is substantially greater when a transsternal surgical approach is used instead of a transcervical approach.[119,120] The patient with myasthenia gravis requiring mechanical ventilation can be one of the most challenging to wean from ventilatory support. Skeletal muscle strength can vary greatly during a short period of time. It is imperative that sustained respiratory muscle strength be confirmed before tracheal extubation and resumption of independent, spontaneous ventilation.

Exacerbation of myasthenia gravis may occur in late pregnancy and the early postpartum period. Consequently, skeletal muscle relaxation produced by regional anesthesia in conjunction with inherent muscle weakness may lead to hypoventilation. Because 15–20% of infants born to myasthenic mothers may exhibit transient neonatal myasthenia within 1–21 days after birth, anticholinesterase therapy and mechanical ventilation may be necessary.

Myasthenic Syndrome (Lambert-Eaton Syndrome)

The myasthenic syndrome is a disorder of neuromuscular transmission associated with carcinomas, particularly small cell carcinoma of the lung (Table 19-6).[121] The onset of the myasthenic syndrome may actually precede discovery of the malignancy by as much as five years. Myasthenic syndrome is an autoimmune disease in which immunoglobulin G (IgG) antibodies against voltage-gated calcium channels (presynaptic) are produced.[122] In those cases associated with carcinoma, the autoantibodies are directed at calcium channels in the tumor; these autoantibodies, however, cross-react with calcium channels at the neuromuscular junction.[123] The result is a decreased release of acetylcholine in response to nerve stimulation. Typically, the patient is a man, 50–70 years old, complaining of proximal extremity weakness that markedly affects gait and the ability to stand and climb stairs. Rarely, the clinical presentation may be respiratory failure.[124,125] Autonomic dysfunction, such as xerostomia, impotence, orthostatic hypotension, constipation, and altered sweating responses, has also been reported.[126]

Treatment of myasthenic syndrome is initially directed at treatment of the underlying neoplasm. The most effective drug for treatment of the myasthenic syndrome is 3,4-diaminopyridine. 3,4-Diaminopyridine improves synaptic transmission by opening voltage-gated potassium channels, which increases transmitter release at the synapse.[127] Side effects of 3,4-diaminopyridine include perioral and digital paresthesias and seizures. Guanidine also enhances acetylcholine release and may be effective for the treatment of myasthenic syndrome.[128] Although the administration of pyridostigmine rarely produces a significant increase in muscle strength, pryridostigmine in combination with guanidine or 3,4-diaminopyridine may be effective. Other therapeutic modalities for myasthenic syndrome include intravenous immunoglobulin and plasmapheresis.[129,130] Like the treatment of myasthenia gravis, effective long-term treatment of the myasthenic syndrome requires an experienced neurologist and an individualized therapeutic regimen.[131]

Management of Anesthesia

Patients with myasthenic syndrome are sensitive to the effects of both depolarizing and nondepolarizing muscle relaxants. Consequently, the doses of these drugs should be reduced, and neuromuscular function should be monitored carefully. Reported experience with anesthesia in patients receiving aminopyridines is limited, but it is recommended that their administration be continued up to the time of surgery.[132] The preanesthetic administration of immunoglobulin may improve muscle strength in the perioperative period.[133]

Because the myasthenic syndrome is difficult to diagnose, a high index of suspicion for this disorder should be maintained if unexpected muscle weakness occurs in patients with malignant tumors. Although myasthenic syndrome is most frequently associated with small cell carcinoma of the lung, muscle weakness can occur with other malignancies as well.

Guillain-Barré Syndrome (Polyradiculoneuritis)

Guillain-Barré syndrome is currently the most common cause of acute, flaccid paralysis. Guillain-Barré syndrome is an autoimmune disease triggered by a bacterial or viral infection. The list of infectious triggers is long and includes campylobacter, mycoplasma, cytomegalovirus, Epstein-Barr virus, hemophilus, parainfluenza, influenza, adenovirus, herpes simplex, and varicella.[134,135] It is likely that the infection triggers an immune response that targets the Schwann cell membrane or myelin, resulting in demyelination and axonal degeneration.[134-136] Most patients have a history of a respiratory tract or gastrointestinal tract infection within 4 weeks of the onset of neurologic symptoms. Guillain-Barré syndrome is characterized by the acute or subacute onset of skeletal muscle weakness or paralysis of the legs. Sensory disturbances such as paresthesias often precede the paralysis. Typically, the paralysis progresses cephalad to include the muscles of the trunk and arms. Difficulty in swallowing and impaired ventilation resulting from intercostal muscle paralysis can occur. Progression usually occurs over 10–12 days, followed by gradual recovery. The most serious immediate problem is ventilatory insufficiency. The vital capacity should be measured frequently. If the vital capacity decreases to less than 15–20 ml · kg^{-1}, mechanical ventilation of the lungs is indicated.[137] The more rapid the onset of quadriplegia, the more likely the need for prolonged ventilatory support. Although 85% of patients with this syndrome achieve a good or full recovery, chronic or recurrent neuropathy develops in 3–5% of patients.[138] Mortality from Guillain-Barré syndrome is between 2 and 12% and occurs primarily in elderly patients with coexisting pulmonary disease.[139]

Table 19-6. COMPARISON OF MYASTHENIC SYNDROME AND MYASTHENIA GRAVIS

	Myasthenic Syndrome	Myasthenia Gravis
Manifestations	Proximal limb weakness (arms > legs)	Extraocular, bulbar, and facial muscle weakness
	Exercise improves with strength	Fatigue with exercise
	Muscle pain common	Muscle pain uncommon
	Reflexes absent or decreased	Reflexes normal
Gender	Male > female	Female > male
Coexisting pathology	Small cell carcinoma of the lung	Thymoma
Response to muscle relaxants	Sensitive to succinylcholine and non-depolarizing muscle relaxants	Resistant to succinylcholine Sensitive to nondepolarizing muscle relaxants
	Poor response to anticholinesterases	Poor response to anticholinesterases

Reprinted with permission from Stoelting RK, Dierdorf SF (eds): Anesthesia and Co-existing Disease, 3d ed. New York, Churchill Livingstone.

Autonomic nervous system dysfunction occurs in many patients with Guillain-Barré syndrome. This dysfunction can produce wide fluctuations in blood pressure, tachycardia, cardiac dysrhythmias, and cardiac arrest.[140] In a manner similar to autonomic hyperreflexia, physical stimulation can precipitate hypertension, tachycardia, and cardiac dysrhythmias. Appropriate α- and β-adrenergic blockade may be required for those patients. Evidence of mild hepatic dysfunction has also been reported in patients with Guillain-Barré syndrome.[141]

In addition to ventilatory support and meticulous general medical care, the most effective treatments are plasmapheresis and high-dose intravenous immunoglobulin.[142,143] Corticosteroids are not beneficial.

Subtypes of Guillain-Barré include acute inflammatory demyelinating polyneuropathy (AIDP), acute motor axonal neuropathy (AMAN), acute motor-sensory axonal neuropathy (AMSAN), and Fisher syndrome. Electrophysiologic studies may be helpful in differentiating among these disorders.[144]

Management of Anesthesia

Autonomic nervous system dysfunction indicates that compensatory cardiovascular responses may be absent, resulting in significant hypotension secondary to postural changes, blood loss, or positive airway pressure. On the other hand, noxious stimuli such as laryngoscopy and tracheal intubation may produce exaggerated increases in heart rate and blood pressure. Direct-acting vasopressors may be required to control blood pressure. Cardiovascular function should be carefully monitored in the perioperative period.

The administration of succinylcholine should be avoided because of the danger of drug-induced potassium release and hyperkalemia. This risk may actually persist after clinical recovery from the disorder.[145] A nondepolarizing muscle relaxant with minimal cardiovascular effects, such as vecuronium, rocuronium, and rapacuronium, would be a useful choice. However, the sensitivity of patients with Guillain-Barré syndrome to nondepolarizing muscle relaxants may vary from extreme sensitivity to resistance, depending on the phase of the disease.[146] It is likely that mechanical ventilation will be required during the immediate postoperative period. Some patients with Guillain-Barré syndrome have pronounced sensory disturbances and may benefit from the use of epidural opioids.[147,148]

It should be remembered that it can be very difficult to differentiate Guillain-Barré syndrome from other neurologic disorders such as anterior spinal artery syndrome or chronic inflammatory demyelinating polyneuropathy. Guillain-Barré syndrome has been reported to occur after surgery.[149,150]

CENTRAL NERVOUS SYSTEM DISEASES
Multiple Sclerosis

Multiple sclerosis is an acquired disease of the central nervous system characterized by central nervous system inflammation and multiple sites of demyelination in the brain and spinal cord. The cause of multiple sclerosis is multifactorial and involves a complex series of immunologic events occurring in genetically susceptible individuals. Viruses have long been implicated as the cause of multiple sclerosis; however, proof of this relationship has been difficult to establish. It is speculated that molecular mimicry of viruses to myelin may serve as the immunologic trigger that causes demyelination. The similarity of the virus to myelin produces immunologic cross-reactivity which sets into motion the immunologic and inflammatory responses in the central nervous system characteristic of multiple sclerosis.[151] Initially myelin is damaged but can be replaced by the oligodendrocytes that synthesize myelin. Ultimately, the oligodendrocytes are destroyed and myelin can no longer be replaced. Demyelination exposes the axon to harmful factors and interferes with neural transmission.[152] The complex interaction between the

immune and inflammatory responses with the inherent reparative processes of the body explains the relapsing nature of multiple sclerosis.[153]

The symptoms of multiple sclerosis depend on the sites of demyelination in the brain and spinal cord. Demyelination of the optic tracts produces visual disturbances, whereas demyelination of the oculomotor pathways results in nystagmus. Lesions of the spinal cord cause limb weakness and paresthesias. The legs are affected more than the arms. Bowel retention and urinary incontinence are frequent complaints. Involvement of the brain stem can produce diplopia, trigeminal neuralgia, cardiac dysrhythmias, and autonomic dysfunction, while alterations in ventilation can lead to hypoxemia, apnea, and respiratory failure.[154–158] The course of multiple sclerosis is characterized by an exacerbation of symptoms at unpredictable intervals over a period of years. Residual symptoms eventually persist during remission and may lead to severe disability. In some patients the course is relatively benign, with frequent periods of demyelination followed by prolonged remission. As is typical in many immune disorders, pregnancy is associated with an improvement in symptoms, but relapse frequently occurs in the first three postpartum months.[159]

The diagnosis of multiple sclerosis is based primarily on clinical determinations. Clinical criteria include age of onset between 10 and 50 years, neurologic signs and symptoms indicative of CNS white matter disease, two or more attacks separated by a month or more, and involvement of two or more noncontiguous anatomic areas.[160] Laboratory confirmation of the diagnosis can be obtained by chemical analysis of the cerebrospinal fluid and cranial magnetic resonance imaging (MRI). An estimated 70% of patients with multiple sclerosis have elevated levels of IgG in the cerebrospinal fluid, and elevated levels of albumin in the CSF are usually indicative of blood–brain barrier dysfunction.[161] MRI has been established as a sensitive diagnostic tool for multiple sclerosis and provides direct evidence of the location of demyelinated plaques in the central nervous system. MRI is also used as a measure of the effectiveness of treatment modalities for multiple sclerosis.[162]

There have been significant advances in recent years in the treatment of multiple sclerosis. Current treatment is directed at modulating the immunologic and inflammatory responses that damage myelin. Corticosteroids (methylprednisolone) are the primary agents for treatment of an acute exacerbation of multiple sclerosis. Corticosteroids have diverse effects that act to suppress cellular immune responses.[163] Corticosteroids may not, however, influence the long term course of the disease. Interferon (B-1a, B-1b) alters the inflammatory response and may augment natural disease suppression mechanisms.[164] Glatiramir (copolymer-1) is a mixture of polypeptides that mimics the structure of myelin and may serve as a decoy for autoantibodies. Nonspecific immunosuppressants such as azathioprine, methotrexate, cyclophosphamide, and cyclosporine have also been used, but with variable success. Although the treatment of multiple sclerosis with intravenous immunoglobulin has been done for many years, this therapy is still experimental.[165] Strategies currently under research are directed at producing remyelination. Symptomatic therapy for some of the complications of multiple sclerosis include diazepam, dantrolene, and baclofen for skeletal muscle spasticity. Painful dysesthesias, tonic seizures, dysarthria, and ataxia may be treated with carbamazepine. Nonspecific therapeutic measures include the avoidance of excessive fatigue, emotional stress, and hyperthermia. Demyelinated nerve fibers are extremely sensitive to increases in temperature. A temperature increase of as little as 0.5°C may block impulse conduction in demyelinated fibers.[166]

Management of Anesthesia

The effect of surgery and anesthesia on the course of multiple sclerosis is controversial. Some reports indicate that symptoms of multiple sclerosis are exacerbated by anesthesia, particularly regional anesthesia.[167,168] Other studies, however, report that anesthesia does not affect the course of the disease.[169] A relatively high proportion of patients with multiple sclerosis who receive spinal anesthesia do have an exacerbation of symptoms after surgery.[170] It could be speculated that demyelinated areas of the spinal cord might be more sensitive to the effects of local anesthetics. This increased sensitivity could explain the exacerbation after spinal anesthesia. Intrathecal morphine in conjunction with spinal and general anesthesia has been used successfully in patients with multiple sclerosis.[171,172] Epidural anesthesia has been used for labor and delivery in women with multiple sclerosis. The neurologic relapse rate, however, was greater if bupivacaine in concentrations higher than 0.25% was used.[173] It is likely that well managed epidural analgesia is associated with minimal risk of a postpartum exacerbation.[174] Certainly, pyrexia and, most likely, metabolic and hormonal changes induced by surgery and anesthesia could produce a neurologic exacerbation independent of the type of anesthesia. Despite the confusion in the medical literature, certain recommendations seem warranted. Before surgery, the patient should be advised that surgery and anesthesia could produce a relapse despite a well managed anesthetic. Ideally, the patient should have a thorough neurologic examination before the operation to document coexisting neurologic deficits. After surgery, the neurologic examination can be repeated so that pre- and postoperative findings can be compared. In view of the fact that spinal anesthesia can cause an unpredictable exacerbation, use of this type of anesthesia should be reserved for special situations. The patient's temperature should be monitored closely during anesthesia and measures employed to reduce alterations in body temperature.

Selection of agents for general anesthesia should take into consideration potential interactions with medications the patient is receiving. For example, patients receiving corticosteroids may need corticosteroid supplementation during the perioperative period. There are no reported adverse interactions between interferon and glatiramir. In theory, succinylcholine could produce an exaggerated release of potassium, although this has not been reported in patients with multiple sclerosis. Anticonvulsants such as carbamazepine and phenytoin can produce resistance to nondepolarizing muscle relaxants.[175] Autonomic dysfunction caused by multiple sclerosis may exaggerate the hypotensive effects of volatile anesthetics. Consequently, careful monitoring of cardiovascular function is indicated. Respiratory muscle weakness and respiratory control dysfunction increase the likelihood of the need for supplemental oxygen and/or mechanical ventilation during the immediate postoperative period.[176,177]

Epilepsy

A seizure disorder is a common manifestation of many types of central nervous system diseases. A seizure results from the excessive discharge of large numbers of neurons that become depolarized in a synchronous fashion. Idiopathic seizures usually begin during childhood. The sudden onset of seizures in a young or middle-aged adult should arouse suspicion of focal brain disease, particularly a tumor. The onset of seizures after 60 years of age is usually secondary to cerebrovascular disease, but can be a result of head injury, brain tumor, or metabolic disturbances.[178] The onset of seizures requires a thorough neurologic evaluation to determine the etiology. Advanced neuroimaging techniques have provided powerful diagnostic tools for the determination of structural causes of epilepsy. Research in molecular biology and genetics has revealed that some forms of epilepsy are caused by mutations in ion channels. Although the current number of epileptic syndromes caused by mutations is small, there is little doubt that more will be identified.[179] The availability of several new antiseizure drugs has increased the therapeutic options for the treatment of epilepsy.[180] Selecting the right drug or drugs for the treatment of epilepsy may require trial and error to balance efficacy with side effects.[181]

Table 19-7. CLASSIFICATION OF SEIZURES

LOCALIZATION-RELATED EPILEPSIES AND SEIZURES

Idiopathic
  Benign childhood epilepsy
  Childhood epilepsy with occipital paroxysms

GENERALIZED EPILEPSIES

Idiopathic
  Absence epilepsy
    Childhood
    Juvenile
  Benign neonatal convulsions
  Myoclonic epilepsy
    Neonatal
    Juvenile
  Grand mal seizures on awakening
Idiopathic and/or symptomatic
  West's syndrome
  Lennox-Gestaut syndrome
  Myoclonic–astatic seizures
  Myoclonic absences
Symptomatic
  Nonspecific etiology

UNDETERMINED EPILEPSIES AND SYNDROMES

With both generalized and focal seizures
  Neonatal seizures
  Severe myoclonic epilepsy of infancy
  Acquired epileptic aphasia

SPECIAL SYNDROMES

Febrile seizures
Alcohol-related seizures

Modified with permission from Riela AR: Management of seizures. Crit Care Clin 5:863, 1989.

There are more than 40 types of epilepsy based on several clinical features. The most common classification system is the International Classification of Epileptic Seizures (Table 19-7). A description of the most frequently encountered types of seizures follows.

Grand Mal Seizure. A grand mal seizure is characterized by generalized tonic–clonic activity. All respiratory activity is arrested and a period of arterial hypoxemia ensues. The tonic phase lasts for 20–40 seconds and is followed by the clonic phase. In the postictal phase, the patient is lethargic and confused. Initial treatment is directed toward maintaining arterial oxygenation and stopping the seizure activity. Diazepam and thiopental are effective drugs for the treatment of acute, generalized seizures. Antiseizure drugs effective for seizure control and prevention are phenytoin, valproate, felbamate, carbamazepine, and lamotrigine (Table 19-8).

Focal Cortical Seizure. Focal cortical seizures, also known as Jacksonian epilepsy, may be sensory or motor, depending on the site of neuronal discharge. There is usually no loss of consciousness, although the seizure activity may spread to produce a grand mal seizure.

Absence Seizure (Petit Mal). Absence seizures, previously called petit mal seizures, are characterized by a brief loss of awareness lasting about 30 seconds. Additional manifestations include staring, blinking, and rolling the eyes. There is an immediate resumption of consciousness. Absence seizures typically occur in children and young adults. Absence seizures without other seizure activity are best treated with ethosuximide. Valproate is the drug of choice for absence seizures associated with other seizure activity.

Akinetic Seizure. Akinetic seizures are characterized by a sudden, brief loss of consciousness and loss of postural tone. These types of seizures usually occur in children and can produce severe head injury from a fall.

Table 19-8. ANTICONVULSANT DRUGS

Drug	Seizure Type	Therapeutic Blood Level (mg · ml^{-1})	Side Effects
Phenobarbital	Generalized	15–35	Sedation, increased drug metabolism
Valproate	Generalized Absence	50–100	Pancreatitis Hepatic dysfunction
Felbamate	Generalized Partial		Insomnia, ataxia, nausea
Phenytoin	Generalized Partial	10–20	Gingival hyperplasia Dermatitis Resistance to NM blockers (nondepolarizers)
Fosphenytoin	Generalized Partial		Paresthesias Hypotension
Carbamazepine	Generalized Partial	6–12	Cardiotoxic, hepatitis Resistance to NM blockers
Lamotrigine	Generalized Partial		Rash Stevens-Johnson syndrome
Topiramate	Generalized Partial		
Gabapentin	Generalized Partial		Fatigue, somnolence
Primidone	Generalized Partial	6–12	Nausea, ataxia
Clonazepam	Absence	0.01–0.07	Ataxia
Ethosuximide	Absence	40–100	Leukopenia Erythema multiforme

Myoclonic Seizure. Myoclonic seizures occur as isolated clonic jerks in response to a sensory stimulus. In most cases a single group of muscles is involved. Myoclonic seizures are often associated with degenerative and metabolic brain diseases.

Psychomotor Seizure. Psychomotor seizures are seen as an impairment of consciousness, inappropriate motor acts, hallucinations, amnesia, and unusual visceral symptoms. This type of seizure is preceded by an aura.

Status Epilepticus. Status epilepticus is defined as two consecutive tonic–clonic seizures without regaining consciousness, or seizure activity that is unabated for 30 minutes or longer.[182] Status epilepticus can include all types of seizure activity. Grand mal status epilepticus is of the greatest concern because mortality can be as high as 20%. Typically, grand mal status epilepticus lasts for 48 hours with a seizure frequency of four to five per hour. As the seizure progresses, skeletal muscle activity diminishes and seizure activity may be evident only on the electroencephalogram (EEG). Respiratory effects of status epilepticus include inhibition of the respiratory centers, uncoordinated skeletal muscle activity that impairs ventilation, and abnormal autonomic activity that produces bronchoconstriction. In addition to the danger of arterial hypoxemia from inadequate airway control, there is a high likelihood of permanent neuronal damage from continued seizures.[183] Diazepam or lorazepam are considered the drugs of choice for the treatment of status epilepticus. Because the effects of the benzodiazepines are transient, a longer-acting anticonvulsant (*e.g.*, phenytoin, phenobarbital) must also be administered. Thiopental is quite effective for the initial treatment of status epilepticus, but the effect is transient. Muscle relaxants may be required to facilitate tracheal intubation if a secured airway is necessary. Although muscle relaxants will terminate the skeletal muscle manifestations of a seizure, there is no effect on seizure activity in the brain. On rare occasions general anesthesia with isoflurane or barbiturates may be required for the treatment of status epilepticus.[184,185]

Management of Anesthesia

Patients receiving antiseizure medications should be maintained on their normal medication regimen until the time of surgery. After the operation, medications should be given parenterally until oral intake can be resumed. In management of anesthesia for the patient with a seizure disorder, the potential influence of anticonvulsants on the response to anesthesia must be considered. Conversely, an anesthesia technique must be used that will not increase the likelihood of seizure activity. Because anticonvulsant drugs affect the liver and neuromuscular systems, the potential for significant drug interaction certainly exists. Stimulation of the hepatic microsomal enzymes by phenobarbital may accelerate and increase the magnitude of biotransformation of anesthetic drugs. Increased biotransformation of volatile halogenated anesthetics may increase the risk of organ toxicity. Other known side effects of anticonvulsants include leukopenia, anemia, and hepatitis from phenytoin; pancreatitis, hepatic failure, and coagulopathy from valproate; aplastic anemia, cardiotoxicity, and hypothyroidism from carbamazepine; leukopenia from felbamate; and rash and hypersensitivity from lamotrigine.[186]

Although most inhaled anesthetics, including nitrous oxide, have been reported to produce seizure activity, such activity during the administration of halothane, isoflurane, desflurane, or sevoflurane is extremely rare. Desflurane produces a dose-dependent depression of EEG activity similar to that of isoflurane.[187] Enflurane predictably produces spike and wave activity on the EEG, particularly when hypocarbia exists. Children seem to be especially susceptible to enflurane-induced seizure activity.[188] It would appear that halothane, isoflurane, sevoflurane, or desflurane are preferable to enflurane for patients with seizure disorders.

The use of ketamine is controversial. Ketamine has been shown to produce seizure activity in patients with known seizure disorders. There are, however, data indicating that ketamine is safe to use in patients with seizure disorders. It would seem reasonable to avoid the use of ketamine for patients with seizure disorders because alternative drugs such as barbiturates, benzodiazepines, and propofol are available.

There is some evidence that propofol may activate the cerebral cortex.[189] Most studies, however, indicate that propofol has a more depressant effect on the EEG than does thiopental, and has been noted to increase the seizure threshold in patients receiving electroconvulsive therapy.[190] Propofol has also been shown to terminate local anesthetic–induced seizures.[191]

Methohexital may produce seizure activity in children.[192] Certainly, methohexital has been used for many patients with seizure disorders without adverse effects. Although methohexital may not be contraindicated in patients with seizures, thiopental or propofol would be useful alternatives.

Seizure activity has also been reported to occur after the administration of fentanyl, sufentanil, and alfentanil; however, other studies have found no seizure activity after the use of these opioids.[193–196] The reported seizure activity may represent myoclonic activity or some form of opioid-induced skeletal muscle rigidity. With the usual clinical doses, seizure activity after fentanyl and sufentanil is not likely.[197] Clinical doses of alfentanil have been reported to produce seizure activity.[198] Prolonged administration of large doses of fentanyl ($200–400$ $\mu g \cdot kg^{-1}$) or sufentanil ($40–160$ $\mu g \cdot kg^{-1}$) may produce seizures and should be used with caution in patients with seizure disorders.[199,200] Patients being chronically treated with anticonvulsants do have an increased fentanyl requirement during surgery, which most likely reflects enhanced metabolism by hepatic enzyme induction. Another potential drug interaction in patients receiving phenytoin and carbamazepine is resistance to nondepolarizing muscle relaxants.[201]

The patient with a seizure disorder should receive his or her normal therapeutic drug regimen up to and including the morning of surgery. After surgery, this regimen should be resumed as quickly as possible. A decline in blood levels of anticonvulsant drugs will increase the likelihood of postoperative seizures.

Parkinson's Disease

Parkinson's disease, one of the more common disabling neurologic diseases, affects 3% of the population older than 65 years. Parkinson's disease is a degenerative disease of the central nervous system caused by loss of dopaminergic fibers in the basal ganglia of the brain. The characteristic pathologic feature is destruction of dopamine-containing nerve cells in the substantia nigra of the basal ganglia. The cause or causes of this selective destruction are not known. Current theories of the etiology include mitochondrial dysfunction with disordered oxidative metabolism, excitotoxicity (persistent activation of glutamatergic receptors), inadequate neurotrophic support, exposure to toxins (herbicides), or viral infection.[202] Other than the well known postencephalitis Parkinson's disease, however, there is little evidence that Parkinson's disease is caused by a virus. It has been conclusively demonstrated that the clinical effects of Parkinson's disease are caused by dopamine deficiency. Dopamine deficiency increases activity of γ-aminobutyric acid (GABA). GABA inhibits thalamic and brainstem nuclei, which suppresses cortical motor function and thereby causes tremor, akinesia, and gait and posture abnormalities.[203]

The most characteristic clinical features of Parkinson's disease are resting tremor, cogwheel rigidity of the extremities, bradykinesia, shuffling gait, stooped posture, and facial immobility. These features are all secondary to diminished inhibition of the extrapyramidal motor system as a result of depletion of dopamine from the basal ganglia. Other features that occur in patients with Parkinson's disease are seborrhea, sialorrhea, orthostatic hypotension, bladder dysfunction, pupillary abnormalities, diaphragmatic spasm, oculogyric crises, and dementia. Mental depression can be severe enough to necessitate the use of antidepressant medications.

The treatment of Parkinson's disease is directed toward increasing dopamine levels in the brain but preventing adverse peripheral effects of dopamine. Levodopa is the single most effective therapy for patients with Parkinson's disease. When administered orally, however, levodopa is converted to dopamine and causes side effects such as nausea, vomiting, and hypotension. Levodopa is administered in combination with a peripheral dopamine decarboxylase inhibitor carbidopa (Sinemet; Merck, Sharp & Dohme, West Point, PA). Side effects of levodopa administration include depletion of myocardial norepinephrine stores, peripheral vasoconstriction, hypovolemia, and orthostatic hypotension. Although levodopa has significantly reduced morbidity and mortality from Parkinson's disease, there is some evidence to suggest that the administration of levodopa may accelerate the pathologic process causing Parkinson's disease. This hypothesis is highly controversial and not universally accepted, but has influenced the early treatment of Parkinson's to include other types of drugs: anticholinergics, amantadine, dopamine receptor agonists, selegiline (MAO-B inhibitor), and COMT inhibitors. The anticholinergics (trihexyphenidyl, benztropine) are effective because they counteract loss of inhibition of cholinergic neurons. Anticholinergics can worsen dementia and are reserved for younger patients in the early phases of Parkinson's disease. Amantadine is a glutamate receptor antagonist and may exert a neuroprotective effect on neurons in the basal ganglia. The dopamine receptor agonists (bromocriptine, pergolide, pramipexole, ropinorole) exert their effect directly on dopamine receptors in the brain. Side effects of the dopamine receptor agonists include pulmonary and retroperitoneal fibrosis, erythromelalgia, and Raynaud's phenomenon. Selegiline is a selective MAO-B inhibitor which decreases the metabolism of dopamine. COMT inhibitors (entacapone, tolcapone) prevent the degradation of levodopa. Many of the aforementioned types of drugs, although not entirely successful as sole agents for the treatment of Parkinson's, are quite effective in combination with levodopa.[204] A variety of surgical techniques for the palliation of Parkinson's have been recommended. Stereotactic pallidotomy and transplantation of neural tissue have demonstrated some efficacy.[205]

Management of Anesthesia

Management of anesthesia is usually determined by potential interaction between anesthesia drugs and anti-Parkinson medications and the severity of neurologic impairment. The patient's therapeutic regimen should be administered on the morning of surgery. The half-life of levodopa is short, and interruption of therapy for more than 6–12 hours can result in severe skeletal muscle rigidity that interferes with ventilation. Phenothiazines and butyrophenones (droperidol) should be avoided because these drugs antagonize the effects of dopamine in the basal ganglia. Alfentanil has been reported to produce acute dystonic reactions in patients with untreated Parkinson's disease.[206] Although ketamine could produce an exaggerated sympathetic nervous system response, with resultant tachycardia and hypertension, it has been used without difficulty in patients with Parkinson's disease. However, the likelihood of coexisting ischemic heart disease in the elderly patient with Parkinson's disease may make the use of ketamine less attractive. In theory, halothane could produce cardiac dysrhythmias in patients receiving levodopa, but this has not been documented. There are no reports of adverse responses to isoflurane, sevoflurane, or desflurane in patients with Parkinson's disease. The choice of muscle relaxants does not seem to be directly influenced by the presence of Parkinson's disease. Although there is one case report of hyperkalemia after the administration of succinylcholine, further investigation has demonstrated that this was an isolated occurrence.[207]

The potential hazards of drug interactions in patients taking MAO inhibitors have been well documented in the medical literature. The interaction between MAO inhibitors and meperidine appears to be the most significant. The use of selegiline for the treatment of the early phases of Parkinson's disease increases the likelihood of having to anesthetize a patient who is receiving MAO-B inhibitors. Although definitive studies of anesthesia for patients receiving selegiline have not been performed, anecdotal reports have indicated that anesthesia is usually uneventful. However, there have been reports of agitation, muscle rigidity, and hyperthermia in patients receiving meperidine and selegiline.[208] The MAO-B enzyme acts on phenylethylamine, benzylamine, tyramine, and dopamine with little effect on epinephrine and norepinephrine.[209] This could explain why there is less risk of massive sympathetic discharge in patients receiving selective MAO-B inhibitors. Patients with Parkinson's disease who are being treated with dopamine agonists may be at increased risk for neuroleptic malignant syndrome.[210]

Autonomic dysfunction is common in Parkinson's disease. Gastrointestinal dysfunction is very common and is manifested by excessive salivation, dysphagia, and esophageal dysfunction. Consequently, the patient with Parkinson's disease should be considered at risk for aspiration pneumonitis. The most consistent cardiovascular abnormality is orthostatic hypotension. The disease process undoubtedly contributes to hypotension, which is further compounded by the tendency of anti-Parkinson drugs to produce peripheral vasodilation.[211] Patients with Parkinson's disease would be more likely to manifest exaggerated decreases in blood pressure in response to inhaled halogenated anesthetics.

Respiratory complications are common in patients with Parkinson's disease. Upper airway obstruction may occur as a result of poor coordination of upper airway muscles secondary to neurotransmitter imbalance caused by the disease process or induced by the administration of antidopaminergic drugs. Some Parkinson's patients with upper airway obstruction may respond to the administration of anti-Parkinson drugs.[212]

In the postoperative period, patients with Parkinson's disease are more susceptible to the development of mental confusion and even hallucinations. These alterations in mental function may not appear until the day after surgery.[213] The precise mechanism of this confusion is not known, but could have significant impact on outpatient surgery in patients with Parkinson's disease.

Huntington's Disease (Huntington's Chorea)

Huntington's disease is a neurodegenerative disease caused by severe neuronal loss in the corpus striatum and later the cortex. Huntington's disease is one of the trinucleotide repeat disorders. The unstable trinucleotide repeat encodes the huntingtin protein. Although the function of the huntingtin protein is not known, intranuclear inclusions of huntingtin and ubiquitin are found in neuronal cells that eventually die.[214,215] Huntington's disease is a heritable disorder that is transmitted as an autosomal dominant trait. The Huntington's gene has been identified and is expressed when the patient is 35–40 years of age. Identification of the Huntington's disease gene has provided a technique for predictive testing; however, the delayed nature of the clinical manifestations of the disease has presented legal and ethical concerns about early predictive testing.[216]

Disordered movement and dementia are the clinical hallmarks of Huntington's disease. Although the chorea is the most common movement disorder, athetosis and dystonia also occur. Movement abnormalities can involve the extremities, trunk, face, eyes, oropharynx, and respiratory muscles.[217] The disease progresses for several years, and accompanying mental depression makes suicide a frequent occurrence. Death usually results from malnutrition and aspiration pneumonitis. The duration of Huntington's disease averages 17 years from the time of diagnosis to death.

There is no specific therapy for Huntington's disease. Pharmacotherapy is directed at relief of mental depression and control of movement disorders. A number of drugs that affect central nervous system neurotransmitter function have been evaluated, but show little promise. Movement disorders such as chorea do not specifically require therapy unless function is significantly diminished. Drugs that reduce dopaminergic transmission, such as phenothiazines, butyrophenones, and thioxanthines, or drugs that deplete dopamine such as tetrabenzamine and reserpine, reduce the severity of chorea.[218] Antidepressants such as the tricyclic antidepressants or serotoninergic antidepressants (fluoxitene) may be effective for improving the patient's mental status.

Management of Anesthesia

Many of the manifestations of Huntington's disease are typical of patients with neurodegenerative disorders. With progression of the disease, the pharyngeal muscles become more dysfunctional and the risk of aspiration pneumonitis increases. Consequently, appropriate anti-aspiration maneuvers must be used. If preoperative and postoperative sedation are necessary, the butyrophenones or phenothiazines are logical choices. There are reported cases of neuroleptic malignant syndrome in patients with Huntington's disease, which is most likely secondary to the administration of neuroleptic drugs rather than intrinsic effects of Huntington's disease.[219] Reported anesthesia experience with patients with Huntington's disease is largely anecdotal. Although there are no specific contraindications to the use of inhaled or intravenous anesthetics, delayed awakening and generalized tonic spasms have been reported after the administration of thiopental.[220] In contrast, a rapid recovery after the administration of propofol has been reported.[221,222] Decreased plasma cholinesterase activity with a prolonged response to succinylcholine has been reported.[223] It has been suggested that patients with Huntington's disease may be sensitive to the effects of nondepolarizing muscle relaxants, although the reported response to atracurium has been normal.[222,224] Spinal anesthesia has been successfully administered to patients with Huntington's disease.[225]

Alzheimer's Disease

Alzheimer's disease is the major cause of dementia in the United States. More than four million people in the United States are afflicted with Alzheimer's disease. The disease affects a large proportion of the population older than 70 years, and is the major reason that patients are admitted to nursing homes. As life expectancy for men and women increases, a larger part of the population will be susceptible to this disease. Although dementia is caused by more than 60 disorders, Alzheimer's disease is responsible for 50–60% of the cases. Dementia is characterized by intellectual and cognitive deterioration that impairs social function. The clinical diagnosis can be made if a patient exhibits loss of memory and deficits in two or more areas of cognition. The mental status examination is central to the diagnosis of Alzheimer's disease. Any systemic cause of dementia, such as cerebral vascular disease, must be eliminated before the diagnosis of Alzheimer's disease is made. Although neuroimaging changes (CT, MRI) and alterations in the EEG are not diagnostic for Alzheimer's disease, these diagnostic techniques are useful for eliminating other causes of dementia. Pathologic changes in the brain include a characteristic cortical atrophy and the presence of neurofibrillary tangles and neuritic plaques in the presence of massive neuronal degeneration. Deposition of β-amyloid appears to be central to the process of degeneration. There is strong evidence that there are four different genetic loci that may predispose to the development of Alzheimer's. These different loci may explain the differences in clinical presentation and age of onset.[214]

Because the precise pathophysiologic mechanism for Alzheimer's is unknown, there is no specific therapy. Most therapy has been directed at increasing neurotransmitter levels, especially acetylcholine. As neuronal systems degenerate, neurotransmitter systems deteriorate. Consequently, therapy has been directed at increasing acetylcholine levels by acetylcholine precursor loading, cholinesterase inhibition, direct cholinergic receptor stimulation, and indirect cholinergic stimulation.[226] Although these therapies have produced clinical improvement in some patients with Alzheimer's disease, the results have not been dramatic. Currently used cholinesterase inhibitors include donepezil, tacrine, velnacrine, and a sustained-release preparation of physostigmine. Tacrine and velnacrine can produce direct hepatotoxicity.[227] Therapy has also been directed at increasing neurotransmitter levels in the noradrenergic and serotoninergic systems as well. Many other drugs, including cerebrovascular vasodilators, vitamins, and antidepressants, are used as adjunctive therapy for Alzheimer's disease.

Management of Anesthesia

Selection of anesthetic drugs and techniques for patients with Alzheimer's disease is guided by the patient's general physiologic condition, the degree of neurologic deterioration, and the potential for interaction between anesthetics and medications that the patient is receiving. Because of dementia, these patients are likely to be disoriented and uncooperative preoperatively. Sedative drugs, such as those used for preoperative medication, should be administered rarely because further mental confusion could result. Anesthetics known to result in rapid postanesthetic recovery, such as propofol, desflurane, and sevoflurane, may be advantageous because they permit a more rapid return to the patient's preoperative state. The possibility of coexisting hepatic dysfunction from tacrine and velnacrine may also influence the choice of a halogenated, volatile anesthetic. If an anticholinergic is required, glycopyrrolate, which does not cross the blood–brain barrier may be preferable to atropine or scopolamine. In theory, an anticholinergic drug that enters the brain could exacerbate the dementia. The patient's preoperative drug list should be reviewed for the possibility of interaction with anesthetics.

Amyotrophic Lateral Sclerosis

Amyotrophic lateral sclerosis (ALS) is a degenerative disease of motor cells (anterior horn cells) throughout the central nervous system. Progression of the disease is relentless, and death usually follows within 3–5 years of diagnosis. Upper and lower motor neurons are involved almost exclusively, although lower motor neurons are affected first.[228] The cause of ALS is unknown, but proposed causes include a slow viral infection, glutamate excitotoxicity, free radical stress, immune dysfunction, impaired neural protein repair, and altered axonal transport.[229] Although the similarity between ALS and poliomyelitis is striking, data indicate that the incidence of ALS in postpoliomyelitis patients is actually decreased.[230]

The signs and symptoms of ALS reflect the upper and lower motor neuron dysfunction. Frequently reported initial manifestations are atrophy, weakness, and fasciculation of skeletal muscles, often beginning in the intrinsic muscles of the hand. Computed tomographic scanning of muscles demonstrates a symmetric atrophy of muscle and replacement of muscle tissue with fat.[231] As the disease progresses, the atrophy and weakness involve most skeletal muscles, including those of the tongue, pharynx, larynx, and chest. Pulmonary function studies demonstrate a decrease in vital capacity, maximal voluntary ventilation, and diminished expiratory muscle function.[232,233] Serial pulmonary function testing may be useful for determination of prognosis and intervention options.[234] In rare instances the initial presentation of ALS may be acute respiratory failure.[235] Eventually, respiratory failure develops in all patients with ALS, and mechanical ventilation of the lungs is necessary. Patients with ALS have evidence of autonomic dysfunction manifested as an increased resting heart rate, orthostatic hypotension, and elevated resting levels of norepinephrine and epinephrine. There is usually a decreased R–R interval variation on the ECG and a decreased heart rate response to the administration of atropine.[236] The cause of death in patients with ALS is usually respiratory failure. Sudden death from circulatory collapse frequently occurs in ventilator-dependent patients with ALS.[237]

Management of Anesthesia

Neuromuscular transmission is markedly abnormal in patients with ALS.[238] Consequently, these patients can be very sensitive to nondepolarizing muscle relaxants. As with other patients with lower motor dysfunction, ALS patients should be considered vulnerable to hyperkalemia in response to the administration of succinylcholine. Bulbar involvement with dysfunction of pharyngeal muscles predisposes patients with ALS to pulmonary aspiration. The need for postoperative ventilatory support is highly likely for these patients. There is no evidence that a specific anesthetic drug or combination of drugs is best for patients with ALS. Subclinical autonomic dysfunction can produce severely exaggerated decreases in cardiovascular function in response to anesthetics.[239]

Creutzfeldt-Jakob Disease

Creutzfeldt-Jakob disease is one of three disorders that constitute the class of diseases known as the human spongiform encephalopathies. The other two diseases in this group are kuru and Gerstmann-Straussler syndrome. Pathologically, these disorders are characterized by vacuolation of brain tissue and neuronal loss. Creutzfeldt-Jakob disease is caused by an unusual infectious agent—a prion. A prion is a small proteinaceous infectious agent. Prions are resistant to alcohol, formalin, ionizing radiation, proteases, and nucleases, but can be inactivated by heat (autoclaving), phenol, detergents, and extremes of pH.[240] Creutzfeldt-Jakob disease is an almost unique disease in that the incubation time is long (years), and there is an absence of fever and inflammation. There has been considerable concern in recent years about the potential transmission of prions from animals (cows) to man. Though much less common, Creutzfeldt-Jakob disease, like multiple sclerosis, is known for its diverse clinical presentations and varied neurologic signs.[241]

The typical clinical characteristics include subacute dementia, myoclonus, and EEG changes. The EEG pattern is relatively characteristic, with diffuse, slow activity, and periodic complexes. Because of the dementia and wide array of presenting symptoms, patients with Creutzfeldt-Jakob disease are often misdiagnosed as having psychiatric disorders. There is no specific therapeutic drug for Creutzfeldt-Jakob disease.

Management of Anesthesia

Creutzfeldt-Jakob disease is transmissible. There are reports of cases developing after accidental inoculation and surgery.[242,243] The transmission of Creutzfeldt-Jakob disease has been linked to contaminated dural graft material, corneal transplants, and administration of pooled human growth hormone.[244,245] Although there have been no documented reports of transmission of Creutzfeldt-Jakob disease by blood transfusion, donor restrictions have been proposed.[246,247] Because of the transmissibility of the disease, appropriate precautions should be taken to protect other patients and health care providers. The Creutzfeldt-Jakob prion is not inactivated by 3–10% formalin and 70% alcohol. Sodium hypochlorite (bleach) 0.05% and sterilization with steam or ethylene oxide will destroy the infectious agent.[248]

Although reported anesthetic experience with patients with Creutzfeldt-Jakob disease is limited, certain speculations and recommendations seem warranted. Patients with degenerative neurologic diseases are prone to aspirate gastric contents because they have impaired swallowing function and decreased activity of laryngeal reflexes. Therefore, appropriate anti-aspiration maneuvers are indicated during anesthesia. Because lower motor neuron dysfunction also occurs in these patients, the use of succinylcholine should be avoided. The autonomic and peripheral nervous systems may also be involved, which may result in abnormal cardiovascular responses to anesthesia and vasoactive drugs.[249,250]

ANEMIAS

The causes of anemia are numerous (Table 19-9). Anemias can be classified as nutritional deficiency anemias, hemolytic anemias, hemoglobinopathies, and hemoglobin deficiency syndromes (thalassemias).

Regardless of the cause of the anemia, compensatory physiologic mechanisms develop to offset the decreased oxygen-carrying capacity of the blood. Typically, in an otherwise healthy person, symptoms do not develop from anemia until the hemoglobin level decreases below 7 g $\cdot$ dl^{-1}. Symptoms are highly variable and depend on other concurrent disease processes. Physiologic compensation includes increased plasma volume, increased cardiac output, and increased levels of red blood cell 2, 3-diphosphoglycerate (Table 19-10). Because elderly patients with chronic anemia have an increased plasma volume, transfusion of whole blood to these patients may result in congestive heart failure. Similarly, the myocardial depressant effects of anesthetics may be exaggerated in patients with increased cardiac output at rest as compensation for anemia.

Concern about the transmission of blood-borne infectious diseases such as human immunodeficiency virus has greatly influenced the perioperative use of blood products and has radically altered recommendations for perioperative blood transfusion not only in normal patients, but also in patients with chronic anemia. Traditional hematocrit levels that previously triggered the need for preoperative blood transfusion have been challenged. Currently, there is no universally accepted hematocrit level that mandates blood transfusion. The patient's physiologic status and coexisting diseases must be factored into a highly subjective decision.[251]

Nutritional Deficiency Anemias

The three primary causes of nutritional deficiency anemia are iron deficiency, vitamin B$_{12}$ deficiency, and folic acid deficiency. Chronic illness, as well as poor dietary intake, can result in nutritional deficiency anemia.

Iron deficiency anemia produces the typical microcytic, hypochromic red blood cell. Iron deficiency anemia may be an absolute deficiency secondary to decreased oral intake or a relative deficiency caused by a rapid turnover of red blood cells (*e.g.*, chronic blood loss, hemolysis). Measuring the hemoglobin and serum ferritin levels is a rapid and effective mechanism for differentiating true iron deficiency anemia from other causes.[252] Severe iron deficiency anemia can result in respiratory distress, congestive heart failure, thrombocytopenia, and neurologic abnormalities.[253-255]

Table 19-9. TYPES OF ANEMIA

NUTRITIONAL

Iron deficiency
Vitamin B$_{12}$ deficiency
Folic acid deficiency

HEMOGLOBINOPATHIES

Hemoglobin S (sickle cell)

HEMOLYTIC

Spherocytosis
Glucose-6-phosphate dehydrogenase deficiency
Pyruvate kinase deficiency
Immune-mediated
Drug-induced ABO incompatibility

THALASSEMIAS

Thalassemia major (Cooley's anemia)
Thalassemia intermedia
Thalassemia minor

Table 19-10. COMPENSATORY MECHANISMS TO INCREASE OXYGEN DELIVERY WITH CHRONIC ANEMIA

Increased cardiac output
Increased red blood cell 2,3-diphosphoglycerate
Increased P-50
Increased plasma volume
Decreased blood viscosity

Megaloblastic anemia can be caused by vitamin B$_{12}$ (cobalamin) deficiency, folate deficiency, or refractory bone marrow disease.[256] Absorption of vitamin B$_{12}$ by the gastrointestinal tract depends on production of intrinsic factor, a glycoprotein produced by gastric parietal cells. Atrophy of the gastric mucosa causes vitamin B$_{12}$ deficiency and megaloblastic anemia. Chronic gastritis and gastric atrophy in some patients are caused by autoantibodies to gastric parietal cells.[257] In addition to megaloblastic anemia, vitamin B$_{12}$ deficiency can interfere with myelination and produce significant nervous system dysfunction.[258] In adults this is usually manifest by a peripheral neuropathy secondary to degeneration of the lateral and posterior columns of the spinal cord. The neuropathy is evidenced by symmetric paresthesias with loss of proprioception and vibratory sensation, especially in the lower extremities. Administration of parenteral vitamin B$_{12}$ reverses both the hematologic and neurologic changes in adults. Congenital vitamin B$_{12}$ deficiency, however, produces severe neurologic changes that can only be partially reversed with therapy. The coexisting neuropathy of vitamin B$_{12}$ deficiency must be considered when regional anesthesia or peripheral nerve blocks might be used. The clinical significance of the effects of nitrous oxide on vitamin B$_{12}$ metabolism is controversial. Nitrous oxide inactivates the vitamin B$_{12}$ component of methionine synthetase; certainly, prolonged exposure to nitrous oxide results in megaloblastic anemia and neurologic changes similar to those that occur with pernicious anemia.[259] Relatively short exposures to nitrous oxide have also been reported to produce megaloblastic changes.[260-262] Whether the duration of exposure to nitrous oxide obtained during the course of a normal anesthetic produces such changes in humans has not been established. The issue of nitrous oxide causing postoperative neurologic dysfunction is extremely controversial and case reports of neuropathy linked to intraoperative nitrous oxide exposure have increased in recent years.[263-266] Whether these reports influence the future use of nitrous oxide is not yet clear.

Folic acid deficiency also produces megaloblastic anemia. Although peripheral neuropathy may occur, it is not as common as with vitamin B$_{12}$ deficiency. The administration of folic acid during early pregnancy markedly reduces the risk of neural tube defects in infants.[267] Causes of folic acid deficiency include alcoholism, pregnancy, and malabsorption syndromes. Methotrexate, phenytoin, and ethanol are among the drugs known to interfere with folic acid absorption.

Hemolytic Anemias

The normal life span of an erythrocyte is 120 days. Abnormalities in the erythrocyte, however, may result in the premature destruction of red blood cells (hemolysis). Causes of hemolytic anemia include structural erythrocyte abnormalities, enzyme deficiencies, and immune hemolytic anemias.

Hereditary Spherocytosis

Spherocytosis, elliptocytosis, pyropoikilocytosis, and stomatocytosis are the four types of hereditary red blood cell membrane defects resulting in abnormally shaped red blood cells.

Hereditary spherocytosis is the most common of the red blood cell membrane defects producing hemolysis. Spherocytosis is a disorder of the proteins (spectrin) of the red blood cell cytoskeleton in which the red blood cell is more rounded, more fragile, and more susceptible to hemolysis than the normal, biconcave red blood cell. As a result of this increased fragility, the spleen destroys the abnormal red blood cells and a chronic anemia ensues. Cholelithiasis from chronic hemolysis and elevation of the serum bilirubin occur frequently in patients with hereditary spherocytosis. Patients with hereditary spherocytosis may have hemolytic crises accompanied by anemia, vomiting, and abdominal pain. These crises may be triggered by infection or folic acid deficiency.[268]

Hereditary spherocytosis is treated by splenectomy, which is usually delayed until the patient is 6 years old or older.[269] Splenectomy before that age is associated with a high incidence of bacterial infections, especially those secondary to pneumococcus. Before splenectomy, most patients require a folic acid supplement owing to excessive utilization of folic acid for red blood cell production. Transfusion is rarely necessary for patients with hereditary spherocytosis.

There are no special considerations during anesthesia for patients with hereditary spherocytosis. Preoperative transfusion is not necessary because adequate compensatory mechanisms for chronic anemia have developed in these patients.

Glucose-6-phosphate Dehydrogenase Deficiency

Glucose-6-phosphate dehydrogenase (G6PD) deficiency is the most common enzymopathy in humans and afflicts 400 million people worldwide.[270] An estimated 1% of the African-American male population in the United States is affected by this disorder. African black, Asian, and Mediterranean populations are also susceptible to G6PD deficiency. In patients with G6PD deficiency, G6PD activity decreases by 50% during the 120-day life span of the red blood cell. G6PD initiates the hexose monophosphate shunt. This shunt produces nicotinamide–adenine dinucleotide phosphate (NADPH). Without NADPH, the red blood cell is susceptible to damage by oxidation. A deficiency of G6PD results in decreased levels of reduced glutathione when the red blood cell is exposed to oxidant compounds. This increases the rigidity of the red blood cell membrane and accelerates clearance of these stiff cells from the circulation. In severe forms of G6PD deficiency, oxidation produces denaturation of globin chains and causes intravascular hemolysis.[271]

There are a number of drugs that accentuate the destruction of erythrocytes in patients with G6PD deficiency, including analgesics, antibiotics, sulfonamides, and antimalarials (Table 19-11). There is considerable variability in the hemolytic response to drugs; many drugs (e.g., aspirin) induce hemolysis only in very high doses.[272] Patients with G6PD deficiency are unable to reduce methemoglobin produced by sodium nitrate; therefore, sodium nitroprusside and prilocaine should not be administered. Characteristically, the crisis begins 2–5 days after drug administration. The hemolytic episode is usually self-limited because only the older red blood cells are affected.[273] Bacterial infections can also trigger hemolytic episodes. Presumably, oxi-

dant compounds produced by active white blood cells may hemolyze susceptible red blood cells.

Glutathione synthetase is another enzyme of the hexose monophosphate shunt, and deficiency of this enzyme may also produce anemia.

Anesthetic drugs have not been implicated as hemolytic agents; however, early postoperative evidence of hemolysis might indicate a G6PD deficiency syndrome.

Pyruvate Kinase Deficiency

Pyruvate kinase is a glycolytic enzyme of the Embden-Meyerhof pathway. This pathway converts glucose to lactate and is the primary pathway for adenosine triphosphate synthesis in the red blood cell. A deficiency of pyruvate kinase produces a potassium leak from erythrocytes, increasing their rigidity and enhancing destruction in the spleen. Pyruvate kinase deficiency is responsible for 95% of the deficiency syndromes in the Embden-Meyerhof pathway, whereas deficiency of glucose phosphate isomerase accounts for 4%. Clinically, these patients exhibit anemia, premature cholelithiasis, and splenomegaly. The degree of anemia varies from a very mild anemia that does not require transfusion to a severe, transfusion-dependent anemia. Splenectomy may be beneficial for patients with severe anemia. The clinical features resemble those of patients with spherocytosis. There are no special considerations for anesthesia other than those for any patient with chronic anemia.

Immune Hemolytic Anemia

The immune hemolytic anemias are characterized by immunologic alteration in the red blood cell membrane and are caused by drugs, disease, or erythrocyte sensitization.

There are three types of immune hemolytic anemia: autoimmune hemolysis, drug-induced immune hemolysis, and alloimmune hemolysis (erythrocyte sensitization).[274] Autoimmune hemolytic anemia includes warm and cold antibody hemolytic anemia. Cold autoimmune hemolytic anemia is of special concern to the anesthesiologist because of the likelihood that the cold operating room environment and hypothermia that are used during cardiopulmonary bypass may initiate a hemolytic crisis. Cold hemagglutinin disease is caused by IgM autoantibodies that react with the I antigen of red blood cells.[275] Maintaining a warm environment is essential for prevention of hemolysis.[276] Plasmapheresis to reduce the titer of cold antibody is recommended before hypothermic procedures such as cardiopulmonary bypass. Collagen vascular diseases, neoplasia, and infections produce immune hemolytic anemias by a variety of mechanisms, including warm and cold antibody-mediated hemolysis.

There are three types of drug-induced immune hemolysis: autoantibody type, hapten-induced type, and immune complex type. Hemolysis induced by a response to α-methyldopa is of the autoimmune type mediated by an IgG antibody that does not fix complement. The hapten-induced type is characteristic of the response to penicillin and other antibiotics. The immune complex type of reaction can occur after the administration of quinidine, quinine, sulfonamides, isoniazid, phenacetin, acetaminophen, cephalosporins, tetracycline, hydralazine, and hydrochlorothiazide.

The classic example of alloimmune hemolysis (erythrocyte sensitization) is hemolytic disease of the newborn produced by Rh sensitization. An Rh-negative mother with Rh antibodies produces hemolysis in an Rh-positive fetus. Differences in fetal and maternal ABO groups may also cause hemolysis. This is, however, unusual because A and B antibodies are of the IgM class and do not readily cross the placenta.

Hemoglobinopathies

There are more than 300 different hemoglobinopathies described in the literature. Fortunately, most are quite rare and

---

Table 19-11. DRUGS THAT PRODUCE HEMOLYSIS IN PATIENTS WITH GLUCOSE-6-PHOSPHATE DEHYDROGENASE DEFICIENCY

Phenacetin	Nalidixic acid
Aspirin (high doses)	Isoniazid
Penicillin	Primaquine
Streptomycin	Quinine
Chloramphenicol	Quinidine
Sulfacetamide	Doxorubicin
Sulfanilamide	Methylene blue
Sulfapyridine	Nitrofurantoin

may never be encountered by an anesthesiologist during his or her career. Of the hemoglobinopathies, the most common in the United States are the sickle cell diseases. An estimated 8–10% of African-Americans have the sickle cell trait, and 1 in 400 has sickle cell anemia.

Sickle Cell Disease

Hemoglobin S is a variant hemoglobin produced by substitution of valine for glutamic acid in the sixth position of the β chain. When hemoglobin S deoxygenates, a gel structure is formed that produces structural changes in the red blood cell. The kinetics of the gel formation by hemoglobin S is complex, and factors such as rapidity of deoxygenation may determine how the gel polymerizes and deforms the red blood cell. Low oxygen tension and acidosis exaggerate sickle cell formation. Consequently, any condition that causes a decrease in oxygen tension (*e.g.*, arterial hypoxemia) or decreased blood flow may produce a sickling of red blood cells. Sickling begins at oxygen tensions less than 50 mm Hg and becomes most pronounced when the arterial oxygen tension decreases to 20 mm Hg. Local factors can also influence sickling. Systemic oxygenation may be adequate, but vascular occlusion may produce stasis with localized hypoxemia and initiate sickling. Similarly, if sickling occurs, increasing systemic oxygenation may not reverse the sickling if arteries supplying the area are occluded. It is certainly better to prevent sickling rather than treat it. The likelihood of sickling is directly related to the amount of hemoglobin S in the blood.

The definitive diagnosis of sickle cell disease is made with hemoglobin electrophoresis. This test not only detects hemoglobin S but also reveals any other type of hemoglobin present. Although there are several variants of hemoglobin S disease, the most common are SS (sickle cell anemia), SA (sickle cell trait), SC, and S-thalassemia. In sickle cell anemia, 70–98% of the hemoglobin is S, and the remainder is hemoglobin F (fetal). In patients with SA, 10–40% of the hemoglobin is hemoglobin S. Red blood cells with hemoglobin S and C are less likely to sickle than those with SS, but more likely to sickle than SA cells.

Clinical Manifestations.   The patient with SA usually has a normal life expectancy and few complications with the hemoglobinopathy. Hemoglobin levels are normal, and sickling occurs only under extreme physiologic conditions. Although the risk of anesthesia is small, there have been some reports of death in the perioperative period. Of the 514 patients with SA who received general anesthesia reported in the literature, there have been 5 deaths.[277,278] Not all of the deaths could be attributed to sickle cell trait, however.

Patients with SS are the most severely affected of those with sickle cell hemoglobinopathies. Clinical manifestations include chronic anemia and chronic hemolysis. Infarction of multiple organs is produced by occlusion of vessels with deformed erythrocytes.

There are two patterns of pulmonary complications in patients with sickle cell disease: sickle cell lung disease and acute chest syndrome. Sickle cell lung disease is characterized by generalized pulmonary fibrosis with hypoxemia and ultimately cor pulmonale, which is a significant cause of mortality in patients with SS disease. Sickle cell patients with acute chest syndrome have fever, chest pain, dyspnea, cough, and tachypnea and may suffer acute pulmonary hypertension and death.[279] Cardiac dysfunction, characterized by decreased ventricular filling and reduced ejection fraction, in conjunction with pulmonary disease produces decreased exercise tolerance.[280] Because of the slow blood flow and decreased local oxygen tension, the renal medulla is particularly vulnerable to infarction and necrosis. Papillary necrosis secondary to medullary ischemia occurs frequently, and there is an inability to concentrate urine. Glomerular filtration declines with age and nephrotic syndrome is common.[281] Renal transplantation may be required.[282] By the time the patient with sickle cell anemia is 6 years old, the spleen

is virtually nonexistent because of repeated infarctions. The absence of splenic function increases the patient's vulnerability to bacterial infection. Chronic hemolysis of erythrocytes produces an elevated serum bilirubin level and results in a high incidence of cholelithiasis in patients with SS disease. Repeated cerebral infarction from large cerebral vessel occlusion and hemorrhage can produce neurologic dysfunction.[283] Priapism also occurs with increased frequency in patients with sickle cell disease.

The clinical manifestations of SC disease are intermediate in severity between SA and SS hemoglobinopathies. Anemia is mild, with hemoglobin concentrations of $10–11 \text{ g} \cdot \text{dl}^{-1}$. Sickle cell crises are less common in patients with SC disease than in those with SS. Pulmonary dysfunction secondary to upper respiratory tract infections, pneumonia, and pulmonary embolization is relatively common in patients with SC disease. There are at least 40 other variants of the S hemoglobinopathy, some of which are quite rare. Hemoglobin SA, SS, and SC are the three most frequently encountered variants (Table 19-12).

Treatment.   Although the exact molecular defect of S hemoglobin has been known for 50 years, no definitive or corrective therapy is available. Supportive therapy has improved, increasing survival, so that many patients with SS disease live until their late 40s.

The best therapy is prevention of sickling. Maintenance of good systemic oxygenation and hydration to ensure good tissue perfusion is essential. Transfusion with normal adult hemoglobin (AA) to dilute the hemoglobin S erythrocytes and decrease blood viscosity may be indicated. A variety of techniques aimed at reversing the sickling process have been attempted, but with little success. Because reversal of the sickling process is so difficult, prevention becomes essential. The administration of hydroxyurea has been shown to increase the production of hemoglobin F, which is a potent inhibitor of polymerization of hemoglobin S. Treatment with hydroxyurea has been shown to decrease the frequency and severity of painful crises, the incidence of acute chest syndrome, and the need for transfusion.[284] Bone marrow transplantation and transplantation of cord blood stem cells have also been efficacious.[285,286]

There are three forms of clinical crises in patients with sickle cell anemia: vaso-occlusive (painful) crises, aplastic crises, and splenic sequestration crises. Vaso-occlusive crises are characterized by sickling, venous thrombosis, organ infarction, and severe pain. Pain may be secondary to infarction of bone and muscle.[287] Pain management is an important aspect of the care of patients during a vaso-occlusive crisis. Aplastic crises produce dramatic decreases in erythropoiesis and hematocrit level. Splenic sequestration crises occur in children less than 6 years of age.[288]

Management of Anesthesia.   Because arterial hypoxemia and vascular stasis are powerful stimuli for sickling, it is imperative that the risk of these be minimized during anesthesia and the postoperative period. Patients with sickle cell anemia are at increased risk for perioperative complications including acute chest syndrome, sickling crises, infection, and intractable pain. Optimal perioperative management requires that the anesthesiologist, surgeon, and hematologist interact closely.[289] Surgical diseases that occur with increased frequency in patients with sickle cell anemia include cholelithiasis, peptic ulceration, ischemic colitis, and leg ulcers. Laparoscopic surgical techniques have reduced morbidity in patients with sickle cell disease.[290,291]

Preoperative sedation should not depress ventilation. During surgery and the postoperative period, the inspired oxygen concentration should be increased to maintain or increase the arterial oxygen tension as reflected by continuous monitoring using pulse oximetry. Although regional anesthesia is often used for these patients, the administration of supplemental oxygen may still be indicated. Regional anesthesia may produce compensatory vasoconstriction and decreased oxygen delivery to nonblocked areas, making red blood cells in those areas

Table 19-12. COMMON HEMOGLOBIN S VARIANTS

	Hemoglobin SS	Hemoglobin SC	Hemoglobin SA
Hemoglobin level (g·dl⁻¹)	7–8	9–12	13–15
Life expectancy (years)	30	Slightly reduced	Normal
Propensity for sickling	++++	++	+
Clinical features	Vaso-occlusive crises	Vaso-occlusive crises	Few, under physiologic conditions
	Splenic infarction	Retinal thrombosis	
	Hepatomegaly	Femoral head necrosis	
	Skin ulceration		

vulnerable to sickling. Circulatory stasis can be minimized with adequate hydration and anticipation of intraoperative volume loss to avoid acute hypovolemia. The use of extremity tourniquets is controversial. There are no definitive studies documenting the safety or danger of tourniquet use. Some authors recommend that a tourniquet not be used for patients with hemoglobin S because of the potential dangers, whereas other authors suggest that a tourniquet can be used if it is critical to the success of the operation.[292] The environmental temperature should be controlled to maintain normothermia. Fever increases the rate of gel formation by S hemoglobin. Although hypothermia retards gel formation, the decreased temperature also produces peripheral vasoconstriction. Consequently, normothermia is desirable. Preoperative transfusion to reduce hemoglobin S levels to 30–40% has been demonstrated to reduce perioperative complications in patients with sickle cell anemia.[293,294] The decision for preoperative transfusion will depend upon the patient's preoperative condition and the extent of the surgical procedure. Precise guidelines for preoperative transfusion of the sickle cell patient have not been developed and consultation with a hematologist is helpful.[295] There is evidence that autotransfusion can be used successfully if an exchange transfusion to dilute the number of hemoglobin S red blood cells is performed before anesthesia.[296]

Although inhaled, halogenated anesthetics accelerate precipitation of hemoglobin S *in vitro*, the clinical significance of this finding is not known. Maintenance of perfusion and oxygenation is more critical than is the type of anesthesia. Because of low peripheral blood flow, hypothermia, and acidosis, cardiopulmonary bypass is especially dangerous for patients with sickle cell disease.[297]

Close monitoring of the sickle cell patient during the postoperative period for pulmonary complications and aggressive treatment with supplemental oxygen are necessary as hypoxemia may be the primary trigger of acute chest syndrome.[298] Acute chest syndrome during the early postoperative period produces significant morbidity and mortality. Pain management of the patient with sickle cell disease during a sickling crisis or in the postoperative period can be challenging. A variety of techniques including opioids (morphine), non-narcotic analgesics, and epidural analgesia have been used.[299,300]

Although patients with SA are at less risk than patients with hemoglobin SS, the same perioperative precautions applied to patients with SS should also be used for those with SA. The patient with SC hemoglobin is also at risk during anesthesia and should be treated accordingly.[301]

Thalassemia

Thalassemia represents a number of inherited disorders that result in the production of abnormal globin chains. Although there are four globin chains ($\alpha, \beta, \gamma, \delta$), the α and β thalassemias are the most common. The abnormal globin chains precipitate in the red blood cell, leading to their destruction in the bone marrow and the peripheral blood. The anemia results in increased erythropoietin production, extramedullary erythropoiesis, and splenomegaly.[302] A wide variety of clinical phenotypes

are manifest, from very mild to very severe anemia.[303] β Thalassemia major, or Cooley's anemia, is usually fatal. β Thalassemia minor produces a mild hemolytic anemia and iron deficiency. β Thalassemia intermedia is an intermediate form of thalassemia but usually does not require transfusion. α Thalassemia produces a mild hemolytic anemia. The incidence of thalassemia is highest in the Mediterranean area, the Middle East, India, and Southeast Asia.

Transfusion therapy is essential but often produces iron toxicity with resultant myocardial siderosis, which can markedly reduce ventricular function. Cardiac iron toxicity is a significant cause of mortality in patients with thalassemia. Treatment consists of the administration of iron chelators such as desferrioxamine and deferiprone.[304,305] Hepatic fibrosis as a result of iron toxicity may also occur.

Management of Anesthesia. Anesthetic considerations depend on the severity of the anemia. If the patient is transfusion-dependent, careful evaluation of hepatic and cardiac function is warranted because of the potential for iron toxicity. When an anesthetic is selected, the likelihood of cardiomyopathy and hepatic dysfunction must be considered in addition to the effects of the anemia. Extramedullary hematopoiesis can produce hyperplasia of the facial bones and make direct laryngoscopic examination difficult.[306] Extradural spinal cord compression and massive hemothorax from extramedullary hematopoiesis have been reported in patients with thalassemia.[307,308]

COLLAGEN VASCULAR DISEASES

A number of diseases are classified as the collagen vascular or connective tissue diseases (Table 19-13). The four most common disorders of this group are rheumatoid arthritis, systemic lupus erythematosus (SLE), scleroderma, and polymyositis. Although many such patients can be categorized as having discrete disease syndromes, many others with collagen vascular diseases are considered to have overlap syndromes (also termed mixed connective tissue diseases) with features of different collagen vascular diseases, and cannot be conveniently classified. The etiology of the collagen vascular diseases is unknown, although

Table 19-13. COLLAGEN VASCULAR DISEASES

Rheumatoid arthritis
Lupus
  Systemic lupus erythematosus
  Drug-induced lupus
  Discoid lupus
Scleroderma
  Progressive systemic sclerosis
  CREST syndrome (calcinosis cutis, Raynaud's phenomenon, esophageal dysfunction, sclerodactyly, telangiectasia)
  Focal scleroderma
Polymyositis/dermatomyositis
Overlap syndromes

current theories have implicated the immune system, with pathologic effects on small blood vessels. Although all of these diseases have localized features involving the joints, each has diffuse systemic effects as well. Both the localized and systemic alterations in these patients are significant in the management of anesthesia.

Rheumatoid Arthritis

Rheumatoid arthritis is a chronic inflammatory disease characterized by a symmetric polyarthropathy and significant systemic involvement. Many theories about the etiology of rheumatoid arthritis have been proposed, but none thoroughly explains all the aspects of rheumatoid arthritis. An inflammatory response with complex cell interactions produces destruction of synovial tissue. The initiator of this destructive process may be an antigen that initiates cellular and humoral responses in genetically susceptible individuals. The presence of rheumatoid factor (IgM) in 75% of patients with rheumatoid arthritis and the type of cellular response to inflammation certainly suggests an autoimmune process. However, the inability to identify a single etiology of rheumatoid arthritis suggests multiple etiologies for rheumatoid arthritis that may also include adrenal cortical dysfunction and infection.[309,310] The pathologic changes of rheumatoid arthritis begin with cellular hyperplasia of the synovium, followed by invasion of the synovium by lymphocytes, plasma cells, and fibroblasts. Ultimately, the cartilage and articular surfaces are destroyed.

The hands and wrists are involved first, particularly the metacarpophalangeal and proximal interphalangeal joints. In the lower extremity the knee is involved most frequently. Compression of lower extremity peripheral nerves by the deformed knee can produce paresis and sensory loss over the lower leg. The upper cervical spine may be affected by the arthritic process in nearly 80% of patients with rheumatoid arthritis. Plain radiographs of the cervical spine demonstrate bony changes such as atlantoaxial subluxation and odontoid fracture.[311,312] MRI, however, demonstrates the impact of these bony changes on the spinal cord. Spinal cord impingement may be clearly demonstrated by cervical MRI. The degree of cord compression does not correlate well with the patient's symptoms, and asymptomatic patients may have a high degree of spinal canal stenosis (Fig. 19-4).[313] Although a very rare event, spinal cord damage after laryngoscopy and tracheal intubation has been reported.[314] Intradural spinal cord compression by a rheumatoid nodule has also been reported.[315] Rheumatoid arthritis commonly affects the joints of the larynx, resulting in limitation of vocal cord movement and generalized erythema and edema of the laryngeal mucosa that may progress to airway obstruction.[316-319] In addition to cervical spine and laryngeal changes, arthritic changes in the temporomandibular joint also occur. All of these abnormalities can seriously complicate laryngoscopy and tracheal intubation.

Extra-articular and systemic manifestations of rheumatoid arthritis are diverse (Table 19-14). Pericarditis occurs in nearly one third of patients with rheumatoid arthritis and can produce chronic constrictive pericarditis or pericardial tamponade.[320] Although cardiac tamponade develops in only a small proportion of patients with rheumatoid arthritis, rheumatoid arthritis is more likely to produce tamponade than SLE. Ventricular dysfunction can result from myocarditis and coronary arteritis. Other cardiovascular effects of rheumatoid arthritis include dysrhythmias secondary to development of rheumatoid nodules in the cardiac conduction system, and aortitis, producing aortic root dilation and aortic insufficiency. Pulmonary changes are common and include pleural effusions, pulmonary nodules, interstitial lung disease, obstructive lung disease, and restrictive lung disease.[321] Several of the antirheumatic drugs cause pulmonary dysfunction as well. Renal failure is a common cause of death in patients with rheumatoid arthritis. There are several

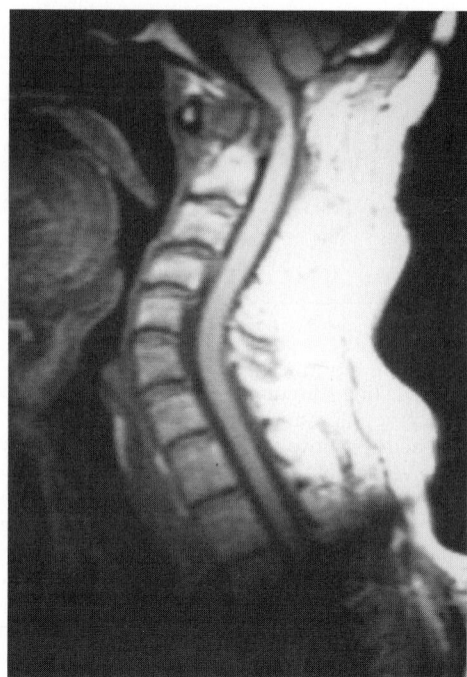

Figure 19-4. Magnetic resonance imaging of the cervical spine in a patient with rheumatoid arthritis. Although the patient had no neurologic symptoms, there is severe spinal stenosis in the upper cervical spine.

causes of renal dysfunction. Renal dysfunction may be secondary to vasculitis, amyloidosis, or drugs used to treat the disease such as analgesics and cyclosporine. There may also be a direct effect of the rheumatoid process that produces subclinical renal dysfunction that is subsequently aggravated by drugs and vasculitis.[322]

Neurologic complications of rheumatoid arthritis include peripheral nerve compression (carpal tunnel syndrome) and cervical nerve root compression. Mononeuritis multiplex is presumed to be caused by deposition of immune complexes in blood vessels supplying the affected nerves. Rheumatoid vasculitis may also affect cerebral blood vessels, producing a cerebral necrotizing vasculitis.[323]

Table 19-14. EXTRA-ARTICULAR MANIFESTATIONS OF RHEUMATOID ARTHRITIS

Skin	**Peripheral Nervous System**
Raynaud's phenomenon	Compression syndromes
Digital necrosis	Mononeuritis
Eyes	**Central Nervous System**
Scleritis	Dural nodules
Corneal ulceration	Necrotizing vasculitis
Lung	**Liver**
Pleural effusion	Hepatitis
Pulmonary fibrosis	
	Blood
Heart	Anemia
Pericarditis	Leukopenia
Cardiac tamponade	
Coronary arteritis	
Aortic insufficiency	
Kidney	
Interstitial fibrosis	
Glomerulonephritis	
Amyloid deposition	

Table 19-15. ADVERSE EFFECTS OF DRUGS USED TO TREAT COLLAGEN VASCULAR DISEASES

Drug	Effects
Corticosteroids	Hypertension
	Osteoporosis
	Fluid retention
	Infection
Aspirin	Platelet dysfunction
	Peptic ulcer
	Hepatic dysfunction
	Hypersensitivity
NSAIDs	Peptic ulcer
	Hypertension
	Hyperglycemia
	Leukopenia
COX-2 inhibitors	Renal dysfunction
Gold	Aplastic anemia
	Dermatitis
	Nephritis
Antimalarials	Myopathy
	Retinopathy
Penicillamine	Glomerulonephritis
	Aplastic anemia
	Myasthenia
Azathioprine	Leukopenia
	Biliary stasis
Cyclophosphamide	Leukopenia
	Hemorrhagic cystitis
	Inhibition of pseudocholinesterase
Cyclosporine	Renal dysfunction
	Hypertension
	Hypomagnesemia
Methotrexate	Hepatotoxicity
	Anemia
	Leukopenia

Mild anemia is present in almost all patients with rheumatoid arthritis. The anemia may be secondary to the rheumatoid process or may result from side effects of drug therapy. Felty's syndrome is the clinical complex of rheumatoid arthritis, leukopenia (<2000 cells $\cdot$ ml^{-1}), and hepatosplenomegaly.

A large number of drugs have been used for the treatment of rheumatoid arthritis. Analgesics and nonsteroidal anti-inflammatory drugs (NSAIDs) such as aspirin, ibuprofen, indomethacin, naproxen, piroxicam, sulindac, and tolmetin have been used extensively. Methotrexate has proved so highly successful as an antirheumatic drug that it is now considered to be a first-line drug. Other drugs known to alter the immune response include hydroxychloroquine, sulfasalazine, azathioprine, penicillamine, cyclosporine, and gold. Newer drugs aimed at modulating the immune response include drugs that inhibit tumor necrosis factor (TNF) (etanercept) and disrupt T-cell proliferation (leflunomide).[324,325] Specific cyclo-oxygenase-2 (COX-2) inhibitors such as celeoxib and rofecoxib have anti-inflammatory and analgesic effects but produce fewer gastrointestinal side effects. Because of the adverse side effects produced by the long-term administration of steroids, treatment with corticosteroids is reserved for those patients who fail to respond to treatment with first- and second-line drugs.[326] Many drugs used for the treatment of rheumatoid arthritis cause anemia, thrombocytopenia, and hepatitis (Table 19-15). Surgical procedures such as synovectomy, tenolysis, and joint replacement are performed to relieve pain and restore joint function.

Management of Anesthesia

Because rheumatoid arthritis is a multisystem disease and the clinical manifestations are so diverse, individualized preoperative evaluation is important in the identification of systems that may be affected.[327]

The joint effects of rheumatoid arthritis, including arthritic changes in the temporomandibular joints, cricoarytenoid joints, and cervical spine can render rigid, direct laryngoscopy and tracheal intubation very difficult.[328] The mobility of these joints should be evaluated before surgery so that a plan for tracheal intubation can be formulated. Because atlantoaxial instability is relatively common, flexion of the neck may compress the spinal cord. Neck pain radiating to the occiput may be the first symptom of cervical spine involvement.[329] Patients with rheumatoid arthritis with symptoms or evidence of cervical cord compression can be fitted with a soft cervical collar preoperatively to minimize the risk of overmanipulation of the neck during surgery.[330] Many patients with rheumatoid arthritis, however, are asymptomatic. Preoperative imaging of the cervical spine (radiography, MRI) may be indicated if the degree of cervical involvement is not known.[331] It is not clear whether routine cervical spine radiography is indicated for elective surgical procedures.[332] Although there have been no documented reports of spinal cord damage in patients with rheumatoid arthritis undergoing tracheal intubation for elective surgery, alleged neurologic damage after laryngoscopy has been the source of litigation against anesthesiologists. Consequently, it is important that any preoperative evidence of neurologic dysfunction be documented before surgery. To minimize the risk of neurologic damage during tracheal intubation, awake fiberoptic laryngoscopy may be the best means of performing tracheal intubation in patients with significant rheumatoid arthritis of the cervical spine. Because many patients with rheumatoid arthritis undergo repeated anesthetics, it is quite helpful if the technique of airway management is clearly documented in the patient's medical record. However, progression of the rheumatoid process may alter joint function to the extent that neck motion may diminish with time and render a previously successful intubation technique useless. Cricoarytenoid arthritis may be recognized by erythema and edema of the vocal cords. Involvement of the cricoarytenoid joints reduces the size of the glottic inlet and necessitates the use of a smaller than predicted tracheal tube. Exaggerated postextubation edema and stridor may also occur.

The degree of cardiopulmonary involvement by the rheumatoid process influences the selection of the type of anesthesia. Functional evaluation of the lungs and heart is necessary if the clinical history suggests dysfunction. It may be difficult to determine if the dysfunction is secondary to rheumatoid arthritis or to more common causes of cardiopulmonary disease such as arteriosclerosis or smoking. The need for postoperative ventilatory support should be anticipated if severe pulmonary disease is present.

Medications that the patient is receiving influence the management of anesthesia. Corticosteroid supplementation may be necessary during the perioperative period. Aspirin and other anti-inflammatory drugs interfere with platelet function, and clotting may be abnormal. Many rheumatoid medications suppress red blood cell formation and anemia is common. Drug-induced hepatic dysfunction may be present, which can influence the choice of anesthesia.

Restriction of joint mobility necessitates careful positioning of the patient during the operation. The extremities should be positioned to minimize the risk of neurovascular compression and additional joint injury. Preoperative evaluation of joint motion helps determine how the extremities should be positioned.

Rheumatoid arthritis is a multisystem disease. The potential joint disabilities have been well documented in the medical literature and are often obvious. More significant and less evident are the effects on the spinal cord, heart, lungs, kidneys, and liver. The type and severity of systemic dysfunction must be considered when planning an anesthetic for the patient with rheumatoid arthritis.[330]

Systemic Lupus Erythematosus

Systemic lupus erythematosus (SLE) is an autoimmune disease with diverse clinical and immunologic manifestations. The precise etiology of SLE is unknown, but appears to be a complex interaction between genetic susceptibility and hormonal and environmental factors.[333] Patients with SLE produce autoantibodies primarily to DNA but also to RNA polymerase, cardiolipin, and ribosomal phosphoproteins.[334] Some of the clinical manifestations of SLE may be a result of the production of an autoantibody highly specific for a single protein within an organ.[335]

The clinical manifestations of SLE are very diverse. The most common presenting features of SLE are polyarthritis and dermatitis. The arthritis is oligoarticular and migratory. The classic malar rash is present in only one third of SLE patients. Renal disease is a common cause of morbidity and mortality in patients with SLE. Proteinuria, hypertension, and decreased creatinine clearance are the usual manifestations of SLE nephritis. Of patients with SLE, 10–20% develop end-stage renal disease and require dialysis or transplantation. Recurrent nephritis in the grafted kidney reduces the success of renal transplant in SLE patients.[336,337] Central nervous system involvement occurs in up to 50% of patients with SLE and is a result of vascular abnormalities. Central nervous system manifestations include seizures, stroke, dementia, psychosis, and peripheral neuropathy.[338] The cranial MRI is an excellent diagnostic technique for SLE brain lesions and may also demonstrate the effects of therapy.[339]

Systemic lupus erythematosus produces a diffuse serositis that manifests as pleuritis and pericarditis. Although 60% of SLE patients have a pericardial effusion, cardiac tamponade is uncommon. Cardiac tamponade may, however, be the presenting symptom of SLE.[340-342] Cardiomyopathy, cardiac conduction abnormalities, reduced ventricular function, and coronary arteritis can occur in patients with SLE.[343] A noninfectious endocarditis (Libman-Sacks endocarditis) often affects mitral valve function and can produce mitral insufficiency. Effective treatment of SLE has improved patient survival, but has increased the likelihood of ischemic heart disease. Pulmonary effects of SLE include pleural effusion, pneumonitis, pulmonary hypertension, and alveolar hemorrhage.[344,345] There is a high correlation of pulmonary hypertension with Raynaud's phenomenon in patients with SLE.[346] Patients with SLE are susceptible to infection, which may present as pneumonitis or adult respiratory distress syndrome. Pulmonary function studies in patients with SLE demonstrate a restrictive lung disease pattern and a decreased diffusion capacity.[347] Patients with SLE may have cricoarytenoid arthritis that can manifest as hoarseness, stridor, or airway obstruction.[348-350]

Nearly one third of patients with SLE have detectable antiphospholipid antibodies and may have thromboembolic complications. Other potentially serious manifestations of SLE include peritonitis, pancreatitis, bowel ischemia, protein-losing enteropathy, and lupoid hepatitis.[351]

There is no specific etiologic therapy for SLE. Despite the diverse effects of SLE and the lack of specific therapy, current regimens have improved survival.[352] Most therapy for SLE is directed at altering T- and B-cell activity with immunosuppressants (corticosteroids) or cytotoxic drugs (cyclophosphamide, azathioprine, cyclosporine). Bone marrow transplantation for the treatment of SLE is under investigation.[353] Nonsteroidal anti-inflammatory drugs (NSAIDs) are the first line treatment for arthritis; however, these drugs can cause renal dysfunction. The antimalarials, hydroxychloroquine and chloroquine, are administered for the treatment of arthritis if treatment with NSAIDs is unsatisfactory. The antimalarials may alter lysosome function and interfere with the induction of autoimmunity.[354] An individual patient's therapy will depend upon the severity of the disease and the specific organ system affected. Therapeutic

regimens for SLE change frequently and continue to develop.[355] The potential for side effects from any of the drugs used for the treatment of SLE is significant and treatment can result in morbidity.[356]

Drug-induced lupus may be caused by procainamide, quinidine, hydralazine, methyldopa, captopril, enalapril, clonidine, isoniazid, or minocycline. Drug-induced lupus may be caused by reactive drug metabolites and autoreactive T cells.[357] The clinical manifestations of drug-induced lupus are generally mild and include arthralgia, fever, anemia, and leukopenia. These effects typically resolve within 4 weeks of discontinuation of the drug, although some patients have significant morbidity.[358]

Management of Anesthesia

Careful preoperative evaluation of the patient with SLE is necessary because of the diverse systemic effects of the disease. Signs and symptoms of cardiopulmonary dysfunction must be recognized preoperatively.[359] Preoperative chest radiography, echocardiography, or pulmonary function testing may be necessary if the clinical history suggests dysfunction. Anesthesia management is influenced not only by the degree of organ dysfunction, but also by the drugs used to treat SLE. Although there are no specific contraindications to a particular type of anesthetic, myocardial dysfunction will certainly influence the choice of anesthetic agents and types of intraoperative monitors. It has been demonstrated that patients with SLE are at risk for postoperative infections and pulmonary complications.[360] Because renal dysfunction is so common in patients with SLE, renal function should be quantified preoperatively if there is any suggestion of a recent change in renal function. Although minor abnormalities in liver function are present in many patients with SLE, these changes are not usually significant. However, a fatal lupoid hepatitis, characterized by prolonged jaundice, hyperglobulinemia, and hepatosplenomegaly, develops in some patients.

Arthritic involvement of the cervical spine is unusual in patients with SLE. Consequently, tracheal intubation is not usually difficult. However, the potential for laryngeal involvement and upper airway obstruction requires clinical evaluation of laryngeal function.[361] Should postextubation laryngeal edema or stridor occur, the intravenous administration of corticosteroids is effective for alleviation of symptoms.

Drugs administered to the patient for treatment of SLE may also influence the management of anesthesia. Patients receiving corticosteroids may require intraoperative administration of corticosteroids. Cyclophosphamide inhibits plasma cholinesterase and may produce a prolonged response to succinylcholine or mivacurium.

Scleroderma

Scleroderma (systemic sclerosis) is an autoimmune collagen vascular disease affecting the skin, joints, and visceral organs. Vascular endothelium is damaged by autoantibodies to endothelial cells or immune mediators, resulting in increased vascular permeability, leakage of serum proteins, lymphatic obstruction, and ultimately tissue fibrosis. The fibrotic process is accelerated by an increase in collagen production.[362,363] This widespread reactivity explains the diverse clinical manifestations of scleroderma. The manifestations are observed most readily in the skin, which becomes thickened and swollen. Eventually, the skin becomes atrophic and small arteries are obliterated. The skin becomes fibrotic and taut and produces severe restriction of joint mobility. Raynaud's phenomenon is the presenting feature of 70% of patients with scleroderma. Vasospasm occurs in blood vessels that are already narrowed by intimal proliferation and fibrosis.[364]

The same pathologic process that affects the vascular system in the skin affects small blood vessels in other organs as well. Lung involvement occurs in 80% of patients with scleroderma and is characterized by interstitial fibrosis, pulmonary hypertension, and an impaired diffusing capacity.[365] These changes, in conjunction with the effects of chronic aspiration pneumonitis, produce a restrictive lung disease. Treatment of the pulmonary effects of scleroderma include supplemental oxygen, vasodilators, captopril, and immunosuppressants.[366] Myocardial fibrosis occurs in 70–80% of patients with scleroderma, although only 25% have clinical symptoms. Patients with clinical cardiac symptoms have a very poor prognosis.[367,368] Degeneration of contractile myocardium and conducting tissue results in decreased contractility and cardiac dysrhythmias.[369] The administration of nifedipine to patients with myocardial involvement from scleroderma may improve myocardial perfusion and performance. Pericarditis with effusion is very common in patients with scleroderma.[370]

Renal dysfunction is relatively common in patients with scleroderma. This dysfunction is secondary to pathologic changes in the renal vasculature similar to the changes in the digital arteries that produce Raynaud's phenomenon. Renal dysfunction can be so severe that a scleroderma renal crisis develops with hypertension, retinopathy, and a rapid deterioration in renal function.

Gastrointestinal motility is decreased and is very pronounced in the esophagus. The frequent episodes of gastroesophageal reflux and aspiration pneumonitis exacerbate pulmonary dysfunction.[371] Cimetidine is very effective for the treatment of epigastric pain secondary to hyperacidity. Although metoclopramide increases esophageal motility, the high incidence of side effects from metoclopramide limits its usefulness for chronic administration. Involvement of the colon and small intestine may result in pseudo-obstruction.[372]

Currently, therapy for scleroderma is limited to the relief of specific organ dysfunction, generalized immunosuppression (cyclophosphamide, cyclosporine, prednisone), and decreasing collagen production (penicillamine, interferon). Although the administration of these drugs may produce some improvement, it also introduces the risk of significant side effects.

Management of Anesthesia

Scleroderma, like other collagen vascular diseases, is a multiorgan disease with many systemic manifestations. Consequently, the altered organ systems must be thoroughly evaluated so that a logical plan for anesthesia can be selected. There are no specific contraindications to the use of any type of anesthesia, although the selection must be guided by the degree of organ dysfunction.

Tracheal intubation can be quite difficult.[373] Fibrotic and taut facial skin can markedly hinder active and passive mouth opening and severely restrict mobility of the temporomandibular joints. Awake flexible fiberoptic laryngoscopy and tracheal intubation may be required; tracheostomy may be necessary in severely affected patients.[374] Orotracheal intubation is preferable to nasotracheal intubation because of the fragility of the nasal mucosa and the propensity for severe nasal hemorrhage.

The patient with scleroderma is at risk for aspiration pneumonitis during the induction of anesthesia owing to the high incidence of gastroesophageal reflux. Appropriate measures to minimize the risk of acid aspiration, such as the use of histamine-2 blockers and oral antacids, may be indicated.

Chronic arterial hypoxemia is often present because of restriction of lung expansion and impaired oxygen diffusion. Consequently, controlled mechanical ventilation with an increased inspired oxygen concentration is usually necessary. Compromised myocardial function and decreased coronary vascular reserve often necessitate the use of invasive cardiovascular monitoring because the response to inhaled anesthetics may be exaggerated. Venous access can be difficult and a venous cutdown or central venous catheterization may be necessary. Muscle involvement may increase the sensitivity to muscle relaxants and short-acting neuromuscular blockers should be used.

Regional anesthesia may be administered to patients with scleroderma, although there are reports of prolonged responses to local anesthetics.[376,377] The anesthesiologist is often consulted as to the efficacy of sympathetic blockade for the treatment of vasospasm secondary to Raynaud's phenomenon. Stellate ganglion block may, however, produce deleterious effects on contralateral blood flow in patients with scleroderma.[378] Long-term intrathecal pain management can be helpful for intractable ischemic limb pain.[379]

Polymyositis/Dermatomyositis

Polymyositis is a noninfectious inflammatory myopathy affecting skeletal muscle. Dermatomyositis is a type of inflammatory myopathy associated with a characteristic skin rash. The other type of inflammatory myopathy is inclusion body myopathy. Pathologically, the myopathic processes in these three diseases are different. Polymyositis is a cell-mediated immune response against muscle fibers. Cytotoxic T cells enter muscle cells and destroy the muscle fiber. Muscle from patients with polymyositis reveals inflammation and fatty replacement. In dermatomyositis, a complement-mediated reaction attacks and destroys endomysial capillaries, resulting in muscle ischemia and muscle cell death.[380]

Common presenting symptoms of polymyositis are muscle pain, tenderness, and proximal muscle weakness. Patients with dermatomyositis have a skin rash characterized by a purplish discoloration of the eyelids (heliotrope rash), periorbital edema, erythematous lesions on the knuckles, and a sun-sensitive erythematous rash on the face, neck, and chest.[381] Although the pathogenic processes of polymyositis and dermatomyositis are different, the changes in the lungs and heart produced by these two diseases are similar. Of patients with polymyositis or dermatomyositis, 50% have evidence of pulmonary disease, including interstitial lung disease, bronchopneumonia, and alveolitis. Aspiration pneumonitis is one of the most common complications of polymyositis and undoubtedly contributes to the pathologic changes in the lungs.[382] These changes produce a restrictive lung disease pattern and decreased diffusing capacity.[383,384] Myocardial fibrosis can result in congestive heart failure and cardiac dysrhythmias.[385–387]

The most effective treatment for polymyositis and dermatomyositis is the administration of corticosteroids. Patients that do not respond to corticosteroids are treated with immunosuppressants such as methotrexate, azathioprine, cyclosporine, or chlorambucil. Antimalarials may be effective for treatment of the skin rash associated with dermatomyositis.[388,389] Immunoglobulin therapy and total body irradiation have been recommended for patients resistant to other forms of therapy.

Management of Anesthesia

Mobility of the temporomandibular joints and cervical spine is usually adequate in patients with polymyositis. However, some patients have restricted mobility that can make direct laryngoscopy difficult. Adequate mouth and neck mobility must be ascertained before induction of anesthesia. Awake flexible fiberoptic laryngoscopy and tracheal intubation may be required for those patients with restricted neck mobility and inadequate mouth opening.

Dysphagia and gastroesophageal reflux are very common and there is an increased likelihood of aspiration pneumonitis.[390] Appropriate precautions to avoid aspiration of gastric contents should be taken during the perioperative period. Gastrointestinal perforations, which necessitate surgery, are relatively common in patients with polymyositis.[391]

Although the typical electromyographic changes of polymyositis suggest the potential for hyperkalemia after succinylcholine, succinylcholine has been administered to patients with polymyositis without complication.[392] Prolonged neuromuscular blockade has been reported after the administration of vecuronium in a patient with polymyositis.[393] This prolonged response may be secondary to the myopathy or an interaction between the nondepolarizing muscle relaxant and immunosuppressants.[394] The reported experience with anesthesia for patients with polymyositis and dermatomyositis is very limited, and generalizations from a few case reports must be interpreted with caution. It should be anticipated that considerable individual variation in response to muscle relaxants will occur. It would seem prudent to avoid the administration of succinylcholine if possible, and to use shorter-acting muscle relaxants such as mivacurium or rapacuronium. Because of the preoperative muscle weakness, postoperative ventilatory support may be necessary.

The degree of cardiopulmonary dysfunction influences the choice of anesthesia and selection of intraoperative monitors. Further preoperative evaluation of cardiopulmonary function may be required if the clinical history suggests a deterioration in cardiac or pulmonary function.

SKIN DISORDERS

Most primary diseases of the skin are localized and cause few systemic effects or complications during the administration of anesthesia. Two skin disorders, however, can result in complications during anesthesia—the blistering diseases, epidermolysis bullosa and pemphigus.

Epidermolysis Bullosa

Epidermolysis bullosa is a rare skin disorder that may be inherited or acquired. Patients with heritable forms have an abnormal collagen that is insufficient in anchoring different skin layers together.[395] The acquired forms are autoimmune disorders in which autoantibodies are produced that destroy the basement membrane of the skin and mucosa.[396] Regardless of the etiology, the end result is the loss or absence of normal intercellular bridges and separation of skin layers (Fig. 19-5). The separation of the skin layers results in intradermal fluid accumulation and bullae formation. Even minor skin trauma produces skin blisters. Lateral shearing forces applied to the skin are especially damaging because of skin separation. Pressure applied perpendicular to the surface of the skin is not as hazardous.

Although there are 25 subtypes of epidermolysis bullosa, these disorders can be conveniently categorized into three groups depending on where the actual skin separation occurs: epidermolytic (epidermolysis simplex), junctional, and dermolytic (epidermolysis bullosa dystrophica).[397] Although serious complications from skin and mucosal loss can occur with any form of epidermolysis, the simplex form is generally benign. Patients with the junctional form rarely survive beyond early childhood. Laryngeal involvement is unusual, but is most likely to occur with the junctional type.[398,399]

Epidermolysis bullosa dystrophica produces severe scarring of the fingers and toes, with pseudosyndactyly formation and underlying bone deformities such as ankylosis of the interphalangeal joints and resorption of the metacarpals and metatarsals (Fig. 19-6). Involvement of the esophageal mucosa is present in most patients, resulting in dysphagia and esophageal strictures that contribute to poor nutrition.[400] Anemia and hypoalbuminemia from chronic infection and malnutrition are common. Secondary infection of bullae with *Staphylococcus aureus* or β-hemolytic streptococci is common. Severe anemia and cardiomyopathy develop as a result of malnutrition.[401,402] Mitral valve prolapse has also been reported in patients with epidermolysis bullosa.[403]

Glomerulonephritis may be secondary to streptococcal infection. Albumin loss secondary to nephritis, in combination with albumin loss into bullous skin lesions, can produce hypovolemia that further impairs renal function.[404] In addition to chronic skin infection, there is an increased propensity to neoplastic degeneration. Hypoplasia of tooth enamel results in carious degeneration of the teeth and the need for extensive dental restorations. Other diseases associated with epidermolysis bullosa include porphyria cutanea tarda, amyloidosis, multiple myeloma, diabetes mellitus, and hypercoagulation. Patients with epidermolysis bullosa rarely survive beyond the third decade of life.

Medical therapy for epidermolysis bullosa has not been very successful. Corticosteroids have been used without much benefit. Phenytoin, which inhibits collagenase, may produce a favorable response in some patients, but long-term studies have not been encouraging.[405] Surgical therapy is directed at preserving and improving hand function.

Management of Anesthesia

It is critical that trauma to the skin and mucous membranes be avoided or minimized in patients with epidermolysis bullosa.

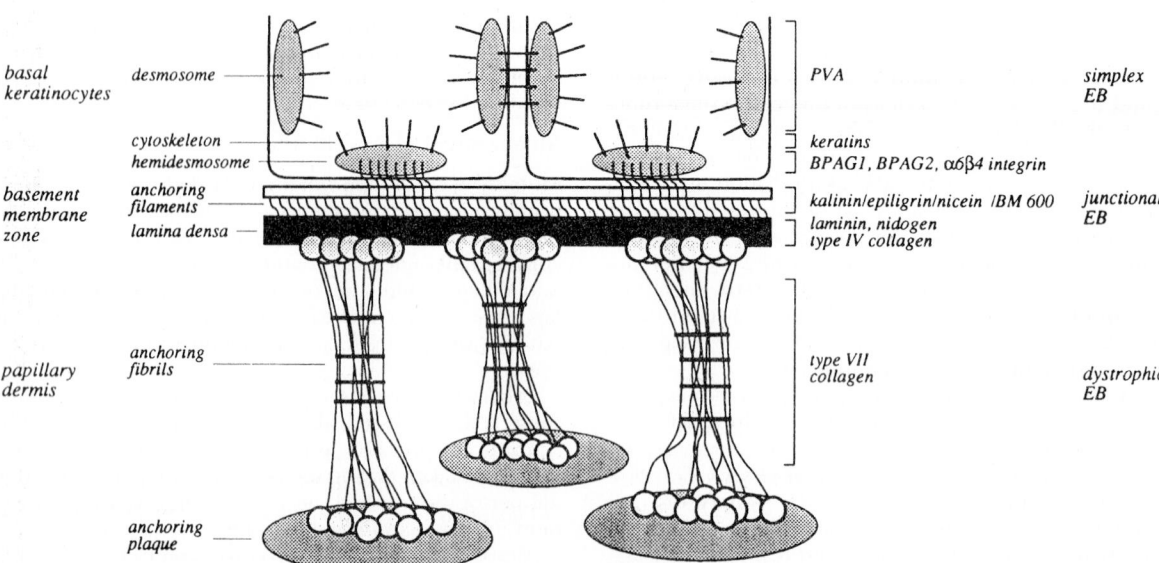

Figure 19-5. The ultrastructure of the zones of the skin. The diagram demonstrates where skin separation occurs in the different types of epidermolysis bullosa. (Reproduced with permission from Uitto J, Christiano AM: Molecular genetics of the cutaneous basement membrane zone. J Clin Invest 90:687, 1992; copyright of the American Society for Clinical Investigation.)

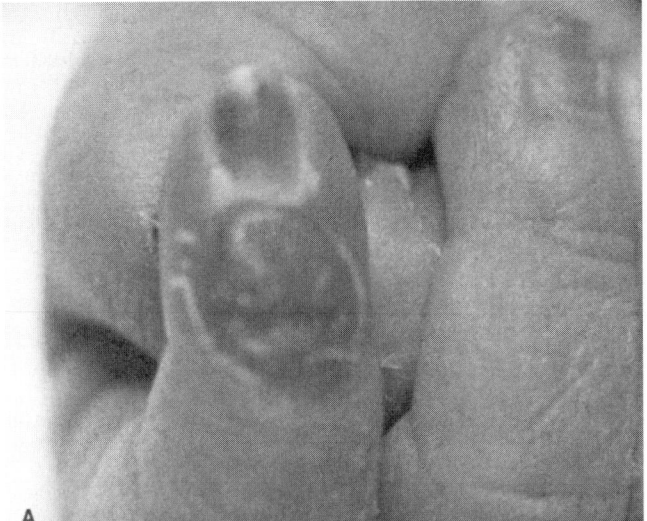

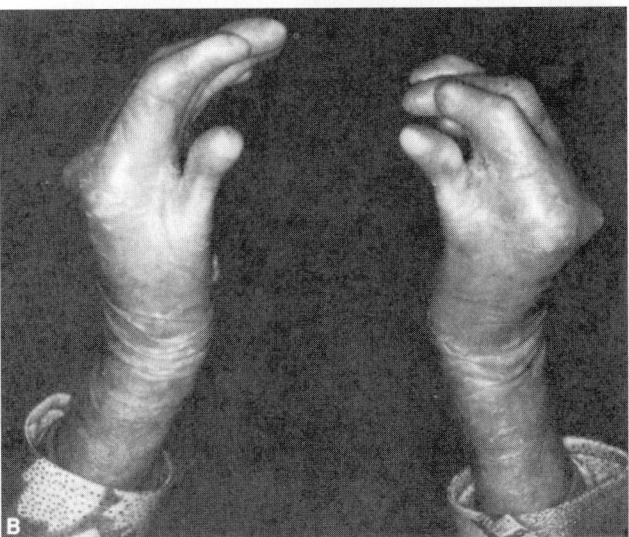

Figure 19-6. Epidermolysis bullosa. (*A*) Bullous lesion of the finger of a neonate with epidermolysis. (*B*) Hands of an older child with epidermolysis showing progression to produce severe scarring and pseudosyndactyly. (Courtesy of James E. Bennett, M.D., Division of Plastic Surgery, Indiana University School of Medicine, Indianapolis, IN.)

Trauma from adhesive tape, blood pressure cuffs, tourniquets, and adhesive ECG electrodes can cause bullae formation.[406] The blood pressure cuff must be padded with a loose cotton dressing. Intravascular catheters should be anchored with sutures or a gauze dressing rather than adhesive tape. Trauma from a face mask may be reduced by gentle application against the skin. Lubrication of the mask and the patient's face can be quite helpful for reducing trauma. Use of upper airway instruments, including oropharyngeal and nasopharyngeal airways, should be kept to a minimum because squamous epithelium lining the oropharynx and esophagus is susceptible to bullous formation. Frictional trauma to the oropharynx may result in formation of large intraoral bullae, airway obstruction, and extensive hemorrhage from denuded mucosa.[407,408]

Laryngeal involvement in patients with epidermolysis bullosa is extremely rare. However, when tracheal intubation is performed, the laryngoscope and tracheal tube should be well lubricated to reduce friction against the oropharyngeal mucosa.[409] Scarring of the oral cavity can produce microstomia and immobility of the tongue, which increases the difficulty of tracheal intubation.[410,411] Flexible, fiberoptic laryngoscopy may be required.[412] Insertion of an esophageal stethoscope should

be avoided because it may lead to the formation of intraoral and esophageal bullae. Although the safety of tracheal intubation has been established for patients with the dystrophic form of epidermolysis bullosa, it has not yet been established for infants with the junctional form. The junctional form affects all mucosa, including the respiratory epithelium.[413] However, the types of surgical procedures (intra-abdominal) required in infants with the junctional form, usually mandate tracheal intubation.

Surgical procedures for patients with epidermolysis bullosa are usually peripheral and involve the hands. Ketamine is very useful for anesthesia for such superficial procedures because it provides good analgesia and usually does not require supplemental inhalation anesthesia. There are, however, no contraindications to inhalation anesthesia. Regional anesthesia, including spinal, epidural, and brachial plexus anesthesia, has been used successfully for patients with epidermolysis bullosa.[414,415]

Porphyria cutanea tarda, often associated with epidermolysis bullosa, does not have the same implications for anesthesia as acute intermittent porphyria.

Despite all the potential complications with anesthesia for patients with epidermolysis bullosa, appropriate intraoperative management is associated with surprisingly few complications.[416]

Pemphigus

Pemphigus is a vesiculobullous disease that may involve extensive areas of the skin and mucous membranes. Pemphigus is an autoimmune disease, as evidenced by the finding that patients with pemphigus have circulating antibodies that bind to the surface of epithelial cells. These autoantibodies are highly specific and result in the excessive production of proteolytic enzymes that disrupt cell adhesion, leading to separation of epithelial layers. Drugs such as penicillamine, captopril, phenobarbital, piroxicam, propranolol, levodopa, and cephalosporins can cause a drug-induced pemphigus.[417]

There are several types of pemphigus including pemphigus vulgaris, pemphigus foliaceus, pemphigus vegetans, pemphigus erythematosus, and paraneoplastic pemphigus. Pemphigus vulgaris is the most common type and the most clinically significant for the anesthesiologist because of the occurrence of oral lesions. Oral lesions occur in 50–70% of patients with pemphigus vulgaris and usually precede the onset of skin lesions. Lesions of the pharynx, larynx, esophagus, conjunctiva, urethra, cervix, and anus can develop.[418] Extensive oropharyngeal lesions may make eating painful to the extent that malnutrition occurs. Skin denudation and bullae formation can result in significant fluid and protein losses and the risk of secondary bacterial infection is great. As with epidermolysis bullosa, lateral shearing forces are more likely to produce bullae than pressure exerted perpendicular to the skin surface. Treatment with corticosteroids and immunosuppressants is highly effective. The administration of immunosuppressants such as azathioprine, cyclophosphamide, methotrexate, and mycophenolate reduces the risk of steroid-induced side effects.[419]

Paraneoplastic pemphigus is an autoimmune disease associated with a number of malignant tumors, especially lymphomas and leukemias. IgG autoantibodies are produced that react with desmosomal proteins. Some patients with paraneoplastic pemphigus develop fatal bronchiolitis obliterans and respiratory failure.[420,421]

Pemphigus foliaceus (superficial pemphigus) is a less severe form of pemphigus in which skin separation occurs near the epidermal surface; the oral mucosa is not affected. Pemphigus foliaceus can be fatal if untreated. Pemphigus vegetans is histologically similar to pemphigus vulgaris and involves the axillae, groin, skin flexures, and the oral cavity. Pemphigus erythematosus (Senear-Usher syndrome) is a superficial form of pemphigus with erythematous hyperkeratotic lesions over the nose and malar areas; the oral cavity is not involved.

Management of Anesthesia

Preoperative drug therapy and the extreme fragility of the mucous membranes are the primary concerns for the management of anesthesia in patients with pemphigus. Corticosteroid supplementation will be necessary during the preoperative period. Management of the upper airway and tracheal intubation should be performed as described for patients with epidermolysis bullosa. Ketamine and regional anesthesia have been used successfully for patients with pemphigus.[422-424]

There are no specific contraindications to the use of any inhaled or intravenous anesthetic; however, potential side effects of treatment drugs and interactions with anesthetics must be considered. For example, methotrexate produces hepatorenal dysfunction and bone marrow suppression, and cyclophosphamide may prolong the effect of succinylcholine and mivacurium by inhibiting cholinesterase activity.

REFERENCES

1. Ozawa E, Hagiwara Y, Yoshida M: Creatine kinase, cell membrane and Duchenne muscular dystrophy. Mol Cell Biochem 190:143, 1999
2. Brown RH: Dystrophin-associated proteins and the muscular dystrophies. Annu Rev Med 48:457, 1997
3. Metzinger L, Blake DJ, Squier MV et al: Dystrophin deficiency at the sarcolemma of patients with muscular dystrophy. Hum Mol Genet 6:1185, 1997
4. Staiano A, Giudice ED, Roman A et al: Upper gastrointestinal tract motility in children with progressive muscular dystrophy. J Pediatr 121:720, 1999
5. Bensen ES, Jaffe KM, Tarr PI: Acute gastric dilatation in Duchenne muscular dystrophy: A case report and review of the literature. Arch Phys Med Rehab 77:512, 1996
6. Backman E, Nylander E: The heart in Duchenne muscular dystrophy: A progressive longitudinal study. Eur Heart J 13:1239, 1992
7. Yotsakura M, Miyagawa M, Tsuya T et al: A 10 year follow-up study by orthogonal Frank lead ECG in patients with progressive dystrophy of the Duchenne type. J Electrocardiol 25:345, 1992
8. Sasaki K, Sakata K, Kachi E et al: Sequential changes in cardiac structure and function in patients with Duchenne type muscular dystrophy: A two-dimensional echocardiographic study. Am Heart J 135:937, 1998
9. Ishikawa Y, Bach JR, Minami R: Cardioprotection for Duchenne's muscular dystrophy. Am Heart J 137:895, 1999
10. Hoogerwaard EM, de Voogt WG, Wilde AAM et al: Evolution of cardiac abnormalities in Becker muscular dystrophy over a 13 year period. J Neurol 244:657, 1997
11. Negri SM, Cowan MD: Becker muscular dystrophy with bundle branch reentry ventricular tachycardia. J Cardiovasc Electrophysiol 9:652, 1998
12. Ducceshi V, Nigro G, Sarubbi B et al: Autonomic nervous system imbalance and left ventricular systolic dysfunction as potential candidates for arrhythmogenesis in Becker muscular dystrophy. Int J Cardiol 59:275, 1997
13. Emery AEH: The muscular dystrophies. Br Med J 317:991, 1998
14. Fishbein MC, Siegel RJ, Thompson CE et al: Sudden death of a carrier of X-linked Emery-Dreifuss muscular dystrophy. Ann Intern Med 119:900, 1993
15. Cartegni L, di Barletta MR, Barresi R et al: Heart specific localization of emerin: New insights into Emery-Dreifuss muscular dystrophy. Hum Mol Gen 6:2257, 1997
16. Duggan DJ, Gorospe JR, Fanin M et al: Mutations in the sarcoglycan genes in patients with myopathy. N Engl J Med 336:618, 1997
17. Van der Kooi AJ, de Voogt WG, Barth PG et al: The heart in limb girdle muscular dystrophy. Heart 79:73, 1998
18. Ng W, Lau C-P: Cardiac arrhythmias as presenting symptoms in patients with limb girdle muscular dystrophy. Int J Cardiol 59:157, 1997
19. Laforet P, de Toma C, Eymard B et al: Cardiac involvement in genetically confirmed facioscapulohumeral muscular dystrophy. Neurology 51:1454, 1998
20. Tiomny E, Khilkevic O, Korczyn AD et al: Esophageal smooth muscle dysfunction in oculopharyngeal muscular dystrophy. Digest Dis Sci 48:1350, 1996
21. Voit T: Congenital muscular dystrophies: 1997 update. Brain Dev 20:65, 1998
22. Larach MG, Rosenberg H, Gronert GA, Allen GC: Hyperkalemic cardiac arrest during anesthesia in infants and children with occult myopathies. Clin Ped 36:9, 1997
23. Kunst G, Graf BM, Scheiner R et al: Differential effects of sevoflurane, isoflurane, and halothane on Ca^{2+} release from the sarcoplasmic reticulum of skeletal muscle. Anesthesiology 91:179, 1999
24. Wang JM, Stanley TH: Duchenne muscular dystrophy and malignant hyperthermia: Two case reports. Can Anaesth Soc J 33:492, 1986
25. Patel V, Dierdorf SF, Krishna G et al: Negative halothane-caffeine contracture test in mdx (dystrophin-deficient) mice. Metabolism 40:883, 1991
26. Mader N, Gilly H, Bittner RE: Dystrophin deficient mdx muscle is not prone to MH susceptibility: An in vitro study. Br J Anaesth 79:125, 1997
27. Ririe DG, Shapiro F, Sethna NF: The response of patients with Duchenne's muscular dystrophy to neuromuscular blockade with vecuronium. Anesthesiology 88:351, 1998
28. Uslu M, Mellinghof H, Diefenbach C: Mivacurium for muscle relaxation in a child with Duchenne's muscular dystrophy. Anesth Analg 89:340, 1999
29. Nitahara K, Sakuragi T, Matsuyama M et al: Response to vecuronium in a patient with facioscapulohumeral muscular dystrophy. Br J Anaesth 83:499, 1999
30. Ptacek LJ, Johnson KJ, Griggs RC: Genetics and physiology of the myotonic muscle disorders. N Engl J Med 328:482, 1993
31. Moxley RT: The myotonias: Their diagnosis and treatment. Comp Ther 22:8, 1996
32. Streib EW: Successful treatment with tocainide of recessive generalized myotonia. Ann Neurol 19:501, 1986
33. Ueda H, Shimokawa M, Yamamoto M et al: Decreased expression of myotonic dystrophy protein kinase and disorganization of sarcoplasmic reticulum in skeletal muscle of myotonic dystrophy. J Neurol Sci 162:38, 1999
34. Fragola PV, Calo L, Luzi M et al: Doppler echocardiographic assessment of diastolic function in myotonic dystrophy. Cardiology 88:498, 1997
35. Phillips MF, Harper PS: Cardiac disease in myotonic dystrophy. Cardiovasc Res 33:13, 1997
36. Merino JL, Carmona JR, Fernandez-Lozano J et al: Mechanisms of sustained ventricular tachycardia in myotonic dystrophy. Circulation 98:541, 1998
37. Streib EW, Meyers DG, Sun SF: Mitral valve prolapse in myotonic dystrophy. Muscle Nerve 8:650, 1985
38. Jammes Y, Pouget J, Grimaud C et al: Pulmonary function and electromyographic study of respiratory muscles in myotonic dystrophy. Muscle Nerve 8:586, 1985
39. Ververs CCM, Van der Meche FGA, Verbraak AFM et al: Breathing pattern awake and asleep in myotonic dystrophy. Respiration 63:1, 1996
40. Fitting J-W, Leuenberger P: Procainamide for dyspnea in myotonic dystrophy. Am Rev Resp Dis 140:1442, 1989
41. Hannon VM, Cunningham AJ, Hutchinson M et al: Aspiration pneumonia and coma: An unusual presentation of dystrophica myotonia. Can Anaesth Soc J 33:803, 1986
42. Fall LH, Young WN, Power JA et al: Severe congestive heart failure and cardiomyopathy as a complication of myotonic dystrophy in pregnancy. Obstet Gynecol 76:481, 1990
43. Cope DK, Miller JN: Local and spinal anesthesia for cesarean section in a patient with myotonic dystrophy. Anesth Analg 65:687, 1986
44. Abe K, Matsuo Y, Kadekawa J et al: Respiratory training for patients with myotonic dystrophy. Neurology 51:641, 1998
45. Sugino M, Ohsawa N, Ito T et al: A pilot study of dehydroepiandrosterone sulfate in myotonic dystrophy. Neurology 51:586, 1998
46. Sermon K, Lissens W, Joris H et al: Clinical application of preimplantation diagnosis for myotonic dystrophy. Prenatal Diagnosis 17:925, 1997
47. Keller C, Reynolds A, Lee B et al: Congenital myotonic dystrophy requiring prolonged endotracheal intubation and noninvasive assisted ventilation: Not a uniformly fatal condition. Pediatrics 101:704, 1998
48. Streib EW: Hypokalemic periodic paralysis in two patients with paramyotonia congenita (PC) and known hyperkalemic/exercise-induced weakness. Muscle Nerve 12:936, 1989

49. Ricker K: Myotonic dystrophy and proximal myotonic myopathy. J Neurol 246:334, 1999
50. Russell SH, Hirsch NP: Anaesthesia and myotonia. Br J Anaesth 72:210, 1994
51. Mitchell MM, Ali HH, Savarese JJ: Myotonia and neuromuscular blocking agents. Anesthesiology 49:44, 1978
52. Nightengale P, Healy TEJ, McGuinness K: Dystrophica myotonia and atracurium. Br J Anaesth 57:1131, 1985
53. Stirt JA, Stone DJ, Weinberg G et al: Atracurium in a child with myotonic dystrophy. Anesth Analg 64:369, 1985
54. Buzello W, Kreig N, Schlickewei A: Hazards of neostigmine in patients with neuromuscular disorders. Br J Anaesth 54:529, 1982
55. Ogawa K, Iranami H, Yoshiyama T et al: Severe respiratory depression after epidural morphine in a patient with myotonic dystrophy. Can J Anaesth 40:968, 1993
56. Aldridge LM: Anaesthetic problems in myotonic dystrophy. Br J Anaesth 57:1119, 1985
57. Mathieu J, Allard P, Gobeil G et al: Anesthetic and surgical complications in 219 cases of myotonic dystrophy. Neurology 49:1646, 1997
58. White DA, Smyth DG: Continuous infusion of propofol in dystrophica myotonia. Can J Anaesth 36:200, 1989
59. Speedy H: Exaggerated physiological responses to propofol in myotonic dystrophy. Br J Anaesth 64:110, 1990
60. Bouly A, Nathan N, Feiss P: Propofol in myotonic dystrophy. Anaesthesia 46:705, 1991
61. Ishizawa Y, Yamaguchi H, Dohi S et al: A serious complication due to gastrointestinal malfunction in a patient with myotonic dystrophy. Anesth Analg 65:1066, 1986
62. Jaffe R, Mock M, Abramowicz J et al: Myotonic dystrophy and pregnancy: A review. Obstet Gynecol Surv 41:272, 1986
63. Paterson RA, Tousignant M, Skene SD: Cesarean section for twins in a patient with myotonic dystrophy. Can Anaesth Soc J 32:418, 1990
64. Cherng Y-G, Wang Y-P, Liu C-C et al: Combined spinal and epidural anesthesia for abdominal hysterectomy in a patient with myotonic dystrophy. Reg Anesth 19:69, 1994
65. Blumgart CH, Hughes DG, Redfern N: Obstetric anaesthesia in dystrophica myotonia. Anaesthesia 45:26, 1990
66. Cannon SC: Sodium channel defects in myotonia and periodic paralysis. Annu Rev Neurosci 19:141, 1996
67. Ptacek L: The familial periodic paralyses and nondystrophic myotonias. Am J Med 104:58, 1998
68. Rosen CA, Thomas JP, Anderson D: Bilateral vocal cord paralysis caused by familial hypokalemic periodic paralysis. Otolaryngol Head Neck Surg 120:785, 1999
69. Ebeid MR, Baquero JL, Gelband H: Periodic paralysis and ventricular tachycardia: Possible role of calcium channel blockers. Pediatr Cardiol 17:31, 1996
70. Dalakas MC, Engel WK: Treatment of "permanent" muscle weakness in familial hypokalemic periodic paralysis. Muscle Nerve 6:182, 1983
71. Links TP, Smit AJ, Molenaar WM et al: Familial hypokalemic periodic paralysis. J Neurol Sci 122:33, 1994
72. Ashwood EM, Russell WJ, Burrow DD: Hyperkalemic periodic paralysis. Anaesthesia 47:579, 1992
73. Walsh F, Kelly D: Anaesthetic management of a patient with familial normokalemic periodic paralysis. Can J Anaesth 43:684, 1996
74. Rooney RT, Shanahan EC, Sun T et al: Atracurium and hypokalemic familial periodic paralysis. Anesth Analg 67:782, 1988
75. Rollman JE, Dickson CM: Anesthetic management of a patient with hypokalemic periodic paralysis for coronary artery bypass surgery. Anesthesiology 63:526, 1985
76. Lema G, Urzua J, Moran S et al: Successful anesthetic management of a patient with hypokalemic periodic paralysis undergoing cardiac surgery. Anesthesiology 74:373, 1991
77. Christensen KS: Hypokalemic periodic paralysis secondary to renal tubular acidosis. Eur Neurol 24:303, 1985
78. Manary MJ, Keating JP, Hirshberg GE: Quadriparesis due to potassium depletion. Crit Care Med 14:750, 1986
79. Hecht ML, Valtysson B, Hogan K: Spinal anesthesia for a patient with a calcium channel mutation causing hypokalemic periodic paralysis. Anesth Analg 84:461, 1997
80. Viscomi CM, Ptacek LJ, Dudley D: Anesthetic management of familial hypokalemic periodic paralysis during parturition. Anesth Analg 88:1081, 1999
81. Lambert C, Blanloeil Y, Horber RK et al: Malignant hyperthermia in a patient with hypokalemic periodic paralysis. Anesth Analg 79:1012, 1994
82. Moslehi R, Langlois S, Yan I et al: Linkage of malignant hyperthermia and hyperkalemic periodic paralysis to the adult skeletal muscle sodium channel (SCN4A) gene in a large pedigree. Am J Med Genet 76:21, 1998
83. Marchiori PE, dos Reis M, Quevedo ME et al: Acetylcholine receptor antibody in myasthenia gravis. Acta Neurol Scand 80:387, 1989
84. Zweiman B, Levinson AI: Immunologic aspects of neurological and neuromuscular diseases. JAMA 268:2918, 1992
85. Marx A, Wilisch A, Schultz A et al: Pathogenesis of myasthenia gravis. Virchows Arch 430:355, 1997
86. Massey JM: Acquired myasthenia gravis. Neurol Clin 15(3):577, 1997
87. Dushay KM, Zibrak JD, Jensen WA: Myasthenia gravis presenting as isolated respiratory failure. Chest 97:232, 1990
88. Osserman KE, Genkins G: Studies on myasthenia gravis. Review of a twenty-year experience in over 1200 patients. Mt Sinai J Med 38:497, 1971
89. Batocchi AP, Majolini L, Evoli A et al: Course and treatment of myasthenia during pregnancy. Neurology 52:447, 1999
90. Plauche WC: Myasthenia gravis. Clin Obstet Gynecol 26:592, 1983
91. Hofstad H, Ohm O, Mork SJ et al: Heart disease in myasthenia gravis. Acta Neurol Scand 70:176, 1984
92. Johannesen K-A, Mygland A, Gilhus NE et al: Left ventricular function in myasthenia gravis. Am J Cardiol 69:129, 1992
93. Thomas CE, Mayer SA, Gungor Y et al: Myasthenic crisis: Clinical features, mortality, complications, and risk factors for prolonged intubation. Neurology 48:1253, 1997
94. Phillips LH, Melnick PA: Diagnosis of myasthenia gravis in the 1990s. Semin Neurol 10:62, 1990
95. Mahalati K, Daeson RB, Collins JO et al: Predictable recovery from myasthenia gravis crisis with plasma exchange: Thirty-six cases and review of current management. J Clin Apheresis 14:1, 1999
96. Howard JF: Intravenous immunoglobulin for the treatment of acquired myasthenia gravis. Neurology 51(suppl 5):S30, 1998
97. Urschel JD, Grewal RP: Thymectomy for myasthenia gravis. Postgrad Med J 74:139, 1998
98. Wilkins KB, Bulkley GB: Thymectomy in the integrated management of myasthenia gravis. Adv Surg 32:105, 1999
99. Iani C, Caramia M, Morosetti FB et al: The treatment of severe forms of myasthenia gravis. Funct Neurol 3:321, 1998
100. Haider-Ali AM, MacGregor FB, Stewart M: Myasthenia gravis presenting with dysphagia and post-operative ventilatory failure. J Laryngol Otol 112:1194, 1998
101. Smith CE, Donati F, Bevan DR: Cumulative dose response curve for atracurium in patients with myasthenia gravis. Can J Anaesth 36:402, 1989
102. Eisenkraft JB, Book WJ, Papatestas AE: Sensitivity to vecuronium in myasthenia gravis: A dose–response study. Can J Anaesth 37:301, 1990
103. Baraka A, Dajani A: Atracurium in myasthenics undergoing thymectomy. Anesth Analg 64:1127, 1984
104. Ramsey FM, Smith GD: Clinical use of atracurium in myasthenia gravis. Can Anaesth Soc J 32:642, 1985
105. Bell CF, Florence AM, Hunter JM et al: Atracurium in the myasthenic patient. Anaesthesia 39:961, 1984
106. Hunter JM, Bell CF, Florence AM et al: Vecuronium in the myasthenic patient. Anaesthesia 40:848, 1985
107. Sanfilippo M, Fierro G, Cavalleti MV et al: Rocuronium in two myasthenic patients undergoing thymectomy. Acta Anaesthesiol Scand 41:1365, 1997
108. Baraka A, Taha S, Yazbeck V et al: Vecuronium block in the myasthenic patient. Anaesthesia 48:588, 1993
109. Abel M, Eisenkraft JB, Patel N: Response to suxamethonium in a myasthenic patient in remission. Anaesthesia 46:30, 1991
110. Vanlinthout LEH, Robertson EN, Booij KHDJ: Response to suxamethonium during propofol-fentanyl-N$_2$O/O$_2$ anaesthesia in a patient with active myasthenia gravis receiving long term anticholinesterase therapy. Anaesthesia 49:509, 1994
111. Baraka A: Suxamethonium block in the myasthenic patient: Correlation with plasma cholinesterase. Anaesthesia 47:217, 1992
112. Baraka A, Baroody M, Yazbeck V: Repeated doses of suxamethonium in the myasthenic patient. Anaesthesia 48:782, 1993
113. Nilsson E, Paloheimo M, Muller K et al: Halothane-induced variability in the neuromuscular transmission of patients with myasthenia gravis. Acta Anaesthesiol Scand 33:395, 1989

114. Rowbottom SJ: Isoflurane for thymectomy in myasthenia gravis. Anaesth Intens Care 17:444, 1989

115. Lorimer M, Hall R: Remifentanil and propofol total intravenous anaesthesia for thymectomy in myasthenia gravis. Anaesth Intens Care 26:210, 1998

116. Akpolal N, Tilgen H, Gursoy F et al: Thoracic epidural anaesthesia and analgesia with bupivacaine for transsternal thymectomy for myasthenia gravis. Eur J Anesthesiol 14:220, 1997

117. Nilsson E, Perttunen K, Kalso E: Intrathecal morphine for post-sternotomy pain in patients with myasthenia gravis: Effects on respiratory function. Acta Anaesthesiol Scand 41:549, 1997

118. Baraka A: Anesthesia and myasthenia gravis. Can J Anaesth 39:476, 1992

119. Eisenkraft JB, Papatestas AE, Kahn CH et al: Predicting the need for postoperative mechanical ventilation in myasthenia gravis. Anesthesiology 65:79, 1986

120. Naguib M, El Dawlatly AA, Ashour M et al: Multivariate determinants of the need for postoperative ventilation in myasthenia gravis. Can J Anaesth 43:1006, 1996

121. Nath U, Grant R: Neurological paraneoplastic syndromes. J Clin Pathol 50:975, 1997

122. Boonyapisit K, Kaminski H, Ruff RL: Disorders of the neuromuscular junction ion channels. Am J Med 106:97, 1999

123. McEvoy KM: Diagnosis and treatment of Lambert-Eaton myasthenic syndrome. Neurol Clin 12:387, 1994

124. Beydouin SR: Delayed diagnosis of Lambert-Eaton myasthenic syndrome in a patient with recurrent refractory respiratory failure. Muscle Nerve 17:689, 1994

125. Nicolle MW, Stewart DJ, Remtulla H et al: Lambert-Eaton myasthenic syndrome presenting with severe respiratory failure. Muscle Nerve 19:1328, 1996

126. O'Suilleabhain P, Low PA, Lennon VA: Autonomic dysfunction in the Lambert-Eaton myasthenic syndrome. Neurology 50:88, 1998

127. Sanders DB: 3,4-Diaminopyridine (DAP) in the treatment of Lambert-Eaton myasthenic syndrome (LEMS). Ann NY Acad Sci 841:811, 1998

128. Oh SJ, Kim DS, Head TC et al: Low dose guanidine and pyridostigmine: Relatively safe and effective long-term symptomatic therapy in Lambert-Eaton myasthenic syndrome. Muscle Nerve 20:1146, 1997

129. Rich MM, Teener JW, Bird SJ: Treatment of Lambert-Eaton syndrome with intravenous immunoglobulin. Muscle Nerve 20:614, 1997

130. Muchnik S, Losavio AS, Vidal A et al: Long term follow-up of Lambert-Eaton syndrome treated with intravenous immunoglobulin. Muscle Nerve 20:674, 1997

131. Newsom-Davis J: A treatment algorithm for Lambert-Eaton myasthenic syndrome. Ann N Y Acad Sci 841:817, 1998

132. Telford RJ, Hollway TE: The myasthenic syndrome. Anaesthesia in a patient treated with 3,4-diaminopyridine. Br J Anaesth 64:363, 1990

133. Biarnes A, Rochera MI: Lambert-Eaton (myasthenic syndrome): Pre-anesthetic treatment with intravenous immunoglobulins. Anaesthesia 51:797, 1996

134. Hahn AF: Guillain-Barré syndrome. Lancet 352:635, 1998

135. Jacobs BC, Rothbarth PH, van der Meche FGA et al: The spectrum of antecedent infections in Guillain-Barré syndrome. Neurology 51:1110, 1998

136. Yuki N: Pathogenesis of axonal Guillain-Barré syndrome: Hypothesis. Muscle Nerve 17:680, 1994

137. Newton-John H: Prevention of pulmonary complications in severe Guillain-Barré syndrome by early assisted ventilation. Med J Aust 142:444, 1985

138. Mendell JR: Chronic inflammatory demyelinating polyradiculoneuropathy. Annu Rev Med 44:211, 1994

139. Lawn ND, Wijdicks EFM: Fatal Guillain-Barré syndrome. Neurology 52:635, 1999

140. Krone A, Reuther P, Fuhrmeister U: Autonomic dysfunction in polyneuropathies: A report of 106 cases. J Neurol 230:111, 1983

141. Oomes PG, van der Meche FGA, Kleyweg RP et al: Liver function disturbances in Guillain-Barré syndrome. Neurology 46:96, 1996

142. Sater RA, Rostami A: Treatment of Guillain-Barré syndrome with intravenous immunoglobulin. Neurology 51(suppl 5):S9, 1998

143. Pascuzzi RM, Fleck JD: Acute peripheral neuropathy in adults. Neurol Clin 15(3):529, 1997

144. Alam TA, Chaudhry V, Cornblath DR: Electrophysiological studies in Guillain-Barré syndrome: Distinguishing subtypes by published criteria. Muscle Nerve 21:1275, 1998

145. Feldman JM: Cardiac arrest after succinylcholine administration in a pregnant patient recovered from Guillain-Barré syndrome. Anesthesiology 72:942, 1990

146. Fiacchino F, Gemma M, Bricchi M et al: Hypo- and hypersensitivity to vecuronium in a patient with Guillain-Barré syndrome. Anesth Analg 78:187, 1994

147. Moulin DE, Hagen N, Feasby TE et al: Pain in Guillain-Barré syndrome. Neurology 48:328, 1997

148. Connelly M, Shagrin J, Warfield C: Epidural opioids for the management of pain in a patient with Guillain-Barré syndrome. Anesthesiology 72:381, 1990

149. Collier CB: Postoperative paraplegia: An unusual case. Anaesth Intens Care 22:293, 1994

150. Rosenberg SK, Stacey BR: Postoperative Guillain-Barré syndrome, arachnoiditis, and epidural analgesia. Reg Anesth 21:486, 1996

151. Noseworthy JH: Progress in determining the causes and treatment of multiple sclerosis. Nature 399(suppl 1):A40, 1999

152. Al-Omaishi J, Bashir R, Gendleman HE: The cellular immunology of multiple sclerosis. J Leukoc Biol 65:444, 1999

153. Rudick RA, Cohen JA, Weinstock-Guttman B et al: Management of multiple sclerosis. N Engl J Med 337:1604, 1997

154. Kuwahira I, Kondo T, Ohto Y et al: Acute respiratory failure in multiple sclerosis. Chest 97:246, 1990

155. Funakawa I, Hara K, Yasuda T et al: Intractable hiccups and sleep apnea syndrome in multiple sclerosis: Report of two cases. Acta Neurol Scand 88:401, 1993

156. Schroth WS, Tenner SM, Rappaport BA et al: Multiple sclerosis as a cause of atrial fibrillation and electrocardiographic changes. Arch Neurol 49:422, 1992

157. Vita G, Fazio MC, Milone S et al: Cardiovascular autonomic dysfunction in multiple sclerosis is likely related to brainstem lesions. J Neurol Sci 120:82, 1993

158. Buyse B, Demedts M, Meekers J et al: Respiratory dysfunction in multiple sclerosis: A prospective analysis of 60 patients. Eur Resp J 10:139, 1997

159. Cook SD, Troiano R, Bansil S et al: Multiple sclerosis and pregnancy. Adv Neurol 64:83, 1994

160. Miller A: Diagnosis of multiple sclerosis. Semin Neurol 18:309, 1998

161. Baum K, Nehring C, Girke W et al: Relations between MRI and CT findings, cerebrospinal fluid parameters and clinical features. Clin Neurol Neurosurg 92:49, 1990

162. Khoury SJ, Weiner HL: Multiple sclerosis. What have we learned from magnetic resonance imaging studies? Arch Intern Med 158:565, 1998

163. Andersson P-B, Goodkin DE: Glucocorticosteroid therapy for multiple sclerosis: A critical review. J Neurol Sci 160:16, 1998

164. Van Oosten BW, Truyen L, Barkhof F, Polman CH: Choosing drug therapy for multiple sclerosis. Drugs 56:555, 1998

165. Arnason BGW: Immunologic therapy of multiple sclerosis. Annu Rev Med 50:291, 1999

166. Eisen A: Neurophysiology in multiple sclerosis. Neurol Clin 1:615, 1983

167. Siemkowicz E: Multiple sclerosis and surgery. Anaesthesia 31:1211, 1976

168. Baskett PJF, Armstrong R: Anaesthetic problems in multiple sclerosis. Anaesthesia 25:397, 1970

169. Kytta J, Rosenberg PH: Anaesthesia for patients with multiple sclerosis. Ann Chir Gynaecol 73:299, 1984

170. Jones RM, Healy TEJ: Anaesthesia and demyelinating disease. Anaesthesia 35:879, 1980

171. Berger JM, Ontell R: Intrathecal morphine in conjunction with a combined spinal and general anesthetic in a patient with multiple sclerosis. Anesthesiology 66:400, 1987

172. Leigh J, Fearnley SJ, Lupprian KG: Intrathecal diamorphine during laparotomy in a patient with advanced multiple sclerosis. Anaesthesia 45:640, 1990

173. Bader AM, Hunt CO, Datta S et al: Anesthesia for the obstetric patient with multiple sclerosis. J Clin Anesth 1:21, 1988

174. Confavreaux C, Hutchinson M, Hours MM et al: Rate of pregnancy-related relapse in multiple sclerosis. N Engl J Med 339:285, 1998

175. Roth S, Ebrahim ZY: Resistance to pancuronium in patients receiving carbamazepine. Anesthesiology 66:691, 1987

176. Tantucci C, Massucci M, Piperno R et al: Control of breathing

and respiratory muscle strength in patients with multiple sclerosis. Chest 105:1163, 1994

177. Foglio K, Clini E, Facchetti D et al: Respiratory muscle function and exercise capacity in multiple sclerosis. Eur Resp J 7:23, 1994

178. Annegers JF: Epidemiology and genetics of epilepsy. Neurol Clin 12:15, 1994

179. McNamera JO: Emerging insights into the genesis of epilepsy. Nature 399(suppl 1):A15, 1999

180. Bazil CW, Pedley TA: Advances in the medical treatment of epilepsy. Annu Rev Med 49:135, 1998

181. Feely M: Drug treatment of epilepsy. Br Med J 318:106, 1999

182. Walsh GO, Delgado-Escueta AV: Status epilepticus. Neurol Clin 11:835, 1993

183. Rawal K, D'Souza BJ: Status epilepticus. Crit Care Clin 1:339, 1985

184. Kofke WA, Young RSK, Davis P et al: Isoflurane for refractory status epilepticus. Anesthesiology 71:653, 1989

185. Mirski MA, Williams MA, Hanley DF: Prolonged pentobarbital and phenobarbital coma for refractory generalized status epilepticus. Crit Care Med 23:400, 1995

186. Tetzlaff JE: Intraoperative defect in haemostasis in a child receiving valproic acid. Can J Anaesth 38:222, 1991

187. Rampil IJ, Lockhart SH, Eger EI et al: The electroencephalographic effects of desflurane in humans. Anesthesiology 74:434, 1991

188. Steen PA, Michenfelder JD: Neurotoxicity of anesthetics. Anesthesiology 50:437, 1979

189. Smith M, Smith SJ, Scott CA et al: Activation of the electrocortigram by propofol during surgery for epilepsy. Br J Anaesth 76:499, 1996

190. Reddy RV, Moorthy SS, Mattice T et al: An electroencephalographic comparison of effects of propofol and methohexital. Electroencephalogr Clin Neurophysiol 83:162, 1992

191. Momota Y, Artu AA, Powers KM: Posttreatment with propofol terminates lidocaine-induced epileptiform electroencephalogram activity in rabbits: Effects on cerebrospinal fluid dynamics. Anesth Analg 87:900, 1998

192. Rockoff MA, Goudsouzian NG: Seizures induced by methohexital. Anesthesiology 54:333, 1981

193. Molbegott LP, Flashburg MH, Karasic HL et al: Probable seizures after sufentanil. Anesth Analg 66:91, 1987

194. Scott JC, Sarnquist FH: Seizure-like movements during a fentanyl infusion with absence of seizure activity in a simultaneous EEG recording. Anesthesiology 62:812, 1985

195. Sebel PS, Bovill JG, Wauquier A et al: Effects of high-dose fentanyl anesthesia on the electroencephalogram. Anesthesiology 55:203, 1981

196. Bovill JG, Sebel PS, Wauquier A et al: Electroencephalographic effects of sufentanil anesthesia in man. Br J Anaesth 54:45, 1982

197. Smith NT, Benthuysen JL, Bickford RG et al: Seizures during opioid anesthetic induction: Are they opioid induced rigidity? Anesthesiology 71:852, 1989

198. Keene DL, Roberts D, Splinter WM et al: Alfentanil mediated activation of epileptiform activity in the electrocortigram during resection of epileptogenic foci. Can J Neurol Sci 24:37, 1997

199. Carlsson C, Smith DS, Keykhah MM et al: The effects of high dose fentanyl on cerebral circulation and metabolism in rats. Anesthesiology 57:375, 1982

200. Young ML, Smith DS, Greenberg J et al: Effects of sufentanil on regional glucose utilization in rats. Anesthesiology 61:564, 1984

201. Ornstein E, Matteo RS, Young WL et al: Resistance to metocurine-induced neuromuscular blockade in patients receiving phenytoin. Anesthesiology 63:294, 1985

202. Lang AE, Lozano AM: Parkinson's disease. First of two parts. N Engl J Med 339:1044, 1998

203. Lang AE, Lozano AM: Parkinson's disease. Second of two parts. N Engl J Med 339:1130, 1998

204. Hingtgen CM, Siemers E: The treatment of Parkinson's disease: Current concepts and rationale. Comp Ther 24:560, 1998

205. Brandabur MM: Current therapy in Parkinson's disease. Surg Neurol 52:318, 1992

206. Mets B: Acute dystonia after alfentanil in untreated Parkinson's disease. Anesth Analg 72:557, 1991

207. Muzzi DA, Black S, Cucchiara RF: The lack of effect of succinylcholine on serum potassium in patients with Parkinson's disease. Anesthesiology 71:322, 1989

208. Zornberg GL, Bodkin JA, Cohen BM: Severe adverse interaction between pethidine and selegiline. Lancet 337:246, 1991

209. Golbe LI, Langston JW, Shoulson I: Selegiline and Parkinson's disease. Drugs 39:646, 1990

210. Ueda M, Hamamoto M, Nagayama H et al: Susceptibility to neuroleptic malignant syndrome in Parkinson's disease. Neurology 52:777, 1999

211. Korczyn AD: Autonomic nervous system disturbance in Parkinson's disease. Adv Neurol 53:463, 1990

212. Lydon AM, Boylan JF: Reversibility of Parkinsonism-induced acute upper airway obstruction by benztropine therapy. Anesth Analg 87:975, 1998

213. Golden WE, Lavender RC, Metzer WS: Acute postoperative confusion and hallucinations in Parkinson disease. Ann Intern Med 111:218, 1989

214. Martin JB: Molecular basis of the neurodegenerative disorders. N Engl J Med 340:1970, 1999

215. Petersen A, Mani K, Brundin P: Recent advances on the pathogenesis of Huntington's disease. Exper Neurol 157:1, 1999

216. Huggins M, Block M, Kanani SH et al: Ethical and legal dilemmas arising during predictive testing for adult-onset disease: The experience of Huntington disease. Am J Hum Genet 47:4, 1990

217. Mochizuki H, Kamakura K, Kumada M et al: A patient with Huntington's disease presenting with laryngeal chorea. Eur Neurol 41:119, 1999

218. Feigin A, Kieburtz K, Shoulson I: Treatment of Huntington's disease and other choreic disorders. In Kurlan R (ed): Treatment of Movement Disorders, p 337. Philadelphia, JB Lippincott, 1995

219. Mateo D, Munoz-Blanco JL, Gimenez-Roldan S: Neuroleptic malignant syndrome related to tetrabenazine introduction and haloperidol discontinuation in Huntington's disease. Clin Neuropharmacol 15:63, 1992

220. Davies DD: Abnormal response to anaesthesia in a case of Huntington's chorea. Br J Anaesth 38:490, 1966

221. Kaufman MA, Erb TL: Propofol for patients with Huntington's chorea? Anaesthesia 45:889, 1990

222. Soar J, Matheson KH: A safe anaesthetic in Huntington's disease? Anaesthesia 48:743, 1993

223. Propert DN: Pseudocholinesterase activity and phenotypes in mentally ill patients. Br J Psychiatry 134:477, 1979

224. Lamont AMS: Brief report: Anaesthesia and Huntington's chorea. Anaesth Intens Care 7:189, 1979

225. Fernandez IG, Sanchez MP, Ugalde AJ et al: Spinal anaesthesia in a patient with Huntington's chorea. Anaesthesia 52:391, 1997

226. Mayeux R, Sano M: Treatment of Alzheimer's disease. N Engl J Med 341:1670, 1999

227. Donepezil (aricept) for Alzheimer's disease. Med Lett Drugs Ther 39:53, 1997

228. Chou SM, Norris FH: Amyotrophic lateral sclerosis: Lower motor neuron disease spreading to upper motor neurons. Muscle Nerve 16:864, 1993

229. Jackson CE, Bryan WW: Amyotrophic sclerosis. Semin Neurol 18:27, 1998

230. Armon C, Daube JR, Windebank AJ et al: How frequently does classic amyotrophic lateral sclerosis develop in survivors of poliomyelitis? Neurology 40:172, 1990

231. Kuther G, Rodiek SO, Struppler A: CT-scanning of skeletal muscles in amyotrophic lateral sclerosis. Adv Exp Med Biol 209:143, 1987

232. Vitacca M, Clini E, Facchetti D et al: Breathing pattern and respiratory mechanics in patients with amyotrophic lateral sclerosis. Eur Resp J 10:1614, 1997

233. Polkey MI, Lyall RA, Green M et al: Expiratory muscle function in amyotrophic lateral sclerosis. Amer J Resp Crit Care Med 158:734, 1998

234. Schiffman PL, Belsh JM: Pulmonary function at diagnosis of amyotrophic lateral sclerosis. Chest 103:508, 1993

235. Kuisma MJ, Saarinen KV, Teirmaa HT: Undiagnosed amyotrophic lateral sclerosis and respiratory failure. Acta Anaesthesiol Scand 37:628, 1993

236. Chida K, Sakamaki S, Takasu T: Alteration in autonomic function and cardiovascular regulation in amyotrophic lateral sclerosis. J Neurol 236:127, 1989

237. Shimizu T, Hayashi H, Kato S et al: Circulatory collapse and sudden death in respirator-dependent amyotrophic lateral sclerosis. J Neurol Sci 124:45, 1994

238. Maselli RA, Wollman RL, Leung C et al: Neuromuscular transmission in amyotrophic lateral sclerosis. Muscle Nerve 16:1193, 1993

239. Jacka MJ, Sanderson F: Amyotrophic lateral sclerosis presenting during pregnancy. Anesth Analg 86:542, 1998

240. Johnson RT, Gibbs CJ: Creutzfeldt-Jakob disease and related transmissible spongiform encephalopathies. N Engl J Med 339:1994, 1998
241. Bendheim PE: The human spongiform encephalopathies. Neurol Clin 2:281, 1984
242. Martinez-Lage JF, Poza M, Sola J et al: Accidental transmission of Creutzfeldt-Jakob disease by dural cadaveric grafts. J Neurol Neurosurg Psychiatry 57:1091, 1994
243. Brown P, Cathala F, Raubertas RF et al: The epidemiology of Creutzfeldt-Jakob disease. Neurology 37:895, 1987
244. Nakamura Y, Aso E, Yanagawa H: Relative risk of Creutzfeldt-Jakob disease with cadaveric dura transplantation in Japan. Neurology 53:218, 1999
245. Marzewski DJ, Towfighi J, Harrington MG et al: Creutzfeldt-Jakob disease following pituitary-derived human growth hormone therapy. Neurology 38:1131, 1988
246. Collinge J: Variant Creutzfeldt-Jakob disease. Lancet 354:317, 1999
247. Manuelidis L: The dimensions of Creutzfeldt-Jakob disease. Transfusion 34:915, 1994
248. DuMoulin GC, Hedley-Whyte J: Hospital-associated viral infection and the anesthesiologist. Anesthesiology 59:51, 1983
249. MacMurdo SD, Jakymec AJ, Bleyaert AL: Precautions in the anesthetic management of a patient with Creutzfeldt-Jakob disease. Anesthesiology 60:590, 1984
250. Sadeh M, Goldhammer Y, Chagnac Y: Creutzfeldt-Jakob disease associated with peripheral neuropathy. Isr J Med 26:220, 1990
251. Salem MR, Manley S, Crystal GJ et al: Perioperative hemoglobin requirements. In Salem MR (ed): Blood Conservation in the Surgical Patient, p 107. Baltimore, Williams & Wilkins, 1996.
252. Provan D: Mechanisms and management of iron deficiency anemia. Br J Haematol 105(suppl 1):19, 1999
253. Hetzel TM, Losek JD: Unrecognized severe anemia in children presenting with respiratory distress. Am J Emerg Med 16:386, 1998
254. Berger M, Brass LF: Severe thrombocytopenia in iron deficiency anemia. Am J Hematol 24:425, 1987
255. Bruggers CS, Ware R, Altman AJ et al: Reversible focal neurologic deficits in severe iron deficiency anemia. J Pediatr 117:430, 1990
256. Beck WS: Diagnosis of megaloblastic anemia. Annu Rev Med 42:311, 1991
257. Toh B-H, van Driel IR, Gleeson PA: Pernicious anemia. N Engl J Med 337:1441, 1997
258. Lovblad K-O, Ramelli G, Remonda L et al: Retardation of myelination due to dietary vitamin B12 deficiency: Cranial MRI findings. Pediatr Radiol 27:155, 1997
259. Nunn JF, Chanarian J: Nitrous oxide inactivates methionine synthetase. In Eger EI (ed): Nitrous Oxide/N2O, p 211, New York, Elsevier-Dutton, 1985
260. Schilling RF: Is nitrous oxide a dangerous anesthetic for vitamin B12 deficient subjects? JAMA 255:1605, 1986
261. Berger JJ, Modell JH, Sypert GW: Megaloblastic anemia and brief exposure to nitrous oxide: A causal relationship? Anesth Analg 67:197, 1988
262. Koblin DD, Tomerson BW, Waldman FM: Disruption of folate and vitamin B12 metabolism in aged rats following exposure to nitrous oxide. Anesthesiology 73:506, 1990
263. Sesso RMCC, Iunes Y, Melo ACP: Myeloneuropathy following nitrous oxide anesthesia in a patient with macrocytic anaemia. Neuroradiology 41:588, 1999
264. Lee P, Smith I, Piesowicz A et al: Spastic paraparesis after anaesthesia. Lancet 353:554, 1999
265. Mayall M: Vitamin B12 deficiency and nitrous oxide. Lancet 353:1529, 1999
266. Shaw ADS, Morgan M: Nitrous oxide: Time to stop laughing? Anaesthesia 53:213, 1998
267. Wickramasinghe SN: The wide spectrum and unresolved issues of megaloblastic anemia. Semin Hematol 36:3, 1999
268. Hain WR, Jones SEF: Disease of blood. In Katz J, Steward DJ (eds): Anesthesia and Uncommon Pediatric Diseases, 2d ed, p 663. Philadelphia, WB Saunders, 1993
269. Marchetti M, Quaglini S, Barosi G: Prophylactic splenectomy and cholecystestomy in mild hereditary spherocytosis: Analyzing the decision in different clinical scenarios. J Int Med 244:217, 1998
270. Ruwende C, Hill A: Glucose-6 phosphate dehydrogenase deficiency and malaria. J Mol Med 76:581, 1998
271. Morse EE: Toxic effects of drugs on erythrocytes. Ann Clin Lab Sci 18:13, 1988
272. Beutler E: Glucose-6-phosphate dehydrogenase deficiency. N Engl J Med 324:169, 1991
273. Tabbara IA: Hemolytic anemias. Med Clin North Am 76:649, 1992
274. Domen RE: An overview of immune hemolytic anemias. Cleve Clin J Med 65:89, 1998
275. Park JV, Weiss CI: Cardiopulmonary bypass and myocardial protection: Management problems in cardiac surgical patients with cold autoimmune hemolytic disease. Anesth Analg 67:110, 1988
276. Bedrosian CL, Simel DL: Cold hemagglutinin disease in the operating room. South Med J 80:466, 1987
277. Luban NLC, Epstein BS, Watson SP: Sickle cell disease and anesthesia. Adv Anesthesiol 1:289, 1984
278. The Anaesthesia Advisory Committee to the Chief Coroner of Ontario: Intraoperative death during cesarean section in a patient with sickle-cell trait. Can J Anaesth 34:67, 1987
279. Knight J, Murphy TM, Browning I: The lung in sickle cell disease. Pediatr Pulmonol 28:205, 1999
280. Balfour IC, Covitz W, Arensman FW et al: Left ventricular filling in sickle cell anemia. Am J Cardiol 61:395, 1988
281. Allon M: Renal abnormalities in sickle cell disease. Arch Intern Med 150:501, 1990
282. Gyasi HK, Zarroug AW, Matthew M et al: Anesthesia for renal transplantation in sickle cell disease. Can J Anaesth 37:778, 1990
283. Adams RJ, Nichols FT, McKie V et al: Cerebral infarction in sickle cell anemia: Mechanism based on CT and MRI. Neurology 38:1012, 1988
284. Bunn HF: Mechanisms of disease: Pathogenesis and treatment of sickle cell disease. N Engl J Med 337:762, 1997
285. Brichard B, Vermylen C, Ninane J et al: Persistence of fetal hemoglobin production after successful transplantation of cord blood stem cells in a patient with sickle cell anemia. J Pediatr 128:241, 1996
286. Reed W: New considerations in the treatment of sickle cell disease. Annu Rev Med 49:461, 1998
287. Mani S, Duffy TP: Sickle myonecrosis revisited. Am J Med 95:525, 1993
288. Stasic AF: Anesthetic implications of sickle cell anemia. Prog Anesthesiol 8:3, 1994
289. Garden MS, Grant RE, Jebraili S: Perioperative complications in patients with sickle cell disease. Am J Orthop 25:353, 1996
290. Meshikhes A-WN, Al-Faraj AA: Sickle cell disease and the general surgeon. J R Coll Surg Edinburgh 43:73, 1998
291. Al-Salem AH, Nourallah H: Sequential endoscopic/laparoscopic management of cholelithiasis and choledocholithiasis in children who have sickle cell disease. J Pediatr Surg 32:1432, 1997
292. Stein RE, Urbaniak J: Use of the tourniquet during surgery in patients with sickle cell hemoglobinopathies. Clin Orthop 151:231, 1980
293. Haberkern CM, Neumayr LD, Orringer EP et al: Cholecystectomy in sickle cell anemia patients: Perioperative outcome of 364 cases from the national preoperative transfusion study. Blood 89:1533, 1997
294. Halvorson DJ, McKie V, McKie K et al: Sickle cell disease and tonsillectomy: Preoperative management and postoperative complications. Arch Otolaryngol Head Neck Surg 123:689, 1997
295. Scott-Connor CEH, Brunson CD: The pathophysiology of the sickle cell hemoglobinopathies and implications for perioperative management. Am J Surg 168:268, 1994
296. Cook A, Hanowell LH: Intraoperative autotransfusion for a patient with homozygous sickle cell disease. Anesthesiology 73:177, 1990
297. Heiner M, Teasdale SJ, David T et al: Aortocoronary bypass in a patient with sickle cell trait. Can Anaesth Soc J 26:428, 1979
298. Stuart MJ, Yamaja Setty BN: Sickle cell acute chest syndrome: Pathogenesis and rationale for treatment. Blood 94:1555, 1999
299. Finer P, Blair J, Rowe P: Epidural analgesia in the management of labor pain and sickle cell crisis—a case report. Anesthesiology 68:799, 1988
300. Yaster M, Tobin JR, Billett C et al: Epidural analgesia in the management of severe vaso-occlusive sickle cell crisis. Pediatrics 93:310, 1994
301. Rockoff AS, Christy D, Zeldis N et al: Myocardial necrosis following general anesthesia in hemoglobin SC disease. Pediatrics 61:73, 1978
302. Weatherall DJ: The thalassemias. Br Med J 314:1675, 1997
303. Higgs DR: The thalassemia syndromes. Q J Med 86:559, 1993
304. Wonke B, Wright C, Hoffbrand AV: Combined therapy with deferiprone and desferrioxamine. Br J Haematol 103:361, 1998

305. Hershko C, Konijn AM, Link G: Iron chelators for thalassemia. Br J Haematol 101:399, 1998

306. Voyagis GS, Kyriakis KP: Homozygous thalassemia and difficult tracheal intubation. Am J Hematol 52:125, 1996

307. Aydingoz U, Oto A, Cila A: Spinal cord compression due to epidural extramedullary haematopoiesis in thalassemia: MRI. Neuroradiology 39:870, 1997

308. Smith PR, Manjoney DL, Teitcher JB et al: Massive hemothorax due to intrathoracic extramedullary hematopoiesis in patients with thalassemia intermedia. Chest 94:658, 1988

309. Arend WP: The pathophysiology and treatment of rheumatoid arthritis. Arthritis Rheum 40:595, 1997

310. Jefferies WM: The etiology of rheumatoid arthritis. Med Hypoth 51:111, 1998

311. Toyama Y, Hirabayashi K, Fukimara Y et al: Spontaneous fracture of the odontoid process in rheumatoid arthritis. Spine 17:S436, 1992

312. Chevalier X, Larget-Piet B: General diseases of the spine in rheumatoid arthritis. Curr Opin Rheumatol 6:311, 1994

313. Fagerlund M, Bjornebrink J, Elelund L et al: Ultra-low field MR imaging of cervical spine involvement in rheumatoid arthritis. Acta Radiol 33:89, 1992

314. Yaszemski MJ, Shepler TR: Sudden death from cord compression associated with atlantoaxial instability in rheumatoid arthritis. Spine 15:338, 1990

315. Kraus E, Klinge H, Rautenberg M: Intradural manifestations of rheumatoid arthritis causing spinal cord compression. Neurochirugia 33(suppl 1):56, 1990

316. Geterund A, Bake B, Berthelsen B et al: Laryngeal involvement in rheumatoid arthritis. Acta Otolaryngol 111:990, 1991

317. Vetter TR: Acute airway obstruction due to arytenoiditis in a child with juvenile rheumatoid arthritis. Anesth Analg 79:1198, 1994

318. Absalom AR, Watts R, Kong A: Airway obstruction caused by rheumatoid cricoarytenoid arthritis. Lancet 351:1099, 1998

319. Bossingham DH, Simpson FG: Acute laryngeal obstruction in rheumatoid arthritis. Br Med J 312:295, 1996

320. Escalant A, Kaufman RL, Quisimoro FP et al: Cardiac compression in rheumatoid pericarditis. Semin Arthritis Rheum 20:148, 1990

321. Tanoue LT: Pulmonary manifestations of rheumatoid arthritis. Clin Chest Med 19:667, 1998

322. Boers M: Renal disorders in rheumatoid arthritis. Semin Arthritis Rheum 20:57, 1990

323. Chang DJ, Paget SA: Neurologic complications of rheumatoid arthritis. Rheum Dis Clin North Am 19:955, 1993

324. Arriola ER, Lee NP: Treatment advances in rheumatoid arthritis. West J Med 170:278, 1999

325. Brooks PM: Treatment of rheumatoid arthritis: From symptomatic relief to potential cure. Br J Rheumatol 37:1265, 1998

326. Drugs for rheumatoid arthritis. Med Lett Drugs Ther 36:101, 1994

327. MacKenzie CR, Sharrock NE: Perioperative medical considerations in patients with rheumatoid arthritis. Rheum Dis Clin North Am 24:1, 1998

328. Crosby ET, Lui A: The adult cervical spine: Implications for airway management. Can J Anaesth 37:77, 1990

329. White RH: Preoperative evaluation of patients with rheumatoid arthritis. Semin Arthritis Rheum 14:287, 1985

330. Matti MV, Sharrock NE: Anesthesia on the rheumatoid patient. Rheum Dis Clin North Am 24:19, 1998

331. Collins DN, Barnes CL, FitzRandolph RL: Cervical spine instability in rheumatoid patients having total hip or knee arthroplasty. Clin Orthop 272:127, 1991

332. Macarthur A, Kleiman S: Rheumatoid cervical joint disease: A challenge to the anaesthetist. Can J Anaesth 40:154, 1993

333. Steinberg AD: Concepts of pathogenesis of systemic lupus erythematosus. Clin Immunol Immunopath 63:19, 1992

334. Hahn BH: Antibodies to DNA. N Engl J Med 338:1359, 1998

335. Mevorach D, Raz E, Shalev O et al: Complete heart block and seizures in an adult with systemic lupus erythematosus. Arthritis Rheum 36:259, 1993

336. Mojcik C, Klippel JH: End-stage renal disease and systemic lupus erythematosus. Am J Med 101:100, 1996

337. Stone JH: End-stage renal disease in lupus: Disease activity, dialysis, and outcome of transplantation. Lupus 7:654, 1998

338. Futrell N, Schultz LR, Millikan C: Central nervous system disease in patients with systemic lupus erythematosus. Neurology 42:1649, 1992

339. Bell CL, Partington C, Robbins M et al: Magnetic resonance imaging of central nervous system lesions in patients with lupus erythematosus. Arthritis Rheum 34:432, 1991

340. Doherty NE, Siegel RJ: Cardiovascular manifestations of systemic lupus erythematosus. Am Heart J 110:1257, 1985

341. Kahl LE: The spectrum of pericardial tamponade in systemic lupus erythematosus. Arthritis Rheum 35:1343, 1992

342. Sturfelt G, Eskilsson J, Nived O et al: Cardiovascular disease in systemic lupus erythematosus. Medicine 71:216, 1992

343. Moder KG, Miller T, Tazelaar HD: Cardiac involvement in systemic lupus erythematosus. Mayo Clin Proc 74:275, 1999

344. Murin S, Wiedemann HP, Matthay RA: Pulmonary manifestations of systemic lupus erythematosus. Clin Chest Med 19:641, 1998

345. Zamora M, Warner ML, Tuder R et al: Diffuse alveolar hemorrhage and systemic lupus erythematosus: Clinical presentation, histology, survival, and outcome. Medicine 76:192, 1997

346. Li EK, Lai-Shan T: Pulmonary hypertension in systemic lupus erythematosus: Clinical association and survival in 18 patients. J Rheumatol 26:1923, 1999

347. Groen H, Terborg EJ, Postma DS et al: Pulmonary function in systemic lupus erythematosus is related to distinct clinical, serologic, and nailfold capillary patterns. Am J Med 93:619, 1992

348. Nossent JC, Berend K: Cricoarytenoiditis in systemic lupus erythematosus. Scand J Rheumatol 27:237, 1998

349. Tsunoda K, Soda Y: Hoarseness as the initial manifestation of systemic lupus erythematosus. J Laryngol Otol 110:478, 1996

350. Martin L, Edworthy SM, Ryan JP et al: Upper airway disease in systemic lupus erythematosus: A report of four cases and a review of the literature. J Rheumatol 19:1186, 1992

351. Mills JA: Systemic lupus erythematosus. N Engl J Med 330:1871, 1994

352. Uramoto KM, Michet CJ, Thumboo J et al: Trends in the incidence and mortality of systemic lupus erythematosus, 1950–1992. Arthritis Rheum 42:46, 1999

353. Bulman PM, Hunder G: New approaches for treatment of systemic lupus erythematosus. Ann Int Med 129:1095, 1998

354. Pisetsky DS, Gilkeson G, St Clair EW: Systemic lupus erythematosus. Med Clin North Am 81:113, 1997

355. Godfrey T, Khamashta MA, Hughes GRV: Therapeutic advances in systemic lupus erythematosus. Curr Opin Rheumatol 10:435, 1998

356. Klippel JH: Systemic lupus erythematosus: Treatment related complications superimposed on chronic disease. JAMA 263:1812, 1990

357. Rubin RL: Etiology and mechanism of drug-induced lupus. Curr Opin Rheumatol 11:357, 1999

358. Christodoulou C, Emmanuel P, Ray RA et al: Respiratory distress due to minocycline-induced pulmonary lupus. Chest 115:1471, 1999

359. Cuenco J, Tzeng G, Wittels B: Anesthetic management of the parturient with systemic lupus erythematosus, pulmonary hypertension, and pulmonary edema. Anesthesiology 91:568, 1999

360. Papa MZ, Shiloni E, Vetto JT et al: Surgical morbidity in patients with systemic lupus erythematosus. Am J Surg 157:295, 1989

361. Dell R, Marsh A: Upper airway obstruction complicating SLE. Can J Anaesth 42:229, 1997

362. Furst DE, Clements PJ: Hypothesis for the pathogenesis of systemic sclerosis. J Rheumatol 24(suppl 48):53, 1997

363. Renaudineau Y, Revelen R, Levy Y et al: Anti-endothelial cell antibodies in systemic sclerosis. Clin Diagn Lab Immunol 6:156, 1999

364. Mitchell H, Bolster MB, LeRoy EC: Scleroderma and related conditions. Med Clin North Am 81:129, 1997

365. Minai OA, Dweik RA, Arroliga AC: Manifestations of scleroderma pulmonary disease. Clin Chest Med 19:713, 1998

366. Battle RW, Davitt MA, Cooper SM et al: Prevalence of pulmonary hypertension in limited and diffuse sclerosis. Chest 110:1515, 1996

367. Ferri C, DiBello V, Martini A et al: Heart involvement in systemic sclerosis: An ultrasonic tissue characterisation study. Ann Rheum Dis 57:296, 1998

368. Murata I, Takenoka K, Shinhoara S et al: Diversity of myocardial involvement in systemic sclerosis: An 8-year study of 95 Japanese patients. Am Heart J 135:960, 1998

369. Rokas S, Mavrikakis M, Agrios N et al: Electrophysiologic abnormalities of cardiac function in progressive systemic sclerosis. J Electrocardiol 29:17, 1996

370. Byers RJ, Marshall DAS, Freemont AJ: Pericardial involvement in systemic sclerosis. Ann Rheum Dis 56:393, 1997

371. Lock G, Pfeifer M, Straub RH et al: Association of esophageal dysfunction and pulmonary function impairment and systemic sclerosis. Amer J Gastroenterol 93:341, 1998

372. Lock G, Holstege A, Lang B *et al:* Gastrointestinal manifestations of progressive systemic sclerosis. Amer J Gastroenterol 92:763, 1997

373. Kanter GJ, Barash PG: Undiagnosed scleroderma in a patient with a difficult airway. Yale J Biol Med 71:31, 1998

374. Thompson J, Conklin KA: Anesthetic management of a pregnant patient with scleroderma. Anesthesiology 59:69, 1983

375. Ringel RA, Brick JE, Brick JF *et al:* Muscle involvement in the scleroderma syndromes. Arch Intern Med 150:2550, 1990

376. Lewis GBH: Prolonged regional analgesia in scleroderma. Can Anaesth Soc J 21:495, 1974

377. Neill RS: Progressive systemic sclerosis. Br J Anaesth 52:623, 1980

378. Omote K, Kawamata M, Namiki A: Adverse effects of stellate ganglion block on Raynaud's phenomenon associated with progressive systemic sclerosis. Anesth Analg 77:1057, 1993

379. Lundborg CN, Nitescu PV, Appelgren LK *et al:* Progressive systemic sclerosis: Intrathecal pain management. Reg Anesth Pain Med 24:89, 1999

380. Dalakas MC: Molecular immunology and genetics of inflammatory muscle diseases. Arch Neurol 55:1509, 1998

381. Amato AA, Barohn RJ: Idiopathic inflammatory myopathies. Neurol Clin 15:615, 1997

382. Dickey BF, Myers AR: Pulmonary disease in polymyositis/dermatomyositis. Semin Arthritis Rheum 14:60, 1984

383. Marie I, Hatron P-Y, Hachulla E *et al:* Pulmonary involvement in polymyositis and in dermatomyositis. J Rheumatol 25:1336, 1998

384. Akira M, Hara H, Sakatani M: Interstitial lung disease in association with polymyositis-dermatomyositis: Long term follow-up CT evaluation in seven patients. Radiology 210:333, 1999

385. Gonzalez-Lopez L, Gamez-Nava JI, Sanchez L *et al:* Cardiac manifestations in dermato-polymyositis. Clin Exp Rheum 14:373, 1996

386. Anders H-J, Wanders A, Rihl M *et al:* Myocardial fibrosis in polymyositis. J Rheumatol 26:1840, 1999

387. Gordon M-M, Madhok R: Fatal myocardial necrosis. Ann Rheum Dis 58:198, 1999

388. Adams-Gandhi LB, Boyd AS, King LE: Diagnosis and management of dermatomyositis. Comp Ther 22:156, 1996

389. Mastaglia FL, Phillips BA, Zilko P: Treatment of inflammatory myopathies. Muscle Nerve 20:651, 1997

390. Shapiro J, Martin S, DeGirolami U *et al:* Inflammatory myopathy causing pharyngeal dysphagia: A new entity. Ann Otol Rhinol Laryngol 105:331, 1996

391. Downey EC, Woolley MM, Hanson V: Required surgical therapy in the pediatric patient with dermatomyositis. Arch Surg 123:1117, 1988

392. Brown S, Shupack RC, Patel C *et al:* Neuromuscular blockade in a patient with active dermatomyositis. Anesthesiology 77:1031, 1992

393. Flusche G, Unger-Sargon J, Lambert DH: Prolonged neuromuscular paralysis in a patient with polymyositis. Anesth Analg 66:188, 1987

394. Crosby E, Robblee JA: Cyclosporine-pancuronium interaction in a patient with a renal allograft. Can J Anaesth 35:300, 1988

395. Marinkovich MP: Update on inherited bullous dermatoses. Dermatol Clin 17:473, 1999

396. Like MC, Darling TN, Hsu R *et al:* Mucosal morbidity in patients with epidermolysis bullosa acquisita. Arch Dermatol 135:954, 1999

397. Pearson RW: Clinicopathologic types of epidermolysis bullosa and their nondermatologic complications. Arch Dermatol 124:718, 1988

398. Berson S, Lin AN, Ward RF *et al:* Junctional epidermolysis bullosa of the larynx. Ann Otol Rhinol Laryngol 101:861, 1992

399. Liu RM, Papsin BC, de Jong AL: Epidermolysis bullosa of the head and neck: A case report of laryngotracheal involvement and 10-year review of cases at The Hospital for Sick Children. J Otolaryngol 28:76, 1999

400. Ergun GA, Lin AN, Dannenberg AJ *et al:* Gastrointestinal manifestations of epidermolysis bullosa. Medicine 71:121, 1992

401. Brook MM, Weinhouse E, Jaren Wattanon M *et al:* Dilated cardiomyopathy complicating a case of epidermolysis bullosa dystrophica. Pediatr Dermatol 6:21, 1989

402. Melville C, Atherton D, Burch M *et al:* Fatal cardiomyopathy in dystrophic epidermolysis bullosa. Br J Dermatol 135:603, 1996

403. Banerjee AK: Mitral valve prolapse in a patient with epidermolysis bullosa. Br J Clin Pract 44:282, 1990

404. Mann JFE, Zeier M, Zilow E *et al:* The spectrum of renal involvement in epidermolysis bullosa dystrophica hereditaria: Report of two cases. Am J Kidney Dis 11:437, 1988

405. Lin AN: Management of patients with epidermolysis bullosa. Dermatol Clin 14:381, 1996

406. Simpson RJ, Gabriel MJ: Defibrillator pad for airway management in epidermolysis bullosa—saving face. Anaesth Intens Care 25:589, 1997

407. Broster T, Placek R, Eggers GWN: Epidermolysis bullosa: Anesthetic management for cesarean section. Anesth Analg 66:341, 1987

408. Fisher CG, Ray DAA: Airway obstruction in epidermolysis bullosa. Anaesthesia 44:440, 1989

409. Broughton R, Crawford MR, Vonwiller JB: Epidermolysis bullosa: A review of 15 years' experience, including experience with combined general and regional anesthetic techniques. Anaesth Intens Care 16:260, 1988

410. Wright JT: Comprehensive dental care and general anesthetic management of hereditary epidermolysis bullosa. Oral Surg Oral Med Oral Pathol 70:573, 1990

411. James I, Wark H: Airway management during anesthesia in patients with epidermolysis bullosa dystrophica. Anesthesiology 56:323, 1982

412. Ishimura H, Minami K, Sata T *et al:* Airway management for an uncooperative patient with recessive dystrophic epidermolysis bullosa. Anaesth Intens Care 26:110, 1998

413. Holzman RS, Worthen HM, Johnson K: Anaesthesia for children with junctional epidermolysis bullosa dystrophica (letalis). Can J Anaesth 34:395, 1987

414. Kaplan R, Strauch B: Regional anesthesia in a child with epidermolysis bullosa. Anesthesiology 67:262, 1987

415. Price T, Katz VT: Obstetrical concerns of epidermolysis bullosa. Obstet Gynecol Surv 43:445, 1988

416. Lin AN, Lateef F, Kelly R *et al:* Anesthetic management of epidermolysis bullosa: Review of 129 anesthetic episodes in 32 patients. J Am Acad Dermatol 30:412, 1994

417. Brenner S, Bialy-Golan A, Ruocco V: Drug-induced pemphigus. Clin Dermatol 16:393, 1998

418. Korman NJ: Pemphigus. Dermatol Clin 8:689, 1990

419. Enk AH, Knop J: Mycophenolate is effective in the treatment of pemphigus vulgaris. Arch Dermatol 135:54, 1999

420. Nousari HC, Deterding R, Wojtczack H *et al:* The mechanism of respiratory failure in paraneoplastic pemphigus. N Engl J Med 340:1406, 1999

421. Hasegawa Y, Shimokata K, Ichiyama S *et al:* Constrictive bronchiolitis obliterans and paraneoplastic pemphigus. Eur Respir J 13:934, 1999

422. Vatashky E, Aronson HB: Pemphigus vulgaris: Anaesthesia in the traumatised patient. Anaesthesia 37:1195, 1982

423. Jeyaram C, Torda TA: Anesthetic management of cholecystectomy in a patient with buccal pemphigus. Anesthesiology 40:600, 1974

424. Abouleish EI, Elias MA, Lopez M *et al:* Spinal anesthesia for cesarean section in a case of pemphigus foliaceus. Anesth Analg 84:449, 1997

Clinical Anesthesia (4/e), edited by
Paul G. Barash, Bruce F. Cullen, and
Robert K. Stoelting. Lippincott Williams &
Wilkins, Philadelphia, © 2001.

CHAPTER 20

MALIGNANT HYPERTHERMIA AND OTHER PHARMACOGENETIC DISORDERS

HENRY ROSENBERG, JEFFREY E. FLETCHER, AND
BARBARA W. BRANDOM

As a result of physiologic, metabolic, or anatomic changes, many inherited disorders have significant implications for anesthetic management. In this chapter we discuss the inherited disorders whose manifestations are enhanced or instigated by drugs usually used by anesthesiologists. In some cases, such as the porphyrias, the manifestations may be induced by agents other than anesthetics. In other enzymatic disorders, such as pseudocholinesterase abnormalities, it would be extremely unlikely for a patient to have any problems until he or she is exposed to the depolarizing neuromuscular blocking agent succinylcholine. Malignant hyperthermia (MH) or malignant hyperpyrexia is perhaps the most significant inherited disorder triggered by exposure to anesthetic drugs.

MALIGNANT HYPERTHERMIA

Malignant hyperthermia was first formally described in 1960 in *Lancet*[1] by Denborough and Lovell and subsequently in *The British Journal of Anaesthesia*.[2] That first case report laid the foundation for much of our understanding of the clinical presentations of MH. The patient was a young man who claimed that several of his relatives had died without apparent cause during anesthesia. He was anesthetized with halothane and developed tachycardia, hot sweaty skin, peripheral mottling, and cyanosis. Early recognition and symptomatic treatment saved the patient. It therefore became apparent that this new syndrome had the following elements: patients were otherwise healthy unless exposed to an anesthetic agent; temperature elevation was a hallmark; a heritable or genetic component was present; and a high mortality rate was likely. In addition, with early recognition and treatment it was possible to abort the malignant effects of the syndrome.

In the 1960s other cases of MH were reported in increasing numbers, and a gene pool for MH was established in certain parts of the world. In addition, the association between porcine stress syndrome (PSS) or "pale soft exudative pork syndrome" and MH was described, thus providing an animal model for MH.[3] Porcine breeds such as the Landrace, Poland China, and Pietrain show the classic presentations of MH on induction of anesthesia with potent inhalation agents and succinylcholine. During the 1970s, many more clinical presentations of MH were reported. The development of an *in vitro* diagnostic test was suggested by Kalow *et al* based on exposure of a skeletal muscle biopsy specimen to caffeine and then halothane.[4] In 1975, Harrison reported that dantrolene could be effective in treating and preventing MH in pigs.[5] By 1979, a sufficient number of cases were described showing that intravenous dantrolene could successfully reverse the human form of MH, and the drug was approved for use by the Food and Drug Administration (FDA). During that decade, studies of the pathophysiology of MH were also performed. By the late 1970s, it was apparent that MH most likely resulted from metabolic alterations in skeletal muscle. In the 1980s, lay organizations in the U.S., Canada, and Great Britain were formed to disseminate information to patients affected by MH as well as to enhance awareness of the syndrome

among physicians. The manifestations of MH and its association with other muscle disorders were studied. Application of the muscle biopsy diagnostic halothane–caffeine contraction test was standardized and a registry for MH was created in the U.S. in the late 1980s. In addition, a variety of other tests for diagnosing MH were introduced, many of which subsequently were found to be of little or no validity.

A major step forward occurred in 1985, when the Lopez group directly demonstrated an increased intracellular concentration of calcium ion in muscle from MH-susceptible pigs and humans.[6] The intracellular calcium concentration dramatically increased during an MH crisis and was reversed by the administration of dantrolene.

In the 1990s sophisticated molecular biologic techniques were first applied to identify the genes associated with MH susceptibility. It is anticipated that better understanding of the genetic substrate of the pathophysiology of MH will result in a less invasive diagnostic test than the contracture tests used at present. In the 1990s epidemiologic information helped to differentiate MH from other life-threatening anesthetic complications. It was appreciated that some deaths in children formerly attributed to MH were really the result of destruction of muscle cells that occurred during anesthesia with volatile agents and succinylcholine in patients with unrecognized myopathies.[7]

Clinical Presentations

As our knowledge of MH has grown, the definition of MH has changed. At first MH was thought in all cases to be a heritable syndrome consisting of an extremely elevated body temperature, skeletal muscle rigidity, and acidosis associated with a high mortality rate. However, we have now begun to concentrate on the definition of MH in terms of its underlying pathophysiologic characteristics. MH is a hypermetabolic disorder of skeletal muscle with varied presentations, depending on species, breed, and triggering agents. An important pathophysiologic process in this disorder is intracellular hypercalcemia. Intracellular hypercalcemia activates metabolic pathways that, if untreated, result in adenosine triphosphate depletion, acidosis, membrane destruction, and cell death. Although a heritable component is present in many cases, it is not invariably apparent from patient family history. In addition, disorders that may have symptoms and signs similar to those of MH, such as neuroleptic malignant syndrome, may not have an inherited basis.

Classic Malignant Hyperthermia

Malignant hyperthermia may present in several ways. In almost all cases, the first manifestations of the syndrome occur in the operating room. However, MH also may occur in the recovery room or (rarely) even on return to the patient floor. In the classic case, the initial signs of tachycardia and tachypnea result from sympathetic nervous system stimulation secondary to underlying hypermetabolism and hypercarbia. Because most patients who receive general anesthesia are paralyzed, tachypnea usually is not recognized. Shortly after the increase in heart rate, an increase in blood pressure occurs, often associated with ventricular dysrhythmias induced by sympathetic nervous system stimulation from hypercarbia or caused by hyperkalemia or catecholamine release. Thereafter, muscle rigidity or increase in muscle tone may become apparent. Increase in body temperature, climbing at a rate of 1–2°C every 5 minutes follows. With the increase in metabolism, the patient may "break through" the neuromuscular blockade. At the same time, the CO_2 absorbent becomes activated and warm to the touch (because the reaction with CO_2 is exothermic). The patient will display peripheral mottling and, on occasion, sweating and cyanosis. Blood gas analysis usually reveals hypercarbia and respiratory and metabolic acidosis without marked oxygen desaturation. Elevation of end-tidal CO_2 is one of the earliest signs of MH. On the other hand, vigorous hyperventilation may mask such hypercarbia and delay the diagnosis.[8] A mixed venous sample will show even more dramatic evidence of CO_2 retention and metabolic acidosis.[9] Hyperkalemia, hypercalcemia, lactacidemia, and myoglobinuria are characteristic. Increase in creatine kinase (CK) levels is dramatic, often exceeding 20,000 units in the first 12–24 hours. Death results unless the syndrome is promptly treated. Even with treatment and survival, the patient is at risk for life-threatening myoglobinuric renal failure and disseminated intravascular coagulation. Another significant clinical problem is recrudescence of the syndrome within the first 24–36 hours.[10]

If succinylcholine is used during induction of anesthesia, an acceleration of the manifestations of MH may occur such that tachycardia, hypertension, marked temperature elevation, and dysrhythmias are seen over the course of 5–10 minutes. However, it is important to note that a completely normal response to succinylcholine may be present in some MH-susceptible patients. A potent inhalation agent apparently is necessary to trigger the syndrome in these cases.

Review of case reports of MH suggests that the syndrome becomes apparent most frequently shortly after anesthesia induction, particularly when succinylcholine is used, and at the end of the procedure as the patient is emerging from anesthesia.

Masseter Muscle Rigidity

Rigidity of the jaw muscles after administration of succinylcholine is referred to as *masseter muscle rigidity* (MMR) or *masseter spasm*. The association of this phenomenon with MH was underlined by many case reports of MMR preceding MH.[11,12] Although MMR probably occurs in patients of all ages, it is distinctly most common in children and young adults. Several studies have shown a peak age incidence at 8–12 years of age. Characteristically, anesthesia is induced by inhalation with halothane or sevoflurane, after which succinylcholine is administered. Snapping of the jaw or rigidity on opening of the jaw is seen. However, this rigidity can be overcome with effort and usually abates within 2–3 minutes. A peripheral nerve stimulator usually reveals flaccid paralysis. However, increased tone of other muscles also may be noted. Repeat doses of succinylcholine do not relieve the problem. Tachycardia and dysrhythmias are not infrequent. Only in rare cases does frank MH supervene immediately after MMR. More commonly (if the anesthetic is continued with a triggering agent), the initial signs of MH appear in 20 minutes or more. If the anesthetic is discontinued, the patient usually recovers uneventfully. However, within 4–12 hours, myoglobinuria occurs and CK elevation is detected.

Muscle biopsy with caffeine–halothane contracture testing has shown that approximately 50% of patients who experience MMR are also susceptible to MH.[13,14] Therefore, most authorities recommend that anesthesia (if elective in nature) be discontinued and surgery postponed after an episode of MMR. With the introduction of end-tidal CO_2 monitoring, the availability of dantrolene, and enhanced understanding of MH, some have questioned the advice that all anesthetics must be discontinued after MMR. Instead, they recommend continuation with non-

triggering anesthetics and the use of end-tidal CO_2 monitoring. The issue of whether to give dantrolene after an episode of MMR is also unresolved. Dantrolene is most useful only when there is a clear diagnosis of MH. When MMR is accompanied by rigidity of chest or limb, MH is more likely to follow than after isolated jaw rigidity.[15,16]

The differential diagnosis of MMR consists of the following: (1) myotonic syndrome, (2) temporomandibular joint dysfunction, (3) underdosing with succinylcholine, (4) not allowing sufficient time for succinylcholine to act before intubation, (5) increased resting tension after succinylcholine in the presence of fever or elevated plasma epinephrine. A variety of reports have shown that succinylcholine increases jaw muscle tone in patients with normal muscle.[17] This normal agonistic effect of succinylcholine, further increased by temperature[18] and epinephrine in the presence of halothane, may account for some cases of MMR. The pathophysiology of jaw muscle tone increase is unknown. One reason for the high incidence of positive biopsy results and the low incidence of clinical MH after MMR may relate to selection of patients with marked muscle rigidity for biopsy. Such patients may be at greater risk for MH.[14]

Signs of temporomandibular dysfunction as well as myotonia should be sought following the MMR episode. If rigidity precluding laryngoscopy occurred without temporomandibular joint dysfunction, the patient should be evaluated by a neurologist for the presence of occult myopathy and counseled regarding the need for a muscle biopsy and diagnostic contracture test to evaluate MH susceptibility. It is incumbent upon the anesthesiologist to alert the patient to the possibility that MH may follow in subsequent procedures.

The incidence of MMR is debatable. This sign may occur in as many as 1 in 100 children anesthetized with halothane and given succinylcholine.[19] A retrospective study based on the information supplied to the Danish Malignant Hyperthermia Registry found that the incidence of MMR was 1 in 12,000 (including adults and children).[20] A prospective study found MMR in 1 of 500 children who received halothane followed by intravenous succinylcholine.[21]

Our advice regarding MMR is as follows:

1. When it occurs, the anesthesiologist should, if at all possible, discontinue the anesthetic and postpone surgery. If end-tidal CO_2 monitoring and dantrolene are available and the anesthesiologist is experienced in managing MH, he or she may elect to continue with a nontriggering anesthetic.
2. After episodes of MMR, the patient should be observed carefully for a period of 12–24 hours for myoglobinuria and signs of MH. Administration of $1–2$ mg $\cdot$ kg^{-1} of dantrolene should be considered.
3. The family should be informed of the episode of MMR and its implications.
4. Creatine kinase levels should be checked 6, 12, and 24 hours after the episode. If the CK level is still grossly elevated at 12 hours, additional samples should be drawn until it begins to return to normal.
5. If the CK level is greater than 20,000 IU in the perioperative period and a concomitant myopathy is not present, the diagnosis of MH is very likely.[22] If contracture test results are within normal limits after an episode of MMR, we currently do not recommend that other family members undergo testing, but advise that succinylcholine be avoided in future anesthetics for that patient.

A study by Littleford et al[23] has shown that acidosis and rhabdomyolysis occur after anesthesia if continued with an inhalation agent after MMR, although fulminant MH may not occur. MMR has been documented most frequently in association with succinylcholine, although it may occur after induction with any anesthetic agent, intravenous or inhalation, before succinylcholine administration.[24] As such, many pediatric anesthesiologists avoid the use of succinylcholine except on specific indication. It is also of interest that a thiobarbiturate induction will greatly decrease the incidence of MMR.[25]

Late Onset of MH and Myoglobinuria

Malignant hyperthermia may occur not only in the operating room, but also in the early postoperative period, usually within the first few hours of recovery from anesthesia. The characteristic tachycardia, tachypnea, hypertension, and dysrhythmias indicate that an episode of MH may be about to follow. Isolated myoglobinuria in the postoperative period should also alert the anesthesiologist that a problem has occurred. Myoglobinuria may occur without an obvious increase in metabolism.[26] Succinylcholine may cause rhabdomyolysis in patients who have other muscle disorders that may not be clinically obvious on cursory examination.[7,27,28] It may result from interactions of succinylcholine with other drugs such as inhibitors of cholesterol formation.[29] The presence of myoglobinuria mandates that the patient be referred to a neurologist for further investigation.

Myodystrophies Exacerbated by Anesthesia: Relation to Malignant Hyperthermia

Patients suffering from *muscular dystrophy* are at risk to develop hyperkalemic cardiac arrest after administration of succinylcholine. In some muscle diseases hyperkalemia has been noted after volatile agents only. These adverse events were first believed to represent a form of MH.[30,31] It now appears that the pathophysiology of the hyperkalemic episodes and MH is different. Case reports collected by the Malignant Hyperthermia Association of the United States (MHAUS) and the North American MH Registry indicate that when an apparently healthy child experiences a sudden unexpected cardiac arrest on induction of anesthesia, once hypoxemia and ventilatory problems are ruled out, hyperkalemia should be considered. Of 29 patients with such a presentation, 60% died. In 50% there was evidence of undiagnosed myopathy (usually muscular dystrophy).[7] The treatment of hyperkalemic arrests includes administration of calcium chloride, glucose, insulin, bicarbonate, and hyperventilation.

In 1993 and in 1994 the package insert for succinylcholine was modified to warn against routine use of succinylcholine in children. Of course, in special circumstances, such as airway emergencies and full stomach, succinylcholine may still be appropriate. Some pediatric anesthesiologists are comfortable with the administration of short-acting nondepolarizing neuromuscular blockers in these situations.

Central core disease is an unusual myopathy characterized by muscle weakness. It is probably inherited in a recessive manner. Many cases of MH have been reported in patients with central core disease. Therefore, precautions regarding MH must be taken for all patients with central core disease.[32,33]

The *myotonias* are a varied set of disorders. Patients with any of these disorders will display muscle contractures after succinylcholine. Only one myotonic disorder (myotonia fluctuans) has been linked to MH susceptibility by the halothane–caffeine contracture test.[34]

King or *King-Denborough* syndrome is a rare myopathy characterized by cryptorchidism, markedly slanted eyes, low-set ears, pectus deformity, scoliosis, small stature, and hypotonia. Several patients with this disorder have been diagnosed as MH-susceptible both clinically and by muscle biopsy.[35,36]

Other Conditions Associated with MH

Skeletal abnormalities such as *osteogenesis imperfecta*[37] and the Schwartz-Jampel[38] syndrome, *myotonia*, have been associated with signs of MH. Metabolism is increased in patients with osteogenesis imperfecta because of the bone disease. Fever during anesthesia is common in these patients. The Schwartz-Jampel syndrome is an autosomal recessive myotonic-like condition

with osteoarticular deformities. In both these conditions, association with MH is sporadic. Despite a few well-documented cases of MH in patients with osteogenesis imperfecta, we (and others[39]) have not confirmed MH susceptibility in three cases of osteogenesis imperfecta tested with the halothane–caffeine contracture test. But we have found typical contractures in one other muscle biopsy from a patient with osteogenesis imperfecta.

Pheochromocytoma may be mistaken for MH because of its presentation by tachycardia, hypertension, and fever during anesthesia. However, pheochromocytoma does not predispose to MH.[40] Thyrotoxicosis could also be mistaken for MH. Carbon dioxide production is lower in these endocrine disorders than in MH. Hypertension is greater in pheochromocytoma than in thyrotoxicosis, and even less in MH. Neither endocrine crisis is associated with as much rigidity as MH. Metabolic acidosis was not present during thyrotoxicosis and not as great during pheochromocytoma as during MH. Thyroid crisis did not trigger MH even in susceptible pigs.[41]

Malignant Hyperthermia Outside the Operating Room

The concern that MH may occur outside the operating room without mediation of drugs in humans has been expressed repeatedly. This concern derives from the often-repeated observation that an MH-like syndrome can occur in certain pig breeds in response to stressful situations. However, documented cases of fulminant MH occurring without drug intervention in humans have not been convincing. Gronert *et al* have described a patient who had episodic fevers and whose muscle biopsies tested positive for MH.[42] The fevers were controlled by dantrolene. Reports have shown that some patients who suffered from heatstroke are MH-susceptible, but many questions still remain.

Concerning the relationship of heat syndromes and MH, some also believe that MH-susceptible patients are likely to die suddenly,[43] but the evidence is not convincing. Detailed information usually is not available regarding the medical history of young people who die suddenly and unexpectedly. Was there evidence of a recent infection? What were the results of previous medical treatments, drug levels, and other tests? Studies of sudden death in young people have found that infection and unrecognized cardiac disease account for more than half the causes of such death. Often, the symptoms of such problems either are mild and unrecognized or are ignored. About 10% of sudden unexpected deaths in healthy young adults result from a cerebral bleed, 25% from asthma and epilepsy, and about 15% from undetermined causes.

A great deal of debate and very few data characterize the discussions regarding sudden death and MH. A more widespread, easier-to-use diagnostic test and a better understanding of the pathophysiologic characteristics of MH are necessary to resolve this issue.

Neuroleptic Malignant Syndrome and Other Disorders

The symptoms and signs of the *neuroleptic malignant syndrome* include fever, rhabdomyolysis, tachycardia, hypertension, agitation, muscle rigidity, and acidosis.[44] The mortality rate is unknown, but may be as high as 20%. Dantrolene is an effective therapeutic modality in many cases of neuroleptic malignant syndrome. Therefore, it is not unusual for an anesthesiologist to be consulted in the management of patients with this disorder.

Although the resemblance of neuroleptic malignant syndrome to MH is striking, there are significant differences between the two. MH is acute, whereas neuroleptic malignant syndrome often occurs after longer term drug exposure. Phenothiazines and haloperidol or any of the newer potent antipsychotic agents alone or in combination are usually triggering agents for neuroleptic malignant syndrome. Sudden withdrawal of drugs used to treat Parkinson's disease may also trigger neuroleptic malignant syndrome. Electroconvulsive therapy (ECT) with succinylcholine does not appear to trigger the syndrome.[45]

Also, neuroleptic malignant syndrome does not seem to be inherited, and there are no case reports of it in family members who have had an episode of MH.

Many believe that the changes in neuroleptic malignant syndrome are a reflection of dopamine depletion in the central nervous system by psychoactive agents. In support of this theory, therapy with bromocriptine, a dopamine agonist, is often useful in treatment of neuroleptic malignant syndrome. Therefore, although there appear to be similarities between MH and neuroleptic malignant syndrome,[46] a common pathophysiology is not readily apparent. From an anesthesiologist's viewpoint, it is best to monitor patients with neuroleptic malignant syndrome as though they were susceptible to MH. However drugs such as succinylcholine have been used for ECT without problems in MH patients.

Drugs That Trigger Malignant Hyperthermia

It is clearly established that the potent inhalation agents, including sevoflurane, desflurane, isoflurane, halothane, methoxyflurane, cyclopropane, and ether, may trigger MH. Succinylcholine and decamethonium are also triggers. The status of many other drugs is less clear. Table 20-1 indicates the drugs we believe to be safe and those that are unsafe.

Local Anesthetics

Based on studies indicating that amide or ester local anesthetics do not trigger MH in susceptible swine and that amide local anesthetics do not trigger MH in susceptible humans, it seems clear that all local anesthetics are safe for MH-susceptible patients.[47,48] Preliminary studies of local anesthetics during an MH crisis (e.g., for dysrhythmia control) do not show an exacerbation of MH by amide local anesthetics.

Catecholamines

Although plasma catecholamine concentration increases during an MH crisis, such an elevation is usually secondary to metabolic and cardiovascular changes. Vasopressors and other catecholamines are not involved in triggering MH.[49] Therefore, these drugs should be used as necessary but only with simultaneous treatment of the MH crisis.

Nondepolarizing Relaxants

Although curare is a suspected trigger of MH,[50] vecuronium, rocuronium, atracurium, pancuronium, and all other nondepolarizing drugs are considered safe to use in patients with MH.

Table 20-1. SAFE VERSUS UNSAFE DRUGS IN MALIGNANT HYPERTHERMIA

Safe Drugs	Unsafe Drugs
Althesin	All inhalation agents (except nitrous oxide)
Antibiotics	Succinylcholine
Antihistamines	Potassium salts
Atracurium	
Barbiturates	
Benzodiazepines	
Droperidol	
Ketamine	
Local anesthetics	
Opioids	
Nitrous oxide	
Pancuronium	
Propofol	
Propranolol	
Vasoactive drugs	
Vecuronium	

Anticholinesterases

Clinical studies have shown that anticholinesterase–anticholinergic combinations are safe for reversal of nondepolarizing relaxants in MH-susceptible patients.[51]

Phenothiazines and Drugs Used to Treat Psychoses

Phenothiazines increase intracellular calcium ion concentration and may cause contractures in vitro in muscle from MH-susceptible patients.[52] Phenothiazines also induce the related neuroleptic malignant syndrome. Therefore, although there have been several reports that phenothiazines are effective in managing temperature fluctuations during recovery from MH, these compounds should be used cautiously in MH-susceptible patients. As of 1999 none of the more than 300 records of fulminant MH in the North American MH Registry included administration of phenothiazines, butyrophenones (droperidol), thioxanthenes, or heterocyclics (haloperidol) prior to the appearance of MH (personal communication from M. G. Larach).

Other Drugs

Digoxin, quinidine, and calcium salts do not induce MH in the swine.[53] Therefore, it is reasonable to assume that they are safe to use in clinical situations. However, potassium salts can trigger MH. This results from a depolarization of the muscle membrane, leading to muscle contracture. Neither ketamine nor propofol is an MH trigger.[54]

Incidence and Epidemiology

Although the incidence of reported episodes of MH has increased, the mortality rate from MH has declined. In part these two trends reflect a greater awareness of the syndrome, earlier diagnosis, and better therapy. The incidence of MH varies from country to country, based on differences in gene pools. In the upper midwest of the United States, for example, there are many families containing large numbers of MH-susceptible people. In contrast, other areas of the country and parts of the world have rarely reported MH. The overall incidence is said to be 1 in 50,000 anesthetics administered in adults and 1 in 15,000 anesthetics administered in children. Results of large-scale studies of operative mortality are in general agreement with this figure. For example, a study in Great Britain revealed 3 cases of MH in 100,000 administered anesthetics.[55] Even now, the best epidemiologic study of MH was done in the mid-1980s by Ording.[20] Based on information supplied to the Danish Malignant Hyperthermia Registry comprising the reported incidence of MH in Denmark (population approximately 5 million), this study revealed fulminant MH in approximately 1 in 250,000 administered anesthetics. However, if the definition of MH is expanded to include abortive cases of MH and is further refined to include only cases in which inhalation anesthetics and succinylcholine were used, the incidence was as high as 1 in 4000 anesthetic administrations![20]

A more recent study by Bachand and colleagues examined the incidence of MH in the province of Quebec, Canada, where many families had been biopsied. They traced the pedigrees of the patients to the original immigrants from France. They found an incidence of MH susceptibility in 0.2% of the population. However, that represented only five extended families.[56]

Currently, the consensus is that the mortality from MH is approximately 10%. However, the epidemiologic characteristics of MH are very difficult to define for the following reasons:

1. Widespread diagnostic testing for MH is difficult to apply.
2. The clinical diagnosis of MH is often questionable.
3. Triggering of MH even in susceptible patients may not occur on an individual anesthetic exposure. In some cases, susceptible patients have received triggering agents for up to 13 anesthetics without any problems, only to have MH

triggered on the subsequent anesthetic. Investigation of the Danish Malignant Hyperthermia Registry found the MH genotype to be expressed in only 34–54% of anesthetic exposures.[57]

4. Registries of MH cases do not capture all data. There is a paucity of data concerning the frequency of use of anesthesia in the general population.

Inheritance of Malignant Hyperthermia

Many of the reasons that limit our understanding of the epidemiologic characteristics of MH also limit our accurate assessment of its inheritance. It would seem that studies of the animal model would clarify the issue of inheritance, but this has not been the case. MH in most pig breeds is inherited in an autosomal recessive fashion.[58] Variabilities in clinical presentation and the fact that MH is not regularly apparent on exposure to triggering agents, even in those who are susceptible, result in great difficulty in assessing the inheritance of MH in humans. The inheritance of MH in humans has been described as autosomal dominant, multifactorial, autosomal dominant with variable penetrance, and multigenetic.[59]

Our studies, as well as anecdotal reports from other diagnostic centers, have supported the concept of autosomal dominant inheritance by a single gene with variable penetrance. Representative examples of such clinical documentation of autosomal dominance are as follows:

1. A 34-year-old man died of the classic MH syndrome. Although his father had a history of ptosis, he had MH-negative results on muscle biopsy. His mother was too ill to have a biopsy performed. A maternal cousin was found to be MH-susceptible on the contracture test, as was his maternal uncle.

2. A 4-year-old child developed masseter rigidity during anesthesia with succinylcholine, with a postepisode CK level of 8000 IU. Her two siblings had negative muscle biopsy results; however, her mother had MH-positive results. None of the children had had anesthesia previously.

3. An 8-year-old boy developed masseter rigidity with CK level elevation after receiving succinylcholine. His father stated that his own father had died of hyperthermia during surgery years previously. The father was MH-susceptible on contracture testing.

Studies of large families have also documented an autosomal dominant pattern.[56] We therefore advise patients that siblings and children of MH-susceptible patients have a 50% risk for this disorder. Although baseline CK determinations may be of no value in screening for MH, relatives of MH-susceptible patients with an elevated CK level (without recent trauma or muscle disorder) have a higher than 80% chance of being susceptible. However, relatives with a normal CK level may also be susceptible.

Diagnostic Tests for Malignant Hyperthermia

Development of the *In Vitro* Contracture Test

In 1970, Kalow *et al* demonstrated that isolated muscle from MH-susceptible patients was unusually sensitive to caffeine when exposed *in vitro*.[4] Shortly thereafter, Ellis and coinvestigators demonstrated that muscle from MH-susceptible patients also had a more sensitive than normal contracture response to halothane.[59] Subsequent studies suggested that specific cutpoints for the halothane and caffeine responses could be adopted for diagnosing MH.[60] The European MH Group (EMHG)[61,62] and North American MH Group (NAMHG)[63–65] separately have standardized protocols for contracture testing. Treatment of muscle biopsy specimens in a tissue bath with either halothane or caffeine has come to be the standard test for diagnosing MH susceptibility.[66–70]

Other tests have been proposed to differentiate patients with MH from those who are normal. Some tests use skeletal muscle biopsy specimens, whereas others employ blood elements such as platelets or white blood cells to determine susceptibility. Most of these tests have been proven to be of either questionable or no value in determining MH status. These tests have been reviewed elsewhere,[66–68,70] and only the currently acceptable or potentially useful tests are addressed in this chapter.

Halothane–Caffeine Contracture Test

The contracture test has also been reviewed elsewhere.[66–68,70] However, this test is constantly undergoing refinement, and the newer developments are emphasized in this chapter. Although some procedures and interpretations differ between the EMHG and NAMHG protocols, the following steps are similar. Skeletal muscle (1–3 g) is usually biopsied from the vastus lateralis muscle. Strips of muscle weighing 100–200 mg and measuring 15–30 mm ($\geq$25 mm preferred) in length by 2–3 mm in width by 2–3 mm in thickness are carefully isolated and mounted in a standard muscle bath apparatus (Fig. 20-1). The tissue bath contains a modified Krebs solution at 37°C bubbled with O_2 and CO_2 (95%/5%), and the resting tension is adjusted to the optimum length for maximal twitch tension (usually about 2 g). The bundles are stimulated supramaximally with pulses of frequency 0.1–0.2 Hz with 2-msec pulses to verify viability. After a 15–60-min equilibration in which the preparation is oxygenated with O_2/CO_2 (95/5%), halothane is added to the gas phase, either as a bolus dose or in incrementally increasing concentrations (Fig. 20-2). The concentration of halothane is verified by gas chromatography. A second set of muscle strips is equilibrated and subsequently exposed to incrementally increasing concentrations of caffeine-free base (see Fig. 20-2). It is recommended that the caffeine strips be tested early in the procedure because they tend to be more sensitive to instability over time.[71] Testing is usually completed within about 5 hours of biopsy to ensure adequate viability of the muscle preparations. Owing to time constraints, it is essential that the biopsy be performed at or within about 1 hour of the testing laboratory. Usually a

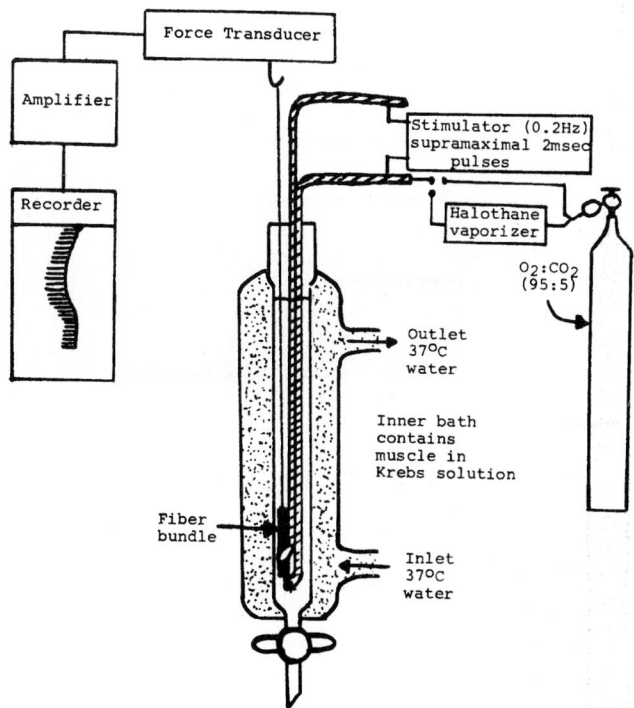

Figure 20-1. Diagram of the muscle bath apparatus used for contracture testing for diagnosing MH susceptibility.

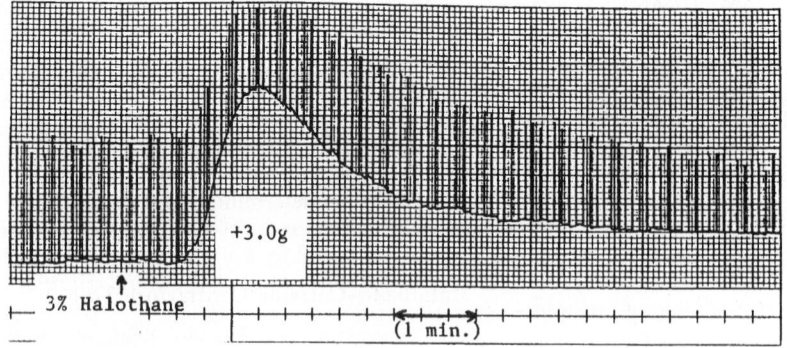

Abnormal Halothane Contracture

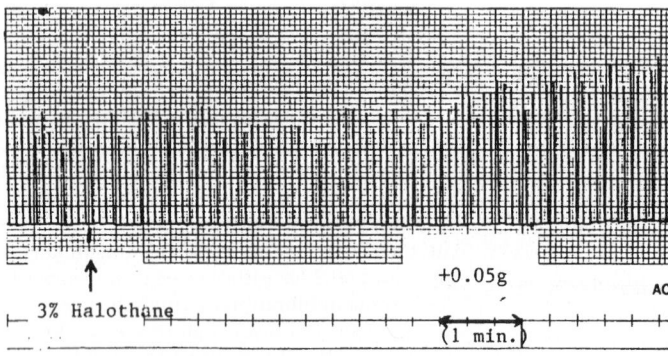

Normal Halothane Contracture

A

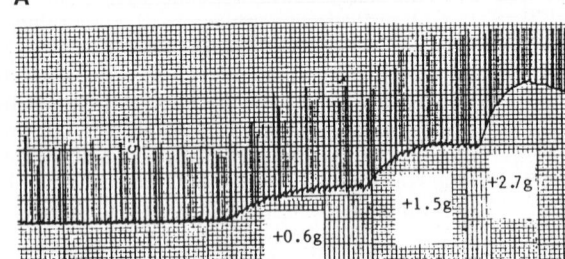

Abnormal Caffeine Dose Response

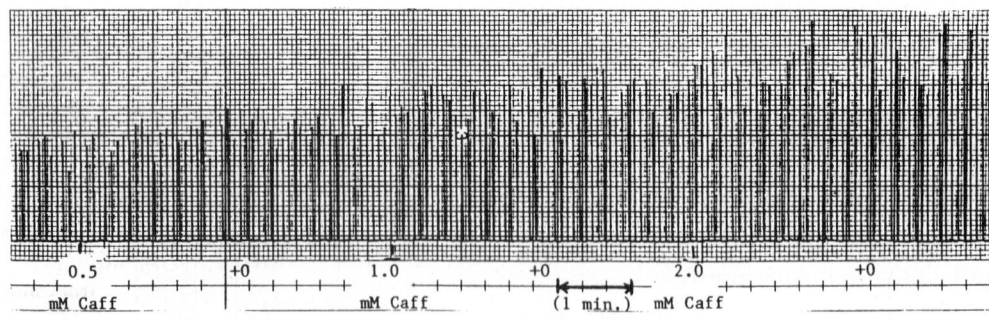

Normal Caffeine Dose Response

B

Figure 20-2. Muscle strips weighing approximately 150 mg and stimulated supramaximally are exposed to 3% halothane or incremental doses of caffeine. (*A*) A 3-g contracture is recorded from this strip from an MHS patient after exposure of the muscle to 3% halothane (*top*); a normal response to 3% halothane (*bottom*). (*B*) Contractures noted after exposure to 0.5, 1, and 2 m*M* caffeine in MHS muscle (*top*); no contracture response to the same caffeine concentrations. Twitch height augmentation is normal following caffeine addition (*bottom*).

histologic evaluation accompanies the contracture test to examine whether the subject has a muscle disorder other than MH.

Interpretation of the Halothane–Caffeine Contracture Test. Two protocols have been adopted for use over the past decade. These protocols were initiated to standardize procedures so that the results from groups of laboratories could be pooled for analysis. Also, a uniform approach was necessary to standardize the phenotype derived from the contracture test for use in genetic analysis.

The EMHG was the first to meet and establish testing standards.[61,62] Halothane is added incrementally by this protocol (0.5, 1.0, 2.0%) with the preparation exposed to each concentration for 3 minutes. In practice, the EMHG requires estimating the time that the expected concentration in the tissue bath is reached (0.11, 0.22, 0.44 mM, respectively) and the 3-minute exposure for each concentration begins after that time is reached. A response indicative of MH susceptibility is based on a contracture threshold (>0.2 g) at a halothane concentration $\leq2\%$ in either of the two muscle strips tested. Caffeine is also added incrementally in concentrations of 0.25, 0.5, 1.0, 1.5, 2.0, 3.0, and 4.0 mM. Each caffeine concentration is maintained until the contracture plateau is reached, or for 3 minutes, whichever is sooner. A positive response is a contracture threshold (>0.2 g) at a concentration of caffeine of 2 mM or less in either of two strips tested.

In the NAMHG protocol[63] a bolus dose of halothane 3% is added to the gas phase for each of three muscle strips and the maximum contracture within 10 minutes is recorded. A positive response is a contracture >0.7 g tension to halothane 3% and a negative response is <0.5 g. An equivocal response to halothane (MH-equivocal, or MHE) is between 0.5 and 0.7 g.[64] As with the EMHG protocol, caffeine is added incrementally, but the concentrations are 0.5, 1.0, 2.0, 4.0, 8.0, and 32 mM; the interval at each concentration is 4 minutes or contracture plateau, whichever is sooner; and three muscle strips are tested. A positive response is a contracture >0.3 g (determined by the specific laboratory) to 2 mM caffeine. The magnitude of contracture at 2 mM caffeine is believed to be more specific and is used as the primary means for interlaboratory comparisons. Also, a response to caffeine 2 mM of <0.2 g is negative, and a response between 0.2 and 0.3 g is MHE.

The interpretations of the outcomes of the halothane and caffeine tests differ between the EMHG and NAMHG protocols. The EMHG protocol requires a positive response to halothane and a positive response to caffeine for a diagnosis of MH-susceptible (MHS). If the outcomes of both tests are negative, then the subject is diagnosed as MH-normal (MHN). If only the caffeine test is abnormal, the patient is considered MHE to caffeine (MHEc). If only the halothane test is abnormal, the patient is considered MHE to halothane (MHEh). The NAMHG protocol differs in that the subject is considered MH positive (MH+ or MHS) if either the response to halothane or the response to caffeine is abnormal. The patient is diagnosed as normal (MH- or MHN) if neither test is positive. As with the EMHG protocol, MHE subjects are treated as positive by the NAMHG.

Sensitivity and Specificity of the Halothane–Caffeine Contracture Test. Three published studies have examined the outcome of the EMHG protocol in patients with a history of fulminant MH. In the first study,[72] of the seven patients with a personal history of fulminant episodes, five were diagnosed as MHS, and two as MHE; all 13 controls (low-risk subjects) were diagnosed as MHN. In a second study[73] the four patients with a personal history of fulminant episodes were all diagnosed as MHS. In the third study, using the combined data from the EMHG,[74] 33 of the 38 patients with a personal history of fulminant MH were MHS and the remaining five were MHE. Sixty-eight of the 73 normal controls were MHN, one was MHEh, and four were MHEc.

The NAMHG protocol was examined in 120 control (low-risk) subjects and 32 patients with a high likelihood of having a fulminant MH episode using data pooled from ten diagnostic centers.[65] Using cutpoints of 0.7 g for halothane (3%) and 0.3 g for caffeine (2 mM), the NAMHG protocol was found to have sensitivity of 88% and specificity of 81% in humans. Lowering the cutpoint for halothane (3%) to 0.5 g with the cutpoint for caffeine (2 mM) of 0.3 g increased the sensitivity to 97% and specificity to 78%.[64,74] Thus, the finding of a positive result by this definition on either or both of the halothane or caffeine contracture tests is the most sensitive definition of MH susceptibility used in North America. In a study specifically using normal vastus lateralis there were no false-positive responses to caffeine (2 mM) or halothane (3%) in 16 patients.[76]

Studies also have been conducted in swine.[77,78] Based on 19 control and 27 MH-susceptible Yorkshire/Duroc swine, the sensitivity of 96% (one false negative) and specificity of 95% (one false positive) were estimated for the NAMHG protocol, using cutpoints of 0.7 g for halothane (3%) and 0.3 g for caffeine (2 mM).[77]

When the outcome of either the NAMHG or EMHG protocols is compared to the outcome of the other in humans, the diagnoses are similar, but not necessarily identical.[73,79] However, in the one study with patients with personal histories of fulminant episodes, all four were diagnosed as MHS by the EMHG protocol and MH+ by the NAMHG protocol.[73] In a comparison of the NAMHG and EMHG halothane testing protocols, the outcomes of the two protocols were identical in nine of ten MH and three of four control pigs.[78] The one negative test to halothane by the EMHG protocol was accompanied by a positive test to caffeine, making the diagnosis MHEc by the EMHG protocol; the pig would be treated as if MH-susceptible. In a study of 84 patients referred for diagnostic testing the two protocols produced similar diagnoses.[79] At a different testing center there was agreement between the diagnoses reached by these two protocols in 87% of 156 patients and 17 controls.[80] The divergence in opinion occurred in patients whose contracture results were near the cutoff rather than in those with strongly positive or unquestionably negative results. Taking the final information conveyed to the patient into account (*e.g.*, for EMHG, MHE is clinically treated as MHS), it is not clear that one protocol is significantly better than another. Both protocols and their interpretations are prone to small numbers of false positives. However, the initial patient selection for diagnostic testing reduces this possibility.[81] The more important function of the test is to decrease the possibility of a false diagnosis that MH exists in families that do not carry the causative gene, as would happen if all relatives of a proband were assumed to be susceptible. The EMHG protocol reduced the number of marginal responders, which may make the remaining diagnoses slightly more accurate for use in genetic studies.[79]

Other Contracture Tests

Ryanodine. An additional contracture test using the plant alkaloid ryanodine was recently proposed for inclusion in the EMHG protocol because the ryanodine receptor (the Ca^{2+} release channel of skeletal muscle) was believed to be the only cause of MH. It was reasoned that this test would afford maximum specificity for MH, and early studies supported this concept.[79,82-85] The NAMHG has adopted the same protocol used by the EMHG to provide a common denominator for data interchange between groups.

The basic testing conditions for ryanodine are similar to those described for halothane and caffeine testing. High-purity ryanodine is employed. A bolus of ryanodine (1 μM) is added to the bath and the time to onset of contracture, time to 0.2-g contracture, time to 1-g contracture, and the time and amplitude of maximum contracture are recorded. Discrimination was improved by using the time to initial contracture and time to development of a 10-mN (1 g) contracture.[86] Variability between laboratories currently prevents recommendation of specific diagnostic guidelines for this test.[86]

4-Chloro-m-cresol. 4-Chloro-*m*-cresol (4-CmC) is a potent activator of ryanodine receptor–mediated Ca^{2+} release. Cumulative administration of 25, 50, 75, 100, 150, and 200 $\mu mol \cdot l^{-1}$ 4-CmC produced concentration-dependent contractures. Contractures developed earlier and to a greater magnitude in muscle from patients identified as MHS by the EMHG protocol than in normal muscle.[87] The accuracy of this test for MHS is 100% compared to the EMHG protocol at a threshold of 75 $\mu mol \cdot l^{-1}$ 4-CmC.[88] However, muscle defined as MHEh by the EMHG protocol reacts to 4-CmC as does normal muscle.[89] Thus the utility of the 4-CmC contracture test is not well defined.

Pitfalls in the Contracture Test

Ideally, each laboratory should derive specimens from patients who are clearly and unequivocally normal and those who are clearly and unequivocally MH-susceptible to verify that cutpoints for MH susceptibility are diagnostic within the laboratory. Unfortunately, because of the variation in presentation of MH and the confusion with signs associated with non-MH causes, it is not always possible to have complete agreement on the MH status of a patient based on a clinical history, even among experts in the field. This problem has made estimates of sensitivity and specificity difficult.

A clinical grading scale has been developed to address concerns for objectively evaluating the clinical episode.[75,90] The scale was developed with the input of 11 internationally recognized experts in the clinical aspects of MH. This scale lacks sensitivity, because incomplete recording of necessary data or early termination of the crisis would not yield scores indicative of MH, even if an episode had occurred. The scoring system also is designed to avoid overweighting duplicative indicators representing the same processes. The value of the grading scale is mainly in identifying those subjects with the most convincing episodes of MH for subsequent evaluation of the sensitivity and specificity of the diagnostic tests. The clinical grading scale is useful in evaluating clinical episodes in those cases in which the subject is rated a 6 (almost certainly MH), but lower scores should not be considered for actual diagnosis. We would even encourage the practice of sending patients rated 6 for diagnostic testing, because these individuals are rare and essential for the continuing evaluation of the sensitivity and specificity of the halothane–caffeine contracture test and the new ryanodine test. Additionally, these subjects may prove to be important for inclusion in the genetic studies of MH.

One of the main problems in MH testing is that, on halothane–caffeine testing, two separate groups may not be discernible; rather, a continuum of responses is observed.[67,91] Susceptibility is determined by a response above or below a certain threshold. Addition of a ryanodine component to the contracture test may improve the specificity of this test for those in whom abnormal function of the ryanodine channel is responsible for MH susceptibility. But this may not be the case for all MH-susceptibles. In addition, there may be variability between individual strips from the same muscle biopsy specimen.[22,67,70,92–94] At present the cause for this variation is not understood, but both protocols require testing multiple muscle strips to halothane and caffeine.

There have been a few incidents in which patients who were diagnosed as nonsusceptible by contracture testing subsequently experienced clinical episodes highly suggestive of MH; and in one case, the estimated false-negative rate was 4 out of 171 subjects (2%).[95,96] The interpretation of these studies is controversial, and not all investigators are convinced that these are valid cases of MH. In contrast, two studies have reported 16 MHN patients receiving triggering agents on 23 occasions[97] and 13 MHN patients receiving triggering agents on 26 occasions,[98] all without complications. Unfortunately, studies like these are difficult to conduct because they require large patient populations and tracking of subjects diagnosed several years before the actual study. Such studies are also rare in the literature because they are negative findings and more difficult to publish than studies of false-negatives. Until more data are gathered, it is difficult to put the occasional false-negative diagnosis into proper perspective.

Variability seems to exist between families in the magnitude of contracture.[99] This may be due to the inheritance of different genetic defects. Although some investigators have suggested using different cutpoints for different families,[100] this would be impractical because of the need for testing large numbers of family members to establish these cutpoints. Because relatively few normal controls exceed the standards established by the two protocols,[65,72,74,76] the larger magnitude of contractures observed in some MH families over others[99] may be of interest more in studies of pathophysiology and genetics than in diagnosis.

Until such time as all the basic biochemical defects of MH are uncovered, the contracture test will always be subject to some differences in interpretation. However, the halothane–caffeine contracture test is currently the only method of MH diagnosis that has been standardized and has had sensitivity and specificity confirmed in any manner by multiple centers throughout the world.

Tests with More Limited Usefulness in Malignant Hyperthermia Diagnosis

Alternative tests that have not gained acceptance within the EMHG or NAMHG have been reviewed elsewhere.[66,67,68,70] These tests include lymphocyte tests, platelet aggregation, skinned fiber tests, adenosine triphosphate depletion, erythrocyte osmotic fragility, and others. The tests discussed below have at least some usefulness in some cases of MH.

Elevated resting CK values are associated with MH susceptibility in a few families. However, many subjects susceptible to MH do not have elevated CK values, making this method of diagnosis relatively insensitive.[68] Also, several muscle disorders are associated with resting CK values, making this test nonspecific.[68] Nevertheless, the only identifiable muscle disorder in many cases of elevated CK levels is MH.[101] The most important application of elevated CK levels is in those families in which at least a few members have undergone diagnostic contracture testing, and in these subjects elevated CK levels cosegregate with MH susceptibility. In this instance, other family members can tentatively be diagnosed by CK levels. We caution that this method of diagnosis is only tentative and should be confirmed by contracture testing. Elevated CK values also may be useful in preliminarily identifying key family members to be referred for contracture testing and in identifying MH in children too young to undergo contracture testing.

The use of resting CK values for general screening for MH is neither sensitive nor specific, but there is a relationship between high postoperative CK values associated with MMR and the probability for diagnosis as MH-susceptible by the contracture test.[14,22,67] Although it is not a perfect indicator of MH susceptibility,[102] the chances are about 80% that a CK value >20,000 after MMR will yield a positive diagnosis by contracture testing.[14,22] A relatively normal CK postoperatively does not rule out the possibility of an acute MH reaction during that anesthetic.[103]

Intracellular pH and levels of inorganic phosphate, phosphocreatine, adenosine triphosphate, phosphomonoesterase, and phosphodiesters can be measured noninvasively by nuclear magnetic resonance (NMR) spectrometry. Alterations in the ratio of inorganic phosphate to phosphocreatine, phosphocreatine recovery rates, and other parameters are observed in MH-susceptible patients using NMR.[104–107] Special equipment and personnel are necessary to perform this test, and diagnosis by this method is restricted to just a few centers. As with elevated CK values, several other muscle disorders would give a false-positive diagnosis of MH, making analysis for muscle disorders mandatory. A negative finding should still be confirmed by the *in vitro* contracture test.

Blood tests using genetic screening are included here not because they are currently useful, but to allow for future developments in genetic screening. Neither we nor other investigators[108] advise genetic testing in its current state. As discussed in greater detail under pathogenesis and etiology, the cause–effect relationships of the defects and MH have not been satisfactorily established.

The utility of genetic tests for diagnosing malignant hyperthermia is discussed in more detail in the section on pathogenesis. In a few families where a specific mutation has been identified in the ryanodine receptor gene that correlates with an abnormal contracture response to halothane or caffeine, it is possible to determine MH susceptibility by screening the DNA of relatives for that mutation. If the mutation is present, the patient may be considered to be at risk to MH. But if it is not present, the patient cannot be presumed to be MH-negative.[109] We believe that, as the molecular genetics of MH are unraveled, molecular genetic testing will replace the more invasive diagnostic tests. At present, however, this prospect is remote.

Treatment of Malignant Hyperthermia

Malignant hyperthermia is a treatable disorder. If it is diagnosed early and treated promptly with proper continuing observation, the mortality rate should be close to zero. All institutions in which anesthetic agents are administered should have dantrolene available [36 ampules (720 mg) is recommended] and have a plan of management.

The Acute Episode

The following steps should be taken immediately when MH is diagnosed:

1. Administration of all inhalation agents and succinylcholine should be discontinued.
2. Hyperventilation with 100% oxygen should be instituted at high flow rates, and assistance should be secured. (It is usually helpful to have a cart available containing the agents for treatment of MH.)
3. Assistance should be obtained in mixing dantrolene. The present preparation of dantrolene is poorly soluble. Each ampule containing 20 mg should be mixed with 50 ml of sterile distilled water (not saline solution). Initial intravenous therapy should be started with a minimum dose of $2.5 \text{ mg} \cdot \text{kg}^{-1}$ with repeat doses as needed.[109] It is often recommended that the maximum dose of dantrolene be $10 \text{ mg} \cdot \text{kg}^{-1}$, but more should be given as dictated by clinical circumstances.
4. Titration of dantrolene and bicarbonate to heart rate, body temperature, and Pa_{CO_2} is the best clinical guideline of therapy.
5. In fulminant cases in which significant metabolic acidosis is present, $2-4 \text{ mEq} \cdot \text{kg}^{-1}$ bicarbonate should be given.
6. If it is not already available, a capnometer should be obtained so that CO_2 excretion can be followed.
7. If at all possible, the anesthesia circuit and CO_2 absorbent should be changed because residual inhalation anesthetics may contaminate the anesthesia circuit. If not, very high flows, $>10 \text{ l} \cdot \text{min}^{-1}$, of oxygen should be used.
8. Dysrhythmia control usually follows hyperventilation, dantrolene therapy, and correction of acidosis. Calcium channel blockers should not be used in the acute treatment of MH. Several studies have shown that verapamil can interact with dantrolene to produce hyperkalemia and myocardial depression.[110,111] Lidocaine can be safely used to treat dysrhythmias during an MH crisis.
9. Body temperature elevation should be managed by packing the patient with external ice packs and by use of gastric, wound, and rectal lavage. Gastric lavage is the quickest, most practical means for rapid temperature

control. Some have recommended peritoneal dialysis and others, cardiopulmonary bypass. Cooling should be stopped when body temperature reaches approximately 38°C to avoid hypothermia.
10. Although arterial blood gas determinations are useful for assessing acidosis, central mixed venous blood gas determinations (or, if not available, femoral venous blood gas readings) serve as a better guideline for therapy.
11. Hyperkalemia should be managed in the usual fashion. If hyperkalemia is associated with significant cardiac effects, calcium should be given. During therapy of MH, hypokalemia frequently results. However, potassium replacement should be undertaken very cautiously, if at all, because potassium may retrigger a MH episode.

Management After the Acute Episode

After the acute episode, the clinician should be concerned about three complications of MH:

1. Recrudescence of MH. Although most cases of MH resolve promptly with therapy, some cases are difficult to control. As many as 25% of patients may experience acute recrudescence within hours of the first episode.[112]
2. Disseminated intravascular coagulation.[113] Disseminated intravascular coagulation has often been described in cases of MH, probably resulting from release of thromboplastins secondary to shock and/or release of cellular contents on membrane destruction. The usual regimen for treatment of disseminated intravascular coagulation should be followed.
3. Myoglobinuric renal failure. CK elevations may not occur for 6–12 hours after a MH episode and should be followed as a rough guide for therapy. However, myoglobinuria classically occurs within 4–8 hours of the episode; therefore, bladder catheterization is recommended.

The guidelines for the dose and duration of dantrolene therapy after resolution of acute MH are empirical. It would seem prudent to continue dantrolene, $1 \text{ mg} \cdot \text{kg}^{-1}$ every 6 hours intravenously, for at least 24–36 hours. Some recommend conversion of dantrolene therapy from intravenous to oral form ($4 \text{ mg} \cdot \text{kg}^{-1}$ per day or more) with continuation for several days.

Significant muscle weakness may follow MH, resulting from muscle destruction along with dantrolene administration; this should be managed symptomatically.

A variety of other electrolyte changes may occur, such as hypocalcemia and hyperphosphatemia. Sodium and chloride changes may occur secondary to fluid shifts during the acute episode. All these changes usually respond to control of the acute episode.

Dantrolene

In 1979, intravenous dantrolene was approved by the FDA for treatment of MH. Until that time, the primary use of dantrolene was in the management of spasticity. Dantrolene is a unique muscle relaxant. Unlike neuromuscular blocking agents (whose site of action is at the nicotinic receptor of the neuromuscular junction) or the nonspecific relaxants (which modulate spinal cord synaptic reflexes), dantrolene acts within the muscle cell itself by reducing intracellular levels of calcium. Most likely, this results from a reduction of calcium release by the sarcoplasmic reticulum or inhibition of excitation contracture coupling at the transverse tubular level. It has now been demonstrated that during a MH episode, dantrolene reduces intracellular calcium levels. Therefore, dantrolene is a specific and effective agent in the treatment of MH. In the usual clinical doses, dantrolene has little effect on myocardial contractility.[114]

Studies have also indicated that doses of neuromuscular blocking agents need not be changed significantly after dantrolene administration. However, the drug should be used cautiously in patients with neuromuscular disease.[115]

The serum level of dantrolene required for prophylaxis against MH is about 2.5 $\mu g \cdot ml^{-1}$. The half-life of intravenous dantrolene, which is the only form recommended, is approximately 12 hours. However, the therapeutic level of dantrolene usually persists for 4–6 hours after a usual intravenous dose of $2.5 \ mg \cdot kg^{-1}$.[116] Therefore, dantrolene should be supplemented at least every 6 hours after a clinical episode. Some muscle weakness may persist for 24 hours after dantrolene therapy is discontinued. Nausea and phlebitis are other complications of acute dantrolene administration. Hepatotoxicity has been demonstrated only with long-term use of oral dantrolene. Prophylaxis for MH should be carried out with intravenous or oral dantrolene ($5 \ mg \cdot kg^{-1}$ per 24 hours) in those *rare* situations where prophylaxis is desired.[117]

Management of the Patient Susceptible to Malignant Hyperthermia

Because of an increasing awareness of MH and more widespread use of diagnostic tests, it is not unusual for an anesthesiologist to be confronted with a MH-susceptible patient or a patient who has a family history of MH. The management of such patients should be carefully planned.

In the preoperative interview, the anesthesiologist should try to obtain sufficient information regarding previous episodes of MH and their documentation. The anesthesiologist should allow adequate time to reassure patients and their families that he or she is familiar with MH and its implications and that appropriate prophylaxis and therapy will be instituted as necessary. It may be worth mentioning that there have been no deaths from MH in previously diagnosed MH-susceptible patients when the anesthesia team was aware of the problem. Some believe that anxiety may predispose a patient to MH and therefore recommend that anxiolytic agents be included in the premedication. Standard premedicant drugs such as opioids, benzodiazepines, ataractics, barbiturates, and antihistamines do not cause problems in MH-susceptible patients when administered in appropriate doses; however, we do not recommend phenothiazines for premedication. Anticholinergics are also used routinely.

Dantrolene need not be given preoperatively if nontrigger agents are used and end-tidal CO_2 and core temperature are monitored. Dantrolene must be immediately available in the operating room, and equipment for rapid measurement of blood gases and electrolytes should be available.

The anesthesia machine is prepared by draining or removing vaporizors, changing tubing and CO_2 absorbent, and flowing oxygen at $10 \ l \cdot min^{-1}$ for 20 minutes.[118] Obviously, iced solutions and adequate supplies of dantrolene must be available in the vicinity of the operating room when MH-susceptible patients are anesthetized.

Exhaled CO_2 should be monitored because the earliest sign of MH is an increase in CO_2 production and excretion.[119] In the absence of capnography, blood gas monitoring is recommended. Arterial and central venous monitoring is recommended for MH-susceptible patients, as dictated by the surgical procedure. Body temperature should be monitored by nasopharyngeal, rectal, or esophageal routes in all patients for all surgical procedures. Skin temperature, although acceptable, is not as desirable because it may lag core temperature.[120]

If possible, a regional, local, or major conduction anesthetic should be used with either amide or ester local anesthetics. If not possible, intravenous induction of anesthesia followed by nitrous oxide, oxygen, and nondepolarizing relaxant with opioid supplementation is recommended. Other induction agents that have not been implicated in MH are midazolam, diazepam, droperidol, and propofol.

Neuromuscular blocking agents such as pancuronium, vecuronium, atracurium and cisatracurium, rocuronium, and miva-

curium are safe, according to animal and human studies. We routinely reverse nondepolarizing relaxants with anticholinesterase and anticholinergic agents.

Many thousands of safe anesthetics have been administered with nitrous oxide in MH-susceptible patients. Two cases have been reported in which early signs of MH have been documented despite the use of a safe anesthetic technique.[121] Therefore, even under the most controlled circumstances, the anesthesiologist should be alert to the early signs of MH.

We do not continue dantrolene after operation if there are no signs of MH. However, the patient must be observed closely for 4–6 hours. MH has not occurred after surgery when dantrolene pretreatment and safe anesthetic techniques were used. The patient may be discharged on the same day as surgery if indicated.

The same precautions should be taken for the obstetric patient as for the routine surgical patient. We are not convinced that the stress of labor may precipitate MH, and we recommend well-conducted epidural anesthesia for labor and delivery without dantrolene pretreatment but with careful monitoring of vital signs. If an emergency cesarean section with general anesthesia is necessary, alternatives to succinylcholine should be used. In the very acute situation, anesthesia should be induced and dantrolene administration should be considered thereafter. The maternal:fetal partition ratio for dantrolene is probably 0.4.[122] Dantrolene has not been reported to produce significant problems for the fetus or newborn, but existing data are very scanty.

Malignant Hyperthermia in Species Other Than Pigs and People

Malignant hyperthermia has been reported sporadically in many species. Clinical episodes have been documented in cats, dogs, and horses. Capture myopathy is a syndrome characterized by temperature elevation, rhabdomyolysis, acidosis, and death in wild animals (*e.g.,* zebra, elk).[123] This also has been suggested to be an MH variant.

Medicolegal Aspects

In this era of malpractice actions, it is not surprising that MH cases have been the subject of malpractice suits. Because MH may be considered an inborn genetic problem with a relatively fixed associated mortality that may go unrecognized before a patient's exposure to triggering agents, it may be used as a "cover" for other problems.

Fever, opisthotonic posturing, and neurologic abnormalities may accompany hypoxic brain injury, and because of their similarity to MH, MH may be incorrectly implicated in the differential diagnosis. Furthermore, after cardiac arrest from any cause, CK and potassium levels may be significantly elevated. We do not know of data concerning the incidence of litigation after the occurrence of MH.

Some have stated that, with the advent of dantrolene, there should be no deaths from MH; this is probably unrealistic because the syndrome may be truly explosive in some cases and impossible to control with current therapy. Also, we are not completely familiar with all factors that lead to MH, including which drugs may trigger it and the proper dose of dantrolene needed to prevent recrudescence. Nevertheless, certain common themes underlie the basis for litigation in MH:

1. Failure to obtain a thorough personal history in regard to anesthetic problems and a family history of any unexplained perioperative problems.
2. Failure to monitor temperature continuously with an electronic temperature monitoring device. Several jury trial cases have been lost by the defense because the patient's temperature was not monitored. Intraoperative tempera-

ture monitoring is now considered a "standard of care" in the U.S. by the legal profession, despite the failure of the American Society of Anesthesiologists to recommend routine temperature monitoring during administration of all general anesthetics.

3. Failure to have adequate supplies of dantrolene on hand with a plan of management of MH.

4. Failure to investigate unexplained increases in body temperature and increased skeletal muscle tone (especially after succinylcholine administration) when associated with increased heart rate and dysrhythmias.

Several examples of medicolegal cases involving these principles are described below:

1. Increased heart rate developed in a 35-year-old man during a bowel resection for regional enteritis. His oral temperature by mercury thermometer was 37°C. The oral thermometer was left in place and the anesthesia continued with halothane and nitrous oxide. Toward the end of the procedure, there was a rapid increase in heart rate followed by an increase in body temperature. Despite cooling and administration of procainamide (this episode occurred in the predantrolene era) and other appropriate medical therapy, disseminated intravascular coagulopathy eventually developed and the patient died. The plaintiff won the case when it was tried by jury primarily because continuous electronic temperature monitoring was available and was not used.

2. A young female patient had shoulder surgery with isoflurane–nitrous oxide–oxygen. Again, temperature was not monitored continuously. At the end of the procedure, premature ventricular beats and increasing end-tidal carbon dioxide were noted. The patient had a cardiac arrest as the dysrhythmia was being treated. As the drapes were being removed, the patient felt warm. A temperature probe revealed a reading of nearly 42°C. The patient was diagnosed as having an acute episode of MH. Dantrolene was administered an hour later. The patient developed DIC over the next day and died. The case was settled out of court.

3. A 26-year-old woman was undergoing a breast augmentation in a plastic surgeon's office using general anesthesia with isoflurane. Toward the end of the procedure, her heart rate increased as did end-tidal carbon dioxide and and skin temperature. Dantrolene was not available and the patient was sent to a nearby emergency room. By the time dantrolene was given, her temperature was about 43°C. She developed DIC and died. The case is under litigation.

4. Symptoms of bowel obstruction developed in a middle-aged man. He was taken to a local hospital, and anesthesia was administered with nitrous oxide–oxygen–halothane and succinylcholine. His temperature was not monitored, but an unexplained tachycardia (140–160 beats·min^{-1}) was present throughout the 2-hour procedure. On arrival in the intensive care unit after the operation, the patient was slightly hypotensive. Invasive monitoring was started. Despite marked metabolic and respiratory acidosis, a Pa_{CO_2} of 100 mm Hg, and a recorded temperature of nearly 42°C, MH was not diagnosed. A cooling blanket and antibiotics failed to arrest the decrease in the patient's blood pressure, which eventually led to cardiac arrest. A judgment against the physicians and hospital of $4.5 million was reached.

There have been several malpractice cases filed against anesthesiologists in which cardiac arrest and death occurred after succinylcholine was used in patients with an undiagnosed myopathy. The usual outcome is an out-of-court settlement.

The message is clear. All facilities where general anesthesia is administered (including hospitals, outpatient surgery centers, physician offices, dental offices) should have a full supply of dantrolene available. All patients undergoing general anesthesia should have standard monitoring, including end-tidal carbon dioxide and, except for brief cases, body temperature.

Patient Support Services

To answer the needs of patients and families who wished to learn more about MH and of those families whose relatives have died from MH, support groups were founded in several countries (*e.g.*, the Malignant Hyperthermia Association [of Canada] and the Malignant Hyperthermia Association of the United States). Both groups serve as a repository of information about MH, provide names of physicians knowledgeable about MH and the location of MH diagnostic centers, and simply lend an ear to those with MH who have questions. Both organizations have an advisory committee of physicians but are run by volunteers who usually have a personal connection with MH. Both organize annual meetings for physicians and nonphysicians. The Malignant Hyperthermia Association of the United States publishes a quarterly newsletter, *The Communicator*, with excerpts from the medical literature, explanatory articles, questions and answers, and related information. In addition, a hotline has been organized so that a physician with an urgent question about MH can be placed in contact with a knowledgeable specialist. Approximately 30–40 calls a month are handled by this hotline.

The address of the Malignant Hyperthermia Association of the United States is 32 S. Main St., P.O. Box 1069, Sherburne, NY 13815. The phone number is 1-800-98MHAUS. The hotline number is 1-800-MHHyper. The Web site address is http://www.mhaus.org.

The address of the Malignant Hyperthermia Association of Canada is Room 314, Elizabeth Wing, Toronto General Hospital, 101 College Street, Toronto, Ontario M5G1L7.

In 1989, the North American MH Registry was formed. Based in Pittsburgh, Pennsylvania (Children's Hospital of Pittsburgh, 412-692-5464), the Registry will eventually be the repository for patient- and family-specific information for MH-susceptible patients. The Registry was merged with MHAUS in 1992.

Physicians who want to provide patient services for MH must prepare for lengthy discussions about the disorder, because patients usually have very limited information.

Pathogenesis and Etiology

With the clinical complexities of MH as a background, the equally complex pathophysiology and etiology can be more easily explored. Several major developments have contributed to the present understanding of MH. The first was the recognition that the syndrome is genetically transmitted.[2] This finding is significant because it suggests that a rigorous application of modern molecular genetics will lead to the identification of mutations in specific proteins causing the disorder. A second finding was a greater sensitivity of biopsied skeletal muscle from MH-susceptible patients to halothane or caffeine.[124] This was the basis for an *in vitro* diagnostic test and studies of the mechanisms underlying MH. The third was the recognition of similarities between human MH and porcine stress syndrome.[125] This animal model was used to elucidate the role of altered Ca^{2+} regulation in MH and led to the finding that a mutation in the ryanodine receptor may be a causative factor in some families with MH.[126] Fourth, MH has been identified as a heterogeneous disorder.[127,128] Heterogeneity may account for some variability in presentation and forces investigators to consider the role of a final common pathway resulting from a mutation in any one of several different proteins. Fifth, the finding that pigs or human subjects with MH do not always trigger in response to adequate triggering agents, has suggested that a modulator influences the expression of the syndrome.[129,130]

Experimental Models for Malignant Hyperthermia

Although MH is rare in humans, breeding pigs for leaner meat and better musculature has resulted in the appearance of the MH gene (or genes) in relatively high frequency in a number of herds (*e.g.*, Poland, China, Landrace, Pietrain). This has been a major concern for breeders because the meat from pigs with MH is not marketable. A syndrome in pigs undergoing anesthesia is similar to the MH syndrome in humans. However, the porcine syndrome can also be elicited in the absence of anesthetics, by factors such as heat and stress. Although pigs administered MH-triggering anesthetics have provided a model for human MH, there is no evidence that a human stress syndrome completely analogous to the porcine stress syndrome (PSS) exists in the majority of patients. However, some evidence is accumulating for an association between exertional heat stroke and MH.[131-133] A single genetic defect in the ryanodine receptor has been associated with porcine MH, and this specific mutation is found in a small percentage of humans with MH. The mode of inheritance in swine (autosomal recessive)[134] is different from that in humans (autosomal dominant). The porcine model has been extensively exploited in studies of MH. Reports of MH exist, but are rare, in horses, dogs, and cats. Of these, only the dog has been proposed as a model of human MH.[135] The pattern of inheritance in the dog appears to be autosomal dominant, yet there are some differences between the anesthesia-elicited canine and human MH syndromes.

Understanding the Malignant Hyperthermia Defect: Necessary Concepts

A hypothesis explaining MH must account for the puzzling clinical observations surrounding this disorder. Most importantly, the large majority of these patients function normally in the absence of anesthetics. Therefore, the defect should not significantly interfere with normal muscle physiology. The defect, at least in humans, appears to be expressed significantly only in skeletal muscle. The expression of the syndrome shows a large variability among individuals. For example, 30% of patients have had up to three uneventful anesthetics.[136,137] A spectrum of presentations can occur, ranging from relatively minor intraoperative complications to rapid temperature rise, muscle rigidity, acidosis, dysrhythmias, and death. Some cases have a greater latency to onset and are not made manifest until several hours postoperatively. MH does not always occur in response to triggering agents. This is a well-established observation in human MH[136,137] and similar observations have been reported in swine. Young PSS-susceptible pigs experience a period of several weeks during which they cannot be triggered.[138,139] Also, while most investigators would agree that PSS is a more consistently triggered syndrome than the human MH syndrome, even adult swine occasionally do not respond to adequate triggering agents in either a barnyard challenge with halothane alone[140] or prolonged halothane,[141] or halothane and succinylcholine challenge.[129] The term "MH" may, in fact, be a misnomer, as sometimes patients show no signs of temperature elevation. Finally, many cases do not exhibit rigidity, which is sometimes incorrectly considered a hallmark sign of the syndrome. The large variability among individuals may be explained by different genes causing MH in different families or by other predisposing factors being expressed differently in different patients or families.[142] The function of many different proteins has been reported to be altered in MH skeletal muscle. Thus, it is reasonable to assume that systems other than those directly involved in Ca^{2+} regulation are secondarily altered in MH and these may play a crucial role in modifying the response to triggering agents. The involvement of secondary systems would explain the high variability in the phenotype.

Skeletal Muscle: Site of the Malignant Hyperthermia Defect

The MH and PSS defects are expressed in skeletal muscle, as evidenced by the *in vitro* contracture test for MH susceptibility. Results regarding other tissues are more controversial, especially in humans, and are not considered in detail in this chapter. The defects are expressed in Type I and Type II fibers.[143] While the distributions and amounts of protein in whole skeletal muscle[144] and in isolated sarcoplasmic reticulum[145] appear to be normal by electrophoretic analysis, down-regulation of specific proteins, including the ryanodine receptor[146] and dihydropyridine receptor,[147] has been reported. Additionally, the expression of subtypes of the sodium channel is altered in MH muscle.[148-150] The gross distribution of lipids in MH muscle is close to normal,[151] but subtle differences have been reported.[152,153] The detection of protein and lipid alterations depends on the methodologies employed and, in some cases, is an artifact of the methodology.

Acidosis is highly characteristic of human MH and the PSS on *in vivo* challenge with triggering agents. These findings are confirmed by a marked decrease in pH in *in vitro* incubates of porcine MH skeletal muscle.[154] However, in human MH skeletal muscle incubated *in vitro*, the pH decrease is much less and is similar for MH and control human muscle. Based on the *in vitro* contracture response to halothane, the MH lesion and possible modifying factors are not uniformly expressed in the skeletal muscle mass.[155]

Altered Calcium Regulation: The Common Final Pathway

Ultimately, the main problem in skeletal muscle is a lack of control of myoplasmic Ca^{2+} concentration during anesthesia,[6,156] which may be manifest clinically as muscle rigidity. Ca^{2+} levels are controlled by a complex interaction of Ca^{2+} release from the terminal cisternae, the adenosine triphosphate-driven Ca^{2+} pumps at the sarcoplasmic reticulum and sarcolemma, Na^+/Ca^{2+} exchange, several Ca^{2+} buffering proteins (calsequestrin, parvalbumin) and mitochondrial Ca^{2+} regulation (Fig. 20-3). Although several of these systems may become involved as the MH syndrome progresses, the difficulty in Ca^{2+} regulation appears to originate in the Ca^{2+} release mechanism in the terminal cisternae. The Ca^{2+} release mechanism could be made sensitive to anesthetics by any of several possibilities, including: a mutation in the skeletal muscle calcium release channel, termed the ryanodine receptor (*ryr*1); a protein directly coupled to *ryr*1 (e.g., dihydropyridine receptor); or an altered modulator of *ryr*1 function (*e.g.*, fatty acids). The target of succinylcholine is not clear at this time, but is presumed to be the acetylcholine receptor. Opening of the acetylcholine receptor depolarizes the muscle by opening the voltage-dependent sodium currents, which have altered function in MH. Depolarization leads to Ca^{2+} release from the sarcoplasmic reticulum. Dantrolene antagonizes Ca^{2+} release from the sarcoplasmic reticulum and can lower elevated Ca^{2+} levels and reverse an episode of MH.[6]

Presence or Absence of a Malignant Hyperthermia-Associated Defect Within Skeletal Muscle Organelles

Sarcolemma. The sarcolemma (Fig. 20-3) maintains the membrane potential of the muscle cell and acts as a permeability barrier to ions, including Na^+, K^+, Cl^-, and Ca^{2+}. Skeletal muscle, in most cases, does not require extracellular Ca^{2+} for nerve- or electrically evoked contractility. In contrast, halothane-induced contractures[155-157] and, to a lesser extent (depending on the species), caffeine-induced contractures[156] require extracellular Ca^{2+}. A loss of integrity in the sarcolemma could cause a large influx of Ca^{2+} from the extracellular medium. Also, opening specific Ca^{2+} channels (*e.g.*, dihydropyridine receptors) in the sarcolemma would allow the entry of extracellular Ca^{2+}. However, the dihydropyridine receptors in skeletal muscle do

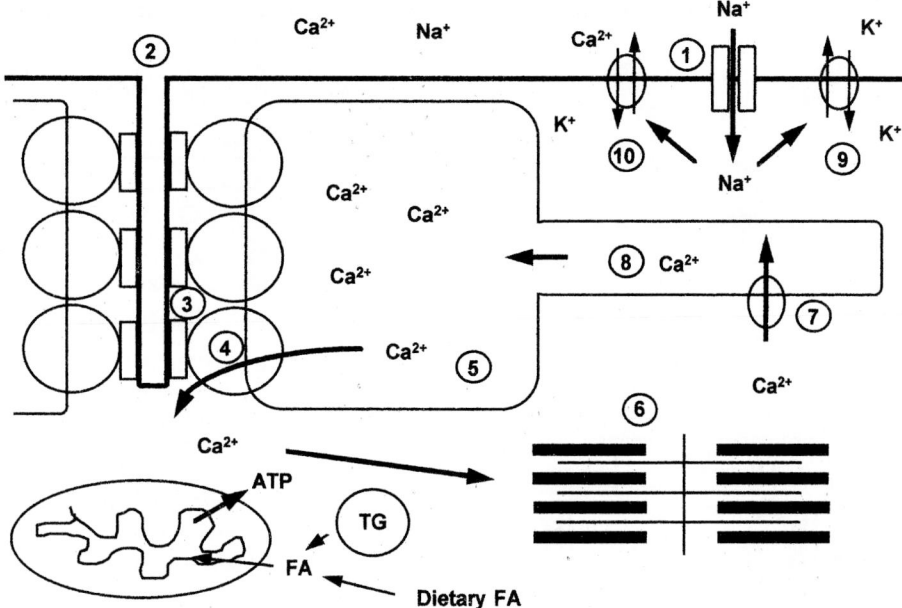

Figure 20-3. Excitation-contraction coupling and MH. The action potential generated at the endplate region of the neuromuscular junction is propagated down the sarcolemma (muscle plasma membrane) by the opening of voltage-dependent Na^+ channels (1). The action potential continues down into the t-tubules (2) to the dihydropyridine receptors (3). The dihydropyridine receptors in skeletal muscle function as voltage sensors and are coupled to the Ca^{2+} release channels (4). Through this coupled signaling process, the Ca^{2+} release channels are opened, some of the available terminal cisternae Ca^{2+} stores (5) are released, and the levels of myoplasmic Ca^{2+} are elevated. The Ca^{2+} then diffuses to the myofibrils (6) and interacts with the troponin/tropomyosin complex associated with actin (thin lines) and allows interaction of actin with myosin (thick lines) for mechanical movement. The Ca^{2+} diffuses away from the myofibrils and this Ca^{2+} signal is terminated by an ATP-driven Ca^{2+} pump (7), which pumps Ca^{2+} into the longitudinal sarcoplasmic reticulum (8). The Ca^{2+} diffuses from the longitudinal sarcoplasmic reticulum to the terminal cisternae, where it is concentrated for release by Ca^{2+} binding proteins. Na^+ entering during the action potential is subsequently extruded from the cell by the Na^+/K^+-ATPase (9) and possibly through Na^+/Ca^{2+} exchange (10). This latter process would elevate intracellular Ca^{2+} and could result from delayed inactivation of Na^+ currents. A major form of energy for supplying cellular ATP for the ion pumps and numerous other energy consuming processes is fatty acids (FA) derived from the serum (dietary FA), or from intramuscular triglyceride (TG) stores. Therefore, a defect in the intracellular Ca^{2+} regulating processes (increased Ca^{2+} release or decreased Ca^{2+} uptake), or a defect in the sarcolemma could account for an increase in myoplasmic Ca^{2+}.

not normally appear to act as Ca^{2+} channels in the same manner that they do in other tissues. There are reports of altered dihydropyridine receptor binding,[146,147] diminished maximum sarcolemmal Ca^{2+} accumulation,[158] and adenosine triphosphate–stimulated Ca^{2+} uptake in PSS.[159] Also, there is an altered Na^+ current and distribution of Na^+ channel subtypes in MH muscle.[148,149]

Terminal Cisternae: Ca^{2+} Release. The terminal cisternae of the sarcoplasmic reticulum are the sites of Ca^{2+} sequestration. They are coupled to the t-tubules through *ryr*1 and the dihydropyridine receptor (see Fig. 20-3). Several investigators have reported a hypersensitive Ca^{2+}-induced Ca^{2+} release in terminal cisternae preparations from porcine MH muscle.[129,160–162] Also observed for PSS Ca^{2+}-induced Ca^{2+} release are an enhanced rate of release from skinned fibers[163] and terminal cisternae preparations.[164,165] The maximum amount of Ca^{2+} released is normal for PSS vesicles.[166] In the human MH population, the Ca^{2+} release process appears to be less dramatically affected than that in PSS muscle. For example, the threshold of Ca^{2+}-induced Ca^{2+} release in terminal cisternae–containing fractions is not altered in a human MH population.[161,167] Although the alterations in Ca^{2+} release reported in swine cannot be observed in isolated heavy sarcoplasmic reticulum preparations from humans, abnormalities in Ca^{2+} release are observed when preparations containing additional cellular components are examined, such as skinned fiber preparations (Fig. 20-4). MH subjects have a greater than normal rate and hypersensitivity of Ca^{2+}-induced Ca^{2+} release[168] and Ca^{2+} release is hypersensitive to caffeine using the skinned fiber preparation.[169]

With respect to anesthetic action, the rate of halothane-induced Ca^{2+} release is abnormally high in PSS-susceptibles.[162,170]

In contrast, in human MH muscle[171] and PSS muscle,[172] the dose–response curves for halothane-induced Ca^{2+} release are normal when the amount of Ca^{2+} release is monitored. The concentration of Ca^{2+} in the assay medium greatly influences the rate and amount of Ca^{2+} release by halothane.[162,163] Therefore, it is believed that the differences observed in halothane-induced Ca^{2+} release in PSS muscle are actually due to an acceleration in Ca^{2+}-induced Ca^{2+} release by halothane. Free calcium was determined (with fura-2) in voltage-clamped human muscle fibers.[173] The kinetics and voltage dependence of calcium release for MH muscle was normal; however, the maximal peak rate of Ca^{2+} release increased about threefold. Although resting Ca^{2+} concentrations are normal, human skeletal muscle cell cultures have a twofold greater than normal sensitivity to halothane.[174] There is no effect of temperature on the rate of halothane-induced Ca^{2+} release.[170,176]

In heavy sarcoplasmic reticulum preparations (containing triads and sarcoplasmic reticulum), halothane at clinically relevant concentrations cannot induce a sustained net Ca^{2+} release if physiologic levels of adenosine triphosphate and Mg^{2+} are included. This ability to overcome the effects of halothane under approximate physiologic conditions is due to the enormous capacity of the Ca^{2+} pumping system.[167] Transient net Ca^{2+} release at lower than clinical concentrations of halothane has been reported for PSS terminal cisternae preparations.[175] The addition of fatty acids, even to vesicles isolated from normal muscle, markedly (~20–30-fold) decreases the concentration of halothane required for the sustained opening of the Ca^{2+} release channel in the presence of adenosine triphosphate and Mg^{2+}.[167] Under these conditions, fatty acids can cause a sustained Ca^{2+} release at clinical concentrations of halothane. Unlike

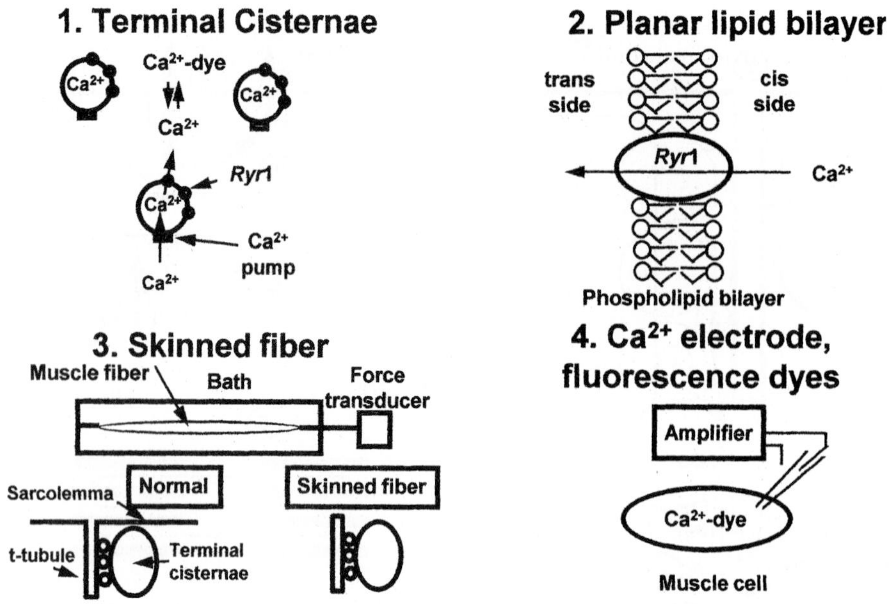

Figure 20-4. Methods to examine Ca^{2+} regulation. (*1*) *Terminal cisternae.* Skeletal muscle can be homogenized and resealed portions of the terminal cisternae containing the Ca^{2+} release channel (*ryr*1) can be recovered by a series of centrifugation steps. These vesicles can take up Ca^{2+} from the bathing medium by means of the ATP-driven Ca^{2+} pump and can subsequently release Ca^{2+} by opening of *ryr*1. Ca^{2+} levels in the extravesicular medium can be monitored spectrophotometrically by a number of dyes (usually metalochrome indicators such as arsenazo III or antipyrylazo III). Alternatively, $^{45}Ca^{2+}$ and filtration of the vesicles can be used. The amount of calcium released is usually determined by the decrease in radioactivity retained on the filters that contain the vesicles. Both the spectrophotometric and radioisotopic approaches allow monitoring of Ca^{2+} uptake and Ca^{2+} release, and these processes can be dissociated pharmacologically with the *ryr*1 blocker, ruthenium red. The terminal cisternae method allows the overall response of a large population of channels to be examined and may best reflect the overall responsiveness of the muscle. (*2*) *Planar lipid bilayers.* It is possible to incorporate *ryr*1 into artificial lipid bilayers (*i.e.*, planar lipid bilayer) and monitor the Ca^{2+} current as electrical charge movement through one to several channels at a time. Although this method can provide very useful, detailed information on the opening and closing of individual *ryr*1s, it does not provide an indication of the overall responsiveness of the muscle in which both Ca^{2+} uptake and Ca^{2+} release are participating and in which many modulating substances are present. (*3*) *Skinned fibers.* A third approach involves skinned fiber preparations in which the sarcolemma is either removed mechanically or made permeable chemically, and the function of the sarcoplasmic reticulum (Ca^{2+} uptake and release) and myofibrils (actin and myosin) monitored by the contractile response of the fiber. This preparation has an interesting advantage in that type I and type II fibers can be distinguished. Also, the t-tubules seal completely, allowing the function of the dihydropyridine receptors and Na^+ channels to be examined. This method only examines one muscle fiber at a time, which might be a slight disadvantage in MH or PSS skeletal muscle, because the defect is not uniformly expressed throughout the tissue. (*4*) *Ca^{2+} electrodes and fluorescence dyes.* The cytoplasmic Ca^{2+} levels can be monitored in intact muscle either with fluorescence dyes or Ca^{2+} electrodes. The former can monitor a muscle mass, while the latter examines individual fibers. Both approaches can be used with muscle fibers or cell culture systems.

studies of Ca^{2+} release in the absence of fatty acids,[176] there is an absolute temperature dependence (occurs at 37°C, not at 25°C) of the fatty acid enhancement of halothane-induced Ca^{2+} release,[130] which is consistent with the temperature dependence of halothane-induced contractures of MH muscle.[155,177]

Mitochondria. Mitochondria oxidize a variety of substrates to generate the form of energy (adenosine triphosphate) most useful for driving cellular reactions. Defects in mitochondrial function do not appear to initiate the MH syndrome. The uncoupling of Ca^{2+}-stimulated, but not adenosine diphosphate-stimulated, mitochondrial succinate oxidation has been demonstrated in muscle from pigs and humans[178] susceptible to MH. It is essential that these studies are conducted at physiologic temperatures (37–40°C), since a defect in uncoupling of Ca^{2+}-stimulated mitochondrial succinate oxidation does not occur at room temperature. This temperature dependence of mitochondrial uncoupling deserves attention.

Longitudinal Sarcoplasmic Reticulum: Ca^{2+} Uptake. The longitudinal sarcoplasmic reticulum (Fig. 20-3) is primarily involved in removing Ca^{2+} from the myoplasm through the adenosine triphosphate–driven Ca^{2+} pump. While earlier studies had suggested a defect in Ca^{2+} uptake might cause the loss of Ca^{2+} regulation associated with MH, subsequent studies have ruled out a role for the Ca^{2+} pump in causing MH.[170]

Myofibrils. Relatively few studies have been conducted on myofibrils in MH. However, there is apparently no defect in

the Ca^{2+} sensitivity of the fast or slow fibers of the contractile system from MH skeletal muscle.

Proteins or Systems Reported Altered in Malignant Hyperthermia Muscle

Calcium Release Channel of Skeletal Muscle (*ryr*1)

Skeletal muscle *ryr*1 is encoded by a different gene (chromosome 19q13.1) than *ryr*2 (chromosome 1), which is the cardiac muscle equivalent of *ryr*1. A third ryanodine receptor (*ryr*3) with a wide tissue distribution is distinct from *ryr*1 and *ryr*2. *Ryr*1 is the primary conduit through which the sarcoplasmic reticulum stores of Ca^{2+} are released to the sarcoplasm.[126] *Ryr*1 is an extremely large homotetramer, having subunits of about 560,000 MW each. *Ryr*1 has binding sites for the contracture-inducing plant alkaloid ryanodine[179] and the preservative 4-chloro-*m*-cresol.[180]

A mutation in *ryr*1 is the hypothesis with the most substantial support to explain human MH. This hypothesis originated with the identification of the Arg615Cys mutation in porcine MH muscle. The *ryr*1 mutation hypothesis is supported by biochemical studies demonstrating abnormal binding of ryanodine to *ryr*1 in human MH muscle under specific nonphysiologic conditions[179] and by physiologic studies showing subtle effects of halothane on isolated *ryr*1 currents in human MH muscle.[181] In theory, the addition of halothane opens a hypersensitive $ryr1$, Ca^{2+} regulation becomes unstable, and this leads to an uncontrolled release of Ca^{2+} to the myoplasm and the MH syndrome. The hypersensitivity of $ryr1$ may be due to a reduced inhibitory effect of Mg^{2+} on $ryr1$, as demonstrated for PSS muscle.[182] The hypothesis in which a defect in $ryr1$ directly leads to the MH syndrome is attractive and simple to understand. In conflict with this hypothesis, the buffering capacity of the Ca^{2+} pump in the presence of adenosine triphosphate is able to sustain normal Ca^{2+} regulation in the presence of halothane in terminal cisternae preparations isolated from MH muscle.[130] It also is difficult to explain the intra- and interindividual variability in human MH and the occurrence of nonrigid MH with this direct cause-and-effect hypothesis. Supporting the notion of $ryr1$'s crucial role in MH, investigators have reported genetic linkage of the locus encoding $ryr1$ with a positive contracture test (see Using Molecular Biology to Understand Malignant Hyperthermia). However, many other genes are encoded in that region that also could be involved in MH.[183] Furthermore, studies have identified genetic linkage to chromosomes other than that encoding $ryr1$, suggesting that MH is a heterogeneous disorder (see Using Molecular Biology to Understand Malignant Hyperthermia).

Unlike the hypersensitive Ca^{2+} release in porcine muscle,[160] Ca^{2+} regulation in human MH heavy sarcoplasmic reticulum fractions appears to be normal.[161] However, using planar bilayer approaches capable of monitoring single $ryr1$ channels, subtle changes in the function of $ryr1$ have been observed in human MH muscle,[181,184] similar in some respects to those in PSS muscle in planar bilayers.[185] These differences relate primarily to an increased probability of the MH $ryr1$'s being in an open state. While differences between normal and PSS-susceptibles have been reported in the absence of halothane or caffeine,[185] human MH muscle requires the presence of caffeine[184] or halothane[181] to detect differences in $ryr1$ function. In human MH muscle two populations of ion channels appear to be present—one halothane-insensitive and the other halothane-sensitive.[181] The halothane-sensitive channels have an increased probability of opening in the presence of clinically relevant concentrations of halothane. The halothane-sensitive channels do not occur in muscle from all MH patients, and both types (or states) of channels can coexist in the same muscle biopsy,[181] is the case with the K_d of ryanodine binding.[179]

Whether these subtle differences in $ryr1$ function in planar bilayers, or the differences in K_d of ryanodine binding, in human muscle reflect a different acylation or phosphorylation state of $ryr1$ should be investigated.

In agreement with the altered function of the PSS $ryr1$, there has been a specific mutation identified (Arg^{615} to Cys^{615}) in $ryr1$ in PSS.[186] The mutation is on the cytoplasmic surface of $ryr1$.[187] The porcine mutation may account for the altered functional states of $ryr1$ and ryanodine binding in PSS swine. However, the porcine mutation does not appear to account directly for the caffeine sensitivity of PSS muscle.[188] Approximately 50% of the families with human MH exhibit linkage to the gene encoding $ryr1$.[127,189–206] In the few (2–4%) MH families in which the human equivalent (Arg^{614} to Cys^{614}) to the PSS $ryr1$ mutation has been identified, the evidence for this mutation as a direct cause–effect is not as compelling as in porcine muscle, as there is discordance between inheriting the mutation and the outcome of the diagnostic test.[197,198] Also, not all subjects known to have the Arg614Cys mutation have exhibited the MH syndrome. A major reason for the attenuated effects of the $ryr1$ mutation in human muscle is likely the dominant mode of inheritance versus recessive inheritance in the pig. Thus, normal copies of $ryr1$ are expressed in human MH muscle, but not PSS muscle. The number of mutations in $ryr1$ reported at scientific meetings to date is about 30, including Arg614Cys, and this number is constantly rising. Each of these mutations commonly is found in only one or two families. None has an overall frequency in MH families of 10% or greater.[33,199,200]

There is a twofold greater than normal sensitivity to halothane in cell cultures from MH muscle.[174] However, a twofold increase in sensitivity to triggering agents in cell culture does not equate to the much greater sensitivity of MH muscle to halothane observed *in vivo*. Transfection of human MH skeletal muscle cell cultures with normal (wild-type) $ryr1$ does not result in the MH-negative phenotype (judged by sensitivity of Ca^{2+} transients to halothane), whereas expression of a mutated $ryr1$ (Arg^{163} to Cys^{163}) in normal muscle cells causes hypersensitivity to halothane.[174] Transfection of nonmuscle cell lines with any one of 19 $ryr1$ mutations increased the sensitivity of the cells to relatively high concentrations of halothane and caffeine.[202,203] Therefore, there is evidence that cell cultures may be useful models for elucidating the mechanisms by which MH mutations enhance the sensitivity of muscle to triggering agents (see also Sodium Channel).

In summary, there are physiologic, biochemical, pharmacologic, and molecular genetic data supporting a mutation in $ryr1$ as an important factor, and perhaps an initiating factor, in about 50% of the families with MH. The effects of the altered $ryr1$ function on Ca^{2+} regulation determined *in vitro* are not as pronounced in humans as in swine, possibly owing to the dominant mode of inheritance in humans. It is highly probable that other systems come into play as modulators of the MH response. This may better explain the extreme intra- and interindividual variability in the human MH syndrome, which is in contrast to the more consistent response in MH swine.

Sodium Channel

Skeletal and cardiac muscle sodium channels are composed of two subunits (α, 220,000 MW; β, 40,000 MW). The α subunit forms the ion pore, allowing Na^+ to enter the cell, and the smaller β subunit can modify the kinetics of the ion flux.[204,205] Sodium channels in skeletal muscle are of two, and possibly three,[150] subtypes. These subtypes can be differentiated by their sensitivity to tetrodotoxin (TTX), a toxin from the puffer fish that blocks the channel pore. The adult sodium channel (SKM1) is 90% blocked by a 100 nM concentration of TTX. The "embryonic" sodium channel (SKM2) in skeletal muscle is identical to the cardiac sodium channel, and is blocked by a 10-μM concentration of TTX in cell culture. A third channel is expressed following denervation, and this subtype is not antagonized by TTX, even at a 100-μM concentration. The adult sodium channel α subunit, encoded on chromosome 17,[204,205] was formerly believed to be the only subtype expressed in normal, mature skeletal muscle. The embryonic sodium channel α subunit appears early in muscle differentiation and is encoded on chromosome 3. Each of the α subunits interacts with the same β subunit (β_1), encoded on chromosome 19.[206] Recently, the sodium channels of normal human skeletal muscle (vastus lateralis) were shown to be composed of approximately 50% SkM1 and 50% SkM2.[150] Specific mutations in the α subunit of SkM1 have been implicated as the cause of other disorders of skeletal muscle, including the myotonic form of hyperkalemic periodic paralysis,[205,207] paramyotonia congenita,[208] and myotonia fluctuans.[209] These disorders are well known to exhibit masseter muscle rigidity and whole body rigidity to agents associated with the MH syndrome,[210] although they lack the signs of acidosis characteristic of MH.

A role for altered sodium channel function is becoming more evident in human MH. The function of the sodium channel is abnormal in primary cultures of human MH skeletal muscle.[211] There are two populations of sodium currents separated by their kinetics of inactivation (*i.e.*, closing of the channel). These are the normally inactivating and delayed inactivating fast sodium currents. There is a greater proportion of the slow inactivation of the Na^+ current in cultured human MH muscle[148] that would keep the sodium current active for a longer time (delayed inactivation). The consequence of this prolonged sodium current in MH muscle is a longer membrane depolarization and increased period of Ca^{2+} release from the terminal cisternae. The increased levels of intracellular Na^+ would have to be removed by Na^+/K^+-adenosine triphosphatase activity. Additionally, the accumulation of Na^+ likely activates Na^+/Ca^{2+} exchange and could account for the need for extracellular Ca^{2+} for *in vitro* halothane-induced contractures. Studies in swine also have suggested that halothane selectively affects either time-dependent Na^+ or K^+ currents in PSS muscle, in agreement with the findings in human MH muscle.[212] A toxin from the sea anemone (ATX II) causing delayed inactivation of the sodium current, as found in human MH muscle cultures, enhances the response of normal muscle to halothane, caffeine, and ryanodine.[213] This finding supports a role for altered Na^+ channel currents in the response of MH muscle to triggering agents. Veratridine, also a sodium channel inhibitor, enhances the response of MH muscle to halothane.[214] Therefore, altered Na^+ currents may be important for at least some of the signs associated with MH. Those patients expressing sodium channel abnormalities may be more likely to exhibit certain signs, such as muscle rigidity.

The expression of sodium channel subtypes is also altered in MH skeletal muscle. SkM2 (embryonic form) appears to be down-regulated in MH, in cell culture systems, or in biopsies of vastus lateralis muscle.[149] This would lead to a predominance of SkM1 in MH muscle. SkM1 is more sensitive to halothane than SkM2.[215] There are immunologically distinct differences between t-tubule Na^+ channels and those on the surface membrane.[216] Therefore, the distribution of sodium channel subtypes within the t-tubules could be altered in MH. Preliminary studies have demonstrated that transfection of muscle cell cultures with cDNA encoding *ryr*1, and containing mutations associated with MH, causes down-regulation of SkM2.[217] Therefore, down-regulation of SkM2 in MH muscle appears to be the result of a sequence of events initiated by the MH mutation. While the significance of altered SkM1 and SkM2 expression is less clear than that of altered sodium channel function, an increase in the SkM1 subtype may increase the sensitivity to triggering agents.

Fatty acid production is elevated in MH (see Elevated Fatty Acid Production). Fatty acids modulate the expression of the skeletal muscle sodium channels from normal patients.[149] Intracellular injection of fatty acids into primary cell cultures of normal human skeletal muscle turns on inactive adult Na^+ currents.[211] In contrast, the adult Na^+ channels in primary cultures of skeletal muscle from MH-susceptible humans are apparently already maximally active, even without injected fatty acid, and the intracellular injection of fatty acids has no further effect.[211] Therefore, the sodium channel in MH cell cultures acts as if fatty acids are elevated, and this may account for the greater proportion of SkM1:SkM2 ratio in MH muscle. Based on the above results, the MH mutation may increase fatty acid production, which then decreases the expression of SkM2.

There also is evidence for linkage of MH to chromosome 17[218,219] at or near the locus encoding the Na^+ channel α subunit.[220] In one family, a Gly1306Ala mutation in the sodium channel known to cause myotonia fluctuans cosegregated with MH susceptibility, as determined by contracture testing.[221] Two of these patients had whole body rigidity and/or masseter muscle rigidity to succinylcholine, although without metabolic acidosis. As with *ryr*1, it is not clear in most cases if the altered function reflects a primary defect in the Na^+ channel protein, or if the function is altered indirectly by processes such as phosphorylation or acylation.[222]

In summary, changes in sodium channel expression or function could be the result of mutations within a sodium channel subtype, or a secondary effect of a primary mutation in another protein (*e.g.*, *ryr*1). Also, second-messenger systems, such as fatty acids, may play a role in altered sodium channel function and expression. These changes in sodium channel function may be essential for the phenotypic expression of certain aspects of the MH syndrome, such as muscle rigidity.

Elevated Fatty Acid Production

Lipids are an important component of a cell, as they provide energy and structure (*e.g.*, membranes) and participate in function. Several lipid metabolites, including fatty acids, serve second-messenger functions.[224] Fatty acids are the major source of energy in the resting state of skeletal muscle and can also contribute up to 65% of the energy during exercise.[224] Fatty acids provide about 70% of the energy in resting muscle. Therefore, fatty acid utilization is likely up-regulated in MH muscle to compensate for the energy consumed by the adenosine triphosphatases attempting to maintain Na^+ and Ca^{2+} homeostasis. Intramuscular triacylglycerides have been reported as utilized during an MH crisis in swine.[225]

In addition to existing in a free form, fatty acids are esterified to phospholipids, triacylglycerides, diacylglycerides, monoacylglycerides, cholesterol esters, and many proteins. Free fatty acids are maintained at very low levels in a cell (since they are not only essential, but very toxic) and most of the "free" fatty acids actually are bound to fatty acid–binding proteins.[226]

Fatty acid production is elevated in mitochondrial fractions[178] and whole muscle homogenates[227] from PSS and MH susceptibles. There is an age-related increase in fatty acid production in skeletal muscle that parallels an age-related increase in susceptibility to the PSS.[138] When only static levels of free fatty acids are examined, they are at normal levels in human MH[151] and PSS muscle. However, the flux of fatty acids through β-oxidation can still be increased to a large extent in MH muscle without increasing the levels of free fatty acids. The fatty acid flux is derived from triacylglycerides, and this likely accounts for the low levels of triacylglycerides (or total neutral lipid) in biopsied MH or PSS skeletal muscle.[167,228] The hormone-sensitive lipase (chromosome 19q13.1) has been suggested to be a gene candidate,[183] as this enzyme liberates fatty acids from triacylglyceride.

The effects of fatty acids on Ca^{2+} release from skeletal muscle sarcoplasmic reticulum are significant, but not dramatic, in the absence of anesthetics,[229,230] and they are not mediated through *ryr*1.[231] However, the fatty acids act in synergy with halothane and decrease the amount of halothane required for sustained Ca^{2+} release by 20–30-fold![130,161] This fatty acid enhancement of halothane-induced Ca^{2+} release, in contrast with all other studies of Ca^{2+} release, exhibits the same temperature dependence (*i.e.*, it occurs only at 37°C, not at 25°C) as halothane-induced contractures of skeletal muscle and is mediated through *ryr*1.[130] While the concentration of fatty acid required for this effect exceeds that of the normal unbound form, halothane can displace fatty acids from fatty acid–binding proteins.[232] Therefore, it is highly likely that sufficient concentrations of fatty acids could be achieved at the site of halothane action. If the production of free fatty acids is sustained by accelerated triacylglyceride breakdown and the fatty acids are shunted toward acylation of *ryr*1 and the sodium channel, then this could lead to greatly elevated myoplasmic Ca^{2+} levels. In the case of *ryr*1, this would lead to a greater sensitivity to halothane [see Calcium Release Channel of Skeletal Muscle (*ryr*1)]. For the sodium channel, this would cause an increase in relative expression of SkM1:SkM2 (see Sodium Channel).

Phospholipase C and Inositol 1,4,5-Trisphosphate

Phosphatidylinositol phospholipids have become of interest in MH since one specific metabolite of phospholipase C action, IP$_3$, has been demonstrated to be elevated in human MH[233] and PSS[234] muscle, but not in MH human blood specimens.[233] This product of the hydrolysis of the phospholipid, phosphatidylinositol 4,5-bisphosphate, causes Ca^{2+} release from intracellular stores.[235] The elevation of all products of phosphatidylinositol hydrolysis is observed,[235] and this suggests that phospholipase C activity may be elevated in MH. Activation of phospholipase C in skeletal muscle also elevates diacylglycerol and indirectly elevates free fatty acids by deacylation of the diacylglycerol.

Diacylglycerol and fatty acids have diverse cell signaling effects.[223,236] In addition to elevated IP_3 production, MH muscle is also hypersensitive to IP_3.[237] Therefore, secondary involvement of this system could have multiple effects that together increase the sensitivity of Ca^{2+} release.

Antioxidant Defense

The antioxidant defense abnormality reported in PSS[238] is especially interesting as it could be either the cause or the effect of accelerated fatty acid production. In either case, it provides a novel target site for prophylactic and therapeutic intervention.[239] Observations supporting an antioxidant defense abnormality in PSS include the production in plasma of excess thiobarbituric acid reactive substances and conjugated dienes, which are nonspecific markers of peroxidation of unsaturated fatty acids.[238,239] Despite an antioxidant defense abnormality, the levels of skeletal muscle antioxidants and antioxidant enzymes examined are normal. Excessive peroxidation could contribute to the loss of Ca^{2+} regulation in MH muscle. These studies have suggested that vitamin E may be an antagonist of the MH episode, although at least one study has suggested otherwise.[239]

Phosphorylation Activity

Higher than normal levels of phosphorylation and altered sensitivity to protein phosphatase inhibition have been reported in porcine MH muscle. Altered phosphorylation could be either a primary or secondary defect in MH. As a secondary defect, perhaps as a result of fatty acid and/or diacylglycerol activation of protein kinase C, such activity could play a modulatory role in MH, as suggested for fatty acids.

Molecular Biology and Malignant Hyperthermia

Modern molecular biology provides powerful approaches for identifying and understanding mutations in genetic disorders. These studies can be conducted with no prior knowledge of the actual proteins involved through a process termed reverse genetics. Using some of the techniques of reverse genetics (restriction fragment length polymorphisms and linkage analysis), it was determined that MH is a heterogeneous disorder.[126,219,240] Linkage of MH (based on contracture test data) has been reported to markers on regions of chromosomes 1q,[242] 3q13.1,[241] 5p,[242] 7q21.1,[240] 17q11.2-q24,[218,219] and 19q13.1.[190,193] The identification of a gene locus is only the first step in the process of reverse genetics. It then becomes much more difficult to narrow the large stretches of DNA identified by linkage down to a single gene and mutation(s) within that gene.

Once the actual genes have been identified, the proteins responsible may be elucidated and the pathophysiology understood. For example, based on the localization of the gene for Duchenne's dystrophy to the X chromosome, it was eventually determined that patients with this disorder did not manufacture a specific protein (dystrophin), which is now believed to be needed for the maintenance of muscle cell integrity. However, for MH the process of identifying the responsible genes could be a far greater task than that for Duchenne's muscular dystrophy for several reasons. First, since there are several chromosomes involved, each presumably with any of a number of specific mutations, we may never know when we have identified all causes of MH. Second, the mutations identified to date have all been point mutations, which are more difficult to identify than the large areas of deletion associated with Duchenne's muscular dystrophy. Third, the only way to phenotype individuals is by the in vitro contracture test, and many family members may choose not to undergo this procedure.

Two genetic findings have been repeatedly demonstrated and seem certain. First, chromosome 19q13.1 is linked to about 50% of the families with MH first demonstrated by the MacLennan[126] and McCarthy[189] groups. Second, more than one gene can cause

MH.[127,243] The number of reported mutations associated with MH in the most studied protein, ryr1, is approaching 30 (21 are published). In addition, four of these mutations (Arg163Cys,[242] Ile403Met,[244] Arg2434His,[245] Tyr522Ser[246]) have been associated with both central core disease (CCD) and MH. While early genetic studies had suggested 100% concordance of MH and CCD,[243,244] other studies have found the relationship to be less clear.[247,248]

A mutation associated with MH has been reported in the α_1 subunit of the human skeletal muscle, dihydropyridine-sensitive, L-type voltage-dependent calcium channel (dihydropyridine receptor). The Arg to His substitution at residue 1086 results from the nucleotide substitution of G3333A.[249] One mutation (Gly1306Ala) has been described in the adult Na^+ channel α subunit associated with myotonia fluctuans that correlates with the diagnosis of MH in a North American family.[221] The same mutation occurring in a German family did not correlate with a positive contracture test for MH.[209] Perhaps coinheritance of a second factor is required for a positive diagnosis in some Na^+ channel mutations.

There have been several reports of discordance between segregation of mutations identified in ryr1 and the outcome of the in vitro contracture test for MH.[197,198,250] This discordance is relatively rare and the reason for it is unknown. However, a study in swine has demonstrated that there is an excellent correlation between the contracture test outcome and the genetic susceptibility for MH. Nonetheless, it is still possible that a false diagnosis may occur, as the sensitivity and specificity of the diagnostic tests are not 100%.[251] Alternatively, the involvement of modulating factors in a positive contracture test, as demonstrated with the sodium channel,[213] may influence the diagnostic outcome.

In summary, none of the ryr1, Na^+ channel, or dihydropyridine receptor mutations has been conclusively demonstrated as the direct cause of the human MH syndrome, while the Arg615Cys mutation in ryr1 is almost certainly the cause of porcine MH. This discrepancy most likely is due to the recessive mode of inheritance in swine and dominant mode of inheritance in humans. The human MH syndrome appears to be highly dependent on modulators that are secondarily affected by the primary mutation. No single mutation accounts for the majority of MH, suggesting that a large percentage of MH may be due to spontaneous mutations. Strong evidence exists for the involvement of mutations in ryr1 in human MH; however, some of the reported mutations could be polymorphisms unrelated to MH. Also, some of the mutations may have an association with MH, but cannot be causative on their own. These mutations may trigger a sequence of events that are dependent on the expression of modulating factors modifying the MH episode.

A Hypothesis to Explain Many Observations in Human Malignant Hyperthermia Muscle

Cause-effect relationships between the primary defect and the human MH syndrome are unclear. It is clear that the function or structure of several proteins is altered in MH skeletal muscle. Skeletal muscle from MH susceptible patients exhibits elevated fatty acid production. Fatty acid production is likely upregulated as an energy source to pump excess Ca^{2+} out of the myoplasm (Fig. 20-4). Fatty acids modify the function of ryr1, especially the response to halothane, and expression of subtypes of the Na^+ channel. These effects of fatty acids may play an important role as a modulator of the syndrome. We postulate that the pathophysiologic change during a MH crisis results from widespread alteration of protein function secondary to elevated utilization of fatty acids. Phospholipase C activity and protein phosphorylation are other systems that affect a wide variety of proteins and could play a role in modifying the expression of the MH syndrome.

The Future of Research in Malignant Hyperthermia

While molecular genetics has dominated the research in MH in recent years, a deeper understanding of the physiology and biochemistry of the interplay among *ryr*1, the Na$^+$ channel, and fatty acid metabolism still is needed. DNA-based linkage analyses are no longer pursued to the same extent as in the early 1990s. Instead, the focus of recent molecular genetic studies has been on identifying new mutations in *ryr*1. Further linkage studies are necessary to identify other chromosomes linked to MH. Molecular genetic approaches may be the only hope for a diagnostic blood test. However, such a test will be restricted to the few families (less than 20% of families to date) in which a specific proven causative mutation is known to exist.

Summary

The defect for MH appears to be expressed only in skeletal muscle in humans, and the consequences of the defect are manifest in virtually all organelles in skeletal muscle. Any one of at least six different genes may cause MH, although the exact proteins remain to be identified in some cases. Mutations have been identified in *ryr*1 and the dihydropyridine receptor. A mutation in a sodium channel subunit may be associated with some signs of MH, but this requires the expression of other factors. A disturbance in fatty acid metabolism, as a secondary effect, alters the function of several organelles and can lead to a hypersensitive *ryr*1 response to halothane and altered Na$^+$ channel subunit expression in skeletal muscle. The MH syndrome is the result of a complex and poorly understood interaction among several systems in skeletal muscle.

OTHER INHERITED DISORDERS

Inherited diseases affect every bodily organ and every physiologic and biochemical process. Some are mild and allow a relatively normal life span, whereas others are incompatible with extrauterine existence even for a few days. Adding to the complexity is a natural variability of genetic penetrance and expressivity even in a single family. All of these disorders have as a common feature an abnormality in one or more genes that affects the function of one or more enzymes. The metabolic basis of inherited diseases is the subject of several well-known books,[252] which may be consulted for an in-depth appreciation of our state of knowledge of many of these disorders.

Disorders of Plasma Cholinesterase

Plasma cholinesterase, pseudocholinesterase, or *nonspecific cholinesterase* is an enzyme with a molecular weight of 320,000 and a tetrahedral structure. It is found in plasma and most tissue but not in red blood cells. Pseudocholinesterase degrades acetylcholine released at the neuromuscular junction, as well as other choline and aliphatic esters.[253] The half-life of pseudocholinesterase has been estimated to be 8–16 hours. It is very stable in serum samples and can be stored for long periods of time at -20°C with little or no activity loss. Cholinesterase is manufactured in the liver. Therefore, decreased plasma cholinesterase activity occurs in advanced cases of hepatocellular dysfunction.

Inherited variants of pseudocholinesterase are of interest to the anesthesiologist because the duration of action of succinylcholine, mivacurium, and (in some cases) ester-linked local anesthetics, as well as the toxicity of cocaine,[254] is a function of the activity of this enzyme system. Prolonged apnea after succinylcholine, or mivacurium, administration occurs in patients who have very low absolute activity of pseudocholinester-

ase or have enzyme variants.[255] These patients otherwise have no symptoms.

Many physiologic, pharmacologic, and pathologic factors can either increase or decrease the activity of this enzyme to a significant extent. However, it is only when there is a >75% decrease in the levels of the normal pseudocholinesterase that there is clinically evident prolongation of succinylcholine activity (see below). Table 20-2 lists some of the causes for variation in plasma cholinesterase activity.

Succinylcholine-Related Apnea

Succinylcholine is hydrolyzed by a two-step process, first to succinylmonocholine and then to succinic acid. It has been estimated that only about 5% of the injected drug reaches the end-plate region because of a combination of both hydrolysis and diffusion from the plasma. Urinary excretion and protein binding play unimportant roles in the disposition of the drug when plasma cholinesterase activity is normal. The rate of metabolism determines the duration of action of succinylcholine.

A variety of assay procedures are available for pseudocholinesterase activity. However, most involve the reaction of a thiocholine (*e.g.,* butyrylthiocholine) with serum or plasma containing

---

Table 20-2. SOME CAUSES OF CHANGES IN CHOLINESTERASE ACTIVITY

Inherited
Cholinesterase variants that may lead to decreased or increased activity (*e.g.,* silent gene or C5 variant)

Physiologic
Decreases in last trimester of pregnancy
Reduced activity of the newborn

Acquired Decreases
Liver diseases
Carcinoma
Debilitating diseases
Collagen diseases
Uremia
Malnutrition
Myxedema

Acquired Increases
Obesity
Alcoholism
Thyrotoxicosis
Nephrosis
Psoriasis
Electroshock therapy

Drugs Related to Diseases
Echothiophate iodide
Neostigmine
Pyridostigmine
Chlorpromazine
Cyclophosphamide
Monoamine oxidase inhibitors
Pancuronium
Contraceptives
Organophosphorus insecticides
Hexafluorenium

Other Causes of Decreased Activity
Plasmapheresis
Extracorporeal circulation
Tetanus
Radiation therapy
Burns

The significance of these factors depends on the severity of disease, drug dosage, and individual variation. Adapted from Whittaker M: Plasma cholinesterase variants and the anesthetist. Anaesthesia 35:174, 1980.

Table 20-3. BIOCHEMICAL CHARACTERISTICS OF SOME CHOLINESTERASE VARIANTS

Genotype	Cholinesterase Activity	Dibucaine Number	Fluoride Number	Chloride Number	Succinylcholine Number
EuEu	677–1860	78–86	55–65	1–12	89–98
EaEa	140–525	18–26	16–32	46–58	4–19
EuEa	285–1008	51–70	38–55	15–34	51–78
EuEf	579–900	74–80	47–48	14–30	87–91
EfEa	475–661	49–59	25–33	31–36	56–59
EfEs	351	63	26	25	81

Eu = normal enzyme gene; Ea = atypical enzyme gene; Ef = fluoride-resistant gene; Es = silent gene.
Reproduced with permission from Viby-Mogensen J: Succinylcholine neuromuscular blockade in subjects homozygous for atypical plasma cholinesterase. Anesthesiology 55:429, 1981.

cholinesterase. The reaction product is coupled with 5,5'-dithiobis(2-nitrobenzoic acid) and forms a colored product that can be followed spectrophotometrically. The use of benzoylcholine, a specific substrate for plasma cholinesterase, avoids contamination of the assay for plasma cholinesterase by the esterase in red blood cells which is released when hemolysis occurs.

Kalow et al were the first to show that qualitative as well as quantitative differences in the pseudocholinesterase enzyme determine the duration of succinylcholine apnea.[256] Kalow found that in certain persons displaying succinylcholine sensitivity, the local anesthetic dibucaine (Nupercaine) inhibited the hydrolysis of a benzylcholine substrate less than it inhibited the reaction in those displaying a normal response to succinylcholine. Thus, this atypical phenotype may be referred to as dibucaine-resistant. The percentage inhibition of the reaction was termed the *dibucaine number*. It was found to be constant for a person and did not depend on the concentration of the enzyme.

A discontinuous distribution of dibucaine numbers suggested an inheritance pattern based on alteration at a single gene locus (Table 20-3). Those with dibucaine numbers in the range of 80 would be homozygous normal with a normal response to succinylcholine, those with dibucaine numbers of 20 would be homozygous atypical with a marked prolongation of succinylcholine activity, and those with dibucaine numbers in the 60 range would be heterozygous and, in general, have a normal response to succinylcholine. This theory was substantiated by other workers.

Over the years, two other major allelic variants were discovered. In one case, the silent gene, the enzyme is not produced. In the other, there is a differential inhibition of cholinesterase activity by fluoride.[257] In those with prolonged duration of succinylcholine activity with this genotype, fluoride ion inhibits the *in vitro* hydrolysis of substrate by the enzyme less than it does in normals. Thus the phenotype may be referred to as fluoride-resistant. A *fluoride number*, similar to a dibucaine number, is thereby created. Other variants exist.

When there is a question of succinylcholine sensitivity, the absolute activity of pseudocholinesterase should be determined as well as the dibucaine and fluoride numbers. In some cases, because of biologic variability or unusual combinations of genotype (*e.g.*, combination of atypical and fluoride genes), it is helpful to use other inhibitors of the cholinesterase reaction in genotyping the patient. Bromide, urea, sodium chloride, and succinylcholine have been used to distinguish the various genotypes (see Table 20-3).

Molecular genetic techniques have been successfully applied to pseudocholinesterase variants. La Du's laboratory has identified a point mutation in the gene for human serum cholinesterase in which a nucleotide change leads to an alteration of a single amino acid (adenine to guanine) in the protein.[258] This change apparently alters the affinity of atypical cholinesterase for choline esters. Other base pair alterations account for other atypical variants, including the K and J silent gene variants,

which, while common, produce little to no clinical prolongation of succinylcholine action (Table 20-4).[259]

The identification of the genetic defect offers the prospect that more accurate and precise diagnostic tests for atypical pseudocholinesterase variants will be offered soon.

The frequencies of occurrence of the various genes vary to some extent with ethnic background. For example, South African blacks[260] and Eskimo populations have the silent gene much more frequently, patients with Huntington's chorea are more likely to have an Ef gene (fluoride-resistant) than are normal controls, and Israelis have a higher chance of having an atypical genotype than Americans. In European studies, the approximate percentages in the population of the genotypes are as follows: EuEu (96%), EuEa (2.5%), EuEf or EuEs (0.3%), EaEf (0.005%), EaEa (0.05%), and EfEf or EfEs (0.006%).[261]

Patients homozygous for atypical, fluoride, or silent genes as well as those with the combination of atypical with fluoride, atypical with silent genes, or fluoride with silent genes should wear safety identification bracelets indicating that succinylcholine administration will lead to prolonged apnea. Relatives should be tested as well. There are only a few cholinesterase research units that investigate families and interpret results: Whittaker's in Great Britain, Hanel and Viby-Mogensen's in Denmark, and La Du's in the U.S. (University of Michigan, Department of Anesthesiology).

Clinical Implications of Pseudocholinesterase Abnormalities

Important questions for the anesthesiologist are: Which patients are at risk for development of an abnormal response to succinylcholine? What are the clinical characteristics of this response? and What are the treatment options?

Significant prolongation of succinylcholine's effects occurs in the following genotypes: EaEa, EfEf, EaEs, EfEa, and EsEs. The more common situations in which homozygote normals and heterozygotes are at risk are as follows: patients who have been receiving echothiophate eyedrops (up to 2 weeks after therapy is discontinued), patients who are undergoing plasmapheresis,[262] patients with severe liver disease, and patients (par-

Table 20-4. STRUCTURAL CHANGES OF BCHE VARIANTS

Atypical	70ASP→GLY
Silent	117 GLY→Frame shift
Fluoride-1	243 THR→MET
Fluoride-2	390 GLY→VAL
K Variant	539 ALA→THR
H Variant	142 VAL→MET
J Variant	497 GLU→VAL

ticularly heterozygotes) who have received succinylcholine after reversal of nondepolarizing blockade with neostigmine.

Viby-Mogensen[263,264] has studied the question of plasma cholinesterase apnea in detail. His cholinesterase unit found that 6.2% of patients who displayed apnea for 50–250 minutes after a "usual" dose of succinylcholine had an acquired deficiency of plasma cholinesterase. He then studied 70 patients who were genotypically normal for pseudocholinesterase and administered 1.0 mg·kg^{-1} of succinylcholine during a 50% nitrous oxide–oxygen–1% halothane anesthetic and followed the depression and return of thumb twitch. He found that there was indeed a relationship between the duration of apnea, the return of a full twitch response, and plasma cholinesterase activity.[269] However, only moderate prolongation of apnea was found when cholinesterase was depressed by as much as 70%. Apnea is significantly prolonged only with extreme depression of cholinesterase activity.

In a second study with a similar protocol, he found that heterozygotes having one normal gene (e.g., EuEa, EuEf) had a normal response to succinylcholine, including typical fasciculations and a depolarizing type of block with train-of-four stimulations.[263] However, heterozygotes without the usual gene (e.g., EaEf) had a prolonged response to succinylcholine, with apnea lasting as long as 24 minutes. Most showed typical fasciculations. Fade with train-of-four stimulations was the rule. It should be noted that others have found that heterozygotes with one normal gene display a prolonged response to succinylcholine under certain conditions. About 1 in 500 heterozygotes is prone to such a response.

Apnea lasts from 120 minutes to more than 300 minutes in homozygous atypical patients (EaEa) when they are given succinylcholine.[264] The onset of neuromuscular block is similar to that in normals; however, there is fade in response to train-of-four stimulation. The other class of patients who regularly display prolonged apnea after succinylcholine administration comprises patients who are homozygous for the silent gene.

Treatment of Succinylcholine Apnea

The safest course of treatment after the patient fails to breathe within 10–15 minutes after succinylcholine administration is to continue mechanical ventilation until adequate muscle tone has returned. Two units of blood may contain adequate amounts of pseudocholinesterase to hydrolyze the succinylcholine,[265] although blood transfusion is not recommended for routine treatment of succinylcholine-induced apnea.

The use of cholinesterase inhibitors in treating succinylcholine apnea is controversial. When given along with blood or plasma, the improvement is rapid and lasting. If they are administered alone before there is evidence of fade with train-of-four stimulation, there may be a transient improvement followed by intensification of the neuromuscular block. Remember that neostigmine inhibits the degradation of succinylcholine by plasma cholinesterase. The best chance for reversal of succinylcholine-related apnea in these situations occurs when no more than 0.03 mg·kg^{-1} of neostigmine is given 90–120 minutes after succinylcholine when a nondepolarizing type of blockade is present.

C5 Variant

An isoenzyme of pseudocholinesterase has been demonstrated whereby the hydrolysis of succinylcholine is increased, and therefore the duration of apnea is decreased after succinylcholine administration. The gene does not appear to be an allele of the Eu and Ea gene and is found infrequently in the population.[266]

Plasma Cholinesterase Abnormalities and the Metabolism of Local Anesthetics

Although the ester-linked local anesthetics (e.g., procaine, tetracaine, 2-chloroprocaine) are metabolized by pseudocholinester-

ase, prolongation of block and/or clinical toxicity of these local anesthetics in homozygous atypical patients has rarely been documented.[267,268] Jatlow et al have shown delayed hydrolysis of cocaine in vitro with plasma from homozygote atypicals.[269] They theorized that such persons may be at risk for toxic reaction from normal doses of cocaine.

Mivacurium Disposition and Plasma Cholinesterase. Despite being a nondepolarizing relaxant, mivacurium is metabolized to a significant extent by pseudocholinesterase. Although it is theoretically possible to reverse neuromuscular block in patients with atypical pseudocholinesterase who receive mivacurium, the few cases so far reported indicate that anticholinesterase agents may not be effective under such situations. These individuals should be managed in a manner similar to patients with the atypical enzyme who received succinylcholine.[270] When abnormal plasma cholinesterase does not metabolize mivacurium as rapidly as expected, the neuromuscular blocker is cleared by the kidneys as curare is. The most rapid adequate recovery from mivacurium-induced block will be obtained when the plasma concentration of mivacurium has decreased to the level at which 3–4 responses to a train-of-four stimulation to the ulnar nerve are palpable. Then neostigmine should induce recovery as it would from blocker that was expected to be long-acting.

THE PORPHYRIAS

All the porphyrias result from a defect in heme synthesis. The heme pigments are tetrapyrroles that are the essential elements in hemoglobin, myoglobin, and the cytochromes, i.e., compounds that are involved in the transport of oxygen, activation of oxygen, and the electron transport chain. Cytochrome P-450 is a hemoprotein intimately involved in the conversion of lipid-soluble nonpolar drugs to soluble polar compounds that may be excreted in the urine.

A complete deficiency of enzymes that are involved in heme synthesis is incompatible with life. However, a partial deficiency may lead to the accumulation of one or more of the molecular intermediates in heme production. Such an accumulation of precursors is responsible for the clinical manifestations of the porphyrias (in an as-yet unexplained manner).

The rate-limiting step in heme synthesis is the conjugation of succinyl-CoA with glycine to form D-aminolevulinic acid (the enzyme is aminolevulinic acid synthetase). In the porphyrias, there is a partial deficiency of enzymes subsequent to this initial step, which results in a stimulation of this reaction to form aminolevulinic acid. The result is overproduction of intermediate products before the deficient step (Fig. 20-5).

The porphyrias generally manifest after puberty. Inheritance is through an autosomal dominant pattern, but congenital erythropoietic porphyria is inherited as an autosomal recessive pattern.

A functional classification for the anesthesiologist is based on a division of the porphyrias into inducible and noninducible forms. The inducible porphyrias are those in which the acute symptoms are precipitated on drug exposure (Table 20-5).[271] These forms are acute intermittent porphyria, variegate porphyria, and hereditary coproporphyria. These porphyrias cause an acute neurologic syndrome and are therefore of interest to the anesthesiologist. Cutaneous manifestations, with particular sensitivity to ultraviolet light exhibited by skin fragility and bleeding, are the chief features of the other porphyrias. About 80% of patients with variegate porphyria are photosensitive. Some patients with hereditary coproporphyria also may have skin lesions. The porphyrias are very difficult to diagnose in the latent phase of the disorder. Direct assay of the intermediates themselves may be used in the acute state to measure the elevated levels of the heme intermediates. The inducible porphyrias are seen as a neurologic syndrome with a variety of presentations.

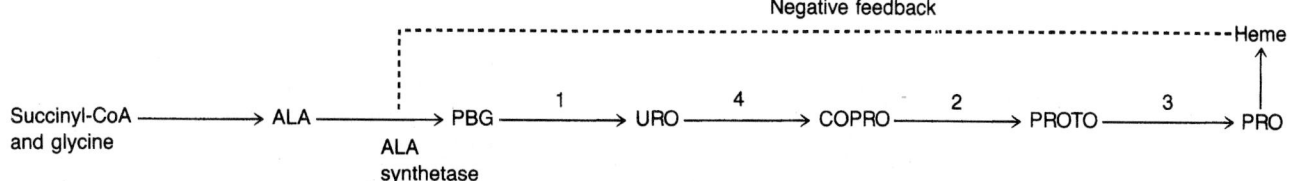

Figure 20-5. Biosynthesis of heme and sites of defects in certain porphyrias. (ALA = aminolevulinic acid; PGB = porphobilinogen; URO = uroporphyrinogen; COPRO = coproporphyrinogen; PROTO = protoporphyrinogen; PRO = protoporphyrin.) In intermittent acute porphyria, there is a partial deficiency of the enzyme at site 1. In hereditary coproporphyria, there is an enzyme deficiency at site 2. In variegate porphyria, the enzyme problem is at site 3. In porphyria cutanea tarda, there is a deficiency at site 4. (Reprinted with permission from Mees DL, Frederickson EL: Anesthesia and the porphyrias. South Med J 68:29, 1975.)

The central, peripheral, and autonomic nervous systems may be involved in the porphyrias. A frequent manifestation is colicky abdominal pain, often with nausea and vomiting, which may suggest the diagnosis of acute abdomen, leading to exploratory laparotomy. Other symptoms are psychiatric disturbance, quadriplegia, hemiplegia, alterations of consciousness, and pain. Hyponatremia and hypokalemia may result from vomiting during the acute attack or may be related to hypothalamic disturbance. Death may result from paralysis of the respiratory muscles. The cause of these changes is unknown; they may be related to metabolites of the intermediates or result from deficiency of the heme pigment in the nerve cell itself.

A number of patients with concurrent human immunodeficiency virus and porphyria cutanea tarda have been recognized. The etiology of the association of these two disorders is unknown at this time.[272]

Because the porphyrias are unusual disorders, there is limited experience with the clinical use of many anesthetic drugs. *In vitro* studies suggest that certain anesthetics or anesthetic adjuvants may be contraindicated, but sufficient clinical experience is lacking (see below).[273]

Management of Patients with Porphyria

It is important to recognize porphyria in patients who are scheduled for surgery. It may become apparent through a careful family history and personal history related to anesthesia. A careful history in the patient with porphyria should concentrate on neurologic background. Laboratory work should include electrolyte and blood urea nitrogen levels. Physical examination includes inspection of cutaneous lesions over the body.

In the anesthetic management of patients with porphyria, the chief concern is to avoid the administration of drugs that can induce a crisis; the drugs that induce cytochrome enzyme production can trigger the syndrome. Chief among those are the barbiturates; therefore, all barbiturates are contraindicated in porphyria. Ethyl alcohol, nonbarbiturate sedatives, hydantoin anticonvulsants, and a variety of other drugs also can induce a crisis (see Table 20-5). Endogenous factors, such as fasting, infection, and estrogens, may also precipitate porphyria. Diagnosis can be especially difficult because attacks may occur at a variable time period after drug administration or they may not occur at all despite administration of inducing drugs.

Propofol appears to be a safe induction agent.[274] Nitrous oxide, muscle relaxants, and opioids are unequivocally safe drugs. Experience with other inhalation agents and reversal agents has been favorable, but *in vitro* studies suggest that they might exacerbate a crisis.

Most experts have advised that regional techniques be avoided to prevent confusion should neurologic signs develop after operation. However, reports of uneventful epidural anesthesia in the parturient with acute intermittent porphyria may indicate that this technique can be safely performed in these patients.[275] Blistered or fragile skin areas should be padded and given special attention. Glucose infusion should be started because starvation may induce an attack.

The acute attack should be treated with glucose infusion, and hyponatremia, hypokalemia, and hypomagnesemia should be treated. Pyridoxine and hematin also have been valuable in some cases. Supportive therapy for respiratory insufficiency and treatment of pain is also suggested.

Table 20-5. DRUGS KNOWN TO PRECIPITATE PORPHYRIA

Sedatives
Barbiturates
Hypnotics such as chlordiazepoxide, glutethimide, diazepam

Analgesics
Pentazocaine, antipyrine, aminopyridine
Lidocaine

Anticonvulsants
Phenytoin, methsuximide

Antibiotics
Sulfonamides, chloramphenicol

Steroids
Estrogens, progesterones

Hypoglycemic sulfonylureas
Tolbutamide, chlorpropramide

Toxins
Lead, ethanol

Miscellaneous
Ergot preparations
Amphetamines
Methyldopa

GLYCOGEN STORAGE DISEASES

The metabolic pathways involving glucose degradation to lactate, glucose conversion to glycogen, and the breakdown of glycogen to glucose are important to the whole body biochemistry as well as to cellular physiology in general. The enzymatic steps involved in glucose metabolism have been studied intensively since the earliest days of modern biochemistry. The glycogen storage diseases are inherited and are characterized by dysfunction of one of the many enzymes involved in glucose metabolism. To date, several different glycogen storage disorders, each based on the deficiency of an enzyme involved in glucose metabolism, have been identified. Some of the glycogen storage diseases are incompatible with life past infancy, whereas others are not. Anesthetic experience with these diseases is limited, but several particular problems have been identified[276]:

Hypoglycemia. Hypoglycemia is a constant risk in these patients. It results from failure to metabolize stored glycogen to glucose.

Acidosis. This is related to fat and protein metabolism because glycogen stores are not metabolically available.

Cardiac and Hepatic Dysfunction. This is secondary to destruction and displacement of normal tissue by the accumulated glycogen.

Detailed descriptions of glucose metabolism are given elsewhere. Figure 20-6 outlines the glycogen–glucose–lactate pathway. There are, of course, multiple enzymatic steps to reach each of the end points.

Defects in Glucose Metabolism

Type I (Von Gierke's Disease; Glucose-6-phosphate Deficiency). Inheritance is autosomal recessive. The prognosis is moderately good, with many patients surviving into adulthood. Short stature and liver enlargement are characteristic. These patients tolerate fasting very poorly. Hypoglycemia, acidosis, and convulsions may be a problem. Prolonged bleeding has been described. Often, preoperative hyperalimentation is used to reduce liver glycogen stores. Portacaval shunt has been performed with limited success in these patients.[277]

Type II (Pompe's Disease). Inheritance of this disease is considered to be autosomal recessive. This is a devastating disease with a very poor prognosis. There is a deficiency of lysosomal acid maltase with an accumulation of glycogen in the lysosomes, especially in the heart, liver, muscle, and central nervous system. Cardiac compromise resulting from outflow obstruction of hypertrophied muscle occurs, as does congestive heart failure secondary to myocardial disruption by glycogen stores. A case report has been described in which halothane was used without incident.[278] In another case, halothane led to prompt hypotension and intractable cardiac failure.[279] A late-onset form with a better prognosis has been described as well.

Type III (Forbes' Disease; Debranching Enzyme Deficiency). Inheritance of this disease is autosomal recessive.

Type IV (Andersen's Disease; Branching Enzyme Deficiency). This is a very rare disorder, characterized by a defect in the synthesis of normal glycogen. Cirrhosis of the liver and death are characteristic before a patient reaches age 2 years.

Type V (McArdle's Disease; Muscle Phosphorylase Deficiency). An autosomal recessive inheritance pattern and cramping with exercise are characteristic of this disorder. Skeletal muscle is not able to mobilize glycogen stores, the usual fuel in muscle, for sustained exercise. Myoglobinuria occurs with overexertion in these patients and may occur after succinylcholine administration as well. Muscle atrophy occurs in adulthood. Tourniquets should not be used in these patients, and frequent automated blood pressure readings should be done with caution. Severe rhabdomyolysis has been observed after bypass for cardiac surgery.[280]

Type VI (Hers' Disease; Reduced Hepatic Phosphorylase). A decreased ability to mobilize hepatic glycogen occurs in this disorder, with normal muscle and cardiac physiology.

Type VII (Muscle Phosphofructokinase Deficiency). This disorder is similar to McArdle's disease and is characterized by muscle cramping. The same enzymatic defect in erythrocytes leads to chronic hemolysis.

Type VIII (Deficient Hepatic Phosphorylase Kinase). This results from a deficiency in the regulatory enzyme controlling the phosphorylase enzyme. A case report has described fever and acidosis during succinylcholine, halothane, and ketamine anesthesia.[281] Liver transplantation has been used with success in the more severe forms of the glycogen storage diseases.

Defects of Fructose Metabolism

Fructose-6-phosphate is converted to fructose-1,6-diphosphate during glucose breakdown to lactate. Conversely, fructose-1,6-diphosphate is converted to fructose-6-phosphate by the enzyme fructose-1,6-diphosphatase during gluconeogenesis.

In fructose-1,6-diphosphatase deficiency, there is an inability to produce glycogen from lactate. Hypoglycemia may result. Acidosis has been reported because lactate is formed preferentially. In errors of fructose metabolism, like those of glucose metabolism, hypoglycemia and acidosis pose the greatest threats to the patient.[282]

The Mucopolysaccharidoses

The mucopolysaccharides are polysaccharides that yield mixtures of monosaccharides and derived products after hydrolysis. The mucopolysaccharides contain N-acetylated hexosamine in a characteristic repeating unit. For example, chondroitin sulfate A is a monosaccharide of d-glucuronic acid and N-acetyl d-galactosamine 4-sulfate. Monopolysaccharides are found in all cells.

The mucopolysaccharidoses are genetically determined diseases in which mucopolysaccharides are stored in tissues in abnormal quantities and excreted in large amounts in the urine. The disorders result from a deficiency of a specific lysosomal enzyme that is required to break down these compounds. As a result, mucopolysaccharides accumulate in tissues, producing specific clinical manifestations. There are seven basic forms of mucopolysaccharidoses and several subgroups. Most of the mucopolysaccharidoses are inherited as autosomal recessive traits. All the mucopolysaccharidoses are progressive, and patients characteristically are marked by coarse facial features (gargoylism); associated skeletal abnormalities such as lumbar lordosis, stiff joints, chest deformity, dwarfing, and hypoplasia of the odontoid process (Morquio's syndrome); corneal opacities; limitation of joint motion; and heart, liver, and spleen enlargement resulting from mucopolysaccharide accumulation. Mental deterioration also occurs frequently.

The Hunter and Hurler syndromes are the best known variants of the mucopolysaccharidoses. The Hunter syndrome is an X-linked recessive disease.[283] Respiratory infection and heart disease, both valvular and ischemic, often lead to death when patients are young. Patients may commonly present for repair of inguinal hernia or ear, nose, and throat or orthopedic procedures. The thick, soft tissues and the copious, thick secretions make perioperative and intraoperative airway management a particular problem.[283] In Leroy and Crocker's series, minor difficulties occurred with anesthesia in patients in more than one

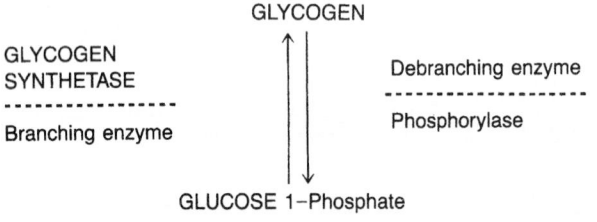

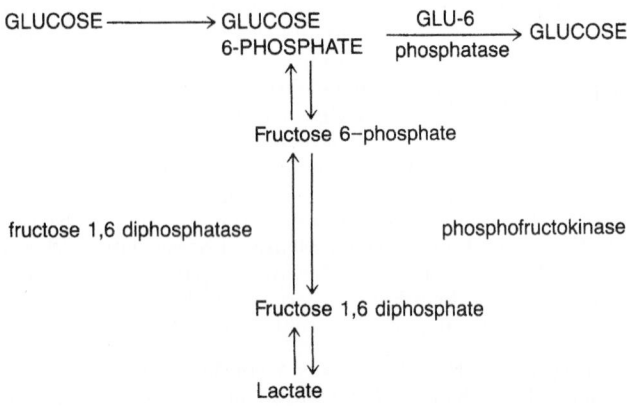

Figure 20-6. The glycogen–glucose–lactate pathway.

third of 60 operations.[284] Postoperative respiratory obstruction was noted in several cases. Because of the underlying heart disease, these patients should have electrocardiograms and echocardiographic tests performed before surgery.

Mucopolysaccharidosis IV (Morquio's syndrome) is associated with perhaps the most significant skeletal deformities. In addition to cardiovascular disorders and respiratory insufficiency from marked chest wall deformity, acute, subacute, or chronic myelopathy is extremely common. This is secondary to severe hypoplasia or absence of the odontoid process of the second cervical vertebra. In anesthesia care, the head should be positioned carefully and precautions such as avoidance of succinylcholine should be taken with patients with spinal cord compromise.

Osteogenesis Imperfecta

Osteogenesis imperfecta is seen in approximately 1 of 50,000 births. Most cases are autosomal dominant; some are autosomal recessive. The pathophysiologic characteristics include decreased collagen synthesis, which leads to osteoporosis, joint laxity, and tendon weakness. The manifestations of osteogenesis imperfecta are small bowed limbs, large head, short neck, blue sclerae, otosclerosis, joint laxity, brittle teeth, and a tendency to fractures. An increased bleeding tendency is also seen resulting from abnormal platelet function, and aortic and mitral valve dysfunction resulting from dilation of the valve ring.

The patient should be handled carefully because minor trauma may lead to fractures. Airway management may also be difficult because of cervical spine involvement with this disorder. Patients have short necks, and mandibular fractures frequently occur. The patient's cardiovascular status should be evaluated, especially mitral and aortic valve function. Kyphoscoliosis may also occur, with pulmonary compromise. Care should be taken to pad the pressure areas, particularly for long procedures. One should be prepared to obtain platelet transfusions. The patient's temperature should be monitored because hyperthermia (possibly resulting from central nervous system dysfunction or excessive metabolism in bone) has been reported.[285] Signs consistent with MH have been observed, but contracture tests for MH susceptibility have not confirmed a constant association between osteogenesis imperfecta and MH.[39]

Prader-Willi Syndrome

The inheritance pattern of Prader-Willi syndrome is debated.[286,287] Its clinical features include hypotonia, obesity, diabetes, hypogonadism, mental deficiency, and dental caries. The problems related to anesthesia are those that are secondary to the patient's hypoglycemia, obesity, and hypotonia. There are possible problems related to the neuromuscular blockade. The airway must be protected during surgery with an endotracheal tube, and the blood glucose level should be monitored during operation. Careful attention must also be paid to maintaining airway patency intraoperatively as well as postoperatively.

Riley-Day Syndrome (Familial Dysautonomia)

A deficiency of dopamine β-hydroxylase that leads to decreased norepinephrine at the nerve endings is thought to be the cause of Riley-Day syndrome.[288] This syndrome is inherited in an autosomal recessive fashion. Patients with Riley-Day syndrome exhibit copious pulmonary secretions, dysphagia, denervation supersensitivity, no sensitivity to pain, no response to histamine, and impairment of temperature control. The impairment of temperature control leads to intermittent fevers.

There are numerous problems related to anesthesia. These include corneal abrasions, excess secretions, pneumonia, labile blood pressure secondary to baroreceptor insensitivity, a decreased vascular volume, possible decreased response to hypoxia and hypercarbia, increased potential for aspiration because of swallowing problems, postural hypotension, and sensitivity to vasopressors.

Anesthesia management is well summarized by Axelrod et al.[289] Perioperative management should include diazepam (0.1-0.2 mg·kg⁻¹ po) without an opioid. Antacid may be given on call. Intraoperative management should include temperature monitoring and careful blood pressure monitoring. Application of regional techniques may result in more stable cardiovascular function. Fresh gases should be humidified. Vasopressors need to be titrated carefully because of the hypersensitivity response. After operation secretions can be managed with chest percussion therapy. Postoperatively, opioids should be used only with great care to minimize the risk of apnea.[290]

REFERENCES

1. Denborough MA, Lovell RRH: Anaesthetic deaths in a family. Lancet 2:45, 1960
2. Denborough MA, Forster JFA, Lovell RRH et al: Anaesthetic deaths in a family. Br J Anaesth 34:395, 1962
3. Nelson TE: Porcine stress syndromes. In Gordon RA, Britt BA, Kalow W (eds): International Symposium on Malignant Hyperthermia, p 191. Springfield, IL, Charles C Thomas, 1973
4. Kalow W, Britt BA, Terreau ME, Haist C: Metabolic error of muscle metabolism after recovery from malignant hyperthermia. Lancet 2:895, 1970
5. Aldrete JA, Britt BA: Second International Symposium on Malignant Hyperthermia. New York, Grune & Stratton, 1978
6. Lopez JR, Allen PD, Alamo L et al: Myoplasmic free [Ca²⁺] during a malignant hyperthermia episode in swine. Muscle Nerve 11:82, 1988
7. Larach MG, Rosenberg H, Gronert GA, Allen GC: Hyperkalemic cardiac arrest during anesthesia in infants and children with occult myopathies. Clin Pediatr 36(1):9, 1997
8. Karan SM, Crowl F, Muldoon SM: Malignant hyperthermia masked by capnographic monitoring. Anesth Analg 78:590, 1994
9. Gronert GA, Ahern CP, Milde JH: Treatment of porcine malignant hyperthermia: Lactate gradient from muscle to blood. Can Anaesth Soc J 33:729, 1986
10. Mathieu A, Bogosian AJ, Ryan JF et al: Recrudescence after survival of an initial episode of malignant hyperthermia. Anesthesiology 51:454, 1979
11. Donlon JV, Newfield P, Sreter I, Ryan JF: Implications of masseter spasm after succinylcholine. Anesthesiology 49:298, 1978
12. Relton JES, Creighton RE, Conn AW, Nabeta S: Generalized muscular hypertonicity associated with general anaesthesia: A suggested anaesthetic management. Can Anaesth Soc J 14:22, 1967
13. Ellis FR, Halsall PJ: Suxamethonium spasm. A differential diagnostic conundrum. Br J Anaesth 56:381, 1984
14. O'Flynn RP, Shutack JG, Rosenberg H, Fletcher JE: Masseter muscle rigidity and malignant hyperthermia susceptibility in pediatric patients: An update on management and diagnosis. Anesthesiology 80:1228, 1994
15. Larach MG, Rosenberg H, Larach DG, Broennle AM: Prediction of malignant hyperthermia susceptibility by clinical signs. Anesthesiology 66:57, 1987
16. Hackl W, Mauritz W, Schemper M et al: Prediction of malignant hyperthermia susceptibility: Statistical evaluation of clinical signs. Br J Anaesth 64:425, 1990
17. Van Der Speck AFL, Fang WB, Ashton-Miller JA et al: The effects of succinylcholine on mouth opening. Anesthesiology 67:459, 1987
18. Storella RJ, Keykhah MM, Rosenberg H: Halothane and temperature interact to increase succinylcholine-induced jaw contracture in the rat. Anesthesiology 79:1261, 1993
19. Schwartz L, Rockoff MA, Koka BV: Masseter spasm with anesthesia: Incidence and implications. Anesthesiology 61:772, 1984
20. Ording H: Incidence of malignant hyperthermia in Denmark. Anesth Analg 64:700, 1985
21. Hannallah RS, Kaplan RF: Jaw relaxation after a halothane/succinylcholine sequence in children. Anesthesiology 81:99, 1994
22. Rosenberg H, Fletcher JE: Masseter muscle rigidity and malignant hyperthermia susceptibility. Anesth Analg 65:161, 1986
23. Littleford JA, Patel LR, Bose D et al: Masseter muscle spasm in children: Implications of continuing the triggering anesthetic. Anesth Analg 72:151, 1991

24. Albrecht A, Wedel DJ, Gronert GA: Masseter muscle rigidity and nondepolarizing neuromuscular blocking agents. Mayo Clin Proc 72:329, 1997

25. Lazzell VA, Carr AS, Lerman J et al: The incidence of masseter muscle rigidity after succinylcholine in infants and children. Can J Anaesth 41:475, 1994

26. Friedman S, Baker T, Gatti M et al: Probable succinylcholine-induced rhabdomyolysis in a male athlete. Anesth Analg 81:422, 1995.

27. Miller ED, Sanders DB, Rowlingson JC et al: Anesthesia-induced rhabdomyolysis in a patient with Duchenne's muscular dystrophy. Anesthesiology 48:146, 1978

28. Sullivan M, Thompson WK, Gill GD: Succinylcholine-induced cardiac arrest in children with undiagnosed myopathy. Can J Anaesth 41:497, 1994

29. Rosenberg AD, Neuwirth MG, Kagen LJ et al: Intraoperative rhabdomyolysis in a patient receiving pravastatin, a 3-hydroxy-3-methylglutaryl coenzyme A (HMG CoA) reductase inhibitor. Anesth Analg 81:1089, 1995

30. Kelfer HM, Singer WD, Reynolds RN: Malignant hyperthermia in a child with Duchenne muscular dystrophy. Pediatrics 71:118, 1983

31. Smith CL, Bush GH: Anaesthesia and progressive muscular dystrophy. Br J Anaesth 57:1113, 1985

32. Frank JP, Harati Y, Butler IJ et al: Central core disease and malignant hyperthermia syndrome. Ann Neurol 7:11, 1980

33. Brandt A, Schleithoff L, Jurkat-Rott K et al: Screening of the ryanodine receptor gene in 105 malignant hyperthermia families: Novel mutations and concordance with the in vitro contracture test. Hum Mol Genet 8:2055, 1999

34. Olckers A, Meyers DA, Meyers S et al: Adult muscle sodium channel α-subunit is a gene candidate for malignant hyperthermia susceptibility. Genomics 14:829, 1992

35. McPherson EW, Taylor CA Jr: The King syndrome: Malignant hyperthermia, myopathy, and multiple anomalies. Am J Med Genet 8:159, 1981

36. Isaacs H, Badenhorst ME: Dominantly inherited malignant hyperthermia (MH) in the King-Denborough syndrome. Muscle Nerve 15:740, 1992

37. Rampton AJ, Kelly DA, Shanahan EC, Ingram GS: Occurrence of malignant hyperpyrexia in a patient with osteogenesis imperfecta. Br J Anaesth 56:1443, 1984

38. Viljoen D, Beighton P: Schwartz-Jampel syndrome (chondrodystrophic myotonia). J Med Gen 29:58, 1992

39. Porsborg P, Astrup G, Bendixen D et al: Osteogenesis imperfecta and malignant hyperthermia. Is there a relationship? Anaesthesia 61:863, 1996

40. Allen GC, Rosenberg H: Phaeochromocytoma presenting as acute malignant hyperthermia—a diagnostic challenge. Can J Anaesth 37:593, 1990

41. Kumar MV, Carr RJ, Komanduri V et al: Differential diagnosis of thyroid crisis and malignant hyperthermia in an anesthetized porcine model. Endocr Res 25:87, 1999

42. Gronert GA, Thompson RL, Onofrio BM: Human malignant hyperthermia: Awake episodes and correction by dantrolene. Anesth Analg 59:377, 1980

43. Ryan JF, Tedeschi LG: Sudden unexplained death in a patient with a family history of malignant hyperthermia. J Clin Anesth 9(1):66, 1997

44. Caroff SN: The neuroleptic malignant syndrome. J Clin Psych 41:79, 1980

45. Addonizio G, Susman VL: ECT as a treatment alternative for patients with symptoms of neuroleptic malignant syndrome. J Clin Psych 48:102, 1987

46. Caroff SN, Rosenberg H, Fletcher JE et al: Malignant hyperthermia susceptibility in neuroleptic malignant syndrome. Anesthesiology 67:20, 1987

47. Wingard DW, Bobko S: Failure of lidocaine to trigger porcine malignant hyperthermia. Anesth Analg 58:99, 1979

48. Berkowitz A, Rosenberg H: Femoral block with mepivacaine for muscle biopsy in malignant hyperthermia patients. Anesthesiology 62:651, 1985

49. Gronert GA, Milde JH, Taylor SR: Porcine muscle responses to carbachol, α and β adrenoreceptor agonist, halothane or hyperthermia. J Physiol 307:319, 1980

50. Britt BA, Webb GE, LeDuc C: Malignant hyperthermia induced by curare. Can Anaesth Soc J 21:371, 1974

51. Ording H, Nielsen VG: Atracurium and its antagonism by neostigmine (plus glycopyrrolate) in patients susceptible to malignant hyperthermia. Br J Anaesth 58:1001, 1986

52. Hon CA, Landers DF, Platts AA: Effects of neuroleptic agents on rat skeletal muscle contracture in vitro. Anesth Analg 72:194, 1991

53. Gronert GA, Ahern CP, Milde JH et al: Effect of CO_2, calcium, digoxin, and potassium on cardiac and skeletal muscle metabolism in malignant hyperthermia susceptible swine. Anesthesiology 64:24, 1986

54. Raff M, Harrison GG: The screening of propofol in MHS swine. Anesth Analg 68:750, 1989

55. Lunn JN, Farrow SC, Fowkes FGR et al: Epidemiology in anaesthesia. Br J Anaesth 54:803, 1982

56. Bachand M, Vachond N, Boisvert M et al: Clinical reassessment of malignant hyperthermia in Abitibi-Temiscamingue. Can J Anaesth 44:696, 1997

57. Bendixen D, Skovgaard LT, Ording H: Analysis of anaesthesia in patients suspected to be susceptible to malignant hyperthermia before diagnostic in vitro contracture test. Acta Anaesthesiol Scand 41:480, 1997

58. Seewald MJ, Eichinger HM, Lehmann-Horn F, Iaizzo PA: Characterization of swine susceptible to malignant hyperthermia by in vivo, in vitro and post-mortem techniques. Acta Anaesthesiol Scand 35:345, 1991

59. Ellis FR, Harriman DGF, Keaney NP et al: Halothane-induced muscle contracture as a cause of hyperpyrexia. Br J Anaesth 43:721, 1971

60. Rosenberg H, Reed S: In vitro contracture tests for susceptibility to malignant hyperthermia. Anesth Analg 62:415, 1983

61. European Malignant Hyperpyrexia Group: A protocol for the investigation of malignant hyperpyrexia. Br J Anaesth 56:1267, 1984

62. European MH Group: Laboratory diagnosis of malignant hyperpyrexia susceptibility (MHS). Br J Anaesth 57:1038, 1985

63. Larach MG: Standardization of the caffeine–halothane muscle contracture test. Anesth Analg 69:511, 1989

64. Larach MG, Landis JR, Bunn JS et al: Prediction of malignant hyperthermia susceptibility in low-risk subjects. An epidemiologic investigation of caffeine–halothane contracture responses. Anesthesiology 76:16, 1992

65. Allen GC, Larach MG, Kunselman AR: The sensitivity and specificity of the caffeine–halothane contracture test: A report from the North American Malignant Hyperthermia Registry. The North American Malignant Hyperthermia Registry of MHAUS. Anesthesiology 88:570, 1998

66. Britt BA: Muscle assessment of malignant hyperthermia susceptible patients. In Britt BA (ed): Malignant Hyperthermia, p 193, Boston, Martinus Nijhoff Publishing, 1987

67. Fletcher JE, Rosenberg H: Laboratory methods for malignant hyperthermia diagnosis. In Williams CH (ed): Experimental Malignant Hyperthermia, p 121. Berlin, Springer-Verlag, 1988

68. Ording H: Diagnosis of susceptibility to malignant hyperthermia in man. Br J Anaesth 60:287, 1988

69. Rosenberg H, Fletcher JE: International Malignant Hyperthermia Workshop and Symposium. Hiroshima, Japan, July 16-19, 1994. Anesthesiology 82:803, 1995

70. Fletcher JE: Current laboratory methods for the diagnosis of malignant hyperthermia susceptibility. In Levitt RC (ed): Anesthesiology Clinics of North America. Temperature Regulation During Anesthesia, p 553. Philadelphia, WB Saunders, 1994

71. Adnet PJ, Krivosic-Horber RM, Adamantidis MM et al: Is resting membrane potential a possible indicator of viability of muscle bundles used in the in vitro caffeine contracture test? Anesth Analg 74:105, 1992

72. Ranklev E, Fletcher R: Investigation of malignant hyperthermia in Sweden. Acta Anaesthesiol Scand 30:693, 1986

73. Ording H, Bendixen D: Sources of variability in halothane and caffeine contracture tests for susceptibility to malignant hyperthermia. Eur J Anaesth 9:367, 1992

74. Ording H: The European MH Group: Protocol for in vitro diagnosis of susceptibility to MH and preliminary results. In Britt BA (ed): Malignant Hyperthermia, p 269. Boston, Martinus Nijhoff Publishing, 1987

75. Larach MG: The North American Malignant Hyperthermia Registry. In Levitt RC (ed): Anesthesiology Clinics of North America. Temperature Regulation During Anesthesia, p 607. Philadelphia, WB Saunders, 1994

76. Melton AT, Martucci RW, Kien ND, Gronert GA: Malignant hyper-

thermia in humans—standardization of contracture testing protocol. Anesth Analg 69:437, 1989

77. Fletcher JE, Calvo PA, Rosenberg H: Phenotypes associated with malignant hyperthermia susceptibility in swine genotyped as homozygous or heterozygous for the ryanodine receptor mutation. Br J Anaesth 71:410, 1993

78. Fletcher JE, Conti PA, Rosenberg H: Comparison of North American and European malignant hyperthermia group halothane contracture testing protocols. Acta Anaesthesiol Scand 35:483, 1991

79. Fletcher JE, Rosenberg H, Aggarwal M: Comparison of European and North American malignant hyperthermia diagnostic protocol outcomes for use in genetic studies. Anesthesiology 90:654, 1999

80. Islander G, Twetman ER: Comparison between the European and North American protocols for diagnosis of malignant hyperthermia susceptibility in humans. Anesth Analg 88:1155, 1999

81. Loke JC, MacLennan DH: Bayesian modeling of muscle biopsy contracture testing for malignant hyperthermia susceptibility. Anesthesiology 88:589, 1998

82. Hopkins PM, Ellis FR, Halsall PJ: Ryanodine contracture: A potentially specific *in vitro* diagnostic test for malignant hyperthermia. Br J Anaesth 66:611, 1991

83. Lenzen C, Roewer N, Wappler F *et al:* Accelerated contractures after administration of ryanodine to skeletal muscle of malignant hyperthermia susceptible patients. Br J Anaesth 71:242, 1993

84. Wappler F, Roewer N, Lenzen C *et al:* High-purity ryanodine and 9,21-dehydroryanodine for *in vitro* diagnosis of malignant hyperthermia in man. Br J Anaesth 72:240, 1994

85. Hopkins PM, Ellis FR, Halsall PJ: Comparison of *in vitro* contracture testing with ryanodine, halothane and caffeine in malignant hyperthermia and other neuromuscular disorders. Br J Anaesth 70:397, 1993

86. Hopkins PM, Hartung E, Wappler F: Multicentre evaluation of ryanodine contracture testing in malignant hyperthermia. The European Malignant Hyperthermia Group. Br J Anaesth 80:389, 1998

87. Wappler F, Scholz J, von Richthofen V *et al:* 4-Chloro-*m*-cresol-induced contractures of skeletal muscle specimen from patients at risk for malignant hyperthermia. Anaesthesiol Intensivmed Notfallmed Schmerzther 32:541, 1997

88. Ording H, Glahn K, Gardi T *et al:* 4-Chloro-*m*-cresol test—a possible supplementary test for diagnosis of malignant hyperthermia susceptibility. Acta Anaesthesiol Scand 41:967, 1997

89. Gilly H, Musat I, Fricker R *et al:* Classification of malignant hyperthermia-equivocal patients by 4-chloro-*m*-cresol. Anesth Analg 85:149, 1997

90. Larach MG, Localio AR, Allen GC *et al:* A clinical grading scale to predict malignant hyperthermia susceptibility. Anesthesiology 80:771, 1994

91. Nelson TE, Flewellen EH, Gloyna DF: Spectrum of susceptibility to malignant hyperthermia—diagnostic dilemma. Anesth Analg 62:545, 1983

92. Nelson TE, Bedell DM, Jones EW: Porcine malignant hyperthermia: Effects of temperature and extracellular calcium concentration on halothane-induced contracture of susceptible skeletal muscle. Anesthesiology 42:301, 1975

93. Allen GC, Fletcher JE, Huggins FJ *et al:* Caffeine and halothane contracture testing in swine using the recommendations of the North American Malignant Hyperthermia Group. Anesthesiology 72:71, 1990

94. Urwyler A, Funk B, Censier K, Drewe J: Effect of halothane equilibration kinetics on *in vitro* muscle contractures for malignant hyperthermia screening. Acta Anaesthesiol Scand 36:115, 1992

95. Isaacs H, Badenhorst M: False-negative results with muscle caffeine–halothane contracture testing for malignant hyperthermia. Anesthesiology 79:5, 1993

96. Wedel DJ, Nelson TE: Malignant hyperthermia—diagnostic dilemma: False-negative contracture responses with halothane and caffeine alone. Anesth Analg 78:787, 1994

97. Allen GC, Rosenberg P, Fletcher JE: Safety of general anesthesia in patients previously tested negative for malignant hyperthermia susceptibility. Anesthesiology 72:619, 1990

98. Ording H, Hedengran AM, Skovgaard LT: Evaluation of 119 anaesthetics received after investigation for susceptibility to malignant hyperthermia. Acta Anaesthesiol Scand 35:711, 1991

99. Urwyler A, Censier K, Kaufmann MA, Drewe J: Genetic effects on the variability of the halothane and caffeine muscle contracture tests. Anesthesiology 80:1287, 1994

100. MacKenzie AE, Allen G, Lahey D *et al:* A comparison of the caffeine–halothane muscle contracture test with the molecular genetic diagnosis of malignant hyperthermia. Anesthesiology 75:4, 1991

101. Weglinski MR, Wedel DJ, Engel AG: Malignant hyperthermia testing in patients with persistently elevated serum creatine kinase levels. Anesth Analg 84:1038, 1997

102. Kaplan RF, Rushing E: Isolated masseter muscle spasm and increased creatine kinase without malignant hyperthermia susceptibility or other myopathies. Anesthesiology 77:820, 1992

103. Antognini JF: Creatine kinase alterations after acute malignant hyperthermia episodes and common surgical procedures. Anesth Analg 81:1039, 1995.

104. Olgin J, Argov Z, Rosenberg H *et al:* Noninvasive evaluation of malignant hyperthermia susceptibility with phosphorus nuclear magnetic resonance spectroscopy. Anesthesiology 68:507, 1988

105. Webster DW, Thompson RT, Gravelle DR *et al:* Metabolic response to exercise in malignant hyperthermia-sensitive patients measured by ^{31}P magnetic resonance spectroscopy. Magnet Res Med 15:81, 1990

106. Olgin J, Rosenberg H, Allen G *et al:* A blinded comparison of noninvasive, *in vivo* phosphorus nuclear magnetic resonance spectroscopy and the *in vitro* halothane/caffeine contracture test in the evaluation of malignant hyperthermia susceptibility. Anesth Analg 72:36, 1991

107. Payen J-F, Bosson J-L, Bourdon L *et al:* Improved noninvasive diagnostic testing for malignant hyperthermia susceptibility from a combination of metabolites determined *in vivo* with ^{31}P-magnetic resonance spectroscopy. Anesthesiology 78:848, 1993

108. Hopkins PM, Halsall PJ, Ellis FR: Diagnosing malignant hyperthermia susceptibility. Anaesthesia 49:373, 1994

109. Brandt A, Schieithoff L, Jurkat-Rott K *et al:* Screening of the ryanodine receptor gene in 105 malignant hyperthermia families: Novel mutations and concordance with the *in vitro* contracture test. Hum Mol Genetics 8:2055, 1999

110. Rubin AS, Zablocki AD: Hyperkalemia, verapamil, and dantrolene. Anesthesiology 66:246, 1987

111. Saltzman LS, Kates RA, Corke BC *et al:* Hyperkalemia and cardiovascular collapse after verapamil and dantrolene administration in swine. Anesth Analg 63:473, 1984

112. Fletcher R, Blennow G, Olsson AK *et al:* Malignant hyperthermia in a myopathic child: Prolonged postoperative course requiring dantrolene. Acta Anaesthesiol Scand 26:435, 1982

113. Jensen AG, Bach V, Werner MU *et al:* A fatal case of malignant hyperthermia following isoflurane anaesthesia. Acta Anaesthesiol Scand 30:293, 1986

114. Britt BA: Dantrolene. Can Anaesth Soc J 31:61, 1984

115. Watson CB, Reierson N, Norfleet EA: Clinically significant muscle weakness induced by oral dantrolene sodium prophylaxis for malignant hyperthermia. Anesthesiology 65:312, 1986

116. Lerman J, McLeod ME, Strong HA: Pharmacokinetics of intravenous dantrolene in children. Anesthesiology 70:625, 1989

117. Allen GC, Cattran CB, Peterson RG, Lalande M: Plasma levels of dantrolene following oral administration in malignant hyperthermia-susceptible patients. Anesthesiology 69:900, 1988

118. Beebe JJ, Sessler DI: Preparation of anesthesia machines for patients susceptible to malignant hyperthermia. Anesthesiology 69:395, 1988

119. Neubauer KR, Kaufman RD: Another use for mass spectrometry: Detection and monitoring of malignant hyperthermia. Anesth Analg 64:837, 1985

120. Vaughan MS, Cork RC, Vaughan RW: Inaccuracy of liquid crystal thermometry to identify core temperature trends in postoperative adults. Anesth Analg 61:284, 1982

121. Ruhland G, Hinkle AJ: Malignant hyperthermia after oral and intravenous pretreatment with dantrolene in a patient susceptible to malignant hyperthermia. Anesthesiology 60:159, 1984

122. Shime J, Gare D, Andrews J, Britt B: Dantrolene in pregnancy: Lack of adverse effects on the fetus and newborn infant. Am J Obstet Gynecol 159:831, 1988

123. Harthoorn AM, Young E: A relationship between acid base balance and capture myopathy in zebra (*Equus burchelli*) and apparent therapy. Vet Rec 95:337, 1974

124. Harrison GG, Biebuyck JF, Terblanche J *et al:* Hyperpyrexia during anaesthesia. Br Med J 3:594, 1968

125. Hall LW, Woolf N, Bradley JW, Jolly DW: Unusual reaction to suxamethonium chloride. Br Med J 2:1305, 1966

126. MacLennan DH, Phillips MS: Malignant hyperthermia. Science 256:789, 1992

127. Levitt RC, Nouri N, Jedlicka AE *et al:* Evidence for genetic heterogeneity in malignant hyperthermia susceptibility. Genomics 11:543, 1991

128. Iles DE, Segers B, Heytens L *et al:* High-resolution physical mapping of four microsatellite repeat markers near the RYR1 locus on chromosome 19q13.1 and apparent exclusion of the MHS locus from this region in two malignant hyperthermia susceptible families. Genomics 14:749, 1992

129. Fletcher JE, Calvo PA, Rosenberg H: Phenotypes associated with malignant hyperthermia susceptibility in swine genotyped as homozygous or heterozygous for the ryanodine receptor mutation. Br J Anaesth 71:410, 1993

130. Fletcher JE, Tripolitis L, Rosenberg H, Beech J: Malignant hyperthermia: Halothane- and calcium-induced calcium release in skeletal muscle. Biochem Mol Biol Int 29:763, 1993

131. Figarella-Branger D, Kozak-Ribbens G, Rodet L *et al:* Pathological findings in 165 patients explored for malignant hyperthermia susceptibility. Neuromuscul Disord 3:553, 1993

132. Hopkins PM, Ellis FR, Halsall PJ: Evidence for related myopathies in exertional heat stroke and malignant hyperthermia. Lancet 338:1491, 1991

133. Kochling A, Wappler F, Winkler G, Schulte am Esch JS: Rhabdomyolysis following severe physical exercise in a patient with predisposition to malignant hyperthermia. Anaesth Intensive Care 26:315, 1998

134. Mabry JW, Christian LL, Kuhlers DL: Inheritance of porcine stress syndrome. J Hered 72:429, 1981

135. Nelson TE: Malignant hyperthermia in dogs. J Am Vet Med Assoc 198:989, 1991

136. Halsall PJ, Cain PA, Ellis FR: Retrospective analysis of anaesthetics received by patients before susceptibility to malignant hyperpyrexia was recognized. Br J Anaesth 51:949, 1979

137. Rosenberg H, Fletcher JE: International Malignant Hyperthermia Workshop and Symposium. Hiroshima, Japan, July 16–19, 1944. Anesthesiology 82:803, 1995

138. Cheah KS, Cheah AM, Waring JC: Phospholipase A2 activity, calmodulin, Ca²⁺ and meat quality in young and adult halothane-sensitive and halothane-insensitive British Landrace pigs. Meat Sci 17:37, 1986

139. Fay RS, Gallant EM: Halothane sensitivity of young pigs *in vivo* and *in vitro.* Am J Physiol 259:R133, 1990

140. Gallant EM, Rempel WE: Porcine malignant hyperthermia: False negatives in the halothane test. Am J Vet Res 48:488, 1987

141. Haggendal J, Jonsson L, Carlsten J: The role of sympathetic activity in initiating malignant hyperthermia. Acta Anaesthesiol Scand 34:677, 1990

142. Urwyler A, Censier K, Kaufmann MA, Drewe J: Genetic effects on the variability of the halothane and caffeine muscle contracture tests. Anesthesiology 80:1287, 1994

143. Ervasti JM, Strand MA, Hanson TP *et al:* Ryanodine receptor in different malignant hyperthermia-susceptible porcine muscles. Am J Physiol 260:C58, 1991

144. Marjanen LA, Denborough MA: Electrophoretic analysis of proteins in malignant hyperpyrexia susceptible skeletal muscle. Int J Biochem 16:919, 1984

145. Sullivan JS, Denborough MA: The isolation and chemical characterization of skeletal muscle microsomes from swine susceptible to malignant hyperpyrexia. Int J Biochem 14:741, 1982

146. Mickelson JR, Ervasti JM, Litterer LA *et al:* Skeletal muscle junctional membrane protein content in pigs with different ryanodine receptor genotypes. Am J Physiol 267:C282, 1994

147. Ervasti JM, Claessens MT, Mickelson JR, Louis CF: Altered transverse tubule dihydropyridine receptor binding in malignant hyperthermia. J Biol Chem 264:2711, 1989

148. Wieland SJ, Fletcher JE, Rosenberg H, Gong QH: Malignant hyperthermia: Slow sodium current in cultured human muscle cells. Am J Physiol 257:C759, 1989

149. Wieland SJ, Gong QH, Fletcher JE, Rosenberg H: Altered sodium current response to intracellular fatty acids in halothane-hypersensitive skeletal muscle. Am J Physiol 271:C347, 1996

150. Fletcher JE, Wieland SJ, Karan SM *et al:* Sodium channel in human malignant hyperthermia. Anesthesiology 86:1023, 1997

151. Fletcher JE, Rosenberg H, Michaux K *et al:* Triglycerides, not phospholipids, are the source of elevated free fatty acids in muscle from patients susceptible to malignant hyperthermia. Eur J Anaesthesiol 6:355, 1989

152. Seewald MJ, Eichinger HM, Iaizzo PA: Malignant hyperthermia: An altered phospholipid and fatty acid composition in muscle membranes. Acta Anaesthesiol Scand 35:380, 1991

153. Hartmann S, Otten W, Kratzmair M *et al:* Influences of breed, sex, and susceptibility to malignant hyperthermia on lipid composition of skeletal muscle and adipose tissue in swine. Am J Vet Res 58:738, 1997

154. Cheah KS, Cheah AM, Fletcher JE, Rosenberg H: Calcium accumulation by sarcoplasmic reticulum in whole muscle homogenate preparations of malignant hyperthermia diagnostic patients and pigs. Acta Anaesthesiol Scand 34:114, 1990

155. Nelson TE, Bedell DM, Jones EW: Porcine malignant hyperthermia: Effects of temperature and extracellular calcium concentration on halothane-induced contracture of susceptible skeletal muscle. Anesthesiology 42:301, 1975

156. Iaizzo PA, Klein W, Lehmann-Horn F: Fura-2 detected myoplasmic calcium and its correlation with contracture force in skeletal muscle from normal and malignant hyperthermia susceptible pigs. Pflugers Arch 411:648, 1988

157. Fletcher JE, Huggins FJ, Rosenberg H: The importance of calcium ions for *in vitro* malignant hyperthermia testing. Can J Anaesth 37:695, 1990

158. Ervasti JM, Mickelson JR, Louis CF: Transverse tubule calcium regulation in malignant hyperthermia. Arch Biochem Biophys 269:497, 1989

159. Mickelson JR, Ross JA, Hyslop RJ *et al:* Skeletal muscle sarcolemma in malignant hyperthermia: Evidence for a defect in calcium regulation. Biochim Biophys Acta 897:364, 1987

160. Nelson TE: Abnormality in calcium release from skeletal sarcoplasmic reticulum of pigs susceptible to malignant hyperthermia. J Clin Invest 72:862, 1983

161. Fletcher JE, Mayerberger S, Tripolitis L *et al:* Fatty acids markedly lower the threshold for halothane-induced calcium release from the terminal cisternae in human and porcine normal and malignant hyperthermia susceptible skeletal muscle. Life Sci 49:1651, 1991

162. Mickelson JR, Ross JA, Reed BK, Louis CF: Enhanced Ca²⁺-induced calcium release by isolated sarcoplasmic reticulum vesicles from malignant hyperthermia susceptible pig muscle. Biochim Biophys Acta 862:318, 1986

163. Carrier L, Villaz M, Dupont Y: Abnormal rapid Ca²⁺ release from sarcoplasmic reticulum of malignant hyperthermia susceptible pigs. Biochim Biophys Acta 1064:175, 1991

164. Mickelson JR, Gallant EM, Litterer LA *et al:* Abnormal sarcoplasmic reticulum ryanodine receptor in malignant hyperthermia. J Biol Chem 263:9310, 1988

165. Mickelson JR, Gallant EM, Rempel WE *et al:* Effects of the halothane-sensitivity gene on sarcoplasmic reticulum function. Am J Physiol 257:C787, 1989

166. Foster PS, White MD, Denborough MA: Characterization of the terminal cisternae and longitudinal tubules of sarcoplasmic reticulum from malignant hyperpyrexia susceptible porcine skeletal muscle. Int J Biochem 21:1119, 1989

167. Fletcher JE, Tripolitis L, Erwin K *et al:* Fatty acids modulate calcium-induced calcium release from skeletal muscle heavy sarcoplasmic reticulum fractions: Implications for malignant hyperthermia. Biochem Cell Biol 68:1195, 1990

168. Endo M, Yagi S, Ishizuka T *et al:* Changes in the Ca-induced Ca release mechanism in the sarcoplasmic reticulum of the muscle from a patient with malignant hyperthermia. Biomed Res 4:83, 1983

169. Takagi A, Sunohara N, Ishihara T *et al:* Malignant hyperthermia and related neuromuscular diseases: Caffeine contracture of the skinned muscle fibers. Muscle Nerve 6:510, 1983

170. Louis CF, Zualkernan K, Roghair T, Mickelson JR: The effects of volatile anesthetics on calcium regulation by malignant hyperthermia-susceptible sarcoplasmic reticulum. Anesthesiology 77:114, 1992

171. McSweeney DM, Heffron JJ: Uptake and release of calcium ions by heavy sarcoplasmic reticulum fraction of normal and malignant hyperthermia-susceptible human skeletal muscle. Int J Biochem 22:329, 1990

172. O'Brien PJ: Porcine malignant hyperthermia susceptibility: Hypersensitive calcium-release mechanism of skeletal muscle sarcoplasmic reticulum. Can J Vet Res 50:318, 1986

173. Struk A, Lehmann-Horn F, Melzer W: Voltage-dependent calcium release in human malignant hyperthermia muscle fibers. Biophys J 75:2402, 1998
174. Censier K, Urwyler A, Zorzato F, Treves S: Intracellular calcium homeostasis in human primary muscle cells from malignant hyperthermia-susceptible and normal individuals. Effect of overexpression of recombinant wild-type and Arg163Cys mutated ryanodine receptors. J Clin Invest 101:1233, 1998
175. Ohnishi ST, Waring AJ, Fang SR et al: Abnormal membrane properties of the sarcoplasmic reticulum of pigs susceptible to malignant hyperthermia: Modes of action of halothane, caffeine, dantrolene, and two other drugs. Arch Biochem Biophys 247:294, 1986
176. Nelson TE: Porcine malignant hyperthermia: Critical temperatures for in vivo and in vitro responses. Anesthesiology 73:449, 1990
177. Sullivan JS, Denborough MA: Temperature dependence of muscle function in malignant hyperpyrexia-susceptible swine. Br J Anaesth 53:1217, 1981
178. Cheah KS, Cheah AM, Fletcher JE, Rosenberg H: Skeletal muscle mitochondrial respiration of malignant hyperthermia-susceptible patients: Ca^{2+}-induced uncoupling and free fatty acids. Int J Biochem 21:913, 1989
179. Hawkes MJ, Nelson TE, Hamilton SL: [^{3}H]ryanodine as a probe of changes in the functional state of the Ca^{2+}-release channel in malignant hyperthermia. J Biol Chem 267:6702, 1992
180. Herrmann-Frank A, Richter M, Sarkozi S et al: 4-Chloro-m-cresol, a potent and specific activator of the skeletal muscle ryanodine receptor. Biochim Biophys Acta 1289:31, 1996
181. Nelson TE: Halothane effects on human malignant hyperthermia skeletal muscle single calcium-release channels in planar lipid bilayers. Anesthesiology 76:588, 1992
182. Owen VJ, Taske NL, Lamb GD: Reduced Mg^{2+} inhibition of Ca^{2+} release in muscle fibers of pigs susceptible to malignant hyperthermia. Am J Physiol 272:C203, 1997
183. Levitt RC, McKusick VA, Fletcher JE, Rosenberg H: Gene candidate. Nature 345:297, 1990
184. Fill M, Stefani E, Nelson TE: Abnormal human sarcoplasmic reticulum Ca^{2+} release channels in malignant hyperthermic skeletal muscle. Biophys J 59:1085, 1991
185. Fill M, Coronado R, Mickelson JR et al: Abnormal ryanodine receptor channels in malignant hyperthermia. Biophys J 57:471, 1990
186. Fujii J, Otsu K, Zorzato F et al: Identification of a mutation in porcine ryanodine receptor associated with malignant hyperthermia. Science 253:448, 1991
187. Mickelson JR, Knudson CM, Kennedy CF et al: Structural and functional correlates of a mutation in the malignant hyperthermia-susceptible pig ryanodine receptor. FEBS Lett 301:49, 1992
188. Shomer NH, Mickelson JR, Louis CF: Caffeine stimulation of malignant hyperthermia-susceptible sarcoplasmic reticulum Ca^{2+} release channel. Am J Physiol 267:C1253, 1994
189. McCarthy TV, Healy JM, Heffron JJ et al: Localization of the malignant hyperthermia susceptibility locus to human chromosome 19q12-13.2. Nature 343:562, 1990
190. MacKenzie AE, Allen G, Lahey D et al: A comparison of the caffeine halothane muscle contracture test with the molecular genetic diagnosis of malignant hyperthermia [see comments]. Anesthesiology 75:4, 1991
191. Ball SP, Dorkins HR, Ellis FR et al: Genetic linkage analysis of chromosome 19 markers in malignant hyperthermia. Br J Anaesth 70:70, 1993
192. Healy SJ, Heffron JJ, Lehane M et al: Diagnosis of susceptibility to malignant hyperthermia with flanking DNA markers. Br Med J 303:1225, 1991
193. Phillips MS, Khanna VK, De Leon S et al: The substitution of Arg for Gly^{2433} in the human skeletal muscle ryanodine receptor is associated with malignant hyperthermia. Hum Mol Genet 3:2181, 1994
194. Wallace AJ, Wooldridge W, Kingston HM et al: Malignant hyperthermia—a large kindred linked to the RYR1 gene. Anaesthesia 51:16, 1996
195. Lynch PJ, Krivosic-Horber R, Reyford H et al: Identification of heterozygous and homozygous individuals with the novel RYR1 mutation Cys35Arg in a large kindred [see comments]. Anesthesiology 86:620, 1997
196. Robinson R, Curran JL, Hall WJ et al: Genetic heterogeneity and HOMOG analysis in British malignant hyperthermia families. J Med Genet 35:196, 1998
197. Deufel T, Sudbrak R, Feist Y et al: Discordance, in a malignant

hyperthermia pedigree, between in vitro contracture-test phenotypes and haplotypes for the MHS1 region on chromosome 19q12-13.2, comprising the C1840T transition in the RYR1 gene Am J Hum Genet 56:1334, 1995 [erratum: Am J Hum Genet 57(2):520, 1995]
198. Fagerlund TH, Ording H, Bendixen D et al: Discordance between malignant hyperthermia susceptibility and RYR1 mutation C1840T in two Scandinavian MH families exhibiting this mutation. Clin Genet 52:416, 1997
199. Fortunato G, Carsana A, Tinto N et al: A case of discordance between genotype and phenotype in a malignant hyperthermia family. Eur J Hum Genet 7:415, 1999
200. Fagerlund T, Ording H, Bendixen D et al: RYR mutation G1021A (Gly341Arg) is not frequent in Danish and Swedish families with malignant hyperthermia susceptibility. Clin Genet 49:186, 1996
201. Stewart SL, Rosenberg H, Fletcher JE: Failure to identify the ryanodine receptor G1021A mutation in a large North American population with malignant hyperthermia. Clin Genet 54:358, 1998
202. Tong J, Oyamada H, Demaurex N et al: Caffeine and halothane sensitivity of intracellular Ca^{2+} release is altered by 15 calcium release channel (ryanodine receptor) mutations associated with malignant hyperthermia and/or central core disease. J Biol Chem 272:26332, 1997
203. Tong J, McCarthy TV, MacLennan DH: Measurement of resting cytosolic Ca^{2+} concentrations and Ca^{2+} store size in HEK-293 cells transfected with malignant hyperthermia or central core disease mutant Ca^{2+} release channels. J Biol Chem 274:693, 1999
204. Lehmann-Horn F, Rudel R: Molecular pathophysiology of voltage-gated ion channels. In: Reviews of Physiology, Biochemistry and Pharmacology, p 195. Berlin, Springer, 1996
205. Cannon SC: Sodium channel defects in myotonia and periodic paralysis. Ann Rev Neurosci 19:141, 1996
206. Kallen RG, Cohen SA, Barchi RL: Structure, function and expression of voltage-dependent sodium channels. Mol Neurobiol 7:383, 1993
207. Rojas CV, Wang JZ, Schwartz LS et al: A Met-to-Val mutation in the skeletal muscle Na^{+} channel α-subunit in hyperkalaemic periodic paralysis. Nature 354:387, 1991
208. Ptacek LJ, George AL Jr, Barchi RL et al: Mutations in an S4 segment of the adult skeletal muscle sodium channel cause paramyotonia congenita. Neuron 8:891, 1992
209. Ricker K, Moxley RT 3rd, Heine R, Lehmann-Horn F: Myotonia fluctuans. A third type of muscle sodium channel disease. Arch Neurol 51:1095, 1994
210. Russell SH, Hirsch NP: Anaesthesia and myotonia. Br J Anaesth 72:210, 1994
211. Wieland SJ, Fletcher JE, Gong QH, Rosenberg H: Effects of lipid-soluble agents on sodium channel function in normal and MH-susceptible skeletal muscle cultures. Adv Exp Med Biol 301:9, 1991
212. Iaizzo PA, Lehmann-Horn F, Taylor SR, Gallant EM: Malignant hyperthermia: Effects of halothane on the surface membrane. Muscle Nerve 12:178, 1989
213. Fletcher JE, Adnet PJ, Reyford H et al: ATX II, a sodium channel toxin, sensitizes skeletal muscle to halothane, caffeine, and ryanodine. Anesthesiology 90:1294, 1999
214. Adnet PJ, Etchrivi TS, Halle I et al: Effects of veratridine on mechanical responses of human malignant hyperthermic muscle fibers. Acta Anaesthesiol Scand 42:246, 1998
215. Ruppersberg JP, Rudel R: Differential effects of halothane on adult and juvenile sodium channels in human muscle. Pflugers Arch 412:17, 1988
216. Schotland DL, Fieles W, Barchi RL: Expression of sodium channel subtypes during development in rat skeletal muscle. Muscle Nerve 14:142, 1991
217. Stewart SL, MacLennan DH, Fletcher JE: Altered calcium regulation in malignant hyperthermia down-regulates a sodium channel transcript. FASEB J 12:A1476, 1998
218. Moslehi R, Langlois S, Yam I, Friedman JM: Linkage of malignant hyperthermia and hyperkalemic periodic paralysis to the adult skeletal muscle sodium channel (SCN4A) gene in a large pedigree. Am J Med Genet 76:21, 1998
219. Levitt RC, Olckers A, Meyers S et al: Evidence for the localization of a malignant hyperthermia susceptibility locus (MHS2) to human chromosome 17q. Genomics 14:562, 1992
220. Olckers A, Meyers DA, Meyers S et al: Adult muscle sodium channel α-subunit is a gene candidate for malignant hyperthermia susceptibility. Genomics 14:829, 1992

221. Vita GM, Olckers A, Jedlicka AE *et al:* Masseter muscle rigidity associated with glycine1306-to-alanine mutation in the adult muscle sodium channel α-subunit gene [see comments]. Anesthesiology 82:1097, 1995

222. Schmidt JW, Catterall WA: Palmitylation, sulfation, and glycosylation of the α subunit of the sodium channel. Role of post-translational modifications in channel assembly. J Biol Chem 262:13713, 1987

223. Graber R, Sumida C, Nunez EA: Fatty acids and cell signal transduction. J Lipid Mediat Cell Signal 9:91, 1994

224. Carroll JE: Myopathies caused by disorders of lipid metabolism. Neurol Clin 6:563, 1988

225. Hall GM, Lucke JN, Orchard C *et al:* Porcine malignant hyperthermia. VIII: Leg metabolism. Br J Anaesth 54:941, 1982

226. Glatz JF, Vork MM, Cistola DP, van der Vusse GJ: Cytoplasmic fatty acid binding protein: Significance for intracellular transport of fatty acids and putative role on signal transduction pathways. Prostaglandins Leukot Essent Fatty Acids 48:33, 1993

227. Fletcher JE, Rosenberg H: *In vitro* muscle contractures induced by halothane and suxamethonium. II: Human skeletal muscle from normal and malignant hyperthermia susceptible patients. Br J Anaesth 58:1433, 1986

228. Duthie GG, Wahle KW, Harris CI *et al:* Lipid peroxidation, antioxidant concentrations, and fatty acid contents of muscle tissue from malignant hyperthermia-susceptible swine. Arch Biochem Biophys 296:592, 1992

229. Cheah AM: Effect of long chain unsaturated fatty acids on the calcium transport of sarcoplasmic reticulum. Biochim Biophys Acta 648:113, 1981

230. Messineo FC, Rathier M, Favreau C, *et al:* Mechanisms of fatty acid effects on sarcoplasmic reticulum. III. The effects of palmitic and oleic acids on sarcoplasmic reticulum function—a model for fatty acid membrane interactions. J Biol Chem 259:1336, 1984

231. Dettbarn C, Palade P: Arachidonic acid-induced Ca^{2+} release from isolated sarcoplasmic reticulum. Biochem Pharmacol 45:1301, 1993

232. Dubois BW, Evers AS: ^{19}F-NMR spin-spin relaxation (T2) method for characterizing volatile anesthetic binding to proteins. Analysis of isoflurane binding to serum albumin. Biochemistry 31:7069, 1992

233. Wappler F, Scholz J, Kochling A *et al:* Inositol 1,4,5-trisphosphate in blood and skeletal muscle in human malignant hyperthermia. Br J Anaesth 78:541, 1997

234. Foster PS, Gesini E, Claudianos C *et al:* Inositol 1,4,5-trisphosphate phosphatase deficiency and malignant hyperpyrexia in swine. Lancet 2:124, 1989

235. Henzi V, MacDermott AB: Characteristics and function of Ca^{2+}- and inositol 1,4,5-trisphosphate-releasable stores of Ca^{2+} in neurons. Neuroscience 46:251, 1992

236. Nishizuka Y: Intracellular signaling by hydrolysis of phospholipids and activation of protein kinase C. Science 258:607, 1992

237. Lopez JR, Perez C, Linares N *et al:* Hypersensitive response of malignant hyperthermia-susceptible skeletal muscle to inositol 1,4,5-triphosphate induced release of calcium. Naunyn Schmiedebergs Arch Pharmacol 352:442, 1995

238. Duthie GG, Arthur JR: Free radicals and calcium homeostasis: Relevance to malignant hyperthermia? Free Radic Biol Med 14:435, 1993

239. Duthie GG, Arthur JR: The antioxidant abnormality in the stress-susceptible pig. Effect of vitamin E supplementation. Ann NY Acad Sci 570:322, 1989

240. Iles DE, Lehmann-Horn F, Scherer SW *et al:* Localization of the gene encoding the α_2/δ-subunits of the L-type voltage-dependent calcium channel to chromosome 7q and analysis of the segregation of flanking markers in malignant hyperthermia susceptible families. Hum Mol Genet 3:969, 1994

241. Sudbrak R, Procaccio V, Klausnitzer M *et al:* Mapping of a further malignant hyperthermia susceptibility locus to chromosome 3q13.1. Am J Hum Genet 56:684, 1995

242. Robinson RL, Monnier N, Wolz W *et al:* A genome wide search for susceptibility loci in three European malignant hyperthermia pedigrees. Hum Mol Genet 6:953, 1997

243. Hogan K: The anesthetic myopathies and malignant hyperthermias. Curr Opin Neurol 11:469, 1998

244. Quane KA, Healy JM, Keating KE *et al:* Mutations in the ryanodine receptor gene in central core disease and malignant hyperthermia. Nat Genet 5:51, 1993

245. Zhang Y, Chen HS, Khanna VK *et al:* A mutation in the human ryanodine receptor gene associated with central core disease. Nat Genet 5:46, 1993

246. Quane KA, Keating KE, Healy JM *et al:* Mutation screening of the RYR1 gene in malignant hyperthermia: Detection of a novel Tyr to Ser mutation in a pedigree with associated central cores. Genomics 23(1):236, 1994

247. Islander G, Henriksson KG, Ranklev-Twetman E: Malignant hyperthermia susceptibility without central core disease (CCD) in a family where CCD is diagnosed. Neuromuscul Disord 5:125, 1995

248. Fagerlund T, Ording H, Bendixen D, Berg K: Search for three known mutations in the RYR1 gene in 48 Danish families with malignant hyperthermia. Clin Genet 46:401, 1994

249. Monnier N, Procaccio V, Stieglitz P, Lunardi J: Malignant-hyperthermia susceptibility is associated with a mutation of the α_1-subunit of the human dihydropyridine-sensitive L-type voltage-dependent calcium-channel receptor on skeletal muscle [see comments]. Am J Hum Genetics 60:1316, 1997

250. Serfas KD, Bose D, Patel L *et al:* Comparison of the segregation of the RYR1 C1840T mutation with segregation of the caffeine/halothane contracture test results for malignant hyperthermia susceptibility in a large Manitoba Mennonite family [see comments]. Anesthesiology 84:322, 1996

251. Allen GC, Larach MG, Kunselman AR: The sensitivity and specificity of the caffeine-halothane contracture test: A report from the North American Malignant Hyperthermia Registry. The North American Malignant Hyperthermia Registry of MHAUS. Anesthesiology 88:579, 1987

252. Stanbury JB, Wyngaarden JB, Frederickson DS: The Metabolic Basis of Inherited Disease, 6th ed. New York, McGraw-Hill, 1989

253. Whittaker M: In Monographs in Human Genetics, Vol. 11. New York, Karger, 1986

254. Xie W, Altamirano CV, Bartels CF *et al:* An improved cocaine hydrolase: The A328Y mutant of human butyrylcholinesterase is 4-fold more efficient. Mol. Pharmacol 55:83, 1999

255. Viby-Mogensen J: Succinylcholine neuromuscular blockade in subjects homozygous for atypical plasma cholinesterase. Anesthesiology 55:429, 1981

256. Kalow W, Genest K: A method for the detection of atypical forms of human serum cholinesterase: Determination of dibucaine numbers. Can J Biochem 35:339, 1957

257. Harris H, Whittaker M: Differential inhibition of serum cholinesterase with fluoride: Recognition of two new phenotypes. Nature (Lond) 191:496, 1961

258. Primo-Parma SL, Bartels CF, Wiersema B *et al:* Characterization of 12 silent alleles of the human butyrylcholinesterase (BCHE) gene. Am J Hum Genet 58:52, 1996

259. McGuire M, Noguiera CG, Bartels CF *et al:* Identification of the structured mutation responsible for the dibucaine-resistant (atypical) variant form of human cholinesterase. Proc Natl Acad Sci USA 86:953, 1989

260. Krause A, Lane AB, Jenkins T: Pseudocholinesterase variation in southern Africa populations. South African Med J 71:298, 1987

261. Hanel HK, Viby-Mogensen J, Schaffalitzky de Muckadell OB: Serum cholinesterase variants in the Danish population. Acta Anaesthesiol Scand 22:505, 1978

262. Patterson JL, Walsh ES, Hall GM: Progressive depletion of plasma cholinesterase during daily plasma exchange. Br Med J 2:580, 1979

263. Viby-Mogensen J: Correlation of succinylcholine duration of action with plasma cholinesterase activity in subjects with normal enzyme. Anesthesiology 53:517, 1980

264. Viby-Mogensen J: Succinylcholine neuromuscular blockade in subjects heterozygous for abnormal plasma cholinesterase. Anesthesiology 55:231, 1981

265. Lovely MJ, Patteson SK, Beuerlein FJ, Chesney JT: Perioperative blood transfusion may conceal atypical pseudocholinesterase. Anesth Analg 70:326, 1990

266. Harris H, Hopkinson DA, Robson EB *et al:* Genetic studies on a new variant of serum cholinesterase detected by electrophoresis. Ann Hum Genet 26:359, 1963

267. Brodsky JB, Campos FA: Chloroprocaine analgesia in a patient receiving echothiophate iodide eye drops. Anesthesiology 48:288, 1978

268. Raj PP, Rosenblatt R, Miller J *et al:* Dynamics of local anesthetic compounds in regional anesthesia. Anesth Analg 56:110, 1977

269. Jatlow P, Barash PG, Van Dyke C *et al:* Cocaine and succinylcholine sensitivity: A new caution. Anesth Analg 58:235, 1979

270. Petersen RS, Bailey PL, Kalameghan R, Ashwood ER: Prolonged neuromuscular block after mivacurium. Anesth Analg 76:194, 1993

271. Murphy PC: Acute intermittent porphyria: The anaesthetic problem and its background. Br J Anaesth 36:801, 1964

272. Lafeuillade A, Dhiver C, Martin I *et al:* Porphyria cutanea tarda associated with HIV infection. AIDS 4:924, 1990

273. Harrison GG, Meissner PN, Hift RJ: Anesthesia for the porphyric patient. Anaesthesia 48:417, 1993

274. McLoughlin C: Use of propofol in a patient with porphyria. Br J Anaesth 62:114, 1989

275. McNeill MJ, Bennet A: Use of regional anaesthesia in a patient with acute porphyria. Br J Anaesth 64:371, 1990

276. Cox JM: Anesthesia and glycogen storage disease. Anesthesiology 29:1221, 1963

277. Casson H: Anesthesia for portacaval bypass in patients with metabolic diseases. Br J Anaesth 47:969, 1975

278. McFarlane HJ, Soni N: Pompe's disease and anesthesia. Anaesthesia 41:1219, 1986

279. Ellis FR: Inherited muscle disease. Br J Anaesth 52:153, 1980

280. Lobato EB, Janelle GM, Urdaneta F, Malias MA: Noncardiogenic pulmonary edema and rhabdomyolysis after protamine administration in a patient with unrecognized McArdle's disease. Anesthesiology 91:303, 1999

281. Edelstein G, Hirshman CA: Hyperthermia and ketoacidosis during anesthesia in a child with glycogen-storage disease. Anesthesiology 52:90, 1980

282. Hashimoto Y, Watanabe H, Satou M: Anesthetic management of a patient with hereditary fructose 1,6-diphosphate deficiency. Anesth Analg 57:503, 1978

283. Leroy JG, Crocker AC: Clinical definition of the Hurler-Hunter phenotypes. Am J Dis Child 112:518, 1966

284. Busoni P, Cognani G: Failure of laryngeal mask to secure the airway in a patient with Hunter's syndrome (mucopolysaccharidosis type II). Paediatr Anaesth 9:153, 1999

285. Oliverio RM: Anesthetic management of intramedullary nailing in osteogenesis imperfecta: Report of a case. Anesth Analg 52:232, 1973

286. Ohta T, Gray TA, Rogan PK *et al:* Imprinting mutation mechanisms in Prader-Willi syndrome. Am J Hum Genet 64:397, 1999

287. Kuslich CD, Kobori JA, Mohapatra G *et al:* Prader-Willi syndrome is caused by disruption of the SNRPN gene. Am J Hum Genet 64:70, 1999

288. Brown BR, Watson PD, Taussig LM: Congenital metabolic diseases of pediatric patients. Anesthesiology 43:197, 1975

289. Axelrod FB, Donenfeld RF, Danzinger F, Turndorf M: Anesthesia in familial dysautonomia. Anesthesiology 68:631, 1988

290. Stubbig K, Schmidt H, Schreckenberger R *et al:* Anaesthesia and intensive therapy in autonomic dysfunction. Anaesthetist 42:316, 1993

Clinical Anesthesia (4/e), edited by
Paul G. Barash, Bruce F. Cullen, and
Robert K. Stoelting. Lippincott Williams &
Wilkins, Philadelphia, © 2001.

CHAPTER 21

PREOPERATIVE MEDICATION

JOHN R. MOYERS AND CARLA M. VINCENT

Anesthetic management for patients begins with preoperative psychological preparation and, if necessary, preoperative medication. Specific pharmacologic actions should be kept in mind when these drugs are administered before operation, and they should be tailored to the needs of each patient. The anesthesiologist should assess the patient's mental and physical condition during the preoperative visit. Because it is part of and the beginning of the anesthetic, choice of preoperative medication is based on the same considerations as the choice of anesthesia, including the patient's medical problems, requirements of the surgery, and the anesthesiologist's skills. Satisfactory preoperative preparation and medication facilitate an uneventful perioperative course. Poor preparation may begin a series of problems and misadventures.

No consensus exists on the choice of preoperative medications. Their use has been dominated by tradition, which has been modified somewhat by the change in anesthetic agents and techniques over the years. Beecher stated that "empirical procedures firmly established in the habits of good doctors have a life, not to say, immortality of their own."[1] Similarly, "the emotional attachment of an anesthesiologist to his own regimen is often more obvious than his objective assessment of its effects."[2] Another reason for lack of consensus may be that several different drugs or combinations of drugs can accomplish the same goals. However, there is general agreement that most patients should enter the operating room after anxiety has been relieved and other specific goals have been met through preoperative preparation and medication. This should be accomplished without undue sedation, which can interfere with patient safety or, given the dramatic increase in the number of outpatient surgical procedures, prolong length of stay in the operating room.

PSYCHOLOGICAL PREPARATION

Psychological preparation of the patient involves the preoperative visit and interview with the patient and family members. The anesthesiologist should explain anticipated events and the proposed anesthetic management in an effort to reduce anxiety and allay apprehension. Patients may perceive the day of surgery as the biggest, most threatening day in their lives; they do not wish to be treated impersonally in the operating room. The anesthesiologist's first direct encounter with the patient may be in the immediate preoperative period. A growing number of outpatients, particularly those in ASA classes I and II, receive their preanesthetic evaluations just prior to surgery. Preoperative visits must be conducted efficiently, but they must also be informative and reassuring, answering all questions. Most of the anesthesiologist's time is spent with an unconscious or sedated patient; therefore, he or she must take time before the operation to earn the trust and confidence of that patient.

Most patients are anxious before surgery. Studies show that, depending on the intensity of inquiry, from 40 to 85% of patients are apprehensive before surgery.[3,4] Preoperative anxiety states are at a high level, and patients expect apprehension to be relieved before they arrive in the operating room.[5] A study by Egbert et al showed that an average of 57% of patients felt anxious before operation.[4] The highest levels of anxiety were noted in patients scheduled for major genitourologic surgery (79%) and for cancer surgery (86%). They found neither age nor gender differences in levels of apprehension among the

study population. In an analysis of 500 adult surgical patients, Norris and Baird found that female patients were more likely than males to experience preoperative anxiety.[3] Furthermore, they noted an increased incidence of anxiety in female patients who weighed more than 70 kg and in patients previously or currently taking sedative drugs. They also documented a trend toward greater levels of anxiety in more ill patients. There was no difference in anxiety with respect to age, social status, nature of the operation, or previous hospital experience.

An informative and comforting preoperative visit may replace many milligrams of depressant medication. The study by Egbert and colleagues showed that more patients were adequately prepared for surgery after a preoperative interview than after 2 $mg \cdot kg^{-1}$ of pentobarbital given intramuscularly 1 hour before surgery (Table 21-1).[4] During ward rounds on the afternoon before surgery, the patients in their preoperative interview group were visited by the anesthesiologist, who discussed each patient's condition, the time of the operation, and the anesthetic. The patient was informed about perioperative events and asked about previous anesthetic experiences. The patients in this study who received pentobarbital for preoperative medication but had no interview appeared and felt drowsy but were not calm. Leigh et al investigated adult preoperative patients using objective tests of anxiety.[6] They found that the anesthesiologist's 10-minute preoperative visit produced lower anxiety levels before operation than no visit at all. Furthermore, they found that the preoperative visit was more effective than a booklet given to the patients the day before surgery, which was specifically designed to reassure them about anesthesia. The booklet was not a substitute for a proper preoperative visit and interview. Likewise, Done and Lee found viewing a preoperative video to increase patients' recall of anesthesia-related information, but stressed the need to provide patient-specific details.[7]

Psychological preparation cannot accomplish everything and will not relieve all anxiety. Besides psychological preparation, there are other goals of preoperative medication. Control of pain and satisfactory levels of amnesia or sedation cannot be achieved with consistent success at the preoperative visit alone. In addition, emergency situations may provide little or no time for a preoperative interview. More seriously ill or elderly patients, conversely, may not tolerate the physiologic effects of sedative medications. Always remember that the substitution of preoperative depressant drugs for a comforting and tactful preoperative visit may compromise patient safety.

PHARMACOLOGIC PREPARATION

The ideal drug or combination of drugs for preoperative pharmacologic preparation is as elusive as is the ideal anesthetic technique. Routine administration of the same drugs to all patients has fallen into disfavor as a selective approach has emerged. In selecting the appropriate drugs for preoperative medication, the patient's psychological condition and physical status must be considered. The patient's age is also important. Is the patient in the pediatric or the geriatric age group? The surgical procedure and its duration are important factors, as well. Is this an outpatient procedure? Is it elective surgery or emergency surgery? The anesthesiologist must know the patient's weight; prior response to depressant drugs, including unwanted side effects; and allergies. Finally, the anesthesio-

Table 21-1. COMPARISON OF PREOPERATIVE VISIT AND PENTOBARBITAL (2 mg · kg⁻¹ im) (PERCENTAGE OF PATIENTS)

	Felt Drowsy	Felt Nervous	Adequate Preparation
Control group	18	58	35
Pentobarbital group	30	61	48
Preoperative visit	26	40	65
Preoperative visit and pentobarbital	38	38	71

Data from Egbert LD, Battit GE, Turndorf H *et al:* The value of the preoperative visit by an anesthestist. JAMA 185:553, 1963.

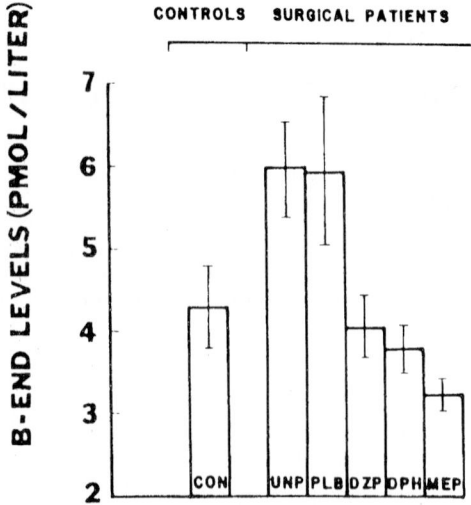

Figure 21-1. Plasma β-endorphin (B-END) concentrations as measured in control (CON) patients or in presurgical patients receiving no premedication (UNP), intramuscular saline (PLB), oral diazepam 10 mg (DZP), intramuscular diphenhydramine 1 mg · kg⁻¹ (DPH), or intramuscular meperidine 1 mg · kg⁻¹ (MEP). Measurements were made 1 hour after treatment. Mean ± SEM. (Reprinted with permission from Walsh J, Puig MM, Lovitz MA *et al:* Premedication abolishes the increase in plasma β-endorphin observed in the immediate preoperative period. Anesthesiology 66:402, 1987.)

gist's experience and familiarity with certain preoperative medications more than others are determinants.

The goals to be achieved for each patient with preoperative medication are intimately involved in the selection process (Table 21-2). The desired goals may be multiple and should be tailored to the needs of each patient. Some of the goals, such as relief of anxiety and production of sedation, apply to almost every patient, whereas others are important only occasionally. Prophylaxis against allergic reactions applies in just a few instances. Prevention of autonomic reflexes mediated through the vagus nerve or an antiemetic effect may be better attempted immediately before the anticipated need rather than achieved at the time of preoperative medication. Most preoperative medication regimens do not produce sufficient obtundation to be clinically significant in reducing anesthetic requirement. But preoperative medication often prevents preoperative elevations of plasma concentrations of β-endorphins that normally accompany the stress response (Fig. 21-1).[8,9]

Some patients should not receive depressant drugs before surgery. Patients with little physiologic reserve, at the extremes of age, with a head injury, or with hypovolemia may be harmed more than helped by many of the medications normally used before operation. In contrast, the conditions of others demand that attempts be made pharmacologically to reduce anxiety, provide analgesia, or dry secretions in the airway to produce a safer perioperative course. For elective surgery, the anesthesiologist will, in most instances, want the patient to enter the operating room free of anxiety and sedated, yet easily arousable and cooperative. The patient should not be overly obtunded or display other unwanted side effects of the preoperative drugs. The patient who asks to be "asleep" before leaving the hospital room should be told that apprehension and sedation may be reduced but it would be unsafe to produce a comatose state. The time and route of administration of the preoperative medi-

cations are important. As a general rule, oral medications should be given to the patient 60–90 minutes before arrival in the operating room. It is acceptable to administer oral drugs with up to 150 ml of water.[10] For full effect, intramuscular medications should be given at least 20 minutes and preferably 30–60 minutes before the patient's arrival in the operating room. Every attempt should be made to have the preoperative medications achieve their full effect before the patient's arrival in the operating room rather than after induction of anesthesia. The drug(s), doses, route of administration, and effects should be recorded on the anesthetic record. A list of common preoperative medications is presented in Table 21-3.

The choice of premedicant drugs is not based on a large body of scientific data that is either definitive or persuasive. The subject is difficult to study. Often, the investigations involve

Table 21-2. VARIOUS GOALS FOR PREOPERATIVE MEDICINE

1. Relief of anxiety
2. Sedation
3. Amnesia
4. Analgesia
5. Drying of airway secretions
6. Prevention of autonomic reflex responses
7. Reduction of gastric fluid volume and increased pH
8. Antiemetic effects
9. Reduction of anesthetic requirements
10. Facilitation of smooth induction of anesthesia
11. Prophylaxis against allergic reactions

Modified from Stoelting RK: Psychological preparation and preoperative medication. In Miller RD (ed): Anesthesia. New York, Churchill Livingstone, 1981.

Table 21-3. COMMON PREOPERATIVE MEDICATIONS, DOSES, AND ADMINISTRATION ROUTES

Medication	Administration Route	Dose (mg)
Diazepam	Oral	5–20
Lorazepam	Oral, im	1–4
Midazolam	im	3–7
	iv	Titration of 1.0–2.5-mg doses
Secobarbital	Oral, im	50–200
Pentobarbital	Oral, im	50–200
Morphine	im	5–15
Meperidine	im	50–150
Cimetidine	Oral, im, iv	150–300
Ranitidine	Oral	50–200
Metoclopramide	Oral, im, iv	5–20
Atropine	im, iv	0.3–0.6
Glycopyrrolate	im, iv	0.1–0.3
Scopolamine	im, iv	0.3–0.6

im = intramuscular; iv = intravenous.
Modified from Stoelting RK, Miller RD (eds): Basics of Anesthesia. New York, Churchill Livingstone, 1984.

only one dose of drug or one dose of a number of drugs given in combination. In some studies drugs are given parenterally, whereas in others they are administered orally or even rectally. Different investigations may study the effect of the drugs at different times after administration. The patients' responses and the investigators' observations of those responses are subjective and difficult to quantify. Also, the studies may involve heterogeneous groups of patients in whom the psychological preoperative preparation has not been standardized.

Sedative Hypnotics and Tranquilizers

Benzodiazepines

Benzodiazepines are among the most popular drugs used for preoperative medication (Table 21-4). They are used to produce anxiolysis, amnesia, and sedation. The anticonvulsant and muscle relaxant effects of the benzodiazepines are not usually important when preoperative medication is considered. Because the site of action of benzodiazepines is on specific receptors in the central nervous system, there is relatively little depression of ventilation or of the cardiovascular system with premedicant doses. Benzodiazepines have a wide therapeutic index and a low incidence of toxicity. Other than central nervous system depression, there are few side effects of this group of drugs. Specifically, nausea and vomiting are not usually associated with administration of benzodiazepines for preoperative medication. These drugs are also used before operation to reduce the unpleasant dreams and delirium that may occur after ketamine administration.

There are some hazards and unwanted side effects of the benzodiazepines. The central nervous system depression they cause is sometimes long and excessive, especially with use of lorazepam. There may be pain at the intramuscular or intravenous injection site with diazepam, as well as the possibility of phlebitis. These drugs are not analgesic agents. Benzodiazepines may not always produce a calming effect but may cause agitation, as evidenced by restlessness and delirium.

The proposed mechanisms of action of the benzodiazepines describe specific receptors and actions within the central nervous system (Fig. 21-2).[11] The sedative action is said to result from a facilitation or enhancement of inhibitory neurotransmission mediated by γ-aminobutyric acid. The anxiolytic effect comes from the action of glycine-mediated inhibition of neuronal pathways in the brain stem and in the brain. The site of action of the benzodiazepines in producing amnesia is unknown.

Diazepam. The calming, amnesic, and sedative effects of diazepam make it a very popular choice for premedication. It

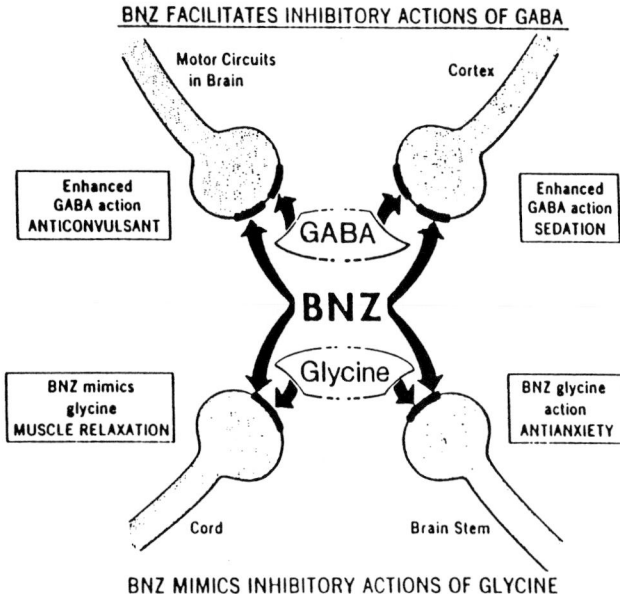

BNZ FACILITATES INHIBITORY ACTIONS OF GABA

BNZ MIMICS INHIBITORY ACTIONS OF GLYCINE

Figure 21-2. Schematic diagram of possible mechanisms for pharmacologic effects of benzodiazepines (BNZs). GABA = γ-aminobutyric acid. (Reprinted from Richter JJ: Current theories about the mechanisms of benzodiazepines and neuroleptic drugs. Anesthesiology 54:66, 1981.)

is the standard against which other benzodiazepines are usually compared. Because diazepam is insoluble in water and must be dissolved in organic solvents (propylene glycol, sodium benzoate), pain may occur on intramuscular or intravenous injection. Phlebitis is often a sequela of intravenous injection. Administration of diazepam orally with up to 150 ml of water is preferable to an intramuscular injection. More than 90% of an oral dose of diazepam is rapidly absorbed. Peak effect after oral administration occurs within 0.5–1 hour in adults and within 15–30 minutes in children (Fig. 21-3).[12] Diazepam does cross the placenta, with fetal concentrations equaling or exceeding maternal levels.[13] Because the drug is highly protein-bound, patients with low serum albumin levels, such as those with cirrhosis of the liver or chronic renal failure, may exhibit an increased effect of the drug. Hepatic microsomal enzymes metabolize the drug via oxidative N-demethylation to metabolites possessing weaker pharmacologic activity. Desmethyldiazepam and oxazepam are the primary metabolites; a smaller amount of the drug is converted to temazepam. Prolonged sedation resulting from active metabolites is usually seen after chronic use of diazepam rather than after the use of a single dose in the preoperative setting. The elimination half-time of diazepam is 21–37 hours in healthy volunteers. It may be prolonged in patients with cirrhosis or in elderly patients. Because absorption is unpredictable after intramuscular injection and because of pain with parenteral administration, many prefer to administer diazepam orally (see Fig. 21-3).[12] It is not as reliable in preventing recall as lorazepam, but the antegrade amnesia effect may be enhanced by scopolamine.[14] There is no evidence for the production of retrograde amnesia after diazepam administration.

There is little effect of diazepam outside the central nervous system. Minimal depression of ventilation, circulation, or hepatic or renal function occurs. Soroker *et al* demonstrated little or no effect on ventilation after diazepam administration.[15] Detectable Pa_{CO_2} increases were demonstrable only after intravenous administration of 0.2 mg $\cdot$ kg^{-1} of diazepam in another study.[16] The increase in carbon dioxide results from a decrease in tidal volume. In another investigation, after intravenous doses of 0.4 mg $\cdot$ kg^{-1}, the slope of the carbon dioxide response curve decreased, but the curve was not shifted to the right.[17] Despite the safety of relatively high intravenous doses of diazepam,

Table 21-4. COMPARISON OF PHARMACOLOGIC VARIABLES OF BENZODIAZEPINES

	Diazepam	Lorazepam	Midazolam
Dose equivalent (mg)	10	1–2	3–5
Time to peak effect after oral dose (hr)	1–1.5	2–4	0.5–1
Elimination half-time (hr)	20–40	10–20	1–4
Clearance (ml $\cdot$ kg^{-1} $\cdot$ min^{-1})	0.2–0.5	0.7–1.0	6.4–11.1
Volume of distribution (l $\cdot$ kg^{-1})	0.7–1.7	0.8–1.3	1.1–1.7

Adapted from Reves JG, Fragen RJ, Vinick HR *et al*: Midazolam: Pharmacology and uses. Anesthesiology 62:310, 1985; and Stoelting RK: Pharmacology and Physiology in Anesthetic Practice. Philadelphia, JB Lippincott, 1987.

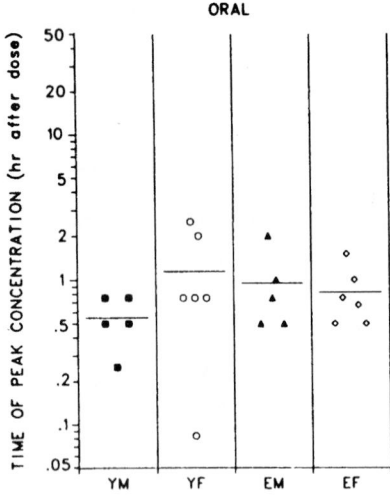
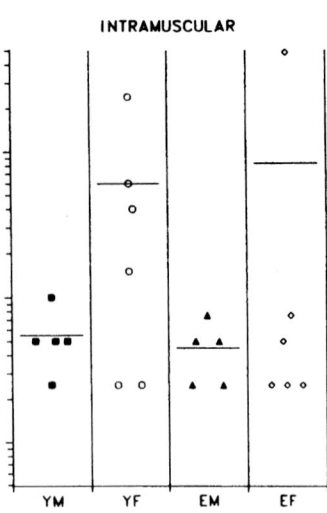

Figure 21-3. Individual and mean (*horizontal bar*) times of peak plasma concentrations after oral or intramuscular (deltoid) administration of diazepam, 5 mg, to adult patients (20–78 years of age) categorized as young male (YM), young female (YF), elderly male (EM), and elderly female (EF) patients. (Reprinted with permission from Divoll M, Greenblatt DJ, Ochs HR *et al:* Absolute bioavailability of oral and intramuscular diazepam: Effects of age and sex. Anesth Analg 62:1, 1983.)

respiratory arrest has been reported with as little as 2.5 mg.[18] Furthermore, ventilatory depression may be compounded by other depressant drugs, especially opioids and alcohol. There is little cardiovascular depression seen after the doses of diazepam used for preoperative medication. Indeed, higher intravenous doses produce little circulatory depression.[16] There is not much clinical effect on the neuromuscular junction after diazepam has been given for preoperative medication. There have been attempts to reduce myalgias and fasciculations produced by succinylcholine with diazepam. The effect on fasciculations has been variable, but myalgias were reduced in one study.[19] Premedication with diazepam does not reliably prevent an increase in intraocular pressure after intubation of the trachea.[20] In animals, diazepam has reduced the seizure threshold for lidocaine, but this effect has not been proved in humans.[21]

Some controversy exists with regard to interaction of diazepam with other drugs. Cimetidine delays the hepatic clearance of diazepam.[22] The proposed mechanism is the inhibition of microsomal enzymes of cimetidine. There is some question as to whether this is clinically significant when diazepam is used as a single dose before operation. Diazepam 0.2 mg · kg^{-1} has been shown to decrease the minimum alveolar concentration for halothane.[23] The magnitude in reduction of anesthetic requirement from premedication doses may or may not be important to the anesthesiologist.

Lorazepam. Lorazepam resembles oxazepam structurally and is 5–10 times as potent as diazepam. Lorazepam can produce profound amnesia, relief of anxiety, and sedation (Fig. 21-4).[24] When lorazepam is compared with diazepam, their ef-

fects are very similar. Although it is insoluble in water and requires a solvent such as polyethylene glycol or propylene glycol, administration of lorazepam, unlike diazepam, is not associated with pain on injection or phlebitis. Prolonged sedation is more likely after lorazepam administration. Even though the elimination half-life of diazepam is longer than that of lorazepam (20–40 hours vs. 10–20 hours), the effect of diazepam may be shorter because it more rapidly dissociates from the benzodiazepine receptor.[25]

Lorazepam is reliably absorbed both orally and intramuscularly. Maximal effect occurs 30–40 minutes after intravenous injection.[26] Bradshaw *et al* demonstrated clinical effects 30–60 minutes after oral administration of lorazepam.[27] A study by Blitt *et al* demonstrated that lack of recall was not produced until 2 hours after intramuscular injection.[28] Peak plasma concentrations may not occur until 2–4 hours after oral administration. Therefore, lorazepam must be ordered well before surgery so that the drug has time to be effective before the patient arrives in the operating room. Lorazepam also may be given sublingually.[29] As stated previously, the elimination half-life is 10–20 hours. The usual dose is about 25–50 μg · kg^{-1}. The dose for an adult should not exceed 4.0 mg.[24,25,30] With recommended doses, anterograde amnesia may be produced for as long as 4–6 hours without excessive sedation. Higher doses lead to prolonged and excessive sedation without more amnesia. Because of its slow onset and length of action, lorazepam is not useful in instances in which rapid awakening is necessary, such as with outpatient anesthesia. There are no active metabolites of lorazepam; and because its metabolism is not dependent on

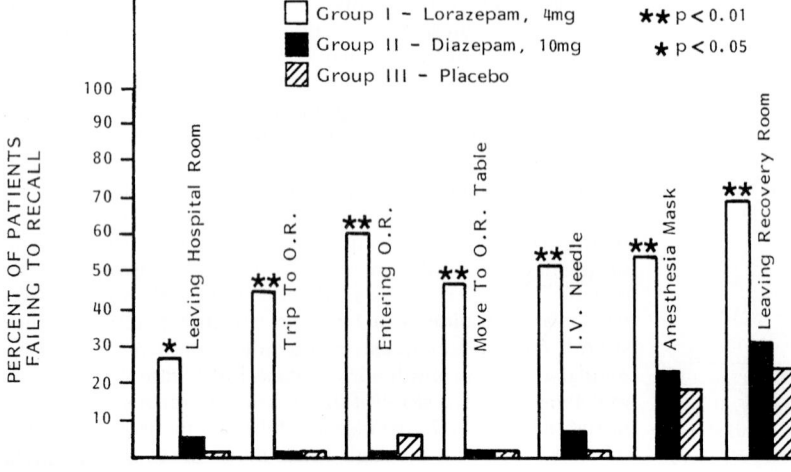

Figure 21-4. Percentage of patients in each group failing to recall specific events of the operative day. Medications were administered intramuscularly. (Reprinted with permission from Fragen RJ, Caldwell N: Lorazepam premedication: Lack of recall and relief of anxiety. Anesth Analg 55:792, 1976.)

microsomal enzymes, there is less influence on its effect from age or liver disease.[31] As with diazepam, little cardiorespiratory depression occurs with lorazepam. However, there is the danger of unwanted respiratory depression in those with lung disease.[32]

Midazolam. Midazolam has predominantly replaced diazepam in its use for preoperative medication and conscious sedation. The physicochemical properties of the drug allow for its water solubility and rapid metabolism. As with other benzodiazepines, midazolam produces anxiolysis, sedation, and amnesia. It is two to three times as potent as diazepam because of its increased affinity for the benzodiazepine receptor. The usual intramuscular dose is $0.05-0.1$ mg $\cdot$ kg^{-1} and titration of $1.0-2.5$ mg at a time intravenously. There is no irritation or phlebitis with injection of midazolam. The incidence of side effects after administration is low, although depression of ventilation and sedation may be greater than expected, especially in elderly patients or when the drug is combined with other central nervous system depressants. There is more rapid onset of action and predictable absorption after intramuscular injection of midazolam than after diazepam. The time of onset after intramuscular injection is $5-10$ minutes, with peak effect occurring after $30-60$ minutes. The onset after intravenous administration of 5 mg would be expected to occur after $1-2$ minutes. In addition to quicker onset, more rapid recovery occurs after midazolam administration compared with diazepam. This is probably the result of the lipid solubility of midazolam and its rapid distribution in the peripheral tissues and metabolic biotransformation. For these reasons, midazolam usually should be given within an hour of induction.[33] Midazolam is metabolized by hepatic microsomal enzymes to essentially inactive hydroxylated metabolites. H$_2$ receptor antagonists do not interfere with its metabolism.[34] The elimination half-life of midazolam is approximately $1-4$ hours and may be extended in the elderly.[35] Tests show that mental function usually returns to normal within 4 hours of administration.[33] After administration of 5 mg, amnesia lasts from 20 to 32 minutes.[36] Intramuscular administration may produce longer periods of amnesia. The lack of recall may be augmented by concomitant administration of scopolamine. The properties of midazolam make it ideal for shorter procedures.

Other Benzodiazepines. Oxazepam, another benzodiazepine that has been used for preoperative medication, is one of the pharmacologically active metabolites of diazepam. It is absorbed slowly after oral administration and has an elimination half-life of $5-15$ hours. Temazepam has been given in oral doses of $20-30$ mg before surgery. It must be given well before surgery because peak plasma levels do not occur until approximately $2-2.5$ hours after administration. Triazolam is a short-acting benzodiazepine. The adult oral dose of the drug is $0.25-0.5$ mg. Peak plasma concentrations occur in about 1 hour and its elimination half-life is $1.7-5.2$ hours. The drug may become long-acting in the elderly. Similarly, a study by Pinnock et al did not show triazolam to be of short duration when compared with diazepam for premedication for minor gynecologic surgery.[37] Alprazolam (1 mg) given to adults has been shown to produce a modest reduction in anxiety before surgery.[38]

Barbiturates

Use of barbiturates for preoperative medication is a time-tested practice with a long record of safety. These drugs are used primarily for their sedative effects. While barbiturate administration for pharmacologic preparation before surgery has been replaced in many instances by the use of benzodiazepines, they may be useful in certain settings. There is little cardiorespiratory depression associated with the usual preoperative doses. The barbiturates may be given orally as well as parenterally, and the drugs are relatively inexpensive. Barbiturates, however, are unlikely to produce sedation in the presence of pain. In fact, disorientation and paradoxical excitation may result. Low doses of barbiturates have been said to lower the pain threshold and

be antianalgesic. The agents lack specificity of action on the central nervous system and have a lower therapeutic index than the benzodiazepines. Barbiturates should not be used in patients with certain kinds of porphyria.

Secobarbital. Secobarbital usually is administered to adults in oral doses of $50-200$ mg when used for preoperative medication. Onset usually occurs $60-90$ minutes after administration, and sedative effects last 4 hours or longer. Indeed, even though secobarbital traditionally has been considered a "short-acting" barbiturate, it may impair performance for as long as $10-22$ hours.[39]

Pentobarbital. Pentobarbital may be administered orally or parenterally. The oral dose used for adults is usually $50-200$ mg. Pentobarbital has a biotransformation half-life of about 50 hours. Therefore, its use is not often suitable for shorter procedures.

Butyrophenones

Intravenous or intramuscular doses of $2.5-7.5$ mg of droperidol produce the appearance of sedation in patients before operation. Calmness and tranquility may be observed, but patients often state that they feel dysphoric and restless and even experience fear of death. Patients' dysphoric feelings have led to refusal of surgery. Because droperidol is a dopamine antagonist, extrapyramidal signs may appear after its administration.[40] This has been reported to occur in about 1% of patients. The butyrophenones also cause mild α-blocking effects. Another butyrophenone, haloperidol, is a long-acting antipsychotic drug that has been used infrequently for preoperative medication.

Currently, droperidol is usually administered for its antiemetic effect rather than its sedative properties (see Antiemetics). Low clinical doses (up to 2.5 mg) of droperidol have been used before operation or just before emergence from anesthesia to prevent nausea and vomiting in the recovery room.

As a dopaminergic receptor blocker, droperidol counters the inhibitory effect of dopamine on the carotid body and the ventilatory response to hypoxia. Consequently, it preserves the carotid body response to hypoxia. For these reasons, it is said that droperidol may be a good premedication for patients who are dependent on the hypoxic ventilatory drive (Fig. 21-5).[41]

Other Sedative Drugs

Hydroxyzine. Hydroxyzine is a nonphenothiazine tranquilizer. It is often given for its proposed additive effects to opioids and does not cause an increase in side effects. Hydroxyzine has sedative action and anxiolytic properties. It has limited analgesic properties and does not produce amnesia. It is an antihistamine and an antiemetic.

Diphenhydramine. Diphenhydramine is a histamine receptor antagonist with sedative and anticholinergic activity. It is also an antiemetic. A dose of 50 mg will last $3-6$ hours in an adult. Diphenhydramine has been used recently in combination with cimetidine, steroids, and other drugs for prophylaxis in patients with chronic atopy and for prophylaxis before chemonucleolysis and dye studies.[42] Diphenhydramine blocks the histamine receptor to prevent effects of histamine peripherally.

Phenothiazines. Promethazine, promazine, and perphenazine are often used in combination with opioids. Phenothiazines have sedative, anticholinergic, and antiemetic properties. These effects, added to the analgesic effects of the opioids, have been used for preoperative medication.

Opioids

Morphine and meperidine were historically the most frequently used opioids for intramuscular preoperative medication. Recently, the use of intravenous fentanyl just before surgery has become popular. Opioids are used when analgesia is needed before operation. It has been stated in the strict sense that "unless there is pain, there is no need for narcotic in preanes-

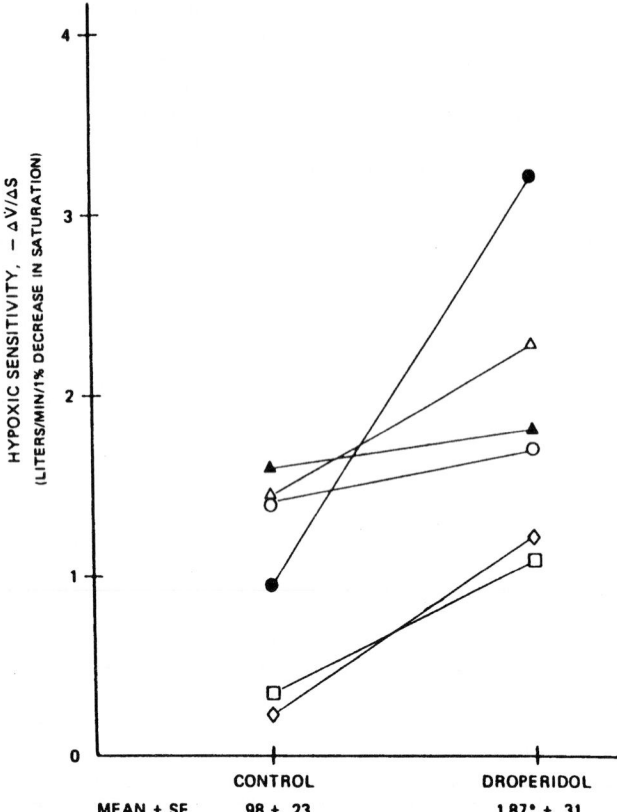

Figure 21-5. Hypoxic sensitivity (change in ventilation for each 1% decrease in oxygen saturation) is increased after intravenous administration of droperidol, 2.5 mg. Solid symbols represent repeated experiments on the same subjects as those represented by the open symbols. (Reprinted from Ward DS: Stimulation of hypoxic ventilatory drive by droperidol. Anesth Analg 63:106, 1984.)

thetic medication.''[43] For the patient experiencing pain before operation, the opioids can produce good analgesia and even euphoria. Opioids have been ordered for patients before operation to ameliorate the discomfort that may occur during regional anesthesia or the insertion of invasive monitoring catheters or large intravenous lines. The dose of opioid may need to be reduced in the debilitated or elderly patient. The elderly patient often exhibits a reduced sensitivity to pain. Furthermore, elderly patients can have an increased analgesic response to opioids. Opioids also have been used before operation in the opioid-dependent patient.

Preoperative administration of opioids in other settings has been controversial. They have been given before surgery prior to a nitrous oxide–opioid anesthetic. This is done in an attempt to have a basal state of anesthesia on board when the patient arrives in the operating room and to get a preview of the patient's response to opioids. Opioids have been given to patients before operation to provide analgesia on their awakening in the recovery room. The other approach is to titrate the opioid intravenously during emergence or on the patient's arrival in the recovery room. Preoperative administration of opioids can lower anesthetic requirements.[44] This may or may not be clinically significant for a specific patient receiving a particular anesthetic technique. Some anesthesiologists use opioids in combination with other drugs before operation to facilitate anesthetic induction by mask. This is popular especially in patients in whom an intravenous route for induction drugs cannot be used. It must be remembered that opioids decrease ventilation during spontaneous breathing and therefore decrease uptake of inhalation drugs. If necessary, the anesthesiologist may want to use

assisted or controlled ventilation of the lungs to overcome the respiratory depressant effects of the opioids. Finally, opioids are not the best drugs to relieve apprehension, produce sedation, or prevent recall.

Administration of opioids has the potential for causing several side effects. They usually exhibit no direct myocardial effects except in the case of very high doses of meperidine. However, opioids do interfere with the compensatory constriction of smooth muscles of the peripheral vasculature. This may lead to orthostatic hypotension. Histamine release after injection of morphine may compound these circulatory effects. As with most preoperative medications, it is probably safest to have the patient remain at bed rest after opioid premedication. The analgesic properties and respiratory depressant effects of opioids go hand in hand. The decrease in the carbon dioxide drive at the medullary respiratory center may be prolonged. Furthermore, there is a decrease in the responsiveness to hypoxia at the carotid body after injection of only low doses of opioids.[45] The anesthesiologist may wish to consider supplemental oxygen for the patient receiving opioid premedication. In general, the opioid agonist-antagonists produce less respiratory depression, but they also produce less analgesia. Rather than euphoria, the opioids may produce dysphoria. When this side effect does occur, it is most commonly seen in a patient who does not have pain before operation and has received the opioid premedication. Nausea and vomiting may result from opioid administration. The effect of opioids on the vestibular apparatus leading to motion sickness or stimulation of the medullary chemoreceptor trigger zone is a postulated reason for nausea and vomiting. Choledochoduodenal sphincter (sphincter of Oddi) spasm has occasionally been noted subsequent to injection of opioids. The opioid produces smooth muscle constriction, which leads to right upper quadrant pain.[46] Pain relief may be achieved with naloxone or possibly glucagon. Occasionally, the pain from biliary tract spasm is difficult to differentiate from the pain of angina pectoris. The administration of nitroglycerin should relieve angina pectoris and pain resulting from biliary tract spasm; an opioid antagonist should relieve only pain resulting from biliary tract spasm. Some question the use of opioid premedication in patients with biliary tract disease. All opioids have the potential to induce choledochoduodenal sphincter spasm. Meperidine is less likely than morphine to produce this side effect. Opioids may produce pruritus. Morphine, possibly through histamine release, often produces itching, especially around the nose. Opioids also may cause flushing, dizziness, and miosis.

Other drugs are often combined with opioids for their additive effects or to overcome the disadvantages of opioid side effects. The sedative-hypnotics and scopolamine are often used with opioids to produce sedation, anxiolysis, and amnesia in addition to analgesia. In selected patients, the combination of morphine and a benzodiazepine or scopolamine may be useful for pharmacologic preoperative preparation.

Morphine

Morphine is well absorbed after intramuscular injection. The onset of effect should occur within 15–30 minutes. The peak effect occurs in 45–90 minutes and lasts as long as 4 hours. After intravenous administration, the peak effect usually occurs within 20 minutes. Morphine is not reliably absorbed after oral administration. As with the other opioids, depression of ventilation and orthostatic hypotension may occur after injection of morphine. The effect of morphine on the chemoreceptive trigger zone may produce nausea and vomiting. Nausea and vomiting may also occur owing to a vestibular component. This has been postulated because the supine patient is less likely to complain of nausea and vomiting. After morphine administration, motility of the gastrointestinal tract is decreased. Also, gastrointestinal secretions may be increased. Inclusion of morphine in the preoperative medication reduces the likelihood that undesirable increases in heart rate will accompany surgical stimulation in the presence of volatile anesthetics.

Meperidine

Meperidine is about one tenth as potent as morphine. It may be given orally or parenterally. A single dose of meperidine usually lasts 2–4 hours. The onset after intramuscular injection is unpredictable, and a great deal of variability in time to peak effect exists. Meperidine is primarily metabolized in the liver. An increase in heart rate may be seen after meperidine administration, as may orthostatic hypotension.

Fentanyl

Fentanyl is a synthetic opioid agonist structurally similar to meperidine. It is 75–125 times more potent than morphine in its analgesic characteristics. The lipid solubility of fentanyl is greater than that of morphine, which contributes to its rapid onset of action. Peak plasma concentrations occur within 6–7 minutes following intravenous administration and its elimination half-time is 3–6 hours. The drug's short duration of action is attributed to redistribution to inactive tissues, such as the lungs, fat, and skeletal muscle. Metabolism occurs primarily by N-demethylation to norfentanyl, which is a less potent analgesic. A decreased clearance rate in the elderly may prolong elimination.

In doses of $1–2\ \mu g \cdot kg^{-1}$ intravenously, fentanyl may be used to provide preoperative analgesia. Oral transmucosal fentanyl preparations of fentanyl are available, delivering $5–20\ \mu g \cdot kg^{-1}$ of the drug. This form has been examined as a premedicant in both adults and children to relieve anxiety and pain. Due to a high incidence of preoperative nausea and vomiting, oral transmucosal fentanyl (in doses greater than $15\ \mu g \cdot kg^{-1}$) is not recommended in children younger than six years of age.[47] Fentanyl causes neither myocardial depression nor histamine release, but may be associated with ventilatory depression and profound bradycardia. Synergistic effects with benzodiazepines warrant close observation when this combination is given in the preoperative period.

Opioid Agonist-Antagonists

Opioid agonist-antagonists have been chosen for preoperative medication in an attempt to reduce the ventilatory side effects of pure opioid agonists. However, there is a ceiling on the analgesia that can be produced by agonist-antagonist drugs. They are similar to the pure opioids with regard to side effects. In addition, dysphoria may be even more likely to occur after their administration. Another issue to remember is that the agonist-antagonist drug can reduce the effectiveness of a pure opioid agonist needed to control postoperative pain. The most commonly used opioid agonist-antagonists are pentazocine, butorphanol, and nalbuphine.

Gastric Fluid pH and Volume

Many patients who come to the operating room are at risk for aspiration pneumonitis. The classic example is the patient with acute pain and a "full stomach" who must have emergency surgery. The pregnant patient, the obese patient, the diabetic, the patient with hiatus hernia or gastroesophageal reflux, all may be at risk for aspiration of gastric contents and subsequent chemical pneumonitis. Although it is not certain, it is believed that in adults aspiration of more than 25 ml of gastric fluid with a pH lower than 2.5 will cause pulmonary sequelae. This has not been, and probably never will be, proved in humans. However, using these guidelines, some have estimated that 40–80% of patients scheduled for elective surgery may be at risk.[48,49] However, clinically significant pulmonary aspiration of gastric contents is very rare in healthy patients having elective surgical procedures, and few anesthesiologists advocate routine prophylaxis.[50,51] An earlier suggestion that gastric fluid volume is greater

and pH lower in outpatients compared with inpatients has not been confirmed.[51,52]

The necessity of prolonged fasting (nothing by mouth after midnight) before induction of anesthesia for elective surgery has been challenged.[53] Some institutions allow ingestion of clear liquids until 3 or even 2 hours before surgery in selected patients. Indeed, gastric fluid volume immediately after induction of anesthesia is not increased by ingestion of 150 ml of water, coffee, or orange juice 2–3 hours earlier.[54] A similar study by Shevde and Trivedi described the administration of 240 ml of water, coffee, or pulp-free orange juice to healthy volunteers. All had gastric volumes of less than 25 ml with a slight decrease in pH within 2 hours of taking one of the three liquids.[55] There is concern about comfort, hypovolemia, and hypoglycemia in the pediatric age group perioperatively after prolonged fasting. An investigation by Splinter and associates concluded that drinking clear fluid up to 3 hours before scheduled surgery does not have a measurable effect on gastric volume and pH of healthy children aged 2–12 years.[56] Other studies in infants, children, and healthy adults scheduled for elective surgery have found similar results.[57] Therefore, fears that ingestion of oral fluid on the morning of surgery will invariably result in a predictable increase in gastric fluid volume are unfounded. It must be appreciated, however, that these data are from healthy patients not "at risk" for aspiration and apply only to ingestion of clear liquids. The American Society of Anesthesiologists has defined and summarized preoperative fasting practices through guidelines adapted in 1998 (see Table 21-5).[51]

Many different kinds of drugs have been used to alter gastric fluid volume and increase the pH of gastric fluid. Anticholinergics, H_2 receptor antagonists, antacids, and gastrokinetic agents have all been used to reduce the possibility of aspiration pneumonitis.

Anticholinergics

Neither atropine nor glycopyrrolate has been shown to be very effective in increasing gastric fluid pH or reducing gastric fluid volume. A study by Stoelting demonstrated that when given intramuscularly 1–1.5 hours before operation, neither atropine (0.4 mg) nor glycopyrrolate (0.2 mg) was successful in altering the gastric fluid pH or volume.[48] A similar study reported that glycopyrrolate ($4–5\ \mu g \cdot kg^{-1}$) given before operation did not reduce the percentage of patients at risk for aspiration pneumonitis.[49] That is, in a significant number of patients the gastric fluid pH remained below 2.5 and the gastric fluid volume was greater than $0.4\ ml \cdot kg^{-1}$. Giving higher doses of glycopyrrolate

---

Table 21-5. SUMMARY OF FASTING RECOMMENDATIONS TO REDUCE THE RISK OF PULMONARY ASPIRATION*

Ingested Material	Minimum Fasting Period (applied to all ages)
Clear liquids†	2 hours
Breast milk	4 hours
Infant formula	6 hours
Nonhuman milk	6 hours
Light meal (toast and clear liquids)	6 hours

* Applies only to healthy patients who are undergoing elective procedures and are not intended for women in labor. Following the guidelines does not guarantee complete gastric emptying.
† Examples of clear liquids include water, fruit juices without pulp, carbonated beverages, clear tea, and black coffee.
Adapted from Practice Guidelines for Preoperative Fasting and the Use of Pharmacologic Agents to Reduce the Risk of Pulmonary Aspiration: Application to Healthy Patients Undergoing Elective Procedures. A Report by the American Society of Anesthesiologists Task Force on Preoperative Fasting. Anesthesiology 90:896, 1999.

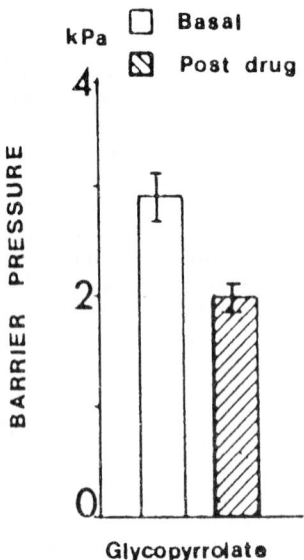

Figure 21-6. Barrier pressure (esophageal sphincter pressure minus gastric pressure) before and after intravenous administration of glycopyrrolate, 0.3 mg, to adult patients. Mean ± SE. (Reprinted with permission from Brock-Utne JG, Welman RS, Moshal MG *et al:* The effect of glycopyrrolate (Robinul) on the lower esophageal sphincter. Can Anaesth Soc J 25:144, 1978.)

(0.3 mg) is not more effective. Furthermore, intravenous doses of anticholinergics may cause relaxation of the gastroesophageal junction (Fig. 21-6). Theoretically, this may also occur after intramuscular doses. Therefore, the risk of aspiration pneumonitis may be increased, but this specific effect of intramuscular administration of anticholinergics for preoperative use has not been proved.

Histamine Receptor Antagonists

The H_2 receptor antagonists, cimetidine, ranitidine, famotidine, and nizatidine reduce gastric acid secretion. They block the ability of histamine to induce secretion of gastric fluid with a high hydrogen ion concentration. Therefore, the H_2 receptor antagonists increase gastric fluid pH. Their antagonism of the histamine receptor occurs in a selective and competitive manner. It is important to remember that these drugs cannot be expected reliably to affect gastric fluid volume or gastric-emptying time. Compared with other premedicants, they have relatively few side effects. Because there are few side effects and because many elective patients are at risk for aspiration pneumonitis, some anesthesiologists have advocated the preoperative use of H_2 receptor antagonists. Multiple-dose regimens may be more effective in increasing gastric pH than a single dose before operation on the day of surgery.[58] An H_2 antagonist also may be used for the allergic patient or in preparing a patient for exposure to a trigger of the allergic response, such as chymopapain or dye.

Cimetidine. Cimetidine usually is administered in 150–300 mg doses orally or parenterally. Administration of 300 mg of cimetidine orally 1–1.5 hours before surgery has been shown to increase the gastric fluid pH above 2.5 in 80% of patients.[59] There was no effect on gastric fluid volume. However, a study by Maliniak *et al* reported that cimetidine (300 mg) given intravenously 2 hours before operation increased gastric fluid pH and decreased gastric fluid volume.[60] Cimetidine can be given intravenously for those unable to take oral medications. It may be necessary to increase the dose for the very obese patient. Cimetidine can cross the placenta, but adverse fetal effects are unproved. In one multicenter investigation, 126 patients were studied who were to have elective cesarean section with general

anesthesia.[61] These patients received either 30 ml of an antacid 1–3 hours before operation or 300 mg of cimetidine orally at bedtime and again intramuscularly 1–3 hours before operation. There was an increase in gastric fluid pH and a reduction in gastric fluid volume in the cimetidine-treated group. Most important for this discussion, there were no differences in the neurobehavioral scores of the neonates between the two groups. The gastric effects of cimetidine last as long as 3 or 4 hours, and therefore this drug is suitable for operations of that duration.

Cimetidine has few side effects, but there are some of note. It inhibits the hepatic mixed-function oxidase enzyme system; therefore, it can prolong the half-life of many drugs, including diazepam, chlordiazepoxide, theophylline, propranolol, and lidocaine. The clinical significance of this after one or two preoperative doses of cimetidine is uncertain. There is also some question of hepatic blood flow reduction by cimetidine and a prolonged effect of the drug in patients with renal failure. Life-threatening cardiac dysrhythmias, hypotension, cardiac arrest, and central nervous system depression have been reported after cimetidine administration. These side effects may be especially likely to occur in critically ill patients after rapid intravenous administration. It has been postulated that airway resistance may increase in asthmatic patients because cimetidine could produce unopposed H_2 receptor–mediated bronchial constriction. As discussed previously, cimetidine does not affect gastric fluid already present.

Ranitidine. Ranitidine is more potent, specific, and longer acting than cimetidine. The usual oral dose is 50–200 mg. Ranitidine, 50–100 mg, given parenterally will decrease gastric fluid pH within 1 hour. It is as effective in reducing the number of patients at risk for gastric aspiration as cimetidine and produces fewer cardiovascular or central nervous system side effects. The effects of ranitidine last up to 9 hours. Thus, it may be superior to cimetidine at the conclusion of lengthy procedures in reducing the risk of aspiration pneumonitis during emergence from anesthesia and extubation of the trachea.

Other Histamine Receptor Antagonists. Famotidine is a third H_2 receptor blocker that has been given preoperatively to raise gastric fluid pH. Its pharmacokinetics are similar to those of cimetidine and ranitidine, with the exception of having a longer serum elimination half-life than the other two drugs.[62] Famotidine in a dose of 40 mg orally 1.5–3 hours preoperatively has been shown to be effective in increasing gastric pH.[63] Nizatidine 150–300 mg orally 2 hours before surgery will similarly decrease preoperative gastric acidity.[64]

Antacids

Antacids are used to neutralize the acid in gastric contents. A single dose of antacid given 15–30 minutes before induction of anesthesia is almost 100% effective in increasing gastric fluid pH above 2.5. The nonparticulate antacid, 0.3 *M* sodium citrate, is commonly given before operation when an increase in gastric fluid pH is desired. The nonparticulate antacids do not produce pulmonary damage themselves if aspiration of gastric fluid containing these antacids should occur. Colloid antacid suspension may be more effective than the nonparticulate antacids in increasing gastric fluid pH. However, aspiration of gastric fluid containing particulate antacids may cause significant and persistent pulmonary damage, despite the increase in gastric fluid pH.[65] The serious pulmonary sequelae have been manifested in the form of pulmonary edema and arterial hypoxemia.

Antacids work at the time given. There is no "lag time," as with the H_2 receptor blockers. Antacids are effective on the fluid already present in the stomach. This makes them especially attractive in emergency situations for those patients who are able to take medications orally.

However, antacids do increase gastric fluid volume, unlike H_2 receptor blockers.[59] The risk of aspiration depends on both the pH and the volume of gastric content. The increase in gastric fluid volume from antacid administration may become readily apparent after repeated doses, such as during labor, during which opioid administration may also contribute to delayed gastric emptying. Withholding antacids because of concern about increasing gastric volume is not warranted, considering animal evidence documenting increased mortality after aspiration of low volumes of acidic gastric fluid (0.3 ml · kg^{-1}, pH 1) compared with aspiration of large volumes of buffered gastric fluid (1–2 ml · kg^{-1}, pH 1.8).[66] Antacids may slow gastric emptying, and complete mixing with all gastric contents may be questionable in the immobile patient. The effect of antacids on food particles within the stomach is unknown.

Omeprazole

Omeprazole suppresses gastric acid secretion in a dose-dependent manner by binding to the proton pump of the parietal cell. For an adult patient intravenous doses of 40 mg 30 minutes before induction have been used. Oral doses of 40–80 mg must be given 2–4 hours before surgery to be effective. Effect on gastric pH may last as long as 24 hours. Much like the other H$_2$ receptor antagonists, investigators have found increases in gastric pH and inconsistent effects on gastric volume with administration of omeprazole.[67-69]

Gastrokinetic Agents

Gastrokinetic agents are useful because of their effectiveness in reducing gastric fluid volume. Metoclopramide is an example of a gastrokinetic agent that may be administered before operation.

Metoclopramide.   Metoclopramide is a dopamine antagonist that stimulates upper gastrointestinal motility, increases gastroesophageal sphincter tone, and relaxes the pylorus and duodenum. It also has antiemetic properties. Metoclopramide speeds gastric emptying but has no known effect on acid secretion and gastric fluid pH. It may be administered orally or parenterally. A parenteral dose of 5–20 mg is usually given 15–30 minutes before induction. When the drug is administered intravenously over 3–5 minutes, it usually prevents the abdominal cramping that can occur from more rapid administration. An oral dose of 10 mg achieves onset within 30–60 minutes. The elimination half-life of metoclopramide is approximately 2–4 hours.

The clinical usefulness of the gastrokinetic agents is found in those patients who are likely to have large gastric fluid volumes, such as parturients, patients scheduled for emergency surgery who have just eaten, obese patients, patients with trauma, outpatients, and those with gastroparesis secondary to diabetes mellitus.

However, the administration of metoclopramide does not guarantee gastric emptying. Significant gastric fluid volume may still be present despite its administration. The effect of metoclopramide on the upper gastrointestinal tract may be offset by concomitant atropine administration or prior injection of opioids. It will not further reduce gastric volume in patients undergoing elective surgery with already small gastric volumes. It may not be effective after administration of sodium citrate.[70-72] In contrast, metoclopramide may be especially effective in reducing the risk of aspiration pneumonitis when combined with an H$_2$ receptor antagonist (for example, ranitidine) before elective surgery.[73]

As mentioned previously, the drugs used to alter gastric fluid pH and volume are relatively free of side effects. The risk–benefit ratio for these drugs in reducing the risk of pulmonary sequelae from aspiration is often very favorable. Indeed, the drugs do decrease the number of patients at risk. However, none of the drugs or combinations of drugs is absolutely reliable in preventing the risk of aspiration pneumonitis in all patients all of the time. Therefore, their use does not eliminate the need for careful anesthetic techniques to protect the airway during induction, maintenance, and emergence from anesthesia.

Antiemetics

There are several groups of patients in whom the antiemetic effects of drugs may be helpful in reducing nausea and vomiting. These are patients scheduled for ophthalmologic surgery, patients with a prior history of nausea and vomiting or motion sickness, patients scheduled for laparoscopic surgery or gynecologic procedures, and patients who are obese. A risk score for predicting postoperative nausea and vomiting after inhalation anesthesia identified four risk factors: female gender, prior history of motion sickness or postoperative nausea, nonsmoking, and the use of postoperative opioids. The investigators suggested prophylactic antiemetic therapy when two or more of the risk factors were present when using volatile anesthetics.[74] Many anesthesiologists prefer not to administer antiemetics as part of a preoperative regimen, but believe that antiemetics should be administered intravenously just before they are needed at the conclusion of surgery.

Droperidol

Droperidol has been administered, usually intravenously, in low clinical doses to prevent postoperative nausea and vomiting. An investigation by Korttila *et al* showed that 1.25 mg of droperidol given intravenously 5 minutes before the conclusion of surgery reduced the incidence of nausea and vomiting after operation.[75] They found the antiemetic effect of droperidol to be better than that of either metoclopramide or domperidone. Another study by Santos and Datta demonstrated the effectiveness of droperidol as an antiemetic for patients having cesarean section with spinal anesthesia (Fig. 21-7).[76] However, low doses of droperidol may not always be effective in preventing nausea and vomiting. Higher doses at the end of surgery may lead to excessive sedation in the recovery room.

Metoclopramide

As mentioned in the section on gastrokinetic agents, metoclopramide does have antiemetic properties. The effect after preoperative administration is controversial and inconsistent, as demonstrated and discussed in the study by Cohen *et al.*[77] This may partially result from the brief duration of action of metoclopramide.

Ondansetron

Ondansetron is a serotonin subtype-3 receptor antagonist. Administered in doses of 4–8 mg intravenously to adults before induction, ondansetron has been shown to be highly effective in preventing postoperative nausea and vomiting.[78] Its use preoperatively is not warranted in most patient populations, but should be reserved for highly selective situations.

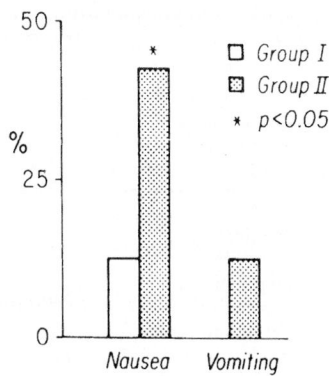

Figure 21-7. Incidence of nausea and vomiting after elective cesarean section after intravenous administration of droperidol, 2.5 mg (Group 1), or saline (Group 2). (Reprinted from Santos A, Datta S: Prophylactic use of droperidol for control of nausea and vomiting during spinal anesthesia for cesarean section. Anesth Analg 63:85, 1984.)

Table 21-6. COMPARISON OF SOME OF THE EFFECTS OF ANTICHOLINERGIC DRUGS

	Atropine	Glycopyrrolate	Scopolamine
Increased heart rate	+++	++	+
Antisialagogue	+	++	+++
Sedation	+	0	+++

0 = no effect; + = small effect; ++ = moderate effect; +++ = large effect.
Adapted from Stoelting RK: Pharmacology and Physiology in Anesthetic Practice. Philadelphia, JB Lippincott, 1991.

Other Antiemetics

Some of the phenothiazines, especially prochlorperazine, have antiemetic action. Hydroxyzine and diphenidol are two other drugs with antiemetic value. Although it has antiemetic properties, domperidone has not been proved effective in reducing postoperative nausea and vomiting.[75]

Anticholinergics

Previously, anticholinergic drugs were widely used when inhalation anesthetics produced copious respiratory tract secretions and intraoperative bradycardia was a frequent danger. The advent of newer inhalation agents has almost completely dispelled the routine use of anticholinergic drugs for preoperative medication. Their routine use has been questioned by several authors, who believe that the same care in selection of anticholinergics should be exhibited as in the choice of other drugs. Specific indications for an anticholinergic before surgery are (1) antisialagogue effect and (2) sedation and amnesia (Table 21-6). Uses that are less firmly established and not universally agreed on include the preoperative prescription of anticholinergics for their vagolytic action or in an attempt to decrease gastric acid secretion.

Antisialagogue Effect

Anticholinergics have been prescribed in a selective fashion when drying of the upper airway is desirable. For example, when endotracheal intubation is contemplated, an anesthesiologist may want to reduce secretions. In the study by Falick and Smiler, conditions were more often rated as satisfactory after endotracheal intubation when an anticholinergic drug had been administered.[29] The antisialagogue effect may be important for intraoral operations and instrumentations of the airway such as bronchoscopic examination. Administration of anticholinergics may be desirable before the use of topical anesthesia for the airway to prevent a dilutional effect of secretions and to allow contact of the local anesthetic with the mucosa.

Scopolamine is a more potent drying agent than atropine. It is less likely to increase heart rate and more likely to produce sedation and amnesia. Glycopyrrolate is a more potent and longer-acting antisialagogue than atropine, with less likelihood of increasing heart rate. Because glycopyrrolate is a quaternary amine, it does not easily cross the blood–brain barrier and does not produce sedation. Anticholinergics are not the only drugs that can dry secretions. As demonstrated by the study of Forrest et al, several other drugs and placebo (presumably a reflection of apprehension) can cause a patient to have a dry mouth before operation[80] (Table 21-7).

Sedation and Amnesia

When sedation and amnesia are desired before operation, scopolamine is frequently the anticholinergic chosen, especially in combination with morphine. Scopolamine and atropine both cross the blood–brain barrier. Scopolamine is a much more potent sedative and amnestic drug than atropine. In a study of patient acceptance of preoperative medication, the combination of morphine and scopolamine was superior to that of morphine and atropine.[81] Scopolamine does not produce amnesia in all patients. It may not be as effective as lorazepam or diazepam in preventing recall. Scopolamine has an additive amnestic effect when combined with benzodiazepines. The study by Frumin et al showed that the combination of diazepam and scopolamine produced amnesia more often than did diazepam alone.[14]

Vagolytic Action

Vagolytic action of the anticholinergic drugs is produced through the blockade of effects of acetylcholine on the sinoatrial node. Atropine given intravenously is more potent than glycopyrrolate and scopolamine in increasing heart rate. The vagolytic action of the anticholinergic drugs is useful in the prevention of reflex bradycardia during surgery. Bradycardia may result from traction on extraocular muscles or abdominal viscera, from carotid sinus stimulation, or after the administration of repeated doses of intravenous succinylcholine. The prevention of reflex bradycardia with intramuscular doses of the anticholinergics is unreliable, given the drug dosages and timing usually involved with preoperative medication administered on the unit. Many anesthesiologists prefer to give atropine or glycopyrrolate intravenously just before surgery and the anticipated bradycardic stimulus. Atropine and glycopyrrolate given intravenously immediately before surgery have been equally effective in preventing bradycardia resulting from repeated doses of succinylcholine.[82]

Elevation of Gastric Fluid pH Level

High doses of anticholinergics often are needed to alter gastric fluid pH. Even then, when given in the preoperative setting, anticholinergics cannot be relied on consistently to decrease gastric hydrogen ion secretion.[49,50] This function has largely

Table 21-7. INCIDENCE OF SIDE-EFFECTS 1 HOUR AFTER PREOPERATIVE MEDICATION (PERCENTAGE OF PATIENTS)

Medication	Dry Mouth	Slurred Speech	Dizzy	Nauseated	Relaxed
Pentobarbital (50–150 mg)	29	27	10	7	2
Secobarbital (50–150 mg)	41	32	8	9	4
Diazepam (5–15 mg)	35	20	10	3	12
Hydroxyzine (50–150 mg)	45	31	6	2	9
Morphine (5–10 mg)	80	33	15	7	20
Meperidine (50–100 mg)	85	45	20	12	25
Placebo	34	21	7	12	4

Modified from Forrest WH, Brown CR, Brown BW et al: Subjective responses to six common preoperative medications. Anesthesiology 47:241, 1977.

been replaced by the use of H_2 receptor antagonists (see Gastric Fluid pH and Volume).

Side Effects in Anticholinergic Drugs

Scopolamine and atropine may cause central nervous system toxicity, the so-called "central anticholinergic syndrome." This is most likely to occur after the administration of scopolamine, but can be seen after high doses of atropine. The symptoms of central nervous system toxicity resulting from anticholinergic drugs include delirium, restlessness, confusion, and obtundation. Elderly patients and patients with pain appear to be particularly susceptible. The central nervous system toxic effect of anticholinergics has been noted to be potentiated by inhalation anesthetics. Some clinicians have successfully treated the syndrome after it occurred with 1–2 mg of physostigmine intravenously.

The anticholinergics relax the lower esophageal sphincter. In theory, after parenteral administration of an anticholinergic drug, the risk of pulmonary aspiration of gastric contents is increased. This has yet to be proved as an important clinical issue.

Mydriasis and cycloplegia from anticholinergic drugs could be unwanted in patients with glaucoma because of resulting increased intraocular pressure. This seems unlikely with the doses used for preoperative medication. Atropine and glycopyrrolate may be less likely to increase intraocular pressure than scopolamine. In patients with glaucoma, most anesthesiologists feel safe in continuing medications for glaucoma up until the time of surgery and using atropine or glycopyrrolate when necessary (see Chapter 34).

Because anticholinergic drugs block vagal activity, relaxation of bronchial smooth muscle occurs and respiratory dead space increases. The magnitude of the increase in dead space depends on prior bronchomotor tone, but increases as large as 25–33% have been reported. Anticholinergic drugs cause secretions to dry and thicken. In theory, a dose of anticholinergic drug given before operation could lead to inspissation of secretions and an increase in airway resistance. This may develop into more than a theoretical issue when patients with diseases such as cystic fibrosis are being considered.

Sweat glands of the body are innervated by the sympathetic nervous system and use cholinergic transmission. Therefore, administration of anticholinergic agents interferes with the sweating mechanism, which may cause body temperature to increase. This side effect of anticholinergic medication must be considered carefully in a child with a fever.

Atropine is more likely than glycopyrrolate or scopolamine to cause an increase in heart rate. Unwanted increases in heart rate are much more likely after intravenous administration than after intramuscular administration. In fact, heart rate may transiently decrease after intramuscular administration as a result of a peripheral agonist effect of the anticholinergic agent.

α_2-Adrenergic Agonists

α_2-Adrenergic agonists have been used as premedicants.[83,84] Clonidine in doses of 2.5–5 $\mu g \cdot kg^{-1}$ has been administered preoperatively to produce sedation, reduce maximum allowable concentration, and prevent hypertension and tachycardia from endotracheal intubation and surgical stimulation. It has even been used as part of anesthetic technique to produce induced hypotension.[85] Dexmedetomidine is another α_2-adrenergic agonist studied for preoperative use to attenuate intraoperative sympathoadrenal responses.[86] After the administration of clonidine preoperatively, one is more likely to see episodes of hypotension and bradycardia during anesthesia when there are periods of little surgical stimulation. Furthermore, some anesthesiologists ask if preoperative α_2-adrenergic agonists are a substitute for a properly conducted anesthetic if appropriate attention is given to depth of anesthesia.

Other Drugs Given with Preoperative Medications

Although they are not preoperative medications in the strict sense, other drugs are often given at the time of preoperative medication. Examples of such drugs are insulin, steroids, antibiotics, and methadone for patients who are addicted to opioids. They may be prescribed by either the anesthesiologist or the surgeon to be given on the ward or in the operating room immediately prior to surgery. Regardless of these factors, their actions may affect the anesthetic, and the anesthesiologist must be knowledgeable about their administration and actions.

Antibiotics

Antibiotics are often administered immediately before operation for contaminated, potentially contaminated, or dirty surgical wounds. Prophylactic antibiotics may be warranted for "clean" surgical procedures when infection would be catastrophic. Other instances for the use of prophylactic antibiotics include in the immunosuppressed patient, in the aged, or in patients taking steroids. Antibiotics given immediately before surgery are also used for the prevention of endocarditis. Patients with valvular heart disease, prosthetic valves, mitral valve prolapse, or other cardiac abnormalities may be endangered by bacteremia produced during surgery.[87] Antibiotic administration comes under the anesthesiologist's purview because of the desire to have such agents given immediately before exposure to pathogens, which is just before the beginning of surgery.

It has been estimated that 60–70% of surgical patients receive antibiotics just before surgery or intraoperatively. Cephalosporins are the most popular. However, no drug or combination of drugs may be relied on to protect against all potential pathogens in all patients for all types of surgery. As with any other medication, the anesthesiologist must know the side effects and complications of the antibiotics to be administered. Some are associated with allergic reactions, hypotension, and bronchospasm (*e.g.,* penicillin and vancomycin). Allergic reactions from cephalosporin administration have been estimated to occur in about 5% of patients. Cross-reactivity of the cephalosporins in patients with a known penicillin allergy has been estimated at anywhere from 5 to 20%. The aminoglycosides, vancomycin, and the polymyxins have been implicated in nephrotoxicity. In addition, ototoxicity has resulted from aminoglycoside and vancomycin administration. Pseudomembranous colitis is a known complication of clindamycin administration. Finally, the aminoglycosides are known to extend the neuromuscular blocking effects of muscle relaxants.

Steroids

Steroid administration may be necessary immediately before surgery in the patient treated for hypoadrenocorticism or in the patient with suppression of the pituitary-adrenal axis owing to present or previous administration of corticosteroids. It is impossible to identify the specific duration of therapy or dose of steroids that produces pituitary and adrenal suppression. Marked variability among patients exists. Certainly, more suppression may be expected the higher the dose and the longer the duration of therapy. A conservative estimate is to consider treatment in any patient who has received corticosteroid therapy for at least 1 month in the past 6–12 months.

Because of disease states of the pituitary-adrenal axis or its suppression from steroid therapy, patients may not be able to respond to the stress of surgery. The dose and duration of supplemental steroid administration depend on an estimate of the stress of the surgical procedure in the perioperative period. One regimen is to administer 25 mg of cortisol preoperatively and then give an intravenous infusion of 100 mg of cortisol over the next 12–24 hours for adult patients.[88] Another method is to administer 100 mg of hydrocortisone intravenously before, during, and after surgery. This dose is meant to equal the estimated maximum amount of steroid that stress could produce in patients perioperatively. When considering whether to administer steroids or a higher dose of steroids, the anesthesiologist should keep in mind that the risk–benefit ratio is usually very small.

Insulin

Anesthesia and surgery may interrupt the regular meal schedule and insulin administration of diabetics (see Chapters 18 and 41). Perioperative stress may increase serum glucose concentrations. A plan for perioperative insulin and glucose management must be agreed on among the anesthesiologist, the surgeon, and the endocrinologist involved in the diabetic patient's care. There are several methods of doing this, none of which has proved superior to the others. One method is to administer one fourth to one half of the usual daily dose of intermediate-acting insulin preoperatively in the morning of surgery and begin an infusion of glucose-containing fluid. A second way is to administer no insulin or no glucose preoperatively and to measure serum glucose levels frequently during anesthesia. Regular insulin or glucose is then administered intraoperatively and postoperatively as needed. A third method is to begin an infusion of insulin and glucose immediately preoperatively and to check serum glucose levels frequently.

Opioid Dependency

Withdrawal produced by drug cessation is a preoperative issue in the patient who is taking methadone or is dependent on other opioids. There should be an attempt to maintain opioid use at the usual level by continuing methadone or substituting other appropriate agents for methodone. The anesthesiologist should be cautioned about using agonist-antagonist drugs in these patients in the preoperative period for fear of producing withdrawal.

DIFFERENCES IN PREOPERATIVE MEDICATION BETWEEN PEDIATRIC AND ADULT PATIENTS

Differences between children and adults with regard to preoperative medication include aspects of psychological preparation, the emphasis on oral medications when pharmacologic preparation is desired, and more frequent use of anticholinergics for their vagolytic activity. What remains the same is the need to assess the needs of each child individually and to tailor the psychological preparation and preoperative medication accordingly (see Chapter 44).

Psychological Factors in Pediatric Patients

Hospital admission and major surgery can produce long-lasting psychological effects in some children. The hospital stay is stressful and full of apprehension over the short term for almost all children. Psychological stress and anxiety are less likely to occur with minor procedures and brief hospitalizations. Repeated hospitalizations have not necessarily been shown to increase the number of pediatric patients manifesting long-lasting psychological trauma.[89,90] The demeanor and communicative efforts of the anesthesiologist can make a difference to the child who is getting ready for a trip to the operating room, anesthesia, and surgery.

Age is probably the most important aspect when psychological preparation of the pediatric patient is considered.[91] A baby younger than 6 months of age is not emotionally upset when separated from his or her mother. Others in the health care team can substitute very easily. Preoperative preparation in this age group is often directed toward other goals, for example, obtundation of vagal reflex responses. However, preschool children are upset when separated from their mothers and fear

the operating room. This is an age when hospitalization may be the most upsetting.[89–93] It is difficult to explain the forthcoming events to children in this age group. It is easier to communicate with patients from age 5 years to adolescence. The anesthesiologist can explain and offer reassurance about such issues as separation from parents and the home, operating room events, and any of the patient's perceived fears of surgery and anesthesia. Adolescent patients may already be anxious and apprehensive. They may also be worried about loss of consciousness, have a fear of death, or be apprehensive about what they will do or say after preoperative sedation or during anesthesia. The more fearful child may be difficult to identify. This is usually the child who is quiet during the preoperative interview and appears nonchalant or even detached. If these patients can be identified before operation, they are often candidates for heavy pharmacologic preparation.

Other important psychological aspects in preoperative preparation include the anxiety level, attitude, and behavior of the parents, the socioeconomic status of the family, the magnitude of the planned surgery, and the hospital environment.

Psychological Preparation

For the above reasons, a good preoperative visit and proper psychological preparation may be even more important in children than adults.[94–96] This is an art that is acquired by the anesthesiologist. The preoperative visit is a time of reassurance and explanation. It is an opportunity to gain the child's trust. Most anesthesiologists will want to involve the parents when possible. The child can then see the parents' acceptance of the anesthesiologist. Some hospitals have found brochures, motion pictures, and slide shows to be helpful in preparing pediatric patients for the operating room.[97] The child may want to bring a personal belonging, such as a stuffed animal or blanket, to the operating room for security. Some children wish to take an active role by doing such things as holding the face mask during inhalation induction of anesthesia. It may be helpful in a case with supportive parents to have them accompany the child to the operating room suite after an examination of events that may occur during induction. It is common in many hospitals for a parent to go into the operating room and stay until induction is complete.

Differences in Pharmacologic Preparation

The discussion of pharmacologic preparation for the pediatric patient presumes proper psychological preparation, a satisfactory operating room environment, and preparation for an efficient and timely induction of anesthesia (see Chapter 44).

Sedative-Hypnotics

As in adults, the sedative-hypnotic medications are used to reduce apprehension and produce sedation and amnesia. They are also used to facilitate smooth induction of anesthesia when an inhalation method is to be used. The use of preoperative medication is controversial in pediatric patients and may not be completely successful in 20% of instances. It has not been proved to reduce unwanted psychological outcome after surgery in anesthesia. It has been shown that the uneventful induction of anesthesia is less likely to produce long-lasting psychological problems in children.[89,92] After 6 months to 1 year of age, the child scheduled for a surgical procedure may benefit from a sedative hypnotic drug before surgery. There is some emphasis on avoiding intramuscular injections in children. The oral route is often used for preoperative medication in the older child, whereas in preschool children drugs may also be given rectally. Many different sedative-hypnotic drugs via different routes (oral, intranasal, and rectal) have been prescribed for children before operation. Midazolam can be given intramuscularly (0.2 mg · kg^{-1}). However, the most effective and acceptable route for midazolam is the oral route, achieved by mixing 0.5–0.75 mg · kg^{-1} with flavored syrup, apple juice, or cola because of its bitter taste.[98] It is effective in producing sedation and compliance, but not usually sleep, in about 15 minutes and lasts for 30–60 minutes. Oral ketamine 5–10 mg has been prescribed 20–30 minutes before induction. Although often allowing smooth separation from parents, oral secretions and preoperative or postoperative delirium can be problems. Both ketamine (3–8 mg · kg^{-1}) and midazolam (0.2 mg · kg^{-1}) can be given using a nasal atomizer, with the caveat that nasal drug administration and bitter aftertaste are disadvantageous. Ketamine (5 mg · kg^{-1}) and midazolam (0.3–1.0 mg · kg^{-1}) have also been given rectally before induction of anesthesia. A further option in the pharmacologic preparation of children is the rectal administration of methohexital (Fig. 21-8). Methohexital (20–30 mg · kg^{-1}) may be given immediately before operation, while the child is still in the parent's arms. The intramuscular route is also possible.

Opioids

There is the occasional need for opioid premedication in children. Methadone has the advantage of oral administration, usually prescribed in the 0.1–0.2 mg · kg^{-1} dose range. Intramuscular morphine and meperidine are used, often in combination with other premedications. Intramuscular morphine is often seen as part of the pharmacologic preparation for the child with congenital heart disease. In many hospitals, opioids have been combined with sedative-hypnotic and anticholinergic drugs to make a "cocktail" that may be given orally for preoperative medication. Transmucosal administration of fentanyl (5–20 μg · kg^{-1}) appears to be effective in producing sedation preoperatively. However, transmucosal fentanyl may increase gastric fluid volume and also increase the incidence of rigidity, respiratory depression, pruritus, nausea, and vomiting.[47,99–101] Fentanyl (2 μg · kg^{-1}) and sufentanil (3.0 μg · kg^{-1}) given by the intranasal route have been shown to calm pediatric patients

preoperatively. Again, postoperative nausea and vomiting, in addition to respiratory complications, have resulted in lack of enthusiasm for this technique.

Anticholinergics

Easily induced vagal reflexes make anticholinergics especially important in children. Bradycardia may result from airway manipulation, surgical manipulation, or anesthetic drugs such as halothane or succinylcholine. Also, the child's cardiac output is more dependent on heart rate than is the adult's. If no contraindication exists, most pediatric patients receive atropine intravenously immediately after induction of anesthesia and placement of an intravenous catheter. If the intramuscular route has been used for atropine, it will often be administered immediately after the patient becomes unconscious during induction of anesthesia. Glycopyrrolate also has been used in children in this setting. Scopolamine has a place in premedication of the pediatric patient to produce sedation, amnesia, and drying of the airways. One must be aware of the hazards of administering an anticholinergic to a child with a fever or when inspissation of secretions is not wanted. Finally, it has been noted that patients with Down syndrome appear to be sensitive to atropine. This is especially evident with the effect on heart rate and mydriasis.

PREOPERATIVE MEDICATION FOR OUTPATIENTS

See Chapter 46.

REFERENCES

1. Beecher HK: Preanesthetic medication. JAMA 157:242, 1955
2. Lyons SM, Clarke RSJ, Vulgaraki K: The premedication of cardiac surgical patients. Anaesthesia 30:459, 1975
3. Norris W, Baird WLM: Pre-operative anxiety: A study of the incidence and aetiology. Br J Anaesth 39:503, 1967
4. Egbert LD, Battit GE, Turndorf H et al: The value of the preoperative visit by the anesthetist. JAMA 185:553, 1963
5. Korttila K, Aromaa U, Tammisto T: Patient's expectations and acceptance of the effects of the drugs given before anaesthesia: Comparison of light and amnesic premedication. Acta Anaesthesiol Scand 25:381, 1981
6. Leigh JM, Walker J, Janaganathan P: Effect of preoperative anesthetic visit on anxiety. Br Med J 2:987, 1977
7. Done ML, Lee A: The use of a video to convey preanesthetic information to patients undergoing ambulatory surgery. Anesth Analg 87:531, 1998
8. Walsh J, Puig MM, Lovitz MA et al: Premedication abolishes the increase in plasma β-endorphin observed in the immediate preoperative period. Anesthesiology 66:402, 1987
9. Pippingskold A, Lehtinen AM, Laatikainen T et al: The effect of orally administered diazepam and midazolam on plasma β-endorphin, ACTH and preoperative anxiety. Acta Anaesthesiol Scand 35:175, 1991
10. Soreide E, Holst-Larsen K, Reite K et al: Effects of giving water 20–450 ml with oral diazepam premedication 1–2 h before operation. Br J Anaesth 71:503, 1993
11. Mohler H, Richards JG: The benzodiazepine receptor: A pharmacologic element of brain function. Eur J Anaesthesiol 2:15, 1988
12. Divoll M, Greenblatt DJ, Ochs HR et al: Absolute bioavailability of oral and intramuscular diazepam: Effect of age and sex. Anesth Analg 62:1, 1983
13. Dawes GS: The distribution and action of drugs on the fetus in utero. Br J Anaesth 45:766, 1973
14. Frumin MJ, Herekar VR, Jarvik ME: Amnesic actions of diazepam and scopolamine in man. Anesthesiology 45:406, 1976
15. Soroker D, Barzilay E, Konichezky S et al: Respiratory function following premedication with droperidol or diazepam. Anesth Analg 57:695, 1978
16. Rao S, Sherbaniuk RW, Prasad K et al: Cardiopulmonary effects of diazepam. Clin Pharmacol 14:182, 1973
17. Gross JB, Smith L, Smith TC: Time course of ventilatory response

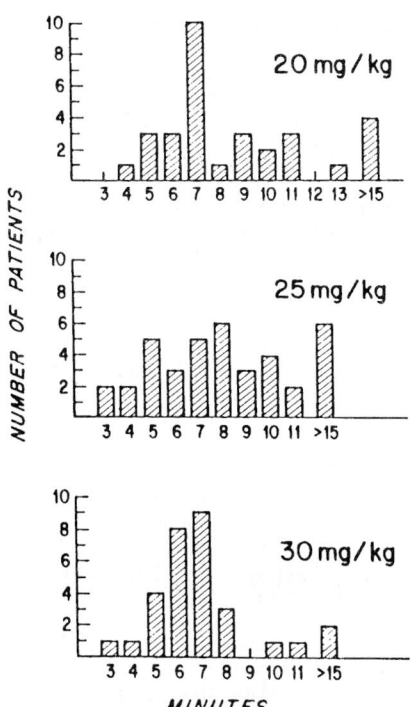

Figure 21-8. Frequency distribution of sleep induction times after rectal instillation of methohexital. Patients averaged 3.3 years in age and 15 kg in body weight. (Reprinted from Liu LMP, Goudsouzian NG, Liu PL: Rectal methohexital premedication in children, a dose-comparison study. Anesthesiology 53:343, 1980.)

to carbon dioxide after intravenous diazepam. Anesthesiology 57:18, 1982

18. Braunstein MC: Apnea with maintenance of consciousness following intravenous diazepam. Anesth Analg 58:52, 1979

19. Davies AO: Oral diazepam premedication reduces the incidence of postsuccinylcholine muscle pains. Can Anaesth Soc J 30:603, 1983

20. Fjeldborg P, Hecht PS, Busted N et al: The effect of diazepam pretreatment on the succinylcholine-induced rise in intraocular pressure. Acta Anaesthesiol Scand 29:415, 1985

21. Moore DC, Balfour RI, Fitzgibbons D: Convulsive arterial plasma levels of bupivacaine and the response to diazepam therapy. Anesthesiology 50:454, 1979

22. Greenblatt DJ, Abernathy DR, Morse DS et al: Clinical importance of the interaction of diazepam and cimetidine. N Engl J Med 310:1639, 1984

23. Perisho JA, Buechel DR, Miller RD: The effect of diazepam (Valium) in minimum alveolar anesthetic requirement (MAC) in man. Can Anaesth Soc J 18:563, 1971

24. Fragen RJ, Caldwell N: Lorazepam premedication: Lack of recall and relief of anxiety. Anesth Analg 55:792, 1976

25. White PF: Pharmacologic and clinical aspects of preoperative medication. Anesth Analg 65:963, 1986

26. Dundee JW, Lilburn JR, Nair SG et al: Studies of drugs given before anaesthesia: XXVI. Lorazepam. Br J Anaesth 49:1047, 1977

27. Bradshaw EG, Ali AA, Mulley BA et al: Plasma concentrations and clinical effects of lorazepam after oral administration. Br J Anaesth 53:517, 1981

28. Blitt CD, Petty WC, Wright WA et al: Clinical evaluation of injectable lorazepam as a premedicant: The effect on recall. Anesth Analg 55:522, 1976

29. Gale GD, Galloon S, Porter WR: Sublingual lorazepam: A better premedication? Br J Anaesth 55:761, 1983

30. Heisterkamp DV, Cohen PT: The effect of intravenous premedication with lorazepam (Ativan), pentobarbital and diazepam on recall. Br J Anaesth 47:79, 1975

31. Kraus JW, Desmond PV, Marshall JP et al: Effects of aging and liver disease on disposition of lorazepam. Clin Pharmacol Ther 24:44, 1978

32. Denaut M, Yernault JC, DeCoster A: Double blind comparison of the respiratory effects of parenteral lorazepam and diazepam in patients with chronic obstructive lung disease. Curr Med Res Opin 2:611, 1975

33. Reves JG, Fragen RJ, Vinick HR et al: Midazolam: Pharmacology and uses. Anesthesiology 62:310, 1985

34. Greenblatt DJ, Locniskar A, Scavone JM et al: Absence of interaction of cimetidine and ranitidine with intravenous and oral midazolam. Anesth Analg 65:176, 1986

35. Greenblatt DJ, Abernathy DR, Locniskar A et al: Effect of age, gender and obesity on midazolam kinetics. Anesthesiology 61:27, 1984

36. Dundee JW, Wilson DB: Amnesic action of midazolam. Anaesthesia 35:459, 1980

37. Pinnock CA, Fell D, Hunt PCW et al: A comparison of triazolam and diazepam as premedication for minor gynaecologic surgery. Anaesthesia 40:324, 1985

38. Franssen C, Hans P, Brichant JF et al: Comparison between alprazolam and hydroxyzine for oral premedication. Can J Anaesth 40:13, 1993

39. Koch-Weser J, Greenblatt DJ: The archaic barbiturate hypnotics. N Engl J Med 291:790, 1974

40. Patton CM: Rapid induction of acute dyskinesis by droperidol. Anesthesiology 43:126, 1975

41. Ward DS: Stimulation of the hypoxic ventilatory drive by droperidol. Anesth Analg 63:106, 1984

42. Beaven MA: Anaphylactoid reactions to anesthetic drugs. Anesthesiology 55:3, 1981

43. Cohen EN, Beecher HK: Narcotics in preanesthetic medication: A controlled study. JAMA 147:1664, 1951

44. Tsunoda Y, Hattori Y, Takatsuko E et al: Effects of hydroxyzine, diazepam and pentazocine on halothane minimum alveolar anesthetic concentration. Anesth Analg 52:390, 1973

45. Weil JV, McCullough RE, Kline JS: Diminished ventilatory response to hypoxia and hypercapnia after morphine in man. N Engl J Med 292:1103, 1975

46. Radnay PA, Brochman E, Mankikar D et al: The effect of equianalgesic doses of fentanyl, morphine, meperidine, and pentazocine on common bile duct pressure. Anesthetist 29:26, 1980

47. Epstein RH, Mendel HG, Witkowski TA et al: The safety and efficacy of oral transmucosal fentanyl citrate for preoperative sedation in young children. Anesth Analg 83:1220, 1996

48. Stoelting RK: Responses to atropine, glycopyrrolate and Riopan on gastric fluid pH and volume in adult patients. Anesthesiology 48:367, 1978

49. Manchikanti L, Roush JR: The effect of preanesthetic glycopyrrolate and cimetidine in gastric fluid pH and volume in outpatients. Anesth Analg 63:40, 1984

50. Warner MA, Warner ME, Weber JG: Clinical significance of pulmonary aspiration during the perioperative period. Anesthesiology 78:56, 1993

51. A Report by the American Society of Anesthesiologists Task Force on Preoperative Fasting: Practice guidelines for preoperative fasting and the use of pharmacologic agents to reduce the risk of pulmonary aspiration: Application to healthy patients undergoing elective procedures. Anesthesiology 90:896, 1999

52. Talke PO, Solanki DR: Dose response study of oral famotidine for reduction of gastric acidity and volume in outpatients and inpatients. Anesth Analg 77:1143, 1993

53. Kallar SK, Everett LL: Potential risks and preventive measures for pulmonary aspiration: New concepts in preoperative fasting guidelines. Anesth Analg 77:171, 1993

54. Hutchinson A, Maltby JR, Reid CRG: Gastric fluid volume and pH in elective inpatients: Part I. Coffee or orange juice versus overnight fast. Can J Anaesth 35:125, 1988

55. Shevde K, Trivedi N: Effects of clear liquids on gastric volume and pH in healthy volunteers. Anesth Analg 72:528, 1991

56. Splinter WM, Schaefer SE, Zunder IH: Clear fluids three hours before surgery do not affect the gastric fluid contents of children. Can J Anaesth 37:498, 1990

57. Litman RS, Wu CL, Quinlivan JK: Gastric volume and pH in infants fed clear liquids and breast milk prior to surgery. Anesth Analg 79:482, 1994

58. Maltby JR, Eliot RH, Warnell I et al: Gastric fluid volume and pH in elective surgical patients: Triple prophylaxis is not superior to ranitidine alone. Can J Anaesth 37:650, 1990

59. Stoelting RK: Gastric fluid pH in patients receiving cimetidine. Anesth Analg 57:675, 1978

60. Maliniak K, Vahil AH: Pre-anesthetic cimetidine and gastric pH. Anesth Analg 58:309, 1979

61. Hodgkinson R, Glassenberg R, Joyce TH et al: Comparison of cimetidine (Tagamet) with antacid for safety and effectiveness in reducing gastric acidity before elective cesarean section. Anesthesiology 59:86, 1983

62. Feldman M, Burton ME: Histamine-2 receptor antagonists. N Engl J Med 323:1672, 1990

63. Escolano F, Castaño J, Lopez R et al: Effects of omeprazole, ranitidine, famotidine and placebo on gastric secretion in patients undergoing elective surgery. Br J Anaesth 69:404, 1992

64. Mikawa K, Nishina K, Maekawa N et al: Gastric fluid volume and pH after nizatidine in adults undergoing elective surgery: Influence of timing and dose. Can J Anaesth 42:730, 1995

65. Bond VK, Stoelting RK, Gupta CD: Pulmonary aspiration syndrome after inhalation of gastric fluid containing antacids. Anesthesiology 51:452, 1979

66. James CF, Modell JH, Gibbs CP et al: Pulmonary aspiration: Effects of volume and pH in the rat. Anesth Analg 63:665, 1984

67. Rocke DA, Rout CC, Gouws E: Intravenous administration of the proton pump inhibitor omeprazole reduces the risk of acid aspiration at emergency cesarean section. Anesth Analg 78:1093, 1994

68. Haskins DA, Jahr JS, Texidor M et al: Single-dose oral omeprazole for reduction of gastric residual acidity in adults for outpatient surgery. Acta Anaesthesiol Scand 36:513, 1992

69. Atanassoff PG, Alon E, Pasch T: Effects of single-dose intravenous omeprazole and ranitidine on gastric pH during general anesthesia. Anesth Analg 75:95, 1992

70. Nimmo WS: Drugs, diseases and altered gastric emptying. Clin Pharmacokinet 1:189, 1976

71. Cohen SE, Jasson J, Talafre M-L et al: Does metoclopramide decrease the volume of gastric contents in patients undergoing cesarean section? Anesthesiology 61:604, 1984

72. Schmidt JF, Jorgensen BC: The effect of metoclopramide on gastric contents after preoperative ingestion of sodium citrate. Anesth Analg 63:841, 1984

73. O'Sullivan G, Sear JW, Bullingham RES et al: The effect of magne-

sium trisilicate, metoclopramide and ranitidine on gastric pH, volume and serum gastrin. Anaesthesia 40:246, 1985

74. Apfel CC, Läärä E, Koivuranta M *et al:* A simplified risk score for predicting postoperative nausea and vomiting. Anesthesiology 91:693, 1999

75. Korttila K, Kauste A, Auvinen J: Comparison of domperidone, droperidol and metoclopramide in the prevention and treatment of nausea and vomiting after balanced general anesthesia. Anesth Analg 58:396, 1979

76. Santos A, Datta S: Prophylactic use of droperidol for control of nausea and vomiting during spinal anesthesia for cesarean section. Anesth Analg 63:85, 1984

77. Cohen SE, Woods WA, Wyner J: Antiemetic efficacy of droperidol and metoclopramide. Anesthesiology 60:67, 1984

78. Khalil SN, Kataria B, Pearson K *et al:* Ondansetron prevents postoperative nausea and vomiting in women outpatients. Anesth Analg 79:845, 1994

79. Falick YS, Smiler BG: Is anticholinergic premedication necessary? Anesthesiology 43:472, 1975

80. Forrest WH, Brown CR, Brown BW: Subjective responses to six common preoperative medications. Anesthesiology 47:241, 1977

81. Conner JT, Bellville JW, Wender R *et al:* Morphine, scopolamine and atropine as intravenous surgical premedicants. Anesth Analg 56:606, 1977

82. Sorensen O, Eriksen S, Hommegaard P *et al:* Thiopental–nitrous oxide–halothane anesthesia and repeated succinylcholine: Comparison of preoperative glycopyrrolate and atropine administration. Anesth Analg 59:686, 1980

83. Abi-Jaoude F, Brusset A, Ceddaha A *et al:* Clonidine premedication for coronary artery bypass grafting under high-dose alfentanil anesthesia: Intraoperative and postoperative hemodynamic study. J Cardiothorac Vasc Anesth 7:35, 1993

84. Segal IS, Jarvis DA, Duncan SR *et al:* Clinical efficacy of oral-transdermal clonidine combinations during the perioperative period. Anesthesiology 74:220, 1991

85. Woodcock TE, Millar RK, Dixon F, Prys-Roberts C: Clonidine premedication for isoflurane induced hypotension. Br J Anaesth 60:388, 1988

86. Jaakola ML, Kanto J, Scheinin H *et al:* Intramuscular dexmedetomidine premedication: An alternative to midazolam–fentanyl combination in elective hysterectomy? Acta Anaesthesiol Scand 38:238, 1994

87. Dajani AS, Taubert KA, Wilson W *et al:* Prevention of bacterial endocarditis Recommendations by the American Heart Association. JAMA 277:1794, 1997

88. Symreng T, Karlberg BE, Kaogedal B *et al:* Physiological cortisol substitution on long-term steroid-treated patients undergoing major surgery. Br J Anaesth 53:949, 1981

89. Vernon DTA, Schulman JL, Foley JM: Changes in children's behavior after hospitalization. Am J Dis Child 111:581, 1966

90. Jessner L, Blom GE, Waldfogel S: Emotional implications of tonsillectomy and adenoidectomy on children. Psychoanal Study Child 7:126, 1952

91. Vetter TR: The epidemiology and selective identification of children at risk for preoperative anxiety reactions. Anesth Analg 77:96, 1993

92. Eckenhoff JE: Relationship of anesthesia to post-operative personality changes in children. Am J Dis Child 86:587, 1953

93. Beeby DG, Hughes JOM: Behaviour of unsedated children in the anaesthetic room. Br J Anaesth 52:279, 1980

94. Booker PD, Chapman DH: Premedication in children undergoing day-care surgery. Br J Anaesth 51:1083, 1979

95. Jackson K: Psychological preparation as a method of reducing the emotional trauma of anesthesia in children. Anesthesiology 12:293, 1981

96. Visintainer MA, Wolfer JA: Psychological preparation for pediatric patients: The effect on children's and parents' stress responses and adjustment. Pediatrics 56:187, 1975

97. Karl HW, Pauze KJ, Heyneman N *et al:* Pre-anesthetic preparation of pediatric outpatients: The role of a videotape for parents. J Clin Anesth 2:172, 1990

98. Weldon BC, Watcha MF, White PF: Oral midazolam in children: Effect of time and adjunctive therapy. Anesth Analg 75:51, 1992

99. Feld LH, Champeau MW, van Steennis CA *et al:* Preanesthetic medication in children: A comparison of oral transmucosal fentanyl citrate versus placebo. Anesthesiology 71:374, 1989

100. Nicolson SC, Betts EK, Jobes DR *et al:* Comparison of oral and intramuscular preanesthetic medication for pediatric inpatient surgery. Anesthesiology 71:8, 1989

101. Goldstein-Dressner MC, Davis PJ, Kretchman E *et al:* Double-blind comparison of oral transmucosal fentanyl citrate with oral meperidine, diazepam, and atropine as preanesthetic medication in children with congenital heart disease. Anesthesiology 74:28, 1991

Clinical Anesthesia (4/e), edited by
Paul G. Barash, Bruce F. Cullen, and
Robert K. Stoelting. Lippincott Williams &
Wilkins, Philadelphia, © 2001.

CHAPTER 22

DELIVERY SYSTEMS FOR INHALED ANESTHETICS

J. JEFFREY ANDREWS AND RUSSELL C. BROCKWELL

An anesthesia system consists of the various components that communicate with each other during the administration of inhalation anesthesia.[1] System components include the anesthesia machine, the vaporizers, the anesthetic circuit, the ventilator, and the scavenging system. A thorough understanding of these parts is essential to the safe practice of anesthesia. Malpractice claims associated with gas delivery equipment are infrequent but severe, and continued to occur throughout the 1990s.[2] This chapter discusses the normal operation, function, and integration of major system components. More importantly, it illustrates some problems and hazards associated with each and describes appropriate preoperative checks.

ANESTHESIA MACHINES

Anesthesia machines have evolved from simple, pneumatic devices to sophisticated, computer-based, fully integrated anesthesia systems (Figs. 22-1 and 22-2). A few years ago, a rudimentary background in pneumatics sufficed; but today, an understanding of pneumatics, electronics, and even computer science is useful. Even though it is more difficult for the anesthesiologist to achieve a thorough understanding of modern anesthesia machines, it is essential to the safe practice of anesthesia. The anesthesiologist must be aware of design differences between manufacturers so that appropriate preoperative checks can be performed.

Anesthesia Machine Standards

Anesthesia machine standards provide guidelines to manufacturers regarding minimum performance, design characteristics, and safety requirements for anesthesia machines. During the past two decades, the progression of anesthesia machine standards has been as follows:

  1979: American National Standards Institute (ANSI) Z79.8-1979[3]

  1988: American Society for Testing and Materials (ASTM) F1161-88[4]

  1994: ASTM 1161-94[5]

  1998: ASTM F1850-98a[6]

To comply with the new 1998 ASTM F1850-98a standard, newly manufactured workstations must have monitors that measure the following parameters: continuous breathing system pressure, exhaled tidal volume, ventilatory carbon dioxide concentration, anesthetic vapor concentration, inspired oxygen concentration, oxygen supply pressure, arterial hemoglobin oxygen saturation, arterial blood pressure, and continuous electrocardiogram. The anesthesia workstation must have a prioritized alarm system that groups the alarms into three categories: high, medium, and low priority. These monitors and alarms may be automatically enabled and made to function by turning on the anesthesia workstation, or the monitors and alarms can be manually enabled and made functional by following a pre-use checklist.[6]

Generic Anesthesia Machine

A diagram of a generic two-gas anesthesia machine is shown in Figure 22-3. Both oxygen and nitrous oxide have two supply sources—a *pipeline supply source* and a *cylinder supply source*. The pipeline supply source is the primary gas source for the anesthesia machine. The hospital piping system provides gases to the machine at approximately 50 pounds per square inch gauge (psig), which is the normal working pressure of most machines. The cylinder supply source serves as a backup if the pipeline fails. The oxygen cylinder source is regulated from 2200 to approximately 45 psig, and the nitrous oxide cylinder source is regulated from 745 to approximately 45 psig.[7-23]

A safety device traditionally referred to as the *fail-safe valve* is located downstream from the nitrous oxide supply source. It serves as an interface between the oxygen and nitrous oxide supply sources. This valve shuts off or proportionally decreases the supply of nitrous oxide (and other gases) if the oxygen supply pressure decreases. Contemporary machines have an alarm device to monitor the oxygen supply pressure. An alarm is actuated at a predetermined oxygen pressure, such as 30 psig.[7,8,18,23]

Most Ohmeda machines have a *second-stage oxygen regulator* located downstream from the oxygen supply source. It is adjusted to a precise pressure level, such as 14 psig.[8,11-17] This regulator supplies a constant pressure to the oxygen flow control valve regardless of fluctuating oxygen pipeline pressures. For example, the flow from the oxygen flow control valve will be constant if the oxygen supply pressure is greater than 14 psig.

The *flow control valves* are an important anatomic landmark because they divide the anesthesia machine into two parts. The *high-pressure circuit* is the part of the machine that is upstream from the flow control valves, and the *low-pressure circuit* is the part of the machine that is downstream from the flow control valves. The operator regulates flow entering the low-pressure circuit by adjusting the flow control valves. The oxygen and nitrous oxide flow control valves are linked mechanically or pneumatically by a *proportioning system* to help prevent delivery of a hypoxic mixture. The flow travels through a *common manifold* and may be directed to a *calibrated vaporizer*. Precise amounts of inhaled anesthetic can be added, depending on the vaporizer setting. The total fresh gas flow travels toward the *common gas outlet*.[7,8]

Many Ohmeda machines have a *machine outlet check valve* between the vaporizers and the common gas outlet.[8-15] Its purpose is to prevent backflow into the vaporizer, thereby minimizing the effects of downstream intermittent pressure fluctuations on inhaled anesthetic concentration (see Vaporizers: Intermittent Back Pressure). The presence or absence of a check valve profoundly influences which preoperative leak test is indicated (see Checking Anesthesia Machines). The *oxygen flush connection* joins the mixed-gas pipeline between the one-way check valve and the machine outlet. Thus, the oxygen flush, when activated, has a "straight shot" to the common gas outlet.[7,8]

Portions of this chapter have appeared with permission in Andrews JJ: Inhaled anesthetic delivery systems. In Miller RD (ed): Anesthesia, 5th ed, p 174. Philadelphia, Churchill Livingstone, 1999.

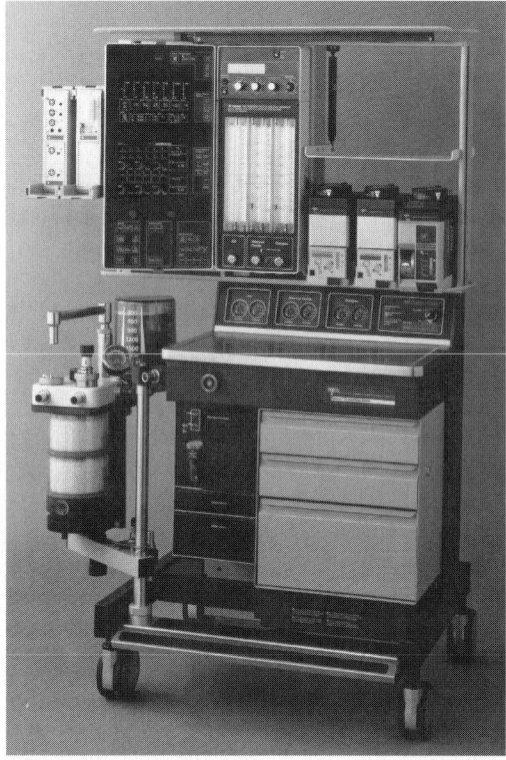

Figure 22-1. Ohmeda CD Anesthesia System. (Permission granted by Ohmeda, a division of BOC Health Care, Inc., Madison, Wisconsin.)

Pipeline Supply Source

The pipeline supply source is the primary gas source for the anesthesia machine. Most hospitals today have a central piping system to deliver medical gases such as oxygen, nitrous oxide,

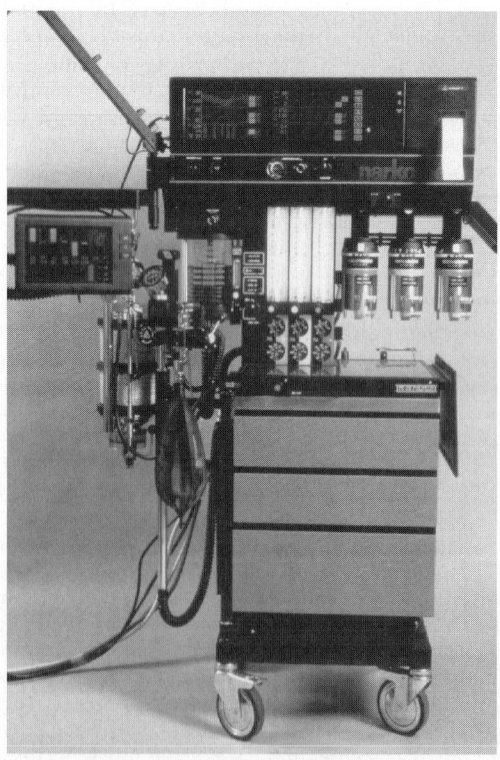

Figure 22-2. North American Dräger Narkomed 4 Anesthesia System. (Courtesy of North American Dräger, Telford, Pennsylvania.)

and air to the operating room. The central piping system must supply the anesthesia machine with the appropriate gas at the appropriate pressure for the machine to function properly. Unfortunately, this does not always occur.

In a survey of approximately 200 hospitals in 1976, 31% reported difficulties with pipeline systems.[24] The most common problem was inadequate oxygen pressure, followed by excessive pipeline pressures. The most devastating reported hazard, however, was accidental crossing of oxygen and nitrous oxide pipelines, which caused several deaths. This problem caused 23 deaths in a newly constructed wing of a general hospital in Sudbury, Ontario, during a 5-month period.[24,25]

The operator must take two actions if a pipeline crossover is suspected. First, the backup oxygen cylinder should be turned on. Then, the pipeline supply must be disconnected. This second step is mandatory because the machine will preferentially use the inappropriate 50-psig pipeline supply source instead of the lower pressure (45 psig) oxygen cylinder source.

Gas enters the anesthesia machine through the pipeline inlet connections (Fig. 22-3; see arrows). The pipeline inlet fittings are gas-specific Diameter Index Safety System (DISS) threaded body fittings. The DISS provides threaded noninterchangeable connections for medical gas lines, which minimizes the risk of misconnection. A check valve is located downstream from the inlet. It prevents reverse flow of gases from the machine to the pipeline or the atmosphere.[6]

Cylinder Supply Source

Anesthesia machines have reserve E cylinders if a pipeline supply source is not available or if the pipeline fails. Color-coded cylinders are attached to the anesthesia machine through the hanger yoke assembly. The hanger yoke assembly orients and supports the cylinder, provides a gas-tight seal, and ensures a unidirectional flow of gases into the machine.[7] Each hanger yoke is equipped with the Pin Index Safety System (PISS). The PISS is a safeguard introduced to eliminate cylinder interchanging and the possibility of accidentally placing the incorrect gas on a yoke designed to accommodate another gas. Two pins on the yoke are arranged so that they project into the cylinder valve. Each gas or combination of gases has a specific pin arrangement.[26]

Gas travels from the high-pressure cylinder source to the anesthesia machine when the cylinder is turned on (Fig. 22-3). A check valve is located downstream from each cylinder if a double-yoke assembly is used. The check valve has several functions. First, it minimizes gas transfer from a cylinder at high pressure to one with lower pressure. Second, it allows an empty cylinder to be exchanged for a full one while gas flow continues from the other cylinder into the machine with minimal loss of gas. Third, it minimizes leakage from an open cylinder to the atmosphere if one cylinder is absent.[7,8] A cylinder supply pressure gauge is located downstream from the check valves. The gauge will indicate the pressure in the cylinder having the higher pressure when two reserve cylinders of the same gas are opened at the same time.[20]

Each cylinder supply source has a pressure-reducing valve known as the cylinder pressure regulator. It reduces the high and variable storage pressure present in a cylinder to a lower, more constant pressure suitable for use in the anesthesia machine. The oxygen cylinder pressure regulator reduces the oxygen cylinder pressure from a high of 2200 psig to approximately 45 psig. The nitrous oxide cylinder pressure regulator receives pressure of up to 745 psig and reduces it to approximately 45 psig.[7,8]

The cylinders should be turned off except during the preoperative machine checking period or when a pipeline source is unavailable. If left on, the reserve cylinder supply can be silently depleted whenever the pressure inside the machine decreases to a value lower than the regulated cylinder pressure. Oxygen

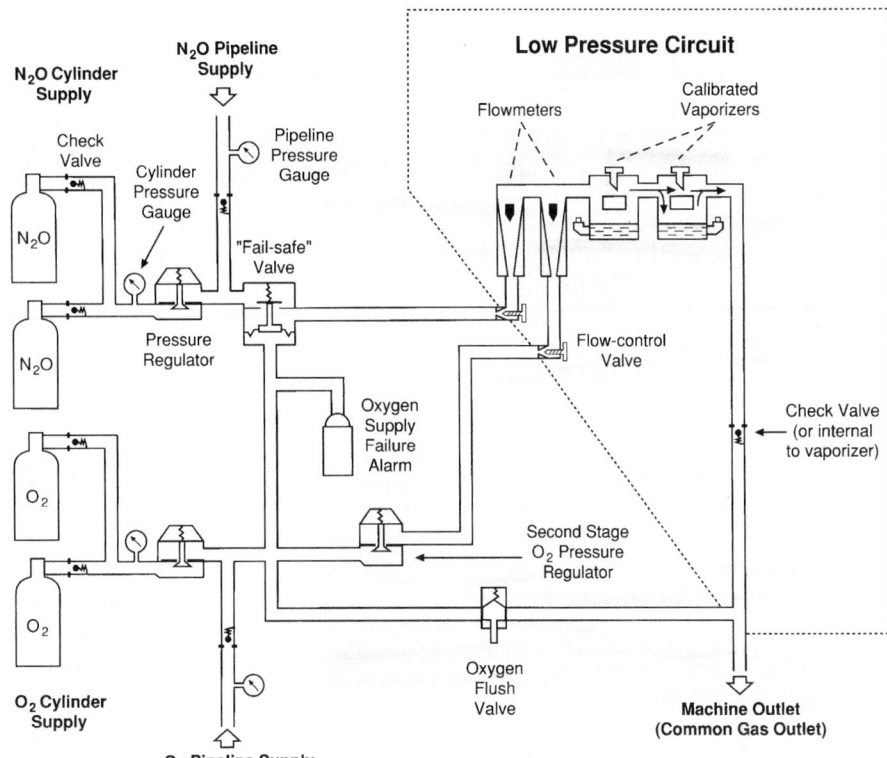

Figure 22-3. Diagram of a generic two-gas anesthesia machine. (Modified with permission from Check-Out, A Guide for Preoperative Inspection of an Anesthesia Machine. American Society of Anesthesiologists, Park Ridge, Illinois, 1987.)

pressure within the machine can decrease below 45 psig with oxygen flushing or with ventilator use, particularly at high peak flow rates. The pipeline supply pressures of all gases can be less than 45 psig if problems exist in the central piping system. If the cylinders are left on, they will eventually become depleted. Then, no reserve supply will be available if there is a pipeline failure.[8,27]

Oxygen Supply Pressure Failure Safety Devices

Oxygen and nitrous oxide supply sources existed as independent entities in older models of anesthesia machines, and they were not pneumatically or mechanically interfaced. Therefore, abrupt or insidious oxygen pressure failure had the potential to lead to the delivery of a hypoxic mixture. The 1998 ASTM F1850-98a standard states that, "The anesthesia gas supply device shall be designed so that whenever oxygen supply pressure is reduced to below the manufacturer specified minimum, the delivered oxygen concentration shall not decrease below 19% at the common gas outlet."[6] Contemporary anesthesia machines have a number of safety devices that act together in a cascade manner to minimize the risk of hypoxia as oxygen pressure decreases. Several of these devices are described below.

Pneumatic and Electronic Alarm Devices

Many older anesthesia machines have a pneumatic alarm device that sounds a warning when the oxygen supply pressure decreases to a predetermined threshold value, such as 30 psig. The 1998 ASTM F1850-98a standard mandates that a medium priority alarm shall be activated within 5 seconds when the oxygen pressure decreases below a manufacturer-specific pressure threshold.[6] Electronic alarm devices are now used to meet this guideline.

Fail-Safe Valves

A fail-safe valve is present in the gas line supplying each of the flowmeters except oxygen. Controlled by oxygen supply pressure, the valve shuts off or proportionally decreases the

supply pressure of all other gases (nitrous oxide, air, carbon dioxide, helium, nitrogen) as the oxygen supply pressure decreases. Unfortunately, the misnomer "fail-safe" has led to the misconception that the device prevents administration of a hypoxic mixture. This is not the case. Machines that are not equipped with a flow proportioning system (see Proportioning Systems) can deliver a hypoxic mixture under normal working conditions. The oxygen flow control valve can be closed intentionally or accidentally. Normal oxygen pressure will keep other gas lines open so that a hypoxic mixture can result.[7,8]

Ohmeda machines are equipped with a fail-safe valve known as the pressure-sensor shut off valve (Fig. 22-4). The valve is threshold in nature, and it is either open or closed. Oxygen supply pressure opens the valve, and the valve return spring closes the valve. Figure 22-4 shows a nitrous oxide pressure-sensor shutoff valve with a threshold pressure of 20 psig.[12,13,15-17] In Figure 22-4A, an oxygen supply pressure greater than 20 psig is exerted upon the mobile diaphragm. This pressure moves the piston and pin upward and the valve opens. Nitrous oxide

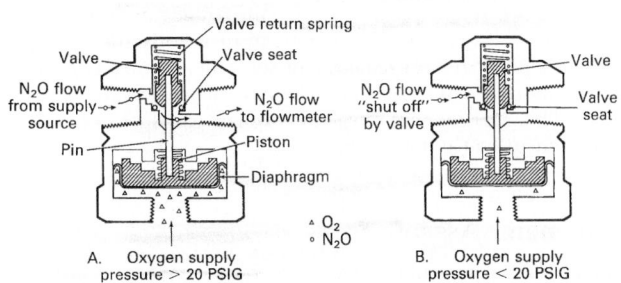

Figure 22-4. Pressure-sensor shutoff valve. The valve is open in *A* because the oxygen supply pressure is greater than the threshold value of 20 psig. The valve is closed in *B* because of inadequate oxygen pressure. (Redrawn with permission from Bowie E, Huffman LM: The Anesthesia Machine: Essentials for Understanding. Madison, WI, Ohmeda, a division of BOC Health Care Inc., 1985.)

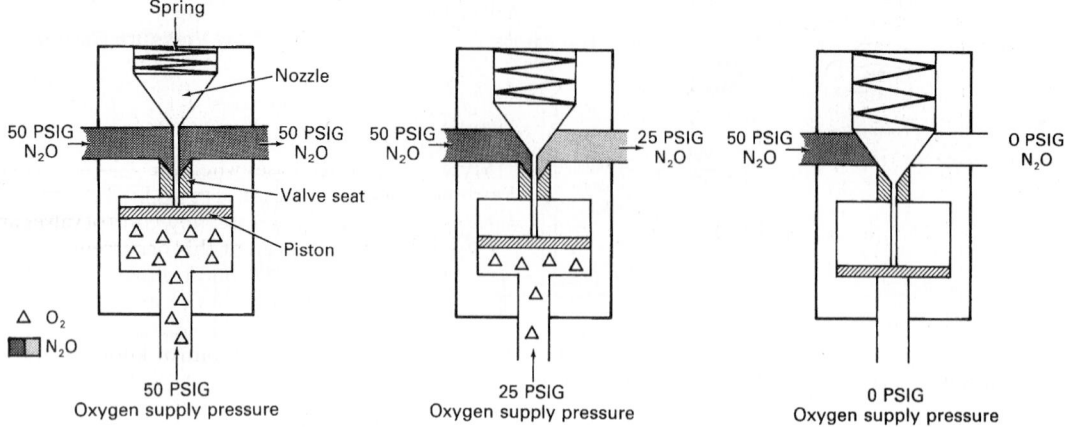

Figure 22-5. Oxygen Failure Protection Device (OFPD), which responds proportionally to changes in oxygen supply pressure. (Redrawn with permission from Narkomed 2A Anesthesia System. Technical Service Manual, 6th ed. Telford, PA, North American Dräger, June 1985.)

flows freely to the nitrous oxide flow control valve. In Figure 22-4B, the oxygen supply pressure is less than 20 psig, and the force of the valve return spring completely closes the valve.[8] Nitrous oxide flow stops at the closed fail-safe valve, and it does not advance to the nitrous oxide flow control valve.

North American Dräger uses a fail-safe valve known as the Oxygen Failure Protection Device (OFPD) that interfaces the oxygen pressure with that of other gases, such as nitrous oxide, air, carbon dioxide, helium, and nitrogen.[18-23] It differs from Ohmeda's oxygen pressure-sensor shutoff valve because the OFPD is based on a proportioning principle rather than a threshold principle. The pressure of all gases controlled by the OFPD will decrease proportionally with the oxygen pressure. The OFPD consists of a seat-nozzle assembly connected to a spring-loaded piston, as shown in Figure 22-5. The oxygen supply pressure in the left panel is 50 psig. This pressure pushes the piston upward, forcing the nozzle away from the valve seat. Nitrous oxide (or other gases) advances toward the flow control valve at 50 psig. The oxygen pressure in the right panel is 0 psig. The spring is expanded and forces the nozzle against the seat, preventing flow through the device. Finally, the center panel shows an intermediate oxygen pressure of 25 psig. The force of the spring partially closes the valve. The nitrous oxide pressure delivered to the flow control valve is 25 psig. There is a continuum of intermediate configurations between the extremes (0–50 psig) of oxygen supply pressure. These intermediate valve configurations are responsible for the proportional nature of the OFPD.[18]

Second-Stage Oxygen Pressure Regulator

Most contemporary Ohmeda machines have a second-stage oxygen pressure regulator set at a specific value ranging from 12 to 19 psig.[12-17] Oxygen flowmeter output is constant when the oxygen supply pressure exceeds the set value. Ohmeda pressure-sensor shutoff valves are set at a higher threshold value (20–30 psig). This ensures that oxygen is the last gas flow to decrease if oxygen pressure fails.

Flowmeter Assembly

The flowmeter assembly (Fig. 22-6) precisely controls and measures gas flow to the common gas outlet. The flow control valve regulates the amount of flow that enters a tapered, transparent flow tube known as a Thorpe tube. A mobile indicator float inside the flow tube indicates the amount of flow passing through the flow control valve. The quantity of flow is indicated on a scale associated with the flow tube.[7,8]

Physical Principles of Flowmeters

Opening the flow control valve allows gas to travel through the space between the float and the flow tube. This space is known as the annular space (Fig. 22-7). The indicator float hovers freely in an equilibrium position where the upward force resulting from gas flow equals the downward force on the float resulting from gravity at a given flow rate. The float moves to a new equilibrium position in the tube when flow is changed. These flowmeters are commonly referred to as *constant pressure*

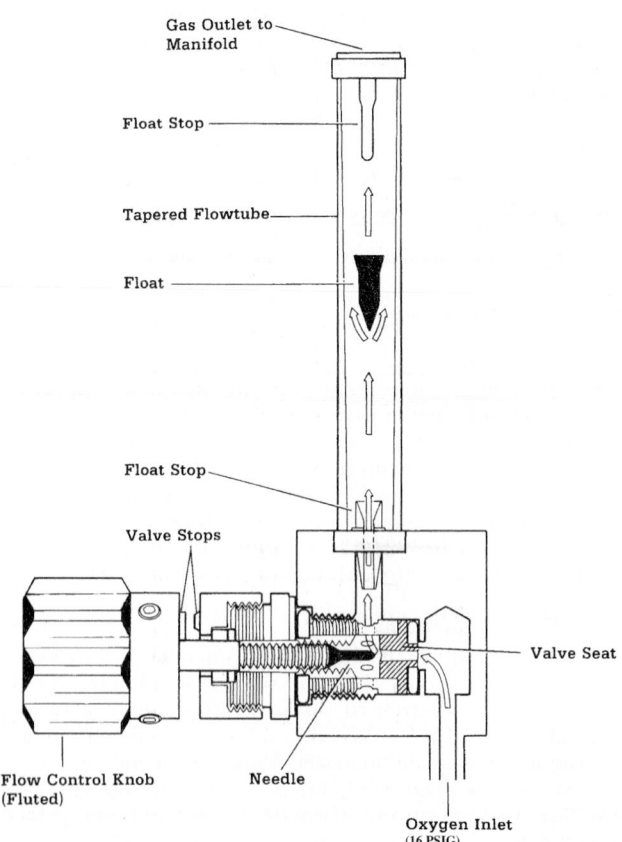

Figure 22-6. Oxygen flowmeter assembly. The oxygen flowmeter assembly is composed of the flow control valve assembly plus the flowmeter subassembly. (Reproduced with permission from Bowie E, Huffman LM: The Anesthesia Machine: Essentials for Understanding. Madison, WI, Ohmeda, a division of BOC Health Care Inc, 1985.)

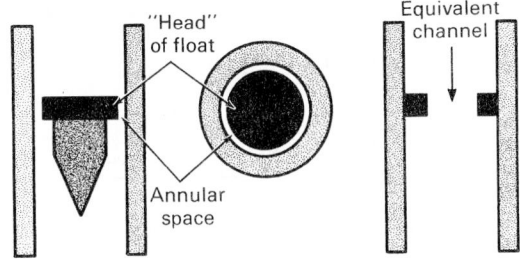

Figure 22-7. The annular space. The clearance between the head of the float and the flow tube is known as the annular space. It can be considered an equivalent to a circular channel of the same cross-sectional area. (Redrawn with permission from Macintosh R, Mushin WW, Epstein HG: Physics for the Anaesthetist, 3rd ed. Oxford, Blackwell Scientific Publications, 1963.)

flowmeters because the pressure decrease across the float remains constant for all positions in the tube.[7,26,28]

Flow tubes are tapered, with the smallest diameter at the bottom of the tube and the largest diameter at the top. The term *variable orifice* designates this type of unit because the annular space between the float and the inner wall of the flow tube varies with the position of the float. Flow through the constriction created by the float can be laminar or turbulent, depending on the flow rate (Fig. 22-8). The characteristics of a gas that influence its flow rate through a given constriction are viscosity (laminar flow) and density (turbulent flow). Because the annular space is tubular at low flow rates, laminar flow is present and viscosity determines the gas flow rate. The annular space simulates an orifice at high flow rates, and turbulent gas flow then depends predominantly on the density of the gas.[7,28]

Components of Flowmeter Assembly

Flow Control Valve Assembly. The flow control valve (see Fig. 22-6) assembly is composed of a flow control knob, a needle

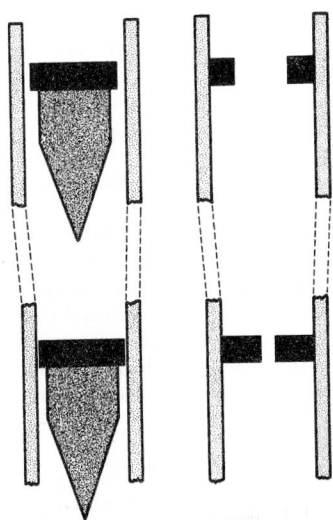

Figure 22-8. Flow tube constriction. The lower pair of illustrations represents the lower portion of a flow tube. The clearance between the head of the float and flow tube is narrow. The equivalent channel is tubular because its diameter is less than its length. Viscosity is dominant in determining gas flow rate through this tubular constriction. The upper pair of illustrations represents the upper portion of a flow tube. The equivalent channel is orificial because its length is less than its width. Density is dominant in determining gas flow rate through this orificial constriction. (Redrawn with permission from Macintosh R, Mushin WW, Epstein HG: Physics for the Anaesthetist, 3rd ed. Oxford, Blackwell Scientific Publications, 1963.)

valve, a valve seat, and a pair of valve stops.[7] The assembly can receive its pneumatic input either directly from the pipeline source (50 psig) or from a second-stage pressure regulator. The location of the needle valve in the valve seat changes to establish different orifices when the flow control valve is adjusted. Gas flow increases when the flow control valve is turned counterclockwise, and it decreases when the valve is turned clockwise. Extreme clockwise rotation results in damage to the needle valve and valve seat. Therefore, flow control valves are equipped with valve "stops" to prevent this occurrence.[8]

SAFETY FEATURES Contemporary flow control valve assemblies have numerous safety features. The oxygen flow control knob is physically distinguishable from other gas knobs. It is distinctively fluted, projects beyond the control knobs of the other gases, and is larger in diameter than the flow control knobs of other gases. All knobs are color-coded for the appropriate gas, and the chemical formula or name of the gas is permanently marked on each. Flow control knobs are recessed or protected with a shield or barrier to minimize inadvertent change from a preset position. If a single gas has two flow tubes, the tubes are arranged in series and are controlled by a single flow control valve.[6]

Flowmeter Subassembly. The flowmeter subassembly (see Fig. 22-6) consists of the flow tube, the indicator float with float stops, and the indicator scale.[7]

FLOW TUBES Contemporary flow tubes are made of glass. Most have a single taper in which the inner diameter of the flow tube increases uniformly from bottom to top. Manufacturers provide double flow tubes for oxygen and nitrous oxide to provide better visual discrimination at low flow rates. A fine flow tube indicates flow from approximately 200 ml · min⁻¹ to 1 l · min⁻¹, and a coarse flow tube indicates flow from approximately 1 l · min⁻¹ to 10–12 l · min⁻¹. The two tubes are connected in series and supplied by a single flow control valve. The total gas flow is that shown on the higher flowmeter.

INDICATOR FLOATS AND FLOAT STOPS Contemporary anesthesia machines use several different types of bobbins or floats, including plumb-bob floats,[11–13,16,17] rotating skirted floats,[14,15] and ball floats.[18–22] Flow is read at the top of plumb-bob and skirted floats and at the center of the ball on the ball-type floats.[7] Flow tubes are equipped with float stops at the top and bottom of the tube. The upper stop prevents the float from ascending to the top of the tube and plugging the outlet. It also ensures that the float will be visible at maximum flows instead of being hidden in the manifold. The bottom float stop provides a central foundation for the indicator when the flow control valve is turned off.[7,8]

SCALE The flowmeter scale can be marked directly on the flow tube or located to the right of the tube.[6] Gradations corresponding to equal increments in flow rate are closer together at the top of the scale because the annular space increases more rapidly than does the internal diameter from bottom to top of the tube. Rib guides are used in some flow tubes with ball-type indicators to minimize this compression effect. They are tapered glass ridges that run the length of the tube. There are usually three rib guides that are equally spaced around the inner circumference of the tube. In the presence of rib guides, the annular space from the bottom to the top of the tube increases almost proportionally with the internal diameter. This results in a nearly linear scale.[7] Rib guides are employed on North American Dräger flow tubes.[18–20,22]

SAFETY FEATURES The flowmeter subassembly for each gas on the Ohmeda Modulus I, Modulus II, Modulus II Plus, and CD is housed in an independent, color-coded, pin-specific module. The flow tubes are adjacent to a gas-specific, color-coded backing. The flow scale and the chemical formula or name of the gas are permanently etched on the backing to the right of the flow tube.[11–13,16,17] Flowmeter scales are individually hand-calibrated using the specific float to provide a high degree of accuracy. The tube, float, and scale make an inseparable unit. The entire set must be replaced if any component is damaged.[11–13,16,17]

North American Dräger does not use a modular system for the flowmeter subassembly. The flow scale, the chemical symbol, and the gas-specific color codes are etched directly onto the flow tube.[18-22] The scale in use is obvious when two flow tubes for the same gas are used.

Problems with Flowmeters

Leaks. Flowmeter leaks are a substantial hazard because the flowmeters are located downstream from all machine safety devices except the oxygen analyzer.[1] Leaks can occur at the O-rings between the glass flow tube and the metal manifold and in the glass flow tubes, the most fragile pneumatic component of the anesthesia machine. Gross damage to glass flow tubes is usually apparent, but subtle cracks and chips may be overlooked, resulting in errors of delivered flows.[29]

Eger *et al* in 1963[30] demonstrated that, in the presence of a flowmeter leak, a hypoxic mixture is less likely to occur if the oxygen flowmeter is located downstream from all other flowmeters.[28] Figure 22-9 is a contemporary version of the figure in Eger's original publication. The unused air flow tube has a large leak. Nitrous oxide and oxygen flow rates are set at a ratio of 3:1. A potentially dangerous arrangement is shown in Figure 22-9A and B because the nitrous oxide flowmeter is located in the downstream position. A hypoxic mixture can result because a substantial portion of oxygen flow passes through the leak, and all nitrous oxide is directed to the common gas outlet. A safer configuration is shown in Figure 22-9C and D. The oxygen flowmeter is located in the downstream position. A portion of the nitrous oxide flow escapes through the leak, and the remainder goes toward the common gas outlet. A hypoxic mixture is less likely because all the oxygen flow is advanced by the nitrous oxide.[30] North American Dräger flowmeters are arranged as in Figure 22-9C, and Ohmeda flowmeters are arranged as in Figure 22-9D.

A leak in the oxygen flow tube can produce a hypoxic mixture even when oxygen is located in the downstream position (Fig. 22-10).[1,29] Oxygen escapes through the leak and nitrous oxide flows toward the common outlet, particularly at high ratios of nitrous oxide to oxygen flow.

Inaccuracy. Flow error can occur even when flowmeters are assembled properly with appropriate components. Dirt or static electricity can cause a float to stick, and the actual flow may be higher or lower than that indicated. Sticking is more common in the low flow range because the annular space is smaller. A damaged float can cause inaccurate readings because the precise relationship between the float and the flow tube is altered. Back pressure from the breathing circuit can cause a float to drop so that it reads less than the actual flow. Finally, if flow-

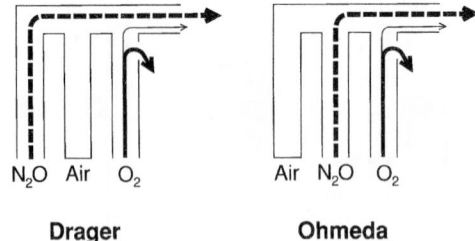

Figure 22-10. Oxygen flow tube leak. An oxygen flow tube leak can produce a hypoxic mixture regardless of flow tube arrangement. (Reproduced with permission from Andrews JJ: Inhaled anesthetic delivery systems. In Miller RD (ed): Anesthesia, 5th ed, p 174. Philadelphia, Churchill Livingstone, 1999.)

meters are not aligned properly in the vertical position, readings can be inaccurate because tilting distorts the annular space.[7,29,31]

Ambiguous Scale. Before the standardization of flowmeter scales and the widespread use of oxygen analyzers, at least two deaths resulted from confusion created by ambiguous scales.[29,31,32] The operator read the float position beside an adjacent but erroneous scale in both cases. Today, this error is less likely to occur because contemporary flowmeter scales are marked either directly onto or to the right of the appropriate flow tube.[6] Confusion is minimized when the scale is etched directly onto the tube.

Proportioning Systems

Manufacturers have equipped newer machines with proportioning systems in an attempt to prevent delivery of a hypoxic mixture. Nitrous oxide and oxygen are interfaced either mechanically or pneumatically so that the minimum oxygen concentration at the common outlet is 25%.

Ohmeda Link-25 Proportion Limiting Control System

Contemporary Ohmeda machines use the Link-25 System. The heart of the system is the mechanical integration of the nitrous oxide and oxygen flow control valves. It allows independent adjustment of either valve, yet automatically intercedes to maintain a minimum 25% oxygen concentration with a maximum nitrous oxide–oxygen flow ratio of 3:1. The Link-25 automatically increases oxygen flow to prevent delivery of a hypoxic mixture.[11-17]

Figure 22-11 shows the Ohmeda Modulus II Link-25 System. The nitrous oxide and oxygen flow control valves are identical. A 14-tooth sprocket is attached to the nitrous oxide flow control valve, and a 28-tooth sprocket is attached to the oxygen flow control valve. A chain physically links the sprockets. When the nitrous oxide flow control valve is turned through two revolutions, or 28 teeth, the oxygen flow control valve will revolve once because of the 2:1 gear ratio. The final 3:1 flow ratio results because the nitrous oxide flow control valve is supplied

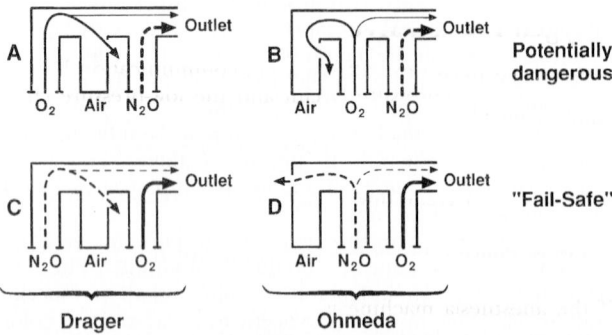

Figure 22-9. Flowmeter sequence—a potential cause of hypoxia. In the event of a flowmeter leak, a potentially dangerous arrangement exists when nitrous oxide is located in the downstream position (*A* and *B*). The safest configuration exists when oxygen is located in the downstream position (*C* and *D*). (Modified with permission from Eger EI II, Hylton RR, Irwin RH *et al*: Anesthetic flowmeter sequence—a cause for hypoxia. Anesthesiology 24:396, 1963.)

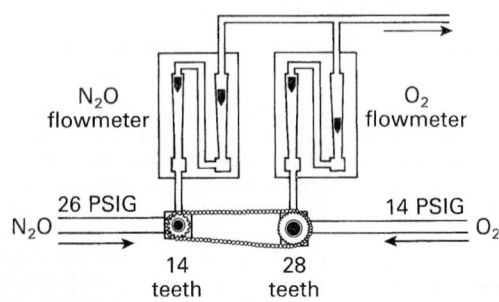

Figure 22-11. Ohmeda Link-25 Proportion Limiting Control System.

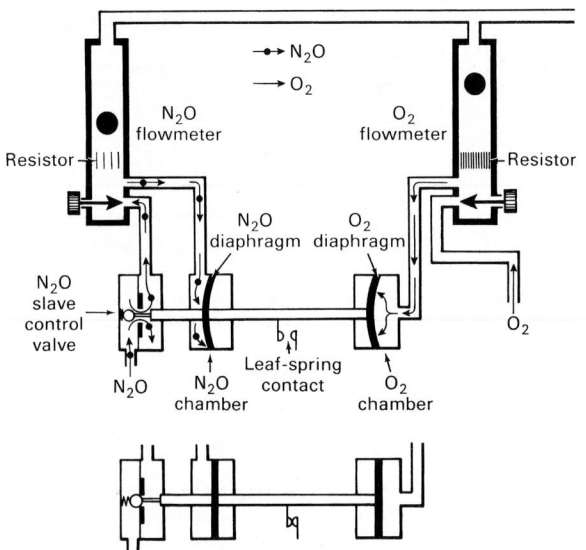

Figure 22-12. North American Dräger Oxygen Ratio Monitor Controller. (Redrawn with permission from Schreiber P: Safety Guidelines for Anesthesia Systems. Telford, PA, North American Dräger, 1984.)

by approximately 26 psig, whereas the oxygen flow control valve is supplied by 14 psig. Thus, the combination of the mechanical and pneumatic aspects of the system yields the final oxygen concentration.[12,13]

North American Dräger Oxygen Ratio Monitor Controller

North American Dräger's proportioning system, the Oxygen Ratio Monitor Controller (ORMC), is used on the North American Dräger Narkomed 2A, 2B, 3, and 4.[18-23] It is a pneumatic oxygen–nitrous oxide interlock system designed to maintain a fresh gas oxygen concentration of at least $25 \pm 3\%$. The device controls the fresh gas oxygen concentration to levels substantially higher than 25% at oxygen flow rates less than $1 \, l \cdot min^{-1}$. The ORMC limits nitrous oxide flow to prevent delivery of a hypoxic mixture.[18-22] This is unlike the Ohmeda Link-25, which actively increases oxygen flow.

A schematic of the ORMC is shown in Figure 22-12. It is composed of an oxygen chamber, a nitrous oxide chamber, and a nitrous oxide slave control valve; all are interconnected by a mobile horizontal shaft. The pneumatic input into the device is from the oxygen and the nitrous oxide flowmeters. These flowmeters are unique because they have specific resistors located downstream from the flow control valves. These resistors create back pressures directed to the oxygen and nitrous oxide chambers. The value of the oxygen flow tube resistor is three to four times that of the nitrous oxide flow tube resistor, and the relative value of these resistors determines the value of the controlled fresh gas oxygen concentration. The back pressure in the oxygen and nitrous oxide chambers pushes against rubber diaphragms attached to the mobile horizontal shaft. Movement of the shaft regulates the nitrous oxide slave control valve, which feeds the nitrous oxide flow control valve.[1,19,23]

If the oxygen pressure is proportionally higher than the nitrous oxide pressure, the nitrous oxide slave control valve opens more widely, allowing more nitrous oxide to flow. As the nitrous oxide flow is increased manually, the nitrous oxide pressure forces the shaft toward the oxygen chamber. The valve opening becomes more restrictive and limits the nitrous oxide flow to the flowmeter.

Figure 22-12 illustrates the action of a single ORMC under different sets of circumstances. The back pressure exerted on the oxygen diaphragm, in the upper configuration, is greater than that exerted on the nitrous oxide diaphragm. This causes the horizontal shaft to move to the left, opening the nitrous oxide slave control valve. Nitrous oxide is then able to proceed to its flow control valve and out through the flowmeter. In the bottom configuration, the nitrous oxide slave control valve is closed because of inadequate oxygen back pressure.[1,18,23]

Limitations

Proportioning systems are not foolproof. Machines equipped with proportioning systems still can deliver a hypoxic mixture under the following conditions.

Wrong Supply Gas. Both the Link-25 and the ORMC will be fooled if a gas other than oxygen is present in the oxygen pipeline. In the Link-25 System, the nitrous oxide and oxygen flow control valves will continue to be mechanically linked, and a hypoxic mixture will proceed to the common outlet. The oxygen rubber diaphragm of the ORMC will recognize adequate "oxygen" pressure, and flow of both the wrong gas plus nitrous oxide will result. The oxygen analyzer is the only machine monitor that will detect this condition in both systems.

Defective Pneumatics or Mechanics. Normal operation of the Ohmeda Link-25 and the North American Dräger ORMC is contingent upon pneumatic and mechanical integrity.[33] Pneumatic integrity in the Ohmeda System depends on properly functioning second-stage regulators. A nitrous oxide-oxygen ratio other than 3:1 will result if the regulators are not precise. The chain connecting the two sprockets must be intact. A 97% nitrous oxide concentration can occur if the chain is cut or broken.[34] In the North American Dräger System, a functional Oxygen Failure Protection Device (OFPD) is necessary to supply appropriate pressure to the ORMC. The mechanical aspects of the ORMC, such as the rubber diaphragms, the flow tube resistors, and the nitrous oxide slave control valve, must likewise be intact.

Leaks Downstream. The ORMC and the Link-25 function at the level of the flow control valves. A leak downstream from these devices, such as a broken oxygen flow tube (see Fig. 22-10), can cause delivery of a hypoxic mixture. Oxygen escapes through the leak, and the predominant gas delivered at the common outlet is nitrous oxide. The oxygen analyzer is the only machine safety device that can detect the problem.[1] North American Dräger recommends a preoperative positive pressure leak test to detect such a leak.[18-22] Ohmeda recommends a preoperative negative pressure leak test because of the check valve located at the common outlet[9-13,15] (see Checking Anesthesia Machines).

Inert Gas Administration. Administration of a third inert gas, such as helium, nitrogen, or carbon dioxide, can cause a hypoxic mixture because contemporary proportioning systems link only nitrous oxide and oxygen.[11-22,35] Use of an oxygen analyzer is mandatory if the operator uses a third inert gas.

Oxygen Flush Valve

The oxygen flush valve allows direct communication between the oxygen high-pressure circuit and the low-pressure circuit (see Fig. 22-3). Flow from the oxygen flush valve enters the low-pressure circuit downstream from the vaporizers and downstream from the Ohmeda machine outlet check valve. The spring-loaded oxygen flush valve stays closed until the operator opens it by depressing the oxygen flush button. Actuation of the valve delivers $35-75 \, l \cdot min^{-1}$ to the breathing circuit.[8]

The oxygen flush valve can provide effective jet ventilation if the anesthesia machine is equipped with a one-way check valve positioned between the vaporizer and the oxygen flush valve. Because the Ohmeda Modulus II has such a valve, the entire oxygen flow of $45-75 \, l \cdot min^{-1}$ is delivered to the common gas outlet at a high pressure of 50 psig. On the other hand, the Ohmeda Modulus II Plus, which does not have the check valve, provides only 7 psig at the common gas outlet because some oxygen flow travels retrograde through an internal relief valve located upstream from the oxygen flush valve. The North American Dräger Narkomed 2A, which also does not have the check valve, provides an intermediate pressure of 18 psig to the common gas outlet because some oxygen flow travels retrograde through a pop-off valve located in the vaporizers.[36]

The oxygen flush valve is associated with several hazards. A defective or damaged valve can stick in the fully open position, causing barotrauma.[37] A valve sticking in a partially open position can result in patient awareness because the oxygen flow from the incompetent valve dilutes the inhaled anesthetic.[38] Improper use of normally functioning oxygen flush valves also can result in problems. Overzealous intraoperative oxygen flushing can dilute inhaled anesthetics. Oxygen flushing during the inspiratory phase of positive pressure ventilation can cause barotrauma. Excess volume cannot be vented from the breathing circuit because the ventilator relief valve is closed and the Adjustable Pressure Limiting (APL) valve is either out-of-circuit or closed.[39] If a machine is equipped with a freestanding vaporizer downstream from the common gas outlet, oxygen flushing can deliver large quantities of inhaled anesthetic to the patient. Finally, inappropriate preoperative use of the oxygen flush to evaluate the low-pressure circuit for leaks can be misleading, particularly on Ohmeda machines with a check valve at the common outlet.[40] Back pressure from the breathing circuit closes the check valve airtight, and major low-pressure circuit leaks can go undetected (see Checking Anesthesia Machines).

VAPORIZERS

Through the years, vaporizers have evolved from rudimentary ether inhalers to copper kettles to the present temperature-compensated, variable bypass vaporizers. With the introduction of the new inhaled anesthetic, desflurane, even more sophisticated vaporizers have been introduced. Before the discussion of variable bypass vaporizers, the Datex-Ohmeda Tec 6 desflurane vaporizer, and the Datex-Ohmeda Aladin cassette vaporizer, certain physical principles are reviewed briefly to facilitate understanding of the operating principles, construction, and design of contemporary vaporizers.

Physics

Vapor Pressure

Contemporary inhaled volatile anesthetics exist in the liquid state below 20°C. When a volatile liquid is in a closed container, molecules escape from the liquid phase to the vapor phase until the number of molecules in the vapor phase is constant. These molecules bombard the wall of the container and create a pressure known as the *saturated vapor pressure*. As the temperature increases, more molecules enter the vapor phase, and the vapor pressure increases (Fig. 22-13). Vapor pressure is independent of atmospheric pressure and is contingent only on the temperature and physical characteristics of the liquid. The boiling point of a liquid is that temperature at which the vapor pressure equals atmospheric pressure.[41-43] At 760 mm Hg, the boiling points for desflurane, isoflurane, halothane, enflurane, and sevoflurane are approximately 22.8, 48.5, 50.2, 56.5, and 58.5°C, respectively. Unlike other contemporary inhaled anesthetics, desflurane boils at temperatures commonly encountered in clinical settings such as pediatric and burn operating rooms. This unique physical characteristic mandates a special vaporizer design to deliver desflurane.

Latent Heat of Vaporization

Energy must be expended to convert a molecule from the liquid to gaseous state because the molecules of a liquid tend to cohere. The *latent heat of vaporization* is defined as the number of calories required to change 1 g of liquid into vapor without a

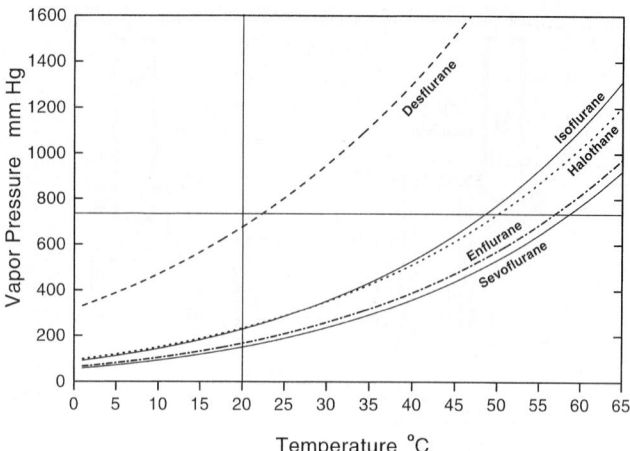

Figure 22-13. Vapor pressure versus temperature curves for desflurane, isoflurane, halothane, enflurane, and sevoflurane. The vapor pressure curve for desflurane is both steeper and shifted to higher vapor pressures when compared with the curves for other contemporary inhaled anesthetics. (From inhaled anesthetic package insert equations; from Susay SR, Smith MA, Lockwood GG: The saturated vapor pressure of desflurane at various temperatures. Anesth Analg 83:864, 1996.)

temperature change. The energy for vaporization must come from the liquid itself or from an outside source. The temperature of the liquid decreases during vaporization in the absence of an outside energy source. Energy loss can lead to significant decreases in temperature of the remaining liquid. This temperature drop will greatly decrease vaporization.[41,43,44]

Specific Heat

The *specific heat* of a substance is the number of calories required to increase the temperature of 1 g of a substance by 1°C.[41,43,45] The substance can be solid, liquid, or gas. The concept of specific heat is important to the design, operation, and construction of vaporizers because it is applicable in two ways. First, the specific heat value for an inhaled anesthetic is important because it indicates how much heat must be supplied to the liquid to maintain a constant temperature when heat is lost during vaporization. Second, manufacturers select vaporizer metals that have a high specific heat to minimize temperature changes associated with vaporization.

Thermal Conductivity

Thermal conductivity is a measure of the speed with which heat flows through a substance. The higher the thermal conductivity, the better the substance conducts heat.[41] Vaporizers are constructed of metals that have relatively high thermal conductivity, which helps maintain a uniform temperature.

Variable Bypass Vaporizers

The Ohmeda Tec 4, the Ohmeda Tec 5, and the North American Dräger Vapor 19.1 are classified as variable bypass, flow-over, temperature-compensated, agent-specific, out-of-circuit vaporizers.[41] *Variable bypass* refers to the method for regulating output concentration. As gas flow enters the vaporizer's inlet, the setting of the concentration control dial determines the ratio of flow that goes through the bypass chamber and through the vaporizing chamber. The gas channeled to the vaporizing chamber flows over the liquid anesthetic and becomes saturated with vapor. Thus, *flow-over* refers to the method of vaporization. The Tec 4, the Tec 5, and the Vapor 19.1 are classified as *temperature-compensated* because they are equipped with an automatic temperature-compensating device that helps maintain a constant vaporizer output over a wide range of temperatures.

These vaporizers are *agent-specific* and *out-of-circuit* because they are designed to accommodate a single agent and to be located outside the breathing circuit. Variable bypass vaporizers are used to deliver halothane, enflurane, isoflurane, and sevoflurane, but not desflurane.

Basic Operating Principles

A diagram of a generic, variable bypass vaporizer is shown in Figure 22-14. Vaporizer components include the concentration control dial, the bypass chamber, the vaporizing chamber, the filler port, and the filler cap. Using the filler port, the operator fills the vaporizing chamber with liquid anesthetic. The maximum safe level is predetermined by the position of the filler port, which is positioned to minimize the chance of overfilling. If a vaporizer is overfilled or tilted, liquid anesthetic can spill into the bypass chamber, causing an overdose. The concentration control dial is a variable restrictor, and it can be located either in the bypass chamber or the outlet of the vaporizing chamber. The function of the concentration control dial is to regulate the relative flow rates through the bypass and vaporizing chambers.

Flow from the flowmeters enters the inlet of the vaporizer. More than 80% of the flow passes straight through the bypass chamber to the vaporizer outlet, and this accounts for the name "bypass chamber." Less than 20% of the flow from the flowmeters is diverted through the vaporizing chamber. Depending on the temperature and vapor pressure of the particular inhaled anesthetic, the flow through the vaporizing chamber entrains a specific flow of inhaled anesthetic. All three flows—flow through the bypass chamber, flow through the vaporizing chamber, and flow of entrained anesthetic—exit the vaporizer at the outlet. The final concentration of inhaled anesthetic is the ratio of the flow of the inhaled anesthetic to the total gas flow.[41,46]

The vapor pressure of an inhaled anesthetic depends on the ambient temperature (Fig. 22-13). For example, at 20°C the vapor pressure of isoflurane is 238 mm Hg, whereas at 35°C the vapor pressure almost doubles (450 mm Hg). Variable bypass vaporizers have an internal mechanism to compensate for different ambient temperatures. The temperature-compensating valve of the Ohmeda Tec 4 is shown in Figure 22-15.[47] At high temperatures, such as those commonly used in pediatric or burn operating rooms, the vapor pressure inside the vaporizing chamber is high. To compensate for this increased vapor pressure, the bimetallic strip of the temperature-compensating valve leans to the right. This allows more flow to pass through the bypass chamber and less flow to pass through the vaporizing

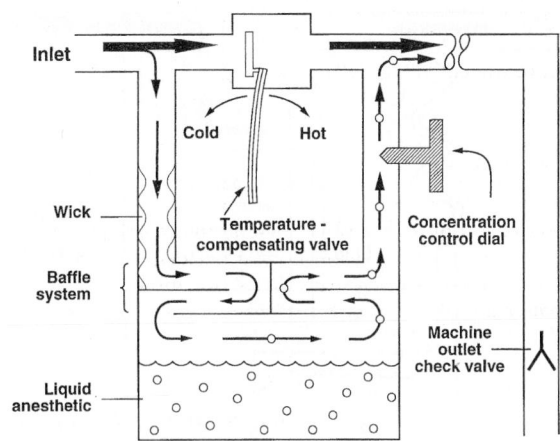

Figure 22-15. Simplified schematic of the Ohmeda Tec 4 vaporizer.

chamber. The net effect is a constant vaporizer output. In a cold operating room environment, the vapor pressure inside the vaporizing chamber decreases. To compensate for this decrease in vapor pressure, the bimetallic strip swings to the left, causing more flow to pass through the vaporizing chamber and less to pass through the bypass chamber. The net effect is a constant vaporizer output.

Factors That Influence Vaporizer Output

The output of an ideal vaporizer with a fixed dial setting would be constant regardless of varied flow rates, temperatures, back pressures, and carrier gases. Designing such a vaporizer is difficult because as ambient conditions change, the physical properties of gases and of vaporizers themselves can change.[46] Contemporary vaporizers approach ideal but still have some limitations. Several factors can influence vaporizer output.

Flow Rate. With a fixed dial setting, vaporizer output varies with the rate of gas flowing through the vaporizer. This variation is particularly notable at extremes of flow rates. The output of all variable bypass vaporizers is less than the dial setting at low flow rates (less than 250 ml · min⁻¹). This results from the relatively high density of volatile inhaled anesthetics. Insufficient turbulence is generated at low flow rates in the vaporizing chamber to upwardly advance the vapor molecules. At extremely high flow rates, such as 15 l · min⁻¹, the output of most variable bypass vaporizers is less than the dial setting. This discrepancy is attributed to incomplete mixing and saturation in the vaporizing chamber. Also, the resistance characteristics of the bypass chamber and the vaporizing chamber can vary as flow increases. These changes can result in decreased output concentration.[46]

Temperature. Because of improvements in design, the output of contemporary temperature-compensated vaporizers is almost linear over a wide range of temperatures. Automatic temperature-compensating mechanisms in bypass chambers maintain a constant vaporizer output with varying temperatures.[8,47,48] A bimetallic strip (Fig. 22-15) or an expansion element (Fig. 22-16) directs a greater proportion of gas flow through the bypass chamber as temperature increases.[46] Wicks are placed in direct contact with the metal wall of the vaporizer to help replace heat used for vaporization. Vaporizers are constructed with metals having relatively high specific heat and high thermal conductivity to minimize heat loss.

Intermittent Back Pressure. Intermittent back pressure associated with positive pressure ventilation or with oxygen flushing can cause higher vaporizer output concentration than the dialed setting. This phenomenon, known as the *pumping effect*,[41,46,49–51] is more pronounced at low flow rates, low dial settings, and low levels of liquid anesthetic in the vaporizing chamber. Additionally, the pumping effect is increased by rapid respiratory rates, high peak inspired pressures, and rapid drops

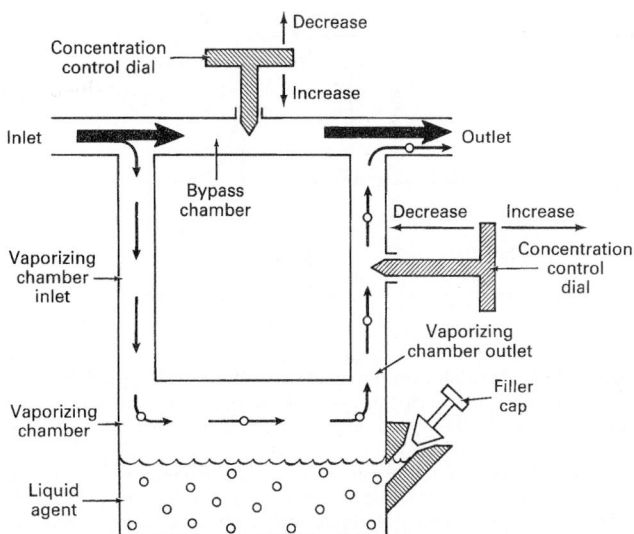

Figure 22-14. Generic variable bypass vaporizer.

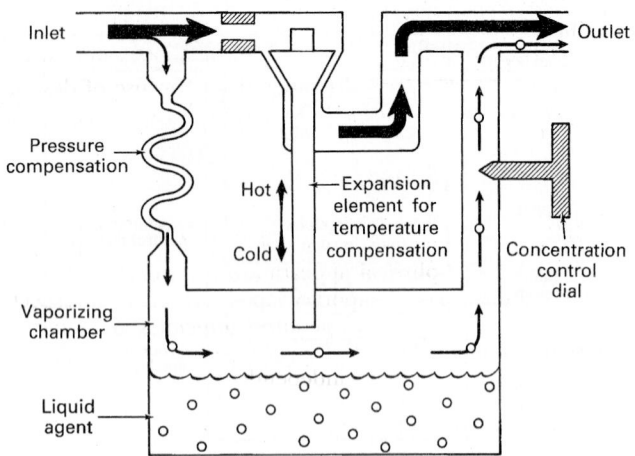

Figure 22-16. Simplified schematic of the North American Dräger Vapor 19.1 vaporizer.

in pressure during expiration.[47-51] The Ohmeda Tec 4 and North American Dräger Vapor 19.1 are relatively immune from the pumping effect.[47,48] One proposed mechanism for the pumping effect is dependent on retrograde pressure transmission from the patient circuit to the vaporizer during the inspiratory phase of positive pressure ventilation. Gas molecules are compressed in both the bypass and vaporizing chambers. When the back pressure is suddenly released during the expiratory phase of positive pressure ventilation, vapor exits the vaporizing chamber via the vaporizing chamber outlet and retrograde through the vaporizing chamber inlet. This occurs because the output resistance of the bypass chamber is lower than that of the vaporizing chamber, particularly at low dial settings. The enhanced output concentration results from the increment of vapor that travels in the retrograde direction to the bypass chamber.[46,49-51]

To decrease the pumping effect, the vaporizing chambers of the Tec 4 and the Vapor 19.1 are smaller than those of older variable bypass vaporizers such as the Fluotec Mark II (750 ml).[47,48,50] Therefore, no substantial volumes of vapor can be discharged from the vaporizing chamber into the bypass chamber during the expiratory phase. The North American Dräger Vapor 19.1 (Fig. 22-16) has a patented, long spiral tube that serves as the inlet to the vaporizing chamber.[48,50] When the pressure in the vaporizing chamber is released, some of the vapor enters this tube but does not enter the bypass chamber because of tube length.[50] The Tec 4 (Fig. 22-15) has an extensive baffle system in the vaporizing chamber, and a one-way check valve has been inserted at the common gas outlet to minimize the pumping effect. This check valve attenuates but does not eliminate the pressure increase because gas still flows from the flowmeters to the vaporizer during the inspiratory phase of positive pressure ventilation.[41,52]

Carrier Gas Composition. Vaporizer output is influenced by the composition of the carrier gas that flows through the vaporizer.[47,48,53-60] When the carrier gas is quickly switched from 100% oxygen to 100% nitrous oxide, there is a rapid transient decrease in vaporizer output followed by a slow increase to a new steady-state value (Fig. 22-17b).[58,59] The transient decrease in vaporizer output is attributed to nitrous oxide's being more soluble than oxygen in halogenated liquid.[58] Therefore, the quantity of gas leaving the vaporizing chamber is transiently diminished until the anesthetic liquid is totally saturated with nitrous oxide.

The explanation for the new steady-state output value is less well understood.[60] With contemporary vaporizers such as the North American Dräger Vapor 19.1 and the Ohmeda Tec 4, the steady-state output value is less when nitrous oxide rather than oxygen is the carrier gas (Fig. 22-17b).[47,48] Conversely, the output of some older vaporizers is enhanced when nitrous oxide is the carrier gas instead of oxygen.[53,55] The steady-state plateau

is achieved more rapidly with increased flow rates, regardless of the ultimate output value.[59] Factors that contribute to the characteristic steady-state response resulting when various carrier gases are used include the viscosity and density of the carrier gas, the relative solubilities of the carrier gas in the liquid anesthetic, the flow splitting characteristics of the specific vaporizer, and the dial setting.[55,58-60]

Safety Features

The North American Dräger 19.1, the Ohmeda Tec 4, and the Ohmeda Tec 5 have many safety features that have minimized or eliminated many hazards once associated with variable bypass vaporizers. Agent-specific, keyed filling devices help prevent filling a vaporizer with the wrong agent. Overfilling of these vaporizers is minimized because the filler port is located at the maximum safe liquid level. Today's vaporizers are firmly secured to the vaporizer manifold, and there is little need to move them. Thus, problems associated with tipping are minimized. Contemporary interlock systems prevent administration of more than one inhaled anesthetic.[47,48,61]

Hazards

Despite many safety features, some hazards are still associated with contemporary variable bypass vaporizers.

Misfilling. Vaporizers not equipped with keyed fillers have occasionally been misfilled with the wrong anesthetic liquid.[62] A potential for misfilling exists even on contemporary vaporizers equipped with keyed fillers.[63-65]

Contamination. Contamination of anesthetic vaporizer contents has occurred by filling an isoflurane vaporizer with a contaminated bottle of isoflurane. A potentially serious incident was avoided because the operator did not use the contaminated vaporizer after detecting an abnormal acrid odor.[66]

Tipping. Tipping can occur when vaporizers are incorrectly "switched out" or moved. However, tipping is unlikely when a vaporizer is attached to a manifold in the upright position. Excessive tipping can cause the liquid agent to enter the bypass chamber and can cause a high output concentration.[67] The Tec 4 is slightly more immune to tipping than is the Vapor 19.1 because of its extensive baffle system. However, if either vaporizer is tipped, it should not be used until it has been flushed for 20-30 minutes at high flow rates with the vaporizer set at a low concentration.[41]

Overfilling. Improper filling procedures combined with failure of the vaporizer sight glass can cause overfilling and overdose. Liquid anesthetic enters the bypass chamber, and up to ten times the intended vapor concentration can be delivered.[68]

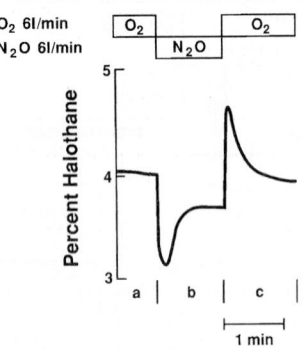

Figure 22-17. Halothane output of a North American Dräger Vapor 19.1 vaporizer with different carrier gases. The initial output concentration is approximately 4% halothane when oxygen is the carrier gas at flows of $6 \ l \cdot min^{-1}$ (*a*). When the carrier gas is quickly switched to 100% nitrous oxide (*b*), the halothane concentration decreases to 3% within 8-10 sec. Then, a new steady-state concentration of approximately 3.5% is attained within 1 min. (Modified with permission from Gould DB, Lampert BA, MacKrell TN: Effect of nitrous oxide solubility on vaporizer aberrance. Anesth Analg 61:939, 1982.)

Simultaneous Inhaled Anesthetic Administration. Two inhaled anesthetics can be administered simultaneously when the center Tec 4 vaporizer is removed from Ohmeda machines equipped with the older style Selectatec® vaporizer manifold. The left or right vaporizer should be moved to the central position if the central vaporizer is removed as indicated by the manifold label. The interlock system will then function properly because the two remaining vaporizers are adjacent.[12-14]

Leaks. Leaks occur often with vaporizers, and vaporizer leaks can cause patient awareness during anesthesia.[41,69-71] A loose filler cap is the most common source of vaporizer leaks. With some key-filled Penlon and Dräger vaporizers, a loose filler screw clamp allows escape of saturated anesthetic vapor.[71] Leaks can occur at the O-ring junction between the vaporizer and its manifold. A vaporizer must be in the "on" position to detect a leak within it. Vaporizer leaks in the North American Dräger System can be detected with a conventional positive pressure leak test because of the absence of check valves. Ohmeda recommends a negative pressure leak testing device (suction bulb) to detect vaporizer leaks in the Modulus I, Modulus II, and the Excel because of the check valve at the machine outlet[11-13,15] (see Checking Anesthesia Machines).

The Datex-Ohmeda Tec 6 Vaporizer for Desflurane

Controlled vaporization of desflurane requires an electrically heated, pressurized vaporizer because of desflurane's unique physical properties.[72,73] The vapor pressure of desflurane is three to four times that of contemporary inhaled anesthetics, and it boils at 22.8°C,[72] which is near room temperature (Fig. 22-13). Desflurane has minimum alveolar anesthetic concentration (MAC) values of 6–7%.[72] Desflurane is valuable because it has a low blood gas solubility coefficient of 0.45 at 37°C, and recovery from anesthesia is more rapid than with most other potent inhaled anesthetics.[74]

Unsuitability of Contemporary Variable Bypass Vaporizers for Controlled Vaporization of Desflurane

Desflurane's high volatility and moderate potency preclude its use with contemporary variable bypass vaporizers such as Ohmeda Tec 4, Tec 5, or the North American Dräger Vapor 19.1 for two reasons[72]:

1. The vapor pressure of desflurane is near one atmosphere. The vapor pressures of sevoflurane, enflurane, isoflurane, halothane, and desflurane at 20°C are 160, 172, 240, 244, and 669 mm Hg,[74] respectively (Fig. 22-13). Normal flow through a traditional vaporizer would vaporize many more volumes of desflurane. For example, at 1 atm and 20°C, 100 ml · min^{-1} passing through the vaporizing chamber entrains 735 ml · min^{-1} desflurane versus 27, 29, 46, and 47 ml · min^{-1} of sevoflurane, enflurane, isoflurane, and halothane, respectively.[72] Under these same conditions, the amount of bypass flow necessary to achieve sufficient distribution of anesthetic vapor to produce 1% desflurane output would be approximately 73 l · min^{-1}, compared to 5 l · min^{-1} or less for the other three anesthetics. Above 22.8°C at 1 atm, desflurane will boil. The amount of vapor produced would be limited only by the heat energy available from the vaporizer owing to its specific heat.[72]

2. Contemporary vaporizers lack an external heat source. Although desflurane has a heat of vaporization approximately equal to that of sevoflurane, enflurane, isoflurane, and halothane, its MAC is 4–9 times higher than that of the other four inhaled anesthetics. Thus, the absolute amount of desflurane vaporized over a given time period is considerably higher than with other anesthetics. Supplying desflurane in higher concentrations would cause excessive cooling of the vaporizer. In the absence of an external

heat source, temperature compensation using traditional mechanical devices would be almost impossible over a broad clinical range of temperatures because of desflurane's steep vapor pressure versus temperature curve (Fig. 22-13).[72]

Operating Principles of the Tec 6

To achieve controlled vaporization of desflurane, Ohmeda has introduced the Tec 6 vaporizer, which is electrically heated and pressurized.[75] The physical appearance and operation of the Tec 6 are similar to contemporary vaporizers, but some aspects of the internal design and operating principles are radically different. A simplified schematic of the Tec 6 is shown in Figure 22-18. The vaporizer has two independent gas circuits arranged in parallel. The fresh gas circuit is shown in gray, and the vapor circuit is shown in white. The fresh gas from the flowmeters enters at the fresh gas inlet, passes through a fixed restrictor (R1), and exits at the vaporizer gas outlet. The vapor circuit originates at the desflurane sump, which is electrically heated and thermostatically controlled to 39°C, a temperature well above desflurane's boiling point. The heated sump assembly serves as a reservoir of desflurane vapor. At 39°C, the vapor pressure in the sump is approximately 1300 mm Hg absolute,[76] or approximately 2 atm absolute (Fig. 22-13). Just downstream from the sump is the shutoff valve. After the vaporizer warms up, the shutoff valve fully opens when the concentration control valve is turned to the on position. A pressure-regulating valve downstream from the shutoff valve down-regulates the pressure to approximately 1.1 atm absolute (74 mm Hg gauge) at a fresh gas flow rate of 10 l · min^{-1}. The operator controls desflurane output by adjusting the concentration control valve (R2), which is a variable restrictor.[72]

The vapor flow through R2 joins the fresh gas flow through R1 at a point downstream from the restrictors. Until this point, the two circuits are physically divorced. They are interfaced pneumatically and electronically, however, through differential pressure transducers, a control electronics system, and a pressure-regulating valve. When a constant fresh gas flow rate encounters the fixed restrictor R1, a specific back pressure proportional to the fresh gas flow rate pushes against the diaphragm of the control differential pressure transducer. The differential pressure transducer conveys the pressure difference between the fresh gas circuit and the vapor circuit to the control electronics system. The control electronics system regulates the pressure-regulating valve so that the pressure in the vapor circuit equals the pressure in the fresh gas circuit. This equalized pressure

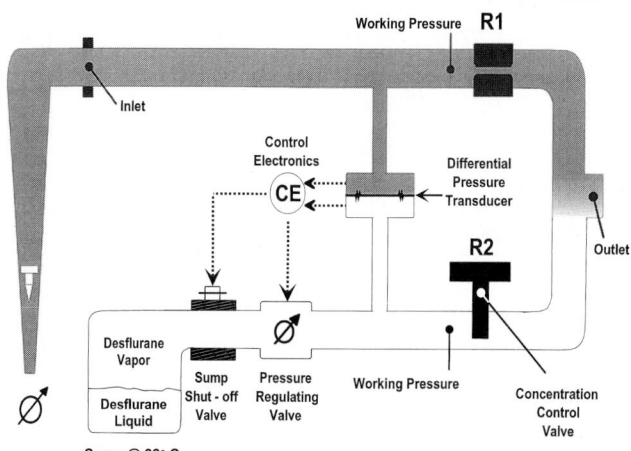

Figure 22-18. Simplified schematic of the Tec 6 desflurane vaporizer. (Modified with permission from Andrews JJ: Operating Principles of the Ohmeda Tec 6 Desflurane Vaporizer: A Collection of Twelve Color Illustrations. Washington, D.C., Library of Congress, 1996.)

Table 22-1. FRESH GAS FLOW RATE VERSUS WORKING PRESSURE

Fresh Gas Flow Rate (l·min⁻¹)	Working Pressure at R1 and R2 (Gauge) (Gas Inlet Pressure)		
	mbar	cm water	mm Hg
1	10	10.2	7.4
5	50	51.0	37.0
10	100	102.0	74.0

Reprinted with permission from Andrews JJ, Johnston RV Jr: The new Tec 6 desflurane vaporizer. Anesth Analg 76:1338, 1993.

supplying R1 and R2 is the working pressure, and the working pressure is constant at a fixed fresh gas flow rate. If the operator increases the fresh gas flow rate, more back pressure is exerted upon the diaphragm of the control pressure transducer, and the working pressure of the vaporizer increases.[72]

Table 22-1 shows the approximate correlation between fresh gas flow rate and working pressure for a typical vaporizer. At a fresh gas flow rate of 1 l·min⁻¹, the working pressure is 10 millibars (mbar), or 7.4 mm Hg gauge. At a fresh gas flow rate of 10 l·min⁻¹, the working pressure is 100 mbar, or 74 mm Hg gauge. Therefore, there is a linear relationship between fresh gas flow rate and working pressure. When the fresh gas flow rate is increased tenfold, the working pressure increases tenfold.[72]

Listed below are two specific examples to demonstrate the operating principles of the Tec 6.[72]

Example A: Constant fresh gas flow rate of 1 l·min⁻¹, with an increase in the dial setting.
With a fresh gas flow rate of 1 l·min⁻¹, the working pressure of the vaporizer is 7.4 mm Hg. That is, the pressure supplying R1 and R2 is 7.4 mm Hg. As the operator increases the dial setting, the opening at R2 becomes larger, allowing more vapor to pass through R2. Specific vapor flow values at different dial settings are shown in Table 22-2.

Example B: Constant dial setting with an increase in fresh gas flow from 1 to 10 l·min⁻¹.
At a fresh gas flow rate of 1 l·min⁻¹, the working pressure is 7.4 mm Hg, and at a dial setting of 6% the vapor flow rate through R2 is 64 ml·min⁻¹ (Tables 22-1 and 22-2). With a tenfold increase in the fresh gas flow rate, there is a concomitant tenfold increase in the working pressure to 74 mm Hg. The ratio of resistances of R2 to R1 is constant at a fixed dial setting of 6%. Because R2 is supplied by 10 times more pressure, the vapor flow rate through R2 increases tenfold to 640 ml·min⁻¹. Vaporizer output is constant because both the fresh gas flow and the vapor flow increase proportionally.

Table 22-2. DIAL SETTING VERSUS FLOW THROUGH RESTRICTOR R2

Dial Setting (vol%)*	Fresh Gas Flow Rate (l·min⁻¹)	Approximate Vapor Flow Rate through R2 (ml·min⁻¹)
1	1	10
6	1	64
12	1	136
18	1	220

* Volume percent = [(vapor flow rate)/(fresh gas flow rate) + (vapor flow rate)] × 100%.
Reprinted with permission from Andrews JJ, Johnston RV Jr: The new Tec 6 desflurane vaporizer. Anesth Analg 76:1338, 1993.

Factors that Influence Vaporizer Output

Varied altitude and carrier gas composition influence Tec 6 output. Each is discussed below:

Varied Altitudes. Unlike contemporary variable bypass vaporizers, the Tec 6 vaporizer requires manual adjustments of the concentration control dial at altitudes other than sea level to maintain a constant partial pressure of anesthetic. The Tec 6 itself works at absolute pressures; therefore, altitude makes no difference to the vaporizer's performance *per se*. It will accurately deliver the dialed volume percent (vol%) of desflurane. However, when this gas is brought to ambient atmosphere at high altitudes, the vol% will represent an absolute decrease in the partial pressure of the anesthetic. This is not the case with contemporary variable bypass vaporizers, which deliver a constant partial pressure of anesthetic. To compensate for the reduction of partial pressure of vapor at altitude, the Tec 6 rotary valve must be advanced to maintain the required anesthetic partial pressure. The required dial setting may be calculated using the following formula:[75]

$$\text{Required dial setting} = \text{Normal dial setting (vol\%)} \times (760 \text{ mm Hg}) / (\text{ambient pressure (mm Hg)})$$

For example, at an altitude of 2000 m (6564 feet), where the ambient pressure is 608 mm Hg, the operator must advance the concentration control dial from 10 to 12.5% to maintain the required anesthetic partial pressure.[75] In hyperbaric settings, the operator must decrease the dial setting to prevent delivery of an overdose.

Carrier Gas Composition. Vaporizer output approximates the dial setting when oxygen is the carrier gas because the Tec 6 vaporizer is calibrated using 100% oxygen.[75] At low flow rates when a carrier gas other than 100% oxygen is used, however, a clear trend toward reduction in vaporizer output emerges. This reduction parallels the proportional decrease in viscosity of the carrier gas. Nitrous oxide has a lower viscosity than oxygen, so the back pressure generated by resistor R1 (see Fig. 22-18) is lower when nitrous oxide is the carrier gas, and the working pressure is reduced. At low flow rates using nitrous oxide as the carrier gas, vaporizer output is approximately 20% less than the dial setting. This suggests that, at clinically useful fresh gas flow rates, the gas flow across resistor R1 is laminar, and the working pressure is proportional to both the fresh gas flow rate and the viscosity of the carrier gas.[77]

Safety Features

Because desflurane's vapor pressure is near 1 atm, misfilling contemporary vaporizers with desflurane can theoretically cause desflurane overdose and hypoxemia.[78] Ohmeda has introduced a unique, anesthetic-specific filling system to minimize occurrence of this potential hazard. The agent-specific filler cap of the desflurane bottle prevents its use with traditional vaporizers. The filling system also minimizes spillage of liquid or vapor anesthetic by maintaining a "closed system" during the filling process. Each desflurane bottle has a spring-loaded filler cap with an O-ring on the tip. The spring seals the bottle until it is engaged in the filler port of the vaporizer. Thus, this anesthetic-specific filling system interlocks the vaporizer and the dispensing bottle, preventing loss of anesthetic to the atmosphere.[75] One case report described misfilling a Tec 6 desflurane vaporizer with sevoflurane, an error made possible by the similarities between the keyed fillers on the bottles of desflurane and sevoflurane. The desflurane vaporizer detected this error and promptly shut off.[65]

Major vaporizer faults cause the shutoff valve located just downstream from the desflurane sump (Fig. 22-18) to close, producing a no-output situation. The valve is closed and a "no output" alarm is activated immediately if any of the following conditions occur: (a) the anesthetic level decreases to below

20 ml; (b) the vaporizer is tilted; (c) a power failure occurs; or (d) there is a disparity between the pressure in the vapor circuit versus the pressure in the fresh gas circuit exceeding a specified tolerance.[75]

Summary

The Tec 6 vaporizer is an electrically heated, thermostatically controlled, constant-temperature, pressurized, electromechanically coupled dual circuit, gas–vapor blender. The pressure in the vapor circuit is electronically regulated to equal the pressure in the fresh gas circuit. At a constant fresh gas flow rate, the operator regulates vapor flow using a conventional concentration control dial. When the fresh gas flow rate increases, the working pressure increases proportionally. At a specific dial setting at different fresh gas flow rates, vaporizer output is constant because the amount of flow through each circuit is proportional.[72]

The Datex-Ohmeda Aladin Cassette Vaporizer

The vaporizer system used in the Datex-Ohmeda Anesthesia Delivery Unit (ADU) is unique, and the electronically controlled vaporizer is designed to deliver five different inhaled anesthetics including halothane, isoflurane, enflurane, sevoflurane, and desflurane. The vaporizer consists of a permanent internal control unit housed within the ADU and an interchangeable Aladin agent cassette which contains anesthetic liquid. The Aladin agent cassettes are color-coded for each anesthetic agent, and they are also magnetically coded so that the Datex Ohmeda ADU can identify which anesthetic cassette has been inserted. The cassettes are filled using agent-specific fillers.[41,79]

The anatomy of the ADU vaporizer (see Fig. 22-19) is very similar to that of the Dräger vapor 19.1 and the Ohmeda Tec 4 vaporizer, and it is made up of the bypass chamber and vaporizing chamber. A fixed restrictor is located in the bypass chamber, and flow measurement units are located in the bypass chamber and in the outlet of the vaporizing chamber. The heart of the ADU vaporizer is the electronically controlled flow control valve located in the vaporizing chamber outlet. This valve is controlled by a central processing unit (CPU). The CPU receives input from multiple sources including the concentration control dial, a pressure sensor located inside the vaporizing chamber, a temperature sensor located inside the vaporizing chamber, a flow measurement unit located in the bypass chamber, and a flow measurement unit located in the outlet of the vaporizing chamber. The CPU also receives input from the flow meters regarding the composition of the carrier gas. Using data from these multiple sources, the CPU is able to precisely regulate the flow control valve to attain the desired vapor concentration. Appropriate electronic control of the flow control valve is essential to the proper function of this vaporizer.[41,79]

A fixed restrictor is located in the bypass chamber, and it causes the vaporizer inlet flow to split into two portions (see Fig. 22-19). One portion passes through the bypass chamber, and the other portion enters the inlet of the vaporizing chamber and passes through a one-way check valve. The one-way check valve protects against back flow of agent into the bypass chamber.[41] A precise amount of carrier gas flow and vapor flow passes through the flow control valve, which is regulated by the CPU. This flow then joins the bypass flow to the outlet of the vaporizer.[41,79]

Vaporization of desflurane presents a unique challenge, particularly when the room temperature is greater than the boiling point of desflurane (22.8°C). At higher temperatures, the pressure inside the sump increases, and the sump becomes pressurized. When the sump pressure exceeds the pressure in the bypass chamber, the one-way check valve located in the vaporizing chamber inlet closes shut, preventing carrier gas from entering the vaporizing chamber. Then, the carrier gas passes straight through the bypass chamber. Under these conditions, the electronically controlled flow control valve simply meters in the appropriate flow of pure desflurane vapor.

When large quantities of anesthetic liquid are vaporized during high fresh gas flow rates and/or high dial settings, the vaporizer cools because of the latent heat of vaporization. To offset this cooling effect, the ADU is equipped with a fan which warms the vaporizer back up toward room temperature. The fan is activated during two common clinical scenarios: (1) desflurane induction and maintenance, and (2) sevoflurane induction.

ANESTHETIC CIRCUITS

Gas exits the anesthesia machine at the common gas outlet and then enters an anesthetic circuit. The function of an anesthetic circuit is not only to deliver oxygen and anesthetic gases to the patient, but also to eliminate carbon dioxide. Carbon dioxide can be removed either by washout with adequate fresh gas

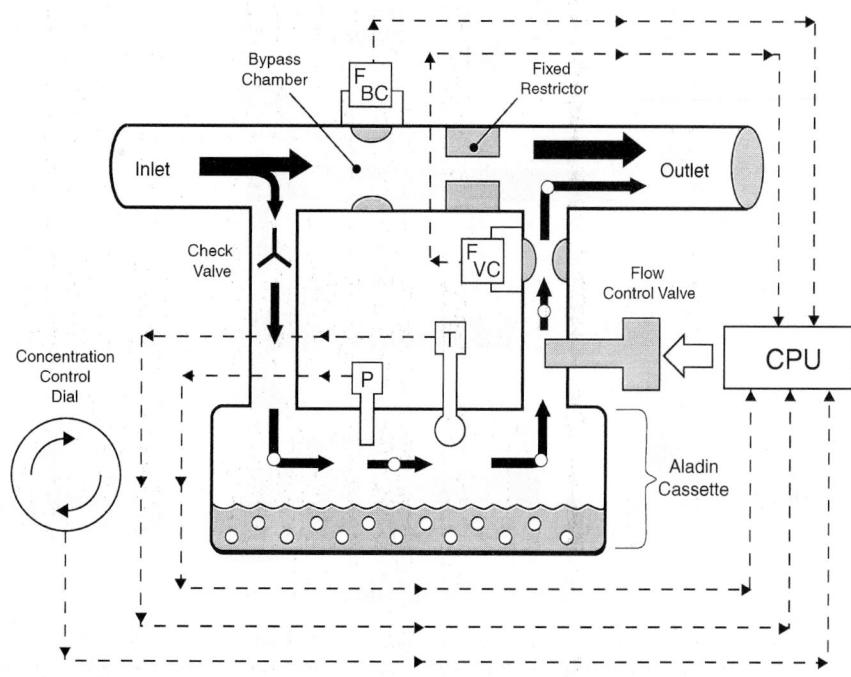

Figure 22-19. Simplified schematic of the Datex-Ohmeda Aladin Cassette Vaporizer. The black arrows represent flow from the flowmeters, and the white circles represent anesthetic vapor. The heart of the vaporizer is the electronically controlled flow control valve located in the outlet of the vaporizing chamber. CPU = central processing unit; F_{BC} = flow measurement unit that measures flow through the bypass chamber; F_{VC} = flow measurement unit that measures flow through the vaporizing chamber; P = pressure sensor; T = temperature sensor. (Modified with permission from Andrews JJ: Operating Principles of the Datex-Ohmeda Aladin Cassette Vaporizer: A Collection of Twelve Color Illustrations. Washington, D.C., Library of Congress, 2000.)

inflow or by soda lime absorption. This discussion is limited to semiclosed rebreathing circuits and the circle system.

Mapleson Systems

In 1954 Mapleson described and analyzed five different semiclosed anesthetic systems; these are now classically referred to as the Mapleson systems, designated A to E.[80] Willis *et al* added the F system to the original five.[81] The Mapleson systems are shown in Figure 22-20. System components can include a face mask, a spring-loaded pop-off valve, reservoir tubing, fresh gas inflow tubing, and a reservoir bag. Three distinct functional groups emerge—the A, the BC, and DEF groups. The Mapleson A, also known as the Magill circuit, has a spring-loaded pop-off valve located near the face mask, and the fresh gas flow enters the opposite end of the circuit near the reservoir bag. In the B and C systems, the spring-loaded pop-off valve is located near the face mask, but the fresh gas inlet tubing is located near the patient. The reservoir tubing and breathing bag serve as a blind limb where fresh gas, dead space gas, and alveolar gas can collect. Finally, in the Mapleson DEF group, or T-piece group, the fresh gas enters near the patient, and excess gas is popped off at the opposite end of the circuit.

Even though the component arrangement and components are simple, functional analysis of the Mapleson systems can be complex.[82,83] The amount of carbon dioxide rebreathing associated with each system is multifactorial, and variables that dictate the ultimate carbon dioxide concentration include the following: (1) the fresh gas inflow rate, (2) the minute ventilation, (3) the mode of ventilation (spontaneous or controlled), (4) the tidal volume, (5) the respiratory rate, (6) the I:E ratio, (7) the duration of the expiratory pause, (8) the peak inspiratory flow rate, (9) the volume of the reservoir tube, (10) the volume of the breathing bag, (11) ventilation by mask, (12) ventilation through an endotracheal tube, and (13) the CO_2 sampling site.

The performance of the Mapleson systems is best understood by studying the expiratory phase of the respiratory cycle (Fig. 22-20).[84] During spontaneous ventilation, the Mapleson A has the best efficiency of the six systems, requiring a fresh gas inflow rate of just 1 times the minute ventilation to prevent rebreathing of carbon dioxide. But it has the worst efficiency during controlled ventilation, requiring a minute ventilation as much as $20 \; 1 \cdot min^{-1}$ to prevent rebreathing. Systems DEF are slightly more efficient than systems BC. To prevent rebreathing CO_2, the DEF systems require a fresh gas inflow rate of approximately 2.5 times the minute ventilation, whereas the fresh gas inflow rates required for BC systems are somewhat higher.[83]

To summarize the relative efficiency of different Mapleson systems with respect to prevention of rebreathing: during spontaneous ventilation, A > DFE > CB; during controlled ventilation, DFE > BC > A.[83,85] The Mapleson A, B, and C systems are

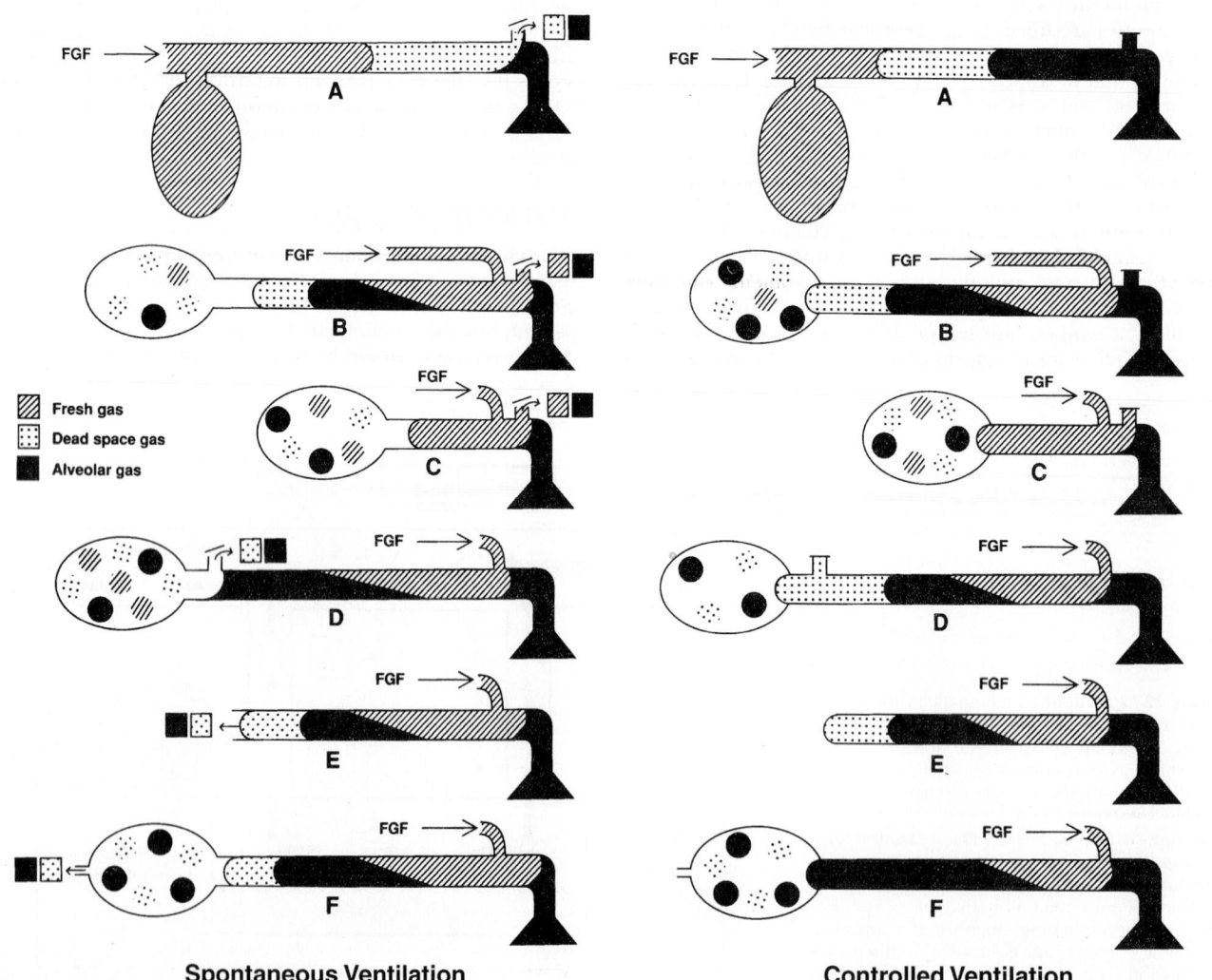

Spontaneous Ventilation   **Controlled Ventilation**

Figure 22-20. Gas disposition at end expiration during spontaneous (*left*) and controlled (*right*) ventilation in circuits A–F. FGF = fresh gas flow. (Modified with permission from Sykes MK: Rebreathing circuits: A review. Br J Anaesth 40:666, 1968.)

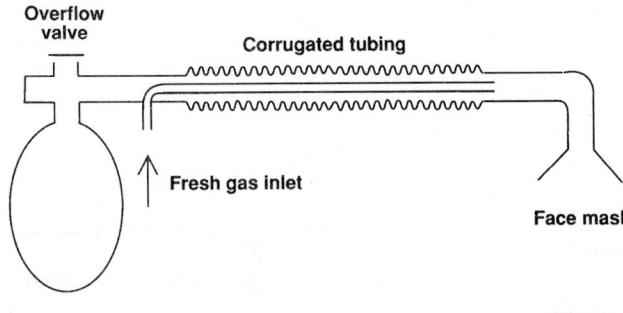

Figure 22-21. The Bain circuit. (Redrawn with permission from Bain JA, Spoerel WE: A streamlined anaesthetic system. Can Anaesth Soc J 19:426, 1972.)

rarely used today, but the DEF systems are commonly employed. In the United States, the most popular representative from the DEF group is the Bain circuit.

Bain Circuit

The Bain circuit is a modification of the Mapleson D system. It is a coaxial circuit in which the fresh gas flows through a narrow inner tube within the outer corrugated tubing.[86] The central tube originates near the reservoir bag, but the fresh gas actually enters the circuit at the patient end (Fig. 22-21). Exhaled gases enter the corrugated tubing and are vented through the expiratory valve near the reservoir bag. The Bain circuit may be used for both spontaneous and controlled ventilation. The fresh gas inflow rate necessary to prevent rebreathing is 2.5 times the minute ventilation.

There are many advantages to this circuit. It is lightweight, convenient, easily sterilized, and reusable. Scavenging of the gases from the expiratory valve is facilitated because the valve is located away from the patient. Exhaled gases in the outer reservoir tubing add warmth to inspired fresh gases. The hazards of the Bain circuit include unrecognized disconnection or kinking of the inner fresh gas hose. These problems can cause hypercarbia from inadequate gas flow or increased respiratory resistance. An obstructed bacterial filter positioned between the Bain circuit and the endotracheal tube can cause hypoxemia and mimic the signs and symptoms of severe bronchospasm.[87]

The outer tube should be transparent to allow inspection of the inner tube. The integrity of the inner tube can be assessed as described by Pethick.[88] High-flow oxygen is fed into the circuit while the patient end is occluded until the reservoir bag is filled. The patient end is opened and oxygen is flushed into the circuit. If the inner tube is intact, the Venturi effect occurs at the patient end. This effect causes a decrease in pressure within the circuit, and the reservoir bag deflates. Conversely, a leak in the inner tube allows the fresh gas to escape into the expiratory limb, and the reservoir bag will remain inflated. This test is recommended as a part of the preanesthesia check if a Bain circuit is used.

Circle System

The circle system is the most popular breathing system in the United States. It is so named because its components are arranged in a circular manner. This system prevents rebreathing of carbon dioxide by soda lime absorption but allows partial rebreathing of other exhaled gases. The extent of rebreathing of the other exhaled gases depends on component arrangement and the fresh gas flow rate.

A circle system can be semiopen, semiclosed, or closed, depending on the amount of fresh gas inflow.[89] A *semiopen system* has no rebreathing and requires a very high flow of fresh gas. A *semiclosed system* is associated with rebreathing of gases and is

the most commonly used system in the United States. A *closed system* is one in which the inflow gas exactly matches that being taken up, or consumed, by the patient. There is complete rebreathing of exhaled gases after absorption of carbon dioxide, and the overflow (pop-off) valve is closed.

The circle system (Fig. 22-22) consists of seven components, including the following: (1) a fresh gas inflow source; (2) inspiratory and expiratory unidirectional valves; (3) inspiratory and expiratory corrugated tubes; (4) a Y-piece connector; (5) an overflow or pop-off valve, referred to as the adjustable pressure-limiting (APL) valve; (6) a reservoir bag; and (7) a canister containing a carbon dioxide absorbent. The unidirectional valves are placed in the system to ensure unidirectional flow through the corrugated hoses. The fresh gas inflow enters the circle by a connection from the common gas outlet of the anesthesia machine.

Numerous variations of the circle arrangement are possible, depending on the relative positions of the unidirectional valves, the pop-off valve, the reservoir bag, the carbon dioxide absorber, and the site of fresh gas entry. However, to prevent rebreathing of carbon dioxide, three rules must be followed: (1) a unidirectional valve must be located between the patient and the reservoir bag on both the inspiratory and expiratory limbs of the circuit; (2) the fresh gas inflow cannot enter the circuit between the expiratory valve and the patient; and (3) the overflow (pop-off) valve cannot be located between the patient and the inspiratory valve. If these rules are followed, any arrangement of the other components will prevent rebreathing of carbon dioxide.[90]

The most efficient circle system arrangement that allows the highest conservation of fresh gases is one with the unidirectional valves near the patient and the pop-off valve just downstream from the expiratory valve. This arrangement conserves dead space gas and preferentially eliminates alveolar gas. A more practical arrangement, used on all contemporary anesthesia machines (Fig. 22-22), is less efficient because it allows alveolar and dead space gas to mix before venting.[90,91]

The advantages of the circle system include relative stability of inspired concentration, conservation of respiratory moisture and heat, and prevention of operating room pollution. Additionally, it can be used for closed-system anesthesia or with low oxygen flows. The major disadvantage of the circle system stems from its complex design. The circle system has approximately 10 connections, and the multiple connection sites set the stage for misconnections, disconnections, obstructions, and leaks. In a closed-claim analysis of adverse anesthetic outcomes arising

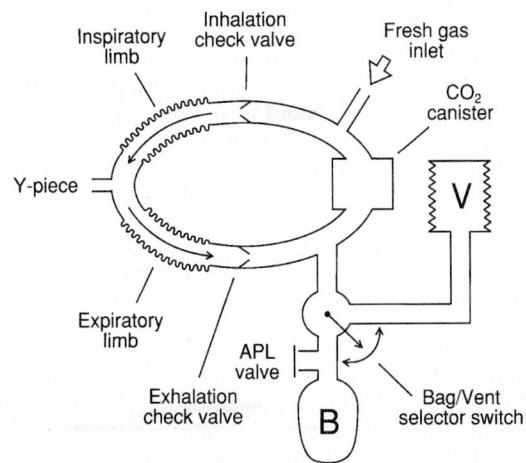

Figure 22-22. Components of the circle system. B = reservoir bag; V = ventilator; APL = adjustable pressure limiting. (Reproduced with permission from Andrews JJ: Inhaled anesthetic delivery systems. In Miller RD (ed): Anesthesia, 5th ed, p 174. Philadelphia, Churchill Livingstone, 1999.)

from gas delivery equipment, a third (25/72) of malpractice claims resulted from breathing circuit misconnections or disconnections.[2] Malfunctioning valves can cause serious problems. Rebreathing can occur if the valves stick in the open position, and total occlusion of the circuit can occur if they are stuck closed. If the expiratory valve is stuck shut, breath stacking and tension pneumothorax can occur. Obstructed filters located in the expiratory limb of the circle breathing system have caused increased airway pressures, hemodynamic collapse, and bilateral tension pneumothorax. Causes of expiratory filter obstruction include defective filters, patient secretions, and albuterol nebulization.[92-94] The Datex-Ohmeda 7900 series Smart Ventilator uses flow transducers on both the inspiratory and expiratory limb of the circle system. Cracked flow transducer tubing can cause a leak in the circle system that is difficult to detect.[95]

CARBON DIOXIDE ABSORPTION

Different anesthesia systems eliminate carbon dioxide with varying degrees of efficiency. The closed and semiclosed circle system both require carbon dioxide absorption. Desirable features of carbon dioxide absorbents include lack of toxicity with common anesthetics, low resistance to air flow, low cost, ease of handling, and efficiency.

The Absorber Canister

On modern anesthesia machines, the absorber canister (see Fig. 22-22) is composed of two clear plastic canisters arranged in series. The canisters can be filled either with bulk absorbent or with absorbent supplied by the factory in prefilled plastic disposable cartridges called prepacks. Free granules from bulk absorbent can create a clinically significant leak if they lodge between the clear plastic canister and the O-ring gasket of the absorber. Leaks have also been caused by defective prepacks which were larger than factory specifications.[96] Prepacks can also cause total obstruction of the circle system if the clear plastic shipping wrapper is not removed prior to use.[97]

Chemistry of Absorbents

Two formulations of carbon dioxide absorbents are commonly used today: These are soda lime and baralyme.

By weight, the approximate composition of "high moisture" soda lime is 80% calcium hydroxide, 15% water, 4% sodium hydroxide, and 1% potassium hydroxide (an activator). Small amounts of silica are added to produce calcium and sodium silicate. This addition produces a hard compound and reduces dust formation. The efficiency of the soda lime absorption varies inversely with hardness; therefore, little silicate is used in contemporary soda lime. Sodium hydroxide is the catalyst for the carbon dioxide absorptive properties of soda lime.[98,99] Baralyme is a mixture of approximately 20% barium hydroxide and 80% calcium hydroxide. It may also contain some potassium hydroxide.

The size of the absorptive granules has been determined by trial and error, which represents a compromise between resistance to air flow and absorptive efficiency.[100] The smaller the granules, the more surface area is available for absorption. However, air flow resistance increases. The granular size of soda lime and baralyme in anesthesia practice is between 4 and 8 mesh, a size at which resistance to air flow is negligible. "Mesh" refers to the number of openings per linear inch in a sieve through which the granular particles can pass. A 4-mesh screen means that there are 4 quarter-inch openings per linear inch. An 8-mesh screen has 8 eighth-inch openings per linear inch.[98]

The absorption of carbon dioxide by soda lime is a chemical process, not a physical process. Carbon dioxide combines with water to form carbonic acid. Carbonic acid reacts with the hy-

droxides to form sodium (or potassium) carbonate and water. Calcium hydroxide accepts the carbonate to form calcium carbonate and sodium (or potassium) hydroxide. The equations are as follows:

1. $CO_2 + H_2O \Leftrightarrow H_2CO_3$
2. $H_2CO_3 + 2NaOH \text{ (KOH)} \Leftrightarrow Na_2CO_3 \text{ (}K_2CO_3\text{)} + 2H_2O + \text{Heat}$
3. $Na_2CO_3 \text{ (}K_2CO_3\text{)} + Ca(OH)_2 \Leftrightarrow CaCO_3 + 2NaOH \text{ (KOH)}$

Some carbon dioxide may react directly with $Ca(OH)_2$, but this reaction is much slower.

The reaction with baralyme differs from that of soda lime because more water is liberated by a direct reaction of barium hydroxide and carbon dioxide:

1. $Ba(OH)_2 + 8H_2O + CO_2 \Leftrightarrow BaCO_3 + 9H_2O + \text{Heat}$
2. $9H_2O + 9CO_2 \Leftrightarrow 9H_2CO_3$

Then by direct reactions and by KOH and NaOH,

3. $9H_2CO_3 + 9Ca(OH)_2 \Leftrightarrow CaCO_3 + 18H_2O + \text{Heat}$

Absorptive Capacity

The maximum amount of carbon dioxide that can be absorbed is 26 l of CO_2 per 100 g of absorbent. However, channeling of gas through granules may substantially decrease this efficiency and allow only 10–20 l of carbon dioxide to actually be absorbed.[101]

Indicators

Ethyl violet, the pH indicator added to both soda lime and baralyme to help assess the functional integrity of the absorbent, is a substituted triphenylmethane dye with a critical pH of 10.3.[99] Ethyl violet changes from colorless to violet when the pH of the absorbent decreases as a result of carbon dioxide absorption. The pH of fresh absorbent exceeds the critical pH, so the dye exists in its colorless form (Fig. 22-23, left). As absorbent becomes exhausted, however, the pH decreases below 10.3, so ethyl violet changes to its violet form (Fig. 22-23, right) through alcohol dehydration. Ethyl violet is not always a reliable indicator of the functional status of absorbent. Fluorescent lights can deactivate the dye so that the absorbent appears white even though it is exhausted.[102]

Interactions of Inhaled Anesthetics with Absorbents

It is important and desirable to have carbon dioxide absorbents that are neither intrinsically toxic nor toxic when exposed to common anesthetics. Soda lime and baralyme generally fit this description, but inhaled anesthetics do interact with absorbents to some extent. Historically speaking, an uncommon anesthetic, trichloroethylene, reacts with soda lime to produce toxic com-

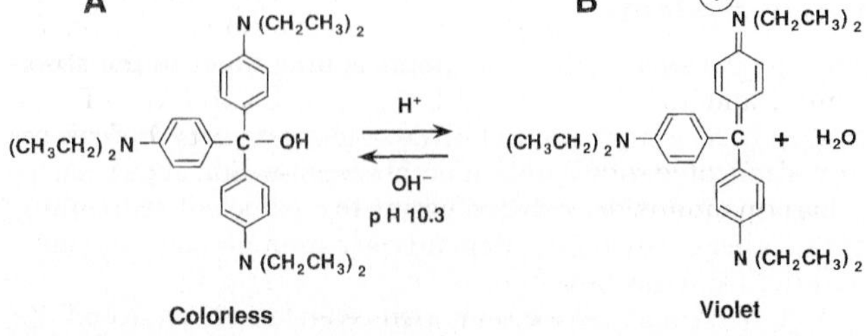

Figure 22-23. (A and B). Ethyl violet. (Reprinted with permission from Andrews JJ, Johnston RV Jr, Bee DE, Arens JF: Photodeactivation of ethyl violet: A potential hazard of sodasorb. Anesthesiology 72:59, 1990.)

pounds. In the presence of alkali and heat, trichloroethylene degrades into dichloroacetylene, which can cause cranial nerve lesions and encephalitis. Phosgene, a potent pulmonary irritant, is also produced, and phosgene can cause adult respiratory distress syndrome (ARDS).[103]

Sevoflurane has been shown to produce degradation products upon interaction with carbon dioxide absorbents.[104] The major degradation product produced is fluoromethyl-2,2-difluoro-1-(trifluoromethyl)vinyl ether, or *Compound A*. During sevoflurane anesthesia, factors apparently leading to an increase in the concentration of Compound A include: (1) low flow or closed-circuit anesthetic techniques; (2) the use of baralyme rather than soda lime; (3) higher concentrations of sevoflurane in the anesthetic circuit; (4) higher absorbent temperatures; and (5) fresh absorbent.[104-106] Baralyme dehydration increases the concentration of Compound A, and soda lime dehydration decreases the concentration of Compound A.[107,108] Apparently, the degradation products do not cause toxic effects in humans even during low-flow anesthesia,[105] but further studies are needed to verify this.[109-111]

Desiccated soda lime and baralyme can degrade contemporary inhaled anesthetics to clinically significant concentrations of carbon monoxide (CO), which in turn can produce carboxyhemoglobin concentrations reaching 30% or more.[112] Higher levels of carbon monoxide are more likely after prolonged contact between absorbent and anesthetics, and after disuse of an absorber for at least two days, especially over a weekend. Thus, case reports describing carbon monoxide poisoning have been most common in patients anesthetized on Monday morning, presumably because continuous flow from the anesthesia machine dehydrated the absorbents over the weekend.[113,114] A fresh gas flow rate of $5\,l\cdot min^{-1}$ or more through absorbent (without a patient) is sufficient to cause critical drying of the absorbent, particularly if the breathing bag is left off the breathing circuit. Absence of the bag facilitates retrograde flow through the circle system (see Fig. 22-22).[112] Because the inspiratory valve leaflet produces some resistance to flow, the fresh gas flow takes the retrograde path of least resistance through the absorbent and out the 22-mm breathing bag terminal.

Several factors appear to increase the production of carbon monoxide and carboxyhemoglobin: (1) the inhaled anesthetic used (for a given MAC multiple, the magnitude of CO production from greatest to least is desflurane ≥ enflurane > isoflurane ≫ halothane = sevoflurane); (2) the absorbent dryness (completely dry absorbent produces more CO than hydrated absorbent); (3) the type of absorbent (at a given water content, baralyme produces more CO than does soda lime); (4) the temperature (an increased temperature increases CO production); (5) the anesthetic concentration (more CO is produced from higher anesthetic concentrations)[115]; (6) low fresh gas flow rates; and (7) reduced animal size.[116]

Interventions have been suggested to reduce the incidence of carbon monoxide exposure in humans undergoing general anesthesia.[114] The interventions include: (1) educating anesthesia personnel regarding the etiology of CO production; (2) turning off the anesthesia machine at the conclusion of the last case of the day to eliminate fresh gas flow which dries the absorbent; (3) changing carbon dioxide absorbent if fresh gas was found flowing during the morning machine check; (4) rehydrating desiccated absorbent by adding water to the absorbent[113]; and (5) changing the chemical composition of soda lime. The elimination of sodium and potassium hydroxides from desiccated soda lime diminishes degradation of desflurane to carbon monoxide and sevoflurane to Compound A, but does not compromise carbon dioxide absorption.[117]

ANESTHESIA VENTILATORS

The anesthesia ventilator can substitute for the breathing bag of the circle system, the Bain circuit, and other breathing systems. Ten years ago, anesthesia ventilators were mere adjuncts to the anesthesia machine. Today, they have attained a prominent central role in newer anesthesia systems. This discussion focuses on the classification, operating principles, and hazards of anesthesia ventilators.

Classification

Ventilators can be classified according to their power source, drive mechanism, cycling mechanism, and bellows type.[118,119] The following section reviews ventilator classification and terminology before the discussion of individual anesthesia machine ventilators.

Power Source

The power source required to operate a mechanical ventilator is provided by compressed gas, electricity, or both. Older pneumatic ventilators required only a pneumatic power source to function properly. Contemporary North American Dräger and Ohmeda electronic ventilators require both an electronic and a pneumatic power source.[16,18-22,120,121]

Drive Mechanism

Most anesthesia machine ventilators are classified as double-circuit, pneumatically driven ventilators. In a double-circuit system, a driving force (compressed gas) compresses a bag or bellows, which in turn delivers gas to the patient. The driving gas in the Ohmeda 7000, 7810, and 7900 is 100% oxygen.[16,120,121] In the North American Dräger AV-E, a Venturi device mixes oxygen and air.[18-22]

Cycling Mechanism

Most anesthesia machine ventilators are time-cycled and provide ventilator support in the control mode. Inspiration is initiated by a timing device. Older pneumatic ventilators use a fluidic timing device. Contemporary electronic ventilators use a solid-state timing device and are thus classified as time-cycled and electronically controlled.

Bellows Classification

The direction of bellows movement during the expiratory phase determines the bellows classification. *Ascending (standing) bellows* ascend during the expiratory phase (Fig. 22-24, *right*), whereas *descending (hanging) bellows* descend during the expiratory phase. Older pneumatic ventilators use weighted descending bellows, while most contemporary electronic ventilators have ascending bellows. Of the two configurations, the ascending bellows is safer. An ascending bellows will not fill if a total disconnection occurs. The bellows of a descending bellows ventilator, however, will continue its up-and-down movement during a disconnection. The driving gas pushes the bellows upward during the inspiratory phase. During the expiratory phase, room air is entrained into the breathing system at the site of the disconnection because gravity acts on the weighted bellows. The disconnection pressure monitor and the volume monitor may be fooled even if a disconnection is complete[1] (see Breathing Circuit Problems).

Operating Principles of Ascending Bellows Ventilators

Contemporary examples of ascending bellows, double-circuit, electronic ventilators include the North American Dräger AV-E and the Ohmeda 7000, 7800, and 7900 series. A generic ascending bellows ventilator is shown in Figure 22-24. It may be viewed as a breathing bag (bellows) located within a clear plastic box. The bellows physically separates the driving gas circuit from the patient gas circuit. The driving gas circuit is located outside the bellows, and the patient gas circuit is inside the bellows. During the inspiratory phase (Fig. 22-24, *left*) the

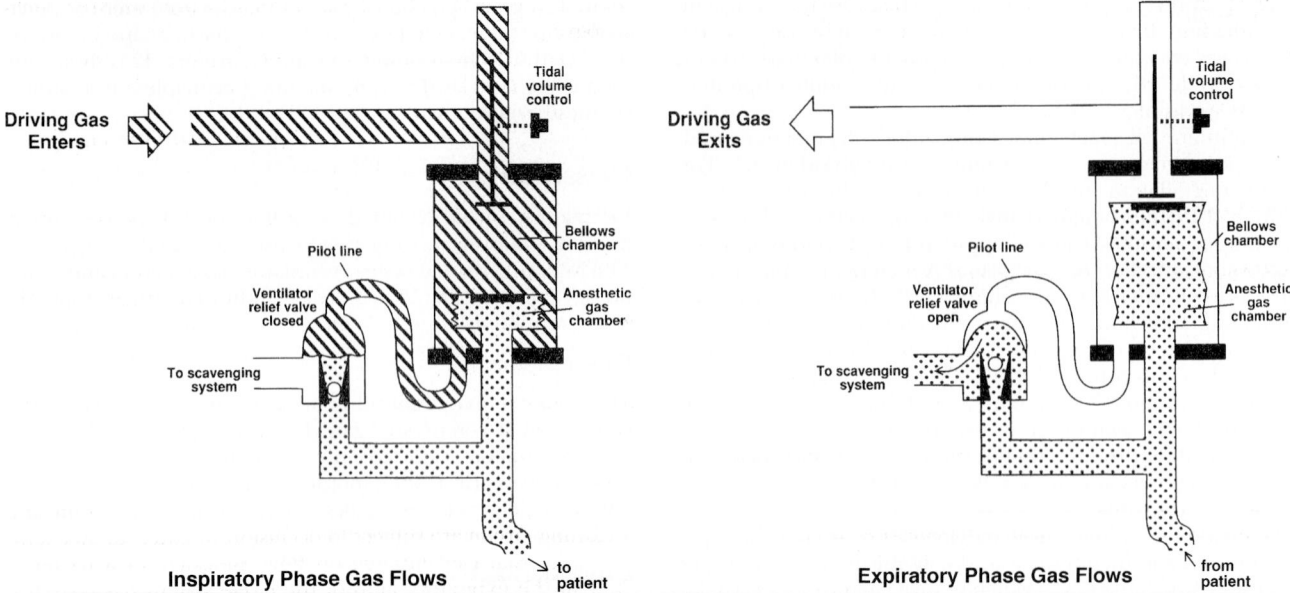

Figure 22-24. Inspiratory and expiratory phase gas flows of a generic ascending bellows anesthesia ventilator. (Reprinted with permission from Andrews JJ: Understanding your anesthesia machine and ventilator. In 1989 Review Course Lectures, p 59. Cleveland, International Anesthesia Research Society, 1989.)

driving gas enters the bellows chamber, causing the pressure within it to increase. This increase in pressure is responsible for two events. First, the ventilator relief valve closes, preventing anesthetic gas from escaping into the scavenging system. Second, the bellows is compressed, and the anesthetic gas within the bellows is delivered to the patient's lungs. This compression action is analogous to the hand of the anesthesiologist squeezing the breathing bag.[39]

During the expiratory phase (Fig. 22-24, *right*), the driving gas exits the bellows chamber. The pressure within the bellows chamber and the pilot line declines to zero, causing the mushroom portion of the ventilator relief valve to open. Exhaled patient gas fills the bellows before any scavenging. This occurs because a weighted ball similar to those used in ball-type positive end expiratory pressure (PEEP) valves is incorporated into the base of the ventilator relief valve. The ball produces 2–3 cm water of back pressure; therefore scavenging occurs only after the bellows fills completely and the pressure inside the bellows exceeds this pressure threshold. This design causes all ascending bellows ventilators to produce 2–3 cm water pressure of PEEP within the breathing circuit. Scavenging occurs only during the expiratory phase, as the ventilator relief valve is open only during expiration.[39]

Gas flow from the anesthesia machine into the breathing circuit is continuous and independent of ventilator activity. During the inspiratory phase of mechanical ventilation, the ventilator relief valve is closed, and the breathing system's APL valve (pop-off valve) is either closed or out of circuit. Therefore, the patient receives volume from the bellows and flowmeters during the inspiratory phase. Factors that influence the correlation between set tidal volume and exhaled tidal volume include the flowmeter settings, the inspiratory time, the compliance of the breathing circuit, external leakage, and the location of the tidal volume sensor.[16,17,120,121] Usually, the volume gained from the flowmeters during inspiration is counteracted by the volume lost to the breathing circuit compliance. The set tidal volume generally approximates the exhaled tidal volume. However, oxygen flushing during the inspiratory phase can result in barotrauma because excess volume cannot be vented.[39]

Problems and Hazards

Numerous hazards are associated with anesthesia ventilators. These include problems with the breathing circuit, the bellows assembly, and the control assembly.

Breathing Circuit Problems

Breathing circuit disconnection is a leading cause of critical incidents in anesthesia.[2,122] The most common disconnection site is at the Y-piece. Disconnections can be complete or partial (leaks). A common source of leaks with older absorbers is failure to close the APL valve (pop-off valve) upon initiation of mechanical ventilation. The bag/ventilator switch on contemporary absorbers helps minimize this problem. Pre-existing undetected leaks can occur in compressed, corrugated, disposable anesthetic circuits. To detect such a leak preoperatively, the circuit must be fully expanded before the circuit is checked for leaks.[123] As mentioned above, disconnections and leaks manifest more readily with the ascending bellows because the bellows will not fill.[1]

Several disconnection monitors exist. The most important monitor is a vigilant anesthesia care provider monitoring breath sounds, chest wall excursion, and mechanical monitors.

Pneumatic and electronic pressure monitors are helpful in diagnosing disconnections. Factors that influence monitor effectiveness include the disconnection site, the pressure sensor location, the threshold pressure alarm limit, the inspiratory flow rate, and the resistance of the disconnected breathing circuit.[124,125] Various anesthesia machines and ventilators have different locations for the pressure sensor and different values for the threshold pressure alarm limit (Table 22-3). The threshold pressure alarm limit may be preset at the factory or adjustable. An audible or visual alarm is actuated if the peak inspiratory pressure of the breathing circuit does not exceed the threshold pressure alarm limit. When an adjustable threshold pressure alarm limit is available, such as on the North American Dräger Narkomed 2A, 2B, 3, and 4, the operator should set the pressure alarm limit to within 5 cm water of the peak inspiratory pressure.[15–19] Figure 22-25 illustrates how a partial disconnection

Table 22-3. DISCONNECTION PRESSURE MONITORS

Machine/ Ventilator	Location of Pressure Sensor	Threshold Pressure Alarm Limit (cm water)
OHMEDA MODULUS II		
GMS Absorber Ohmed 7000 Vent	Patient side of expiratory valve	6
OHMEDA MODULUS II PLUS		
GMS Absorber Ohmeda 7810	Patient side of inspiratory valve	Δ4–9 PEEP compensated
NAD NARKOMED 2A		
NAD AV-E	CO_2 absorber or Y-piece	8, 12, 26
NAD NARKOMED 2B,3		
NAD AV-E	CO_2 absorber or Y-piece	5→30 (12 default)

Data from Ohmeda[12,13,16,120,121] and North American Dräger.[18–21]

(leak) may be unrecognized by the low-pressure monitor if the threshold pressure alarm limit is set too low or if the factory preset value is relatively low.

Respiratory volume monitors are useful in detecting disconnections. Volume monitors sense exhaled tidal volume, minute volume, or both. The user should bracket the high and low threshold volumes slightly above and below the exhaled volumes. For example, if the exhaled minute volume of a patient is $10 \, l \cdot min^{-1}$, reasonable alarm limits would be $8–12 \, l \cdot min^{-1}$. Some Datex-Ohmeda ventilators are equipped with volume monitor sensors that use infrared light/turbine technology. The volume sensor is located in the expiratory limb of the breathing circuit. Exposure of the sensor clip to a direct beam of overhead surgical lighting can cause erroneous volume readings

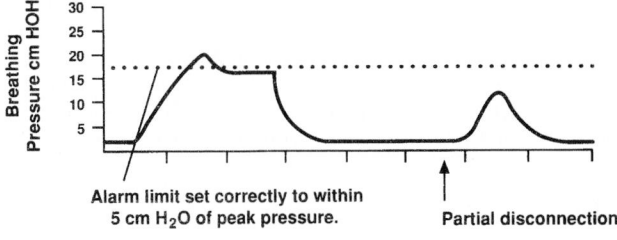

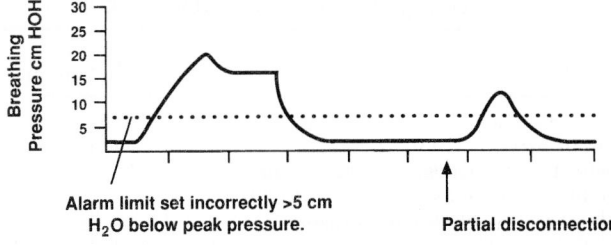

Figure 22-25. Threshold pressure alarm limit. (*Top*) The threshold pressure alarm limit (*dotted line*) has been set appropriately. An alarm is actuated when a partial disconnection occurs (*arrow*) because the threshold pressure alarm limit is not exceeded by the breathing circuit pressure. (*Bottom*) A partial disconnection is unrecognized by the pressure monitor because the threshold pressure alarm limit has been set too low. (Redrawn with permission from Baromed Breathing Pressure Monitor. Operator's Instruction Manual. Telford, PA, North American Dräger, 1986.)

because the surgical beam interferes with the infrared technology.[126]

Carbon dioxide monitors are probably the best devices for revealing patient disconnections. Carbon dioxide concentration is measured near the Y-piece either directly or by aspiration of a gas sample to the instrument. A drastic change in the differences between the inspiratory and end-tidal carbon dioxide concentration or the absence of carbon dioxide indicates a disconnection, a nonventilated patient, or other problems.[1]

Misconnections of the breathing system are not uncommon, despite efforts by standards committees to eliminate this problem by assigning different diameters to various hoses and terminals. Anesthesia machines, breathing systems, ventilators, and scavenging systems incorporate a multitude of hose terminals. Hoses have been connected to inappropriate terminals and even to various solid cylindrically shaped protrusions of the anesthesia machine.[1]

Occlusion (obstruction) of the breathing circuit may occur. Tracheal tubes can become kinked. Hoses throughout the breathing circuit are subject to occlusion by external mechanical forces that can impinge on flow. Blockage of a bacterial filter in the expiratory limb of the circle system has caused a bilateral tension pneumothorax.[93] Incorrect insertion of flow direction–sensitive components can result in a no-flow state.[1] Examples of these components include some PEEP valves and cascade humidifiers. Depending on the location of the occlusion and the pressure sensor, a high-pressure alarm may alert the anesthesiologist to the problem.

Excess inflow to the breathing circuit from the anesthesia machine during the inspiratory phase can cause barotrauma. The best example of this phenomenon is oxygen flushing. Excess volume cannot be vented from the system during inspiration because the ventilator relief valve is closed and the APL valve is either out of circuit or closed.[39] A high-pressure alarm, if present, may be activated when the pressure becomes excessive. In the North American Dräger System, both audible and visual alarms are actuated when the high-pressure threshold is exceeded.[18–22] In the Modulus II Plus System, the Ohmeda 7810 ventilator automatically switches from the inspiratory to the expiratory phase when the adjustable peak pressure threshold is exceeded.[16] This minimizes the possibility of barotrauma if the peak pressure threshold is set appropriately by the anesthesiologist.

Bellows Assembly Problems

Leaks can occur in the bellows assembly. Improper seating of the plastic bellows housing can result in inadequate ventilation because a portion of the driving gas is vented to the atmosphere. A hole in the bellows can lead to alveolar hyperinflation and possibly barotrauma in some ventilators because high-pressure driving gas can enter the patient circuit. The value on the oxygen analyzer may increase when the driving gas is 100% oxygen, or it may decrease if the driving gas is composed of an air–oxygen mixture.[127]

The ventilator relief valve can cause problems. Hypoventilation occurs if the valve is incompetent because anesthetic gas is delivered to the scavenging system during the inspiratory phase instead of to the patient. Gas molecules preferentially exit into the scavenging system because it represents the path of least resistance, and the pressure within the scavenging system can be subatmospheric. Ventilator relief valve incompetency can result from a disconnected pilot line, a ruptured valve, or from a damaged flapper valve.[128,129] A ventilator relief valve stuck in the closed position can produce barotrauma. Excessive suction from the scavenging system can draw the ventilator relief valve to its seat and close the valve during both the inspiratory and expiratory phases.[1] Breathing circuit pressure escalates because excess anesthetic gas cannot be vented.

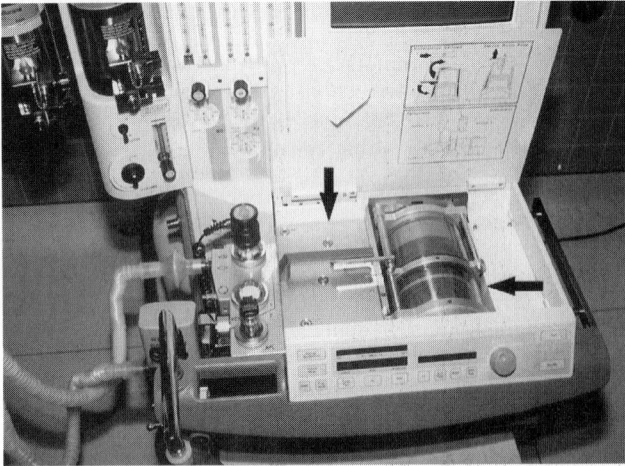

Figure 22-26. The Narkomed 6000. The horizontal arrow indicates the piston cylinder unit. The vertical arrow indicates a rectangular manifold that houses the valves for fresh gas decoupling.

Control Assembly Problems

The control assembly can be the source of both electrical and mechanical problems. Electrical failure can be total or partial; the former is the more obvious. Some mechanical problems include leaks within the system, faulty regulators, and faulty valves. An occluded muffler on the North American Dräger AV-E can cause barotrauma. Obstruction of driving gas outflow closes the ventilator relief valve, and excess patient gas cannot be vented.[130]

Narkomed 6000 Piston Ventilator

The Narkomed 6000 ventilator may be classified as an electrically powered, piston-driven, single-circuit, electronically controlled ventilator with fresh gas decoupling. Unlike traditional double-circuit operating room ventilators that use compressed gas to drive the bellows, the 6000 uses a piston. The piston cylinder unit (see Fig. 22-26) consists of an outer cylinder and an internal piston that is controlled by a precise motor gear unit. The piston is sealed by two membranes, and patient gas is contained inside the piston unit. With volume-controlled IPPV or SIMV, the piston stops during plateau time in the end position. When the maximum airway pressure is reached in the volume-controlled or pressure-controlled ventilation, inspiratory flow will be reduced so that the pressure is held at a constant level.[131]

With traditional ascending bellows ventilators during the inspiratory phase, the patient receives flow from the bellows and flow from the anesthesia machine (which can include flow from the oxygen flush valve) because the ventilator relief valve is closed shut. As mentioned earlier, the combination of these two flows can cause barotrauma. The Narkomed 6000 avoids this potential hazard by using fresh gas decoupling technology. During the inspiratory phase, fresh gas flow from the anesthesia machine and flow from the oxygen flush valve are diverted to the circle system reservoir bag using a series of pneumatic valves. This safety feature minimizes the potential hazard of barotrauma since the patient receives flow only from inside the piston unit.

SCAVENGING SYSTEMS

Scavenging is the collection and subsequent removal of vented gases from the operating room.[132] The amount of gas used to anesthetize a patient commonly far exceeds the patient's needs. Therefore, scavenging minimizes operating room pollution. In 1977, the National Institute for Occupational Safety and Health (NIOSH) prepared a document entitled "Criteria for a Recommended Standard: Occupational Exposure to Waste Anesthetic Gases and Vapors."[133] Although it was maintained that a safe level of exposure could not be defined, the NIOSH recommendations are shown in Table 22-4.[133] In 1991 the American Society for Testing and Materials (ASTM) released the ASTM F1343-91 standard entitled "Standard Specification for Anesthetic Equipment—Scavenging Systems for Anesthetic Gases."[134] The document provided guidelines for devices that safely and effectively scavenge excess anesthetic gas to reduce contamination in anesthetizing areas. In 1999, the American Society of Anesthesiology (ASA) Task Force on Trace Anesthetic Gases developed a booklet entitled "Waste Anesthetic Gases: Information for Management in Anesthetizing Areas and the Postanesthesia Care Unit." This publication addresses analysis of the literature, the role of regulatory agencies, scavenging and monitoring equipment, and recommendations.[135]

The two major causes of waste gas contamination in the operating room are the anesthetic technique employed and equipment issues.[135,136] Regarding the anesthetic technique, the following factors cause operating room contamination: failure to turn off gas flow control valves at the end of an anesthetic; poorly fitting masks; flushing the circuit; filling anesthetic vaporizers; use of uncuffed endotracheal tubes; and use of breathing circuits such as the Jackson-Rees, which is difficult to scavenge. Equipment failure or failure to understand the equipment can cause operating room contamination. Leaks can occur in the high-pressure hoses, the nitrous oxide tank mounting, the high-pressure and low-pressure circuits of the anesthesia machine, or in the circle system, particularly the carbon dioxide canister. The anesthesia care provider must be certain that the scavenging system is operational and adjusted properly to ensure adequate scavenging. If side-stream carbon dioxide or multigas analyzers are used, the analyzed gas (50–250 ml · min⁻¹) must be directed to the scavenging system or returned to the breathing system.[135,136]

Components

Scavenging systems have five components (Fig. 22-27): (1) the gas collecting assembly, (2) the transfer means, (3) the scavenging interface, (4) the gas disposal assembly tubing, and (5) an active or passive gas disposal assembly.[134] An active system uses a central vacuum to eliminate waste gases. The pressure of the waste gas itself produces flow through a passive system.

Table 22-4. NIOSH RECOMMENDATIONS, 1977[133]

Anesthetic Gas	Maximum TWA* Concentration (ppm)
Halogenated agent alone	2
Nitrous oxide	25
Combination of halogenated agent plus nitrous oxide:	
Halogenated agent	0.5
Nitrous oxide	25
Dental facilities (nitrous oxide alone)	50

* TWA = Time-weighted average. Time-weighted average sampling, also known as time-integrated sampling, is a sampling method that evaluates the average concentration of anesthetic gas over a prolonged period of time, such as 1 to 8 hours.

Reprinted with permission from US Department of Health, Education, and Welfare: Criteria for a recommended standard: Occupational exposure to waste anesthetic gases and vapors. March ed, Washington DC, 1977.

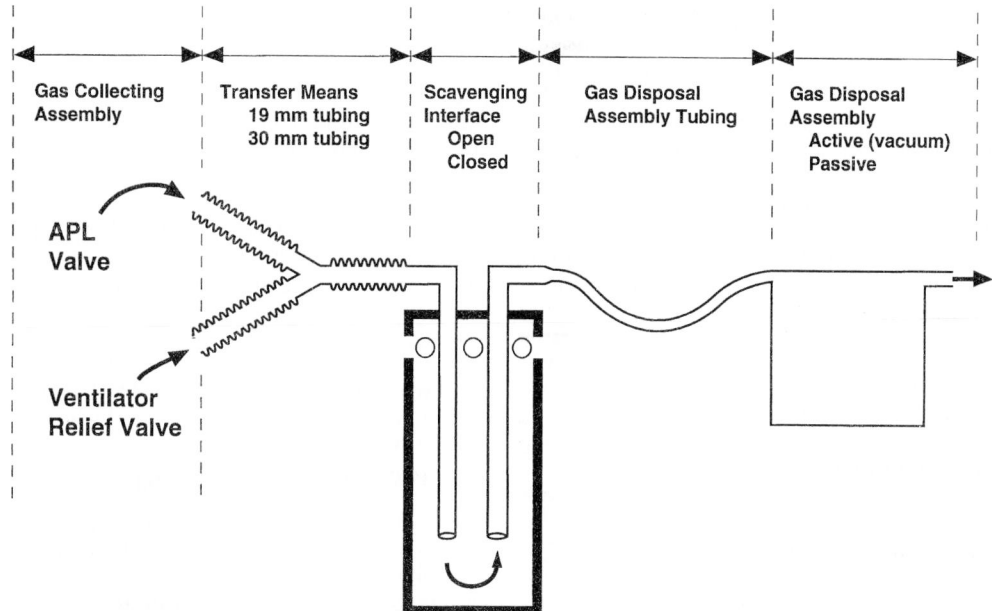

Figure 22-27. Components of a scavenging system. APL = adjustable pressure limiting valve.

Gas Collecting Assembly

The gas collecting assembly captures excess anesthetic gas and delivers it to the transfer tubing.[134] Excess gas is vented from the anesthesia system either through the APL valve or through the ventilator relief valve. All excess gas passes through these valves, accumulates in the gas collecting assembly, and is directed to the transfer means.

Transfer Means

The transfer means carries excess gas from the gas collecting assembly to the scavenging interface. The tubing must be either 19 or 30 mm, as specified by the ASTM F1343-91 standard.[134] The tubing should be sufficiently rigid to prevent kinking, and as short as possible to minimize the chance of occlusion. Some manufacturers color-code the transfer tubing with yellow bands to distinguish it from 22-mm breathing system tubing. Many machines have separate transfer tubes for the APL valve and for the ventilator relief valve. The two tubes frequently merge into a single hose before they enter the scavenging interface. Occlusion of the transfer means can be particularly problematic since it is upstream from the pressure-buffering scavenging interface. If the transfer means is occluded, breathing circuit pressure will increase, and barotrauma can occur.

Scavenging Interface

The scavenging interface is the most important component of the system because it protects the breathing circuit or ventilator from excessive positive or negative pressure.[132] The interface should limit the pressures immediately downstream from the gas collecting assembly to between −0.5 and +10 cm water with normal working conditions.[134] Positive pressure relief is mandatory, irrespective of the type of disposal system used, to vent excess gas in case of occlusion downstream from the interface. If the disposal system is active, negative pressure relief is necessary to protect the breathing circuit or ventilator from excessive subatmospheric pressure. A reservoir is highly desirable with active systems, since it stores excess waste gas until the evacuation system can eliminate it. Interfaces can be open or closed, depending on the method used to provide positive and negative pressure relief.[132]

Open Interfaces.   An open interface contains no valves and is open to the atmosphere, allowing both positive and negative pressure relief. Open interfaces should be used only with active disposal systems that use a central vacuum system. Open interfaces require a reservoir because waste gases are intermittently discharged in surges, whereas flow to the active disposal system is continuous.[132]

Many contemporary anesthesia machines are equipped with open interfaces like those in Figure 22-28A and B.[137] An open canister provides reservoir capacity. The canister volume should be large enough to accommodate a variety of waste gas flow rates. Gas enters the system at the top of the canister and travels through a narrow inner tube to the canister base. Gases are stored in the reservoir between breaths. Positive and negative pressure relief is provided by holes in the top of the canister. The open interface shown in Figure 22-28A differs somewhat from the one shown in Figure 22-28B. The operator can regulate the vacuum by adjusting the vacuum control valve shown in Figure 22-28B.[137]

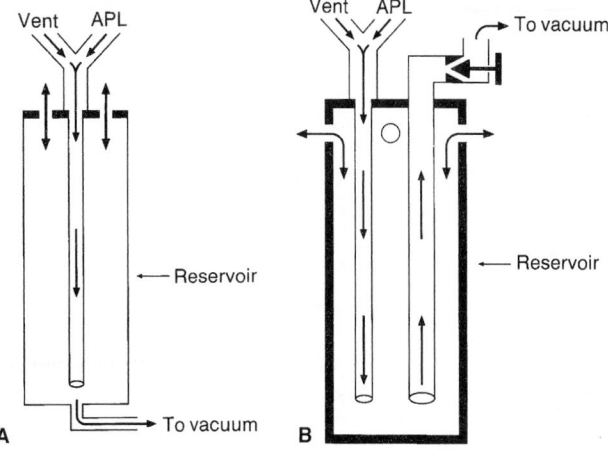

Figure 22-28.   (*A and B*). Two open scavenging interfaces. Each requires an active disposal system. APL = adjustable pressure limiting valve. (Modified with permission from Dorsch JA, Dorsch SE: Controlling trace gas levels. In Dorsch JA, Dorsch SE (eds): Understanding Anesthesia Equipment, 4th ed, p 355. Baltimore, Williams & Williams, 1999.)

The efficiency of an open interface depends on several factors. The vacuum flow rate per minute must equal or exceed the minute volume of excess gases to prevent spillage. The volume of the reservoir and the flow characteristics within the interface are important. Spillage will occur if the volume of a single exhaled breath exceeds the capacity of the reservoir. Leakage can occur long before the volume of waste gas delivered to the reservoir equals the reservoir volume if large-scale turbulence occurs within the interface.[138]

Closed Interfaces. A closed interface communicates with the atmosphere through valves. All closed interfaces must have a positive pressure relief valve to vent excess system pressure if obstruction occurs downstream from the interface. A negative pressure relief valve is mandatory to protect the breathing system from subatmospheric pressure if an active disposal system is used.[132] Two types of closed interfaces are commercially available. One has positive pressure relief only; the other has both positive and negative pressure relief.

POSITIVE PRESSURE RELIEF ONLY   This interface (Fig. 22-29, *left*) has a single positive pressure relief valve and is designed to be used only with passive disposal systems. Waste gas enters the interface at the waste gas inlets. Transfer of the waste gas from the interface to the disposal system relies on the pressure of the waste gas itself since a vacuum is not used. The positive pressure relief valve opens at a preset value such as 5 cm water if an obstruction between the interface and the disposal system occurs.[139] A reservoir bag is not necessary.

POSITIVE AND NEGATIVE PRESSURE RELIEF   This interface has a positive pressure relief valve, at least one negative pressure relief valve, and a reservoir bag. It is used with active disposal systems. Figure 22-29 (*right*) is a schematic of North American Dräger's closed interface for suction systems. A variable volume of waste gas intermittently enters the interface through the waste gas inlets. The reservoir stores transient excess gas until the vacuum system eliminates it. The operator should adjust the vacuum control valve so that the reservoir bag is properly inflated (*A*) and not overdistended (*B*) or completely deflated (*C*). Gas is vented to the atmosphere through the positive pressure relief valve if the system pressure exceeds +5 cm water. Room air is entrained through the negative pressure relief valve if the system pressure is more negative than −0.5 cm water. A backup negative pressure relief valve opens at −1.8 cm water if the primary negative pressure relief valve becomes occluded.[18]

The effectiveness of a closed system in preventing spillage depends on the inflow rate of excess gas, the vacuum flow rate, and the volume of the reservoir. Leakage of waste gases into the atmosphere occurs only when the reservoir bag becomes fully inflated and the pressure increases sufficiently to open the positive pressure relief valve. In contrast, the effectiveness of an open system to prevent spillage depends not only on the volume of the reservoir but also on the flow characteristics within the interface.[138]

Gas Disposal Assembly Tubing

The gas disposal assembly tubing (Fig. 22-27) conducts waste gas from the scavenging interface to the gas disposal assembly. It should be collapse-proof and should run overhead, if possible, to minimize the chance of occlusion.[134]

Gas Disposal Assembly

The gas disposal assembly ultimately eliminates excess waste gas (Fig. 22-27). There are two types of disposal systems: active and passive.

The most common method of gas disposal is the active assembly, which uses a central vacuum. The vacuum is a mechanical flow-inducing device that removes the waste gases. An interface with a negative pressure relief valve is mandatory because the pressure within the system is negative. A reservoir is very desirable, and the larger the reservoir, the lower the suction flow rate needed.[132,138]

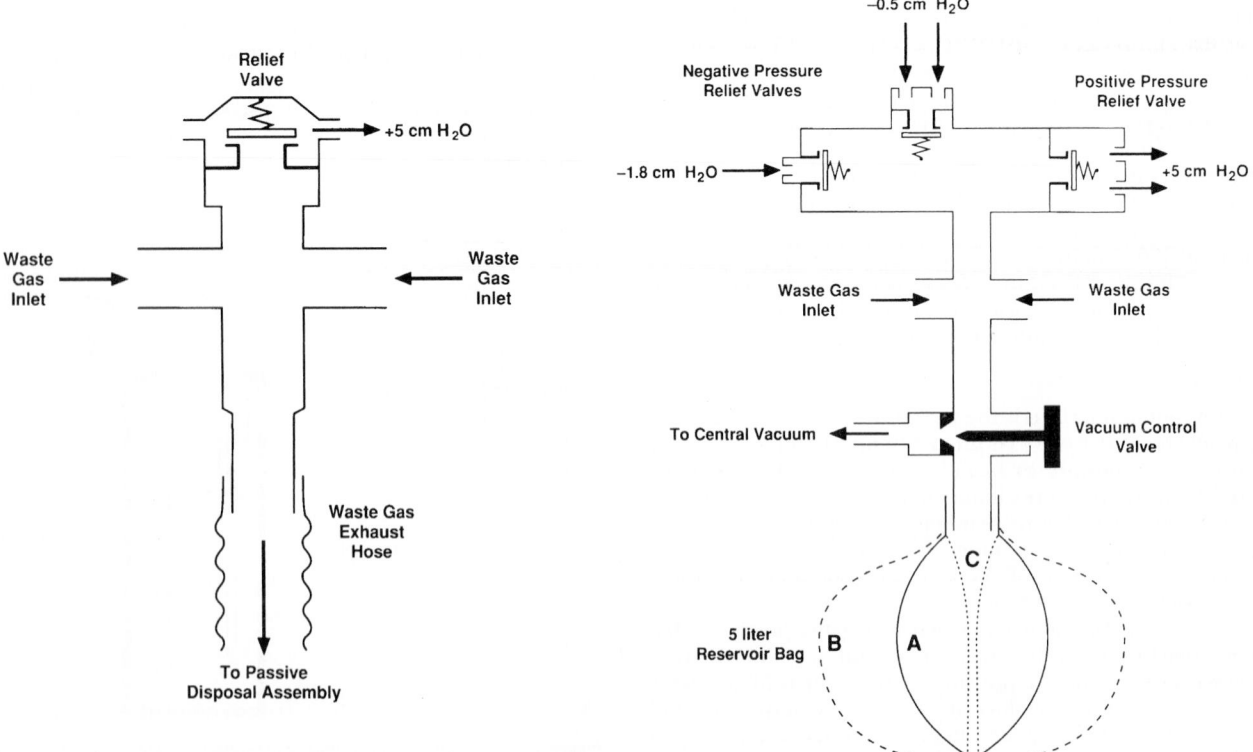

Figure 22-29. Closed scavenging interfaces. (*Left*) Interface used with a passive disposal system. (*Right*) Interface with an active system. (*Left:* Modified with permission from Scavenger Interface for Air Conditioning. Instruction Manual. Telford, PA, North American Dräger, October 1984. *Right:* Modified with permission from Narkomed 2A Anesthesia System. Technical Service Manual. Telford, PA, North American Dräger, October 1985.)

A passive disposal system does not use a mechanical flow-inducing device. Instead, the pressure of the waste gas itself produces flow through the system. Positive pressure relief is mandatory, but negative pressure relief and a reservoir are unnecessary. Excess waste gas can be eliminated in a number of ways. Some include venting through the wall, ceiling, floor, or to the room exhaust grill of a nonrecirculating air conditioning system.[132,138]

Hazards

Scavenging systems minimize operating room pollution, yet they add complexity to the anesthesia system. A scavenging system extends the anesthesia circuit all the way from the anesthesia machine to the ultimate disposal site. This extension increases the potential for problems. Obstruction of scavenging pathways can cause excessive positive pressure in the breathing circuit, and barotrauma can occur. Excessive vacuum applied to a scavenging system can cause negative pressures in the breathing system.

CHECKING ANESTHESIA MACHINES

A complete anesthesia apparatus checkout procedure should be performed each day before the first case. An abbreviated version should be performed before each subsequent case. Several checkout procedures exist, but the 1993 FDA Anesthesia Apparatus Checkout Recommendations (Appendix A) is the most popular.[140-144] The FDA checkout procedures serve only as generic guidelines because the designs of different machines vary considerably. Also, many machines have been modified in the field. Therefore, specific checks must be performed on specific machines. The user must refer to the operator's manual for special procedures or precautions.

The three most important preoperative checks are (1) oxygen analyzer calibration, (2) the low-pressure circuit leak test, and (3) the circle system test.

Oxygen Analyzer Calibration

The oxygen analyzer is the most important machine monitor because it is the only machine safety device that evaluates the integrity of the low-pressure circuit. Other machine safety devices, such as the fail-safe valve, the oxygen supply failure alarm, and the proportioning system, are all upstream from the flow control valves (Fig. 22-3). The only machine monitor that detects problems downstream from the flow control valves is the oxygen analyzer. Calibration of this monitor is described in Appendix A: Anesthesia Apparatus Checkout Recommendations, 1993, #9.

Low-Pressure Circuit Leak Test

The low-pressure leak test checks the integrity of the anesthesia machine from the flow control valves to the common outlet. It evaluates the portion of the machine that is downstream from all safety devices except the oxygen analyzer. The components located within this area are *precisely* the ones most subject to breakage and leaks. Leaks in the low-pressure circuit can cause hypoxia or patient awareness.[71,145] Flow tubes, the most delicate pneumatic component of the machine, can crack or break. A typical three-gas anesthesia machine has 16 O-rings in the low-pressure circuit. Leaks can occur at the interface between the glass flow tube and the manifold, and at the O-ring junction between the vaporizer and its manifold. Loose filler caps on vaporizers are a common source of leaks, and these leaks can cause patient awareness under anesthesia.[71,146]

Several different methods have been used to check the low-pressure circuit for leaks. They include the oxygen flush test, the common gas outlet occlusion test, the traditional positive-pressure leak test, the North American Dräger positive-pressure leak test, the Ohmeda 8000 internal-positive pressure leak test, the Ohmeda negative-pressure leak test, the 1993 FDA universal negative-pressure leak test, and others. One reason for the large number of methods is that the internal design of various machines differs considerably. The most notable example is that most Ohmeda machines have a check valve near the common gas outlet whereas North American Dräger machines do not. The presence or absence of the check valve profoundly influences which preoperative check is indicated.

Several mishaps have resulted from application of the wrong leak test to the wrong machine.[31,69,147] Therefore, it is mandatory to perform the appropriate low-pressure leak test before every case. To do this, it is essential to understand the exact location and operating principles of the Ohmeda check valve. Most Ohmeda anesthesia machines have a machine outlet check valve located in the low-pressure circuit (see Table 22-5). The check valve is located downstream from the vaporizers and upstream from the oxygen flush valve (Fig. 22-3). It is open (Fig. 22-30, *left*) in the absence of back pressure. Gas flow from the manifold moves the rubber flapper valve off its seat and allows gas to proceed freely to the common outlet. The valve closes (Fig. 22-30, *right*) when back pressure is exerted on it.[8] Back pressure sufficient to close the check valve may occur with the following conditions: oxygen flushing, peak breathing circuit pressures generated during positive-pressure ventilation, or use of a positive-pressure leak test.

Generally speaking, machines without check valves can be tested using a positive-pressure leak test, and machines with check valves must be tested using a negative-pressure leak test. When performing a positive-pressure leak test, the operator

---

Table 22-5. CHECK VALVES AND RECOMMENDED LEAK TEST

| Anesthesia Machine | Machine Outlet Check Valve | Vaporizer Outlet Check Valve | Leak Test Recommended by Manufacturer | |
			Positive Pressure	*Negative Pressure (Suction Bulb)*
North American Dräger				
Narkomed 2A, 2B, 3, & 4	No	No	X	
Ohmeda Unitrol	Yes	Variable		X
Ohmeda 30/70	Yes	Variable		X
Ohmeda Modulus I	Yes	Variable		X
Ohmeda Modulus II	Yes	No		X
Ohmeda Excel series	Yes	No		X
Ohmeda Modulus II Plus	No	No		X
Ohmeda CD	No	No		X

Data from Ohio Medical Products,[9,11] Ohmeda,[10,12,13,15–17] and North American Dräger.[18–22]

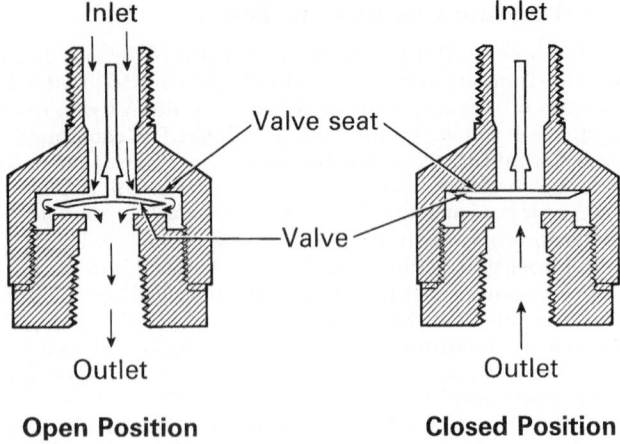

Open Position   **Closed Position**

Figure 22-30. Machine outlet check valve. (Reproduced with permission from Bowie E, Huffman LM: The Anesthesia Machine: Essentials for Understanding. Madison, WI, Ohmeda, a division of BOC Health Care, Inc., 1985.)

generates positive pressure in the low-pressure circuit using flow from the anesthesia machine or from a positive-pressure bulb to detect a leak. When performing a negative-pressure leak test, the operator creates negative pressure in the low-pressure circuit using a suction bulb to detect leaks. Two different low-pressure circuit leak tests are described below.

Oxygen Flush Positive-Pressure Leak Test

Historically, older anesthesia machines did not have check valves in the low-pressure circuit. Therefore, it was common practice to pressurize the breathing circuit and the low-pressure circuit with the oxygen flush valve to test for internal anesthesia machine leaks. Because many modern Ohmeda machines now have check valves in the low-pressure circuit; however, application of a positive-pressure leak test to these machines can be misleading or even dangerous (Fig. 22-31). Inappropriate use of the oxygen flush valve to evaluate the low-pressure circuit for leaks can lead to a false sense of security despite the presence of huge leaks.[31,40,69,147] Positive pressure from the patient circuit closes the check valve, and the value on the airway pressure gauge does not decline. The system appears to be tight, but in actuality, only the circuitry downstream from the check valve is leak-free.[27] Thus, a vulnerable area exists from the check valve back to the flow control valves because this area is not tested by a positive-pressure leak test.

1993 FDA Universal Negative-Pressure Leak Test

The 1993 FDA universal negative-pressure leak test[144] (Appendix A, Section #5) is named "universal" because it can be used to check all contemporary anesthesia machines, regardless of the presence or absence of check valves in the low-pressure circuit. It can be applied to Ohmeda machines, North American Dräger machines, and others. The 1993 FDA check is based upon the Ohmeda negative-pressure leak test (Fig. 22-32). It is performed using a negative-pressure leak testing device, which is a simple suction bulb. The machine master switch, the flow control valves, and vaporizers are turned off. The suction bulb is attached to the common fresh gas outlet and squeezed repeatedly until it is fully collapsed. This action creates a vacuum in the low-pressure circuitry. The machine is leak-free if the hand bulb remains collapsed for at least 10 seconds. A leak is present if the bulb reinflates during this period. The test is repeated with each vaporizer individually turned to the on position because internal vaporizer leaks can be detected only with the vaporizer turned on.

The FDA universal negative-pressure low-pressure circuit leak test has several advantages.[145] It will help eliminate the present confusion regarding exactly which specific check should be performed on specific machines. The universal test is quick and simple to perform. It has an obvious end point, and it isolates the problem. For example, if the bulb reinflates in less than 10 seconds, a leak is present somewhere in the low-pressure circuit. Therefore, it differentiates between breathing-circuit leaks and leaks in the low-pressure circuit. The universal negative-pressure leak test is the most sensitive of all contemporary leak tests because it is not volume-dependent; that is, it does not involve a compliant breathing bag or corrugated hoses. It can detect leaks as small as 30 ml · min[-1]. Finally, the operator does not need a detailed or in-depth knowledge of proprietary design differences. If the operator performs the universal test correctly, the leak will be detected.

Circle System Test

The circle system test (Appendix A, Sections #11–12) evaluates the integrity of the circle breathing system, which spans from the common gas outlet to the Y-piece (Fig. 22-22). It has two parts—the *leak test* and the *flow test*. To thoroughly check the circle system for leaks, valve integrity, and obstruction, both tests must be performed preoperatively. The *leak test* is performed by closing the pop-off valve, occluding the Y-piece, and pressurizing the circuit to 30 cm water pressure using the oxygen flush valve. The value on the pressure gauge will not decline if the circle system is leak-free, but this does not assure valve integrity. The value on the gauge will read 30 cm water if the unidirectional valves are stuck shut or if the valves are incompetent.

The *flow test* checks the integrity of the unidirectional valves, and it detects obstruction in the circle system. It can be performed by removing the Y-piece from the circle system and breathing through the two corrugated hoses individually. The

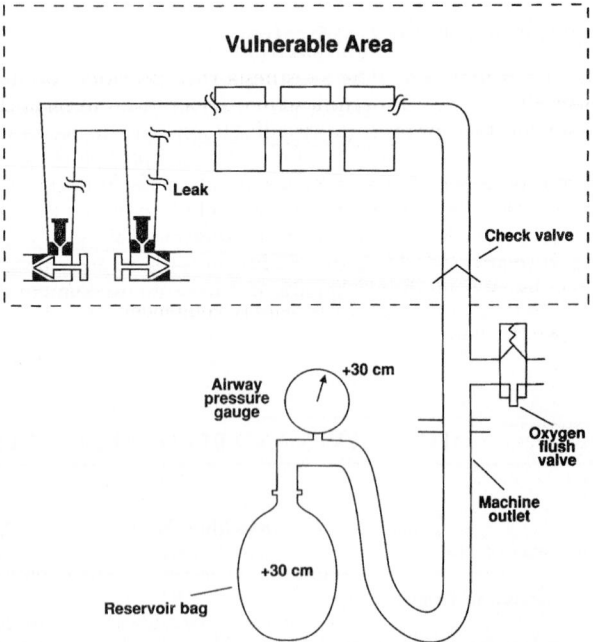

Figure 22-31. Inappropriate use of the oxygen flush valve to check the low-pressure circuit of an Ohmeda machine equipped with a check valve. The area within the rectangle is not checked by the inappropriate use of the oxygen flush valve. The components located within this area are precisely the ones most subject to breakage and leaks. Positive pressure within the patient circuit closes the check valve, and the value on the airway pressure gauge does not decline despite leaks in the low-pressure circuit.

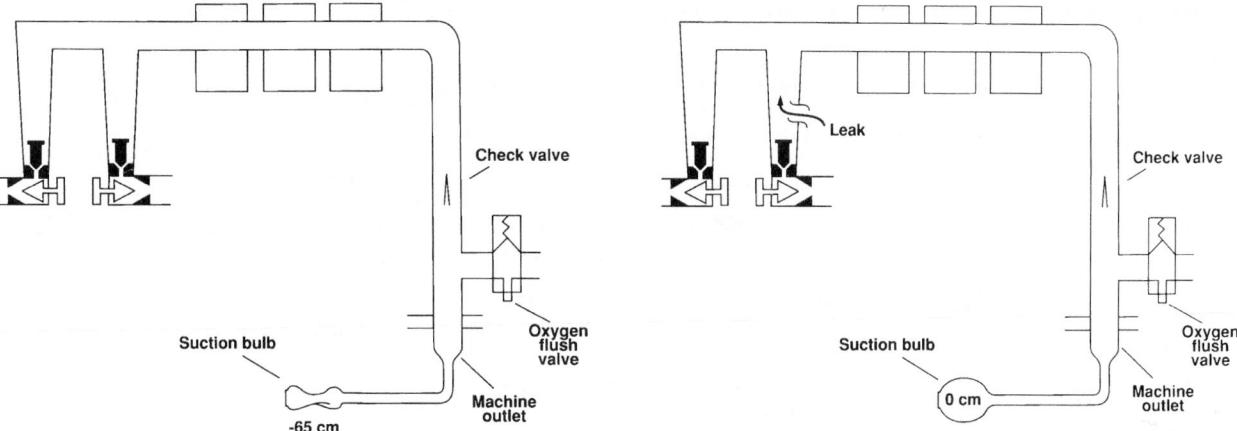

Figure 22-32. FDA negative-pressure leak test. (*Left*) A negative-pressure leak testing device is attached directly to the machine outlet. Squeezing the bulb creates a vacuum in the low-pressure circuit and opens the check valve. (*Right*) When a leak is present in the low-pressure circuit, room air is entrained through the leak and the suction bulb inflates. (Reprinted with permission from Andrews JJ: Understanding anesthesia machines. In 1988 Review Course Lectures, p 78. Cleveland, International Anesthesia Research Society, 1988.)

valves should be present, and they should move appropriately. The operator should be able to inhale but not be able to exhale through the inspiratory limb. The operator should be able to exhale but not inhale through the expiratory limb. The flow test can also be performed by using the ventilator and a breathing bag attached to the Y piece as described in the 1993 FDA Anesthesia Apparatus Checkout Recommendations (Appendix A, Section #12).[144]

SUMMARY

Rapid advances in the anesthesia industry make it increasingly difficult for the anesthesia care provider to keep up with anesthesia system technology. Nevertheless, a thorough understanding of the anesthesia machine, ventilator, circuit and monitors is mandatory for the safe practice of anesthesia. Anesthesia systems are equipped with dozens of safety features, yet none of them is foolproof. The anesthesia care provider still must check all components of the system preoperatively using appropriate checkout procedures.

REFERENCES

1. Schreiber P: Safety Guidelines for Anesthesia Systems. Telford, PA, North American Dräger, 1984
2. Caplan RA, Vistica MF, Posner KL, Cheney FW: Adverse anesthetic outcomes arising from gas delivery equipment. Anesthesiology 87:741, 1997
3. American National Standards Institute: Minimum Performance and Safety Requirements for Components and Systems of Continuous Flow Anesthesia Machines for Human Use (ANSI Z79.8-1979). New York, American National Standards Institute, 1979
4. American Society for Testing and Materials: Standard Specification for Minimum Performance and Safety Requirements for Components and Systems of Anesthesia Gas Machines (ASTM F1161-88). Philadelphia, American Society for Testing and Materials, 1988
5. American Society for Testing and Materials: Standard Specification for Minimum Performance and Safety Requirements for Components and Systems of Anesthetic Gas Machines (ASTM 1161-94). Philadelphia, American Society for Testing and Materials, 1994
6. American Society for Testing and Materials: Standard Specification for Particular Requirements for Anesthesia Workstations and Their Components (ASTM F1850-98a). Philadelphia, American Society for Testing and Materials, 1998
7. Dorsch JA, Dorsch SE: The anesthesia machine. In Dorsch JA, Dorsch SE (eds): Understanding Anesthesia Equipment, 4th ed, p 75. Baltimore, Williams & Wilkins, 1999
8. Bowie E, Huffman LM: The Anesthesia Machine: Essentials for Understanding. Madison, WI, Ohmeda, The BOC Group, Inc, 1985
9. 30/70 Proportionate Anesthesia Machine (Canadian version): Madison, WI, Ohio Medical Products, 1982
10. Ohmeda Unitrol Anesthesia System: Operation and Maintenance Manual. Madison, WI, Ohmeda, The BOC Group, Inc, 1985
11. Modulus Anesthesia Gas Machine: Operation Maintenance. Madison, WI, Ohio Medical Products, The BOC Group, Inc, 1981
12. Modulus II Anesthesia System: Operation and Maintenance Manual. Madison, WI, Ohmeda, The BOC Group, Inc, 1985
13. Modulus II Anesthesia System: Service Manual. Madison, WI, Ohmeda, The BOC Group, Inc, 1985
14. Ohmeda 8000 Anesthesia Machine: Operation and Maintenance Manual. Madison, WI, Ohmeda, The BOC Group, Inc, 1985
15. Ohmeda Excel 110 and 210: Operation and Maintenance Manual. Madison, WI, Ohmeda, The BOC Group, Inc, 1987
16. Modulus II Plus Anesthesia System: Operation and Maintenance Manual. Madison, WI, Ohmeda, The BOC Group, Inc, 1988
17. Ohmeda CD Anesthesia System: Operation and Maintenance Manual. Madison, WI, Ohmeda, The BOC Group, Inc, 1990
18. Narkomed 2A Anesthesia System: Technical Service Manual, 6th ed. Telford, PA, North American Dräger, 1985
19. Narkomed 2A Anesthesia System: Instruction Manual, 7th ed. Telford, PA, North American Dräger, 1985
20. Narkomed 2B Anesthesia System: Operator's Manual. Telford, PA, North American Dräger, 1988
21. Narkomed 3 Anesthesia System: Operator's Instruction Manual. Telford, PA, North American Dräger, 1986
22. Narkomed 4 Anesthesia System: Operations Instruction Manual. Telford, PA, North American Dräger, 1990
23. Cicman JH, Jacoby MI, Skibo VF *et al:* Anesthesia systems. Part 1: Operating principles of fundamental components. J Clin Monit 8:295, 1992
24. Feeley TW, Hedley-Whyte J: Bulk oxygen and nitrous oxide delivery systems: Design and dangers. Anesthesiology 44:301, 1976
25. Pelton DA: Non-flammable medical gas pipeline systems. In Wyant GM (ed): Mechanical Misadventures in Anesthesia, p 8. Toronto, University of Toronto Press, 1978
26. Adriani J: Clinical application of physical principles concerning gases and vapors to anesthesiology. In Adriani J (ed): The Chemistry and Physics of Anesthesia. 2nd ed, p 58. Springfield, IL, Charles C. Thomas, 1962
27. Dorsch JA, Dorsch SE: Equipment checking and maintenance. In Dorsch JA, Dorsch SE (eds): Understanding Anesthesia Equipment, 4th ed, p 937. Baltimore, Williams & Wilkins, 1999
28. Macintosh R, Mushin WW, Epstein HG: Flowmeters. In Macintosh R, Mushin WW, Epstein HG (eds): Physics for the Anaesthetist, 3rd ed, p 196. Oxford, Blackwell Scientific Publications, 1963
29. Eger EI II, Epstein RM: Hazards of anesthetic equipment. Anesthesiology 24:490, 1964
30. Eger EI II, Hylton RR, Irwin RH *et al:* Anesthetic flowmeter sequence—a cause for hypoxia. Anesthesiology 24:396, 1963

31. Rendell-Baker L: Problems with anesthetic and respiratory therapy equipment. Int Anesthesiol Clin 20:1, 1982

32. Mazze RI: Therapeutic misadventures with oxygen delivery systems: The need for continuous in-line oxygen monitors. Anesth Analg 51:787, 1972

33. Richards C: Failure of a nitrous oxide–oxygen proportioning device. Anesthesiology 71:997, 1989

34. Abraham ZA, Basagoitia B: A potentially lethal anesthesia machine failure. Anesthesiology 66:589, 1987

35. Neubarth J: Another hazardous gas supply misconnection (letter). Anesth Analg 80:206, 1995

36. Gaughan SD, Benumof JL, Ozaki GT: Can an anesthesia machine flush valve provide for effective jet ventilation? Anesth Analg 76:800, 1993

37. Anderson CE, Rendell-Baker L: Exposed O$_2$ flush hazard. Anesthesiology 56:328, 1982

38. Anonymous: Internal leakage from anesthesia unit flush valves. Health Devices 10:172, 1981

39. Andrews JJ: Understanding your anesthesia machine and ventilator. In International Anesthesia Research Society: 1989 Review Course Lectures, p 59. Cleveland, 1989

40. Dodgson BG: Inappropriate use of the oxygen flush to check an anaesthetic machine. Can J Anaesth 35:336, 1988

41. Dorsch JA, Dorsch SE: Vaporizers (anesthetic agent delivery devices). In Dorsch JA, Dorsch SE (eds): Understanding Anesthesia Machines, 4th ed, p 121. Baltimore, Williams & Wilkins, 1999

42. Macintosh R, Mushin WW, Epstein HG: Vapor pressure. In Macintosh R, Mushin WW, Epstein HG (eds): Physics for the Anaesthetist, 3rd ed, p 68. Oxford, Blackwell Scientific Publications, 1963

43. Adriani J: Principles of physics and chemistry of solids and fluids applicable to anesthesiology. In Adriani J (ed): The Chemistry and Physics of Anesthesia, 2nd ed, p 7. Springfield, IL, Charles C. Thomas, 1962

44. Macintosh R, Mushin WW, Epstein HG: Vaporization. In Macintosh R, Mushin WW, Epstein HG (eds): Physics for the Anaesthetist, 3rd ed, p 26. Oxford, Blackwell Scientific Publications, 1963

45. Macintosh R, Mushin WW, Epstein HG: Specific heat. In Macintosh R, Mushin WW, Epstein HG (eds): Physics for the Anaesthetist, 3rd ed, p 17. Oxford, Blackwell Scientific Publications, 1963

46. Schreiber P: Anaesthetic Equipment: Performance, Classification, and Safety. New York, Springer-Verlag, 1972

47. Tec 4 Continuous Flow Vaporizer: Operator's Manual. Steeton, England, Ohmeda, The BOC Group, Inc, 1987

48. Dräger Vapor 19.n Anaesthetic Vaporizer: Instructions for Use, 14th ed. Lubeck, Federal Republic of Germany, Drägerwerk, 1990

49. Hill DW, Lowe HJ: Comparison of concentration of halothane in closed and semi-closed circuits during controlled ventilation. Anesthesiology 23:291, 1962

50. Hill DW: The design and calibration of vaporizers for volatile anaesthetic agents. In Scurr C, Feldman S (eds): Scientific Foundations of Anaesthesia, 3rd ed, p 544. London, William Heineman Medical Books, 1982

51. Hill DW: The design and calibration of vaporizers for volatile anaesthetic agents. Br J Anaesth 40:648, 1968

52. Morris LE: Problems in the performance of anesthesia vaporizers. Int Anesthesiol Clin 12:199, 1974

53. Stoelting RK: The effects of nitrous oxide on halothane output from Fluotec Mark 2 vaporizers. Anesthesiology 35:215, 1971

54. Diaz PD: The influence of carrier gas on the output of automatic vaporizers. Br J Anaesth 48:387, 1976

55. Nawaf K, Stoelting RK: Nitrous oxide increases enflurane concentrations delivered by ethrane vaporizers. Anesth Analg 58:30, 1979

56. Prins L, Strupat J, Clement J: An evaluation of gas density dependence of anaesthetic vaporizers. Can Anaesth Soc J 27:106, 1980

57. Lin CY: Assessment of vaporizer performance in low-flow and closed-circuit anesthesia. Anesth Analg 59:359, 1980

58. Gould DB, Lampert BA, MacKrell TN: Effect of nitrous oxide solubility on vaporizer aberrance. Anesth Analg 61:938, 1982

59. Palayiwa E, Sanderson MH, Hahn CEW: Effects of carrier gas composition on the output of six anaesthetic vaporizers. Br J Anaesth 55:1025, 1983

60. Scheller MS, Drummond JC: Solubility of N$_2$O in volatile anesthetics contributes to vaporizer aberrancy when changing carrier gases. Anesth Analg 65:88, 1986

61. Tec 5 Continuous Flow Vaporizer: Operation and Maintenance Manual. Steeton, England, Ohmeda, The BOC Group, Inc, 1990

62. Karis JH, Menzel DB: Inadvertent change of volatile anesthetics in anesthesia machines. Anesth Analg 61:53, 1982

63. Riegle EV, Desertspring D: Failure of the agent-specific filling device (letter): Anesthesiology 73:353, 1990

64. George TM: Failure of keyed agent-specific filling devices. Anesthesiology 61:228, 1984

65. Broka SM, Gourdange PA, Joucken KL: Sevoflurane and desflurane confusion. Anesth Analg 88:1194, 1999

66. Lippmann M, Foran W, Ginsburg R et al: Contamination of anesthetic vaporizer contents. Anesthesiology 78:1175, 1993

67. Munson WM: Cardiac arrest: A hazard of tipping a vaporizer. Anesthesiology 26:235, 1965

68. Sinclair A: Vaporizer overfilling. Can J Anaesth 40:77, 1993

69. Peters KR, Wingard DW: Anesthesia machine leakage due to misaligned vaporizers. Anesth Rev 14:36, 1987

70. Meister GC, Becker KE Jr: Potential fresh gas flow leak through Dräger vapor 19.1 vaporizer with key-index fill port. Anesthesiology 78:211, 1993

71. Lewis SE, Andrews JJ, Long GW: An unexpected Penlon sigma elite vaporizer leak. Anesthesiology 90:1221, 1999

72. Andrews JJ, Johnston RV Jr: The new Tec 6 desflurane vaporizer. Anesth Analg 76:1338, 1993

73. Weiskopf RB, Sampson D, Moore MA: The desflurane (Tec 6) vaporizer: Design, design considerations and performance evaluation. Br J Anaesth 72:474, 1994

74. Eger EI: New inhaled anesthetics. Anesthesiology 80:906, 1994

75. Tec 6 Vaporizer: Operation and Maintenance Manual. Steeton, England, The BOC Group, Inc, 1993

76. Susay SR, Smith MA, Lockwood GG: The saturated vapor pressure of desflurane at various temperatures. Anesth Analg 83:864, 1996.

77. Johnston RV Jr, Andrews JJ: The effects of carrier gas composition on the performance of the Tec 6 desflurane vaporizer. Anesth Analg 79:548, 1994

78. Andrews JJ, Johnston RV Jr, Kramer GC: Consequences of misfilling contemporary vaporizers with desflurane. Can J Anaesth 40:71, 1993

79. Datex-Ohmeda AS/3 Anesthesia Delivery Unit: User's Reference Manual. Tewksbury, MA, Datex-Ohmeda, 1998

80. Mapleson WW: The elimination of rebreathing in various semiclosed anaesthetic systems. Br J Anaesth 26:323, 1954

81. Willis BA, Pender JW, Mapleson WW: Rebreathing in a T-piece: Volunteer and theoretical studies of the Jackson-Rees modification of Ayre's T-piece during spontaneous respiration. Br J Anaesth 47:1239, 1975

82. Rose DK, Froese AB: The regulation of Pa$_{CO_2}$ during controlled ventilation of children with a T-piece. Can Anaesth Soc J 26(2):104, 1979

83. Froese AB, Rose DK: A detailed analysis of T-piece systems. In Steward (ed): Some Aspects of Paediatric Anaesthesia, p 101. Elsevier North-Holland Biomedical Press, 1982

84. Sykes MK: Rebreathing circuits: A review. Br J Anaesth 40:666, 1968

85. Dorsch JA, Dorsch SE: The breathing system II. The Mapleson systems. In Dorsch JA, Dorsch SE (eds): Understanding Anesthesia Equipment, 2nd ed, p 182. Baltimore, Williams & Wilkins, 1984

86. Bain JA, Spoerel WE: A streamlined anaesthetic system. Can Anaesth Soc J 19:426, 1972

87. Aarhus D, Holst-Larsen E, Holst-Larsen H: Mechanical obstruction in the anaesthesia delivery-system mimicking severe bronchospasm. Anaesthesia 52:992, 1997

88. Pethick SL: Letter to the editor. Can Anaesth Soc J 22:115, 1975

89. Moyers J: A nomenclature for methods of inhalation anesthesia. Anesthesiology 14:609, 1953

90. Eger EI II: Anesthetic systems: Construction and function. In Eger EI II (ed): Anesthetic Uptake and Action, p 206. Baltimore, Williams & Wilkins, 1974

91. Eger EI II, Ethans CT: The effects of inflow, overflow and valve placement on economy of the circle system. Anesthesiology 29:93, 1968

92. Smith CE, Otworth JR, Kaluszyk GSW: Bilateral tension pneumothorax due to a defective anesthesia breathing circuit filter. J Clin Anesth 3:229, 1991

93. McEwan AI, Dowell L, Karis JH: Bilateral tension pneumothorax caused by a blocked bacterial filter in an anesthesia breathing circuit. Anesth Analg 76:440, 1993

94. Walton JS, Fears R, Burt N, Dorman BH: Intraoperative breathing circuit obstruction caused by albuterol nebulization. Anesth Analg 89:650, 1999

95. Dhar P, George I, Sloan P: Flow transducer gas leak detected after induction. Anesth Analg 89:1587, 1999

96. Kshatri AM, Kingsley CP: Defective carbon dioxide absorber as a cause for a leak in a breathing circuit. Anesthesiology 84:475, 1996

97. Norman PH, Daley MD, Walker JR, Fusetti S: Obstruction due to retained carbon dioxide absorber canister wrapping. Anesth Analg 83:425, 1996.

98. Adriani J: Carbon dioxide absorption. In Adriani J (ed): The Chemistry and Physics of Anesthesia, 2nd ed, p 151. Springfield, IL, Charles C. Thomas, 1962

99. Dewey & Almy Chemical Division: The Sodasorb Manual of CO_2 Absorption. New York, WR Grace and Company, 1962

100. Hunt HE: Resistance in respiratory valves and canisters. Anesthesiology 16:190, 1955

101. Brown ES: Performance of absorbents: Continuous flow. Anesthesiology 20:41, 1959

102. Andrews JJ, Johnston RV Jr, Bee DE et al: Photodeactivation of ethyl violet: A potential hazard of sodasorb. Anesthesiology 72:59, 1990

103. Case History 39: Accidental use of trichloroethylene (Trilene, Trimar) in a closed system. Anesth Analg 43:740, 1964

104. Morio M, Fujii K, Satoh N et al: Reaction of sevoflurane and its degradation products with soda lime. Anesthesiology 77:1155, 1992

105. Frink EJ Jr, Malan TP, Morgan SE et al: Quantification of the degradation products of sevoflurane in two CO_2 absorbents during low-flow anesthesia in surgical patients. Anesthesiology 77:1064, 1992

106. Fang ZX, Kandel L, Laster MJ et al: Factors affecting production of Compound A from the interaction of sevoflurane with Baralyme® and soda lime. Anesth Analg 82:775, 1996

107. Eger EI II, Ion P, Laster MJ, Weiskopf RB: Baralyme dehydration increases and soda lime dehydration decreases the concentration of Compound A resulting from sevoflurane degradation in a standard anesthetic circuit. Anesth Analg 85:892, 1997

108. Steffey EP, Laster MJ, Ionescu P et al: Dehydration of Baralyme® increases compound A resulting from sevoflurane degradation in a standard anesthetic circuit used to anesthetize swine. Anesth Analg 85:1382, 1997

109. Eger EL II, Koblin DD, Bowland T et al: Nephrotoxicity of sevoflurane versus desflurane anesthesia in volunteers. Anesth Analg 84:160, 1997

110. Kharasch ED, Frink EJ Jr, Zager R et al: Assessment of low-flow sevoflurane and isoflurane effects on renal function using sensitive markers of tubular toxicity. Anesthesiology 86:1238, 1997

111. Bito H, Ikeuchi Y, Ikeda K: Effects of low-flow sevoflurane anesthesia on renal function: Comparison with high-flow sevoflurane anesthesia and low-flow isoflurane anesthesia. Anesthesiology 86:1231, 1997

112. Berry PD, Sessler DI, Larson MD: Severe carbon monoxide poisoning during anesthesia. Anesthesiology 90:613, 1999

113. Baxter PJ, Kharasch ED: Rehydration of desiccated Baralyme prevents carbon monoxide formation from desflurane in an anesthesia machine. Anesthesiology 86:1061, 1997

114. Woehlck HJ, Dunning M, Connolly LA: Reduction in the incidence of carbon monoxide exposures in humans undergoing general anesthesia. Anesthesiology 87:228, 1997

115. Fang ZX, Eger EI, Laster MJ et al: Carbon monoxide production from degradation of desflurane, enflurane, isoflurane, halothane, and sevoflurane by soda lime and Baralyme®. Anesth Analg 80:1187, 1995

116. Bonome C, Belda J, Alvarez-Refojo F et al: Low-flow anesthesia and reduced animal size increase carboxyhemoglobin levels in swine during desflurane and isoflurane breakdown in dried soda lime. Anesth Analg 89:909, 1999

117. Neumann MA, Laster MJ, Weiskopf RB et al: The elimination of sodium and potassium hydroxides from desiccated soda lime diminishes degradation of desflurane to carbon monoxide and sevoflurane to compound A but does not compromise carbon dioxide absorption. Anesth Analg 89:768, 1999

118. Spearman CB, Sanders HG: Physical principles and functional designs of ventilators. In Kirby RR, Smith RA, Desautels DA (eds): Mechanical Ventilation, p 59. New York, Churchill Livingstone, 1985

119. McPherson SP, Spearman CB: Introduction to ventilators. In McPherson SP, Spearman CB (eds): Respiratory Therapy Equipment, 3rd ed, p 230. St Louis, CV Mosby, 1985

120. 7000 Electronic Anesthesia Ventilator: Operation Maintenance. Madison, WI, Ohmeda, The BOC Group, Inc, 1985

121. 7000 Electronic Anesthesia Ventilator: Service Manual. Madison, WI, Ohmeda, The BOC Group, Inc, 1985

122. Cooper JB, Newbower RS, Kitz RJ: An analysis of major errors and equipment failures in anesthesia management. Considerations for prevention and detection. Anesthesiology 60:34, 1984

123. Reinhart DJ, Friz R: Undetected leak in corrugated circuit tubing in compressed configuration. Anesthesiology 78:218, 1993

124. Raphael DT, Weller RS, Doran DJ: A response algorithm for the low-pressure alarm condition. Anesth Analg 67:876, 1988

125. Slee TA, Pavlin EG: Failure of low pressure alarm associated with use of a humidifier. Anesthesiology 69:791, 1988

126. Sattari R, Reichard PS, Riddle RT: Temporary malfunction of the Ohmeda modulus CD series volume monitor caused by the overhead surgical lighting. Anesthesiology 91:894, 1999

127. Feeley TW, Bancroft ML: Problems with mechanical ventilators. Int Anesthesiol Clin 20:83, 1982

128. Khalil SN, Gholston TK, Binderman J: Flapper valve malfunction in an Ohio closed scavenging system. Anesth Analg 66:1334, 1987

129. Sommer RM, Bhalla GS, Jackson JM: Hypoventilation caused by ventilator valve rupture. Anesth Analg 67:999, 1988

130. Roth S, Tweedie E, Sommer RM: Excessive airway pressure due to a malfunctioning anesthesia ventilator. Anesthesiology 65:532, 1986

131. Dorsch JA, Dorsch SE: Anesthesia ventilators. In Dorsch JA, Dorsch SE (eds): Understanding Anesthesia Equipment, 4th ed, p 309. Baltimore, Williams & Wilkins, 1999

132. Dorsch JA, Dorsch SE: Controlling trace gas levels. In Dorsch JA, Dorsch SE (eds): Understanding Anesthesia Equipment, 4th ed, p 355. Baltimore, Williams & Wilkins, 1999

133. US Department of Health, Education, and Welfare: Criteria for a Recommended Standard: Occupational Exposure to Waste Anesthetic Gases and Vapors. March ed. Washington, DC, 1977

134. American Society for Testing and Materials: Standard Specification for Anesthetic Equipment—Scavenging Systems for Anesthetic Gases (ASTM F1343-91). Philadelphia, American Society for Testing and Materials, 1991

135. ASA Task Force on Trace Anesthetic Gases (McGregor DG, Chair): Waste Anesthetic Gases: Information for Management in Anesthetizing Areas and the Postanesthesia Care Unit (PACU), p 3. Park Ridge, IL, American Society of Anesthesiologists, 1999

136. Kanmura Y, Sakai J, Yoshinaka H, Shirao K: Causes of nitrous oxide contamination in operating rooms. Anesthesiology 90:693, 1999

137. Open Reservoir Scavenger: Operator's Instruction Manual. Telford, PA, North American Dräger, 1986

138. Gray WM: Scavenging equipment. Br J Anaesth 57:685, 1985

139. Scavenger Interface for Air Conditioning: Instruction Manual. Telford, PA, North American Dräger, 1984

140. Cooper JB: Toward prevention of anesthetic mishaps. Int Anesthesiol Clin 22:167, 1984

141. Spooner RB, Kirby RR: Equipment related anesthetic incidents. Int Anesthesiol Clin 22:133, 1984

142. Emergency Care Research Institute: Avoiding anesthetic mishaps through pre-use checks. Health Devices 11:201, 1982

143. Food and Drug Administration: Anesthesia Apparatus Checkout Recommendations, 8th ed. Rockville, MD, Food and Drug Administration, 1986

144. Food and Drug Administration: Anesthesia Apparatus Checkout Recommendations. Rockville, MD, Food and Drug Administration, 1993

145. Myers JA, Good ML, Andrews JJ: Comparison of tests for detecting leaks in the low-pressure system of anesthesia gas machines. Anesth Analg 84:179, 1997

146. Dorsch JA, Dorsch SE: Hazards of anesthesia machines and breathing systems. In Dorsch JA, Dorsch SE (eds): Understanding Anesthesia Equipment, 4th ed, p 399. Baltimore, Williams & Wilkins, 1999

147. Comm G, Rendell-Baker L: Back pressure check valves a hazard. Anesthesiology 56:227, 1982

APPENDIX A

Anesthesia Apparatus Checkout Recommendations, 1993

This checkout, or a reasonable equivalent, should be conducted before administration of anesthesia. These recommendations are only valid for an anesthesia system that conforms to current and relevant standards and includes an ascending bellows ventilator and at least the following monitors: Capnograph, pulse oximeter, oxygen analyzer, respiratory volume monitor (spirometer) and breathing system pressure monitor with high- and low-pressure alarms. This is a guideline which users are encouraged to modify to accommodate differences in equipment design and variations in local clinical practice. Such local modifications should have appropriate peer review. Users should refer to the operator's manual for the manufacturer's specific procedures and precautions, especially the manufacturer's low-pressure leak test (step #5).

Emergency Ventilation Equipment

*1. Verify Back-up Ventilation Equipment Is Available & Functioning

High-Pressure System

*2. Check Oxygen Cylinder Supply
  a. Open O_2 cylinder and verify at least half full (about 1000 psi).
  b. Close cylinder.
*3. Check Central Pipeline Supplies
  a. Check that hoses are connected and pipeline gauges read about 50 psi.

Low-Pressure System

*4. Check Initial Status of Low-Pressure System
  a. Close flow control valves and turn vaporizers off.
  b. Check fill level and tighten vaporizers' filler caps.
*5. Perform Leak Check of Machine Low-Pressure System
  a. Verify that the machine master switch and flow control valves are OFF.
  b. Attach "Suction Bulb" to common (fresh) gas outlet.
  c. Squeeze bulb repeatedly until fully collapsed.
  d. Verify bulb stays *fully* collapsed for at least 10 seconds.
  e. Open one vaporizer at a time and repeat 'c' and 'd' as above.
  f. Remove suction bulb, and reconnect fresh gas hose.
*6. Turn on Machine Master Switch and all other necessary electrical equipment.
*7. Test Flowmeters
  a. Adjust flow of all gases through their full range, checking for smooth operation of floats and undamaged flow tubes.
  b. Attempt to create a hypoxic O_2/N_2O mixture and verify correct changes in flow and/or alarm.

Scavenging System

*8. Adjust and Check Scavenging System
  a. Ensure proper connections between the scavenging system and both APL (pop-off) valve and ventilator relief valve.
  b. Adjust waste gas vacuum (if possible).
  c. Fully open APL valve and occlude Y-piece.
  d. With minimum O_2 flow, allow scavenger reservoir bag to collapse completely and verify that absorber pressure gauge reads about zero.
  e. With the O_2 flush activated, allow the scavenger reservoir bag to distend fully, and then verify that absorber pressure gauge reads < 10 cm H_2O.

Breathing System

*9. Calibrate O_2 Monitor
  a. Ensure monitor reads 21% in room air.
  b. Verify low O_2 alarm is enabled and functioning.

  c. Reinstall sensor in circuit and flush breathing system with O_2.
  d. Verify that monitor now reads greater than 90%.
10. Check Initial Status of Breathing System
  a. Set selector switch to "Bag" mode.
  b. Check that breathing circuit is complete, undamaged and unobstructed.
  c. Verify that CO_2 absorbent is adequate.
  d. Install breathing circuit accessory equipment (*e.g.*, humidifier, PEEP valve) to be used during the case.
11. Perform Leak Check of the Breathing System
  a. Set all gas flows to zero (or minimum).
  b. Close APL (pop-off) valve and occlude Y-piece.
  c. Pressurize breathing system to about 30 cm H_2O with O_2 flush.
  d. Ensure that pressure remains fixed for at least 10 seconds.
  e. Open APL (pop-off) valve and ensure that pressure decreases.

Manual and Automatic Ventilation Systems

12. Test Ventilation Systems and Unidirectional Valves
  a. Place a second breathing bag on Y-piece.
  b. Set appropriate ventilator parameters for next patient.
  c. Switch to automatic ventilation (Ventilator) mode.
  d. Turn ventilator ON and fill bellows and breathing bag with O_2 flush.
  e. Set O_2 flow to minimum, other gas flows to zero.
  f. Verify that during inspiration bellows delivers appropriate tidal volume and that during expiration bellows fills completely.
  g. Set fresh gas flow to about $5 \; l \cdot min^{-1}$.
  h. Verify that the ventilator bellows and simulated lungs fill *and empty* appropriately without sustained pressure at end expiration.
  i. *Check for proper action of unidirectional valves.*
  j. Exercise breathing circuit accessories to ensure proper function.
  k. Turn ventilator OFF and switch to manual ventilation (Bag/APL) mode.
  l. Ventilate manually and assure inflation and deflation of artificial lungs and appropriate feel of system resistance and compliance.
  m. Remove second breathing bag from Y-piece.

Monitors

13. Check, Calibrate and/or Set Alarm Limits of all Monitors
  Capnometer
  Oxygen Analyzer
  Pressure monitor with High and Low Airway Pressure Alarms
  Pulse Oximeter
  Respiratory Volume Monitor (Spirometer)

Final Position

14. Check Final Status of Machine
  a. Vaporizers off.
  b. APL valve open.
  c. Selector switch to "Bag."
  d. All flowmeters to zero (or minimum).
  e. Patient suction level adequate.
  f. Breathing system ready to use.

---

* If an anesthesia provider uses the same machine in successive cases, these steps need not be repeated or may be abbreviated after the initial checkout.

Reproduced from Anesthesia Apparatus Checkout Recommendations, FDA. Rockville, MD, Food and Drug Administration, 1993.

Clinical Anesthesia (4/e), edited by
Paul G. Barash, Bruce F. Cullen, and
Robert K. Stoelting. Lippincott Williams &
Wilkins, Philadelphia, © 2001.

CHAPTER 23

AIRWAY MANAGEMENT

WILLIAM H. ROSENBLATT

PERSPECTIVES ON AIRWAY MANAGEMENT

Perhaps the most important job of the anesthesiologist is the management of the patient's airway. Though many medical disciplines deal with airway management on an emergency basis, few others are responsible for the routine, deliberate, and usually elective ablation of the patient's intrinsic controls of respiration. Published morbidity and mortality data demonstrate that airway difficulties and mismanagement are responsible for a significant proportion of adverse anesthetic outcomes in clinical practice. Keenan and Boyan reported that failure to provide adequate ventilation was responsible for 12 of 27 cardiac arrests during the operative period.[1] The single largest source of unfavorable outcome in the American Society of Anesthesiologists (ASA) closed-claims study was for adverse respiratory episodes, which accounted for 34% of 1541 liability claims.[2] Three mechanisms of injury accounted for 75% of these undesirable events: inadequate ventilation (38%), esophageal intubation (18%), and difficult tracheal intubation (17%). Death and brain damage occurred in nearly 85% of the cases studied. In their analysis of 300 liability claims for less frequent, but important categories of ventilation-related undesirable outcomes, Cheney et al identified recurrent themes of management error or patterns of injury: airway trauma, pneumothorax, airway obstruction, aspiration, and bronchospasm.[3] Given these statistics, it is clear that management of the airway is paramount to safe perioperative care and the following steps become necessary to favorably affect outcome: (1) a thorough airway history and physical examination; (2) a management plan for use of a supraglottic means of ventilation (e.g., face mask, Laryngeal Mask Airway [LMA]); (3) a management plan for intubation and extubation techniques; (4) an alternative plan of action should emergencies arise.

Review of Airway Anatomy

The term "airway," refers to the upper airway—consisting of the nasal and oral cavities, pharynx, larynx, trachea, and principal bronchi. The airway in humans is primarily a conducting pathway. Because the oroesophageal and nasotracheal passages cross each other, anatomic and functional complexities have evolved for protection of the sublaryngeal airway against aspiration of food that passes through the pharynx. Anatomically complex, the airway undergoes growth and development and significant changes in its size, shape, and relation to cervical spine between infancy and childhood.[4] Similar to other systems in the body, it is not immune from the influence of genetic, nutritional, and hormonal factors. Table 23-1 illustrates the anatomic differences in the larynx between the infant and adult.

The laryngeal skeleton consists of nine cartilages (three paired and three unpaired); together, these house the vocal folds, which extend in an anterior–posterior plane from the thyroid cartilage to the arytenoid cartilages. The shield-shaped thyroid cartilage acts as the anterior "protective housing" of the vocal mechanism (Fig. 23-1). Movements of the laryngeal structures are controlled by two groups of muscles: the extrinsic muscles, which move the larynx as a whole, and the intrinsic muscles, which move the various cartilages in relation to one another. The larynx is innervated bilaterally by two branches of

each vagus nerve: the superior laryngeal nerve and the recurrent laryngeal nerve. Because the recurrent laryngeal nerves supply all of the intrinsic muscles of the larynx (with the exception of cricothyroid), trauma to these nerves can result in vocal cord dysfunction. As a result of unilateral nerve injury, airway function is usually unimpaired, but the protective role of larynx in preventing aspiration may be compromised.

The cricothyroid membrane, provides coverage to the cricothyroid space. The membrane, which is typically 9 mm in height and 3 cm in width, is composed of a yellow elastic tissue that lies directly subcutaneous to the skin and a thin facial layer. It is located in the anterior neck between the thyroid cartilage superiorly and the cricoid cartilage inferiorly. It can be identified 1–1.5 fingerbreadths below the laryngeal prominence (thyroid notch, or Adam's apple). It is often crossed horizontally in its upper third by the anastomosis of the left and right superior cricothyroid arteries. The membrane has a central portion known as the conus elasticus and two lateral portions, which are thinner and located directly over the laryngeal mucosa. Because of anatomic variability in the course of veins and arteries and its proximity to the vocal folds (which are 0.9 cm above the ligaments' upper border), it is suggested that any incisions or needle punctures to the cricothyroid membrane be made in its inferior third and be directed posteriorly.

At the base of the larynx, suspended by the underside of the cricothyroid membrane, is the signet ring–shaped cricoid cartilage. This cartilage is approximately 1 cm in height anteriorly, but almost 2 cm in height in its posterior aspect as it extends in a cephalad direction, behind the cricothyroid membrane and the thyroid cartilage (Fig. 23-1). The trachea is suspended from the cricoid cartilage by the cricotracheal ligament. The trachea measures ~15 cm in adults and is circumferentially supported by 17–18 C-shaped cartilages, with a posterior membranous aspect overlying the esophagus (Fig. 23-2).

The first tracheal ring is anterior to the sixth cervical vertebrae. The tracheal cartilages are interconnected by fibroelastic tissue, which allows for expansion of the trachea both in length and diameter with inspiration/expiration and flexion/extension of the thoracocervical spine. The trachea ends at the carina at the level of the fifth thoracic vertebra, where it bifurcates into the principal bronchi (Fig. 23-3). The right principal bronchus is larger in diameter than the left, and deviates from the plane of the trachea at a less acute angle. Because it is therefore a fairly direct continuation of the trachea, aspirated materials, as well as a deeply inserted tracheal tube, tend to gain entry into the right principal bronchus. Cartilaginous rings support the first seven generations of the bronchi.

Patient History and Physical Exam

Preoperative evaluation of the patient should elicit a thorough history of airway-related untoward events as well as related symptoms. If feasible, a search for documentation to confirm or elucidate these problems should be conducted. Signs and symptoms related to the airway should be elicited, such as snoring (e.g., obstructive sleep apnea), chipped teeth, changes in voice, dysphagia, stridor, cervical spine pain or limited range of motion, upper extremity neuropathy, temporomandibular joint pain or dysfunction, and significant or prolonged sore throat/mandible after a previous anesthetic. Many congenital and ac-

Table 23-1. ANATOMIC DIFFERENCES BETWEEN THE PEDIATRIC AND ADULT AIRWAYS

Proportionately smaller infant/child larynx

Narrowest portion: Cricoid cartilage in infant/child; vocal folds in adult

Relative vertical location: C3, C4, C5 in infant/child; C4, C5, C6 in adult

Epiglottis: Longer, narrower, and stiffer in infant/child

Aryepiglottic folds closer to midline in infant/child

Vocal folds: Anterior angle with respect to perpendicular axis of larynx in infant/child

Pliable laryngeal cartilage in infant/child

Mucosa more vulnerable to trauma in infant/child

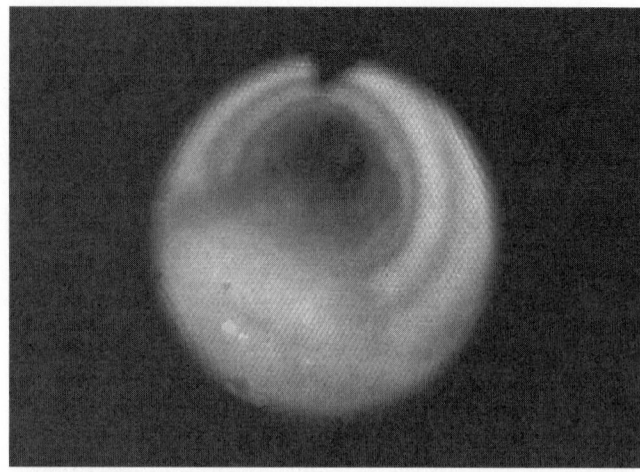

Figure 23-2. Bronchoscopic view of the adult trachea. The cartilaginous, C-shaped tracheal rings are seen anteriorly, and the membranous portion, overlying the esophagus, is posterior.

quired syndromes are associated with difficult airway management (Table 23-2).

Of course, some pathology will only present on the induction of anesthesia and/or attempts at laryngoscopy (Fig. 23-4). In one landmark case, a patient who was an impossible mask ventilation, laryngoscopy, and LMA placement had an unsuspected airway mass.[5]

In general, tracheal intubation is difficult under the following conditions: (1) the presence of equally important priorities to the management of the airway ("full stomach," "open globe," etc.), (2) abnormal airway anatomy, (3) an emergency, or (4) direct injury to the larynx and/or trachea. Physical examination should focus on the state of dentition, the presence of a beard, mouth size, submandibular soft tissue compliance, atlanto-occipital extension, identification of the cricothyroid membrane, and the presence of pharyngeal pathology. Although the finding of abnormal anatomy is not necessarily synonymous with the difficult airway, it should kindle a heightened level of suspicion. Several investigators have identified anatomic features as having unfavorable influences on the mechanics of direct laryngoscopy; these are explainable on the basis of disproportion, distortion, decreased mobility of joints, and dental overbite. In the earliest attempt to describe anatomic correlates of difficult intubation, Cass *et al* placed emphasis on a short muscular neck with a full dentition, a receding mandible with

obtuse mandibular angles, protruding maxillary incisor teeth, decreased mobility at temporomandibular joints, a long high arched palate, and increased alveolar-mental distance.[6] Early radiographic studies showed that the posterior depth of the mandible (the distance between the bony alveolus immediately behind the third molar tooth and the lower border of mandible) was an important factor in determining the ease or difficulty of laryngoscopy.[7] Later, the "thyromental distance," the distance from the tip of the mentum to the thyroid notch, was described as being a crucial measure to be evaluated.[8] A distance of less than 6 cm was determined to be predictive of a difficult laryngoscopy. This concept was expanded upon by Savva,[9] who measured the sternomental distance with maximal head extension. This measure functionally "added" the atlanto-occipital joint into the evaluation. A measure of less than 12 cm was proposed to

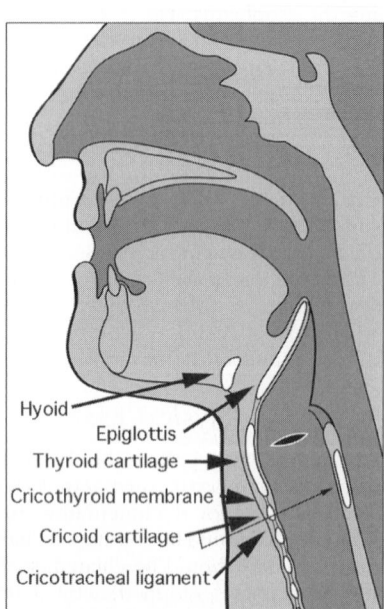

Figure 23-1. The major landmarks of the airway mechanism. Note that the cricoid cartilage is less than 1 cm in height in its anterior aspect, but may be 2 cm in height posteriorly (*small arrow*).

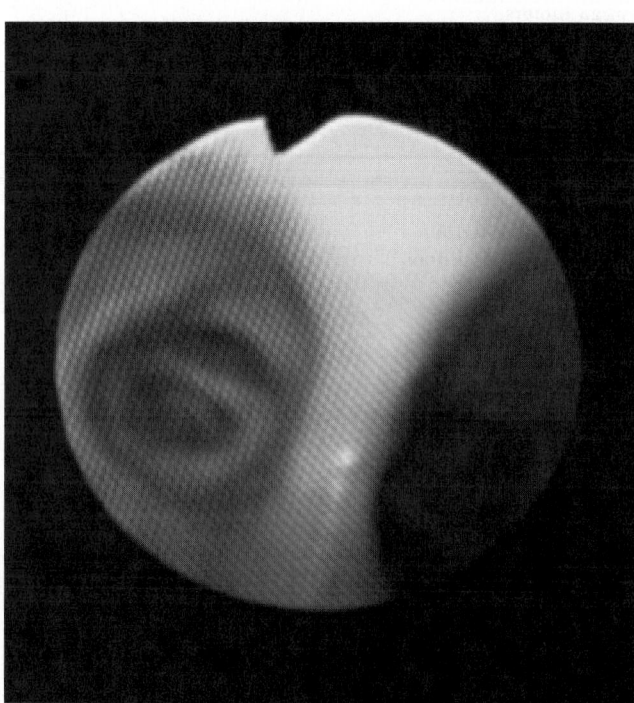

Figure 23-3. The adult tracheal carina. The cartilaginous rings of the principal bronchi are easily visualized beyond the carina.

Table 23-2. SYNDROMES ASSOCIATED WITH DIFFICULT AIRWAY MANAGEMENT

Pathologic Condition	Principal Pathologic Clinical Features Pertaining to Airway
CONGENITAL	
Pierre Robin syndrome	Micrognathia, macroglossia, glossoptosis, cleft soft palate
Treacher Collins syndrome (mandibulofacial dysostosis)	Auricular and ocular defects; malar and mandibular hypoplasia, microstomia, choanal atresia
Goldenhar's syndrome (oculo-auriculo-vertebral syndrome)	Auricular and ocular defects; malar and mandibular hypoplasia; occipitalization of atlas
Down's syndrome (mongolism)	Poorly developed or absent bridge of the nose; macroglossia, microcephaly, cervical spine abnormalities
Klippel-Feil syndrome	Congenital fusion of a variable number of cervical vertebrae; restriction of neck movement
Alpert's syndrome (acrocephalosyndactyly)	Maxillary hypoplasia, prognathism, cleft soft palate, tracheobronchial cartilaginous anomalies
Beckwith's syndrome (infantile gigantism)	Macroglossia
Cherubism	Tumorous lesion of mandibles and maxillae with intraoral masses
Cretinism (congenital hypothyroidism)	Absent thyroid tissue or defective synthesis of thyroxine; macroglossia, goiter, compression of trachea, deviation of larynx/trachea
Cri du chat syndrome	Chromosome 5-P abnormal; microcephaly, micrognathia, laryngomalacia, stridor
Meckel's syndrome	Microcephaly, micrognathia, cleft epiglottis
von Recklinghausen disease (neurofibromatosis)	Increased incidence of pheochromocytoma; tumors may occur in the larynx and right ventricle outflow tract
Hurler's syndrome (mucopolysaccharidosis I)	Stiff joints, upper airway obstruction due to infiltration of lymphoid tissue; abnormal tracheobronchial cartilages; frequent upper respiratory infections
Hunter's syndrome (mucopolysaccharidosis II)	Same as in Hurler's syndrome, but less severe; pneumonias
Pompe's disease (glycogen storage II)	Muscle deposits, macroglossia
ACQUIRED	
Infections	
Supraglottitis	Laryngeal edema
Croup	Laryngeal edema
Abscess (intraoral, retropharyngeal)	Distortion and stenosis of the airway and trismus
Papillomatosis	Chronic viral infection forming obstructive papillomas, primarily supraglottic. Frequent surgical removals. May be spread subglottic, especially after tracheostomy
Ludwig's angina	Distortion and stenosis of the airway and trismus
Arthritis	
Rheumatoid arthritis	Temporomandibular joint ankylosis, cricoarytenoid arthritis, deviation of larynx, restricted mobility of cervical spine
Ankylosing spondylitis	Ankylosis of cervical spine; less commonly ankylosis of temporomandibular joints; lack of mobility of cervical spine
Benign tumors	
Cystic hygroma, lipoma, adenoma, goiter	Stenosis or distortion of the airway
Malignant tumors	
Carcinoma of tongue, carcinoma of larynx, carcinoma of thyroid	Stenosis or distortion of the airway; fixation of larynx or adjacent tissues secondary to infiltration or fibrosis from irradiation
Trauma	
Head injury, facial injury, cervical spine injury	Cerebrospinal rhinorrhea, edema of the airway; hemorrhage; unstable fracture(s) of the maxillae and mandible; intralaryngeal damage; dislocation of cervical vertebrae
Miscellaneous conditions	
Morbid obesity	Short, thick neck and large tongue are likely to be present
Acromegaly	Macroglossia; prognathism
Acute burns	Edema of airway

be a positive finding. Turning attention to the intraoral cavity, Mallampati suggested that when the tongue base is disproportionately large, it renders laryngoscopy and intubation difficult; difficulty arises not only from the anatomic overshadowing of the larynx but also from the acuity of the angle between the tongue base and larynx.[10] This anatomic relationship does not allow easy exposure of the glottis. In contrast, it is logical to deduce that a proportionate tongue would not hinder exposure of laryngeal inlet, provided there are no associated factors that impede axis alignment or restrict the mobility of joints. A massive tongue not only overshadows the larynx but also masks the visibility of pharyngeal space and other structures, including

soft palate, uvula, and faucial pillars. For elicitation of this clinical sign, the patient remains seated with his or her head in the neutral position, opens the mouth as widely as possible, and protrudes the tongue to the maximum extent. The Mallampati classification is based on the extent to which the base of tongue is able to mask the visibility of pharyngeal structures (Fig. 23-5). Samsoon and Young modified the Mallampati classification to include a fourth class, representing an extreme form of Mallampati's Class III, in which the soft palate is totally masked by the tongue.[11] In this "Class IV," only the hard palate is visible. Significant correlation was found between airway class and degree of ease or difficulty of exposure of glottis by direct laryngos-

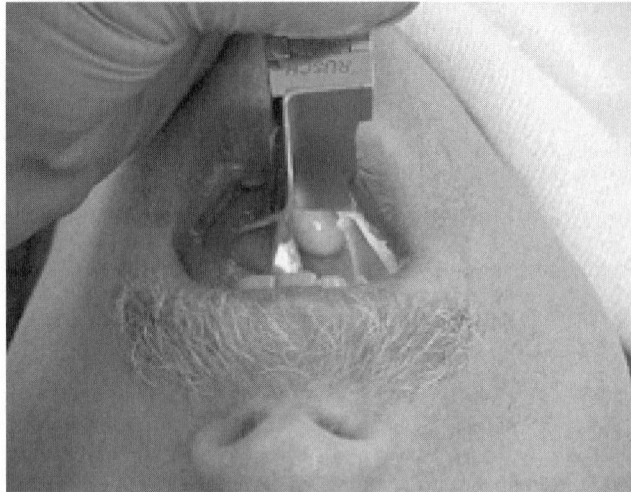

Figure 23-4. A 40-year-old male whose epiglottic cyst was discovered at laryngoscopy.

copy. The practical value of this method lies in its ease of application. Unfortunately, this index, as with most others, has not proven to be sensitive or specific in identifying difficult-to-intubate patients. In a trial of 675 patients, this index detected only 5 of 12 difficult airways, and gave 139 false positives.[12]

It should be noted that the traditional examinations of the airway, including the Mallampati/Samsoon and Young classes, the thyromental distance, and the sternomental distance, may reveal much about the ability to perform direct laryngoscopy, but say little about the ability to use supraglottic ventilatory devices (*e.g.*, Laryngeal Mask Airway, Cuffed Oropharyngeal Airway [COPA], Tracheal Esophageal Combitube), or indirect vision guides (*e.g.*, the fiberoptic bronchoscope, the Bullard laryngoscope).

CLINICAL MANAGEMENT OF THE AIRWAY
Preoxygenation

Preoxygenation (also commonly termed "denitrogenation") should be practiced in all cases when time permits.[13] This procedure entails the replacement of the nitrogen volume of the

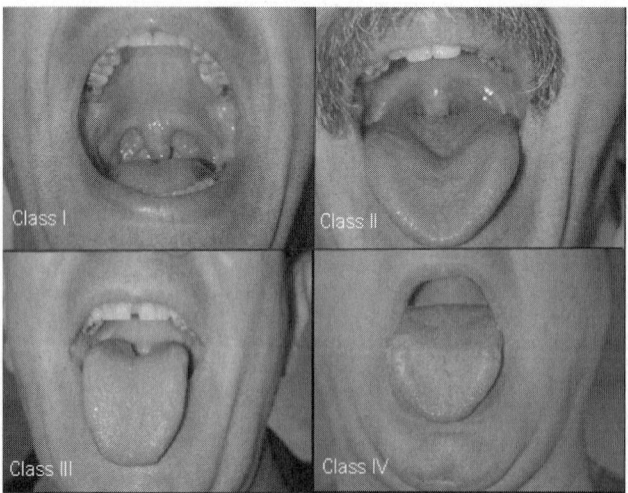

Figure 23-5. Mallampati/Samsoon–Young classification of the oropharyngeal view.[10] *Class I:* uvula, faucial pillars, soft palate visible; *Class II:* faucial pillars, soft palate visible; *Class III:* soft and hard palate visible; *Class IV:* hard palate visible only (added by Samsoon and Young).

lung (upwards of 69% of the functional residual capacity [FRC]) with oxygen to provide a reservoir for diffusion into the alveolar capillary blood after the onset of apnea.[14] Preoxygenation with 100% O_2 and spontaneous ventilation with a tight-fitting face mask for 5 minutes can furnish up to 10 minutes of oxygen reserve following apnea (in a patient without significant cardiopulmonary disease and a normal oxygen consumption).[15] In one study of healthy, nonobese patients who were allowed to breathe 100% O_2 preoperatively, subjects sustained an oxygen saturation of greater than 90% for 6 ± 0.5 min, whereas obese patients experienced oxyhemoglobin desaturation to under 90% in 2.7 ± 0.25 min.[16] The patient breathing room air (21% O_2) will experience oxyhemoglobin desaturation to a level of under 90% after approximately 2 min under ideal conditions. Patients in respiratory failure, or with conditions affecting metabolism or lung volumes, frequently evidence desaturation sooner owing to increased O_2 extraction, decreased FRC, or right-to-left transpulmonary shunting. The most common reason for not achieving a maximum alveolar F_{IO_2} during preoxygenation is a loose-fitting mask, allowing the entrainment of room air.[13] Less time-consuming methods of preoxygenation have also been described. Using a series of 4 vital capacity breaths of 100% O_2 over a 30-sec period, a high arterial Pa_{O_2} (339 torr) can be achieved, but the time to desaturation is consistently shorter as compared to techniques of breathing 100% O_2 for 5 min.[17] A modified vital capacity technique, wherein the patient is asked to take eight deep breaths in a 60-sec period, shows promise in terms of prolonging the time to desaturation.[13,18] I prefer the technique of applying a tight-fitting mask for 5 min or more of tidal volume breathing; the mask is placed immediately after the patient has been made comfortable on the operating room table, and remains in place during intravenous catheter insertion and application of monitors. Pharyngeal insufflation of oxygen is a technique that has been described to prolong the duration that an apneic patient sustains an oxyhemoglobin saturation of >90%. In this technique, oxygen is insufflated at a rate of $3\,1 \cdot min^{-1}$ via a catheter passed through the nares. This technique relies upon the phenomenon of apneic oxygenation, a process by which gases are entrained into the alveolar space during apnea, as long as there is a patent airway.[19] This entrainment can provide enough oxygen to sustain hemoglobin saturation for prolonged periods. It is based upon the decrease in intrathoracic pressure, relative to atmospheric pressure, produced as approximately 210 cm³ of oxygen diffuses into the alveolar capillary bed each minute while as little as 12 cm³ of carbon dioxide diffuses into the alveolar space (the remainder of the carbon dioxide being buffered in the blood or tissues). The alveolar carbon dioxide is not removed in this situation, limiting the duration of this technique of oxygenation.

Support of the Airway with the Induction of Anesthesia

With the induction of anesthesia and the onset of apnea, ventilation and oxygenation are supported by the anesthesiologist. Traditional methods include the anesthesia face mask, and the tracheal tube. Recently, a number of supralaryngeal airway support devices have been introduced into worldwide clinical practice. Of these, the Laryngeal Mask Airway (LMA) has gained significant acceptance among anesthesiologists in the United States, with use rates as high as 35% of all general anesthesia cases, in some settings.[20] This device, and others that have evolved from it, are reviewed here extensively, since they represent a significant change in airway management practice.

The Anesthesia Face Mask

The anesthesia face mask is the device most commonly used to deliver anesthetic gases and oxygen as well as to ventilate the patient who has been made apneic.

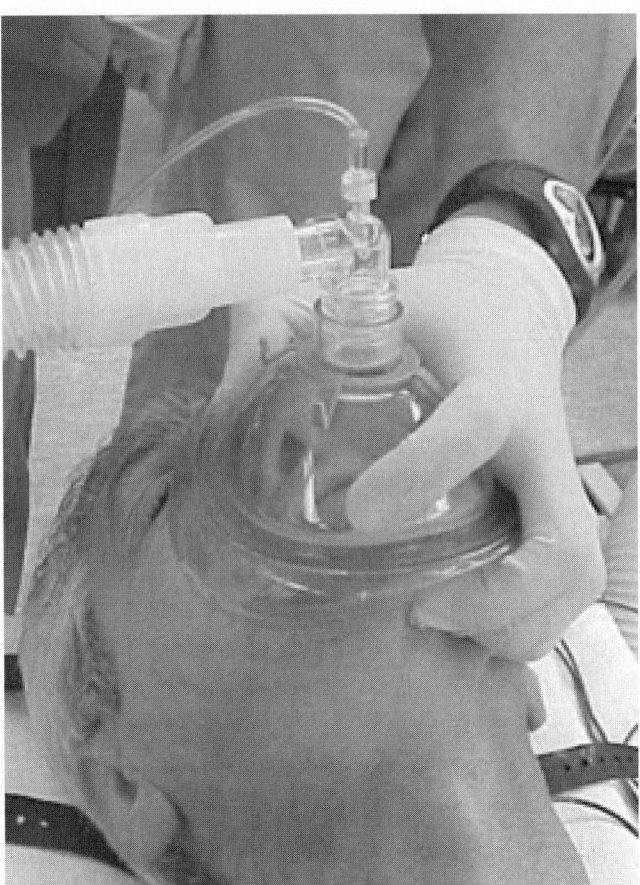

Figure 23-6. Holding the anesthesia mask on the face. The thumb and the first finger grip the mask in such a fashion that the anesthesia circuit (or ambu bag) connection abuts the web between these digits. This allows the palm of the hand to apply pressure to the left side of the mask, while the tips of these three digits apply pressure over the right. The third finger helps to secure under the mentum, while the forth finger is under the angle of the mandible or along the lower mandibular ridge. Mask straps (on pillow) may be used to complement the hand grip by securing the right side of the mask.

The skillful use of a face mask is challenging and, despite the many advances in airway management, remains a mainstay in the delivery of anesthesia and resuscitation. When the induction of anesthesia commences, the patient's level of consciousness changes from the awake state, with a competent and protected airway, to the unconscious state, with an unprotected and potentially obstructed airway. This is drug-induced central ventilatory drive depression with a relaxation of the musculature of the upper airway that can rapidly lead to hypercapnea and hypoxia. Thus, ventilation by face mask becomes critical to management of the airway.

Appropriate positioning of the patient is paramount to successful mask ventilation. With the patient in the supine position, the head and neck are placed in the *sniffing* position, which is discussed extensively below. Not only does this position improve mask ventilation by anteriorizing the base of the tongue and the epiglottis, but also aligns the axes of the oral cavity, pharynx, and trachea in preparation for laryngoscopy.

The mask is gently held over the patient's face with the left hand, leaving the right hand free for other uses (Fig. 23-6). Elastic "mask straps" may be used to help secure the mask in the awake or anesthetized patient who is breathing spontaneously and without obstruction, or to complement the left-hand grip. The mask straps can be particularly helpful for the clinician with short fingers. However, prolonged use of tight-fitting mask straps has been associated with motor and sensory neuropraxias.

After induction of anesthesia, a tight fit of the face mask is achieved by downward displacement of the mask between the thumb and first/second fingers with concurrent upward displacement of the mandible with the remaining fingers. This latter maneuver, commonly known as a *jaw thrust*, raises the soft tissues of the anterior airway off of the pharyngeal wall and allows for improved ventilation. In those patients who are obese, edentulous, or bearded, two hands or a mask strap may be required to ensure a tight fitting mask seal. When two hands are required for holding the face mask, a second operator will obviously be required to ventilate the patient (Fig. 23-7). If need be, the second operator can lend a third hand to the mask fitting.

It must be noted that the patient with normal lung compliance should require no more than 20–25 cm H_2O pressure to inflate the lungs. If more pressure than this is required, the clinician should reevaluate the adequacy of the airway, then adjust the mask fit, seek the aid of a second operator in order to perform two- or three-handed mask holds, and/or consider other devices that aid in the creation of a open passage for air flow through the upper airway. Both rigid oral airways and soft nasal airways create an artificial passage between the roof of the mouth, tongue, and the posterior pharyngeal wall (Fig. 23-8).

Oral airways, which come in a wide variety of sizes, can stimulate the semiconscious patient and provoke coughing, vomiting, and/or laryngospasm. The level of anesthesia must be assessed before they are inserted. Likewise, a LMA or COPA may be used at this juncture if the anesthetic is adequate. Nasal airways, less stimulating to the patient, can cause significant nasal trauma and bleeding and should be used with extreme caution in patients with known coagulopathy or nasal deformities. These devices are contraindicated in the patient with a basilar skull fracture.

Obstruction to mask ventilation may be caused by laryngospasm, an intrinsic closure of the vocal folds. Laryngospasm occurs as a result of foreign body (*e.g.,* oral or nasal airway), saliva, blood, or vomitus touching the glottis, or even a light plane of anesthesia. Hypoxia as well as noncardiogenic pulmonary edema can result if there is continued spontaneous ventilation against closed vocal cords. Treatment of laryngospasm includes removal of an offending stimulus (if it can be identified), continuous positive airway pressure, deepening of the anesthetic state, and the use of a rapid-acting muscle relaxant.

If there are no contraindications (*e.g.,* a "full stomach" or other aspiration risk), mask ventilation can be the technique employed for the duration of anesthesia maintenance. Otherwise, it is commonly used to administer anesthetic gases until the anesthetic state is adequate for use of another means of airway support (*e.g.,* tracheal tube). This decision is made after careful consideration of the patient's coexisting diseases and surgical requirements.

The Laryngeal Mask Airway

The LMA was introduced into clinical practice in the 1980s, and was approved as a substitute for the face mask during elective anesthesia by the U.S. Food and Drug Administration in 1991 (Fig. 23-9). It also was recommended as a substitute for the tracheal tube in cases where tracheal intubation was not necessary. Though initially the LMA enjoyed limited acceptance among anesthesiologists, its role has expanded in recent years, so that practicing anesthesiologists report that 23% of all cases are being managed with the LMA.[20]

LMA Design. The LMA is composed of a small "mask" designed to sit in the hypopharynx, with an anterior surface aperture overlying the laryngeal inlet. The rim of the mask is composed of an inflatable silicone cuff which fills the hypopharyngeal space, creating a seal that allows positive pressure ventilation with up to 20 cm H_2O pressure.[21] The adequacy of the seal is dependent on correct placement and appropriate size. It is less dependent on the cuff filling pressure. Attached to the

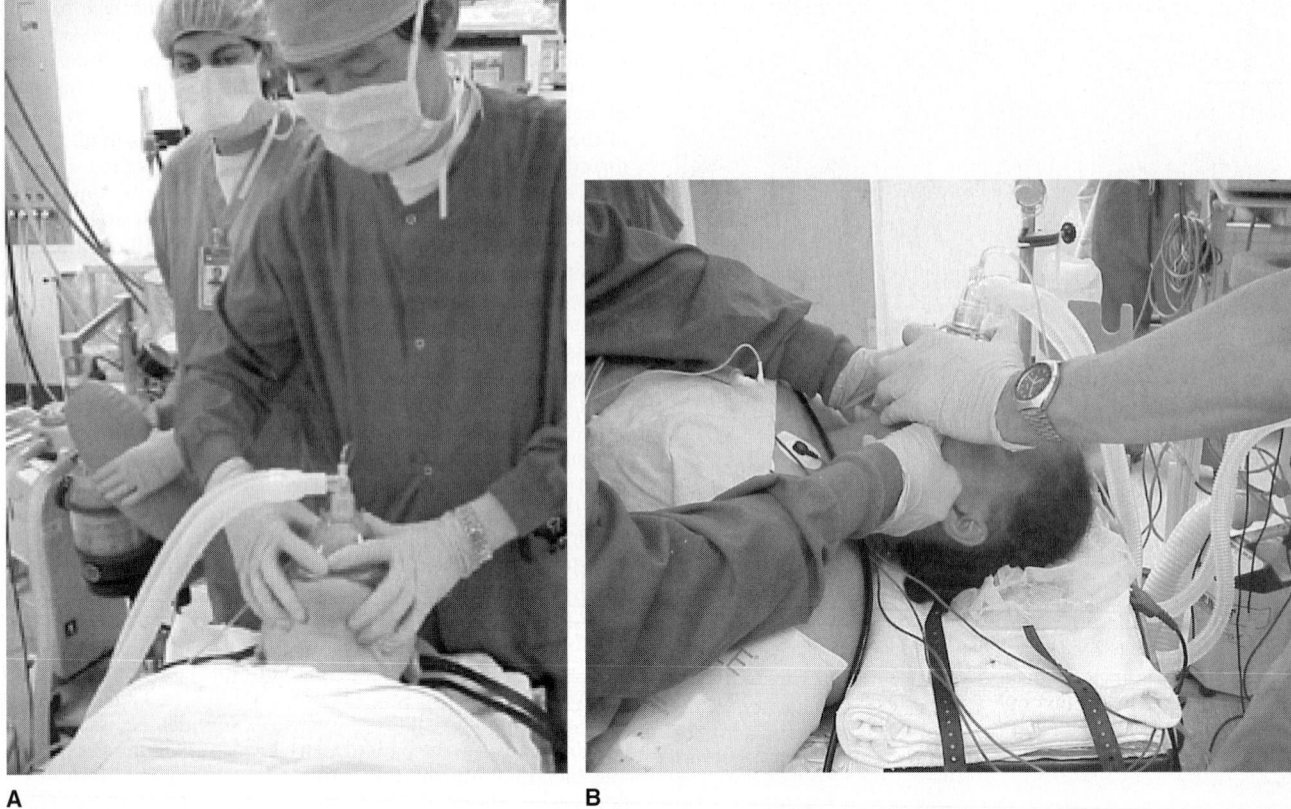

A   B

Figure 23-7. When mask ventilation is difficult owing to upper airway obstruction, a second operator may be required so that (*A*) two or (*B*) three hands can be used in a jaw thrust maneuver.

posterior surface of the mask is a barrel (airway tube) which extends from the mask's central aperture through the mouth and can be connected to an ambu bag or anesthesia circuit.

A range of sizes are available for use in neonates through adults. LMA size selection is critical to its successful use, and to the avoidance of minor as well as more significant complications. Table 23-3 gives the recommended size for patient weight and the maximum inflation volumes.

The manufacturer recommends that the clinician choose the largest size that will comfortably fit in the oral cavity, then inflate to the minimum pressure that allows ventilation to 20 cm H_2O without an air leak. The intracuff pressure should never exceed 60 cm H_2O (and should be periodically monitored if nitrous oxide is used as part of the anesthetic). When an adequate seal cannot be obtained with 60 cm H_2O cuff pressure, the LMA may be malpositioned and/or sizing should be reevaluated.

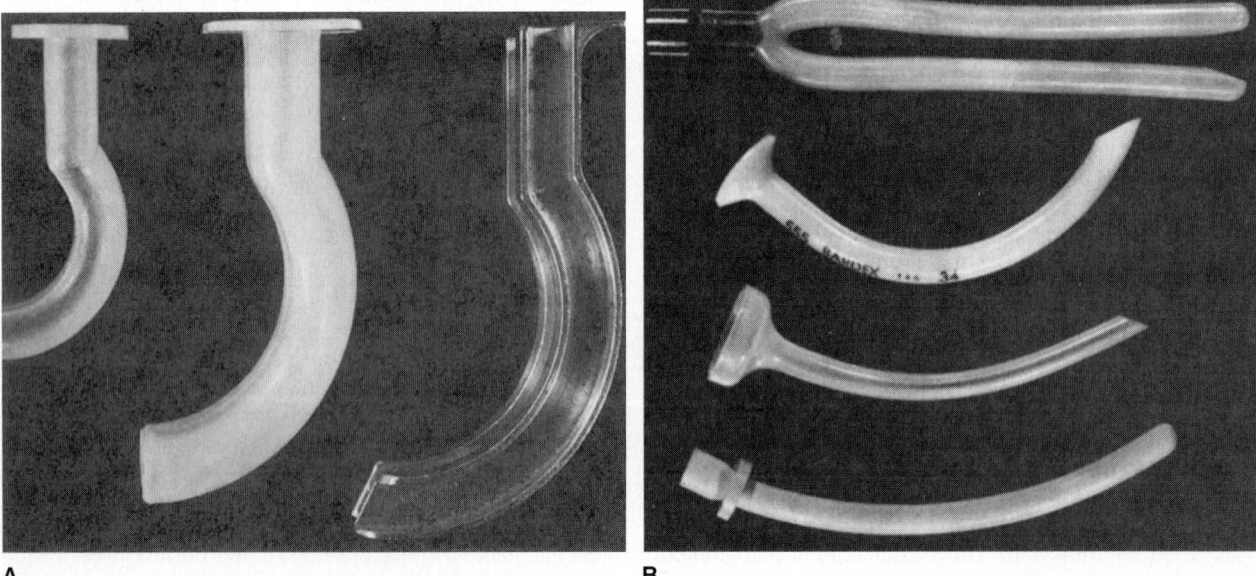

A   B

Figure 23-8. A variety of oral (*A*) and nasal (*B*) airways are available. The goal of these devices is to hold the base of the tongue forward to create an air passage.

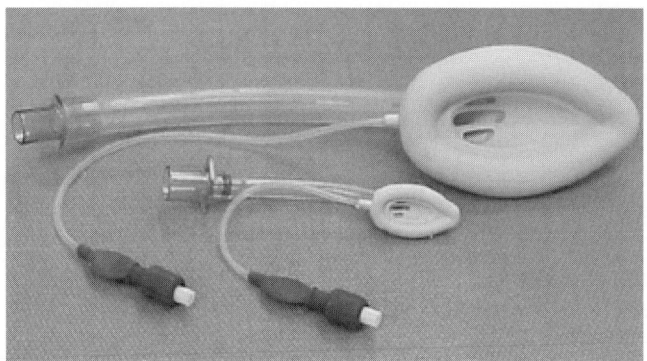

Figure 23-9. The original LMA design: a size 1 and size 6 LMA-Classic. The two bars over the airway aperture prevent the epiglottis from obstructing the LMA barrel.

Light anesthesia may also contribute to poor seal or partial or complete laryngospasm.

LMA Insertion. The insertion of the LMA as described by its inventor, Dr. Archie J. I. Brain, has been modified by a number of writers. Discussion of these various alternatives is beyond the scope of this text. Dr. Brain's initial contemplations of this unique airway considered routine and natural placement of a "foreign body" in the hypopharynx—food. It was Dr. Brain's intent to mimic the placement of food into the hypopharynx and thereby establish the placement of a device, which could then serve as an airway.

In order to understand the insertion technique, we must therefore review the processes of deglutination: lubrication with saliva; formation of a flat oval food bolus by the tongue; initiation of the swallowing reflex by stimulation of the palate; upward pressure by the tongue flattening the food bolus against the palate; directing of the food bolus toward the posterior pharyngeal wall and into the hypopharynx by the shape of the palate and pharyngeal wall; head extension and neck flexion opening the space behind the larynx to allow passage of the food bolus into the hypopharynx; and finally, opening of the upper esophageal sphincter to allow esophageal entry of the food bolus. These functions allow the food bolus to reach its mark blindly, while avoiding the anterior pharyngeal structures and avoiding reflex responses meant to protect the airway.

Prototype insertion methods involved rotation through 180° and the early use of an introducer to prevent down-folding of the epiglottis. The currently recommended, technique illustrated in Figure 23-10 has been found to be less traumatic and have a 98% success rate. In this technique the mask is lubricated with a non-silicone, non-local anesthetic–containing lubricant (simulating the saliva), and is fully deflated to form a thin, flat wedge shape (*cf.* masticated food bolus). The operator's nondominant hand is placed under the occiput to flex the neck on the thorax

and extend the head at the atlanto-occipital joint (creating a space behind the larynx; this action also tends to open the mouth). The index finger of the dominant hand is placed in the cleft between the mask and barrel. The hard palate is visualized and the superior (nonaperture) surface of the mask is placed against it. Force is applied by the index finger in an upward direction toward the top of the patient's head. This will cause the mask to flatten out against the palate and follow the shape of the palate as it slides into the pharynx and hypopharynx. The index finger continues along this arc, always applying an outward pressure until the resistance of the upper esophageal sphincter is met. The most common error made by clinicians is applying pressure with a posterior vector. This tends to catch the tip of the LMA on the posterior pharyngeal wall, causing folding with resultant misplacement and trauma.

Once insertion is complete, removal of the inserting hand is facilitated by gentle stabilization of the LMA barrel with the nondominant hand. Prior to attachment of the anesthesia circuit, the LMA is inflated with the minimum amount of gas to form an effective seal. Though it is difficult to suggest a particular volume of gas to be used, the operator should be accustomed to the feel of the pilot bulb when it is inflated to 60 cm H_2O pressure, the maximum suggested seal pressure. Accompanying the inflation, one should be able to observe a rising of the cricoid and thyroid cartilage and lifting of the barrel out of the mouth by approximately 1 cm as the mask is lifted off the upper esophageal sphincter. The mask is fixed in position by bringing the barrel down against the chin and taping in the midline while a gentle upward pressure is exerted against the hard palate. If a midline position is not possible owing to the nature of the patient position or surgical procedure, a flexible LMA (discussed below) should be considered. A bite block is recommend to prevent biting and occlusion of the LMA barrel.[22]

The LMA and Gastroesophageal Reflux. Although the distal tip of the LMA's mask sits in the esophageal inlet, it does not reliably seal it. A predominant clinical perception is that the LMA does not protect the trachea from regurgitated gastric contents. As of December 1999, just 20 cases of suspected pulmonary aspiration have been reported (with an estimated 100,000,000 uses of the LMA worldwide). Of these, only 12 were verified as true aspiration events and none resulted in death, though five patients required positive-pressure ventilation. There were predisposing factors in most of the cases, including obesity, dementia, emergency surgery, upper abdominal surgery, Trendelenburg position, intraperitoneal insufflation, or a difficult airway.[23–33] Indeed when used in patients at low risk for regurgitation, the rate of aspiration during LMA use is similar to that in all non-LMA general anesthetics (~2 in 10,000 cases), though the incidence of gastroesophageal reflux may be increased when compared to use of the face mask.[34–40]

Some evidence suggests that there may be more gastroesophageal reflux during LMA use with a patient in the Trendelenburg

Table 23-3. LMA SIZING AND INFLATION VOLUMES

LMA Size	Patient Weight	Increase in Size (%)	Maximum Inflation Volume (ml)	Test Inflation Volume (ml)
1	Neonates/infants up to 5 kg	—	4	6
1.5	5–10 kg	21	7	10
2	10–20 kg	21	10	15
2.5	20–30 kg	18	14	21
3	>30 kg	15.7	20	30
4	Small adults	14.4	30	45
5	Normal adults	13.8	40	60
6	Large adults	8.1		

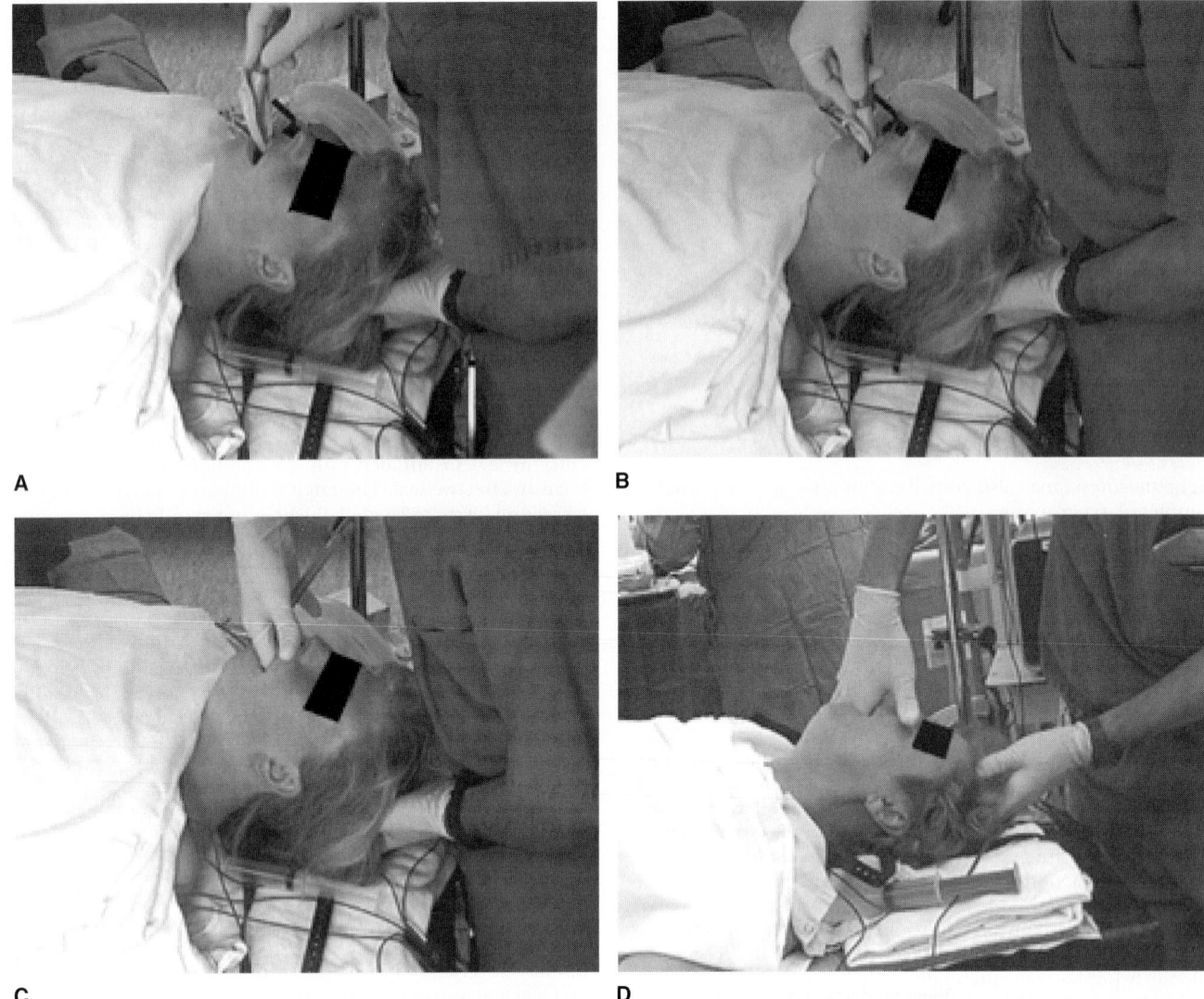

Figure 23-10. Insertion of the LMA. The LMA is inserted with the index finger of the dominant hand pressing with a force vector against the hard palate (*A* and *B*). The outward force vector is continued from the hard palate to the pharynx and hypopharynx (*C*) until the index finger meets resistance against the upper esophageal sphincter (*D*).

or lithotomy position.[39,41] If regurgitated gastric contents are noted in the LMA barrel, maneuvers similar to those applied when using an ETT should be instituted: Trendelenburg position, administer 100% oxygen, leave the LMA in place and use a flexible suction device down the barrel, deepen anesthetic if necessary.

When populations of patients considered to have a full stomach are studied (in controlled trials, prospective series, or anecdotally), there is a very low incidence of aspiration noted with elective or emergency LMA use. Reports have included patients who are morbidly obese or experience frequent gastroesophageal reflux and those undergoing elective cesarean section or airway rescue during labor and those presenting to emergency departments or paramedic crews.[42–51]

During cardiopulmonary resuscitation, the incidence of gastroesophageal regurgitation is four times greater with a bagvalve mask than with the LMA.[52]

Unconventional Use of the LMA. Since its introduction, a wealth of clinical data has indicated that the LMA can be safely used in the operating room in a variety of clinical situations. A large number of clinical situations traditionally managed with tracheal intubation and mechanical ventilation have been per-

formed with the LMA. Table 23-4 presents a number of these clinical situations, describes some of the advantages and precautions of LMA use, and provides appropriate references. A few of these clinical scenarios are discussed in the text.

LMA and Positive-Pressure Ventilation. Though first introduced for use with spontaneous ventilation, the LMA has proved useful for cases in which positive-pressure ventilation is either desired or preferred.[53,54] Contrary to initial impression, positive-pressure ventilation can be safely accomplished with the LMA.[55–60] There is no difference found in gastric inflation with positive pressure (<17 cm H_2O) when comparing the LMA and the ETT.[61,62] When using the LMA, one should limit tidal volumes to 8 ml · kg^{-1} and airway pressure to 20 cm H_2O since this is the sealing pressure of the device under normal circumstances. The clinician should also auscultate over the throat in order detect leak, or over the stomach to detect gastric insufflation. LMA use has been described with the supine, prone, lateral, oblique, Trendelenburg, and lithotomy positions.[63]

Duration of LMA Use. Duration of LMA use has also been a controversial issue. Though the manufacturer recommends use for a maximum of 2–3 hours, reports of use lasting more than 24 hours can be found.[64]

Table 23-4. REPORTED UNCONVENTIONAL USE OF THE LMA

Clinical Situation	Proposed Advantages	Precautions	Citations*
Ear and nose	O₂ saturation Airway protection Head movement	Dislodgement and blood/pus aspiration	A1–A9
Dental	As above Reduced dysrhythmias Reduced bleeding Reduced epistaxis	Increased vigilance during extraction	A10–A18
Laryngeal	Vocal cord biopsy		A19
Oral, mandible, tongue	Many cases of rescue after failed face mask or laryngoscopy		A20–A30
Adenotonsillectomy	Reduced tracheal soiling Better recovery Less postoperative stridor and laryngeal spasm Less bronchospasm	Flexible LMA should be used May be difficult to insert LMA	A21, A31–A44
Laser surgery		Laser precautions: mask will rupture	A45–A55
Major head and neck surgery	Has been used in a difficult airway	Laryngospasm may occur LMA may be displaced Surgical mask puncture	A56–A58
Carotid endarterectomy	Reduced cardiovascular stimulation Smooth emergence	Distortion of surgical anatomy	A43, A59
Tracheostomy	Difficult airway Observe percutaneous procedures (LMA has been used as a tracheostomy mask)		A60–A65
Microlaryngeal surgery	Unobstructed glottis		A66–A68
Tracheal/carina surgery	Unobstructed glottis Safe laser use below LMA		A47, A69–A73
Thyroid/parathyroid	Dynamic observation during nerve stimulation	Laryngospasm LMA displacement No tracheal support if weakened cartilage	A56, A69–A79
Ophthalmic surgery	Improved intraocular pressure control Cough-free emergence (LMA has been used as an eye irrigator)	Valsalva can occur	A44, A69, A80–A104
Gynecologic laparoscopy		Possible increased regurgitation with Trendelenburg	A105–A113
Bronchoscopy	Easy access to glottis Continued oxygenation/ventilation View of glottis/upper trachea Large bore for foreign body extraction		A114–A140
Endoscopy			A141
Neurosurgery	Smooth emergence Smooth "wakeup" test		A142–A146
Cardiopulmonary resuscitation	As first airway Drug delivery		A147–A148
Lower abdominal surgery		Adequate depth of anesthesia must be assured	A149–A151
Upper abdominal surgery		Generally considered contraindicated, though has been safely used	A149, A152–A154
Cardiothoracic surgery	Reduced cardiovascular response	Generally considered unusable due to the high airway pressures often required (see Proseal)	A155–A157

* Citations appear in Appendix A at the end of this chapter.

The LMA-flexible. The advent of the LMA-flexible (Fig. 23-11) has permitted extension of LMA use to a variety of cases in which the airway is shared with the surgical team (*e.g.*, otolaryngologic surgery).[65] The LMA-flexible differs from the original design by virtue of a thin-walled, small-diameter, wire-reinforced (kink-resistant) barrel, which can be positioned out of the midline without affecting the hypopharyngeal position of the mask. It was designed to be used with a tonsillar mouth gag, as employed in surgery on the mouth and pharynx.[66,67] The LMA-flexible has also proved useful when heavy drapes are placed over the head and airway, when there is movement of the head position during surgery (*e.g.*, typanostomy tubes), or when the LMA barrel cannot be secured in the midline (*e.g.*,

mid or lateral facial surgery). The use of this mask in surgery above the level of the hypopharynx affords a number of clinically important advantages over tracheal intubation (Table 23-5).

When correctly placed, the LMA mask serves as a superb block of the airway from blood, secretions, and surgical debris above the level of the mask, as compared to the tracheal tube, which is known not to protect the trachea from liquids instilled into the pharynx[68-71] (Fig. 23-12).

The LMA and Bronchospasm. As a supraglottic airway, the LMA appears to be well suited to the patient with a history of extrinsic asthma. The LMA presents a unique opportunity for the clinician to conveniently and effectively control the airway

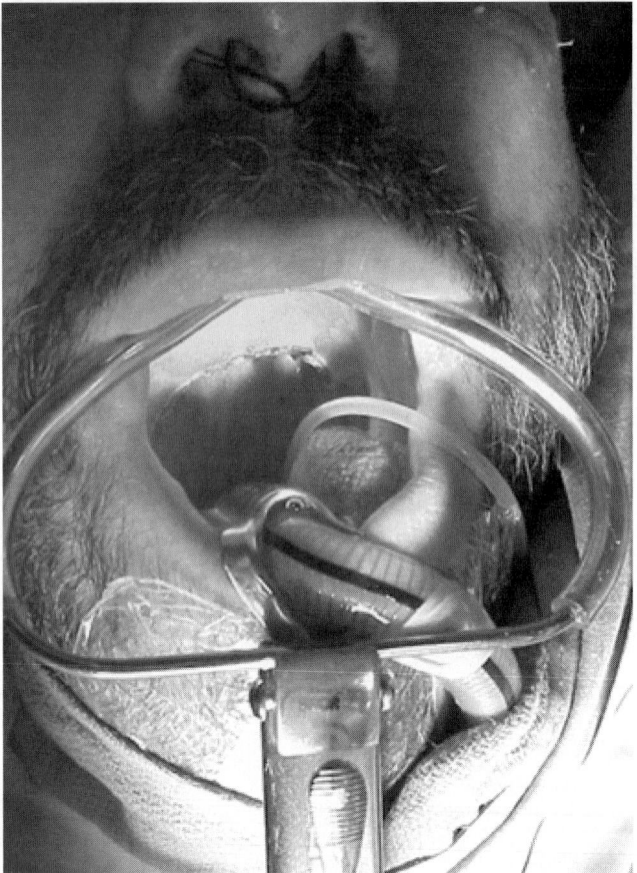

Figure 23-11. An LMA-flexible in place with a Crow-Davis mouth gag during a tonsillectomy and uvulopharyngopalatoplasty. The uvula has been removed. The LMA mask is not visible to the surgeon when correctly placed.

without having to introduce a foreign body into the trachea. Thus, it may be an ideal airway tool in the asthmatic patient who is not at risk for reflux and aspiration.[72-75] Because the halogenated inhaled anesthetics are potent bronchodilators, it is at the time of emergence when they are discontinued that the patient at risk for bronchospasm is most likely to wheeze. In the patient managed with the LMA, there is no foreign body in the sensitive broncho-respiratory tree and the patient can be fully emerged prior to removal of the device. In the event that uncontrollable bronchospasm does occur intraoperatively (*e.g.*, from vagal stimuli such as traction on the peritoneum), intubation can be performed through the LMA or after its removal.[76]

LMA Removal. Timing of the removal of the LMA at the end of surgery is also critical.[77-79] The LMA should be removed either when the patient is deeply anesthetized or after protective reflexes have returned and the patient is able to open the mouth

Table 23-5. ADVANTAGES OF THE LMA IN SUPRAGLOTTIC SURGERY

Improved protection of the airway from blood and surgical debris
Reduced cardiovascular responses
Reduced coughing on emergence
Reduced laryngospasm after airway device removal
Improved oxygen saturation after airway device removal
Ability to administer oxygen until complete restoration of airway reflexes

on command. Removal during excitation stages of emergence can be accompanied by coughing and/or laryngospasm. Many clinicians remove the LMA fully inflated; thus, it acts as a "scoop" for secretions above the mask, bringing them out of the airway. This has been particularly useful in otolaryngologic surgery (Fig. 23-12).

Contraindications to LMA Use. The primary contraindication to elective use of the LMA is a risk of gastric-contents aspiration (*e.g.*, full stomach, hiatus hernia with significant gastroesophageal reflux, morbid obesity, intestinal obstruction, delayed gastric emptying, poor history). Other contraindications include poor lung compliance or high airway resistance, glottic or subglottic airway obstruction, and limited mouth opening (<1.5 mm).[63]

LMA Use Complications. Apart from gastroesophageal reflux and aspiration, reported complications have included laryngospasm, coughing, gagging, retching, bronchospasm, and other events characteristic of airway manipulation. The incidence of sore throat is approximately 10%, as compared to 30% with tracheal intubation, but has been reported as 0–70%.[63] Also reported are hoarseness (4–47%) and dysphagia (4–24%). The LMA may cause transient changes in vocal cord function.[80] This is possibly related to cuff overinflation during prolonged procedures.

There have been several reports of nerve injury associated with LMA use. As of April 1999, 11 cases of nerve palsy have been reported: recurrent (7), hypoglossal (2), and lingual (2).[81] All but one of these resolved spontaneously. In all cases, size 3 and 4 LMAs were in use and nitrous oxide was one of the inhalation agents (which can increase cuff pressures by 9–38%).[82] Cuff pressures were not monitored in any of the cases. It is hypothesized that lingual nerve injuries occur as the nerve is trapped between the mandible and the LMA barrel lying lateral to the tongue. The hypoglossal nerve runs rostral and lateral to the hyoid bone, and may be pressed up against the bone. The recurrent nerve may be compressed between the LMA cuff and the cricoid or thyroid cartilage. Unmonitored increases in pressure due to N_2O diffusion, light anesthesia with constriction of pharyngeal musculature, tissue edema and venous engorgement from a head-down position, and lidocaine gel lubricant have been blamed for nerve injury.[83] To prevent such injury, the cuff of the LMA should be inflated to no more than 60 cm H_2O and should be monitored if N_2O is in use. The use of a larger LMA, with less pressure, has also been recommended.[84]

One death has been associated with an LMA device. An elderly woman suffered a tear of her esophagus after use of the intubating LMA (LMA-Fastrach®), dying 9 weeks later from septic shock after a series of related complications.[85] Interestingly, the actual complication was most likely a small esophageal tear from an inadvertent esophageal intubation. Therefore this complication was more of a misadventure of "blind intubation" not inherently attributable to the LMA-Fastrach itself. No other deaths due to complication of LMA use have been reported in the literature. It has been estimated, though, that 600 deaths occur each year in the developed world because of complications of difficult tracheal intubation.[86]

The LMA-Proseal®. Although the original LMA and the LMA-flexible have been used successfully for positive-pressure ventilation, they are not ideally suited to this task for two reasons: first, if poorly seated in the hypopharynx, gastric inflation may occur; second, the seal pressure is limited to approximately 20 cm H_2O. In 1994 an LMA prototype that includes a gastric drain was described.[87] It was believed that such a design would reduce both the risk of gastric inflation (by providing a low-resistance pathway for pressure transmitted to the esophagus) and the risk of aspiration of refluxed gastric contents. Subsequently, it was found that the design, which also incorporates a second, posterior cuff, could reliably allow positive-pressure ventilation with 40 cm H_2O pressure. A prototype of this mask, termed the

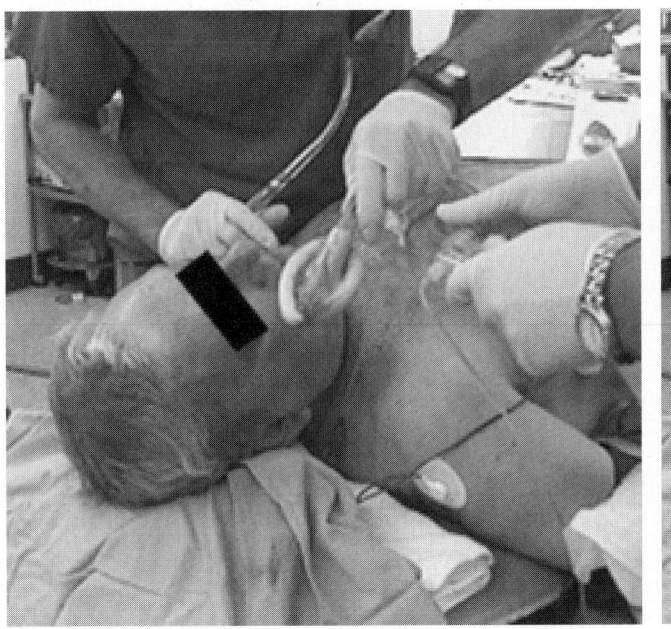
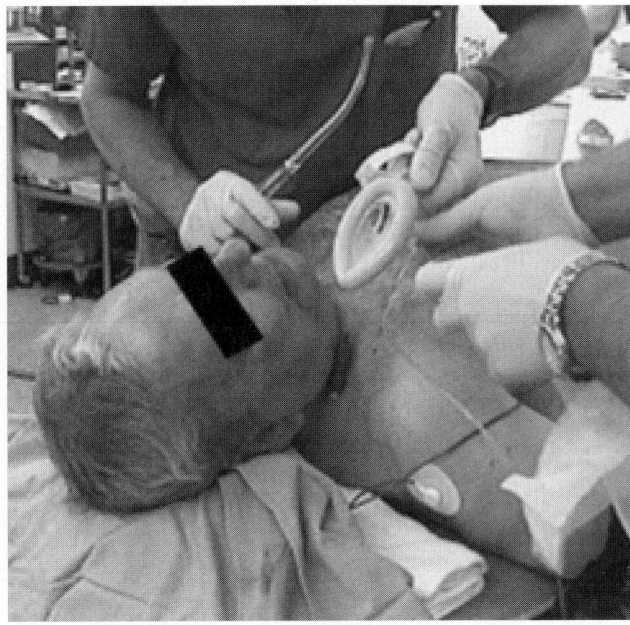

A   **B**

Figure 23-12. Following endoscopic sinus surgery, (*A*) the superior, pharyngeal surface of the LMA is blood-stained whereas (*B*) the laryngeal surface remains clean.

LMA-Proseal (Fig. 23-13), has been used in patients and is now undergoing multicenter trials (personal communication with Archie Brain).[88]

Another advantage of this design is that the gastric drain can be an aid in determining correct positioning of the mask, since malpositions (*e.g.,* nasopharynx, intratracheal) are accompanied by an air leak via this lumen.[87–90] This can be accentuated by filling the proximal few centimeters of the lumen with a water-soluble surgical lubricant and observing for bubbles or movement of the meniscus (Fig. 23-13d).

The design of the LMA-Proseal also makes use of the flexible, wire-reinforced barrel pioneered with the LMA-flexible, making it less prone to displacement with head movement. The second, gastric drain is also constructed of soft silicone, mounted lateral to the airway tube. A small gastric tube can be inserted into the stomach via this lumen. A silicone bite block is cemented between the two tubes. Because of the array of components at the level of the teeth (*e.g.,* airway barrel, gastric drain, bite block), the LMA-Proseal may be more difficult to insert into the airway. For this reason, the inventor included a surgical stainless steel insertion device which replicates the insertion technique of the LMA-Fastrach. After placement, the insertion device is removed. It is expected that this new design will improve the clinician's ability and comfort in safely using the LMA with positive-pressure ventilation and in patients at risk for gastric-contents aspiration.

The LMA and the Difficult Airway. Apart from its role as a routine anesthetic airway device, the LMA has a history of being a valuable tube in the care of the patient with the anticipated, or the unanticipated, difficult airway. This will be considered later in this chapter.

The Cuffed Oropharyngeal Airway

Another supraglottic airway device now available is the Cuffed Oropharyngeal Airway, or COPA (Mallinckrodt Medical, Athlone, Ireland). This device (Fig. 23-14) resembles a Guedel airway with an inflatable cuff along the distal half of its length and a 15-mm circuit adapter at the proximal end. The inflated cuff fills the pharynx and displaces the epiglottis and base of the tongue anteriorly. An unobstructed, sealed airway is provided. A flange around the circuit adapter has two posts for the attachment of a stabilizing head strap. The COPA was designed for airway maintenance during anesthesia with spontaneous ventilation and is in many ways comparable to the LMA in this population.[91,92] It has been used in the difficult-to-intubate patient, also.

Tracheal Intubation

Routine Laryngoscopy

PREPARING FOR LARYNGOSCOPY AND THE "BEST ATTEMPT." Whether laryngoscopy is undertaken with the patient in an awake or unconscious state, repeated attempts often result in edema and bleeding of the anterior upper airway structures (tongue, vallecula, epiglottis, laryngeal structures), hindering subsequent attempts at visualization and causing increased airway obstruction. It is therefore important to assure that the first attempt at laryngoscopy is a "best attempt."

First, when faced with the critically ill patient, the most skilled laryngoscopist available should be positioned to perform the laryngoscopy. In less acute situations, it is not inappropriate for a trainee, clinician extender, or other skilled personnel to assume this role. Second, the availability of all the materials needed to perform laryngoscopy and intubation should be assured, as should the availability of materials needed to manage a failed intubation. When devices are fashioned in a variety of sizes, the operator should have at hand the presumed correct size, as well as one size smaller and one size larger of each item (Table 23-6).

Other devices that complete the equipment list, but may not be uniformly available, include: end-tidal CO_2 monitoring (*e.g.,* capnography or colorimetric device [*e.g.,* Easy Cap II, Mallinckrodt]), pulse oximetry, LMA, transtracheal jet ventilation catheter, and a high-pressure oxygen source.

The height of the supine patient surface should be at the level of the laryngoscopist's xyphoid cartilage, with the bed or operating room table in a nonmovable mode (*e.g.,* wheels locked). The clinician performing the intubation must have unobstructed access to the head.

DIRECT LARYNGOSCOPY. Successful laryngoscopy involves the distortion of the normal anatomic planes of the supralaryngeal

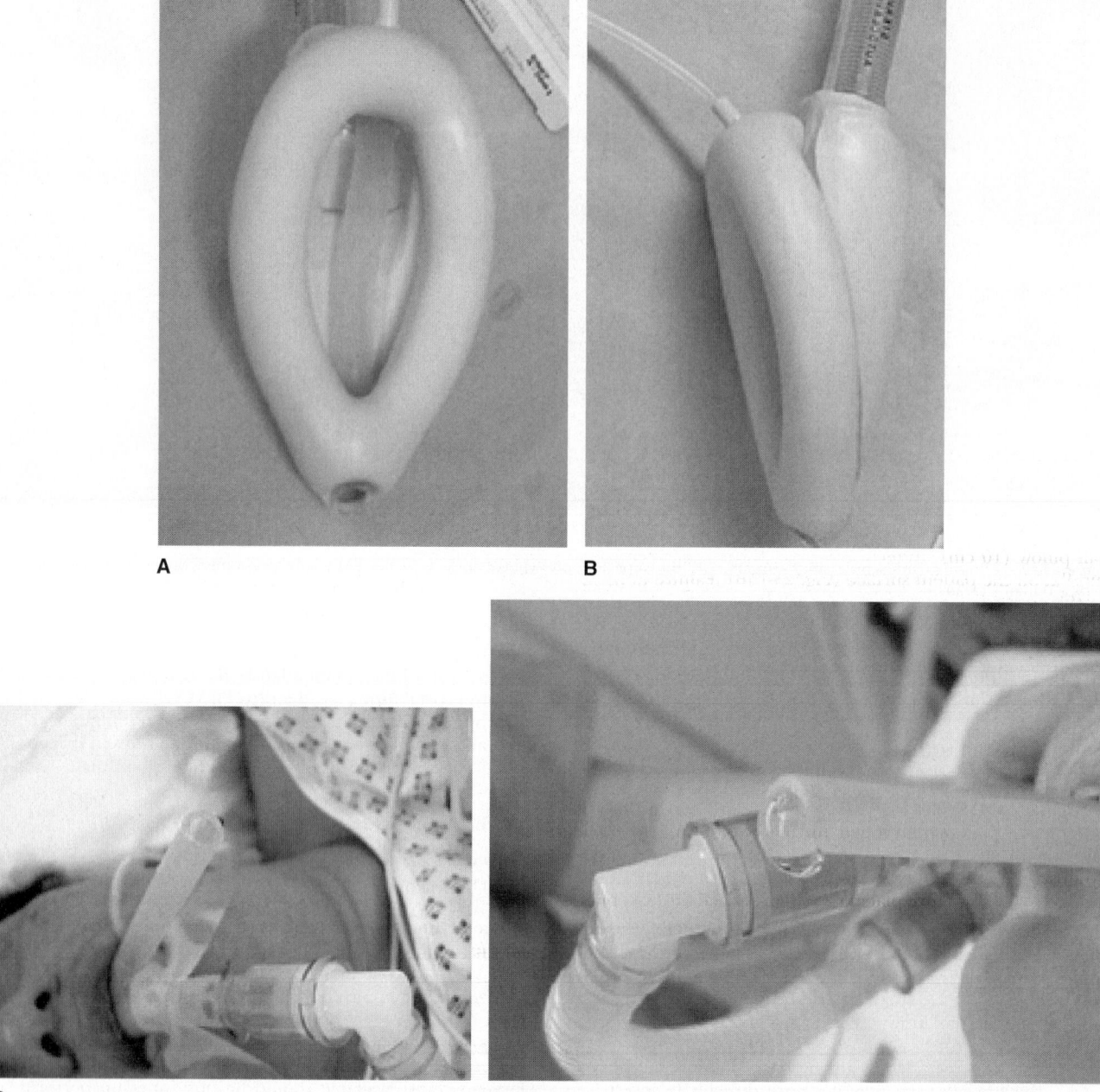

Figure 23-13. The LMA-Proseal: (*A*) Anterior view showing gastric drain passing through the bowl. (*B*) Lateral view showing the circumferential and posterior mask cuffs. (In the photograph, the view of the esophageal lumen is obscured by the airway lumen.) (*C*) The airway lumen and gastric drain, separated by an integral bite block, emerge from the patient. (*D*) A drop of water-soluble lubricant has been placed in the proximal aperture of the esophageal lumen in order to monitor for gas leak, which should not be present.

airway to produce a line of direct visualization from the operator's eye to the larynx: this requires alignment of the oral, pharyngeal, and laryngeal axes. A number of criteria must be met if this is to occur:

The oral aperture has to be adequate to allow visualization (and instrumentation).

The tongue must be small (relative to the oral cavity and mandibular space) and pliable enough to allow its distortion.

The mandibular space (the area between the mentum and the hyoid bone) must be able to accommodate the tongue as it is displaced by the laryngoscope.

With the head in a neutral position—that is, with the base of the occiput on the same plane as the lower thoracic spine,

the face pointed directly upward—there is no overlap of the three axes, and direct visualization cannot occur (Fig. 23-15A). To remedy this, an optimal "sniff" or Magill position should be achieved. This position, which entails a slight flexion of the neck on the thorax (35°) and severe extension of the head on the neck (an 80–85° angle between the sagittal axis of head at level of nose, and the long axis of neck) at the atlanto-occipital joint, accomplishes the best possible alignment of the oral, pharyngeal, and laryngeal axes (Fig. 23-15B).[93] The sniff position may be simulated by imagining or assuming the head and neck position of the long-distance runner.[94] This position maximally opens the airway, moves the epiglottis out of the visual line, and maximally reduces airway resistance.[95] The Magill position can be accomplished in the clinical setting by placing a

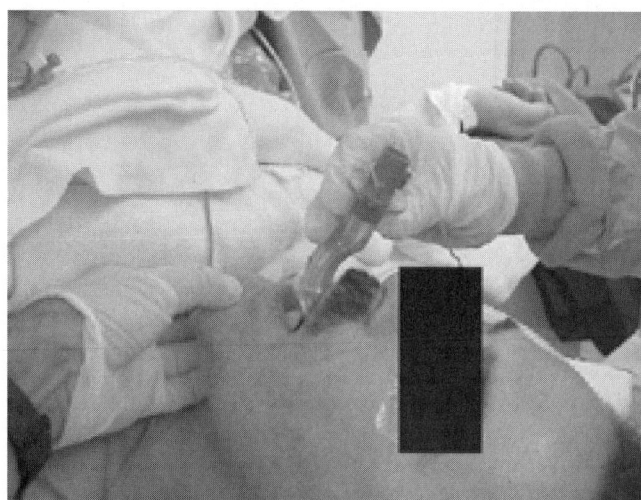

Figure 23-14. The COPA is inserted with the concavity in an cephalad direction. Once in the oral cavity, it is rotated into position, and inflated. A strap is used to keep the device in place.

small pillow (10 cm) under the head, while the shoulders remain flat on the patient surface (Fig. 23-15B). Failure to maintain this position during laryngoscopy is one of the most common reasons for a poor-grade laryngoscopic view.[96]

A sniff position pillow (Dupaco, Oceanside, CA) that is comfortable for the awake patient, but easily reconfigured after anesthetic induction to provide an ideal sniff position, has been developed by Dr. Kaiduan Pi (Fig. 23-16).

Overextension of the head on the neck and/or anterior movement of the mandible after the administration of neuromuscular relaxation can hinder the laryngeal view by moving the thyroid cartilage and larynx anteriorly.

The obese patient may need further positioning to move the mass of the chest away from the plane across which the laryngoscope handle will sweep as it is manipulated into the mouth. This may require placing a wedge-shaped lift (*e.g.*, blankets, pillows) under the scapula, shoulders, and nape of neck, raising the head and neck above the thorax and providing a grade in order to allow gravity to take the mass away from the airway (Fig. 23-17).

If, during the laryngoscopy, a satisfactory laryngeal view is not achieved the backward-upward-rightward pressure (BURP) maneuver may aid in improving the view. In this maneuver, a second operator displaces the larynx (*a*) backward against the

---

Table 23-6. EQUIPMENT FOR LARYNGOSCOPY*

Oxygen source and self-inflating ventilation bag (*e.g.*, ambu bag)
Face mask†
Oropharyngeal and nasopharyngeal airways†
Tracheal tubes†
Tracheal tube stylet
Syringe for tracheal tube cuff inflation
Suction apparatus
Laryngoscope handle (2), tested for working order and battery freshness
Laryngoscope blades: Common blades include the curved (Macintosh) and straight (Miller)†
Pillow, towel, blanket, or foam for head positioning
Stethoscope

---

* Equipment that should be immediately available in the ideal clinical setting.
† Presumed size as well as one larger and one smaller should be immediately available.

cervical vertebrae, (*b*) superiorly as possible and (*c*) slightly laterally to the right, using external pressure over the cricoid cartilage. The BURP maneuver has been shown to improve the laryngeal view, decreasing the rate of difficult intubation in 1993 patients from 4.7% to 1.8%.[97,98] When a left-handed operator is using a left-handed laryngoscope blade, the lateral external pressure should displace the larynx to the left. Similarly, Benumof describes "optimal external laryngeal manipulation," which consists of pressing posteriorly and cephalad over the thyroid, hyoid, and cricoid, as improving laryngeal view by at least one Cormack and Lehane grade.[99,100]

Once alignment has been achieved, the mouth is opened by one of two techniques (Fig. 23-18). The first accomplishes hyperextension of the atlanto-occipital joint head by the use of the dominant hand under the occiput. This maneuver tends to open the mouth, and can be accentuated by using the fifth finger of the nondominant hand (holding the laryngoscope) to apply pressure over the chin in a caudad direction (Fig. 23-18a). In the second technique, which tends to be more effective but requires contact of the (gloved) hand with the teeth and/or gum, caudad pressure is applied with the thumb of the dominant hand on the mandibular molars on the patient's same side while the first finger, crossed above or below the thumb, applies cephalad pressure to the ipsilateral maxillary molars (Fig. 23-18b). The ultimate goal of both techniques is rotation and translation of the temporomandibular joint in order to achieve the widest interincisor gap. The patient, whether conscious or not, is now ready for laryngoscopy.

USE OF THE LARYNGOSCOPE BLADE. Proper use of the laryngoscope blade is vital to the success of this basic airway management technique. Two blade types are commonly available and each is applied in a unique manner (Fig. 23-19). The curved (Macintosh) blade is used to pull the epiglottis out of the line of sight by tensing the glossoepiglottic ligament, whereas the straight blade (Miller) compresses the epiglottis against the base of the tongue. Both blades include a flange along the left side of their length which is used to sweep the tongue to the left side of the mouth. Blades with a right-side flange are available for the left-handed practitioner, but they are not commonly found in practice.

In most available systems the flange incorporates the light source, either a bulb placed near the distal blade aspect or a rigid fiberoptic cable that transmits light produced within the handle. In either case, these blades must be long enough to achieve their respective applications. Therefore, blade size needs to be chosen appropriately and, on occasion, exchanged after a failed attempt. As a generalization, the Macintosh blade is regarded as better wherever there is little room to pass an endotracheal tube (*e.g.*, small mouth), whereas the Miller blade is considered better in the patient who has a small mandibular space, large incisor teeth or a large epiglottis.[94]

With the left hand holding the laryngoscope handle, the blade is inserted into the right side of the mouth, with care taken not to compress the upper lip against the teeth. As the blade is advanced toward the epiglottis, it is swept leftward, using the flange to displace the tongue to the left as the blade compresses it into the mandibular space. Once reaching the base of the tongue (the Macintosh blade tip in the vallecula, or the Miller blade compressing the epiglottis against the base of the tongue), the operator's arm and shoulder lift in an anterior and caudad direction (Fig. 23-20).

Importantly, the laryngoscopist must strive to avoid rotating the wrist and laryngoscope handle in a cephalad direction, bringing the blade against the upper incisor teeth. Extending either blade style too deeply can bring the tip of the blade to rest under the larynx itself, so that forward pressure lifts the entire airway from view (Fig. 23-21).

Special considerations apply to the technique of laryngoscopy and intubation in the infant and child. Because of the relatively larger size of the occiput in children, producing an anatomic

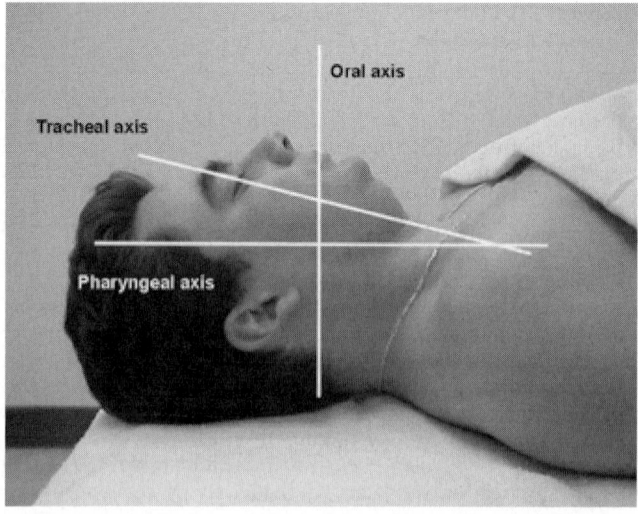
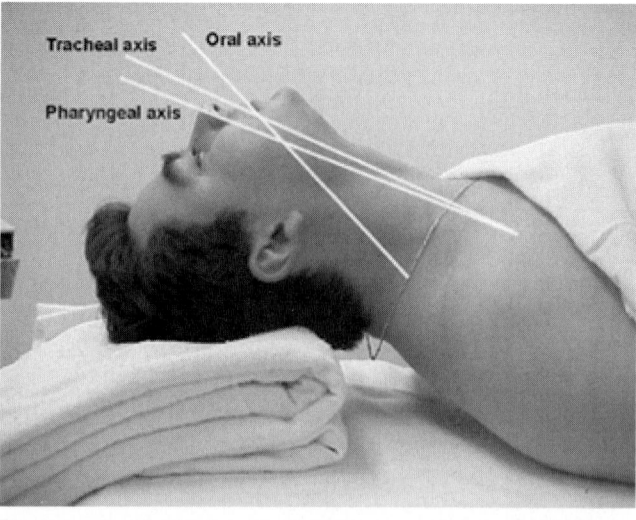

A   **B**

Figure 23-15. (*A*) With the patient supine and no head support, the oral, pharyngeal, and tracheal axes do not overlap. (*B*) The "sniff" position maximally overlaps the three axes.

sniffing position, elevation of the head (as done in the adult) is not needed.[101] On occasion, one may need to elevate the thorax instead. The relatively short neck gives the impression of an anterior position of the larynx. Posterior cricoid pressure is often required to place the laryngeal inlet into view. A straight blade is more helpful in displacing the stiff, omega-shaped, and high epiglottis. Since the cricoid cartilage is the narrowest aspect of the airway until 6 to 8 years of age, the intubator must be sensitive to resistance to advancement of the ETT that has easily passed the vocal folds. Hyperextension at the atlanto-occipital joint, as done in adult, may cause airway obstruction due to the relative pliability of the trachea. In the child, there is a higher risk of endobronchial intubation or extubation with head movement owing to the short length of the trachea.

With laryngoscopy, the view of the larynx may be complete, partial, or impossible. A laryngeal view scoring system that has won general acceptance was developed by Cormack and Lehane, who described four grades of laryngeal view:[100] Grade I includes visualization of the entire glottic aperture; Grade II

includes visualization of only the posterior aspects of the glottic aperture; Grade III is visualization of the tip of the epiglottis; Grade IV is visualization of no more than the soft palate (Fig. 23-22). This system has proved useful not only as a means of recording the laryngeal view on individual patients, but also as a clinical endpoint in the evaluation of the predictive value of preoperative airway assessments tools.

Once the larynx is visualized with a left side–flanged blade, the tracheal tube is inserted from the right-hand side, care being taken not to obstruct the view of the vocal folds. Whenever possible, the action of the endotracheal tube passing through the vocal folds should be witnessed by the laryngoscopist. The tracheal tube should be inserted to a depth of at least 2 cm after the disappearance of the tracheal tube cuff past the vocal folds in order to approximate placement in the mid trachea. This should present the 21-cm and 23-cm external markings at the teeth for the typical adult female and male, respectively.[102] Choice of adult tracheal tube size may be made by the generalization that for women, size

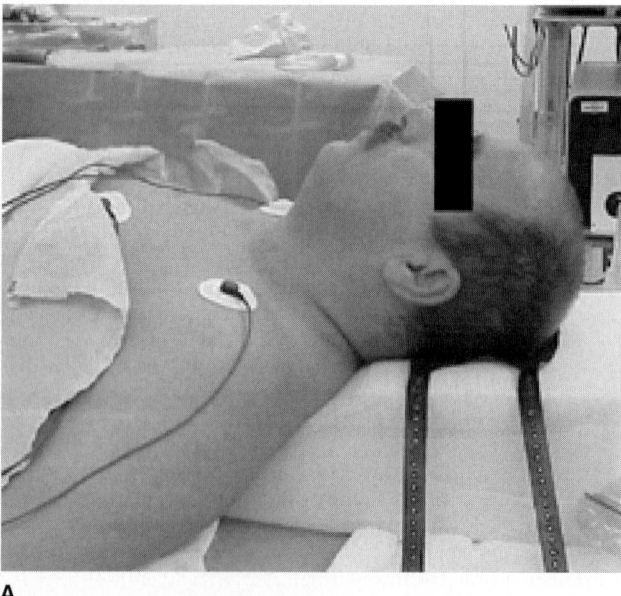
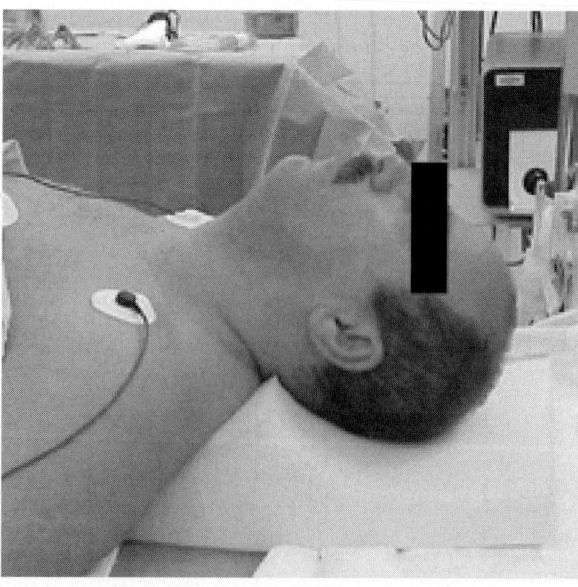

A   **B**

Figure 23-16. (*A*) Pi's pillow (Dupaco, Oceanside, CA) places the patient in a comfortable position prior to the induction of anesthesia and (*B*) in an ideal "sniff" position during airway management.

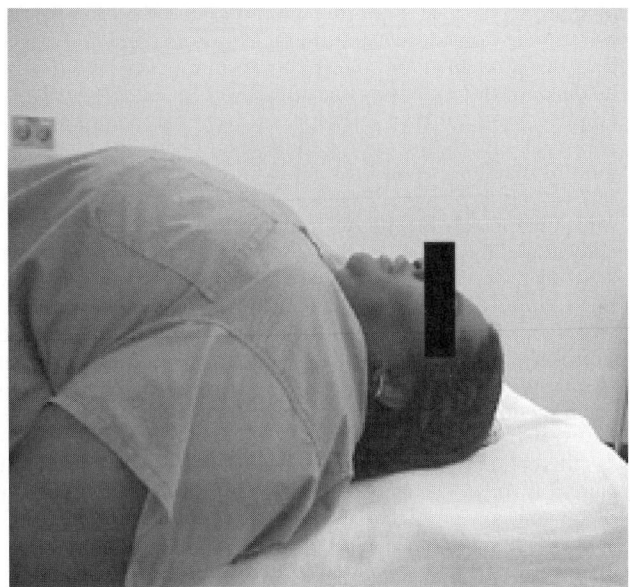
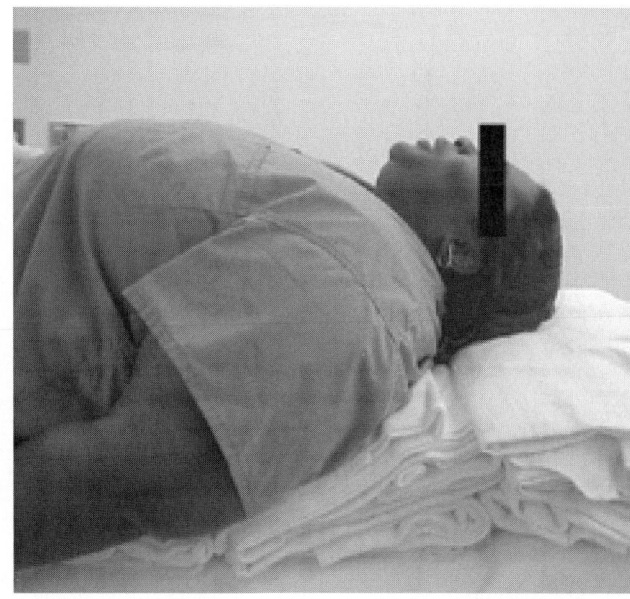

A   B

Figure 23-17. (*A*) With the morbidly obese patient, a 10-cm pillow may not provide a position adequate for laryngoscopy. (*B*) A wedge-shaped lift is used to move the mass of the morbidly obese patient's chest away from the area of laryngoscopy and to improve the compliance of the thoracic cavity.

7–8 id (internal diameter) may be used, and for a man, size 8–9 id. The larger tracheal tubes may be desirable if pulmonary toilet or diagnostic or therapeutic bronchoscopy is to be part of the clinical course. Pediatric laryngoscope blades and tracheal tube sizes are discussed in detail elsewhere in this chapter (Table 23-7).

Verification of successful tracheal tube placement is made by a variety of methods. The gold standard for confirmation of placement includes visualization of placement through the vocal folds and sustained detection of exhaled carbon dioxide as measured with capnography or a disposable chemical colorimetric device such as the Easy Cap II (Mallinckrodt). Other portable techniques include auscultation over the chest and abdomen, visualization of the chest excursion, observation of condensation in the ETT, use of a self-inflating bulb (Tubechek-B, Ambu, Linthicum, MD), lighted stylets (Trachlight, Laerdal Medical, Armonk, NY; SURCH-LITE, Aaron Medical Industries, St. Petersburg, FL), fiberoptic bronchoscope identification of the tracheal rings, chest x-ray, and a device called the SCOTI that detects the patency of the tracheal tube–tracheal lumen using a sonographic technique.[103,104]

NPO Status and the Rapid-Sequence Induction. Induction of anesthesia in patients who have "full stomachs" or incompetent gastroesophageal sphincters can result in regurgitation and pulmonary aspiration. Individuals at risk include the morbidly obese, pregnant women, diabetics with gastroparesis, those who require emergency operations, patients with gastroesophageal reflux disease, and patients who have recently eaten. Individuals experiencing emotional stress have increased gastric acid secretions and are also at an increased risk for aspiration.[105] Threshold values of a $pH < 2.5$ or gastric volume >25 ml are widely accepted as placing the patient at risk of sequelae should aspiration occur. Although few cases occur in modern anesthetic practice, the consequences of developing an aspiration syndrome can be devastating; hence, all efforts to avoid its development should be made. Therapeutic interventions are directed toward maintaining NPO status and administering gastric antisecretory agents, including histamine-2 (H_2) blockers, prostaglandin E_1 analogs, and omeprazole. Common anesthetic practice

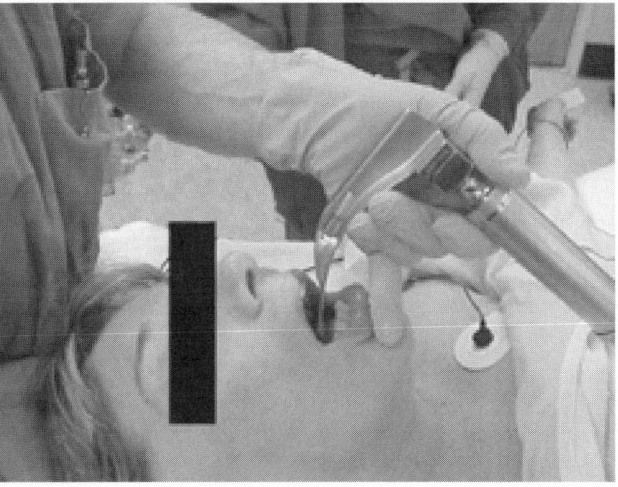
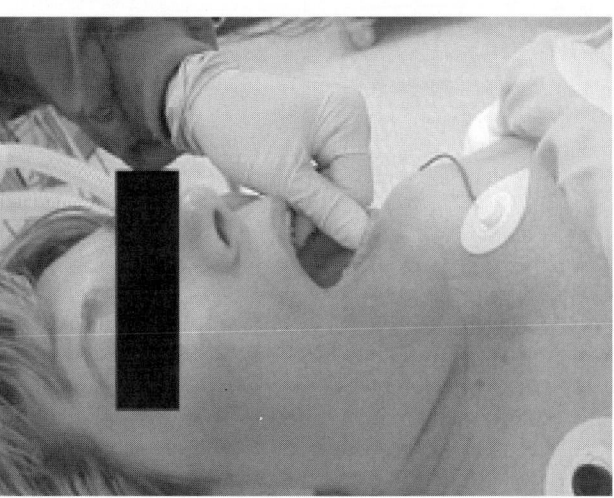

A   B

Figure 23-18. Techniques of opening the mouth in preparation for laryngoscopy. (*A*) Hyperextension of the atlanto-occipital joint and use of the fifth finger of the dominant hand; (*B*) the thumb–first finger "scissors" technique.

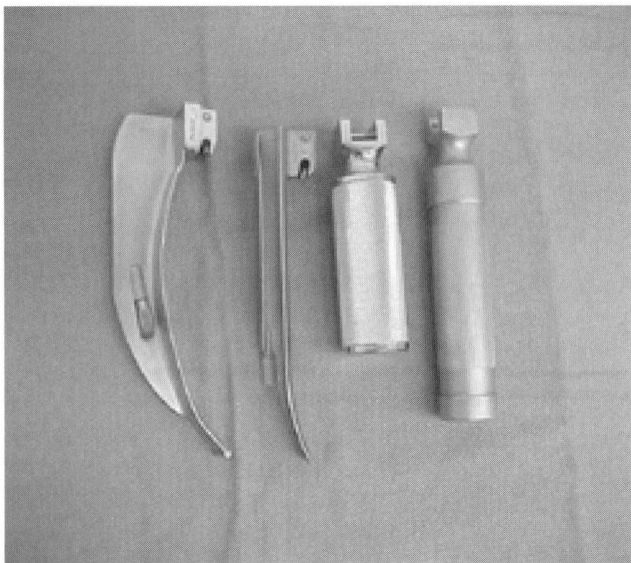

Figure 23-19. Macintosh and Miller laryngoscope blades with small and regular-sized handles.

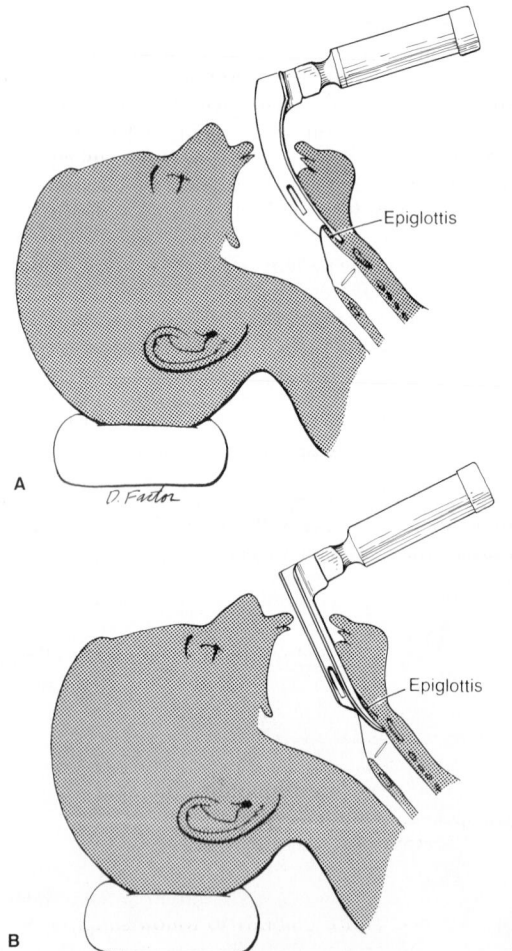

Figure 23-20. (*A*) When a curved laryngoscope blade is used, the tip of the blade is placed in the vallecula, the space between the base of the tongue and the pharyngeal surface of the epiglottis. (*B*) The tip of a straight blade is advanced beneath the epiglottis.

dictates a policy of "nothing by mouth" orders for 8 hours prior to the induction of anesthesia. However, controversy exists over this guideline, and many centers allow clear liquids to be taken until hours before the operation unless delayed gastric emptying is a concern. H_2 blockers help maintain gastric pH above 2.5, thereby decreasing the severity of any chemical pneumonitis that may occur. Prostaglandin E_1 analogs (*i.e.,* misoprotol) act directly on gastric parietal cells to increase gastric pH, while omeprazole blocks the final step in the secretion of hydrochloric acid by parietal cells.[106] The use of metaclopramide (for its gastropropulsive effects) and nasogastric suction may reduce the volume of gastric content. The use of a nonparticulate antacid may decrease the acidity of any residual contents of the stomach by serving as a buffer. The combination of cimetidine and metoclopramide given to ambulatory patients during the preinduction phase is better than either drug alone for increasing gastric pH and decreasing gastric volume.[107]

The technique of rapid-sequence induction is performed to gain control of the airway in the least amount of time after the ablation of protective airway reflexes with the induction of anesthesia. In the rapid-sequence technique, the administration of an intravenous anesthetic induction agent is immediately followed by a rapidly acting neuromuscular blocking drug. Direct laryngoscopy and intubation are performed as soon as muscle relaxation is confirmed. Cricoid pressure (Sellick's maneuver) is applied by an assistant from the beginning of induction until confirmation of endotracheal tube placement. Cricoid pressure entails the downward displacement of the cricoid cartilage against the vertebral bodies (Fig. 23-23). In this manner, the lumen of the esophagus is ablated, while the completely circular nature of the cricoid cartilage maintains the tracheal lumen. Early cadaveric studies showed that correctly applied cricoid pressure was effective in preventing gastric fluids, under 100 cm H_2O pressure, from leaking into the pharynx. Cricoid pressure is contraindicated with active vomiting (risk of esophageal rupture), cervical spine fracture, and laryngeal fracture.

If during rapid-sequence induction there are difficulties in securing the airway and oxyhemoglobin desaturation occurs, gentle positive pressure ventilation may be used while maintaining cricoid pressure. This positive pressure should require <25 cm H_2O pressure. If more positive pressure is used, there is a risk of gastric distention and regurgitation.

The Intubating Laryngeal Mask Airway. Blind, fiberoptic aided, stylet-guided, and laryngoscopy-directed intubation via the LMA has been widely reported in adults and children.[76,108–114] There are several limitations to this procedure including the maximal size ETT that can be used, the minimal length of the ETT required to ensure that its cuff is within the larynx and not wedged between or above the vocal folds, and the difficulty in removing the LMA after intubation.[76,115] In an effort to overcome these limitations, Brain introduced a version of the LMA with a large-diameter (13 mm id), short-length (14 cm) rigid stainless steel barrel curved to align the mask aperture to the glottic vestibule (Fig. 23-24).[116–118]

The mask incorporates a vertically oriented semirigid bar, fixed at the proximal end of the bowl aperture and positioned to sit beneath the epiglottis in the average adult. A handle at the proximal end of the barrel is used for insertion, repositioning, and removal. A secondary advantage of the handle is that the operator need never reach into the patient's mouth. This new device, the LMA-Fastrach, can accommodate up to an 8.0-mm id cuffed ETT, which can be inserted blindly or over a fiberscope. The LMA-Fastrach is designed to be used with a straight, armored, silicone tracheal tube (Euromedics, Malaysia), although standard polyvinyl chloride tracheal tubes have been used.[119] To date, the LMA-Fastrach has been distributed in adult sizes with cuffs equivalent to the size 3, 4, and 5 LMAs. Experience has suggested that most adults between 40 and 70 kg are best managed with a size 4 LMA-Fastrach, larger persons requiring the size 5. Pediatric sizes are not yet available.

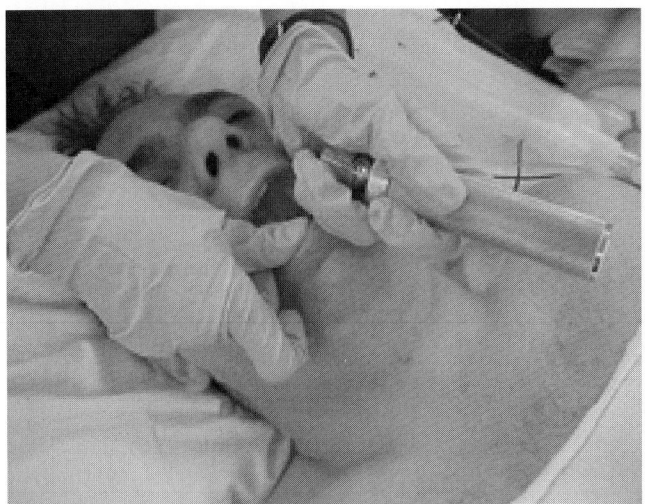
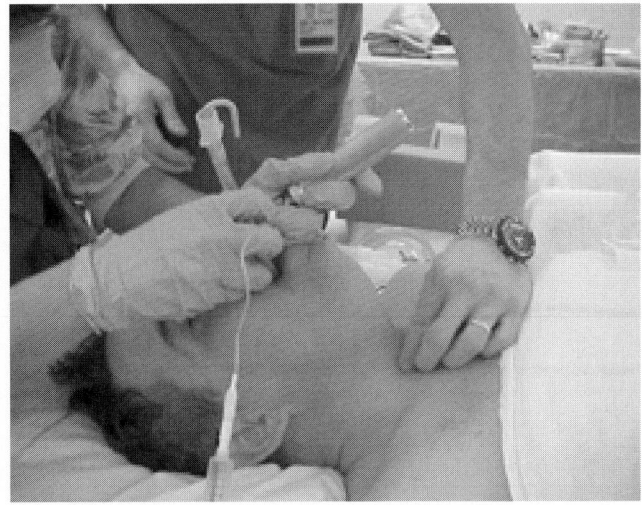

A   **B**

Figure 23-21. The sequence of routine laryngoscopy. (*A*) With the mouth maximally opened, the laryngoscope is held in the left hand and the blade inserted on the right side of the mouth. Using the blade flange, the tongue is swept to the left as the wrist pulls in a caudad direction. (*B*) While visualizing the laryngeal inlet, the tracheal tube is inserted.

The LMA-Fastrach is indicated for routine, elective intubation and for anticipated and unanticipated difficult intubation. Since it was designed to facilitate blind tracheal intubation, the presence of airway secretions, blood, or edema (*e.g.,* from previous intubation attempts or trauma) does not interfere with its use. Because the design of the barrel is based upon the normal adult palate-to-glottis relationship, patients who are evaluated as being manageable with tracheal intubation based on external exam, but subsequently are found to have a high Cormack–Lehane score (due to lingual tonsil hyperplasia or cervical spine immobility, for example) should be successfully managed with the LMA-Fastrach.[100] In the largest trial of the LMA-Fastrach to date, ventilation was satisfactory in 95% and unsatisfactory in 1% of 500 uses, and 96% were intubated within three attempts (79.8% on first, 12.4% on second, 4% on third).[120] Patients who are assessed as grossly abnormal on preoperative airway exam may often still be managed with the LMA-Fastrach.[121] The LMA-Fastrach has been demonstrated to be useful as a ventilatory and intubating device after failed rapid sequence intubation.[119]

The contraindications to the LMA-Fastrach are similar to those of the LMA. Since the goal of the LMA-Fastrach is tracheal intubation, it may prove useful for management of patients at moderate risk for gastroesophageal regurgitation and aspiration, or for high-risk patients on whom other techniques have failed.

The LMA-Fastrach is inserted with the head in a neutral position. It can be used in the unconscious or awake patient (with the use of topical anesthetics). The mask of the LMA-Fastrach is tested, deflated, and lubricated as described for the LMA. It is inserted into the mouth, with the handle held parallel to the chest, so the mask lies flat against the palate. Gentle pressure on the handle and barrel, toward the chin, reproduces the palatal pressure described for insertion of the LMA. A smooth backward rotation of the handle toward the top of the head seats the tip of the mask in the hypopharynx, posterior to the cricoid cartilage. Once seated, the LMA-Fastrach's mask is inflated via the pilot cuff. An ambu bag or anesthesia circuit is attached to the proximal end of the LMA-Fastrach barrel and ventilation is attempted. By using the LMA-Fastrach handle, the position of the device can be optimized by lateral and anterior–posterior manipulation. A seemingly common cause of airway obstruction is the downfolding of the epiglottis. This can be relieved with a smooth rotational movement of the inflated LMA-Fastrach out of the airway (6 cm along the axis of the insertion) and immediate re-placement.

After adequate ventilation is achieved, the ETT is advanced though the barrel. As the ETT exits the bowl aperture of the LMA-Fastrach, the semirigid elevating bar is pushed anteriorly, carrying the epiglottis out of the way of the airway. If positioned correctly, the ETT can freely enter the glottis.

Once intubation is achieved and confirmed (*e.g.,* by auscultation or capnography), the ETT circuit adapter is removed and the LMA-Fastrach is withdrawn over the ETT. During this removal procedure, the ETT is stabilized by one of two methods. A silicone stabilizing rod can be held against the ETT as the LMA-Fastrach is retreated out of the mouth. The advantage of this technique is that the operator's hands do not have to enter the oral cavity. The disadvantage is that in the mid-removal position, the operator loses direct contact with the ETT. In the second technique, described by Rosenblatt and Murphy, a Magill forceps is used to hold the proximal tip of the ETT while the LMA-Fastrach is removed.[119] In the mid-removal position, a finger is placed in the mouth to identify and stabilize the ETT, while the Magill forceps is removed and the LMA-Fastrach is fully retreated. This technique requires the hand to be placed in the mouth, but allows more control of the ETT.

Extubation of the Trachea

Though a wealth of literature is focused on the field of tracheal intubation, few reviews have well contemplated the area of extubation after completion of surgery, or prolonged ventilatory support.[122] Indeed, the period of extubation may be far more treacherous than that of intubation (Table 23-8A).

Routine Extubation. Extubation of the trachea must not be considered a benign procedure. It is not simply the elimination or reversal of tracheal intubation. Extubation is fraught with its own set of potential complications (Table 23-8B). Appropriately trained personnel and equipment should be immediately available at the time of extubation. This may range from a postanesthetic care unit nurse or respiratory therapist with a set of laryngoscopes to a surgeon prepared to perform an emergency tracheostomy.

Most adult patients are extubated after the return of consciousness and spontaneous respiration, the resolution of neuromuscular block, and the ability to follow simple commands (Table 23-9). The patient is asked to open the mouth and a suction catheter is used to remove excessive secretions and/or blood. The airway pressure is allowed to rise to 5–15 cm of H_2O to allow for a "passive cough," and the endotracheal tube is removed after the cuff (if present) is deflated.[122] If coughing

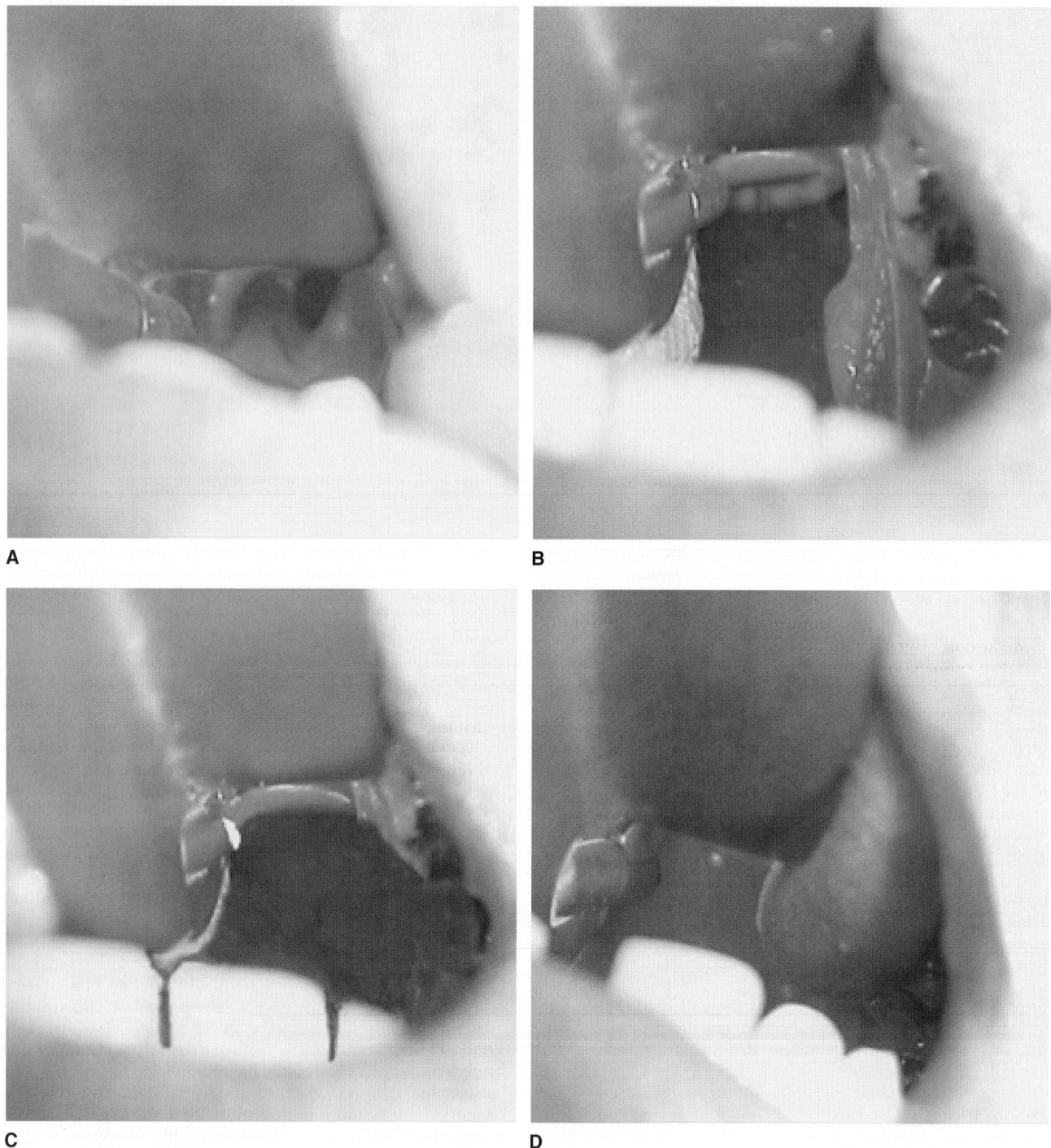

A

B

C

D

Figure 23-22. The Cormack–Lehane laryngeal view scoring system: (*A*) Grade 1, (*B*) Grade 2, (*C*) Grade 3, (*D*) Grade 4.

or straining is contraindicated or hazardous (*e.g.*, increased intracranial pressure), extubation may be performed while the patient is in a surgical plane of anesthesia. In patients at risk for gastric contents aspiration (*e.g.*, full stomach) or upper airway obstruction, the clinician needs to assess the relative risk of each potential morbidity. For the latter risk, and possibly the former, a maneuver has been described in which an LMA is placed posterior to the ETT, which is then removed. This obviates the problem of upper airway obstruction, and may offer some protection against regurgitation and aspiration.[123–125] Because of the risks of atelectasis and diffusion hypoxia, the ability to administer oxygen should be available at the time of extubation.

Difficult Extubation.   The patient who presented as a difficult

airway at the time of anesthetic induction must be considered a difficult airway at the time of extubation, even when corrective surgery was performed in the interim (*e.g.*, uvulopharyngoplasty in the obstructive sleep apnea patient).

As a cause of ventilatory compromise, laryngospasm deserves special attention because of it prevalence in children and because it accounts for 23% of all critical postoperative respiratory events in adults.[122] Laryngospasm may be triggered by respiratory secretions, vomitus, or blood in the airway; pain in any part of the body; and pelvic or abdominal visceral stimulation. The cause of airway obstruction during laryngospasm is the contraction of the lateral cricoarytenoids, the thyroarytenoid, and the cricothyroid muscles. Management of laryngospasm

Table 23-7. SIZE AND LENGTH OF TRACHEAL TUBES RELATIVE TO AIRWAY ANATOMY

Age	Internal Diameter (mm)	Distance from Lips to Mid-trachea* (cm)	Diameter of Trachea (mm)	Length of Trachea (cm)	Distance from Lips to Carina (cm)
Premature	2.5	8			
Full term	3.0	10			
1–6 mo	3.5	11	5	6	13
6–12 mo	4.0	12			
2 yr	4.5	13			
4 yr	5.0	14			
6 yr	5.5	15			
8 yr	6.5	16	8	8	18
10 yr	7.0	17–18			
12 yr	7.5	18–20			
14 yr	8.0–9.0	20–22	20† 15‡	14† 12‡	28† 24‡

* Add 2–3 cm for nasal tubes.
† Males.
‡ Females.

consists of the immediate removal of the offending stimulus (if identifiable), administration of oxygen with continuous positive airway pressure, and, if other maneuvers are unsuccessful, the use of a small dose of short-acting muscle relaxants.[122]

Negative-pressure pulmonary edema may result from any airway obstruction in a patient who continues to have a voluntary respiratory effort. Negative intrathoracic pressure is transmitted to the alveoli, which are unable to expand owing to the more proximal obstruction. Fluid is entrained from the pulmonary capillary bed. Negative-pressure pulmonary edema is treated as any other form of noncardiogenic edema.

IDENTIFICATION OF PATIENTS AT RISK AT EXTUBATION. A number of well known clinical situations may place patients at increased risk for complication at the time of extubation. Table 23-10 lists the risk factors for extubation complications. However, the clinician should evaluate every patient in terms of potential problems, in the same manner that they are prepared for the unanticipated difficult intubation.

APPROACH TO THE DIFFICULT EXTUBATION. When there is a suspicion that a patient may have difficulty with oxygenation or ventilation after tracheal extubation, the clinician may choose from a number of management strategies. These may range from the preparation of standby reintubation equipment to the active establishment of a route or guide for reintubation and/or oxygenation. When the patient's intubation is without difficulty and there is no substantial reason to believe that an interim insult to the airway has occurred, extubation may be accom-

plished in a routine fashion, with a heightened state of readiness for reintubation. When there has been difficulty with intubation or there is a clinical suspicion that reintubation will be difficult, extubation over a guiding stylet may be a successful technique. Any number of devices can be used as a stylet (Table 23-11).

A popular test to predict airway patency after extubation is the detection of a leak upon deflation of the ETT cuff.[126] Recent investigations have cast doubt on the reliability of this test. In this study no patient with a positive leak test (no leak around the ETT cuff) developed problems after extubation.

When using an FOB, the tracheal structures can be observed during the removal of the ETT. If extubation is tolerated, the FOB can be slowly withdrawn into the subglottic region. If secretions do not obstruct the objective lens, the vocal folds and other structures may be visualize and evaluated.

A number of obturators are available for use in trial extubation (where they may be left in place in the airway for extended periods) or endotracheal tube exchange (e.g., failure of the ETT cuff).[127] It is beyond the scope of this text to describe all the commercially available catheters. The Cook airway exchange catheters (Cook Critical Care, Bloomington, IN) are manufactured with external diameters of 2.7, 3.7. 4.7, and 6.33 mm (Fig. 23-25a). The smallest diameter catheter (which can fit within a 3.0-mm id ETT) is 45 cm long, whereas the others are 83 cm in length). They all have a central lumen and rounded, atraumatic ends. The catheters are graduated from the distal end. The proximal end is fitted with either a 15-mm or a Luer-lock Rapi-Fit adapter, which can be quickly removed and replaced for ETT removal or change. With these adapters an oxygen source can be used to provide insufflated or jet-ventilated oxygen if the patient fails extubation and/or if reintubation over the catheter fails.

The Patil two-part intubation catheter (Cook Critical Care, Bloomington, IN) is a 6.0-mm od (outer diameter), 3.4-mm id, 63-cm catheter composed of two interlocking lengths. One half can be used as a malleable stylet for blind intubation or intubation through an LMA. The second length, and/or a Rapi-fit adapter, can be added for use in oxygen insufflation or as an ETT exchange catheter.

The Cardiomed endotracheal ventilation catheter (Gromley, Ontario, Canada) designed by Richard Cooper, M.D., a Canadian anesthesiologist, is 85 cm in length, and has inner and outer diameters of 3 and 4 mm, respectively. An integral Luer-lock fitting adapter is found at the proximal end, whereas the blunted distal end incorporates eight helically arranged side holes in addition to the distal end hole (Fig. 23-25b). The arrangement of these holes is meant to center the catheter during oxygen insufflation, and prevent traumatic "whip-

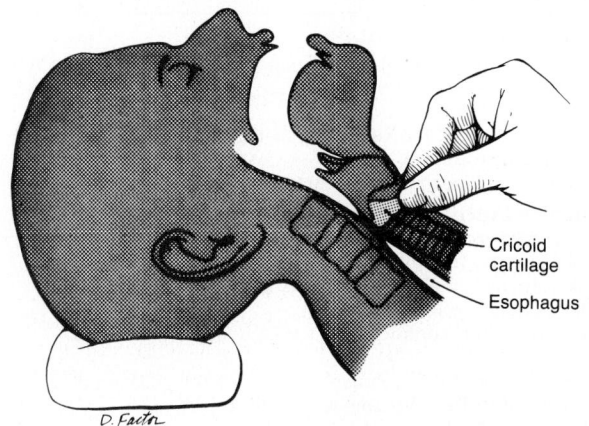

Figure 23-23. Cricoid pressure (Sellick's maneuver) is applied to occlude the esophagus and prevent aspiration of gastric contents.

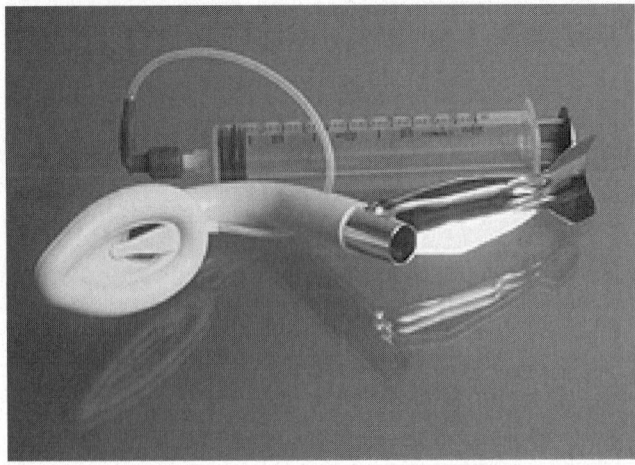
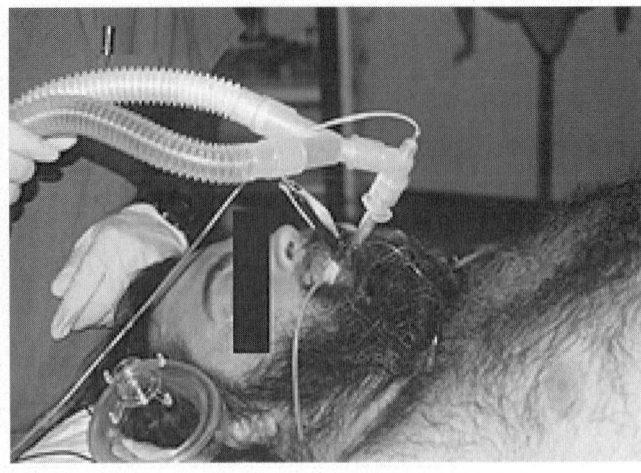

A   **B**

Figure 23-24. (*A*) The LMA-Fastrach; (*B*) The LMA-Fastrach used for intubation in a patient outside the operating room.

ping"within the trachea. The use of this catheter for ETT exchange, tracheal reintubation, oxygen insufflation, jet ventilation, and end-tidal CO_2 detection after extubation has been documented by the inventor.[122]

THE DIFFICULT AIRWAY
The Difficult Airway Algorithm

In 1993, the American Society of Anesthesiologists' (ASA) Task Force on the Difficult Airway published an algorithm that has become a staple of management for clinicians (Fig. 23-26).[128]

Table 23-8. TRACHEAL EXTUBATION

A. Causes of Ventilatory Compromise During Tracheal Extubation

Residual anesthetic
Poor central respiratory effort
Decreased respiratory rate
Decreased respiratory drive in response to CO_2
Decreased respiratory drive in response to O_2
Reduced tone of upper airway musculature
Reduced gag and swallow reflex
Decreased threshold to laryngospasm
Surgical airway compromise
Surgical airway edema
Vocal cord paralysis
Arytenoid cartilage dislocation
Supraglottic edema with airway obstruction by the epiglottis
Retroarytenoid edema with limited vocal fold abduction
Subglottic edema
Tracheomalacia (from long-standing tracheal intubation)
Bronchospasm

B. Complications of Tracheal Extubation

Respiratory drive failure
Hypoxia (*e.g.,* atelectasis)
Upper airway obstruction (*e.g.,* edema, residual anesthetic)
Vocal fold–related obstruction (*e.g.,* vocal cord paralysis)
Tracheal obstruction (*e.g.,* subglottic edema)
Bronchospasm
Aspiration
Hypertension
Increased intracranial pressure
Increased pulmonary artery pressure
Increased bronchial stump pressure (*e.g.,* after pulmonary resection)
Increased ocular pressure
Increased abdominal wall pressure (*e.g.,* risk of wound dehiscence)

The ASA defines the difficult airway as the situation in which the "conventionally trained anesthesiologist experiences difficulty with mask ventilation (*e.g.,* the unassisted anesthesiologist . . . unable . . . to maintain S_pO_2 greater than 90% using 100% oxygen), difficulty with tracheal intubation (*e.g.,* unable to properly place an ETT with conventional laryngoscopy . . . with more than three attempts or more than 10 minutes), or both." Based on available data, the incidence of failed intubation is 0.05–0.35%, whereas the incidence of failed intubation/inability to perform mask ventilation is 0.01–0.03%.[11,129,130]

When writing in 1993, the Task Force was not able anticipate the advent of new devices and techniques that would alter the basic nature of airway management. The addition of such devices as the LMA, LMA-Fastrach, COPA, and lighted stylet to routine as well as difficult airway management armamentarium has required a re-evaluation of the algorithm.[58,131]

The ASA algorithm stands as a model for the approach to the difficult airway for nurse anesthetists, emergency medicine physicians, and prehospital personnel, as well as for anesthesiologists. Although the algorithm largely speaks for itself, its salient features are discussed here.

Entry into the algorithm is with the evaluation of the airway. Although there is some debate as to the value of particular evaluation methods and indices, the clinician must use all avail-

---

Table 23-9. CRITERIA FOR ROUTINE "AWAKE" EXTUBATION

Subjective Clinical Criteria:

Follows commands
Clear oropharynx/hypopharynx (e.g., no active bleeding, secretions cleared)
Intact gag reflex
Sustained head lift for 5 seconds, sustained hand grasp
Adequate pain control
Minimal end expiratory concentration of inhaled anesthetics

Objective Criteria:

Vital Capacity: $\geq$10 ml/kg
Peak voluntary negative inspiratory pressure: >20 cm H_2O
Tidal Volume >6 cc/kg
Sustained tetanic contraction (5 sec)
T_1/T_4 ratio >0.7
Alveolar-Arterial PaO_2 gradient (on FIO_2 of 1.0): <350 mm Hg*
Dead Space to Tidal Volume ratio: $\leq$0.6*

---

*Used during weaning from mechanical ventilation in the intensive care setting.

Table 23-10. CLINICAL SITUATIONS PRESENTING INCREASED RISK FOR COMPLICATIONS AT EXTUBATION[122]

Paradoxical vocal cord motion (pre-existing)	Poorly understood mechanism
Thyroid surgery	4.3% recurrent laryngeal nerve injury Local edema Tracheomalacia (from long-standing goiter)
Laryngoscopy (diagnostic)	Edema, laryngospasm, especially with biopsy
Uvulopalatoplasty	Palatal and oropharyngeal edema
Obstructive sleep apnea syndrome (uncorrected)	
Carotid endarterectomy	Wound hematoma, glottic edema, nerve palsies
Maxillofacial trauma	Laryngeal fracture, reduced level of consciousness, requirements for mandibular/maxillary wires
Cervical vertebrae decompression	Supraglottic and hypopharyngeal edema
Parkinson's disease	
Rheumatoid arthritis	
Generalized edema	Laryngotracheal narrowing
Angioneurotic edema	Laryngotracheal narrowing
Anaphylaxis	Laryngotracheal narrowing
Hypopharyngeal infections	Laryngotracheal narrowing
Hypoventilation syndromes*	
Hypoxemic syndromes†	
Inadequate airway protective reflexes	Aspiration risk

* Residual anesthetic or preoperative medications (including alcohol and illicit drugs), central sleep apnea, carotid endarterectomy, poliomyelitis, Guillain-Barré syndrome, myasthenia gravis, botulism, thoracic skeletal deformity, severe pain (with diaphragmatic splinting), morbid obesity, severe chronic obstructive pulmonary disease.

† Hypoventilation, ventilation-perfusion mismatch, intracardiac or intrapulmonary shunting, increased oxygen consumption, severe anemia, impaired alveolar oxygen diffusion.

able data to reach a general impression as to the difficulty of the patient's airway in terms of laryngoscopy and intubation, supraglottic ventilation techniques, and ability of the patient to cooperate with awake procedures. Incorporated into this process are the history regarding previous airway management and other airway-related symptoms (*e.g.*, snoring), the findings on physical exam, and the clinician's personal level of comfort with the situation. Paramount to the decision process is the patient's relative aspiration risk—when there is no or minimal aspiration risk (absence of recent ingestion, obesity, gastroesophageal reflux symptoms, ascites, pregnancy, excessive opioid administration). Many difficult airways may be managed with anesthesia mask or LMA ventilation, either in lieu of or during tracheal intubation or tracheostomy. If there is a significant risk of gastric regurgitation or foreign body aspiration, the patient judged to be a difficult intubation should be managed in an awake state whenever possible. The exception to this is the patient who is unable to cooperate owing to mental retardation, intoxication, anxiety, depressed level of consciousness, or age.[94]

Preparation of the patient for awake intubation is discussed below. In most instances, awake intubation is successful if approached with care and patience. When awake intubation fails,

the clinician has a number of options. First, one can consider cancellation of the surgical case. In this situation, specialized equipment or personnel can be assembled for a return to the operating room. Where cancellation is not an option, regional anesthetic techniques can be considered, or, if demanded by the situation, a surgical airway may be called for.

The decision to proceed with regional anesthesia because the airway has been assessed, or proven to be difficult to manage, must be considered in terms of risks and benefits (Table 23-12).

The algorithm truly becomes useful in the unanticipated difficult airway. When induction agents (with or without muscle relaxants) have been given and the airway cannot be controlled, vital management decisions must be made rapidly. This section of the algorithm may also be applied to the uncooperative patient who is recognized to have a difficult airway. Typically, the clinician has attempted direct laryngoscopy and intubation after successful or failed anesthesia mask ventilation (unless a rapid-sequence induction is being performed). Even if the patient's oxygen saturation remains adequate throughout these efforts, the number of laryngoscopy attempts should be limited to three. As discussed earlier, significant soft tissue trauma can result from multiple laryngoscopies, thereby worsening the situation. First, mask ventilation should be reinstituted if it had been successful previously. The clinician may then turn to the most convenient and/or appropriate technique for establishing tracheal intubation, if needed. This might include, but is not limited to, blind oral or nasal intubation; intubation facilitated by a fiberoptic bronchoscope, LMA, LMA-Fastrach, bougie, lighted stylet, or a retrograde wire; or a surgical airway. (The most widely regarded of these procedures will be discussed with clinical scenarios, below.) When mask ventilation fails, the algorithm suggests two noninvasive, supraglottic ventilation and oxygenation techniques (the LMA and Combitube), a minimally invasive technique (transtracheal jet ventilation), or a surgical airway. At this point, the patient can be awakened, various intubation techniques can be attempted in a stable situation, or a surgical airway can be performed if needed.

Table 23-11. DEVICES USED AS EXTUBATING STYLETS

Device	Advantage	Disadvantage
Fiberoptic bronchoscope	Visualize structures Oxygen can be insufflated through working channel	ETT cannot be exchanged
Eschmann catheter or similar device	Inexpensive, semirigid	Cannot visualize or oxygenate
Exchange/ventilatory catheter	Oxygen can be insufflated through central lumen	Cannot visualize, may be too flexible

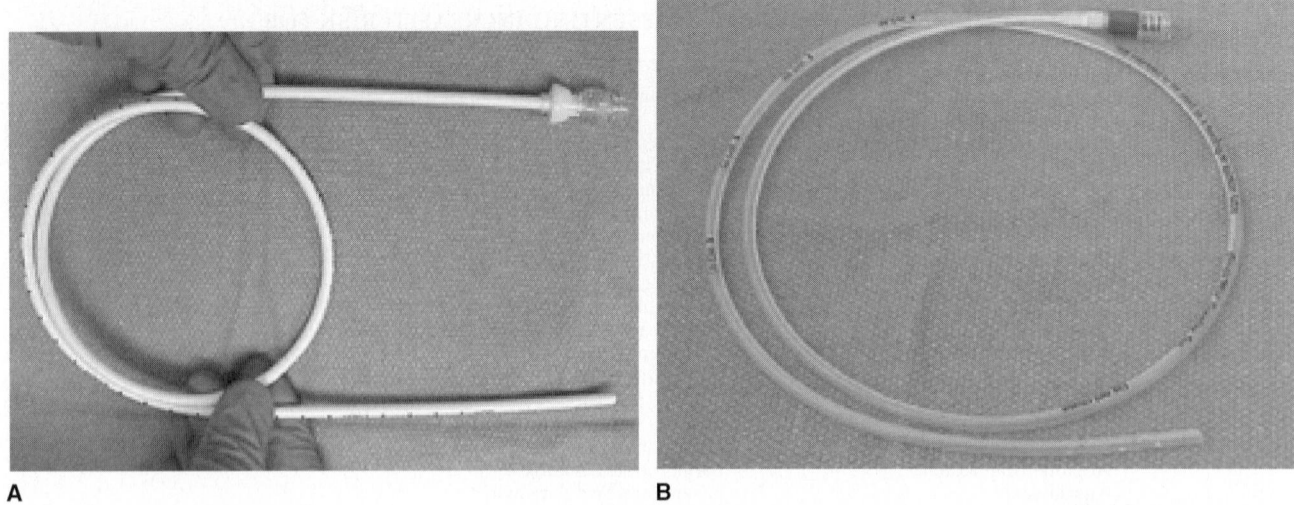

Figure 23-25. (*A*) The Cook airway exchange catheter fitted with a Rapifit Luer-lock adapter (Cook Critical Care, Bloomington, IN). A 15-mm Rapifit adapter for attachment to an anesthesia circuit or ambu bag is also available. (*B*) The Cardiomed endotracheal ventilation catheter.

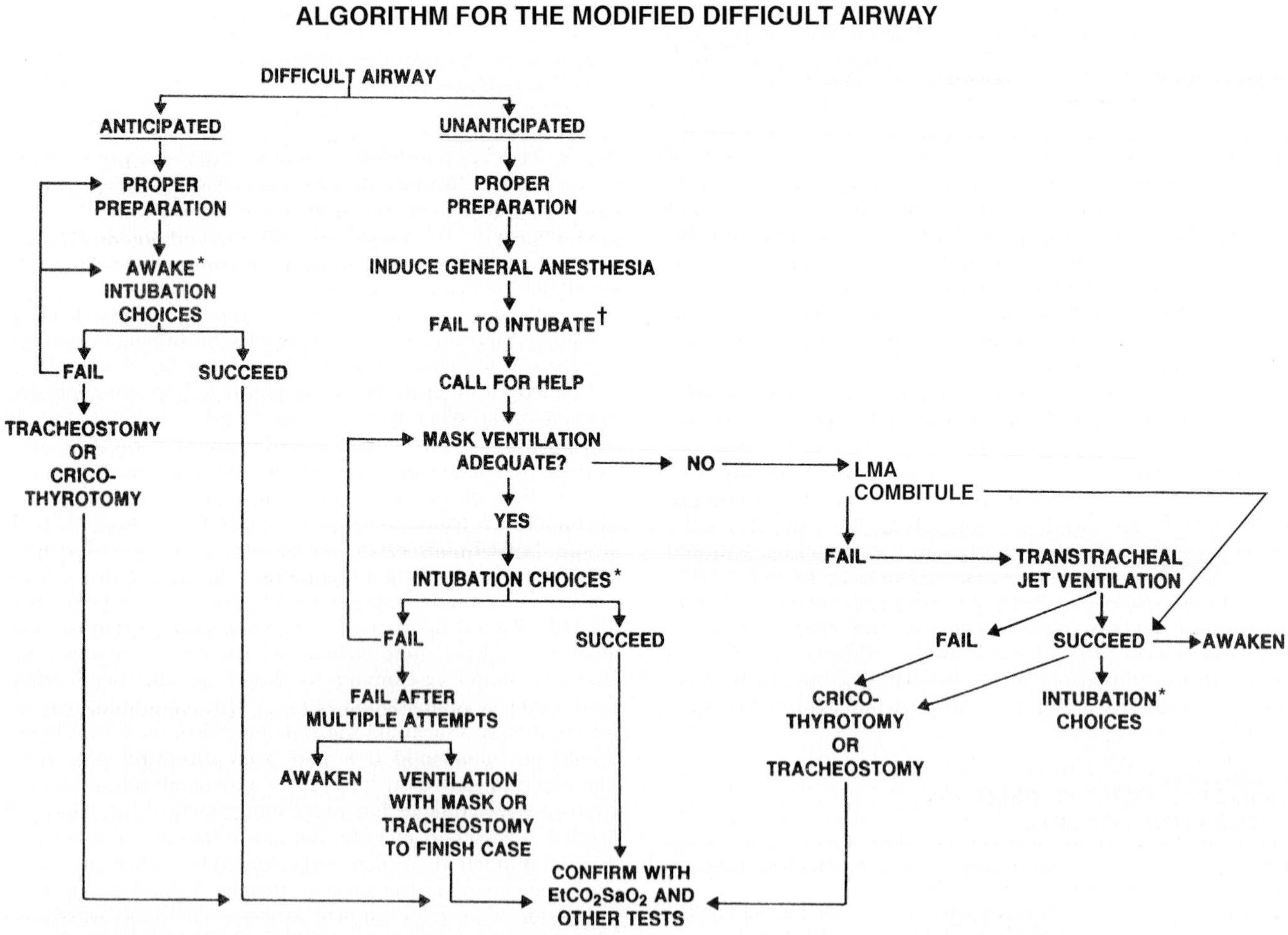

ALGORITHM FOR THE MODIFIED DIFFICULT AIRWAY

* *E.g.*, Blind nasal, FOB-aided, LMA-Fastrach, Retrograde, etc.
† Consider: return to spontaneous ventilation; awaken patient.

Figure 23-26. Algorithm for managing the patient with a difficult airway. (Modified from the algorithm prepared by the American Society of Anesthesiologists' Task Force on Airway Management[94,128].)

Table 23-12. FACTORS TO CONSIDER IN PROCEEDING WITH REGIONAL ANESTHESIA (RA) AFTER THE PATIENT HAS BEEN JUDGED TO HAVE A DIFFICULT AIRWAY

May Consider RA	Should Not Consider RA
Superficial surgery	Cavity-invading surgery
Minimal sedation needed	Significant sedation needed
Anesthetic may be provided with local infiltration	Extensive neuroaxial local anesthetic administration will be required, or risk of intravascular injection/absorption is high
Access to the airway is good	Access to the airway is poor
Surgery can be halted at any time	Surgery cannot be stopped once started

Awake Airway Management

Awake airway management remains a mainstay of the ASA's Difficult Airway Algorithm. If, after a thorough exam of the airway and review of previous anesthetics or other emergency airway events, the ability to safely control ventilation and oxygenation, without the risk of gastric content aspiration is in doubt, awake management is indicated. Airway management is not synonymous with intubation: anesthesia mask, LMA, COPA, tracheal esophageal Combitube, and other devices may provide alternatives to tracheal intubation, depending on the clinical situation. Awake intubation provides many advantages over the anesthetic state, including maintenance of spontaneous ventilation in the event that the airway cannot be secured rapidly, increased size and patency of the pharynx, relative forward placement of the base of the tongue, posterior placement of the larynx, and patency of the retropalatal space.[132,133] The effect of sedatives and general anesthetics on airway patency may be secondary to direct effects on motoneurons and on the reticular activating system.[134] The sleep apnea patient may be particularly prone to obstruction with minimal sedation. Additionally, the awake state confers some maintenance of upper and lower esophageal sphincter tone, thus reducing the risk of reflux. In the event that reflux occurs, the patient can close the glottis and/or expel aspirated foreign bodies by cough to the extent that these reflexes have not been obtunded by local anesthesia.[135] Lastly, patients at risk for neurologic sequelae (*e.g.,* patients with unstable cervical spine pathology) may undergo sensory-motor monitoring after tracheal intubation. In an emergent situation, there may be cautions (*e.g.,* cardiovascular stimulation in the presence of cardiac ischemia or ischemic risk, bronchospasm, increased intraocular pressure, increased intracranial pressure)[136] but no absolute contraindications to awake intubation. Contraindications to elective awake intubation include patient refusal or inability to cooperate (*e.g.,* child, profound mental retardation, dementia, intoxication) or allergy to local anesthetics.

Once the clinician has decided to proceed with awake airway management, the patient must be prepared both physically and psychologically. Most adult patients will appreciate an explanation of the need for an awake airway exam and will be more cooperative once they realize the importance of and rationale for any uncomfortable procedures. The full extent of the procedures need not be explained in total, or all at once. The clinician might explain that he or she is going to "examine" the airway in order to plan a course of action. This can include nasal endoscopy. Once the airway has been prepared and examined, patients will realize that they should experience no further discomfort during the intubation, which may then be discussed.

Apart from appropriate explanation, medication can also be used to allay anxiety. If sedatives are to be used, the clinician must keep in mind that producing obstruction or apnea in the difficult airway patient can be devastating and an overly sedated patient may not be able to protect the airway from regurgitated gastric contents, or cooperate with procedures. Small doses of benzodiazepines (diazepam, midazolam, lorazapam) are commonly used to alleviate anxiety without producing significant respiratory depression. These drugs may be given in iv or oral forms (when available) and may be reversed with specific antagonists (*e.g.,* flumazenil). Opioid receptor agonists (*e.g.,* fentanyl, alfentanil, remifentanil) can also be used in small, titrated doses for their sedative and antitussive effects, although caution must be exercised. A specific antagonist (*e.g.,* naloxone) should always be immediately available. Ketamine and droperidol have also been popular among clinicians.

Administration of antisialagogues is important to the success of awake intubation techniques. As will be discussed below, clearing of airway secretions is essential to the use of indirect optical instruments (*e.g.,* fiberoptic bronchoscope, rigid fiberoptic laryngoscope) because small amounts of any liquid can obscure the objective lens. The commonly used drugs atropine (0.5–1 mg im or iv) and glycopyrrolate (0.2–0.4 mg, im or iv) have other significant effects: by reducing saliva production, these drugs increase the effectiveness of topically applied local anesthetics by removing a barrier to mucosal contact and reducing drug dilution. Vasoconstriction of the nasal passages is needed if there is to be instrumentation of this part of the airway. If the patient is at risk for gastric regurgitation and aspiration, prophylactic measures should be undertaken. Often, it is also prudent to supply supplemental oxygen to the patient by nasal cannula (which can be placed over the nose or mouth).

Local anesthetics are a cornerstone of awake airway control techniques. The airway, from the base of the tongue to the bronchi, comprises an undeniably sensitive series of tissues. Topical anesthesia and injected nerve block techniques have been developed to blunt the protective airway reflexes as well as to provide analgesia. As is well known to the anesthetic practitioner, local anesthetics are both effective and potentially dangerous drugs. The clinician should have a thorough understanding of the mechanism of action, metabolism, toxicities, and acceptable cumulative doses of the drugs that he or she chooses to employ in the airway. Because much of the agent used will be within the tracheal-bronchial tree and will travel to the alveoli, there will be significant and rapid intravascular absorption.

Despite the availability of myriad local anesthetics, only those most commonly used in airway preparation will be discussed here.

Among otolaryngologists, cocaine is a popular topical agent. Not only is it a highly effective local anesthetic, but also it is the only local anesthetic that is a potent vasoconstrictor. It is commonly available in a 4% solution. The total dose applied to the mucosa should not exceed 200 mg in the adult. Cocaine should not be used in patients with a known cocaine hypersensitivity, hypertension, ischemic heart disease, pre-eclampsia, or those taking monoamine oxidase inhibitors.[137] Since cocaine is metabolized by pseudocholinesterase, it is contraindicated in patients deficient in this enzyme.

Lidocaine, an amide local anesthetic, is available in a wide variety of preparations and doses (Table 23-13). Topically applied, peak onset is within 15 minutes. Toxic plasma levels are

Table 23-13. AVAILABLE LIDOCAINE PREPARATIONS

Preparation	Doses
Injectable/topical solution	1%, 2%, 4%
Viscous solution	1%, 2%
Ointment	1%, 5%
Aerosol	10%

not impossible to achieve but are not commonly reported in airway management.

Tetracaine is an amide local anesthetic with a longer duration of action than either cocaine or lidocaine. Solutions of 0.5%, 1%, and 2% are available. Absorption of this drug from the respiratory and GI tracts is rapid, and toxicity after nebulized application has been reported with doses as low as 40 mg, although the acceptable safe dose in adults is 100 mg.[138]

Benzocaine is popular among some clinicians because of its very rapid onset (<1 minute) and short duration (~10 minutes). It is available in 10%, 15%, and 20% solutions. It has been combined with tetracaine (Hurricaine®, Beutlich Pharmaceuticals) to prolong the duration of action. A 0.5-second aerosol administration of Hurricaine delivers 30 mg of benzocaine, the toxic dose being 100 mg. Another common preparation is Cetacaine spray, which combines benzocaine with tetracaine, butyl aminobenzoate, benzalkonium chloride, and cetyldimethylethyl ammonium bromide. Benzocaine may produce methemoglobinemia, which is treated by the administration of methylene blue.

There are three anatomic areas to which the clinician directs local anesthetic therapy: the nasal cavity/nasopharynx, the pharynx/base of tongue, and the larynx/trachea. The nasal cavity is innervated by the greater and lesser palantine nerves (innervating the nasal turbinates and most of the nasal septum) and the anterior ethmoid nerve (innervating the nares and anterior third of the nasal septum). The two palantine nerves arise from the sphenopalantine ganglion, located posterior to the middle turbinate. Two techniques for nerve block have been described. The ganglion can be approached through a noninvasive nasal approach: cotton-tipped applicators soaked in local anesthetic are passed along the upper border of the middle turbinate until the posterior wall of the nasopharynx is reached. They are left in place for 5–10 minutes. In the oral approach, a needle is introduced into the greater palantine foramen, which can be palpated in the posterior lateral aspect of the hard palate, 1 cm medial to the second and third maxillary molars. Anesthetic solution (1–2 ml) is injected with a spinal needle inserted in a superior/posterior direction at a depth of 2–3 cm. Care must be taken not to inject into the sphenopalantine artery. The anterior ethmoid nerve can be blocked by cotton-tipped applicators soaked in local anesthetic placed along the dorsal surface of the nose until the anterior cribiform plate is reached. The applicator is left in place for 5–10 minutes.

The oropharynx is innervated by branches of the vagus, facial, and glossopharyngeal nerves. The glossopharyngeal nerve (GPN) travels anteriorly along the lateral surface of the pharynx, its three branches supplying sensory innervation to the posterior third of the tongue, the vallecula, the anterior surface of the epiglottis (lingual branch), the walls of the pharynx (pharyngeal branch), and the tonsils (tonsillar branch). A wide variety of techniques may be used to anesthetize this part of the airway. The simplest techniques involve aerosolized local anesthetic solution, or a voluntary "swish and swallow." As long as the clinician has developed a plan to anesthetize all relevant structures, has allowed enough time for drying agents to work, and remains continually cognizant of the total dose of local anesthetics administered, most patients will be adequately anesthetized in this way.

Some patients may require a GPN block, especially when topical techniques do not adequately block the gag reflex. The branches of this nerve are most easily accessed as they transverse the palatoglossal folds. These folds are seen as soft tissue ridges which extend from the posterior aspect of the soft palate to the base of the tongue, bilaterally (Fig. 23-27).

A noninvasive technique employs anesthetic-soaked cotton-tip applicators which are positioned against the inferiormost aspect of the folds, being left in place for 5–10 minutes. When the noninvasive technique proves inadequate, local anesthetic

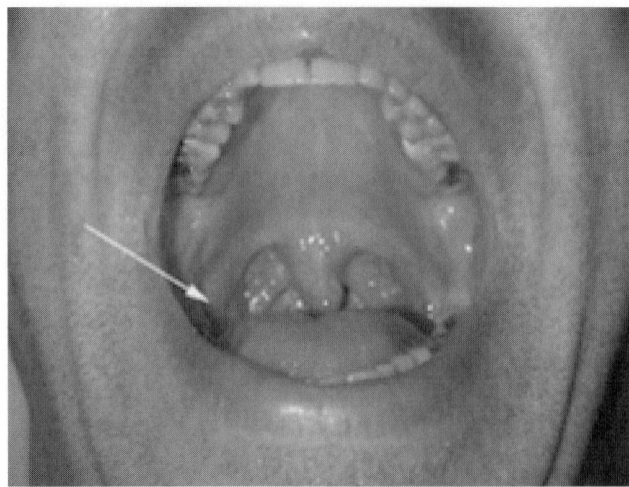

Figure 23-27. The palatoglossal arch (*arrow*) is a soft tissue fold which is a continuation from the posterior edge of the soft palate to the base of the tongue. A local anesthetic–soaked swab placed in the gutter along the base of the tongue is left in contact with the fold for 5–10 minutes.

can be injected. Standing on the side contralateral to the side to be blocked, the operator displaces the extended tongue to the contralateral side and a 25G spinal needle is inserted into the membrane near the floor of the mouth. An aspiration test is performed. If air is aspirated, the needle has passed through-and-through the membrane. If blood is aspirated, the needle is redirected more medially. The lingual branch is most readily blocked in this manner, but retrograde tracking of the injectate has also been demonstrated.[135] Though providing a reliable block, this technique is reported to be painful and may result in a bothersome persistent hematoma.[139] A posterior approach to the GPN has been described in the otolaryngologic literature (for tonsillectomy). It may be difficult to visualize the site of needle insertion, which is behind the palatopharyngeal arch where the nerve is in close proximity to the carotid artery. Because of the risk for arterial injection and bleeding, the technique will not be described here; however, the reader is referred to a more authoritative text.[140]

The internal branch of the superior laryngeal nerve (SLN), which is a branch of the vagus nerve, provides sensory innervation to the base of the tongue, epiglottis, aryepiglottic folds, and arytenoids. The branch originates from the SLN lateral to the cornu of the hyoid bone. It then pierces the thyrohyoid membrane and travels under the mucosa in the pyriform recess. The remaining portion of the SLN, the external branch, supplies motor innervation to the cricothyroid muscle. Several blocks of this nerve have been described. In many instances topical application of anesthetics in the oral cavity will provide adequate analgesia. An external block is performed with the patient supine with the head extended and the clinician standing on the side ipsilateral to the nerve to be blocked. Beneath the angle of the mandible the clinician identifies the superior cornu of the hyoid bone (Fig. 23-28). Using one hand, medially directed pressure is applied to the contralateral hyoid cornu, displacing the ipsilateral hyoid cornu toward the clinician. Caution must be taken to locate the carotid artery and displace it if necessary. The needle can be inserted directly over the hyoid cornu and then "walked" off the cartilage in an anterior-caudad direction until it can be passed through the ligament to a depth of 1–2 cm (Fig. 23-29A). Before the injection of local anesthetic, an aspiration test should be performed to ensure that one has not entered the pharynx or a vascular structure. Local anesthetic with epinephrine (1.5–2 ml) is injected in the space between the thyrohyoid membrane and the pharyngeal mucosa. The superior laryngeal nerve can also be blocked with a noninvasive

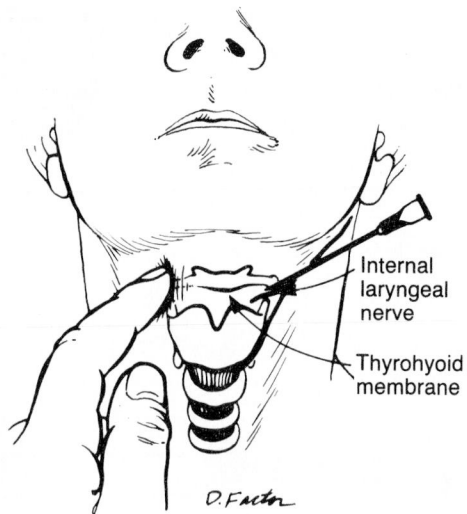

Figure 23-28. When a superior laryngeal nerve block is performed, pressure is applied to the contralateral greater cornu of the hyoid to facilitate identification of anatomic landmarks. The needle is inserted at the level of the thyrohyoid membrane just inferior to the greater cornu of the thyroid cartilage.

block internal technique. The patient is asked to open the mouth widely, and the tongue is grasped using a gauze pad or tongue blade. A right-angle forceps (*e.g.,* Jackson-Krause forceps) with anesthetic-soaked cotton swabs is slid over the lateral tongue and into the pyriform sinuses bilaterally. The cotton swabs are held in place for 5 minutes.

Sensory innervation of the vocal folds and the trachea is provided by the recurrent laryngeal nerve. Transtracheal injection of local anesthetic can easily be performed to produce adequate analgesia, and the technique is described in detail below (see Retrograde Intubation) (Fig. 23-29B). Lidocaine, 4 ml of 2% or 4% solution, is injected.

An effective and noninvasive technique of tracheal and vocal cord topical analgesia utilizes the working channel of the fiberoptic bronchoscope. A disadvantage of this technique is that solutions leaving the working channel can obscure the objective lens. This can be overcome by use of an epidural catheter, inserted through the working channel, as described by Ovassapian.[141] Not only does this prevent the obscuring of the view, but also it allows specific "aiming" of the anesthetic stream.

Clinical Difficult Airway Scenarios

The clinician approaching the patient with a difficult airway has a vast armamentarium of techniques and instruments that can be applied to securing and maintaining oxygenation and ventilation. Although this array can be confusing, textbook authors cannot dictate specific approaches in every situation;[142] moreover, the variability of patient presentation makes specific recommendations difficult. Thus, in order to discuss management, the following section presents a number of brief clinical scenarios and the author's own approach. The major alternative airway management techniques are discussed in this manner. All the clinical cases described herein have been managed by the author or a colleague. Other techniques that might be applied in each situation are also discussed, together with the author's own "decision tree" regarding their applicability. In these cases, as in actual practice, the first technique applied may not have been the best one. The principle of flexibility (and a keen eye to the need to change course quickly) will be emphasized repeatedly. In view of the critical importance of the act of airway control, the clinician must be prepared to alter his or her approach as the situation demands.

Case 1: Flexible Fiberoptic-Aided Intubation

A 50-year-old man with symptomatic cervical vertebrae disk herniation presents for disk resection and spinal fixation. He has a history of tobacco use, alcohol consumption, and gastroesophageal reflux. In the preoperative holding area 0.4 mg of glycopyrrolate is administered. Fifteen minutes later, when the patient states that his oral secretions are minimized, topical anesthesia is administered to the airway. The patient receives 4 mg of intravenous midazolam. An intubating oral airway is placed without eliciting a gag reflex and a flexible fiberoptic bronchoscope is advanced into the airway. The vocal ligaments are visualized, and 4 ml of 4% lidocaine solution is injected through the fiberscope's working channel, being seen to bathe the laryngeal and sublaryngeal structures. The distal end of the fiberscope is advanced into the larynx, and a 7.0-id endotracheal

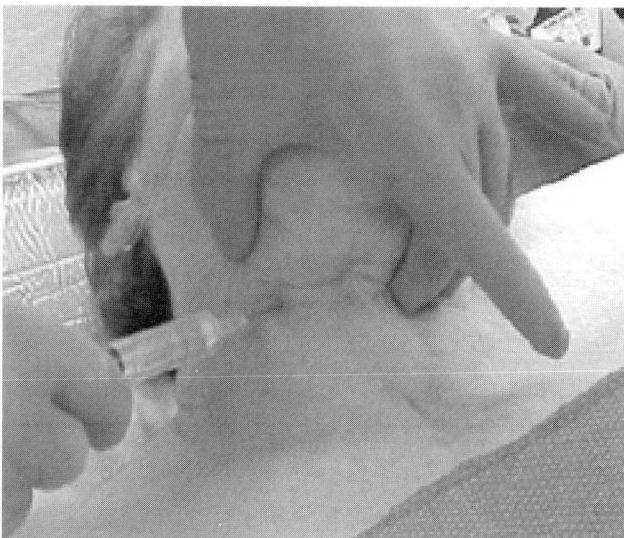

A

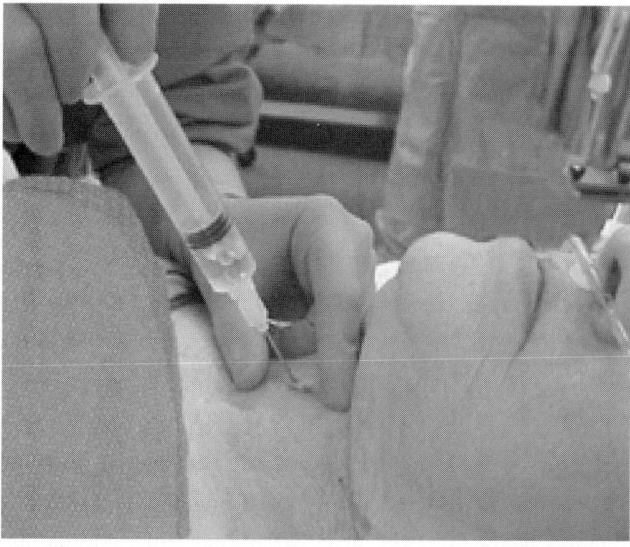

B

Figure 23-29. (*A*) Superior laryngeal nerve block; (*B*) transtracheal aspiration and injection of local anesthetic (note bubble of aspirated tracheal air).

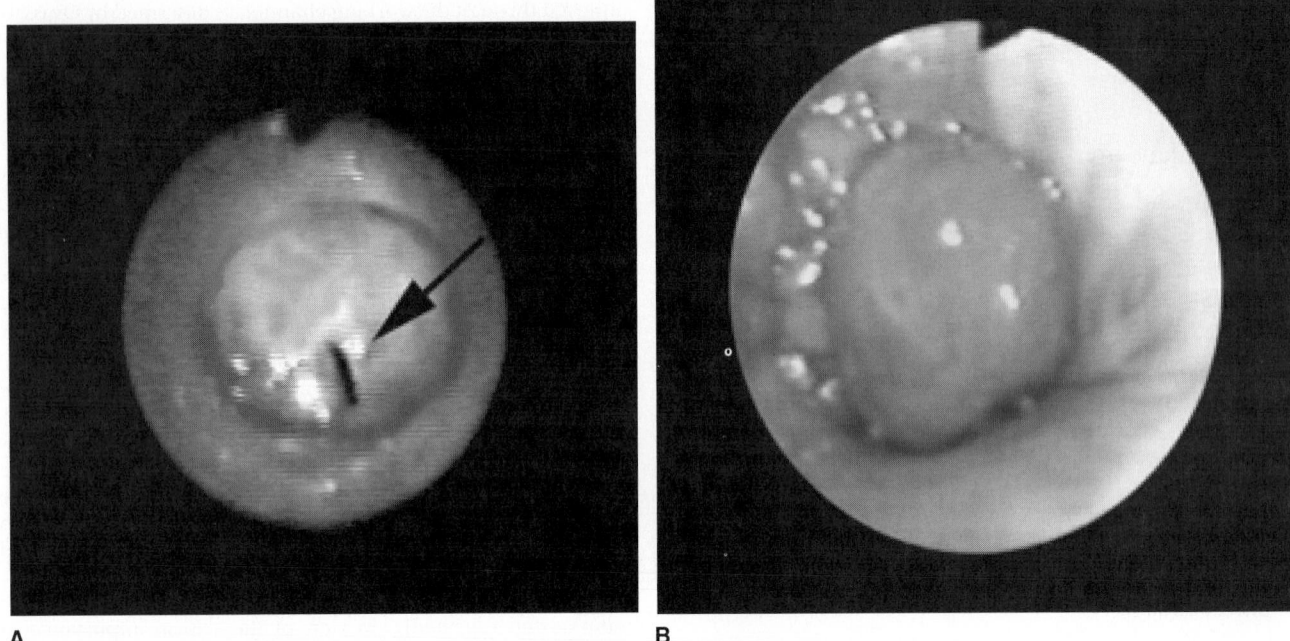

A   B

Figure 23-30. The fiberoptic bronchoscope may be useful for diagnosis and therapy below the level of the vocal ligaments including bronchial segments exam and toilet (see Fig. 23-3). (*A*) Laryngeal web; (*B*) bronchial tumor.

tube, which had been threaded onto the fiberscope's insertion shaft, is advanced into the trachea. The fiberscope is removed while the structures of the carina, trachea, and, finally, the tracheal tube are observed. The anesthesia circuit is attached to the tracheal tube and a steady output of carbon dioxide is detected by capnography. A brief sensory and motor neurologic exam is performed by the attending surgeon and general anesthesia is induced.

Use of the Fiberoptic Bronchoscope in Airway Management.   The fiberoptic bronchoscope (FOB) is a ubiquitous instrument in anesthesia, being available to 99% of surveyed active ASA members.[142] The technique of fiberoptic-aided intubation was first performed using a choledochoscope in a patient with Still's disease.[143] By the late 1980s it was recognized that the use of the flexible FOB represented such a great advancement in the management of the patient with a difficult airway that experts stated that no anesthesiologist could afford not to be facile with this technique.[144] It is now generally accepted that for a variety of clinical situations, the FOB is a critical tool in the armamentarium of the anesthesiologist dealing with the awake or unconscious patient who is, or appears to be, difficult to intubate.[145] The FOB has proven to be the most versatile tool available in this regard.[141]

There is no true or firm indication for FOB-aided intubation, as there might be with direct laryngoscopy (*e.g.,* rapid-sequence induction for the full-stomach patient). There are, however, many clinical situations where the FOB can be of unparalleled aid in securing the airway, especially if the clinician has made an effort to master the necessary skills by using it in routine intubations.[141] These include anticipated difficult intubation due to historical or physical exam findings, unanticipated difficult intubation (where other techniques have failed), lower and upper airway obstruction, unstable or fixed cervical spine disease, mass effect in the upper or lower airways, dental risk or damage, and awake intubation.[141] Unlike the other devices used to intubate the trachea, the FOB can also serve to visualize structures below the level of the vocal folds. For example, it can identify the placement of the tracheal tube or aid in placement of a double lumen tracheal tube. It may be helpful in

diagnosis within the trachea and bronchial tree, or in pulmonary toilet (Fig. 23-30).

Contraindications to FOB-aided intubation are relative, and revolve about the limitations of the device (Table 23-14).

Because the optical elements are small (the objective lens is typically 2 mm in diameter or smaller), minute amounts of airway secretions, blood, or traumatic debris can hinder visualization. Care must be taken to remove these obstacles from the airway beforehand: application of intramuscular or intravenous antisialagogues (*e.g.,* glycopyrrolate, 0.2–0.4 mg; atropine, 0.5–1 mg) will produce a drying effect within 15 minutes, but caution should be taken in patients who may not be able to tolerate an increase in heart rate. Vasoconstriction of the nose using topical oxymetazoline, phenylephrine, or cocaine reduces the chances of bleeding should this route be chosen. If an awake intubation is planned using the FOB, the patient must be able to cooperate—a "quiet" airway, with little motion of the head, neck, tongue, and larynx, is vital to success. Finally, because FOB-aided intubation of the trachea can require significant time, especially if the clinician is not facile with the device, hypoxia or impending hypoxia is a contraindication, and a more rapid method of securing an airway (*e.g.,* LMA or surgical airway) should be considered.

Elements of the Fiberoptic Bronchoscope.   The FOB is a fragile device with optical and nonoptical elements. The fundamental element consists of a glass-fiber bundle. Each fiber is 8–12 μm in diameter, and is coated with a secondary glass layer, the

Table 23-14. CONTRAINDICATIONS TO FIBEROPTIC BRONCHOSCOPY

Hypoxia
Heavy airway secretions not relieved with suction or antisialagogues
Bleeding from the upper or lower airway not relieved with suction
Local anesthetic allergy (for awake attempts)
Inability to cooperate (for awake attempts)

cladding. The cladding aids in maintaining the image within each fiber as the light is reflected off the sidewall at a rate of 10,000 times per meter as it moves from the objective lens to the eyepiece lens in the operator's handle. The typical intubating FOB has 10,000–25,000 such fibers encased in a 60-cm, water-impermeable insertion cord, marked every 10 cm. Though the fibers are allowed to rotate over each other throughout the length of the cord, they are fused together at the two ends in a coherent pattern; that is, the arrangement of the fibers at the eyepiece end is identical to the arrangement at the objective lens, where a diopter ring allows focusing. Therefore, one might envision that the image before the objective lens (*i.e.,* the objective) is divided into 10,000 individual and unique pictures, which independently travel down an unwieldy cord, to be reassembled in front of the eyepiece lens. Broken fibers, which may occur because of bending of the insertion cord, entrapping the cord in other equipment, and dropping the FOB, are readily apparent and are generally no more than a nuisance until the number of broken fibers interferes with the visual field.

The insertion cord also contains a working channel: a lumen, up to 2 mm in diameter, which travels from the distal tip to the handle. It can be used for applying suction, or oxygen, and instilling lavaging fluids or drugs (*e.g.,* local anesthetics). There is one report of gastric rupture attributed to the insufflation of oxygen through the working channel when the FOB was within the esophagus.[146] In general, FOBs <2 mm in external diameter (*e.g.,* pediatric) do not have a working channel.

Two wires traveling from a lever in the handle down the length of the insertion cord control movement of the distal tip in the sagittal plane. The entire insertion cord is protected by a metal "wrap" until the level of the distal tip, which is hinged for movement. Coronal plane movement is accomplished by a combined use of the control lever and rotation of the entire FOB from handle to distal end. Because the fibers are able to move over one another, except for where they are fused at the extreme ends of the optic cord, rotational control is maximized by reducing any curves in the FOB shaft (Fig. 23-31).

The final element of the FOB is the light source. Illumination of the objective is provided by one or two noncoherent bundles of glass fibers which transmit light from the handle to the distal tip. The light is provided either by a "universal" cord which emerges from the handle and is inserted into a medical-grade endoscopic light source, or may be provided by a battery-operated light source on the handle.

Preparation of the Fiberoptic Bronchoscope. When approaching the FOB-aided intubation, one must ensure that the device is in working order. A series of inspections are made, as listed in Table 23-15.

Use of the Fiberoptic Bronchoscope. The FOB is held in the nondominant hand, the thumb over the control lever and the index finger poised over the working channel valve (see Fig. 23-31). The dominant hand will be used to steady and hold the insertion cord as it is manipulated in the patient. Many operators are tempted to "switch" hands, but the thumb of the nondominant hand should be well able to control the gross movement of the control level. Any experienced endoscopist will recognize that the fine control required to hold the shaft of the endoscope steady and make adjustments is where the art of endoscopy lies.

The insertion shaft is lubricated with a water-soluble lubricant, and it is threaded through the lumen of an ETT, the objective end emerging from the main ETT orifice. A clinically appropriate ETT should be chosen, but the larger the ratio between the internal diameter of the ETT and the external diameter of the insertion shaft, the greater the risk of "hangup" on airway structures, as occurs in 20–30% of attempts (Fig. 23-32).[141] Hangup occurs when a cleft exists between these two devices because of the differential sizes. Hangup may involve

entrapment of the epiglottis, corniculate/arytenoid cartilages, the aryepiglottic folds, or the vocal folds.[147] A variety of methods have been described for overcoming hangup, including use of a small ETT, rotation of the plane of the ETT bevel 90 clockwise and/or counterclockwise, the use of soft-tipped ETTs, asking the patient to inspire deeply during the ETT advancement, and the "double setup" ETT, which uses a small ETT (*e.g.,* 5.0 id) within a clinically adequate ETT (*e.g.,* 7.5 id) to overcome the clefts caused by size differentials.[147,148]

The clinician chooses the route of intubation, either oral or nasal, based on clinical requirements, surgical needs, operator experience, and other intubation techniques available should FOB-aided intubation fail. This last factor is important because should an attempt at nasal intubation fail, there may be significant bleeding hindering other indirect visualization techniques. The nasal route is considered easier by many clinicians. The differences between oral and nasal FOB-aided intubation are discussed in Table 23-16.

A variety of intubating oral airways (IOA) are commercially available. Their chief function is to provide a clear visual path from the oral aperture to the pharynx, keep the bronchoscope in the midline, prevent the patient from biting the insertion cord, and provide a clear airway for the spontaneously or mask-ventilated patient. The common characteristic of all IOAs is a channel along the length of the airway large enough to allow the passage of the endotracheal tube. The Ovassapian airway (Fig. 23-33) provides two sets of semicircular, incomplete flexible flanges which stabilize the ETT (up to size 9.0 id) in the midline but allow its removal from the airway after intubation has been accomplished so that the IOA can be removed from the mouth. The flat lingual surface of the airway gives it good lateral and rotational stability. The Patil-Syracuse endoscopic airway and the Luomanen oral airway (Fig. 23-33) were also designed for fiberoptic-aided intubation. Each has a central groove, open at the lingual (Patil-Syracuse) or palatal (Luomanen) aspect, which allows easy removal of the ETT. The flat lingual surface provides good stability. Though this style of IOA provides superb access to the pharynx, it is larger than other airways and is often uncomfortable for the patient. The Williams airway (Fig. 23-33) and the Berman airway were both designed for blind oral intubation. It is often difficult to manipulate the tip of the fiberscope when it is within these narrow airways. Both are molded plastic with a complete circular internal lumen which guides the ETT toward the larynx. These airways have a small profile and are often better tolerated by the awake patient, but tend to be less stable on the tongue. Because the internal lumen is a complete circle, the Williams airway must be retreated off the ETT if it is going to be removed after intubation. This may pose difficulty if the ETT in use has a fused circuit adapter. The Berman airway solves this problem by being split along the length of one side. The plastic of the opposite side is thin and malleable. If the interincisor gap is adequate, the airway can be opened laterally to allow removal from the ETT.

After successful navigation through the supraglottic airway, the endoscopist visualizes the vocal folds. If glottic closure, gag, or coughing occur as the FOB distal tip stimulates the structures of the larynx, the operator can choose to apply local anesthetic through the working channel, administer more sedation, or withdraw the scope and reinforce preparatory procedures. The clinician might also decide to advance the FOB into the larynx without further preparation. The actions taken must be dictated by the individual clinical situation; in the elective scenario, for example, there may be time for reinforced airway analgesia, whereas in the face of impending respiratory arrest patient discomfort may need to be tolerated. Once the larynx is entered, the operator may choose a structure, such as the tracheal carina, to serve as an identifying landmark as the ETT is advanced. Simply because the FOB has entered the trachea, there is no guarantee that the intubation will be successful. As noted above,

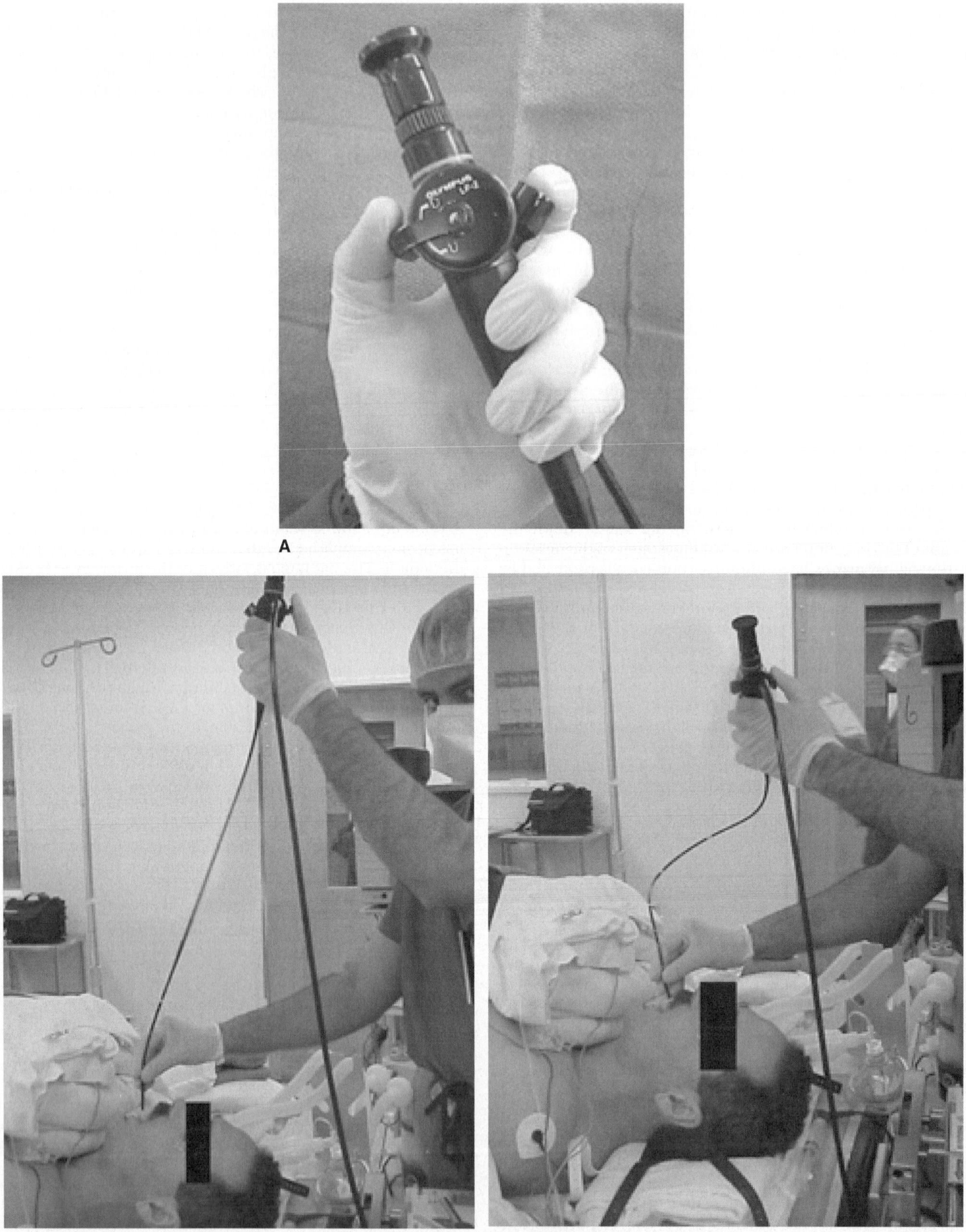

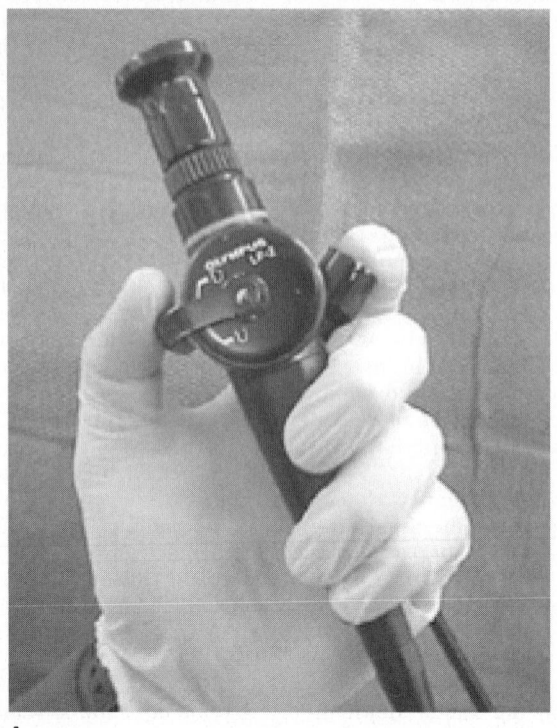

A

B

C

Figure 23-31. Handling of the fiberoptic bronchoscope. (*A*) The handle is held in the nondominant hand with the tip of thumb over the sagittal plane control lever. The index finger can be used to control the working channel (*e.g.,* suction, oxygen insufflation). The dominant hand is used for fine manipulation at the distal end. (*B*) The operator's two hands should be kept maximally apart so as to keep the insertion shaft as straight as possible, maximizing coronal plane rotational control. (*C*) Curves introduced along the shaft reduce coronal plane rotational control.

Table 23-15. PREPARATION OF THE FIBEROPTIC BRONCHOSCOPE

Procedure	Finding	Significance and Action
Inspect passive angulation: Allow FOB to hang from the hand.	Observer deviations from "plum"	Angulation may signify damage to the insertion shaft. If lever controls are operative, the FOB may be usable. Excessive angulation or curvature may make manipulation difficult, disorienting the operator, so the scope should not be used.
Active angulation: The control lever is used to manipulate the distal tip	Does the lever control move the tip in the sagittal plane smoothly and to the extent stated by the manufacturer?	There may be a damaged or entrapped control wire. The device should be repaired by the manufacturer.
Apply suction to the working channel.	No or minimal suction at distal aperture.	Caking of secretions within channel may require cleaning by the manufacturer. Crimping of insertion cord requires repair.
Picture clarity: Observe printed writing a few millimeters in front of the objective lens	Foggy or dirty picture	The objective lens and eyepiece lens can be cleaned with a lint-free cloth. Use a commercial defogger. Prior to placing in the patient, warm water may prevent further fogging by equalizing the lens and patient temperatures. Suction or oxygen insufflation If these are unsuccessful, the FOB may need cleaning by the manufacturer.

20–30% of ETT advancements are accompanied by hangup. Therefore, a patient with a critical airway should not be induced with a general anesthetic with the assumption that the ETT will be easy to pass.

Once the ETT enters the trachea, the clinician may choose to view the ETT and a chosen anatomic landmark simultaneously (*e.g.*, the tracheal carina) to assure correct ETT placement before the FOB is withdrawn.

There have been a number of variations and adjuncts to FOB-aided intubation. The reader is referred to the primary literature listed in Table 23-17, which is not meant to be exhaustive.

Although FOB-aided intubation is a versatile and vital technique, there are several pitfalls, most of which have been discussed. Table 23-18 lists the most common reasons for failure of FOB-aided intubation.

Rigid Fiberoptic Intubation Devices. Rigid fiberoptic devices allow indirect views of the larynx and act as an ETT guide for intubation. More than one third of all anesthesiologists have access to these devices.[142] The most commonly available of these devices include the Bullard (Circon ACMI, Stanford, CT), Wu, and Upsher laryngoscopes (Fig. 23-34). Although these laryngoscopes may be used in routine clinical situations, they are particularly useful when movement of the patient's head and neck is impossible or contraindicated, (*e.g.*, atlanto-occipital joint disease and the spine-injured patient). They are also applicable when there is a limited oral aperture (0.64 cm in the case of the Bullard). These devices consist of a rigid, stainless steel laryngoscope-like blade which encases a fiberoptic cable with a proximal eyepiece and distal objective lens. The blades have an anatomic curve to match the neutral position of the human oral cavity:pharynx:hypopharynx relationship. Alignment of the oral, pharyngeal, and tracheal axes is not required. Illumination is provided by a second fiberoptic cable transmitting light from a battery or free-standing light source.

The Bullard scope, which comes in adult and pediatric sizes, has been the best investigated. It features a fixed fiberoptic cable located on the posterior aspect of the blade. The eyepiece lens has an adjustable diopter. A working channel also runs the length of the blade. Once the larynx is visualized, the ETT is advanced using a detachable stylet, although other techniques have been described.[149] Recently, the advantages of the Bullard scope over traditional laryngoscope blades in managing the spine-injured patient and the obese patient have been investigated.[150-152]

The Upsher scope (Mercury Medical, Clearwater, FL) is available in an adult size as of this writing. Instead of a stylet, the ETT is held and advanced through a C-shaped lumen in the blade. There is no working channel in this scope. The eyepiece is focusable.

The Wu scope (Pentax) differs from the other devices in that a flexible fiberoptic endoscope is fitted into a passage within a three-part stainless steel handle and blade. A second, larger lumen accepts the ETT. A working channel is positioned alongside the endoscope lumen. Two adult sizes are manufactured. Once the larynx is visualized and the ETT advanced into the trachea, the two stainless steel pieces of the laryngoscope blade are disassembled and removed from the mouth. Unlike the other two devices, the Wu scope can also be used for nasal intubation by assembling only the anterior blade portion and the handle. An ETT, previously placed in the pharynx via the nares, can be fitted into the anterior portion of the blade.

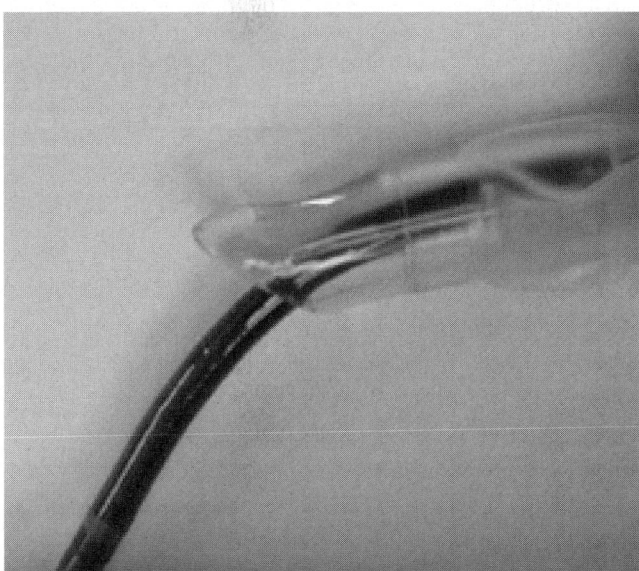

Figure 23-32. The size discrepancy between the fiberoptic bronchoscope and the tracheal tube that has been threaded onto it can create a cleft that can entrap anterior anatomic structures, hindering advancement of the tracheal tube into the larynx (hang-up).

TABLE 23-16. TECHNIQUES OF NASAL AND ORAL FOB-AIDED INTUBATION

	Nasal	Oral
Preparation	Antisialagogues, topical decongestant, serial dilations with soft and lubricated nasal trumpets*	Antisialagogue, intubating oral airway (IOA)
ETT	Softened by placing in warm water. May be kept either on proximal insertion cord (near handle) or inserted† into the nose so that it is felt to turn the bend from the nasal cavity into the nasopharynx.	Kept either on proximal insertion cord (near handle) or inserted 4–5 cm into the IOA
Structures seen	Floor of nose, nasal turbinates, superior aspect of the soft palate, nasopharyngeal posterior wall, base of tongue, epiglottis (distal tip),‡ arytenoid cartilages, vocal folds, tracheal rings, carina	IOA (anterior or anterior/posterior depending on IOA) Soft palate/uvula Epiglottis (distal tip),‡ arytenoid cartilages, vocal folds, tracheal rings, carina

* Although phenylephrine and cocaine have been used to decongest the nose, evidence suggests that oxymetazoline may be the best agent.

† The bevel of the ETT should follow along the nasal septum, away from the turbinates. If the ETT will not turn into the nasopharynx, it may be rotated 90° in a clockwise or counterclockwise direction and readvanced.

‡ An obstructing base of tongue or epiglottis can be moved by extension at the atlanto-occipital joint, jaw thrust, chin lift, or assistant pulling tongue forward.

Case 2: Retrograde Wire Intubation

A 65-year–old female with a 60-pack/year history of smoking and advanced rheumatoid arthritis presents to the emergency department (ED) in respiratory distress. Her oxygen saturation with a nonrebreather oxygen mask is 85%. She has a limited oral aperture (~2.5 cm) and a thyromental distance of 6 cm. Although the cricothyroid membrane can be palpated, there is limited access to it and the tracheal rings owing to a significant cervical kyphosis. The sputum is noted to be blood-tinged and contains thickened bronchial secretions. Awake blind nasal intubation is attempted twice by the emergency department physicians, is unsuccessful, and results in epistaxis. Retrograde intubation of the airway is performed with the patient in a sitting position by percutaneous placement of an 18-gauge catheter through the cricothyroid using a saline-filled 10-ml syringe to detect bubbles associated with tracheal entry (after initial local anesthetic infiltration of the skin over the membrane). The needle is advanced over the mid-cricothyroid membrane at a angle of 45° to the chest. After the free aspiration of air is noted, the Teflon sheath of the catheter is advanced into the trachea. A 0.035-inch radiologic guide wire 110 inches in length is ad-

vanced via the catheter until the proximal end emerges from the mouth. A 7.0 ETT is placed over the wire and is guided into the trachea. The wire is removed by pushing it into the percutaneous puncture site and retrieving it from the proximal end of the tracheal tube. Breath sounds are auscultated over the lung fields as ventilation is assisted with positive pressure. Once improved oxygen saturation is noted, the patient receives sedation with intravenous midazolam.

Use of the Retrograde Wire Intubation in Airway Management. Retrograde wire intubation (RWI) involves the antegrade pulling or guiding of an ETT into the trachea using a wire or catheter which has been passed into the trachea via a percutaneous puncture through the cricothyroid membrane or the cricotracheal membrane, and blindly passed retrograde into the larynx, hypopharynx, and pharynx and out of the mouth or nose. Retrograde intubation was first described in 1960 by Butler and Cirillo, with the placement a red rubber urethral catheter

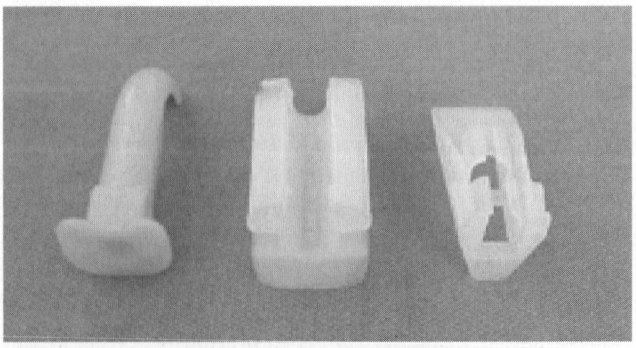

Figure 23-33. (*A*) Williams airway, (*B*) Luomanen airway, and (*C*) Ovassapian fiberoptic intubating airway.

Table 23-17. AIDS TO FIBEROPTIC AIDED INTUBATION

Technique	Advantage
Endoscopy mask	Control ventilation maintained during or between attempts at FOB-aided intubation
Laryngeal mask	Excellent view of the larynx and ability to ventilate during or between attempts at FOB-aided intubation
Fiberoptic-aidedretrograde intubation	Guiding of the FOB with a wire known to be entering the trachea
Retrograde fiberoptic intubation	Changing a tracheostomy to an oral or nasal tracheal tube when antegrade intubation is difficult or impossible
FOB-aided intubation with the aid of a rigid laryngoscope	Helpful with an obstructing mass or large epiglottis

Table 23-18. COMMON REASONS FOR FAILURE DURING FIBEROPTIC-AIDED INTUBATION

Lack of experience: Not practicing on routine intubations
Failure to adequately anesthetize the airway of the awake patient: Secretions not dried; rushed technique
Failure to adequately dry the airway: Underdose or rushed technique
Nasal cavity bleeding: Inadequate vasoconstriction; rushed technique; forcible ETT insertion
Obstructing base of tongue or epiglottis: Poor choice of intubating airway; require chin lift/jaw thrust
Inadequate sedation of the awake patient
Hangup: ETT too large
Fogging of the FOB: Suction or oxygen not attached to working channel; cold bronchoscope

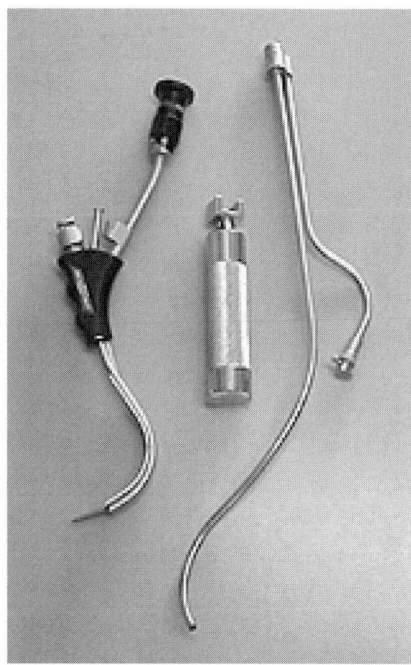

Figure 23-34. The Bullard laryngoscope, battery handle, and stylet.

via a previous tracheostomy up through the larynx and out of the mouth.[153] The percutaneous technique used today was first described by Waters in 1963, using an epidural catheter.[154] In 1993 the technique was include in the ASA's Difficult Airway Algorithm.[128]

The basic equipment used in the retrograde intubation technique is listed in Table 23-19.

Retrograde wire intubation has been described in a number of clinical situations as a primary intubation technique (elective or urgent) and after failed attempts at direct laryngoscopy, fiberoptic-aided intubation, and LMA-guided intubation.[155] The most common indications are inability to visualize the vocal folds owing to blood, secretions, or anatomic variations, unstable cervical spine, upper airway malignancy, and mandibular fracture. Contraindications include lack of access to the cricothyroid membrane or the cricotracheal ligament (due to severe neck deformity, obesity, mass), laryngotracheal disease (stenosis, malignancy, infection), coagulopathy, and skin infection.

The anatomic relationships to be considered in RWI have been described elsewhere in this chapter. Typically, the procedure requires 5 minutes to perform.[156] Because most clinicians are not facile with the technique, it may take several minutes in inexperienced hands; therefore, RWI is relatively contraindicated in the hypoxic patient. RWI has been used in elective and emergent situations, in adults and infants, in the operating room, ED, and the prehospital environment. Complications reported with RWI are listed in Table 23-20.

In the current patient (as in Case 1), RWI was chosen in a setting where the patient was not apneic and was therefore supporting her own ventilation and oxygenation, albeit poorly. The two cases differ in impending respiratory failure (Case 2) versus FOB-aided intubation undertaken in an stable situation (Case 1). In many situations, where awake intubation is an obvious initial approach to securing the airway, there is little time for patient preparation (*e.g.*, the administration of antisial-

agogues, topical anesthetics, and/or sedation). In this regard, RWI does not require a clear visual field or significant patient cooperation and can often be performed with little analgesia of the airway.

Performing Retrograde Wire Intubation (Fig. 23-35). RWI is generally performed with the patient in a supine position, although the sitting position is often used for patients in respiratory distress. Extension of the head or the neck displaces the cricoid and tracheal cartilages anteriorly and displaces the sternocleomastoid muscles laterally, though, as in Case 2, this may not always be possible. The skin should be prepared. If the patient is conscious, a local anesthetic skin wheel is made over the puncture site. Local anesthesia of the airway should be administered to prevent discomfort and airway reflexes as time permits. In general, topical anesthesia of the trachea, larynx, pharynx, and nasal passages is desirable. Translaryngeal anesthesia is a particularly convenient technique since a percutaneous entry of the trachea is required during the RWI. Structures above and below the vocal folds are anesthetized during the ensuing patient cough if a local anesthetic–filled syringe is used to facilitate the recognition of appropriate placement (with tracheal air bubbles) and then is injected to provide airway anesthesia[157] (see Fig. 23-33).

As noted earlier, the cricothyroid membrane (CTM) and cricotracheal ligament (CTL) are both potential sites for translaryngeal puncture. Although the CTM has the advantage of being directly anterior to the large posterior surface of the cricoid cartilage, thereby protecting the esophagus from a punc-

Table 23-19. EQUIPMENT FOR RETROGRADE WIRE INTUBATION

18G or larger angiocatheter
Luer-lock syringe, 3 ml or larger
Guide wire:
• Preferably J-type end
• Length: at least 2.5 times the length of a standard ETT (typically 110–120 cm)
• Diameter: capable of passing via angiocatheter being chosen
Other: Scalpel blade, nerve hook, Magill forceps, 30″ silk suture, epidural catheter

Table 23-20. COMPLICATIONS ASSOCIATED WITH RETROGRADE WIRE INTUBATION

Bleeding (11)
Subcutaneous emphysema (4)
Pneumomediastinum (1)
Breath-holding (1)
Catheter traveling caudad (2)
Trigeminal nerve trauma (1)
Pneumothorax (1)

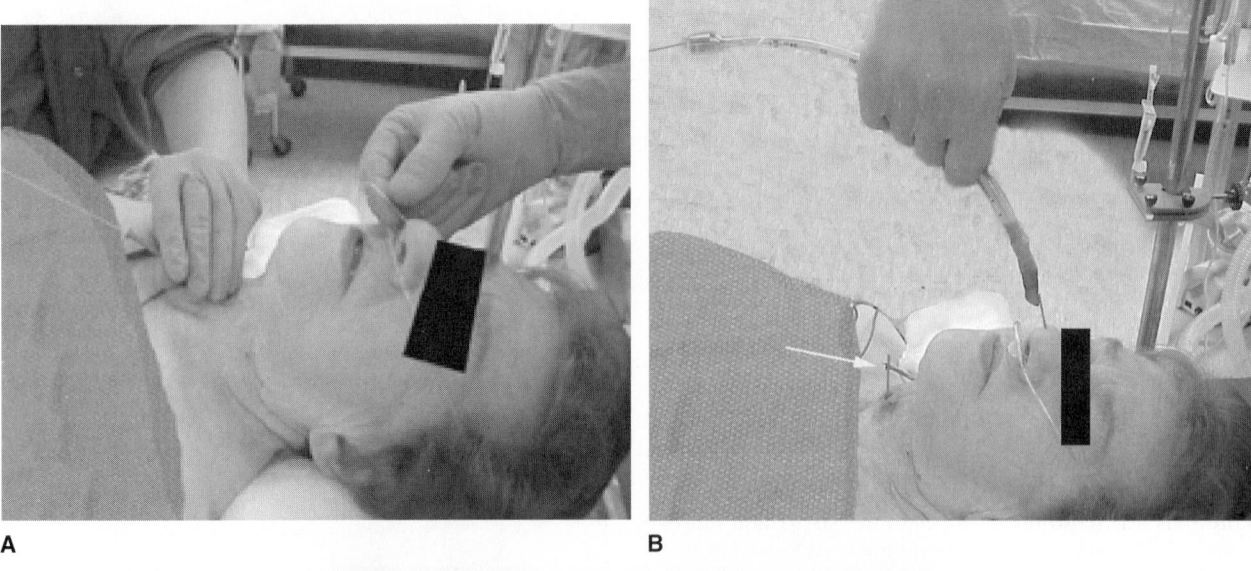

A   B

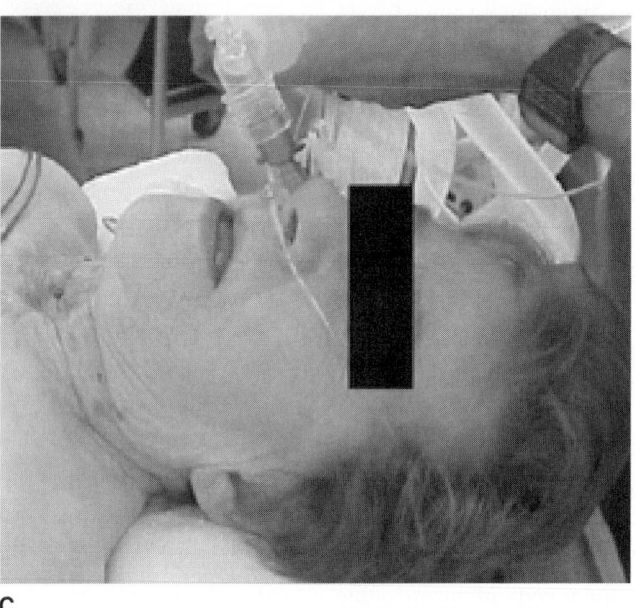

C

Figure 23-35. The sequence of retrograde wire intubation after the cricothyroid or cricotracheal ligament is identified and a percutaneous puncture is performed with air aspiration (see Fig. 23-29B). (*A*) The retrograde device (twisted wire, Cook Critical Care) is advanced until it emerges from the mouth or nose. (*B*) The wire is clamped at the entrance site (*arrow*) and the endotracheal tube is advanced over the wire in an antegrade fashion. [In the picture, the wire has been threaded through the ETT Murphy eye (see Table 23-21).] (*C*) The wire is removed, leaving the tracheal tube in place.

turing needle, it places the needle in close proximity (0.9–1.5 cm) to the vocal folds and hence allows for a somewhat smaller margin of error at the time of the intubation.

Although classically performed with a Tuohy needle and epidural catheter, the advent of smaller-diameter, stiffer wires with atraumatic "J" tips has made the guidewire modification popular. These guidewires are typically 0.032–0.038 inches in diameter, being able to pass though an 18G intravenous catheter. The typical length is between 110 and 120 cm. The only requirement for length is that the wire be more than twice as long as the tracheal tube to be used, so that no matter where in its course along the wire the tracheal tube should be, both ends of the wire are always accessible to the operator. Kits that conveniently incorporate all the necessary equipment are available (Cook Critical Care).

The needle/catheter approaches the trachea at 90° to the coronal and sagittal planes if possible (as it was not in Case 2). In this orientation, the needle is likely to impact the posterior

aspect of the cricoid cartilage if advanced too far, and not puncture the esophagus. Additionally, this angle will help to avoid trauma to the near-lying vocal folds.

After the percutaneous puncture is made and the trachea identified by free air aspiration, the catheter is angled cephalad and the wire is advanced (J-tip) into the trachea until it emerges from the mouth or nose. The wire may need to be retrieved from the mouth with a "sweeping" finger, Magill forceps, or nerve hook. Any obstruction to advancement of the wire should prompt re-evaluation of the angle of the catheter and the position of the head and neck (*e.g.*, catheter directed posterior and/ or caudad, neck flexed). Coughing typically heralds caudad traveling of the wire. If the wire is retracted and found to be bent, it is prudent to procure a new one. When complaints of pain are encountered above the level of the larynx, it is typically due to the wire passing into an inadequately prepared nasal cavity. Options include retracting the wire modestly and asking the patient to open the mouth and maximally protrude the

Table 23-21. TECHNIQUES OF ETT ADVANCEMENT OVER A RETROGRADE WIRE

Technique	Advantage	Disadvantage
Wire travels through entire main lumen of the ETT	Standard technique	Margin of error* equals distance from vocal folds to puncture site No stylet after removal of wire "Railroading"† can occur
Wire placed into ETT lumen via Murphy eye	Increased margin of error Decreased railroading	Cannot use stylet (below)
Wire enters distal end of ETT and exits via Murphy eye	Decreased railroading	Margin of error equals distance from vocal folds to puncture site Cannot use stylet (below)
ETT "exchange" stylet is placed over wire, prior to placement of ETT	Decreased railroading Can use stylet to vastly increase margin of error once wire is removed	Cost
Fiberoptic bronchoscope is placed over wire prior to placement of ETT	Decreased railroading Can use stylet to vastly increase margin of error once wire is removed Visualization	Cost
Silk suture	No railroading Margin of error issues reduced	May be difficult to place silk suture
Small ETT	Reduced railroading	May not be clinically adequate

* *Margin of error* refers to the distance below the vocal folds that the endotracheal tubes extends at the time that the guidewire is removed. If this distance is not adequate, there is a risk of immediate extubation.
† *Railroading* refers to the differential size of the guidewire and the tracheal tube. A large discrepancy in size allows for a cleft which may entrap the epiglottis, arytenoid cartilages, aryepiglottic folds, or vocal folds, hindering intubation attempts.

tongue during the readvancement, reaching into the oropharynx to retrieve the wire, or patiently repreparing the nasal passages. Once the wire is satisfactorily retrieved, placement of the tracheal tube may be performed using the wire in a number of fashions, depending on the operator's preference and previous experience. Table 23-21 lists common techniques, together with their advantages and disadvantages. Details of these techniques have been described elsewhere.[158]

In the case reported, other techniques may have been considered. Although indirect visual devices (flexible fiberoptic bronchoscope, rigid fiberoptic laryngoscope) may have also been helpful in this case, three elements worked against their use: (1) tissue trauma from repeated attempts at blind nasal intubation produced a bloody airway, frustrating the use of these devices; (2) the patient was unable to cooperate owing to her respiratory distress; (3) because of the impending respiratory failure, there was little time for adequate airway analgesia. A coughing, gagging, conscious patient makes fiberoptic techniques nearly impossible. Straining and coughing during fiberoptic intubation attempts have resulted in Mallory-Weiss tears of the esophagus, resulting in significant hemorrhage.

Blind nasal intubation was the first technique attempted in this patient. Until recently, blind nasal intubation has been a staple of airway control, especially in the emergency department, where it has been largely supplanted by rapid-sequence intubation.[159] This technique requires significant analgesia of the nasal passages in the awake patient. Success is far more likely in the spontaneously breathing patient. With the head in the Magill position, the ETT is advanced into the nares, nasal passage (keeping the ETT bevel alongside the nasal septum), and into the pharynx. Breath sounds are auscultated from the ETT, and its position adjusted keep them maximized. The patient's head and larynx can be manipulated externally as necessary.

Case 3: Esophageal Tracheal Combitube

A 55-year-old male with a history of cirrhosis and esophageal varices requires airway control due to acute, recurrent upper gastrointestinal bleeding. Apart from fresh blood in the airway, physical exam of his external airway is consistent with a routine laryngoscopy. Furthermore, he had been intubated for similar events in the past. After a rapid sequence induction, the larynx cannot be visualized on three laryngoscopies owing to fresh blood emanating from the esophagus. On all three attempts, the ETT is advanced blindly, and the absence of breath sounds over the thorax together with the presence of copious blood in the ETT leads to the diagnosis of esophageal intubation. A large adult-sized esophageal tracheal Combitube (Kendall, Mansfield, NY) is requested, blindly inserted into the airway, and the pharyngeal and distal cuffs are inflated. Ventilation through the pharyngeal perforations lumen (blue) produces bilateral breath sounds to auscultation, and the oxygen saturation increases to >90%. Copious blood is suctioned from the esophageal lumen. The patient is transported to the angiography suite where his esophageal varices are embolized. The esophageal tracheal Combitube is removed and the patient is intubated with direct laryngoscopy.

History of the Tracheal Esophageal Combitube. The tracheal esophageal Combitube was developed from the concept of the esophageal operator airway (ESO), which was introduced in 1968.[160] The ESO consisted of a tracheal-like tube, 34 cm in length, with an inflatable cuff at its sealed, distal end. It was inserted blindly into the esophagus, so that the cuff lay at a level caudad and posterior to the tracheal carina. Sixteen holes communicating with the central lumen were positioned so as to be in the hypopharynx when inserted to the proper depth. A face mask at the proximal end was used to "seal" the airway. Ventilation was achieved by applying positive pressure to the proximal open aperture, where it emerged from the face mask. Unfortunately, significant problems/complications became apparent as the ESO came into common practice (Table 23-22).

These shortcomings of the ESO were addressed by Dr. Michael Frass, a critical care physician in Vienna, Austria in 1986.[161]

Table 23-22. PROBLEMS ASSOCIATED WITH THE ESOPHAGEAL OBTURATOR AIRWAY

Difficulty in obtaining a tight face mask fit, especially during prehospital transportation. Often, two hands were needed to produce an adequate fit, especially in the bearded or edentulous.
Inadvertent or unrecognized tracheal intubation with the blind/cuffed distal end, resulting in complete airway obstruction
Esophageal or gastric rupture, possibly due to the length

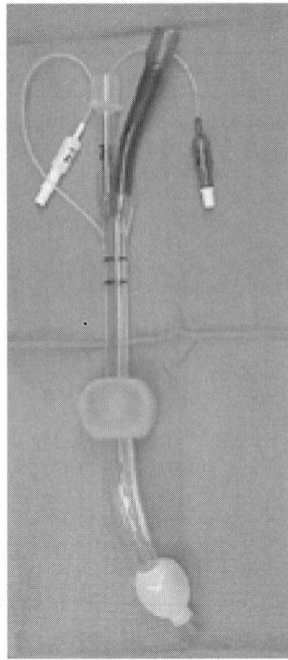

Figure 23-36. The esophageal tracheal Combitube.

The face mask of the ESO was replaced by an oropharyngeal balloon, sealing the upper airway and anchoring the device against the hard palate. As with the ESO, perforations at the hypopharyngeal level allowed egress of air near the level of the larynx, while the distal (esophageal) tip remained occluded and was still included in a cuff. These modifications of the ESO did not solve the problem of complete airway obstruction if the device was accidentally introduced into the trachea. To solve this problem Dr. Frass's final modification included a second lumen, patent from proximal to distal end, without perforations. This design, named the tracheal esophageal Combitube, is functional if introduced into the esophagus (ventilation being achieved through the esophageal lumen, via the hypopharyngeal perforations) or in the trachea (ventilation being achieved through the tracheal lumen, via distal aperture). In either case, the proximal balloon seals both the oral and nasal passages, and the distal conventional tracheal tube cuff isolates the respiratory system from the gastrointestinal system. The device is available in two sizes: the 41Fr size is used for larger adults (height > 5.5 feet) and the 37Fr size is used for adults 4–6 feet tall (Fig. 23-36).

Use of the Esophageal Tracheal Combitube. The esophageal tracheal Combitube is inserted blindly. The operator lifts the lower jaw and tongue anteriorly with one hand, and the esophageal tracheal Combitube is inserted with a downward, caudad-curved motion until the proximal depth indicator (two black rings printed on the double lumen tube) come to rest at the level of the teeth. The oropharyngeal balloon is inflated with 100 ml of air through a blue plastic pilot balloon (85 ml in the small adult size) while the distal cuff is inflated with 5–15 ml (via a white pilot balloon). An ambu bag or anesthesia circuit is attached to the proximal end of the esophageal lumen (constructed of blue polyvinyl chloride), and ventilation is confirmed by auscultation or other means. Because 90% of esophageal tracheal Combitube placements result in an esophageal position, ventilation occurs via this lumen's hypopharyngeal perforations. If no breath sounds are auscultated and/or gastric inflation is noted, the esophageal tracheal Combitube has been positioned in the trachea. Without repositioning, ventilation is changed to the distal end of tracheal lumen (clear polyvinyl chloride). If no maneuver improves ventilation, the device is most likely in the esophagus, but has been advanced too deeply,

with the oropharyngeal cuff obstructing the airway.[162] In this case, the cuffs should be deflated, the device withdrawn 2 cm and the ventilation sequence repeated.

Advantages of the esophageal tracheal Combitube include rapid airway control, airway protection from regurgitation, ease of use by the inexperienced operator, no requirement to visualize the larynx, and being able to maintain the neck in a neutral position. It has been shown to be useful in the patient with massive upper gastrointestinal bleeding or vomiting, cervical spine injury or deformity (though the presence of a rigid cervical collar may make insertion difficult or impossible), and as a rescue device in failed rapid-sequence induction or unanticipated difficult intubation. It is also useful in the grossly obese, in acute bronchospasm, during cardiopulmonary resuscitation, and for prolonged ventilation after airway rescue.[163–174] Several series have demonstrated the esophageal tracheal Combitube's value in prehospital management of the airway.[175–177]

Techniques for exchange of the esophageal tracheal Combitube for an endotracheal tube have been described.[178]

Contraindications to esophageal tracheal Combitube use include esophageal obstruction or other abnormality, ingestion of caustic agents, upper airway foreign body or mass, lower airway obstruction, height less than 4 feet, and an intact gag reflex. Since the esophageal tracheal Combitube includes latex in its construction, it should not be used in patients with latex allergy.

Complications associated with the esophageal tracheal Combitube have included lacerations to the pyriform sinus and esophageal wall resulting in subcutaneous emphysema, pneumomediastinum, pneumoperitoneum, and esophageal rupture.[179–181]

Case 4: Failed Rapid-Sequence Induction and the LMA

A 39-year-old male presents for elective uvulopharyngopalatoplasty. He has no previous surgical history. His maximal incisor gap is 5 cm, thyromental distance is 7 cm, and his oropharyngeal view is a Samsoon–Young Class 2. There is no limitation in head and neck flexion and extension. During a sleep apnea study, he had had 15 apneic events each hour. The patient has a significant history of gastroesophageal reflux, and rapid-sequence induction is planned. After the administration of pentothal, succinylcholine, and cricoid pressure (Sellick maneuver), direct laryngoscopy with a Macintosh number 3 laryngoscope blade reveals a large epiglottis obscuring the view of the vocal folds (Cormack–Lehane Grade 3).[100] Significant hyperplasia of the base of the tongue, which prevents its full displacement, is also noted. The BURP maneuver does not improve the view.[97] A Macintosh 4 and Miller 3 blades are used and do not improve the view. Oxygen saturation, which was 100% prior to induction, is now 92%, and face-mask ventilation is initiated with the Sellick maneuver in place. Complete obstruction to ventilation is encountered, despite chin and/or jaw lift, two-person ventilation, and a reduction in the degree of cricoid pressure. The oxygen saturation falls to 85% and a size 5 LMA (which had been prepared prior to the induction of anesthesia) is inserted with the technique as described by the inventor. Immediately, a clear airway is established, and the Sellick pressure remains in place. A second dose of pentothal is administered, and the patient is intubated by the blind passage of a 7.0-id ETT via the LMA. The LMA is then removed using a Cook airway exchange catheter (Cook Critical Care, Bloomington, IN) as a stylet, and the surgical case proceeds.

The LMA in the Failed Airway. One clear advantage of LMA use is in the failed airway. There have been many reported (and unreported) cases of failed intubation and failure to ventilate by mask in which the airway was rescued with an LMA.[182,183] Parmet *et al* estimate that 1:800,000 patients cannot be managed with an LMA, providing an 80-fold increase in margin of safety over the oft-noted 1:10,000 patients who cannot be ventilated by mask nor intubated by traditional means.[184] Likewise, a wealth of literature describes the use of the LMA in elective difficult airway management in awake and unconscious patients, in anticipated and unanticipated situations, in cervical spine injury, and in pediatric dysmorphic syndromes.[183-199] The characteristics of the LMA that underlie its superiority as a tool in the difficult airway armamentarium are that it is well tolerated by the patient, simulating the natural distension of the hypopharyngeal tissues by food, and that its insertion follows an intrinsic pathway, requiring no tissue distortion (as with laryngoscopy), which may not be possible in all patients. Finally, it is a blind technique not hindered by blood, secretions, debris, and edema from previous attempts at laryngoscopy.[200] Because the LMA's ease of insertion is not dependent on anatomy that can be assessed on routine physical exam, typical airway assessment measures do not apply to its application.[201] The major disadvantage of the LMA in resuscitation is the lack of mechanical protection from regurgitation and aspiration. Lower rates of regurgitation during CPR (3.5%) than with the bag-valve mask ventilation (12.4%) have been shown.[52,202-205] Even in the face of regurgitation, pulmonary aspiration is a rare event with the LMA.[205-207] Unfortunately, the use of the Sellick maneuver may prevent proper seating of the LMA in a minority of instances.[208-210] This may require the brief removal of the cricoid pressure until the LMA has been properly seated. Cricoid pressure is effective with an LMA *in situ*. Had it been available, the Fastrack-LMA would also have been an ideal device in this scenario.

Case 5: Deviation from the Difficult Airway Algorithm

Thirteen hours after admission to the intensive care unit, a 76-year-old female who had sustained trauma to the face, head, and neck in a motor vehicle accident is noted to have progressive decline in her consciousness and respiratory effort. On examination, there appears to be an adequate interincisor gap and thyromental distance. The oropharyngeal view and range of motion of the head and neck cannot be evaluated. Owing to the inability to fully evaluate the airway with respect to ease of intubation, an awake procedure is chosen. Fiberoptic devices are not considered usable because of the presence of fresh and clotted blood in the mouth as a result of continued epistaxis. Other airway techniques that require significant patient preparation are not considered because of the rapid progression of the patient's respiratory failure. Additionally, the presence of fresh blood in the oral and pharyngeal cavities will hinder adequate drying and analgesia. Blind nasal intubation is considered contraindicated based upon the obvious facial trauma and the risk of cribiform plate disruption. Neither equipment for retrograde intubation nor the tracheal esophageal Combitube is readily available. A lighted stylet intubation guide is available, but no clinician present is experienced with this technique. Although the mental status change is believed to reflect an intracranial process (*e.g.,* intracranial hypertension), the risk of complete loss of the airway is judged to be the primary clinical hazard. Awake direct laryngoscopy is attempted with manual in-line stabilization of the neck. After clearing fresh blood from the pharynx with a Yankauer suction catheter, a Cormack–Lehane Grade 3 laryngeal view is obtained; but because of patient resistance (biting on the laryngoscope and movement), tracheal intubation is not achieved. The decision is made to proceed with rapid-sequence induction and intubation, with preparations made for an emergency tracheostomy. After surgical preparation of the neck and preoxygenation, intravenous succinylcholine and etomidate are administered, direct laryngoscopy is undertaken, the larynx is easily visualized, and the trachea is intubated.

Muscle Relaxants and Direct Laryngoscopy. In the case described above, the use of muscle relaxants significantly improved the ability to visualize the larynx.[211-213] In a recent study, the use of muscle relaxants during a direct laryngoscopy increased the success rate of intubation and was associated with fewer incidents of airway trauma, intubation attempts, esopha-

geal intubations, aspiration, and even death.[214] Intubating conditions with and without muscle relaxation have been investigated in few well controlled trials because the superior intubating conditions achieved with muscle relaxants has discouraged inclusion of control groups.[215] Muscle relaxation actions that improve laryngoscopic view include allowing complete temporomandibular joint relaxation and opening, anterior movement of the epiglottis, and widening of the laryngeal vestibule and laryngeal sinus.[95] In addition, the finding that laryngoscopic stimulation of the pharyngeal musculature causes the upper airway lumen to appear small is offset by the use of relaxants.

Leaving the Algorithm. The situation described in Case 5 is unusual in that rapid-sequence induction was attempted because the clinical situation had deviated from the ASA Difficult Airway Algorithm owing to the progressive nature of the airway compromise. The situation was more akin to the "crash" airway described by Walls *et al.*[159] In this case, the institution of muscle relaxation, which might be considered contraindicated in the apparently difficult-to-intubate patient, allowed for full visualization of the larynx. Knowing that failure to intubate in this case would result in probable loss of the airway, the clinician was prepared for cricothyroidotomy. Although the ASA's Difficult Airway Algorithm is a valuable tool in the process of approaching the difficult airway, the clinician must always be prepared for the case that does not fit the mold. As stated earlier, adaptability in a rapidly changing clinical situation is critical to the success of airway management. Also of interest in this case was the availability of a lighted stylet for use in similar difficult airway scenarios. Although this device may have been useful in the current case, no clinician present was familiar with its operation. A critical situation is not an occasion for trying an unfamiliar technology.

Other Devices

An ever increasing number of airway management devices are commercially available. Although encyclopedic coverage of these tools is beyond the scope of this chapter, a review of the more established of this equipment follows.

Lighted Stylets

These devices rely on transillumination of the airway. A light source introduced into the trachea will produce a well circumscribed glow of the tissues over the larynx and trachea. The same light placed in the esophagus will produce no or a diffuse light. A number of devices have become available, including disposable, partly disposable, and fully reusable systems. Although there are many reports of successful intubation using these devices, some common problems have been noted: In general, the operating theater lights must be dimmed to best appreciate the circumscribed glow; a stylet tip successfully placed in the trachea, but not pointing in an anterior direction, may give a false-negative impression; it is often difficult to remove the semirigid stylet from the ETT after intubation.

Airway Bougie

These encompass a series of solid or hollow, semimalleable stylets that maybe be blindly manipulated in to the trachea. An ETT is then "threaded" over the bougie and into the trachea. These bougies are generally low in cost and highly portable. The Eschmann introducer (Eschmann Health Care, Kent, England) was introduced in 1949. It is 60 cm long, 15Fr-gauge, and angled 40 degrees 3.5 cm from its distal end (Fig. 23-37). It is constructed from a woven polyester base, which is malleable. It can be very helpful when the larynx cannot be visualized with laryngoscopy. The introducer (also known as the gum elastic bougie) can be manipulated under the epiglottis, its angled segment directed anteriorly towards the larynx. Once it has

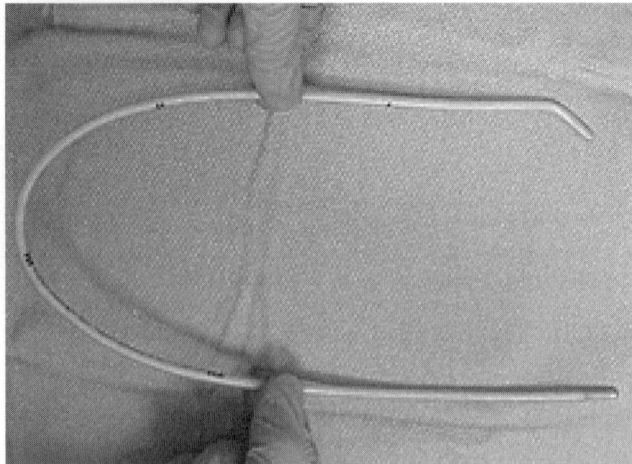

Figure 23-37. The Eschmann introducer.

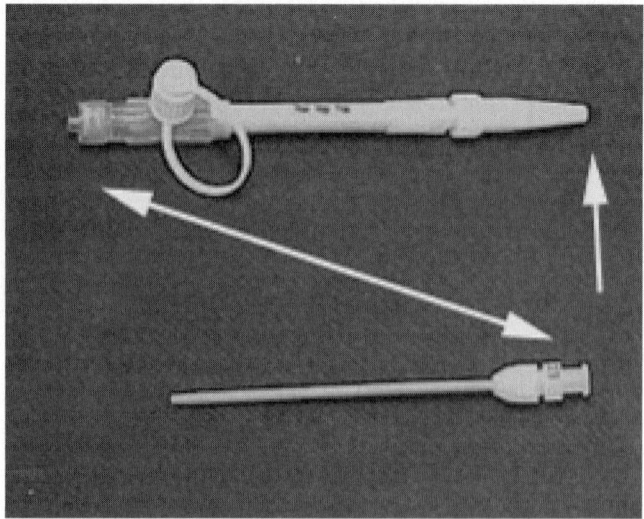

Figure 23-38. The Cook Critical Care transtracheal ventilation catheter with Luer-locking end (*two-headed arrow*) and oxygen hose friction fitting (*single-headed arrow*).

entered the larynx and trachea, a distinctive "clicking" feel is elicited as the tip passes over the cartilaginous structures.

Minimally Invasive Transtracheal Procedures

When access to the airway from the mouth or nose fails or is unavailable (*e.g.,* maxillofacial, pharyngeal, or laryngeal trauma, pathology, or deformity), emergency access via the extrathoracic trachea is a feasible route to the airway. The clinician must be familiar with these alternative techniques of oxygenation and ventilation. The decision to proceed with an invasive procedure can be difficult, and most clinicians will hesitate at potentially grave risk to the patient. One should consider becoming facile with at least one of these techniques in elective situations, such as transtracheal aspiration for airway analgesia or elective retrograde intubation. (Consider, for example, assisting a surgical colleague on a tracheostomy). Although tracheostomy and cricothyroidotomy are beyond the scope of this chapter, percutaneous techniques will be considered.

Cricothyroidotomy, cricothyrotomy, coniotomy, and minitracheostomy are synonyms for establishing an air passage through the cricothyroid membrane. The anatomy of this structure and those surrounding it was discussed earlier in this chapter. Although cricothyrotomy is the procedure of choice in an emergency situation, it may also apply to an elective situation when there is limited access to the trachea (*e.g.,* severe cervical kyphoscoliosis). Cricothyrotomy is contraindicated in neonates and children under 6 years of age, and in patients with laryngeal fractures.

Percutaneous Transtracheal Jet Ventilation (TTJV)

Percutaneous transtracheal jet ventilation (TTJV), as a form of cricothyroidotomy, is the most familiar to anesthesiologists.[216] The ASA Difficult Airway Algorithm lists transtracheal jet ventilation as an option in the cannot-mask ventilate, cannot-intubate situation.[128] TTJV is a simple and relatively safe means to sustain the patient's life in this critical situation.[217] An intravenous catheter of 12, 14, or 16 gauge, attached to a 5-ml or larger, empty or partially fluid-filled (saline or local anesthetic) syringe, should be used to enter the airway. The patient is positioned supine, with the head midline or extended on the neck and thorax (if not contraindicated by the clinical situation). After aseptic preparation, local anesthetic is injected over the cricothyroid membrane (if the patient is awake and time permits). The right-handed clinician stands on the right side of the patient, facing the head. The clinician can use his or her nondominant hand to stabilize the larynx. The catheter-needle is advanced at right angles to all planes in the caudad third of the

membrane. From the moment of skin puncture there should be constant aspiration on the syringe plunger. Free aspiration of air confirms entrance into the trachea. Unless there is significant pulmonary fluid (*e.g.,* blood, aspirated gastric contents, or water from drowning), the aspiration of tracheal air should be incontrovertible. The needle-catheter assembly should be advanced slightly, and subsequently the catheter advanced fully into the airway alone. Although this technique has been described with common angiocatheters, dedicated devices made of kink-resistant materials and with accessory ports are available (Fig. 23-38).

Once the catheter has been successfully placed in the airway, an oxygen source is attached. The clinician may have several options in this regard. If a high-pressure system is available—for example, a metered and adjustable oxygen source with a hand-controlled valve (Fig. 23-39) and a Luer-lock connector—25–30 psi of oxygen (central hospital supply or regulated tank) can be delivered directly through the catheter, with insufflations of 1–1.5 seconds at a rate of 12 insufflations per minute. If a 16-gauge catheter has been placed, this system will deliver a tidal volume of 400–700 ml. Manual closure of the mouth and nose may be needed during the insufflation (but *not* exhalation)

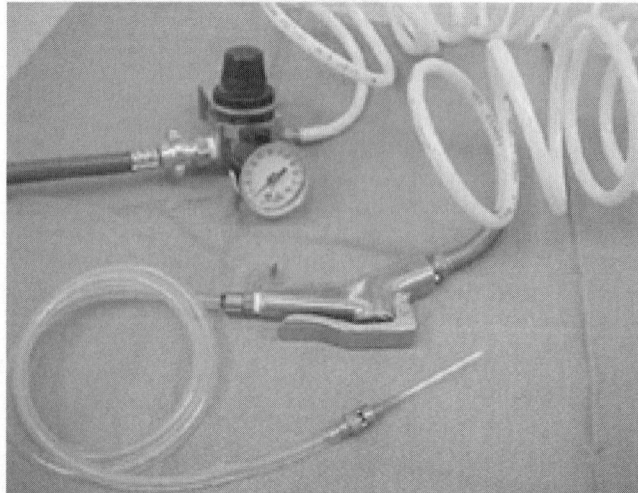

Figure 23-39. System for regulation of a high-pressure oxygen source for transtracheal jet ventilation.

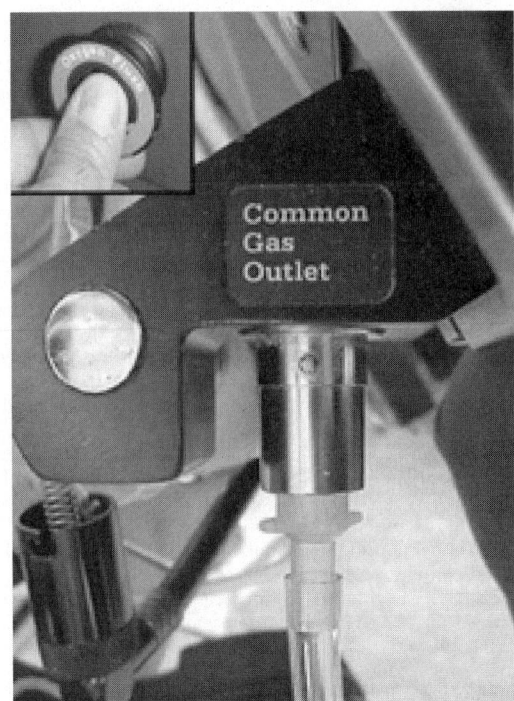

Figure 23-40. When a dedicated system is not available, the fresh gas flow outlet (15-mm diameter) of the anesthesia machine can be fitted with a tracheal tube adapter and oxygen tubing. The Oxygen Flush button is used to deliver "breaths" (*inset*).

phase if there is significant air leak through the upper airway. If such a system has not been preassembled, the fresh gas outlet of the anesthesia machine (15-mm internal-diameter female adapter) can also be used to provide high pressure (Fig. 23-40).

Low-pressure systems cannot provide enough flow to expand the chest adequately to allow for ventilation, but should be able

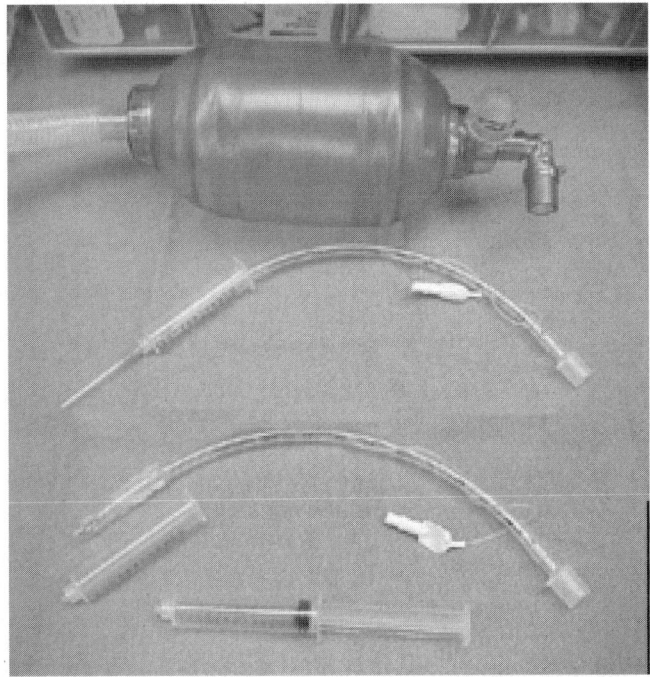

Figure 23-41. A simple system for low-pressure transtracheal oxygenation can be rapidly constructed using an angiocatheter, a syringe, and a cuffed tracheal tube.

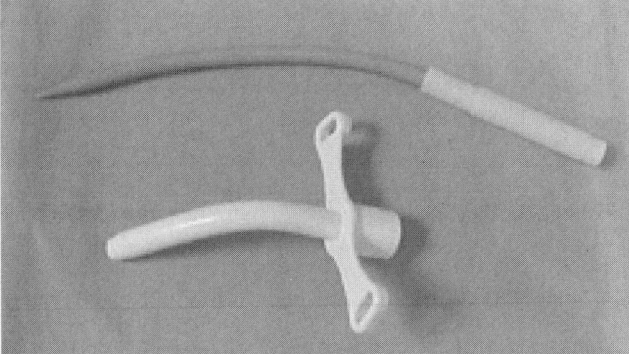

Figure 23-42. The Melker cricothyroidotomy cannula and curved dilator (Cook Critical Care, Bloomington, IN). The guidewire is not shown.

to provide oxygen while a more definitive airway is secured. A simple connection to the tracheal catheter can be achieved by placing a cuffed ETT into the barrel of a 5–10-ml syringe, inflating the cuff to provide a seal, using the distal end of the syringe to engage the catheter, while the 15-mm adapter of the ETT is fitted to an anesthesia circuit or ambu bag (Fig. 23-41).

Specialized percutaneous cricothyroidotomy systems have been developed which improve the ease of this technique while providing all necessary equipment. These devices generally provide a large-bore access which is adequate for oxygenation and ventilation with low-pressure systems. The Melker emergency cricothyroidotomy catheter set (Cook Critical Care, Bloomington, IN) uses a Seldinger—a catheter-over-a-wire technique—familiar to most anesthesia practitioners (Fig. 23-42). The set comes in a variety of cannula sizes (3.5-, 4-, and 6-mm internal diameter). Preparation and positioning of the patient are the same as with needle cricothyroidotomy. A 1–1.5-cm vertical incision of the skin only is made over the lower third of the cricothyroid membrane. Aiming 45° caudad, a percutaneous puncture of the subcutaneous tissue and cricothyroid membrane is made with the provided 18-gauge needle-catheter assembly and syringe. After air is aspirated, the catheter is advanced into the trachea. The provided guidewire is inserted through the catheter and into the trachea. The catheter is removed and the tracheal cannula, fitted internally with a curved dilator, is threaded onto the wire. The dilator is advanced through the membrane using firm pressure. Significant resistance to its advancement may indicate that the skin incision needs to be extended. Once the cannula-dilator has been fully inserted, the dilator and wire are removed. The 15-mm circuit adapter end of the cannula is now attached to an ambu bag or anesthesia circuit.

Other percutaneous systems include Nu-Trake (Weiss Emergency Airway System; International Medical Devices) and the QuickTrach® transtracheal catheter (VBM Medizintechnik GMBH). Non-needle puncture techniques are beyond the current discussion.

CONCLUSION

Apart from monitoring, the management of the routine patient airway is the most common task of the anesthesiologist—even during the administration of regional anesthesia, the airway must be monitored and possibly supported. Unfortunately, routine tasks often become neglected tasks in terms of the care and vigilance that is afforded each event. But the consequences of a lost airway are so devastating that the clinician can never afford a lackadaisical approach.

Although the ASA's Task Force on the Difficult Airway has given the medical community an immensely valuable tool in the approach to the patient with the difficult airway, the Task Force's algorithm must be viewed as a starting point only. Judgment, experience, the clinical situation, and available resources all affect the appropriateness of the chosen pathway through, or divergence from, the algorithm. The clinician need not be expert in all the equipment and techniques currently available. Rather, a broad range of approaches should be mastered, so that the failure of one does not present a road block to success.

Similarly, the medical manufacturing community, and the far-sighted clinicians who supply it with concepts for airway management products, has supplied a vast array of devices. Many represent redundancy in concept, and each has its supporters and detractors. No one device can be considered superior to another when considered in isolation. It is the clinician and his or her resources (both equipment and personnel) and judgment that determine the effectiveness of any technique.

Acknowledgments. The author would like to thank Cephas Swamidoss, M.D., for his contributions to the chapter, and Annette Forte, whose tireless effort are responsible for the chapter's completion.

REFERENCES

1. Keenan RL, Boyan CP: Cardiac arrest due to anesthesia: A study of incidence and causes. JAMA 253:2373, 1985
2. Caplan RA, Posner KL, Ward RJ et al: Adverse respiratory events in anesthesia: A closed claims analysis. Anesthesiology 72:828, 1990
3. Cheney FW, Posner KL, Caplan RA: Adverse respiratory events infrequently leading to malpractice suits. A closed claims analysis. Anesthesiology 75:932, 1991
4. Westhorpe RN: The position of the larynx in children and its relationship to the ease of intubation. Anaesth Intens Care 15:384, 1987
5. Patel SK, Whitten CW, Ivy R 3rd et al: Failure of the laryngeal mask airway: An undiagnosed laryngeal carcinoma. Anesth Analg 86:438, 1998
6. Cass NM, James NR, Lines V: Difficult direct laryngoscopy complicating intubation for anesthesia. Br Med J 1:488, 1956
7. White A, Kander: Anatomical factors in difficult direct laryngoscopy. Br J Anaesth 47:468, 1975
8. Matthew M, Hanna LS, Aldretre JA: Preoperative indices to anticipate the difficult intubation. Anesth Analg 68:S187, 1989
9. Savva D: Prediction of difficult tracheal intubation. Br J Anaesth 73:149, 1994
10. Mallampati SR, Gatt SP, Gugino LD et al: A clinical sign to predict difficult tracheal intubation: A prospective study. Can Anaesth Soc J 32:429, 1985
11. Samsoon GL, Young JR: Difficult tracheal intubation: A retrospective study. Anaesthesia 42:487, 1987
12. Oates JD, Macleod AD, Oates PD et al: Comparison of two methods for predicting difficult intubation. Br J Anaesth 66:305, 1991
13. Benumof JL: Preoxygenation: Best method for both efficacy and efficiency (editorial). Anesthesiology 91:603, 1999
14. Wilson WC: Emergency airway management on the ward. In Hannowell LA, Waldron RJ (eds): Airway Management, p 443, Lippincott-Raven Publishers, 1996
15. Gambee AM, Hertzka RE, Fisher DM: Preoxygenation techniques: Comparison of three minutes and four breaths. Anesth Analg 66:468, 1987
16. Jense HG, Dubin SA, Silverstein PI, O'Leary-Escolas U: Effect of obesity on safe duration of apnea in anesthetized humans. Anesth Analg 72:89, 1991
17. Gold MI, Duarte I, Muravchick S: Arterial oxygenation in conscious patients after 5 minutes and after 30 seconds of oxygen breathing. Anesth Analg 60:313, 1981
18. Baraka AS, Taha SK, Aouad MT et al: Preoxygenation: Comparison of maximal breathing and tidal volume breathing techniques. Anesthesiology 91:612, 1999
19. Frumin MJ, Epstein RM, Cohen G: Apneic oxygenation in man. Anesthesiology 20:789, 1959
20. Rosenblatt WH, Ovassappian A, Eige S: Use of the laryngeal mask airway in the United States: A randomized survey of ASA members. ASA Annual Meeting, Orlando, Florida, 1998
21. Keller C, Brimacombe J: Mucosal pressure, mechanism of seal, airway sealing pressure, and anatomic position for the disposable versus reusable laryngeal mask airways. Anesth Analg 88:1418, 1999
22. Keller C, Sparr HJ, Brimacombe JR: Laryngeal mask bite blocks—rolled gauze versus Guedel airway. Acta Anaesthesiol Scand 41:1171, 1997
23. Brain AIJ: The laryngeal mask and the oesophagus. Anaesthesia 46:701, 1991
24. Wilkinson PA, Cyna AM, MacLeod DM et al: The laryngeal mask: Cautionary tales. Anaesthesia 45:167, 1990
25. Nanji GM, Maltby JR: Vomiting and aspiration pneumonitis with the laryngeal mask airway. Can J Anaesth 38:69, 1992
26. Brimacombe J, Berry A: Aspiration and the laryngeal mask airway—a survey of Australian intensive care units. Anaesth Intens Care 20:534, 1992
27. Griffin RM, Hatcher IS: Aspiration pneumonia and the laryngeal mask airway. Anaesthesia 45:1039, 1990
28. Koehli N: Aspiration and laryngeal mask airway. Anaesthesia 46:419, 1991
29. Alexander R, Arrowsmith JE, Frossard JR: The layrngeal mask airway: Safe in the x ray department. Anaesthesia 48:734, 1993
30. Maroof M, Khan RM, Siddique MS: Intraoperative aspiration pneumonitis and the laryngeal mask airway. Anesth Analg 77:405, 1993
31. Langer A, Hempel V, Ahlhelm T et al: Die Kehlkopfmaske bei 1900 allgeneinanasthesien-Erfahrungsbericht. Anaesthesiol Intensivmed Notfalmed Schmerzther, 28:156, 1993
32. Lussman RF, Gerber HR: Severe aspiration pneumonia with the laryngeal mask. Anaesthesiol Intensivmed Notfalmed Schmerzther 32:194, 1997
33. Ismail-Zade IA, Vanner RG: Regurgitation and aspiration of gastric contents in a child during general anaesthesia using the laryngeal mask airway. Paediatr Anaesth 6:325, 1996
34. Lopez-Gil M, Brimacombe J, Alvarez M: Safety and efficacy of the laryngeal mask airway. A prospective survey of 1400 children. Anaesthesia 51:969, 1996
35. Brimacombe JR, Berry A: The incidence of aspiration associated with the laryngeal mask airway: A meta-analysis of published literature. J Clin Anesth 7:297, 1995
36. Kallar SK, Everett LL: Potential risks and preventive measures for pulmonary aspiration: New concepts in preoperative fasting guidelines. Anesth Analg 77:171, 1993
37. Warner MA, Warner ME, Weber JG: Clinical significance of pulmonary aspiration during the perioperative period. Anesthesiology 78:62, 1993
38. Owens TM, Robertson P, Twomey C et al: The incidence of gastroesophageal reflux with the laryngeal mask: A comparison with the face mask using esophageal lumen pH electrodes. Anesth Analg 80:980, 1995
39. McCrory CR, McShane AJ: Gastroesophageal reflux during spontaneous respiration with the laryngeal mask airway. Can J Anaesth 46:268, 1999
40. Joshi GP, Morrison SG, Okonkwo NA, White PF: Continuous hypopharyngeal pH measurements in spontaneously breathing anesthetized outpatients: Laryngeal mask airway versus tracheal intubation. Anesth Analg 82:254, 1996
41. el Mikatti N, Luthra AD, Healy TE, Mortimer AJ: Gastric regurgitation during general anaesthesia in different positions with the laryngeal mask airway. Anaesthesia 50:1053, 1995
42. Hong S-Y, Byung-Te S: Laryngeal Mask Airway for Cesarean Section. World Congress of Anaesthesiologists D770, 1996
43. Liew E, Chan-Liao M: Experience of Using Laryngeal Mask Anesthesia for Cesarean Section. World Congress of Anaesthesiologists D771.14, 1996
44. Dysart R: The Laryngeal Mask Airway in Pregnancy and Postpartum (Abstract). New Zealand Society of Anaesthetists & Australia College of Anaesthetists, 1993
45. Pennant JH, Walker MB: Comparison of the endotracheal tube and laryngeal mask in airway management by paramedical personnel. Anesth Analg 74:531, 1992
46. Hayes A, McCarrol SM: Airway management in unskilled personnel—a comparison of laryngeal mask airway, pocket mask and bag valve mask techniques. Anesthesiology 83:A223, 1995
47. Grantham H, Phillips G: The laryngeal mask in prehospital emergency care. Emerg Med 7:57, 1995
48. Tanigawa K, Shigematsu A: Choice of airway devices for 12,020 cases of nontraumatic cardiac arrest in Japan. Prehosp Emerg Care 2:96, 1998
49. Atherton GL, Johnson JC: Ability of paramedics to use the Combitube in prehospital cardiac arrest. Ann Emerg Med 22:1263, 1993

50. Haden RM, Pinnock CA, Scott PV: Incidence of aspiration with the laryngeal mask airway. Br J Anaesth 72:496, 1994

51. Yardy N, Hancox D, Strang TSO: A comparison of two airway aids for emergency use by unskilled personnel: The Combitube and laryngeal mask. Anaesthesia 54:181, 1999

52. Stone BJ, Chantler PJ: The incidence of regurgitation during cardiopulmonary resuscitation: A comparison between the bag valve mask and laryngeal mask airway. Resuscitation 38:3, 1998

53. Verghese C, Brimacombe J: Survey of laryngeal mask airway usage in 11,910 patients: Safety and efficacy for conventional and non-conventional usage. Anesth Analg 82:129, 1996

54. Graziotti PJ: Intermittent positive pressure ventilation through a laryngeal mask airway. Is a nasogastric tube useful? Anaesthesia 47:1088, 1992

55. Ho BY, Skinner HJ, Mahajan RP: Gastro-oesophageal reflux during day case gynaecological laparoscopy under positive pressure ventilation: Laryngeal mask vs. tracheal intubation. Anaesthesia 54:93, 1999

56. Voyagis GS, Papakalou EP: A comparison of the laryngeal mask and tracheal tube for controlled ventilation. Acta Anaesthesiol Belg 47:81, 1996

57. Ruiz J, Lansiaux S, Beauvoir-Bonnard C et al: Mechanical ventilation using a laryngeal mask airway in children. Anesthesiology 89(3A):A1274, 1998

58. Brimacombe JR: Positive pressure ventilation with the size 5 laryngeal mask. J Clin Anesth 9:113, 1997

59. André E, Capdevila X, Vialles N et al: Pressure-controlled ventilation with a laryngeal mask airway during general anaesthesia. Br J Anaesth 80(suppl 1):244, 1998

60. Gursoy F, Algren JT, Skjonsby BS: Positive pressure ventilation with the laryngeal mask airway in children. Anesth Analg 82:33, 1996

61. Latorre F, Eberle B, Weiler N et al: Laryngeal mask airway position and the risk of gastric insufflation. Anesth Analg 86:867, 1998

62. Brimacombe JR, Brain AI, Berry AM et al: Gastric insufflation and the laryngeal mask. Anesth Analg 86:914, 1998

63. Brimacombe JR, Brain AIJ: The Laryngeal Mask Airway. A Review and Practical Guide. London, WB Saunders, 1997

64. Brimacombe J, Shorney N: The laryngeal mask airway and prolonged balanced regional anaesthesia. Can J Anaesth 40:360, 1993

65. Brimacombe J, Keller C: Comparison of the flexible and standard laryngeal mask airways. Can J Anaesth 46:558, 1999

66. Williams PJ, Bailey PM: Comparison of the reinforced laryngeal mask airway and tracheal intubation for adenotonsillectomy. Br J Anaesth 70:30, 1993

67. Brimacombe JR, Keller C, Gunkel AR et al: The influence of the tonsillar gag on efficacy of seal, anatomic position, airway patency, and airway protection with the flexible laryngeal mask airway: A randomized, cross-over study of fresh adult cadavers. Anesth Analg 89:181, 1999

68. John RE, Hill S, Hughes TJ: Airway protection by the laryngeal mask: A barrier to dye placed in the pharynx. Anaesthesia 46:366, 1991

69. Cork RC, Depa RM, Standen JR: Prospective comparison of use of the laryngeal mask and endotracheal tube for ambulatory surgery. Anesth Analg 79:719, 1994

70. Webster AC, Morley-Forster PK, Watson J et al: Evaluation of the flexible reinforced laryngeal mask airway (FRLMA) for intranasal surgery (abstract). Anesthesiology 87:A30, 1997

71. Young PJ, Basson C, Hamilton D et al: Prevention of tracheal aspiration using the pressure-limited tracheal tube cuff. Anaesthesia 54:559, 1999

72. Kim ES, Bishop MJ: Endotracheal intubation, but not laryngeal mask airway insertion, produces reversible bronchoconstriction. Anesthesiology 90:391, 1999

73. Berry A, Brimacombe J, Keller C et al: Pulmonary airway resistance with the endotracheal tube versus laryngeal mask airway in paralyzed anesthetized adult patients. Anesthesiology 90:395, 1999

74. Groudine SB, Lumb PD, Sandison MR: Pressure support ventilation with the laryngeal mask airway: A method to manage severe reactive airway disease post-operatively. Can J Anaesth 42:341, 1995

75. Ferrari LR, Goudsouzian NG: The use of the laryngeal mask airway in children with bronchopulmonary dysplasia. Anesth Analg 81:310, 1995

76. Benumof JL: Laryngeal mask airway and the ASA difficult airway algorithm. Anesthesiology 84:686, 1996

77. Asai T, Morris S: The laryngeal mask airway: Its features, effects and role. Can J Anaesth 41:930, 1994

78. Erskine RJ, Rabey PG: The laryngeal mask airway in recovery. Anaesthesia 47:354, 1992

79. Kitching AJ, Walpole AR, Blogg CE: Removal of the laryngeal mask airway in children: Anaesthetized compared with awake (abstract). Br J Anaesth 76:874, 1996

80. Beckford NS, Mayo R, Wilkinson A 3d et al: Effects of short-term endotracheal intubation on vocal function. Laryngoscope 100:331, 1990

81. Lowinger D, Benjamin B, Gadd L: Recurrent laryngeal nerve injury caused by a laryngeal mask airway. Anaesth Intens Care 27:202, 1999

82. Lumb AB, Wrigley MW: The effect of nitrous oxide on laryngeal mask cuff pressure: In vitro and in vivo studies. Anaesthesia 47:320, 1992

83. Lowinger D, Benjamin B, Gadd L: Recurrent laryngeal nerve injury caused by a laryngeal mask airway. Anaesth Intens Care 27:202, 1999

84. Brain AI: Pressure in laryngeal mask airway. Anaesthesia 51:603, 1996

85. Branthwaite MA: An unexpected complication of the intubating laryngeal mask. Anaesthesia 54:166, 1999

86. Bellhouse CP, Dore C: Criteria for estimating likelihood of difficulty of endotracheal intubation with the Macintosh laryngoscope. Anaesth Intens Care 16:329, 1988

87. Brain AI: The oesophageal vent-laryngeal. Br J Anaesth 72:727, 1994

88. Agro F, Agro F, Brimacombe J et al: Awake use of a new laryngeal mask prototype in a non-fasted patient requiring urgent peripheral vascular surgery. Resuscitation 40:187, 1999

89. Molloy AR: Unexpected position of the laryngeal mask airway. Anaesthesia 46:592, 1991

90. Goudsouzian NG, Denman W, Cleveland R et al: Radiologic localization of the laryngeal mask airway in children. Anesthesiology 77:1085, 1992

91. Greenberg RS, Kay NH: Cuffed oropharyngeal airway (COPA) as an adjunct to fibreoptic tracheal intubation. Br J Anaesth 82:395, 1999

92. Greenberg RS, Brimacombe J, Berry A et al: A randomized controlled trial comparing the cuffed oropharyngeal airway and the laryngeal mask airway in spontaneously breathing anesthetized adults. Anesthesiology 88:970, 1998

93. Horton WA, Fahy L, Charters P: Defining a standard intubating position using "angle finder." Br J Anaesth 62:6, 1989

94. Benumof JL: The American Society of Anesthesiologists' management of the difficult airway algorithm and explanation-analysis of the algorithm. In Benumof, JL (ed): Airway Management: Principles and Practice. St Louis, Mosby, 1996

95. Sivarajan M, Joy JV: Effects of general anesthesia and paralysis on upper airway changes due to head position in humans. Anesthesiology 85:787, 1996

96. Salem MR, Mathrubhutham M, Bennett EJ: Difficult intubation. N Engl J Med 295:879, 1976

97. Ulrich B, Listyo R, Gerig HJ et al: The difficult intubation: The value of BURP and 3 predictive tests of difficult intubation. Anaesthesist 47:45, 1998

98. Takahata O, Kubota M, Mamiya K et al: The efficacy of the "BURP" maneuver during a difficult laryngoscopy. Anesth Analg 84:419, 1997

99. Benumof JL, Cooper SD: Quantitative improvement in laryngoscopic view by optimal external laryngeal manipulation. J Clin Anesth 8:136, 1996

100. Cormack RS, Lehane J: Difficult tracheal intubation in obstetrics. Anaesthesia 39:1105, 1984

101. Wheeler M: The difficult pediatric airway. In Hagberg C (ed): Handbook of Difficult Airway Management, Philadelphia, Churchill Livingston, 2000

102. Benumof JBL: Conventional (laryngoscopic) orotracheal and nasotracheal intubation (single-lumen tube). In Benumof JBL (ed): Airway Management: Principles and Practice, p 261. St Louis, Mosby, 1996

103. Salem MR, Wafai Y, Joseph NJ et al: Efficacy of the self-inflating bulb in detecting esophageal intubation. Does the presence of a nasogastric tube or cuff deflation make a difference? Anesthesiology 80:42, 1994

104. Cardoso MM, Banner MJ, Melker RJ et al: Portable devices used to detect endotracheal intubation during emergency situations: A review. Crit Care Med 26:957, 1998

105. Bresnick WH, Rask-Madsen C, Hogan DL et al: The effect of acute emotional stress on gastric acid secretion in normal subjects and duodenal ulcer patients. J Clin Gastroenterol 17:117, 1993

106. Haskins DA, Jahr JS, Texidor M et al: Single-dose oral omeprazole for reduction of gastric residual acidity in adults for outpatient surgery. Acta Anaesthesiol Scand 36:513, 1992

107. Dimich I, Katende R, Singh PP et al: The effects of intravenous cimetidine and metoclopramide on gastric pH and volume in outpatients. J Clin Anesth 3:40, 1991

108. Rabb MF, Minkowitz HS, Hagberg CA: Blind intubation through the laryngeal mask airway for management of the difficult airway in infants. Anesthesiology 84:1510, 1996

109. Heard CMB, Caldicott LD, Fletcher JE et al: Fiberoptic-guided endotracheal intubation via the laryngeal mask airway in pediatric patients: A report of a series of cases. Anesth Analg 82:1287, 1996

110. Brimacombe J, Agro F, Carassiti M et al: Use of a lighted stylet for intubation via the laryngeal mask airway (abstract). Can J Anaesth 45:556, 1998

111. Atherton DP, O'Sullivan E, Lowe D et al: A ventilation-exchange bougie for fibreoptic intubations with the laryngeal mask airway. Anaesthesia 51:1123, 1996

112. Gajraj NM: Tracheal intubation through the laryngeal mask using a gum elastic bougie. Anaesthesia 51:796, 1996

113. Gabbott DA, Sasada MP: Tracheal intubation through the laryngeal mask using a gum elastic bougie in the presence of cricoid pressure and manual in-line stabilisation of the neck. Anaesthesia 51:389, 1996

114. Elwood T, Cox RG: Laryngeal mask insertion with a laryngoscope in paediatric patients. Can J Anaesth 43:435, 1996

115. Bahk JH, Kim CS: A method for removing the laryngeal mask airway after using it as an intubation guide. Anesthesiology 86:1218, 1997

116. Brain AIJ, Verghese C, Addy EV et al: The intubating laryngeal mask. I: Development of a new device for intubation of the trachea. Br J Anaesth 79:699, 1997

117. Kapila A, Addy EV, Verghese C et al: The intubating laryngeal mask airway: An initial assessment of performance. Br J Anaesth 79:710, 1997

118. Brain AIJ, Verghese C, Addy EV et al: The intubating laryngeal mask. II: A preliminary clinical report of a new means of intubating the trachea. Br J Anaesth 79:704, 1997

119. Rosenblatt WH, Murphy M: The intubating laryngeal mask: Use of a new ventilating intubating device in the emergency department. Ann Emerg Med 33:234, 1999

120. Baskett PJ, Parr MJ, Nolan JP: The intubating laryngeal mask: Results of a multicentre trial with experience of 500 cases. Anaesthesia 53:1174, 1998

121. Monrigal JP, Tesson B, Granry JC: Evaluation of the efficiency of the LMA Fastrach in case of difficult intubation. Anesthesiology 9:A1359, 1999

122. Cooper RM: Extubation and changing the endotracheal tube. In Benumof JL (ed): Airway Management: Principles and Practice, p 864. St Louis, Mosby, 1996

123. Asai T: Use of the laryngeal mask during emergence from anaesthesia. Eur J Anaesthesiol 15:379, 1998

124. Asai T, Shingu K: Use of the laryngeal mask during emergence from anesthesia in a patient with an unstable neck. Anesth Analg 88:469, 1999

125. Nair I, Bailey PM: Use of the laryngeal mask for airway maintenance following trachea extubation [letter]. Anaesthesia 50:174, 1995

126. Engoren M: Evaluation of the cuff-leak test in a cardiac surgery population. Chest 116:1029, 1999

127. Loudermilk EP, Hartmannsgruber M, Stoltzfus DP et al: A prospective study of the safety of tracheal extubation using a pediatric airway exchange catheter for patients with a known difficult airway. Chest 111:1660, 1997

128. Practice guidelines for management of the difficult airway: A report by the American Society of Anesthesiologists Task Force on Management of the Difficult Airway. Anesthesiology 78:597, 1993

129. Rocke DA, Murry WB, Rout CC et al: Relative risk analysis factors associated with with difficult intubation in obstetric anesthesia. Anesthesiology 77:597, 1993

130. Lyons G: Failed intubation. Anaesthesia 40:759, 1985

131. Benumof JL: ASA difficult airway algorithm: New thoughts and considerations. In Hagberg C (ed): Handbook of Difficult Airway Management, p 31. New York, Churchill Livingstone, 2000

132. Nandi PR, Charlesworth CH, Taylor SJ et al: Effect of general anaesthesia on the pharynx. Br J Anaesth 66:157, 1991

133. Hudgel DW, Hendricks C: Palate and hypopharynx—sites of inspiratory narrowing of the upper airway during sleep. Am Rev Resp Dis 138:1542, 1988

134. Iscoe SD: Central control of the upper airway. In Mathew OP, Sant' Ambrogio G (eds): Respiratory function of the upper airway. New York, Marcel Dekker, 1988

135. Benumof JL: Management of the difficult adult airway: With special emphasis on awake tracheal intubation Anesthesiology 75:1087, 1991

136. McLeskey CH, Cullen BF, Kennedy RD et al: Control of cerebral perfusion pressure during induction of anesthesia in high-risk neurosurgical patients. Anesth Analg 53:985, 1974

137. Fleming JA, Byck R, Barash P: Pharmacology and therapeutic application of cocaine. Anesthesiology 73:518, 1990

138. Weisel W, Tella RA: Reaction to tetracaine used as topical anesthetic in bronchoscopy: A study of 1000 cases. JAMA 147:218, 1951

139. Sitzman BT, Rich GF, Rockwell JJ et al: Local anesthetic administration for awake direct laryngoscopy. Are glossopharyngeal nerve blocks superior? Anesthesiology 86:34, 1997

140. Sanchez A, Trivedi NS, Morrison DE: Preparation of the patient for awake intubation. In Benumof JL (ed): Airway Management: Principles and Practice, p 159. St Louis, Mosby, 1996

141. Ovassapian A: Fiberoptic Endoscopy and the Difficult Airway, 2nd ed. Philadelphia, Lippincott-Raven, 1996

142. Rosenblatt WH, Wagner PJ, Ovassapian A et al: Practice patterns in managing the difficult airway by anesthesiologists in the United States. Anesth Analg 87:153, 1998

143. Murphy P: A fibre-optic endoscope used for nasal intubation. Anaesthesia 22:489, 1967

144. Ovassapian A, Yelich SJ, Dykes MH et al: Learning fibreoptic intubation: Use of simulators v. traditional teaching. Br J Anaesth 61:217, 1988

145. Benumof JL: Management of the difficult airway. Anesthesiology 75:1087, 1991

146. Hershey MD, Hannenberg AA: Gastric distention and rupture from oxygen insufflation during fiberoptic intubation. Anesthesiology 85:1479, 1996

147. Rosenblatt WH: Overcoming obstruction during bronchoscope-guided intubation of the trachea with the double setup endotracheal tube. Anesth Analg 83:175, 1996

148. Brull SJ, Wiklund R, Ferris C et al: Facilitation of fiberoptic orotracheal intubation with a flexible tracheal tube. Anesth Analg 78:746, 1994

149. Gorback MS: Management of the challenging airway with the Bullard laryngoscope. J Clin Anesth 3:473, 1991

150. Hastings RH, Vigil AC, Hanna R et al: Cervical spine movement during laryngoscopy with the Bullard, Macintosh, and Miller laryngoscopes. Anesthesiology 82:859, 1995

151. Cohn AI, McGraw SR, King WH: Awake intubation of the adult trachea using the Bullard laryngoscope. Can J Anaesth 42:246, 1995

152. Cohn AI, Hart RT, McGraw SR et al: The Bullard laryngoscope for emergency airway management in a morbidly obese parturient. Anesth Analg 81:872, 1995

153. Butler FS, Cirillo AA: Retrograde tracheal intubation. Anesth Analg 39:333, 1960

154. Waters DJ: Guided blind endotracheal intubation. Anaesthesia 18:158, 1963

155. Sanchez A, Pallares V: Retrograde intubation technique. In Benumof JL (ed): Airway Management: Principles and Practice. St Louis, Mosby, 1996

156. Barriot P, Riou B: Retrograde technique for tracheal intubation in trauma patients. Crit Care Med 16:712, 1988

157. Reynaud J, Lacour M, Diop L et al: Intubation tracheale guidee a bouche fermee (technic de D.J. Waters). Bull Soc Med Afr Noire Lang Fr 12774, 1967

158. Sanchez A, Pallares V: Retrograde intubation technique. In Benumof JL (ed): Airway Management: Principles and Practice. St Louis, Mosby, 1996

159. Walls RM: Management of the difficult airway in the trauma patient. Emerg Med Clin North Am 16:45, 1998

160. Don Michael TL, Lambert EH, Mehran A: Mouth to lung airway for cardiac resuscitation. Lancet 2:1329, 1968

161. Frass M, Frenzer R, Zahler J: Respiratory tube or airway, U.S. patent no. 4, 688,568

162. Green-KS, Beger-TH SO: Proper use of the Combitube (letter). Anesthesiology 81:513, 1994

163. Klauser R, Roggla G, Pidlich J et al: Massive upper airway bleeding after thrombolytic therapy: Successful airway management with the Combitube. Ann Emerg Med 21:431, 1992

164. Kulozik U, Georgi R, Krier C: Intubation with the Combitube-TM in massive hemorrhage from the locus Kieselbachii. Anasthesiol Intensivmed Notfallmed Schmerzther 31:191, 1996

165. Hofbauer R, Roggla M, Staudinger T et al: Emergency intubation with the Combitube in a patient with persistent vomiting. Anasthesiol Intensivmed Notfallmed Schmerzther 29:306, 1994

166. Deroy R, Ghoris M: The Combitube elective anesthetic airway management in a patient with cervical spine fracture. Anesth Analg 87:1441, 1998

167. Mercer MH, Gabbott DA: Insertion of the Combitube airway with the cervical spine immobilized in a rigid cervical collar. Anaesthesia 53:971, 1998

168. Banyai M, Falger S, Roggla M et al: Emergency intubation with the Combitube in a grossly obese patient with bull neck. Resuscitation 26:271, 1993

169. Liao D, Shalit M: Successful intubation with the Combitube in acute asthmatic respiratory distress by a paramedic. J Emerg Med 14:561, 1996

170. Blostein PA, Koestner AJ, Hoak S: Failed rapid sequence intubation in trauma patients: Esophageal tracheal Combitube is a useful adjunct. J Trauma 44:534, 1998

171. Crosby ET, Cooper RM, Douglas et al: The unanticipated difficult airway with recommendations for management. Can J Anaesth 45:757, 1998

172. Sofferman RA, Johnson DL, Spencer RF: Lost airway during anesthesia induction: Alternatives for management. Laryngoscope 107:1476, 1997

173. Brugger S, Staudinger T, Frottier P et al: Successful intubation with the Combitube of two patients with bull neck. Acta Med Aust 20:78, 1993

174. Frass M, Frenzer R, Mayer G et al: Mechanical ventilation with the esophageal tracheal combitube (ETC) in the intensive care unit. Arch Emerg Med 4:219, 1987

175. Rumball CJ, MacDonald D: The PTL, Combitube, laryngeal mask, and oral airway: A randomized prehospital comparative study of ventilatory device effectiveness and cost-effectiveness in 470 cases of cardiorespiratory arrest. Prehosp Emerg Care 1:1, 1997

176. Tanigawa K, Shigematsu A: Choice of airway devices for 12,020 cases of nontraumatic cardiac arrest in Japan. Prehosp Emerg Care 2:96, 1998.

177. Atherton GL, Johnson JC: Ability of paramedics to use the Combitube in prehospital cardiac arrest. Ann Emerg Med 22:1263, 1993

178. Gaitini LA, Vaida SJ, Somri M et al: Fiberoptic-guided airway exchange of the esophageal-tracheal Combitube in spontaneously breathing versus mechanically ventilated patients. Anesth Analg 88:193, 1999

179. Richards CF: The pyriform sinus perforation during Esophageal Tracheal Combitube. J Emerg Med 16:37, 1998

180. Vezina D, Lessard MR, Bussieres J et al: Complications associated with the use of the Esophageal Tracheal Combitube. Can J Anaesth 45:76, 1998

181. Klein H, Williamson M, Sue Ling HM et al: Esophageal rupture associated with the use of the Combitube. Anesth Analg 85:937, 1997

182. Martin SE, Ochsner MG, Jarman RH et al: Laryngeal mask airway in air transport when intubation fails: Case report. J Trauma Injury Infect Crit Care 42:333, 1997

183. Brimacombe JR, De Maio B: Emergency use of the laryngeal mask airway during helicopter transfer of a neonate. J Clin Anesth 7:689, 1995

184. Parmet JL, Colonna-Romano P, Horrow JC et al: The laryngeal mask airway reliably provides rescue ventilation in cases of unanticipated difficult tracheal intubation along with difficult mask ventilation. Anesth Analg 87:661, 1998

185. Bahk JH, Kim JK, Kim CS: Use of the laryngeal mask airway to preoxygenate in a paediatric patient with Treacher-Collins syndrome. Paediatr Anaesth 8:274, 1998

186. Daum REO, O'Reilly BJ: The laryngeal mask airway in ENT surgery. J Laryngol Otol 106:28, 1992

187. Bing J: Masque laryngé pour réduction de fracture du nez. Ann Fr Anesth Réanim 10:494, 1991

188. Williams PJ, Thompsett C, Bailey PM: Comparison of the reinforced laryngeal mask airway and tracheal intubation for nasal surgery. Anaesthesia 50:987, 1995

189. Rheineck Leyssius AT, Vos RJ, Blommesteijn R et al: Use of the laryngeal mask airway versus orotracheal intubation to secure a patent airway in rhinoplastic surgery. ASA Abstr A293, 1994

190. Dain SL, Webster AC, Morley-Forster P et al: Propofol for insertion of the laryngeal mask airway for short ENT procedures in children. Abstract presented at IARS Meeting, March 1995

191. Johnston DF, Wrigley SR, Robb PJ et al: The laryngeal mask airway in paediatric anaesthesia. Anaesthesia 45:924, 1990

192. Watcha MF, Garner FT, White PF et al: Laryngeal mask airway vs face mask and Guedel airway during pediatric myringotomy. Arch Otolaryngol Head Neck Surg 120:877, 1994

193. Terada H et al: Airway obstruction due to pus from sinusitis during the use of the LM. J Japan Soc Clin Anesth 17:673, 1993

194. Quinn AC, Samaan A, McAteer EM et al: The reinforced laryngeal mask airway for dento-alveolar surgery. Br J Anaesth 77:185, 1996

195. Young T M: The laryngeal mask in dental anaesthesia. Eur J Anaesthesiol 4:53, 1991

196. George JM, Sanders GM: The reinforced laryngeal mask in paediatric outpatient dental surgery. World Congress of Anaesthesiologists, D884, 1996

197. Goodwin A, Ogg T, Lamb W, Adlam D: The reinforced laryngeal mask in dental day surgery. Ambulat Surg 1:31, 1993

198. Morrison AG, O'Donnell NG: Laryngeal mask insertion, cricoid pressure and manual in-line stabilisation. Anaesthesia 51:285, 1996

199. Asai T, Neil J, Stacey M: Ease of placement of the laryngeal mask during manual in-line neck stabilization. Br J Anaesth 80:617, 1998

200. Asai T, Latto P: Role of the laryngeal mask in patients with difficult tracheal intubation and difficult ventilation. In Latto IP, Vaughan RS (eds): Difficulties in Tracheal Intubation, p 177. London, WB Saunders, 1997

201. Brimacombe JR, Berry AM: Mallampati grade and laryngeal mask placement. Anesth Analg 82:1112, 1996

202. Baskett PJF: The use of the laryngeal mask airway by nurses during cardiopulmonary resuscitation: Results of a multicentre trial. Anaesthesia 49:3, 1994

203. Verghese C, Prior Willeard PFS: Immediate management of the airway during cardiopulmonary resuscitation in a hospital without a resident anaesthesiologist. Eur J Emerg Med 1:123, 1994

204. Samarkandi AH, Seraj MA: The role of the laryngeal mask airway in cardiopulmonary resuscitation. Resuscitation 2:103, 1994

205. Brimacombe J: Does the laryngeal mask airway have a role outside the operating theatre? Can Anaesth J 42:258, 1995

206. Oxer HF: The laryngeal mask airway in prehospital emergency care. Emerg Med 7:56, 1995

207. Leach A, Alexander CA: The laryngeal mask in cardiopulmonary resuscitation in a district general hospital: A preliminary communication. Resuscitation 25:245, 1993

208. Aoyama K, Takenaka I: Cricoid pressure impedes positioning and ventilation through the laryngeal mask. Can J Anaesth 43:1035, 1996

209. Strang TI: Does the laryngeal mask airway compromise cricoid pressure? Anaesthesia 47:829, 1992

210. Asai T, Barcklay K: Cricoid pressure impedes placement of the laryngeal mask airway and subsequent tracheal intubation through the mask. Br J Anaesth 72:47, 1994

211. Baumgarten RK, Carter CE, Reynolds WJ et al: Priming with nondepolarizing relaxants for rapid tracheal intubation: A double-blind evaluation. Can J Anaesth 35:5, 1988

212. Cicala R, Westbrook L: An alternative method of paralysis for rapid-sequence induction. Anesthesiology 69:983, 1988

213. Gnauck K, Lungo JB, Scalzo A et al: Emergency intubation of the pediatric medical patient: Use of anesthetic agents in the emergency department. Ann Emerg Med 23:1242, 1994

214. Li J, Murphy-Lavoie H, Bugas C et al: Complications of emergency intubation with and without paralysis. Am J Emerg Med 17:141, 1999

215. Sosis M: Modified rapid sequence induction I. Anesthesiology 70:1031, 1989

216. Benumof JL, Gaughan SD: Concerns regarding barotrauma during jet ventilation (letter). Anesthesiology 76:1072, 1992

217. Benumof JL: Transtracheal jet ventilation via percutaneous catheter and high-pressure source, In Benumof JL (ed): Airway Management: Principles and Practice. St Louis, Mosby—Year Book, 1996

APPENDIX A: Citations from Table 23-4

Because the LMA has had a significant impact on the practice of routine and difficult airway management, a list of pertinent references is included.

A1. Ebata T, Nishiki S, Masuda A *et al:* Clinical reports: Anaesthesia for Treacher Collins syndrome using a laryngeal mask airway. Can J Anaesth 38:1043, 1992

A2. Daum REO, O'Reilly BJ: The laryngeal mask airway in ENT surgery. J Laryngol Otol 106:28, 1992

A3. Bing J: Masque laryngé pour réduction de fracture du nez. Ann Fr Anesth Réanim 10:494, 1991

A4. Williams PJ, Thompsett C, Bailey PM: Comparison of the reinforced laryngeal mask airway and tracheal intubation for nasal surgery. Anaesthesia 50:987, 1995

A5. Rheineck Leyssius AT, Vos RJ, Blommesteijn R *et al:* Use of the laryngeal mask airway versus orotracheal intubation to secure a patent airway in rhinoplastic surgery. 1994 ASA Abstr A293, 1994

A6. Dain SL, Webster AC, Morley-Forster P *et al:* Propofol for insertion of the laryngeal mask airway for short ENT procedures in children. Abstract presented at IARS Meeting, March 1995

A7. Johnston DF, Wrigley SR, Robb PJ *et al:* The laryngeal mask airway in paediatric anaesthesia. Anaesthesia 45:924, 1990

A8. Watcha MF, Garner FT, White PF *et al:* Laryngeal mask airway vs. face mask and Guedel airway during pediatric myringotomy. Arch Otolaryngol Head Neck Surg 120:877, 1994

A9. Terada H *et al:* Airway obstruction due to pus from sinusitis during the use of the LM. J Japan Soc Clin Anesth 17:673, 1993

A10. Quinn AC, Samaan A, McAteer EM *et al:* The reinforced laryngeal mask airway for dento-alveolar surgery. Br J Anaesth 77:185, 1996

A11. Young TM: The laryngeal mask in dental anaesthesia. Eur J Anaesthesiol 4:53, 1991

A12. George JM, Sanders GM: The reinforced laryngeal mask in paediatric outpatient dental surgery. World Congress of Anaesthesiologists, D884, 1996

A13. Goodwin A, Ogg T, Lamb W, Adlam D: The reinforced laryngeal mask in dental day surgery. Ambulatory Surg 1:31, 1993

A14. Noble H, Wooler DJ: Laryngeal masks and chair dental anaesthesia. Anaesthesia 46(7):591, 1991

A15. Bailie R, Barnett MB, Fraser JF: The Brain laryngeal mask: A comparative study with the nasal mask in paediatric dental outpatient anaesthesia. Anaesthesia 46(5):358, 1991

A16. Wat LI, Handysides EA: The reinforced laryngeal mask is a safe, effective airway for pediatric dental anesthesia. Anesthesiology 89:A44, 1998

A17. Porcelijn T, Veerkamp JSJ: Ambulatory anaesthesia with propofol and a laryngeal mask airway for dental treatment of toddlers. International Congress of the Israel Society of Anesthesiologist, May 1996

A18. Christie IW: A means of stabilising laryngeal mask airways during dental procedures. Anaesthesia 51:604, 1996

A19. Brimacombe J, Sher M, Laing D, Berry A: The laryngeal mask airway (LMA) for vocal cord biopsy. World Congress of Anaesthesiologists, P1269, 1996

A20. Brain AI, McGhee TD, McAteer EJ *et al:* The laryngeal mask airway: Development and preliminary trials of a new type of airway. Anaesthesia 40:356, 1985

A21. Mason DG, Bingham RM; The laryngeal mask airway in children. Anaesthesia 45(9):760, 1990

A22. Zagnoev M, McCloskey J, Martin T: Fiberoptic intubation via the laryngeal mask airway. Anesth Analg 78:813, 1994

A23. Allen JG, Flower EA: The Brain laryngeal mask: An alternative to difficult intubation. Br Dent J 168:202, 1990

A24. Judkins KC: When the chips are down: The laryngeal mask in anger (letter). Anaesthesia 48:353, 1993

A25. Stott SA: Use of the laryngeal mask in the developing world. Anaesthesia 48(5):450, 1993

A26. Kadota Y, Oda T, Yoshimura N: Application of a laryngeal mask to a fiberoptic bronchoscope-aided tracheal intubation. J Clin Anesth 4:503, 1992

A27. Mecklem D, Brimacombe JR, Yarker J: Glossopexy in Pierre Robin sequence using the laryngeal mask airway. J Clin Anesth 7:267, 1995

A28. Brimacombe J, Berry A: Use of a size 2 LMA to relieve life-threatening hypoxia in an adult with quinsy. Anaesth Intens Care 21:475, 1993

A29. Sher M, Brimacombe J, Laing D: Anaesthesia for laser pharyngoplasty: A comparison of the tracheal tube with the reinforced laryngeal mask airway. Anaesth Intens Care, 23(2):149, 1995

A30. Nakata Y, Goto T, Uezono S *et al:* Anesthetic duration with sevoflurane for acceptable cuffed oropharyngeal airway or laryngeal mask airway placement. Anesthesiology 89:A550, 1998

A31. Williams PJ, Bailey PM: Comparison of the reinforced laryngeal mask airway and tracheal intubation for adenotonsillectomy. Br J Anaesth 70:30, 1993

A32. Webster AC, Morley-Forster PK, Ganapathy S *et al:* Anaesthesia for adenotonsillectomy: A comparison between tracheal intubation and the armoured laryngeal mask airway. Can J Anaesth 40(12):1171, 1993

A33. Dubreuil M, Cros AM, Boudey C *et al:* Is adenoidectomy in children safer with laryngeal mask than with facial mask or with endotracheal intubation? Bordeaux International Congress, July 1992

A34. Fiani N, Scandella C, Giolitto N, Prudhomme G: Comparison of reinforced laryngeal mask vs. endotracheal tube in tonsillectomy. Anesthesiology 85:A491, 1994

A35. Williams PJ, Bailey PM: The reinforced laryngeal mask airway for adenotonsillectomy. Br J Anaesth 72:729, 1994

A36. Puig C, Parizot P, Hayem C *et al:* Masque laryngé pour adenoidectomie chez l'enfant. SFAR Conference, September 1992

A37. Alexander CA: A modified Intavent laryngeal mask for ENT and dental anaesthesia. Anaesthesia 45(10):892, 1990

A38. van Heerden PV, Kirrage D: Large tonsils and the laryngeal mask airway. Anaesthesia 44(8):703, 1991

A39. Venn PJH: Use of laryngeal mask during tonsillectomy. Br J Anaesth 81:298, 1998

A40. Brimacombe JR, Berry AM: Use of the laryngeal mask airway in otolaryngology. J Otolaryngol 24(2):125, 1995

A41. Porter H, Bailey PM: Laryngeal mask and tonsillectomy. Reply to 1430. Br J Anaesth 81:996, 1998

A42. Howard-Griffin RM, Driver IK: Laryngeal mask airway in adenotonsillectomy in children. Anaesthesia 51(4):409, 1996

A43. Tait AR, Pandit UA, Voepel-Lewis T *et al:* Use of the laryngeal mask airway in children with upper respiratory tract infections: A comparison with endotracheal intubation. Anesth Analg 86:706, 1998

A44. Watcha MF, White P, Tychsen L, Stevens JL: Comparative effects of laryngeal mask airway and endotracheal tube insertion on intraocular pressure in children. Anesth Analg 75:355, 1992

A45. Garbin GS, Bogetz MS, Grekin RC, Frieden IJ: ASA Abstracts: The laryngeal mask as an airway during laser treatment of port wine stains. Anesthesiology 75(3A):953, 1991

A46. Epstein RH, Halmi W: Oxygen leakage around the laryngeal mask airway during laser treatment of port wine stains in children. Anesthesiology 79(3A):A1154, 1993

A47. Brimacombe J, Sher M, Berry A: The reinforced laryngeal mask airway for laser pharyngoplasty. Anaesthesia 48:1105, 1993

A47. Divatia JV, Sareen R, Upadhye SM *et al:* Anaesthetic management of tracheal surgery using the laryngeal mask airway. Anaesth Intens Care 22:69, 1994

A48. McCulloch T, Jones MR, O'Neill A: Safety of the laryngeal mask airway with the flash-pumped dye laser. World Congress of Anaesthesiologists, Abstract P130014, 1996

A49. Sosis MB: Evaluation of five metallic tapes for protection of endotracheal tubes during CO$_2$ laser surgery. Anesth Analg 68:392, 1989

A50. Sosis MB, Dillon F: Prevention of CO$_2$ laser-induced endotracheal tube fires with the Laser-Guard protective coating. J Clin Anesth 4:25, 1992

A51. Brimacombe J: The incendiary characteristics of the laryngeal and reinforced laryngeal mask airway to CO$_2$ laser strike: A comparison with two polyvinyl chloride tracheal tubes. Anaesth Intens Care 22:694, 1994

A52. Lumb AB, Wrigley MW: The effect of nitrous oxide on laryngeal mask cuff pressure. Anaesthesia 47:320, 1992

A53. Biro P: Damage to laryngeal masks during sterilization. Anesth Analg 77:1079, 1993

A54. Pennant JH, Gajraj NM: Lasers and the laryngeal mask airway. Anaesthesia 49(5):448, 1994

A55. Brimacombe J, Sher M: The laryngeal mask for laser surgery to the pharynx. Anaesthesia 49(11):1009, 1994

A56. Tanigawa K, Inoue Y, Iwata S: Protection of recurrent laryngeal nerve during neck surgery: A new combination of neutracer, laryngeal mask airway and fibreoptic bronchoscope. Anesthesiology 74:966, 1991

A57. Kalapac S, Donald A, Brimacombe J: Laryngeal mask biopsy. Anaesth Intens Care 24(2):283, 1996

A58. Maltby JR, Loken RG, Beriault MT, Archer DP: Laryngeal mask airway with mouth opening less than 20 mm. Can J Anaesth 42(12):1140, 1995

A59. Costa e Silva L, Brimacombe J: The laryngeal mask for carotid endarterectomy. J Cardiothorac Vasc Anesth 10:972, 1996

A60. Brimacombe J, Clarke G, Simons S: The laryngeal mask airway and endoscopic guided percutaneous tracheostomy. Anaesthesia 49(4):358, 1994

A61. Dexter TJ: The laryngeal mask airway: A method to improve visualisation of the trachea and larynx during fibreoptic assisted percutaneous tracheostomy. Anaesth Intens Care 22(1):35, 1994

A62. Dexter TJ: Laryngeal oedema, a marker of an "at risk" airway? Anaesthesia 49(8):826, 1994

A63. Ip-Yam P, Shaw S: The laryngeal mask airway and endoscopic guided percutaneous tracheostomy. Anaesthesia 49(8):733, 1994

A64. Verghese C, Rangasami J, Kapila A, Parke T: Airway control during percutaneous dilatational tracheostomy: Pilot study with the intubating laryngeal mask airway. Br J Anaesth 81:608, 1998

A65. Morita Y, Takenoshita M: Laryngeal mask airway fitted over a tracheotomy orifice: A means to ventilate a tracheotomized patient during induction of anesthesia. Anesthesiology 89:1295, 1998

A66. Brimacombe J, Sher M, Laing D, Berry A: The laryngeal mask airway: A new technique for fiberoptic guided vocal cord biopsy. J Clin Anesth 8:273, 1996

A67. Lee SK, Hong KH, Choe H, Song HS: Comparison of the effects of the laryngeal mask airway and endotracheal intubation on vocal function. Br J Anaesth 71:648, 1993

A68. Wilson IG, Fell D, Robinson SL, Smith G: Cardiovascular responses to insertion of the laryngeal mask. Anaesthesia 47:300, 1992

A69. Slinger P, Robinson R, Shennib H et al: Alternative technique for laser resection of a carinal obstruction. J Cardiothorac Vasc Anesth 6(6):749, 1992

A69. Akhtar TM, Shankar RK, Street MK: Is Guedel's airway and face mask dead? Today's Anaesthetist 9:56, 1994

A70. Greatorex RA, Denny NM: Application of the laryngeal mask airway to thyroid surgery and the preservation of the recurrent laryngeal nerve. Ann Roy Coll Surg 73:352, 1991

A70. Benumof JL: The rigid bronchoscope: Gold standard technique for laser resection of a carinal tumour. J Cardiothoracic Anesth 6:753, 1992

A71. Akhtar TM: LMA and visualisation of vocal cords during thyroid surgery. Can J Anaesth 38:140, 1991

A71. Catala JC, Garcia-Pedrajas F, Carrera J, Monedero P: Placement of an endotracheal device via the laryngeal mask airway in a patient with tracheal stenosis. Anesthesiology 84:239, 1996

A72. Eckhardt WF III, Forman S, Denman W et al: Another use of the laryngeal mask airway—as a blocker during tracheoplasty. Anesth Analg 80:622, 1995

A72. Premachandra DJ: Application of the laryngeal mask airway to thyroid surgery and the preservation of the recurrent laryngeal nerve. Ann Roy Coll Surg Engl 74:226, 1992

A73. Goldik Z, Lazarovici H, Baron E et al: Continuous fibreoptic video laryngoscopy through the laryngeal mask during thyroidectomy. Br J Anaesth 74:13(abstr), 1995

A73. Uchiyama M, Yoshino A: Insertion of the Montgomery T-tube. Anaesthesia 50(5):476, 1995

A74. Hobbiger HE, Allen JG, Greatorex RG et al: The laryngeal mask airway for thyroid and parathyroid surgery. Anaesthesia 51:972, 1996

A75. Ready AR, Barnes J: Complications of thyroidectomy. Br J Anaesth 81:1555, 1994

A76. Marthensson H, Terins J: Recurrent laryngeal nerve palsy in thyroid gland surgery related to operations and nerves at risk. Arch Surg 120:475, 1985

A78. Charters P, Cave-Bigley D: Application of the laryngeal mask airway to thyroid surgery and the preservation of the recurrent laryngeal nerve. Ann Roy Coll Surg Engl 74:225, 1992

A79. Charters P, Cave-Bigley D, Roysam CS et al: Should a laryngeal mask be routinely used in patients undergoing thyroid surgery? Anesthesiology 75:918, 1991

A80. Denny NM, Gadelrab R: Complications following general anaesthesia for cataract surgery: A comparison of the laryngeal mask airway with tracheal intubation. J Roy Soc Med 86:521, 1993

A81. Holden R, Morsman CDG, Butler J et al: Intra-ocular pressure changes using the laryngeal mask airway and tracheal tube. Anaesthesia 46:922, 1991

A82. Akhtar TM, McMurray P, Kerr WJ et al: A comparison of laryngeal mask airway with tracheal tube for intra-ocular ophthalmic surgery. Anaesthesia 47:668, 1992

A83. Verghese C, Smith TGC, Young E: Prospective survey of the use of the laryngeal mask airway in 2359 patients. Anaesthesia 48:58, 1993

A84. Daum REO, Downes RN, Vardy S: Day-stay cataract surgery under general anaesthesia. Today's Anaesthesia 7(2):24, 1992

A85. Nathanson MH, Ferguson C, Nancekievill DG: Airway maintenance for short ophthalmological procedures in children. Anaesthesia 47:542, 1992

A86. Thomson KD: The effect of the laryngeal mask airway on coughing after eye surgery under general anaesthetic. Ophthal Surg 23:630, 1992

A87. Thomson JPS: Eye movement during cataract surgery. Anaesth Intens Care 21:376, 1993

A88. Lamb K, James MFM, Janicki PK: The laryngeal mask airway for intraocular surgery: Effects of intraocular pressure and stress responses. Br J Anaesth 69:143, 1992

A89. Ripart J, Cohendy R, Eledjam J: The laryngeal mask and intraocular surgery. Br J Anaesth 70:704, 1993

A90. Barclay K, Wall T, Wareham K et al: Intra-ocular pressure changes in patients with glaucoma: Comparison between the laryngeal mask airway and tracheal tube. Anaesthesia 49(2):159, 1994

A91. Balog CC, Bogetz MS, Good WH et al: The laryngeal mask airway is an ideal airway for many outpatient pediatric ophthalmologic procedures. Anesth Analg 78(suppl 2):S17, 1994

A92. Myint Y, Singh AK, Peacock JE et al: Changes in intra-ocular pressure during general anaesthesia: A comparison of spontaneous breathing through a laryngeal mask with positive pressure ventilation through a tracheal tube. Anaesthesia 50:126, 1995

A93. Wainwright AC: Positive pressure ventilation and the laryngeal mask airway in ophthalmic anaesthesia. Br J Anaesth 75:249, 1995

A94. Langenstein H, Moller F, Krause R et al: Die Handhabung der Larynxmaske bei Augenoperationen. Congress on Anaesthesia in Eye Surgery, Congress-Centrum Stadtpark, Hannover, 10 May 1996 (Abstract).

A95. Janke EL, Fletcher JE, Lewis IH: Anaesthetic management of the Kenny-Caffey syndrome using the laryngeal mask. Paediatr Anaesth 6:235, 1996

A96. Fuchs K, Kukule I, Knoch M et al: Larynxmaske versus Intubation bei erschwerten Intubationsbedingungen beim Franceschetti-Zwahlen-Klein-Syndrom (Treacher-Collins syndrome). Anaesthesiol Intensivmed Notfallmed Schmerzther 28:190, 1993

A98. Alexander R: The laryngeal mask airway and ocular injury. Can J Anaesth 40:901, 1993

A99. Milligan KA: Laryngeal mask in the prone position. Anaesthesia 49(5):449, 1994

A100. McCartney CA, Wilkinson DJ, Rabey PG et al: The laryngeal mask airway and intra-ocular surgery. Anaestheaia 47(5):445, 1992

A101. Brimacombe J, Berry A: The laryngeal mask airway and intra-ocular surgery. Anaesthesia 48:827, 1993

A102. Brimacombe J, Aebersold R, Smith J: Laryngeal mask for ophthalmic splash injuries. Today's Anaesthetist 11(2):52, 1996

A103. Handysides EA, Wat LI: A prospective comparison of the reinforced laryngeal mask airway and tracheal intubation for orofacial and ophthalmologic surgery. Anesthesiology 89:A569, 1998

A104. Jalowiecki PO, Krawczyk LM, Karpel EK et al: Use of laryngeal mask in ophthalmic surgery: Comparison with endotracheal intubation. Abstract from meeting of European Society of Anaesthesiologists, Lausanne, 3 May. Br J Anaesth 78:A27, 1997

A105. Gynaecological laparoscopy: The report of the working party of the confidential enquiry into gynaecological laparoscopy. London, Royal College of Obstetricians and Gynaecologists, 1978

A106. Dingley J, Asai T: Insertion methods of the laryngeal mask airway: A survey of current practice in Wales. Anaesthesia 51:596, 1996

A107. Verghese C, Brimacombe J: Survey of laryngeal mask airway usage in 11,910 patients: Safety and efficacy for conventional and nonconventional usage. Anesth Analg 82:129, 1996

A108. Akhtar TM, Street MK: Risk of aspiration with the laryngeal mask. Br J Anaesth 72:447, 1994

A109. Wilkinson PA, Cyna AM, MacLeod DM et al: The laryngeal mask: Cautionary tales. Anaesthesia 45:167, 1990; 73:518, 1990

A110. Goodwin APL, Rowe WL, Ogg TW: Day case laparoscopy: A comparison of two anaesthetic techniques using the laryngeal mask during spontaneous breathing. Anaesthesia 47:892, 1992

A111. Swann DG, Spens H et al: Anaesthesia for gynaecological laparoscopy: A comparison between the laryngeal mask and tracheal intubation. Anaesthesia 48:431, 1993

A112. Brimacombe J: Laparoscopy and the laryngeal mask airway (letter). Br J Anaesth 73:121, 1994

A113. Malins AF, Cooper GM: Laparoscopy and the laryngeal mask airway. Br J Anaesth 73:121, 1994

A114. Darling JR, Keohane M, Murray JMA: Split laryngeal mask as an aid to training in fibreoptic tracheal intubation. Anaesthesia 48:1079, 1993

A115. Maroof M, Khan RM, Khan H et al: Evaluation of modified laryngeal mask airway as an aid to fiber optic intubation. Anesthesiology 77:A1062, 1992

A116. Brimacombe J, Newell S, Swainston R: A potential new technique for awake fibreoptic bronchoscopy: Use of the laryngeal mask airway. Med J Aust 156:876, 1992

A117. Brimacombe J, Tucker P, Simons S: The laryngeal mask airway in awake diagnostic bronchoscopy: A retrospective study of 200 consecutive patients. Eur J Anaesthesiol 12:357, 1995

A118. Alberge MC, Rabarijoana A, Macchi P et al: Use of the laryngeal mask airway for bronchoscopy in awake patients with respiratory insufficiency (abstract). Anesthesiology 81:A1462, 1994

A119. Walker RWM, Murrell D: Yet another use for the laryngeal mask airway (letter). Anaesthesia 46:591, 1991

A120. McNamee CJ, Meyns B, Pagliero KM: Flexible bronchoscopy via the laryngeal mask: A new technique. Thorax 46:141, 1991

A121. Maroof M, Siddique M, Khan RM: Difficult diagnostic laryngoscopy and bronchoscopy aided by the laryngeal mask airway (abstract). J Laryngol Otol 106:722, 1992

A122. Smith TGC, Whittet H, Heyworth T: Laryngomalacia—a specific indication for the laryngeal mask? (letter). Anaesthesia 47:910, 1992

A123. Dich-Nielson JO, Nagel P: Flexible fibreoptic bronchoscopy via the laryngeal mask (abstract). Acta Anaesthesiol Scand 37:17, 1993

A124. Cortés J, Franco M, Cid M et al: Uso de la mascarilla laringea para broncoscopia fibroptica en un neonato con malformaciones faciales. Rev Española 39:324, 199.

A125. Du Plessis MC, Marshall Barr A, Verghese C et al: Fibreoptic bronchoscopy under general anaesthesia using the laryngeal mask airway. Eur J Anaesthesiol 10:363, 1993

A126. Lawson R, Lloyd-Thomas AR: Three diagnostic conundrums solved using the laryngeal mask airway. Anaesthesia 48:790, 1993

A127. Buzzetti V, Cigada M, Solca M, Iapichino G: Use of the laryngeal mask airway during fibreoptic bronchoscopy. Intens Care World 13:72, 1996

A128. Tatsumi K, Furuya H, Nagahata T et al: Removal of a bronchial foreign body in a child using the laryngeal mask. Masui Jap J Anesth 42:441, 1993

A129. Yahagi N, Kumon K, Tanigami H: Bronchial lavage with a fibreoptic bronchoscope via a laryngeal mask airway in an infant (letter). Anaesthesia 49:450, 1994

A130. Credle WFJ, Smiddy JF, Elliot RC: Complications of fiberoptic bronchoscopy. Am Rev Resp Dis 109:67, 1974

A131. Suratt PM, Smiddy JF, Gruber B: Deaths and complications associated with fiberoptic bronchoscopy. Chest 69:747, 1976

A132. Pereira W, Kovnat DM, Snider GL: A prospective comparative study of complications following fiberoptic bronchoscopy. Chest 73:813, 1978

A133. Dresin RB, Albert RK, Talley PA et al: Flexible fibreoptic bronchoscopy in the teaching hospital. Chest 74:144, 1978

A134. Lukowsky GI, Ovchinnikov AA, Bilal A: Complications of rigid bronchoscopy under general anaesthesia and flexible fibreoptic bronchoscopy under topical anaesthesia. Chest 79:316, 1981

A135. Harrison BDW: Guidelines for care during bronchoscopy. Thorax 48:584, 1993

A136. Wrigley SR, Black AE, Sidhu VS: A fibreoptic laryngoscope for paediatric anaesthesia. A study to evaluate the use of the 2.2 mm Olympus (LF-P) intubating fibrescope. Anaesthesia 50:709, 1995

A137. Brimacombe J, Berry A: Laryngeal mask size selection and the sixth LMA (letter). J Clin Anesth 7:265, 1995

A138. Ferson DZ, Nesbitt JC, Nesbitt K et al: The laryngeal mask airway: A new standard for airway evaluation in thoracic surgery. Ann Thorac Surg 63:768, 1997

A139. Llagunes J, Rodriguez-Hesles C, Catala JC et al: Therapeutic fibreoptic bronchoscopy in critically ill patients via laryngeal mask. Anaesth Intens Care 24:396, 1996

A140. Mizikov V, Variushina T, Kirimov U: The laryngeal mask for fibreoptic bronchoscopy in children (abstract). Br J Anaesth A73:78, 1997

A141. Brimacombe J: Laryngeal mask airway for access to the upper gastrointestinal tract. Anesthesiology 84:1009, 1996

A142. Hagberg C, Berry J, Haque S: The laryngeal mask airway for awake craniotomy in pediatric patients (abstract). Anesthesiology 83:A184, 1995

A143. Costa E, Silva L, Brimacombe J: Tracheal tube/laryngeal mask exchange for emergence. Anesthesiology 85:218, 1996

A144. Conci F, Arosio M, Gramegna M et al: La maschera laringea in neurochirurgia, neuroradiologia e neurorianimazione. Minerva Anestesiol 61:17, 1995

A145. Brimacombe JR, Brimacombe JC, Berry AM et al: A comparison of the laryngeal mask airway and cuffed oropharyngeal airway in anesthetized adult patients (abstract). Anesth Analg 87:147, 1998

A146. Silva LCE, Brimacombe JR: The laryngeal mask airway for stereotactic implantation of fetal hypophysis. Anesth Analg 82:430, 1996

A147. Bryden DC, Gwinnutt CL: Tracheal intubation via the laryngeal mask airway: A viable alternative to direct laryngoscopy for nursing staff during cardiopulmonary resuscitation. Resuscitation 36:19, 1998

A148. Brain AIJ: Use of the laryngeal mask airway as a face-mask substitute in cardio-pulmonary resuscitation (abstract). Minerva Anestesiol 61:7, 1995

A149. Verghese C, Brimacombe J: Survey of laryngeal mask airway usage in 11,910 patients: Safety and efficacy for conventional and nonconventional usage. Anesth Analg 82:129, 1996

A150. Brimacombe J: The laryngeal mask airway for abdominal surgery. J Clin Exp Med 171:949, 1994

A151. Brimacombe J: Airway protection with the new laryngeal mask prototype (letter). Anaesthesia 51:602, 1996

A152. Waite K, Filshie J: The use of a laryngeal mask airway for CT radiotherapy planning and daily radiotherapy. Anaesthesia 45:894, 1990

A153. Okazaki H: Use of the laryngeal mask for adult patient. J Clin Exp Med 12:869, 1992

A154. Lauretti GR, Garcia LV, De Mattos AL et al: anestesia epidural continua e máscara laringea para transplante renal. Rev Brasil Anestesiol 44:CBA203, 1994

A155. Hattamer SJ, Dodds TM: Use of the laryngeal mask airway in managing a patient with a large anterior mediastinal mass: A case report. J Amer Assoc Nurse Anesthetists 64:497, 1996

A156. Polaner DM: The use of heliox and the laryngeal mask airway in a child with an anterior mediastinal mass. Anesth Analg 82:208, 1996

A157. Langenstein H, Möller F: Erste Erfahrungen mit der Intubationslarynxmaske. Anaesthesist 47:311, 1998

Clinical Anesthesia (4/e), edited by
Paul G. Barash, Bruce F. Cullen, and
Robert K. Stoelting. Lippincott Williams &
Wilkins, Philadelphia, © 2001.

CHAPTER 24

PATIENT POSITIONING

MARK A. WARNER AND JOHN T. MARTIN

Positioning a patient for a surgical procedure is frequently a compromise between what the anesthetized patient can tolerate, both structurally and physiologically, and what the surgical team requires for access to their anatomic targets.[1,2] Physiologic instability resulting from disease or injury may be magnified by rapidly moving a seriously ill patient from bed to transport cart, through corridors and elevators, and onto the operating table. Induction of anesthesia and positioning may need to be delayed until that patient is hemodynamically stable, or establishment of the intended surgical posture may need to be modified to match the patient's tolerance. This chapter presents the physiologic significance of various positions in which a patient may be placed during an operation, briefly describes the techniques of establishing the positions, and discusses the potential complications of each posture.

It is very important for clinicians to understand the physiologic and potential pathologic consequences of patient positioning. Although considerable information is available on the physiologic effects of various positions, there is a paucity of information on the complications of positioning. Until recently, there have been few studies, either retrospective or prospective, that provided epidemiologic evidence of the frequency and natural history of many of the perioperative positioning complications. Why? In decades preceding the 1990s, catastrophic perioperative outcomes, such as death or hypoxic brain injury from either the delivery of inadequate oxygen or failure adequately to ventilate patients, were infrequent but potentially avoidable consequences of the delivery of anesthesia. The development of pulse oximetry and end-tidal respiratory monitoring in the 1980s, and the subsequent acceptance of monitoring standards of care by the anesthesia community, contributed to a dramatic decline in the frequency of these major events. Less catastrophic, yet still disabling, perioperative complications, such as neuropathies, consequently increased in importance and priority for study.

In the 1990s, a number of studies of large surgical populations provided new information on the frequency and natural history of rare perioperative events such as neuropathies and vision loss. These studies occasionally provided sufficient data to allow speculation on potential mechanisms of injury. Based on the findings of these studies, investigators are seeking to confirm mechanisms of injury and the efficacy of novel interventions to decrease the frequency of or to prevent these perioperative events. For now, however, the mechanism and even the onset of many potential positioning-related complications often are unknown.

The lack of solid scientific information on basic mechanisms of positioning-related complications often leads to medicolegal entanglements. Attempts to determine the etiology of complications alleged to be caused by patient positioning are often unconscionably biased. Notations on anesthesia and operating room records may be absent or uninformative. On some occasions, medicolegal conclusions have been shaped by assumptions and assertions made by people having no understanding of the case in question and no personal familiarity with proceedings in an operating room. Careful, but laconic, descriptive notations about positions used during anesthesia and surgery, as well as brief comments about special protective measures such as eye care and pressure-point padding, are useful information to include on the anesthesia record. In potentially complicated or contentious circumstances, a brief resume in the progress notes is advisable. Only in this manner can subsequent inquiries be properly answered on behalf of either the patient or the anesthesiologist. When credible, expanded knowledge that further delineates mechanisms of positioning-related complications is available, these issues and the care of patients will be improved.

DORSAL DECUBITUS POSITIONS

Physiology

Circulatory

In the horizontal supine position (Fig. 24-1*A*), the influence of gravity on the vascular system is minimal. Intravascular pressures from head to foot vary little from mean pressures at the level of the heart; therefore, almost no perfusion gradient exists between the heart and arteries in either the head or the lower extremities. Similarly, venous gradients from the periphery to the right atrium consist principally of the cyclic intrathoracic pressure changes that occur with respiration.

If the patient in the dorsal decubitus position is tilted head high or head low, the effects of gravity on blood flow in the head or the feet can become quite significant as the gradient to or from the heart increases. Pressures have been shown to change by 2 mm Hg for each 2.5 cm that a given point varies in vertical height above or below the reference point at the heart.[3]

When the lower extremities are below the level of the heart, blood pools in distensible dependent vessels, causing a reduction in effective circulating volume, cardiac output, and systemic perfusion. If the head is high and blood pressure measured at the level of the heart is low, the blood pressure in the brain is decreased further according to the magnitude of the head elevation.

The *tilt test,* which is the cardiovascular response to a head-up tilt of 75 degrees maintained for 3 minutes, can be a useful indicator of the magnitude of acute blood loss.[4] If sustained tilt causes an increase in heart rate of more than 25 beats · min^{-1} but does not produce hypotension or syncope, the blood volume deficit is 9–14 ml · kg^{-1}. If syncope occurs on tilting, the deficit is likely to be as much as 20 ml · kg^{-1}. Hypotension without tilting indicates a deficit in excess of 20 ml · kg^{-1}.

If the head is tilted down (see Fig. 24-1*B*), pressure in the cerebral veins increases in proportion to the gradient upward to the heart. Many alert patients so positioned complain of a rapidly occurring, pounding vascular headache. Congestion develops in the nasal mucosa and conjunctivae. In the presence of an intracranial pathologic process, such as a head injury or a stroke, elevations of cerebral venous pressure resulting from head-down tilt can provoke or intensify cerebral edema and dangerously raise intracranial pressure. Head-down tilt also increases cerebrospinal fluid pressure in the cranial vault, adding its effect to the total intracranial pressure elevation.

Kubal *et al*[5] have shown that myocardial oxygen consumption can increase in awake patients scheduled for coronary artery bypass grafting when they are placed in mild degrees of head-down tilt as a means of distending jugular vessels and facilitating the percutaneous introduction of pulmonary artery catheters. Measurements suggested that an acute volume loading of the heart had occurred with the onset of the head-down tilt. Angina recurred in some patients, and one showed electrocardiographic changes indicative of myocardial ischemia.

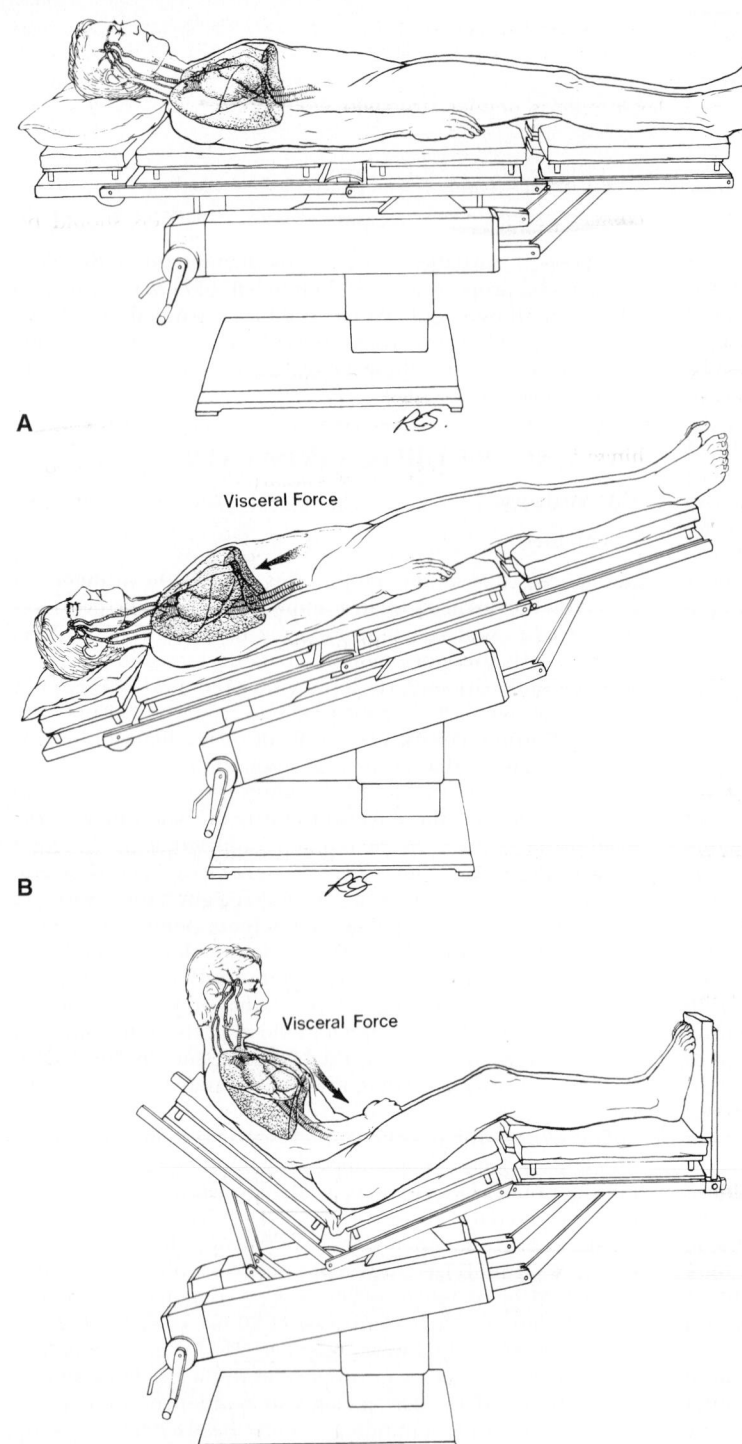

A

Visceral Force

B

Visceral Force

C

Figure 24-1. (*A*) Supine adult with minimal gradients in the horizontal vascular axis. Pulmonary blood volume is greatest dorsally. Viscera displace the dorsal diaphragm cephalad. Cerebral circulation is slightly above heart level if the head is on a small pillow. (*B*) Head-down tilt aids blood return from lower extremities but encourages reflex vasodilation, congests vessels in the poorly ventilated lung apices, and increases intracranial blood volume. (*C*) Elevation of the head shifts abdominal viscera away from the diaphragm and improves ventilation of the lung bases. According to the gradient above the heart, pressure in arteries of the head and neck decreases; pressure in accompanying veins may become subatmospheric.

Head-down tilt has been used to treat hypotension. A well entrenched practice that was based on the suggestions of physiologist Walter Cannon during World War I,[6] this maneuver has been shown to be counterproductive.[7] Although it does increase central blood volume by recovering pooled blood from caudad portions of the body, and although cardiac output is increased transiently, the enlarged central blood mass activates baroreceptors on the great vessels of the chest and neck.[8] The result is rapid peripheral vasodilation, unchanged or reduced cardiac output, and decreased organ perfusion. In a study of patients in intensive care units, Sibbald *et al*[7] found that head-down tilt caused an unpredictable further decrease in mean arterial pressure in a significant number of patients who were already hypotensive.

In the microcirculation, natural and spontaneous fluctuations in blood flow serve the nutritive requirements of the tissues.[9] When an awake human is supine and motionless, the spontaneous fluctuations weaken progressively until they disappear in approximately 1 hour. The subject then becomes uncomfortable. Although tissue blood flow continues to decrease if immobility is enforced, a normal flow pattern returns if the subject becomes restless and moves about.[10]

In the absence of hypocarbia, hypovolemia, or hypothermia, a similar impairment of changes in microcirculatory distribution of blood flow occurs after the induction of anesthesia, despite early augmentation of tissue flow owing to the vasodilative properties of the anesthetic agents. Normal tissue perfusion is re-established by awakening movements of the patient at the end of anesthesia.[10]

West *et al*[11] have identified three separate perfusion zones in the pulmonary circulation, based on the interrelationship among pressures in the alveoli, arterioles, and venules.

In Zone 1, alveolar pressure exceeds either arterial or venous pressure and perfusion of the lung unit is prevented. Although it is rarely present in a normal lung, Zone 1 can be produced by pulmonary hypotension, excessive positive end-expiratory pressure, or overdistention of alveolar units from large tidal volumes during positive-pressure ventilation.

In Zone 2, arterial pressure exceeds alveolar pressure, whereas alveolar pressure remains higher than venous pressure. This relationship is found in nondependent portions of the lung, and perfusion is the result of a fluctuating balance between arterial and alveolar pressures.

In Zone 3, hydrostatic forces in the dependent portion of the lung produce venous congestion, and perfusion is determined by the difference between arterial pressure and venous pressure.

In the dorsal recumbent positions, the pulmonary circulation tends to be most congested along the dorsal body wall and least congested substernally. When the patient is tilted head high, Zone 3 moves toward the lung bases as better ventilatory mechanics improve gas exchange. If the tilt is head down, Zone 3 shifts cephalad into the poorly ventilated lung apices, and abnormal ventilation–perfusion ratios can be expected to intensify.

Respiratory

In the supine position, mobile abdominal viscera gravitate toward the dorsal body wall and press the dorsal parts of the diaphragm cephalad. The displacement lengthens muscle fibers in that portion of the diaphragm and increases the strength and effectiveness of its contractions during spontaneous ventilation. The benefit is improved aeration of the congested, compacted, and less compliant lung bases. With head-up tilt (see Fig. 24-1 *C*), the visceral weight shifts away from the diaphragm and ventilation is enhanced. In the head-down position, the visceral mass, its weight potentially increased by the presence of abdominal fat, fluid, or tumors, can cause significant respiratory embarrassment by impeding caudad excursions of the contracting diaphragm and preventing adequate expansion of the lung bases.

In the supine position, gravity-induced vascular congestion forces the dorsal portions of the lung to function as a Zone 3.[11] Consequently, the compliance of the area is reduced, and passive ventilation tends to distribute gas preferentially to more easily distensible substernal units where pulmonary blood volume is less. To prevent development of a clinically significant ventilation–perfusion imbalance during use of controlled ventilation, tidal volumes must be used that are greater than the average amount that is sufficient for the spontaneously breathing, conscious patient.[12]

Variations of the Dorsal Decubitus Position

Supine

Horizontal. In the traditional horizontal supine position (dubbed "lying-at-attention"), the patient lies on the back with a small pillow beneath the head (see Fig. 24-1*A*). The arms are either comfortably padded and restrained alongside the trunk or abducted on well padded arm boards. Either arm (or both) may be extended ventrally and the flexed forearm secured to

an elevated frame in such a way that perfusion of the hand is not compromised, no skin-to-metal contact exists to cause electrical burns if a cautery is used, and the brachial neurovascular bundle is neither stretched nor compressed at the axilla (see the left arm arrangement in Fig. 24-15). The lumbar spine may need padded support to prevent a postoperative backache (see Complications of the Dorsal Decubitus Positions). Bony contact points at the occiput, elbows, and heels should be padded.

Although the horizontal supine posture has a long history of widespread use, it does not place hip and knee joints in neutral positions and is poorly tolerated for any length of time by an immobilized, awake patient.

Contoured. A contoured supine posture (Fig. 24-2*C*) has been termed the *lawn chair position*.[13] It is established by arranging the surface of the operating table so that the trunk–thigh hinge is angulated approximately 15 degrees and the thigh–knee hinge is angulated a similar amount in the opposite direction. The patient of average height then lies comfortably with hips and knees flexed gently. Quite often a person who has been required to lie motionless on a rigid horizontal table and then is changed to the contoured supine position offers an almost involuntary expression of relief and appreciation.

As in the horizontal supine position, the patient should have a pad or pillow beneath the occiput, elbows, and heels. Arms can be positioned as described for the horizontal supine posture.

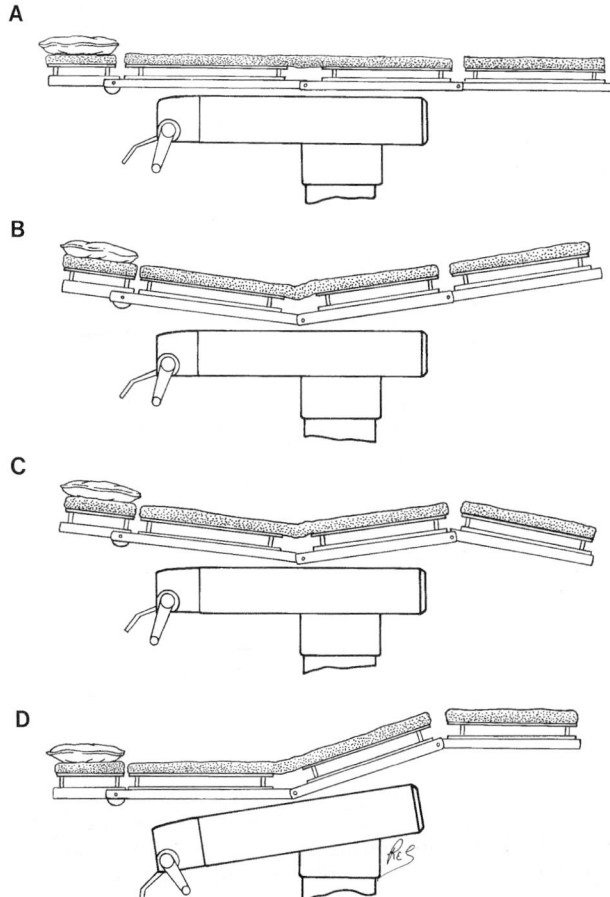

Figure 24-2. Establishment of the contoured supine ("lawn chair") position. (*A*) Traditional flat supine table top. (*B*) Thighs flexed on trunk. (*C*) Knees gently flexed in final body position. (*D*) Trunk section leveled to stabilize floor-supported arm board. (Reproduced with permission from Martin JT, Warner MA [eds]: Positioning in Anesthesia and Surgery, 3rd ed. Philadelphia, WB Saunders, 1997.)

Frog-Leg. On occasion, a pelvic surgeon may wish to place a supportive hand or instrument in the patient's vagina at some point during a laparotomy or laparoscopy. Placing the patient supine with the knees bent and the soles of the feet together (the frog-leg position, Fig. 24-3) separates the thighs sufficiently to permit access to the perineum and vagina for the surgeon standing at the patient's flank. If the patient's skeleton is stiff, lateral spread of the knees may seriously stress the hips or stretch branches of the obturator nerves; a pad of sufficient size should be used to support each knee (1) to minimize the opportunity for postoperative hip and back pain, and (2) to prevent a dislocated hip or fracture of an osteoporotic femur during the operation.

Lateral Uterine Displacement. With a patient in the supine position, a mobile abdominal mass, such as a very large tumor or a pregnant uterus, can rest on the great vessels of the abdomen and compromise circulation. This is known as the *aortocaval syndrome* or the *supine hypotensive syndrome*. A significant degree of perfusion can be restored if the compressive mass is rolled toward the left hemiabdomen by manual compression, by a mechanical device producing leftward displacement, by leftward tilt of the table top, or by a wedge under the right hip.[14] In some quarters, this modification of the dorsal decubitus position is referred to as *semisupine.*

Lithotomy

Standard. In the standard lithotomy position (Fig. 24-4), the patient lies supine with arms crossed on the trunk or with one or both arms extended laterally to less than 90 degrees on arm boards. Each lower extremity is flexed at the hip and knee, and both limbs are simultaneously elevated and separated so that the perineum becomes accessible to the surgeon. For most gynecologic procedures, the patient's thighs are flexed approximately 90 degrees on the trunk and the knees are bent sufficiently to maintain the lower legs nearly parallel to the floor. More acute flexion of the knees or hips can threaten to angulate and compress major vessels at either joint.

Numerous devices are available to hold legs that are elevated during delivery or operation. Each should be fitted to the stature of the individual patient. Care should be taken to ensure that angulations or edges of the padded holder do not compress the popliteal space or the upper dorsal thigh. Compartment syndromes of one or both lower extremities have resulted from prolonged use of the lithotomy position with some types of support devices.[15]

When the legs are to be lowered to the original supine position at the end of the procedure, they should first be brought together at the knees and ankles in the sagittal plane and then lowered slowly together to the table top. This minimizes torsion

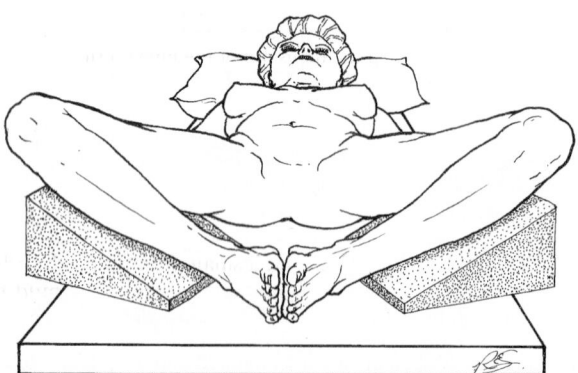

Figure 24-3. The frog-leg position for simultaneous access to the abdomen and vagina. See text. (Reproduced with permission from McLeskey CH [ed]: Geriatric Anesthesiology. Baltimore, Williams & Wilkins, 1997.)

stress on the lumbar spine that would occur if each leg were lowered independently. It also permits gradual accommodation to the increase in circulatory capacitance, thereby avoiding sudden hypotension.[16]

Low. For most urologic procedures and for many procedures that require simultaneous access to the abdomen and perineum, the degree of thigh elevation in the lithotomy position is only approximately 30–45 degrees (Fig. 24-5). This reduces perfusion gradients to and from the lower extremities and improves access to a perineal surgical site for members of the operating team who may need to stand at the lateral aspect of either leg.

High. Some surgeons prefer to improve access to the perineum by suspending the patient's feet from high poles. The effect is to have the patient's legs almost fully extended on the thighs (Fig. 24-6) and the thighs flexed 90 degrees or more on the trunk. The posture produces a significant uphill gradient for arterial perfusion into the feet, requiring careful avoidance of systemic hypotension. Less mobile patients may tolerate this posture poorly because of angulation and compression of the contents of the femoral canal by the inguinal ligament (see Fig. 24-6A), or stretch of the sciatic nerve (see Fig. 24-6B), or both.

Exaggerated. Transperineal access to the retropubic area requires that the patient's pelvis be flexed ventrally on the spine, the thighs almost forcibly flexed on the trunk, and the lower legs aimed skyward so as to be out of the way (Fig. 24-7). The result places the long axis of the symphysis pubis almost parallel to the floor. This exaggerated lithotomy position stresses the lumbar spine, produces a significant uphill gradient for perfusion of the feet, and may restrict ventilation because of abdominal compression by bulky thighs. It can be tolerated under anesthesia but can rarely be assumed by an awake patient. Control of ventilation is usually necessary. If painful lumbar spine disease exists, an alternative surgical position may need to be chosen beforehand to avoid severely accentuating the lumbar distress after surgery. This position has been associated with a very high frequency of lower extremity compartment syndrome.[17] Maintenance of adequate perfusion pressure in the legs is important.

Tilted. Frequently, some degree of head-down tilt is added to one of the lithotomy positions. If the tilt is great enough, and particularly in the instance of the exaggerated lithotomy position, the patient may slide cephalad. Care must be taken to avoid this situation; there are several anecdotes from medicolegal actions involving patients who slid off operating tables with resulting head injuries.

Depending on the degree of head depression, the addition of tilt to the lithotomy position combines the worst features of both the lithotomy and the head-down postures. The weight of abdominal viscera on the diaphragm adds to whatever abdominal compression is produced by the flexed thighs of an obese patient or of one placed in an exaggerated lithotomy position. Ventilation should be assisted or controlled. Because elevation of the lower extremities above the heart produces an uphill perfusion gradient, systemic hypotension and compressive leg wrapping should be avoided because they are potential contributors to the development of compartment syndromes in the legs of lithotomized patients.[15] This perfusion gradient often is unpredictable and exaggerated, potentially increasing the risk of compartment syndrome.[18]

Head-Down Tilt—The Trendelenburg Position. Sometime during the mid-1800s, Bardenhauer, an innovative German surgeon in Cologne, began to elevate the hips of patients to gravitate the viscera cephalad and help expose lesions deep within the pelvis.[19] Others may have used the posture at about the same time. That unique maneuver, tilting a patient 30–45 degrees head down (Fig. 24-8), was adopted and popularized by Friedrich Trendelenburg of Bonn and Leipzig before 1870. However, its publication apparently awaited an article by Meyer, an American pupil of Trendelenburg, in 1885.[20]

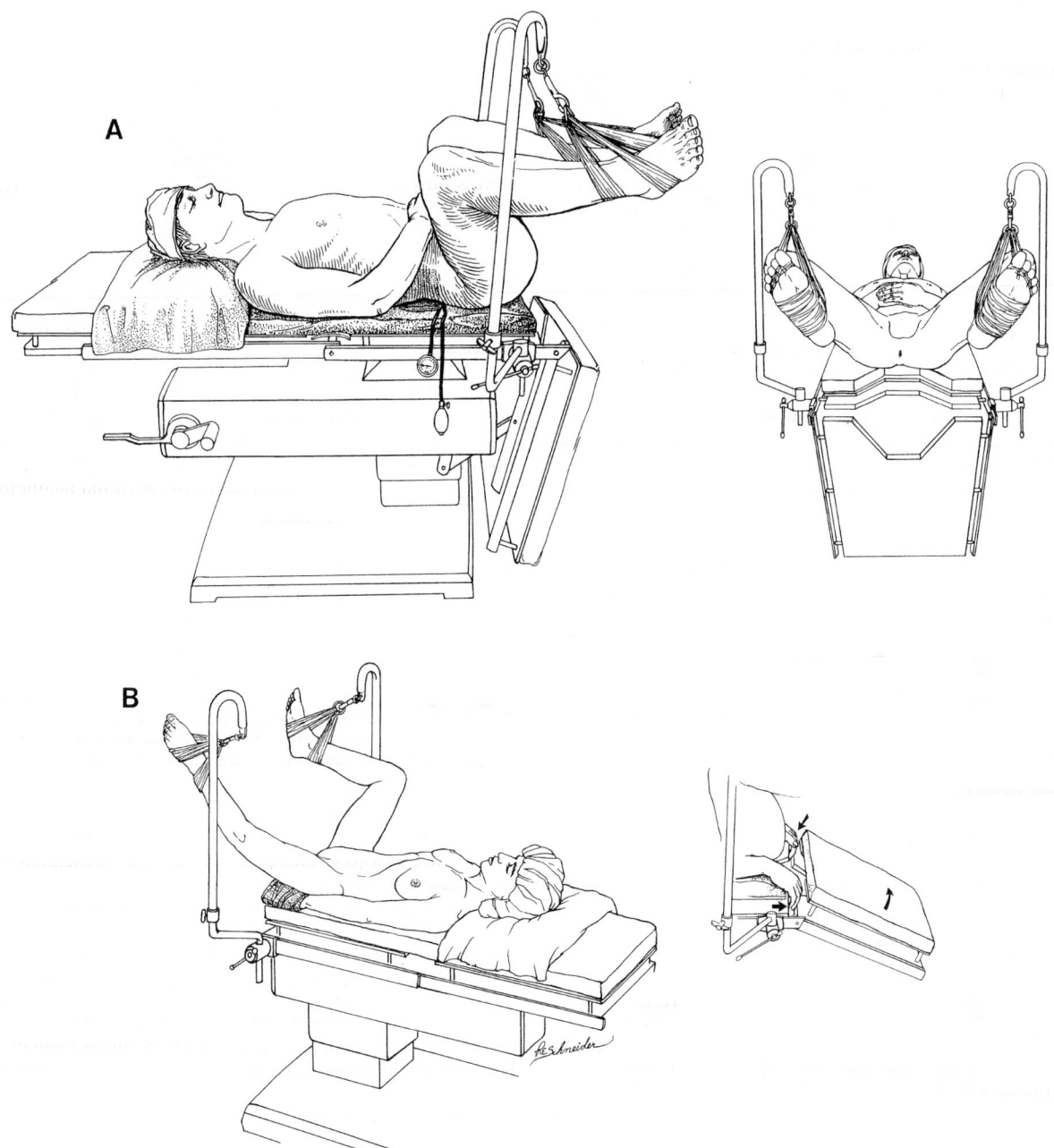

Figure 24-4. Standard lithotomy position with "candy cane" extremity support. (*A*) Thighs are flexed approximately 90 degrees on abdomen; knees are flexed enough to bring lower legs grossly parallel to the torso section of the table top. Arms are retained on boards, crossed on the abdomen, or snugged at the sides of patient. An inflatable bladder (blood pressure cuff bulb and manometer visible) placed under the lumbar spine helps retain lumbar curvature and may minimize postoperative backache. (*B*) Note the possibility for a scissoring injury to fingers as the leg section of the angulated table top is returned to horizontal. Towel-wrapping the hands helps keep the digits out of the hinge. (Modified with permission from Figures 6-5, 6-14, and 6-15 of Martin JT, Warner MA [eds]: Positioning in Anesthesia and Surgery, 3rd ed. Philadelphia, WB Saunders, 1997.)

During World War I, Walter Cannon, the eminent physiologist, espoused the notion that the Trendelenburg position was advantageous in the treatment of shock. He believed that it improved circulatory return from the lower extremities and improved cerebral circulation.[6] Although he repudiated that opinion in 1923,[21] the use of the "Trendelenburg" position to treat shock remained a common practice for many years. Reports of Cole in 1952,[22] Weil in 1957,[23] Guntheroth *et al* in 1964,[24] Taylor and Weil in 1976,[25] and Sibbald's group in 1979[7] have carefully detailed the disadvantages of the Trendelenburg position as a means of treating shock.

An alternate position that is useful for treating supine patients with perfusion deficits, such as moderate hypovolemia from blood loss or vasodilation from spinal anesthesia, is mild elevation of the lower extremities with the trunk remaining horizontal (see Fig. 24-2*D*). The blood volume in the legs is thought to be "autotransfused" into the central circulation by the maneuver. With the thorax level and a small pillow placed under the patient's head, changes in pulmonary function should be minimal and cerebral blood volume should be relatively unchanged.

Because of vasocompensation, whatever increase in mean arterial pressure accompanies elevation of the legs may be transient. In most instances, however, the rational therapy for the perfusion deficits described earlier is volume infusion rather than postural adjustment.

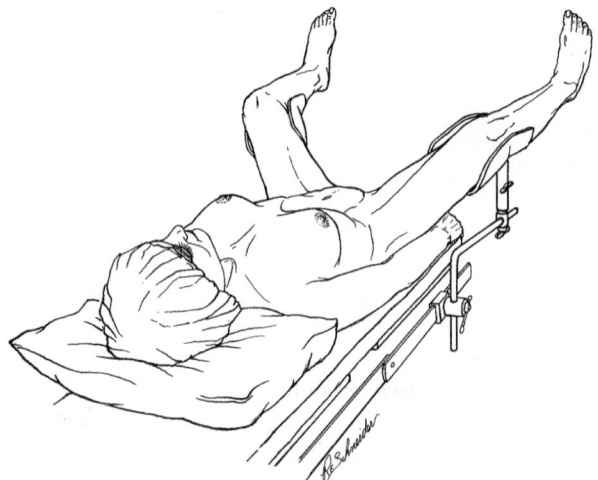

Figure 24-5. Low lithotomy position for perineal access, transurethral instrumentation, or combined abdominoperineal procedures.

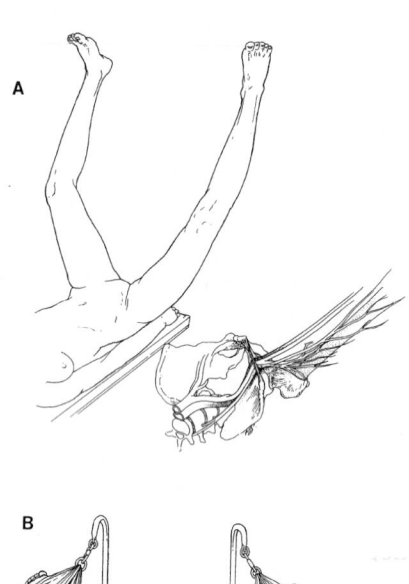

A

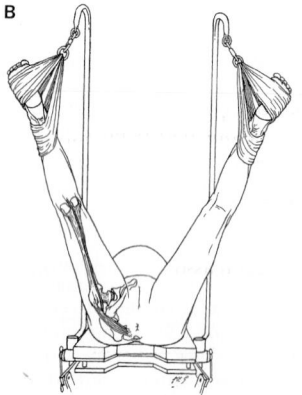

B

Figure 24-6. High lithotomy position. Note potential for angulation and compression/obstruction of contents of femoral canal (*A, insert*) or stretch of sciatic nerve (*B*). (*A* reproduced with permission from McLeskey CH [ed]: Geriatric Anesthesiology. Baltimore, Williams & Wilkins, 1997. *B* reproduced with permission from Martin JT, Warner MA [eds]: Positioning in Anesthesia and Surgery, 3rd ed. Philadelphia, WB Saunders, 1997.)

Reich and associates,[26] studying well instrumented, anesthetized patients, have compared circulatory variables in the level supine position with those recorded after 3 minutes of marked (60-degree) elevation of the lower extremities or after 3 minutes of 20 degrees of head-down tilt. They found that head-down tilt only minimally increased cardiac output and mean arterial pressure, whereas leg raising slightly increased mean arterial

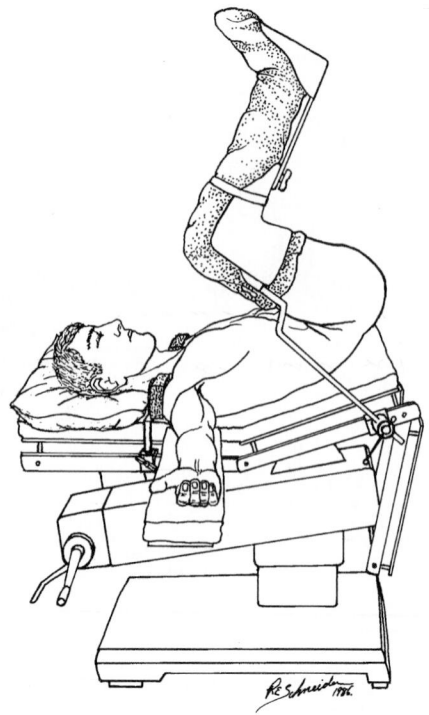

Figure 24-7. The exaggerated lithotomy position. Shoulder braces, usually needed to stabilize the torso, are placed over the acromioclavicular area to minimize compression of the brachial plexus and adjacent vessels. (Reprinted with permission from Martin JT, Warner MA [eds]: Positioning in Anesthesia and Surgery, 3rd ed. Philadelphia, WB Saunders, 1997.)

pressure without affecting cardiac output. In each posture, there was evidence of deteriorating pulmonary function and right ventricular stress. They urged caution in the use of either maneuver in patients with pulmonary disease or right ventricular compromise.

Cephalad displacement of the diaphragm and obstruction of its caudad inspiratory stroke accompany the Trendelenburg position because of gravity-shifted abdominal viscera. Consequently, the work of spontaneous ventilation is increased for an anesthetized patient in a posture that already worsens the ventilation–perfusion ratio by gravitational accumulation of blood in the poorly ventilated lung apices. During controlled ventilation, higher inspiratory pressures are needed to expand the lung.

Intracranial vascular congestion and increased intracranial pressure can be expected to result from head-down tilt. For patients with known or suspected intracranial disease, the position should be used only in those rare instances in which a surgically useful alternate posture cannot be found. Maintenance of the position should then be as brief as possible, and the need for postoperative neurologic intensive care should be anticipated.

The classic Trendelenburg position used 30–45 degrees of head-down tilt and required some means of preventing the patient from sliding cephalad out of position. Anklets and bent knees are a satisfactory method of retaining the tilted patient in position (see Fig. 24-8) if the anklets are not excessively tight and if the flexed knee joints are placed sufficiently caudad of the leg–thigh hinge of the table top so that the adjacent firm edge of the depressed leg section of the table cannot indent either proximal calf. Should indentation occur, compressive ischemia and phlebitis or a compartment syndrome are likely to result.

Historically, shoulder braces also have been used to prevent cephalad sliding. These braces are best tolerated if placed over the acromioclavicular joints, but care must be taken to see

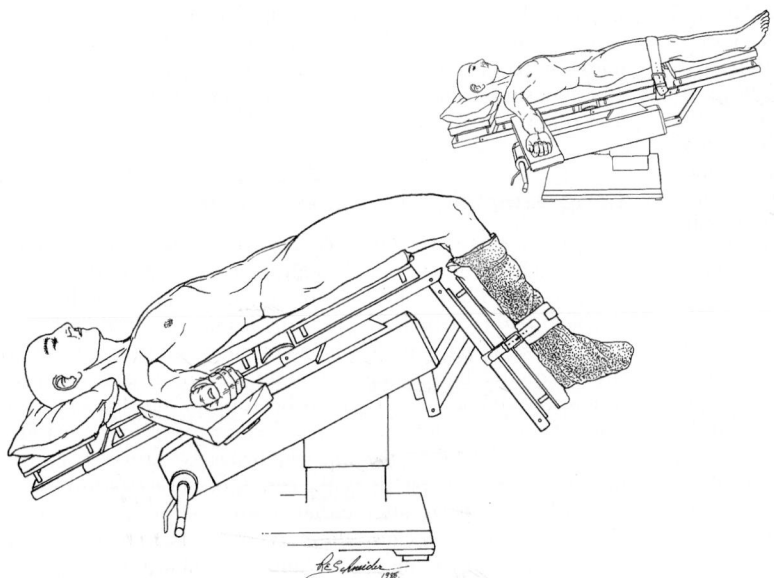

Figure 24-8. Head-down tilt. *Foreground* figure shows traditional steep (30- to 45-degree) tilt described by Trendelenburg. Leg restraints and knee flexion stabilize the patient, avoiding the need for wristlets or shoulder braces that threaten the brachial plexus. *Upper* figure shows 10 to 15 degrees of head-down tilt (the Scultetus position), which is more common in modern surgical procedures. (Reprinted with permission from Martin JT, Warner MA [eds]: Positioning in Anesthesia and Surgery, 3rd ed. Philadelphia, WB Saunders, 1997.)

that the shoulder is not forced sufficiently caudad to trap and compress the subclavian neurovascular bundle between the clavicle and the first rib. If the braces are placed medially against the root of the neck, they may easily compress neurovascular structures that emerge from the area of the scalene musculature.

Head-Down Tilt—The Scultetus Position. The usual amount of head-down tilt now used in most surgical suites is probably approximately 10–15 degrees (see Fig. 24-8, *insert*). This corresponds not to the position of Trendelenburg (see Fig. 24-8), but to one referred to as the Scultetus position. The name appears to be derived from that of the German surgeon, Johann Schultes (1595–1645), who was known as Scultetus.

Although the Scultetus position does not threaten to dislodge the patient cephalad, its minimal head-down tilt has been shown to cause an increase in myocardial oxygen consumption in spontaneously ventilating patients.[5] The use of head-down tilt as a method of increasing the caliber of veins in the superior caval circuit to assist in the insertion of central catheters should be seriously questioned in patients with impaired myocardial perfusion. It should be avoided in the presence of increased intracranial pressure.

In a study of 34 premedicated adults whose hearts were initially in sinus rhythm, Keusch and associates[27] compared the electrocardiographic effects of introducing a pulmonary artery catheter with a self-sealing diaphragm through the right internal jugular vein with each patient first in 5–10 degrees of head-down tilt (posture A) and then in 5 degrees of head-up tilt with right tilt (posture B, semisupine). Access to the pulmonary artery was equally swift in either position. Although the overall incidence of dysrhythmias was similar in both groups (A: 29/34, B: 26/34), during head-up right tilt the patients had only half as many malignant dysrhythmias (8/26) as they did when head down (17/29). In most instances, head-down tilt malignant dysrhythmias changed to benign ones when the patient was placed in the head-up right tilt position, further confirming the head-down position as an unnecessary choice to facilitate pulmonary artery catheter insertion.

Complications of the Dorsal Decubitus Positions

Postural Hypotension

Depending on the resilience of the patient's vasocompensatory mechanisms, postural hypotension may be seen when a head-elevated position is being established. On a statistical basis, it can be presumed to be the most frequent complication of a head-elevated posture. If mean arterial pressure at the circle of Willis remains above 60 mm Hg in a patient who is not hypertensive, the postural hypotension may require little treatment other than to appropriately decrease the concentration of anesthetic drugs to preserve compensatory reflexes. If the degree of hypotension encountered is more severe, further head elevation should be delayed until the level of anesthetic is decreased; in addition, judicious use of fluids and vasopressors can re-establish effective perfusion.

Postural hypotension may also appear in the presence of inadequately replaced blood loss when the intravascular space has been functionally increased either by lowering the legs to horizontal at the termination of the lithotomy position or by returning a head-down tilt to horizontal. Volume repletion is the indicated therapy, although judiciously small doses of vasopressors may sometimes be needed initially.

Pressure Alopecia

Prolonged compression of hair follicles can produce hair loss. Abel and Lewis[28] described patients who had pain, swelling, and exudation where the occiput had been supporting the weight of the head for long periods in the Trendelenburg position. Alopecia occurred between the 3rd and 28th postoperative day; regrowth was complete within 3 months. Use of tight head straps to hold anesthetic face masks and prolonged hypotension and hypothermia have also been associated with compression alopecia.[29] Frequently turning the patient's head during long operations[30] and use of padded, soft head supports are recommended to reduce the risks of this complication.

Pressure Point Reactions

Weight-bearing bony prominences can produce ischemic necrosis of overlying tissue unless proper padding is applied. Hypothermia and vasoconstrictive hypotension may enhance the process. The heels, the elbows, and the sacrum are particularly vulnerable and should be carefully padded as a prophylactic routine. This is particularly important when patients are thin or when the operation will be prolonged.

BRACHIAL PLEXUS AND UPPER EXTREMITY INJURIES
Brachial Plexus Neuropathy

Root Injuries. Shoulder braces placed tight against the base of the neck can compress and injure the roots of the brachial plexus. Braces, if needed at all, are considered less harmful when placed more laterally over the acromioclavicular joint.

The dorsal decubitus positions do not usually threaten structures in the patient's neck unless considerable lateral displacement of the head occurs. In that position, the roots of the brachial plexus on the side of the obtuse head–shoulder angle can be stretched and damaged. If the upper extremity is fixed at the wrist, the stretch injury of the plexus can be accentuated as the head moves laterally away from the anchoring point of the wrist. Similarly, exaggerated rotation of the head away from an extended arm can be associated with a brachial plexus injury.

Sternal Retraction.   Frequently, the patient undergoing a median sternotomy has both arms padded and secured alongside the torso. An alternative is to have both arms abducted.[31] Vander Salm et al[32,33] described first rib fractures and brachial plexus injuries associated with median sternotomies. They related the extent of the injury to the amount of retractor displacement of the rib, with the most severe injury being caused by displacement sufficient to produce a first rib fracture. Roy and associates,[34] in a study of 200 consecutive adults scheduled for cardiac surgery *via* a median sternotomy, positioned the left arm either abducted and padded on an arm board with the palm supinated or secured by a draw sheet alongside the trunk; the right arm was always placed alongside the trunk. They found a 10% incidence of upper extremity nerve injury that was not influenced by internal mammary artery harvest, internal jugular vein catheterization, or left arm position. Surgical manipulation was more contributory than extremity positioning in producing trauma to the brachial plexus. Jellish et al[31] reported that there is less slowing of somatosensory evoked potentials (SSEPs) of the ulnar nerve during sternotomy when both arms are abducted instead of tucked at the sides. However, they found no differences in perioperative symptoms between patients in the arm-abducted *vs.* arm-at-side groups.

Compromised Retroclavicular Space.   If the shoulder is allowed to move dorsally, or if the supine patient shifts cephalad while the shoulder mechanism is anchored at the levels of the hip or shoulder, the retroclavicular space is diminished or obliterated and the clavicle may be pressed forcibly against the underlying first rib. In the process, the subclavian neurovascular bundle can be compressed and its structures injured. Occasionally, a dampened pulse at the wrist identifies this situation in the sitting position; support under the elbow is required to lift the shoulder and relieve the obstruction.

Long Thoracic Nerve Dysfunction

Several lawsuits have centered on postoperative serratus anterior muscle dysfunction and winging of the scapula (Fig. 24-9) alleged to be the result of position-related injuries to the long thoracic nerve of Bell, which arises from nerve roots C5, C6, and C7. Because C5 and C6 fibers of the nerve course through the middle scalene muscle and emerge from its lateral border to join the fibers from C7, it has been proposed that neuropathies of the long thoracic nerve are traumatic in origin.[35] Johnson and Kendall[36] described the widely variable etiology of serratus anterior muscle paralysis in a review of 111 cases and found only 13% occurring after either a surgical procedure or an obstetric delivery. Because the nerve is not routinely involved in a stretch injury of the brachial plexus and because the plexus is not routinely involved when long thoracic nerve dysfunction occurs, the relationship between postoperative long thoracic nerve palsy and patient positioning remains speculative. Based on evidence of Foo and Swann[37] plus data from litigations, Martin[38] concluded that in the absence of demonstrable trauma, postoperative dysfunctions of the long thoracic nerve were quite likely the result of coincidental neuropathies, possibly of viral origin.

Axillary Trauma from the Humeral Head

Excessive abduction of the arm on an arm board may thrust the head of the humerus into the axillary neurovascular bundle. The bundle is stretched at that point and its neural structures may be damaged. In the same manner, vessels can be compressed or occluded and perfusion of the extremity can be jeopardized.

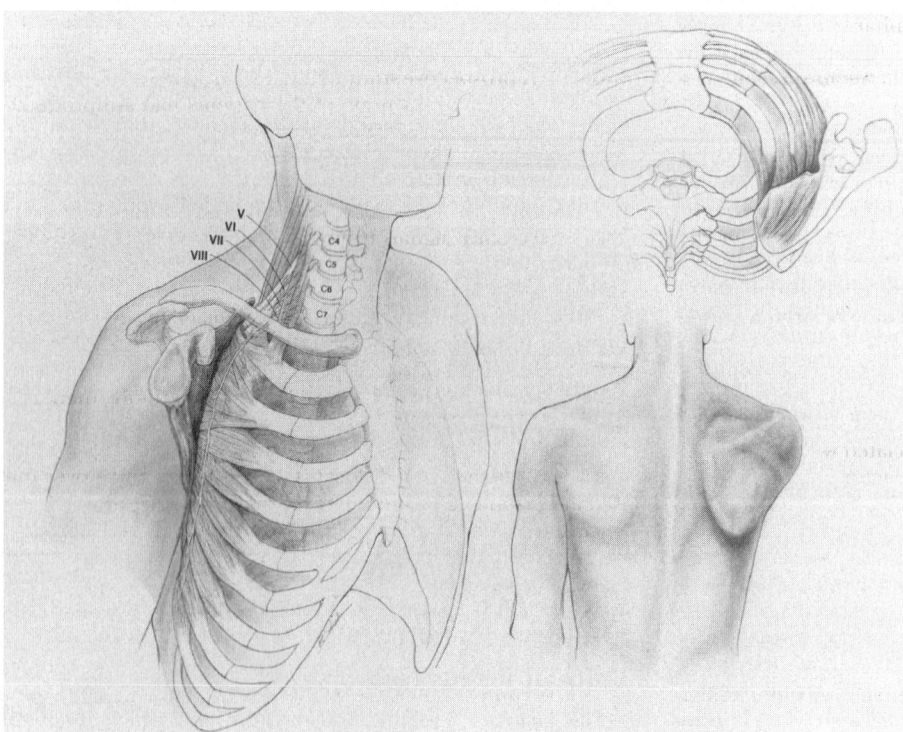

Figure 24-9. Scapular winging. The serratus anterior muscle (*upper right*) is supplied solely by the long thoracic nerve that branches immediately from C5, C6, C7, and sometimes C8 (*left figure*). Arising on the lateral ribs and inserting on the deep surface of the scapula, the muscle keeps the shoulder girdle approximated to the dorsal rib cage. Long thoracic nerve palsy allows dorsal protrusion of the scapula (*lower right*). See text. (Reproduced with permission from Martin JT: Postoperative isolated dysfunction of the long thoracic nerve: A rare entity of uncertain etiology. Anesth Analg 69:614, 1989.)

Radial Nerve Compression

The radial (musculospiral) nerve, arising from roots C6–8 and T1, passes dorsolaterally around the middle and lower portions of the humerus in the musculospiral groove. At a point on the lateral aspect of the arm, approximately three fingerbreadths proximal to the lateral epicondyle of the humerus, the nerve can be compressed against the underlying bone and injured. Pressure from the vertical bar of an anesthesia screen or a similar device against the lateral aspect of the arm[39] and excessive cycling of an automatic blood pressure cuff[40] have been implicated in causing damage to the radial nerve. Postoperative radial nerve dysfunction is a relatively rare reason for malpractice litigation.[41,42]

Clinical manifestations of a radial nerve lesion include wrist drop, weakness of abduction of the thumb, inability to extend the metacarpophalangeal joints, and loss of sensation in the web space between the thumb and index finger.[43] Radial nerve function can be rapidly assessed by noting the patient's ability actively to extend the distal phalanx of the thumb.

Median Nerve Dysfunction

Isolated injuries to the median nerve allegedly owing to positioning are uncommon and the mechanism is obscure.[41,42] A more likely source of injury is iatrogenic trauma to the nerve during access to vessels in the antecubital fossa, as might occur during venipuncture. Anecdotally, this problem appears to occur primarily in men 20–40 years of age who cannot easily extend their elbows completely. Forced elbow extension after administration of muscle relaxants and while positioning the arms has been suggested as one potential mechanism for this problem. A quick check of sensation over the dorsal and palmar surfaces of the distal phalanges of the first and second fingers identifies an acute injury.

Ulnar Neuropathy

Improper anesthetic care and patient malpositioning have been implicated as causative factors in the development of ulnar neuropathies since reports by Budinger[44] and Garriques[45] in the 1890s. These factors likely play an etiologic role for this problem in some surgical patients. Other factors, however, may contribute to the development of postoperative ulnar neuropathies. In a series of 12 inpatients with newly acquired ulnar neuropathy, Wadsworth and Williams[46] determined that external compression of an ulnar nerve during surgery was a factor in only 2 patients. A prospective study at Mayo Clinic found that ulnar neuropathies develop in medical as well as surgical patients during inpatient and outpatient care.[47] It is clear that ulnar neuropathies may develop in both surgical and medical patients during or after an episode of care. The mechanisms of the neuropathy, however, are unclear.

Typically, anesthesia-related ulnar nerve injury is thought to be associated with external nerve compression or stretch caused by malpositioning during the intraoperative period. Although this implication may be true for some patients, three findings suggest that other factors may contribute. First, a retrospective study found male sex, high body mass index (≥38), and prolonged postoperative bed rest to be associated with these ulnar neuropathies.[48] Of these, male sex is the factor most commonly associated with perioperative ulnar neuropathy. Various reports suggest that 70–90% of patients who have this problem are male.[41,42,46–48] Second, many patients with perioperative ulnar neuropathies have a high frequency of contralateral ulnar nerve conduction dysfunction.[49] This finding suggests that many of these patients likely have asymptomatic but abnormal ulnar nerves before their anesthetics, and these abnormal nerves may become symptomatic during the perioperative period. Finally, many patients do not notice or complain of ulnar nerve symptoms until more than 48 hours after their surgical proce-

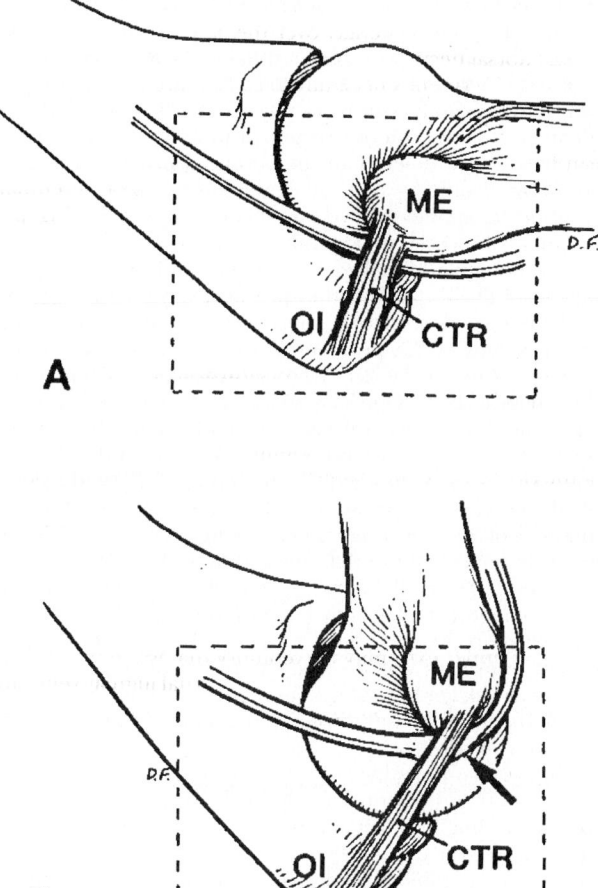

Figure 24-10. Medial-to-lateral view of right elbow. The cubital tunnel retinaculum (CTR) is lax in extension (*A*) as it stretches from the medial epicondyle (ME) to the olecranon (Ol). The retinaculum tightens in flexion (*B*) and can compress the ulnar nerve (*arrow*). (Reprinted with permission from O'Driscoll SW, Horii E, Carmichael SW et al: The cubital tunnel and ulnar neuropathy. J Bone Joint Surg Am 73:613, 1991.)

dures.[48,49] A prospective study of ulnar neuropathy in 1502 surgical patients found that none of the patients had symptoms of the neuropathy during the first 2 postoperative days.[50] It is not clear whether onset of symptoms indicates the time that an injury has occurred to the nerve. Prielipp et al[51] found that 8 of 15 awake volunteers who had notable alterations in their ulnar nerve SSEP signals from direct ulnar nerve pressure did not perceive a paresthesia, even when the SSEP waveforms decreased as much as 72%.

Elbow flexion can cause ulnar nerve damage by several mechanisms. In some patients, the ulnar nerve is compressed by the aponeurosis of the flexor carpi ulnaris muscle and cubital tunnel retinaculum when the elbow is flexed by more than 110 degrees[52,53] (Fig. 24-10). In other patients, this fibrotendinous roof of the cubital tunnel is poorly formed and can lead to anterior subluxation or dislocation of the ulnar nerve over the medial epicondyle of the humerus during elbow flexion. This displacement has been observed in approximately 16% of cadavers in whom the flexor muscle aponeurosis and supporting tissues have not been dissected.[54,55] Ashenhurst[55] has speculated that the ulnar nerve may be chronically damaged by recurrent mechanical trauma as the nerve subluxates over the medial epicondyle.

External compression in the absence of elbow flexion also may damage the ulnar nerve.[56] Although compression within the medial epicondylar groove may be possible if the groove is shallower than normal, the bony groove usually is deep and the nerve is well protected from external compression.[57] More likely, external compression may occur distal to the medial epicondyle, where the nerve and its associated artery are relatively superficial. In an anatomic study, Contreras et al[58] observed that the ulnar nerve and posterior recurrent ulnar artery pass posteromedially to the tubercle of the coronoid process, where they are covered only by skin, subcutaneous fat, and a thin distal band of the aponeurosis of the flexor carpi ulnaris.

Patients in whom perioperative ulnar neuropathies develop are predominantly male.[41,42,46–48] Alvine and Schurrer[49] found that 15 of the 17 patients they prospectively identified to have perioperative ulnar neuropathies were men. In an earlier retrospective study of this problem, Warner et al[48] found the male-to-female ratio to be 2:1. Why are men more likely to have this complication? One can speculate that there are several anatomic differences between men and women that increase the likelihood of perioperative ulnar neuropathy developing in men. First, two anatomic differences may increase the chance of ulnar nerve compression in the region of the elbow. The tubercle of the coronoid process is approximately 1.5 times larger in men than women.[58] In addition, there is less adipose tissue over the medial aspect of the elbow of men compared with women of similar body fat composition.[58–60] Second, men may be more likely to have a well developed cubital tunnel retinaculum than women, and the retinaculum, if present, is thicker. A thicker cubital tunnel retinaculum may increase the risk of ulnar nerve compression in the cubital tunnel when the elbow is flexed.

Clinical manifestations of ulnar nerve dysfunction vary with the location and extent of the lesion.[61] Nearly all patients have numbness, tingling, or pain in the sensory distribution of the ulnar nerves once they become symptomatic. However, there can be considerable ulnar nerve dysfunction before symptoms appear. Prielipp et al[51] found that only 8 of 15 male volunteers with significant ulnar nerve conduction slowing noted any symptoms. More studies are needed to understand better the mechanism and natural history of ulnar neuropathy.

Ulnar nerve injury is relatively common.[41,42,50] Also, a significant proportion of patients have symptoms of bilateral ulnar nerve dysfunctions both before and after surgery.[49] Therefore, some have speculated it might be helpful during the preanesthetic interview to inquire about a history of ulnar neuropathies ("crazy bone" problems) or previous surgery at the elbow. If such a history is indicated, the finding must be recorded and a discussion with the patient or family should present the possibility of a postoperative recurrence despite special precautions of padding and positioning.

The time of recognition of digital anesthesia associated with ulnar nerve dysfunction may be quite important in establishing the origin of the postoperative syndrome. If ulnar hypesthesia or anesthesia is noted promptly after the end of anesthesia, as in the recovery facility, the condition is likely to be associated with events that occurred during anesthesia or surgery. If the recognition is delayed for many hours, the likelihood of cause shifts from the intra-anesthetic period to postoperative events. In a review of closed claims, Kroll and associates[41] commented that postoperative ulnar dysfunction can occur as a result of events in the postanesthetic period and that nerve injury may develop in certain susceptible patients "despite conventionally accepted methods of positioning and padding."

Opioids may mask postoperative dysesthesias and pain, but even strong analgesics cannot mask a loss of sensation due to nerve dysfunction. It may be helpful to assess ulnar nerve function and record these observations before discharging the patient from the recovery room.

Carpal Tunnel Syndrome Mimicking Ulnar Neuropathy

The prospective study of ulnar neuropathy from Mayo Clinic found 47 of 1502 patients had symptoms of numbness and tingling in the fourth and fifth fingers during the perioperative period.[50] On close assessment, 38 of these patients had transient carpal tunnel syndrome mimicking ulnar neuropathy. In 36 of these 38 patients, the symptoms resolved within 5 days of onset. Why does this syndrome develop in patients after procedures? The authors speculate that interstitial edema from perioperative fluid administration and decreased mobility may transiently increase pressure in a limited wrist compartment. As patients begin to use their arms, ambulate, and diurese in the days after their procedures, this edema and pressure in the wrist compartment may decrease and the symptoms should resolve. Further study is needed to determine the true cause for this phenomenon. Transient carpal tunnel syndrome should be considered, however, when evaluating postoperative patients for possible ulnar neuropathy.

Arm Complications

An arm that is hyperabducted, whether intentionally or by inadvertent pressure from the hip of a surgical assistant, can force the head of the humerus into the axillary neurovascular bundle and damage nerves and vessels to the arm. Abduction of the arm to more than 90 degrees from the trunk should be avoided. An arm board should be securely attached to the operating table to prevent its accidental release. An arm that is not properly secured can slip over the edge of the table or arm board, resulting in injury to the capsule of the shoulder joint by excessive dorsal extension of the humerus, fracture of the neck of an osteoporotic humerus, or injury to the ulnar nerve at the elbow. Conversely, in the unlikely event that the retaining strap is excessively tight across the supinated forearm (Fig. 24-11), the potential exists for pressure to compress the anterior interosseous nerve, a branch of the median nerve in the upper forearm that courses with its artery along the volar surface of the tough interosseous membrane. The result is an ischemic injury to the distribution of the nerve and artery that resembles a compartment syndrome in the lower extremity and may require prompt surgical decompression.[62]

Backache

Lumbar backache can be worsened by the ligamentous relaxation that occurs with general, spinal, or epidural anesthesia. Loss of normal lumbar curvature in the supine position is apparently the issue. Several folded towels or an inflatable bladder of a blood pressure cuff (see Fig. 24-4A) placed under the lumbar spine before the induction of anesthesia may help retain lordosis and make a patient with known lumbar distress more comfortable. An exception to this is the patient with palpable tender points in the lumbar area; the pressure of the pad may create enough distress for the patient to object strongly to its presence.

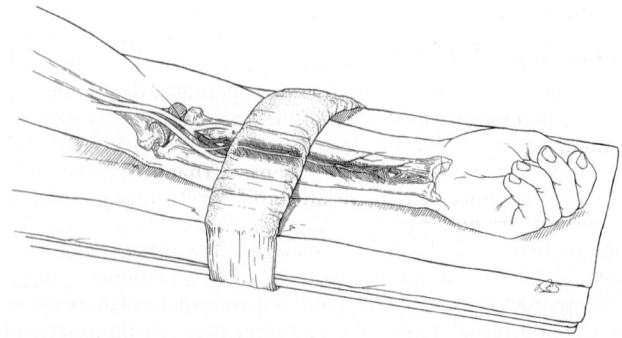

Figure 24-11. Arm restraint, if excessively tight, can compress the anterior interosseous nerve and vessel against the interosseous membrane in the volar forearm to produce an ischemic neuropathy. (Reproduced with permission from McLeskey CH [ed]: Geriatric Anesthesiology. Baltimore, Williams & Wilkins, 1997.)

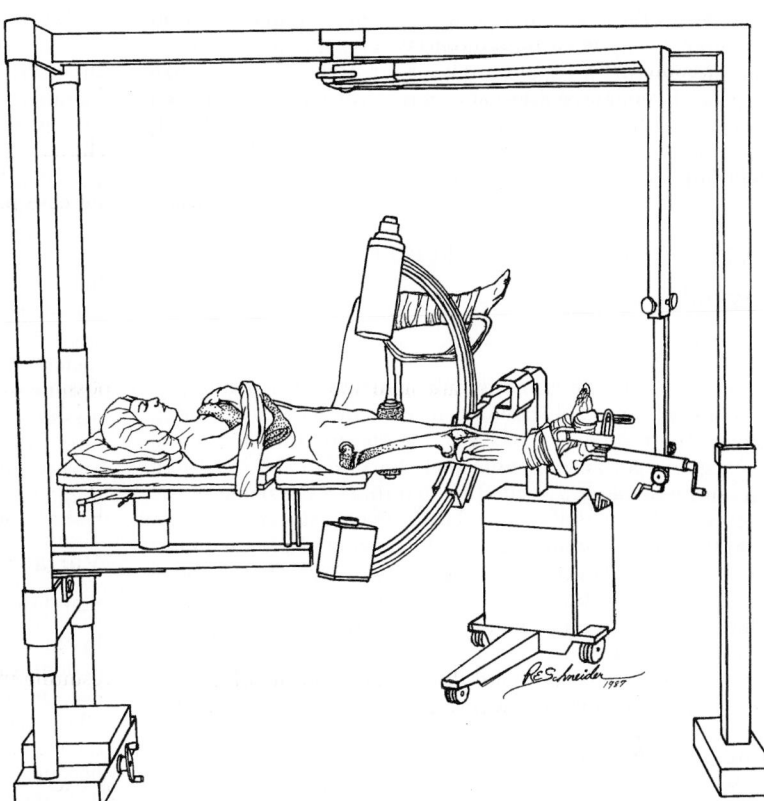

Figure 24-12. Traction table with perineal post stabilizing patient while leg is elongated to reposition bone ends. Elevated leg risks hypoperfusion; pelvic post threatens genitalia. (Reproduced with permission from Martin JT, Warner MA [eds]: Positioning in Anesthesia and Surgery, 3rd ed. Philadelphia, WB Saunders, 1997.)

Elevation of the legs can worsen the pain of a herniated nucleus pulposus. When the lithotomy position is contemplated for a patient with a history of low back pain or a herniated lumbar disk, gentle passive attempts to have the patient assume the posture before anesthesia may be helpful in determining whether the position can be tolerated.

Perineal Crush Injury

The supine patient who is placed on a fracture table for repair of a fractured femur usually has the pelvis retained in place by a vertical pole at the perineum (Fig. 24-12), with the foot of the injured extremity fixed to a mobile rest. A worm gear on the rest lengthens the distance between the foot and the pelvis so that the bone fragments can be distracted and realigned. Unless the pole is well padded, severe pressure can be exerted on the pelvis, and damage can occur to the genitalia and the pudendal nerves. Complete loss of penile sensation has been reported after use of the fracture table.[63,64] The correct position for the pole is against the pelvis between the genitalia and the uninjured limb.[63]

Compartment Syndrome

If, for whatever reason, perfusion to an extremity is inadequate, a compartment syndrome may develop. Characterized by ischemia, hypoxic edema, elevated tissue pressure within fascial compartments of the leg, and extensive rhabdomyolysis, the syndrome produces extensive and potentially lasting damage to the muscles and nerves in the compartment. Because the pathologic process is at tissue level, distal pulses and capillary refill may remain intact while a compartment syndrome is developing in an extremity; thus, they are not useful indicators of the ongoing process. Ferrihemate, resulting from myoglobin destruction, exerts a direct toxic effect on renal tubular epithelium, and renal failure is likely.[65] Circulating debris from infections in the involved extremities is apt to be filtered by pulmonary microvasculature with injurious consequences for the lung.

Causes of a compartment syndrome while a patient is in any of the dorsal decubitus positions include (1) systemic hypotension and loss of driving pressure to the extremity (augmented by elevation of the extremity); (2) vascular obstruction of major leg vessels by intrapelvic retractors, by excessive flexion of knees or hips, or by undue popliteal pressure from a knee crutch; and (3) external compression of the elevated extremity by straps or leg wrappings that are too tight, by the inadvertent pressure of the arm of a surgical assistant, or by the weight of the extremity against a poorly supportive leg holder.[15,66] A tight strap on an arm board has been alleged to have compressed the anterior interosseous neurovascular bundle and created a forearm compartment syndrome.

Several clinical characteristics seem to be associated with perioperative compartment syndrome. Prolonged lithotomy posture in excess of 5 hours has been a common factor in literature anecdotes of postlithotomy compartment syndromes. For lengthy procedures in the lithotomy position, well padded holders that immobilize the limb by supporting the foot without compressing the calf or popliteal fossa seem to be the least threatening choice. There is considerable variability in the perfusion pressure of the lower extremity in elevated legs. Halliwill *et al*[18] found significant blood pressure variation at the ankle in volunteers placed in various lithotomy positions. Several volunteers had mean pressures of less than 20 mm Hg when positioned in the high lithotomy position. This pressure is less than intracompartment pressures commonly measured in many lithotomy positions.

Usually, decompressive fasciotomies are the only means of terminating the cycle of ischemia and compartment edema. Alkalinizing the urine and promoting diuresis may reduce the degree of renal damage.

Finger Injury

In 1968, Courington and Little[67] described the amputation of a young woman's fingers that were caught between the leg and thigh sections of the operating table as the leg section was returned to the horizontal position at the termination of an operation during which the patient was in the lithotomy position (see Fig. 24-4*B*). A towel used to create a boxing-glove–like wrap on the hands of lithotomized patients may prevent such a tragic misadventure.[68] Carefully removing the patient's hands from the risky position before raising the foot of the table is less troublesome and probably as safe.

LATERAL DECUBITUS POSITIONS
Physiology

Circulatory

In the lateral decubitus position, the patient is turned onto one side of the trunk and stabilized to prevent accidental rolling toward either the supine or the prone posture. It is of practical and legal importance to note that the side of the body that rests on the table is the side that determines the name of the position (left side down = left lateral decubitus position).

If the legs are maintained in the long axis of the body, almost no pressure gradients exist along the great vessels from head to foot. Small hydrostatic differences are detected between the values recorded simultaneously by blood pressure cuffs placed on the two arms.

If the lower extremities are flexed laterally at the hips and allowed to remain below the level of the heart, blood pools in the distensible vessels of the dangling legs because of gravity-induced increases in venous pressure and resultant venous stasis. Wrapping the legs and thighs in compressive bandages is a common method to combat venous pooling. Marked flexion of the lower extremities at knees and hips can partially or completely obstruct venous return to the inferior vena cava either by angulation of vessels at the popliteal space and inguinal ligament or by thigh compression against an obese abdomen. A small support should be placed just caudad of the down-side axilla to lift the thorax enough to relieve pressure on the axillary neurovascular bundle and prevent disturbed blood flow to the arm and hand.

In the low-pressure pulmonary circuit, hydrostatic gradients occur between the two hemithoraces. Although the degree of gravity-induced lateral displacement of the heart is different in the two lateral decubitus positions, it is generally true that most of the down-side lung lies below the level of the atrium and that the up-side lung lies above it. Vascular congestion of the down-side lung resembles a Zone 3 of West *et al*,[11] whereas the relative hypoperfusion of the up-side lung resembles a Zone 2. Kaneko *et al*[69] found that the transition between Zone 3 and Zone 2 occurred at approximately 18 cm above the most dependent part of the lung.

If the cervical spine of the patient who is placed in a horizontal lateral decubitus position is carefully maintained in alignment with the thoracolumbar spine, almost no gradient occurs between pressures in the mediastinum and those in the head. However, if the head is improperly supported and sufficient lateral angulation of the neck occurs in either direction, obstruction of jugular flow may be produced.

Respiratory

In the presence of a supple chest, the lateral decubitus position can decrease the volume of the down-side hemithorax. The weight of the chest may force the down-side rib cage into a less expanded conformation. Gravity-induced shifts of mediastinal structures toward the down-side chest wall tend further to reduce the volume of the dependent lung. Abdominal viscera force the down-side diaphragm cephalad if the long axis of the trunk is horizontal or head down.

Spontaneous ventilation can partially compensate for the diaphragmatic stretching in the dependent hemithorax because the contractile efficiency of the elongated diaphragmatic mus-

cle fibers is increased. The compacted lung base and Zone 3 vascular congestion decrease compliance and interfere with the distribution of gas during positive-pressure ventilation. An elevated kidney rest placed against either the down-side rib margin or flank, or that migrates into that position as the patient shifts on it, further interferes with movement of the down-side hemidiaphragm and passive ventilation of the dependent lung.

The up-side hemithorax is much less compressed than the dependent side, and because the lung lies above the level of the atria, it has less vascular congestion than the down-side lung. As a result, unless contralateral flexion has stretched the up-side flank muscles to the point of rigidity and limited excursions of the costal margin, positive-pressure ventilation is directed preferentially to the more compliant up-side lung. The result can easily be excessive ventilation of the underperfused up-side lung and hypoventilation of the congested down-side lung. The potential for a clinically significant ventilation–perfusion mismatch is obvious, particularly in the presence of pulmonary disease.

Variations of the Lateral Decubitus Positions

Standard (Horizontal) Lateral Position

In the horizontal lateral decubitus position (Fig. 24-13), the patient is rolled onto one side on a flat table surface and stabilized in that posture by flexing the down-side thigh to almost 90 degrees on the trunk. The down-side knee is bent to retain the leg on the table and improve stabilization of the trunk. The peroneal nerve of that side is padded to minimize compression damage caused by the weight of the legs. The up-side thigh and leg are extended comfortably, and pillows are placed between the lower extremities. The head is supported by pillows or a head rest so that the cervical and thoracic spines are properly aligned. A small pad (usually referred to incorrectly as an axillary roll), thick enough to raise the thorax and prevent excessive compression of the shoulder, is placed just caudad to and out of the down-side axilla. It should ensure adequate perfusion of the down-side hand and minimize circumduction of the dependent shoulder, which might stretch its suprascapular nerve.

Arms may be extended ventrally and retained on a single arm board with suitable padding between them, or they may be individually retained on a padded two-level arm support that can also help to stabilize the thorax (Fig. 24-14*A*). An alternate

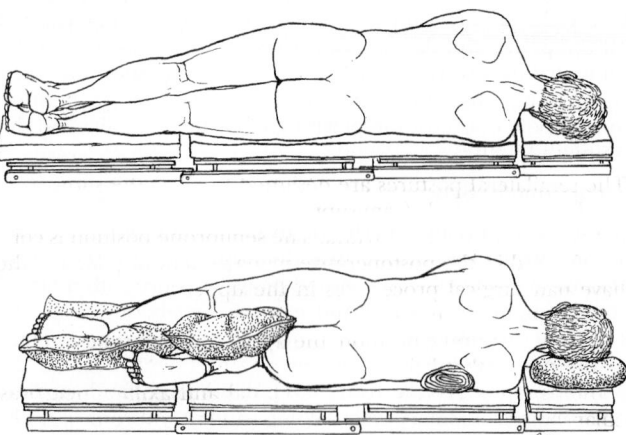

Figure 24-13. The standard lateral decubitus position. Proper head support, axillary roll, and leg pillow arrangement are shown on lower figure. Down-side leg is flexed at hip and knee to stabilize torso. Retaining straps and pad for down-side peroneal nerve are not shown. (Reproduced with permission from Martin JT, Warner MA [eds]: Positioning in Anesthesia and Surgery, 3rd ed. Philadelphia, WB Saunders, 1997.)

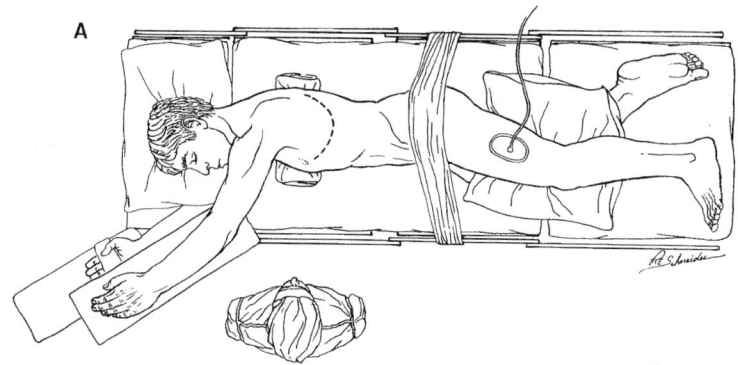

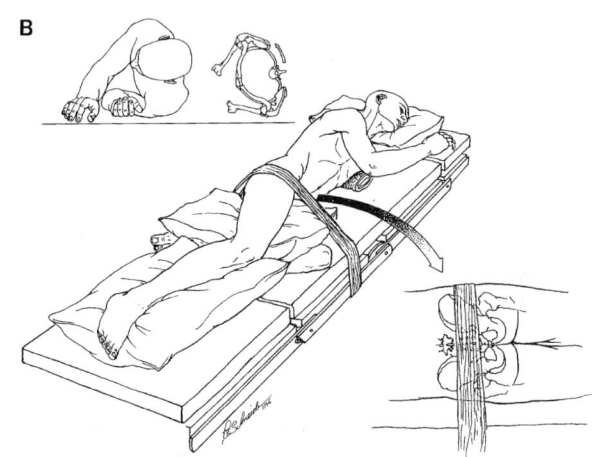

Figure 24-14. Lateral position with arms (*A*) arranged on two-tiered arm supports or (*B*) positioned in front of the patient's head either on pillows or on the table surface. Note the location of the stabilizing strap(s) between the iliac crest and the head of the up-side femur (*B, lower right*) rather than on the head of the femur. Potential ventral relocation of the torso can threaten the down-side axillary neurovascular bundle (*B, upper left*). (Reproduced with permission from Martin JT, Warner MA [eds]: Positioning in Anesthesia and Surgery, 3rd ed. Philadelphia, WB Saunders, 1997.)

method of arm arrangement is to flex each elbow and place the arms on suitable padding on the table in front of the patient's face (see Fig. 24-14*B*).

The patient is stabilized in the lateral position by the use of one or more retaining tapes stretched across the hip and fixed to the underside of the table top. Care must be taken to see that the hip tapes lie safely between the iliac crest and the head of the femur rather than over the head of the femur in a compressive manner that could result in its aseptic necrosis (see Fig. 24-14*B, lower insert*). An additional restraining tape may be used across the thorax if needed; it is functional and safe if placed just caudad of the axilla, where it has little effect on thoracic expansion, but it can be dangerous if placed across the costal margins, where it inevitably restricts ventilation.

Semisupine and Semiprone

The semilateral postures are designed to allow the surgeon to reach anterolateral (semisupine) and posterolateral (semiprone) structures of the trunk. The semiprone position is commonly used in the postoperative management of patients who have had surgical procedures in the upper airway and in the postanesthesia care of children.

In the semisupine position, the up-side arm must be carefully supported so that it is not hyperextended and no traction or compression is applied to the brachial and axillary neurovascular bundles (Fig. 24-15). The supporting bar should be well wrapped to prevent electrical grounding contact (see Fig. 24-15*A*). Sufficient noncompressible padding should be placed under the dorsal torso (see Fig. 24-15, *large figure*) and hip to prevent the patient from rolling supine and stretching the anchored extremity. The pulse of the restrained wrist should be checked to ensure adequate circulation in the elevated arm and hand (Fig. 24-15*B*).

If the patient in the semiprone position is rolled more than approximately halfway between lateral and prone positions, the down-side arm is usually placed dorsal to the torso to avoid stress on that shoulder (Fig. 24-16). The down-side lower extremity is straight, whereas the up-side lower extremity is flexed at the hip and knee to prevent further pronation.

Sims' Position

In 1857, the prominent New York City gynecologist J. Marion Sims began to use a modification of the lateral position for operations on the perineum, rectum, vagina, and bladder[70] (Fig. 24-17). Subsequently, it became widely used as a birthing posture. It resembles the semiprone position in that the down-side lower extremity is extended, the up-side is flexed at the hip and knee to expose the perineum, and the patient rolls slightly ventrad.

Flexed Lateral Positions

Lateral Jackknife. The lateral jackknife position places the down-side iliac crest over the hinge between the back and thigh sections of the table (Fig. 24-18). The table top is angulated at that point to flex the thighs on the trunk laterally. After the patient has been suitably positioned and restrained, the chassis of the table is tipped so that the uppermost surface of the patient's flank and thorax becomes essentially horizontal. As a result, the feet are below the level of the atria, and significant amounts of blood may pool in distensible vessels in each leg.

The lateral jackknife position is usually intended to stretch the up-side flank and widen intercostal spaces as an asset to a thoracotomy incision. However, in terms of lumbar stress, restriction by the taut flank of up-side costal margin motion, and pooling of blood in depressed lower extremities, its physiologic

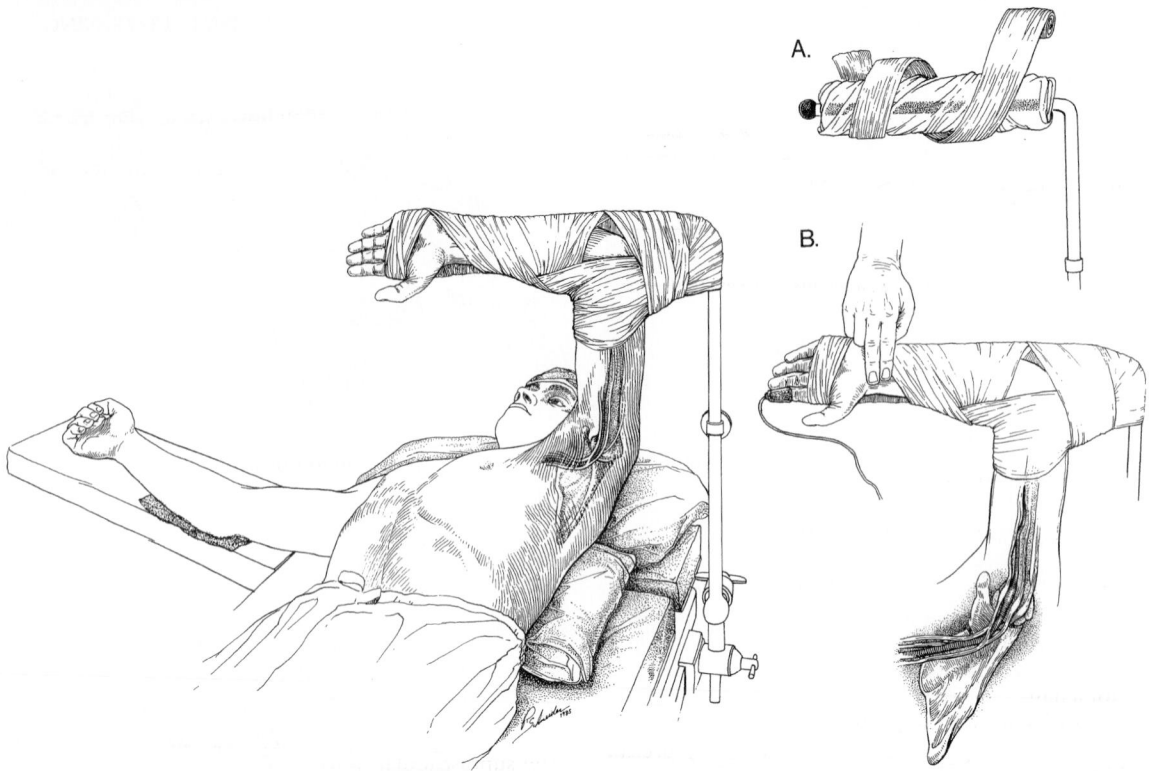

Figure 24-15. The semisupine position with dorsal pads supporting the torso, the extended arm padded at the elbow, and the elevated arm restrained on a well cushioned, adjustable overhead bar (*A*). Axillary contents (*B*) are not under tension and are not compressed by the head of the humerus, and a pulse oximeter ensures that the digital circulation is not compromised. The position is safe only if the arm does not become a hanging mechanism to support the torso. (Reproduced with permission from Collins VJ [ed]: Principles of Anesthesiology, 3rd ed. Philadelphia, Lea & Febiger, 1993.)

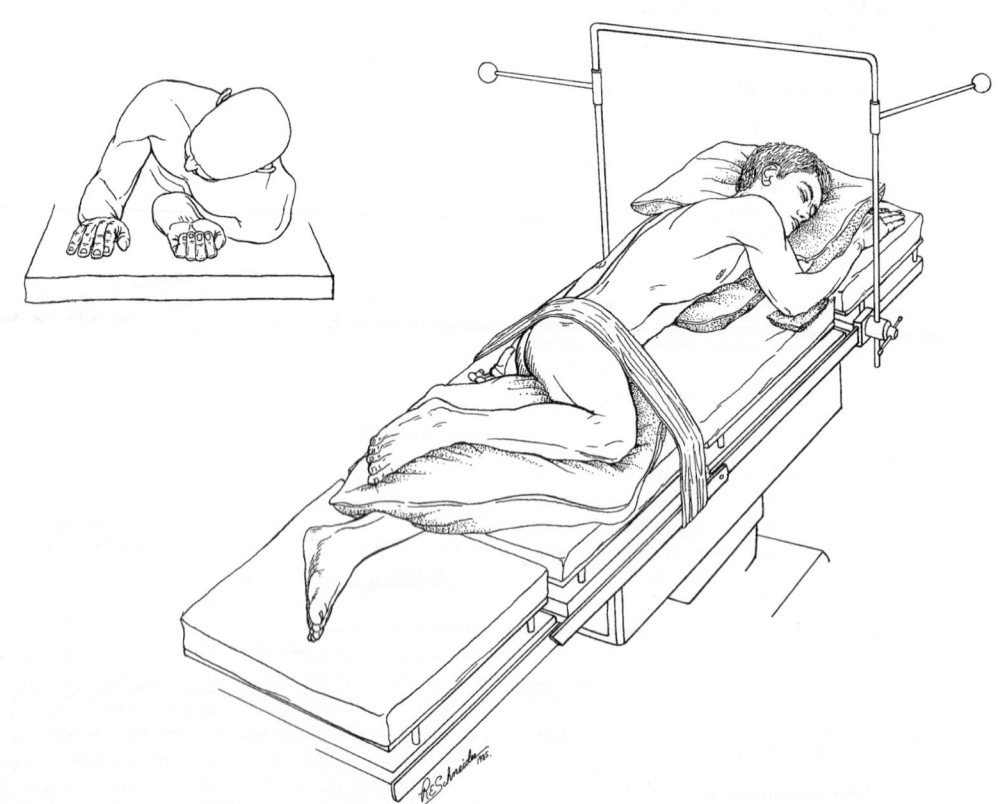

Figure 24-16. The semiprone position with the down-side leg extended and the up-side leg flexed at the knee, permitting moderate ventral rotation of the trunk. The down-side arm should be just behind the trunk to prevent axillary compression, as shown in the inset. (Reproduced with permission from Martin JT, Warner MA [eds]: Positioning in Anesthesia and Surgery, 3rd ed. Philadelphia, WB Saunders, 1997.)

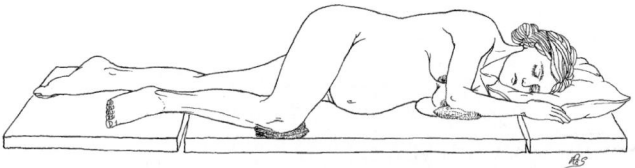

Figure 24-17. The Sims position, used as a means of access to the structures of the perineum. (Reproduced with permission from Martin JT, Warner MA [eds]: Positioning in Anesthesia and Surgery, 3rd ed. Philadelphia, WB Saunders, 1997.)

price is high. Actually, its usefulness to the surgeon is brief, and its use should be limited. Once the rib-spreading retractor is placed in the incision, the position is of no value for the rest of the operation.[71]

Kidney. The kidney position (Fig. 24-19) resembles the lateral jackknife position, but it adds the use of an elevated rest (the "kidney rest") under the down-side iliac crest to increase the amount of lateral flexion and improve access to the up-side kidney under the overhanging costal margin. Unlike the lateral jackknife position, the kidney position does not have a useful alternative for a flank approach to the kidney. Thus, the physiologic insults associated with the posture need to be limited by vigilant anesthesia and rapid surgery. Strict stabilizing precautions should be taken to prevent the patient from subsequently shifting caudad on the table in such a manner that the elevated rest relocates into the down-side flank and becomes a severe impediment to ventilation of the dependent lung.

Complications of the Lateral Decubitus Positions

Eyes and Ears

Injuries to the dependent eye are unlikely if the head is properly supported during and after the turn from the supine to the lateral position. If the patient's face turns toward the mattress, however, and the lids are not closed or the eyes otherwise protected, preventable abrasions of the ocular surface can oc-

cur. Direct pressure on the globe can displace the crystalline lens or, particularly if systemic hypotension is present, cause retinal ischemia.

In the lateral position, the weight of the head can press the down-side ear against a rough or wrinkled supporting surface. Careful padding with a pillow or a foam sponge is usually sufficient protection against contusion of the ear. The external ear should also be palpated to ensure that it has not been folded over in the process of placing support beneath the head.

Neck

Lateral flexion of the neck is possible when the head of a patient in the lateral position is inadequately supported. If the cervical spine is arthritic, postoperative neck pain can be troublesome. Pain from a symptomatic protrusion of a cervical disk can be intensified unless the head is carefully positioned so that lateral or ventral flexion, extension, or rotation is avoided. Patients with unstable cervical spines can be intubated while awake and turned gently into the operative position while repeated neurologic checks, with which the patient cooperates and responds, are accomplished to detect the development of a positioning injury.[72]

Suprascapular Nerve

Ventral circumduction of the dependent shoulder can rotate the suprascapular notch away from the root of the neck (Fig. 24-20). Because the suprascapular nerve is fixed both paravertebrally and at the notch, circumduction can stretch the nerve and produce troublesome, diffuse, dull shoulder pain. The diagnosis is established by blocking the nerve at the notch and producing pain relief. Treatment may require resecting the ligament over the notch to decompress the nerve. A supporting pad placed under the thorax just caudad of the axilla and thick enough to raise the chest off the shoulder should prevent a circumduction stretch injury to the nerve.

Long Thoracic Nerve

Instances of postoperative winging of the scapula (see Fig. 24-9) have followed use of the lateral decubitus position.[38] Although coincidental viral neuropathies of the long thoracic nerve may

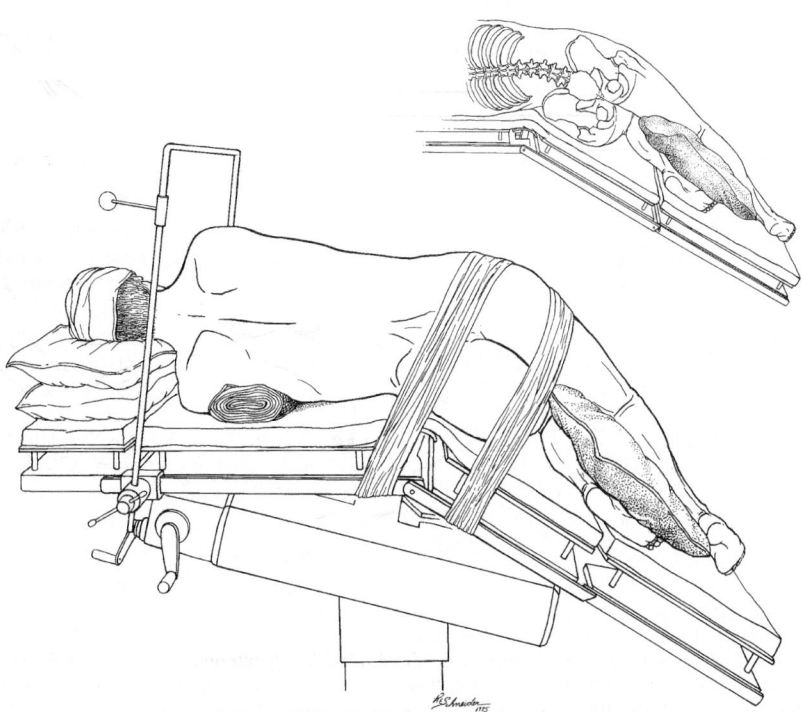

Figure 24-18. The lateral jackknife position, intended to open intercostal spaces. Note the properly placed restraining tapes (*large figure*) thrusting cephalad to retain the iliac crest at the flexion point of the table and prevent caudad slippage, which compresses the down-side flank (*insert*). (Reproduced with permission from Martin JT, Warner MA [eds]: Positioning in Anesthesia and Surgery, 3rd ed. Philadelphia, WB Saunders, 1997.)

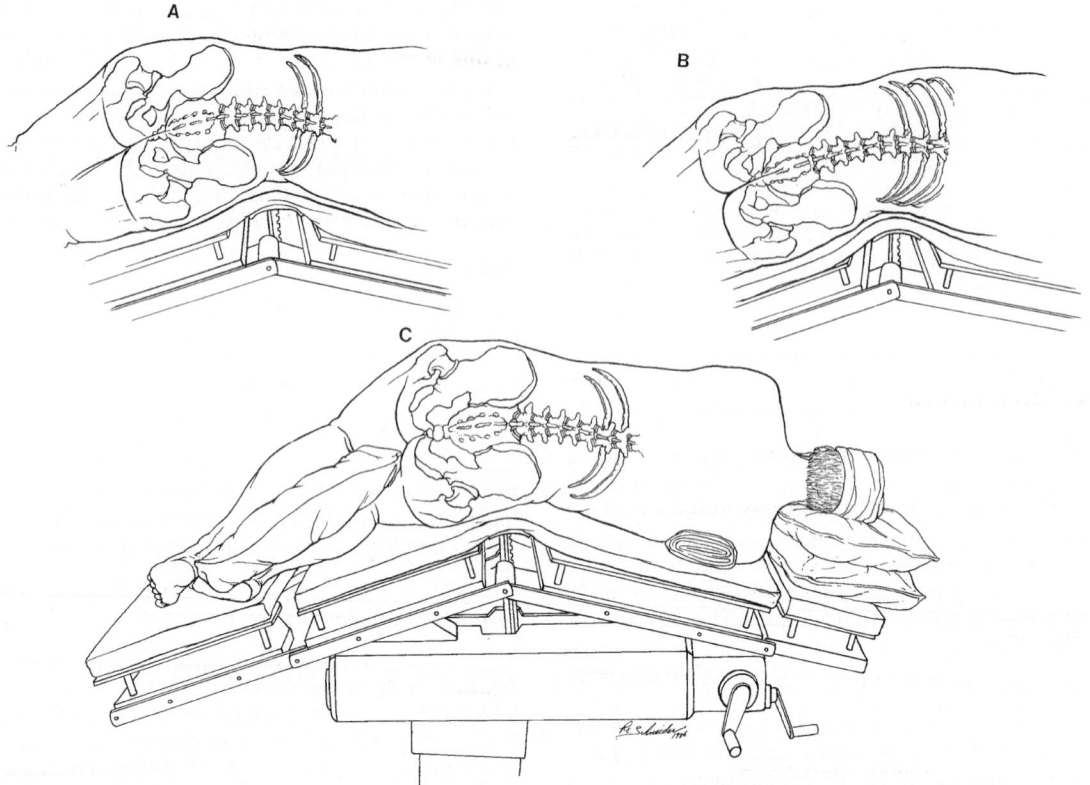

Figure 24-19. The flexed lateral (kidney) position. Upper panels show improper locations of the elevated transverse rest, the flexion point of the table, in the flank (*A*) or at the lower costal margin (*B*) to impede ventilation of the down-side lung. The iliac crest at the proper flexion point (*C*), allowing the best possible expansion of the down-side lung. Restraining tapes deleted for clarity. (Reproduced with permission from Martin JT, Warner MA [eds]: Positioning in Anesthesia and Surgery, 3rd ed. Philadelphia, WB Saunders, 1997.)

play a major etiologic role in postoperative appearances of scapular winging in patients for whom only a dorsal decubitus position was used, the possibility of trauma to the nerve while establishing the lateral position is difficult to refute. Lateral flexion of the neck may stretch the long thoracic nerve in the obtuse angle of the neck. A firm head pillow pressed firmly against the down-side thoracic outlet in theory can traumatize either the long thoracic nerve or the root of the brachial plexus.

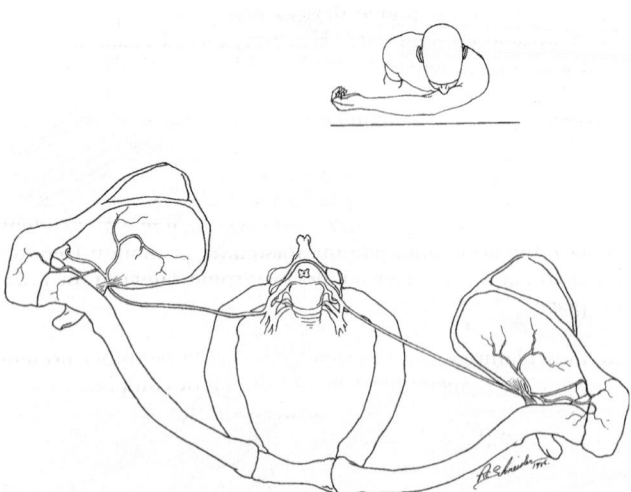

Figure 24-20. Circumduction of the arm displacing the scapula and stretching the suprascapular nerve between its anchoring points at the cervical spine and the suprascapular notch. (Reproduced with permission from Martin JT, Warner MA [eds]: Positioning in Anesthesia and Surgery, 3rd ed. Philadelphia, WB Saunders, 1997.)

Aseptic Necrosis of the Up-side Femoral Head

Compression of the head of the femur into the acetabulum by pressure from a misplaced restraining tape in the lateral decubitus position can result in aseptic necrosis of the hip. Obstruction of the nutrient artery to the femoral head is the assumed cause, and the incidence of the complication is not known. Nevertheless, the tapes that stabilize the patient should be carefully placed across the up-side hip on the soft tissue in the space between the head of the femur and the crest of the ilium to avoid direct pressure on the femoral head (see Fig. 24-18).

Unstable Spine

Turning a patient with an unstable vertebral column into the lateral position requires careful teamwork and a sufficient number of personnel to ensure gentle handling. Bivalve frames such as the Foster and Stryker are rarely used. If the trachea is intubated while the patient is awake, neurologic evaluations can be accomplished while the slow turn is in progress as well as after the final position is established.[72] Use of SSEP recordings before and after the turn may also be helpful. Having the responsible surgeon present and involved in establishing the desired position is prudent. Final support of the head and extremities should be accomplished before release of the patient by members of the turning team. Resumption of the supine position and movement of the patient to a bed or a transport cart require equally meticulous attention.

Peroneal Nerve

Pressure from weight of the down-side knee against the mattress may compress the common peroneal nerve as it courses laterally around the neck of the fibula. The patient's inability to dorsiflex the foot and loss of sensation over the dorsum of the foot indicate dysfunction of the nerve.[73] Padding the area of the head of the fibula is usually a sufficient precautionary measure.

VENTRAL DECUBITUS (PRONE) POSITIONS
Physiology

Circulatory

In the prone position, the circulatory dynamics vary according to the postural modification in use. If the legs remain essentially horizontal, pressure gradients in the blood vessels are minimal. If the patient is kneeling, or if the table chassis is rotated head high, significant pooling of venous blood in distensible dependent vessels is likely to occur.

With the patient lying on the soft abdominal wall, pressure of compressed viscera is transmitted to the dorsal surface of the abdominal cavity. Mesenteric and paravertebral vessels are compressed, causing engorgement of veins within the spinal canal. Obstruction of the inferior vena cava can produce immediate, visible distention of vertebral veins.[74] Because bleeding from incised vessels about the spine is increased under these circumstances, numerous modifications of the prone position have been created to free the abdomen from pressure, reduce the congestion of intraspinal veins, and facilitate surgical hemostasis.[74]

If the head of a prone patient is below the level of the heart, venous congestion of the face and neck becomes evident. Turning the patient's head can alter arterial perfusion and venous drainage in both extracranial and intracranial vessels. Conjunctival edema is usual and reflects the influence of gravity on accumulation of extravascular fluid.

If the head is above the level of the heart, mean vascular pressures are decreased according to the distance above the heart, air entrainment in open veins is possible, and conjunctival edema is less evident or absent.

Kaneko et al[69] described the perfusion of the entire lung of prone subjects in terms that subsequently fit the Zone 3 of West et al.[11] Backofen and Schauble[75] found that even the carefully established and supported prone position caused a significant fall in stroke volume and cardiac index, despite the development of increased vascular resistance in both the systemic and pulmonary circuits. No significant changes were detected in mean arterial pressure, right atrial pressure, or pulmonary artery occlusion pressure. On the basis of these observations, they recommend that, in patients whose cardiovascular status is precarious, invasive hemodynamic monitors be introduced to detect otherwise unrecognizable deterioration of cardiac function caused by positioning.

Respiratory

Using computed tomography, Gattinoni's group[76] found a dramatic redistribution of computed tomographic densities from the dorsal (paravertebral supine) to the ventral (substernal) portions of the lungs when subjects were turned from the supine to the prone position. The original areas of compression atelectasis reopened when those parts of the lung became nondependent, whereas fresh areas of compression atelectasis formed rather promptly in newly dependent areas of the lung. In their study group, they found no change in oxygenation or shunting when pronation occurred.

If the thorax is supple or compliant, the body weight of an anesthetized, prone patient compresses the anteroposterior diameter of the relaxed chest to a degree that is real but poorly defined. If the particular prone posture in use allows the pressure of the abdominal viscera to be sufficient to force the diaphragm cephalad, the lung is shortened along its long axis. With both the dorsoventral and the cephalocaudad dimensions of the lung decreased, and in the presence of the relative vascular congestion of a Zone 3 of West et al,[11,69] the compliance of the compacted prone lung can be anticipated to decrease. The result of decreased pulmonary compliance in a poorly positioned, prone, anesthetized patient is either an increased work of spontaneous ventilation or the need for higher inflation pressures during positive-pressure ventilation.

Proper positioning can retain more nearly normal pulmonary compliance by minimizing the cephalad shift of the diaphragm caused by compressed abdominal viscera. If the patient is arranged so that the abdomen hangs free, the loss of functional residual capacity is less in the prone position than in either the supine or the lateral position.[77] Rehder et al[78] noted that the weight of the freed abdominal contents had an "inspiratory effect on the diaphragm" when the pronated patient was properly supported by pads under the shoulder girdle and pelvis.

Variations of the Ventral Decubitus Position

Full (Horizontal) Prone

In the so-called *full* or *horizontal prone position* (Fig. 24-21), the requirement to elevate the trunk off the supporting surface so that the ventral abdominal wall is freed of compression almost always results in the head and lower extremities being below the level of the spine. If the table top is angulated at the trunk–thigh hinge to remove the lumbar lordosis and separate the lumbar spinous processes, and if the chassis is then rotated head-up sufficiently to level the patient's back, a significant perfusion gradient may develop between the legs and the heart. Wrapping the legs in compressive bandages, or the use of full-length elastic hosiery, minimizes pooling of blood in distensible vessels and supports venous return.

Various ventral supports, including parallel rolls of tightly packed sheets, padded and adjustable metal frames, and four-pillar frames, have been devised to free the abdomen from compression.[73,74] Each has merit, and no specific unit is unquestionably superior to all others. The choice is based on the physique of the patient, the requirements of the surgical procedure, and the available equipment.

Pronated patients with limited mobility of the neck, a history of postural neck pain, or a history suggesting a symptomatic cervical disk should have their heads retained in the sagittal plane, either with a skull-pin head clamp[79] or with a rocker-based face rest. If the neck is pain free and its mobility is satisfactory, the head can be turned laterally and supported on one of several soft sponge devices that prevents pressure on the down-side eye and ear.[80] However, forced rotation of the pronated head should be carefully avoided lest it induce postoperative neck pain.

When a patient is scheduled to be pronated after induction of anesthesia, it is worthwhile during the preanesthetic interview to obtain and record information about any limitations that may exist in his or her ability to raise the arms overhead during work or sleep.[74] If the patient is symptomatic, it may be prudent to place the arms alongside the torso after pronation (see the discussion of the Thoracic Outlet Syndrome, later). If the arms are placed alongside the head (i.e., extended ventrally at the shoulder, flexed at the elbow, and abducted onto arm boards), the musculature about the shoulders should be under no tension, neither humeral head should stretch or compress its axillary neurovascular bundle, ulnar nerves at the elbow should be padded, and the pulses at the wrists should remain full.

Prone Jackknife

The prone jackknife posture is used to provide access to the sacral, perianal, and perineal areas as well as to the lower alimentary canal (Fig. 24-22). The thighs are flexed on the trunk more than is usual in the full prone position, with the table surface hinges determining the degree of flexion achievable.[74]

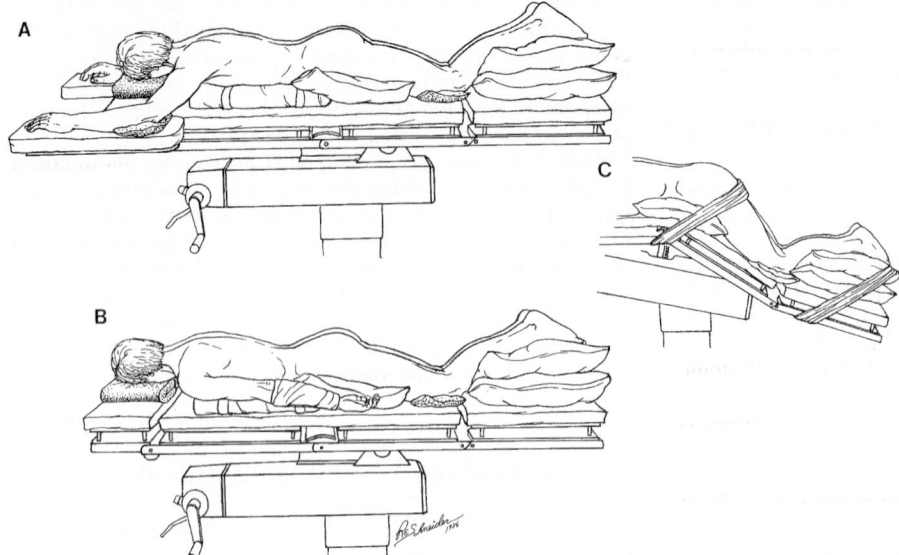

Figure 24-21. The classic prone position. (*A*) Flat table with relaxed arms extended alongside patient's head. Parallel chest rolls extended from just caudad of clavicle to just beyond inguinal area, with pillow over pelvic end. Elbows and knees are padded, and legs are bent at the knees. Head is turned onto a C-shaped foam sponge that frees the down-side eye and ear from compression. (*B*) Same posture with arms snugly retained alongside torso. (*C*) Table flexed to reduce lumbar lordosis; subgluteal area straps placed after the legs are lowered to provide cephalad thrust and prevent caudad slippage. (Reproduced with permission from Martin JT [ed]: Positioning in Anesthesia and Surgery, 3rd ed. Philadelphia, WB Saunders, 1997.)

Prone Kneeling

Kneeling positions have been used to improve operative conditions in the lumbar and cervico-occipital areas (Fig. 24-23). Numerous frames have been constructed to support the weight of a kneeling patient, and their usefulness again depends on local use and the physique of the patient. If the vertebral column is unstable, kneeling frames are not as useful as parallel longitudinal supports because kneeling risks application of shearing forces at the fracture site, with the potential for damage of the contents of the spinal canal. In massively obese patients who

must be operated on in the prone position, kneeling frames tend to prevent pressure on the abdomen more successfully than longitudinal frames.

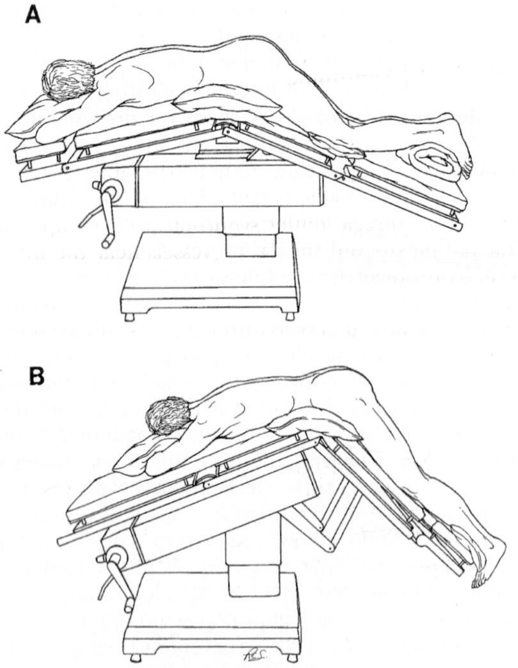

Complications of the Ventral Decubitus Positions

Eyes and Ears

The eyes and ears are at risk in the prone position even when the head is turned to one side. The eyelids should be closed, and each eye should be protected in some manner so that the lids cannot be accidentally separated and the cornea scratched. Instillation of lubrication in the eyes should be considered. Lightweight protective goggles have proved effective in this circumstance, although pressure injury from the goggle rims can occur. The eyes should also be protected against the head turning medially after positioning as well as against pressure being exerted on the globe. Monitoring wires and intravenous tubing should be checked after pronation to see that none has migrated underneath the head. If the head is retained in the sagittal plane, the eyes should be checked after positioning to ensure that they are safe from compression by the head rest.

Figure 24-22. The prone jackknife positions. (*A*) Low jackknife position with the trunk–thigh hinge of the table used as the flexion position and augmented by a pillow under the pelvis. (*B*) Full jackknife position with the thigh–leg hinge of the table used as the flexion point to achieve more acute angulation of the hips on the torso. (Reproduced with permission from Martin JT, Warner MA [eds]: Positioning in Anesthesia and Surgery, 3rd ed. Philadelphia, WB Saunders, 1997.)

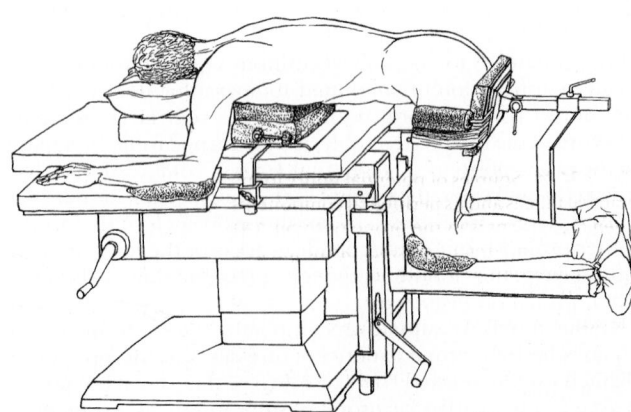

Figure 24-23. The Andrews kneeling frame with Wiltse's thoracic jack in use. (Reproduced with permission from Martin JT, Warner MA [eds]: Positioning in Anesthesia and Surgery, 3rd ed. Philadelphia, WB Saunders, 1997.)

Conjunctival edema usually occurs in the eyes of the pronated patient if the head is at or below the level of the heart. It is usually transient, inconsequential, and requires only reestablishment of the normal tissue perfusion gradients of the supine position, or of a slight amount of head-up tilt, to be redistributed.

Blindness. Permanent loss of vision can occur after nonocular surgical procedures, especially those performed in a ventral decubitus position.[81-90] Visual loss after neurovascular and cardiopulmonary bypass procedures is well recognized and may be related to embolic events produced by the surgical intervention itself.[91-93] Visual loss after noncardiac, non-neurovascular procedures may initially be noticed by a loss of acuity (implying a pathologic process of the optic nerve or retina), a loss of visual field (implying a cortical, or, less likely, optic nerve pathologic process), or both. Although permanent postoperative visual loss is thought to be unusual under such circumstances, there is little information beyond anecdotal speculation regarding the frequency of this event.

Reported causes of significant permanent postoperative visual loss usually involve compromise of oxygen delivery to elements of the visual pathway and include ischemic optic neuropathy (anterior or posterior), retinal artery occlusion (central or branch), and cortical blindness.[94] No case series exists to provide information regarding the frequency of these events after nonocular, noncardiac surgery in a general surgical population. Roth et al[83] surveyed approximately 61,000 patients undergoing nonocular surgery (including cardiac surgery) over a 4-year period and identified 34 ocular injuries (mostly corneal abrasions), including one case of permanent postoperative visual loss from ischemic optic neuropathy after lumbar spinal fusion. In a review of 3450 spinal surgeries, Stevens et al[89] identified 3 patients who had permanent postoperative visual loss. Brown et al[95] identified three patients in whom postoperative ischemic optic neuropathy developed after noncardiac surgery over a 10-year period in one institution.

Positioning appears to be a risk factor for some of these events. Studies noting a relative high frequency of postoperative visual loss in spinal surgery patients have implicated positioning as one causative factor.[84-87,90,93] Use of the knee–chest position,[84] the prone position,[85,90,96] and the horseshoe head rest[86] have been cited as potential causes of visual loss, perhaps by direct pressure on the globe increasing the intraocular pressure beyond the perfusion pressure of the retina. Other reports, including those of spinal surgery patients, describe visual loss after intraoperative hypotension and massive blood loss,[81-83,88,89] which may prevent adequate oxygen delivery to the visual apparatus. For example, all patients with ischemic optic neuropathy in the series of Brown et al[95] experienced periods of significant anemia (hemoglobin concentration <8 g/dl) and intraoperative hypotension. It is possible that venous congestion in the

head associated with the prone position may be a contributing factor.

Neck Problems

Anesthesia impairs reflex muscle spasm that protects the skeleton against motion that would be painful if the patient were alert. Lateral rotation of the head and neck of an anesthetized, pronated patient, particularly one with an arthritic cervical spine, can stretch relaxed skeletal muscles and ligaments and injure articulations of cervical vertebrae. Postoperative neck pain and limitation of motion can result. The arthritic neck is usually best managed by keeping the head in the sagittal plane when the patient is prone.

Extremes of head and neck rotation can also interfere with flow in either the ipsilateral or contralateral vessels to and from the head. Excessive head rotation can reduce flow in both the carotid[97] and vertebral systems.[98] Impaired cerebral perfusion is the obvious consequence.

Brachial Plexus Injuries

Stretch injuries to the roots of the brachial plexus (Fig. 24-24A) on the side contralateral to the turned face are possible if the contralateral shoulder is held firmly caudad by a wrist restraint. If an arm is placed on an arm board alongside the head, care must be taken to ensure that the head of the humerus is not stretching and compressing the axillary neurovascular bundle (see Fig. 24-24B,C).

When an arm is placed on an arm board alongside the head, the forearm naturally pronates. As a result, the ulnar nerve, lying in the cubital tunnel (the groove between the olecranon process and the medial epicondyle of the humerus), is vulnerable to being compressed by the weight of the elbow (see Fig. 24-24D). Consequently, the medial aspect of the elbow must be well padded and its weight borne principally on the medial epicondyle.

Repetitious and prolonged inflations of automated blood pressure cuffs may result in injurious compression of either the radial nerve in the musculospiral groove above the elbow or the ulnar nerve before it enters the cubital tunnel[10] (see Fig. 24-24E).

Thoracic Outlet Syndrome

Some patients complain of paresthesias in their arms after working with items on an overhead shelf, changing an overhead light bulb, or sleeping with one or both arms elevated alongside the head. The most likely explanation for the distress is the presence of a thoracic outlet syndrome with compression of the brachial plexus and subclavian vessels near the first rib.

As noted previously, it is recommended that all patients scheduled to be pronated should be questioned in the preanesthetic interview about their ability to work or sleep with arms elevated

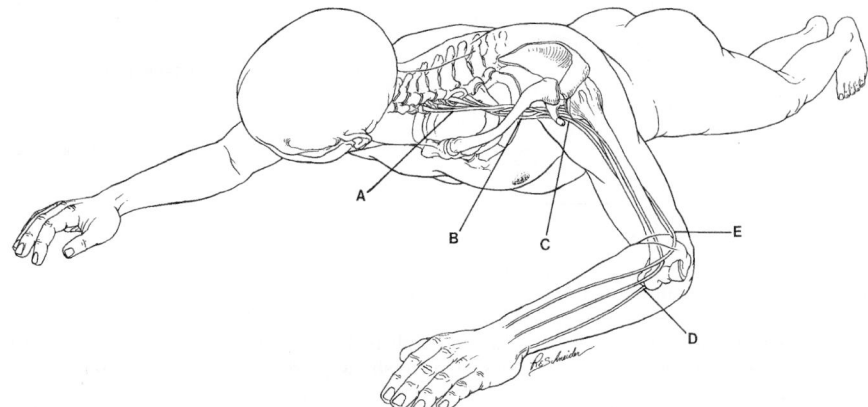

Figure 24-24. Sources of potential injury to the brachial plexus and its peripheral components when the patient is in the prone position. (*A*) Neck rotation stretching roots of the plexus. (*B*) compression of the plexus and vessels between the clavicle and first rib. (*C*) Injury to the axillary neurovascular bundle from the head of the humerus. (*D*) Compression of the ulnar nerve before, beyond, and within the cubital tunnel. (*E*) Area of vulnerability of the radial nerve to lateral compression proximal to the elbow. (Reproduced with permission from Martin JT, Warner MA [eds]: Positioning in Anesthesia and Surgery, 3rd ed. Philadelphia, WB Saunders, 1997.)

overhead, and their responses should be recorded on the charts.[74] A useful technique of inquiry if the history is in question is to have the patient clasp hands behind the occiput during the interview (Fig. 24-25). If the patient describes dysesthesias caused by having the arms overhead, or if dysesthesias occur while the patient is clasping hands on his or her occiput during the interview, it may be prudent to keep the arms alongside the trunk in the prone position. Agonizing, debilitating, and unremitting postoperative pain has been known to follow overhead arm placement in pronated patients who have had prior discomfort in their arms in that position.[74]

Breast Injuries

Average-sized breasts of a pronated woman, if forced laterally by ventral chest supports, can be stretched and injured along their sternal borders. Medial and cephalad displacement seems better tolerated. Massive breasts of a very large patient, if forced laterally, may not cause distress to the patient; however, if the arms are retained alongside of the torso, the huge breasts may force each arm far enough laterally to cause the surgical team difficulty in reaching the depths of an incision in the dorsal midline. Direct pressure on breasts containing enhancement prostheses can rupture the prosthesis. Tense skin grafts over mastectomy sites require considerable soft padding to prevent pressure necrosis and loss of the graft during a lengthy procedure in the prone position. No information has been located that pertains to gynecomastia and the prone position.

Coronary Artery Grafts

Mediastinal contents shift somewhat ventrad when a patient assumes the prone position. Apparently, the degree to which the ventrodorsal dimension of a stable chest is compressed by pronation can vary with the patient and the type of ventral supporting system used. Weinlander et al[99] reported a patient

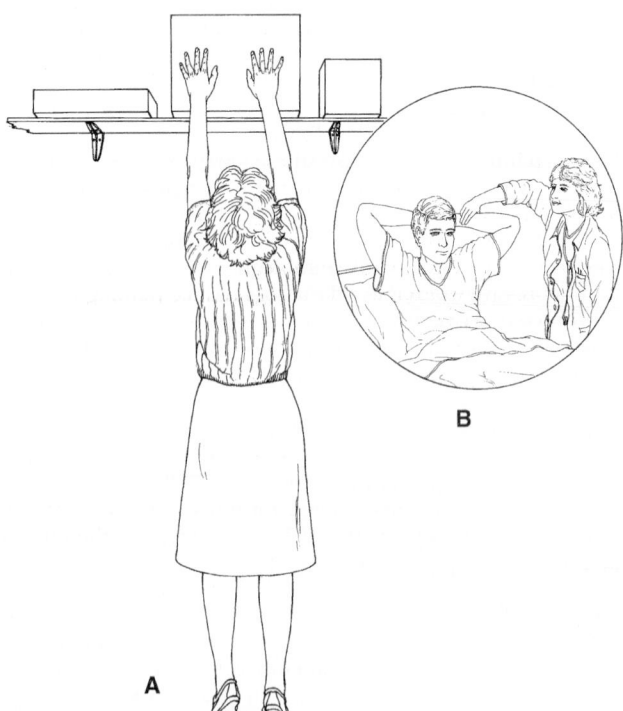

Figure 24-25. Assessment of a potential thoracic outlet syndrome. (*A*) The patient has a history of distress when trying to work or sleep with arms over head. (*B*) Interview was carried out with patient's hands clasped on occiput and radial pulses checked for damping. (Reproduced with permission from McLeskey CH [ed]: Geriatric Anesthesiology. Baltimore, Williams & Wilkins, 1997.)

who had received a coronary artery bypass graft 8 years previously and who had, in the interim, been successfully anesthetized for a lumbar laminectomy done in the prone position on longitudinal chest rolls. For a repeat laminectomy, he was anesthetized and placed on a kneeling frame. The sternum was elevated by a pad to relieve venous congestion of the head and neck. Electrocardiographic evidence of myocardial ischemia followed placement of the sternal pad, was not relieved by drug therapy, and necessitated intra-aortic balloon pump support for emergency coronary artery revascularization after the laminectomy. Although a number of questions remain unanswerable, Weinlander's group believed that sternal compression resulting from the pad adversely affected the previously functional coronary artery grafts and probably caused the ischemia. The implication that a sternal pad compresses the chest more than does a longitudinal frame is interesting, but further proof is needed.

The Unstable Spine

Pronating the patient whose spine is unstable requires skillful teamwork. (See also the previous discussion of lateral decubitus positions.) Enough people should be part of the turning team to control the weight being lifted without allowing sudden shifts of the patient's posture. Participation of the principal surgeon should be a requirement if stabilizing traction must be removed during positioning. Keeping the patient sedated but awake during tracheal intubation in the supine position permits multiple neurologic evaluations during pronation and final positioning to ensure that the maneuvers caused no new deficits.[72]

Use of bivalve nursing frames, such as the Foster or Stryker, allows anesthesia and intubation to be accomplished with the patient on the dorsal shell of the frame while traction is unchanged. Depending on the position of the neck in traction and the mobility of the mandible, fiberoptic or "blind" techniques may be needed for tracheal intubation. Addition of the ventral shell to the frame provides firm fixation of the patient during pronation. Removal of the dorsal shell after the turn permits the operation to be carried out on the remaining ventral shell without further risk from positioning torsion and without removing the corrective traction. Once the patient is pronated, care must be taken to ensure the stability of transoral anesthesia devices and the safety of the eyes and face.

Abdominal Compression

Compression of the abdomen by the weight of the prone patient's trunk can cause viscera to force the diaphragm cephalad enough to impair ventilation. If intra-abdominal pressure approaches or exceeds venous pressure, return of blood from the pelvis and lower extremities is reduced or obstructed. Because the vertebral venous plexuses communicate directly with the abdominal veins, increased intra-abdominal pressure is transmitted to the perivertebral and intraspinal surgical field in the form of venous distention and increased difficulty with hemostasis. All of the various supportive pads and frames, when properly used, are designed to remove pressure from the abdomen and avoid these problems.[74]

Viscerocutaneous Stomata

Stomata that drain visceral contents into containers affixed to the abdominal wall are at risk in the prone position if they lie against a part of the ventral supporting frame or pad (Fig. 24-26). Compressive ischemia of the stomal orifice can cause it to slough.

Knee Injuries

Extremely heavy patients, or those who have a pathologic condition of the knees, can have their knee joints injured in the kneeling position if the supportive ledges are not heavily padded (see Fig. 24-23). Often there is no suitable alternative position for these patients, and the possibility of postoperative knee

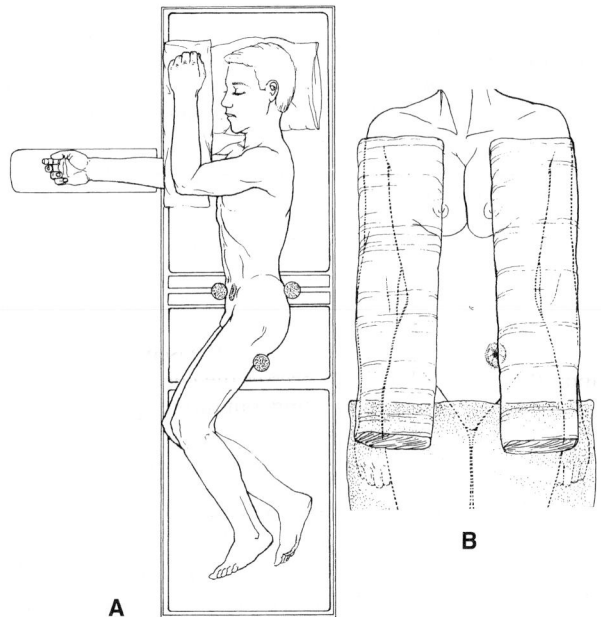

Figure 24-26. Postural supports compromising visceral stoma. Both the vertical abdominal support of a device designed to maintain a patient in the lateral position (*A*) and the longitudinal chest rolls supporting a pronated patient (*B*) can cause ischemic compression of a viscerocutaneous anastomosis and subsequent necrosis. Surgical repair of the stoma may be needed. (Reproduced with permission from McLeskey CH [ed]: Geriatric Anesthesiology. Baltimore, Williams & Wilkins, 1997.)

problems caused by the kneeling prone position should be carefully discussed in the preanesthetic interview.

HEAD-ELEVATED POSITIONS
Physiology
Circulatory

Coonan and Hope[100] have reviewed circulatory changes that occur in alert humans with the change from the supine to the erect position. As the head is raised above the level of the heart, pressure gradients develop and increase with the degree of elevation. Blood shifts from the upper body toward the feet. Atrial filling pressures decrease, sympathetic tone increases, parasympathetic tone decreases, the renin-angiotensin-aldosterone system is activated, and fluid and electrolytes are retained by the kidneys.[101,102] Intrathoracic blood volume decreases as much as 500 ml, pulmonary vascular resistance can double, and left atrial pressure falls more than right atrial pressure.[103] Cardiac output decreases 20–40%, and stroke volume falls by as much as 50%. Heart rate can increase by 30%. The arterial tree constricts, and systemic vascular resistance increases 30–60% to maintain a steady or increased mean arterial pressure, but the venous capacitance system is essentially unaffected.[104,105] Oxygen consumption by the tissues is unchanged; therefore, the reduced oxygen supply (reduced cardiac output) causes an increased arteriovenous oxygen content difference.[106]

Cerebral blood flow decreases by approximately 20% with high head elevation. Renal blood flow decreases as much as 30% (as much as 76% in massively obese patients in the sitting position), glomerular filtration decreases, and reduced secretion of antidiuretic hormone and aldosterone results in retention of water and sodium.[107]

Albin *et al*[108,109] and Dalrymple[110] noted similar alterations in cardiovascular parameters when the head-elevated position was established after patients were anesthetized. Although signifi-

cant changes were not encountered with less than 60 degrees of head-up tilt, the magnitude of changes was often greater than the awake patient values presented previously. The alterations increased progressively for more than 1 hour after the final posture was achieved. The question arose as to whether an impaired circulatory system could or should adjust to these stresses.

The presence of an intracranial pathologic process can be expected to exacerbate potentially harmful reductions in cerebral blood flow associated with head elevation.[111] In the anesthetized, seated patient, mean arterial pressure should be measured at the level of the circle of Willis because that site is more reliable as an indicator of cerebral perfusion pressure in the head-elevated posture than is measurement at the level of the arm or wrist.[100]

Respiratory

As the patient becomes more upright in the head-elevated dorsal decubitus position, the inspiratory stroke of the diaphragm becomes less impeded by the bulk of abdominal viscera. Spontaneous chest wall motion requires less effort, and less pressure is needed to inflate the lungs during passive inspiration. Functional residual capacity increases in the head-elevated positions.[112] Age-related increases in shunting are less in the head-elevated position than in the supine position.[112] Gurtner[113] found that the diffusing capacity for oxygen was reduced in the sitting position as a result of the gravity-related decreases in perfusion of the upper portions of the lungs. Slutsky *et al*,[114] however, found no difference between the supine position and the sitting position when measuring the ventilatory responses to hypoxia in volunteers.

Variations of the Head-Elevated Positions
Sitting

The full sitting position, characterized by the patient sitting upright in a chair, is uncommon in current practice. In the past it was used for instillation of air in the lumbar spine before pneumoencephalography, but now it is rarely chosen as a surgical position. It has disappeared as well in modern dental offices.

The classic sitting position for surgery places the patient in a semireclining posture on an operating table, with the legs elevated to approximately the level of the heart and the head flexed ventrally on the neck (Fig. 24-27). Head flexion should not be sufficient to force the chin into the suprasternal notch (see section on Midcervical Tetraplegia, later). Elastic stockings or compressive wraps around the legs reduce pooling of blood in the lower extremities. The head is held in place by some type of a face rest or by a three-pin skull fixation frame.

Supine—Tilted Head Up

A dorsal recumbent position with the head of the patient elevated somewhat is used for many operations involving the ventral and lateral aspects of the head (Fig. 24-28) and neck and occasionally, with the neck flexed, for transcranial access to the top of the brain. Its purpose is to improve access to the surgical target for the operating team as well as to drain blood and irrigation solutions away from the wound. The back section of the surgical table can be elevated as needed to produce a low sitting position (see Fig. 24-28*A*), or the entire table can be rotated head-high with the patient's extended legs supported by a foot rest (see Fig. 24-28*B*). Although the degree of tilt involved is not great, small pressure gradients are created along the vascular axis that can pool blood in the lower extremities or entrain air in patulous vessels that are incised above the level of the heart.

Vidabaek[115] has described a position (Fig. 24-29) that uses a modest degree of head elevation along with a carefully arched thoracolumbar spine to improve access to the organs of the

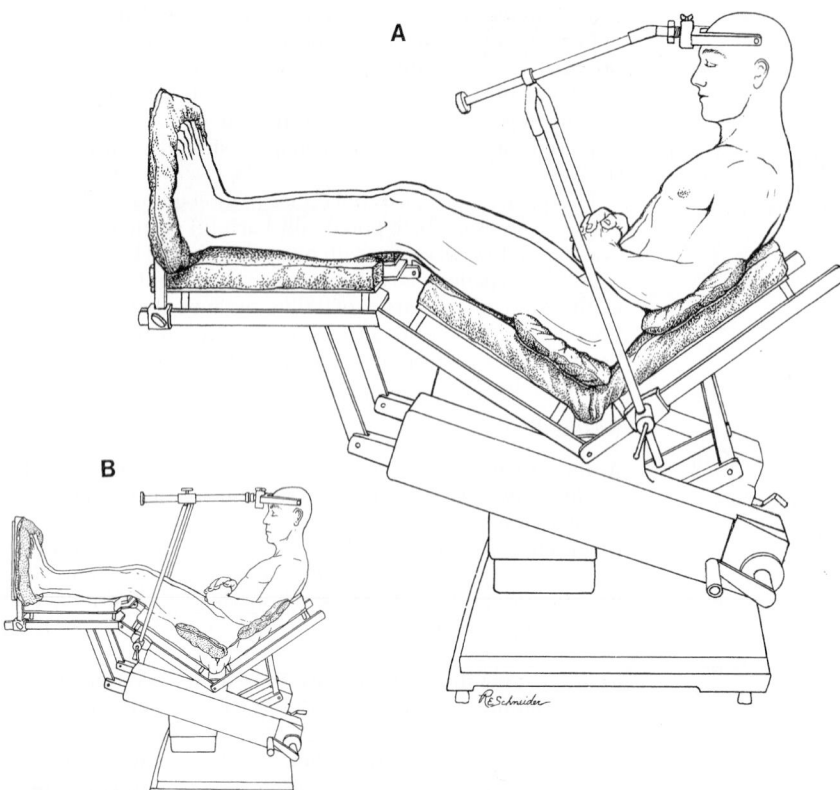

Figure 24-27. (*A*) Conventional neurosurgical sitting position. The legs are at approximately the level of the heart and gently flexed on the thighs; the feet are supported at right angles to the legs; subgluteal padding protects the sciatic nerve. The frame of the head holder is *properly* clamped to the side rails of the back section in the event of hemodynamically significant air embolism. (*B*) *Improper* attachment of the head frame to the table side rails at the thigh section. In this position, the patient's head could not be quickly lowered because it would require disengaging the skull clamp. (Reproduced with permission from Martin JT, Warner MA [eds]: Positioning in Anesthesia and Surgery, 3rd ed. Philadelphia, WB Saunders, 1997.)

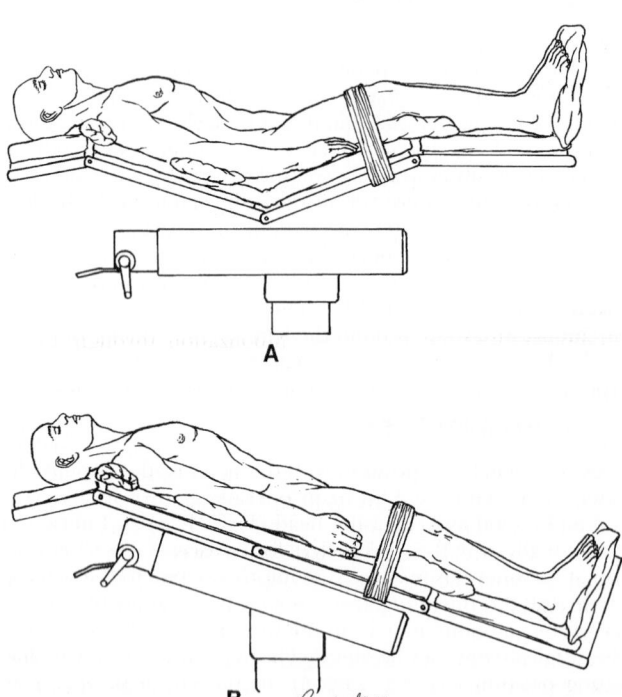

Figure 24-28. Head-elevated positions often used for operations about the ventral and ventrolateral aspects of the head, face, neck, and cervical spine. (*A*) The legs are at approximately heart level and the gradient into the head is appreciable but slight. (*B*) The flat table and foot rest are useful when a thyroidectomy is planned under regional anesthesia. (Reproduced with permission from Martin JT, Warner MA [eds]: Positioning in Anesthesia and Surgery, 3rd ed. Philadelphia, WB Saunders, 1997.)

upper abdomen. In a small series, he noted its usefulness to the surgeon as well as its associated difficulties for patients with precarious cardiovascular systems.

For operations around the shoulder joint, the patient is often placed in a head-elevated semisupine position, with the upper torso rotated toward the nonsurgical shoulder and supported by a firm roll or pad (Fig. 24-30). The upper trunk is moved laterally until the raised surgical shoulder extends beyond the edge of the operating table. The torso is supported so that the hips are on the table, the surgical shoulder is off and above the table edge, and the head rests on either a pillow (see Fig. 24-30A) or a horseshoe head rest (see Fig. 24-30B). Access is thereby provided to both the dorsal and ventral aspects of the shoulder girdle. The surgical arm remains on the ventral torso and is prepared and draped to be mobile in the surgical field.

Lateral—Tilted Head Up

The lateral decubitus position with the head somewhat elevated, a means of access to occipitocervical lesions, has also been referred to as the *park bench position*.[116] All the stabilizing requirements needed for the usual lateral decubitus position apply. The head is held firmly in a three-pin skull fixation holder, which can be readjusted as needed during surgery. Although the degree of head elevation used is mild, the position does not completely remove the threat of air embolization. The anesthesiologist has good access to the patient's face and ventral thorax for purposes of monitoring, manipulation, and resuscitation. Considerable attention should be directed to avoiding compression of neck veins, which can lead to an increase in intracranial pressure and to edema of the tongue.

Prone—Tilted Head Up

The ventral decubitus posture with the table rotated head high (Fig. 24-31) has become a widely used replacement for the sitting position as a means of access to dorsal structures of the head and neck. Usually the perceived advantage of the position

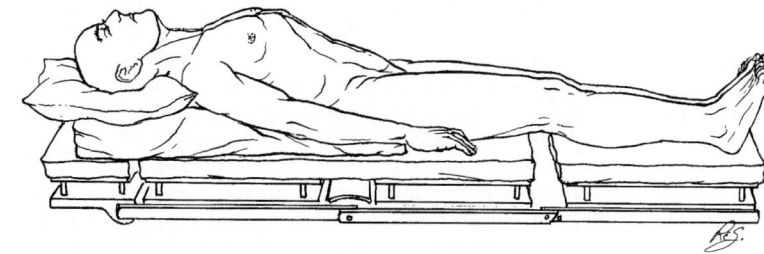

Figure 24-29. The xiphoid-high posture of Vidabaek used to gain access to the upper abdomen. (Reproduced with permission from Martin JT, Warner MA [eds]: Positioning in Anesthesia and Surgery, 3rd ed. Philadelphia, WB Saunders, 1997.)

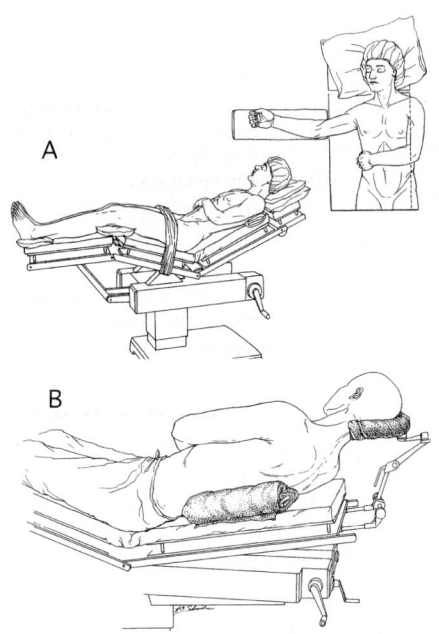

Figure 24-30. (A) The barber chair position for surgery around the shoulder joint. (B) The upper torso is rotated toward the nonsurgical shoulder and supported with a firm roll or pad. (Reproduced with permission from Martin JT, Warner MA [eds]: Positioning in Anesthesia and Surgery, 3rd ed. Philadelphia, WB Saunders, 1997.)

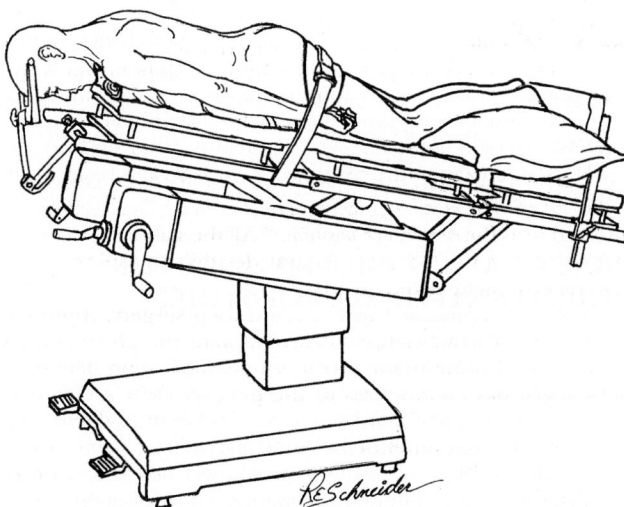

Figure 24-31. The skull-pin head rest used to stabilize a patient in the head-elevated prone position. Note the chest rolls used to free the abdomen from compression and the gluteal strap to minimize caudad slippage after head-up tilt. (Reproduced with permission from Martin JT, Warner MA [eds]: Positioning in Anesthesia and Surgery, 3rd ed. Philadelphia, WB Saunders, 1997.)

is the avoidance of air embolization. Although the pressure gradients for air entrainment into patulous veins are less than in the full sitting position, the hazard is not eliminated. As a result of the positive-pressure inflation cycle of passive ventilation, a bothersome recurrent flux of cerebrospinal fluid into and out of the exposed wound may be encountered. The posture also severely restricts resuscitative access to the ventral thorax.

Complications of the Head-Elevated Positions

Postural Hypotension

In the anesthetized patient, establishing any of the head-elevated positions is frequently accompanied by some degree of reduction in systemic blood pressure. The normal protective reflexes are inhibited by drugs used during anesthesia. Measuring mean arterial pressures at the level of the circle of Willis is recommended to assess cerebral perfusion pressures more accurately. Treatment of hypotension consists of temporarily delaying the elevation of the head as the patient is positioned; reducing the concentration of anesthetic drugs; infusing crystalloids or colloids to increase effective circulating volume; and using appropriately small amounts of a vasopressor as a temporary expedient.

Air Embolus

Air embolization is potentially lethal. In the bloodstream, air migrates to the heart, where it creates a compressible foam that destroys the propulsive efficiency of ventricular contraction and irritates the conduction system. Air can also move into the pulmonary vasculature, where bubbles obstruct small vessels and compromise gas exchange, or it can cross through a patent foramen ovale to the left side of the heart and the systemic circulation.

Opportunities for venous air embolization through an incised vein in a surgical wound located above the heart increase with the degree of elevation of the operative site. Although the occurrence of air emboli is a relatively frequent phenomenon in head-elevated positions, most of the emboli are small in volume, clinically silent, and recognizable only by sophisticated detection techniques. Nevertheless, the potential for continuing, dangerous accumulations of entrained air requires immediate detection of the embolization, a careful search for its portal of entry, and prompt treatment of its clinical effects.

Air embolism may be diagnosed by the presence of one or several of the following, in any order: a change in heart sounds noted by a parasternal Doppler probe; a cardiac murmur; cardiac dysrhythmias; hypotension; a decrease in expired carbon dioxide; the appearance of nitrogen in the expired air; and the sudden appearance of vigorous spontaneous ventilation despite continuing mechanical ventilation. Air bubbles in the central circulation can also be recognized with transesophageal echocardiography.

Approximately 20–35% of the population[117] has a residual foramen ovale that is functionally closed as long as pressure in the left atrium exceeds that in the right. However, in the sitting position, right atrial pressure can be higher than left. That gradient, augmented by (1) the presence of air in the right side of the heart, (2) positive-pressure ventilation, and (3) positive end-expiratory pressure, may be sufficient to reopen an existing probe-patent, but functionally closed, foramen ovale. Air in the right atrium thereby gains paradoxical access to the coronary, cerebral, and systemic circulations.[118] In anesthetized and newly positioned patients, Perkins-Pearson et al[119] suggest that, when pulmonary artery occlusion pressures are found to be lower than right atrial pressures, the head-elevated posture should be abandoned in favor of a position in which the head is level with the heart.

Cucchiara and associates[120] have injected agitated saline through a right-sided heart catheter and used transesophageal echocardiography to detect paradoxical passage of fluid across the atrial septum. Positive-airway pressure aided in determining paradoxical flow in 3 of their 20 patients.

Pneumocephalus

In the usual craniotomy, most of the brain lies subjacent to the incision. After the dura is incised, cerebrospinal fluid is removed to improve working conditions, and the surgical field is open to the air. During closure of the craniotomy, most of the intracranial air escapes from the wound and any residual pneumocephalus is of little consequence. However, when an incision is made through the dura in the posterior fossa or cervical spine of a seated patient, the bulk of the brain lies above the incision. Cerebrospinal fluid drains downward out of the wound, and tissue retraction can allow air to bubble up over the surfaces of the brain to become trapped in the upper reaches of the cranium.[121] When brain mass is decreased by ventricular drainage, steroids, and diuresis, the space available to a pneumocephalus is enlarged. Diffusion of nitrous oxide into the accumulated air, or the warming of trapped gas, can produce a tension pneumocephalus with signs of increased intracranial pressure and delayed awakening from anesthesia.

Toung et al[122] found postoperative pneumocephalus in all of a group of seated patients and in most of those who had been in the prone or the park bench position. Intraventricular air was present in most of the seated patients and was rare in those in the other positions. None of their group of 100 patients had neurologic changes attributable to the trapped intracranial air. Standefer et al[123] reported a 3% incidence of symptomatic (tension) pneumocephalus in seated, anesthetized patients whose duras were opened.

Ocular Compression

Pressure from a padded head rest on the eyes of a patient who has been placed in a head-elevated position can dislocate a crystalline lens or render the globe ischemic. Unilateral blindness has been reported as a result (see section on Blindness, earlier).[124] Modern skull-pin head clamps that grip firmly when properly applied have made ocular compression in the sitting position a rarity. In the head-elevated lateral decubitus or prone position, the threats to the eyes are those described in the preceding discussions of those nonelevated postures.

Edema of the Face, Tongue, and Neck

McAllister[125] has encountered severe postoperative macroglossia, apparently due to venous and lymphatic obstruction caused by prolonged, marked neck flexion. The patient's chin was firmly against the chest and an oral airway was in place to protect the endotracheal tube. Ellis et al[126] reported a similar patient who needed a tracheostomy because of massive swelling of the tongue, lips, pharynx, and epiglottis occurring shortly after extubation at the end of administration of a lengthy anesthetic in the sitting position that involved deliberate hypotension. Extremes of neck flexion, with or without head rotation, have been widely used to gain access to structures in the posterior fossa and cervical spine, but their potential for damage should be understood and excessive flexion–rotation avoided

if possible. Moore and associates[127] have described five cases of macroglossia in patients with posterior fossa disease and have suggested that the primary mechanism is neurologically determined rather than being the result of either vascular obstruction or local trauma.

Midcervical Tetraplegia

This devastating injury occurs after marked flexion of the neck, with or without rotation of the head, and is attributed to stretching of the spinal cord with resulting compromise of its vasculature in the midcervical area. An element of spondylosis or a spondylotic bar may be involved.[128,129] The result is paralysis below the general level of the fifth cervical vertebra. Although most reports in the literature have described the condition as occurring after the use of the sitting position, midcervical tetraplegia has also occurred after prolonged, nonforced head flexion for intracranial surgery in the supine position. The role of a tethered cord in the production of the syndrome has not been established. No useful preoperative evaluation can as yet establish the potential for this complication.

Reversible changes in SSEPs elicited by stimulation of the median nerve have been found to occur after neck flexion.[130,131] However, in studies with monkeys, Cottrell et al[132] have shown that SSEPs may not be sensitive enough to detect midcervical tetraplegia, and Levy and associates[133] have suggested using motor evoked potentials for this purpose.

Sciatic Nerve

Stretch injuries of the sciatic nerve can occur in some seated patients if the hips are markedly flexed without bending the knees. Prolonged compression of the sciatic nerve as it emerges from the pelvis is possible in a thin, seated patient if the buttocks are not suitably padded. Foot drop may be the result of injuries to either the sciatic nerve or the common peroneal nerve and can be bilateral.

AMERICAN SOCIETY OF ANESTHESIOLOGISTS ADVISORY ON PREVENTION OF PERIOPERATIVE PERIPHERAL NEUROPATHIES

The American Society of Anesthesiologists approved an advisory on peripheral neuropathies in 1999.[134] This advisory includes pertinent literature and a summary of the opinions of anesthesia providers on a variety of positioning and peripheral neuropathy issues. The paucity of literature related to these issues limited the advisory to recommendations based on opinions and current practices of a broadly representative group of anesthesia providers from around the United States. Additional input and opinions were obtained from consultants from around the world. A summary of the findings of the advisory is shown in Table 24-1.

PRACTICAL CONSIDERATIONS FOR PERIOPERATIVE NEUROPATHIES

Efforts to prevent perioperative neuropathies are frequently debated, and there often is confusion over how to manage a neuropathy once it has occurred. In general, there are no data to support recommendations on any of these issues. Therefore, the following opinions have been formulated by personal experience, guided by advice from neurologists who primarily care for patients with peripheral neuropathies, and seasoned or supported by speculation derived from anecdotal case reports.

Padding Exposed Peripheral Nerves

Many types of padding materials are advocated to protect exposed peripheral nerves. They often consist of cloth (e.g., blan-

Table 24-1. SUMMARY OF TASK FORCE CONSENSUS

Preoperative assessment: When judged appropriate, it is helpful to ascertain that patients can comfortably tolerate the anticipated operative position.

Upper extremity positioning:
- Arm abduction should be limited to 90 degrees or less in supine patients. Patients who are positioned prone may comfortably tolerate arm abduction of 90 degrees or more.
- Arms should be positioned to decrease pressure on the postcondylar groove of the humerus (ulnar groove). When arms are tucked at the side, a neutral forearm position is recommended. When arms are abducted on arm boards, either supination or a neutral forearm position is acceptable.
- Prolonged pressure on the radial nerve in the spiral groove of the humerus should be avoided.
- Extension of the elbow beyond a comfortable range may stretch the median nerve.

Lower extremity positioning:
- Lithotomy positions that stretch the hamstring muscle group beyond a comfortable range may stretch the sciatic nerve.
- Prolonged pressure on the peroneal nerve at the fibular head should be avoided.
- Neither extension nor flexion of the hip increases the risk of femoral neuropathy.

Protective padding:
- Padded armboards may decrease the risk of upper extremity neuropathy.
- The use of chest rolls in laterally positioned patients may decrease the risk of upper extremity neuropathies.
- Padding at the elbow and at the fibular head may decrease the risk of upper and lower extremity neuropathies, respectively.

Equipment:
- Properly functioning automated blood pressure cuffs on the upper arms do not affect the risk of upper extremity neuropathies.
- Shoulder braces in steep head-down positions may increase the risk of brachial plexus neuropathies.

Postoperative assessment: A simple postoperative assessment of extremity nerve function may lead to early recognition of peripheral neuropathies.

Documentation: Charting specific positioning actions during the care of patients may result in improvements of care by (1) helping practitioners focus attention on relevant aspects of patient positioning, and (2) providing information that continuous improvement processes can use to lead to refinements in patient care.

kets and towels), foam sponges (*e.g.*, "eggcrate" foam), and gel pads. There are no data to suggest that any of these materials is more effective than any other, or that any is better than no padding at all. A good rule of thumb would be to position and pad exposed peripheral nerves to (1) prevent their stretch beyond normally tolerated limits while awake; (2) avoid their direct compression, if possible; and (3) distribute over as large an area as possible any compressive forces that must be placed on them.

Prolonged Duration in One Position

Prolonged duration in one position appears to increase the risk of neuropathy and other integumentary damage. For example, prolonged duration in lithotomy positions greatly increases the risk of lower extremity neuropathy.[135,136] When possible, it would appear prudent to limit as much as practical the time any patient spends in one position. However, intermittent movement of the limbs or head during the intraoperative period may increase the opportunity for a number of different problems, including but not limited to dislodging an endotracheal tube, abrading a cornea, or moving an extremity into a suboptimal position. Practitioners must judge the benefits *vs.* risks of any intraoperative changes in a patient's position.

Course of Action for the Patient With a Neuropathy

Although each situation is unique and requires careful assessment, the following guidelines may suggest a basic course of action that will lead to appropriate care:

- Is the neuropathy sensory or motor? Sensory lesions are more frequently transient than motor lesions. If the symptoms are numbness or tingling only, it may be appropriate to inform the patient that many of these neuropathies can be expected to resolve during the first 5 days.[50] The patient should be instructed to avoid postures that might compress or stretch the involved nerve. Arrangements should be made for frequent contact with the patient. A call to alert a neurologist is appropriate, and if the symptoms still persist on postoperative day 5, the neurologist should be consulted.
- If the neuropathy has a motor component, a neurologist should be consulted immediately. Electromyographic studies may be needed to assess the location of any acute lesion. This knowledge may direct an appropriate treatment plan. The studies may also demonstrate chronic abnormalities of the nerve or, if applicable, the contralateral nerve.

REFERENCES

1. Martin JT, Warner MA (eds): Positioning in Anesthesia and Surgery, 3rd ed. Philadelphia, WB Saunders, 1997
2. Anderton JM, Keen RI, Neave R (eds): Positioning the Surgical Patient. London, Butterworths, 1988
3. Enderby GEH: Postural ischemia and blood pressure. Lancet 1:185, 1954
4. Green DM, Metheny D: Estimation of acute blood loss by tilt test. Surgical Gynecology and Obstetrics 84:1045, 1947
5. Kubal K, Komatsu T, Sanchala V *et al:* Trendelenburg position used during venous cannulation increases myocardial oxygen demands. Anesth Analg 63:239, 1984
6. Porter WT: Shock at the front. Boston Medical and Surgical Journal 175:874, 1916
7. Sibbald WJ, Patterson NAM, Holliday RL *et al:* The Trendelenburg position: Hemodynamic effects in hypotensive and normotensive patients. Crit Care Med 7:218, 1979
8. Dripps RD, Comroe JH Jr: Circulatory physiology: The adjustments to blood loss and postural changes. Surg Clin North Am 26: 1368, 1946
9. Burch GE: Method for recording simultaneously the time course of digital rate and of digital volume of inflow and outflow during a single pulse cycle in man. J Appl Physiol 7:99, 1954
10. Coonan TJ, Hope CE: Cardiorespiratory effects of changes of body position. Canadian Anaesthetists Society Journal 30:424, 1983
11. West JB, Dollery CT, Naimark A: Distribution of blood flow in isolated lung: Relations to vascular and alveolar pressures. J Appl Physiol 19:713, 1964
12. Froese AB, Bryan AC: Effects of anesthesia and paralysis on diaphragmatic mechanics in man. Anesthesiology 41:242, 1974
13. Warner MA: Supine positions. In Martin JT, Warner MA (eds): Positioning in Anesthesia and Surgery, 3rd ed, p 39. Philadelphia, WB Saunders, 1977
14. Smith BE: Obstetrics. In Martin JT, Warner MA (eds): Positioning in Anesthesia and Surgery, 3rd ed, p 267. Philadelphia, WB Saunders, 1997
15. Martin JT: 1992–Compartment syndromes: Concepts and perspectives for the anesthesiologist. Anesth Analg 75:275, 1992
16. Little DM: Posture and anesthesia. Canadian Anaesthetists Society Journal 7:2, 1960
17. Angermeier KW, Jordan GH: Complications of the exaggerated lithotomy position: A review of 177 cases. J Urol 151:866, 1994
18. Halliwill JR, Hewitt SA, Joyner MJ *et al:* Effects of various lithotomy positions on lower extremity blood pressures. Anesthesiology 89:1373, 1999
19. Wilcox S, Vandam LD: Alas, poor Trendelenburg and his position! A critique of its uses and effectiveness. Anesth Analg 67:574, 1988
20. Meyer W: Ueber die Nachbehandlung des hohen Steinschnittes sowie ueber Verwenbarkeit desselben zur Operation von Blasenscheidenfisteln. Archiv für Klinische Chiruque 31:494, 1885

21. Cannon WB: Traumatic Shock. New York, Appleton and Co, 1923
22. Cole F: Head lowering in the treatment of hypotension. JAMA 150:273, 1952
23. Weil MH: Current concepts in the management of shock. Circulation 16:1097, 1957
24. Guntheroth WG, Abel FL, Mullins GL: The effect of Trendelenburg's position on blood pressure and carotid flow. Surgical Gynecology and Obstetrics 119:354, 1964
25. Taylor J, Weil MH: Failure of the Trendelenburg position to improve circulation during clinical shock. Surgical Gynecology and Obstetrics 124:1005, 1976
26. Reich DL, Konstadt SN, Hubbard M, Thys DM: Do Trendelenburg and passive leg raising improve cardiac performance? Anesth Analg 67:S184, 1988
27. Keusch DJ, Winters S, Thys DM: The patient's position influences the incidence of dysrhythmias during pulmonary artery catheterization. Anesthesiology 70:582, 1989
28. Abel RR, Lewis GM: Postoperative alopecia. Arch Dermatol 81:72, 1960
29. Gormley T, Sokoll MD: Permanent alopecia from pressure of a headstrap. JAMA 199:157, 1967
30. Lawson NW, Mills NL, Ochsner JL: Occipital alopecia following cardiopulmonary bypass. J Thorac Cardiovasc Surg 71:342, 1976
31. Jellish WS, Blakeman B, Warf P, Slogoff S: Hands-up positioning during asymmetric sternal retraction for internal mammary artery harvest: A possible method to reduce brachial plexus injury. Anesth Analg 84:260, 1997
32. Vander Salm TJ, Cereda J-M, Cutler BS: Brachial plexus injury following median sternotomy. J Thorac Cardiovasc Surg 80:447, 1980
33. Vander Salm TJ, Cutler BS, Okike ON: Brachial plexus injury following median sternotomy: Part II. J Thorac Cardiovasc Surg 83:914, 1982
34. Roy RC, Stafford MA, Charlton JE: Nerve injury and musculoskeletal complaints after cardiac surgery: Influence of internal mammary artery dissection and left arm position. Anesth Analg 67:277, 1988
35. Gregg JR, Labosky D, Harty M et al: Serratus anterior paralysis in the young athlete. J Bone Joint Surg Am 61:825, 1979
36. Johnson JTH, Kendall HO: Isolated paralysis of the serratus anterior muscle. J Bone Joint Surg Am 37:567, 1955
37. Foo CL, Swann M: Isolated paralysis of the serratus anterior. J Bone Joint Surg Br 65:552, 1983
38. Martin JT: Postoperative isolated dysfunction of the long thoracic nerve: A rare entity of uncertain etiology. Anesth Analg 69:614, 1989
39. Britt BA, Gordon RA: Peripheral nerve injuries associated with anesthesia. Canadian Anaesthetists Society Journal 11:514, 1964
40. Bickler PE, Schapera A, Bainton CR: Acute radial nerve injury from use of an automatic blood pressure monitor. Anesthesiology 73:186, 1990
41. Kroll DA, Caplan RA, Posner K et al: Nerve injury associated with anesthesia. Anesthesiology 73:202, 1990
42. Cheney FW, Domino KB, Caplan RA et al: Nerve injury associated with anesthesia. Anesthesiology 90:1062, 1999
43. Chusid JG: Correlative Neuroanatomy and Functional Neurology, p 145. Los Altos, CA: Lange Medical Publications, 1985
44. Büdinger K: Ueber Lähmungen nach Chloroform-Narkosen. Archiv für Klinische Chiruque 47:121, 1894
45. Garriques HJ: Anaesthesia-paralysis. Am J Med Sci 133:81, 1897
46. Wadsworth TG, Williams JR: Cubital tunnel external compression syndrome. BMJ 1:662, 1973
47. Warner MA, Warner DO, Harper CM et al: Ulnar neuropathy in medical patients. Anesthesiology 92:613, 2000
48. Warner MA, Warner ME, Martin JT: Ulnar neuropathy: Incidence, outcome, and risk factors in sedated or anesthetized patients. Anesthesiology 81:1332, 1994
49. Alvine FG, Schurrer ME: Postoperative ulnar-nerve palsy: Are there predisposing factors? J Bone Joint Surg 69:255, 1987
50. Warner MA, Warner DO, Matsumoto JY et al: Ulnar neuropathy in surgical patients. Anesthesiology 90:54, 1999
51. Prielipp RC, Morell RC, Walker FO et al: Ulnar nerve pressure: Influence of arm position and relationship to somatosensory evoked potentials. Anesthesiology 91:345, 1999
52. Campbell WW, Pridgeon RM, Riaz G et al: Variations in anatomy of the ulnar nerve at the cubital tunnel: Pitfalls in the diagnosis of ulnar neuropathy at the elbow. Muscle Nerve 14:733, 1991

53. O'Driscoll SW, Horii E, Carmichael SW et al: The cubital tunnel and ulnar neuropathy. J Bone Joint Surg Am 73:613, 1991
54. Childress HM: Recurrent ulnar nerve dislocation at the elbow. J Bone Joint Surg 38:978, 1956
55. Ashenhurst EM: Anatomical factors in the etiology of ulnar neuropathy. CMAJ 87:159, 1962
56. Macnicol MF: Extraneural pressures affecting the ulnar nerve at the elbow. Hand 14:5, 1982
57. Pechan J, Julis I: The pressure measurement in the ulnar nerve: A contribution to the pathophysiology of the cubital tunnel syndrome. J Biomech 8:75, 1975
58. Contreras MG, Warner MA, Charboneau WJ et al: The anatomy of the ulnar nerve at the elbow: Potential relationship of acute ulnar neuropathy to gender differences. Clin Anat 11:372, 1998
59. Shimokata H, Tobin JD, Muller DC et al: Studies in the distribution of body fat: I. Effects of age, sex, and obesity. J Gerontol 44:66, 1989
60. Hattori K, Numata N, Ikoma M et al: Sex differences in the distribution of subcutaneous and internal fat. Hum Biol 63:53, 1991
61. Chusid JG: Correlative Neuroanatomy and Functional Neurology, p 149. Los Altos, CA: Lange Medical Publications, 1985
62. Hill NA, Howard FM, Huffer BR: The incomplete anterior interosseous nerve syndrome. J Hand Surg [Am] 10:4, 1985
63. Hofmann A, Jones RE, Schoenvogel R: Pudendal nerve neuropraxia as a result of traction on the fracture table. J Bone Joint Surg Am 64:136, 1982
64. Lindenbaum SD, Fleming LL, Smith DW: Pudendal nerve palsies associated with closed intramedullary femoral fixation. J Bone Joint Surg Am 64:934, 1982
65. Orken DE: Modern concepts of the role of nephrotoxic agents in the pathogenesis of acute renal failure. Prog Biochem Pharmacol 7:219, 1972
66. Matsen FA III: Compartmental syndrome: A unified concept. Clin Orthop 113:8, 1975
67. Courington FW, Little DM Jr: The role of posture in anesthesia. Clinical Anesthesia 3:24, 1968
68. Martin JT: Lithotomy positions. In Martin JT, Warner MA (eds): Positioning in Anesthesia and Surgery, 3rd ed, p 47. Philadelphia, WB Saunders, 1997
69. Kaneko K, Milic-Emily J, Dolovich MB et al: Regional distribution of ventilation and perfusion as a function of body position. J Appl Physiol 21:767, 1966
70. Sims JM: In Silver Suture in Surgery: The Anniversary Discourse Before the New York Academy of Medicine. Nov. 18, 1857. New York, Samuel S. and William Wood, 1858
71. Lawson NW, Meyer DJ Jr: The lateral decubitus position: Anesthesiologic considerations. In Martin JT, Warner MA (eds): Positioning in Anesthesia and Surgery, 3rd ed, p 127. Philadelphia, WB Saunders, 1997
72. Lee C, Barnes A, Nagel EL: Neuroleptanalgesia for awake pronation of surgical patients. Anesth Analg 56:276, 1977
73. Chusid JG: Correlative Neuroanatomy and Functional Neurology, p 157. Los Altos, CA: Lange Medical Publications, 1985
74. Martin JT: The ventral decubitus (prone) positions. In Martin JT, Warner MA (eds): Positioning in Anesthesia and Surgery, 3rd ed, p 155. Philadelphia, WB Saunders, 1997
75. Backofen JE, Schauble JR: Hemodynamic changes with prone positioning during general anesthesia. Anesth Analg 64:194, 1985
76. Gattinoni L, Pelosi P, Vitale G et al: Body position changes redistribute lung computed-tomographic density in patients with acute respiratory failure. Anesthesiology 74:15, 1991
77. Douglas WW, Rehder K, Beynen FM et al: Improved oxygenation in patients with acute respiratory failure: The prone position. American Review of Respiratory Disease 115:559, 1977
78. Rehder K, Knopp TJ, Sessler AD: Regional intrapulmonary gas distribution in awake and anesthetized-paralysed prone man. J Appl Physiol 45:528, 1978
79. Reid SA, Grundy BL: The head-elevated positions: Surgical aspects: The neurosurgical skull clamp. In Martin JT, Warner MA (eds): Positioning in Anesthesia and Surgery, 3rd ed, p 71. Philadelphia, WB Saunders, 1997
80. Gravenstein N, Grundy BL, Lobato EB: The central nervous system. In Martin JT, Warner MA (eds): Positioning in Anesthesia and Surgery, 3rd ed, p 291. Philadelphia, WB Saunders, 1997
81. Johnson MW, Kincaid MC, Trobe JD: Bilateral retrobulbar optic nerve infarctions after blood loss and hypotension. Ophthalmology 94:1577, 1987

82. Rizzo JF, Lessell L: Posterior ischemic optic neuropathy during general surgery. Am J Ophthalmol 103:808, 1987

83. Roth S, Thisted RA, Erickson JP et al: Eye injuries after nonocular surgery. Anesthesiology 85:1020, 1996

84. Stambough JL, Cheeks ML: Central retinal artery occlusion: a complication of the knee-chest position. J Spinal Disord 5:363, 1992

85. Bekar A, Türeyen K, Aksoy K: Unilateral blindness due to patient positioning during cervical syringomyelia surgery: Unilateral blindness after prone position. J Neurosurg Anesthesiol 8:227, 1996

86. Myers MA, Hamilton SR, Bogosian AJ et al: Visual loss as a complication of spinal surgery. Spine 22:1325, 1997

87. Katz DM, Trobe JD, Cornblath WT et al: Ischemic optic neuropathy after lumbar spine surgery. Arch Ophthalmol 112:925, 1994

88. Katzman SS, Moschonas CG, Dzioba RB: Amaurosis secondary to massive blood loss after lumbar spine surgery. Spine 19:468, 1994

89. Stevens WR, Glazer PA, Kelley SD et al: Ophthalmic complications after spinal surgery. Spine 22:1319, 1997

90. Levin H, Ben-David B: Transient blindness during hysteroscopy: A rare complication. Anesth Analg 81:880, 1995

91. Sweeny PJ, Breuer AC, Selshorst JB et al: Ischemic optic neuropathy: A complication of cardiopulmonary bypass surgery. Neurology 32:560, 1982

92. Shaw PJ, Bates D, Cartlidge NEF, et al: Neurologic and neuropsychologic morbidity following major surgery: Comparison of coronary artery bypass and peripheral vascular surgery. Stroke 18:700, 1987

93. Shapira OM, Kimmel WA, Lindsey PS, et al: Anterior ischemic optic neuropathy after open heart operations. Ann Thorac Surg 61:660, 1996

94. Roth S, Gillesberg I: Injuries to the visual system and other sense organs. In Benumof JL, Saidman LJ (eds): Anesthesia and Perioperative Complications, 2nd ed. St. Louis, Mosby, 1999

95. Brown RH, Schauble JF, Miller NR: Anemia and hypotension as contributors to perioperative vision loss. Anesthesiology 80:222, 1994

96. Connolly SE, Gordon KB, Horton JC: Salvage of vision after hypotension-induced ischemic optic neuropathy. Am J Ophthalmol 117:235, 1994

97. Sherman DD, Hart RG, Easton JD: Abrupt change in head position and cerebral infarction. Stroke 12:2, 1981

98. Toole JF: Effects of change of head, limb and body position on cephalic circulation. N Engl J Med 279:307, 1968

99. Weinlander CM, Coombs DW, Plume SK: Myocardial ischemia due to obstruction of an aortocoronary bypass graft by intraoperative positioning. Anesth Analg 64:933, 1985

100. Coonan TJ, Hope CE: Cardio-respiratory effects of change of body position. Canadian Anaesthetists Society Journal 30:424, 1983

101. Sonkodi S, Agabiti-Rosei E, Fraser R et al: Response of the renin-angiotensin-aldosterone system to upright tilting and to intravenous furosemide: Effect of prior metoprolol and propranolol. Br J Clin Pharmacol 13:341, 1982

102. Williams GH, Cain JP, Dluly RG et al: Studies on the control of plasma aldosterone concentration in normal man: 1. Response to posture, acute and chronic volume depletion and sodium loading. J Clin Invest 51:1731, 1972

103. Fournier P, Mensch-Dechene J, Ranson-Bitker B et al: Effect of sitting up on pulmonary blood pressure, flow and volume in man. J Appl Physiol 46:36, 1979

104. Gauer OH, Thron HL: Postural changes in the circulation. In Hamilton WF, Dow P (eds): Handbook of Physiology, Section 2, Vol 3, p 2409. Washington, DC, American Physiological Society, 1965

105. Ward RJ, Danziger F, Bonica JJ et al: Cardiovascular effects of change of posture. Aerospace Med 37:257, 1966

106. Bevegard S, Holmgren A, Jonsson B: The effect of body position on the circulation at rest and during exercise, with special reference to the influence on the stroke volume. Acta Physiol Scand 49:279, 1960

107. Rhodes JM, Graham-Brown RAC, Sarkany I: Reversible renal failure in an obese patient: Hazard of sitting with feet continuously elevated. Lancet 2:96, 1979

108. Albin MS, Janetta PJ, Maroon JC et al: Anaesthesia in the sitting position. In Recent Progress in Anaesthesiology and Resuscitation. Amsterdam, Excerpta Medica International Congress Series No. 347:775, 1975

109. Albin MS, Babinski M, Wolf S: Cardiovascular response to the sitting position (letter). Br J Anaesth 52:961, 1980

110. Dalrymple DG: Cardiorespiratory effects of the sitting position in neurosurgery. Br J Anaesth 51:1079, 1979

111. Shenkin HA, Scheuerman EB, Spitz EB et al: Effect of change of posture upon cerebral circulation of man. J Appl Physiol 2:317, 1949

112. Don HF: The measurement of trapped gas in the lungs at functional residual capacity and the effects of posture. Anesthesiology 35:582, 1971

113. Gurtner GH: Interrelationships of factors affecting pulmonary diffusing capacity. J Appl Physiol 30:619, 1979

114. Slutsky AS, Goldstein RG, Rebuck AS: The effect of posture on ventilatory response to hypoxia. Canadian Anaesthetists Society Journal 27:445, 1980

115. Vidabaek F: Posture with elevated and extended thorax. Acta Anaesthesiol Scand 24:458, 1980

116. Gilbert RGB, Brindle F, Galindo A: Anesthesia for Neurosurgery, p 126. Boston, Little, Brown, 1966

117. Hagen PT, Scholz DG, Edwards WD: Incidence and size of patent foramen ovale during the first ten decades: A necropsy study of 965 normal hearts. Mayo Clin Proc 59:17, 1984

118. Gronert GA, Messick JM, Cucchiara RF et al: Paradoxical air embolism from a patent foramen ovale. Anesthesiology 50:548, 1979

119. Perkins-Pearson NAK, Marshall WK, Bedford RF: Atrial pressures in the seated position: Implications for paradoxical air embolism. Anesthesiology 57:493, 1982

120. Cucchiara RF, Seward JB, Nishimura RA et al: Identification of patent foramen ovale during sitting position craniotomy by transesophageal echocardiography with positive airway pressure. Anesthesiology 63:107, 1985

121. Kitahata LM, Katz JD: Tension pneumocephalus after posterior fossa craniotomy, a complication of the sitting position. Anesthesiology 44:448, 1976

122. Toung TKJ, McPherson RW, Ahn H: Pneumocephalus: Effects of patient position on incidence of aerocele after posterior fossa and upper cervical cord surgery. Anesth Analg 65:65, 1986

123. Standefer M, Bay JW, Trusso R: The sitting position in neurosurgery: A retrospective analysis of 488 cases. Neurosurgery 14:649, 1984

124. Hollenhorst RW, Svein HJ, Benoit CF: Unilateral blindness occurring during anesthesia for neurosurgical operations. Arch Ophthalmol 52:819, 1954

125. McAllister RG: Macroglossia: A positional complication. Anesthesiology 40:199, 1974

126. Ellis SC, Bryan-Brown CW, Hyderally H: Massive swelling of the head and neck. Anesthesiology 42:102, 1975

127. Moore JK, Chaudhri S, Moore AP, Easton J: Macroglossia and posterior fossa disease. Anaesthesia 43:382, 1988

128. Hitselberger WE, House WF: A warning regarding the sitting position for acoustic tumor surgery. Archives of Otolaryngology 106:69, 1980

129. Wilder BL: Hypothesis: The etiology of midcervical quadriplegia after operation with the patient in the sitting position. Neurosurgery 11:530, 1982

130. McCallum JE, Bennett MH: Electrophysiologic monitoring of spinal cord function during intraspinal surgery. Surgical Forum 26:469, 1975

131. McPherson RW, Szymanski J, Rogers MC: Somatosensory evoked potential changes in position-related brain stem ischemia. Anesthesiology 61:88, 1984

132. Cottrell JE, Hassan NF, Hartung J et al: Hyperflexion and quadriplegia in the seated position. Anesthesiology Review 5:34, 1985

133. Levy WJ, York OH, McCaffrey M et al: Motor evoked potentials from transcranial stimulation of the motor cortex in humans. Neurosurgery 15:287, 1984

134. American Society of Anesthesiologists Task Force on Prevention of Perioperative Peripheral Neuropathies: Practice advisory for the prevention of perioperative peripheral neuropathies. Anesthesiology 92:1168, 2000

135. Warner MA, Martin JT, Schroeder DR et al: Lower extremity motor neuropathy associated with surgery performed on patients in a lithotomy position. Anesthesiology 81:6, 1994

136. Warner MA, Warner DO, Harper CM et al: Lower extremity neuropathies associated with the lithotomy position. Anesthesiology (in press)

Clinical Anesthesia (4/e), edited by
Paul G. Barash, Bruce F. Cullen, and
Robert K. Stoelting. Lippincott Williams &
Wilkins, Philadelphia, © 2001.

CHAPTER 25

MONITORING THE ANESTHETIZED PATIENT

GLENN S. MURPHY AND JEFFERY S. VENDER

Monitoring represents the process by which anesthesiologists recognize and evaluate potential physiologic problems in a timely manner. The term is derived from *monere,* which in Latin means to warn, remind, or admonish. In perioperative care, monitoring implies the following four essential features: observation and vigilance, instrumentation, interpretation of data, and initiation of corrective therapy when indicated.

Monitoring is an essential aspect of anesthesia care. Patient safety is enhanced when appropriate monitoring is operational and clinical judgments are proper. Effective monitoring reduces the potential for poor outcomes that may follow anesthesia by identifying derangements before they result in serious or irreversible injury. Electronic monitors improve a physician's ability to respond because they are able to make repetitive measurements at higher frequencies than humans, and do not fatigue or become distracted. Monitoring devices increase the specificity and precision of clinical judgments. At no time in the history of anesthesia have practitioners had the capability routinely to monitor so many diverse physiologic variables in real time, often noninvasively, as they do today. Our understanding of the physiologic effects of anesthesia and its inherent risks is enhanced by using appropriate intraoperative physiologic monitoring.

This chapter discusses the methods by which anesthesiologists monitor organ function during anesthesia care. The descriptions of the technologic and scientific principles used in monitoring devices have been simplified for clarity.

Cost containment has been raised as a reason to discourage the use of expensive, technologically advanced monitoring systems. The value of a given monitor depends on the clinical expertise of the anesthesiologist, the clinical setting, the anesthetic technique, and the performance of the specific equipment in question. Monitoring devices should not be denied solely on the basis of expense.[1] Although it is appropriate for society to demand cost containment, anesthesiologists have a responsibility to assess how monitoring should be used. Professional societies, regulatory agencies, and the legal profession have played important roles in establishing current monitoring practices.

Standards for basic anesthetic monitoring have been established by the American Society of Anesthesiologists (ASA). Since 1986, these standards have emphasized the evolution of technology and practice. Today's standards (last amended on October 25, 1995) emphasize the importance of regular and frequent measurements, integration of clinical judgment and experience, and the potential for extenuating circumstances that can influence the applicability or accuracy of monitoring systems.[2]

Standard I requires qualified personnel to be present in the operating room, to monitor the patient continuously and modify anesthesia care based on clinical observations and the responses of the patient to dynamic changes resulting from surgery or drug therapy. Standard II focuses attention on continually evaluating the patient's oxygenation, ventilation, circulation, and temperature. Standard II specifically mandates the following:

1. Using an oxygen analyzer with a low concentration limit alarm during general anesthesia.

2. Quantitative assessment of blood oxygenation during any anesthesia care.
3. Continuously ensuring the adequacy of ventilation by physical diagnostic techniques during all anesthesia care. Quantitative monitoring of tidal volume and capnography are encouraged in patients undergoing general anesthesia.
4. Ensuring the adequacy of circulation by the continuous display of the electrocardiogram (ECG), and determining the arterial blood pressure at least at 5-minute intervals. During general anesthesia, circulatory function is to be continually evaluated by assessing the quality of the pulse, either electronically or by palpation or auscultation.
5. Endotracheal intubation requires qualitative identification of carbon dioxide in the expired gas. During general anesthesia, capnography and end-tidal carbon dioxide analysis are encouraged.
6. During all anesthetics, the means for continuously measuring the patient's temperature must be available. When changes in body temperature are intended or anticipated, temperature should be continuously measured and recorded on the anesthesia record.

The ASA standards emphasize the melding of physical signs with instrumentation. Electronic monitoring, no matter how sophisticated or comprehensive, does not necessarily reduce the need for clinical skills such as inspection, palpation, and auscultation. Although the authors believe that electronic monitors augment clinical judgments when properly used, there is little evidence that electronic monitors, by themselves, reduce mortality or morbidity. Moreover, there is considerable controversy regarding the need to apply specific monitors in unique clinical situations, particularly those that may add significant cost. Monitoring can be classified as invasive, minimally invasive, or noninvasive. Invasive monitors place patients at risk for complications related to their application and use. Anesthesiologists must balance the potential risk of instituting invasive monitoring with the presumed benefits derived from its application.

The variety of devices available for patient monitoring is expansive and changing as advances in biomedical engineering find their way into the marketplace. The Association for the Advancement of Medical Instrumentation has been effective in promoting design guidelines to ensure patient and operator safety and reduce stress and distractions often associated with medical monitoring.[3]

The proliferation of alarm tones during anesthesia care can be disturbing and may paradoxically impair clinical vigilance. Monitoring systems may be insufficiently sensitive to reject errors. During routine anesthesia care, a minimum of five alarms (inspired oxygen, airway pressure, oximetry, blood pressure, and heart rate) should be operational. Unfortunately, spurious warnings occur with high frequency during routine anesthesia monitoring. The integration of alarm signals is an important area in need of continuing evaluation. Loeb[4] reported that anesthesia providers have difficulty in accurately recognizing the source of an alarm tone. Alarm annunciators using unique sound and visual prompts are being incorporated into anesthesia equipment. Warning signals for ventilation, oxygenation, drug administration, temperature, and cardiovascular parameters need to be designed so that problem identification is fast, simple, and relevant.

INSPIRATORY AND EXPIRED GAS MONITORING: OXYGEN

The concentration of oxygen in the anesthetic circuit must be measured. Measuring inspired oxygen does not guarantee the adequacy of arterial oxygenation.[5] Gas machine manufacturers place oxygen sensors on the inspired limb of the anesthesia circuit to ensure that hypoxic gas mixtures are never delivered to patients. Oxygen monitors require a fast response time (2–10 seconds), accuracy (±2%), and stability when exposed to humidity and inhalation agents.

Paramagnetic Oxygen Analysis

Oxygen is a highly paramagnetic gas. Paramagnetic gases are attracted to magnetic energy because of unpaired electrons in their outer shell orbits. Differential paramagnetic oximetry has been incorporated into a variety of operating room monitors (Datex Medical Instruments, Inc. Tewksbury, Massachusetts). These instruments detect the change in sample line pressure resulting from the attraction of oxygen by switched magnetic fields. Signal changes during electromagnetic switching correlate with the oxygen concentration in the sample line.

Galvanic Cell Analyzers

Galvanic cell analyzers meet the performance criteria necessary for operative monitoring. These analyzers measure the current produced when oxygen diffuses across a membrane and is reduced to molecular oxygen at the anode of an electrical circuit. The electron flow (current) is proportional to the partial pressure of oxygen in the fuel cell. Galvanic cell analyzers require regular replacement of the galvanic sensor capsule. In the sensor, the electric potential for the reduction of oxygen results from a chemical reaction. Over time, the reactants require replenishment.[6]

Polarographic Oxygen Analyzers

Polarographic oxygen analyzers are commonly used in anesthesia monitoring. In this electrochemical system, oxygen diffuses through an oxygen-permeable polymeric membrane and participates in the following reaction: $O_2 + 2H_2O + 4e \rightarrow 4 OH^-$. The current change is proportional to the number of oxygen molecules surrounding the electrode. Polarographic oxygen sensors are versatile and are important components of gas machine oxygen analyzers, blood gas analyzers, and transcutaneous and transconjunctival oxygen analyzers.

MONITORING OF EXPIRED GASES
Carbon Dioxide

Expiratory CO_2 monitoring (PE_{CO_2}) has evolved as an important physiologic and safety monitor. CO_2 is usually sampled near the endotracheal–gas delivery interface. Alterations in ventilation, cardiac output (CO), distribution of pulmonary blood flow, and metabolic activity influence PE_{CO_2} and the capnograph display obtained during quantitative expired gas analysis.

Capnometry is the measurement and numeric representation of the CO_2 concentration during inspiration and expiration. A *capnogram* is a continuous concentration–time display of the CO_2 concentration sampled at a patient's airway during ventilation. *Capnography* is the continuous monitoring of a patient's

capnogram. The capnogram is divided into four distinct phases (Fig. 25-1). The first phase (A–B) represents the initial stage of expiration. Gas sampled during this phase occupies the anatomic dead space and is normally devoid of CO_2. At point B, CO_2-containing gas presents itself at the sampling site, and a sharp upstroke (B–C) is seen in the capnogram. The slope of this upstroke is determined by the evenness of ventilation and alveolar emptying. Phase C–D represents the alveolar or expiratory plateau. At this phase of the capnogram, alveolar gas is being sampled. Normally, this part of the waveform is almost horizontal. Point D is the highest CO_2 value and is called the end-tidal CO_2 (ET_{CO_2}). ET_{CO_2} is the best reflection of the alveolar CO_2 (PA_{CO_2}). As the patient begins to inspire, fresh gas is entrained and there is a steep downstroke (D–E) back to baseline. Unless rebreathing of CO_2 occurs, the baseline approaches zero.

The utility of capnography depends on an understanding of the relationship between arterial CO_2 (Pa_{CO_2}), alveolar CO_2 (PA_{CO_2}), and ET_{CO_2}. This concept assumes that ventilation and perfusion are appropriately matched, that CO_2 is easily diffusible across the capillary–alveolar membrane, and that no sampling errors occur during measurement. If these conditions are met, changes in ET_{CO_2} reflect changes in Pa_{CO_2} even if it is assumed that all alveoli do not empty at the same time. If one assumes an idealized mathematical model of ventilation–perfusion, $ET_{CO_2} \approx PA_{CO_2} \approx Pa_{CO_2}$. If the Pa_{CO_2}–PA_{CO_2} gradient is constant and small, capnography provides a noninvasive, continuous, real-time reflection of ventilation. During general anesthesia, the ET_{CO_2}–Pa_{CO_2} gradient typically is 5–10 mm Hg. A maldistribution of ventilation and perfusion ($\dot{V}/\dot{Q}$) or problems in gas sampling may result in a widening of the ET_{CO_2}–Pa_{CO_2} gradient. $\dot{V}/\dot{Q}$ maldistribution is a common cause of an increased Pa_{CO_2}–PA_{CO_2} gradient. Other patient factors that may influence the accuracy of ET_{CO_2} monitoring by widening the Pa_{CO_2}–ET_{CO_2} gradient include shallow tidal breaths, prolongation of the expiratory phase of ventilation, or uneven alveolar emptying.

Dead space (wasted) ventilation is the extreme example of $\dot{V}/\dot{Q}$ mismatch where a complete absence of perfusion in the presence of adequate alveolar ventilation occurs. Because only perfused alveoli can participate in gas exchange, the nonperfused alveoli have a Pa_{CO_2} of zero. The ventilation-weighted average of the perfused and nonperfused alveoli determines the ET_{CO_2}. Therefore, conditions resulting in an increase of dead space ventilation lower the ET_{CO_2} measurement and increase the Pa_{CO_2}–ET_{CO_2} gradient. The common clinical causes associated with a widened Pa_{CO_2}-ET_{CO_2} gradient include embolic phenomena (thrombus, fat, air, amniotic fluid), hypoperfusion states with reduced pulmonary blood flow, and chronic obstructive pulmonary disease. In contrast, conditions that increase pulmonary shunt (perfusion in the absence of ventilation) result in minimal changes in the Pa_{CO_2}–ET_{CO_2} gradient.

Capnography is an essential element in determining the appropriate placement of endotracheal tubes. The presence of a stable ET_{CO_2} for three successive breaths indicates that the tube is not in the esophagus. A continuous, stable CO_2 waveform

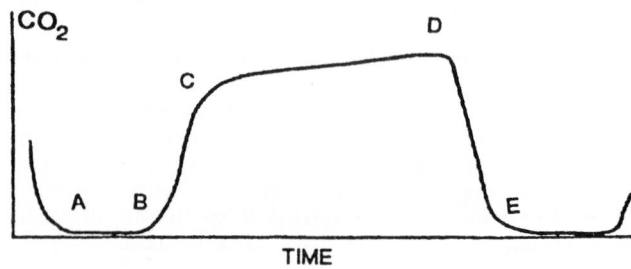

Figure 25-1. The normal capnogram. Point D delineates the end-tidal CO_2. ET_{CO_2} is the best reflection of the alveolar CO_2 tension.

ensures the presence of alveolar ventilation but does not necessarily indicate that the endotracheal tube is properly positioned in the trachea. For example, the tip of the tube could be located in a mainstem bronchus. Capnography is also a monitor of potential changes in perfusion or dead space, is a very sensitive indicator of anesthetic circuit disconnects and gas circuit leaks, and is a method to detect the quality of CO_2 absorption. Increases in ET_{CO_2} can be expected when CO_2 production exceeds ventilation, such as in hyperthermia or when an exogenous source of CO_2 is present. Table 25-1 summarizes the common elements that may be reflected by changes in ET_{CO_2} during anesthesia care.

A sudden drop in ET_{CO_2} to near zero followed by the absence of a CO_2 waveform is a potentially life-threatening problem that could indicate malposition of an endotracheal tube into the pharynx or esophagus, sudden severe hypotension, pulmonary embolism, a cardiac arrest, or an artifact resulting from disruption of sampling lines. When a sudden drop of the ET_{CO_2} occurs, it is essential quickly to verify that there is pulmonary ventilation and to identify physiologic and mechanical factors that might account for a zero line capnogram. During life-saving cardiopulmonary resuscitation, the generation of adequate perfusion can be assessed by the restoration of the CO_2 waveform.

Whereas abrupt decreases in the ET_{CO_2} are often associated with an altered cardiopulmonary status (*e.g.*, embolism or hypoperfusion), gradual reductions in ET_{CO_2} more often reflect decreases in Pa_{CO_2} that occur after increases in minute ventilation where ventilation overmatches CO_2 production.

Gas sampling errors also affect the Pa_{CO_2}–ET_{CO_2} gradient. With sidestream analyzers, the tidal sample can be diluted with fresh gas, producing a falsely low ET_{CO_2}. This can be particularly significant in neonates, infants, and small children with small tidal volumes. The site of sampling can affect accuracy. The best site for sampling is immediately adjacent to the endotracheal tube connector. Sampling errors resulting from loose connections or system leaks also may dilute the expiratory sample and reduce the estimate of ET_{CO_2}.

The size and shape of the capnogram waveform can be informative.[7] A slow rate of rise of the second phase (B–C) is suggestive of either chronic obstructive pulmonary disease or acute airway obstruction as from bronchoconstriction (asthma). A normally shaped capnogram with an increase in ET_{CO_2} suggests alveolar hypoventilation or an increase in CO_2 production. Transient increases in ET_{CO_2} are often observed during tourniquet release, aortic unclamping, or the administration of bicarbonate.

Several methods for the quantification of CO_2 have been applied to patient monitoring systems. One of the most commonly used methods is based on infrared absorption spectrophotometry (IRAS).

Table 25-1. FACTORS THAT MAY CHANGE END-TIDAL CO_2 (ET_{CO_2}) DURING ANESTHESIA

Increases in ET_{CO_2}	Decreases in ET_{CO_2}
ELEMENTS THAT CHANGE CO_2 PRODUCTION	
Increases in metabolic rate	Decreases in metabolic rate
Hyperthermia	Hypothermia
Sepsis	Hypothyroidism
Malignant hyperthermia	
Hyperthyroidism	
Shivering	
ELEMENTS THAT CHANGE CO_2 ELIMINATION	
Hypoventilation	Hyperventilation
Rebreathing	Hypoperfusion
	Pulmonary embolism

Infrared Absorption Spectrophotometry

Asymmetric, polyatomic molecules like CO_2 absorb infrared light at specific wavelengths. Operating room IRAS devices can detect CO_2, N_2O, and the potent inhaled anesthetic agents. Operating room instruments are designed to measure the unique energy absorbed by the gases and vapors of interest when a sample of the inspired and expired gas is placed into the optical path of an infrared beam.[8] The mixtures complicate the analysis because of interactions between the gases and vapors and the closeness of absorption spectra for the gases of interest. All anesthetic vapors absorb infrared light at 3.6 μm. Therefore, manufacturers using this signature cannot display with certainty the concentration of a specific anesthetic agent of interest. Optical filters and unique detection systems enhance the sensitivity of IRAS monitoring and permit estimation of CO_2, N_2O, and the specific potent inhalational agent present in the measurement chamber. IRAS devices have five components: an infrared light source, a gas sampler, an optical path, a detection system, and a signal processor. The light source produces the infrared energy. The light is focused and filtered so that the quality of the photons with respect to the energy and frequency is stable over time. Narrow wavelengths are then presented to the gas stream. Most instruments in common use continuously withdraw a small sample of gas from the airway. Sample rates vary from 50 to 300 ml · min^{-1}. The sample stream can be scavenged or returned to the breathing circuit. Water vapor must be removed before the sample is placed into the measurement chamber; liquid contamination of the sample stream affects the performance of IRAS devices. Once the sample has entered the measurement chamber, a detection system calibrated to determine the concentration of a specific gas or agent over time is activated. Changes in temperature, pressure, and acoustic characteristics in the detection chamber can be used to determine the concentration of the gas or agents of interest. Signal detectors create electrical currents analyzed by the signal processor, which transforms the current change to a measurement. The capnogram or agent waveform is an oscilloscopic representation of the electrical current changes over time. The signal-processing section of an IRAS instrument has a memory section that correlates the absorbed energy with a concentration as predicted by the Lambert-Beer law.

Multiple Expired Gas Analysis

Most operating room gas analyzers incorporate methods so that they can monitor concentrations of at least O_2, CO_2, and the inhaled anesthetic agents. Intraoperative breath-by-breath analysis of respiratory and anesthetic gases requires stand-alone monitors or a single instrument that is multiplexed to a collecting system, which permits the sampling of the gas stream from multiple locations. Currently, multiroom *mass spectrometry systems* are the only systems that use multiplexing for respiratory gas monitoring. Mass spectrometers bombard the gas mixture with electrons, creating ion fragments of a predictable mass and charge. These fragments are accelerated in a vacuum. A sample of this mixture enters a measurement chamber, where the fragment stream is subjected to a high magnetic field. The magnetic field separates the fragments by their mass and charge. The fragments are deflected onto a detector plate, and each gas has a specific landing site on the detector plate. The ion impacts are proportional to the concentration of the parent gas or vapor. The processor section of the mass spectrometer system calculates the concentration of the gases of interest and sends the information to the respective location of the original sample.

Another unique approach to monitor respiratory gases is based on *Raman scattering*. Raman scattering results when photons generated by a high-intensity argon laser collide with gas molecules. After impact, the gases are momentarily excited to

Table 25-2. DETECTION OF CRITICAL EVENTS BY IMPLEMENTING GAS ANALYSIS

Event	Monitoring Modality
Error in gas delivery	O_2, N_2, CO_2, agent analysis
Anesthesia machine malfunction	O_2, N_2, CO_2, agent
Disconnection	CO_2, O_2, agent analysis
Vaporizer malfunction or contamination	Agent analysis
Anesthesia circuit leaks	N_2, CO_2 analysis
Endotracheal cuff leaks	N_2, CO_2
Poor mask or LMA fit	N_2, CO_2
Hypoventilation	CO_2 analysis
Malignant hyperthermia	CO_2
Airway obstruction	CO_2
Air embolism	CO_2, N_2
Circuit hypoxia	O_2 analysis
Vaporizer overdose	Agent analysis

LMA = laryngeal mask airway.
Modified with permission from Knopes KD, Hecker BR: Monitoring anesthetic gases. In Lake CL (ed): Clinical Monitoring, p 24. Philadelphia, WB Saunders, 1990.

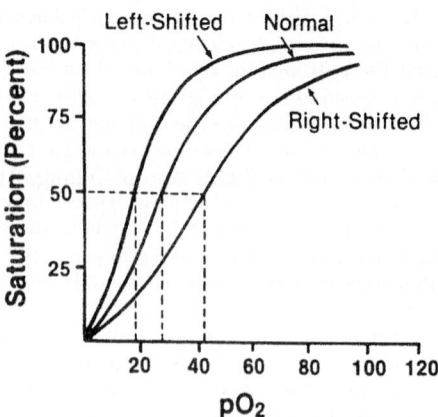

Figure 25-2. The oxyhemoglobin dissociation curve. The relationship between arterial saturation of hemoglobin and oxygen tension is represented by the sigmoid-shaped oxyhemoglobin dissociation curve. When the curve is left-shifted, the hemoglobin molecule binds oxygen more tightly. (Reproduced with permission from Brown M, Vender JS: Noninvasive oxygen monitoring. Crit Care Clin 4:493, 1988.)

unstable vibrational and rotatory states. When the gases return to their normal state, photons of a characteristic frequency are emitted. The scattered photons are measured as peaks in a spectrum that determines the concentration and composition of respiratory gases and inhaled vapors. Advances in laser technology have made Raman spectroscopic monitors available for clinical use. The instrument is fast and easy to calibrate. O_2, N_2, N_2O, CO_2, and H_2O vapor are all measurable using Raman scattering technology.

The clinical indications for routine CO_2 and O_2 gas monitoring are well documented. Monitors equipped to measure anesthetic gases are also prevalent and desirable. Nitrogen monitoring provides quantification of washout during preoxygenation. A sudden rise in N_2 in the exhaled gas indicates either introduction of air from leaks in the anesthesia delivery system or venous air embolism. Critical events that can be detected by the analysis of respiratory gases and anesthetic vapors are listed in Table 25-2.

OXYGENATION MONITORING

The assessment of oxygenation is an integral part of anesthesia practice. Early detection and prompt intervention may limit serious sequelae of hypoxemia. The clinical signs associated with hypoxemia (*e.g.*, tachycardia, altered mental status, cyanosis) are often masked or difficult to appreciate during anesthesia. The mechanisms responsible for hypoxemia are multifactorial. Oxygen analyzers assess oxygen delivery to the patient. Other noninvasive technologies detect the presence of arterial hypoxemia. Arterial oxygen monitors do not ensure adequacy of oxygen delivery to, or utilization by, the tissues and should not be considered a replacement for arterial blood gas measurements when more definitive information regarding oxygenation is desired.

Pulse Oximetry

Pulse oximetry is the standard of care for monitoring oxygenation during anesthesia. Pulse oximeters measure pulse rate and oxygen saturation of hemoglobin (Hb) (SpO_2) on a noninvasive, continuous basis. Figure 25-2 displays the oxyhemoglobin dissociation curve that defines the relationship of hemoglobin saturation and oxygen tension. On the steep part of the curve, a predictable correlation exists between SaO_2 and PO_2. In this range, the SaO_2 is a good reflection of the extent of hypoxemia

and the changing status of arterial oxygenation. Shifts in the oxyhemoglobin dissociation curve to the right or to the left define changes in the affinity of Hb for oxygen. At a PO_2 of >75 mm Hg, the SaO_2 plateaus and loses its ability to reflect changes in PaO_2.

Pulse oximetry is based on several premises:

1. The color of blood is a function of oxygen saturation.
2. The change in color results from the optical properties of Hb and its interaction with oxygen.
3. The ratio of O_2Hb and reduced Hb can be determined by absorption spectrophotometry.

Pulse oximetry combines the technology of plethysmography and spectrophotometry. Plethysmography produces a pulse trace that is helpful in tracking circulation. Oxygen saturation is determined by spectrophotometry, which is based on the Beer-Lambert law. At a constant light intensity and Hb concentration, the intensity of light transmitted through a tissue is a logarithmic function of the oxygen saturation of Hb. Two wavelengths of light are required to distinguish O_2Hb from reduced Hb. Light-emitting diodes in the pulse sensor emit red (660 nm) and near infrared (940 nm) light. The percentage of O_2Hb and reduced Hb is determined by measuring the ratio of infrared and red light sensed by a photodetector. Pulse oximeters perform a plethysmographic analysis to differentiate the pulsatile "arterial" Hb saturation from the nonpulsatile signal resulting from "venous" absorption and other tissues such as skin, muscle, and bone. The absence of a pulsatile waveform during extreme hypothermia or hypoperfusion limits the ability of a pulse oximeter to calculate the SpO_2.

The SpO_2 measured by pulse oximetry is not the same as the arterial saturation (SaO_2) measured by a laboratory co-oximeter. Pulse oximetry measures the "functional" saturation, which is defined by the following equation:

$$\text{Functional } SaO_2 = O_2Hb/(O_2Hb + \text{reduced Hb}) \times 100$$

Laboratory co-oximeters use multiple wavelengths to distinguish other types of Hb by their characteristic absorption. Co-oximeters measure the "fractional" saturation, which is defined by the following equation:

$$\text{Fractional } SaO_2 = O_2Hb/(O_2Hb + \text{reduced Hb} + COHb + MetHb) \times 100$$

In clinical circumstances where other Hb moieties are present, the SpO_2 measurement is higher than the SaO_2 reported by the blood gas laboratory. In most patients, MetHb and COHb are present in low concentrations so that the functional saturation approximates the fractional value.

Pulse oximetry has been used in all patient age groups to detect and prevent hypoxemia. The clinical benefits of pulse oximetry are enhanced by its simplicity. Modern pulse oximeters are noninvasive, continuous, and autocalibrating. They have quick response times and their battery backup provides monitoring during transport. The clinical accuracy is typically reported to be $\pm 2-3\%$ at $70-100\%$ saturation and $\pm 3\%$ at $50-70\%$ saturation. Published data from numerous investigations support accuracy and precision reported by instrument manufacturers.

The appropriate use of pulse oximetry necessitates an appreciation of both physiologic and technical limitations. Despite the numerous clinical benefits of pulse oximetry, other factors affect its accuracy and reliability. Factors that may be present during anesthesia care and that affect the accuracy and reliability of pulse oximetry include dyshemoglobins, vital dyes, nail polish, ambient light, light-emitting diode variability, motion artifact, and background noise. Electrocautery can interfere with pulse oximetry if the radiofrequency emissions are sensed by the photodetector. Reports of burns or pressure necrosis exist but are infrequent. These complications can be reduced by inspecting the digits during monitoring.

Recent developments in pulse oximetry technology permit more accurate measurements of Spo_2 during patient movement or low-perfusion conditions. These instruments use complex signal processing of the two wavelengths of light to improve the signal-to-noise ratio and reject artifact. Studies in volunteers suggest that the performance of pulse oximeters incorporating this technology is superior to conventional oximetry during motion of the hand.[9]

There is overwhelming evidence supporting the capability of pulse oximetry for detecting desaturation before it is clinically apparent. Pulse oximetry has wide applicability in many hospital and nonhospital settings. However, there are no definitive data demonstrating a reduction in morbidity or mortality associated with the advent of pulse oximetry. An older large, randomized trial did not detect a significant difference in postoperative complications when routine pulse oximetry was used.[10] However, there was a sense that use of Spo_2 provided early warning of hypoxemia, and anesthesiologists using Spo_2 felt a greater level of comfort than those who did not use Spo_2. A reduction of anesthesia mortality, as well as fewer malpractice claims for respiratory events, coincident with the introduction of pulse oximeters suggests that the routine use of these devices may have been a contributing factor. Pulse oximetry is an inexpensive, essential tool for anesthesia care.

BLOOD PRESSURE MONITORING

Perioperative measurement of arterial blood pressure is an important indicator of the adequacy of circulation. Systemic blood pressure monitoring is commonly performed indirectly using extremity-encircling cuffs or directly by inserting a catheter into an artery and transducing the arterial pressure trace. Today, anesthesiologists have a variety of techniques available for measuring changes in systolic, diastolic, and mean arterial pressure (MAP).

Arterial Pressure Wave

The size, shape, and transmission of the pressure wave throughout the arterial circulation are related to the dynamics of pulsatile flow, the acceleration and deceleration of blood, the elasticity of the large conducting arteries, and a modulated impedance that controls regional blood flow. Factors contributing to the propagation and character of the pressure pulse include the energy content imparted by ventricular systole (1–600 watts), contour transformation by the vascular tree, and reflective waves

that are produced at the periphery. Arterial pressure is created by the interaction of myocardial and vascular factors that impart both potential and kinetic energy to a dynamic arterial blood volume.

Estimates of pressure recorded in the ascending aorta are different from those measured in a peripheral artery because of the aforementioned factors. Figure 25-3 demonstrates that whereas MAP decreases from the aorta to distal arteries, systolic pressure increases. This is due to the tapering of peripheral arteries, which confines the pressure trace energy. Arterial blood pressure represents the lateral pressure exerted on arteries by blood flow. During the cardiac cycle, an arterial pulse wave results as the left ventricular stroke volume is ejected into the blood-filled arterial vascular tree. The elasticity of the aorta and conducting arteries, blood volume, stroke volume, CO, and peripheral vascular resistance determine the beat-to-beat arterial blood pressure.

Direct and indirect measurements of arterial blood pressure depend to a great extent on our ability to evaluate the quality and character of the arterial pulse wave. Many factors influence the accuracy of blood pressure monitoring. Monitoring techniques, no matter how simple or sophisticated, are often constrained by the natural properties of fluid motion and physiologic alterations that often influence accuracy and precision. Blood pressure measurements rely on devices (transducers) that convert pressure (force/unit area) into another form of energy. For example, the Riva-Rocci auscultatory methodology uses the character of sound energy produced when blood flow is restored in the brachial artery after its occlusion.

Discrepancies between indirect methods of estimating systemic blood pressure and intra-arterial pressure measurements occur frequently. Indirect measurements depend on changes in flow or volume and are frequently lower than simultaneously recorded intra-arterial pressure measurements. Although some of the differences are related to the constraints of hydraulically coupled transducing systems, it is probable that real differences exist because intra-arterial transducers respond to force displacement rather than transformations in flow or volume.

Indirect Measurement of Arterial Blood Pressure

The simplest method of blood pressure determination estimates systolic blood pressure by palpating the return of the arterial

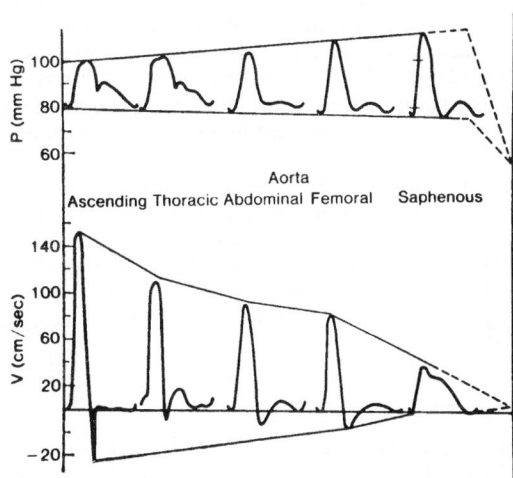

Figure 25-3. Blood pressure and velocity measurements in normal arteries of dogs. As measurements are made farther away from the ascending aorta, estimates of systolic pressure increase while the blood velocity decreases. The apparent increases in blood pressure occur as a result of reflected waves. (Reproduced with permission from Milnor WR: Hemodynamics. Baltimore, Williams & Wilkins, 1989.)

pulse while an occluding cuff is deflated. Modifications of this technique include the observance of the return of Doppler sounds, the transduced arterial pressure trace, or a photoplethysmographic pulse wave as produced by a pulse oximeter.

Auscultation of the Korotkoff sounds permit estimation of both systolic (SP) and diastolic (DP) blood pressures. MAP can be calculated using an estimating equation (MAP = DP + 1/3 [SP–DP]). Korotkoff sounds result from turbulent flow within an artery created by the mechanical deformation from the blood pressure cuff. Systolic blood pressure is signaled by the appearance of the first Korotkoff sound. Disappearance of the sound or a muffled tone signals the diastolic blood pressure.

The detection of sound changes is subjective and prone to errors based on deficiencies in sound transmission or hearing. Cuff deflation rate also influences accuracy. Quick deflations underestimate blood pressure. Palpation and auscultatory techniques require pulsatile blood flow and are unreliable during conditions of low flow. These techniques are reasonably accurate when aneroid gauges are within calibration, the encircling cuff is appropriately sized and positioned, the inflation is above the true systolic pressure, and the Korotkoff sounds or pulse is properly identified.

The American Heart Association recommends that the bladder width for indirect blood pressure monitoring should approximate 40% of the circumference of the extremity. Bladder length should be sufficient to encircle at least 60% of the extremity. Falsely high estimates result when cuffs are too small, when cuffs are applied too loosely, when the extremity is below heart level, or when uneven compression is transmitted to the underlying artery. Falsely low estimates result when cuffs are too large, when the extremity is above heart level, or after quick deflations.

Doppler sphygmomanometry is based on the detection of the Doppler shift using an ultrasonic transceiver to sense the restoration of blood flow during cuff deflation. Some instruments sense the velocity of erythrocytes, whereas others detect arterial wall motion distal to the occlusive blood pressure cuff. These instruments are more sensitive than palpatory or auscultative techniques and are clinically useful when the peripheral pulse is faint. Compact battery-operated devices are helpful to assess the blood pressure when routine indirect methods fail.

Since 1976, microprocessor-controlled oscillotonometers have replaced auscultatory and palpatory techniques for routine perioperative blood pressure monitoring. Standard oscillometry measures mean blood pressure by sensing the point of maximal fluctuations in cuff pressure produced while deflating a blood pressure cuff. Most current instruments use oscillometric techniques to measure systolic, diastolic, and mean blood pressures by determining parameter identification points during cuff deflation. Substantial differences exist among the many devices designed for clinical use with respect to their method of operation.

In a generic noninvasive oscillometric monitor (*noninvasive blood pressure,* or NIBP), cuff pressure is sensed by a pressure transducer whose output is digitalized for processing. After the cuff is inflated by an air pump, cuff pressure is held constant while oscillations are sampled. If no oscillations are sensed by the pressure transducer, the microprocessor switches open a deflation valve, and the next lower pressure level is sampled for the presence of oscillations. Artifact-rejection algorithms are implemented during the stepwise deflation sequence at parameter identification points. The microprocessor controlling the operation of the NIBP compares the amplitude of oscillation pairs and numerically displays the blood pressure estimate. Figure 25-4 depicts how a typical NIBP is obtained. In this example, the effect of respiratory variation, a premature ventricular complex, and cuff movement is demonstrated.

Automated oscillometry has been demonstrated to correlate well with direct intra-arterial measurement of MAP and diastolic blood pressure. Automated oscillometry may underestimate systolic blood pressure, with mean errors reported from −6.9 to −8.6 mm Hg compared with direct radial artery pressure measurements.

Oscillometry requires the careful evaluation of several cardiac cycles at each increment of deflation to smooth out pronounced respiratory variations or motion artifacts. Cuff movement or erratic pulse transmission influences accuracy. In the anesthetized patient, automated oscillometry is usually accurate and versatile. A variety of cuff sizes makes it possible to use oscillometry in all age groups. Modern instruments incorporate a faster access mode, which can be useful in situations in which rapid changes in arterial blood pressure are anticipated.

Problems With Noninvasive Blood Pressure Monitoring

Cuff-based pressure monitoring continues to be the standard method used in the perioperative period. When clinical circumstances require frequent blood pressure readings for a prolonged period, it is advisable periodically to move the cuff to alternative sites. Failure to deflate the cuff increases venous pressure. Hematomas have been described both beneath and distal to the cuff. Tremors or shivering can delay cuff deflation and prolong the deflation cycle. A compartment syndrome attributed to a prolonged inflation cycle has been described. Ulnar neuropathy has been reported after the use of automated cycled blood pressure cuffs. Compression of the ulnar nerve can be avoided by applying the encircling cuff proximal to the ulnar groove. Automated sequencing may alter the timing of intravenous drug administration when the access site is located in the same extremity. Hydrostatic errors result when blood pressure cuffs are placed on extremities that are above or below

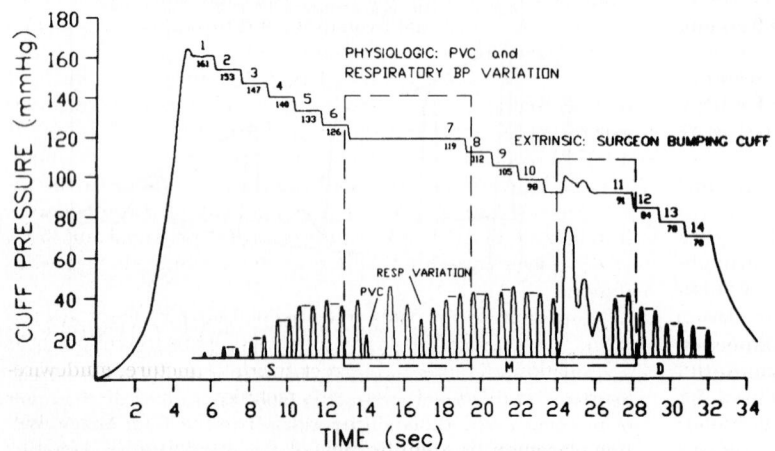

Figure 25-4. Diagram illustrating motion artifact, a premature ventricular contraction, and respiratory artifact as sensed by a Dinamap noninvasive blood pressure monitor. (Reproduced with permission from Ramsey M: Blood pressure monitoring: Automated oscillometric devices. Journal of Clinical Monitoring 7:56, 1991.)

the level of the right atrium. The hydrostatic offset can be mathematically corrected by adding or subtracting 0.7 mm Hg for each centimeter that the cuff is off the horizontal plane of the heart.

Indirect Continuous Noninvasive Techniques

Several methods for monitoring blood pressure continuously and noninvasively have been designed and evaluated for intraoperative blood pressure surveillance. These techniques provide clinicians with a continuous blood pressure estimate and an accurate display of the arterial blood pressure trace. *Indirect continuous noninvasive techniques* (ICNTs) continue to be evaluated because it is desirable to enhance beat-to-beat blood pressure monitoring while reducing the inherent risks and costs of direct intra-arterial monitoring. Clinical studies suggest that accuracy and precision of ICNTs are satisfactory, even under conditions of rapidly changing hemodynamics.[11–13] At present, however, ICNTs are not considered substitutes for direct arterial pressure monitoring in critically ill patients in the operating room.

Invasive Measurement of Vascular (Arterial Blood) Pressure

Indwelling arterial cannulation permits the opportunity to monitor arterial blood pressure continuously and to have vascular access for arterial blood sampling. Intra-arterial blood pressure monitoring uses saline-filled tubing to transmit the force of the pressure pulse wave to a pressure transducer that converts the displacement of a silicon crystal into voltage changes. These electrical signals are amplified, filtered, and displayed as the arterial pressure trace. Intra-arterial pressure transducing systems are subject to many potential errors based on the physical properties of fluid motion and the performance of the catheter-transducer-amplification system used to sense, process, and display the pressure pulse wave.

The behavior of transducers, fluid couplings, signal amplification, and display systems can be described by a complex second-order differential equation. Solving the equation predicts the output and characterizes the fidelity of the system's ability faithfully to display and estimate the arterial pressure over time. The fidelity of fluid-coupled transducing systems is constrained by two properties: damping (ζ) and natural frequency (Fo). Zeta (ζ) describes the tendency for saline in the measuring system to extinguish motion. Fo describes the tendency for the measuring system to resonate. The fidelity of the transduced pressure depends on optimizing ζ and Fo so that the system can respond appropriately to the range of frequencies contained in the pressure pulse wave. Analysis of high-fidelity recordings of arterial blood pressure indicate that the pressure trace contains frequencies from 1 to 30 Hz.

The performance of a transducing system is often described by its bandwidth. The bandwidth contains the frequencies in which the transducing system faithfully reproduces the frequencies contained in the pulse pressure wave. Conventional disposable, saline-coupled transducers with 60 inches of pressure tubing have an acceptable bandwidth and commonly have frequency responses approaching 30 Hz. If the system begins to resonate (ringing) or becomes damp (inertia), the fidelity of the system is impaired and estimates of blood pressure become less accurate. Measuring the bandwidth of transducer systems requires complicated equipment. Estimates of ζ and Fo can be obtained at the bedside.

Studies have demonstrated that system fidelity is optimized when catheters and tubing are stiff, the mass of the fluid is small, the number of stopcocks is limited, and the connecting tubing is not excessive. Damping lowers the effective bandwidth of the transducer system, which promotes the potential for resonance. Figure 25-5 demonstrates the effect of damping on the character of the arterial pressure trace. In clinical practice,

underdamped catheter-transducer systems tend to overestimate systolic pressure by 15–30 mm Hg and amplify artifact (catheter whip). Likewise, excessive increases in ζ reduce fidelity and underestimate systolic pressure. The presence of air bubbles in the coupling fluid reduces the natural frequency of the transducing system. Dynamic calibration can determine the fidelity of the pressure recording system. For clinical use, it is sufficient to place the transducer at the level of the right atrium, open the stopcock to atmosphere, and balance the electronic amplifying system to display "zero." Periodic checks of the zero reference point ensures that transducer drift is eliminated.

Gardner[14] suggested using the "fast flush" test to determine the natural frequency and damping characteristics of the transducing system. This test examines the characteristics of the resonant waves recorded after the release of a flush. Damping is estimated by the amplitude ratio of the first pair of resonant waves and the natural frequency is estimated by dividing the paper speed by the interval cycle. Kleinman et al[15] have confirmed the utility of the fast flush test. Because many therapeutic decisions are based on changes in arterial blood pressure, it is imperative that anesthesiologists understand the physical limitation imposed by fluid-filled pressure transducer systems. Significant exaggeration of pressure measurements occur when the transducer system has a resonant frequency in the range of the pressure wave frequencies. Systolic pressure is underestimated when measured with overdamping systems and overestimated by underdamping or resonating systems. Mean pressure estimates are typically less affected even when damping and resonance are not optimal.

Arterial Cannulation

Multiple arteries can be used for direct measurement of blood pressure, including the radial, brachial, axillary, femoral, and dorsalis pedis arteries. The radial artery remains the most popular site for cannulation because of its accessibility and the presence of a collateral blood supply. In the past, assessment of the patency of the ulnar circulation by performance of an Allen's test has been recommended before cannulation. Allen's test is performed by compressing both radial and ulnar arteries while the patient tightens his or her fist. Releasing pressure on each respective artery determines the dominant vessel supplying blood to the hand. The prognostic value of the Allen's test in assessing the adequacy of the collateral circulation has not been confirmed.[16,17]

Radial artery cannulation and blood pressure monitoring have been associated with several problems. The radial artery pulse pressure wave is subject to inaccuracies inherent to its distal location. After separation from cardiopulmonary bypass, large pressure gradients between aortic and radial arteries have been described.

Complications of Invasive Arterial Monitoring

Traumatic cannulation has been associated with median nerve dysfunction, hematoma formation, and thrombosis. Abnormal radial artery blood flow after catheter removal occurs frequently. Studies suggest that blood flow normalizes in 3–70 days. Radial artery thrombosis can be minimized by avoiding polypropylene-tapered catheters and reducing the duration of arterial cannulation. Flexible guidewires may reduce the potential trauma associated with catheters negotiating tortuous vessels. During cannula removal, the potential for thromboembolism may be diminished by compressing the proximal and distal arterial segment while aspirating the cannula during withdrawal.

Many cannulation sites have been used for direct arterial blood pressure monitoring (Table 25-3). Three techniques for cannulation are common: direct arterial puncture, guidewire-assisted cannulation (Seldinger's technique), and the transfixion–withdrawal method. A necessary condition for percutaneous placement is identification of the arterial pulse. Doppler

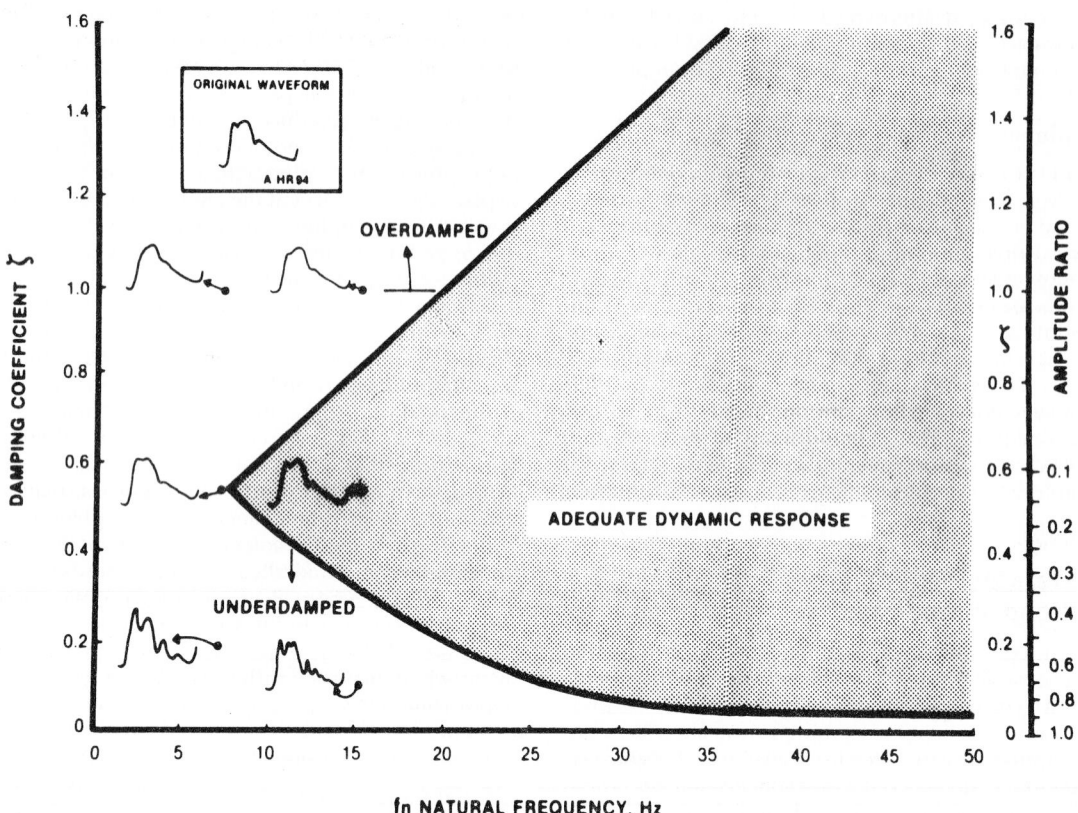

Figure 25-5. The relationship between the frequency of fluid-filled transducing systems and damping. The shaded area represents the appropriate range of damping for a given natural frequency (Fn). The size of the wedge also depends on the steepness of the arterial pressure trace and heart rate. (Reproduced with permission from Gardner RM: Direct blood pressure measurement: Dynamic response requirements. Anesthesiology 54:231, 1981.)

flow probes are helpful in situations in which the location of the arterial pressure pulse is difficult to palpate.

Arterial cannulation is regarded as an invasive procedure with a documented morbidity. Ischemia after radial artery cannulation resulting from thrombosis, proximal emboli, or prolonged shock has been described.[18] Contributing factors include severe atherosclerosis, diabetes, low CO, and intense peripheral vasoconstriction. Ischemia, hemorrhage, thrombosis, embolism, cerebral air embolism (retrograde flow associated with flushing), aneurysm formation, arteriovenous fistula formation, skin necrosis, and infection have occurred as the direct result of arterial cannulation, arterial blood sampling, or high-pressure flushing.

Continuous-flush devices are incorporated into disposable transducer kits and infuse at 3–6 ml·h⁻¹. In neonates, the infusion volume may contribute to fluid overload. Continuous-flush devices have little effect on the blood pressure measurement. However, pressurized flush systems may serve as a source of an air embolism. Removing air from the pressurized infusion bag, stopcocks, and tubing minimizes the potential for air embolism.

Arterial sampling is an important source of bacterial contamination of transducer systems. Shinozaki and colleagues[19] found that the stopcocks are an important source of contamination. The longer the transducer system is in place, the greater the incidence of nosocomial contamination. Guidelines published by the Centers for Disease Control[20] (CDC) recommend that intravascular catheters should be routinely changed every 48 or 72 hours to reduce the risk of catheter-associated infection.

Direct arterial pressure monitoring requires constant vigilance. The data displayed must correlate with clinical conditions before therapeutic interventions are initiated. Sudden increases in the transduced blood pressure may represent a hydrostatic error because the position of the transducer was not adjusted after change in the operating room table's height. Sudden decreases often result from kinking of the tubing. Before initiating therapy, the transducer system should be "rezeroed" and the patency of the arterial cannula verified. This ensures the accuracy of the measurement and avoids a potentially dangerous medication error.

Table 25-3. ARTERIAL CANNULATION AND DIRECT BLOOD PRESSURE MONITORING

Arterial Cannulation Site	Clinical Points of Interest
Radial artery	Preferred site for monitoring
	Nontapered catheters preferred
Ulnar artery	Complication similar to radial
	Primary source of hand blood flow
Brachial artery	Insertion site medial to biceps tendon
	Median nerve damage is potential hazard
	Can accommodate 18-gauge cannula
Axillary artery	Insertion site at junction of pectoralis and deltoid muscle
	Specialized kits available
Femoral artery	Easy access in low flow states
	Potential for local and retroperitoneal hemorrhage
	Longer catheters preferred
Dorsalis pedis artery	Collateral circulation = posterior tibial artery
	Higher systolic pressure estimates

Central Venous and Pulmonary Artery Monitoring

Central venous cannulas are important portals for intraoperative vascular access and for the assessment of changes in vascular volume. Percutaneous insertion of central venous pressure (CVP) catheters is a skill that every anesthesiologist needs to acquire. CVP portals permit the rapid administration of fluids, insertion of pulmonary artery catheters (PACs), insertion of transvenous electrodes, monitoring of CVP, and a site for observation and treatment of venous air embolism.

The right internal jugular vein is the preferred site for cannulation because it is accessible from the head of the operating table, has a predictable anatomy, and has a high success rate in both adults and children.[21] The left-sided internal jugular vein is also available but is less desirable because of the potential for damaging the thoracic duct or difficulty in maneuvering catheters through the jugular–subclavian junction. Accidental carotid artery puncture is a potential problem with either location.

Three techniques (posterior, central, and anterior) have been described for internal jugular cannulation. Each insertion point is referenced to the triangle formed by the sternal and clavicular heads of the sternocleidomastoid muscle and the clavicle. Venipuncture using a 22-gauge "seeker" needle minimizes trauma to adjacent structures. When the location of the internal jugular vein is difficult to ascertain, ultrasonography can assist in identifying the proximity of internal jugular vein and the carotid artery. Alternatives to the internal jugular vein include the external jugular, subclavian, antecubital, and femoral veins.

Central Venous Pressure Monitoring

The benefit of CVP monitoring has been the subject of considerable debate. Proponents of CVP monitoring believe that CVP pressures are essentially equivalent to right atrial pressures and serve as a reflection of right ventricular preload.[22] Conditions that affect right atrial pressure also influence the CVP pressure trace. The normal CVP waveform consists of three peaks (a, c, and v waves) and two descents (x, y), each resulting from the ebb and flow of blood in the right atrium (Fig. 25-6). Corresponding events occur in the left atrium and similar pressure contours are observed during monitoring of pulmonary artery pressure when the PAC is placed in the occluded position.

The character of the CVP trace depends on many factors, including heart rate, conduction disturbances, tricuspid valve function, normal or abnormal intrathoracic pressure changes, and changes in right ventricular compliance. In patients with atrial fibrillation, a waves are absent. When resistance to the emptying of the right atrium is present, large a waves are often observed. Examples include tricuspid stenosis, right ventricular

hypertrophy due to pulmonic stenosis, or acute or chronic lung disease associated with pulmonary hypertension. Large a waves are often observed when right ventricular compliance is impaired.

Tricuspid regurgitation typically produces giant v waves that begin immediately after the QRS complex. Large v waves are often observed when right ventricular ischemia or failure is present or when ventricular compliance is impaired by constrictive pericarditis or cardiac tamponade. Diagnosis of right ventricular ischemia is often difficult. A prominent v wave during CVP monitoring may suggest right ventricular papillary muscle ischemia and tricuspid regurgitation. When right ventricular compliance decreases, the CVP often increases with prominent a and v waves fusing to form an *m* or *w* configuration.

Central venous pressure monitoring is helpful in the diagnosis and treatment of pericardial tamponade, where equalization of diastolic filling pressures typically occurs. As the CVP tracing becomes monophasic, the y descent is lost. Equalization of diastolic filling pressures of the CVP, right ventricle, pulmonary artery, and pulmonary artery occlusion pressure is a characteristic of hemodynamically significant pericardial constriction and cardiac tamponade. After treatment, a dramatic drop in filling pressures, restoration of systemic blood pressure, and a normalization of the CVP waveform should occur.

Central venous pressure monitoring is often unreliable for estimating left ventricular filling pressures, especially when cardiopulmonary disease processes alter the normal cardiovascular pressure–volume relationships. CVP monitoring is less invasive and less costly than pulmonary artery monitoring and offers unique understanding of right-sided hemodynamic events and the status of vascular volume.

Pulmonary Artery Monitoring

The development of the flow-directed, balloon flotation PAC was a major advance in hemodynamic monitoring, and it has become an important tool in the quantitative assessment of cardiopulmonary function. The original indication for PAC monitoring was for the management of complicated myocardial infarction. Because right-sided heart pressures are often unreliable determinants of left ventricular filling pressures, pulmonary artery monitoring is commonly used in the perioperative period when caring for patients with pre-existing cardiopulmonary or renal disease or shock, or when surgical interventions or ongoing disease processes are associated with excessive blood or fluid losses or cardiopulmonary dysfunction. Numerous articles have reviewed the various applications and benefits of pulmonary artery monitoring.[23] Use should be guided by the information needed for enhanced diagnosis and therapy.[24] Today, PAC monitoring is commonly used in surgical patients to help evaluate and treat hemodynamic alterations, which contribute significantly to the morbidity and mortality inherent to the surgical care of high-risk patients.

The ASA established a task force to examine the evidence supporting the clinical effectiveness of PAC monitoring. Issues such as the timing of PAC monitoring, its effect on treatment decisions, patient selection and case mix, and evidence regarding PAC monitoring contribution to positive or negative outcomes were evaluated using stringent evidence-based methodology. This effort identified many flaws in the body of evidence, which made it difficult to draw meaningful conclusions regarding the effectiveness of PAC monitoring to reduce morbidity or mortality. The consensus opinion implies that PAC monitoring may reduce perioperative complications if critical hemodynamic data obtained during appropriate PAC monitoring are accurately interpreted and appropriate treatment is tailored to the conditions as they change over time.[25] Monitoring the hemodynamic status of high-risk patients may reduce cardiac complications (*e.g.*, myocardial ischemia, congestive heart failure, dysrhythmias), renal insufficiency, brain injury, and pulmonary complications.

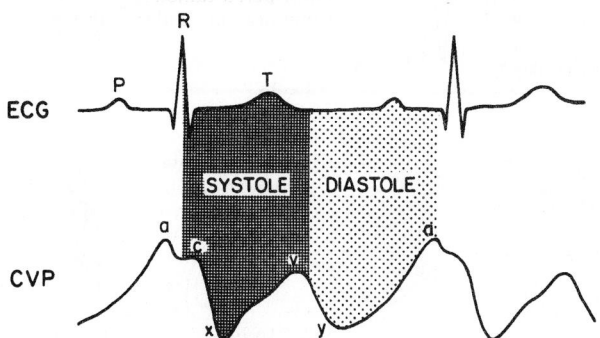

Figure 25-6. The normal central venous pressure trace. (Redrawn with permission from Mark JB: Central venous pressure monitoring: Clinical insights beyond the numbers. J Cardiothorac Vasc Anesth 5:163, 1991.)

Table 25-4. DERIVED HEMODYNAMIC VARIABLES

Name	Abbreviation	Calculation	Units
Cardiac index	CI	CO/BSA	$1 \cdot min^{-1} \cdot m^{-2}$
Systemic vascular resistance	SVR	(MAP-CVP/CO) × 80	$dyne\text{-}cm \cdot s^{-5}$
Pulmonary vascular resistance	PVR	(MPAP-PCWP/CO) × 80	$dyne\text{-}cm \cdot s^{-5}$
Stroke index	SI	CI/heart rate	$cc \cdot beat^{-1} \cdot m^{-2}$
Left ventricular stroke work index	LVSWI	SI × (MAP-PCWP) × 0.0136	$g\text{-}m \cdot beat^{-1} \cdot m^{-2}$
Right ventricular stroke work index	RVSWI	SI × (MPAP-CVP) × 0.0136	$g\text{-}m \cdot beat^{-1} \cdot m^{-2}$

BSA = body surface area; MAP = mean arterial pressure; CVP = central venous pressure; MPAP = mean pulmonary arterial pressure; PCWP = pulmonary capillary wedge pressure.

Pulmonary artery catheters permit the measurement of intracardiac pressures, thermodilution CO (TCO), mixed venous oxygen saturation, intracavitary electrograms, and lung water. This information can help define clinical problems, monitor the progression of hemodynamic dysfunctions, and guide the response of corrective therapy.

The measurement of intracardiac pressures can indirectly assess left ventricular preload, diagnose the existence of pulmonary hypertension, or differentiate cardiac and noncardiac causes of pulmonary edema. PACs allow for the rapid and reproducible measurements of TCO, calculation of oxygen delivery (CO × arterial O_2 content), and assessment of cardiac work. Hemodynamic measurements are often predicated on the manipulation of preload, afterload, and contractility. Several derived indices of hemodynamic function necessitate measurements commonly obtained from PAC monitoring (Table 25-4).

Access to mixed venous blood from the pulmonary artery port provides an indirect assessment of the balance between O_2 delivery and O_2 utilization. Mixed venous oxygen saturation ($S\bar{v}o_2$) measurements are needed to calculate mixed venous oxygen content ($C\bar{v}o_2$). $C\bar{v}o_2$ is an important variable used for calculating intrapulmonary (Eqn. 25-1) or intracardiac shunts (Eqn. 25-2).

$$\frac{Cco_2 - Cao_2}{Cco_2 - C\bar{v}o_2} = \frac{\dot{Q}s}{\dot{Q}t} \qquad (25\text{-}1)$$

$$\frac{Sao_2 - SRAo_2}{Sao_2 - S\bar{v}o_2} = \frac{\dot{Q}p}{\dot{Q}s} \qquad (25\text{-}2)$$

Where Cco_2 = capillary O_2 content, Cao_2 = arterial O_2 content, $C\bar{v}o_2$ = mixed venous O_2 content, $\dot{Q}s/\dot{Q}t$ = shunt fraction, Sao_2 = arterial O_2 saturation, $SRAo_2$ = right atrial O_2 saturation, $S\bar{v}o_2$ = mixed venous O_2 saturation, and $\dot{Q}p/\dot{Q}s$ = pulmonary-to-systemic shunt.

The validity of PAC monitoring depends on a properly functioning pressure monitoring system, correctly identifying the "true" *pulmonary capillary wedge pressure* (PCWP), and integration of the various factors that affect the relationship of PCWP, and the other cardiac pressures and volumes that are determinants of ventricular function. Figure 25-7 depicts the transduced pressure waves observed as a PAC is floated to the wedged position. Catheter placement is most commonly performed by observing the pressure waves as the catheter is floated from the CVP position through the right heart chambers into the pulmonary artery.

Pulmonary artery catheter monitoring necessitates an appreciation of the various physiologic determinants of CO and oxygen delivery. The PAC is used to continuously monitor the pulmonary artery pressure and intermittently monitor pulmonary wedge pressure. PCWP is used to assess left ventricular preload indirectly by reflecting changes in left ventricular end-diastolic pressure (LVEDP). Figure 25-8 depicts the relationship between the various pressures in the cardiopulmonary system.

It has been well demonstrated that right-sided pressures often are poor indicators of left ventricular filling, either as absolute numbers or in terms of the direction of change in response to therapy. The correlation of these pressures as estimates of LVEDP (or left ventricular end diastolic volume [LVEDV]) is directly related to their proximity to the left ventricle and the status of ventricular compliance. Assuming an open conduit from the catheter tip to the left ventricle, when the PAC is occluded ("wedged"), the right-sided heart chambers and valves are bypassed. During end-diastole, there is cessation of forward blood flow, and a static fluid column is presumed to exist from the left ventricle to the PAC tip. Ideally, changes in LVEDP are reflected by all proximal pressures (left atrial, pulmonary venous, pulmonary artery end-diastolic pressure [PAEDP], and PCWP). Alterations of internal or external forces applied to the open conduit during PCWP measurements may invalidate the PCWP-LVEDP-LVEDV relationship.

Factors Affecting the Accuracy of Pulmonary Artery Catheter Data

Pulmonary Vascular Resistance.   Any disease process or condition that increases pulmonary vascular resistance has the potential to reduce pulmonary blood flow and alter the relationship between PCWP and PAEDP. Pathologic conditions such as acute or chronic lung disease, pulmonary emboli, alveolar hypoxia, acidosis, and hypoxemia, and many vasoactive drugs increase pulmonary vascular resistance and have the potential to modify

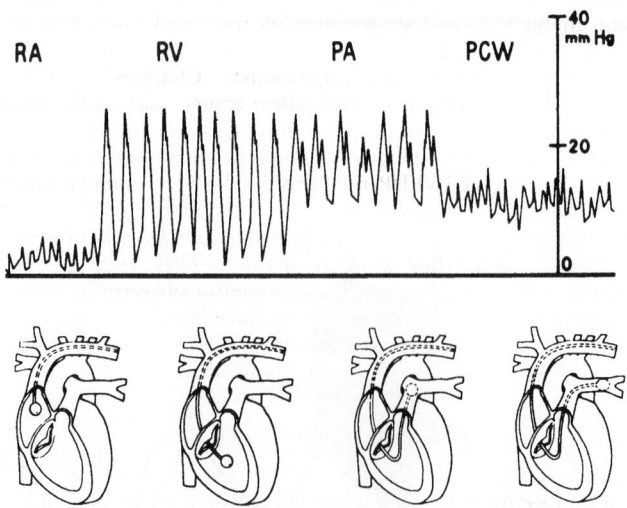

Figure 25-7. Pressure tracing observed during the flotation of a pulmonary artery catheter. (Reproduced with permission from Dizon CT, Barash PG: The value of monitoring pulmonary artery pressure in clinical practice. Conn Med 41:622, 1979.)

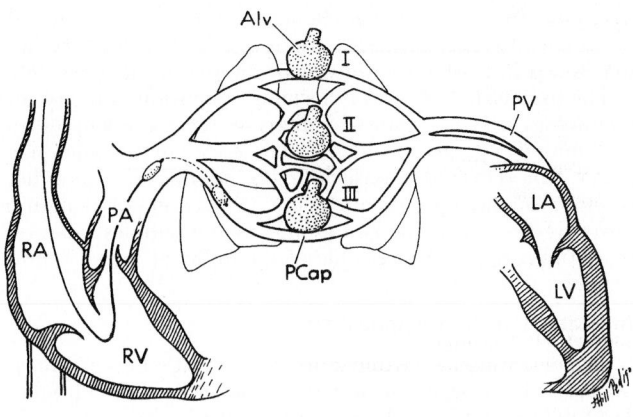

PAEDP ⟷ PWP ⟷ PVP ⟷ LAP ⟷ LVEDP

Figure 25-8. The anatomic position of a pulmonary artery catheter in the pulmonary artery. The dashed line positions the inflated balloon in the "wedged" position. (RA = right atrium; RV = right ventricle; PA = pulmonary artery; Alv = alveolus; Pcap = pulmonary capillary; PV = pulmonary vein; LA = left atrium; LV = left ventricle.) I, II, and III characterize the relationship of $P_{aveolar}$, $P_{arterial}$, and P_{venous} as described by West. The bottom of the figure shows a progressive correlation of vascular pressures. (Reproduced with permission from Vender JS: Invasive cardiac monitoring. Crit Care Clin 4:455, 1988.)

the PCWP-PAEDP relationship. Tachycardia shortens ventricular diastole and also increases pulmonary vascular resistance.

Alveolar–Pulmonary Artery Pressure Relationships. West *et al*[26] described a gravity-dependent difference between ventilation and perfusion in the lung. The variability in pulmonary blood flow is a result of differences in pulmonary artery (PA), alveolar (Palv), and venous pressures (PV) and is categorized into three distinct zones. Only Zone III (PA > PV > Palv) meets the criteria for uninterrupted blood flow and a continuous communication with distal intracardiac pressures. Increases in alveolar pressure, decreases in perfusion, or changes in positioning can convert areas of Zone III into either Zone II or I. Flow-directed PACs usually advance to gravity-dependent areas of highest blood flow.

The location of a PAC can be confirmed by a lateral chest film to ascertain that the catheter tip is below the level of the left atrium. The following characteristics suggest that the PAC tip is not in Zone III: PCWP > PAEDP, nonphasic PCWP tracing, and inability to aspirate blood from the distal port when the catheter is wedged.

Respiratory Pattern and Airway Pressure. Changes in intrathoracic and intrapleural pressure affect transmural cardiac pressures. Transmural pressure is defined as the net distending pressure of the left ventricle. Changes in intrathoracic pressure affect the PCWP-LVEDP relationship. Positive end-expiratory pressure (PEEP) therapy can induce changes in both intravascular and intrapleural pressures. PEEP increases alveolar pressure, potentially converting Zone III areas to Zone II. If PEEP is transmitted across the alveoli, intrapleural pressure increases. Pulmonary compliance determines the extent of this effect. PEEP alters ventricular distensibility and decreases venous return. This causes a disproportionate increase in PCWP (and LVEDP) compared with changes in LVEDV.

The effect of PEEP therapy is minimal if the levels of PEEP are low (≤10 cm) and the PAC is located in Zone III. Higher levels of PEEP influence the PCWP-LVEDP relationship. During high PEEP therapy, esophageal pressure measurements can be made to determine intrapleural pressure. Alternatively, subtracting 1–2 mm Hg from the displayed "wedge" pressure for each 5 cm H_2O of PEEP therapy gives an estimate when PEEP is above 10 cm H_2O.

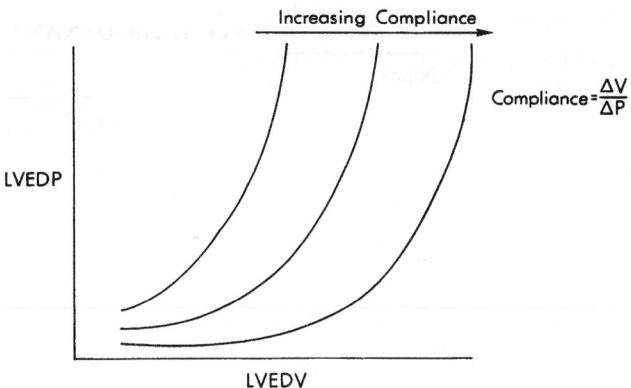

Figure 25-9. Typical ventricular compliance curve. (Reproduced with permission from Vender JS: Invasive cardiac monitoring. Crit Care Clin 4:455, 1988.)

Intracardiac Factors. Pathologic obstruction at the mitral valve secondary to mitral stenosis, atrial myxoma, or clot can interfere with the ability of left atrial pressure to reflect LVEDP. Similarly, mitral regurgitation, a noncompliant left atrium, or left-to-right intracardiac shunting often is associated with large v waves.

Decreases in left ventricular compliance, aortic regurgitation, or premature closure of the mitral valve may reverse the left atrial pressure–LVEDP pressure gradient. When this occurs, PCWP is not a valid reflection of LVEDV.

Figure 25-9 graphically depicts the relationship between LVEDP and LVEDV. The LVEDP–LVEDV relationship is not linear. A family of LVEDP–LVEDV compliance curves characterizes the effect of changing the stiffness of the left ventricle. Ventricular compliance is a dynamic factor influenced by many physiologic and pathologic variables. The LVEDP-LVEDV compliance curves suggest that at low preloads, larger increases in LVEDV produce smaller changes in LVEDP. Conversely, at higher preloads, a similar change in LVEDV produces a greater pressure change. For a given LVEDV, any decrease in ventricular compliance results in an increase in LVEDP. This explains the development of hydrostatic pulmonary edema at normal LVEDV. Factors that are associated with changes in ventricular compliance are listed in Table 25-5.

Adverse Effects of Pulmonary Catheter Monitoring

Complications from PAC monitoring can result during central venous access, the catheterization procedure, or any time after PAC placement. Central venous access represents an invasive process with inherent risks, some of which are potentially life threatening.

Unintentional puncture of nearby arteries, bleeding, neuropathy, and pneumothorax may result from needle insertion into adjacent structures. Air embolism may occur if a cannula is open to the atmosphere and air is entrained during or after CVP placement. Dysrhythmias are common during the catheterization procedure, with a reported incidence of 4.7–68.9%. Ventricular tachycardia or fibrillation may be induced during catheter advancement. Catheter advancement has been associ-

Table 25-5. DECREASED LEFT VENTRICULAR COMPLIANCE: COMMON ETIOLOGIES

Myocardial ischemia	Cardiac tamponade
Restrictive myopathies	Myocardial fibrosis
Right-to-left intraventricular shunts	Inotropic drugs
Aortic stenosis	Hypertension

Table 25-6. ADVERSE EFFECTS ASSOCIATED WITH PULMONARY ARTERY MONITORING

Complication	Reported Incidence (%)
Central venous access	
Arterial puncture	1.1–13
Postoperative neuropathy	5.3
Pneumothorax	0.3–1.1
Air embolism	0.3–4.5
Flotation of pulmonary artery catheter	
Minor dysrhythmias	4–68.9
Ventricular tachycardia or fibrillation	0.3–62.7
Right bundle branch block	0.1–4.3
Complete heart block (prior left bundle-branch block)	0–8.5
Complications associated with catheter residence	
Pulmonary artery rupture	0.1–1.5
Positive cultures from catheter tip	1.4–34.8
Sepsis secondary to catheter resistance	0.7–11.4
Thrombophlebitis	6.5
Venous thrombosis	0.5–66.7
Pulmonary infarction	0.1–5.6
Mural thrombus	28–61
Valvular or endocardial vegetations	2.2–100
Deaths attributed to pulmonary artery catheter	0.02–1.5

Reproduced with permission from the Task Force on Guidelines for Pulmonary Artery Monitoring of the American Society of Anesthesiologists. Anesthesiology 78:380, 1993.

ated with right bundle-branch block and, in patients with pre-existing left bundle-branch block, may precipitate complete heart block. Table 25-6 summarizes the adverse effects as reported by the ASA task force on pulmonary artery catheterization.[25]

The rate of iatrogenic deaths associated with PAC monitoring is uncertain. The most dreaded complication associated with PAC monitoring is pulmonary artery rupture. Pulmonary hypertension, coagulopathy, and heparinization are often present in patients who have died of pulmonary artery rupture. Perforations and subsequent hemorrhage can be avoided by restricting "overwedging," minimizing the number of balloon inflations, and using proper technique during balloon inflations. Sepsis is a potential complication of the continued use of PACs. Although cultures of PAC tips are often positive, the exact incidence of catheter-related sepsis is uncertain. Catheter-related sepsis has a reported incidence of 0.7–11.4%.

Since the advent of PACs, several modifications have been integrated into the design that enhance their monitoring capabilities. The first significant design modification incorporated a thermistor at the tip, permitting the measurement of CO. Other features have been introduced for clinical use or evaluation. These include mixed venous oximetry, measurement of right ventricular ejection fraction, pacing options, and continuous CO monitoring (CCOM).

Mixed Venous Oximetry

Continuous estimates of $S\bar{v}O_2$ provide a reflection of total tissue oxygen balance. Oxygen delivery ($\dot{D}O_2$) equals the arterial oxygen content multiplied by the CO ($\dot{D}O_2 = [Hb \times 13.8] \times CO$), where 13.8 represents the volume of oxygen carried by Hb converted to grams per liter. Oxygen consumption ($\dot{V}O_2$) is determined by the difference between arterial and venous oxygen delivery. The relationship between $S\bar{v}O_2$, $\dot{V}O_2$, and $\dot{D}O_2$ is demonstrated in the following equation derived from the Fick relationship:

$$S\bar{v}O_2 = SaO_2 - \frac{\dot{V}O_2}{Hb \times 13.8} \times CO$$

This equation indicates that changes in $S\bar{v}O_2$ vary directly with changes in CO, Hb, and SaO_2 and inversely with $\dot{V}O_2$. The normal $S\bar{v}O_2$ is 75%, which denotes tissue oxygen extraction = 25%.

The oximetric PAC uses reflectance spectrophotometry and technology similar to pulse oximetry. Several wavelengths are transmitted through optical fibers embedded in the pulmonary artery. The reflected intensity of light identifies the saturation of blood surrounding the tip of the PAC. Three-wavelength *in vivo* systems correlate well with simultaneous samples measured by co-oximetry.[27,28] An example of the utility of mixed venous oximetry is depicted in Figure 25-10.

Indicator Dilution Applications

Indicator dilution determination of CO is based on a concept proposed by Stewart and tested by Hamilton and colleagues. TCO determination is the most widely used adaptation of the indicator dilution principle, which was first described by Fegler in 1954.[29] Today, cooled 5% dextrose or 0.9% saline is used as the indicator. A thermistor located at the PAC tip records the decrease in temperature as the bolus of cooled injectate passes through the pulmonary artery. Computers contend with the complexity of the TCO equation, which includes the following factors: specific heat of the blood and the indicator fluid, the volume of injectate, catheter size, specific gravity of the blood and indicator, the volume of the injectate, and the area of the blood temperature curve. Unlike dye dilution techniques, in which the concentration of indicator increases with each determination, the effect of adding cold injectate on core temperature is insignificant. Comparison studies suggest that using either room-temperature or iced injectates provides accurate estimates of CO. Iced injectate is preferred because it produces a more exacting curve with a better signal-to-noise ratio.[30]

When properly performed, TCO measurements correlate well with direct Fick or dye dilution estimates of CO. In clinical practice, triplicate determinations are averaged to increase precision. Differences in values of 12–15% are not of clinical significance. TCO estimates vary with the respiratory cycle. This variability can be reduced by performing measurements at peak inspiration or end-expiration. Precision is enhanced by ensuring that the rate of injection and the volume are constant. Most CO computers delay the repeat measurement 30–90 seconds to stabilize the thermal environment of the pulmonary thermistor.

Observation of the thermal curve is helpful. Low-amplitude curves result when the injectate volume is too small, the temperature differential between injectate and blood temperature is

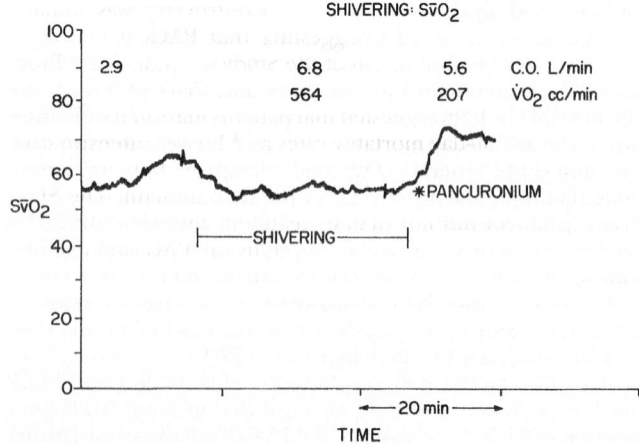

Figure 25-10. This $S\bar{v}O_2$ recording in a postcoronary artery bypass patient demonstrates the effects of shivering and its treatment, and the relationship between $S\bar{v}O_2$, cardiac output (CO), and metabolic rate ($\dot{V}O_2$). (Reproduced with permission from Vender JS: Invasive cardiac monitoring. Crit Care Clin 4:455, 1988.)

small, or when the thermistor is improperly positioned. Tricuspid or pulmonic regurgitation and intracardiac shunts may produce recirculation errors and a falsely elevated TCO.

Adaptations for Continuous Cardiac Output Monitoring

Continuous CO monitoring offers the potential to identify acute changes in ventricular performance as they occur. A properly positioned PAC provides access to the right atrium, right ventricle, and pulmonary artery outflow tract. These locations provide many options for assessment of CCOM. Several thermal techniques are currently used. Pulsed thermodilution uses a coiled right ventricular filament that is randomly heated. A thermistor at the tip of the PAC detects changes in blood temperature and sends the temperature information to a microcomputer that uses stochastic analysis to create a thermodilution curve. CO is computed continuously from a conservation of heat equation.[31]

Another technique applies heat to a thermistor located at the tip of a PAC. The right ventricular outflow subsequently cools the tip. The temperature changes registered are proportional to the decreased temperature produced by right ventricular blood flow. Both of these systems require calibration using standard thermodilution before initiating the CCOM mode. CCOM compares favorably with bolus CO measurements, even under conditions of varying patient temperature and CO.[32]

Doppler PAC methodology measures the blood flow velocity in the pulmonary artery. If the diameter of the pulmonary artery can be measured or estimated, then continuous monitoring of the CO is possible.[33]

Right Ventricular Ejection Fraction

Calculation of right ventricular ejection fraction and end-diastolic volume may be performed with a special PAC that uses a rapid response thermistor and a sophisticated computer system. This system analyzes the exponential decay of the pulmonary artery temperature over several cardiac cycles and calculates the ejection fraction by subtracting the mean residual fraction from the CO. Studies have demonstrated good correlation with *in vitro* techniques and clinical utility for detecting intraoperative right ventricular ischemia.[34-36] Right ventricular ejection fraction monitoring has been recommended when impairment of right ventricular function is suspect. Accuracy requires proper placement. Atrial fibrillation and tricuspid regurgitation can affect the accuracy of the thermal decay methodology.

Clinical Benefits of Pulmonary Artery Monitoring

The debate regarding the clinical benefit of PAC monitoring has persisted since the mid-1980s. Controversy was initially stimulated by two articles suggesting that PACs may worsen outcome.[37,38] The publication of the Study to Understand Prognosis and Preferences for Outcomes and Risks of Treatment (SUPPORT) in 1996 suggested that patients managed with PACs had increased 30-day mortality rates and longer intensive care unit and hospital stays.[39] This study design had several limitations that make interpretation of the data difficult. The SUPPORT protocol did not define treatment interventions to be used in response to the data provided by the PAC, and patients who received PACs were more critically ill than those who did not. The SUPPORT study illustrates the need for a large-scale prospective trial, in which patients are randomized to a control or PAC group, to determine the clinical benefits of PAC monitoring.

Inadequate understanding and application by physician users have been implicated as conditions that limit the benefit of PAC monitoring. To optimize clinical outcome and reduce complications, the care provider must be able to interpret and use the data provided by the PAC. A questionnaire that measured physician knowledge of the technical and theoretical aspects of PAC monitoring was administered to critical care specialists

in the United States and Europe. These surveys revealed knowledge of pulmonary artery catheterization is not uniformly good among intensive care unit physicians, with only half of respondents able to read the PCWP correctly from a clearly marked tracking.[40,41] Changes in training and credentialing have been proposed to improve these deficiencies in knowledge.[42,43] In experienced and knowledgeable hands, the PAC can add valuable information with limited risk.

NONINVASIVE TECHNIQUES FOR CARDIAC OUTPUT

The quest for technically simple, noninvasive methods for accurately estimating CO continues. Two methods are available for clinical use.

Impedance Plethysmography

Impedance plethysmography is based on determining the pulsatile changes in resistance occurring during ventricular ejection. Four electrodes are applied to the neck and thorax and a small electric current is applied. Impedance measurements (dZ/dT) are made using two thoracic electrode pairs. Changes in impedance correlate with stroke volume. CO is estimated by determining stroke volume and ventricular ejection time.[44] Electrode placement is an important source of error. Other factors influencing bioimpedance measurements include intrathoracic fluid shifts and changes in hematocrit. More than 150 validation studies have been published, and both poor and good correlations between impedance plethysmography and a reference method have been reported.[45] Although impedance plethysmography has not gained wide acceptance, the technique offers clinicians a simple, quick method to determine CO with minimal direct patient risk.

Doppler Ultrasonography

Continuous-wave or pulsed-wave Doppler ultrasonography can measure the velocity of blood in the ascending or descending aorta or outflow tract of the pulmonary artery. CO is calculated by multiplying the time-weighted average velocity of blood flow by an estimate of aortic or pulmonary artery cross-sectional area that can be directly measured or predicted from a nomogram. Accuracy and precision depend on the estimate of the vessel diameter and the alignment of the Doppler probe. Velocity measurements are most accurate when the Doppler probe and the blood flow are parallel. If the alignment exceeds 25 degrees, velocity measurements lose precision. Suprasternal, transtracheal, and transesophageal probes have been designed for clinical use.[46,47] The development of esophageal Doppler probes allows for continuous, minimally invasive estimation of CO, and may allow for optimization of intravascular volume status without the use of a CVP or PAC.[48]

TRANSESOPHAGEAL ECHOCARDIOGRAPHY

The use of transesophageal echocardiography (TEE) in the perioperative period has increased significantly since its first application in humans was reported by Frazen in 1976. Rapid technological advances have occurred since then, including a reduction in transducer size, the development of biplane and multiplane probes, and the use of pulsed-wave, continuous-wave, and color flow Doppler. Improvements in computer design and image acquisition have allowed for a more comprehensive examination of the heart and surrounding structures. TEE appears to offer distinct advantages over other monitors of cardiovascular function, and can provide the anesthesiologist with unique diagnostic information in the operating room.

Ultrasound transducers use piezoelectric crystals to transmit and receive high-frequency sound waves. As emitted ultrasound waves are propagated through the surrounding tissues, the energy is absorbed, scattered, or reflected back to the transducer. The amount of ultrasound energy reflected back to the transducer depends on differences in acoustic impedance between two tissues. The greater the difference in density, the greater the reflection. Because sound waves travel through soft tissue at a constant velocity, the time delay for the ultrasound beam to be reflected back to the transducer can be used to calculate the precise distance between the transducer and the object being interrogated.

Modern TEE machines offer a number of imaging techniques. In *M-mode*, or motion mode, all of the structures along a narrow ultrasound beam are plotted on the *x*-axis vs. time on the *y*-axis. M-mode allows only a few millimeters of the heart to be visualized at any one time. *Two-dimensional (2-D) mode* uses multiple scanning lines to create a two-dimensional image of a cross-section of the heart. This image is updated 30–60 times per second, which produces a real-time display of cardiac motion.

Doppler technology provides information about blood flow in the heart and major vessels. The *Doppler effect* is based on the principle that moving objects (red blood cells) change the frequency of the emitted ultrasound beam. If an object is moving toward the transducer, the ultrasound beam is compressed, which increases the frequency of the transmitted signal. An object moving away from the transducer lowers the frequency of the transmitted ultrasound beam. This information allows the calculation of blood flow velocity within the cardiovascular system. Current TEE machines use three Doppler systems: pulsed-wave, continuous-wave, and color flow Doppler. *Pulsed-wave Doppler* uses a single crystal to emit and receive short bursts of ultrasound at a known frequency (pulse repetition frequency). By measuring the time required for the transmitted ultrasound bursts to return to the transducer, the velocity of blood flow at precise locations in the heart can be measured. A major limitation of pulsed-wave Doppler is that high-velocity flows cannot be accurately quantified. The maximal velocity that can be measured is limited to one half of the pulse repetition frequency; this is known as the Nyquist limit. *Continuous-wave Doppler* uses two crystals (one to transmit, one to receive) to measure blood flow velocity continuously. This allows for accurate measurement of high-velocity flows, but does not permit precise localization. *Color flow Doppler* uses pulsed-wave technology to measure blood flow velocity at multiple sites. Blood flow toward the transducer is coded red and flow away from the transducer is coded blue. Rapidly accelerating or turbulent flow is coded green. By superimposing this color map on a 2-D image of the heart, the direction and velocity of blood flow in the heart can be easily imaged.

Monitoring Applications

There are a number of important monitoring applications for TEE in the perioperative period. In 1996, the ASA and the Society of Cardiovascular Anesthesiologists published practice guidelines to define the proper indications for performing TEE in the operative setting.[49] Indications were divided into three categories.

Category I indications are supported by the strongest evidence or expert opinion; TEE frequently is useful in improving clinical outcomes and is often indicated, depending on patient risk and practice setting. Category II indications are supported by weaker evidence and expert consensus; TEE may be useful in improving clinical outcomes, depending on individual circumstances. Category III indications have little current scientific or expert support, and TEE is infrequently useful in improving clinical outcomes. These indications are summarized in Table 25-7.

Transesophageal echocardiography is used extensively as a monitor of ventricular function. TEE appears to provide more accurate estimates of left ventricular preload than pulmonary artery catheterization. In echocardiography, preload is determined by measuring end-diastolic area. Studies in patients undergoing cardiac or vascular surgery revealed that end-diastolic area calculated by TEE correlated well with left ventricular preload, whereas pulmonary artery diastolic pressure correlated poorly with left ventricular preload.[50,51] Left atrial and left ventricular pressures may also be calculated using Doppler measurements of flow across the mitral valve, or from the pulmonary veins into the left atrium. TEE estimates of intracardiac filling pressures correlate well with data obtained from PACs.[52] Left ventricular contractility can be estimated using a variety of techniques. Ejection fraction can be determined by measuring left ventricular end-diastolic area (EDA) and end-systolic area (ESA):

$$\text{ejection fraction area} = \frac{\text{EDA} - \text{ESA}}{\text{EDA}} \times 100.$$

Stroke volume can be calculated by measuring the Doppler velocity of flow across an area of the heart (aortic valve, pulmonary artery, left ventricular outflow tract) and multiplying this value times the area through which the flow occurs. The stroke volume times heart rate yields CO. The use of biplane or multiplane probes appears to increase the accuracy of CO measurements.[53]

Transesophageal echocardiography may provide a more meaningful reference standard for myocardial ischemia than ECG. Within seconds of the onset of myocardial ischemia, abnormal inward motion and thickening of the affected myocardial segment occurs. Wall motion abnormalities precede changes in the ECG or PAC. Clinical studies suggest that many episodes of ischemia detected by TEE are missed by standard intraoperative ECG monitoring.[54,55] However, not all wall motion abnormalities are due to ischemia. Ventricular pacing, conduction abnormalities, translational motion of the heart, stunned myocardium, and changes in loading conditions can all mimic myocardial ischemia on TEE.

Transesophageal echocardiography is the only intraoperative monitor that provides information on the structure and function of the mitral, aortic, tricuspid, and pulmonic valves. The severity of stenotic or regurgitant valvular disease can be determined using Doppler studies. One of the most important indications for TEE in the operating room is in the assessment of patients requiring valvular surgery. The use of TEE before cardiopulmonary bypass provides new information or prompts changes in valve surgery in 9–13% of cases.[49] In patients undergoing mitral valve repair, postcardiopulmonary bypass TEE revealed persistent valvular dysfunction in 6–11% of patients, leading to second pump runs in 3–10% of cases.[49]

Transesophageal echocardiography may be used to determine the etiology of acute hypotension in the perioperative period. Left ventricular failure or dysfunction can be differentiated from other common causes of severe hypotension, such as hypovolemia or decreased systemic vascular resistance. Unusual causes of acute hypotension, including pericardial tamponade, pulmonary embolism, and aortic dissection, can be rapidly diagnosed with TEE. The early detection of the cause of hemodynamic instability allows for the appropriate therapy to be instituted (volume expansion, inotropes, vasopressors).

Transesophageal echocardiography is moderately invasive and is associated with major and minor complications. Major complications (esophageal trauma, dysrhythmias, hemodynamic instability) occur in 0.2–0.5% of examinations.[49] Minor complications (lip injuries, dental injuries, hoarseness, dysphagia) occur in 0.1–13% of cases, and may be related to endotracheal intubation rather than TEE.[49] Complication rates may be reduced when examinations are performed by experienced practitioners. Most complication rates have been reported from studies in awake patients; some complications may be less frequent in anesthetized surgical patients.

Table 25-7. INDICATIONS FOR PERIOPERATIVE TRANSESOPHAGEAL ECHOCARDIOGRAPHY

Category I indications: Supported by the strongest evidence or expert opinion; TEE is frequently useful in improving clinical outcomes in these settings and is often indicated, depending on individual circumstances (*e.g.*, patient risk and practice setting).
  Intraoperative evaluation of acute, persistent, and life-threatening hemodynamic disturbances in which ventricular function and its determinants are uncertain and have not responded to treatment
  Intraoperative use in valve repair
  Intraoperative use in congenital heart surgery for most lesions requiring cardiopulmonary bypass
  Intraoperative use in repair of hypertrophic obstructive cardiomyopathy
  Intraoperative use for endocarditis when preoperative testing was inadequate or extension of infection to perivalvular tissue is suspected
  Preoperative use in unstable patients with suspected thoracic aortic aneurysms, dissection, or disruption who need to be evaluated quickly
  Intraoperative assessment of aortic valve function in repair of aortic dissections with possible aortic valve involvement
  Intraoperative evaluation of pericardial window procedures
  Use in intensive care unit for unstable patients with unexplained hemodynamic disturbances, suspected valve disease, or thromboembolic problems (if other tests or monitoring techniques have not confirmed the diagnosis or patients are too unstable to undergo other tests)
Category II indications: Supported by weaker evidence and expert consensus; TEE may be useful in improving clinical outcomes in these settings, depending on individual circumstances, but appropriate indications are less certain.
  Perioperative use in patients with increased risk of myocardial ischemia or infarction
  Perioperative use in patients with increased risk of hemodynamic disturbances
  Intraoperative assessment of valve replacement
  Intraoperative assessment of repair of cardiac aneurysms
  Intraoperative evaluation of removal of cardiac tumors
  Intraoperative detection of foreign bodies
  Intraoperative detection of air emboli during cardiotomy, heart transplantation operations, and upright neurosurgical procedures
  Intraoperative use during intracardiac thrombectomy
  Intraoperative use during pulmonary embolectomy
  Intraoperative use for suspected cardiac trauma
  Preoperative assessment of patients with suspected acute thoracic aortic dissections, aneurysms, or disruption
  Intraoperative use during repair of thoracic aortic dissections without suspected aortic valve involvement
  Intraoperative detection of aortic atheromatous disease or other sources of aortic emboli
  Intraoperative evaluation of pericardectomy or pericardial effusions, or evaluation of pericardial surgery
  Intraoperative evaluation of anastomotic sites during heart or lung transplantation
  Monitoring placement and function of assist devices
Category III indications: Little current scientific or expert support; TEE is infrequently useful in improving clinical outcomes in these settings, and appropriate indications are uncertain.
  Intraoperative evaluation of myocardial perfusion, coronary artery anatomy, or graft patency
  Intraoperative use during repair of cardiomyopathies other than hypertrophic obstructive cardiomyopathy
  Intraoperative use for uncomplicated endocarditis during noncardiac surgery
  Intraoperative monitoring for emboli during orthopedic procedures
  Intraoperative assessment of repair of thoracic aortic injuries
  Intraoperative use for uncomplicated pericarditis
  Intraoperative evaluation of pleuropulmonary diseases
  Monitoring placement of intra-aortic balloon pumps, automatic implantable cardiac defibrillators, or pulmonary artery catheters
  Intraoperative monitoring of cardioplegia administration

TEE = transesophageal echocardiography.
Reproduced with permission from American Society of Anesthesiologists and Society of Cardiovascular Anesthesiologists Task Force on Transesophageal Echocardiography: Practice guidelines for perioperative transesophageal echocardiography. Anesthesiology 84:96, 1996.

MONITORING NEUROLOGIC FUNCTION

The best assessment of neurologic function is a thorough neurologic examination that evaluates the integration of brain and spinal cord function. However, anesthesia, sedation, and muscle relaxants, as well as existing neuropathology or trauma, may significantly impair the sensitivity or even the ability to perform a standard neurologic examination in the operating room. Therefore, monitoring neurologic function has become an important component of anesthesia care. Intraoperative neurologic monitoring often guides anesthesia and surgical decision making. Many intraoperative factors have the potential to influence spontaneous or evoked neural activity. General anesthesia can influence synaptic transmission and neural activity directly or by altering physiologic factors such as blood flow or blood pressure.

Intracranial Pressure Monitoring

Intracranial pressure (ICP) monitoring was initially used in trauma, where the relationship between uncontrolled ICP elevation and fatality has been firmly established.[56] ICP can be monitored by insertion of a subarachnoid bolt, a ventricular catheter, or an epidural transducer, or by insertion of a fiberoptic sensor in the cranial cavity. Each of these techniques requires a burr hole for intracranial access.

The cerebrospinal fluid (CSF) pressure wave is pulsatile and oscillates with the cardiac and respiratory cycle. Normal ICP is less than 15 mm Hg. Continuous recordings of the ICP in neurotrauma victims demonstrate three distinct pathologic waveforms. A waves (plateau waves) are found in patients with elevated baseline ICP and consist of a further elevation of ICP for periods from 5–20 minutes; A waves result from abrupt increases in regional cerebral blood volume where cerebral blood flow is decreased due to brain swelling, venous obstruction, or obstruction of CSF flow. B and C waves are of lesser magnitude and are related to respiratory pattern and blood pressure. Unlike A waves, they are not thought to be useful in guiding therapy or predicting outcome.

Intracranial pressure monitoring assumes that *cerebral perfusion pressure* (CPP = MAP − ICP) is uniformly distributed and that intracranial hypertension results in ischemia, displacement, compression, or herniation of the brain. ICP monitoring does not measure neural function or neural recovery.

Subarachnoid Devices

It is possible to monitor ICP using hollow stainless steel bolts or intraventricular catheters that are connected to a fluid-filled transducer system or a gravity manometer. Both methods are associated with the potential for infection or inaccuracy due to damping. Although the subarachnoid bolt is easiest to place and has a lower infection rate, the ventricular catheter allows CSF removal or insertion of a small volume of fluid to test the compliance of the cranial cavity.

Epidural Devices

Epidural sensors reduce the potential for infection because the dura is not breached. Two systems for epidural monitoring of ICP are in common use. The Ladd epidural transducer system uses a pressure-sensitive pneumatic switch that deforms as the dura changes conformation. Similarly, a fiberoptic system for ICP monitoring has been designed, which can be inserted epidurally or passed through an intraventricular catheter to sense ICP changes. Fiberoptic ICP monitoring is accurate and versatile.[57]

Electroencephalogram

The electroencephalogram (EEG) represents the spontaneous electrical activity of the superficial cerebral cortex as recorded from either the scalp or surface electrodes. The EEG signal originates from postsynaptic excitatory and inhibitory potentials produced by the pyramidal cells located in the outer cerebral cortex. In the operating room, the EEG signal can often be recorded to assess cortical activity. Signal processing requires the amplification of small voltages (10–100 mV), which are 1000 times smaller than ECG signals. Conventional EEG analysis uses scalp electrodes positioned at standardized points referenced to cranial dimensions. The voltage difference between a pair of EEG electrodes is amplified and compared with measurements using a reference electrode. This method, differential amplification, reduces artifacts. The resulting signal is then passed through electronic filters, which reduce or remove unwanted frequencies, and is then displayed as voltage over time. The EEG is usually characterized by activity in four frequency bands: beta (>12 Hz), alpha (8–12 Hz), theta (4–8 Hz), and delta (<4 Hz).

In unanesthetized patients, the EEG trace demonstrates background rhythms regulated by "pacemaker neurons" of the lower brain structures and the local electrical activity resulting from cortical neurons underlying the active electrode. During anesthesia, the background alpha rhythm predominates. With deeper anesthesia or during ischemia, EEG activity generally decreases in both amplitude and frequency. A total of 50% of the brain's oxygen consumption has been attributed to the energy requirement for the generation of EEG activity.

Electroencephalographic monitoring has been advocated for the intraoperative detection of cerebral ischemia during carotid endarterectomy; during deliberate hypotension; for the intraoperative or perioperative assessment of pharmacologic interventions; for identification of epileptic foci; or for the assessment of coma or brain death.[58]

Deep anesthesia, cerebral ischemia, or other pathologic states abolish or reduce normal neural EEG activity (alpha and beta rhythms), and slower frequencies (delta and theta) predominate. Sleep or surgical anesthesia typically increases amplitude (synchronization), whereas arousal characteristically decreases amplitude (desynchronization). Deep anesthesia may depress the EEG by directly effecting the cortical activity or by depression of pacemaker regulation. High concentrations of isoflurane or desflurane can cause periods of electrical silence interspersed with brief episodes of activity. Similar effects are seen by many intravenous sedative drugs such as barbiturates. This pattern is termed *burst suppression*. Increasing depth of anesthesia often results in EEG slowing with increases in amplitude, leading to burst suppression. At the highest levels of anesthesia, the EEG can become isoelectric, mimicking the effect of hypothermia or brain hypoxia. EEG interpretation requires experienced observers and the ability to integrate the changes with anesthetic, physiologic, and surgical events.

Processing Electroencephalographic Data

Several signal-processing techniques have been used to improve the ability of clinicians to interpret changes in the EEG and evaluate trends. The EEG signal is usually digitized, processed, and then graphically displayed for interpretation. Real-time analysis using Fourier transformation to identify amplitudes and frequencies of interest or a periodic analysis are often performed to convert voltage / time data to power spectral information, where power *vs.* frequency information is graphically displayed over epochs (*e.g.*, the *compressed spectral array*).

The *spectral edge frequency* is often calculated and displayed to summarize the changes in the power spectrum. The spectral edge is the frequency that is just above 95% of the power contained in the raw EEG. Monitoring the spectral edge has been considered useful in detection of cerebral ischemia and anesthetic depth.[59] Other descriptors such as the peak power frequency or the median power frequency have been used to describe EEG data under anesthesia.[60]

Today, there are many instruments that process EEG data to create graphic displays of brain electrical function. Instrumentation and software for mapping the frequency spectrum of the standard 16 EEG leads can produce pictorial images of brain electrical activity over time. Brain mapping may provide insight into the distribution of electrical activity associated with the administration of anesthetic agents. Intraoperative brain mapping remains controversial because of the potential for mapping artifact.[61]

Bispectral Index

The bispectral index (BIS) is a variable derived from the EEG that is a measure of the hypnotic effect of anesthetic agents. The BIS is the first processed EEG descriptor that predicts depth of consciousness. Previous EEG parameters, such as the spectral edge frequency, do not change in a linear manner with increasing depth of anesthesia. Furthermore, different anesthetic agents have differing effects on the processed EEG.

The calculation of the BIS integrates four different processed EEG descriptors into a single variable. These four parameters were selected on the basis of EEG data collected from thousands of anesthetics. The EEG data were correlated with the clinical state of the patient (level of consciousness, response to surgical incision). Each parameter has a particular stage of anesthesia where it performs most accurately. The BetaRatio parameter reflects light sedation, the SynchFastSlow detects surgical levels of anesthesia, and the burst suppression ratio (BSR) and QUAZI predominate during deep levels of anesthesia.[62] The parameters are then ranked and combined to yield a single number, the BIS. The range of valves for the BIS is from 0 to 100, with decreasing numbers indicating deeper levels of sedation or anesthesia. BIS valves of less than 60 appear to predict absence of consciousness.

Clinical studies have demonstrated that the BIS can reliably predict the level of sedation, loss of consciousness, and the probability of recall using a variety of anesthetic agents (thiopental, propofol, midazolam, isoflurane, and sevoflurane).[63–66] The BIS does not appear to be as reliable in predicting movement in response to a noxious stimulation. Motor responses to painful stimuli may be mediated by subcortical structures, which are not measured by the BIS monitor. The use of the BIS can facilitate faster emergence and improved recovery from general anesthesia by allowing more precise titration of anesthetic effect.[67]

Evoked Potential Monitoring

Stimulation of neural structures to evoke responses is useful for monitoring the functional integrity of brain stem, visual, auditory, or peripheral neural pathways. Evoked potentials (EPs) represent small electrical signals generated in neural pathways after periodic stimulation. In the cortex and subcortex, EPs are smaller than the background EEG, and it is necessary to remove the random background electrical activity to record EP data. Computer signal averaging and filtering permits display of the EP voltages over time. EPs are usually quantitated by the time from stimulation (latency) and the amplitude of the peaks generated by the neural structures of interest. Three sensory pathways are available for intraoperative monitoring.[68]

Brain stem auditory evoked responses (BAERs) are monitored by stimulation of the cochlea using pulsed sound waves in the ear. Three to five waves are usually recorded using electrodes placed near the ear and cortex. BAERs are useful in assessing brain stem function in comatose patients and during surgical procedures of the cerebellopontine angle, floor of the fourth ventricle, or procedures in proximity to the fifth, seventh, or eighth cranial nerves.[69] Unlike other EPs, the BAERs are relatively resistant to the effects of anesthesia.

Visual evoked potentials (VEPs) are produced by flashing light to stimulate the retina and recording the EPs over the occipital cortex. VEPs assess the integrity of the visual pathway and have been used during resection of pituitary tumors, craniopharyngiomas, or surgery in the vicinity of the optic tracts. Unlike BAERs, VEPs are technically difficult to obtain during anesthesia, and questions have arisen about their usefulness in surgery.

Somatosensory evoked potentials (SSEPs) are produced by stimulating peripheral nerves and recording responses from electrodes monitoring the transmission of the EPs through the sensory pathway. The nerves usually stimulated are the median, ulnar, peroneal, or posterior tibial. Surface electrodes are placed to record the signal from peripheral nerves, plexuses, nerve roots, the dorsal columns, the brain stem lemniscal pathways to the thalamus, and the sensory cortex.

Median nerve SSEPs have been used to monitor cerebral function in patients undergoing neurosurgical procedures or those with cerebral ischemia. In these patients, examination of the timing and amplitude of the response measured over the contralateral scalp at 20 milliseconds (N20) represents the cortical response to stimulation. Similarly, examination of the negative waves occurring 11–14 milliseconds interrogates spinal roots, spinal cord, and brain stem.

Monitoring the responses of upper or lower extremity nerves may assist in evaluating spinal cord function during instrumentation of the spine or during thoracoabdominal surgery, where spinal cord ischemia is a possible risk factor. Deterioration of spinal cord function decreases the amplitude and increases the latency of the SSEP waveform. Monitoring of SSEPs is thought to be a sensitive indicator of the spinal cord's functional integrity. Despite the fact that SSEP monitoring does not evaluate the function of the motor pathway, it appears to be useful during spinal surgery, notably for correction of scoliosis.[70] Intraoperative SSEPs should be regarded as an extension of the sensory neurologic examination during anesthesia care, but may not totally replace the "wake-up" test. During anesthesia, monitoring both the area of risk and the contralateral pathways helps identify changes resulting from surgery as opposed to those due to other global variables, such as the effect of anesthesia.

Motor evoked potentials (MEPs) provide a means of assessing descending motor pathways during neurosurgical, orthopedic, or vascular procedures. MEPs can be obtained by transcranial electrical stimulation, transcranial magnetic stimulation, or direct spinal cord stimulation.[71] Attenuation of transcranially elicited MEPs by commonly used anesthetic techniques has limited their usefulness during surgery. Further investigation with MEPs is needed to define fully their use during surgery.[72]

Facial nerve stimulation is commonly performed during procedures in the posterior fossa. Intentional stimulation or surgical irritation of the facial nerve can be evaluated visually or by evaluating the electromyogram. Although facial nerve function is rather insensitive to anesthetic influences, muscle relaxants need to be limited to provide adequate monitoring conditions.

Noninvasive Monitoring of Cerebral Hemodynamics

Transcranial Doppler monitoring of cerebral blood velocity offers anesthesiologists the potential to assess alterations in regional cerebral perfusion in patients at risk for cerebral ischemia or cerebral emboli. Low-frequency ultrasound can penetrate areas of the cranium and detection of the reflected Doppler signal can permit estimation of blood flow velocity. The Doppler signals are transformed by computer to calculate and display systolic, diastolic, and mean blood velocity (Vbf). Vbf serves as an index of cerebral blood flow in the region interrogated.

Three interrogation sites have been described. The temporal bone is used to determine the Vbf of the middle, anterior, and posterior cerebral arteries. The orbit permits measurement from the ophthalmic artery and portions of the internal carotid artery. The foramen magnum portal interrogates Vbf in the intracranial vertebral and basilar arteries. Transcranial Doppler can detect intracranial air or particulate embolism, and monitoring beat-to-beat changes in Vbf correlates with changes in regional cerebral blood flow.[73] Interest in using transcranial Doppler as an early warning of critical reductions in cerebral perfusion during anesthesia has been reported.[74] Unfortunately, the methodology cannot be used in all patients, and the instrumentation requires training with respect to insonation technique and interpretation of the sonograms displayed.

Similarly, *infrared spectroscopy* has been adapted to monitor cerebral oxygen delivery. This methodology is possible because infrared light (650–1100 nm) penetrates the scalp and skull so that reflective pulse oximetry is feasible. In the brain, venous oximetry signals predominate over arterial signals and the output of these instruments correlates best with cerebral $S\bar{v}O_2$. Cerebral $S\bar{v}O_2$ and the regional cerebral Hb oxygen saturation monitored by near-infrared cranial spectroscopy are sensitive indicators of changing regional cerebral oxygen saturation resulting from systemic hypoxia, regional cerebral oligemia, or anemia.[75,76] These devices are still being investigated for general clinical applications.

TEMPERATURE MONITORING

The ability to monitor body temperature is a standard of anesthesia care. The continual observation of temperature changes in anesthetized patients allows for the detection of accidental heat loss or malignant hyperthermia. Humans maintain their core temperature by balancing heat production from metabolism and the many environmental factors that supply heat or cool the body. Regional temperature information from skin, muscle, the body cavities, spinal cord, and brain are integrated in the central nervous system. Conceptually, thermoregulation involves the integration of "set points," which, when exceeded, trigger temperature-dissipating, temperature-conserving, or heat-producing mechanisms. Both general and regional anesthesia inhibit afferent and efferent control of thermoregulation.[77,78] In addition, the operating room environment and surgical exposure often contribute to excessive heat losses. Heat loss is common during surgery because the surgical environment transfers heat from the patient and anesthesia reduces heat production and diminishes the capability of patients to monitor and maintain thermoregulation.

Heat is produced as a consequence of cellular metabolism. In adults, thermoregulation involves the control of basal metabolic rate, muscular activity, sympathetic arousal, vascular tone, and hormone activation balanced against exogenous factors that determine the need for the body to create heat or to adjust the transfer of heat to the environment.

Heat losses may result from radiation, conduction, convection, and evaporation. Radiation refers to the infrared rays emanating from all objects above absolute temperature. Conduction refers to the transfer of heat from contact with objects. Convection refers to the transfer of heat from air passing by objects. Evaporation represents the heat loss resulting when water vaporizes. For every gram of water evaporated, 0.58 kcal of heat is lost.

Perioperative hypothermia predisposes patients to increases in metabolic rate (shivering) and cardiac work, decreases in drug metabolism and cutaneous blood flow, and impairments of coagulation. Clinical studies have demonstrated that patients in whom intraoperative hypothermia develops are at a higher risk for development of postoperative myocardial ischemia and wound infection compared with patients who are normothermic in the perioperative period.[79,80] Anesthesiologists frequently monitor temperature and attempt to maintain central core temperature at near-normal values in all patients undergoing anesthesia.

Central core temperatures can be estimated using probes that can be placed into the bladder, distal esophagus, ear canal, trachea, nasopharynx, or rectum.[81] Pulmonary artery blood temperature is also a good estimate of central core temperature.

Temperature is usually measured using electrical probes containing calibrated thermistors or thermocouples that serve as temperature transducers. Thermistors respond to temperature changes by changing their electrical resistance. Thermocouples are constructed by passing current through a circuit where the electrodes are made of two dissimilar metals. The current measured is directly proportional to the temperature difference between the two metal junctions. Thermocouple temperature probes maintain one junction at a known temperature and place the second junction on the temperature probe tip. Skin temperature can also be monitored using liquid crystal thermometry. Although convenient, temperature strips do not correlate with core temperature measurements.[82]

Thermoregulatory responses are based on a physiologically weighted average reflecting changes in the mean body temperature. Mean body temperature is estimated by the following equation:

$$\text{Mean temperature} = 0.85 \text{ T core} + 0.15 \text{ T skin}$$

Skin temperature monitoring has been advocated to identify peripheral vasoconstriction, but is not adequate to determine alterations in mean body temperature that may occur during surgery. Core temperature sites have been established as reliable indicators of changes in mean temperature. During routine noncardiac surgery, temperature differences between these sites are small. When anesthetized patients are being cooled, changes in rectal temperature often lag behind those of other probe locations, and the adequacy of rewarming is best judged by measuring temperature at several locations.

FUTURE TRENDS IN MONITORING

Diagnostic and therapeutic advances in medicine have had a great impact on the strategies and techniques available for intraoperative monitoring. Today's anesthesia practice has narrowed the distinction between laboratory medicine and patient monitoring. Technologic advances in instrument design, computerization, and engineering have made it possible to have ready access to serum chemistries, hematologic profiles, assessment of coagulation, and arterial blood gas measurements. Modern monitoring systems have the potential to transfer processed and raw data from the operating room to information management systems, which offer the potential for creating meaningful paperless anesthesia records and enhanced archiving of the conduct of anesthesia care as depicted by real-time monitoring trends.

The U.S. Department of Health and Human Services proposed implementation of patient record systems in 1996.[83] Proprietary systems for automated anesthesia records are now in the marketplace. These offer file sharing so that information that is traditionally viewed as patient monitoring can also be used for billing, ordering supplies, and quality improvement. Although computerization of the hospital environment has direct and indirect costs, the benefits to physicians, patients, insurers, and hospital administrators indicate that, like in other business environments, information management is coming to operating room monitoring and anesthesiology.[84,85] The clinical and administrative data that can be obtained from anesthesia work stations integrated with hospital information systems should enhance the quality of care and improve the intraoperative monitoring of anesthetized patients.

REFERENCES

1. Roizen MF, Schreider B, Austin W et al: Pulse oximetry, capnography, and blood gas measurements: Reducing cost and improving the quality of care with technology. Journal of Clinical Monitoring 9:237, 1993
2. American Society of Anesthesiologists: The Standards for Intraoperative Monitoring: Directory of Members, p 477. Park Ridge, Illinois, American Society of Anesthesiologists, 2000
3. Association for the Advancement of Medical Instrumentation: Human Factors, Engineering Guidelines and Preferred Practices for the Design of Medical Devices. Arlington, Virginia, Association for the Advancement of Medical Instrumentation, 1988
4. Loeb RG: A measure of intraoperative attention to monitor displays. Anesth Analg 76:337, 1993
5. Barker L, Webb RK, Runiciman EB et al: The Australian Incident Monitoring Study. The oxygen analyzer: Applications and limitations—an analysis of 200 incident reports. Anaesth Intensive Care 21:570, 1993
6. Mayer RM: Oxygen analyzers: Failure rates and life-spans of galvanic cells. Journal of Clinical Monitoring 6:196, 1990
7. Williamson JA, Webb RK, Cockings J et al: The Australian Incident Monitoring Study: The capnograph applications and limitations—an analysis of 2000 incident reports. Anaesth Intensive Care 21:551, 1993
8. Walder B, Lauber R, Zbinden AM: Accuracy and cross-sensitivity of 10 different anesthetic gas monitors: Journal of Clinical Monitoring 9:364, 1993
9. Barker SH, Shah WK. The effects of motion on the performance of pulse oximeters in volunteers. Anesthesiology 86:101, 1997
10. Moller JT, Pederson T, Rasmussen LS et al: Randomized evaluation of pulse oximetry in 20,802 patients: II. Perioperative events and postoperative complications. Anesthesiology 78:445, 1993
11. Langewouters GJ, Settels JJ, Roelandt R et al: Why use Finapres or Pertapres rather than intra-arterial or intermittent non-invasive techniques of blood pressure measurement? J Med Eng Technol 22:37, 1998
12. Vogel AJ, Van Montfrans GA: Reproducibility of twenty-four hour finger arterial blood pressure, variability and systemic hemodynamics. J Hypertens 15:1761, 1997
13. Hirschl MM, Binder M, Harken H, et al: Accuracy and reliability of noninvasive continuous finger blood pressure measurement in critically ill patients. Crit Care Med 24:1684, 1996
14. Gardner RM: Direct blood pressure measurement: Dynamic response requirements. Anesthesiology 54:227, 1981
15. Kleinman B, Powell S, Kumar P, Gardner RM: The fast flush test measures the dynamic response for the entire pressure monitoring system. Anesthesiology 77:1215, 1992
16. Slogoff S, Keats AS, Arlund C: On the safety of radial artery cannulation. Anesthesiology 59:42, 1983
17. McGregor AD: The Allen test: An investigation of its accuracy by fluorescein angiography dye. J Hand Surg Br 12:82, 1987
18. Vender JS, Watts RD: Differential diagnosis of hand ischemia in the presence of an arterial cannula. Anesth Analg 61:465, 1982

19. Shinozaki T, Dean RS, Mazuzan JE *et al:* Bacterial contamination of arterial lines: A prospective study. JAMA 249:233, 1983

20. Simmons BP: Guidelines for the Prevention of Intravascular Infection. Atlanta, GA: Centers for Disease Control, 1981

21. Sanford TJ: Internal jugular vein cannulation versus subclavian vein cannulation. An anesthesiologist's view: The right internal jugular vein. Journal of Clinical Monitoring 1:58, 1985

22. Mark JB: Central venous pressure monitoring: Clinical insights beyond the numbers. Journal of Cardiothoracic Anesthesia 5:163, 1991

23. Vender JS: Pulmonary artery catheter monitoring. Anesthesiology Clinics of North America 6:743, 1988

24. Tuman KJ, Carroll GC, Ivankovich AD: Pitfalls of interpretation of pulmonary artery catheter data. Journal of Cardiothoracic Anesthesia 3:625, 1989

25. American Society of Anesthesiologists Task Force: Practice guidelines for pulmonary artery catheterization. Anesthesiology 78:380, 1993

26. West JB, Dollery CT, Naimark A: Distribution of blood flow in isolated lung: Relation to vascular and alveolar pressures. J Appl Physiol 19:713, 1984

27. Gettinger A, Glass D: In vivo comparison of two mixed venous saturation catheters. Anesthesiology 66:373, 1987

28. Scuderi PE, MacGregor DA, Bowton DL *et al:* A laboratory comparison of three pulmonary artery oximetry catheters. Anesthesiology 81:245, 1994

29. Fegler G: Measurement of cardiac output in anesthetized animals by thermodilution method. Quarterly Journal of Experimental Physiology 39:153, 1954

30. Pearl RGB, Rosenthal MH, Mielson L *et al:* Effect of injectate volume and temperature on thermodilution cardiac output determination. Anesthesiology 64:798, 1986

31. Yelderman ML, Ramsey MA, Quinn MD *et al:* Continuous thermodilution cardiac output measurement in intensive care unit patients. J Cardiothorac Vasc Anesth 6:270, 1992

32. Mihm FG, Gettinger A, Hanson CW *et al:* A multicenter evaluation of a new continuous cardiac output pulmonary artery catheter system. Crit Care Med 26:1346, 1998

33. Iberti TJ, Silverman JH: Continuous cardiac output measurements in critically ill patients. J Cardiothorac Vasc Anesth 6:267, 1992

34. Hines R, Barash PG: Intraoperative right ventricular dysfunction detected with a right ventricular ejection fraction catheter. Journal of Clinical Monitoring 2:206, 1986

35. Mukherjee R, Spinale FG, VonRecum AF *et al:* In vitro validation of right ventricular thermodilution ejection fraction system. Ann Biomed Eng 19:165, 1991

36. Dennis JW, Menawat S, Sobowale O *et al:* Superiority of end-diastolic volume and ejection fraction measurements over wedge pressure in evaluating cardiac function during aortic reconstruction. J Vasc Surg 16:372, 1992

37. Robin ED: Death by pulmonary artery flow-directed catheter. Chest 92:727, 1987

38. Gore JM, Goldberg RJ, Spodick DH *et al:* A community wide assessment of the use of pulmonary artery catheters in patients with acute myocardial infarctions. Chest 92:721, 1987

39. Connor AF, Speroff T, Dawson NV *et al:* The effectiveness of right heart catheterization in the initial care of critically ill patients. JAMA 276:889, 1996

40. Iberti TJ, Fischer EP, Leibowitz AB *et al:* A multicenter study of physician's knowledge of pulmonary artery catheter. JAMA 264:2928, 1990

41. Gnaegi A, Feihl F, Perret C: Intensive care physicians insufficient knowledge of right-heart catheterization at the bedside: Time to act? Crit Care Med 25:213, 1997

42. Papadakos PJ, Vender JS: Training requirement for pulmonary artery catheter utilization in adult patients. New Horiz 5:287, 1997

43. Ginosar Y, Thijs LG, Sprung CL: Raising the standard of hemodynamic monitoring: Targeting the practice or practitioner? Crit Care Med 25:209, 1997

44. Young JD, McQuillan P: Comparison of thoracic electrical bioimpedance and thermodilution for the measurement of cardiac index in patients with severe sepsis. Br J Anaesth 70:58, 1993

45. Raaijmakers E, Faes TJ, Scholten RJ, *et al:* A meta-analysis of three decades of validating thoracic impedance cardiography. Crit Care Med 27:1203, 1999

46. Perrino AC, Fleming J, LaMantia KR: Transesophageal Doppler cardiac output monitoring: Performance during aortic reconstructive surgery. Anesth Analg 73:705, 1991

47. Perrino AC, O'Connor T, Luther M: Transtracheal Doppler cardiac output monitoring: Comparison to thermodilution during noncardiac surgery. Anesth Analg 78:1060, 1994

48. Sinclair S, James S, Singer M: Intraoperative intravascular volume optimization and length of hospital stay after repair of proximal femoral fracture: Randomized controlled trial. BMJ 315:909, 1997

49. American Society of Anesthesiologists and Society of Cardiovascular Anesthesiologists Task Force on Transesophageal Echocardiography: Practice guidelines for perioperative transesophageal echocardiography. Anesthesiology 84:96, 1996

50. Harpole DH, Clements FM, Quill T *et al:* Right and left ventricular performance during and after abdominal aortic aneurysm repair. Ann Surg 209:356, 1989

51. Cheung AT, Savino JS, Weiss SJ *et al:* Echocardiographic and hemodynamic indexes of left ventricular preload in patients with normal and abnormal ventricular function. Anesthesiology 81:376, 1994

52. Kuecherer HF, Muhiuden IA, Kusumoto FM: Estimation of mean left atrial pressure from transesophageal pulsed Doppler echocardiography of pulmonary venous flow. Circulation 81:1488, 1990

53. Hozumi T, Shakudo M, Applegate R *et al:* Accuracy of cardiac output estimation with biplane transesophageal echocardiography. J Am Soc Echocardiogr 6:62, 1993

54. Hauser AM, Gangadharen F, Ramos RG *et al:* Sequence of mechanical, electrocardiographic, and clinical effects of repeated coronary artery occlusion in human beings: Echocardiographic observations during coronary angioplasty. J Am Coll Cardiol 5:193, 1980

55. Smith JS, Cahalan MK, Benefiel DJ *et al:* Intraoperative detection of myocardial ischemia in high-risk patients: Electrocardiography versus two-dimensional transesophageal echocardiography. Circulation 72:1015, 1985

56. Saul TG, Druker TB: Effect of intracranial pressure monitoring and aggressive treatment on mortality in severe head injury. J Neurosurg 56:498, 1982

57. Crutchfield JS, Narayan RK, Robertson CS *et al:* Evaluation of a fiberoptic intracranial pressure monitor. J Neurosurg 72:482, 1990

58. Nuwer MR: Intraoperative electroencephalography. J Clin Neurophysiol 10:437, 1993

59. Rampil I, Correll JW, Rosenbaum SH *et al:* Computerized electroencephalogram monitoring and carotid artery shunting. Neurosurgery 13:276, 1983

60. Sidi A, Halimi P, Cotev S: Estimating anesthetic depth by electroencephalography during anesthetic induction and intubation in patients undergoing cardiac surgery. J Clin Anesth 2:101, 1990

61. Deleon MG: Electrical source analysis by brain mapping techniques. Physiol Meas 14:A95, 1993

62. Rampil IJ: A primer for EEG signal processing in anesthesia. Anesthesiology 89:980, 1998

63. Lui J, Singh H, White PF: Electroencephalographic bispectral index correlates with intraoperative recall and depth of propofol-induced sedation. Anesth Analg 84:185, 1997

64. Glass PS, Bloom M, Kearse L *et al:* Bispectral analysis measures sedation and memory effects of propofol, midazolam, isoflurane, and alfentanil in healthy volunteers. Anesthesiology 86:836, 1997

65. Sebel PS, Lang E, Rampil IJ *et al:* A multicenter study of bispectral electroencephalogram analysis for monitoring anesthetic effect. Anesth Analg 84:891, 1997

66. Kearse LA, Rosow C, Zaslavski A *et al:* Bispectral analysis of the electroencephalogram predicts conscious processing of information during propofol sedation and hypnosis. Anesthesiology 88:25, 1998

67. Song D, Joshi GP, White PF: Titration of volatile anesthetics using bispectral index facilitates recovery after ambulatory anesthesia. Anesthesiology 87:847, 1997

68. American Electroencephalographic Society: Guidelines on evoked potentials. J Clin Neurophysiol 11:40, 1994

69. Nagao S, Roccaforte P, Moody RA: Acute intracranial hypertension and auditory brain-stem responses: II. The effect of posterior fossa mass lesions on brain-stem function. J Neurosurg 52:351, 1980

70. Forbes HJ, Allen PW, Waller CS *et al:* Spinal cord monitoring in scoliosis surgery: Experience with 1168 cases. J Bone Joint Surg Br 73:487, 1991

71. Adams DC, Emerson RG, Heyer EJ *et al:* Monitoring of intraoperative motor-evoked potentials under conditions of controlled neuromuscular blockade. Anesth Analg 77:913, 1993

72. Zentner J, Albrech T, Heuser D: Influence of halothane, enflurane,

and isoflurane on motor evoked potentials. Neurosurgery 31: 298, 1992

73. Doblar DD, Frenett L, Lim YC *et al:* Immediate detection of carotid arterial thrombosis by transcranial Doppler monitoring. Anesthesiology 80:209, 1994

74. Lam AM, Newell DW: Intraoperative use of transcranial Doppler ultrasonography. Neurosurg Clin N Am 7:709, 1996

75. McCormick PW, Stewart M, Goetting MG *et al:* Noninvasive cerebral optical spectroscopy for monitoring oxygen delivery and hemodynamics. Crit Care Med 19:89, 1991

76. Williams IM, Picton AJ, Hardy SC *et al:* Cerebral hypoxia detected by near infrared spectroscopy. Anaesthesia 49:762, 1994

77. Sessler DI: Central thermoregulatory inhibition by general anesthesia. Anesthesiology 75:557, 1991

78. Ozaki M, Kurz A, Sessler DI *et al:* Thermoregulatory thresholds during epidural and spinal anesthesia. Anesthesiology 81:282, 1994

79. Kurz A, Sessler DJ, Lenhardt R: Perioperative normothermia to reduce the incidence of surgical wound infection and shorten hospitalization. N Engl J Med 334:1209, 1996

80. Frank SM, Fleisher LA, Breslow MJ *et al:* Perioperative maintenance of normothermic reduces the incidence of morbid cardiac events: A randomized clinical trial. JAMA 277:1127, 1997

81. Yamakage M, Kawanna S, Watanabe H *et al:* The utility of tracheal temperature monitoring. Anesth Analg 76:795, 1993

82. Vaughan MS, Cork RD, Vaughan RW: Inaccuracy of liquid crystal thermometry to identify core temperature trends in postoperative adults. Anesth Analg 61:284, 1982

83. U.S. Department of Health and Human Services: Initiatives Toward the Electronic Health Care System of the Future. Washington, DC, U.S. Department of Health and Human Services, 1992

84. Smith NT: The M-15: A truly different workstation. Journal of Clinical Monitoring 10:352, 1994

85. Gibby GL: Anesthesia information-management systems: Their role in risk-versus cost assessment and outcomes research. J Cardiothorac Vasc Anesth 11(2 suppl 1):2, 1997

FIVE

MANAGEMENT OF ANESTHESIA

Clinical Anesthesia (4/e), edited by
Paul G. Barash, Bruce F. Cullen, and
Robert K. Stoelting. Lippincott Williams &
Wilkins, Philadelphia, © 2001.

CHAPTER 26

EPIDURAL AND SPINAL ANESTHESIA

CHRISTOPHER M. BERNARDS

There are no absolute indications for spinal or epidural anesthesia. However, there are clinical situations in which patient preference, patient physiology, or the surgical procedure makes central neuraxial block the technique of choice. There is also growing evidence that these techniques may improve outcome in selected situations. Spinal and epidural anesthesia have been shown to blunt the "stress response" to surgery,[1] to decrease intraoperative blood loss,[2,3] to lower the incidence of postoperative thromboembolic events,[2–5] and to decrease morbidity and mortality in high-risk surgical patients.[6] In addition, both spinal and epidural techniques can be used to extend analgesia into the postoperative period or to provide analgesia to nonsurgical patients. Thus, these techniques are an indispensable part of modern anesthetic practice, and every anesthesiologist should be adept at performing them.

ANATOMY

Proficiency in spinal and epidural anesthesia requires a thorough understanding of the anatomy of the spine and spinal cord. The anesthesiologist must be familiar with the surface anatomy of the spine but must also develop a mental picture of the three-dimensional anatomy of deeper structures. In addition, one must appreciate the relationship between the cutaneous dermatomes, the spinal nerves, the vertebrae, and the spinal segment from which each spinal nerve arises.

Vertebrae

The spine consists of 33 vertebrae (7 cervical, 12 thoracic, 5 lumbar, 5 fused sacral, and 4 fused coccygeal) (Fig. 26-1). With the exception of C1, the cervical, thoracic, and lumbar vertebrae consist of a body anteriorly, two pedicles that project posteriorly from the body, and two laminae that connect the pedicles (Fig. 26-2). These structures form the vertebral canal, which contains the spinal cord, spinal nerves, and epidural space. The laminae give rise to the transverse processes that project laterally and the spinous process that project posteriorly. These bony projections serve as sites for muscle and ligament attachments. The pedicles contain a superior and inferior vertebral notch through which the spinal nerves exit the vertebral canal. The superior and inferior articular processes arise at the junction of the lamina and pedicles and form joints with the adjoining vertebrae. The first cervical vertebra differs from this typical structure in that it does not have a body or a spinous process.

The five sacral vertebrae are fused together to form the wedge-shaped sacrum, which connects the spine with the iliac wings of the pelvis (Fig. 26-1). The 5th sacral vertebra is not fused posteriorly, giving rise to a variably shaped opening known as the sacral hiatus. Occasionally other sacral vertebrae do not fuse posteriorly, giving rise to a much larger sacral hiatus. The sacral cornu are bony prominences on either side of the hiatus and aid in identifying it. The sacral hiatus provides an opening into the sacral canal, which is the caudal termination of the epidural space. The four rudimentary coccygeal vertebrae are fused together to form the coccyx, a narrow, triangular bone that abuts the sacral hiatus and can be helpful in identifying it. The tip of the coccyx can often be palpated in the proximal gluteal cleft, and by running one's finger cephalad along its

smooth surface, the sacral cornu can be identified as the first bony prominence encountered.

Identifying individual vertebrae is important for correctly locating the desired interspace for epidural and spinal blockade. The spine of C7 is the first prominent spinous process encountered while running the hand down the back of the neck. The spine of T1 is the most prominent spinous process and immediately follows C7. The 12th thoracic vertebra can be identified by palpating the 12th rib and tracing it back to its attachment to T12. A line drawn between the iliac crests crosses the body of L5 or the L4–L5 interspace.

Ligaments

The vertebral bodies are stabilized by five ligaments that increase in size between the cervical and lumbar vertebrae (Fig. 26-2). From the sacrum to T7, the supraspinous ligament runs between the tips of the spinous processes. Above T7 this ligament continues as the ligamentum nuchae and attaches to the occipital protuberance at the base of the skull. The interspinous ligament attaches between the spinous processes and blends posteriorly with the supraspinous ligament and anteriorly with the ligamentum flavum. The ligamentum flavum is a tough, wedge-shaped ligament composed of elastin. It consists of right and left portions that span adjacent vertebral laminae and fuse in the midline to varying degrees.[7,8] The ligamentum flavum is thickest in the midline measuring 3–5 mm at the L2–L3 interspace of adults. This ligament is also farthest from the spinal meninges in the midline, measuring 4–6 mm at the L2–L3 interspace.[7] As a result, midline insertion of an epidural needle is least likely to result in unintended meningeal puncture. The anterior and posterior longitudinal ligaments run along the anterior and posterior surfaces of the vertebral bodies.

Epidural Space

The epidural space is the space that lies between the spinal meninges and the sides of the vertebral canal (Fig. 26-3). It is bounded cranially by the foramen magnum, caudally by the sacrococcygeal ligament covering the sacral hiatus, anteriorly by the posterior longitudinal ligament, laterally by the vertebral pedicles, and posteriorly by both the ligamentum flavum and vertebral lamina. The epidural space is not a closed space but communicates with the paravertebral space by way of the intervertebral foramina. The epidural space is shallowest anteriorly where the dura may in some places fuse with the posterior longitudinal ligament. The space is deepest posteriorly, although the depth varies because the space is intermittently obliterated by contact between the dura mater and the ligamentum flavum or vertebral lamina. Contact between the dura mater and the pedicles also interrupts the epidural space laterally. Thus, the epidural space is composed of a series of discontinuous compartments that become continuous when the potential space separating the compartments is opened up by injection of air or liquid (Fig. 26-3).[8]

The most ubiquitous material in the epidural space is fat, which is principally located in the posterior and lateral epidural space. A rich network of valveless veins (Batson's plexus) courses through the anterior and lateral portions of the epidural space,

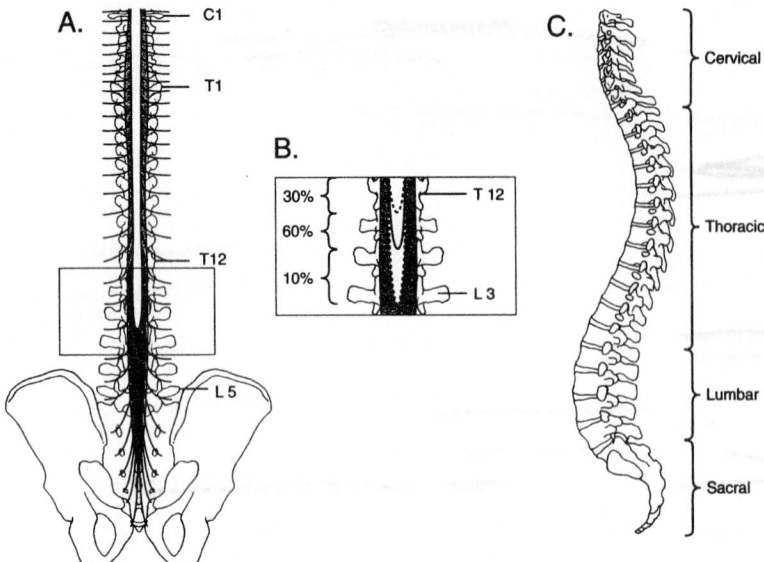

Figure 26-1. Posterior (*A*) and lateral (*C*) views of the human spinal column. Note the inset (*B*), which depicts the variability in vertebral level at which the spinal cord terminates.

with few if any veins present in the posterior epidural space (Fig. 26-2).[9, 10] The epidural veins anastomose freely with extradural veins including the pelvic veins, the azygos system, and the intracranial veins. The epidural space also contains lymphatics and segmental arteries running between the aorta and the spinal cord.

Meninges

The spinal meninges consist of three protective membranes (dura mater, arachnoid mater, and pia mater) that are continuous with the cranial meninges (Fig. 26-4).

Dura Mater

The dura mater is the outermost and thickest meningeal tissue. The spinal dura mater begins at the foramen magnum, where it fuses with the periosteum of the skull, forming the cephalad border of the epidural space. Caudally, the dura mater ends at approximately S2 where it fuses with the filum terminale. The dura mater extends laterally along the spinal nerve roots and becomes continuous with the connective tissue of the epineurium at approximately the level of the intervertebral foramina. The dura mater is composed of randomly arranged collagen fibers and elastin fibers arranged longitudinally and circumferentially.[11] The dura mater is largely acellular except for a layer of cells that forms the border between the dura and arachnoid mater.

There is controversy regarding the existence and clinical significance of a midline connective tissue band, the plica medianis dorsalis, running from the dura mater to the ligamentum flavum. Anatomic studies using epiduroscopy[12] and epidurography[13] have demonstrated the presence of the plica medianis dorsalis and have led to speculation that this tissue band may on occasion be responsible for difficulty in inserting epidural catheters and for unilateral epidural block. However, using cryomicrotome sections to investigate the epidural space, Hogan failed to find evidence of a substantial connection between

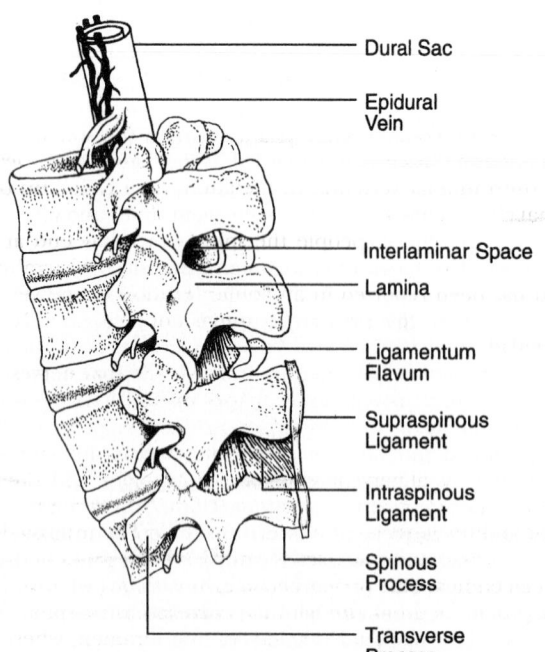

Figure 26-2. Detail of the lumbar spinal column and epidural space. Note that the epidural veins are largely restricted to the anterior and lateral epidural space.

Labels on Figure 26-2:
- Dural Sac
- Epidural Vein
- Interlaminar Space
- Lamina
- Ligamentum Flavum
- Supraspinous Ligament
- Intraspinous Ligament
- Spinous Process
- Transverse Process

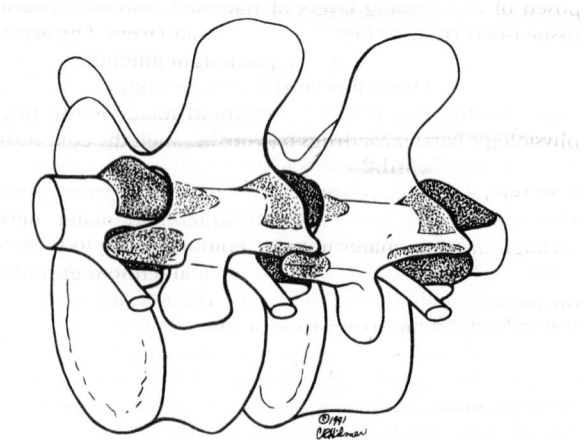

Figure 26-3. The compartments of the epidural space (*stippled areas*) are discontinuous. Areas where no compartments are indicated represent a potential space where the dura mater normally abuts the sides of the vertebral canal. (Reprinted with permission from Hogan Q: Lumbar epidural anatomy: A new look by cryomicrotome section. Anesthesiology 75:767, 1991.)

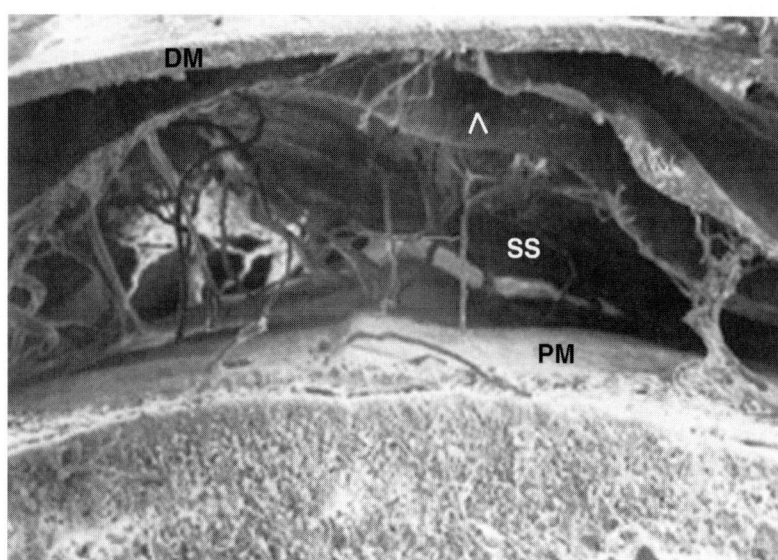

Figure 26-4. The spinal meninges of the dog demonstrating the pia mater (PM) in apposition to the spinal cord, the subarachnoid space (SS), the arachnoid mater (AM), trabeculae (*arrow*), and the dura mater (DM). The separation between the arachnoid mater and the dura mater demonstrates the subdural space. The subdural space is only a potential space *in vivo* but is created here as an artifact of preparation. (Reprinted with permission from Peters A, Palay SL, Webster H [eds]: The Fine Structure of the Nervous System: The Neurons and Supporting Cells. Philadelphia, WB Saunders, 1976.)

the dura mater and the ligamentum flavum.[8] He speculated that the injection of either air or contrast required for the earlier studies may have compressed epidural contents (*e.g.*, fat) and produced an artifact mimicking a connective tissue band. In addition, Hogan has shown in a clinical study that there is no significant impediment to spread of injectate across the midline.[14] Thus, the plica medianis dorsalis does not appear to be clinically relevant with respect to clinical epidural anesthesia.

The inner surface of the dura mater abuts the arachnoid mater. There is a potential space between these two membranes called the subdural space (Fig. 26-4). Occasionally, drug intended for either the epidural space or the subarachnoid space is injected into the subdural space.[15] Subdural injection has been estimated to occur in 0.82% of intended epidural injections.[16] The radiology literature suggests that the incidence of subdural injection during intended subarachnoid injection may be as high as 10%.[17]

Arachnoid Mater

The arachnoid mater is a delicate, avascular membrane composed of overlapping layers of flattened cells with connective tissue fibers running between the cellular layers. The arachnoid cells are interconnected by frequent tight junctions and occluding junctions. These specialized cellular connections likely account for the fact that the arachnoid mater is the principal physiologic barrier for drugs moving between the epidural space and the spinal cord.[18]

In the region where the spinal nerve roots traverse the dura and arachnoid membranes, the arachnoid mater herniates through the dura mater into the epidural space to form arachnoid granulations. As with the cranial arachnoid granulations, the spinal arachnoid granulations serve as a site for material in the subarachnoid space to exit the central nervous system (CNS). Although some have postulated that the arachnoid granulations are a preferred route for drugs to move from the epidural space to the spinal cord, the available experimental data suggest that this is not the case.[19]

The subarachnoid space lies between the arachnoid mater and the pia mater and contains the cerebrospinal fluid (CSF). The spinal CSF is in continuity with the cranial CSF and provides an avenue for drugs in the spinal CSF to reach the brain. In addition, the spinal nerve roots and rootlets run in the subarachnoid space.

Pia Mater

The spinal pia mater is adherent to the spinal cord and is composed of a thin layer of connective tissue cells interspersed with collagen. Trabeculae connect the pia mater with the arachnoid mater and the cells of these two meninges blend together along the trabeculae. Unlike the arachnoid mater, the pia mater is fenestrated in places so that the spinal cord is in direct communication with the subarachnoid space. The pia mater extends to the tip of the spinal cord where it becomes the filum terminale, which anchors the spinal cord to the sacrum. The pia mater also gives rise to the dentate ligaments, which are thin connective tissue bands extending from the side of the spinal cord through the arachnoid mater to the dura mater. These ligaments serve to suspend the spinal cord within the meninges.

Spinal Cord

In the first-trimester fetus, the spinal cord extends from the foramen magnum to the end of the spinal column. Thereafter, the vertebral column lengthens more than the spinal cord so that at birth the spinal cord ends at approximately the level of the third lumbar vertebra. In the adult, the caudad tip of the spinal cord typically lies at the level of the first lumbar vertebra. However, in 30% of people the spinal cord may end at T12, whereas in 10% it may extend to L3 (Fig. 26-1).[20] A sacral spinal cord has been reported in an adult.[20] Flexion of the vertebral column causes the tip of the spinal cord to move slightly cephalad.

The spinal cord gives rise to 31 pairs of spinal nerves, each composed of an anterior motor root and a posterior sensory root. The nerve roots are in turn composed of multiple rootlets. The portion of the spinal cord that gives rise to all of the rootlets of a single spinal nerve is called a cord segment. The skin area innervated by a given spinal nerve and its corresponding cord segment is called a dermatome (Fig. 26-5). The intermediolateral gray matter of the T1–L2 spinal cord segments contains the cell bodies of the preganglionic sympathetic neurons. These sympathetic neurons run with the corresponding spinal nerve to a point just beyond the intervertebral foramen, where they exit to join the sympathetic chain ganglia.

The spinal nerves and their corresponding cord segments are named for the intervertebral foramen through which they run. In the cervical region, the spinal nerves are named for the

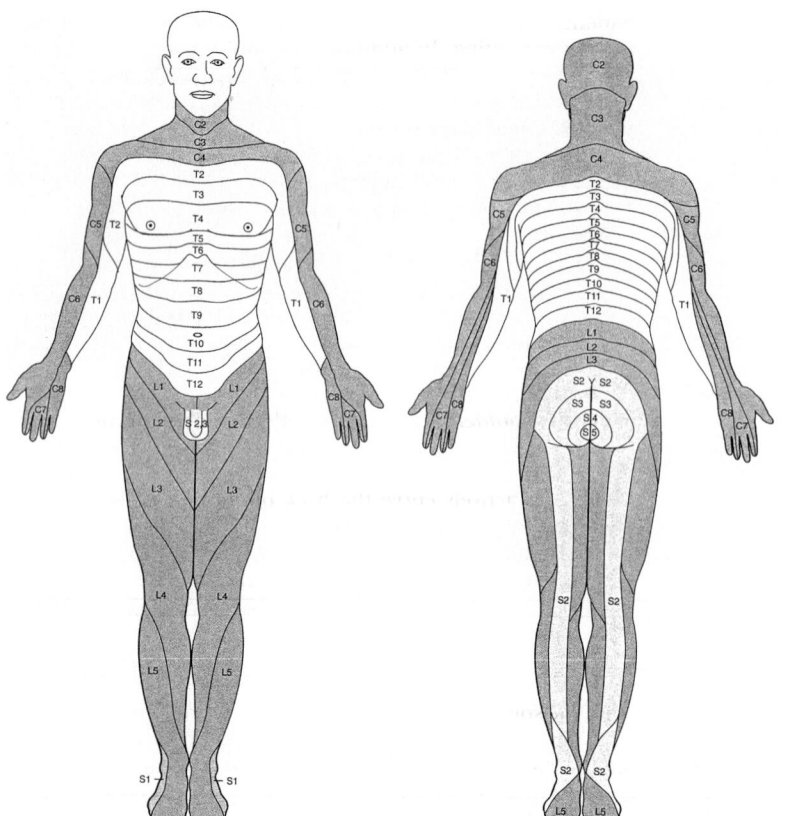

Figure 26-5. Human sensory dermatomes.

vertebra forming the caudad half of the intervertebral foramen; for example, C4 emerges through an intervertebral foramen formed by C3 and C4. In the thoracic and lumbar regions, the nerve roots are named for the vertebrae forming the cephalad half of the intervertebral foramen; for example, L4 emerges through an intervertebral foramen formed by L4 and L5. Because the spinal cord ends between L1 and L2, the thoracic, lumbar, and sacral nerve roots run increasingly longer distances in the subarachnoid space to get from their spinal cord segment of origin to the intervertebral foramen through which they exit. Those nerves that extend beyond the end of the spinal cord to their exit site are collectively known as the cauda equina (Fig. 26-1).

TECHNIQUE

Spinal and epidural anesthesia should be performed only after appropriate monitors are applied and in a setting where equipment for airway management and resuscitation are immediately available. Before positioning the patient, all equipment for spinal block should be ready for use (*e.g.*, local anesthetics mixed and drawn up, needles uncapped, prep solution available). Preparing all equipment ahead of time minimizes the time required to perform the block and thereby enhances patient comfort.

Needles

Spinal and epidural needles are named for the design of their tips (Fig. 26-6). The Whitacre and Sprotte spinal needles have a "pencil-point" tip with the needle hole on the side of the shaft. The Greene and Quincke needles have beveled tips with cutting edges. The pencil-point needles require more force to insert than the bevel-tip needles but provide a better tactile "feel" of the various tissues encountered as the needle is in-

serted. In addition, the bevel has been shown to cause the needle to be deflected from the intended path as it passes through tissues, whereas pencil-point needles are not deflected.[21]

Epidural needles have a larger diameter than spinal needles to facilitate the injection of fluid or air when using the "loss-of-resistance" technique to identify the epidural space. In addition, the larger diameter allows for easier insertion of catheters into the epidural space. The Tuohy epidural needle has a curved tip to help control the direction the catheter moves in the epidural space. The Hustead needle tip is also curved, although somewhat less than the Tuohy needle. The Crawford needle tip is straight, making it less suitable for catheter insertion.

The outside diameter of both epidural and spinal needles is used to determine their gauge. Larger-gauge (*i.e.*, smaller-diameter) spinal needles are less likely to cause postdural puncture headaches (PDPH), but are more readily deflected than smaller-gauge needles. Epidural needles are typically sized 16–19 gauge and spinal needles 22–29 gauge. Spinal needles smaller than 22 gauge are often easier to insert if an introducer needle is used. The introducer is inserted into the interspinous ligament in the intended direction of the spinal needle and the spinal needle is then inserted through the shaft of the introducer. The introducer prevents the spinal needle from being deflected or bent as it passes through the interspinous ligament.[21] Needles of the same outside diameter may have different inside diameters. This is important because inside diameter determines how large a catheter can be inserted through the needle and determines how rapidly CSF appears at the needle hub during spinal needle insertion.

All spinal and epidural needles come with a tight-fitting stylet. The stylet prevents the needle from being plugged with skin or fat and, importantly, prevents dragging skin into the epidural or subarachnoid spaces, where the skin may grow and form dermoid tumors.

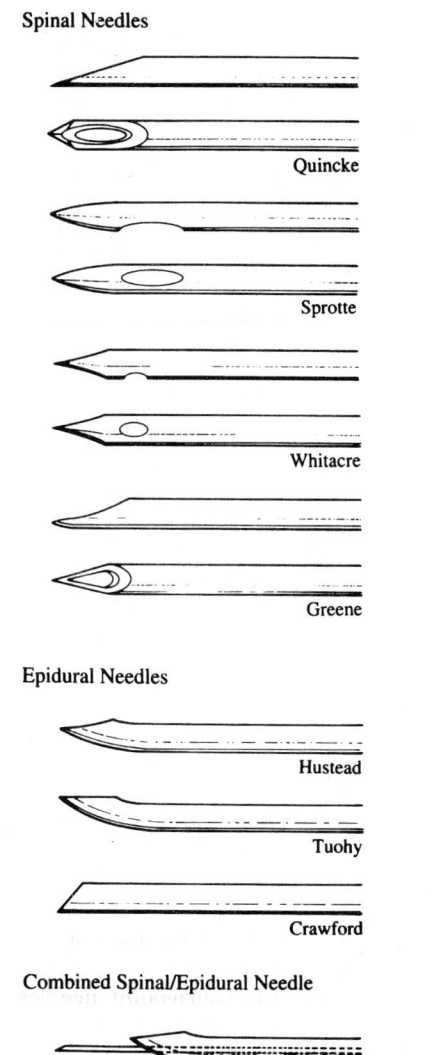

Spinal Needles

Quincke

Sprotte

Whitacre

Greene

Epidural Needles

Hustead

Tuohy

Crawford

Combined Spinal/Epidural Needle

Figure 26-6. Some of the commercially available needles for spinal and epidural anesthesia. Needles are distinguished by the design of their tips.

Sedation

If the patient desires, light sedation is appropriate before placement of spinal or epidural block. In general, the patient should not be heavily sedated because successful spinal and epidural anesthesia requires patient participation to maintain good position, evaluate block height, properly evaluate an epidural test dose, and indicate paresthesias to the anesthesiologist if the needle contacts neural elements. Once the block is placed and adequate block height assured, the patient can be sedated as deemed appropriate.

Spinal Anesthesia

Position

Careful attention to patient positioning is critical to successful spinal puncture. Poor positioning can turn an otherwise easy spinal anesthetic into a challenge for both the anesthesiologist and the patient. Spinal needles are most often inserted with the patient in the lateral decubitus position, and this technique is described in detail in this section. However, both the prone jackknife and sitting positions offer advantages under specific circumstances. The sitting position is sometimes used in obese

patients because it is often easier to identify the midline with the patient sitting. In addition, the sitting position allows the anesthesiologist to restrict spinal block to the sacral dermatomes (saddle block) when using hyperbaric local anesthetic solutions. Usually, spinal block is performed in the prone jackknife position only when this is the position to be used for surgery. The use of hypobaric local anesthetic solutions with the patient in the prone jackknife position produces sacral block for perirectal surgery.

In the lateral decubitus position, the patient lies with the operative side down when hyperbaric local anesthetic solutions are used and with the operative side up when hypobaric solutions are used, thus ensuring that the earliest and most dense block occurs on the operative side. The back should be at the edge of the table so that the patient is within easy reach. The patient's shoulders and hips are both positioned perpendicular to the bed to help prevent rotation of the spine. The knees are drawn to the chest, the neck is flexed, and the patient is instructed to actively curve the back outward. This spreads the spinous processes apart and maximizes the size of the interlaminar foramina. It is useful to have an assistant who can help the patient maintain this position. Using the iliac crests as a landmark, the L2–L3, L3–L4, and L4–L5 interspaces are identified and the desired interspace chosen for needle insertion. Interspaces above L2–L3 are avoided to decrease the risk of hitting the spinal cord with the needle. Some find it helpful to mark the spinous processes flanking the desired interspace with a skin marker obviating the need to reidentify the intended interspace after the patient is prepared and draped.

The patient is prepared with an appropriate antiseptic solution and draped. All antiseptic solutions are neurotoxic, and care must be taken not to contaminate spinal needles or local anesthetics with the preparation solution. How the patient is draped is a matter of personal preference, but the author finds that preparing and draping out a large area (*e.g.,* T12–S1) with towels is preferable to using a commercial one-piece drape with a limited center hole. Draping a large area permits easier identification of a rotated or inadequately flexed back and allows the anesthesiologist to move readily to another interspace if this becomes necessary.

Midline Approach

For the midline approach to the subarachnoid space, the skin overlying the desired interspace is infiltrated with a small amount of local anesthetic to prevent pain when inserting the spinal needle. The anesthesiologist should avoid raising too large a skin wheal because this can obscure palpation of the interspace, especially in obese patients. Additional local anesthetic (1–2 ml) is then deposited along the intended path of the spinal needle to a depth of 1–2 inches. This deeper infiltration provides additional anesthesia for spinal needle insertion and helps identify the correct path for the spinal needle.

The spinal needle or introducer needle is inserted in the middle of the interspace with a slight cephalad angulation of 10–15 degrees (Fig. 26-7). The needle is then advanced, in order, through the subcutaneous tissue, supraspinous ligament, interspinous ligament, ligamentum flavum, epidural space, dura mater, and finally arachnoid mater. The ligaments produce a characteristic "feel" as the needle is advanced through them, and the anesthesiologist should develop the ability to distinguish a needle that is advancing through the high-resistance ligaments from one that is advancing through lower-resistance paraspinous muscle. This allows early detection and correction of needles that are not advancing in the midline. Penetration of the dura mater produces a subtle "pop" that is most easily detected with the pencil-point needles. Detection of dural penetration prevents inserting the needle all the way through the subarachnoid space and contacting the vertebral body. In addition, learning to detect dural penetration allows the practitioner to insert the spinal needle quickly without hav-

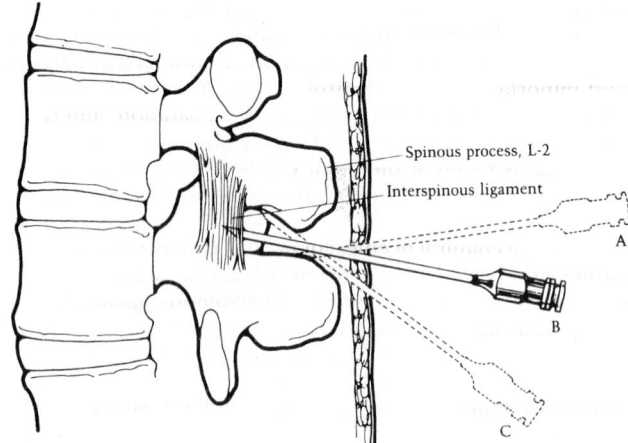

Figure 26-7. Midline approach to the subarachnoid space. The spinal needle is inserted with a slight cephalad angulation and should advance in the midline without contacting bone (*B*). If bone is contacted, it may be either the caudad (*A*) or the cephalad spinous process (*C*). The needle should be redirected slightly cephalad and reinserted. If bone is encountered at a shallower depth, then the needle is likely walking up the cephalad spinous process. If bone is encountered at a deeper depth, then the needle is likely walking down the inferior spinous process. If bone is repeatedly contacted at the same depth, then the needle is likely off the midline and walking along the lamina. (Reprinted with permission from Mulroy MF: Regional Anesthesia: An Illustrated Procedural Guide. Boston, Little, Brown, 1989.)

ing to stop every few millimeters and remove the stylet to look for CSF at the needle hub.

Once the needle tip is believed to be in the subarachnoid space, the stylet is removed to see if CSF appears at the needle hub. With small-diameter needles (26–29 gauge), this usually requires 5–10 seconds, but may require ≥1 min in some patients. Gentle aspiration may speed the appearance of CSF. If CSF does not appear, the needle orifice may be obstructed by a nerve root, and rotating the needle 90 degrees may result in CSF flow. Alternatively, the needle orifice may not be completely in the subarachnoid space, and advancing an additional 1–2 mm may result in brisk CSF flow. This is particularly true of pencil-point needles, which have their orifice on the side of the needle shaft proximal to the needle tip. Finally, failure to obtain CSF suggests that the needle orifice is not in the subarachnoid space and the needle should be reinserted.

If bone is encountered during needle insertion, the anesthesiologist must develop a reasoned, systematic approach to redirecting the needle. Simply withdrawing the needle and repeatedly reinserting it in different directions is not appropriate. When contacting bone, the depth should be immediately noted and the needle redirected slightly cephalad. If bone is again encountered at a greater depth, then the needle is most likely walking down the inferior spinous process and should be redirected more cephalad until the subarachnoid space is reached. If bone is encountered again at a shallower depth, then the needle is most likely walking up the superior spinous process and should be redirected more caudad. If bone is repeatedly encountered at the same depth, then the needle is likely off the midline and walking along the vertebral lamina (Fig. 26-7).

When redirecting a needle, it is important to withdraw the tip into the subcutaneous tissue. If the tip remains embedded in one of the vertebral ligaments, attempts at redirecting the needle will simply bend the shaft and not reliably change needle direction. If an introducer needle is used, it also must be withdrawn into the subcutaneous tissue before being redirected. Changes in needle direction should be made in small incre-

ments because even small changes in needle angle at the skin may result in fairly large changes in position of the needle tip when it reaches the spinal meninges at a depth of 4–6 cm. Care should be exercised when gripping the needle to ensure that it does not bow. Insertion of a curved needle causes it to veer off course.

If the patient experiences a paresthesia, it is important to determine whether the needle tip has encountered a nerve root in the epidural space or in the subarachnoid space. When the paresthesia occurs, immediately stop advancing the needle, remove the stylet, and look for CSF at the needle hub. The presence of CSF confirms that the needle encountered a cauda equina nerve root in the subarachnoid space and the needle tip is in good position. Given how tightly packed the cauda equina nerve roots are, it is surprising that all spinal punctures do not produce paresthesias. If CSF is not visible at the hub, then the paresthesia probably resulted from contact with a spinal nerve root traversing the epidural space. This is especially true if the paresthesia occurs in the dermatome corresponding to the nerve root that exits the vertebral canal at the same level that the spinal needle is inserted. In this case, the needle has most likely deviated from the midline and should be redirected toward the side opposite the paresthesia. Occasionally, pain experienced when the needle contacts bone may be misinterpreted by the patient as a paresthesia, and the anesthesiologist should be alert to this possibility.

Once the needle is correctly inserted into the subarachnoid space, it is fixed in position and the syringe containing local anesthetic is attached. CSF is gently aspirated to confirm that the needle is still in the subarachnoid space and the local anesthetic slowly injected (≤0.5 ml · s^{-1}). After completing the injection, a small volume of CSF is again aspirated to confirm that the needle tip remained in the subarachnoid space while the local anesthetic was deposited. This CSF is then reinjected and the needle, syringe, and any introducer removed together. If the surgical procedure is to be performed in the supine position, the patient is helped onto his or her back. To prevent excessive cephalad spread of hyperbaric local anesthetic, care should be taken to ensure that the patient's hips are not raised off the bed as he or she turns.

Once the block is placed, strict attention must be paid to the patient's hemodynamic status with blood pressure or heart rate supported as necessary. Block height should also be assessed early by pin-prick or temperature sensation. Temperature sensation is tested by wiping the skin with alcohol and may be preferable to pin prick because it is not painful. If, after a few minutes, the block is not rising high enough or is rising too high, the table may be tilted as appropriate to influence further spread of hypobaric or hyperbaric local anesthetics.

Paramedian Approach

The paramedian approach to the epidural and subarachnoid spaces is useful in situations where the patient's anatomy does not favor the midline approach (*e.g.*, inability to flex the spine or heavily calcified interspinous ligaments). This approach can be used with the patient in any position and is probably the best approach for the patient in the prone jackknife position.

The spinous process forming the lower border of the desired interspace is identified. The needle is inserted ~1 cm lateral to this point and is directed toward the middle of the interspace by angling it ~45 degrees cephalad with just enough medial angulation (~15 degrees) to compensate for the lateral insertion point. The first significant resistance encountered should be the ligamentum flavum. Bone encountered before the ligamentum flavum is usually the vertebral lamina of the cephalad vertebra and the needle should be redirected accordingly. An alternative method is to insert the needle perpendicular to the skin in all planes until the lamina is contacted. The needle is then walked off the superior edge of the lamina and into the subarachnoid space. The lamina provides a valuable landmark that facilitates correct needle placement; however, repeated needle contact with the periosteum can be painful.

Lumbosacral Approach

The lumbosacral (or Taylor) approach to the subarachnoid and epidural spaces is simply a paramedian approach directed at the L5–S1 interspace, which is the largest interlaminar space. This approach may be useful when anatomic constraints make other approaches unfeasible. The patient may be positioned laterally, prone or sitting, and the needle inserted at a point 1 cm medial and 1 cm inferior to the posterior superior iliac spine. The needle is angled cephalad 45–55 degrees and just medial enough to reach the midline at the level of the L5 spinous process. As with the paramedian approach, the interspinous ligament is bypassed and the first significant resistance felt should be the ligamentum flavum.

Continuous Spinal Anesthesia

Inserting a catheter into the subarachnoid space increases the utility of spinal anesthesia by permitting repeated drug administration as often as necessary to extend the level or duration of spinal block. A common and reasonable recommendation for subsequent dosing or "topping up" of continuous spinal blocks is to administer half the original dose of local anesthetic when the block has reached two-thirds of its expected duration.

The technique is similar to that described for "single shot" spinal anesthesia except that a needle large enough to accommodate the desired catheter must be used. After inserting the needle and obtaining free-flowing CSF, the catheter is simply threaded into the subarachnoid space a distance of 2–3 cm. It is often easier to insert the catheter if it is directed cephalad or caudad instead of lateral. If the catheter does not easily pass beyond the needle tip, rotating the needle 180 degrees may be helpful or another interspace may be used. The catheter should never be withdrawn back into the needle shaft because of the risk of shearing the catheter off into the subarachnoid space.

A variety of catheters and needles are available for continuous spinal anesthesia. Commonly, 18-gauge epidural needles and 20-gauge catheters are used. However, needles and catheters this size carry a higher risk of causing PDPH, especially in young patients. Because of this risk, smaller needle and catheter combinations have been developed with catheters ranging in size from 24 to 32 gauge. Although smaller catheters decrease the risk of PDPH, they have also been associated with multiple reports of neurologic injury, specifically, cauda equina syndrome (see section on Complications). For this reason, the U.S. Food and Drug Administration has advised against using any catheter smaller than 24 gauge for continuous spinal anesthesia.

Epidural Anesthesia

For the novice, correct placement of an epidural needle can be technically more challenging than spinal needle placement because there is less room for error. However, with experience, epidural needle placement is often easier than spinal needle placement because the larger-gauge needles used for epidural anesthesia are less likely to be deflected from their intended path and they produce much better tactile feel of the interspinous and flaval ligaments. In addition, the loss-of-resistance technique provides a much clearer end point when entering the epidural space than does the subtle "pop" of a spinal needle piercing the dura mater.

Patient preparation, positioning, monitors, and needle approaches for epidural anesthesia are the same as for spinal anesthesia. Unlike spinal anesthesia, epidural anesthesia may be performed at any intervertebral space. However, at vertebral levels above the termination of the spinal cord, the epidural needle may accidentally puncture the spinal meninges and damage the underlying spinal cord. To prevent accidental menin-

geal puncture, the anesthesiologist must learn to identify the interspinous ligaments and the ligamentum flavum by their feel. In addition, epidural needles must be advanced slowly and, most importantly, under control.

After proper positioning, sterile skin preparation, and draping, the desired interspace is identified and a local anesthetic skin wheal is raised at the point of needle insertion. Because epidural needles are relatively blunt, it is sometimes helpful to pierce the skin with a $\geq$18-gauge hypodermic needle before inserting the epidural needle. For epidural anesthesia using the midline approach, the epidural needle is inserted through the subcutaneous tissue and into the interspinous ligament. The interspinous ligament has a characteristic "gritty" feel, much like inserting a needle into a bag of sand. This is especially true of younger patients. If the interspinous ligament is not clearly identified, the needle may not be in the midline. After engaging the interspinous ligament, the needle is advanced slowly through it until an increase in resistance is felt. This increased resistance represents the ligamentum flavum.

The epidural needle must now traverse the ligamentum flavum and stop within the epidural space before puncturing the spinal meninges. Numerous techniques for identifying the epidural space have been used successfully; however, the loss of resistance to fluid has the advantage of simplicity, reliability, and speed. In addition, use of fluid instead of air for loss of resistance decreases the risk of PDPH in the event of accidental meningeal puncture.[22]

A glass syringe or a specially designed low, resistance plastic syringe is filled with 2–3 ml of saline and a small (0.1–0.3 ml) air bubble. The syringe is attached to the epidural needle and the plunger pressed until the air bubble is visibly compressed. If the needle tip is properly embedded within the ligamentum flavum, it should be possible to compress the air bubble without injecting fluid. In this way, the air bubble serves as a gauge of the appropriate amount of pressure to exert on the syringe plunger. If the air bubble cannot be compressed without injecting fluid, then the needle tip is most likely not in the ligamentum flavum. In this case, the needle tip may still be in the interspinous ligament, or it may be off the midline in the paraspinous muscles. To differentiate between these possibilities, the anesthesiologist can carefully advance the needle and syringe a few millimeters in an effort to engage the ligamentum flavum. If it is still not possible to compress the air bubble, the needle should be withdrawn into the subcutaneous tissue, and reinserted.

Once the ligamentum flavum is identified, the needle is slowly advanced with the nondominant hand while the dominant hand maintains constant pressure on the syringe plunger (Fig. 26-8). As the needle tip enters the epidural space, there is a sudden and dramatic loss of resistance as the saline is rapidly injected. Saline injection into the epidural space can be moderately painful, and patients should be forewarned. If the needle is advancing obliquely through the ligamentum flavum, it is possible to enter into the paraspinous muscles instead of the epidural space. In this case the loss of resistance is less dramatic. To help verify that the needle has entered the epidural space, 0.5 ml of air can be drawn into the syringe and injected. In the epidural space there is virtually no resistance to air injection, whereas in the paraspinous muscles air injection encounters demonstrable resistance.

After entering the epidural space, the needle is advanced no further. Because the dura mater abuts the ligamentum flavum, the dura will now be tented over the needle tip, and advancing the needle any more than necessary heightens the risk of accidental meningeal puncture (i.e., "wet tap"). When the syringe is disconnected from the needle, it is common to have a small amount of fluid flow from the needle hub. This is usually the saline flowing back out of the epidural space, but could be CSF if the needle accidentally entered the subarachnoid space. CSF can often be distinguished by the fact that it is warm, whereas the

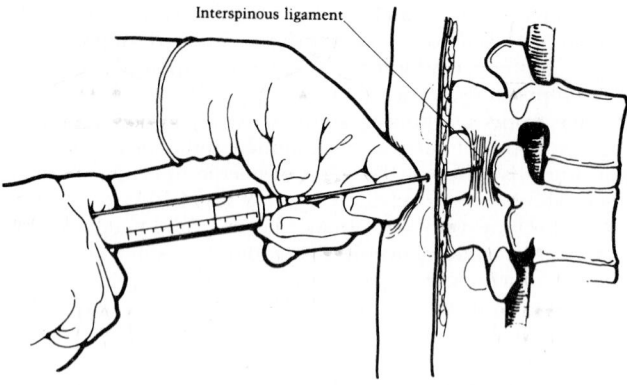

Figure 26-8. Proper hand position when using the loss-of-resistance technique to locate the epidural space. After embedding the needle tip in the ligamentum flavum, a syringe with 2–3 ml saline and an air bubble is attached. The left hand rests securely on the back and the fingers of the left hand grasp the needle firmly. The left hand advances the needle slowly and under control by rotating at the wrist. The fingers of the right hand maintain constant pressure on the syringe plunger but do not aid in advancing the needle. If the needle tip is properly engaged in the ligamentum flavum, it should be possible to compress the air bubble without injecting the saline. As the needle tip enters the epidural space, there will be a sudden loss of resistance and the saline is suddenly injected. (Reprinted with permission from Mulroy MF: Regional Anesthesia: An Illustrated Procedural Guide. Boston, Little Brown, 1989.)

saline is room temperature. CSF also tests positive for glucose. In addition, accidental meningeal puncture usually results in much larger volumes of CSF rapidly escaping from the epidural needle.

If a single-shot technique is to be used, a local anesthetic test dose should be administered to help rule out undetected subarachnoid or intravenous (iv) needle placement. After a negative test dose, the desired volume of local anesthetic should be administered in small increments (*e.g.*, 5 ml) at a rate of $0.5–1 \; ml \cdot s^{-1}$. Slow, incremental injection decreases the risk of pain during injection and allows detection of adverse reactions to accidental iv or subarachnoid placement before the entire dose is administered.

Continuous Epidural Anesthesia

Use of a catheter for epidural anesthesia affords much greater flexibility than the single-shot technique because the catheter can be used to prolong a block that is too short, extend a block that is too low, or provide postoperative analgesia. Potential disadvantages include catheter migration into an epidural vein or the subarachnoid space, or out an intervertebral foramen. Catheter use is also more likely to result in unilateral epidural block, a clinical fact that has been shown to result from catheter tips ending up in the anterior epidural space or migrating out an intervertebral foramen.[14, 23]

An ever-changing selection of epidural catheters is commercially available. They differ in diameter, stiffness, location of injection holes, presence or absence of a stylet, construction material, and so forth. Whichever catheter is chosen, it is important to verify that it passes easily through the epidural needle before the needle is placed in the epidural space. Epidural catheters are usually inserted through either Tuohy or Hustead needles because their curved tips help direct the catheter away from the dura mater. The needle bevel should be directed either cephalad or caudad, although the direction of the bevel does not guarantee that the catheter will travel in that direction. The catheter typically encounters resistance as it reaches the curve at the tip of the needle, but steady pressure usually results in passage into the epidural space. If the catheter will not pass

beyond the needle tip, it is possible that the needle opening is not completely in the epidural space, or that some structure in the epidural space is preventing catheter insertion (*e.g.*, epidural fat). In this instance, the needle can be carefully advanced 1–2 mm more or rotated 180 degrees and the catheter reinserted. Although either of these maneuvers may result in successful catheter placement, they also increase the risk of accidental meningeal puncture. Alternatively, the procedure can be repeated at another interspace or with a different needle approach (*e.g.*, paramedian). Occasionally, a catheter will advance only a short distance past the needle tip. This raises the possibility that the needle tip is not in the epidural space and needs to be repositioned. In this case, the catheter should not be withdrawn back into the epidural needle because of the risk that the catheter tip will be sheared off by the bevel's sharp edge. Rather, the needle and catheter should be pulled out in tandem and the procedure repeated.

The catheter should be advanced only 3–5 cm into the epidural space. Placing a longer length of catheter in the epidural space increases the risk that it will enter an epidural vein, puncture the spinal meninges, exit an intervertebral foramen, wrap around a nerve root, or end up in some other disadvantageous location. Once the catheter is appropriately positioned in the epidural space, the needle is slowly withdrawn with one hand as the catheter is stabilized with the other. After the needle is removed, the length of catheter in the epidural space is confirmed by subtracting the distance between the skin and the epidural space from the length of catheter below the skin. Documenting this distance is important when trying to determine if catheters used in the postoperative period have been dislodged.

An epidural test dose must be administered through the catheter to test for iv or subarachnoid placement before incrementally delivering the entire epidural drug dose. In addition, because of the risk of undetected iv or subarachnoid migration of the catheter over time, additional test doses must be administered before each additional therapeutic ("top-up") dose is given through the catheter. As with continuous spinal anesthesia, a reasonable guideline for top-up doses is to administer half the initial local anesthetic dose at an interval equal to two-thirds the expected duration of the block.

Epidural Test Dose

The epidural test dose is designed to identify epidural needles or catheters that have entered an epidural vein or the subarachnoid space. Failure to do so may result in intravascular injection of toxic doses of local anesthetic or total spinal block. Aspirating the catheter or needle to check for blood or CSF is helpful if positive, but the incidence of false-negative aspirations is too high to rely on this technique alone.[24]

The most common test dose is 3 ml of local anesthetic containing $5 \; \mu g \cdot ml^{-1}$ epinephrine (1 : 200,000). The dose of local anesthetic should be sufficient that subarachnoid injection results in clear evidence of spinal anesthesia. Intravenous injection of this dose of epinephrine typically produces an average 30 $beats \cdot min^{-1}$ heart rate increase between 20 and 40 seconds after injection.[25, 26] Heart rate increases may not be as evident in patients taking β-adrenergic blockers; reflex bradycardia usually occurs in these patients.[25, 27] In β-blocked patients, systolic blood pressure increases of ≥20 mm Hg may be a more reliable indicator of intravascular injection.[25, 27]

Isoproterenol has also been used to detect intravascular injection.[28] In addition, air injection combined with precordial Doppler ultrasonography to detect the characteristic murmur has been used successfully to test for iv placement of epidural catheters.[24] These techniques have been developed for use in laboring women where the sensitivity of epinephrine as a test dose is disturbingly low because maternal heart rate increases during contractions are often as large as those produced by epinephrine.[29] The clinical indications for these alternative tests of intravascular injection await additional, larger studies.

Combined Spinal-Epidural Anesthesia

Combined spinal-epidural anesthesia (CSEA) is a useful technique by which a spinal block and an epidural catheter are placed simultaneously. This technique is growing in popularity because it combines the rapid onset, dense block of spinal anesthesia with the flexibility afforded by an epidural catheter. There are special epidural needles with a separate lumen to accommodate a spinal needle available for CSEA (Fig. 26-6). However, the technique is easily performed by first placing a standard epidural needle in the epidural space and then inserting an appropriately sized spinal needle through the shaft of the epidural needle and into the subarachnoid space. The desired local anesthetic is injected into the subarachnoid space, the spinal needle removed, and a catheter placed in the epidural space via the epidural needle. The catheter can then be used to extend the height or duration of intraoperative block or to provide postoperative epidural analgesia.

An interesting pharmacologic aspect of CSEA is the observation that after the peak spinal block height is established, both saline and local anesthetic injected into the epidural space are effective at pushing the block level higher.[30-32] This observation has been interpreted to indicate that the mechanism by which the epidural top-up increases block height is due to a volume effect (*i.e.*, compression of the spinal meninges forcing CSF cephalad) as well as a local anesthetic effect.

A potential risk of this technique is that the meningeal hole made by the spinal needle may allow dangerously high concentrations of subsequently administered epidural drugs to reach the subarachnoid space. Anecdotal case reports and *in vitro* animal studies suggest that this may be a legitimate concern.[29, 33-35] Although CSEA shows great promise, additional, prospective studies are necessary to identify the relative risks and limitations of the technique.

PHARMACOLOGY

Successful spinal or epidural anesthesia requires a block that is high enough to block sensation at the surgical site and lasts for the duration of the planned procedure. However, because interindividual variability is considerable (Figs. 26-9 and 26-10), reliably predicting the height and duration of central neuraxial block that will result from a particular local anesthetic dose is difficult. Thus, recommendations regarding local anesthetic choice and dose must be viewed as approximate guidelines. The clinician must understand the factors governing spinal and epidural block height and duration to individualize local anesthetic choice and dose for each patient and procedure.

Spinal Anesthesia

Block Height

Table 26-1 lists some common surgical procedures that are readily performed under spinal anesthesia, and the block height that is usually sufficient to ensure patient comfort. Also listed are techniques appropriate to achieve the desired block height. The rationales for these recommendations are detailed in the following sections.

Baricity and Patient Position. The height of spinal block is thought to be determined by the cephalad spread of local anesthetic in the CSF. Table 26-2 lists some of the many variables that have been proposed to influence the spread of local anesthetics in the subarachnoid space. Many of these variables have been shown to be of negligible clinical importance. Of those factors that do exert significant influence on local anesthetic spread, the baricity of the local anesthetic solution relative to

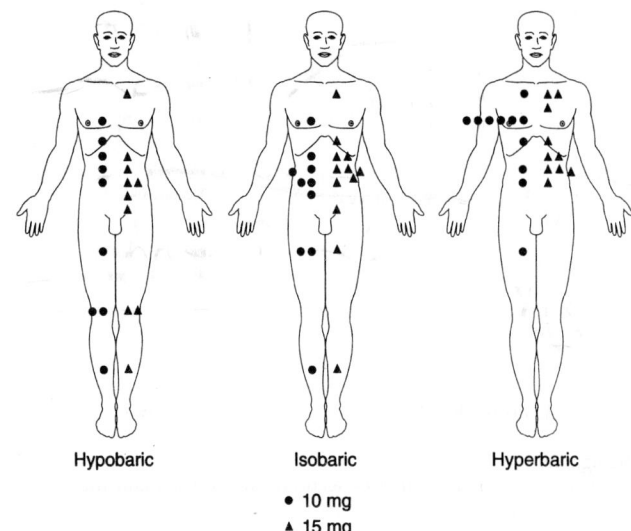

Hypobaric   Isobaric   Hyperbaric

● 10 mg
▲ 15 mg

Figure 26-9. Peak spinal block height following 10- and 15-mg doses of hypobaric, isobaric, and hyperbaric tetracaine solutions injected at L3–L4 with patients in the lateral horizontal position. Note that dose has no influence on block height and that there is considerable interindividual variability in peak block height, especially with the hypobaric solution. (Adapted with permission from Brown DT, Wildsmith JA, Covino BG, Scott DB: Effect of baricity on spinal anaesthesia with amethocaine. Br J Anaesth 52:589, 1980.)

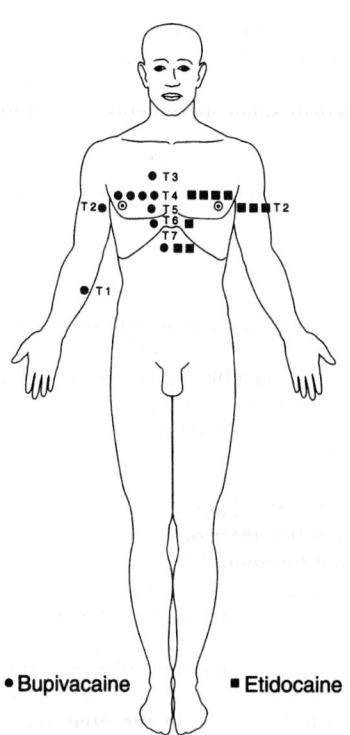

● Bupivacaine   ■ Etidocaine

Figure 26-10. Peak epidural block height following 20 ml of 0.75% bupivacaine and 1.5% etidocaine injected via a catheter at the L1–L2 interspace. Note that despite a well controlled technique, the interindividual variability in block height is considerable and demonstrates the difficulty in accurately predicting block height in an individual patient. (Adapted with permission from Sinclair CJ, Scott DB: Comparison of bupivacaine and etidocaine in extradural blockade. Br J Anaesth 56:147, 1984.)

Table 26-1. REPRESENTATIVE SURGICAL PROCEDURES APPROPRIATE FOR SPINAL ANESTHESIA

Surgical Procedure	Suggested Block Height	Technique	Comments
Perianal Perirectal	L1–L2	Hyperbaric solution/sitting position Hypobaric solution/jack knife position Isobaric solution/horizontal position	Patients must remain in relative head up or head down position when using hypobaric and hyperbaric solutions to maintain restricted spread during the procedure
Lower extremity Hip Transurethral resection of the prostate Vaginal/cervical	T10	Isobaric solution	Hypobaric and hyperbaric solutions are also suitable but may produce higher blocks than necessary
Herniorrhaphy Pelvic procedures Appendectomy	T6–T8	Hyperbaric solution/horizontal position	Isobaric solutions injected at L2–L3 interspace may also be suitable
Abdominal Cesasean section	T4–T6	Hyperbaric solution/horizontal position	Upper abdominal procedures usually require concomitant general anesthesia to prevent vagal reflexes and pain from traction on diaphragm, esophagus, and the like

patient position is probably the most important. Baricity is defined as the ratio of the density (mass/volume) of the local anesthetic solution divided by the density of CSF, which averages $1.0003 \pm 0.0003 \text{ g} \cdot \text{ml}^{-1}$ at 37°C. Solutions that have the same density as CSF have a baricity of 1.0000 and are termed *isobaric*. Solutions that are more dense than CSF are termed *hyperbaric*, whereas solutions that are less dense than CSF are termed *hypobaric*.

Table 26-3 lists the baricity of local anesthetic solutions commonly used for spinal anesthesia. For practical purposes, solutions with a baricity <0.9990 can be expected reliably to behave hypobarically in all patients. Hypobaric solutions are typically prepared by mixing the local anesthetic solution in distilled water. Solutions with a baricity of ≥1.0015 can be expected reliably to behave hyperbarically. Hyperbaric solutions are typically prepared by mixing the local anesthetic in 5–8% dextrose. The baricity of the resultant solution depends upon the amount of dextrose added; however, dextrose concentrations between 1.25% and 8% result in equivalent block heights.[36, 37] Lower dextrose concentrations have been shown to have a concentration-dependent effect on block height with 0.33% producing a block to T9.5 on average, 0.83% producing a block to T7.2, and 8% producing a block to T3.6.[38]

Table 26-2. FACTORS THAT HAVE BEEN SUGGESTED AS POSSIBLE DETERMINANTS OF SPREAD OF LOCAL ANESTHETIC SOLUTIONS WITHIN THE SUBARACHNOID SPACE

CHARACTERISTICS OF THE LOCAL ANESTHETIC SOLUTION

Baricity
Local anesthetic dose
Local anesthetic concentration
Volume injected

PATIENT CHARACTERISTICS

Age
Weight
Height
Gender
Pregnancy
Patient position

TECHNIQUE

Site of injection
Speed of injection
Barbotage
Direction of needle bevel
Addition of vasoconstrictors

DIFFUSION

Adapted with permission from Greene NM: Distribution of local anesthetic solutions within the subarachnoid space. Anesth Analg 64:715, 1985.

Table 26-3. BARICITY OF SOLUTIONS COMMONLY USED FOR SPINAL ANESTHESIA

	Baricity*
HYPERBARIC	
Tetracaine: 0.5% in 5% dextrose	1.0133
Bupivacaine: 0.75% in 8.25% dextrose	1.0227
Lidocaine: 5% in 7.5% dextrose	1.0265
Procaine: 10% in water	1.0104
ISOBARIC†	
Tetracaine: 0.5% in normal saline	0.9997
Bupivacaine: 0.75% in saline	0.9988
Bupivacaine: 0.5% in saline	0.9983
Lidocaine: 2% in saline	0.9986
HYPOBARIC	
Tetracaine: 0.2% in water	0.9922
Bupivacaine: 0.3% in water	0.9946
Lidocaine: 0.5% in water	0.9985

* Measured at 37°C, except for hypobaric 0.5% lidocaine measured at 25°C. At 37°C, this solution's baricity is less.
† These solutions are slightly hypobaric but are used clinically as if they were isobaric.
Data from Horlocker TT, Wedel DJ: Density, specific gravity, and baricity of spinal anesthetic solutions at body temperature. Anesth Analg 76:1015, 1993; Lambert D, Covino B: Hyperbaric, hypobaric and isobaric spinal anesthesia. Resident Staff Physician 33:79 1987; Greene NM: Distribution of local anesthetic solutions within the subarachnoid space. Anesth Analg 64:715, 1985; and Bodily N, Carpenter R, Owens B: Lidocaine 0.5% spinal anaesthesia: A hypobaric solution for short-stay perirectal surgery. Can J Anaesth 39:770, 1992.

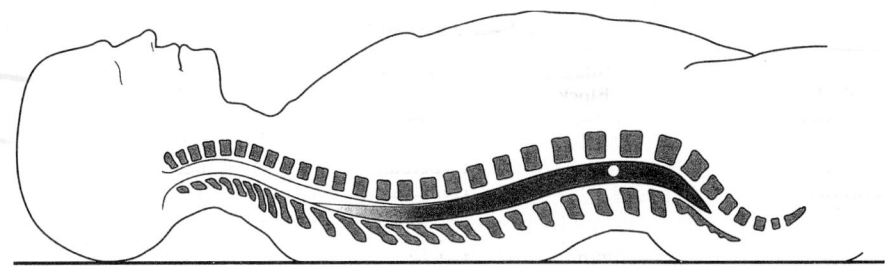

Figure 26-11. In the horizontal supine position, hyperbaric local anesthetic solutions injected at the height of the lumbar lordosis (*circle*) flow down the lumbar lordosis to pool in the sacrum and in the thoracic kyphosis. Pooling in the thoracic kyphosis is thought to explain the fact that hyperbaric solutions produce blocks with an average height of T4–T6.

Baricity is important in determining local anesthetic spread and thus block height because gravity causes hyperbaric solutions to flow downward in CSF to the most dependent regions of the spinal column, whereas hypobaric solutions tend to rise in CSF. In contrast, gravity has no effect on the distribution of truly isobaric solutions. Thus, the anesthesiologist can exert considerable influence on block height by choice of anesthetic solution and proper patient positioning. Spinal block can be restricted to the sacral and low lumbar dermatomes ("saddle block") by administering a hyperbaric local anesthetic solution with the patient in the sitting position[39] or by administering a hypobaric solution with the patient in the prone jackknife position. Similarly, high thoracic to midcervical levels of anesthesia can be reached by administering hyperbaric solutions with the patient in the horizontal and Trendelenburg positions[40, 41] or by administering hypobaric solutions with the patient in a semisitting position. However, this use of hypobaric solutions is not recommended because the high block achieved and the diminished venous return associated with the upright posture can lead to significant cardiovascular compromise.

The sitting, Trendelenburg, and jackknife positions have marked influences on the distribution of hypobaric and hyperbaric solutions because these positions accentuate the effect of gravity. However, most spinal anesthetics are administered as hyperbaric solutions injected while patients are in the horizontal lateral position, after which they are turned to the horizontal supine position. In this situation the influence of gravity is more subtle because the dependent areas of the spinal column do not deviate as much from the horizontal. While the patient is turned laterally, gravity has a small but measurable effect on local anesthetic distribution in that hyperbaric solutions produce a denser, longer-lasting block on the dependent side whereas hypobaric solutions will have the opposite effect.[42] This makes hypobaric solutions ideal for unilateral procedures performed in the lateral position (*e.g.,* hip surgery). Hyperbaric solutions can be used to advantage for unilateral procedures performed in the supine position if the operative side is dependent during drug injection and the patient is left in the lateral position for at least 6 minutes.[42] Despite differences in block density and duration, peak block height will be comparable between the dependent and nondependent sides.

When the patient is turned supine after hyperbaric drug injection in the lateral position, the normal spinal curvature influences subsequent movement of the injected solution. Hyperbaric solutions injected at the height of the lumbar lordosis will tend to flow cephalad to pool in the thoracic kyphosis and caudad to pool in the sacrum (Fig. 26-11). Pooling of hyperbaric local anesthetic solutions in the thoracic kyphosis has been evoked to explain the clinical observation that hyperbaric solutions tend to produce blocks with an average height in the midthoracic region (Fig. 26-9). In addition, hyperbaric solutions have also been observed to produce blocks with a bimodal distribution, that is, one group of patients with blocks centered in the low thoracic region and a second group of patients with blocks centered in the high thoracic region.[43, 44] The presumed explanation for this observation is that the lumbar lordosis produces "splitting" of the local anesthetic solution with some

portion flowing caudad toward the sacrum and the remainder flowing cephalad into the thoracic kyphosis. The cephalad extent of the block then depends on what fraction of the injected drug flows cephalad. Consistent with this hypothesis, eliminating the lumbar lordosis by maintaining the hips flexed has been shown to significantly reduce[44] or eliminate[43] the bimodal distribution of blocks without affecting maximal block height.

Obviously, gravity influences the distribution of hyperbaric and hypobaric solutions only until they are sufficiently diluted in CSF so that they become isobaric. At this point, the local anesthetic solution no longer moves in response to changes in patient position and the block is said to be "fixed." The time required for a local anesthetic solution to become fixed may be considerable. Povey *et al* showed that hyperbaric bupivacaine injected in the sitting position produces a saddle block that is restricted to the lumbar segments for as long as the subjects remained sitting.[39, 40] However, even 60 minutes after bupivacaine injection, the block spread to midthoracic levels after the patients were turned supine. Similarly, Bodily *et al*[45] found that hypobaric lidocaine administered in the jackknife position rose as many as six dermatomes when patients were allowed to sit upright in the recovery room as long as 60 minutes after lidocaine injection. Whether it is also possible to affect spread so long after injecting hyperbaric or hypobaric solutions in the horizontal position is unclear. Nonetheless, these findings demonstrate that in some situations it may be possible to exert influence on block height by adjusting patient position for at least 60 minutes after local anesthetic injection.

In contrast to the situation with hyperbaric solutions, patient position has no effect on the distribution of isobaric solutions because these solutions are not influenced by gravity. Consequently, isobaric solutions tend not to spread as far from the site of injection and produce blocks with an average height in the low thoracic region[37,46] (Fig. 26-9). The obvious caveat is that the local anesthetic solution must be truly isobaric in the patient in whom it is used. Because of the interindividual variability in CSF density, it is difficult reliably to produce isobaric local anesthetic solutions. Nonetheless, as indicated in Table 26-3, several local anesthetic solutions are used as if they were isobaric. It is noteworthy that whereas isobaric solutions produce an average block height that is lower than that of comparable hyperbaric solutions,[37, 46–48] the "isobaric" solutions produce blocks with a much greater variability in height.[49–51] Logan *et al* have termed plain bupivacaine "an unpredictable spinal anesthetic agent."[49] The greater variability in spread may stem in part from the fact that these solutions are actually slightly hypobaric, and their spread has been shown to be affected by patient position.[52, 53] Temperature-related changes in baricity may also play a role in the variability in distribution of these nearly isobaric solutions. For example, Stienstra and van Poorten[54] have shown that the distribution of plain bupivacaine is significantly altered by changes in temperature of the injected solution. In addition, McClure *et al*[55] have shown that increasing the volume and decreasing the concentration of isobaric tetracaine also increases the variability in block height. These and other unknown factors may play a role in the unpredictability of these nearly isobaric solutions. Although unpredictability is cause for concern, the lower average block height achieved offers potential advantages for surgical procedures below the umbilicus because of the decreased incidence of cardiovascular side effects associated with lower blocks. The isobaric solution that most reliably produces a low thoracic block is 10 mg of tetracaine crystals diluted in 1 or 2 ml room temperature saline and injected in the horizontal position.[55]

Dose, Volume, and Concentration. Studies aimed at determining the effect of these three interdependent variables on block height, are difficult to conduct and interpret because it is not possible to change one variable without simultaneously changing another. Nonetheless, it is possible to draw some conclusions regarding the effect of these variables on block height. Several studies with isobaric tetracaine and bupivacaine solutions have found that neither injected volume nor drug concentration affects block height when dose is held constant.[55–59] Drug dose does appear to play a small role in determining block height with isobaric bupivacaine. Two studies have found that 10 mg of isobaric bupivacaine results in significantly lower blocks than does 15 or 20 mg, but there is no difference in block height between the two higher doses.[60, 61] In contrast, two studies that examined the effect of different doses of isobaric tetracaine found that doses between 5 and 15 mg had no effect on block height, producing blocks with an average height of T9–T10.[46, 62]

Drug dose and volume appear to be relatively unimportant in predicting the spread of hyperbaric local anesthetic solutions injected in the horizontal position. Increasing the dose and volume of hyperbaric tetracaine while holding concentration constant does not affect block height when doses between 7.5 and 15 mg are used.[46, 62, 63] Similarly, increasing the dose and volume of hyperbaric 0.5% bupivacaine does not increase block height when doses between 10 and 20 mg are used.[64,65] However, doses of hyperbaric 0.5% bupivacaine <10 mg have been shown to result in blocks that are ~2.5 dermatomes lower than those achieved with doses >10 mg.[64] The fact that bupivacaine dose affects block height only at the extreme low end of the usual dose range is consistent with the experience with isobaric bupivacaine reported previously. The fact that drug dose is relatively unimportant in determining block height with hyperbaric solutions likely results from an overwhelming effect of baricity and patient position in determining spread of these solutions.

Injection Site. The site of injection can have an important effect on block height in some situations. In particular, sensory block height resulting from isobaric 0.5% bupivacaine is reduced by 2 dermatomes per interspace when comparing different groups of patients who received injections at the L2–L3, L3–L4, or L4–L5 interspaces.[66,67] In an even more convincing study, this group of investigators performed repeated blocks in the same patient and found that by moving from the L3–L4 to the L4–L5 interspace mean block height could be reduced from T6 to T10 when using isobaric 0.5% bupivacaine.[68] In contrast, Sundnes *et al*[64] found no relationship between injection site and block height when using a hyperbaric bupivacaine solution, presumably because of the overwhelming effect of gravity and patient position on distribution of hyperbaric local anesthetics. Whether isobaric and hyperbaric solutions of other local anesthetics behave similarly is not clear.

Patient Characteristics. Data from Carpenter and colleagues suggest that the most important patient variable governing block height may be lumbosacral CSF volume.[69] In their study, the correlation coefficient for linear regression of lumbosacral CSF volume and peak block height was a compelling 0.91, with larger CSF volumes resulting in lower blocks. This study was performed in young adults (age 33 ± 4 years) using hyperbaric lidocaine, thus, it is unclear if the findings can be extrapolated to other local anesthetics or patient ages. Also, although they are mechanistically important, the clinical application of these data will be limited unless and until a simple method is developed to predict accurately lumbosacral CSF volume.

Patient age, weight, and height have all been suggested to

have an effect on block height; however, none of these variables is an important or reliable predictor of block height.[70] Studies investigating the effect of age on block height in adults are conflicting, with some studies indicating that age does not correlate with block height[71] and others that it does.[51,72] However, even in the studies that reported a correlation between age and block height, the correlation was not strong enough to serve as a reliable predictor of block height in the clinical setting. For example, the range of block heights reported by Cameron *et al*[51] for spinal block with isobaric bupivacaine was the same for patients in their seventh decade (T11-T2) as it was for patients in their ninth decade.

Patient height and vertebral column length are also poor predictors of the extent of sensory blockade in adults, at least within the range of heights commonly encountered.[73–75] It is possible that extremes in height might decrease cephalad spread of sensory block. Similarly, weight is a poor predictor of block height in nonobese adults, although block height does appear to be somewhat higher in obese patients receiving isobaric local anesthetics.[66,76,77]

Onset

Most patients can sense the onset of spinal block within a very few minutes after drug injection regardless of the local anesthetic used. However, there is a significant difference among drugs in the time to reach peak block height. Lidocaine and mepivacaine tend to reach peak block height between 10 and 15 minutes, whereas tetracaine and bupivacaine may require >20 minutes before peak block height is reached.

Duration

Spinal blocks do not end abruptly after a fixed time. Rather, they recede gradually from the most cephalad dermatome to the most caudad. As a result, surgical anesthesia lasts significantly longer at sacral levels than at thoracic levels. Therefore, when discussing the duration of spinal block it is necessary to distinguish between duration at the surgical site and the time required for the block to resolve completely. The former is important for providing adequate surgical anesthesia, and the latter for ensuring a timely recovery. A thorough understanding of the factors that govern block duration is necessary if the clinician is to choose techniques that result in an appropriate duration of spinal blockade.

Local Anesthetic. The principal determinant of spinal block duration is the local anesthetic drug used. Procaine is the shortest-acting local anesthetic for subarachnoid use, lidocaine and mepivacaine are agents of intermediate duration, and bupivacaine and tetracaine are the longest-acting drugs available for use in the United States. Table 26-4 lists the range of times required for sensory block to regress two dermatomes and to resolve completely with the local anesthetics most commonly used for spinal anesthesia. Although drug choice is the principal determinant of block duration, the factors discussed in the following sections can be used to alter block duration as necessary for a particular clinical situation. These variables are responsible for the wide range of block duration found in Table 26-4.

Drug Dose. Increasing local anesthetic dose clearly increases the duration of spinal block.[60,61,63,78,79] For example, Brown *et al*[46] demonstrated that duration of sensory block at L1 after 15 mg tetracaine was ~20% greater than after 10 mg. Sheskey *et al*[61] demonstrated a ~40% increase in block duration at L2 when comparing 10 mg bupivacaine with 15 mg. Similarly, Axelsson *et al*[78] found that duration of sensory block at L2 was nearly doubled when comparing 10 mg bupivacaine with 20 mg.

Block Height. If drug dose is held constant, higher blocks tend to regress faster than lower blocks.[79] Consequently, isobaric local anesthetic solutions usually produce longer blocks than hyperbaric solutions using the same dose. The conventional wisdom is that greater cephalad spread results in relatively lower drug concentration in the CSF and spinal nerve roots. As a

Table 26-4. DOSE AND DURATION OF LOCAL ANESTHETICS USED FOR SPINAL ANESTHESIA

Drug	Dose (mg)*	Duration of Sensory Block†		
		Two-Dermatome Regression (min)	Complete Resolution (min)	Prolongation by Adrenergic Agonists (%)‡
Procaine	50–200	30–50	90–120	30–50
Lidocaine	25–100	40–100	140–240	20–50
Bupivacaine	5–20	90–140	240–380	20–50
Tetracaine	5–20	90–140	240–380	50–100

* The lowest doses are used primarily for very restricted blocks (*e.g.*, saddle block), lest they become too dilute to be effective.
† Duration is influenced by dose and block height. The duration of surgical anesthesia obviously depends on the surgical site.
‡ The effect of adrenergic agonists depends on the dose and choice of agonist. Prolongation is greatest at lumbar and sacral dermatomes and least at thoracic dermatomes.

result, it takes less time for local anesthetic concentration to decrease below the minimally effective concentration.

Adrenergic Agonists. Adrenergic agonists, such as epinephrine, phenylephrine, and more recently, clonidine, are added to local anesthetics in an effort to prolong the duration of spinal anesthesia. Their effectiveness depends upon the local anesthetic with which they are combined. In addition, they are more effective at prolonging block in the lumbar and sacral dermatomes than in thoracic dermatomes.

Epinephrine is typically administered in doses of 0.2–0.3 mg and phenylephrine in doses of 2–5 mg. There is evidence to suggest a relationship between the dose of vasoconstrictor added and the duration of spinal anesthesia; however, the relationship is not strong.[80-83] At the maximal doses used clinically, phenylephrine (5 mg) prolongs spinal block to a greater degree than epinephrine (0.5 mg).[84, 85] At lower doses, epinephrine (0.2–0.3 mg) and phenylephrine (2–3 mg) appear to be equally effective in prolonging spinal block.[83, 86] Thus, both choice of adrenergic agonist and dose administered appear to play a role in determining block duration.

Clonidine has been added to intrathecal local anesthetics in a dose of 75–150 mg.[87, 88] At this dose, it is at least as effective as moderate doses of phenylephrine and epinephrine at prolonging sensory block, but has been associated with greater decreases in blood pressure in some,[87] but not all studies.[88] Clonidine also prolongs spinal block when administered orally.[89-91]

Tetracaine is the local anesthetic whose effects are most dramatically prolonged by addition of adrenergic agonists. The duration of tetracaine spinal block may be increased 70–100% at lumbar and sacral dermatomes by addition of phenylephrine. Epinephrine may prolong tetracaine spinal anesthesia by 40–60%. Clonidine prolongs tetracaine spinal block by 50–70%, with the larger effect occurring at lumbar dermatomes.

Bupivacaine spinal block is also prolonged by adrenergic agonists, although the effect is somewhat less than that seen with tetracaine (Table 26-4). Epinephrine in doses of 0.2 mg prolongs bupivacaine spinal block by 20–30%, but only in lumbar dermatomes. Larger doses of epinephrine (0.3–0.5 mg) prolong sensory block in thoracic dermatomes as well by 30–50%. Clonidine prolongs bupivacaine spinal block by 30–50%.

The effect of adrenergic agonists on the duration of lidocaine spinal block is controversial. Some clinical studies have demonstrated that adrenergic agonists clearly prolong lidocaine spinal block,[81,92-94] whereas others have concluded that adrenergic agonists do not produce clinically useful prolongation.[95,96] This discrepancy may be explained, in part, by the fact that spinal block duration is so variable that studies using small numbers of patients may lack sufficient statistical power to detect real differences in mean block duration between groups. This problem was obviated in an interesting study by Chiu et al.,[97] who used a crossover study design to demonstrate that 0.2 mg of epinephrine significantly prolonged lidocaine sensory block in lumbar and sacral dermatomes. Thus, the available data suggest that adding epinephrine to lidocaine will result in a somewhat longer block, at least in lumbar and sacral dermatomes, than would be achieved if epinephrine were not added.

The mechanism by which adrenergic agonists prolong spinal block is not clear. Originally, epinephrine and phenylephrine were added to local anesthetics with the intent of reducing local spinal cord blood flow and thereby slowing the rate of drug elimination from the spinal cord and CSF. There are animal studies that support this mechanism[98,99] and others that do not.[100,101] Animal studies with clonidine indicate that it does reduce regional spinal cord blood flow.[102] There are no human studies that have investigated the effect of intrathecal adrenergic agonists on spinal cord blood flow. However, there are human studies that demonstrate that epinephrine decreases the rate of local anesthetic clearance from the CSF[103,104] and also slows the rate at which subarachnoid local anesthetic appears in the plasma.[92] These findings are consistent with a vasoconstrictor-mediated decrease in drug clearance from the spinal cord; however, they are not proof that this is the only or even the principal mechanism by which adrenergic agonists prolong spinal anesthesia.

Adrenergic agonists are potent analgesic agents in their own right when administered into the subarachnoid space.[105] Analgesia results from inhibition of nociceptive afferents, an effect that is mediated by stimulation of α-adrenergic receptors in the spinal cord dorsal horn. In addition, large intrathecal doses of α-adrenergic agonists have been shown to produce flaccidity in animal models by hyperpolarizing motor neurons.[106] Thus, prolongation of motor and sensory block by adrenergic agonists may be due, in part, to direct inhibitory effects of these drugs on sensory and motor neurons.

Epidural Anesthesia

Any procedure that can be performed under spinal anesthesia can also be performed under epidural block, and requires the same block height (Table 26-1). As with spinal anesthesia, there is a great deal of individual variability in spread (Fig. 26-10) and duration of epidural block (Table 26-5). Therefore, to choose the most appropriate local anesthetic and dose for a particular clinical situation, the anesthesiologist must be familiar with the variables that affect spread and duration of epidural anesthesia.

Table 26-5. LOCAL ANESTHETICS USED FOR SURGICAL EPIDURAL BLOCK

Drug*	Duration of Sensory Block		
	Two-Dermatome Regression (min)	Complete Resolution (min)	Prolongation by Epinephrine (%)
Chloroprocaine 3%	45–60	100–160	40–60
Lidocaine 2%	60–100	160–200	40–80
Mepivacaine 2%	60–100	160–200	40–80
Ropivacaine 0.5–1.0%	90–180	240–420	No
Etidocaine 1–1.5%	120–240	300–460	No
Bupivacaine 0.5–0.75%	120–240	300–460	No

* These concentrations are recommended for surgical anesthesia; more dilute concentrations are appropriate for epidural analgesia.

Block Spread

Injection Site. Unlike spinal anesthesia, epidural anesthesia produces a segmental block that spreads both caudally and cranially from the site of injection (Fig. 26-12). Thus, injection site is arguably the most important determinant of the spread of epidural block.

Caudal epidural blocks are largely restricted to sacral and low lumbar dermatomes. Low thoracic levels can be reached with caudal injections if large volumes are used (*e.g.,* 30 ml). However, the block at thoracic dermatomes tends to be patchy and short-lived following caudal injection.[107] Lumbar local anesthetic injections with volumes of 10 ml often extend caudad to include all sacral dermatomes, although the onset of block in the L5 and S1 roots is often delayed and may be patchy.[108] Twenty-milliliter volumes produce better-quality sacral anesthesia following lumbar injection. The slow onset at L5 and S1 is thought to result from their larger diameter and consequent slower drug penetration. Lumbar injections can be extended to midthoracic levels (T4–T6) when 20-ml volumes of local

anesthetic are used. Thoracic injections produce a symmetric segmental band of anesthesia, the width of which depends on the dose of local anesthetic administered. When using a mid- to upper thoracic injection site, it is prudent to reduce the local anesthetic doses by ~30–50% relative to lumbar doses to prevent excessive cephalad spread. It is generally not feasible to produce surgical anesthesia in low lumbar and sacral dermatomes with midthoracic or higher injection sites. Thoracic epidural block is ideally suited for anesthesia of the chest and abdomen.

Dose, Volume, and Concentration. Within the range typically used for surgical anesthesia, drug concentration is relatively unimportant in determining block spread. However, drug dose and volume are important variables determining both spread and quality of epidural block. If drug concentration is held constant, increasing the volume of local anesthetic (and thereby the dose) results in significantly greater average spread and greater block density. However, the relationship is nonlinear. For example, doubling the volume and dose of 1.5% lidocaine

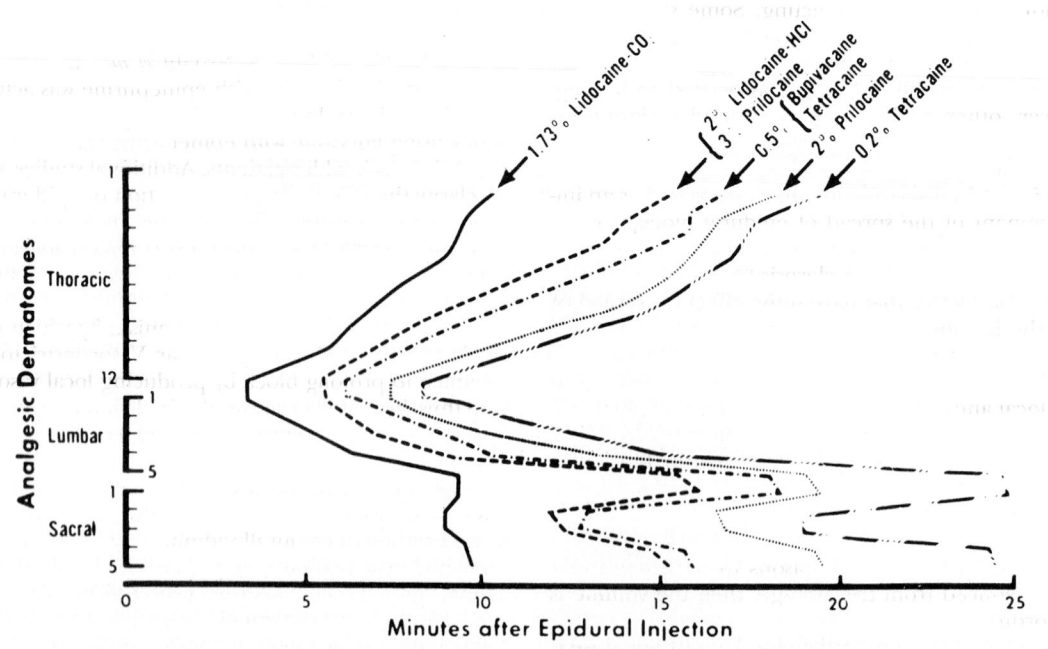

Figure 26-12. Spread of epidural sensory block over time after injection of various local anesthetic solutions at the L2–L3 interspace. All solutions contained epinephrine 1:200,000. Sensory block spreads both cephalad and caudad from the site of injection with time. Note the delay in onset of block at the L5 and S1 dermatomes with all solutions tested. (Reprinted with permission from Bromage PR: Epidural Analgesia. Philadelphia, WB Saunders, 1978.)

or 0.75% bupivacaine from 10 to 20 ml has been shown to increase spread by only three to four spinal segments.[108, 109]

Volume appears to be important in determining block spread independent of drug dose, but again the relationship is nonlinear. Erdemir *et al* showed that tripling the injected volume of lidocaine from 10 to 30 ml, while holding dose constant (300 mg) increased the cephalad extent of block by only 4.3 dermatomes.[110] This tendency toward greater spread is thought to be explained by the observation that increasing the volume of solution injected into the epidural space increases cephalad distribution.[111]

Position. When a single-shot technique is used, maintaining patients in the lateral position during and after epidural injection of surgical doses of local anesthetics does not seem to have a clinically important effect on spread of the block from side to side.[112] Similarly, studies examining the effect of patient position on cephalad spread of epidural block have found that the effect of posture on spread is not clinically important.[113] Ponhold *et al*,[114] however, demonstrated that maintaining a 30-degree head-up position significantly increased the frequency of adequate block at the L5 and S1 nerve roots even though there was no effect on the cephalad extent of anesthesia.

Patient Characteristics

Age. Most,[108, 109, 115-118] but not all[119] studies that have examined the effect of age on epidural block have demonstrated greater spread in older patients. However, the effect of age is probably clinically significant only when comparing adults whose ages differ by three or more decades. Even so, the difference in block height is not likely to be more than three or four dermatomes.

Greater spread in older patients is thought to be related to a less compliant epidural space and diminished ability for epidural solutions to leak out of intervertebral foramina.[111, 120] Both of these age-related changes would be expected to result in more extensive spread of solutions in the epidural space.

Height and Weight. The correlation between patient height[108, 109, 118, 119] or weight[118, 119] and spread of epidural block is weak and of little clinical significance except perhaps in patients who are extremely tall, extremely short, or morbidly obese.

Pregnancy. Studies examining the effect of pregnancy on spread of epidural block are conflicting. Some studies have demonstrated greater spread at term[121] and during early pregnancy,[122] suggesting that greater spread during pregnancy is not simply the result of anatomic changes associated with pregnancy. However, other studies have not found a significant difference in spread of epidural block between pregnant and nonpregnant women.[123, 124]

Atherosclerosis. Atherosclerosis has been suggested as an important determinant of the spread of epidural block.[121] However, subsequent studies have failed to find any relationship between block spread and atherosclerosis.[109, 115, 125]

Given the myriad factors that have some effect on spread of epidural anesthesia, how should anesthesiologists choose an appropriate local anesthetic dose for a single-shot epidural block? A useful recommendation is to assume that a 20-ml volume of all local anesthetics intended for surgical anesthesia will produce a midthoracic block on average after lumbar injection. If there are multiple reasons to expect that the block may spread excessively in an individual patient (*e.g.*, advanced age, obesity, very short stature, high injection site) or if the procedure does not require a high block, then the dose is reduced accordingly. If there are multiple reasons to expect that the spread may be reduced from the average, then the volume is increased accordingly.

Obviously, choice of the appropriate local anesthetic dose is obviated if an epidural catheter is used. In this situation, the anesthesiologist should begin with a lower dose than he or she anticipates will be needed and administer additional local anesthetic as necessary to extend the block to the desired level.

Onset

The onset of epidural block with all local anesthetics can usually be detected within 5 minutes in the dermatomes immediately surrounding the injection site. The time to peak effect differs somewhat among local anesthetics. Shorter-acting drugs usually reach their maximum spread in 15–20 minutes, whereas longer acting drugs require 20–25 minutes. Increasing the dose of local anesthetic speeds the onset of both motor and sensory block.

Duration

Local Anesthetic. As with spinal anesthesia, choice of local anesthetic is the most important determinant of the duration of epidural block. Chloroprocaine is the shortest-duration drug used for epidural anesthesia, lidocaine and mepivacaine provide blocks of intermediate duration, and bupivacaine, ropivacaine, and etidocaine produce the longest-lasting epidural blocks. Table 26-5 lists local anesthetics commonly used for epidural block and approximate duration of surgical anesthesia. Of note, tetracaine and procaine are not generally used for epidural block because of the poor-quality block they produce.

When used epidurally, some local anesthetics exhibit considerable separation in both the intensity and duration of sensory and motor block. Etidocaine produces the most intense motor block and is unusual among local anesthetics in that motor block may considerably outlast sensory block.[126] The phenomenon of the postoperative patient who is in pain yet still unable to move his legs has led some anesthesiologists to abandon etidocaine for epidural use. This is unfortunate, because etidocaine's superior muscle relaxation is sometimes beneficial during surgery. Bupivacaine has the opposite sensorimotor profile in that low concentrations of bupivacaine produce sensory block that is relatively more intense than motor block. This separation of sensory and motor block underlies the common practice of using dilute bupivacaine solutions for epidural analgesia since the laboring patient may be comfortable yet still able to move about.

Dose. Increasing the dose of local anesthetic administered results in increased duration[108, 127-129] and density[108, 128, 129] of epidural block.

Age. Studies that have evaluated the effect of age on epidural block duration are inconclusive. Veering *et al*[117] found that duration of epidural block with plain bupivacaine was not significantly affected by age. Nydahl *et al*[116] found that epidural block using bupivacaine with epinephrine was actually shorter in older patients. In contrast, Park *et al*[115] found that epidural block using lidocaine with epinephrine was slightly but significantly longer in older patients. Additional studies are necessary to clarify the effect of age on duration of epidural block.

Adrenergic Agonists. Epinephrine, in a concentration of 5 $m\mu \cdot ml^{-1}$ (1 : 200,000) is the most common adrenergic agonist added to epidural local anesthetics. It has been shown to prolong the duration of lidocaine and mepivacaine epidural block by as much as 80%.[130] The mechanism by which epinephrine prolongs epidural block is not clear. Vasoconstrictors have been assumed to prolong block by producing local vasoconstriction and thus decreased local anesthetic clearance from the epidural space. The fact that epinephrine reduces peak plasma concentrations of some local anesthetics after epidural injection is considered to be supportive evidence of this mechanism. However, iv infusion of epinephrine also decreases peak plasma concentration of epidurally administered local anesthetics, presumably by increasing their volume of distribution.[131] Thus, it is unclear what role local vasoconstriction plays in epinephrine's ability to prolong epidural block. As discussed earlier for spinal anesthesia, prolongation of motor and sensory block may be due, in part, to direct inhibitory effects of epinephrine on sensory and motor neurons.

Epinephrine does not significantly prolong the duration of anesthesia when added to the concentrated solutions of bupivacaine,[132,133] etidocaine,[128,133] or ropivacaine[134] that usually are used for surgical anesthesia. However, epinephrine does appear to prolong analgesia and improve the quality of block when added to more dilute solutions of these local anesthetics, such as those used for labor analgesia.[135-137]

Summary

The extent and duration of both spinal and epidural block are influenced by a number of variables, some of which are under the control of the anesthesiologist. Understanding the impact of these variables will allow the anesthesiologist rationally to select the most appropriate drug and dose for any clinical situation. However, even the most experienced anesthesiologist will still have blocks that are not adequate for the planned procedure. The frequency of failed blocks can be kept to a minimum if the clinician aims to produce blocks that are a little higher and a little longer than seems necessary. It is often easier to deal with a block that is too high or too long than to cover up for a block that is too low or too brief.

PHYSIOLOGY
Neurophysiology

The physiology of local anesthetic neural blockade is discussed in detail in Chapter 17. This section briefly presents aspects of the physiology of neural blockade that are unique to spinal and epidural anesthesia.

Site of Action

The site of action of spinal and epidural anesthesia is not precisely known. After epidural administration, local anesthetic is found in the spinal nerves within the epidural space, in spinal nerve rootlets within the CSF, and in the spinal cord. Similarly, after intrathecal administration in animals, local anesthetic is found in all sites between the spinal nerve rootlets and the interior of the spinal cord.[138, 139] Thus, neural blockade can potentially occur at any or all points along the neural pathways extending from the site of drug administration to the interior of the spinal cord.

In an interesting study in humans, Boswell *et al* demonstrated that patients are able to feel paresthesias during direct electrical stimulation of the spinal cord under spinal anesthesia.[140] Cortical evoked potentials from direct spinal cord stimulation were also maintained under spinal anesthesia, although amplitudes were decreased. In contrast, paresthesias and cortical evoked potentials from tibial nerve stimulation were abolished by spinal anesthesia. These investigators concluded that neural pathways in the spinal cord were largely intact during spinal anesthesia and that the spinal nerve rootlets were the principal site of neural blockade.

The site of epidural block is less well localized. Monkey studies suggest that epidural block occurs largely at sites in the spinal meninges, including the cauda equina nerve roots, dorsal root entry zone, and the long tracts of spinal cord white matter.[141] However, these findings are not entirely consistent with the segmental onset of epidural anesthesia (Fig. 26-12) or with the limited segmental blocks that can be produced with small doses of lumbar epidural local anesthetics in humans. These clinical observations are most readily explained by block of the segmental spinal nerves as they traverse the epidural or paravertebral spaces. In reality, epidural block likely occurs at both extradural and subdural sites with extradural radicular block predominating early and subdural spinal block predominating later. This supposition is consistent with human studies by Urban who rigorously examined the anatomic pattern of analgesia that occurred during onset and regression of epidural block.[142] He concluded that local anesthetics initially acted upon radicular structures, followed later by actions within the spinal cord.

Human studies demonstrate that somatosensory evoked potentials are maintained during epidural anesthesia, although amplitudes are decreased and latencies increased. This contrasts with spinal block, in which evoked potentials are completely eliminated, and supports the clinical impression that epidural block is generally less dense than that achieved with spinal anesthesia.

Differential Nerve Block

Differential block refers to a clinically important phenomenon in which nerve fibers subserving different functions display varying sensitivity to local anesthetic blockade. *In vivo* sympathetic nerve fibers appear to be blocked by the lowest concentration of local anesthetic, followed in order by fibers responsible for pain, touch, and motor function. This observation has led to the widely held belief that differences in sensitivity to local anesthetic blockade are explained solely by differences in fiber diameter, with smaller-diameter neurons exhibiting greater sensitivity than larger-diameter neurons. Although the mechanism for differential block in spinal and epidural anesthesia is not known, it is clear that fiber diameter is not the only, or perhaps even the most important factor contributing to differential block.[143, 144]

Differential block occurs with both peripheral nerve blocks and central neuraxial blocks. In the peripheral nervous system, differential block is a temporal phenomenon, with sympathetic block occurring first, followed in time by sensory and motor block. In contrast, with spinal and epidural anesthesia, differential block is manifest as a spatial separation in the modalities blocked. This is seen most clearly with spinal anesthesia, where the level of sympathetic block may extend to as many as two to six dermatomes higher than the level at which pin-prick sensation is absent,[145] which in turn extends two to three dermatomes higher than the level of motor block. This spatial separation is believed to result from a gradual decrease in local anesthetic concentration within the CSF as a function of distance from the site of injection. With epidural anesthesia, similar zones of differential sensory and sympathetic block are found.[146]

Perhaps the most troublesome consequence of differential block is the occasional patient who has intact touch and proprioception at the surgical site despite adequate blockade of pain sensation. Even the most stoic patients are likely to find this unpleasant and may lie in fear that the procedure will soon become painful. In no instance should the anesthesiologist downplay the distress this may cause patients. Reassurance and judicious sedation as necessary are usually sufficient to overcome this problem.

Central Effects of Neuraxial Block

Another important neurophysiologic aspect of central neuroaxial block is that it produces sedation,[147] potentiates the effect of sedative, hypnotic drugs[148-150] and markedly decreases anesthetic requirement.[151] The mechanisms underlying these effects are not known, but "deafferentation," (*i.e.*, the loss of ascending sensory input to the brain) is commonly invoked as causative.

Cardiovascular Physiology

Cardiovascular side effects, principally hypotension and bradycardia, are arguably the most important and common physiologic changes during spinal and epidural anesthesia. Understanding the homeostatic mechanisms responsible for control of blood pressure and heart rate is essential for understanding and treating the cardiovascular changes associated with spinal and epidural anesthesia.

Spinal Anesthesia

Blockade of sympathetic efferents is the principal mechanism by which spinal anesthesia produces cardiovascular derangements. As would be expected, the incidence of significant hypotension or bradycardia is related in general to the extent of sympathetic blockade, which in turn parallels block height.[152, 153] However, the severity of cardiovascular changes has been shown not to correlate with peak block height in one study[154] and to correlate poorly in another (Fig. 26-13).[152] Additional risk factors associated with hypotension include age >40–50 years, concurrent general anesthesia, obesity, hypovolemia, and addition of phenylephrine to the local anesthetic.[152, 155]

Hypotension during spinal anesthesia is the result of both arterial and venodilation. Venodilation increases volume in capacitance vessels, thereby decreasing venous return and right-sided cardiac filling pressures.[154, 156–158] This fall in preload is thought to be the principal cause of decreased cardiac output during high spinal anesthesia. Arterial dilation during spinal anesthesia results in significant decreases in total peripheral resistance (Fig. 26-14).[157, 159] Thus, the hypotension that accompanies 30-40% of spinal anesthetics may be the result of reductions in afterload, reductions in cardiac output, or both (Fig. 26-14).

Heart rate does not change significantly during spinal anesthesia in most patients (Fig. 26-14). However, clinically significant bradycardia occasionally occurs, with a reported incidence of 10–15%. As with hypotension, the risk of bradycardia increases with increasing block height.[152] Additional risk factors associated with bradycardia include age <50 years, American Society of Anesthesiologists Class 1 physical status, and concurrent use of β blockers.[152, 155] The mechanism responsible for bradycardia is not clear. Blockade of the sympathetic cardioaccelerator fibers originating from T1–T4 spinal segments is often suggested as the cause. The fact that bradycardia is more common with high blocks supports this mechanism. However, significant bradycardia sometimes occurs with blocks that are seemingly too low to block cardioaccelerator fibers. Diminished venous return has also been proposed as a cause of bradycardia during spinal anesthesia. Intracardiac stretch receptors have been shown reflexively to decrease heart rate when filling pressures fall.[160] Consistent with this mechanism, Jacobsen et al demonstrated a significant reduction in left ventricular volumes and heart rate during hypotensive episodes in two patients during epidural anesthesia.[161] They concluded that central volume depletion elicited a vagally mediated reflex slowing of heart rate. Similarly, Baron et al demonstrated that vagal activity is enhanced by decreased venous return during epidural anesthesia.[162] However, this mechanism does not operate at all times in all patients. Anzai and Nishikawa demonstrated significant heart rate increases in 40 patients who had their filling pressures suddenly decreased by body tilt during spinal anesthesia.[158] In reality, both blockade of cardioaccelerator fibers and decreased filling pressures as well as other unrecognized factors likely contribute to bradycardia during spinal anesthesia.

Although bradycardia is usually of moderate severity and well tolerated, there have been reports of sudden, unexplained, severe bradycardia and asystole during both spinal and epidural anesthesia.[163, 164] In addition, multiple case reports document that spinal anesthesia can also produce second- and third-degree heart block[165–167] and that pre-existing first-degree block may be a risk factor for progression to higher-grade blocks during spinal anesthesia.[165] These reports document the need for careful and continued vigilance of patients with central neuraxial blockade. Prompt, and occasionally aggressive, treatment of the cardiovascular changes that accompany the blockade may be required.

Epidural Anesthesia

The hemodynamic changes produced by epidural anesthesia depend largely on whether or not epinephrine is added to the local anesthetic solution (Fig. 26-14).[168] High epidural block with non-epinephrine-containing solutions results in decreased stroke volume, cardiac output, total peripheral resistance, and arterial pressure. The magnitude of these changes is usually less than that seen with comparable levels of spinal block.[168] As with spinal anesthesia, these hemodynamic changes are believed to result from venous and arterial dilation induced by sympathetic blockade. In contrast, when epinephrine-containing solutions are used for epidural anesthesia, stroke volume and cardiac output increase significantly (Fig. 26-14).[168] However, peripheral resistance falls dramatically, resulting in a decrease in arterial pressure greater than that seen with non-epinephrine-containing solutions. β_2-Adrenergic–mediated vasodilatation produced by low doses of absorbed epinephrine accounts for the greater decrease in peripheral vascular resistance and blood pressure. Decreased peripheral resistance may also contribute to the marked increase in cardiac output. However, epinephrine-induced venoconstriction with a resultant increase in venous return may also play an important role in increasing cardiac output.[169]

Treating Hemodynamic Changes

Treatment of hypotension secondary to spinal and epidural block must be aimed at the root causes: decreased cardiac output, decreased peripheral resistance, or both. Bolus crystalloid administration has often been advocated as a means of restoring venous return and thus cardiac output during central neuraxial blockade. However, the effectiveness of this therapy in normovolemic patients is controversial. Prehydrating patients with 500–1500 ml of crystalloid does not reliably prevent hypotension, but it has been shown to decrease the incidence of hypotension during spinal anesthesia in some,[170,171] but not all[153] studies. Similarly, prehydration with crystalloid has been shown not to be effective in preventing hypotension during spinal anesthesia for cesarean section.[172] Thus, although judicious crystalloid preloading of patients before central neuraxial blocks may benefit some patients, this practice cannot be relied on to prevent clinically significant hypotension in all or even most patients. The reason for this is that increasing preload can only increase stroke volume, which has limited ability to restore blood pressure if heart rate or systemic vascular resistance remains low. In this regard, colloids offer an interesting alternative to crystalloids for preloading before placing central neuraxial blocks. Marhofer et al have shown that 500 ml 6% hetastarch actually increases the systemic vascular resistance index in el-

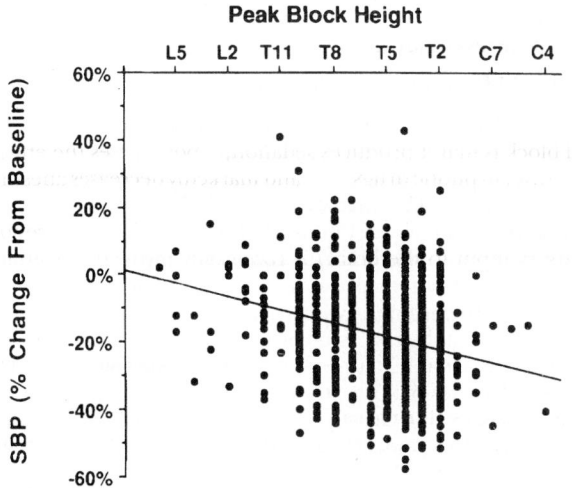

Figure 26-13. The relationship between peak block height and change in systolic blood pressure (SBP) during spinal anesthesia. Although there is a statistically significant correlation between block height and decrease in systolic blood pressure, the interindividual variability is so great that the relationship has little predictive value. This is reflected in the R^2 of 0.07 for the linear regression line. (Reprinted with permission from Carpenter RL, Caplan RA, Brown DL et al: Incidence and risk factors for side effects of spinal anesthesia. Anesthesiology 76:906, 1992.)

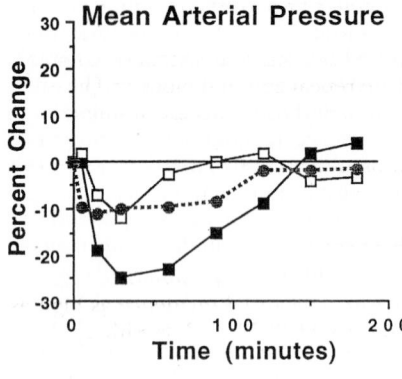

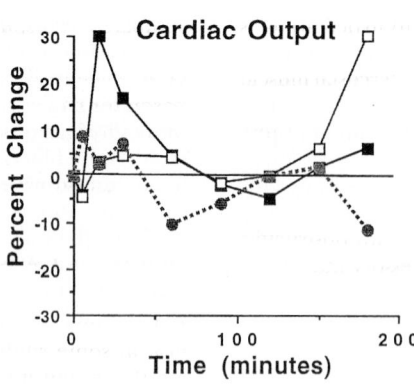

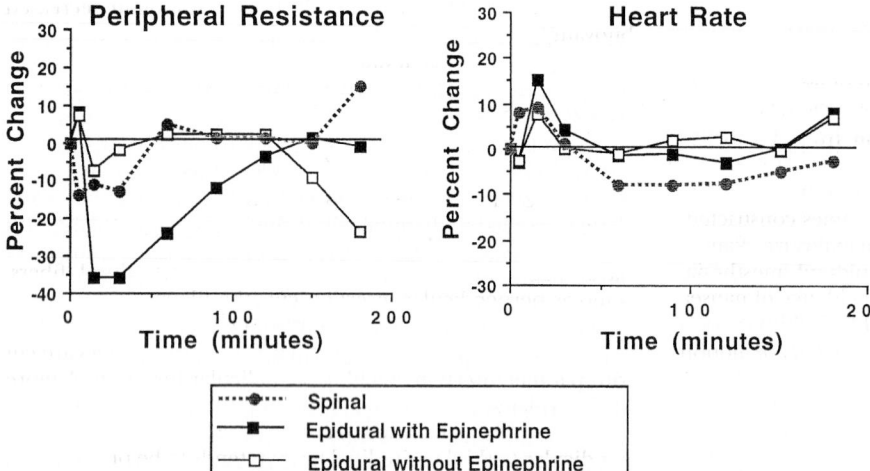

Figure 26-14. The cardiovascular effects of spinal and epidural anesthesia in volunteers with T5 blocks. The effects of spinal anesthesia and epidural anesthesia without epinephrine were generally comparable and are both qualitatively and quantitatively different from the effects of epidural anesthesia with epinephrine. (Modified and reprinted with permission from Bonica JJ, Kennedu WF Jr, Ward RJ, Tolas AG: A comparison of the effects of high subarachnoid and epidural anesthesia. Acta Anaesthesiol Scan [Suppl] 23:429, 1966.)

derly patients having spinal anesthesia, 1500 ml crystalloid significantly decreases the systemic vascular resistance index.[173]

Vasopressors are a more reliable approach to treating hypotension secondary to central neuraxial blockade. Drugs with both α- and β-adrenergic activity have been shown to be superior to pure α agonists for correcting the cardiovascular derangements produced by spinal and epidural anesthesia.[174,175] Ephedrine is the drug most commonly used to treat hypotension. Ephedrine boluses of 5–10 mg increase blood pressure by restoring cardiac output and peripheral vascular resistance. Dopamine, in low to moderate doses, has also been shown to correct the hemodynamic changes induced by central neuraxial block.[176,177] Dopamine may be preferable to ephedrine for long-term infusion because tachyphylaxis can develop to repeated ephedrine boluses. Pure α-adrenergic agonists, most commonly phenylephrine, are also used to correct hypotension during spinal anesthesia. However, α agonists increase blood pressure largely by increasing systemic vascular resistance, sometimes at the expense of a further decrease in cardiac output.[175] In addition, phenylephrine boluses have been shown to produce transient left ventricular dysfunction during epidural anesthesia with non-epinephrine-containing local anesthetics.[178] A potential, but as yet unstudied, role for α agonists may be to treat hypotension that occurs during epidural anesthesia with epinephrine-containing local anesthetics. Because the principal derangement in this situation is a marked decrease in systemic

vascular resistance, α agonists may be an appropriate choice for treating hypotension in this setting.

Deciding when to treat hemodynamic derangements during spinal and epidural anesthesia is perhaps more difficult than deciding how to treat them. There are no studies that clearly define the lower limit of acceptable blood pressure or heart rate for any group of patients. In the absence of such data, several authors have recommended treating blood pressure if it decreases more than 25–30% below baseline or, in normotensive patients, if systolic pressure falls below 90 mm Hg. Recommendations regarding bradycardia suggest initiating treatment if heart rate falls below 50–60 beat · min^{-1}. These recommendations are reasonable, although not universally applicable. Ultimately, anesthesiologists must decide what is an acceptable blood pressure and heart rate for an individual patient based on that patient's underlying medical condition.

Respiratory Physiology

Spinal and epidural blocks to midthoracic levels have little effect on pulmonary function in patients without pre-existing lung disease. Drugs used perioperatively for sedation during spinal or epidural block likely have a larger impact on pulmonary function than the block *per se*. In particular, lung volumes, resting minute ventilation, dead space, arterial blood gas tensions, and shunt fraction show little or no change during spinal or epidural anesthesia. Interestingly, the ventilatory response to hypercapnia is actually increased by spinal and epidural block.[179, 180]

High blocks associated with abdominal and intercostal muscle paralysis can impair ventilatory functions requiring active exhalation. For example, expiratory reserve volume, peak expiratory flow, and maximum minute ventilation may be significantly reduced by high spinal and epidural blocks. The negative impact of high blocks on active exhalation suggests caution when using spinal or epidural anesthesia in patients with obstructive pulmonary disease who may rely on their accessory muscles of respiration to maintain adequate ventilation.

Patients with high spinal or epidural blocks may complain of dyspnea despite normal or elevated minute ventilation. This likely results from the patient's inability to feel the chest wall move while breathing. This is understandably frightening to the patient, but reassurance is usually effective in alleviating their fear. The anesthesiologist must also be alert to the possibility that the complaint of dyspnea stems from incipient respiratory failure secondary to respiratory muscle paralysis. A normal speaking voice, as opposed to a faint gasping voice, suggests ventilation is normal.

Gastrointestinal Physiology

The gastrointestinal effects of spinal and epidural anesthesia are largely the result of sympathetic blockade. The abdominal organs derive their sympathetic innervation from T6 to L2. Blockade of these fibers results in unopposed parasympathetic activity by way of the vagus nerve. Consequently, secretions increase, sphincters relax, and the bowel becomes constricted. Some surgeons believe this improves surgical exposure. Nausea is a common complication of spinal and epidural anesthesia. The etiology is unknown, but an increased incidence of nausea during spinal anesthesia is associated with blocks higher than T5, hypotension, opioid administration, and a history of motion sickness.[152, 155]

Endocrine-Metabolic Physiology

Surgery produces numerous endocrine and metabolic changes, including increased protein catabolism and oxygen consumption as well as increases in circulating concentrations of catecholamines, growth hormone, renin, angiotensin, thyroid-stimulating hormone, β-endorphin, glucose, and free fatty acids, among others.[1] These endocrine–metabolic changes have collectively been termed the *surgical stress response.*

The mechanisms responsible for the stress response are complex and incompletely understood. However, afferent sensory information from the surgical site plays an important role in initiating and maintaining these changes.[1] Not surprisingly, spinal and epidural anesthesia have been shown to inhibit many of the endocrine–metabolic changes associated with the stress response. The inhibitory effect is greatest with lower abdominal and lower extremity procedures and least with upper abdominal and thoracic procedures.[1] The salutary effect of spinal and epidural anesthesia is believed to result from blockade of the afferent sensory information that helps initiate the stress response.

Although some aspects of the surgical stress response may be beneficial, it is generally viewed as maladaptive and possibly a contributor to postoperative morbidity and mortality.[1] Despite the ability of central neuraxial block to decrease the stress response, there is as yet no clear evidence that this results in decreased morbidity or mortality.

COMPLICATIONS

Backache

Although postoperative backache occurs after general anesthesia, it is more common after epidural and spinal anesthesia.[181]

Compared with spinal anesthesia, back pain after epidural anesthesia is more common (11% vs. 30%) and of longer duration.[182] Back pain has been cited in one study as the most common reason for patients to refuse repeat epidural block.[182] The etiology of backache is not clear, although needle trauma, local anesthetic irritation, and ligamentous strain secondary to muscle relaxation have been offered as explanations.

Postdural Puncture Headache

Postdural puncture headache (PDPH) is a common complication of spinal anesthesia, with a reported incidence as high as 25% in some studies. The risk of PDPH is less with epidural anesthesia, but it occurs in up to 50% of young patients after accidental meningeal puncture with large-diameter epidural needles. The headache is characteristically mild or absent when the patient is supine, but head elevation rapidly leads to a severe fronto-occipital headache, which again improves upon returning to the supine position. Occasionally cranial nerve symptoms (*e.g.,* diplopia, tinnitus) and nausea and vomiting are also present. The headache is believed to result from the loss of CSF through the meningeal needle hole, resulting in decreased buoyant support for the brain. In the upright position, the brain sags in the cranial vault, putting traction on pain-sensitive structures. Traction on cranial nerves is believed to cause the cranial nerve palsies occasionally seen.

The incidence of PDPH decreases with increasing age (Fig. 26-15) and with the use of small-diameter spinal needles with noncutting tips.[183, 184] Inserting cutting needles with the bevel aligned parallel to the long axis of the meninges has also been shown to decrease the incidence of PDPH.[184, 185] Some authors have suggested that parallel insertion spreads dural fibers, whereas perpendicular insertion cuts the fibers, resulting in a larger meningeal hole. However, the collagen fibers of the dura mater are arranged randomly; therefore, as many fibers are cut with parallel insertion as with perpendicular insertion. A more likely explanation arises from the fact that the dura mater is under longitudinal tension. Thus, a slit-like hole oriented perpendicular to this longitudinal tension tends to be pulled open, whereas a hole oriented parallel to this tension is pulled closed. Some studies have suggested that women are at greater risk of development of PDPH. However, if age differences are accounted for, there does not appear to be a sex difference in the incidence of PDPH.[184] Folklore aside, remaining supine after meningeal puncture does not decrease the incidence of

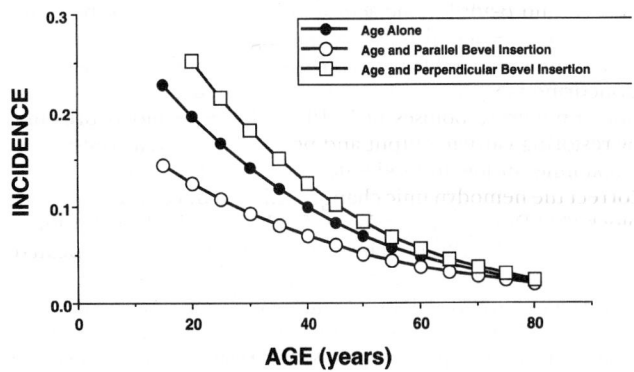

Figure 26-15. The incidence of postdural puncture headache decreases as patient age increases. When using beveled needles, the incidence is higher than average at any given age if the needle is inserted perpendicular to the spinal meninges and lower if inserted parallel to the spinal meninges. (Modified and reprinted with permission from Lybecker H, Møller JT, May O, Nielsen HK: Incidence and prediction of post-dural puncture headache: A prospective study of 1021 spinal anesthesias. Anesth Analg 70:389, 1990.)

PDPH. Finally, use of fluid instead of air for loss of resistance during attempted epidural anesthesia does not alter the risk of accidental meningeal puncture, but does markedly decrease the risk of subsequent development of PDPH.[22]

Postdural puncture headache usually resolves spontaneously in a few days to a week for most patients. However, there are reports of PDPH persisting for months after meningeal puncture. Initial treatment is appropriately conservative if this meets the patient's needs. Bed rest and analgesics as necessary are the mainstay of conservative treatment. Caffeine has also been shown to produce short-term symptomatic relief.[186]

Epidural blood patch is an alternative for patients who are unable or unwilling to await spontaneous resolution of PDPH. It is believed that a clot forms over the meningeal hole, thereby preventing further CSF leak while the meningeal rent heals. Ten to 20 milliliters of autologous blood is aseptically removed and injected into the epidural space at or near the interspace at which the meningeal puncture occurred. This is effective in relieving symptoms within 1–24 hours in 85–95% of patients; ~90% of patients who fail an initial blood patch respond to a second patch. The most common side effects of blood patch are backache and radicular pain, although transient bradycardia and cranial nerve palsies have also been reported.

The timing of epidural blood patch has been controversial. Early studies suggested that prophylactic blood patch in patients at high risk for PDPH was ineffective.[168] This led several authors to suggest that blood patch should not be performed before symptoms of PDPH develop. Subsequent studies that used larger volumes of blood in the epidural space (15–20 ml) have shown that prophylactic blood patch is effective in preventing PDPH in patients in whom the meninges were accidentally punctured during attempted epidural anesthesia.[187,188] Prophylactic blood patch is not appropriate for most patients, but is worth considering in high-risk outpatients for whom a return trip to the hospital for epidural blood patch would be difficult.

Epidurally administered fibrin glue has also been shown to be an effective alternative to blood administration for treatment of PDPH.[189] Whether it is superior to blood requires further study, but it may be an attractive alternative for some patients. In the future, it may be necessary to drop the term *blood patch* in favor of *meningeal patch*.

Hearing Loss

Lamberg *et al* demonstrated that a transient (1–3 days) mild decrease in hearing acuity (>10 dB) is common after spinal anesthesia patients with an incidence of roughly 40% and a 3:1 female:male predominance.[190] Similarly, Gültekin *et al*[191] demonstrated a 45% incidence of hearing impairment in patients undergoing prilocaine spinal anesthesia, but a much lower incidence (18%) in patients having bupivacaine spinal anesthesia. The mechanism of hearing loss in these studies is unclear, but the marked female predominance, the absence of PDPH, and the difference in incidence between prilocaine and bupivacaine suggests that CSF leak is not the cause.

Systemic Toxicity

The toxicity of local anesthetics is discussed in detail in Chapter 17. Systemic toxicity does not occur with spinal anesthesia because the drug doses used are too low to cause toxic reactions even if injected intravenously. Both CNS and cardiovascular toxicity may occur during epidural anesthesia. CNS toxicity may result from local anesthetic absorption from the epidural space, but more commonly occurs after accidental intravascular injection of local anesthetic. Because the plasma concentrations of local anesthetics required to produce serious cardiovascular toxicity are very high, this complication likely results only from accidental intravascular local anesthetic injection. An adequate iv test dose and incremental injection of local anesthetics are the most important methods to prevent both CNS and cardiovascular toxicity during epidural anesthesia.

Total Spinal

Total spinal anesthesia occurs when local anesthetic spreads high enough to block the entire spinal cord and occasionally the brain stem during either spinal or epidural anesthesia. Profound hypotension and bradycardia are common secondary to complete sympathetic blockade. Respiratory arrest may occur as a result of respiratory muscle paralysis or dysfunction of brain stem respiratory control centers. Management includes vasopressors, atropine, and fluids as necessary to support the cardiovascular system, plus oxygen and controlled ventilation. If the cardiovascular and respiratory consequences are managed appropriately, total spinal block will resolve without sequelae.

Neurologic Injury

Serious neurologic injury is a rare but widely feared complication of epidural and spinal anesthesia. Multiple large series of spinal and epidural anesthesia report that neurologic injury occurs in ~0.03–0.1% of all central neuraxial blocks, although in most of these series the block was not clearly proven to be causative.[192] Persistent paresthesias and limited motor weakness are the most common injuries, although paraplegia and diffuse injury to cauda equina roots (cauda equina syndrome) do occur rarely. Injury may result from direct needle trauma to the spinal cord or spinal nerves, from spinal cord ischemia, from accidental injection of neurotoxic drugs or chemicals, from introduction of bacteria into the subarachnoid or epidural space, or very rarely from epidural hematoma.[192]

Local anesthetics intended for epidural and intrathecal use can themselves be neurotoxic in concentrations used clinically.[193] In particular, hyperbaric 5% lidocaine has been implicated as a cause of multiple cases of cauda equina syndrome after subarachnoid injection through small-bore ("microspinal") catheters during continuous spinal anesthesia.[194] Hyperbaric solutions injected through these high-resistance catheters have been shown to produce very little turbulence and thus poor mixing of the local anesthetic with CSF.[195] Nerve injury is believed to result from pooling of toxic concentrations of undiluted lidocaine around dependent cauda equina nerve roots. Consequently, the U.S. Food and Drug Administration has banned the use of these small-gauge catheters for continuous spinal anesthesia. Although the combination of microspinal catheters and high concentrations of lidocaine has clearly been implicated in causing cauda equina syndrome, this complication has also occurred when larger (20-gauge) catheters,[194] 2% lidocaine,[196] and 0.5% tetracaine were used.[194] A common thread in all of these reports has been the apparent maldistribution of the local anesthetic in the CSF. Maldistribution should be suspected whenever spinal block is unexpectedly restricted, and maneuvers, such as altering patient position or drug baricity, should be used to improve drug distribution before additional drug is injected through a continuous spinal catheter. If these maneuvers fail to improve drug distribution, an alternative anesthetic technique should be used.

The mechanism by which local anesthetics produce cauda equina syndrome is not yet clear; however, *in vitro* evidence suggests that local anesthetics produce excitotoxic damage by depolarizing neurons and increasing intracellular calcium concentrations.[197] It is also unclear as yet whether adjuncts, such as epinephrine, added to local anesthetics contribute to cauda equina syndrome. However, based on animal studies, it has been argued that epinephrine should not be added to intrathecal lidocaine.[198] Rather, if prolonged duration of spinal anesthesia is necessary, a longer-acting drug like bupivacaine should be used.

Transient Radicular Irritation. In addition to cauda equina syndrome, transient radicular irritation (TRI) has emerged as a concern after central neuraxial blockade. TRI is defined as pain, dysesthesia, or both in the legs or buttocks after spinal anesthesia, and was first proposed as a recognizable entity by Schneider *et al.*[199] All local anesthetics have been shown to cause TRI, although the risk appears to be greater with lidocaine than other local anesthetics.[200-206]

In a large epidemiologic study of nearly 2000 patients, Freedman *et al* characterized the clinical picture of TRI.[207] They found that patients receiving lidocaine were significantly more likely to have TRI than patients receiving spinal tetracaine or bupivacaine, although TRI did occur with these latter drugs as well. Additional risk factors for TRI included surgery in the lithotomy position (with lidocaine, but not bupivacaine or tetracaine), outpatient status, and obesity. Variables shown not to increase the risk of TRI included lidocaine dose, type of spinal needle, addition of epinephrine to lidocaine, paresthesia, hypotension, and blood-tinged CSF. In a separate study, Sakura *et al* has shown that the addition of phenylephrine is a risk factor for TRI when 0.5% tetracaine is used for spinal anesthesia.[208]

Pain from TRI is not trivial with most patients rating it as moderate (visual analogue scale = 4–7/10). The pain usually resolved spontaneously within 72 hours, but a very few patients required 6 months.[207]

The mechanism responsible for TRI is unknown, but it would be inappropriate to conclude that TRI is simply a milder manifestation of cauda equina syndrome. Differences in clinical presentation, risk factors, and the like suggest that these are not simply two points along a continuum of the same process.

Spinal Hematoma

Spinal hematoma is a rare but potentially devastating complication of spinal and epidural anesthesia, with an incidence estimated to be <1 in 150,000. Patients most commonly present with numbness or lower extremity weakness, a fact that can make early detection difficult in patients receiving perioperative spinal local anesthetics for pain control. Early detection is critical since a delay of more than 8 hours in decompressing the spinal cord reduces the odds of good recovery.[209]

Coagulation defects are the principal risk factor for epidural hematoma. This raises the legitimate question as to how to treat patients who are or who will be anticoagulated. This issue has been addressed in a Consensus Statement from the American Society for Regional Anesthesia (www.asra.com/consensus/intro.shtml). In brief, patients taking antiplatelet drugs (*e.g.,* nonsteroidal anti-inflammatory drugs [NSAIDS]) or receiving subcutaneous unfractionated heparin for deep vein thrombosis prophylaxis are not viewed as being at increased risk of spinal hematoma. Patients receiving fractionated low–molecular-weight heparin (*e.g.,* enoxaprin) are considered to be at increased risk of spinal hematoma. Patients who are "fully anticoagulated" (*i.e.,* have an elevated prothrombin time or partial thromboplastin time) at the time of block placement or epidural catheter removal are considered to be at increased risk of spinal hematoma. Similarly, patients receiving thrombolytic or fibrinolytic therapy are at increased risk of neuraxial bleeding. For those patients who may have an epidural or intrathecal catheter placed, its removal is nearly as great a risk for spinal hematoma as its insertion, and the timing of removal and anticoagulation should be coordinated. In addition, drugs and regimens not considered to put patients at increased risk for neuraxial bleeding when used alone (*e.g.,* mini dose unfractionated heparin and NSAIDs) may in fact increase the risk when combined.

CONTRAINDICATIONS

The only absolute contraindication to spinal or epidural anesthesia is patient refusal. However, several pre-existing conditions increase the relative risk of these techniques, and the anesthesiologist must carefully weigh the expected benefits before proceeding. Some conditions that increase the apparent risk of central neuraxial block include the following:

1. Hypovolemia or shock increases the risk of hypotension.
2. Increased intracranial pressure increases the risk of brain herniation when CSF is lost through the needle, or if a further increase in intracranial pressure follows injection of large volumes of solution into the epidural or subarachnoid spaces.
3. Coagulopathy or thrombocytopenia increase the risk of epidural hematoma.
4. Sepsis increases the risk of meningitis.
5. Infection at the puncture site increases the risk of meningitis.

Pre-existing neurologic disease, particularly diseases that wax and wane (*e.g.,* multiple sclerosis), have been considered a contraindication to central-neuraxial block by some authors. However, there is no evidence to suggest that spinal or epidural anesthesia alters the course of any pre-existing neurologic disease. Recommendations to avoid regional anesthesia in these patients stem largely from a medicolegal concern that the anesthetic may be incorrectly blamed for any subsequent worsening of the patient's pre-existing condition. Although this is a legitimate concern, it is not a reason to avoid central-neuraxial block if this is an otherwise appropriate choice.

SPINAL OR EPIDURAL ANESTHESIA?

Spinal and epidural anesthesia each have advantages and disadvantages that may make one or the other technique better suited to a particular patient or procedure. Controlled studies comparing both techniques for surgical anesthesia have consistently found that spinal anesthesia takes less time to perform, produces more rapid onset of better-quality sensorimotor block, and is associated with less pain during surgery.[182] Despite these important advantages of spinal anesthesia, epidural anesthesia offers advantages, too. Chief among them are the lower risk of PDPH, less hypotension if epinephrine is not added to the local anesthetic, the ability to prolong or extend the block using an indwelling catheter, and the option of using an epidural catheter to provide postoperative analgesia.

REFERENCES

1. Kehlet H: The stress response to surgery: Release mechanisms and the modifying effect of pain relief. Acta Chir Scand Suppl 550:22, 1988
2. Modig J, Borg T, Karlström G et al: Thromboembolism after total hip replacement: role of epidural and general anesthesia. Anesth Analg 62:174, 1983
3. Thornburn J, Louden J, Vallance R: Spinal and general anesthesia in total hip replacement: Frequency of deep vein thrombosis. Br J Anaesth 52:1117, 1980
4. Christopherson R, Beattie C, Frank S et al: Perioperative morbidity in patients randomized to epidural or general anesthesia for lower extremity vascular surgery. Anesthesiology 79:422, 1993
5. Rosenfeld B, Beattie C, Christopherson R et al: The effects of different anesthetic regimens on fibrinolysis and the development of postoperative arterial thrombosis. Anesthesiology 79:435, 1993
6. Yeager M, Glass D, Neff R, Brinck-Johnsen T: Epidural anesthesia and analgesia in high-risk surgical patients. Anesthesiology 66: 729, 1987
7. Zarzur E: Anatomic studies of the human lumbar ligamentum flavum. Anesth Analg 63:499, 1984
8. Hogan Q: Lumbar epidural anatomy: A new look by cryomicrotome section. Anesthesiology 75:767, 1991
9. Gershater F, St. Louis EL: Lumbar epidural venography: Review of 1,200 cases. Radiology 131:409, 1979
10. Meijenhorst GC: Computed tomography of the lumbar epidural veins. Radiology 145:687, 1982

11. Fink BR, Walker S: Orientation of fibers in human dorsal lumbar dura mater in relation to lumbar puncture. Anesth Analg 69:768, 1989

12. Blomberg R: The dorsomedian connective tissue band in the lumbar epidural space of humans: An anatomical study using epiduroscopy in autopsy cases. Anesth Analg 65:747, 1986

13. Savolaine ER, Pandya JB, Greenblatt SH, Conover SR: Anatomy of the human lumbar epidural space: New insights using CT-epidurography. Anesthesiology 68:217, 1988

14. Hogan Q: Epidural catheter tip position and distribution of injectate evaluated by computed tomography. Anesthesiology 90(4): 964, 1999

15. Manchada V, Murad S, Shilyansky G, Mehringer M: Unusual clinical course of accidental subdural local anesthetic injection. Anesth Analg 62:1124, 1983

16. Lubenow T, Keh-Wong E, Kristof K et al: Inadvertent subdural injection: A complication of epidural block. Anesth Analg 67: 175, 1988

17. Jones M, Newton T: Inadvertent extra-arachnoid injections in myelography. Radiology 80:818, 1963

18. Bernards C, Hill H: Morphine and alfentanil permeability through the spinal dura, arachnoid and pia mater of dogs and monkeys. Anesthesiology 73:1214, 1990

19. Bernards C, Hill H: The spinal nerve root sleeve is not a preferred route for redistribution of drugs from the epidural space to the spinal cord. Anesthesiology 75:827, 1991

20. Reiman A, Anson B: Vertebral level of termination of the spinal cord with report of a case of sacral cord. Anat Rec 88:127, 1944

21. Drummond G, Scott D: Deflection of spinal needles by the bevel. Anaesthesia 35:854, 1980

22. Aida S, Taga K, Yamakura T et al: Headache after attempted epidural block: The role of intrathecal air. Anesthesiology 88(1): 76, 1998

23. Asato F, Goto F: Radiographic findings of unilateral epidural block. Anesth Analg 83(3):519, 1996

24. Leighton BL, Norris MC, DeSinome CA et al: The air test as a clinically useful indicator of intravenously placed epidural catheters. Anesthesiology 73:610, 1990

25. Mackie K, Lam A: Epinephrine-containing test dose during beta-blockade. J Clin Monit 7:213, 1991

26. Moore D, Batra M: The components of an effective test dose prior to epidural block. Anesthesiology 55:693, 1981

27. Guinard J, Mulroy M, Carpenter R, Knopes K: Test doses: Optimal epinephrine content with and without acute beta-adrenergic blockade. Anesthesiology 73:386, 1990

28. Leighton B, DeSimone C, Norris M, Chayen B: Isoproterenol is an effective marker of intravenous injection in laboring women. Anesthesiology 71:206, 1989

29. Leighton BL, Norris MC, Sosis M et al: Limitations of epinephrine as a marker of intravascular injection in laboring women. Anesthesiology 66:688, 1987

30. Takiguchi T, Okano T, Egawa H et al: The effect of epidural saline injection on analgesic level during combined spinal and epidural anesthesia assessed clinically and myelographically [see Comments]. Anesth Analg 85(5):1097, 1997

31. Stienstra R, Dahan A, Alhadi BZ et al: Mechanism of action of an epidural top-up in combined spinal epidural anesthesia. Anesth Analg 83(2):382, 1996

32. Stienstra R, Dilrosun-Alhadi BZ, Dahan A et al: The epidural "top-up" in combined spinal-epidural anesthesia: The effect of volume versus dose. Anesth Analg 88(4):810, 1999

33. Myint Y, Bailey P, Milne B: Cardiorespiratory arrest following combined spinal epidural anaesthesia. Anaesthesia 48:684, 1993

34. Bernards C, Kopacz D, Michel M: Effect of needle puncture on morphine and lidocaine flux through the spinal meninges of the monkey. Anesthesiology 80:853, 1994

35. Hodgkinson R, Husain FJ: Obesity, gravity, and spread of epidural anesthesia. Anesth Analg 60:421, 1981

36. Lee A, Ray D, Littlewood D, Wildsmith J: Effect of dextrose concentration on the intrathecal spread of amethocaine. Br J Anaesth 61:135, 1988

37. Chambers WA, Edstrom HH, Scott DB: Effect of baricity on spinal anaesthesia with bupivacaine. Br J Anaesth 53:279, 1981

38. Bannister J, McClure JH, Wildsmith JA: Effect of glucose concentration on the intrathecal spread of 0.5% bupivacaine. Br J Anaesth 64:232, 1990

39. Povey HM, Jacobsen J, Westergaard-Nielsen J: Subarachnoid anal-

gesia with hyperbaric 0.5% bupivacaine: Effect of a 60-min period of sitting. Acta Anaesthesiol Scand 33:295, 1989

40. Povey HM, Olsen PA, Pihl H: Spinal analgesia with hyperbaric 0.5% bupivacaine: Effects of different patient positions. Acta Anaesthesiol Scand 31:616, 1987

41. Sinclair CJ, Scott DB, Edström H: Effect of the Trendelenberg position on spinal anaesthesia with hyperbaric bupivacaine. Br J Anaesth 54:497, 1982

42. Martin-Salvaj G, Van Gessel E, Forster A et al: Influence of duration of lateral decubitus on the spread of hyperbaric tetracaine during spinal anesthesia: A prospective time-response study. Anesth Analg 79:1107, 1994

43. Smith T: The lumbar spine and subarachnoid block. Anesthesiology 29:60, 1968

44. Logan MR, Drummond GB: Spinal anesthesia and lumbar lordosis. Anesth Analg 67:338, 1988

45. Bodily M, Carpenter R, Owens B: Lidocaine 0.5% spinal anaesthesia: A hypobaric solution for short-stay perirectal surgery. Can J Anaesth 39:770, 1992

46. Brown DT, Wildsmith JA, Covino BG, Scott DB: Effect of baricity on spinal anesthesia with amethocaine. Br J Anaesth 52:589, 1980

47. Cummings GC, Bamber DB, Edstrom HH, Rubin AP: Subarachnoid blockade with bupivacaine. A comparison with cinchocaine. Br J Anaesth 56:573, 1984

48. Møller IW, Fernandes A, Edström HH: Subarachnoid anaesthesia with 0.5% bupivacaine: Effects of density. Br J Anaesth, 56: 1191, 1984

49. Logan MR, McClure JH, Wildsmith JA: Plain bupivacaine: An unpredictable spinal anaesthetic agent. Br J Anaesth 58:292, 1986

50. McKeown DW, Stewart K, Littlewood DG, Wildsmith JA: Spinal anesthesia with plain solutions of lidocaine (2%) and bupivacaine (0.5%). Regional Anesth 11:68, 1986

51. Cameron AE, Arnold RW, Ghorisa MW, Jamieson V: Spinal analgesia using bupivacaine 0.5% plain: Variation in the extent of the block with patient age. Anaesthesia 36:318, 1981

52. Kalso E, Tuominen M, Rosenberg PH: Effect of posture and some c.s.f. characteristics on spinal anaesthesia with isobaric 0.5% bupivacaine. Br J Anaesth 54:1179, 1982

53. Tuominen M, Kalso E, Rosenberg P: Effects of posture on the spread of spinal anaesthesia with isobaric 0.75% or 0.5% bupivacaine. Br J Anaesth 54:313, 1982

54. Stienstra R, van Poorten JF: The temperature of bupivacaine 0.5% affects the sensory level of spinal anesthesia. Anesth Analg 67: 272, 1988

55. McClure JH, Brown DT, Wildsmith JA: Effect of injected volume and speed of injection on the spread of spinal anaesthesia with isobaric amethocaine. Br J Anaesth 54:917, 1982

56. Van Zundert AA, De Wolf AM: Extent of anesthesia and hemodynamic effects after subarachnoid administration of bupivacaine with epinephrine. Anesth Analg 67:784, 1988

57. Nielsen TH, Kristoffersen E, Olsen KH et al: Plain bupivacaine: 0.5% or 0.25% for spinal analgesia? Br J Anaesth 62:164, 1989

58. Bengtsson M, Malmqvist LA, Edström HH: Spinal analgesia with glucose-free bupivacaine: Effects of volume and concentration. Acta Anaesthesiol Scand 28:583, 1984

59. Blomqvist H, Nilsson A, Arwestrôm E: Spinal anaesthesia with 15mg bupivacaine 0.25% and 0.5%. Regional Anesth 13:165, 1988

60. Mukkada TA, Bridenbaugh PO, Singh P, Edström HH: Effects of dose, volume, and concentration of glucose-free bupivacaine in spinal anesthesia. Regional Anesth 11:98, 1986

61. Sheskey MC, Rocco AG, Bizzarri-Schmid M et al: A dose-response study of bupivacaine for spinal anesthesia. Anesth Analg 62:931, 1983

62. Wildsmith J, McClure J, Brown D, Scott D: Effects of posture on the spread of isobaric and hyperbaric amethocaine. Br J Anaesth 53:273, 1981

63. Pflug AE, Aasheim GM, Beck HA: Spinal anesthesia: Bupivacaine versus tetracaine. Anesth Analg 55:489, 1976

64. Sundnes KO, Vaagenes P, Skretting P et al: Spinal analgesia with hyperbaric bupivacaine: Effects of volume of solution. Br J Anaesth 54:69, 1982

65. Chambers WA, Littlewood DG, Scott DB: Spinal anesthesia with hyperbaric bupivacaine: Effect of added vasoconstrictors. Anesth Analg 61:49, 1982

66. Taivainen T, Tuominen M, Rosenberg PH: Influence of obesity on the spread of spinal analgesia after injection of plain 0.5%

bupivacaine at the L3-4 or L4-5 interspace. Br J Anaesth 64: 542, 1990

67. Tuominen M, Kuulasmaa K, Taivainen T, Rosenberg PH: Individual predictability of repeated spinal anaesthesia with isobaric bupivacaine. Acta Anaesthesiol Scand 33:13, 1989

68. Tuominen M, Taivainen T, Rosenberg PH: Spread of spinal anaesthesia with plain 0.5% bupivacaine: Influence of the vertebral interspace used for injection. Br J Anaesth 62:358, 1989

69. Carpenter RL, Hogan QH, Liu SS et al: Lumbosacral cerebrospinal fluid volume is the primary determinant of sensory block extent and duration during spinal anesthesia [see Comments]. Anesthesiology 89:24, 1998

70. Pargger H, Hampl KF, Aeschbach A et al: Combined effect of patient variables on sensory level after spinal 0.5% plain bupivacaine. Acta Anaesthesiol Scand 42(4):430, 1998

71. Veering BT, Burm AG, van Kleef JW et al: Spinal anesthesia with glucose-free bupivacaine: Effects of age on neural blockade and pharmacokinetics. Anesth Analg 66:965, 1987

72. Pitkänen M, Haapaniemi L, Tuominen M, Rosenberg PH: Influence of age on spinal anaesthesia with isobaric 0.5% bupivacaine. Br J Anaesth 56:279, 1984

73. Norris M: Height, weight, and the spread of subarachnoid hyperbaric bupivacaine in the term parturient. Anesth Analg 67: 555, 1988

74. Norris MC: Patient variables and the subarachnoid spread of hyperbaric bupivacaine in the term parturient. Anesthesiology 72: 478, 1990

75. Wildsmith JA, Rocco AG: Current concepts in spinal anesthesia. Reg Anesth 10:119, 1985

76. McCulloch WJ, Littlewood DG: Influence of obesity on spinal analgesia with isobaric 0.5% bupivacaine. Br J Anaesth 58: 610, 1986

77. Pitkänen MT: Body mass and spread of spinal anesthesia with bupivacaine. Anesth Analg 66:127, 1987

78. Axelsson KH, Edström HH, Sundberg AE, Widman GB: Spinal anaesthesia with hyperbaric 0.5% bupivacaine: Effects of volume. Acta Anaesthesiol Scand 26:439, 1982

79. Bengtsson M, Edström HH, Löfström JB: Spinal analgesia with bupivacaine, mepivacaine and tetracaine. Acta Anaesthesiol Scand 27:278, 1983

80. Racle J, Benkhadra A, Poy J, Gleizal B: Effect of increasing amounts of epinephrine during isobaric bupivacaine spinal anesthesia in elderly patients. Anesth Analg 66:882, 1987

81. Vaida GT, Moss P, Capan LM, Turndorf H: Prolongation of lidocaine spinal anesthesia with phenylephrine. Anesth Analg 65: 781, 1986

82. Egbert LD, Deas TC: Effect of epinephrine upon the duration of spinal anesthesia. Anesthesiology 21:345, 1960

83. Concepcion M, Maddi R, Francis D et al: Vasoconstrictors in spinal anesthesia with tetracaine: A comparison of epinephrine and phenylephrine. Anesth Analg 63:134, 1984

84. Meagher RP, Moore DC, DeVries JC: Phenylephrine: The most effective potentiator of tetracaine spinal anesthesia. Anesth Analg 45:134, 1966

85. Caldwell C, Nielsen C, Baltz T et al: Comparison of high-dose epinephrine and phenylephrine in spinal anesthesia with tetracaine. Anesthesiology 62:804, 1985

86. Park WY, Balingit PE, Macnamara TE: Effects of patient age, pH of cerebrospinal fluid, and vasopressors on onset and duration of spinal anesthesia. Anesth Analg 54:455, 1975

87. Fukuda T, Dohi S, Naito H: Comparisons of tetracaine spinal anesthesia with clonidine or phenylephrine in normotensive and hypertensive humans. Anesth Analg 78:106, 1994

88. Bonnet F, Brun-Buisson V, Saada M et al: Dose-related prolongation of hyperbaric tetracaine spinal anesthesia by clonidine in humans. Anesth Analg, 68:619, 1989

89. Dobrydnjov I, Samarutel J: Enhancement of intrathecal lidocaine by addition of local and systemic clonidine. Acta Anaesthesiol Scand 43(5):556, 1999

90. Ota K, Namiki A, Ujike Y, Takahashi I: Prolongation of tetracaine spinal anesthesia by oral clonidine. Anesth Analg 75:262, 1992

91. Ota K, Namiki A, Iwasaki H, Takahashi I: Dosing interval for prolongation of tetracaine spinal anesthesia by oral clonidine in humans. Anesth Analg 79:1117, 1994

92. Axelsson K, Widman B: Blood concentration of lidocaine after spinal anaesthesia using lidocaine and lidocaine with adrenaline. Acta Anaesthesiol Scand 25:240, 1981

93. Leicht CH, Carlson SA: Prolongation of lidocaine spinal anesthesia with epinephrine and phenylephrine. Anesth Analg 65:365, 1986

94. Moore D, Artru A, Kelly W, Jenkins D: Use of computed tomography to locate a sheared epidural catheter. Anesth Analg 66: 795, 1987

95. Chambers WA, Littlewood DG, Logan MR, Scott DB: Effect of added epinephrine on spinal anesthesia with lidocaine. Anesth Analg 60:417, 1981

96. Spivey DL: Epinephrine does not prolong lidocaine spinal anesthesia in term parturients. Anesth Analg 64:468, 1985

97. Chiu AA, Liu S, Carpenter RL et al: The effects of epinephrine on lidocaine spinal anesthesia: A cross-over study. Anesth Analg 80(4):735, 1995

98. Kozody R, Swartz J, Palahniuk RJ et al: Spinal cord blood flow following subarachnoid lidocaine. Can Anaesth Soc J 32:5:472, 1985

99. Kozody R, Palahniuk RJ, Cumming MO: Spinal cord blood flow following subarachnoid tetracaine. Can Anaesth Soc J 32:1: 23, 1985

100. Kozody R, Ong B, Palahniuk RJ et al: Subarachnoid bupivacaine decreases spinal cord blood flow in dogs. Can Anaesth Soc J 32:3:216, 1985

101. Denson DD, Bridenbaugh PO, Turner PA et al: Neural blockade and pharmacokinetics following subarachnoid lidocaine in the rhesus monkey. I. Effects of epinephrine. Anesth Analg 61:746, 1982

102. Crosby G, Russo M, Szabo M, Davies K: Subarachnoid clonidine reduces spinal cord blood flow and glucose utilization in conscious rats. Anesthesiology 73:1179, 1990

103. Converse JG, Landmesser CM, Harmel MH: The concentration of pontocaine hydrochloride in the cerebrospinal fluid during spinal anesthesia, and the influence of epinephrine in prolonging the sensory anesthetic effect. Anesthesiology 15:1, 1954

104. Mörch ET, Rosenberg MK, Truant AT: Lidocaine for spinal anesthesia. A study of the concentration in the spinal fluid. Acta Anaesthesiol Scand 1:105, 1957

105. Reddy SV, Maderdrut JL, Yaksh TL: Spinal cord pharmacology of adrenergic agonist-mediated antinociception. J Pharmacol Exp Ther 213:525, 1980

106. Phillis J, Tebecis A, York D: Depression of spinal motoneurons by noradrenalin, 5-hydroxytryptamine and histamine. Eur J Pharmacol 4:471 1968

107. Park W, Massengale M, Macnamara T: Age, height, and speed of injection as factors determining caudal anesthetic level and occurrence of severe hypertension. Anesthesiology 51:81, 1979

108. Park WY, Hagins FM, Rivat EL, Macnamara TE: Age and epidural dose response in adult men. Anesthesiology 56:318, 1982

109. Grundy EM, Ramamurthy S, Patel KP et al: Extradural analgesia revisited. Br J Anaesth 50:805, 1978

110. Erdemir HA, Soper LE, Sweet RB: Studies of factors affecting peridural anesthesia. Anesth Analg 44:400, 1965

111. Burn JM, Guyer PB, Langdon L: The spread of solutions injected into the epidural space. Br J Anaesth 45:338, 1973

112. Apostolou GA, Zarmakoupis PK, Mastrokostopoulos GT: Spread of epidural anesthesia and the lateral position. Anesth Analg 60: 584, 1981

113. Park WY, Hagins FM, Massengale MD, Macnamara TE: The sitting position and anesthetic spread in the epidural space. Anesth Analg 63:863, 1984

114. Ponhold H, Kulier A, Rehak P: 30 degree trunk elevation of the patient and quality of lumbar epidural anesthesia: Effects of elevation in operations on the lower extremities. Anaesthetist 42:788, 1993

115. Park WY, Massengale M, Kim SI et al: Age and the spread of local anesthetic solutions in the epidural space. Anesth Analg 59:768, 1980

116. Nydahl PA, Philipson L, Axelsson K, Johansson JE: Epidural anesthesia with 0.5% bupivacaine: Influence of age on sensory and motor blockade. Anesth Analg 73:780, 1991

117. Veering BT, Burm AG, van Kleef JW et al: Epidural anesthesia with bupivacaine: Effects of age on neural blockade and pharmacokinetics. Anesth Analg 66:589, 1987

118. Hirabayashi Y, Saitoh K, Fukuda H, Shimizu R: Effect of age on dose requirement for lumbar epidural anesthesia. Masui 42:808 1993

119. Duggan J, Bowler GM, McClure JH, Wildsmith JA: Extradural

block with bupivacaine: Influence of dose, volume, concentration and patient characteristics. Br J Anaesth, 61:324, 1988

120. Hirabayashi Y, Shimizu R, Matsuda I, Inoue S: Effect of extradural compliance and resistance on spread of extradural analgesia. Br J Anaesth 65:508, 1990

121. Bromage P: Spread of analgesic solutions in the epidural space and their site of action: A statistical study. Br J Anaesth 34:161, 1962

122. Fagraeus L, Urban BJ, Bromage PR: Spread of epidural analgesia in early pregnancy. Anesthesiology 58:184, 1983

123. Grundy EM, Zamora AM, Winnie AP: Comparison of spread of epidural anesthesia in pregnant and nonpregnant women. Anesth Analg 57:544, 1978

124. Kalas DB, Senfield RM, Hehre FW: Continuous lumbar peridural anesthesia in obstetrics. IV: Comparison of the number of segments blocked in pregnant and nonpregnant subjects. Anesth Analg 45:848, 1966

125. Sharrock NE: Lack of exaggerated spread of epidural anesthesia in patients with arteriosclerosis. Anesthesiology 47:307, 1977

126. Axelsson K, Nydahl PA, Philipson L, Larsson P: Motor and sensory blockade after epidural injection of mepivacaine, bupivacaine, and etidocain: A double-blind study. Anesth Analg 69:739, 1989

127. Kerkkamp HE, Gielen MJ, Wattwil M et al: An open study comparison of 0.5%, 0.75% and 1.0% ropivacaine, with epinephrine, in epidural anesthesia in patients undergoing urologic surgery. Reg Anesth 15:53, 1990

128. Buckley FP, Littlewood DG, Covino BG, Scott DB: Effects of adrenaline and the concentration of solution on extradural block with etidocaine. Br J Anaesth 50:171, 1978

129. Scott DB, McClure JH, Gaisi RM et al: Effects of concentration of local anaesthetic drugs in extradural block. Br J Anaesth 52:1033, 1980

130. Bromage PR, Burfoot MF, Crowell DE, Pettigrew RT: Quality of epidural blockade. I: Influence of physical factors. Br J Anaesth 36:342, 1964

131. Sharrock NE, Go G, Mineo R: Effect of i.v. low-dose adrenaline and phenylephrine infusions of plasma concentrations of bupivacaine after lumbar extradural anaesthesia in elderly patients. Br J Anaesth 67:694, 1991

132. Kier L: Continuous epidural analgesia in prostatectomy: Comparison of bupivacaine with and without adrenaline. Acta Anaesthesiol Scand 18:1, 1974

133. Sinclair CJ, Scott DB: Comparison of bupivacaine and etidocaine in extradural blockade. Br J Anaesth 56:147, 1984

134. Cederholm I, Anskär S, Bengtsson M: Sensory, motor, and sympathetic block during epidural analgesia with 0.5% and 0.75% ropivacaine with and without epinephrine. Reg Anesth 19:18, 1994

135. Abboud T, Sheik-ol-Eslam A, Yanagi T et al: Safety and efficacy of epinephrine added to bupivacaine for lumbar epidural analgesia in obstetrics. Anesth Analg 64:585, 1985

136. Eisenach JC, Grice SC, Dewan DM: Epinephrine enhances analgesia produced by epidural bupivacaine during labor. Anesth Analg 66:447, 1987

137. Finucane B, McCraney J, Bush D: Double-blind comparison of lidocaine and etidocaine during continuous epidural anesthesia for vaginal delivery. South Med J 71:667, 1978

138. Cohen E: Distribution of local anesthetic agents in the neuroaxis of the dog. Anesthesiology 29:1002, 1968

139. Post C, Freedman J, Ramsay C, Bonnevier A: Redistribution of lidocaine and bupivacaine after intrathecal injection in mice. Anesthesiology 63:410 1985

140. Boswell M, Iacono R, Guthkelch A: Sites of action of subarachnoid lidocaine and tetracaine: Observations with evoked potential monitoring during spinal cord stimulator implantation. Reg Anesth 17:37, 1992

141. Cusick J, Myklebust J, Abram S: Differential neural effects of epidural anesthetics. Anesthesiology 53:299, 1980

142. Urban B: Clinical observations suggesting a changing site of action during induction and recession of spinal and epidural anesthesia. Anesthesiology 39:496, 1973

143. Fink BR: Mechanisms of differential axial blockade in epidural and subarachnoid anesthesia. Anesthesiology 70:851, 1989

144. Fink BR, Cairns AM: Lack of size-related differential sensitivity to equilibrium conduction block among mammalian myelinated axons exposed to lidocaine. Anesth Analg 66:948, 1987

145. Chamberlain D, Chamberlain B: Changes in skin temperature of the trunk and their relationship to sympathetic block during spinal anesthesia. Anesthesiology 65:139, 1986

146. Brull SJ, Greene NM: Zones of differential sensory block during extradural anaesthesia. Br J Anaesth 66:651, 1991

147. Gentili M, Huu PC, Enel D et al: Sedation depends on the level of sensory block induced by spinal anaesthesia. Br J Anaesth 81(6):970, 1998

148. Ben-David B, Vaida S, Gaitini L: The influence of high spinal anesthesia on sensitivity to midazolam sedation [see Comments]. Anesth Analg 81(3):525, 1995

149. Tverskoy M, Shagal M, Finger J, Kissin I: Subarachnoid bupivacaine blockade decreases midazolam and thiopental hypnotic requirements. J Clin Anesth 6(6):487, 1994

150. Tverskoy M, Shifrin V, Finger J et al: Effect of epidural bupivacaine block on midazolam hypnotic requirements. Reg Anesth 21(3):209, 1996

151. Hodgson P, Liu S, Gras T: Does epidural anesthesia have general anesthetic effects? A prospective, randomized, double-blind, placebo-controlled trial. Anesthesiology 91:1687, 1999

152. Carpenter RL, Caplan RA, Brown DL et al: Incidence and risk factors for side effects of spinal anesthesia. Anesthesiology 76:906, 1992

153. Coe AJ, Revanäs B: Is crystalloid preloading useful in spinal anaesthesia in the elderly? Anaesthesia 45:241, 1990

154. Phero JC, Bridenbaugh PO, Edström HH et al: Hypotension in spinal anesthesia: A comparison of isobaric tetracaine with epinephrine and isobaric bupivacaine without epinephrine. Anesth Analg 66:549, 1987

155. Tarkkila P, Isola J: A regression model for identifying patients at high risk of hypotension, bradycardia and nausea during spinal anesthesia. Acta Anesthesiol Scand 36:554, 1992

156. Shimosato S, Etsten BE: The role of the venous system in cardiocirculatory dynamics during spinal and epidural anesthesia in man. Anesthesiology 30:619, 1969

157. Kennedy WF, Jr., Bonica JJ, Akamatsu TJ et al: Cardiovascular and respiratory effects of subarachnoid block in the presence of acute blood loss. Anesthesiology 29:29, 1968

158. Anzai Y, Nishikawa T: Heart rate responses to body tilt during spinal anesthesia. Anesth Analg 73:385, 1991

159. Ward RJ, Bonica JJ, Freund FG et al: Epidural and subarachnoid anesthesia: Cardiovascular and respiratory effects. JAMA, 191:275, 1965

160. Pathak CL: Autoregulation of chronotropic response of the heart through pacemaker stretch. Cardiology 58:45, 1973

161. Jacobsen J, Søfelt S, Brocks V et al: Reduced left ventricular diameters at onset of bradycardia during epidural anaesthesia. Acta Anaesthesiol Scand 36:831, 1992

162. Baron JF, Decaux-Jacolot A, Edouard A et al: Influence of venous return on baroreflex control of heart rate during lumbar epidural anesthesia in humans. Anesthesiology 64:188, 1986

163. Caplan RA, Ward RJ, Posner K, Cheney FW: Unexpected cardiac arrest during spinal anesthesia: A closed claims analysis of predisposing factors. Anesthesiology 68:5, 1988

164. Mackey DC, Carpenter RL, Thompson GE et al: Bradycardia and asystole during spinal anesthesia: A report of three cases without morbidity. Anesthesiology 70:866, 1989

165. Bernards CM, Hymas NJ: Progression of first degree heart block to high-grade second degree block during spinal anaesthesia. Can J Anaesth 39(2):173, 1992

166. Jordi EM, Marsch SC, Strebel S: Third degree heart block and asystole associated with spinal anesthesia. Anesthesiology 89(1):257, 1998

167. Shen CL, Hung YC, Chen PJ et al: Mobitz type II AV block during spinal anesthesia. Anesthesiology 90(5):1477, 1999

168. Bonica JJ, Kennedy WF Jr, Ward RJ, Tolas AG: A comparison of the effects of high subarachnoid and epidural anesthesia. Acta Anaesthesiol Scand 23:429, 1966

169. Kerkkamp HE, Gielen MJ: Hemodynamic monitoring in epidural blockade: Cardiovascular effects of 20ml 0.5% bupivacaine with and without epinephrine. Reg Anesth 15:137, 1990

170. Graves CL, Underwood PS, Klein RL, Kim YI: Intravenous fluid administration as therapy for hypotension secondary to spinal anesthesia. Anesth Analg 47:548, 1968

171. Venn PJ, Simpson DA, Rubin AP, Edstrom HH: Effect of fluid preloading on cardiovascular variables after spinal anaesthesia with glucose-free 0.75% bupivacaine. Br J Anaesth 63:682, 1989

172. Rout CC, Rocke DA, Levin J et al: A reevaluation of the role of crystalloid preload in the prevention of hypotension associated

with spinal anesthesia for elective cesarean section. Anesthesiology 79:262, 1993

173. Marhofer P, Faryniak B, Oismuller C et al: Cardiovascular effects of 6% hetastarch and lactated Ringer's solution during spinal anesthesia [In Process Citation]. Reg Anesth Pain Med 24(5):399, 1999

174. Butterworth J, Piccione W, Berrizbeitia L et al: Augmentation of venous return by adrenergic agonists during spinal anesthesia. Anesth Analg 65:612, 1986

175. Ward RJ, Kennedy WF, Bonica J et al: Experimental evaluation of atropine and vasopressors for the treatment of hypotension of high subarachnoid anesthesia. Anesth Analg 45:621, 1966

176. Lundberg J, Norgren L, Thomson D, Werner O: Hemodynamic effects of dopamine during thoracic epidural analgesia in man. Anesthesiology 66:641, 1987

177. Butterworth JF IV, Austin JC, Johnson MD et al: Effect of total spinal anesthesia on arterial and venous responses to dopamine and dobutamine. Anesth Analg 66:209, 1987

178. Goertz AW, Seeling W, Heinrich H et al: Effect of phenylephrine bolus administration of left ventricular function during high thoracic and lumbar epidural anesthesia combined with general anesthesia. Anesth Analg 76:541, 1993

179. Sakura S, Saito Y, Kosaka Y: Effect of lumbar epidural anesthesia on ventilatory response to hypercapnia in young and elderly patients. J Clin Anesth 5:109, 1993

180. Steinbrook R, Concepcion M, Topulos G: Ventilatory responses to hypercapnia during bupivacaine spinal anesthesia. Anesth Analg 67:247, 1988

181. Dahl JB, Schultz P, Anker-Møller E et al: Spinal anaesthesia in young patients using a 29-gauge needle: Technical considerations and an evaluation of postoperative complaints compared with general anaesthesia. Br J Anaesth 64:178, 1990

182. Seeberger MD, Lang ML, Drewe J et al: Comparison of spinal and epidural anesthesia for patients younger than 50 years of age. Anesth Analg 78:667, 1994

183. Halpern S, Preston R: Postdural puncture headache and spinal needle design. Anesthesiology 81:1376, 1994

184. Lybecker H, Møller JT, May O, Nielsen HK: Incidence and prediction of postdural puncture headache. A prospective study of 1021 spinal anesthesias. Anesth Analg 70:389, 1990

185. Flaatten H, Thorsen T, Askeland B et al: Puncture technique and postural postdural puncture headache: A randomised, double-blind study comparing transverse and parallel puncture. Acta Anaesthesiol Scand 42(10):1209, 1998

186. Camann WR, Murray RS, Mushlin PS, Lambert DH: Effects of oral caffeine on postdural puncture headache. A double-blind, placebo-controlled trial. Anesth Analg 70:181, 1990

187. Cheek TG, Banner R, Sauter J, Gutsche BB: Prophylactic extradural blood patch is effective. Br J Anaesth 61:340, 1988

188. Colonna-Romano P, Shapiro BE: Unintentional dural puncture and prophylactic epidural blood patch in obstetrics. Anesth Analg 69:522, 1989

189. Crul BJ, Gerritse BM, van Dongen RT, Schoonderwaldt HC: Epidural fibrin glue injection stops persistent postdural puncture headache. Anesthesiology 91(2):576, 1999

190. Lamberg T, Pitkanen MT, Marttila T, Rosenberg PH: Hearing loss after continuous or single-shot spinal anesthesia. Reg Anesth 22(6):539, 1997

191. Gültekin S, Yilmaz N, Ceyhan A et al: The effect of different anaesthetic agents in hearing loss following spinal anaesthesia. Eur J Anaesthesiol 15(1):61, 1998

192. Kane R: Neurologic deficits following epidural or spinal anesthesia. Anesth Analg 60:150, 1981

193. Lambert LA, Lambert DH, Strichartz GR: Irreversible conduction block in isolated nerve by high concentrations of local anesthetics. Anesthesiology 80:1082, 1994

194. Rigler M, Drasner K, Krejcie T et al: Cauda equina syndrome after continuous spinal anesthesia. Anesth Analg 72:275, 1991

195. Ross B, Coda B, Heath C: Local anesthetic distribution in a spinal model: a possible mechanism of neurologic injury after continuous spinal anesthesia. Reg Anesth 17:69, 1992

196. Drasner K, Rigler M, Sessler D, Stoller M: Cauda equina syndrome following intended epidural anesthesia. Anesthesiology 77:582, 1992

197. Gold MS, Reichling DB, Hampl K et al: Lidocaine toxicity in primary afferent neurons from the rat. J Pharmacol Exp Ther 285(2):413, 1998

198. Drasner K: Lidocaine spinal anesthesia: A vanishing therapeutic index? [Editorial; Comment]. Anesthesiology 87(3):469, 1997

199. Schneider M, Ettlin T, Kaufmann M et al: Transient neurologic toxicity after hyperbaric subarachnoid anesthesia with 5% lidocaine [see Comments]. Anesth Analg 76(5):1154, 1993

200. Hiller A, Rosenberg PH: Transient neurological symptoms after spinal anaesthesia with 4% mepivacaine and 0.5% bupivacaine. Br J Anaesth 79(3):301, 1997

201. Liguori GA, Zayas VM, Chisholm MF: Transient neurologic symptoms after spinal anesthesia with mepivacaine and lidocaine [see Comments]. Anesthesiology 88(3):619, 1998

202. Martinez-Bourio R, Arzuaga M, Quintana JM et al: Incidence of transient neurologic symptoms after hyperbaric subarachnoid anesthesia with 5% lidocaine and 5% prilocaine [see Comments]. Anesthesiology 88(3):624, 1998

203. Hampl KF, Heinzmann-Wiedmer S, Luginbuehl I et al: Transient neurologic symptoms after spinal anesthesia: A lower incidence with prilocaine and bupivacaine than with lidocaine [see Comments]. Anesthesiology 88(3):629, 1998

204. Salmela L, Aromaa U: Transient radicular irritation after spinal anesthesia induced with hyperbaric solutions of cerebrospinal fluid-diluted lidocaine 50 mg/ml or mepivacaine 40 mg/ml or bupivacaine 5 mg/ml. Acta Anaesthesiol Scand 42(7):765, 1998

205. Axelrod EH, Alexander GD, Brown M, Schork MA: Procaine spinal anesthesia: A pilot study of the incidence of transient neurologic symptoms. J Clin Anesth 10(5):404, 1998

206. Bergeron L, Girard M, Drolet P et al: Spinal procaine with and without epinephrine and its relation to transient radicular irritation. Can J Anaesth 46(9):846, 1999

207. Freedman JM, Li DK, Drasner K et al: Transient neurologic symptoms after spinal anesthesia: An epidemiologic study of 1,863 patients [published erratum appears in Anesthesiology 89(6):1614, 1998]. Anesthesiology 89(3):633, 1998

208. Sakura S, Sumi M, Sakaguchi Y et al: The addition of phenylephrine contributes to the development of transient neurologic symptoms after spinal anesthesia with 0.5% tetracaine [see Comments]. Anesthesiology 87(4):771, 1997

209. Vandermeulen EP, Van Aken H, Vermylen J: Anticoagulants and spinal-epidural anesthesia. Anesth Analg 79:1165, 1994

Clinical Anesthesia (4/e), edited by
Paul G. Barash, Bruce F. Cullen, and
Robert K. Stoelting. Lippincott Williams &
Wilkins, Philadelphia, © 2001.

CHAPTER 27

PERIPHERAL NERVE BLOCKADE

MICHAEL F. MULROY

GENERAL PRINCIPLES

Regional anesthesia of the extremities and of the trunk is a useful alternative to general anesthesia in many situations. Peripheral nerve blocks have attracted renewed interest because of their salutary role in reducing postoperative pain[1] and shortening outpatient recovery.[2]

Local Anesthetic Drug Selection and Doses

The pharmacology of local anesthetics is reviewed at length in Chapter 17. Although high concentrations of drug are needed to produce rapid onset of anesthesia in the epidural space, lower concentrations (*e.g.*, 1% lidocaine, 0.25% or 0.5% bupivacaine) are more appropriate on peripheral nerves because of concerns about local and systemic toxicity. Local toxicity of these anesthetics appears to be concentration dependent.[3,4] Lower concentrations are also indicated because larger volumes are often required to anesthetize poorly localized peripheral nerves or to block a series of nerves. The use of a high-concentration solution presents the patient with a high total-milligram dose of local anesthetic, which may produce toxic blood levels.

The absorption of drug and the duration of anesthesia vary with the dose, drug, location injected, and presence of vasoconstrictors. The highest blood levels of local anesthetic occur after intercostal blockade, followed by epidural, caudal, and brachial plexus blockade. Similarly, the duration depends on the blood supply of the area of injection. Equivalent doses of local anesthetic may produce only 3–4 hours of anesthesia when placed in the epidural space, but 24–36 hours when placed on the sciatic nerve. In general, the addition of epinephrine 1 : 200,000 is advantageous in prolonging the duration of blockade and in reducing the systemic blood levels of local anesthetic. Its use is not appropriate in the vicinity of "terminal" blood vessels, such as in the digits or penis, or when using an intravenous (iv) regional technique. The recommended doses and drugs in this chapter assume the addition of epinephrine to the solution.

Nerve Localization

The blockade techniques associated with reliable proximity of nerves to bones or arteries are the easiest technically to perform (*e.g.*, epidural, intercostal, axillary). Less reliable landmarks, such as the psoas compartment or obturator foramen, require either large volumes of local anesthetic solution or the establishment of a distinct localization of the desired nerve to provide adequate anesthesia. Paresthesias are the traditional sign of successful localization. There is potential for intraneural injection if paresthesias are obtained. This is usually signaled by a complaint from the patient of a "cramping" or "aching" pain during the initial injection. If this occurs, the needle should be immediately withdrawn by a few millimeters and a small test injection repeated. Even without intraneural injection, residual neuropathy of peripheral nerves appears more likely if paresthesias are obtained. Selander *et al*[5] have reported a 2.8% incidence of residual ulnar neuropathy when paresthesias were used to locate nerves, compared with a 0.8% incidence with the transar-

terial technique of axillary blockade. Other larger series have reported a much lower incidence of dysesthesia since short bevel needles have been used,[6] and it appears premature to abandon the paresthesia technique.[7] A third problem with this technique is the inevitable discomfort associated with it; patient education and sedation must be handled appropriately (see later).

The use of a nerve stimulator is an alternative nerve localization technique. A low-current electrical impulse applied to a peripheral nerve produces stimulation of motor fibers and identifies the proximity of the nerve without actual needle contact or patient discomfort (or cooperation). This technique is particularly suited to the patient who is uncooperative as a result of inebriation or heavy sedation. Because the nerve stimulator does not actually contact the nerve, its use may reduce the chance for nerve injury, although it still may occur.[7] Its use does not improve the success rate of regional anesthesia, at least in a training program,[8] because a familiarity with the anatomy and technique is necessary to bring the needle into proximity with the nerve. Nevertheless, this is a useful adjunct to regional anesthesia, and some comments about appropriate use of this device are warranted.

The ideal stimulator should have a variable-amperage output. This allows a high current to be delivered in the exploration phase and then a progressively lower current to document proximity of the nerve. Whereas 1 mA can be used to produce the first motor twitch, actual injection of anesthetic should be delayed until stimulation is produced by as little as 0.3–0.5 mA. At that point, 2–3 ml of local anesthetic should be sufficient to abolish motor twitch, indicating that it is appropriate to inject the remainder of the proposed dose. The accuracy of the localization can be improved by the use of insulated needles. A plastic sheath along the shaft allows the current flow to be concentrated at the tip and is more likely to produce stimulation only when the tip is near the nerve fiber rather than after the tip has moved past its target. Current flow can also be improved by using the positive (red) pole of the stimulator as the ground (or reference) electrode and the negative (black) lead as the connection to the needle itself. Despite these steps, the stimulator is still only an adjunct to nerve localization and not a reliable substitute for good technique.

Equipment

Although reusable syringes and needles can be manufactured to a higher standard, their cost and concern about infection generally lead to a preference for disposable equipment. There are a large number of high-quality disposable kits available on the market, and many of the major manufacturers customize their packages at the request of large institutions willing to commit to purchasing a sufficient volume. The use of disposable trays places the burden of sterilization on the manufacturer, although the liability for checking the sterility of contents always remains with the user.

Needles used for regional techniques are often modified from standard injection needles (Fig. 27-1). For peripheral blockade, the "short bevel" or "B bevel" is often used. This shorter angulation of the bevel (16–20 degrees versus conventional 12–13 degrees) was introduced by Selander *et al*[9] and has been shown in animals to produce less injury to nerves, perhaps by pushing the nerve away rather than piercing it when contact is made. Other modifications, such as the "pencil-point" insulated needle, have been introduced in attempts to reduce nerve injury. Another feature of regional blockade needles is the addition of a "security bead" to the shaft. This small bead is added approximately 6 mm from the juncture of the shaft and the hub and prevents the shaft of the needle from retracting below the skin in the event that it becomes separated from the hub. These two modifications are useful features for peripheral nerve blockade.

Special syringes are also useful for performing peripheral nerve blockades. Plastic and glass are equally useful. With respect to size, a 10-ml syringe is usually a good compromise. Large volumes are usually required for peripheral nerve blockade, so that 3- and 5-ml syringes are rarely adequate. Larger than 10-ml volume often presents such bulk and weight that fine control is hampered. If a larger syringe is used, it is usually advisable to have an assistant manipulate the syringe and have it attached to the needle by a short length of extension tubing. The use of finger rings (the "control syringe") is helpful in controlling injection, facilitating aspiration, and allowing the operator to refill the syringe with one hand (Fig. 27-2). Luer-Lok adapters for the syringe-hub connection are also advantageous. Although friction fittings produce tight seals, the amount of force required for attaching or removing the syringe may displace a needle that has been meticulously maneuvered into the appropriate close contact with a nerve.

The selection of antiseptic solutions is usually a local preference. Organic iodine preparations are the current standard for skin asepsis. They are usually nonirritating to tissues and carry the added advantage of a distinct color. Colorless preparation solutions are dangerous because of the possibility of confusion with (or contamination of) local anesthetic solutions. Colored alcohol solutions are acceptable skin cleansers for many of the simple infiltrations that do not require extensive preparation. For major deep blockade, a wide area of skin preparation is more desirable, and the borders of the clean area can be extended by draping on four sides with sterile towels. Regional anesthesia does not require the same degree of sterile preparation and gowning as indicated for surgery, but strict attention to asepsis is desirable to reduce the chance of infection.

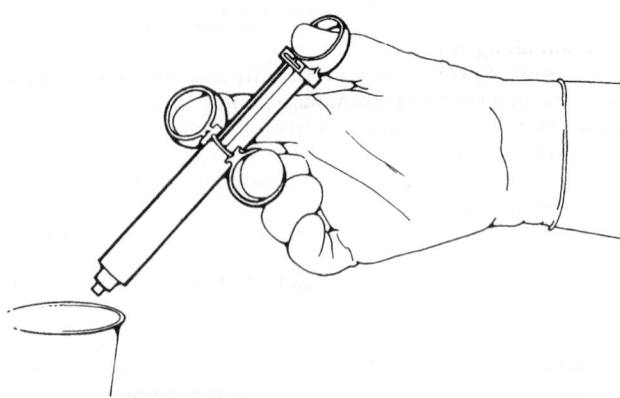

Figure 27-2. The three-ring ("control") syringe. Use of this adaptation to the plunger of a standard 10-ml syringe allows greater control of injection, easier aspiration, and the opportunity to refill the syringe with one hand. Plastic adapters are available for disposable syringes as demonstrated; glass syringes are supplied with a metal plunger and ring attached. (Reproduced with permission from Mulroy M: Handbook of Regional Anesthesia. Boston, Little, Brown, 1996.)

Common Complications

Systemic toxicity of local anesthetics is the most serious concern.[10] This syndrome and the problems of allergy and other unique toxicities are addressed in Chapter 17. Central nervous system excitation and myocardial depression are the two most common hazards associated with high blood levels of local anesthetics. No peripheral nerve blockade using significant quantities of local anesthetic should be performed without oxygen and appropriate resuscitation equipment immediately available. This includes blockades using small quantities of anesthetic but near cerebral vessels, such as stellate ganglion or cervical plexus blockade. With peripheral nerve blockade, careful use of a test dose and small incremental injections are appropriate if intravascular injection is a risk. Toxicity can also occur owing to slow absorption of high doses. Patients should be observed carefully for 20–30 minutes following injection because peak levels occur at this time.

Peripheral neuropathy usually results from intraneural local anesthetic injection or needle trauma, although there are other causes.[11] Careful attention should be paid to positioning the patient with numb extremities. Postoperative follow-up is important in confirming that neurologic function has returned to normal. If a deficit is detected, early neurologic assessment is critical in determining whether a pre-existing neuropathy was involved. Fortunately, most of these syndromes resolve uneventfully, but full recovery of some peripheral injuries requires several months as a result of slow regeneration of injured peripheral nerves. Sympathetic concern and involvement of the anesthesiologist in arranging physical therapy during recovery help reduce patient dissatisfaction.

Other minor complications such as pain at the site of injection and local hematoma formation are not uncommon but are usually of short duration and respond to reassurance by the anesthesiologist. Hematoma around a peripheral nerve is not of the same significance as that in the epidural or subarachnoid space. Again, expressed concern and help with local therapy and analgesics alleviate patient dissatisfaction.

PATIENT PREPARATION
Patient Selection

In general, all patients scheduled for extremity, thoracic, abdominal, or perineal surgery should be considered candidates for a regional anesthetic technique. This can be used as the only

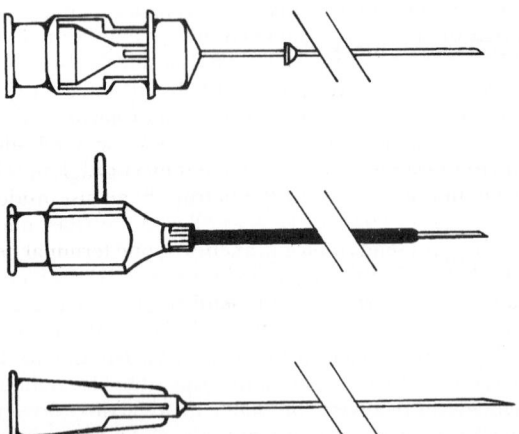

Figure 27-1. Regional anesthesia needles. Characteristic features of needles used for peripheral nerve blockade include the "security bead" on the shaft just below its juncture with the hub (*top*) and the shorter bevel angle compared with standard Quincke-type needle points (*bottom*). Further modifications to enhance the use of a nerve stimulator include the attachment prong for the electrode and the insulated shaft (*middle*).

anesthetic, as a supplement to provide analgesia and muscle relaxation along with general anesthesia, or as the initial step for provision of prolonged postoperative analgesia such as with intercostal blockade or continuous epidural anesthesia. Patient refusal can be an impediment to regional anesthesia, although this is frequently a "relative" refusal. Often, the patient's real objections to "being awake" or "being aware" can be managed by the use of sedatives and amnestic drugs. True, unwavering refusal of "any needles" is a contraindication to regional anesthesia, although gentle attempts at patient education should be offered. Other contraindications include local infection and severe systemic coagulopathy. The presence of pre-existing neurologic disease is often discussed. Some data are available in the case of spinal anesthesia, but the use of peripheral nerve blockade in this situation is unclear. A classic example is whether an arm blockade should be used for a scheduled ulnar nerve transposition at the elbow. Although some physicians avoid any procedure that may confuse the picture of postoperative neuropathy, others believe that if there is a clear difference in the potential injury and the pre-existing disease, regional techniques are appropriate. There are no clear answers in this regard, and full patient education and cooperation are most appropriate. Finally, the level of patient anxiety is an important consideration. Extreme apprehension regarding surgery necessitates heavy sedation, and the advantages of regional anesthesia in providing rapid recovery, alertness, and protection of airway reflexes may be negated. The use of regional anesthesia in these situations is a matter of judgment and experience.

Premedication and Sedation

The best preparation for a regional technique is careful patient education. Calm, gentle explanation of the technique as it is performed reduces most patient anxiety to a manageable level. In most cases, however, supplemental medication is also useful. In addition to the general comments about premedication discussed in earlier chapters, regional anesthesia techniques have some special requirements. First, sedation must be adjusted to the required level of patient cooperation. If paresthesias are to be sought, medication must be light enough to allow the patient to identify and report nerve contact. Although a mild dose of opioid (50–100 μg of fentanyl or equivalent) will help ease the discomfort of nerve localization, patient responsiveness must be maintained. This does not preclude the use of an amnestic agent. Small doses of propofol or midazolam may provide excellent amnesia at levels of consciousness that still allow cooperation. They are also excellent supplements in the outpatient setting, where short duration of effect is desired. If paresthesias are not needed, as in intercostal blockade, heavy sedation may allow greater patient tolerance of the injections. Although intramuscular premedication was common with hospitalized patients, careful titration of iv drugs at the time of the blockade has essentially replaced this practice as the most effective way to adjust the level of sedation to individual patient needs and sensitivities.

Monitoring

Although current discussions of "monitoring" typically include mechanical and electrical devices, repetitive assessment of the patient's mental status when receiving local anesthetics is of paramount importance. The anesthesiologist must maintain frequent verbal contact with these patients and ideally have an uninvolved assistant available to assess the level of consciousness at all times. There are no electrical or mechanical devices that detect rising blood levels of local anesthetic; close observation for peak levels owing to iv (within 2 minutes) and subcutaneous (~20 minutes) absorption is essential. An electrocardiogram is appropriate to detect the pulse rise seen with epinephrine when it is included in a test dose. It is also useful if systemic toxicity

occurs with bupivacaine. Other pulse counters such as mechanical meters and pulse oximeters are also useful when monitoring the pulse rate change with epinephrine. Blood pressure monitoring should be performed, as with use of any anesthetic. A baseline pressure should be obtained whenever any sympathetic blockade is performed and at frequent intervals thereafter. Beyond these specific comments, the standards for monitoring and record keeping on any patient undergoing regional anesthesia are the same as for patients undergoing any general anesthetic.

Discharge Criteria

Concern is occasionally expressed about discharging patients from postanesthesia care units when an extremity is still anesthetized. If regional anesthesia is administered to provide prolonged analgesia, numbness may be expected to persist for 10 (with intercostal anesthesia) to 24 (with sciatic blockade) hours after bupivacaine or ropivacaine administration. Patients with numb extremities have been successfully discharged from the postanesthesia care unit to the floors as long as their mental alertness is adequate. Outpatients may be discharged home with numb arms or legs as long as the patient is reliable and adequate instruction about care of the insensitive extremity is provided.

SPECIFIC TECHNIQUES

The remainder of this chapter is devoted to the details of the performance of specific types of blockade, arranged by sections of the body. No attempt has been made to describe every regional technique practiced, but to focus on those of clinical usefulness to the anesthesiologist. The common methods are described, in recognition that several alternative approaches have been advocated in each case.

Head and Neck

Regional anesthesia of the head and neck has limited surgical application. Concern about control and maintenance of the airway makes many anesthesiologists uncomfortable with regional techniques when intraoperative airway intervention is awkward. Trigeminal nerve blockade and occipital nerve blockade are used for diagnostic or neurolytic blockade for chronic pain syndromes. Cervical plexus blockade is useful for some surgical procedures on the neck, and topical-regional airway anesthesia is effective in reducing the subjective discomfort and hemodynamic responses to tracheal intubation.

Trigeminal Nerve Blockade

Sensory and motor nerve function of the face is provided by the branches of the fifth cranial (trigeminal) nerve. The roots of this nerve arise from the base of the pons and send sensory branches to the large gasserian (or semilunar) ganglion, which lies on the superior margin of the petrous bone just inside the skull above the foramen ovale. A smaller motor fiber nucleus lies behind it and sends motor branches to one terminal nerve, the mandibular. The three major branches of the trigeminal each have a separate exit from the skull (Fig. 27-3). The uppermost ophthalmic branch passes through the sphenoidal fissure into the orbit. The main terminal fibers of this nerve, the frontal nerve, bifurcate into the supratrochlear and supraorbital nerves. These two branches traverse the orbit along the superior border and exit on the front of the face in the easily palpated supraorbital notch for the former and along the medial border of the orbit for the latter.

The two major branches of the trigeminal nerve are the middle (maxillary) and lower (mandibular). The maxillary nerve contains only sensory fibers and exits the skull through the foramen rotundum. It passes beneath the skull anteriorly through the sphenomaxillary fossa. At this point, it lies medial

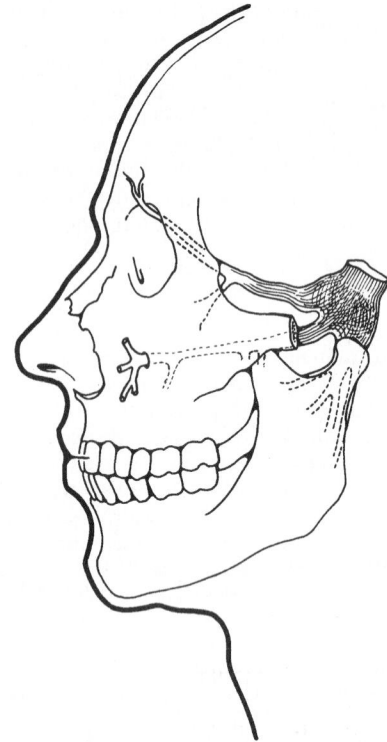

Figure 27-3. Lateral view of major branches of the trigeminal nerve. Each major branch exits the skull by a separate foramen. The ophthalmic branch travels in the orbit. The maxillary and mandibular branches emerge from the skull medial to the lateral pterygoid plate, which serves as the landmark for their identification. (Reproduced with permission from Mulroy M: Handbook of Regional Anesthesia. Boston, Little, Brown, 1996.)

to the lateral pterygoid plate on each side. At the anterior end of this channel, it again moves superiorly to re-enter the skull in the infraorbital canal in the floor of the orbit. In the spheno-maxillary fossa, it branches to form the sphenopalatine nerves and to give off the posterior dental branches. The anterior dental nerves arise from the main trunk as it passes through the infraorbital canal. The terminal infraorbital nerve emerges from the foramen of the same name just below the eye and lateral to the nose and gives off the terminal palpebral, nasal, and labial nerves. The mandibular nerve is the third and largest branch of the trigeminal, and the only one to receive motor fibers. It exits the skull posterior to the maxillary nerve through the foramen ovale. At this point, it is just posterior to the lateral pterygoid plate of the sphenoid bone. The motor nerves separate into an anterior branch immediately below the foramen ovale. The main branch continues as the inferior alveolar nerve medial to the ramus of the mandible. This nerve curves anteriorly to follow the mandible and exits as a terminal branch through the mental foramen. The mental nerve provides sensation to the lower lip and jaw.

Gasserian Ganglion Blockade

Ideally, the simplest blockade of the trigeminal nerve is performed in the central ganglion, which includes all three branches, and it is frequently recommended for treatment of disabling trigeminal neuralgia. This blockade is technically the most difficult and has the most undesirable potential for the complications of subarachnoid injection of anesthetic after neurolytic blockade. Residual numbness of the face is sometimes unpleasant, and a neuritis may be as unpleasant as the original condition. Protective corneal sensation may also be lost, and special care of the eye may be needed. Nevertheless, it is a technique useful in severe cases of trigeminal neuralgia that

are unresponsive to more peripheral blockade. Alcohol injection has been performed in the past, although radiofrequency ablation by neurosurgeons is now more common. The procedure for blockade follows:

1. Three landmarks are needed to help locate the foramen ovale. First, a skin wheal is raised 3 cm lateral to the corner of the mouth on the involved side. A second mark is made on the skin 1 cm anterior to the midpoint of the zygoma (the midpoint lies just above the deepest part of the sigmoid notch of the mandible). The third landmark is the pupil of the eye on the ipsilateral side.
2. A 12.5-cm needle is introduced through the skin wheal on the cheek. The needle is advanced posteriorly in the sagittal plane formed by an imaginary line between the pupil and the point of insertion. As it moves posteriorly, it is angled superiorly toward the third point (anterior to the midpoint of the zygomatic arch). If advanced properly, the needle will pass through the muscles of the cheek without entering the oral cavity and will contact the base of the skull medial to the mandible and the zygoma. If it has remained in the plane of the pupil, it will be near the foramen ovale.
3. Once bone is contacted, the needle is withdrawn and reinserted to angle slightly more posteriorly until the foramen is entered. At this point, paresthesias of the maxillary branch are sought. The needle should not be advanced more than 1 cm beyond the opening of the foramen. If there is any question about localization, biplanar fluoroscopy is useful in confirming position.
4. After localization of the nerve, careful aspiration is performed to detect unwanted subarachnoid placement of the needle. Two ml of 1% lidocaine injected slowly usually produces anesthesia of all three sensory branches. If alcohol is used, the anesthesia is preceded by a severe burning sensation; this can be reduced by prior injection of a few drops of local anesthetic.

Superficial Trigeminal Nerve Branch Blockade

Fortunately, most anesthetic applications of trigeminal blockade can be more easily performed by injection of the individual terminal superficial branches. This is relatively simple because the three superficial branches and their associated foramina all lie in the same sagittal plane on each side of the face (Fig. 27-4). Each of these foramina are readily palpable, and these nerves can be easily blocked with superficial injections of small quantities of local anesthetic. Although the bony landmarks are usually sufficient themselves, paresthesias are desirable before alcohol injection. Each of these blocks can be performed with the patient in the supine position. The procedure for blockade follows:

1. The supraorbital notch is easily palpated along the medial superior rim of the orbit, usually 2.5 cm from the midline. Two to three ml of local anesthetic injected immediately in the vicinity of the notch produces anesthesia of the ipsilateral forehead. Anesthesia of the supratrochlear nerve by superficial infiltration of the medial aspect of the orbital rim is needed if the band of anesthesia is to cross the midline.
2. The infraorbital foramen lies below the inferior orbital rim in the same plane at approximately the same distance from the midline as the supraorbital notch (usually 2.5 cm). If the foramen cannot be palpated directly, it can be sought by gently probing with a small-gauge needle. This needle should be introduced through a skin wheal approximately 0.5 cm below the expected opening, because the canal angles cephalad from this point toward the orbital floor. Again, injection of a small quantity of local anesthetic immediately in the vicinity of the foramen produces anesthesia of the middle third of the ipsilateral face.

cephalad and slightly anterior. This direction should be toward the imagined posterior border of the globe of the eye.
3. The needle should contact the pterygoid plate. It is then withdrawn and redirected slightly anterior until it succeeds in passing beyond the pterygoid plate. At this point, the nerve should lie approximately 1 cm deeper. A paresthesia in the nose or the upper teeth confirms the nerve localization.
4. Anesthesia can be achieved by injecting 5 ml into the fossa, either on obtaining the paresthesia or blindly by advancing 1 cm beyond the plate.

The major complication of concern is spread of the anesthetic to adjacent structures, especially to the nerves in the orbit.

Mandibular Nerve Blockade

This nerve can also be blocked for inferior dental pain. It is the only branch where anesthesia carries the risk of loss of motor (mastication) function (Fig. 27-6). The procedure for blockade follows:

1. Head position and landmarks are the same as those described for the maxillary nerve blockade.
2. A 2-inch needle is introduced through the skin wheal and directed medially but slightly posterior and without the cephalad angulation required for maxillary nerve anesthesia. This leaves the needle approximately perpendicular to the skin in all planes.
3. When the pterygoid plate is contacted, the needle is redirected posteriorly until it passes beyond the plate. It should contact the nerve 0.5–1 cm deep to this point.
4. Paresthesia of the jaw or cheek confirms identification of the nerve. Five to ten ml of solution injected incrementally at this point should produce anesthesia of the terminal branches. If paresthesias are essential, exploration should be carried gently cephalad and caudad from the initial point where the needle passes posterior to the plate. As with maxillary blockade, paresthesias can be painful to the patient, and the use of an assistant to secure the head is occasionally necessary.

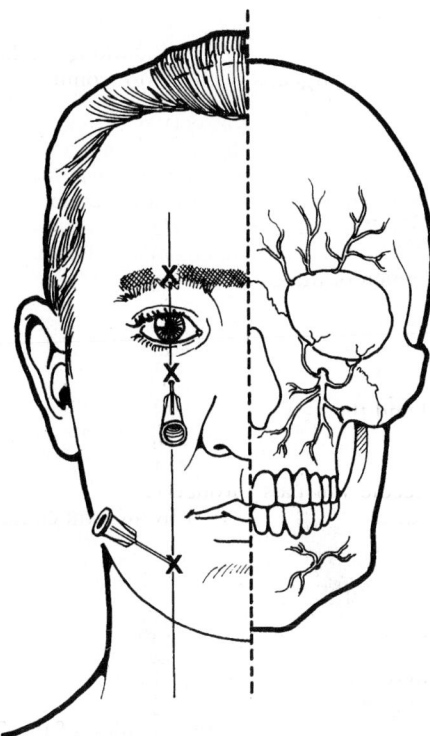

Figure 27-4. Terminal branches of the trigeminal nerve. Each of the three terminal branches (the supraorbital, infraorbital, and mental) exits its respective bony canal in the same sagittal plane, approximately 2.5 cm from the midline. The infraorbital canal is angled slightly cephalad, while the mental canal can be entered if the needle is directed medially and slightly caudad. (Reproduced with permission from Mulroy M: Handbook of Regional Anesthesia. Boston, Little, Brown, 1996.)

3. The mental nerve also emerges approximately 2.5 cm from the midline, usually midway between the upper and lower borders of the mandible. The mental canal angles medially and inferiorly so that, in this case, needle insertion should start approximately 0.5 cm above and 0.5 cm lateral to the anticipated location of the orifice if it cannot be palpated directly. In older patients, resorption of the superior margin of the mandibular bone will make the foramen appear to lie more superiorly along the ramus. Again, 2 ml of local anesthesia injected into the canal produces anesthesia of the mandibular area.

Maxillary Nerve Blockade

If anesthesia in superior dental nerves is also required or if superficial infraorbital nerve blockade does not produce adequate anesthesia, proximal block of the maxillary nerve is required. This can be performed by a lateral approach to the sphenopalatine fossa (Fig. 27-5). The procedure for blockade follows:

1. The patient lies supine with a small towel under the occiput and the head turned slightly away from the side to be blocked. The zygomatic arch is marked along its course, and the patient is asked to open and close the mouth slowly so that the curved upper border of the mandible can be identified. The lowest point of the mandibular notch is palpated, and an "X" is marked at this spot, which is usually at the midpoint of the zygoma. A skin wheal is raised at the "X" after the appropriate skin preparations.
2. With the patient's jaw in the open position, a 7.5-cm needle is introduced through the "X" and directed 45 degrees

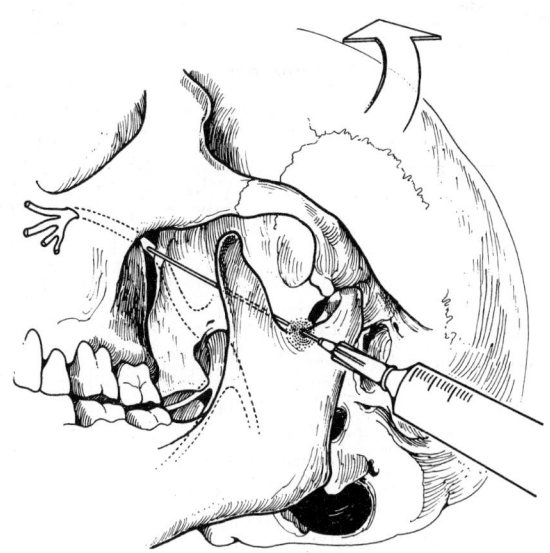

Figure 27-5. Lateral approach to the maxillary nerve. The needle is introduced through the skin just over the notch of the mandible and directed anteriorly and cephalad to identify the pterygoid plate. As the needle is advanced anteriorly off the plate, the maxillary nerve is encountered before it re-enters the skull in the infraorbital canal in the base of the orbit. (Reproduced with permission from Mulroy M: Handbook of Regional Anesthesia. Boston, Little, Brown, 1996.)

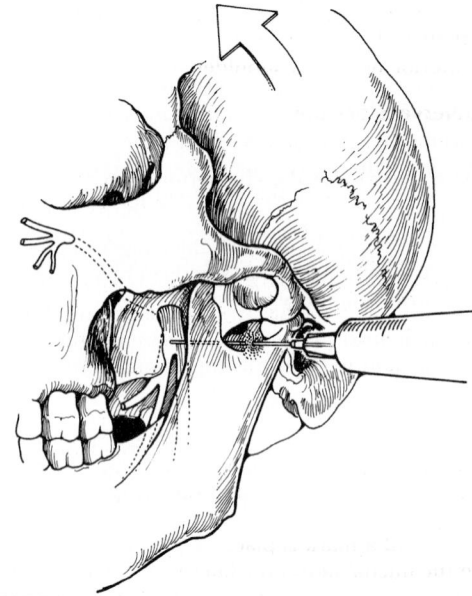

Figure 27-6. Lateral approach to the mandibular nerve. The needle is introduced in the same manner as for the maxillary nerve block, but directed posteriorly. After contacting the pterygoid plate, it is directed farther posteriorly until it passes behind the plate, where it should encounter the nerve. (Reproduced with permission from Mulroy M: Handbook of Regional Anesthesia. Boston, Little, Brown, 1996.)

Facial nerve anesthesia can occasionally be seen when large volumes are injected to block the mandibular nerve. This is of little consequence unless neurolytic agents are used. A more serious complication is the possibility of intravascular injection in this highly vascularized area. Injection should be performed incrementally with small quantities and constant observation for signs of central toxicity.

Cervical Plexus Blockade

Sensory and motor fibers of the neck and posterior scalp arise from the nerve roots of the second, third, and fourth cervical nerves. This cervical plexus is unique in that the sensory fibers separate from the motor fibers early in their course and can be blocked separately. Classic plexus anesthesia along the tubercles of the vertebral body produces both motor and sensory blockade. The transverse processes of the cervical vertebrae form peculiar elongated troughs for the emergence of their nerve roots. These troughs lie immediately lateral to a medial opening for the cephalad passage of the vertebral artery. The trough at the terminal end of the transverse process divides into an anterior and a posterior tubercle, which can often be easily palpated. These tubercles also serve as the attachments for the anterior and middle scalene muscles, which thus form a compartment for the cervical plexus as well as for the brachial plexus immediately below. The compartment at this level is less developed than the one formed around the brachial plexus. The motor branches (including the phrenic nerve) curl anteriorly around the lateral border of the anterior scalene and proceed caudad and medially toward the muscles of the neck. They give anterior branches to the sternocleidomastoid muscle as they pass behind it. The sensory fibers, as mentioned, also emerge behind the anterior scalene muscle but separate from the motor branches and continue laterally to emerge superficially under the posterior border of the sternocleidomastoid muscle. They provide sensory anesthesia to the anterior and posterior skin of the neck and shoulder.

Anesthesia of either the superficial cervical nerves or the cervical plexus itself can be used for operations on the lateral or anterior neck. Thyroidectomy and carotid endarterectomy

fall into this category, although supplemental local infiltration of the thyroid gland may occasionally be necessary because of sensory innervation from cranial nerves. In carotid surgery, local infiltration of the carotid bifurcation may be necessary to block reflex hemodynamic changes associated with glossopharyngeal stimulation. Cervical plexus anesthesia alone is rarely adequate for shoulder surgery. It is preferable to perform interscalene anesthesia of the brachial plexus for these procedures because the likelihood of adequate motor relaxation is greater and the cervical plexus is blocked coincidentally. The procedure for deep cervical plexus blockade follows:

1. The patient is placed supine with a small towel under the head, with the head turned slightly to the side opposite the one to be blocked.
2. The mastoid process is identified and marked. The transverse processes can often be palpated. If not, the most prominent tubercle, that of C6, is marked, and a line is drawn between it and the mastoid process (Fig. 27-7).
3. The cervical processes should be felt approximately 0.5 cm posterior to the line drawn between the mastoid and the sixth cervical tubercle. The second vertebral process should lie approximately 1.5 cm below the mastoid itself. (There is no process for the first vertebra.)
4. The third and fourth processes lie approximately 1.5 cm below their respective superior neighbors.
5. Skin wheals are raised at the three "X" marks that have been placed over the transverse processes.
6. A 3.75-cm needle is introduced perpendicular to the skin and directed posterior and slightly caudad at each "X" until it rests on the transverse process. It is important to maintain a caudad direction to avoid entry directly into the intervertebral foramina. The needle is walked caudad. It should slip off the bone if it is truly on the process rather than continuing to contact bone if it is on the vertebral body. It is important to contact the transverse process as far laterally as possible to avoid any contact of the needle with the vertebral artery (Fig. 27-8).
7. Paresthesias are usually not necessary. A syringe is connected to the needle, and 5 ml of local anesthetic solution is deposited along the transverse process. Anesthesia in the distribution of the nerve should follow within 5 minutes.

The major potential complication of this procedure is intravascular injection into the vertebral artery. Again, injection should be made in small increments, with frequent observation of the patient's mental status and frequent aspiration to detect intravascular placement. If the needle is advanced too far medially into the vertebral foramen, epidural or even subarachnoid anesthesia may be produced. This is more likely in the cervical region because of longer sleeves of dura that accompany these nerve branches. Again, frequent aspiration and careful lateral placement of the needle are important.

Phrenic nerve blockade occurs with deep cervical plexus anes-

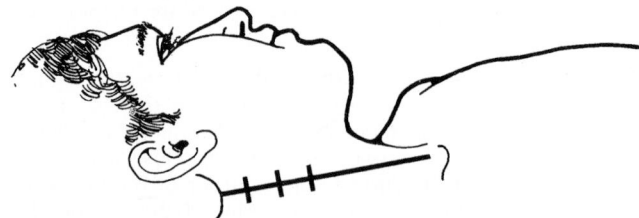

Figure 27-7. Superficial landmarks for cervical plexus blockade. A line is drawn from the mastoid process to the prominent tubercle of C6. The transverse processes of C2, C3, and C4 lie 0.5 cm posterior to this line and at 1.5-cm intervals below the mastoid. (Reproduced with permission from Mulroy M: Handbook of Regional Anesthesia. Boston, Little, Brown, 1996.)

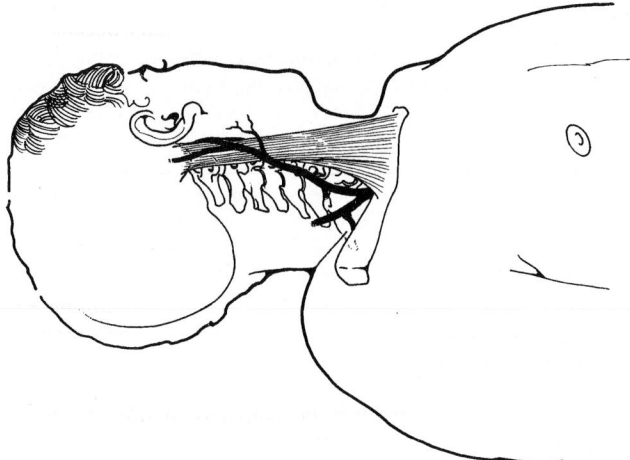

Figure 27-8. Anatomy of deep cervical plexus blockade. The transverse processes lie under the lateral border of the sternocleidomastoid muscle, each with a distal trough or sulcus that defines the path of nerve exit. (Reproduced with permission from Mulroy M: Handbook of Regional Anesthesia. Boston, Little, Brown, 1996.)

thesia. This blockade is not indicated in any patient who depends on the diaphragm for tidal ventilation, nor is bilateral blockade desirable in most patients. Recurrent laryngeal nerve or vagal blockade can also occur because of diffusion of the local anesthetic. This is a troublesome but not serious complication. It may interfere with the ability to evaluate vocal cord function following thyroid surgery.

Superficial Cervical Plexus Blockade. This is performed in the same position as deep cervical plexus blockade and results in anesthesia only of the sensory fibers of the plexus. The procedure for blockade follows:

1. An "X" is made along the posterior border of the sternocleidomastoid muscle at the level of C4. This usually corresponds with the junction of the external jugular vein as it crosses the posterior border of the muscle (Fig. 27-9).
2. A skin wheal is raised at this mark, and superficial local anesthetic infiltration is performed along the posterior border of the sternocleidomastoid muscle 4 cm above and

below the level of the "X." Ten to twelve ml of local anesthetic solution usually provides sensory anesthesia of the anterior neck and shoulder.

Occipital Nerve Blockade

The ophthalmic branch of the trigeminal nerve provides sensory innervation of the forehead and anterior scalp, but the remainder of the scalp is innervated by fibers of the greater and lesser occipital nerves, terminal branches of the cervical plexus. These nerves can be blocked by superficial injection at the point on the posterior skull where they emerge from below the muscles of the neck (Fig. 27-10). Anesthesia is rarely used for surgical procedures; it is more often applied as a diagnostic step in evaluating head and neck pain complaints. The procedure for blockade follows:

1. The block is performed in the sitting position, with the patient leaning the head forward to expose the prominent nuchal ridge of bone at the posterior base of the skull.
2. The external occipital protuberance is identified in the midline, and a mark is placed lateral to this prominence along the nuchal line at the lateral border of the insertion of the erector muscles of the neck, usually 2.5 cm from the midline. The branches of the greater occipital nerve usually pass laterally from behind the muscle to cross the nuchal line at this point.
3. After skin preparation, a small needle is introduced through the mark to the depth of the skull itself. A ridge of 1–4 ml of local anesthetic (1% lidocaine or equivalent) is then deposited across the path of the emerging nerves just above the level of the bone. Paresthesias are occasionally encountered but are not essential for obtaining simple skin anesthesia.
4. If more anterior anesthesia of the scalp is required, the lesser occipital nerve branches are also blocked by advancing the needle subcutaneously from this point in an anterior direction toward the mastoid process. A band of anesthetic solution is deposited along the line between the skin entry and the mastoid. A larger volume (6–8 ml) is required.

Complications of this technique are rare. Care must be taken not to advance the needle anteriorly under the skull, as the foramen magnum might be entered unintentionally with a long

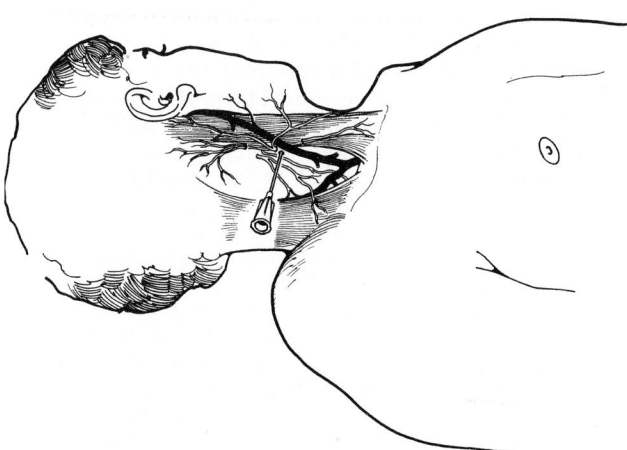

Figure 27-9. Superficial cervical plexus blockade. The sensory fibers of the plexus all emerge from behind the lateral border of the sternocleidomastoid muscle. A needle inserted at its midpoint, usually where the external jugular vein crosses the muscle, can be directed superiorly and inferiorly to block all these terminal branches. (Reproduced with permission from Mulroy M: Handbook of Regional Anesthesia. Boston, Little, Brown, 1996.)

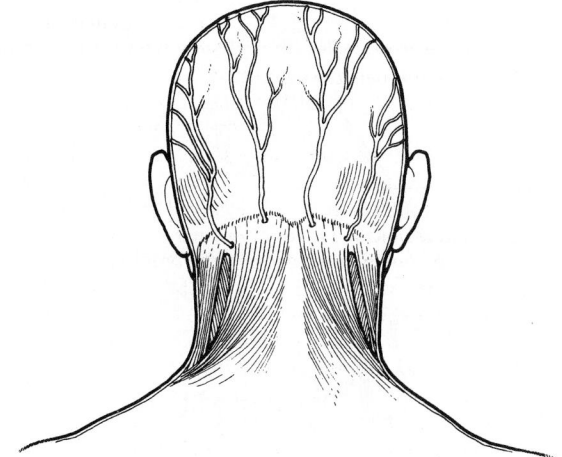

Figure 27-10. Occipital nerve blockade. The greater and lesser branches of the occipital nerve emerge from under the muscles at the level of the nuchal ridge on the posterior scalp. They can be easily blocked by a subcutaneous ridge of anesthetic solution. (Reproduced with permission from Mulroy M: Handbook of Regional Anesthesia. Boston, Little, Brown, 1996.)

needle. Local hematoma may be produced with the superficial injection, but this is only a temporary problem.

Airway Anesthesia

Manipulation of the airway either during laryngoscopy or during tracheal intubation is often associated with laryngospasm, coughing, and undesirable cardiovascular reflexes (see also Chapter 23). The anesthesiologist can abolish or blunt these reflexes by anesthetizing one or all of the sensory pathways involved. The nasal mucosa is innervated by fibers of the sphenopalatine ganglion, a branch of the middle division of the fifth cranial nerve. These branches lie on the lateral wall of the nasal passages on each side, under the mucosa just posterior to the middle turbinate (Fig. 27-11). The branches of these fibers continue caudad to provide sensory innervation to the superior portion of the pharynx, uvula, and tonsils. Anesthesia of the maxillary branch of the trigeminal nerve is possible but not a practical solution for airway anesthesia. Transmucosal topical application of local anesthetic is more appropriate. Below the sphenopalatine fiber distribution, sensory innervation of the oral pharynx and supraglottic regions is provided by branches of the glossopharyngeal nerve. These nerves lie laterally on each side of the pharynx submucosally in the region of the posterior tonsillar pillar. Direct submucosal injection can be performed but carries the risk of unintentional intravascular injection into several blood vessels in this area. Topical anesthesia of the terminal branches in the mouth and throat is again an easier approach, but deep injection of the glossopharyngeal nerve may be required to block the gag reflex completely. The larynx itself is innervated by the superior laryngeal branch of the vagus nerve in the area above the vocal cords. This branch leaves the main vagal trunk in the carotid sheath and passes anteriorly. Its internal branch penetrates the thyrohyoid membrane and divides to provide the sensory fibers to the cords, epiglottis, and arytenoids.

The recurrent laryngeal nerve provides innervation to the areas below the vocal cords, including motor innervation for all but one of the intrinsic laryngeal muscles. The trachea itself is also innervated by the recurrent laryngeal nerve. Topical anesthesia is again the simplest approach to this nerve.

Airway anesthesia can be performed by anesthetizing one or all of these sensory distributions. Full anesthesia facilitates procedures such as nasal intubation or fiberoptic laryngoscopy.

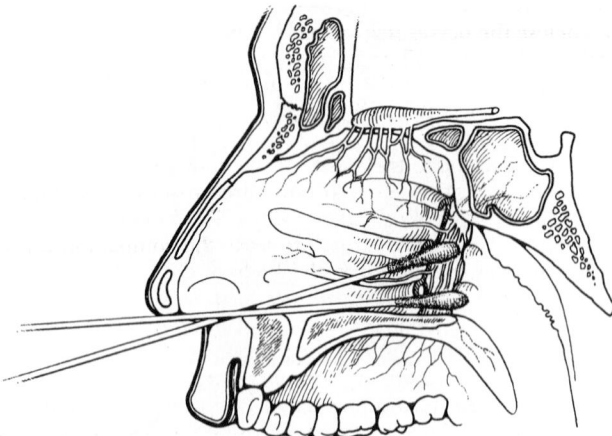

Figure 27-11. Nasal airway anesthesia. Cotton pledgets soaked with anesthetic are inserted along the inferior and middle turbinates to produce anesthesia of the underlying sphenopalatine ganglion by transmembrane diffusion of the solution. Wide pledgets also are needed to provide maximal topical anesthesia and vasoconstriction of the nasal mucosa. (Reproduced with permission from Mulroy M: Handbook of Regional Anesthesia. Boston, Little, Brown, 1996.)

Airway anesthesia below the vocal cords is best avoided if there is concern about potential aspiration, as this may blunt the reflex cough reaction to the presence of foreign bodies in the trachea. Topical postpharyngeal anesthesia may also ablate protective laryngeal reflexes.

In the performance of airway anesthesia, the patient can be anesthetized in the supine position, although many patients find it more comfortable to be semiupright or sitting when topical anesthesia is sprayed into the posterior pharynx. These positions allow them greater ease in swallowing excess solutions and may reduce gagging. In whatever position chosen, there should be a firm support behind the head to reduce involuntary withdrawal motions by the patient, which might dislocate needles being used for injections.

1. For nasal mucosal anesthesia, cotton pledgets soaked with anesthetic solution are introduced through the nares and passed along the turbinates all the way to the posterior end of the nasal passage (see Fig. 27-11). A second set of pledgets is introduced with a cephalad angulation to follow the middle turbinate back to the mucosa overlying the sphenoid bone. This pledget is the more critical one because anesthesia in this mucosal area is most likely to anesthetize the branches of the sphenopalatine ganglia as they pass along the lateral wall of the airway. Bilateral anesthesia is preferable, even if a nasal tube is to be inserted only on one side; bilateral blockade of the sphenopalatine fibers also produces posterior pharyngeal anesthesia caudad to this level. The pledgets should be allowed to remain in contact with the nasal mucosa for at least 2–3 minutes to allow adequate diffusion of local anesthetic.

   Cocaine in a 4% solution has been the traditional topical anesthetic for this application because of its unique vasoconstrictive properties. Cocaine produces shrinkage of the mucosa and reduces the chance of bleeding. Because of the toxicity of cocaine and a significant abuse problem in the United States, alternate solutions have been recommended, primarily a mixture of 3–4% lidocaine and 0.25–0.5% phenylephrine.

2. Topical anesthesia to the posterior pharynx can be performed while the nasal applicators are in place. This can be done with a commercial spray or with an atomizer filled with a 4% solution of lidocaine. (A higher concentration of local anesthetic is required to penetrate mucosal membranes.) For effective anesthesia in the posterior pharyngeal wall, topical application is performed in two stages. First, the tongue itself is sprayed with a local anesthetic, and the patient is encouraged to gargle and swallow the residual liquid in the mouth. The numb tongue is then grasped with a gauze pad with one hand while the spray device is inserted into the mouth with the other. The patient is then encouraged to take rapid deep breaths ("pant like a puppy") while the spray is applied on inspiration. The inspiratory flow of gases should be enough to draw the lidocaine solution into the posterior pharynx and even to the vocal cords themselves. If superior laryngeal nerve blockade has been performed before this, it is likely that the aerosol will be carried into the trachea itself. Again, a few minutes are needed for adequate onset of topical anesthesia in the pharynx. Topical anesthesia is less effective if there are copious secretions. Premedication with an anticholinergic is frequently beneficial.

3. Superior laryngeal nerve blockade can also be performed while the nasal pledgets are in place (Fig. 27-12). This nerve is blocked bilaterally by identifying the superior ala of the thyroid cartilage, which usually lies just inferior to the posterior portion of the hyoid bone on each side. A 5-ml syringe with a 1% lidocaine solution with a 23-gauge, 1.75-cm needle is used. The index finger of one hand

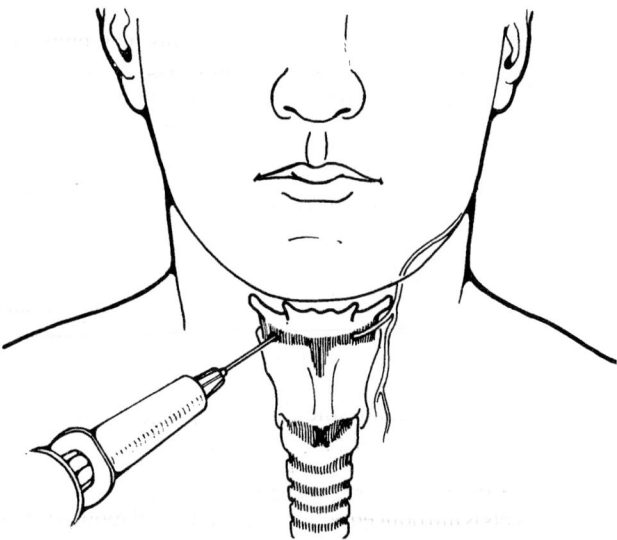

Figure 27-12. Superior laryngeal nerve blockade. The needle is advanced superiorly off the lateral wing of the thyroid cartilage to drop through the thyrohyoid membrane. (Reproduced with permission from Mulroy M: Handbook of Regional Anesthesia. Boston, Little, Brown, 1996.)

larynx, and posterior pharynx, without the need for either steps 2 or 3.

6. After each of these steps has been completed, the pledgets can be removed from the nasal passages and nasal intubation performed. If tracheal or laryngeal anesthesia has been omitted because of concern about aspiration, there should be some pharmacologic intervention to reduce the cardiovascular response to the passage of the tube into the trachea. This can be facilitated by pretreatment with iv β-adrenergic blocking drugs, by administration of sedation, or by administration of rapid-acting thiobarbiturates immediately after the airway is secured.

Complications of these techniques are rare. Systemic toxicity from the local anesthetics is a distinct possibility because of the large quantities of drug required to produce sufficient mucosal anesthesia. If all four stages of airway anesthesia are undertaken, the total milligram doses applied usually exceed the maximal recommended dose for peripheral injection. Fortunately, the mucosal absorption is less than the peripheral absorption, but close attention to the patient's mental status and preparation for treatment of toxicity are necessary. Aspiration of gastric contents is also a possibility when the protective reflexes of the airway are interrupted. Precautions should be taken in the form of the usual prophylaxis to reduce stomach acidity as well as provision for suction and adequate oxygenation if emesis or regurgitation occurs.

retracts the skin of the neck caudad down over the thyroid cartilage; the needle is inserted until it rests on the superior margin of the cartilage. The tension on the skin is then released and the needle is withdrawn slightly and allowed to walk superiorly off the cartilage. The needle is then reinserted and passed through the thyrohyoid membrane, which is perceived as a discernible resistance. After careful aspiration, 2.5 ml of solution is injected into the space below the membrane. This procedure is repeated on the opposite side. This blockade can be performed as part of total airway anesthesia or it can be used independently to provide increased acceptance of indwelling endotracheal tubes in the intensive care unit.

4. The glossopharyngeal nerve can be blocked by a direct injection into the base of the anterior tonsillar pillar if persistent gagging is a problem. The tongue is retracted medially with a gloved finger or a tongue blade to expose the base of the anterior pillar. A long 25-gauge (spinal) needle is inserted 0.5 cm subcutaneously into the base of the pillar 0.5 cm lateral to the base of the tongue. After careful aspiration, 2 ml of 1.5% lidocaine is injected, and the procedure is repeated on the opposite side. This produces anesthesia of the lingual branch (base of the tongue), and may even anesthetize the pharyngeal and tonsillar branches by diffusion. This allows laryngoscopy with less gagging and hemodynamic response.

5. Tracheal anesthesia can be performed by a direct transcricoid ("transtracheal") injection. This is accomplished by raising a small skin wheal over the cricothyroid membrane. A 20-gauge iv catheter is then inserted gently through this skin wheal and through the membrane. Entry into the trachea can be confirmed by the ability to aspirate air through the catheter. The steel stylet is then removed, and the plastic catheter is left in the trachea. A syringe with 4 ml of 4% lidocaine is attached to the catheter, and the local anesthetic is sprayed into the trachea during inspiration. The flow of air usually carries the local anesthetic distally; the resultant cough continues to spread the anesthetic more proximally up to the underside of the vocal cords and the larynx. Not uncommonly, if the local anesthetic is injected while the patient forcibly exhales, it is possible to obtain adequate anesthesia of the trachea,

Upper Extremity

The innervation of the upper extremity is conveniently derived from five closely approximated nerve roots, extending from C5 to T1 (the brachial plexus). These roots undergo a series of mergers and divisions that produce the terminal nerves of the arm and hand. The plexus branches are close enough to each other to allow reliable anesthesia to be achieved at several points associated with consistent bony or vascular landmarks.

In their proximal course, the nerve roots lie in a well demarcated fascial envelope formed by the anterior fascia of the middle scalene muscle and the posterior fascia of the anterior scalene. These muscles attach to the posterior and anterior tubercles of the transverse processes of the cervical vertebrae from which the nerves emerge. The tubercle can be used as a faithful landmark to guide localization of the nerve, and the fascial planes serve to keep anesthetic solution injected between them close to the nerve bundle. The fascia extends outward for a variable distance from the lateral border of the muscles to enclose the nerves in a "sheath," which can extend into the axilla. This enclosed bundle passes over the first rib just behind the midpoint of the clavicle (and just posterior to the insertion of the anterior scalene on the rib), where it is joined by the subclavian artery, which rises from the mediastinum to cross the rib and pass into the axilla. At the midpoint of the rib, the plexus has consolidated into only three trunks; these rapidly subdivide into the terminal branches. The musculocutaneous nerve is the first major branch to leave the companionship of its partners as it passes into the body of the coracobrachialis muscle high in the axilla. As the individual nerves form, separate compartments in the sheath are formed by developing septa, and reliable blockade of all the nerves with a single injection is not practical distal to the axilla.

Although many techniques of approach to the brachial plexus have been described, there are basically three anatomic locations where anesthetics are placed: (1) the interscalene groove near the transverse processes, (2) the subclavian sheath at the first rib, and (3) surrounding the axillary artery in the axilla. Because of the specific configuration of the nerves at each of these levels, the anesthesia produced is significantly different with each approach and applicable to different situations.[12] Interscalene injection at the level of the sixth cervical transverse process produces extension of the blockade to the lower fibers of the cervical plexus and therefore is ideally suited for shoulder operations and upper arm procedures. It frequently spares the lowest branches of the plexus, the C8 and T1 fibers, which innervate the caudad (ulnar) border of the forearm. Blockade at the level of the first rib is most reliable in producing anesthesia of all four terminal nerves of the forearm and hand. The axillary technique is simpler but carries the risk of missing the musculocutaneous and medial antebrachial cutaneous nerves that depart the sheath high in the axilla, and thus might produce inadequate anesthesia of the forearm. The choice of the appropriate approach depends not only on the patient's anatomy but also on the site of surgery.

The terminal branches can also be anesthetized by local anesthetic injection along their peripheral courses as they cross the joint spaces, or by the injection of a dilute local anesthetic solution intravenously below a pneumatic tourniquet on the upper arm ("intravenous regional", or Bier block).

Brachial Plexus Blockade: Interscalene Approach

This technique was first popularized by Winnie,[13] who stressed the advantages of the fascial sheath provided by the "envelope" of muscles that surround the origins of the brachial plexus in the neck. Localization of the nerves uses a combination of the muscular and bony landmarks surrounding the nerves.

1. The patient is positioned supine with the head turned to the side opposite that to be blocked. A small towel is placed under the occiput. The arm on the side to be blocked is held at the side, and the patient is asked to hold the shoulder down by pretending to reach for the hip or knee.

2. The lateral border of the sternocleidomastoid muscle is identified and marked, and the patient is then asked to raise the head slightly into a "sniffing" position. This tenses the scalene muscle behind the sternocleidomastoid muscle, and the groove between the anterior and middle scalene is palpated by rolling the fingers posteriorly off the lateral border of the sternocleidomastoid muscle. This groove is marked along its entire extent, as high up as possible. The patient then relaxes the muscles of the neck, and the level of the cricoid cartilage is marked. The index finger then gently palpates in the groove at the level of the cricoid (Fig. 27-13). The prominent transverse process of C6 can often be felt directly.

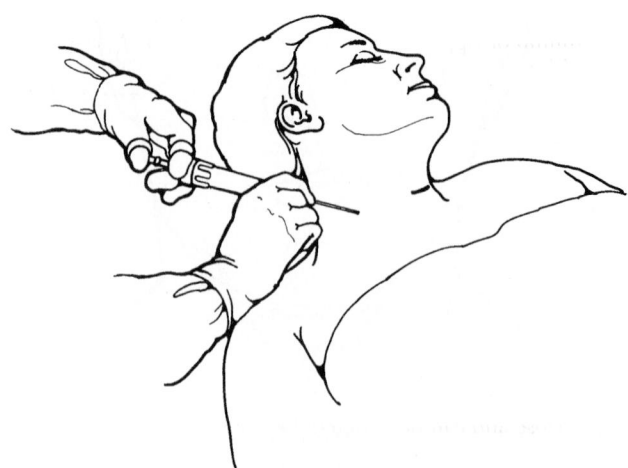

Figure 27-14. Hand position for interscalene blockade. The needle is directed medially and caudad into the interscalene groove while one hand exerts constant control of the depth by resting on the clavicle. (Reproduced with permission from Mulroy M: Handbook of Regional Anesthesia. Boston, Little, Brown, 1996.)

3. After aseptic skin preparation, a skin wheal is raised in the groove at the level of the cricoid. A 22-gauge, 3.75-cm needle is introduced through the wheal perpendicular to the skin in all planes so that it is directed medially, caudad, and slightly posteriorly. Resting one hand on the clavicle allows better control of the syringe (Fig. 27-14).

4. The needle is advanced until the tubercle is contacted or a paresthesia is elicited (or a motor twitch is obtained with a nerve stimulator; Fig. 27-15). If bone is contacted before nerve, the needle is withdrawn and redirected in small steps in an anteroposterior plane until the nerves are identified.

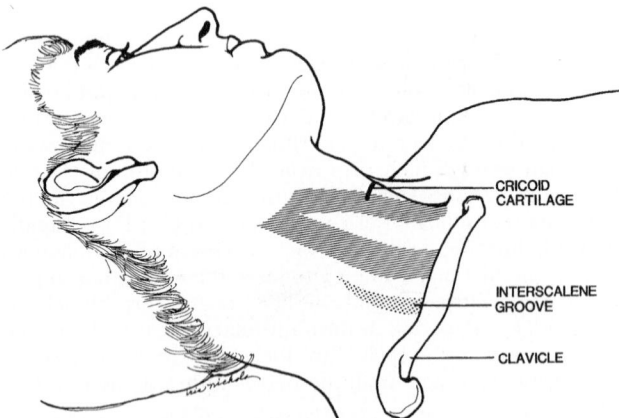

Figure 27-13. Superficial landmarks for interscalene brachial plexus blockade. The sternocleidomastoid muscle is identified, and the anterior scalene muscle is found by moving the fingertips over the lateral border of the larger muscle while it is slightly tensed. The groove between the anterior and middle scalene muscles can usually be felt easily, along with the tubercle of the 6th cervical vertebra, which lies at the level of the cricoid cartilage. (Reproduced with permission from Mulroy M: Handbook of Regional Anesthesia. Boston, Little, Brown, 1996.)

CRICOID CARTILAGE

INTERSCALENE GROOVE

CLAVICLE

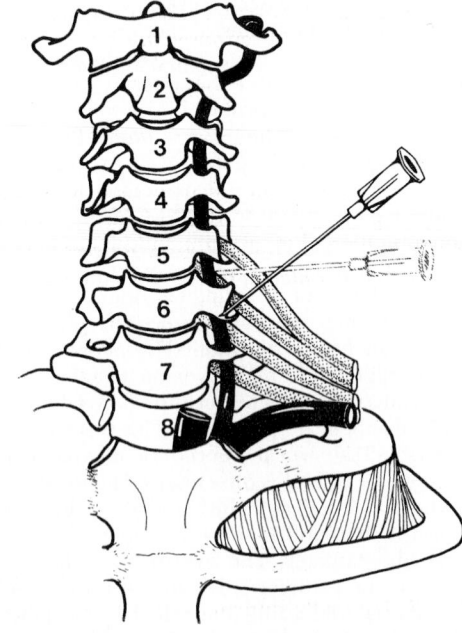

Figure 27-15. Needle direction for interscalene blockade. The needle is always kept in a caudad direction; medial insertion allows the point to pass into the intervertebral foramen and produces epidural, spinal, or intra-arterial injection of anesthetic. Note the relation of the vertebral artery and the nerve roots to the transverse processes. (Reproduced with permission from Mulroy M: Handbook of Regional Anesthesia. Boston, Little, Brown, 1996.)

5. Once the nerve is located (usually a paresthesia to the thumb or upper arm), the needle is fixed in this position with one hand while 25–30 ml of local anesthetic solution is injected. Careful aspiration is performed first, and the initial injection is performed in small increments to detect intraneural or intra-arterial placement of the needle. A larger volume (30–40 ml) is required if greater spread is desired, such as to the cervical plexus or inferiorly to the C8 to T1 fibers.

6. If arm surgery requiring a tourniquet is planned, a subcutaneous ring of anesthetic across the axilla is usually required to block the superficial intercostobrachial fibers crossing from the chest wall into the axilla.

Complications from this approach are related to the structures located in the vicinity of the tubercle. The cupola of the lung is close and can be contacted if the needle is directed too far inferior. Pneumothorax should be considered if cough or chest pain is produced while exploring for the nerve. If the needle is allowed to pass directly medially, it may enter the intervertebral foramina, and injection of local anesthetic may produce spinal or epidural anesthesia. The vertebral artery passes posteriorly at the level of the sixth vertebra to lie in its canal in the transverse process; direct injection into this vessel can rapidly produce central nervous system toxicity and convulsions. Careful aspiration and incremental injections are helpful in avoiding both of these potential problems.

Even with appropriate injection, the local anesthetic solution spread to contiguous nerves. This produces cervical plexus blockade with high volumes, which may be desirable if shoulder surgery is contemplated. The involvement of the motor fibers of the cervical roots also produces diaphragmatic paralysis,[14] which may be a problem in patients with respiratory insufficiency. A Horner's syndrome is common because of spread to the sympathetic chain on the anterior vertebral body.

Neuropathy of the C6 root is a potential problem because the needle may unintentionally pin the nerve root against the tubercle and predispose to intraneural injection. The needle should be withdrawn slightly if the first injection produces the characteristic "crampy" pain sensation.

Inadequate anesthesia is most likely to occur in the ulnar distribution. As mentioned previously, this can be reduced by the use of higher volumes. Supplemental local anesthesia of the ulnar nerve may also be helpful.

Brachial Plexus Blockade: Supraclavicular Approach

The description of the approach to the brachial plexus at this level is originally attributed to Kulenkampff, but the classic technique is based on the modifications recommended by Moore[15] and Winnie and Collins.[16] Current techniques avoid the originally described medial direction of the needle, which may contact the pleura.

1. The patient lies in the same position as for interscalene blockade, with the ipsilateral arm held at the side and pulled downward to exaggerate the landmarks of the clavicle and the neck muscles.

2. The outline of the clavicle is drawn on the skin, as well as the interscalene groove (as described previously). The midpoint of the clavicle is marked. An "X" is placed posterior to this midpoint in the interscalene groove, usually 1 cm behind the clavicle. The groove ideally extends all the way to the first rib, where the muscles insert, but palpation of the rib is usually difficult. On the thin patient, the pulsation of the subclavian artery can be appreciated in the groove or just anterior to it.

3. After aseptic preparation, a skin wheal is raised at the mark, and a 3.75-cm, 22-gauge needle attached to a 10-ml syringe is introduced in the sagittal plane and advanced caudad until the first rib is contacted (Figs. 27-16 to 27-18). It is important that the direction of the needle remain

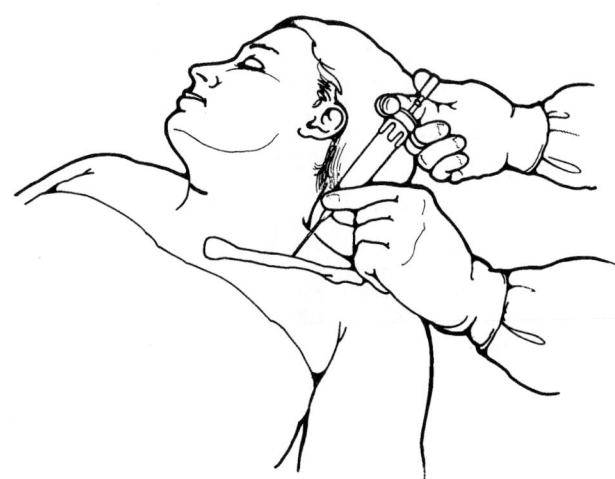

Figure 27-16. Hand position for supraclavicular blockade. The needle is directed caudad behind the midpoint of the clavicle in the interscalene groove. Again, control of depth is maintained by the hand resting on the clavicle. The syringe is kept in the sagittal plane parallel to the patient's head to prevent medial angulation, which would increase the chance of pneumothorax. (Reproduced with permission from Mulroy M: Handbook of Regional Anesthesia. Boston, Little, Brown, 1996.)

perpendicular to the rib, which usually requires that the syringe remain parallel to the axis of the head and neck. If the rib is not contacted, careful exploration should be carried out first laterally to the mark and, last of all, medially. The greatest danger of contacting the pleura occurs when probing medially.

4. An alternate approach is to introduce the needle just above the clavicle from the anterior surface of the body, and advance it directly posterior, following a line that would be traversed by a plumb bob toward the floor (assuming the patient is supine).[17] If no paresthesia is encountered, the syringe and needle are withdrawn and rotated in small increments caudad and advanced again. Theoretically, the needle will encounter the nerves before contacting the rib or the pleura.

5. If a paresthesia is produced during the course of explora-

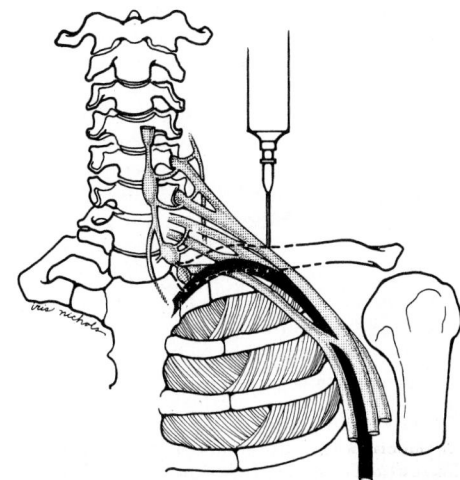

Figure 27-17. Needle direction for supraclavicular blockade (anteroposterior view). The needle is directed downward onto the first rib, where it can be expected to contact the three trunks of the brachial plexus as they cross over the rib. The rib at this point lies along the anteroposterior plane of the body. (Reproduced with permission from Mulroy M: Handbook of Regional Anesthesia. Boston, Little, Brown, 1996.)

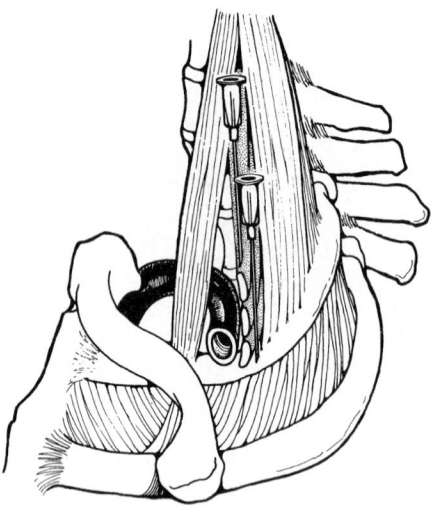

Figure 27-18. Needle direction for supraclavicular blockade (lateral view). The subclavian artery rises from the chest to join the three trunks of the brachial plexus in crossing over the first rib. The nerves usually lie posterior to the artery at this point, although they rapidly encircle it as it becomes the axillary artery. Note that once the needle contacts the rib, it should be withdrawn almost completely to the skin before redirection because short steps along the bone may simply "push" the nerves ahead of the needle. (Reproduced with permission from Mulroy M: Handbook of Regional Anesthesia. Boston, Little, Brown, 1996.)

tion, the anesthetic solution is injected while the needle is fixed in position. Twenty-five to 40 ml of 1% lidocaine or 0.25% bupivacaine may produce adequate analgesia; higher concentrations will produce anesthesia and profound motor blockade. Multiple paresthesias are not usually required because there are only three trunks at this level and the sheath that encloses them is well defined.

6. If a paresthesia is not obtained on needle insertion, exploration is continued until the rib is identified. A 5-cm needle may be needed to reach the rib in the heavier patient. Once the rib is contacted, the needle is walked in an anteroposterior plane until a paresthesia is found. Again, the needle is kept in the sagittal plane on the dorsal surface of the rib during exploration. If the needle advances beyond the anterior or posterior border of the rib as it curves medially at these two points, it is simply redirected in the opposite direction until the rib is found again. Medial direction is avoided. While exploring along the direction of the rib, the needle should be withdrawn almost to the skin before redirection for each pass. If it is lifted only a few millimeters from the rib, it may simply push the nerve bundle ahead of it without making contact.

7. If no paresthesia is obtained, the artery can be used as a landmark. Once it is entered with the needle, a series of injections posterior to it can be used to produce a "wall" of 40 ml of anesthetic solution in this area.

8. If a tourniquet is to be used, a ring of subcutaneous anesthesia should be infiltrated along the axilla to block the sensory fibers from the chest wall that cross here to innervate the inner aspect of the upper arm.

Pneumothorax is the most serious complication of this technique. Although it is rare in experienced hands, it does occur more frequently with this approach to the brachial plexus than with any other approach. This may limit the use of this technique, particularly in outpatients, in whom the insertion of a chest tube would then require hospitalization. The other complications of peripheral blockade do not occur with any greater frequency with this blockade than with other methods of blockade.

Axillary Technique

The axillary technique carries the least chance of pneumothorax and thus may be ideal for the outpatient. The nerves are anesthetized around the axillary artery, where they have regrouped into their terminal branches. Because of the observation that the single sheath may be broken up into separate compartments by fascial septa surrounding individual nerves in the axilla, there are several approaches to blockade at this level. Although the septa do not limit diffusion of drug in every case,[18] Thompson and Rorie[19] have identified several patients in whom the development of these divisions has limited the spread of anesthetic to other nerves. This has led to the recommendation that local anesthetic be injected at multiple sites in the axilla in contrast to the single injections possible with the proximal approaches. Another obstacle to the single-injection technique at this level is the early departure of the musculocutaneous branch from the sheath high in the axilla. In light of these controversies, several techniques are described.

1. The patient lies supine with the arm extended 90 degrees from the side and flexed at the elbow. Extension beyond 90 degrees potentially compresses the axillary artery because of the pressure from the head of the humerus and may make identification of the landmarks more difficult. A pillow under the forearm also reduces rotation of the shoulder joint, which can obscure the pulse.

2. The axillary artery is marked as high in its course in the axilla as is practical. It is usually felt in the intramuscular groove between the coracobrachialis and the triceps muscles. It also passes between the insertions of the pectoralis major and the latissimus dorsi muscles on the humerus.

3. After aseptic preparation, a skin wheal is raised over the proximal portion of the artery. The index and middle fingers of the nondominant hand straddle the artery just below this point, both localizing the pulsation and compressing the sheath below the intended site of injection (Fig. 27-19).

4. Common Approaches
   A) *Eliciting paresthesia.* A three-ring syringe with a 2.5-cm short bevel needle is held in the other hand, and the needle is introduced alongside the artery seeking a paresthesia. Ideally, the nerves serving the area of proposed surgery are sought first. The median and the

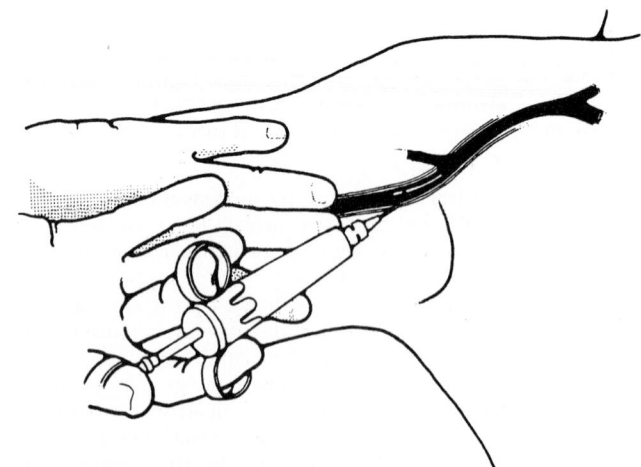

Figure 27-19. Hand position for axillary blockade. Two fingers of equal length straddle the artery while the needle is introduced along its long axis with a central angulation. The palpating fingers serve not only to identify the vessel but also to compress the perivascular sheath and encourage the spread of anesthetic solution centrally. (Reproduced with permission from Mulroy M: Handbook of Regional Anesthesia. Boston, Little, Brown, 1996.)

musculocutaneous nerves lie on the superior aspect of the artery (as viewed by the operator), whereas the ulnar and radial nerves lie below and behind the vessel (Fig. 27-20).

When a paresthesia is obtained, the contents of the syringe are injected, taking precautions to avoid intraneural injection. Firm pressure is maintained on the distal sheath to encourage the solution to move centrally from the point of injection, hopefully to include the point of origin of the musculocutaneous nerve. If a 10-ml syringe is used, the anesthesiologist may elect to fix the needle in position, refill the syringe, and inject a total dose of 25–40 ml of anesthetic solution near this single paresthesia. (A larger bolus may be injected without the need for refilling if a 50-ml syringe is attached to the needle by an iv extension tube.) If multiple injections are planned, and other paresthesias are desired, they should be elicited within 5 minutes of the original injection. Beyond this time, spread of the solution may produce hypesthesia of the other nerves, which prevents their identification. A second paresthesia should be sought on the side of the artery opposite the original one. With this approach, 15–20 ml of solution is injected following elicitation of each paresthesia.

B) *Perivascular infiltration.* Using the same approach with a shorter, smaller-gauge needle, 5–10 ml of local anesthetic is injected closely on each side of the artery, using multiple passes with a moving needle *not* seeking paresthesias, producing a "wall" of solution that intercepts the paths of each of the branches. After initial infiltration, sensation or motor function is tested in the peripheral nerve distribution within 5 minutes. If anesthesia is not present, reinjection of the area is again performed with multiple passes. This approach may reduce nerve injury.[20]

C) *Transarterial.* Again, preparation and landmarks are the same, but the artery is deliberately entered directly with the needle. The needle is advanced through the vessel until aspiration confirms that it has passed just posterior; at this point, half the anesthetic solution is injected incrementally with careful attention to avoid intravascular placement. The needle is then withdrawn back through the vessel until aspiration confirms that

it is just anterior to the artery. The other half of the solution is injected. This technique is simple and effective and should be kept in mind as an alternative if the vessel is unintentionally entered during either of the aforementioned techniques.

D) *Nerve stimulator.* The nerve stimulator can be used to identify the nerves in the axilla using the same approach, with injection of anesthetic in the area of one or more responses. If a single injection is made near one of the nerves in the perivascular area at the axillary crease, a separate stimulation of the musculocutaneous nerve may be required. Alternatively, all four major peripheral nerves may be stimulated and anesthetized lower in the arm, at the junction of the upper and middle third of the humerus (midhumeral approach[21]). At this point, the median nerve is stimulated subcutaneously near the artery, the ulnar nerve is deeper and medial to the artery, the musculocutaneous nerve is under the biceps and 2–4 cm away from the artery, and the radial nerve is behind the humerus.

5. If forearm anesthesia is required with higher axillary techniques, supplementary anesthesia of the musculocutaneous nerve may be obtained by injecting an additional 5–10 ml of anesthetic solution into the body of the coracobrachialis muscle. This muscle can be easily grasped between the thumb and forefinger, and the entry into its fascial compartment is readily identified. This step may be required even if 40 ml of solution is used in the perivascular injection because the musculocutaneous nerve may be spared as often as 25% of the time even with this or larger volumes. A supplemental injection of 5 ml subcutaneously inferior to the artery is also required to anesthetize the medial antebrachial cutaneous nerve.

The complications of the axillary approaches to the brachial plexus are minimal compared with those of the more proximal approaches. The problem of neuropathy is the foremost consideration, and the relative risk with various techniques remains controversial. Hematoma can occur if the vessel is punctured, but this is rarely a problem. The use of small-gauge needles may reduce this possibility. The advantages of any one technique in reducing complications remains unclear, and the success rate of the various techniques is variable and appears to depend on personal familiarity.[20]

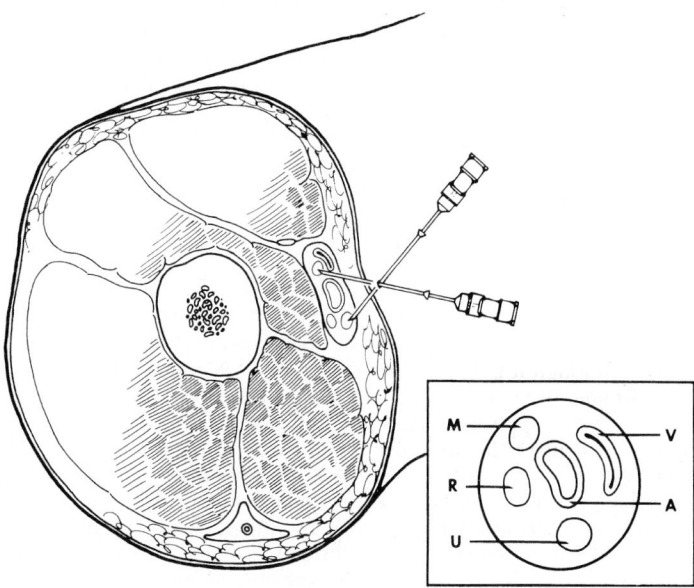

Figure 27-20. Needle position for axillary injection. The median (M) and musculocutaneous nerves lie on the superior side of the artery (A), although the latter may have already departed the axillary sheath at the level of injection. The ulnar nerve (U) lies inferior, and the radial nerve (R) is inferior and posterior. V, vein.

Intravenous Regional Anesthesia

The simplest technique of arm anesthesia is the injection of local anesthetic into the venous system below an occluding tourniquet (Bier block).

1. A small-gauge (20 or 22) iv plastic catheter is inserted in the arm to be blocked on the dorsum of the hand. It is taped firmly in place, and a heparin port or small syringe is attached and saline is injected to maintain patency. A pneumatic tourniquet is applied over the upper arm.
2. The arm is elevated to promote venous drainage. An elastic bandage may be applied to produce further exsanguination. After exsanguination, the tourniquet is inflated to 300 mm Hg or 2.5 times the patient's systolic blood pressure and is tested for adequate occlusion of the radial pulse.
3. The arm is returned to the horizontal position, a 50-ml syringe with 0.5% lidocaine is attached to the previously inserted cannula, and the contents are injected. The forearm discolors, and the patient perceives a transient "pins and needles" sensation as anesthesia ensues over the following 5 minutes. Epinephrine should not be added to the local anesthetic solution.
4. For short procedures, the cannula can be removed at this point. If surgery may extend beyond 1 hour, the cannula can be left in place and reinjected after 90 minutes.
5. Beyond 45 minutes of surgery, many patients experience discomfort at the level of the tourniquet. Special "double-cuff" tourniquets are available for this blockade to alleviate this problem. The proximal cuff is inflated first, allowing anesthesia to be induced in the area under the distal cuff. If discomfort ensues, the distal cuff is inflated over the anesthetized area of skin, and the uncomfortable proximal cuff is released. This step is critical because the major risk of this procedure is premature release of solution into the circulation. If a double cuff is used, both cuffs should be tested before starting and the proper sequence for inflation and deflation meticulously followed. The potential for leakage of anesthetic into the circulation is greater with these narrower cuffs used in the double setup. Because the shifting process also increases the potential for unintentional release of anesthetic, the use of a single, wider cuff may be better for short procedures.
6. If surgery is completed in less than 20 minutes, the tourniquet is left inflated for at least that total period of time. If 40 minutes has elapsed, the tourniquet can be deflated as a single maneuver. Between 20 and 40 minutes, the cuff can be deflated, reinflated immediately, and finally deflated after 1 minute to delay the sudden absorption of anesthetic into the systemic circulation, although this may not lower the eventual peak levels achieved.
7. The duration of anesthesia is minimal beyond the time of tourniquet release. Although bupivacaine may produce a slight prolongation of analgesia, the advantage is short. Furthermore, the cardiotoxicity of bupivacaine makes this drug an unwise choice for a Bier block.

The simplicity of this technique is offset by the significant risk of systemic local anesthetic toxicity if the tourniquet fails or is released prematurely. Careful testing of the tourniquet and slow injection of solution into a peripheral (not antecubital) vein will reduce the chance of leakage under the tourniquet.[22] Systemic blood levels are time dependent, and careful attention should be paid to the sequence of tourniquet release and to patient monitoring during this period. A separate iv site for injection of resuscitation drugs is needed as well as ready availability of all appropriate resuscitative equipment. With careful attention to these details, this technique is one of the most effective and reliable available to the anesthesiologist.

Distal Upper Extremity Blockade

As in the leg, the nerves to the hand can be blocked at the point where they cross the two major joints, the elbow and the wrist (Fig. 27-21). At these two levels, the overlying muscles are thinned and the bony landmarks are more prominent, allowing easier identification of the nerves. Peripheral blockade is usually not as dense as central blockade but may be useful in anesthetizing one branch that was missed with a central blockade or in providing localized anesthesia on the hand. Because the sensory branches to the forearm from the musculocutaneous nerve and the internal cutaneous nerve have already branched so extensively that adequate anesthesia of the forearm is not easily obtained, blockade at the elbow really produces no greater anesthesia than blockade at the wrist.

Blockade at the Elbow. Two nerves to the hand cross this joint on the inner aspect, whereas the ulnar travels posteriorly in its well known superficial groove. The procedure for blockade follows:

1. The ulnar nerve is blocked by injection of 1–4 ml of local anesthetic proximal to the groove formed by the medial condyle of the humerus and the olecranon. This is easily done with the joint flexed at approximately 30 degrees. Further flexion may cause the nerve to roll medially and anterior to the condyle. Paresthesias can usually be readily obtained, but direct injection on a paresthesia or directly into the groove under pressure is not advised because of the risk of damage to the nerve. If the injection is made deep to the fascia, anesthesia should commence within 5 minutes.
2. The median nerve crosses the joint in the company of the brachial artery. A line is drawn between the two condyles on the inner aspect of the joint, and a skin wheal is raised at the point where this line crosses the pulsation of the brachial artery, usually 1 cm to the ulnar side of the biceps tendon. A needle is introduced perpendicularly at this

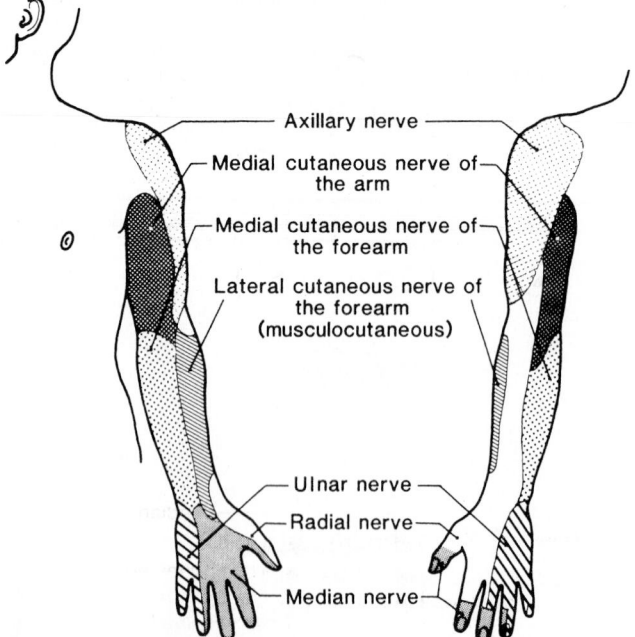

Figure 27-21. Sensory dermatomes of the arm. Sensation is provided by the terminal nerves, as identified. This pattern is different from the classic dermatomal distribution of the nerve roots. Different patterns of anesthesia develop if the blockade is performed at the root level (interscalene blockade) versus the terminal nerve level (axillary blockade). (Reproduced with permission from Mulroy M: Handbook of Regional Anesthesia. Boston, Little, Brown, 1996.)

point, and paresthesias are sought immediately adjacent to the artery. Five ml of solution is sufficient to produce anesthesia, and, again, intraneural injection is carefully avoided.

3. The radial nerve is identified along the same intracondylar line, approximately 2 cm lateral to the biceps tendon. Another skin wheal is raised here, and, again, a needle is inserted to search for paresthesias in a fan-shaped pattern. If paresthesias are not obtained, a "wall" of anesthetic solution can be deposited here but with less chance of reliable anesthesia.

Blockade at the Wrist. The nerves lie more superficially at this joint and are closely associated with easily identified landmarks (Fig. 27-22). For this reason, blockade at this level is usually preferred to other distal approaches. The procedure for blockade follows:

1. The ulnar nerve lies between the ulnar artery and the flexor carpi ulnaris. A skin wheal is raised at the level of the styloid process on the palmar side of the forearm between these two landmarks. A small-gauge needle is inserted, and 3 ml of solution is injected into the area, with or without paresthesias.
2. At the same level on the forearm, the median nerve lies between the tendons of the palmaris longus and the flexor carpi radialis. If only the palmaris longus can be felt, the nerve is just to the radial side of this tendon. A skin wheal is raised, and a needle is inserted until it pierces the deep fascia. Three milliliters of solution produces anesthesia.
3. The radial nerve requires a broader injection because it has already started to ramify as it crosses the wrist. The anatomic "snuffbox" formed by the tendons of the extensor pollicis longus and extensor pollicis brevis tendons is located, and 3 ml of solution is injected here. A subcutaneous wheal is then raised from this point, extending over the dorsum of the wrist 3–4 cm onto the back of the hand.

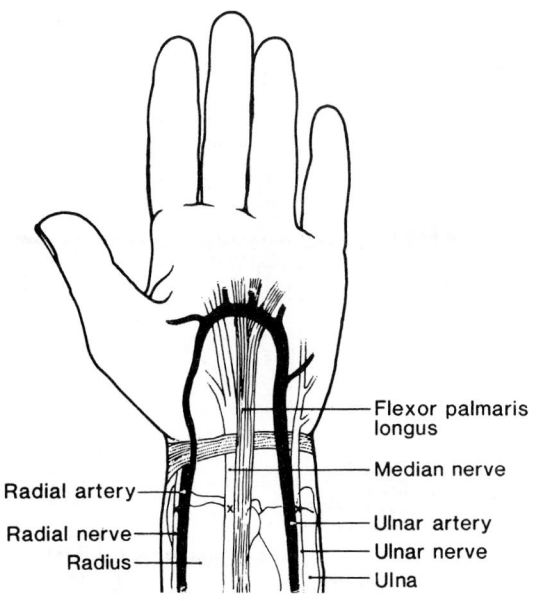

Figure 27-22. Terminal nerves at the wrist. The median nerve lies just to the radial side of the flexor palmaris longus. The ulnar and radial nerves lie just "outside" their respective arteries. The radial nerve has already begun branching at this level and must be blocked by a wide subcutaneous ridge of anesthetic. (Reproduced with permission from Mulroy M: Handbook of Regional Anesthesia. Boston, Little, Brown, 1996.)

Suprascapular Block

The suprascapular nerve is another terminal branch of the brachial plexus that can be anesthetized by a separate injection. Anesthesia of this nerve has become popular for providing postoperative pain relief following shoulder arthroscopy or reconstructive surgery. The nerve arises from the superior trunk of the brachial plexus in the neck, courses through the suprascapular notch, and then passes behind the lateral border of the spine of the scapula to the infraspinatus fossa. It has two terminal branches, a sensory articular branch to the shoulder joint and a motor branch to the supraspinatus muscle. The technique for nerve blockade is as follows:

1. The patient is placed in the upright sitting position, leaning forward so that the scapulae are accentuated. The spine of the scapula is identified and marked along its entire length. The inferior tip of the scapula is then identified, and the original line of the spine is bisected at a point immediately superior to this inferior tip.
2. A skin wheal is raised approximately 1 cm superior and 1 cm lateral from this midpoint of the scapular spine, and a 1.5 inch needle is advanced through the skin until contact is made with the superior surface of the scapula. The needle is then withdrawn and redirected cephalad and medially towards the midline until the edge of the suprascapular notch is encountered. At this point, the patient may perceive a paresthesia into the shoulder joint, or the nerve stimulator may produce an internal rotation of the arm itself.
3. Once the nerve is localized, 10 ml of local anesthetic is injected. Even in the absence of nerve localization, this volume of solution injected into the notch should produce adequate anesthesia of the shoulder joint.

Trunk

Anesthesia of the abdomen and chest is most simply obtained with spinal and epidural injections of local anesthetics, as discussed in Chapter 26. In some situations, a narrower band of intercostal or paravertebral anesthesia is preferable, or epidural injection may be hazardous because of infection or coagulopathy. In many clinical situations, it may also be desirable to separate the anesthesia of the somatic and sympathetic fibers that occurs in combination when axial blockades are performed. The sympathetic nerves separate from their somatic counterparts early in their course, which makes independent somatic and sympathetic blockade a practical consideration. Sympathetic blockade is most commonly performed at the major ganglia, particularly the stellate, celiac, and lumbar plexus. These blockades often require multiple injections and are technically more difficult than axial anesthesia, but they do offer advantages in certain clinical situations.

The somatic nerves of the chest emerge from their respective intervertebral foramina and pass through the narrow, triangular-shaped paravertebral space. In this triangle, they give off the sympathetic branch and also a small dorsal branch, which provides sensation to the midline of the back. The main trunks then pass into the intercostal groove along the ventral caudad surface of each rib. An artery and vein travel along with each of these nerves in the groove under the protection of the overhanging external edge of the rib. The fasciae of the internal and external intercostal muscles provide interior and external borders of this intercostal groove. As the nerves travel beyond the midaxillary line, they give off a lateral sensory branch while the main trunk continues on to the anterior abdominal wall to provide sensory and motor innervation for the trunk and abdomen down to the level of the pubis. The intercostal groove becomes much less well defined anterior to the midaxillary line, and the nerve begins to move away from its protected position. The lowermost intercostal nerve (the 12th) is much less closely applied to its accompanying rib and is not as easy to identify and anesthetize using a classic intercostal blockade technique. The upper lumbar roots form the ilioinguinal nerves, which pass laterally within the muscles of the abdominal wall at the level of the iliac crest and eventually move anteriorly to provide innervation of the groin region as the ilioinguinal nerves.

The anatomic basis for separate sympathetic anesthesia is the early separation of sympathetic fibers from their somatic roots in the form of the white rami communicantes, which separate from the somatic nerves shortly after their emergence from the intervertebral foramina and join the sympathetic ganglia, which lie anteriorly on each side of the vertebral bodies. These preganglionic fibers of the sympathetic system usually arise only from the first thoracic through the second lumbar segments. The spinal ganglia formed by these fibers constitute the sympathetic trunks, which extend upward into the neck and caudad along the lumbar spine. They give terminal sympathetic branches to all the areas of the body. The sympathetic innervation of the head and the lower extremities is derived from fibers that originate from the spinal cord, join sympathetic trunks, and then pass cephalad or caudad along the chain of ganglia before reaching their target organs. Segmental sympathetic innervation of the body from the cervical to the sacral roots is provided by postganglionic nerves departing from the chains (the gray rami communicantes), which rejoin the somatic nerves early in their course. In the head (where motor and sensory innervation is by cranial nerves), the sympathetic fibers reach their end organs by traveling with the arterial vascular supply. The sympathetic ganglia in the neck lie along the lateral border of the relatively flat vertebral bodies. In the chest, the vertebral bodies become more rounded, and the chain of ganglia lies more posteriorly on the lateral side of the vertebral body near the head of each rib. In the abdomen and pelvis, the sympathetic chains begin to move anteriorly and lie on the ventral surface of the vertebral bodies, and thus are more widely separated from their respective somatic nerves.

Intercostal Nerve Blockade

Anesthesia of the intercostal nerves provides both motor and sensory anesthesia of the entire abdominal wall from the xiphoid to the pubis. The 6th to 11th ribs are usually easily identified, and their accompanying nerves are reliably blocked by injections along the easily palpated sharp posterior angulation of the ribs, which occurs between 5 and 7 cm from the midline in the back. Ribs above the fifth are difficult to palpate because of the overlying scapula and paraspinous muscles and are therefore most easily blocked using the paravertebral technique. Establishing five or six levels of intercostal nerve blockade is a useful anesthetic procedure for providing analgesia and motor relaxation for upper abdominal procedures such as cholecystectomy and gastric surgery. This form of anesthesia usually requires supplementation with light general anesthesia or an additional sympathetic blockade because much of the intraperitoneal and subdiaphragmatic sensation is carried by other nerve trunks. This form of anesthesia for upper abdominal surgery offers the advantages of muscle relaxation without the necessity of an accompanying sympathetic blockade (unless celiac plexus blockade is chosen as an optional supplement). Intercostal blockade with long-acting amide local anesthetics also provides postoperative analgesia for 8–12 hours, which may greatly facilitate patient satisfaction and immediate recovery.[23] Unilateral blockade of these nerves is a useful treatment for the pain of rib fracture and also serves to reduce postoperative analgesia requirements in patients with subcostal incisions. Several segments must be blocked in each of these applications because of the overlap of the intercostal nerves. This technique is also useful in reducing the pain associated with the insertion of chest tubes or percutaneous biliary drainage procedures. The procedure for blockade follows:

1. For the performance of intercostal blockade, the patient may be in the lateral, sitting, or prone position. For operative anesthesia, the prone position is most practical. A pillow is placed under the abdomen to provide slight flexion of the thoracic spine. The arms are draped over the edge of the stretcher or operating table so that the scapula falls away laterally from the midline. The anesthesiologist stands at the patient's side. Most anesthesiologists prefer to stand on the side that allows their dominant hand to hold the syringe at the caudad end of the patient.

2. The spinous processes in the midline from T6 through T12 are marked (Fig. 27-23). The ribs are then identified along the line of their most extreme posterior angulation. For the 12th rib, this is usually 7 cm from the midline. At the level of the sixth rib, this posterior angulation is best appreciated somewhat more medially, usually 5 cm from the midline. These two ribs are marked first at their inferior borders, and a line is drawn between these two points. The rest of the ribs between them are identified, and a mark is placed on the inferior border of each rib along the angled parasagittal plane identified by the first line between the 6th and 12th ribs.

3. After aseptic preparation, sedation and analgesia are provided for the patient, and a skin wheal is raised at each mark.

4. The ribs are usually blocked starting with the lowermost and moving upward. The 12th rib is not closely associated with its intercostal nerve, and a reliable blockade is not usually possible. For upper abdominal procedures, block-

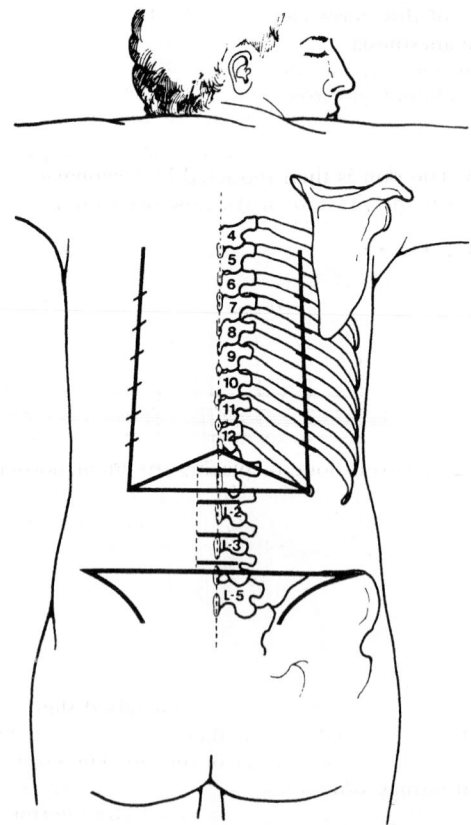

Figure 27-23. Landmarks for intercostal blockade. The inferior borders of the ribs are identified at their most prominent points on the back. The marks then usually lie along a line that angles slightly medially from the 12th to the 6th rib. The triangle drawn between the 12th ribs and their spinous processes is used for the celiac plexus blockade. (Reproduced with permission from Mulroy M: Handbook of Regional Anesthesia. Boston, Little, Brown, 1996.)

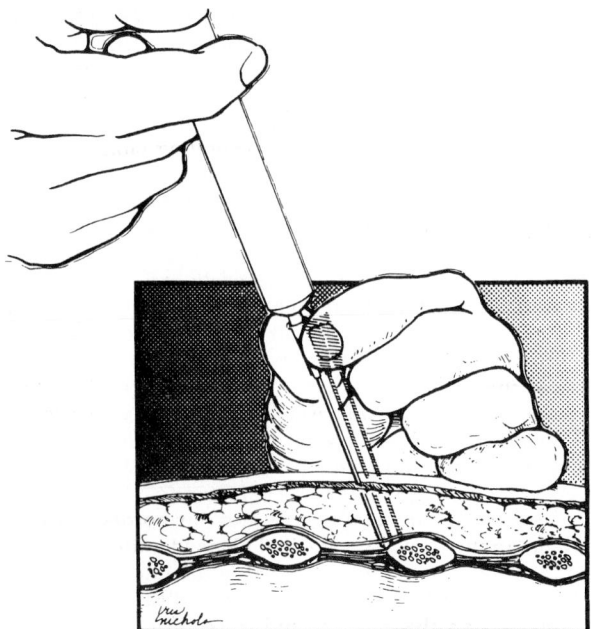

Figure 27-24. Hand and needle positions for intercostal blockade. The depth of the needle is controlled by the hand resting on the back. The other hand injects solution when the needle is under the rib, but that is the only function performed while the needle is near the pleura. (Reproduced with permission from Mulroy M: *Handbook of Regional Anesthesia.* Boston, Little, Brown, 1996.)

ade of this nerve can be omitted without jeopardizing the anesthesia.

5. Starting with the lowest rib on the side closest to the anesthesiologist, the index finger of the cephalad hand is placed on the skin above the identifying mark; this finger should lie immediately over the midpoint of the rib. The skin is then retracted in a cephalad direction, so that the previous mark now lies over the rib itself, somewhat toward the inferior side. The anesthesiologist's other hand inserts a 22-gauge, 3.75-cm needle directly onto the rib. This needle is attached to a 10-ml syringe filled with local anesthetic. The syringe and needle are held in such a way that they maintain a constant 10-degree cephalad angulation.

6. Once the needle is safely "parked" on the dorsal surface of the rib, the cephalad hand releases the tension on the skin and takes control of the needle and syringe (Fig. 27-24). This is done by placing the ulnar border of the hand firmly against the skin and grasping the hub of the needle firmly between the thumb and index finger. The middle finger of this hand rests along the shaft of the needle to provide guidance. Once the syringe is firmly gripped by the cephalad hand, the fingers of the caudad hand are placed in an "injection" position, either in the rings of a three-ring syringe or on the plunger of a straight syringe.

7. The needle and syringe are then raised slightly off the bone and walked in a caudad direction until they pass below the inferior border of the rib. The entire needle and syringe unit is kept at a 10-degree cephalad angle to the rib at all times. As it passes the inferior border, the needle is advanced 4–6 mm under the rib, with the needle actually pointing slightly cephalad into the intercostal groove.

8. Once in the groove, aspiration is performed, and 3–5 ml of local anesthetic solution is injected. Generally, 0.25% bupivacaine produces good sensory anesthesia, whereas 0.5% bupivacaine is required for prolonged anesthesia

with motor blockade. Ropivacaine 0.5% also provide motor blockade, but for a shorter duration. Aspiration is not reliable in preventing intravascular injection of the anesthetic; a slight jiggling motion of the needle during the injection will reduce this chance by ensuring that the needle is in a vessel only transiently if it does occur.

9. As soon as the injection is complete, the needle is withdrawn from the groove and moved cephalad and "parked" again on the safe dorsal surface of the rib. The fingers of the caudad hand are then removed from the injection position and assume control of the syringe again. The cephalad hand now relinquishes control and is moved up to the next rib to repeat this cyclic process.

10. The six or seven designated ribs on each side are blocked in this process by progressively moving up the back, with control of the syringe alternating between the cephalad and caudad hands at the time of injection. The ribs on the opposite side are blocked in a similar manner. This can be done with the anesthesiologist standing on the same side and reaching across the back, or by moving to the opposite side of the patient. If the contralateral blockades are performed from the opposite side of the bed, an attempt should be made to switch hands, so that the functions of the cephalad and caudad hands remain the same even though the right and left hands have changed roles. It is sometimes more difficult for operators to control the syringe with their nondominant hand, but attempting to hold the syringe in the cephalad hand often makes maintenance of the proper cephalad angulation difficult. The syringe often ends up being rotated along its long axis as it is moved to the caudad edge of the rib, with the result that the needle is pointed in a caudad rather than a cephalad direction.

11. If the intercostal nerve blockades are to be supplemented by a number of somatic paravertebral nerve blockades or sympathetic blockade of the celiac plexus, these are performed at the completion of intercostal anesthesia. Care should be taken to adjust the total dose of drug in such combinations of techniques so that the maximal recommended amounts are not exceeded.

Despite frequent concern about the incidence of pneumothorax with intercostal blockade, this complication is rare in experienced hands. This depends primarily on maintaining strict safety features of the described technique. Emphasis should be placed on absolute control of the syringe and needle at all times, particularly during the injection. The cephalad hand, which is securely resting on the back, is the one that controls the depth of needle insertion. The needle rests on the safe dorsal side surface of the rib at all other times except for the brief moment of injection.

A common complication is related to the sedation required to perform this blockade in the prone position. The 12–14 needle insertions are uncomfortable, and patients usually require opioid and amnestic sedation. Overdose can lead to airway obstruction and respiratory depression in the prone position. Attention must also be paid to the patient's mental status because this blockade produces the highest blood levels of local anesthetics when compared with any other regional anesthetic technique. Because this blockade is frequently supplemented by a light general anesthetic for surgery, signs of systemic toxicity are rarely seen. When the blockade is performed for postoperative pain relief, the dose should be reduced to 0.25% bupivacaine or ropivacaine to minimize the chance for toxicity.

It is possible to produce partial spinal or epidural anesthesia if the injection is made close to the midline and the anesthetic tracks along a dural sleeve to the epidural or subarachnoid space. This appears to be more likely if intrathoracic injection is performed intraoperatively by a surgeon. Hypotension may result in this situation. Hypotension has also been observed rarely when this blockade is used for postoperative pain relief in a patient who has received generous doses of opioids. Once the local anesthetic succeeds in relieving the pain, the patient's intrinsic sympathetic response is reduced, and the respiratory depressant effect of previously injected opioids is unmasked. Patients should be observed for at least 20–30 minutes after performance of intercostal blockade. Respiratory insufficiency can also be seen if the intercostal muscles are blocked in a patient who depends on them for ventilation. Patients with chronic obstructive disease with ineffective diaphragm motion are not good candidates for this technique.

Paravertebral Blockade

The upper five ribs are more difficult to palpate laterally, and blockade of their associated intercostal nerves is best performed with a paravertebral injection. This approach is technically more difficult and has slightly greater potential for complications because of the proximity of the lung and of the intervertebral foramina. Anatomically, the injection is made into the triangle formed by the intervertebral body, the pleura, and the plane of the transverse processes (Fig. 27-25). The intervertebral foramina at each level lie between the transverse processes and approximately 2 cm anterior to the plane formed by the transverse processes in their associated fasciae. At this point, the sympathetic ganglia lie close to the somatic nerves, and coincidental sympathetic blockade is usually attained. This is also related to the injection of larger volumes of local anesthetic, which is required because location of the nerve is less reliable with this technique. Nevertheless, it is a useful technique for segmental anesthesia, particularly of the upper thoracic segments. It is also useful if a more proximal blockade is needed, such as to relieve the pain of herpes zoster or of a proximal rib fracture. Paravertebral nerve blockade has been used successfully for outpatient surgery. In the upper chest, it is effective for providing intraoperative anesthesia and postoperative analgesia for breast surgery.[24] It has also been used successfully for outpatient hernia operations, providing significant postoperative analgesia.

The paravertebral approach varies somewhat, depending on the spinal level. In the upper thoracic spine, the transverse process is located lateral to the spinous process of the vertebral body above it. In the lower thoracic spine, the spinous processes are less steeply angled, so that the 11th and 12th spinous processes lie between the associated transverse processes. In the lumbar region, the spinous processes are straight, and the transverse processes lie opposite their own respective spinous process. Thus, paravertebral blockade in the upper thoracic region is performed at each level by identifying the spinous process of the vertebra above the level to be blocked; in the lumbar region, the spinous process of the level to be blocked is used to locate the transverse process.

1. This blockade is also performed in the prone position, with a pillow under the patient's abdomen to produce flexion of the thoracic and lumbar spine. The spinous processes in the region to be blocked are marked. These can be identified by counting upward from the fourth lumbar process (which usually lies just at or above the line joining the two iliac crests) or by counting down from the seventh cervical process (which is the most prominent in the cervical region).

2. Transverse lines are drawn across the cephalad border of the spinous processes and extended laterally to overlie the transverse process (~1–4 cm). In the lumbar region, the lines overlie the transverse process of the associated vertebra. In the thoracic region, they indicate the transverse process of the vertebral body immediately below the associated spinous process. Finally, a vertical line is drawn parallel to the spine 3–4 cm lateral to it joining the transverse lines from the spinous processes. For a diagnostic blockade, a single nerve may need to be anesthetized. For pain control, several levels must be identified. The injection of at least three segments (as in intercostal blockade) is required to produce reliable segmental blockade because of sensory overlap.

3. After aseptic skin preparation, skin wheals are raised at the intersections of the vertical and transverse lines.

4. A 22-gauge needle is introduced through the skin wheal in the sagittal plane and directed slightly cephalad to contact the transverse process. A 7.5-cm needle is usually required in the average patient, and the transverse process lies between 3 and 5 cm from the skin. Gentle cephalad or caudad exploration may be required to identify the bone. The depth of the transverse process is carefully noted on the needle shaft.

5. The needle is now withdrawn from the transverse process and walked inferiorly to pass below its caudad edge. This usually requires more perpendicular direction relative to the skin. The needle is advanced 2 cm below the transverse process and angled slightly medial to attempt to contact the vertebral body. Paresthesias are not sought unless a neurolytic injection is planned. When the needle has entered the paravertebral space, 5–10 ml of local anesthetic solution is injected after careful aspiration.

The complication of pneumothorax is more likely in the thoracic region with a paravertebral technique than with intercostal blockade.[25] The needle should be directed medially as it passes below the transverse process and never more than 2 cm beyond the transverse process (see Fig. 27-25). If cough or chest pain occurs, a chest radiograph should be performed to rule out pneumothorax. Subarachnoid injection is also more likely in the thoracic area because of the extension of the dural sleeves to the level of the intervertebral foramina. Careful aspiration is important but may not prevent the unintentional injection of local anesthetic into a subdural pocket. Total spinal anesthesia can result with a 5–10-ml injection. Systemic toxicity is also a possibility because of the need for relatively large volumes of local anesthetic. Attention must be paid to the total milligram dose injected. The volume required for each level obviously limits the concentrations that can be used and the total number of levels that can be blocked. If lumbar paravertebral injections

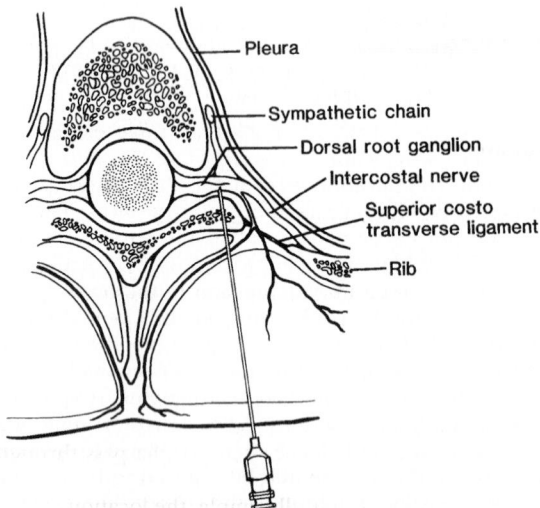

Figure 27-25. Paravertebral blockade. As it exits the intervertebral foramen, the thoracic somatic nerve enters a small triangular space formed by the vertebral body, the plane of the transverse process, and the pleura. Medial direction of the needle is obviously important in reducing the chance of a pneumothorax.

are combined with intercostals, the concentration and total volume for both blockades may have to be reduced.

Intrapleural Anesthesia

Upper abdominal analgesia can also be obtained by inserting an epidural catheter into the intrapleural space for injection or infusion of local anesthetic. The anesthetic appears to diffuse through the parietal pleura onto the intercostal nerves and produce anesthesia similar to that provided by injection of multiple intercostal nerve blocks. It may also act upon the sympathetic nerves by diffusion to the ganglia lying along the anterior vertebral borders.

1. As with intercostal block, the technique can be performed with the patient in the prone, lateral, or sitting position.
2. The seventh or eighth intercostal space is identified 8–10 cm from the midline and marked at the upper border of the lower rib.
3. A skin wheal is made at this site, and a blunt-tipped epidural needle (*e.g.,* Touhy) is inserted with the bevel directed cephalad and advanced over the inferior rib in a slightly medial and cephalad angle through the intercostal muscles. Once in the intercostal layers, the stylet is removed, and an air-filled 5-ml glass syringe is attached.
4. The needle is advanced farther until the parietal pleura is punctured, signaled by a negative pressure that moves the plunger of the syringe forward. The syringe is removed, and a standard epidural catheter is threaded 5–6 cm beyond the tip. Aspiration is performed to exclude perforation of the lung or a blood vessel.
5. Twenty ml of 0.5% bupivacaine with epinephrine is injected into the pleural space, and the catheter is carefully taped to the skin. Reinjection is required every 3–6 hours, or a constant infusion of 0.25% bupivacaine (0.125 ml·kg^{-1}·h^{-1}) can be initiated.

There have been several enthusiastic reports of success with this technique,[26] but limitations have been described. Pain relief is usually reliable, and respiratory depression is not a problem. However, the duration is short enough that large quantities of local anesthetic are required to maintain analgesia, and systemic toxicity has been reported in 1.3% of patients.[27] The incidence of pneumothorax (averaging 2%) is not inconsequential, especially with first attempts. Puncture of the lung also occurs, apparently with a higher incidence if a loss-of-resistance technique is used rather than the passive identification process described earlier. A major limitation is the unilateral analgesia, which limits this technique to procedures such as cholecystectomy and nephrectomy, rib fracture, and treatment of herpetic pain. Loss of local anesthetic solution to thoracostomy drainage makes this technique less reliable for thoracotomy pain.

Ilioinguinal Blockade

The L1 nerve root (occasionally joined by a branch of the T12 root) provides sensory innervation to the lowermost portion of the abdominal wall and the groin by means of its superior iliohypogastric branch and its inferior ilioinguinal branch. These nerves travel in a path similar to that of the intercostal nerves, but without the convenient bony landmark of a rib to identify them. Nevertheless, they can be anesthetized relatively easily in the groin because of their relationship to the anterosuperior iliac spine. Anesthesia of these two nerves is useful in providing lower abdominal wall anesthesia to supplement intercostal blockade. It is more commonly used to produce field anesthesia for hernia repair surgery. Anesthesia of these nerves alone is not sufficient for hernia repair, and subcutaneous infiltration is also necessary. The procedure for blockade follows:

1. The patient lies in a supine position, and the anterosuperior iliac spine is identified. An "X" is placed on the skin 2.5 cm medial to the spine and slightly cephalad.
2. After aseptic preparation, a skin wheal is raised at the "X."
3. A 2.5-cm, 22-gauge needle is introduced through the "X" and directed perpendicular to the skin until it reaches the fascia of the external oblique muscle. A "wall" of local anesthetic solution is then laid down between this point and the iliac spine and also opposite the mark on an imaginary line extending toward the umbilicus. Injections are made at and below the level of the external oblique, with some solution injected at the level of the internal oblique. A total of 10–15 ml of anesthetic is usually required. A solution of 1% lidocaine, 0.25% bupivacaine, or an equivalent is adequate.
4. If field anesthesia for inguinal hernia repair is required, further subcutaneous infiltration of anesthetic is performed along the skin crease of the groin and along the imaginary line extending to the umbilicus. This produces a triangular-shaped area of skin anesthesia. For hernia operations, further anesthesia of the spermatic cord is required. This is usually performed by local injections in the area of the cord and the internal ring. Although epinephrine is useful in the subcutaneous and ilioinguinal blockade, it should be avoided in solutions used to anesthetize the base of the penis or the spermatic cord. Further anesthesia of the groin area and below can be obtained by blockade of the femoral and lateral femoral cutaneous nerves (see Penile Blockade), but this may result in unwanted weakness of the leg musculature, which may prevent ambulation.

Complications of this procedure are extremely rare. Hematoma formation and unwanted motor blockade of the femoral nerve are possible, but rare. More commonly, anesthesia produced by this technique is inadequate for hernia repair because the patient is still able to perceive the discomfort of peritoneal traction. Administration of local anesthesia by the surgeon or systemic opioids may be required.

Penile Blockade

If surgery is confined to the penis (*e.g.,* circumcision, urethral procedures), the organ should be blocked with simple local infiltration. Two skin wheals are raised at the dorsal base of the penis, one on each side just below and medial to the pubic spine. A 22-gauge, 3.75-cm needle is introduced on each side, and 5 ml of anesthetic is deposited superficially and deep along the lower border of the pubic ramus to anesthetize the dorsal nerve. An additional 5 ml is infiltrated in the subcutaneous tissue around the underside of the shaft to produce a complete ring of anesthetic. A larger needle or a second injection site may be needed to complete the ring. Twenty to 25 ml of 0.75% lidocaine or 0.25% bupivacaine usually suffices. Epinephrine is strictly avoided.

Sympathetic Blockade

Stellate Ganglion

Separate blockade of the sympathetic fibers of the upper extremity and head can be achieved by a single injection of a local anesthetic on the stellate ganglion. The ganglion is the large fusion of the first thoracic sympathetic ganglion with the lower cervical ganglion on each side, and it lies on the generally flat lateral border of the vertebral body of C7. All the fibers to the middle and superior cervical ganglia pass through this lowermost collection and thus can be anesthetized with a single injection. Although technically simple, the location of this ganglion near the carotid artery, the vertebral artery, and the pleura makes this a challenging blockade. It is useful in providing pain relief for sympathetic dystrophies of the upper arm. Stellate ganglion blockade may relieve the pain of acute herpes zoster infection of the head or neck region. It has also been advocated as a means of reducing post-thoracotomy pain by blocking the sympathetic sensory fibers to the pleural cavity. The procedure for blockade follows:

1. The patient is placed in a supine position with a small towel or pillow under the neck, and the arms are held at the side.
2. The medial border of the sternocleidomastoid muscle on the involved side is marked with a pen, as is the level of the cricoid cartilage. Gentle palpation approximately 2 cm lateral to the cartilage often reveals the anterior tubercle of the transverse process of the sixth cervical vertebra (Chassaignac's tubercle). A circle is marked over this tubercle, and an "X" is placed 1.5–2 cm caudad to this mark at the same distance from the midline. This "X" should overlie the tubercle of the seventh cervical vertebra and should fall at the medial border of the sternocleidomastoid muscle body and approximately two fingerbreadths above the clavicle itself.
3. A skin wheal is made at the "X" after aseptic skin preparation.
4. With the index and middle finger of one hand, the sternocleidomastoid muscle and the carotid sheath are retracted laterally (Fig. 27-26). A 22- or 25-gauge, 3.75-cm needle is introduced through the "X" and passed directly posterior until it rests on bone. Paresthesia of the brachial plexus implies that the needle is too far laterally and has passed beyond the transverse process. It may have to be readjusted slightly more medially and perhaps more cephalad or caudad.
5. Once bone is contacted, the needle is withdrawn a few millimeters, and very careful aspiration is performed to rule out contact with the vertebral artery. A 2-ml test dose is injected to evaluate further an unrecognized intravascular position. The patient's mental status must be closely observed.
6. If no change occurs, a total of 10 ml of local anesthetic can be injected incrementally with frequent aspiration.

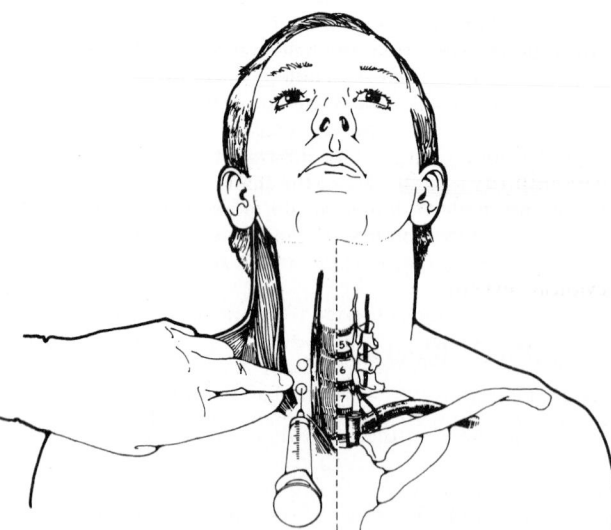

Figure 27-26. Stellate ganglion blockade. The sternocleidomastoid muscle and the carotid sheath are retracted laterally with one hand while the needle is introduced directly onto the lateral border of the seventh vertebral body, just medial to the transverse process. The vertebral artery passes posteriorly at this level to enter its canal in the transverse process, but here it lies near the level of intended injection. After contacting bone, the needle is withdrawn slightly and careful aspiration is performed before incremental injection. (Reproduced with permission from Mulroy M: Handbook of Regional Anesthesia. Boston, Little, Brown, 1996.)

One percent lidocaine or 0.25% bupivacaine or their equivalents are more than adequate to produce anesthesia of the sympathetic nerves.

7. Onset of sympathectomy is usually, but not reliably, indicated by the appearance of a Horner's syndrome on the ipsilateral side. Ptosis, miosis, and anhydrosis usually develop within 10 minutes, as well as vasodilatation in the arm. Nasal congestion is another common sign usually associated with Horner's syndrome.

As implied, there are several potential complications of stellate ganglion blockade related to the surrounding anatomy. The pleura can be punctured, with resulting pneumothorax. Intravascular injection is the most serious complication because of the proximity of the vertebral artery to the site of injection. Careful aspiration and incremental injections are essential. Only a few milligrams of local anesthetic is required to produce cerebral symptoms when injected directly into the vertebral circulation. Cardiovascular changes are possible with the loss of the cardiac accelerator fibers from the cervical sympathetic ganglia. This is particularly a problem if bilateral blockade is performed, a procedure rarely indicated. Hoarseness from recurrent laryngeal nerve paralysis is a minor but troublesome side effect. Somatic anesthesia of the brachial plexus nerves can be produced by injection behind the level of the tubercle, and phrenic nerve paralysis has also been reported. Subarachnoid injection is also a possibility if the needle is misplaced. The close association of so many vital structures has discouraged the use of neurolytic agents in the region of the stellate ganglion.

Celiac Plexus

The thoracic sympathetic ganglia send branches anteriorly that merge as greater and lesser splanchnic nerves to pass below the diaphragm and around the aorta to coalesce in a diffuse periaortic supplementary sympathetic ganglion known as the celiac plexus. This extensive network is usually located at the level of the first lumbar vertebra in the retroperitoneal space, along the aorta at the level of the origin of the celiac artery. Fibers from this ganglion send postganglionic innervation to all the intra-abdominal organs and appear to carry pain sensation from many of the intraperitoneal organs such as the pancreas and liver. Injection into this retroperitoneal space allows anesthetic solution to diffuse around the ganglia and the splanchnic nerves to provide blockade of these fibers. This blockade produces supplementary intra-abdominal anesthesia when used in conjunction with intercostal blockade or general anesthesia. It is more commonly applied as a neurolytic sympathetic blockade for the relief of pain from malignancy of the pancreas, liver, or other upper abdominal organs.[28] The procedure for blockade follows:

1. As with intercostal blockade, the patient is placed in the prone position with the thoracic spine flexed by the use of a pillow under the abdomen.
2. The spinous processes of the 12th thoracic and the 1st lumbar vertebral bodies are identified and marked along their entire extent. The 12th rib is likewise identified and marked 7 cm from the midline. A line is drawn between the 12th ribs on each side, usually crossing the midline at the level of the spinous process of the L1 vertebra. Lines are also drawn from the spinous process of the 12th thoracic vertebra to the points on these ribs on both sides. The net result is a shallow triangle, with the spinous process of the 12th vertebra at its apex (see Fig. 27-23).
3. Skin wheals are raised bilaterally at the marks along the ribs after aseptic skin preparation. Deeper infiltration of local anesthetic with a 22-gauge needle is often helpful in improving patient tolerance of this procedure.
4. On each side, a 12.5-cm, 22- or 20-gauge needle is intro-

duced through the skin wheals and advanced anteriorly and medially and cephalad along the two lines of the triangle that was previously drawn (Fig. 27-27). The needle should be passed at approximately a 45-degree angle anteriorly so that it will contact the lateral border of the vertebral body of L1 at a depth of approximately 5 cm from the skin. (The 12th spinous process partially overlies the L1 vertebral body.)

5. When contact with a vertebral body is made, the needle is withdrawn several centimeters, and the angle of insertion is steepened so that it advances more anteriorly with subsequent passage, in the hope that it will walk off the anterior border of the vertebral body. The periosteum may be encountered several times during this attempt and should always be palpated gently because of the associated discomfort. Intravenous sedation may be required for tolerance of this blockade, although it must be kept to a minimum if evaluation of a diagnostic pain blockade is desired.

6. Once the anterior border of the vertebral body is reached, the needle is advanced 2–3 cm beyond this, and careful aspiration is performed. On the left side, advancement should be halted whenever aortic pulsation is appreciated. If the artery is unintentionally punctured, the needle should be withdrawn slightly and cleared immediately of blood. On the right side, the needle can often be advanced 1–2 cm further than the needle on the left side.

7. If radiologic confirmation is desired, it is obtained at this point, before injection of the anesthetic. The bony landmarks themselves are usually sufficient to identify the retroperitoneal space anterior to the first lumbar vertebral body. If neurolytic agents are to be used or if the anatomy is difficult, radiographic confirmation may be desirable. Although simple flat-plate radiographs are usually sufficient, fluoroscopy may be indicated in difficult cases. The use of a computed tomographic scan is not economically justified except in the most difficult of anatomic localizations.

8. Careful aspiration is performed, and a test dose is injected on each side to rule out subarachnoid or intravascular injection.

9. A large volume of local anesthetic solution is required. Twenty to 25 ml of 0.75% lidocaine or 0.25% bupivacaine is usually adequate, but a large volume is needed to diffuse in the retroperitoneal space to reach the ganglia.

10. The most reliable sign of successful anesthesia is the disappearance of pain in patients or the appearance of hypotension in normal patients. Patients with pain must remain supine for several hours and should have appropriate iv fluid supplementation to avoid orthostatic hypotension. Gradual ambulation is mandatory.

Hypotension is the most common complication of celiac plexus blockade. As mentioned previously, it can be reduced by the administration of 1 liter of balanced salt solution before performing the blockade. The most serious complication is the development of paralysis from unrecognized subarachnoid injection of a neurolytic drug. Radiographic confirmation of needle location is advisable before injection of any neurolytic drug. Even with correct placement of neurolytic drugs, back pain is common and patients may require iv opioids. This pain can be reduced by diluting the alcohol solution with an equal volume of local anesthetic such that a total volume of 50 ml is injected, consisting of 25 ml of alcohol and 25 ml of anesthetic. Even with this approach, diaphragmatic irritation (manifested as shoulder pain) is not uncommon. The duration of pain relief in the patient with chronic pain is unpredictable but is often 2–6 months. The blockade can be repeated as often as necessary, although a trial diagnostic blockade with a local anesthetic agent is indicated before each use of neurolytic drugs. One minor side effect of celiac plexus blockade is the increased peristalsis of the gut that is produced by the shift in the balance of the parasympathetic and sympathetic innervations. This may produce diarrhea within the first 12 hours after the blockade and may be a source of relief to patients on chronic opioid therapy for cancer pain.

Lumbar

Lumbar sympathetic blockade combines some of the anatomic considerations for stellate ganglion blockade and paravertebral anesthesia. As with the sympathetic innervation of the head and arm, the sympathetic nerves to the lower extremities all exit the cord above L2 and all pass through a common "gateway" ganglion in the sympathetic chain at the L2 level. Thus, as in the neck, sympathetic blockade of the lower extremity can be achieved by a single injection of one ganglion. The approach to this ganglion is similar to paravertebral anesthesia, as discussed previously, except that in the lumbar region, the sympathetic chain lies much more anterior from the somatic nerves, and thus a clean separation of sympathetic blockade from somatic blockade can be attained more easily.

As in the upper extremity, lumbar sympathectomy can be used in the treatment of sympathetic dystrophies or herpes zoster in an early stage. It is also occasionally used in patients with severe vascular disease in the lower extremities to give some indication of whether the patient would profit from permanent chemical or surgical sympathectomy. The procedure for blockade follows:

1. The patient position is similar to that for celiac plexus blockade. The patient lies prone with a pillow under the lumbar spine.

2. The spinous processes of L2 and L3 are identified and marked over their entire course. A horizontal line is drawn through the midpoint of the L2 spinous process and extended 5 cm to either side of the midline. An "X" is placed at this point, which should overlie the space between the

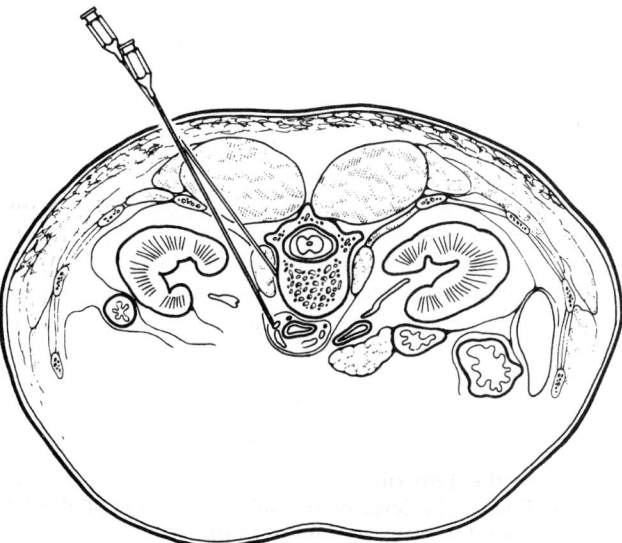

Figure 27-27. Celiac plexus blockade. The surface landmarks are described in Figure 27-23. The needles are advanced medially and superiorly to contact the lateral aspect of the vertebral body. They are then advanced more anteriorly to pass beyond the vertebra to the prevertebral space, where the greater and lesser splanchnic nerves and their subsequent celiac plexus lie. No attempt is made to advance the needles to the anterior aspect of the vessels. (Reproduced with permission from Mulroy M: Handbook of Regional Anesthesia. Boston, Little, Brown, 1996.)

transverse process of the second and third vertebrae or the caudad edge of the second transverse process.

3. A skin wheal is raised after aseptic skin preparation at each "X."

4. A 10-cm needle is introduced on each side through the "X," angled 30–45 degrees cephalad, and advanced until it contacts the transverse process (Fig. 27-28).

5. The depth of the needle insertion is marked, and the needle is then withdrawn slightly, angled caudad, and walked inferiorly off the transverse process (usually in a direction perpendicular to the skin). A slight medial angulation is used in the hope of contacting the vertebral body below the transverse process. The needle is advanced 5 cm below the depth of the transverse process. If it encounters a vertebral body, it is angled slightly more anteriorly to walk off that body at the desired depth.

6. Once the needle is in position, careful aspiration is performed, and a test dose is injected on both sides. Ten ml of local anesthetic solution injected on each side should produce sympathetic blockade. Again, 1% lidocaine, 0.25% bupivacaine, or an equivalent concentration is more than sufficient to produce sympathetic nerve blockade. If a neurolytic drug such as phenol is used, confirmation of needle position by radiography should be obtained. A slightly more caudad site of injection may be more effective for neurolytic blockade;[29] injection of smaller quantities at several levels may be more appropriate for neurolytic drugs.

7. Care is taken not to inject anesthetic solution as the needle is withdrawn, because this may produce a somatic nerve blockade as the needle passes the course of the L2 nerve root.

8. Vasodilatation and increase in skin temperature should be noted within the leg in 5–10 minutes. This can be quantitated objectively if a skin temperature probe is placed on the foot before the start of the blockade.

Complications with this technique are unusual, but, again, intravascular or subarachnoid injection can be a potential problem. The most troublesome and frequent complication is simultaneous blockade of the L2 somatic nerve root. This produces a band of anesthesia across the lateral and anterior thigh, which may confuse the evaluation of a diagnostic sympathetic blockade.

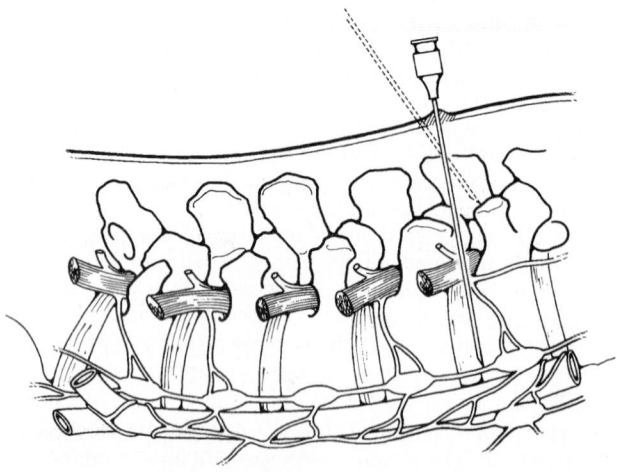

Figure 27-28. Lumbar sympathetic blockade. The needle is first placed on the transverse process of L2 and then advanced below it to pass 5 cm deeper. The needle can be angled slightly medially to contact the body of the vertebra; the sympathetic chain lies along the anterior margin of these bodies. (Reproduced with permission from Mulroy M: Handbook of Regional Anesthesia. Boston, Little, Brown, 1996.)

Hypogastric Plexus

At the terminal end of the prevertebral sympathetic chain is the superior hypogastric plexus, which extends from the lower one third of the fifth lumbar vertebral body to the upper third of the first sacral vertebral body. Fibers passing through this ganglion provide visceral sensation to the pelvic organs. Malignancies in the pelvis often produce chronic pain syndromes that involve transmission of nociception through this ganglion plexus, and significant relief can be obtained by the performance of neurolytic blocks in this area.[30]

1. The patient is placed in the prone position with a pillow under the pelvis to reduce the lumbar lordosis.

2. The L4–5 intervertebral space is identified and marked, and a line drawn at the midline of this space. An "X" is then placed on the skin 5–7 cm lateral to this interspace on both sides.

3. Aseptic skin preparation is performed, and a skin wheal raised at the "X" marks at each side.

4. Fifteen cm, 22-gauge needles are then introduced through the skin wheals and direct medially. Both needles are advanced at approximately a 45-degree angle with a 30-degree caudad deflection to approach the anterolateral body of the L5–S1 space. If the L5 vertebral body is encountered, the needle is redirected more anteriorly. The use of fluoroscopy and contrast dye can document the correct placement of the needles just anterior to the L5–S1 intervertebral space.

5. After careful aspiration to exclude intervascular placement, anesthesia can be obtained with 8 ml of 0.25% bupivacaine for a diagnostic block. For neurolytic procedures, an equal volume of 10% phenol can be used on each side.

The major risk of this block is intervascular placement of the drug. The side effects and complications of neurolytic agents apply here if they are used.

Lower Extremity

The nerves to the lower extremity are most easily blocked by the spinal, caudal, or epidural techniques described in Chapter 26. There are occasions when anesthesia by these routes is contraindicated because of systemic sepsis or coagulopathy, or when selective anesthesia of one leg or foot is needed. Peripheral nerve blockade is possible because the motor and sensory fibers to the lower extremities are somewhat similar to those of the upper extremities in that they form a series of intertwined branching roots and divisions that are enclosed in a fascial sheath before they emerge as the terminal nerves to the extremity. They can also be successfully blocked by a single injection in one plane, although the anatomic landmarks identifying this fascial sheath are not as clearly defined as those in the upper extremity. Because of this, the majority of lower extremity blockades are performed more distally, where the nerves have already separated into terminal branches. Thus, in addition to the fascial compartment approach (psoas blockade), there are peripheral approaches described at the hip, knee, and ankle.

The nerves to the legs emerge from the roots of L2 through the third sacral spinal segments (Fig. 27-29). The upper nerve roots from L2 to L4 form the lumbar plexus, which then ramifies eventually to form the lateral femoral cutaneous, femoral, and obturator nerves. These primarily provide sensorimotor innervation of the upper leg, although a branch of the femoral nerve commonly extends along the medial side of the knee as far down as the big toe. A branch of this lumbar plexus, the lumbosacral trunk of L4 and L5, joins the sacral fibers to form the major trunks of the large nerve of the posterior thigh and lower leg, the sciatic. The sciatic nerve is made up of two main trunks, the tibial and the common peroneal, which divide just

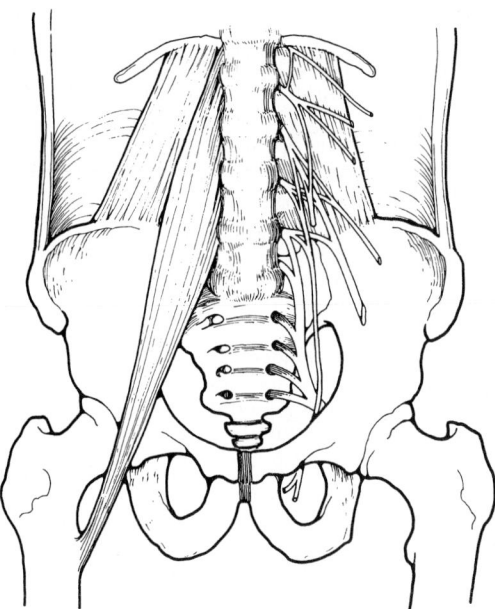

Figure 27-29. Psoas compartment anatomy. The roots of the lumbar plexus emerge from their foramina into a fascial plane between the quadratus lumborum muscle posteriorly and the psoas muscle anteriorly. The origin of the lumbosacral plexus is broader than the corresponding brachial plexus in the neck, and the lower sacral roots cannot be easily reached by a single injection. (Reproduced with permission from Mulroy M: Handbook of Regional Anesthesia. Boston, Little, Brown, 1996.)

above the knee. As in the brachial plexus, the upper nerve roots emerge from their foramina into a compartment lined by the fasciae of muscles anterior and posterior to it. In this case, the quadratus lumborum is posterior, whereas the posterior fascia of the psoas muscle provides the anterior border of the compartment. The sacral roots have a similar envelope except that the posterior border is the bone of the ilium, which prevents approach with a needle.

The lumbar plexus branches form their three terminal nerves early. Each of these passes anteriorly and laterally to circle around the pelvis and emerge anteriorly in the groin. The femoral nerve is the only one to continue in the fascial compartment formed by the psoas fascia as it passes into the groove between the psoas and the iliac muscles. The femoral nerve becomes associated with the femoral artery in the area of the groin and passes under the inguinal ligament just lateral to the artery. The lateral femoral cutaneous nerve migrates laterally early and passes under the inguinal ligament near the anterosuperior iliac spine. The third branch of the lumbar plexus, the obturator, remains somewhat medial and posterior in the pelvis and emerges under the superior ramus of the pubis through the obturator foramen to supply motor and sensory fibers to the medial thigh and medial border of the knee.

The branches of the sacral plexus also travel laterally within the pelvis before exiting posteriorly through the sciatic notch as the sciatic nerve. This largest nerve of the body is actually the conjunction of two trunks. The lateral trunk forms from the roots of L4 through S2 and eventually emerges as the common peroneal nerve. Other branches of L4 through S3 form the medial trunk, eventually becoming the tibial nerve. These combined nerves exit through the sciatic notch and pass anteriorly to the piriformis muscle between the ischial tuberosity and the greater trochanter of the femur. They curve caudad and descend the posterior thigh immediately behind the femur. After their bifurcation high in the popliteal fossa, the peroneal nerve provides the motor and sensory fibers to the anterior calf and

dorsum of the foot, whereas the tibial nerve remains posterior and provides sensation to the calf and sole of the foot. Thus, there are three major branches that cross the knee: the femoral, tibial, and peroneal. By the time these nerves reach the ankle, there are five branches that cross this joint to provide innervation for the skin and muscles of the foot.

Psoas Compartment Blockade

As described previously, the roots of the lumbar plexus lie in an envelope similar to the interscalene fascial compartment in the neck (see Fig. 27-29). Unfortunately, this fascial compartment is more difficult to identify in the lower than in the upper extremity and lies much deeper beneath the skin than its equivalent in the neck. Nevertheless, psoas compartment blockade is useful if single-injection anesthesia of the leg is desired.[31] The procedure for blockade follows:

1. The patient is placed in the prone or the lateral position. The spinous processes of the lumbar vertebrae are identified, and an "X" is placed on the skin 5 cm lateral to the spinous process of L3. This is similar to the technique described for lumbar paravertebral blockade.
2. After aseptic preparation, a skin wheal is raised at the "X." A 10-cm needle is advanced perpendicular to the skin in all planes and passed through the muscles of the back. The nerve roots should lie at a depth of between 7 and 10 cm. Although in some patients the well demarcated fascial planes can identify the entry into the perineural sheath, anesthesia is much more reliable if paresthesias are obtained. If they are not obtained at a 10-cm depth, probing with the needle in a fan-like manner should be performed in a cephalad-caudad plane (which is perpendicular to the known paths of the emerging nerves).
3. When a paresthesia is obtained, the needle is fixed in position and careful aspiration and administration of a test dose are used to rule out intravascular or subarachnoid placement. Forty ml of local anesthetic solution is usually required to fill the sheath. Lidocaine 1.5% or bupivacaine 0.5% is adequate to provide sensory and motor anesthesia. Lower concentrations provide adequate sensory anesthesia with less profound motor blockade. Fifteen to 20 minutes may be required for spread of the anesthetic to all the roots of the lumbosacral plexus. It may take longer to produce anesthesia of the caudad branches (the lower sacral fibers that form the tibial nerve), or they may not be anesthetized at all.[32]

Complications of this technique are rare, although hematoma in the muscle sheath and neuropathy of the nerves are possible. Inadequate anesthesia of some of the branches may occur more frequently than these rare complications.

Anesthesia at the Level of the Hip

Many anesthesiologists feel more confident when administering regional anesthesia in the hip region when paresthesias are sought for each of the major nerves. This technique is cumbersome and usually requires the patient to assume at least two separate positions for the injections. The anesthesia is more reliable but also requires a larger volume of anesthetic drug. Each of the four nerves may be blocked selectively on an individual basis. Anesthesia of the lateral femoral cutaneous nerve is occasionally used to provide sensory anesthesia for obtaining a skin graft from the lateral thigh. It can also be blocked as a diagnostic tool to identify cases of meralgia paresthetica. A sciatic nerve blockade alone provides adequate anesthesia for the sole of the foot and lower leg. Procedures on the knee require anesthesia of the femoral and the obturator nerves. Anesthesia of the lateral femoral cutaneous is also required if a tourniquet is to be placed on the thigh during foot surgery. Femoral nerve block provides significant postoperative analgesia for the first 18 hours after total knee arthroplasty,[33] and the use of a continuous technique can facilitate rehabilitation.[1]

Sciatic Nerve Blockade, Classic Posterior Approach

1. The patient lies with the side to be blocked uppermost and rolls slightly anterior, flexing the knee so that the ankle of the involved side rests on top of the knee of the opposite side (Fig. 27-30). This position rotates the femur so that the trochanter is more easily palpated and the muscles overlying the sciatic nerve become stretched.
2. The superior aspect of the greater trochanter of the hip is marked with a circle. A similar circle is placed on the posterosuperior iliac spine, and a line is drawn between these two points.
3. A perpendicular line is drawn from the midpoint of this original line and extended 5 cm in the caudad direction. An "X" is marked at this point. A third line drawn between the greater trochanter and the sacral hiatus should intersect this "X." In the taller patient, the original perpendicular may need to be extended caudad to intersect with the third line, and the nerve may lie closer to the intersection of the second and third lines than to the original "X."
4. A skin wheal is raised at the "X" after aseptic skin preparation.
5. A 10-cm needle is introduced perpendicular to the skin in all planes, and paresthesias or motor responses of the lower leg and foot are sought. If they are not obtained at the full depth of the needle, the needle is withdrawn to the skin and reintroduced in a fanwise fashion in a path perpendicular to the imagined course of the nerve in the hip. This path can usually be visualized by following the muscular groove on the back of the thigh up and into the imagined position of the sciatic notch. The bony edges of the sciatic notch itself may be encountered. These should be noted, and the search continued. The nerve should lie at approximately this depth as it emerges from

inside the pelvis. Nerve localization is critical because blind infiltration of a large quantity of local anesthetic rarely produces adequate anesthesia. If localization cannot be obtained in the first 10 minutes, the landmarks should be reassessed.

6. When a paresthesia or motor response in the foot is obtained, the needle is held immobile, and 25 ml of local anesthetic is injected. Again, 1.5% lidocaine, 0.5% bupivacaine, or the equivalent is adequate. A lower concentration may be needed if several nerves are to be blocked, which requires a large total volume of anesthetic in several locations.

Sciatic Nerve Blockade, Supine Approach (Lithotomy).
If a patient is uncomfortable in the lateral position or cannot be turned to the side because of a fracture or pain, the nerve can be blocked with the patient in the supine position. An assistant is required to elevate the leg into a lithotomy-type position so that the posterior aspect can be reached. The procedure for blockade follows:

1. With the patient supine, the hip is flexed by an assistant so that the upper leg is at a 90-degree angle to the torso.
2. The greater trochanter is identified as well as the ischial tuberosity, and a line is drawn between these two. An "X" is marked on the midpoint of this line.
3. A skin wheal is raised at the "X" after aseptic skin preparation. A 10-cm needle is introduced, and paresthesias are sought in a direction along the length of this line (which is perpendicular to the course of the nerve).
4. When a paresthesia or motor response in the foot is obtained, 25 ml of local anesthetic is injected.

Lateral Femoral Cutaneous Nerve Blockade.
The other three nerves of the leg can be blocked at the level of the hip with the patient in the supine position. If no paresthesias are sought, the patient can be sedated more heavily than was used for the sciatic nerve blockade.

1. In the supine position, the anterosuperior iliac spine is identified and marked. An "X" is placed on the skin 2.5 cm below and 2.5 cm medial to the spine.
2. A skin wheal is raised at the "X" after aseptic preparation.
3. A 3.75-cm, 22-gauge needle is introduced through the wheal and directed laterally until a "pop" is felt as it pierces the fascia lata. Three to 5 ml of local anesthetic solution is injected as the needle is withdrawn slowly. The needle is then reinserted slightly medially, and the procedure is repeated until a "wall" of anesthesia has been spread over a 5-cm area above and below the fascia lata extending medially from the level of the anterosuperior spine. A total of 15–20 ml of local anesthetic may be required. No paresthesias are sought.

Femoral Nerve Blockade.
This blockade can be performed blindly, or paresthesias or nerve stimulation can be sought for a "three-in-one" blockade [see Lumbar Plexus ("Three-in-One") Blockade]. The procedure for blockade follows:

1. In the supine position, a line is drawn from the anterosuperior iliac spine to the pubic tubercle. The femoral artery is identified as it passes below this line, and an "X" is marked on the skin lateral to the artery 2.5 cm below the line.
2. After aseptic preparation, a skin wheal is raised at the mark.
3. A 5-cm, 22-gauge needle is introduced through the "X" and passed perpendicular to the skin until it lies next to the artery and slightly deep to it (Fig. 27-31). Entry into the vessel is not sought, but the needle should be easily perceived to be moving with pulsation of the vessel if it is in sufficient proximity.

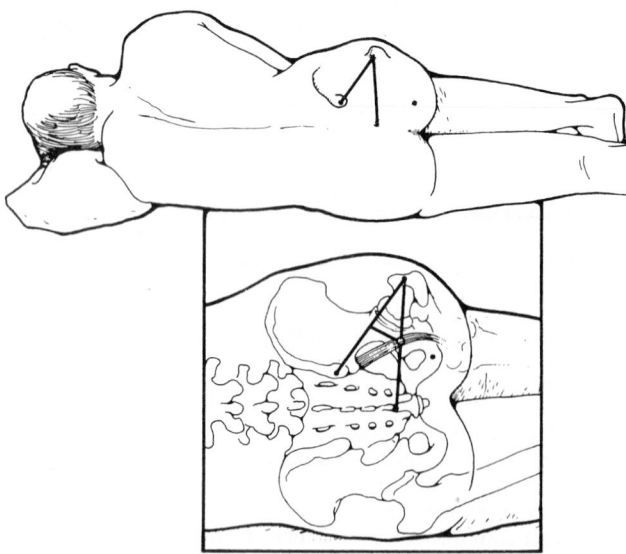

Figure 27-30. Sciatic nerve blockade, classic posterior approach. With the patient in the lateral position and the hip and knee flexed, the muscles overlying the sciatic nerve are stretched to allow easier identification. The nerve lies beneath a point 5 cm caudad along the perpendicular line that bisects the line joining the posterosuperior iliac spine and the greater trochanter of the femur. This is also usually the intersection of that perpendicular line with another line joining the greater trochanter and the sacral hiatus. (Reproduced with permission from Mulroy M: Handbook of Regional Anesthesia. Boston, Little, Brown, 1996.)

4. The needle is then reinserted slightly more laterally, and the process is repeated again until 20 ml of anesthetic solution has been injected to form another "wall" along the presumed path of the obturator nerve (see Fig. 27-31).

Lumbar Plexus ("Three-in-One") Blockade. Winnie *et al*[34] have popularized the concept of a single-injection blockade for the lumbar plexus, utilizing the fascial plane that the femoral nerve travels in as it crosses the pelvis. The object of this blockade is to inject a large quantity of local anesthetic solution in this plane so that it will spreads upward into the pelvis and anesthetize the obturator and lateral femoral cutaneous nerves at the point where they still travel in conjunction with the femoral nerve. Unfortunately, the obturator is frequently missed with this technique.[32] Because it is essential to have the needle exactly in the plane of the nerve, eliciting paresthesias or use of nerve stimulation is critical for this approach. The procedure for blockade follows:

1. Preparation for femoral nerve blockade is made as described previously.
2. The needle is inserted in a cephalad manner rather than in a perpendicular angle recommended previously. It is advanced alongside the artery angled at about 45 degrees so that it passes under the inguinal ligament. A paresthesia is sought, recognizing that the nerve lies slightly posterior to and occasionally partially under the femoral artery. When the paresthesia is obtained, the needle is fixed and the fingers of an assistant are used to compress the femoral artery and the neural sheath below the inguinal ligament while the operator injects 40 ml of anesthetic solution. The injection is performed incrementally after careful aspiration.

Complications of these techniques are rare. Hematomas can occur in any of the areas of injection and are annoying but rarely serious. The problem of systemic toxicity is a major one because of the large volumes of anesthetic solution required. As mentioned previously, careful attention must be paid to the total-milligram dose involved when multiple injections are used. Neuropathy is a possibility. Intraneural injection must be avoided by watching for signs of any discomfort at the time of actual injection. If the technique is used for analgesia following outpatient surgery, quadriceps weakness may limit ambulation, and crutches may be needed to enable patient discharge home.

Popliteal Fossa Blockade

The nerves of the lower leg can also be anesthetized by injections at the level of the knee.[35] The success of this technique depends on locating the sciatic nerve near its bifurcation into the tibial and peroneal branches high in the popliteal fossa (Fig. 27-32). Supplemental anesthesia of the femoral nerve is needed to block its terminal saphenous branch, which serves the medial anterior calf and the dorsum of the foot. The procedure for blockade follows:

Classical Approach

1. The patient is placed in a prone position. The triangular borders of the popliteal fossa are outlined by drawing the borders of the biceps femoris and the semitendinosus muscles. The base of the triangle is the skin crease behind the knee. The patient can help identify the muscles by slightly flexing the lower leg.
2. After the triangle is drawn, a perpendicular line is drawn from the midpoint of the base to the apex of the triangle. Six centimeters from the base, an "X" is drawn 1 cm lateral to this bisecting line.
3. After aseptic skin preparation, a skin wheal is raised at the "X."
4. A 7.5- or 10-cm needle is introduced through the "X" and directed 45 degrees cephalad along the middle of the

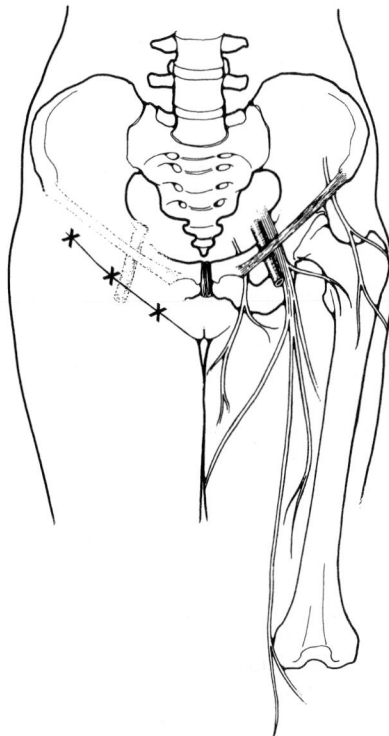

Figure 27-31. Blockade of the anterior lumbosacral branches in the groin. The lateral femoral cutaneous nerve emerges approximately 2.5 cm medial to the anterosuperior iliac spine and is best blocked 2.5 cm caudad to this point. The femoral nerve emerges alongside and slightly posterior to the femoral artery and is again easily approached approximately 2.5 cm below the inguinal ligament. On that same line, the obturator nerve emerges from the obturator canal but is deeper and less reliably located. (Reproduced with permission from Mulroy M: Handbook of Regional Anesthesia. Boston, Little, Brown, 1996.)

4. Five ml of local anesthetic is injected slowly as the needle is withdrawn. The needle is then reinserted slightly more laterally, and the process is repeated again until another "wall" of anesthesia has been laid down lateral to and slightly deep to the femoral artery.
5. Anesthesia of the medial thigh should ensue within 5–10 minutes.

Obturator Nerve Blockade. This nerve is more difficult to locate because of its depth, but anesthesia is essential for operations in the area of the knee. The procedure for blockade follows:

1. In the supine position, the pubic tubercle is identified and an "X" is placed 1.5 cm below and 1.5 cm lateral to this structure. This should lie medial to the femoral artery, and a line drawn between the three "X's" used for these three nerve blockades should be parallel to the line between the superior spine and the pubic tubercle.
2. After aseptic skin preparation, a skin wheal is raised at the "X," and a 7.5-cm, 22-gauge needle is introduced through the "X" perpendicular to the skin.
3. The needle is advanced until it contacts bone, which should be the inferior ramus of the pubis. The needle is withdrawn slightly and redirected laterally and slightly caudad to enter the obturator foramen. It is advanced another 2-3 cm, and 5 ml of anesthetic is injected as the needle is withdrawn through the presumed depth of the obturator foramen.

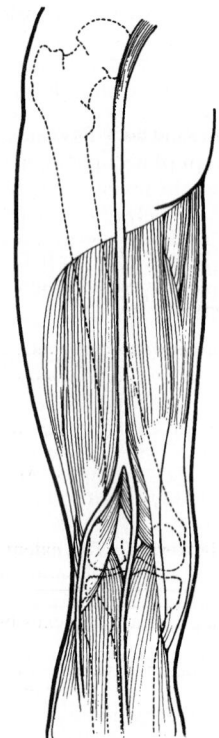

Figure 27-32. Popliteal fossa blockade. The two major trunks of the sciatic bifurcate in the popliteal fossa 7–10 cm above the knee. A triangle is drawn using the heads of the biceps femoris and the semitendinosus muscles and the skin crease of the knee; a long needle is inserted 1 cm lateral to a point 5 cm cephalad on the line from the skin crease that bisects this triangle. (Reproduced with permission from Mulroy M: Handbook of Regional Anesthesia. Boston, Little, Brown, 1996.)

triangle (Fig. 27-33). The nerves should be passing down the back of the leg parallel to the bisecting line of the triangle. A fanwise search is conducted perpendicular to this line until the nerve is contacted. If the femur is contacted by the needle, the depth is noted. The nerve should lie midway between the skin and the femur.

5. Once a paresthesia or response to a stimulator is obtained, the needle is fixed in position and 30–40 ml of local anesthetic solution is injected.

6. The femoral branches can be injected in the same position

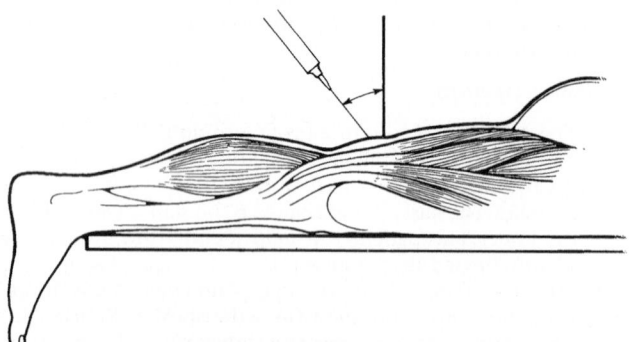

Figure 27-33. Popliteal fossa blockade, needle direction. The needle is inserted at the point described in Figure 27-32 and angled 45 degrees cephalad. The nerves usually are contacted halfway between the skin and the femur. (Reproduced with permission from Mulroy M: Handbook of Regional Anesthesia. Boston, Little, Brown, 1996.)

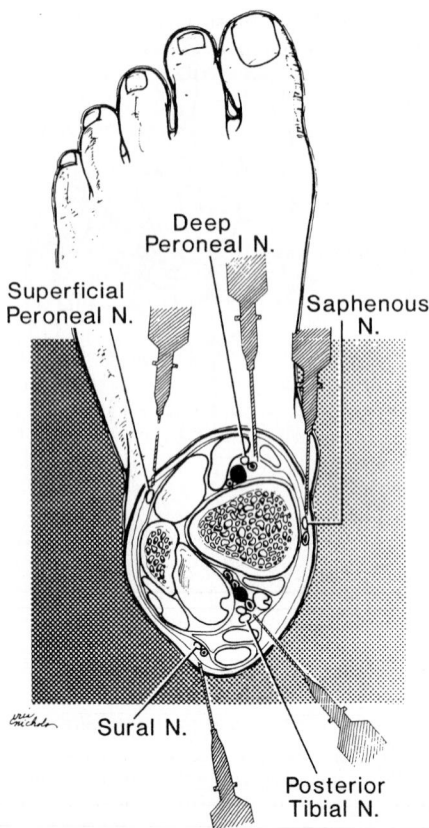

Figure 27-34. Ankle blockade. Injections are made at five separate nerve locations. The superficial peroneal nerve, sural nerve, and saphenous nerve are usually blocked simply by subcutaneous infiltration because they may have already generated many superficial branches as they cross the ankle joint. Paresthesias can be sought in the posterior tibial or the deep peroneal nerve, but the bony landmarks usually suffice to provide adequate localization for the deeper injections. (Reproduced with permission from Mulroy M: Handbook of Regional Anesthesia. Boston, Little, Brown, 1996.)

by raising a subcutaneous wheal of 5–10 ml of local anesthetic along the medial tibial head just below the knee.

Lateral Approach. An alternative approach to the block of the popliteal fossa is from the lateral side while the patient is lying supine.[36]

1. On the lateral side of the knee, the groove between the biceps femoris tendon and the vastus lateralis muscle is identified and marked. An "X" is placed 7 cm cephalad to the lateral femoral epicondyle.

2. A 22 gauge, 10-cm needle is inserted at this mark at a horizontal plane. The shaft of the femur is usually contacted within about 5 cm. The needle is then redirected 30 degrees posteriorly to search for the sciatic nerve or its divisions at approximately the same depth of the femur. A paresthesia or motor response to nerve stimulation in the foot identify the nerve, usually the common peroneal nerve which lies laterally. A second stimulation or paresthesia of the tibial nerve may be sought. 10–15 ml of anesthesia injected around each nerve provides adequate anesthesia.

Ankle Blockade

All the nerves of the foot can be blocked at the level of the ankle.[37] Although this approach is ideal in producing the least amount of immobility of the lower extremity, it is technically more difficult because at least five nerves must be anesthetized (Fig. 27-34). Several of these nerves can be blocked by simple infiltration of a "wall" of anesthesia, but increased reliability can be produced by seeking paresthesias of the major branches. If paresthesias are not sought, this blockade may actually be less time consuming than other techniques, even though five separate injections are required. The procedure for blockade follows:

1. Posterior tibial nerve. The posterior tibial nerve is the major nerve to the sole of the foot. It can be approached with the patient either in the prone position or with the hip and knee flexed so that the foot rests on the bed. The medial malleolus is identified, along with the pulsation of the posterior tibial artery behind it. A needle is introduced through the skin just behind the posterior tibial artery and directed 45 degrees anteriorly, seeking a paresthesia in the sole of the foot. Five ml of a local anesthetic produce anesthesia if a paresthesia is identified. If not, a fan-shaped injection of 10 ml can be performed in the triangle formed by the artery, the Achilles tendon, and the tibia itself.

2. Sural nerve. With the foot in the same position, the other posterior nerve of the ankle can be blocked by injection on the lateral side. The subcutaneous injection of a ridge of anesthesia behind the lateral malleolus, filling the groove between it and the calcaneus, produces anesthesia of the sural nerve. This will require another 5 ml of local anesthetic.

3. Saphenous nerve. The last three branches of the ankle lie anteriorly. The patient is either turned supine, or the leg can now be extended so that the anesthesiologist's attention is turned to the anterior surface. The saphenous nerve is anesthetized by infiltrating 5 ml of local anesthetic around the saphenous vein at the level where this vein passes anterior to the medial malleolus. A wall of anesthesia between the skin and the bone itself suffices to block the nerve.

4. Deep peroneal nerve. This is the major nerve to the dorsum of the foot and lies in the deep plane of the anterior tibial artery. Pulsation of the artery is sought at the level of the skin crease on the anterior midline surface of the ankle. If it can be felt, 5 ml of local anesthetic is injected just lateral to this. If the artery is not palpable, the tendon of the extensor hallucis longus can be identified by asking the patient to extend the big toe. Injection can be made into the deep planes below the fascia using either one of these landmarks.

5. Superficial peroneal branches. Finally, a subcutaneous ridge of anesthetic solution is laid along the skin crease between the anterior tibial artery and the lateral malleolus. This subcutaneous ridge will overlies the previous subfascial injection for the deep peroneal nerve. Another 5–10 ml of local anesthetic may be required to cover this area.

Anesthesia of the foot should ensue within 10 minutes after performance of these five injections. Complications of this blockade are rare, although neuropathy can be produced. Care should be taken not to pin any of the deep nerves against the bone at the time of injection, and intraneural injection should be avoided as usual.

REFERENCES

1. Singelyn FJ, Deyaert M, Joris D *et al:* Effects of intravenous patient-controlled analgesia with morphine, continuous epidural analgesia, and continuous three-in-one block on post-operative pain and knee rehabilitation after unilateral total knee arthroplasty. Anesth Analg 87:88, 1998
2. Pavlin DJ, Rapp SE, Polissar NL *et al:* Factors affecting discharge time in adult outpatients. Anesth Analg 87:816, 1998
3. Selander D, Brattsand R, Lundborg G *et al:* Local anesthetics: Importance of mode of application, concentration, and adrenaline for the appearance of nerve lesions. Acta Anaesthesiol Scand 23:127, 1979
4. Ready LB, Plummer MH, Haschke RH *et al:* Neurotoxicity of intrathecal local anesthetics in rabbits. Anesthesiology 63:364, 1985
5. Selander D, Edshage S, Wolff T: Paresthesiae or no paresthesiae? Acta Anaesthesiol Scand 23:27, 1979
6. Winchell SW, Wolfe R: The incidence of neuropathy following upper extremity nerve blocks. Regional Anaesthesia 10:12, 1985
7. Moore DC, Mulroy MF, Thompson GE: Peripheral nerve damage and regional anaesthesia. Br J Anaesth 73:435, 1994
8. Smith BL: Efficacy of a nerve stimulator in regional anesthesia: Experience in a resident training programme. Anaesthesia 31:778, 1976
9. Selander D, Dhuner KG, Lundborg G: Peripheral nerve injury due to injection needles used for regional anesthesia. Acta Anaesthesiol Scand 21:182, 1977
10. Brown DL, Ransom DM, Hall JA *et al:* Regional anesthesia and local anesthetic-induced systemic toxicity: seizure frequency and accompanying cardiovascular changes. Anesth Analg 81:321, 1995
11. Stoelting RK: Postoperative ulnar nerve palsy: Is it a preventable complication? Anesth Analg 76:7, 1993
12. Lanz E, Theiss D, Jankovic D: The extent of blockade following various techniques of brachial plexus block. Anesth Analg 62:55, 1983
13. Winnie AP: Interscalene brachial plexus block. Anesth Analg 49:455, 1970
14. Urmey WF, Talts KH, Sharrock NE: One hundred percent incidence of hemidiaphragmatic paresis associated with interscalene brachial plexus anesthesia as diagnosed by ultrasonography. Anesth Analg 72:498, 1991
15. Moore DC: Regional Block. Springfield, Illinois, Charles C Thomas, 1954
16. Winnie AP, Collins VJ: The subclavian perivascular technique of brachial plexus anesthesia. Anesthesiology 25:353, 1964
17. Brown DL, Cahill DR, Bridenbaugh DL: Supraclavicular nerve block: Anatomic analysis of a method to prevent pneumothorax. Anesth Analg 76:530, 1993
18. Partridge BL, Katz J, Benirschke K: Functional anatomy of the brachial plexus sheath: Implications for anesthesia. Anesthesiology 66:743, 1987
19. Thompson GE, Rorie DK: Functional anatomy of the brachial plexus sheaths. Anesthesiology 59:117, 1983
20. Selander D: Axillary plexus block: Paresthetic or perivascular (editorial). Anesthesiology 66:726, 1987
21. Bouaziz H, Narchi P, Mercier FJ *et al:* Comparison between conventional axillary block and a new approach at the midhumeral level. Anesth Analg 84:1058, 1997
22. Grice SC, Morell RC, Balestrieri FJ *et al:* Intravenous regional anesthesia: Evaluation and prevention of leakage under the tourniquet. Anesthesiology 65:316, 1986
23. Bridenbaugh PO, DuPen SL, Moore DC *et al:* Postoperative intercostal nerve block analgesia versus narcotic analgesia. Anesth Analg 52:81, 1973
24. Coveney E, Weltz CR, Greengrass R *et al:* Use of paravertebral block anesthesia in the surgical management of breast cancer: Experience in 156 cases. Annals of Surg 227:496, 1998
25. Eason MJ, Wyatt R: Paravertebral thoracic block a reappraisal. Anaesthesia 34:638, 1979
26. Reiestad F, Stromskag KE: Intrapleural catheter in the management of postoperative pain. Regional Anaesthesia 11:89, 1986
27. Stromskag KE, Minor B, Steen PA: Side effects and complications related to intrapleural analgesia: An update. Acta Anaesthesiol Scand 34:473, 1990
28. Brown DL, Bulley K, Quiel EL: Neurolytic block for pancreatic cancer pain. Anesth Analg 66:869, 1987
29. Umeda S, Arai T, Hatano Y *et al:* Cadaver anatomic analysis of the best site for chemical lumbar sympathectomy. Anesth Analg 66:643, 1987
30. Plancarte R., de Leon-Casasola OA, El-Helaly M *et al:* Neurolytic superior hypogastric plexus block for chronic pelvic pain associated with cancer. Regional Anesthesia 22:562, 1997
31. Chayen D, Nathan H, Chayen M: The psoas compartment block. Anesthesiology 45:95, 1976
32. Parkinson SK, Mueller JB, Little WL, Bailey SL: Extent of blockade with various approaches to the lumbar plexus. Anesth Analg 68:243, 1989

33. Allen HW, Liu SS, Ware PD *et al:* Peripheral nerve blocks improve analgesia after total knee replacement surgery. Anesth Analg 87:93, 1998

34. Winnie AP, Ramamurthy S, Durrani Z: The inguinal paravascular technique of lumbar plexus anesthesia: "The 3-in-1 block." Anesth Analg 52:989, 1973

35. Rorie DK, Byer DE, Nelson DO *et al:* Assessment of block of the sciatic nerve in the popliteal fossa. Anesth Analg 59:371, 1980

36. Zetlaoui PJ, Bouaziz H: Lateral approach to the sciatic nerve in the popliteal fossa. Anesth Analg 87:79, 1998

37. Schurman DJ: Ankle block anesthesia for foot surgery. Anesthesiology 44:342, 1976

Clinical Anesthesia (4/e), edited by
Paul G. Barash, Bruce F. Cullen, and
Robert K. Stoelting. Lippincott Williams &
Wilkins, Philadelphia, © 2001.

CHAPTER 28

ANESTHESIA FOR NEUROSURGERY

AUDRÉE A. BENDO, IRA S. KASS, JOHN HARTUNG,
AND JAMES E. COTTRELL

NEUROPHYSIOLOGY AND NEUROANESTHESIA

To understand how anesthetics act on the nervous system and how these actions may affect the practice of neuroanesthesia, one first needs to understand the basic principles of neurophysiology. The following description of cellular neurophysiology provides background information only; greater detail may be sought elsewhere.[1-5]

Membrane Potentials

Neurons have an electrical potential across their cell membrane owing to different intra- and extracellular ion concentrations. These concentration differences lead to an opposing voltage called the *equilibrium potential*. The Nernst equation calculates the equilibrium potential for a single ion. The Nernst or equilibrium potential for potassium (E_K) at 37°C can be calculated using the following equation:

$$E_K = -61 \log(K_i / K_o)$$

where K_i is the potassium concentration inside the cell and K_o is its concentration outside the cell.[4] This value is approximately −90 mV, yet the membrane potential for most neurons at rest is closer to −70 mV. This is because both sodium and potassium ions contribute to the resting membrane potential. An ion's contribution to the membrane potential of a neuron is determined by its conductance, which is proportional to the membrane's permeability for that ion. Because the conductance to potassium (g_K) is much higher than the sodium conductance (g_{Na}) in an unexcited neuron, the resting membrane potential is nearer to the potassium equilibrium potential than the sodium equilibrium potential ($E_{Na} = +45$ mV). The following equation can be used to calculate a cell's membrane potential:

$$E_m = [g_K(E_K) + g_{Na}(E_{Na}) + g_X(E_X)] / (g_K + g_{Na} + g_X)$$

where X refers to any other ion.[4]

The conductance of ions across the cell membrane is through channels, which are proteins that span the membrane and have a hydrophilic pore. Many channels are predominantly permeable to one ion type. The sodium channel (Fig. 28-1) is highly selective for sodium and lets very little potassium pass through it; the potassium channel is likewise selective for potassium. These channels are controlled by gates that open and close. During rest, most of the sodium channels have their gates closed, and more of the potassium channels' gates are in the open position. The opening and closing of the ion channel's gates controls the conductance of the cell membrane for that ion.

Neurons signal over long distances by propagating action potentials, which are rapid depolarizations of the membrane, along their axons. The action potential is caused by a fast increase in the sodium conductance (because of the opening of the sodium activation gate) and a slower increase in the potassium conductance. These conductance changes are triggered by a depolarization of the cell membrane, and therefore the channels that open in response to the depolarization are described as voltage-sensitive channels. When the neuron depolarizes past a threshold voltage level, an action potential is generated. The peak voltage of the action potential is approximately +20 mV; this level is attained because, at the peak, the sodium conductance is much greater than the potassium conductance. The voltage during the action potential returns rapidly to resting levels (repolarizes) because of the following:

1. The sodium conductance shuts itself off by closing a second gate (inactivation gate) in the channel (see Fig. 28-1).
2. The potassium conductance increases due to the opening of potassium channels.

A detailed description of membrane potentials, ion channels, gating, and action potentials can be found in Aidley,[1] Hille,[2] and Kandel and Schwartz.[4]

Synaptic Transmission

Neurons communicate using chemical synapses. The chemical, called a transmitter, is released from the presynaptic neuron, diffuses across the synaptic cleft, and combines with a receptor molecule on the postsynaptic neuron. The release of the neurotransmitter is initiated by an action potential traveling down the axon of the presynaptic neuron, causing the depolarization of the presynaptic terminal. This depolarization leads to the opening of voltage-dependent calcium channels and the entry of calcium from the extracellular fluid into the terminal. Vesicles containing the neurotransmitter then fuse with the terminal membrane, releasing the neurotransmitter into the synaptic cleft. The combination of the neurotransmitter with its receptor located on the postsynaptic cell alters ion channels associated with the receptor. These channels are described as ligand-gated channels. The opening of these ion channels leads to a change in the membrane potential of the postsynaptic neuron. If the transmitter is excitatory, this postsynaptic neuron is depolarized and therefore is more likely to generate an action potential. If the transmitter is inhibitory, the neuron is hyperpolarized and is less likely to generate an action potential.

In addition to opening ion channels, neurotransmitters work through intracellular second messengers. One example of a second messenger is cyclic AMP, which activates protein kinases to phosphorylate proteins and change their activity. Ion channels may be phosphorylated, which may change their conductance. A group of proteins that bind guanosine triphosphate, called G proteins, are activated when a transmitter binds a specific receptor molecule. In some cases these G proteins activate ion channels directly, but in other cases they can either stimulate (G_s) or inhibit (G_i) adenylate cyclase, the enzyme that converts adenosine triphosphate (ATP) into cyclic AMP[1] (Fig. 28-2). G proteins can also activate the phosphatidylinositol second-messenger system; in this case, a transmitter binds to a receptor, which causes another G protein (G_p) to activate phospholipase C (Fig. 28-3). This membrane-bound enzyme breaks down a membrane phospholipid into diacylglycerol and inositol trisphosphate, both of which are second messengers. Diacylglycerol activates protein kinase C, which will then phosphorylate other proteins, whereas inositol trisphosphate increases cytosolic calcium by releasing it from intracellular stores (endoplasmic reticulum).[6]

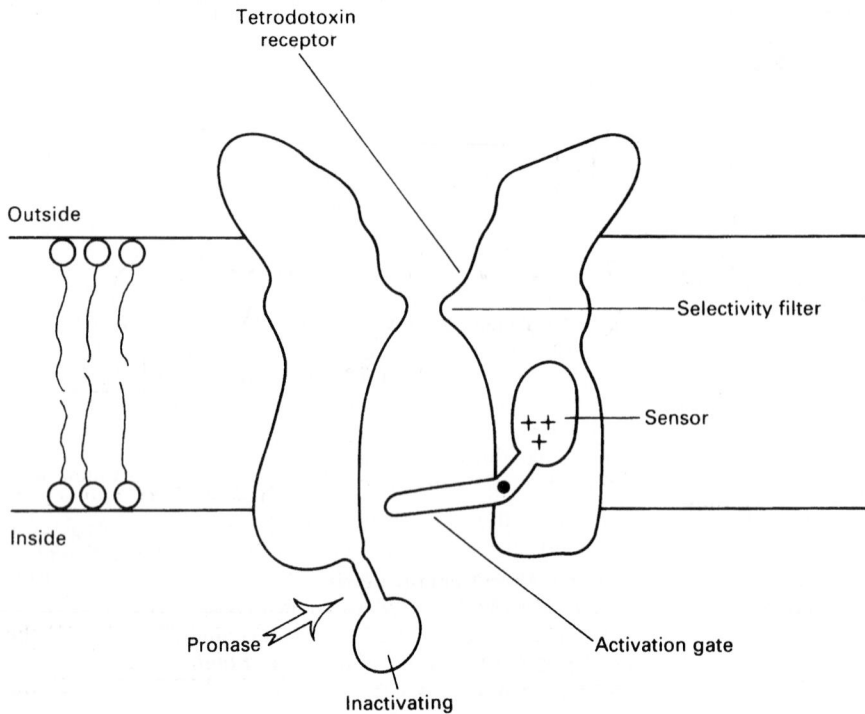

Figure 28-1. Sodium channel. The selectivity filter allows sodium but not potassium to pass through. The channel is open and allows sodium through when both the activation gate and the inactivation gate, which is also called the inactivating particle, are in the open position. Closing either gate will block the passage of ions. (Reprinted with permission from Aidley DJ: The Physiology of Excitable Cells. New York, Cambridge University Press, 1989.)

There are many neurotransmitters in the brain. In this chapter two common neurotransmitters and their receptors will be examined.

γ-Aminobutyric acid (GABA) is a major inhibitory amino acid transmitter that is active throughout the brain and reduces the excitability of neurons by hyperpolarizing them. There are two major GABA receptors. Activation of the $GABA_A$ receptor opens chloride channels[7]; this activity is enhanced by benzodiazepines and barbiturates. The $GABA_B$ receptor acts via a second messenger either to open potassium channels or to close calcium channels, but does not affect chloride channels.[8] The response to $GABA_B$ receptor activation has a slower onset and a more prolonged activation than the response to the $GABA_A$ receptor. Both receptors may be present on the same neuron, providing a mechanism for rapid and prolonged inhibition.

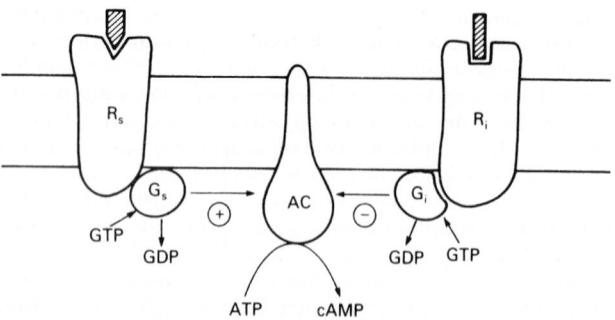

Figure 28-2. G proteins and adenylate cyclase. Different transmitters bind to either a stimulatory receptor (R_s) or an inhibitory receptor (R_i). Both are coupled to GTP-binding proteins (G proteins). G_s stimulates adenylate cyclase to increase cAMP levels; G_i inhibits adenylate cyclase and decreases cAMP levels. (Reprinted with permission from Aidley DJ: The Physiology of Excitable Cells. New York, Cambridge University Press, 1989.)

Glutamate is the major excitatory transmitter in the brain. Its activation depolarizes neurons, making it more likely that they will fire action potentials. There are three main inotropic glutamate receptors, which have been named for their preferential pharmacologic agonists. The AMPA and kainate receptors allow sodium and potassium but not calcium through their channels.[9,10] These channels are responsible for the normal excitatory responses seen with glutamate. The third glutamate receptor, the N-methyl-D-aspartate receptor (NMDA), is activated when neurons are depolarized; the channels associated with this receptor are not opened by glutamate at normal resting membrane potentials. These channels allow passage of calcium as well as sodium and potassium. NMDA receptor activation is important in changing a neuron's excitability over a period of hours and days (long-term potentiation); this has been correlated with learning in animals.[10] Glutamate receptors have also been associated with neuronal injury after anoxia.[11] In addition to inotropic effects, glutamate activates metabotropic receptors, which act via a second messenger. Inositol trisphosphate, one second messenger, releases calcium from intracellular stores (see Fig. 28-3); this can affect the excitability of the neuron.[6]

The above is a simple description of how synapses operate to convey information from one neuron to another. This process is finely controlled; there are neurotransmitters that act on presynaptic terminals to regulate the amount of transmitter the terminal releases.[3] Indeed, some neurons have receptors on their presynaptic terminals, called *autoreceptors,* that reduce the amount of transmitter that terminal releases in response to the buildup of that same transmitter in the synapse. This is a way of controlling the concentration of transmitter in the synaptic cleft. There are compounds called *neuromodulators* that, when applied to a neuron alone, have no observable effect on the excitability of that neuron but alter the effect of other excitatory or inhibitory inputs to that neuron. These neuromodulators are released in the same manner as neurotransmitters; indeed, it is possible for the same substance to be a neuromodulator at one synapse and a neurotransmitter at another. Furthermore,

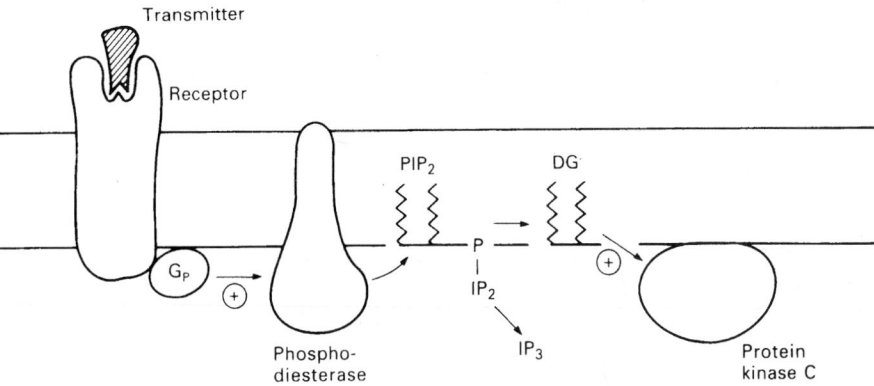

Figure 28-3. G proteins and phosphodiesterase. A transmitter binds to a receptor activating a G protein (G_p), which activates the membrane-bound enzyme phosphodiesterase. This enzyme converts phosphatidylinositol-4,5-bisphosphate (PIP_2) into inositol 1,4,5-trisphosphate (IP_3), which is water-soluble and causes the release of calcium from endoplasmic reticulum, and diacylglycerol, which is lipid-soluble and remains in the membrane to activate protein kinase C. Protein kinase C will in turn phosphorylate certain other proteins, altering their activity. (Reprinted with permission from Aidley DJ: The Physiology of Excitable Cells. New York, Cambridge University Press, 1989.)

some synapses have been shown to release two neuroactive compounds from the same presynaptic terminal; these cotransmitters can have synergistic actions on the postsynaptic terminal. Many of the peptide neurotransmitters, such as enkephalin and substance P, are released as cotransmitters with a nonpeptide transmitter (*e.g.*, norepinephrine and serotonin).

Brain Metabolism

The main substance used for energy production in the brain is glucose.[12] When oxygen levels are sufficient, glucose is metabolized to pyruvate in the glycolytic pathway (Fig. 28-4). This biochemical process generates ATP from adenosine diphosphate and inorganic phosphate and produces NADH from nicotinamide adenine dinucleotide (NAD). Pyruvate from this reaction then enters the citric acid cycle, which, with regard to energy production, primarily generates NADH from NAD. The mitochondria use oxygen to couple the conversion of NADH back to NAD with the production of ATP from ADP and inorganic phosphate. This process, called *oxidative phosphorylation,* forms three ATP molecules for each NADH converted. The process of aerobic metabolism yields 38 ATP molecules for each glucose molecule metabolized.[13]

This pathway requires oxygen; if oxygen is not present, the mitochondria can neither make ATP nor regenerate NAD from NADH. The metabolism of glucose requires NAD as a cofactor and is blocked in its absence. Thus, in the absence of oxygen, glycolysis proceeds by a modified pathway termed *anaerobic glycolysis;* this modification involves the conversion of pyruvate to lactate, regenerating NAD. There is a net hydrogen ion production, which lowers the intracellular pH. A major problem with anaerobic glycolysis, in addition to lowering pH, is that only two molecules of ATP are formed for each molecule of glucose metabolized.[13] This level of ATP production is insufficient to meet the brain's energy needs.

When the oxygen supply to a neuron is reduced, mechanisms that reduce and/or slow the fall in ATP levels include: (1) the utilization of phosphocreatine stores (a high-energy phosphate that can donate its energy to maintain ATP levels), (2) the production of ATP at low levels by anaerobic glycolysis, and (3) a rapid cessation of spontaneous electrophysiologic activity.

Pumping ions across the cell membrane is the largest energy requirement in the brain (Table 28-1). The sodium, potassium, and calcium concentrations of a neuron are maintained against large electrochemical differences with respect to the outside of the cell. When a neuron is not excited (firing action potentials), there is a slow leak of potassium out of the cells and of sodium into the cells. Neuronal activity markedly increases the flow of potassium, sodium, and calcium; this increases the rate of ion pumping required to maintain the neuron's ion concentration. Because ion pumping uses ATP as an energy source, the ATP requirement of active neurons is greater than that for resting neurons. If energy production does not meet the demand of energy use in the brain, the neurons first become unexcitable and then are irreversibly damaged.[14,15]

Neurons require energy to maintain their structure and internal function. The cell's membranes, internal organelles, and cytoplasm are made of carbohydrates, lipids, and proteins, which require energy for their synthesis. Ion channels, enzymes, and cell structural components are important protein molecules that are continuously formed, modified, and broken down in the cell. If ATP is not available, protein synthesis cannot continue and the neuron will die. Carbohydrates and lipids are also continuously synthesized and degraded in normally functioning neurons; their metabolism also requires energy. Most cellular synthesis takes place in the cell body; thus, energy is required for the transport of components down the axon to the nerve terminal. The importance of this transport is illustrated by the death of the distal end of an axon when it is severed from its cell body. Thus, energy is required to maintain the integrity of neurons even in the absence of electrophysiologic activity.

The overall metabolic rate for the brain of a young adult man (mean age, 21 years) is 3.5 ml $O_2 \cdot min^{-1} \cdot 100\ g^{-1}$ brain tissue or 5.5 mg glucose $\cdot min^{-1} \cdot 100\ g^{-1}$.[12] This rate is virtually

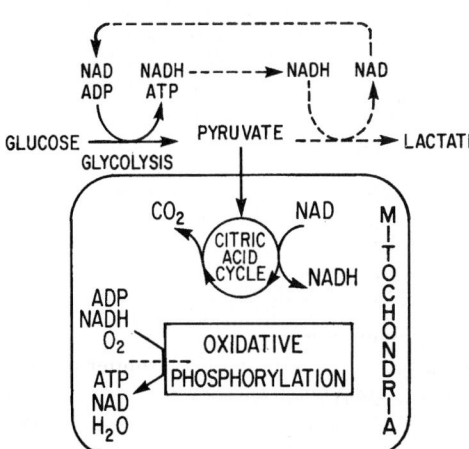

Figure 28-4. Energy metabolism in the brain. Dotted lines indicate reactions that occur during ischemia. The dotted line across the oxidative phosphorylation reaction indicates that this reaction is blocked during ischemia.

Table 28-1. CELLULAR PROCESSES THAT REQUIRE ENERGY

Pumping ions across membranes
Metabolism of proteins, lipids, carbohydrates, and other molecules
Transporting of molecules within cells

---

the same in elderly men (mean age, 71 years). Children (mean age, 6 years) have a markedly higher metabolic rate of 5.2 ml $O_2 \cdot min^{-1} \cdot 100 \ g^{-1}$ brain tissue. Although the reasons for this high metabolic rate are unknown, it may reflect extra energy requirements for the growth and development of the nervous system.[12]

Cerebral Blood Flow

The brain receives approximately 15% of cardiac output, yet makes up only 2% of total body weight.[12] The disproportionately large blood flow is due to the high metabolic rate of the brain. Global blood flow and metabolic rate remain fairly stable. Regional blood flow and metabolic rate of the brain can change dramatically; when metabolic rate goes up in a region of the brain, the blood flow to that region also increases. The mechanism of this coupling of blood flow and metabolism is not known; however, an increase in either potassium or hydrogen ion concentrations in the extracellular fluid surrounding arterioles may lead to dilatation and increased flow. Other agents that may mediate the coupling are calcium, adenosine, nitric oxide and the eicosanoids (*e.g.*, prostaglandins).[14] None of these mechanisms need be exclusive, and more than one or all of them may contribute to this exquisite coupling of flow and metabolism.

Increasing carbon dioxide level causes vasodilatation and increased blood flow (Fig. 28-5). Increasing the carbon dioxide tension from 40 to 80 mm Hg doubles the flow; reducing the carbon dioxide from 40 to 20 mm Hg halves the flow.[16,17] These changes are transient, and blood flow returns to normal in 6–8 hours, even if the altered carbon dioxide levels are maintained. These effects may be related to hydrogen ion concentration. High carbon dioxide levels increase the extracellular hydrogen ion concentration and blood flow, whereas low carbon dioxide levels decrease the extracellular hydrogen ion concentration and reduce blood flow. The bicarbonate concentration in the extracellular fluid of the brain adjusts, bringing the pH back to normal, even though the carbon dioxide levels remain altered.[18] This has important clinical implications in patients hyperventilated for prolonged periods. If normocarbia is rapidly re-established, brain interstitial fluid pH will decrease and cerebral blood flow (CBF) will increase dramatically, perhaps increasing intracranial pressure (ICP).

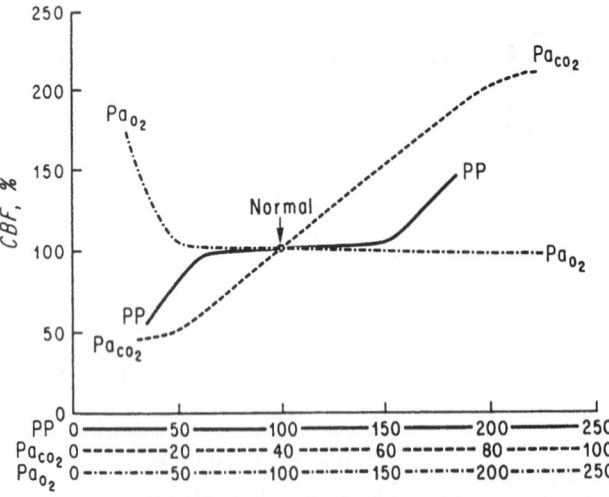

Figure 28-5. The effect of perfusion pressure (PP), arterial carbon dioxide pressure (Pa_{CO_2}), and arterial oxygen pressure (Pa_{O_2}) on cerebral blood flow. Each parameter on the abscissa is varied independently while the other parameters are held at their normal levels. (Reprinted with permission from Michenfelder JD: Anesthesia and the Brain, pp 6, 94–113. New York, Churchill Livingstone, 1988.)

If a patient is hypoventilated, carbon dioxide increases, pH decreases, and blood flow increases throughout the brain. The arterioles could become maximally dilated throughout the brain, impeding the ability to direct flow to areas of high metabolic demand. Thus, this luxury flow caused by high carbon dioxide levels throughout the brain could "steal" blood flow from areas that require extra oxygen and produce metabolites. This is particularly important during focal ischemia with the blockage of an intracerebral artery. The vessels supplying collateral flow to the area of the blocked artery would already be maximally dilated due to the metabolic demands of the ischemic tissue, and high Pa_{CO_2} would cause blood flow to be shunted away to areas of less demand.[19] The blood flow to the brain can be manipulated to advantage during focal ischemia. Reducing carbon dioxide with hyperventilation or reducing metabolism with agents such as thiopental would reduce blood flow to most areas of the brain, and the vessels in the ischemic area would be maximally dilated because of low pH. These manipulations, which are sometimes called *inverse steal* or the *Robin Hood effect* (rob from the rich, give to the poor), could have the effect of maximizing blood flow to compromised areas.[19] The clinical relevance of flow redistribution due to hypocarbia has been questioned.[20]

The CBF autoregulates with respect to pressure changes. In normotensive individuals, mean arterial pressure (MAP) can vary from 50 to 150 mm Hg and CBF will be maintained constant because of an adjustment of the cerebral vascular resistance (see Fig. 28-5). This phenomenon is a myogenic response of the arterioles due to their ability to constrict in response to an increased distending pressure. This response takes a few minutes to develop; therefore, after a rapid increase in MAP, there is a short period (about 1–3 min) of increased blood flow.[21,22] If mean blood pressure falls below 50 mm Hg, CBF is reduced; at a pressure of 40 mm Hg, mild symptoms of cerebral ischemia occur.[22,23] Patients who are hypertensive demonstrate a shift of autoregulation to a higher blood pressure.[24] Their lower limit of autoregulation could be well above 50 mm Hg; their upper limit of autoregulation is also increased. This shift, due to hypertrophy of the vessel wall, takes 1 or 2 months to become established.[23] Autoregulation can be abolished by trauma, hypoxia, and certain anesthetic and adjuvant anesthetic drugs. When blood pressure exceeds the autoregulated range, it can cause a disruption of the blood–brain barrier and cerebral edema.

The cerebral vasculature is also regulated by neurogenic factors that seem to have their greatest influence on the larger cerebral vessels. They control flow to large areas of the brain and play less of a role in the regulation of local CBF.[22] The innervation includes cholinergic, adrenergic, and serotonergic systems. Sympathetic activation leads to increased MAP and shifts the autoregulatory curve to the right, increasing the pressure at which the breakthrough of autoregulation occurs.[23]

Cerebrospinal Fluid

The neurons in the brain are exquisitely sensitive to changes in their environment. Small alterations in extracellular ion levels can profoundly alter neuronal activity. Substances that circulate in the blood, such as catecholamines, if not sequestered from direct contact with the brain, might also disrupt brain function. Thus the composition of the fluid surrounding the brain is tightly regulated and distinct from extracellular fluid in the rest of the body (Table 28-2).[25] There are two barriers, the blood–brain barrier and the blood–cerebrospinal fluid barrier, that maintain the difference between blood and cerebrospinal fluid (CSF) composition.

Brain capillary endothelial cells (the blood–brain barrier) have tight junctions that prevent extracellular passage of substances between the endothelial cells. They also have a low level of pinocytotic activity, which reduces the transport of large

Table 28-2. COMPOSITION OF CEREBROSPINAL FLUID AND SERUM IN MAN

	CSF	Serum
Sodium (mEq · l^{-1})	141	140
Potassium (mEq · l^{-1})	2.9	4.6
Calcium (mEq · l^{-1})	2.5	5.0
Magnesium (mEq · l^{-1})	2.4	1.7
Chloride (mEq · l^{-1})	124	101
Bicarbonate (mEq · l^{-1})	21	23
Glucose (mg · 100 ml^{-1})	61	92
Protein (mg · 100 ml^{-1})	28	7000
pH	7.31	7.41
Osmolality (mOsm · kg^{-1} H$_2$O)	289	289

Adapted with permission from Artru AA: Cerebrospinal fluid. In Cottrell JE, Smith DS (eds): Anesthesia and Neurosurgery, p 95. St Louis, CV Mosby, 1994.

molecules across the cells. Processes of astrocyte glial cells are interposed between the neurons of the brain and the capillaries. The functional importance of the astrocytes to the blood–brain barrier is currently unknown; however, they are located wherever the blood–brain barrier is present and appear to be necessary for the development and perhaps the maintenance of the barrier. The blood–brain barrier impedes the flow of ions such as potassium, calcium, magnesium, and sodium; polar molecules such as glucose, amino acids, and mannitol; and macromolecules such as proteins.[25] Lipid-soluble compounds, water, and gases such as carbon dioxide, oxygen, and volatile anesthetics pass rapidly through the blood–brain barrier. Many substances that do not cross the blood–brain barrier are required for brain function; these substances are transported across the capillary endothelial cell by carrier-mediated processes. These processes consist of either active transport, which requires the expenditure of energy, or passive transport, which does not. Passive transport, also referred to as *facilitated diffusion,* can move molecules into the brain only if their concentration in the blood is higher than their concentration in the brain. Glucose is an example of a molecule that enters the brain by passive transport. All of these transport processes have a limited capacity. The blood–brain barrier can become disrupted by acute hypertension, osmotic shock, disease, tumor, trauma, irradiation, and ischemia.

Cerebrospinal fluid is primarily formed in the choroid plexus of the cerebral ventricles. The capillaries of the choroid plexus have fenestrations and intercellular gaps that allow free movement of molecules across the endothelial cells; however, they are surrounded by choroid plexus epithelial cells, which have tight junctions and form the basis of the blood–CSF barrier. It is these cells that secrete the CSF. The CSF volume in the brain is between 100 and 150 ml; it is formed and reabsorbed at a rate of 0.3–0.4 ml · min^{-1}. This allows a complete replacement of the CSF volume three or four times a day. The blood–CSF barrier is similar to the blood–brain barrier in that it allows the free movement of water, gases, and lipid-soluble compounds but requires carrier-mediated active or passive transport processes for glucose, amino acids, and ions. Proteins are largely excluded from the CSF. The CSF is primarily formed by the transport of sodium, chloride, and bicarbonate with the osmotic movement of water. Two clinically used substances that reduce CSF formation are furosemide, which inhibits the combined transport of sodium and chloride, and acetazolamide, which reduces bicarbonate transport by inhibiting carbonic anhydrase.[26] The CSF flows from the lateral ventricles to the third and fourth ventricles and then to the cisterna magna. It then flows around the brain and spinal cord in the cerebral and spinal subarachnoid space. The fluid in the subarachnoid space provides cushioning for the brain, reducing the effect of head

Table 28-3. THE THREE MAJOR COMPONENTS THAT OCCUPY SPACE IN THE SKULL

The brain, which includes neurons and glia
The cerebrospinal fluid and extracellular fluid
The blood perfusing the brain

trauma. The CSF is absorbed into the venous system of the brain by the villi in the arachnoid membrane. These arachnoid villi allow one-way flow of CSF from the subarachnoid space into the venous sinuses when CSF pressure is greater than the pressure in these sinuses. Owing to the high rate of CSF formation and its absorption into the venous system, proteins and other matter released into the brain extracellular fluid are removed. If the foramina connecting the ventricles or the arachnoid villi are blocked, pressure builds and hydrocephalus develops.

Intracranial Pressure

The brain is enclosed in the cranium, which has a fixed volume; therefore, if any of the components located in the cranial vault increase in volume, the ICP will increase (Table 28-3). An increase in volume of one of these components can increase ICP and result in two major deleterious effects on the organism. The first is to reduce blood flow to the brain. The cerebral perfusion pressure (CPP) is determined by the MAP minus the ICP. If ICP increases to a greater extent than MAP, CPP is reduced. If ICP rises sufficiently, the brain can become ischemic. The second important effect of increased ICP is its ability to induce brain herniation. This herniation could be across the meninges, down the spinal canal, or through an opening in the skull. Herniation can rapidly lead to neurologic degeneration and death.

The ICP in humans is normally less than 10 mm Hg.[27] Under normal circumstances, a small increase in intracranial volume will not greatly increase ICP because of the elastance of the components located in the cranium (Fig. 28-6). After a certain point, however, the capacity of the system to adjust to increased volume is exceeded and even a small increase in volume will

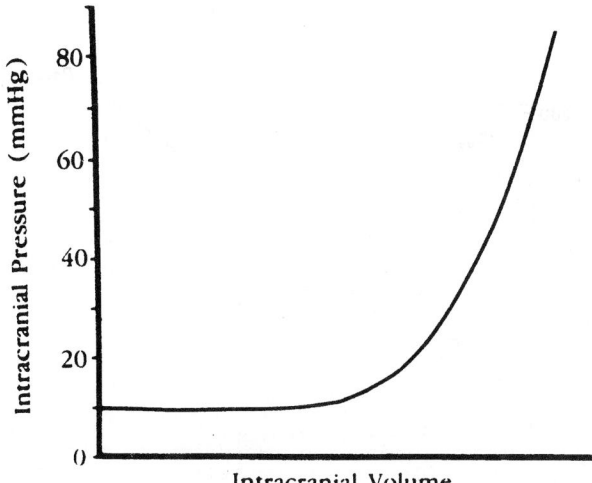

Figure 28-6. The effect of increasing volume on intracranial pressure. At first, as volume is increased, pressure does not increase, owing to the elastance of intracranial structures. This elastance is exceeded and then a small increase in volume can cause a large increase in intracranial pressure. (Modified from Miller JD, Garibi J, Pickard JD: The effects of induced changes of cerebrospinal fluid volume during continuous monitoring of ventricular pressure. Arch Neurol 28:265, 1973.)

increase ICP.[28] Increases in ICP can be caused by the following: (1) increased CSF volume due to blockage of the circulation or absorption of the CSF, as described above; (2) increased blood volume from vasodilatation or hematoma; and (3) increased brain tissue volume caused by a tumor or edema.

Brain edema is typically classified as cytotoxic or vasogenic.[29] The former is due to neuronal damage, which leads to increased sodium and water in the brain cells, and therefore an increase in intracellular volume. Vasogenic edema is caused by a breakdown of the blood–brain barrier and the movement of protein from the blood into the brain's extracellular space. Water moves osmotically with the protein, increasing the extracellular fluid volume in the brain.

Pathophysiology

The brain is the organ most sensitive to ischemia; therefore, when the blood supply to the brain is limited, ischemic damage to neurons can occur.[14] To understand the rationale for treatments used to protect the brain against ischemic damage, one needs an appreciation of the pathophysiologic mechanisms that may lead to this damage. The central event precipitating damage is reduced energy production due to blockage of oxidative phosphorylation. This causes ATP production per molecule of glucose to be reduced by 95%. At this rate of production, ATP levels fall, leading to the loss of energy-dependent homeostatic mechanisms. (Complete ischemia would block all ATP production.) The activity of ATP-dependent ion pumps is reduced and the intracellular levels of sodium and calcium increase, while intracellular potassium levels decrease (Fig. 28-7). These ion changes cause the neurons to depolarize and release excitatory amino acids such as glutamate. High levels of glutamate further depolarize the neurons and allow more calcium to enter through the NMDA receptor channel. The high intracellular calcium level is thought to trigger a number of events that could lead to the anoxic or ischemic damage. These include increasing the activity of proteases and phospholipases.[30] The latter would increase the levels of free fatty acids and free radicals. Free radicals are known to damage proteins and lipids, whereas free fatty acids interfere with membrane function. In addition, there is a buildup of lactate and hydrogen ions. All of these processes, coupled with the reduced ability to synthesize

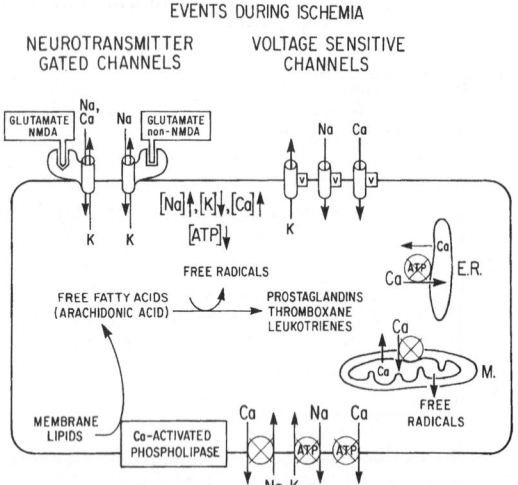

Figure 28-7. The effect of ischemia on ion and metabolite levels in neurons. For clarity, ion channels are shown on the top membrane and ion pumps on the bottom membrane; their actual location can be on any membrane surface. Circles indicate energy-driven pumps, and a crossed-through circle indicates that this pump is blocked or has reduced activity during ischemia. V indicates a voltage-dependent channel.

Table 28-4. PROCEDURES THAT MAY PROTECT AGAINST ISCHEMIC DAMAGE

Maintaining ATP levels by reducing the metabolic rate
Blocking sodium or calcium influx
Scavenging free radicals
Blocking receptors for excitatory amino acids
Maintaining blood flow

proteins and lipids due to the reduced ATP levels, may lead to irreversible damage with ischemia. In addition, phospholipase activation leads to the production of excess arachidonic acid, which, on reoxygenation, can form eicosanoids, including thromboxane, prostaglandins, and leukotrienes. Thromboxane can cause intense vasoconstriction and reduced blood flow in the postischemic period, while leukotrienes can increase edema. Thus, procedures that may protect against ischemia should interfere with these damaging mechanisms (Table 28-4). Specific agents that might accomplish these objectives will be detailed in the section on brain protection later in the chapter.

Ischemia can be either global or focal in nature; an example of the former would be cardiac arrest; of the latter, a localized stroke. The mechanisms leading to neuronal damage are probably similar for both, but there are important distinctions between the two. In focal ischemia there are three regions. The first receives no blood flow and responds the same as globally ischemic tissue; the second, called the *penumbra*, receives collateral flow and is partially ischemic; the third is normally perfused. If the insult is maintained for a prolonged period, the neurons in the penumbra will die. More neurons in the penumbra will survive if collateral blood flow is increased. Mechanisms such as inverse steal (described under Cerebral Blood Flow) will enhance collateral blood flow, and hence neuron survival, in focal but not global ischemia.

Epileptic activity is sudden, excessive, and synchronous discharges of large numbers of neurons. Aside from those patients with established epilepsy, this massive increase in activity is seen in patients with ionic and electrolyte imbalances, disorders of brain metabolism, infection, brain tumor, brain trauma, or elevated body temperature.[31] The electroencephalogram (EEG) shows spikes, which are rapid changes in voltage corresponding to excess activity in many neurons. During the epileptiform activity, sodium and calcium ions enter the cells and potassium leaves. Thus the cells use more energy (ATP) for ion pumping. High extracellular potassium may be responsible for the large and progressive depolarization of the neurons that is commonly found. The mechanisms that lead to permanent neuronal damage with epilepsy may be similar to those that damage cells during ischemia. Intracellular calcium levels rise, which may precipitate the damage. It is clear that during epileptiform activity the energy demand, and hence the cerebral metabolic rate (CMR) and blood flow, increases greatly. Thus, in conditions in which blood flow to the brain may be compromised, it is imperative to avoid excess brain activity. Anticonvulsant medications increase neuronal inhibition or reduce excitatory processes in the brain. Epileptic activity may be accompanied by systemic lactic acidosis, reduced arterial oxygenation, and increased carbon dioxide; therefore, it is important to maintain ventilation, oxygenation, and blood pressure. Prolonged or recurring epileptic activity can lead to profound brain damage.

Brain trauma can directly lead to permanent physical neuronal damage. Primary damage can also be caused by brain herniation or severing of blood vessels in the brain, resulting in direct ischemia. Reversal of the primary damage is not possible; however, much of the brain injury in trauma patients is secondary and occurs following the initial insult.[32] Calcium influx resulting from the trauma has been implicated as a trigger for the damage.[33] It is important to prevent the secondary ischemia that frequently follows brain trauma and is possibly due to the release of vasoconstrictive substances during reperfusion.[34] In addition, hemorrhage may increase intracranial blood volume and ICP, reducing CPP. The intracranial blood can be damaging by directly promoting free-radical formation using the iron in hemoglobin. Secondary damage may be reduced with proper monitoring and treatment. Treatment includes reducing ICP, maintaining blood flow, reducing vasospasm, removing blood from the subarachnoid space, and perhaps using pharmacologic agents that interfere with the cascade of events that lead to neuron damage.

Brain tumors are expanding, space-occupying lesions that may significantly increase ICP and lead to reduced CPP or brain herniation. Frequently, the blood vessels supplying the tumor have a leaky blood–brain barrier which may contribute to vasogenic brain edema and elevated ICP.

Thus, for several pathophysiologic events in the brain, ionic imbalance (particularly high intracellular calcium levels) has been implicated as a possible cause of brain damage. A common mechanism of neuronal cell death for various pathophysiologic events may exist.

NEUROANESTHESIA

Effects of Anesthetics and Other Adjunctive Drugs on Brain Physiology

Volatile Anesthetics

Halothane, enflurane, sevoflurane, desflurane, and isoflurane have direct vasodilatory effects that increase CBF (Table 28-5). Halothane with nitrous oxide (1.5 MAC) has been shown to increase blood flow almost 65%, whereas enflurane and isoflurane have a lesser effect at equal anesthetic potency.[35] Enflurane increased blood flow approximately 35%; isoflurane caused an even smaller increase. The increase in CBF returns to baseline levels approximately 3 hours after the initial exposure to 1.3 MAC of anesthetic.[36] Sevoflurane and desflurane appear similar to isoflurane with respect to CBF.[37–39] The importance of increased CBF is its influence on ICP. Increasing blood flow would tend to increase the amount of blood in the head, which could lead to increases in ICP under conditions of abnormal intracranial elastance. The volatile anesthetics reduce the CMR; isoflurane reduces the metabolic rate to a greater extent than halothane.[40] Sevoflurane and desflurane are similar to isoflurane. It is thought that isoflurane's metabolic effect, which reduces

CBF, competes with its direct vasodilatory action to limit the net increase in CBF with this agent. Enflurane has been shown to induce seizure-type discharges; this effect is potentiated by hypocapnia. Seizures induced with 1.5 MAC enflurane, hypocapnia, and an auditory stimulus increased CMR and blood flow by 50%.[41] The main advantage of desflurane over isoflurane is a faster onset and recovery from anesthesia. Studies have indicated that it can cause greater ICP increases than isoflurane in patients with altered intracranial elastance.[42] Therefore, it is not recommended for patients with space-occupying lesions. Desflurane has also been shown to cause sympathetic hyperactivity in healthy volunteers.[43] Sevoflurane has the potential for toxicity, since it can be converted to toxic agents; however, the concentration of these agents is normally below the toxic threshold.[44] Sevoflurane has been shown to be a useful alternative to halothane for pediatric induction if given with nitrous oxide.[45] Sevoflurane demonstrated cerebral protection during incomplete ischemia in rats when compared to fentanyl with nitrous oxide.[46] These considerations make sevoflurane and isoflurane the volatile anesthetics of choice for neuroanesthesia. However, both of these agents are vasodilators and have the potential to increase ICP under certain circumstances.[47,48]

Nitrous oxide can increase CBF and ICP.[49,50] Barbiturates and hypocapnia in combination may prevent these increases. There are indications that, even when given independently, barbiturates, benzodiazepines, and morphine are effective in blunting nitrous oxide's effect on CBF and ICP.[51,52] In contrast, a volatile anesthetic may add to the increases in CBF obtained with nitrous oxide.[53] Although the data on nitrous oxide's effect on brain metabolism are far from unequivocal, the evidence seems to indicate that there can be a substantial increase in CMR if nitrous oxide is administered alone.[49] Although nitrous oxide is commonly used in neuroanesthesia, its use should be carefully considered given its potential effects on CBF, CMR, and ICP.[54]

Intravenous Anesthetics

Barbiturates decrease the CMR and CBF.[55,56] A major problem with barbiturates is that they can substantially reduce MAP, which, if not controlled, can reduce CPP. At high doses (10–55 mg · kg^{-1}), thiopental can produce an isoelectric EEG and decrease the CMR by 50%.[56] This direct metabolic effect of thiopental leads to constriction of the cerebral vasculature and thereby reduces CBF. Barbiturates are also effective in reducing elevated ICP and controlling epileptiform activity.[57] Methohexital is an exception with regard to epileptiform activity; it can activate some seizure foci in patients with temporal lobe epilepsy.[58]

Etomidate, like the barbiturates, reduces CMR and CBF.[59–61] In addition to the indirect effect of reduced cerebral metabolism on blood flow, etomidate is also a direct vasoconstrictor even before metabolism is suppressed.[60] Its advantage over the barbiturates is that it does not produce clinically significant cardiovascular depression. Prolonged use of etomidate may suppress the adrenocortical response to stress.[62]

Propofol is a rapidly acting intravenous anesthetic that, like etomidate and the barbiturates, reduces the CMR and CBF.[63–65] It is able to reduce ICP; however, because it also reduces MAP, its effect on CPP must be carefully monitored.[66] Propofol demonstrated longer-lasting ventilatory depression when compared with barbiturates.[67]

Benzodiazepines have been shown to reduce CMR and CBF;[68,69] however, this effect is not as pronounced as that with the barbiturates. As with the barbiturates, the blood flow reduction by benzodiazepines is thought to be secondary to a reduction in CMR. Benzodiazepines may reduce ICP owing to their effect on CBF. Flumazenil is a benzodiazepine antagonist that has been shown to reverse the CMR, CBF, and ICP lowering effects of the benzodiazepine midazolam.[70] Thus, flumazenil should be used cautiously, if at all, in patients with high ICP or abnormal intracranial elastance.

Table 28-5. EFFECTS OF ANESTHETICS ON CBF/CMRO₂

	CBF	CMRO$_2$	Direct Cerebral Vasodilation
Halothane	↑ ↑ ↑	↓	Yes
Enflurane	↑ ↑	↓	Yes
Isoflurane	↑	↓ ↓	Yes
Desflurane	↑	↓ ↓	Yes
Sevoflurane	↑	↓ ↓	Yes
N₂O alone	↑	↑	—
N₂O with volatile anesthetics	↑ ↑	↑	—
N₂O with intravenous anesthetics	0	0	—
Thiopental	↓ ↓ ↓	↓ ↓ ↓	No
Etomidate	↓ ↓ ↓	↓ ↓ ↓	No
Propofol	↓ ↓ ↓	↓ ↓ ↓	No
Midazolam	↓ ↓	↓ ↓	No
Ketamine	↑ ↑	↑	Yes
Fentanyl	↓ /0	↓ /0	No

The opioid anesthetics, morphine and fentanyl, cause either a minor reduction or no effect on CBF and CMR when compared with conditions in the unstimulated brain;[71,72] however, if the patient is aroused or in pain, they can cause a modest reduction in these parameters.[73] There is controversy concerning the effects of sufentanil: some studies demonstrate a reduction in CBF and metabolism,[74,75] whereas others report an increase in blood flow and ICP.[76,77] The latter study found no increase in ICP with fentanyl.[77] The duration of the increased blood flow and ICP effects of sufentanil in the above studies was short and could be overcome by hypocapnia. In animal studies, alfentanil decreased CBF and metabolism after 35 minutes and had no significant effect on ICP.[78] In patients with brain tumors, alfentanil increased CSF pressure.[79] Its effect on CSF pressure was less than that found with sufentanil but greater than that found with fentanyl. Alfentanil had the greatest effect on MAP and CPP.[77] Remifentanil, a rapidly metabolized opioid, had similar effects to fentanyl on CBF; both agents maintained CO_2 reactivity.[80] Remifentanil's main advantage is that it allows a more rapid neurologic assessment of the patient.

Ketamine, a dissociative anesthetic, activates certain areas in the brain and can increase CBF and CMR.[81-83] It is therefore not commonly used in neuroanesthesia.

Barbiturates, propofol, and benzodiazepines are intravenous agents recommended for neuroanesthesia; opioids, particularly fentanyl and remifentanil, have also proved useful.

BRAIN PROTECTION

Morbidity and mortality rates for elective neurosurgery are so low that detecting a decrease in mortality is virtually out of the question and daunting sample sizes would be required to detect even a 30% improvement in major morbidity. Accordingly, we are limited to drawing inferences from the laboratory, from clinical trials of therapies that are instituted subsequent to ischemic injury—primarily in stroke and head trauma patients—and from a small number of trials that test for prophylactic neuroprotection.

Mild Hypothermia

Laboratory results have demonstrated since 1956[84] that the beneficial attributes of mild hypothermia are likely to outweigh its real but manageable untoward effects when neurosurgical procedures are high risk and/or protracted. Berntman *et al* found that one degree of hypothermia (to 36°C) maintains ATP at normoxic levels during a hypoxic insult that depletes ATP by half at normothermia (37°C), and three degrees of hypothermia (to 34°C) more than doubled preservation of phosphocreatine.[85] These results suggest that the initial decline of cerebral metabolic rate (CMR) during hypothermia is greater than has been previously assumed.[86,87]

The protection afforded by intra-ischemic mild hypothermia has been attributed to reduction of calcium entry, reduction of glutamate release, reduction of glycine and dopamine release, recovery of ubiquitin synthesis, inhibition of protein kinase C, and reduction of free-radical–triggered lipid peroxidation. However, the protection afforded by intra-ischemic mild hypothermia is likely to be attributable to diminution of all the deleterious consequences of ischemia and the consequent relative preservation or restoration of favorable conditions, because the reduction in CMR that occurs during mild hypothermia retards and diminishes the primary synergists of the ischemic cascade.[86,87]

A survey conducted in 1993–1994 indicates that more than 40% of neuroanesthesiologists already use mild (33–35°C) to moderate (28–32°C) intraoperative hypothermia, 26% use hypothermia in every patient, and 14% think it is unethical to continue to use normothermia.[88] A multi-institutional clinical trial of intraoperative mild hypothermia for elective neurosurgical cases is underway, with encouraging preliminary data.[89] Until those results are available, mild hypothermia remains a neurosurgical option rather than a standard of care. In contrast, the data are available on mild hyperthermia. A few bouts of postoperative hyperthermia can undo all of the advantages of intraoperative hypothermia, and/or degrade the condition of normothermic patients.[90-94]

Our guess is that the future of intraoperative mild hypothermia is quite promising. Likewise, for head injury patients, moderate hypothermia in the ambulance may be within the window of opportunity for neuroprotection.

Anesthetic and Adjuvant Drugs

Clinically verified pharmacologic brain protection is even more elusive than the benefits of mild hypothermia. Nevertheless, as with hypothermia, reducing CMR is the mainstay of cerebral protection.

Barbiturates

Some of the proximate mechanisms by which barbiturates lower CMR include reduction of calcium influx, sodium channel blockade, inhibition of free-radical formation, potentiation of GABAergic activity, and inhibition of glucose transfer across the blood–brain barrier. All of these mechanisms are consistent with Goodman and coauthors' report that pentobarbital coma markedly reduces lactate, glutamate, and aspartate in the extracellular space of head-injured patients with severely increased ICP.[95] An *in vitro* investigation suggests that thiopental also delays the loss of transmembrane electrical gradients caused by application of NMDA and AMPA. This stands in marked contrast to the effect of propofol, which can aggravate glutamate excitotoxicity and increase neuronal damage.[96] Unfortunately, the only clinical trial providing evidence of barbiturate protection remains that of Nussmeier and coauthors.[97]

Calcium Channel Blockers

Several clinical trials and two meta-analyses suggest that calcium channel blockers—nimodipine, nicardipine, and AT877—reduce the frequency of vasospasm subsequent to subarachnoid hemorrhage and/or improve outcome.[98,99] The most favorable finding of the most recent meta-analysis suggests that nimodipine improves outcome, on average, by preventing one poor outcome in 1 of every 13 patients treated.[99] Whether the reduction in blood pressure that accompanies these Ca blockers improves outcome relative to hypertensive, hypervolemic hemodilution remains controversial. Neither meta-analysis was able to detect a statistically significant reduction in mortality.

Magnesium loading for cerebral protection is receiving renewed enthusiasm,[100] and more than 600 patients have been randomized in an ongoing study designed to test efficacy in 2700 patients.[101] Magnesium blocks both ligand- and voltage-dependent Ca entry and has shown considerable promise in *in vivo* experiments.[102,103] The fact that magnesium is also powerfully protective *in vitro* suggests that it may critically reduce calcium influx, as distinct from primarily improving CBF subsequent to cerebrovascular dilation, as may be the case with nimodipine.[104] Nelson and Grether's retrospective finding that *in utero* exposure to $MgSO_4$ was more frequent in very low–birthweight children without cerebral palsy than in low–birth-weight children with cerebral palsy also implies a potential for broad spectrum efficacy.[105]

Steroids

Clinical application of the 21-amino steroid tirilazad has also shown tentative promise.[106] Unfortunately, recent results from a North American trial of tirilazad subsequent to subarachnoid hemorrhage failed to reach statistical significance.[107] This discrepancy may be due to the preponderant use of phenytoin in the NA trial (80% of patients), as phenytoin has been shown to increase clearance of tirilazad by 50% in healthy volunteers.[108] Tirilazad did not compare favorably with methylprednisolone in a recent clinical trial for acute spinal cord injury.[109]

Additional Clinical Trials

Remacemide reduces glutamate release, and hence excitotoxicity, by blocking NMDA channels. Evidence for a prophylactic beneficial effect of this NMDA blocker was gleaned by combining scores from nine neuropsychological tests in coronary artery bypass patients. Those data allow the inference ($p < 0.03$) that in exchange for a higher risk of dizziness during nine days of drug administration, patients in the treatment group retained more of their ability to learn.[110]

Piracetam,[111] a nootropic agent that may increase compromised cerebral blood flow; ebselen,[112] an antioxidant that may reduce exotoxicity; and cerebrolysin,[113] a porcine brain tissue hydrolysate containing a mixture of 85% free amino acids and 15% small peptides, have all shown encouraging results in preliminary clinical stroke trials. Similarly promising results have been obtained with neurotrophic insulin-like growth factor (IGF-I) in a subset of head injury patients.[114]

Sodium Channel Blockers—From the Laboratory

Sodium channel blockers have shown particular promise in laboratory investigations.[115] Like barbiturates, riluzole reduces Na influx and also reduces glutamate release during ischemia.[116] Riluzole has shown protective effects in gerbils after global ischemia and in rats after focal ischemia when administered subsequent to initiation of the cerebral insult.[117,118] Most recently, riluzole has demonstrated neuroprotective effects in a rabbit model of experimental spinal cord ischemia.[119] Riluzole also appears to be efficacious in the treatment of amyotrophic lateral sclerosis in humans.[120]

Lamotrigine, an anticonvulsant that blocks voltage-gated sodium channels, has also shown cerebroprotective properties after experimental middle cerebral artery occlusion[121] and after transient global ischemia.[122] An even more promising use-dependent sodium channel blocker, BW619C89, has demonstrated efficacy against experimental focal ischemia, global ischemia, subdural hematoma, middle cerebral artery occlusion, and traumatic brain injury. A single oral dose of BW619C89 given prior to permanent middle cerebral artery occlusion provided substantial long-term protection in rats.[123]

What to Avoid

The evidence against some current practices and anesthetics is stronger than the evidence in their favor.

Post-Injury Hypothermia

Overenthusiasm and extension of hypothermia beyond where laboratory evidence indicates a window of opportunity is a real concern. Although hypothermia may be the most potent technique at our disposal for prophylactic cerebral protection, Dietrich and coauthors' experimental results,[124] and more recently those of Yubo *et al*,[125] indicate that hypothermia administered after an ischemic event only delays neuronal death. Recent clinical trials of moderate hypothermia after head injury are encouraging, but none of them has shown a statistically significant improvement in outcome,[126–129] and reported trends are of a magnitude that could be expected from the elimination of bouts of hyperthermia in the hypothermic groups in combination with comparatively lax temperature control in "normothermic" groups.

The authors of the largest published study of moderate hypothermia interpreted their findings to "suggest an improved outcome 12 months after the injury" in a subgroup of patients with initial Glasgow Coma Scale scores (GCS) of 5–7.[129] Unfortunately, that inference ignored the authors' own logistic regression analysis, which shows that this result may have been an artifact of initial differences in the computed tomographic classes of patients assigned to the hypothermic vs. normothermic groups.[130] Another recent report draws an encouraging inference about mild postischemic hypothermia; even though there was no normothermic control group, 10 out of 25 patients contracted pneumonia, and 9 patients died.[131] Results from a recent multicenter trial of moderate hypothermia in head-injured patients are yet to be published, but the trial was terminated after enrollment of 392 patients because morbidity and mortality were higher in the hypothermic group and suggestive improvements in outcome within subgroups of patients were not sufficient to meet pre-established continuation criteria.[132]

Despite this lack of empirical support, a 1998 survey indicates that 34% of today's neurosurgeons advocate the use of moderate hypothermia for 24 hours in the ICU after head trauma.[133] One worries that the desire to help head-injured patients is interfering with the objective analysis of data.[134]

Etomidate

EEG burst suppression with etomidate prior to temporary vessel occlusion gained prominence 11 years ago on the basis of a clinical trial for which there was no control group, no alternative drug tested, and no historical standard for comparison.[135] Despite the absence of supportive clinical evidence and the presence of troubling laboratory results,[136] etomidate remains the standard regimen for cerebral protection at several institutions.[137] We now have clinical evidence that the standard propylene glycol formulation of etomidate[138] induces more cerebral tissue hypoxia, tissue acidosis, and neurologic deficits than does an EEG-equivalent dose of desflurane.[139]

Nitrous Oxide and Ketamine

In 1938, C. D. Courville published "The pathogenesis of necrosis of the cerebral gray matter following nitrous oxide anesthesia"—an article that presented photographs of vacuolated cortical neurons from patients who died subsequent to administration of nitrous oxide (N_2O).[140] Sixty years later, Jevtovic-Todorovic and coauthors published compelling evidence that N_2O causes vacuolation of both the endoplasmic reticulum and mitochondria of neurons in the posterior cingulate and retrosplenial cortices of rats.[141] Are we on our way to where we might have been if Courville's work had received more sustained attention?

Nitrous oxide's mechanism of action appears to be NMDA receptor antagonism, and like other NMDA antagonists, N_2O has been shown to reduce damage from excessive glutamate release. Also like other NMDA antagonists, including "angel dust" and MK-801, N_2O can cause neural damage in and of itself.[141,142] In patients with folic acid deficiency, a single exposure to N_2O has caused spinal cord degeneration.[143] Less direct, but also less rare, brief exposure to N_2O causes a substantial increase in plasma homocysteine,[144] which can increase coagulation[145] and decrease flow-mediated vasodilation[146]—either of which could complicate recovery in a neurosurgical ICU patient. Prolonged hyperhomocysteinemia is an independent risk factor for cerebrovascular disease.[147]

In comparison to the highly variable degree of cerebral protection probably provided by all anesthetics whose primary mechanism of action is activation of GABA receptors, N_2O is likely to be deleterious. This has been shown experimentally in reference to isoflurane[148,149] and methohexital;[150] but in defense of clinical N_2O use, it has been argued that "co-administration of agents that are known to activate or potentiate the GABA receptor appears to block the neurotoxic effects of NMDA antagonists."[151] Accordingly, Jevtovic-Todorovic *et al* found that pretreatment with pentobarbital nearly eliminated the toxic effect of N_2O in rats—but that was not under the condition of cerebral ischemia.[141]

While neuroanesthesiologists are familiar with the ability of barbiturates to reduce ischemic damage, the question is whether

N_2O diminishes the protective effect of primary anesthetics in the event of cerebral ischemia. That question has been inadvertently addressed by investigations of barbiturate neuroprotection. For example, in 1966 Goldstein *et al* found substantial prophylactic barbiturate protection using a well controlled and highly regarded experimental model[152]; but when Steen *et al* tried to replicate that finding in 1979, they changed the experimental protocol to include administration of N_2O and failed to find cerebral protection.[153]

In a 1984 report that also used N_2O and failed to find cerebroprotection in a primate model, Gisvold *et al* did not proffer an explanation for the Goldstein–Steen discrepancy, but did comment that: "Although N_2O may not be as indifferent as hitherto believed, it is most unlikely that it should offset a beneficial effect of the barbiturate."[154] This prevailing assumption prompted examination of 32 published investigations of barbiturate protection. Twenty-one of 24 papers that used little or no N_2O found protection while 6 of 8 papers that co-administered substantial N_2O failed to find protection ($p < 0.01$).[155]

The question of N_2O's effect on the neuroprotective effect of primary anesthetics has been addressed more directly by several investigations. Following Arnfred and Secher's demonstration that thiopental more than doubles survival time in mice subjected to hypoxia[156] while N_2O used alone reduces survival,[157] we found that co-administration of N_2O virtually eliminates the protective effect of thiopental in the same model.[155,158,159] Two years later, Baughman and coauthors found that 0.5 MAC N_2O added to either 1 MAC or 0.5 MAC isoflurane cut the protective effect of isoflurane in half relative to the effect of 0.5 MAC N_2O alone during moderate forebrain ischemia.[149] More recently, Sugaya and Kitani reported that N_2O attenuates the protective effect of isoflurane on preservation of a critically important neuronal cytoskeletal protein during forebrain ischemia in the rat.[160] Most recently, Jevtovic-Todorovic and coauthors found that the adverse effects of ketamine are multiplied 5-fold in the presence of what would otherwise be an ineffective dose of N_2O in their rat model.[161]

Evidence that the above clinical and *in vivo* laboratory findings resulted in part from a direct neurotoxic effect of N_2O is provided by findings in the hippocampal slice model, where nitrous oxide markedly reduced electrophysiologic recovery from severe hypoxia without affecting fundamental biochemical parameters like ATP concentration, Ca influx, K efflux, and Na influx.[162]

Direct neurotoxicity aside, N_2O has been repeatedly shown to increase cerebral metabolic rate (CMR), cerebral blood flow (CBF), and intracranial pressure (ICP) when used alone; but these effects are variable when N_2O is used as an adjunct anesthetic, with or without hypocapnia and with or without EEG burst suppression. The CBF/CMR issue presented by N_2O has been articulated in reference to barbiturates and midazolam: "If N_2O elevates cerebral metabolism without causing a concomitant increase in CBF during barbiturate anesthesia, as it has been shown to do during midazolam anesthesia, the resulting mismatch between CBF and $CMRO_2$ could be critical during O_2 deprivation."[163]

Prospects

Until evidence is sufficient to warrant a standard-of-care recommendation for prophylactic cerebral protection, each clinician must proceed on a best-guess basis. Our guess is that mild hypothermia is useful, that magnesium loading is promising, and that etomidate, nitrous oxide, ketamine, and post-injury hypothermia should be avoided.

MONITORING

Electroencephalogram

The EEG can be used to monitor cerebral function during general anesthesia. The primary use of intraoperative EEG mon-

itoring is the detection of cerebral ischemia during carotid endarterectomy, cerebral aneurysmectomy with temporary clip application, cardiopulmonary bypass, and extracranial–intracranial bypass procedures. EEG monitoring is also used for intraoperative or perioperative assessment of pharmacologic interventions, such as barbiturate-induced burst suppression, during deliberate hypotension, and for the assessment of coma or brain death. Another important intraoperative application of EEG is in the diagnosis and management of intractable epilepsy.

The EEG waves recorded on the surface of the scalp are spontaneous electrical potentials generated by the pyramidal cells of the granular cortex. The EEG signal consists of graded summations of inhibitory and excitatory postsynaptic potentials that create dipole fields in the dendrites of the pyramidal cells.[164] When a number of dipoles develop at once, the summation creates electrical potentials large enough to produce detectable voltage on the scalp.

The EEG waveforms are interpreted by pattern recognition and quantification. Specific complexes are described in terms of morphology, spatial and temporal distribution, and reactivity of the waveforms. Quantification involves measuring frequency and amplitude. Frequency is measured in Hertz (Hz) and is defined as the number of times per second the wave crosses the zero voltage line. Amplitude, which is measured in microvolts (μV), is the electrical height of the wave. The frequency bands are divided into delta (0–3 Hz), theta (4–7 Hz), alpha (8–13 Hz), and beta (>13 Hz) rhythms (Table 28-6).

The traditional EEG is a plot of voltage against time. Sixteen channels are usually recorded, allowing analysis of activity of different regions of the brain. EEG waveform changes associated with anesthetic drugs, Pao_2, $Paco_2$, and temperature are described in Table 28-7.

The EEG response to anesthetic agents can vary from cortical excitation through depression to isoelectricity. Usually, anesthetic induction produces a decrease in alpha and an increase in beta activity. As the depth of anesthesia increases, EEG frequency decreases until theta and delta activity predominate. By further increasing the dose of anesthesia, the EEG changes to a burst suppression pattern, which coincides with near-maximal depression of cerebral metabolic activity. Complete electrical silence or isoelectricity follows an additional increase in anesthesia. Anesthesia-induced burst suppression is used to provide cerebral protection by metabolic suppression. EEG monitoring verifies burst suppression and electrical silence, and is valuable when determining the dose of drug required to induce and maintain the coma.

Efforts to use the EEG as a monitor of depth of anesthesia have been problematic because of the variety of agents used during an anesthetic and because some anesthetic agents do not follow the general pattern described above (Fig. 28-8).[41,165] Current techniques using processed EEG in combination with facial muscle activity show promise for the assessment of anesthetic depth and detection of conditions that may reduce intraoperative awareness.[166]

Intraoperative EEG monitoring allows early detection of cere-

Table 28-6. EEG FREQUENCY RANGES

Delta rhythm (0–3 Hz)	Deep sleep, deep anesthesia, or pathologic states (*e.g.*, brain tumors, hypoxia, metabolic encephalopathy)
Theta rhythm (4–7 Hz)	Sleep and anesthesia in adults, hyperventilation in awake children and young adults
Alpha rhythm (8–13 Hz)	Resting, awake adult with eyes closed; predominantly seen in occipital leads
Beta rhythm (>13 Hz)	Mental activity, light anesthesia

Table 28-7. EEG CHANGES ASSOCIATED WITH ANESTHETIC DRUGS, Pao₂, Paco₂, AND TEMPERATURE

Increased Frequency
Barbiturates (low dose)
Benzodiazepines (low dose)
Etomidate (low dose)
Propofol (low dose)
Ketamine
N_2O (30–70%)
Inhalation agents (<1 MAC)
Hypoxia (initially)
Hypercarbia (mild)
Seizures

**Decreased Frequency/
   Increased Amplitude**
Barbiturates (moderate dose)
Etomidate (moderate dose)
Propofol (moderate dose)
Opioids
Inhalation agents (>1 MAC)
Hypoxia (mild)
Hypocarbia (moderate to extreme)
Hypothermia

**Decreased Frequency/
   Decreased Amplitude**
Barbiturates (high dose)
Hypoxia (mild)
Hypercarbia (severe)
Hypothermia (<35°C)

Electrical Silence
Barbiturates (coma dose)
Etomidate (high dose)
Propofol (high dose)
Desflurane (2 MAC)
Isoflurane (2 MAC)
Sevoflurane (2 MAC)
Hypoxia (severe)
Hypothermia (<15–20°C)
Brain death

bral hypoxia and ischemia. Inadequate Pao₂ or insufficient CBF is reflected within seconds in the EEG.[167,168] Hypoxia may initially produce EEG activation, which is followed by slowing and eventually electrical silence.[168]

Other physiologic parameters that affect EEG waveforms are Paco₂, temperature, and sensory stimulation. Hypocarbia causes EEG slowing. Mild hypercarbia causes increased frequency, and severe hypercarbia produces a decrease in frequency and amplitude. When body temperature falls below 35°C, hypothermia causes a progressive slowing of activity. Complete electrical silence occurs at 15–20°C. Sensory stimulation is associated with EEG activation.

When monitoring an EEG during anesthesia, the changes resulting from hypoxia or ischemia must be distinguished from the drug and physiologic effects that also may influence the EEG. Because of this, the EEG must always be interpreted within the clinical context in which it is observed.

A specific intraoperative application of the EEG, called *electrocorticography* (EcoG), is the localization of epileptic foci during surgery for intractable epilepsy. For these procedures, recording electrodes are applied on or in the brain. The craniotomy can be performed under local anesthesia with conscious sedation (typically using propofol or fentanyl and droperidol) or under a light general anesthetic. The anesthetic administered must avoid pharmacologic cortical depression, which would prevent provocative seizure activity. Provocative techniques and agents, such as hyperventilation, low-dose barbiturates (methohexital 10–50 mg, thiopental 25–50 mg), propofol 10–20 mg, or etomidate 2–4 mg, have been used to activate the foci.[169] If the patient is under general anesthesia, alfentanil 20–50 $\mu g \cdot kg^{-1}$ and enflurane can be used.

Computerized EEG Processing

The development of the computer-processed EEG has facilitated intraoperative EEG monitoring. The most widely used and best validated technique is *power-spectrum analysis,* which uses a computer to perform a Fourier transformation. A given epoch of EEG (usually 2–8 seconds) is converted from a plot of voltage against time to a plot of power (amplitude squared) against frequency. With this technique, data are displayed in one of three formats: the compressed spectral array, the density spectral array, and the band spectral array or power bands. For example, to generate the compressed spectral array format, the Fourier transformation converts the irregular EEG waves to equivalent sine waves of known frequency and power (Fig. 28-9).[167] This display shows time and power as one axis (vertical) and frequencies on the horizontal axis. The Fourier spectral data from successive segments are stacked one on top of the other, creating a pseudo three-dimensional display; that is, the plot is shifted vertically with time and compressed. A major advantage of power-spectrum analysis is that it retains almost all the information in the original EEG. Power-spectrum analysis has documented value as a monitor of cerebral ischemia and possible value in the determination of anesthetic depth.[166,170,171] The main disadvantages of this analysis technique are lack of detection of spike activity, inclusion of artifact within frequency bands, and limited review of raw EEG data to determine reliability of the ongoing input.

An early method used for processing the EEG was the zero-cross analysis. The zero-cross frequency, or mean frequency, of the EEG is estimated by counting the number of times the EEG waveform crosses the zero-voltage axis.[166] Aperiodic analysis is a variant of the zero-cross method. With this technique, each waveform is analyzed in relation to its frequency, amplitude, and time of occurrence. Aperiodic analysis does not rely on averaging many waveforms over a given epoch. The signal is broken into the four component frequencies, with the amplitudes at each frequency in each hemisphere displayed. Aperiodic analysis of the EEG can be used quite effectively to detect the presence of intraoperative cerebral ischemia (Fig. 28-10).[172]

Several technical matters must be considered to effectively implement intraoperative electrophysiologic monitoring. Awake controls should be obtained before induction of general anesthesia. Monitoring should be continuous throughout anesthesia and continue until the patient is awake. Bilateral data must be obtained, especially during cerebrovascular procedures. For example, during a carotid endarterectomy, bilateral changes may indicate anesthetic or systemic effects, whereas ipsilateral changes on the operated side are more likely consistent with surgical trauma or ischemia. Marked changes in anesthetic depth, systemic blood pressure, Paco₂, and brain temperature must be avoided in order to distinguish between anesthetic and physiologic effects on the EEG and those due to hypoxia or ischemia.

Evoked Potentials

Evoked potentials are used intraoperatively to monitor the integrity of specific sensory and motor pathways. Sensory evoked potentials (SEPs) evaluate the functional integrity of ascending

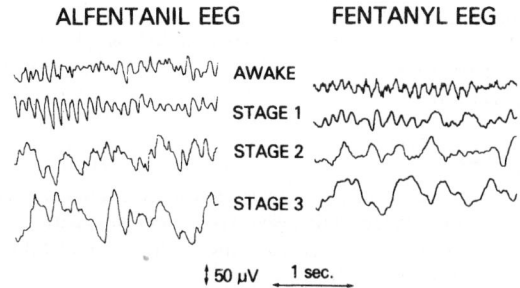

Figure 28-8. EEG changes with increasing doses of fentanyl and alfentanil. *Awake:* mixed alpha (8–13 Hz) and beta (>13 Hz) activity; *Stage 1:* slowing with alpha spindles; *Stage 2:* more slowing, theta activity present (4–7 Hz); *Stage 3:* maximal slowing, delta waves present (<4 Hz) with high amplitude. (Reprinted with permission from Scott JC, Ponaganis KV, Stanski DR: EEG quantification of narcotic effect: The comparative pharmacodynamics of fentanyl and alfentanil. Anesthesiology 62:234, 1985.)

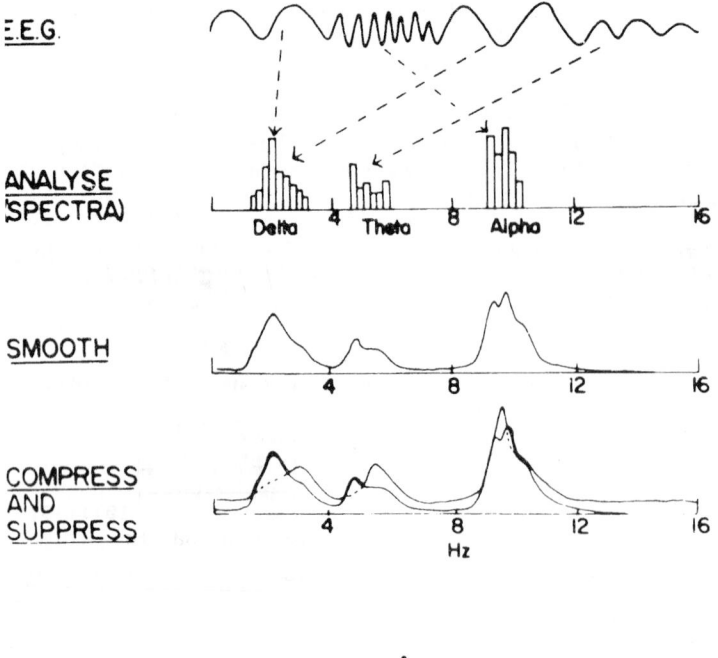

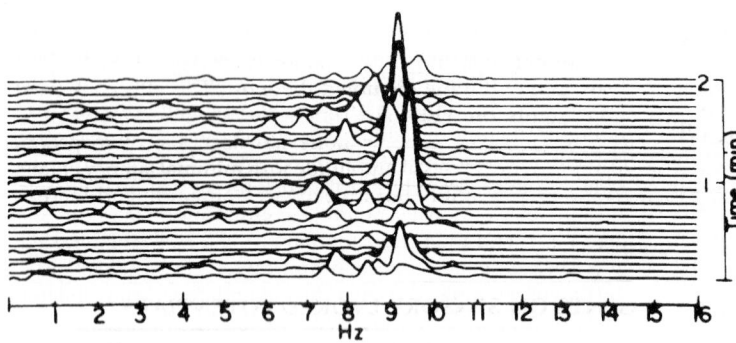

Figure 28-9. Schematic diagram of technique used to generate compressed spectral array. Below the diagram is an example of compressed spectra of the alpha rhythm from a normal subject. (Reprinted with permission from Stockard JJ, Bickford RG: The neurophysiology of anesthesia. In Gordon E [ed]: A Basis and Practice of Neuroanesthesia, 2nd ed, pp 3–49. Amsterdam, Elsevier, 1981.)

sensory pathways, whereas motor evoked potentials (MEPs) test the functional integrity of descending motor pathways.

There are major differences between evoked potentials and the EEG. The EEG is a recording of spontaneous, random electrical activity that has a nonspecific function and generates a relatively large signal, *e.g.,* 50 μV or more. Evoked potentials are comparatively small-amplitude responses (0.1–20 μV) to a specific stimulus that are pathway-specific.

Sensory Evoked Potentials

The application of a sensory stimulus—a click, a flash, a shock—results in an afferent nerve impulse that can be detected by appropriately placed surface electrodes as transient potential differences. The amplitude of these evoked potentials is very small and obscured by normal background bioelectric activity from the EEG, electrocardiogram (ECG), muscle activity, and other extraneous electrical activity. Signal averaging is required to extract the evoked responses from this background noise. The background noise is random and is eliminated by the averaging process.

Three SEP modalities are employed clinically: *somatosensory* (SSEP), *auditory* (BAEP), and *visual* (VEP). The waves of the evoked potential are thought to represent potentials from specific neural generators. The individual peaks in the waveform are described in terms of polarity (negative, positive), post-stimulus latency (msec), and peak-to-peak amplitude (μV or nV). They are also described by the distance separating the neural generators and recording electrodes (near-field, far-field).

Anesthetic Considerations for Sensory Evoked Potential Recording. Compromise or injury of a neurologic pathway is manifested as an increase in the latency and/or a decrease in the amplitude of evoked potential waveforms. For SSEPs, a 50% reduction in amplitude from baseline in response to a specific surgical maneuver is considered to be a significant change warranting action to avert potential damage. For BAEPs, an increase in latency of more than 1 millisecond is considered clinically significant. Accordingly, anesthetic, physiologic, and environmental factors capable of producing this pattern of alteration must be controlled when recording evoked potentials. All anesthetics that have been studied influence evoked potentials to some extent. Table 28-8 summarizes the known effects of intravenous and inhaled agents.[173–197] The sensitivity of evoked potentials to drug effects varies with the sensory modality being monitored. Evoked potentials of cortical origin (*i.e.,* the cortical component of the somatosensory evoked potentials [SSEP] and visual evoked potentials [VEP]) are more vulnerable to anesthetic influences than brain stem potentials (*e.g.,* brain stem auditory evoked potentials [BAEP] and the subcortical components of SSEP). In general, to obtain satisfactory intraoperative SEP recordings, it is important to maintain constant anesthetic drug levels. Specifically, bolus administration of intravenous agents and step changes in inspired inhalation agent concentration must be avoided, especially at times when neurologic injury might occur. When recording cortical evoked potentials (SSEPs or VEPs), one should employ intravenous techniques. High concentrations of volatile agents essentially eliminate cortical evoked potentials. However, end-tidal concentrations of 0.5

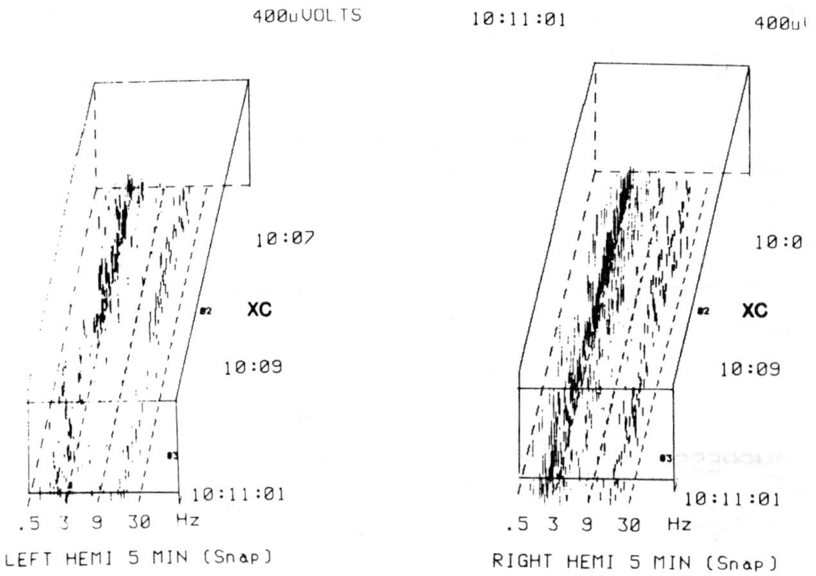

400uVOLTS   10:11:01   400u

10:07

XC

10:09

10:11:01

.5 3 9 30 Hz

LEFT HEMI 5 MIN (Snap)

10:0

XC

10:09

10:11:01

.5 3 9 30 Hz

RIGHT HEMI 5 MIN (Snap)

Figure 28-10. EEG as displayed by a Lifescan™ monitor using aperiodic analysis. This photograph was obtained approximately 3 minutes after occlusion (marked "XC") of the left carotid artery. Frequency is displayed on the *x* axis. The amplitude of each mapped EEG wave is a vertical "pole." Time is displayed on the diagonal axis, with the most recent time at the bottom front of the box. This display shows attenuation of activity on the left with occlusion that is more apparent in the higher frequency range. The regional cerebral blood flow with occlusion was 9 ml · 100 g⁻¹ · min⁻¹. (Reprinted with permission from Spackman TN, Faust RJ, Cucchiara RF *et al:* A comparison of aperiodic analysis of the EEG with standard EEG and cerebral blood flow for detection of ischemia. Anesthesiology 66:229, 1987.)

MAC of a volatile agent are compatible with satisfactory recordings in patients who are neurologically normal.

In general, volatile agents cause a dose-dependent increase in latency and a decrease in amplitude of the cortical SSEP or VEP.[173–177] As exemplified in a study by Peterson *et al* (Fig. 28-11), reductions in SSEP amplitude greater than 50% were observed with 1 MAC halothane, 0.5 MAC enflurane, and 0.5 MAC

isoflurane, all administered with 60% nitrous oxide in oxygen.[173] The authors concluded that halothane disrupted the SSEP the least, and enflurane disrupted the most. The effects of inhalation agents on VEPs are similar to the effects on cortical SSEPs.[175–177] Nitrous oxide alone has been shown to produce significant decreases in amplitude with minimal latency changes in the cortical SSEP, but it decreases amplitude and increases

Table 28-8. EFFECTS OF INTRAVENOUS AND INHALED AGENTS ON SENSORY EVOKED POTENTIALS

	BAEPs		cSSEPs		VEPs	
	Lat	*Amp*	*Lat*	*Amp*	*Lat*	*Amp*
INTRAVENOUS AGENTS						
Thiopental						
4–6 mg · kg⁻¹	0	0	0	0	—	—
20 mg · kg⁻¹	↑	0	↑	↓	↑	↓
75 mg · kg⁻¹	↑	↓	↑	↓	↑	↓
Pentobarbital						
9–18 mg · kg⁻¹	↑	↓	↑	↓	↑	↓
Droperidol						
0.1 mg · kg⁻¹	—	—	↑	↓		
Diazepam						
0.1 mg · kg⁻¹	0	0	↑ /0	↓ /0	0	↓
Midazolam	0	0	↑ /0	↓ /0	—	—
Morphine	—	—	↑	↓ /0	—	—
Fentanyl	0	0	↑ /0	↓ /0	0	↓
Sufentanil	0	0	↑ /0	↓ /0	—	—
Alfentanil	0	0	↑ /0	↓ /0	—	—
Etomidate						
0.05–0.3 mg · kg⁻¹ · min⁻¹	0	0	↑	↑	↑	0
Propofol						
2–6 mg · kg⁻¹	↑	0	↑	↓ /0	—	—
Ketamine	↑	0	↑ /0	↑	↑	↑
INHALATION AGENTS						
Desflurane	↑	0	↑	↓	—	—
Enflurane	↑	0	↑	↑ *	↑	↓
Halothane	↑	0	↑	↓ *	↑	↓
Isoflurane	↑	0	↑	↓ *	↑	↓
Sevoflurane	↑	0	↑	↓	—	—
Nitrous oxide	0	↓	0	↓	↑	↓

BAEPs = brain stem auditory evoked potentials; cSSEPs = cortical somatosensory evoked potentials; VEPs = visual evoked potentials; ↑ = increased; ↓ = decreased; 0 = no change; — = no data; Lat = latency; Amp = amplitude.
* 1.5 MAC enflurane and isoflurane (but not halothane) will occasionally abolish the cortical evoked response to median nerve stimulation.

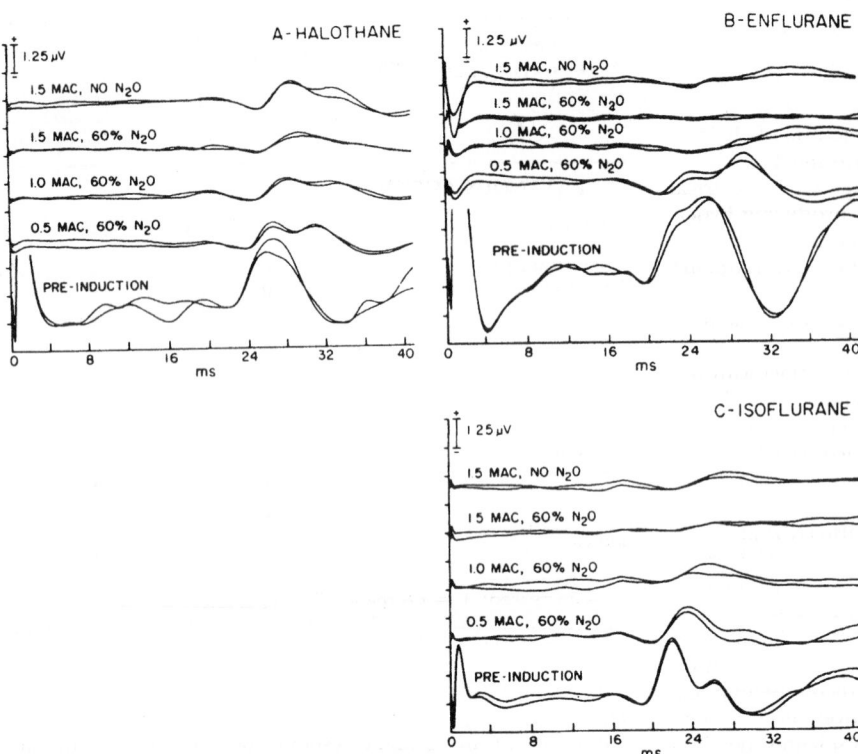

Figure 28-11. The responses of cortical somatosensory evoked potentials to various minimal alveolar concentrations (MACs) of halothane, enflurane, and isoflurane. A marked alteration of evoked potentials occurs at 1 MAC and higher levels of inhaled agents, and a modest improvement of the response occurs when N_2O is withdrawn. (Reprinted with permission from Peterson DO, Drummond JC, Todd MM: Effects of halothane, enflurane, isoflurane, and nitrous oxide on multilevel somatosensory evoked potentials. Anesthesiology 65:35, 1986.)

latency in the VEP.[178-180] When nitrous oxide is administered in combination with a volatile anesthetic, it produces a profound depressant effect on SSEPs or VEPs.

Brain stem responses are considerably more resistant to anesthetic influences than are cortical responses. For example, clinically used concentrations of the inhaled agents tend to increase the latencies of early or subcortical peaks of the BAEP with minimal amplitude effects.[181-183] Most anesthetic regimens are compatible with recording of brain stem responses. However, as with the other evoked potential modalities, large step changes (greater than 0.5 MAC) in inspired inhalation agent concentration should be avoided during critical periods.

Studies on the effects of intravenous agents demonstrate that induction doses of thiopental, etomidate, and fentanyl preserve SSEP recordings.[184] Increasing doses of thiopental result in dose-dependent increases in latency and decreases in amplitude in cortical SSEPs and progressive increases in latency in BAEPs.[185] Very high doses of thiopental, exceeding that which produce an isoelectric EEG, alter SSEPs and BAEPs predictably, but waveforms are preserved.[186] VEPs are more sensitive than the other sensory modalities to the effects of barbiturates with only the early potentials persisting at low doses and increasing in latency at higher doses.[186] Either bolus administration or intravenous infusion of etomidate causes increases in latency and increases in amplitude of cortical SSEPs and slight decreases in amplitude of cervical potentials.[187] Etomidate produces minimal changes in the early or subcortical peaks of the BAEP, but causes a dose-dependent attenuation and prolongation of the middle latency cortical peaks.[188] Etomidate alone does not change VEP amplitudes (P100 or N70), but increases latency (P60, N70, and P100).[189] During fentanyl–nitrous oxide anesthesia, etomidate causes decreases in amplitude and increases in latency of VEPs. The benzodiazepines produce minimal SSEP and VEP changes and no changes in BAEPs.[187,190-192] Propofol increases the latency and decreases the amplitude of cortical SSEPs.[193] Propofol (2 mg · kg^{-1} iv followed by an infusion) increases the BAEP latency of I, III, and V waves without changing the amplitudes.[194] Propofol completely suppresses middle-latency auditory potentials.

The opioids produce minimal changes in SEP waveforms. For example, fentanyl and morphine cause minimal latency prolongation and amplitude depression of the SSEP waveforms,[184,195] and high-dose opioid administration has been shown to be compatible with reproducible recordings of SSEPs.[196] Opioids also produce minimal to no effect on BAEP recordings.[197] Furthermore, low-dose continuous infusions of opioids tend to depress SEPs less than intermittent bolus injections.[195]

Because opioids preserve SEP recordings even in relatively high doses, they are recommended for use as infusions during intraoperative monitoring. As with all intravenous agents used, bolus administration should be avoided during critical times when neurologic injury might occur.

Physiologic factors such as temperature, systemic blood pressure, PaO_2, and $PaCO_2$ can alter SEPs and must be controlled during intraoperative recordings. Both hypothermia and hyperthermia alter all SEPs.[198-200] In addition, fluids used to irrigate the brain or spinal cord can cause marked changes in recordings despite normal core temperature measurement. Therefore, body-temperature irrigating fluids should be used. Systemic hypotension below levels of cerebral autoregulation produces progressive decreases in amplitude of cortical SSEPs until the waveform is lost.[198,201,202] During scoliosis surgery, SSEP changes have been observed that resolved with increases in systemic blood pressure, suggesting that spinal cord manipulation during "safe" levels of hypotension may cause significant ischemia.[203] Changes in PaO_2 and $PaCO_2$ also alter SEPs, probably reflecting changes in blood flow or oxygen delivery to neural structures.[198,202,204]

Motor Evoked Potentials

A motor evoked potential (MEP) can be produced by direct (epidural) or indirect (transosseous) stimulation of the brain or spinal cord. Following transcranial stimulation, the signal descends through both the dorsolateral and ventral spinal cord. It is primarily localized in the pyramidal tracts, and can be recorded from spinal cord (epidural space), peripheral nerve, and muscle using conventional electromyographic and evoked potentials averaging techniques. Stimulation of the motor cortex elicits contralateral peripheral nerve signals, electromyographic signals, or limb movements.

Transosseous activation of motor neurons is accomplished by either electrical or magnetic stimulation. Transcranial electrical stimulation of the motor cortex is a reliable method of eliciting intraoperative MEPs. It is achieved by delivering brief high-voltage pulses through scalp electrodes. Percutaneous electrical stimulation can be uncomfortable, however, producing hypertension and tachycardia in awake and anesthetized patients.[205] These cardiovascular responses may be minimized by reducing the rate and duration of stimulation.

Transcranial magnetic stimulation is produced by placing a magnetic coil over the motor cortex.[206] This technique is painless, noninvasive, and does not require direct contact with the scalp. Because high-resistance tissues such as bone and skin are transparent to magnetic fields, smaller voltages can be used to stimulate neural elements below the surface. Despite these advantages, it is more difficult to perform in the operating room because the stimulating coils are cumbersome and tend to overheat with repeated stimulation. There also is the problem of movement of ferromagnetic objects that lie within the magnetic field.

With either electrical or magnetic stimulation, there is concern that repetitive cortical stimulation can induce epileptic activity, neural damage, and cognitive or memory dysfunction. Guidelines for transcranial MEP stimulation recommend intermittent rather than continuous stimulation over several hours and cautious use in patients with a history of seizures, possible skull fractures, or implanted metallic devices.[207] Disruptions of the calvarium—*i.e.*, a skull fracture—could focus the current toward certain regions of the brain and potentially cause neural damage. Other situations of concern are patients with cardiac pacemakers and central venous or pulmonary artery catheterization. Transcranial MEP stimulation should probably be avoided in these patients.

There are several indications for intraoperative monitoring of MEPs. They are especially useful in preserving motor function during procedures in which surgically induced damage may be specific to the motor system. For example, surgical removal of intramedullary tumors can result in selective damage to corticospinal tracts, and MEPs are used to guide surgical resection. During scoliosis surgery, a direct monitor of motor pathway function obviates the need for the intraoperative wake-up test and provides continuous information about motor function throughout the surgical procedure. During cerebrovascular procedures and resection of cerebral tumors involving the motor cortex or subcortical motor pathways, the ability to guide the surgical resection by monitoring motor function may prevent postoperative motor deficits. Paralysis is an unpredictable complication that can occur after aortic aneurysm surgery. Although SSEPs have been used to identify intraoperative spinal cord dysfunction during aortic cross-clamping, a monitor of motor function would provide more specific information. In all of these procedures, MEPs should be monitored in conjunction with SSEPs to fully evaluate the functional integrity of both motor and sensory pathways.

Motor evoked potentials are extremely sensitive to depression by anesthetics. Table 28-9 summarizes the known effects of intravenous and inhaled agents.[208-215] Increasing N_2O concentration gradually attenuates and abolishes MEPs at concentrations between 60 and 70%.[208,209] However, N_2O concentration of 50% is reported to cause a minimal response alteration and appears to be compatible with monitoring.[208] The volatile agents are powerful depressants of myogenic MEPs.[210] During nitrous oxide–opioid anesthesia, even low concentrations of isoflurane are reported to abolish MEP responses.[211] Benzodiazepines, barbiturates, and propofol also produce marked depressed of the myogenic MEP.[209,212] Fentanyl, etomidate, and ketamine have little or no effect on myogenic MEP and are compatible with intraoperative recording.[212-214] Muscle relaxants affect the re-

Table 28-9. EFFECTS OF INTRAVENOUS AND INHALED AGENTS ON MOTOR EVOKED POTENTIALS

	Latency	Amplitude
INTRAVENOUS AGENTS		
Thiopental	↑	↓
Diazepam	↑	↓
Midazolam	0	↓
Fentanyl	0	0
Etomidate	0	↓/0
Propofol	0	↓
Ketamine*	↑	↓
INHALED AGENTS		
Desflurane	↑	↓
Enflurane	↑	↓
Halothane	↑	↓
Isoflurane	↑	↓
Sevoflurane	↑	↓
Nitrous oxide	↑	↓

↑ = increased; ↓ = decreased; 0 = no change.
* Latency delay in doses ≥35–40 mg · kg^{-1}, amplitude depression in doses ≥15–20 mg · kg^{-1}.

corded electromyographic response by depressing myoneural transmission. By adjusting a continuous infusion of muscle relaxant to maintain one or two twitches in a train of four, reliable MEP responses have been recorded.[215] Although it appears that MEPs are more sensitive to the effects of anesthetic agents, reliable responses can be recorded with a nitrous oxide–narcotic technique and with agents such as ketamine or etomidate. It appears that agents with central nervous system (CNS) inhibitory action (*e.g.*, thiopental and midazolam) produce profound changes in MEP responses and should be avoided. As with SEPs, hypothermia, hypoxia, and hypotension will alter MEPs under anesthesia.

Cranial Nerve Monitoring

Potential injury to the cranial nerves can occur during posterior fossa and lower brain stem procedures. The integrity of these cranial nerves can be preserved by monitoring the electromyographic (EMG) potential of cranial nerves with motor components (V, VII, IX, X, XI, XII).[216] Both spontaneous and triggered muscle activity can be recorded. Recordings can be obtained by placing two wire electrodes within the muscle or using surface electrodes. Simultaneous spontaneous EMG and compound muscle action potential (CMAP) recordings can be obtained by using intramuscular wire and surface electrodes. Intramuscular wire electrodes increase the sensitivity for detecting spontaneous EMG activity, while surface electrodes allow for more reliable monitoring of CMAP amplitude and morphology. With accidental surgical trespass, spontaneous neural activity changes into phasic "bursts" or "train" activity, which suggests injury potential. Evoking the nerves with electrical stimulation facilitates identification and hence preservation of the cranial nerve. Although it is possible to record EMG potentials during partial neuromuscular blockade, it is recommended that muscle relaxants not be administered during cranial nerve monitoring.

Intracranial Pressure Monitoring

Since Lundberg's[217] report in 1960, continuous ICP monitoring has been used to guide the perioperative management of patients with head injury, large brain tumor, ruptured intracranial aneurysm, cerebrovascular occlusive disease, and hydrocephalus. With continuous ICP monitoring, it is possible to optimize CPP (MAP-ICP) in critically ill neurosurgical patients. It also allows early detection and prompt treatment of brain hemorrhage, swelling, and herniation. An important intraoperative indication for ICP monitoring is to detect intracranial hypertension in the multiple trauma patients during a non-neurosurgical procedure.

Techniques used to monitor ICP include ventricular catheters, subdural-subarachnoid bolts or catheters, various epidural transducers, and intraparenchymal fiberoptic devices (Fig. 28-12). The intraventricular catheter is the standard method of monitoring ICP. This technique requires a small scalp incision and a burr hole through the skull. A soft, nonreactive plastic catheter is introduced into the lateral ventricle and connected by sterile tubing filled with saline solution to an external transducer. The intraventricular catheter measures CSF pressures reliably. It allows therapeutic CSF drainage and can also be used for compliance testing. There are, however, several potential problems with this technique. This device depends on the transmission of ICP through fluid-filled tubing that can occlude, thus damping or obliterating the recording. In a patient with severe brain swelling or a large mass lesion and small ventricles, it may be technically difficult to locate the lateral ventricle. Besides not being able to pass the catheter into the CSF, there is a possibility of brain tissue damage, hematoma, and infection. Studies report a low infection rate for the first 4 days after catheter placement.[218–220] Because of this, catheter removal is recommended on or before the fifth day, with replacement at a different site if continued ICP monitoring is necessary.[219]

The subdural-subarachnoid bolt usually consists of some type of hollow screw fixed to the calvarium, with the tip passing through the incised dura.[221] The advantages of the bolt are that it does not require brain tissue penetration or knowledge of ventricular position, and can be placed in any skull location that avoids major venous sinuses. There are several disadvantages to use of this technique. The bolt cannot be used to lower ICP by CSF drainage or to test compliance reliably. As with the intraventricular catheter, the bolt is connected to a transducer with tubing filled with sterile saline. Not only can the tubing block, but also brain substance can obstruct the tip of the bolt; in either situation, the recording may be damped or lost. Drilling side holes just proximal to the tip of the bolt compensates for this problem to some extent. Subdural devices are easily inserted, but can malfunction if they are not coplanar to the brain surface or if they become loose. The major complication of this procedure is infection, commonly meningitis, osteomyeli-

tis, or a localized infection.[218] Epidural bleeding and focal seizures, if the bolt is inserted too deeply, can also occur.

Two primary types of epidural transducers have been developed. One uses a device that has a pressure-sensitive membrane mounted close to or contacting the dura; the other type, known as the Ladd epidural transducer, is based on the principle of the Numoto pressure switch.[222] Although the risk of infection to the brain is lower because of the extradural placement, there are several disadvantages associated with using these devices. Placement in this potential space is more difficult, and there is a risk of bleeding. Technical problems in positioning and calibrating the transducer in situ can also occur. Another shortcoming of the epidural transducer is that intracranial compliance testing and therapeutic CSF drainage cannot be performed.

A relatively recent development in ICP monitoring has been that of a miniaturized fiberoptic device. This sensing device is mounted at the end of a 4-French fiberoptic bundle and can be inserted through a 2-mm burr hole. It senses changes in the amount of light reflected off a pressure-sensitive diaphragm located at the tip of a fiberoptic catheter. Mean pressure can be displayed digitally or as a pressure waveform. With this device, it is possible to insert the tip of the catheter into the subdural, intraparenchymal, or intraventricular compartments. Because it is a solid-state monitor, the problems of infection, leaks, catheter occlusion, and drift that attend fluid- or air-filled systems are minimized or avoided. Animal and human studies show that pressure recordings obtained with the fiberoptic catheter are accurate and reliable.[223,224] The main disadvantage of this device is that it cannot be recalibrated in situ. Because cumulative drift becomes significant with long-term use (i.e., 5 days or more), it is suggested that the monitor be replaced after 5 days.[224] Another limitation of the fiberoptic device is that it cannot be used for CSF drainage or compliance testing unless used in conjunction with a ventriculostomy.

Intraparenchymal ICP monitoring techniques allow direct measurement of brain tissue pressure, which may be important in edema formation and regional capillary blood flow. Intraparenchymal devices use a fiberoptic catheter that is inserted within cortical gray matter. In comparison to ventriculostomies, these monitors are easier to insert, have a smaller diameter, and are less disruptive of brain tissue.[225] Because there is no fluid column, the risk of infection is probably smaller.

New generations of fiberoptic ICP monitors allow simultaneous measurement of ICP, local CBF using laser Doppler flowmetry,[226] brain tissue oxygen pressure (Po_2), carbon dioxide pressure (Pco_2), and pH.[227] By simultaneously monitoring ICP, local CBF, and brain tissue oxygenation, early signs of ischemia can be identified and the effectiveness of therapeutic maneuvers more fully determined. The various ICP monitors are seldom used intraoperatively. They are most valuable in managing critically ill neurosurgical patients in the intensive care unit.

All of the clinically available monitors have recognized advantages and disadvantages. Despite the problems associated with these devices, ICP monitoring provides useful information for evaluating the patient's condition, progress, and need for therapy. Research efforts continue to improve monitoring techniques in terms of reliability, accuracy, and safety.

Cerebral Oxygenation/Metabolism Monitors

Brain Tissue Oxygenation

A multiparameter sensor is available for measuring brain tissue Po_2, Pco_2, pH, and temperature using a combined electrode–fiberoptic system.[227] The sensor was originally designed for continuous intra-arterial blood gas monitoring. It is supplied as a sterile, disposable device comprising two modified optical fibers for the measurements of Pco_2 and pH, a miniaturized

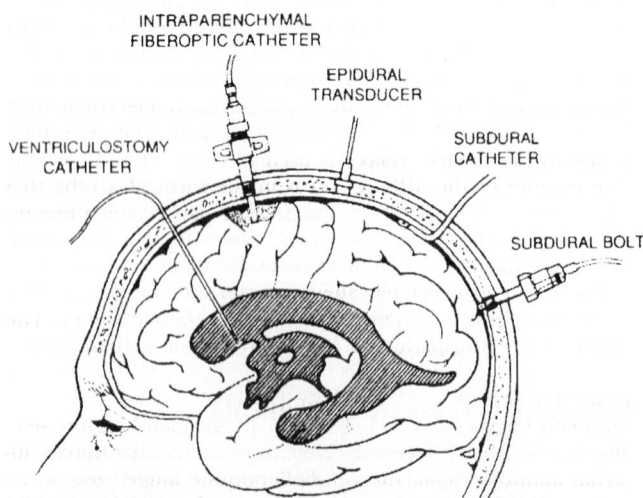

Figure 28-12. Techniques used to measure intracranial pressure.

Clark electrode for Po_2 measurement, and a thermocouple for determining temperature. Coupled with a dialysis catheter, the device permits measurement of other metabolic markers, including lactate, glucose, and excitotoxic amino acids. This sensor is invasive, requiring insertion into the cortex tissue of interest under direct visualization. The measurements obtained are limited to the parenchyma where the electrode is inserted.

Jugular Bulb Venous Oximetry

Continuous or intermittent estimation of the global balance between cerebral oxygen demand and supply can be achieved by jugular bulb venous oximetry. This is done by measuring the oxygen saturation of jugular venous blood ($Sjvo_2$) through percutaneous retrograde cannulation of the internal jugular vein with an intravascular catheter with embedded optical fibers. Normal $Sjvo_2$ is 60–70%. In the absence of anemia and any change in oxygen saturation, increases in $Sjvo_2$ to above 75% are indicative of absolute or relative hyperemia; that is, supply is in excess of metabolic requirement. This can occur as a result of reduced metabolic need (*e.g.*, a comatose or brain-dead patient) or from excessive flow (*e.g.*, severe hypercapnia). A value less than 50% reflects increased oxygen extraction and indicates a potential risk of ischemic injury. This may be due to increased metabolic demand (*e.g.*, fever or seizure) not matched by an equivalent increase in flow, or it may be due to an absolute reduction in flow. Changes in the oxygenation of systemic blood also influence the saturation of blood in the jugular bulb.

This monitor is used intraoperatively and postoperatively to diagnose cerebral ischemia from inadequate perfusion pressure or excessive hyperventilation. Its major limitation is that it does not detect focal ischemia.

Transcranial Oximetry

Near-infrared spectroscopy (NIRS) is a noninvasive optical method for monitoring cerebral regional oxygenation.[228,229] It is based on the principle that light in the near-infrared range (700–900 nm) readily penetrates skin and bone, but reflects off certain chromophores in the brain, such as, oxy- and deoxyhemoglobin and cytochrome AA^3. Therefore, by monitoring the absorption of light at several wavelengths in the near-infrared range, brain tissue concentrations of oxy- and deoxyhemoglobin, total hemoglobin, and hemoglobin oxygen saturation can be measured. The tissue field beneath the sensor contains capillaries, arteries and veins, reflecting a mixed vascular saturation, which NIRS monitors. Cerebral oximetry may prove useful in monitoring ischemia in several clinical neurosurgical conditions, including carotid endarterectomy, head injury, and subarachnoid hemorrhage. Its major limitations include inter-subject variability, variable optical path length, potential contamination from extracranial blood, and lack of a definable threshold. At present, it is considered a trend monitor, with each patient acting as his/her own control. In situations of potential regional ischemia, for example, carotid endarterectomy and temporary clip application during intracranial aneurysm surgery, bilateral monitoring should be used.

NEURORADIOLOGY

Common neuroradiology procedures are computed tomography (CT), magnetic resonance imaging (MRI), angiography, and myelography, although a variety of invasive interventional procedures are becoming common as well. These require the patient's total immobility. Therefore, in uncooperative patients, specifically children, fearful adults, and retarded or obtunded patients, general anesthesia will be required. All the standard equipment and monitors required for the administration of a general anesthetic and possible cardiopulmonary resuscitation must be present.

Computed Tomography Scan

The CT scan produces a series of cross-sectional images by computerized processing of X-ray absorption measurements (photon attenuation data as measured by sodium iodide crystals rotating about the patient's head).[230] Performance of a brain scan requires that the patient lie on a table with his or her head inside a rotating gantry that makes a 180° arc, producing one axial slice or cut. Depending on the generation of the scanner, the rotation may take from a few seconds to 4.5 minutes per cut. Eight cuts are usually required for a complete examination of the head. When contrast enhancement is indicated, the dye may be infused intravenously and the scan repeated. The patient must remain supine and immobile throughout the entire scan.

CT scanning is an excellent modality for detecting skull fractures and acute subarachnoid hemorrhage. It is relatively insensitive for viewing structures within the posterior fossa because image degradation results from artifact produced by the interface of bone and brain parenchyma. For trauma patients, spiral acquisition CT is becoming more popular. Larger anatomic regions can be imaged as the patient is moved at a continuous, constant speed through the scanning field with the X-ray tube rotating continuously.

Most CT examinations are performed without an anesthesiologist present. Oral or intravenous sedation is used for many pediatric examinations and is usually administered by radiology personnel.[231] Iodinated contrast medium, which is particularly valuable in studies of vascular malformations, vascularized tumors, and blood–brain defects, may also be administered orally or intravenously. When general anesthesia is requested, the patient's "nothing-by-mouth" status must be determined. Other issues that need to be resolved before the administration of general anesthesia are remote access to the patient and the establishment of monitoring and equipment that meets the same standard of care that exists in the operating room.

The CT scanner uses ionizing radiation. The radiation exposure during CT is similar to that of a conventional skull X-ray (1.0–2.5 rad).[232] Exposure values for personnel attending the patient are minimal (*e.g.*, 1–2 $mrad \cdot hr^{-1}$ for the anesthesiologist positioned next to the scan). However, radiation monitoring badges and lead aprons should be worn by personnel who participate in CT scanning on a regular basis.

Magnetic Resonance Imaging

Magnetic resonance imaging is a noninvasive diagnostic technique that is superior to CT in many CNS disorders.[233] This technique employs a strong magnetic field and pulsed radiofrequency energy to generate images. When a biologic specimen is placed within a static magnetic field, certain atomic nuclei (nuclei with an odd number of protons, such as ^1H nuclei) act like magnets and are aligned. The atoms are then subjected to a radiofrequency pulse that deflects their orientation. When the radiofrequency pulse is discontinued, the nuclei rotate back into alignment with the static magnetic field. The energy released as the nuclei "relax" is used to create the MR image. The magnet of the MRI system is in the form of a tube that can accommodate the human body. The patient must remain still during investigation, which may last 1 hour, to prevent imaging artifacts.

The MRI is an extremely valuable diagnostic tool that provides excellent contrast between gray and white brain matter. The images can be displayed in axial, coronal, or sagittal planes. Because there is no dental or bony artifact, the MRI is superior to the CT scan in examining the posterior fossa. Other areas optimally imaged by MRI include the pineal gland region, sella and parasellar structures, the limbic system, cranial nerves, internal auditory canal, the cerebellopontine angle, and leptomeninges. Magnetic resonance angiography (MRA) provides images of arterial and dural sinus blood flow. Magnetic resonance spectroscopy provides noninvasive biochemical measurements of specific brain metabolites and can be helpful in the early detection of stroke.

The intense magnetic field creates unique challenges for the anesthesiologist. The high-static magnetic field (0.12–2.00 tesla [T]) and the radiofrequency energy transmitted during image acquisition may damage or cause malfunction of electrical, electronic, or mechanical life support and monitoring equipment. Conversely, the radiofrequency energy generated by these devices can interfere with MR signal detection, producing artifacts that degrade the image. Another problem unique to MRI is that ferromagnetic substances placed within the magnetic field are propelled toward the scanner. A list of MRI-compatible equipment and monitors has been published.[234]

Laryngoscopes are not magnetic, but the batteries are. Therefore, to use a laryngoscope within the scanning room, plastic- or paper-coated batteries must be used. A prebent RAE tube is recommended owing to limited vertical space within the scanner. Very long breathing tubes are required, and either pipeline gases or a remotely placed anesthesia machine can be used. Aluminum cylinders can be used safely within the scanning room. MRI-compatible anesthesia machines and ventilators are available.[234] The anesthesia machine can be bolted to the wall or modified by removal of ferromagnetic components. The ventilators are pneumatically driven, volume-cycled, and have fluidic controls. The ventilator is completely powered by high-pressure oxygen delivered by a wall source or from large cylinders placed outside the imaging room, and electronic parts have been replaced with plastic, aluminum, or nonmetallic alloys.

The implementation of monitoring during MRI is difficult because of remote access to the patient and the interactions between various monitoring devices and the MR scanner, as previously described. For example, standard ECG monitors produce problems with image degradation from wire leads acting as antennas and with artifact produced by radiofrequency pulses and static magnetic fields. Burns under ECG electrodes have been reported. MR-compatible ECG monitors, cables, fasteners, and electrodes have been developed.[234] However, this ECG provides only heart rate and rhythm and cannot be used to monitor ischemia. Additional suggestions for improving ECG monitoring include placing electrodes close together near the three-dimensional center of the imager and twisting the leads. Both noninvasive and invasive pressure monitoring have been successfully used during MRI. Blood pressure is easily measured with an ordinary cuff and long pressure tubing without metal connections. The blood pressure dial must be kept away from the magnetic field. Automated blood pressure devices without metal connectors have also been used. Using nonmetallic components, pressure transducers connected to intravascular catheters for central venous, pulmonary artery, and arterial pressure monitoring can function near the magnet. Transducers are affixed along the side of the magnet at its midpoint to minimize artifact. Shielded electric extension cables couple the transducers to the monitors located outside the scanning room. There have been reports of image degradation with the pulse oximeter. Placing the oximeter a distance from the magnet and the probe on the patient's toe, which is usually outside the magnet, and using a fiberoptic cable may improve image quality. Monitoring of heart rate and respiration can be achieved using nonmetallic precordial or esophageal stethoscopes; however, the drum-like noise of the scanner may obscure auscultated heart and breath sounds. A standard vascular Doppler has also been used to monitor heart rate. Capnography is possible with long tubing and high-powered suction. Changes in respiratory rate are easily observed, but the end-tidal CO_2 reading may be less than the actual value. Although temperature monitoring is particularly important in the cold MRI suite, especially in pediatric patients, it has been difficult to implement. The wires conducting the signal from the thermistor may function as an antenna for radiofrequency signals and produce imaging

artifact and burns. Nonferromagnetic disposable temperature strips may be used. All efforts to minimize patient heat loss should be implemented: using bags of warmed intravenous fluids, heating pads, airway humidification, and covering the patient.

Guidelines for using the MRI have been issued by the National Radiological Protection Board.[235] It is recommended that women in the first trimester of pregnancy not be scanned because of possible developmental consequences. Patients with demand pacemakers should not be scanned because the varying magnetic field can induce electric currents in the pacemaker wires, which may be mistaken for the natural electrical activity of the heart, inhibiting pacemaker output. Metallic objects such as vascular clips or shrapnel can move and become displaced when exposed to the magnetic field. Patients who have a large metallic implant or prosthesis can be scanned until the heat at the site of the implant or prosthesis becomes uncomfortable. There is a possibility that induced currents can affect myocardial contractility or produce arrhythmias. Full resuscitation facilities should be available.

Positron Emission Tomography

Biochemical or physiologic processes involved in cerebral metabolism can be imaged with positron emission tomography (PET). After receiving intravenous radionuclide, such as fluorodeoxyglucose (FDG), the patient is scanned in a specialized detector system. This system detects the positron energy emitted from the radionuclide. Computerized reconstruction procedures produce tomographic images. The information from PET can be overlaid on CT or MR images to improve anatomic localization of detected activity. When the MRI is normal in a patient with seizures, PET might provide localizing information prior to focal resection treatment. The injection of FDG renders the patient radioactive for 24 hours. The usual protocol involves two initial scans lasting 15–20 minutes followed by another scan in 2–3 hours. PET scanners do not require nonferromagnetic monitors and equipment.

Cerebral Angiography

Angiography is used to delineate the vasculature of the brain. Catheters are usually introduced through the common femoral artery, which has replaced direct carotid artery puncture. Digital subtraction angiography reduces the required volume of intra-arterial contrast and the overall duration of the procedure.

There are several risks and problems associated with angiography, including an incidence of neurologic problems related to angiography itself. In addition, arterial spasm, hematoma, and local infection can occur at the site of needle puncture. Subintimal dissection or occlusion of the vessel may result from injection into the vessel wall. Iodine-containing contrast media produce vasodilation and a burning sensation in the distribution of the injected vessel. Septicemia, cerebral embolism, anaphylactic reactions to the iodinated contrast material, and, rarely, seizures or death are all potential complications of cerebral angiography.

The introduction of low-ionic and nonionic contrast material has reduced both the discomfort and toxicity associated with angiography. Because of this, patients usually do not require general anesthesia and are able to tolerate the procedure with minimal or no sedation. When general anesthesia is requested for children or uncooperative adults, the angiogram quality may be enhanced by hyperventilation. Hypocarbia is thought to improve study quality by slowing the cerebral circulation and improving delineation of tumor blood vessels, perhaps through an inverse steal phenomenon.

Myelography

Myelography requires spinal lumbar puncture, the injection of contrast material, and the prone position. It is uncommon for the anesthesiologist to be involved in myelography except for studies in children or uncooperative adults. Metrizamide is a water-soluble contrast agent that has been used for myelograms. Because of its rapid absorption from the CSF, metrizamide does not require aspiration at the end of the procedure, but it is associated with allergic reactions and mental changes, ranging from headache to confusion to convulsions. Any drug that lowers the epileptogenic threshold (*e.g.,* phenothiazines or ketamine) should be avoided in patients receiving metrizamide. Other nonionic contrast media such as iohexol and iopamidol may be used instead of metrizamide because they are associated with a lower osmotic load and a reduced incidence of adverse reactions. However, these agents are much more expensive than standard contrast media.[236]

Interventional Neuroradiology

Interventional neuroradiology has developed from traditional neuroradiology and neurosurgery to procedures that treat CNS disease by endovascular access.[237] Procedures such as therapeutic embolization and superselective angiography of vascular malformations, balloon angioplasty of occlusive cerebrovascular disease or cerebral vasospasm, therapeutic carotid occlusion for giant aneurysms and brain tumors, and others may be performed. Because these procedures are inherently dangerous, anesthesiologists can help prevent and manage morbidity and mortality.

Most interventional neuroradiology procedures are accomplished with conscious sedation. General anesthesia may be used for small children, uncooperative adult patients, and for certain procedures. The agents chosen for conscious sedation must alleviate pain and discomfort and provide anxiolysis, patient immobility, and a rapid return to consciousness for neurologic testing. Both neuroleptanesthesia (*e.g.,* titration of $2-4~\mu g \cdot kg^{-1}$ fentanyl, 2.5–5 mg droperidol, and 3–5 mg midazolam iv) and a propofol infusion technique have been used successfully. The goal of drug titration is to render the patient unconscious with a patent airway.

Before initiating sedation, the patient is made comfortable with padding under head, neck, and body. Two large-bore intravenous catheters are inserted, and all standard monitoring is applied. Oxygen ($2-4~l \cdot min^{-1}$) is delivered by nasal cannula with the capability of monitoring end-tidal carbon dioxide. Arterial pressure can be monitored through the cannulated femoral artery for intracranial and spinal cord procedures and whenever blood pressure manipulation is required. Awake neurologic assessment and other CNS monitors (*e.g.,* EEG, evoked potentials, or transcranial Doppler) may be used. During and after these procedures, careful management of coagulation is required to prevent thromboembolic complications. Special techniques such as deliberate hypotension or hypertension and hypercapnia may be requested for selective procedures.

Complications during instrumentation of the cerebral vasculature can be sudden and dramatic. Simultaneous with airway maintenance, it is important to determine whether the problem is hemorrhagic or occlusive. Hemorrhagic disasters require immediate heparin reversal and low normal blood pressure. Occlusive disasters require deliberate hypertension, titrated to neurologic examination, with or without direct thrombolysis. Other resuscitative measures that might be initiated include rapid fluid infusion, 15° head-up position, hyperventilation, diuretics, anticonvulsants, hypothermia (33–34°C), and thiopental infusion titrated to EEG burst suppression.

Adverse Reactions From Contrast Media

Most contrast media are radiopaque, iodine-containing salts that may be administered orally or, more commonly, injected intravascularly, lymphatically, or directly into the CSF. (Para-magnetic contrast material, typically not iodinated, is available for MR studies.) Neurotoxic, nephrotoxic, and allergic reactions have been reported after administration.[238,239] Neurotoxic reactions are more likely to complicate angiographic investigations and include dizziness, convulsions, unconsciousness, hemiplegia, blindness, and aphasia.[238] These effects are related to the hyperosmolality of the contrast agent. Contrast media may temporarily impair the blood–brain barrier or cross it during disease, causing CNS damage by a direct necrotizing effect.[240] A critical factor appears to be the concentration of the agent. If slurring of speech or confusion is observed, the procedure should be terminated. The occurrence and persistence of more serious CNS problems may require therapy with steroids, low–molecular-weight dextran, or vasopressor-induced elevation of systemic blood pressure to improve blood flow to areas that may be ischemic. The use of low-osmolality, nonionic contrast agents reduces the risk of CNS toxicity during angiography. Iodinated contrast agents are also nephrotoxic. After an initial mild vasodilation, the renal vascular tree vasoconstricts. Therefore, patients with pre-existing renal insufficiency, diabetes mellitus, and low cardiac output are at risk for developing contrast agent–induced nephrotoxicity.

Allergic reactions to contrast media vary from pruritus, burning on injection, and mild skin rashes to wheezing, dyspnea, syncope, and cardiovascular collapse.[239] These reactions most likely result from nonimmunologic release of histamine and other vasoactive mediators from mast cells and basophils. A prospective study conducted by the International Society of Radiologists Committee on Contrast Media[241] reported an approximate 5% incidence of systemic reactions to intravascular contrast media administration. Nineteen fatal reactions (0.006% of 302,082 studies) were reported in this group. In patients with a history of allergy (particularly to iodine or seafood), the incidence of reaction increases to 10–15%. In patients with a history of previous reaction to iodinated contrast agents, the risk of subsequent reaction increases to 17–35%.[239]

Prophylaxis with steroids and antihistamines is recommended in patients with a history of allergies or specific reaction to contrast media. These patients should be evaluated by an allergist and medicated before injection of contrast. Several regimens have been proposed, all including a corticosteroid (*e.g.,* prednisone) and an antihistamine (diphenhydramine) in various combinations and doses before, during, and after the investigation.[239,242] One regimen suggests the administration of prednisone (50 mg po) beginning the evening before (for a total of three doses, 6 hours apart) and diphenhydramine (50 mg iv) immediately before exposure.[242]

Mild allergic reactions require little more than reassurance and perhaps intravenous diphenhydramine. More severe reactions (*e.g.,* respiratory distress, hypotension, or syncope) can be treated initially with subcutaneous epinephrine. Be prepared, however, for all degrees of resuscitation, because emergent therapy for bronchospasm, laryngeal edema, hypotension, arrhythmias, and full cardiopulmonary arrest may be required.

ANESTHETIC MANAGEMENT OF NEUROSURGICAL PATIENTS

The administration of anesthesia to neurosurgical patients requires an understanding of the basic principles of neurophysiology and the effects of anesthetic agents on intracranial dynamics, as reviewed in the previous sections of this chapter.

Preoperative Evaluation

During the preoperative evaluation, the patient's overall medical condition must be considered and integrated into the formulation of an anesthetic management plan. Neurosurgical procedures tend to be lengthy, requiring unusual positioning of the patient and the institution of special techniques such as hyperventilation, cerebral dehydration, and deliberate hypotension. Not all patients can tolerate the position desired by the surgeon; this must be addressed and, if possible, evaluated preoperatively. Furthermore, in patients with cardiac disease, routine institution of osmotherapy or hyperventilation may compromise organ function. Such patients must be medically optimized and, when indicated, cardiac monitoring should be instituted. Except for neurosurgical emergencies (*e.g.,* head trauma or impending herniation), most neurosurgical procedures can be delayed to treat medically unstable conditions.

The preoperative evaluation must include a complete neurologic examination with special attention to the patient's level of consciousness, presence or absence of increased ICP, and extent of focal neurologic deficits. The signs and symptoms frequently associated with intracranial hypertension are headache, nausea, papilledema, unilateral pupillary dilation, and oculomotor or abducens palsy. With advanced stages of intracranial hypertension, the patient exhibits a depressed level of consciousness and irregular respiration. The clinical signs do not reliably indicate the level of ICP. Only a direct CSF pressure measurement can be used to quantitate the pressure; however, indirect evidence of elevated ICP can be determined by evaluating the MRI or CT scan for a mass lesion accompanied by a midline shift of 0.5 cm or greater and/or encroachment of expanding brain on CSF cisterns.

The location of the lesion in the supratentorial or infratentorial compartment will determine the clinical presentation and anesthetic management. Supratentorial disease is usually associated with problems in the management of intracranial hypertension, whereas infratentorial lesions cause problems related to mass effects on vital brain stem structures and elevated ICP due to obstructive hydrocephalus.

Fluid and electrolyte abnormalities are common in patients with reduced levels of consciousness. Patients are usually dehydrated and develop electrolyte abnormalities because of decreased fluid intake, iatrogenic water restriction, neuroendocrine abnormalities, and diuresis from diuretics, steroid-related hyperglycemia, and radiographic contrast agents. Fluid and electrolyte abnormalities must be corrected before induction of anesthesia to prevent cardiovascular instability.

COMMON INTRACRANIAL PATHOLOGY
Supratentorial Intracranial Tumors

Supratentorial tumors (meningiomas, gliomas, and metastatic lesions) change intracranial dynamics predictably. Initially, when the lesion is small and slowly expanding, volume-spatial compensation occurs by compression of the CSF compartment and nearby cerebral veins, which prevents increases in ICP. As the lesion grows, however, compensatory mechanisms are exhausted and further increases in tumor mass cause progressively greater increases in ICP. Primary or metastatic tumors or chronic subdural hematomas can present as chronic mass lesions. Because of the ability of the intracranial compartment to compensate up to a point, patients may exhibit minimal neurologic dysfunction despite the presence of a large mass, elevated ICP, and shifts in the position of brain structures.

Significant changes in ICP can occur with supratentorial tumors if they develop a central area of hemorrhagic necrotic tissue or a wide border of brain edema. As the tumor enlarges, it can outstrip its blood supply, developing a central hemorrhagic area that may expand rapidly, increasing ICP. Brain edema surrounding the tumor increases the effective bulk of the tumor and represents an additional portion of the brain that is not autoregulating. In such situations of compromised intracranial compliance, small increases in arterial pressure may produce large increases in CBF, which can markedly increase intracranial volume and ICP with the attendant complications.

Anesthetic Techniques and Drugs

The goal of neuroanesthetic care for patients with supratentorial tumors is to maximize therapeutic modalities that reduce intracranial volume. ICP must be controlled before the cranium is opened, and optimal operating conditions obtained by producing a slack brain that facilitates surgical dissection. Various maneuvers and pharmacologic agents have been used to reduce brain bulk (Table 28-10). For example, administration of diuretics or steroids, hyperventilation, and systemic blood pressure control may be implemented preoperatively to reduce cerebral edema and brain bulk, thereby reducing ICP. The application of these methods selectively or together, when necessary, is often accompanied by marked clinical improvement. In acute intracranial hypertensive states, adequate oxygenation with mechanical ventilation and hyperventilation provide the foundation for neuroresuscitative care.

Clinical Control of Intracranial Hypertension. Rapid brain dehydration and ICP reduction can be produced by administering diuretics. Two diuretics are employed: the osmotic diuretic mannitol and the loop diuretic furosemide. Mannitol is given as an intravenous infusion in a dose of $0.25–1.0 \ g \cdot kg^{-1}$. Its action begins within 10–15 minutes and is effective for approximately 2 hours. Larger doses produce a longer duration of action but do not necessarily reduce ICP more effectively. Furthermore, larger doses and repeated administration can result in metabolic derangement. Mannitol is effective when the blood–brain barrier is intact. By increasing the osmolality of blood relative to the brain, mannitol pulls water across an intact blood–brain barrier from brain to blood to restore the osmolar balance. When the blood–brain barrier is disrupted, mannitol may enter the brain and increase osmolality. Mannitol could pull water into the brain as the plasma concentration of the agent declines and cause a rebound increase in ICP. This rebound increase in ICP may be prevented by maintaining a mild fluid deficit. Mannitol has been shown to cause vasodilation of vascular smooth muscle, which is dependent on dose and administration rate.[243,244] Mannitol-induced vasodilation affects intracranial and extracranial vessels and can transiently increase cerebral blood volume and ICP while simultaneously decreasing systemic blood pressure.[245,246] Because mannitol may initially increase ICP, it should be given slowly (≥10 minute infusion) and in conjunction with maneuvers that decrease intracranial volume (*e.g.,* steroids or hyperventilation).

Hypertonic agents such as mannitol should be administered cautiously in patients with pre-existing cardiovascular disease. In these patients, the transient increase in intravascular volume may precipitate left ventricular failure. Furosemide may be a better agent to reduce ICP in patients with impaired cardiac reserve. Prolonged use of mannitol may produce dehydration, electrolyte disturbances, hyperosmolality, and impaired renal function.

The loop diuretic furosemide reduces ICP by inducing a systemic diuresis, decreasing CSF production, and resolving cerebral edema by improving cellular water transport.[245,246] Furosemide lowers ICP without increasing cerebral blood volume or blood osmolality; however, it is not as effective as mannitol

Table 28-10. CLINICAL CONTROL OF INTRACRANIAL HYPERTENSION

Diuretics: Osmotic, tubular
Corticosteroids
Hyperventilation on demand
Optimize hemodynamics (MAP, CVP, PCWP, HR)
Avoid overhydration, target normovolemia
Position to improve cerebral venous return
Anesthetic agents (thiopental, propofol)
Mild hypothermia

in reducing ICP.[245] Furosemide can be given alone as a large initial dose (0.5–1 mg · kg^{-1}) or as a lower dose with mannitol (0.15–0.30 mg · kg^{-1}). A combination of mannitol and furosemide diuresis has been shown to be more effective than mannitol alone in reducing ICP and brain bulk, but causes more severe dehydration and electrolyte imbalances.[245,246] With combined therapy, it is necessary to monitor electrolytes intraoperatively and replace potassium as indicated.

Corticosteroids reduce edema around brain tumors;[29,247] however, steroids require many hours or days before a reduction in ICP becomes apparent. The administration of steroids preoperatively frequently causes neurologic improvement that can precede the ICP reduction. One explanation for this is that the neurologic improvement is accompanied by partial restoration of the previously abnormal blood–brain barrier. Postulated mechanisms of action for steroidal reduction in brain edema are brain dehydration, blood–brain barrier repair, prevention of lysosomal activity, enhanced cerebral electrolyte transport, improved brain metabolism, promotion of water and electrolyte excretion, and inhibition of phospholipase A$_2$ activity.[248] The potential complications of continuous perioperative steroid administration are hyperglycemia, glucosuria, gastrointestinal bleeding, electrolyte disturbances, and increased incidence of infection. Therefore, the potential risks and benefits of continuous steroid administration need to be evaluated in these patients.

Hyperventilation has been the mainstay of acute and subacute management of intracranial hypertension. As discussed previously, hyperventilation reduces brain volume by decreasing CBF through cerebral vasoconstriction. For every 1 mm Hg change in PaCO_2, CBF changes by 1–2 ml · 100 g^{-1} · min^{-1}. The duration of effectiveness of hyperventilation for lowering ICP may be as short as 4–6 hours, depending on the pH of the CSF. Hyperventilation is only effective when the CO_2 reactivity of the cerebrovasculature is intact. Impaired responsiveness to changes in CO_2 tension occurs in areas of vasoparalysis, which are associated with extensive intracranial disease such as ischemia, trauma, tumor, and infection.

The typical target PaCO_2 is 30–35 mm Hg. A PaCO_2 below 20 mm Hg (or 25–30 mm Hg in some pathologic conditions) may be associated with ischemia due to extreme cerebral vasoconstriction. By monitoring global cerebral oxygenation with, say, jugular venous oxygen saturation (SjO_2), the therapeutic effectiveness of hyperventilation can be determined and more safely applied.[249]

The autoregulation of CBF has been discussed, as has the relationship between blood pressure and ICP when autoregulation is disturbed. The therapeutic goals are to maintain CPP and to control intracranial dynamics so that cerebral ischemia, edema, hemorrhage, and herniation are avoided. Severe hypotension results in cerebral ischemia and should be treated with volume replacement, inotropes, or vasopressors as dictated by clinical need. Severe hypertension, conversely, can worsen cerebral edema and cause intracranial hemorrhage and herniation. The β-adrenergic blockers, propranolol and esmolol, and the combined α- and β-adrenergic blocker, labetalol, are effective in reducing systemic blood pressure in patients with raised ICP with minimal or no effect on CBF or ICP.

Restricted fluid intake was a traditional approach to intracranial decompression therapy, but is now rarely used to lower ICP. Severe fluid restriction over several days is only modestly effective in reducing brain water content[250] and can cause hypovolemia, resulting in hypotension, inadequate renal perfusion, electrolyte and acid–base disturbances, hypoxemia, and reductions in CBF. In patients who are dehydrated preoperatively, intravascular volume must be restored to normovolemia before induction of anesthesia to prevent hypotension in response to anesthetic agents and positive-pressure ventilation. Fluid resuscitation and maintenance fluids in the routine neurosurgical patient are provided with glucose-free iso-osmolar crystalloid solutions to prevent increases in brain water content. For routine craniotomy, the patient receives hourly maintenance fluids and replacement of urine output. Blood loss is replaced at approximately a 3:1 ratio (crystalloid:blood) down to a hematocrit of approximately 25–30% depending on the patient's physiologic status.

Solutions containing glucose are avoided in all neurosurgical patients with normal glucose metabolism, since these solutions exacerbate ischemic damage and cerebral edema.[251–253] Hyperglycemia augments ischemic damage by promoting neuronal lactate production, which worsens cellular injury. Intravenous fluids containing glucose and water (D$_5$W$_{0.45\%}$ NaCl or D$_5$W) are particularly problematic because the glucose is metabolized and the free water remains in the intracranial fluid compartment, resulting in brain edema. Brain water can interfere with surgical exposure and, after closure of the skull, can compromise cerebral perfusion. In normal patients, both preoperative dexamethasone treatment and general anesthesia–induced gluconeogenesis may elevate resting glucose levels. Therefore, blood glucose levels should be monitored during craniotomy and maintained at near low-normal range.[251] This should be accomplished mainly by withholding glucose.

For most neurosurgical patients, a neutral head position, elevated 15–30°, is recommended to decrease ICP by improving venous drainage. Flexing or turning of the head may obstruct cerebral venous outflow, causing a dramatic ICP elevation that has been shown to resolve with resumption of a neutral head position. Lowering the head impairs cerebral venous drainage, which can quickly result in an increase in brain bulk and ICP.

The application of positive end-expiratory pressure (PEEP) to mechanically ventilated patients can potentially increase ICP. This effect occurs when PEEP increases mean intrathoracic pressure, impairing cerebral venous outflow and cardiac output. When PEEP is required to maintain oxygenation, it should be applied cautiously and with appropriate monitoring to minimize decreases in cardiac output and increases in ICP. PEEP levels of 10 cm H$_2$O or less have been used without significant increases in ICP or decreases in CPP.[254] When higher levels of PEEP are required to optimize the PaO_2-PEEP–CPP relationship, both central venous pressure and ICP monitoring are indicated.

The administration of pharmacologic agents that increase cerebral vascular resistance can acutely reduce ICP. Thiopental, propofol, and etomidate are potent cerebral vasoconstrictors that can be used for this purpose. The effects of these agents on CBF, cerebral metabolic rate for oxygen (CMRO$_2$), ICP, and CPP are reviewed in this chapter. These agents are usually administered during induction of anesthesia but may also be administered in anticipation of noxious stimuli or to treat persistently elevated ICP in the intensive care unit.

Although rarely used to reduce ICP, hypothermia does this by decreasing brain metabolism, CBF, cerebral blood volume, and CSF production.[127,128] Drugs that centrally suppress shivering, muscle relaxants, and mechanical ventilation are required when hypothermic techniques are employed. Intraoperatively, a modest degree of hypothermia, approximately 34°C, is recommended as a way to confer neuronal protection during focal ischemia.[255] Hypothermic techniques are also employed to cool febrile neurosurgical patients. Hyperthermia is particularly dangerous in neurosurgical patients because it increases brain metabolism, CBF, and the propensity for cerebral edema.

Premedication

Lethargic patients do not receive premedication. Patients who are alert and anxious may receive an anxiolytic (*e.g.*, midazolam 5 mg po) before coming to the operating room. If there is any doubt about the patient's level of consciousness, the patient may be given sedation or analgesics in the operating room after an intravenous route is established. For the preinduction insertion of invasive monitoring devices in an awake, conversant patient, premedicants (*e.g.*, small doses of opioids) should be considered to alleviate the discomfort from needle punctures.

Monitoring

In addition to the routine monitors, measurement of intraarterial blood pressure, arterial blood gases, central venous pressure, and urine output is recommended for all major neurosurgical procedures. An arterial cannula is inserted before induction of anesthesia to continuously monitor blood pressure and to estimate CPP. When the arterial pressure transducer is at midhead level (usually the level of the external auditory meatus), MAP approximates the MAP at the level of the circle of Willis. Cerebral perfusion pressure is calculated as the difference between MAP and central venous pressure in patients without intracranial hypertension or the ICP in those with intracranial hypertension. When the cranium is open, ICP equals atmospheric pressure and CPP equals MAP. With direct arterial pressure monitoring, the hemodynamic consequences of the pharmacologic agents administered during anesthesia are recognized instantly. In addition, the arterial catheter provides ready access for intraoperative measurement of arterial blood gases, hematocrit, serum electrolytes, glucose, and osmolality. Arterial blood gas measurement is necessary to verify the adequacy of hyperventilation. In the elderly and those with ventilation/perfusion mismatch, end-tidal CO_2 may correlate poorly with the $Paco_2$. Therefore, the difference between $Paco_2$ and end-tidal CO_2 must be determined for a given patient in a given position. Radial, femoral, or brachial arteries are suitable for short-term cannulation; however, after ulnar artery collateral blood flow is tested, cannulation of the radial artery is preferred.

Because most neurosurgical patients are dehydrated preoperatively and then subjected to intraoperative diuresis, the measurement of cardiac preload and urine output is important. A right atrial catheter reflects cardiac preload and is used to determine the preoperative fluid deficit and rate of intraoperative fluid infusion. When possible, the central venous pressure catheter should be inserted through an antecubital vein instead of the jugular or subclavian veins. This avoids increased ICP from both the head-down position and decreased cerebral venous outflow. The position of the antecubital central venous pressure can be verified by chest X-ray, transducer pressure waveform, or p-wave configuration on the ECG.

Urine output is also measured as an indicator of perioperative fluid balance. During craniotomy, a diuresis occurs initially following the administration of osmotic or loop diuretics. Reduced urine output may reflect either hypovolemia or release of antidiuretic hormone.

Preoperative ICP monitoring is rarely used in patients for elective supratentorial tumor operations. ICP monitoring is an invasive procedure that can cause bleeding or infection. When performed with local anesthesia before induction, the procedure can be uncomfortable to the patient.

Muscle Relaxants

An increase in ICP has been reported after administration of succinylcholine in animals and humans.[256–258] Intravenous administration of succinylcholine is reported to produce activation of the EEG and increases in CBF and ICP in dogs with normal brains.[257] These cerebral effects have been attributed to succinylcholine-induced increases in muscle afferent activity that produce cerebral stimulation. In many, but not all, patients with compromised intracranial compliance, succinylcholine has been shown to increase ICP.[258,259] This increase can be blocked with a full, paralyzing dose of vecuronium or a pretreatment (defasciculating) dose of metocurine.[258,259] The nondepolarizing agent apparently eliminates the massive afferent input to the brain after succinylcholine.

To achieve muscle relaxation for intubation of the trachea, succinylcholine is not recommended for elective neurosurgical cases; however, succinylcholine remains the best agent for achieving total paralysis for the rapid-sequence intubation of

the trachea. Therefore, in an emergency room or ICU setting, when there is a risk of aspiration or a need for immediate reassessment of neurologic status, succinylcholine should be used. Simultaneously, an effort should be made to control anesthetic depth to protect against the ICP-elevating effects of such noxious stimuli as laryngoscopy, intubation, or tracheal suctioning. In the hemiplegic (or paraplegic) patient, succinylcholine is avoided because of the risk of hyperkalemia.[260] Succinylcholine-induced hyperkalemia has also been reported after closed head injury and ruptured cerebral aneurysms in patients who were not hemiplegic or paraplegic.[261,262]

Nondepolarizing muscle relaxants are used during induction and maintenance of anesthesia in neurosurgical patients. Agents that release histamine are avoided, however. Histamine alone may lower blood pressure and increase ICP, thus lowering CPP. When the blood–brain barrier is disrupted, histamine can produce cerebrovasodilation and increases in CBF.[263] Depending on the dose and rate of administration, most of the benzylisoquinolinium compounds (d-tubocurarine, metocurine, atracurium, mivacurium) have the potential to release histamine and thus increase ICP. Doxacurium and cisatracurium[264] produce minimal to no histamine release over a wide dose range. Atracurium in intubating doses is reported to have no significant effect on ICP, blood pressure, or CPP in neurosurgical patients.[265] The release of laudanosine by atracurium does not appear to have clinical significance in humans. Laudanosine has been reported to produce seizure activity in animals.[266]

The steroidal compounds (pancuronium, pipecuronium, vecuronium, and rocuronium) may be better relaxants for neurosurgical patients because they do not directly affect ICP. Pancuronium does not produce an increase in CBF, CMRO$_2$, or ICP in dogs.[267] However, pancuronium's vagolytic effects can cause increases in heart rate and blood pressure, which may elevate ICP in patients with disturbed autoregulation. Pipecuronium, another long-acting agent, is reported to have no significant effect on ICP or CPP in patients with intracranial tumors[268] and no hemodynamic side-effects. In patients with elevated ICP, vecuronium is currently the agent of choice for intubation and surgical paralysis. Vecuronium has no effect on ICP, heart rate, or blood pressure in neurosurgical patients.[269] To achieve relatively rapid airway control (within 90 seconds), a priming dose of vecuronium (0.01 mg·kg^{-1}) can be administered followed by a higher dose (0.10 mg·kg^{-1}), or high doses of vecuronium (to 0.4 mg·kg^{-1}) can be safely administered without hemodynamic consequence.[270] Rocuronium also has no effect on ICP in neurosurgical patients, but may have some mild vagolytic activity in higher doses (0.9 mg·kg^{-1}).[271]

Induction, Maintenance, and Emergence

When the patient is brought into the operating room, a gross neurologic examination should be repeated and documented because changes in the patient's neurologic status can occur overnight. In patients with elevated ICP by clinical exam, CT scan and/or ICP measurement, osmotherapy may be indicated before induction of anesthesia. After appropriate monitoring devices are applied, the cooperative patient is asked to hyperventilate while preoxygenation is provided. Before laryngoscopy and intubation of the trachea, the patient is smoothly and deeply anesthetized with agents that reduce ICP. In the presence of elevated ICP, thiopental is commonly used to induce anesthesia; however, alternative agents such as propofol, etomidate, or midazolam can be used depending on the patient's medical condition. The following induction sequence is suggested: The intravenous administration of thiopental (3–5 mg·kg^{-1}) or propofol (1.25–2.5 mg·kg^{-1}) is followed by an opioid (fentanyl, 3–5 μg·kg^{-1}) and muscle relaxant. If no airway difficulties are anticipated, vecuronium (0.1 mg·kg^{-1}) is administered while controlled hyperventilation with 100% oxygen is instituted. In patients who have been vomiting because of elevated ICP, cricoid pressure is applied during mask ventilation. To deepen the anesthetic, fentanyl is administered in 50-μg increments to a total dose of 10 μg · kg^{-1}, depending on the blood pressure response. Lidocaine (1.5 mg · kg^{-1}) is also administered intravenously 90 seconds before intubation to suppress laryngeal reflexes.[272] When the peripheral muscle twitch response disappears, an additional 2–3 mg · kg^{-1} bolus of thiopental is administered, and endotracheal intubation is performed as rapidly and smoothly as possible. An esmolol infusion or bolus may also be used to reduce the heart rate and blood pressure response to laryngoscopy and intubation. After induction of anesthesia, ventilation of the lung is controlled mechanically and adjusted to maintain Paco$_2$ between 30 and 35 mm Hg. Arterial blood gases are measured after intubation to establish the arterial end-tidal CO$_2$ gradient.

The most commonly administered maintenance anesthetics for patients with supratentorial tumors are nitrous oxide–opioid and nitrous oxide–volatile inhalation agents. In practice, the opioid most frequently employed is fentanyl, and the volatile agent most frequently employed is isoflurane. Nitrous oxide, 50–70% in oxygen, is typically administered to decrease the total dose of intravenous agent or the required concentration of volatile agent. The cerebrovascular effects of nitrous oxide are not benign,[49,50] and studies report that at equipotent doses, isoflurane has less adverse effects on ICP[273] and CBF[274] than nitrous oxide.

In patients with elevated ICP or low compliance, some clinicians avoid the administration of either nitrous oxide or high concentrations of isoflurane (i.e., greater than 1.0%). Alternatively, an opioid–thiopental or propofol anesthetic technique may be employed with midazolam or low-dose isoflurane added for amnesia. When severe intracranial hypertension exists and the brain is tight despite adequate hyperventilation and the administration of steroids and diuretics, a totally intravenous technique is recommended, e.g., a thiopental infusion (2–3 mg · kg^{-1} · hr^{-1}) and fentanyl boluses or infusion (1–4 μg · kg^{-1} · hr^{-1}).

Emergence from anesthesia should be as smooth as possible, avoiding straining or bucking on the endotracheal tube. Bucking can cause arterial hypertension and elevated ICP during termination of anesthesia, which can lead to postoperative hemorrhage and cerebral edema. To avoid bucking during emergence, muscle relaxants are not reversed until the head dressing is applied. Intravenous lidocaine (1.5 mg · kg^{-1}) can be administered 90 seconds before suctioning and extubation to minimize cough, straining, and hypertension. Antihypertensive agents such as labetalol and esmolol are also administered during emergence to control systemic hypertension.

In the usual craniotomy for excision of a supratentorial tumor, the conduct of the anesthetic is aimed at awakening and extubating the patient at the end of the procedure. The removal of a large tumor improves the patient's intracranial compliance, and hypercarbia required to drive ventilation in the emerging patient is usually well tolerated. The patient is extubated only when fully reversed from paralysis, and when he or she is awake and following commands. If the patient is not responsive, the endotracheal tube remains in place until the patient is awake and following commands. A brief neurologic examination is performed before and after extubation of the trachea. The patient is positioned with the head elevated 30° and transferred to the recovery room with oxygen by mask and oxygen saturation monitoring. Close monitoring and care, including frequent neurologic examinations, are continued in the recovery room.

Infratentorial Intracranial Tumors

The perioperative management of infratentorial tumors poses significant surgical and anesthetic challenges because of the relatively confined space within the posterior fossa. The posterior fossa contains the medulla, pons, cerebellum, major motor and sensory pathways, primary respiratory and cardiovascular centers, and lower cranial nerve nuclei. Because of the posterior fossa's small size, a localized tumor can significantly compromise these vital brain stem structures and cranial nerves. Consequently, when evaluating patients with infratentorial tumors, the anesthesiologist should be aware that these patients have the potential to develop profound neurologic damage. Patients may exhibit depressed levels of consciousness secondary to increased ICP from obstructive hydrocephalus and/or exhibit signs of brain stem compression with depressed respiration and cranial nerve palsies. Preoperative endotracheal intubation and respiratory support may be required.

Special Anesthetic Considerations

Patient Position. A major challenge of infratentorial surgery is preventing further neurologic damage from the position of the patient and exploration. There is considerable controversy among neurosurgeons as to the best position for infratentorial surgery.

Exploration of the posterior fossa has been traditionally performed in the sitting position because it provides excellent surgical exposure and facilitates venous and CSF drainage. From the standpoint of the anesthesiologist, the sitting position provides better ventilation and easier access to the chest, airway, endotracheal tube, and extremities. Furthermore, facial and conjunctival edema is reduced. However, the sitting position is associated with significant risks. In older or debilitated patients, the sitting position can produce cardiovascular instability, resulting in hypotension with cerebral and cardiovascular compromise. A significant risk of venous air embolism occurs in patients operated on in the sitting position, and an attendant risk of paradoxical air embolism may also occur in patients with a patent foramen ovale or other right-to-left shunt.

Other problems associated with the sitting position are peripheral nerve injury, pneumocephalus, jugular venous obstruction, and quadriplegia. Peripheral nerve injuries to the ulnar, sciatic, or lateral peroneal nerves can result if care is not taken in positioning and padding the respective pressure points. Pneumocephalus occurs frequently in patients who have surgery performed in the sitting position.[275] Pneumocephalus may develop into tension pneumocephalus postoperatively, producing serious neurologic dysfunction. Nitrous oxide has been implicated in the genesis of tension pneumocephalus.[276] Because of this, when used, nitrous oxide should be discontinued before dural and cranial closure and avoided if surgery recurs within 7 days. Jugular venous obstruction causing swelling of the face and tongue may result from hyperflexion of the neck. To avoid this, head flexion should be limited by placing two fingers between the mandible and sternum. Paraplegia, triplegia, and quadriplegia have been reported following surgery in the sitting position. This complication has been attributed to mechanical compression of the cervical spinal cord or vertebrobasilar blood vessels and stretching of spinal cord blood vessels, causing ischemia during head flexion.[277] If hypotension occurs, the brainstem and cervical spinal cord are rendered even more vulnerable to an ischemic insult. During positioning for posterior fossa exploration, cases of position-related brain stem and cervical spinal cord ischemia have been reported.[278,279] Therefore, flexion of the head on the cervical spine may be hazardous in some patients with large posterior fossa tumors and in elderly or arthritic patients. A preoperative examination of the mobility of the cervical spine, including a review of radiologic studies to determine the width of the cervical canal, should be performed to establish whether the patient can tolerate the position required for surgery. In addition, the application of SEP monitoring during positioning for surgery may be used to detect position-related ischemia.

Other positions used for posterior fossa exploration are the lateral, prone, and "park bench" or three-quarters prone positions. These alternative positions have been advocated because of the lower incidence of air emboli and greater cardiovascular stability associated with them. Potential disadvantages of these positions are malignant cerebellar edema and venous hemorrhage. To date, there is no evidence that operative position affects postoperative outcome. In a study that reviewed 579 posterior fossa craniectomies, patients in the sitting position had less blood loss and postoperative cranial nerve dysfunction than patients operated on in the horizontal position (supine, prone, lateral, and park bench), and there was no difference in the incidence of hypotension and postoperative cardiopulmonary complications between groups.[280] The incidence of venous air embolism in this series of patients was significantly greater in sitting versus horizontal patients (45% vs. 12%), but it was not associated with a significantly increased morbidity or mortality.[280] The authors concluded that there are significant advantages and disadvantages to both sitting and horizontal positions and that these positions can be used safely.

Because of various advantages and disadvantages to both sitting and horizontal positions, no one best position exists for all patients requiring exploration of the posterior fossa. The selection of the most appropriate position for an individual patient should be based on the location of the tumor, surgical exposure, the patient's medical condition, and consideration of the risks and benefits.

Monitoring.   During posterior fossa exploration, surgical retraction or manipulation of the brain stem or cranial nerves can cause significant cardiac dysrhythmia or alterations in blood pressure. Adequate warning of brain stem compromise is obtained by monitoring the ECG for alterations in cardiac rate and rhythm. In addition, direct arterial pressure monitoring provides continuous information on sudden changes in systemic blood pressure and an estimate of CPP. (To estimate CPP in the sitting position, the arterial transducer should be zeroed to the highest point on the skull.) The hemodynamic consequences of dysrhythmias or air embolism are also instantly recognized with direct arterial pressure monitoring.

Electrophysiologic monitoring of SEPs is used to detect ischemia and compromise of the brain stem or cranial nerves. For example, BAEPs are monitored during surgery for acoustic neuroma to help preserve function of cranial nerve VIII or during posterior fossa procedures to monitor brain stem ischemia. Depending on the tumor's location, SSEPs may also be used to detect brain stem compromise. Position-related ischemia has been observed during monitoring with either BAEPs or SSEPs.[278,279] Electromyography is used during resection of acoustic neuromas and microvascular decompression to test seventh nerve function when the face is not accessible to palpation or visual assessment.

Venous Air Embolism.   Venous air embolism may occur whenever the operative field is elevated 5 cm or more above the right atrial level. Whereas the incidence of air embolism is on average 40–45% in patients operated on in the sitting position, entrainment of air also occurs during operations performed in the lateral, supine, or prone positions. The primary pathophysiologic event in venous air embolism is intense vasoconstriction of the pulmonary circulation, which results in ventilation/perfusion mismatch, interstitial pulmonary edema, and reduced cardiac output as pulmonary vascular resistance increases.

Air may also pass directly through the pulmonary circulation or through right-to-left intracardiac shunts (*e.g.*, probe-patent foramen ovale) to the coronary and cerebral circulation when right atrial pressure exceeds left atrial pressure. A patent foramen ovale exists in 20–30% of the population on autopsy study.[281] In the sitting position, a reported 50% of patients develop right atrial pressure greater than left atrial pressure and thus have the potential for paradoxical air embolism.[282] The calculated risk of paradoxical air embolism is 5–10%. Preoperative screening with precordial two-dimensional contrast echocardiography during a Valsalva maneuver and cough has been suggested as a method to identify patients with patent foramen ovale.[283,284] If a patent foramen ovale is detected preoperatively,

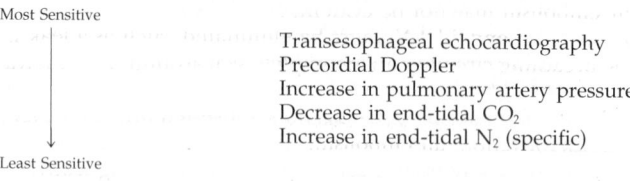

Table 28-11. MONITORS FOR DETECTION OF VENOUS AIR EMBOLISM

Most Sensitive	
↓	Transesophageal echocardiography
	Precordial Doppler
	Increase in pulmonary artery pressure
	Decrease in end-tidal CO_2
Least Sensitive	Increase in end-tidal N_2 (specific)

a position other than sitting is recommended for surgery because of the risk of paradoxical air embolism.

Monitors used for detecting venous air embolism are listed in Table 28-11. The two-dimensional transesophageal echocardiogram detects air bubbles with an echocardiographic probe placed behind the heart. The transesophageal echocardiogram is slightly more sensitive than the precordial Doppler,[285] but is invasive and cumbersome. The transesophageal echocardiogram has the advantage of monitoring air in the right and left cardiac chambers and the aorta, and thus can be used to detect both venous and arterial air embolism.

The precordial Doppler ultrasound transducer is the most sensitive noninvasive monitor of venous air embolism. It detects amounts of air as small as 0.25 ml. The transducer is positioned along the right parasternal border between the third and sixth intercostal spaces to maximize audible signals from the right atrium. Proper placement is confirmed by rapid injection of 5–10 ml of saline into a right atrial catheter. The resultant turbulent flow changes the Doppler sounds to a high-pitched noise similar to the sounds produced by intravascular air.

Pulmonary artery (PA) catheterization has been advocated for patients who undergo surgery in the sitting position. Passage of air into the pulmonary circulation leads to mechanical obstruction and reflex vasoconstriction from local hypoxemia. The PA catheter detects the resultant hypertension. (The change in pulmonary artery pressure correlates with the hemodynamic significance of the embolus because pulmonary artery pressure increases proportionally with the volume of air entering the pulmonary arteries.) Pulmonary artery pressure measurement is slightly more sensitive than capnography for detecting venous air embolism, but it is invasive. The PA catheter lumen is poorly designed for air aspiration. In addition, the fixed distance between the PA catheter tip and the right atrial port makes it difficult to position for both pulmonary capillary wedge pressure measurement and air aspiration. The catheter can be used to identify patients at risk for paradoxical air embolism, *i.e.*, patients who develop right atrial pressure greater than pulmonary capillary wedge pressure. When this occurs, measures to elevate pulmonary capillary wedge pressure, such as volume loading or repositioning, are undertaken.

In the operating room, exhaled gases are measured by infrared analysis, mass spectrometers, and analyzers based on Raman scattering. The infrared absorption technique is the most popular method of measuring the concentration of CO_2 in the airway. The capnograph is very useful for diagnosing venous air embolism. Small volumes of intravascular air produce a ventilation/perfusion mismatch, which is reflected in a reduced end-tidal CO_2. The capnograph complements the capabilities of the precordial Doppler by differentiating hemodynamically insignificant emboli that are heard with the Doppler from significant emboli. Doppler sounds without reduction in end-tidal CO_2 usually indicate insignificant amounts of air.

End-tidal N_2 monitoring is specific for detecting air but is slightly less sensitive than end-tidal CO_2 in detecting subclinical air embolism.[286] As intravascular air in the pulmonary circulation crosses the capillary–alveolar membrane, it is exhaled, increasing the end-tidal N_2 concentration. The advantage of knowing the value of the end-expired N_2 is the ability to calculate the volume of air entrained. When a patient is ventilated with an air–oxygen mixture, the increase in end-tidal N_2 with venous air embolism may not be evident. In addition, other causes of increases in end-tidal N_2 must be eliminated, such as a leak in the breathing circuit or an incomplete seal around the endotracheal tube cuff.

A central venous pressure catheter is inserted whenever there is a risk for venous air embolism. When the catheter is correctly positioned, entrained air can be aspirated from the right atrium. It is suggested that the optimal position for the tip of a single orifice catheter is 3.0 cm above the superior vena cava and the right atrial junction.[287] The position of the right atrial catheter may be confirmed by a chest film, by using a saline-filled catheter as a unipolar lead and following the configuration of the P waves on the ECG, or by transducing a venous waveform. Multi-orifice right atrial catheters are more effective than single-orifice catheters in aspirating air from the circulation.

Early diagnosis of air embolism is essential for successful treatment. The precordial Doppler unit is considered the basic monitoring device for detection of air embolism and is most effective when used in conjunction with end-tidal monitoring. The clinical significance of air embolism detected by Doppler ultrasonography can be assessed by a decrease in end-expired CO_2 or an increase in pulmonary artery pressure. A Doppler in conjunction with either a capnograph or a PA catheter usually detects air before physiologic alteration begins. Treatment is directed at preventing further influx of air. Whenever air embolism is suspected, the surgeon is notified immediately. The surgical field is flooded with saline and packed, and bone edges are waxed. Nitrous oxide, if present, is discontinued to prevent further expansion of embolized air. Neck veins are compressed as a means of increasing jugular venous pressure, which prevents further air entry and helps to localize the source of air. Aspiration of air from the right atrial catheter is attempted. With significant air embolism, patient position should be changed to lower the head to heart level when possible. If necessary, vasopressors and volume infusion are administered to treat hypotension. Positive end-expiratory pressure or Valsalva maneuver are avoided because they increase right atrial pressure and the likelihood of paradoxical embolus from venous air embolism.

Anesthetic Management. When selecting an anesthetic technique for patients in the sitting position, conditions of particular concern are cardiovascular stability and risk of air embolism. In changing an anesthetized patient from the supine to sitting position, a mild transient postural hypotension occurs in about one third of cases and marked hypotension in about 2–5% of cases.[288,289] General anesthesia with positive-pressure ventilation is associated with a reduction in blood pressure mainly caused by a decrease in cardiac output. As patients are placed into the sitting position, venous return is impeded, causing further reductions in cardiac output and blood pressure.[288,289] Therefore, efforts are directed at promoting venous return and maintaining cardiac output during the anesthetic management of these patients. An anesthetic technique that causes the least impairment of cardiovascular performance should be administered when patients are placed in the sitting position. Measures to avoid hypotension are also instituted. These include adequate preoperative hydration, wrapping the legs with elastic bandages, and flexing the patient's hips and knees at heart level. The patient's position is slowly changed, titrating position against systemic blood pressure. Administration of fluids (balanced salt solutions) and small amounts of vasopressors may be necessary.

Because nitrous oxide expands embolized air, some have advocated general anesthesia without nitrous oxide for anesthetizing patients in the sitting position. This, however, would necessitate the use of a volatile anesthetic agent. In some patients, the use of a volatile agent may increase the risk of focal or generalized ischemia from an increase in ICP and an anesthetic-

induced reduction in blood pressure. Therefore, the risks and benefits of using nitrous oxide versus a volatile agent for neurosurgical procedures with an increased potential for air embolism should be discussed and individualized. Nitrous oxide (50%) administration to patients undergoing surgery in the sitting position is reported to have no significant effect on the incidence or severity of venous air embolism, provided nitrous oxide is discontinued immediately on Doppler detection of air.[290] In general, a balanced anesthetic technique (nitrous oxide–oxygen–opioid–muscle relaxant) combined with controlled hyperventilation is recommended for maximal cardiovascular stability and control of intracranial hypertension. If air embolism occurs, nitrous oxide is discontinued. Nitrous oxide may be reintroduced cautiously with concurrent Doppler monitoring to determine whether the embolized air remains a threat.

Postoperative Concerns. The potential for significant cardiorespiratory and neurologic deterioration exists in the immediate postoperative period following posterior fossa exploration. Therefore, direct arterial pressure and ECG monitoring should be continued for the first 24–48 hours postoperatively, and neurologic examinations should be performed frequently.

Central apnea requiring postoperative ventilatory support may result from damage to respiratory centers caused by extensive posterior fossa exploration. If respiratory centers have been manipulated but not destroyed, respiratory impairment is temporary. Postoperative impairment of swallowing and pharyngeal sensation may occur secondary to stretch or manipulation of cranial nerves IX, X, and XII. These patients are at increased risk for aspiration pneumonia or hypoxia and therefore should remain intubated until airway protective reflexes return.

Systemic hypertension frequently occurs after posterior fossa surgery and requires immediate treatment to prevent brain edema and hematoma formation. Postoperative hypertension usually resolves within the first 24 hours. Atrial and ventricular ectopic beats may also occur within the first 24 hours.

Because of the proximity of respiratory and cardiovascular centers, any edema, hematoma, or infarction of the brain stem and cerebellum can produce serious compromise. When a patient fails to awaken satisfactorily from anesthesia, bleeding or acute swelling of the structures in the posterior fossa must be suspected. In addition, patients who are awake and talking may become unresponsive secondary to obstructive hydrocephalus or brain stem compression. Decreased level of consciousness is an early reliable sign of brain stem compression. More serious signs are systemic hypertension, bradycardia, and irregular or absent respirations. Reintubation and prompt surgical intervention to relieve pressure on the brain stem are necessary.

The preoperative level of consciousness and intraoperative conditions will determine whether the patient is extubated at the end of the procedure. A patient with a depressed level of consciousness preoperatively should not be expected to improve immediately after surgery. In general, patients who require preoperative mechanical ventilation usually require postoperative mechanical ventilation. Furthermore, if the surgical procedure is extensive, producing an engorged, swollen brain, postoperative mechanical ventilation is usually necessary.

Pituitary Tumors

The pituitary gland is located at the base of the skull in the sella turcica, a bony cavity within the sphenoid bone, and it is divided into anterior (adenohypophysis) and posterior (neurohypophysis) lobes. A fold of dura (the diaphragma sella) on the superior surface of the sella is pierced by the infundibular stalk, which connects the posterior lobe of the pituitary gland to the hypothalamus. The hypothalamus regulates hormone release from the anterior pituitary through regulatory peptides (hypothalamic releasing and inhibiting factors) that reach the anterior pituitary by a complex portal vascular system. Control of hypothalamic secretion is complex and occurs from neuronal and chemical influences, including feedback from target organ hormones. The large glandular anterior pituitary secretes at least seven hormones. The smaller posterior pituitary stores and secretes two hormones, antidiuretic hormone and oxytocin, which are synthesized in specialized hypothalamic neurons and transported as granules in axons down the pituitary stalk to the posterior pituitary gland. The anterior and posterior pituitary hormones are listed in Table 28-12.

Pituitary tumors can be divided into two general categories, nonfunctioning and hypersecreting. Nonfunctioning pituitary tumors are usually diagnosed when they become large and produce symptoms related to mass effects by impinging on adjacent structures. Headache, impaired vision, cranial nerve palsies, increased ICP, and hypopituitarism may result. The most common nonfunctioning tumors are chromophobe adenomas, craniopharyngiomas, and meningiomas. As these tumors enlarge, they can cause selective or global impairment of pituitary function by compressing the normal gland. A sudden enlargement of the pituitary caused by spontaneous hemorrhage or infarction into the tumor produces a symptom complex known as pituitary apoplexy, a life-threatening condition characterized by acute neurologic deficits and a rapid decline in pituitary function. Therapy includes rapid administration of corticosteroids and emergency surgical decompression.

Functioning pituitary adenomas produce an excess of one or more of the anterior pituitary hormones, and therefore are usually diagnosed when the tumors are small. The most frequently occurring are prolactinomas followed by growth hormone- and adrenocorticotropin-secreting adenomas. Adenomas secreting thyrotropin or follicle-stimulating hormone and luteinizing hormone are rare. Adenomas secreting both growth hormone and prolactin are common, however. Prolactinomas may produce the amenorrhea-galactorrhea syndrome in females and decreased libido and impotence in males. Excessive production of growth hormone before puberty results in gigantism; after puberty, in acromegaly. Cushing's disease develops from an adrenocorticotropin-secreting adenoma that causes bilateral adrenal hyperplasia.

Special Anesthetic Considerations

Preoperative Evaluation. The preoperative evaluation of patients with pituitary tumors requires an assessment of endocrine function and associated medical disorders. Endocrine tests are performed in the basal state and are supplemented by appropriate provocative tests (Table 28-13). These tests diagnose hyperfunctioning or hypofunctioning tumors, the extent of endocrine disturbance, and the adequacy of treatment. A thorough discussion of endocrinologic testing can be found elsewhere.[291]

In Cushing's disease, the increased corticotropin and cortisol can produce multiple systemic effects such as diabetes mellitus with insulin-resistant hyperglycemia, hyperaldosteronism with hypokalemia and metabolic alkalosis, hypertension, mild congestive heart failure, and obesity. These patients require preoperative evaluation and management of hypertension, diabetes, and electrolyte imbalances, as well as a cardiovascular evaluation for ischemic heart disease and congestive heart failure.

Table 28-12. PITUITARY GLAND HORMONES

Anterior Pituitary	Posterior Pituitary
Growth hormone	Antidiuretic hormone
Prolactin	Oxytocin
Gonadotropins:	
Follicle-stimulating hormone	
Luteinizing hormone	
Adrenocorticotropin (ACTH)	
β-Lipotropin	
Thyrotropin (TSH)	

Table 28-13. PREOPERATIVE ENDOCRINE STUDIES FOR PITUITARY TUMORS

ANTERIOR PITUITARY FUNCTION TESTS

Basal levels of pituitary hormones: GH, prolactin, ACTH, TSH, FSH, LH
Serum levels: cortisol (AM and PM), thyroxine, testosterone, estradiol
Urinary levels: 17-ketosteroids, 17-hydroxycorticosteroids, free cortisol, estrogens
Provocative and suppression tests as indicated:
  GH reserve—glucagon stimulation
  GH suppression—glucose suppression (acromegaly)
  Prolactin reserve—chlorpromazine or thyrotropin-releasing hormone provocative testing
  Low- and high-dose dexamethasone suppression (Cushing's syndrome)
  Metyrapone test (Cushing's syndrome)

POSTERIOR PITUITARY FUNCTION TESTS

ADH reserve: Serum and urine osmolality before and after 8–12 hours' water deprivation.

Patients with acromegaly exhibit a general overgrowth of skeletal, connective, and soft tissues. Hands and feet become markedly enlarged and facial features become coarse. All major organs increase in size, including the heart, lungs, liver, and kidneys. These patients also require an evaluation for systemic hypertension, diabetes, ischemic heart disease, cardiomegaly, and congestive heart failure, with appropriate medical management instituted before surgery. Significant anatomic airway changes can occur in acromegalics, making airway management difficult. Facial bone hypertrophy, particularly of the mandible and nose, thick tongue and lips, and hypertrophy of nasal turbinates, soft palate, tonsils, epiglottis, and larynx create difficulties with mask fit and visualization of the larynx. Glottic stenosis caused by soft tissue overgrowth may cause preoperative hoarseness and dyspnea. These patients usually require a smaller endotracheal tube than anticipated based on the size of the patient's facial features, and may be predisposed to postextubation edema. Stretching or compression of the recurrent laryngeal nerves from laryngeal soft tissue or thyroid gland enlargement may result in vocal cord paralysis. Because of these anatomic changes, a thorough preoperative airway examination is required. Patients complaining of hoarseness, dyspnea, or inspiratory stridor should undergo indirect laryngoscopy and X-ray examination of the neck to analyze airway conformation and lumen diameter. Based on this evaluation, preparations for difficult airway management and intubation should be anticipated. For patients with difficult airways and glottic abnormalities, an awake fiberoptic intubation is recommended. This obviates the need for a tracheostomy in all but the most severe cases. Patients without upper airway or vocal cord involvement can be managed in the routine manner.

Pressure effects on the normal pituitary gland from parasellar tumors or other lesions can cause panhypopituitarism. Patients who have panhypopituitarism require replacement therapy with appropriate hormones. These patients should be euthyroid before surgery. Glucocorticoid replacement is required when thyroxine replacement is begun to avoid stressing the insufficient adrenocortical axis. Because glucocorticoids are also necessary to facilitate renal excretion of a water load, diabetes insipidus is usually not observed in the patient with pituitary insufficiency until cortisol replacement therapy is instituted. Preoperatively, the patient with panhypopituitarism will be receiving oral steroid and thyroxine therapy and, when indicated, intranasal instillation of synthetic vasopressin.

During the preanesthetic evaluation, the size and location of the tumor and its effect on intracranial dynamics should be determined. Pituitary microadenomas do not produce mass effects. Pituitary tumors with suprasellar extension, craniopharyngiomas, and other suprasellar tumors may exert a mass effect. In these patients, the CT scan or MRI and the neurologic examination are evaluated for signs of increased ICP. All patients scheduled for pituitary surgery are given supplemental short-acting glucocorticoid therapy perioperatively. Because the surgery involves manipulation or removal of the anterior pituitary, transient or permanent deficiency of adrenocorticotropin and cortisol secretion may result. To assess function of the optic nerves and chiasm, a visual examination, including examination of the visual fields, is performed. When transsphenoidal surgery is planned, an otolaryngologic examination of the nasal passages and nasopharynx is also performed, and a nasal culture is obtained to guide antibiotic therapy in the event of postoperative infection.

Surgical Considerations. Since the introduction of the operating microscope, transsphenoidal excision has been recommended for all pituitary tumors that do not have marked suprasellar extension. Advantages of the transsphenoidal approach include the following: lower morbidity and mortality rates with decreased incidence and severity of diabetes insipidus; elimination of frontal lobe retraction and external scars; magnified visualization and removal of small tumors, which spares normal tissue; decreased frequency of blood transfusions; and shorter hospitalization. Relative disadvantages include the possibility of CSF leakage and meningitis (which is rare with the use of antibiotics), inability to visualize neural structures adjacent to a large tumor, inaccessibility of tumors extending into middle and anterior fossae, and the possibility of bleeding from cavernous sinuses or carotid arteries (which can lead to intracranial hemorrhage, brain stem compression, and significant blood loss). The transcranial approach to the sella permits direct visualization of suprasellar structures: the vascular sinus ring, optic chiasm, hypothalamus, and pituitary stalk. This approach is recommended for pituitary tumors of uncertain diagnosis and those that have significant suprasellar extension with optic nerve or hypothalamic involvement. With this approach, there is potential for damage to the olfactory nerves, frontal lobe vasculature, and optic nerves and chiasm. In addition, the incidence of permanent diabetes insipidus and anterior pituitary insufficiency is increased.

Anesthetic Considerations. The anesthetic management of patients undergoing pituitary surgery is not fundamentally different from that of patients undergoing other craniotomies. Basic neuroanesthetic principles apply whether the transsphenoidal or transcranial approach is used. With the transcranial approach, however, intraoperative measures to control ICP are instituted because of pressure effects, the necessity for brain retraction, and the potential for greater blood loss.

During transsphenoidal procedures, central venous pressure is not routinely monitored. When the patient is positioned with a significant head-up tilt, however, air embolism may occur during this procedure. Therefore, precordial Doppler monitoring and right atrial catheterization are recommended for detection and treatment of air embolism when a significant surgical site–cardiac gradient (15° or more) exists.

Evoked potential monitoring of VEPs may be used during pituitary surgery to monitor direct compression or compromise of blood supply to optic nerves and chiasm. Technical difficulties that cause intraoperative recording problems include changes in pupil size, deviation of eyes, goggle size and bulkiness, and stimulus delivery (light flashes). Because VEPs are entirely cortical in origin, they are also more vulnerable to the effects of general anesthetics.

For transsphenoidal procedures, a sublabial incision and dissection through the nasal septum is performed; therefore, oral endotracheal intubation is required. The nasal septum is usually prepared with 4% cocaine pledgets placed in the nares, followed by injection of 2% lidocaine with epinephrine 1:200,000 to the submucosa. This combination develops a dissection plane, decreases bleeding, and buffers the hypertensive response to nasal dissection. Initially, the cocaine and epinephrine may cause hypertension, tachycardia, and dysrhythmias, and drugs to treat these responses should be available. After oral endotracheal intubation with a RAE tube, the oropharynx is packed with saline-soaked gauze to minimize blood pooling in the glottis, esophagus, and stomach. Intraoperative C-arm fluoroscopy of the skull (lateral views) is used during this procedure, rendering the patient's head and arms relatively inaccessible once the patient is draped.

Potential intraoperative complications during transsphenoidal procedures relate to the anatomic landmarks surrounding the sella turcica. The cavernous sinuses occupy the lateral walls of the sella and contain venous structures, the internal carotid artery, and cranial nerves III, IV, V, and VI. The optic chiasm, with its associated optic nerves and tracts, lies directly above the diaphragma sella in front of the pituitary stalk. Surgical manipulation in the region surrounding the sella can result in the following: hemorrhage from the venous sinuses or internal carotid artery, arterial spasm or thrombotic occlusion secondary to arterial manipulation, venous air embolism if head-up tilt is excessive, cranial nerve weakness secondary to trauma or stretching, and visual complications secondary to damage of the optic nerve or chiasm.[292]

The chosen anesthetic technique should permit gross visual acuity examination before patient extubation. If vision is the same or improved, extubation can proceed. If acuity is worse, futher diagnostic studies and emergent decompressive surgery may be required. After transsphenoidal surgery, the patient will awaken with nasal packing, necessitating mouth-breathing postoperatively. Therefore, these patients must be fully awake and following commands before extubation of the trachea.

Postoperative Concerns. In the immediate postoperative period after either transsphenoidal or transcranial procedures, the primary concerns are corticosteroid coverage and fluid balance. Dexamethasone followed by prednisone is given for 5 days after surgery or until postoperative testing shows an intact pituitary–adrenal axis. Fluid balance is assessed by strict attention to hourly fluid intake and output and urine specific gravity. Development of diabetes insipidus is uncommon during surgery but may occur early in the postoperative course. Diabetes insipidus is commonly seen during the first 12 hours postoperatively and usually lasts for 2–4 days. Diagnosis is based on the following: polyuria (2–15 l · day^{-1}), hypernatremia, high serum osmolality ($\geq$300 mOsm · kg^{-1}), decreased urine osmolality (200 mOsm · kg^{-1}), and decreased urine specific gravity (1.005 or less). Therapy includes replacement of urine losses with intravenous fluids. When urine volumes are excessive, exogenous vasopressin is given, *e.g.*, aqueous vasopressin (5–10 IU, iv or im, q 6 hr) or the synthetic analog of ADH, desmopressin acetate (0.5–2 μg, iv, q 8 hr; 1–4 mg, sc q 6–12 hr; or nasal inhalation 10–20 μg).

Other complications of pituitary tumor surgery include CSF rhinorrhea, hypothalamic injury or stroke, cerebral ischemia, and meningitis. After transsphenoidal surgery, patients must be carefully monitored in the recovery room for airway obstruction caused by bleeding and secretions in the pharynx. Frequent neurologic examinations are performed to note any changes in mental status. Patients who have had an uncomplicated hospital course after transsphenoidal surgery are often discharged within 5–6 days.

CEREBROVASCULAR MALFORMATIONS

Intracranial Aneurysms

Subarachnoid hemorrhage (SAH) from rupture of an aneurysm arising from the circle of Willis produces significant morbidity and mortality.[293,294] Of the estimated 28,000 victims each year in North America, 10,000 die before they can receive medical attention. Of the 18,000 patients who survive to receive medical attention, about half will die or become severely disabled. Only one third of all patients will be functional survivors. The peak age-related incidence for rupture is in the fifth decade of life, and the incidence for females is slightly higher than that for males. Potential risk factors for the development and rupture of aneurysms have been identified. Hypertension, a risk factor for aneurysm formation, is also a significant factor in aneurysm rupture.[295]

A patient with aneurysmal SAH may be classified according to one of several grading systems: Botterell's original classification,[296] the modification by Hunt and Hess[297] (Table 28-14), or the more recent World Federation of Neurosurgeons (WFNS) SAH scale[298] (Table 28-15). These classifications are used by neurosurgeons to estimate surgical risk and outcome. Higher grades, or patients who are clinically more impaired, are associated with the presence of cerebral vasospasm, intracranial hypertension, and increased surgical mortality. In general, the poorer the grade on hospital admission, the worse the prognosis.

The management of unruptured intracranial aneurysms is controversial. In a report from the International Study of Unruptured Intracranial Aneurysms, it was revealed that surgery did not reduce the rate of disability and death in patients with unruptured aneurysms smaller than 10 mm in diameter and no history of SAH.[299]

The presence of blood in the subarachnoid space causes an abrupt, marked rise in ICP, which often results in systemic hypertension and dysrhythmias. The abrupt increase in ICP accounts for the acute onset of a sudden, severe headache. The classic presentation of aneurysmal SAH is that of severe headache associated with stiff neck, photophobia, nausea, vomiting, and often transient loss of consciousness. With this presentation, the diagnosis of SAH is obvious. In about 50% of patients, a small bleed or "warning leak" precedes a major aneurysmal rupture.[300] Warning symptoms and signs tend to be mild and nonspecific (headache, dizziness, orbital pain, slight motor or sensory disturbance) and are generally ignored or misdiagnosed by both patient and physician.

The diagnosis of SAH is made by the combination of clinical findings and a CT scan. This is followed by angiography of both carotid and vertebral arteries to define the cause. Aneurysms are classified according to location and size. They arise at a branch or bifurcation, usually at a point where a major vessel makes a turn changing the axial flow of blood.

There are several potential complications of SAH and surgical treatment of aneurysms. The most important of these are intracranial hypertension, rebleeding, vasospasm, and hydrocephalus. *Intracranial hypertension* is present to some degree in most

Table 28-14. HUNT AND HESS CLASSIFICATION OF PATIENTS WITH SUBARACHNOID HEMORRHAGE

Grade	Criteria
0	Unruptured aneurysm
I	Asymptomatic, or minimal, headache and slight nuchal rigidity
II	Moderate to severe headache, nuchal rigidity, no neurologic deficit other than cranial nerve palsy
III	Drowsiness, confusion, or mild focal deficit
IV	Stupor, moderate to severe hemiparesis, early decerebration, vegetative disturbance
V	Deep coma, decerebrate rigidity, moribund

Adapted from Hunt WE, Hess RM: Surgical risk as related to time of intervention in the repair of intracranial aneurysms. J Neurosurg 28:14, 1968.

Table 28-15. WORLD FEDERATION OF NEUROSURGEONS (WFNS) SAH SCALE

WFNS Grade	GCS Scale*	Motor Deficit
I	15	Absent
II	13–14	Absent
III	13–14	Present
IV	7–12	Present or absent
V	3–6	Present or absent

SAH = subarachnoid hemorrhage; GCS = Glasgow Coma Scale.
* Refer to Table 28-18 for definition of scale.
Adapted from Drake CG, Hunt WE, Sank K *et al*: Report of World Federation of Neurological Surgeons Committee on a universal subarachnoid hemorrhage grading scale. J Neurosurg 68:985, 1988.

patients following a SAH. In the uncomplicated case, intracranial hypertension does not require specific treatment. Intracranial pressure gradually returns to normal by the end of the first week. If an intracerebral hemorrhage, intraventricular hemorrhage, vasospasm, or hydrocephalus develops, intracranial hypertension may be severe and require treatment. Patients may require emergency ventriculostomy, steroids, diuretics, or intubation and hyperventilation. Intracranial pressure should be lowered gradually, especially in patients with unclipped aneurysms. Abrupt lowering of ICP by lumbar puncture, ventricular drainage, or rapid infusion of mannitol can induce rebleeding.

Rebleeding occurs most commonly during the first 24 hours following initial SAH. The chance of rebleeding is about 4% within the first day; after 48 hours, it is 1.5% per day, with a cumulative rebleeding rate of 19% by the end of 2 weeks.[301] Recurrent aneurysmal hemorrhage is a devastating complication associated with increased morbidity and mortality.

Because of the incidence of rebleeding with conservative management of SAH, early aneurysm clipping (days 0–3) is currently recommended for patients who are alert on admission. The debate over "early versus late" surgery was largely resolved following the report of The International Cooperative Study on the Timing of Aneurysm Surgery (ICSTAS).[295,302] In this trial, overall management results demonstrated a similar mortality (20%) and good outcome (60%) for patients with surgery planned for early (0–3 days) and late (11–14 days) intervals. The least favorable outcome and highest mortality occurred in patients with planned surgery for days 7–10 after SAH. Patients who were alert on admission did best with early surgery. When only the North American patients were analyzed, early surgery (days 0–3) provided the best results in lower grade patients.[303] There was no difference in the incidence of intraoperative rupture between early and late surgery, and although there was a relationship between "tightness" of the brain during surgery and the interval from SAH to operation, aneurysm dissection was no more difficult in early than in late surgery.[302] The timing of surgery does not influence the risk for cerebral vasospasm.[304]

Cerebral vasospasm is a major cause of morbidity and mortality in SAH patients.[295,305] Angiographic evidence of vasospasm can be detected in up to 70% of patients. However, clinical vasospasm with ischemic deficits is observed in approximately 30% of patients, most often between days 4 and 12, with a peak at 6–7 days following SAH.[295] The clinical syndrome of vasospasm is often heralded by worsening headache and increasing blood pressure. It is characterized by progressive symptoms of confusion and lethargy, followed by focal motor and speech impairments corresponding to the arterial territory involved. The syndrome may resolve gradually or progess to coma and death within a period of hours to days. The diagnosis of vasospasm is confirmed by angiography. The transcranial Doppler (TCD) is a safe, repeatable, noninvasive method to identify and quantify vasospasm, and can be used to evaluate the effectiveness of various therapies.

The mechanism responsible for vasospasm is unknown; however, structural and pathologic changes have been demonstrated in the vessel wall.[306] There is also evidence that vasospasm after SAH correlates with the amount of blood in the subarachnoid space, and removal of extravasated blood decreases the occurrence and severity of ischemic deficits.[305,306] The component in blood implicated in causing cerebral arterial vasospasm is oxyhemoglobin.

Many drugs have been investigated for prevention or treatment of vasospasm, but most are ineffective. The calcium channel blocker nimodipine has become standard prophylactic therapy. However, the efficacy of prophylactic nimodipine after SAH has been seriously challenged.[307] A recent meta-analysis showed a reduction in vasospasm in nimodipine groups, but a corresponding reduction in mortality was slight and not statistically significant compared to control groups. "Triple-H" therapy—hypervolemia, hypertension, and hemodilution—has become the mainstay of treatment for ischemic neurologic deficits caused by cerebral vasospasm.[308-310] To improve cerebral blood flow to areas of impaired autoregulation, cerebral perfusion pressure is increased by intravascular volume expansion and induced hypertension. Intravascular volume expansion is accomplished with infusion of crystalloid, colloid, or blood to a pulmonary capillary wedge pressure of 12–18 mm Hg or a central venous pressure of 10–12 mm Hg. If this regimen does not reverse the deficit, a vasopressor (e.g., dopamine, dobutamine) is introduced to raise systemic blood pressure until the neurologic deficits subside or reverse. This therapy can worsen cerebral edema, increase ICP, and cause hemorrhagic infarction. Systemic complications include pulmonary edema and cardiac failure in patients at risk. Hemodilution, the last component of triple-H therapy, decreases blood viscosity and improves cerebral blood flow. The optimal hematocrit thought to maximize the oxygen delivery to tissues has been estimated at 33%, but may be higher in ischemic brain.

Another method for treating symptomatic vasospasm is cerebral angioplasty. Transluminal angioplasty can be used to dilate constricted major cerebral vessels in patients who are refractory to conventional treatment.[311,312] Superselective intra-arterial infusion of papaverine dilates distal vessels not accessible to angioplasty.[313] These procedures are usually performed under general anesthesia to minimize movement and permit accurate placement of the intra-arterial balloon used to dilate the cerebral vessels. The risks of angioplasty include aneurysm rupture, intimal dissection, vessel rupture, ischemia, and infarction.

Special Anesthetic Considerations

Preoperative Evaluation. When the neurologic examination is performed, the patient's clinical grade is noted (see Table 28-15). The patient's CT scan or MR image is evaluated to assess the presence and severity of intracranial hypertension. The severity, acuteness, and stage of the SAH as well as the presence of intracranial hypertension and the timing of surgery will determine the anesthetic management. Because the circle of Willis is proximal to the hypothalamus, a SAH in this area can cause a variety of disturbances related to hypothalamic dysfunction (e.g., ECG changes, temperature instability, various changes in endocrine [pituitary] function, various electrolyte disturbances).[314] Sympathetic overactivity and overstimulation of both adrenal cortex and medulla can contribute to hypertension and diabetes, requiring treatment with insulin.

Electrolyte abnormalities frequently occur secondary to the *syndrome of inappropriate antidiuretic hormone* (SIADH) secretion or diabetes insipidus. Hyponatremia is the most common electrolyte disturbance detected and is often associated with a high urinary sodium and osmolality, which is expected with SIADH. Unlike a patient with SIADH, however, the patient with SAH usually has a contracted intravascular volume despite hypona-

tremia. This cerebral salt-wasting syndrome may be caused by release of atrial natriuretic factor from damaged brain. The recommended therapy is to maintain normovolemia with isotonic saline solutions. Other factors contributing to intravascular volume contraction in these patients are supine diuresis secondary to increased thoracic blood volume, negative nitrogen balance, decreased erythropoiesis, increased catecholamine levels, and iatrogenic blood loss. Fluid balance and electrolyte abnormalities should be corrected prior to surgery.

Most aneurysm surgery requires significant intravascular volume shifts (diuresis followed by volume loading) and extensive systemic blood pressure manipulations (deliberate hypotension or hypertension). Therefore, patients with a history of hypertension, ischemic heart disease, and/or congestive heart failure must be in optimal condition to tolerate the hemodynamic changes required for this surgery. Depending on the degree of cardiovascular disease, inadvertent or deliberate hypotension may be poorly tolerated. When patients have significant hypertension, the blood pressure should be lowered gradually to normotensive levels to avoid cerebral ischemia. Agents such as propranolol, labetalol, or esmolol are used in neurosurgical patients because these agents do not affect cerebral blood volume or ICP. When the systemic blood pressure is lowered, a critical level below which neurologic deficits occur may be observed. Systemic blood pressure below this level should be avoided intraoperatively.

Electrocardiographic abnormalities are commonly associated with ruptured cerebral aneurysms.[315] The ECG changes include ST-segment depression or elevation, T-wave inversion or flattening, U waves, prolonged Q-T intervals, and dysrhythmia. The ECG changes are not necessarily associated with increased operative morbidity and mortality or consistent increases in serum myoglobin or creatine kinase. They usually resolve within 10 days following SAH and require no special treatment. When indicated, troponin levels should be drawn to determine the clinical significance of these abnormalities. When cardiac dysrhythmia and occasional frank subendocardial ischemia result in cardiac failure, appropriate treatment must be instituted.

Anesthetic Management. The anesthetic goals for intracranial aneurysm surgery are to avoid aneurysm rupture, maintain cerebral perfusion pressure and transmural aneurysm pressure, and provide a "slack" brain. Patients in WFNS scale I or II who appear anxious should receive premedication. Cerebral perfusion pressure is maintained by using drugs in doses that avoid sudden or profound decreases in systemic blood pressure or increases in ICP. Similarly, transmural pressure, which is defined as the difference between mean arterial pressure and ICP, must be maintained. (The pressure within an aneurysm is equal to the systemic blood pressure.) The relationship between transmural pressure and wall stress or tension of the aneurysm is linear. An increase in mean arterial pressure or fall in ICP will increase transmural pressure, wall stress, and risk of aneurysm rupture. Methods to control brain volume and ICP, such as hyperventilation, diuretics, spinal drainage, and head position, facilitate surgical exposure and minimize the retraction pressure that can cause tissue injury.

Standard monitoring plus an arterial pressure catheter is routinely used. A CVP or PA catheter is recommended in WFNS scale III or higher to provide a more accurate measure of the patient's volume status and cardiac function intraoperatively and postoperatively in the prevention or management of cerebral vasospasm. Electrophysiologic monitoring with the EEG or SSEPs may be used to monitor the adequacy of cerebral perfusion during induced hypotension or temporary/permanent aneurysm clip application. When barbiturates are administered for brain protection, the EEG is used to guide the dose required to achieve a burst suppression pattern.

To minimize the risk of hypertension and aneurysmal rupture during induction of anesthesia, intravenous lidocaine and the β-adrenergic antagonist, esmolol, or labetalol are recommended.

Following induction, ventilation is mechanically controlled to maintain normocarbia if ICP is normal. If intracranial hypertension is present, the $Paco_2$ can be lowered to 25–30 mm Hg. A deep plane of anesthesia must be established prior to insertion of head pins, scalp incision, turning the bone flap, and opening the dura in order to avoid a hypertensive response. When intracranial hypertension is present, anesthesia should be deepened with additional doses of thiopental and fentanyl until the skull is opened. Several techniques can be instituted during aneurysm surgery to provide a "slack" brain and facilitate dissection. These are hyperventilation of the lungs, osmotic diuresis, barbiturate administration, and CSF drainage during the procedure. A lumbar subarachnoid catheter or spinal needle is inserted after induction to allow CSF drainage during the procedure. Excessive loss of CSF must be avoided during insertion of the lumbar drain because it can decrease ICP, thus increasing aneurysmal transmural pressure and the potential for rupture. Removal of CSF after opening the dura is done cautiously with guidance by the surgeons.

The drugs most frequently used to maintain anesthesia during aneurysm surgery are fentanyl and thiopental (bolus dosing or infusions) in conjunction with isoflurane in oxygen. A propofol infusion instead of thiopental may also be used for these procedures. In conditions of poor intracranial compliance, a continuous infusion of thiopental ($1–3 \ mg \cdot kg^{-1} \cdot hr^{-1}$ following a bolus dose of $5 \ mg \cdot kg^{-1}$) is recommended as the primary anesthetic for aneurysm surgery in conjunction with a fentanyl infusion ($1–4 \ \mu g \cdot kg^{-1} \cdot hr^{-1}$) and 0.5 MAC concentration of isoflurane in oxygen. The total dose of fentanyl should not exceed $10–12 \ \mu g \cdot kg^{-1}$, unless postoperative ventilation is planned. Potential disadvantages to using thiopental are blood pressure instability and prolonged recovery from anesthesia. With this technique, a pulmonary artery catheter should be inserted to monitor and optimize cardiovascular performance and intravascular volume. Following an uneventful aneurysm clip application, the thiopental infusion is discontinued to prevent a delay in recovery.

Prior to aneurysm clipping, isotonic crystalloid solutions without glucose are administered to replace overnight fluid losses and provide hourly maintenance fluid requirements. When the aneurysm is secured, intraoperative fluid deficits are replaced and additional volume is administered. At the time of aneurysm dissection, blood is available for transfusion in case the aneurysm ruptures. A bolus of thiopental ($3–5 \ mg \cdot kg^{-1}$) may be given before temporary occlusion of a major intracranial vessel and before aneurysm clipping. If temporary occlusion lasts longer than 10 minutes, recirculation should be established, and additional thiopental administered before reapplying the temporary clip. Following aneurysm clipping, the central venous pressure and pulmonary capillary wedge pressure are raised to 10–12 mm Hg or 12–18 mm Hg, respectively, with crystalloid, colloid, or blood. A postoperative hematocrit of 30–35% is desirable. As discussed previously, intravascular volume expansion with hemodilution is recommended to reduce the risk of postoperative cerebral vasospasm.

When considering the use of deliberate hypotension during aneurysm dissection, the risk–benefit ratio must be assessed for each patient. The potential benefit of hypotension must be weighed against the risk of causing cerebral ischemia or ischemia to other organs. Patients with a history of cardiovascular disease, occlusive cerebrovascular disease, intracerebral hematoma, fever, anemia, and renal disease are not good candidates for induced hypotension. Such patients should only be subjected to moderate reductions in systemic blood pressure (20–30 mm Hg), if at all. The most commonly used agents to induce hypotension are sodium nitroprusside, isoflurane, and esmolol. Overall, induced hypotension has declined in use and has been replaced by temporary clipping.[316,317] The temporary occlusion of a feeding artery produces an acute reduction in focal blood flow and a slack aneurysm, thus eliminating the need

for induced hypotension and its systemic effects. Depending on the location of the aneurysm, either somatosensory evoked potentials or brain stem auditory evoked potentials can be used to monitor the safety of temporary occlusion.[316]

The major intraoperative complication of aneurysm surgery is hemorrhage. When an aneurysm ruptures intraoperatively, there is potential for major ischemic damage from hypotension and the surgical efforts to control bleeding. Hemorrhagic death is also possible. When the leak is small and the dissection is complete, it may be possible for the surgeon to gain control with suction and then apply the permanent clip to the neck of the aneurysm. Alternatively, temporary clips can be applied proximal and distal to the aneurysm to gain control. Thiopental may be given to provide some protection prior to the placement of the temporary clip. During temporary occlusion, normotension should be maintained to maximize collateral perfusion. If temporary occlusion is not planned or not possible and blood loss is not significant, the mean arterial pressure may be transiently decreased to 50 mm Hg or lower to facilitate surgical control. When bleeding is excessive, aggressive fluid resuscitation and blood transfusion must commence immediately. Administration of cerebroprotective agents may not be possible because of associated hemodynamic effects. Under these conditions, induced hypotension is not advised as the intravascular volume must be restored first.

Intraoperative Cerebral Protection. Thiopental has been the drug of choice for intraoperative cerebral protection during aneurysm surgery. In animal models, barbiturates have shown protection during incomplete focal ischemia, but not during global ischemia.[318] Barbiturates are the only agents shown to be useful in humans.[97,318]

Many practitioners institute mild intraoperative hypothermia (32–34°C) during aneurysm surgery[88] to enhance the brain's ability to tolerate ischemia. Its value is unproven, and its use may produce harmful side effects.[319,320] A large multi-institutional study is underway to determine whether mild intraoperative hypothermia will benefit this patient population.

The primary goals at the conclusion of surgery are to avoid coughing, straining, hypercarbia, and hypertension. For patients in Grades I and II who have no intraoperative complications, the endotracheal tube should be removed in the operating room and a neurologic examination performed. Patients who have intraoperative complications or have depressed consciousness preoperatively (Grades III–V) should remain intubated and receive mechanical ventilation until their neurologic status improves.

Postoperative Concerns. Variation in systemic blood pressure is common postoperatively and contributes significantly to morbidity and mortality in patients following aneurysm repair. Causes of hypertension include preexisting hypertension, pain, and CO_2 retention from residual anesthesia. The treatment of postoperative hypertension is critical to prevent the formation of cerebral edema or hematoma. Antihypertensive drugs should be administered after respiratory depression and pain are eliminated as causes. The hypertensive response usually subsides within 12 hours. When indicated, preoperative antihypertensive drugs are reinstituted and maintained.

After clipping of the aneurysm, cerebral vasospasm continues to pose a threat to neurologic integrity. Postoperative hypotension must be avoided, and the patient's intravascular volume must be accurately assessed with either a central venous pressure or pulmonary artery catheter. As previously discussed, a higher than normal intravascular fluid volume should be maintained.

Arteriovenous Malformations

An arteriovenous malformation (AVM) of the brain consists of a tangle of congenitally malformed blood vessels that forms an abnormal communication between the arterial and venous systems. The arterial afferents flow directly into venous efferents without the usual resistance of an intervening capillary bed; thus, oxygenated blood is shunted directly into the venous system, leaving surrounding brain tissue transiently or permanently ischemic. These lesions predominate in males over females (2:1), with the onset of complaints between the ages of 10 and 40. The chief clinical features are parenchymal hemorrhage or SAH, focal epilepsy, and progressive focal neurologic sensory-motor deficits occurring in a child or young adult. A vein of Galen AVM in infants may present with hydrocephalus and/or high-output cardiac failure. The natural history of AVMs is not completely understood.[321,322] The risk of hemorrhage is approximately 1–3% per year. The rate of rebleeding is 6% in the first year after a hemorrhage and about 2% per year thereafter.[321,322] Mortality from initial hemorrhage is high, with reports between 10 and 30%. Recurrence of hemorrhage with a fatal outcome is a constant danger. There are several options for the management of AVMs, including surgical excision, embolization, stereotactic radiosurgery (proton beams, gamma rays, or linear accelerator), a combination of the above, and leaving AVMs alone. Arteriovenous malformations of suitable size and location can be managed successfully with surgical excision. Surgical mortality ranges from 0.6% to 14% and correlates with size, location, and pattern of involvement of the AVM.[322] Early postoperative morbidity ranges from 17% to 28%; however, outcome studies report improvement in morbidity over time.[323] To avoid intraoperative or postoperative massive brain swelling or hemorrhage of large AVMs, operations may be staged or follow preoperative embolization.

Special Anesthetic Considerations

In addition to providing anesthesia for craniotomy and resection of the AVM, anesthesia may be required for radiologic embolization of the AVM. Closed embolization of cerebral AVMs is uncomfortable and invasive. This procedure may be performed under local anesthesia with sedation or under general anesthesia. It has been performed successfully with various combinations of sedative drugs (fentanyl, droperidol, midazolam, or propofol) that allow neurologic examinations during the procedure and permit immediate diagnoses of complications.[237,322] Children, uncooperative patients, and those with intracranial hypertension or airway problems usually require general anesthesia. General anesthesia does not allow direct neurologic assessment. Potential complications of embolization procedures are embolic or ischemic stroke and hemorrhage from the AVM, either acute or delayed. New onset or pre-existing seizures may occur during the embolization procedure, requiring treatment with benzodiazepines or barbiturates.

The anesthetic management of patients with AVMs is similar to the management of patients for aneurysm surgery. Depending on the presentation, the anesthetic approach is modified. For example, a large bleed may present with symptoms relating to mass effects and require maneuvers to reduce ICP. High flow through a large intact AVM may cause a "steal" with resulting cerebral ischemia and require different techniques to improve CPP. With more extensive lesions, hypothermia and high-dose barbiturates have been recommended for brain protection. Induced hypotension may also be required to reduce lesion size and blood flow.

Hyperemic complications, defined as perioperative edema or hemorrhage, may occur after removal of the AVM. Although the mechanism is unclear, one theory proposes that breakthrough cerebral edema and hemorrhage result when blood flow from the surgically obliterated AVM is diverted to the surrounding brain. The smaller vessels in the brain surrounding the AVM are not accustomed to the higher pressure-flow state, and autoregulation is exceeded, resulting in severe brain swelling, edema, and hemorrhage. The clinical syndrome of cerebral hyperperfusion with normal CPP has been called *normal perfusion pressure breakthrough*.[324] Other studies report information that is not consistent with this theory.[325,326] Immediate treatment

should include the simultaneous application of high-dose barbiturates, osmotic diuretics, hyperventilation, and maintenance of a low-normal MAP. Hypothermia may also be instituted. When marked brain swelling occurs intraoperatively, the patient should remain intubated, hyperventilated, and sedated postoperatively. Hypertension during emergence and postoperatively must be controlled, preferably with β-blockers, to prevent bleeding into the bed of the AVM.

DELIBERATE HYPOTENSION

With the exception of profound acute hypotension for AVM embolization,[327] more effort is currently being directed toward avoiding the need to induce hypotension during neurosurgery than toward developing new hypotensive drugs and pharmacologic combinations. That trend is likely to continue until substantial intraoperative brain protection becomes practical, at which time the popularity of induced hypotension may swing back to its former status as a routine procedure during neurosurgery. Meanwhile, "for urgent and rational indication in the carefully selected case,"[328] a clinician's best choice among the better known agents is probably the drug or drug combination with which he or she has the most experience. (See Table 28-16 for clinical information on frequently used agents.)

Commonly Used Drugs

Sodium Nitroprusside

Sodium nitroprusside [$Na_2Fe(CN)_5NO \cdot 2H_2O$] continues to be the most widely used drug for intravenous induction of hypotension. Like all nitrovasodilators, sodium nitroprusside decreases peripheral vascular resistance by metabolic or spontaneous reduction to nitric oxide.[329] Recent laboratory evidence suggests that sodium nitroprusside preferentially increases CBF to the ischemic penumbra and may offer a protective effect in that regard.[330] Adequate blood flow to vital organs is maintained at perfusion pressures above 50 mm Hg. Sodium nitroprusside has rapid onset, a short half-life, and primarily dilates resistance vessels without affecting cardiac output.

Adverse effects may result from sodium nitroprusside infusion. These include cyanide and thiocyanate toxicity, rebound hypertension, intracranial hypertension, blood coagulation abnormalities, increased pulmonary shunting, and hypothyroidism. In addition, myocardial, liver, and skeletal muscle oxygen reserves are decreased by sodium nitroprusside and mitochondria may be damaged.[331] Death from sodium nitroprusside-induced severe acidosis has occurred after infusion of 750 mg over a 5-hour period.[332]

Cyanide is produced when sodium nitroprusside is metabolized (see Fig. 28-13); 1 mg of sodium nitroprusside contains 0.44 mg of cyanide. Toxic blood levels (>100 mg · dl^{-1}) occur when >1 mg · kg^{-1} sodium nitroprusside is administered within 2 hours or when >0.5 mg · kg^{-1} · hr^{-1} is administered within 24 hours. The presenting signs of cyanide toxicity include elevated mixed venous O_2, (Pvo$_2$), requirements for increasing dose (tachyphylaxis and metabolic acidosis. Death from sodium nitroprusside secondary to cyanide has been reported in a pediatric patient when blood cyanide level was 400 mg · dl^{-1}.[333] Greater risk of cyanide toxicity exists in patients who are nutritionally deficient in cobalamine (vitamin B$_{12}$ compounds) or in dietary substances containing sulfur. Measurement of blood cyanide and *p*H will enable detection of abnormalities in high-risk patients for whom larger than recommended amounts of sodium nitroprusside have been used. Treatment should consist of intravenous thiosulfate except in those patients with abnormal renal function, for whom hydroxocobalamin is recommended (see Fig. 28-14). A cyanide antidote kit is commercially available. Circulating levels of thiocyanate increase when renal function is compromised, and CNS abnormalities result when thiocyanate

Table 28-16. DOSAGE, MECHANISM OF ACTION, ADVANTAGES, AND DISADVANTAGES OF COMMONLY USED AGENTS FOR INDUCING HYPOTENSION

Drug	Dosage	Mechanism of Action	Advantages	Disadvantages
Sodium nitro-prusside	$0.5–10\ \mu g \cdot kg^{-1} \cdot min^{-1}$	Nitric oxide-mediated direct vasodilatation	Rapid onset/offset titration control	Cyanide toxicity ↑ ICP Rebound hypertension Coagulation abnormalities ↑ Pulmonary shunting
Nitroglycerin	$1–10\ \mu g \cdot kg^{-1} \cdot min^{-1}$	Nitric oxide–mediated direct vasodilatation	Rapid onset/offset titration control	↑ ICP Rebound hypertension Coagulation abnormalities ↑ Pulmonary shunting
Trimethaphan	$1–5\ mg \cdot min^{-1}$	Ganglionic blockade	Rapid onset/offset	Histamine release Cerebral compromise below MAP 55 mm Hg ↓ Pseudocholinesterase
Esmolol	$0.2–0.5\ mg \cdot kg^{-1} \cdot min^{-1}$ loading dose $50–200\ \mu g \cdot kg^{-1} \cdot min^{-1}$	β-Adrenergic blockade	Rapid onset/offset	Limited efficacy Cardiac depression Bronchospasm
Labetalol	20 mg test dose $0.5–2\ mg \cdot min^{-1}$ (total 300 mg)	α- and β-adrenergic blockade	Reduced probability of adverse effects	Limited efficacy Bronchospasm
Prostaglandin E₁	$0.1–0.65\ \mu g \cdot kg^{-1} \cdot min^{-1}$	Direct vasodilation	Rapid onset ↓ Reflex tachycardia Stable CBF	Slow offset Bradycardia Hyperthermia
Nicardipine	Begin $5\ mg \cdot h^{-1}$ infusion, max $15\ mg \cdot h^{-1}$	Coronary and peripheral vasodilation	Rapid onset ↓ Reflex tachycardia	Slow offset Resists antihypotensive therapy ↑ Pulmonary shunting
Inhalation anesthetics	Titrate by inspired concentration	Vasodilation and myocardial depression	Provides surgical anesthesia	↑ ICP ↑ Cerebral edema ↓ Vital organ blood flow

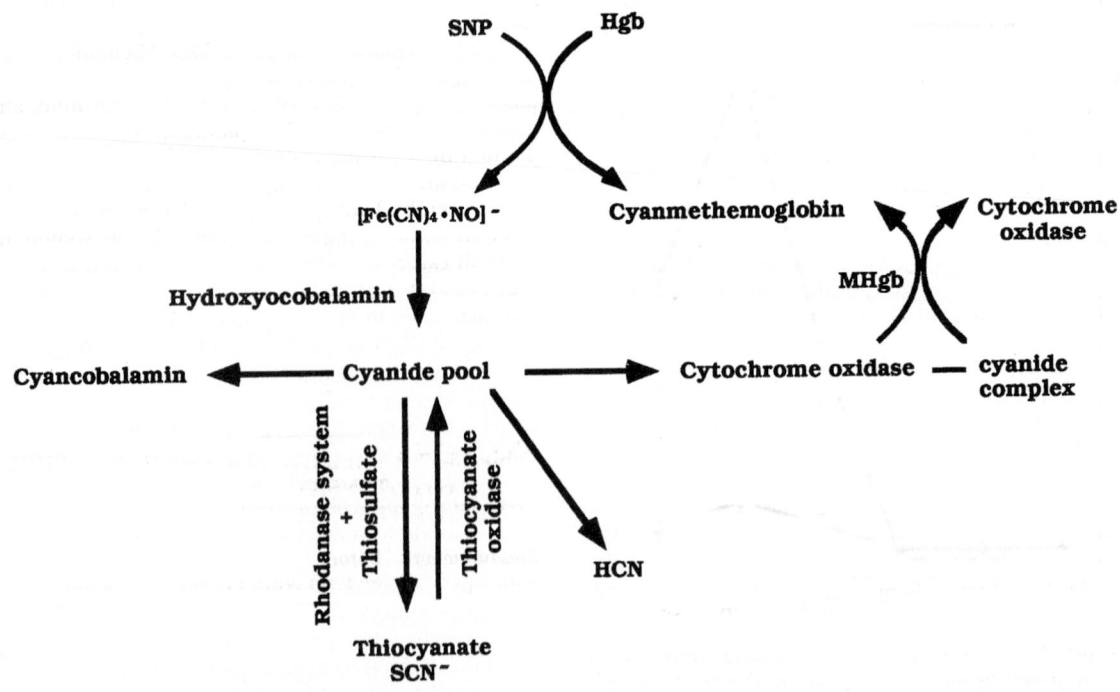

Figure 28-13. Red blood cell biotransformation of sodium nitroprusside. SNP = sodium nitroprusside; Hgb = hemoglobin; mHgb = methemoglobin; SCN = thiocyanate; HCN = hydrogen cyanide.

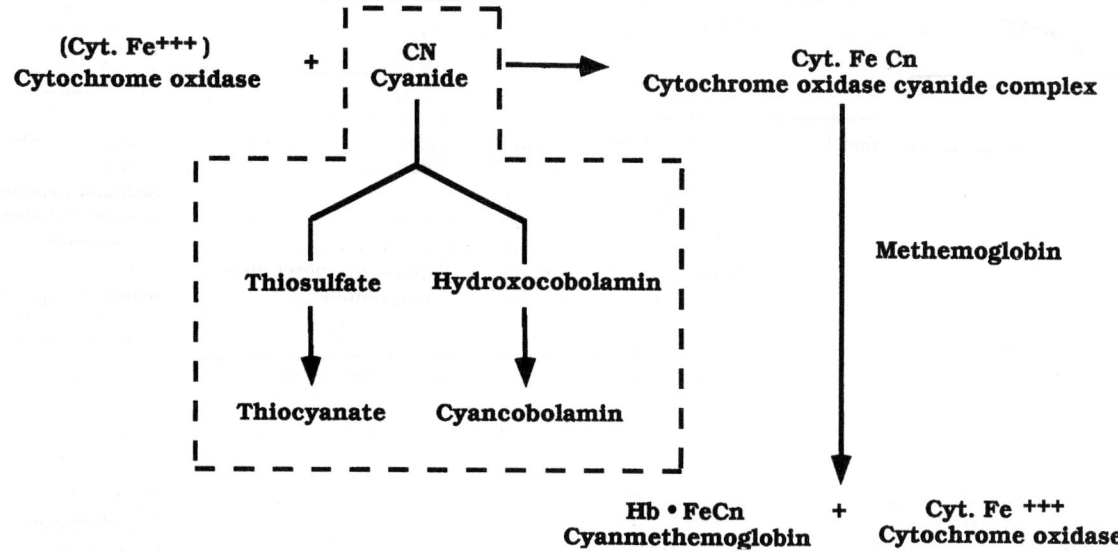

Figure 28-14. Tissue cytochrome oxidase combines with cyanide to form cytochrome oxidase–cyanide complex. Methemoglobin frees cyanide from the complex, forming cyanmethemoglobin. Other potential pathways to prevent toxicity include the addition of thiosulfate or hydroxocobalamin. The dashed line indicates treatment of cyanide toxicity.

levels reach 5–10 mg · dl^{-1}. Fortunately, captopril can be used to lower the dose requirement of sodium nitroprusside and thereby reduce the consequent buildup of cyanide (see Fig. 28-15).[334,335] Another recently advocated strategy for reducing the potential for cyanide toxicity is to maintain sodium nitroprusside–like pharmacodynamics while greatly reducing so-

dium nitroprusside dosage in a 1:10 mixture with trimethaphan.[336,337] Diltiazem,[338] metoprolol,[339] and esmolol have also been shown to effectively reduce sodium nitroprusside requirements, but esmolol does so at the cost of dose-dependent reductions in left ventricular contactility.[340]

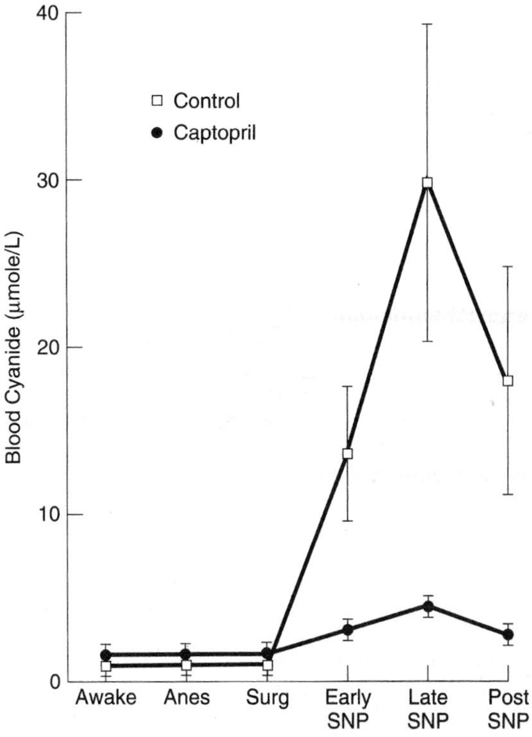

Systemic and pulmonary hypertension occur after abrupt discontinuance of sodium nitroprusside.[341] This results from increased plasma renin activity caused either by ischemic or dilated renal vessels. Gradual sodium nitroprusside discontinuance, preoperative propranolol, and converting enzyme inhibitors (captopril) will attenuate this response until increased plasma renin activity returns to normal (plasma half-life 30 minutes).

Based on results obtained in dogs, Michenfelder and Milde have argued that sodium nitroprusside dilates cerebral capacitance vessels regardless of anesthetic background, and dilates cerebral resistance vessels in addition when autoregulation is blunted by a volatile agent.[342, cf. 343] More recently, Stånge et al have found evidence in pigs that sodium nitroprusside directly impairs cerebral autoregulation.[344] Under either circumstance, if venous return is impeded by a mass lesion, sodium nitroprusside will cause an increase in cerebral blood volume. Accordingly, sodium nitroprusside causes increased ICP in patients with decreased intracranial compliance[345] (see Table 28-17). In the closed cranium an increase in ICP can cause hemispheric

Figure 28-15. Blood cyanide in two groups of patients whose blood pressure was decreased by sodium nitroprusside. Patients pretreated with captopril (3 mg · kg^{-1}) had significantly less cyanide than those not treated, even though a similar degree of hypotension was obtained. Total sodium nitroprusside infused was significantly less in patients treated with captopril. (From Woodside J Jr, Garner L, Bedford RJ: Captopril reduces the dose requirement for sodium nitroprusside-induced hypotension. Anesthesiology 60:413, 1984.)

Table 28-17. CEREBRAL PERFUSION PRESSURE AFTER HYPOTENSION INDUCED BY SODIUM NITROPRUSSIDE

Measurement (mm Hg)	Before Sodium Nitro Prusside	After Sodium Nitro Prusside
MAP	104 ± 2.55	70.0 ± 3.61*
ICP	14.58 ± 1.76	27.61 ± 3.16
CPP	89.32 ± 3.57	43.23 ± 4.60

* Mean arterial pressure (MAP) reduced by 33%; ICP, intracranial pressure; CPP, cerebral perfusion pressure.
From Cottrell JE, Patel KD, Turndorf H, Ransohoff J: Intracranial pressure changes induced by sodium nitroprusside in patients with intracranial mass lesions. J Neurosurg 48:329, 1978.

reductions in CBF due to regional reductions in cerebral perfusion pressure[346] (CPP = MAP − ICP). In the open cranium with open dura, sodium nitroprusside–induced cerebral vasodilatation is not likely to affect regional CBF,[346] but may cause brain swelling and disturb local perfusion, especially in areas under retraction and areas that are distant from the site of small to moderate size craniotomies.

Sodium nitroprusside can cause platelet disintegration and inhibition of platelet aggregation; however, recent evidence indicates that this complication is reversible and transitory.[347] Nevertheless, sodium nitroprusside-induced abnormalities in blood coagulation can exacerbate increased intraoperative bleeding caused by vasodilation.[348]

Increased pulmonary shunting occurs in patients with normal pulmonary function after sodium nitroprusside–induced hypotension, but fibrosed pulmonary vessels of patients with chronic obstructive lung disease show little response to sodium nitroprusside, and shunting increases are not significant.[349] Subsequent work has demonstrated a significant relationship between age and sodium nitroprusside sensitivity, with lower doses capable of inducing equally profound hypotension in older patients.[350] It is possible that further elucidation of this age–dose relationship will allow more appropriate age-specific administration of sodium nitroprusside with a consequent amelioration of sodium nitroprusside–related complications.

Nitroprusside is obtained in a 5-ml amber rubber-stoppered vial containing 50 mg of sodium nitroprusside dihydrate. It can be dissolved in 5% dextrose in water (D_5W) to the concentration desired; 50 mg of sodium nitroprusside in 250, 500, or 1000 ml of D_5W makes a concentration of 200, 100, or $50 \text{ mg} \cdot \text{ml}^{-1}$, respectively. Once dissolved, sodium nitroprusside deteriorates in the presence of light. The container, therefore, should be wrapped in aluminum foil. An unstable sodium nitroprusside ion in aqueous solution reacts with a variety of substances within 3–4 hours, forming colored salts. Other drugs should not be infused in the same solution as sodium nitroprusside.

Because vascular response to sodium nitroprusside can be dramatic, it should be administered with an infusion pump. The usual dose of sodium nitroprusside is $0.5–10 \text{ }\mu\text{g} \cdot \text{kg}^{-1} \cdot \text{min}^{-1}$. The infusion should begin at $1 \text{ }\mu\text{g} \cdot \text{kg}^{-1} \cdot \text{min}^{-1}$ and increased to achieve the desired MAP. If adequate reduction of blood pressure is not obtained with $10 \text{ }\mu\text{g} \cdot \text{kg}^{-1} \cdot \text{min}^{-1}$ within 10–15 minutes, the infusion should be stopped to avoid cyanide toxicity. Direct arterial pressure monitoring should be used during sodium nitroprusside infusion.

Nitroglycerin

Nitroglycerin directly dilates capacitance vessels and has a short half-life and no clinically significant toxic metabolites. As with sodium nitroprusside, decreased intracranial compliance contraindicates nitroglycerin use before dural opening unless steroids, diuretics, or sedatives have improved compliance. Even with the dura open, both nitrates entail some risk of increased cerebral blood volume and significant brain swelling.[341,351] Also similar to sodium nitroprusside, after nitroglycerin-induced hypotension, pulmonary shunting increases in patients with normal pulmonary function in contrast to those with chronic obstructive pulmonary disease. One research report indicates that nitroglycerin reduces cardiac index compared with sodium nitroprusside at MAP of 40 mm Hg.[352]

Nitroglycerin is supplied in a variety of formulations from various manufacturers, some of which require dilution. As obtained from the manufacturer, nitroglycerin is relatively stable when exposed to light and can be kept up to 2 years without refrigeration. The drug is administered continuously for deliberate hypotension or to control increased blood pressure, using a direct intravenous infusion without dilution. Nitroglycerin is adsorbed by plastic bags and should be infused from glass bottles or from high-density polyethylene syringes and tubings. An infusion pump is best for infusion at a beginning rate of $1–2 \text{ }\mu\text{g} \cdot$

$\text{kg}^{-1} \cdot \text{min}^{-1}$, with increases to achieve the desired blood pressure level. Good hypotensive response is usually seen at $2 \text{ }\mu\text{g} \cdot \text{kg}^{-1} \cdot \text{min}^{-1}$. Upper limits of infusion have not been set, since toxic effects have not been described, but the concentration of the infused solution should not exceed $400 \text{ }\mu\text{g} \cdot \text{ml}^{-1}$.

Trimethaphan

Trimethaphan blocks sympathetic ganglia, resulting in resistance and capacitance vessel relaxation, which usually decreases arterial pressure. Trimethaphan's short plasma half-life makes for easy control, but histamine release has been reported to cause bronchospasm[353] and potential ICP increases.[354] The speed of infusion and altered autoregulation may also influence trimethaphan's effect on ICP.[355] Myoneural blockade has been reported after administration of trimethaphan, probably due to its chemical resemblance to neuromuscular blocking agents.

Trimethaphan is not recommended for hypotension below 55 mm Hg MAP because EEG suppression occurs below this level,[356] though that effect may be less frequent when isoflurane is used as a background anesthetic.[357] Laboratory results show that cortical CBF and tissue oxygenation are reduced during profound trimethaphan-induced hypotension (MAP 30–35 mm Hg) relative to sodium nitroprusside-induced hypotension,[358] and that trimethaphan hypotension below MAP 50 mm Hg causes increased brain lactate concentrations.[359] These findings accord well with recent evidence that trimethaphan reduces local CBF during neuroleptanalgesia in humans, even when MAP is maintained at 70 mm Hg.[360] When these cerebral effects are considered in light of experimental evidence that trimethaphan-induced hypotension reduces arterial baroreflex response to rapid blood loss from exsanguination,[361] it seems reasonable to conclude that trimethaphan should not be used as a sole agent for producing hypotension during neurosurgical procedures.

Esmolol and Labetalol

Esmolol, an ultrashort-acting cardioselective β-adrenergic blocker with an estimated half-life of approximately 9 minutes, has been used to decrease blood pressure by itself[362,363] or in combination with other drugs.[364] Esmolol's cardiac depressant properties indicate caution in attempting to use it as a primary hypotensive agent.

Labetalol, a combined α- and β-adrenergic blocker, has also been used as a sole hypotensive agent in humans.[365,366] Like esmolol, labetalol is probably better used in combination therapies[367,368] when inducing hypotension, not only because of bradycardia, but also because of its lack of potency.[364] Both esmolol and labetalol have properties that make them appropriate for reduction of hypotension in neurosurgical patients (they do not dilate cerebral vessels, increase heart rate, cause rebound hypotension, or produce toxic metabolites under laboratory conditions),[369] but neither is adequate when used alone for induction of surgical hypotension.

Prostaglandin E_1

Prostaglandin E_1 (PGE) is a naturally occurring substance that induces rapid hypotension by dilating vascular smooth muscle via a specific PGE receptor. Unlike other direct vasodilators, PGE does not cause reflex tachycardia, but its hypotensive effects have been reported to persist for up to an hour following discontinuation.[370] Cerebral blood flow and carbon dioxide reactivity remain stable during PGE hypotension. Kadoi and coauthors have provided evidence that cerebral flow/metabolism coupling and regional cerebral oxygenation are maintained during PGE-induced hypotension to MAP 67 mm Hg.[371]

Nicardipine

Nicardipine induces hypotension by selectively blocking calcium channels in the musculature of coronary, peripheral, and, to a lesser degree, cerebral vasculature. Like PGE, nicardipine reduces the risk of reflex tachycardia[372] and has a prolonged duration of action.[373] Unlike PGE, nicardipine is as potent as nitroprusside. Caution must be exercised when titrating nicardipine for deliberate hypotension because its effect is difficult to reverse.

Halothane, Enflurane, Isoflurane, Desflurane, and Sevoflurane

The volatile anesthetics induce hypotension when their respective inspired concentrations are increased. Decreased blood pressure results from varying degrees of myocardial depression and peripheral vascular dilatation. Potential adverse effects include autoregulatory loss of vital organ blood flow, reduction in CPP as MAP decreases, ICP increase in patients with intracranial masses, increased cerebral edema, and accumulation of anaerobic metabolites.

Halothane-induced hypotension entails the risk of adverse myocardial depression,[374] loss of autoregulation,[375] and increases in ICP that cannot be resolved through hyperventilation.[376,377] In addition to reducing cardiac output, high-dose or prolonged enflurane anesthesia has been shown to increase CSF production in the laboratory[378] and induce seizures in some patients, especially during hypocapnia.

Laboratory evidence suggests that desflurane hypotension causes substantial reduction in CPP and CBF with a concomitant decrease in $CMRO_2$.[379] Recent results derived from humans indicated that the blood pressure response to changes in inspired concentration of sevoflurane is more rapid than the response to changes in concentrations of isoflurane.[380]

The only inhalation agent currently recommended for deliberate hypotension is isoflurane.[381] MacNab et al have determined that, relative to sodium nitroprusside, isoflurane blunts the stress response to induced hypotension.[382] The hypotension that results from isoflurane is primarily a consequence of peripheral vascular dilation, with maintenance of cardiac output except at higher inspired concentrations. Reports of worsening of ST-segment changes and shunting of blood from collateral-dependent regions in the myocardium have caused concern about using isoflurane in patients with myocardial disease.[383] Pulmonary shunting and dead space are not increased during isoflurane-induced hypotension.

Because of isoflurane's ability to reduce $CMRO_2$ while maintaining CBF,[384] cerebral protection seemed likely. However, Bendo et al[385] have found that isoflurane is not as protective as thiopental in the in vitro hippocampal slice model, and Nehls et al[386] have demonstrated that isoflurane does not afford protection after focal ischemia. Gelb et al have tested the hypothesis that isoflurane-induced hypotension provides a measure of protection relative to sodium nitroprusside-induced hypotension during middle cerebral artery occlusion in monkeys.[387] Unfortunately, they found no difference in neurologic scores or lesion size between the isoflurane and sodium nitroprusside groups. These results are consonant with Sano and coauthors' laboratory finding that isoflurane does not provide more cerebral protection than halothane,[388] and Bendo and coauthors' finding that isoflurane-induced hypotension in dogs causes more cerebral edema than does equivalent hypotension induced with labetalol.[389]

In a nonhuman primate, Van Aken et al[390] have demonstrated loss of autoregulation for 60 minutes after discontinuance of isoflurane and increases in CBF, which could worsen edema and ischemia and increase neurologic deficits. Endlund and coauthors have found that adenylate kinase, a marker of brain cell injury, increased 400% in the CSF of patients in whom hypotension was induced by isoflurane to MAP 50–65 mm Hg for 20–170 minutes.[391] Although high-dose isoflurane per se is not implicated by this result due to lack of a control or alternative hypotensive regimen, recent evidence indicates that equivalent degrees of hypotension can be obtained with less than 1% isoflurane if either labetalol[392] or the angiotension-converting enzyme enalapril[393] is used in conjunction.

HEAD INJURY

Head injury is a leading cause of disability and death in young people. The annual incidence of head injury in the United States is approximately 200 per 100,000 of the population.[394] Approximately 500,000 people each year sustain severe head injury, which includes those requiring hospitalization (450,000) and those who die before reaching the hospital (50,000). Of the 450,000 admitted to the hospital, significant residual disability remains in about 100,000 people each year. Head injury occurs most frequently in young adults aged 15–24 years. Males are affected two to three times more often than females in all age groups and are more likely to sustain severe head injury. More than 50% of patients with severe head injury have multiple injuries resulting in significant blood loss, systemic hypotension, and hypoxia.[395] Causes of head injury include motor vehicle accidents, falls, physical assault, firearm accidents, domestic accidents, birth trauma, and work-related and sports injuries. Motor vehicle accidents cause more than 50% of all head injuries and more than 70% of all fatal head injuries.[394]

Classification of severe head injury is based on the Glasgow Coma Scale (Table 28-18), which defines neurologic impairment in terms of eye opening, speech, and motor function.[396,397] The total score that can be obtained is 15, and severe head injury is determined by a score of 8 or less persisting for 6 hours or more. The Glasgow Coma and Glasgow Outcome Scales permit comparison between series of traumatically head-injured patients based on initial clinical presentation and eventual outcome.[394,398] The prognosis after head injury depends on the type of lesion sustained, the age of the patient, and the severity of the injury as defined by the Glasgow Coma Scale. In general, mortality is closely related to the initial score on the coma scale. For any given lesion and score, however, the elderly have a poorer outcome than do younger patients.[394]

Following head trauma, the primary injury results from the biomechanical effect of forces applied to the skull and brain at the time of the insult and is manifested within milliseconds. Currently, there is no treatment for the primary injury. Secondary injury occurs minutes to hours after the impact and represents complicating processes initiated by the primary injury, such as ischemia, brain swelling and edema, intracranial hemorrhage, intracranial hypertension, and herniation. Factors that

Table 28-18. MODIFIED GLASGOW COMA SCALE

EYE OPENING

Spontaneously	4
To verbal command	3
To pain	2
None	1

BEST VERBAL RESPONSE

Oriented, conversing	5
Disoriented, conversing	4
Inappropriate words	3
Incomprehensible sounds	2
No verbal response	1

BEST MOTOR RESPONSE

Obeys verbal commands	6
Localizes to pain	5
Flexion / withdrawal	4
Abnormal flexion (decorticate)	3
Extension (decerebrate)	2
No response (flaccid)	1

Mild head injury = 13–15; moderate = 9–12; severe = ≤8.
Adapted from Teasdale G, Jennett B: Assessment of coma and impaired consciousness: A practical scale. Lancet 2:81, 1974; and Jennett B: Assessment of the severity of head injury. J Neurol Neurosurg Psychiatry 39:647, 1976.

aggravate the initial injury include hypoxia, hypercarbia, hypotension, anemia, and hyperglycemia. These contributing factors to secondary injury are preventable. Seizures, infection, and sepsis that may occur hours to days after injury will further aggravate brain damage and must also be prevented or treated promptly.

Secondary insults complicate the course of more than 50% of head-injured patients.[395,399] An outcome study using data from the Traumatic Coma Data Bank revealed that hypotension occurring after head injury is profoundly detrimental, with greater than 70% of patients experiencing significant morbidity and mortality (Table 28-19).[400] Furthermore, the combination of hypoxia and hypotension is significantly more detrimental than that of hypotension alone (>90% of patients with severe outcome or death). These findings confirm the importance of avoiding hypovolemic shock in head-injured patients. The management goal in head-injured patients is to initiate timely and appropriate therapy to prevent secondary brain injury. When the initial injury is not fatal, subsequent neurologic damage and systemic complications should be preventable in most patients.

Primary injury or biomechanical trauma to brain parenchyma includes concussion, contusion, laceration, and hematoma. Not all severely head-injured patients require surgery. Generalized brain injury with edema or contusion is a common finding in patients, whether or not a surgically correctable mass lesion is present. Diffuse cerebral swelling occurs because of sudden intracerebral congestion and hyperemia. Twenty-four hours or more after the initial insult, cerebral edema develops in the extracellular spaces of the white matter. Nonoperative treatment of diffuse cerebral swelling includes hyperventilation, diuresis with mannitol and furosemide, and barbiturates in conjunction with ICP monitoring.

Depressed skull fractures and acute epidural, subdural, and intracerebral hematomas usually require craniotomy. Chronic subdural hematomas are often evacuated through burr holes. Depressed skull fractures under lacerations should be elevated and debrided within 24 hours to minimize the risk of infection. Bony fragments and penetrating objects should not be manipulated in the emergency room, because they may be tamponading a lacerated vessel or dural sinus. Traumatic epidural hematoma is an infrequent complication of head injury, usually the result of a motor vehicle accident. The initial injury tears middle meningeal vessels or dural sinuses and causes unconsciousness. When a spasm and clot occur in the vessel(s), the bleeding stops and the patient recovers, experiencing a lucid interval. Over the next several hours, the vessel bleeds and the patient rapidly deteriorates (especially with arterial bleeding). In rapidly deteriorating conditions, treatment should not be delayed pending radiologic evaluation. Emergency evacuation is necessary. Venous epidural hematomas develop more slowly, and there may be time for diagnostic testing. The clinical presentation of acute subdural hematomas ranges from minimal deficits to unconsciousness and signs of a mass lesion (hemiparesis, unilateral decerebration, and pupillary enlargement). A lucid interval may occur. The most common cause of subdural hematoma is trauma, but it may occur spontaneously and is associated with coagulopathies, aneurysms, and neoplasms. It is considered acute if the patient becomes symptomatic within 72 hours, subacute between 3–15 days, and chronic after 2 weeks. Subacute and chronic subdural hematoma are usually observed in patients over age 50 years. There may be no history of head trauma. The clinical presentation in these patients may vary from focal signs of brain dysfunction to a depressed level of consciousness or development of an organic brain syndrome. Intracranial hypertension is usually associated with acute subdural hematoma. Intensive medical therapy to correct elevated ICP and control brain edema and swelling may be required before, during, and after hematoma evacuation. With intracerebral hematomas, the clinical picture may vary from minimal neurologic deficits to deep coma. Large, solitary intracerebral hematomas should be evacuated. Lesions causing delayed neurologic deterioration from fresh hemorrhage are also evacuated but carry a poor prognosis. Depending on the degree of cerebral injury, patients with intracerebral hematomas may require intensive medical therapy to control intracranial hypertension and cerebral edema. Coup and contracoup injuries usually cause cerebral contusion and intracerebral hemorrhage. In general, contused brain tissue is not removed; occasionally, however, contused tissue over the frontal or temporal poles may be removed to control edema formation and prevent herniation.

Emergency Therapy

Emergency therapy should begin at the site of the accident, in the ambulance, and most certainly, in the emergency room. The first step is to secure an open airway and ensure adequate ventilation to prevent secondary injury from hypoxia and hypercarbia. Before securing the airway in a head-injured patient, a quick assessment of the patient's neurologic status and concomitant injuries should be made.

The incidence of cervical spine injuries in surviving head injury victims is 1–3% in adults and 0.5% in children.[401,402] Victims of head-first falls or high-speed motor vehicle accidents have a 10% or greater chance of cervical spine fractures. Radiographic evaluation with a cross-table lateral view can miss 20% of cervical spine fractures.[402] To increase the reliability of radiographic evaluation, anteroposterior and odontoid views, in addition to a lateral view, have been recommended. Reportedly, this combination misses only 7% of fractures.[402] When a cervical spine fracture has not been excluded by radiographic evaluation, cervical alignment with in-line stabilization* is recommended during emergent intubation. (Axial traction is no longer recommended because of the risk of distraction injury to the spinal cord.[401]) If facial fractures and soft tissue edema prevent direct visualization of the larynx, a fiberoptic intubation or intubation with an illuminated stylet may be attempted. In the presence of severe facial and/or laryngeal injuries, a cricothyrotomy may be required. Nasal intubations are avoided in the presence of a suspected basal skull fracture, severe facial fractures, and bleeding diathesis.

For patients without facial injuries, the simplest and most expeditious approach to intubation is preoxygenation followed by rapid-sequence induction with cricoid pressure and maintenance of in-line stabilization. All head-injured patients are as-

Table 28-19. IMPACT OF HYPOXIA AND HYPOTENSION* ON OUTCOME AFTER SEVERE HEAD INJURY (GCS ≤ 8)

| Secondary Insults | Number of Patients | Outcome Percentage | | |
		Good or Moderate	Severe or Vegetative	Dead
Total cases	699	43	21	37
Neither	456	51	22	27
Hypoxia	78	45	22	33
Hypotension	113	26	14	60
Both	52	6	19	75

Hypoxia = PaO_2 < 60 mm Hg; hypotension = SBP < 90 mm Hg; GCS = Glasgow Coma Scale.
* At time of hospital arrival.
Data adapted from the Traumatic Coma Data Bank.[400]

* In-line stabilization requires an assistant to stabilize the patient's head by positioning his or her hands along the side of the head with fingertips on the mastoid holding the occiput down on a backboard.

sumed to have a full stomach. Awake, oral intubation without anesthetic agents may be possible in the severely injured patient, but this is difficult in the awake or uncooperative, combative patient. Depending on the patient's cardiovascular status, virtually any of the intravenous induction agents, except ketamine, can be used. The choice of muscle relaxants is controversial. Succinylcholine can increase ICP. In the setting of acute airway compromise, full stomach, and need to perform subsequent neurologic examinations, the benefits of rapid onset and elimination of succinylcholine may outweigh the risk of transiently increasing ICP.

Following control of the airway in the head-injured patient, attention should focus on resuscitation of the cardiovascular system. Transient hypotension after head injury is not uncommon, but sustained hypotension usually results from hemorrhage secondary to other systemic injuries. These injuries must be sought and aggressively treated.

When multiple trauma complicates head injury, there is no ideal crystalloid resuscitation fluid. A major concern during resuscitation is the development of cerebral edema. Animal investigations reveal that total serum osmolality is a key factor in brain edema formation.[403,404] When serum osmolality is reduced, cerebral edema develops in normal and abnormal brain. This occurs because the blood–brain barrier is relatively impermeable to sodium. Solutions containing sodium in concentrations lower than that in serum cause water movement into the brain, increasing brain water. Thus, hypoosmolar solutions (0.45% NaCl and lactated Ringer's solution) are more likely than isoosmolar fluids (0.9% saline) to increase brain water content. Large-volume fluid resuscitation with isoosmolar crystalloids reduces colloid oncotic pressure and increases peripheral tissue edema. However, in animal investigations, the brain behaves differently than other tissues, and profound lowering of colloid oncotic pressure with maintenance of serum osmolality does not result in edema in normal brain[403] and in some head-injury models.[404,405] These results can be explained by the unique structure of the blood–brain barrier and the fact that colloid oncotic pressure gradients generate weak forces in comparison with osmolar gradients.[403] Some doubt has been cast on the applicability of these laboratory findings to clinical practice. The cryogenic-injury model used in these experiments may not be equivalent to head injury in patients. In head-injured patients, brain capillary permeability may be rendered similar to that of peripheral tissues when the blood–brain barrier is damaged. In addition, the time course of these experiments did not allow observation of edema developing 24–48 hours after initial resuscitation, which occurs in head-injured patients. A recent investigation using the percussive head injury model in rats has shown that reduction in colloid pressure can aggravate cerebral edema under certain conditions.[406] Therefore, it seems reasonable to avoid a profound reduction in colloid oncotic pressure in clinical practice. Iso-osmolar colloid solutions, such as 5% albumin or 6% hetastarch, can be administered to maintain oncotic pressure and intravascular volume. Fresh whole blood, when available, is the ideal colloid resuscitation fluid for hypovolemic patients with ongoing blood loss.

Hypertonic saline solutions may be very useful for volume resuscitation in head-injured patients because they lower ICP and may improve regional CBF.[407,408] Hypertonic saline produces an osmotic diuretic effect on the brain that is similar to that of other hyperosmolar solutions (e.g., mannitol). With long-term use, however, there is concern over the physiologic implications of elevated serum sodium, such as a depressed level of consciousness and/or seizures.

During fluid resuscitation of the head-injured patient, the goals are to maintain serum osmolality, avoid profound reduction in colloid oncotic pressure, and restore circulating blood volume. Immediate therapy is directed at preventing hypotension and maintaining CPP above 70 mm Hg.[409] When indicated, an ICP monitor is inserted to guide fluid resuscitation and

prevent severe elevations in ICP. Iso-osmolar crystalloid solutions, colloid solutions, or both are administered acutely to restore circulating blood volume. Glucose-containing solutions should not be administered because of a significant association between plasma glucose levels and worse neurologic outcome in head-injured patients.[410] Substantial blood loss requires transfusion with crossmatched or fresh whole blood. A minimal hematocrit between 30 and 33% is recommended to maximize oxygen transport.

Hypertension, tachycardia, and increased cardiac output often develop in patients with isolated head trauma, especially young adults.[411] ECG abnormalities and fatal arrhythmias have been reported. The hyperdynamic circulatory responses and ECG changes may result from a surge in epinephrine that accompanies head injury.[412] Either labetalol or esmolol can be used to control hypertension and tachycardia in this situation.

In some patients, severe intracranial hypertension precipitates reflex arterial hypertension and bradycardia (Cushing's triad). A reduction in systemic blood pressure in these patients can further aggravate cerebral ischemia by reducing CPP. Systemic blood pressure must be lowered cautiously when intracranial hypertension is severe. In such cases, a reduction of ICP may interrupt this reflex response.

After stabilization of head-injured patients, including control of airway and systemic blood pressure, therapeutic interventions to control intracranial hypertension are instituted. The head is elevated 15° and maintained in a neutral position without rotation or flexion. Hyperventilation to a $Paco_2$ of 30–35 mm Hg is instituted as a very rapid and effective intervention. Mannitol, 0.25–1 g · kg^{-1}, is given to lower ICP acutely, or a combination of furosemide and mannitol may be administered. Barbiturates are used to control ICP when other measures have failed.[413] Appropriate monitoring must be instituted and hypotension avoided.

Mechanical hyperventilation to a $Paco_2$ 25–30 mm Hg has been routinely employed in head-injured patients based on an assumption that hyperventilation, by reducing CBF, will reduce ICP, thereby preserving CPP and CBF. Clinical investigations, using CBF and jugular bulb oxygen saturation monitoring, have reported a subset of head-injured patients with markedly reduced CBF in relation to their metabolic requirements.[414,415] In these patients hyperventilation may further decrease CBF and aggravate cerebral ischemia.[416]

The 1995 Brain Trauma Foundation algorithm (Table 28-20) for the treatment of intracranial hypertension no longer recom-

---

Table 28-20. SEVERE HEAD INJURY: TREATMENT OF INTRACRANIAL HYPERTENSION

· Insert ICP monitor
· Maintain CPP > 70 mm Hg
· Intracranial hypertension
  First-tier therapy:
    Ventricular drainage (if available)
    Mannitol 0.25–1 g · kg^{-1} iv (may repeat if serum osmolarity < 320 mOsm · l^{-1} and patient euvolemic)
    Hyperventilation to $Paco_2$ 30–35 mm Hg
  Second-tier therapy:
    Hyperventilation to $Paco_2$ < 30 mm Hg (Sjo_2, $AVDO_2$, and/or CBF monitoring recommended)
    High-dose barbiturate therapy
    Consider hypothermia
    Consider hypertensive therapy
    Consider decompressive craniectomy

ICP = intracranial pressure; CPP = cerebral perfusion pressure; Sjo_2 = jugular bulb oxyhemoglobin saturation; $AVDO_2$ = arteriovenous difference in oxygen content; CBF = cerebral blood flow.
Adapted from 1995 Brain Trauma Foundation Guidelines for the Management of Severe Head Injury. J Neurotrauma 13:641, 1996.

mends hyperventilation to a Pa$_{CO_2}$ of 25–30 mm Hg as a first-tier therapy.[417,418] When hyperventilation is initiated for the control of intracranial hypertension, the Pa$_{CO_2}$ should be maintained in the range of 30–35 mm Hg in order to accomplish ICP control while minimizing the associated risk of ischemia. Hyperventilation to Pa$_{CO_2}$ values less than 30 mm Hg should be considered only when secondary therapy of refractory intracranial hypertension is required.

Continuous measurement of jugular bulb oxygen saturation can be used in clinical practice to determine which patients will receive benefit or harm from hyperventilation.[249,419] In emergency situations, we should continue to hyperventilate patients in whom the clinical control of intracranial hypertension is the primary concern. However, when the clinical situation no longer requires it or there is evidence of cerebral ischemia, normocapnic ventilation should be instituted.

Anesthetic Management

The patient is evaluated by CT scan and taken directly to the operating room. There is usually minimal time available for resuscitation and preanesthetic assessment. Information that should be obtained preoperatively is described in Table 28-21. The anesthetic management is a continuation of the initial resuscitation, including airway management, fluid and electrolyte balance, and ICP control. The routine monitors for major neurosurgical procedures are applied. Anesthetic management is directed at avoidance of secondary brain injury. Intraoperative hypotension secondary to blood loss or precipitated by anesthetic drugs should be avoided by appropriate volume expansion. Maintenance of ventilation (Pa$_{CO_2}$ between 30 and 35 mm Hg) and oxygenation (Pa$_{O_2}$ > 60 mm Hg) is extremely important. Positive end-expiratory pressure may be used, if necessary (5–10 cm H_2O does not adversely affect ICP).

Intraoperative brain swelling or herniation from the operative site may complicate hematoma decompression. Such causes as improper patient positioning, contralateral intracerebral hematoma, venous drainage obstruction from packing, and acute hydrocephalus from intraventricular hemorrhage must be eliminated. In this setting, the adequacy of hyperventilation must also be verified. A large alveolar-arterial CO_2 gradient may exist, so that end-tidal CO_2 may not reflect arterial CO_2. The respiratory system and equipment should be reviewed to ensure normal peak inspiratory and expiratory pressures. Hemopneumothorax, high intra-abdominal pressures, a kinked endotracheal or expiratory tube, or a stuck expiratory valve can produce marked peak inspiratory or expiratory pressures as well as hypoxemia and hypercarbia. Fluid and electrolyte balance must be reevaluated in patients with cerebral swelling. Mannitol loses its effect after 1–3 hours, and it may be necessary to repeat the mannitol bolus to increase osmolarity. Volume overload and hyponatremia may also cause cerebral swelling and must be corrected. If cerebral swelling persists, the anesthetic should be converted

to opioid and thiopental infusions with oxygen and air. Thiopental may be given in a series of boluses over 5–10 minutes to a total dose of 5–25 mg · kg^{-1}, followed by an infusion of 4–10 mg · kg^{-1} · h^{-1}. To avoid barbiturate-induced myocardial depression and hypotension, it may be necessary to increase preload and add a vasopressor such as dopamine. Malignant brain swelling may require removal of brain tissue and a temporary scalp closure with a loose dural patch to minimize ICP after closure.

Emergence from anesthesia usually involves transporting an intubated, ventilated, and anesthetized patient to the intensive care unit. Even in an uncomplicated craniotomy for evacuation of hematoma, a period of postoperative ventilation is recommended because brain swelling is maximal 12–72 hours after injury. Hypertension and coughing or bucking on the endotracheal tube should be avoided because it can lead to significant intracranial bleeding. Labetalol or esmolol can be used to treat hypertension, and supplemental barbiturates are given to sedate the patient. Current guidelines for the perioperative treatment of intracranial hypertension resulting from severe head injury are shown in Table 28-20.[418]

Systemic Sequelae

The systemic effects of head injury are diverse and can complicate management.[420] These include cardiopulmonary problems (airway obstruction, hypoxemia, shock, adult respiratory distress syndrome, neurogenic pulmonary edema, ECG changes), hematologic problems (disseminated intravascular coagulation), endocrinologic problems (pituitary dysfunction, i.e., diabetes insipidus, SIADH), metabolic problems (nonketotic hyperosmolar hyperglycemic coma), and gastrointestinal problems (stress ulcers, hemorrhage). Conditions not discussed elsewhere in this chapter will be reviewed.

Aspiration, pneumonia, fluid overload, and trauma-related adult respiratory distress syndrome are common causes of pulmonary dysfunction in head-injured patients. A fulminant pulmonary edema may also occur. Neurogenic pulmonary edema is characterized by marked pulmonary vascular congestion, intraalveolar hemorrhage, and a protein-rich edema fluid. Specific features of this syndrome are its rapid onset, its relationship to hypothalamic lesions, and the ability to prevent or attenuate it by α-blockers and CNS depressants. Neurogenic pulmonary edema is thought to result from massive sympathetic discharge from injured brain secondary to intracranial hypertension. Traditional therapy for pulmonary edema of cardiac origin is ineffective, and the outcome is frequently fatal. Therapy consists of immediate pharmacologic or surgical relief of intracranial hypertension, supportive respiratory care, and careful fluid management.

In head-injured patients, several clotting abnormalities may be present. Disseminated intravascular coagulation has been reported after mild and severe brain trauma and anoxic brain damage, and it presumably develops after release of brain tissue thromboplastin into the systemic circulation.[421] Treatment of the underlying disease process usually results in spontaneous recovery of the coagulation defects. Occasionally, administration of cryoprecipitate, fresh frozen plasma, platelet concentrates, and blood may be required.

Anterior pituitary insufficiency after head injury is a rare occurrence. However, patients exhibiting post-traumatic diabetes insipidus may develop a delayed impairment of anterior pituitary hormones, requiring replacement therapy. Posterior pituitary dysfunction occurs more frequently after head trauma. Diabetes insipidus may occur after craniofacial trauma and basal skull fracture. Its clinical presentation includes polyuria, polydipsia, hypernatremia, high-serum osmolality, and dilute urine. Frequently, post-traumatic diabetes insipidus is transient, and treatment is based on water replacement. If the patient cannot maintain fluid balance, exogenous vasopressin

---

Table 28-21. PREANESTHETIC ASSESSMENT OF THE HEAD-INJURED PATIENT

Airway (cervical spine)
Breathing: ventilation and oxygenation
Circulatory status
Associated injuries
Neurologic status (Glasgow Coma Scale)
Pre-existing chronic illness
Circumstances of the injury:
    Time of injury
    Duration of unconsciousness
    Associated alcohol or drug use

may be administered. The syndrome of inappropriate antidiuretic hormone (SIADH) secretion is associated with hyponatremia, serum and extracellular fluid hypoosmolality, renal excretion of sodium, urine osmolality greater than serum osmolality, and normal renal and adrenal function. The patient develops symptoms and signs of water intoxication (anorexia, nausea, vomiting, irritability, personality changes, and neurologic abnormalities). SIADH secretion usually begins 3–15 days after trauma, lasting no more than 10–15 days with appropriate therapy. Treatment includes water restriction with or without hypertonic saline.

Many factors in neurosurgical patients predispose to nonketotic hyperosmolar hyperglycemic coma, such as steroids, prolonged mannitol therapy, hyperosmolar tube feedings, phenytoin, and limited water replacement.[420] Diagnostic criteria for nonketotic hyperosmolar hyperglycemic coma are hyperglycemia, glucosuria, absence of ketosis, plasma osmolality > 330 $mOsm \cdot kg^{-1}$, dehydration, and CNS dysfunction. Hypovolemia and hypertonicity are the immediate threats to life. Serum sodium may be high, normal, or low, depending on the state of hydration. Serum potassium is low. Serial laboratory tests are essential. Once sodium deficits are replaced and blood pressure and urine output are stable, water deficits are replaced with 0.45% saline. Hyperglycemia usually responds to relatively small doses of insulin. Intermittent furosemide therapy may be given for cerebral edema prophylaxis in the elderly, the adult-onset diabetic, or the patient with compromised renal function.

REFERENCES

1. Aidley DJ: The Physiology of Excitable Cells. New York, Cambridge University Press, 1989
2. Hille B: Ionic Channels of Excitable Membranes. Sunderland, Sinauer Associates, 1992
3. Cooper JR, Bloom FE, Roth RH: The Biochemical Basis of Neuropharmacology. New York, Oxford University Press, 1991
4. Kandel ER, Schwartz JH, Jessel TM: Principles of Neural Science. New York, McGraw-Hill, 2000.
5. Prys RC, Strunin L: Symposium on cellular and molecular aspects of anesthesia. Br J Anaesth 71:1, 1993
6. Berridge MJ: Regulation of ion channels by inositol trisphosphate and diacylglycerol. J Exp Biol 124:323, 1986
7. Brunn-Meyer SE: The GABA/benzodiazepine receptor-chloride ionophore complex: Nature and modulation. Prog Neuropsychopharmacol Biol Psychiatry 11:365, 1987
8. Bormann J: Electrophysiology of GABA$_A$ and GABA$_B$ receptor subtypes. TINS 11:112, 1988
9. Watkins JC, Evans RH: Excitatory amino acid transmitters. Annu Rev Pharmacol Toxicol 21:165, 1981
10. MacDermott AB, Dale N: Receptors, ion channels and synaptic potentials underlying the integrative actions of excitatory amino acids. TINS 10:280, 1987
11. Kass IS, Chambers G, Cottrell JE: The N-methyl-D-aspartate antagonists aminophosphonovaleric acid and MK-801 reduce anoxic damage to dentate granule and CA 1 pyramidal cells in the rat hippocampal slice. Exp Neurol 103:116, 1989
12. Clark DD, Sokoloff L: Circulation and energy metabolism of the brain. In Siegel G, Agranoff B, Albers RW, Molinoff P (eds): Basic Neurochemistry, p 645. New York, Raven Press, 1994
13. Lehninger AL: Principles of Biochemistry. New York, Worth Publishers, 1982
14. Siesjo BK: Cell damage in the brain: A speculative synthesis. J Cereb Blood Flow Metab 1:155, 1981
15. Hansen AJ: Effect of anoxia on ion distribution in the brain. Physiol Rev 65:101, 1985
16. Michenfelder JD: Anesthesia and the Brain, p 23. New York, Churchill Livingstone, 1988
17. Smith AL, Wollman H: Cerebral blood flow and metabolism: Effects of anesthetic drugs and techniques. Anesthesiology 36:378, 1972
18. Plum F, Siesjo BK: Recent advances in CSF physiology. Anesthesiology 42:708, 1975
19. Mihm FG, Cottrell JE, Hartung J et al: Cerebral damage and phar-

20. Michenfelder J: Cerebral blood flow and metabolism. In Cucchiara RF, Michenfelder JD (eds): Clinical Neuroanesthesia, p 1. New York, Churchill Livingstone, 1990
21. Greenfield JC, Rembert JC, Tindall GT: Transient changes in cerebral vascular resistance during the Valsalva maneuver in man. Stroke 15:76, 1984
22. Young WL, Ornstein E: Cerebral and spinal cord blood flow. In Cottrell JE, Smith DC (eds): Anesthesia and Neurosurgery, p 17. St Louis, CV Mosby, 1994
23. Strandgaard S, Olesen J, Skinhoj E et al: Autoregulation of brain circulation in severe arterial hypertension. Br Med J 1:507, 1973
24. Bill A, Linden J, Linden M: Sympathetic effect on cerebral blood vessels in acute arteriole hypertension. Acta Physiol Scand 96:27A, 1976
25. Artru AA: Cerebrospinal fluid. In Cottrell JE, Smith DS (eds): Anesthesia and Neurosurgery, p 95. St. Louis, CV Mosby, 1994
26. Artru AA: Cerebrospinal fluid dynamics. In Cucchiara RF, Michenfelder JD (eds): Clinical Neuroanesthesia, p 41. New York, Churchill Livingstone, 1990
27. Lundberg N: Monitoring of the intracranial pressure. In Critchley M, O'Leary JL, Jennett B (eds): Scientific Foundations of Neurology, p 356. Philadelphia, FA Davis, 1972
28. Miller JD, Garibi J, Pickard JD: The effects of induced changes of cerebrospinal fluid volume during continuous monitoring of ventricular pressure. Arch Neurol 28:265, 1973
29. Fishman RA: Brain edema. N Engl J Med 293:706, 1975
30. Siesjo BK: Cerebral circulation and metabolism. J Neurosurg 60:883, 1984
31. Meldrum B: Epileptic seizures. In Siegel G, Agranoff RW, Albers BW, Mulinoff PB (eds): Basic Neurochemistry, p 885. New York, Raven Press, 1994
32. Gopinath SP, Robertson CS: Management of severe head injury. In Cottrell JE, Smith DS (eds): Anesthesia and Neurosurgery, p 661. St. Louis, CV Mosby, 1994
33. Young W, Koreh I: Potassium and calcium changes in injured spinal cords. Brain Res 365:42, 1986
34. Hall ED, Wolf DL: A pharmacological analysis of the pathophysiologic mechanisms of posttraumatic spinal cord ischemia. J Neurosurg 64:951, 1986
35. Eintrei C, Leszniewski W, Carlson C: Local application of xenon for measurement of regional cerebral blood flow during halothane, enflurane, and isoflurane anesthesia in humans. Anesthesiology 63:391, 1985
36. Boarini DJ, Kassel NF, Sprowell JA et al: Comparison of systemic and cerebrovascular effects of isoflurane and halothane. J Neurosurg 15:400, 1984
37. Ornstein E, Young WL, Fleischer LH et al: Desflurane and isoflurane have similar effects on cerebral blood flow in patients with intracranial mass lesions. Anesthesiology 79:498, 1993
38. Mielck F, Stephan H, Buhre W et al: Effects of 1 MAC desflurane on cerebral metabolism, blood flow and carbon dioxide reactivity in human. Br J Anaesth 81:155, 1998
39. Scheller MS, Tateishi A, Drummond JC et al: The effects of sevoflurane on cerebral blood flow, cerebral metabolic rate for oxygen, intracranial pressure, and the electroencephalogram are similar to those of isoflurane in the rabbit. Anesthesiology 68:548, 1988
40. Todd MM, Drummond JC: A comparison of the cerebrovascular and metabolic effects of halothane and isoflurane in the cat. Anesthesiology 60:276, 1984
41. Michenfelder JD, Cucchiara RF: Canine cerebral oxygen consumption during enflurane anesthesia and its modification during induced seizures. Anesthesiology 40:575, 1974
42. Muzzi DA, Losasso TJ, Dietz NM et al: The effect of desflurane and isoflurane on cerebrospinal fluid pressure in humans with supratentorial mass lesions. Anesthesiology 76:720, 1992
43. Ebert TJ, Perez F, Uhrich TD, Deshur MA: Desflurane-mediated sympathetic activation occurs in humans despite preventing hypotension and baroreceptor unloading. Anesthesiology 88:1227, 1998
44. Nuscheler M, Conzen P, Peter K: Sevoflurane: Metabolism and toxicity. Anaesthetist 47(suppl 1):S24, 1998
45. Sarner JB, Levine M, Davis PJ et al: Clinical characteristics of

sevoflurane in children: A comparison with halothane. Anesthesiology 82:38, 1995

46. Werner C, Kochs E, Hoffman WE *et al:* The effects of sevoflurane on neurological outcome from incomplete ischemia in rats. J Neurosurg Anesth 3:237, 1991

47. Bundgaard H, von Oettingen G, Larsen KM *et al:* Effects of sevoflurane on intracranial pressure, cerebral blood flow and cerebral metabolism. A dose–response study in patients subjected to craniotomy for cerebral tumors. Acta Anaesthesiol Scand 42:621, 1998

48. Artru AA, Lam AM, Johnson JO *et al:* Intracranial pressure, middle cerebral artery flow velocity, and plasma inorganic fluoride concentrations in neurosurgical patients receiving sevoflurane or isoflurane. Anesth Analg 85:587, 1997

49. Pellegrini DA, Miletich DJ, Hoffman WE *et al:* Nitrous oxide markedly increases cerebral cortical metabolic rate and blood flow in the goat. Anesthesiology 60:405, 1984

50. Moss E, McDowall DG: ICP increases with 50 percent nitrous oxide in oxygen in severe head injuries during controlled ventilation. Br J Anaesth 51:757, 1979

51. Phirman JR, Shapiro HM: Modification of nitrous oxide induced intracranial hypertension by prior induction of anesthesia. Anesthesiology 46:150, 1977

52. Hoffman WE, Miletich DJ, Albrecht RF: The effects of midazolam on cerebral blood flow and oxygen consumption and its interaction with nitrous oxide. Anesth Analg 65:729, 1986

53. Sakabe T, Kuramoto T, Kumagae S *et al:* Cerebral responses to the addition of nitrous oxide to halothane in man. Br J Anaesth 48:957, 1975

54. Baughman VL: N$_2$O: Of questionable value. J Neurosurg Anesth 7, 1995

55. Pierce EC, Lambertsen CJ, Deutsch S *et al:* Cerebral circulation and metabolism during thiopental anesthesia and hyperventilation in man. J Clin Invest 41:1664, 1964

56. Michenfelder JD: The interdependency of cerebral function and metabolic effects following massive doses of thiopental in the dog. Anesthesiology 41:231, 1974

57. Shapiro HM, Galindo A, Wyte SR *et al:* Rapid intraoperative reduction of intracranial pressure with thiopentone. Br J Anaesth 45:1057, 1973

58. Rockoff MA, Goudsouzian NG: Seizures induced by methohexital. Anesthesiology 54:333, 1981

59. Renou AM, Vernhiet J, Macrez P *et al:* Cerebral blood flow and metabolism during etomidate anesthesia in man. Br J Anaesth 50:1047, 1978

60. Milde LN, Milde JH, Michenfelder JD: Cerebral functional, metabolic, and hemodynamic effects of etomidate in dogs. Anesthesiology 63:371, 1985

61. Davis DW, Mans AM, Biebuyck JF *et al:* Regional brain glucose utilization in rats during etomidate anesthesia. Anesthesiology 64:751, 1986

62. Fragen KJ, Shanks CA, Molteni A *et al:* Effects of etomidate on hormonal responses to surgical stress. Anesthesiology 61:652, 1984

63. Dam M, Ori C, Pizzolato G *et al:* The effects of propofol anesthesia on local cerebral glucose utilization in the rat. Anesthesiology 73:499, 1990

64. Lagerkranser M, Stange K, Sollevi A: Effects of propofol on cerebral blood flow, metabolism, and cerebral autoregulation in the anesthetized pig. J Neurosurg Anesthesiol 9:188, 1997

65. Cavazzuti M, Porro CA, Barbieri A *et al:* Brain and spinal cord metabolic activity during propofol anesthesia. Br J Anaesth 66:490, 1991

66. Pinaud M, Lelausque J-N, Chetanneau A *et al:* Effects of propofol on cerebral hemodynamics and metabolism in patients with brain trauma. Anesthesiology 73:404, 1990

67. Blouin RT, Conard PF, Gross JB: Time course of ventilatory depression following induction doses of propofol and thiopental. Anesthesiology 75:940, 1991

68. Nugent M, Artru AA, Michenfelder JD: Cerebral metabolic, vascular, and protective effects of midazolam maleate: Comparison to diazepam. Anesthesiology 56:172, 1982

69. Forster A, Juge O, Morel D: Effects of midazolam on cerebral blood flow. Anesthesiology 56:453, 1982

70. Fleischer JE, Milde JH, Moyer TP *et al:* Cerebral effects of high-dose midazolam and subsequent reversal with RO-1788 in dogs. Anesthesiology 68:234, 1988

71. Jobes DR, Kennell EM, Bush GL *et al:* Cerebral blood flow and metabolism during morphine-nitrous oxide anesthesia in man. Anesthesiology 47:16, 1977

72. Vernhiet J, Renou AM, Orgogozo JM *et al:* Effects of diazepam fentanyl mixture on cerebral blood flow and oxygen consumption in man. Br J Anaesth 50:165, 1978

73. Drummond JC, Shapiro HM: Cerebral physiology. In Miller RD (ed): Anesthesia. New York, Churchill Livingstone, 1990

74. Young WL, Prohovnik I, Correll JW *et al:* A comparison of the cerebral hemodynamic effects of sufentanil and isoflurane in humans undergoing carotid endarterectomy. Anesthesiology 71:863, 1989

75. Hanel F, Werner C, von Knobelsdorff G *et al:* The effects of fentanyl and sufentanil on cerebral hemodynamics. J Neurosurg Anesthesiol 9:223, 1997

76. Milde LN, Milde JH, Gallagher WJ: Effects of sufentanil on cerebral circulation and metabolism in dogs. Anesth Analg 70:138, 1990

77. Marx W, Shah N, Long C *et al:* Sufentanil, alfentanil, and fentanyl: Impact on cerebrospinal fluid pressure in patients with brain tumors. J Neurosurg Anesth 1:3, 1989

78. Lutz LJ, Milde JH, Milde LN: Cerebral effects of alfentanil in dogs with reduced intracranial compliance. J Neurosurg Anesth 1:169, 1989

79. Jung R, Free K, Shah N *et al:* Cerebrospinal fluid pressure in anesthetized patients with brain tumors: Impact of fentanyl vs alfentanil. J Neurosurg Anesth 1:136, 1989

80. Ostapkovich ND, Baker KZ, Fogarty-Mack P *et al:* Cerebral blood flow and CO$_2$ reactivity is similar during remifentanil/N$_2$O and fentanyl/N$_2$O anesthesia. Anesthesiology 89:358, 1998

81. Davis DW, Mans AM, Biebuyck JF *et al:* The influence of ketamine on regional brain glucose use. Anesthesiology 69:199, 1988

82. Takeshita H, Okuda Y, Sari A: The effects of ketamine on cerebral circulation and metabolism in man. Anesthesiology 36:69, 1972

83. Cavazzuti M, Porro CA, Biral GP *et al:* Ketamine effects on local cerebral blood flow and metabolism in the rat. J Cereb Blood Flow Metab 7:806, 1987

84. Rosonoff HL: Hypothermia and cerebral vascular lesions: 1. Experimental interruption of the middle cerebral artery during hypothermia. J Neurosurg 13:332, 1956

85. Berntman L, Welsh FA, Harp JR *et al:* Cerebral protective effect of low-grade hypothermia. Anesthesiology 55:495, 1981

86. Hartung J, Cottrell JE: Mild hypothermia and cerebral metabolism. J Neurosurg Anesth 6:1, 1994

87. Hartung J, Cottrell JE: In response to: Effects of hypothermia on cerebral metabolic rate for oxygen [letter]. J Neurosurg Anesth 6:222, 1994

88. Craen RA, Gelb AW, Eliasziw M *et al:* Current anesthetic practices and use of brain protective therapies for cerebral aneurysm surgery at 41 North American centers [Abstract]. J Neurosurg Anesth 6:303, 1994

89. Hindman BJ, Todd MM, Gelb AW *et al:* Mild hypothermia as a protective therapy during intracranial aneurysm surgery: A randomized prospective pilot trial. Neurosurgery 44:23, 1999

90. Azzimondi G, Bassein L, Nonino F *et al:* Fever in acute stroke worsens prognosis: A prospective study. Stroke 26:2040, 1996

91. Reith J, Jorgensen HS, Pedersen PM *et al:* Body temperature in acute stroke: Relation to stroke severity, infarct size, mortality, and outcome. Lancet 347:422, 1996

92. Castillo J, Davalos A, Moya M: Progression of ischaemic stroke and excitotoxic amino acids. Lancet 349:79, 1997

93. Becker KJ, McCarron RM, Hallenbeck JM: Magnitude of fever predicts outcome after transient middle cerebral artery occlusion. Stroke 29:328, 1998

94. Nazir HS, Fabling JM: Postcraniotomy temperature: A retrospective analysis of trends within the first 24 hours. J Neurosurg Anesth 11(Abstr 604):4, 1999

95. Goodman JC, Valadka AB, Gopinath SP *et al:* Lactate and excitatory amino acids measured by microdialysis are decreased by pentobarbital coma in head-injured patients. J Neurotrauma 13:549, 1996

96. Zhu H, Cottrell JE, Kass IS: The effect of thiopental and propofol on NMDA- and AMPA-mediated glutamate excitotoxicity. Anesthesiology 87(4):944, 1997

97. Nussmeier NA, Arlund C, Slogoff S: Neuropsychiatric complications after cardiopulmonary bypass: Cerebral protection by a barbiturate. Anesthesiology 64:165, 1986

98. Barker FG, Ogilvy CS: Efficacy of prophylactic nimodipine for

delayed ischemic deficit after subarachnoid hemorrhage: A meta-analysis. J Neurosurg 84:405, 1996

99. Feigin VL, Rinkel GJ, Algra A et al: Calcium antagonists in patients with aneurysmal subarachnoid hemorrhage: A systematic review. Neurology 50:876, 1998

100. Muir KW: New experimental and clinical data on the efficacy of pharmacological magnesium infusions in cerebral infarcts. Magnesium Res 11:43, 1998

101. Muir KW, Bradford APJ, Lees KR: Therapeutic potential of parenteral magnesium for ischemic stroke and preliminary clinical trial results. Poster. Glasgow: IMAGES Trial Group, 1999 (Available from apjb@clinmed.gla.ac.uk)

102. Hallak M: Effect of parenteral magnesium sulfate administration on excitatory amino acid receptors in the rat brain. Magnesium Res 11:117, 1998

103. Heath DL, Vink R: Neuroprotective effects of $MgSO_4$ and $MgCl_2$ in closed head injury: A comparative phosphorus NMR Study. J Neurotrauma 15:183, 1998

104. Kass IS, Cottrell JE, Chambers G: Magnesium and cobalt, not nimodipine, protect against anoxic damage in the rat hippocampal slice. Anesthesiology 69:710, 1989

105. Nelson KB, Grether JK: Can magnesium sulfate reduce the risk of cerebral palsy in very low birth weight infants? Pediatrics 94:263, 1995

106. Kassell NF, Haley EC Jr, Apperson-Hansen C et al: Randomized, double-blind vehicle controlled trial of tirilazad mesylate in patients with aneurysmal subarachnoid hemorrhage: A cooperative study. J Neurosurg 84:221, 1996

107. Haley EC, Kassell NF, Apperson-Hansen C et al: A randomized double-blind, vehicle-controlled trial of tirilazad mesylate in patients with aneurysmal subarachnoid hemorrhage: A cooperative study in North America. J Neurosurg 86:467

108. Fleishaker JC, Hulst LK, Peters GR: The effect of phenytoin on the pharmacokinetics of tirilazad mesylate in healthy male volunteers. Clin Pharm Therapeut 56:389, 1995

109. Bracken MB, Shepard MJ, Holford TR et al: Methylprednisolone or tirilazad mesylate administration after acute spinal cord injury: 1-year follow up. Results of the Third National Acute Spinal Cord Injury randomized controlled trial. J Neurosurg 89:699, 1998

110. Arrowsmith JE, Harrison MJ, Newman SP et al: Neuroprotection of the brain during cardiopulmonary bypass: A randomized trial of remacemide during coronary artery bypass in 171 patients. Stroke 29:2357, 1998

111. De Deyn PP, Reuck JD, Deberdt W et al: Treatment of acute ischemic stroke with piracetam. Stroke 28:2347, 1997

112. Yamaguchi T, Keiji S, Kintomo T et al: Ebselen in acute ischemic stroke. A placebo-controlled, double-blind clinical trial. Stroke 29:12, 1998

113. Koppi S, Barolin GS: Hemodilution therapy with neuron metabolism specific therapy in ischemic stroke—encouraging results of a comparative study. Wiener Med Wochens 146:41, 1996

114. Hatton J, Rapp RP, Kudsk KK et al: Intravenous insulin-like growth factor-I (IGF-I) in moderate-to-severe head injury: A Phase II safety and efficacy trial. J Neurosurg 86:779, 1997

115. Taylor CP, Narasimhan LS: Sodium channels and therapy of central nervous system diseases. Adv Pharmacol 39:47, 1997

116. Benoit E, Escande D: Riluzole specifically blocks inactivated Na channels in myelinated nerve fiber. Pflugers Arch Eur J Physiol 419:603, 1991

117. Pratt J, Rataud J, Bardot F et al: Neuroprotective actions of riluzole in rodent models of global and focal cerebral ischaemia. Neurosci Lett 140:225, 1992

118. Wahl F, Allix M, Plotkine M et al: Effect of riluzole on focal cerebral ischemia in rats. Eur J Pharmacol 230:209, 1993

119. Lips J, Kalkman CJ, deHaan P: Neuroprotective effects of riluzole in a rabbit of experimental spinal ischemia. SNACC abstract # 1001, JNA 11:4, 1999

120. Bensimon G, Lacomblez L, Meininger V: A controlled trial of riluzole in amyotrophic lateral sclerosis. ALS/Riluzole Study Group. N Engl J Med 330:585, 1994

121. Smith SE, Meldrum BS: Cerebroprotective effect of lamotrigine after focal ischemia in rats. Stroke 26:117, 1995

122. Wiard RO, Dickerson MC, Beek BS: Neuroprotective properties of the novel antiepileptic lamotrigine in a gerbil model of global cerebral ischemia. Stroke 26:466, 1995

123. Smith SE, Hodges H, Sowinski P et al: Long-term beneficial effects of BW619C89 on neurological deficit, cognitive deficit and brain damage after middle cerebral artery occlusion in the rat. Neurosci 77:1123, 1997

124. Dietrich WD, Busto R, Alonso et al: Intraischemic but not postischemic brain hypothermia protects chronically following global forebrain ischemia in rats. J Cereb Blood Flow Metab 13:541, 1993

125. Yubo R, Nowak TS Jr: Therapeutic window for hypothermia after transient focal ischemia in spontaneously hypertensive rats. Stroke 29:327, 1998

126. Clifton GL, Allen S, Barodale OH et al: A phase II study of moderate hypothermia in severe brain injury. J Neurotrauma 10:263, 1993

127. Marion DW, Obrist WD, Carlier PM et al: The use of moderate therapeutic hypothermia for patients with severe head injuries: A preliminary report. J Neurosurg 18:700, 1993

128. Shiozaki T, Sugimoto H, Taneda M et al: Effect of mild hypothermia on uncontrollable intracranial hypertension after severe head injury. J Neurosurg 79:363, 1993

129. Marion DW, Penrod LE, Kelsey SF et al: Treatment of traumatic brain injury with moderate hypothermia. N Engl J Med 336:540, 1997

130. Hartung J, Cottrell JE: Statistics and hypothermia [editorial]. J Neurosurg Anesth 10:1, 1998

131. Schwab S, Schwarz EK, Bertram M et al: Moderate hypothermia in the treatment of patients with severe middle cerebral artery (MCA) territory infarction: A pilot study. Stroke 29:305, 1998

132. Clifton GL: First results of the North American multicenter trial on the usage of hypothermia in head injury patients. Oral presentation, 2nd International Symposium on Therapeutic Hypothermia, Vienna, 1999

133. Marion DW: Response to "Statistics and Hypothermia." J Neurosurg Anesth 10:120, 1998

134. Hartung J, Cottrell JE: In reply: Response to "Statistics and Hypothermia." J Neurosurg Anesth 10:122, 1998

135. Batjer HH, Frankfurt AI, Purdy PD et al: Use of etomidate, temporary arterial occlusion, and intraoperative angiography in surgical treatment of large and giant cerebral aneurysms. J Neurosurg 68:234, 1988

136. Amadeu ME, Abramowicz AE, Chambers G et al: Etomidate does not alter recovery after anoxia of evoked population spikes recorded from the CA1 region of rat hippocampal slices. Anesthesiology 88:1274, 1998

137. Samson D, Batter HH, Bowman G et al: A clinical study of the parameters and effects of temporary arterial occlusion in the management of intracranial aneurysms. Neurosurgery 34:22, 1994

138. Doenicke A, Roizen MF, Hoernecke R et al: Haemolysis after etomidate: Comparison of propylene glycol and lipid formulations. Br J Anaesth 79:386, 1997

139. Hoffman WE, Charbel FT, Edelman G et al: Comparison of the effect of etomidate and desflurane on brain tissue gases and pH during prolonged middle cerebral artery occlusion. Anesthesiology 88:1188, 1998

140. Courville CD: The pathogenesis of necrosis of the cerebral gray matter following nitrous oxide anesthesia. Ann Surg 107:371, 1938

141. Jevtovic-Todorovic V, Todorovic SM, Mennerick S et al: Nitrous oxide (laughing gas) is an NMDA antagonist, neuroprotectant and neurotoxin. Nature Med 4:460, 1998

142. Jevtovic-Todorovic V, Benshoff N, Olney JW: Prolonged nitrous oxide kills neurons in the adult rat brain. J Neurosurg Anesth 10:257, 1998

143. Hadzic A, Glab K, Sauborn KC et al: Severe neurologic deficit after nitrous oxide anesthesia. Anesthesiology 83:863, 1995

144. Badner NH, Drader K, Freeman D et al: The use of intraoperative nitrous oxide leads to postoperative increases in plasma homocysteine. Anesth Analg 87:711, 1998

145. Mayer EL, Jacobsen DW, Robinson K: Homocysteine and coronary atherosclerosis. J Am Coll Cardiol 27:517, 1996

146. Chambers JC, McGregor A, Jean-Marie J et al: Acute hyperhomocysteinemia and endothelial dysfunction. Lancet 351:36, 1998

147. Clarke R, Daly L, Robinson K et al: Hyperhomocysteinemia: An independent risk factor for vascular disease. N Engl J Med 324:1149, 1991

148. Baughman VL, Hoffman WE, Miletich DJ et al: Neurologic outcome in rats following incomplete cerebral ischemia during halothane, isoflurane or N2O. Anesthesiology 69:192, 1988

149. Baughman VL, Hoffman WE, Thomas C et al: The interaction of nitrous oxide and isoflurane with incomplete cerebral ischemia in the rat. Anesthesiology 70:767, 1989

150. Baughman VL, Hoffman WE, Thomas C *et al:* Comparison of methohexital and isoflurane on neurologic outcome and histopathology following incomplete ischemia in rats. Anesthesiology 72:85, 1990

151. Franks NP, Lieb WR: A serious target for laughing gas. Nature Med 4:383, 1998

152. Goldstein A, Wells BA, Keats AS: Increased tolerance to cerebral anoxia by pentobarbital. Arch Int Phamacodyn Ther 161:138, 1966

153. Steen PA, Milde JH, Michenfelder JD: No barbiturate protection in a dog model of complete cerebral ischemia. Ann Neurol 5:343, 1979

154. Gisvold SE, Safar P, Hendrickx HHL *et al:* Thiopental treatment after global brain ischemia in pigtailed monkeys. Anesthesiology 60:88, 1984

155. Hartung J, Cottrell JE: Nitrous oxide reduces thiopental-induced prolongation of survival in hypoxic and anoxic mice. Anesth Analg 66:47, 1987

156. Arnfred I, Secher O: Anoxia and barbiturates: Tolerance to anoxia in mice influenced by barbiturates. Arch Int Pharmacodyn 139:67, 1962

157. Wilhjelm BJ, Arnfred I: Protective action of some anaesthetics against anoxia. Acta Pharmacol 22:93, 1965

158. Milde LN: The hypoxic mouse model for screening cerebral protective agents: A reexamination. Anesth Analg 67:917, 1988

159. Hartung J, Cottrell JE: On hot mice, cold facts and would-be replication. Anesth Analg 69:408, 1989

160. Sugaya T, Kitani Y: Nitrous oxide attenuates the protective effect of isoflurane on microtubule-associated protein 2 degradation during forebrain ischemia in the rat. Brain Res Bull 44:307, 1997

161. Jevtovic-Todorovic V, Benshoff N, Olney JW: Nitrous oxide augments the neurotoxic side effects of ketamine in the adult rat brain. J Neurosurg Anesthesiol 11:4, 1999

162. Amorim P, Chambers G, Cottrell J, Kass IS: Nitrous oxide impairs electrophysiologic recovery after severe hypoxia in rat hippocampal slices. Anesthesiology 87:642, 1997

163. Hoffman WE, Miletich DJ, Albrecht RF: The effects of midazolam on cerebral blood flow and oxygen consumption and its interaction with nitrous oxide. Anesth Analg 65:729, 1986

164. Kiloh LG, McComas AJ, Osselton JW *et al:* The neural basis of the EEG. In Kiloh LG, McComas AJ, Osselton JW (eds): Clinical Electroencephalography, 4th ed, p 24. London, Butterworth, 1981

165. Scott JC, Ponaganis KV, Stanski DR: EEG quantification of narcotic effect: The comparative pharmacodynamics of fentanyl and alfentanil. Anesthesiology 62:234, 1985

166. Rampil IJ: A primer for EEG signal processing in anesthesia. Anesthesiology 89:980, 1998

167. Stockard JJ, Bickford RG: The neurophysiology of anesthesia. In Gordon E (ed): A Basis and Practice of Neuroanesthesia, 2nd ed, p 3. Amsterdam, Elsevier, 1981

168. Trojaborg W, Boysen G: Relation between EEG, regional cerebral blood flow and internal carotid artery pressure during carotid endarterectomy. Electroencephalogr Clin Neurophysiol 34:61, 1973

169. Kofke WA, Tempelhoff R, Dasheiff RM: Anesthetic implications of epilepsy, status epilepticus, and epilepsy surgery. J Neurosurg Anesthesiol 9:349, 1997

170. Tempelhoff R, Modica PA, Grubb RL Jr *et al:* Selective shunting during carotid endarterectomy based on two-channel computerized electroencephalographic/compressed spectral array analysis. Neurosurgery 24:339, 1989

171. Schwilden H, Stoeckel H: Effective therapeutic infusions produced by closed-loop feedback control of methohexital administration during total intravenous anesthesia with fentanyl. Anesthesiology 73:225, 1990

172. Spackman TN, Faust RJ, Cucchiara RF *et al:* A comparison of aperiodic analysis of the EEG with standard EEG and cerebral blood flow for detection of ischemia. Anesthesiology 66:229, 1987

173. Peterson DO, Drummond JC, Todd MM: Effects of halothane, enflurane, isoflurane and nitrous oxide on somatosensory evoked potentials in humans. Anesthesiology 65:35, 1986

174. Schindler E, Muller M, Zickmann B *et al:* Modulation of somatosensory evoked potentials under various concentrations of desflurane with and without nitrous oxide. J Neurosurg Anesthesiol 10:218, 1998

175. Uhl RR, Squires KC, Bruce DL, Starr A: Effects of halothane anesthesia on the human cortical visual evoked response. Anesthesiology 53:273, 1980

176. Chi OZ, Field C: Effects of isoflurane on visual evoked potentials in humans. Anesthesiology 65:328, 1986

177. Chi OZ, Field C: Effects of enflurane on visual evoked potentials in humans. Br J Anaesth 64:163, 1990

178. Sloan TB, Koht A: Depression of cortical somatosensory evoked potentials by nitrous oxide. Br J Anaesth 57:849, 1985

179. Sebel PS, Flynn PJ, Ingram DA: Effect of nitrous oxide on visual, auditory and somatosensory evoked potentials. Br J Anaesth 56:1403, 1984

180. Lam AM, Sharar SR, Mayberg TS *et al:* Isoflurane compared with nitrous oxide anesthesia for intraoperative monitoring of somatosensory-evoked potentials. Can J Anaesth 41:295, 1994

181. Manninen PH, Lam AM, Nicholas JP: The effects of isoflurane and isoflurane-nitrous oxide anesthesia on brain stem auditory evoked potentials in humans. Anesth Analg 64:43, 1985

182. Schwender D, Conzen P, Klasing S *et al:* The effects of anesthesia with increasing end-expiratory concentrations of sevoflurane on midlatency auditory evoked potentials. Anesth Analg 81:817, 1995

183. Schwender D, Klasing S, Conzen P *et al:* Midlatency auditory evoked potentials during anesthesia with increasing end-expiratory concentrations of desflurane. Acta Anaesthesiol Scand 40:171, 1996

184. McPherson RW, Sell B, Traystman RJ: Effects of thiopental, fentanyl and etomidate on upper extremity somatosensory evoked potentials in humans. Anesthesiology 65:584, 1986

185. Drummond JC, Todd MM, Sang H: The effect of high dose sodium thiopental on brain stem auditory and median nerve somatosensory evoked responses in humans. Anesthesiology 63:249, 1985

186. Sutton LN, Frewen T, Marsh R *et al:* The effects of deep barbiturate coma on multimodality evoked potentials. J Neurosurg 57:178, 1982

187. Koht A, Schütz W, Schmidt G *et al:* Effects of etomidate, midazolam, and thiopental on median nerve somatosensory evoked potentials and the additive effects of fentanyl and nitrous oxide. Anesth Analg 67:435, 1988

188. Thornton C, Heneghan CPH, Navaratnarajah M *et al:* Effect of etomidate on the auditory evoked response in man. Br J Anaesth 57:554, 1985

189. Chi OZ, Subramoni J, Jasaitis D: Visual evoked potentials during etomidate administration in humans. Can J Anaesth 37:452, 1990

190. Grundy BL, Brown RH, Greenberg BA: Diazepam alters cortical potentials. Anesthesiology 51:538, 1979

191. Loughnan BL, Sebel PS, Thomas D *et al:* Evoked potentials during diazepam or fentanyl. Anaesthesia 42:95, 1987

192. Sloan TB, Fugina ML, Toleikis JR: Effects of midazolam on median nerve somatosensory evoked potentials. Br J Anaesth 64:590, 1990

193. Maurette P, Simeon F, Castagnera L *et al:* Propofol anaesthesia alters somatosensory evoked cortical potentials. Anaesthesia 43:44, 1988

194. Chassard D, Joubaub A, Colson A *et al:* Auditory evoked potentials during propofol anaesthesia in man. Br J Anaesth 62:522, 1989

195. Pathak KS, Brown RH, Cascorbi HF *et al:* Effects of fentanyl and morphine on intraoperative somatosensory cortical-evoked potentials. Anesth Analg 63:833, 1984

196. Kalkman CJ, Rheineck-Leyssius AT, Bovill JG: Influence of high-dose opioid anesthesia on posterior tibial nerve somatosensory cortical evoked potentials: Effects of fentanyl, sufentanil, and alfentanil. J Cardiothorac Anesth 2:758, 1988

197. Samra SK, Lilly DJ, Rush NL *et al:* Fentanyl anesthesia and human brain stem auditory evoked potentials. Anesthesiology 61:261, 1984

198. Browning JL, Heizer ML, Baskins DS *et al:* Variations in corticomotor and somatosensory evoked potentials: Effects of temperature, halothane anesthesia, and arterial partial pressure of CO_2. Anesth Analg 74:643, 1992

199. Doyle WJ, Fria TJ: The effects of hypothermia on the latencies of the auditory brain stem response (ABR) in the rhesus monkey. Clin Neurophysiol 60:258, 1985

200. Dubois M, Coppola R, Buchsbaum MS: Somatosensory evoked potentials during whole body hyperthermia in humans. Electroencephalogr Clin Neurophysiol 52:157, 1981

201. Haghighi SS, Oro JJ: Effects of hypovolemic hypotensive shock on somatosensory and motor evoked potentials. Neurosurgery 24:246, 1989

202. Ranganathan K, Bendo AA, Cottrell JE *et al:* SSEP latencies are prolonged by reductions in MAPs and hypocapnia in cats. J Neurosurg Anesthesiol 6:A332, 1994

203. Grundy BL, Nash CL, Brown RH: Arterial pressure manipulation

alters spinal cord function during correction of scoliosis. Anesthesiology 54:249, 1981

204. Haghighi SS, Oro JJ, Gibbs SR et al: Effect of graded hypoxia on cortical and spinal somatosensory evoked potentials. Surg Neurol 37:350, 1992

205. Levy WJ, York DH, McCaffrey M et al: Motor evoked potentials from transcranial stimulation of the motor cortex in humans. Neurosurgery 15:287, 1984

206. Maccabee PJ, Amassian VE, Cracco RQ et al: Stimulation of the human nervous system using the magnetic coil. J Clin Neurophysiol 8:38, 1991

207. Agnew WF, McCreery DB: Considerations for safety in the use of extracranial stimulation for motor evoked potentials. Neurosurgery 20:143, 1987

208. Ghaly RF, Stone JL, Levy WJ et al: The effect of nitrous oxide on transcranial magnetic-induced electromyographic responses in the monkey. J Neurosurg Anesthesiol 2:175, 1990

209. Zentner J, Kiss I, Ebner A: Influence of anesthetics—nitrous oxide in particular—on electromyographic response evoked by transcranial electrical stimulation of the cortex. Neurosurgery 24:253, 1989

210. Haghighi SS, Madsen R, Green KD et al: Suppression of motor evoked potentials by inhalation anesthetics. J Neurosurg Anesthesiol 2:73, 1990

211. Kalkman CJ, Drummond JC, Ribberink AA: Low concentrations of isoflurane abolish motor evoked responses to transcranial electrical stimulation during nitrous oxide/opioid anesthesia in humans. Anesth Analg 73:410, 1991

212. Kalkman CJ, Drummond JC, Ribberink AA et al: Effects of propofol, etomidate, midazolam and fentanyl on motor evoked responses to transcranial electrical or magnetic stimulation in humans. Anesthesiology 76:502, 1992

213. Ghaly RF, Stone JL, Aldrete A et al: Effects of incremental ketamine hydrochloride doses on motor evoked potentials (MEPs) following transcranial magnetic stimulation: A primate study. J Neurosurg Anesthesiol 2:79, 1990

214. Ghaly RF, Stone JL, Levy WJ et al: The effect of etomidate on motor evoked potentials induced by transcranial magnetic stimulation in the monkey. Neurosurgery 27:936, 1990

215. Kalkman CJ, Drummond JC, Kennelly NA et al: Intraoperative monitoring of tibialis anterior muscle motor evoked responses to transcranial electrical stimulation during partial neuromuscular blockade. Anesth Analg 75:584, 1992

216. Yingling CD: Intraoperative monitoring of cranial nerves in skull base surgery. In Jackler RK, Brackmann DE (eds): Neurotology, p 967. St. Louis, Mosby, 1994

217. Lundberg N: Continuous recording and control of ventricular fluid pressure in neurosurgical practice. Acta Psychiatr Neurol Scand 36(suppl 149):1, 1960

218. Rosner MJ, Becker DP: ICP monitoring: Complications and associated factors. Clin Neurosurg 23:494, 1976

219. Mayhall CG, Archer NH, Lamb V et al: Ventriculostomy-related infections. A prospective epidemiologic study. N Engl J Med 310:553, 1984

220. Aucoin PJ, Kotilainen HR, Gantz NM et al: Intracranial pressure monitors. Epidemiologic study of risk factors and infections. Am J Med 80:369, 1986

221. Mollman HD, Gaylan LR, Ford SE: A clinical comparison of subarachnoid catheters to ventriculostomy and subarachnoid bolts: A prospective study. J Neurosurg 68:737, 1988

222. Roberts P, Fullenwider C, Stevens F et al: Experimental and clinical experience with a new solid state intracranial pressure monitor with in vivo zero capability. In Ishii S, Nagai H, Brock M (eds): Intracranial Pressure V, p 104. Berlin, Springer Verlag, 1983

223. Ostrup RC, Luerssen TG, Marshall LF et al: Continuous monitoring of intracranial pressure with a miniaturized fiberoptic device. J Neurosurg 67:206, 1987

224. Crutchfield JS, Narayan RK, Robertson CS et al: Evaluation of a fiberoptic intracranial pressure monitor. J Neurosurg 72:482, 1990

225. Sundbarg G, Nordstrom CH, Messeter K et al: A comparison of intraparenchymatous and intraventricular pressure recording in clinical practice. J Neurosurg 67:841, 1987

226. Bolognese P, Miller JI, Heger IM, Milhorat TH: Laser-Doppler flowmetry in neurosurgery. JNA 5:151, 1993

227. Hoffman WE, Charbel FT, Edelman G: Brain tissue oxygen, carbon dioxide, and pH in neurosurgical patients at risk for ischemia. Anesth Analg 82:582, 1996

228. McCormick PW, Steward M, Goelting MG et al: Noninvasive cerebral optical spectroscopy for monitoring cerebral oxygen delivery and hemodynamics. Crit Care Med 19:89, 1991

229. Kurth CD, Wher B: Cerebral hemoglobin and optical path length influence near-infrared spectroscopy measurement of cerebral oxygen saturation. Anesth Analg 84:1297, 1997

230. Hounsfield GN: Computerized transverse axial scanning (tomography): Part I. Description of system. Br J Radiol 46:1016, 1973

231. Frush DP, Bisset GS III, Hall SC: Pediatric sedation in radiology: The practice of safe sleep. Am J Roentgenol 167:1381, 1996

232. Perry BJ, Bridges C: Computerized transverse axial scanning (tomography): Part III. Radiation dose considerations. Br J Radiol 46:1048, 1973

233. Stark DD, Bradley WG: Magnetic Resonance Imaging. St. Louis, CV Mosby, 1988

234. Patteson SK, Chesney JT: Anesthetic management for magnetic resonance imaging: Problems and solutions. Anesth Analg 74:121, 1992

235. Saunders RF, Smith H: Safety aspects of NMR clinical imaging. Br Med Bull 40:148, 1984

236. Caro JJ, Trindade E, McGregor M: The cost-effectiveness of replacing high-osmolality with low-osmolality contrast media. Am J Roentgenol 159:869, 1992

237. Young, WL, Pile-Spellman J, Hacein-Bey L et al: Invasive neuroradiologic procedures for cerebrovascular abnormalities: Anesthetic considerations. Anesth Clin North Am 15:631, 1997

238. Junck L, Marshall WH: Neurotoxicity of radiologic contrast agents. Ann Neurol 13:469, 1983

239. Goldberg M: Systemic reactions to intravascular contrast media: A guide for the anesthesiologist. Anesthesiology 60:46, 1984

240. Numaguchi Y, Fleming MS, Hasao K et al: Blood–brain barrier disruption due to cerebral arteriography: CT findings. J Comput Assist Tomogr 8:936, 1984

241. Shehadi WH, Toniolo G: Adverse reactions to contrast media: A report from the Committee on Safety of Contrast Media for the International Society of Radiology. Radiology 137:299, 1980

242. Greenberger PA, Patterson R, Tapio CM: Prophylaxis against repeated radiocontrast media reactions in 857 cases. Arch Intern Med 145:2197, 1985

243. Ravussin P, Abou-Madi M, Archer D et al: Changes in CSF pressure after mannitol in patients with and without elevated CSF pressure. J Neurosurg 69:869, 1988

244. Domaingue CM, Nye DH: Hypotensive effect of mannitol administered rapidly. Anaesth Intens Care 13:134, 1985

245. Cottrell JE, Robustelli A, Post K et al: Furosemide and mannitol-induced changes in intracranial pressure and serum osmolality and electrolytes. Anesthesiology 47:28, 1977

246. Schettini A, Stahurski B, Young HF: Osmotic and osmotic loop diuresis in brain surgery: Effects on plasma and CSF electrolytes and ion excretion. J Neurosurg 56:679, 1982

247. Miller JD, Sakalas R, Ward JD et al: Methylprednisolone treatment in patients with brain tumors. Neurosurgery 1:114, 1977

248. Ohnishi T, Sher PB, Posner JB et al: Capillary permeability factor secreted by malignant brain tumor. Role in peritumoral brain edema and possible mechanism for antiedema effect of glucocorticoids. J Neurosurg 72:245, 1990

249. Matta BF, Lam AM, Mayberg TS et al: A critique of the intraoperative use of jugular venous bulb catheters during neurosurgical procedures. Anesth Analg 79:745, 1994

250. Jelsma LF, McQueen JD: Effect of experimental water restriction on brain water. J Neurosurg 26:35, 1967

251. Sieber FE, Smith DS, Traystman RJ et al: Glucose: A reevaluation of its intraoperative use. Anesthesiology 67:72, 1987

252. Pulsinelli WA, Waldman S, Rawlinson D et al: Moderate hyperglycemia augments ischemic brain damage: A neuropathologic study in the rat. Neurology 32:1239, 1982

253. Pulsinelli WA, Levy DE, Sigsbee B et al: Increased damage after ischemic stroke in patients with hyperglycemia with or without established diabetes mellitus. Am J Med 74:540, 1983

254. Cooper KR, Boswell PA, Choi SC: Safe use of PEEP in patients with severe head injury. J Neurosurg 63:552, 1985

255. Boris-Moller F, Smith ML, Siesjo BK: Effects of hypothermia on ischemic brain damage: A comparison between pre-ischemic and post-ischemic cooling. Neurosci Res Comm 5:87, 1989

256. Cottrell JE, Hartung J, Giffin JP et al: Intracranial and hemodynamic changes after succinylcholine administration in cats. Anesth Analg 62:1006, 1983

257. Lanier WL, Iaizzo PA, Milde JH: Cerebral function and muscle

afferent activity following IV succinylcholine in dogs anesthetized with halothane: The effects of pretreatment with defasciculating doses of pancuronium. Anesthesiology 71:87, 1989

258. Minton MD, Grosslight, KR, Stirt JA *et al:* Increases in intracranial pressure from succinylcholine: Prevention by prior nondepolarizing blockade. Anesthesiology 65:165, 1986

259. Stirt JA, Grosslight KR, Bedford RF *et al:* "Defasciculation" with metocurine prevents succinylcholine-induced increases in intracranial pressure. Anesthesiology 67:50, 1987

260. Cooperman LH, Strobel GE, Kennal EM: Massive hyperkalemia after administration of succinylcholine. Anesthesiology 32:161, 1970

261. Stevenson PH, Birch AA: Succinylcholine-induced hyperkalemia in a patient with a closed head injury. Anesthesiology 51:89, 1979

262. Iwatsuki N, Kuroder H, Ameha K *et al:* Succinylcholine-induced hyperkalemia in patients with ruptured cerebral aneurysm. Anesthesiology 53:64, 1980

263. Vesely R, Hoffman WE, Gil KS *et al:* The cerebrovascular effects of curare and histamine in the rat. Anesthesiology 66:519, 1987

264. Schramm WM, Papousek A, Michalek-Sauberer A *et al:* The cerebral and cardiovascular effects of cisatracurium and atracurium in neurosurgical patients. Anesth Analg 86:123, 1998

265. Rosa G, Orfei P, Sanfilippo M *et al:* The effects of atracurium besylate (Tracrium®) on intracranial pressure and cerebral perfusion pressure. Anesth Analg 65:381, 1986

266. Hennis PJ, Fahey MR, Canfell PC *et al:* Pharmacology of laudanosine in dogs. Anesthesiology 65:56, 1986

267. Lanier WL, Milde JH, Michenfelder JD: The cerebral effects of pancuronium and atracurium in halothane-anesthetized dogs. Anesthesiology 63:589, 1985

268. Rosa G, Sanfilippo M, Orfei P *et al:* The effects of pipecuronium bromide on intracranial pressure and cerebral perfusion pressure. J Neurosurg Anesthesiol 3:253, 1991

269. Stirt JA, Maggio W, Haworth C *et al:* Vecuronium: Effect on intracranial pressure and hemodynamics in neurosurgical patients. Anesthesiology 67:570, 1987

270. Ginsberg B, Glass PS, Quill T *et al:* Onset and duration of neuromuscular blockade following high-dose vecuronium administration. Anesthesiology 71:201, 1989

271. Mirakhur RK: Safety aspects of non-depolarizing neuromuscular blocking agents with special reference to rocuronium bromide. Eur J Anaesthesiol 11:133, 1994

272. Hammil JF, Bedford RDF, Weaver DC *et al:* Lidocaine before endotracheal intubation: Intravenous or laryngotracheal. Anesthesiology 55:578, 1981

273. Jung R, Reinsel R, Marx W *et al:* Isoflurane and nitrous oxide: Comparative impact on cerebrospinal fluid pressure in patients with brain tumors. Anesth Analg 75:724, 1992

274. Lam AM, Mayberg TS, Eng CC *et al:* Nitrous oxide-isoflurane anesthesia causes more cerebral vasodilation than an equipotent dose of isoflurane in humans. Anesth Analg 78:462, 1994

275. Toung TJK, McPherson RW, Ahn H *et al:* Pneumocephalus: Effects of patient position on the incidence and location of aerocele after posterior fossa and upper cervical cord surgery. Anesth Analg 65:65, 1986

276. Artru AA: Nitrous oxide plays a direct role in the development of tension pneumocephalus intraoperatively. Anesthesiology 57:59, 1982

277. Wilder BL: Hypothesis: The etiology of midcervical quadriplegia after operation with the patient in the sitting position. Neurosurgery 11:530, 1982

278. McPherson RW, Szymanski T, Rogers MC: Somatosensory evoked potential changes in position related brain stem ischemia. Anesthesiology 61:88, 1984

279. Grundy BL, Procopio PT, Janetta PJ: Evoked potential changes produced by positioning for retromastoid craniectomy. Neurosurgery 10:766, 1982

280. Black S, Ockert DB, Oliver WC *et al:* Outcome following posterior fossa craniectomy in patients in the sitting or horizontal positions. Anesthesiology 69:49, 1988

281. Hagen PT, Scholz DG, Edward WD: Incidence and size of patent foramen ovale during the first 10 decades of life: An autopsy study of 965 normal hearts. Mayo Clin Proc 59:17, 1984

282. Perkins-Pearson NAK, Marshall WK, Bedford RF: Atrial pressures in the seated position: Implications for paradoxical air embolism. Anesthesiology 57:493, 1982

283. Guggiari M, Lechat P, Garen-Colonne C *et al:* Early detection of patent foramen ovale by two-dimensional contrast echocardiography for prevention of paradoxical air embolism during sitting position. Anesth Analg 67:192, 1988

284. Schwarz G, Fuchs G, Weihs W *et al:* Sitting position for neurosurgery: Experience with preoperative contrast echocardiography in 301 patients. J Neurosurg Anesthesiol 6:83, 1994

285. Muzzi DA, Losasso TJ, Black S *et al:* Comparison of a transesophageal and precordial ultrasonic Doppler sensor in the detection of venous air embolism. Anesth Analg 70:103, 1990

286. Matjasko J, Petrozza P, MacKenzie CF: Sensitivity of end-tidal nitrogen in venous air embolism detection in dogs. Anesthesiology 63:418, 1985

287. Bunegin L, Albin MS, Helsel PE *et al:* Positioning the right atrial catheter: A model for reappraisal. Anesthesiology 55:343, 1981

288. Albin MS, Babinski M, Wolf S: Cardiovascular responses to the sitting position. Br J Anaesth 52:1961, 1980

289. Marshall WK, Bedford RF, Miller ED: Cardiovascular responses in the seated position: Impact of four anesthetic techniques. Anesth Analg 62:648, 1983

290. Losasso TJ, Muzzi DA, Dietz NM *et al:* Fifty percent nitrous oxide does not increase the risk of venous air embolism in neurosurgical patients operated upon in the sitting position. Anesthesiology 77:21, 1992

291. Grossman A: Clinical Endocrinology. Oxford, Boston, Blackwell Scientific, 1992

292. Ciric I, Ragin A, Baumgartner C *et al:* Complications of transsphenoidal surgery: Results of a national survey, review of the literature, and personal experience. Neurosurgery 40:225, 1997

293. Kassell NF, Torner JC: Epidemiology of intracranial aneurysms: Anesthetic considerations in the surgical repair of intracranial aneurysms. In Varkey GP (ed): International Anesthesiology Clinics, vol 20, p 89. Boston, Little, Brown, 1982

294. Guy J, McGrath BJ, Borel CO *et al:* Perioperative management of aneurysmal subarachnoid hemorrhage: Part I. Operative management. Anesth Analg 81:1060, 1995

295. Kassell NF, Torner JC, Haley EC *et al:* The International Cooperative Study on the Timing of Aneurysm Surgery. Part I: Overall management results. J Neurosurg 73:18, 1990

296. Botterell EH, Longhead WM, Scott JW *et al:* Hypothermia and interruption of the carotid or carotid and vertebral circulation in the surgical management of intracranial aneurysms. J Neurosurg 13:1, 1956

297. Hunt WE, Hess RM: Surgical risk as related to time of intervention in the repair of intracranial aneurysms. J Neurosurg 28:14, 1968

298. Drake CG, Hung WE, Sank K *et al:* Report of World Federation of Neurological Surgeons Committee on a universal subarachnoid hemorrhage grading scale. J Neurosurg 68:985, 1988

299. Unruptured intracranial aneurysms—Risk of rupture and risks of surgical intervention. International Study of Unruptured Intracranial Aneurysms Investigators. N Engl J Med 339:1725, 1998

300. Sekhar LN, Heros RC: Origin, growth, and rupture of saccular aneurysms. A review. Neurosurgery 8:248, 1981

301. Kassell NF, Torner JC: Aneurysmal rebleeding: A preliminary report from the Cooperative Aneurysm Study. J Neurosurg 13:479, 1983

302. Kassell NF, Torner JC, Jane JA *et al:* The International Cooperative Study on the Timing of Aneurysm Surgery. Part II: Surgical results. J Neurosurg 73:37, 1990

303. Haley EC Jr, Kassell NF, Torner JC: The International Cooperative Study on the Timing of Aneurysm Surgery. The North American experience. Stroke 23:205, 1992

304. MacDonald RL, Wallace MC, Coyne TJ: The effect of surgery on the severity of vasospasm. J Neurosurg 80:433, 1992

305. Kassell NF, Sasaki T, Colohan ART *et al:* Cerebral vasospasm following aneurysmal subarachnoid hemorrhage. Stroke 16:562, 1985

306. McGrath BJ, Guy J, Borel CO *et al:* Perioperative management of aneurysmal subarachnoid hemorrhage: Part 2. Postoperative management. Anesth Analg 81:1295, 1995

307. Barker FG II, Ogilvy CS: Efficacy of prophylactic nimodipine for delayed ischemic deficit after subarachnoid hemorrhage: A meta-analysis. J Neurosurg 84:405, 1996

308. Awad IA, Carter LP, Spetzler RF *et al:* Clinical vasospasm after subarachnoid hemorrhage: Response to hypervolemia, hemodilution and arterial hypertension. Stroke 18:365, 1987

309. Origitano TC, Wascher TM, Reichman OH *et al:* Sustained increased cerebral blood flow with prophylactic hypertensive hyper-

volemic hemodilution ("triple-H" therapy) after subarachnoid hemorrhage. Neurosurgery 27:729, 1990

310. Medlock MD, Dulebohn SC, Elwood PW: Prophylactic hypervolemia without calcium channel blockers in early aneurysm surgery. Neurosurgery 30:12, 1992

311. Newell DW, Eskridge JM, Mayberg MR et al: Angioplasty for the treatment of symptomatic vasospasm following subarachnoid hemorrhage. Neurosurgery 71:654, 1989

312. Zubkov YN, Nikiforov BM, Shustin VA: Balloon catheter technique for dilatation of constricted cerebral arteries after aneurysmal SAH. Acta Neurochirurg 70(1-2):65, 1984

313. Kaku Y, Yonekawa Y, Tsukahara T et al: Superselective intra-arterial infusion of papaverine for the treatment of cerebral vasospasm after subarachnoid hemorrhage. J Neurosurg 77:842, 1992

314. Eng CC, Lam AM: Cerebral aneurysms: Anesthetic considerations. In Cottrell JE, Smith DS (eds): Anesthesia and Neurosurgery, 3rd ed, p 376. St. Louis, Mosby-Yearbook, 1994

315. Davis TP, Alexander J, Lesch M: Electrocardiographic changes associated with acute cerebrovascular disease: A clinical review. Prog Cardiovasc Dis 36(3):245, 1993

316. Mizoi K, Yoshimoto T: Permissible temporary occlusion time in aneurysm surgery as evaluated by evoked potential monitoring. Neurosurgery 33:434, 1993

317. Ogilvy CS, Carter BS, Kaplan S et al: Temporary vessel occlusion for aneurysm surgery: Risk factors for stroke in patients protected by induced hypothermia and hypertension and intravenous mannitol administration. J Neurosurg 84:785, 1996

318. Cottrell JE: Brain Protection. ASA Annual Refresher Course Lectures. Lecture 153, 1997

319. Todd MM et al and I HAST Study Group: A pilot trial of hypothermia during aneurysm surgery. JNA 8:323, 1996

320. Sessler DI: Mild perioperative hypothermia. N Engl J Med 336:1730, 1997

321. Brown RJ, Wiebers DO, Forbes G et al: The natural history of unruptured intracranial arteriovenous malformations. J Neurosurg 68:352, 1988

322. Dodson BA: Interventional neuroradiology and the anesthetic management of patients with arteriovenous malformations. In Cottrell JE, David DS (eds): Anesthesia and Neurosurgery, 3rd ed, p 407. St. Louis, Mosby-Yearbook, 1994

323. Heros RC, Korosue K, Diebold PM: Surgical excision of cerebral arteriovenous malformations: Late results. Neurosurgery 26:570, 1990

324. Batjer HH, Devous MD, Meyer YJ et al: Cerebrovascular hemodynamics in arteriovenous malformation complicated by normal perfusion pressure breakthrough. Neurosurgery 22:503, 1988

325. Young WL, Prohovnik I, Ornstein E et al: Pressure autoregulation is intact after arteriovenous malformation resection. Neurosurgery 32:491, 1993

326. Young WL, Kader A, Ornstein E et al: Cerebral hyperemia after arteriovenous malformation resection is related to "breakthrough" complications but not to feeding artery pressure. Neurosurgery 38:1085, 1996

327. Hashimoto T, Young WL, Christopher C et al: Cardiac pause for deliberate systemic hypotension: Dose–response characteristics of adenosine. Anesthesiology 91:A191, 1999

328. Little DM Jr: Induced hypotension during anesthesia and surgery. Anesthesia 16:320, 1955

329. Johns RA: Endothelium-derived relaxing factor. Basic review and clinical implications. J Cardiothorac Vasc Anesth 5:69, 1991

330. Zhang F, White JG, Iadecola C: Nitric oxide donors increase blood flow and reduce brain damage in focal ischemia: Evidence that nitric oxide is beneficial in the early stages of cerebral ischemia. J Cereb Blood Flow Metab 14:217, 1994

331. Endrich B, Franke N, Peter K et al: Induced hypotension: Action of sodium nitroprusside and nitroglycerin on the microcirculation. A micropuncture investigation. Anesthesiology 66:605, 1987

332. Merrifield AJ, Blundell MD: Toxicity of sodium nitroprusside [letter]. Br J Anaesth 46:324, 1974

333. Davies DW, Kadar D, Steward DJ et al: A sudden death associated with the use of sodium nitroprusside for induction of hypotension during anesthesia. Can Anaesth Soc J 22:547, 1975

334. Woodside J Jr, Garner L, Bedford RJ: Captopril reduces the dose requirement for sodium nitroprusside-induced hypotension. Anesthesiology 60:413, 1984

335. Thomsen LJ, Riisager S, Jensen KA et al: Cerebral blood flow and

336. Miller R, Toth C, Silva DA: Nitroprusside vs. a nitroprusside-trimethaphan mixture: A comparison of dosage requirements and hemodynamic effects during induced hypotension for neurosurgery. Mt Sinai J Med (NY) 54:308, 1987

337. Nakazawa K, Taneyama C, Benson KT et al: Mixtures of sodium nitroprusside and trimethaphan for induction of hypotension. Anesth Analg 73:59, 1991

338. Bernard J-M, Moren J, Demeure D et al: Diltiazem reduces the nitroprusside doses for deliberate hypotension [Abstract]. Anesthesiology 77:A427, 1992

339. Bemann S, Jensen KA, Riisager S et al: Cerebral blood flow and metabolism during hypotension induced with sodium nitroprusside and metoprolol. Eur J Anaesthesiol 8:197, 1991

340. Shah N, Del Valle O, Edmondson R et al: Esmolol infusion nitroprusside-induced hypotension: Impact on hemodynamics, ventricular performance, and venous admixture. J Cardiothorac Vasc Anesth 6:196, 1992

341. Cottrell JE, Ilner P, Kittary MJ et al: Rebound hypertension after sodium nitroprusside-induced hypotension. Clin Pharmacol Ther 27:32, 1980

342. Michenfelder JD, Milde JH: The interaction of sodium nitroprusside, hypotension, and isoflurane in determining cerebral vascular effects. Anesthesiology 69:870, 1988

343. Rogers AT, Prough DS, Gravlee GP et al: Sodium nitroprusside does not dilate cerebral resistance vessels during hypothermic cardiopulmonary bypass. Anesthesiology 74:820, 1991

344. Stånge K, Lagerkranser M, Solevi A: Nitroprusside-induced hypotension and cerebrovascular autoregulation in the anesthetized pig. Anesth Analg 73:745, 1991

345. Cottrell JE, Patel KP, Ransohoff JR: Intracranial pressure changes induced by sodium nitroprusside in patients with intracranial mass lesions. J Neurosurg 48:329, 1978

346. Pinaud M, Souron R, Lelausque JN et al: Cerebral blood flow and cerebral oxygen consumption during nitroprusside-induced hypotension to less than 50 mm Hg. Anesthesiology 70:255, 1989

347. Harris SN, Escobar A, Rinder C et al: Nitroprusside-induced platelet dysfunction: A reversible phenomenon? [Abstract]. Anesthesiology 3A:145, 1992

348. Hines R, Barash PG: Infusion of sodium nitroprusside induces platelet dysfunction in vitro. Anesthesiology 70:611, 1989

349. Casthely PA, Lear S, Cottrell JE et al: Intrapulmonary shunting during induced hypotension. Anesth Analg 61:231, 1982

350. Wood M, Hyman S, Wood AJJ: A clinical study of sensitivity to sodium nitroprusside during controlled hypotensive anesthesia in young and elderly patients. Anesth Analg 66:132, 1987

351. Cottrell JE, Gupta B, Rappaport H et al: Intracranial pressure during nitroglycerin-induced hypotension. J Neurosurg 53:309, 1980

352. Maktabi M, Warner D, Sokoll M: Comparison of nitroprusside, nitroglycerin, and deep isoflurane for induced hypotension. J Neurosurg 19:350, 1986

353. Ivankovitch AD, Miletich DJ, Tinker JH: Nitroprusside and other short-acting hypotensive agents. Int Anesth Clin 16:132, 1978

354. Stoyka WW, Schutz H: The cerebral response to sodium nitroprusside and trimethaphan-controlled hypotension. Can Anaesth Soc 22:275, 1975

355. Karlin AD, Hartung J, Cottrell JE: Rate of induction of hypotension with trimethaphan modifies the intracranial pressure response in cats. Br J Anaesth 61:161, 1988

356. Thomas WA, Cole PV, Etherington NJ et al: Electrical activity of the cerebral cortex during induced hypotension in man. Br J Anesth 57:134, 1985

357. Lloyd-Thomas AR, Cole PV, Prior PF: Isoflurane prevents EEG depression during trimethaphan-induced hypotension in man. Br J Anaesth 65:313, 1990

358. Maekawa T, McDowall DG, Okuda Y: Brain surface oxygen tension and cerebral cortical blood flow during hemorrhagic and drug-induced hypotension in the cat. Anesthesiology 51:313, 1979

359. Michenfelder JD, Theye RA: Canine systemic and cerebral effects of hypotension induced by hemorrhage, trimethaphan, halothane or nitroprusside. Anesthesiology 46:188, 1977

360. Abe K, Demizu A, Kamada K et al: Local cerebral blood flow with prostaglandin E1 or trimethaphan during cerebral aneurysm clip ligation. Can J Anaesth 38:831, 1991

361. Taneyama C, Goto H, Goto K et al: Attenuation of arterial barore-

ceptor reflex response to acute hypovolemia during induced hypotension. Anesthesiology 73:433, 1990

362. Orenstein E, Matteo RS, Wienstein JA *et al:* A controlled trial of esmolol for the induction of deliberate hypotension. J Clin Anesth 1:31, 1988

363. Orenstein E, Young WL, Ostapkovich N *et al:* Deliberate hypotension in patients with intracranial arteriovenous malformations: Esmolol compared with isoflurane and sodium nitroprusside. Anesth Analg 72:639, 1991

364. Edmonson R, Del Valle O, Shah N *et al:* Esmolol for potentiation of nitroprusside-induced hypotension: Impact on the cardiovascular, adrenergic, and renin-angiotensin systems in man. Anesth Analg 69:202, 1989

365. Cot DHP, Drummond JC, Shapiro HM *et al:* Labetalol in controlled hypotension. Br J Anaesth 51:1, 1979

366. Goldberg ME, McNulty SE, Azad SS *et al:* A comparison of labetalol and nitroprusside for inducing hypotension during major surgery. Anesth Analg 70:537, 1990

367. Toivonen J, Virtanen H, Kaukinen S: Plasma renin, catecholamines, vasopressin and aldosterone during hypotension induced by labetalol with isoflurane. Acta Anaesthesiol Scand 35:496, 1988

368. Okasha AS, el-Attar AM, el-Gamal NA: Hemodynamic changes and glucose utilization during controlled hypotensive anesthesia with labetalol and sodium nitroprusside. ME J Anesth 9:395, 1988

369. Van Aken H, Puchstein C, Schweppe ML *et al:* Effect of labetalol on intracranial pressure in dogs with and without intracranial hypertension. Acta Anaesthesiol Scand 26:615, 1982

370. Abe K, Demizu A, Mima T *et al:* Carbon dioxide reactivity during prostaglandin E_1 induced hypotension for cerebral aneurysm surgery. Can J Anaesth 39:253, 1992

371. Kadoi Y, Saito S, Kunimoto F *et al:* Cerebral oxygenation during prostaglandin E_1 induced hypotension. Can J Anaesth 45:860, 1998

372. The IV Nicardipine Study Group. Efficacy and safety of intravenous nicardipine in the control of postoperative hypertension. Chest 99:393, 1991

373. Hersey SL, O'Dell NE, Lowe S *et al:* Nicardipine versus nitroprusside for controlled hypotension during spinal surgery in adolescents. Anesth Analg 84:1239, 1997

374. Prys-Roberts C, Lloyd JW, Fisher A *et al:* Deliberate profound hypotension induced with halothane: Studies of hemodynamics and pulmonary gas exchange. Br J Anaesth 46:105, 1974

375. Keaney NP, Pickerodt VWA, McDowall DG: CBF, autoregulation, CSF acid base parameters and deep halothane hypotension. Stroke 4:324, 1973

376. Jennett WB, Barker J, Fitch W *et al:* Effects of anesthesia on intracranial pressure in patients with space occupying lesions. Lancet 1:61, 1969

377. Jennett WB, McDowall DG, Barker J: The effect of halothane on intracranial pressure in cerebral tumors: Report of two cases. J Neurosurg 26:270, 1967

378. Artru AA: Enflurane causes a prolonged and reversible increase in the rate of CSF fluid in the dog. Anesthesiology 57:255, 1982

379. Milde LN, Milde JH: Cerebral and systemic hemodynamic and metabolic effects of desflurane-induced hypotension in dogs. Anesthesiology 74:513, 1991

380. Philip JH, Ji XB, Calalang BS *et al:* Sevoflurane controls blood pressure faster than isoflurane [Abstract]. Anesthesiology 3A:A384, 1992

381. Lam AM, Gelb AW: Cardiovascular effects of isoflurane-induced hypotension for cerebral aneurysm surgery. Anesth Analg 62:742, 1983

382. MacNab MSP, Manninen PH, Lam AM *et al:* The stress response to induced hypotension for cerebral aneurysm surgery: A comparison of two hypotensive techniques. Can Anaesth Soc J 35:111, 1988

383. Reiz S, Balfors E, Bredgaard M: Coronary hemodynamic effects of general anesthesia and surgery. Regional Anesth 7(suppl):S8, 1982

384. Haraldsted VY, Asmussen J, Herlevsen P *et al:* Cerebral arteriovenous difference of oxygen during gradual and sudden increase of the concentration of isoflurane for induction of deliberate hypotension. Acta Anaesthesiol Scand 36:142, 1992

385. Bendo AA, Kass IS, Cottrell JE: Comparison of the protective effect of thiopental and isoflurane against damage in the rat hippocampal slice. Brain Res 403:136, 1987

386. Nehls DG, Todd MM, Spetzler RF *et al:* A comparison of the

cerebral protective effects of isoflurane and barbiturates during temporary focal ischemia in primates. Anesthesiology 66:453, 1987

387. Gelb AW, Boisvert DP, Tang C *et al:* Primate brain tolerance to temporary focal cerebral ischemia during isoflurane or sodium nitroprusside-induced hypotension. Anesthesiology 70:678, 1989

388. Sano T, Drummond JC, Patel PM *et al:* A comparison of the cerebral protective effects of isoflurane and mild hypothermia in a model of incomplete forebrain ischemia in the rat. Anesthesiology 76:221, 1992

389. Bendo AA, Kozlowski PB, Capuano C *et al:* Cerebral edema formation in dogs following hypotension induced with isoflurane and labetalol. Acta Anaesthiol Belg 44:103, 1993

390. Van Aken H, Fitch W, Graham DI: Cardiovascular and cerebrovascular effects of isoflurane-induced hypotension in the baboon. Anesth Analg 65:565, 1986

391. Enlund M, Ahlstedt B, Revenas B *et al:* Adverse effects of the brain in connection with isoflurane-induced hypotensive anaesthesia. Acta Anaesthesiol Scand 33:413, 1989

392. Toivonen J, Virtanen H, Kaukinen S: Labetalol attenuates the negative effects of deliberate hypotension induced by isoflurane. Acta Anaesthesiol Scand 36:84, 1992

393. Van Aken J, Leusen I, Lacroix E *et al:* Influence of converting enzyme inhibition on isoflurane-induced hypotension for cerebral aneurysm surgery. Anesthesia 47:261, 1992

394. Kraus JF: Epidemiology of head injury. In Cooper PR (ed): Head Injury, 3rd ed, p 1. Baltimore, Williams & Wilkins, 1993

395. Miller JD: Assessing patients with head injury. Br J Surg 77:241, 1990

396. Teasdale G, Jennett B: Assessment of coma and impaired consciousness: A practical scale. Lancet 2:81, 1974

397. Jennett B: Assessment of the severity of head injury. J Neurol Neurosurg Psychiatry 39:647, 1976

398. Jennett B, Bond MR: Assessment of outcome after severe brain damage: A practical scale. Lancet 1:480, 1975

399. Chesnut RM, Marshall LF, Marshall SB: Medical management of intracranial pressure. In Cooper PR (ed): Head Injury, 3rd ed, p 225. Baltimore, Williams & Wilkins, 1993

400. Chesnut RM, Marshall LF, Klauber MR *et al:* The role of secondary brain injury in determining outcome from severe head injury. J Trauma 34:216, 1993

401. Hastings RH, Marks JD: Airway management for trauma patients with potential cervical spine injuries. Anesth Analg 73:471, 1991

402. Crosby ET, Lui A: The adult cervical spine: Implications for airway management. Can J Anaesth 37:77, 1990

403. Zornow MH, Todd MM, Moore SS: The acute cerebral effects of changes in plasma osmolality and oncotic pressure. Anesthesiology 67:936, 1987

404. Kaieda R, Todd MM, Cook LN *et al:* Acute effects of changing plasma osmolality and colloid oncotic pressure on the formation of brain edema after cryogenic injury. Neurosurgery 24:671, 1989

405. Kaieda R, Todd MM, Warner DS: Prolonged reduction in colloid oncotic pressure does not increase brain edema following cryogenic injury in rabbits. Anesthesiology 72:554, 1989

406. Drummond JC, Patel PM, Cole DJ *et al:* The effect of the reduction of colloid oncotic pressure, with and without reduction of osmolality, on post-traumatic cerebral edema. Anesthesiology 88:993, 1998

407. Smerling A: Hypertonic saline in head trauma: A new recipe for drying and salting. J Neurosurg Anesth 4:1, 1992

408. Prough DS, Whitley JM, Taylor CL *et al:* Regional cerebral blood flow following resuscitation from hemorrhagic shock with hypertonic saline. Anesthesiology 75:319, 1991

409. Chan KH, Dearden NM, Miller JD *et al:* Multimodality monitoring as a guide to treatment of intracranial hypertension after severe brain injury. Neurosurg 32:547, 1993

410. Lam AM, Winn HR, Cullen BF *et al:* Hyperglycemia and neurologic outcome in patients with head injury. J Neurosurg 75:545, 1991

411. Clifton GL, Robertson CS, Kyper K *et al:* Cardiovascular response to severe head injury. J Neurosurg 59:447, 1983

412. Clifton GL, Ziegler M, Grossman R: Circulating catecholamines and sympathetic activity after head injury. Neurosurgery 8:10, 1981

413. Eisenberg HM, Frankowski RF, Contant CF *et al:* High dosage barbiturate control of elevated intracranial pressure in patients with severe head injury. J Neurosurg 69:15, 1988

414. Obrist WD, Langfitt TW, Jaggi JL *et al:* Cerebral blood flow and metabolism in comatose patients with acute head injury. Relationship to intracranial hypertension. J Neurosurg 61:241, 1984
415. Muizelaar JP, Marmarou A, Ward JD *et al:* Adverse effects of prolonged hyperventilation in patients with severe head injury: A randomized clinical trial. J Neurosurg 75:731, 1991
416. Stringer WA, Hasso AN, Thompson JR *et al:* Hyperventilation-induced cerebral ischemia in patients with acute brain lesions: Demonstration by xenon-enhanced CT. AJNR 14:475, 1993
417. Chesnut RM: Medical management of severe head injury. Present and future. New Horizons 3:581, 1995
418. Guidelines for the Management of Severe Head Injury. Brain Trauma Foundation, American Association of Neurologic Surgery, Joint Section on Neurotrauma and Critical Care. J Neurotrauma 13:641, 1996
419. Robertson CS, Gopinath SP, Goodman JC *et al:* SjVO$_2$ monitoring in head-injured patients. J Neurotrauma 12:891, 1995
420. Matjasko MJ: Multisystem sequelae of severe head injury. In Cottrell JE, Smith DS (eds): Anesthesia and Neurosurgery, 3rd ed, p 685. St. Louis, Mosby-Yearbook, 1994
421. Miner ME, Kaufman HH, Graham SH *et al:* Disseminated intravascular coagulation fibrinolytic syndrome following head injury in children: Frequency and prognostic implications. J Pediatr 100: 687, 1982

Clinical Anesthesia (4/e), edited by
Paul G. Barash, Bruce F. Cullen, and
Robert K. Stoelting. Lippincott Williams &
Wilkins, Philadelphia, © 2001.

CHAPTER 29

RESPIRATORY FUNCTION IN ANESTHESIA

M. CHRISTINE STOCK

Anesthesiologists directly manipulate pulmonary function to a greater extent than any other organ system. Thus, a sound and thorough working knowledge of applied pulmonary physiology is essential to the safe conduct of anesthesia. This chapter discusses pulmonary anatomy, the control of ventilation, oxygen and carbon dioxide transport, ventilation-perfusion relationships, lung volumes and pulmonary function testing, abnormal physiology and anesthesia, the effect of smoking on pulmonary function, and postoperative pulmonary function and complications.

FUNCTIONAL ANATOMY OF THE LUNGS

Volumes by Gray[1] and Netter[2] illustrate the basic anatomy of the lungs well and give a complete and fully detailed description of human lung anatomy. This chapter emphasizes functional lung anatomy, with structure described as it applies to the mechanical and physiologic function of the lungs.

Thorax

The thoracic cage is shaped like a truncated cone, with small superior and large inferior openings and diaphragms attached at the base. The thoracic vertebral column provides major vertical support for the thorax. Anteriorly, the sternum renders support and is so named because of its sword-like appearance. The sternal angle, an important anatomic landmark, is formed by the junction of the manubrium and the sternal body with the second rib. The sternal angle is located in the horizontal plane that passes through the vertebral column at the T4 or T5 level. This plane separates the superior from the inferior mediastinum. The predominant ventilatory changes in thoracic diameter occur in the anteroposterior direction in the upper thoracic region and in the lateral or transverse direction in the lower portion of the thorax.[3]

Muscles of Ventilation

The ventilatory musculature has been the focus of considerable scientific attention. The ventilatory muscles are endurance muscles. Poor nutrition, chronic obstructive pulmonary disease (COPD) with gas trapping, and increased airway resistance predispose to the development of ventilatory failure due to ventilatory muscle fatigue.[4] The ventilatory muscles include the diaphragm, intercostal muscles, abdominal muscles, cervical strap muscles, sternocleidomastoid muscles, and the large back and intervertebral muscles of the shoulder girdle. The primary ventilatory muscle is the diaphragm, with minor contributions from the intercostal muscles. Normally, at rest, inspiration requires work and expiration is passive. As ventilatory effort increases, abdominal muscles assist with rib depression and increase intra-abdominal pressure to facilitate forced exhalation. With a further increase in effort, the cervical strap muscles help to elevate the sternum and upper portions of the chest. Finally, the large back and paravertebral muscles of the shoulder girdle become important during maximum ventilatory effort. Generally, muscles that raise the ribs are functionally inspiratory, whereas muscles that lower the ribs are important primarily during forced expiration. In a person with normal lung parenchyma, both breathing and coughing can be performed exclusively by the diaphragm.

Ventilatory muscles must create sufficient force to lift the ribs to create subatmospheric pressure in the intrapleural space. Breathing is an endurance phenomenon—something that is done repetitively over a long period of time. The type of muscle fiber correlates with fatigability and oxidative capacity.[5] Fatigue-resistant fibers are characterized by a slow-twitch response to electrical stimulation. They comprise approximately 50% of the diaphragmatic fibers and, because of their high oxidative capacity, function mostly as endurance units.[6] Fast-twitch muscle fibers, which are susceptible to fatigue, have rapid responses to electrical stimulation. Fast-twitch fibers impart strength; they allow the muscle to produce greater force over a short period of time. Thus, fast-twitch fibers are useful during brief periods of maximal ventilatory effort and slow-twitch fibers provide endurance.[7]

The electrical activity of the ventilatory muscles reflects the function of the muscles during different types of ventilatory effort.[8] During breathing at rest, the electrical activity of the diaphragm gradually and progressively rises during the early portion of inspiration and gradually falls to zero by late inspiration.[9] However, during forced exhalation or expulsive efforts such as coughing, diaphragmatic electrical activity remains high even throughout expiration.[10] The intercostal muscles are active primarily during inspiration, and debate continues as to their significance during expiration. The muscles of the abdominal wall, the most powerful muscles of expiration, are important for expulsive efforts such as coughing.[11]

To perform work, a muscle must be firmly anchored at both its origin and insertion. The diaphragm is unique because its insertion is mobile—an untethered central tendon that originates from fibers directly attached to the vertebral bodies and the costal portions of the lower ribs and sternum. Diaphragmatic contraction results in descent of the diaphragmatic dome and expansion of the thoracic base. These changes result in decreased intrathoracic and intrapleural pressure, with a corresponding increase in intra-abdominal pressure.

The cervical strap muscles elevate and fix the first two ribs. They are active even during spontaneous ventilation at rest. The cervical strap muscles are the most important inspiratory accessory muscles. Their importance is magnified if diaphragmatic function is impaired, as in patients with cervical spinal cord transection. The primary function of the sternocleidomastoid muscle is to elevate the sternum, thereby increasing the anteroposterior diameter of the chest wall. The large back muscles, such as the pectoralis major and minor, the latissimus dorsi, and the serratus anterior, are used to augment inspiration by enlarging the rib cage during high levels of ventilatory activity.

Lung Structures

With an intact respiratory system, the expandable lung tissue completely fills the pleural cavity. The visceral and parietal pleurae are constantly in contact with each other, creating a potential intrapleural space in which pressure decreases when the diaphragm descends and the rib cage expands. The resultant subatmospheric intrapleural pressure is a reflection of the

Table 29-1. MAJOR DIVISIONS OF THE LUNG

Lung Side/Lobe	Bronchopulmonary Segment
RIGHT	
Upper	Apical
	Anterior
	Posterior
Middle	Medial
	Lateral
Lower	Superior
	Medial basal
	Lateral basal
	Anterior basal
	Posterior basal
LEFT	
Upper	Apical posterior
	Anterior
Lingula	Superior
	Inferior
Lower	Superior
	Posterior basal
	Anteromedial basal
	Lateral basal

opposing and equal forces between the lung tissue and chest wall structures. These equal and opposing forces create the functional residual capacity (FRC), the volume of gas in the lungs at passive end-expiration. The intrapleural space normally has a slightly subambient pressure (-2 to -3 mm Hg) at FRC. With inspiration, the intrapleural pressure becomes more negative as the chest wall expands. When the thorax is opened, healthy lung retracts because pressures within both the alveolar spaces and along the visceral pleurae are ambient.

Both the right and left lungs contain oblique fissures that separate the upper from the lower lobes. In addition, the right lung has a horizontal fissure separating the middle and lower lobes. Major divisions of the right and left lung are listed in Table 29-1. Working knowledge of the bronchopulmonary segments is important for localizing lung pathology, interpreting lung radiographs, identifying lung regions during bronchoscopy, and operating on the lung. Each bronchopulmonary segment is separated from its adjacent segments by well-defined connective tissue planes. Therefore, pulmonary pathology initially tends to remain segmental.

The lung parenchyma can be subdivided into three airway categories based on functional lung anatomy (Table 29-2). The conductive airways provide basic gas transport, but no gas exchange takes place in them. The next group of airways, which have smaller diameters, are transitional airways. They are conduits for gas movement, and additionally perform limited gas diffusion and exchange. Finally, the smallest respiratory airways' primary function is gas exchange. Ventilation–perfusion ($\dot{V}_A/\dot{Q}$) relationships are defined by the function of the respiratory airways.

Conventionally, airways with diameters of >2 mm are considered large airways and create 90% of total airway resistance.

By the seventh airway generation, the internal diameter has decreased to approximately 2 mm and the cumulative cross-sectional area is 5.0 cm². The number of alveoli increases progressively with age, starting at approximately 24 million at birth and reaching the final adult count of 300 million by the age of 8–9 years. The alveoli are associated with about 250 million precapillaries and 280 billion capillary segments, resulting in a surface area of ~70 m² for gas exchange.

Conductive Airways

In the adult, the trachea is a fibromuscular tube ~10–12 cm long with an outside diameter of ~20 mm. Structural support is provided by 20 U-shaped hyaline cartilages, with the open part of the U facing posteriorly. The cricoid membrane tethers the trachea to the cricoid cartilage at the level of the sixth cervical vertebral body. The trachea enters the superior mediastinum and bifurcates at the sternal angle (the lower border of the fourth thoracic vertebral body). Normally, half of the trachea is intrathoracic and half is extrathoracic. Both ends of the trachea are attached to mobile structures. Thus, the carina can move superiorly as much as 5 cm from its normal resting position. Airway "motion" becomes important in the intubated patient. In the adult, the tip of an orotracheal tube moves an average of 3.8 cm with flexion and extension of the neck but can travel as far as 6.4 cm.[12] In infants and children, tracheal tube movement with respect to the trachea is even more critical: displacement of even 1 cm can move the tube out of the trachea or below the carina.

The tracheal wall includes several cellular structures that are important in removing mucus from the lungs.[13] The tracheal epithelial layer is composed primarily of pseudostratified columnar ciliated epithelium. Interspersed between the cells are goblet cells and brush cells. Chronic exposure to irritants such as tobacco smoke increases the number of mucus-producing goblet cells and decreases the number of ciliated cells,[14] resulting in an increased volume of secretions and reduced ability to remove them. The cilia beat in an organized and coordinated manner, creating metachronal wave movement of the superficial "gel" mucus layer toward the mouth. Brush cells appear to be the source of low-viscosity fluid for the serous layer. The histologic structures of other larger airways are similar to those in the trachea.

The next airway generation is composed of the right and left main-stem bronchi. The diameter of the right bronchus is generally greater than that of the left. In the adult, the right bronchus leaves the trachea at ~25° from the vertical tracheal axis, whereas the angle of the left bronchus is ~45°. Thus, inadvertent endobronchial intubation or aspiration of foreign material is more likely to occur in the right lung than the left. Furthermore, the right upper lobe bronchus dives almost directly posterior at ~90° from the right main bronchus. Foreign bodies and fluid aspirated by a supine subject usually fall into the right upper lobe. In children less than 3 years old, the angles created by the right and left main-stem bronchi are approximately equal, with takeoff angles of about 55°.

The right main bronchus is ~2.5 cm long before its initial branching into lobar bronchi. However, in 10% of adults, the right upper lobe bronchus departs from the right main-stem

Table 29-2. FUNCTIONAL AIRWAY DIVISIONS

Type	Function	Structure
Conductive	Bulk gas movement	Trachea to terminal bronchioles
Transitional	Bulk gas movement	Respiratory bronchioles
	Limited gas exchange	Alveolar ducts
Respiratory	Gas exchange	Alveoli
		Alveolar sacs

Table 29-3. DIMENSIONS AND NUMBERS OF AIRWAYS

Airway Generation	Airway Name	Diameter (cm)	Cumulative Cross-Sectional Area (cm²)
0	Trachea	1.80	2.54
1	Main-stem bronchi	1.22	2.33
2	Lobar bronchi	0.83	2.13
3	Segmental bronchi	0.56	2.00
4	Subsegmental bronchi 1	0.45	2.48
8	Subsegmental bronchi 5	0.18	6.59
16	Terminal bronchiole	0.06	180
17	Respiratory bronchiole 1	0.05	300
20	Alveolar duct 1	0.045	1600
23	Alveolar sac	0.041	11,800

Based on data from Weibel ER: Morphometrics of the lung. In Fenn WO, Rahn H (eds): Handbook of Physiology, Section 3, vol 1, p 285. Washington DC, American Physiological Society, 1964.

bronchus 2.5 cm from the carina. Furthermore, in ~2–3% of adults, the right upper lobe bronchus opens into the trachea, above the carina. Patients with these anomalies require special consideration when placing double-lumen tracheal tubes, especially if one contemplates inserting a right-sided endobronchial tube. After the right upper and middle lobe bronchi divide from the right main bronchus, the main channel becomes the right lower lobe bronchus.

The left main bronchus is ~5 cm long prior before its initial branching point to the left upper lobe and the lingula, then continues on as the left lower lobe bronchus.

Eighteen segmental bronchi form the next generation of airways (see Table 29-1). Their anatomic positions are important for normal clearance of secretions and for postural drainage. Each successive generation beyond the segmental bronchi undergoes progressive and significant increases in total cross-sectional area (Table 29-3). Bronchi, defined as airways containing cartilaginous elements, become as small as 1 mm in diameter.

The bronchioles typically have diameters of 1 mm. They are devoid of cartilaginous support and have the highest proportion of smooth muscle in the wall. There are approximately three to four bronchiolar generations. The final bronchiolar generation is the terminal bronchiole, which is the last airway component that is not directly involved in gas exchange.

Transitional Airways

The respiratory bronchiole, which follows the terminal bronchiole, is the first site in the tracheobronchial tree where gas exchange occurs. Respiratory bronchioles are characterized by intermittent alveolar outpockets, and histologically by a gradual change from cuboidal epithelium to squamous cells. In adults, two or three generations of respiratory bronchioles eventually lead to alveolar ducts. There are usually four to five generations of alveolar ducts, each with multiple openings into alveolar sacs. The final divisions of alveolar ducts terminate in alveolar sacs that open into alveolar clusters.

Respiratory Airways and the Alveolar–Capillary Membrane

Intact alveoli range between 100 and 300 μm in diameter. The intra-alveolar septa form the supportive latticework and are composed of elastic, collagenous, and reticular fibers. The pulmonary capillaries also are incorporated into and supported by this fibrous lattice. The pulmonary capillary beds are the densest capillary networks in the body. The calculated diameter for pulmonary capillaries is between 10 and 14 μm. This extensive vascular branching system starts with pulmonary arterioles in the region of the respiratory bronchioles. Each alveolus is closely associated with ~1000 short capillary segments.

The alveolar–capillary interface is complicated but well designed to facilitate gas exchange. Viewed with electron microscopy, the alveolar wall consists of a thin capillary epithelial cell, a basement membrane, a pulmonary capillary endothelial cell, and a surfactant lining layer. The flattened, squamous Type I alveolar cells cover ~80% of the alveolar surface. Type I cells contain flattened nuclei and extremely thin cytoplasmic extensions that provide the surface for gas exchange. The volume of a Type I cell is twice that of a Type II alveolar cell, but its surface is 50 times greater.[15] Type I cells are highly differentiated and metabolically limited, which makes them highly susceptible to injury. When Type I cells are damaged severely (during acute lung injury or adult respiratory distress syndrome), Type II cells replicate and modify to form new Type I cells.[16]

Type II alveolar cells are interspersed among Type I cells, primarily at alveolar-septal junctions. These polygonal cells have vast metabolic and enzymatic activity and manufacture surfactant.[17] The enzymatic activity required to produce surfactant is only 50% of the total enzymatic activity present in Type II alveolar cells.[18] The remaining enzymatic activity modulates local electrolyte balance and endothelial and lymphatic cell functions.[19] Both Type I and Type II alveolar cells have tight intracellular junctions, thus providing a relatively impermeable barrier to fluids.

Type III alveolar cells, alveolar macrophages, are an important element of lung defense. Their migratory and phagocytic activities result in the ingestion of foreign materials within alveolar spaces.[20]

Finally, numerous finger-like projections of the capillary endothelial cells greatly increase their surface area. They also provide intimate contact between the capillary endothelial cell and the entire circulating blood volume. Capillary endothelial cells are ideally suited for metabolism of circulating substances. Thus, the alveolar–capillary membrane has two primary functions: transport of respiratory gases (oxygen and carbon dioxide) and the widely varied metabolic activities of local and humoral substances.

Collateral Ventilation

Airways ≤1 mm in diameter are susceptible to blockage, resulting in accumulation of fluids and secretions and inhibition of gas exchange, especially oxygen transport. The pores of Kohn were the first structures described that provide collateral ventilation. Located in the interspaces between the alveolar–capillary networks, they provide intra-alveolar communication.[21] Conduits that afford direct communication between small respiratory bronchioles and neighboring alveoli also create collateral ventilation and may be more important. These communications are of larger diameter than the pores of Kohn, 30 μm versus

8–10 μm, and their anatomic position allows access to a greater number of alveoli.[22]

Pulmonary Vascular Systems

Two major circulatory systems supply blood to the lungs: the pulmonary and bronchial vascular networks. The pulmonary vascular system delivers mixed-venous blood from the right ventricle to the pulmonary capillary bed via the pulmonary arteries. After gas exchange occurs in the pulmonary capillary bed, oxygen-rich and carbon dioxide-poor blood is returned to the left atrium via the pulmonary veins. The pulmonary veins run independently along the intralobar connective tissue planes. The pulmonary arteries contain a specialized connective tissue that maintains blood vessel patency despite changes in lung volume and intrathoracic pressure during breathing or a change in body position. The pulmonary capillary system adequately provides for the metabolic and oxygen needs of the alveolar parenchyma. However, the bronchial arterial system must provide oxygen to the conductive airways and pulmonary vessels. Anatomic connections between the bronchial and pulmonary venous circulations create an absolute shunt of ~2–5% of the total cardiac output, and represents "normal" shunt.

LUNG MECHANICS

Lung movement is entirely passive and responds to forces external to the lungs. During spontaneous ventilation, the external forces are produced by ventilatory muscles. The lungs' response is governed by the impedance of the chest wall and by the airways. This impedance, or hindrance, falls mainly into two categories: (1) elastic recoil of the lung and gas–liquid interface and (2) resistance to gas flow.

Elastic Work

The lungs' natural tendency is to collapse; thus, normal expiration at rest is passive because gas flows out of the lungs when they elastically recoil. The thoracic cage exerts an outwardly directed force and the lungs exert an inwardly directed force that together result in a subatmospheric intrapleural pressure. Because the outward force of the thoracic cage exceeds the inward force of the lung, the overall tendency of the lung is to remain inflated when it resides within the thoracic cage. At FRC, the outward and inward forces on the lung are equal. Thus, at passive end-exhalation, the respiratory muscles are relaxed and the lung returns to its resting volume within the relaxed thorax: FRC. Gravitational forces create a more subatmospheric pressure in nondependent areas of the lung than in dependent areas. In the upright adult, the difference in intrapleural pressure from the top to the bottom of the lung is ~7 cm H_2O.

Surface tension at an air-fluid interface produces forces that tend to further reduce the area of interface. The gas pressure within a bubble is always higher than the surrounding gas pressure because of the bubble's surface tension. Thus, the bubble remains inflated. The alveoli resemble bubbles in this respect, although alveolar gas communicates with the atmosphere via the airways, unlike a bubble. The Laplace equation describes this phenomenon: P = 2T/R, where P is the pressure within the bubble (dyn · cm^{-2}), T is the surface tension of the liquid (dyn · cm^{-1}), and R is the radius of the bubble (cm).

During inspiration, the surface tension of the liquid in the lung increases to 40 mN · m^{-1}, a value close to that of plasma. During expiration, this surface tension falls to 19 mN · m^{-1}, a value lower than that of any other known fluid. The alveoli experience hysteresis, that is, different pressure–volume relationships during inspiration and expiration. In contrast to a bubble, the pressure within an alveolus decreases as the radius of curvature decreases. Thus, gas tends to flow from larger to smaller alveoli and thereby maintain stability and prevent lung collapse.

The alveolar transmural pressure gradient, or transpulmonary pressure, is the difference between intrapleural and alveolar pressure and is directly proportional to lung volume. Intrapleural pressure can be safely measured with a percutaneously inserted catheter,[23] but clinicians rarely perform this technique. Esophageal pressure can be used as a reflection of intrapleural pressure, but the esophageal balloon must reside in the midesophagus to avoid inaccurate measurement.[24] Commercially available esophageal pressure monitors increase the ease and accuracy of measuring esophageal pressure as a reflection of intrapleural pressure.[25] These monitors are useful for estimating the elastic work performed by the patient during spontaneous ventilation, mechanical ventilation, or a combination of spontaneous and mechanical ventilation. By estimating intrapleural pressure on a real-time basis, it is possible to quantitate the patient's work of breathing as one intervenes. For example, if one changes the level of ventilatory support or changes the patient's breathing apparatus, one can assess the alterations in the patient's contribution to the total work of breathing, or to changes in the work of breathing imposed by the breathing apparatus.[26-31]

Total ventilatory work is a combination of physiologic work and imposed work of breathing. Physiologic work includes elastic work (inspiratory work required to overcome the elastic recoil of the pulmonary system) and resistive work (work to overcome resistance to gas flow in the airway). For a patient in whom breathing apparatus is employed, the concept of total work of breathing encompasses physiologic work plus imposed ventilatory work: the (usually resistive) work performed by the patient to overcome the resistance imposed by the breathing apparatus. Examples of imposed work include the resistance imposed by tracheal tubes and demand valves.[32]

If the lungs are slowly inflated and deflated, the pressure–volume curve during inflation differs from that obtained during deflation. The two curves form a hysteresis loop that becomes progressively broader as the tidal volume is increased (Fig. 29-1). A greater pressure than anticipated is required during inflation, and recoil pressure is less than expected during deflation. Thus, the lung accepts deformation poorly, and, once deformed, assumes its original shape slowly and with effort. This phenomenon, another example of elastic hysteresis, is important for the maintenance of normal lung compliance. However, for the purposes of the following discussion, it will be ignored.

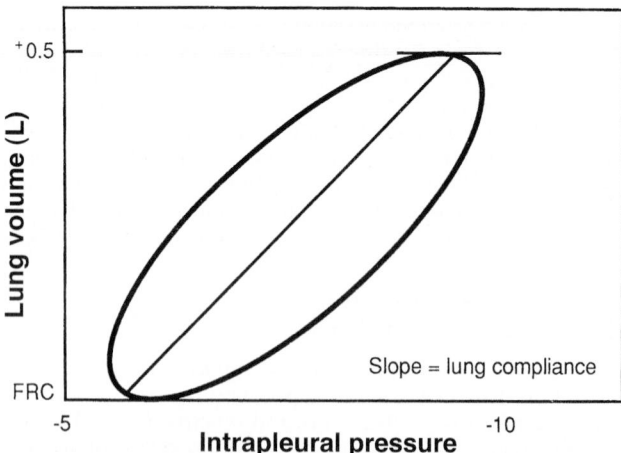

Figure 29-1. Dynamic pressure–volume loop of resting tidal volume. Quiet, normal breathing is characterized by hysteresis of the pressure–volume loop. The lung is more resistant to deformation than expected and returns to its original configuration less easily than expected. The slope of the line connecting the zenith and nadir lung volumes is lung compliance, ~500 ml per 3 cm H_2O = 167 ml per cm H_2O.

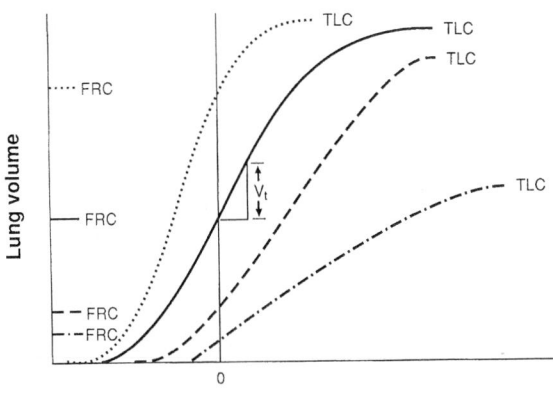

Figure 29-2. Pulmonary pressure–volume relationships at different values of total lung capacity, ignoring hysteresis. The solid line depicts the normal pulmonary pressure–volume relationships. Humans normally breathe on the linear, steep part of this sigmoidal curve, where the slope, which is equal to compliance, is greatest. The vertical line at zero defines FRC, regardless of the position of the curve on the graph. Mild restrictive lung disease, indicated by the dashed line, shifts the curve to the right with little change in slope. However, with restrictive disease, the patient breathes on a lower FRC, at a point on the curve where the slope is less. Severe restrictive pulmonary disease profoundly depresses the FRC and diminishes the slope of the entire curve (*dashed-dotted line*). Obstructive disease (*dotted line*) elevates both FRC and compliance. (FRC = functional residual capacity; TLC = total lung capacity.)

The sum of the pressure–volume relationships of the thorax and lung results in a sigmoidal curve (Fig. 29-2). The vertical line drawn at end-expiration coincides with FRC. Normally, humans breathe on the steepest part of the sigmoidal curve, where compliance is highest. The compliance of the curve is represented by the slope of the curve ($\Delta V / \Delta P$). In restrictive diseases, the curve shifts to the right, the slope is depressed, or both. These changes result in smaller FRCs and lower lung compliance. When lung compliance is small, larger changes in intrapleural pressure are needed to create the same tidal volume; that is, one has to suck harder to get the same volume of gas into the lungs. The body, being a smart organism, prefers to move less gas with each breath rather than sucking harder to achieve the same tidal volume. Thus, patients with low lung compliance typically breathe with smaller tidal volumes at more rapid rates. Spontaneous ventilatory rate is one of the most sensitive indices of lung compliance. Continuous positive airway pressure (CPAP) will shift the vertical line to the right, thus allowing the patient to breathe on a steeper and more favorable portion of the volume–pressure curve, resulting in a slower ventilatory rate with a larger tidal volume. However, patients with diseases that increase lung compliance experience larger than normal FRC (gas trapping) and their pressure–volume curves shift to the left and steepen. These patients expend less elastic work to inspire, but elastic recoil is reduced significantly. Chronic obstructive lung disease and acute asthma are the most common examples of diseases with high lung compliance. If lung compliance and FRC are sufficiently high that elastic recoil is minimal, the patient must use ventilatory muscles to actively expire. The difficulty these patients experience in emptying the lungs is compounded by the increased airway resistance.

Both compliance and inspiratory elastic work can be measured for a single breath by measuring airway (Paw) and intrapleural (Ppl) pressures and tidal volume. If esophageal pressure is measured carefully, the esophageal pressure values can be substituted for Ppl values (see above). Lung compliance, C_L, the slope of the volume–pressure curve, is given by the equation

$$C_L = \frac{\Delta V}{\Delta P_L} + \frac{Vt}{P_{Li} - P_{Le}} = \frac{Vt}{(Paw_i - Ppl_i) - (Paw_e - Ppl_e)} \quad (1)$$

where P_L is transpulmonary pressure, Vt is tidal volume, Paw_e and Paw_i are expiratory and inspiratory airway pressures, and Ppl_e and Ppl_i are expiratory and inspiratory intrapleural pressures.

Elastic work (W_{el}) is performed during inspiration only, expiration being passive during normal breathing. The area within the triangle in Figure 29-2 describes the work required to inspire. The equation that yields elastic work (and the area of the triangle) is

$$W_{el} = \tfrac{1}{2}(Vt)(P_{Li} - P_{Le})$$
$$= \tfrac{1}{2}(Vt)[(Paw_i - Ppl_i) - (Paw_e - Pple)] \quad (2)$$

Resistance to Gas Flow

Both laminar and turbulent flow exist within the respiratory tract, usually in mixed patterns. The physics of each, however, is significantly different and worth consideration.

Laminar Flow

Below critical flows, gas proceeds through a straight tube as a series of concentric cylinders that slide over one another. Thus, fully developed flow has a parabolic profile with a velocity of zero at the cylinder wall and a maximum velocity at the center of the advancing "cone." Peripheral cylinders tend to be stationary and the central cylinder moves fastest. This type of streamlined flow is usually inaudible. The advancing conical front means that some fresh gas reaches the end of the tube before the tube has been completely filled with fresh gas. That is, significant alveolar ventilation can occur when the tidal volume (Vt) is less than anatomic dead space; this fact, noted by Rohrer in 1915,[33] is important in high-frequency ventilation. Gas flowing in a straight, unbranched tube meets resistance that can be calculated by the following equation:

$$R = \frac{8 \times length \times viscosity}{\pi \times (radius)^4} = \frac{P_B - P_A}{flow} \quad (3)$$

where P_B and P_A are barometric and alveolar pressures. The inverse relationship between resistance and the fourth power of the radius explains the critical importance of narrowed air passages. Viscosity is the only physical gas property that is relevant under conditions of laminar flow. Helium has a low density, but its viscosity is close to that of air. Helium will not improve gas flow if the flow is laminar; usually, however, flow is turbulent when there is critical airway narrowing or abnormally high airway resistance.

Turbulent Flow

High flow rates, particularly through branched or irregularly shaped tubes, disrupt the orderly flow of laminar gas. Turbulent flow is usually audible and is almost invariably present when high resistance to gas flow is problematic. Turbulent flow usually presents with a square front so that no fresh gas will reach the end of the tube until the amount of gas entering the tube is almost equal to the volume of the tube. Thus, turbulent flow effectively purges the contents of a tube. Four conditions that will change laminar flow to turbulent flow are high gas flows, sharp angles within the tube, branching in the tube, and a change in the tube's diameter.

During turbulent flow, the driving pressure is proportional to the square of the required gas flow rate, proportional to gas density, independent of viscosity, and inversely proportional to the fifth power of the radius of the tube.

Resistance during laminar flow is inversely proportional to gas flow rate. Conversely, during turbulent flow, resistance increases in proportion to the flow rate. A detailed description

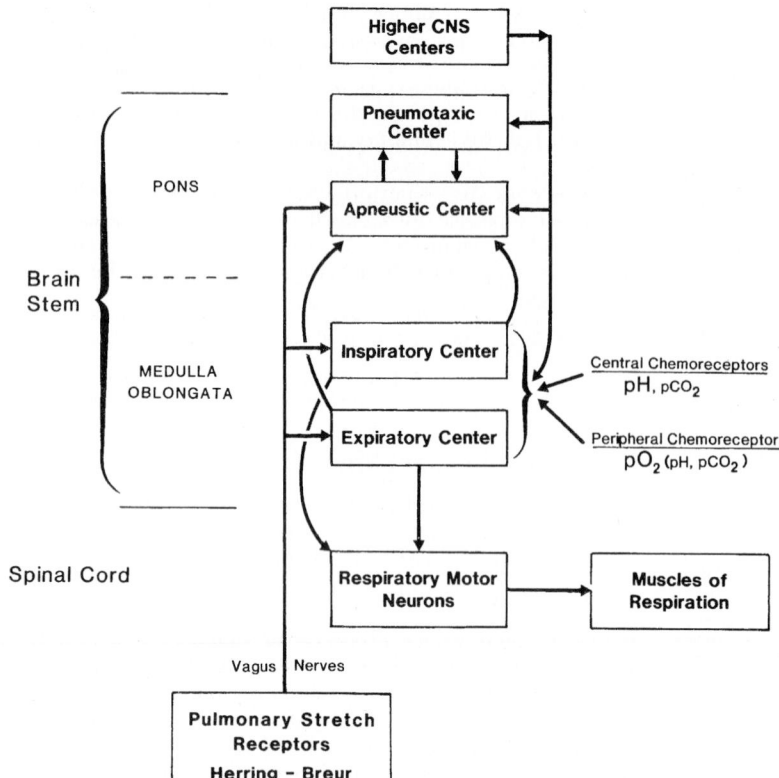

Figure 29-3. Classic CNS respiratory centers. Diagram illustrates major respiratory centers, neurofeedback circuits, primary neurohumoral sensory inputs, and mechanical outputs.

of these phenomena is beyond the scope of this chapter, but the reader is referred to descriptions by Nunn.[34]

Increased Airway Resistance

Bronchiolar smooth muscle hyper-reactivity (true broncho-spasm), mucosal edema, mucous plugging, epithelial desquamation, tumors, and foreign bodies all increase airway resistance. The normal response to increased inspiratory resistance is increased inspiratory muscle effort, with little change in FRC.[35] Accessory muscles act according to the degree of resistance.

There are two principal compensatory mechanisms for high inspiratory resistance. The muscle spindles' afferent discharge augments the activity in the motor neuron pool of the anterior horn. The conscious subject can detect small increases in inspiratory resistance.[36] Additional compensatory increases in effort are driven by an elevated partial pressure of carbon dioxide in arterial blood (Pa_{CO_2}).[37]

Emphysematous patients retain remarkable ability to preserve an adequate alveolar ventilation, even with gross airway obstruction. In patients with preoperative FEV_1 values <1 l, there was no correlation between FEV_1 and Pa_{CO_2}, which was normal in most patients. Furthermore, asthmatic patients compensate well for increased airway resistance and also keep the mean Pa_{CO_2} in the lower end of normal range.[38] Thus, an increased Pa_{CO_2} in the setting of increased airway resistance deserves serious attention.

Mild expiratory resistance does not result in activation of the expiratory muscles in conscious or anesthetized subjects. The initial work to overcome expiratory resistance is performed by augmenting inspiratory force until a sufficiently high lung volume is achieved, so that elastic recoil overcomes expiratory resistance.[39] The immediate effects of excessive expiratory resistance are to use accessory muscles to force gas from the lungs. This response is useful during acute increases in expiratory resistance. However, patients who chronically use accessory muscles to expire are at risk for ventilatory muscle fatigue if they experience an acute worsening of ventilatory work, most commonly precipitated by pneumonia or heart failure.

CONTROL OF VENTILATION

Mechanisms that control ventilation are extremely complex, requiring integration with many parts of the central and peripheral nervous systems (see Fig. 29-3). LeGallois, who localized the respiratory centers in the brainstem in 1812, demonstrated that breathing does not depend on an intact cerebrum. Rather, breathing depends on a small region of the medulla near the origin of the vagus nerves.[40] Countless studies in the past two centuries have greatly increased our knowledge and understanding of the anatomic components of ventilatory control. However, experimental work performed in animals is difficult to apply to humans because of interspecies variation.

Generation of Ventilatory Pattern

Please refer to Table 29-4 for definitions of terms used in this section. A *respiratory center* is a specific area in the brain that integrates any neural traffic resulting in spontaneous ventilation. Within the pontine and medullary reticular formations there are several discrete respiratory centers that function as the control system (Fig. 29-3).[41]

Initial descriptions of brain stem respiratory functions are based on classic ablation and electrical stimulation studies.[42-45] Another method for localizing respiratory centers entails recording action potentials from different areas of the brain stem with microelectrodes. This method is based on the assumption that local brain activity that occurs in phase with respiratory activity is evidence that the area under study has "respiratory neurons."[46] These techniques are imperfect for precisely localizing discrete respiratory centers.

Medullary Centers

The medulla oblongata contains the most basic ventilatory control centers in the brain. Specific medullary areas are active primarily during inspiration or during expiration, with many neural inspiratory or expiratory interconnections. The inspiratory centers that reside in the dorsal respiratory group (DRG) are located in the dorsal medullary reticular formation. The DRG is the source of elementary ventilatory rhythmicity[47,48] and serves as the "pacemaker" for the respiratory system.[49] Whereas resting lung volume occurs at end-expiration, the electrical activity of the ventilatory centers is at rest at end-inspiration. The rhythmic activity of the DRG persists even when all incoming peripheral and interconnecting nerves are sectioned or blocked completely. Isolating the DRG in this manner results in ataxic, gasping ventilation with frequent maximum inspiratory efforts: apneustic breathing.

The ventral respiratory group (VRG), which is located in the ventral medullary reticular formation, serves as the expiratory coordinating center. The inspiratory and expiratory neurons function by a system of reciprocal innervation, or negative feedback.[46] When the DRG creates an impulse to inspire, inspiration occurs, and then the DRG impulse is quenched by a reciprocating VRG impulse. This VRG transmission prohibits further use of the inspiratory muscles, thus allowing passive expiration to occur.

Pontine Centers

The pontine centers process information that originates in the medulla. The apneustic center is located in the middle or lower pons. With activation, this center sends impulses to inspiratory DRG neurons and is designed to sustain inspiration. Electrical stimulation results in inspiratory spasm.[50] The middle and lower pons contain specific areas for phase-spanning neurons.[51] These neurons assist with the transition between inspiration and expiration and do not exert direct control over ventilatory muscles.

The pneumotaxic respiratory center is in the rostral pons. A simple transection through the brain stem that isolates this portion of the pons from the upper brain stem reduces ventilatory rate and increases tidal volume. If both vagus nerves are additionally transected, apneusis results.[52] Thus, the primary function of the pneumotaxic center is to limit the depth of inspiration. When maximally activated, the pneumotaxic center secondarily increases ventilatory frequency. The pneumotaxic center performs no pacemaking function and has no intrinsic rhythmicity.

Higher Respiratory Centers

Many higher brain structures clearly affect ventilatory control processes. In the midbrain, stimulation of the reticular activating system increases the rate and amplitude of ventilation.[53] The cerebral cortex also affects breathing pattern, although precise neural pathways are not known.[54] Occasionally, the ventilatory control process becomes subservient to other regulatory centers. For example, the respiratory system plays an important role in the control of body temperature because it supplies a large surface area for heat exchange. This is especially important in animals in which panting is a primary means of dissipating heat. Then, ventilatory pattern is influenced by neural input

from descending pathways from the anterior and posterior hypothalamus to the pneumotaxic center of the upper pons.

Vasomotor control and certain respiratory responses are closely linked. Stimulation of the carotid sinus not only decreases vasomotor tone but also inhibits ventilation. Alternatively, stimulation of the carotid body chemoreceptors (see Chemical Control of Ventilation) results in an increase in both ventilatory activity and vasomotor tone.[55,56]

Reflex Control of Ventilation

Reflexes that directly influence ventilatory pattern usually do so to prevent airway obstruction. *Deglutition*, or swallowing, involves the glossopharyngeal and vagus nerves. Stimulation of the anterior and posterior pharyngeal pillars of the posterior pharynx induces swallowing. During swallowing, inspiration ceases momentarily, is usually followed by a single large breath, and briefly increases ventilation. The ventilatory centers that coordinate breathing and deglutition have not been identified.[57]

Vomiting significantly modifies normal ventilatory activity.[58] Swallowing, salivation, gastrointestinal reflexes, rhythmic spasmodic ventilatory movements, and significant diaphragmatic and abdominal muscular activity must be coordinated over a very brief interval. Because of the obvious risk of aspirating gastric contents, it is advantageous to inhibit inspiration during vomiting. Input into the respiratory centers occurs from both cranial and spinal cord nerves.

Coughing results from stimulation of the tracheal subepithelium, especially along the posterior tracheal wall and carina.[59] Coughing also requires coordination of both airway and ventilatory muscle activity. An effective cough requires deep inspiration, then forced exhalation against a momentarily closed glottis to increase intrathoracic pressure, thus allowing an expulsive expiratory maneuver.

Proprioception in the pulmonary system, the qualitative knowledge of the gas volume within the lungs, probably arises from smooth muscle spindle receptors. These proprioceptors, which are located within the smooth muscle of all airways, are sensitive to pressure changes.[60] Airway stretch reflexes can be demonstrated during distention of isolated airways, so that airway pressure, rather than volume distention, appears to be the primary stimulation.[61] Clinical conditions in which pulmonary airway stretch receptors are stimulated include pulmonary edema and atelectasis. Certain drugs, such as acetylcholine, pilocarpine, and histamine, which are administered in doses large enough to decrease lung compliance, also enhance the stretch reflex.[62] In contrast, airway stretch receptors are inhibited by inhalation of vaporized water, intravenously administered antihistamines, and topically administered local anesthetics.

Golgi tendon organs (tendon spindles), which occur in series arrangements within ventilatory muscles, facilitate proprioception. The intercostal muscles are rich in tendon spindles,

Table 29-4. DEFINITION OF RESPIRATORY PATTERN TERMINOLOGY

Word	Definition
Eupnea	"Good breathing": Continuous inspiratory and expiratory movement without interruption
Apnea	"No breathing": Cessation of ventilatory effort at passive end-expiration (lung volume = FRC)
Apneusis	Cessation of ventilatory effort with lungs filled at TLC
Apneustic ventilation	Apneusis with periodic expiratory spasms
Biot	Ventilatory gasps interposed between periods of ventilation apnea; *also* "agonal ventilation"

whereas the diaphragm has a limited number. Thus, the pulmonary stretch reflex primarily involves the intercostal muscles but not the diaphragm.[63] When the lungs are full and the chest wall is stretched, these receptors send signals to the brain stem that inhibit further inspiration.

In 1868, Hering and Breuer reported that lightly anesthetized, spontaneously breathing animals would cease or decrease ventilatory effort during sustained lung distention.[64] This response was blocked by bilateral vagotomy. The *Hering–Breuer reflex* is prominent in lower-order mammals such as rabbits but is only weakly present in humans. The Hering–Breuer reflex is sufficiently active in lower mammals that even 5 cm H_2O CPAP will induce apnea. In humans, however, the reflex is only weakly present, as evidenced by the fact that humans will continue to breathe spontaneously with CPAP in excess of 40 cm H_2O. This inflation reflex is associated with inspiratory muscle inhibition, as documented by marked reductions in electrical activity of both the phrenic nerve and the diaphragmatic muscle itself. The second component of the Hering–Breuer reflex, the deflation reflex, produces increased ventilatory muscle activity following sustained lung deflation. This reflex is not significant in humans. Both pulmonary and airway stretch reflexes operate secondarily to the pacemaking and modulating effects of the brain stem ventilatory control centers.

Chemical Control of Ventilation

Peripheral Chemoreceptors

In a simplistic view of chemical ventilatory control, the peripheral chemoreceptors primarily respond to lack of oxygen, and the central nervous system (CNS) receptors primarily respond to changes in P_{CO_2}, pH, and acid–base disturbances.

The peripheral chemoreceptors are composed of the carotid and aortic bodies.[65,66] The carotid bodies, located at the bifurcation of the common carotid artery, have predominantly ventilatory effects. The aortic bodies, which are scattered about the aortic arch and its branches, have predominantly circulatory effects. The neural output from the carotid body reaches the central respiratory centers via the afferent glossopharyngeal nerves. Output from the aortic bodies travels to the medullary centers via the vagus nerve. Both carotid and aortic bodies are stimulated by decreased Pa_{O_2}, but not by decreased Sa_{O_2} or Ca_{O_2}. When Pa_{O_2} falls below 100 mm Hg, neural activity from these receptors begins to increase. However, it is not until the Pa_{O_2} reaches 60–65 mm Hg that neural activity increases sufficiently to substantially augment minute ventilation. Thus, patients who depend on hypoxic ventilatory drive have Pa_{O_2} values in the mid-60s. Once these patients' Pa_{O_2} values exceed 60–65 mm Hg, ventilatory drive diminishes and Pa_{O_2} falls until ventilation is again stimulated by arterial hypoxemia. When we withdraw mechanical ventilation from the patient who depends on hypoxic ventilatory drive, the Pa_{O_2} must fall below 65 mm Hg so that the patient will regain hypoxic ventilatory drive.

The carotid bodies are also sensitive to decreased pH_a, but this response is minor. Similarly, changes in Pa_{CO_2} do not stimulate these receptors sufficiently to alter minute ventilation. Increases in blood temperature, hypoperfusion of the carotid bodies themselves, and some chemicals will stimulate these receptors. Sympathetic ganglion stimulation by nicotine or acetylcholine will stimulate the carotid and aortic bodies; this effect is blocked by hexamethonium. Blockade of the cytochrome electron transport system by cyanide will prevent oxidative metabolism and thus stimulate these receptors also.

Ventilatory effects resulting from stimulation of these receptors cause increased ventilatory rate and tidal volume. Hemodynamic changes resulting from stimulation of these receptors include bradycardia, hypertension, increases in bronchiolar tone, and increases in adrenal secretion. The carotid body chemical receptors have been termed *ultimum moriens* ("last to die"). The peripheral receptor's response to hypoxemia is resistant to the influences of anesthesia and tissue hypoxia that may depress central responses. However, the peripheral receptor's response is not sufficiently robust to reliably increase ventilatory rate or minute ventilation to herald the onset of arterial hypoxemia during general anesthesia or recovery from anesthesia.

Central Chemoreceptors

Approximately 80% of the ventilatory response to inhaled carbon dioxide originates in the central medullary centers. Acid–base regulation involving carbon dioxide, H^+, and bicarbonate is related primarily to chemosensitive receptors located in the medulla close to or in contact with the cerebrospinal fluid (CSF). The chemosensitive areas of the brain stem are in the infralateral aspects of the medulla near the origin of cranial nerves IX and X. The area just beneath the surface of the ventral medulla is exquisitely sensitive to the extracellular fluid H^+ concentration.[67] Although the central response is the major factor in the regulation of breathing by carbon dioxide, carbon dioxide has little direct stimulating effect on these chemosensitive areas. These receptors are primarily sensitive to changes in H^+ concentration. Carbon dioxide has a potent but indirect effect by reacting with water to form carbonic acid, which dissociates into hydrogen and bicarbonate ions.[68]

Increased Pa_{CO_2} is a more potent ventilatory stimulus than increased arterial H^+ concentration from a metabolic source. Carbon dioxide, but not H^+, passes readily through the blood–brain and blood–CSF barriers. Local buffering systems immediately neutralize H^+ in arterial blood and body fluids. In contrast, the CSF has minimal buffering capacity. Thus, once carbon dioxide crosses into the CSF, H^+ are created and trapped in the CSF, resulting in a CSF H^+ concentration considerably greater than that found in the blood. Because carbon dioxide crosses the blood–brain barrier readily, the P_{CO_2} values in the CSF, cerebral tissue, and jugular venous blood rise quickly and to the same degree as the Pa_{CO_2}, although the central values are ~10 mm Hg above those measured in arterial blood.

The ventilatory response to changes in Pa_{CO_2} (increased V_t, increased respiratory rate) is rapid and peaks within 1–2 minutes after the change in Pa_{CO_2}. With the same level of carbon dioxide stimulation, the resultant increase in ventilation declines over a period of several hours, probably as a result of bicarbonate ions that are actively transported from the blood into the CSF through the arachnoid villi.[69] Central medullary chemoreceptors also respond to temperature change. Cold CSF (with normal pH) or local anesthetic applied to the medullary surface will depress ventilation.

Ventilatory Response to Altitude

Ventilatory response and adaptation to high altitude are good examples of the integration of peripheral and central chemoreceptor control of ventilation. The following mechanism of acclimatization was proposed by Severinghaus and co-workers in 1963 and has since been confirmed.[70]

Following ascent from sea level to 4000 m, acute exposure to high altitude and low Pi_{O_2} results in arterial hypoxemia. This decrease in Pa_{O_2} activates the peripheral hypoxemic ventilatory drive by stimulating the carotid and aortic bodies, and causes increased minute ventilation. As minute ventilation increases, Pa_{CO_2} and CSF P_{CO_2} decrease, causing concomitant increases in pH_a and CSF pH. The alkaline shift of the CSF decreases ventilatory drive via medullary chemoreceptors, partially offsetting hypoxemic drive. A temporary equilibrium is attained within minutes, with Pa_{CO_2} only 2–5 mm Hg below normal and Pa_{O_2} approximately 45 mm Hg. This initially profound hypoxemia probably causes the acute respiratory distress and other associated symptoms (headache, diarrhea) associated with rapid ascent. However, the CNS is able to restore CSF pH to normal (7.326) by pumping bicarbonate ions out of the CSF over 2–3 days. In 2–3 days, CSF bicarbonate concentration decreases approximately 5 mEq·l⁻¹ and restores CSF pH to within 0.01 pH unit of values at sea level. Then, centrally mediated ventilatory drive returns to normal, and hypoxic drive and stimulation of peripheral receptors can proceed unopposed. Thus, after 3 days' exposure to 4000 m altitude, ventilatory adaptation would result in a new equilibrium, with Pa_{CO_2} approximately 30 mm Hg and Pa_{O_2} approximately 55 mm Hg. Following descent to sea level, the low CSF bicarbonate concentration persists for several days, and the climber "overbreathes" until CSF bicarbonate and pH values return to normal.

Breath-holding

Most adults with normal lungs and gas exchange can hold their breath for ~1 minute when breathing room air without previously hyperventilating. After 1 minute of breath-holding under these circumstances, Pa_{O_2} decreases to ~65–70 mm Hg and Pa_{CO_2} increases by ~12 mm Hg. In the absence of supplemental oxygen and hyperventilation, the "breakpoint" at which normal people feel compelled to breathe is remarkably constant at a Pa_{CO_2} of 50 mm Hg.[71,72] However, if the individual breathes 100% oxygen prior to breath-holding, he should be able to hold his breath for 2–3 minutes, or until Pa_{CO_2} rises to 60 mm Hg. Hyperventilation sufficient to reduce Pa_{CO_2} to 20 mm Hg can lengthen the period of breath-holding to 3–4 minutes.[74] Hyperventilation with 100% oxygen prior to breath-holding should extend the apneic period to 6–10 minutes. The Pa_{CO_2} rate of rise in awake, preoxygenated adults with normal lungs who hold their breath without previous hyperventilation is 7 mm Hg·min⁻¹ in the first 10 seconds, 2 mm Hg·min⁻¹ in the next 10 seconds, and 6 mm Hg·min⁻¹ thereafter.[72]

The duration of voluntary breath-holding is directly proportional to lung volume at onset. This is probably related both to oxygen stores in the alveoli and to the rate at which Pa_{CO_2} rises. With smaller lung volumes, the same amount of carbon dioxide is emptied into a smaller volume during the apneic period, thus increasing the carbon dioxide concentration more rapidly than occurs with larger lung volumes. Of note, apneic patients during general anesthesia actually "breath-hold" at FRC rather than at vital capacity, which would tend to accelerate the rate of rise of carbon dioxide. Despite this difference in lung volume, the rate of rise of Pa_{CO_2} in apneic anesthetized patients is 12 mm Hg during the first minute and 3.5 mm Hg·min⁻¹ thereafter, significantly lower than in the awake state.[74,75] During anesthesia, metabolic rate and carbon dioxide production are significantly less than during ambulatory wakefulness, which probably accounts for the different rates of rise in carbon dioxide levels.

Hyperventilation with room air prior to prolonged breath-holding during exercise is inadvisable. During underwater swimming after poolside hyperventilation, the urge to breathe is first stimulated by a rising Pa_{CO_2}. Swimmers who hyperventilate with room air prior to swimming long distances underwater frequently lose consciousness from arterial hypoxemia before the Pa_{CO_2} is sufficiently increased to stimulate the "need" to breathe.

Hyperventilation rarely is followed by an apneic period in awake humans, despite a markedly depressed Pa_{CO_2}. However, minute ventilation may decrease significantly. Aggressive intermittent positive pressure breathing treatments for patients with COPD can depress minute ventilation sufficiently to create arterial hypoxemia if they breathe room air after cessation of therapy.[76] In contrast, even mild hyperventilation during general anesthesia will produce prolonged apneic periods.[77]

Quantitative Aspects of Chemical Control of Breathing

The ventilatory responses to oxygen and carbon dioxide can be assessed quantitatively. Unfortunately, the quantitative indices of hypoxemic sensitivity are not clinically useful because the normal range is wide. The reader is referred to more comprehensive sources for a discussion of the quantitative indices of hypoxemic sensitivity.[78]

Ventilatory responses to Pa_{CO_2} changes are measured in several ways, provided that carbon dioxide production remains constant. When subjects voluntarily increase minute ventilation to a prescribed level, the Pa_{CO_2} decreases hyperbolically. The plot of minute ventilation (independent variable) and Pa_{CO_2} (dependent variable) is the metabolic hyperbola (Fig. 29-4). The metabolic hyperbola is cumbersome to evaluate and difficult to use clinically.

The curve more commonly used is the Pa_{CO_2} ventilatory response curve (see Fig. 29-4). It describes the effect of changing Pa_{CO_2} on the resultant minute ventilation. Usually, subjects inspire carbon dioxide to raise Pa_{CO_2}, and the effect on minute ventilation is measured. Creating these curves and observing how they change in a variety of circumstances allows quantitative study of factors that affect the chemical carbon dioxide control of ventilation. The carbon dioxide response curve approaches linearity in the range most often encountered in life: at Pa_{CO_2} values between 20 and 80 mm Hg. Once the Pa_{CO_2} exceeds 80 mm Hg, the curve becomes parabolic, with its peak ventilatory response at a Pa_{CO_2} between 100 and 120 mm Hg. Increasing the Pa_{CO_2} above 100 mm Hg allows carbon dioxide to act as a ventilatory and CNS depressant, the origin of the term "carbon dioxide narcosis," with 1 MAC being approximately 200 mm Hg.

The slope of the carbon dioxide response curve is considered to represent carbon dioxide sensitivity. Normal carbon dioxide sensitivity ranges from 0.5–0.7 l·min⁻¹·mm Hg⁻¹ CO_2. When Pa_{CO_2} reaches 100 mm Hg, carbon dioxide sensitivity is at its peak and normally reaches as high as 2.0 l·min⁻¹·mm Hg⁻¹ CO_2. The *setpoint*, the point of intersection of the carbon dioxide response curve and the metabolic hyperbola, defines normal resting Pa_{CO_2}. Extrapolation of the carbon dioxide response curve to the x-intercept (where minute ventilation is 0) defines the apneic threshold. In awake, normal adults, the apneic threshold normally occurs at a Pa_{CO_2} of ~32 mm Hg, although adults usually continue to breathe when they achieve the apneic

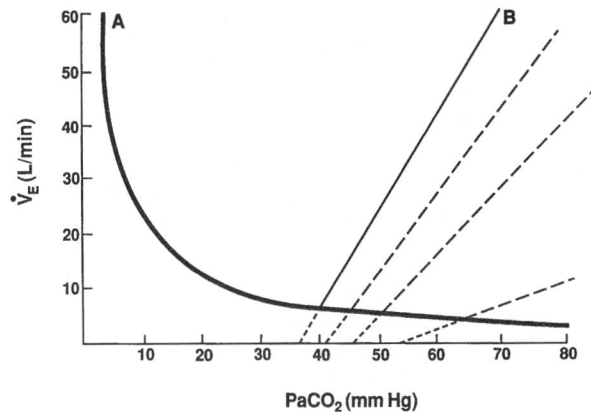

Figure 29-4. Carbon dioxide–ventilatory response curve. The metabolic hyperbola, curve *A*, is generated by varying $\dot{V}E$ and measuring changes in carbon dioxide concentration. The hyperbolic configuration makes it cumbersome for clinical use. The carbon dioxide–ventilatory response curve, *B*, is linear between approximately 20 and 80 mm Hg. It is generated by varying Pa_{CO_2} (usually by controlling inspired carbon dioxide concentration) and measuring the resultant $\dot{V}E$. This is the most commonly used test of ventilatory response. The slope defines "sensitivity"; the setpoint, or resting Pa_{CO_2}, occurs at the intersection of the metabolic hyperbola and the carbon dioxide–ventilatory response curve; and the apneic threshold can be obtained by extrapolating the carbon dioxide–ventilatory response curve to the x-intercept. In the absence of surgical stimulation, increasing doses of potent inhaled anesthesia or opioids will shift the curve to the right and eventually depress the slope (*dashed lines*). Painful stimulation will reverse these changes to varying and unpredictable degrees.

threshold because the sensation of apnea is disturbing to awake adults. The slope of the curve is a measure of the response of the entire ventilatory mechanism to carbon dioxide stimulation.

Once Pao_2 exceeds 100 mm Hg, it no longer influences the carbon dioxide response curve. When the Pao_2 is between 65 and 100 mm Hg, its effect on the carbon dioxide response curve is small. However, when Pao_2 falls below 65 mm Hg, the carbon dioxide response curve shifts to the left and its slope increases, probably as a result of increased ventilatory drive stimulated by the peripheral chemoreceptors. Thus, during measurements of carbon dioxide ventilatory response, the subject should breathe supplemental oxygen.

The carbon dioxide response curve can be generated rapidly by increasing the fraction of inspired carbon dioxide ($Fico_2$) by requiring the subject to rebreathe exhaled gas. The results obtained with this technique are less pure because the $Fico_2$ is not controlled.

Three clinical states result in a left shift and/or a steepened slope of the carbon dioxide response curve. These same three situations are the only causes of true hyperventilation, *i.e.,* an increase in minute ventilation such that the decreased $Paco_2$ creates respiratory alkalemia (either primary or compensatory). The three causes of hyperventilation (enhanced carbon dioxide response) are arterial hypoxemia, metabolic acidemia, and central etiologies. Examples of central etiologies that cause hyperventilation include drug administration, intracranial hypertension, hepatic cirrhosis, and nonspecific arousal states such as anxiety and fear. Aminophylline, salicylates, and norepinephrine stimulate ventilation independent of peripheral chemoreceptors. Opioid antagonists, given in the absence of opioids to presumably normal people, do not stimulate ventilation. However, when given after opiate administration, they do reverse the effects of opioids on the carbon dioxide response curve.

Ventilatory depressants displace the carbon dioxide response curve to the right or decrease its slope or both. Changes in physiology that depress ventilation include metabolic alkalemia, denervation of peripheral chemoreceptors, normal sleep, and drugs. During normal sleep, the carbon dioxide response curve is displaced to the right, with the degree of displacement depending on the depth of sleep. Usually, $Paco_2$ increases up to 10 mm Hg during deep sleep. Hypoxemic responses are not impaired by sleep, which is convenient for continued survival at high altitude.

Opioids displace the carbon dioxide response curve to the right with little change in slope at sedative doses. With higher, "anesthetic" doses, the curve shifts farther to the right and its slope is depressed, simulating the effect of potent inhalation agents on the carbon dioxide response curve (see Fig. 29-4). Opioids induce pathognomonic changes in ventilatory patterns: a decreased ventilatory rate with an increased tidal volume. Not until opioids nearly induce apnea is tidal volume decreased. Large narcotic doses usually result in apnea before consciousness is lost. Like sex, breathing requires both ability and desire.

Barbiturates in sedative or light hypnotic doses have little effect on the carbon dioxide response curve. In doses adequate to allow skin incision, barbiturates shift the carbon dioxide response curve to the right. The ventilatory pattern resulting from barbiturate administration is characterized by decreased tidal volume and increased ventilatory rate. Potent inhaled anesthetics displace the carbon dioxide response curve to the right and decrease the slope, the degree depending on the anesthetic dose and the level of surgical stimulation. As the inhaled anesthetic dose increases, the carbon dioxide response curve eventually becomes horizontal (slope = 0), resulting in essentially no ventilatory response to $Paco_2$ changes.

Potent inhaled anesthetics and opioids displace the setpoint to the right, implying that the resting, steady-state $Paco_2$ is higher and minute ventilation lower. Furthermore, when the carbon dioxide response curve shifts to the right, the apneic threshold also increases (see Fig. 29-4). Surgical stimulation

reverses the ventilatory response changes induced by inhaled anesthetics and opioids, but the degree of reversal is not predictable. Enflurane, halothane, and isoflurane all produce qualitatively similar carbon dioxide ventilatory responses. At equipotent doses, when administered with oxygen, the greatest to least ventilatory depression occurs with enflurane, halothane, and isoflurane.

OXYGEN AND CARBON DIOXIDE TRANSPORT

This chapter discusses only external respiration, in which oxygen moves from the ambient environment into the pulmonary capillaries and carbon dioxide leaves the pulmonary capillaries to enter the atmosphere. The movement of gas across the alveolar–capillary membrane depends on the integrity of the pulmonary and cardiac systems. Unless it is otherwise stated, the reader should assume that the ventilation and perfusion of alveolar–capillary units are normal. Abnormal distribution of ventilation or perfusion of the lungs is discussed later (see Ventilation–Perfusion Relationships).

Bulk Flow of Gas (Convection)

Convection, in which all gas molecules move in the same direction, is the primary mechanism responsible for gas flow in large and most small airways, down to the bronchi and bronchiolar airways of the 14th or 15th generation. Because the cross-sectional area of the airways progressively increases as gas moves toward the lung periphery, the average velocity of gas particles decreases as they travel toward the alveoli. As a result, the greatest part of airway resistance occurs in the larger airways, where gas molecules travel more quickly. During normal quiet ventilation, gas flow within convective airways is mainly laminar, thus reducing resistance to gas flow (see Resistance to Gas Flow).

Gas Diffusion

Diffusion within a gas-filled space is random molecular motion that results in complete mixing of all gases. In the lung, diffusion gradually becomes the predominant mode of gas transport, beginning with the terminal bronchioles (16th airway generation). Once gas reaches the small alveolar ducts, alveolar sacs, and alveoli, both diffusion and regional $\dot{V}/\dot{Q}$ relationships influence gas transport. Historically, clinicians assumed that defects in gas diffusion were responsible for arterial hypoxemia. However, the most frequent cause of arterial hypoxemia is physiologic shunt (see Ventilation–Perfusion Relationships).[80]

The other usage of "diffusion" refers to the passive movement of molecules across a membrane that is governed primarily by concentration gradient. In this sense, carbon dioxide is 20 times more diffusible across human membranes than is oxygen; therefore, carbon dioxide crosses membranes easily. As a result, hypercarbia is never the result of defective diffusion; rather, it is the result of inadequate alveolar ventilation with respect to carbon dioxide production.

True diffusion defects that create arterial hypoxemia are rare. The most common reason for a measured decrease in diffusing capacity (see Pulmonary Function Testing) is mismatched ventilation and perfusion, which functionally results in a decreased surface area available for diffusion.

Distribution of Ventilation and Perfusion

The efficiency with which oxygen and carbon dioxide exchange at the alveolar–capillary level highly depends on the matching of capillary perfusion and alveolar ventilation. At this level, the marriage between the lung and the circulatory system must be well-matched and intimate.

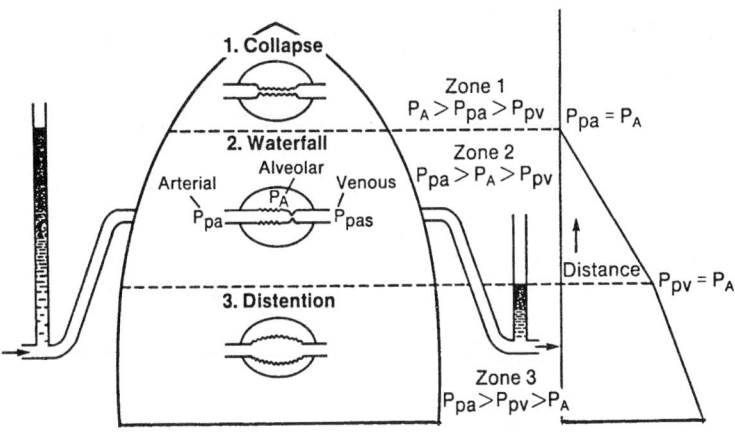

Figure 29-5. Distribution of blood flow in the isolated lung. In Zone 1, alveolar pressure (P_A) exceeds pulmonary artery pressure (Ppa), and no flow occurs because the vessels are collapsed. In Zone 2, arterial pressure exceeds alveolar pressure, but alveolar pressure exceeds pulmonary venous pressure (Ppv̄). Flow in Zone 2 is determined by the arterial–alveolar pressure difference (Ppa − P_A), which steadily increases down the zone. In Zone 3, pulmonary venous pressure exceeds alveolar pressure, and flow is determined by the arterial–venous pressure difference (Ppa − Ppv̄), which is constant down this pulmonary zone. However, the pressure across the vessel walls increases down the zone, so that their caliber increases, as does flow. (Reproduced with permission from West JB, Dollery CT, Naimark A: Distribution of blood flow in isolated lung: Relation to vascular and alveolar pressures. J Appl Physiol 19:713, 1964.)

Distribution of Blood Flow

Blood flow within the lung is mainly gravity-dependent. Because the alveolar–capillary beds are not composed of rigid vessels, the pressure of the surrounding tissues can influence the resistance to flow through the individual capillaries. Thus, blood flow depends on the relationship between pulmonary artery pressure (Ppa), alveolar pressure (P_A), and pulmonary venous pressure (Ppv̄) (Fig. 29-5). West created a lung model that divides the lung into three zones.[80,81] Zone 1 conditions occur in the most gravity-independent part of the lung above the level where pulmonary artery pressure is equal to alveolar pressure. Because alveolar pressure is approximately equal to atmospheric pressure, pulmonary artery pressure in Zone 1 is subatmospheric but necessarily greater than pulmonary venous pressure (P_A > Ppa > Ppv̄). Alveolar pressure that is transmitted to the pulmonary capillaries promotes their collapse, with a consequent theoretical blood flow of zero to this lung region. Thus, Zone 1 receives ventilation in the absence of perfusion and creates alveolar dead space ventilation. Normally, Zone 1 areas exist only to a limited extent. However, in conditions of decreased pulmonary artery pressure, such as hypovolemic shock, Zone 1 enlarges.

Zone 3 occurs in the most gravity-dependent areas of the lung where Ppa > Ppv̄ > P_A and blood flow is primarily governed by the pulmonary arterial to venous pressure difference. Because gravity also increases pulmonary venous pressure, the pulmonary capillaries become distended. Thus, perfusion in Zone 3 is lush, resulting in capillary perfusion in excess of ventilation, or physiologic shunt.

Finally, Zone 2 occurs from the lower limit of Zone 1 to the upper limit of Zone 3, where Ppa > P_A > Ppv̄. The pressure difference between pulmonary artery and alveolar pressure determines blood flow in Zone 2. Pulmonary venous pressure has little influence. Well-matched ventilation and perfusion occur in Zone 2, which contains the majority of alveoli.

Distribution of Ventilation

Alveolar pressure is the same throughout the lung; therefore, the more negative intrapleural pressure at the apex (or the least gravity-dependent area) results in larger, more distended apical alveoli than in other areas of the lung. The transpulmonary pressure (Paw − Ppl), or distending pressure of the lung, is greater at the top and lower at the bottom, where intrapleural pressure is less negative. Despite the smaller alveolar size, more ventilation is delivered to dependent pulmonary areas. The decrease in intrapleural pressure at the base of the lungs during inspiration is greater than at the apex because of diaphragmatic proximity. Thus, more gas is sucked into dependent areas of the lung.

Ventilation–Perfusion Relationships

As discussed above, the majority of blood flow is distributed to the gravity-dependent part of the lung. During a spontaneous breath, the largest portion of the tidal volume also reaches gravity-dependent lung. Thus, the nondependent area of the lung receives a lower proportion of both ventilation and perfusion, and dependent lung receives greater proportions of ventilation and perfusion. Nevertheless, ventilation and perfusion are not matched perfectly, and a variety of $\dot{V}_A/\dot{Q}$ ratios result throughout the lung. The ideal $\dot{V}_A/\dot{Q}$ ratio of 1 is believed to occur at approximately the level of the third rib. Above this level, ventilation occurs slightly in excess of perfusion, whereas below the third rib the $\dot{V}_A/\dot{Q}$ ratio becomes less than 1 (Fig. 29-6).

In a simplified model, gas exchange units can be divided into normal ($\dot{V}_A/\dot{Q}$ = 1:1), dead space ($\dot{V}_A/\dot{Q}$ = 1:0), shunt ($\dot{V}_A/\dot{Q}$ = 0:1), or a silent unit ($\dot{V}_A/\dot{Q}$ = 0:0) (Fig. 29-7). Although this model is helpful in understanding $\dot{V}_A/\dot{Q}$ relationships and their influences on gas exchange,[82] $\dot{V}_A/\dot{Q}$ really occurs as a continuum. In the lungs of a healthy, upright, spontaneously breathing individual, the majority of alveolar–capillary

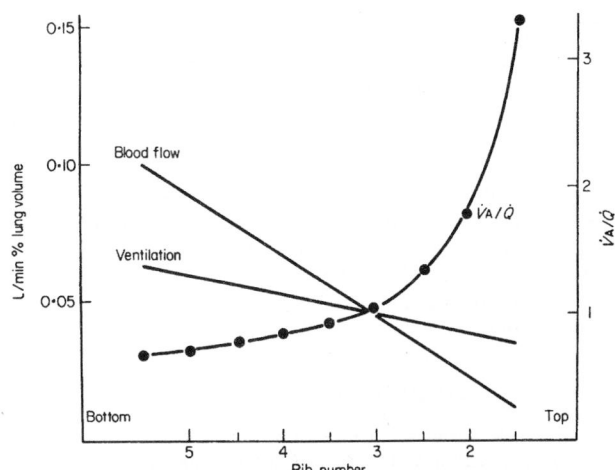

Figure 29-6. Distribution of ventilation, blood flow, and ventilation–perfusion ratio in the normal, upright lung. Straight lines have been drawn through the ventilation and blood flow data. Because blood flow falls more rapidly than ventilation with distance up the lung, ventilation–perfusion ratio rises, slowly at first, then rapidly. (Reproduced with permission from West JB: Ventilation/Blood Flow and Gas Exchange, 4th ed. Oxford, England, Blackwell Scientific Publications, 1985.)

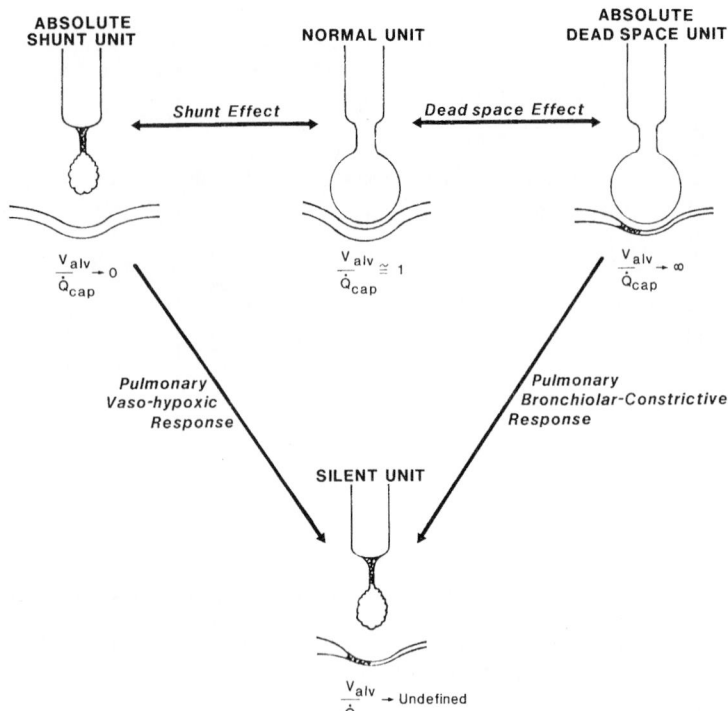

Figure 29-7. Continuum of ventilation–perfusion relationships. Gas exchange is maximally effective in normal lung units and only partially effective in shunt and dead space effect units. It is totally absent in silent units, absolute shunt, and deadspace units.

units are normal gas exchange units. The $\dot{V}A/\dot{Q}$ ratio varies between absolute shunt (in which $\dot{V}A/\dot{Q} = 0$) to absolute dead space (in which $\dot{V}A/\dot{Q} = \infty$). Rather than absolute shunt, most units with low $\dot{V}A/\dot{Q}$ mismatch receive a small amount of ventilation relative to blood flow. Similarly, most dead space units are not absolute, but rather are characterized by low blood flow relative to ventilation.

Hypoxic pulmonary vasoconstriction, stimulated by alveolar hypoxia, severely decreases blood flow. Thus, poorly ventilated alveoli also receive minuscule blood flow. Furthermore, decreased regional pulmonary blood flow results in bronchiolar constriction and diminishes the degree of dead space ventilation.[83,84] When either of these phenomena occurs, the shunt or dead space units effectively become silent units in which little ventilation or perfusion occurs.

Many pulmonary diseases result in both physiologic shunt and dead space abnormalities. However, most disease processes can be characterized as producing either primarily shunt or dead space in their early stages. Increases in dead space ventilation primarily affect carbon dioxide elimination and have little influence on arterial oxygenation until dead space ventilation exceeds 80–90% of minute ventilation ($\dot{V}E$). Similarly, physiologic shunt primarily affects arterial oxygenation with little effect on carbon dioxide elimination until the physiologic shunt fraction exceeds 75–80% of the cardiac output. Defective to absent gas exchange can be the net effect of either abnormality in the extreme.[85]

Physiologic Dead Space

Each inspired breath is composed of gas that contributes to alveolar ventilation (V_A) and gas that becomes dead space ventilation (V_D). Thus, tidal volume (V_t) = $V_A + V_D$. In the normal, spontaneously breathing person, the ratio of alveolar to dead space ventilation for each breath is 2:1. Conveniently, the rule of "1, 2, 3" applies to normal, spontaneously breathing persons. For each breath, 1 ml·lb^{-1} (lean body weight) becomes V_D, 2 ml·lb^{-1} becomes V_A, and 3 ml·lb^{-1} constitutes the V_t.

Physiologic dead space consists of anatomic and alveolar dead space. Anatomic dead space ventilation, approximately 2 ml·kg^{-1} ideal body weight, accounts for the majority of physiologic dead space.[86] It arises from ventilation of structures that do not exchange respiratory gases: the oronasopharynx to the terminal and respiratory bronchioles. Clinical conditions that modify anatomic dead space include tracheal intubation, tracheostomy, and large lengths of ventilator tubing between the tracheal tube and the ventilator Y-piece.

Alveolar dead space ventilation arises from ventilation of alveoli where there is little or no perfusion. Because disease changes anatomic dead space little, physiologic dead space is primarily influenced by changes in alveolar dead space. Rapid changes in physiologic dead space ventilation most often arise from changes in pulmonary blood flow, resulting in decreased perfusion to ventilated alveoli. The most common etiology of acutely increased physiologic dead space is an abrupt decrease in cardiac output.[87] Another pathologic condition that interferes with pulmonary blood flow is pulmonary embolism, whether due to thrombus or to fat, air, or amniotic fluid.

Chronic pulmonary diseases create dead space ventilation by irreversibly changing the relationship between alveolar ventilation and blood flow; this alteration is especially prominent in patients with COPD. Furthermore, acute diseases such as adult respiratory distress syndrome can cause an increase in dead space ventilation owing to intense pulmonary vasoconstriction. Finally, therapeutic or supportive manipulations such as positive-pressure ventilation or positive airway pressure therapy can increase alveolar dead space because depressed venous return to the right heart will decrease cardiac output.[88] Intravenous fluid administration will usually overcome this problem.

Assessment of Physiologic Dead Space

Because the lung receives nearly 100% of the cardiac output, assessment of physiologic dead space ventilation in the acute setting yields valuable information about pulmonary blood flow and, ultimately, about cardiac output. If pulmonary blood flow decreases, the most likely cause is a decreased cardiac output. Thus, it is clinically useful to be able to readily assess the degree of physiologic dead space ventilation.

There are two easy and several difficult ways to assess dead space ventilation. A comparison of minute ventilation and $Paco_2$ allows a gross qualitative assessment of physiologic dead space ventilation. The $Paco_2$ is determined only by alveolar ventilation and $\dot{V}co_2$. If $\dot{V}co_2$ remains constant, $Paco_2$ also will remain constant as long as minute ventilation supplies the same degree of alveolar ventilation. If the spontaneously breathing individual must increase minute ventilation to maintain the same $Paco_2$, he or she has experienced an increase in dead space ventilation because less of the minute ventilation is contributing to alveolar ventilation. Alternatively, a mechanically ventilated patient with a fixed minute ventilation and no increase in $\dot{V}co_2$ also experiences an increased dead space ventilation if the $Paco_2$ rises. Hence, when $Paco_2$ in a mechanically ventilated patient increases, it is necessary to determine if the cause is increased dead space ventilation or an increased $\dot{V}co_2$.

The mechanically ventilated patient with normal lungs has a dead space to alveolar ventilation ratio (V_D/V_A) of 1:1 rather than 1:2, as during spontaneous ventilation. If mechanical V_T is 1000 ml, 500 ml contributes to V_A and 500 ml contributes to V_D. At rest, the required $\dot{V}_A$ with normal $\dot{V}co_2$ is approximately 60 ml $\cdot$ kg^{-1} $\cdot$ min^{-1}. A 70-kg man would then require a $\dot{V}_A$ of 4200 ml $\cdot$ min^{-1}. During spontaneous breathing, the required $\dot{V}_E$ would be 6300 ml $\cdot$ min^{-1}, but during mechanical ventilation $\dot{V}_E$ would have to be 8400 ml $\cdot$ min^{-1}. Using this calculation, if a 70-kg resting patient requires $\dot{V}_E$ much in excess of 8400 ml $\cdot$ min^{-1}, either V_D or $\dot{V}co_2$ is increased. A rule of thumb for mechanically ventilated patients is that doubling baseline minute ventilation decreases $Paco_2$ from 40 to 30 mm Hg, and quadrupling minute ventilation decreases $Paco_2$ from 40 to 20 mm Hg.

The $Paco_2$ will be greater than or equal to end-tidal $Paco_2$ ($Petco_2$) unless the patient inspires carbon dioxide. The difference between $Petco_2$ and $Paco_2$ is due to dead space ventilation. Measurement of this difference—which is simple, readily obtainable, and fairly inexpensive—yields reliable information relative to the degree of dead space ventilation. Clinical situations that change pulmonary blood flow sufficiently to increase dead space ventilation can be detected by comparing $Petco_2$ with temperature-corrected $Paco_2$. Yamanaka and Sue[89] found that the $Petco_2$ in ventilated patients varied linearly with the dead space to tidal volume ratio (V_D/V_T), and that $Petco_2$ correlated poorly with $Paco_2$. Thus, in the critically ill, mechanically ventilated patient and in anesthetized patients, monitoring $Petco_2$ gives far more information about ventilatory efficiency or dead space ventilation than it does about the absolute value of $Paco_2$.

Anesthesiologists commonly measure $Petco_2$ to detect venous air embolism during anesthesia. A lowered cardiac output alone, in the absence of venous air embolism, may sufficiently decrease pulmonary perfusion so that dead space ventilation increases and $Petco_2$ falls. Thus, a depressed $Petco_2$ is a sensitive but nonspecific monitor. Air in the pulmonary arteries mechanically interferes with blood flow and also causes pulmonary arterial constriction, further decreasing pulmonary blood flow. A decreased $Petco_2$ suggests that a physiologically significant air embolism has occurred. The same physiologic considerations apply to detecting pulmonary thromboembolism.

Depressed cardiac output is the most common cause of acutely decreased pulmonary blood flow and increased physiologic dead space ventilation in the operating room and intensive care unit. Weil et al[90] observed a correlation between $Petco_2$ and cardiac output during resuscitation in pigs when $Paco_2$ was kept constant ($r = 0.79$). They concluded that the increase in $P\bar{v}co_2$ and the concurrent decrease in $Petco_2$ reflected a critical reduction in cardiac output, which diminished alveolar blood flow to the extent that carbon dioxide clearance by the lung failed to keep pace with systemic carbon dioxide production.

Some clinicians use the divergence of $Petco_2$ from $Paco_2$ as a reflection of pulmonary blood flow for other applications. During intentional pharmacologic or surgical manipulation of pulmonary blood flow, the difference between $Paco_2$ and $Petco_2$ serves as a useful physiologic monitor of the effectiveness of these interventions. Furthermore, regarding $Petco_2$ as a reflection of pulmonary perfusion is a useful tool for studying and monitoring the effectiveness of closed-heart massage during resuscitation efforts. Murray and Modell[91] suggested that an appropriate positive end-expiratory pressure (PEEP) level could be chosen based on the difference between $Paco_2$ and $Petco_2$. However, extrapolating their canine findings to humans has been unsuccessful.

The most quantitative technique used to measure physiologic dead space utilizes a modification of the Bohr equation:

$$\frac{V_D}{V_T} = \frac{Paco_2 - P\bar{E}co_2}{Paco_2} \qquad (4)$$

where $P\bar{E}co_2$ is the Pco_2 from the mixture of all expired gases over the period of time during which measurements are made. This calculation estimates the fraction of each breath that does not contribute to gas exchange. In spontaneously breathing patients, normal V_D/V_T is between 0.2 and 0.4, or ~0.33. In patients receiving positive-pressure ventilation, V_D/V_T becomes ~0.5. The major limitation of performing this calculation is the difficulty in collecting exhaled gas for $P\bar{E}co_2$ measurement. Exhaled gases, collected in cumbersome 8-l bags, can easily be contaminated with inspired air or supplemental oxygen. The measurement also will be inaccurate if the patient does not maintain a steady ventilatory pattern. Therefore, extreme care must be taken to ensure that all measurements are performed accurately. In practice, this measurement is rarely performed.

Physiologic Shunt

Whereas physiologic dead space ventilation applies to areas of the lung that are ventilated but poorly perfused, physiologic shunt occurs in lung that is perfused but poorly ventilated. The physiologic shunt ($\dot{Q}_{SP}$) is that portion of the total cardiac output ($\dot{Q}_T$) that returns to the left heart and systemic circulation without receiving oxygen in the lung. When pulmonary blood is not exposed to alveoli or when those alveoli are devoid of ventilation, the result is *absolute shunt*, in which $\dot{V}_A/\dot{Q} = 0$. *Shunt effect*, or *venous admixture*, is the more common clinical phenomenon and occurs in areas where alveolar ventilation is deficient compared to the degree of perfusion: $0 < \dot{V}_A/\dot{Q} < 1$.

Because blood passing through areas of absolute shunt receives no oxygen, arterial hypoxemia resulting from absolute shunt is not reversed with supplemental oxygen. Alternatively, supplemental oxygen supplied to patients with arterial hypoxemia due to venous admixture will increase the Pao_2. Although ventilation to these alveoli is deficient, they do carry a small amount of oxygen to the capillary bed.

A small percentage of venous blood normally bypasses the right ventricle and empties directly into the left atrium. This anatomic, absolute shunt arises from the venous return from the pleural, bronchiolar, and thebesian veins. This venous drainage accounts for 2–5% of total cardiac output and explains the small shunt that normally occurs. Anatomic shunts of greatest magnitude usually are associated with congenital heart disease that causes right-to-left shunt. Intrapulmonary anatomic shunts can also cause anatomic shunt. For example, the arterial hypoxemia associated with advanced hepatic failure is due to arteriovenous malformations.[92] Diseases that may cause absolute shunt include acute lobar atelectasis, extensive acute lung injury, advanced pulmonary edema, and consolidated pneumonia. Disease entities that tend to produce venous admixture include mild pulmonary edema, postoperative atelectasis, and chronic obstructive pulmonary disease.

Assessment of Arterial Oxygenation and Physiologic Shunt

The simplest assessment of oxygenation is qualitative comparison of the patient's F_{IO_2} and Pa_{O_2}. The highest possible Pa_{O_2} for any given F_{IO_2} (and Pa_{CO_2}) can be calculated from the alveolar gas equation:

$$P_{AO_2} = F_{IO_2}(P_B - P_{H_2O}) - \frac{P_{ACO_2}}{R} \qquad (5)$$

where P_{AO_2} and P_{ACO_2} are alveolar P_{O_2} and P_{CO_2}, P_{H_2O} is water vapor pressure at 100% saturation and 37°C, and R is respiratory quotient. Assuming that one makes the calculation for a well-perfused alveolus, the alveolar and arterial P_{CO_2} are equal. Therefore, Pa_{CO_2} can be substituted for P_{ACO_2}. Respiratory quotient (R) in the ratio of O_2 consumed ($\dot{V}_{O_2}$) to CO_2 produced ($\dot{V}_{CO_2}$):

$$\frac{\dot{V}_{CO_2}}{\dot{V}_{O_2}} = \frac{200 \text{ ml} \cdot \text{min}^{-1}}{250 \text{ ml} \cdot \text{min}^{-1}} = 0.8 \qquad (6)$$

Oxygen tension–based indices do not reflect mixed venous contribution to arterial oxygenation and can be misleading.[93] Even if venous admixture is small, mixed venous blood with very low oxygen content will magnify the effect of a small shunt. Oxygen tension–based indices, for example, Pa_{O_2}/F_{IO_2}, alveolar to arterial P_{O_2} difference (DA-a_{O_2}), and ratio Pa_{O_2}/P_{AO_2}, do not take into account the influence of $C\bar{v}_{O_2}$ on the arterial oxygenation process. Therefore, in critically ill patients who are hypoxemic, the insertion of a pulmonary artery catheter to assess shunt and to measure cardiac output may be essential to understanding the influence of cardiac function on arterial oxygenation.

DA-a_{O_2} is a useful quantitative assessment of arterial oxygenation mainly when arterial hemoglobin is well saturated. When Pa_{O_2} is below 150 mm Hg (and certainly when it is below 100 mm Hg), the relationship between oxygen content and oxygen tension is nonlinear. Normal DA-a_{O_2} is <5 mm Hg when hemoglobin is well saturated with oxygen.

The assessment of arterial oxygenation requires knowledge, at least, of F_{IO_2} and either Pa_{O_2} or Sa_{O_2}. Oxygen tension–based indices of oxygenation are useful, but they do not take into account the contribution of mixed venous blood to arterial oxygenation. Mixed venous blood can become extremely desaturated in the critically ill patient owing to inadequate cardiac output, anemia, arterial hypoxemia, or increased $\dot{V}_{O_2}$. The best knowledge of the efficiency with which the lungs oxygenate the arterial blood can be obtained only by calculating shunt fraction or ventilation–perfusion ratio (VQI) (see below).

Physiologic Shunt Calculation

The clinical reference standard for the calculation of physiologic shunt fraction is derived from a two-compartment pulmonary blood flow model where one compartment performs ideal gas exchange and contains perfectly married alveolar–capillary units. The other compartment is the shunt compartment and contains pulmonary capillaries that enjoy no exposure to ventilated alveoli. Using the Fick relationship, the following equation can be derived:

$$\frac{\dot{Q}_{SP}}{\dot{Q}_T} = \frac{Cc'_{O_2} - Ca_{O_2}}{Cc'_{O_2} - C\bar{v}_{O_2}} \qquad (7)$$

where Cc'_{O_2} and $C\bar{v}_{O_2}$ are end-capillary and mixed-venous oxygen contents, respectively. Normal intrapulmonary shunt is approximately 5%. Because this equation is based on an artificial two-compartment model, the absolute value is physically meaningless. A calculated $\dot{Q}_{SP}/\dot{Q}_T$ of 25% means that if the lung existed in two compartments, 25% of the cardiac output would travel through the shunt compartment. Because the lung does

not exist in two compartments, this equation only grossly estimates pulmonary oxygen exchange defects. Nevertheless, it remains our best tool for clinically evaluating the efficiency with which the lungs oxygenate arterial blood. Observing shunt fraction change with therapeutic intervention or with the progress of disease is more valuable than knowing the absolute value *per se*.

Because hemoglobin concentration is uniform throughout the vascular system, the oxygen contents in the shunt equation are determined primarily by oxyhemoglobin saturation. Thus, the shunt equation can be approximated by substituting saturation values for each term; the new value, called *ventilation–perfusion ratio* (VQI),[93] is determined as follows:

$$VQI = \frac{Sc'_{O_2} - Sa_{O_2}}{Sc'_{O_2} - S\bar{v}_{O_2}} \cong \frac{1 - Sa_{O_2}}{1 - S\bar{v}_{O_2}} \qquad (8)$$

If the patient is neither breathing a hypoxic gas mixture nor has a methemoglobin or carboxyhemoglobin value in excess of 5–6%, Sc'_{O_2} must equal 1 because the model requires a perfect alveolar–capillary interface. This substitution results in the final expression in the equation above. The absolute values of VQI are meaningless, although "normal" should be 0–4%. Like $\dot{Q}_{SP}/\dot{Q}_T$, the importance of these values lie in their trend as disease and treatment progress.

Sa_{O_2} and $S\bar{v}_{O_2}$ can be estimated continuously with pulse oximetry and by using a pulmonary artery catheter with oximetry capability. By interfacing the outputs of these two devices with a computer, VQI can be calculated continuously. The greatest advantage of calculating $\dot{Q}_{SP}/\dot{Q}_T$ or VQI to assess arterial oxygenation is that these values include the contribution of mixed venous blood.

PULMONARY FUNCTION TESTING

Anesthesiologists frequently care for patients with significant pulmonary dysfunction. It is important for the anesthesiologist to be able to interpret tests of pulmonary function intelligently and to know which tests will help to define dysfunction if the patient's history and physical are suggestive of disease. This section discusses lung volumes, tests of pulmonary mechanics, and diffusing capacity.

Lung Volumes and Capacities

Known, reproducible pulmonary gas volumes and capacities provide a reliable basis for comparison between normal and abnormal measurements.[94] Because normal measurements vary with size, height is most frequently used to define "normal." Lung capacities are composed of two or more lung volumes. Lung volumes and capacities are schematically illustrated in Figure 29-8.

Tidal volume is the volume of gas that moves in and out of the lungs during quiet breathing and is ~6–8 ml · kg^{-1}. Tidal volume falls with decreased lung compliance or when the patient has reduced ventilatory muscle strength.

Vital capacity is usually ~60 ml · kg^{-1}, but may vary as much as 20% from normal in healthy individuals. Vital capacity correlates well with the capability for deep breathing and effective coughing. It usually is decreased by restrictive pulmonary disease such as pulmonary edema or atelectasis. Vital capacity also may be reduced by the mechanically induced restriction that occurs with problems such as pleural effusion, pneumothorax, pregnancy, large ascites, or ventilatory muscle weakness.

The *inspiratory capacity* is the largest volume of gas that can be inspired from the resting expiratory level and frequently is decreased in the presence of significant extrathoracic airway obstruction. This measurement is one of the few simple tests that can detect extrathoracic airway obstruction. Most routine pulmonary function tests measure only exhaled flows and volumes, which may be relatively unaffected by extrathoracic ob-

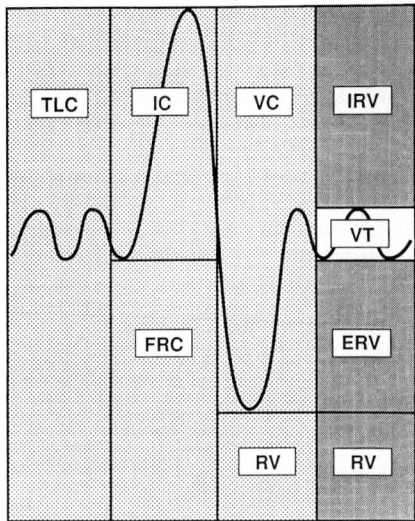

Figure 29-8. Lung volumes and capacities. The darkest bar on the far right depicts the four basic lung volumes that sum to create TLC. Other lung capacities are composed of two or more lung volumes. The overlying spirographic tracing orients the reader to the relationship between the lung volumes and capacities and the spirogram. ERV = expiratory reserve volume; FRC = functional residual capacity; IC = inspiratory capacity; IRV = inspiratory reserve volume; RV = residual volume; VT = tidal volume; TLC = total lung capacity; VC = vital capacity.

struction until it is severe. Changes in the absolute volume of inspiratory capacity usually parallel changes in vital capacity. *Expiratory reserve* volume is not of great diagnostic value.

Functional residual capacity (FRC) is the volume of gas remaining in the lungs at passive end-expiration. *Residual volume* is that gas remaining within the lungs at the end of forced maximal expiration. The FRC serves two primary physiologic functions. It determines the point on the pulmonary volume–pressure curve for resting ventilation (see Fig. 29-2). The tangent defined by the midportion pulmonary volume–pressure curve at FRC defines lung compliance. Thus, FRC determines the elastic pressure–volume relationships within the lung. Furthermore, FRC is the resting expiratory volume of the lung. As such, it greatly influences ventilation–perfusion relationships within the lung. When FRC is reduced, venous admixture (low $\dot{V}_A/\dot{Q}$) increases and results in arterial hypoxemia (see sections Oxygen and Carbon Dioxide Transport and Lung Mechanics.)

The FRC also may be used to quantify the degree of pulmonary restriction. Disease processes that reduce FRC and lung compliance include acute lung injury, pulmonary edema, pulmonary fibrotic processes, and atelectasis. Mechanical factors also reduce FRC, for example, pregnancy, obesity, pleural effusion, and posture. The FRC decreases 10% when a healthy subject lies down. Ventilatory muscle weakness or paralysis also will decrease FRC. In contrast, patients with chronic obstructive pulmonary disease have excessively compliant lungs that recoil less forcibly. Their lungs retain an abnormally large volume at the end of passive expiration, a phenomenon called *gas trapping*.

FRC Measurement

The FRC and residual volume must be measured indirectly because residual volume cannot be removed from the lung. The multiple-breath nitrogen washout test is performed by having the subject breathe 100% oxygen for several minutes so that alveolar nitrogen is gradually "washed out." With each breath, the volume of gas and the concentration of nitrogen in the exhaled gas are measured. A rapid nitrogen analyzer coupled to a spirometer or pneumotachometer provides a breath-by-breath analysis of nitrogen washout. Electronic signals proportional to nitrogen concentrations and exhaled volumes

(or flow, if a pneumotachometer is used) are integrated to derive the exhaled volume of nitrogen for each breath. Then, the values for all breaths are summed to provide a total volume of nitrogen washed out of the lungs. The test proceeds until the alveolar nitrogen concentration is reduced to less than 7%, usually requiring 7–10 minutes. FRC is calculated using the equation:

$$FRC = N_2 \text{ volume} \times \frac{[N_2]_f}{[N_2]_i} \qquad (9)$$

where $[N_2]_i$ and $[N_2]_f$ are the fractional concentrations of alveolar nitrogen at the beginning and end of the test, respectively.

Pulmonary Function Tests

Forced Vital Capacity (FVC)

The FVC is the volume of gas that can be expired as forcefully and rapidly as possible after maximal inspiration. Normally, FVC is equal to vital capacity. Because forced expiration significantly increases intrapleural pressures but changes airway pressure little, bronchiolar collapse, obstructive lesions, and gas trapping are exaggerated. Thus, FVC may be reduced in chronic obstructive diseases even when the vital capacity appears near normal. FVC is nearly always decreased by restrictive diseases. FVC values $<15 \text{ ml} \cdot \text{kg}^{-1}$ are associated with an increased incidence of postoperative pulmonary complications, probably because these patients cough ineffectively.[95] FVC reduced to this level represents a profound defect, most commonly seen in quadriplegics or severe neuromuscular disease. Finally, FVC is largely dependent on patient effort and cooperation.

Forced Expiratory Volume (FEV)

FEV_T is the volume of gas expired over a given time interval during the FVC maneuver. The interval, described by the subscript T, is the time elapsed in seconds from the onset of expiration. Because FEV_T records a volume of gas expired over time, it is actually a measure of flow. By measuring expiratory flow at specific intervals, the severity of airway obstruction can be ascertained. Decreased FEV_T values are common in both obstructive and restrictive disease patterns. The most important application of FEV_T is its comparison with the patient's FVC. Normal subjects can expire at least three quarters of FVC within the first second of the forced expiratory maneuver. The FEV_1, the most frequently employed value, is normally greater than or equal to 75% of the FVC, or $FEV_1/FVC \geq 0.75$.

Normally, an individual can expire 50–60% of FVC in 0.5 sec, 75–85% in 1 sec, 94% in 2 sec, and 97% in 3 sec. Cooperative patients with obstructive disease will exhibit a reduced FEV_1/FVC in most cases. However, patients with restrictive disease usually have normal FEV_1/FVC ratios. The validity of the evaluation of the FEV_1/FVC is highly dependent on patient cooperation and effort. It is possible to deliberately produce an artificially low FEV_1/FVC.

Forced Expiratory Flow (FEF)

$FEF_{25-75\%}$ is the average flow during the middle half of the FEV maneuver. This test is also called maximum midexpiratory flow rate (MMFR). The length of time required for a subject to expire the middle half of the FVC is divided into 50% of the FVC. The spirogram in Figure 29-9 marks the place from 25% to 75% of FVC, constituting the middle 50% of FVC. The straight line connecting the 25% and 75% volumes has a slope approximately equal to average flow. A normal value for a healthy 70-kg man is approximately $4.7 \text{ l} \cdot \text{sec}^{-1}$ (or $280 \text{ ml} \cdot \text{min}^{-1}$). Normally, both the absolute value and the percentage of predicted value for the individual being studied are recorded. A normal value is $100 \pm 25\%$ of predicted. Decreased flow rates indicate medium-sized airway obstruction. This value is typically normal in restrictive diseases. This test is fairly sensitive in the

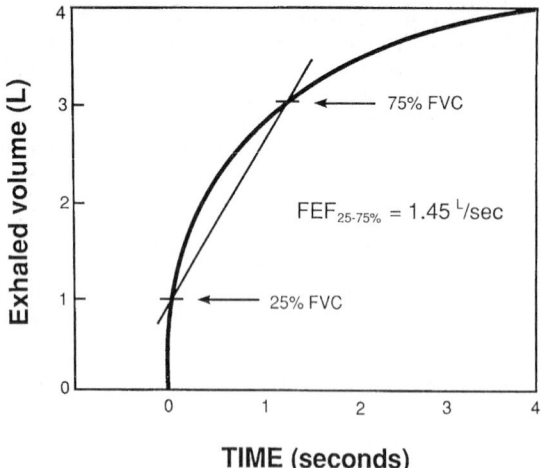

Figure 29-9. $FEF_{25-75\%}$. The spirogram depicts a 4 l FVC on which the points representing 25% and 75% FVC are marked. The slope of the line connecting these points is the $FEF_{25-75\%}$.

early stages of obstructive airway disease. Decreased $FEV_{25-75\%}$ frequently will be observed before other obstructive manifestations occur. Although somewhat effort-dependent, the test is much more reliable and reproducible than FEV_1/FVC.

Maximum Voluntary Ventilation

Maximum voluntary ventilation (MVV) is the largest volume of gas that can be breathed in 1 minute by voluntary effort. The MVV is measured by having the subject breathe as deeply and as rapidly as possible for 10, 12, or 15 seconds. The results are extrapolated to 1 minute. The subject is instructed to set his or her own ventilatory rate and move more than tidal volume but less than vital capacity in each breath.

MVV measures the endurance of the ventilatory muscles and indirectly reflects lung–thorax compliance and airway resistance. MVV is the best ventilatory endurance test that can be performed in the laboratory. Values that vary by as much as 30% from predicted values may be normal, so that only large reductions in MVV are significant. Healthy, young adults average ~ 170 $l \cdot min^{-1}$. Values are lower in women and decrease with age in both sexes. Because this maneuver exaggerates air trapping and exerts the ventilatory muscles, MVV is decreased greatly in patients with moderate to severe obstructive disease. MVV is usually normal in patients with restrictive disease.

Flow–Volume Loops

The flow–volume loop graphically demonstrates the flow generated during a forced expiratory maneuver followed by a forced inspiratory maneuver, plotted against the volume of gas expired (Fig. 29-10). The subject forcefully exhales completely, then immediately and forcefully inhales to vital capacity. The expired and inspired volumes are plotted on the abscissa and flow is plotted on the ordinate. Although a variety of numbers can be generated from the flow–volume loop, the configuration of the loop itself is probably the most informative part of the test.

Significant decreases in flow or volume are evident in a single graphical display. Obstructive diseases are accompanied by decreased flows and restrictive processes by decreased volumes. The shape of the expiratory curve is largely independent of patient effort, with flow determined mainly by the elastic recoil properties of the lungs (from 75% of TLC down to residual volume). Normally, the flow decreases linearly with volume over most of the vital capacity range, so that the expiratory curve is linear (Fig. 29-10A). In those with obstructive lung disease, flow decreases particularly at lower lung volumes, and the flow-

volume loop takes on a scooped-out appearance (Fig. 29-10B). Obstruction of the upper airway and trachea is accompanied by characteristic limitations to expiratory and inspiratory flow that result in a flat, ovoid loop. Thus, the flow–volume loop is useful in the diagnosis of large airway and extrathoracic airway obstruction (Fig. 29-10C).

Restrictive disease usually results in relatively normal peak expiratory flows and a linear decrease in flow, but the lung volume itself is decreased (Fig. 29-10D). Moderate to severe restriction results in equal flows at all lung volumes and appears as a miniature flow–volume loop.

Carbon Monoxide Diffusing Capacity

Because P_{O_2} in the pulmonary capillary blood varies with time as it moves through the pulmonary capillary bed, oxygen cannot be used to assess diffusion capacity. A gas mixture containing carbon monoxide is the traditional diagnostic gas used to measure diffusing capacity. Its partial pressure in the blood is nearly zero, and its affinity for hemoglobin is 200 times that of oxygen.[96] Carbon monoxide diffusing capacity (DL_{CO}) collectively measures all the factors that affect the diffusion of gas across the alveolar–capillary membrane. The DL_{CO} is recorded in mL $CO \cdot min^{-1} \cdot mm Hg^{-1}$ at STPD.

In persons with normal hemoglobin concentrations and normal $\dot{V}_A/\dot{Q}$ matching, the main factor limiting diffusion is the alveolar–capillary membrane. Small amounts of carbon dioxide and inspired gas can produce measurable changes in the concentration of inspired gas compared to expired gas. There are several methods for determining DL_{CO}, but all methods measure diffusing capacity according to the equation

$$DL_{CO} = \frac{ml\ CO\ transferred \cdot min^{-1}}{mean\ P_{A CO_2} - mean\ capillary\ P_{CO_2}} \quad (10)$$

The average value for resting subjects when the single-breath method is used is 25 ml $CO \cdot min^{-1} \cdot mm Hg^{-1}$. DL_{CO} values can increase to two or three times normal during exercise.

The DL_{O_2} may be estimated from the DL_{CO} by multiplying DL_{CO} by 1.23, although the DL_{CO} is usually the reported value. DL_{CO} can be divided by the lung volume at which the measurement was made to obtain an expression of diffusing capacity per unit lung volume.

Some of the other factors that can influence DL_{CO} are as follows:

1. hemoglobin concentration: decreased hemoglobin concentration decreases the DL_{CO};
2. alveolar P_{CO_2}: an increased $P_{A CO_2}$ raises DL_{CO};
3. body position: the supine position increases DL_{CO};
4. pulmonary capillary blood volume.

Diffusing capacity is decreased in alveolar fibrosis associated with sarcoidosis, asbestosis, berylliosis, oxygen toxicity, and pulmonary edema. These states are frequently categorized as diffusion defects, but low DL_{CO} is probably more closely related to loss of lung volume or capillary bed perfusion. DL_{CO} is decreased in obstructive disease because of the decreased alveolar surface area, loss of capillary bed, the increased distance from the terminal bronchiole to the alveolar–capillary membrane, and $\dot{V}_A/\dot{Q}$ mismatching. Space-occupying lesions and lung resection also decrease diffusing capacity. In short, the decrease in measured DL_{CO} actually is caused by abnormal $\dot{V}_A/\dot{Q}$ matching in most cases. Very few disease states truly inhibit oxygen diffusion across the alveolar–capillary membrane.

Pulmonary Function Tests Summary

Although we have a host of pulmonary function tests from which to choose, spirometry is the most useful, cost-effective, and commonly used test.[97] Screening spirometry yields VC, FVC, and FEV_1. From these values, two basic types of pulmonary

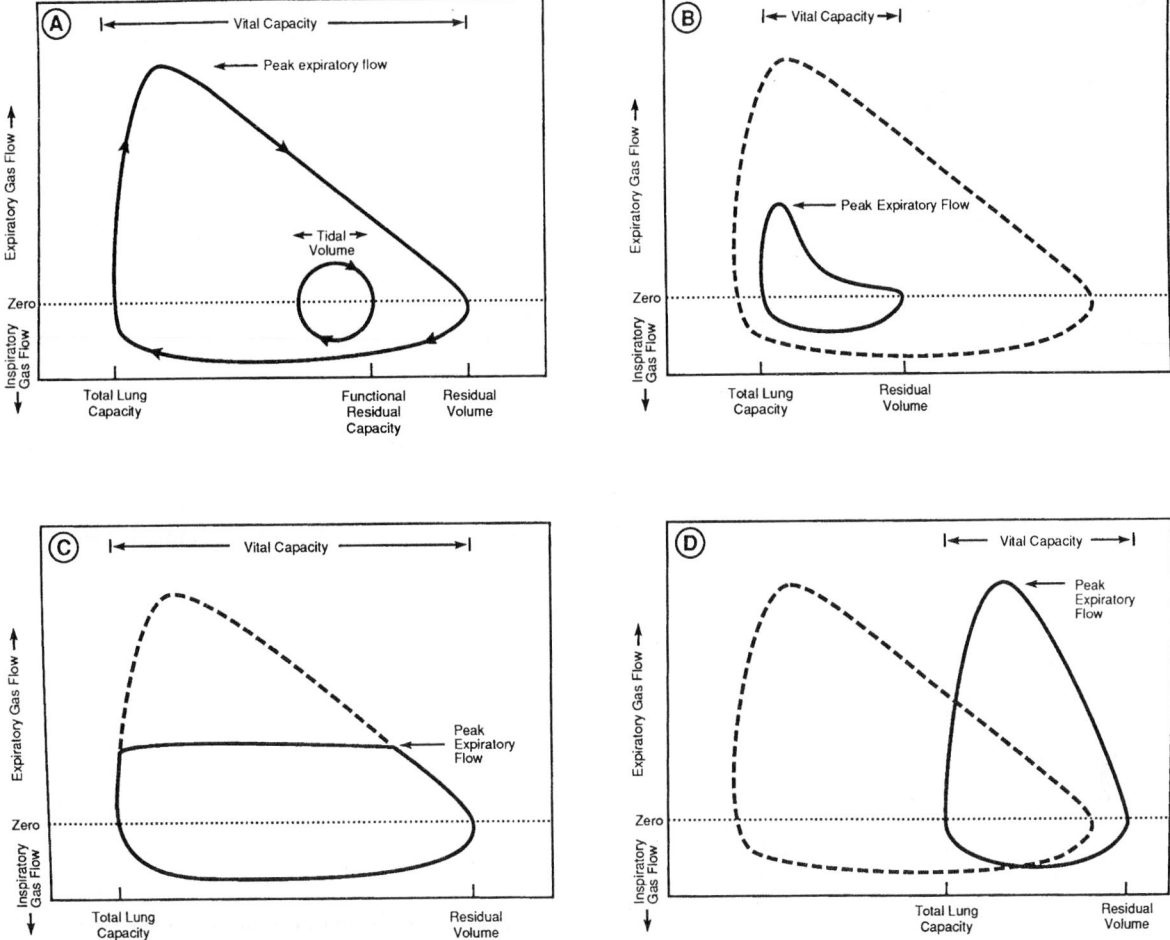

Figure 29-10. Flow–volume loops. Curve *A* is a normally configured adult flow–volume loop. The slope of the loop after the subject reaches peak expiratory flow is nearly linear. Obstructive pulmonary disease, caused by increased air resistance in the bronchial tree, results in curve *B*, with markedly decreased peak expiratory flow and a "scooped-out" appearance for the remainder of expiration. Residual volume is larger and vital capacity is smaller than normal. Curve *C* results from upper airway (extrathoracic) airway obstruction. A flattened expiratory curve with decreased peak expiratory flow is pathognomonic of upper airway obstruction. Curve *D* is found in restrictive lung disease that results in a miniature flow–volume loop with normal peak expiratory flows and a normally shaped curve. However, residual volume, total lung capacity, and vital capacity are all proportionally reduced.

dysfunction can be identified and quantitated: obstructive defects and restrictive defects. The primary criterion for airflow obstruction is decreased FEV_1/FCV ratio. Other measurements, such as $FEF_{25-75\%}$, can be used to support the diagnosis of an obstructive defect, or assist in making decisions (*e.g.*, whether to institute bronchodilation). A restrictive defect is a proportional decrease in all lung volumes; thus, VC, FVC, and FEV_1 all are reduced, but FEV_1/FVC remains normal. When there is a question about whether a decreased VC is due to restriction, TLC should be measured. Reduced TLC defines a restrictive defect, but is not necessary to perform unless VC on screening spirometry is reduced. The American Thoracic Society published an experts' consensus concerning interpretations of lung function tests.[98] Table 29-5 summarizes the distinction between pulmonary function results obtained from those with restrictive and obstructive defects.

ANESTHESIA AND OBSTRUCTIVE PULMONARY DISEASE

Patients with marked obstructive pulmonary disease are at increased risk for both intraoperative and postoperative pulmonary complications. For example, patients with reduced FEV_1/FVC or reduced midexpiratory flow not only suffer airway obstruction but usually exhibit increased airway reactivity. Because of the hazard of provoking reflex bronchoconstriction during laryngoscopy and tracheal intubation, patients with COPD or asthma should receive aggressive bronchodilator therapy preoperatively. High alveolar concentrations of potent inhalational anesthetics will blunt airway reflexes and reflex bronchoconstriction[99] but require a fairly robust cardiovascular system. Adjunctive iv administration of opioids and lidocaine prior to airway instrumentation will decrease airway reactivity. Furthermore, a single dose of corticosteroids may help to prevent postoperative increases in airway resistance.

Spontaneous ventilation during general anesthesia in patients with severe obstructive disease is more likely to result in hypercarbia than in patients with normal pulmonary function.[100] Preoperative FEV_1 reduction is related to the $Paco_2$ increase. Therefore, controlled mechanical ventilation with ventilatory rates <10 breaths · min^{-1} should prevent hypercarbia, minimize $\dot{V}A/\dot{Q}$ mismatch, and allow time for exhalation. Low ventilatory rates necessitate larger tidal volumes, which may predispose the patient to pulmonary barotrauma because of high peak airway pressures. Tidal volume and inspiratory flows should be adjusted to keep peak airway pressure below 40 cm H_2O[101,102] if possible. Higher inspiratory flows produce a shorter inspiratory time and, usually, a high peak airway pressure. Thus, a balance that avoids

Table 29-5. PULMONARY FUNCTION TESTS IN RESTRICTIVE AND OBSTRUCTIVE LUNG DISEASE

Value	Restrictive Disease	Obstructive Disease
Definition	Proportional decreases in all lung volumes	Small airway obstruction to expiratory flow
FVC	↓↓↓	Normal or slightly ↑
FEV_1	↓↓↓	Normal or slightly ↓
FEV_1/FVC	Normal	↓↓↓
$FEF_{25-75\%}$	Normal	↓↓↓
FRC	↓↓↓	Normal or ↑ if gas trapping
TLC	↓↓↓	Normal or ↑ if gas trapping

↓↓↓,↑↑↑ = large decrease or increase, respectively; ↓,↑ = small/moderate decrease or increase, respectively.

high peak airway pressure yet allows the longest possible expiratory time should be sought.

Ideally, depending on the procedure and the duration of anesthesia, one would extubate the patient's trachea at the end of the operation. The irritating tracheal tube increases both airway resistance and reflex bronchoconstriction, limits the ability of the patient to clear secretions effectively, and increases the risk of iatrogenic infection. For some patients with obstructive disease (for example, the young asthmatic), many advocate tracheal extubation during deep anesthesia at the conclusion of the operation.

ANESTHESIA AND RESTRICTIVE PULMONARY DISEASE

Restrictive disease is characterized by proportional decreases in all lung volumes. The decreased FRC produces low lung compliance, and also results in arterial hypoxemia because of low $\dot{V}_A/\dot{Q}$ mismatching. These patients typically breathe rapidly and shallowly.

Positive-pressure ventilation of patients with restrictive disease is fraught with high peak airway pressures because more pressure is required to expand stiff lungs. Lower mechanical tidal volumes at more rapid rates reduce the risk of barotrauma but augment ventilation-induced cardiovascular depression and increase the chances of developing atelectasis. Larger tidal volumes and lower rates result in less cardiovascular compromise, but the higher peak airway pressure increases the risk of barotrauma.[103] A variety of ventilatory schemes have been developed to ventilate patients with profound restrictive lung disease (see Chapter 56). The use of PEEP will increase FRC and reverse arterial hypoxemia and will not, by itself, cause barotrauma.[104] During controlled mechanical ventilation, the cardiovascular effects of PEEP can be profound, although most cardiovascular changes can be reversed by allowing spontaneous ventilation or by iv fluid administration. Inotropes or pressors are rarely required when cardiovascular function is depressed as a consequence of increased mean airway pressure.

Because the FRC is small, a lower oxygen store is available during apneic periods. Even preoxygenation with an F_{IO_2} of 1.0 can result in arterial hypoxemia seconds after the cessation of breathing. Patients with severe restrictive diseases tolerate apnea poorly. Because arterial hypoxemia develops so rapidly, transportation of these patients within the hospital should be performed with a pulse oximeter.

FRC decreases 10–15% when healthy, spontaneously breathing individuals lie supine. Controlled ventilation further reduces FRC only slightly.[105] General anesthesia consistently decreases FRC by a further 5–10%,[106] which usually results in decreased lung compliance.[107] The FRC reaches its nadir within the first 10 minutes of anesthesia[106,108,109] and is independent of whether ventilation is spontaneous or controlled. The diminished FRC persists in the postoperative period[110] but may be restored postoperatively by the use of PEEP or CPAP.[106,111,112]

However, once positive airway pressure is removed, FRC plummets to previously diminished levels, which reach a new postoperative nadir 12 hours after operation.[113]

EFFECTS OF CIGARETTE SMOKING ON PULMONARY FUNCTION

Smoking affects pulmonary function in many ways. The irritant smoke decreases ciliary motility and increases sputum production. Thus, these patients have a high volume of sputum and decreased ability to clear it effectively. As smoking habits persist, airway reactivity and the development of obstructive disease become problematic. Studies of the pathogenesis of COPD suggest that smoking results in an excess of pulmonary proteolytic enzymes which directly cause damage to the lung parenchyma.[114] Exposure to smoke increases synthesis and release of elastolytic enzymes from alveolar macrophages—cells instrumental in the genesis of COPD due to smoking.[115,116] Further damage to the lung tissue is probably caused by reactive metabolites of oxygen, such as hydroxyl radicals and hydrogen peroxide, which are usually used by the macrophages to kill microorganisms. The immunoregulatory function of the macrophages is also changed by cigarette smoking, with changes occurring in the presentation of antigens and interaction with T lymphocytes.[117] Other direct effects on lung tissue caused by smoking include increased epithelial permeability[118] and changed pulmonary surfactant.[119] The airway irritation or small airway reactivity evoked by inhaling cigarette smoke is the result of activation of sensory endings located in the central airways, which is primarily caused by nicotine.[120]

Early in the disease, mild $\dot{V}_A/\dot{Q}$ mismatch, bronchitic disease, and airway hyper-reactivity are primary problems. Later, these problems are accompanied by gas trapping, flattened diaphragmatic configuration (which decreases the efficiency with which the diaphragm functions), and barrel chest deformity. Lung compliance increases significantly, so that limited elastic recoil prevents complete passive emptying. As a result, many patients exhale forcibly to reduce gas trapping.

Smoking also affects gas exchange. With gas trapping, ventilation and perfusion become increasingly mismatched. Large areas of dead space ventilation and venous admixture occur. Carbon dioxide elimination is inefficient because of dead space ventilation. The typical minute ventilation for patients with advanced obstructive lung disease can be 1.5–2 times normal. In addition, venous admixture produces arterial hypoxemia that is exquisitely sensitive to low concentrations of supplemental oxygen. Gas exchange is further impaired by the increased carboxyhemoglobin concentration that results from inspiring smoke. Normal carboxyhemoglobin concentration in nonsmokers is approximately 1%; in smokers, however, it can be as high as 8–10%. Cessation of smoking, even for 12–24 hours preoperatively, can decrease CO concentration to near normal. Although normalization of mucociliary function requires 2–3 weeks of abstinence from smoking, several months of smoking abstinence is required to return sputum clearance to normal.[121] Smokers are at increased risk for developing head and neck cancers, which may influence airway management.

Smoking is one of the main and most prevalent risk factors associated with postoperative morbidity.[122] COPD patients who smoke have a two-[123] to sixfold[124] risk of developing postoperative pneumonia compared to nonsmokers.[125,126] Further, smokers' relative risk of PPC is doubled, even if they do not have evidence of clinical pulmonary disease or abnormal pulmonary function.[127] The incidence of PPC in smokers can be reduced by abstinence from smoking, although there is no consensus on the minimal or optimal duration of preoperative abstinence.[128-130] Smokers who decrease, but do not stop, cigarette consumption without the aid of nicotine replacement therapy, continue to acquire equal amounts of nicotine from fewer cigarettes by changing their technique of smoking to maximize nicotine intake.[131] Levels of serum nicotine and cotinine and urinary mutagenesis levels remain unchanged. Thus, "cold turkey" reduction in the number of cigarettes smoked has much less effect than expected on all aspects of pulmonary function, including PPCs. Use of properly dosed nicotine supplements and antidepressants (e.g., sustained-released bupropion [Zyban®]) can safely achieve abstinence in as many as 40–50% of subjects during the medication administration. These patients may be converted from "partial quitters," who are at high risk for PPC,[124] to "former smokers," whose risk is reduced after 4 weeks.[132] Smoking patients should be advised to *stop* smoking 2 months prior to elective operations to maximize the effect of smoking cessation,[130] or for at least 4 weeks to gain some benefit from improved mucociliary function, and some reduction in PPC rate. If patients cannot stop smoking for these periods of time, they should be advised to stop smoking for at least 24 hours prior to the operation so that carboxyhemoglobin levels will approach normal.

PULMONARY FUNCTION POSTOPERATIVELY

Risk of Postoperative Pulmonary Complications

Preoperative Pulmonary Assessment

Markedly impaired pulmonary function is likely in patients who have the following:

1. Any chronic disease that involves the lung
2. Smoking history, persistent cough, and/or wheezing
3. Chest wall and spinal deformities
4. Morbid obesity
5. Requirement for single lung anesthesia or lung resection
6. Severe neuromuscular disease

Preoperative pulmonary evaluation must include history and physical examination, and may include chest radiograph, arterial blood gas analysis, and screening spirometry, depending on the patient's history. A history of sputum production, wheezing or dyspnea, exercise intolerance, or limited daily activities may yield more practical information than does formal testing. Arterial blood analysis, which should be sampled while the patient breathes room air, adds information regarding gas exchange and acid–base balance. Arterial blood gas sampling is primarily useful if the patient's history suggests that s/he may be chronically hypoxemic or may "retain" CO_2—i.e., a patient with a chronic, compensated arterial acidemia.

Preoperative assessment of pulmonary function may alert the anesthesiologist to the special needs of a patient with respiratory disease and may allow improvement of pulmonary function before an elective operation. There are published data[133] and published opinions[134,135] concerning guidelines that select patients who should undergo pulmonary function testing preoperatively and whether the tests have any predictive value.[136] The goals one might *hope* to achieve through preoperative pulmo-

nary function would be to predict the likelihood of pulmonary complications, to obtain quantitative baseline information concerning pulmonary function, and to identify patients who may benefit from therapy to improve pulmonary function preoperatively. For patients who will have lung resections, pulmonary function testing does provide some predictive benefit.[137] For all other patients, however, overwhelming evidence suggests that preoperative pulmonary function testing does *not* predict or assign risk for PPCs.[138,139]

The need to obtain baseline pulmonary function data should be reserved for those patients with severely impaired preoperative pulmonary function, such as quadriplegics or myasthenics, so that assessment for weaning from mechanical ventilation and/or tracheal extubation might be based on the patient's baseline pulmonary function. Ideally, tests should be chosen to quantify specific pulmonary problems.

Postoperative Pulmonary Function

The changes in pulmonary function that occur postoperatively are primarily restrictive, with proportional decreases in all lung volumes and no change in airway resistance. The decrease in FRC, however, is the yardstick by which the severity of the restrictive defect is gauged. This defect is generated by abdominal contents that impinge on and prevent normal movement of the diaphragm, and by an abnormal respiratory pattern devoid of sighs and characterized by shallow, rapid respirations. The normal resting respiratory rate for adults is 12 breaths per minute, whereas the postoperative patient in the ward usually breathes approximately 20 breaths per minute. Furthermore, most (but not all) of the factors that tend to make the restrictive defect worse are also those factors associated with a higher risk of postoperative pulmonary complications.

The operative site is the single most important determinant of both the degree of pulmonary restriction and the risk of postoperative pulmonary complications.[138] Nonlaparoscopic upper abdominal operations cause the most profound restrictive defect, precipitating a 40–50% decrease in FRC compared to preoperative levels, when conventional postoperative analgesia is employed. Lower abdominal and thoracic operations cause the next most severe change in pulmonary function, with decreases in FRC to 30% of preoperative levels. Most other operative sites—intracranial, peripheral vascular, otolaryngologic—have approximately the same effect on FRC, with reductions to 15–20% of preoperative levels.[140]

Postoperative Pulmonary Complications

Two problems confound interpretation of the literature examining postoperative pulmonary complications. First, there is no clear definition of what constitutes a postoperative pulmonary complication. For example, some series include only pneumonia, while others add atelectasis and/or ventilatory failure. Thus, to interpret data concerning rates of postoperative pulmonary complications, it is important to discern what complications are specifically being addressed. Second, the criteria by which to make the diagnosis of postoperative pneumonia or atelectasis vary from study to study. For the purposes of this discussion, postoperative pulmonary complications include atelectasis and pneumonia only. Reasonable, well-accepted diagnostic criteria for these diagnoses include: change in the color and quantity of sputum, oral temperature exceeding 38.5°C, and a new infiltrate on chest X-ray.

The operative site is the single most important determinant of both the degree of pulmonary restriction and postoperative pulmonary complications.[138] Nonlaparoscopic upper abdominal operations increase risk for PPC at least twofold,[138] with rates of occurrence varying from 20–70%.[141] Lower abdominal and intrathoracic operations are associated with slightly less risk, but still higher risk than extremity, intracranial, and head/neck operations.

Other patients at risk for PPC are those with COPD. These patients' risk can be minimized by ensuring that they do not have an active pulmonary infection and that any increased resistance associated with reactive airways disease is minimized by the use of therapeutic bronchodilation. Interestingly, those with asthma are not at increased risk for atelectasis or pneumonia. However, exacerbation of asthma in the postoperative period can be problematic. Careful attention must be given to assuring bronchodilating regimens and steroid administration in the perioperative period.

There are several strategies by which it is possible to reduce risk of PPC: the use of lung-expanding therapies postoperatively, choice of analgesia,[142] and cessation of smoking. After upper abdominal operations, which are associated with the highest incidence of postoperative pulmonary complications, FRC recovers over 3–7 days. With the use of intermittent CPAP by mask, FRC will recover within 72 hours.[143] Patients use incentive spirometers correctly only 10% of the time unless therapy is supervised.[144] Stir-up regimens are as effective as incentive spirometry at preventing postoperative pulmonary complications,[143] and they are less expensive than supervised incentive spirometry; thus, they are preferred over incentive spirometry therapy.

After median sternotomy for cardiac operations, FRC does not return to normal for several weeks, regardless of postoperative pulmonary therapy.[145] The persistently low FRC in this population probably is due to mechanical factors such as a widened mediastinum, intrapleural fluid, and altered chest wall compliance. The single most important aspect of postoperative pulmonary care is getting the patient out of bed, preferably walking.

The choice of anesthestic technique for intraoperative anesthesia does not change the risk for PPC independent of the operative site. However, choice of postoperative analgesia strongly influences the risk of PPC.[138] The advent of postoperative epidural analgesia, particularly for abdominal and thoracic operations, has markedly decreased the risk of PPC and appears to contribute to decreased length of stay in the hospital postoperatively.

Although obesity is associated with marked restrictive defects, some studies demonstrate that obesity does not independently increase the risk of PPC while others do demonstrate increased independent risk for PPCs in the obese population.[146] Similarly, there are data both to support[146] and refute advanced age as an independent risk factor for PPCs.

Several authors have attempted to assess the influence of overall health on PPC risk. The use of indices that weight and score various aspects of physiology and health shows that all are associated with increased risk of PPC.[139] That is, patients who are in a poor state of health preoperatively tend to be at higher risk of PPC.

Patients with obstructive airway disease and decreased expiratory flows may benefit from preoperative bronchodilator therapy and formal pulmonary toilet.[147] High-risk patients with COPD who receive bronchodilation, chest physical therapy, deep breathing, forced oral fluids ($>3\,l\cdot day^{-1}$), and preoperative instruction in postoperative respiratory techniques, and those who stop smoking experience postoperative pulmonary complications at a rate approximately equal to that observed in normal patients.[148–150] Interestingly, although a regimen of this nature significantly reduces the incidence of postoperative pulmonary complications,[151] airway obstruction and arterial hypoxemia are not measurably reversed during the 48–72 hours of preoperative therapy.[152] It is possible that the reduced complication rate results from the additional attention that these patients receive rather than from the specific regimen employed.

REFERENCES

1. Goss CM (ed): Gray's Anatomy of the Human Body, 29th ed. Philadelphia, Lea & Febiger, 1966

2. Netter FH: Respiratory System. In Divertic MB, Brass A (eds): Ciba Collection of Medical Illustrations, vol 7. Newark, NJ, Ciba, 1979

3. Wade OL: Movements of thoracic cage and diaphragm in respiration. J Physiol (Lond) 124:193, 1954

4. Gillespi DJ, Marsh HMM, Divertie MB et al: Clinical outcome of respiratory failure in patients requiring prolonged (>24 hours) mechanical ventilation. Chest 90:364, 1986

5. Burke RE, Levine DN, Zojas FE et al: Mammalian motor units: Physiologic histochemical correlation in these types of cat gastrocnemius. Science 174:709, 1971

6. Lieberman DA, Falkner JA, Craig AB Jr et al: Performance and histochemical composition of guinea pig and human diaphragm. J Appl Physiol 34:233, 1973

7. Roussos C, Macklin PT: Diaphragmatic fatigue in man. J Appl Physiol 43:189, 1977

8. Murphy AJ, Koepec GH, Smith EM et al: Sequence of action of diaphragm and intercostal muscles during respiration: II. Expiration. Arch Phys Med 40:337, 1959

9. Petit JM, Milic-Emili G, Delhez L: Role of the diaphragm in breathing in conscious normal man: An electromyographic study. J Appl Physiol 15:1101, 1960

10. Coryllos PN: Action of the diaphragm in cough: Experimental and clinical study on the human. Am J Med Sci 194:523, 1937

11. Campbell EJM, Green JH: The behavior of the abdominal muscles and intra-abdominal pressure during quiet breathing and increased pulmonary ventilation: A study in man. J Physiol (Lond) 127:423, 1955

12. Conrardy PA, Goodman CR, Lainge F et al: Alteration of endotracheal tube position: Flexion and extension of the neck. Crit Care Med 4:8, 1976

13. Rhodin JAG: An Atlas of Ultrastructure. Philadelphia, WB Saunders, 1963

14. Auerbach O, Stout AP, Hammond EC et al: Changes in bronchial epithelium in relation to cigarette smoking and in relation to lung cancer. N Engl J Med 265:253, 1961

15. Gail DB, L'Enfant CJM: Cells of the lung: Biology and clinical implications. Am Rev Respir Dis 127:366, 1983

16. Bachoven M, Weibel ER: Basic pattern of tissue repair in human lungs following unspecific injury. Chest 65:145, 1974

17. Kikkawa Y, Yoneda K, Smith F: The type II epithelial cells of the lung: Chemical composition and phospholipid synthesis. Lab Invest 32:295, 1975

18. Fishman AP: Non-respiratory function of lung. Chest 72:84, 1977

19. Mason RJ, Williams MC, Widdicombe JH: Secretion and fluid transport by alveolar type II epithelial cells. Chest 81(suppl):61, 1982

20. Hocking WG, Golden DW: The pulmonary-alveolar macrophage. N Engl J Med 301:580, 1979

21. Macklin CC: Alveolar pores and their significance in the human lung. Arch Pathol 21:202, 1936

22. Lambert MW: Accessory bronchio-alveolar channels. Anat Rec 127:472, 1957

23. Downs JB: A technique for direct measurement of intrapleural pressure. Crit Care Med 4:207, 1976

24. Baydur A, Behrakis P, Zin WA: A simple method for assessing the validity of the esophageal balloon technique. Am Rev Resp Dis 126:788, 1982

25. Blanch MJ, Kirby RR, Gabrielli A et al: Partially and totally unloading the respiratory muscles based on real time measurements of work of breathing. Chest 106:1835, 1994

26. Brochard L, Rua F, Lorino H: Inspiratory pressure support compensates for the additional work of breathing caused by the endotracheal tube. Anesthesiology 75:739, 1991

27. Brochard L, Rau F, Lorino H: Inspiratory pressure support prevents diaphragmatic fatigue during weaning from mechanical ventilation. Am Rev Respir Dis 139:513, 1989

28. Sassoon CS, Giron AE, Ely EA: Inspiratory work of breathing on flow-by and demand-flow continuous positive airway pressure. Crit Care Med 17:1108, 1989

29. Van de Graff WB, Gordey K, Dornseif SE: Pressure support: Changes in ventilatory pattern and components of the work of breathing. Chest 100:1082, 1991

30. Marini JJ: Breathing effort and work of breathing during mechanical ventilation: Positive pressure ventilation. Probl Crit Care 4:184, 1990

31. Banner MJ, Blanch PB, Kirby RR: Imposed work of breathing and

methods of triggering a demand-flow, continuous positive airway pressure system. Crit Care Med 21:183, 1993

32. Banner MJ: Respiratory muscle function and the work of breathing: Clinical implications. Crit Care Updates 2:1, 1995

33. Rohrer F: Der Strömungswiderstand in den menschlichen Atemwegen. Pflugers Arch 162:225, 1915

34. Nunn JF: Resistance to gas flow and airway closure. In Applied Respiratory Physiology, p 50. Boston, Butterworths, 1987

35. Fink BR, Ngai SH, Holiday DA: Effect of air flow resistance on ventilation and respiratory muscle activity. JAMA 168:2245, 1958

36. Campbell EJM, Freedman S, Smith PS, Taylor ME: The ability of man to detect added elastic loads to breathing. Clin Sci 20:223, 1961

37. Nunn JF, Ezi-Ashi TI: The respiratory effects of resistance to breathing in anesthetized man. Anesthesiology 22:174, 1961

38. Palmer KNV, Diament ML: Effect of aerosol isoprenaline on blood-gas tensions in severe bronchial asthma. Lancet 2:1232, 1967

39. Campbell EJM: The effects of increased resistance to expiration on the respiratory behavior of the abdominal muscles and intraabdominal pressure. J Physiol 136:556, 1957

40. LeGallois CJJ: Expériences sur le Principe de la Vie, p 325. Paris, D'Hautel, 1812

41. Brodie DA, Borison HL: Evidence for a medullary inspiratory pacemaker: Functional concept of central regulation of respiration. Am J Physiol 188:347, 1957

42. Comroe JH Jr: The effects of direct chemical and electrical stimulation of the respiratory center in the cat. Am J Physiol 139:490, 1943

43. Ngai SH, Wang SC: Organization of central respiratory mechanisms in the brainstem of the cats: Localization by stimulation and destruction. Am J Physiol 190:343, 1957

44. Pitts RF: The differentiation of respiratory centers. Am J Physiol 134:192, 1941

45. Pitts RF, Magoun HW, Ranson SW: Localization of the medullary respiratory centers in the cat. Am J Physiol 126:673, 1939

46. Salmoiraghi GC, Burns BD: Localization and patterns of discharge of respiratory neurons in the brainstem of a cat. J Neurophysiol 23:2, 1960

47. Cohen MI: Neurogenesis of respiratory rhythm in the mammal. Physiol Rev 51:1105, 1979

48. Guz A: Regulation of respiration in man. Ann Resp Physiol 37:303, 1975

49. Pitts RF, Magoun HW, Ranson SW: The origin of respiratory rhythmicity. Am J Physiol 127:654, 1939

50. Lumsden TL: Observations on the respiratory centers in the cat. J Physiol (Lond) 57:153, 1923

51. Cohen MI, Wang SC: Respiratory neuronal activity in the pons of the cat. J Neurophysiol 22:33, 1959

52. Stella G: On the mechanism of production and the physiologic significance of "apneusis." J Physiol (Lond) 93:10, 1938

53. Kabat H: Electrical stimulation of points in the forebrain and midbrain: The resultant alterations in respiration. J Comp Neurol 64:187, 1936

54. Kaada BR: Somato-motor, autonomic and electrocorticographic responses to electrical stimulation of "rhinencephalic" and other structures in primates, cat and dog: A study of responses from the limbic, subcallosal, orbito-insular, piriform and temporal cortex, hippocampus-fornix and amygdala. Acta Physiol Scand 24(suppl 83):1, 1951

55. Chai CY, Wang SC: Localization of central cardiovascular control mechanism in lower brainstem of the cat. Am J Physiol 202:25, 1962

56. Uvnas B: Central cardiovascular control. In Handbook of Physiology, Section I, vol II: Neurophysiology, p 1131. Washington DC, American Physiological Society, 1960

57. Bosma JF: Deglutition: Pharyngeal stage. Physiol Rev 37:275, 1957

58. Wang SC, Borison HL: The vomiting center: A critical experimental analysis. Arch Neurol Psychiatry 63:928, 1950

59. Gaylor JB: The intrinsic nervous mechanisms of the human lung. Brain 57:143, 1934

60. von Euler C: On the role of proprioceptors in perception and execution of motor acts with special reference to breathing. In Pengelly LD, Rebuck AS, Campbell JBL (eds): Loaded Breathing, p 139. Ontario, Canada, Longman, Don Mills, 1974

61. Davis HL, Fowler WS, Lambert EH: Effect of volume and rate of inflation and deflation on transpulmonary pressure and response of pulmonary stretch receptors. Am J Physiol 187:558, 1956

62. Dawes GS, Comroe JH Jr: Chemoreflexes from the heart and lungs. Physiol Rev 34:167, 1954

63. Jung-Caillot MC, Duron B: Number of neuromuscular spindles and electrical activity of the respiratory muscles. In Durm B (ed): Respiratory Centers and Afferent Systems, p 165. Paris, INSERM, 1976

64. Hering E, Breuer J: Die Sebsteuerung der Atmung durch den Nervus vagus. Stizber Akad Wiss Wien 57:672, 1868

65. Biscoe TJ: Carotid body: Structure and function. Physiol Rev 58:604, 1978

66. Coleridge HM: Thoracic chemoreceptors in the dog: A histological and electrophysiologic study of the location, innervation and blood supply of the aortic bodies. Circ Res 26:235, 1970

67. Leusen I: Regulation of cerebrospinal fluid composition with reference to breathing. Physiol Rev 52:1, 1972

68. Cohen MI: Discharge patterns of brainstem respiratory neurons in relation to carbon dioxide tension. J Neurophysiol 31:142, 1968

69. Heinemann HO, Golaring RM: Bicarbonate and the regulation of ventilation. Am J Med 57:361, 1974

70. Severinghaus JW, Mitchell RA, Richardson BW et al: Respiratory control at high altitude suggesting active transport regulation of CSF pH. J Appl Physiol 18:1155, 1166, 1963

71. Ferris EB, Engel GL, Stevens CD, Webb J: Voluntary breath holding. J Clin Invest 25:734, 1946

72. Stock MC, Downs JB, McDonald JS et al: The carbon dioxide rate of rise in awake apneic man. J Clin Anesth 1:96, 1988

73. Engle GL, Ferris EB, Webb JP et al: Voluntary breathholding: II. The relation of the maximum time of breathholding to the oxygen tension of the inspired air. J Clin Invest 23:734, 1946

74. Eger EI, Severinghaus JW: The rate of rise of $Paco_2$ in the apneic anesthetized patient. Anesthesiology 22:419, 1961

75. Stock MC, Schisler JQ, McSweeney TD: The $Paco_2$ rate of rise in anesthetized patients with airway obstruction. J Clin Anesth 1:328, 1989

76. Wright FG, Foley MF, Downs JB et al: Hypoxemia and hypocarbia following intermittent positive-pressure breathing. Anesth Analg 55:555, 1976

77. Fink BR: The stimulant effect of wakefulness on respiration: Clinical aspects. Br J Anaesth 33:97, 1961

78. Berger AJ, Mitchell RA, Severinghaus JW: Regulation of respiration: III. N Engl J Med 297:194, 1977

79. West JB: Ventilation/Blood Flow and Gas Exchange, 4th ed. Oxford, England, Blackwell Scientific Publications, 1985

80. West JB, Dollery CT, Naimark A: Distribution of blood flow in isolated lung: Relation to vascular and alveolar pressures. J Appl Physiol 19:713, 1964

81. West JB, Dollery CT: Distribution of blood flow and the pressure-flow relations of the whole lung. J Appl Physiol 20:175, 1965

82. Bendixen HH, Egbert LD, Hedley-Whyte J et al: Respiratory Care. St Louis, CV Mosby, 1965

83. Benumof JL, Pirla AF, Johanson I et al: Interaction of Pvo_2 with Pao_2 on hypoxic pulmonary vasoconstriction. J Appl Physiol 51:871, 1981

84. Swenson EW, Finley TN, Guzman SV: Unilateral hypoventilation in man during temporary occlusion of one pulmonary artery. J Clin Invest 40:828, 1961

85. West JB: Ventilation–perfusion relationships. Am Rev Respir Dis 116:919, 1977

86. Fowler WS: Lung function studies: II. The respiratory deadspace. Am J Physiol 154:405, 1948

87. Freeman J, Nunn JF: Ventilation–perfusion relationships after hemorrhage. Clin Sci 24:135, 1963

88. Bergman NA: Effect of varying respiratory waveforms on distribution of inspired gas during artificial ventilation. Am Rev Respir Dis 100:518, 1969

89. Yamanaka MK, Sue DY: Comparison of arterial-end-tidal Pco_2 difference and deadspace/tidal volume ratio in respiratory failure. Chest 92:832, 1987

90. Weil MH, Bisera J, Trevino RP et al: Cardiac output and end-tidal carbon dioxide. Crit Care Med 13:907, 1985

91. Murray IP, Modell JH: Early detection of endotracheal tube accidents by monitoring carbon dioxide concentration in respiratory gas. Anesthesiology 59:344, 1983

92. Meler C, Naeije R, Delchamps P et al: Pulmonary and extrapulmonary contributions and hypoxia in liver cirrhosis. Am Rev Respir Dis 139:632, 1989

93. Räsänen J, Downs JB, Malec DJ, Oates K: Oxygen tensions and oxyhemoglobin saturations in the assessment of pulmonary gas exchange. Crit Care Med 15:1058, 1987

94. Christi RV: Lung volume and its subdivisions. J Clin Invest 11:1099, 1932

95. Tisi GM: Preoperative evaluation of pulmonary function. Am Rev Respir Dis 119:293, 1979

96. Apthorp GH, Marshall R: Pulmonary diffusing capacity: A comparison of breath-holding and steady-state methods using carbon monoxide. J Clin Invest 40:1775, 1961

97. Crapo RO: Pulmonary function testing. N Engl J Med 331:25, 1994

98. American Thoracic Society: Lung function testing: Selection of reference values and interpretive strategies. Am Rev Respir Dis 144:1202, 1991

99. Yakaitas RW, Blitt CP, Anguillo JP: End-tidal halothane concentration for endotracheal intubation. Anesthesiology 47:386, 1977

100. Pietak W, Weenig CS, Hickey RF et al: Anesthetic effects on ventilation in patients with chronic obstructive pulmonary disease. Anesthesiology 42:160, 1975

101. Connors AF, McAferee D, Gray BA: Effect of inspiratory flow rate on gas exchange during mechanical ventilation. Am Rev Respir Dis 124:537, 1981

102. Tuxen DV, Lane S: The effects of ventilatory pattern on hyperinflation, airway pressures, and circulation in mechanical ventilation of patients with severe airflow obstruction. Am Rev Respir Dis 136:872, 1987

103. Petersen GW, Baier H: Incidence of pulmonary barotrauma in a medical ICU. Crit Care Med 11:67, 1983

104. Pepe PE, Hudson LD, Carrico CJ: Early application of positive end-expiratory pressure in patients at risk for the adult respiratory distress syndrome. N Engl J Med 311:281, 1984

105. Bergofsky EH: Ions and membrane permeability in the regulation of the pulmonary circulation. In Fishman AP, Hect H (eds): The Pulmonary Circulation and Interstitial Space, p 269. Chicago, University of Chicago Press, 1969

106. Brisner B, Hedenstierna G, Lundquist H et al: Pulmonary densities during anesthesia with muscular relaxation: A proposal of atelectasis. Anesthesiology 62:422, 1985

107. Don HF, Robson JG: The mechanics of the respiratory system during anesthesia. Anesthesiology 26:168, 1965

108. Don HF, Wahba M, Cuadrado L et al: The effects of anesthesia and 100 percent oxygen on the functional residual capacity of the lungs. Anesthesiology 32:251, 1970

109. Westbrook PR, Stubbs SE, Sessler AD et al: Effects of anesthesia and muscle paralysis on respiratory mechanics in normal man. J Appl Physiol 34:81, 1973

110. Alexander JI, Spence AA, Parikh RK et al: The role of air-way closure in postoperative hypoxemia. Br J Anaesth 45:34, 1975

111. Wyche MQ, Teichner RL, Kallost T et al: Effects of continuous positive-pressure breathing on functional residual capacity and arterial oxygenation during intra-abdominal operation. Anesthesiology 38:68, 1973

112. Rose DM, Downs JB, Heenen TJ: Temporal responses of functional residual capacity and oxygen tension to changes in positive end-expiratory pressure. Crit Care Med 9:79, 1981

113. Craig DB: Postoperative recovery of pulmonary function. Anesth Analg 60:46, 1981

114. Diamond L, Lai YL: Augmentation of elastase-induced emphysema by cigarette smoke: Effects of reducing tar and nicotine content. J Toxicol Environ Health 20:287, 1987

115. Janoff A, Raju L, Dearing R: Levels of elastase activity in bronchoalveolar lavage fluids of healthy smokers and non-smokers. Am Rev Resp Dis 127:540, 1983

116. Rodriguez FJ, White RR, Senior RM, Levine EA: Elastase release from human alveolar macrophages: Comparison between smokers and non-smokers. Science 198:313, 1977

117. Deshazo RD, Banks DE, Diem JE et al: Broncho-alveolar lavage cell–lymphocyte interactions in normal nonsmokers and smokers. Am Rev Resp Dis 127:545, 1983

118. Hogg JC: The effect of smoking on airway permeability. Chest 83: 1, 1983

119. Clements JA: Smoking and pulmonary surfactant. N Engl J Med 286: 261, 1972

120. Lee L-Y, Gerhardstein DC, Wang AL, Burki NK: Nicotine is responsible for airway irritation evoked by cigarette smoke inhalation in men. J Appl Physiol 75:1955, 1993

121. Beckers S, Camu F: The anesthetic risk of tobacco smoking. Acta Anaesth Belg 42:45, 1991

122. Warner MA, Divertie MB, Tinker JH: Preoperative cessation of smoking and pulmonary complications in coronary artery bypass patients. Anesthesiology 60:380, 1984

123. Garibaldi RA, Britt MR, Coleman ML et al: Risk factors for postoperative pneumonia. Am J Med 70:677, 1981

124. Bluman LG, Mosca L, Newman N, Simon DG: Preoperative smoking habits and postoperative pulmonary complications. Chest 113:883, 1998

125. Morton HTJ: Tobacco smoking and pulmonary complications after operation. Lancet 1:368, 1944

126. Dales RE, Dionne G, Leech JA et al: Preoperative prediction of pulmonary complications following thoracic surgery. Chest 104:155, 1993

127. Chalon J, Tayyab MA, Ramanathan S: Cytology of respiratory complications after operation. Chest 67:32, 1975

128. Lillington GA, Sachs DPL: Preoperative smoking reduction: All or nothing at all? Chest 113:856, 1998

129. Celli BR: Perioperative care of patients undergoing upper abdominal surgery. Clin Chest Med 14:227, 1993

130. Waner MA, Offord KP, Warner ME et al: Role of postoperative cessation of smoking and other factors in postoperative pulmonary complications: A blinded prospective study of coronary artery bypass patients. Mayo Clin Proc 64:609, 1989

131. Benowitz NL, Jacob P, Kozlowski LT et al: Influence of smoking fewer cigarettes on exposure to tar, nicotine and carbon monoxide. N Engl J Med 3115:1310, 1986

132. Hurt RD, Sachs DPL, Gover ED et al: A comparison of sustained-release bupropion and placebo of smoking cessation. N Engl J Med 337:1195, 1997

133. American College of Physicians: Preoperative pulmonary function testing. Ann Intern Med 112:793, 1990

134. Dunn WF, Scanlon PD: Preoperative pulmonary function testing for patients with lung cancer. Mayo Clin Proc 68:371, 1993

135. Celli BR: What is the value of preoperative pulmonary function testing? Med Clin North Am 77:309, 1993

136. Mitchell CK, Smoger SH, Pfeifer MP et al: Multivariate analysis of factors associated with postoperative pulmonary complications following general elective surgery. Arch Surg 133:194, 1998

137. Kearney DJ, Lee TH, Reilly JJ et al: Assessment of operative risk in patients undergoing lung resection: Importance of predicted pulmonary function. Chest 105:753, 1994

138. Ferguson MK: Preoperative assessment of pulmonary risk. Chest 115:58S, 1999

139. Lawrence VA, Dhanda R, Hilsenbeck SG, Page CP: Risk of pulmonary complications after elective abdominal surgery. Chest 110:744, 1996

140. Ali J, Gana TJ: Lung volumes 24 h after laparoscopic cholecystectomy—justification for early discharge. Can Respir J 5:109, 1998

141. Hall JC, Tarala RA, Hall JL et al: A multivariate analysis of the risk of pulmonary complications after laparotomy. Chest 99:923, 1991

142. Gust R, Pecher S, Gust A et al: Effect of patient-controlled analgesia on pulmonary complications after coronary artery bypass grafting. Crit Care Med 27:2218, 1999

143. Stock MC, Downs JB, Gauer PK et al: Prevention of postoperative pulmonary complications with CPAP, incentive spirometry and conservative therapy. Chest 87:151, 1985

144. Lyager S, Wernberg M, Rajani N et al: Can postoperative pulmonary complications be improved by treatment with Bartlett-Edwards incentive spirometer after upper abdominal surgery? Acta Anaesthesiol Scand 23:312, 1979

145. Stock MC, Downs JB, Cooper RB et al: Comparison of continuous positive airway pressure, incentive spirometry, and conservative therapy after cardiac operations. Crit Care Med 12:969, 1984

146. Brooks-Brunn JA: Predictors of postoperative pulmonary complications following abdominal surgery. Chest 111:564, 1997

147. Chumillas S, Pace JL, Delgado F et al: Prevention of postoperative pulmonary complications through respiratory rehabilitation: A controlled clinical trial. Arch Phys Med Rehab 79:5, 1998

148. Stein M, Cassara EL: Preoperative pulmonary evaluation and therapy for surgery patients. JAMA 211:787, 1970

149. Brooks-Brunn JA: Validation of a predictive model for postoperative pulmonary complications. Heart Lung 27:151, 1998

150. Williams CD, Brenowitz JB: "Prohibitive" lung function and major surgical procedures. Am J Surg 132:703, 1976

151. Gracey DR, Divertie MB, Didier EP: Preoperative pulmonary preparation of patients with chronic obstructive pulmonary disease: A prospective study. Chest 76:123, 1979

152. Petty TL, Brink GA, Miller NW, Corsello PR: Objective functional improvement in chronic airway obstruction. Chest 57:216, 1970

Clinical Anesthesia (4/e), edited by
Paul G. Barash, Bruce F. Cullen, and
Robert K. Stoelting. Lippincott Williams &
Wilkins, Philadelphia, © 2001.

CHAPTER 30

ANESTHESIA FOR THORACIC SURGERY

JAMES B. EISENKRAFT, EDMOND COHEN, AND
STEVEN M. NEUSTEIN

The number of noncardiac thoracic surgical operations has dramatically increased in recent years and is expected to increase further in the future. A report using data from the National Center for Health Statistics in the United States showed that in 1979, approximately 53,000 procedures on the lung and bronchus were performed; this number had grown to 73,000 by 1983.[1] Mediastinoscopies increased from 33,000 in 1979 to 44,000 in 1983. Most recently, there has been an increase in the number of video-assisted thoracoscopic procedures. The increase in this type of surgery has been associated with and sometimes has been made possible by advances in anesthesia care. Indeed, thoracic anesthesia is developing into a subspecialty in its own right, with reference texts devoted exclusively to this subject.[2, 3]

The physiologic, pharmacologic, and clinical considerations for the patient undergoing pulmonary surgery are reviewed, followed by sections on anesthesia for diagnostic and therapeutic procedures, high-frequency ventilation, and special situations, including bronchopleural fistula (BPF) and tracheal reconstruction. A discussion of myasthenia gravis is included because of the relationship between the thymus gland and myasthenia and because thymectomy is one of the most commonly performed surgical procedures in these patients. The chapter concludes with a review of the postoperative management of the thoracic surgical patient.

PREOPERATIVE EVALUATION

In addition to the routine assessment for major surgery, the preoperative evaluation of the patient for thoracic surgery should focus on the extent and severity of pulmonary disease and of cardiovascular involvement.

History

Dyspnea. Dyspnea occurs when the requirement for ventilation is greater than the patient's ability to respond appropriately. Dyspnea is quantitated as to the degree of physical activity required to produce it, the level of activity possible (*e.g.*, ability to walk on level ground or climb stairs), and management of daily activities. Severe exertional dyspnea usually implies a significantly diminished ventilatory reserve and a forced expiratory volume in 1 second (FEV_1) of less than 1500 ml, with possible need for postoperative ventilatory support.

Cough. Recurrent productive cough for 3 months of the year for 2 consecutive years is necessary to make the diagnosis of chronic bronchitis. Cough indirectly increases airway irritability. If the cough is productive, the volume, consistency, and color of the sputum should be assessed. Sputum should be cultured to rule out infection and to establish whether there is a need for preoperative antibiotic therapy. Blood-stained sputum or episodes of gross hemoptysis should alert the anesthesiologist to the possibility of a tumor invading the respiratory tract (*e.g.*, the mainstem bronchus), which might interfere with endobronchial intubation.

Cigarette Smoking. Cigarette smoking increases the risk of chronic lung disease and malignancy as well as the incidence of postoperative pulmonary complications. The number of pack-years (packs smoked per day multiplied by the number of years) is directly related to measurable changes in respiratory gas flow and closing capacity, making these patients prone to postoperative atelectasis and arterial hypoxemia.

Physical Examination

The physical examination of the patient should address in particular the following aspects.

Respiratory Pattern

The presence of cyanosis and clubbing, the breathing pattern, and the type of breath sounds should be noted.

Cyanosis. The presence of peripheral cyanosis (in the fingers, toes, or ears) should be distinguished from causes of poor circulation (acrocyanosis). The presence of central cyanosis (in the buccal mucosa) is usually secondary to arterial hypoxemia. If cyanosis is present, the arterial saturation is 80% or less (Pao_2 <50–52 mm Hg), which indicates a limited margin of respiratory reserve.

Clubbing. Clubbing is often seen in patients with chronic lung disease, malignancies, or congenital heart disease associated with right-to-left shunt.

Respiratory Rate and Pattern. A patient's inability to complete a normal sentence without pausing for breath is an indication of severe dyspnea. Inspiratory paradox, the abdomen moving in while the chest moves out, suggests diaphragmatic fatigue and respiratory dysfunction. The patient should be assessed for paroxysmal retraction (Hoover's sign), limited diaphragmatic movement because of hyperinflation, asymmetry of chest movement secondary to phrenic nerve involvement, hemothorax, pleural effusion, and pneumothorax. The pattern and rate of breathing have important roles in distinguishing between obstructive and restrictive lung disease. For a constant minute ventilation, the work done against air flow resistance decreases when breathing is slow and deep. Work done against elastic resistance decreases when breathing is rapid and shallow (*e.g.*, as in pulmonary infarct or pulmonary fibrosis).

Breath Sounds. Wet sounds (crackles) are usually caused by excessive fluid in the airways and indicate sputum retention or edema. Dry sounds (wheezes) are produced by high-velocity gas flow through bronchi and are a sign of airway obstruction. Distant sounds are an indication of emphysema and possibly bullae. The trachea should be in the midline. Displacement of the trachea may be secondary to a number of causes, including mediastinal mass, and should alert the anesthesiologist to a potentially difficult intubation of the trachea or airway obstruction on induction of anesthesia.

Evaluation of the Cardiovascular System

One of the most important factors in the evaluation of a patient scheduled for thoracic surgery is the presence of an increase in pulmonary vascular resistance secondary to a fixed reduction in the cross-sectional area of the pulmonary vascular bed. The pulmonary circulation is a low-pressure, high-compliance system capable of handling an increase in blood flow by recruitment of normally underperfused vessels. This acts as a compensatory mechanism, which normally prevents an increase in pulmonary arterial pressure. In chronic obstructive pulmonary disease (COPD), there is distention of the pulmonary capillary bed with reduced ability to tolerate an increase in blood flow (reduced compliance). Such patients demonstrate an increase in pulmonary vascular resistance when cardiac output increases because of a reduced ability to compensate for an increase in pulmonary blood flow. This results in pulmonary hypertension, signs of which include a narrowly split second heart sound, increased intensity of the pulmonary component of the second heart sound, and right ventricular and atrial hypertrophy.

An increase in pulmonary vascular resistance is of significance in the management of the patient during anesthesia because several factors, such as acidosis, sepsis, hypoxia, and application of positive end-expiratory pressure (PEEP), all further increase the pulmonary vascular resistance and increase the likelihood of right ventricular failure.

In patients with ischemic or valvular heart disease, the function of the left side of the heart should also be carefully evaluated. This is discussed elsewhere in this volume (see Chapter 32).

Electrocardiogram

A patient with COPD may present with electrocardiographic features of right atrial and ventricular hypertrophy and strain. These include a low-voltage QRS complex due to lung hyperinflation and poor R-wave progression across the precordial leads. An enlarged P wave ("P pulmonale") in standard lead II is diagnostic of right atrial hypertrophy. The electrocardiographic changes of right ventricular hypertrophy are an R/S ratio of greater than 1.0 in lead V_1 (i.e., R-wave voltage exceeds S-wave voltage).

Chest Radiography

Hyperinflation and increased vascular markings are usually present with COPD. Prominent lung markings often occur in bronchitis, whereas they are decreased in emphysema, particularly at the bases, where actual bullae may be present in severe cases. Hyperinflation, with an increased anteroposterior chest diameter, may be present, together with an enlarged retrosternal air space of greater than 2 cm in diameter seen in a lateral chest radiograph.

The location of the lung lesion should be assessed by posteroanterior and lateral projections on chest radiography. In addition to tracheal or carinal shift, a mediastinal mass may indicate a difficult intubation, a difficult and bloody dissection, difficulty in using a double-lumen tube (because of deviation of the mainstem bronchus), or a collapsed lobe owing to bronchial obstruction with possible sepsis. Review of a computed tomographic study is also useful and often provides more information about tumor size and location than the chest radiograph.

Arterial Blood Gases

A common finding in arterial blood gas analysis of patients with COPD is hypoventilation and CO_2 retention. The "blue bloaters" (chronic bronchitics) are cyanotic, hypercarbic, hypoxemic, and usually overweight. They are in a state of chronic respiratory failure and have a reduced ventilatory response to CO_2. In these patients, the high Pa_{CO_2} increases cerebrospinal fluid bicarbonate concentration, the medullary chemoreceptors become reset to a higher level of CO_2, and sensitivity to CO_2 is decreased. Such patients hypoventilate when given high oxygen concentrations because of a decreased hypoxic drive.

The "pink puffers" (patients with emphysema) typically are thin, dyspneic, and pink, with essentially normal blood gas values. They present with an increase in minute ventilation to maintain their normal Pa_{CO_2}, which explains the increase in work of breathing and dyspnea.

Pulmonary Function Testing and Evaluation for Lung Resectability

There are three goals in performing pulmonary function tests in patients scheduled for lung resection. The first is to identify those patients at risk of increased postoperative morbidity and mortality. In thoracic surgery for lung cancer, the specific question is: How much lung tissue may be safely removed without making the patient a pulmonary cripple? This should be weighed against the 1-year mean survival rate of the patient with surgically untreated lung carcinoma. The second goal is to identify those patients who will need short- or long-term postoperative ventilatory support. The third goal is to evaluate the beneficial effect and reversibility of airway obstruction with the use of bronchodilators.

Effects of Anesthesia and Surgery on Lung Volumes

Anesthesia and postoperative medications can cause changes in lung volumes and ventilatory pattern (see Chapter 29). Total lung capacity (TLC) decreases after abdominal surgery but not after surgery on an extremity. Vital capacity is decreased by 25–50% within 1–2 days after surgery and generally returns to normal after 1–2 weeks. Residual volume (RV) increases by 13%, whereas expiratory reserve volume decreases by 25% after lower abdominal surgery and 60% after upper abdominal and thoracic surgery. Tidal volume (V_T) decreases by 20% within 24 hours after surgery and gradually returns to normal after 2 weeks. Pulmonary compliance decreases by 33% with similar reductions in functional residual capacity (FRC) secondary to small airway closure. Most of the patients who undergo lung resection are smokers with a certain degree of COPD and are prone to postoperative complications in direct relation to the amount of lung to be resected (lobectomy or pneumonectomy) and to the severity of the preoperative lung disease.

Spirometry

Forced vital capacity (FVC), forced expired volume in one second (FEV_1), and peak expiratory flow can be measured at the patient's bedside using a spirometer. The measurement can be recorded as a volume–time trace or as a flow–volume loop.

A vital capacity of at least three times the V_T is necessary for an effective cough. A vital capacity of less than 50% of predicted or less than 2 l is an indicator of increased risk.[4] An abnormal preoperative vital capacity can be identified in 30–40% of postoperative deaths. A patient with an abnormal vital capacity has a 33% chance of complications and a 10% risk of postoperative mortality.

FEV_1 is a more direct indication of airway obstruction. An FEV_1 of less than 800 ml in a 70-kg male is probably incompatible with life and is an absolute contraindication to lung resection. Mortality in patients with an FEV_1 greater than 2 l is 10%, and in patients below 1 l is between 20% and 45%.[5]

The ratio FEV_1/FVC is useful in differentiating between restrictive and obstructive disease. It is normal in restrictive disease because both decrease, whereas in obstructive disease the ratio usually is low because the FEV_1 is markedly decreased.

Maximum voluntary ventilation is a nonspecific test and is an indicator of both restriction and obstruction. Although maximum voluntary ventilation has not been systematically evaluated as a predictor of morbidity, it is generally accepted that a maximum voluntary ventilation below 50% of predicted value is an indication of high risk.

A ratio of RV to TLC (RV/TLC) of greater than 50% is generally indicative of a high-risk patient for pulmonary resection. Mittman[6] found that an RV/TLC ratio of greater than 40% was associated with a 30% mortality rate, compared with a 7% mortality when RV/TLC was less than 40% (normal range 20–25%).

Flow–Volume Loops

The flow–volume loop displays essentially the same information as a spirometer but is more convenient for measurement of specific flow rates (Fig. 30-1). The shape and peak air flow rates during expiration at high lung volumes are effort dependent but indicate the patency of the larger airways. Effort-independent expiration occurs at low lung volumes and usually reflects small airways resistance, best measured by forced expiratory flow during the middle half of the FVC ($FEF_{25-75\%}$).

In general, patients with obstructive airways disease (Fig. 30-2), such as asthma, bronchitis, and emphysema, have grossly reduced FEV_1/FVC ratios because of increased airways resistance and a reduction in FEV_1. Peak expiratory flow rate and maximum voluntary ventilation are usually reduced, whereas total lung capacity increases secondary to increases in RV. In these patients, the effort-independent portion of the flow–volume curve is markedly depressed inward, with reduction of the flow rate at 25–75% of FVC.

In patients with restrictive disease (see Fig. 30-2), such as pulmonary fibrosis and scoliosis, there is a reduction in FVC with a relatively normal FEV_1. Because the airways resistance is normal, FEV_1/FVC is also normal. TLC is markedly reduced, whereas maximum voluntary ventilation and $FEF_{25-75\%}$ are usually normal. The flow–volume curves of these patients are normal in shape, but the lung volumes and peak flow rates are lower (see Fig. 30-2).

Significance of Bronchodilator Therapy. Pulmonary function tests are usually performed before and after bronchodilator therapy to assess the reversibility of the airways obstruction. This is useful in the assessment of the degree of airways obstruction and the patient's effort ability. After treatment with bronchodilators, increases in peak expiratory flow compared with a baseline indicate reversibility of airways obstruction (often seen in asthmatic patients). A 15% improvement in pulmonary function tests may be considered a positive response to bronchodilator therapy and indicates that this therapy should be initiated before surgery. The overall prognosis of COPD is better related to the level of spirometric function after bronchodilator therapy than to a baseline function.

Split-Lung Function Tests

Regional lung function studies serve to predict the function of the lung tissue that would remain after lung resection. A whole

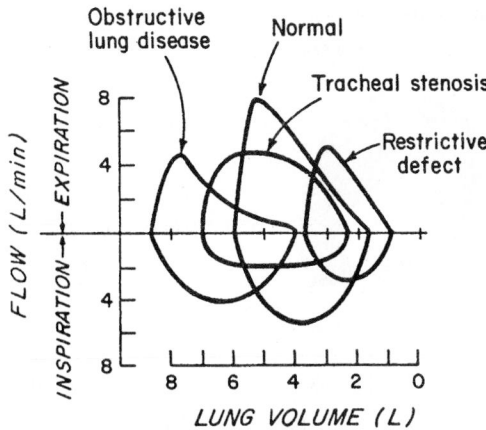

Figure 30-2. Flow–volume loops relative to lung volumes (1) in a normal subject, (2) in a patient with chronic obstructive pulmonary disease (COPD), (3) in a patient with fixed obstruction (tracheal stenosis), and (4) in a patient with pulmonary fibrosis (restrictive defect). Note the concave expiratory form in the patient with COPD and the flat inspiratory curve in the patient with a fixed obstruction. (Reproduced with permission from Goudsouzian N, Karamanian A: Physiology for the Anesthesiologist, 2nd ed. Norwalk, Appleton-Century-Crofts, 1984.)

(two)-lung test may fail to estimate whether the amount of postresection lung tissue will allow the patient to function at a reasonable level of activity without disabling dyspnea or cor pulmonale.

Regional Perfusion Test. This involves the intravenous injection of insoluble radioactive xenon (^{133}Xe). The peak radioactivity of each lung is proportional to the degree of perfusion of each lung.

Regional Ventilation Test. Using an inhaled, insoluble radioactive gas, the peak radioactivity over each lung is proportional to the degree of ventilation. Combining radiospirometry with whole lung testing (FEV_1, FVC, maximal breathing capacity) has resulted in a fair degree of correlation between predicted volumes and pulmonary function tests measured after pneumonectomy. It is generally held that a FEV_1 of 800 ml is the minimum accepted volume for postresection survival.

Regional Bronchial Balloon Occlusion Test. This test basically simulates the postresection condition preoperatively by using balloon occlusion of the bronchus to the segment of the lung to be resected. Spirometry and arterial blood gas analysis are then performed with the remaining functional lung.

Pulmonary Artery Balloon Occlusion Test

The postoperative stress on the right ventricle and remaining pulmonary vascular bed can be simulated by occluding the pulmonary artery of the lung to be resected using a specially designed balloon-tipped pulmonary artery (PA) catheter that has a pressure-sensing port just proximal to the balloon. This test may be performed with or without exercise. If, on balloon occlusion of the pulmonary artery of the lung to be resected, the mean pulmonary artery pressure increases above 40 mm Hg, Pao_2 is less than 60 mm Hg, or $Paco_2$ is greater than 45 mm Hg, it is unlikely that the patient will be able to tolerate pneumonectomy without experiencing postoperative respiratory failure or cor pulmonale.

The preoperative pulmonary evaluation of patients considered for lung resection is summarized as follows. First, a whole-lung test with spirometry and arterial blood gases should be done. If any of the following values—$Paco_2 > 40$ mm Hg, $FEV_1 < 50\%$, FVC < 21, maximal breathing capacity < 50%, or RV/TLC > 50%—is found to be outside these limits, a second level of split-lung function testing should be done to estimate the exact contribution of the resected portion of the lung to either ventilation or perfusion. Conventional spirometry should yield

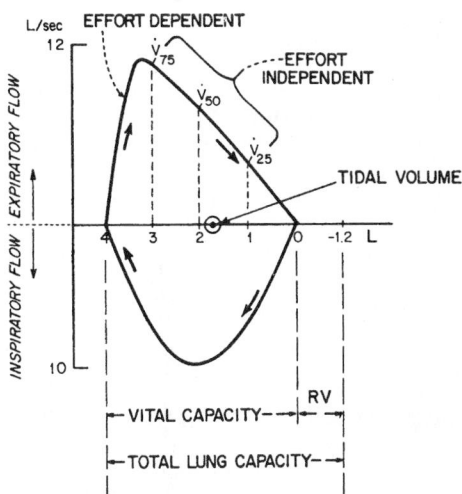

Figure 30-1. Flow–volume loop in a normal subject. $\dot{V}_{75}$, $\dot{V}_{50}$, and $\dot{V}_{25}$ represent flow at 75, 50, and 25% of vital capacity, respectively. (RV = residual volume). (Reproduced with permission from Goudsouzian N, Karamanian A: Physiology for the Anesthesiologist, 2nd ed. Norwalk, Appleton-Century-Crofts, 1984.)

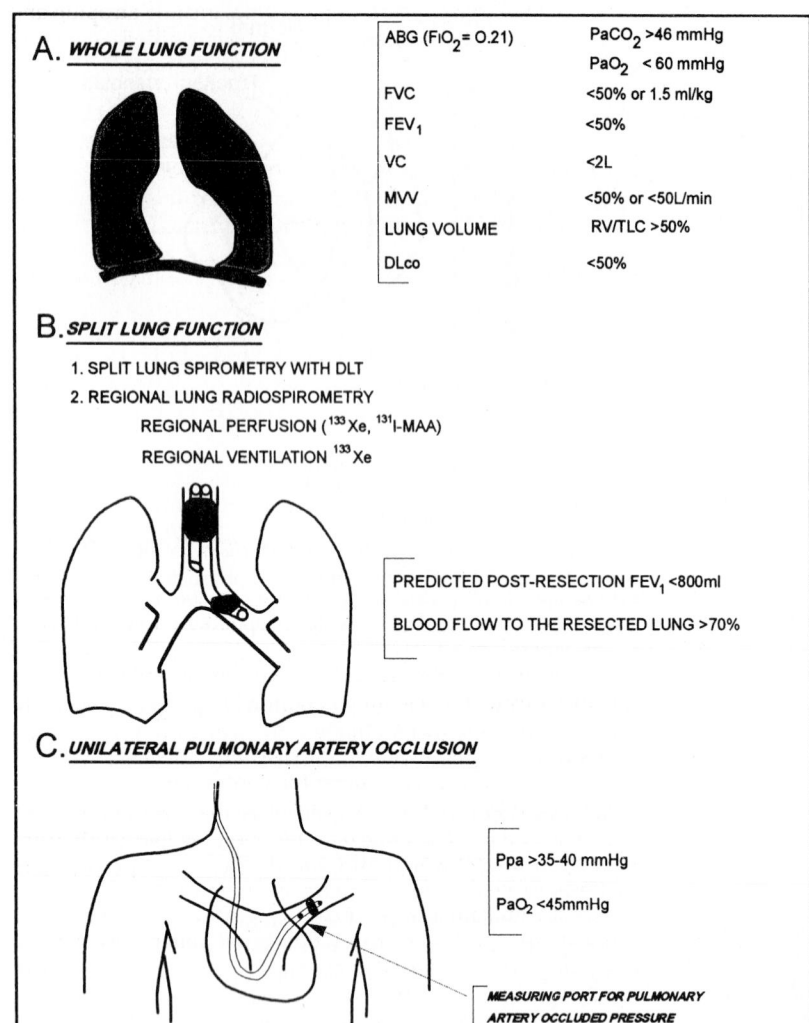

A. **WHOLE LUNG FUNCTION**

ABG (FiO₂ = 0.21)	PaCO₂ >46 mmHg
	PaO₂ < 60 mmHg
FVC	<50% or 1.5 ml/kg
FEV₁	<50%
VC	<2L
MVV	<50% or <50L/min
LUNG VOLUME	RV/TLC >50%
DLco	<50%

B. **SPLIT LUNG FUNCTION**

1. SPLIT LUNG SPIROMETRY WITH DLT
2. REGIONAL LUNG RADIOSPIROMETRY
  REGIONAL PERFUSION (¹³³Xe, ¹³¹I-MAA)
  REGIONAL VENTILATION ¹³³Xe

PREDICTED POST-RESECTION FEV₁ <800ml

BLOOD FLOW TO THE RESECTED LUNG >70%

C. **UNILATERAL PULMONARY ARTERY OCCLUSION**

Ppa >35-40 mmHg

PaO₂ <45mmHg

MEASURING PORT FOR PULMONARY ARTERY OCCLUDED PRESSURE

Figure 30-3. The order of tests to determine the cardiopulmonary status of the patient and the extent of lung resection that would be tolerated. (*A*) The whole-lung function test is a basic screening test. (*B*) The split-lung function tests are regional tests to determine the involvement of the diseased lung to be removed. (*C*) Tests that mimic the postoperative cardiopulmonary function are the decisive tests to determine if the patient will be able to tolerate the planned resection. (Adapted with permission from Neustein SM, Cohen E: Preoperative evaluation of thoracic surgical patients. In Cohen E [ed]: The Practice of Thoracic Anesthesia, p 187. Philadelphia, JB Lippincott, 1995.)

a predicted postresection FEV₁ greater than 800 ml. If these criteria cannot be met, surgery is usually contraindicated. A postoperative simulation of ventilation or perfusion by bronchial or pulmonary artery occlusion can produce additional information, and risk–benefit ratio must be considered for each individual patient. The preoperative evaluation of the patient for lung resection is summarized in Figure 30-3.

PREOPERATIVE PREPARATION

The wide spectrum of physiologic changes occurring during thoracic surgery puts patients at great risk of developing postoperative complications. Morbidity and mortality increase when these changes are superimposed on an acutely or chronically compromised patient. Several conditions, including infection, dehydration, electrolyte imbalance, wheezing, obesity, cigarette smoking, cor pulmonale, and malnutrition, show particular correlations with postoperative complications. Proper, vigorous preoperative preparation can improve the patient's ability to face the surgery with a reduced risk of morbidity and mortality. It is important that conditions predisposing to postoperative complications be effectively treated before surgery.

Smoking

Approximately 33% of adult patients presenting for surgery are smokers, and there is extensive evidence that they are at increased risk for development of postoperative respiratory

complications.[7] Smoking increases airway irritability, decreases mucociliary transport, and increases secretions. Smoking also decreases FVC and FEF₂₅–₇₅%, thereby increasing the incidence of postoperative pulmonary complications. On the other hand, cessation of smoking for a period of longer than 4–6 weeks before surgery is associated with a decreased incidence of postoperative complications.[8] Furthermore, cessation of smoking for 48 hours before surgery has been shown to decrease the level of carboxyhemoglobin, to shift the oxyhemoglobin dissociation curve to the right, and to increase tissue oxygen availability. It should be emphasized that most of the beneficial effects of cessation of smoking, however, such as improvement in ciliary function, improvement in closing volume, increase in FEF₂₅–₇₅%, and reduction in sputum production, usually occur 2–3 months after the cessation of smoking.

Infection

Acute or chronic infection should be vigorously treated before surgery. Broad-spectrum antibiotics are commonly used. Treatment of the acutely ill patient depends on the results of the Gram stain of the sputum and on blood culture findings. In one prospective study, the incidence of mortality was lower (9%) in the group treated with prophylactic antibiotics compared with the untreated patients (17%), and a lower incidence of postoperative pulmonary infection was shown as well.[9] Although not all surgeons administer antibiotics prophylactically to their patients, infection, when present before surgery, should be vigorously treated.

Hydration and Removal of Bronchial Secretions

Correction of hypovolemia and electrolyte imbalance should be accomplished before surgery because hydrating the patient decreases the viscosity of the bronchial secretions and facilitates their removal from the bronchial tree. Humidification is extremely useful. The use of mucolytic drugs, such as acetylcysteine (Mucomyst), or of oral expectorants (potassium iodide) can be of benefit to patients with viscous secretions. Commonly used methods for removing the secretions from the bronchial tree include postural drainage, vigorous coughing, chest percussion, deep breathing, and the use of an incentive spirometer. These often require patient cooperation and frequent verbal encouragement to maximize the beneficial effect.

Wheezing and Bronchodilation

The presence of acute wheezing represents a medical emergency, and elective surgery should be postponed until effective proper treatment has been instituted. Chronic wheezing is often seen in patients with COPD and is attributable to the presence of gas flow obstruction secondary to smooth muscle contraction, accumulation of secretions, and mucosal edema. Smooth muscle contraction may occur in small airways only (detectable by changes in $FEF_{25-75\%}$) or may be widespread, with a large reduction of FEV_1 and FVC. The efficacy of bronchodilators in reversing the bronchospastic component is extremely important. A trial of bronchodilators and measurement of their effects on pulmonary function should be performed in any patient who shows evidence of air flow obstruction. Several classes of bronchodilators are available.

Sympathomimetic Drugs. Sympathomimetic drugs increase the formation of $3'5'$-cyclic adenosine monophosphate (cAMP). The balance between cAMP, which produces bronchodilation, and cyclic guanosine monophosphate, which produces bronchoconstriction, determines the state of contraction of the bronchial smooth muscle. Thus, increasing cAMP production causes relaxation of the bronchial tree. Sympathomimetic drugs, such as epinephrine, isoproterenol, isoetharine, and ephedrine, all have mixed β_1 and β_2 sympathetic agonist effects. The β_1 (cardiac effects) of these drugs are often undesirable in treating patients with COPD. Selective β_2 sympathomimetic drugs, such as albuterol, terbutaline, and metaproterenol, given as inhaled aerosols, are the preferred drugs in the treatment of bronchospasm, particularly in patients with cardiac disease.

Phosphodiesterase Inhibitors. Phosphodiesterase inhibitors inhibit the breakdown of cAMP by cytoplasmic phosphodiesterase. The methylxanthines, such as aminophylline, increase the level of cAMP, resulting in bronchodilation. In addition, aminophylline improves diaphragmatic contractility and increases the patient's resistance to fatigue. Therapeutic blood levels of aminophylline are $5-20~\mu g \cdot ml^{-1}$ and can be achieved by giving a loading dose of $5-7~mg \cdot kg^{-1}$ infused over 20 minutes, followed by a continuous intravenous (iv) infusion of $0.5-0.7~mg \cdot kg^{-1} \cdot h^{-1}$. Aminophylline may cause ventricular arrhythmias, and this side-effect should be borne in mind when treating patients who have myocardial ischemia.

Steroids. Although they are not true bronchodilators, steroids are traditionally considered to decrease mucosal edema and may prevent the release of bronchoconstricting substances. They are of questionable benefit in acute bronchospasm. Steroids may be given orally, parenterally, or in aerosol form, such as beclomethasone by inhaler.

Cromolyn Sodium. Cromolyn sodium stabilizes mast cells and inhibits degranulation and histamine release. It is useful in the prevention of bronchospastic attacks but is of little value in the treatment of the acute situation.

Parasympatholytics. Parasympatholytics include atropine and ipratropium. In the past, atropine has been avoided in patients with COPD and bronchitis because of the concern regarding increases in the viscosity of mucus produced by this agent. However, atropine blocks the formation of cyclic guanosine monophosphate and therefore has a bronchodilator effect. Marini *et al*[10] found that inhaled atropine alone improved FEV_1 in 85% of patients with COPD. When atropine was given together with terbutaline, the FEV_1 improved in 93% of patients, whereas terbutaline alone improved FEV_1 in only 56% of patients. Therefore, the antimuscarinic drugs such as atropine potentiate the bronchodilator effect of the sympathomimetic agents.

In conclusion, the preoperative preparation of the patient for thoracic surgery should focus on those conditions that are treatable before surgery so that the patient is in optimal condition at the time of surgery.

INTRAOPERATIVE MONITORING

All patients undergoing thoracic surgical procedures require monitoring with an electrocardiogram (lead II and, if possible, V_5), chest or esophageal stethoscopes for heart and breath sound auscultation, and a temperature probe. A chest stethoscope should be placed over the dependent hemithorax to assess dependent lung ventilation. Pulse oximetry is a standard of care during the administration of anesthesia and is especially valuable during thoracic surgery because hypoxemia may occur during one-lung ventilation.

Dysrhythmias occur commonly both during and after thoracic surgery, making the usual need for continuous electrocardiographic monitoring even more important. Intraoperative supraventricular tachyarrhythmias may be caused by cardiac manipulation. Dysrhythmias occurring during one-lung ventilation may be a sign of inadequate oxygenation or ventilation. Postoperative dysrhythmias may be related to sympathetic nervous system stimulation from pain or to a reduced pulmonary vascular bed from the lung resection. Patients presenting for lung resection often have COPD owing to cigarette smoking, have right-sided heart strain, and are prone to multifocal atrial tachydysrhythmias.

The axis of electrocardiogram lead II parallels that of the P wave, making this lead useful for arrhythmia detection. The simultaneous monitoring of lead V_5 also allows for monitoring of anterolateral wall myocardial ischemia. The use of multiple leads facilitates a greater sensitivity of ischemia detection.[11] The following types of invasive monitoring are also indicated and have led to markedly improved patient care.

Direct Arterial Catheterization

Peripheral arterial catheterization has become an essential tool for the anesthesiologist in the management of patients undergoing major thoracic surgical procedures. It allows for continuous beat-to-beat measurement of blood pressure as well as frequent sampling for the determination of arterial blood gases. The risk, when utilizing a 20-gauge Teflon catheter in the radial artery, is extremely low, and any risk can be further decreased by ensuring patency of the ulnar artery. This can be done by the use of a modified Allen test, digital plethysmography, or Doppler ultrasonography. Although the modified Allen test is a commonly performed technique, its usefulness has been challenged. Permanent ischemic complications have been reported in patients with normal Allen test results, and catheterization in patients with abnormal Allen test findings has not resulted in ischemic sequelae. The incidence of ischemic complications after radial artery catheterization has been reported to be 0.01%.

Continuous blood pressure readings are critical during thoracic surgery because surgical manipulations or intravascular volume shifts can cause sudden major changes in the blood pressure. Immediate recognition of the change allows time for proper identification of the etiology and the institution of appropriate treatment.

Serial blood gas determinations are performed as needed in the management of patients undergoing one-lung anesthesia or during cases in which part of the lung may be "packed away" for a period. Arterial hypoxemia may occur because of shunting through the collapsed lung and inadequate hypoxic pulmonary vasoconstriction (HPV). Significant changes in acid–base status as well as hyperventilation or hypoventilation can also be determined.

A radial artery catheter can be placed in either extremity during thoracic surgery. For a mediastinoscopic examination, it is useful to place the catheter in the right arm and to use it to monitor for compression of the innominate artery by the mediastinoscope.[12] This can help to avoid central nervous system complications resulting from inadequate cerebral blood flow through the right carotid artery (see the section on Mediastinoscopy). During thoracotomy, the radial artery catheter is often placed in the dependent arm to aid in stabilizing the catheter. However, a roll must be placed under the patient to protect the axilla and avoid compression of the axillary artery and brachial plexus in this arm. In rare cases, the arterial catheter can be placed in the brachial, femoral, or dorsalis pedis artery if the ulnar collateral circulation is thought to be inadequate.

Central Venous Pressure Monitoring

Central venous pressure (CVP) is usually measured as an indication of right atrial and right ventricular pressures. It is a useful monitor if the factors affecting it are realized and its limitations are understood. The CVP reflects the patient's blood volume, venous tone, and right ventricular performance; however, it is also affected by central venous obstructions and alterations of intrathoracic pressure (e.g., PEEP). Serial measurements are more useful than an individual number, and the response of the CVP to a volume infusion is a useful test of right ventricular function. The CVP reflects right-sided heart function and not left ventricular performance. The combination of the CVP as a monitor of right atrial pressure and the esophageal stethoscope to "monitor" left atrial pressure (e.g., rales, S_3) is still a useful technique in patients with good left ventricular function. A CVP catheter is often used in patients with good left ventricular function during thoracic surgical procedures for either monitoring or infusion/insertion applications. CVP monitoring is needed when there may be large volume shifts (e.g., pneumonectomy) or the patient is hypovolemic. Uses of CVP catheter or large-bore introducer include: (1) insertion of a transvenous pacemaker where necessary; (2) infusion of vasoactive drugs; and (3) insertion of a PA catheter, which may subsequently be required during surgery or in the postoperative period.

The CVP catheter can be placed centrally from either the external or the internal jugular vein, from the subclavian veins, or from one of the arm veins. The success rate is highest using the right internal jugular vein, and a pacemaker or PA catheter can be inserted most easily from this vein. The major disadvantage of using the external jugular vein during thoracotomy is that the catheter often kinks when the patient is turned to the lateral decubitus position. The subclavian technique leads to a high incidence of pneumothorax, which can be disastrous if it occurs in the dependent lung during one-lung ventilation.

Pulmonary Artery Catheterization

The use of the PA catheter allows measurements of left-sided filling pressures, the determination of cardiac output by thermodilution, calculation of derived hemodynamic and respiratory parameters (e.g., systemic vascular resistance and intrapulmonary shunt, respectively), and clinical use of Starling function curves. In addition, advanced versions of the basic catheter allow measurement of mixed venous oxygen saturation or right ventricular ejection fraction as well as the application of atrial or ventricular pacing. The PA catheter is indicated during thoracic surgery in specific situations (Table 30-1).

In the past, CVP catheters were used to monitor patients with left-sided heart disease or pulmonary disease; however, the CVP has been shown to have a poor correlation with the left atrial pressure in these types of patient. Many studies have shown the disparity between left- and right-sided pressures owing to the many factors separating the CVP reading from the true left ventricular preload.

The PA catheter is most reliably inserted through the right internal jugular vein using a modified Seldinger technique. Insertion of the PA catheter through either the external jugular vein or the subclavian vein often leads to obstruction of the catheter when the patient is placed in the lateral decubitus position. Complications of PA catheter insertion and use can be divided into immediate and long term. Immediate complications include the development of supraventricular and ventricular dysrhythmias during insertion, onset of a right bundle-branch block or complete heart block in patients with a pre-existing left bundle-branch block, and all the potential complications of inserting a needle into a central vein (e.g., arterial puncture, hematoma formation, pneumothorax, nerve damage, Horner's syndrome, air embolization, or thoracic duct injury). The incidence of dysrhythmias is decreased by changing the position of the patient from Trendelenburg to a head-up right lateral tilt position before flotation of the PA catheter. Long-term complications of use of the PA catheter include balloon rupture and gas embolization, pulmonary infarction, pulmonary artery rupture, knotting of the catheter in the right ventricle, infection, vascular obstruction, and erroneous diagnosis from misinterpretation of data.[13]

Pulmonary artery rupture is the most serious complication associated with the use of the PA catheter. Risk factors for this complication include hypothermia, pulmonary hypertension, anticoagulation, and being elderly or female. Pulmonary artery perforation most commonly manifests as hemoptysis.

Management of pulmonary artery rupture and massive airway hemorrhage includes protecting the nonbleeding lung by placement of a double-lumen endotracheal tube. This allows suctioning and application of continuous positive airway pressure (CPAP) to the bleeding lung, which is not possible if the single-

---

Table 30-1. INDICATIONS FOR PULMONARY ARTERY CATHETERIZATION IN THORACIC SURGERY

1. Patients with known cardiovascular disease, with or without heart failure
2. Surgery in which cross-clamping of the thoracic aorta is anticipated
3. Patients with respiratory failure
4. Patients with suspected or diagnosed pulmonary emboli
5. Patients who have undergone previous cardiac surgery
6. When a pneumonectomy is anticipated
7. When significant shifts of intravascular volume are anticipated
8. When sepsis is present
9. Patients who receive continuous infusions of inotropes or vasodilators
10. Patients with pulmonary hypertension or elevated pulmonary vascular resistance
11. When cor pulmonale is present
12. Patients treated with bleomycin

Adapted with permission from Noback CR: Intraoperative monitoring. In Kaplan JA (ed): Thoracic Anesthesia, p 231. New York, Churchill Livingstone, 1983.

lumen tube is merely advanced into the bronchus of the non-bleeding lung. If a single-lumen tube is already in place, another alternative is the placement of a bronchial blocker alongside the tracheal tube after the site of bleeding has been identified. The bleeding most often comes from the right side because the PA catheter usually floats to the right side. Bronchoscopy may allow identification of the bleeding site. Other treatment modalities include the use of PEEP, inflation of the PA catheter balloon to tamponade the bleeding, and the administration of protamine, if possible, if the patient has been anticoagulated with heparin. Fluid resuscitation is essential, and if the bleeding continues, surgical exploration and lung resection may be necessary.

Misinterpretation of data from a PA catheter is a real risk in a patient with cardiac and pulmonary disease undergoing thoracic surgery with one-lung ventilation. These errors can be produced by altered ventilatory modes, the location of the PA catheter tip, ventricular compliance changes, or ventricular interdependence.[13] A major limitation of the PA catheter is the assumption that the pulmonary capillary wedge pressure is a good approximation of left ventricular end-diastolic volume. The use of pulmonary capillary wedge pressure directly to assess preload assumes a linear relationship between ventricular end-diastolic volume and ventricular end-diastolic pressure. However, alterations in ventricular compliance affect this pressure-volume relationship during surgery. Reductions in ventricular compliance can be seen with myocardial ischemia, shock, right ventricular overload, or pericardial effusion. Numerous investigators have demonstrated a poor correlation between pulmonary capillary wedge pressure and left ventricular end-diastolic volume in acutely ill patients.[14] This correlation is further worsened by the application of PEEP. Therefore, whenever pulmonary capillary wedge pressure is used to estimate left ventricular preload, the number must be interpreted in light of the clinical situation. The interdependence of the right and left ventricles must also be remembered when interpreting pulmonary capillary wedge pressure. Ventricular interdependence can cause misdiagnosis when the interventricular septum encroaches on the left ventricular cavity, leading to increased values of pulmonary capillary wedge pressure. An increased pulmonary capillary wedge pressure associated with a decreased cardiac output can be interpreted as left ventricular failure, when, in fact, left ventricular end-diastolic volume may not be increased but decreased because of compression of the left ventricle by a distended right ventricle (Fig. 30-4). This situation can occur with acute respiratory failure and high levels of PEEP. Techniques such as echocardiography, which directly measure ventricular dimensions, are necessary to resolve this complex situation.

Because most of the pulmonary blood flow is to the right lower lobe, the tip of a flow-directed PA catheter is usually located in the right lower lobe. During a left thoracotomy with one-lung ventilation, the catheter tip would then be in the dependent lung and should provide accurate hemodynamic measurements. However, during a right thoracotomy with one-lung ventilation, the catheter tip should be in the nondependent lung. Cohen et al[15] reported that during right thoracotomies with the tip of the PA catheter in a West zone 1 or 2 region of the right lung, hemodynamic measurements may be inaccurate. These authors found that cardiac output measurements were lower during right thoracotomies than left thoracotomies, and the derived parameters of stroke volume index and oxygen delivery were also inappropriately low. Therefore, hemodynamic data derived from a PA catheter in the nondependent collapsed lung must be carefully evaluated.

Assessment of right ventricular function is made difficult by the complex geometry and shape of the right ventricle. The thermodilution technique used to measure cardiac output with the PA catheter can also be used to determine right ventricular ejection fraction if a fast-response thermistor is used. There are numerous situations during thoracic surgery when decreased right ventricular function precludes adequate right-sided heart output to a normal left ventricle. Because the right ventricle is very sensitive to increases in afterload, right ventricular function can be evaluated by comparing right ventricular ejection fraction with a measure of right ventricular afterload, such as pulmonary vascular resistance. Right ventricular function curves may be even more useful than left ventricular function curves in patients with chronic pulmonary disease undergoing thoracic surgical procedures.

The multipurpose PA catheter, with five pacing electrodes, is now widely available. This catheter can be used for atrial, ventricular, or atrioventricular sequential pacing in patients who require a PA catheter for hemodynamic monitoring. Another design of PA catheter incorporates a channel through which a pacing wire may be inserted (Paceport Catheter). Indications for a pacing PA catheter are (1) intermittent third-degree heart block, (2) second-degree heart block, (3) left bundle-branch block, (4) digitalis toxicity, and (5) severe bradycardia.

A PA catheter capable of monitoring $S\bar{v}O_2$ is also available. Four mechanisms can account for a decreased $S\bar{v}O_2$: (1) decreased SaO_2, (2) decreased cardiac output, (3) increased oxygen consumption, and (4) decreased hemoglobin concentration. $S\bar{v}O_2$ represents a measure of global tissue oxygen extraction and consumption and is in general directly related to cardiac output via the Fick formula. The monitoring of $S\bar{v}O_2$ has been evaluated in patients undergoing one-lung anesthesia.[16] Changes in $S\bar{v}O_2$ were mainly dependent on changes in SaO_2.

Transesophageal Echocardiography

Transesophageal echocardiography is a useful intraoperative monitor for ventricular function, valvular function, and wall motion changes that might reflect ischemia. Its use in thoracic surgical patients has been limited. In one study, central lung tumors were seen with transesophageal echocardiography in nine of nine patients, peripheral lung tumors in one of three patients, and an anterior mediastinal mass in one of one patient.[17] In this study, transesophageal echocardiography revealed pulmonary artery compression in five patients and pulmonary artery infiltration in two patients.

In another study investigating echocardiographic recognition of mediastinal tumors, transesophageal echocardiography revealed that the tumors were often adjacent to the heart and identified those patients in whom there was compression of the innominate vein or pulmonary artery or infiltration of the heart.[18]

Intraoperative transesophageal echocardiography has also revealed tumor invasion of the heart, indicating that a resection by thoracotomy without cardiopulmonary bypass was not feasible.[19] In another case report, transesophageal echocardiography monitoring during an attempted resection of a tumor invading the left atrium showed embolization of the tumor.[20] Fragments

	PCWP	Cardiac Output	LVEDV
LV failure	↑	↓	↑
Ventricular interdependence	↑	↓	↓

Figure 30-4. Comparison of left ventricular failure and ventricular interdependence. (PCWP = pulmonary capillary wedge pressure; LVEDV = left ventricle end-diastolic volume.) (Reproduced with permission from Keefer JR, Barash PG: Pulmonary artery catheterization. In Blitt CD [ed]: Monitoring in Anesthesia and Critical Care Medicine, p 213. New York, Churchill Livingstone, 1985.)

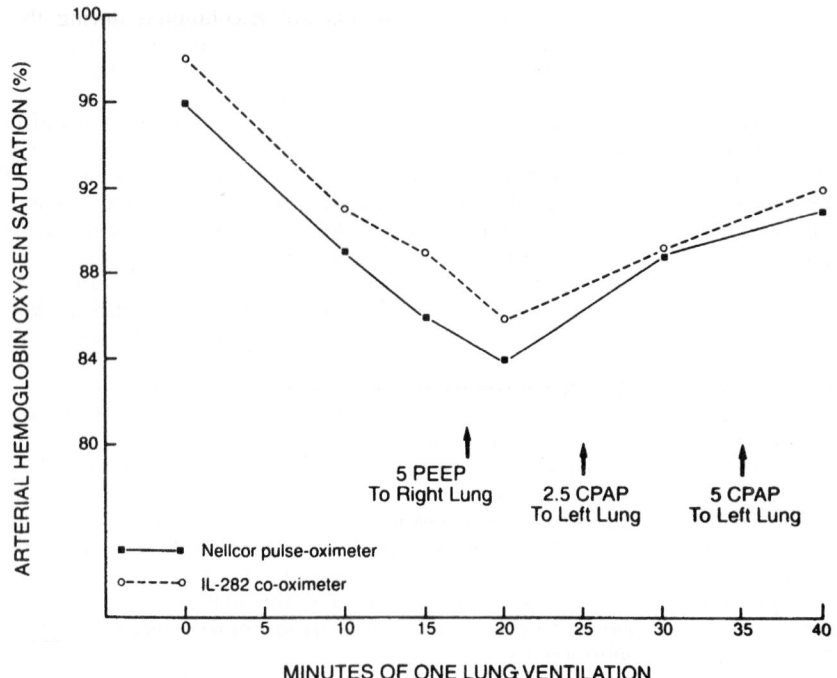

Figure 30-5. Changes in hemoglobin oxygen saturation during one-lung ventilation. Early detection of hypoxemia with pulse oximetry facilitates prompt treatment with positive end-expiratory pressure (5 cm H₂O) and incremental continuous positive airway pressure (2.5–5 cm H₂O) until arterial saturation is returned to an acceptable level. (PEEP = positive end-expiratory pressure; CPAP = continuous positive airway pressure.) (Reproduced with permission from Brodsky JB, Shulman MS, Swan M: Pulse oximetry during one-lung ventilation. Anesthesiology 65:213, 1985.)

of the tumor were seen to pass through the aortic valve. This patient subsequently died of disseminated metastases. In an exploratory thoracotomy for hemothorax, intraoperative transesophageal echocardiography revealed the presence of a subcute aortic dissection, which was believed to be the etiology of the hemothorax.[21]

Monitoring of Oxygenation and Ventilation

Oxygenation

During the administration of all thoracic surgical anesthetics, the concentration of oxygen in the breathing system must be measured using an oxygen analyzer with a low oxygen concentration limit alarm. Such analyzers vary in sophistication from fuel cells, polarographic and paramagnetic analyzers, to mass and Raman spectrometers that can monitor all the gases used during anesthesia. Adequacy of blood oxygenation must also be ensured, and adequate illumination and exposure of the patient are necessary to assess the color of shed blood or the presence of cyanosis of the lips, nail beds, or mucous membranes. Most patients undergoing thoracic surgical or diagnostic procedures have an arterial catheter in place for continuous monitoring of blood pressure and sampling of arterial blood for arterial blood gas determinations. In such cases, baseline arterial blood gas values should be obtained with an $F_{IO_2} = 0.21$ (room air) before starting the procedure and repeated regularly and/or whenever indicated during surgery. Arterial blood is usually analyzed for oxygen tension (Pa_{O_2}), and saturation is calculated from the oxyhemoglobin dissociation curve, correcting for temperature, pH, and Pa_{CO_2}.

The oxygen content of arterial blood can be assessed using a bench co-oximeter, such as the IL482 (Instrumentation Laboratory, Lexington, MA), which uses spectrophotometric principles to measure the total hemoglobin (Hb_{TOT}), which represents 100% (g · dl⁻¹), and the percentages of oxyhemoglobin (HbO_2), methemoglobin, and carboxyhemoglobin. Deoxygenated (reduced) hemoglobin (RHb) is the difference between 100% and the sum of carboxyhemoglobin, methemoglobin, and HbO_2.

The oxyhemoglobin percentage* (HbO_2%, previously termed *fractional concentration*) is the more important index for assessing oxygen content. The oxygen saturation of available hemoglobin* (total amount of hemoglobin available to bind oxygen, or Sa_{O_2}%, and previously known as functional saturation) differs from HbO_2% depending on the amount of dyshemoglobins (carboxyhemoglobin, methemoglobin) present. Thus, if the hemoglobin concentration is 15 g · dl⁻¹, and 1 g of hemoglobin combines with 1.34 ml O_2 when fully saturated, the formula (15 × HbO_2% × 1.34) provides the more accurate estimate of ml O_2 · dl⁻¹ of blood than using (15 × Sa_{O_2}% × 1.34) or using the calculated saturation from a saturation nomogram based on Pa_{O_2}.†

Pulse oximetry is now a standard of care for noninvasive assessment of oxygenation. Pulse oximeters are fairly accurate in estimating hemoglobin saturation with oxygen over the range of 60–100%. Their value has also been demonstrated during one-lung ventilation, when rapid assessment of oxygenation is extremely important, and when blood gas analysis may involve some delay[22] (Fig. 30-5). Pulse oximetry does not, however, eliminate the need for arterial blood gas analysis during thoracic surgery. A low Sp_{O_2} reading provides the clinician with an indication for sampling and laboratory analysis of arterial blood, but an erroneously high Sp_{O_2} reading may also occur.[23]

The monitoring of transcutaneous oxygen tension (Ptc_{O_2}) has also been used during thoracic surgery and one-lung ventilation. Although these monitors are noninvasive and continuous, a warm-up time is required before use, and the skin underlying the sensor must be heated to 45°C to arterialize the blood. Generally, Ptc_{O_2} is approximately 80% of actual arterial oxygen tension (Pa_{O_2}) and is accurate only when the patient is hemodynamically stable with a cardiac index in excess of 2.2 l · min⁻¹ · m⁻². During periods of hypotension, Ptc_{O_2} does not follow Pa_{O_2} but decreases. Thus, a low Ptc_{O_2} may be misleading

---

* National Committee for Clinical Laboratory Standards, Villanova, Pennsylvania. Vol 2, no 10, p 342, 1982.

† HbO_2% (fractional saturation) = HbO_2/Hb_{TOT}. Sa_{O_2}% (functional saturation) = $HbO_2/(HbO_2 + RHb)$.

in the presence of an adequate Pao_2 and poor tissue perfusion. For these reasons, pulse oximetry is usually preferred over transcutaneous oxygen monitoring during thoracic surgery.

Another device that has been reported for continuous monitoring of oxygenation is the *optode*, a fiberoptic probe for continuous intra-arterial measurement of Pao_2. It consists of a single optical fiber with a luminescent dye coating at the tip. It is heparin coated, less than 0.5 mm in diameter, and passes easily through a 20-gauge arterial cannula. It does not appear to interfere with the arterial pressure waveform, and blood samples can easily be withdrawn from the cannula with the optode in place. A flash lamp emits light that excites the molecules of the luminescent dye. The excited electrons of the dye can either decay to a lower energy level by emitting light or react with oxygen without light emission. Thus, the light emitted is inversely proportional to the amount of oxygen. This device has been evaluated, but further improvements in accuracy are required for use at a low Pao_2.[24] Once the problems of accuracy and reliability have been adequately addressed, the optode would likely be useful in thoracic surgical patients because it also permits simultaneous arterial pressure monitoring and arterial blood sampling.

Ventilation

All patients must be continually monitored to ensure adequacy of ventilation. Monitoring includes qualitative signs such as chest excursion (visual observation of the lungs when the chest is open), observation of the reservoir bag, and auscultation of breath sounds. An esophageal or precordial stethoscope should be used routinely. In addition, during one-lung ventilation, a stethoscope should be placed on the chest wall under the ventilated dependent lung. During controlled ventilation, circuit low- and high-pressure alarms with an audible signal must be used. The respiratory rate, V_T, minute volume, and inflation pressures should be observed.

Adequacy of ventilation should be confirmed by monitoring arterial blood gases, $Paco_2$ in particular. This may be estimated continuously and noninvasively by using a capnometer. The end-tidal CO_2 concentration represents alveolar CO_2 ($Paco_2$), which approximates $Paco_2$. There is normally a small arterial-to-alveolar CO_2 gradient (4–6 mm Hg), depending on alveolar dead space. The capnogram waveform is also helpful in diagnosing airway obstruction, incomplete relaxation, and even malposition of the double-lumen tube. In the latter application, a capnograph is coupled with each port of the double-lumen tube (one or two capnographs may be used), and the correct position of the double-lumen tube is identified by simultaneous and synchronous CO_2 readings on each of the two analyzers. The waveforms from each lung are examined for shape, height, and rhythm, depending on the correct position of the tube as well as on the ventilation/perfusion ($\dot{V}/\dot{Q}$) ratio for each lung.[25] A decrease in end-tidal CO_2 in the gas from one lumen of the double-lumen tube suggests malposition of the tube. During one-lung ventilation, systemic hypoxemia is usually a greater problem than hypercarbia.[26] This is because CO_2 is some 20 times more diffusible than oxygen and $Paco_2$ is more dependent on ventilation compared with Pao_2, which is more dependent on perfusion.

Sidestream Spirometry. Using a patented airway sampling adapter that incorporates a Pitot tube flowmeter system (D-Lite; Datex-Ohmeda, Tewksbury, MA), volume–pressure and flow–volume loops may be displayed from patients who are tracheally intubated and whose lungs are being mechanically ventilated.[27] This technique of continuous spirometry has been used as a monitor of ventilation as well as a means to detect displacement of a double-lumen tube.[28]

Physiology of the Lateral Decubitus Position. Ventilation and blood flow in the upright position have been discussed in a previous chapter (see Chapter 24). These variables will now be considered as they pertain to the lateral decubitus position

under six circumstances that are encountered during thoracic surgery.

LATERAL POSITION, AWAKE, BREATHING SPONTANEOUSLY, CHEST CLOSED. In the lateral decubitus position, the distribution of blood flow and ventilation is similar to that in the upright position but turned by 90 degrees (Fig. 30-6). Blood flow and ventilation to the dependent lung are significantly greater than to the nondependent lung. Good $\dot{V}/\dot{Q}$ matching at the level of the dependent lung results in adequate oxygenation in the awake patient breathing spontaneously. There are two important concepts in this situation. First, because perfusion is gravity dependent, the vertical hydrostatic gradient is smaller in the lateral than in the upright position; therefore, zone 1 is usually less extended. Second, in regard to ventilation, the dependent hemidiaphragm is pushed higher into the chest by the abdominal contents compared with the nondependent lung hemidiaphragm. During spontaneous ventilation, the conserved ability of the dependent diaphragm to contract results in an adequate distribution of V_T to the dependent lung. Because most of the perfusion is to the dependent lung, the $\dot{V}/\dot{Q}$ matching in this position is maintained similar to that in the upright position.

LATERAL POSITION, AWAKE, BREATHING SPONTANEOUSLY, CHEST OPEN. Controlled positive-pressure ventilation is the most common way to provide adequate ventilation and ensure gas exchange in an open chest situation. Frequently, thoracoscopy is performed using intercostal blocks with the patient breathing spontaneously to allow proper lung examination. The thoracoscope provides an adequate seal of the open chest to prevent a "free" open-chest situation. Two complications can arise from the patient breathing spontaneously with an open chest. The first is mediastinal shift, usually occurring during inspiration (Fig. 30-7). The negative pressure in the intact hemithorax, compared with the less negative pressure of the open hemithorax, can cause the mediastinum to move vertically downward and push into the dependent hemithorax. The mediastinal shift can create circulatory and reflex changes that may result in a clinical picture similar to that of shock and respiratory distress. Sometimes, depending on the severity of the distress, the patient needs to be tracheally intubated immediately, with initiation of positive-pressure ventilation, and the anesthesiologist must be prepared to intubate in this position without disturbing the

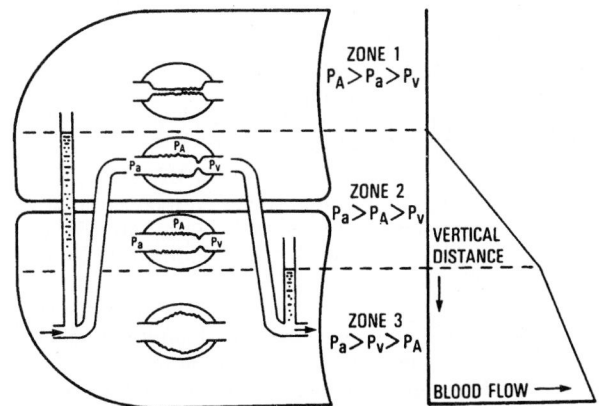

Figure 30-6. Schematic representation of the effects of gravity on the distribution of pulmonary blood flow in the lateral decubitus position. Vertical gradients in the lateral decubitus position are similar to those in the upright position and cause the creation of zones 1, 2, and 3. Consequently, pulmonary blood flow increases with lung dependency and is largest in the dependent lung and least in the nondependent lung. (P_a = pulmonary artery pressure; P_A = alveolar pressure; P_v = pulmonary venous pressure.) (Reproduced with permission from Benumof JL: Physiology of the open-chest and one lung ventilation. In Kaplan JA [ed]: Thoracic Anesthesia, p 288. New York, Churchill Livingstone, 1983.)

EXPIRATION

Pneumothorax

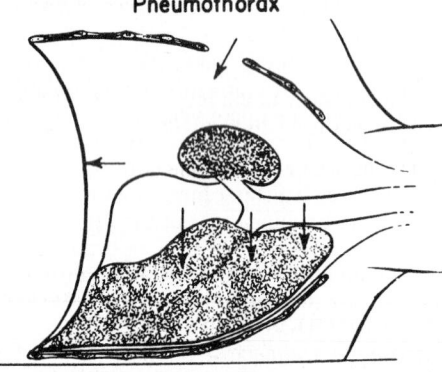

INSPIRATION

Pneumothorax

Figure 30-7. Schematic representation of mediastinal shift in the spontaneously breathing, open-chested patient in the lateral decubitus position. During inspiration, negative pressure in the intact hemithorax causes the mediastinum to move downward. During expiration, relative positive pressure in the intact hemithorax causes the mediastinum to move upward. (Reproduced with permission from Tarhan S, Moffitt EA: Principles of thoracic anesthesia. Surg Clin North Am 53:813, 1973.)

surgical field. The second phenomenon is paradoxical breathing (Fig. 30-8). During inspiration, the relatively negative pressure in the intact hemithorax compared with atmospheric pressure in the open hemithorax can cause movement of air from the nondependent into the dependent lung. The opposite occurs during expiration. This gas movement reversal from one lung to the other represents wasted ventilation and can compromise the adequacy of gas exchange. Paradoxical breathing is increased by a large thoracotomy or by an increase in airways resistance in the dependent lung. Positive-pressure ventilation or adequate sealing of the open chest eliminates paradoxical breathing.

LATERAL POSITION, ANESTHETIZED, BREATHING SPONTANEOUSLY, CHEST CLOSED.   The induction of general anesthesia does not cause significant change in the distribution of blood flow but has an important impact on the distribution of ventilation. Most of the VT enters the nondependent lung, and this results in a significant $\dot{V}/\dot{Q}$ mismatch. Induction of general anesthesia causes a reduction in the volumes of both lungs secondary to a reduction in FRC. Any reduction in volume in the dependent lung is of a greater magnitude than that in the nondependent lung for several reasons. First, the cephalad displacement of the dependent diaphragm by the abdominal contents is more pronounced and is increased by paralysis. Second, the mediastinal structures pressing on the dependent lung or poor positioning of the dependent side of the operating table prevents the

lung from expanding properly. The aforementioned factors will move lungs to a lower volume on the S-shaped volume–pressure curve (Fig. 30-9). The nondependent lung moves to a steeper position on the compliance curve and receives most of the VT, whereas the dependent lung is on the flat (noncompliant) part of the curve.

LATERAL POSITION, ANESTHETIZED, BREATHING SPONTANEOUSLY, CHEST OPEN.   Opening the chest has little impact on the distribution of perfusion. However, the upper lung is now no longer restricted by the chest wall and is free to expand, resulting in a further increase in $\dot{V}/\dot{Q}$ mismatch as the nondependent lung is preferentially ventilated owing to a now increased compliance.

LATERAL POSITION, ANESTHETIZED, PARALYZED, CHEST OPEN.   During paralysis and positive-pressure ventilation, diaphragmatic displacement is maximal over the nondependent lung, where there is the least amount of resistance to diaphragmatic movement caused by the abdominal contents (Fig. 30-10). This further compromises the ventilation to the dependent lung and increases the $\dot{V}/\dot{Q}$ mismatch.

ONE-LUNG VENTILATION, ANESTHETIZED, PARALYZED, CHEST OPEN.   During two-lung ventilation in the lateral position, the mean blood flow to the nondependent lung is assumed to be 40% of cardiac output, and 60% of cardiac output goes to the dependent lung (Fig. 30-11). Normally, venous admixture (shunt) in the lateral position is 10% of cardiac output and is equally

EXPIRATION

Pneumothorax

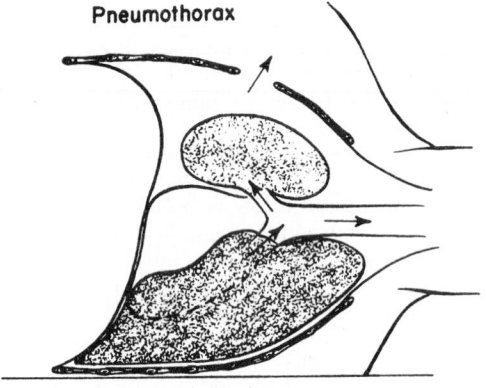

INSPIRATION

Pneumothorax

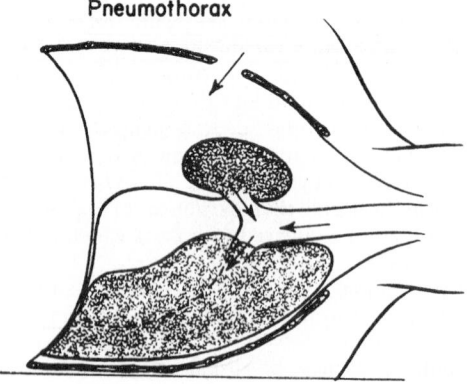

Figure 30-8. Schematic representation of paradoxical respiration in the spontaneously breathing, open-chested patient in the lateral decubitus position. During inspiration, movement of gas from the exposed lung into the intact lung and movement of air from the environment into the open hemithorax cause collapse of the exposed lung. During expiration, the reverse occurs, and the exposed lung expands. (Reproduced with permission from Tarhan S, Moffitt EA: Principles of thoracic anesthesia. Surg Clin North Am 53:813, 1973.)

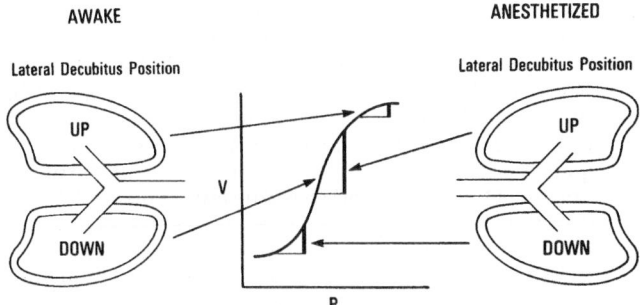

Figure 30-9. The left-hand side of the schematic shows the distribution of ventilation in the awake patient (closed chest) in the lateral decubitus position, and the right-hand side shows the distribution of ventilation in the anesthetized patient (closed chest) in the lateral ducubitus position. The induction of anesthesia has caused a loss in lung volume in both lungs, with the nondependent (up) lung moving from a flat, noncompliant portion to a steep, compliant portion of the pressure–volume curve, and the dependent (down) lung moving from a steep, compliant part to a flat, noncompliant part of the pressure–volume curve. Thus, the anesthetized patient in the lateral decubitus position has most tidal ventilation in the nondependent lung (where there is the least perfusion) and less tidal ventilation in the dependent lung (where there is the most perfusion). (V = volume; P = pressure.) (Reproduced with permission from Benumof JL: Physiology of the open-chest and one lung ventilation. In Kaplan JA [ed]: Thoracic Anesthesia, p 294. New York, Churchill Livingstone, 1983.)

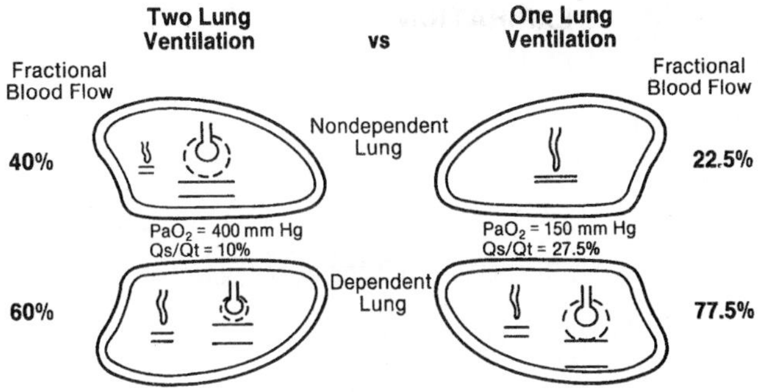

Figure 30-11. Schematic representation of two-lung ventilation versus one-lung ventilation. Typical values for fractional blood flow to the nondependent and dependent lungs, as well as PaO_2 and $\dot{Q}s/\dot{Q}t$ for the two conditions, are shown. The $\dot{Q}s/\dot{Q}t$ during two-lung ventilation is assumed to be distributed equally between the two lungs (5% to each lung). The essential difference between two-lung and one-lung ventilation is that, during one-lung ventilation, the nonventilated lung has some blood flow and therefore an obligatory shunt, which is not present during two-lung ventilation. The 35% of total flow perfusing the nondependent lung, which was not shunt flow, was assumed to be able to reduce its blood flow by 50% by hypoxic pulmonary vasoconstriction. The increase in $\dot{Q}s/\dot{Q}t$ from two-lung to one-lung ventilation is assumed to be due solely to the increase in blood flow through the nonventilated, nondependent lung during one-lung ventilation. (Reproduced with permission from Benumof JL: Anesthesia for Thoracic Surgery, p 112. Philadelphia, WB Saunders, 1987.)

divided as 5% in each lung. Therefore, the average percentage of cardiac output participating in gas exchange is 35% in the nondependent lung and 55% in the dependent lung.

One-lung ventilation creates an obligatory right-to-left transpulmonary shunt through the nonventilated, nondependent lung because the $\dot{V}/\dot{Q}$ ratio of that lung is zero. In theory, an additional 35% should be added to the total shunt during one-lung ventilation. However, assuming active HPV, blood flow to the nondependent hypoxic lung will be reduced by 50% and therefore is $(35/2) = 17.5\%$. To this must be added 5%, which is the obligatory shunt through the nondependent lung. The shunt through the nondependent lung is therefore 22.5% (see Fig. 30-11). Together with the 5% shunt in the dependent lung, total shunt during one-lung ventilation is $22.5\% + 5 = 27.5\%$. This results in a PaO_2 of approximately 150 mm Hg ($FiO_2 = 1.0$).[29]

Because 72.5% of the perfusion is directed to the dependent lung during one-lung ventilation, the matching of ventilation in this lung is important for adequate gas exchange. The dependent lung is no longer on the steep (compliant) portion of the

volume–pressure curve because of reduced lung volume and FRC. There are several reasons for this reduction in FRC, including general anesthesia, paralysis, pressure from abdominal contents, compression by the weight of mediastinal structures, and suboptimal positioning on the operating table. Other considerations that impair optimal ventilation to the dependent lung include absorption atelectasis, accumulation of secretions, and the formation of a fluid transudate in the dependent lung. All of these create a low $\dot{V}/\dot{Q}$ ratio and a large $P(A-a)O_2$ gradient.

ONE-LUNG VENTILATION

Absolute Indications for One-Lung Ventilation

Separation of the lungs to prevent spillage of pus or blood from an infected or bleeding source is an absolute indication for one-lung ventilation (Table 30-2). Life-threatening complications, such as massive atelectasis, sepsis, and pneumonia, can result from bilateral contamination. Bronchopleural and bronchocutaneous fistulae both represent low-resistance pathways for the

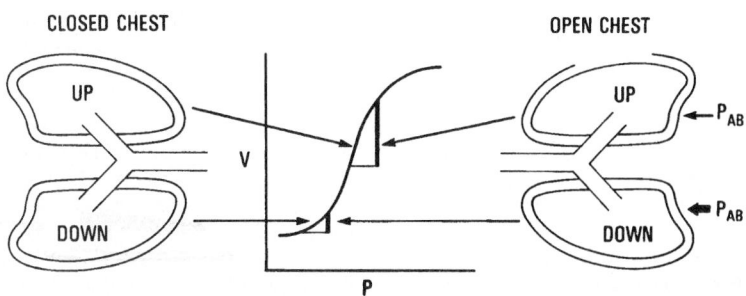

Figure 30-10. This schematic of a patient in the lateral decubitus position compares the closed-chested anesthetized condition with the open-chested anesthetized and paralyzed condition. Opening the chest increases nondependent lung compliance and reinforces or maintains the larger part of the tidal ventilation going to the nondependent lung. Paralysis also reinforces or maintains the larger part of tidal ventilation going to the nondependent lung because the pressure of the abdominal contents (P_{AB}) pressing against the upper diaphragm is minimal, and it is therefore easier for positive-pressure ventilation to displace this less resisting dome of the diaphragm. (V = volume; P = pressure.) (Reproduced with permission from Benumof JL: Physiology of the open-chest and one lung ventilation. In Kaplan JA [ed]: Thoracic Anesthesia, p 295. New York, Churchill Livingstone, 1983.)

Modified from Benumof JL: Physiology of the open-chest and one lung ventilation. In Kaplan JA (ed): Thoracic Anesthesia, p 299. New York, Churchill Livingstone, 1983.

V_T delivered by positive-pressure ventilation, and both prevent adequate alveolar ventilation. Giant cysts or unilateral bullae may rupture under positive-pressure ventilation. This can be avoided by selective lung ventilation. During bronchopulmonary lavage, an effective separation of the lungs is mandatory to avoid accidental spillage of fluid from the lavaged lung to the nondependent ventilated lung. Video assisted thoracoscopic surgery requires lung separation and is becoming the most common indication for one-lung ventilation.

Relative Indications for One-Lung Ventilation

In clinical practice, a double-lumen tube is commonly used for a lobectomy or pneumonectomy; these represent relative indications for lung separation. Upper lobectomy, pneumonectomy, and thoracic aortic aneurysm repair are relatively high-priority indications. These procedures are technically difficult, and optimal surgical exposure and a quiet operative field are highly desirable. Lower or middle lobectomy and esophageal resection are of lower priority. Nevertheless, many surgeons are accustomed to operating with the lung collapsed, which minimizes lung trauma from retractors and manipulation, improves visualization of lung anatomy, and facilitates identification and separation of anatomic structures and lung fissures. Thoracoscopy, if not performed with an intercostal block in the spontaneously breathing patient, is greatly facilitated by collapse of the lung under examination.

Methods of Lung Separation

Bronchial Blockers

Bronchial Blocker. Lung separation can be achieved with a reusable bronchial blocker. Magill described an endobronchial blocker that is placed using a bronchoscope and directed to the nonventilated lung. Inflation of the cuff at the distal end of the blocker serves to block ventilation to that lung. The lumen of the blocker permits suctioning of the airway distal to the catheter tip. Depending on the clinical circumstance, oxygen can be insufflated through the catheter lumen. A conventional endotracheal tube is then placed in the trachea. This technique can be useful in achieving selective ventilation in children younger than 12 years of age. However, because the blocker balloon requires a high distending pressure, it easily slips out of the bronchus into the trachea, obstructing ventilation and losing the seal between the two lungs. This displacement can be secondary to changes in position or to surgical manipulation. The loss of lung separation can be a life-threatening situation if it was performed to prevent spillage of pus, blood, or fluid from bronchopulmonary lavage. For this reason, bronchial blockers are rarely used in current practice.

Arterial Embolectomy Catheter. Selective airway occlusion can be achieved by the use of a Fogarty catheter designed for embolectomy procedures. Placement of the embolectomy catheter is best performed under direct vision with the aid of a fiberoptic bronchoscope. A conventional endotracheal tube is then placed alongside the catheter after withdrawing the bronchoscope. Alternatively, the bronchial blocker may be inserted through the lumen of a standard tracheal tube if the rubber diaphragm in a swivel connector is first perforated for passage of the blocker. The swivel connector is then placed between the tracheal tube and the Y-piece of the breathing circuit. A fiberscope can be inserted through the lumen of the tracheal tube to facilitate positioning of the blocker under direct vision.

Univent Tube. The Univent is a single-lumen endotracheal tube with a movable endobronchial blocker. In this tube, the bronchial blocker is housed in a small channel bored in the endotracheal tube wall. After intubation of the trachea, the movable blocker is manipulated into the desired mainstem bronchus with the aid of a fiberoptic bronchoscope.[30] Disadvantages of the Univent tube are that correct positioning of the blocker may be difficult to achieve or maintain. The Univent tube may be ideal for cases in which changing tubes (*e.g.,* from single- to double-lumen) may be difficult (*e.g.,* mediastinoscopy followed by thoracotomy), or in cases of bilateral lung transplantion.

Double-Lumen Endobronchial Tubes

These tubes are currently the most widely used means of achieving lung separation and one-lung ventilation. There are several different types of double-lumen tube, but all are essentially similar in design in that two catheters are bonded together. One lumen is long enough to reach a mainstem bronchus, and the second lumen ends with an opening in the distal trachea. Lung separation is achieved by inflation of two cuffs, the proximal tracheal cuff and the distal bronchial cuff located in the mainstem bronchus (see Positioning Double-Lumen Tubes). The endobronchial cuffs of right-sided tubes are slotted or otherwise designed to allow ventilation of the right upper lobe because the right mainstem bronchus is too short to accommodate both the right lumen tip and a right bronchial cuff.

Robertshaw Tube. This double-lumen tube is available in left- and right-sided forms without a carinal hook, which makes insertion easier (Fig. 30-12). This tube has the advantages of having D-shaped, large-diameter lumina that allow easy suctioning and offer low resistance to gas flow and a fixed curvature to facilitate proper positioning and to reduce the possibility of kinking. The original red rubber tubes are available in three sizes: small, medium, and large. Clear, polyvinyl chloride disposable Robertshaw-design double-lumen tubes are now in wide use. These tubes are available in a right or left design and in French sizes 35, 37, 39, and 41. A French size 28 has been made available for use in pediatric cases. The advantages of the disposable tubes include relative ease of insertion, proper positioning, easy recognition of the blue color of the endobronchial cuff when fiberoptic bronchoscopy is used, confirmation of position on a chest radiograph using the radioopaque lines in the wall of the tube, and continuous observation of tidal gas exchange and of respiratory moisture through the clear plastic. The right-sided endobronchial tube is designed to minimize occlusion of the right upper lobe. The right endobronchial cuff

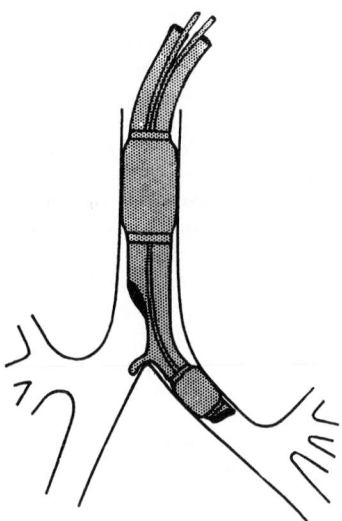

Figure 30-12. Left mainstem endobronchial intubation using a Carlens tube. Note carinal ''hook'' used for correct positioning. (Reproduced with permission from Hillard EK, Thompson PW: Instruments used in thoracic anaesthesia. In Mushin WW [ed]: Thoracic Anaesthesia, p 315. Oxford, Blackwell Scientific, 1963.)

is doughnut shaped and allows the right upper lobe ventilation slot to ride over the right upper lobe orifice. The tube is also suitable for use in long-term ventilation in the intensive care unit because it has a high-volume low-pressure cuff. These are now considered the tubes of choice for achieving lung separation and one-lung ventilation.

Despite the availability of disposable double-lumen tubes, many centers continue to use the red rubber Robertshaw tubes. There are several reasons for this. First, the cost of reusable tubes is significantly less than that of the disposable tubes. Second, some anesthesiologists believe that although the red rubber tubes may be more difficult to insert, they are less likely to dislocate during patient positioning and surgical manipulation. Third, during insertion of the double-lumen tube, the tracheal cuff often directly rubs against the patient's upper teeth. If these teeth are prominent and sharp, the thin-walled tracheal cuffs of the disposable tubes are much more likely to tear as compared with the thicker-walled cuffs of the red rubber tubes. Fourth, if the wrong size of disposable tube is selected and insertion is attempted, the tube cannot be reused because sterility is compromised. This does not apply to the red rubber tubes, which withstand repeated sterilization.[31]

Positioning Double-Lumen Tubes. This section concentrates on the insertion of Robertshaw-design double-lumen tubes (both disposable and nondisposable), because they are the most widely used. Before insertion, the double-lumen tube should be prepared and checked. The tracheal cuff (high-volume, low-pressure) can accommodate up to 20 ml of air, and the bronchial cuff should be checked using a 3-ml syringe. The tube should be coated liberally with water-soluble lubricant ointment and the stylet should be withdrawn, lubricated, and gently placed back into the bronchial lumen without disturbing the tube's preformed curvature. The Macintosh 3 blade is preferred for intubation of the trachea because it provides the largest area through which to pass the tube. The insertion of the tube is performed with the distal concave curvature facing anteriorly. After the tip of the tube is past the vocal cords, the stylet is removed and the tube is rotated through 90 degrees. A left-sided tube is rotated 90 degrees to the left and a right-sided tube is rotated to the right. Advancement of the tube ceases when moderate resistance to further passage is encountered, indicating that the tube tip has been firmly seated in the mainstem bronchus. It is important to remove the stylet before rotat-

ing and advancing the tube to avoid tracheal or bronchial lacerations. Rotation and advancement of the tube should be performed gently and under continuous direct laryngoscopy to prevent hypopharyngeal structures from interfering with proper positioning. Once the tube is thought to be in the proper position, a sequence of steps should be performed to check its location.

First, the tracheal cuff should be inflated and equal ventilation of both lungs established. If breath sounds are not equal, the tube is probably too far down and the tracheal lumen opening is in a mainstem bronchus or is lying at the carina. Withdrawal of the tube by 2–3 cm usually restores equal breath sounds. The second step is to clamp the right side (in the case of the left-sided tube) and remove the right cap from the connector. Then the bronchial cuff is slowly inflated to prevent an air leak from the bronchial lumen around the bronchial cuff into the tracheal lumen. This ensures that excessive pressure is not applied to the bronchus and helps avoid laceration. Inflation of the bronchial cuff rarely requires more than 2 ml of air. The third step is to remove the clamp and check that both lungs are ventilated with both cuffs inflated. This ensures that the bronchial cuff is not obstructing the contralateral hemithorax, either totally or partially. The final step is to clamp each side selectively and watch for absence of movement and breath sounds on the ipsilateral (clamped) side; the ventilated side should have clear breath sounds, chest movement that feels compliant, respiratory gas moisture with each tidal ventilation, and no air leak. If peak airway pressure during two-lung ventilation is 20 cm H_2O, it should not exceed 40 cm H_2O for the same V_T during one-lung ventilation.

Other methods that have been used for ensuring the correct placement of a double-lumen tube include fluoroscopy, chest radiography, selective capnography, and the use of an underwater seal. Determination of the presence of air leaks when positive pressure is applied to one lumen of a double-lumen tube is easily done in the operating room. If the bronchial cuff is not inflated and positive pressure is applied to the bronchial lumen of the double-lumen tube, gas leaks past the bronchial cuff and returns through the tracheal lumen. If the tracheal lumen is connected to an underwater seal system, gas will be seen to bubble up through the water. The bronchial cuff can then be gradually inflated until no gas bubbles are seen and the desired cuff seal pressure can be attained. This test is of extreme importance when absolute lung separation is needed, such as during bronchopulmonary lavage.

The most important advance in checking the proper position of a double-lumen tube is the introduction of the pediatric flexible fiberoptic bronchoscope. Smith *et al*[32] showed that when the disposable double-lumen tube was thought to be in correct position by auscultation and physical examination, subsequent fiberoptic bronchoscopy showed that 48% of tubes were, in fact, malpositioned. Such malpositions, however, are usually of no clinical significance.[33] When using a left-sided double-lumen tube, the bronchoscope is usually first introduced through the tracheal lumen. The carina is visualized; no bronchial cuff herniation should be seen. The upper surface of the blue endobronchial cuff should be just below the tracheal carina. The bronchial cuff of the disposable double-lumen tube is easily visualized because of its blue color. The bronchoscope should then be passed through the bronchial lumen and the left upper lobe orifice should be identified. When a right-sided double-lumen tube is used, the carina should be visualized through the tracheal lumen but, more important, the orifice of the right upper lobe bronchus should be identified when the bronchoscope is passed through the right upper lobe ventilating slot of the double-lumen tube. Pediatric fiberoptic bronchoscopes are available in several sizes: 5.6, 4.9, and 3.6 mm in external diameter. The 4.9-mm diameter bronchoscopes can be passed through double-lumen tubes of French sizes 37 and larger. The 3.6-mm diameter bronchoscope is easily passed through all sizes of double-lumen tube. In general, it is recommended that the largest size that can pass through the lumen of a double-lumen tube be used because it provides better visualization and facilitates identification of the bronchial anatomy.

Problems of Malposition of the Double-Lumen Tube. The use of a double-lumen tube is associated with a number of potential problems, the most important of which is malposition. There are several possibilities for tube malposition. The double-lumen tube may be accidentally directed to the side opposite the desired mainstem bronchus. In this case, the lung opposite the side of the connector clamped will collapse. Inadequate separation, increased airway pressures, and instability of the double-lumen tube usually occur. In addition, because of the morphology of the double-lumen tube curvatures, tracheal or bronchial lacerations may result. If a left-sided double-lumen tube is inserted into the right mainstem bronchus, it obstructs ventilation to the right upper lobe. It is therefore essential to recognize and correct such a malposition as soon as possible.

Second, the double-lumen tube may be passed too far down into either the right or the left mainstem bronchus. In this case, breath sounds are very diminished or not audible at all over the contralateral side. This situation is corrected when the tube is withdrawn until the opening of the tracheal lumen is above the carina.

Third, the double-lumen tube may not be inserted far enough, leaving the bronchial lumen opening above the carina. In this position, good breath sounds are heard bilaterally when ventilating through the bronchial lumen, but no breath sounds are audible when ventilating through the tracheal lumen because the inflated bronchial cuff obstructs gas flow arising from the tracheal lumen. The cuff should be deflated and the double-lumen tube rotated and advanced into the desired mainstem bronchus.

Fourth, a right-sided double-lumen tube may occlude the right upper lobe orifice. The mean distance from the carina to the right upper lobe orifice is 2.3 ± 0.7 cm in men and 2.1 ± 0.7 cm in women.[34] With right-sided double-lumen tubes, the ventilatory slot in the side of the bronchial catheter must overlie the right upper lobe orifice to permit ventilation of this lobe. The margin of safety, however, is extremely small, and varies from 1 to 8 mm.[34] It is, therefore, difficult to ensure proper ventilation to the right upper lobe and to avoid dislocation of the double-lumen tube during surgical manipulation. When right endobronchial intubation is required, a disposable right-sided double-lumen tube is perhaps the best choice because of the slanted doughnut shape of the bronchial cuff, which allows the ventilation slot to ride off the right upper lobe ventilation orifice and increases the margin of safety.

Fifth, the left upper lobe orifice may be obstructed by a left-sided double-lumen tube. Traditionally, it was believed that the take-off of the left upper lobe bronchus was at a safe distance from the carina and that it would not be obstructed by a left-sided double-lumen tube. However, the mean distance between the left upper lobe orifice and the carina is 5.4 ± 0.7 cm in men and 5.0 ± 0.7 cm in women.[34] The average distance between the openings of the right and left lumens on the left-sided disposable tubes is 6.9 cm.[34] Therefore, an obstruction of the left upper lobe is possible while the tracheal lumen is still above the carina. There is also a 20% variation in the location of the blue endobronchial cuff on the disposable tubes because this cuff is attached at the end of the manufacturing process.

Finally, bronchial cuff herniation may occur and obstruct the bronchial lumen if excessive volumes are used to inflate the cuff. The bronchial cuff has also been known to herniate over the tracheal carina, and in the case of a left-sided double-lumen tube, to obstruct ventilation to the right mainstem bronchus.

Another rare complication with double-lumen tubes is tracheal rupture. Overinflation of the bronchial cuff, inappropriate positioning, and trauma owing to intraoperative dislocation

that resulted in bronchial rupture have been described in association with the Robertshaw tube and the disposable double-lumen tube.[35] Therefore, the pressure in the bronchial cuff should be assessed and decreased if the cuff is found to be overinflated. If absolute separation of the lungs is not needed, the bronchial cuff should be deflated and then reinflated slowly to avoid excessive pressure on the bronchial walls. The bronchial cuff should also be deflated during any repositioning of the patient unless lung separation is absolutely required during this time.

Contraindications to Use of the Double-Lumen Tube. Use of a double-lumen tube to achieve lung separation is relatively contraindicated in situations in which there is a lesion in the airway itself or a difficult upper airway that results in poor laryngeal visualization. It is also relatively contraindicated in some critically ill patients in whom short periods of apnea or hypoxemia, which may occur during insertion of a double-lumen tube, may be life-threatening. In patients requiring rapid intubation (*e.g.*, with a full stomach), a double-lumen tube is not necessarily contraindicated because the disposable tubes with stylets are as easily inserted as single-lumen tubes in most cases.

Lung Separation in the Patient with a Tracheostomy

Occasionally a patient with permanent tracheotomy is scheduled for surgery on the lung that requires lung separation. Examples of such patients include those who have undergone resection of a tumor in the floor of the mouth or of the base of the tongue, followed by extensive reconstructive surgery with creation of a permanent tracheal stoma. Routine follow-up may reveal a lung lesion that requires a diagnostic procedure. Conventional double-lumen endobronchial tubes are designed to be inserted through the mouth, not through a tracheal stoma. The standard double-lumen tubes are usually too stiff to negotiate the curve required for insertion through a tracheal stoma, and are difficult to position.[36]

A separately inserted bronchial blocker, either within or alongside a single-lumen tube that has been placed through the tracheostomy, may permit adequate lung separation.[37] Compared with an orotracheal or nasotracheal single-lumen tube, passing a Fogarty catheter (to function as a bronchial blocker) through a tracheostomy into a mainstem bronchus may be easier because of the shorter distances involved.

Saito *et al*[38] have described a spiral, wire-reinforced, double-lumen endobronchial tube made of silicone (Koken Medical, Tokyo, Japan) that is designed for placement through a tracheostomy.[38] The middle section of the tube consists of two thin-walled silicone catheters with an internal diameter of 5 mm, glued together and reinforced with a stainless steel spiral wire and covered in a silicone coating with two pilot balloons. The distal section, which contains the bronchial lumen and the bronchial cuff, is made of wire-reinforced silicone to avoid excessive flexibility. The dimensions are based on the Mallinckrodt double-lumen tube. The bronchial cuff is located 1.2 cm from the tip, and the distance between the tip orifice and the tracheal orifice is 4.9 cm. In a clinical trial in patients with permanent tracheal stomas, the tubes functioned well in achieving lung separation, with no sign of kinking or movement, and permitted easy passage of a suction catheter.

Lung Separation in the Patient with a Difficult Airway

When separation of the lungs is required and the patient has a clearly recognized difficult airway, then awake intubation using a flexible fiberoptic bronchoscope can be planned to place a double-lumen, Univent or a single-lumen tube. The single-lumen tube may then be exchanged for a double-lumen or Univent tube using a tube exchanger plus laryngoscopy, or a Fogarty embolectomy catheter may be passed through the lumen of the single-lumen tube to act as an independent bronchial blocker. Furthermore, depending on the expected extent and the duration of the surgical procedure and the degree of fluid shift, an airway not initially classified as difficult may become difficult secondary to facial edema, secretions, and laryngeal trauma from the initial intubation.

The indications for one-lung ventilation were discussed earlier in this chapter. Recently, the popularity of the VAT procedure has increased. The improvements in video-endoscopic surgical equipment and a growing enthusiasm for minimally invasive surgical approaches have popularized VAT in the practice of surgery for diagnostic and therapeutic procedures. Most of these procedures require a well collapsed lung and should be considered as absolute indications for one-lung ventilation. The lung must be well collapsed to allow the surgeon an optimal view of the surgical field and to palpate the lesion in the lung parenchyma. In addition, it is difficult to place the stapler on a lung that is not completely collapsed, and there is an increase in incidence of postoperative air leaks in these circumstances. Because of its widespread use today, VAT significantly increases the number of cases with a potentially difficult airway that require lung separation. In the past, before the era of VAT, most open thoracotomies were for surgical exposure. Most of the patients were intubated with a double-lumen tube. However, when faced with a difficult intubation, the anesthesiologist often managed these cases with a single-lumen tube, intermittent ventilation, compressing the operated lung with lap pads, or the use of low V_T with a high ventilatory rate to allow the surgeon to proceed with the lung resection. Only rarely was there an absolute need for lung separation in a patient with a difficult airway.

Methods of Lung Separation in the Patient with a Difficult Airway

An airway may be recognized initially as difficult when conventional laryngoscopy reveals a Grade III or IV view. Sometimes, depending on the type and duration of surgery and the degree of fluid shift, an airway that initially was not classified as difficult may become difficult secondary to facial edema, the presence of secretions, and laryngeal trauma from the initial intubation.[39,40]

A logical approach to lung separation is shown in Figure 30-13. When lung separation is mandated, and the patient has a recognized difficult airway, awake intubation using flexible fiberoptic bronchoscopy can be attempted using a double-lumen tube, Univent, or a single-lumen tube. The same approach may be used for the patient with an unrecognized difficult airway and a failure to intubate with conventional laryngoscopy. When using a double-lumen tube over a fiberoptic bronchoscope, the anesthesiologist should keep in mind that it is a bulky tube with a large external diameter, and because of the length of the double-lumen tube, only a limited part of the fiberoptic bronchoscope is available for manipulation. In addition, the mismatch between the flexibility of the fiberoptic bronchoscope and the rigidity of the double-lumen tube makes the tube harder to advance over the fiberoptic bronchoscope. The Univent tube has the same bulky external diameter and is also often hard to pass between the vocal cords, particularly in a patient who is awake.

Single-Lumen Tube Can Be Successfully Placed. If a failure to provide lung separation could result in a life-threatening situation, there are two possibilities to provide one-lung ventilation when a single-lumen tube is already in place. First, depending on the indication for lung isolation, a tube exchanger can be used to switch to a double-lumen or a Univent tube. The second possibility is to direct a bronchial blocker through the single-lumen tube into the selected mainstem bronchus. These two methods, however, offer limited protection or an inadequate seal in cases such a lung lavage, pulmonary abscess, or hemoptysis, where a double-lumen tube would be the tube of choice.

USE OF A TUBE EXCHANGER. Several tube exchangers are commercially available (Cook Critical Care, Bloomington, IN; Sheridan Catheter Corporation, Argyle, NY). On all of these tube exchangers, the depth is marked in centimeters, and they are available in a wide range of external diameters and easily adapted for either oxygen insufflation or jet ventilation.

The size of the tube exchanger and the size of the tube to be inserted should be tested *in vitro* before use in a patient. The French size 11 tube changer will pass through a 35–41 French size double-lumen tube, while the French size 14 tube exchanger does not pass through a French size 35. To prevent lung laceration, the tube exchanger should never be inserted against resistance. Finally, when passing any tube over an airway guide, a laryngoscope should be used to facilitate passage of the tube over the airway guide past supraglottic tissues.

USE OF A BRONCHIAL BLOCKER. The use of a bronchial blocker has been discussed earlier in this chapter. An independently passed bronchial blocker may be used with a single-lumen tube to obtain lung isolation, thereby avoiding the use of a double-lumen or Univent tube in a patient with a difficult airway. The

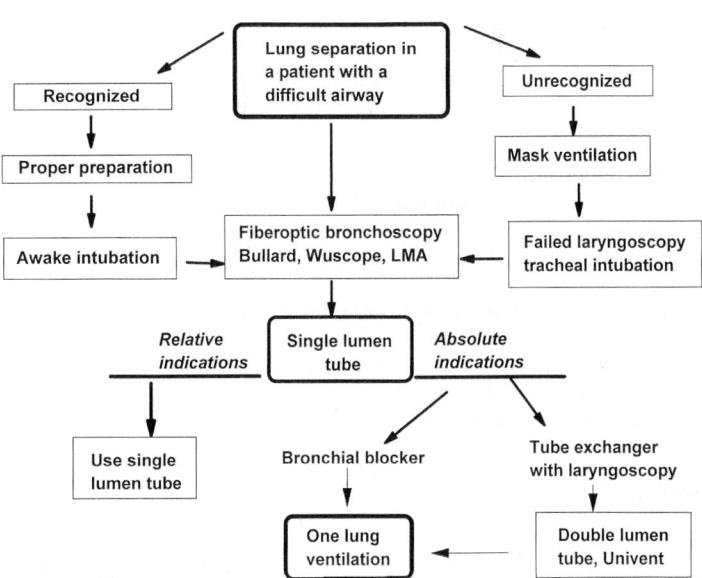

Figure 30-13. Lung separation in a patient with a difficult airway.

most commonly used independent bronchial blocker is a number 7.0 Fogarty embolectomy catheter, which has an occlusion balloon that can range in volume from 5.0–8.0 ml. The balloon should be inflated to a volume sufficient to occlude the lumen of the mainstem bronchus and to hold the catheter in place. The fiberoptic bronchoscope is passed through a bronchoscopy elbow, down a single-lumen tube to visualize the carina, and past the Fogarty balloon-tipped catheter into the appropriate mainstem bronchus. The Fogarty catheter is supplied with a wire stylet in place, which can be curved at the distal end to facilitate passage through the bronchoscopy elbow and down the single-lumen tube. The catheter balloon is then inflated, under direct vision using the bronchoscope, with enough volume to occlude the main bronchus. The balloon of the Fogarty catheter is a high-pressure, low-volume device and can exert significant pressure on the mucosa of the bronchial wall.

Drawbacks to the use of bronchial blockers include difficulty in directing the blocker into the desired bronchus, even with help of a fiberscope, and the inability to effectively suction the airway distal to the blocker; also during the surgical manipulation, the blocker may slip into the trachea, resulting in life-threatening airway obstruction.

In an attempt to overcome these potential problems, a snare-guided bronchial blocker has been introduced (Cook Critical Care, Bloomington, IN). A fiberscope is passed through the loop of the bronchial blocker and then guided into the desired bronchus. The blocker is then slid distally over the fiberscope into the selected bronchus. Bronchoscopic visualization confirms blocker placement and bronchial occlusion. The string (snare) is then removed through the blocker and the 1.8-mm diameter lumen may then be used as a suction port or for insufflation of oxygen. Disadvantages of this new device are its high cost and the inability to reinsert the snare (string) once it has been pulled out, making it impossible to redirect the blocker should it become necessary. Finally, the external diameter is somewhat larger, which requires it to be passed through a single-lumen tube of at least 7.5–8 mm in internal diameter.

Single-Lumen Tube Cannot Be Successfully Placed. If a single-lumen tube cannot be placed with the aid of a fiberscope, and the patient's condition is stable, the clinician may use some alternative devices to assist in placement of the single-lumen tube. There are several commercially available laryngoscopes that can facilitate endobronchial intubation. The two best known are the Bullard laryngoscope (Circon, ACMI, Stamford, CT) and the Wu laryngoscope (Achi Corp., Dublin, CA). The Bullard laryngoscope is an anatomically shaped, rigid instrument that uses a fiberoptic bundle to obtain a view of the larynx. Thus, the oral, pharyngeal, and tracheal axes do not have to

be aligned in order to view the larynx. The Wu laryngoscope uses a similar concept but consists of a rigid blade portion and a separate, flexible fiberoptic portion. Successful use of these devices is associated with a relatively lengthy learning curve, and the clinician facing a difficult airway should not be using these laryngoscopes for the first time.

Finally, the Fastrach (Gensia, Inc., San Diego, CA), a new version of the conventional LMA, is a reasonable alternative. First, it permits ventilation of the patient during the airway manipulation, and second, this new form of the laryngeal airway mask permits insertion of a large-diameter (8 mm) single-lumen tube. In rare cases, when none of these methods results in a successful intubation, the plan to perform the procedure should be re-evaluated, or a Combitube (Kendall-Sheridan Catheter Corp., Argyle, NY) can be inserted to allow ventilation, if not lung separation.

Conclusion of the Surgical Procedure

Depending on the extent and the duration of the procedure and the degree of fluid shift, an airway, initially not classified as difficult may become difficult secondary to facial edema, secretions, and laryngeal trauma from the original intubation. In these cases, when planning to provide lung separation, the postoperative period should be considered and the appropriate tube placed. Many procedures that are not considered to represent absolute indications for lung separation are lengthy and complex. Complex lung resection, with or without chest wall resection, thoracoabdominal esophagogastrectomy, thoracic aortic aneurysm resection with or without total circulatory arrest, or an extensive vertebral tumor resection, may result in facial edema, secretion, and hemoptysis, requiring postoperative ventilatory support. Other indications for postoperative ventilatory support are marginal respiratory reserve, unexpected blood loss or fluid shift, hypothermia, and inadequate reversal of neuromuscular blockade.

If a Univent tube was used to provide one-lung ventilation the blocker may be fully retracted and the Univent tube can function as a single-lumen tube. If an independent bronchial blocker was used, then the blocker is removed, leaving the single-lumen tube in place. The problem arises when a double-lumen tube was inserted for lung separation. In a patient with a difficult airway and subsequent facial edema, the double-lumen tube may be left in place after surgery.

If the decision to leave the double-lumen tube in place is made, it is important to keep in mind that the intensive care unit staff is usually less experienced in managing such a tube, which may easily become dislocated. In addition, it is more difficult to suction through the lumen, and a longer, narrower

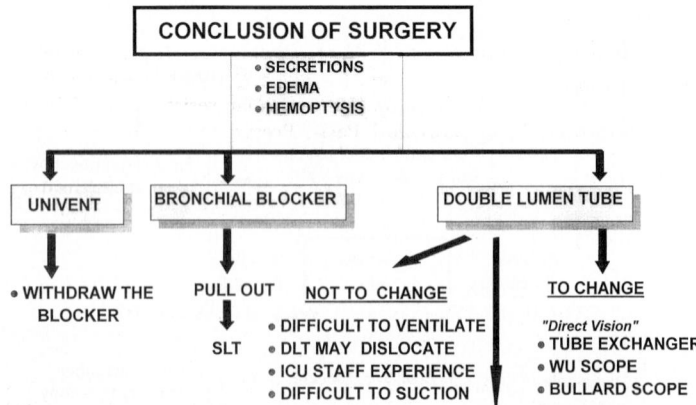

Figure 30-14. Conclusion of the surgical procedure. See text for discussion. (DLT = double-lumen tube; SLT = single-lumen tube.)

suction catheter is needed to reach the tip of the endobronchial lumen. Another possibility is to withdraw the double-lumen tube to place the 19–20-cm mark at the teeth, so that the endobronchial lumen is above the carina and both lungs can be ventilated. Tracheal extubation from the double-lumen tube should be considered after diuresis and steroid therapy to allow reduction of the facial and airway edema.

If it is decided to change the double-lumen to a single-lumen tube, the decision should not be accomplished blindly. A tube exchanger must be used to maintain access to the airway, as previously discussed. Tube exchange may be performed under direct vision using a Bullard or Wu laryngoscope. With these laryngoscopes, the tube exchanger or a stylet can be placed under direct vision through the vocal cords alongside the existing tube to permit passage of a single-lumen tube (Fig. 30-14).

In summary, the clinician should be able to master different methods of lung separation and make him/herself familiar with the devices available to provide one-lung ventilation and optimal, and safe management of the patient. In addition, one should always plan in advance for the postoperative period when choosing the method of lung separation. Finally, in these cases, a close dialog with the surgical team is of vital importance.

MANAGEMENT OF ONE-LUNG VENTILATION

This section discusses the management of one-lung ventilation in a paralyzed patient in the lateral decubitus position with an open chest. Inspired oxygen fraction (FIO_2), V_T and respiratory rate, dependent lung, PEEP, and nondependent lung CPAP are reviewed and an approach to the management of one-lung ventilation is presented.

Inspired Oxygen Fraction

An FIO_2 of 1.0 is usually used during one-lung ventilation. This high oxygen concentration serves to protect against hypoxemia during the procedure. In many studies, an FIO_2 of 1.0 has been used and resulted in a shunt of 25–30% and mean PaO_2 values between 150 and 210 mm Hg during one-lung ventilation.[41] In addition to a higher margin of safety, high FIO_2 values cause vasodilatation of the vessels in the dependent lung, which increases the capability of this lung to accept blood flow redistribution due to nondependent lung HPV. A high FIO_2 may, however, cause absorption atelectasis and potentially further increase the degree of shunt because of the collapsed alveoli. The risk can be reduced by using a lower FIO_2, by the application of positive-pressure ventilation, or by the use of a high V_T and PEEP. Theoretically, a high FIO_2 can also cause lung injury owing to oxygen toxicity, although this complication is unlikely to occur in the time frame of a surgical operation. Lower FIO_2 values (0.25–0.50) have also been used, with resulting mean PaO_2 values between 62 and 87 mm Hg.[42,43]

The use of an FIO_2 less than 1.0 during one-lung ventilation offers the benefits of reducing the risk of absorption atelectasis and may permit use of lower concentrations of potent inhaled anesthetics, which in higher concentrations might be more depressant to the myocardium, particularly in high-risk patients. An FIO_2 of less than 1.0 may also be indicated in patients with bleomycin toxicity. The combination of N_2O/O_2 with pulse oximetry monitoring may represent an optimal solution in such cases. However, the risk–benefit ratio for each patient should always be carefully considered.

Tidal Volume and Respiratory Rate

During one-lung ventilation, the dependent lung should be ventilated with a V_T of 10–12 ml·kg^{-1}. V_Ts ranging between 8 and 15 ml·kg^{-1} produced no significant effect on transpulmo-

nary shunt or PaO_2.[44] A V_T of less than 8 ml·kg^{-1} can result in a decrease in FRC and enhanced formation of atelectasis in the dependent lung. A V_T of greater than 15 ml·kg^{-1} can increase the pulmonary vascular resistance of the dependent lung (similar to the application of PEEP) and divert blood flow into the nondependent lung. The value of 10–12 ml·kg^{-1} is a middle range between 8 and 15 ml·kg^{-1} and appears to have the smallest effect on PaO_2 and percentage shunt.

The respiratory rate should be adjusted to maintain a $PaCO_2$ of 35 ± 3 mm Hg. Elimination of CO_2 is usually not a problem during one-lung ventilation if the double-lumen tube is positioned correctly. The shunt during one-lung ventilation has little influence on $PaCO_2$ values because the arteriovenous PCO_2 difference is normally only 6 mm Hg. Furthermore, CO_2 is 20 times more diffusible than O_2 and will be eliminated faster. It is also important not to hyperventilate the patient's lungs because hypocapnia increases vascular resistance in the dependent lung, inhibits nondependent lung HPV, increases shunt, and decreases PaO_2. Hypocarbia is thought to inhibit HPV secondary to a vasodilator effect. Because hypocarbia can only be achieved only by hyperventilating the dependent lung, it raises the mean intra-alveolar pressure and therefore increases the vascular resistance in that lung. Finally, one-lung ventilation decreases the deadspace-to-tidal volume (V_D/V_T) ratio and enhances CO_2 elimination.[45]

Positive End-Expiratory Pressure to the Dependent Lung

The beneficial effect of selective PEEP 10 cm H_2O ($PEEP_{10}$) to the dependent lung is caused by an increased lung volume at end-expiration (FRC), which improves the $\dot{V}/\dot{Q}$ relationship in the dependent lung. The increase in FRC prevents airway and alveolar closure at end-expiration. Therefore, it is not surprising that attempts have been made to improve oxygenation during one-lung ventilation by the application of PEEP to the dependent lung. However, the results were somewhat disappointing. Most of the studies showed either no change in PaO_2, a decrease, or a slight increase in PaO_2,[41,45] probably owing to the PEEP inducing an increase in lung volume that caused compression of the small interalveolar vessels and increased pulmonary vascular resistance. If this increase in resistance is limited to the dependent lung, blood flow can be diverted only to the nondependent (nonventilated) lung, increasing percentage shunt and futher decreasing PaO_2.

The studies of PEEP cited previously used an FIO_2 of 1.0 with a mean PaO_2 during one-lung ventilation of between 150 and 200 mm Hg, at which further improvement in PaO_2 is clinically unnecessary. The possibility that the application of PEEP can improve PaO_2 in a diseased dependent lung (low lung volume and low $\dot{V}/\dot{Q}$ ratio) with a low PaO_2 (<80 mm Hg) during one-lung ventilation has been addressed by Cohen et al.[46] They found that application of $PEEP_{10}$ during one-lung ventilation in patients with a low PaO_2 may increase FRC to normal values, resulting in a lower pulmonary vascular resistance and in an improved $\dot{V}/\dot{Q}$ ratio and PaO_2. Presumably, patients with a higher PaO_2 had a dependent lung with an adequate FRC, and the application of PEEP had the negative effect of redistributing blood flow away from the dependent ventilated lung (Fig. 30-15).

Continuous Positive Airway Pressure to the Nondependent Lung

The single most effective maneuver to increase PaO_2 during one-lung ventilation is the application of CPAP to the nondependent lung. This has been clearly demonstrated in several studies.[41,43,47] A lower level of CPAP (5–10 cm H_2O) maintains the patency of the nondependent alveoli, allowing some oxygen uptake to occur in the distended alveoli. CPAP should be applied after delivering a V$_T$ to the nondependent lung to keep it slightly expanded. CPAP, applied by insufflation of oxygen under positive pressure, keeps this lung "quiet" and prevents it from collapsing completely. Inflation of oxygen without maintaining a positive pressure failed to improve Pao$_2$,[41] although some improvement in Pao$_2$ occurred after 45 minutes of one-lung ventilation (from 140 ± 107 to 206 ± 76 mm Hg) with oxygen insufflation only.[48] Intermittent reinflation of the collapsed (nondependent) lung with oxygen also resulted in a significant improvement in Pao$_2$.[49] The beneficial effects of CPAP 10 cm H$_2$O (CPAP$_{10}$) are not attributable solely to the effect of positive pressure in diverting blood flow away from the collapsed lung because (in dogs) the hyperinflation of nitrogen into the nondependent lung under 10 cm H$_2$O failed to improve Pao$_2$.

The application of high-level CPAP (15 cm H$_2$O) is not beneficial. At this pressure, the lung becomes overdistended, which interferes with surgical exposure. Also, this level of CPAP might have hemodynamic consequences, whereas CPAP$_{10}$ has been shown to have no significant hemodynamic effects.[43]

Continuous positive airway pressure can be applied to the nondependent lung using a number of simple systems, all of which have essentially the same features: an oxygen source, tubing to connect the oxygen source to the nonventilated lung, a pressure relief valve, and a pressure gauge.[3] The catheter to the nondependent lung is usually insufflated with 5 l·min^{-1} of oxygen using a modified Ayre T-piece pediatric circuit, and the valve on the expiratory limb is adjusted to the desired pressure as read on the attached gauge (Fig. 30-16). Instead of a pressure gauge or manometer inserted into the circuit, a weighted pop-off valve, such as a ball or spring-loaded PEEP valve, can be used.

High-frequency ventilation with oxygen to the nondependent lung and conventional ventilation to the dependent lung has also been used to improve Pao$_2$ during one-lung ventilation (see High-Frequency Ventilation, later).

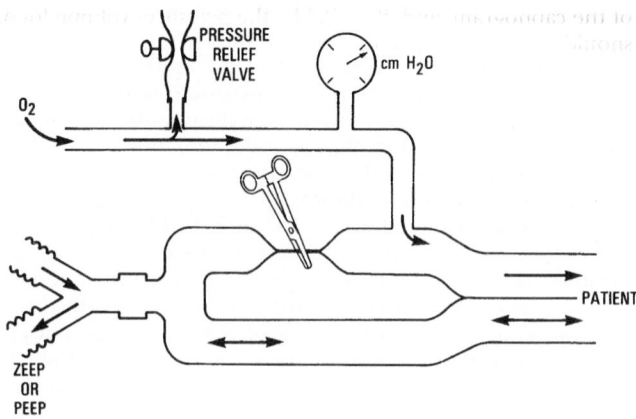

Figure 30-16. Schematic of a simple, selective up-lung continuous positive airway pressure system. The fresh inflow of oxygen is restricted or limited by a pressure release valve, and therefore a constant distending airway pressure to the nonventilated lung occurs. The dependent lung can be ventilated with positive end-expiratory pressure (PEEP) or zero end-expiratory pressure (ZEEP). (Reproduced with permission from Benumof JL: Physiology of the open-chest and one lung ventilation. In Kaplan JA [ed]: Thoracic Anesthesia, p 310. New York, Churchill Livingstone, 1983.)

Clinical Approach to Management of One-Lung Ventilation

Once the patient is in the lateral position, the position of the double-lumen tube should be rechecked. Two-lung ventilation should be maintained for as long as possible, and when one-lung ventilation needs to be instituted, it is generally recommended that an Fio$_2$ of 1.0 be used. The lungs should be ventilated using a V$_T$ of 10–12 ml · kg^{-1} at a rate adjusted to maintain Paco$_2$ at 35 ± 3 mm Hg. This is usually monitored with the use of a capnometer or other multigas analyzer.

After initiation of one-lung ventilation, Pao$_2$ can continue to decrease for up to 45 minutes.[44] Frequent monitoring of arterial blood gases and use of a pulse oximeter continue throughout the operative period. It is also essential to work closely with the surgeon. If there are any questions concerning the position of the double-lumen tube, and if fiberoptic bronchoscopy is not available, the surgeon can palpate the tube and help to manipulate it into the correct position with direct digital guidance.

If hypoxemia occurs during one-lung ventilation, the position of the double-lumen tube should be rechecked using a fiberoptic bronchoscope. If the dependent lung is not severely diseased, a satisfactory Pao$_2$ on two-lung ventilation should not decrease to dangerously hypoxic levels on one-lung ventilation. If a left thoracotomy is being performed using a right-sided double-lumen tube, ventilation to the right upper lobe should be ensured. After the tube position has been confirmed as correct, CPAP$_{10}$ should be applied to the nondependent lung after a V$_T$ that expands the lung. In most cases, the Pao$_2$ increases to a safe level. During thoracoscopy, application of CPAP is usually not possible because it impedes the surgeon. This is especially so during VAT surgical procedures. In this case, PEEP to the ventilated lung may be tried.

In the very rare case in which the Pao$_2$ remains low despite all of these maneuvers, intermittent two-lung ventilation can be reinstituted with the surgeon's cooperation. Also, depending on the stage of surgical dissection, if a pneumonectomy is being performed, ligation of the pulmonary artery eliminates the shunt.

During one-lung ventilation, the peak airway pressure, the effective V$_T$ delivered (measured by a spirometer), the shape

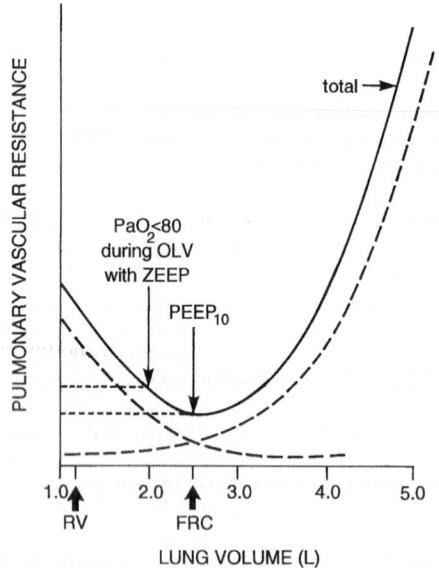

Figure 30-15. Effect of 10 cm H$_2$O PEEP on FRC. It is postulated that, in patients having Pao$_2$ < 80 mm Hg with ZEEP, FRC is low. PEEP$_{10}$ increases FRC and thereby increases Pao$_2$. (PEEP$_{10}$ = positive end-expiratory pressure [10 cm H$_2$O]; OLV = one-lung ventilation; FRC = functional residual capacity; RV = residual volume; ZEEP = zero end-expiratory pressure.)

of the capnogram, and, if available, the pressure–volume loop, should be checked continuously. A sudden increase in peak airway pressure may be secondary to tube dislocation because of surgical manipulation, resulting in impaired ventilation. In addition, the ability to auscultate by a stethoscope over the dependent lung is extremely important.

If any questions arise about the stability of the patient, or if the patient becomes hypotensive, dusky, or tachycardic, two-lung ventilation should be resumed until the problem has been resolved. Because of pericardial manipulation (during left thoracotomy in particular) and pulling on the great vessels, cardiac arrhythmias and hypotension are not uncommon. Cardiotonic drugs should be prepared and kept available for use during any thoracic surgical procedure. Most thoracic surgical procedures represent only relative indications for one-lung ventilation, and the benefits of one-lung ventilation should always be weighed against the risks to the patient.

CHOICE OF ANESTHESIA FOR THORACIC SURGERY

The choice of anesthesia technique for a thoracic surgical procedure must take into account the patient's cardiovascular and respiratory status and the particular effects of anesthetic drugs on these and other organ systems.

Thoracic surgical patients are more likely than others to have increased airway reactivity and a propensity to develop bronchoconstriction. This is because many of these patients are cigarette smokers and have chronic bronchitis or COPD. In addition, surgical manipulation of the airways and bronchial tree by instruments, a double-lumen tube, or the surgeon makes bronchoconstriction more likely to occur. Halothane, enflurane, and isoflurane have all been shown to decrease airways reactivity and bronchoconstriction provoked by hypocapnia or inhaled or irritant aerosols. Their mechanism of action is probably a direct one on the airway musculature itself, and these agents are therefore the drugs of choice in patients with reactive airways. For an inhalation induction, halothane might be preferable because it is the least pungent of the three drugs, although once the patient is asleep isoflurane may be the preferred drug because it raises the cardiac dysrhythmia threshold and provides greater cardiovascular stability. Fentanyl does not appear to influence bronchomotor tone, but morphine may increase tone by a central vagotonic effect and by releasing histamine.

In most patients, anesthesia is safely induced with thiopental, thiamylal, or propofol. In patients with reactive airways, ketamine may be the drug of choice for induction of anesthesia because it has a bronchodilator effect and has been successfully used in the treatment of asthma. Thiopental has been associated with bronchospasm in asthmatic patients, although the reactivity in such cases may be related to inadequate levels of anesthesia before instrumentation of the airway.

The muscle relaxants of choice for thoracic procedures are those that lack a histamine-releasing or vagotonic effect and that have some sympathomimetic effect. In this respect, pancuronium, vecuronium, rocuronium, and cisatracurium probably represent the drugs of choice. Succinylcholine is useful to provide rapid profound relaxation for intubation of the trachea and is not associated with an increase in airways reactivity.

Intravenous lidocaine ($1–1.5\ mg\cdot kg^{-1}$) can be used before manipulations of the airway to prevent reflex bronchospasm. It has also been given by infusion to depress airway reactivity in patients who have poor cardiovascular function and cannot tolerate normal doses of the potent inhaled agents. Intravenous lidocaine has also been used to treat bronchospasm occurring during anesthesia. Lidocaine nebulized and administered *via* the airways has a similar salutary effect on bronchial tone.

Atropine may be used to block the antimuscarinic effects of acetylcholine and thereby protect against cholinergically induced bronchoconstriction. It may be administered intravenously or in nebulized form (see Bronchoscopy).

HYPOXIC PULMONARY VASOCONSTRICTION

General anesthesia may impair pulmonary gas exchange, and arterial hypoxemia may occur as a result. In patients undergoing halothane–oxygen anesthesia with spontaneous two-lung ventilation, Nunn[50] found a calculated shunt of 14% of pulmonary blood flow as compared with a calculated shunt of 1% in normal, conscious, supine patients measured using the same techniques. He suggested that the large shunt observed was probably due to perfusion of totally unventilated parts of the lung. Marshall et al[51] confirmed this and concluded that postoperative hypoxemia may also be a result of the residual effects of the anesthetic on venous admixture. With this background, many investigators have studied the regulation of the pulmonary circulation through a homeostatic mechanism called hypoxic pulmonary vasoconstriction (HPV), which normally diverts blood away from hypoxic regions of the lung and thereby optimizes the gas exchange function of the lung.

Hypoxic pulmonary vasoconstriction was first described by Von Euler and Liljestrand in 1946.[52] They were studying changes in the pulmonary circulation of the cat in response to changes in inspired gas mixtures and found that 10.5% inspired O_2 (in N_2) mixtures caused an increase in pulmonary artery pressure. Breathing 100% O_2 caused a decrease in pulmonary artery pressure. They concluded that the increased pressure during hypoxia was caused by a direct effect on the pulmonary vessels. Whereas they delivered hypoxic gas mixtures to both lungs, others have studied the effects of the size of the hypoxic segment and the size of the hypoxic stimulus on perfusion pressure and on flow diversion. Pulmonary perfusion pressure (in dogs) increased with the size of the hypoxic segment from zero (smallest hypoxic segment) to approximately 2.2 times baseline for the hypoxic whole lung. Flow diversion, as a percentage of flow to the test segment under normoxic conditions, decreased with increasing size of the hypoxic test segment from a maximum of 75% for very small segments to zero when the whole lung was made hypoxic. Flow diversion increased linearly as PaO_2 was decreased over the range of 128–28 mm Hg. In both flow diversion and changes in perfusion pressure, the response to HPV was predictable, continuous, and maximal at a predicted PaO_2 of 30 mm Hg (4% oxygen). Thus, HPV causes a rise in both perfusion (pulmonary artery) pressure and flow diversion.[53]

The choice of anesthetic technique for one-lung ventilation must take into consideration the effects on oxygenation and therefore on HPV. Normally, collapse of the nonventilated, nondependent lung results in activation of reflex HPV in this lung. This causes local increases in pulmonary vascular resistance and diversion of blood flow to other, better oxygenated parts of the pulmonary vascular bed (*i.e.*, the dependent oxygenated and ventilated lung). The stimulus to HPV appears to be a function of both PaO_2 and $P\bar{v}O_2$ in isolated rat lungs ventilated with hypoxic mixtures, but in the atelectatic lung the stimulus is the $P\bar{v}O_2$.[54] A decrease in cardiac output may potentiate HPV by lowering $S\bar{v}O_2$. The response is believed to be accounted for by each smooth muscle cell in the pulmonary arterial wall responding to the oxygen tension in its vicinity. Because HPV causes flow diversion, PaO_2 should be higher than if there were no HPV. The relationship between PaO_2 and the size of the hypoxic segment (Fig. 30-17) shows that, when little of the lung is hypoxic, HPV has little effect on PaO_2 because shunt is small in this situation. When most of the lung is hypoxic, there is no significant normoxic region to which the hypoxic region

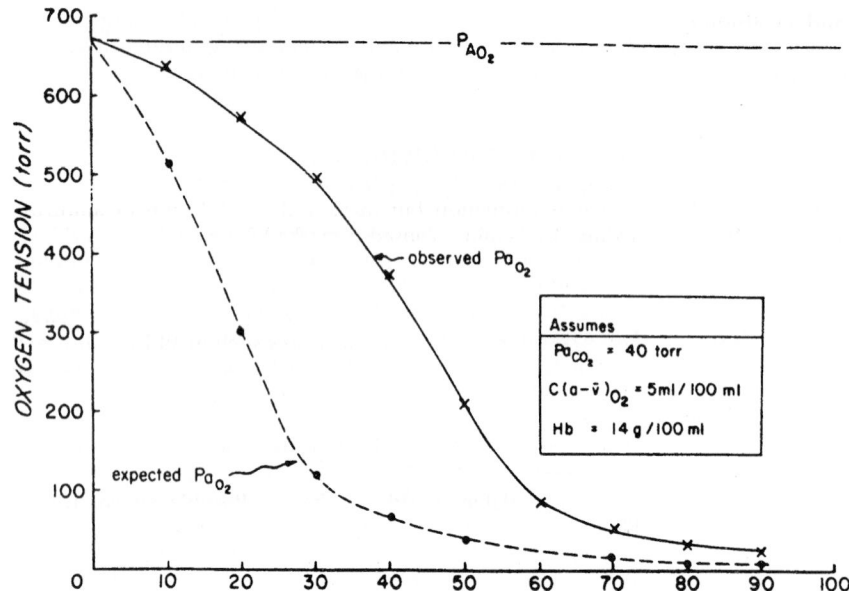

Figure 30-17. Role of hypoxic vasoconstriction in preserving Pa_{O_2} (in dogs). Assumptions are shown in insert. Lung is ventilated with $Fi_{O_2} = 1.0$, while increasing portions of lung are subjected to hypoxia or atelectasis. In the absence of hypoxic pulmonary vasoconstriction, the expected Pa_{O_2} would follow the broken line, whereas in the presence of an active hypoxic pulmonary vasoconstriction response, observed Pa_{O_2} is maintained close to the solid line. ($PA_{O_2} = $ alveolar Po_2; $Pa_{O_2} = $ arterial Po_2.) (Adapted with permission from Marshall BE, Marshall C, Benumof JL *et al:* Hypoxic pulmonary vasoconstriction in dogs: Effects of lung segment size and alveolar oxygen tension. J Appl Physiol 51:1543, 1981.)

can divert flow, and then it does not matter, in terms of Pa_{O_2}, whether the hypoxic region has active HPV or not. When the amount of lung made hypoxic is 30–70%, such as occurs during one-lung ventilation, there may be a large difference between the Pa_{O_2} to be expected with normal HPV compared with that expected in its absence. HPV can raise Pa_{O_2} from potentially dangerous levels to higher and safer ones. Conversely, inhibition of HPV may cause or contribute to hypoxemia during anesthesia.

Effects of Anesthetics on Hypoxic Pulmonary Vasoconstriction

All of the inhalation anesthetics and many of the intravenous drugs used in anesthesia have been studied for their effects on HPV. The results have not always been consistent. Benumof[55] has classified the preparations used to study these effects as *in vitro, in vivo* nonintact, *in vivo* intact, and human studies. Based on the results of these three types of preparation, it is generally believed that inhaled agents inhibit HPV, whereas intravenous drugs do not have this effect.[56]

Human studies are perhaps the most significant because of their applicability to the clinical situation. Bjertnaes[57] used perfusion scans (scintigraphy) to assess the effect of anesthetics on human HPV. In his patients, lung separation was achieved using a double-lumen tube. One lung could then be ventilated with 100% O_2 and the other with 100% nitrogen. HPV was assessed in the presence and absence of ether, halothane, and intravenous drugs (thiopental and fentanyl). Based on his scintigraphic findings, Bjertnaes[57] concluded that the inhaled agents, in clinically useful concentrations, inhibited HPV in humans.

Jolin Carlsson *et al*[58] used separate lung ventilation and a triple-gas washout technique to study HPV in eight patients. They demonstrated the presence of HPV in response to 8% O_2 in 92% nitrogen in the test lung but found no further change with the addition of 1.0% or 1.5% end-tidal isoflurane, and blood gas readings remained essentially unaltered. Attempts to use higher concentrations caused unacceptable hypotension. These authors concluded that isoflurane might be indicated for anesthesia in the presence of lung disease or during one-lung ventilation because arterial oxygenation might be better preserved than would be the case with an anesthetic that more effectively inhibited HPV. Thus, although it is possible that higher concentrations of isoflurane might have caused a clear change in the differential blood flow distribution, at clinically

used concentrations the effect of HPV in their subjects was all but unmeasurable.

Weinreich *et al*[59] used a ketamine infusion and found a lower incidence of hypoxemia (defined as Pa_{O_2} <70 mm Hg) than other studies reporting the use of halothane for one-lung ventilation. Rees and Gaines[60] compared a ketamine–oxygen technique with an enflurane (1–3% inspired)–oxygen technique for one-lung ventilation and found no differences between the groups in Pa_{O_2} or shunt. These findings suggested that ketamine afforded no advantage over enflurane during one-lung ventilation.

Rogers and Benumof[61] compared the effects of inhaled (isoflurane and halothane) with intravenous (methohexital and ketamine) anesthesia during one-lung ventilation and concluded that the inhaled anesthetics at approximately 1 minimum alveolar concentration (MAC) do not significantly affect HPV in humans, as evidenced by a lack of significant differences in Pa_{O_2} between use of the two techniques. The conclusions of this study have been questioned because the period of clinical exposure to the potent inhaled agents was very short. Thus, clinically relevant tissue concentrations of anesthetic may not have been achieved.

In a subsequent study, Benumof *et al*[62] investigated the changes in Pa_{O_2} and shunt that occurred after conversion from 1 MAC halothane or isoflurane anesthesia to intravenous anesthesia (fentanyl, diazepam, and sodium thiopental) during one-lung ventilation for thoracic surgery in 12 patients. In this study, they found that during one-lung atelectasis, 1 MAC halothane anesthesia slightly but significantly increased shunt and decreased Pa_{O_2} (compared with intravenous anesthesia), whereas 1 MAC isoflurane anesthesia very slightly but nonsignificantly increased shunt and decreased Pa_{O_2} (compared with intravenous anesthesia). Fundamental differences between the two studies[61,62] were in the duration of the periods of one-lung ventilation with the potent inhaled agent and in the MAC multiples of the drugs used. In the earlier study,[61] end-tidal concentrations of halothane and isoflurane were kept constant for approximately 20 minutes at 1.45 and 1.15 MAC, respectively. In the later study,[62] patients were maintained on one-lung anesthesia with the potent inhaled agent (1 MAC) for 40 minutes before final measurements under these conditions were taken. The authors also concluded that halothane and isoflurane had only a small inhibitory effect on the one-lung HPV response.[62] A randomized crossover study during one-lung ventilation with an Fi_{O_2} of 1.0 found that 1 MAC isoflurane anesthesia was associated with greater Pa_{O_2} values than was 1 MAC enflurane.[63]

Shimizu *et al* compared the effects of isoflurane and sevoflurane on Pao_2 during one-lung ventilation in 20 patients undergoing thoracotomy and found no significant difference between the groups in Pao_2, concluding that both agents can be used safely.[64] In an *in vitro* study Loer *et al* showed that desflurane inhibits HPV, with an ED_{50} of 1.6 MAC.[65]

Thus, overall, the potent inhaled anesthetics are the drugs of choice during thoracic surgery. The technique chosen should, however, always be dictated by the needs of the particular patient, so that in the presence of cardiovascular instability or poor oxygenation when depression of HPV is a possibility, a balanced technique may be chosen. Propofol in doses of 6–12 $mg \cdot kg^{-1} \cdot hr^{-1}$ does not abolish HPV during one-lung ventilation in humans.[66]

Other Determinants of Hypoxic Pulmonary Vasoconstriction

Aside from potent inhaled agents, other drugs and maneuvers used during anesthesia may also have an inhibitory effect on regional or whole-lung HPV. Factors associated with an increase in pulmonary artery pressure antagonize the effect of increased resistance caused by HPV and result in increased flow to the hypoxic region. Such indirect inhibitors of HPV include mitral stenosis, volume overload, thromboembolism, hypothermia, vasoconstrictor drugs, and a large hypoxic lung segment. Direct inhibitors of HPV include infection; vasodilator drugs, such as nitroglycerin and nitroprusside; hypocarbia; and metabolic alkalemia. All of these potential inhibitors should be considered when evaluating a patient for hypoxemia during thoracic surgery.

Potentiators of Hypoxic Pulmonary Vasoconstriction

Whereas in the past most research effort has been directed to studying inhibition of HPV, more recent research has investigated substances that may potentiate it. Almitrine, a respiratory stimulant drug, has been found to improve Pao_2 in patients with COPD and to have this effect in the absence of ventilatory stimulation. Indirect evidence suggested that it may potentiate HPV in intact dogs, although a subsequent and more extensive study with dogs concluded that almitrine caused nonspecific pulmonary vasoconstriction that was greater in the 100% oxygen-ventilated lung than in the hypoxic lung regions, thus causing a reduction of the HPV response.[67]

It has been suggested that prostaglandins may play a role in HPV inhibition, and therefore prostaglandin inhibitors have been investigated as potentiators of HPV. Ibuprofen, a cyclooxygenase inhibitor, has been found to potentiate HPV in hypoxic isolated rat lung preparations and to reverse the inhibition of HPV caused by halothane. In an animal model, lidocaine has also been found to have salutary effects in terms of reversing depression of HPV. The value, if any, of such potentiators in humans undergoing one-lung anesthesia has not yet been reported.

Nitric Oxide and One-Lung Ventilation

Nitric oxide is an endothelial-derived relaxing factor that appears to be an important mediator for smooth muscle relaxation.[68] HPV is inhibited by inhaled nitric oxide. Inhibition of nitric oxide synthase (NOS) improved, but did not completely restore, HPV in dogs suffering from sepsis.[69] Frostell *et al*[70] showed that inhalation of nitric oxide selectively induced vasodilation and reversed HPV in healthy humans without causing systemic vasodilatation. It was theorized that intravenous administration of almitrine (to increase HPV) causing vasoconstriction throughout the lung together with inhalation of nitric oxide

to inhibit HPV locally and cause increased flow in the ventilated regions, would improve $\dot{V}/\dot{Q}$ matching and Pao_2 in patients with $\dot{V}/\dot{Q}$ mismatching or during one-lung ventilation.[71]

Moutafis *et al*[72] studied the effects of inhaled nitric oxide in combination with almitrine infusion during one-lung ventilation in 40 patients undergoing thoracoscopic procedures. They found that inhaled nitric oxide alone did not affect Pao_2 during one-lung ventilation but the additional infusion of almitrine 16 $mg \cdot kg^{-1} \cdot min^{-1}$ caused a marked increase in Pao_2. These authors suggested that this nonventilatory technique should be of value during special thoracic procedures, such as thoracoscopy, where there is a need to manipulate the pulmonary circulation to improve Pao_2 but measures such as PEEP and CPAP cannot be used. Moutafis *et al*[73] have also reported the use of almitrine infusion/nitric oxide inhalation to improve Pao_2 during one-lung ventilation for bronchopulmonary lavage.

While the use of almitrine appears to be attractive, this drug is not without side effects.[74] Also, the manufacturer has not made it available outside of France. Possible alternatives to almitrine might be phenylephrine[75] and prostaglandin $F_{2\alpha}$.[76]

ANESTHESIA FOR DIAGNOSTIC PROCEDURES

Bronchoscopy

Early bronchoscopes were of the rigid type, but in 1966 the Machida and Olympus Companies introduced the first practical bronchofiberscopes. Since then, these have been improved dramatically and have simplified many otherwise complicated bronchoscopies. The indications for bronchoscopy are shown in Table 30-3 and the instruments of choice in Table 30-4. Operator preferences and experience may play a major role in the choice of instrument.

Before bronchoscopy is performed, the patient must be evaluated for chronic lung disease, respiratory obstruction, bronchospasm, coughing, hemoptysis, and infectivity of secretions. Medications should be reviewed, and the need for a more major procedure should always be anticipated. Thus, bronchoscopy may lead to thoracotomy or sternotomy. The planned technique for bronchoscopy should be discussed with the surgeon before the operation, and all equipment and connectors should be checked for compatibility. Monitoring during bronchoscopy should include an electrocardiogram, a blood pressure cuff, a precordial stethoscope, and a pulse oximeter. If thoracotomy is planned, an arterial cannula should also be

Table 30-3. INDICATIONS FOR BRONCHOSCOPY

Diagnostic	Therapeutic
Cough	Foreign bodies
Hemoptysis	Accumulated secretions
Wheeze	Atelectasis
Atelectasis	Aspiration
Unresolved pneumonia	Lung abscess
Diffuse lung disease	Reposition endotracheal tubes
Preoperative evaluation	Placement of endobronchial
Rule out metastases	tubes
Abnormal chest radiograph	Laser surgery of the airway
Assess local disease recurrence	
Recurrent laryngeal nerve palsy	
Diaphragm paralysis	
Acute inhalation injury	
Exclude tracheoesophageal fistula	
During mechanical ventilation	
Selective bronchography	

Adapted from Landa JF: Indications for bronchoscopy. Chest 73(suppl): 686, 1978, with permission of author and publisher.

Table 30-4. INSTRUMENTS OF CHOICE FOR BRONCHOSCOPY

RIGID
Foreign bodies
Massive hemoptysis
Vascular tumors
Small children
Endobronchial resections

FIBEROPTIC/FLEXIBLE
Mechanical problems of neck
Upper lobe and peripheral lesions
Limited hemoptysis
During mechanical ventilation
Pneumonia, for selective cultures
Positioning of double-lumen tubes
Difficult intubation
Checking position of endotracheal tube
Bronchial blockade

COMBINATION
Positive cytologic findings with negative chest radiographic results

Adapted from Landa JF: Indications for bronchoscopy. Chest 73(suppl): 686, 1978, with permission of author and publisher.

placed as well as other monitors (*e.g.*, PA or CVP catheters) that may be indicated by the patient's condition. Many anesthetic techniques are useful for bronchoscopy.

Local Anesthesia

The patient should first be pretreated with a drying agent. The local anesthetics most commonly used are lidocaine and tetracaine. In all cases, the total dose of anesthetic must be considered and the potential for toxicity recognized. A nebulizer can be used to spray the oropharynx and base of the tongue, or the patient may gargle viscous lidocaine. The tongue is then held forward, and pledgets soaked in local anesthetic are held in each piriform fossa using Krause forceps to achieve block of the internal branch of the superior laryngeal nerve. Tracheal anesthesia is achieved by a transtracheal injection of local anesthetic, or by spraying the vocal cords and trachea under direct vision using a laryngoscope or through the suction channel of the bronchofiberscope. Alternatively, a superior laryngeal nerve block can be performed by an external approach, and a glossopharyngeal block can be used to depress the gag reflex. These blocks cause depression of airway reflexes, so that patients must be kept on nothing by mouth for several hours after the examination. If fiberoptic bronchoscopy is to be performed transnasally, the nasal mucosa should be pretreated topically with 4% cocaine, or viscous lidocaine may be administered through the nares. Local anesthesia for bronchoscopy has the advantages of a patient who is awake, cooperative, and breathing spontaneously. Sedatives may be added to make the patient more comfortable. Disadvantages of local anesthesia include poor tolerance of any bleeding by the patient and the occasional lack of patient cooperation.

General Anesthesia

General anesthesia for bronchoscopy is often combined with topical laryngeal anesthesia so that less general anesthesia is needed. A balanced technique uses N_2O/O_2, incremental doses of an intravenous drug such as thiopental, an opioid, and a muscle relaxant. A potent inhaled anesthetic technique is also satisfactory, although the use of N_2O may cause some optical distortion for the surgeon because of changes in the refractive index of the gas mixture. In addition, the use of N_2O and potent inhaled agents creates an operating room contamination problem for the waste anesthesia gases, but limited scavenging

may be possible by placing a suction catheter in the patient's oropharynx. Unless there is some contraindication, ventilation of the lungs is usually controlled. In any patient undergoing a thoracic diagnostic procedure for a suspected malignancy, the possibility of the myasthenic syndrome with sensitivity to nondepolarizing muscle relaxants must always be considered. Muscle relaxant doses should be titrated to effect using a neuromuscular monitoring system.

Rigid Bronchoscopy

A modern rigid ventilating bronchoscope is essentially a hollow tube with a blunted, beveled tip. Various sizes and designs are available, but in all a side arm is provided for connection to an anesthesia source. A number of techniques have been described for maintaining ventilation and oxygenation during rigid bronchoscopic examination.

Apneic Oxygenation. After preoxygenation and induction of general anesthesia, skeletal muscle paralysis and cessation of intermittent positive-pressure breathing, the $Paco_2$ increases. During the first minute the increase is ~6 mm Hg · min^{-1}. Subsequently, the average rate of increase is 3 mm Hg · min^{-1}. Oxygen is insufflated at 10–15 l · min^{-1} through a small catheter placed above the carina. If the patient has been adequately denitrogenated, this technique can provide adequate oxygenation for more than 30 minutes.[77] The apneic period should not be allowed to extend beyond 5 minutes, however, because the technique is limited by buildup of CO_2, respiratory acidosis, and cardiac dysrhythmias.

Apnea and Intermittent Ventilation. Oxygen and anesthesia gases are delivered to the bronchoscope *via* the anesthesia circuit. Ventilation is possible only when the eyepiece is in place, which limits the period for instrumentation by the surgeon. Intermittent ventilation of the lungs is achieved by squeezing the reservoir bag. In this way, assuming a good bronchoscope fit in the airway, compliance is constantly monitored, the risk of barotrauma is reduced, and Vt may be estimated. The disadvantage of this technique is that with prolonged bronchoscopies, poor levels of arterial blood gases, and in particular hypercarbia, may result. This may lead to cardiac arrhythmias.

Sanders Injection System. Sanders applied the Venturi principle to provide ventilation of the lungs by attaching a jet ventilator to the bronchoscope.[78] Oxygen from a high-pressure source (50 psig) is delivered, using a controllable pressure-reducing valve and toggle switch, to a 2.5–3.5-cm 18- or 16-gauge needle inside and parallel to the long axis of the bronchoscope. When the toggle switch is depressed, the jet of oxygen entering the bronchoscope entrains air, and the air–oxygen mixture resulting at the distal tip of the bronchoscope emerges at a pressure to provide adequate ventilation and oxygenation. The intraluminal tracheal pressure depends on the driving pressure from the reducing valve, the size of the needle jet, and the length, internal diameter, and design of the bronchoscope. Increasing the size of the needle jet increases the total gas flow for any given driving pressure. For each combination of gas driving pressure, jet orifice, and bronchoscope diameter, only one inflation pressure can be attained, regardless of the volume or compliance of the lung. As long as the proximal end of the bronchoscope is open, the system is strictly pressure limited, and the pressure does not increase because of obstruction at the distal end. Pressure varies inversely with the cross-sectional area of the bronchoscope, so that insertion of a suction catheter or biopsy forceps into the lumen causes the intratracheal pressure to increase. Provided there is not a tight fit between the bronchoscope and the airway, the risk of barotrauma is low. If the fit is tight, driving pressure should be decreased.

The advantages of the Sanders system are that because continuous ventilation is possible (because the presence of an eyepiece is not necessary for ventilation of the lungs), the duration of the bronchoscopy procedure is minimized, but the efficiency also permits extended bronchoscopy. A disadvantage is that entrainment of air by the oxygen jet results in a variable F_{IO_2} at the distal end of the bronchoscope, ventilation of the lungs may be inadequate if compliance is poor, and adequacy of ventilation may be difficult to assess. A comparison between the intermittent ventilation and Sanders techniques found that Pa_{O_2} was satisfactory with either method but was higher in the intermittent ventilation group.[79] Pa_{CO_2} was lower and arterial pH higher in the Sanders group, indicating superiority of this method, particularly for long procedures.

The basic Sanders technique has been modified to increase F_{IO_2} and to deliver N_2O and potent inhaled anesthetics. The 16-gauge oxygen jet has been replaced with a longer jet (Carden side arm) that allows ventilation with 100% oxygen and the development of much higher pressures at the tracheal end of the bronchoscope, while using a driving pressure of 50 psig. The Sanders injector system may also be used with a ventilating bronchoscope, the side arm of which is connected to a supply of anesthesia gases, so that the injection jet entrains the anesthesia gases.[80]

Mechanical Ventilator. Ventilation of the lungs may be achieved by connecting a mechanical ventilator to an anesthesia circuit that is connected to the bronchoscope side arm.

High-Frequency Positive-Pressure Ventilation. High-frequency positive-pressure ventilation (HFPPV) has been used in conjunction with rigid bronchoscopy and has been compared with the Sanders injector in patients with tracheobronchial stenosis. With HFPPV of up to 150 breaths · min^{-1}, blood gases were identical with both techniques. At a frequency of 500 breaths · min^{-1}, oxygenation deteriorated and CO_2 was not removed effectively. HFPPV has the advantage that the tracheobronchial wall remains perfectly immobilized during ventilation.[81]

Other Techniques. Cuirass ventilation, external chest compression, and a ventilating catheter or endotracheal tube placed alongside the bronchoscope have also been used to provide ventilation during bronchoscopy.

Fiberoptic Bronchoscopy

The new generations of fiberscopes, with their improved optics and smaller diameters, have revolutionized bronchoscopy. Examination of the fifth order of bronchial branching is now possible, and the diagnostic potential of this instrument is thereby enhanced. The flexibility has also been applied in preoperative assessment of the airway, management of difficult tracheal intubations, endotracheal tube positioning and change, bronchial toilet, correct positioning of double-lumen tubes, bronchial blockade, and evaluation of the larynx and trachea.

Nasal fiberoptic bronchoscopy under topical anesthesia is well tolerated by most awake patients. A suction catheter in the mouth is useful to remove oral secretions. Oral insertion is also possible in both awake and asleep patients and should be performed *via* a specially designed airway, which guides the fiberscope over the back of the tongue and prevents potential damage to it by the patient's teeth.

Physiologic Changes Associated with Fiberoptic Bronchoscopy. In all patients, insertion of the fiberoptic bronchoscope is associated with hypoxemia. The average decline in Pa_{O_2} is 20 mm Hg and lasts for 1–4 hours after the procedure. By 24 hours, the blood gas tensions are usually back to normal. It is therefore recommended that if the initial Pa_{O_2} is 70 mm Hg (F_{IO_2} = 0.21), bronchoscopy should be performed only with the administration of supplemental oxygen. This can be provided using mouth-held nasal prongs, a special face mask with a diaphragm through which the fiberscope can be passed, or an endotracheal tube with a T-piece diaphragm adapter.

During and after fiberoptic bronchoscopy, patients experience increased airway obstruction. Thus, in 35 patients, insertion of the bronchoscope was associated with an increase in FRC (17–30%) and decreases in Pa_{O_2}, vital capacity, FEV$_1$, and forced inspiratory flow.[82] All had returned to baseline by 24 hours. These changes are thought to be secondary to direct mechanical activation of irritative reflexes in the airway and, possibly, to mucosal edema. They may be avoided if atropine, either intramuscular or aerosolized into the airway, is administered before the procedure. Isoproterenol has a similar salutary effect on lung function but is associated with an increased incidence of cardiac arrhythmias. Overall, atropine is recommended as premedication for fiberoptic bronchoscopy. Concern that atropine may have an overall undesirable effect by increasing viscosity of secretions in patients with COPD is unsubstantiated.

The standard adult fiberoptic bronchoscope has an external diameter of 5.7 mm and a 2-mm diameter suction channel. If suction at 1 atm is applied to the fiberscope, air is removed at a rate of 14 l · min^{-1}. If the fiberscope is in the airway, this causes decreases in F_{IO_2}, Pa_{O_2}, and FRC, leading to decreased Pa_{O_2}. Suctioning should therefore be kept brief. The adult fiberscope passes through endotracheal tubes of 7 mm or greater internal diameter. Clearly, passage through an endotracheal tube decreases the cross-sectional area available for ventilating the patient, so that if fiberoscopy is planned, an endotracheal tube of the largest possible diameter should be used.

Insertion of the bronchoscope also causes a significant PEEP effect, that may result in barotrauma in ventilated patients. If PEEP is already being used, it should be discontinued before passage of the fiberscope. A postendoscopy chest radiograph is advisable to exclude the presence of mediastinal emphysema or pneumothorax. In patients whose tracheas are intubated with endotracheal tubes of less than 8 mm internal diameter, use of pediatric fiberscopes, which have smaller diameters, would be more appropriate.

The suction channel of the adult fiberoptic bronchoscope has been used to oxygenate and ventilate the lungs of patients. By attaching a jet ventilation system (similar to that used to drive the Sanders injector for rigid bronchoscopy) to the suction connection at the head of a fiberoptic bronchoscope, successful ventilation of the lungs of patients undergoing gynecologic procedures was achieved.[83] A driving pressure of 50 psig of oxygen was used with a ventilatory rate of 18–20 breaths · min^{-1}. This technique permitted adequate ventilation of patients with normally compliant lungs and chest walls. Ventilation of the lungs should be performed only with the tip of the instrument in the trachea because a more peripheral location may produce barotrauma.

Neodymium-yttrium-aluminum garnet (Nd-YAG) lasers are used for the resection of obstructing and endobronchial lesions. This procedure is performed under general anesthesia. The lasers may be introduced into the bronchial tree through a fiberoptic bundle passed *via* the suction port of the fiberoptic bronchoscope. During laser resection, F_{IO_2} should be kept to a minimum and titrated against oxygen saturation (as continuously monitored by pulse oximeter) to make endotracheal fire less likely. Laser therapy of bronchial tumors is also possible using a rigid bronchoscope. HFPPV through a rigid bronchoscope provides satisfactory operating conditions for laser resection of tracheal tumors and has the advantage of producing airway immobility.

Complications of Bronchoscopy

Complications of rigid bronchoscopy include mechanical trauma to the teeth, hemorrhage, bronchospasm, loss of a sponge, bronchial or tracheal perforation, subglottic edema, and barotrauma. The incidence of complications is much lower with fiberoptic bronchoscopy. Nevertheless, complications may arise owing to overdose with topical anesthetic, insertion trauma, local trauma, hemorrhage, upper airway obstruction related to passage of the instrument through an area of tracheal stenosis, hypoxemia, and bronchospasm. In most cases, it is best to intubate the trachea with an endotracheal tube after bronchoscopy under general anesthesia. This permits avoidance or treatment of some of these problems, particularly the increased airway irritability. Intubation also facilitates effective suctioning of the trachea and bronchi and allows the patient to recover more gradually from general anesthesia.

DIAGNOSTIC PROCEDURES FOR MEDIASTINAL MASSES

Patients with an anterior mediastinal mass present a special problem for the anesthesiologist. Although such masses may cause obvious superior vena cava obstruction, they may also cause obstruction of major airways and cardiac compression, which are less obvious and may become apparent only on induction of anesthesia. Three cases of anterior mediastinal mass were described,[84] in two of which airway obstruction occurred after induction of anesthesia and onset of paralysis. In the first case, total occlusion of the trachea starting 2–3 cm above the carina and extending to both mainstem bronchi was observed, and a bronchoscope was passed through the obstruction. In the second case, extrinsic compression of the left mainstem bronchus occurred on inspiration during recovery from anesthesia. In the third case of anterior mediastinal mass, flow–volume studies were performed with the patient in the upright and supine positions and demonstrated marked reductions in FEV_1 and peak expiratory flow in the latter position. These findings suggested potential obstruction with onset of anesthesia; radiation therapy to the mediastinum was commenced, after which the flow–volume studies showed improved function. The planned surgical procedure was then performed under local anesthesia.

One potential disadvantage of preoperative radiation therapy is that it may affect tissue histologic appearance, thereby preventing an accurate diagnosis. Furthermore, if the patient is a child, it may be difficult to obtain tissue samples under local anesthesia. In a series of 44 patients ages 18 years of age or younger with anterior mediastinal masses who underwent general anesthesia before radiation or chemotherapy, no fatalities occurred. However, seven patients had airway compromise.[85] This report concluded that general anesthesia may be safely induced before radiation therapy and that the benefits of obtaining an accurate tissue diagnosis outweighed the risks.[85] Others have disagreed with these conclusions, stating that anesthesia is not safe when the reported rate of life-threatening complications is 16–20%.

Airway obstruction caused by an anterior mediastinal mass has been attributed to changes in lung and chest wall mechanics associated with changes in position or to onset of paralysis in muscles that previously maintained airway patency. Preoperative evaluation of a patient with an anterior mediastinal mass in order to avoid life-threatening total airway obstruction is shown in Figure 30-18.[84] It is important to determine in the history if the patient has dyspnea in the supine position and to examine the computed tomographic scan to determine the extent of the tumor and its effect on surrounding structures. If such obstruction occurs, it may be relieved by passage of a rigid bronchoscope or anode tube past the obstruction, by direct laryngoscopy,[86] or by changing the position of the patient.

In a situation in which the biopsy procedure cannot be performed under local anesthesia and there is concern that muscle paralysis may result in airway compression, fiberoptic intubation of the awake patient followed by general anesthesia with spontaneous ventilation has been described for thoracotomy. Thus, during spontaneous inspiration, the normal transpulmonary pressure gradient distends the airways and helps to maintain their patency, even in the presence of extrinsic compression.

Mediastinoscopy

Mediastinoscopy was introduced as a means of assessing spread of carcinoma of the bronchus. The lymphatics of the lung drain

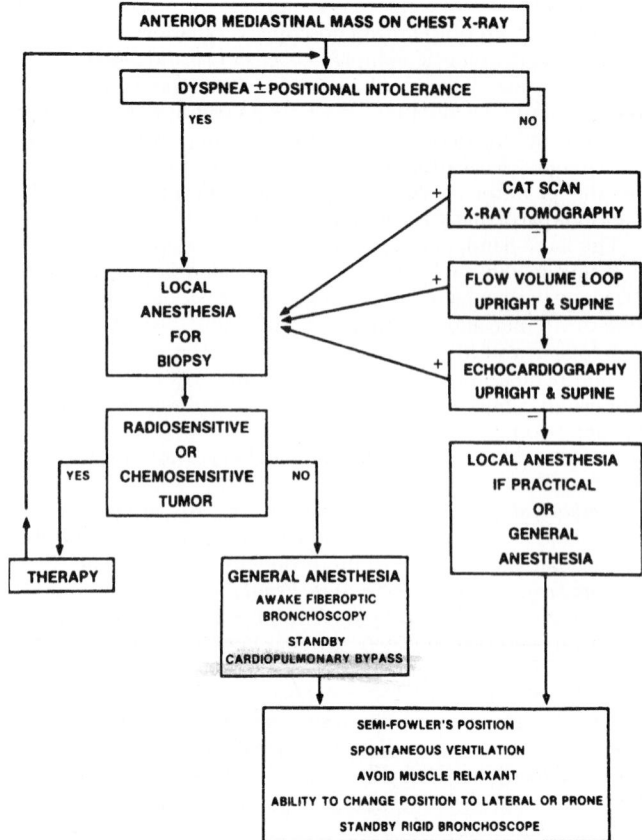

Figure 30-18. Flow chart describing the preoperative evaluation of the patient with an anterior mediastinal mass. (+ indicates positive finding; − indicates negative work-up.) (Reproduced with permission from Neuman GC, Weingarten AE, Abramowitz RM *et al:* Anesthetic management of the patient with an anterior mediastinal mass. Anesthesiology 60:144, 1984.)

first to the subcarinal and paratracheal areas and then to the sides of the trachea, the supraclavicular areas, and the thoracic duct. Examination of these nodes has provided a tissue diagnosis and greater selectivity of patients for thoracotomy. It is most useful in right-lung tumors because left-lung cancers tend to spread to subaortic nodes that are more accessible by an anterior mediastinoscopy in the second or third interspace (Chamberlain procedure). Apart from diagnostic uses, mediastinoscopy has also been used to place electrodes for atrial-triggered pacing. The transcervical approach to the thymus is an adaptation of mediastinoscopy.

The anesthetic considerations for mediastinoscopy follow naturally from an understanding of the anatomy of this procedure and its potential complications. For cervical mediastinoscopy, the patient is placed in a reverse Trendelenburg position, and the mediastinoscope is inserted into the superior mediastinum through a transverse incision just above the suprasternal notch. The instrument is advanced along the anterior aspect of the trachea and passes behind the innominate vessels and the aortic arch (Fig. 30-19). The left recurrent nerve is vulnerable as it loops around the aortic arch, and any of these structures may be traumatized. Because of scarring, previous mediastinoscopy is a contraindication to a repeat examination. Relative contraindications include superior vena cava obstruction, tracheal deviation, and aneurysm of the thoracic aorta.

Preoperative evaluation should include a search for airway obstruction or distortion. Review of a computed tomographic scan is very helpful in this regard. Evidence of impaired cerebral circulation, history of stroke, or signs of the Eaton-Lambert syndrome resulting from oat cell carcinoma should be sought.

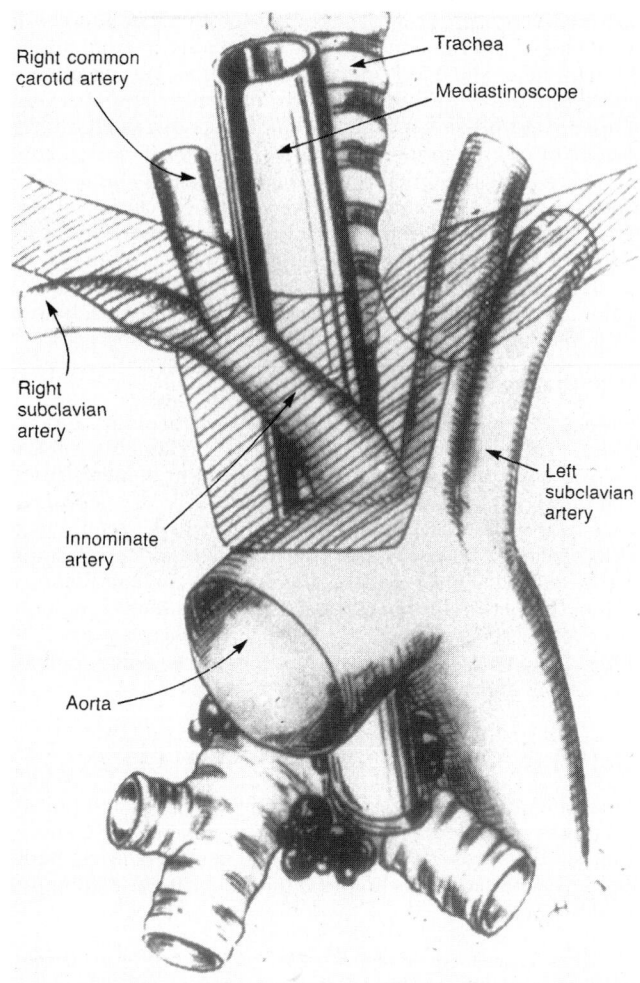

Figure 30-19. Anatomic relationships during mediastinoscopy. Note the position of the mediastinoscope behind the right innominate artery and aortic arch and anterior to the trachea. (Reproduced with permission from Carlens E: Mediastinoscopy: A method for inspection and tissue biopsy in the superior mediastinum. Dis Chest 36:343, 1959.)

Blood must be available for the procedure because hemorrhage is a real risk and may be life threatening.

Mediastinoscopy may be performed under local anesthesia, and this approach is claimed to offer greater simplicity and safety in patients with limited pulmonary reserve or in those with cerebrovascular disease. However, most surgeons and anesthesiologists prefer general anesthesia using an endotracheal tube and continuous ventilation because this offers a more controlled situation and greater flexibility in terms of surgical manipulation. The anesthetic technique should include a muscle relaxant to prevent the patient from coughing because this may produce venous engorgement in the chest or trauma by the mediastinoscope to surrounding structures.

The incidence of morbidity with mediastinoscopy has been reported as 1.5–3.0%, and that of mortality, 0.09%. The most common complication is hemorrhage (0.73%) because of the proximity of major vessels and the vascularity of certain tumors. Tamponade may be the only recourse, and thoracotomy or median sternotomy may be required to achieve hemostasis. Needle aspiration of any structure is essential before any biopsy is taken. If severe bleeding occurs, induced arterial hypotension may be helpful in reducing the size of the tear in a vessel. If bleeding is venous, fluids given *via* an upper limb vein may enter the mediastinum, in which case a large-bore catheter should be placed in a lower limb vein. A venous laceration may

also result in air embolism, particularly if the patient is breathing spontaneously. Some recommend the use of a precordial Doppler probe if the risk of air embolism is likely.

Pneumothorax is the second most common complication (0.66%). It is usually right-sided, often recognized at the time of the occurrence, and is treated according to size. A symptomatic pneumothorax should be treated by chest tube decompression.

Recurrent laryngeal nerve injury occurred in 0.34% of cases and was permanent in 50% of these cases. The nerve may be damaged by the mediastinoscope or be involved in tumor. Such injury is not a problem unless both nerves are damaged, in which case upper airway obstruction may result. Autonomic reflexes may be initiated by manipulation of the trachea or the aorta, the latter having pressor receptors located in the arch. Vagally mediated reflexes may be blocked by atropine.

"Apparent" cardiac arrest has been reported when the right radial pulse was monitored using a plethysmograph, and the tracing suddenly disappeared in the presence of a normal electrocardiogram. A normal pulse returned after the mediastinoscope was removed, and the cause of the apparent arrest was pressure on the innominate artery by the instrument. Decreases in right arm as compared to left arm blood pressure have been reported in cases undergoing mediastinoscopy. Duration was 15–360 seconds. This is of particular significance if there is a history of impaired cerebral circulation or transient ischemic attacks, or if a carotid bruit is present, because transient left hemiparesis may occur after mediastinoscopy. It is therefore recommended that blood pressure be monitored in the left arm and that the right radial pulse be monitored continuously during mediastinoscopy. A decrease in the right radial pulse amplitude is an indication for repositioning the mediastinoscope, especially in a patient with a history of cerebrovascular disease.

Other reported complications include acute tracheal collapse, tension pneumomediastinum, mediastinitis, hemothorax, and chylothorax. A chest radiograph taken in the immediate postoperative period is a useful precaution in all patients after mediastinoscopy.

Thoracoscopy

Thoracoscopy involves the insertion of an endoscope into the thoracic cavity and pleural space. It is used for the diagnosis of pleural disease, effusions, and infectious disease (especially in immunosuppressed patients and those with acquired immunodeficiency syndrome) and for staging procedures, chemical pleurodesis, and lung biopsy. It is also used in therapeutic procedures such as CO_2 laser treatment of spontaneous pneumothorax or bullous emphysema[87] and Nd-YAG laser vaporization of malignant pleural tumors. A small incision is made in the lateral chest wall, and with the insertion of the instrument, fluid, and biopsy specimens are easily obtained.

This procedure may be performed using local, regional, or general anesthesia, the choice depending on the expected duration of the procedure and the physical status of the patient. The most common methods are local anesthetic infiltration or intercostal nerve blocks two spaces above and below the usual sixth intercostal space. Intercostal blocks also anesthetize the parietal pleura. The addition of a stellate ganglion block helps to suppress the cough reflex that is sometimes provoked during manipulation of the hilum of the lung.

When air enters the pleural cavity under inspection, a partial pneumothorax occurs, permitting good surgical visualization. Changes in Pao_2, $Paco_2$, and electrocardiographic rhythm are usually minimal when the procedure is performed using local or regional anesthesia. (The physiology of this situation was discussed in the section on Lateral Position, Awake, Breathing Spontaneously, Chest Open.)

With local anesthesia, the spontaneous pneumothorax is usually well tolerated because the skin and chest wall form a seal around the thoracoscope and limit the degree of lung collapse. Occasionally, however, the procedure is poorly tolerated, and general anesthesia must be induced. The insertion of a double-lumen tube with the patient in the lateral position may be difficult, in which case the patient may be temporarily placed in the supine position for the intubation.

If general anesthesia is required, either a single- or a double-lumen tube may be used. Positive-pressure ventilation interferes with endoscopic visualization, however, and therefore a double-lumen tube is preferable. In addition, if pleurodesis is being performed, general anesthesia through a double-lumen tube allows for complete re-expansion of the lung and avoids the pain associated with instillation of talc for recurrent pneumothorax. To overcome the pathophysiologic effects of the pneumothorax, although small, a high FIO_2 is recommended for either local or general anesthesia.

Video-Assisted Thoracoscopic Surgery

Video-assisted thoracoscopy (VAT) (see Chapter 38) entails making small incisions in the chest wall, which allows the introduction of a video camera and surgical instruments into the thoracic cavity.[88] While the first thoracoscopy was performed by Jacobeus in 1910, using what was at that time a cystoscope, in recent years the surgical techniques, instruments, and video technology have been improved to permit a wide variety of procedures to be performed using VAT. These now include diagnostic procedures for evaluation of pleural disease and effusions, staging of lung cancer, and the identification of parenchymal disease, including nodules, mediastinal tumors and pericardial disease. They also include therapeutic procedures such as operations for pleural disease, including pleurodesis, decortication and drainage of emphysema, resection of lung tissue or bullae, pericardial window or stripping, and esophageal surgery.

Anesthesia Considerations

As with a traditional thoracotomy, for VAT the patient needs to be positioned in the lateral decubitus position, and lung collapse is needed for adequate surgical exposure. This generally mandates use of lung separation. VAT is most commonly performed under general anesthesia with one-lung ventilation. The need for one-lung ventilation is much greater with VAT than with open thoracotomy because it is not possible to retract the lung during a VAT as it is during an open thoracotomy. The operated lung should be deflated as soon as possible after tracheal intubation and positioning, because it may take as much as 30 minutes for complete lung collapse to occur. Also the surgeon enters the thoracic cavity much sooner during a VAT than with open thoracotomy. Suction applied to the airway can help facilitate a more rapid deflation of the lung. In some cases, carbon dioxide is insufflated into the pleural cavity to facilitate visualization by the surgeon. Insufflation pressures should be as low as possible and the CO_2 inflow rate kept less than $2l \cdot min^{-1}$. Higher pressures can cause mediastinal shift, hemodynamic compromise, increases in airway pressure and increases in end-tidal CO_2. Hemodynamic compromise presents a picture similar to that due to tension pneumothorax. Significant hemodynamic changes can be produced when pressures of as little as 5 mm Hg are used to insufflate CO_2 into the chest cavity.[89]

Continuous positive airway pressure (CPAP) is commonly used for the treatment of hypoxemia during one-lung ventilation for thoracotomy and is usually very effective. However, during VAT, CPAP interferes with the surgical procedure, and is only used as a last resort. PEEP to the nonoperated (dependent) lung should be used, rather than CPAP to the operated lung during VAT, and a lower PaO_2 may have to be tolerated during a VAT compared with a thoracotomy.

When a diagnostic VAT is being performed, it is possible to perform the procedure under epidural anesthesia or intercostal nerve blocks. The patient continues to breathe spontaneously, although he or she may require some sedation. During spontaneous respiration, the lung to be operated on collapses because of open chest physiology. If a pneumothorax is created during placement of intercostal nerve blocks, it is not of clinical concern because a pneumothorax occurs as part of the surgical procedure and a chest tube is placed at the conclusion of surgery. For procedures done under local or regional anesthesia techniques, an ipsilateral stellate ganglion block is often placed to inhibit the cough reflex due to manipulation of the hilum of the lung. Anesthesia of the visceral pleura can be achieved using instillation of topical local anesthetic solutions.

Postoperative Concerns

There is less pain after VAT than open thoracotomy and an epidural catheter is usually placed before surgery only if there is a likelihood that a thoracotomy will need to be performed, even though the procedure is starting as a VAT. After a positive biopsy during VAT, an open thoracotomy may be required to perform a lobectomy or pneumonectomy. The patient's respiratory function is better preserved after VAT, and the recovery is faster. However, postoperative arrhythmias, which commonly occur after thoracotomy, have also been reported after VAT. Other complications that may occur include bleeding, pulmonary edema and pneumonia.

ANESTHESIA FOR SPECIAL SITUATIONS

Management of patients with BPFs, empyema, cysts, and bullae, and those requiring tracheal reconstruction is considered here. Many of these cases are appropriately managed using high-frequency ventilatory techniques; therefore, these techniques are described first.

High-Frequency Ventilation

With conventional positive-pressure ventilation, VT and rates usually exceed or approach those in the normal, spontaneously breathing patient. Gas transport to the alveoli occurs by convection in the larger airways and then by convection and molecular diffusion in the more distal airways and alveoli. High-frequency ventilation differs from conventional positive-pressure ventilation in that smaller VT and more rapid rates are used. Gas transport may depend more on molecular diffusion, high-velocity flow, and coaxial gas flow in the airways, with gas in the center moving distally and that in the periphery moving proximally.

There are three different types of high-frequency ventilation. *High-frequency positive-pressure ventilation* (HFPPV) uses small VT at rates of 60–120 breaths $\cdot min^{-1}$ (1–2 Hz). The ventilator used (*e.g.,* Bronchovent) has a negligible internal compliance, so that the VT generated, which usually approximates the dead space volume, equals the volume set on the ventilator and represents all fresh gas. The high instantaneous gas flows generated facilitate gas exchange and movement in the conducting airways.

HFPPV may be delivered by an open or a closed system. An example of the former is the percutaneous placement of a transtracheal catheter or placement of a catheter through the nose or mouth with its distal end above the carina. Inflow is intraluminal and outflow is extraluminal. This technique has been used during bronchoscopy, tracheal resection, and reconstructive surgery. When open systems are used, the gas outflow pathway is not established mechanically and depends on natural airway patency. It is therefore subject to compromise. Also, aspiration is a potential complication with open systems.

The closed system is superior because it integrates both airway patency and outflow protection. A closed system is represented by a catheter placed in a short segment of an endotracheal tube for delivery of the HFPPV, whereas the remainder of the tube lumen represents the exit pathway for gas. A quadruple-lumen endotracheal tube (Hi-Lo Jet Tracheal Tube; Mallinckrodt, Inc., Argyle, NY) has been designed specifically for delivery of HFPPV. One lumen is for the HFPPV delivery, one for gas outflow, one for cuff inflation, and one for measuring airway pressures at the distal end of the tube. The use of a closed system also permits application of PEEP, a situation not possible with an open arrangement.

High-frequency jet ventilation (HFJV) uses a pulse of a small jet of fresh gas introduced from a high-pressure source (50 psig) into the airway through a small catheter or additional lumen in an endotracheal tube. Rates used are usually 100–400 breaths · min^{-1}. The fresh gas jet entrains gas from an injection cannula side-port reservoir. This system is somewhat analogous to the Sanders injector system described in the section on Bronchoscopy, and FIO_2 is similarly variable. The jet and entrained gas flows cause forward motion of the mass of gas in the airways. HFJV can be used with an open system or with a closed arrangement, as described earlier. In the latter, PEEP may be added to enhance oxygenation. Also, with use of high fresh gas flows from an anesthesia circuit, inhaled anesthetics may be delivered as an entrained gas mixture.

High-frequency oscillation ventilation uses a mechanism that oscillates gas at rates of 400–2400 breaths · min^{-1}. It has not been described in association with thoracic surgical procedures. In this system, VT is small (50–80 ml), and gas exchange occurs through enhanced molecular diffusion and coaxial airway flow.

The potential advantages offered by HFPPV during thoracic anesthesia are that lower VT and inspiratory pressures result in a quiet lung field for the surgeon, with minimal movements of airway, lung tissue, and mediastinum. Thus, HFPPV has been used to ventilate both the nondependent and the dependent lung during thoracic surgical procedures, with adequate arterial blood gas measurements obtained throughout. At high frequencies (>6 Hz), however, CO_2 retention may become a problem.

High-frequency jet ventilation has been used to ventilate the nondependent lung to improve PaO_2 during one-lung anesthesia while the dependent lung was ventilated with conventional intermittent positive-pressure ventilation. PaO_2 increased compared with that obtained during simple collapse of the nondependent lung. A study comparing HFJV with CPAP to the nondependent lung during conventional intermittent positive-pressure ventilation to the dependent lung found that both improved PaO_2 significantly during both closed and open stages of the surgery. When the chest was open, HFJV maintained satisfactory cardiac output, whereas CPAP usually decreased cardiac output, but there were no significant differences in $PaCO_2$ between HFJV and CPAP. Because similar increases in PaO_2 may be obtained using selective CPAP to the nondependent lung and while using much simpler equipment than that necessary to deliver high-frequency ventilation, the use of CPAP would seem preferable to high-frequency ventilation to increase PaO_2 during most one-lung anesthesia situations.

In certain situations, HFJV to the nondependent lung may offer some advantage. Thus, combined unilateral HFJV and contralateral intermittent positive-pressure ventilation in the management of a patient who required a right lower lobectomy for bronchial carcinoma associated with emphysema, pneumoconiosis, and a previous thoracoplasty for pulmonary tuberculosis is reported. This technique has been recommended in any patient requiring partial lung resection in the presence of severe pulmonary impairment.[90]

The lower pressures and VTs associated with high-frequency ventilation result in a small leak through BPFs, and HFJV is now generally considered the conservative treatment of choice in this condition. Another advantage of high-frequency ventila-

tion is that the rapid rate small VT can be delivered through small tubes or catheters, so that if an airway has to be divided, the passage of a small tube across the surgical field permits ventilation of the distal airway and lung tissue. This use has been applied during sleeve resection of the lung, tracheal reconstruction, and surgery for tracheal stenosis. In all three situations, the surgeon is able to work easily around the small catheter used to provide the high-frequency ventilation.

Conventional intermittent positive-pressure ventilation (650 ml × 14 breaths · min^{-1}) to the dependent lung has been compared to HFJV (150–200 breaths · min^{-1}; minute volume 10–15 l) to the dependent lung during one-lung ventilation using an FIO_2 of 0.5. There were no significant differences between the groups in PaO_2, $PaCO_2$, or hemodynamic indices, although shunt fraction was higher in the HFJV group. A significant PEEP effect was also noted in this group, but not in the intermittent positive-pressure ventilation group. The unintentional generation of PEEP during HFJV is well known and is thought to be due to expiratory flow limitation. The PEEP to the dependent lung increases pulmonary vascular resistance in this lung and causes diversion of blood flow to the nondependent, nonventilated lung, thereby increasing shunt fraction (32.9% versus 42.4%). It was concluded that the theoretical benefits of HFJV on the cardiovascular system are outweighed by the effects of mean airway pressure increasing shunt to the nonventilated lung during one-lung anesthesia. Although adequate gas exchange was maintained with HFJV during one-lung anesthesia with FIO_2 of 0.5, it was found to be more difficult to assess the adequacy of ventilation during HFJV. Its routine use during one-lung anesthesia is therefore not recommended.

Bronchopleural Fistula and Empyema

A BPF is an abnormal communication between the bronchial tree and the pleural cavity. Occasionally, there is an additional communication to the surface of the chest, a cutaneous BPF. A BPF occurs most commonly after pulmonary resection for carcinoma. Other causes include traumatic rupture of a bronchus or bulla (sometimes caused by barotrauma or PEEP), penetrating chest wound, or spontaneous drainage into the bronchial tree of an empyema cavity or lung cyst. The incidence of BPF is higher after pneumonectomy than following other types of lung resection. The problems associated with BPF and empyema are that positive-pressure ventilation may result in contamination of healthy lung, loss of air, decreased alveolar ventilation leading to CO_2 retention, and the development of a tension pneumothorax.

If an empyema is present, it should be drained under local anesthesia before any surgery to close the BPF. Drainage is performed with the patient sitting up and leaning toward the affected side. Empyemas are often loculated and complete drainage is not always possible. A drain to an underwater seal system is left in the cavity before administration of anesthesia for surgery of the BPF, and after drainage of an empyema a chest radiograph should be obtained to determine the efficacy of the procedure.

The priorities in the anesthetic management of BPF are the isolation of the affected side in terms of contamination and ventilation. The ideal approach is intubation of the trachea while the patient is awake using a double-lumen tube with the patient breathing spontaneously. Supplemental oxygen should be administered, and the patient should be constantly reassured. Neuroleptanalgesia is satisfactory in providing a suitably cooperative patient, and the airway is then pretreated with topical anesthesia. The endobronchial tube selected should be such that the bronchial lumen is on the side opposite the BPF. Selection of the largest possible tube provides a close fit in the trachea, which helps to stabilize the tube. Once the tube is adequately positioned in the trachea, there may be a considerable outpouring of pus from the tracheal lumen if an empyema is present, and therefore this lumen should be immediately suctioned using a large-bore suction catheter. The healthy and, possibly, the affected lung may then be ventilated; adequacy of oxygenation and ventilation is assessed by pulse oximetry and arterial blood gas analysis.

An alternative technique is to insert the double-lumen tube under general anesthesia, with the patient breathing spontaneously to avoid a tension pneumothorax. With either technique, the chest drainage tube must be left unclamped to avoid any bouts of coughing and to prevent the buildup of a tension pneumothorax in the event that a predisposing valvular mechanism exists. In patients who do not have an empyema, use of a single-lumen tube has been described and may be satisfactory if the BPF and air leak are small. A rapid-sequence induction with ketamine or thiopental followed by a relaxant has also been described but is associated with considerable risk of contamination and tension pneumothorax.

Bronchopleural fistula may also be treated conservatively using various ventilatory techniques. Thus, the bronchus of the normal lung may be intubated and ventilated, allowing the BPF to rest and heal. This approach may result in an intolerable shunt, however, and PEEP may be necessary to maintain Pao_2. Differential lung ventilation using a double-lumen tube has also been described, the healthy lung being ventilated with normal V_T, while the affected lung is exposed to a smaller V_T or to CPAP with oxygen at pressures just below the critical opening pressure of the fistula. The critical opening pressure of the BPF can be assessed by determining the lowest level of CPAP that must be applied to the bronchus on the affected side to produce continuous bubbling through the underwater seal chest drain.

For a large BPF, HFJV may be the nonsurgical treatment of choice. The use of small V_T results in minimal gas loss through the fistula, which may heal more quickly. In addition, hemodynamic effects are usually minimal and spontaneous efforts at ventilation are usually abolished, thereby decreasing the work of breathing and eliminating the need for relaxants or excessive sedation.

High-frequency jet ventilation may not always be superior to conventional ventilation in the conservative management of BPF. Thus, HFJV is less effective in reducing the ventilatory leak through a BPF when the peripheral leak is combined with severe injury and decreased compliance in the remainder of the lung than when only an airway is disrupted. In one series,[78] HFJV was compared with controlled ventilation of the lungs, and it was found that adequate gas exchange could not be achieved at comparable mean airway pressures with HFJV, although peak airway pressures decreased. Indeed, in some patients, flow through the BPF actually increased with HFJV. Thus, HFJV should be used selectively in patients with BPF.[91]

Lung Cysts and Bullae

Air-filled cysts of the lung are usually bronchogenic, postinfective, infantile, or emphysematous. They may be associated with COPD or be an isolated finding. A bulla is a thin-walled space filled with air that results from the destruction of alveolar tissue. The walls are, therefore, composed of visceral pleura, connective tissue septa, or compressed lung tissue. In general, bullae represent an area of end-stage emphysematous destruction of the lung.

Patients may be considered for surgical bullectomy when dyspnea is incapacitating, when the bullae are expanding, when there are repeated pneumothoraces owing to rupture of bullae, or if the bullae compress a large area of normal lung. Most of these patients have severe COPD and CO_2 retention and little functional respiratory reserve. The first consideration in management is maintenance of a high Fio_2. If the bulla or cyst communicates with the bronchial tree, positive-pressure ventilation may cause it to expand or even to rupture if it is compliant, producing a situation analogous to tension pneumothorax. If

the bulla is very compliant, most of the applied V_T may be wasted in this additional dead space. Nitrous oxide should be avoided because it causes expansion of any air spaces in the body, including bullae. Once the chest is open, even more of the V_T may enter the compliant bulla, which is no longer limited by chest wall integrity, and an increase in ventilation is needed until the bulla is controlled.

The anesthetic management of these patients is challenging, particularly if the disease is bilateral. Ideally, a double-lumen tube is inserted with the patient awake or under general anesthesia but breathing spontaneously. The avoidance of positive-pressure ventilation (when possible) helps to decrease the likelihood of the potential problems described previously, although oxygenation may be precarious with spontaneous ventilation. Once the endotracheal tube is in place, each lung may be controlled separately, and adequate ventilation can be applied to the healthy lung if bilateral disease is not present. Gentle positive-pressure ventilation with rapid, small V_T and pressures not to exceed 10 cm H_2O may be used during the induction and maintenance of anesthesia, especially if the bullae have been shown to have no or only poor bronchial communication by preoperative ventilation scanning. While the surgery is being performed, as each bulla is resected, the operated lung can be separately ventilated to check for air leaks and the presence of additional bullae.

If positive-pressure ventilation is to be applied before the chest is opened, the possibility of a tension pneumothorax must be kept in mind, and treatment should be readily available. The diagnosis of pneumothorax may be made by a unilateral decrease in breath sounds (this may be difficult to distinguish in a patient with bullous disease), increase in ventilatory pressure, progressive tracheal deviation, wheezing, or cardiovascular changes. Treatment of a pneumothorax involves the rapid placement of a chest tube. An added risk of chest tube placement is the creation of a cutaneous BPF, which causes problems for ventilation. Alternatively, general anesthesia is induced only after the surgeon has prepared the operative field and draped the patient. In the event of sudden deterioration in the patient's condition during induction, the surgeon may perform an immediate median sternotomy. In any event, the time from induction of anesthesia to sternotomy must be kept to a minimum. Thoracoscopic laser ablation of bullae has also been described.[88]

To avoid these problems in a patient with known bullae, HFJV has been used in a patient with a large bulla undergoing coronary artery bypass graft and in another patient undergoing bilateral bullectomy. If bilateral bullectomy is to be performed, a median sternotomy usually is used. Benumof[92] has described the use of sequential one-lung ventilation using a double-lumen tube in the management of a patient needing bilateral bullectomy. The side with the largest bulla and least lung function, as assessed before surgery by ventilation and perfusion scans, should be operated on first. In this way, the lung with the better function should support gas exchange first. If hypoxemia develops during this one-lung situation, application of CPAP to the nonventilated lung during the deflation phase of a tidal breath should increase Pao_2.

In an extreme situation in which no respiratory reserve exists, it may not be possible to maintain an adequate Pao_2 on one-lung ventilation, and in such a situation it may be necessary to use an extracorporeal oxygenator and femorofemoral bypass may be needed. Heparinization is an additional surgical problem in such cases. Such a severe situation may also be well suited to surgery in a hyperbaric chamber. Oxygenation can be ensured, and the cyst or bulla shrinks under hyperbaric conditions.

Unlike most cases of pulmonary resection, patients after bullectomy are left with a greater amount of functional lung tissue than was previously available to them, and the mechanics of respiration are improved. At the end of the procedure, the double-lumen tube is replaced by a single-lumen tube, and the

Table 30-5. SURGICAL TREATMENT OF END-STAGE EMPHYSEMA

Unproven Efficacy	Proven Efficacy
Costochondrectomy	Transtracheal oxygen catheter
Transverse sternotomy	Tracheostomy
Thoracoplasty	Needle aspiration of bullae
Phrenic nerve resection	Tube thoracostomy
Pneumoperitoneum	Bullectomy
Abdominal belting	Lung volume reduction
Talc pleurodesis	Lung transplantation
Sympathectomy	
Vagotomy	

patients generally require several days to be weaned from the respirator. During this time, the positive airway pressure used should be minimized to avoid causing a pneumothorax owing to rupture of suture or staple lines or of residual bullae.

Lung Volume Reduction Surgery

Emphysematous changes are common in the general population, occasionally resulting in pneumothoraces; a significant number of these patients require surgical intervention. Many surgical procedures have been performed to alleviate the dyspnea in severely emphysematous patients, some with beneficial effect and others without any proven beneficial outcome. (Table 30-5). Recently, laser and videoscopic technology has been used to ablate small bullae.[87,93-95]

In 1959, Brantigan, from the University of Maryland, reported on the surgical management of diffuse emphysema. "In patients with distended lungs caused by severe COPD, the normal outward circumferential pull on the bronchioles had been lost, causing their collapse during expiration. Reducing overall lung volume, by means of multiple wedge excisions or plications, would restore the elastic pull on the small airways and reduce expiratory airway obstruction."[96]

He suggested that, in these patients with severe dyspnea, a distended chest, and a flattened diaphragm, surgical excision of a functionless but nonbullous area by multiple wedge resection, can relieve the dyspnea. He proposed an operation ". . . directed at restoration of a physiologic principle . . . and not concerned with the removal of pathologic tissue." Thus, lung volume reduction results in the use of "bilateral multiple wedge excisions of bullous and nonbullous areas of the lung in patients with diffuse emphysema to improve pulmonary mechanics."

Lung volume reduction surgery (LVRS) should not be confused with excision of bullous emphysema or of giant bullae. In these cases, the presumed mechanism of improvement in lung function, exercise tolerance, and oxygenation is secondary to re-expansion of more normal, underlying compressed lung.[97]

The Brantigan procedure did not receive wide acceptance. In the absence of an automated stapler, surgery was performed with a hand-sutured line of resection, which resulted in a high incidence of persistent air leak and an 18–20% mortality rate. The procedure was resurrected by Cooper et al[98] after their experience with lung transplantation in patients with severe emphysema. The critical issue was to determine the optimal size of donor lungs for emphysematous recipients. The TLC of the recipient is much larger than that of the donor lung. If the lung does not fill the recipient chest, complications such as prolonged air leak and pleural effusion will persist. To their surprise, "the distended thorax and the flattened diaphragms in the recipient immediately assumed a more normal configuration postoperatively."[98] This ability of the chronically distended chest to configure to a smaller volume gave credence to the notion that downsizing the lungs in an emphysematous

patient might improve respiratory mechanics by alleviating the overdistention. This is the basis of a resurgence of interest in the Brantigan proposal as to the surgical options for diffuse bullous emphysema (e.g., lung volume reduction).

Outcome of Lung Volume Reduction Surgery

Lung volume reduction surgery (LVRS) gained popularity rapidly.[99-101] Because of the possible dramatic increase in the number of procedures without sufficient evidence of beneficial outcome, the National Institutes of Health and the Health Care Finance Agency concluded in 1995 that "although initial results were promising, LVRS was often being performed with insufficient evaluation and a randomized study should be undertaken to evaluate the procedure critically."[102] The National Emphysema Treatment Trial (NETT) was established as a randomized, multicenter, prospective clinical trial of medical versus surgical therapy (LVRS) for treatment of patients with severe bilateral emphysema. Although the outcome of the randomized NETT study is not yet known, there is evidence of beneficial effect of LVRS (at least in the short term). It is beyond the scope of this chapter to review all the published data on LVRS, and the reader is referred to excellent reviews of the subject.[103-105] In brief, Brenner et al, in 256 consecutive patients with LVRS reported an 85% survival rate at 1 year and 81% at 2 years.[106] However, there is evidence that the initial improvement in FEV_1, as an indicator of pulmonary function and improvement in airflow, peaks at 6 months and subsequently deteriorates. Alternatively, Gelb et al reported that 2 years after LVRS, relief of dyspnea remained improved in 110 out of 112 patients with decrease in TLC as a result of reduction in RV and air trapping.[107]

Patient Selection

The patient selection criteria are summarized in Table 30-6. Indications for a good outcome include age younger than 75 years, FEV_1 greater than 0.5 l (FEV_1 of 15–20% of predicted is less useful as a predictor of postoperative respiratory support), Pao_2 greater than 55 mmHg, $Paco_2$ 40–45 mmHg (>50 mmHg is of concern).

Lung-Volume Measurement. Body plethysmography (BP) versus inert gas technique (IG) provides some information on the degree of trapped gas in the emphysematous lung (trapped gas index = IG/BP).

Table 30-6. LUNG VOLUME REDUCTION SURGERY

PATIENT SELECTION

Progressive emphysema
Severe, symptomatic dyspnea
Radiographic evidence of diffuse emphysema
Identifiable distention and hyperinflated lung tissue
FEV_1 < 40%, RV > 150%, TLC > 120% predicted
No previous chest surgery
Smoking cessation
Acceptable cardiac function

CONTRAINDICATIONS

Age >75 years
Uniformly destroyed lungs
   FEV_1 < 15% of predicted
   $Paco_2$ > 55 mm Hg
   O_2 > 6 l/min
Pulmonary hypertension
Severe kyphoscoliosis
Predominance of chronic bronchitis, asthma
Active infection
Inability to complete preoperative rehabilitation program

FEV_1 = forced expiratory volume in 1 second; RV = residual volume; TLC = total lung capacity.

Ventilation–Perfusion Scan. The ideal candidate presents with 30–40% reduction in perfusion to the upper lobes. In case of α_1-antitrypsin deficiency, decreased perfusion also is evident in the lower lobes. The least favorable candidates by scanning are those with a patchy, mottled pattern, uniformly affecting the lung.[108]

Anesthetic Management

Bronchodilator therapy is continued until the morning of surgery. Morphine and atropine premedication is administered to facilitate insertion of bronchoscopes and tracheal intubation. In addition to steroids, intraoperative bronchodilators are commonly used.

During induction of anesthesia, increases in intrathoracic pressure after neuromuscular blockade should be avoided. These patients are intravascularly depleted and have large wasted muscle mass. They commonly present with polycythemia, which may give a false impression of adequate hydration. Therefore, hydration, stable hemodynamic induction with an agent such as etomidate, and gentle ventilation may attenuate the increase in intrathoracic pressure and the degree of hypotension. Patients who have undergone surgery for emphysematous conditions are best managed with spontaneous respiration as soon as possible after the procedure. Therefore, short-acting neuromuscular blocking agents (rocuronuim, atracurium, vecuronium) are indicated. Opioid analgesia can be achieved with fentanyl or remifentanil infusion.[109,110]

Pain relief must be optimal as soon as possible because it enables early tracheal extubation and early mobilization, which is crucial to the recovery of these patients. A thoracic epidural catheter is best placed before induction of anesthesia in the sitting position at T3–T4 level.[111,112] In case of technical difficulty in placing the thoracic catheter, lumbar epidural catheters are used; however, the doses of medication should be increased for effective analgesia.

One-lung ventilation is an absolute requirement, whether the procedure is performed by sternal split or bilateral thoracoscopy.[113] The author (EC) prefers using a double-lumen tracheal tube over a Univent for complete and reliable isolation and rapid lung deflation. However, whichever tube is used in these patients with a marginal respiratory reserve, perfect isolation and confirmation with fiberoptic bronchoscopy is mandatory.

In the PACU, it is important to recognize the early signs of tension pneumothorax and dynamic hyperinflation as possible complications. Adequate analgesia, chest physiotherapy, incentive spirometry, and early ambulation are all important for a successful outcome. The most commonly used medications with the epidural catheter are opioids and low-dose bupivacaine combinations, often with a patient-controlled analgesia mode.[112]

Anesthesia for Resection of the Trachea

Tracheal resection and reconstruction are technically difficult for the surgeon and challenging for the anesthesiologist. Indications for this type of procedure include congenital lesions (agenesis, stenosis), neoplasia (primary or secondary), injuries (direct or indirect), infections, and postintubation injuries (caused by an endotracheal tube or tracheotomy). For the surgical team, the major problems are maintenance of ventilation to the lungs while the airway is being operated on and postoperative integrity of the anastomoses. In this respect, the presence of lung disease sufficiently severe to require postoperative ventilatory support is a relative contraindication to tracheal resection or reconstruction.

Monitoring of these patients should include placement of an arterial cannula in the left radial artery to permit continuous measurement of blood pressure during periods of innominate artery compression. Steroids should be administered to help reduce any tracheal edema, and a high FiO_2 should be used throughout the procedure to ensure an adequate oxygen reserve at all times in the FRC, so that temporary interruptions of ventilation are less likely to produce hypoxemia.

Numerous methods have been reported to provide oxygenation and ventilation of the lungs during these procedures. A small-bore anode tube may be pushed through and distal to an upper lesion, so that resection may occur around the tube. This technique is useful only in mild stenoses. Alternatively, an endotracheal tube may be passed through the glottis to above the stenosis, and a sterile endotracheal or bronchial tube may later be inserted into the trachea opened distal to the site of stenosis, with the sterile anesthesia tubing being led across the surgical field. After resection of the lesion, the sterile and distally placed endotracheal tube is withdrawn, and the upper tube (originally passed through the glottis) is advanced across the anastomosis. With low tracheal or bronchial lesions, resection and reconstruction may be performed around an endobronchial or double-lumen tube. During these procedures, the patient is kept in a head-down position to minimize aspiration of blood and debris into the alveoli, and ventilation must be carefully monitored throughout.

Clearly, the presence of large-bore tubes in the airway may make these resections technically difficult, and the use of high-frequency ventilation techniques may improve surgical access. Thus, a small-diameter catheter or catheters may be placed across or through the stenotic lesion or transected airway(s) and ventilation to the distal airways and lungs maintained using HFPPV or HFJV. Potential disadvantages of these high-frequency ventilation techniques are that, by necessity, the system is "open" (see High-Frequency Ventilation), and egress of gas during exhalation may be compromised if the stenosis is tight. Also, the catheter may become occluded by blood and become displaced, and distal aspiration of debris or blood may occur. With complex resections, two anesthesia teams with two machines and anesthesia circuits or sets of ventilating equipment may be necessary to ensure adequate ventilation of the two distal airway segments, although during carinal resections, HFPPV to the left lung alone usually provides adequate oxygenation and ventilation.

In very difficult cases, cardiopulmonary bypass has been used to provide oxygenation and carbon dioxide removal during the period of resection; after resection, anesthesia can be maintained using a standard endotracheal tube. Cardiopulmonary bypass carries an attendant risk of massive hemorrhage as a result of the necessary heparinization.

After tracheal resection or reconstructive surgery, patients should be kept with their neck and head flexed to reduce tension on the anastomotic suture lines. In some cases, this is maintained by using sutures between the chin and the anterior chest wall. Extubation of the trachea is performed as early as possible to minimize tracheal trauma due to the endotracheal tube and cuff.

Bronchopulmonary Lavage

This procedure involves irrigation of the lung and bronchial tree and is used as a treatment for alveolar proteinosis, radioactive dust inhalation, cystic fibrosis, bronchiectasis, and asthmatic bronchitis. Lung lavage is performed under general anesthesia using a double-lumen tube, so that one lung may be ventilated while the other is being treated with lavage fluid.[114]

The preoperative assessment of these patients should include ventilation–perfusion scans so that lavage can be performed first on the more severely affected lung (*i.e.,* the one with the least ventilation). If involvement is equal, the left lung is generally lavaged first because gas exchange should be better through the larger, right lung. Patients are premedicated and supplied with supplemental oxygen *en route* to the operating room.

Anesthesia is induced with an intravenous drug and maintained with an inhaled agent in oxygen to maintain the highest possible F_{IO_2}. Muscle relaxation facilitates placement of the double-lumen tube, and the cuff seal should be checked to maintain perfect separation at a pressure of 50 cm H_2O to prevent leakage of lavage fluid around the cuff. A fiberoptic bronchoscope is useful to check the position of the bronchial cuff of the double-lumen tube. Monitoring should include an arterial catheter, and a stethoscope should be placed over the ventilated lung to check for rales, the presence of which may indicate leakage of lavage fluid into this lung.

The patient is maintained on an F_{IO_2} of 1.0 throughout the procedure. Before lavage this serves to denitrogenate the lungs, so that only oxygen and carbon dioxide remain. Instillation of fluid then allows these gases to be absorbed, resulting in greater access by the fluid to the alveolar spaces than if the more insoluble nitrogen bubbles remained.

Once the trachea is intubated, the patient is turned so that the side to be lavaged is lowermost, and the double-lumen tube position and seal are checked once again. With the patient in a head-up position, warmed heparinized isotonic saline is infused by gravity from a reservoir 30 cm above the midaxillary line into the catheter to the dependent lung, while the nondependent lung is ventilated. When fluid ceases to flow in (usually after 700–1000 ml in an adult), the patient is placed in a head-down position and fluid is allowed to drain out. The lavage is continued until the effluent is clear (as opposed to the milky fluid that drains initially when lavage is being performed for alveolar proteinosis), at which point the lung is suctioned and ventilation is re-established with large V_T (and pressures), because compliance is decreased owing to loss of surfactant. With each lavage, inflow and outflow volumes are monitored so that the patient is not "drowned" in fluid and there is no excessive absorption or leakage to the ventilated side. At least 90% of the saline volume should be recovered with each lavage. Two-lung ventilation is re-established and, as compliance improves, an air–oxygen mixture (addition of nitrogen) may be introduced to help maintain alveolar patency. After a further period of ventilation, most patients' tracheas can be extubated in the operating room. In the post-treatment period, patients are encouraged to cough and engage in breathing exercises to fully re-expand the treated lung. From 3 days to 1 week after lavage of the first lung, the patient may return to the operating room for lavage of the other lung.

Problems sometimes encountered with this procedure include spillage of lavage fluid from the treated to the ventilated lung. This must be managed by stopping the lavage and ensuring functional separation of the lungs before continuing. Double-lumen tube positioning is critical. Spillage may cause profound decreases in oxygenation, which may necessitate terminating the procedure and maintaining two-lung ventilation with oxygen and PEEP.

During periods when lavage fluid is being instilled into the dependent lung, oxygenation usually improves because the increased intra-alveolar pressure caused by the fluid produces diversion of the pulmonary blood flow to the nondependent, ventilated lung. Conversely, when the fluid is drained out of the dependent lung, hypoxemia may occur.[114] In some cases in which severe hypoxemia was anticipated during right lung lavage, the risk has been reduced by passing a balloon-tipped catheter into the right main pulmonary artery (checked by radiography) and inflating the balloon during periods of right lung drainage. In this way, blood flow to the dependent, right, nonventilated lung is minimized during periods of drainage. This technique is not without risk (*e.g.*, pulmonary artery rupture) and is reserved for those patients considered to be at greatest risk for hypoxemia during lavage. Almitrine by infusion and nitric oxide by inhalation have also been reported to improve oxygenation during bronchopulmonary lavage.[73]

If the patient has recently had a diagnostic open lung biopsy, a BPF may be present. If this is a possibility, a chest tube should be inserted on the side of the BPF, and this side should be lavaged first. The chest drain is removed several days later.

Limitations in the sizes of available double-lumen tubes preclude their use for lavage in patients weighing less than 40 kg. In such cases, cardiopulmonary bypass may be required to provide oxygenation during lavage.

Myasthenia Gravis

The thoracic anesthesiologist will most likely have to manage patients with myasthenia gravis (MG) for thymectomy, which is now considered the treatment of choice in most cases of MG. MG is a disorder of the neuromuscular junction, the function of which is altered routinely in the modern practice of anesthesia. The worldwide prevalence of the disease is 1 per 20,000 to 30,000 of the population; it is more common in women than men in 6:4 ratio. People of any age may be affected, but peaks of incidence occur in the third decade for women and the fifth decade for men. MG is a chronic disorder characterized by weakness and fatigability of voluntary muscles with improvement following rest.[115] Onset usually is slow and insidious, any skeletal muscle or group of muscles may be affected, and the condition is associated with relapses and remissions. The most common onset is ocular; if the disease remains localized to the eyes for 2 years, the likelihood of progression to generalized MG is low. In some cases, the disease is generalized and may involve the bulbar musculature, causing problems with breathing and swallowing. Peripheral muscle involvement may cause weakness, clumsiness, and difficulty in holding up the head or in walking. The most commonly used clinical classification of MG is shown in Table 30-7.

In MG there is a decrease in the number of postsynaptic acetylcholine receptors at the end plates of affected muscles. This causes a decrease in the margin of safety of neuromuscular transmission. MG is an autoimmune disorder, and most of the affected patients have circulating antibodies to the acetylcholine receptors. These antibodies may cause complement-mediated lysis of the postsynaptic membrane or direct blockade of the receptors,

---

Table 30-7. CLINICAL CLASSIFICATION OF MYASTHENIA GRAVIS

I	Ocular myasthenia—Involvement of ocular muscles only. Mild with ptosis and diplopia. Electrophysiologic testing of other musculature is negative for MG.
IA	Ocular myasthenia with peripheral muscles showing no clinical symptoms but showing a positive electromyogram for MG.
II	Generalized myasthenia
IIA	Mild—Slow onset, usually ocular, spreading to skeletal and bulbar muscles. No respiratory involvement. Good response to drug therapy. Low mortality rate.
IIB	Moderate—As IIA but progressing to more severe involvement of skeletal and bulbar muscles. Dysarthria, dysphagia, difficulty chewing. No respiratory involvement. Patient's activities limited. Fair response to drug therapy.
III	Acute fulminating myasthenia—Rapid onset of severe bulbar and skeletal weakness with involvement of muscles of respiration. Progression usually within 6 months. Poor response to therapy. Patient's activities limited. Low mortality rate.
IV	Late severe myasthenia—Severe MG developing at least 2 years after onset of Group I or Group II symptoms. Progression of disease may be gradual or rapid. Poor response to therapy and poor prognosis.

MG = myasthenia gravis.
Adapted from Osserman KE, Genkins G: Studies in myasthenia gravis—a review of a 20-year experience in over 1200 patients. Mt Sinai J Med 38:497, 1971.

or may modulate the receptor turnover such that the degradation rate exceeds the resynthesis rate. Studies of the end plate area show loss of synaptic folds and a widening of the synaptic cleft.

The diagnosis of MG is suspected from the history and confirmed by pharmacologic, electrophysiologic, or immunologic testing. Patients cannot sustain or repeat muscular contraction. The electrical counterpart of this is a decrement in the muscle action potentials evoked by repetitive stimulation of a motor nerve. Mechanical and electrical (electromyography) decrements improve with 2–10 mg of intravenous edrophonium (Tensilon test). Myasthenic patients characteristically are sensitive to *d*-tubocurarine. When the routine electromyographic results are equivocal, a regional curare test may be performed using a tourniquet to isolate the limb and to limit the action of the drug. In the regional curare test, electromyograms are performed before and after the administration of 0.2 mg of curare. In equivocal cases, a positive result of a test for anti-acetylcholine receptor antibodies is considered diagnostic.

Medical Therapy

Anticholinesterases are used to prolong the action of acetylcholine at the postsynaptic membrane and may also exert their own agonist effect at the acetylcholine receptors. They are the most commonly used therapy in MG (Table 30-8). Myasthenic patients learn to regulate their medication and titrate dose against optimum effect. Overdosage causes the muscarinic effects of acetylcholine and may cause a cholinergic crisis. Underdosage causes weakness or a myasthenic crisis. In a patient with weakness, distinction between the two types of crisis may be made by performing a Tensilon test or by examining pupillary size, which will be large (mydriatic) in a myasthenic but small (miotic) in a cholinergic crisis. Muscarinic side effects are treatable with atropine.

The immunologic basis of MG has led to the use of immunosuppressive drugs such as steroids, azathioprine, cyclophosphamide and, most recently, cyclosporine. Steroids often produce initial deterioration before an improvement. The usual regimen is prednisone 1 mg · kg⁻¹ on alternate days. The other drugs mentioned represent third and fourth lines of treatment.

Plasma exchange or plasmapheresis may produce dramatic but transient improvements in muscle strength with decreases in anti-acetylcholine receptor antibody titers. Usually reserved for severe MG, plasma exchange has been shown to improve respiratory function in both operated and nonoperated patients with MG. Plasmapheresis causes a decrease in plasma cholinesterase levels that may prolong the effect of drugs such as succinylcholine that are normally broken down by this enzyme system.

Abnormalities are found in 75% of thymus glands removed from patients with MG (85% show hyperplasia; 15% thymoma). After thymectomy, approximately 75% of patients either go into remission or are improved. Thymectomy is now considered the treatment of choice in most patients with MG, except for those in Osserman Class I.

Table 30-8. ANTICHOLINESTERASE DRUGS USED TO TREAT MYASTHENIA GRAVIS

| Drug | Dose (mg) | | | Efficacy |
	Oral	iv	im	
Pyridostigmine (Mestinon)	60	2.0	2.0–4.0	1
Neostigmine (Prostigmine)	15	0.5	0.7–1.0	1
Ambenonium (Mytelase)	6	NA	NA	2.5

iv = intravenous; im = intramuscular; NA = not available.

Table 30-9. DISORDERS ASSOCIATED WITH MYASTHENIA GRAVIS

Thymoma	Multiple sclerosis
Thyroid disease	Ulcerative colitis
Hyperthyroidism	Leukemia
Hypothyroidism	Lymphoma
Thyroiditis	Convulsive disorders
Idiopathic thrombocytopenic	Extrathymic neoplasia
purpura	Polymyositis
Rheumatoid arthritis	Sjögren's syndrome
Systemic lupus erythema-	Scleroderma
tosus	
Anemias	
Pernicious	
Hemolytic	

Management of General Anesthesia

When possible, patients with MG should be admitted for elective surgery while in remission. On admission, the patient's physical and emotional states should be optimized. Other diseases occasionally associated with MG should be excluded (Table 30-9). The patient's current drug therapy should be reviewed and possible drug interactions considered. Because patients are less active while in the hospital, their anticholinesterase dosage may need to be decreased. If the patient has a history of respiratory disease or bulbar involvement, preoperative evaluation should include respiratory function studies. Breathing exercises and instruction in the use of incentive spirometers may be indicated. Patients should be told of the possible need for postoperative intubation of the trachea and ventilation of the lungs. Ideally, patients with MG should be scheduled to be the first case of the day in the operating room. Patients receiving steroid therapy should receive perioperative coverage.

Because the trachea is to be intubated and the lungs ventilated for the planned procedure in the patient with MG, anticholinesterase therapy should be withheld on the morning of surgery so that the patient is weak on arrival at the operating room. This avoids interactions with other drugs used in the operating room. Anticholinesterase therapy may be continued if the patient is physically or psychologically dependent on it. Premedication is satisfactorily achieved with a benzodiazepine or barbiturate. Opioids are usually avoided because of the risk of producing respiratory depression.

Monitoring should be dictated by the patient's state and planned surgical procedure, but should include an assessment of neuromuscular transmission (mechanomyogram/twitch monitor or integrated electromyographic monitor) if agents affecting neuromuscular transmission are to be used.[116]

Induction of anesthesia is readily achieved with a short-acting barbiturate or propofol. In elective cases, intubation of the trachea, maintenance, and relaxation are readily achieved using potent inhaled anesthetics. Anesthesia may be deepened using a potent inhaled agent and the trachea intubated under its effect. Myasthenic patients are more sensitive than normal patients to the neuromuscular depressant effects of the potent inhaled agents. In patients with MG, isoflurane at 1.9 MAC end-tidal concentration induced a neuromuscular block of 30–50%, whereas halothane at 1.8 MAC induced a block of 10–20%. Both agents produced fade in the train-of-four ratio of 41% and 28%, respectively.[117] Because these drugs are easily administered and withdrawn, they are the most commonly used anesthetic drugs for patients with MG. At the end of the procedure, the drug is discontinued and recovery of neuromuscular function begins.

Nondepolarizing Relaxants. In some cases, patients with MG cannot tolerate the cardiovascular depressant effects of the potent inhaled anesthetics, in which case muscle relaxants may be used, titrating dose against monitored effect. Patients with MG are sensitive to the nondepolarizing relaxants. A usual defasciculating dose in a normal patient may represent an ED_{90} in a patient with MG.[116] All of the nondepolarizing relaxants have been successfully and uneventfully used, with careful monitoring, in patients with MG. They should be titrated in 1/10 to 1/20 of the usual dose. Atracurium is probably the preferred agent because of its short elimination half-life (20 minutes), small volume of distribution, lack of cumulative effect, and high clearance. The Hofmann elimination pathway results in atracurium having very reproducible pharmacodynamics and kinetics, and most patients do not require reversal if monitored carefully. The ED_{90} of atracurium in patients with MG is approximately one-fifth of that in normal patients.[118] Relaxation is readily maintained thereafter using an atracurium infusion, and recovery time is not prolonged with this drug. Cisatracurium is also an appropriate choice.[119]

Although other short- or intermediate-duration nondepolarizing agents may be used, they do have cumulative effects, which may represent a potential disadvantage. Long-acting relaxants are probably best avoided in patients with MG. Myasthenic patients show increased sensitivity to mivacurium. Because mivacurium is metabolized by cholinesterase, anticholinesterase drugs prolong the recovery from this relaxant.[120] If necessary, the other nondepolarizers may be reversed by increments of anticholinesterase drugs while neuromuscular transmission is carefully monitored to obtain maximum antagonism yet avoid a cholinergic crisis. All anticholinesterases have been safely used. Edrophonium may be the drug of choice because its onset of action is rapid and higher doses have a prolonged duration of action. Because of the risk of cholinergic crisis with anticholinesterase agents, the rapid, predictable, spontaneous recovery from atracurium (or cisatracurium) may represent an additional advantage in that reversal may not be necessary.[116]

The sensitivity of patients with MG to nondepolarizing relaxants is very variable, depending on the individual patient, the severity of MG, and the treatment. There are conflicting reports as to the sensitivity of patients with MG in remission. All such patients should be considered sensitive to nondepolarizers until proved otherwise.

Succinylcholine. Myasthenic patients are resistant to the neuromuscular blocking effects of succinylcholine. The ED_{95} is 2.6 times normal in these patients.[121] Clinically, however, the use of succinylcholine has been without incident, with normal clinical doses producing adequate relaxation for endotracheal intubation and a normal recovery time, despite the occasionally reported early onset of Phase II block. Doses of 0.2–1.0 mg·kg^{-1} have been used in a number of patients with MG, and most did not show fasciculation before becoming paralyzed. Fade in response to train-of-four stimulation was observed in some patients during recovery, but recovery was not delayed. Prior administration of an anticholinesterase may complicate the response to succinylcholine by delaying its metabolism.

When a rapid-sequence intubation of the trachea is required, rapid onset of muscle relaxation may be achieved with succinylcholine or with moderate doses of a nondepolarizer in the latter case, with an associated prolongation of effect. A succinylcholine (1.5 mg·kg^{-1})–vecuronium (0.01 mg·kg^{-1}) sequence has been safely used in three patients with MG for thymectomy. The authors suggested that this technique may be particularly advantageous when rapid-sequence induction of anesthesia is indicated.[122]

Other Drug Interactions. Medications with neuromuscular blocking properties should be used with caution in patients with MG, particularly if relaxants are being used concurrently. Such drugs include antiarrhythmics (quinidine, procainamide, calcium channel blockers), diuretics (by causing hypokalemia), nitrogen mustards, quinine, and aminoglycoside antibiotics. Dantrolene has been used safely in a patient with MG.

Recovery from Anesthesia. Recovery from anesthesia must be carefully monitored in these patients. Extubation of the trachea should be performed when the patients are responsive and able to generate negative inspiratory pressures of greater than −20 cm H_2O. After extubation of the trachea, patients are carefully observed in the recovery area or the intensive care unit. As soon as possible, patients should resume their usual pyridostigmine regimen. Cases of mild respiratory depression may be treatable with parenteral anticholinesterase; more severe cases may require reintubation of the trachea and mechanical ventilation of the lungs. In the immediate postoperative period, post-thymectomy patients often show a marked improvement in their condition and a decreased need for anticholinesterase therapy.

Postoperative Respiratory Failure

Myasthenic patients are at increased risk for development of postoperative respiratory failure. There have been several attempts to predict before surgery which patients with MG will require prolonged postoperative ventilation of the lungs.[123] For patients who underwent trans-sternal thymectomy, positive predictors were a duration of MG greater than 6 years; history of chronic respiratory disease, other than that directly caused by MG; pyridostigmine dosage greater than 750 mg·day^{-1}; and a preoperative vital capacity of less than 2.9 l. This predictive system was not found useful when applied in patients with MG undergoing trans-sternal thymectomy at other centers, and of no value in patients with MG undergoing other types of surgical procedure.[123] Each patient should therefore be treated on his or her own merits.

A study of patients undergoing trans-sternal thymectomy suggested that the need for postoperative mechanical ventilation correlated best with preoperative maximum static expiratory pressure. It was concluded that expiratory weakness, by reducing cough efficacy and ability to clear secretions, was the main predictive determinant. Adequate clearance of secretions is essential in these patients and may occasionally necessitate bronchoscopy.

In general, the postoperative morbidity in terms of respiratory failure is lower after transcervical rather than trans-sternal thymectomy.[123] Techniques described that may be useful in reducing postoperative ventilatory failure include preoperative plasma exchange and high-dose perioperative steroid therapy. If the anticipated duration of the surgical procedure is 1–2 hours, preoperative oral anticholinesterase therapy may be of value because the peak effect of the drug coincides with the conclusion of the surgical procedure and attempts at tracheal extubation.

Postoperative Care

In the immediate postoperative period, pain relief for patients with MG is usually provided by opioid analgesics, such as meperidine, but in reduced doses. The analgesic effect of morphine and other opioid analgesics has been reported to be increased by anticholinesterases, which has led to the recommendation that the dose of opioid analgesics be reduced by one third in patients receiving anticholinesterase therapy. Combined regional and general anesthesia techniques have also been used to provide good surgical conditions and improved postoperative analgesia in patients with MG undergoing thymectomy. Combined epidural–general anesthesia has been reported to provide excellent intraoperative and postoperative conditions for both surgeon and patient.[124,125]

Myasthenic Syndrome (Eaton-Lambert Syndrome)

The myasthenic syndrome is a very rare disorder of neuromuscular transmission that is sometimes associated with small cell carcinoma of the lung. Complaints of weakness may be mistaken for MG, but in Eaton-Lambert syndrome, symptoms do not respond to administration of anticholinesterases or steroids, and activity improves strength. The defect in this condition is thought to be prejunctional, associated with diminished release of acetylcholine from nerve terminals, and improved by agents such as 4-aminopyridine, guanidine, and germine that increase repetitive firing. Affected patients are particularly sensitive to the effects of all muscle relaxants, which should be used with great caution or avoided entirely. The possibility of Eaton-Lambert syndrome should be considered in all patients with known malignant disease and those patients undergoing diagnostic procedures for suspected carcinoma of the lung. Anesthesia considerations in these patients are essentially the same as in those with MG.[126]

POSTOPERATIVE MANAGEMENT AND COMPLICATIONS

Atelectasis

Patients who require thoracotomy often have pre-existing pulmonary disease that, when combined with the operative procedure, is likely to result in significant pulmonary dysfunction and possibly pneumonia. Atelectasis, the most significant cause of postoperative morbidity, has been reported to occur in up to 100% of patients undergoing thoracotomy for pulmonary resection. It occurs more commonly in the basal lobes than in the middle or upper lung regions. It may be secondary to reduction of normal respiratory effort due to splinting from pain, obesity, intrathoracic blood and fluid accumulation, and decreased compliance, all of which lead to rapid, shallow, constant V_T. Such a respiratory pattern produces small airway closure and obstruction with inspissated secretions, resulting ultimately in alveolar air resorption and terminal airway collapse. A poor cough and limited clearance of secretions add to the problem. Other sources of atelectasis include mucus plugging, which can obstruct a lobe or even an entire lung, and incomplete re-expansion of the remaining lung tissue after one-lung anesthesia. The diagnosis of atelectasis can be made by clinical findings, chest radiography, or arterial blood gas analysis. This problem is best resolved by increasing resting lung volume or FRC. FRC can be increased by an increase in transpulmonary pressure (difference between airway pressure and intrapleural pressure) or in lung compliance.

The tracheas of many patients can be extubated shortly after brief thoracic surgical procedures using standard extubation criteria. However, most patients with COPD undergoing extensive thoracic surgical procedures require postoperative ventilation to avoid atelectasis and other pulmonary complications. Mechanical ventilation increases airway pressure and, to a lesser extent, intrapleural pressure; therefore, transpulmonary pressure increases. Most postoperative thoracotomy patients are ventilated using intermittent mandatory ventilation and PEEP. Ventilation settings include: $V_T = 12$ ml·kg^{-1}, rate = 8 breaths·min^{-1}, $F_{IO_2} = 0.5$, and PEEP = 5–20 cm H_2O. The goal is to keep the Pao_2 between 80 and 100 mm Hg and the $Paco_2$ and pH normal. The intermittent mandatory ventilation rate is decreased as tolerated to 2 breaths·min^{-1}, and then the PEEP level is reduced to 5 cm H_2O. When arterial blood gases are adequate at these settings and the vital capacity is greater than 10 ml·kg^{-1}, inspiratory force is greater than −20 cm H_2O, and the level of consciousness is adequate, the patient's trachea is ready for extubation.

In addition to the use of incentive spirometry and bronchodilators, coughing and clearance of secretions, and mobilizing the patient, adequate analgesia is essential to the prevention and treatment of atelectasis. Atelectasis caused by collapse of lung tissue distal to a mucus plug can be treated by positioning the patient in the lateral decubitus position with the fully expanded lung in the dependent position. This improves $\dot{V}/\dot{Q}$ matching and facilitates clearance of mucus from the nondependent obstructed lung. However, the patient should not be placed with the operative side in the dependent position after a pneumonectomy because of the risk of cardiac herniation.

Postoperative Pain Control

After extubation of the trachea, respiratory therapy and pain management become critical components of postoperative care. Adequate postoperative pain control is necessary to ensure a good respiratory effort.[115] Administration of intravenous opioids has been the standard form of pain management for years. These drugs may improve pulmonary function slightly or allow respiratory therapy maneuvers; however, meperidine (50 mg) has been shown to be relatively ineffective at allowing patients to increase their ability to cough. Advantages of intravenous opioids are the ease of administration, relatively low toxicity, and the lack of a need for close medical supervision. The key disadvantage is the inadequate pain relief leading to postoperative atelectasis and great discomfort on the part of the patient. The administration of sufficient opioid to treat pain adequately is likely to cause sedation and respiratory depression.

Patient-controlled analgesia has been reported to decrease the amount of postoperative pain, drug use, sedation, and pulmonary complications.[127] Patient-controlled analgesia also eliminates the delays associated with personnel-administered medications and in general is very well accepted by patients. Subcutaneous patient-controlled analgesia with hydromorphone has been reported to be as effective as intravenous patient-controlled analgesia. Complications related to the use of patient-controlled analgesia are presented elsewhere in this volume (see Chapter 54).

Many clinicians have suggested the use of intercostal nerve blocks before, during, or after thoracic surgery to decrease pain and improve postoperative respiratory function. Studies have documented a decrease in requirements for postoperative opioids, improved respiratory function, and some decrease in time of hospital stay. The intercostal block can be performed externally before or after surgery using a standard technique. However, the easiest method during thoracic surgery is to have the surgeon perform the block under direct vision from inside the thorax while the chest is open. Bupivacaine 0.5%, in doses of 2–3 ml, can be placed in the five intercostal spaces around the incision and in intercostal spaces where chest tubes will be placed. This provides 6–24 hours of moderate pain relief, but patients still complain of diaphragmatic and shoulder discomfort caused by the chest tubes. Higher volumes of local anesthetic (e.g., 5–10 ml) should not be used in the intercostal space because of the high absorption rate and attendant systemic toxicity that can be produced, as well as the possibility of pushing the drug centrally and producing a paravertebral sympathetic or epidural block with central sympatholysis and severe hypotension. The intraoperative placement of catheters in intercostal grooves allows for a continuous postoperative intercostal nerve block. The technique reduces pain and improves pulmonary function. Although bupivacaine has been used in most reports, lidocaine has also been used.

A prolonged intercostal nerve block may be obtained by cryoanalgesia, a technique of freezing the nerve under direct vision at the time of thoracotomy. A cryoprobe is applied directly to the nerve to disrupt the axon but not the support structures. In this way, conduction is interrupted until the nerve regenerates over the next 1–6 months, by which time full structure and function are usually restored. Hypoesthesia in the scar and adjacent skin is a common late finding. During the postoperative period, the patients are numb in the segments thus treated. Ideally, any drains or chest tubes should be located within the area made analgesic with the cryoprobe to minimize immediate postoperative discomfort. Cryoanalgesia provides excellent analgesia when supplemented with other pain treatments. Because cryoanalgesia is of prolonged duration, it is not used routinely after thoracotomy but rather in cases in which prolonged analgesia would be necessary, such as after surgery for chest trauma.

Another approach to postoperative pain control after thoracic surgery is the use of epidural or intrathecal opioids. Epidural morphine produces profound analgesia lasting from 16–24 hours after thoracotomy and does not cause a sympathetic block or sensory or motor loss. These are significant advantages over other methods of administering opioids or local anesthetics. The opioids have been successfully used by both the thoracic and lumbar epidural routes. Morphine, in a dose of 5–7 mg diluted in 15–20 ml of fluid, has been used in the lumbar epidural technique. This technique has led to a 30% increase in postoperative expiratory flow rates without significant side effects, even in patients with chronic lung disease.

Epidural morphine has been shown to decrease pain and improve respiratory function in post-thoracotomy patients.[128] The successful use of lumbar epidural sufentanil or fentanyl diluted to 20 ml has also been reported. There have been reports of severe respiratory depression with epidural fentanyl and several reports with sufentanil. The addition of epinephrine, 5 mg · ml^{-1}, to sufentanil administered in the thoracic epidural space decreases the plasma concentration of sufentanil and increases the duration of block. Lumbar epidural hydromorphone (1.25–1.5 mg) has been reported to provide excellent analgesia, with fewer side effects than epidural morphine. Severe respiratory depression was reported in one patient who received hydromorphone *via* a thoracic epidural catheter. A prophylactic low-dose infusion of naloxone, or nalbuphine, an agonist–antagonist drug, can reduce the incidence of respiratory depression.

Subarachnoid (intrathecal) morphine, in a dose of 10–12 $\mu g \cdot kg^{-1}$, has been successfully used after thoracic surgery.[129] With this technique, the drug acts directly on the spinal cord, and analgesia can be produced with a lower dose than by the epidural or intravenous routes. When morphine is given intrathecally before the induction of anesthesia, a decrease in the dose of anesthetic drugs required may occur. All patients who have received intrathecal or epidural opioids must be closely observed for potential side effects, including delayed respiratory depression, urine retention, pruritus, nausea, and vomiting. These effects appear to be dose related and may be reversed with naloxone.

Noxious stimuli, including surgical incision, may lead to changes in the central nervous system that exacerbate postoperative pain. The administration of analgesic agents before surgery is termed *pre-emptive analgesia* and may prevent these neuroplastic changes, thereby decreasing postoperative pain. The administration of lumbar epidural fentanyl before thoracotomy incision reduced postoperative pain scores and use of patient-controlled analgesia morphine by a small but significant amount, compared with administration of lumbar epidural fentanyl after skin incision.[130]

Interpleural analgesia is another technique for postoperative pain treatment. Although the mechanism has not been fully elucidated, the injection of local anesthetic between the pleural layers is thought to block multiple intercostal nerves or the pain fibers traveling with the thoracic sympathetic chain. The surgeon can place the catheter under direct vision while the chest is open. Catheter malposition has been documented after percutaneous placement, especially if the patient is not breathing spontaneously. The chest tubes should not be suctioned for approximately 15 minutes after injection of local anesthetic to avoid loss of the anesthetic into the drainage. The efficacy of interpleural blockade for post-thoracotomy pain relief has been reported to be both poor and good.[127]

Respiratory Therapy Techniques

Physiotherapy is one of the oldest forms of therapy for the prevention and treatment of respiratory complications. Techniques include postural drainage, breathing exercises, vibration, deep breathing, coughing, and percussion. Many clinicians feel that chest physiotherapy is useful despite the sparse data to support its physiologic benefits. Decades ago, it was also felt that forced exhalation against resistance would create increased airway pressures and inflation of the lungs. Thus, water-filled blow bottles were designed for postoperative use. However, studies subsequently showed that a forced exhalation decreases the expiratory transpulmonary pressure and lung volumes and should be avoided in postoperative patients. It was suggested that the blow bottles were useful only because of the large inspiration that preceded the forced exhalation.

Intermittent positive-pressure breathing has also been used extensively in the postoperative period to prevent and treat respiratory insufficiency. Most of the studies demonstrated little physiologic benefit and, in fact, some authors showed that intermittent positive-pressure breathing could be harmful after thoracotomy because of the hypoventilation that subsequently occurred after the forced hyperventilation. The hyperventilation led to decreased FRC and Pa_{CO_2} secondary to the decreased expiratory transpulmonary pressure.

Incentive spirometry is the most widely used postoperative respiratory care device. This device, producing a long, deep breath, has been shown to cause fewer complications and less atelectasis than intermittent positive-pressure breathing, blow bottles, or chest physiotherapy. Patients with a decreased FRC and decreased Pa_{O_2} experience a reduction of atelectasis on chest radiography and improved arterial oxygenation. The technique produces an increase in inspiratory transpulmonary pressure but not an increase in expiratory pressure. Expiratory transpulmonary pressure can best be increased by the use of CPAP by mask. A comparison of mask CPAP with chest physiotherapy, postural drainage, and endotracheal suction in the treatment of postoperative atelectasis found that 15 cm H_2O CPAP applied once an hour for 25–35 breaths led to clinically significant improvement within 12 hours, whereas the other techniques produced little change. This technique appears to be very useful in the treatment of atelectasis to avoid reintubation of the trachea in patients after surgery. Gastric distention, regurgitation, and pulmonary aspiration are the potential dangers of mask CPAP.

Other Complications After Thoracic Surgery

The other major complications after thoracic surgery can be grouped into cardiovascular, pulmonary, and related problems. The cardiovascular complications are often the most difficult to manage in patients with associated respiratory insufficiency. The low cardiac output syndrome and postoperative cardiac arrhythmias are the most common and life-threatening of these problems. In the postoperative period, advanced hemodynamic monitoring is used to make the differential diagnosis of left or right ventricular failure and the low output syndrome. A key monitor is the PA catheter, which facilitates the construction of Starling function curves. Other diagnostic modalities, such as echocardiography, may be required to rule out the presence of pericardial effusions or tamponade after opening the pericardium during certain types of thoracic surgical procedure. The low cardiac output syndrome must be differentiated from hypovolemia resulting from intrathoracic hemorrhage, tamponade, pulmonary emboli, or the effects of mechanical ventilation with PEEP. Postoperative fluid administration can lead to pulmonary edema resulting from the resection of lung tissue and the concomitant reduction of the pulmonary vascular bed. A postoperative pulmonary embolism can originate from the remaining pulmonary artery stump or tumor tissue. Therapeutic interventions for postoperative myocardial dysfunction include inotropic drugs, vasodilators, and combinations of these drugs, as needed, to improve ventricular function. The goal is to shift the Starling function curve up and to the left by reducing preload of either the left or right side of the heart and increasing cardiac output. Vasodilators are very effective at decreasing right ventricular afterload and improving right ventricular function because this side of the heart is especially afterload dependent. Combinations of inotropes and vasodilators, such as isoproterenol and nitroglycerin, or combined drugs, such as amrinone, can be especially useful in the treatment of right-sided heart failure.

Postoperative cardiac dysrhythmias are common after thoracic surgery. Patients undergoing pulmonary resection have postoperative supraventricular tachycardias with a frequency and severity proportional to both their age and the magnitude of the surgical procedure. Many factors contribute to these arrhythmias, including underlying cardiac disease, degree of surgical trauma, intraoperative cardiac manipulation, stimulation of the sympathetic nervous system by pain, a reduced pulmonary vascular bed, effects of anesthetics and cardioactive drugs, and metabolic abnormalities.

In a series of 300 thoracotomies for lung resection, it was found that atrial fibrillation occurred in 20% of patients with malignant disease but in only 3% with benign disease. A 22% incidence of dysrhythmias has been reported after pneumonectomies.[90] Multifocal atrial tachycardia often occurs in patients with COPD and concomitant right-sided cardiac dysfunction. The right side of the heart may be further strained by the reduction in the size of the pulmonary vasculature from the lung resection, and especially after right pneumonectomy. The prophylactic use of digitalis in thoracic surgical patients is controversial, particularly in patients with signs of congestive heart failure. Factors against its use include the potential toxic effects of the drug and the difficulty in assessing adequacy of digitalization in the absence of heart failure. A prospective, placebo-controlled, randomized study demonstrated no advantage to prophylactic digitalization of patients undergoing thoracic surgery.[131] A factor in favor of its use is the drug's efficacy in reducing the incidence of potentially fatal complications in older patients. In some studies it has been reported to reduce the incidence of perioperative dysrhythmias. If digitalis is to be instituted, normokalemia should be ensured to reduce the likelihood of digitalis toxicity.

Supraventricular tachycardias can also be treated with either β blocking or calcium channel blocking drugs after ruling out underlying reversible physiologic abnormalities, such as hypoxia. Verapamil has been the standard treatment for these problems until the introduction of the ultrashort-acting β blocker, esmolol. Esmolol has been shown to be equally effective in controlling the ventricular rate in patients with postoperative atrial fibrillation or flutter and in increasing the conversion rate to regular sinus rhythm from 8 to 34%. Owing to its short duration of action (β elimination half-life of 9 minutes) and β_1-cardioselectivity, it is the drug of choice in the postoperative period to control these dysrhythmias. Esmolol, in an iv loading dose of 500 $\mu g \cdot kg^{-1}$ given over one minute followed by an infusion of 50–200 $\mu g \cdot kg^{-1} \cdot min^{-1}$ has been shown to be effective in the control of supraventricular tachycardias.

Hemorrhage and pneumothorax are always major concerns after intrathoracic surgery. Because of these problems, interpleural thoracostomy tubes with an underwater seal system are routinely used after thoracic surgery. Slippage of a suture on any major vessel or airway in the chest can lead to the slow or rapid development of hypovolemic shock or a tension pneumothorax. Drainage of more than 200 $ml \cdot hr^{-1}$ of blood is an indication for surgical re-exploration for hemorrhage. Management of the pleural drainage system is fraught with confusion. The chest bottles must be kept below the level of the chest, and the tubes should not be clamped during patient transport. These tubes can be life saving, but errors in technique can lead to serious complications. The creation of a pneumothorax in the nonoperative chest by central venous catheter placement is very hazardous because this lung is essential both intraopera-

tively during one-lung anesthesia and postoperatively after contralateral lung resection. Dehiscence of the bronchial stump may lead to the formation of a BPF, which carries a mortality rate of 20%. Surgical treatment may be needed, in which case ventilation of the patient may be difficult because of loss of VT through the fistula. A double-lumen endobronchial tube positioned in the contralateral mainstem bronchus or the use of HFJV may be required for safe management. HFJV allows ventilation with lowered peak airway pressures. However, there have been reports in which ventilation by HFJV was difficult. If a double-lumen endobronchial tube is placed, the lung with the fistula can be ventilated independently with either CPAP or HFJV.

Both central and peripheral neurologic injuries can occur during intrathoracic procedures. Such injuries often result in serious and disabling loss of function and are very distressing to the patient. Peripheral nerves can be injured, either in the chest or in other parts of the body, by pressure or stretching. It has been recognized for years that most of these postoperative neuropathies are caused by malpositioning of the patient on the operating table, with subsequent stretching or compression of the nerves. The nerve injury may be apparent immediately after surgery or may not become obvious until several days later. These patients often complain of a variety of unpleasant sensations, including paresthesias, cold, pain, or anesthesia in the area supplied by the affected nerves. The brachial plexus is especially vulnerable to trauma during thoracic surgery owing to its long superficial course in the axilla between two points of fixation, the vertebrae above and the axillary fascia below. Stretching is the chief cause of damage to the brachial plexus, with compression playing only a secondary role. Branches of the brachial plexus may also be injured lower in the arm by compression against objects such as an ether screen or other parts of the operating table. Intrathoracic nerves can be directly injured during a surgical procedure by being transected, crushed, stretched, or cauterized. The intercostal nerves are the ones most frequently injured during intrathoracic surgical procedures. The recurrent laryngeal nerve can become involved in lymph node tissue and injured at the time of a node biopsy, especially when the biopsy is performed through a mediastinoscope. This nerve can also be injured during tracheostomy or radical pulmonary dissections. The phrenic nerve is frequently injured during pericardiectomy, radical pulmonary hilar dissections, division of the diaphragm during esophageal surgery, or dissection of mediastinal tumors.

Prevention is the treatment of choice for all these intraoperative nerve injuries. Analgesics may be necessary to control postoperative pain in the distribution of the nerve injury and to aid in maintaining joint mobility during the healing phase. Subsequent surgical procedures may be necessary to move a swollen ulnar nerve at the elbow or to stent a partially paralyzed vocal cord.

REFERENCES

1. Rutkow IM: Thoracic and cardiovascular operations in the United States, 1979 to 1984. J Thorac Cardiovasc Surg 92:181, 1986
2. Cohen E (ed.): The Practice of Thoracic Anesthesia. Philadelphia, JB Lippincott, 1995
3. Benumof JL: Anesthesia for Thoracic Surgery, 2nd ed. Philadelphia, WB Saunders, 1995
4. Gass GD, Olsen GN: Clinical significance of pulmonary function tests. Preoperative pulmonary function testing to predict postoperative morbidity and mortality. Chest 89:127, 1986
5. Lockwood P: Lung function test results and the risk of post-thoracotomy complications. Respiration 30:529, 1973
6. Mittman C: Assessment of operative risk in thoracic surgery. Am Rev Respir Dis 84:197, 1961
7. Jones RM, Rosen M, Seymour L: Smoking and anaesthesia (editorial). Anaesthesia 42:1, 1987
8. Pearce AC, Jones RM: Smoking and anesthesia: Preoperative abstinence and preoperative morbidity. Anesthesiology 61:576, 1984

9. Cooper DKL: The incidence of postoperative infection and the role of antibiotic prophylaxis in pulmonary surgery: A review of 221 consecutive patients undergoing thoracotomy. Br J Dis Chest 75:154, 1981

10. Marini JJ, Lakshmimara Y, Kradyan WA: Atropine and terbutaline aerosols in chronic bronchitis. Chest 80:285, 1981

11. London MJ, Hollenberg M, Wong MG et al: Intraoperative myocardial ischemia: Localization by continuous 12-lead electrocardiography. Anesthesiology 69:232, 1988

12. Petty C: Right radial artery pressure during mediastinoscopy. Anesth Analg 58:428, 1979

13. Iberti TJ, Fischer EP, Leibowitz AB et al: A multicenter study of physician's knowledge of the pulmonary artery catheter. JAMA 264:2928, 1990

14. Raper R, Sibbald WJ: Misled by the wedge. Chest 89:427, 1986

15. Cohen E, Eisenkraft JB, Thys D et al: Hemodynamics and oxygenation during OLA: Right vs left. Anesthesiology 63:3A, A566, 1985

16. Thys DM, Cohen E, Eisenkraft J: Mixed venous oxygen saturation during thoracic anesthesia. Anesthesiology 69:1005, 1988

17. Pothoft G, Curtius JM, Wassermann K et al: Transesophageal echography in staging of bronchial cancers. Pneumologie 446:111, 1992

18. Manguso L, Pitrolo F, Bond F et al: Echocardiographic recognition of mediastinal masses. Chest 93:144, 1988

19. Neustein SM, Cohen E, Reich DL, Kirschner PA: Transesophageal echocardiography and the intraoperative diagnosis of left atrial invasion by carcinoid tumor. Can J Anaesth 40:664, 1993

20. Suriani RJ, Konstadt SN, Camunas J, Goldman M: Transesophageal echocardiographic detection of left atrial involvement in a lung tumor. J Cardiothorac Vasc Anesth 7:73, 1993

21. Neustein SM, Narang J: Spontaneous hemothorax due to subacute aortic dissection. J Cardiothorac Vasc Anesth 7:79, 1993

22. Brodsky JB, Shulman MS, Swan M et al: Pulse oximetry during one-lung ventilation. Anesthesiology 63:212, 1985

23. Van Norman G, Cheney FW: Falsely elevated oximeter reading dangerous on one lung. Park Ridge, Illinois, Anesthesia Patient Safety Foundation Newsletter 4:23, 1989

24. Barker SJ, Hyatt J: Continuous measurement of intra-arterial pH, $PaCO_2$, and PaO_2 in the operating room. Anesth Analg 73:43, 1991

25. Shafieha MA, Sit J, Kartha R et al: End-tidal CO_2 analyzers in proper positioning of double-lumen tubes. Anesthesiology 64:844, 1986

26. Yam PCI, Innes PA, Jackson M et al: Variation in the arterial to end-tidal PCO_2 difference during one-lung thoracic anaesthesia. Br J Anaesth 72:21, 1994

27. Merilainen P, Hanninen H, Tuomaala L: A novel sensor for routine continuous spirometry of intubated patients. J Clin Monit 9:374, 1993

28. Bardoczky GI, Levarlet M, Engelman E, deFrancoquen P: Continuous spirometry for detection of double-lumen endobronchial tube displacement. Br J Anaesth 70:499, 1993

29. Benumof JL: Isoflurane anesthesia and arterial oxygenation during one-lung ventilation. Anesthesiology 64:419, 1986

30. MacGillivay RG: Evaluation of a new tracheal tube with a movable bronchus blocker. Anaesth 43:687, 1988

31. Hurford WE, Alfille PH: A quality improvement study of the placement and complications of double-lumen endobronchial tubes. J Cardiothorac Vasc Anesth 7:517, 1993

32. Smith G, Hirsch, N, Ehrenwerth J: Sight and sound: Can double-lumen endotracheal tubes be placed accurately without fiberoptic bronchoscopy? Br J Anaesth 58:1317, 1987

33. Cohen E, Neustein SM, Goldofsky S, Camunas J: Incidence of malposition of PVC and red rubber left-sided double lumen tubes and clinical sequelae. J Cardiothorac Vasc Anesth 9:122, 1995

34. Benumof JL, Partridge BL, Salvatierra C et al: Margin of safety in positioning modern double-lumen endotracheal tubes. Anesthesiology 67:729, 1987

35. Wagner DL, Gammage GW, Wong ML: Tracheal rupture following the insertion of a disposable double-lumen endotracheal tube. Anesthesiology 63:698, 1985

36. Andros TG, Lennon PF: One-lung ventilation in a patient with a tracheostomy and severe tracheobronchial disease. Anesthesiology 79:1127, 1993

37. Bellver J, Garcia-Aguado A, Andres JD et al: Selective bronchial intubation with the Univent system in patients with a tracheostomy. Anesthesiology 79:1453, 1993

38. Saito T, Naruke T, Carney E, et al: New double-lumen intrabron-

chial tube (Naruke tube) for tracheostomized patients Anesthesiology 89:1038, 1998

39. Cohen E, Benumof J: Lung separation in the patient with a difficult airway: Current Opinion in Anesthesiology 12:29, 1999

40. Benumof J: Difficult tubes and difficult airways. J Cardiothorac Vasc Anesth 12:131, 1998

41. Capan LM, Turndorf H, Patel K et al: Optimization of arterial oxygenation during one-lung anesthesia. Anesth Analg 59:847, 1980

42. Lunding M, Fernandes A: Arterial oxygen tensions and acid-base status during thoracic anaesthesia. Acta Anaesthesiol Scand 11:43, 1967

43. Cohen E, Eisenkraft JB, Thys DM et al: Oxygenation and hemodynamic changes during one-lung ventilation. J Cardiothorac Anesth 2:34, 1988

44. Katz JA, Larlane RG, Fairly HB et al: Pulmonary oxygen exchange during endobronchial anesthesia: Effect of tidal volume and PEEP. Anesthesiology 56:164, 1982

45. Tarhan S, Lundborg RO: Effects of increased expiratory pressure on blood gas tensions and pulmonary shunting during thoracotomy with use of the Carlens catheter. Can Anaesth Soc J 17:4, 1970

46. Cohen E, Thys DM, Eisenkraft JB et al: PEEP during one-lung anesthesia improves oxygenation in patients with low PaO_2. Anesth Analg 64:200, 1985

47. Hogue CW: Effectiveness of low levels of nonventilated lung continuous positive airway pressure in improving arterial oxygenation during one-lung ventilation. Anesth Analg 79:364, 1994

48. Rees DI, Wansbrough SR: One-lung anesthesia and arterial oxygen tension during continuous insufflation of oxygen to the non-ventilated lung. Anesth Analg 61:501, 1982

49. Malmkvist G: Maintenance of oxygenation during one lung ventilation. Effect of intermittent reinflation of the collapsed lung with oxygen. Anesth Analg 68:763, 1989

50. Nunn JF: Factors influencing the arterial oxygen tension during halothane anesthesia with spontaneous respiration. Br J Anaesth 36:327, 1964

51. Marshall BE, Cohen PJ, Klingenmaier CH et al: Pulmonary venous admixture before, during and after halothane: Oxygen anesthesia in man. J Appl Physiol 27:653, 1967

52. Von Euler US, Liljestrand G: Observations on the pulmonary arterial blood pressure in the cat. Acta Physiol Scand 12:301, 1946

53. Marshall BE, Marshall C, Benumof JL et al: Hypoxic pulmonary vasoconstriction in dogs: Effects of lung segment size and alveolar oxygen tensions. J Appl Physiol 51:1543, 1981

54. Domino KB, Wetstein L, Glasser SA et al: Influence of mixed venous oxygen tension (PvO_2) on blood flow to atelectatic lung. Anesthesiology 59:428, 1983

55. Benumof JL: One-lung ventilation and hypoxic pulmonary vasoconstriction: Implications for anesthetic management. Anesth Analg 64:821, 1985

56. Eisenkraft JB: Effects of anesthetics on the pulmonary circulation. Br J Anaesth 65:63, 1990

57. Bjertnaes LJ: Hypoxia-induced pulmonary vasoconstriction in man: Inhibition due to diethyl ether and halothane anaesthesia. Acta Anaesthesiol Scand 22:578, 1978

58. Jolin Carlsson A, Bindslev L, Hedenstierna G: Hypoxia-induced pulmonary vasoconstriction in the human lung: The effect of isoflurane anesthesia. Anesthesiology 66:312, 1987

59. Weinreich AI, Silvay G, Lumb PD: Continuous ketamine infusion for one-lung ventilation. Can Anaesth Soc J 27:485, 1980

60. Rees DI, Gaines GY: One-lung anesthesia: A comparison of pulmonary gas exchange during anesthesia with ketamine or enflurane. Anesth Analg 63:521, 1984

61. Rogers SM, Benumof JL: Halothane and isoflurane do not decrease PaO_2 during one-lung ventilation in intravenously anesthetized patients. Anesth Analg 64:946, 1985

62. Benumof JL, Augustine SD, Gibbons JA: Halothane and isoflurane only slightly impair arterial oxygenation during one-lung ventilation in patients undergoing thoracotomy. Anesthesiology 67:910, 1987

63. Slinger P, Scott WAC: Arterial oxygenation during one-lung ventilation: A comparison of enflurane and isoflurane. Anesthesiology 82:940, 1995

64. Shimizu T, Abe K, Kinovchik, Yoshiya I: Arterial oxygenation during one-lung ventilation. Can J Anaesth 44:1162, 1997

65. Loer SA, Scheeren TWL, Tarnow J: Desflurane inhibits HPV in isolated rabbit lungs. Anesthesiology 83:552, 1995

66. Van Keer L, Van Aken H, Vandermeersch E, Vermaut G: Propofol does not inhibit HPV in humans. J Clin Anesth 1:284, 1989

67. Chen L, Miller FL, Malmkvist G et al: High-dose almitrine bimesylate inhibits hypoxic pulmonary vasoconstriction in closed-chest dogs. Anesthesiology 67:534, 1987

68. Furchgott RF, Vanhoutte PM: Endothelium derived relaxing and contracting factors. FASEB J 3:2007, 1989

69. Fischer SR, Deyo DJ, Bone HG et al: Nitric oxide synthase inhibition restores HPV in sepsis. Am J Respir Crit Care Med 156:833, 1997

70. Frostell CG, Blomqvist H, Hedenstierna G et al: Inhaled nitric oxide selectively reverses human HPV without causing systemic vasodilation. Anesthesiology 78:427, 1993

71. Troncy E, Francoeur M, Blaise G: Inhaled nitric oxide: clinical applications, indications and toxicology. Can J Anaesth 44: 973, 1997

72. Moutafis M, Liu N, Dalibon N, et al: The effects of inhaled nitric oxide and its combination with intravenous almitrine on PaO_2 during one-lung ventilation in patients undergoing thoracoscopic procedures. Anesth Analg 85:1130, 1997

73. Moutafis M, Dalibon N, Colchen A, Fischler M: Improving oxygenation during bronchopulmonary lavage using nitric oxide inhalation and almitrine infusion. Anesth Analg 89:302, 1999

74. B'chir A, Mebassa A, Losserm MR et al: Intravenous almitrine bimesylate reversibly inhibits lactic acidois and hepatic dysfunction in patients with lung injury. Anesthesiology 89:823, 1998

75. Doering EB, Hanson CW, Reily D et al: Improvement in oxygenation by phenylephrine and nitric oxide in patients with adult respiratory distress syndrome. Anesthesiology 87:18, 1997

76. Scherer R, Vigfusson G, Lawin P: Pulmonary blood flow reduction by prostaglandin $F_2\alpha$ and pulmonary artery balloon manipulation during one-lung ventilation in dogs. Acta Anaesth Scand 30:2, 1986.

77. Frumin MJ, Epstein R, Cohen G: Apneic oxygenation in man. Anesthesiology 20:789, 1959

78. Sanders RD: Two ventilating attachments for bronchoscopes. Del Med J 39:170, 1967

79. Giesecke AH, Gerbershagen H, Dortman C et al: Comparison of the ventilating and injection bronchoscopes. Anesthesiology 38:298, 1973

80. Carden E: Recent improvements in anesthetic techniques for use during bronchoscopy. Otology, Rhinology, and Laryngology 83: 777, 1974

81. Vourc'h G, Fishler M, Michon F et al: Manual jet ventilation vs high-frequency jet ventilation during laser resection of tracheobronchial stenosis. Br J Anaesth 55:973, 1983

82. Matsushima Y, Jones RL, King EG et al: Alterations in pulmonary mechanics and gas exchange during routine fiberoptic bronchoscopy. Chest 86:184, 1984

83. Satyanarayana T, Capan L, Ramanathan S et al: Bronchofiberscopic jet ventilation. Anesth Analg 59:350, 1980

84. Neuman G, Weingarten AE, Abramowitz RM et al: The anesthetic management of the patient with an anterior mediastinal mass. Anesthesiology 60:144, 1984

85. Ferrari LR, Bedford RF: General anesthesia prior to treatment of anterior mediastinal masses in pediatric cancer patients. Anesthesiology 72:991, 1990

86. DeSoto H: Direct laryngoscopy as an aid to relieve airway obstruction in a patient with a mediastinal mass. Anesthesiology 67: 116, 1987

87. Barker SJ, Clarke C, Trivedi N et al: Anesthesia for thoracoscopic laser ablation of bullous emphysema. Anesthesiology 78:44, 1993

88. Brodsky JB, Cohen E: Videoassisted thoracscopic surgery. Current Opinion in Anaesthesiology 13:41, 2000

89. Plummer S, Hartley M, Vaughan RS: Anaesthesia for telescopic procedures in the thorax. Br J Anaesth 80:223, 1998

90. Capan LM, Miller S, Patel KP: Pro: Application of CPAP to the non-dependent lung is preferable to HFV for optimal oxygenation during pulmonary surgery. J Cardiothorac Anesth 1:584, 1987

91. Bishop MJ, Benson MS, Sato P et al: Comparison of high-frequency jet ventilation with conventional ventilation for bronchopleural fistula. Anesth Analg 66:833, 1987

92. Benumof JL: Sequential one-lung ventilation for bilateral bullectomy. Anesthesiology 67:268, 1987

93. Conacher D: Lung volume reduction. Br J Anaesth 79:530, 1997

94. Mets B: Current status of lung volume reduction. Current Opinion in Anaesthesiology 13:61, 2000

95. Argenziano M, Moazami N, Thomashow B et al: Extended indications for lung volume reduction surgery in advanced emphysema. Ann Thorac Surg 62:1588, 1996

96. Brantigan OC, Mueller E, Kress MB: A surgical approach to pulmonary emphysema. American Review of Respiratory Disease 80:194, 1959

97. Cohen E, Kirshner PA, Benumof JL: Case conference: Anesthesia for bullectomy. Journal of Cardiothoracic Anesthesia 4:119, 1990

98. Cooper JD, Trulock EP, Triantafillou AN et al: Bilateral pneumonectomy (volume reduction) for chronic obstructive pulmonary disease. J Thorac Cardiovac Surg 109:106, 1995

99. Benfield JR, Cree Em, Pellet JR et al: Current approach to the surgical management of emphysema. Arch Surg 93:59, 1966

100. Davies L, Calverley PMA: Lung volume reduction surgery in chronic obstructive pulmonary disease. Thorax 51 (suppl 2): S29, 1996

101. Deslauriers J: History of surgery for emphysema. Semin Thorac Cardiovasc Surg 8:43, 1996

102. National Emphysema Treatment Trial Research Group: Rationale and design of the National Emphysema Treatment Trial: A prospective randomized trial of lung volume reduction surgery. The National Emphysema Treatment Trial Research Group. Chest 116:1750, 1999

103. Fessler HE, Wise RA: Lung volume reduction surgery: Is less really more? Am J Respir Crit Care Med 159:1031, 1999

104. Young J, Fry-Smith A, Hyde C: Lung volume reduction surgery for chronic obstructive pulmonary disease (COPD) with underlying severe emphysema. Thorax 54:779, 1999

105. Zollinger A, Thomas P: Anesthesia for lung volume reduction surgery. Current Opinion in Anaesthesiology 11:45, 1998

106. Brenner M, McKenna RJ, Chen JC, et al: Survival following bilateral staple lung volume reduction surgery for emphysema. Chest, 118: 390, 1999

107. Gelb AF, Brenner M, McKenna RJ et al: Serial lung function and elastic recoil 2 years after lung volume reduction surgery for emphysema. Chest 113: 1497, 1998

108. Gaissert HA, Trulock EP, Cooper JD et al: Comparison of early functional results after volume reduction or lung transplantation for chronic obstructive pulmonary disease. J Thorac Cardiovasc Surg 111:296, 1996

109. Krucylak PE, Naunheim KS, Keller CA, Baudendistal LJ: Anesthetic management of patients undergoing thoracoscopic lung reduction for treatment of end-stage emphysema. Anesth Analg 80:SCA80, 1995

110. Bussières JS: Anesthesia for patients undergoing surgery for emphysema. Chest Surg Clin N Am 5:869, 1995

111. Triantafillou AN: Anesthetic management for bilateral volume reduction surgery. Semin Thorac Cardiovasc Surg 8:94, 1996

112. Hurford WE, Dutton RP, Alfille PH et al: Comparison of thoracic and lumbar epidural infusions of bupivacaine and fentanyl for post-thoracotomy analgesia. J Cardiothorac Vasc Anesth 5:521, 1993

113. Wakabayashi A: Thoracoscopic technique for management of giant bullous disease. Ann Thorac Surg 56:708, 1993

114. Cohen E, Eisenkraft JB: Bronchopulmonary lavage: Effects on oxygenation and hemodynamics. J Cardiothorac Anesth 4:119, 1990

115. Drachman DB: Myasthenia gravis: Review article. N Engl J Med 330:1797, 1994

116. Eisenkraft JB, Neustein SM: Anesthesia for esophageal and mediastinal surgery. In Kaplan JA (ed): Thoracic Anesthesia, 2nd ed, p 389. New York, Churchill-Livingstone, 1991

117. Nilsson E, Muller K: Neuromuscular effects of isoflurane in patients with myasthenia gravis. Acta Anaesthesiol Scand 34:126, 1990

118. Smith CE, Donati F, Bevan DR: Cumulative dose-response curves for atracurium in patients with myasthenia gravis. Can J Anaesth 36:402, 1989

119. Baraka A, Siddik S, Kawkabani N: Cisatracurium in a myasthenic patient undergoing thymectomy. Can J Anaesth 46:779, 1999

120. Seigne RD, Scott RPF: Mivacurium chloride and myasthenia gravis. Br J Anaesth 72:468, 1994

121. Eisenkraft JB, Book WJ, Papatestas AE, Hubbard M: Resistance to succinylcholine in myasthenia gravis: A dose-response study. Anesthesiology 69:760, 1988

122. Baraka A, Tabboush Z: Neuromuscular response to succinylcholine-vecuronium sequence in three myasthenic patients undergoing thymectomy. Anesth Analg 72:827, 1991

123. Eisenkraft JB, Papatestas AE, Kahn CH *et al:* Predicting the need for postoperative mechanical ventilation in myasthenia gravis. Anesthesiology 65:79, 1986
124. Burgess FW, Wilcosky B: Thoracic epidural anesthesia for transsternal thymectomy in myasthenia gravis. Anesth Analg 69:529, 1989
125. Gorback MS: Analgesic management after thymectomy. Anesthesiol Rep 2:262, 1990
126. Telford RJ, Hollway TE: The myasthenic syndrome: Anesthesia in a patient treated with 3.4 diaminopyridine. Br J Anaesth 64:363, 1990
127. Kavanagh BP, Katz J, Sandler AN: Pain control after thoracic surgery: A review of current techniques. Anesthesiology 81:737, 1994
128. Whiting WG, Sandler AN, Lau LC *et al:* Analgesic and respiratory effects of epidural sufentanil in post-thoracotomy patients. Anesthesiology 69:36, 1988
129. Cohen E, Neustein SM: Intrathecal morphine during thoracotomy. J Thorac Cardiovasc Anesth 7:154, 1993
130. Katz J, Kavanagh BP, Sandler AN *et al:* Preemptive analgesia. Anesthesiology 77:439, 1992
131. Ritchie J, Bowe P, Gibbons JRP: Prophylactic digitalization for thoracotomy: A reassessment. Ann Thorac Surg 50:86, 1990

Clinical Anesthesia (4/e), edited by
Paul G. Barash, Bruce F. Cullen, and
Robert K. Stoelting. Lippincott Williams &
Wilkins, Philadelphia, © 2001.

CHAPTER 31

CARDIOVASCULAR ANATOMY AND PHYSIOLOGY

CAROL L. LAKE

The perioperative management of patients during either cardiac or noncardiac surgery requires an extensive knowledge of cardiovascular anatomy and physiology.

ANATOMY

Heart

Transesophageal echocardiography[1] (Fig. 31-1) visualizes the functional anatomy of the four cardiac chambers, four valves, and great vessels.

Right Atrium

Systemic veins drain into the right atrium (RA) via the superior vena cava (SVC), inferior vena cava (IVC), and the coronary sinus. The ostium of the IVC is guarded by the eustachian valve while the ostium of the coronary sinus is guarded by the thebesian valve. The right and left atria are separated by the interatrial septum with its central ovoid portion, the fossa ovalis, the remnant of the fetal foramen ovale.

Blood leaving the RA passes through the tricuspid valve, which consists of three leaflets—anterior, posterior, and medial—comprising an area of 8–11 cm^2 (Fig. 31-2). The anterior leaflet, the largest, is attached to the crista supraventricularis (described below) and controlled by the anterior papillary muscle (APM). The APM originates from a prominent intraventricular muscle, the moderator band, and the anteriolateral ventricular wall. Connecting the papillary muscles to the valve leaflets are strong, fibrous structures known as the chordae tendineae.

Right Ventricle

The right ventricle (RV) is a pocket wrapped around one third of the left ventricle (LV). Its muscle fibers are continuous with those of the LV. Anatomically, it consists of inferoposterior inflow (sinus) and anterosuperior outflow (infundibular) portions divided by the crista supraventricularis. The inflow portion contains prominent muscle bands (moderator, septal, and parietal) and muscle bundles known as trabeculae carneae. The crista supraventricularis also joins the interventricular septum and LV to the right ventricular free wall and may help to integrate right and left ventricular function.[2]

Pulmonary Artery and Peripheral Pulmonary Circulation

The pulmonic valve separates the right ventricular infundibulum from the main pulmonary artery (PA). It is a trileaflet valve (right, left, and anterior cusps), normally about 4 cm^2 in area (see Fig. 31-2). As it originates from the superior portion of the RV, the PA passes under the aorta before it bifurcates into the right and left pulmonary arteries. The remnant of the fetal ductus arteriosus, the ligamentum arteriosum, connects the upper aspect of the bifurcation to the inferior aortic surface.

The pulmonary arteries and veins of the lower lobes are normally larger and more prominent than those of the upper lobes. Pulmonary arteries branch into arterioles and thence into capillaries, which spread over the alveolar surfaces between two alveolar endothelial layers. The size of the peripheral pulmonary vessels indicates pulmonary blood volume and flow. With left-to-right cardiac shunts, the main pulmonary artery

and hilar vessels are prominent. With pulmonary hypertension, however, dilation of the main pulmonary artery and abrupt tapering of the peripheral pulmonary vessels are noted.

Left Atrium

The left atrium (LA) is slightly larger than the right and receives one or two pulmonary veins on its left and two or three on its right side. Leaving the LA, blood traverses the mitral valve consisting of two major anteromedial and posterolateral leaflets, papillary muscles, and chordae tendineae. The normal adult mitral valve is about 6–8 cm^2 in area. Valves of less than 1 cm^2 are severely stenotic. The blood supply to the mitral chordae and papillary muscles is often quite tenuous.[3]

Left Ventricle

Normally, the LV is thicker (8–15 mm) and more densely trabeculated than the right. Its internal dimension is also greater, about 4.5 cm compared with 3.5 cm for the RV.[4] The interventricular septum, with its membranous superior portion near the aortic valve and muscular inferior portion, divides the RV from the LV. Both ventricles consist of an inner layer, the endocardium covered with endothelium, the myocardium or muscle layer, and the outer layer, the epicardium.

Aorta and Its Branches

The aortic valve is adjacent to the mitral valve, separated only by the fibrous tissue framework that comprises the annuli of both valves (see Fig. 31-2). Three pocket-like structures of unequal size, the right and left (coronary) and posterior (noncoronary) cusps, form the aortic valve. A normal aortic valve is about 3–4 cm^2 in area. The aorta at the level of the valve dilates to form the sinuses of Valsalva in which the coronary ostia are located.

The ascending aorta, just beyond the aortic valve, has no branches. Major branches of the aorta, the innominate, left carotid, and left subclavian arteries, arise from the aortic arch. The innominate artery subdivides into the right subclavian and right carotid arteries.

Arterial Circulation

The anatomy of many peripheral arteries is important to anesthesiologists, for direct arterial cannulation, as targets to be avoided during venous cannulation, and in prevention of complications arising from certain surgical procedures. Among these are the coronary, carotid, cerebral, renal, bronchial, and spinal cord circulations (Fig. 31-3A).

Coronary Circulation

Two coronary arteries, right and left, originate from the sinuses of Valsalva in the aortic valve to supply blood to the myocardium. The left coronary artery usually has a short common or left main coronary artery before bifurcation into anterior descending and circumflex branches. The anterior descending artery courses downward over the anterior left ventricular wall and supplies the interventricular groove through its diagonal and septal perforator branches. Occlusive disease in the anterior

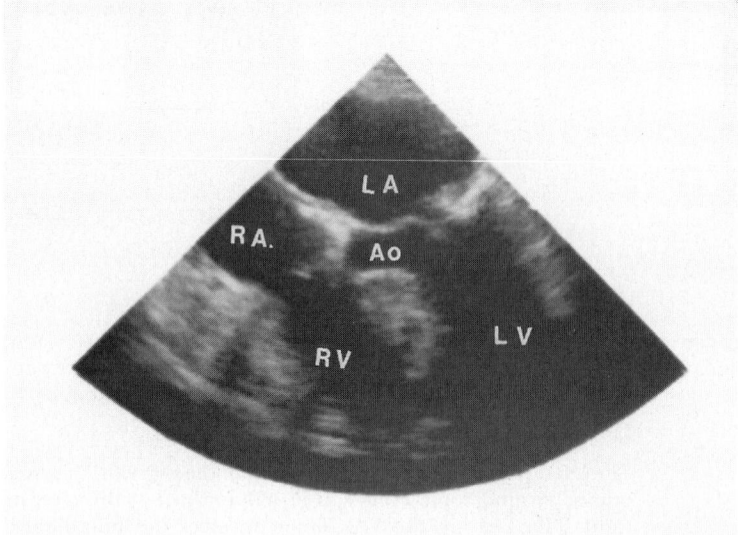

Figure 31-1. The functional anatomy of all four cardiac chambers, atrioventricular valves, aortic outflow track, and inter-atrial and inter-ventricular septa are easily visualized using either transthoracic or transesophageal echocardiography.

descending distribution produces ischemic electrocardiographic changes in leads V_3–V_5. The circumflex branch follows the atrioventricular groove, giving off the obtuse marginal branch and supplying all the posterior LV and part of the right ventricular wall.[5] Electrocardiographic (ECG) changes resulting from circumflex coronary artery disease are seen in leads I and a V_L (Fig. 31-4 and Table 31-1).

The sinus node and atrioventricular nodal arteries originate from the right coronary artery. The right atrial myocardium is also supplied by the sinus node artery. The right coronary artery terminates on the diaphragmatic surface of the heart as the posterior descending artery[6] (Fig. 31-4). The blood supply to the atrioventricular node and common bundle of His is the atrioventricular branch of the right coronary artery (in 90% of hearts) and the septal perforating branches of the left anterior descending coronary artery (in 10% of hearts).[7] Branches to the interatrial septum and posterior interventricular septum also arise from the atrioventricular nodal artery. The right bundle branch and the left anterior fascicle are supplied by branches of the left anterior descending artery but can be supplied by the atrioventricular nodal artery.[7] Both the left anterior and posterior descending coronary arteries supply the posterior fascicle.[7] Significant right coronary artery occlusion causes ischemic changes in ECG leads II, III, and a V_F as well as conduction abnormalities. However, the amount of myocardium jeopar-

dized by a clinically significant coronary stenosis cannot be completely determined from angiographic evaluation.

Coronary Dominance. Descriptions of the coronary circulation often refer to the dominance of one or the other coronary artery. Dominance is determined by which artery crosses the crux or junction between atria and ventricles to supply the posterior descending coronary branch. In about 50% of humans, the right coronary artery is dominant, in 20%, the left, and in 30%, a balanced pattern exists. Areas of the myocardium affected by stenosis or occlusion of individual coronary arteries are listed in Table 31-1. Collateral vessels may develop between the major coronary arteries in response to myocardial ischemia.[8]

Cerebral Circulation

The cerebral circulation consists of the anterior communicating arteries, the internal carotid arteries, the posterior communicating arteries, and the vertebral arteries. Together these vessels form the circle of Willis (Fig. 31-5). The external carotid arteries supply the face and neck but not the brain.

Arteries of the Upper Extremity

In the upper extremity the subclavian artery gives rise to the axillary, brachial, radial, and ulnar arteries (see Fig. 31-3). Because the brachial artery is beneath the basilic vein, it may be

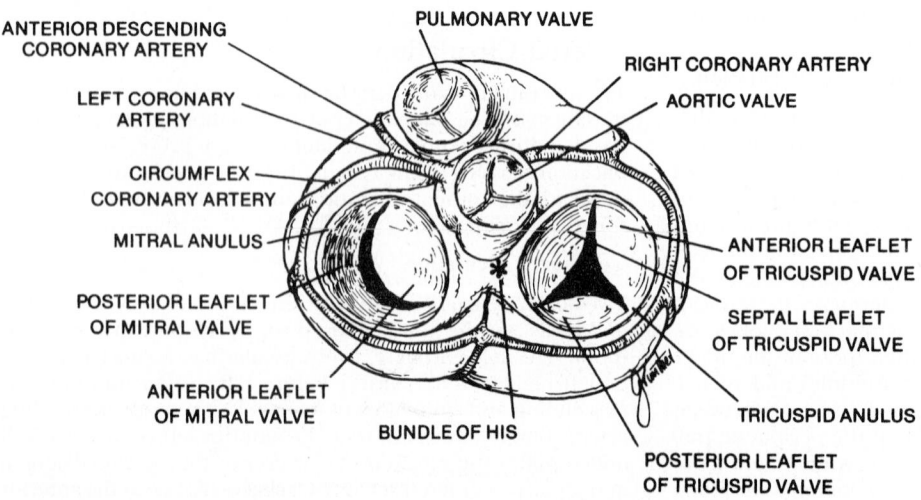

Figure 31-2. A coronal section of the heart at the level of the valves. The close proximity of all four cardiac valves is easily recognized. (Reprinted with permission from Lowe DA: Abnormalities of the atrioventricular valves. In Lake CL (ed): Pediatric Cardiac Anesthesia, 3rd ed. Norwalk, CT, Appleton & Lange, 1998.)

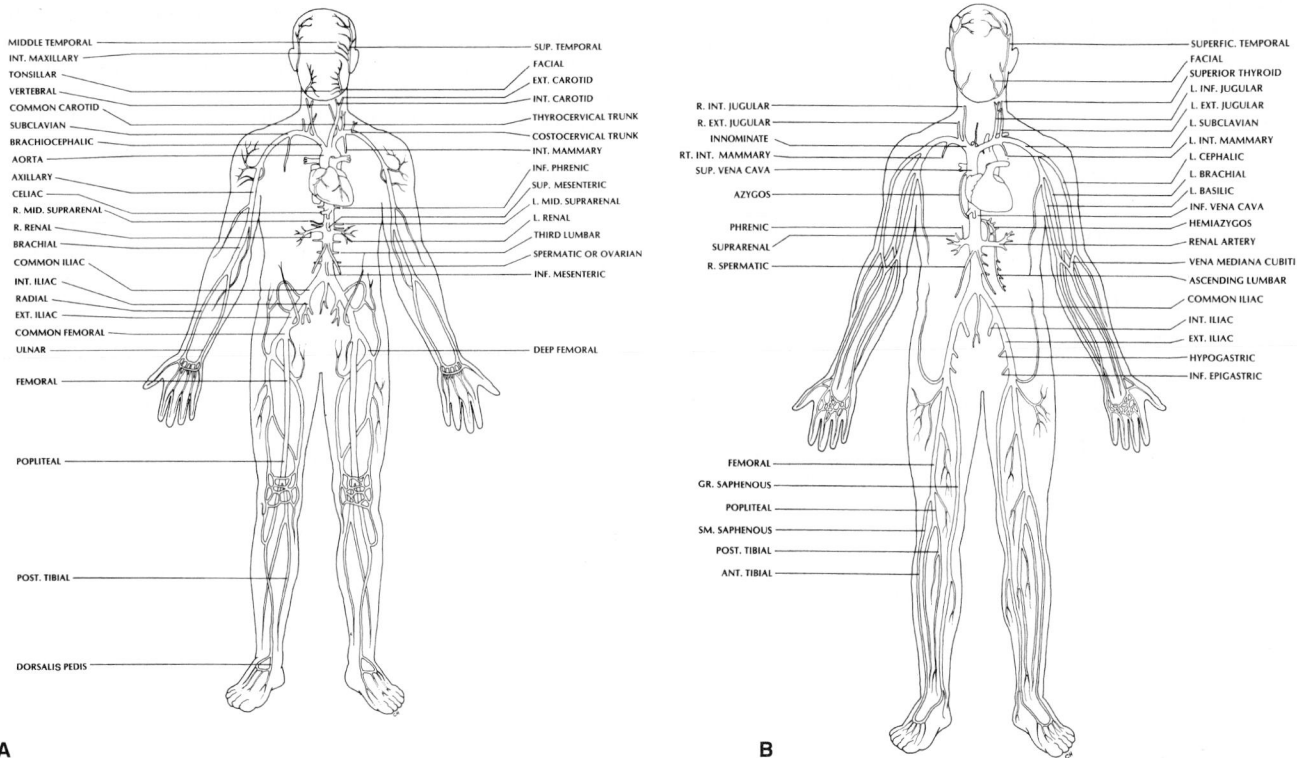

A   B

Figure 31-3. (*A*) The major arteries of the human body used by anesthesiologists to directly monitor arterial pressure include the radial, ulnar, femoral, brachial, axillary, dorsalis pedis, and superficial temporal. (*B*) The major veins of the human body accessible for cannulation include the internal and external jugular, subclavian, femoral, basilic, cephalic, median cubital, and saphenous.

punctured during attempted basilic vein cannulation in the antecubital fossa. Aberrant radial arteries often traverse the radial styloid process to enter the thenar webbed space. Attempted cannulation of veins over the anatomic "snuffbox" may result in cannulation of an aberrant radial artery.

Intra-abdominal and Lower Extremity Arteries

The abdominal branches of the aorta include the superior mesenteric, inferior mesenteric, and celiac arteries, principally supplying the gastrointestinal tract (see Fig. 31-3). The kidneys are

perfused via the renal arteries, receiving about 20% of the cardiac output. The aorta bifurcates into right and left iliac arteries in the lower torso. At the level of the inguinal ligament, the iliacs bifurcate into superficial and deep femoral arteries. The femoral artery can be easily cannulated just below the inguinal ligament. Just below the knee, the femoral artery bifurcates into anterior and posterior tibial arteries. In the foot, the superficial arteries are the dorsalis pedis, located just lateral to the extensor hallucis longus tendon and the posterior tibial artery behind the medial malleolus of the ankle.

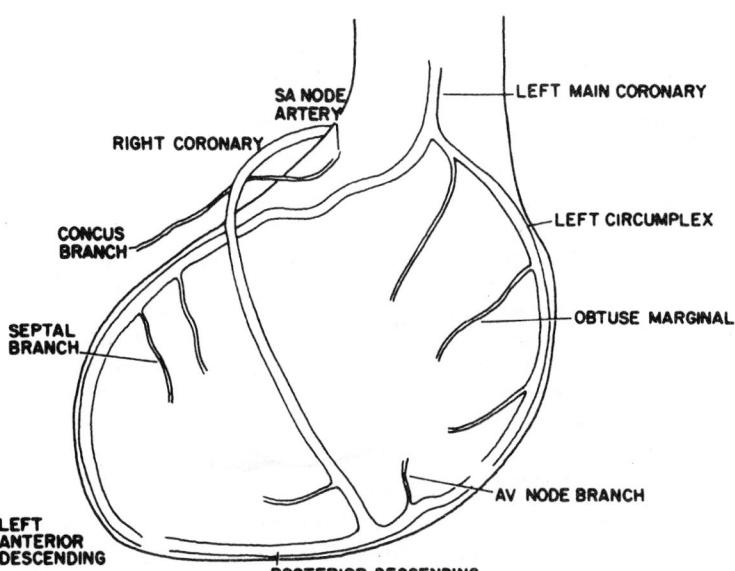

Figure 31-4. In this lateral view, the normal left coronary artery divides into the anterior descending (LAD) and circumflex (CFX) coronary arteries. The right coronary artery usually gives off the arteries to the sinus and atrioventricular nodes before terminating on the inferior surface of the heart as the posterior descending artery.

Table 31-1. CORONARY ARTERY DISTRIBUTION

LEFT CORONARY ARTERY
Anterior descending branch
Right bundle branch
Left bundle branch
Anterior and posterior papillary muscles (mitral)
Anterolateral left ventricle

CIRCUMFLEX BRANCH
Lateral left ventricle

RIGHT CORONARY ARTERY
SA and AV nodes
Right atrium and ventricle
Posterior interventricular septum
Posterior fascicle of left bundle branch
Interatrial septum

Spinal Cord

The major blood supply (75%) to the spinal cord consists of the anterior spinal arteries which traverse the length of the cord and arise from the vertebral arteries. Only the posterior parts of the posterior columns and posterior horns are supplied by the posterior spinal artery (25%), originating from the terminal portion of the anterior spinal arteries. Anastomoses between the anterior and posterior spinal arteries (circumflex arteries) are inconstant and insufficient to sustain adequate cord circulation. In addition, there are radicular arteries that are branches of the intercostal and lumbar arteries; these arteries anastomose with the anteroposterior spinal artery system (Fig. 31-6). There are usually eight (varying from four to ten) radicular branches, at least one in the cervical, two in the thoracic, and one in the lumbar region. The largest of these is the arteria radicularis magna, or artery of Adamkiewicz, in the lower thoracic or upper lumbar region. When this vessel originates from the suprarenal aorta in the lower thoracic or upper lumbar region, it is generally the only significant radicular artery. However, if the origin of the arteria radicularis magna is infrarenal (lumbar segments 2–4), the segmental blood supply to the cord is usually good and there is another major radicular vessel in the thoracic area. Precise radiologic verification of the spinal cord blood supply can be difficult.[9]

Bronchial Circulation

Three bronchial arteries (two for the left lung and one for the right lung) originate from the thoracic aorta at T5 and T6 or intercostal arteries to provide nutrients to the lung and heat and water exchange in the airways. The bronchial circulation, normally small, can enlarge in response to injury, tumor growth, and inadequate pulmonary blood flow (as in cyanotic congenital heart disease) and function in gas exchange.[10]

Hepatic and Portal Circulations

Surgery for hepatic transplantation or portal hypertension requires a knowledge of the blood supply to the liver. The liver is supplied by the hepatic artery and portal vein. Total hepatic blood flow is about 20% of the cardiac output and averages $100 \ ml \cdot min^{-1} \cdot 100 \ g^{-1}$ of tissue. Portal venous flow supplies about 65–80% of the total hepatic blood flow, with the remainder coming from the hepatic arterial system. The portal vein, which carries nutrients from the gut to the liver, arises from the superior mesenteric, splenic, and renal veins.

Peripheral Venous Circulation

Major veins follow a course similar to that of the arteries. From the head, the internal and external jugular veins join the subclavian veins of either side (see Fig. 31-3B). The course of the external jugular vein is often tortuous and variable, and it has two sets of valves, one at the entrance to the subclavian vein and the other about 4 cm superior to the clavicle. From the arms, the basilic (medial aspect) and cephalic veins join as the brachial vein. This vein becomes the axillary vein in the axilla and thence the subclavian. Normally, subclavian veins from both sides unite to form the SVC.

Cardiac veins, the great and middle cardiac veins and the posterior left ventricular vein, drain into the coronary sinus. Near the orifice of the great cardiac vein, the oblique vein of Marshall (vein of the left atrium) enters the coronary sinus. Anterior cardiac veins and the small cardiac vein may enter the right atrium independently of the coronary sinus. Thebesian veins, which traverse the myocardium, drain into various cardiac chambers. Thebesian venous flow, coupled with bronchial and pleural venous flows, contributes the normal 1–3% arteriovenous shunt.

In the legs there are both superficial and deep veins. The greater and lesser saphenous veins are the principal superficial veins. The greater saphenous vein, overlying the medial malleolus, is frequently used as a conduit during aortocoronary bypass grafting. The lesser saphenous vein is located in the posterior aspect of the calf. The saphenous vein joins the femoral vein in the thigh to enter the pelvis as the iliac vein. Right and left iliac veins unite to form the IVC. Veins leaving the liver, the right, left and middle hepatic veins, enter the IVC.

Bronchial veins from the extrapulmonary portions of the proximal tracheobronchial tree drain via the azygos and hemiazygos veins into the SVC. The azygos vein also drains the perispinal areas and the esophagus. These veins assume greater importance if the IVC is occluded. Bronchial venous drainage from the intrapulmonary branches is to the pulmonary veins (left side of the heart).

Cardiac Conduction System

The system for electrical activation of the heart, the conduction system, consists of the sinoatrial (SA) node, the atrioventricular (AV) node, the bundle of His, right and left bundle branches, and the Purkinje system. Pacemaker cells found in these areas include the P cells or round cells and transitional or T cells.[11] The SA node is in the right atrial wall at the junction of the RA with the SVC. The SA and AV nodes are connected via the internodal conduction system, which consists of three tracts:

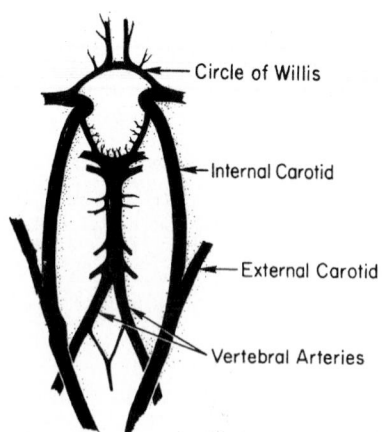

Figure 31-5. The cerebral circulation includes the internal carotid and the vertebral arteries. Together with the anterior communicating and posterior communicating arteries, the carotid arteries from both sides join to form the circle of Willis, which provides collateral circulation to the brain in the event of stenosis or occlusion of one carotid artery. (Modified with permission from Lake CL: Cardiovascular Anesthesia, p 411. New York, Springer-Verlag, 1985.)

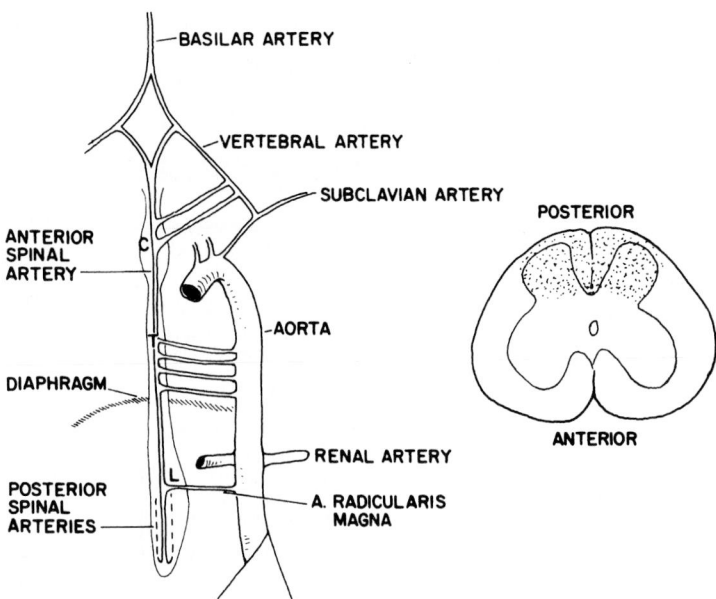

Figure 31-6. The circulation to the spinal cord is often tenuous. It consists of anterior and posterior spinal arteries which arise from the vertebral arteries and radicular arteries which originate from the intercostal and lumbar arteries. However, the radicular branches are quite variable and ligation of a significant radicular branch causes spinal cord ischemia. In the cross section of the spinal cord (*right*), the stippled portion indicates the posterior spinal artery distribution to the posterior columns and horns. C, T, and L are cervical, thoracic, and lumbar portions of the spinal cord.

the anterior (Bachmann's bundle), middle, and posterior internodal systems.[12] Conduction also spreads rapidly through the atrial musculature to the left atrium via Bachmann's bundle. In human hearts, the AV node is located in the floor of the right atrium, near the ostium of the coronary sinus.[7] The AV node consists of three areas, the A-N transitional zone containing cells smaller than normal atrial cells, the N region of round or P cells similar to those in the SA node, and the N-H region, a transitional zone near the bundle of His. The fibers forming the common bundle of His pass along the superior edge of the membranous interventricular septum to the apex of the muscular portion of the septum (see Fig. 31-2). Here the bundle divides into right and left bundle branches, which extend subendocardially along the surfaces of both ventricles. The right bundle branch emerges in the right ventricular endocardium near the moderator band at the base of the anterior papillary muscle. It usually extends for some distance without dividing, but one branch passes through the moderator band and the other passes over the right ventricular endocardial surface. Subdivision of the left bundle into anterior and posterior fascicles occurs shortly after its origin. There is also a small collection of short medial fascicles that originate from the left bundle just after the anterior fascicle and activate the septal myocardium. The posterior fascicle terminates in the posterior papillary muscle.

Peripherally, the fascicles of both right and left bundle branches subdivide to form the Purkinje network. The left bundle branch fascicles make their initial functional contact with the endocardium of the interventricular septum below the aortic valve. Right bundle branch fascicles contact ventricular subendocardium near the base of the anterior papillary muscle.

Cardiac and Vascular Nerves

Sympathetic System

Nerves to the heart and blood vessels originate from sympathetic neurons of the thoracolumbar region and parasympathetic nerves originate from the cervical region. Sympathetic fibers come from the stellate ganglion and the caudal cervical sympathetic trunks. From these trunks arise the right dorsal medial and dorsal lateral cardiac nerves, which frequently unite to form one large nerve that follows the course of the left main coronary

artery. It further separates into branches along the anterior descending and circumflex coronary arteries.

Parasympathetic System

Parasympathetic preganglionic neurons arise in the medulla oblongata in the dorsal vagal nucleus and the nucleus ambiguus. These fibers enter the thorax as branches from the recurrent laryngeal and thoracic vagus nerve. The dorsal and ventral cardiopulmonary plexuses between the aortic arch and the tracheal bifurcation receive both sympathetic and parasympathetic branches. From the plexuses emerge three large cardiac nerves, the right and left coronary cardiac nerves and the left lateral cardiac nerve. Ganglia occur within the heart, usually close to the structures innervated by the short postganglionic neurons. Postganglionic transmission occurs from stimulation of nicotinic cholinergic receptors at the postganglionic junction by acetylcholine. Release of acetylcholine at the neuroeffector junction activates muscarinic receptors in the heart.

Cerebral Vasomotor Center

Afferent nerves from the heart ascend via the 10th cranial nerve (vagus) and spinal cord to the nucleus tractus solitarius and the dorsal vagal nucleus and nucleus ambiguus to form the parasympathetic motor efferent system of the medullary vasomotor center. Sympathetic activation of heart and vasculature originates in the rostral ventrolateral (RVL) medulla, ventromedial rostral medulla, and the parvocellular region of the paraventricular nucleus. The RVL neurons receive multiple inputs from other medullary nuclei and modulate sympathetic output.[13] Although the vasomotor center independently regulates arterial pressure, blood flow distribution, and cardiac contractility, higher centers such as the cerebral cortex, hypothalamus, and pons also influence cardiovascular responses (see Fig. 31-7).

Cardiac Receptors. Vagal receptors located in various cardiac chambers are sensitive to changes in heart rate or chamber pressure. Vagal innervation affects the atrial musculature, the SA and AV nodes, and the ventricular myocardium.[14] The greatest concentrations of parasympathetic nerves are in the SA node, with lesser numbers in the AV node, RA, LA, and ventricles. Parasympathetic α_1 but not α_2 receptors have been identified.

Sympathetic fibers extend to all portions of the atria, ventricles, and conduction system. α_1, α_2, β_1, and β_2 subtypes of

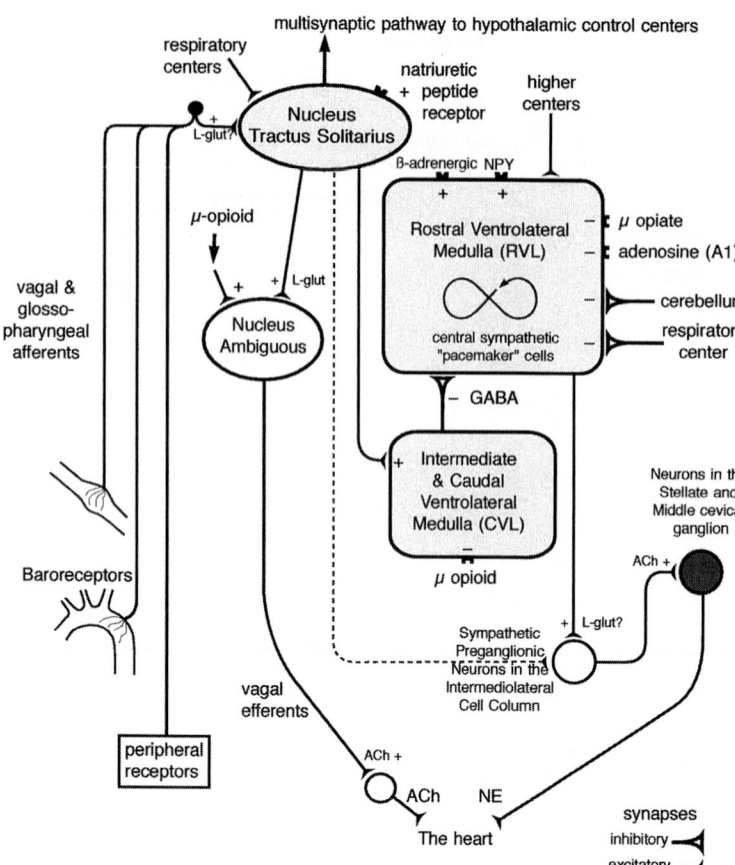

Figure 31-7. The central nervous system exerts considerable control over the heart and circulation via the rostral ventrolateral medulla (RVL), nucleus tractus solitarius, and intermediate and caudal ventrolaterial medulla. The RVL contains neurons that provide regular output to sympathetic preganglionic neurons like a pacemaker. The baroreceptor pathway, effects of GABAergic input, and opioid effects on RVL are also depicted. (Reprinted with permission from Lynch C, Lake CL: Cardiovascular anatomy and physiology. In Youngberg J, Lake C, Roizen M *et al:* Cardiac, Vascular and Thoracic Anesthesia, p 136. Philadelphia, Churchill Livingstone, 2000.)

adrenergic receptors are present. Human RA contains about 74% β_1 and 26% β_2 receptors.[15] The proportions of β receptors differ in the ventricle, with 86% β_1 and 14% β_2.

Neural Supply of the Peripheral Vasculature

Innervation of the peripheral circulation, with the exception of the cerebral and coronary vasculature, originates from the thoracolumbar sympathetic fibers. Vasodilation results from reduced sympathetic tone or activation of vasodilatory receptors. Stimulation of α-adrenergic fibers causes constriction in the arterial vascular beds of the skin, skeletal muscle, splanchnic organs, kidneys, and systemic veins. Stimulation of β_2 receptors dilates systemic veins and arteries of the muscle, splanchnic, and renal circulations.

Pericardium

The normal pericardium consists of thick fibrous and serous visceral layers. It has certain anatomic functions, among which

are the isolation of the heart from other mediastinal structures, maintenance of the heart in optimal functional shape and position, minimization of cardiac dilatation, and prevention of adhesions.[16] The pericardium also contains vagal nerve branches.

CARDIOVASCULAR CATHETERIZATION AND ANGIOGRAPHY

Abnormalities of both the anatomy and physiology of the cardiovascular system are diagnosed by invasive catheterization when noninvasive procedures such as echocardiography insufficiently define the defects.

Catheterization

In all age groups, cardiac catheterization is usually performed via the femoral vessels. Occasionally, the brachial vessels are used in adults if the femoral vessels cannot be entered or catheters cannot be manipulated through the abdominal aorta.[17]

Table 31-2. NORMAL CATHETERIZATION DATA

Site	Pressure (mm Hg)	Oxygen Saturation (%)
Inferior vena cava	0–8	80 ± 5
Superior vena cava	0–8	70 ± 5
Right atrium	0–8	75 ± 5
Right ventricle	15–30/0–8	75 ± 5
Pulmonary artery	15–30/4–12	75 ± 5
Pulmonary wedge	5–12 (mean)	75 ± 5
Left atrium	12 (mean)	95 ± 1
Left ventricle	100–140/4–12	95 ± 1
Aorta	100–140/60–90	95 ± 1

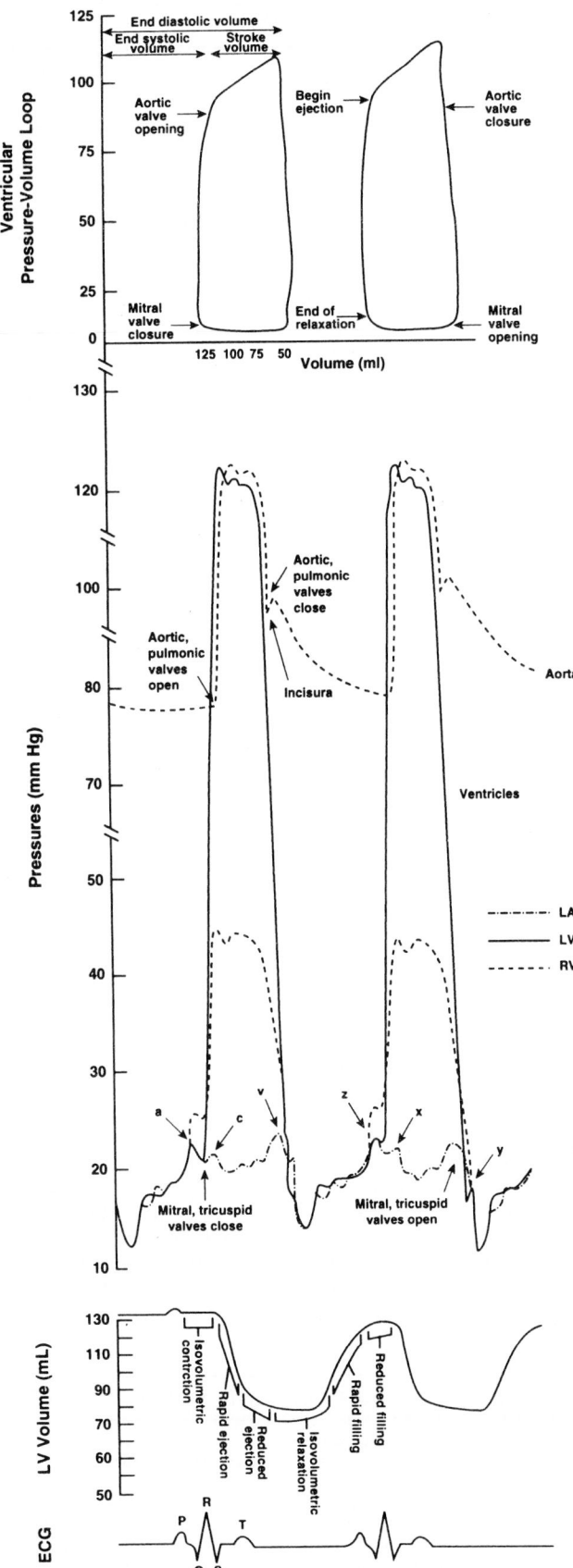

Figure 31-8. The events of the cardiac cycle from filling of the atria to ventricular emptying are demonstrated using waveforms from the aorta, pulmonary artery, right and left ventricles, and central veins. The relationship between the electrocardiogram and the phases of the cardiac cycle shows that ventricular systole occurs immediately following the QRS complex. The changes in ventricular pressure–volume waveform coincide with ventricular ejection and filling.

Table 31-3. MEASUREMENTS DURING CARDIAC CATHERIZATION

<table>
<tr><th colspan="2">Fick Principle Cardiac Output</th></tr>
</table>

Cardiac Output (Q) (L/min) $= \dfrac{\dot{V}_{O_2}}{CaO_2 - CvO_2} \times 100$

$\dot{V}_{O_2}$ = oxygen consumption

CaO_2 = arterial oxygen content

CvO_2 = venous oxygen content

Oxygen Content $= \alpha\, pO_2 + 1.34\, Hb \times \%Hb$ saturation

$(\alpha = .0031)$

Indicator—Dilution Cardiac Output

$$\dfrac{60 \times \text{indicator dose (mg)}}{\text{average concentration} \times \text{time (sec)}}$$

Example: thermodilution (Stewart-Hamilton equation)

$$Q = \dfrac{V_I (T_B - T_I) K_1 K_2}{T_B(t)\, dt}$$

V_I = injectate volume

T_B = blood temperature

T_I = injectate temperature

K_1 = density factor
(specific heat) (specific gravity) injectate
(specific heat) (specific gravity) blood

K_2 = computation constant for deadspace of catheter, heat change in transit, injection rate

$T_B(t)\, dt$ = change in blood temperature as a function of time

Shunt Flows

Qp = Qs = 1   No shunt
           Bidirectional Shunt

$Qpe = \dfrac{\dot{V}_{O_2}}{CPV_{O_2} - CMV_{O_2}}$

CPV_{O_2} = pulmonary venous oxygen content

CMV_{O_2} = mixed venous oxygen content

Qp − Qpe = L → R shunt

Qs − Qpe = R → L shunt

Qpe = effective pulmonary flow

Qp = pulmonary flow

Qs = systemic flow

Valve Areas

Aortic

Valve Area $= \dfrac{\text{Aortic Valve Flow (AVF)}}{1 \times 44.5 \sqrt{AVG_{(systolic)}}}$

AVF = CO/SEP$_{minute}$

SEP $= \dfrac{\text{Systolic ejection period}}{\text{beat}} \times HR$

Mitral

Valve Area $= \dfrac{\text{Mitral Valve Flow}}{0.7 \times 44.5 \sqrt{MVG_{(diastolic)}}}$

MVF = CO/DFP$_{minute}$

DFP $= \dfrac{\text{Diastolic filling period}}{\text{beat}} \times HR$

Direct vascular cutdowns are rarely necessary because the Seldinger technique, with various sizes of sheaths and introducers, provides adequate access in most patients.[18] The passage of catheters through either the venous or the arterial system is guided by fluoroscopy. Pressure measurements are made in each cardiac chamber or great vessel, their pressure waveforms recorded, and vascular or ventricular angiography performed. Normal pressure values and oxygen saturations are presented in Table 31-2. Oxygen saturation is greater in the IVC than in the SVC owing to the contribution of blood from the renal veins. Normal pressure waveforms are seen in Figure 31-8. Measurements commonly made or calculated during cardiac cathe-

Table 31-4. HEMODYNAMIC VARIABLES: CALCULATIONS AND NORMAL VALUES

Variable	Calculation	Normal Values
Cardiac index (CI)	CO/BSA	2.5–4.0 $l \cdot min^{-1} \cdot m^{-2}$
Stroke volume (SV)	CO/HR	60–90 $ml \cdot beat^{-1}$
Stroke index (SI)	SV/BSA	40–60 $ml \cdot beat^{-1} \cdot m^{-2}$
Mean arterial pressure (MAP)	Diastolic pressure + one third pulse pressure	80–120 mm Hg
Systemic vascular resistance (SVR)	MAP − CVP/CO × 79.9	1200–1500 $dyn \cdot cm \cdot s^{-5}$
Pulmonary vascular resistance (PVR)	PAP − PWP/CO × 79.9	100–300 $dyn \cdot cm \cdot s^{-5}$
Right ventricular stroke work index (RVSWI)	0.0136(PAP − CVP)SI	5–9 $g \cdot m \cdot beat^{-1} \cdot m^{-2}$
Left ventricular stroke work index (LVSWI)	0.0136(MAP − PWP)SI	45–60 $g \cdot m \cdot beat^{-1} \cdot m^{-2}$

CVP = mean central venous pressure; BSA = body surface area; CO = cardiac output; PAP = mean pulmonary artery pressure; PWP = pulmonary wedge pressure; MAP = mean arterial blood pressure.

terization are detailed in Tables 31-3 and 31-4. These include cardiac output (Fick, dye dilution or thermodilution), measurement of valve areas,[19] and calculation of shunt flows.

Angiography

Cineangiography with iodinated dyes is performed to quantitate ventricular contractility, to evaluate shunting between cardiac chambers, to demonstrate valvular regurgitation, or to delineate vascular outlines (*e.g.*, pulmonary venous return, aortic dissection, pulmonary embolism). Angiography assesses the amount of valvular regurgitation by grading the amount of contrast agent re-entering the chamber preceding the valve. For instance, in the case of aortic regurgitation, 1+ regurgitation is a small amount of contrast material entering the left ventricle during diastole but clearing with each systole. The left ventricle is faintly opacified during diastole and fails to clear with systole with 2+ regurgitation. In 3+ aortic regurgitation, the left ventricle is progressively opacified during diastole and eventually completely opacified, whereas in 4+ aortic regurgitation, the left ventricle is completely opacified on the first diastole and remains opacified for several beats.

Coronary Arteriography

Selective coronary angiography using either the retrograde brachial technique of Sones or the percutaneous femoral approach of Amplatz or Judkins selectively evaluates each coronary artery for the presence and extent of coronary occlusive disease, aneurysm formation, or congenital anomalies (see Fig. 31-4). Coronary arteriography occasionally causes ventricular ectopy, the Bezold–Jarisch reflex, ventricular asystole, or fibrillation. More common are T-wave changes, bradycardia, and mild hypotension. Even in normal coronary arteries, injection of the right coronary artery produces T-wave inversion in lead II and injection of the left artery produces T-wave peaking in lead II.[20] These changes revert to normal when the catheter is removed from the coronary ostia or the blood pressure is increased by having the patient cough.

Determination of Shunts

A shunt exists when arterial and venous blood mix at either an intracardiac or an extracardiac location, usually as a result of a congenital cardiac malformation. The site of a shunt can be determined by measurement of oxygen saturations in various cardiac chambers. A 10% step-up in oxygen saturation at the atrial level indicates left-to-right shunting into the right atrium. A 5% step-up at the ventricular or aorticopulmonary level indicates shunting at that site.

PHYSIOLOGY

Cardiac Cycle

The cardiac cycle begins with the filling of the right and left atria while the tricuspid and mitral valves are closed (see Fig. 31-8). For a complete discussion of the events of the cardiac cycle in normal and abnormal hearts, the reader should consult Pagel *et al.*[21,22] The V wave on the venous pressure waveform represents the gradual increase in atrial blood volume as blood returns from the periphery. Once the aortic valve has closed but ventricular pressure still exceeds atrial pressure, the ventricle undergoes isovolumetric relaxation. About 0.02–0.04 sec after closure of the aortic valve, atrial and ventricular pressures equalize, and a small gradient develops across the AV valves as ventricular pressure decreases further. The AV valve cusps bulge into the ventricle and separate slightly. After cross-over of the atrial and ventricular pressure waves, the AV valves open completely. The V wave of the atrial pressure waveform crests when the atria are filled, and the tricuspid and mitral valves open to initiate ventricular filling. The Y wave results from opening of

the AV valves combined with ventricular relaxation. Effective atrial systole at resting heart rates contributes about 5–20% of the stroke volume. Acute atrial fibrillation increases atrial pressures, reduces atrial compliance, increases atrial oxygen consumption, and eliminates the contribution of the atria to ventricular filling.[23]

During initial ventricular filling, ventricular volume increases rapidly, the rapid filling phase, during which time the ventricular pressure continues to decrease because ventricular expansion exceeds filling. Peak ventricular filling in early diastole occurs at $500–700 \ ml \cdot sec^{-1}$ as ventricular relaxation actually produces a negative intracavitary pressure (diastolic suction). The elastic recoil of the heart and great vessels during diastole contributes to the accelerated filling phase of the ventricle, particularly during tachycardia.

A period of reduced ventricular filling follows the rapid filling phase. The third heart sound, S_3, occurs at the point of transition from rapid ventricular filling to reduced filling. The nadir of the ventricular pressure curve at the end of the rapid filling phase probably marks the end of ventricular relaxation and the beginning of elastic distention of the ventricle. The upswing in the ventricular pressure abolishes forward movement of blood and can force the AV valves into a semiclosed position unless venous return is great. The previous ventricular contraction provides much of the energy for the subsequent diastolic expansion through the energy expenditure of the gross movement and deformation of the heart during systole.[24] Atrial systole, the A wave on the venous pressure waveform, which coincides with the P wave on the ECG, concludes ventricular filling.

Right atrial pressure, a guide to right atrial and right ventricular function, is indirectly assessed by observation of the level of jugular venous pressure, the end-expiratory peak pulsation of the internal jugular vein above the sternal angle with the subject in a 30° reverse Trendelenburg position. Normally, the level is <4 cm. A sustained increase in the level of more than 1 cm during abdominal compression (hepatojugular reflux) indicates abnormal right ventricular function. Only when biventricular function is normal can the central venous pressure be used as a guide to left ventricular function.

There are three phases of activity in the left atrium: (1) the reservoir phase of inflow during ventricular diastole; (2) a conduit phase of passive emptying during ventricular end diastole; (3) contraction and active emptying during ventricular end diastole.[25] All of these left atrial functions are affected by atrial relaxation, stiffness, and contractility.[25]

In hearts with poorly functioning ventricles, atrial contraction is important and a fourth heart sound, S_4, which occurs 0.04 sec after the P wave, results from vibrations of left ventricular muscle and mitral valve. The S_4 is most likely to occur with vigorous atrial contraction. The adequacy of ventricular filling is determined by the distensibility (compliance) of the ventricles, the filling time, and the effective filling pressure. The effective filling pressure is the transmural ventricular pressure. Tachycardia also decreases the time available for ventricular filling, decreasing filling time from 400–500 ms at a heart rate of 60 beats per minute to 10 ms or less at 160 beats per minute. Mitral stenosis, ischemic heart disease, and hypertrophic cardiomyopathy slow ventricular filling and alter ventricular distensibility. The intraventricular pressure just prior to the beginning of ventricular contraction is end-diastolic pressure (see Table 31-2). However, normal end-diastolic pressures do not imply normal ventricular function. Increased end-diastolic pressures occur with hypervolemia or changes in ventricular compliance as well as decreased contractility.

The period just before the sudden increase in ventricular pressure is presystole, which includes atrial systole and the time just before isovolumetric ventricular contraction. The Z point on the venous pressure waveform is the period when atrial and ventricular pressures are essentially equal immediately preceding ventricular systole. The isovolumetric phase of ventricular

Table 31-5. CARDIAC ION CHANNELS

Channel		Activation Kinetics	Inactivation Kinetics
Sodium ("fast")	I_{Na}	Very fast	Fast, except for a fraction that reopen
Calcium ("slow")			
L-type (or high-voltage activated [HVA])	$I_{Ca.t}$	Fast	Variable, Ca^{2+}-dependent component
T-type	$I_{Ca.T}$	Fast	Moderate
Potassium			
Inward rectifier	I_{KI}	Instantaneous	Mg^{2+} and polyamine block of outward current
Plateau or background	$I_{K.pt?TWIKj}$	Instantaneous or fast	None?
Delayed rectifier	$I_{K.s}$	Slow	None
	$I_{K.t}$	Moderate	Slight
	I_{RAK}, I_{HK2}	Very rapid activation	None
Transient outward	I_{to1}	Fast	Moderate
	$I_{K(Ca)}$, $I_{to2?}$	Fast	Moderate
ACh, adenosine, PAF-activated	$I_{K(ACh.Ado)}$	Instantaneous, activated via G_i protein	Mg^{2+} and polyamine block of outward current
ATP-sensitive	$I_{K(AIP)}$	Instantaneous if active	Mg^{2+} block of outward current
Na-activated	$I_{K(Na)}$	Instantaneous if active	
Fatty acid–activated	$I_{K.AA}$, $I_{K.PC}$	Instantaneous if active	
Pacemaker (nonspecific)	I_f	Slow	Slow
Chloride			
Transient outward	$I_{Cl(Ca)}$, I_{to2*}	Fast	Fast
CFTR rest and stretch-activated	$I_{CL.cAMP}$	Instantaneous if active	None

contraction is marked by the C wave on the venous waveform. Isovolumetric contraction is the period between closure of the AV valves and opening of the semilunar (aortic, pulmonic) valves. Intraventricular pressure increases, but there is no change in intraventricular volume. After this point, the AV valves close, atrial diastole begins, the ventricles begin to contract, and ventricular pressure soon exceeds atrial pressure. Ventricular systole occurs immediately after the QRS complex on the electrocardiogram, about 0.12–0.20 sec after atrial contraction. AV valve closure is facilitated by the increased ventricular pressure and the cessation of atrial systole. Closure of the AV valves is noted clinically by the normally split first heart sound, S_1.

The aortic and pulmonic valves open at the summit of the C wave. The atrial pressure decreases, resulting in the X descent, because blood goes into the aorta and pulmonary artery. Once the ventricular pressure exceeds the aortic pressure, the aortic and pulmonic valves open. The majority of ventricular ejection occurs during the rapid ejection phase. The pressure in the aorta is slightly lower, whereas ventricular pressure increases rapidly. Initially the output into the aorta exceeds the runoff into the peripheral circulation. Peak aortic pressure occurs slightly after peak aortic blood flow. As aortic runoff and ventricular output equilibrate, the period of reduced ventricular ejection occurs. Forward flow continues until the end of ventricular diastole, protodiastole, when a brief period of retrograde flow initiates aortic and pulmonic valve closure. On pressure waveforms, semilunar valve closure is marked by a notch or incisura. The second heart sound, S_2, results from rapid deceleration of blood causing vibration of the outflow tracks and great vessels and closure of the semilunar valves.

Cardiac Electrophysiology

Cellular Electrophysiology

Cardiac pacemaker cells have an intracellular ionic composition which differs from that found in the extracellular fluid. The most important ions are calcium, sodium, and potassium. An active transport system in the cell membrane, the sodium–potassium pump, maintains normal concentration gradients for sodium and potassium by pumping sodium ions out of the cell and potassium ions into the cell. Extracellular ions cross the cell membrane through specialized membrane proteins, the ion channels, which are characterized by their conductance, selectivity, gating, and density. Conductance is the rate (ions · ms^{-1}) at which ions pass through the channel. In a given channel, each ion has a particular conductance. Channels are named for the ion most rapidly transferred since some ions, but not others, are transported. Density is described as the number of channels per square micrometer. However, density may be variable over the cellular sarcolemma. Gating is the property of the channel that allows it to be activated or inactivated in response to voltage changes or binding of an agonist. Examples of these channels, which directly or indirectly control cardiac function, are given in Table 31-5.

β Receptors, consisting of the receptor, the G protein (guanosine triphosphate binding protein) system,[26] and adenylate cyclase are also located in the cell membrane. Receptors recognize and bind agonists, activating the G protein Gs, which, in turn, activates adenylate cyclase to stimulate hydrolysis of adenosine triphosphate to cyclic adenosine monophosphate. Cyclic adenosine monophosphate opens the calcium channel, permitting calcium influx. The entire complex forms a transmembrane signaling system (see Fig. 31-8).

The SA node is normally the dominant pacemaker because, in it, automaticity is most highly developed and impulses are initiated at the fastest rate. In SA nodal cells, when the internal membrane potential reaches −50 mV, the depolarization rate increases to 1–2 V · sec^{-1}, causing a slowly depolarizing action potential. Automaticity decreases in order from SA node, AV node, His bundle, proximal Purkinje fibers, and distal Purkinje fibers. The rate of Phase 4 depolarization is faster in the SA node than in the AV node and faster in the AV node than in the terminal Purkinje fibers, causing less highly developed pacemakers to be depolarized by the propagated wave from above before they spontaneously depolarize. Interactions between sympathetic and parasympathetic innervations also affect the intrinsic depolarization rate.

The compound action potential in cells results from local ionic transmembrane fluxes or currents through the channels (Fig. 31-9). Ionic transfer is facilitated by the energy released from the hydrolysis of adenosine triphosphate. Pacemaker cells in the unexcited state are maintained at a resting potential of -80 mV by the inward (anomalous) rectifier current I_{K1}. As the slow spontaneous depolarization of Phase 4 proceeds, there is an increase in the permeability of the membrane, which permits positively charged sodium ions to move across the cell membrane into the cell, resulting in depolarization. This sodium influx (fast sodium current, I_{Na}) reverses the transmembrane potential from -80 mV to $+20-30$ mV and initiates the rapid depolarization (Phase 0) of the action potential in a cardiac pacemaker cell (Fig. 31-9). During Phase 0 there is also a decrease in permeability to potassium. At about -30 mV, inward calcium transfer (I_{Ca}) begins through the L-type (long-lasting, high-threshold) channels which require greater than -40 mV to activate for opening. The spread of depolarization throughout the atrial and ventricular muscle results in the P wave and the QRS complex of the electrocardiogram, respectively. After excitation, the cell membrane undergoes an initial period of rapid repolarization (Phase 1), followed by a variable period when the membrane potential is close to 0, the plateau of the action potential. The plateau is caused by decreasing sodium and calcium influx (through the L-type calcium channel) and increasing potassium efflux. Four K^+ currents participate in repolarization, including I_{to}, the transient outward current during the initial phase of repolarization; the I_K plateau and delayed K current (I_K) during the plateau; and I_{K1} or inward rectifier during final repolarization.[27] The duration of the action potential is rate-dependent owing to enhanced calcium entry. Phase 3, the repolarization phase that results from "delayed outward" potassium current I_{x1}, corresponds to the T wave of the electro-

cardiogram. During Phase 4, the resting membrane potential is generated by active exchange of intracellular sodium for potassium through the sodium–potassium ATPase or sodium pump. The resting potassium conductance that maintains the resting potential is G_{K1}, the inward (anomalous) rectifier. In the latter part of Phase 4, the resting membrane potential is stable in ventricular muscle cells until the cell is excited again. In automatic cells such as the SA and AV nodes, slow, spontaneous depolarization occurs during Phase 4 as a result of the pacemaker currents calcium I_f and I_{K2}.

During depolarization, the cell membrane is absolutely refractory to other stimuli because almost all of the sodium channels inactivate. The end of the absolute refractory period is signaled by the earliest transient depolarization that can be elicited because sufficient numbers of activatable sodium channels are present. The absolute refractory period ends at the beginning of the T wave of the electrocardiogram. Once repolarization reaches the threshold potential, the cell is relatively refractory, since an unusually strong stimulus can produce depolarization. This period is marked by the T wave of the ECG. The earliest propagated action potential defines the end of the effective or functional refractory period.

Action Potential Alterations

Changes in the action potential itself or factors that affect the action potential alter the rate of firing of an automatic cell. The rate of an automatic cell depends on the slope of Phase 4 depolarization, the maximum diastolic potential (the maximum level of resting membrane potential achieved at the end of

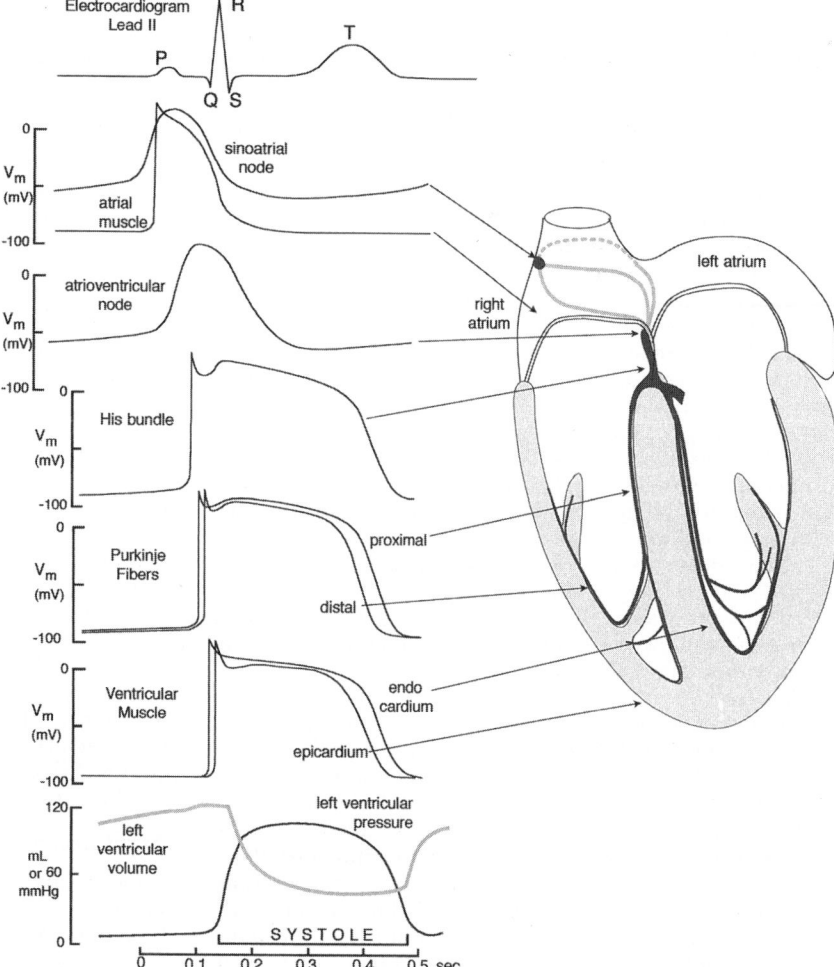

Figure 31-9. The action potential of an automatic cell such as the sinoatrial node differs from that of the ventricular muscle cell in that the cell slowly depolarizes spontaneously during Phase 4. The action potential in a Purkinje cell has the most rapid rate of depolarization, 400–800 $V \cdot sec^{-1}$. When the cell is stimulated, an action potential occurs due to a rapid influx of sodium ions into the cell (Phase 0). Phase 1 includes a notch caused by the "early outward current", I_{eo}, which is a transient K efflux, probably activated by an intracellular calcium increase. Phase 2 is the plateau of the action potential resulting principally from calcium entry through the slow channel of the cell membrane. During Phase 3, repolarization of the cell occurs while during Phase 4, the sodium entering during Phase 0 is actively pumped out of the cell. In a ventricular muscle cell, unlike the automatic cells, there is no spontaneous Phase 4 depolarization. (Reprinted with permission from Lynch C, Lake CL: Cardiovascular anatomy and physiology. In Youngberg J, Lake C, Roizen M *et al* (eds): Cardiac, Vascular, and Thoracic Anesthesia, p 87. Philadelphia, Churchill Livingstone, 2000.)

Table 31-6. ACTION POTENTIAL ALTERATIONS[28-31]

EFFECTS ON PHASE 4

Hypothermia ↓ slope
Hypothermia ↑ rate
Hypoxia ↑ slope
Ischemia ↑ slope
Hyperkalemia ↓ rate
Hypokalemia ↑ rate
Hyponatremia ↓ slope
Hypercarbia ↑ slope
Increased pH ↑ slope

EFFECTS ON ACTION POTENTIAL DURATION

Hypercalcemia ↓
Hypocalcemia ↑

EFFECTS ON DIASTOLIC DEPOLARIZATION

Hypoxia ↓ max diastolic potential
Hyperkalemia ↓ max diastolic potential
Hypercarbia ↓ max diastolic potential (Purkinje only)
Hypercarbia ↓ diastolic depolarization
Increased pH ↓ diastolic depolarization

repolarization), the RMP, and the threshold potential.[28] The variable expression of the previously described ion channels in different parts of the heart produces the characteristic electrophysiology of the pacemakers, conduction tissue, atria, and ventricles. Factors affecting the action potential are listed in Table 31-6.[28-31] In addition to effects on the action potential, alterations in potassium current affect membrane electrical stability. Low extracellular K^+ reduces conductance through the inward rectifier channel (G_{K1}). Thus, there is greater cellular excitability and tendency for ectopy. With increased extracellular K, more potassium current escapes from the cell and the membrane is relatively stable.

Clinical Electrophysiology

The first wave of the normal electrocardiogram is the P wave, which is produced by atrial depolarization resulting from an action potential in the SA node. It is usually upright, except in lead aV_R, and 0.11 sec in duration. Sinus node rate exhibits a circadian rhythm, decreasing nocturnally. Sinus node recovery time is also prolonged at night.[32]

An electrical impulse travels from the SA node to the AV node in 0.04 sec via atrial tissue, specialized atrial conducting tissue, or the anterior, middle, and posterior tracts of the right atrium. Transmission is further delayed in the AV node because its conduction velocity is about $0.2 \text{ m} \cdot \text{sec}^{-1}$. The effective refractory period of the AV node demonstrates circadian rhythm and is increasingly prolonged at night.[32] The PR interval (normally 0.2 ms or less), which occupies the time between atrial and ventricular depolarization, is nearly isoelectric, because atrial repolarization is not recordable. Significant interactions between the parasympathetic and sympathetic nervous systems control the conduction through the AV node with predominantly sympathetic activity.[33]

Ventricular depolarization begins ~0.12-0.20 sec in adults and 0.15-0.18 sec in children after depolarization of the SA node to produce the QRS complex.[34] The entire QRS complex should be <10 sec. The first negative wave of the QRS complex is the Q wave, which should be ≤0.04 s in duration and less than one fourth of the subsequent R wave in amplitude. The first positive wave in the QRS is the R wave, and the second negative wave is the S wave. The right and left branches of the bundle of His connecting with the Purkinje fibers conduct the depolarizing impulse rapidly over the endocardial surface of the heart. Normally in sinus rhythm the earliest area of ventricular

activation is the trabecular area on the anterior right ventricular surface about 18-25 ms after the surface QRS complex. Activation then spreads toward the apex and base of the heart, with the latest activation at the cardiac base. Electrical activation also spreads from endocardium to epicardium.

On the electrocardiogram the time from the end of ventricular depolarization to the beginning of repolarization, the ST segment, is isoelectric. More than 1 mm of elevation in the standard leads or 2 mm of elevation in the precordial leads is abnormal in this segment. No more than 0.5 mm of depression should be seen in any lead. The J point, the junction between the QRS complex and the ST segment, is depressed or elevated with the ST segment. Ventricular repolarization results in the T wave. T waves are normally upright in leads I, II, and V_3-V_6, inverted in lead aV_R, and variable in leads II, aV_L, aV_F, V_1, and V_2. The T wave should not exceed 5 mm in height in the standard leads or 10 mm in the precordial leads. The QT interval, varying inversely with heart rate, should be slightly less than one half of the RR interval.[35] The U wave, a small upright deflection after the T wave, is usually nondetectable.

Physiology of the Cardiac Nerves

Neural Regulation

Neural regulation of the heart is complex. The dominance of either the sympathetic or the parasympathetic system varies with age and physical condition, but the inhibitory parasympathetic system usually predominates.[36,37] Parasympathetic stimulation, particularly of the right vagus nerve, decreases heart rate by slowing the SA node. Lower pacemakers such as the AV node or His bundle may take over, causing "nodal rhythm." Vagal stimulation tends to suppress ventricular automaticity, which may facilitate termination of ventricular dysrhythmias. Intense vagal stimulation depresses both atrial and ventricular contractility by stimulation of cardiac muscarinic receptors that alter the myocyte cyclic adenosine monophosphate level, by inhibition of norepinephrine release from nearby sympathetic nerve terminals by acetylcholine, and by inhibition of adrenergic receptor activation. One of the G proteins, Gi, which inhibits adenylcyclase, lowering the levels of cyclic adenosine monophosphate, is coupled with the muscarinic receptor to control potassium channels and decrease heart rate (Fig. 31-10).

Stimulation of the stellate ganglion or other sympathetic cardiac fibers increases heart rate, contractility, and ejection fraction. The right stellate ganglion has a greater effect on heart rate, whereas the left has more effect on contractility. Abnormalities of sympathetic cardiac nerve tone occur in long QT interval syndromes.[38]

The role of the cardiac α receptors is unclear, but their action is modulated by G protein signal transduction. β_1 Receptors of the heart have positive chronotropic, inotropic, and lusitropic effects on the heart by stimulation of adenylcyclase. Action potentials may be restored by β_1 stimulation owing to increased numbers of activatable calcium channels in sufficient density to permit regenerative ionic flux along a fiber. Activation of cardiac β_2 receptors also increases rate and contractility, particularly in end-stage heart failure. The effects of norepinephrine on contractility are mediated by increased calcium entry through more active calcium channels and increased sarcoplasmic reticular uptake of calcium. Increased sarcoplasmic uptake of calcium has a lusitropic effect while making the increased calcium (in the sarcoplasmic reticulum) available for subsequent contractions (see Fig. 31-10).

Atrial Receptors

Parasympathetic receptors Type A, Type B, and receptors innervated by Group C fibers reflexly alter intravascular volume or heart rate. The primary locations of Types A and B receptors are the cavoatrial junction, pulmonary venous–atrial junction,

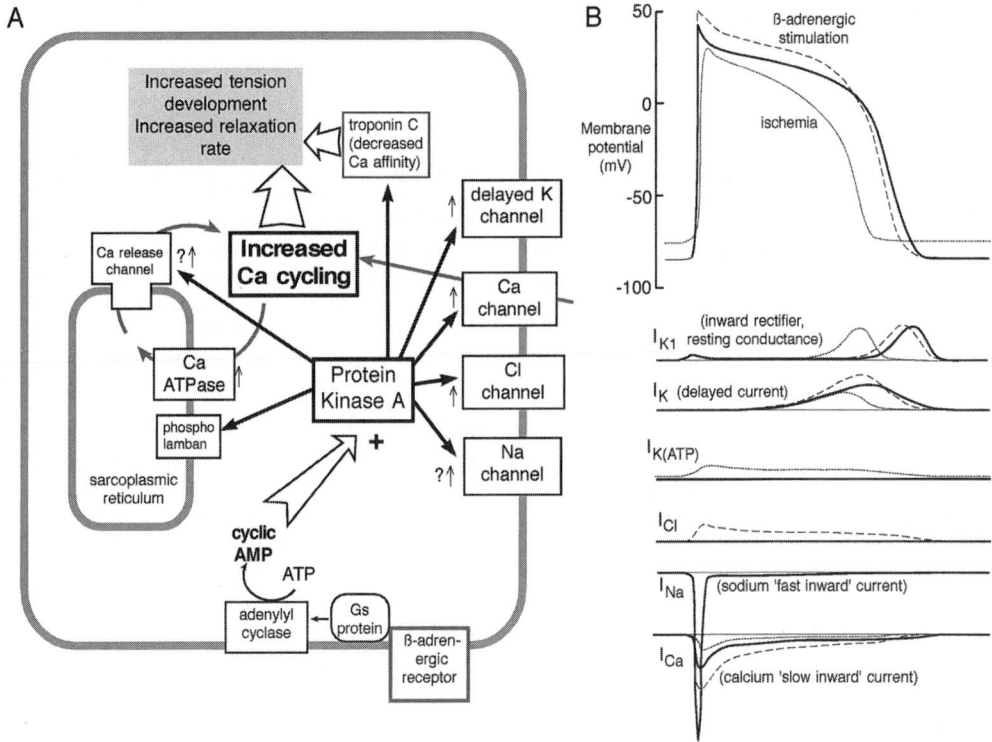

Figure 31-10. Effects of adrenergic stimulation on the heart. β-Adrenergically stimulated protein phosphorylation occurs owing to activation of protein kinase A and increased cyclic adenosine monophosphate (cAMP) production. Increased cycling of Ca^{2+} and phosphorylation of multiple ion channels (Ca, Cl, Na, and delayed K) occurs. (Reprinted with permission from Lynch C, Lake CL: Cardiovascular anatomy and physiology. In Youngberg J, Lake C, Roizen M *et al* (eds): Cardiac, Vascular, and Thoracic Anesthesia, p 100. Philadelphia, Churchill Livingstone, 2000.)

atrial appendage, and atrial body.[39] Type A receptors may actually respond to heart rate rather than atrial pressure.[39] Type B receptors are stretch receptors whose discharge is closely related to atrial volume and varies with the rate of atrial pressure increase.

Ventricular Receptors

Stimulation of ventricular receptors causes either cardiovascular excitation or depression. Types of ventricular receptors include the pressure-sensitive coronary baroreceptors, mechanoreceptors (innervated by nonmyelinated vagal afferent fibers), and sympathetic mechanosensitive or chemosensitive receptors.[39]

The Bainbridge reflex, described below, is mediated by the parasympathetic receptors. Myocardial ischemia increases discharge of both vagal and sympathetic receptors. The sympathetic afferent fibers may transmit the pain sensation associated with coronary occlusion. Postcardiotomy hypertension results from a cardiogenic reflex transmitted through the sympathetic afferent fibers of the stellate ganglion.[39] Finally, opiate receptors of the K type, found in vagus, cardiac, and sympathetic ganglia, may mediate dysrhythmias, particularly during ischemia and reperfusion.[40,41]

Both cardiac contraction and conduction are modulated through the β-adrenergic receptors and guanine nucleotide binding proteins or G proteins. G protein molecules consist of seven transmembrane α-helical segments, which create a central cleft to which various ligands can bind. When binding occurs, the receptor undergoes a conformational change. An example of the G protein signaling system in the heart is the binding of catecholamines to the β-adrenergic receptor, which in turn, activates the stimulatory G protein and adenyl cyclase, increasing intracellular cyclic AMP, cardiac contractility, and heart rate. However, a detailed discussion of the G proteins is beyond the scope of the chapter and may be found in other sources.[42]

Coronary Circulatory Physiology

About 5% of the cardiac output, or $250 \text{ ml} \cdot \text{min}^{-1}$, perfuses the coronary arteries of a 70-kg person. Physiologically, the coronary circulation consists of large, low-resistance epicardial vessels and higher-resistance intramyocardial arteries and arterioles. Myocardial flow, pressure, and oxygen consumption are integrally related. Coronary blood flow is locally regulated by metabolic, mechanical, anatomic, and possibly myogenic factors.[43] Numerous methods to measure human myocardial blood flow have been described.[44] Coronary flow is determined by the duration of diastole and the difference between diastolic aortic pressure and left ventricular end-diastolic pressure. During systole about 15–25% of the coronary flow distends and is stored in the extramural coronary arteries. Only a small amount actually perfuses the myocardium. During diastole, this stored blood perfuses the myocardium[45] (Fig. 31-11). The majority of left

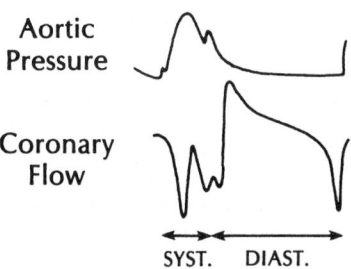

Figure 31-11. This diagrammatic relationship between aortic pressure and coronary flow demonstrates that little coronary flow occurs during systole while the majority occurs during diastole. This relationship is particularly true to the left coronary artery which supplies the left ventricle. The right ventricle, being thinner and developing less pressure, produces less impediment to systolic coronary flow.

coronary artery flow occurs in diastole because intramyocardial pressure is lowest at that time.[46] Right coronary artery flow occurs in both systole and diastole because intramyocardial pressure is lower in the thinner right ventricle. Intramyocardial pressure affects coronary flow to a small extent because of the varying stiffness of ventricular muscle over the cardiac cycle.[46] Coronary flow also decreases from epicardium to endocardium as a consequence of extravascular pressure.

The zero flow pressure, normally about 12–50 mm Hg, is a minimum coronary pressure required to initiate flow. The source of this pressure is the collapsed intramyocardial coronary microvessels when tissue pressures exceed intraluminal pressures and intracavitary back pressure. At least half of coronary vascular resistance results from vessels larger than 100 μm in diameter, whereas 10% results from coronary veins.[47] Coronary flow ceases completely at 20 mm Hg, the critical closure or critical flow pressure.[48]

Myocardial oxygen consumption is high; therefore, coronary venous blood is only 30% saturated and its Po_2 of 18–20 mm Hg is the lowest anywhere in the body. Because oxygen extraction cannot be increased further, coronary flow must increase if the heart requires additional oxygen.

Coronary Autoregulation

Coronary perfusion is autoregulated to maintain a constant flow over a range of perfusion pressures (usually between 50 and 120 mm Hg) at any given myocardial oxygen demand.[49] Above and below these limits, coronary flow varies with perfusion pressure. The term *autoregulation* refers strictly to pressure-dependent changes in coronary resistance unrelated to changes in myocardial metabolism.[49] The principal site of coronary autoregulation is the coronary arteriole, a <150-μm–diameter vessel, although small coronary arteries (>150 μm) can be recruited to increase flow during hypoperfusion.[50] Nevertheless, the coronary arterioles are not fully dilated even during hypoperfusion states.[51]

However, changes in myocardial oxygen demand alter autoregulation. The involved metabolite, therefore, is oxygen (specifically, myocardial oxygen tension, Po_2) acting through mediators such as adenosine.[45] Adenosine-induced vasodilation is inversely related to arterial diameter, with the greatest dilation occurring in smaller vessels.[50] Hyperoxia decreases, and a low Po_2 of 49 mm Hg increases coronary blood flow and myocardial oxygen consumption independently of changes in oxygen content or delivery.[52] The threshold oxygen tension for autoregulation is 32 mm Hg.[53] Coronary autoregulation is also closely coupled with coronary venous Po_2, particularly at Po_2 < 25 mm Hg.[45,53] Decreased heart rate attenuates autoregulation, whereas pharmacologic coronary constriction augments it.[53]

The autoregulatory mechanism may even extend into different myocardial layers.[45] Autoregulation is greater in the subepicardium than in the subendocardium, possibly because of the transmural gradient to which the subendocardial vessels are exposed.[49] Autoregulation in the right coronary artery may be less than in the left coronary artery. Pressure and flow-dependent changes in myocardial oxygen consumption in the right ventricle explain these differences.[49]

Immediately after occlusion of a coronary artery, reperfusion flow increases beyond preocclusion levels, a process termed *reactive hyperemia*. In a related process, *reactive dilation*, large coronary arteries dilate after relief of occlusion; but unlike in reactive hyperemia, the onset is delayed to 60 sec and sustained for 150 sec after relief of occlusion.[54]

The most important regulators of coronary vascular tone are metabolic and involve multiple pathways. Modulation of basal tone and normal autoregulation is mediated by glybenclamide-sensitive K_{ATP} channels, which are enhanced by adenosine receptor activation.[55,56] Other mediators and pathways such as oxygen, potassium, pH, carbon dioxide, endothelium-derived relaxing factor, prostaglandins, prostacyclin, histamine, and adenosine triphosphate may also be involved in regulating coronary tone.[43] Prostaglandin E_1 dilates the coronary arteries, probably acting through adenosine as a mediator. Prostaglandin E_2, however, is a coronary vasoconstrictor.[57] Acetylcholine increases coronary flow. Acting through the H_1 receptor, histamine contracts epicardial coronary arteries, provoking spasm, but the H_2 receptor mediates vasodilation.[58] Histamine also promotes production of prostaglandin in the heart.[58] Although norepinephrine (or sympathetic cardiac nerve stimulation) causes coronary constriction through its α effects, the associated increase in myocardial contractility increases coronary flow. Similarly, vagal stimulation may directly produce coronary vasodilation, but the associated decrease in heart rate and contractility causes secondary coronary vasoconstriction.

Coronary Flow Reserve

Coronary flow increases during maximal dilation of the coronary arteries. The difference between resting and maximal coronary flow is the coronary flow reserve. Coronary flow is heterogeneous throughout the myocardium, although there is correlation between regional flow in neighboring myocardial areas.[59] Although coronary vasodilation occurs in response to ischemia or other endogenous stimuli, maximal flow, which is normally unavailable to the heart, may be achieved with pharmacologic agents. Exhaustion of autoregulatory vasodilator reserve does not necessarily mean that exhaustion of pharmacologic vasodilator reserve has occurred. Coronary flow reserve can be decreased by (1) decreased maximal flow and (2) increased regulated coronary flow.[60] Maximal coronary flow is decreased by tachycardia, increased blood viscosity, increased myocardial contractility, and myocardial hypertrophy.[45]

As epicardial coronary artery stenosis occurs, so does arteriolar vasodilation in order to maintain flow at normal levels. Once the vasodilator reserve is exhausted (usually at stenoses of >90%), however, an increase in the stenosis of the coronary artery will decrease flow. Administration of a vasodilator to a vascular bed served by a normal and a stenotic coronary artery connected by collaterals will dilate the normal arterioles but produce little change in the arterioles served by the stenotic artery, since they are maximally dilated. The increased flow to the normal arterioles is termed "coronary steal."

Endocardial/Epicardial Flow Ratio

The distribution of coronary flow is as important as total flow. The ratio of flow in the endocardium to that in the epicardium, the endo/epi ratio, is used to assess flow distribution. Subepicardial flow is usually adequate; thus, if the endo/epi ratio remains constant, adequate subendocardial blood flow is inferred.[60] However, with maximal coronary vasodilation, the endo/epi ratio varies with the coronary perfusion pressure.[45] The ratio is minimally affected by changes in afterload but reduced by increased left ventricular preload. The latter results either from a disproportionate increase in subendocardial diastolic tissue pressure or an increase in coronary sinus pressure.[45] However, increased right ventricular preload decreases right ventricular blood flow without altering its intramyocardial distribution.[61]

Transient subendocardial ischemia accompanies the onset of severe exercise. Although anemia increases coronary blood flow by autoregulation, severe anemia decreases the endo/epi ratio, indicating subendocardial ischemia.[45] Hypoxia, on the other hand, increases both coronary blood flow and the endo/epi ratio.

Neural Influences

Coronary arteries are also responsive to neural stimuli.[62] Parasympathetic and sympathetic nerves extend to the precapillary coronary vessels. Parasympathetic stimulation directly activates coronary muscarinic receptors, inducing dilation.

Sympathetic stimulation causes coronary dilatation as a result of the metabolic factors produced by increased Mvo_2 and direct β receptor stimulation. α_2 Adrenoceptors or muscarinic receptors are present in the sympathetic nerve endings of coronary arteries. Activation of α-adrenergic receptors by norepinephrine and acetylcholine (via the vagus nerve) reduces sympathetic neurotransmitter output, which would reduce the dilation of these vessels causing coronary vasoconstriction. α_2 Agonists also mediate release of endothelial-derived relaxing factor in coronary arteries. β_1-Adrenergic receptors predominate over α_1 receptors in canine circumflex coronary artery.[63] Termination of the sympathetic cardiac effects results from extensive neuronal uptake of norepinephrine.[64] Only small amounts of the norepinephrine released by the heart enter the systemic circulation.[64]

Coronary artery spasm may result from unopposed α_1-adrenoceptor stimulation in the presence of β-adrenergic blockade or when a pure α agonist is given. Acute coronary occlusion attenuates the baroreflex responses of heart rate and systemic vascular resistance.[51]

Cardiac Output

Cardiac output is the volume of blood pumped by the heart each minute. It is the product of the heart rate and the volume of each beat (stroke volume) but is determined by preload, afterload, heart rate, contractility, and ventricular compliance. Cardiac output measurements are usually corrected for the size of the patient by dividing the output by the body surface area to give the cardiac index. A normal cardiac index is 2.5–3.5 $l \cdot min^{-1} \cdot m^{-2}$ and may be determined by Fick principle or indicator-dilution methods (Fig. 31-12 and Table 31-4). Cardiac output increases with increased heart rate, preload, or contractility and decreased afterload.

Determinants

Preload. Preload is defined as the end-diastolic stress on the ventricle (end-diastolic fiber length or end-diastolic volume). The determinants of preload are blood volume, venous tone, ventricular compliance, ventricular afterload, and myocardial contractility. The distribution of the blood volume between intrathoracic and extrathoracic compartments also affects preload. Extrathoracic blood volume increases with standing, whereas the negative intrathoracic pressure during inspiration increases intrathoracic blood volume.

Stroke volume is determined by the volume of blood in the heart at the beginning of systole (end-diastolic volume or EDV) and the amount of blood remaining in the ventricle at closure of the aortic valve at the end of systole (end-systolic volume

or ESV). The degree of stretch of the left ventricular fibers, influenced by the amount of blood in the ventricle, determines the amount of work the ventricle can do.[65] An increase in preload increases end-diastolic volume and wall tension.

End-diastolic volume is not synonymous with end-diastolic pressure; nor are the two linearly related. The ejection fraction, normally 0.6–0.7, is the ratio of the stroke volume to the end-diastolic volume:

$$\text{Ejection fraction} = \text{EDV} - \text{ESV}/\text{EDV}$$

Severe impairment of ventricular function is present when the ejection fraction is <0.4.

Afterload. Afterload is the wall stress or tension faced by the myocardium during ventricular ejection. It is the force opposing ventricular fiber shortening during ejection. Left ventricular afterload depends upon the shape, size, radius, and wall thickness of the ventricle, the principal factors being the radius (related to preload and chamber volume) and aortic impedance (controlled by arterial compliance and systemic vascular resistance). Other factors involved in afterload include arterial wall stiffness (aortic), blood viscosity, and the mass of blood in the aorta. Usually, the ejection phase stress is implied in discussions of afterload, although there are wall stresses during the isovolumetric contraction phase.

Clinically, systemic vascular resistance is frequently used as an estimate of afterload (see Table 31-4). However, systemic vascular resistance reflects only peripheral arteriolar tone rather than left ventricular systolic wall tension. A true measure of left ventricular afterload, such as left ventricular end-systolic wall stress, which incorporates left ventricular chamber pressure, ventricular dimensions, wall thickness, and peripheral loading conditions, should be used to accurately assess afterload.[66] However, these measurements require direct intraventricular pressure determination and echocardiographic evaluation of wall thickness and ventricular dimensions. Compared with left ventricular end-systolic wall stress, systemic vascular resistance underestimates afterload when afterload is increased or decreased or contractility is improved.[66]

When afterload is reduced, the ventricle shortens more quickly and completely.[67] An increase in afterload decreases the extent and velocity of shortening and increases active tension and the time to peak tension in cardiac muscle. Wall tension, ventricular radius, and end-diastolic volume are also increased to maintain stroke volume. In the poorly contractile heart, acute increases in afterload severely reduce stroke volume. Hypertrophy occurs in ventricles facing a chronic increase in afterload, so that wall stress and shortening characteristics return toward normal.

Heart Rate. Heart rate is primarily determined by the automaticity of the sinus node. However, its intrinsic rate depends upon neural and humoral influences. An increase in heart rate increases cardiac output, even if the stroke volume remains constant, by increasing the extent and velocity of shortening and dP/dt.[68] The increase of dP/dt with heart rate is even more pronounced if end-diastolic dimensions are maintained by volume infusion.[68] At heart rates between 120 and 160 beats · min^{-1}, cardiac output increases but not as much as at more optimal heart rates (Fig. 31-13). An increase in heart rate shortens the filling time between beats, reducing end-diastolic volume. Because most cardiac filling occurs during the first half-second of the rapid filling phase, cardiac output decreases at heart rates >160 beats · min^{-1} because of inadequate filling time.

Cardiac output is also increased during the heartbeat after a ventricular extrasystole. This extrasystolic potentiation results from increased ejection fraction, decreased left ventricular end-diastolic volume, and enhanced diastolic filling. The mechanism is probably increased availability of calcium to the contractile mechanism.[69]

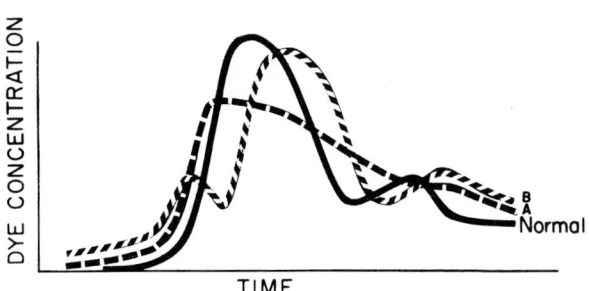

Figure 31-12. A normal dye dilution curve has an uninterrupted buildup slope, a steep disappearance slope with a short disappearance time, and a prominent recirculation peak. In right-to-left shunts (*A*), there is a deformity on the buildup slope by the abnormal early appearance of the dye in the arterial circulation. Left-to-right (*B*) shunting causes a decreased peak dye concentration, absence of the recirculation peak, and a prolongation of the disappearance time. (Reprinted with permission from Lake CL: Cardiovascular Anesthesia. New York, Springer-Verlag, 1985.)

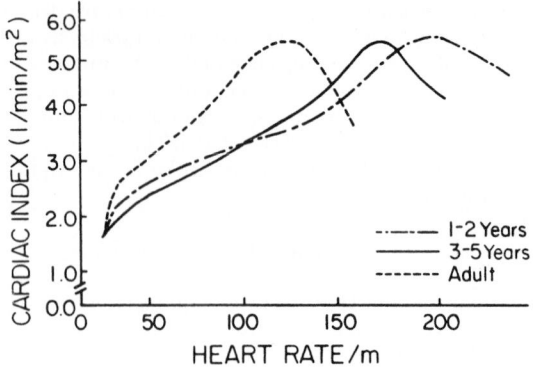

Figure 31-13. The effect of heart rate on cardiac output varies with age. In children, an increase in heart rate increases cardiac output because the immature heart is relatively noncompliant and does not increase its stroke volume in response to increased demands. In the adult, however, an increase in heart rate beyond 120 beats/min^{-1} does not increase cardiac index. (Reprinted with permission from Wetsel RC: Critical Care State of the Art, 1981.)

Contractility. Contractility is the inotropic state independent of changes in preload, afterload, or heart rate.

Cardiac Systole. Myocardial contraction begins when the action potential, acting through the T-(tubule) system of the sarcoplasmic reticulum, results in calcium release into the sarcoplasm. A cyclic adenosine monophosphate-dependent protein kinase in the heart stimulates calcium transport by the vesicles of the sarcoplasmic reticulum (see Fig. 31-14). Intracellular cyclic adenosine monophosphate protein kinase is activated and transfers the terminal phosphate of adenosine triphosphate to troponin I, phospholamban, or other intracellular proteins. Troponin has three components: troponin I, the inhibitory factor inhibiting the magnesium-stimulated adenosine triphosphatase of actomyosin; troponin C, which is the calcium-sensitive factor; and troponin T, the tropomyosin-binding subunit.

The actin and myosin filaments forming the myofibrils of the cardiac myocyte are functionally divided into sarcomeres. The sarcomere is further divided into three major subdomains, the electron-lucent I band composed primarily of actin; the Z line, where actin filaments from adjacent sarcomeres meet and sarcoplasmic reticulum is juxtaposed to the t-tubule system (junctional SR); and the electron-dense A band composed of myosin thick filaments (further subdivided by the M band into two symmetric bundles). Junctional SR is characterized by a larger lumen containing calsequestrin, a protein that provides extra "releasable" calcium and has low calcium-binding affinity. Calcium entering the myocyte through the L-type calcium channels primarily activates release of SR calcium, a process called calcium-induced calcium release (CICR). A portion of the entering calcium binds to calcium release channels (CaRC) to activate their opening, permitting rapid efflux of stored calcium from the SR lumen into the myoplasm to bind to troponin C.

Phospholamban, a membrane-bound protein that modulates the activity of calcium-stimulated magnesium adenosine triphosphatase, permits increased calcium uptake and calcium release by the SR in its phosphorylated state.[70] Adenosine triphosphatase from the calcium pump, which couples hydrolysis of one molecule of adenosine triphosphate with the active transport of two calcium ions, is the channel through which the activator calcium is released to initiate systole. The increased free calcium is bound to troponin C, releasing the inhibition of actin–myosin interaction by the troponin–tropomyosin complex. Contraction of actin and myosin occurs (see Fig. 31-13). The strength of contraction depends upon the length of the sarcomere and the amount of activator calcium because cardiac contractility is controlled by the degree of activation of the myocytes. Likewise, relaxation depends upon the rate of calcium delivery to troponin, the quantity of available calcium, and the rate of calcium removal from troponin.[71]

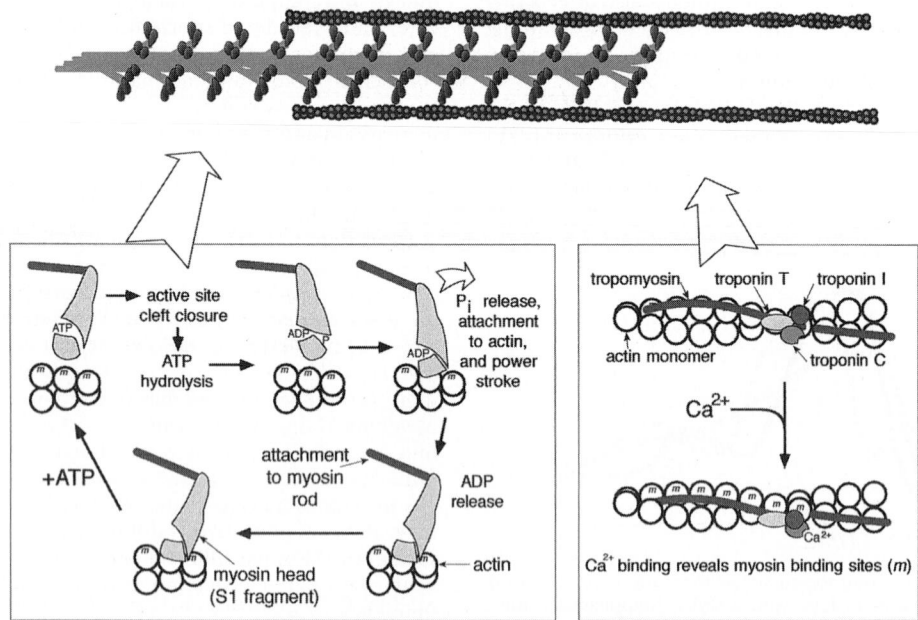

Figure 31-14. (*Left*) A schematic diagram of the actin filament with its individual monomers and active myosin binding site (m). The myosin head (S1 fragment) is dissociated from actin by binding with ATP. Subsequent ATP hydrolysis and release of inorganic phosphate (P$_i$) "cocks" the head group into a tension-generating conformation. Attachment of the myosin head to actin allows the head to apply tension to the myosin rod and to the actin filament. (*Right*) Calcium binding to troponin C causes troponin I, the inhibitory subunit, to decrease its affinity for actin. Via tropomyosin, seven m sites on actin monomers are revealed. (Adapted from Rayment I, Holden HM, Whitaker M *et al:* Structure of the actin–myosin complex and implications for muscle contraction. Science 261:58, 1993; reproduced with permission of C. Lynch III.)

Diastole. Myocardial relaxation occurs as a result of reuptake of or binding of calcium ion by the SR, a lusitropic or relaxing effect of cyclic adenosine monophosphate.[72] Relaxation is a load-dependent process. In the relaxing heart, load is the premature lengthening of cardiac muscle. Myocardial relaxation depends upon internal restoring forces such as cardiac fibers, hemodynamic loading such as the impedance of the arterial system, and external restoring forces resulting from deformation of the wall of the intact heart.[73]

Alterations in Contractility. Cardiac output is increased by increasing load, either volume or pressure (heterometric autoregulation); by the Anrep effect (homeometric autoregulation); the treppe phenomenon; or by a change in the inotropic state independent of the above mechanisms.

The Anrep effect improves ventricular performance several beats after the initial stretching of the myocardial fibers owing to abruptly increased aortic or left ventricular pressure. It results from increased contractility with more rapid activation of the contractile process, increased developed force, and increased velocity of shortening. Homeometric autoregulation is operative for only a few minutes as the initially increased ventricular end-diastolic volume and circumference decrease with recovery of stroke work.[73]

The treppe phenomenon (force–frequency relation, staircase effect, or Bowditch's phenomenon) is a progressive increase in contractile force associated with a sudden increase in heart rate. It results from a variation in myofibril calcium sensitivity and an alteration in activator calcium. A long pause between beats also increases the force of contraction; this is known as the Woodworth phenomenon or reverse (negative) staircase effect.[74] Increasing contractility increases the ejection fraction if end-systolic volume decreases while end-diastolic volume remains the same. Contractility is decreased by hypoxia, cardiomyopathy, myocardial ischemia, or infarction.

Compliance. Compliance is the nonlinear change in ventricular end-diastolic volume/change in end-diastolic pressure. The rapidity of diastolic filling is a major determinant of cardiac output, which is reduced by decreased compliance. Although

ventricular contractility may be normal, reduced relaxation from coronary artery disease, hypertrophic cardiomyopathy, cardiac tamponade, and hypertensive heart disease impairs diastolic filling which, in turn, limits cardiac output.

Myocardial Mechanics

The mechanical function of the heart is evaluated by *ejection phase indices* (Starling stroke volume vs. end-diastolic pressure curves, stroke work vs. end-diastolic pressure, force–velocity curves, ejection fraction, velocity of circumferential fiber shortening), *preload recruitable stroke work, isovolumic phase indices* (rate of left ventricular pressure development at 40 mm Hg pressure, $[dP/dt]P_{40}$; maximum dP/dt; maximal velocity of contractile element shortening, V_{max}; point of maximum, $dP/dt/P$ or Vpm), and *end-systolic indices* (pressure–volume or pressure–length relationship at end-systole). Many of these measurements are complicated and affected by preload or afterload as noted in Table 31-7.

Starling (Ventricular Function) Curve

If the cardiac muscle is stretched, it develops greater contractile tension because of changes in myofibril calcium sensitivity and alterations in the amount of activator calcium. This observation is the basis of Starling's law: "The law of the heart is therefore the same as that of skeletal muscle, namely, that the mechanical energy set free on passage from the resting to the contracted state depends . . . on the length of the muscle fibers."[75] Atrial as well as ventricular muscle obeys Starling's law. Increased preload or initial fiber length increases resting tension, velocity of tension development, and peak tension. An increase in venous return stretches the muscle fibers to increase contractility and improve cardiac output. However, this process occurs only at subnormal filling pressures. In the upright position, ventricular filling pressures decrease to ~4 mm Hg, and the normal heart operates on the ascending limb of the ventricular function curve. Peak ventricular output occurs at filling pressures of ~10 mm Hg in normal humans.[76] Whether the heart can fall

---

Table 31-7. MEASURES OF MYOCARDIAL CONTRACTILITY

Indices	Usefulness
EJECTION PHASE INDICES	
Stroke volume versus EDP	Useful for acute contractility if ventricular function curve obtained
	Afterload-sensitive
Stroke work versus EDP	Not useful for basal contractility
Ejection fraction (EF)	Useful for basal contractility when EDV is known
	Afterload-dependent
Maximum acceleration of aortic blood flow	Afterload-dependent
Mean velocity of circumferential fiber shortening (V_{cf})	Afterload-dependent
	More sensitive for basal contractility than EF
Mean normalized systolic ejection rate	Afterload-dependent
	Less useful than mean V_{cf}
Maximum chamber elastance	Useful for acute contractility changes
	Nonlinear behavior complicates interpretation
ISOVOLUMIC PHASE INDICES	
$dP/dt/P_{40}$ mm Hg pressure	Useful in acute contractility changes
	Not useful for basal contractility
Maximum dP/dt	Dependent on timing of aortic valve opening
V_{pm}	Useful in acute contractility changes
	Most reliable measure for acute contractility changes
	Dependent upon preload/afterload if increased
V_{max}	Not as useful as $dP/dt/P_{40}$
	Decreases with increased preload or afterload
	Useful for basal contractility

P = intraventricular pressure; V = velocity of shortening of contractile elements.
Prepared by C. Lynch with data from Strobeck JE, Sonnenblick EH: Pathophysiology of heart failure: Deficiency in cardiac contraction. In Cohn JN (ed): Drug Treatment in Heart Failure, p 13. Secaucus, NJ, Advanced Therapeutics Communications International, 1988.

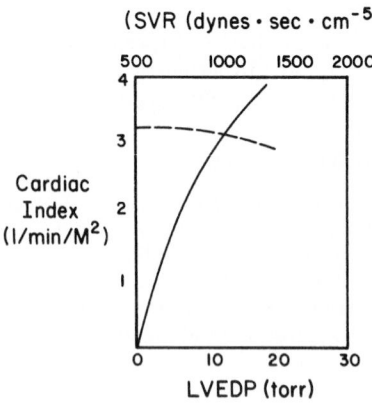

(SVR (dynes · sec · cm^{-5})

Figure 31-15. The ventricular function (Starling) curve of the normal left ventricle (*solid line*) is affected much more by changes in preload (left ventricular end-diastolic pressure) than it is by an increase in afterload (*dotted line*). The failing heart moves to a curve downward and to the right of the normal heart. Venodilator therapy decreases preload without increasing cardiac index (the heart moves to the left on the curve) while reduction of afterload increases cardiac index without a change in preload. Combined preload and afterload reduction decreases filling pressure and increases cardiac index.

onto a descending limb of the length–stroke volume curve like skeletal muscle is unclear.[76] On the descending limb, the heart decompensates and further increases in end-diastolic volume decrease stroke volume, but disengagement of actin and myosin does not occur. In all probability, the heart moves to a different curve.

Ventricular function curves are influenced by afterload, although they incorporate the effects of preload alterations (Fig. 31-15). Starling curves are used clinically when weaning patients from cardiopulmonary bypass, to assess the effects of anesthetic agents on the heart, and to guide fluid and pharmacologic therapy in the perioperative period. The increased stretch and end-diastolic length produced by atrial (atrial kick) or early contracting ventricular fibers (idioventricular kick) increase ventricular stroke volume. Both of these effects are manifestations of Starling's law.

Pressure–Volume Loops

Another index of contractility that is less affected by preload, afterload, or other conditions is the pressure–volume loop, an end-systolic index (Fig. 31-16). At end-systole, ejection ceases, and the aortic valve closes with the ventricle at minimum dimension and volume.

In such loops, the height and width of the loop are determined by the ventricular systolic pressure and stroke volume. The area subtended by the systolic portion of the curve provides a measure of stroke work during ejection, whereas the area of the diastolic limb is a measure of diastolic work performed during ventricular filling and distention. The volume between the systolic and diastolic portions of the loop is the stroke volume. Cardiac work, the product of pressure and volume, is the area of the pressure–volume loop, which is linearly related to myocardial oxygen consumption under various hemodynamic conditions.[77] In a given ventricle, all the end-systolic points are positioned on the same line, which represents the elastance of that ventricle (the change in end-systolic pressure / change in end-systolic volume, although elastance is actually the linear relationship between length and force). Contractility is directly proportional to elastance, with its slope becoming steeper with increased contractility and flatter with decreased contractility. The slope of the end-systolic pressure–volume relation is linear and correlates well with the ejection fraction.[78]

Pressure–volume loops also reveal information about ventric-

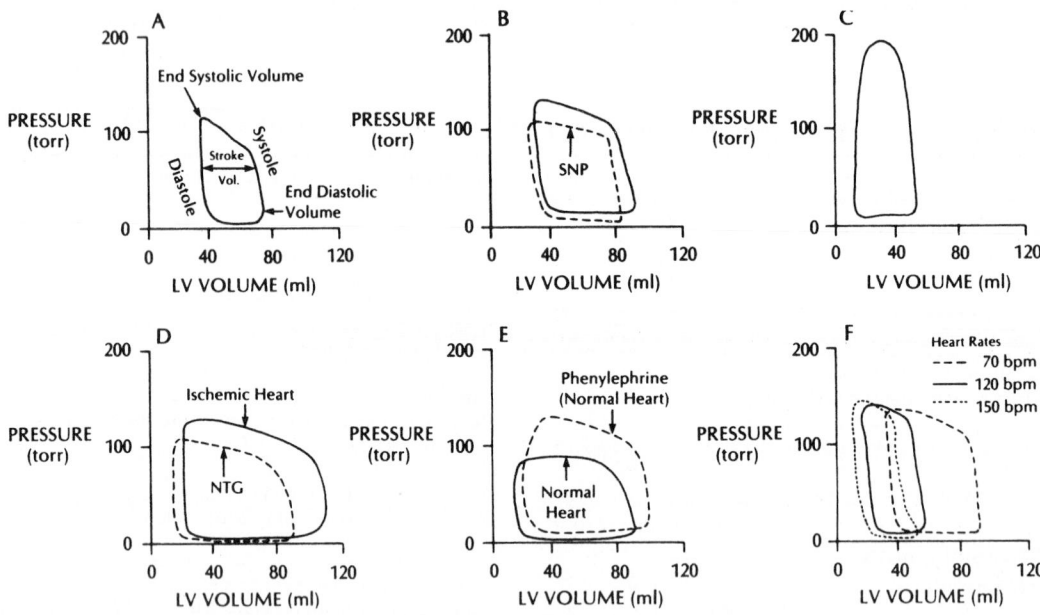

Figure 31-16. Pressure–volume loops. (*A*) The relationship of ventricular pressure and volume over the entire cardiac cycle. The loop begins on the bottom left with opening of the mitral valve and filling of the ventricle to end diastolic volume. When multiple pressure–volume loops are created, the slope of the individual end-systolic pressure–volume relations indicates myocardial contractility. An extension of the bottom portion of the loop (without ventricular systole) would give a diastolic pressure–volume relation for the ventricle. Isovolumetric contraction begins at the lower right portion of the curve with closure of the mitral valve. The aortic valve opens at the upper right portion of the loop and ventricular ejection begins. At the upper left of the loop, the aortic valve closes (end-systolic volume) and isovolumetric relaxation returns the loop to the starting point. Stroke volume is the difference between the volume at the end of diastole and the end of systole. The area of the loop is stroke work. (*B*) The effects of afterload reduction with sodium nitroprusside (SNP) on the pressure–volume loop. (*C*) The changes in the pressure–volume loop in a patient with aortic stenosis with a high peak systolic pressure and steep diastolic slope representing reduced ventricular compliance. (*D*) An ischemic heart has its pressure–volume shifted upward and to the right. (*E*) The effects of increasing the afterload of a normal heart with phenylephrine. (*F*) In a normal heart, an increase in heart rate markedly reduces left ventricular volume. See also Figure 31-17.

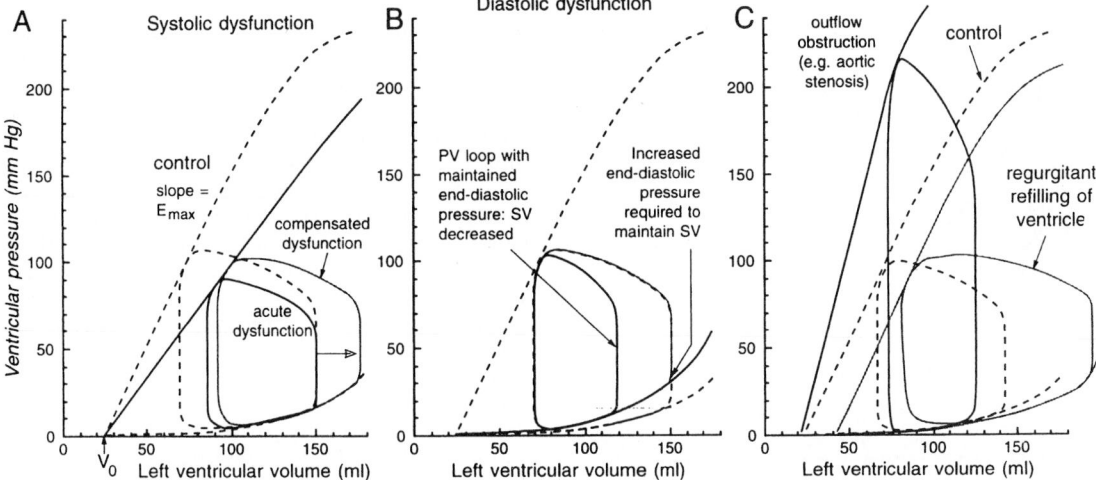

Figure 31-17. (*A*) The ventricular pressure–volume relationship in systolic dysfunction demonstrates depressed E_{max} and decreased stroke volume. With compensation, the stroke volume is restored by an increased end-diastolic volume. (*B*) With diastolic dysfunction, stroke volume is decreased unless end-diastolic pressure increases to maintain it. As in Figure 31-16C, ventricular outflow obstruction usually enhances systolic function because of ventricular hypertrophy, but associated diastolic dysfunction decreases stroke volume while increasing total ventricular work. With regurgitant ventricular filling, a compensatory increase in stroke volume occurs. (Reprinted with permission from Lynch C, Lake CL: Cardiovascular anatomy and physiology. In Youngberg J, Lake C, Roizen M *et al* (eds): Cardiac, Vascular, and Thoracic Anesthesia, p 119. Philadelphia, Churchill Livingstone, 2000.)

ular compliance. Compliance actually changes during each contraction. The normal relationship between diastolic pressure and volume is curvilinear. There is a relatively gentle slope at low end-diastolic pressures (*e.g.*, little change in pressure for large changes in volume). At end-diastolic pressures at the upper limits of normal ($\geq$ 12 mm Hg), the curve becomes steeper, and pressure is almost exponentially related to end-diastolic volume. Ventricular compliance decreases under such conditions. The ventricular end-systolic pressure/volume relationship may be dependent on the type of loading intervention but can be used to assess left ventricular performance under various conditions.[79] (Figs. 31-16 and 31-17). However, one limitation of pressure–volume loops is that pressure may inaccurately reflect end-systolic afterload. The ratio of pressure to volume at end-systole can also be used as an index of contractile function. However, this assumes that at higher pressures there are larger volumes at a given inotropic state.

Pressure–Length Loops

Measurement of a pressure–length loop is a reproducible and sensitive method to evaluate total or regional systolic and diastolic myocardial function. However, it requires direct measurement of changes in myocardial length and intraventricular pressure. Ventricular segment length is plotted on the *x*-axis and ventricular pressure on the *y*-axis (Fig. 31-18). Normal loops are rectangular and include four segments: isovolumic contraction (*right*), ejection (*top*), isovolumic relaxation (*left*), and filling (*bottom*). The area of the loop represents ventricular stroke work.[80] Pressure–length loops are altered by changes in preload, afterload, inotropic state, and ischemia. Ischemia increases postsystolic shortening and systolic lengthening, as depicted in Figure 31-18 (*inset*).[81]

Force–Velocity Curve

Myocardial contractility can also increase when the myocardial fibers increase their developed force or velocity of shortening without a change in fiber length. Force–velocity curves evaluate contractility (velocity of shortening) at constant fiber length in a passively stretched muscle (preloaded), which is stimulated to contract against either no load or an afterload. Force–velocity curves are much more sensitive indicators of contractility than

Starling curves and are based on the Hill model of isolated muscle.

As afterload is increased, the initial rate of shortening follows a hyperbolic relationship (Fig. 31-19). The force or tension developed during contraction is measured by dP/dt_{max}, the maximum rate of rise of intraventricular pressure during the isometric phase of ventricular contraction. The point of the curve where no shortening occurs, although the muscle develops maximal force, is termed P_0. Extrapolation of the curve back to zero load where the maximal velocity of shortening occurs is termed V_{max}. Both preload and afterload affect dP/dt_{max}. As preload increases, the maximum isometric tension that the muscle develops increases, but the maximal velocity of shortening is unchanged. An increase in myocardial contractility increases both the developed tension and the maximum velocity of shortening, shifting the force–velocity curve upward and to the right.

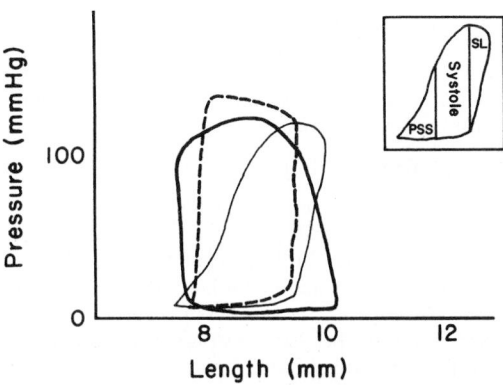

Figure 31-18. The normal pressure–length loop (*thick black line*) is a rectangle whose area indicates total ventricular work. Ischemia (*thin solid line*) causes the loop to lean toward the right because of increased systolic lengthening and postsystolic shortening (*inset*). Increased afterload (*dotted line*) causes the loop to become taller at a similar preload. (Reprinted with permission from Lake CL (ed): Clinical Monitoring for Anesthesia and Critical Care. Philadelphia, WB Saunders, 1994.)

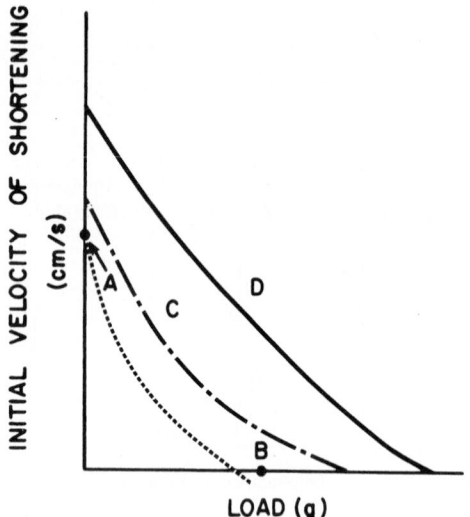

Figure 31-19. A force velocity curve of cardiac muscle shows the point of maximal shortening with no load or V_{max} (point A). Point B is P_0 where no shortening occurs although tension development is maximal. Curve C is a force–velocity curve with increased preload. Curve D demonstrates increased myocardial contractility. On any curve, load (afterload) increases from left to right. (Reprinted with permission from Lake CL: Cardiovascular Anesthesia, p 10. New York, Springer-Verlag, 1985.)

Preload Recruitable Stroke Work (PRSW)

Stroke work is linearly related to left ventricular end-diastolic volume. A plot of end-diastolic volume against stroke work demonstrates that stroke work increases with increased preload and decreases with unloading. Thus, the PRSW is determined by plotting stroke work from successive pressure–volume loops during alterations in preload.

Cardiac Work

Because of the difficulties in obtaining the data for pressure–volume loops or force–velocity curves under clinical conditions, cardiac work is often measured as a substitute. Cardiac work describes pump function in terms of the load carried and the distance moved. Calculation of cardiac work standardized to body surface area (left and right ventricular stroke work indexes) is shown in Table 31-4. Using cardiac work instead of cardiac output or stroke volume to describe pump function has several advantages: (1) calculation includes heart rate, preload, and afterload—the major variables affecting cardiac function; (2) the stroke work index defines the area of the pressure–volume loop; and (3) the stroke work index measures both systolic and diastolic performance.[82]

Right Ventricular Function

The functional significance of the RV in normal circulatory homeostasis is minimal. Although the right ventricular spiral muscles contract during systole, direct left ventricular assistance to right ventricular contraction has been demonstrated.[83] Compared to the LV, intraventricular pressure develops more gradually in the RV and declines more slowly during diastole. Right ventricular pumping capability depends on (1) pressure against which it ejects, (2) filling volume, and (3) right ventricular contractility.[84] The RV obeys Starling's law except that its curve is upward and to the left of the left ventricular curve. At higher end-diastolic pressures, the RV response is flatter than that of the LV. Increases in filling volume increase right ventricular stroke volume up to the limit imposed by the restraint of the pericardium (normally, ~20% acute increase in cardiac volume).[85] The contractility of the RV depends upon sympathetic

tone, myocardial structural integrity, and the chemical content of the coronary perfusate.[84] Normal right ventricular systolic pressures are only 30–40 mm Hg because the recruitable vasculature of the pulmonary circulation allows between 5 and 20 l of blood to flow within it. Peak ejection occurs later than in the LV and the ejection fraction is only 0.4. This difference in function results because the right ventricular free wall is flattened by the pull of the interventricular septum toward the LV during systole, giving a bellows-like action for expulsion of blood.[85] Because of this mechanism, right ventricular function is less likely to be impaired during right coronary arterial occlusion.[85]

During systole, right ventricular stroke volume is more sensitive to afterload than left ventricular stroke volume. Factors that oppose blood flow from the RV (afterload) include the resistance of the pulmonary vascular bed, pulmonary arterial impedance, the mass of the pulmonary blood, blood viscosity, and pulse wave reflection altering pulmonary artery pressure. In diastole the RV is twice as distensible (more compliant) as the LV.[84]

Under conditions of pressure overload, such as increased pulmonary vascular resistance or left ventricular failure, the RV hypertrophies to generate systemic pressures. Although acute right ventricular failure is compatible with life, the symptoms caused by increased venous pressure suggest that right ventricular function is important for maintenance of normal venous pressures.[85]

Ventricular Interdependence

Because the ventricles are anatomically associated, alterations of volume and pressure in one ventricle affect these parameters in the other.[86] During normal respiration with negative intrathoracic pressure, increased venous return increases right ventricular end-diastolic volume during inspiration, pulmonary vascular capacitance increases, left ventricular diastolic volume decreases, and left ventricular stroke volume increases but left ventricular transmural pressure is unchanged. Important factors in ventricular interdependence are septal position and deformability, pulmonary venous capacitance, right ventricular distensibility, the trans-septal pressure gradient, and the presence of the pericardium.

In vitro experimental animal models confirm that when left ventricular pressure increases, diastolic compliance and systolic ventricular function decrease in the RV and *vice versa*. The mechanisms are (1) the Frank–Starling effect caused by decreased ventricular diastolic volume and (2) decreased systolic ventricular function.[87] The etiology of the depressed systolic function is unclear.[87] Computer models confirm that hypertrophy from right ventricular pressure overload, which increases septal thickness and decreases septal compliance, decreases transfer of pressure and volume between the ventricles, limiting ventricular interdependence.

Myocardial Metabolism

An understanding of myocardial metabolism is essential to the preservation of the heart during conditions of stress, cardiac arrest, or elective asystole during cardiac surgery. Metabolism includes both substrate utilization and oxygen consumption.

Sources of Energy

The energy supply of the heart is derived primarily from lactate and fatty acids delivered by the coronary blood. Free or nonesterified fatty acids (palmitic and oleic acids) are the preferred fuel. Myocardial uptake of fatty acids is almost linear, with the plasma concentration above the threshold of 345 μmol $\cdot$ l^{-1}.[88] Fatty acid uptake by the heart from either fatty acid–albumin complexes or lipoprotein triglyceride occurs by passive diffusion or carrier-mediated transport. During fasting, free fatty acids are always used as fuel. The heart has a limited ability to synthesize fatty acids from acetyl coenzyme A, except for the formation of structural lipids. The oxidation of fatty acids and ketone bodies inhibits uptake of glucose, pyruvate oxidation, and glycolysis while facilitating glycogen synthesis.[88] Oxidation of nonesterified fatty acids accounts for 90% of myocardial oxygen consumption.

Fuel selection by the heart probably depends on regulatory enzymes controlled by factors other than substrate availability and product removal. Myocardial lactate utilization is regulated by the arterial lactate concentrations and pyruvate oxidation in the Krebs tricarboxylic acid cycle. Glucose, pyruvate, acetate, and triglycerides can also be used by the heart as energy sources. Utilization of glucose by the myocardium depends on the arterial glucose and insulin concentrations. Glucose is normally used postprandially. However, glucose use by the myocardium as the primary energy source occurs only with high glucose levels, insulin secretion, or hypoxia. Glucose is the only substrate used by the heart anaerobically. As long as the entry of acetyl coenzyme A into the Krebs cycle is not inhibited, the heart will use as much pyruvate as it is given. Substrates such as fructose, glycogen, or proteins are used for energy only during special circumstances, such as starvation, diabetic ketoacidosis, or anoxia.

Myocardial Oxygen Consumption

The heart has one of the highest metabolic rates of any organ. At rest it uses 8–10 ml of oxygen per 100 g of myocardium per minute. The subendocardium requires about 20% more oxygen than the epicardium. Myocardial oxygen consumption (MVo_2) is determined by heart rate, wall tension, and myocardial contractility. The relative importance of each of these factors is difficult to evaluate because they are interrelated through wall tension.[89] Less important factors include the oxygen costs of shortening of muscle fibers, electrical activation, and catecholamines as well as the basal oxygen requirements and the level of arterial oxygenation. Tension development constitutes about 50% of MVo_2 (Table 31-8).

Myocardial wall tension is related to the tension–time index, left ventricular end-diastolic pressure, and ventricular size. Wall tension can be divided into its components: the rate of force development, the magnitude of force development, the interval during which force is generated and maintained for each contraction, and the frequency with which force is developed per unit time.[89] Wall tension is measured according to Laplace's law:

$$T = Pr/2h$$

where radius (r) is cardiac radius, T is cardiac tension, P is interventricular pressure, and h is ventricular muscle thickness. Increases in ventricular chamber pressure or volume increase both the magnitude of force development and the force maintained during ejection.

Table 31-8. FACTORS INVOLVED IN MYOCARDIAL OXYGEN SUPPLY AND DEMAND

MYOCARDIAL OXYGEN CONSUMPTION (DEMAND)
Heart rate
Contractile state
Myocardial wall tension
Arterial oxygen content
Basal oxygen requirements
Oxygen cost of muscle fiber shortening
Oxygen cost of electrical activation

MYOCARDIAL OXYGEN SUPPLY
Aortic diastolic pressure
Left ventricular end-diastolic pressure
Coronary artery diameter
Arterial oxygen content

Myocardial Supply–Demand Ratio

A balance must always exist between oxygen consumption (demand) and myocardial oxygen supply if ischemia is to be avoided. Factors important to this relationship are shown in Table 31-8. Myocardial oxygen supply is dependent upon the diameter of the coronary arteries, left ventricular end-diastolic pressure, aortic diastolic pressure, and arterial oxygen content. In the normal heart, the coronary perfusion pressure is the difference between the aortic diastolic pressure and the left ventricular end-diastolic pressure. Myocardial blood flow is determined by the blood pressure at the coronary ostia, arteriolar tone, intramyocardial pressure or extravascular resistance, coronary occlusive disease, heart rate, coronary collateral development, and blood viscosity.

Myocardial blood flow is reduced by a low aortic diastolic pressure, increased pulmonary wedge pressure (both of which increase subendocardial tissue pressure), and tachycardia, which shortens diastole, reducing the duration of blood flow. Increasing preload or intracavitary pressure increases wall tension and oxygen demand while decreasing subendocardial perfusion.

Myocardial oxygen supply is also affected by the level of arterial oxygenation. Oxygen content resulting from Pao_2, hemoglobin, 2,3-diphosphoglycerate (DPG), and pH, Pco_2, or temperature effects on the oxyhemoglobin dissociation curve can be an important factor in patients with obstructive lung disease or severe anemia. Normal oxygen extraction by the heart is 60–70% and changes very little with increased cardiac work because coronary vascular resistance decreases. However, if the coronary vascular resistance response is limited, oxygen extraction can be increased to more than 90%.[89] An increase in oxygen extraction and coronary vasodilation constitutes the metabolic reserve of the heart in the case of increased demand.

Heart rate and diastolic ventricular volume are the two factors most likely to produce ischemia if either or both are increased. Increased myocardial contractility or afterload, by increasing arterial pressure and myocardial oxygen supply, offsets their tendency to increase myocardial oxygen consumption.

Distribution of Cardiac Output

The cardiac output is distributed to the systemic circulation as follows: brain 12%, heart 4%, liver 24%, kidneys 20%, muscle 23%, skin 6%, and intestines 8%. About 15% of the blood volume remains in the heart and pulmonary circulation, with the remainder in the systemic circulation. Of the blood in the systemic circulation, about 64% is in the veins. The total tissue blood flow in a given vascular bed is a function of the effective perfusion pressure and vascular resistance. Effective perfusion pressure is the difference between arterial and venous pressure across the vascular bed. Autoregulation maintains a constant blood flow in the face of changes in perfusion pressure in the cerebral, renal, coronary, hepatic arterial, intestinal, and muscle circulations. Reflexes that alter circulatory distribution are in Table 31-9.[90–97] The carotid sinus, a dilated portion of the common carotid artery just before its bifurcation, contains two types of receptors that sense pressure in the carotid sinus, providing the most important aspect of reflex circulatory control.

Peripheral Circulatory Physiology

The peripheral circulation consists of resistance and capacitance vessels. The majority of the resistance is in the arterial circulation, which consists of the Windkessel vessels, the precapillary resistance vessels, and the capillary exchange vessels. The Windkessel vessels are distensible elastic arteries such as the aorta and large muscular arteries that damp the pulsatile output of the ventricle. The arterioles, the precapillary resistance vessels, are muscular vessels that provide more than 60% of the

Table 31-9. CARDIOVASCULAR REFLEXES

REFLEX-CAROTID SINUS (PRESSORECEPTOR, BARORECEPTOR)[90,91]

Anatomy:	Carotid-afferent nerve of Hering (glossopharyngeal)
	Aortic-vagus
	Cardiovascular centers in medulla
Stimulus:	Increased blood pressure
Response:	Inhibition of sympathetic and increase in parasympathetic activity, causing decreased cardiac contractility, heart rate, and vasoconstrictor tone
Other:	Gain determined by pulse pressure
	Reduces arterial pressure fluctuation to one third of expected threshold 60 torr, limits 175–300 torr

REFLEX-VALSALVA MANEUVER

Anatomy:	Same as pressoreceptor reflex
Stimulus:	Forced expiration against closed glottis
Response:	Increased venous pressure in head, upper extremities, with decreased right heart venous return causing decreased blood pressure and cardiac output and reflex increase in heart rate
Other:	Glottic opening increases venous return to right heart, resulting in forceful right and then left ventricular contraction, followed by transient bradycardia

REFLEX-MÜLLER MANEUVER

Anatomy:	Decreased pleural pressure increasing left ventricular volume through afterload reduction
Stimulus:	Inspiratory effort against a closed airway
Response:	Right ventricular end-diastolic volume and left ventricular end-diastolic pressure increase, while left ventricular end-diastolic volume is unchanged or decreased, and ejection fraction is unchanged
Other:	Net effect on left ventricular function depends on ventricular interdependence, heart rate, and contractility (position of the heart on diastolic pressure–volume curve)
	Müller maneuver may cause ventricular akinesis due to increased wall stress, increasing myocardial oxygen demand, or increased left ventricular transmural pressure, decreasing motion in nonfunctional ventricular myocardium

REFLEX-BEZOLD–JARISCH[93–95]

Anatomy:	Left ventricular mechanoreceptors with afferent pathway in nonmyelinated vagal C fibers
Stimulus:	Noxious stimuli to the ventricular wall
Response:	Hypotension, bradycardia, and parasympathetically induced coronary vasodilation
Other:	Reperfusion of previously ischemic tissue elicits reflex

REFLEX-CARDIOGENIC HYPERTENSIVE CHEMOREFLEX[96]

Anatomy:	Chemoreceptors located between the aorta and pulmonary artery and supplied by the left coronary artery
	Afferent reflex pathway is intrathoracic vagal branches and the efferent path is via phrenic, vagal, and sympathetic routes
Stimulus:	Serotonin
Response:	Arterial pressure increases markedly in 4–6 sec owing to increased inotropy and peripheral vasoconstriction
Other:	Reflex may be responsible for hypertension during angina, myocardial infarction, and after coronary bypass grafting and is abolished by vagotomy, atropine, or local anesthesia of the intertruncal space

REFLEX-CUSHING'S REFLEX

Anatomy:	Increased cerebrospinal fluid (CSF) pressure compresses cerebral arteries
Stimulus:	Cerebral ischemia secondary to increased CSF pressure
Response:	An increase in arterial pressure sufficient to reperfuse the brain
	Intense sympathetic activity causes severe peripheral vasoconstricion as a result of this reflex

REFLEX-BAINBRIDGE ATRIAL REFLEX[39,97]

Anatomy:	Primarily mediated through vagal myelinated afferent fibers; activation of sympathetic afferent fibers may also occur[39]
	Increased right atrial pressure directly stretches the SA node and enhances its automaticity, increasing the heart rate
Stimulus:	Increased vagal tone and distention of the right atrium or central veins
Response:	Depends upon the pre-existing heart rate
	With pre-existing tachycardia, there is no effect
	Volume loading at a slow heart rate causes progressive tachycardia
	Global atrial distention in response to high pressures causes bradycardia, hypotension, and decreased systemic vascular resistance
Other:	Experimental distention of the cavoatrial junctions or other small portions of the atria increases heart rate, but clinical conditions such as heart failure usually do not produce such locally increased atrial pressure[97]

REFLEX-CHEMORECEPTOR

Anatomy:	Carotid and aortic bodies chemoreceptors whose nerve fibers pass through the nerve of Hering and the vagus nerve to the medullary vasomotor centers
Stimulus:	Decreasing oxygen tension or increased hydrogen ion concentrations
Response:	Increased pulmonary ventilation and blood pressure with decreased heart rate (carotid body chemoreceptors)
	Stimulation of the aortic bodies causes tachycardia
Other:	Normally, the peripheral chemoreceptors are minimally active

REFLEX-OCULOCARDIAC

Anatomy:	Afferent fibers run with the short or long ciliary nerves to the ciliary ganglion and then with the ophthalmic division of the trigeminal nerve to the gasserian ganglion
Stimulus:	Traction on the extraocular muscles (more especially the medial rather than the lateral rectus) or pressure on the globe
Response:	Bradycardia and hypotension as a consequence of this reflex
Other:	Demonstrated in 30–90% of patients undergoing ophthalmic surgery and attenuated by intravenous atropine

(continued)

Table 31-9. CARDIOVASCULAR REFLEXES (*continued*)

REFLEX-CELIAC (VAGOVAGAL)

Anatomy: Vagal stimulation via mesenteric traction, rectal distention, traction on gallbladder, respiratory tract receptors
Response: Bradycardia, apnea, hypotension with narrowed pulse pressure
Other: Traction on the mesentery or gallbladder, stimulation of vagal nerve fibers in the respiratory tract, or rectal distention stimulates afferent vagal nerve endings to cause bradycardia, apnea, and hypotension (vagovagal reflex)
              Manipulation around the celiac plexus decreases systolic pressure, narrows pulse pressure, and slightly decreases heart rate

peripheral resistance. At the most distal portion of the terminal arterioles are precapillary sphincters that regulate the flow of blood into specific capillary beds. The capillary exchange vessels contribute about one fourth of the total peripheral resistance, although most capillaries consist of a single endothelial cell layer without any surrounding smooth muscle. The systemic veins are the capacitance system.

Arterial Pulses and Blood Pressure

Arterial Pulse

The arterial pulse is a wave of vascular distention resulting from the impact of the stroke volume of each beat being ejected into a closed system. The wave of distention begins at the base of the aorta and passes over the entire arterial system with each heart beat. The pulse is not caused by the passage of the blood itself. The pulse waveform is the result of the combined effects of the forward-propagating pressure wave and its reflectance back toward the heart from various parts of the vasculature. Wave reflection may occur in high-resistance arterioles, branching points, or sites of changes in arterial distensibility, but the major source is the arteriole.[98] The velocity of the pulse wave depends on the elasticity of the vessel. The pulse wave velocity is most rapid in the least distensible arteries. In the aortic arch, the pulse wave travels 3–5 m · sec^{-1}, and the aortic pulse waveform precedes the brachial waveform by about 0.05 sec. In large distensible arteries such as the subclavian, the pulse wave travels 7–10 m · sec^{-1}, whereas in the small nondistensible peripheral arteries it travels about 15–30 m · sec^{-1}. Such differences become important when timing the counterpulsation of an intra-aortic balloon.

The arterial pressure waveform changes as it moves peripherally (Fig. 31-20). In central aortic waveforms, the closure of the aortic valve is indicated by a notch or incisura on the descending limb. By contrast, peripheral pulse waveforms have a greater amplitude, more pronounced diastolic wave, and lower mean pressure, and the foot of the wave is delayed.[98] The dicrotic notch, corresponding to the incisura, is more prominent. Systolic pressure is higher, whereas mean and diastolic pressures are slightly lower in the periphery. Such changes are best explained by a tubular model of the vascular system. In such a system, the contour of the pressure wave depends on the velocity of the pressure wave, the duration of the pulse, and the length of the tube.[98]

Pulse contour also changes with hemodynamic conditions. In children, wave reflection facilitates cardiac performance by a relative decrease in arterial pressure during systole and a relative increase during diastole. As aging occurs, wave reflection occurs earlier in the cardiac cycle, increasing systolic pressure and decreasing diastolic pressure. In shock, the pulse wave velocity is reduced by hypotension, increased heart rate reduces the duration of cardiac systole, and peripheral vasoconstriction increases the peripheral reflection coefficient. Pulse waveforms vary in atrial fibrillation, beats with short systolic durations demonstrating diastolic waves and those with long durations having accentuated systolic peaks. Patients with hypertrophic cardiomyopathy have double systolic pulse waveforms because the initial systolic wave of ventricular ejection occurs during the first half of systole and the reflected wave returns during the same systole.[98]

Blood Pressure

Arterial pressure is the lateral pressure exerted by the contained blood on the walls of the vessels. Mean arterial pressure is the product of the cardiac output and the systemic vascular resistance. If a normal arterial waveform is present, mean pressure is about one third the difference between the systolic and diastolic pressures. However, mean pressure remains constant, whereas pulse pressure and systolic pressure increase as blood moves peripherally in the circulation.

Arterial pressure varies with the respiratory cycle. It normally decreases 6 mm Hg or less during inspiration because pulmonary venous capacitance increases during inspiration to a greater extent than the increase in right-sided heart venous return and output, thus causing a decrease in left ventricular stroke output and pressure. These changes are exaggerated in pericardial tamponade, causing pulsus paradoxus. Clinically, pulsus paradoxus is measured by auscultation of the blood pressure until the first heart sound is heard intermittently. Further deflation of the cuff to the pressure where all beats are heard yields the difference known as the paradoxical pulse.

Factors Controlling Peripheral Vascular Tone

Factors controlling blood pressure include central and autonomic nervous function, cardiac output, peripheral vascular resistance, and hormonal mechanisms including antidiuretic hormone, catecholamines, the renin–angiotensin system, and atrial natriuretic peptide.[99] Three medullary centers—the nucleus tractus solitarius, the caudal ventrolateral medulla, and the

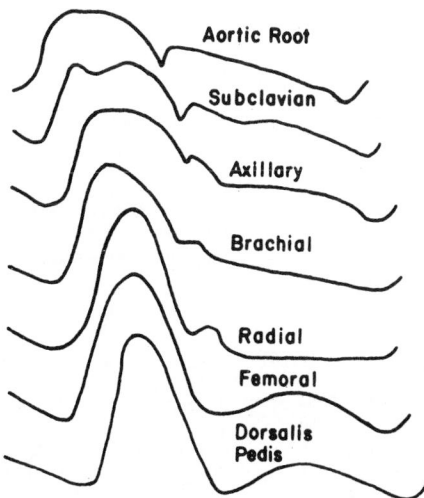

Figure 31-20. The change in the pulse waveform as it moves from the aortic root to the dorsalis pedia artery is dramatic. These changes result from both forward wave propagation and wave reflection at branch points in the circulation. The waveform has a greater amplitude, higher systolic pressure, lower diastolic pressure, and reduced mean pressure in the peripheral circulation. (Reprinted with permission from Bedford RF: Invasive blood pressure monitoring. In Blitt CD (ed): Monitoring in Anesthesia and Critical Care Medicine, p 100. New York, Churchill Livingstone, 1995.)

rostal ventrolateral medulla—are important in blood pressure control. Arteriolar tone is regulated by intrinsic and extrinsic mechanisms. The intrinsic mechanism is the inherent myotonic activity of vascular smooth muscle cells and vascular endothelial cells. Extrinsic factors include neural (sympathetic) and humoral factors. Sympathetic neural activity provides rapid alteration of tone in response to a need for greater blood flow. Figure 31-21 details the intracellular mechanisms for peripheral vasodilation and vasoconstriction. Nitric oxide and prostacyclin production and endothelin release from endothelial cells will produce vasodilation and vasoconstriction, respectively, in vascular smooth muscle cells.

Humoral factors such as endothelial-derived relaxing factor, antidiuretic hormones, or atrial natriuretic factors are less important in overall circulatory regulation.

Endothelium-Derived Relaxing Factor

Nitric oxide (NO), the endothelium-derived relaxing factor (EDRF), is a short-lived substance that activates soluble guanylate cyclase to increase intracellular cyclic guanosine 3',5'-monophosphate, causing relaxation of vascular smooth muscle. It is formed from L-arginine by the enzyme nitric oxide synthase (NOS) in various mammalian tissues, particularly vascular endothelium (Fig. 31-22). NOS is activated when intracellular calcium increases as a result of extracellular calcium entry or intracellular calcium release. Basal release of EDRF occurs in all except cerebral and coronary vessels. Atherosclerosis impairs endothelium-dependent relaxation. Decreased production of EDRF may also contribute to both systemic and pulmonary hypertension. Hypoxia impairs endothelium-dependent vasodilation owing to inhibition of EDRF production and decreased

half-life.[100] Endothelium-derived relaxing factor also inhibits platelet adhesion and aggregation.

Natriuretic Peptides

Atrial natriuretic peptide (ANP) is a peptide stored in the perinuclear granules of human atrial myocytes and to a lesser extent in the ventricle.[101] Brain or B-type natriuretic peptide (BNP) is also produced in primarily in atrium, while natriuretic peptide C is localized in the central nervous system. Natriuretic peptide receptors A, B, and C are receptor guanylyl cyclases, consisting of intracellular and extracellular domains. Atrial natriuretic peptide is released in response to increased vascular volume (atrial distention), epinephrine, vasopressin, morphine, and increased atrial pressure.[101] Normal circulating plasma levels are $25-100\ \mu g \cdot ml^{-1}$.[102]

The primary effects of ANP are direct peripheral vasodilation, suppression of antidiuretic hormone (ADH) release when the ADH is elevated by hemorrhage or dehydration, inhibition of aldosterone release, and direct renal effects such as increased glomerular filtration, natriuresis, and diuresis. Factors such as renal perfusion pressure and renal sympathetic nerve activity in conjunction with physiologic plasma concentrations of ANF produce natriuresis.[103] Kaliuresis does not occur. Atrial natriuretic factor affects not only blood pressure (by decreasing cardiac output and vascular resistance) but also water and electrolyte balance and blood volume. It has no direct inotropic or chronotropic properties.

Renin–Angiotensin System

Renin is a proteolytic enzyme produced in the granular juxtaglomerular cells of the kidney. Its release is governed by the

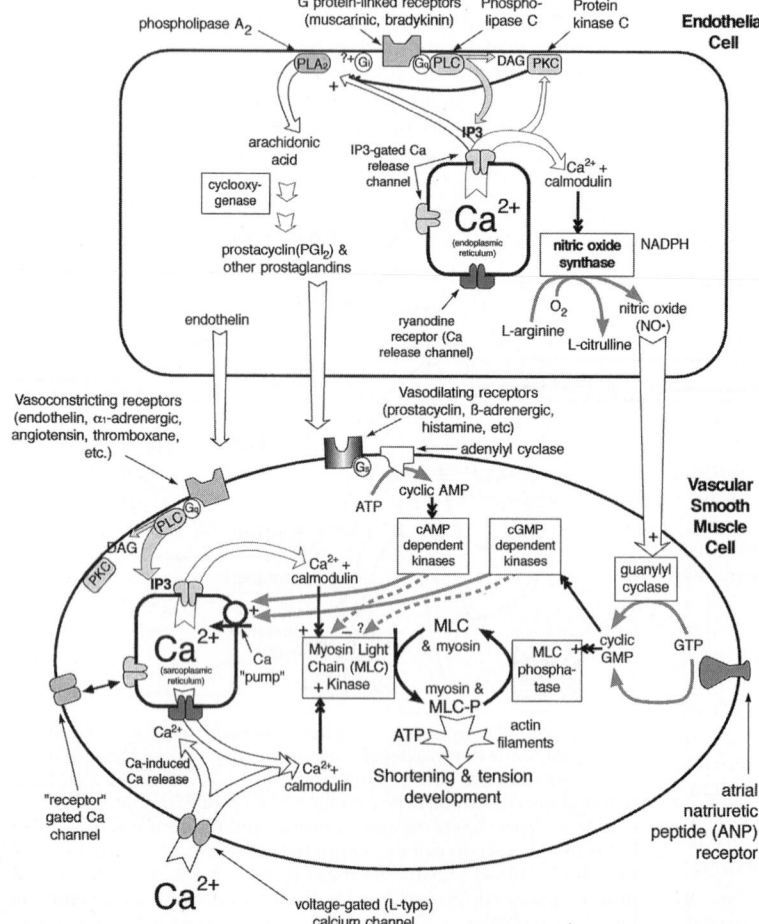

Figure 31-21. Vascular smooth muscle and endothelial function. Both endothelial cells and vascular smooth muscle cells have intracellular stores of calcium which can be released by the production of inositol triphosphate (IP₃). In both types of cells, agonist binding to specific receptors results in activation of phospholipase C (PLC) via guanine protein Gq (α). In the vascular smooth muscle cell, PLC activation results in IP₃ formation and release of intracellular calcium. Calcium binds to calmodulin, activating myosin light chain kinase (MLC), which then phosphorylates, causing myosin to interact with actin, producing shortening or tension generation. In contrast, in the endothelial cell, calcium binds to calmodulin to activate nitric oxide synthase, producing nitric oxide. Nitric oxide can diffuse to the vascular smooth muscle and modulate its behavior via activation of guanylate cyclase. Phospholipase A can be activated by G protein–linked pathways or by phosphokinase C and calcium, resulting in production of arachidonic acid. Arachidonic acid generates prostacyclin via the cyclooxygenase system, allowing relaxation of vascular smooth muscle. (Reprinted with permission from Lynch C, Lake CL: Cardiovascular anatomy and physiology. In Youngberg J, Lake C, Roizen M *et al* (eds): Cardiac, Vascular, and Thoracic Anesthesia, p 126. Philadelphia, Churchill Livingstone, 2000.)

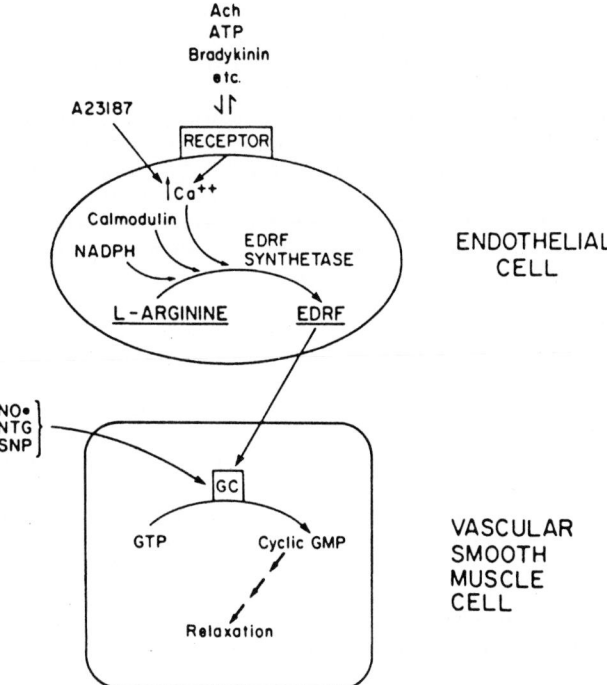

Figure 31-22. Endothelium-derived relaxing factor (EDRF) is produced from L-arginine by a process requiring calcium, calmodulin, nicotinamide adenine dinucleotide phosphate–dependent enzyme (NADPH), and EDRF synthetase. Increases in cytosolic calcium produced by agonists such as the calcium ionophore (A23187) or receptor-mediated agonists (acetylcholine, adenosine triphosphate [ATP], bradykinin) activate EDRF synthetase to produce EDRF. EDRF or other substances such as sodium nitroprusside (SNP), nitroglycerin (NTG), or nitric oxide (NO) produce vascular smooth muscle (VSM) relaxation by activation of adenylate cyclase. (Reprinted with permission from Johns RA: Endothelium-derived relaxing factor: Basic review and clinical implications. J Cardiothorac Vasc Anesth 5:71, 1991.)

macula densa, an intrarenal stretch-type receptor, circulating potassium, angiotensin II, epinephrine, and concentrations of antidiuretic hormone, and by the renal sympathetic nerves. Renin secretion is also inversely related to renal perfusion.[104] The half-life of renin is 4–15 min, during which it initiates the formation of angiotensin I from angiotensinogen, which is synthesized in the liver. Angiotensin I is biologically inactive until it is cleaved by angiotensin-converting enzyme in lung and other tissues to angiotensin II.[105] Angiotensin II and angiotensin III, formed by hydrolysis of angiotensin II, stimulate the secretion of aldosterone and inhibit renin release through a negative-feedback loop. The half-life of angiotensin II is about 30 sec.

Sympathetic Nervous System

Norepinephrine is the important agonist at the α_1 receptor mediating smooth muscle vasoconstriction in arteries and veins independently of neural supply. Epinephrine is more potent as a β_2 receptor agonist than is norepinephrine. β_2 receptors, located in both pre- and postsynaptic regions, dilate arteries by stimulation of adenylcyclase.

Specific Peripheral Circulations

Pulmonary Circulation

The pulmonary circulation is a low-pressure, high-flow system that has five principal functions: (1) metabolic transport of humoral substances and drugs[106]; (2) transport of blood through the lungs; (3) reservoir for the left ventricle; (4) filtration of venous drainage; and (5) transport of gas, fluid, and solutes

across the walls of exchanging vessels. Normally, all circulating blood passes through the pulmonary circulation at least once each minute, but only 500 ml is present at a given time.

Metabolic Transport

The pulmonary vascular endothelium is important for removal, biosynthesis, and release of various vasoactive hormones, including biogenic amines, prostaglandins, leukotrienes, and peptides. Norepinephrine is removed by the lung by a carrier-mediated, temperature- and drug-sensitive transport process. Epinephrine, histamine, vasopressin, and dopamine, however, are unaltered by transpulmonary passage.[106] Almost complete removal of 5-hydroxytryptamine, adenosine triphosphate, and monophosphate occurs in the lungs. Acetylcholine and bradykinin are inactivated by the lungs. Prostaglandins of the E and F series are also removed either by a carrier-mediated, energy-requiring process or by rapid degradation by 15-hydroxyprostaglandin dehydrogenase. Prostacyclin (PGI_2) is not inactivated in the lung. Many drugs such as propranolol, lidocaine, bupivacaine, captopril, and fentanyl are removed extensively during transpulmonary passage.

Intravascular Transport

The passage of blood and its distribution to various segments of the lung depend upon pulmonary blood flow, pulmonary vascular resistance or impedance, left atrial pressure, the transmural distending pressure, and the distensibility of the pulmonary vessel walls. Blood flow to the lung apex is less than that to the base because of regional differences in pulmonary venous, alveolar, and arterial pressures. However, the pulmonary circulation accommodates a large increase in flow with little change in pressure by a substantial decrease in resistance. Pulmonary resistance is about one fifth systemic and pulmonary impedance is about one half systemic; pulse wave reflections are stronger in the pulmonary beds—although the reflecting sites are similar, the vascular bed is smaller. Abundant vascular smooth muscle is present in pulmonary vessels, distributed evenly between arteries and veins. Muscular arterioles are absent in the lung.

Capillary endothelium, endothelial basement membrane, interstitial space, epithelial basement membrane, and alveolar epithelium form the alveolocapillary membrane, which separates the blood and gas phases in the lung. The pulmonary veins perform primarily a reservoir function, preventing pulmonary edema in the event of reduced left ventricular compliance.[107]

Measurements of Pulmonary Tone

Measurements of pulmonary tone are essential to therapeutic investigations. However, the available measurement methods are either difficult or have significant limitations. Normal values for pulmonary vascular resistance are given in Table 31-4.

Pulmonary artery pressures are clinically measured using flow-directed catheters. Wedging of the tip of these catheters in a small branch of the pulmonary artery measures the pulmonary artery wedge pressure or occluded pressure (PAoP) (see Table 31-2). As the pressure of the column of blood from the tip of the catheter (beyond the point of balloon occlusion) equilibrates with left atrial pressure, PAoP is achieved. Normally, left atrial pressure is similar to left ventricular end-diastolic pressure in the absence of mitral valvular stenosis. Other reasons for a PAoP that is greater than left ventricular end-diastolic pressure include increased airway pressures or the presence of an intra-atrial mass. Normally, the PAoP is 1–4 mm Hg lower than pulmonary end-diastolic pressure. However, with tachycardia or increased pulmonary resistance, the pulmonary wedge pressure may be the same or slightly higher than pulmonary end-diastolic pressure.

Pulmonary artery pressure is not linearly related to either flow or left atrial pressure. An increase in pulmonary flow or left atrial pressure is unaccompanied by a proportional increase in pulmonary arterial pressure. Therefore, calculated pulmonary vascular resistance decreases when either pulmonary flow or left atrial pressure increases. The nonlinearity results from distention or recruitment of vessels when flow or pressure increases. However, in Zone 3 of the lung (where left atrial pressure is greater than airway pressure), pulmonary artery pressure is the most important factor determining pulmonary blood flow.[108] Therefore, regardless of the effect on the pulmonary vascular tone, agents or manipulations that change pulmonary flow or left atrial pressure will change calculated pulmonary vascular resistance. Only if a particular intervention does not change pulmonary flow or left atrial pressure, or if the changes in pulmonary resistance can be explained only by active changes in pulmonary tone (e.g., a decrease in pulmonary artery pressure accompanied by an increase in pulmonary blood flow), is pulmonary vascular resistance unchanged. Even in these circumstances, however, reflex effects caused by the drug or maneuver cannot be eliminated.[109]

Another major factor affecting indirect measurements is airway pressure, because the degree of lung inflation and the ventilatory pressure directly influence pulmonary pressure–flow relationships. Either increases or decreases in lung volume beyond normal functional residual capacity increase pulmonary resistance because of compression of small intra-alveolar vessels.

Effects of Drugs and Maneuvers on Pulmonary Tone

Baseline pulmonary tone, stimulation of pulmonary chemoreceptors, autonomic influences, bronchospasm, and other physiologic or nonphysiologic conditions actively or passively affect the pulmonary vasculature or modify its response to drugs. These factors are summarized in Table 31-10.

Alveoli in a poorly ventilated area of lung that contains hypoxic gas cause the precapillary arterial vessels supplying that area to constrict in order to divert blood away from the area.

Table 31-10. ALTERATIONS IN PULMONARY VASCULAR RESISTANCE

Factors	Changes
ACTIVE CHANGES	
Sympathetic stimulation	Increased or unchanged
Parasympathetic stimulation	Unchanged
Catecholamines	Increased
Angiotensin	Increased
Acetylcholine	Decreased
Histamine	Increased/decreased
Bradykinin	Decreased
Serotonin	Increased
Prostaglandin E$_1$	Decreased
Prostaglandin F	Increased
Hypoxia	Increased
Hypercarbia	Increased or unchanged
Acidemia	Increased
PASSIVE CHANGES	
Pulmonary hypertension	Decreased
Left atrial hypertension	Decreased
Increased pulmonary interstitial pressure	Increased
Increased blood viscosity	Increased
Increased pulmonary blood volume	Decreased

Data from Murray JP: The Normal Lung, p 128. Philadelphia, WB Saunders, 1976; Perloff WH: Physiology of the heart and circulation. In Swedlow DB, Raphaely RC (eds): Cardiovascular Problems in Pediatric Critical Care, p 1. New York, Churchill Livingstone, 1986; Stalcup A *et al*: Inhibition of angiotensin-converting enzyme activity in cultured endothelial cells by hypoxia. J Clin Invest 63:966, 1979; Hyman AL *et al*: Autonomic regulation of the pulmonary circulation. J Cardiovasc Pharmacol 7(suppl 3)S80, 1985.

This process is termed hypoxic pulmonary vasoconstriction. Pulmonary hypertension does not occur because the hypoxia is localized. If hypoxia is generalized, pulmonary hypertension ensues.[110] Metabolic acidosis slightly enhances hypoxic pulmonary vasoconstriction, whereas respiratory acidosis has no effect.[111] Metabolic and respiratory alkalosis decreases it.[111] Drugs such as nitroprusside, nitroglycerin, and the inhalation anesthetics decrease hypoxic pulmonary vasoconstriction, resulting in worsening of venous admixture and arterial Po$_2$.[112] However, increased pulmonary artery pressure from whatever mechanism inhibits hypoxic pulmonary vasoconstriction.

Bronchial Circulation

Bronchial flow depends upon the cardiac output and blood pressure and ceases at aortic pressures <40 mm Hg.[113] It is increased by positive airway pressure and increased by hypoxia and hypercarbia.[10] Sympathetic stimulation or epinephrine decreases bronchial flow, whereas parasympathetic or vagal stimulation increases it.[113] Bronchial veins are more responsive to autonomic influences than are bronchial arteries.[113] Histamine also increases bronchial flow, but prostaglandins decrease it.

Renal Circulation

Renal blood flow is well in excess of the amount needed for renal perfusion. It is autoregulated so that glomerular filtration remains relatively constant despite changes in arterial pressure between 70 and 180 mm Hg. Theories proposed to explain renal autoregulation include the juxtaglomerular theory (vasoactive hormonal release from the juxtaglomerular apparatus in response to the quantity or quality of filtrate reaching the macula densa) and the myogenic theory (changes in afferent arteriole tone provide the autoregulation). Of these, the myogenic theory seems most likely.[114]

The main purpose of the excessive renal flow is to provide energy for active renal tubular reabsorption of sodium. Renal oxygen consumption is high, and the arteriovenous oxygen content difference is low. Of the blood delivered to the glomeruli, about 20% is filtered to form an ultrafiltrate of plasma. The main driving force is the glomerular hydrostatic pressure, which is essentially the systemic arterial pressure modified by the renal vasculature. Glomerular capillary pressure, about two thirds of systemic pressure, is increased by dilation of the afferent arteriole or constriction of the efferent arteriole.[114] Renal arteriolar tone is also influenced by sympathetic stimulation, catecholamines, kinins, prostaglandins, and other vasoactive substances. Other factors affecting glomerular filtration include the total surface area available for filtration and the permeability of the glomerular membrane. The ultrafiltrate collects in Bowman's space before passing into the renal tubular system.

Hepatic Circulation

Hepatic arterial flow increases in response to decreased portal venous flow. The mechanisms for this alteration (the arterial "buffer response") include myogenic, metabolic, and neural controls as well as the quantity of the portal venous blood and the washout of some endogenous substance, probably adenosine, generated by hepatic tissue.[115] Portal flow is controlled by preportal arterioles in the splanchnic organs from which the portal vein originates. Precapillary sphincters (presinusoidal) adjust portal flow to maintain an even distribution throughout the liver. The major site of resistance to portal flow is postsinusoidal, regulated by α-sympathetic receptors affecting venous smooth muscle.[115] Normally, the liver contains about 15% of the blood volume. Sympathetic neural activation can mobilize one half of the hepatic blood volume. Like the systemic vasculature, the hepatic arteriole is the major site of resistance.

Physiology of the Venous System

Systemic veins have a conduit and a reservoir function. Since the smallest postcapillary venules lack muscular layers, and venules and small veins have only small amounts of muscle, the postcapillary resistance is usually small. However, postcapillary resistance is important because the ratio of precapillary to postcapillary resistance determines the capillary filtration pressure. The major capacitance vessels include medium and large veins as well as the venae cavae. About 60% of the systemic blood volume is in small veins and venules whose diameters range from 20 μm to 2 mm.[116]

The term *vascular capacitance* is used for the vascular pressure–volume relationship at a given level of venous tone. Venous tone is normally at 70% of maximum in the erect human. Venodilation to accommodate as much as 70–75% of the systemic blood volume buffers sudden increases in arterial blood pressure by allowing sequestration of blood in systemic veins. The compliance of the venous system is regulated by venomotor tone, which is controlled by cerebral autonomic impulses. Sympathetically mediated venoconstriction adds about 1 l of blood to the circulation, but passive constriction from a reduction in venous pressure contributes about two thirds of the total volume mobilized. Individual organs contribute about 30–50% of their blood volume by sympathetically mediated venoconstriction.

Venous return (VR), the rate of flow of blood from the periphery to the heart, is a major determinant of cardiac preload. In a steady state, cardiac output is equal to venous return. It is determined by the pressure gradient from the peripheral vascular beds (P_{MS} or mean systemic pressure) to the right side of the heart (P_{RA}) and the resistance to venous return (R_V).[116,117] This gradient is described by P_{MS}–P_{RA} and the formula for venous return becomes

$$VR = (P_{MS} - P_{RA})/R_V$$

The upstream driving pressure from the peripheral tissue to the right atrium is the mean circulatory filling pressure or mean systemic pressure. The term *mean systemic pressure* should not be confused with *mean arterial pressure*. The mean circulatory filling pressure, which is an equalization of pressures between the venous and arterial beds when flow is 0, is usually about 10 mm Hg, similar to the mean systemic filling pressure. It is increased by catecholamines or increased sympathetic activity.[116] An increase in right atrial pressure decreases the pressure gradient and venous return. The resistance to venous return is primarily determined by large veins, such as the venae cavae and peripheral large and medium-sized veins, which are responsive to autonomic influences or vasoactive mediators. Factors which increase VR include redistribution of blood from vascular beds with low volume and high flows to those with high volume and low flow, polycythemia or conditions increasing blood viscosity, and venous constriction.[117] Cutaneous venous tone is determined by thermoregulatory mechanisms rather than systemic pressure regulatory mechanisms.

Loss of venous tone, as in autonomic neuropathy or during anesthesia, limits the normal compensatory increases in venous tone to changes in posture, positive airway pressure, or decreased blood volume. If these factors are excessive, ventricular preload is adversely affected. Venoconstriction induced by hypovolemia, anxiety, or exercise augments intrathoracic blood volume and preload.

Physiology of the Pericardium

The pericardium has limited but important physiologic functions in the maintenance of biventricular systolic and diastolic function.[118] As dilatation of the left ventricle occurs, intrapericardial pressure limits right ventricular filling and reduces forward flow to the lungs, possibly preventing pulmonary edema. Shifts of the left ventricular diastolic pressure–volume relationship are equal to changes in pericardial pressure and volume. During cardiac tamponade, increased intrapericardial fluid causes hypotension, decreased cardiac output, myocardial ischemia, and tachycardia. However, a vagally mediated depressive reflex is also operative, contributing further to the decreased

cardiac output resulting from the presence of pericardial fluid.[119] Increased intrapericardial pressure results in an underfilled ventricle, which operates on the ascending limb of Starling's curve.

REFERENCES

1. Stumper O, Fraser AG, Anderson RH *et al:* Transesophageal echocardiography in the longitudinal axis: Correlation between anatomy and images and its clinical implications. Br Heart J 64:282, 1990
2. James TN: Anatomy of the crista supraventricularis: Its importance for understanding right ventricular function, right ventricular infarction and related conditions. J Am Coll Cardiol 6:1083, 1985
3. Lam JHS, Ranganathan N, Wigle ED, Silver MD: Morphology of the human mitral valve. I. Chordae tendineae. Circulation 41:449, 1970
4. Byrd BF, Schiller NB, Botvinick EH, Higgins CB: Normal cardiac dimensions by magnetic resonance imaging. Am J Cardiol 55:1440, 1985
5. James TN: Blood supply of the human interventricular septum. Circulation 17:391, 1958
6. Nerantzis CE, Toutouzas P, Avgoustakis D: The importance of the sinus node artery in the blood supply of the atrial myocardium. Acta Cardiol 38:35, 1983
7. James TN: Morphology of the human atrioventricular node, with remarks pertinent to its electrophysiology. Am Heart J 62:756, 1961
8. Fujita M, Sasayama S, Ohno A *et al:* Importance of myocardial ischemia for coronary collateral development in conscious dogs. Int J Cardiol 27:179, 1990
9. Williams GM, Perler BA, Burdick JF *et al:* Angiographic localization of spinal cord blood supply and its relationship to postoperative paraplegia. J Vasc Surg 13:23, 1991
10. Deffebach ME, Charan NB, Lakshminarayan S, Butler J: The bronchial circulation. Am Rev Respir Dis 135:463, 1987
11. Lowe JE, Hartwich T, Takla M, Schaper J: Ultrastructure of electrophysiologically identified human sinoatrial nodes. Basic Res Cardiol 83:401, 1988
12. Bachmann G: The inter-auricular time interval. Am J Physiol 41:309, 1916
13. Brown DL, Guyenet PG: Electrophysiological study of cardiovascular neurons in the rostral ventrolateral medulla in rats. Circ Res 56:359, 1985
14. De Geest H, Levy MN, Zieske H, Lipman RI: Depression of ventricular contractility by stimulation of the vagus nerves. Circ Res 17:222, 1965
15. Stiles GL, Taylor S, Lefkowitz RJ: Human cardiac b adrenergic receptors: Subtype heterogeneity delineated by direct radiological binding. Life Sci 33:467, 1983
16. Spodick DH: The normal and diseased pericardium: Current concepts of pericardial physiology, diagnosis and treatment. J Am Coll Cardiol 1:240, 1983
17. Kennedy JW: Registry Committee of the Society for Cardiac Angiography: Complications associated with cardiac catheterization and angiography. Cathet Cardiovasc Diagn 8:5, 1982
18. Seldinger SI: Catheter replacement of the needle in percutaneous arteriography. Acta Radiol 39:368, 1953
19. Cannon SR, Richards KL, Crawford M: Hydraulic estimation of stenotic orifice area: A correction of the Gorlin formula. Circulation 71:1170, 1985
20. Conti CR: Coronary arteriography. Circulation 55:227, 1977
21. Pagel PS, Grossman W, Haering JM, Warltier DC: Left ventricular diastolic function in the normal and diseased heart. Anesthesiology 79:836, 1993
22. Pagel PS, Grossman W, Haering JM, Warltier DC: Left ventricular diastolic function in the normal and diseased heart. Anesthesiology 79:1104, 1993
23. White CW, Holida MD, Marcus ML: Effects of acute atrial fibrillation on the vasodilator reserve of the canine atrium. Cardiovasc Res 20:683, 1986
24. Robinson TF, Factor SM, Sonnenblick EH: The heart as a suction pump. Sci Am 254:84, 1986
25. Barbier P, Solomon SB, Schiller NB, Glantz SA: Left atrial relaxation and left ventricular systolic function determine left atrial reservoir function. Circulation 100:427, 1999
26. Birnbaumer L, Brown AM: G proteins and the mechanism of

action of hormones, neurotransmitters, and autocrine and paracrine regulatory factors. Am Rev Respir Dis 141:S106, 1990

27. Carmeliet E: Mechanisms and control of repolarization. Eur Heart J 14(suppl H):3, 1993
28. Wendt DJ, Martin JB: Autonomic neural regulation of intact Purkinje system of dogs. Am J Physiol 258:H1420, 1990
29. Coraboeuf E, Weidman S: Temperature effects on the electrical activity of Purkinje fibers. Helv Physiol Pharmacol Acta 12:32, 1954
30. Kohlhardt M, Mnich Z, Maier G: Alteration of the excitation process of the sinoatrial pacemaker cell in the presence of anoxia and metabolic inhibitors. J Mol Cell Cardiol 9:477, 1977
31. Fisch C, Knoebel SB, Feigenbaum H, Greenspan K: Potassium and the monophasic action potential, electrocardiogram, conduction, and arrhythmias. Prog Cardiovasc Dis 8:387, 1966
32. Cinca J, Morja A, Figueras J et al: Circadian variations in the electrical properties of the human heart assessed by sequential bedside electrophysiologic testing. Am Heart J 112:315, 1986
33. Urthaler F, Neely BH, Hageman GR, Smith LR: Differential sympathetic–parasympathetic interactions in sinus node and AV junction. Am J Physiol 250:H43, 1986
34. Hoffman BF, Moore EN, Stuckey JH et al: Functional properties of the atrioventricular conduction system. Circ Res 13:308, 1963
35. Kovacs SJ: The duration of the QT interval as a function of heart rate: A derivation based on physical principles and comparison to measured values. Am Heart J 110:876, 1985
36. de Marneffe M, Jacobs P, Haardt R, Englert M: Variations of normal sinus node function in relation to age: Role of autonomic influence. Eur Heart J 7:662, 1986
37. Evans JM, Randall DC, Funk JN, Knapp CF: Influence of cardiac innervation on intrinsic heart rate in dogs. Am J Physiol 258:H1132, 1990
38. Medak R, Benumof JL: Perioperative management of prolonged Q-T interval syndrome. Br J Anaesth 55:361, 1983
39. Longhurst JC: Cardiac receptors: Their function in health and disease. Prog Cardiovasc Dis 27:201, 1984
40. Wong TM, Lee AY-S, Tai KK: Effects of drugs interacting with opioid receptors during normal perfusion or ischemia and reperfusion in the isolated rat heart. An attempt to identify cardiac opioid receptor subtypes involved in arrhythmogenesis. J Mol Cell Cardiol 22:1167, 1997
41. Lee AY-S: Endogenous opioid peptides and cardiac arrhythmias. Int J Cardiol 27:145, 1990
42. Lynch C, Jaeger JM: The G protein cell signaling system. In Lake CL, Barash PG, Sperry RJ: Advances in Anesthesia, vol 11 p 65. Chicago, Mosby–Year Book, 1994
43. Feigl EO, Neat GW, Huang AH: Interrelations between coronary artery pressure, myocardial metabolism and coronary blood flow. J Mol Cell Cardiol 22:375, 1990
44. White CF, Wilson RF, Marcus ML: Methods of measuring myocardial blood flow in humans. Prog Cardiovasc Dis 31:79, 1988
45. Hoffman JIE: Determinants and prediction of transmural myocardial perfusion. Circulation 58:381, 1978
46. Westerhof N: Physiological hypotheses—intramyocardial pressure. A new concept, suggestions for measurement. Basic Res Cardiol 85:105, 1990
47. Marcus ML, Chilian WM, Kanatsuka H et al: Understanding the coronary circulation through studies at the microvascular level. Circulation 82:1, 1990
48. Rubio P, Berne RM: Regulation of coronary blood flow. Prog Cardiovasc Dis 43:105, 1975
49. Dole WP: Autoregulation of the coronary circulation. Prog Cardiovasc Dis 29:293, 1987
50. Chilian WM, Layne SM: Coronary microvascular responses to reductions in perfusion pressure. Circ Res 66:1227, 1990
51. Trimarco B, Ricciardelli B, Cuocolo A et al: Effects of coronary occlusion on arterial baroreflex control of heart rate and vascular resistance. Am J Physiol 252:H749, 1987
52. Baron JF, Vicaut E, Hou X, Duvelleroy M: Independent role of arterial O2 tension in local control of coronary blood flow. Am J Physiol 258:H1388, 1990
53. Dole WP, Nuno DW: Myocardial oxygen tension determines the degree and pressure range of coronary autoregulation. Circ Res 59:202, 1986
54. Vatner SF: Regulation of coronary resistance vessels and large coronary arteries. Am J Cardiol 56:16E, 1985
55. Samaha FF, Heineman W, Ince C et al: ATP-sensitive potassium channel is essential to maintain basal coronary vascular tone in vivo. Am J Physiol 31:C1220, 1992
56. Narishige T, Egashira K, Akatsuka Y et al: Glibenclamide, a putative ATP-sensitive K+ channel blocker, inhibits coronary autoregulation in anesthetized dogs. Circ Res 73:771, 1993
57. Karmazyn M, Dhalla NS: Physiological and pathophysiological aspects of cardiac prostaglandins. Can J Physiol Pharmacol 61:1207, 1983
58. Marone G, Triggiani M, Cirillo R et al: Chemical mediators and the human heart. Prog Biochem Pharmacol 20:38, 1985
59. Austin RE, Aldea GS, Coggins DL et al: Profound spatial heterogeneity of coronary reserve. Circ Res 67:319, 1990
60. Hoffman JIE: Transmural myocardial perfusion. Prog Cardiovasc Dis 29:429, 1987
61. Dyke CM, Brunsting LA, Salter DR et al: Preload dependence of right ventricular blood flow. I. The normal right ventricle. Ann Thorac Surg 43:478, 1987
62. Vatner SF: a-Adrenergic regulation of the coronary circulation in the conscious dog. Am J Cardiol 52:15A, 1983
63. Shepherd JT, Vanhoutte PM: Mechanisms responsible for coronary vasospasm. J Am Coll Cardiol 8:50A, 1986
64. Goldstein DS, Brush JE, Eisenhofer G et al: In vivo measurement of neuronal uptake of norepinephrine in the human heart. Circulation 78:41, 1988
65. Little RC, Little WC: Cardiac preload, afterload, and heart failure. Arch Intern Med 142:819, 1982
66. Lang RM, Borow KM, Neumann A, Janzen D: Systemic vascular resistance: An unreliable index of left ventricular afterload. Circulation 74:1114, 1986
67. Prewitt RM, Wood LDH: Effect of altered resistive load on left ventricular systolic mechanics in dogs. Anesthesiology 56:195, 1982
68. Schaeffer S, Taylor AL, Lee HR et al: Effect of increasing heart rate on left ventricular performance in patients with normal cardiac function. Am J Cardiol 61:617, 1988
69. Wisenbaugh T, Nissen S, DeMaria A: Mechanics of postextrasystolic potentiation in normal subjects and patients with valvular heart disease. Circulation 74:10, 1986
70. Hathaway DR, March KL, Lash JA et al: Vascular smooth muscle. A review of the molecular basis of contractility. Circulation 83:382, 1991
71. Braunwald E, Sonnenblick EH, Ross J: Contraction of the normal heart. In Braunwald E (ed): Textbook of Cardiovascular Medicine, 2nd ed, p 409. Philadelphia, WB Saunders, 1983
72. Katz AM: Cyclic adenosine monophosphate effects on the myocardium: A man who blows hot and cold with one breath. J Am Coll Cardiol 2:143, 1983
73. Brutsaert DL, Rademakers FE, Sys SU et al: Analysis of relaxation in the evaluation of ventricular function of the heart. Prog Cardiovasc Dis 28:143, 1985
74. Woodworth RS: Maximal contraction, "staircase" contraction, refractory period, and compensatory pause of the heart. Am J Physiol 8:213, 1902
75. Starling EH: The Lineacre lecture on the law of the heart. In Chapman CB, Mitchell JH (eds): Starling on the Heart, p 119. London, Pall Mall, 1965
76. Parker JO, Case RB: Normal left ventricular function. Circulation 60:4, 1979
77. Chung N, Wu X, Bailey KR, Ritman EL: LV pressure–volume area and oxygen consumption. Evaluation in intact dog by fast CT. Am J Physiol 258:H1208, 1990
78. Jacob R, Kissling G: Ventricular pressure–volume relations as the primary basis for evaluation of cardiac mechanics. Return to Frank's diagram. Basic Res Cardiol 84:227, 1989
79. Van der Linden LP, Van der Wilde ET, Bruschke AVG, Baan J: Comparison between force–velocity and end-systolic pressure volume characterization of intrinsic LV function. Am J Physiol 259:H1419, 1990
80. Foex P, Francis CM, Cutfield GR, Leone B: The pressure–length loop. Br J Anaesth 60:65S, 1988
81. Safwat A, Leone BJ, Norris RM, Foex P: Pressure–length loop area: Its components analyzed during graded myocardial ischemia. J Am Coll Cardiol 17:790, 1991
82. Barash PG, Kopriva CJ: Cardiac monitoring. In Thomas SJ, Kramer JL (eds): Manual of Cardiac Anesthesia, 2nd ed, p 23. New York, Churchill Livingstone, 1993
83. Damino RJ, Cox JL, Lowe JE, Santamore WP: Left ventricular

pressure effects on right ventricular pressure and volume outflow. Cathet Cardiovasc Diagn 19:269, 1990

84. Weber KT, Janicki JS, Shroff SG *et al:* The right ventricle: Physiologic and pathophysiologic considerations. Crit Care Med 11:323, 1983

85. Barnard D, Alpert JS: Right ventricular function in health and disease. Curr Prob Cardiol 12:423, 1987

86. Santamore WP, Shaffer T, Papa L: Theoretical model of ventricular interdependence: Pericardial effects. Am J Physiol 259:H181, 1990

87. Maruyama Y, Nunokawa T, Kiowa T *et al:* Mechanical interdependence between the ventricles. Basic Res Cardiol 78:544, 1983

88. Berne RM (ed): Handbook of Physiology. The Cardiovascular System, p 873. Baltimore, Williams & Wilkins, 1979

89. Weber KT, Janicki JS: The metabolic demand and oxygen supply of the heart: Physiologic and clinical considerations. Am J Cardiol 44:722, 1979

90. Shoukas AA: Overall systems analysis of the carotid sinus baroreceptor reflex control of the circulation. Anesthesiology 79:1402, 1993

91. Hering HE: Der karotisdruckversuch. Munch Med Wochenschr 70:1287, 1923

92. Schmidt RM, Kumada M, Sagewa K: Cardiovascular responses to various pulsatile pressures in the carotid sinus. Am J Physiol 223:1, 1972

93. Von Bezold A, Hirt L: Uber die physiologischen wirkungen des essigsauren veratrins. Physiol Lab Wuerzburg Untersuchungen 1:75, 1867

94. Mark AL: The Bezold–Jarisch reflex revisited: Clinical implications of inhibitory reflexes originating in the heart. J Am Coll Cardiol 1:90, 1983

95. Jarisch A, Richter H: Die afferenten bahnen des veratrine effektes in den herznerven. Arch Exp Pathol Pharmacol 193:355, 1939

96. James TN: A cardiogenic hypertensive chemoreflex. Anesth Analg 69:633, 1989

97. Ledsome JR, Linden RJ: A reflex increase in heart rate from distention of the pulmonary vein–atrial junction. J Physiol 170:456, 1964

98. O'Rourke MF, Yaginuma T: Wave reflections and the arterial pulse. Arch Intern Med 144:366, 1984

99. Burnstock G: Integration of factors controlling vascular tone. Anesthesiology 79:1368, 1993

100. Johns RA: Endothelium-derived relaxing factor: Basic review and clinical implications. J Cardiothorac Vasc Anesth 5:69, 1991

101. Ferrari R, Agnoletti G: Atrial natriuretic peptide: Its mechanism of release from the atrium. Int J Cardiol 25:S3, 1989

102. de Bold AJ: Atrial natriuretic factor. A hormone produced by the heart. Science 230:767, 1985

103. Blaine EH: Atrial natriuretic factor plays a significant role in body fluid homeostasis. Hypertension 15:2, 1990

104. Reid IA: The renin–angiotensin system and body function. Arch Intern Med 145:1475, 1985

105. Ryan J, Smith U, Niemeyer R: Angiotensin I: Metabolism by plasma membrane of lung. Science 176:64, 1972

106. Said SI: Metabolic functions of the pulmonary circulation. Circ Res 50:325, 1982

107. Goto M, Arakawa M, Suzuki T *et al:* A quantitative analysis of reservoir function of the human pulmonary "venous" system for the left ventricle. Jpn Circ J 50:222, 1986

108. Thorvaldson J, Ilebekk A, Loraand S, Kiil F: Determinants of pulmonary blood volume. Effects of acute changes in pulmonary vascular pressure and flow. Acta Physiol Scand 121:45, 1984

109. Rich S, Martinez J, Lam W *et al:* Reassessment of the effects of vasodilator drugs in primary pulmonary hypertension. Guidelines for determining a pulmonary vasodilator response. Am Heart J 105:119, 1983

110. Rudolph AM, Yuan S: Response of the pulmonary vasculature to hypoxia and H^+ ion concentration changes. J Clin Invest 45:399, 1966

111. Brimioulle S, Lejeune P, Vachiery J-L *et al:* Effects of acidosis and alkalosis on hypoxic pulmonary vasoconstriction in dogs. Am J Physiol 258:347, 1990

112. Marshall BE, Marshall C: Anesthesia and the pulmonary circulation. In Covino BG, Fozzard HA, Strichartz G (eds): Effects of Anesthesia, p 121. Bethesda, American Physiological Society, 1985

113. Baier H: Functional adaptations of the bronchial circulation. Lung 164:247, 1986

114. Fried TA, Stein JH: Glomerular dynamics. Arch Intern Med 143:787, 1983

115. Kang YG, Gelman S: Liver transplantation. In Gelman S (ed): Organ Transplantation, p 142. Philadelphia, WB Saunders, 1987

116. Rothe CF: Physiology of venous return. Arch Intern Med 146:977, 1986

117. Jacobsohn E, Chorn R, O'Connor M: The role of the vasculature in regulating venous return and cardiac output: Historical and graphical approach. Can J Anaesth 44:849, 1997

118. Lake CL: Anesthesia and pericardial disease. Anesth Analg 62:431, 1983

119. Friedman HS, Lajam F, Gomes JA *et al:* Demonstration of a depressor reflex in acute cardiac tamponade. J Thorac Cardiovasc Surg 73:278, 1977

Clinical Anesthesia (4/e), edited by
Paul G. Barash, Bruce F. Cullen, and
Robert K. Stoelting. Lippincott Williams &
Wilkins, Philadelphia, © 2001.

CHAPTER 32

ANESTHESIA FOR CARDIAC SURGERY

SERLE K. LEVIN, W. CHASE BOYD, PETER T. ROTHSTEIN, AND STEPHEN J. THOMAS

Anesthetizing patients for open heart surgery is exciting, intellectually challenging, and emotionally rewarding. Competent and skillful clinical management requires a thorough understanding of normal and altered cardiac physiology; an intimate knowledge of the pharmacology of anesthetic, vasoactive, and cardioactive drugs; and a familiarity with the physiologic derangements associated with cardiopulmonary bypass and the surgical procedures themselves. This chapter presents a brief overview of the subject to familiarize the reader with the critical physiologic and technical considerations when caring for cardiac surgical patients. The initial discussions concerning coronary artery and valvular heart disease lay the physiologic and some of the pharmacologic groundwork upon which anesthetic planning and therapeutic decisions are based. First, we describe the balance of myocardial oxygen supply and demand, with particular reference to the patient with coronary artery disease. Next, we focus on those variables that regulate myocardial performance, specifically myocardial contractility, heart rate, and loading conditions (both preload and afterload). We then discuss the bells, whistles, and mechanics of cardiopulmonary bypass. Following this, we describe anesthetic considerations relevant to all adults undergoing cardiac surgery either with or without cardiopulmonary bypass (CPB), including preoperative evaluation, choice of monitoring techniques, selection of anesthetic drugs, and the actual conduct of the anesthetic before, during, and after bypass. The chapter concludes with some special topics as well as a brief introduction to the child with congenital heart disease. Some of the issues discussed are controversial because the field is continuously evolving. We have tried, whenever possible, to suggest what is the consensus about these topics, but, inevitably, our own preferences will be apparent. For the sake of brevity, numerous tables are included that summarize data and provide readily accessible guidelines for the various phases of the operative procedure. Many monographs are available for those who desire more detailed analysis of any aspect of cardiac anesthesia.[1,2]

CORONARY ARTERY DISEASE

The prevention or treatment of ischemia before cardiopulmonary bypass in patients undergoing coronary artery bypass graft surgery reduces the incidence of perioperative myocardial infarction.[3,4] The hemodynamic profile during the prebypass period, how the anesthetic is managed, and who does the managing are also important because the avoidance or treatment of factors known to increase myocardial oxygen demand ($M\dot{V}O_2$) reduces the frequency of precardiopulmonary bypass ischemic episodes.[5] In addition, not only is control of $M\dot{V}O_2$ critical, but it is well recognized that many, if not most, ischemic events occur with minimal or no change in $M\dot{V}O_2$, suggesting that a primary reduction in oxygen supply is a major etiologic factor in intraoperative ischemia.[5-7] Therefore, successful management of patients with coronary artery disease requires control of the factors determining $M\dot{V}O_2$ and, insofar as possible, optimizing oxygen delivery to the myocardium. The determinants of myocardial oxygen supply and demand are listed in Table 32-1 and are also discussed in Chapter 31.

Myocardial Oxygen Demand

Wall tension and contractility are the principal determinants of $M\dot{V}O_2$.[8] Laplace's law states that wall tension is directly proportional to both developed intracavitary pressure and ventricular radius and inversely proportional to wall thickness. Therefore, preventing or promptly treating ventricular distention is desirable in helping to control or reduce $M\dot{V}O_2$. Because contractility is also of major importance, myocardial depression is often beneficial so long as such depression does not result in an increase in wall tension, which itself may produce ischemia.

Myocardial Oxygen Supply

Any increase in myocardial oxygen requirements can be met only by raising coronary blood flow. Blood oxygen content (hemoglobin concentration × O_2 saturation × 1.34) is obviously important, as is oxygen extraction by the myocardium, but these are infrequently the basis of intraoperative ischemia. Oxygenation and blood volume are usually well maintained during anesthesia. Coronary sinus PO_2 is about 27 mm Hg (50% saturation), and although extraction can be increased somewhat under conditions of stress, this is inadequate to meet the continuously changing levels of demand. Therefore, the principal mechanism for matching oxygen supply to alterations in $M\dot{V}O_2$ is exquisite regulation and control of coronary blood flow.

Coronary Blood Flow

The critical factors that modify coronary blood flow are diastolic time available for perfusion (namely, heart rate), coronary perfusion pressure, coronary vascular tone, and the presence and severity of intraluminal obstructions. We are most concerned with flow to the subendocardial region of the left ventricle, the area most vulnerable to ischemia, because metabolic requirements are greater owing to greater systolic shortening and also because flow is restricted during systole.[9]

Perfusion of the left ventricular subendocardium takes place almost entirely during diastole, whereas the majority of right ventricular flow occurs during systole (in the absence of pulmonary hypertension) (Fig. 32-1). This temporal disparity is explained by the differences in intracavitary pressures during systole. Because left ventricular flow is diastolic, it is evident that not only is diastolic pressure important but duration of diastole is also critical in determining the volume of left ventricular subendocardial flow. The time available for diastole decreases with increasing heart rate.

Coronary perfusion pressure for the left ventricle is often defined as aortic diastolic pressure (AoDP) minus left ventricular end-diastolic pressure (LVEDP). This is an oversimplification because there is no single AoDP. Rather, it is likely that there is a range of pressures that drive blood to the subendocardium. In the presence of intraluminal obstruction or increased vascular tone, this pressure is reduced, as depicted in Figure 32-2. The precise degree of reduction is unknown to the clinician. Although the pressure at the end of the circuit is unknown and the subject of controversy, it is convenient and useful to consider ventricular filling pressure as this end pressure. Therefore, a low

Table 32-1. MYOCARDIAL OXYGEN BALANCE

Demand	Supply
Wall tension	Coronary blood flow
Preload	Driving pressure (DBP − LVEDP)
Afterload	Diastolic time
Contractility	Coronary resistance
Heart rate	Collaterals
	Arterial O_2 content
	Myocardial O_2 extraction

DBP = diastolic blood pressure; LVEDP = left ventricular end-diastolic pressure.

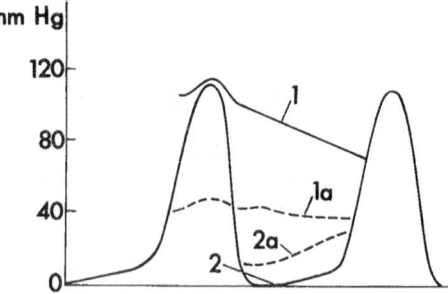

Figure 32-2. The pressure relationships between the aorta (1) and the left ventricle (2) determine coronary perfusion pressure. In coronary artery disease, myocardial perfusion may be compromised by decreased pressure distal to a significant stenosis (1a) (not quantifiable clinically) and/or by an increase in left ventricular end-diastolic pressure (2a). (Reprinted with permission from Gorlin R: Coronary Artery Disease, p 75. Philadelphia, WB Saunders, 1976.)

ventricular filling pressure is ideal both in terms of improving perfusion (higher pressure gradient) and of reducing $M\dot{V}O_2$ (decreased ventricular volume and wall tension). The consequences of altering systemic pressure are more difficult to predict because the cost of increasing perfusion pressure (afterload) is increased $M\dot{V}O_2$. It has been shown experimentally that at any given heart rate, hypotension is more likely to induce ischemia than is hypertension.[10]

Alterations in tone of the small intramyocardial arterioles regulate diastolic vascular resistance in the absence of flow, limiting obstructions in the epicardial vessels. These adjustments allow matching of oxygen supply and metabolic demand over a wide range of perfusion pressures. The difference between autoregulated supply and the amount available under conditions of maximal vasodilation is coronary vascular reserve, which is normally three to five times basal flow. As epicardial

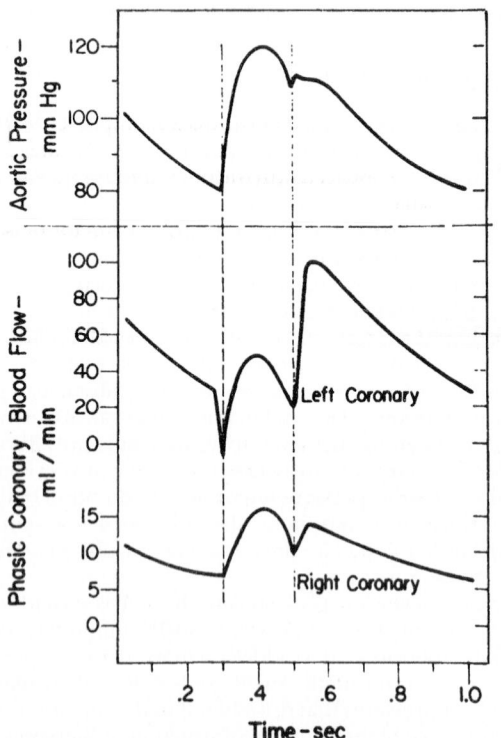

Figure 32-1. Coronary artery blood flow during a single cardiac cycle. Left ventricular flow *via* the left coronary artery occurs primarily during diastole, whereas right ventricular perfusion is predominantly systolic. (Reprinted with permission from Berne FM, Levy MN: Cardiovascular Physiology, 5th ed, p 200. St. Louis, CV Mosby, 1986.)

stenosis becomes more pronounced, progressive vasodilation of these resistance vessels allows preservation of basal flow, but at the cost of reduced reserve. Whenever demand increases above available reserve, signs, symptoms, and metabolic evidence of ischemia develop (Fig. 32-3).

Prinzmetal *et al*[11] first described angina and myocardial infarction in patients with angiographically normal coronary vessels. Subsequently, Maseri *et al* and others have emphasized repeatedly the frequency with which primary reductions in oxygen supply cause ischemia (Fig. 32-3).[12,13] Small adjustments in coronary vascular tone at the site of previous obstructions can cause substantial reductions in luminal cross-sectional area. Alterations in stenosis diameter are possible because at least two thirds of plaques or atheroma are not concentric. Therefore, a certain portion of normal vessel wall, or at least reactive vessel wall, is present in the stenosis. It is now apparent that anesthesia is not protective against "supply" ischemia, which occurs frequently during surgery (Fig. 32-4).[7] The etiology of this is unclear, but it may be caused by circulating catecholamines, local effects of blood components such as platelets at areas of atherosclerosis, or other as yet undetermined factors. It is not uncommon during anesthesia for a patient to show signs of ischemia without any change in heart rate, blood pressure, or ventricular filling pressure. Most ischemic episodes are unaccompanied by hemodynamic changes.[7,14] Drugs such as nitroglycerin and the calcium entry blockers may be used to prevent and/or treat such episodes of coronary spasm[15] although prophylactic use of these agents is usually ineffective.

Hypotension, vasospasm, and acute thrombosis all decrease coronary perfusion pressure, reduce coronary blood flow, and limit oxygen delivery to the myocardium. Unstable angina pectoris and/or acute coronary thrombosis is a result of plaque rupture with ensuing platelet activation and thrombus formation. The presence of potentially hyper-reactive normal vessel wall adjacent to the thrombus may result in vasospasm and total occlusion of the vessel lumen in the presence of a previously nonocclusive eccentric plaque or thrombus. This type of acute thrombosis is thought to be the cause of acute myocardial infarction and sudden death (generally ischemia-induced cardiac dysrhythmias).

Hemodynamic Goals

Although the precise relationship between intraoperative ischemia and postoperative myocardial infarction remains controversial,[16,17] there is consensus that a primary goal of a successful anesthetic is the prevention of myocardial ischemia.[18] Failing that, the prompt identification and treatment of new episodes

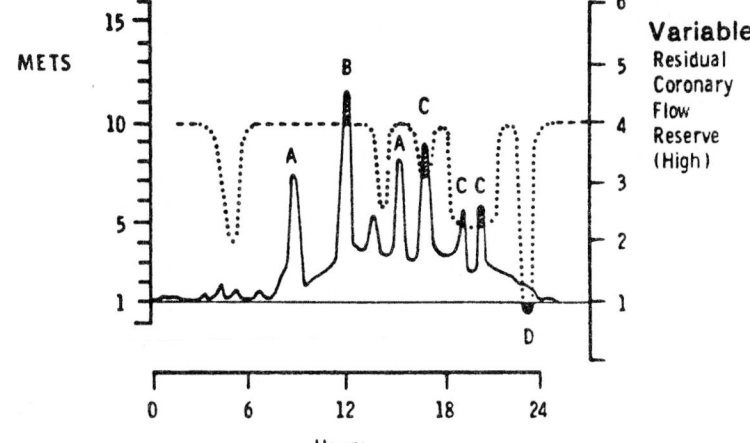

Figure 32-3. Schematic illustration of mechanisms producing myocardial ischemia. Myocardial oxygen demand is plotted on the left (as multiples of basal oxygen consumption) and oxygen supply on the right. In this example, maximal coronary flow reserve is reduced from 6 to 4 times basal levels by fixed intraluminal obstruction. As long as myocardial oxygen demand remains below this maximal limit, no ischemia occurs (*A*). Ischemia will develop, however, whenever oxygen demand exceeds maximal supply (*B*) or when supply is further compromised by coronary vasoconstriction (*C*). More pronounced coronary vasospasm may produce ischemia at rest (*D*). (Reprinted with permission from Maseri A, Chierchia S, Kaski JC: Mixed angina pectoris. Am J Cardiol 56:30E, 1985.)

are essential. As is evident from the previous discussion and from the summary in Table 32-2, anesthetic decisions are designed to reduce and control those factors that increase myocardial oxygen demand, specifically, heart rate, contractility, and wall tension. At the same time, every attempt is made to optimize coronary blood flow, notably, maintaining coronary perfusion pressure and increasing diastolic time. The buzz words for patients with coronary artery disease are "slow, small, and well perfused." Combinations of anesthetics, sedatives, muscle relaxants, and vasoactive drugs are selected to provide this hemodynamic milieu. Techniques to effectively prevent or treat alterations in coronary vascular tone—antiplatelet drugs, specific bradycardic agents, etc.—are still evolving and await further clinical trial before definitive recommendations can be made.[18]

Monitoring for Ischemia

Electrocardiogram

The ideal monitoring technique is not yet available. ST segment analysis in multiple leads (most commonly leads II and V_5) is currently the standard. Patients likely to develop right ventricular ischemia[19] or those with disease of the right coronary artery might benefit from monitoring of leads V_{4R} or V_{5R}. Computerized ST segment trending and interactive monitors that alarm when the ST segment deviates from the programmed algorithm aid in the detection of intraoperative events overlooked by even the most astute observer.

Heart Rate and Blood Pressure

Multiple attempts have been made to determine ischemic thresholds using commonly measured hemodynamic variables. Among the earliest of these was the rate–pressure product, obtained by multiplying heart rate by peak systolic pressure. For each patient, ischemia developed when a particular rate–pressure product was reached. The rate–pressure product was considered an easily determined index of $M\dot{V}O_2$. Although rate–pressure product may correlate with oxygen demand, especially during exercise, it is not a sensitive or specific indicator of intraoperative ischemia. Kissin et al[20] point out that identical rate–pressure products are possible from multiple combinations of heart rate and blood pressure. Improved conditions for oxygen balance are likely with a low heart rate and high blood pressure compared with the opposite, that is, hypotension and tachycardia.

In an effort to produce a more reliable predictor of ischemia, Buffington[10] devised the pressure–rate ratio. Using a canine model, he observed the effects of 20 combinations of various blood pressures and heart rates and found that no single value of either blood pressure or heart rate or the rate–pressure

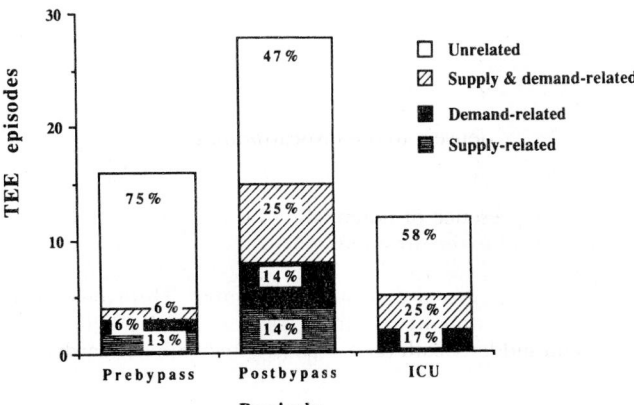

Figure 32-4. Association of transesophageal echocardiographic (TEE) wall motion changes with hemodynamic indices of supply and demand from continuous monitoring of 50 patients undergoing coronary artery bypass surgery. (Reproduced with permission from Leung JM, O'Kelly BV, Mangano DT *et al:* Relationship of regional wall motion abnormalities to hemodynamic indices of myocardial oxygen supply and demand in patients undergoing CABG surgery. Anesthesiology 73:802, 1990.)

Table 32-2 CORONARY ARTERY DISEASE—HEMODYNAMIC GOALS

P	Keep the heart small; ↓ wall tension; ↑ perfusion pressure
A	Maintain; hypertension is better than hypotension
C	Depression is beneficial when LV function is adequate
R	Slow, slow, slow
Rhy	Usually sinus
$M\dot{V}O_2$	Control of oxygen demand is frequently not enough; monitor for and treat "supply" ischemia
CPB	Elevated VFP is usually not needed after CABG

P = preload; A = afterload; C = contractility; R = rate; Rhy = rhythm; $M\dot{V}O_2$ = myocardial oxygen balance; CPB = postcardiopulmonary bypass; CABG = coronary artery bypass graft; VFP = ventricular filling pressure; LV = left ventricle.

product was predictive of ischemia. The ischemia threshold was mutually dependent on both the heart rate and coexisting blood pressure. No ischemia occurred if mean arterial pressure (MAP) exceeded heart rate, that is, if the pressure–rate ratio exceeded unity.

Leung et al,[7] using transesophageal echocardiography to detect regional wall motion abnormalities suggestive of ischemia, found that neither the rate–pressure product nor the MAP/heart rate ratio was a sensitive predictor of ischemic changes and questioned their clinical usefulness. Furthermore, most (73%) of the ischemic episodes (detected by transesophageal echocardiography) in 50 patients undergoing coronary artery bypass graft surgery were not associated with acute changes in heart rate, blood pressure, or pulmonary arterial pressure, suggesting that most intraoperative ischemic episodes are related to decreased oxygen supply. Gordon et al, using the electrocardiogram as a monitor of ischemia, also demonstrated the lack of sensitivity and specificity of the pressure–rate ratio.[21]

Pulmonary Artery Catheter

Sudden elevations in pulmonary artery or capillary wedge pressure indicating systolic and/or diastolic dysfunction, large A waves reflecting decreased ventricular compliance, and V waves signaling the development of ischemia-induced papillary muscle dysfunction and mitral regurgitation are purported signs of ischemia that may be detected with a pulmonary artery catheter. Several studies contradict this long-held dogma and demonstrate that the pulmonary artery catheter is of little value as a monitor of myocardial ischemia. Leung et al[22] found that only 10% of all regional wall motion abnormalities were associated with an acute rise in pulmonary capillary wedge pressure in 40 patients undergoing elective coronary artery bypass graft surgery. Haggmark et al[23] investigated 53 patients with coronary artery disease undergoing vascular surgery and compared several indicators of ischemia. They found that neither an increase in the pulmonary capillary wedge pressure nor the occurrence of an abnormal pulmonary capillary wedge pressure waveform was a sensitive indicator for myocardial ischemia. Van Daele et al[24] similarly found in 98 anesthetized patients prior to undergoing coronary artery bypass graft surgery that elevation of the pulmonary capillary wedge pressure was neither a sensitive nor a reliable indicator of ischemia. Furthermore, a large prospective study (1094 patients) by Tuman et al[25] showed that even high-risk cardiac surgical patients may be safely managed without routine use of a pulmonary artery catheter, and if a clinical need develops intraoperatively, delayed placement of a pulmonary artery catheter does not change outcome. Fontes et al assessed the limitations of pulmonary artery catheters in the management of critically ill patients in the intensive care unit. Comparing PA catheters to transesophageal echocardiography, the PA catheters predicted normal left ventricular function well, but performed poorly in judging preload and ventricular dysfunction.[26] Although pulmonary capillary wedge pressure changes are no longer considered a sensitive or reliable indicator of ischemia, the pulmonary artery catheter provides information regarding the patient's volume status and cardiac output.

Intraoperative Transesophageal Echocardiography

Since its introduction in the 1980s, two-dimensional transesophageal echocardiography (TEE) has become a vital, invaluable diagnostic and monitoring tool during cardiac surgery. TEE permits assessment of ventricular volume and regional wall motion, measurement of valve gradients, estimation and quantitation of valvular regurgitation, and visualization of the thoracic aorta as well as intracardiac air. It is of inestimable value in intraoperative decision making.

Basics.   The TEE image is a two-dimensional slice of a three-dimensional object. Reconstructing the three-dimensional image requires the integration of anatomic references with the multiple image planes available in today's omniplane transdu-

cers. The American Society of Echocardiography (ASE)/Society of Cardiovascular Anesthesiologists (SCA) task force for intraoperative echocardiography has published guidelines for performing a comprehensive intraoperative echocardiographic examination.[27] These recommendations describe a series of 20 standard tomographic views of the heart and great vessels that should be included in all intraoperative echocardiographic examinations. With experience, a thorough examination can be completed in less than 10 minutes.

Evaluation of Ventricular Function.   A variety of techniques have been employed in an attempt to quantify ventricular function with echocardiography. Nevertheless, qualitative assessment currently predominates in the clinical arena. The midpapillary short axis view of the left ventricle is the standard initial view for ventricular evaluation (Fig. 32-5). The presence of the papillary muscles assures that the same view is observed on repeated examinations. Because the left ventricle lies obliquely in the chest, its apex is directed away from the esophagus. The resulting image is a foreshortened ventricular long axis and the apex may not be well visualized.[28]

Qualitative assessment of left ventricular function is based on visual assessment of segmental excursion and myocardial thickening throughout the left ventricle. Segmental excursion is the systolic inward movement of a ventricular segment along an imaginary radius toward the center of the cavity.[15] Evaluation of both excursion and thickening is necessary to account for the heart's normal systolic translation (lateral motion of the entire heart in the chest) and rotation (circular motion of the heart around the long axis of the left ventricle). Furthermore, an infarcted segment of myocardium will not thicken but may undergo excursion due to surrounding normal myocardium. This represents a segment of abnormal regional wall motion.

Ischemia.   Although segmental wall motion abnormalities (SWMA) complicate both quantitative and qualitative assessment of global systolic ventricular function,[29] they provide information regarding coronary artery disease. The anatomy of the coronary blood supply to the ventricle is relatively constant; therefore, the location of segmental wall motion abnormalities often reflects the involved coronary artery. The level of the segmental wall motion abnormality (basal, midpapillary, or apical) often correlates with location of the coronary lesion on cardiac catheterization (proximal, mid, and distal). The ventricular distribution of the three main coronary arteries is depicted

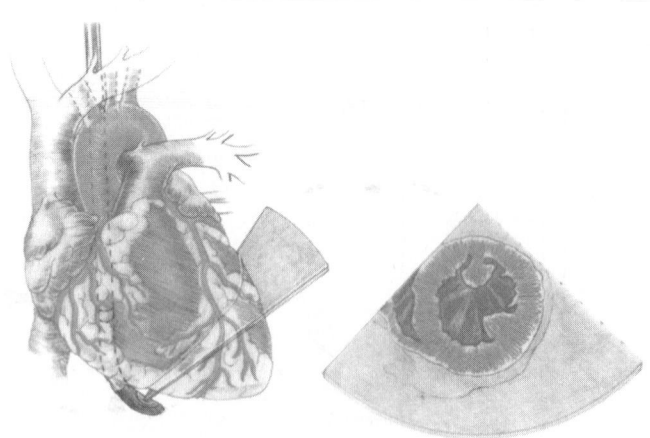

Figure 32-5. The echo probe is advanced to obtain the transgastric midpapillary short axis view of the left ventricle. The illustration on the left depicts the anatomic relationship between the echo probe, the heart, and the ultrasound plane. The right side depicts the two-dimensional image of the ultrasound plane. (Reproduced with permission from Cahalan MK: Intraoperative Transesophageal Echocardiography: An Interactive Text and Atlas. New York, Churchill Livingstone, 1996.)

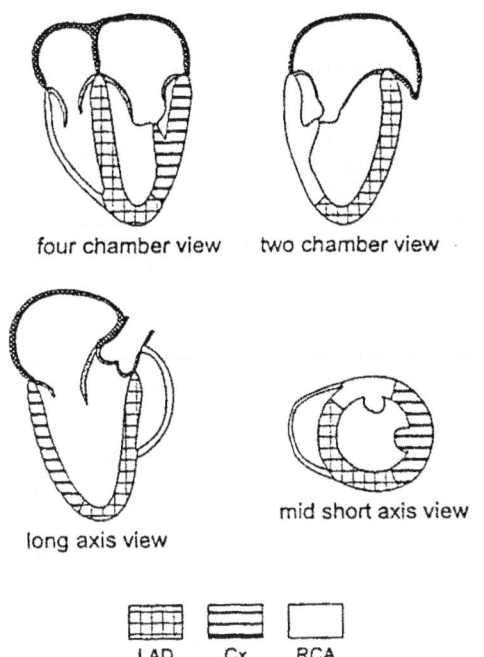

four chamber view   two chamber view

long axis view

mid short axis view

LAD   Cx   RCA

Figure 32-6. The distribution of the three main coronary arteries in relation to various two-dimensional TEE images. (Reproduced with permission from Thomas SJ (ed): Manual of Cardiac Anesthesia, 3rd ed. New York, Churchill Livingstone, 2001 [in press].)

Table 32-3. DEFINITIONS FOR CHANGES IN REGIONAL WALL MOTION

Class of Motion	Wall Thickening	Change in Radius
1. Normal	Marked	>30% decrease
2. Mild hypokinesis	Moderate	10–30% decrease
3. Severe hypokinesis	Minimal	<10% decrease
4. Akinesis	None	None
5. Dyskinesis	Thinning	Increase

ability to attain the required images and to recognize new SWMA in real time.[16]

Although ventricular wall motion is clearly very sensitive to coronary blood flow, the definition of ischemia is difficult. There is little agreement on a "gold standard" for the diagnosis of ischemia. Most studies have compared SWMA to changes in ST segments recorded on ECG. The concordance between SWMA and ECG evidence of ischemia is variable, ranging from 30% to 100%.[31,32] This discrepancy may exist for a number of reasons. SWMAs are more sensitive to compromised coronary blood flow than are ECG changes. Animal models have demonstrated that a 50% decrease in coronary blood flow will produce a new SWMA on TEE, whereas ECG evidence of ischemia requires a 75% decrease in coronary blood flow.[33] In a similar study, when progressive coronary occlusion did generate ECG changes, they always occurred minutes after the appearance of SWMAs.[34] Thus, SWMAs on TEE can appear when the compromise in coronary flow is insufficient to produce ECG changes. If the compromise in coronary flow is enough to produce ECG evidence of ischemia, TEE SWMAs precede these ECG changes.

Not all SWMAs are indicative of ischemia. Nonischemic myocardium adjacent to ischemic or infarcted myocardium may be interpreted as SWMAs, a phenomenon known as "tethering." SWMAs also occur with pacing, bundle branch blocks, and myocarditis.[35] Tachycardia and hypovolemia may elicit new SWMAs. Although controversial, increased afterload has also been implicated as a cause for new SWMAs.[36,37] Differentiating stunned myocardium from ischemia as the etiology for new SWMAs is important because treatment differs. Stunned myocardium requires supportive measures such as an inotropic infusion until function returns, while inadequate revascularization with ongoing ischemia requires a reassessment of graft patency and consideration of further revascularization. In the future, echocardiographic contrast agents that delineate coronary perfusion territories may refine this evaluation.[38,39]

in Figure 32-6. Note that all three coronary arteries supply segments of the ventricle at the transgastric midpapillary short axis level, enhancing the utility of this view as a monitoring plane. The wall motion in these segmental ventricular wall segments is described as normal, hypokinetic, akinetic, or dyskinetic and assigned a corresponding numeric grade (Fig. 32-7; Table 32-3).

The diagnosis of a new SWMA requires a change of two classes in the qualitative segmental level of function. The use of cine loop (side-by-side comparison of the ventricle over time) with the midpapillary short axis view of the ventricle improves the ability to recognize new wall motion abnormalities. In one study, however, the short axis midpapillary view detected only 17% of all SWMAs, emphasizing the importance of evaluating the ventricle in multiple planes with careful standardization of location and edge definition.[30] Training will increase the operator's

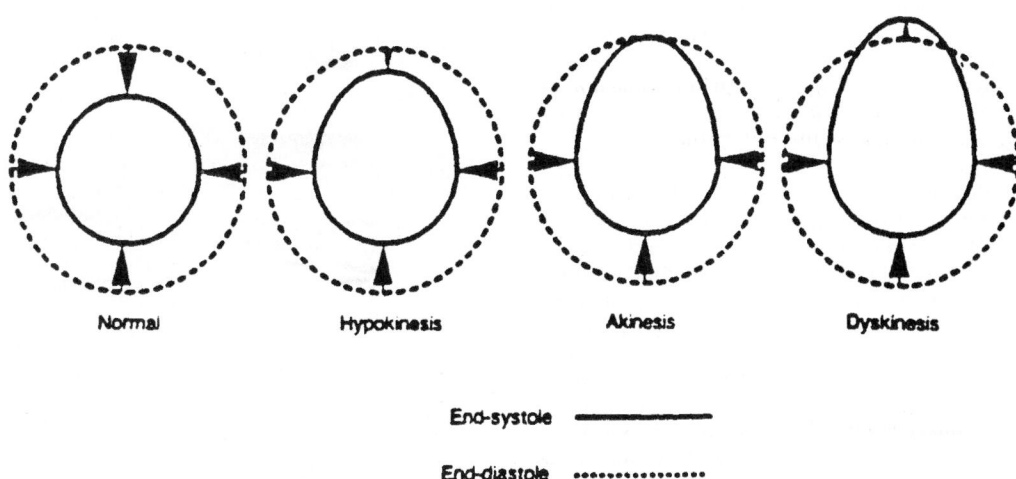

Normal   Hypokinesis   Akinesis   Dyskinesis

End-systole ——————

End-diastole ··············

Figure 32-7. Segmental ventricular wall motion is evaluated for both excursion and thickening.

Quantification of Ventricular Function. Attempts to quantify global ventricular function have utilized linear measurements, geometric estimates of ventricular volume, and Doppler measurements of blood flow. Although useful, these methods all have clinical shortcomings.

LINEAR MEASUREMENTS. Fractional shortening (FS) and fractional area of change (FAC) are linear parameters that utilize the observation that the systolic decrease in ventricular volume occurs primarily along the short axis of the ventricle. Fractional shortening is the percentage change in the diameter of the ventricle from diastole to systole measured in M mode:

$$FS = \% \; \Delta Diameter = [(LVID_d - LVID_s)/LVID_d] \times 100$$

where LVID is left ventricular internal diameter, s is systole, and d is diastole.

TEE substitutes the percentage change in area obtained from planimetry (FAC = fractional area change) for the linear M-mode measurement. Both FS and FAC have demonstrated a linear correlation with ejection fraction (EF) determined by radionuclide angiography and cineangiography.[40,41] Nevertheless, FAC still demonstrates an intraobserver variability of 10% and an interobserver variability of 6–23%.[42–44]

Part of this variability may be attributed to difficulty in defining the endocardial border. The endocardial border is clearly delineated when it is perpendicular to the ultrasound beam. However, as the endocardial border becomes parallel to the ultrasound beam, the image becomes broad, blurred, and may even drop out. In the short axis midpapillary view, this occurs along the septal and lateral walls of the ventricle. Finally, the papillary muscles have been included as part of the endocardial border in some studies and as part of the chamber volume in other studies. Because the FAC method assesses global left ventricular function with a single short axis view, it is inherently inaccurate in the setting of an asymmetric ventricle. Such variability, coupled with the time required to manually trace the endocardial border, limits the clinical utility of the FAC method.

Automated border detection (ABD) overcomes some of these limitations. Improved computer software with ABD can provide real-time measurements of FAC.[46,47] The FAC determined by ABD has been clinically correlated with EF determined by radionuclide angiography.[48] Furthermore, the system remains accurate with serial changes in ventricular area.[42] About 80% of the ABD values for EDA, ESA, and FAC are within the limits of expert offline analysis. A limitation of the ABD is that it cannot extrapolate the endocardial border.[42]

Although EF has traditionally been used as an indicator of left ventricular function, it is dependent on preload, afterload, and contractility.[43] In an attempt to isolate and quantify left ventricular performance, the left ventricular area measurements obtained with ABD have been combined with left ventricular pressure measurements to generate pressure–area loops (Fig. 32-8). These pressure–area loops have been used to derive indices of contractility that are independent of the ventricle's loading conditions.[44–46] Routine application of this system is limited by its complexity and the necessity of a left ventricular pressure catheter.

GEOMETRIC QUANTIFICATION. A more sophisticated and complex approach to determining ventricular function has utilized assumptions about ventricular shape to determine ventricular volume. The end-diastolic volume and end-systolic volume can then be used to calculate the EF. The simplest method assumes that the ventricle is a prolate ellipsoid (two short axes of equal diameter and a long axis that is twice the diameter of the short axis) (Fig. 32-9). The formula $V = D^3$ assumes that the ventricular volume can then be calculated from the measurement of the short axis midpapillary diameter. Measurements are made in systole and diastole and the corresponding values applied to a nomogram to obtain the EF (Table 32-4). Although a linear relationship of minor axis length to chamber volume has been demonstrated,[47] the "cubed formula" significantly

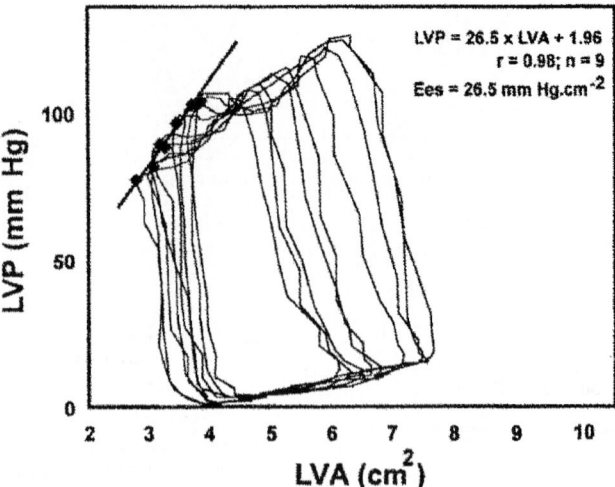

Figure 32-8. Continuous pressure–area loops generated during preload reduction. The end-systolic points are shown as black diamonds. The slope of the line connecting these points, the end-systolic pressure–area relationship, is a measure of contractility. (Reproduced with permission from Declerck C, Hillel Z, Shih H *et al:* A comparison of left ventricular performance indices measured by transesophageal echocardiography with automated border detection. Anesthesiology 89:341, 1998.)

overestimates ventricular volume in large ventricles. As a ventricle dilates, it becomes more spherical, dilating primarily along the minor axes.[35,48] This increases the error associated with the assumptions of the cubed formula. In an attempt to account for this error, Teichholz[49] utilized regression formulas to modify the formula:

$$Volume = [7.0/(2.4 + D)] \times D^3$$

The area–length ellipsoid formula and the modified Simpson's rule are more sophisticated geometric models that have been used in an attempt to increase the accuracy of the calculated EF. The ASE recommends that ventricular volumes be calculated with a modification of Simpson's rule. Simpson's rule states that the ventricular volume is equal to the summation of a series of disks from the ventricular apex to the base (Fig. 32-10). The intraoperative utility of these formulas is limited by the time required to perform the neccesary measurments, the complexity of the calculations, and the inability of TEE to accurately measure the ventricular long axis.[28] Estimating ventricular volume with three-dimensional reconstruction from two-dimensional image planes is currently being evaluated.[50]

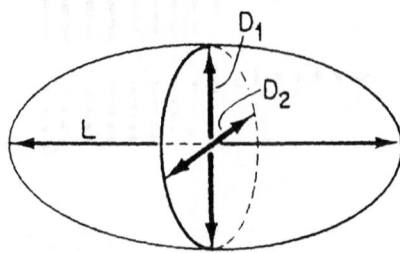

Figure 32-9. A prolate ellipsoid model of the left ventricle with the two short axes (D1, D2) of equal diameter and the long axes (L) twice the diameter of the short axes. (Reproduced with permission from Weyman A: Principles and Practice of Echocardiography, 2nd ed. Philadelphia, Lea & Febiger, 1994.)

Table 32-4. A NORMOGRAM CALCULATING EJECTION FRACTION FROM THE FRACTIONAL SHORTENING MEASUREMENTS

LVIDs → LVIDd ↓	20	22	24	26	28	30	32	34	36	38	40	42	44	46	48	50	52	56	58	60	62	64	66	68	70	72	74	76
40		83	78	73	66	58	49	39	27	14																		
41		85	80	74	68	61	52	43	32	20	7																	
42			81	76	70	64	56	47	37	26	14																	
43			83	78	72	66	59	51	41	31	20	7																
44			84	79	74	68	62	54	45	36	25	13																
45			85	81	76	70	64	57	49	40	30	19	7															
46				82	77	72	66	60	52	44	34	24	12															
47				83	79	74	68	62	54	46	37	28	17	8														
48				84	80	76	70	63	57	49	40	31	21	9														
49				84	81	76	71	63	59	51	43	34	24	14	5													
50				85	81	77	72	67	61	54	46	37	28	18	9													
51					82	78	74	68	62	56	48	40	31	21	13	4												
52					83	79	75	70	64	58	51	43	34	25	17	9												
53					84	80	76	71	66	59	53	45	37	28	21	13	4											
54					84	81	77	72	67	61	55	48	40	33	24	16	8											
55					85	82	78	73	68	63	57	50	42	34	27	20	12	4										
56						82	79	74	70	64	58	52	45	37	30	23	16	8										
57						83	80	75	71	66	60	54	47	39	33	26	19	12	4									
58						84	80	76	72	67	62	56	49	42	35	29	22	15	8									
59						84	81	77	73	68	63	57	51	44	38	32	25	18	11	4								
60						83	82	78	74	70	64	59	53	46	40	34	28	21	15	7								
61							82	79	75	71	66	60	54	48	42	37	31	24	18	11	4							
62							83	80	76	72	67	62	56	50	45	39	33	27	21	14	7							
63							84	80	77	73	68	63	58	52	47	41	36	30	24	17	11	4						
64							84	81	78	74	69	64	59	53	48	43	38	32	26	20	14	7						
65							85	82	78	75	70	66	61	55	50	45	40	35	29	23	17	10	3					
66							85	82	79	75	71	67	62	56	52	47	42	37	31	26	20	13	7					
67								83	80	76	72	68	63	58	54	49	44	39	34	28	22	16	10	3				
68								84	80	77	73	69	64	59	55	51	46	41	36	30	25	19	13	7				
69								84	81	78	74	70	66	61	57	52	48	43	38	33	27	22	16	10	3			
70								85	82	79	75	71	67	62	58	54	49	45	40	35	30	24	18	12	6			
71								85	82	79	76	72	68	63	59	55	51	46	42	37	32	26	23	15	9	3		
72									83	80	76	73	69	64	60	57	52	48	44	39	34	29	23	18	12	6		
73									83	80	77	74	70	65	62	58	54	50	45	41	36	31	26	20	15	9	3	

(From Kessler KM. Cathet Cardiovasc Diagn 5(3):295, 1979.)

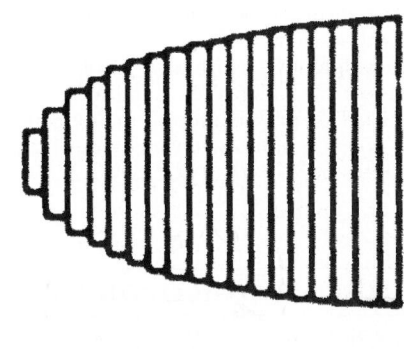

SIMPSON'S RULE

Figure 32-10. Simpson's Rule: The ventricular volume is equal to the summation of a series of disks from the ventricular apex to the base. (Reproduced with permission from Weyman A: Principles and Practice of Echocardiography, 2nd ed. Philadelphia, Lea & Febiger, 1994.)

DOPPLER QUANTIFICATION. Stroke volume can be quantified using two-dimensional echocardiography with Doppler measurements of blood velocity:

$$\text{Stroke volume} = \text{CSA} \times \text{VTI}$$

$$\text{CSA} = \pi r^2$$

where CSA is cross-sectional area, r is the radius of the cylinder [r = (diameter of the cylinder)/2], and VTI is velocity time integral.

Pulse wave Doppler (PWD) displays the velocity profile of blood at a specific location within the heart. It assumes that blood flow at this location is laminar and parallel to the ultrasound beam. Any deviation in the angle between the ultrasound beam and the blood flow will underestimate the VTI and consequently the stroke volume. Using a cursor, the VTI is calculated by tracing the PWD profile (Fig. 32-11). The CSA is then determined by measuring the diameter at this same location. Usually, these measurements are made at the left ventricle outflow tract, aortic annulus, or ascending aorta. These sites are assumed to be cylindrical so that the CSA can be calculated by the πr^2 formula. It is important that the diameter be accurately measured as any error in this measurement is subsequently squared.

Currently there is no echocardiographic measurement of global ventricular function that is both quick and accurate.

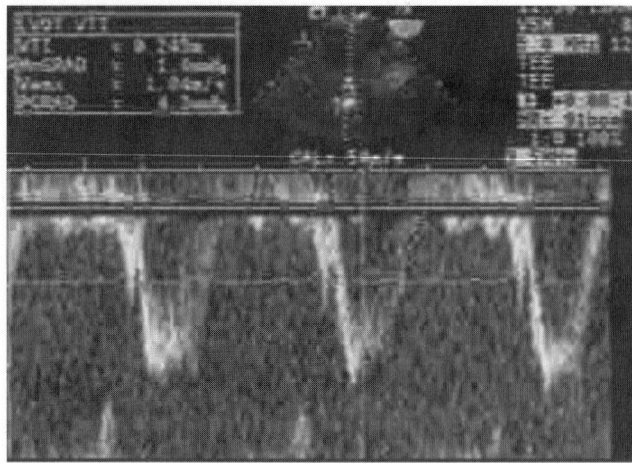

Figure 32-11. The illustrated velocity profile is obtained by placing the sample volume of the pulse wave Doppler in the LVOT and then manually traced with the cursor. The computer integrates this to generate the velocity time integral of the LVOT. Multiplying this by the CSA of the LVOT will estimate the stroke volume of the LVOT. (LVOT = left ventricular outflow tract, CSA = cross-sectional area.)

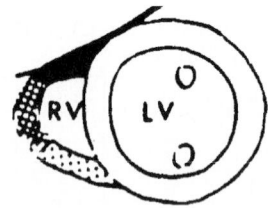

◫ anterior wall of the RV

▦ lateral wall of the RV

■ inferior wall of the RV

Figure 32-12. Nomenclature of the right ventricle as seen in the transverse short axis at the level of the papillary muscles. (Reproduced with permission from Weyman A: Principles and Practice of Echocardiography, 2nd ed. Philadelphia, Lea & Febiger, 1994.)

Therefore qualitative assessment remains the most frequently used modality. With good endocardial definition and integration of the various cross sections of the ventricle, an experienced observer can reasonably estimate ejection fraction. One study found that 75% of the time qualitative estimates of ejection fraction were within 10% of offline quantified values.[29] Qualitative estimates of ejection fraction have also been found to be in agreement with ejection fraction determined by radionuclide angiography and contrast ventriculography.[43,51]

Right Ventricle. The right ventricle is a complex anatomic structure draped over the anteriomedial portion of the left ventricle. There are no accepted three-dimensional representations of the right ventricle. Geometric models that have been employed include prism, triangular-based pyramid, and three-dimensional parallelogram.[35] In the transgastric short axis mid-papillary view, the right ventricle appears crescent-shaped, with the septum forming the medial wall. The right ventricular border is irregular due to trabeculae carneae. Contraction of the right ventricle is also complex. It involves a shortening of the long axis and an inward movement of the free wall, which is primarily responsible for the ejection of blood. Collectively, these properties make it difficult to accurately evaluate right ventricular function.[52]

The ability to qualitatively assess the right ventricle has been limited owing to its asymmetries and its decreased muscle mass relative to the left ventricle. For descriptive purposes, the right ventricle can be divided into three walls: anterior, lateral, and inferior (Fig. 32-12). The diagnosis of right ventricular infarct requires a change in right ventricular function from normal to akinesis or dyskinesis.[53-55] Quantitative measurements of the right ventricle with linear parameters have not been found to accurately reflect right ventricular function.[35] ABD has been applied to normovolemic right ventricles to generate pressure–area loops in order to evaluate right ventricular contractility.[56] It is not clear if this method is accurate with hypervolemic ventricles.[57] In the future, three-dimensional reconstruction of the right ventricle may allow improved evaluation.[58]

If the right ventricle appears dilated, this should trigger an evaluation for an appropriate lesion such as an atrial septal defect, tricuspid regurgitation, or pulmonic regurgitation. Long-standing right ventricular pressure overload can result in right ventricular dilation; however, hypertrophy is more common. Right ventricular hypertrophy is diagnosed with a diastolic right ventricular free wall thickness greater than 0.5 cm.

Aorta. Neurologic dysfunction in cardiac surgical patients continues to be a devastating complication.[59,60] Stroke, defined as a fixed neurologic deficit lasting longer than 24 hours, occurs with an incidence of 2–5% in patients undergoing CABG with CPB while more subtle neurologic dysfunction occurs in 30–60% of these patients.[59,61] Risk factors that have been identified include a history of neurologic disease, older age, and the presence of aortic atherosclerosis.[62-64] Detecting aortic atherosclerotic disease allows surgical modifications that may decrease a patient's morbidity and mortality.[65-67] Prior to echocardiography, detection of aortic atherosclerotic disease relied on surgical palpation or radiographic evidence of its presence. Although successful for detection of severe aortic calcification, these techniques do not reliably predict aortic atheromas.[63,68] TEE can accurately detect the presence of both aortic calcification and atherosclerosis.[68,69] Because TEE is easy to perform, reproducible, quantifiable, and carries minimum risk, it has become the diagnostic method of choice for detecting aortic atheromas. The severity of aortic atherosclectic disease is graded according to the scale depicted in Table 32-5.

TEE completely and accurately images the descending thoracic aorta. However, owing to the interposition of the trachea and/or the right mainstem bronchus between the esophagus and the ascending aorta, the distal ascending aorta and proximal aortic arch are much more difficult. Complete and accurate examination of this segment of the aorta requires direct examination with an epiaortic probe. The presence of a grade 3, 4, or 5 descending thoracic aorta is associated with an increased incidence of postoperative morbidity (stroke) and mortality.[62,63,70] In a series of 189 patients who underwent a CPB/CABG and intraoperative TEE examination of the descending aorta, no strokes were noted in individuals with grades 1 and 2 aortas, whereas stroke rates of 5.5% (5/11), 10.5% (2/19), and 45%

Table 32-5. AORTIC ATHEROSCLEROTIC GRADING

Aortic Atherosclerotic Grade	Description
1	Normal intimal thickening
2	Extensive intimal thickening
3	Sessile atheroma < 0.5 cm
4	Protruding atheroma > 0.5 cm
5	Mobile atheroma of any size

Mild to moderate: grades 1–3; severe: grades 4–5.

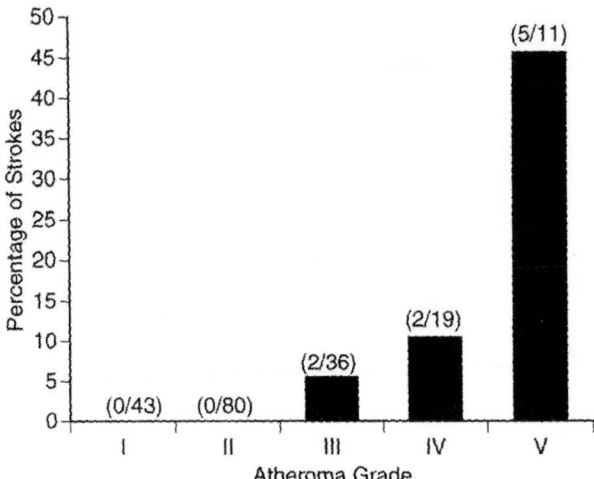

Figure 32-13. Risk of perioperative stroke versus descending thoracic aortic grade. Numbers in parentheses represents the number of patients who suffered a stroke out of the total number of patients with that descending aortic grade. (Reproduced with permission from Hartman GS, Yao FS, Bruefach M *et al*: Severity of aortic artheromatous disease diagnosed by transesophageal echocardiography predicts stroke and other outcomes associated with coronary artery surgery: A prospective study. Anesth Analg 83:701, 1996.)

(5/11) were documented for descending aortas grades 3, 4, and 5[62] (Fig. 32-13). In a subsequent study, an epiaortic examination of the ascending aorta was performed in all patients with a grade 4 or 5 descending thoracic aorta. If a grade 5 ascending thoracic aorta was documented, there was a 71% (5/7) incidence of stroke. It has been shown that if a complete TEE examination of the thoracic aorta is negative for atheromatosis, it is highly unlikely that there is significant atherosclerotic disease in the ascending aorta and proximal aortic arch. If the TEE examination reveals significant atheromatosis (>3 mm) in the aorta, there is a 34% chance of significant disease in the ascending aorta, and epiaortic scanning is applicable.[64] Thus, TEE is a very sensitive but only mildly specific method of determining the extent of atherosclerosis in the thoracic aorta.

Despite TEE's shortcomings in imaging the thoracic aorta for atherosclerosis, it remains a primary tool for rapid and accurate evaluation of patients with suspected thoracic aortic pathology, especially aortic dissections. TEE has consistently demonstrated a 95–100% sensitivity and specificity in diagnosing an acute aortic dissection[71] (Fig. 32-14). It is important to recognize that artifacts may appear as an aortic dissection.[72,73] These artifacts can be classified as linear artifacts or mirror-image artifacts.[74] Linear artifacts may mimic intimal flaps. They frequently occur in the ascending aorta when the aortic diameter is greater than the left atrial diameter. Mirror-image artifacts are more common in the transverse and descending aorta and appear as a double-barrel aorta. These are produced by the aortic–lung tissue interface.[74] A number of methods can be used to decrease the risk of interpreting an artifact as a dissection. Performing a complete two-dimensional assessment of the aorta in multiple image planes will eliminate the majority. Applying color flow Doppler to the aorta may also distinguish a dissection from an artifact. Dissections will disrupt the blood flow pattern to produce a mosaic color flow image, a pattern not seen with artifacts. Finally, M-mode echocardiography can be used to demonstrate independent movement of the true aortic flap, a property not consistent with an artifact. Epiaortic evaluation of the ascending aorta should be performed if an acute dissection is suspected secondary to surgical cannulation of the aorta.

Selection of Anesthetic

Numerous reports documenting the pattern of prebypass hemodynamics and the frequency of prebypass ischemia support the conclusion that there is no one "ideal" anesthetic for patients with coronary artery disease. Two large prospective outcome studies in coronary artery bypass graft patients addressed the question of anesthetic choice. Slogoff and Keats,[75] in a prospective randomized study using various anesthetics in 1012 patients, found a perioperative incidence of myocardial infarction of 4.1% and a mortality of 1.7%. Tuman *et al*,[76] in a prospective nonrandomized study of five anesthetic techniques in 1094 patients, similarly found a perioperative incidence of myocardial infarction of 4.1% and a mortality of 3.1%. In neither study did anesthetic choice influence outcome. Nearly every combination of anesthetic and vasoactive drug has both favorable studies and ardent zealots promoting its use. However, the choice of anesthetic should depend primarily upon the extent of preexisting myocardial dysfunction and the pharmacologic properties of the drugs themselves. The fit patient who has angina only on heavy exertion and good ventricular function profits from having MVo_2 decreased with a volatile-based technique. Conversely, the patient with severe congestive heart failure and a scarred myocardium might be better served by a less depressant technique. Clearly, there are patients who fall all along this spectrum. These examples illustrate the point that myocardial depression is harmful only in the patient whose heart cannot be further depressed without fear of precipitating overt heart failure. Most patients with mild or even moderate dysfunction may benefit from some degree of myocardial depression, decreasing oxygen demand and alleviating or at least decreasing episodes of ischemia.

Cost Containment

Cost containment permeates the practice of medicine today, and cardiac surgery and anesthesia have not been excluded. The high cost of cardiac surgery is due in part to the traditional modes of postoperative ICU care of these patients. Improvements in anesthetic, surgical, and perfusion techniques have reduced the need for prolonged ICU stays in many cardiac surgical patients. Thus, both clinical and economic factors have resulted in an evolving emphasis on "fast-track" recovery, which involves early postoperative awakening and extubation with an abbreviated ICU stay and a shortened overall hospitalization.[77-79]

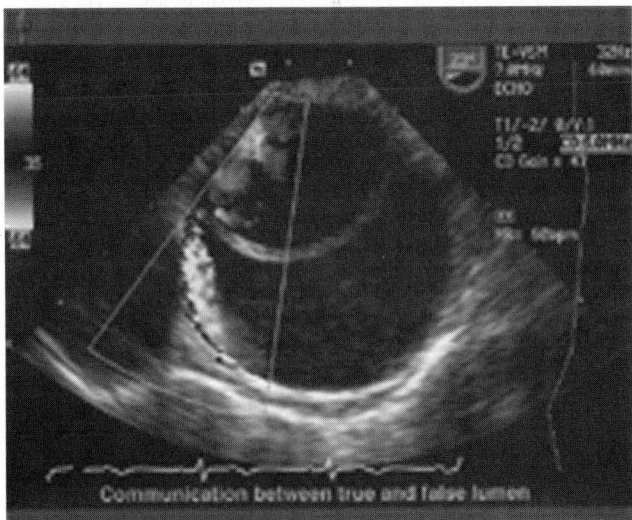

Figure 32-14. Color flow Doppler of the ascending aorta in a patient with aortic dissection. The turbulent color flow represented by the mosaic pattern illustrates blood flow between the true and false lumen.

Early extubation (1–8 hours) is only one of many components that contribute to the success of such an approach. Other key elements include appropriate patient selection, patient education, accelerated rehabilitation, a designated coordinator who maintains daily telephone contact, and adequate follow-up postoperative visits (at 1 week and 1 month). The fast-track recovery protocol has not been associated with an increase in either early or late morbidity or mortality.[80]

There are multiple approaches to achieve early extubation in the cardiac surgical patient. The choice of anesthetic should be based on the known hemodynamic, pharmacologic, and pharmacokinetic effects of each drug as they apply to the particular patient, the experience of the anesthesiologist, and the relative cost–benefit of each agent. Volatile anesthetics with low-dose narcotics[81] and total intravenous (iv) anesthesia with short-acting drugs (e.g., midazolam, alfentanil, remifentanil, propofol) have been utilized to effect early extubation. Another interesting approach is the combination of the opiates, sufentanil and morphine, instilled intrathecally before induction. This reduces postoperative analgesic requirements and, when combined with an appropriate anesthetic technique, allows extubation within 8 hours.[82]

Opioids

The primary advantages of opioids are lack of myocardial depression, maintenance of a stable hemodynamic state, and reduction of heart rate (except for meperidine). Problems include hypertension and tachycardia during surgical stimulation (sternotomy and aortic manipulation), especially in patients with good ventricular function, predictable hypotension when combined with benzodiazepines, lack of titratability when used in high doses, and a low incidence of intraoperative recall. A primary opioid technique may be of value in the patient with severe myocardial dysfunction; in patients with normal ventricles, this may be inadequate as an anesthetic and may need to be combined with other anesthetics or vasoactive drugs. The planned time of extubation is now one of the major factors determining the selection and dosage of opioid.

Inhalation Anesthetics

The desirable features of volatile anesthetics include dose dependency, easy reversibility, titratable myocardial depression, amnesia, and suppression of sympathetic responses to surgical stress and cardiopulmonary bypass. Disadvantages include myocardial depression, systemic hypotension (whether induced by decreased contractility or vasodilation), and lack of postoperative analgesia. Combinations of opioids and volatile anesthetics may produce the advantages of each with minimal untoward effects. It is likely that any volatile anesthetic agent could be used as an adjuvant anesthetic if appropriate doses are used that minimize adverse cardiovascular effects. The known cardiovascular effects of a particular agent may be used to their advantage. For example, the vasodilation produced by isoflurane may be beneficial in reducing the afterload in a patient with a high systemic vascular resistance, or the myocardial depressant effect of enflurane—or, dare we say it, halothane—may be of value in a patient with hypertrophic cardiomyopathy. The use of any volatile agent in a patient with cardiac disease is predicated upon the anesthesiologist's knowledge of the dose-dependent cardiovascular side-effects, the understanding of how such effects will affect a particular patient, and his/her experience in administering these agents.

Isoflurane is a coronary vasodilator, as are the other volatile anesthetics, although to a lesser degree.[83] This effect is dose-related and is clinically insignificant in doses less than 1 minimum alveolar concentration (MAC). Clinical studies using isoflurane to clinical rather than pharmacologic endpoints do not show increased episodes of ischemia or a worsened outcome.[84]

Desflurane and sevoflurane have the advantage of faster recovery compared with the other volatile anesthetic agents. Desflurane has a rapid uptake and distribution, allowing it to be useful in cases where hemodynamic swings are dramatic. It has a cardiac profile similar to that of isoflurane. Of concern is the fact that a sudden increase in inspired concentration can lead to a marked increase in heart rate, mean arterial pressure, and plasma epinephrine levels, making it riskier for use in patients with coronary artery disease.[85,86] Data relating the use of desflurane with myocardial performance have shown that its cardiac depressant effects and vasodilating properties are similar to those of isoflurane.[87,88] In patients undergoing noncardiac surgery, desflurane does increase pulmonary artery pressure, wedge pressure, and pulmonary vascular resistance compared to isoflurane.[88,90] Studying sympathetic nervous system activity, Helman et al found an increase in sympathetic activity and myocardial ischemia in patients anesthetized with desflurane as the sole anesthetic agent for coronary artery bypass surgery compared to patients anesthetized with sufentanil.[90] In contrast, Parsons et al found that a combination of low-dose fentanyl and desflurane had a similar incidence of ischemia when compared to midazolam–fentanyl as the anesthetic choice for coronary artery bypass surgery.[91] The hemodynamic profile of sevoflurane also resembles that of isoflurane.[92] Compared to isoflurane in a technique combining fentanyl with the inhalational anesthetic, sevoflurane had an acceptable cardiovascular profile prior to cardiopulmonary bypass and had similar outcome data to isoflurane.[93]

Intravenous Sedative Hypnotics

An alternative adjuvant anesthetic to a reduced opioid technique is a titratable iv infusion of a short-acting sedative, such as midazolam or propofol, which can be continued postoperatively in the ICU and, after discontinuation, afford a predictable and fairly rapid awakening. Bell et al compared a propofol infusion with a low-dose fentanyl (15 μg · kg^{-1}) technique to a high-dose fentanyl (60 μg · kg^{-1}) anesthetic in cardiac surgical patients with a low cardiac output state.[94] They found that the patients in the propofol/reduced-dose fentanyl group awakened sooner and were extubated earlier than the patients in the high-dose fentanyl group. Comparison between the two sedatives shows both drugs to be effective and safe as anesthetics used in coronary artery bypass surgery with good control of intraoperative and postoperative ischemia.[95,96]

Treatment of Ischemia

The use of anesthetics or vasoactive drugs that will enable the heart to return to the slow, small, perfused state is frequently required during anesthesia. The principal vasoactive drugs are nitrates, β blockers, peripheral vasoconstrictors, and calcium entry blockers. Clinical scenarios for their use are given in Table 32-6. These drugs are discussed extensively in Chapter 12 and are reviewed only briefly here. Volatile anesthetics can also be used to control blood pressure and reduce contractility.

Nitrates

Nitroglycerin is a venodilator and reduces venous return, lessening wall tension and $M\dot{V}O_2$, and also a coronary arterial dilator, effective in coronary stenoses and in collateral beds.[97,98] Nitroglycerin is the drug of choice for the acute treatment of coronary vasospasm. The evidence for the prophylactic use of nitroglycerin is unconvincing for the prevention of either intraoperative ischemic episodes or postoperative cardiac complications. Although nitroglycerin is primarily a systemic venodilator, it does dilate arterial beds and may cause systemic hypotension at higher doses.

Table 32-6. TREATMENT OF INTRAOPERATIVE ISCHEMIA

Demand

↑ BP ± ↑ PCWP	NTG, ↑ anesthetic depth
↑ HR	Treat usual causes, then β blocker

Supply

↓ BP	Vasoconstrictor, ↓ anesthetic depth
↓ BP and ↑ PCWP	Phenylephrine + NTG, inotrope
NL hemodynamics	NTG, CCB

BP = blood pressure; PCWP = pulmonary capillary wedge pressure; HR = heart rate; NL = normal; NTG = nitroglycerin; CCB = calcium channel blocker.

Vasoconstrictors

Vasoconstrictors are useful adjuncts in the prevention and treatment of ischemia owing to their ability to increase systemic blood pressure. Administration of an α-adrenergic agent such as phenylephrine improves coronary perfusion pressure, albeit at the expense of increasing afterload and MVO_2. In addition, concomitant venoconstriction increases venous return and left ventricular preload. In most situations, the increase in coronary perfusion pressure more than offsets any increase in wall tension. Peripheral vasoconstriction is indicated during episodes of systemic hypotension, especially those caused by reduced surgical stimulation or drug-induced vasodilation. Nitroglycerin is sometimes added to counteract any increase in preload. Similarly, phenylephrine can be administered to patients in whom nitroglycerin results in decreased ventricular filling pressures but unacceptably low arterial pressure.

Beta Blockers

β-Adrenergic blockade is often useful in improving myocardial oxygen balance by preventing or treating tachycardia as well as decreasing contractility. The use of atenolol has been shown to improve long-term survival in patients with heart disease undergoing noncardiac surgery.[99,100] Myocardial depression can result in increased ventricular volume and wall tension; clinically, this is not usually a problem. Indications for β blockers include treatment of sinus tachycardia not resulting from the usual causes (e.g., light anesthesia, hypovolemia), slowing the ventricular response to supraventricular dysrhythmias, decreasing heart rate and contractility in hyperdynamic states, and control of ventricular dysrhythmias. Intravenous preparations include propranolol, metoprolol, labetalol, and esmolol. Propranolol is a nonselective β blocker with an elimination half-life of 4–6 hours. Metoprolol is similar to propranolol but has the purported advantage of $β_1$ selectivity. Labetalol combines α-blocking properties with those of β blockade and is useful in treating hyperdynamic situations and in controlling hypertension. Esmolol is a short-acting β blocker that is cardioselective, with a half-life of only 9.5 minutes. It is often useful in treating momentary increases in heart rate owing to episodic sympathetic stimulation.

Calcium Channel Blockers

Calcium channel blockers are useful in slowing the ventricular response in atrial fibrillation and flutter, as coronary vasodilators, and in the treatment of postoperative hypertension. In vitro, all calcium entry blockers depress contractility, reduce coronary and systemic vascular tone, decrease sinoatrial node firing rate, and impede atrioventricular conduction. Unlike the β blockers, which are similar both in structure and pharmacodynamic effect, the calcium entry blockers vary remarkably in their predominant pharmacologic action. The negative inotropic effect is greatest with verapamil and less with nifedipine, diltiazem, and isradipine (in decreasing order).[101] Verapamil is

useful in the treatment of supraventricular tachycardia and slowing the ventricular response in atrial fibrillation and/or flutter; however, its myocardial depressant effects may limit its usefulness in some patients. In patients with reduced myocardial function, iv diltiazem is effective in the treatment of atrial fibrillation and flutter by slowing atrioventricular conduction with minimal myocardial depression. It is also useful in decreasing sinus rate. Nifedipine and diltiazem are coronary vasodilators and are used as anti-anginal agents and in the prevention of coronary vasospasm. It has been shown that continuous infusion of diltiazem during coronary bypass surgery is associated with fewer ischemic episodes, a lower incidence of atrial fibrillation and preservation of myocardial function.[15]

Nifedipine, isradipine, amlodipine, and nicardipine are prominent peripheral vasodilators. Owing to their systemic vasodilatory effects, intravenous isradipine and nicardipine have been shown to be effective in the treatment of postoperative hypertension in cardiac surgical patients, with minimal side-effects.[102,103] Magnesium has use in the treatment of myocardial ischemia. It has coronary artery vasodilating properties, reduces the size of myocardial infarction in the setting of acute ischemia, and decreases mortality associated with infarction.[104–107] Additionally, it is an anti-arrhythmic and minimizes myocardial reperfusion injury.[108,109]

VALVULAR HEART DISEASE

Alterations in loading conditions are the initial physiologic burdens imposed by valvular heart lesions, both stenotic and regurgitant. For example, the left ventricle is pressure-overloaded in aortic stenosis and volume-overloaded in aortic insufficiency and mitral regurgitation. In mitral stenosis, however, the left ventricle is both volume- and pressure-underloaded, whereas the right ventricle faces progressively increasing left atrial and pulmonary artery pressure. The mechanisms used to compensate for these additional stresses consist of chamber enlargement, myocardial hypertrophy, and variations in vascular tone and the level of sympathetic activity. These mechanisms in turn induce secondary alterations, including altered ventricular compliance, development of myocardial ischemia, chronic cardiac dysrhythmias, and progressive myocardial dysfunction. Myocardial contractility is often transiently depressed but may progress to irreversible impairment even in the absence of clinical symptoms. This is especially true in mitral regurgitation and aortic insufficiency, in which markedly reduced afterload favors ejection and forward flow.[110] Conversely, the patient with aortic stenosis may complain of dyspnea, not because of impaired systolic function, but because of reduced ventricular compliance, increased left ventricular end-diastolic pressure, and increased pulmonary pressures.

When a decision for valve replacement or repair is made, the anesthesiologist is often presented with a patient with pulmonary hypertension, severe ventricular dysfunction, and chronic rhythm disorders. Anesthetic management is predicated on understanding the altered loading conditions, preserving the compensatory mechanisms, maintaining circulatory homeostasis, and anticipating problems that may arise during and after valve surgery. In this section, we briefly describe the pathophysiology, the desirable hemodynamic profile, and other pertinent anesthetic considerations for each valvular lesion.

TEE has become the standard of care in the perioperative management of patients undergoing valve surgery.[110] TEE can further refine the preoperative diagnosis, identify valvular pathology and the mechanism of disease, and quantify the degree of stenosis and/or regurgitation. Studies have shown a change in the perioperative plan regarding valve surgery in as many as 19% of cases as a result of the prebypass echocardiographic exam.[110–113] TEE's ability to immediately evaluate the surgical results also affects the operative course. Depending on the surgical intervention, 5–18% of the time TEE reveals findings that result in an immediate return to CPB.[113,114] However, detailed assessment of valve function pre- and post-CPB is complex. Two-dimensional echocardiography and color flow Doppler can provide a gross evaluation of valve function, but complete assessment requires Doppler evaluation of blood flow velocities. Comprehensive reviews of these topic can be found in standard textbooks of echocardiography. Ultimately, the decision to intervene surgically for valve pathology is clinical and must take account of the patient's individual situation. Both valve replacement and repair result in a level of valve pathology that may or may not be in the best interest of the patient.

Aortic Stenosis

Pathophysiology

Progressive calcification and narrowing of the aortic valve orifice are degenerative processes affecting a normal or congenitally bicuspid valve. This results in chronic obstruction to left ventricular ejection. Increased intraventricular systolic pressure with concomitant increase in wall tension is required to maintain forward flow. "Concentric" ventricular hypertrophy, in which the wall gradually thickens but the chamber size remains unchanged, is the compensatory response normalizing wall tension. Contractility is preserved and ejection fraction is maintained at a normal range until late in the disease process (Fig. 32-15). The normal valve area is about 3 cm²; signs and symptoms of aortic stenosis occur when this is reduced to 0.8 cm².

The cost of this concentric hypertrophy is decreased diastolic compliance and a precarious balance between myocardial oxygen supply and $M\dot{V}O_2$. The clinical implications of the low-compliance ventricle are summarized in Table 32-7. Because the ventricle is so stiff, atrial contraction is often critical for maintaining ventricular filling and stroke volume. The "atrial kick" may account for up to 30–40% of left ventricular end-diastolic volume. Hypertrophy-induced impairment of diastolic relaxation can further impede left ventricular filling. Ventricular filling pressure, as reflected by pulmonary capillary wedge pressure, is sometimes difficult to interpret, because it may vary widely yet reflect only small changes in ventricular volume.

Hypertrophied myocardium is susceptible to ischemia, even in the absence of concurrent coronary artery disease. The enlarged muscle mass increases basal myocardial oxygen require-

Table 32-7. CLINICAL AND PHYSIOLOGIC IMPLICATIONS OF A LOW-COMPLIANCE VENTRICLE

Sensitive to volume depletion
Dependent upon atrial kick for adequate ventricular filling
Wide swings in ventricular filling pressure
PCWP underestimates LVEDP
↑ LVEDP reduces coronary perfusion pressure

PCWP = pulmonary capillary wedge pressure; LVEDP = left ventricular end-diastolic pressure.

ments while demand per beat rises owing to the elevated intraventricular systolic pressure. Simultaneously, supply may be impaired, perfusion pressure is reduced (aortic diastolic pressure is decreased, ventricular filling pressure is increased), capillary density is often inadequate in the hypertrophic muscle, and total vasodilator reserve may be impaired.[115] This situation is compounded in the presence of coronary obstruction.

Anesthetic Considerations

The ideal hemodynamic environment for the patient with aortic stenosis is summarized in Table 32-8. Maintenance of adequate ventricular volume and sinus rhythm is crucial. Hypotension must be prevented if at all possible and treated early if it develops. Anticipation of likely hemodynamic changes is essential (e.g., expected decreases in blood pressure following spinal anesthesia). Coronary perfusion pressure must be maintained to prevent the catastrophic cycle of hypotension-induced ischemia, subsequent ventricular dysfunction, and worsening hypotension. Bradycardia is a common clinical etiology for hypotension in the patient with aortic stenosis. Slowing the heart rate and increasing diastolic time will not increase stroke volume. Therefore, bradycardia will induce a fall in total cardiac output and systemic arterial pressure. This is especially pertinent in the elderly patient, in whom sinus node disease and reduced sympathetic responses may predispose to significant bradycardia. Tachycardia must be avoided.

Ischemia may be difficult to detect because the characteristic changes are often obscured by the electrocardiographic signs of left ventricular hypertrophy and strain. Unfortunately, an ideal alternative is not available. Elevated left ventricular filling pressures, although not necessarily reflecting increased volume, often require treatment to optimize coronary perfusion pressure. Nitroglycerin is useful in this regard, but it must be remembered that minimal reductions in ventricular volume are re-

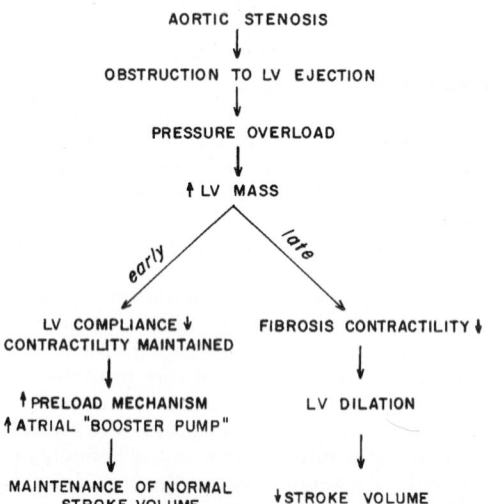

AORTIC STENOSIS
↓
OBSTRUCTION TO LV EJECTION
↓
PRESSURE OVERLOAD
↓
↑ LV MASS

early ↙   ↘ *late*

LV COMPLIANCE ↓   FIBROSIS CONTRACTILITY ↓
CONTRACTILITY MAINTAINED   ↓
↓   LV DILATION
↑ PRELOAD MECHANISM   ↓
↑ ATRIAL "BOOSTER PUMP"
↓   ↓ STROKE VOLUME
MAINTENANCE OF NORMAL
STROKE VOLUME

Figure 32-15. The physiologic consequences of aortic stenosis. (Reprinted with permission from Thomas SJ, Lowenstein E: Anesthetic management of the patient with valvular heart disease. Int Anesthesiol Clin 17:67, 1979.)

Table 32-8. AORTIC STENOSIS— HEMODYNAMIC GOALS

P	Full; adequate intravascular volume to fill noncompliant ventricular chamber
A	Already elevated, but relatively fixed; coronary perfusion pressure must be maintained
C	Usually not a problem; inotropes may be helpful; preinduction in end-stage aortic stenosis with hypotension
R	Not too slow (↓ CO), not too fast (ischemia)
Rhy	Sinus ! Cardioversion if hemodynamic instability from supraventricular dysrhythmia
$M\dot{V}O_2$	Ischemia is an ever-present risk; tachycardia and hypotension must be avoided

Abbreviations are defined in Table 32-2.

quired; therefore, very low doses of nitroglycerin should be used and titrated to effect.

TEE in Aortic Stenosis

In a normal adult the aortic valve is composed of three semilunar cusps attached to the wall of the aorta. The normal annular diameter is 1.9–2.3 cm with an aortic valve area (AVA) of 2–4 cm². The outpouchings of the aortic wall immediately above the valve cusps define the sinuses of Valsalva. The cusps and the corresponding sinuses are named according to their relation with the coronary ostia: left, right, and noncoronary. The sinuses of Valsalva should be symmetric, with a diameter that is 0.2–0.3 cm greater than the aortic valve annular diameter. On the ventricular side of the aortic valve is the cylindrical outflow tract. Its borders are the inferior surface of the anterior leaflet of the mitral valve, the interventricular septum, and the left ventricular free wall. The normal diameter of the left ventricular outflow tract (LVOT) is 2.2 cm ± 0.2 cm.

The short axis view of the aortic valve during systole can provide both a diagnosis and the mechanism of aortic stenosis. All three cusps of the aortic valve should be identified during systolic excursion. In degenerative calcification, the systolic orifice becomes smaller as the leaflet cusps become calcified, thickened, and deformed, resulting in a decreased ability to separate (Fig. 32-16). In contrast, rheumatic valve calcification is along the commissures, resulting in fusion and a progressive decrease in the valve orifice area. Although the rheumatic process usually involves the mitral valve, it can simultaneously or in isolation affect the aortic valve. A bicuspid aortic valve occurs in 2% of the population and predisposes the individual to aortic stenosis as well as aortic regurgitation and endocarditis. Frequently, the bicuspid valves have a raphe in the large cusp, which may be mistaken as a commissure during diastole. Trileaflet valves, if heavily calcified and fibrotic, may be indistinguishable from biscuspid valves.

The systolic aortic valve arc (AVA) can be accurately estimated by planimetry. In the midesophageal aortic valve long axis view, a systolic leaflet separation >1.3 cm reliably excludes severe aortic stenosis.[116] Associated two-dimensional findings with aortic stenosis may include concentric hypertrophy of the left ventricle, left ventricular diastolic dysfunction, and a post-stenotic aortic root dilatation that can become severe enough to require surgical correction.

Doppler interrogation across the stenotic aortic valve permits determination of the pressure gradient and AVA. Color flow Doppler across a stenotic aortic valve will show a mosaic of aliased turbulant flow. In about 90% of patients, the deep trans-

Table 32-9. GRADING FOR AORTIC STENOSIS

	Normal	Mild	Moderate	Severe
AVA (cm²)	3.0–5.0	1.2–2.0	1.1–0.8	<0.8
Peak gradient (mm Hg)	<10	16–34	35–75	>75

AVA = aortic valve area.

gastric long axis view allows excellent alignment of the ultrasound beam with aortic blood flow (angle < 30°).[117,118] If this view cannot be obtained, rotation to an angle between 60° and 90° from the transgastric midpapillary short axis view may align the ultrasound beam with the aortic blood flow. Utilizing the modified Bernoulli equation, the peak and mean aortic valve gradients can be determined from the peak and mean blood flow velocities across the stenotic valve. It is important to note that the cardiac catheterization data frequently report the left ventricular peak to aortic peak pressure gradient. These pressures occur at different times in the cardiac cycle and the gradient is consistently less than the peak instantaneous gradient measured by Doppler.[119] However, the mean gradients measured by echocardiography and catheterization should be the same. The pressure gradient is dependent on the flow through the orifice. The severity of the stenosis may be underestimated if the cardiac output is reduced; conversely, it is overestimated if flow is increased from aortic regurgitation or inotropic support. If one of these scenarios is suspected, the AVA should be calculated utilizing the continuity equation. The continuity equation assumes that the flow across any two orifices is the same. In this case, left ventricular outflow tract flow equals aortic valve (AV) flow. Doppler-derived flow measurements are the product of the VTI and the area of the orifice. The VTI of the LVOT is measured with pulsed Doppler, while the LVOT diameter is measured with two-dimensional echocardiography. Continuous-wave Doppler can measure the peak velocity through the stenotic lesion. The AVA is then calculated from the continuity equation:

$$VTI_{AV} \times area_{AV} = VTI_{LVOT} \times area_{LVOT}$$

$$Area_{AV} = VTI_{LVOT} \times area_{LVOT} / VTI_{AV}$$

The severity of aortic stenosis can be estimated by employing these echocardiographic modalities and the grading criteria outlined in Table 32-9.

Hypertrophic Cardiomyopathy

Hypertrophic cardiomyopathy, also known as idiopathic hypertrophic subaortic stenosis or asymmetric septal hypertrophy, is a genetically determined disease characterized by histologically abnormal myocytes and myocardial hypertrophy developing *a priori* and not in response to pressure or volume overload in a nondilated chamber.[120]

Pathophysiology

The physiologic consequences of hypertrophic cardiomyopathy are depicted in Figure 32-17. Some degree of subvalvular obstruction is present in 20–30% of patients. During systole, the left ventricular outflow tract is narrowed by apposition of the hypertrophic interventricular septum to the anterior leaflet of the mitral valve (Fig. 32-18). Blood is ejected rapidly through this area, creating a Venturi effect, pulling the mitral valve leaflet even closer to the septum (SAM, systolic anterior motion).[121] The timing and duration of septal–leaflet contact determine the severity and clinical significance of the obstruction. Early prolonged contact can generate pressure gradients of 100 mm Hg. If the apposition occurs later, although a pressure gradient may exist, it is of little importance because most of

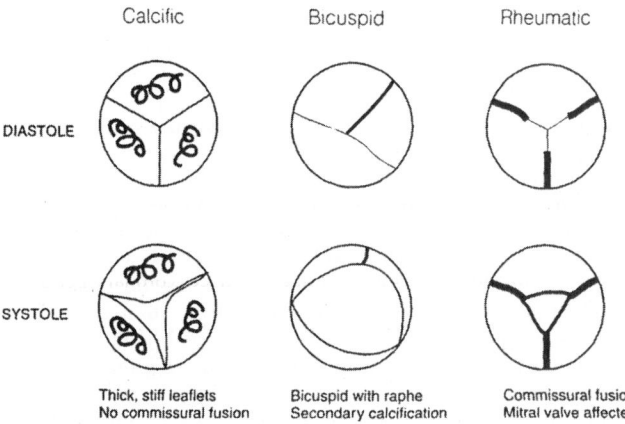

Figure 32-16. Diagram illustrating the three most common causes of aortic stenosis. See text for further discussion. (Reproduced with permission Otto MC, Pearlman AS: Textbook of Clinical Echocardiography. Philadelphia, WB Saunders, 1994.)

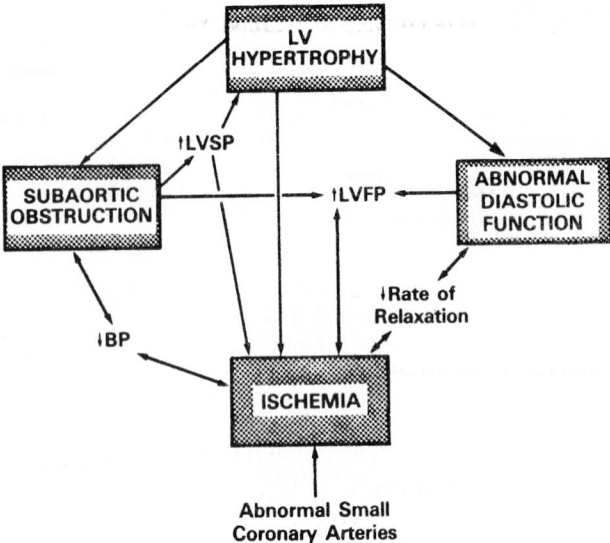

Figure 32-17. The physiologic interrelationships of primary left ventricular hypertrophy in hypertrophic cardiomyopathy. (LVSP = left ventricular systolic pressure; LVFP = left ventricular filling pressure.) (Reprinted with permission from Maron BJ, Bonow RO, Cannon RO *et al:* Hypertrophic cardiomyopathy: Interrelations of clinical manifestations, pathophysiology, and therapy. N Engl J Med 316:344, 1987.)

Table 32-10. HYPERTROPHIC CARDIOMYOPATHY—HEMODYNAMIC GOALS

P	Full, full, full; volume is first prescription for hypotension
A	Up, up, up; a pure vasoconstrictor is next prescription for hypotension
C	Depression is fine
R	Not too slow, not too fast
Rhy	Sinus, sinus, sinus; consider pacing pulmonary artery catheter to better control atrial mechanism
MV̇O₂	Usual precautions apply
CPB	Avoid inotropes post-CPB; the myocardial disease is still present; try vasoconstrictors first

Abbreviations are defined in Table 32-2.

the stroke volume has already been ejected. This obstruction is dynamic and is accentuated by any intervention that reduces ventricular size, facilitating septal–leaflet contact. Therefore, increases in contractility or heart rate or decreases in either preload or afterload are detrimental in this regard. Another hypothesis proposed for systolic anterior motion of the mitral valve is abnormally displaced mitral apparatus.[122]

The histologically abnormal muscle demonstrates impaired diastolic relaxation and reduced ventricular compliance. The clinical and hemodynamic implications are similar to those detailed for aortic stenosis.

The ventricles are hypertrophic, even in the absence of a pressure gradient. In addition, there is evidence of alterations

in the small intramyocardial vessels. Therefore, as expected, myocardial oxygen balance is tenuous, and the development of ischemia is an ever-present possibility.

Anesthetic Considerations

Anesthetic management focuses on maintenance of ventricular filling and reduction in the factors predisposing to outflow tract obstruction or ischemia (Table 32-10). Myocardial depression is desirable, and volatile anesthetics are useful, although their tendency to cause junctional rhythm is of some concern. Because of the exquisite sensitivity of preload to atrial contraction, these patients will benefit from atrial pacing if junctional rhythm occurs. Methods to achieve this include transesophageal pacing or use of a pulmonary artery catheter with pacing capability. This permits the administration of volatile anesthetics without fear of compromising sinoatrial conduction. In addition, control of atrial rate and rhythm is beneficial during the prebypass period.

Although infrequent, hypertrophic cardiomyopathy occasionally coexists with valvular aortic stenosis and may explain unanticipated difficulties in separating from bypass following seemingly uncomplicated aortic valve replacement. If this is suspected, measurement of the gradient between the left ventricle and the outflow tract will resolve the dilemma. In addition, dynamic left ventricular outflow obstruction is occasionally observed following mitral valve repair. Anterior septal motion of the mitral valve is observed echocardiographically. Pharmacologic management of hypotension is with volume replacement and vasoconstrictors rather than inotropes and vasodilators.

Aortic Insufficiency

Rheumatic disease, endocarditis, or processes that dilate the aortic root such as ascending aortic aneurysms or collagen vascular diseases are the primary causes of aortic insufficiency.

Pathophysiology

The fundamental physiologic derangement is chronic volume overload (Fig. 32-19). Chamber size increases gradually, sometimes to massive proportions, increasing wall stress and inducing mural hypertrophy. This pattern of chamber enlargement and increasing ventricular wall thickness is termed *eccentric hypertrophy*. Despite these enormous increases in end-diastolic volume, end-diastolic pressures are usually within the normal range, evidence of a significant increase in chamber diastolic compliance. In contrast to aortic stenosis, considerable alterations in left ventricular volume can occur with only minimal changes in left ventricular filling pressure. Although the ventricle may pump three to four times the normal cardiac output, MV̇O₂ does not increase extraordinarily because the oxygen cost for muscle shortening is low. The contractile state of the myocardium is often difficult to discern from clinical signs and symptoms. Ventricular afterload is chronically reduced because of

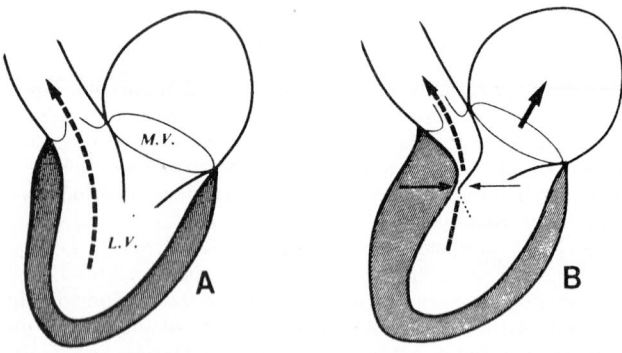

Figure 32-18. Proposed mechanism for outflow tract obstruction in hypertrophic cardiomyopathy. (*A*) The normal outflow tract is ample and offers no impedance to ejection. (*B*) The outflow tract is narrowed by the hypertrophic ventricular septum in hypertrophic cardiomyopathy. A Venturi effect is produced as blood is ejected rapidly through this area, drawing the anterior mitral leaflet toward the septum. Obstruction to forward flow (owing to mitral–septal contact) as well as mitral regurgitation can occur. (Reprinted with permission from Wigle ED, Sasson Z, Henderson ME *et al:* Hypertrophic cardiomyopathy: The importance of the site and the extent of hypertrophy. A review. Prog Cardiovasc Dis 28:1, 1985.)

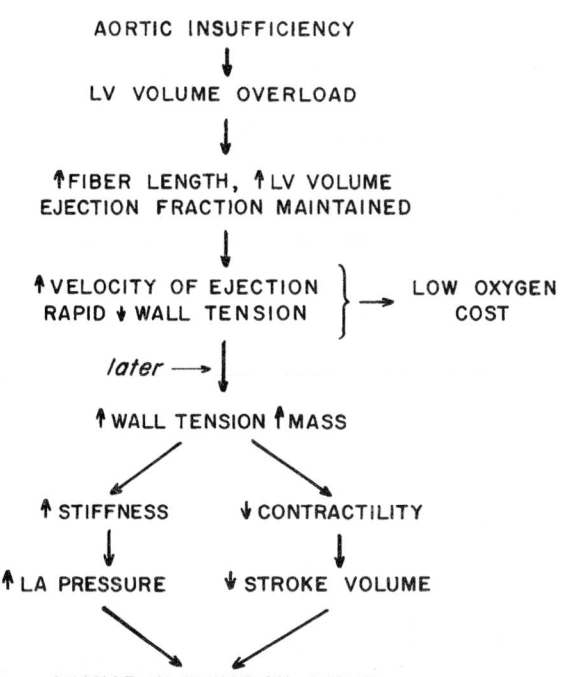

AORTIC INSUFFICIENCY

↓

LV VOLUME OVERLOAD

↓

↑FIBER LENGTH, ↑LV VOLUME
EJECTION FRACTION MAINTAINED

↓

↑VELOCITY OF EJECTION   }   → LOW OXYGEN
RAPID ↓WALL TENSION   }   COST

later → ↓

↑WALL TENSION ↑MASS

↙   ↘

↑STIFFNESS   ↓CONTRACTILITY

↓   ↓

↑LA PRESSURE   ↓STROKE VOLUME

↘   ↙

CHANGE IN FUNCTION CURVE

Figure 32-19. The physiologic consequences of aortic insufficiency. (Reprinted with permission from Thomas SJ, Lowenstein E: Anesthetic management of the patient with valvular heart disease. Int Anesthesiol Clin 17:67, 1979.)

the low diastolic pressure, reflecting continuing diastolic runoff as well as a moderately vasodilated state. This will allow patients to be relatively symptom-free even in the presence of reduced contractility. This is important in terms of planning the anesthetic, but perhaps even more so with respect to timing of aortic valve replacement. Ideally, the valve should be replaced just prior to the onset of irreversible myocardial damage. Therefore, continued follow-up of these patients emphasizes repeated noninvasive measurements of contractility, usually after some form of afterload stress, either pharmacologic- or exercise-induced.

In contrast to chronic aortic insufficiency, acute aortic insufficiency subjects a ventricle with normal diastolic function to sudden volume overload; severe congestive heart failure dominates the clinical picture. The previously normal-sized left ventricle, with limited distensibility, is presented with large regurgitant volumes, rapidly elevating left ventricular end-diastolic pressure (along the steep portion of the diastolic pressure–volume relation). Left ventricular end-diastolic pressure increases to alarming levels, and myocardial contractility becomes impaired. Compensatory mechanisms include tachycardia and peripheral vasoconstriction, but occasionally hypotension and low cardiac output ensue (Table 32-11). Some patients are so

Table 32-11. ACUTE VERSUS CHRONIC AORTIC INSUFFICIENCY

	Chronic	Acute
Left ventricular size	↑	—
Left ventricular compliance	↑	—
Left ventricular end-diastolic pressure	—	↑
Effective cardiac output	Normal	↓
Systemic vascular resistance	—	↑
Pulmonary edema	No	Yes
Pulse pressure	↑	↑/—
Heart rate	—	↑

Table 32-12. AORTIC INSUFFICIENCY— HEMODYNAMIC GOALS

P	Normal to slightly ↑
A	Reduction beneficial with anesthetics or vasodilators; increases augment regurgitant flow
C	Usually adequate
R	Modest tachycardia reduces ventricular volume, raises aortic diastolic pressure
Rhy	Usually sinus; not a problem
M$\dot{V}O_2$	Not usually a problem
CPB	Observe for ventricular distention (↓ HR, ↑ VFP) when going onto CPB

Abbreviations are defined in Table 32-2.

acutely ill that emergency aortic valve replacement is required, whereas in less severe circumstances, mild systemic vasodilation and inotropic support can return hemodynamics toward normal.

Anesthetic Considerations

Full, mildly vasodilated, and modestly tachycardic describe the optimal cardiovascular state for patients with aortic insufficiency (Table 32-12). Vasodilation promotes forward flow, although additional intravascular volume may be necessary to maintain preload. The ideal heart rate is somewhat controversial.[124] It is likely that changes in rate alone will not alter net forward or regurgitant flow; each will be proportionately reduced. Tachycardia does reduce diastolic ventricular volume and wall tension, and also increases diastolic blood pressure, which should improve coronary perfusion and offset the increase in oxygen demand secondary to an increased heart rate. Bradycardia should be avoided because it predisposes to ventricular distention, which causes elevations in left atrial pressure and pulmonary congestion.

Ventricular distention may occur with the onset of cardiopulmonary bypass if the heart slows or if there is unexpected ventricular fibrillation. Monitoring of the appearance of the heart, the rate and rhythm, and ventricular filling pressure if available are especially important in these patients. If distention occurs, the insertion of a left ventricular vent or the immediate application of an aortic crossclamp should relieve the problem.

TEE in Aortic Insufficiency

Annular dilatation or abnormal leaflet motion are the mechanisms that result in aortic insufficiency. Annular dilatation can occur with ascending aortic aneurysms, aortic dissections, and eccentric hypertrophy of the left ventricle. Because the aortic cusp area is 40% greater than the cross-sectional area of a normal aortic root, small increases in the diameter of the aortic annulus can be accommodated before the valve becomes incompetent. Abnormal leaflet motion and coaptation can be noted with calcific degeneration, rheumatic disease, and bicuspid aortic valves. Postinflammatory disease of the aorta is the most common cause of isolated aortic regurgitation. Other two-dimensional echocardiographic findings associated with aortic regurgitation include fluttering and reverse doming of the anterior mitral leaflet, premature closure of the mitral valve, aortic vegetations, leaflet perforations, and eccentric hypertrophy of the left ventricle.

Application of color flow Doppler will identify the aortic regurgitant jet, localize the site of regurgitation, and help grade the severity of the aortic insufficiency.[125] Unlike mitral regurgitation, neither the length nor area of the regurgitant jet correlates with the angiographic grade of aortic insufficiency.[126] Rather, the severity of aortic insufficiency is most reliably graded by comparing the diameter of the regurgitant jet at the level of the aortic valve with the diameter of the LVOT.[127] As in mitral

Table 32-13. GRADING FOR AORTIC INSUFFICIENCY

	Mild	Moderate	Severe
Jet width at origin (mm)	<2	3–5	>5
Jet width/LVOT width	<30%	30–60%	>60%
Jet length (cm)	<2	3–5	>5

LVOT = left ventricle outflow track.

regurgitation, it is important to recall that the size and shape of the color flow jet are dependant on the Nyquest limit. Continuous-wave Doppler across an aortic regurgitant jet will typically demonstrate a pandiastolic flow signal. The peak velocity in early diastole corresponds to the peak aortic to left ventricular diastolic pressure gradient as defined by the modified Bernoulli equation. The slope of the decay in this pressure gradient reflects the severity of aortic insufficiency. With severe aortic insufficiency, there is a rapid equilibration of pressure between the aorta and the left ventricle. This results in a steep slope of decay and a short presure half-time (PHT). If the aortic insufficiency is mild, there is a slow equilibration of the pressure between the aorta and the left ventricle that results in a relatively flat slope of decay and a long PHT. Interpretation of the slope of decay as an index of regurgitation is complicated by factors that increase the equilibration of the pressure gradient between the aorta and left ventricle. These factors include the compliance of the left ventricle and the filling from the mitral valve. The severity of aortic insufficiency (AI) can be graded by employing these echocardiographic modalities and the criteria outlined in Table 32-13.

The presence of moderate to severe AI affects the surgeon's approach to cardiopulmonary bypass. An incompetent aortic valve may prevent the delivery of cardioplegia to the coronary system to produce the diastolic arrest of the heart. After application of the aortic crossclamp, the cardioplegia is normally injected into the aortic root, delivering this solution to the coronary system, producing a diastolic arrest of the heart. If moderate to severe aortic insufficiency is present, the cardioplegia will fill and distend the left ventricle, increasing the ischemic insult incurred during cardiopulmonary bypass. As a result, in the presence of aortic insufficiency the surgeon may elect to arrest the heart by injecting cardioplegia directly into the coronary ostia or into the coronary sinus.

Accurate evaluation of aortic insufficiency is essential in determining the feasibility of performing an aortic repair. Successful aortic valve repairs are routinely performed with aortic dissections, and have been reported with aneurysms and bicuspid aortic valves.[128–131] About 70% of type A dissections lend themselves to repair with an 80–90% freedom from valve replacement 10 years out from the surgery. Repairing aortic valves in patients with bicuspid valves or aortic aneurysms secondary to tissue disorders is controversial.

Mitral Stenosis

Stenosis of the mitral valve is usually of rheumatic origin, with clinical disease becoming manifest within 3–5 years following initial infection. Debilitating symptoms such as fatigue and dyspnea on exertion do not begin for another decade or two.

Pathophysiology

The spectrum of physiologic disruption in patients with mitral stenosis is presented in Figure 32-20. This complicated pathophysiologic profile may be simplified by grouping the changes as either proximal or distal to the obstructing mitral valve.

In mitral stenosis, unlike other valvular lesions, the left ventricle is not subject to either pressure or volume overload. It is often relatively underloaded owing to the obstruction preventing left ventricular filling. The left ventricle may be small,

but ventricular function is usually maintained, although one third of patients may demonstrate contractile abnormalities on angiography, presumably as a result of rheumatic carditis or involvement of the subvalvular apparatus.[132] The diminished ventricular volume precludes effective use of vasodilators to improve left ventricular flow.

Increased left atrial pressure (LAP) and volume overload are inevitable consequences of the narrowed mitral orifice. The relationship between left atrial pressure and the size of the valve orifice is expressed in the formula derived by Gorlin and Gorlin:

$$\text{Valve area} = \text{flow} / K \cdot \sqrt{(\text{pressure gradient})}$$

where flow = (cardiac output) / (diastolic filling time); pressure gradient = (left atrial pressure) − (left ventricular end-diastolic pressure), or LAP − LVEDP; and K is the hydraulic pressure constant. This calculation assumes no regurgitant flow. If we assume a constant valve area, rearrange terms, and eliminate the constant, we have a more useful expression of the clinical variables determining atrial and ventricular pressures:

$$\text{LAP} - \text{LVEDP} = [(\text{cardiac output}) / (\text{diastolic time})]^2$$

Therefore, whenever cardiac output increases or the diastolic filling period decreases, the gradient across the mitral valve is altered by the square of the original changes. This explains why tachycardia or increases in forward flow, seen classically with pregnancy, thyrotoxicosis, or infection, can precipitate pulmonary edema. As LAP increases, left ventricular filling pressure may actually decrease. Thus, the development of atrial fibrillation causes hemodynamic embarrassment, not so much because of the loss of atrial kick but because of the rapid rate that ensues. We are left with the paradoxical situation of a patient in pulmonary edema with a relatively empty left ventricle. The treatment in this situation is therefore not inotropic or vasodilator therapy, but rather attempts to reduce the heart rate or diagnose and treat the cause responsible for the increased flow. The pulmonary capillary wedge pressure can be used as an index of left ventricular filling, keeping in mind that it is higher than the true left ventricular end-diastolic pressure, at least by the amount of the pressure gradient. During episodes of tachycardia or increased flow, the wedge pressure continues to reflect left atrial pressure; however, this is no longer indicative of left ventricular filling pressure.

Persistent elevations in LAP are reflected back through the pulmonary circulation, leading to right ventricular pressure overload with compensatory right ventricular hypertrophy and strain. The progression and severity of pulmonary hypertension are variable and reflect further narrowing of the valve orifice and irreversible reactive changes in the pulmonary vasculature. Right ventricular dysfunction may develop in response to the

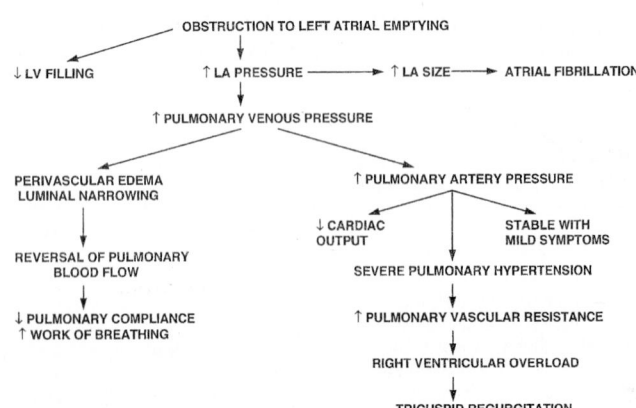

Figure 32-20. The cardiovascular and pulmonary effects of mitral stenosis.

**Table 32-14. MITRAL STENOSIS—
HEMODYNAMIC GOALS**

P	Enough to maintain flow across stenosis
A	Avoid ↑ right ventricular afterload (pulmonary vasoconstrictors) ? inotropes for systemic hypotension
C	LV usually OK until after CPB; right ventricle may be impaired if there is long-standing pulmonary hypertension
R	Slow to allow time for ventricular filling
Rhy	Often atrial fibrillation; control ventricular response
MVo₂	Not a problem
CPB	Vasodilators may help post-CPB right ventricular failure; control of ventricular response may be difficult

Abbreviations are defined in Table 32-2.

afterload stress. Tricuspid annular dilatation and insufficiency may climax this hemodynamic nightmare.

Chronically elevated left atrial pressure causes perivascular edema in the lung, increased vascular pressure in the dependent portions of the lung, redistribution of blood to the upper lung fields, and a somewhat increased work of breathing.

Anesthetic Considerations

Preventing trouble is the cornerstone of prebypass anesthetic management (Table 32-14) because treatment of hemodynamic derangements is sometimes difficult. Avoiding tachycardia precludes episodes of left atrial and pulmonary hypertension with potential right ventricular dysfunction as well as inadequate left ventricular filling with concomitant systemic hypotension. Preoperative maintenance of digitalis and β-blocking drugs, selection of anesthetics with no propensity to increase heart rate, and attainment of anesthetic levels deep enough to suppress autonomic responses are methods to achieve these goals. Episodes of pulmonary hypertension and potential right-sided heart failure stemming from pulmonary vasoconstriction must also be prevented. Hypoxia, hypercarbia, and acidosis are the classic offenders. It is wise, then, to follow the ancient internist's classic nostrum: Avoid them.

Treatment of hypotension in patients with mitral stenosis can present a challenging dilemma. Although these patients normally take diuretics, hypovolemia is not usually the cause; hence the response to volume administration is often disappointing. Use of a vasoconstrictor to offset mild peripheral vasodilation is acceptable, bearing in mind the risk of pulmonary vasoconstriction and possible accentuation of right ventricular dysfunction. It is often prudent to select a drug with some inotropic effect such as ephedrine or epinephrine instead of relying on a pure vasoconstrictor. In separating from cardiopulmonary bypass, much is made of right ventricular failure (discussed subsequently); more commonly, however, it is the left ventricle that is dysfunctional. This may be because intraoperative injury or sudden increase in flow to and distention of the chronically underloaded left ventricle. After bypass, prominent V waves may be present in the left atrial pressure curve. This almost always reflects increased left atrial filling from the right side rather than mitral regurgitation because cardiac output is increased after bypass when compared with preinduction values.

TEE in Mitral Stenosis

The mitral valve area in a normal adult ranges from 4 to 6 cm². It is composed of the funnel-shaped atrioventricular membrane, which is divided into two leaflets (anterior, posterior), and the suspensory tensor structures. The anterior mitral leaflet is triangular, covering about 60% of the valve orifice. It occupies about 40% of the annular circumference and is contiguous with the noncoronary and left coronary cusps of the aortic valve. The broad, crescent-shaped posterior leaflet comprises three scal-

lops. Although equal in surface area, the posterior leaflet occupies about 60% of the annulus and, as a result, is shorter and less mobile (Fig. 32-21). The leaflets are tethered like parachutes by the subvalvular tensor apparatus, which consists of chordae tendineae and their muscular insertions into the anterolateral and posteromedial papillary muscles. Both leaflets receive chordae from each papillary muscle. These fibrous tendons, along with the coordinated contraction of the supporting muscles, prevent the leaflets from prolapsing into the left atrium when high pressures are exerted on the leaflets during left ventricular systole. Doppler interrogation across a normal mitral valve reveals a biphasic filling pattern composed of two waves. Early passive filling of the ventricle during diastole is represented by the E wave while the atrial contribution to ventricular filling generates the A wave (Fig. 32-22). Normal blood flow velocities measured at the tips of the mitral valve leaflets are between 0.50 and 0.80 m · sec⁻¹.[114]

Mitral stenosis results from insufficient opening of the valve leaflets during diastole. The valve leaflets become fibrous and thick while the chordae are shortened. The diastolic excursion of the leaflets is limited, resulting in a characteristic doming or hockey stick deformity of the anterior mitral leaflet that is best seen in the midesophageal four-chamber or long axis view. Calcium deposits begin in the valve commissures and extend to the leaflet bodies, the valve annulus, and the subvalvular apparatus. The extent of calcification is variable and inversely related to the size of the stenotic orifice. Planimetry of the cross-sectional area of the narrowest opening in a two-dimensional short axis view of the mitral valve can be used to directly measure the orifice area. Although reproducible and accurate for transthoracic echocardiography, it has not yet been validated for TEE. Associated two-dimensional findings with mitral stenosis may include an enlarged left atrium (>4 cm) with bowing of the interatrial septum toward the right atrium, occurrence of spontaneous echocontrast, and the presence of atrial thrombi. Spontanous echo contrast is the result of blood cell aggregation and occurs in areas of low flow. It is seen in more than 50% of patients with mitral stenosis and is associated with an increased risk of thromboembolism.[97]

Doppler interrogation across the stenotic mitral valve permits determination of the pressure gradient and the mitral valve area (MVA). Color flow Doppler across a stenotic mitral valve reveals laminar flow acceleration into the stenotic orifice and a turbulent jet emerging into the ventricle. Bernoulli's equation explains the relationship between a pressure drop across a stenotic valve and the corresponding velocity of flow. Simplification of his formula assumes negligible contributions from blood viscosity, viscous friction, and flow acceleration. With these assumptions, a peak instantaneous transvalvular pressure gradient can be estimated. The peak blood flow velocity is measured and applied to the following equation:

$$P = 4V^2$$

where P is pressure, and V is velocity.

The mean pressure gradient can be determined by tracing and integrating the diastolic spectral blood flow velocity profile. The pressure half-time (PHT) method is utilized to calculate the MVA. The PHT is generated from the rate of decline of the E wave of the diastolic spectral blood flow profile. This permits calculation of the MVA by the following equation:

$$MVA(cm^2) = 220/PHT$$

where PHT is the time interval (milliseconds) between the maximum early diastolic transmitral pressure gradient and the time point where the pressure gradient is one half the maximum value. This number is calculated by the computer when the slope of the E wave is entered (Fig. 32-23). When analyzing the transvalvular blood flow velocity profile, one must recall that it is a function not only of the size of the mitral valve orifice, but also of the amount of flow through the orifice, the chamber

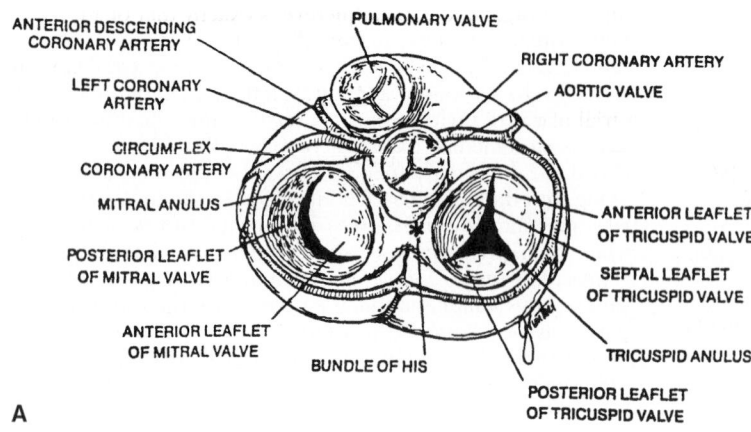

A

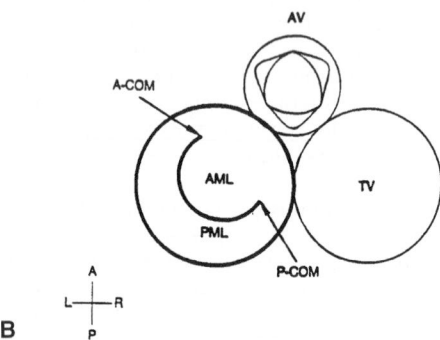

B

Figure 32-21. (*A*) Diagram illustrating the anatomic position of the mitral valve within the heart as viewed in cross-section looking inferiorly toward the cardiac apex. (*B*) Note that the anterior mitral leaflet originates from only 40% of the annular circumference but accounts for 60% of the orifice. (Reproduced with permission from Oka Y, Goldiner PL: Transesophageal Echocardiography. Philadelphia, JB Lippincott, 1992.)

compliance, and the presence of aortic regurgitation.[134] These are variables that affect the transvalvular pressure gradient. Aortic regurgitation results in a rapid equalization of pressure between the left atrium and the left ventricle. This generates a rapid PHT which overestimates the MVA by the PHT equation. The severity of mitral stenosis can be estimated by employing these echocardiographic modalities and the criteria outlined in Table 32-15.

Mitral Regurgitation

Mitral valve prolapse, chronic ischemic heart disease, rheumatic heart disease, endocarditis, and annular dilation are causes of mitral regurgitation. Acute mitral regurgitation occurs with papillary muscle dysfunction or chordal rupture following myocardial infarction and may require emergency surgical repair.

Pathophysiology

Chronic volume overload similar to that described with aortic insufficiency is the cardinal feature of mitral regurgitation. The left atrium acts as a low-pressure vent for left ventricular ejection. Total stroke volume consists of the forward flow *via* the aorta and backward flow into the left atrium. There is no period of isovolumetric contraction because blood is immediately

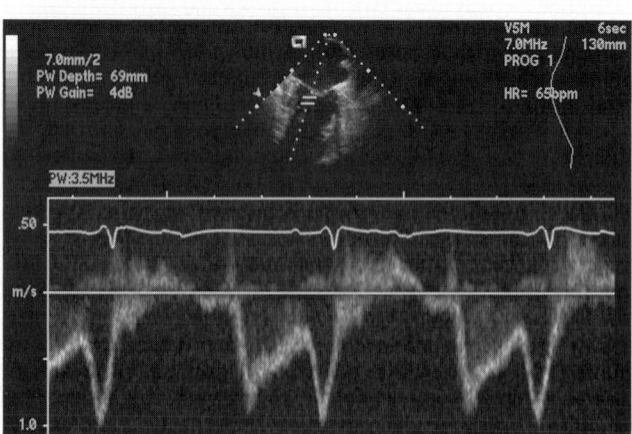

Figure 32-22. Normal Doppler flow velocity profile across the mitral valve. Early passive filling of the ventricle during diastole is represented by the E wave while the atrial contribution to ventricular filling generates the A wave. Normal blood flow velocities measured at the tips of the mitral valve leaflets range between 0.50 and 0.80 m · sec⁻¹.

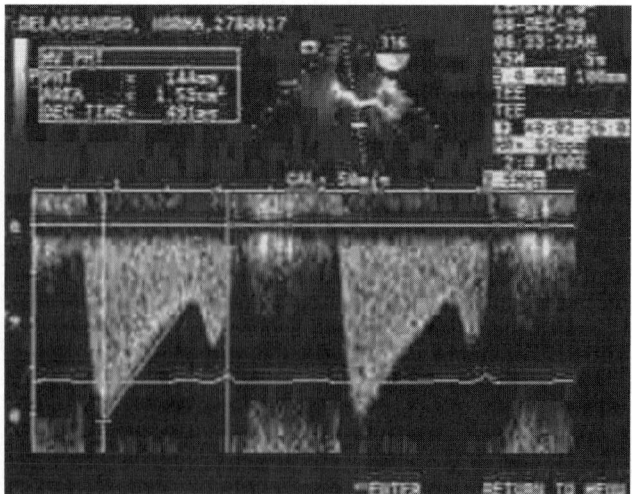

Figure 32-23. The MVA is calculated by the pressure half-time method. Note the decreased slope of the deceleration of the E wave as a result of the prolonged presence of a pressure gradient between the left atrium and left ventricle secondary to the stenotic mitral valve.

Table 32-15. GRADING FOR MITRAL STENOSIS

	Normal	Mild	Moderate	Severe
MVA (cm²)	4.0–6.0	1.5–2.0	1.0–1.5	>1.0
PHT (ms)	<100	100–150	150–200	>220
Mean gradient	<2	2–6	6–12	>12

MVA = mitral valve area; PHT = pressure half-time.

ejected retrograde with the onset of ventricular systole. Despite decreased contractility, patients may be minimally symptomatic despite progressive myocardial damage because of this reduced afterload. The additional oxygen cost is low, needed only for additional muscle shortening because there is little pressure development. Ventricular compliance increases; thus, the large end-diastolic volume does not cause striking increases in left ventricular end-diastolic pressure. Atrial and ventricular chamber enlargement, ventricular wall hypertrophy, and increased blood volume are the compensatory responses. The volume of regurgitant flow is related to the size of the regurgitant orifice, the time available for retrograde flow, and the pressure gradient across the valve. Regurgitant orifice size, in turn, is dependent upon ventricular size. Therefore, both increases in heart rate and preload reduction decrease the amount of regurgitant flow by diminishing ventricular volume. Arteriolar dilators, in contrast, are effective by reducing the ventriculoatrial pressure gradient.

Other similarities of mitral regurgitation to aortic insufficiency include increases in ventricular chamber compliance and difficulty in evaluating left ventricular contractile function. The latter is particularly troublesome because in mitral regurgitation the left ventricle is maximally unloaded. The incompetent valve acts as a low-pressure vent for left ventricular ejection. There is no period of isovolumic contraction because blood is immediately ejected retrograde with the onset of ventricular systole. This explains why many patients have minimal symptoms despite progressive myocardial damage. This reduced afterload also explains why ejection fraction, a measure heavily afterload-dependent, can be misleading in patients with mitral regurgitation. Normal or minimally reduced ejection fractions can be present even with severe impairment of contractile function.[110] Repairing or replacing the valve increases afterload, and often the dysfunctional myocardium becomes apparent. Administration of inotropes and/or vasodilators may be necessary to successfully separate from bypass.

When mitral regurgitation is of acute onset, the hemodynamic picture is different. Volume overload of the left atrium and ventricle occurs in the absence of compensatory ventricular enlargement. Ventricular filling pressures increase dramatically, as do pulmonary pressures. Cardiac output decreases, and pulmonary edema develops. If this occurs in the setting of acute myocardial infarction, cardiac performance may be inadequate despite pharmacologic support. Intra-aortic balloon assistance as well as emergency surgery may be lifesaving.

Anesthetic Considerations

Selection of anesthetics that promote vasodilation and tachycardia is ideal in the patient with mitral regurgitation (Table 32-16). Active pharmacologic intervention is usually unnecessary because most patients are not teetering on the brink of myocardial failure. However, in some patients, especially those with acute myocardial regurgitation, aggressive pharmacologic management may be required. In the absence of acute deterioration, difficulties in management are usually limited to the postbypass period.

The problem of unmasking depressed myocardial contractility has already been discussed. Paradoxically, after the administration of vasodilators and inotropes, a patient occasionally deteriorates even further. As mentioned earlier, in these patients,

the physiologic and clinical picture is exactly that of hypertrophic cardiomyopathy. It is seen after valve repair, not replacement. Systolic anterior motion of the anterior mitral leaflet is demonstrable by echocardiography. If this scenario is suspected, a trial of volume expansion and vasoconstrictors is indicated.

TEE in Mitral Regurgitation

The presence and severity of mitral regurgitation are major determinants of outcome in cardiac surgical patients. If the mitral regurgitation is severe enough to require surgical intervention, a decision must be made regarding the feasibility of performing a mitral valve repair as opposed to replacement. The etiology of the regurgitation and accurate localization of the site of mitral regurgitation are two important factors in this decision. In the suitable patient population, a repair has become the treatment of choice. It avoids the morbidity associated with valvular prostheses and long-term anticoagulation while providing significantly lower hospital mortality, late valve-related events, and better long-term survival.[135-139] Mitral disease localized to the posterior leaflet or to a focal portion of the anterior leaflet is most amenable to repair. Conversely, mitral repair is more difficult when there is heavy calcification of the annulus or extensive disease of the anterior leaflet of the mitral valve. This has resulted in the desire for increasingly sophisticated TEE evaluation of mitral regurgitation.

Mitral regurgitation results from incomplete coaptation of the mitral leaflets, permitting blood to flow from the left ventricle to the left atrium during systole. Mechanical etiologies of mitral regurgitation include (1) annular dilatation, (2) leaflet prolapse, (3) restricted leaflet motion, (4) and leaflet perforation.

1. *Annular dilatation:* The mitral annulus is contiguous with the fibrous skeleton of the heart anteriorly, while the posterior portion of the annulus is composed of the atrioventricular membrane of the free wall of the heart. It is the posterior portion of the mitral valve annulus that is susceptible to the dilatation that can occur with myocardial infarctions and myopathies. In this setting leaflet appearance and motion are frequently normal. Since normal mitral valve coaptation occurs on the left atrial surface of the leaflets, small increases in the diameter of the mitral annulus are possible before the mitral valve becomes incompetent.

2. *Leaflet prolapse:* Redundant leaflet tissue and chordae may be present when there are connective tissue disorders or myxoid degeneration of the mitral valve. This results in excessive leaflet motion with coaptation occurring in the left atrium beyond the plane of the mitral valve annulus. Occasionally, there is complete rupture of the chorda or papillary muscle that anchor the mitral valve leaflets. This

Table 32-16. MITRAL REGURGITATION— HEMODYNAMIC GOALS

P	Usually pretty full; may need to keep that way, although preload reduction may reduce regurgitant flow
A	Decreases are beneficial; increases augment regurgitant flow
C	Unrecognized myocardial depression possible; titrate myocardial depressants carefully
R	A faster rate decreases ventricular volume
Rhy	Atrial fibrillation is occasionally a problem
MV̇O₂	Only if mitral regurgitation is a complication of coronary artery disease; then be careful
CPB	Newly competent valve post-CPB increases afterload; vasodilators may be helpful; inotropes are frequently required

Abbreviations are defined in Table 32-2.

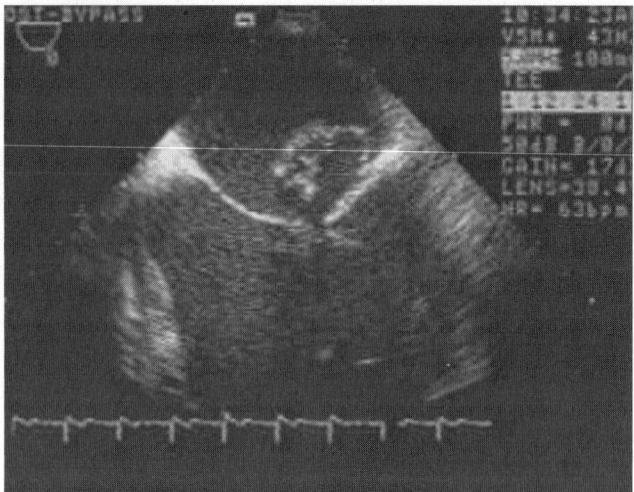

Figure 32-24. Mitral regurgitation due to "flail" posterior leaflet of the mitral valve.

can produce extreme leaflet mobility known as a "flail leaflet" where the tip of the flail leaflet is freely mobile in the left atrium (Fig. 32-24).

3. *Restricted leaflet motion:* Tethering of the leaflets, calcification of the chordae, and scarring of the papillary muscles can restrict leaflet mobility, resulting in an incompetent mitral valve owing to a failure of the leaflets to adjoin.

4. *Leaflet perforation:* Leaflet perforation can occur with endocarditis.

A systematic approach is necessary for accurate localization of the site of mitral regurgitation.[135,136] Maintaining spatial orientation is crucial. The mitral valve lies posterior, inferior, and lateral to the aortic valve. The posterior leaflet forms the lateral edge of the mitral valve and contains three scallops labeled P1, P2, and P3, with P1 located anterior and lateral while P3 is inferior and medial. The anterior leaflet is the medial portion of the valve; although not clearly scalloped, it is likewise subdivided into sections A1, A2, and A3, with A1 anterior and A3 posterior (Fig. 32-25). In the four-chamber view at a rotational angle of 0°, the image plane transects the mitral valve across the middle

scallops (A2, P2). If the probe is withdrawn and/or flexed, the most anterior portion of the mitral valve will be imaged (A1, P1). However, if the TEE is advanced and/or retroflexed from the four-chamber view, the posterior medial portion of the mitral valve will be transected (A3, P3) (Fig. 32-26). If the image plane is rotated 45–90° from the four-chamber view, it will align with the major axis of the mitral valve. Clockwise rotation (toward the patient's right) will place the image plane across the anterior leaflet, and counterclockwise rotation will allow complete transection of the posterior leaflet by the image plane. These views can be used to confirm the location of valve pathology delineated at a rotational angle of 0°. Agreement of the location of mitral regurgitation with TEE and direct surgical observation is excellent.[135,136] Other two-dimensional echocardiographic findings associated with mitral regurgitation include an enlarged left atrium (>4 cm) and eccentric hypertrophy of the left ventricle. The left atrium will be akinetic if atrial fibrillation is present; however, when mitral regurgitation is severe, spontaneous contrast and atrial thrombi are not likely to be present owing to a lack of blood stasis.

Application of color flow Doppler will identify the mitral regurgitant jet and can be used to help localize the site of regurgitation[140] (Fig. 32-27). It is important to recall that the size and shape of the color flow jet are dependent on the Nyquest limit. The Nyquest limit is a color visualization of blood flow velocity which is determined by a number of machine variables including sector scan width, depth of the sector, and density of the scan lines. If the Nyquest limit is low (<40 cm·s^{-1}), color Doppler can overestimate the extent of regurgitation. The type of regurgitatant jet also affects the extent of the color flow area depicted. Eccentric jets, common with isolated individual leaflet abnormalities, frequently impinge on the atrial wall and produce smaller color Doppler areas than central jets of similar regurgitant volumes.[108–110]

The effect of mitral regurgitation on left atrial pressure and the pulmonary circulation is evaluated by analysis of the pulse wave Doppler pattern in the pulmonary veins. Mitral regurgitation increases the left atrial pressure during systole. As mitral regurgitation increases in severity, the pressure gradient from the pulmonary vein to the left atrium decreases. This results in attenuation of the systolic component of the pulmonary vein flow pattern. If severe mitral regurgitation is present, the left atrial pressure may exceed the pulmonary vein pressure during systole, resulting in reversal of the S wave. This is illustrated in

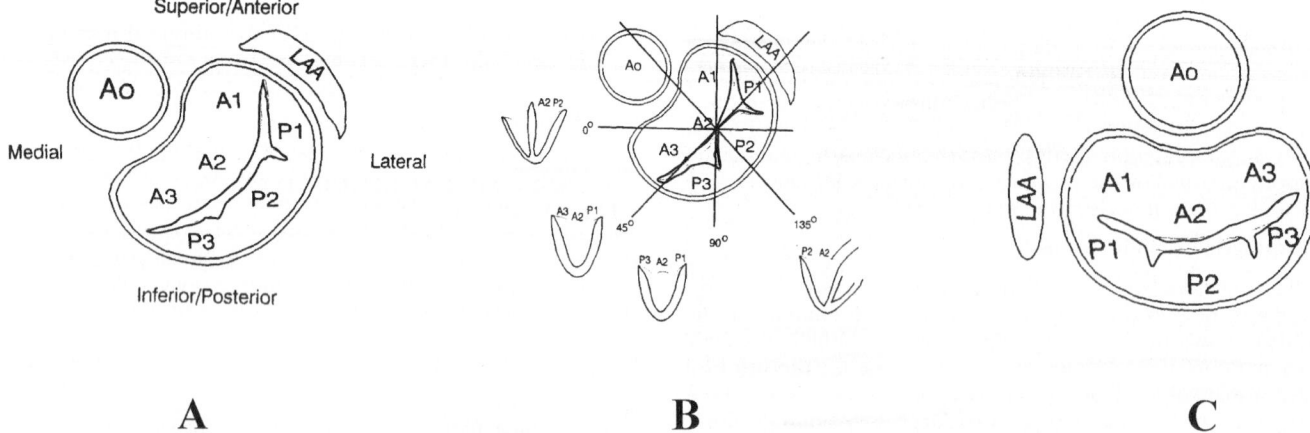

A   **B**   **C**

Figure 32-25. (*A*) View from the left ventricular apex demonstrating the anatomic relationship of the mitral valve to the aorta (Ao) the left atrial appendage (LAA). (*B*) Reference view demonstrating the relationship of the transesophageal echocardiographic imaging planes (0, 45, 90, and 135 degrees) to the mitral valve with the probe positioned in the standard midesophageal position. (*C*) Surgical view of the mitral valve as seen from left atrium. A1, A2, A3 = anterior leaflets sections; P1, P2, P3, = posterior leaflet sections. (Reproduced with permission from Foster GP, Isselbacher EM, Rose GA *et al:* Accurate localization of mitral regurgitant defects using multiplane transesophageal echocardiography. Ann Thorac Surg 65:1025, 1998.)

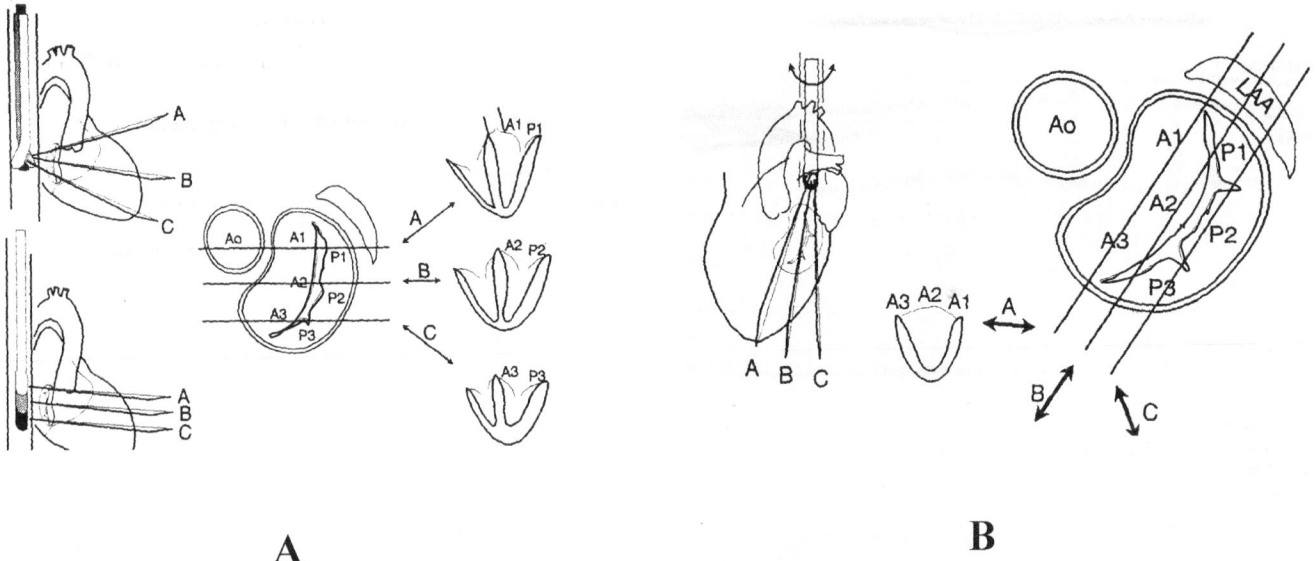

A   **B**

Figure 32-26. (*A*) Effect of flexion and retroflexion (*top left*) or advancement of the TEE probe tip with no flexion (*bottom left*) on the imaging plane in relation to the mitral valve. The transducer rotational angle is 0°. (*B*) Effect of clockwise and counterclockwise probe rotation on the imaging plane in relation to the mitral valve. The transducer rotational angle is adjusted to the major axis of the mitral orifice (typically 45–90°). Ao = aorta; A1, A2, A3 = anterior leaflet sections; P1, P2, P3 = posterior leaflet sections. (Reproduced with permission from Foster GP, Isselbacher EM, Rose GA *et al:* Accurate localization of mitral regurgitant defects using multiplane transesophageal echocardiography. Ann Thorac Surg 65:1025, 1998.)

Figure 32-28. Although systolic reversal of pulmonary vein blood flow is a marker of severe mitral regurgitation, eccentric jets of moderate grade may produce isolated systolic reversal in a pulmonary vein blood flow.[97]

The pulmonary vein flow pattern is one measure that has been used to grade mitral regurgitation. Other commonly used criteria to grade mitral regurgitation are outlined in Table 32-17. When grading mitral regurgitation, a thorough examination with multiple techniques is essential. The severity of mitral regurgitation is very dependent on afterload. If moderate mitral regurgitation is present, the afterload should be increased and the severity reassessed.

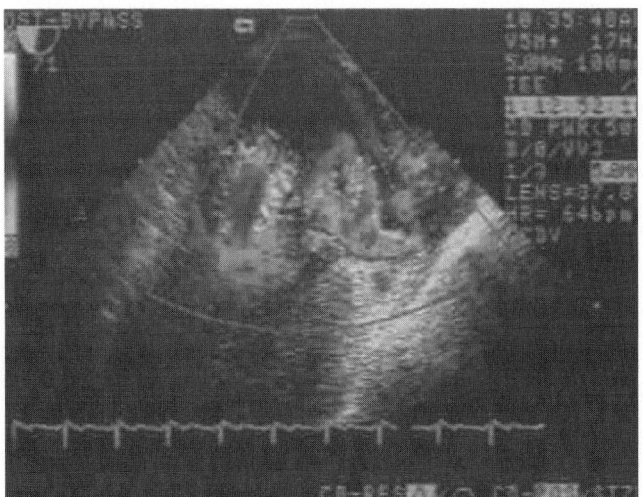

Figure 32-27. The application of color flow Doppler to a regurgitant mitral valve. Note the mosaic pattern in the left atrium during systole.

CARDIOPULMONARY BYPASS
Circuits

Although there are multiple configurations used for cardiopulmonary bypass, they all incorporate essential components, including large catheters for venous drainage, an oxygenator/heat exchanger, and a pump and tubing and cannula for arterial return (Fig. 32-29). In many institutions, additional components are added to this elementary circuit. These include a filter on the arterial return cannula and often on the suction catheters, alarms to detect low levels of blood in the oxygenator to prevent pumping of air, in-line pressure and/or blood gas monitors, and a separate circuit for infusion of crystalloid or blood cardioplegia. Vaporizers can be positioned in the gas inflow circuit so that volatile anesthetics can be administered during the bypass period.

Blood is drained into a reservoir from either a large single two-stage cannula (drains the right atrium and the inferior vena cava) inserted into the right atrium or from two separate smaller cannulas placed in the superior and inferior vena cavae. The rate of venous return is dependent upon intravascular volume, the height of the patient above the reservoir, and proper placement of the cannulas. Flow can be reduced by partially or completely clamping these lines either by the surgeon or the perfusionist. Additional blood is carried to the venous reservoir from the operative field with suction generated by two small roller pumps. The first is the coronary suction that scavenges blood from the operative field, and the other is the vent suction used either to decompress the left ventricle or as an additional "coronary sucker." When used to decompress the left ventricle, this suction line is connected to a catheter inserted across the mitral valve *via* the left superior pulmonary vein, to a metal or plastic tube inserted directly into the apex of the left ventricle, or to the aortic cardioplegic cannula. Many surgeons choose not to routinely vent the left ventricle during coronary artery bypass operations.

A.

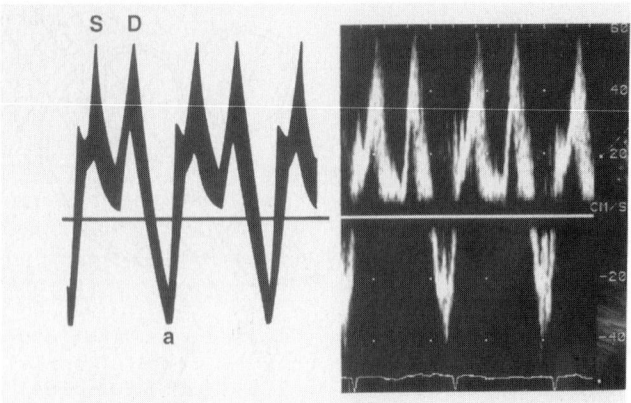

B.

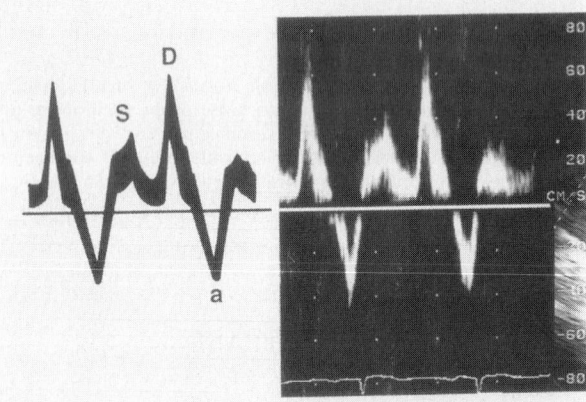

C.

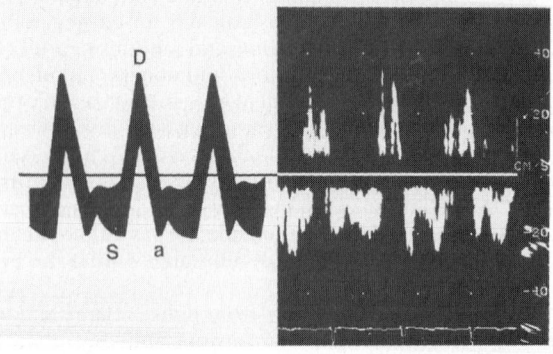

Figure 32-28. The change in the left upper pulmonary vein Doppler flow velocity profile as the left atrial pressure increases. (*A*) Normal profile; note that a normal pulmonary vein flow pattern should have the peak of the S-phase (systolic) wave at least equal to the peak of the D-phase (diastolic) waveform. (*B*) Blunted systolic filling; note the pronounced blunting of the peak of the S-phase waveform relative to the D-phase waveform. (*C*) Systolic reversal; note the inversion of the S-phase waveform. (Reproduced with permission from Rafferty TD: Basics of Transesophageal Echocardiography. New York, Churchill Livingstone, 1995.)

Most commonly, oxygenated blood is returned to the patient through a cannula placed in the ascending aorta. If this proves technically difficult, if emergency cannulation is necessary, or if partial bypass is used during surgery on the descending thoracic aorta, the femoral artery is usually selected. The axillary artery is also an acceptable site for arterial inflow.

Table 32-17. GRADING FOR MITRAL REGURGITATION

	Mild	Moderate	Severe
Jet width at origin (mm)	<2	3–5	>5
Jet area/LA area	<30%	30–60%	>60%
Jet length/LA length	2–6	6–12	>12
Pulmonary vein doppler	Blunting S wave	S wave < D wave	Systolic reversal of flow

LA = left atrium.

Oxygenators

Bubble

Bubble oxygenators utilize direct contact between fresh gas and blood to affect transfer of oxygen (O_2) and carbon dioxide (CO_2). It is far more difficult to transfer O_2 than CO_2 because the solubility ratio is 1:25. Foaming is an extremely efficient method of oxygenation and, in combination with high oxygen tensions, alleviates this problem. Gas is passed through a ceramic manifold to create bubbles small enough to provide sufficient total surface area for gas exchange but not so small as to preclude easy removal. The smaller the bubbles, the greater the surface-to-volume ratio and the greater the oxygen transfer. In bubble oxygenators, CO_2 transfer is proportional to total gas flow, whereas oxygen transport is chiefly dependent upon bubble size. Gas flows do affect oxygen transport, and, at higher flows, CO_2 is sometimes added to the gas mixture to prevent unacceptable levels of hypocarbia. Critical to the function of the bubble oxygenator is the ability to reconstitute the perfusate ("defoaming") by passage through spongy polypropylene mesh impregnated with a charged silicon-containing polymer.

Bubble oxygenators are associated with time-dependent trauma to blood because of the direct blood–gas interface. Hemolysis develops with potential capillary plugging and organ damage from red blood cell debris. Platelet activity is impaired secondary to platelet destruction, induction of aggregation, and adherence to parts of the oxygenator. Decreases in leukocyte counts have also been reported. Additional problems associated with bubble oxygenators include activation of complement *via* the alternate pathway, formation of particulate and gaseous microemboli, and denaturation of blood proteins (including those of the coagulation cascade).[144]

Membrane

To eliminate or attenuate the problems associated with the blood–gas interface, the membrane oxygenator separates the two phases by a thin, gas-permeable membrane of silicon, Teflon, or polypropylene. Blood flows in a thin film along the membrane while gas slowly diffuses across it. The oxygen tension

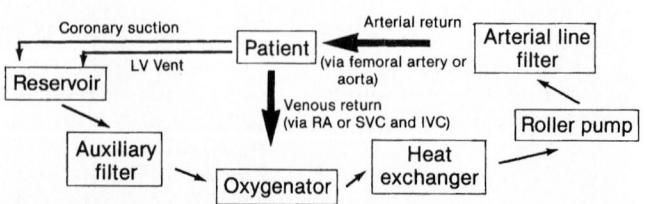

Figure 32-29. The basic circuit for cardiopulmonary bypass. (Reprinted with permission from Thomson IR: Technical aspects of cardiopulmonary bypass. In Thomas SJ [ed]: Manual of Cardiac Anesthesia, 2nd ed, p 480. New York, Churchill Livingstone, 1993.)

is controlled by the F_{IO_2} of the inspired gas, and CO_2 is regulated by total gas flow.

Studies comparing membrane with bubble oxygenators demonstrate less blood trauma with membranes and, in some cases, improved postoperative hemostasis.[145] However, other investigators report that these differences are clinically insignificant as long as perfusion time is less than 2 hours. Differences in performance of the two types of oxygenators are also obscured by the amount of blood scavenged from the operative field because these cells are the most severely damaged from direct mechanical trauma as well as from the turbulent blood–gas interface.

Pumps

Roller

Two types of pumps are used to generate the pressure required to return the perfusate to the patient (or, in the case of a membrane, to drive blood through the oxygenator and then to the patient). The first is a roller pump. A roller pump consists of a central housing with two arms extending 180° in opposite directions with smooth-faced rollers on each end. Flow is generated by compression of a heavy walled section of Silastic tubing by the rollers. Contact between one arm of the roller and the tubing begins where contact between the second roller ends, thus preventing retrograde flow. Shearing forces that would disrupt cells are minimized by ensuring that contact between the roller and tubing is nonocclusive. The roller pump head is driven by an electric motor designed to maintain constant speed, and therefore flow, despite variations in arterial inflow line resistance or power line voltage. If the motor or its power supply fails, the pump can be hand-cranked to provide adequate flow rates and systemic pressures. In many centers, the roller pump has been replaced with the centrifugal pump as the primary pump driving blood to the patient. It is still universally used for cardiotomy and vent suction and for delivering cardioplegia.

Centrifugal

Centrifugal pumps are conical, hardened-plastic housings containing rapidly rotating cones that impart momentum to the blood. This mechanism is pressure-sensitive, and flow is determined by both inflow and outflow pressures as well as by pump head speed. An in-line electromagnetic flow meter is necessary to indicate forward flow because, in contrast to a roller pump, direct conversion from revolutions per minute (rpm) to flow rate is inaccurate. The maximal pressure generated with this pump is lower than that with a roller pump, and the likelihood of disconnects following inadvertent cannula obstruction is reduced.

Pulsatile Flow

Roller pumps generate a sine wave pattern of flow, which, after damping during transit through the inflow tubing and cannulas, results in a nonpulsatile arterial pressure wave. Selection of a different pump or insertion of additional components into a circuit allows the production of a pulsatile waveform. This is both theoretically attractive and intuitively more physiologic, but whether or not it is beneficial is controversial.[146] Pulsatile flow is thought to provide improved perfusion at the capillary level and is associated with lower systemic vascular resistance during bypass, improved oxygen extraction, and lower production of pyruvate and lactate. A decrease in the need for pharmacologic or mechanical support after bypass has also been reported, as well as improved mortality. Some investigators advocate converting to pulsatile perfusion, especially in patients with severe preoperative impairment of ventricular function. Until noncontroversial studies demonstrate beyond doubt the superiority of pulsatile flow, the convenience and simplicity of

nonpulsatility continue to make it the overwhelming choice for almost all procedures requiring cardiopulmonary bypass, even though some suggest that pulsatile perfusion is beneficial in high-risk patients.[147]

Heat Exchanger

A heat exchanger adjusts the temperature of the perfusate to provide moderate systemic hypothermia during the period of cardiac repair. Metabolic requirements are reduced approximately 8% per degree centigrade decrease in body temperature (about 50% of normal at 28°C). Deliberate hypothermia provides protection during periods of hypoperfusion and potential tissue ischemia. In addition, adequate tissue oxygenation is achieved at lower flow rates, reducing trauma to the blood. Lower systemic flow also decreases flow to the heart *via* noncoronary collaterals (vessels arising from pericardial reflections), diminishing the rewarming and the rate of washout of cardioplegic solution. Also, by cooling the tissues surrounding the heart, reducing the rate of cardiac rewarming, hypothermia acts as an adjunct to myocardial protection.

Prime

The prime for most adult perfusions contains a balanced salt solution because such a solution resembles plasma in terms of osmolality and electrolyte composition. Individual recipes add albumin or hetastarch (to increase oncotic pressure), mannitol (to promote diuresis), additional heparin, bicarbonate, calcium, and so on. Although albumin is commonly added to prime solutions to increase oncotic pressure, it has not been shown to provide any clinical benefit in terms of outcome. Blood is infrequently used except in neonates, children, and adults with significant preoperative anemia in whom profound hemodilution might decrease oxygen-carrying capacity below acceptable levels. After mixing of the patient's blood volume with 1500–2500 ml (depending upon oxygenator and circuitry) of prime, acute normovolemic hemodilution to hematocrits of 20–30% is normal. This offsets the increase in viscosity associated with systemic hypothermia. Retrograde arterial prime allows for part of the asanguinous prime to be siphoned off in favor of autologous blood that is slowly bled back into the circuit. Not only can this reduce the incidence of red cell transfusion, it can also minimize the hemodynamic changes associated with the abrupt change in viscosity at the beginning of cardiopulmonary bypass.[148]

Anticoagulation

Prior to cannulation, systemic anticoagulation is mandatory to prevent catastrophic thrombus formation triggered by contact between the blood and oxygenator. Heparin, a polyanionic mucopolysaccharide extracted from bovine lung or porcine intestinal mucosa, accelerates the velocity of the reaction between antithrombin III and the activated forms of Factors II, X, XI, XII, and XIII, effectively neutralizing these factors. A tertiary complex is formed between heparin, antithrombin III, and these serine proteases. The half-life of heparin's anticoagulant effect is approximately 90 minutes in a normothermic patient, the rate of decay decreasing with hypothermia.

Anticoagulant activity varies among samples of commercially prepared heparin, as does patient response to a given dose. Patients receiving heparin in the period immediately prior to surgery and those with reduced levels of antithrombin III are notably resistant to normal precardiopulmonary bypass doses. It seems prudent to assess the adequacy of heparinization prior to starting cardiopulmonary bypass because of the lack of correlation among heparin dosage, blood levels, and clinical effect, as well as to ensure that heparin has in fact been given and distributed. Controversy exists as to whether this is best done by measuring heparin levels or the effect of heparin on the coagulation process. The former utilizes a manual or automated protamine titration test or other assays for heparin level; the latter utilizes a thrombin time (not usually available) or an activated clotting time. Because heparin levels do not always correlate with effect, many centers choose the more functional test, especially since it is easier and less costly. The activated clotting time is the most commonly used test for the adequacy of anticoagulation. It is performed either manually or automatically and indicates the time required for thrombus formation, detected visually or magnetically, when blood is mixed with one of a variety of clotting accelerators. The exact activated clotting time value necessary before initiation of cardiopulmonary bypass to ensure absolute anticoagulation remains controversial. Many use 400 s, a value derived from a study in primates that found no fibrin monomer, an indicator of coagulation, as long as activated clotting time was above that level.[149]

The interpatient relationship between heparin concentration and activated clotting time is not linear, nor is the sensitivity of the activated clotting time (i.e., the change in activated clotting time per unit increase in heparin level). However, the association between the dose of heparin administered and activated clotting time in an individual patient before cardiopulmonary bypass is somewhat linear. There are advocates of such a dose–response curve to determine heparin and protamine requirements.[150] However, this is often too time-consuming; moreover, it overestimates protamine needs because hemodilution and hypothermia alter intrapatient activated clotting time sensitivity.[151] Heparin is usually given in an initial dose of 300–400 U · kg^{-1}; an activated clotting time is measured 5 minutes later, and additional heparin is given as required. The activated clotting time should be rechecked periodically, especially if the interval following initial administration is unduly protracted or if the rewarming period on cardiopulmonary bypass is prolonged. The rate of heparin decay increases during rewarming.

In patients allergic to heparin, alternative anticoagulants can be administered. They range from snake venom derivatives to platelet inhibitors.[152–154] Occasionally, patients exhibit resistance to the anticoagulating effects of heparin resulting from antithrombin III deficiency. FFP or antithrombin III concentrate can be administered to achieve the needed level of anticoagulation from heparin administration. Additionally, bypass circuits can be heparin-coated or bonded to minimize the amount of heparin required to accomplish CPB successfully.[155–157]

Myocardial Protection

A wide variety of methods are used to maintain myocardial cell integrity and energy stores while the coronary circulation is interrupted. Although techniques utilizing cold cardioplegia are the most common, other techniques used include hypothermic fibrillation,[158] intermittent crossclamping interspersed with periods of reperfusion, and continuous warm blood cardioplegia. The two critical elements with respect to cold cardioplegia are hypothermia (10–15°C) and hyperkalemia to ensure diastolic electrical arrest. Individual formulas add a variety of other ingredients, including, but not limited to, glucose as an energy substrate, buffering agents, albumin or mannitol for osmotic activity, citrate to reduce the calcium concentration, and nitroglycerin to improve distribution of the cardioplegic mixture. This solution is mixed with either crystalloid or oxygenated blood and is infused into the aortic root after the crossclamp is applied. The cardioplegia may be injected via a separate circuit on the bypass machine or manually, using a pneumatic infusion device. Direct injection into the aortic root is not feasible in patients with aortic insufficiency. The aorta must be opened and the cardioplegia injected directly into the coronary ostia with small perfusion cannulas. Cardioplegia can also be injected retrograde via the coronary sinus. This is particularly

helpful in patients with severe coronary ostial stenosis or multiple severe lesions preventing adequate distribution, but is often used routinely in both coronary and valve operations. An additional site of cardioplegic injection is directly down newly constructed bypass grafts. During the period of cardioplegic arrest, the anesthesiologist should monitor the electrocardiogram for return of electrical activity, the pulmonary artery pressure (if available) and/or the appearance of the heart for evidence of ventricular distention, and the operative field for return of contraction. The atria are often first to show return of contractile activity. Depending upon the duration of ischemia necessary, periodic reinjection may be necessary to maintain hypothermia and diastolic arrest and to wash out metabolic products. The variations of cardioplegic recipes and techniques are staggering. Several reviews discuss the physiologic and technologic details of cardioplegia; the interested reader is urged to consult them.[159–162]

Blood Conservation in Cardiac Surgery

Postoperative bleeding contributes to the morbidity, mortality, and economic costs of cardiac surgery. Cardiopulmonary bypass itself results in platelet activation and coagulation defects. Given the inherent risks and costs associated with blood transfusions and the general public's fear of receiving blood, considerable attention is being paid to perioperative blood conservation techniques. Such techniques include intraoperative autologous hemodilution, administration of antifibrinolytics, red blood cell scavenging, and attention to surgical hemostasis. Intraoperative hemodilution, which involves the removal of one or more units of whole blood prebypass, is used in those patients who are stable with an adequate initial hematocrit. The autologous blood, which has thus been spared the damaging effects of the bypass circuit, is then reinfused postbypass for volume and red blood cell replacement. Red blood cells may also be salvaged from the field and bypass tubing, washed, and retransfused throughout the procedure.

Pharmacologic measures include antifibrinolytics (ε-aminocaproic acid, tranexamic acid, aprotinin, and desmopressin (DDAVP).[163–166] Aprotinin, an antifibrinolytic and serine protease inhibitor with platelet protective effects, has been shown to significantly decrease blood loss in high-risk patients (e.g., reoperation, known coagulopathy, Jehovah's Witness, sepsis) with a low incidence of adverse events. It inhibits trypsin, kallikrein, and activation of complement, thereby acting as an anti-inflammatory agent as well. Disadvantages of aprotinin include a risk of anaphylaxis on re-exposure (because it is an animal-derived protein, from bovine lung) and its high cost. However, the added direct cost of the drug may be offset by the cost savings owing to the reduction in transfusion requirement, operating room time, and the need for mediastinal re-exploration. ε-Amino caproic acid and tranexamic acid are other antifibrinolytics, which have also been shown to decrease blood loss in cardiac surgery patients. These agents should be administered both before and during bypass to afford optimal results, i.e., to mitigate the effects of the systemic inflammatory response due to the initiation of cardiopulmonary bypass. DDAVP has been shown to benefit a subgroup of cardiac surgical patients who have abnormal platelet function.[167–169]

PREOPERATIVE EVALUATION

The preoperative visit appropriately concentrates on the cardiovascular system but should also focus on the assessment of pulmonary, renal, hepatic, neurologic, endocrine, and hematologic functions. Equally important is a discussion with the patient of the projected events on the day of surgery, including transport to the operating room, preoperative routines (O$_2$ mask, vascular cannulation, anesthetic induction), and, finally, the awakening process in the recovery room or intensive care

Table 32-18. PREOPERATIVE FINDINGS SUGGESTIVE OF VENTRICULAR DYSFUNCTION

History

History of MI, intermittent or chronic CHF
Symptoms of CHF: fatigue, DOE, orthopnea, PND, ankle swelling

Physical Examination

Hypotension/tachycardia (severe CHF)
Prominent neck veins, laterally displace apical impulse, S_3, S_4, rales, pitting edema, pulsatile liver, ascites (tricupsid regurgitation)

Electrocardiogram

Ischemia/infarction, rhythm, or conduction abnormalities

Chest X-ray

Cardiomegaly, pulmonary vascular congestion/pulmonary edema, pleural effusion, Kerley B lines

Cardiac Testing

Catheterization data—LVEDP > 18, EF < 0.4, CI < 2.0 $L \cdot min^{-1} \cdot m^{-2}$
Echocardiography—low EF, multiple regional wall motion abnormalities
Ventriculography—low EF, multiple areas of hypokinesis, akinesis, or dyskinesis

---

MI = myocardial infarction; CHF = congestive heart failure; DOE = dyspnea on exertion; PND = paroxysmal nocturnal dyspnea; LVEDP = left ventricular end-diastolic pressure; EF = ejection fraction; CI = cardiac index.

---

unit. The importance of communicating to the anesthesiologist any symptoms such as chest pain, shortness of breath, or the need for nitroglycerin during transport or the preinduction period should be stressed. The depth and detail of the explanation depend upon the patient's emotional state and desire to know.

Data from the history, physical examination, and laboratory investigations are used to delineate cardiovascular anatomy and functional state. Of critical importance is the assessment of severity of left and/or right ventricular failure. Pertinent findings suggestive of dysfunction are described in Table 32-18. Increases in the severity or frequency of anginal attacks or the presence of ischemia-induced ventricular dysfunction suggest that there are large areas of myocardium at risk. A history of previous arrhythmias should be obtained, including the type, severity, associated symptoms, prior intervention, and successful treatment. Integration of this information leads to appropriate selection of monitoring devices and anesthetic techniques.

Conditions commonly associated with heart disease such as hypertension, diabetes mellitus, and cigarette smoking must also be evaluated. The last is extremely important and may be useful in differentiating whether episodes of intraoperative pulmonary hypertension are caused primarily by pulmonary or cardiac factors. Higher systemic arterial pressures may be desirable throughout surgery in patients with a history or other evidence of carotid artery disease. Evidence for renal dysfunction must be sought because the most common cause of postoperative renal failure is pre-existing renal insufficiency. If renal reserve is reduced, intraoperative measures such as diuretics or dopamine may be used, although no data showing an improved outcome are available.

Current Drug Therapy

Almost without exception, cardiovascular drugs, including cardiac antidysrhythmics, beta or calcium channel blockers, and nitrates are continued until the time of surgery. Interactions between these drugs and anesthetics are rarely detrimental; rather, they are more often beneficial in maintaining hemodynamic control during periods of surgical stress.

The β-blocking drugs are similar in structure and differ in degree of cardioselectivity, mode of excretion, and duration of action. The calcium entry blockers have shorter elimination half-lives and somewhat different pharmacologic actions. Concern about intraoperative hypotension and increased requirement for vasopressor support seems unwarranted. In patients receiving calcium channel blockers without concomitant β blockade, increases in heart rate and contractility may occur during surgical stimulation. Indeed, it has been shown that such patients have more perioperative ischemic electrocardiographic changes than patients receiving β-blocking drugs alone or in combination with calcium channel-blocking drugs. Vasodilation following CPB has been observed in patients taking ACE inhibitors.

Digoxin is prescribed to suppress cardiac dysrhythmias, control the ventricular response to atrial fibrillation, and improve contractility in patients with congestive heart failure. The efficacy of this last indication is sometimes difficult to discern clinically, so that discontinuation of digoxin to avoid digitoxic dysrhythmias seems appropriate. However, in those patients in whom it is being used for rate or rhythm control, continuation until the time of surgery seems advisable. Signs or symptoms of digoxin excess, including ventricular ectopy, atrial tachydysrhythmias, and variable degrees of atrioventricular block, should be sought. The latter is typically manifested by slowing and regularization of the ventricular response to atrial fibrillation. This represents digoxin-induced atrioventricular blockade with a regular junctional escape rhythm. Noncardiac symptoms include gastrointestinal distress or visual disturbances. Toxicity is more common in patients concomitantly receiving drugs that increase digoxin levels (*e.g.*, nifedipine, verapamil, amiodarone) or reduce potassium levels (*e.g.*, diuretics). Most cardiac antidysrhythmics should also be continued to the time of surgery. Their pharmacology is well known (see Chapters 12 and 21), and they usually present little problem with anesthetic management.

Physical Examination

As mentioned previously, the physical examination seeks to elicit signs of cardiac decompensation such as an S_3 gallop, rales, jugular venous distention, or pulsatile liver. Routes for vascular access should be assessed, and the status of peripheral arteries should be evaluated. As always, the airway should be carefully evaluated with respect to ease of mask ventilation and intubation of the trachea. Other pertinent points are described in Table 32-19.

Premedication

Even the most thorough preoperative psychological preparation is often inadequate to assuage the anxieties and apprehensions of a patient facing cardiac surgery. Premedication will assist in providing a calm, anxiety-free, but arousable and hemodynamically stable patient who is prepared for surgery. Selection of drug and dosage is predicated on the patient's age, cardiovascular state, and level of anxiety. Heavy premedication is ideal for the fit person scheduled for coronary artery bypass grafting. Inadequate sedation may predispose to hypertension, tachycardia, or coronary vasospasm, all potential causes of myocardial ischemia. The frail, 50-kg cachetic patient with severe valvular dysfunction fares better with light premedication to avoid possible respiratory depression or loss of endogenous catecholamine support. Additional sedation can always be given in the operating room under direct observation by the anesthesiologist.

Premedication for cardiac surgery often combines the sedative and analgesic properties of an opioid (morphine, 0.1–0.2 $mg \cdot kg^{-1}$) with the sedative and amnestic properties of scopolamine (0.006 $mg \cdot kg^{-1}$) or a benzodiazepine (diazepam 0.05– 0.1 $mg \cdot kg^{-1}$, midazolam 0.03–0.05 $mg \cdot kg^{-1}$, or lorazepam 0.04

Table 32-19. PREOPERATIVE PHYSICAL EXAMINATION

Vital Signs
Current values and range while hospitalized

Height, Weight
For calculation of drug dosages, pump flows, cardiac index

Airway
Anatomic features that could make mask ventilation or intubation difficult

Neck
Jugular venous distention (CHF)
Carotid bruit (cerebrovascular disease)
Landmarks for jugular vein cannulation

Heart
Murmurs characteristic of valve lesions
S_3 (increased LVEDP)
S_4 (decreased compliance)
Click (MVP) or rub (pericarditis)
Lateral PMI displacement (cardiomegaly)
Precordial heave, lift (hypertrophy, wall motion abnormality)

Lungs
Rales (CHF)
Rhonchi, wheezes (COPD, asthma)

Vasculature
Sites for venous and arterial access
Peripheral pulses

Abdomen
Pulsatile liver (CHF, tricuspid regurgitation)

Extremities
Peripheral edema (CHF)

Nervous System
Motor or sensory deficits

CHF = congestive heart failure; LVEDP = left ventricular end-diastolic pressure; MVP = mitral valve prolapse; PMI = point of maximal impulse; COPD = chronic obstructive pulmonary disease.

$mg \cdot kg^{-1}$). The possibility of oversedation, hypercarbia, or hypoxia following premedication is always of concern. However, Hensley et al[170] have shown that morphine and scopolamine, when administered in standard doses, do not produce hypoxia. Rather, if hypoxia does occur after this combination, it is secondary to the additional supplementation administered in the operating room.

The choice of premedication may also affect the hemodynamic response to anesthetics. Thomson et al[171] administered a standard high-dose fentanyl anesthetic to patients premedicated with either morphine and scopolamine or lorazepam. In general, the patients receiving lorazepam were hemodynamically less responsive in that they had less hypertension, more hypotension, and a greater requirement for vasoactive drugs. This suggests that premedication may have a previously unappreciated but profound effect on intraoperative hemodynamics. Clonidine has also been used as a premedication with similar intraoperative effects. The difficulty with premedication currently is that the patients arrive in the operating room after just getting off the bus! Same-day admission does make the job more difficult.

Monitoring

We will emphasize only those aspects of monitoring particularly relevant to cardiac surgery. The subject is discussed extensively in Chapter 25, and we have already reviewed techniques for identification of myocardial ischemia and for evaluation of valve function.

Pulse Oximeter

The need for multiple vascular cannulations and applications of numerous monitoring devices often prolongs the preinduction period. The pulse oximeter should be positioned prior to catheter insertion to detect clinically unsuspected episodes of hypoxemia, especially if additional iv sedation has been administered. Attention must be focused on the entire patient, even during the hunt for successful vascular access.

Electrocardiogram

Simultaneous observation of both a precordial lead V_5 and an inferior lead II or lead III for the presence and location of ischemia has been emphasized. Regional ischemia may be localized by appropriate lead monitoring. Lead II can be monitored to interpret arrhythmias and detect ischemia in the inferior wall of the left ventricle (leads II, III, AVF = right coronary artery). Lead V_5 is monitored to detect ischemia in the anterior wall of left ventricle (left anterior descending artery). Leads I and AVL can be monitored to detect ischemia in the lateral wall of the left ventricle (circumflex artery). If the standard leads prove inadequate for cardiac dysrhythmia detection and analysis, esophageal or epicardial leads may be used. Occasionally, intraoperative myocardial injury causes substantial reductions in QRS voltage. Monitoring an electrocardiogram via a surgically placed ventricular pacing wire provides adequate voltage to facilitate dysrhythmia analysis or to trigger an intra-aortic balloon pump, if this is necessary. A strip-chart recorder documents and facilitates detailed analysis of both ST segment alterations and complex dysrhythmias.

Temperature

Central temperature can be measured with esophageal, tympanic, or Foley catheter probes or with a thermistor from a pulmonary artery catheter. Obviously, this last method is not reliable during the period of aortic crossclamping when there is no flow through the heart. Rectal and toe probes record peripheral temperatures, which lag behind central measurements during both cooling and rewarming.

Arterial Blood Pressure

Systemic arterial pressure is always monitored invasively. The radial or femoral artery is usually cannulated, although the brachial and axillary arteries may also be used. The exact site is often a matter of personal or institutional preference. Criteria include convenience, selection of the fullest or most bounding pulse, and avoidance of the dominant hand. In addition, during dissection of the internal mammary artery, the ipsilateral radial or brachial artery pulse may be transiently occluded; therefore, an artery opposite a planned internal mammary artery is selected. Occasionally, the site of surgery dictates appropriate placement; for example, the right radial artery should be used for any procedure involving the descending thoracic aorta because the left subclavian artery may be included in the proximal aortic clamp. Following cardiopulmonary bypass, radial artery pressure is often misleading and may be as much as 30 mm Hg lower than central aortic pressure.[172] The mechanism is thought to be peripheral vasodilation during rewarming. Whenever such a discrepancy is suspected, aortic pressure can be estimated by palpation by the surgeon, or if direct measurement is needed, a needle may be placed directly into the aorta. The gradient between aortic and radial pressure usually disappears within 45 minutes of separation from bypass.

Central Venous Pressure/Pulmonary Artery Catheter

Access to the central circulation is mandatory for infusion of cardioactive drugs. In addition, right atrial or central venous pressure accurately reflects right ventricular filling pressure and is of critical importance whenever right ventricular dysfunction is suspected. In patients with unimpaired left ventricular function, transduced right atrial pressure is often assumed to be a reliable guide of left-sided filling. This relationship is less predictable in the presence of severe left ventricular dyssynergy, pulmonary hypertension, or reduced left ventricular compliance. In these instances, insertion of a pulmonary artery catheter for measurement of pulmonary capillary wedge pressure provides a somewhat better index of left ventricular filling. In addition, determination of cardiac output and calculation of derived hemodynamic indices offer additional information to guide hemodynamic and anesthetic management.

Indications for pulmonary artery catheterization vary greatly among institutions. In some, these catheters are used routinely, whereas in others, they are limited to patients with specific disease states such as severe left ventricular dysfunction or pronounced pulmonary hypertension. Additional indications include combined procedures (valvular plus coronary) or those that require prolonged intraoperative time (cardiac reoperations or use of one or both internal mammary arteries). Insertion of a pacing pulmonary artery catheter can be helpful whenever exact control of rate and rhythm is desirable, for example, in patients with hypertrophic cardiomyopathy or those with significant bradycardia secondary to β blockade.

When pulmonary artery catheters are used, disagreement still exists as to whether they should be placed before or after the induction of anesthesia. In some patients, early insertion of the catheter and determination of baseline hemodynamic values can beneficially influence anesthetic selection and guide the induction sequence. However, the anxious and uncomfortable hypertensive patient is better served by a smooth induction of anesthesia followed by catheter placement. Incremental sedation followed by preinduction placement is a suitable alternative associated with minimal, if any, hemodynamic change.

It must be remembered that the catheter often migrates toward the periphery of the lung with cardiac manipulation before and during cardiopulmonary bypass. Therefore, it seems prudent to pull the catheter back a few centimeters prior to the initiation of bypass to prevent permanent wedging or possible pulmonary artery rupture. Despite the controversy concerning the routine use of these catheters, there is no disagreement that the capability to measure both cardiac output and ventricular filling pressures must be available in any institution performing cardiac surgery. Whether this is done with a pulmonary artery catheter, direct cannulation of the left atrium and dye dilution techniques, or TEE is immaterial. The critically ill patient requires these measurements to determine the effectiveness of vasoactive drugs, to adjust dosage, and to evaluate the need for further pharmacologic or mechanical intervention.

Echocardiography

Two-dimensional transesophageal echocardiograph (TEE) is the newest, most complex, and most expensive diagnostic device. Detection of ischemia by on-line evaluation of new regional wall motion abnormalities and its utility in assessing valvular lesions, both before and after repair, and the ascending aorta have been mentioned. Other applications specific to cardiac surgical patients are also useful. It is well known that, following cardiopulmonary bypass, ventricular filling pressure, irrespective of site of measurement (left ventricular end-diastolic pressure, left atrium, pulmonary capillary wedge pressure), is a poor and often misleading indicator of ventricular volume status.[173,174] Direct estimation of left ventricular volume with two-dimensional TEE more appropriately directs fluid infusion and selection of vasoactive drugs in patients who are difficult to wean from bypass. In addition, residual valve lesions, intracardiac air, or new areas of ischemia are readily identified. Global dysfunction suggesting residual crossclamp effect, inadequate cardioplegia, or reperfusion injury can be detected.

Central Nervous System Function and Complications

Monitoring of the brain during extracorporeal bypass is difficult, with a lack of standardized equipment or criteria. Neurologic complications after cardiac surgery can be devastating to patients and their families, significantly affecting their quality of life while exponentially increasing the economic cost of recovery after cardiac surgery. Thus, many investigators have recently focused on methods to determine the etiology and improve the detection, prevention, and treatment of postoperative neurologic complications in patients undergoing cardiac surgery.

The incidence of stroke after coronary artery bypass graft (CABG) surgery is approximately 3% (1–5%). There is a much higher incidence (60–70%) of subtle cognitive deficits that can be elicited by detailed neuropsychometric testing. It is known that the neuropsychiatric deficits do improve over the initial 2–6 months after cardiac surgery; however, a significant percentage of patients (13–39%) have residual impairment. The etiology of perioperative neurologic complications is thought to be predominantly secondary to emboli (air, atheroma, other particulate matter) and less importantly to hypoperfusion in susceptible patients (e.g., pre-existing cerebrovascular disease). Most overt strokes after cardiac surgery are focal and likely due to macroemboli, whereas the cognitive changes are subtle and probably result from microemboli (e.g., air, platelet aggregates).

Risk factors for neurologic complications include advanced age (70 years), pre-existing cerebrovascular disease (e.g., carotid artery stenosis 80%), history of prior stroke, peripheral vascular disease, ascending aortic disease, and diabetes. Operative factors include the duration of CPB and intracardiac procedure (e.g., valve replacement). Intraoperative hyperglycemia, which could theoretically result in worsened neurologic damage, has not been associated with poorer neurologic outcome.[175]

Historically, intracardiac (e.g., valvular) procedures are associated with a greater risk of neurologic complications (presumably secondary to greater risk of air emboli) than closed cardiac (i.e., CABG) procedures. As discussed earlier, TEE has given both anesthesiologists and surgeons an appreciation for the adequacy of the de-airing process after intracardiac procedures. From studies using transcranial Doppler to detect cerebral emboli, it is now known that the time points of maximal risk for embolization are at aortic cannulation, onset of CPB, weaning from CPB, and decannulation.[176]

The role of TEE in evaluating the ascending and descending aorta is described above. There are several management options undergoing investigation for patients with severely diseased aortas, especially those with mobile atheromas who are at increased risk of stroke. These include hypothermic fibrillatory arrest with left ventricular vent and no crossclamp, single crossclamp (i.e., distal and proximal grafts performed during same crossclamp), relocation of proximal grafts to area of nondiseased aorta, no proximal grafts (internal mammary arteries only), and hypothermic ischemic arrest with resection and graft replacement of diseased aorta, off bypass if possible.

Cerebral protection is rather limited. Hypothermia is excellent in that it decreases cerebral metabolic rate and prolongs ischemic tolerance; however, profound hypothermia is not practical for routine cardiac surgery. Unfortunately, during routine CPB the patient is normothermic at most points when there is the highest risk of embolization. There is some laboratory evidence that mild hypothermia (34–36°C) may confer some benefit.[177,178] Thus, patients at increased risk for neurologic complications may benefit from remaining mildly hypothermic upon separation from CPB and in the immediate postoperative period. Sodium thiopental has been shown to be cerebroprotective in intracardiac procedures,[179] but not in CABG surgery.[180] This difference may be a result of the "reversible" neurologic impairment secondary to gas emboli, which is more likely during intracardiac procedures than CABG surgery.

Selection of Anesthetic Drugs

The task confronting the anesthesiologist is to render the patient undergoing cardiac surgery analgesic, amnesic, and unconscious while simultaneously suppressing the endocrine and autonomic responses to intraoperative stress. Equally important is preservation of compensatory cardiovascular mechanisms and prevention of perioperative episodes of myocardial ischemia. Although these goals are not unique to the cardiac surgical patient, they are sometimes a bit more difficult to accomplish because of the severity of ischemic and/or valvular disease. Notwithstanding institutional and personal bias with respect to choice of anesthetic, there are no data that document superiority of any anesthetic for either coronary or valvular surgery. The large outcome studies of Tuman *et al* and Slogoff and Keats indicate that the choice of anesthetic has no effect on outcome in CABG patients. As was previously emphasized, the most critical factor governing anesthetic selection is the degree of ventricular dysfunction. Anticipated difficulties during the tracheal intubation sequence, the expected length of surgery, and the anticipated time until extubation of the trachea also influence choice of anesthetic. It is desirable to be able to alter anesthetic depth to accommodate the varying intensity of surgical stress. During intubation of the trachea, incision, sternotomy, pericardiotomy, and manipulation of the aorta, there is intense stimulation and sympathetic response. The period of prepping and draping following intubation of the trachea requires minimal levels of anesthetic, as does the period of hypothermic bypass.

There is no one best technique. Familiarity with all anesthetics and their physiologic and pharmacologic effects in the patient with severe cardiac disease allows great flexibility in anesthetic selection. In addition, it provides numerous options applicable to the cardiac patient undergoing noncardiac surgery.

Potent Inhalation Anesthetics

These drugs are useful both as primary anesthetic drugs and as adjuvants to treat or prevent "breakthrough" hypertension associated with high-dose opioid techniques. The balance of myocardial oxygen supply and $M\dot{V}O_2$ is usually altered favorably by reduction in contractility and afterload. Deleterious declines in perfusion must be prevented or treated, and the possibilities of increases in wall tension must be considered. These agents have been used successfully in all types of valve surgery without untoward effects, although they are sometimes associated with more hemodynamic variability than is seen with opioids. Use of these drugs involves no more hemodynamic intervention than upfront loading with opioids, and the ability to rapidly increase and decrease concentrations permits easy adjustment to variable levels of surgical stimulation. Volatile anesthetics can be administered during bypass through a vaporizer mounted on the pump; they are also appropriate in the postbypass period, assuming that cardiac function is adequate. Volatile anesthetics seem to be more important now, in combination with short-acting opiates or hypnotics, since the volume of off-bypass procedures is increasing and the urge to fast-track continues.

Opioids

The opiods lack negative inotropic effects in the doses used clinically and have thus found widespread use as the primary agents for cardiac surgery. This era began in 1969 when high doses of morphine were used to anesthetize patients for aortic valve replacement.[181] However, hypotension, histamine release, increased fluid requirements, and, often, inadequate anesthesia resulted in a decline in the use of morphine in favor of the more potent fentanyl derivatives. Aside from bradycardia, fentanyl and its analogs are relatively devoid of cardiovascular effects and have proved to be effective anesthetics. As a primary anesthetic agent, fentanyl ($50–100 \ \mu g \cdot kg^{-1}$) or sufentanil ($10–20 \ \mu g \cdot kg^{-1}$) and oxygen provide hemodynamic stability, although they do not consistently prevent a hypertensive response to periods of increased surgical stimulation. In patients with good ventricular function, although high doses of opioids produce unconsciousness and characteristic electrocardiographic slowing, patient recall of intraoperative events remains a potential problem. Adjuvant agents are frequently used to supplement the opioids—benzodiazepines to provide amnesia, and volatile anesthetics or vasodilators to control hypertension. Superiority of any one opioid has not been demonstrated for either coronary or valvular surgery. The use of high-dose opioids prolongs the time until emergence and extubation when compared with techniques primarily based on volatile anesthetics and is no longer in fashion. Alfentanil, with an elimination half-life shorter than that of fentanyl or sufentanil, is suitable for infusion techniques and may provide optimal conditions for early extubation of the trachea. Remifentanil, an ultrashort-acting opioid, is 30 times more potent than alfentanil and undergoes hydrolysis by nonspecific esterases in minutes.[182] Its predictable and rapid elimination is unaffected by hepatic or renal disease, making it an optimal drug for infusion techniques.

Combinations of the fentanyl-type drugs and benzodiazepines, whether given concomitantly or as premedication, result in hypotension secondary to a fall in systemic vascular resistance.[183] The use of any opioid in high doses can produce excessive bradycardia. Vecuronium or cisatracurium may magnify this problem, whereas pancuronium is often useful in preventing it. Abdominal and chest wall rigidity commonly occurs with rapid injection of high doses of opioids and can be severe enough to render ventilation impossible. A low-dose (priming) of nondepolarizing muscle relaxant should be given prior to opioid administration.

Nitrous Oxide

In many centers, nitrous oxide is not used at all during cardiac surgery. Increases in pulmonary vascular resistance associated with nitrous oxide have been demonstrated, with the greatest response in patients with pre-existing pulmonary hypertension.[184] The drug is also a mild myocardial depressant and elicits a compensatory sympathetically mediated increase in systemic vascular resistance.[185] These minimal changes may not be well tolerated in patients with minimal cardiovascular reserve.

It is well known that nitrous oxide increases the size of any air-filled cavity. The possibility of expansion of air introduced into the circulation either before or during bypass should preclude its use immediately before, during, or after bypass.

Induction Drugs

The benzodiazepines, the barbiturates, and etomidate can be used as supplements to either inhalation or opioid anesthetics and, more importantly, are excellent as sole induction drugs in patients with cardiac disease. Obviously, dosage requirements must be altered to fit the clinical situation, but these are excellent drugs with which to begin an anesthetic.

Neuromuscular Blocking Drugs

Muscle relaxants are part of an anesthetic plan for cardiac surgery. Although they are not essential to surgical exposure of the heart, muscle paralysis facilitates intubation of the trachea, prevents shivering, and attenuates skeletal muscle contraction during defibrillation. In addition, muscle relaxants are necessary to prevent or treat opioid-induced truncal rigidity. The chief criteria for selection are the hemodynamic and pharmacokinetic properties associated with each relaxant, the patient's myocardial function, presence of coexisting disease, current pharmacologic regimen, and anesthetic technique. This translates into what is a desirable heart rate and blood pressure for any particular patient.

Intraoperative Management

In this section, we describe the anesthetic management of a patient undergoing a cardiac surgical procedure from the time of arrival in the operating room until care is transferred to intensive care unit personnel. Because the physiologic and pharmacologic rationales for anesthetic selection have previously been discussed, this is rather a sequential description of what happens and what is required during surgery. Anticipation of needs specific to each stage of the procedure and ready availability of necessary equipment and drugs prevent untoward hemodynamic aberrations as well as last-minute scrambling and potentially avoidable delays.

Preparation

The operating room must be readied prior to arrival of the patient. Check the anesthesia machine, and have available all supplies necessary for management of a normal airway or any additional equipment if a difficult intubation of the trachea is anticipated. Anesthetic drugs, emergency drugs, and medicated infusions should be prepared and ready for use. Heparin must be drawn up prior to induction of anesthesia in the unlikely event of the need to "crash" onto bypass. All monitoring equipment should be switched on, working, and calibrated. Confirm that typed and cross-matched blood is available in the operating suite. Table 32-20 is a checklist to aid in proper preoperative preparation of the operating room.

Table 32-20. ANESTHETIC PREPARATION FOR CARDIAC SURGERY

Anesthesia Machine
Routine checkout

Airway Management
Nasal cannula for oxygen supplementation
Laryngoscope/blades, endotracheal tubes, airways, etc.
Suction apparatus
Special equipment if difficult airway is anticipated
Inspired gas humidifier/warmer

Circulatory Access
Intravenous fluids/infusion tubing
Proper catheters for peripheral/central sites
Infusion pumps
Blood/fluid warmers

Monitoring
ECG leads, blood pressure cuff
Pulse oximeter
Esophageal stethoscope
Temperature probes (esophageal, rectal, bladder, tympanic membrane)
Central venous and/or pulmonary artery catheters
Transducers calibrated and zeroed
Strip-chart recorder
Cardiac output computer
Heparin monitoring equipment
Neuromuscular block monitor

Medications
Anesthetic and related
  Opioids
  Barbiturates, benzodiazepines
  Muscle relaxants
Heparin (must be drawn up prior to starting case)
Cardioactive drugs

Syringe:	Infusion:
Calcium chloride	Nitroglycerin/nitroprusside
Nitroglycerin	Inotrope
Phenylephrine or ephedrine	
Epinephrine	

Antibiotics

Miscellaneous
Pacemaker (standard and atrioventricular sequential)
Compatible blood in operating room suite

Preinduction Period

A brief conversation outside the operating room serves to evaluate the patient's general status and level of anxiety and to assess the effectiveness of premedication. Remind the patient to inform you if chest pain, shortness of breath, or other symptoms occur. Angina should be promptly treated with oxygen, sublingual or iv nitroglycerin, additional sedation, or perhaps if related to anxiety-induced hypertension or tachycardia, the prompt induction of general anesthesia. Supplemental oxygen via nasal cannula should be given to all patients once they have been transferred to the operating table, and peripheral oxygen saturation should be monitored with a pulse oximeter during line placement. Electrocardiographic leads and blood pressure cuff are placed, and initial vital signs are recorded.

One or two large-bore iv cannulas are inserted following local anesthesia (additional routes for infusion are desirable in patients undergoing repeat cardiac surgery). In some centers, anesthesia is then induced, and following intubation of the trachea, arterial and central venous cannulas are inserted. In other centers, however, these additional lines are inserted prior to anesthesia. Preinduction or postinduction insertion of central venous or pulmonary artery catheters has been discussed previously. Once they are inserted, however, initial values for all pressures and cardiac output should be recorded, and baseline determinations of arterial blood gases, hematocrit, and activated coagulation time should be obtained.

Throughout the preinduction period, the anesthesiologist must never let preoccupation with placement of iv and pressure monitoring catheters divert his or her attention from the patient. In addition to continuously monitoring vital signs, careful observation of the patient with periodic verbal contact facilitates detection of increased anxiety, excessive response to iv sedation, and hemodynamic or electrocardiographic abnormality.

Induction and Intubation

The exact choice and sequence of drugs are a subtle combination of art and science. The dose, speed of administration, and specific agents selected (e.g., sedative, opioid, volatile drug, muscle relaxant) depend primarily on the patient's cardiovascular reserve and desired cardiovascular profile. A smooth transition from consciousness to blissful sleep is desired without untoward airway difficulties (e.g., coughing, laryngospasm, truncal rigidity) or hemodynamic responses (either hypotension, too much drug, loss of sympathetic tone, myocardial depression; or hypertension, insertion of airway, "tugging" on the jaw). A "slow cardiac induction" sometimes creates rather than alleviates these potential problems. However, a slow, sedated, awake intubation of the trachea may be most appropriate in a bull-necked, obese patient who appears difficult to intubate and ventilate. These examples re-emphasize the necessity for an individual approach to each patient.

Deep planes of anesthesia, brief duration of laryngoscopy, and innumerable pharmacologic regimens have been proposed for eliminating the hypertension and tachycardia associated with intubation of the trachea. None is uniformly successful, and all drug interventions carry some degree of risk, small though they may be. In addition, in some patients, especially those with a slow heart rate prior to induction of anesthesia, the reflex response to intubation of the trachea is primarily vagal, and severe bradycardia and rarely sinus arrest can occur. Furthermore, recent evidence suggests that intubation of the trachea is a strong stimulus for coronary vasoconstriction irrespective of the anesthetic, because left ventricular blood flow is dramatically altered in the absence of hemodynamic changes. Therefore, the response to tracheal intubation may be varied, although it is usually short-lived. Nevertheless, evidence for persistently abnormal hemodynamics or ischemia should be sought and treated.

After documented successful intubation of the trachea, the tube is then secured, an esophageal stethoscope is inserted, and the eyes and all pressure points are protected. The importance of frequent checks of all monitors during these busy minutes cannot be overemphasized.

Preincision Period

The period of time from intubation of the trachea until skin incision is one of minimal stimulation as the surgical team attends to insertion of a bladder catheter, temperature probe, positioning, prepping, and draping. Hypotension often occurs during this period, regardless of the anesthetic technique used. It may be necessary to reduce anesthetic depth or alternatively support systemic pressure with a vasoconstrictor. The potential risks of vasoconstriction in patients with poor left or right ventricular performance must be remembered. Deeper planes of anesthesia are obviously necessary immediately prior to incision and sternotomy.

Incision to Bypass

As previously emphasized, the prebypass period is characterized by periods of intense surgical stimulation that may cause hypertension, tachycardia, or ischemia. Anticipating these events and deepening the anesthetic may be effective, but often a vasodilator or other adjuvant is required. This is particularly true in patients with good ventricular function when an opioid-oxygen technique is used. Hypotension can occur during the less stressful moments before bypass, but it is more commonly associated with cardiac manipulation in preparation for and during atrial cannulation. This may interfere with venous return or produce episodic ectopic beats or sustained supraventricular dysrhythmias. Atrial fibrillation is not uncommon. Depending upon the blood pressure and heart rate response, appropriate treatment may range from nothing at all to vasoconstrictors, cardioversion, or rapid cannulation and institution of bypass. Maintenance of adequate intravascular volume may attenuate the extent of blood pressure decrease. This is a critical time; continual observation of the surgical field is essential.

Prebypass, ST segment analysis is extremely important in identifying and localizing new ischemia, and if it does occur, it should be treated appropriately and the surgeon notified. During all cardiac procedures (perhaps more so than with any other type of surgery), hemodynamic change must be immediately correlated with events in the surgical field. Retracting, lifting, and in general, "mugging" the heart are sometimes necessary; the hemodynamic consequences are unpredictable. This is particularly true following cardiopulmonary bypass when grafts and suture lines are inspected and repaired if necessary. This is also true during reoperations, when dissection may be difficult, tedious, and time-consuming and when continuous retraction of the heart is often necessary. Bleeding, sometimes unexpectedly profuse, will compound the problem. In rare cases in which a cardiac chamber is entered and bleeding is uncontrollable, heparin is administered, the femoral vessels are cannulated, and cardiopulmonary bypass is begun using coronary suction from the field as a major source of venous return. Communication between the anesthesiologist and the surgeon is necessary to keep both apprised of the situation and to ensure that the heart gets a periodic "rest."

Cardiopulmonary Bypass

After heparin has been administered, the cannulas are inserted, and adequate levels of anticoagulation are checked to ensure that the patient is ready for the institution of cardiopulmonary bypass (Table 32-21). Attention is focused on adequacy of venous drainage, oxygenation, unobstructed arterial return, and provision of necessary anesthetics and muscle relaxants. Anesthetic requirements decrease if systemic hypothermia is used.

Once full cardiopulmonary bypass is established, it is no longer necessary to continue ventilation of the lungs. There is complete agreement on this point. However, there is no such consensus about what exactly to do with the lungs during the

period of bypass. Some anesthesiologists completely disconnect the patient from the anesthesia machine; others maintain the lungs slightly inflated with low levels of positive end-expiratory pressure using 100% oxygen or various mixtures of room air. No specific method is associated with superior postoperative pulmonary function.

During the initial minutes of bypass, systemic pressure initially drops to 30–40 mm Hg as pulsatile flow ceases and the effect of the dilute prime becomes apparent. Once adequate mixing is obtained, blood pressure increases to levels primarily determined by flow rate (Table 32-22). There is no consensus as to what constitutes the ideal blood pressure or flow rate during bypass for maintenance of adequate vital organ perfusion, especially of the brain. Commonly, flow rates are maintained at approximately 50–60 ml·kg^{-1}, with systemic blood pressures in the 50–60 mm Hg range. Alternatively, some institutions believe that lower flows are beneficial (less hematologic damage, less rewarming of the heart through noncoronary collaterals) and that the need for higher flows or pressures has not been conclusively demonstrated. Some surgeons believe that a higher perfusion pressure affords better myocardial protection when surgery is performed on the cold fibrillating heart rather than with cardioplegia.

Monitoring and Management During Bypass

The common etiologies of blood pressure changes during cardiopulmonary bypass are listed in Table 32-22. Of primary importance is continuous observation of the surgical field and cannulas to ensure that nothing mechanical is awry. Attention can then be directed to other causes of hypotension or hypertension and their appropriate treatment. Other areas that require periodic monitoring and occasional intervention during bypass are also described in Table 32-22. Maintenance of adequate depths of anesthesia is obviously important during the bypass run, although clinical signs are few. Anesthetic requirements are decreased during the period of hypothermia but return toward normal when the patient is rewarmed.

Table 32-21. CHECKLIST BEFORE INITIATING CARDIOPULMONARY BYPASS

Laboratory Values
ACT or measure of adequate heparinization
Hematocrit

Anesthesia/Machine
Adequate anesthetic and muscle relaxant given
Nitrous oxide off (if used)

Monitor
Arterial pressure—initial hypotension and then return
CVP—indication of inadequate venous drainage
PCWP—LV distention—inadequate drainage, AI—pull back pulmonary artery catheter 1–2 cm

Patient/Field
Cannulas in place: no air locks, clamps, or kinks; no bubbles in arterial cannula
Facial appearance
  Suffusion (inadequate SVC drainage)
  Unilateral blanching (innominate artery cannulation)
Heart
  Signs of distention (especially in AI, ischemia)

Support
Usually not required

The major categories for this table and Tables 32-15 and 32-16 are organized using the mnemonic LAMPS.
ACT = activated clotting time; CVP = central venous pressure; PCWP = pulmonary capillary wedge pressure; LV = left ventricle; SVC = superior vena cava; AI = aortic insufficiency.

Table 32-22. CHECKLIST DURING CARDIOPULMONARY BYPASS

Laboratory Values

ACT or measure of adequate heparinization
ABGs (uncorrected)—acidosis
Hematocrit, sodium, potassium, ionized calcium, glucose levels

Anesthesia/Machine

Discontinue ventilation

Monitor

Arterial pressure
  Hypotension
    Venous cannula—kink, malposition, clamp, air lock
    Inadequate venous return (bleeding, hypovolemia, IVC obstruction, table too low)
    Pump—poor occlusion, low flows
    Arterial cannula—misdirected, kinked, partially clamped, dissection
    Vasodilation—anesthetics, hemodilution, idiopathic
    Transducer or monitor malfunction; radial artery cannula malpositioned/damped waveform
  Hypertension
    Pump—high flow
    Arterial cannula—misdirected
    Vasoconstriction—light anesthesia, response to temperature changes
    Transducer or monitor malfunction; radial artery cannula malpositioned/kinked
Venous pressure—above level of atrium—obstruction to return LV filling pressure—LA, PCWP (if available)—any elevation?
ECG—electrical quiescence (if cardioplegia used)
EEG
Adequacy of perfusion?
  Flow and pressure?
  Acidosis
  Mixed venous oxygen saturation
Urine output
Temperature

Patient/Field

Conduct of the operation
Heart—distention, fibrillation
Cyanosis, venous engorgement, skin temperature
Movement
Breathing, diaphragmatic movement (hypercarbia, light anesthesia)

Support

Vasodilators, anesthetics, or constrictors to control blood pressure when flow is appropriate

ACT = activated clotting time; ABG = arterial blood gas; IVC = inferior vena cava; LV = left ventricle; LA = left atrium; PCWP = pulmonary capillary wedge pressure.

Arterial pH and mixed venous oxygen saturation are often used to assess the adequacy of perfusion. Urine output is also monitored, but so many variables influence this, such as arterial and venous pressure, flow rate, temperature, and diuretic history, that it is difficult to draw meaningful conclusions from this measurement. In addition, postoperative renal failure develops from either aggravation of pre-existing renal dysfunction or persistent low cardiac output following bypass. Although many institutions administer diuretics routinely, they are just as assiduously avoided elsewhere.

Rewarming

When surgical repair is nearly complete, gradual rewarming of the patient begins. A gradient of approximately 10°C is maintained between the patient and the perfusate to prevent formation of gas bubbles. Patient awareness becomes a possibility as the potentiation of anesthetic effects due to hypothermia dissipates. Volatile anesthetics are often avoided because of

residual myocardial depression present at the time of separation from bypass. If adequate doses of anesthetics have not been given, administration during rewarming should be considered to prevent recall of intraoperative events. Upon completion of the surgical repair, a variety of maneuvers are performed to remove any residual air in the ventricles. The anesthesiologist is called upon to vigorously inflate the lungs to remove air from the pulmonary veins and aid in filling the cardiac chambers. TEE is particularly useful in assessing the effectiveness of the de-airing process. The heart is defibrillated and allowed to beat and replace some of its oxygen debt. The field is tidied up, and preparations are made to separate from cardiopulmonary bypass.

Discontinuation of Cardiopulmonary Bypass

Prior to discontinuing cardiopulmonary bypass, the patient should be warmed, the surgical field dry, appropriate laboratory values checked, pulmonary compliance evaluated, and ventilation of the lungs begun (Table 32-23). If necessary, heart rate and rhythm can be regulated either pharmacologically or electrically with appropriate pacing. The venous cannulas are then incrementally occluded as bypass flow is slowly decreased and sufficient pump volume is transfused into the patient. During this time, cardiac function is continually evaluated from monitoring data and direct inspection of the heart; the need for vasoactive or cardioactive drugs is assessed. The potential disparity, previously alluded to, between radial artery and aortic pressures must be kept in mind. Contractility, rhythm, and ventricular filling can all be estimated by careful observation of the beating heart. For example, a low blood pressure but a vigorously contracting, relatively empty ventricle suggests that volume and perhaps a vasoconstrictor are all that is needed to wean the patient from bypass, whereas adequate blood pressure in the presence of a sluggish and overdistended heart may be treated with a vasodilator and/or a small dose of an inotrope.

Table 32-23. CHECKLIST BEFORE SEPARATION FROM CARDIOPULMONARY BYPASS

Laboratory Values

Hematocrit, ABGs
Potassium (? ↑ 2° cardioplegia)
Ionized calcium

Anesthesia/Machine

Lung compliance evaluated
Lungs ventilated (mechanical or manual)
Vaporizers off
Alarms on

Monitor

Temperature (37°C nasopharyngeal, esophageal; 35°C rectal)
ECG—rate, rhythm, ST segment analysis
Monitors zeroed and recalibrated
Arterial pressure, ventricular filling pressures
Strip-chart recorder on (if available)

Patient/Field

Look at the heart, look at the heart
De-aired—aspiration, ballotment of heart
Contractility, size, rhythm, rate
Assess vascular resistance: pump flow $\propto \dfrac{\text{MAP}}{\text{resistance}}$
LV vent out, caval snares released
No major bleeding sites—grafts, suture lines, LV vent site

Support

As needed

ABG = arterial blood gas; LV = left ventricle; MAP = mean arterial pressure.

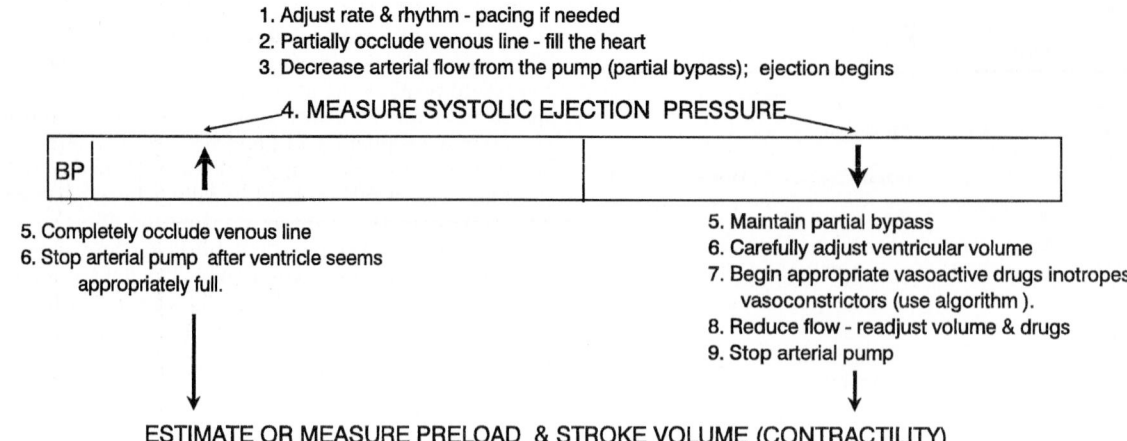

1. Adjust rate & rhythm - pacing if needed
2. Partially occlude venous line - fill the heart
3. Decrease arterial flow from the pump (partial bypass); ejection begins

4. MEASURE SYSTOLIC EJECTION PRESSURE

BP	↑	↓

5. Completely occlude venous line
6. Stop arterial pump after ventricle seems appropriately full.

5. Maintain partial bypass
6. Carefully adjust ventricular volume
7. Begin appropriate vasoactive drugs inotropes, vasoconstrictors (use algorithm).
8. Reduce flow - readjust volume & drugs
9. Stop arterial pump

ESTIMATE OR MEASURE PRELOAD & STROKE VOLUME (CONTRACTILITY)

Figure 32-30. General approach to the termination of CPB. (Modified with permission from Amado WJ, Thomas SJ: Cardiac surgery: Intraoperative management. In Thomas SJ [ed]: Manual of Cardiac Anesthesia, 2nd ed. New York, Churchill Livingstone, 1993.)

See Figure 32-30 for a general approach to termination of cardiopulmonary bypass.

Inadequate cardiac performance must prompt a search for possible etiologies (Table 32-24); structural defects require more than mere regulation of inotropes or vasodilators. If the clinical picture is suggestive of coronary air emboli with diffuse ST segment elevation and a hypocontractile heart, continuous support on cardiopulmonary bypass with a high perfusion pressure and an empty ventricle is indicated.

If pharmacologic support is required, an integration of cardiac physiology (Chapter 31) and pharmacology (Chapter 12) will lead to the rational selection of an appropriate drug or drugs. Numerous algorithms are available to guide decision-making; one is described in Figure 32-31. This algorithm uses arterial pressure, ventricular filling pressure (central venous pressure, pulmonary artery pressure, direct left atrial measurement), and cardiac output. After integrating available data, a diagnosis is made and appropriate treatment is begun. Continual reassessment of the situation is necessary to document the efficacy of treatment or to suggest new diagnoses and therapeutic approaches.

Table 32-24. ETIOLOGY OF RIGHT OR LEFT VENTRICULAR DYSFUNCTION AFTER CARDIOPULMONARY BYPASS

Ischemia

Inadequate myocardial protection
Coronary spasm
Technical difficulties
Emboli (air, thrombus, calcium)
Intraoperative infarction
Reperfusion injury

Uncorrected Structural Defects

Nongraftable vessels, diffuse distal coronary disease
Kinked or clotted grafts
Residual valve gradient
Hypertrophic cardiomyopathy
Shunts

Intraoperative Factors

Excess cardioplegia
Unrecognized ventricular distention

Pre-existing Dysfunction

Cardiomyopathy

Our approach to patients with inadequate cardiac output is summarized in Table 32-25. Heart rate is adjusted as much as possible. Ventricular filling is then optimized by transfusing blood from the pump. It is important not to overdistend the heart by transfusing to an arbitrary level of filling pressure; this may result in further myocardial dysfunction. Looking at the heart to monitor the response to small incremental volume infusions is helpful. The ratio of systemic to pulmonary artery pressure is helpful. They should change in the same direction. If, for example, pulmonary pressures increase and systemic pressure decreases, this is suggestive of ventricular failure. If cardiac output is low and systemic pressure is adequate, an arteriolar dilator may improve forward flow by decreasing afterload. If pressure is too low, precluding use of vasodilators, an inotrope should be selected. Each inotropic drug has a distinct profile with respect to its effects on rate, contractility, systemic and pulmonary vascular resistance, and cardiac dysrhythmogenic potential. By first defining the hemodynamic problem and then deciding what needs treatment and in what order, the most suitable drug for that situation may be selected rather than always selecting the standard "institutional inotrope." If these initial therapies are insufficient to promote adequate forward flow, various combinations of drugs may be tested. If systemic perfusion is still inadequate, mechanical circulatory support is required.

A therapeutic approach to right ventricular failure is outlined in Table 32-26. When pulmonary arterial pressure is normal or decreased, the etiology is usually severe right ventricular ischemia owing to intraoperative damage or to air. Initially, treatment is aimed at improving perfusion on bypass and awaiting recovery and improvement in contractility. If this does not occur, inotropic therapy and vasodilator therapy are indicated. Patients who have right ventricular failure secondary to high pulmonary vascular resistance are approached differently. The mainstay of therapy is reduction of pulmonary vascular resistance with vasodilators such as prostaglandin E_1 (PGE_1)[186] or nitric oxide and inotropic support. The phosphodiesterase III inhibitors, amrinone and milrinone, are particularly useful in that they significantly decrease pulmonary vascular resistance and increase contractility. Overdistention of the ventricle must be assiduously avoided. Combination therapy refers to the infusion of inotropes with vasoconstrictive properties into the left side of the circulation to maintain systemic perfusion but avoid increasing resistance in the pulmonary circulation. Persistent right ventricular failure precluding separation from cardiopulmonary bypass may require the insertion of a right ventricular assist device.

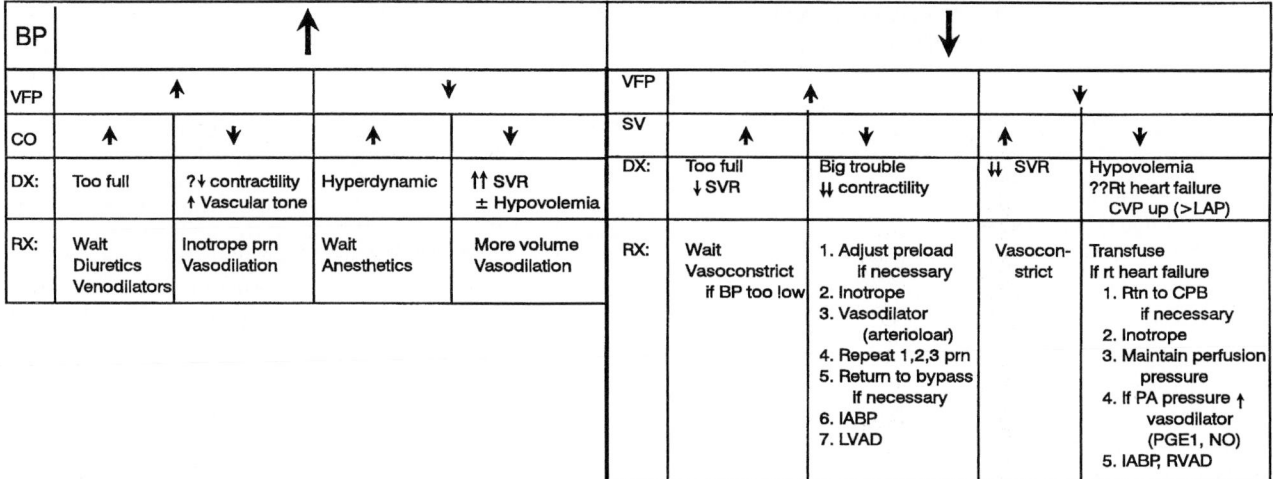

BP	↑					↓			
VFP	↑		↓		VFP	↑		↓	
CO	↑	↓	↑	↓	SV	↑	↓	↑	↓
DX:	Too full	?↓ contractility ↑ Vascular tone	Hyperdynamic	↑↑ SVR ± Hypovolemia	DX:	Too full ↓SVR	Big trouble ↓↓ contractility	↓↓ SVR	Hypovolemia ??Rt heart failure CVP up (>LAP)
RX:	Wait Diuretics Venodilators	Inotrope prn Vasodilation	Wait Anesthetics	More volume Vasodilation	RX:	Wait Vasoconstrict if BP too low	1. Adjust preload if necessary 2. Inotrope 3. Vasodilator (arteriolar) 4. Repeat 1,2,3 prn 5. Return to bypass if necessary 6. IABP 7. LVAD	Vasocon-strict	Transfuse If rt heart failure 1. Rtn to CPB if necessary 2. Inotrope 3. Maintain perfusion pressure 4. If PA pressure ↑ vasodilator (PGE1, NO) 5. IABP, RVAD

Figure 32-31. Algorithm for the diagnosis and treatment of hemodynamic abnormalities at the termination of cardiopulmonary bypass (CPB). (BP = systemic blood pressure; VFP = ventricular filling pressure; CO = cardiac output; DX = diagnosis; RX = treatment; SVR = systemic vascular resistance; CVP = central venous pressure; LAP = left atrial pressure; IABP = intra-aortic balloon pump; LVAD = left ventricular assist device; RVAD = right ventricular assist device; PA = pulmonary artery; PGE_1 = prostaglandin E_1; NO = nitric oxide; RV = right ventricle.) (Modified with permission from Amado WJ, Thomas SJ: Cardiac surgery: Intraoperative management. In Thomas SJ [ed]: Manual of Cardiac Anesthesia, 2nd ed. New York, Churchill Livingstone, 1993.)

Intra-aortic Balloon Pump

The simplest and most readily available mechanical support device is the intra-aortic balloon pump. It consists of a 25-cm sausage-shaped balloon composed of nonthrombogenic polyurethane mounted on a 90-cm stiff vascular catheter. It is usually inserted into the femoral artery, either percutaneously or, after surgical exposure, through a graft sutured directly to the artery, and advanced so that the tip is distal to the left subclavian artery (to prevent emboli to the upper arterial circulation). Occasionally, peripheral vascular disease prevents passage of the balloon via the femoral artery and it must be placed into the ascending aorta. The intra-aortic balloon pump is the only method that decreases myocardial oxygen demand while increasing supply.

The intra-aortic balloon pump does not pump blood. Rather, it utilizes the principle of synchronized counterpulsation to assist a beating, ejecting heart. Aortic blood volume is moved in a direction "counter" to normal flow. Immediately prior to systole, the intra-aortic balloon pump deflates, "removing blood," precipitously reducing blood pressure (afterload reduction), enhancing forward flow, and reducing $M\dot{V}o_2$. Proper timing of balloon deflation is necessary to reduce end-diastolic pressure as much as possible to maximally off-load the ventricle. This blood is then "returned" during diastole as the balloon inflates, elevating aortic diastolic blood pressure (diastolic augmentation), increasing the gradient for coronary perfusion.

The indications and contraindications for intra-aortic balloon pump placement are listed in Table 32-27. The primary indications for intra-aortic balloon pump in the cardiac surgical patient are inability to separate from cardiopulmonary bypass, poor hemodynamic function, and ongoing ischemia following cardiopulmonary bypass despite increasing drug support. Myocardial function often improves with the use of the intra-aortic balloon pump, and systemic perfusion and vital organ function are preserved.[187] It is crucial to control heart rate and suppress atrial and ventricular dysrhythmias to ensure proper balloon timing. As cardiac function returns, the assist ratio is gradually weaned from every beat to every other beat and so on and, assuming no further cardiac deterioration, then removed.

Complications associated with the intra-aortic balloon pump are primarily related to ischemia distal to the site of balloon insertion. Direct trauma to the vessel, arterial obstruction, and thrombosis are most common, although aortic perforation and balloon rupture occur rarely. Platelet destruction and thrombocytopenia may also occur.

Ventricular Assist Device

Infrequently (1%), the heart is unable to meet systemic metabolic demands despite maximal pharmacologic therapy and insertion of the intra-aortic balloon pump. Under these circumstances, devices that actually pump blood and bypass either the

---

Table 32-25. STEPS FOR IMPROVING SYSTEMIC FLOW

1	Appropriate heart rate (pacing—A, V, A/V) and rhythm
2	Optimize ventricular filling
3 or 4	Reduce afterload if blood pressure is acceptable (arteriolar dilators)
4 or 3	Improve contractility (inotrope)
5	Recheck adequacy of ventricular filling
6	Combination therapy
7	IABP
8	VAD

A = atrial; V = ventricular; IABP = intra-aortic balloon pump; VAD = ventricular assist device.

Table 32-26. RIGHT VENTRICULAR FAILURE

PAP	Increased	Normal or Decreased
Diagnosis	? Poor right ventricular	Air, ischemia
Prescription	protection	Volume
	Do not ↑ preload	Support on CPB
	Inotropes	High perfusion
	Afterload reduction	pressure
	(PGE_1, etc.)	? CABG
	? Differential infusions	
	RVAD	

RVAD = right ventricular assist device; PAP = pulmonary artery pressure; CPB = cardiopulmonary bypass; CABG = coronary artery bypass graft.

Table 32-27. INTRA-AORTIC BALLOON PUMP INDICATIONS AND CONTRAINDICATIONS

Indications

Complications of Myocardial Infarction
Hemodynamic—cardiogenic shock
Mechanical—mitral regurgitation, ventricular septal defect
Intractable dysrhythmias
Extension—postinfarction angina
? Limitation of infarct size

Acute Cardiac Instability
Unstable angina—preinfarction angina
PTCA misadventure
Pretransplantation
Cardiac contusion
? Septic shock

Open Heart Surgery
Separation from cardiopulmonary bypass
Right or left ventricular failure
Increasing inotropic requirement
Progressive hemodynamic deterioration
Refractory ischemia

Contraindications
Irreversible brain damage
Severe aortic insufficiency
Inability to insert
Irreversible cardiac disease (if not a candidate for transplant)

left or right ventricle are required. These devices are effective because the injury producing myocardial dysfunction takes place intraoperatively and, more important, is often reversible. Markedly impaired cardiac function after bypass is not necessarily synonymous with cell death but, rather, may represent temporary "stunning" of the myocardium. Survival ranges from 20% to 30%, many with minimal or no decline in cardiac function.

A second group of patients who have shown benefit from assist devices are those with chronic heart failure. These devices allow for hemodynamic support as a temporizing measure prior to heart transplantation.[188] In the failing heart, it is important to make decisions promptly, progress through the therapeutic options, and, if repaired, move swiftly to an assist device. Very often, mechanical support for one ventricle unmasks previously unrecognized failure in the other ventricle, necessitating additional pharmacologic or mechanical intervention.

Postcardiopulmonary Bypass

The procedure is not over when the patient is safely "off pump." Continued vigilance is mandatory during decannulation, protamine administration, "drying up," and chest closure. Anesthetics are administered when clinically indicated. Although removal of the atrial cannulas may trigger cardiac dysrhythmias, they are usually transient. Atrial or junctional dysrhythmias often disappear once the cannulas are out. Heparin is reversed with protamine following removal of the atrial cannulas; the arterial return remains in place for continued transfusion of pump contents. When this is completed and bleeding is controlled, the arterial cannula is removed and the chest is closed. During decannulation, the possibility exists for unexpected bleeding from the atrial or aortic suture lines, which sometimes requires rapid transfusion. Continued vigilance for new ischemia (manifested by ST segment changes, ectopy, atrial arrhythmia, regional wall motion abnormalities) is important because it may indicate a correctable problem with the grafts. Valve patients should have the adequacy of the repair or replacement (*i.e.*, perivalvular leak) assessed by TEE.

Reversal of Anticoagulation

Protamine, a polycationic protein derived from salmon sperm, is used to neutralize heparin. The initial and total doses administered vary widely. Some use a fixed ratio of protamine to heparin, others use $2-4 \text{ mg} \cdot \text{kg}^{-1}$, and still others look to automated protamine titrations to suggest the initial dose. Regardless of the method selected, further requirements are assessed by repeated measures of the activated coagulation time or other clotting assay, as well as the appearance of the surgical field.

Protamine administration is associated with a broad spectrum of hemodynamic effects.[189,190] Idiosyncratic responses include Type I anaphylactic reactions and both immediate and delayed anaphylactoid responses. True anaphylaxis, mercifully rare, is characterized by increased airway pressure, decreased systemic vascular resistance with systemic hypotension, and skin flushing.[191] An increased incidence of reactions has been reported in patients sensitized to protamine from previous cardiac catheterization, hemodialysis, cardiac surgery, or exposure to neutral protamine Hagedorn (NPH) insulin. Perhaps the most devastating complication associated with protamine is sudden and profound pulmonary hypertension accompanied by an elevated central venous pressure, a flaccid distended right ventricle, and systemic hypotension. This complication, which may occur in approximately 1% of patients, is mediated by release of thromboxane and C5a anaphylatoxin.[192,193] The reaction is extremely short-lived; and although reinstitution of bypass is required on rare occasions, it is usually not necessary. Whether protamine is administered via the right atrium, left atrium, or aorta or peripherally probably makes no difference. However, slow administration into a peripheral venous site is advisable.[193] Monitoring of the effectiveness of anticoagulation and its reversal is the subject of a recent review.[194]

Postbypass Bleeding

Persistent oozing following heparin reversal is not uncommon. The usual causes include inadequate surgical hemostasis and reduced platelet count or function, neither of which is identified by a prolonged activated coagulation time. Insufficient doses of protamine, dilution of coagulation factors, and, very rarely, "heparin rebound" are also in the differential diagnosis.

After adequate hemostasis is obtained, the chest is closed. This is occasionally associated with transient decreases in blood pressure, which usually respond to volume infusion. If hypotension persists, the chest should be reopened to rule out cardiac tamponade, a kinked graft, or other serious problems.

As the surgeon completes skin closure, the anesthesiologist prepares for an orderly, unhurried transfer of the patient from the operating room to the recovery room or intensive care unit. Medicated infusions must be regulated with portable infusion pumps. Additional syringes with emergency cardiac medications and necessary equipment for airway management should be carried. Blood pressure and electrocardiograms are monitored, and adjustments of infusions are made as clinically indicated.

MINIMALLY INVASIVE CARDIAC SURGERY

Economics, combined with patient comfort, is the driving force behind the latest innovations in cardiac surgery. The initial changes were centered on avoidance of median sternotomy and the complications associated with it. Minimally invasive direct coronary artery bypass (MIDCAB) and port-access surgery were born from this shift in focus. As surgical skill and equipment improved, the off-pump coronary artery bypass (OPCAB) with sternotomy, a complete coronary vascularization without CPB, emerged.

Improvements in interventional cardiology had all but eliminated the need for single-vessel coronary bypass. Initially, MIDCAB was introduced as an alternative to angioplasty for single left anterior descending coronary artery lesions. Patient comfort and speed of recovery, as well as the expense and complications from CABG, have favored treatment of a single coronary lesion with interventional rather than surgical options. An internal mammary artery anastamosis to the LAD, however, has been shown to have better long-term patency than angioplasty. The first attempts with MIDCAB approached the heart through a left minithoracotomy, allowing surgical access to both the internal mammary artery and the LAD.

Other less invasive approaches have been developed that allow the patient to avoid the major drawbacks of a full sternotomy—a large midline scar, a 6–8-week recovery period to regain use of the upper extremities, and possible complications including sternal wound infection, rib fractures, and brachial plexus injuries. Parasternal incision, minithoracotomy, inframammary incision, and partial sternotomy all improve the speed of recovery without compromising surgical outcome.[195] However, the accessibility of the heart and great vessels is significantly compromised, and hence these approaches remain of limited use.

Without support of the pump, coronary anastamoses were performed on a beating heart. Pharmacologic manipulation of heart rate and myocardial contractility were initially an important part of a successful operation. The slower the heart rate and the less vigorous the contractility, the lower the myocardial oxygen consumption during graft placement. More importantly, it was technically easier for the surgeon to operate on a slow-moving target. Adenosine, β-blocking drugs, and anticholinesterases were used to accomplish the appropriate degree of bradycardia. Heart rates of 40–50 beats $\cdot$ min^{-1} were considered desirable. As surgical retractors improved and other equipment was developed for these cases, the need for pharmacologically induced bradycardia has all but disappeared.

Anesthetic management adapted to this change in surgical focus. Anesthesiologists had to ensure stable hemodynamic conditions during isolation of the coronary artery and suturing of the bypass graft without the support of CPB. To ensure that the anastamosis could be accomplished without terrible alterations in the patient's circulatory status, test occlusions of the coronary artery were performed prior to graft placement. The occlusions simulated the conditions that would be present during the anastamosis and also provided time to 'precondition' the myocardium. The benefit of preconditioning lies in the assumption that brief periods of ischemia allow the myocardium to better tolerate longer periods of ischemia later in the procedure.[196–198] After acceptable hemodynamic conditions were established and preconditioning was completed, the graft was sewn in place on the beating heart. Anesthetic management and patient positioning vary with the surgical approach. One-lung ventilation is necessary with thoracotomies. The ability to pace, cardiovert or defibrillate the heart externally becomes essential because of the inaccessibility of the heart through smaller incisions.

Monitoring concerns for MIDCAB are similar to those in standard coronary surgery. ECG and TEE are important in assessing ischemia prior to and after graft placement. Arterial and central access is necessary to identify and treat major hemodynamic alterations. Although certainly not required, a pulmonary artery catheter can provide information that is useful in treating patients with poor cardiac function or major coexisting disease states. Temperature regulation plays a larger role in MIDCAB management than in conventional heart surgery. Without the pump to warm patients, the downward drift in temperature during surgery can be significant. Normothermia facilitates normal coagulation and permits early extubation; conversely, mild hypothermia may offer a neuroprotective effect.

Variable doses of heparin are used for anticoagulation. The range has been from 100 to 300 U $\cdot$ kg^{-1}, depending on whether or not cardiopulmonary bypass is needed. The appropriate dose of heparin for patients undergoing MIDCAB off-bypass is undetermined.

The choice of anesthetic drugs, as with most minimally invasive procedures, is oriented toward early extubation. Neuraxial narcotics have been used as alternatives to larger doses of parenteral narcotics. Shorter-acting muscle relaxants might be of benefit in plans for early extubation.

As more MIDCAB surgeries were completed without complication, specialized equipment was developed specifically for this technique. The single-vessel bypass was gradually expanded to include more vessels, and eventually the off-pump CABG emerged.

Off-Pump Coronary Artery Bypass (OPCAB)

Complete coronary revascularization without CPB is a worthwhile goal. CPB induces a marked inflammatory response. In addition, it is associated with fluid and electrolyte shifts, potential renal dysfunction in patients with pre-existing renal disease, coagulation abnormalities, and neurologic injury. MIDCAB plus angioplasty is one alternative; OPCAP is another. Avoiding cardiopulmonary bypass, especially in elderly patients, is a reachable goal. CPB is partially responsible for inflammatory, renal, coagulation, and neurologic complications that appear postoperatively. Additionally, the incidence of perioperative stroke is related to the severity of aortic atheromatous disease. Manipulation of an atheromatous aorta for cannulation and crossclamping increases the opportunity for an embolic event. OPCAB attempts to avoid both CPB and aortic manipulation. OPCAB is full myocardial revascularization accomplished through a median sternotomy without CPB.

An understanding of the underlying coronary anatomy and the lesions to be bypassed is vital to the planning and management of these patients. The sequence of graft placement must take into account the hemodynamic disturbances associated with the obligatory ischemia during graft placement and positioning of the heart. The most critical lesions are bypassed last so blood flow can be re-established to the remainder of the heart prior to the greatest ischemic insult. Grafting less vital lesions first allows for a smaller area of ischemia during the critical anastomosis and can help with collateral flow as well. As with a MIDCAB, the anastomosis must be accomplished on a beating heart. The artery to be bypassed is surgically occluded above and below the site of anastamosis. The myocardium distal to the surgical site may become ischemic and dysfunctional. The tighter the initial coronary lesion and the greater the collateral flow distal to it, the better tolerated are the surgical occlusion and ensuing ischemia. A variety of hemodynamic alterations can be anticipated during temporary occlusion and reperfusion. Anastamosis of a right coronary lesion might lead to atrial arrhythmias or bradycardia. Preparations for external cardioversion or epicardial pacing are important. Occasionally, left-sided lesions can be accompanied by severe LV dysfunction, requiring resuscitation with drugs, volume, and an intra-aortic balloon pump, or institution of full CPB.

Monitoring these patients is important, but presents heretofore unseen problems. Because of the surgical manipulation of the heart, methods for evaluating cardiac function or ischemia can be unreliable. The placement of lap pads or traction sutures and rotation of the heart into the right chest to reach the circumflex artery or its branches can make ECG and TEE difficult to interpret. The diagnosis of wall motion abnormalities may have to await return of the heart to its normal position in the chest.

Hemodynamic changes also accompany cardiac retraction. Arterial pressure monitoring is required to immediately identify and treat episodes of hypertension. Central access is also important to facilitate rapid infusion of vasoactive drugs and volume, if needed. Trendelenburg positioning assists in surgical exposure and in maintaining adequate ventricular preload. Many of the same issues discussed for MIDCAB apply to OPCAB—degree of anticoagulation, temperature management, and selection of anesthetic plan with early extubation as a primary goal.

Bleeding can be considerable during the procedure and in the intensive care unit. The bleeding is not a result of a pump-induced coagulopathy, but can still be of sufficient degree to merit blood transfusion. It has been suggested that this type of surgery can actually promote a hypercoagulable state.[199]

The outcome for OPCAB and MIDCAB in comparison to cardiac surgery with the use of cardiopulmonary bypass is still unknown. The crucial question of the long-term patency of grafts sewn onto the beating heart remains to be answered.

Port-Access Surgery

Port-access surgery requires full CPB but without the need for median sternotomy. Full CPB, including cardioplegia-induced cardiac arrest, is achieved by cannulation of the femoral artery and veins. Additionally, a balloon-type catheter ("endovascular clamp") is positioned above the aortic valve to effect aortic crossclamping.[200,201] Removing the cannulas and crossclamp from the surgical field has allowed surgery to be performed through different and less invasive incisions, including inframammary and parasternal approaches.

Both coronary artery and valve procedures can be performed with the port-access technique.[202] Data from a variety of sources have shown that the port-access technique offers similar or better results when compared with conventional bypass via median sternotomy.[203,204] The benefits described include decreased blood loss, infection, sepsis, and length of hospital stay. Reported complications include aortic dissection, aortic catheter migration, arrhythmias, poor cardiac protection, perforation of the inferior vena cava and right ventricle, damage to the femoral artery, and stroke.[205–208] Additionally, it is difficult to "de-air" after mitral and aortic valve replacements. Several contraindications to port access are described—a small adult patient, peripheral vascular disease, and an atheromatous aorta.

The anesthetic implications for port-access surgery are numerous. Monitoring is similar to that required for routine cardiac surgery. It is the responsibility of the anesthesiologist to place both a coronary sinus (to deliver retrograde cardioplegia) and pulmonary artery (to effect LV drainage) catheter via the right internal jugular vein. Initially, fluoroscopy was used to assist in coronary sinus catheter placement, although it has been almost completely superseded by TEE. The aortic cannula can migrate into the aortic arch during surgery, resulting in inadequate cerebral blood flow through the right carotid artery. Continuous TEE monitoring is essential.[209] The placement of bilateral arterial lines simplifies diagnosis of this event when a loss of right radial artery pressure is detected. The choice of anesthetic agent should be oriented toward early awakening and extubation if possible.

Port-access cardiac surgery has proved to be an effective option in the move to noninvasive cardiac surgery. Still, it is used in only a few centers, and the question of its universal adoption remains open.

POSTOPERATIVE CONSIDERATIONS
Bring Backs

Postoperative re-exploration is needed in 4–10% of cases. The indications are persistent bleeding, excessive blood loss, cardiac tamponade, and, infrequently, unexplained poor cardiac performance (rule out tamponade). Surgery is usually required within the first 24 hours but may be later in cases of delayed tamponade. The possibility of cardiac tamponade must always be included in the differential diagnosis of the postoperative

Table 32-28. CARDIAC TAMPONADE— CLINICAL FEATURES

Dyspnea, orthopnea, tachycardia
Beck's triad
  Muffled heart sounds
    ↑ Venous pressure (distended neck veins)
    ↓ Arterial pressure
Paradoxical pulse
Equalization of diastolic pressures
  RAP = RVEDP = PAEDP = LAP = LVEDP
ECG—ST segment change, electrical alternans
Chest x-ray—silhouette normal or slightly enlarged
Echocardiography—best diagnostic tool

RAP = right atrial pressure; RVEDP = right ventricular end-diastolic pressure; PAEDP = pulmonary artery end-diastolic pressure; LAP = left atrial pressure; LVEDP = left ventricular end-diastolic pressure.

"dwindles" because the classic symptoms and signs (Table 32-28) are often absent.

Tamponade

Cardiac tamponade exists when intrapericardial pressure, not intravascular volume and venous pressure, determines venous return. The ventricle is small and underloaded despite elevations in right and left ventricular filling pressures. These increases occur because pressures are routinely measured using atmospheric pressure as the zero reference point. Normally, this is acceptable because the pressure surrounding the heart is within 1–3 mm Hg of atmospheric. With tamponade, this pressure is increased, transmural pressure (inside minus outside) is actually decreased, and intracardiac chamber pressures are deceptively elevated. Classically, there is equilibration of diastolic pressures across the heart. Stroke volume is limited and fixed, and cardiac output and blood pressure become dependent upon heart rate. Compensatory mechanisms include peripheral vasoconstriction to preserve venous return and systemic blood pressure and tachycardia. Also noteworthy is the potential for concurrent myocardial ischemia because of the tachycardia and reduced coronary perfusion pressure.

Clinically, patients present with dyspnea, orthopnea, tachycardia, and hypotension. The intubated, sedated, mechanically ventilated patient in the postanesthesia care unit following cardiac surgery may manifest only hypotension. Ventricular filling pressures are usually elevated but not consistently so. In postoperative cardiac patients, the pericardium is no longer intact, and loculated areas of clot may compress only one chamber, causing isolated increases in filling pressure (*i.e.,* mimicking right and/or left ventricular dysfunction). Urine output is usually diminished. Serial chest films typically show progressive mediastinal widening. The diagnosis of tamponade may be confirmed by transthoracic or transesophageal echocardiography. Owing to its often atypical presentation in the cardiac surgical patient, the diagnosis of tamponade should be considered whenever hemodynamic deterioration or signs of low output failure occur in these patients.

The cure for cardiac tamponade is surgical; anesthetics can only further depress cardiac function. Therefore, drugs are selected that will preserve the compensatory mechanisms sustaining forward flow. Drugs with vasodilator (either venous or arteriolar) or myocardial depressant properties should be avoided in patients with serious hemodynamic compromise; dosages of induction agents should be appropriately reduced. Ketamine, because of its sympathomimetic effects, may be helpful in preserving heart rate and blood pressure response. It is not, however, a panacea and can induce hypotension in patients under maximal sympathetic stress. If, upon reopening the chest, there is minimal fluid or if the patient shows little improvement, a thorough search for other causes of inadequate cardiac performance, such as clotted or kinked grafts, myocardial ischemia, or valve malfunction, is indicated.

Postoperative Pain Management

Early awakening and extubation have brought the problem of postoperative pain management in cardiac surgery into focus. The standard practice has been iv opioids given as needed followed by conversion to oral pain medications. However, the quest is on to find an ideal postoperative pain management technique to complement the goal of early extubation and maximize patient satisfaction. Several studies have shown the benefits of intrathecal administration of opioids. The addition of nonsteroidal anti-inflammatory agents may play an increasing role. In cardiac patients with severe pain associated with sternal fractures due to the sternal retraction device during internal mammary harvest, epidural analgesia has been shown to be safe and effective and results in improved postoperative pulmonary function.

ANESTHESIA FOR CHILDREN WITH CONGENITAL HEART DISEASE

The child with congenital heart disease primarily suffers from structural defects of the heart and large blood vessels. Blood flow to, and oxygenation of, the myocardium is usually not a central issue in pediatric heart disease. This is in contrast to the adult, in whom the major defect is in the small myocardial vessels, resulting in ischemia. Anesthetic management of the child with congenital heart disease requires that one understand how a given anesthetic agent or combination of agents will affect myocardial function, pulmonary and systemic vascular resistance, and sympathetic tone.

Congenital defects cause either too much blood flow to a cardiac chamber (or vessel) or obstruction of flow to a chamber (or vessel). One can classify pediatric cardiac lesions by their primary effect on blood flow (Table 32-29). This classification

***

Table 32-29. EFFECT OF PEDIATRIC CARDIAC LESIONS ON BLOOD FLOW

Volume Overload of the Ventricle or Atrium Resulting in Increased Pulmonary Blood Flow

Atrial septal defect (high flow, low pressure)
Ventricular septal defect (high flow, high pressure)
Patent ductus arteriosus (high flow, high pressure)
Endocardial cushion defect (high flow, high pressure)

Cyanosis Resulting From Obstruction to Pulmonary Blood Flow

Tetralogy of Fallot
Tricuspid atresia
Pulmonary atresia

Pressure Overload on the Ventricle

Aortic stenosis
Coarctation of the aorta
Pulmonary stenosis

Cyanosis Due to a Common Mixing Chamber

Total anomalous venous return
Truncus arteriosus
Double outlet right ventricle
Single ventricle

Cyanosis Due to Separation of the Systemic and Pulmonary Circulations

Transposition of the great vessels

***

covers most congenital defects. One must remember that there is often more than one defect present.

The best way to understand the impact of a congenital defect and how anesthetic agents will interact with this defect is to envision the path blood must follow to maintain flow to the pulmonary arteries and aorta. For example, in the presence of tricuspid atresia, there must be an associated atrial septal defect so that blood may exit the right atrium. In addition, for blood to reach the pulmonary artery there must be either a ventricular septal defect, so that blood may enter the right ventricle, or a patent ductus arteriosus, to allow for pulmonary blood flow if a ventricular septal defect is not present.

When blood can flow to either the pulmonary or systemic circulation from a given chamber or vessel (e.g., endocardial cushion defect, patent ductus arteriosus), relative flow to each circulation will be determined by the vascular resistance of each of the two beds. Decreasing pulmonary vascular resistance relative to the systemic vascular resistance will lead to increased pulmonary blood flow; conversely, increased pulmonary vascular resistance will lead to decreased pulmonary blood flow and increasing cyanosis. A variation on this theme is found in the infant with tetralogy of Fallot who has had a shunt placed to provide flow to the lungs from the subclavian artery (Blalock shunt). If the shunt is large (decreased resistance to flow), pulmonary blood flow will be large; and it is possible to have a child who is both cyanotic, due to intracardiac mixing of systemic and pulmonary venous blood, and in congestive failure, due to increased left ventricular output and increased pulmonary blood flow secondary to a large, low-resistance shunt.

Whereas congestive heart failure in the adult is most often due to ischemic insults or overt infarcts, in the child, congestive failure is most often due to enlarged ventricular dimensions secondary to tremendously increased ventricular output (e.g., ventricular septal defect or patent ductus arteriosus) or to increased afterload (e.g., coarctation of the aorta, aortic stenosis).

Preoperative Evaluation

It is essential that the anesthesiologist understand the functional implications of a child's defect(s). Valve stenosis may be mild or critical. Tetralogy of Fallot may be asymptomatic or accompanied by frequent cyanotic episodes. The severity of a lesion is best evaluated by the child's level of activity—in the newborn and infant, by the ability to feed. Slow feeding, tachypnea, sweating, increasing cyanosis, agitation, or easy fatigability indicate severe congestive failure and/or cyanosis. Infants with an anomalous left coronary artery, arising from the pulmonary artery, will often become agitated during feeding, and have associated ECG changes associated with ischemia. Failure to gain weight is an important marker of the infant with severe cardiac disease. In the older child, activity level must be related to what is normal for a child of a similar age. Rather than asking parents if the child's activity is "normal," one should ask more probing questions about what the child is actually capable of doing.

Children who have a flattening of a growth curve or increasing hematocrit have lesions that are increasing in severity. Syncopal episodes are indicative of critical left ventricular obstruction at the aortic valve. The child with tetralogy of Fallot, with a labile pulmonary outflow tract, may have a history of squatting or acute cyanotic episodes ("Tet spells"). Infants with aortic arch anomalies may also have an absent thymus (DiGeorge syndrome). In the absence of a thymus gland, it is possible for an infant to suffer a graft-versus-host reaction if they are exposed to foreign lymphocytes during transfusion. In the absence of a thymus gland, blood should be irradiated prior to administration to destroy donor lymphocytes.

Children who present for cardiac transplantation are usually in severe congestive failure and may be severely hypoxemic, since the indications for most transplant procedures in children

Table 32-30. NORMAL HEART RATE IN CHILDREN

Age	Beats per Minute
Premature	150 ± 20
Term newborn	130 ± 20
1–6 months	120 ± 20
6–12 months	115 ± 40
1–2 years	110 ± 40
2–4 years	105 ± 35
4–6 years	105 ± 35
6–8 years	95 ± 30
8–10 years	95 ± 30
12–16 years	82 ± 25

Table 32-32. NORMAL RESPIRATORY RATE IN CHILDREN

Age	Respiratory Rate (breaths·min⁻¹)
Birth	40–60
1 year	30
2 years	26
4 years	22
8 years	20
10 years	20

are cardiomyopathies, irreversible pulmonary hypertension (combined heart and lung transplantation procedure), and unreconstructable heart disease.

A resting heart rate, respiratory rate, and blood pressure should be obtained. Normal values for these variables are shown in Tables 32-30, 32-31, and 32-32. Peripheral pulses should be palpated to help decide where to place an arterial catheter.

Preoperatively, digoxin and diuretics are withheld on the day of surgery, unless the digoxin is being administered for control of arrhythmias. Similarly, propranolol, used either as an antiarrhythmic or for control of infundibular spasm in tetralogy of Fallot, is continued until the time of surgery, as are calcium channel blocking agents. If an infant is receiving intravenous PGE_1 to maintain ductal patency, it is crucial that this infusion not be interrupted until a shunt is constructed or cardiopulmonary bypass is established.

Anesthetic plans—including premedication, induction sequence, use of anesthetic agents, placement of arterial and venous catheters, and possibility for postoperative ventilation—should be discussed with the parents, and with the child when appropriate. In almost all cases, vascular catheters can be placed after the induction of anesthesia. A number of children will voice a common fear of waking up during the operative procedure. The anesthesiologist needs to discuss this with the child.

Adolescents, as a group, tend to be anxious patients. The adolescent facing cardiac surgery must deal with special issues of dependence owing to their cardiac defect and physical limitations, and must cope with the possibility of a visually apparent scar. This is happening while the adolescent is normally struggling with issues of independence, body image, and their place in their peer group. Adolescents may be quite distant during preoperative interviews. They may need more reassurance and explanations of procedures than do other children.

The parents should be given information about anesthetic risk and outcome.[210] An estimate of risk is based on the child's

Table 32-31. NORMAL BLOOD PRESSURE IN CHILDREN

Age	Systolic/Diastolic Blood Pressure (mm Hg)
Premature	60/30
Term newborn	75/45
1–6 months	89/60
6–12 months	99/65
1–2 years	100/60
2–4 years	100/60
4–6 years	100/60
6–8 years	105/60
8–10 years	110/60
12–16 years	120/65

underlying condition. As discussed below, the greatest period of anesthetic risk is during induction.

Premedication

Children with cardiac lesions coming to the operating room are treated no differently than children for other surgical procedures. Oral administration of midazolam or ketamine or rectal administration of methohexital are just some of the choices for preoperative sedation.[211-213] In some cases, an inhalation induction in the presence of the child's parents is appropriate. The choice of premedicant drugs should be based on the child's physiology and the presence or absence of confounding factors such as gastroesophageal reflux. The use of an intramuscular injection of a combination of narcotic, a barbiturate, and atropine or scopolamine is rare now.

Small infants, particularly those scheduled later in the day, should not be kept without fluids while awaiting surgery. Clear fluids can be offered to infants until 2–3 hours before induction of anesthesia.[214]

Children who have had long or repeated hospitalizations and previous surgery may be apprehensive prior to surgery. Such children may benefit from sedation on the day of surgery prior to going to the operating room, particularly if they may be waiting for the conclusion of earlier cases.

Induction

In the presence of significant congestive heart failure, an intravenous induction with ketamine, fentanyl, or etomidate or an intramuscular induction with ketamine may be appropriate. In the presence of compensated congestive heart failure, nitrous oxide and low-dose inhalation agent, either sevoflurane or halothane, can be administered until an intravenous route is established. Despite the theoretical argument that a right-to-left intracardiac shunt would delay the uptake of inhalation agents, clinically, this is not a problem.[215] In the child with a cyanotic lesion, in the absence of congestive failure, induction can be carried out with a variety of agents.[216,217] The effect of an anesthetic agent(s) on peripheral oxygenation is the net result of: (1) pulmonary capillary oxygen content, which is in turn dependent on inspired oxygen concentration and hemoglobin concentration; (2) intrapulmonary and intracardiac shunt flow; (3) cardiac output; and (4) oxygen consumption.[218]

In the cyanotic child, sevoflurane, halothane, ketamine, thiopental, or fentanyl are all possible induction choices. With each agent, oxygen saturation usually rises once anesthetic induction is accomplished. Despite much discussion about the ratio of systemic to pulmonary vascular resistance in the management of the child with cyanotic congenital heart disease, there is no evidence that anesthetic agents have a selective effect on one vascular bed versus the other.

In the child with increased or obstructed flow on the left side of the heart, choice of induction agent depends on the state of the ventricle. Thus, in a neonate with coarctation of the aorta, left ventricular failure, and significant metabolic acidosis, fentanyl would be a likely choice. Conversely, an 8-year-old with coarctation, left ventricular hypertrophy, and no congestive failure might be best induced with sevoflurane or halothane. In the child with severe congestive failure, a narcotic or ketamine should probably be used.

The most critical part of the induction sequence is the maintenance of a patent airway. An obstructed airway can lead to hypercarbia and decreased oxygenation. This can lead, in turn, to increased pulmonary vascular resistance, further decreases in oxygenation, and ventricular compromise.

Maintenance

The choice of anesthetic agents following induction is governed by ventricle function (presence or absence of congestive failure), the use of cardiopulmonary bypass, and the anticipation of tracheal extubation at the end of the case, or mechanical ventilation in the postoperative period. The interaction of various anesthetic agents with the circulation in children with congenital heart disease is presented below.

Halothane

Cardiac output and blood pressure are depressed in a dose-dependent manner by halothane.[219] Myocardial contractility and left ventricular stroke work are depressed with minimal change in systemic vascular resistance. Halothane decreases sympathetic activity, resulting in reduced catecholamine release from adrenergic nerve endings and from the adrenal medulla. Hypotension (30% decrease in systolic blood pressure compared with awake values) associated with halothane is common in neonates and infants. At 1 MAC halothane the incidence of hypotension has been reported at 33% (neonates) and 44% (infants).[220] Halothane must be used cautiously in children with severe left ventricular failure or severe cyanosis because the myocardial depression from the drug may further compromise the already poorly contractile ventricle.

There is a decreased threshold for arrhythmias with halothane in the presence of exogenous catecholamines such as epinephrine. It should be remembered, however, that the most common cause for arrhythmias in the prebypass period is manipulation of the heart. In the postbypass period, the most common cause of arrhythmias is the surgical repair.

Sevoflurane, halothane, or isoflurane are the agents of choice for procedures such as thoracotomy for coarctation of the aorta or patent ductus arteriosus in the older child. During these procedures, the lung is retracted to expose the aorta, and high concentrations of oxygen may be needed to compensate for the intrapulmonary shunt that is created.

Hepatic dysfunction following halothane is almost unheard of in the prepubescent child, and it is possible to use halothane repeatedly at short intervals, if needed.

Isoflurane

Isoflurane causes a decrease in blood pressure that appears to be similar in magnitude to that caused by halothane when administered at equipotent doses. However, with isoflurane, myocardial function appears to be better preserved than with halothane.[221] Whereas isoflurane is associated with a rise in heart rate in adults, in many children heart rate will decrease. Isoflurane has the propensity to provoke laryngospasm during an inhalation induction and is best used only after induction has been carried out with another agent.

Sevoflurane

Sevoflurane use may be associated with a decrease in blood pressure. The incidence of hypotension (defined as >30% decrease from baseline) at 1 MAC is highest in neonates and infants under 1 year of age. With incision, blood pressure tends to return toward baseline in all groups except neonates.[222] As with isoflurane, most of the decrease in blood pressure is due

to a decrease in systemic vascular resistance.[223,224] Sevoflurane use is associated with a lower incidence of arrhythmias than is halothane.[225] The ability to use sevoflurane for an inhalation induction, together with its lack of significant myocardial depression, makes it a good choice for induction when an inhalation agent is used.

When tracheal extubation is planned at the termination of surgery or shortly thereafter, an inhalation agent (halothane, isoflurane, or sevoflurane) can be used. Isoflurane can be used during cardiopulmonary bypass as the sole anesthetic agent. A vaporizer can be connected to the oxygenator of the cardiopulmonary bypass circuit for administration of isoflurane during bypass, for example, during repair of an atrial septal defect. Because a number of children anesthetized with halothane will develop junctional rhythm, it is best to avoid this agent following cardiopulmonary bypass when it might not be clear if the nonsinus rhythm is due to the anesthetic agent or is a consequence of the surgery.

Nitrous Oxide

Nitrous oxide can be used in conjunction with one of the potent inhalation agents, morphine, or low-dose fentanyl. Pulmonary artery pressures do not increase in children when they are given nitrous oxide.[226] The drug should be discontinued before initiating cardiopulmonary bypass to avoid an increase in size in any gas bubbles in the circulation.

Ketamine

Ketamine has enjoyed some popularity as an induction agent in children with cyanotic lesions. Its popularity stems from its hemodynamic effects, combined with the facts that it can be given intramuscularly and that spontaneous respiration is maintained while intravenous and arterial cannulas are placed.

Hemodynamic changes associated with ketamine have been examined in the catheterization laboratory and in patients following cardiac surgery. In children given ketamine at the time of cardiac catheterization, the mean heart rate, blood pressure, pulmonary artery and wedge pressure, pulmonary to systemic flow ratios ($\dot{Q}_p/\dot{Q}_s$), and PaO$_2$ were essentially unchanged before and after drug administration.[227] (These children had previously been given thiamylal, which might have modified some of the pressor responses). Large changes in $\dot{Q}_p/\dot{Q}_s$ were seen in a small number of individual patients and occurred in an unpredictable fashion. In children studied postoperatively, ketamine was shown to have no significant effects on pulmonary vascular resistance as long as ventilation was maintained.[228] Should airway obstruction occur with ketamine, pulmonary vascular resistance will increase, but will drop when the obstruction is relieved.

Ketamine may be given intramuscularly (7–10 mg · kg^{-1}) or intravenously (1–2 mg · kg^{-1}). With intramuscular administration, the onset of anesthesia/analgesia occurs within 3–5 minutes. Ketamine, 6 mg · kg^{-1}, can be used as an oral premedication.[212] It requires approximately 20 minutes to achieve a sedative effect. Onset of drug action is heralded by the development of nystagmus. Anesthetic action is variable with ketamine. The interindividual variation in dose–response curves is large. When used as an agent for maintenance of anesthesia with additional use of muscle relaxants, dose intervals may be difficult to determine.

Very small infants are those most likely to develop airway obstruction following ketamine administration, although this is an uncommon event. Too rapid venous administration of ketamine in small infants may cause apnea. Emergence reactions seen in adults and adolescents are not a problem in young infants.

Atropine or scopolamine should be used in conjunction with ketamine to avoid pooling of secretions in the pharynx and resultant laryngospasm. Scrupulous attention must still be paid to the airway when ketamine is used. When oral ketamine is used as a premedicant drug, atropine or scopolamine can be omitted.

Ketamine is the agent of choice for induction of anesthesia in patients with cardiac tamponade. Ketamine usually produces a tachycardia and rise in blood pressure. Oxygenation is usually not impaired.

Etomidate

Etomidate can be used for intravenous induction. Its use through small peripheral veins is associated with pain.

Propofol

Propofol has been used both as an induction agent in the operating room and as the primary anesthetic in the cardiac catheterization laboratory. Data on the hemodynamic effects of propofol in the presence of congenital heart disease have been generated in the cardiac catheterization laboratory.[229] Propofol decreased both arterial pressure and systemic vascular resistance, while cardiac output increased. Notably, however, pulmonary vascular resistance was unchanged. Thus, in children with left-to-right shunts, the shunt was diminished, whereas in children with right-to-left shunts, the shunt was increased. It should be noted that children in this study were premedicated with midazolam or methohexital and received intravenous thiopental prior to propofol administration. In addition, all children breathed room air during the study.

Propofol may have advantages over other agents for anesthesia for radiofrequency ablation for tachyarrhythmias, although a recent report describes the suppression of ectopic atrial tachycardia by propofol.[230,231]

Fentanyl

When used in large doses, fentanyl has little effect on the circulation.[232] As the dose of fentanyl is increased, it becomes long-acting. In doses of 30–50 $\mu g \cdot kg^{-1}$, combined with oxygen and a muscle relaxant, its use was advocated for patent ductus arteriosus ligation in the newborn.[233] Given the variability of development in premature infants, it is not surprising that in a group of premature infants (postconceptional age 29–43 weeks, mean weight 1100 g), the elimination half-life of the drug varied from 6 to 32 hours.[234] There appears to be poor correlation between fentanyl plasma concentration and respiratory depression following the drug's use for patent ductus arteriosus ligation. When combined with nitrous oxide, fentanyl can be used in lower doses. When 10 $\mu g \cdot kg^{-1}$ was administered with nitrous oxide 50% for patent ductus arteriosus ligation in a group of infants at approximately 30 weeks postconception, stress responses to surgery (as measured by plasma concentration of epinephrine, norepinephrine, insulin, glucagon, and glucocorticoids) were blocked compared with a group of infants operated on without fentanyl.[235] No studies are available in children comparing fentanyl to other narcotics with respect to ability to block vascular and hormonal reactions to surgery. Depending on the age and condition of the child, doses of fentanyl up to 100 $\mu g \cdot kg^{-1}$ may be used.

Morphine

Fentanyl and its analogs have largely supplanted morphine in pediatric cardiac anesthesia. But morphine's lack of current popularity in no way diminishes its usefulness. In combination with nitrous oxide, morphine can provide excellent anesthesia in the child with congestive failure and/or cyanosis without depressing myocardial contractility. The sympathetic nervous system is not depressed by this combination of agents. When used alone, morphine increases venous capacitance and decreases peripheral vascular resistance. When morphine is combined with nitrous oxide, peripheral vascular resistance is increased. Hypotension from histamine release is not usually a problem in children. Occasionally, one will see red tracks along the course of the vein where morphine is injected. This is a

transient phenomenon. Morphine does not lower the threshold for arrhythmias when catecholamines are present. The use of morphine in doses of 1 mg · kg^{-1} does commit the patient to a period of postoperative ventilation. The transition from the operating room to the ICU is a smooth one without a sudden decrease in the level of analgesia. Morphine used without supplementation either with nitrous oxide or other intravenous agents cannot be relied upon to produce amnesia or hypnosis. The usual dose of morphine is 1 mg · kg^{-1}, administered over 15 minutes.

Succinylcholine

Succinylcholine has often been used to facilitate tracheal intubation. Because infants have an increased extracellular fluid space compared with adults and succinylcholine is distributed throughout this fluid space, a dose of 2 mg · kg^{-1} is required to provide muscle relaxation for intubation in infants. The drug's major side effects are bradycardia and, very infrequently, asystole. These events are more common with repeated doses. Because of the potential for bradycardia and the ability to use other agents, succinylcholine should have little place in pediatric cardiac anesthesia.

Nondepolarizing Relaxants

A nondepolarizing relaxant can be used both to facilitate tracheal intubation and to provide muscle relaxation during the operative procedure. The choice among nondepolarizing relaxants is based on their hemodynamic effects and duration of action. When an increased heart rate would be beneficial, as in the case of a small infant, pancuronium is the preferred agent. The popularity of the intermediate-acting agents atracurium and vecuronium has spilled over into cardiac anesthesia. For procedures in which the child will be ventilated postoperatively, there is little reason to use these agents.

Neuromuscular blocking agents should be titrated to effect. This is especially important in the case of a reoperation, in which the phrenic nerve may be encased in scar tissue. If excessive relaxants have been given and the diaphragm does not respond to electrical stimulation of the phrenic nerve, it is possible to transect the phrenic nerve with the electrocautery. In the small infant, loss of diaphragmatic activity can cause respiratory failure.

Cardiopulmonary Bypass

Prior to the initiation of cardiopulmonary bypass, agents such as aprotinin are administered to reduce bleeding. The infusion is continued until the end of surgery. Aprotinin has the ability to provoke an antibody response in the recipient, and children who are having repeat procedures are at risk for anaphylaxis, when aprotinin has been used in previous operations.[236–238]

During the course of cardiopulmonary bypass, vasodilating agents are employed to promote uniform cooling and rewarming. Sodium nitroprusside is most commonly used, although phentolamine can be employed as well. The adequacy of flow during cardiopulmonary bypass can be assessed by the difference between esophageal and rectal temperatures. If deep hypothermia is planned (temperature <20°C), a tympanic temperature probe may be placed as well.

Separation from cardiopulmonary bypass will require pharmacologic support in some patients. Hypocalcemia is readily detected by measurement of ionized calcium concentration and is easily treatable. A number of children will require inotropic and/or chronotropic support. Dopamine or dobutamine is generally chosen as the first drug to augment ventricular function. In lesions where the presence of increased pulmonary vascular resistance is known or suspected, dobutamine, amrinone, or milrinone may be useful. Isoproterenol will provide both chronotropic and inotropic support. Pacing should be employed in

Table 32-33. MEDICATIONS GIVEN BY CONTINUOUS INFUSION

Drug	Usual Initial Dose ($\mu g \cdot kg^{-1} \cdot min^{-1}$)	Usual Dose Range ($\mu g \cdot kg^{-1} \cdot min^{-1}$)
Amrinone*	2–5	2–20
Dopamine	2–5	2–20
Dobutamine	2–5	2–20
Epinephrine	0.01	0.01–0.1
Isoproterenol†	0.05–1	0.1–1
Lidocaine	20	20–50
Milrinone	50 $\mu g \cdot kg^{-1}$ (over 3 min)	0.3–0.7
Nitroglycerin	0.5	0.5–5
Nitroprusside	0.5	0.5–5
Norepinephrine	0.1	0.1–1
Phentolamine	0.1–1	0.5–5
Phenylephrine	1	1–3
Prostaglandin E_1	0.05–0.1	0.05–0.2
Trimethaphan	5	5–10
Vasopressin	(1 μg–4 U)	0.004

* Requires initial bolus of 750 $\mu g \cdot kg^{-1}$ over 3 minutes before start of infusion.
† For chronotropic effect following cardiac transplantation, doses of 0.005–0.010 $\mu g \cdot kg^{-1} \cdot min^{-2}$ are used.

the presence of a heart rate that is slow for age. Drugs that are useful in the postbypass period are given in Table 32-33.

Noncardiac Surgery in the Child with Heart Disease

Children with cyanotic disease usually have an uncompromised left ventricle. An inhalation agent can be used in the presence of cyanotic disease for noncardiac surgery such as for extensive dental restorations in a young child. In the presence of congestive heart failure, intravenous agents should be titrated slowly to effect, as in the case of a child with a cardiomyopathy who is awaiting transplant and having a Broviac catheter placed.

Regional Anesthesia

Regional anesthetic techniques can be used to supplement intraoperative anesthesia and for postoperative analgesia. For example, caudal (epidural) opioids can be used for coarctation of the aorta in the older child or ligation of a patent ductus arteriosus. Some physicians have used caudal or intrathecal morphine for cases involving cardiopulmonary bypass (and concomitant heparin administration), although this is not a universal practice.[239–241] The recommendation has been made that one allow 60 minutes to elapse between the placement of a neuraxial block and the administration of heparin, although there is no evidence to support this time interval. Procedures involving a thoracotomy can be supplemented with intercostal nerve blocks if, for some reason, epidural (caudal) or spinal drug administration is not possible or desired.[242] Because of the extremely variable drug absorption from the intercostal space in neonates, this route should be avoided in this population.[243]

Tracheal Extubation and Postoperative Ventilation

Children with simple lesions who have undergone a cardiopulmonary bypass (atrial septal defect, ventricular septal defect without failure repaired across the tricuspid valve) that does not involve ventricular incisions can often have tracheal tubes removed at the conclusion of surgery, or shortly thereafter in the intensive care unit.[244–246] Children having more complex

repairs, or those with ventricular impairment, may benefit from mechanical ventilation in the postoperative period. Mechanical ventilation tends to restore lung volumes and, in the presence of worsening failure or pulmonary edema, will prevent the child from becoming hypoxemic, which would in turn lead to arrhythmias or ventricular impairment.[247]

Children most at risk for ventilatory failure following cardiac surgery are as follows:

1. Infants less than 6 months of age, high O_2 consumption, compliant chest wall, poor nutrition.
2. Infants with pulmonary to systemic flow ratios, $\dot{Q}_p / \dot{Q}_s \geq$ 4:1. The increased pulmonary blood flow will decrease lung compliance and cause airway compression. The left ventricle will also be failing, causing increased left atrial pressures, and pulmonary edema.
3. Pre-existing lung disease. There is often a history of preoperative lung disease (pneumonia, atelectasis) due to airway compression.[248]

A thoracotomy incision in a young infant, for ligation of a patent ductus arteriosus or placement of a Blalock shunt, has been shown to decrease functional residual capacity in this population, and postoperative respiratory support is indicated.[249] In some cases, nasal continuous positive airway pressure (NCPAP) can be employed instead of mechanical ventilation.

Criteria for tracheal extubation following complex repairs are as follows: (1) ability to maintain oxygenation during spontaneous ventilation; (2) coordination of thoracic and abdominal components of respiration; (3) chest x-ray without significant atelectasis, effusions, or infiltrates; (4) short period of time without caloric input, or supplementation with enteral or intravenous feeding for patients requiring ventilation for a long period; and (5) stable inotropic support.

The effects of mechanical ventilation on cardiac performance can be judged by changes in arterial oxygenation and right atrial (central venous) or mixed venous oxygenation. Despite not having a ventricle to supply pulmonary blood flow, children who have had a Fontan procedure have been shown to tolerate mechanical ventilation with end-expiratory pressure.[250]

REFERENCES

1. Kaplan J (ed): Cardiac Anesthesia, 4th ed. Philadelphia, WB Saunders, 1999
2. Thomas SJ (ed): Manual of Cardiac Anesthesia, 3rd ed. New York, Churchill Livingstone, 2001 (in press)
3. Slogoff S, Keats AS: Does perioperative myocardial ischemia lead to postoperative myocardial infarction? Anesthesiology 62:107, 1985
4. Slogoff S, Keats AS: Further observations on perioperative myocardial ischemia. Anesthesiology 65:539, 1986
5. Leung JM, Goehner P, O'Kelly BF et al: Isoflurane anesthesia and myocardial ischemia: Comparative risk versus sufentanil anesthesia in patients undergoing coronary artery bypass graft surgery. Anesthesiology 74:838, 1991
6. Mangano DT, Hollenberg M, Fegert G et al: Perioperative myocardial ischemia in patients undergoing noncardiac surgery: I. Incidence and severity during the 4 day perioperative period. J Am Coll Cardiol 17:843, 1991
7. Leung JM O'Kelly BF, Mangano DT et al: Relationship of regional wall motion abnormalities to hemodynamic indices of myocardial oxygen supply and demand in patients undergoing CABG surgery. Anesthesiology 73:802, 1990
8. Weber KT, Janicki JS: The metabolic demand and oxygen supply of the heart: Physiologic and clinical considerations. Am J Cardiol 44: 22, 1979
9. Hoffman J: Transmural myocardial perfusion. Prog Cardiovasc Dis 29:429, 1987
10. Buffington C: Hemodynamic determinants of ischemic myocardial dysfunction in the presence of coronary stenosis in dogs. Anesthesiology 63:651, 1985
11. Prinzmetal M, Kennamer R, Merliss R: Angina pectoris: A variant form of angina pectoris. Am J Med 27:375, 1959
12. Deanfield JE, Maseri A, Selwyn A: Myocardial ischemia during

daily life in patients with stable angina: Its relation to symptoms and heart rate changes. Lancet 2:753, 1983

13. Maseri A, Chierchia S: Coronary artery spasm, definition, diagnosis and consequences. Prog Cardiovasc Dis 25:169, 1982

14. Urban MK, Gordon MA, Harris SN et al: Intraoperative hemodynamic changes are not good indicators of myocardial ischemia. Anesth Analg 76:942, 1993

15. Seitelberger R, Hannes W, Gleichauf M et al: Effects of diltiazem on perioperative ischemia, arrhythmias, and myocardial function in patients undergoing elective coronary bypass grafting. J Thorac Cardiovasc Surg 107:811, 1994

16. Thomson I: Con: Intraoperative myocardial ischemia is not benign. J Cardiothorac Vasc Anesth 8:593, 1994

17. Nathan H: Pro: Perioperative ischemia is benign. J Cardiothorac Vasc Anesth 8:589, 1994

18. Warltier DC, Pagel PS, Versten JR: Approaches to prevention of perioperative myocardial ischemia. Anesthesiology 92:253, 2000

19. Hines R: Monitoring for right ventricular ischemia: Is it necessary? J Cardiothorac Anesth 1:95, 1987

20. Kissin I, Reves JG, Mardes M: Is the rate pressure product a misleading guide? Anesthesiology 52:373, 1980

21. Gordon MA, Urban MK, O'Connor T, Barash PG: Is the pressure rate quotient a predictor or indicator of myocardial ischemia as measured by ST-segment changes in patients undergoing coronary artery bypass surgery. Anesthesiology 74:848, 1991

22. Leung JM, O'Kelly B, Browner WS et al: Prognostic importance of postbypass regional wall-motion abnormalities in patients undergoing coronary artery bypass graft surgery. Anesthesiology 71:16, 1989

23. Haggmark S, Hohner P, Ostman M et al: Comparison of hemodynamic, electrocardiographic, mechanical, and metabolic indicators of intraoperative myocardial ischemia in vascular surgical patients with coronary artery disease. Anesthesiology 70:19, 1989

24. Van Daele MERM, Sutherland GR, Mitchell MM et al: Do changes in pulmonary capillary wedge pressure adequately reflect myocardial ischemia during anesthesia? A correlative preoperative hemodynamic, electrocardiographic, and transesophageal echocardiographic study. Circulation 81:865, 1990

25. Tuman KJ, McCarthy RJ, Spiess BD et al: Effect of pulmonary artery catheterization on outcome in patients undergoing coronary artery surgery. Anesthesiology 70:199, 1989

26. Fontes ML et al: Assessment of ventricular function in critically ill patients: limitations of pulmonary artery catheterization. J Cardiothorac Vasc Anesth 13:521, 1999

27. Shanewise JS, Cheung AT et al: ASE/SCA guidelines for performing a comprehensive intraoperative multiplane transesophageal echocardiographic examination: Recommendations of the American Society of Echocardiography council for intraoperative echocardiography and the Society of Cardiovascular Anesthesiologists task force for certification in perioperative transesophageal echocardiography. Anesth Analg 89:870, 1999

28. Smith MD, MacPhail B et al: Value and limitations of transesophageal echocardiography in determination of left ventricular volumes and ejection fraction. J Am Coll Cardiol 19:1213, 1992

29. Bergquist BD, Leung JM et al: Transesophageal echocardiography in myocardial revascularization: I. Accuracy of intraoperative real-time interpretation. Anesth Analg 82:1132, 1996

30. Shah PM, Kyo S, Matsumura M et al: Utility of biplane transesophageal echocardiography in left ventricular wall motion analysis. J Cardiothorac Vasc Anesth 5:316, 1991

31. Wohlgelernter D, Jaffe C, Cabin HS et al: Silent ischemia during coronary occlusion produced by balloon inflation: Relation to regional myocardial dysfunction. J Am Coll Cardiol 10:491, 1987

32. Hauser AM, Gangadharan V, Ramos RG et al: Sequence of mechanical, electrocardiographic and clinical effects of repeated coronary artery occlusion in human beings: Echocardiographic observations during coronary angioplasty. J Am Coll Cardiol 5:193, 1985

33. Waters DD, da Luz P, Wyatt HL: Early changes in regional and global left ventricular function induced by graded reductions in regional coronary perfusion. Am J Cardiol 39:37, 1979

34. Battler A, Froelicher VF, Gallagher KP et al: Dissociation between regional myocardial dysfunction and ECG changes during ischemia in the conscious dog. Circulation 62:735, 1980

35. Weyman A: Principles and Practice of Echocardiography, 2nd ed. Philadelphia, Lea & Febiger, 1994

36. Lowenstein E, Haering JM, Douglas PS: Acute ventricular wall

37. motion heterogeneity. A valuable but imperfect index of myocardial ischemia. Anesthesiology 75:385, 1991 [No abstract available]

37. Buffington CW, Coyle RJ: Altered load dependence of postischemic myocardium. Anesthesiology 75:464, 1991

38. Aronson S, Lee BK, Wiencek JG et al: Assessment of myocardial perfusion during CABG surgery with two-dimensional transesophageal contrast echocardiography. Anesthesiology 75:433, 1991

39. Sabia PJ, Powers ER, Ragosta M et al: An association between collateral blood flow and myocardial viability in patients with recent myocardial infarction. N Engl J Med 327:1825, 1992

40. Lewis RP, Sandler H: Relationship between changes in left ventricular dimension and the ejection fraction in man. Circulation 44:548, 1971

41. Urbanowicz JH, Shaaban MJ, Cohen NH et al: Comparison of transesophageal echocardiographic and scintigraphic estimates of left ventricular end-diastolic volume index and ejection fraction in patients following coronary artery bypass grafting. Anesthesiology 72:607, 1990

42. Liu N, Darmon PL, Saada M et al: Comparison between radionuclide ejection fraction and fractional area changes derived from transesophageal echocardiography using automated border detection. Anesthesiology 85:468, 1996

43. Robotham JL, Takata M, Berman M, Harasawa Y: Ejection fraction revisted. Anesthesiology 74:172, 1991

44. Gorcsan J, Gasior TA, Mandarino WA et al: Assessment of the immediate effects of cardiopulmonary bypass on left ventricular performance by on-line pressure–area relations. Circulation 89:80, 1994

45. Declerck C, Hillel Z, Shih H et al: A comparison of left ventricular performance indices measured by transesophageal echocardiography with automated border detection. Anesthesiology 89:341, 1998

46. Gorcsan J, Denault A, Gasior TA et al: Rapid estimation of left ventricular contractibility from end-systolic relations by echocardiographic automated border detection and femoral arterial pressure. Anesthesiology 81:553, 1994

47. Feigenbaum H, Popp RL, Wolfe SB et al: Ultrasound measurements of the left ventricle. A correlative study with angiocardiography. Arch Intern Med 129:461, 1972

48. Gibson DG: Estimation of left ventricular size by echocardiography. Br Heart J 35:128, 1973

49. Teichholz LE, Kreulen T, Herman MV, Gorlin R: Problems in echocardiographic volume determinations: Echocardiographic–angiographic correlations in the presence of absence of asynergy. Am J Cardiol 37:7, 1976

50. Nosir YF, Lequin MH, Kasprzak JD et al: Measurements and day-to-day variabilities of left ventricular volumes and ejection fraction by three-dimensional echocardiography and comparison with magnetic resonance imaging. Am J Cardiol 82:209, 1998

51. Rich S, Sheikh A, Gallastegui J et al: Determination of left ventricular ejection fraction by visual estimation during real-time two-dimensional echocardiography. Am Heart J 104:603, 1982

52. Aebischer N, Meuli R, Jeanrenaud X et al: An echocardiographic and magnetic resonance imaging comparative study of right ventricular volume determination. Int J Card Imaging 14:271, 1998

53. Dell-Italia LJ et al: Right ventricular infarction: Identification by hemodynamic measurements before and after volume loading and correlation with noninvasive techniques. J Am Coll Cardiol 4:931, 1984

54. D'Arcy B, Nanda NC: Two-dimensional echocardiographic features of right ventricular infarction. Circulation 65:167, 1982

55. Lopez-Sendon J et al.: Segmental right ventricular function after acute myocardial infarction: Two-dimensional echocardiographic study in 63 patients. Am J Cardiol 51:390, 1983

56. Ochiai Y, Morita S, Tanoue Y et al: Use of transesophageal echocardiography for postoperative evaluation of right ventricular function. Ann Thorac Surg 67:146, 1999

57. Rafferty T: Invited commentary regarding use of transesophageal echocardiography for postoperative evaluation of right ventricular function. Ann Thorac Surg 67:153, 1999

58. Ota T, Fleishman CE, Strub M et al: Real-time, three-dimensional echocardiography: Feasibility of dynamic right ventricular volume measurement with saline contrast. Am Heart J 137:958, 1999

59. Roach GW et al: Adverse central nervous system outcomes following coronary artery bypass graft surgery in a multicenter study: Incidence, predictors and resource utilization. 335:1857, 1996

60. CASS Principal Investigators: Myocardial infarction and mortality

in the Coronary Artery Surgery Study (CASS) randomized trial. N Engl J Med 310:750, 1984

61. Mangano DT, Mangano CT: Perioperative stroke encephalopathy and CNS dysfunction. J Intens Care Med 1997.

62. Hartman GS, Yao FS, Bruefach M *et al:* Severity of aortic artheromatous disease diagnosed by transesophageal echocardiography predicts stroke and other outcomes associated with coronary artery surgery: A prospective study. Anesth Analg 83:701, 1996

63. Katz ES, Tunick PA, Rusinek H *et al:* Protruding aortic atheromas predict stroke in elderly patients undergoing cardiopulmonary bypass: Experience with intraoperative transesophageal echocardiography. J Am Coll Cardiol 20:70, 1992

64. Konstadt SN, Reich DL, Kahn R, Viggiani RF: Transesophageal echocardiography can be used to screen for ascending aortic atherosclerosis. Anesth Analg 81:225, 1995

65. Subramanian VA, McCabe JC, Geller CM: Minimally invasive direct coronary artery bypass grafting: Two-year clinical experience. Ann Thorac Surg 64:1648, 1997

66. Buffolo E, de Andrade JCS, Branco JNR *et al:* Coronary artery bypass grafting without cardiopulmonary bypass. Ann Thorac Surg 61:63, 1996

67. Tasdemir O, Vural KM, Karagoz H, Bayazit K: Coronary artery bypass grafting on the beating heart without the use of extracorporeal circulation: Review of 2052 cases. J Thorac Cardiovasc Surg 116:68, 1998

68. Royse C, Toyse A, Blake D, Grigg L: Screening the thoracic aorta for atheroma: A comparison of manual palpation, transesophageal and epiaortic ultrasonography. Ann Thorac Cardiovasc Surg 4:347, 1998

69. Konstadt SN, Reich DL, Quintana C, Levy M: The ascending aorta: How much does transesophageal echocardiography see? Anesth Analg 78:240, 1994

70. Paul D, Hartman GS, Barbut MD *et al:* Neurologic risk associated with severe aortic atheromatosis is based on the distribution of disease within the three regions of the thoracic aorta. Anesthesiology 87:A127, 1997

71. Nienaber CA, Spielmann RP, VonKodolitsch Y *et al:* Diagnosis of thoracic aortic dissection: Magnetic resonance imaging versus transesophageal echocardiography. Circulation 85:434, 1992

72. Keren A, Kim CB, Hu BS *et al:* Accuracy of biplane and multiplane transesophageal echocardiography in diagnosis of typical acute aortic dissection and intramural hematoma. J Am Coll Cardiol 28:627, 1996

73. Evangelista A, Garcia-del-Castillo H, Gonzalea-Alujas T *et al:* Diagnosis of ascending aortic dissection by transesophageal echocardiography: Utility of M-mode in recognizing artifacts. J Am Coll Cardiol 27:102, 1996

74. Appelbe AF, Walker PG, Yeoh JK *et al:* Clinical significance and origin of artifacts in transesophageal echocardiography of the thoracic aorta. J Am Coll Cardiol 21:754, 1993

75. Slogoff S, Keats AS: Randomized trial of primary anesthetic agents on outcome of coronary artery bypass operations. Anesthesiology 70:179, 1989

76. Tuman KJ, McCarthy RJ, Spiess BD *et al:* Does choice of anesthetic agent significantly affect outcome after coronary artery surgery? Anesthesiology 70:189, 1989

77. Engelman RM, Rousou JA, Flack JE III *et al:* Fast-track recovery of the coronary bypass patient. Ann Thorac Surg 58:1742, 1994

78. Cheng DC: Fast-track cardiac surgery: Economic implications in postoperative care. J Cardiothorac Vasc Anesth 12:72, 1998

79. Cheng DC, Karski J, Peniston C *et al:* Early tracheal extubation after coronary artery bypass graft surgery reduces costs and improves resource use: A prospective, randomized, controlled trial. Anesthesiology 85:1300, 1996

80. Cheng DC, Karski J, Peniston C *et al:* Morbidity outcome in early versus conventional tracheal extubation after coronary artery bypass grafting: A prospective randomized controlled trial. J Thorac Cardiovasc Surg 112:755, 1996

81. Shapiro BA, Lichtenthal R: Inhalation-based anesthetic techniques are the key to early extubation of the cardiac surgical patient. J Cardiothorac Vasc Anesth 7:135, 1993

82. Swenson JD, Hullander RM, Wingler K, Leivers D: Early extubation after cardiac surgery using combined intrathecal sufentanil and morphine. J Cardiothorac Vasc Anesth 8:509, 1994

83. Pagel S, Kampine JP, Sccchmeling WT, Warltier DC: Comparison of the systemic and coronary hemodynamic actions of desflurane,

isoflurane, halothane, and enflurane in the chronically instrumented dog. Anesthesiology 74:539, 1991

84. Ramsay JG, DeLima LG, Wynands JE *et al:* Pure opioid versus opioid volatile anesthesia for coronary artery bypass graft surgery: A prospective, randomized, double-blind study. Anesth Analg 78:867, 1994

85. Weiskopf R *et al:* Repetitive rapid increases in desflurane concentration blunt transient cardiovascular stimulation in humans. Anesthesiology 81(4):843, 1994

86. Ebert TJ, Muzi M: Sympathetic hyperactivity during desflurane anesthesia in healthy volunteers. Anesthesiology 79:444, 1993

87. Rodig G *et al:* Effects of desflurane and isoflurane on systemic vascular resistance during hypothermic cardiopulmonary bypass. J Cardiothorac Vasc Anesth 11(1):54, 1997

88. Pagel S *et al:* Desflurane and isoflurane produce similar alterations in systemic and pulmonary hemodynamics and arterial oygenation in patients undergoing one-lung ventilation during thoracotomy. Anesth Analg 87:800, 1998

89. Grundmann U *et al:* Cardiovascular effects of desflurane and isoflurane in patients with coronary artery disease. Acta Anaesthesiol Scand 40:1101, 1996

90. Helman JD *et al:* The risk of myocardial ischemia in patients receiving desflurane versus sufentanil anesthesia for coronary artery bypass graft surgery. Anesthesiology 77(1):47, 1992

91. Parsons RS *et al:* Comparison of desflurane and fentanyl-based anesthetic techniques for coronary artery bypass surgery. Br J Anaesth 72:430, 1994

92. Graf BM *et al:* The comparative effects of equimolar sevoflurane and isoflurane in isolated hearts. Anesth Analg 81:1026, 1995

93. Searle N *et al:* Comparison of sevoflurane/fentanyl and isoflurane/fentanyl during elective coronary artery bypass surgery. Can J Anaeth 43(9):890, 1996

94. Bell J, Sartain J, Wilkinson GA, Sherry KM: Propofol and fentanyl anesthesia for patients with low cardiac output state undergoing cardiac surgery: Comparison with high-dose fentanyl anaesthesia. Br J Anaesth 73:162, 1994

95. Jain U *et al:* Multicenter study of target-controlled infusion of propofol-sufentanil or sufentanil-midazolam for coronary artery bypass graft surgery. Anesthesiology 85:522, 1996

96. Wahr JA *et al:* Cardiovascular responses during sedation after coronary revascularization. Anesthesiology 84:1350, 1996

97. Brown BG, Bolson EL, Petersen RB *et al:* The mechanisms of nitroglycerin action: Stenosis vasodilation as a major component of the drug response. Circulation 64:1089, 1981

98. Feldman RL, Joyal M, Conti CR *et al:* Effect of nitroglycerin on coronary collateral flow and pressure during acute coronary occlusion. Am J Cardiol 54:958, 1984

99. Mangano DT, Layug EL, Wallace A, Tateo I: Effect of atenolol on mortality and cardiovascular morbidity after noncardiac surgery. Multicenter study of perioperative ischemia research group [see comments]. N Engl J Med 335:1713, 1996

100. Warltier DC: β-Adrenergic-blocking drugs: Incredibly useful, incredibly underutilized [editorial comment]. Anesthesiology 88:2, 1998

101. Schwinger RH, Bohm M, Erdmann E: Negative inotropic activity of the calcium antagonists isradipine, nifedipine, diltiazem, and verapamil in diseased human myocardium. Am J Hypertens 4:185S, 1991

102. Brister NW, Barnette RE, Schartel SA *et al:* Isradipine for treatment of acute hypertension after myocardial revascularization. Crit Care Med 19:334, 1991

103. Kaplan J: Clinical considerations for the use of intravenous nicardipine in the treatment of postoperative hypertension. Am Heart J 119:443, 1990

104. England MR *et al:* Magnesium administration and dysrhythmias after cardiac surgery. JAMA 268:2395, 1992

105. Caspi J *et al:* Effects of magnesium on myocardial function after coronary artery bypass grafting. Ann Thorac Surg 59:942, 1995

106. Baxter GF, Sumeray MS, Walker JM: Infarct size and magnesium: Insights into LIMIT-2 and ISIS-4 from experimental studies. Lancet 348:1424, 1996

107. Schecter M *et al:* The rationale of magnesium as alternative therapy for patients with acute myocardial infarction without thrombolytic therapy. Am Heart J 132:483, 1996

108. Garcia LA *et al:* Magnesium reduces free radicals in an *in vivo* coronary occlusion-reperfusion model. J Am Coll Cardiol 32:536, 1998

109. Casthely P *et al:* Magnesium and arrythmias after coronary artery bypass surgery. J Cardiothorac Vasc Anesth 8:188, 1994
110. Ross J: Afterload mismatch in aortic and mitral valve disease: Implications for surgical therapy. J Am Coll Cardiol 5:811, 1985
111. Grimm RA, Stewart WJ: The role of intraoperative echocardiography in valve surgery. Cardiol Clin 16:477, 1998 [ix, Review]
112. Sheikh KH, de Bruijn NP, Rankin JS *et al:* The utility of transesophageal echocardiography and Doppler color flow imaging in patients undergoing cardiac valve surgery. J Am Coll Cardiol 15:363, 1990
113. Sheikh KH, Bengtson JR, Rankin JS *et al:* Intraoperative transesophageal Doppler color flow imaging used to guide patient selection and operative treatment of ischemic mitral regurgitation. Circulation 84:594, 1991
114. Ungerleider RM, Greeley WJ, Sheikh KH *et al:* Routine use of intraoperative epicardial echocardiography and Doppler color flow imaging to guide and evaluate repair of congenital heart lesions. A prospective study. J Thorac Cardiovasc Surg 100:297, 1990
115. Marcus ML, Doty DB, Hiratzka LF *et al:* Decreased coronary reserve: A mechanism for angina in patients with aortic stenosis and normal coronary arteries. N Engl J Med 307:1362, 1982
116. Godley RW, Green D, Dillon JC *et al:* Reliability of two-dimensional echocardiography in assessing the severity of valvular aortic stenosis. Chest 79:657, 1981
117. Blumberg FC, Pfeifer M, Holmer SR *et al:* Transgastric Doppler echocardiographic assessment of the severity of aortic stenosis using multiplane transesophageal echocardiography. Am J Cardiol 79:1273, 1997
118. Blumberg FC, Pfeifer M, Holmer SR *et al:* Quantification of aortic stenosis in mechanically ventilated patients using multiplane transesophageal Doppler echocardiography. Chest 114:94, 1998
119. Smith MD, Dawson PL, Elion JL *et al:* Systematic correlation of continuous-wave Doppler and hemodynamic measurements in patients with aortic stenosis. Am Heart J 111:245, 1986
120. Maron BJ, Bonow RO, Cannon RO III *et al:* Hypertrophic cardiomyopathy: Interrelations of clinical manifestations, pathophysiology, and therapy (1). N Engl J Med 316:780, 1987
121. Wigle ED, Sasson Z, Henderson MA *et al:* Hypertrophic cardiomyopathy: The importance of the site and the extent of hypertrophy. A review. Prog Cardiovasc Dis 28:1, 1985
122. Levine RA, Vlahakes GJ, Lefebvre X *et al:* Papillary muscle displacement causes systolic anterior motion of the mitral valve: Experimental validation and insights into the mechanism of subaortic obstruction. Circulation 91:1189, 1995
123. Maron BJ, Wolfson JK, Epstein SE *et al:* Intramural ("small vessel") coronary artery disease in hypertrophic cardiomyopathy. J Am Coll Cardiol 8:545, 1986
124. Firth BG, Dehmer GJ, Nicod P *et al:* Effect of increasing heart rate in patients with aortic regurgitation: Effect of incremental pacing on scintigraphic, hemodynamic, and thermodilation measurements. Am J Cardiol 49:1860, 1982
125. Cohen GI, Duffy CI, Klein AL *et al:* Color Doppler and two-dimensional echocardiographic determination of the mechanism of aortic regurgitation with surgical correlation. J Am Soc Echocardiogr 9:508, 1996
126. Perry GJ, Helmcke F, Nanda NC *et al:* Evaluation of aortic insufficiency by Doppler color flow mapping. J Am Coll Cardiol 9:952, 1987
127. Willems TP, Steyerberg EW, van Herwerden LA *et al:* Reproducibility of color Doppler flow quantification of aortic regurgitation. J Am Soc Echocardiogr 10:899, 1997
128. Fraser CD Jr, Wang N, Mee RB *et al:* Repair of insufficient bicuspid aortic valves. Ann Thorac Surg 58:386, 1994
129. Cosgrove DM, Rosenkranz ER, Hendren WG *et al:* Valvuloplasty for aortic insufficiency. J Thorac Cardiovasc Surg 102:571, 1991
130. Simon P, Mortiz A, Moidl R *et al:* Aortic valve resuspension in ascending aortic aneurysm repair with aortic insufficiency. Ann Thorac Surg 60:176, 1995
131. David TE: Aortic valve-sparing operations in patients with ascending aortic aneurysms. Curr Opin Cardiol 12:391, 1997
132. Heller SJ, Carleton RA: Abnormal left ventricular contraction in patients with mitral stenosis. Circulation 42:1099, 1970
133. Savino JS: Transesophageal echocardiographic evaluation of native valvular disease and repair. Crit Care Clin 12:321, 1996
134. Thomas JD, Wilkins GT, Choong CY *et al:* Inaccuracy of mitral pressure half-time immediately after percutaneous mitral valvo-

tomy. Dependence on transmitral gradient and left atrial and ventricular compliance. Circulation 78:980, 1988
135. Foster GP, Isselbacher EM, Rose GA *et al:* Accurate localization of mitral regurgitant defects using multiplane transesophageal echocardiography. Ann Thorac Surg 65:1025, 1998
136. Lambert AS, Miller JP, Merrick SH *et al:* Improved evaluation of the location and mechanism of mitral valve regurgitation with a systematic transesophageal echocardiography examination Anesth Analg 88:1205, 1999
137. Enriquez-Sarano M, Schaff HV, Orszulak TA *et al:* Valve repair improves the outcome of surgery for mitral regurgitation. A multivariate analysis. Circulation 91:1022, 1995
138. Dalrymple-Hay MJ, Bryant M, Jones RA *et al:* Degenerative mitral regurgitation: When should we operate? Ann Thorac Surg 66:1579, 1998
139. Akins CW, Hilgenberg AD, Buckley MJ *et al:* Mitral valve reconstruction versus replacement for degenerative or ischemic mitral regurgitation. Ann Thorac Surg 58:668, 1994
140. Stewart WJ, Currie PJ, Salcedo EE *et al:* Evaluation of mitral leaflet motion by echocardiography and jet direction by Doppler color flow mapping to determine the mechanisms of mitral regurgitation. J Am Coll Cardiol 20:1353, 1992
141. Cape EG, Yoganathan AP, Weyman AE, Levine RA: Adjacent solid boundaries alter the size of regurgitant jets on Doppler color flow maps. J Am Coll Cardiol 17:1094, 1991
142. Chen CG, Thomas JD, Anconina J *et al:* Impact of impinging wall jet on color Doppler quantification of mitral regurgitation. Circulation 84:712, 1991
143. Thomas JD, Liu CM, Flachskampf FA *et al:* Quantification of jet flow by momentum analysis. An *in vitro* color Doppler flow study. Circulation 81:247, 1990
144. Cavarocchi NC, Pluth JR, Schaff HV *et al:* Complement activation during cardiopulmonary bypass: Comparison of bubble and membrane oxygenators. J Thorac Cardiovasc Surg 91:252, 1986
145. van den Dungen JJ, Karliczek GF, Brenken U *et al:* Clinical study of blood trauma during perfusion with membrane and bubble oxygenators. J Thorac Cardiovasc Surg 83:108, 1982
146. Philbin DM, Hickey R, Buckley MJ: Should we pulse? J Thorac Cardiovasc Surg 84:805, 1982.
147. Hornick P, Taylor K: Pulsatile and nonpulsatile perfusion: The continuing controversy. J Cardiothorac Vasc Anesth 11:310, 1997
148. Rosengart TK *et al:* Retrograde autologous priming for cardiopulmonary bypass: A safe and effective means of decreasing hemodilution and transfusion requirements. J Thorac Cardiovasc Surg 115(2):426, 1998
149. Young JA, Kisker CT, Doty DB: Adequate anticoagulation during cardiopulmonary bypass determined by activated clotting time and the appearance of fibrin monomer. Ann Thorac Surg 26:231, 1978
150. Bull BS, Korpman RA, Huse WM: Heparin therapy during extracorporeal circulation: I. Problems inherent in existing heparin protocols. J Thorac Cardiovasc Surg 69:674, 1975
151. Culliford AT, Gitel SN, Starr N *et al:* Lack of correlation between activated clotting time and plasma heparin during cardiopulmonary bypass. Ann Surg 193:105, 1981
152. Zulys VJ *et al:* Ancrod (Arvin) as an alternative to heparin anticoagulation for cardiopulmonary bypass. Anesthesiology 71(6):870, 1989
153. Teasdale SJ *et al:* Ancrod anticoagulation for cardiopulmonary bypass in heparin-induced thrombocytopenia and thrombosis. Ann Thorac Surg 48(5):712, 1989
154. Bichler J, Fritz H: Hirudin, a new therapeutic tool? Ann Hematol 63(2):67, 1991
155. Despotis GJ, Joist JH: Anticoagulation and anticoagulation reversal with cardiac surgery involving cardiopulmonary bypass: An update. J Cardiothorac Vasc Anesth 13(4; suppl 1):18, 1999
156. Gravlee G: Heparin-coated cardiopulmonary bypass circuits. J Cardiothorac Vasc Anesth. 8(2):213, 1994
157. Weiss BM *et al:* Pro and con of heparin-bonded circuits for cardiopulmonary bypass. J Cardiothorac Vasc Anesth 13(5):646, 1999
158. Akins C: Noncardioplegic myocardial preservation for coronary revascularization. J Thorac Cardiovasc Surg 88:174, 1984
159. Silverman NA, Levitsky S: Intraoperative myocardial protection in the context of coronary revascularization. Prog Cardiovasc Dis 29:413, 1987
160. Buckberg G: Warm versus cold blood cardioplegia: A self-imposed and counterproductive dilemma. Ann Thorac Surg 56:1007, 1993
161. Lell W: Myocardial protection during cardiopulmonary bypass. In

Kaplan JA (ed): Cardiac Anesthesia, p. 103. Philadelphia, WB Saunders, 1993

162. Guyton R: Warm blood cardioplegia: Benefits and risks. Ann Thorac Surg 55:1071, 1993
163. Mannucci PM: Hemostatic drugs. N Engl J Med 339:245, 1998
164. Dunn CJ, Goa KL: Tranexamic acid: A review of its use in surgery and other indications. Drugs 57:1005, 1999
165. Rich JB: The efficacy and safety of aprotinin use in cardiac surgery. Ann Thorac Surg 66:S6, 1998
166. Royston D: Aprotinin versus lysine analogues: The debate continues. Ann Thorac Surg 65:S9, S27, 1998
167. Murkin JM: Cardiopulmonary bypass and the inflammatory response: A role for serine protease inhibitors? J Cardiothorac Vasc Anesth 11(suppl 2):19, 1997
168. Royston D: Preventing the inflammatory response to open-heart surgery: The role of aprotinin and other protease inhibitors. Int J Cardiol 53:S11, 1996
169. Mongan PD, Hosking MP: The role of desmopressin acetate in patients undergoing coronary artery bypass surgery. Anesthesiology 77:38, 1992
170. Hensley FA, Dodson DL, Martin DE et al: Oxygen saturation during preinduction placement of monitoring catheters in the cardiac surgical patient. Anesthesiology 66:834, 1987
171. Thomson IR, Bergstrom RG, Rosenbloom M et al: Premedication and high-dose fentanyl anesthesia for myocardial revascularization: A comparison of lorazepam versus morphine–scopolamine. Anesthesiology 68:194, 1988
172. Bazaral MG, Welch M, Golding LAR et al: Comparison of brachial and radial artery pressure monitoring in patients undergoing coronary artery bypass surgery. Anesthesiology 73:38, 1990
173. Douglas PS, Edmunds LH, Sutton MS et al: Unreliability of hemodynamic indexes of left ventricular size during cardiac surgery. Ann Thorac Surg 44:31, 1987
174. Hansen RM, Viquerat CE, Matthy MA et al: Poor correlation between pulmonary arterial wedge pressure and left ventricular end-diastolic volume after coronary artery bypass graft surgery. Anesthesiology 64:764, 1986
175. Metz S, Keats AS: Benefits of a glucose-containing priming solution for cardiopulmonary bypass. Anesth Analg 72:428, 1991
176. van der Linden J, Casimir-Ahn H: When do cerebral emboli appear during open heart operations? A transcranial Doppler study. Ann Thorac Surg 51:237, 1991
177. Minamisawa H, Nordstrom CH, Smith MJ, Siesjo BK: The influence of mild body and brain hypothermia on ischemic brain damage. J Cereb Blood Flow Metab 10:365, 1990
178. Zhang RL, Chapp M, Chen H et al: Postischemic (1 hour) hypothermia significantly reduces ischemic cell damage in rats subjected to two hours of middle cerebral artery occlusion. Stroke 24:1235, 1993
179. Nussmeier NA, Arlund C, Slogoff S: Neuropsychiatric complications after cardiopulmonary bypass: Cerebral protection by a barbiturate. Anesthesiology 64:165, 1986
180. Zaidan JR, Klochany A, Martin WN et al: Effect of thiopental on neurologic outcome of coronary artery bypass grafting. Anesthesiology 74:406, 1991
181. Lowenstein E, Hallowell P, Levine FH et al: Cardiovascular response to large doses of intravenous morphine in man. N Engl J Med 281:1389, 1969
182. Sebel S et al: Histamine concentrations and hemodynamic responses after remifentanil. Anesth Analg 80:990, 1995
183. Tomicheck RC, Rosow CE, Philbin DM et al: Diazepam–fentanyl interaction: Hemodynamic and hormonal effects in coronary artery surgery. Anesth Analg 62:881, 1983
184. Schulte Sasse U, Hess W, Tarnow J: Pulmonary vascular responses to nitrous oxide in patients with normal and high pulmonary vascular resistance. Anesthesiology 57:9, 1982
185. Pagel PS, Kampine JP, Schmeling WT et al: Effects of nitrous oxide on myocardial contractility as evaluated by the preload recruitable stroke work relationship in chronically instrumented dogs. Anesthesiology 73:1148, 1990
186. D'Ambra MN, Laraia PJ, Philbin DM et al: Prostaglandin E1: A new therapy for refractory right heart failure and pulmonary hypertension after mitral valve replacement. J Thorac Cardiovasc Surg 89:567, 1985
187. Buckley MJ, Craver JM, Gold HK et al: Intra-aortic balloon pump assist for cardiogenic shock after cardiopulmonary bypass. Circulation 48(suppl 3):90, 1973

188. Piccione WJ: Mechanical circulatory assistance: Changing indications and options. J Heart Lung Transplant 16(6):S25, 1997
189. Horrow J: Protamine: A review of its toxicity (review). Anesth Analg 64:348, 1997
190. Jobes DR: Safety issues in heparin and protamine administration for extracorporeal circulation. J Cardiothorac Vasc Anesth 12(2; suppl 1):17, 1998
191. Moorthy SS, Pond W, Rowland RG: Severe circulation shock following protamine (and anaphylactic reaction). Anesth Analg 59:77, 1980
192. Morel DR, Zapol WM, Thomas SJ et al: C5a and thromboxane generation associated with pulmonary vaso- and broncho-constriction during protamine reversal of heparin. Anesthesiology 66:597, 1987
193. Morel DR, Costabella PMM, Pittet JF: Adverse cardiopulmonary effects and increased plasma thromboxane concentrations following the neutralization of heparin with protamine in awake sheep are infusion rate-dependent. Anesthesiology 73:415, 1990
194. Despotis GJ, Gravlee G et al: Anticoagulation monitoring during cardiac surgery: A review of current and emerging techniques. Anesthesiology 91:1122, 1999
195. Doty DB, DiRusso G, Doty JR: Full-spectrum cardiac surgery through a minimal incision: Mini-sternotomy (lower half) technique. Ann Thorac Surg 65(2):573, 1998
196. Hawaleshka A, Jacodsohn E: Ischaemic preconditioning: Mechanisms and potential applications. Can J Anaesth 45(7):670, 1995
197. Perrault L et al: Preconditioning: Can nature's shield be raised against surgical ischemic-reperfusion injury? Ann Thorac Surg 68(5):1988, 1999
198. Riedel BJ: Ischemic injury and its prevention. J Cardiothorac Vasc Anesth 12(6; suppl 2):20, 41, 1998
199. Mariani MA et al: Procoagulant activity after off-pump coronary operation: Is current anticoagulation adequate? Ann Thorac Surg 67(5):1370, 1999
200. Stevens JH et al: Port-access coronary artery bypass grafting: A proposed surgical method. J Thorac Cardiovasc Surg 111:567, 1996
201. Groh MA et al: Port-access coronary artery bypass grafting: Technique and comparative results. Ann Thorac Surg 68(4):1506, 1999
202. Galloway AC et al: Port-access coronary artery bypass grafting: Technical considerations and results. J Card Surg 13(4):281, 1998
203. Colvin SB et al: Port-access mitral valve surgery: Summary of results. J Cardiovasc Surg 13(4):286, 1998
204. Chaney MA et al: An institution's initial experience with port-access minimally invasive cardiac surgery [see comments]. J Cardiothorac Vasc Anesth 12(6):617, 1998
205. Hesselvik JF et al: Intraoperative rupture of the endoaortic clamp balloon in a patient undergoing port-access mitral valve repair. J Cardiothorac Vasc Anesth 13(4):462, 1999
206. Glower DD et al: Comparison of direct aortic and femoral cannulation for port-access cardiac operations. Ann Thorac Surg 68(4):1529, 1999
207. Abramson DC, Gianotti AG: Perforation of the right ventricle with a coronary sinus catheter during preparation for minimally invasive cardiac surgery. Anesthesiology 89(2):519, 1998
208. Grocott H et al: Endovascular aortic balloon clamp migration during minimally invasive cardiac surgery: Detection by transcranial Doppler monitoring. Anesthesiology 88(5):1396, 1998
209. Applebaum RM et al: Utility of transesophageal echocardiography during port-access minimally invasive cardiac surgery. Am J Cardiol 82:183, 1998
210. Hickey PR, Hansen DD, Norwood WI, Castaneda AR: Anesthetic complications in surgery for congenital heart disease. Anesth Analg 63:657, 1984
211. Levine NF, Spahr-Schopfer IA, Hartley E et al: Oral midazolam premedication in children: The minimum time interval for separation from parents. Can J Anaesth 40:726, 1993
212. Gutstein HB, Johnson KL, Heard MB, Gregory GA: Oral ketamine preanesthetic medication in children. Anesthesiology 76:28, 1992
213. Liu LMP, Gaudreault P, Friedman PA et al: Methohexital plasma concentration in children following rectal administration. Anesthesiology 62:567, 1985
214. Cote CJ: NPO after midnight for children: A reappraisal. Anesthesiology 72:589, 1990
215. Tanner GE, Angers DG, Barash PG et al: Effect of left-to-right, mixed left-to-right, and right-to-left shunts on inhalational anesthetic induction in children: A computer model. Anesth Analg 64:101, 1985

216. Greeley WJ, Bushman GA, Davis DP, Reves JG: Comparative effects of halothane and ketamine on systemic arterial oxygen saturation in children with cyanotic heart disease. Anesthesiology 65:666, 1986

217. Laishley RS, Burrows FA, Lerman J, Roy WL: Effect of anesthetic induction regimens on oxygen saturation in cyanotic congenital heart disease. Anesthesiology 65:673, 1986

218. Lister G, Pitt BR: Cardiopulmonary interactions in the infant with congenital heart disease. In Mathay RA, Mathay MA, Dantzker DR (eds): Symposium on Cardiovascular–Pulmonary Interaction in Normal and Diseased Lungs. Clinics in Chest Medicine. Philadelphia, WB Saunders, 1983

219. Barash PG, Glanz S, Katz JD et al: Ventricular function in children during halothane anesthesia: An echocardiographic evaluation. Anesthesiology 49:79, 1979

220. Lerman J, Robinson S, Willis W, Gregory GA: Anesthetic requirements for halothane in young children 0–1 month and 1–6 months of age. Anesthesiology 59:421, 1983

221. Wolf WJ, Neal MB, Peterson MD: The hemodynamic and cardiovascular effects of isoflurane and halothane anesthesia in children. Anesthesiology 64:328, 1986

222. Lerman J, Sikich N, Kleinman S, Yentis S: The pharmacology of sevoflurane in infants and children. Anesthesiology 80:814, 1994

223. Wodey E, Pladys P, Copin C et al: Comparative hemodynamic depression of sevoflurane versus halothane in infants: An echocardiographic study. Anesthesiology 87(4):795, 1997

224. Holzman RS, van der Velde ME, Kaus SJ et al: Sevoflurane depresses myocardial contractility less than halothane during induction of anesthesia in children. Anesthesiology 85:1260, 1996

225. Viitanen H, Baer G, Koivu H, Annila P: The hemodynamic and holter-electrocardiogram changes during halothane and sevoflurane anesthesia for adenoidectomy in children aged one to three years. Anesth Analg 87:1423, 1999

226. Hickey PR, Hansen DD, Strafford K et al: Pulmonary and systemic hemodynamic effects of nitrous oxide in infants with normal and elevated pulmonary vascular resistance. Anesthesiology 65:374, 1986

227. Morray JP, Lynn AK, Stamm SJ et al: Hemodynamic effects of ketamine in children with congenital heart disease. Anesth Analg 63:895, 1984

228. Hickey PR, Hansen DD, Cramolini GM et al: Pulmonary and systemic hemodynamic responses to ketamine in infants with normal and elevated pulmonary vascular resistance. Anesthesiology 62:287, 1985

229. Williams GD, Jones TK, Hanson KA, Morray JP: The hemodynamic effects of propofol in children with congenital heart disease. Anesth Analg 89:1411, 1999

230. Lavoie J, Walsh, EP, Burrows FA et al: Effects of propofol or isoflurane anesthesia on cardiac conduction in children undergoing radiofrequency catheter ablation for tachyarrhythmias. Anesthesiology. 82:884, 1995

231. Lai LP, Lin JL, Wu MH et al: Usefulness of intravenous propofol anesthesia for radiofrequency catheter ablation in patients with tachyarrhythmias: Infeasibility for pediatric patients with ectopic atrial tachycardia. Pacing Clin Electrophysiol. 22:1358, 1999

232. Hickey PR, Hansen DD, Wessel DL et al: Pulmonary and systemic hemodynamic responses to fentanyl in infants. Anesth Analg 64:483, 1985

233. Robinson S, Gregory GA: Fentanyl–air–oxygen anesthesia for ligation of patent ductus arteriosus in preterm infants. Anesth Analg 60:331, 1981

234. Collins C, Koren G, Crean P et al: Fentanyl pharmacokinetics and hemodynamic effects in preterm infants during ligation of patent ductus arteriosus. Anesth Analg 64:1078, 1985

235. Anand KJS, Sippell WG, Aynsley-Green A: Randomised trial of fentanyl anaesthesia in preterm babies undergoing surgery: Effects on the stress response. Lancet 1(8564):62, 1987

236. Dietrich W, Späth P, Ebell A, Richter JA: Prevalence of anaphylactic reactions to aprotinin: Analysis of two hundred forty-eight reexposures to aprotinin in heart operations. J Thorac Cardiovasc Surg. 113:194, 1997

237. Scheule AM, Beierlein W, Wendel HP et al: Fibrin sealant, aprotinin, and immune response in children undergoing operations for congenital heart disease. J Thorac Cardiovasc Surg. 115:883, 1998

238. Cohen DM, Norberto J, Cartabuke R, Ryu G: Severe anaphylactic reaction after primary exposure to aprotinin. Ann Thorac Surg. 67:837, 1999

239. Rosen KR, Rosen DA: Caudal epidural morphine for control of pain following open heart surgery in children. Anesthesiology 70:418, 1989

240. Shayevitz JR, Merkel S, O'Kelly SW et al: Lumbar epidural morphine infusions for children undergoing cardiac surgery. J Cardiothorac Vasc Anesth. 10:217, 1996

241. Hammer GB: Regional anesthesia for pediatric cardiac surgery. J Cardiothorac Vasc Anesth 13:210, 1999

242. Rothstein P, Arthur GR, Feldman HS et al: Bupivacaine for intercostal nerve blocks in children: Blood concentrations and pharmacokinetics. Anesth Analg 65:625, 1986

243. Bricker SRW, Telford RJ, Booker PD: Pharmacokinetics of bupivacaine following intraoperative intercostal nerve block in neonates and in infants aged less than 6 months. Anesthesiology 70:942, 1989

244. Burrows FA, Taylor RH, Hillier S: Early extubation of the trachea after repair of secundum-type atrial septal defects in children. Can J Anaesth. 39:1041, 1992

245. Laussen PC, Reid RW, Stene RA et al: Tracheal extubation of children in the operating room after atrial septal defect repair as part of a clinical practice guideline. Anesth Analg 82:988, 1996

246. Heinle JS, Diaz LK, Fox LS: Early extubation after cardiac operations in neonates and young infants. J Thorac Cardiovasc Surg. 114(3):413, 1997

247. Jenkins J, Lynn A, Edmonds J, Barker G: Effects of mechanical ventilation on cardiopulmonary function in children after open-heart surgery. Crit Care Med 13:77, 1985

248. Downes JJ, Nicodemus HF, Pierce WS, Waldhausen JA: Acute respiratory failure in infants following cardiovascular surgery. J Thorac Cardiovasc Surg 59:21, 1970

249. Gregory GA, Edmunds LH, Kitterman JA et al: Continuous positive airway pressure and pulmonary and circulatory function after cardiac surgery in infants less than three months of age. Anesthesiology 43:426, 1975

250. Williams DB, Kiernan PD, Metke W et al: Hemodynamic response to positive end-expiratory pressure following right atrium–pulmonary artery bypass (Fontan procedure). J Thorac Cardiovasc Surg 87:856, 1984

Clinical Anesthesia (4/e), edited by
Paul G. Barash, Bruce F. Cullen, and
Robert K. Stoelting. Lippincott Williams &
Wilkins, Philadelphia, © 2001.

CHAPTER 33

ANESTHESIA FOR
VASCULAR SURGERY

JOHN E. ELLIS, MICHAEL F. ROIZEN, SRINIVAS MANTHA,
GARY TZENG, AND TINA DESAI

GOALS OF ANESTHESIA

The goals of anesthesia for vascular surgery are similar to those for any procedure: to minimize patient morbidity and maximize surgical benefit. In the current environment, we must also achieve these goals in the most cost-effective manner. The increasing age of the population in Western societies and our desire to restore functional status to the elderly will likely increase the number of vascular procedures performed in the United States. The morbidity from these procedures has decreased rapidly, from a 6-day mortality of >25% for major aortic reconstruction in the mid-1960s to a 5% mortality today. We believe that advances in preoperative preparation and anesthetic management are responsible for much of these improvements. The anesthesiologist may have a greater influence in reducing the morbidity and costs of vascular surgery than in any other surgical procedure.

This chapter discusses the pathophysiology of atherosclerotic vascular disease and the general medical problems common in patients with peripheral vascular disease, particularly coronary artery disease. We believe the heart should be the major focus of the anesthesiologist's attention insofar as myocardial dysfunction remains the single most important cause of morbidity following vascular surgery[1-9] (Table 33-1). Recent studies have identified and emphasized the stressful nature of the postoperative period, while other workers have begun to refine preoperative risk-stratification and risk-reducing strategies. However, preservation of other organ systems (particularly renal and central nervous) is also crucial. Thus this chapter reviews current controversies in the selection of anesthetic techniques, monitoring modalities, and organ protection strategies. The specific surgical goals, anatomy, and complications for cerebrovascular, thoracic aortic, visceral, abdominal aortic, and lower extremity revascularization are placed in the context of optimal anesthetic management. New surgical techniques such as angioplasty, endovascular repair, and the placement of stent grafts, promise to further reduce morbidity and mortality.[10] The anesthetic implications of these new techniques are discussed. The different scenarios that lead to emergency surgery for these conditions and their appropriate management are also discussed.

VASCULAR DISEASE: EPIDEMIOLOGIC, MEDICAL, AND SURGICAL ASPECTS
Pathophysiology of Atherosclerosis

Atherosclerosis is a generalized inflammatory disorder of the arterial tree with associated endothelial dysfunction.[11] It has a number of recognized predisposing risk factors, including advanced age, altered serum lipid and lipoprotein profiles, hypertension, cigarette smoking, obesity and physical inactivity, male gender, diabetes mellitus, hyperhomocysteinemia,[12] and sedentary lifestyle. It is an inflammatory and degenerative process characterized by the formation of intimal plaques composed of oxidized lipid accumulation, inflammatory cells, smooth muscle cells, connective tissue fibers, and calcium deposits. Putative etiologies are endothelial damage caused by hemodynamic shear stress, inflammation from chronic infec-

tions such as gingivitis and chlamydia, hypercoagulability resulting in thrombosis, and the destructive effects of oxidized low-density lipoproteins. Disruption of the fibrous cap over a lipid deposit can lead to plaque rupture and ulceration. Vasoactive influences can result in spasm and acute thrombosis.

Morbidity associated with atherosclerosis arises from plaque enlargement and lumen obstruction (*e.g.*, lower extremity arterial occlusion with limb ischemia) or plaque ulceration, embolization, and thrombus formation (*e.g.*, transient ischemic attacks in patients with carotid disease). Alternatively, atrophy of the media due to atherosclerotic disease may weaken the artery wall, producing aneurysmal dilatation. The clinical expression of atherosclerosis tends to be focal, with clinical symptoms caused by localized interference with circulation occurring in several critical sites. Major arterial sites that are particularly prone to the development of advanced atherosclerotic lesions include the coronary arteries, carotid bifurcation, infrarenal abdominal aorta, and iliofemoral vessels.

Natural History of Patients with Peripheral Vascular Disease

Elderly patients with symptomatic or even asymptomatic peripheral vascular disease have greatly increased mortality rates, particularly from cardiovascular causes (6–15-fold increases).[13] The prevalence of claudication is ~2% among older adults, but 10 times as many elderly patients have asymptomatic lower extremity atherosclerosis. The prevalence of >25% carotid stenosis in patients over 65 years was 43% in men and 34% in women in one of the Framingham studies.[14] The incidence of atherosclerotic disease in one system increases the incidence in other areas.

Approximately 583,000 patients in the United States underwent vascular surgical procedures in 1992.[15] Increasingly, randomized clinical trials are demonstrating the benefits of revascularization surgery. In the United States, for example, more carotid endarterectomies are being performed, presumably because trials have shown that the procedure reduces stroke in symptomatic and asymptomatic patients.[16] Unfortunately, some studies have suggested that subgroups of patients, such as African Americans, women, Medicaid recipients, and diabetics, are more likely to have amputations rather than limb-salvage procedures (angioplasty or bypass surgery) performed for peripheral arterial disease.[17] Abdominal aortic aneurysms occur predominantly in white men.

The goals of vascular surgery are to provide an enduring restoration of normal perfusion, so as to prevent stroke, improve functional status, or prevent death from aneurysm rupture. Current challenges remain: to create a long-lasting arterial substitute for small-caliber vessels[18] and to perform revascularization less invasively and with less morbidity.

An explosion of less invasive procedures is changing vascular surgery. Radiologists, cardiologists, and vascular surgeons, working alone or in combination, place endovascular stents to treat patients with thoracic and abdominal aortic aneurysms. Other new treatment options include lasers, angioplasty, atherectomy (rotary and directional devices), gene therapy to help prevent restenosis and to promote angiogenesis, and thrombolysis, at times with concomitant or secondary surgery. Outcome studies

Table 33-1. PERIOPERATIVE MORTALITY ASSOCIATED WITH CARDIAC EVENTS IN AORTIC RECONSTRUCTION SERIES

Aortic Reconstruction References, Year	Deaths/Total No. of Patients (%)	% Mortality Caused by Cardiac Dysfunction
Szilagyi et al,[1] 1966	59/401 (14.7%)	48
Whittemore et al,[2] 1980	1/110 (0.9%)	100
Crawford et al,[3] 1981	41/860 (4.8%)	54
Johnston KW,[4] 1989	32/666 (4.8%)	69
Golden et al,[5] 1990	8/500 (1.6%)	75
Suggs et al,[6] 1993	3/247 (1.2)	66
Baron et al,[7] 1994	22/457 (4.4)	50
L'Italien et al,[8] 1995	16/322 (5.0)	62
Lloyd et al,[9] 1996	24/1000 (2.4)	50

for many of these procedures are now being published; they appear to be associated with less short-term risk and lower cost than traditional surgery.[19] Less invasive approaches will invariably lead to procedures being performed in patients with such severe comorbidities that they would previously have been denied surgery. The practice of anesthesia for vascular surgery will surely change as the interventional strategies evolve, but the challenges of providing diligent care for these patients will remain.

Medical Therapy for Atherosclerosis

The goals of medical therapy for atherosclerotic peripheral vascular disease are to improve functional status, prevent stroke, prevent limb loss, and reduce potential atherosclerotic progression and cardiovascular morbidity.[20,21] Prevention, including meticulous foot care in diabetic patients, is important to avoid infections and tissue loss. Lifestyle changes such as weight loss and exercise can forestall claudication. The use of statin drugs may reduce progression or even cause regression of atherosclerotic plaques, improve endothelial function, and reduce cardiovascular events in high-risk patients.[22] The use of antioxidant vitamins such as C and E may also improve endothelial function, and folate supplementation may be of benefit for patients with hyperhomocysteinemia.[12] Exercise programs improve vascular endothelial function[23] and may delay the need for vascular surgery in those with claudication. Cessation of smoking is by far the most effective "medical" therapy. While acute smoking cessation before surgery may not reduce perioperative respiratory complications,[24] patients should be encouraged to stop smoking. Cessation rates are approximately 25% after major surgery.[25] Despite the low success rates, the benefits of smoking cessation are so great that such programs are probably very cost-effective. Our recommendations for management of concomitant medical therapy in the perioperative period are listed in Table 33-2.[20]

Antiplatelet therapy is a mainstay of medical therapy for peripheral vascular disease. Chronic therapy with aspirin or other anti-inflammatory drugs may retard the progression of atherosclerosis and prevent morbid cardiovascular events. Therefore, many patients presenting for vascular surgery will be taking aspirin, COX-2 inhibitors, ticlopidine, or clopidogrel. Clopidogrel irreversibly inhibits ADP-induced platelet aggregation, and reduces formation of both arterial and venous thrombi. Oral platelet glycoprotein IIb/IIIa inhibitors may also be used acutely during percutaneous coronary intervention and as adjunctive treatment of acute coronary syndromes.[26] Considerations of the adverse effects of aspirin, including increased bleeding tendency, gastritis, and renal vasoconstriction, as well as thrombotic thrombocytopenic purpura and neutropenia from

ticlopidine[27,28] must be weighed against potential benefits. In general, we recommend that patients continue to take aspirin until the day of surgery for carotid and lower extremity surgery, and individualize the choice for larger operations. When patients develop acute ischemia, systemic anticoagulation may be instituted. The agents used may range from dextran (to enhance microcirculatory blood flow) to heparin, coumadin, or thrombolytics. Therefore, when patients present to us for urgent surgery to reverse acute ischemia, we specifically ask them and their surgeons about recent or planned anticoagulation. If the answer is "yes," we almost always forgo regional anesthesia. The implications of new antiplatelet agents on the use of regional anesthesia are unclear. However, the use of low–molecular-weight heparins is clearly dangerous when combined with regional anesthesia, as discussed below.

A primary concern with the use of anticoagulation and antiplatelet therapy is the risk of spinal hematoma after spinal–epidural anesthesia.[29] Therapeutic anticoagulation with intravenous heparin is routine during vascular surgery and may be continued into the postoperative period as well. Guidelines have been proposed to improve safety in such situations. Spinal and epidural anesthesia may be safely performed in a patient undergoing subsequent therapeutic heparinization provided heparinization occurs a minimum of 60 min after the needle placement. In addition, heparin effect is monitored and maintained within acceptable levels (activated clotting time or activated partial thromboplastin time 1.5–2 times baseline), and indwelling catheters are removed at a time when heparin activity is low or completely reversed.[30] Recently, concern has been growing about the use of low–molecular-weight heparins and the occurrence of spinal and epidural hematoma.[31] From May 1993 through February 1998, the Food and Drug Administration (FDA) received reports of 43 patients in the United States who had spinal or epidural hematoma or bleeding after receiving enoxaparin. Emergency decompressive laminectomy to evacuate the hematoma was required in 28 patients (65%). Permanent paraplegia, often with delay in diagnosis or surgical treatment, occurred in 16 patients (37.2%). Factors suspected of predisposing patients to epidural hematoma include a dose of enoxaparin that exceeds the recommended dose (30 mg every 12 hours), use of epidural catheters, administration of concomitant medications known to increase bleeding, presence of vertebral column abnormalities, older age, and female gender. Because plasma half-life and bioavailability are higher for low–molecular-weight heparins as compared to conventional unfractioned heparin, the guidelines for spinal and epidural anesthesia are different. A single-dose spinal anesthetic may be the safest neuraxial technique in patients receiving preoperative low–molecular-weight heparins. Needle placement should occur at least 10–12 hr after the last dose of low–molecular weight heparin. Subsequent dosing of the anticoagulant should be delayed for at least 2 hr after the needle placement. Presence of blood during needle placement may warrant an additional delay in initiation of postoperative therapy. If a continuous technique is selected, the epidural catheter should be left indwelling overnight and removed the following day, with the first dose of low–molecular weight heparin administered 2 hr after catheter removal.[32]

In patients who have previously undergone procedures during which heparin was administered, heparin antibodies may be present.[33] When suspected, platelet aggregation tests may be performed with heparin in vitro before surgery. When undiagnosed patients with heparin antibodies receive heparin, platelet counts may drop following surgery. In the most severe cases, thrombosis may occur due to platelet activation. Heparin-induced thrombocytopenia (HIT) is one of the most common immune-mediated adverse drug reactions. HIT is caused by IgG antibodies that recognize complexes of heparin and platelet factor 4, leading to platelet activation via platelet Fc gamma IIa receptors. Procoagulant, platelet-derived microparticles, and

Table 33-2. CONCOMITANT MEDICAL THERAPY, SIDE-EFFECTS OF POTENTIAL CONCERN PERIOPERATIVELY, AND THE AUTHORS' CURRENT RECOMMENDATIONS[20]

Medication or Drug Class	Side-Effect of Potential Concern in the Perioperative Period	Recommendation for Perioperative Use
Aspirin	Platelet inhibition may increase bleeding; decreased GFR	Continue until day before surgery; monitor fluid and urine status
HMG CoA reductase inhibitors	Liver function test abnormalities	Assess liver function tests and continue through morning of surgery
β-Blockers	Bronchospasm	Continue through perioperative period
ACE inhibitors	Induction hypotension, cough	Continue through perioperative period; consider 1/2 dose on day of surgery
Diuretics	Hypovolemia, electrolyte abnormalities	Continue through morning of surgery; monitor fluid and urine status
Oral hypoglycemics	Hypoglycemia pre- and intraoperatively	Monitor glucose status perioperatively

GFR = glomerular filtration rate; HMG = 3-hydroxy-3-methylglutaryl–coenzyme A reductase; ACE = angiotension-converting enzyme.

possibly the activation of endothelium cause thrombin generation *in vivo*.[34] The central role of thrombin generation in this syndrome provides a rationale for the use of anticoagulants that reduce thrombin generation (danaparoid) or inhibit thrombin (lepirudin). These drugs may be given to provide anticoagulation during surgery instead of heparin; however, their half-lives are longer than those of heparin, their metabolism depends on renal function, and their interactions with regional anesthesia are unclear.

Chronic Medical Problems and Risk Prediction in Peripheral Vascular Disease Patients

Many disorders are associated with vascular disease; however, diabetes, smoking and its sequelae, chronic pulmonary disease, hypertension, renal insufficiency, and ischemic heart disease are the most common. Understanding the end-organ effects of these diseases can guide appropriate perioperative therapy.[35] It would be suboptimal to administer anesthesia to patients with uncontrolled medical conditions such as severe hypertension, a recent myocardial infarction, uncontrolled diabetes and hyperglycemia, or untreated pulmonary infections. However, an expanding aneurysm, crescendo transient ischemic attacks, or threatened limb loss can force one's hand. In such situations, attempts to rapidly control chronically deranged blood pressure (which could precipitate cerebral ischemia) or electrolytes (which could, for example, result in accidental administration of a bolus of potassium) may be more hazardous than leaving the condition untreated or trying to control the abnormality slowly. The National Veterans Affairs Surgical Risk Study found that low serum albumin values and high ASA physical classification were among the best predictors of morbidity and mortality after vascular surgery[36,37] (Table 33-3).

Whereas chronic medical conditions increase the likelihood of postoperative morbidity and mortality, postoperative complications have even greater predictive value for adverse outcomes (Table 33-4).[38] Other causes of morbidity following vascular surgery include bleeding, pulmonary infections, graft infections, renal insufficiency and failure, hepatic failure, cerebrovascular accidents, and spinal cord ischemia resulting in paraplegia. The incidence of these other causes of morbidity has declined substantially in the past 20 years; in particular, death from renal failure after abdominal aortic reconstruction has declined from 25% to <1% at present. Much of the decline in renal failure has been the result of better perioperative fluid management.[39] While multisystem organ failure may account for an increasing proportion of deaths after vascular surgery, we believe that maintaining adequate cardiac function and perfusion of vital organs remains a vital aspect of reducing perioperative mortality. The factors that limit patient prognosis after vascular surgery remain primarily related to the heart (see Table 33-1). We will therefore examine more closely the effects of known or suspected coronary artery disease on patient management before, during, and after vascular surgery.

Coronary Artery Disease in Patients with Peripheral Vascular Disease

Hertzer *et al*[40] performed coronary angiography in 1000 consecutive patients presenting for vascular surgery and identified severe correctable coronary artery disease in 25% of the entire series. The incidence of significant coronary artery disease (stenosis >70%) detected by angiography was 78% in those with clinical indications of coronary artery disease and 37% in patients without any clinical indications. However, subsequent analysis demonstrated that clincal risk factors still predicted the severity of coronary artery disease (Fig. 33-1).[41] The absence of severe coronary stenoses can be predicted with a positive predictive value of 96% for patients who had none of the following risk factors: history of diabetes, prior angina, previous myocardial infarction, or congestive heart failure.

Short-term postoperative morbidity and mortality after vascular surgery is higher than after other types of noncardiac surgery. Outcome after vascular surgery is determined essentially by

Table 33-3. THE 10 MOST IMPORTANT PREOPERATIVE PREDICTORS OF POSTOPERATIVE 30-DAY MORTALITY AFTER VASCULAR SURGERY IN VETERAN'S AFFAIRS MEDICAL CENTERS

Predictor	Odds Ratio
Ventilator-dependent	2.71
ASA class	1.89
Emergency operation	2.40
DNR status	2.96
BUN >40 mg · dL^{-1}	1.47
Albumin	0.61
Age	1.03
Creatinine >1.2 mg · dL^{-1}	1.48
Esophageal varices	4.30
Operative complexity score	1.32

DNR = do not resuscitate; BUN = blood urea nitrogen.
All variables are statistically significant ($p < 0.05$) and were selected after stepwise multivariable analysis.
Modified from Khuri SF, Daley J, Henderson W *et al*: Risk adjustment of the postoperative mortality rate for the comparative assessment of the quality of surgical care: Results of the National Veterans Affairs Surgical Risk Study. J Am Coll Surg 185(4):315, 1997.

Table 33-4. DEMOGRAPHICS, HOSPITAL CHARACTERISTICS, PREOPERATIVE CHRONIC MEDICAL CONDITIONS, AND POSTOPERATIVE COMPLICATIONS AND THEIR CONTRIBUTIONS TO MORTALITY PREDICTION[38]

Variable	Prevalence (%)	Odds Ratio (mortality)	p Value
DEMOGRAPHIC			
Higher income		0.93/octile	0.0001
Older age		1.03/year	0.0001
African American	5.0	0.62	0.0001
Hispanic	1.9	0.62	0.0012
Other insurance	1.5	1.35	0.0005
Through emergency room	10.8	1.94	0.0001
Transfer from another hospital	1.6	1.80	0.0001
Emergency admit	13.9	2.44	0.0001
Urgent admission	21.4	1.78	0.0001
HOSPITAL			
Urban	90.6	0.82	0.0339
Investor	12.5	0.75	0.0009
Midwest	21.3	1.34	0.0063
South	40.0	1.27	0.0038
CHRONIC MEDICAL			
Dysrhythmias	13.6	2.84	0.0001
Chronic renal failure	1.3	2.60	0.0001
CHF	7.9	1.89	0.0001
Cerebrovascular disease	12.6	1.38	0.0001
Conduction defects	2.8	1.30	0.0404
Coronary obstructive pulmonary disease	3.1	1.20	NS
Diabetes	21.1	1.01	NS
Coronary disease	30.2	0.82	0.0006
Hypertension	44.5	0.65	0.0001
POSTOPERATIVE COMPLICATIONS			
Respiratory failure	7.9	6.19	0.0001
Acute renal failure	3.5	5.60	0.0001
Myocardial infarction	1.4	5.22	0.0001
Stroke	1.0	3.03	0.0001
Peripheral vascular complications	0.8	3.03	0.0001
Postop cardiac failure	5.1	2.50	0.0001

NS = not significant; CHF = chronic heart failure.
From Ellis JE: Health sciences research and large database analysis in vascular surgery and anesthesia: Confirming common sense? Prob Anesth 11:238, 1999.

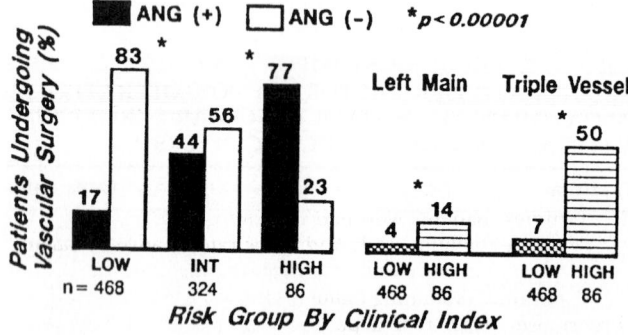

Figure 33-1. Clinical risk factors predict severe (left main or triple vessel) coronary artery disease. A preoperative clinical index (diabetes mellitus, prior myocardial infarction, angina, age >70 years, congestive heart failure) was used to stratify patients. INT = intermediate; ANG(+) = angiogram positive for coronary artery disease; ANG(−) = angiogram negative for coronary artery disease. (Based on data from Paul SD, Eagle KA, Kuntz KM *et al:* Concordance of preoperative clinical risk with angiographic severity of coronary artery disease in patients undergoing vascular surgery. Circulation 94(7):1561, 1966; secondary analysis of data from Hertzer NR, Beven EG, Young JR *et al:* Coronary artery disease in peripheral vascular patients: A classification of 1000 coronary angiograms and results of surgical management. Ann Surg 199:223, 1984.)

patient factors, surgical factors, and institution-specific factors. Cardiac-related death, myocardial infarction (MI), cardiogenic pulmonary edema, unstable angina, and dysrhythmias may occur after vascular surgery. The rates of cardiac-related death range from 0–8% and the infarction rate ranges from 0–15.3%.[42] Complications after carotid endarterectomy are generally less frequent, regardless of the presence or absence of known coronary artery disease; but even after carotid surgery, cardiac causes produce 50–100% of the mortality encountered. Patients undergoing lower extremity revascularization often have more severe medical conditions as a group than patients undergoing abdominal aortic surgery, resulting in equal aggregate risks for cardiac complications in one series.[43]

Long-term morbidity and mortality following vascular surgery are also greatly influenced by the presence of coronary artery disease. The presence of uncorrected coronary artery disease appears to double 5-year mortality after vascular surgery. Coronary artery bypass graft (CABG) is associated with improved survival in peripheral vascular disease patients who have triple-vessel, but not single- or double-vessel coronary artery disease.[44] Previous percutaneous transluminal coronary angioplasty (PTCA) may or may not protect against perioperative cardiac events after vascular surgery.[45–47] The prevalence of asymptomatic coronary artery disease and the substantial short-term and long-term cardiac morbidity and mortality in patients undergoing vascular surgery have led investigators and clinicians to propose and undertake extensive preoperative workups to detect underlying coronary artery disease.

Controversy persists as to whether preoperative identification of patients most likely to have perioperative cardiovascular events related to myocardial ischemia benefits patients. Invasive interventions may benefit patients with vascular disease but are generally more risky than in other groups of patients.[48] Many believe that preparatory coronary revascularization may be "survival tests" that are accompanied by increased short-term morbidity; others believe that these procedures lead to better long-term survival. Patients who have survived coronary revascularization have fewer cardiac complications after vascular surgery.[49]

Three essential purposes are served by preoperative cardiac risk stratification. The first would be to forgo surgery or perform a more conservative surgical procedure in those at high risk. The second goal would be to determine which patients should undergo myocardial revascularization. This goal requires that we identify patients with left main coronary artery disease and those with triple-vessel coronary artery disease and poor left ventricular function, as these patients are most likely to benefit from coronary revascularization in the long run.[44] Finally, because most perioperative myocardial ischemia and infarction occur early in the postoperative period, a third rationale for preoperative segregation of high-risk patients is to target those who might benefit from aggressive therapy in the first 24–72 hr after surgery. Risk-reducing interventions may include invasive monitoring, forced-air warming, stress-reducing anesthetic techniques, perioperative β blockade, or prolonged intensive care unit (ICU) stay. These attempts to reduce morbidity vary widely in cost and their effectiveness is controversial. The choice of risk-reducing strategies depends upon the surgical procedures, the discretion of the anesthesiologists and surgeons, and institutional protocols (clinical pathways).[50]

The patient's history and bedside examination before vascular surgery serve not only to predict coronary anatomy, but also to provide important prognostic information. Studies have consistently identified congestive heart failure, previous myocardial infarction, advanced age, severely limited exercise tolerance, chronic renal insufficiency, and diabetes as risk factors for the development of perioperative cardiac morbidity.[49,51,52] The need for emergency or urgent surgery identifies a group of patients at greatly increased risk for cardiac complications.[53]

Previous work has suggested that risk of reinfarction depends primarily on the amount of time passed since infarction. In the modern era, however, risk stratification with specialized testing (as described below) may identify patients who are at relatively low risk despite a recent infarction. In addition, studies using aggressive hemodynamic monitoring and intensive postoperative care suggest that the rate of reinfarction after a recent infarction is currently much lower in some centers.[54]

Exercise tolerance may also be a useful prognostic indicator, although claudication, orthopedic problems, and frailty may limit a patient's capabilities. Patients with limited exercise capacity have greatly increased perioperative risk.[51] We believe that if patients can walk briskly for two blocks with neither angina nor dyspnea, and have no other indicators of coronary artery disease, they are very unlikely to have left main disease, triple-vessel disease, or severe left ventricular dysfunction. Such patients can probably undergo surgery without specialized noninvasive testing because they are unlikely to be at risk for adverse perioperative outcomes. However, one prospective study with consecutive patient selection of all types of vascular surgery found that clinical parameters and clinical scoring systems failed to reliably and consistently predict adverse cardiac outcomes.[55] Therefore, many investigators have proposed that specialized preoperative tests, such as stress echocardiography or thallium scintigraphy, are more accurate than clinical indicators for predicting perioperative cardiac complications.

Many patients undergo noninvasive testing to evaluate cardiovascular risk before vascular surgery. Routine coronary angiography is impractical to use routinely before vascular surgery because of the costs and risks involved.[56] The use of screening tests has remained controversial, with most recent studies showing great prognostic value[57–61] (Table 33-5), but others showing that these tests do not perform better than the basic clinical evaluation.[62] Given such abundant data and controversies, how can one summarize recommendations for preoperative risk stratification in a patient presenting for vascular surgery? In 1996, the American Heart Association and American College of Cardiology (AHA/ACC) published guidelines for perioperative cardiovascular evaluation before noncardiac surgery.[63] The algorithm incorporates clinical history, exercise tolerance, and surgical procedure in the decision to perform further evaluation. Table 33-6 summarizes some of those guidelines suited for vascular surgery patients. Semiquantitative interpretation (high-risk, intermediate-risk, or low-risk results) of both dipyridamole-thallium scintigraphy and dobutamine stress echocardiography may allow us to refer only high-risk patients for cardiac catheterization. Less severe cases of coronary artery disease (CAD) identified by weakly positive (low-risk) results on these tests may benefit from current state-of-the-art perioperative care and risk reduction. However, these less severe cases will still require careful follow-up after surgery to look for progression of coronary artery disease. Bartels et al[64] followed the AHA/ACC guidelines in 203 patients scheduled for aortic surgery and evaluated the short-term benefits. Cardiac-related mortality was 1% and cardiac morbidity was 12.4%. The authors concluded that the protocol was a safe strategy for preoperative evaluation before vascular surgery.

Dipyridamole-thallium scintigraphy is based on the principle of coronary steal. Dipyridamole is an antiplatelet drug and a coronary artery vasodilator. At rest, coronary arteries supplying the normal myocardium have a great vasodilatory reserve and are able to increase blood flow up to 10 times the normal to meet any extra demand. In the areas of critical stenosis, however, the coronary arteries are vasodilated in nonstressed state and have diminished reserve. Therefore, dipyridamole can vasodilate normal coronary arteries but cannot vasodilate those in areas with stenosis. When thallium radioisotope is injected, stenotic areas of myocardium will have lower concentration of the isotope (cold spot) after dipyridamole administration. When the effect of dipyridamole wears off, the isotope redistributes to ischemic zones. These areas with redistribution are considered ischemic but viable zones whereas those with persistent defects with no redistribution are indicative of infarction. Both redistribution (reversible) and persistent (fixed) defects may be abnormal test results. The early experience with dipyridamole-thallium scintigraphy yielded two important observations: an old myocardial infarction ("fixed" defect) is not a risk factor in itself, and an area of redistribution (i.e., myocardium at risk) is associated with an adverse outcome. Dipyridamole-thallium scintigraphy was most helpful in the risk stratification of patients whose risks were intermediate based on clinical evaluation. In these studies, patients who had low clinical risk or a negative dipyridamole-thallium study had a low rate of adverse cardiac events after vascular surgery.[65] When we analyzed the studies in the literature evaluating thallium scintigraphy before vascular surgery, we found that a positive scan increased a patient's chances of having a postoperative cardiac event by a factor of 4.6.[66]

Congestive heart failure is a strong predictor of morbid postoperative events. Determination of systolic left ventricular function may therefore provide prognostic information. Radionuclide ventriculography can be used to define systolic and diastolic function. Our meta-analysis showed that patients who have an ejection fraction <35% by radionuclide ventriculography are 3.7 times more likely to have a postoperative cardiac event.[66] However, radionuclide ventriculography has generally been supplanted by echocardiography, which can define myocardial structure as well as function, and can also be combined

Table 33-5. NONINVASIVE TESTS TO PREDICT CARDIAC DEATH AND MYOCARDIAL INFARCTION AFTER VASCULAR SURGERY (PUBLISHED AFTER 1994)

Author (year) Reference	Test	Pts (n)	Quality of Study*	Cardiac— Death or MI (%)	Positivity Criterion	Relative Risk	Odds Ratio	Likelihood Ratio Pos	Likelihood Ratio Neg
Marshall (1995)[57]	Adenosine thallium scanning	117	Weak	10.2	>1 reversible defect at least in one segment	3.15	3.67	2.11	0.58
Poldermans (1995)[58]	DSE	300	Fair	5.7	New RWMA at least in one segment	109.8†	144.1†	5.15	0
Vanzetto (1996)[59]	SPECT-DTS	134	Strong	9	>1 reversible defect at least in one segment	19.7	25.3	3.02	0.12
Landesberg (1997)[60]	Preoperative 12-lead EKG	405	Fair	4.7	LVH by voltage criteria or ST-segment depression	7.6	8.4	2.56	0.30

DSE = dobutamine stress echocardiography, RWMA = regional wall motion abnormalities, SPECT-DTS = single-photon emission computed tomographic dipyridamole-thallium scintigraphy
* As defined by American College of Physicians for studies related to preoperative evaluation of cardiac risk for noncardiac surgery.[61]
† Computed after adding 0.5 to all the cells because of zero event in those with negative test result. Without such correction, the relative risk and odds ratio will be infinite.

with exercise or pharmacologic stress. Dobutamine (5–30 μg · kg^{-1} · min^{-1}) stress echocardiography can produce changes in regional wall motion in patients with underlying coronary artery disease. In our meta-analysis, we found that a positive dobutamine stress test increased the risk of a postoperative cardiac event by 6.2-fold.[66]

In the past, some clinicians would place a pulmonary artery catheter preoperatively to measure hemodynamics and perform risk stratification. This approach is rarely used today because catheter placement requires preoperative admission to an ICU, and most patients are now admitted on the day of surgery. Additionally, echocardiography can provide noninvasive preoperative evaluation of cardiac function. Pulmonary artery catheterization may still occasionally prove useful for preoperative optimization of unstable patients who require relatively urgent surgery.

Raby et al found that of the 18% of patients who had ischemia detected by Holter ECG monitoring before vascular surgery, approximately one-third had cardiac complications, while only 1% of patients without ischemia had complications.[67] Our meta-analysis for Holter monitoring of preoperative ischemia suggests that an ischemic Holter recording before surgery increases the risk of a postoperative cardiac event by 2.7-fold.[66] The biggest limitation of ambulatory ECG for preoperative risk stratification is the high percentage (at least one-fourth in our practice) of patients with baseline ECG abnormalities that obscure the diagnosis of new myocardial ischemia. These abnormalities include left ventricular hypertrophy with "strain," bundle branch block, pacemakers, and the effects of digoxin. Also, nonspecific ST-segment changes may occur owing to changes in body temperature, serum electrolytes, ventilation, or body position.

One limitation of specialized testing, including coronary angiography, is the fact that myocardial infarction and cardiac-related mortality need not necessarily be due to severely nar-

Table 33-6. CARDIAC RISK STRATIFICATION AND INTERVENTIONS IN PATIENTS SCHEDULED FOR ELECTIVE VASCULAR SURGERY

Presentation	Interventions	Strength of Recommendation
Any one of major clinical predictors (unstable angina, recent MI,† decompensated CHF, significant arrhythmias)	Coronary angiography (CATH)	Class I*
One or two of intermediate clinical predictors (mild angina pectoris, prior MI, compensated CHF or prior CHF, diabetes mellitus)	Noninvasive test by DTS or DSE	Class I
Strongly positive (high-risk results) on DTS or DSE results	CATH	Class I *
Intermediate-risk results on DTS or DSE results	CATH	Class II *
High-risk anatomic subgroups ("critical" CAD or left main disease, EF < 35%)	Coronary artery bypass grafting (CABG)	Class I*
Documented CAD by clinical or noninvasive testing, CATH, and proceeding for surgery without CABG	Perioperative risk reducing strategies (perioperative atenolol therapy or additional thermal care or both)	Class I

* Recommendations based on American Heart Association / American College of Cardiology guidelines for perioperative cardiovascular evaluation for noncardiac surgery.[63]
† Recent MI = recent myocardial infarction (>7 days but ≤1 month).
Class I: Conditions for which there is evidence and or general agreement that a procedure be performed or a treatment is of benefit; Class II: conditions for which there is a divergence of evidence and/or opinion about the treatment; Class III: conditions for which there is evidence and/or general agreement that the procedure/treatment is not necessary.
CHF = congestive heart failure; DSE = dobutamine stress echocardiography; DTS = dipyridamole-thallium scintigraphy; CAD = coronary artery disease; EF = ejection fraction.

rowed coronary arteries. Recent evidence suggests that the rupture of previously nonocclusive lipid-laden, macrophage-rich coronary plaques can cause spasm and initiate unstable angina, acute myocardial infarction, and sudden death.[68] Therefore, testing that attempts to induce ischemia will miss some patients who have nonobstructive plaques that can rupture and cause transmural infarction.

Clinicians who read the often-conflicting studies in the literature may be perplexed about choosing the best test or pathway for their patients. According to Bayes' theorem, as the prior probability of a disease in a population increases, the predictive value of a positive test increases and predictive value of a negative test decreases. (These concepts are reviewed in more detail in Chapter 18.) The ideal clinical trial to help resolve these controversies would be prospective, collect data over a relatively short period of time, select patients consecutively, and would blind clinicians caring for the patients to the test results. Ethical concerns about not making test results available to clinicians have precluded large-scale randomized trials.

Meta-analysis combines evidence from multiple studies to evaluate the effectiveness of therapies or other interventions. Our meta-analysis of preoperative cardiac testing strategies allows the following conclusions.[66] Tests often demonstrate a bias for better predictive value in earlier studies. This may be due to pretest referral bias in early studies where patients were not recruited consecutively (sicker patients were chosen for earlier studies). Improvement in perioperative care over time may also explain the phenomenon of decreasing predictive value. All four tests (dipyridamole-thallium scanning, radionuclide ventriculography, Holter monitoring, and dobutamine stress echocardiography) are "effective" (the 95% confidence intervals for relative risk are >1.0) in predicting cardiac death or myocardial infarction following vascular surgery. We believe that dobutamine stress echocardiography appears to be the best among these four tests and Holter monitoring the least effective. This conclusion is subject to revision because the 95% confidence intervals for relative risk overlap.

Decision analysis is an explicit analytic tool designed to facilitate complex clinical decisions in which many variables must be considered simultaneously. The optimal decision, which is the course of action with the highest overall expected survival rate and lowest cost, is then calculated. Fleisher et al[69] used decision analysis to examine the effect of preoperative screening with dipyridamole-thallium scans before abdominal aortic surgery on 30-day cardiac-related mortality. The authors suggested that in patients with low prior probability of coronary artery disease, vascular surgery should be performed without cardiac screening. Their analysis demonstrates the importance of local institutional factors (particularly the institution's mortality rates for myocardial revascularization versus those for vascular surgery) in determining the optimal preoperative strategy. The outcomes of different testing strategies must be compared with their costs. Bry et al[70] calculated that dipyridamole-thallium scanning for screening before aortic and infrainguinal surgical procedures cost $392,253 per life saved and $181,039 per MI averted. They suggested that these figures may not be justifiable to society given the current trends of health care reform.

Preoperative Coronary Revascularization

Myocardial revascularization may have long-term benefits in patients with triple-vessel coronary disease or poor left ventricular function.[44] The range of options for preparatory coronary revascularization continues to expand rapidly. These include traditional surgical revascularization (CABG), transmyocardial laser therapy, percutaneous transluminal coronary angioplasty (PTCA), coronary stent placement, excimer laser, rotoblader, and endoscopic CABG. However, mortality rates associated with CABG are 2.4-fold higher in patients with peripheral vascular disease (7.7% versus 3.2%) compared with those without.[71] Higher complication rates can be anticipated for the newer

revascularization techniques when performed in patients with peripheral vascular disease.[48]

Initial observational studies of PTCA performed before major noncardiac surgery suggest that patients who survive successful PTCA do well.[47] Anticoagulation may be continued after these procedures and may preclude the use of regional anesthesia. Advances in the medical management of atherosclerosis include the use of statin drugs, which restore endothelial function, reduce ambulatory myocardial ischemia, may cause plaque regression, and may be equivalent or superior to PTCA in patients with stable angina.

Once the patient has recovered from successful coronary revascularization (1 week after angioplasty and 6–8 weeks after CABG, typically), peripheral vascular surgery is usually then performed. In some cases, CABG can be combined with vascular surgery, most commonly with carotid endarterectomy. However, patients with both symptomatic coronary and carotid disease are at high risk of both cardiac and neurologic complications following surgery, whether combined or staged; their management remains controversial.[72] Elective abdominal aortic aneurysm repair should probably be performed before, simultaneously, or within 2 weeks of CABG because of increased risk of aneurysm rupture seen after this period.[73]

Perioperative Cardiac Monitoring

The goals of perioperative cardiac monitoring are to detect myocardial ischemia and to identify abnormalities of preload, afterload, and ventricular function. Such monitoring may prevent myocardial infarction and allow better perfusion and preservation of other organs such as the liver, kidney, gut, and spinal cord.

Detection of Perioperative Myocardial Ischemia

ECG monitoring remains the mainstay of perioperative detection of myocardial ischemia. ECG evidence of ST-segment depression is a more common indicator of myocardial ischemia in vascular surgery patients than is ST-segment elevation. ST-segment depression occurs in 20–50% of patients undergoing vascular surgery. London et al[74] showed that in patients with risk factors for significant coronary artery disease, the greatest sensitivity for the detection of myocardial ischemia was achieved by intraoperative use of either lead V_5 (sensitivity 75%) or lead V_4 (sensitivity 61%). Simultaneous viewing of leads V_4 and V_5 had a sensitivity of 90% compared with a sensitivity of 80% for the combination of leads II and V_5. Because clinicians often fail to detect intraoperative ischemic ECG changes when viewing oscilloscopes, automated ST-segment monitors promise to increase the detection of such ECG changes. We have documented that the sensitivity of ST-segment monitors for transesophageal echocardiography (TEE)–diagnosed myocardial ischemia is 40%, and 75% for ECG-diagnosed ischemia.[75] Although these monitors are not always accurate, we believe they are useful as alarms for busy clinicians.

Perioperative Holter monitoring has shown that the intraoperative period may be the least stressful for patients with coronary artery disease. Patients undergoing vascular surgery are most likely to manifest myocardial ischemia in the immediate postoperative period, with its associated pain, adrenergic stress, hypothermia, hypercoagulability, anemia, shivering, and sleep deprivation. Several studies have shown that postoperative myocardial ischemia begins earlier than has previously been thought, usually on the day of vascular surgery or the next day (Table 33-7).[76–80] At present, our clinical practice is to obtain a 12-lead ECG once or twice in the first 24 hours following surgery in high-risk patients, and then daily for the next 2–3 days. We believe that such a strategy will detect most ischemia that is severe and protracted enough to represent a prodrome to infarction. Unfortunately, approximately one-fourth of vascular surgery patients will have baseline ECG abnormalities (left bun-

Table 33-7. INCIDENCE AND PROGNOSIS OF POSTOPERATIVE MYOCARDIAL ISCHEMIA DETECTED BY CONTINUOUS ECG MONITORING

Study (year)	No. of Patients	Patient Group	Incidence of Postoperative Myocardial Ischemia	Incidence of Complications
Mangano[76] (1990)	474	Veterans; noncardiac surgery; known or suspected coronary artery disease	194/474 = 41%	15/194 = 8% 2 deaths 8 infarctions 1 unstable angina
Ouyang[77] (1989)	24	Vascular surgery; known coronary artery disease	15/24 = 62%	7/15 = 47% 2 infarctions 5 unstable angina
McCann[78] (1989)	50	Lower extremity vascular surgery	19/50 = 38% (overall periop ischemia)	4/19 = 21% 2 deaths 2 infarctions
Pasternack[79] (1989)	200	Vascular surgery	57/200 = 28%	11/57 = 19% 2 deaths 9 infarctions
Landesberg[80] (1993)	151	Vascular surgery	88/151 = 58% (overall perioperatve ischemia)	8/88 = 9% 6 infarctions 2 unstable angina

dle branch block, paced rhythm, digoxin effect, left ventricular hypertrophy with strain) that preclude the detection of myocardial ischemia.

Other monitoring devices for detecting myocardial ischemia have been proposed. Pulmonary capillary wedge pressure (PCWP) monitoring in patients undergoing vascular surgery has low sensitivity and specificity (~40%) in detecting ischemia; most elevations in PCWP appear to be associated with tachycardia and hypertension, which suggests inadequate anesthesia.[81,82] Our own group found that 90% of patients developed wall motion abnormalities on TEE when the aorta was cross-clamped above the celiac artery. However, the PCWP remained normal in >80% of these episodes.[83] We therefore do not routinely use PCWP as a monitor for myocardial ischemia but believe the pulmonary artery catheter provides useful information about a patient's intravascular volume status, myocardial performance, and organ perfusion.

TEE has also been proposed as a monitor for intraoperative myocardial ischemia. In animal studies and in models of coronary angioplasty during balloon inflation, mechanical dysfunction precedes surface ECG changes when myocardial ischemia is produced. Supporting these observations, Smith et al[84] found that regional wall motion abnormalities were more sensitive than ST-segment change on the ECG in detecting intraoperative ischemia in patients with coronary artery disease undergoing major vascular and coronary surgery. However, Eisenberg et al concluded that ischemia monitoring with TEE during noncardiac surgery appeared to have little incremental clinical value over preoperative clinical data and Holter monitoring in predicting perioperative ischemic outcomes.[85]

Traditionally, creatine kinase myocardial band (CK-MB) isoenzyme determination has been used to document myocardial damage after vascular surgery. Limitations of this method include false-positive results owing to skeletal muscle damage during surgery. The cardiac troponins appear to offer increased sensitivity, primarily because of their prolonged diagnostic window, and may offer enhanced specificity in patients with surgical skeletal muscle damage. In a recent study of 96 vascular surgery patients, all eight patients who received a diagnosis of perioperative infarction (based on new echocardiographic abnormalities in segmental wall motion) had elevations of cardiac troponin I. This study showed that most postoperative myocardial infarctions (PMI) occurred and could be detected on the first postoperative day.[86] Badner et al confirmed these findings; 18 of 323 patients with known CAD undergoing major surgery (5.6%) had a PMI, of which 3 (17%) were fatal. Only 3 of 18 patients

had chest pain, whereas 10 of 18 patients (56%) had other clinical findings. The PMIs occurred on the day of operation in nearly half of the cases.[87]

Management of Perioperative Myocardial Ischemia and Infarction in Vascular Patients

In the modern era, rates of myocardial infarction in patients undergoing major vascular surgery can be reduced to <10%, but the rates are significantly lower for patients undergoing elective vascular repair. PMIs are much more likely to occur in patients undergoing urgent or emergent surgery, who presumably are sicker and do not have the luxury of undergoing extensive preoperative evaluation and preparation.[53]

Stable coronary ischemic syndromes presumably occur with increased oxygen demand by the myocardium in a setting of fixed coronary plaques. Unstable syndromes are thought to be the result of active lesions caused by plaque rupture with local thrombus and vasoreactivity that produce intermittent critical decreases in coronary oxygen supply.[68] The period following vascular surgery is characterized by adrenergic stress (Fig. 33-2).[88] The postoperative adrenergic response can predispose

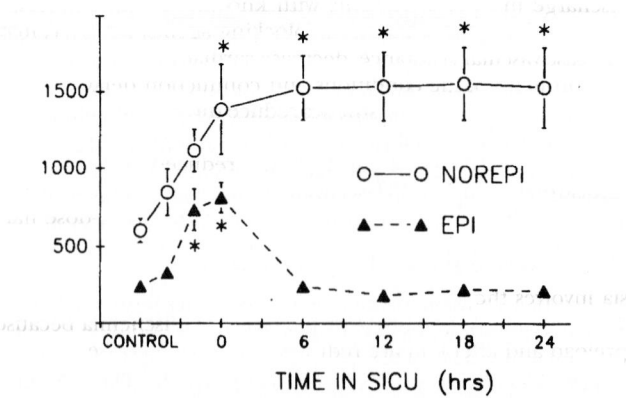

Figure 33-2. Aortic reconstructive surgery is associated with markedly elevated adrenergic tone. Epinephrine levels (pg · mL⁻¹) rise with emergence from anesthesia but begin to fall by 6 hr after surgery. Norepinephrine levels (pg · mL⁻¹) remain elevated for at least a day following surgery. (Reprinted with permission from Breslow MJ: The role of stress hormones in perioperative myocardial ischemia. Int Anesthesiol Clin 30:81, 1992.)

to myocardial ischemia in numerous ways, including tachycardia and decreased diastolic time, coronary vasoconstriction, and platelet aggregation. Factors increasing the likelihood of postoperative myocardial ischemia that the anesthesiologist can control include tachycardia, hypertension, hypotension, anemia, hypothermia, shivering, endotracheal suctioning, and less than optimal analgesia. Other factors, such as postoperative hypercoagulability, rapid eye movement (REM) sleep rebound, and mild postoperative hypoxemia are more speculative culprits.

Postoperative myocardial ischemia confers increased risk to vascular surgical patients (see Table 33-7). Landesberg et al found that patients experienced twice as much ischemia after vascular surgery than before or during.[80] Ischemia that lasted >2 hr was associated with a 32-fold increase in the risk of postoperative morbid cardiac events. In this study, postoperative MI was usually preceded by long periods of severe ST-segment depression. Aggressive efforts at prevention or treatment of ischemia during these periods may improve patient outcome. We refer patients with documented severe postoperative myocardial ischemia (>2 hr; 2 mm ST-segment depression) to a cardiologist because 70% of all adverse cardiac outcomes in a two-year follow-up program were preceded by in-hospital postoperative ischemia.[89]

Various strategies have been proposed to reduce cardiac morbidity during and after vascular surgery, including the prophylactic use of antianginal drugs, and special anesthetic techniques. It is crucial that patients continue to receive their chronic antianginal and antihypertensive medications before and after surgery. Often, the parenteral route for administration of these medications may be necessary following surgery. Recent reports suggest that chronic administration of the calcium entry blocker nifedipine may increase mortality[90]; we are less likely to use nifedipine as first-line therapy. Prophylactic intravenous (iv) nitroglycerin $0.9\ \mu g \cdot kg^{-1} \cdot min^{-1}$ failed to reduce the incidence of perioperative myocardial ischemia (30% in control group versus 32% in nitroglycerin group) in patients with known or suspected coronary artery disease undergoing noncardiac surgery.[91] In this study, the preponderance of myocardial ischemia occurred during emergence from anesthesia, which is associated with acute increases in heart rate.

β-Adrenergic blocking drugs, through their ability to suppress perioperative tachycardia, appear more efficacious than other anti-ischemic drugs in preventing myocardial ischemia and perhaps infarction after vascular surgery. New studies suggest that β-adrenergic blocking drugs suppress ischemia (esmolol)[92] and reduce cardiac events (bisoprolol)[93] after vascular surgery. Mangano et al have suggested that perioperative β blockade (atenolol)[94] reduced mortality at 6 and 24 months after hospital discharge in surgical patients with known or suspected CAD. Side-effects of the β-adrenergic blocking agents, however, may increase vascular resistance, decrease cardiac output, and aggravate bronchospastic conditions and conduction delays.

High-dose narcotic anesthetics reduce the stress response and may improve overall outcome after major surgery. Postoperative infusion of sufentanil $1\ \mu g \cdot kg^{-1} \cdot h^{-1}$ reduced the severity of myocardial ischemia (ST-segment changes) following CABG, although clinical outcome was not improved.[95] High-dose narcotics may mandate overnight ventilation, which may not be a cost-effective therapy. Another approach using intensive analgesia involves the use of epidural analgesia. Epidural local anesthetics may reduce perioperative myocardial ischemia because preload and afterload are reduced, the postoperative adrenergic and coagulation responses are reduced, and, with thoracic administration, the coronary arteries are dilated. Despite these effects on intermediate variables, improvement in cardiac outcomes has generally not been demonstrated.[96] Concerns about respiratory depression, neuroaxis hematomas, and the expense and reimbursement for surveillance have limited the use of peridural narcotics in greater numbers of patients. Although epidural anesthesia may improve outcome in other organ sys-

tems, especially the lungs, its ability to reduce myocardial infarction remains speculative.

Given the prominent role of coronary thrombosis in causing acute coronary syndromes and the hypercoagulable state after vascular surgery, future development in the treatment of postoperative myocardial ischemia may include drugs with antiplatelet or anticoagulant effects, such as aspirin and newer platelet inhibitors, warfarin, or heparin. Increased postoperative hemorrhage, however, makes the use of anticoagulant therapy problematic in surgical patients. At present, we do not know how to balance these risks and benefits, or which patients might benefit most from such therapy.

α_2-Adrenergic agonists decrease noradrenergic central nervous system transmission and produce sedation, anxiolysis, and analgesia. Clonidine premedication reduces hypertension, tachycardia, norepinephrine levels, and the incidence of intraoperative myocardial ischemia in patients undergoing vascular reconstruction.[97] However, prophylactic use of the α_2-adrenergic agonist dexmedetomidine in vascular surgery patients may require greater intraoperative pharmacologic intervention to support blood pressure and heart rate.[98] Another α_2-adrenergic agonist, mivazerol, has recently been shown to reduce perioperative cardiac event and cardiac death rates in patients with known coronary heart disease undergoing vascular surgery.[99]

Anemia (hematocrit <28%) may increase the incidence of postoperative myocardial ischemia and cardiac events in high-risk patients undergoing noncardiac surgery.[100,101] Therefore, we are more likely to transfuse high-risk patients or those who demonstrate myocardial ischemia with packed red blood cells to augment the hematocrit to 30%. Hypothermia is also associated with increased adrenergic tone and postoperative myocardial ischemia and events in vascular surgery patients.[102] We therefore aggressively warm patients and conserve heat during and after such surgery. Suctioning, extubation, and weaning from mechanical ventilation may also produce myocardial ischemia. Therefore, we attempt to extubate patients in the operating room with the same attention to the control of hemodynamics as during induction. If patients require postoperative ventilation, we provide adequate sedation, analgesia, and occasionally even paralysis (which can prevent shivering and its attendant increases in oxygen consumption). We treat tachycardia aggressively, often with β-adrenergic blocking agents, after we have corrected other potential causes such as fever, pain, anemia, and hypovolemia.

Occasionally, in patients with evolving myocardial infarction, we have resorted to using an intra-aortic balloon pump (IABP) to improve coronary blood flow while decreasing workload. Definitive studies of its effectiveness are lacking, and IABP placement can be difficult and risky in patients with peripheral vascular disease.[103] We have also referred some patients to interventional cardiologists immediately after surgery for emergent cardiac catheterization, selective thrombolysis, and PTCA for unstable angina or evolving postoperative myocardial infarction.[104]

Other Medical Problems in Vascular Surgery Patients

Hypertension occurs in the majority of vascular surgery patients and may produce end-organ damage to the heart and kidneys. The hypertrophied left ventricle is at risk for subendocardial ischemia, even in the absence of obstructive coronary artery disease. Hypertrophied hearts may be more prone to diastolic dysfunction, which can result in "flash" pulmonary edema in the postoperative period. Therefore, antihypertensive medication should be continued in the vast majority of cases through the morning of surgery. β-Adrenergic blocking drugs are well tolerated in patients with claudication, despite theoretical concerns about peripheral vasoconstriction and bronchospasm. Calcium channel antagonists are also frequently used, as are

ACE inhibitors. The ACE inhibitors may contribute to prerenal azotemia in patients with renal artery stenosis, while diuretics may produce hypokalemia. ACE inhibitors reduce central sympathetic tone and heart rate[105]; they may be associated with an increased incidence of hypotension following induction of anesthesia if normal doses of induction agents are used.[106]

One benefit of the modern system of same-day admission is that it allows us to interview many patients in a preanesthesia clinic a week or so before surgery. At that time, if hypertension is poorly controlled, we consult with the patient's internist or cardiologist and adjust or begin the antihypertensive regimen. Lowering blood pressure gradually in this way before surgery allows for restoration of normal intravascular volume and results in a more stable perioperative course.

Diabetic patients have a greatly increased risk for peripheral vascular disease. Aggressive treatment (home glucose monitoring program) to maintain euglycemia has recently been shown to promote wound healing and to forestall retinopathy and the development of proteinuria, but its effects on the progression of large vessel peripheral vascular disease and coronary artery disease are unknown. Coronary disease is ubiquitous in diabetic patients requiring vascular surgery. Diabetic patients generally have higher risks of myocardial infarction (5.2% versus 2.1%) and wound infection (2.6% versus 0.6%) compared with nondiabetics undergoing abdominal aortic aneurysm.[107] The dramatic increase in the risk of postoperative death (7%) in diabetic patients with autonomic neuropathy suggests that simple tests to identify such patients might be part of the preoperative workup.[108] Patients with diabetes and severe coronary artery disease may live longer if they undergo CABG rather than PTCA. We typically give our diabetic patients one-third to one-half of their usual insulin dose on the morning of surgery, begin an iv infusion of glucose-containing fluid, and check a "fingerstick" glucometer reading before commencing with an anesthetic. We attempt to maintain intraoperative euglycemia by frequently monitoring and guiding plasma glucose levels. We are especially fastidious about glucose management during carotid and thoracic aortic procedures, where hyperglycemia may exacerbate neurologic injury.

Patients with peripheral vascular disease may have hypercoagulable states.[109] Hypercoagulable states are more common in younger patients presenting for vascular surgery and in those with vascular thrombosis in unusual locations. Hypercoagulable responses to surgery may also predispose patients to vascular graft occlusion after surgery. Postoperative abnormalities include elevated fibrinogen levels, antithrombin III deficiency, impaired fibrinolysis, protein C deficiency, and protein S deficiency. Heparin-induced thrombosis (HIT) can occur paradoxically on an immunologic basis (IgG) after several days of exposure to heparin. This problem, which can be fatal, appears to be increasing in incidence, particularly in patients who have had previous vascular or cardiac surgery and heparin exposure. Patients typically present with thrombocytopenia, a normal prothrombin time, and normal fibrinogen levels. Mortality and complications resulting from HIT are reported to be about 20–30% each. Discontinuation of heparin (including in the flush solution of invasive monitors) is a simple and essential maneuver, and anticoagulation has to be continued by alternative drugs. Low–molecular-weight heparins are associated with a reduced, but still significant incidence of HIT. The heparinoid danaparoid-sodium and the thrombin inhibitor recombinant hirudin have been used successfully for anticoagulation of patients with HIT.[34] However, these have longer half-lives than heparin, have prolonged kinetics in renal failure, and cannot be reversed with protamine.

Patients with peripheral vascular disease have frequently abused tobacco. Preoperative spirometry may help identify patients likely to have postoperative pulmonary complications.[110] In one study of vascular surgery patients, the incidence of postoperative pulmonary complications (pneumonia, ventilator dependence >48 hr, or the adult respiratory distress syndrome) was 12.9%. Patients with forced expiratory volume in 1 s (FEV_1) <2.0 $L \cdot s^{-1}$ had a much higher incidence of pulmonary complications (22.5% versus 5.8% for FEV_1 2.0 $L \cdot s^{-1}$). Not surprisingly, respiratory failure was much more common in patients undergoing repair of aortic aneurysm (~30%) than surgery for lower extremity occlusive disease (8%) or for carotid procedures (5%).[111]

Renal insufficiency or failure exists in many patients who present for arterial reconstruction. Patients with pre-existing renal insufficiency have an increased risk of postoperative renal failure, as well as cardiac complications and death. Postoperative renal failure markedly increases the chance of death.[39] If patients receive chronic dialysis treatments, we prefer that they receive dialysis on the day before or the same day as surgery. Some patients will actually be hypovolemic as a result, which can contribute to hypotension upon induction of general or regional anesthesia. Many dialysis patients receive recombinant erythropoietin, which normally increases the hematocrit to ~30%. Left ventricular hypertrophy and mitral annular calcification are more common in dialysis patients and may predispose to pulmonary edema in the perioperative period; electrocardiography and echocardiography may help the clinician to make these diagnoses. In addition, we usually seek laboratory and electrocardiographic evidence of hyperkalemia and avoid succinylcholine when possible if we suspect hyperkalemia. We are careful when positioning patients to avoid putting pressure on the arm used for hemodialysis; we also do not measure blood pressure in that arm. Vascular access may be difficult in patients who have had multiple arteriovenous fistulae placed for hemodialysis. We also anticipate a more difficult abdominal dissection in some patients who have received peritoneal dialysis.

CAROTID ENDARTERECTOMY

The most common cause of carotid artery occlusive disease is atherosclerosis. Carotid disease is bilateral in about half of all cases. Atherosclerotic plaque usually develops at the lateral aspect of the carotid artery bifurcation (where shear stress is lowest) and commonly extends into the internal and external carotid arteries. The embolization of thrombotic material or debris from the plaque can result in stroke or transient neurologic symptoms. Risk factors for carotid disease include advanced age, hypertension, and tobacco abuse. Elevated serum lipid levels and a history of diabetes mellitus are less powerful predictors. Patients with left main coronary artery disease and other peripheral vascular disease are more likely to have carotid disease as well.[112]

Carotid disease may manifest itself only as an asymptomatic bruit, or as amaurosis fugax (transient attacks of monocular blindness) when embolization is to the ophthalmic artery. Other patients may experience episodes of paresthesias, clumsiness of the extremities, or speech problems, which resolve spontaneously after a short period of time. These are the classic transient ischemic attacks (TIAs). The differentiation between a TIA and a reversible ischemic neurologic deficit (RIND) is one of degree and somewhat arbitrary. A TIA resolves within 24 hr, whereas a RIND will last longer than 24 hr before complete resolution. Unfortunately, in some patients the first manifestation of carotid artery disease may be a stroke. One of two pathophysiologic mechanisms is thought to be responsible for the development of neurologic symptoms: embolism or hypoperfusion. A high-grade (preocclusive) obstruction of the carotid lumen may reduce distal blood flow below a critical level, especially when systemic blood pressure is low.

Patients who present with TIAs have a ~10% risk of stroke during the subsequent year. Of the patients who do have a stroke after the onset of TIAs, ~20% will have the stroke within the first month and ~50% within 1 year of symptoms. In subsequent years the stroke risk decreases to ~5% per year. In asymptomatic patients with a stenosis of >75%, the stroke risk is ~5% per year; but if the asymptomatic stenosis is <75%, the risk is 1–2% per year.[113] Patients with ulcerated soft plaques seem to have a higher risk of stroke that approaches 7–8% per year. The serious nature of cerebrovascular disease is underscored by the fact that about one-third of all acute strokes are fatal and another third result in significant residual functional deficit.

An isolated, cervical bruit in asymptomatic patients also seems to be associated with a higher risk of stroke, but the correlation between the location of the bruits and the type of subsequent stroke is poor. A bruit *per se* does not define the presence of a critical carotid lesion, nor are critical carotid lesions always associated with bruits. Therefore, we use the results of auscultation of a bruit to prompt further testing. The most common noninvasive test is the duplex scan, which combines B-mode anatomic imaging and pulse Doppler spectral analysis of blood flow velocity. The presence of high velocities and turbulent flow is used to predict the extent of carotid stenosis. The accuracy of duplex scanning reaches 95% in experienced hands when compared with angiography. Angiography provides measurements of the size and morphology of the atheromatous plaque and can also document aortic arch or intracranial disease, which may occur in conjunction with carotid disease and can cause strokes that are not prevented by carotid endarterectomy. Increasingly, given the risk and expense of angiography (1% rate of neurologic deficits in some studies), some surgeons will operate on the basis of duplex scanning or magnetic resonance angiography without a contrast angiogram.

There are pharmacologic and surgical treatments for carotid artery disease. Combined administration of aspirin and dipyridamole, when compared with placebo, reduces the incidence of TIAs. Therefore, most patients presenting for carotid endarterectomy will be taking aspirin; we confirm this when taking a history and continue aspirin throughout and beyond the perioperative period, unless there are clear contraindications to its use, in order to decrease morbid cardiovascular events.[114] In contrast, carotid endarterectomy, in conjunction with aspirin therapy, has proven superior to medical therapy alone in a large trial of symptomatic patients with a stenosis >70% in the North American trial (NASCET).[115] In this trial, major or fatal ipsilateral stroke was significantly reduced from 13.1% in the medical group to 2.5% in the surgical group. Estimates of the cumulative risk of any ipsilateral stroke at two years were 26% in the medical patients and 9% in the surgical patients. For asymptomatic patients with a stenosis of >60%, the Asymptomatic Carotid Atherosclerosis (ACAS) study also detected a substantial outcome benefit. However, the overall risk of stroke was lower in both medical and surgical groups than for symptomatic patients in NACSET. In ACAS, ipsilateral stroke and any perioperative stroke or death was estimated to be 11.0% for patients treated medically and 5.1% for surgical patients after 5 years.[116] Of course, carotid endarterectomy is justifiable only if the operative morbidity and mortality are lower than the natural risk for ischemic events in the untreated patient. The number of asymptomatic patients who need to undergo CEA to prevent 1 stroke is approximately 20–40, leading some investigators to question its cost-effectiveness in this setting. For a thorough review of this area, the reader is referred to the guidelines published for carotid endarterectomy by the American Heart Association.[117] Less invasive techniques using balloon dilatation and stenting of carotid stenoses are being used;[118] randomized trials have begun to compare the outcomes of these procedures to traditional CEA.

Factors that consistently predict neurologic and cardiac morbidity and mortality after carotid endarterectomy include the following: age ≥75 years, experience of the surgeon, preoperative neurologic symptoms or previous stroke, history of angina, diastolic blood pressure >110 mm Hg, carotid endarterectomy performed in preparation for CABG, internal carotid artery thrombus, stenosis near the carotid siphon, or contralateral

carotid occlusion. Patients undergoing CEA for lesions of the left carotid artery may suffer stroke more often, possibly due to technical difficulties, because most surgeons are right-handed.

Preoperative Evaluation and Preparation

Although the most common cause of TIAs is occlusive carotid disease, other neurologic disease such as intracerebral tumor or cerebrovascular malformation may produce similar symptoms. Cardiac diseases also may produce neurologic symptoms, including atrial fibrillation, valvular heart disease, dilated cardiomyopathy, or a myocardial infarction with akinetic ventricular segments leading to intracardiac thrombus formation and cerebral embolization. Coronary artery disease is common in patients presenting for carotid endarterectomy.[40] We are less likely to request special studies (dobutamine stress echocardiography or dipyridamole-thallium scintigraphy) or cardiac catheterization before carotid endarterectomy than for other major vascular procedures. Our rationale is that carotid endarterectomy can prevent stroke, is less stressful, and does not result in death as frequently as other vascular operations. Indeed, it has been proposed that preoperative risk can be based not only on the presence of coronary artery disease but also on the basis of exercise tolerance and extent of the surgical procedure.[56]

In the North American trial, the 30-day results were as follows: death, 1.1%; disabling stroke, 1.8%; nondisabling stroke, 3.7%, cardiac death 0.3%.[119] These values are clearly lower than those reported for CABG, even in patients free of significant carotid disease. Therefore, it is difficult to recommend a CABG procedure to a patient with symptomatic carotid disease and stable coronary disease because the combined mortality and stroke rate after CABG may be higher than that of an expertly performed carotid endarterectomy. Cerebrovascular disease is associated with increased mortality after CABG. On the other hand, patients who have had previous CABG may have lower mortality following CEA.[119]

We therefore usually undertake carotid endarterectomy in patients for whom the operation offers benefits even if they have stable coronary artery disease. Our classification of stable coronary artery disease is based on a thorough history, physical examination, and review of basic laboratory tests, not specialized testing. We do not delay urgent surgery that might prevent a stroke for extensive cardiac evaluation in the patient with stable cardiac disease. However, the long-term risks of adverse cardiac events after carotid endarterectomy are related to progression of coronary artery disease. Identification and coronary revascularization of patients with triple-vessel or left main coronary artery disease and those with very low ejection fractions may prolong their lives.[44]

The approach to patients with both severe coronary artery disease and carotid occlusive disease is controversial.[120] The risk of stroke in patients with symptomatic carotid disease undergoing CABG surgery can range from 8.7–17%. In patients with asymptomatic carotid disease, CABG may entail a stroke risk ranging from 0.3–9.2%; equally important, the perioperative mortality may be as high as 13%.[121] Options include either a concurrent (performed under one anesthetic) operation or two separate, staged procedures. Concurrent carotid and coronary revascularization procedures have been performed with an operative mortality rate as low as 2% and a neurologic complication rate as low as 3%, but other series have reported much higher rates of complications (combined perioperative mortality and stroke rates ranging from 8–40%). Operative strategies used in concurrent operations vary among surgeons. Some surgeons will begin with a simultaneous carotid endarterectomy and a saphenous vein harvest. After these procedures have been completed, coronary artery bypass is initiated. This technique avoids the potential threats posed to the brain by pump-associated hypotension, fluctuations in perfusion pressure, and nonpulsatile blood flow. This strategy presumes that hypoperfusion is the dominant mechanism of stroke after CABG. However, studies suggest that embolic events may predominate. Emboli may occur when the ascending aorta is cannulated or occluded with a cross-clamp and protruding aortic arch atheromas are dislodged; mobile atheroma are seen using TEE in 15% of patients with severe carotid artery disease.[122] Therefore, other surgeons will perform a simultaneous correction of both the coronary and carotid arteries during the aortic cross-clamp period. They seek to protect the brain with systemic hypothermia of 20–25°C. With this strategy, several investigators have reported extremely low rates of perioperative strokes. Although these reports are encouraging, rigorous scientific proof for a preferred operative strategy in patients with severe coronary and carotid disease is not yet available.

Monitoring and Preserving Neurologic Integrity

The two main goals of intraoperative management are to protect the brain and to protect the heart, yet these two goals often conflict. For example, increasing arterial blood pressure to augment cerebral blood flow can increase afterload or myocardial contractility, thereby increasing the oxygen demand of the heart. Also, while hypothermia may provide effective cerebral protection, it also poses a significant challenge to myocardial well-being if patients wake up shivering. General approaches to myocardial protection have been summarized above. Our approaches to neurologic and myocardial protection during carotid endarterectomy involve compromises that must be made if both organs are to be protected.

Routine aspects of anesthetic care that may affect cerebral outcome if hemispheric ischemia occurs during carotid endarterectomy include blood pressure augmentation, manipulation of $Paco_2$, glucose management, and choice of intraoperative fluid administration. Whether further interventions to reduce cerebral metabolism and cerebral oxygen requirements are neuroprotective is controversial. Recent research suggests that the outcome of cerebral ischemia may be improved by antagonizing or modifying processes that normally occur after reperfusion rather than during ischemia. Shunts may be used if cerebral hypoperfusion is suspected. Percutaneous approaches using carotid stenting are no panacea; neurologic events occur during and after these procedures as well.[123]

The rationale behind maintaining a stable, high-normal blood pressure throughout the procedure is based on the assumption that blood vessels in ischemic or hypoperfused areas of brain have lost normal autoregulation. Flow in such areas is believed to be mainly pressure-dependent. Under these circumstances, prolonged, severe hypotension may jeopardize the brain. Consequently, we maintain blood pressure in the patient's high-normal range. Nonetheless, hypotension and hypoperfusion may not be the precipitating or sole cause of stroke after carotid endarterectomy; embolic events may be just as or even more important, and often occur postoperatively (Fig. 33-3).[119] In addition, blood pressure augmentation with sympathomimetic drugs is not without risk to the heart. Indiscriminate use of phenylephrine to raise blood pressure during deep general anesthesia with a volatile anesthetic increases the incidence of intraoperative segmental wall abnormalities detected by TEE compared with light anesthesia without the use of phenylephrine.[124] However, the judicious use of phenylephrine to raise blood pressure only in specific instances of EEG-detected reversible cerebral ischemia seems to be without detriment to the heart.[125] While phenylephrine lowers ejection fraction measured with TEE and causes cardiac dilatation in patients with CAD, norepinephrine maintains cardiac function while raising blood pressure.[126] Phenylephrine and norepinephrine both raise cerebral blood flow velocities to a similar extent, and the increase is proportional to increases in systemic blood pressure.[127] Whatever the choice of vasopressor, we believe that one benefit of EEG or other neurophysiologic monitoring is that it allows the

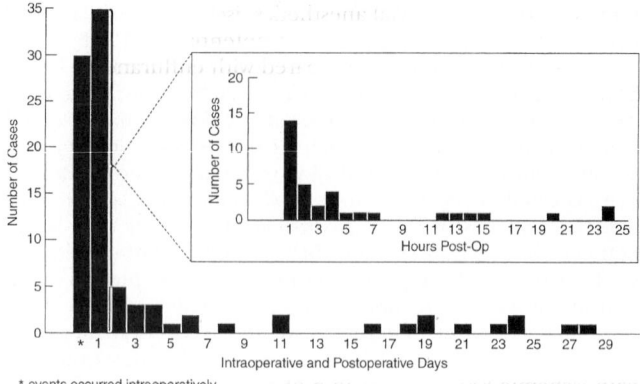

Figure 33-3. Data from the North American Symptomatic Carotid Trial (NASCET). Of the perioperative strokes, 35% (30/85) occurred intraoperatively, while 65% (55/85) occurred after the patient left the operating room (delayed events). The figure illustrates the time of onset of the 92 surgical outcome events.[119]

anesthesiologist to use less vasopressor and to maintain a lower blood pressure during the period of temporary carotid occlusion than would be otherwise feasible. Thus, as long as the patient is without new neurologic deficits or the EEG or other neurophysiologic monitor is unchanged, the anesthesiologist may decrease the afterload in the patient who is at risk for myocardial ischemic events. Based on these studies, then, limited vasopressor use during hypotensive episodes associated with a change in neurophysiologic monitoring appears defensible, allowing the clinician to treat only those patients who might benefit most, and sparing other patients from its risks.

Hypercapnia dilates cerebral blood vessels and thus increases cerebral blood flow. However, hypercapnia during carotid endarterectomy may be detrimental if it dilates vessels in normal areas of the brain while vessels in ischemic brain areas that are already maximally dilated cannot respond. The net effect, then, is a "steal" phenomenon, *i.e.,* a diversion of blood flow from hypoperfused brain regions to normally perfused brain regions. Most authorities recommend the maintenance of normocarbia or moderate hypocarbia at best.

Moderate hyperglycemia may worsen ischemic brain injury. Increased cerebral lactic acidosis resulting from the anaerobic glycolysis of increased brain glucose stores is postulated to be directly or indirectly responsible for the adverse effect. Because of the neuroendocrine response to surgery, with its resultant breakdown of glycogen, and the relatively high incidence of diabetes in this patient population, blood sugar levels will often already be mildly elevated during carotid endarterectomy. The administration of dextrose-containing iv fluid may exacerbate hyperglycemia. A similar effect may result from lactated solutions because lactate is metabolized to dextrose. Although there is no proof that the focal neurologic injury that may follow carotid endarterectomy is actually augmented by hyperglycemia, we nonetheless prefer normal saline for intraoperative fluid substitution. Isovolemic hemodilution with dextran or hetastarch may be beneficial in cases of cerebral ischemia because blood viscosity is reduced and attendant microcirculatory disturbances are thus ameliorated.

Virtually all commonly used anesthetic agents reduce cerebral metabolism and thereby decrease the brain's requirements for oxygen. It has been assumed that under anesthesia the brain's tolerance of temporary ischemia is enhanced. However, the notion that reduced cerebral metabolism is associated with cerebral protection has been challenged.[128] Nonetheless, we believe that as long as this method of pharmacologic brain protection is not clearly refuted, there is no good justification to deny its potential benefits to a patient. The following section reviews the putative benefits of inhalational and iv anesthetic agents as well as hypothermia in reducing cerebral metabolism.

Among the inhalational anesthetics, isoflurane has emerged as the volatile agent with the most potential protective effect against cerebral ischemia. Compared with enflurane and halothane, isoflurane decreased the frequency of EEG-detected cerebral ischemic changes during carotid endarterectomy.[129] Nonetheless, clinical neurologic outcome was not different among the anesthetic groups. However, isoflurane's protective effects are maximal only at ~2 minimal alveolar concentrations (MAC). At this MAC level systemic hypotension will occur in many patients; therefore, maximal protection may not be clinically achievable. Desflurane and sevoflurane also reduce cerebral oxygen requirements at MAC values comparable to those with isoflurane and result in faster emergence and recovery than isoflurane. Sevoflurane anesthesia for CEA was associated with ischemic EEG changes in 5 of 52 patients at an estimated $rCBF_{50}$ of 11.5 ± 1.4 mL $\cdot$ 100 g$^{-1} \cdot$ min^{-1}.[130] This value of critical cerebral blood flow is lower than values during halothane anesthesia, and slightly higher than values for isoflurane.[131] Desflurane's propensity to cause tachycardia may detract from its use in a patient group in which coexisting coronary artery disease is exceedingly common.

Barbiturates may offer a degree of brain protection during periods of regional ischemia. Thiopental decreases cerebral metabolic oxygen requirements to about 50% of baseline. These maximally achievable reductions in oxygen requirements correspond to a silent, *i.e.*, isoelectric, EEG. Beyond this point additional doses of barbiturates are neither necessary nor helpful. In cases of massive global ischemia where basal cellular metabolism has already deteriorated, even high doses of barbiturates will not improve neurologic outcome. Therefore, some clinicians use thiopental not only for induction of anesthesia but also for continuous infusion and/or as a 4–6 mg $\cdot$ kg^{-1} bolus just before carotid occlusion. The cardiac depressant effects of the barbiturates may require inotropic support. Unfortunately, no rigorous proof is available that the use of barbiturates in the described manner can improve neurologic outcome after carotid endarterectomy. Excellent results have been obtained for CEA using high doses of barbiturates during carotid occlusion, without neurophysiologic monitoring or shunt placement; on average, tracheal extubation was delayed until 2 hr after surgery was completed.[132]

Both etomidate and propofol decrease brain electrical activity and thus decrease cellular oxygen requirements. Etomidate preserves cardiovascular stability and may be beneficial in a patient population whose cardiac reserves are often limited. Propofol also allows rapid awakening of the patient and neurologic assessment at the end of surgery. Propofol may also be associated with a lower incidence of myocardial ischemia than is an isoflurane-based anesthetic.[133] While the available evidence for the protective effects of etomidate or propofol during carotid endarterectomy is inconclusive, a small series in patients undergoing temporary ischemia for intracranial aneurysm clipping suggests that etomidate, propofol, or barbiturate use prolongs tolerable ischemia and reduces brain infarction.[134] Some animals studies have supported, and others refuted, the utility of α_2 agonists in reducing cerebral infarction in animal models.

Hypothermia can depress neuronal activity sufficiently to decrease cellular oxygen requirements below the minimum levels normally required for continued cell viability. In theory, hypothermia represents the most effective method of cerebral protection. Even a mild decrease in temperature of about $2-3°C$ at the time of arterial hypoxemia may reduce ischemic damage to the brain. The first reported carotid endarterectomy was performed with the patient's head covered by ice packs. Unfortunately, this method is cumbersome, unpredictable, and rarely used. We allow patients to cool passively in the operating room and avoid warming the operating suite, iv fluids, or inspired gases until the carotid repair has been completed. Afterward, forced-air warming may counteract the adrenergic response and increased incidence of myocardial ischemia associated with hypothermia in vascular surgery patients.[102]

Effective pharmacologic brain protection is still theoretical. The outcome of cerebral ischemia may be improved by preventing activation of the neuron's excitatory amino acid (EAA) receptor after reperfusion. However, to date no conclusive data exist for use of this method in humans. Ischemia also leads to neuronal calcium overload, which in turn sets off a series of harmful biochemical intracellular events. Given early after the onset of stroke symptoms, nimodipine, a calcium channel blocker, may confer some benefit to patients. Nitric oxide synthesis inhibitors and free-radical scavengers may also have important therapeutic roles. Some centers still use iv steroids to protect the brain from the effects of hypoxia.

Temporary occlusion ("cross-clamping") of the carotid artery acutely disrupts blood flow, even if flow to the ipsilateral hemisphere of the brain was already markedly diminished by severe stenosis. Continued blood supply to the brain will depend entirely on adequate collateral blood flow through the circle of Willis if no shunt is used. If carotid stenosis has worsened gradually before carotid endarterectomy is performed, collaterals from the circle of Willis may have had time to develop, and the cerebral circulation may not be compromised by carotid occlusion during surgery. However, if collateral flow is compromised because of occlusive disease of the contralateral carotid artery and/or the vertebral arteries, the chances are greater that marked hypoperfusion of the brain will occur during carotid clamping. Indeed, patients with bilateral carotid disease have a higher risk of perioperative stroke after carotid endarterectomy than patients with unilateral disease only. The need for shunts in carotid surgery remains a controversial issue. Some surgeons never use shunts, others use them routinely, and still others use them only selectively. Surgeons who never use shunts usually rely on expedient surgery to avoid neurologic problems and do not report worse overall outcome statistics than those who do.

The routine use of shunts is not risk-free. Placement of a shunt is associated with an embolism-related stroke rate of at least 0.7% from the dislodgement and embolization of atheroma. The technical problems of shunting include air embolism, kinking of the shunt, shunt occlusion against the side of the vessel wall, and injury or disruption of the distal internal carotid artery. Patients with shunts in may still develop EEG abnormalities; in these situations, we alert surgeons that shunt adjustments may be necessary. The shunt may impair surgical access to the artery, thereby increasing cross-clamp time. Most importantly, the use of a shunt is beneficial only if the cause of neurologic dysfunction is inadequate blood flow. However, the majority of studies suggest that as many as 65–95% of all neurologic deficits during carotid endarterectomy may be caused by thromboembolic events (Fig. 33-3), which may occur when the carotid artery is dissected, at which point insertion of a shunt will not prevent a deficit. Not surprisingly, there is no rigorous proof that the routine insertion of a shunt reduces the incidence of postoperative neurologic deficits. In the NASCET trial, shunting (used in 41% of patients) was not associated with a change in risk of stroke.[119]

Surgeons who use shunts selectively will need a monitoring device of cerebral perfusion to help them decide when to place the shunt. To this end, a variety of cerebral perfusion monitors are used.[135] Some surgeons simply palpate the distal end of the clamped carotid artery between their thumb and forefinger. If a pulse is detected, collateral flow is presumed to be adequate and they proceed to occlude the carotid artery. Conversely, if there is no pulse, a shunt will be placed. More commonly, however, the mean blood pressure distal to the carotid clamp (also referred to as "stump pressure") is evaluated invasively. Under halothane anesthesia a mean stump pressure above 60 mm Hg is sufficient to prevent ischemia in most cases. If a nitrous oxide/opioid-based anesthetic is undertaken, the stump pressure must be higher than 60 mm Hg for blood flow to be adequate because cerebrovascular resistance is increased with this anesthetic technique.[136] The major criticism of stump pres-

FREQUENCY BAND

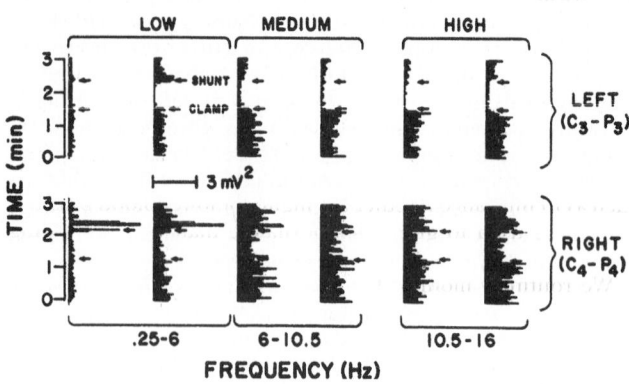

Figure 33-4. Acute cerebral ischemia following left carotid artery occlusion detected with processed EEG; the placement of a shunt in this case promptly reversed the ischemic changes. (Courtesy of Dr. Bruce L. Gewertz.)

sure measurement is the large number of false-positive results; that is, a stump pressure of <60 mm Hg when regional cerebral blood flow (rCBF) is >24 mL · min^{-1} · 100 g^{-1} brain. Such results occur in about 30% of patients. Thus, a shunt may be placed when none is needed. In other cases, a false-negative result may be obtained, when an "adequate" stump pressure is measured, yet the patient has stenosis of the middle cerebral artery distal to the arteries that provide "back-bleeding." In this situation, cerebral ischemia could occur despite a stump pressure >60 mm Hg. Despite these limitations, stump pressure monitoring has the advantages of being inexpensive and readily available; however, its overall value in terms of outcome improvement has not yet been proved.

The interpretation of the information gained from the scalp-recorded EEG has been simplified by the use of computerized data reduction methods. The EEG reflects the spontaneous electrical activity of cortical (surface) neurons. Increasing levels of ischemia lead to a decrease in recorded electrical activity. EEG deterioration begins usually below a cerebral blood flow rate of about 15 mL · min^{-1} · 100 g^{-1} brain tissue, but cellular metabolic failure does not seem to occur until blood flow falls below 10–12 mL · min^{-1} · 100 g^{-1} brain tissue.[137] Under conditions of focal cortical ischemia, the frequency of the recorded EEG waves over the affected area of the brain will slow significantly, *i.e.,* >50%. In addition, the amplitude of the waves may decrease (attenuate) to a comparable extent. The appearance of a disorganized background rhythm may also be a sign of ischemia. Finally, as ischemia becomes severe, the EEG will become isoelectric. Ischemic EEG changes occur in 28% of all monitored patients during carotid endarterectomy.[138] When they occur, they define a patient subgroup with a significantly increased risk of perioperative stroke. The most common manifestations of EEG ischemia during carotid endarterectomy are ipsilateral attenuation, ipsilateral slowing with attenuation, and ipsilateral slowing without attenuation.

In practice, the EEG can be obtained using a 16-channel strip-chart recording or a processed EEG monitor with 2 or 4 channels. A 16-channel strip-chart EEG generally requires a technician to set up the monitor and to monitor and interpret the large amount of (unprocessed) data generated. In contrast, a 2- or 4-channel processed EEG monitor provides less data but can be monitored more easily. Figure 33-4 shows a processed EEG reflecting acute cerebral ischemia following left carotid artery occlusion; the placement of a shunt in this case promptly reversed the ischemic changes.

However, EEG monitoring has several limitations.[135] For one, deep brain structures are not monitored by EEG. Also, in pa-

tients with pre-existing or fluctuating neurologic deficits the EEG may be false negative; *i.e.,* these patients can develop perioperative strokes despite the absence of major intraoperative EEG changes. In these patients there may be cell populations that are electrically silent or immediately adjacent to regions of infarction and therefore not monitored by the EEG. The still viable regions may progress to irreversible deterioration in the course of the operative procedure. Furthermore, the EEG may not be an ischemia-specific monitor because decreases in temperature and blood pressure as well as increases in the depth of anesthesia produce EEG changes that mimic ischemic changes. However, EEG changes secondary to anesthetics or hypothermia are more likely to be bilateral, whereas hemispheric ischemia is more likely to affect the electrical activity of only one side of the brain. Thus, we are compulsive in informing the encephalographer about adjustments to the anesthetic regimen.

Intraoperative false-positive results, that is, changes in the EEG without accompanying demonstrable deficits, may be related to several factors. The brain can tolerate relatively brief periods of ischemia without infarction. Thus, temporary, reversible EEG changes should not be expected to produce postoperative deficits routinely. The flow threshold for electrical failure is higher than the flow threshold for metabolic failure. Although the EEG may be viewed as an early-warning system for cerebral ischemia, not all EEG changes indicate that irreversible ischemia is taking place. Finally, focal embolic events may not be detected by the EEG.

Most importantly, the value of relatively costly EEG monitoring has not been rigorously established. Even if the advanced warning of an EEG can prevent some strokes, it would presumably do so only in the minority of patients who suffer strokes from intraoperative hypoperfusion (Fig. 33-3).

Evaluation of the cost-effectiveness of EEG monitoring can be thought of as a comparison of the cost of monitoring with the cost of the deficits that monitoring may prevent. Let us assume that 100,000 carotid endarterectomies are performed each year with a deficit rate of 3% (3000 new deficits each year) and that the use of monitoring devices might prevent one-sixth of these deficits (500 deficits per year). Assume that an additional 15% of patients would undergo temporary shunting of carotid flow because of EEG monitoring and that 0.7% would experience shunt insertion–associated neurologic deficits. This assumption would result in an additional 106 deficits related to monitoring, or a net of 394 deficits preventable by monitoring. If each deficit cost $100,000, on average, in medical care, loss of wages and productivity, and quality-adjusted years of life, the deficits preventable by monitoring would cost $39,400,000 per year. The breakeven point for monitoring costs would be $394 per patient: at that price, the cost of monitoring would equal the cost of the deficits that monitoring would prevent. If monitoring could be provided for less than $394, it would be cost-effective. This analysis neglects the benefit that EEG monitoring may have in preserving myocardial function (by allowing the anesthesiologist to decrease the afterload in the patient who is at risk for myocardial ischemic events), permitting an unhurried and technically superior endarterectomy, identifying delayed ischemia, and aiding in the detection of shunt malfunction. Unfortunately, there are no data showing that EEG demonstration of neurologic dysfunction during carotid endarterectomy results in better patient outcome than does any other method.

Somatosensory evoked potential (SSEP) monitoring is based on the detection of cortical potentials after electrical stimuli are presented to a peripheral nerve. Detecting the potentials requires computer-assisted mathematical analysis and considerable expertise. In contrast to the EEG, which interrogates only cortical function, SSEP monitoring also evaluates deep brain structures. Any damage to these neural structures results in characteristic changes in the SSEP, usually in a decrease in amplitude and/or an increase in latency. If neural damage is severe, the cortical-evoked potential is completely abolished. Severe damage occurs at about one-third of normal cerebral blood flow, *i.e.*, at 15 mL · min^{-1} · 100 g^{-1} brain tissue.

Whereas some studies have been optimistic about the value of SSEP monitoring in the detection of cerebral ischemia, other investigators have concluded that SSEP is neither sensitive nor specific for the detection of ischemic injury during carotid endarterectomy.[139] Virtually all commonly used anesthetics lead to SSEP changes that mimic changes produced by cerebral hypoxia. Therefore, a constant light plane of anesthesia needs to be maintained if increased latencies and decreased amplitudes of evoked potentials are to be ascribed to inadequate cerebral perfusion. False-negative results may also occur. Based on the available data, we conclude that this monitoring system cannot yet be considered essential for a safe carotid endarterectomy.

Transcranial Doppler (TCD) techniques measure the mean blood flow velocity in the middle cerebral artery. A 40% decrease in flow velocity corresponds with major EEG changes during carotid endarterectomy.[140] Middle cerebral artery flow velocities are significantly lower in patients with stump pressures below 30 mm Hg. TCD can detect acute thrombotic occlusion during carotid endarterectomy, as well as microemboli that occur during initial carotid dissection. In the latter case, the surgeon might be warned to modify his or her technique in the hope of avoiding a significant embolic stroke. In addition, TCD may help in identifying patients who are at risk of developing postoperative hyperperfusion syndrome. TCD flow velocity measurements correlate well with the measurement of regional oxyhemoglobin saturation (rsO$_2$) by infrared cerebral spectroscopy.[135] Whether cerebral spectroscopy alone or in conjunction with TCD will play a role in carotid endarterectomy in the future remains to be determined. Thus, although all these data are certainly encouraging, definitive proof that the use of TCD or tissue spectroscopy will lead to improved outcome is not available.

Cerebral blood flow can also be measured intraoperatively by the intravenous or intracarotid injection of radioactive xenon or krypton. However, the expense and expertise required to collect and interpret the data have limited the use of this method to only a few research centers. Jugular venous oxygen saturation has been proposed to monitor global cerebral blood flow and oxygen consumption. But because of interhemispheric mixing of venous blood, jugular venous oxygen saturation is not capable of reflecting focal cerebral perfusion and is probably of limited use during carotid endarterectomy.

In the North American trial, 93% of patients underwent CEA with general anesthesia; 51% of patients had intraoperative cerebral monitoring (31% EEG, 14% stump pressure, 7% evoked potentials, and 3% transcranial Doppler). However, the use of monitoring was not associated with reduced risk of stroke.[119] In summary, none of the above procedures or neurophysiologic monitors has been shown to improve outcome. Because embolism, not hypoperfusion, is probably the most common cause of perioperative stroke, the real value of cerebral monitoring may lie in the avoidance of interventions such as the placement of shunts (which can cause stroke) and blood pressure augmentation (with its detrimental effects on the heart).

Anesthetic and Monitoring Choices for Elective Surgery

General discussions of cardiac function and myocardial ischemia monitoring can be found earlier in this chapter. Our practice with patients undergoing carotid endarterectomy, summarized below, is somewhat different. Our intraoperative monitors include the usual monitors employed during all major, general, or regional anesthetics: precordial stethoscope, temperature probe, blood pressure cuff, pulse oximeter, and an end-tidal carbon dioxide tension monitor. We routinely place an intra-arterial catheter for blood pressure monitoring, so that beat-to-beat changes in pressure are detected and treated promptly. However, in some patients, particularly elderly females, cannulation of the radial artery may be difficult. Before surgery, we also measure the blood pressures noninvasively in both arms because generalized peripheral vascular disease in this patient population can produce striking differences between the two upper extremities.[141] However, it is not clear in such a circumstance whether the higher or lower blood pressure should be used to guide hemodynamic management during carotid occlusion.

We routinely monitor leads II and V$_5$ of the ECG for ST-T segment changes because of the high incidence of perioperative myocardial ischemia after carotid reperfusion.[142] In high-risk patients, we may use TEE as an additional monitor. Rarely is it necessary to use a central venous or pulmonary artery catheter, even if TEE is not available. We seek to avoid central venous or pulmonary artery catheterization because of the risk of an accidental carotid artery puncture during cannulation of the internal jugular vein. We restrict the use of central venous access to the rare patient with uncompensated congestive heart failure undergoing urgent carotid endarterectomy, and then may insert it from the contralateral brachial or subclavian vein. Finally, in our experience, iv access for volume administration can be limited to one well secured, well running medium-bore iv catheter because major blood loss or fluid shifts during carotid endarterectomy are rare.

Maintaining intraoperative hemodynamic stability begins with the preoperative visit. For most patients, the assurance provided by the preoperative interview obviates the need for sedative drugs to prevent anxiety-induced myocardial ischemia. If sedatives are deemed indispensable, a "light" short-acting premedication is chosen to facilitate early perioperative neurologic assessment. Equally importantly, we obtain blood pressure and heart rate determinations from the preoperative clinic, other hospital or clinic visits, and at the time of admission, thus determining the range of a patient's acceptable values. We seek to maintain hemodynamics within this range intraoperatively. Chronic antianginal, antihypertensive, and aspirin medications are generally continued on the day of surgery. Patients who come to the hospital the same day as surgery must be reminded to take their medications at home. When patients forget to take their medications, we give them readily available oral or parenteral substitutes.

In the past, we would routinely administer iv normal saline the night before surgery at a rate of 100 mL · hr^{-1} for a 70-kg patient. This amount of saline attenuates preoperative hypovolemia and reduces the incidence of severe hypotension after we induce general anesthesia in hypertensive patients. Today, however, because almost all of our patients present to the hospital on the same day as surgery, we encourage patients to drink clear fluids until midnight, and attempt to perform their surgery as the first case of the day; otherwise clear fluids are encouraged up until 4 hr before surgery. In the operating room, we generally avoid administering more than 10 mL · kg^{-1} of crystalloid in a typical 2-hour operation because fluid overload may contribute to postoperative hypertension.

For procedures performed under general anesthesia, we typically use propofol[133] for induction, although thiopental or etomidate may be used. If thiopental is used, esmolol is particularly valuable to blunt hypertensive and tachycardic responses to intubation. However, when a patient has a diastolic blood pressure >100 mm Hg in the operating room or is not well hydrated (often, both conditions exist simultaneously), induction of general anesthesia may result in hypotension. The clinician can anticipate this possibility and induce general anesthesia slowly, being prepared to use pharmacologic blood pressure augmentation if blood pressure decreases excessively. Because the respiratory depression and sedation caused by opioids may persist into the postoperative period and may confound the results of early neurologic assessment, we generally restrict the use of opioids whenever possible (*e.g.,* fentanyl ≤3–5 mg · kg^{-1}) or use remifentanil.

In essence, our approach represents a "combined technique." We provide patients with a "light" general anesthetic that permits EEG monitoring and results in blood pressures in the high range of normal. We spray the trachea with 100 mg lidocaine to minimize stimulation by the endotracheal tube during surgery, and often perform a superficial cervical block before incision to decrease anesthetic requirements, postoperative pain, and the need for analgesics. Others have described the use of the laryngeal mask airway (LMA) during carotid endarterectomy. Compared to patients managed with endotracheal intubation, a reduced incidence of hypertensive and tachycardic episodes requiring interventional drug therapy was found in the group whose airway was managed by LMA.[143] Anesthesia is maintained with 50% nitrous oxide in oxygen and light levels of isoflurane because of its salutary effects on the incidence of cerebral ischemia.[129] The newer volatile agents, desflurane and sevoflurane, may be used to faciltate rapid awakening and assessment of neurologic status. We do not routinely use continuous infusions of vasopressors (such as phenylephrine) to augment blood pressure, but rely on a patient's endogenous pressure-sustaining responses. Vasopressors are used to treat hypotension or EEG changes. Because sudden onset of bradycardia and hypotension may be caused by activation of baroreceptor reflexes with surgical irritation of the carotid sinus, we ask our surgeons to infiltrate the carotid bifurcation with 1% lidocaine to attenuate this response. However, this practice may result in more postoperative hypertension. We typically use vecuronium or another medium-duration relaxant to provide muscle relaxation, although the choice of muscle relaxant depends on the heart rate we wish to obtain. One of us administers no muscle relaxant except as necessary for intubation. The other usually gives an additional dose of muscle relaxant immediately before carotid occlusion when the concentration of isoflurane is decreased to allow the blood pressure to rise. One limitation of this technique is that it lessens the potential neuroprotective effects of isoflurane because the cerebral metabolic depression it produces is dose-dependent. Passive hypothermia may provide some cerebral protection; therefore, we do not actively warm patients until after carotid reperfusion, at which time forced-air warming may be used for patients who are hypothermic. Our patients are almost always extubated at the end of the surgical procedure after we confirm neurologic integrity. Our overall institutional results are good (mortality of 1%; stroke and myocardial infarction, both 0.76%).[144] Others have achieved similar results using a nitrous oxide/opioid technique or a continuous infusion of thiopental. There is no proof that any one general anesthetic technique provides a superior outcome.

Regional anesthesia is used by many centers for carotid endarterectomy.[145] The necessary sensory blockade of the C2 to C4 dermatomes can be achieved by superficial or deep cervical block or by subcutaneous infiltration of the surgical field. Superficial and deep plexus blocks appear to be equivalent in providing good surgical conditions and patient satusfaction; deep plexus blocks are more effective when a paresthesia is obtained.[146] Proponents of regional anesthetic techniques claim the following advantages: greater stability of blood pressure during surgery, inexpensive and easy cerebral monitoring, avoidance of tracheal intubation in patients with chronic obstructive lung disease, and avoidance of negative inotropic anesthetic agents in patients with limited cardiac reserves. In addition, overall hospital costs associated with the use of regional anesthesia may be lower.

Disadvantages of regional anesthesia are that potential pharmacologic brain protection with anesthetics cannot be provided and that, in the case of panic, sudden loss of consciousness, or

onset of seizures, control of the airway may be difficult. While emergent intubation is uncommon, it may be difficult under these circumstances and complicate surgical management. Regional anesthesia requires that the patient remain highly cooperative throughout the operation, and sedation can be provided only to a limited extent during carotid occlusion. In a study of nearly 400 patients who had regional anesthesia for carotid endarterectomy, one-fourth of the patients had neurologic changes with carotid occlusion. These patients were six times more likely (6.6% versus 1.1%) to have permanent neurologic impairment, often due to carotid thrombosis.[147] To date, evidence for the above cited advantages of regional anesthesia remains limited. Others have found no difference in neurologic or cardiac complications or hospital stay between patients receiving regional or general anesthesia for carotid endarterectomy. The NASCET study found no difference in event rate between regional and general anesthesia, although only 7% of the 1415 patients received a regional anesthetic. Based on the currently available evidence, the choice of anesthetic technique should take into account the preference of the surgeon and the experience and expertise of the anesthesiologist.

Initially, the internal carotid artery is isolated where the plaque or ulcerative lesion has been identified radiographically (usually starting near the bifurcation). Heparin is typically given in a dose of 50–100 U · kg^{-1}. The surgeon isolates the diseased carotid segment with clamps or ties placed on the proximal and distal internal carotid artery and on the external carotid artery. After a period of test occlusion during which the adequacy of cerebral blood flow may be assessed with the modalities previously described, an incision is made into the artery. A shunt may be inserted at this time.

The surgeon then endarterectomizes the ulcerated or plaque-containing area. Occasionally, a long or tortuous region is shortened by resection and reanastomosis; or if the remaining portion of the intima is too thin, a vein (often from the leg) or a Dacron patch is used. The use of a patch may also improve long-term patency rates. Because suturing of the patch requires more time than suturing of the native vessel, an internal shunt is used more often during these procedures. Time is of the essence to help prevent neurologic deficits. If the shunt has been placed, it is then removed and, in all cases, the arteriotomy is closed, usually with a running suture. Shunt placement and removal rarely take less than 1 minute or more than 4 minutes, and the total occlusion time rarely exceeds 40 minutes.

Postoperative Management

Common problems arising after carotid endarterectomy include the onset of new neurologic dysfunction, hemodynamic instability during emergence from general anesthesia, and respiratory insufficiency.[145] Patients who have undergone general anesthesia may be awakened while still on the operating table to permit early neurologic evaluation. A new neurologic deficit may demand immediate re-exploration, or at least arteriography. A few surgeons routinely perform arteriography after restoring blood flow, but most believe that the complications of routine arteriography (emboli, allergic reactions, vasospasm, bleeding from the puncture hole, and stroke) are greater than its benefits (the detection of inadequate repairs, suture lines, or flow). With another method, duplex ultrasonography, the resutured vessel may be imaged at the end of surgery. The risks of arteriography are avoided, but the benefits have not yet been established by randomized controlled trials. Before or soon after we extubate the trachea, we ask the patient to move his extremities to exclude acute thrombosis of the endarterectomy site. The examination should also seek to identify cranial nerve (hypoglossal and facial) injuries arising from surgical manipulation.

Hyperperfusion syndrome is thought to result from blood flow to the brain that is greatly in excess of its metabolic needs following carotid endarterectomy. It often does not occur until several days after surgery, when patients present with severe ipsilateral headache and can progress to develop signs of increased cerebral excitability or frank seizures. Some clinicians have recommended that patients with a high-grade stenosis or previous stroke who develop severe ipsilateral headache following carotid endarterectomy should be started on phenytoin for seizure prophylaxis.

The incidence of both hypertensive and hypotensive episodes after carotid endarterectomy may be >60%. Hypertension is more common than hypotension; left untreated, about 30% of patients will develop severe hypertension with systolic blood pressure >200 mm Hg. Severe hypertension seems to occur more often in patients with poorly controlled preoperative hypertension. Both acute tachycardia and hypertension may precipitate acute myocardial ischemia and failure, and hypertension may lead to cerebral edema and/or hemorrhage. Post-CEA hypertension is significantly associated with adverse events (stroke or death, with a statistical trend towards reduced cardiac complications), while postoperative hypotension and bradycardia do not correlate with primary or secondary outcomes.[148] We therefore routinely treat hypertension, if only to reduce the work of the heart. Thus, having excluded and/or treated other causes of hypertension such as bladder distention, pain, hypoxemia, and hypercarbia, we lower systolic pressures of >160 mm Hg and diastolic pressures of >95 mm Hg to within the range of a patient's perioperative values. Hyperdynamic responses accompanying emergence and extubation may be attenuated by prophylactic administration of iv lidocaine, esmolol, labetolol, or nitroglycerin. We prefer to use drugs with short half-lives that can be titrated to avoid undue hypotension. We believe that by supplementation with a regional anesthetic and tracheal lidocaine spray these responses are suppressed. The incidence of myocardial ischemia is high in the first few hours after carotid endarterectomy, even in patients who have been "awake" during carotid endarterectomy with a deep cervical block and prophylactic nitroglycerin infusions.[142] Patients who undergo carotid artery stenting also manifest intra- and postprocedural hemodynamic abnormalities similar to surgical patients.[149] The causes of postoperative hypertension are unclear. Overzealous administration of iv fluid or surgical or chemical denervation of the baroreceptors of the carotid sinus nerve may be responsible. Postoperative hypertension may be associated with an increased incidence of neurologic deficits. Usually, the hypertensive episode has its peak 2–3 hr after surgery, but in individual cases it may persist for 24 hr.

Postoperative hypotension and bradycardia after carotid endarterectomy are less frequent than hypertension. Surgical removal of the atheroma re-exposes the baroreceptors of the carotid sinus nerve to higher levels of transmural pressure and causes brain stem-mediated vagal bradycardia and hypotension. Chemical denervation of the carotid baroreceptors with a local anesthetic by the surgeon results in fewer hypotensive patients but increases the incidence of postoperative hypertension. Over time, the baroreceptors seem to adjust and the hypotensive phase resolves within 12–24 hr. For patients who are hypotensive, some argue against any treatment as long as the ECG is unchanged and the patient's neurologic status is stable. Other clinicians, however, typically administer iv fluids and/or vasopressors such as ephedrine, dopamine, or phenylephrine to restore blood pressure to the low range of normal. Because significant hypertension and hypotension can be due to or caused by myocardial ischemia or infarction, we routinely obtain a 12-lead ECG in the recovery room.

Postoperative respiratory insufficiency may be caused by bilateral recurrent laryngeal nerve injury, a massive hematoma, or deficient carotid body function. Injury to the recurrent laryngeal nerve must be suspected in patients with a history of contralateral carotid endarterectomy or thyroid resection. In such patients, preoperative evaluation of vocal cord function may be considered. Whereas unilateral recurrent laryngeal nerve injury may only manifest as transient hoarseness, bilateral injury of the nerves may lead to paralysis of both vocal cords and hence acute airway obstruction.

Wound hematomas develop in up to 2% of patients after carotid endarterectomy. Whereas small hematomas caused by venous oozing usually can be treated by reversing residual heparin with protamine or by applying gentle digital compression for a few minutes, an expanding hematoma must be carefully and immediately evaluated because tracheal compression and loss of the airway may ensue rapidly. In some cases, evacuation of the hematoma may not relieve the airway obstruction if lymphatic obstruction has produced massive pharyngolaryngeal edema.[150] Indeed, four patients (0.3%) in the NACSET trial died directly due to neck hematomas.[119] Risk factors for neck hematoma may also include failure to reverse heparin and the presence of an endotracheal tube beyond the end of surgery.[151] Hematomas are more common and delayed if a patch angioplasty has been performed. Therefore, some clinicians routinely reverse heparin with protamine in patients who have had a patch angioplasty. Some studies, however, have suggested that protamine may contribute to postoperative stroke.[152] However, in the NASCET trial, heparin reversal using protamine (used in 40% of patients) was not associated with a change in risk of stroke.[119]

Surgical manipulation may also damage the nerve supply to the carotid body. While unilateral loss of carotid body function is unlikely to be significant, a bilateral loss may prevent the patient from increasing ventilation in response to a decrease in Pao_2. Therefore, supplemental oxygen should be routinely used in the recovery area. Similarly, drugs that depress respiratory drive should be avoided as much as possible in postoperative pain management. It is our experience that administration of acetaminophen constitutes effective pain relief in most patients when skin infiltration or plexus block with local anesthetic was performed in the operating room.

In experienced centers, carotid endarterectomy causes only minor postoperative physiologic derangements in most patients. As a consequence, routine postoperative intensive care is unusual in our practice and has been questioned. In one study, postoperative intensive care surveillance was necessary only for patients with four or more of the following risk factors: stroke, congestive heart failure, chronic kidney failure, hypertension, arrhythmia, and MI. Equally important, all patients requiring interventions or with adverse outcomes could be identified by the eighth postoperative hour.[153] We believe that routine admission of all patients to the ICU is probably not necessary and that intensive care surveillance can be limited to high-risk patients. Certain complications of carotid endarterectomy, such as hyperperfusion syndrome or bleeding after a patch angioplasty, may not occur until several days after carotid endarterectomy.

Management of Emergent Carotid Surgery

The patient who awakens with a major new neurologic deficit or who develops a suspected stroke in the immediate postoperative period represents a surgical emergency and requires immediate consultation with a surgeon. Although postoperative neurologic deficits may be due to inadequate collateral flow, carotid thrombosis may cause postoperative stroke and prompt surgical re-exploration can produce significant neurologic improvement. If a new neurologic deficit occurs in the postanesthesia recovery unit, most surgeons believe that immediate re-exploration is indicated, and logic would dictate utilization of pharmacologic methods of "cerebral protection"; but this "logic" is controversial. Alternatively, if the deficit is deemed only focal and minor, it is most commonly due to microembolization. Consequently, noninvasive assessment of internal carotid flow and anticoagulation after exclusion of a hemorrhagic brain lesion usually constitute indicated treatment.

A patient undergoing emergency carotid endarterectomy may have a full stomach and thus may require protection against aspiration of gastric contents. The main goal is to minimize the hemodynamic stress of a rapid-sequence induction while maintaining adequate perfusion pressure across the stenotic lesion. General anesthesia is maintained with any of a variety of techniques aimed at attenuating hemodynamic fluctuations, achieving normocarbia (or a carbon dioxide level slightly below normal, as in elective operations), and maintaining adequate carotid artery perfusion pressure. An anesthetic technique similar to one for elective situations is used.

For patients undergoing neck exploration for a wound hematoma following carotid endarterectomy, oxygen is given at high concentration by face mask with a reservoir bag or Ayre's T-piece. In the event of acute airway obstruction, a high concentration of oxygen in the functional residual volume of the lung may provide additional protection against hypoxemia until the airway is secured by intubation or until the hematoma is evacuated surgically. A tracheostomy or cricothyroidotomy tray should be immediately available, as well as other devices for management of the difficult airway. It may be difficult to visualize the trachea because of edema or because of deviation away from the hematoma, caused by pressure of the hematoma.

If the hematoma does not obstruct the airway and the patient is not having difficulty breathing spontaneously, induction may be accomplished as in an elective procedure. If the airway appears compromised, topical anesthesia of the lips, tongue, posterior pharynx, and epiglottis is provided. The larynx may then be visualized traditionally or with fiberoptic laryngoscopy. Esmolol is particularly useful to control hyperdynamic cardiovascular responses during awake intubation. If no difficulty with tracheal intubation is anticipated, induction is performed as described previously. However, if difficulty is expected, the wound is opened and drained externally, and tracheal intubation is performed before general anesthesia is induced.

AORTIC RECONSTRUCTION

In vascular surgery, understanding the pathophysiology of the disease and anticipating the surgical approach and techniques allow the anesthesiologist to serve the patient most effectively. The surgical goal in these operations is to create an enduring restoration of the normal circulation while minimizing the duration of ischemia to viscera, especially to the renal circulation. This goal is difficult to achieve: each of the possible surgical approaches compromises some aspects while optimizing others. Surgery may be undertaken to correct aneurysmal or occlusive disease; sometimes the two coexist.

Aneurysmal Disease

Aneurysms pose an ever-present threat to life because of their unpredictable tendency to rupture or embolize.[154,155] Mortality from rupture may be as high as 85% and even patients who receive emergent surgery have mortality rates one-half that. Therefore, early recognition and aggressive surgical management are warranted, even in the absence of symptoms. Thoracoabdominal aneurysms occur in patients with hypertension or other risk factors for atherosclerotic disease. Abdominal aortic aneurysms are not uncommonly detected in elderly patients undergoing coincidental ultrasound scan of the urinary tract.[156]

The size of the aneurysm is the most important predictor of subsequent rupture and mortality. A prospective study followed 300 consecutive patients (mean age 70 years; 70% men) who presented with abdominal aortic aneurysm (average size, 4.1 cm) and were initially managed nonoperatively. The diameter of the aneurysm increased by a median of 0.3 cm per year. The 6-year cumulative incidence of rupture was 1% among patients with aneurysms <4.0 cm and 2% for aneurysms 4.0–4.9 cm in diameter. By comparison, the 6-year cumulative incidence of rupture was 20% among patients with aneurysms >5.0 cm in diameter.[157] Larger aneurysms expand even more rapidly. Patients with aneurysms of the abdominal aorta that do not undergo operation have an 80% 5-year mortality, predominantly owing to rupture.

Should these patients therefore undergo surgery for asymptomatic aneurysms? This question was answered by Szilagyi et al[1] in 1966 when they showed that, for aneurysms >6 cm in diameter, surgery approximately doubled a patient's life expectancy. Since then, perioperative mortality has declined from 18–25% in the mid-1960s, to 8–12% in the early 1970s, to 2–4% today. The outcome after aortic reconstructive surgery has improved dramatically over the past four decades. Perioperative mortality from supraceliac aneurysms still exceeds 4%. Most morbidity is myocardial, and most myocardial morbidity occurs postoperatively. Also, mortality in patients having repair of small abdominal aortic aneurysm is less than mortality for those having larger aneurysms resected. Consequently, even patients with abdominal aortic aneurysms larger than 6 cm in diameter are considered candidates for aortic reconstructive surgery. This change has resulted from three factors: (1) the lower morbidity associated with elective repair today, (2) the persistently higher mortality (45–90%) associated with emergency aortic reconstruction, and (3) the unpredictability of aneurysm enlargement and rupture.

Although patients undergoing open surgery for aneurysmal disease have higher perioperative morbidity and mortality (by a factor of 2) and a lower median survival time (5.8 versus 10.7 years) than do patients undergoing aortic reconstruction for occlusive disease, successful surgical repair of an abdominal aortic aneurysm is associated with prolonged life expectancy. Still, life expectancy after successful abdominal aortic aneurysm repair is diminished (62% versus 85% expected at 5 years). This suggests that in addition to resection of small aneurysms, attention to coronary artery disease, the cause of most of the late deaths, is probably required to prolong life in these patients. The diagnosis, treatment, and prognosis of coronary artery disease in patients with peripheral vascular disease have already been discussed.

Occlusive Disease

The pathologic conditions that give rise to chronic visceral ischemia include atherosclerotic occlusive disease, fibromuscular dysplasia, inflammatory arteriopathies, external compression, and aneurysmal atherosclerotic disease. They occur more commonly in the elderly, who often are hypertensive, and in persons who have abused tobacco. In most cases, symptomatic disease of the mesenteric artery is due to atherosclerotic narrowing of the origins of the three major visceral vessels: the celiac, superior mesenteric, and inferior mesenteric arteries. The extensive collateral network of the gut is usually sufficient to maintain an adequate intestinal blood supply if only one of these vessels is occluded. However, single-vessel lesions may be important when previous intra-abdominal surgery has interrupted collateral pathways. When there is occlusive disease in the celiac and superior mesenteric arteries, the major mesenteric supply often comes from the inferior mesenteric artery via the marginal artery. If the inferior mesenteric artery is not revascularized during infrarenal aortic grafting, the risk of bowel ischemia is present, with a reported incidence of colonic infarction after aortic operations of 1–2% and that of small bowel infarction of 0.15%, and with a mortality of up to 90% after the occurrence of such infarction.

Acute mesenteric occlusion can be of either embolic or thrombotic origin. If embolic, it commonly has a cardiac source and may follow a recent myocardial infarction. If thrombotic, it may occasionally be due to aortic dissection or trauma but is usually the result of progressing atherosclerosis. Sudden occlusion of the superior mesenteric artery without the previous development of collateral vessels can lead to bowel infarction within a few hours. The diagnosis must be strongly suspected in patients with cardiac disease who suddenly develop severe central abdominal pain, with minimal physical signs. If surgical intervention occurs in the first 4–6 hr before gangrene of the bowel develops, revascularization will reduce the otherwise high mortality and morbidity.

Occlusive disease of the abdominal aorta tends to be progressive, with compromise of the distal circulation leading to disabling claudication or limb-threatening ischemia. In the case of aortoiliac occlusive disease, surgical intervention is indicated only for the relief of disabling symptoms. Compared with abdominal aortic aneurysm surgery, the mean age of patients undergoing aortoiliac reconstruction is ~10 years younger, the surgical mortality is lower, and life expectancy after surgery is higher.

In setting out to correct occlusive disease of the aortoiliac segment, the surgeon endeavors to return to near normal the inflow to the limbs at the groin while maintaining flow to the internal iliac and visceral branches. Patients who have critical limb ischemia and stenotic aortoiliac disease also commonly have occlusive lesions of the femoral, popliteal, or tibial vessels. While the prevalence of distal femoral-popliteal occlusive disease in patients undergoing repair of an abdominal aortic aneurysm is only ~11%, the prevalence is almost 50% in patients presenting for occlusive aortoiliac procedures. The long-term patency of the aortobifemoral bypass depends on adequate "run-off," that is, the status of distal occlusive disease in the femoral segment. The need for subsequent femoral-popliteal bypass can be reduced greatly if the profunda femoris artery is opened by profundoplasty performed concomitantly with the aortobifemoral bypass. This may prolong surgery but is beneficial to the patient. Despite profundoplasty, some patients will still require subsequent distal revascularization.

Pathophysiology of Aortic Occlusion and Reperfusion

Occlusion of the aorta, particularly at the supraceliac level, has consequences for many organ systems, including the cardiovascular system and visceral organs to which blood flow may be impaired. Supraceliac aortic occlusion carries higher risk for patients, particularly when concomitant renal or visceral revascularization is required. Visceral organ ischemia is usually responsible for mortality rates that can approach 25%, although institutions where these procedures are performed routinely have reported substantially lower mortality rates. Prolonged cross-clamp times are associated with increased risks of visceral ischemia. Complications include renal failure, mesenteric/colonic ischemia, hepatic ischemia with coagulopathy, and spinal cord ischemia.

Arterial hypertension routinely occurs after aortic occlusion. The mechanisms of this response have remained controversial. Beyond increased afterload, etiologies proposed include changes in preload, blood volume distribution, myocardial performance, and activation of the sympathetic nervous system. The pathophysiology of aortic clamping and unclamping has been extensively summarized by Gelman.[158]

The level at which the aorta is occluded affects the degree of hemodynamic response. Blood volume shifts from the lower to upper half of body during high aortic cross-clamp owing to lower splanchnic venous capacitance (Fig. 33-5). Edema of the head and neck often follows supraceliac clamping, and may preclude early extubation. Shifted blood volume results in increased left ventricular preload. Our work using TEE has demonstrated a 28% increase in left ventricular end-diastolic area with supraceliac aortic occlusion (Table 33-8).[159] Most studies concur that cardiac output decreases with supraceliac occlusion,

especially in patients with underlying coronary disease, despite compensatory mechanisms that seek to augment contractility in the setting of elevated preload and afterload (Fig. 33-6). Although elevated systemic arterial pressure may also be helpful by increasing coronary perfusion, increased preload and afterload associated with high thoracic aortic occlusion also increase myocardial oxygen demand and can produce myocardial ischemia. Renin activity increases with suprarenal or infrarenal aortic occlusion and may contribute to hypertension. Epinephrine and norepinephrine levels consistently increase after aortic occlusion. These changes may help the myocardium increase contractility to adapt to elevated afterload and preload, but our work suggests that these responses are associated with postoperative cardiac and renal dysfunction.

Our work with TEE has shown that myocardial dysfunction is routine in patients undergoing supraceliac aortic occlusion. In these patients, mean arterial pressure rises 54%, PCWP rises 38%, and ejection fraction decreases by 38% (Table 33-8). Additionally, 92% of the patients studied had myocardial ischemia, as evidenced by abnormal wall motion and thickening.[159] Abnormal wall motion generally persists despite aggressive nitrate therapy, but usually resolves promptly after aortic unclamping. Therefore, nitrates can also be used to treat increases in preload, but they will not prevent all wall motion abnormalities. Care must be taken when using vasodilators so that decreased blood flow distal to supraceliac aortic occlusion does not promote visceral ischemia (Fig. 33-7). This sets up two competing goals, similar to the conflicts in hemodynamic management for carotid endarterectomy, because a higher blood pressure may be good for vital organ perfusion, but bad for the heart. In general, we tolerate arterial pressures up to 200 mm Hg during supraceliac occlusion, unless other means (discussed below) are used to perfuse the lower part of the body or prolong the tolerable period of visceral ischemia.

Hemodynamic and echocardiographic changes are much more modest in patients undergoing infraceliac or infrarenal aortic occlusion (Table 33-8). The neuroendocrine changes are also less severe in patients undergoing infrarenal aortic occlusion compared with supraceliac occlusion. With infrarenal aortic occlusion, blood volume from the infrasplanchnic vasculature may shift to the compliant splanchnic vasculature, producing relatively small changes in cardiac preload (Fig. 33-5). The hemodynamic responses to cross-clamping and unclamping are further attenuated in patients undergoing aortic occlusion for reconstruction of occlusive disease compared with those having aneurysm repair. Patients with occlusive disease likely have developed collateral circulation, which can continue to perfuse the lower body during aortic cross-clamping.

Unclamping of the thoracic aorta can result in severe hypotension (Fig. 33-8). Reactive hyperemia after reperfusion may be attenuated by aggressive fluid loading just before reperfusion and gradual release of the aortic clamp. Hypotension may also be due to humoral factors. Tissues distal to aortic occlusion become acidotic; however, treatment with bicarbonate does not reliably prevent hypotension upon reperfusion. Treatment with bicarbonate does result in hypercarbia, and ventilation must be increased proportionally.

Humoral factors that may contribute to organ dysfunction after aortic occlusion include acidosis, the renin-angiotensin system, the sympathetic nervous system, oxygen free radicals, prostaglandins, platelet, and neutrophil sequestration, complement activation, and cytokine release. Tissue hypoxia leads to metabolism of ATP, producing adenosine, hypoxanthiane, xanthine oxidase, and oxygen free radicals. Some workers have recommended the use of mannitol before aortic clamping and unclamping because it functions as a hydroxyl free radical scavenger and may prevent tissue injury. Mannitol decreases the production of thromboxane after aortic unclamping, possibly decreasing leukocyte deposition in the lung after aortic surgery.[160] Prostaglandins are increased with aortic occlusion, but

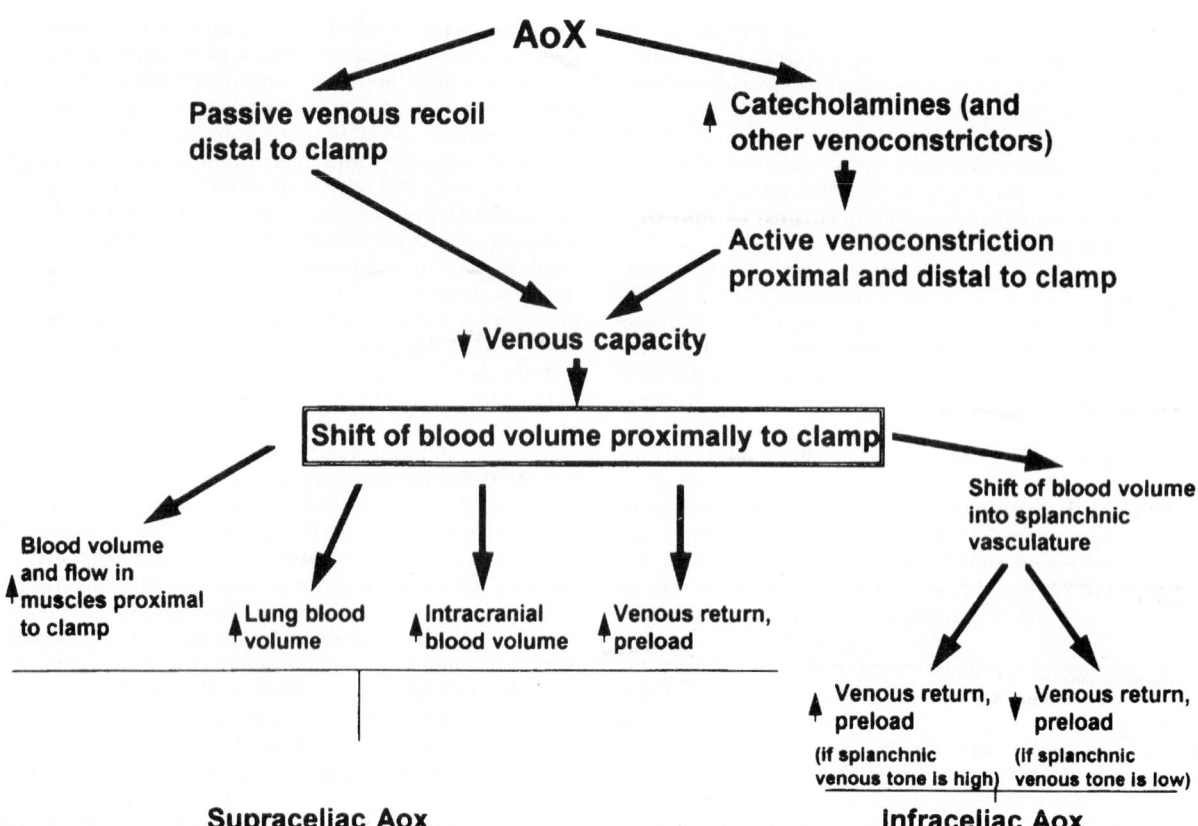

Figure 33-5. Blood volume redistribution during aortic cross-clamping. This schedule depicts the reason for the decrease in venous capacity, which results in blood volume redistribution from the vasculature distal to aortic occlusion to the vasculature proximal to aortic occlusion. If the aorta is occluded above the splanchnic system, the blood volume travels to the heart, increasing preload and blood volume in all organs and tissues proximal to the clamp. However, if the aorta is occluded below the splanchnic system, blood volume may shift into the splanchnic system or into the vasculature of other tissues proximal to the clamp. The distribution of this blood volume between the splanchnic and nonsplanchnic vasculature determines changes in preload. AoX = aortic cross-clamping; ↑ and ↓ = increase and decrease, respectively. (Reprinted with permission from Gelman S: The pathophysiology of aortic cross-clamping and unclamping. Anesthesiology 82:1026, 1995.)

studies are hampered by confounding factors, such as prosta-cyclin release, which can result from mesenteric traction. The response to mesenteric traction can cause profound vasodila-tion and facial flushing, which can be treated with α agonists or nonsteroidal anti-inflammatory drugs (NSAIDs).[161] We ask our surgeons to release mesenteric traction while we restore intravascular volume and provide pharmacologic support of afterload; we generally prefer not to use NSAIDs because of

their effects on platelet function. C3a and C5a increase during abdominal aortic aneurysm surgery and can produce smooth muscle contraction and pulmonary hypertension. Sludging in tissues distal to aortic occlusion may produce microaggregates, which can exacerbate pulmonary and other tissue injury. Hy-poxic insult to the intestines during aortic occlusion and increased gut permeability can produce endotoxemia during aortic reconstruction. After thoracoabdominal aortic recon-

Table 33-8. EFFECT OF LEVEL OF AORTIC OCCLUSION ON CHANGES IN CARDIOVASCULAR VARIABLES

Cardiovascular Variable	% Change in Variable, by Level of Aortic Occlusion		
	Supraceliac	Suprarenal–infraceliac	Infrarenal
Mean arterial blood pressure	54	5*	2*
Pulmonary capillary wedge pressure	38	10*	0*
End-diastolic area	28	2*	9*
End-systolic area	69	10*	11*
Ejection fraction	−38	−10*	−3*
Abnormal motion of wall, % of patients	92	33	0
New myocardial infarctions, % of patients	8	0	0

* Statistically different ($p < 0.05$) from group undergoing supraceliac aortic occlusion.
Adapted with permission from Roizen MF, Ellis JE, Foss JF *et al:* Intraoperative management of the patient requiring supraceliac aortic occlusion. In Veith FJ, Hobson RW, Williams RA, Wilson SE (eds): Vascular Surgery, 2nd ed, p 256. New York, McGraw-Hill, 1994.

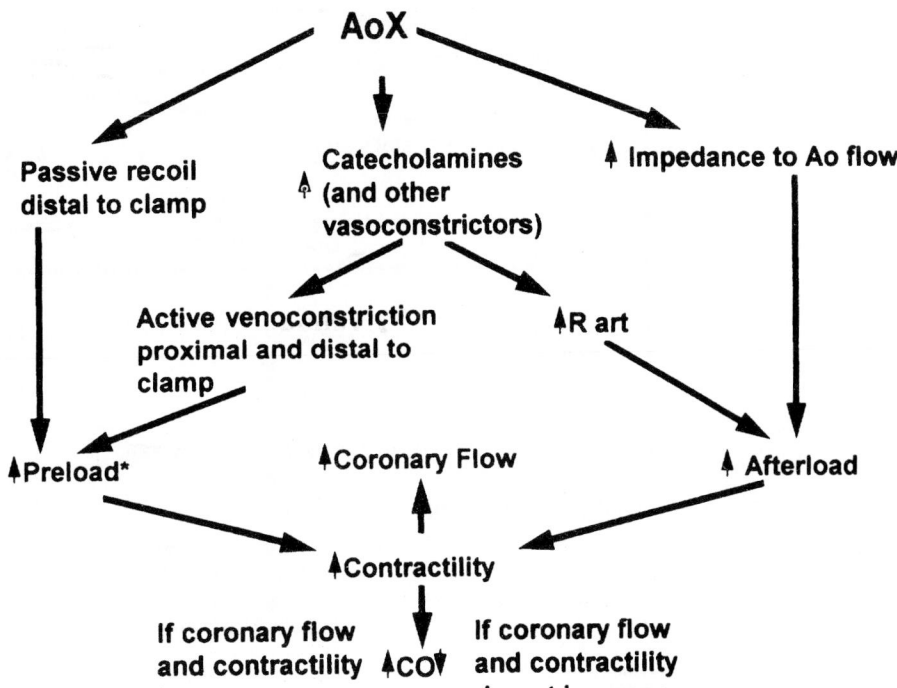

Figure 33-6. Systemic hemodynamic response to aortic cross-clamping. Preload does not necessarily increase. If during infrarenal aortic cross-clamping blood volume shifts into the splanchnic vasculature, preload does not increase (Fig. 33-5). AoX = aortic cross-clamping; Ao = aortic; Rart = arterial resistance; ↑ and ↓ = increase and decrease, respectively; * = different patterns are possible (see Fig. 33-5). (Reprinted with permission from Gelman S: The pathophysiology of aortic cross-clamping and unclamping. Anesthesiology 82:1026, 1995.)

struction, activation of polymorphonuclear leukocytes (PMNs) is highly correlated with plasma endotoxin levels; PMN activation may better predict renal and respiratory failure than aortic cross-clamp times or transfusion requirements.[162]

Aortic aneurysm repair is associated with endotoxin, proinflammatory, and an almost coincidental anti-inflammatory cytokine release.[163] High tumor necrosis factor (TNF) levels may be associated with adverse outcome; however, some studies have suggested that impaired TNF responses are associated with higher APACHE scores and poor outcomes.[164] After open aortic

aneurysm repair, peak plasma concentrations of TNF and interleukin-6 (IL-6) are significantly higher in hypotensive patients and in those who die.[165] During endovascular repair, the release of IL-6 from the aneurysmal thrombus can cause leukocyte stimulation and production of TNF-α.[166] With endovascular repair, intestinal ischemia seems less profound, with different cytokine activation patterns (increased IL-6 in conventional surgery and increased TNF-α in endovascular repair), and less dramatic compared to open techniques.[167] Anesthetic techniques appear to minimally influence inflammatory cytokine stress responses; rather, cytokine responses are greatest with prolonged operative times.[168] Therefore, further research is needed to determine if pharmacologic therapy of the inflammatory response to surgery can reduce morbidity and mortality after aortic reconstruction. High-dose methylprednisolone may be effective in reducing the inflammatory response and its mediators, improving pulmonary function, reducing pain and fatigue, and shortening hospital stay after aneurysm resection. Methylprednisolone also decreases C-reactive protein concentration and suppresses T-cell activation.[169]

Spinal cord ischemia occurs in 1–11% of operations involving repair of the distal descending thoracic aorta.[170] An understanding of the spinal cord blood supply explains this dreaded complication (Fig. 33-9).[171] The two posterior arteries, which together supply only 25% of the blood to the cord, are formed from the anastomoses of the posterior branch of the vertebral artery and the ascending branch of the bifurcation of the second posterior radicular artery. The anterior spinal artery, which supplies blood to the anterolateral 75% of the cord, is formed throughout by a series of radicular arteries. The mid-thoracic region, supplied by the anterior spinal artery, usually receives only one afferent vessel, which arises from a left or right intercostal vessel. The afferent arteries to the posterior spinal cord from T2 to T8 are also poor in collateralization. The blood supply to the thoracolumbar cord (from T8 to the conus terminalis) is derived from the radicular artery known as the artery of Adamkiewicz. It arises from the left side in 60% of cases. In 75% of cases it joins the anterior spinal artery between T8 and T12, and in 10% of cases it joins between L1 and L2. Although other radicular arteries supply this third section, much of the blood

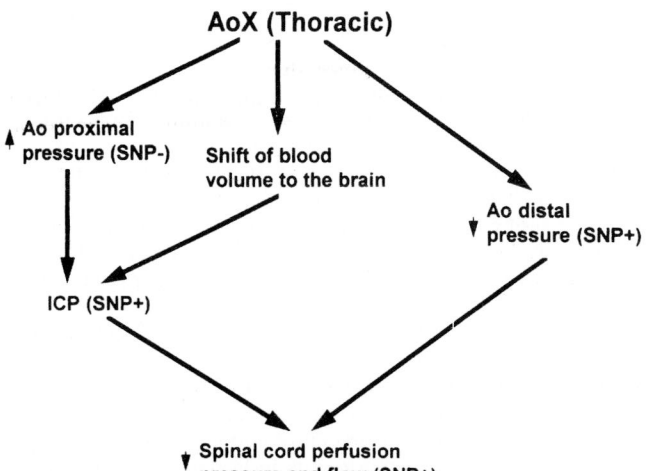

Figure 33-7. Spinal cord blood flow and perfusion pressure during thoracic aortic occlusion, with or without sodium nitroprusside (SNP) infusion. The changes (*arrows*) represent the response to aortic cross-clamping *per se*. SNP+ = SNP aggravates the effect of cross-clamping; SNP– = SNP counteracts the effect of cross-clamping; AoX = aortic cross-clamping; Ao = aortic; ICP = intercranial pressure; ↑ and ↓ = increase and decrease, respectively. (Reprinted with permission from Gelman S: The pathophysiology of aortic cross-clamping and unclamping. Anesthesiology 82:1026, 1995.)

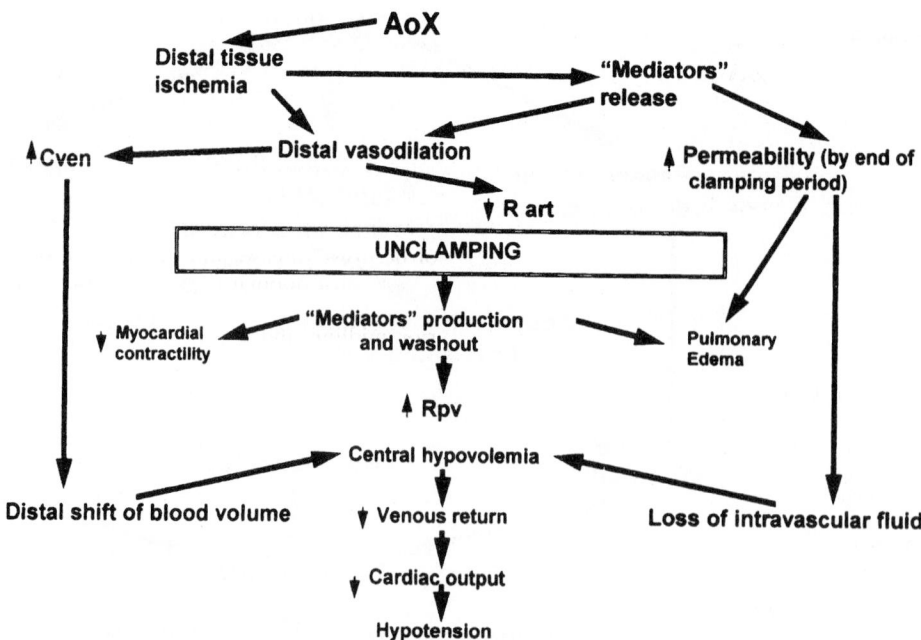

Figure 33-8. Systemic hemodynamic response to aortic unclamping. Preload does not necessarily increase. AoX = aortic cross-clamping; Cven = venous capacitance; Rart = arterial resistance; Rpv = pulmonary vascular resistance; ↑ and ↓ = increase and decrease, respectively. (Reprinted with permission from Gelman S: The pathophysiology of aortic cross-clamping and unclamping. Anesthesiology 82:1026, 1995.)

flow in the anterior spinal artery is dependent on the artery of Adamkiewicz.[172] Because the flow in the spinal arteries is dependent on collateralization and is often bidirectional, the blood supply to the spinal cord can be "stolen" and "given" to the rest of the body when pressures there are lower. Such a situation may arise when a single high aorta-occluding clamp is applied. Spinal cord ischemia is a devastating complication and much energy is spent trying to prevent it. To date, the only definitive preventive methods are fast surgery and maintenance of normal cardiac function.

Infrarenal aortic reconstruction may be associated with a 3% incidence of renal failure, while the rates for supraceliac occlusion may be five times as great. With suprarenal occlusion, renal blood flow decreases by >80%. These significant reductions in renal perfusion are not improved by dopamine or mannitol infusion.[173] Even when the aorta is occluded below the renal arteries, renal hypoperfusion may result. In one study, infrarenal aortic cross-clamping decreased renal blood flow by 38%, increased renal vascular resistance by 75%, and redistributed blood flow from the renal cortex. These changes persisted for at least 1 hr after release of the aortic clamp, but early signs of renal tubular damage, such as the appearance of lysozyme in the urine, were never observed.[174] In one series of patients undergoing thoracoabdominal aneurysm resection, 13% required dialysis; this complication occurred more frequently in patients with preoperative renal dysfunction or a greater extent of the aortic replacement, and in those who developed coagulopathy, paraplegia, or paraparesis. We believe that the incidence of renal failure is related both to the amount of aorta involved and to preoperative renal dysfunction.[39]

Patients undergoing thoracoabdominal aneurysm resection have a particularly high incidence of pulmonary complications. Aortic reperfusion may result in pulmonary sequestration of microaggregates and neutrophils, which may contribute to postoperative respiratory dysfunction. Pulmonary vascular resistance routinely rises after reperfusion; increased permeability and pulmonary edema are not uncommon. As noted above, mannitol may attenuate these responses.[160]

Surgical Procedures for Aortic Reconstruction

In vascular surgery, anesthesiologists serve the patient most effectively by understanding the pathophysiology of the disease and anticipating the surgical approach and techniques. The surgical goal in these operations is to create an enduring restoration of the normal circulation to the viscera while minimizing the duration of ischemia to viscera, especially to the renal circulation.

Generous exposure of the thoracic and abdominal aorta and its major branches can be obtained with a left thoracoabdominal incision and retroperitoneal dissection. The thoracoabdominal approach is favored for complex thoracoabdominal aortic replacement in the presence of stenotic or aneurysmal disease. The visceral branches are often excised from the parent aorta with a button of aortic wall. If the patient also has mesenteric occlusive disease (approximately one-fourth of patients undergoing thoracoabdominal aortic aneurysm surgery), endarterectomy of these branch vessels is performed before they are attached to small openings cut in the graft at appropriate positions. If only mesenteric revascularization is to be performed and aortic replacement is not used, endarterectomy of any or all the major branches of the aorta may be performed with this exposure.

Elective surgery for asymptomatic mesenteric occlusive disease is generally not justified because the risks of surgery often outweigh the possible gains. Perioperative mortality ranges from 7.5–18%. Cardiac disorders, postoperative hemorrhage, and early graft occlusion with bowel infarction are the major causes of perioperative death. Surgery is indicated for symptomatic patients and for a small group of asymptomatic patients with proven major occlusive disease of mesenteric vessels who are to undergo a concomitant intra-abdominal procedure that is likely to interrupt collateral pathways. Such procedures include aortic reconstruction for occlusive or aneurysmal disease and colonic, small bowel, or gastric resections. Surgery may be performed for acute or chronic visceral ischemia. Better long-term results of surgery for chronic visceral ischemia may be obtained in elective procedures by performing as complete a revasculari-

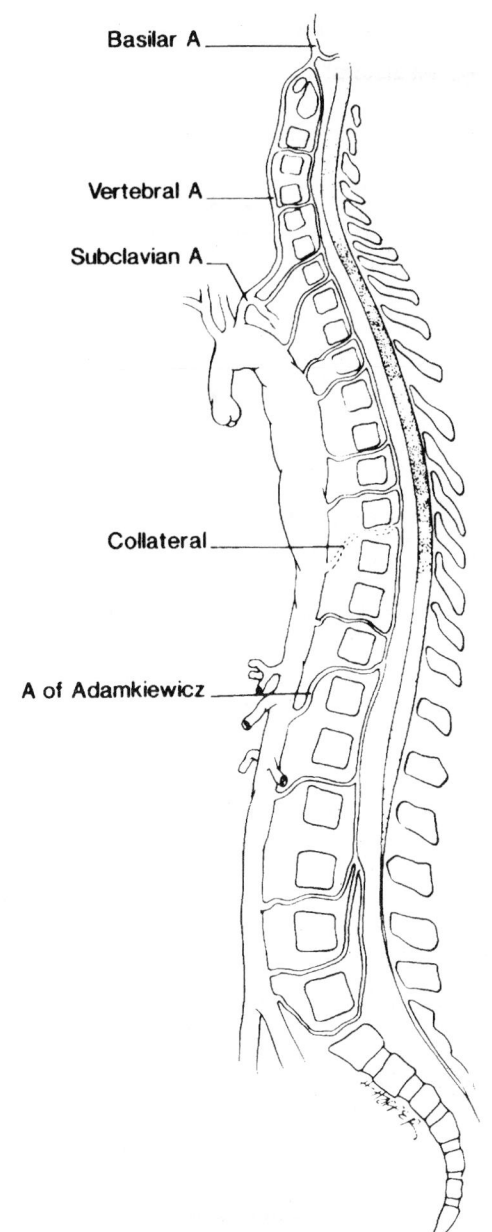

Figure 33-9. The artery of Adamkiewicz usually arises at the T11–12 level and provides the blood supply to the lower spinal cord. Its variable location and the uncertainty of additional collateral blood supply explain, in part, the unpredictability of paraplegia following descending aortic surgery. (Reprinted with permission from Piccone W, DeLaria GA, Najafi H: Descending thoracic aneurysms. In Bergan JJ, Yao JST (eds): Aortic Surgery, p 249. Philadelphia, WB Saunders, 1989.)

Labels in figure: Basilar A, Vertebral A, Subclavian A, Collateral, A of Adamkiewicz

zation as possible. If single-vessel endarterectomy is performed, it may be carried out for either the celiac axis or the superior mesenteric artery. To overcome the problem of kinking from the infrarenal location, surgeons have used externally supported Gore-Tex grafts. A transabdominal approach is satisfactory for most procedures, including supraceliac grafting. A left thoracoretroperitoneal approach, as used for thoracoabdominal aneurysms, may be advantageous for transaortic endarterectomy of the celiac axis and the superior mesenteric artery.

Reconstruction of the infrarenal aorta is performed either to replace a segment in the presence of aneurysmal degenerative disease or to increase inflow to and outflow from a vessel with stenosing occlusive disease. Although the natural history of the two diseases is different, the segmental nature of the disease

processes, with relatively normal vessels above and below the lesion, provides the basis for reconstruction in each. Recommended preoperative evaluations of the patient's anatomy include palpation alone, ultrasonography, computed tomography, digital subtraction angiography, aortography, and magnetic resonance imaging. Aortography exposes the patient to risks and increases costs but allows determination of the presence of iliac occlusive or aneurysmal disease, juxtarenal or suprarenal extension of the aneurysm, renal artery aneurysmal or occlusive disease, and visceral artery lesions.

The most popular surgical exposure for either occlusive or aneurysmal abdominal aortic disease is through a vertical anterior midline abdominal incision, with a transperitoneal approach to the retroperitoneal structures. Another approach gaining favor is a retroperitoneal one anterior to the kidney. In a randomized, prospective trial that compared the transabdominal with the retroperitoneal approach to the aorta for routine infrarenal aortic reconstruction, there was no difference in pulmonary complications. The retroperitoneal approach was associated with less ileus and small bowel obstruction, shorter stays in the hospital and ICU, and lower hospital costs. It was accompanied, however, by an increase in long-term incisional pain.[173]

After the relevant portions of the aorta and the iliac arteries are exposed, the aneurysmal segment of the aorta is replaced with a graft. Before aortic occlusion, heparin is commonly administered systemically to reduce the risk of thromboembolic complications. It is now recognized that distal ischemia complicating aortic surgery is not generally due to thrombosis, but rather to dislodgement of atheroemboli from the diseased aorta. The recognition of the embolic nature of distal ischemic problems suggests that in the absence of major distal occlusive disease, systemic heparinization may be unnecessary in the repair of abdominal aortic aneurysms.

A tube graft (*i.e.,* end-to-end anastomoses on both sides) in which the graft is covered with old aorta is often used for aneurysmal resection. When the iliac vessels are not aneurysmal or stenotic, a tube graft may be used as replacement for the diseased aorta, thus making the procedure faster with less blood loss. The standard graft material, in use since the late 1950s, has been Dacron, in either knitted or woven form. Dacron grafts appear to be associated with rare episodes of anaphylactic reactions, which may be related to the stabilizers used in their manufacture.[175] More recently, polytetrafluoroethylene grafts, which are less porous, have become available.

Arterial reconstruction surgery has been developed on the basis of the principle of anatomic correctness. Although this is usually the easiest and best option, situations do occur that require less advantageous revascularization procedures. Such situations include repeat surgery, surgery for graft infection, the presence of contraindications to transabdominal surgery (*e.g.,* sepsis, adhesions, radiation therapy, malignancy), as well as less traumatic alternatives in frail, elderly, high-risk patients. In general, the price paid when alternative techniques such as axillofemoral bypass are used is reduced long-term patency (~50% at 3 years). Temporary axillofemoral bypass may also be performed to decompress the upper half of the body during surgery requiring thoracic aortic occlusion. Another option for reconstruction in the presence of unilateral iliac occlusive disease is femorofemoral bypass, either alone or in combination with axillo-unifemoral or aorto-unifemoral bypass. These procedures also have lower long-term patency rates than anatomically correct revascularization.

Several situations may cause the surgeon to change from an infrarenal procedure, which is less risky to the heart and other organs, to a suprarenal procedure. Aneurysms of the abdominal aorta involve the pararenal aorta in up to 20% of cases. Also, significant stenosis of the renal artery may coexist and require repair. Significant stenosis of the celiac trunk or superior mesenteric artery may be repaired at the time of abdominal aortic reconstruction. The patient who has previously undergone aortic surgery, para-aortic lymph node dissection, or radiotherapy will frequently require anastomosis to a higher graft origin. Ruptured aneurysms often must be controlled initially by supraceliac clamping. In these cases, great care must be taken so that material is not dislodged into the renal arteries during operative manipulation and clamping.

Endovascular Surgery of Aortic Aneurysms

Endovascular repair has exploded recently.[10] It is associated with less hemodynamic changes,[176] reduced stress responses, lower mortality, and shorter hospital length of stay compared to open surgery.[19] With experience, many centers report an evolution from general anesthetics to regional anesthetics to local with sedation. However, complications can occur, particularly during the early experience ("learning curve") in an institution. A large European registry found that 2.5% of patients underwent a conversion to an open AAA repair; 10% had device-related or procedure-related complications; and 3% had arterial complications.[177] Thirty-day mortality was 2.6% overall, and higher with higher ASA physical classification. Older patients (>75 years), patients with impaired cardiac status, and those considered too "sick" for open surgery had more complications. Myocardial ischemia, angina, and dysrhythmias may result from the fever and tachycardia that routinely occur after endovascular repair. Endoleak (failure to completely exclude the aneurysm sac from the systemic circulation) occurred in 16% immediately after the procedure and in 9% at 30 days, and may require subsequent open operation. We conclude that endovascular procedures show great promise, but their long-term viability remains unknown. These procedures will continue to challenge anesthesiologists, especially when performed in patients who would not have been considered surgical candidates in the past.

Protecting the Spinal Cord and Visceral Organs

Thoracic aortic occlusion reduces distal blood flow tremendously (see Fig. 33-7). In 1–11% of operations involving repair of the distal descending thoracic aorta, spinal cord ischemia does occur. Various strategies have been used to protect the spinal cord from ischemia, including maintenance of proximal hypertension during cross-clamping, local or systemic hypothermia, magnesium, cerebrospinal fluid drainage, papaverine, and a variety of other drugs to protect the brain and spinal cord during resection of abdominal or thoracoabdominal aneurysms or coarctation repairs.[170] Spinal cord sensory-evoked or motor-evoked potentials may prove useful in predicting patients at risk for spinal cord ischemia and in gauging spinal cord protection, but there has not been much experience in the use of the techniques. Spinal cord metabolism can be reduced by moderate hypothermia and high-dose barbiturates. Local hypothermia achieved by infusion of cold saline into the epidural space, when combined with CSF drainage, has been reported to signficantly reduce paraplegia rate.[178] Alternatively, femoral-femoral bypass and deep hypothermic cardiac arrest may be used in patients at high risk of paraplegia.[179] Reperfusion injury may be addressed by the use of mannitol, steroids, calcium channel blockers, and avoidance of hyperglycemia. The multitude of proposed pharmacologic and surgical maneuvers to reduce spinal cord ischemia and neurologic deficits after thoracic aortic occlusion highlights the serious nature of this complication and the lack of consensus on its prevention. Table 33-9 summarizes some of these approaches.[170] We still believe that short cross-clamp times are the common element of successful regimens.

Some surgeons place a Gott shunt, a heparinized tube that can decompress the heart and also provide distal perfusion. The Gott shunt can be placed proximally into the ascending

Table 33-9. METHODS OF SPINAL CORD PROTECTION DURING DESCENDING THORACIC AORTIC SURGERY[170]

Limitation of cross-clamp duration
Distal circulatory support
Reattachment of critical intercostal arteries
CSF drainage
Hypothermia
  Moderate systemic (32–34°C)
  Epidural cooling
  Circulatory arrest
Maintenance of proximal blood pressure
  Pharmacotherapy:
    Systemic:
      Corticosteroids, barbiturates, naloxone, calcium channel antagonists, O₂ free radical scavengers, NMDA antagonists, mannitol, magnesium, vasodilators (adenosine papaverine, prostacyclin), perfluorocarbons, colchicine
    Intrathecal:
      Papaverine, magnesium, tetracaine, perfluorocarbons
Avoidance of postoperative hypotension
Sequential aortic clamping
Enhanced monitoring for spinal cord ischemia
  Somatosensory evoked potentials (SSEP)
  Motor evoked potentials (MEP)
  Hydrogen saturated saline
  Avoidance of hyperglycemia

aorta (the most common site), the aortic arch, the descending aorta, or the left ventricle, and inserted distally into the descending aorta (most commonly), the femoral artery, or the abdominal aorta. Even with a Gott shunt or partial bypass, there is an obligatory time of visceral ischemia when the visceral blood supply arises from a point between the proximal and distal clamps. Placement of a shunt may result in atheroembolism, which can produce rather than prevent ischemic injury and death. Other surgeons may place a temporary *ex vivo* right axillofemoral bypass graft before positioning for thoracotomy. After the thoracic aortic surgery is completed, the axillofemoral graft is removed. The placement of a shunt or distal perfusion attenuates the hemodynamic response to aortic unclamping, reduces acidosis, and could conceivably ameliorate the hormonal and metabolic changes that accompany aortic occlusion.

Other groups have chosen to use partial bypass, either from the left atrium or ascending aorta, to the iliac or femoral artery to provide distal perfusion and decompress the heart. A heat exchanger may be used to induce hypothermia, which may be neuroprotective. Segmental sequential surgical repair may minimize the duration of ischemia to any given vascular bed.[180] Intercostal artery reattachment in hopes of preserving blood flow to the anterior spinal cord may also be beneficial. After reperfusion, the heat exchanger can be used to warm the patient. Other potential advantages of left atrial–left femoral artery shunt with centrifugal pump support are better operative field exposure, afterload reduction, avoidance of clamp injury, and maintenance of stable distal aortic perfusion without heparin.

Using rapid autotransfusion, some surgeons repair aneurysms of the descending thoracic and thoracoabdominal aorta by using an "open" technique, in which a single cross-clamp is placed proximal to the aneurysm to exsanguinate the lower body.[181] A low incidence of spinal cord injury (8.5%) and renal insufficiency (5.6% dialysis) using this technique may result from the free draining of the intercostal and lumbar arteries during aortic occlusion, which decreases cerebrospinal fluid and central venous pressures and increases spinal cord perfusion gradients. A markedly reduced incidence of neurologic deficits has been reported when distal aortic perfusion is combined with drainage of cerebrospinal fluid.[182] Cerebrospinal fluid drainage is used

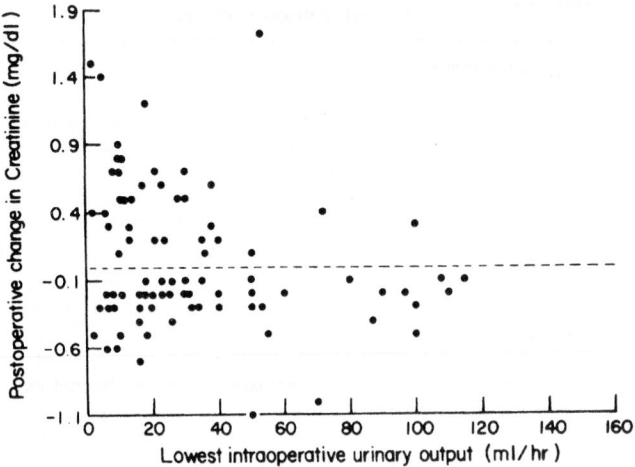

Figure 33-10. Lowest hourly intraoperative urinary output and maximal adverse change in renal function as assayed by change in creatinine from preoperatively to 7 days postoperatively; there was no correlation between lowest intraoperative urinary output and change in renal function postoperatively. (Modified with permission from Alpert RA, Roizen MF, Hamilton WK *et al:* Intraoperative urinary output does not predict postoperative renal function in patients undergoing abdominal aortic revascularization. Surgery 95:707, 1984.)

in the hope of improving the pressure gradient, allowing spinal cord blood flow as aortic occlusion lowers distal arterial pressures and increases the central venous pressure. As in almost all other successful series, patients with short cross-clamp times (<30 min) had fewer neurologic deficits.[170] The new endovascular techniques represent an alternative therapy when anatomy permits; lower paraplegia rates have been reported compared to open surgery.[183]

The development of acute renal failure after aortic reconstruction is associated with a high morbidity and a mortality exceeding 30%.[39] This complication is most frequent in patients with ruptured aneurysms who have significant hypotensive episodes and in those for whom suprarenal aortic clamping is required. Approximately one-fourth of patients undergoing thoracoabdominal aortic aneurysm repair have occlusive visceral disease, which may also be corrected to reduce the risk of renal failure without increasing the risk of gastrointestinal complications. As in the preservation of other organ function, we believe that maintenance of cardiac function represents the best prophylaxis against renal failure.

Previous work from our group has shown that intraoperative urinary output is not predictive of postoperative renal function. In 137 patients undergoing aortic reconstruction (38 at the supraceliac level), we found no significant correlation between intraoperative mean urinary output, or lowest hourly urinary output, and changes from preoperative to postoperative levels of creatinine or blood urea nitrogen (Fig. 33-10).[184] Thus, urinary output, which is believed to be an index of perfusion and is therefore monitored routinely during surgery, was not predictive of postoperative renal function in normovolemic patients. When patients who underwent aortic occlusion at the suprarenal level were compared with those who underwent occlusion at the infrarenal level, there was no difference in postoperative renal function. Rather, preoperative renal dysfunction was the most powerful predictor of postoperative renal dysfunction.

The use of mannitol, furosemide, dopamine, or fenoldopam, however, has not been clearly shown to prevent renal failure.[39] We believe that preoperative renal function and the maintenance of an appropriate intravascular volume and normal myocardial function are the most important determinants of postoperative renal function. Recent work in patients with diabetes

and chronic renal insufficiency undergoing coronary angiography has shown that maintaining intravascular volume is superior to the use of furosemide or mannitol in preventing dye-associated tubular necrosis.[185] These results may be particularly applicable to vascular surgery patients who frequently undergo angiography shortly before surgery.

If prolonged renal ischemia is anticipated, selective profound hypothermia and the direct intra-arterial infusion of mannitol into the kidneys may decrease the incidence of postoperative renal impairment. Our management, however, is biased by the results of our own studies. Thus, when intraoperative urinary output is $<0.125 \text{ mL} \cdot \text{kg}^{-1} \cdot \text{h}^{-1}$, we exclude mechanical problems in urine collection and ensure the adequacy of left-sided cardiac filling volumes or pressures. We then continue to monitor but do not usually treat. Urinary output usually returns to acceptable levels within 2 hr. If it does not, or if we are uneasy about low urinary output, 2–5 mg of furosemide or mannitol $0.25 \text{ g} \cdot \text{kg}^{-1}$ is administered intravenously to stimulate urine production. Dopamine at $3–5 \text{ }\mu\text{g} \cdot \text{kg}^{-1} \cdot \text{min}^{-1}$ may be used, but its prophylactic value has not been proven in patients undergoing aortic surgery.[186] It may even result in visceral hypoperfusion.[187] Thus, virtually all investigators have concluded that maintenance of adequate intravascular volume and myocardial function largely prevents renal insufficiency.

Monitoring and Anesthetic Choices for Aortic Reconstruction

We routinely place arterial catheters in patients undergoing aortic reconstruction. In patients undergoing thoracic aortic clamping with distal perfusion, we may measure distal pressure as well. We also routinely place a pulmonary artery catheter (PAC) in patients undergoing suprarenal aortic cross-clamp, but not in patients when the clamp will be infrarenal. Placement of the PAC can usually wait until induction of anesthesia is completed. In some relatively healthy patients, the risk of pulmonary artery catheterization probably exceeds the benefit.[188,189] However, we do place PACs routinely in patients with a history of congestive heart failure, diabetes with end-organ damage, cor pulmonale, renal insufficiency, or poor left ventricular function on preoperative or intraoperative echocardiography.

For patients undergoing thoracic or thoracoabdominal aortic resection, we may place a dialysis catheter in a femoral or subclavian vein. This large catheter provides two very large-bore sites for transfusion and facilitates postoperative hemodialysis in the unfortunate cases in which renal failure occurs. For a patient undergoing an infrarenal procedure, we are generally satisfied with a 9 French introducer in the right internal jugular vein (with a triple-lumen central venous catheter or a PAC) and a large-bore peripheral iv catheter.

If we elect to drain cerebrospinal fluid, we use two regular epidural trays and place catheters into the intrathecal space at L3–4 and L4–5. We use two catheters because one may kink. We allow cerebrospinal fluid to drain passively, typically removing 50 mL before aortic cross-clamp and another 50 mL during aortic occlusion. Catheters with a one-way pressure valve allow drainage only when the cerebrospinal fluid pressure exceeds 5–10 mm Hg. Some clinicians have used larger needles made specifically for lumbar cerebrospinal fluid drainage[180]; these are placed the night before surgery in case a "bloody tap" results, so that clotting may be assured. We generally wait until coagulopathy, which is common after thoracoabdominal repair, has resolved to remove cerebrospinal fluid drains, usually on the first or second postoperative day.

Virtually all anesthetic techniques and drugs have been used for aortic reconstructive surgery. We believe that our ability to maintain hemodynamic equilibrium and attend to detail is more crucial to outcome than is the choice of drugs.

Halogenated agents produce vasodilation that has advantages and disadvantages. It provides an additional means of controlling afterload and preload but can lead to an increased need for intravascular volume. An increase in intravascular volume can be detrimental at the end of the procedure by causing relative hypervolemia and even pulmonary edema. To prevent this problem, we simulate the increase in central blood volume that occurs with awakening for the 30–45 min of closure by tilting the patient (head lower than feet). Tilting allows one to predict the patient's postanesthetic volume status and make appropriate adjustments. Volatile drugs also permit careful, deliberate induction, manipulation of hemodynamic variables, and adjustment of dose. They can also be used to treat stress-induced increases in left ventricular filling pressures.[190] They provide a moderate degree of muscle relaxation, decreasing the need for muscle relaxants, and increasing the ease of reversing paralysis. Volatile anesthetics also facilitate tracheal extubation at the end of surgery. Thus, the stressful stimuli and hypertension associated with continued intubation of the trachea after surgery are avoided. Also, this approach permits early assessment of neurologic function and the presence of angina (although the vast majority of episodes of postoperative myocardial ischemia are "silent").

Since isoflurane was introduced, we have avoided using halothane; occlusion of the aorta at the supraceliac level tends to make the liver hypoxic for a time during which halothane can, in theory, create a hepatitis-like condition. Isoflurane may be a coronary vasodilator, but it does not appear to place patients at increased risk for myocardial ischemia, infarction, or cardiac death compared with halothane anesthetics.[191] Current FDA labeling suggests that "sevoflurane should be used with caution in patients with renal insufficiency (creatinine >1.5 mg · dL^{-1}). . . . While a level of compound A exposure at which clinical nephrotoxicity might be expected to occur has not been established, it is prudent to consider all of the factors leading to compound A exposure in humans, especially duration of exposure, fresh gas flow rate, and concentration of sevoflurane. . . . Sevoflurane may be associated with glycosuria and proteinuria when used in long procedures at low flow rates."[192]

All commonly used opioids produce similar cardiovascular effects unless they are administered rapidly in large doses. Induction of anesthesia with opioids, which can be accomplished quickly, decreases the cardiac index by a small amount. In sufficient doses, opioids produce analgesia and hypnosis, with only slight decreases in cardiac contractility and blood pressure. Higher doses predictably decrease peripheral vascular resistance, especially when administered after benzodiazepines. With continual infusion of opioids or other drugs, anesthesia can be maintained throughout the surgical procedure. Surgical stimulation after opioid induction significantly increases the heart rate, arterial blood pressure, and systemic vascular resistance. Nitroglycerin, nitroprusside, or a volatile anesthetic can be added to the opioid for manipulation of the circulation during cross-clamping and unclamping.

Nitrous oxide can be used with opioids or with the inhalational drugs. However, it increases afterload and myocardial work while depressing myocardial inotropic performance and output. In one study of patients undergoing abdominal aortic surgery, nitrous oxide increased the need for nitroglycerin to treat elevated PCWP and myocardial ischemia, although clinical outcome was not affected.[193] Nitrous oxide may decrease renal and splanchnic blood flows[194] and may have long-lasting toxic effects by causing nutritional, neurologic, and immunologic deficits. It can also contribute to bowel distention.

Our work[195] suggests that large doses of the synthetic narcotic sufentanil improve patient outcome after aortic reconstruction. In a prospective, controlled study, patients were randomly assigned to receive either an isoflurane- or sufentanil-based anesthetic for aortic reconstruction. Intraoperatively and postoperatively, systemic and pulmonary capillary blood pressures and heart rates were kept within 20% of mean preoperative (baseline) values. Sufentanil anesthesia alone was associated with less major (cardiac and renal) morbidity than isoflurane anesthesia (Table 33-10).[195] Sufentanil may have a protective effect because of its superior blockade of the adrenergic stress response. Further study is needed to determine whether all opioids are protective. A disadvantage of the opioids is that most linger into the postoperative period. However, in >50% of the patients who received a high-dose, opioid–nitrous oxide anesthetic technique (sufentanil 15–20 μg · kg^{-1}) for suprarenal aortic reconstruction, tracheal extubation was accomplished in the operating room. High-dose opioid anesthetics also produce excellent postoperative analgesia.

Combined general-epidural and general-spinal anesthetics have been used successfully for aortic reconstruction.[32,196] A detailed description of the advantages and disadvantages of regional anesthetics can be found below in Lower Extremity Revascularization. For patients requiring thoracotomy, the analgesia provided by thoracic epidural infusion of narcotics and/or local anesthetics may be particularly helpful in improving spirometric function. Thoracic epidural local anesthetics can also dilate coronary arteries[197] and help to prevent stress-induced elevations in PCWP. Some clinicians are reluctant to use epidural anesthesia for supraceliac aortic reconstruction because of concerns about concurrent heparinization and the associated incidence of paraplegia. In such patients, the use of peridural narcotics without local anesthetics can preserve sensory and motor function and can allow early assessment of neurologic integrity. Because urinary catheters are typically left in place for at least 36 hr after aortic reconstruction surgery, urinary retention is not a major issue. We often use intrathecal or epidural narcotics after supraceliac aortic occlusion. Animal studies have shown that intrathecal naloxone improves neurologic function after thoracic aortic occlusion, but results in humans have been inconclusive. Another disadvantage of epidural local anesthetics is that although patients must receive increased amounts of iv fluids, they are still likely to become hypotensive after reperfusion.[198] Therefore, we are prepared for the possibility of fluid overload toward the end of the procedure. Alternatively, infusions of dopamine or dobutamine may be used to maintain systemic vascular resistance and contractility in the presence of the sympathectomy induced by the use of local anesthetics for regional block.[199]

We believe that prophylaxis of stress and pain by any mechanism (epidural anesthetics, opiate infusion, or α_2 agonists) may result in lower morbidity in those least able to tolerate the myocardial and cardiovascular demands of stress.

The choices of muscle relaxants for use today are many. We choose an agent based primarily on the hemodynamic goals, the patient's renal function, and on whether or not the patient's trachea will be extubated in the operating room. We typically use an intermediate-duration relaxant with lower doses of narcotics (or remifentanil) supplemented with volatile anesthetics, propofol, β-adrenergic blocking drugs, or α_2 agonists in patients to be extubated in the operating room. For patients whose lungs will be ventilated postoperatively and who have received high doses of narcotics, we may take advantage of pancuronium's vagolytic effects to prevent severe bradycardia.

Management of Elective Aortic Surgery

We believe that prehydration reduces variations in blood pressure on induction of anesthesia. After the patient's preoperative condition has been optimized, the range of hemodynamic variables for that patient is determined. The anesthetic management is then planned to keep the patient within 20% of this range, as long as the PCWP does not exceed 15 mm Hg, the heart rate does not exceed 80–90 beats · min^{-1}, and signs of organ ischemia are absent. We typically provide premedication with the patient's usual medications and fentanyl 1–2 μg · kg^{-1} iv and 1–2 mg midazolam iv in the holding area (these dosages are reduced for old age, debility, or pulmonary disease). Anti-

Table 33-10. MORBIDITY AFTER AORTIC RECONSTRUCTION WITH EITHER OF TWO DIFFERENT ANESTHETIC AGENTS

Morbidity	Isoflurane-Based Anesthetic ($n = 50$)	Sufentanil-Based Anesthetic ($n = 46$)
Renal insufficiency	16	4*
Congestive heart failure	13	4*
Ventilation > 24 hr	9	4
Pneumonia	2	1
Renal failure	3	1
Stroke	2	0
Myocardial ischemia	0	1
Death	2	1
Important or severe complications	20	9*
Important or severe complications and failure	17	7*

* $p < 0.05$ by Fisher's exact test.
Modified with permission from Benefiel DJ, Roizen MF, Lampe GH et al: Morbidity after aortic surgery with sufentanil versus isoflurane anesthesia. Anesthesiology 65:A516, 1986.

cholinergic drugs are usually avoided because they produce dry mouth and tachycardia, which increases myocardial oxygen consumption. The patient should be given antihypertensive medication, including diuretics, before being brought to the operating room. Many diabetic patients who require insulin are given an insulin infusion throughout surgery. Preoperative considerations and drug therapy for diabetic patients have already been described earlier in this chapter.

In the preoperative holding area or in the operating room, the monitors and catheters that are needed for induction of anesthesia are placed, usually a radial artery catheter in the nondominant hand, a manual blood pressure cuff, pulse oximeter, ECG (leads II and V_5), ST-segment trend monitor, precordial stethoscope, a 16-gauge iv line, and, occasionally, a central venous or pulmonary artery catheter.

Our anesthetic technique using sufentanil is as follows. After 3 mg of d-tubocurarine is given, an infusion of 750 μg of sufentanil in 100 mL of saline is begun at a rate of about 15–50 μg $\cdot$ min^{-1} $\cdot$ 70 kg^{-1}, and the patient is coached to breathe 100% oxygen from a face mask. After about 3 min, 75 mg of thiopental iv is administered, and 0.1 mg $\cdot$ kg^{-1} pancuronium or vecuronium is given over 3–5 min. When the depth of anesthesia is judged adequate by the lack of response to Foley catheter insertion or by pinpoint pupils, and when muscle relaxation is adequate, the trachea is intubated and mechanical ventilation begun with 0–60% nitrous oxide in oxygen. The remainder of the pre-cross-clamping phase is devoted to meticulous attention to the details of maintaining temperature homeostasis (unless hypothermia is desired for its potential spinal cord protection): maintaining volume homeostasis as judged by heart rate, blood pressure, pulmonary capillary pressure, or central venous pressure; maintaining left ventricular end-diastolic volume as assessed by echocardiography; ensuring absence of organ ischemia; monitoring (but usually not treating) urine output; and keeping systemic and pulmonary blood pressures and heart rate in the patient's usual range. Every increase in blood pressure or heart rate is either anticipated or treated as soon as it occurs with 25–50 μg of sufentanil. Further increases are treated with repeated doses, or with the addition of nitroglycerin or nitroprusside, volatile anesthetic, esmolol, or propranolol, depending on the event and the suspected cause.

For the half hour immediately before cross-clamping and aortic occlusion, the patient is kept slightly hypovolemic by examining the ventricular volume by means of echocardiography or by keeping PCWP at 5–15 mm Hg. At the time of occlusion we are prepared to give a vasodilating drug through an iv catheter placed specifically for that purpose to avoid hypotension from an accidental bolus of vasodilator. This catheter site is often the third lumen of a triple-lumen central venous catheter or pulmonary artery catheter. The difference in our management of aortic occlusion at different levels (e.g., supraceliac versus infrarenal) is that we rigorously and meticulously plan the management and execute the procedure for all occlusions at renal vessels or above.

Without evidence to the contrary, it is assumed that a little hypertension is just as harmful as a little hypotension. For example, in extreme cases, we might permit the systolic blood pressure of a patient whose preoperative range is 110–170 mm Hg to decrease to as low as 90 mm Hg, or to increase to as high as 190 mm Hg. If values approach or exceed these limits, we execute our contingency treatment plan. Hypertension may be treated by increasing the amount of anesthetic, infusing nitroprusside, or tilting the patient head-up. Hypotension may be treated by placing the patient in a head-down position, infusing more fluid, or beginning a dilute infusion of phenylephrine at a rate that restores systolic blood pressure to ~100 mm Hg.

Our accepted range for the patient's heart rate is similarly based on preoperative determinations. If a normal range of 60–90 beats $\cdot$ min^{-1} is established preoperatively, we initiate treatment once these limits are exceeded intraoperatively. Bradycardia is better tolerated than tachycardia during these operations, because minimizing myocardial oxygen demand is one of our primary concerns. If the intravascular fluid volume is acceptable, we treat tachycardia aggressively, by increasing the level of anesthesia with more opioid or volatile agent, or with an iv infusion of a β-adrenergic receptor blocking drug. Imaging with TEE allows some latitude in the range of acceptable values before intervention must be undertaken. However, PCWPs are not allowed to remain abnormal—i.e., <5 mm Hg or >15 mm Hg—during this procedure, assuming that these values correlate with the echocardiographic values. Increases in pulmonary artery pressures are treated aggressively with more anesthetic, nitroglycerin, or nitroprusside. For low filling pressures, more fluid is infused, except in the 1- or 2-min interval immediately before application of the aortic cross-clamp.

Our approach is different when we are concerned about spinal cord perfusion in patients whose aorta will be occluded at the thoracic level without distal perfusion. In these instances, we will accept some proximal hypertension while the aorta is occluded in the hope of obtaining higher distal perfusion pressures and preventing distal ischemia. This choice may come at the expense of myocardial well-being.

The application of a cross-clamp to the supraceliac aorta probably produces the greatest hemodynamic stress ever experienced by a patient. In fact, 92% of the patients we studied had ischemia, as evidenced by abnormal motion and thickening of the left ventricle (see Table 33-8).[159] More distal levels of temporary occlusion are less stressful hemodynamically. Stabilizing pulmonary and systemic arterial pressures by administering vasodilating drugs before and during suprarenal cross-clamping may not be sufficient to normalize myocardial performance. We have used phosphodiesterase inhibitors, which increase contractility and reduce afterload, before application of the aortic cross-clamp, but we still see myocardial dysfunction with supraceliac occlusion.

Another technique for maintaining normal volumes during cross-clamping is controlled volume depletion, that is, the removal of a specific amount of blood from the patient just before or during application of the cross-clamp for a short period of time. During the minutes remaining just before the cross-clamp is removed, this amount of blood is replaced. Although we have used this technique, we do not advocate its routine use. A third technique for maintaining normal hemodynamic values is the use of volatile anesthetics, rather than nitroglycerin or nitroprusside, as the vasodilating agent. This technique is usually effective, but close observation is necessary to ensure that myocardial dilation and dysfunction do not occur. The kinetics of desflurane may make it suitable for use in this manner with infrarenal aortic occlusion.

Administration of exogenous vasoconstrictors is avoided if possible. In patients undergoing carotid endarterectomy, phenylephrine doubles the incidence of wall motion abnormalities observed by echocardiography in patients whose blood pressure is maintained simply by light anesthesia and endogenous vasoconstrictors.[84] Phenylephrine causes the heart to dilate in patients with coronary artery disease, whereas norepinephrine raises blood pressure without causing myocardial depression.[126]

To ensure adequate volume at the time of cross-clamp removal, blood lost during occlusion is replaced with crystalloid or colloid, warmed cell-saver blood or banked blood to keep the hematocrit slightly above 30%, because it will decrease to 30% in the postocclusion period. We believe that this is the minimal acceptable value for patients in this risk group.[100] Guided by filling pressures or echocardiographic estimates of volume, we are careful not to dilate the left ventricle to an abnormal size.

We routinely use autotransfusion devices and prefer to have a second person (usually a technician) to operate them. We continue to do this even though a recent trial suggests that autotransfusion devices do not reduce transfusion of allogenic blood.[200] After the sixth unit of blood has been given and if more blood loss is anticipated, or after 8 units of blood has been administered, 10 units of platelets is requested for the patient (and occasionally 2 units of fresh frozen plasma). After giving 8–10 units of packed cells, we routinely administer 1 unit of fresh frozen plasma for each unit of packed cells. When no more blood is at hand, and if it is absolutely necessary (i.e., when colloid or crystalloid cannot be used), the best available type-specific, washed packed cells are administered.

Because a large part of the vascular tree is excluded from circulation during temporary aortic occlusion, blood loss can be considerable during supraceliac cross-clamping without the onset of hypotension or tachycardia. Therefore, if we find ourselves decreasing the concentration of volatile anesthetic or the infusion rate of vasodilators, or worse, find ourselves giving vasopressors while the aorta is still occluded, we order more blood and seek to correct what is now severe hypovolemia. Observation of the surgical field and close communication between anesthesiologist and surgeon are of key importance. Evisceration of bowel, often necessary for optimal exposure of the thoracoabdominal aorta, further depletes intravascular volume. Blood loss into the pleural or retroperitoneal cavity may not be readily detected. Watching the volumes in the suction bottles supplements the data, as does observation of left ventricular cavity size on echocardiography.

Thus, immediately before and during removal of the cross-clamp, we stop infusing vasodilators. We allow blood pressure, PCWP, and filling volumes to go as high as possible without

the occurrence of myocardial ischemia. The surgeon then opens the aorta gradually to ensure that severe hypotension does not develop and that there is not too much bleeding from the suture line. Pathophysiologic events on removal of the aortic cross-clamp are associated with inadequate preload. We therefore infuse crystalloid, colloid, or blood; usually, 2 units of banked or cell-saver blood is pressured into venous access sites just before reperfusion. Guided by filling pressures or echocardiographic estimates of volume, or both, we are careful not to dilate the left ventricle.

Moderate hypotension (i.e., a decrease in systolic pressure of 40–60 mm Hg) typically accompanies removal of the aortic cross-clamp, regardless of whether the clamp is replaced infrarenally or so that blood flow to only one leg is obstructed. Our observations of the echocardiogram lead us to believe that hypotension is caused mainly by relative volume depletion. If hypotension persists for more than 4 min after removal of the clamp and does not return toward normal after blood deficits have been replaced, we search for other causes, including hidden blood loss or myocardial dysfunction. Myocardial dysfunction may be caused by inadequate metabolism of the citrate present in replacement blood; such blood has not yet gone to the liver, where citrate is metabolized. This problem can be treated by administration of calcium, which is chelated by citrate. If necessary, the surgeon can reclamp or occlude the aorta, preferably below the renal arteries. Thus, volume replacement and maintenance are mainstays of therapy before, during, and immediately after removal of the aortic cross-clamp. At this point in the procedure, pulmonary artery pressures may not be low on the oscilloscope because reperfusion of ischemic tissues is associated with the release of lactic acid and other unknown mediators that can cause pulmonary vasoconstriction. Mannitol prophylaxis may prevent part of this response, and we frequently give mannitol 0.5-1.0 $g \cdot kg^{-1}$ immediately before release of the clamp.[160] Removal of the clamp from the second leg usually causes fewer hemodynamic effects, presumably because of collateral blood vessels across the pelvis.

During closure, we again ensure adequate organ perfusion as well as hemodynamic and temperature homeostasis, and we reverse the effects of muscle relaxants. Reversal is easier when patients are warm. Hypothermia after aortic reconstruction is associated with other complications, including coagulopathy, low cardiac output states, and significantly higher incidences of organ dysfunction and death. Whether hypothermia causes these problems or is a marker for sicker patients who undergo more extensive operations is unclear. We routinely use forced-air warming on the upper portion of the body in these patients, although their lateral position and extensive exposure during thoracic procedures make maintaining normothermia difficult.

During emergence from anesthesia, we use infusions of nitroglycerin and esmolol or another β-adrenergic blocking agent to prevent hemodynamic variations outside the patient's normal range. If ventilation is adequate (as is common 6 hr after an initial dose of sufentanil), the trachea is extubated; otherwise, controlled ventilation is maintained until spontaneous ventilation is judged adequate. If we elect to use a predominantly inhalational anesthetic technique, we often place an epidural catheter and administer epidural local anesthetics and opioids for postoperative analgesia. When the sufentanil-based technique described above is used, rarely is much additional pain therapy needed for 24 hr. Continuing care into the postoperative period is important for patient outcome.

Anesthesia for Emergency Aortic Surgery

The most common cause of emergency aortic reconstruction is a leaking or ruptured aortic aneurysm. Ruptured aneurysms can be atherosclerotic, mycotic, syphilitic, or inflammatory, or may occur in patients with the marfanoid syndrome. Ruptured aneurysms carry associated mortality roughly ten times greater than elective repair.[201] Therefore, efforts should be made to increase the number of elective operations performed for aortic aneurysms before they rupture, as urgent/emergent surgery is associated with increased mortality even in the absence of frank rupture.

Symptoms of ruptured abdominal aortic aneurysms include pain, faintness or frank collapse, and vomiting. Pain in the back, abdomen, or both is almost always present. Therefore, many surgeons believe that pain in combination with a known abdominal aortic aneurysm or pulsatile abdominal mass indicates dissection or rupture and the immediate need for surgical exploration until proved otherwise. Ruptures most commonly occur into the retroperitoneum. This site permits tamponade of the hemorrhage; however, retroperitoneal hemorrhage and subsequent hematoma can displace the left renal vein, inferior vena cava, and intestine, possibly leading to damage to these structures during the surgical approach. Venous hemorrhage is often much more difficult to control than arterial hemorrhage.

Approximately 25% of aneurysms rupture into the peritoneal cavity, a site associated with a great degree of exsanguination. Other sites of rupture include adjacent structures after formation of fistulae with the inferior vena cava, iliac veins, or renal veins. Aortoenteric fistulae most commonly rupture into the fixed third position of the duodenum. These fistulae usually occur between the overlying bowel and a portion of the aorta that has previously undergone resection and grafting for an existing aneurysm. The mortality from these fistulae is high, often exceeding 50%. In rare cases, an abdominal aortic aneurysm may dissect proximally, resulting in hemopericardium. The overall mortality rates vary in published series from 15–90%, and the time from the onset of symptoms to control of bleeding appears to be the key to determining outcome. The importance of controlling bleeding gives credence to the inescapable sense of urgency that accompanies such events. Other factors that adversely affect outcome are a history of chronic hypertension, age >80 years, heart disease, renal insufficiency, a hematocrit <32.5% at diagnosis, hypotension at diagnosis, surgery lasting >400 min, hypotension lasting >110 min, a systolic blood pressure <100 mm Hg at the end of the operation, and blood loss >11,000 mL.[202]

Management of hemodynamically unstable patients is challenging. Shock frequently accompanies rupture. However, the absence of hypotension does not rule out the possibility of rupture, and shock may occur suddenly. Patients with dissection may have severe hypertension, which must be controlled immediately if rupture is to be prevented. Rapid diagnosis with immediate laparotomy and control of the proximal aorta are of the highest priority. If systolic blood pressure is <90 mm Hg, some clinicians advocate the administration of oxygen by face mask, with tracheal intubation performed only after proximal control of the aorta has been achieved. Because experienced anesthesia personnel can usually intubate the trachea rapidly, and because of the substantial threat of aspiration pneumonitis, we prefer an awake intubation or a rapid-sequence tracheal intubation after small doses of etomidate (0.1 mg · kg^{-1}) and a steroid. We believe that this method causes little morbidity, creates only a slight delay, and prevents a potentially serious complication. However, if the patient has lost consciousness or has marked hypotension unresponsive to rapid volume infusion, the probability of rupture into the free peritoneal cavity is high. In this case, the trachea is immediately intubated in a rapid-sequence fashion, usually with the aid of muscle relaxants and perhaps a small dose of etomidate; ventilation with 100% oxygen is also started. Almost simultaneously, laparotomy is begun so that the surgeon can clamp the aorta.

We attempt to replace volume to normalize systemic blood pressure (at this time, often the only guide to volume replacement in the patient with an uncontained rupture). However, when rupture is suspected, rapid control of the proximal portion of the aorta is probaby more important than is optimizing

the patient's preoperative condition. A difference from elective surgery is that heparin is not administered before aortic cross-clamping.

The patient is resuscitated quickly (before induction of anesthesia, if possible) with type-specific non–cross-matched blood and crystalloid administered via large-bore venous catheters by roller pumps or pressured bags. If type-specific blood is not available, O-negative washed red blood cells may be given. We emphasize the importance of large-bore catheters placed in the most easily accessible vein. A 14-gauge catheter placed in each antecubital fossa is more useful for rapid volume expansion than are attempts at placement of a pulmonary artery catheter. We recommend the use, when possible, of fluid warmers that deliver rapid volumes of normothermic fluids.

Once the aorta is controlled with a cross-clamp and blood pressure and perfusion are restored, additional venous access and a radial, brachial, or axillary arterial line are secured. It is often necessary to have a second anesthesiologist secure vascular access while the first is securing the airway, monitoring blood pressure, and administering volume. Attention may be turned to placing a pulmonary artery catheter once blood pressure is adequate. Even more quickly, an echocardiographic probe can be inserted for rapid assessment of left ventricular volume and contractility. At this point, volume administration is guided by means of PCWP or by the echocardiogram (left ventricular end-diastolic area). High-normal filling pressures are desirable for attenuation of hypotension after removal of the aortic clamp. Some patients with hemorrhagic shock will require infusions of dopamine, epinephrine, or norepinephrine to sustain an adequte blood pressure even after restoration of normal blood volume. Recent work suggests that vasopressin may be particularly effective in restoring blood pressure when hemorrhagic shock is resistant to catecholamines.[203] These patients are often profoundly acidotic; if we administer sodium bicarbonate, we increase ventilation to help eliminate the extra carbon dioxide produced. Augmentation of cardiac output with dopexamine increases oxygen delivery perioperatively, with only limited increase in total body or myocardial oxygen demand, and may improve survival.[204] However, similar studies with dobutamine have yielded opposite conclusions.[205] At the present time, given the high incidence of cardiac-related morbidity, we restrict our use of inotropic support to patients with hypotension or low cardiac output (cardiac index <2 L · min^{-1} · m^{-2}) despite adequte filling pressures. We do not hesitate to paralyze and administer propofol, midazolam, and/or opioids to these patients if they are hemodynamically stable, because they usually require postoperative mechanical ventilation of the lungs and sedation to minimize cardiovascular stress. The acute respiratory distress syndrome (ARDS) develops frequently in patients who survive surgery for a ruptured aneurysm. Recent advances in ventilation strategies for patients with the ARDS may include permissive hypercapnea, "open lung" (high PEEP to optimize lung compliance) ventilation, noninvasive ventilation, and aggressive CPAP trials. These approaches may reduce the length of postoperative ventilation, reduce cytokine release,[206] and even reduce mortality.[207]

Hemodynamically stable patients constitute a second group of patients in whom shock is reversible with volume administration. In such patients, it may be assumed that hemorrhage has been at least partially contained. However, because rapid exsanguination can occur at any time, patients are transported immediately to the operating room for emergency laparotomy, and the same urgency is maintained. Venous access is then ensured. If the blood pressure and heart rate are stable when the patient arrives, sterile preparation of the abdomen is begun. The intravascular volume status may be assessed by observation of the patient for a decrease in systemic blood pressure or an increase in the heart rate when the head is raised 10–15 degrees. Administration of a 25-mg bolus of thiopental iv may also aid in the assessment of volume. Normally, induction of anesthesia is delayed until the patient's abdomen is prepared and draped and the surgeon is ready. Thus, in this situation, minimal extra time is spent on inserting and attaching monitors.

Preoxygenation is followed by rapid-sequence induction of anesthesia with small doses of a narcotic and an induction agent, often etomidate, a rapidly acting muscle relaxant, application of cricoid pressure, and tracheal intubation. To blunt the hemodynamic effects of laryngeal visualization and tracheal intubation, one may administer an iv bolus of lidocaine or esmolol, or an additional narcotic or an induction agent. However, hypotension may easily occur following induction, in which case we administer 100% oxygen, elevate the patient's legs, and rapidly administer blood and fluids. If these measures fail to restore adequate blood pressure and perfusion, we infuse phenylephrine or dopamine until the aorta can be occluded.

Because of hypothermia from massive fluid resuscitation and the aortic occlusion above the hepatic artery, replacement blood may not pass through the liver in amounts adequate to allow for metabolism of citrate. Therefore, if either hypotension due to poor myocardial contractility (which may be easily assessed with echocardiography) or coagulopathy develops, administration of calcium may be therapeutic. It has been suggested that the aggressive fluid resuscitation of trauma patients in the emergency room before transport to the operating room may result in increased mortality, perhaps by causing hypothermia or dilutional coagulopathy, or by raising blood pressure and increasing bleeding.[208] At present, however, we cannot recommend allowing patients to remain hypotensive but believe that attention should be paid to maintaining temperature, adequate hematocrit, and coagulation in addition to simply normalizing intravascular volume.

We routinely use autotransfusion in patients with actual or suspected rupture of an aortic aneurysm, even though a recent study questions its effectiveness in reducing transfusion requirements.[200] This device can be operated by a separate team, allowing the primary anesthesiologist to direct all of his or her attention to the patient's volume status, gas exchange, and depth of anesthesia. Our mnemonic for treatment of such patients is "wovcath," for wonder what (if any) anesthetic to give, oxygen, vecuronium, coagulation, acid-base change, temperature change, and hemodynamic change. This mnemonic lists, in reverse order, the important aspects of patient care that we try to remember when everything about these patients invites disorganization.

After successful surgery for ruptured abdominal aortic aneurysm, the survival rate is about 50% at one month and 33% at 3 years, much lower than survival rates after elective operation. Survival is highest if intraoperative urine output is >200 mL and respiratory failure or myocardial infarction does not occur. The decision to repair a ruptured abdominal aortic aneurysm can be made on clinical grounds. However, after surgery (when information on intraoperative and postoperative variables is also available), these prognostic variables assist clinical judgment and guide discussions of prognosis with the family.[202]

The complications that occur during aortic occlusion can usually be linked to the heart, central nervous system, or kidneys. Organ dysfunction can be minimized by maintaining intraoperative values for hemodynamic variables within the normal preoperative range, ensuring that cardiac dilation does not occur at any point, and minimizing episodes of tachycardia. Attention to the details of preoperative drug therapy, preoperative hydration, and temperature homeostasis may also promote an improved outcome. Further, vigilance must continue into the postoperative period if morbidity and mortality are to be minimized. As opposed to elective aortic reconstruction, in which preserving myocardial function is the primary goal, in emergency resection the crucial factor for patient survival is first rapid control of blood loss and reversal of hypotension, and then preservation of myocardial function.

LOWER EXTREMITY REVASCULARIZATION

The number of patients undergoing lower extremity revascularization has increased as surgeons attempt to improve functional status in elderly patients. In our institution, many vascular patients undergo revision or repeat operations. They often have complex medical histories and diseases of multiple organ systems. Their coexisting diseases present additional challenges beyond those of routine anesthetic management. Despite this fact, patients are now frequently admitted to the hospital on the day of surgery. For others, surgery is emergent or urgent. In all of these situations, the primary goal of anesthetic management is to prevent the development of perioperative complications. These patients are at particularly high risk for perioperative cardiac complications including myocardial ischemia and infarction, low cardiac output (forward failure), and pulmonary edema (backward failure). Krupski et al[43] have shown that the incidence of cardiac morbidity after infrainguinal procedures may exceed that associated with abdominal aortic procedures because patients scheduled for distal procedures often have more preoperative cardiac risk factors than patients scheduled for aortic procedures. Patients undergoing lower extremity revascularization may also receive less attentive care than patients undergoing "major" procedures.

In addition to maintaining adequate cardiac function, another goal of our anesthetic and perioperative care is to assure adequate perfusion and prevent hypercoagulable responses to surgery so as to maintain graft patency in the immediate postoperative period. Pulmonary, renal, neurologic, and hepatic dysfunction may occur following vascular surgery; proper intraoperative and postoperative management may help to prevent these adverse outcomes as well. Vascular surgery represents a tremendous stress to patients whose reserve is already marginal, as suggested by the increased mortality of patients who receive surgery rather than thrombolytic therapy for acute limb ischemia.[209] Anesthetic techniques that reduce the stress response may improve outcome. We believe that ideal anesthetic management of these patients may decrease morbidity and mortality and hasten recovery and hospital discharge. These combined effects should increase the cost-effectiveness of lower extremity revascularization.

The number of patients undergoing arterial reconstruction with angioplasty as well as surgically is increasing in the United States, while the rate of amputation has remained stable.[210] Because some patients may undergo multiple procedures, an anesthesiologist may become cynical about the effectiveness of lower extremity revascularization; but long-term patency and limb-salvage rates are good, demanding that anesthesiologists do all they can to optimize outcome in these procedures (Fig. 33-11).[211] The typical cost of a limb-salvage procedure approaches $20,000, which may be less than the costs of amputation when rehabilitation and the loss of independence are considered.

There are three clinical indications for elective surgery for chronic peripheral occlusive disease: (1) claudication, (2) ischemic rest pain or ulceration, and (3) gangrene. Patients with claudication have symptoms on walking that are relieved by rest. Such patients are not at significant risk for imminent limb loss. Patients with rest pain, ulceration, or gangrene are at variable risk for imminent limb loss and may have severe progressive ischemia. Thus, reconstruction for such patients is semiurgent or urgent. When a patient presents with a gangrenous (black) or pregangrenous (blue) toe, several causes other than progression of chronic arteriosclerotic occlusive disease must be considered. Local infection is particularly common in diabetic patients. Emboli may originate from the heart, a proximal aneurysm, or any proximal atherosclerotic lesion. Intra-arterially administered lytic agents, particularly urokinase, may have been administered, precluding regional anesthesia.[32]

Vascular reconstruction procedures are generally categorized

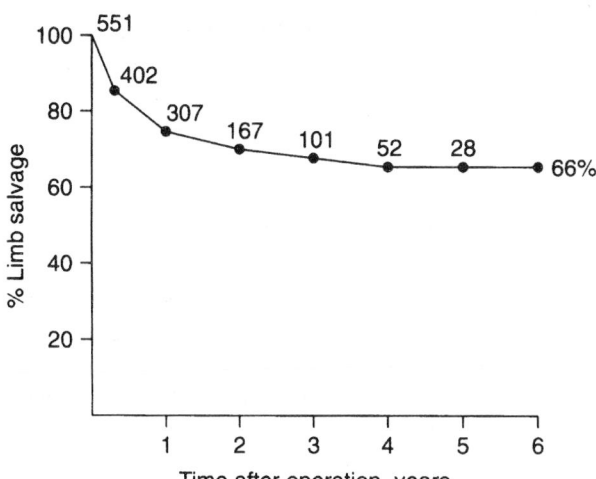

Figure 33-11. Cumulative life-table of limb salvage rates of all patients undergoing reconstructive arterial operations for limb-threatening infrainguinal arteriosclerosis. The number with each point indicates the number of cases observed with intact limbs for that length of time. (Reprinted with permission from Veith FJ, Panetta TF, Wengerter KR *et al:* Femoro-popliteal-tibial occlusive disease. In Veith FJ, Hobson RW, Williams RA, Wilson SE (eds): Vascular Surgery, 2nd ed, p 421. New York, McGraw-Hill, 1994.)

as either inflow or outflow procedures. Inflow reconstruction involves bypass of the obstruction in the aortoiliac segment, whereas outflow procedures are those performed distal to the inguinal ligament for bypass of femoral-popliteal or distal obstructions. The most common inflow reconstruction procedure for obstructions in the aortoiliac segment is aortofemoral bypass. The usual vascular reconstruction below the inguinal ligament is a bypass graft that originates in the common femoral artery and extends to the popliteal or tibial artery. Such a bypass may be performed with a reversed saphenous vein, the saphenous vein *in situ,* or a prosthetic graft.

The complexity of femoral-popliteal and femorotibial bypass varies widely. The site for distal anastomosis and the quality of the outflow vessels are assessed by preoperative angiography. Prosthetic bypasses can be performed more quickly and require less dissection than the saphenous vein bypass, because it is not necessary to make multiple incisions for vein harvest. Prosthetic bypasses, however, have significantly lower patency rates than saphenous vein bypasses, particularly when they extend below the knee. The best short- and long-term results are achieved with the saphenous vein, but this technique requires longer operative time and greater technical expertise than are needed for prosthetic grafts. The duration and complexity of the operation are usually determined by the quality of the saphenous vein and the quality and size of the distal outflow vessels.

In a reversed saphenous vein bypass, the vein is dissected, all branches are ligated and divided, and the vein is excised. The direction of the saphenous vein is reversed to permit blood flow in the direction of the valves, and the vein is tunneled from the femoral artery to the distal vessel. The use of the vein *in situ* offers significant advantages over the reversed-vein bypass; because the vein is not removed from its bed, it is subjected to little trauma; twisting or kinking is unlikely. These advantages have improved patency rates. The use of intraluminal angioscopy is reported to result in better vein preparation, smaller incisions, improved patency, and shorter hospital stay.[212] The quality of the repair is determined from the pulse quality, Doppler ultrasound studies, or completion angiography.

The surgeons' concerns for patients with peripheral vascular insufficiency include not only those problems involving the cardiovascular system but also specific problems related to the operative repair. Tunneling of the graft between the incisions may be more stimulating than other parts of the procedure and may cause hypertension under general anesthesia. The patient is usually given heparin during the procedure. In most cases, the heparin effect is not antagonized because bleeding problems are rare and graft reocclusion is a concern. Graft patency is evaluated carefully in the recovery room. Most surgeons believe that the patient's feet should be kept warm and that the patient should be well hydrated so that peripheral vasoconstriction, which may limit outflow from the new graft, is prevented. If graft thrombosis develops early in the postoperative period, the patient is promptly returned to the operating room for graft thrombectomy and for evaluation and correction of the cause of the thrombosis. It can be anticipated that, during graft thrombectomy, significant blood loss will occur with flushing of the graft.

Anesthetic Management of Elective Lower Extremity Revascularization

There is perhaps no other disease entity about which the anesthesiologist can be misled so easily than vascular disease of the lower extremity. One is apt to hear, "Oh, it's just a local procedure," or "Just put a spinal in and let's get on with it; you don't have to read the chart." However, the morbidity and mortality following distal operations approach those following infra-aortic reconstruction and are mainly of cardiac origin.[43] Thus, although we often use epidural or spinal anesthetics and opioids for pain relief, we pay as close attention to body temperature, oxygen delivery, and hemodynamic homeostasis during peripheral vascular procedures as during aortic procedures that involve much greater hemodynamic fluctuations. The devices and the concerns previously described apply, with special attention to the postoperative period. It is during the postoperative period that most cardiac problems arise and pain relief and correction of hemodynamic and fluid disequilibria are most likely to be needed. Care must be taken not to allow overhydration to occur intraoperatively in support of blood pressure, and then to cause congestive heart failure as the epidural sympathectomy wears off. Dye loads given for "completion angiography" also contribute to fluid shifts; thus, monitoring of cardiac preload is important for a successful outcome.

We routinely monitor hemodynamic variables invasively in patients undergoing lower extremity revascularization. Our preference is to place a radial arterial line in almost all patients, because the associated morbidity is low. An arterial line provides real-time information on blood pressure that can guide pharmacologic therapy for the rapid hemodynamic fluctuations that accompany induction of, and emergence from, anesthesia. Arterial cannulation also facilitates blood drawing in the crucial first 24 hr after surgery. Arterial catheterization is difficult in ~10% of patients, most of whom are women. Guide wire techniques may improve the rate of success. If radial artery catheterization is impossible, we usually forgo placement in other arteries or surgical placement ("cut-down"), relying instead on noninvasive blood pressure measurement.

We also commonly place central venous pressure catheters for a variety of reasons. Blood loss may be insidious and unrecognized during prolonged, revision, infrapopliteal, or *in situ* procedures. Rapid blood loss or hemodynamic changes are not usually encountered with distal reconstruction, but the procedure tends to be lengthy, making intraoperative urinary drainage advisable. Our experience is that blood loss is generally underestimated, and we routinely measure the central venous pressure and obtain a hematocrit every 2 hr in patients undergoing below-knee procedures. Because the major morbidity and mortality with this procedure are related to the cardiovascular system, with rates above 8% and 2%, respectively, the noninvasive nature and the absence of hemodynamic alterations should not lull the anesthesiologist into a casual attitude.

Table 33-11. REGIONAL ANESTHESIA VS. GENERAL ANESTHESIA

Anesthetic Technique	Advantages	Disadvantages
REGIONAL	Effective blockade of stress response Patient as monitor (dyspnea, angina) Improved graft blood flow Possible prevention of postoperative hypercoagulability Postoperative analgesia Possible prevention or improvement of chronic pain syndromes (RSD) Possible improved cardiopulmonary morbidity	Time-consuming May be technically difficult May be inadequate for the surgery Patient discomfort during long cases Sympathectomy requires volume loading Respiratory depression (from sedation or high level of blockade) Rare neurologic sequelae Precludes thrombolytic therapy
GENERAL	Controlled airway Hemodynamics easily controlled Reliable Patient comfort ensured for long cases	Hyperdynamic state after surgery Large fluctuations in catecholamine levels Postoperative hypercoagulability not inhibited Greater perturbation of respiratory mechanics

From Tzeng GF: Hemostatic interventions and regional anesthesia for vascular surgery. Prob Anesth 11:207, 1999.

Cardiac preload is reduced by epidural and spinal anesthesia due to the venodilation caused by their sympatholytic properties. Later, as the spinal or epidural anesthetic recedes, the patient's blood volume is distributed back to the central circulation. This "autotransfusion" can lead to elevated filling pressures, which may precipitate congestive heart failure if not recognized and treated appropriately. In our experience, central venous pressure monitoring is helpful in diagnosing and treating postoperative hypovolemia. The early diagnosis and treatment of even subtle hypovolemia are thought to be important in preventing postoperative renal dysfunction and early graft thrombosis. In some patients (for example, the female octogenarian with poor venous access), the placement of a triple-lumen catheter allows for concurrent volume loading, multiple drug infusions, and central venous pressure monitoring. Triple-lumen central venous catheters are also useful in the patient who will have vein harvested from the upper extremities. The risks associated with central catheter placement can be minimized by attention to strict aseptic technique during placement by an experienced or closely supervised practitioner. The risks associated with an indwelling catheter can be minimized by inserting a single- or double-lumen catheter where feasible and removing the catheter as soon as it is no longer needed.

We do not believe that the information obtained from a PAC justifies the additional risks (including heart block, dysrhythmia, pulmonary artery rupture, and pulmonary infarction)[189] associated with routine use of this monitor in this patient population. Berlauk et al[213] found that patients who were monitored during lower extremity revascularization with PACs had a lower incidence of early graft occlusion than did patients with central venous pressure monitoring. This study has been criticized because patients in the PAC group received nitroglycerin and volume loading (which have been previously shown to reduce morbidity from vascular surgery),[214] whereas those in the central venous pressure group did not. Also, the investigators and practitioners were not blinded to the randomization groups, so the potential for introduction of bias during diagnosis and treatment was very high. We believe that the prophylactic use of nitrates and volume loading in this study may have contributed more to the observed improved outcome than did the use of PACs. Therefore, we do not routinely use PACs, but rather restrict their use to the ~10–20% of patients with the most severe co-morbidity. These conditions include severe left ventricular dysfunction, renal failure, diabetes mellitus with autonomic neuropathy, and severe cor pulmonale and pulmonary hypertension. Further discussions about invasive monitoring can be found earlier in the chapter.

The choice of anesthetic for lower extremity revascularization is individualized for each patient. Table 33-11 summarizes advantages and disadvantages of regional versus general anesthesia for this procedure. The patient may have a preference for one technique over another based on previous experiences. Technical factors may contribute to the decision: obesity, previous laminectomy, or severe kyphoscoliosis may make it difficult to establish regional blockade. Septicemia, local infection, anticoagulation, and certain neurologic diseases provide varying degrees of relative and absolute contraindications to regional anesthetic techniques. Regional anesthesia may be poorly tolerated by patients who are orthopneic, uncomfortable lying still for many hours, or demented and uncooperative. Indeed, failed regional anesthesia (11% of spinals and 16% of epidurals) is associated with a 9% mortality, compared to 2% for successful regional or general anesthesia for femoral bypass.[215] Sedation allows patients to better tolerate a regional anesthetic for a long procedure, but we administer sedation judiciously as these patients are often frail or at risk for pulmonary aspiration. The combination of a high level of regional blockade and sedation may rarely produce cardiovascular collapse.[216] The patient with rest pain who has received narcotic premedication may become very sedated or even apneic when the pain is suddenly relieved by a regional anesthetic. The argument that regional anesthesia allows the patient to be a monitor for myocardial ischemia, by being able to complain of angina, may be specious, as the vast majority of episodes of perioperative myocardial ischemia are painless. Regional anesthesia may offer several advantages, however, including avoidance of hyperdynamic responses to tracheal intubation and extubation, reduced incidences of postoperative respiratory and infectious complications, and reduced postoperative hypercoagulability and graft thrombosis (Table 33-11).[32] Other studies refute any effects of regional anesthesia on thrombotic outcomes,[217,218] and suggest only higher costs for postoperative surveillance.[219] In some cases, the combination of regional and general anesthesia may provide patients with the benefits of each technique. To reduce the incidence of pruritus and respiratory depression from epidural narcotic analgesia, some anesthesiologists routinely infuse naloxone or place partial opiate agonists into the epidural space.

The operative procedure may also dictate the choice of anesthetic. Prolonged in situ and/or repeat procedures are usually not amenable to a single-shot spinal technique; catheter spinal or continuous epidural techniques may be useful in these situations. The use of microcatheters for continuous spinal anesthesia was abandoned after reports of cauda equina syndrome, but the use of continuous spinal anesthesia through a larger catheter (such as those intended for use in the epidural space) does not appear to be a problem as they permit better dispersal and dilution of local anesthetic in the cerebrospinal fluid. The incidence of postdural puncture headache is low in elderly

Table 33-12. ANTICOAGULATION THERAPIES AND NEURAXIAL BLOCKADE RECOMMENDATIONS

Anticoagulant	Neuraxial Blockade Recommendations
Low-dose (subQ) UH	Appears safe for regional anesthesia.
Intravenous UH	Acceptable, but return of aPTT to near baseline is imperative prior to blockade. Concomitant administration of iv UH and continuous epidural blockade appears relatively safe as long as catheter is removed 2–4 hours after the last dose of UH.
LMWH	Blockade should occur no earlier than 10–12 hours after last LMWH dose. LMWH should not be initiated until a minimum of 2 hours after catheter removal.
NSAIDs	Appears safe for regional anesthesia. However, combination therapy with other anticoagulants may increase the risk of neuraxial bleeding. There are no data on newer antiplatelet agents.
Oral anticoagulants	Single-dose prophylaxis appears to be safe for institution of block. Chronic therapy requires cessation of therapy and measurement of PT (INR) prior to blockade. No definitive recommendations for removing catheters in therapeutically anticoagulated patients. Clinical judgment should be made on an individual basis.
Thrombolytic drugs	Appears to have high risk for adverse neuraxial bleeding and should be cautioned against blockade "except in highly unusual circumstances."

subQ = subcutaneous; UH = unfractionated heparin; aPTT = activated partial thromboplastin time; iv = intravenous; LMWH = low-molecular-weight heparin; NSAIDs = nonsteroidal antiinflammatory drugs; PT (INR) = prothrombin time (international normalized ratio).
From Tzeng GF: Hemostatic interventions and regional anesthesia for vascular surgery. Prob Anesth 11:207, 1999.

patients. At times, we have combined spinal and epidural anesthesia for lengthy procedures. A standard epidural needle is placed into the lumbar epidural space, and through it, a longer spinal needle is advanced into the subarachnoid space. Long-acting local anesthetics (often supplemented with 0.1–0.2 mg of preservative-free morphine) are injected into the subarachnoid space, the spinal needle is removed, and an epidural catheter is passed. The spinal anesthetic provides the rapid onset of a reliable, dense, and long-lasting anesthetic. If the procedure takes longer than the 4–6 hr, the spinal anesthetic is effective; then the epidural catheter can be used to supplement surgical anesthesia and to provide postoperative analgesia.

The formation of an epidural hematoma is a dreaded complication of any neuraxial anesthetic technique. We try to ensure that every health care provider who participates in the care of patients who have had epidural or spinal anesthesia is vigilant for the signs of an epidural hematoma and is aware of the need for its emergent operative evacuation. Severe back pain or pressure is the earliest symptom of epidural hematoma formation. The pain often develops a radicular component and the patient may develop focal neurologic findings that correlate with injury to the spinal cord or nerve root. Both CT and MRI are acceptable imaging modalities for the diagnosis of a lumbar epidural hematoma. Time is of the essence, for if the spinal cord compression persists for longer than 6–12 hr, catastrophic paralysis may result. One must realize that if the patient is recovering from a general or a regional anesthetic, the spinal

cord may have been compressed long before the patient started to complain. If a hematoma is diagnosed by CT, MRI, or myelography, the patient must have an emergent laminectomy and decompression if the risk of paralysis is to be minimized.[32]

Coagulopathy therefore represents a relative contraindication to regional anesthesia. The degree of coagulopathy at which it becomes unsafe to perform regional anesthesia is unknown, is highly controversial, and must be part of the risk–benefit calculation in each patient. Use of NSAIDs such as aspirin and the use of subcutaneous heparin before surgery do not seem to be problematic,[220] while anecdotal reports suggest that thrombolytic therapy is a contraindication for the use of regional anesthesia.[32,221] The placement of epidural catheters with subsequent systemic heparinization before arterial occlusion appears to be safe. However, the authors of the most often quoted study (with ~3100 patients) in support of such practice postponed surgery for a day for patients who had a "bloody tap" during attempted epidural catheterization.[222] The surgery was then subsequently performed under general anesthesia. Beginning oral coumadin after surgery also appears safe in patients who have a pre-established epidural catheter.[32] Many practitioners do not feel comfortable removing an epidural catheter from a patient who is coagulopathic or is receiving a heparin infusion. Some clinicians advocate the cessation of the heparin infusion and the correction of coagulopathy before catheter removal. Table 33-12 summarizes some suggestions for management of regional anesthetics and anticoagulation therapy.[32]

General anesthesia for lower extremity revascularization has the advantage of obviating patient discomfort and lack of cooperation (Table 33-11). It allows for adequate oxygenation and ventilation and facilitates hemodynamic manipulation. Its use is virtually mandated in patients who are to have vein harvested from an arm (unless spinal and brachial plexus blocks are performed coincidentally). General anesthesia has been associated with a higher incidence of postoperative respiratory complications in some studies.[223] However, while reduction in cardiac complications is often a stated reason for avoiding general anesthesia, recent series (Table 33-13) have been unable to show such an effect in patients undergoing lower extremity revascularization.[215] Regional anesthetics may or may not reduce postoperative thrombotic complications (Table 33-13). We do not feel that the evidence favoring regional anesthesia is so overwhelming that we would withhold a general anesthetic from most patients to whom we have offered a regional anesthetic.

Specific types of general anesthetic may be preferred for patients undergoing vascular surgery. High-dose narcotic anesthetics may be associated with less renal insufficiency and congestive heart failure after aortic reconstruction than are volatile

Table 33-13. MYOCARDIAL ISCHEMIA AND MYOCARDIAL INFARCTION (MI) AFTER DIFFERENT ANESTHETIC TECHNIQES FOR LOWER EXTREMITY REVASCULARIZATION

Authors Reference	Anesthetic Technique		
	General	Epidural	Spinal
Christopherson et al[96] (n = 100)	45% ischemia 3.9% MI	35% ischemia 4.1% MI	—
Bode et al[215] (n = 326)	3.6% MI	6.3% MI	3.7% MI

* The choice of anesthetic technique does not seem to influence rates of perioperative myocardial ischemia or infarction after lower extremity revascularization. In the first study, myocardial ischemia was diagnosed by continuous ambulatory electrocardiography (Holter monitoring).

anesthetics.[195] This effect may be attributed to the superior ability of narcotics to blunt the adrenergic response to surgery. Despite these findings, we usually provide general anesthesia with doses of narcotics, which, although generous, still permit extubation in the operating room. Whether the benefits of prolonging anesthesia justify the risks and costs incurred by patients undergoing lower extremity revascularization remains to be studied.

Patients who receive general anesthesia can have a carefully controlled emergence and extubation, whether in the operating room or later in the ICU. We prefer to perform tracheal extubation at the end of surgery in the operating room, with the same intense monitoring of hemodynamics used during induction of anesthesia. We believe it important to appreciate the complex physiology of the anesthetic emergence. This period is punctuated by large increases in catecholamine levels (see Fig. 33-2) and a high incidence of myocardial ischemia.[224] Emergence is a period of careful titration: opiates are infused to control pain and blunt sympathetic discharge while still allowing the patient to ventilate effectively. Therefore, while still intubated and breathing spontaneously, patients receive incremental doses of narcotics titrated to adequate respiration (respiratory rate 8–16 min^{-1}; end-tidal PC_{O2} <50 mm Hg). The anesthesiologist does not have the luxury of administering large amounts of opiates to blunt this response during the anesthetic emergence if he or she wishes to extubate the patient in the operating room. Therefore, additional iv drugs are often required to control hemodynamics during emergence. Our usual practice is to titrate iv labetalol, metoprolol, or esmolol for extubation to keep heart rate below 80 beats · min^{-1} in the vast majority of patients who can tolerate β-adrenergic receptor blockade.

Anesthesia for Emergency Surgery for Peripheral Vascular Insufficiency

Emergency surgery for peripheral vascular insufficiency is required when acute arterial occlusion results in severe ischemia and threatens the viability of a limb. Immediate operation and restoration of blood flow are needed if limb loss is to be avoided. Depending on the etiology of the occlusion, the patient may or may not be at very high risk. Although this problem may appear to be localized to an extremity, the occluding material may originate in the heart or in major arteries. Therefore, peripheral vascular occlusion may be the result of a more serious cardiovascular problem. In fact, some patients with peripheral vascular occlusion are the sickest patients we have ever anesthetized.

With acute arterial occlusion, the involved extremity suddenly becomes cold and pulseless. Patients usually complain of coldness, pain, numbness, and paresthesias, and they may lose motion and sensation. Abnormal sensation in the toes, feet, and legs in response to light touch and pinprick, as well as abnormal proprioception and loss of motor function in the feet and toes, are hallmarks of acute ischemia and nonviability. If the ischemia is not reversed in a matter of hours, irreversible loss of viability is likely to result.

Acute arterial occlusion may develop in patients with preexisting peripheral occlusive or aneurysmal disease caused by thrombosis of a stenotic or ulcerated atherosclerotic artery. Acute arterial occlusion can also occur in patients with normal peripheral arteries that contain emboli. Such embolism is usually of cardiac origin in patients with cardiac dysrhythmias, recent MIs, or ventricular aneurysms.

The cause is important in planning operative treatment. If the cause is an arterial embolus, Fogarty embolectomy through a groin incision, angioscopy, or laser atherectomy under local anesthesia may suffice. However, if the cause is thrombosis of severely diseased atherosclerotic arteries, bypass reconstruction will be required. Although preoperative angiography may be of help in the differential diagnosis, often the cause is not uncovered until the vessel is opened. Thus, the anesthesiologist must be prepared for either a simple procedure or a complex, extended procedure. An incision in the groin is usually made for exposure of the femoral artery. Attempts to pass Fogarty catheters proximally and distally are made in the effort to establish flow and extract the thrombus. If flow is not restored in this manner, more complex reconstructive procedures such as aortofemoral, axillofemoral, or femoral-popliteal bypass may be required. Femoral venous drainage on restoration of flow to the femoral artery can aid in management by washing the initial venous effluent from an acutely ischemic extremity. Drainage may entail significant blood loss. Significant fluid losses can also be anticipated when the artery is flushed during thrombectomy and fluid is sequestered in edematous revascularized tissue. Serum potassium levels can change quickly because cell death and release of intracellular potassium into the circulation can be anticipated. Venous drainage into the autotransfusion suction with subsequent washing before reinfusion has been used to prevent the complications of hyperkalemia. Myoglobin may also be released into the circulation, and the development of a compartment syndrome is a possibility. Skill and intensive care as meticulous as that given patients with visceral ischemia may also benefit patients with peripheral vascular insufficiency.

Anticoagulants are commonly administered to patients suspected of having peripheral vascular occlusion. If a patient has received anticoagulants, the appropriateness of using a major conduction block (subarachnoid or epidural block with or without catheter placement) is controversial. We believe that regional anesthesia should be avoided when patients have received thrombolytic therapy.[32]

CONCLUSIONS

Patients undergoing vascular reconstruction are generally elderly. Vascular disease is a generalized process; thus, patients having surgery for a specific vascular disorder are likely to have atherosclerotic disease elsewhere in the vascular system. Most of the patients have coronary artery disease. The skills of the anesthesiologist can therefore greatly influence outcome in vascular surgery. The considerations for preoperative patient evaluation are the same as for patients with cardiac disease undergoing other noncardiac procedures. Many have a history of smoking, and chronic obstructive pulmonary disease, renal insufficiency, and lipid abnormalities are frequently present. The major morbidity in each of the operations relates to myocardial well-being; therefore, the heart should be the major focus of the anesthesiologist's attention. Attempts to segregate patients who have significant coronary artery disease by use of preoperative testing are controversial. The benefits of coronary revascularization are likely to persist long after vascular surgery in patients with triple-vessel coronary artery disease.

In cerebrovascular surgery, the goals in anesthesia management, *i.e.,* ensuring adequate myocardial and brain perfusion and a rapidly arousable patient, may be facilitated with the use of neurophysiologic monitoring as a guide to afterload reduction. In aortic reconstruction, ensuring intact myocardial function is probably the best way of making certain that spinal cord, visceral, and renal perfusion will be adequate.

In the case of peripheral occlusive disease, the absence of hemodynamic changes should not lull the anesthesiologist into loss of vigilance with regard to myocardial well-being. In addition, vigilance in ensuring routine prehydration and use of a warming device are probably more important to outcome than is occasional brilliance. We prefer the diligent, compulsive practitioner to the occasionally brilliant one. Nowhere is such diligence needed more than in the postoperative period, when most morbidity related to the heart occurs. Perhaps it is most important to remember that the best patient results are achieved when intraoperative vigilance is extended to the preoperative and postoperative periods as well.

REFERENCES

1. Szilagyi DE, Smith RF, Derusso FJ *et al:* Contribution of abdominal aortic aneurysmectomy to prolongation of life. Ann Surg 164:678, 1966
2. Whittemore AD, Clowes AW, Hechtman HB *et al:* Aortic aneurysm repair: Reduced operative mortality associated with maintenance of optimal cardiac performance. Ann Surg 192:414, 1980
3. Crawford ES, Saleh SA, Babb JW III *et al:* Infrarenal abdominal aortic aneurysm: Factors influencing survival after operation performed over a 25-year period. Ann Surg 193:699, 1981
4. Johnston KW: Multicenter prospective study of nonruptured abdominal aortic aneurysm: II. Variables predicting morbidity and mortality. J Vasc Surg 9:437, 1989
5. Golden MA, Whittemore AD, Donaldson MC, Mannick JA: Selective evaluation and management of coronary artery disease in patients undergoing repair of abdominal aortic aneurysms: A 16-year experience. Ann Surg 212:415, 1990
6. Suggs WD, Smith RB III, Weintraub WS *et al:* Selective screening for coronary artery disease in patients undergoing elective repair of abdominal aortic aneurysms. J Vasc Surg 18:349, 1993
7. Baron JF, Mundler O, Bertrand M *et al:* Dipyridamole-thallium scintigraphy and gated radionuclide angiography to assess cardiac risk before abdominal aortic surgery. N Engl J Med 330:663, 1994
8. L'Italien GJ, Cambria RP, Cutler BS *et al:* Comparative early and late cardiac morbidity among patients requiring different vascular surgery procedures. J Vasc Surg 21:935, 1995
9. Lloyd WE, Paty PS, Darling RC 3rd *et al:* Results of 1000 consecutive elective abdominal aortic aneurysm repairs. Cardiovasc Surg 4:724, 1996
10. Baker B: Anesthesia for endovascular surgery. Prob Anesth 11:179, 1999
11. Ross R: Atherosclerosis—an inflammatory disease. N Engl J Med 340:115, 1999
12. Hankey GJ, Eikelboom JW: Homocysteine and vascular disease. Lancet 354:407, 1999
13. Criqui MH, Langer RD, Fronek A *et al:* Mortality over a period of 10 years in patients with peripheral arterial disease. N Engl J Med 326:381, 1992
14. Fine-Edelstein JS, Wolf PA, O'Leary DH *et al:* Precursors of extracranial carotid atherosclerosis in the Framingham study. Neurology 44:1046, 1994
15. Stanley JC, Barnes RW, Ernst CB *et al:* Vascular surgery in the United States: Workforce issues. Report of the Society for Vascular Surgery and the International Society for Cardiovascular Surgery, North American Chapter, Committee on Workforce Issues. J Vasc Surg 23:172, 1996
16. Tu JV, Hannan EL, Anderson GM *et al:* The fall and rise of carotid endarterectomy in the United States and Canada. N Engl J Med 339(20):1441, 1998
17. Tunis SR, Bass EB, Klag MJ, Steinberg EP: Variation in utilization of procedures for treatment of peripheral arterial disease: A look at patient characteristics. Arch Intern Med 153:991, 1993
18. Niklason LE, Gao J, Abbott WM *et al:* Functional arteries grown *in vitro.* Science 284(5413):489, 1999
19. Quinones-Baldrich WJ, Garner C, Caswell D *et al:* Endovascular, transperitoneal, and retroperitoneal abdominal aortic aneurysm repair: Results and costs. J Vasc Surg. 30(1):59, 1999
20. Sorrentino MJ, Roizen MF: Secondary prevention of coronary artery disease: Implications for the patient with peripheral vascular disease. Prob Anesth 11:157, 1999
21. Cooke JP, Ma A: Medical therapy of peripheral arterial occlusive disease. Surg Clin North Am 75:569, 1995
22. Pitt B, Waters D, Brown WV *et al:* Aggressive lipid-lowering therapy compared with angioplasty in stable coronary artery disease. Atorvastatin versus revascularization treatment investigators. N Engl J Med 341(2):70, 1999
23. Hambrecht R, Wolf A, Gielen S *et al:* Effect of exercise on coronary endothelial function in patients with coronary artery disease. N Engl J Med 342(7):454, 2000
24. Warner MA, Offord KP, Warner ME *et al:* Role of preoperative cessation of smoking and other factors in postoperative pulmonary complications: A blinded prospective study of coronary artery bypass patients. Mayo Clin Proc 64(6):609, 1989
25. Simon JA, Browner WS, Mangano DT: Predictors of smoking relapse after noncardiac surgery. Study of Perioperative Ischemia (SPI) Research Group. Am J Pub Health 82(9):1235, 1992
26. White HD: Newer antiplatelet agents in acute coronary syndromes. Am Heart J 138(6 Pt 2):S570, 1999
27. Bennett CL, Davidson CJ, Green D *et al:* Ticlopidine and TTP after coronary stenting. JAMA. 282(18):1717, 1999
28. Harker LA, Boissel JP, Pilgrim AJ, Gent M: Comparative safety and tolerability of clopidogrel and aspirin: Results from CAPRIE. CAPRIE Steering Committee and Investigators. Clopidogrel versus aspirin in patients at risk of ischaemic events. Drug Saf. 21(4):325, 1999
29. Vandermeulen EP, Van Aken H, Vermylen J: Anticoagulants and spinal-epidural anesthesia. Anesth Analg 79:1165, 1994
30. Horlocker TT, Heit JA: Low molecular weight heparin: Biochemistry, pharmacology, perioperative prophylaxis regimens, and guidelines for regional anesthetic management. Anesth Analg 85:874, 1997
31. Wysowski DK, Talarico L, Bacsanyi J, Botstein P: Spinal and epidural hematoma and low-molecular-weight heparin [letter]. N Engl J Med 338:1774, 1998
32. Tzeng GF: Hemostatic interventions and regional anesthesia for vascular surgery. Prob Anesth 11:207, 1999
33. Ananthasubramaniam K, Shurafa M, Prasad A: Heparin-induced thrombocytopenia and thrombosis. Prog Cardiovasc Dis 42(4):247, 2000
34. Warkentin TE: Heparin-induced thrombocytopenia: A ten-year retrospective. Annu Rev Med 50:129, 1999
35. Roizen MF: Anesthetic implications of concurrent diseases. In Miller RD (ed): Anesthesia, 5th ed, vol 1, p 903. Philadelphia, Churchill Livingstone, 2000
36. Khuri SF, Daley J, Henderson W *et al:* Risk adjustment of the postoperative mortality rate for the comparative assessment of the quality of surgical care: Results of the National Veterans Affairs Surgical Risk Study. J Am Coll Surg. 185(4):315, 1997
37. Daley J, Khuri SF, Henderson W *et al:* Risk adjustment of the postoperative morbidity rate for the comparative assessment of the quality of surgical care: Results of the National Veterans Affairs Surgical Risk Study. J Am Coll Surg. 185(4):328, 1997
38. Ellis JE: Health sciences research and large database analysis in vascular surgery and anesthesia: Confirming common sense? Prob Anesth 11:238, 1999
39. Garwood S, Aronson S: Renal protection in vascular surgery. Prob Anesth 11:247, 1999
40. Hertzer NR, Beven EG, Young JR *et al:* Coronary artery disease in peripheral vascular patients: A classification of 1000 coronary angiograms and results of surgical management. Ann Surg 199:223, 1984
41. Paul SD, Eagle KA, Kuntz KM *et al:* Concordance of preoperative clinical risk with angiographic severity of coronary artery disease in patients undergoing vascular surgery. Circulation 94(7):1561, 1996
42. Mangano DT: Perioperative cardiac morbidity. Anesthesiology 72:153, 1990
43. Krupski WC, Layug EL, Reilly LM *et al:* Comparison of cardiac morbidity rates between aortic and infrainguinal operations: Two-year follow-up. Study of Perioperative Ischemia Research. J Vasc Surg 18:609, 1993
44. Rihal CS, Eagle KA, Mickel MC *et al:* Surgical therapy for coronary artery disease among patients with combined coronary artery and peripheral vascular disease. Circulation 91:46, 1995
45. Huber KC, Evans MA, Bresnahan JF *et al:* Outcome of noncardiac operations in patients with severe coronary artery disease successfully treated preoperatively with coronary angioplasty. Mayo Clin Proc 67:15, 1992
46. Posner KL, Van Norman GA, Chan V: Adverse cardiac outcomes after noncardiac surgery in patients with prior percutaneous transluminal coronary angioplasty. Anesth Analg 89(3):553, 1999
47. Gottlieb A, Banoub M, Sprung J *et al:* Perioperative cardiovascular morbidity in patients with coronary artery disease undergoing vascular surgery after percutaneous transluminal coronary angioplasty. J Cardiothorac Vasc Anesth 12(5):501, 1998
48. Muller DW, Shamir KJ, Ellis SG, Topol EJ: Peripheral vascular complications after conventional and complex percutaneous coronary interventional procedures. Am J Cardiol 69:63, 1992
49. L'Italien GJ, Paul SD, Hendel RC *et al:* Development and validation of a Bayesian model for perioperative cardiac risk assessment in a cohort of 1,081 vascular surgical candidates. J Am Coll Cardiol 27(4):779, 1996

50. Klock PA, Ellis JE: Clinical pathways for vascular anesthesia and surgery. Prob Anesth 11:224, 1999

51. Detsky AS, Abrams HB, Forbath N et al: Cardiac assessment for patients undergoing noncardiac surgery: A multifactorial clinical risk index. Arch Intern Med 146:2131, 1986

52. Lee TH, Marcantonio ER, Mangione CM et al: Derivation and prospective validation of a simple index for prediction of cardiac risk of major noncardiac surgery. Circulation 100(10):1043, 1999

53. Taylor LM Jr, Yeager RA, Moneta GL et al: The incidence of perioperative myocardial infarction in general vascular surgery. J Vasc Surg 15(1):52, 1992

54. Shah KB, Kleinman BS, Sami H et al: Reevaluation of perioperative myocardial infarction in patients with prior myocardial infarction undergoing noncardiac operations. Anesth Analg 71:231, 1990

55. Lette J, Waters D, Lassonde J et al: Multivariate clinical models and quantitative dipyridamole-thallium imaging to predict cardiac morbidity and death after vascular reconstruction. J Vasc Surg 14:160, 1991

56. Fleisher LA: Preoperative cardiac evaluation before major vascular surgery. Prob Anesth 11:167, 1999

57. Marshall ES, Raichlen JS, Forman S et al: Adenosine radionuclide perfusion imaging in the preoperative evaluation of patients undergoing peripheral vascular surgery. Am J Cardiol 76:817, 1995

58. Poldermans D, Arnese M, Fioretti PM et al: Improved cardiac risk stratification in major vascular surgery with dobutamine-atropine stress echocardiography. J Am Coll Cardiol 26:648, 1995

59. Vanzetto G, Machecourt J, Blendea D et al: Additive value of thallium single-photon emission computed tomography myocardial imaging for prediction of perioperative events in clinically selected high cardiac risk patients having abdominal aortic surgery. Am J Cardiol 77:143, 1996

60. Landesberg G, Einav S, Christopherson R et al: Perioperative ischemia and cardiac complications in major vascular surgery: Importance of the preoperative twelve-lead electrocardiogram. J Vasc Surg 26:570, 1997

61. Palda VA, Detsky AS: Perioperative assessment and management of risk from coronary artery disease. Ann Intern Med 127:313, 1997

62. Mangano DT, London MJ, Tubau JF et al: Dipyridamole thallium-201 scintigraphy as a preoperative screening test: A reexamination of its predictive potential. Study of Perioperative Ischemia Research Group. Circulation 84:493, 1991

63. Eagle KA, Brundage BH, Chaitman BR et al: Guidelines for perioperative cardiovascular evaluation for noncardiac surgery. Report of the American College of Cardiology/American Heart Association Task Force on Practice Guidelines. Committee on Perioperative Cardiovascular Evaluation for Noncardiac Surgery. Circulation 93:1278, 1996

64. Bartels C, Bechtel JF, Hossmann V, Horsch S: Cardiac risk stratification for high-risk vascular surgery. Circulation 95:2473, 1997

65. Eagle KA, Singer DE, Brewster DC et al: Dipyridamole-thallium scanning in patients undergoing vascular surgery: Optimizing preoperative evaluation of cardiac risk. JAMA 257: 2185, 1987

66. Mantha S, Roizen MF, Barnard J et al: Relative effectiveness of four preoperative tests for predicting adverse cardiac outcome after vascular surgery: A meta-analysis. Anesth Analg 79:422, 1994

67. Raby KE, Goldman L, Creager MA et al: Correlation between preoperative ischemia and major cardiac events after peripheral vascular surgery. N Engl J Med 321:1296, 1989

68. Gutstein DE, Fuster V: Pathophysiology and clinical significance of atherosclerotic plaque rupture. Cardiovasc Res 41(2):323, 1999

69. Fleisher LA, Skolnick ED, Holroyd KJ, Lehmann HP: Coronary artery revascularization before abdominal aortic aneurysm surgery: A decision analytic approach. Anesth Analg 9:661, 1994

70. Bry JD, Belkin M, O'Donnell TF Jr: An assessment of the positive predictive value and cost-effectiveness of dipyridamole myocardial scintigraphy in patients undergoing vascular surgery. J Vasc Surg 19:112, 1994

71. Birkmeyer JD, O'Connor GT, Quinton HB et al: The effect of peripheral vascular disease on in-hospital mortality rates with coronary artery bypass surgery: Northern New England Cardiovascular Disease Study Group. J Vasc Surg 21:445, 1995

72. Giangola G, Migaly J, Riles TS et al: Perioperative morbidity and mortality in combined vs. staged approaches to carotid and coronary revascularization. Ann Vasc Surg 10(2):138, 1996

73. Blackbourne LH, Tribble CG, Langenburg SE et al: Optimal timing of abdominal aortic aneurysm repair after coronary artery revascularization. Ann Surg 219:693, 1994

74. London MJ, Hollenberg M, Wong MG et al: Intraoperative myocardial ischemia: Localization by continuous 12-lead electrocardiography. Anesthesiology 69:232, 1988

75. Ellis JE, Shah MN, Briller JE et al: A comparison of methods for the detection of myocardial ischemia during noncardiac surgery: Automated ST-segment analysis systems, electrocardiography, and transesophageal echocardiography. Anesth Analg 75:764, 1992

76. Mangano DT, Browner WS, Hollenberg M et al: Association of perioperative myocardial ischemia with cardiac morbidity and mortality in men undergoing noncardiac surgery. N Engl J Med 323:1781, 1990

77. Ouyang P, Gerstenblith G, Furman WR et al: Frequency and significance of early postoperative silent myocardial ischemia in patients having peripheral vascular surgery. Am J Cardiol 64:1113, 1989

78. McCann RL, Clements FM: Silent myocardial ischemia in patients undergoing peripheral vascular surgery: Incidence and association with perioperative cardiac morbidity and mortality. J Vasc Surg 9:583, 1989

79. Pasternack PF, Grossi EA, Baumann FG et al: Beta blockade to decrease silent myocardial ischemia during peripheral vascular surgery. Am J Surg 158:113, 1989

80. Landesberg G, Luria MH, Cotev S: Importance of long-duration postoperative ST-segment depression in cardiac morbidity after vascular surgery. Lancet 341:715, 1993

81. Haggmark S, Hohner P, Ostman M et al: Comparison of hemodynamic, electrocardiographic, mechanical, and metabolic indicators of intraoperative myocardial ischemia in vascular surgical patients with coronary artery disease. Anesthesiology 70:19, 1989

82. Van Daele ME: Do changes in pulmonary capillary wedge pressure adequately reflect myocardial ischemia during anesthesia? A correlative preoperative hemodynamic, electrocardiographic and transesophageal echocardiographic study. Circulation 81:865, 1990

83. Roizen MF, Beaupre PN, Alpert RA et al: Monitoring with two-dimensional transesophageal echocardiography: Comparison of myocardial function in patients undergoing supraceliac, suprarenal-infraceliac, or infrarenal aortic occlusion. J Vasc Surg 1:300, 1984

84. Smith JS, Cahalan MK, Benefiel DJ et al: Intraoperative detection of myocardial ischemia in high-risk patients: Electrocardiography versus two-dimensional transesophageal echocardiography. Circulation 872:1015, 1985

85. Eisenberg MJ, London MJ, Leung JM et al: Monitoring for myocardial ischemia during noncardiac surgery: A technology assessment of transesophageal echocardiography and 12-lead electrocardiography. The Study of Perioperative Ischemia Research Group. JAMA 268:210, 1992

86. Adams JE III, Sicard GA, Allen BT et al: Diagnosis of perioperative myocardial infarction with measurement of cardiac troponin I. N Engl J Med 330:670, 1994

87. Badner NH, Knill RL, Brown JE et al: Myocardial infarction after noncardiac surgery. Anesthesiology. 88(3):572, 1998

88. Breslow MJ: The role of stress hormones in perioperative myocardial ischemia. Int Anesthesiol Clin 30:81, 1992

89. Mangano DT, Browner WS, Hollenberg M et al: Long-term cardiac prognosis following noncardiac surgery. JAMA 268:233, 1992

90. Furberg CD, Psaty BM, Meyer JV: Nifedipine: Dose-related increase in mortality in patients with coronary heart disease. Circulation 92:1326, 1995

91. Dodds TM, Stone JG, Coromilas J et al: Prophylactic nitroglycerin infusion during noncardiac surgery does not reduce perioperative ischemia. Anesth Analg 76:705, 1993

92. Raby KE, Brull SJ, Timimi F et al: The effect of heart rate control on myocardial ischemia among high-risk patients after vascular surgery. Anesth Analg 88(3):477, 1999

93. Poldermans D, Boersma E, Bax JJ et al: The effect of bisoprolol on perioperative mortality and myocardial infarction in high-risk patients undergoing vascular surgery. Dutch Echocardiographic Cardiac Risk Evaluation Applying Stress Echocardiography Study Group. N Engl J Med 341(24):1789, 1999

94. Mangano DT, Layug EL, Wallace A, Tateo I: Effect of atenolol on mortality and cardiovascular morbidity after noncardiac surgery. Multicenter Study of Perioperative Ischemia Research Group. N Engl J Med 335(23):1713, 1996

95. Mangano DT, Siliciano D, Hollenberg M et al: Postoperative myo-

cardial ischemia: Therapeutic trials using intensive analgesia following surgery. Anesthesiology 76:342, 1992

96. Christopherson R, Beattie C, Frank SM et al: Perioperative morbidity in patients randomized to epidural or general anesthesia for lower extremity vascular surgery: Perioperative Ischemia Randomized Anesthesia Trial Study Group. Anesthesiology 79:422, 1993

97. Ellis JE, Drijvers G, Pedlow S et al: Premedication with oral and transdermal clonidine provides safe and efficacious postoperative sympatholysis. Anesth Analg 79:1133, 1994

98. Talke P, Li J, Jain U et al: Effects of perioperative dexmedetomidine infusion in patients undergoing vascular surgery: The Study of Perioperative Ischemia Research Group. Anesthesiology 82:620, 1995

99. Oliver MF, Goldman L, Julian DG, Holme I: Effect of mivazerol on perioperative cardiac complications during non-cardiac surgery in patients with coronary heart disease: The European Mivazerol Trial (EMIT). Anesthesiology 91(4):951, 1999

100. Nelson AH, Fleisher LA, Rosenbaum SH: Relationship between postoperative anemia and cardiac morbidity in high-risk vascular patients in the intensive care unit. Crit Care Med 21:860, 1993

101. Hogue CW Jr, Goodnough LT, Monk TG: Perioperative myocardial ischemic episodes are related to hematocrit level in patients undergoing radical prostatectomy. Transfusion 38(10):924, 1998

102. Frank SM, Fleisher LA, Breslow MJ et al: Perioperative maintenance of normothermia reduces the incidence of morbid cardiac events. A randomized clinical trial. JAMA 277(14):1127, 1997

103. Miller JS, Dodson TF, Salam AA, Smith RB III: Vascular complications following intra-aortic balloon pump insertion. Am Surg 58:232, 1992

104. Roth S, Shay J, Chua KG: Coronary angioplasty following acute perioperative myocardial infarction. Anesthesiology 71:300, 1989

105. Ligtenberg G, Blankestijn PJ, Oey PL et al: Reduction of sympathetic hyperactivity by enalapril in patients with chronic renal failure. N Engl J Med 340(17):1321, 1999

106. Coriat P, Richer C, Douraki T et al: Influence of chronic angiotensin-converting enzyme inhibition on anesthetic induction. Anesthesiology 81(2):299, 1994

107. Treiman GS, Treiman RL, Foran RF et al: The influence of diabetes mellitus on the risk of abdominal aortic surgery. Am Surg 60:436, 1994

108. Charlson ME, MacKenzie CR, Gold JP: Preoperative autonomic function abnormalities in patients with diabetes mellitus and patients with hypertension. J Am Coll Surg 179:1, 1994

109. Donaldson MC, Weinberg DS, Belkin M et al: Screening for hypercoagulable states in vascular surgical practice: A preliminary study. J Vasc Surg 11:825, 1990

110. Smetana GW: Preoperative pulmonary evaluation. N Engl J Med 340(12):937, 1999

111. Kispert JF, Kazmers A, Roitman L: Preoperative spirometry predicts perioperative pulmonary complications after major vascular surgery. Am Surg 58:491, 1992

112. Berens ES, Kouchoukus NT, Murphy SF et al: Preoperative carotid artery screening in elderly patients undergoing cardiac surgery. J Vasc Surg 15:313, 1992

113. Chambers BR, Norris JW: Outcome in patients with asymptomatic neck bruits. N Engl J Med 315:860, 1986

114. Mayo Asymptomatic Carotid Endarterectomy Study Group: Results of a randomized controlled trial of carotid endarterectomy for asymptomatic carotid stenosis. Mayo Clin Proc 67:513, 1989

115. North American Symptomatic Carotid Endarterectomy Trial Collaborators: Beneficial effect of carotid endarterectomy in symptomatic patients with high grade stenosis. N Engl J Med 325:445, 1991

116. Executive Committee for the Asymptomatic Carotid Atherosclerosis Study: Endarterectomy for asymptomatic carotid artery stenosis. JAMA 273:1421, 1995

117. Moore WS, Barnett HJM, Beebe HG et al: Guidelines for carotid endarterectomy: A multidisciplinary consensus statement from the Ad Hoc committee. American Heart Association. Circulation 91:566, 1995

118. Mathur A, Roubin GS, Iyer SS et al: Predictors of stroke complicating carotid artery stenting. Circulation 97(13):1239, 1998

119. Ferguson GG, Eliasziw M, Barr HW et al: The North American Symptomatic Carotid Endarterectomy Trial: Surgical results in 1415 patients. Stroke 30(9):1751, 1999

120. Rizzo RJ, Whittemore AD, Couper GS: Combined carotid and coronary revascularization: The preferred approach to the severe vasculopath. Ann Thorac Surg 54:1099, 1992

121. Schwartz LB, Bridgman AAAH, Kieffer RW et al: Asymptomatic carotid stenosis and stroke in patients undergoing cardiopulmonary bypass. J Vasc Surg 21:146, 1995

122. Ostoic T, Helgason C, Hoff J et al: Determining the source of stroke: Evaluation of the findings with transesophageal echocardiography in the context of coexisting carotid artery disease. Circulation 88:18, 1993

123. Qureshi AI, Luft AR, Janardhan V et al: Identification of patients at risk for periprocedural neurological deficits associated with carotid angioplasty and stenting. Stroke 31(2):376, 2000

124. Smith JS, Roizen MF, Cahalan MK et al: Does anesthetic technique make a difference? Augmentation of systolic blood pressure during carotid endarterectomy: Effects of phenylephrine versus light anesthesia and of isoflurane versus halothane on the incidence of myocardial ischemia. Anesthesiology 69:846, 1988

125. Modica PA, Tempelhoff R, Rick KM et al: Computerized electroencephalographic monitoring and selective shunting: Influence on intraoperative administration of phenylephrine and myocardial infarction after general anesthesia for carotid endarterectomy. Neurosurgery 30:842, 1992

126. Goertz AW, Lindner KH, Seefelder C et al: Effect of phenylephrine bolus administration on global left ventricular function in patients with coronary artery disease and patients with valvular aortic stenosis. Anesthesiology 78(5):834, 1993

127. Strebel SP, Kindler C, Bissonnette B et al: The impact of systemic vasoconstrictors on the cerebral circulation of anesthetized patients. Anesthesiology 89(1):67, 1998

128. Todd MM, Warner DS: A comfortable hypothesis reevaluated: Cerebral metabolic depression and brain protection during ischemia (editorial). Anesthesiology 76:161, 1992

129. Michenfelder JD, Sundt TM, Fode N et al: Isoflurane when compared to enflurane and halothane decreases the frequency of cerebral ischemia during carotid endarterectomy. Anesthesiology 67:336, 1987

130. Grady RE, Weglinski MR, Sharbrough FW, Perkins WJ: Correlation of regional cerebral blood flow with ischemic electroencephalographic changes during sevoflurane–nitrous oxide anesthesia for carotid endarterectomy. Anesthesiology 88(4):892, 1998

131. Messick JM Jr, Casement B, Sharbrough FW et al: Correlation of regional cerebral blood flow (rCBF) with EEG changes during isoflurane anesthesia for carotid endarterectomy: Critical rCBF. Anesthesiology 66(3):344, 1987

132. Frawley JE, Hicks RG, Horton DA et al: Thiopental sodium cerebral protection during carotid endarterectomy: Perioperative disease and death. J Vasc Surg 19:732, 1994

133. Mutch WA, White IW, Donen N et al: Haemodynamic instability and myocardial ischaemia during carotid endarterectomy: A comparison of propofol and isoflurane. Can J Anaesth 42(7):577, 1995

134. Lavine SD, Masri LS, Levy ML, Giannotta SL: Temporary occlusion of the middle cerebral artery in intracranial aneurysm surgery: Time limitation and advantage of brain protection. J Neurosurg 87(6):817, 1997

135. McKinsey JF, Davidovitch R, Gewertz BL: Intraoperative monitoring for cerebral ischemia during carotid endarterectomy. Prob Anesth 11:193, 1999

136. McKay RD, Sundt TM, Michenfelder JD et al: Internal carotid artery stump pressure and cerebral blood flow during carotid endarterectomy: Modification by halothane, enflurane and Innovar. Anesthesiology 45:390, 1976

137. Sundt TM Jr, Sharbrough FW, Piepgras DG et al: Correlation of cerebral blood flow and electroencephalographic changes during carotid endarterectomy: With results of surgery and hemodynamics of cerebral ischemia. Mayo Clin Proc 56:533, 1981

138. Kearse LA Jr, Lopez-Bresnahan M, McPeck K, Zaslavsky A: Preoperative cerebrovascular symptoms and electroencephalographic abnormalities do not predict cerebral ischemia during carotid endarterectomy. Stroke 26(7):1210, 1995

139. Kearse LA Jr, Brown EN, McPeck K: Somatosensory evoked potentials sensitivity relative to electroencephography for cerebral ischemia during carotid endarterectomy. Stroke 23:498, 1992

140. Jansen C, Vrins EM, Eikelboom BC et al: Carotid endarterectomy with transcranial Doppler and electroencephalographic monitoring. A prospective study in 130 operations. Stroke 24:665, 1993

141. Frank SM, Beattie C, Christopherson R: Right and left arm blood

pressure discrepancies in vascular surgery patients. Anesthesiology 75:457, 1991

142. Landesberg G, Erel J, Anner H *et al:* Perioperative myocardial ischemia in carotid endarterectomy under cervical plexus block and prophylactic nitroglycerin infusion. J Cardiothorac Vasc Anesth 7:259, 1993

143. Marietta DR, Lunn JK, Ruby EI, Hill GE: Cardiovascular stability during carotid endarterectomy: Endotracheal intubation versus laryngeal mask airway. J Clin Anesth 10(1):54, 1998

144. McKinsey JF, Desai TR, Bassiouny HS *et al:* Mechanisms of neurologic deficits and mortality with carotid endarterectomy. Arch Surg 131(5):526, 1996

145. Wilke HJ 2nd, Ellis JE, McKinsey JF: Carotid endarterectomy: Perioperative and anesthetic considerations. J Cardiothorac Vasc Anesth 10(7):928, 1996

146. Stoneham MD, Doyle AR, Knighton JD *et al:* Prospective, randomized comparison of deep or superficial cervical plexus block for carotid endarterectomy surgery. Anesthesiology 89(4):907, 1998

147. Davies MJ, Mooney PH, Scott DA *et al:* Neurologic changes during carotid endarterectomy under cervical block predict a high risk of postoperative stroke. Anesthesiology 78:829, 1993

148. Wong JH, Findlay JM, Suarez-Almazor ME: Hemodynamic instability after carotid endarterectomy: Risk factors and associations with operative complications. Neurosurgery 41(1):35, 1997

149. Qureshi AI, Luft AR, Sharma M *et al:* Frequency and determinants of postprocedural hemodynamic instability after carotid angioplasty and stenting. Stroke (10):2086, 1999

150. O'Sullivan JC, Wells DG, Wells GR: Difficult airway management with neck swelling after carotid endarterectomy. Anaesth Intens Care 14:464, 1986

151. Carmichael FJ, McGuire GP, Wong DT *et al:* Computed tomographic analysis of airway dimensions after carotid endarterectomy. Anesth Analg 83(1):12, 1996

152. Mauney MC, Buchanan SA, Lawrence WA *et al:* Stroke rate is markedly reduced after carotid endarterectomy by avoidance of protamine. J Vasc Surg 22(3):264, 1995; discussion 269

153. Lipsett PA, Tierney S, Gordon TA *et al:* Carotid endarterectomy: Is intensive care unit care necessary? J Vasc Surg 20:403, 1994

154. Lawrence PF, Gazak C, Bhirangi L *et al:* The epidemiology of surgically repaired aneurysms in the United States. J Vasc Surg 30(4):632, 1999

155. Ernst CB: Abdominal aortic aneurysm. N Engl J Med 328(16):1167, 1993

156. Davies AJ, Winter RK, Lewis MH: Prevalence of abdominal aortic aneurysms in urology patients referred for ultrasound. Ann R Coll Surg Engl 81(4):235, 1999

157. Guirguis EM, Barber GG: The natural history of abdominal aortic aneurysms. Am J Surg 162:481, 1991

158. Gelman S: The pathophysiology of aortic cross-clamping and unclamping. Anesthesiology 82:1026, 1995

159. Roizen MF, Ellis JE, Foss JF *et al:* Intraoperative management of the patient requiring supraceliac aortic occlusion. In Veith FJ, Hobson RW, Williams RA, Wilson SE (eds): Vascular Surgery, 2nd ed, p 256. New York, McGraw-Hill, 1994

160. Paterson IS, Klausner JM, Goldman G *et al:* Pulmonary edema after aneurysm surgery is modified by mannitol. Ann Surg 210:796, 1989

161. Latson TW, Reinhart DJ, Allison PM *et al:* Ketorolac tromethamine may be efficacious in treating hypotension from mesenteric traction. J Cardiothorac Vasc Anesth 6:456, 1992

162. Foulds S, Cheshire NJ, Schachter M *et al:* Endotoxin related early neutrophil activation is associated with outcome after thoracoabdominal aortic aneurysm repair. Br J Surg 84(2):172, 1997

163. Holzheimer RG, Gross J, Schein M: Pro- and anti-inflammatory cytokine-response in abdominal aortic aneurysm repair: A clinical model of ischemia-reperfusion. Shock 11(5):305, 1999

164. Ziegenfuss T, Wanner GA, Grass C *et al:* Mixed agonistic-antagonistic cytokine response in whole blood from patients undergoing abdominal aortic aneurysm repair. Intensive Care Med 25(3):279, 1999

165. Froon AH, Greve JW, Van der Linden CJ, Buurman WA: Increased concentrations of cytokines and adhesion molecules in patients after repair of abdominal aortic aneurysm. Eur J Surg 162(4):287, 1996

166. Swartbol P, Truedsson L, Norgren L: Adverse reactions during endovascular treatment of aortic aneurysms may be triggered by interleukin 6 release from the thrombotic content. J Vasc Surg 28(4):664, 1998

167. Syk I, Brunkwall J, Ivancev K *et al:* Postoperative fever, bowel ischaemia and cytokine response to abdominal aortic aneurysm repair—a comparison between endovascular and open surgery. Eur J Vasc Endovasc Surg 15(5):398, 1998

168. Norman JG, Fink GW: The effects of epidural anesthesia on the neuroendocrine response to major surgical stress: A randomized prospective trial. Am Surg 63(1):75, 1997

169. Nagelschmidt M, Fu ZX, Saad S *et al:* Preoperative high dose methylprednisolone improves patients outcome after abdominal surgery. Eur J Surg 165(10):971, 1999

170. O'Connor CJ: Thoracic and thoracoabdominal aortic aneurysm repair. Prob Anesth 11:266

171. Piccone W, DeLaria GA, Najafi H: Descending thoracic aneurysms. In Bergan JJ, Yao JST (eds): Aortic Surgery, p 249. Philadelphia, WB Saunders, 1989

172. Williams GM, Perler BA, Burdick JF *et al:* Angiographic localization of spinal cord blood supply and its relationship to postoperative paraplegia. J Vasc Surg 13:23, 1991

173. Pass LJ, Eberhart RC, Brown JC *et al:* The effect of mannitol and dopamine on the renal response to thoracic aortic cross-clamping. J Thorac Cardiovasc Surg 95:608, 1988

174. Gamulin Z, Forster A, Morel D *et al:* Effects of infrarenal aortic cross-clamping on renal hemodynamics in humans. Anesthesiology 61:394, 1984

175. Roizen MF, Rodgers GM, Valone FH *et al:* Anaphylactoid reactions to vascular graft material presenting with vasodilation and subsequent disseminated intravascular coagulation. Anesthesiology 71:331, 1989

176. Kahn RA, Moskowitz DM, Manspeizer HE *et al:* Endovascular aortic repair is associated with greater hemodynamic stability compared with open aortic reconstruction. J Cardiothorac Vasc Anesth 13(1):42, 1999

177. Buth J, Laheij RJ: Early complications and endoleaks after endovascular abdominal aortic aneurysm repair: Report of a multicenter study. J Vasc Surg 31(1 Pt 1):134, 2000

178. Cambria RP, Davison JK, Zannetti S *et al:* Thoracoabdominal aneurysm repair: Perspectives over a decade with the clamp-and-sew technique. Ann Surg 226(3):294, 1997

179. Safi HJ, Miller CC 3rd, Subramaniam MH *et al:* Thoracic and thoracoabdominal aortic aneurysm repair using cardiopulmonary bypass, profound hypothermia, and circulatory arrest via left side of the chest incision. J Vasc Surg 28(4):591, 1998

180. Frank SM, Parker SD, Rock P *et al:* Moderate hypothermia, with partial bypass and segmental sequential repair for thoracoabdominal aortic aneurysm. J Vasc Surg 19:687, 1994

181. Scheinin SA, Cooley DA: Graft replacement of the descending thoracic aorta: Results of "open" distal anastomosis. Ann Thorac Surg 58:19, 1994

182. Safi HJ, Bartoli S, Hess KR *et al:* Neurologic deficit in patients at high risk with thoracoabdominal aortic aneurysms: The role of cerebral spinal fluid drainage and distal aortic perfusion. J Vasc Surg 20:434, 1994

183. Greenberg R, Resch T, Nyman U *et al:* Endovascular repair of descending thoracic aortic aneurysms: An early experience with intermediate-term follow-up. J Vasc Surg 31(1 Pt 1):147, 2000

184. Alpert RA, Roizen MF, Hamilton WK *et al:* Intraoperative urinary output does not predict postoperative renal function in patients undergoing abdominal aortic revascularization. Surgery 95:707, 1984

185. Solomon R, Werner C, Mann D *et al:* Effects of saline, mannitol, and furosemide to prevent acute decreases in renal function induced by radiocontrast agents. N Engl J Med 331:1416, 1994

186. Baldwin L, Henderson A, Hickman P: Effect of postoperative low-dose dopamine on renal function after elective major vascular surgery. Ann Intern Med 120(9):744, 1994

187. Soong CV, Halliday MI, Hood JM *et al:* Effect of low-dose dopamine on sigmoid colonic intramucosal pH in patients undergoing elective abdominal aortic aneurysm repair. Br J Surg 82(7):912, 1995

188. Valentine RJ, Duke ML, Inman MH *et al:* Effectiveness of pulmonary artery catheters in aortic surgery: A randomized trial. J Vasc Surg 27(2):203, 1998

189. ASA Task Force on Guidelines for Pulmonary Artery Catheterization: Practice guidelines for pulmonary artery catheterization: A report by the American Society of Anesthesiologists Task Force on Pulmonary Artery Catheterization. Anesthesiology 78:380, 1993

190. Eyraud D, Benmalek F, Teugels K *et al:* Does desflurane alter left

ventricular function when used to control surgical stimulation during aortic surgery? Acta Anaesthesiol Scand 43(7):737, 1999

191. Stuhmeier KD, Mainzer B, Sandmann W, Tarnow J: Isoflurane does not increase the incidence of intraoperative myocardial ischaemia compared with halothane during vascular surgery. Br J Anaesth 69:602, 1992

192. Summary of safety-related drug labeling changes approved by FDA. December 1997. http://www.fda.gov/medwatch/safety/1997/dec97.htm#ultane

193. Hohner P, Backman C, Diamond G et al: Anaesthesia for abdominal aortic surgery in patients with coronary artery disease: II. Effects of nitrous oxide on systemic and coronary haemodynamics, regional ventricular function and incidence of myocardial ischaemia. Acta Anaesthesiol Scand 38:793, 1994

194. Seyde WC, Ellis JE, Longnecker DE: The addition of nitrous oxide to halothane decreases renal and splanchnic flow and increases cerebral blood flow in rats. Br J Anaesth 58:63, 1986

195. Benefiel DJ, Roizen MF, Lampe GH et al: Morbidity after aortic surgery with sufentanil versus isoflurane anesthesia. Anesthesiology 65:A516, 1986

196. Breslow MJ, Jordan DA, Christopherson R et al: Epidural morphine decreases postoperative hypertension by attenuating sympathetic nervous system hyperactivity. JAMA 261:3577, 1989

197. Blomberg S, Emanuelsson H, Kvist H et al: Effects of thoracic epidural anesthesia on coronary arteries and arterioles in patients with coronary artery disease. Anesthesiology 73:840, 1990

198. Lunn JK, Dannemiller FJ, Stanley TH: Cardiovascular responses to clamping of the aorta during epidural and general anesthesia. Anesth Analg 58:372, 1979

199. Raner C, Biber B, Lundberg J et al: Cardiovascular depression by isoflurane and concomitant thoracic epidural anesthesia is reversed by dopamine. Acta Anaesthesiol Scand 38:136, 1994

200. Clagett GP, Valentine RJ, Jackson MR et al: A randomized trial of intraoperative autotransfusion during aortic surgery. J Vasc Surg 29(1):22, 1999

201. Manheim LM, Sohn MW, Feinglass J et al: Hospital vascular surgery volume and procedure mortality rates in California, 1982–1994. J Vasc Surg 28(1):45, 1998

202. Wakefield TW, Whitehouse WM Jr, Shu-Chen W et al: Abdominal aortic aneurysm rupture: Statistical analysis of factors affecting outcome of surgical treatment. Surgery 91:586, 1982

203. Morales D, Madigan J, Cullinane S et al: Reversal by vasopressin of intractable hypotension in the late phase of hemorrhagic shock. Circulation 100(3):226, 1999

204. Wilson J, Woods I, Fawcett J et al: Reducing the risk of major elective surgery: Randomised controlled trial of preoperative optimisation of oxygen delivery. Br Med J 318:1099, 1999

205. Hayes MA, Timmins AC, Yau EH et al: Elevation of systemic oxygen delivery in the treatment of critically ill patients. N Engl J Med 330:1717, 1994

206. Ranieri VM, Suter PM, Tortorella C et al: Effect of mechanical ventilation on inflammatory mediators in patients with acute respiratory distress syndrome: A randomized controlled trial. JAMA 282:54, 1999

207. National Institutes of Health/National Heart, Lung, and Blood Institute ARDS Network. Available at: http://hedwig.mgh.harvard.edu/ardsnet/nih.html.

208. Bickell WH, Wall MJ Jr, Pepe PE et al: Immediate versus delayed fluid resuscitation for hypotensive patients with penetrating torso injuries. N Engl J Med 331:1105, 1994

209. Ouriel K, Shortell CK, DeWeese JA et al: A comparison of thrombolytic therapy with operative revascularization in the initial treatment of acute peripheral arterial ischemia. J Vasc Surg 19:1021, 1994

210. Tunis SR, Bass EB, Steinberg EP: The use of angioplasty, bypass surgery, and amputation in the management of peripheral vascular disease. N Engl J Med 325:556, 1991

211. Veith FJ, Panetta TF, Wengerter KR et al: Femoro-popliteal-tibial occlusive disease. In Veith FJ, Hobson RW, Williams RA, Wilson SE (eds): Vascular Surgery, 2nd ed, p 421. New York, McGraw-Hill, 1994

212. Harward TR, Govostis DM, Rosenthal GJ et al: Impact of angioscopy on infrainguinal graft patency. Am J Surg 168:107, 1994

213. Berlauk JF, Abrams JH, Gilmour IJ et al: Preoperative optimization of cardiovascular hemodynamics improves outcome in peripheral vascular surgery: A prospective, randomized clinical trial. Ann Surg 214:289, 1991

214. Bush HL Jr, LoGerfo FW, Weisel RD et al: Assessment of myocardial performance and optimal volume loading during elective abdominal aortic aneurysm resection. Arch Surg 112:1301, 1977

215. Bode RH Jr, Lewis KP, Zarich SW et al: Cardiac outcome after peripheral vascular surgery. Comparison of general and regional anesthesia. Anesthesiology 84(1):3, 1996

216. Caplan RA, Ward RJ, Posner K, Cheney FW: Unexpected cardiac arrest during spinal anesthesia: A closed claims analysis of predisposing factors. Anesthesiology 68:5, 1988

217. Schunn CD, Hertzer NR, O'Hara PJ et al: Epidural versus general anesthesia: Does anesthetic management influence early infrainguinal graft thrombosis? Ann Vasc Surg 12(1):65, 1998

218. Pierce ET, Pomposelli FB Jr, Stanley GD et al: Anesthesia type does not influence early graft patency or limb salvage rates of lower extremity arterial bypass. J Vasc Surg 25(2):226, 1997

219. Ammar AD: Postoperative epidural analgesia following abdominal aortic surgery: do the benefits justify the costs? Ann Vasc Surg 2(4):359, 1998

220. Horlocker TT, Wedel DJ, Offord KP: Does preoperative antiplatelet therapy increase the risk of hemorrhagic complications associated with regional anesthesia? Anesth Analg 70:631, 1990

221. Dickman CA, Shedd SA, Spetzler RF et al: Spinal epidural hematoma associated with epidural anesthesia: Complications of systemic heparinization in patients receiving peripheral vascular thrombolytic therapy. Anesthesiology 72:947, 1990

222. Rao TLK, El-Etr AA: Anticoagulation following placement of epidural and subarachnoid catheters: An evaluation of neurologic sequelae. Anesthesiology 55:618, 1981

223. Yeager MP, Glass DD, Neff RK et al: Epidural anesthesia and analgesia in high-risk surgical patients. Anesthesiology 66:729, 1987

224. Breslow MJ, Parker SD, Frank SM et al: Determinants of catecholamine and cortisol responses to lower extremity revascularization: The PIRAT Study Group. Anesthesiology 79:1202, 1993

Clinical Anesthesia (4/e), edited by
Paul G. Barash, Bruce F. Cullen, and
Robert K. Stoelting. Lippincott Williams &
Wilkins, Philadelphia, © 2001.

CHAPTER 34

ANESTHESIA AND THE EYE

KATHRYN E. McGOLDRICK

Anesthesia for ophthalmic surgery presents many unique challenges (Table 34-1). In addition to possessing technical expertise, the anesthesiologist must have detailed knowledge of ocular anatomy, physiology, and pharmacology. It is essential to appreciate that ophthalmic drugs may significantly alter the reaction to anesthesia and that, concomitantly, anesthetic drugs and maneuvers may dramatically influence intraocular dynamics. Patients undergoing ophthalmic surgery may represent extremes of age and coexisting medical diseases (*e.g.,* diabetes mellitus, coronary artery disease, essential hypertension, chronic lung disease), but they are likely to be in the elderly age group. Apprehension is predictable in blind or potentially blind patients awaiting surgery.

It is mandatory to be knowledgeable about the numerous surgical procedures unique to the specialty of ophthalmology. Whereas the list of ocular surgical interventions is lengthy, these procedures may, in general, be classified as extraocular or intraocular. This distinction is critical because anesthetic considerations are different for these two major surgical categories. For example, with intraocular procedures, profound akinesia (relaxation of recti muscles) and meticulous control of intraocular pressure (IOP) are requisite. However, with extraocular surgery, the significance of IOP fades, whereas concern about elicitation of the oculocardiac reflex assumes prominence.

OCULAR ANATOMY

The anesthesiologist should be knowledgeable about ocular anatomy to enhance his or her understanding of surgical procedures and to aid the surgeon in the performance of regional blocks when needed[1,2] (Fig. 34-1). Salient subdivisions of ocular anatomy include the orbit, the eye itself, the extraocular muscles, the eyelids, and the lacrimal system.

The orbit is a bony box, or pyramidal cavity, housing the eyeball and its associated structures in the skull. The walls of the orbit are composed of the following bones: frontal, zygomatic, greater wing of the sphenoid, maxilla, palatine, lacrimal, and ethmoid. A familiarity with the surface relationships of the orbital rim is mandatory for the skilled performance of regional blocks.

The optic foramen, located at the orbital apex, transmits the optic nerve and the ophthalmic artery, as well as sympathetic nerves from the carotid plexus. The superior orbital fissure transmits the superior and inferior branches of the oculomotor nerve, the lacrimal, frontal, and nasociliary branches of the trigeminal nerve, as well as the trochlear and abducens nerves and the superior and inferior ophthalmic veins. The inferior orbital or sphenomaxillary fissure contains the infraorbital and zygomatic nerves and a communication between the inferior ophthalmic vein and the pterygoid plexus. The infraorbital foramen, located about 4 mm below the orbital rim in the maxilla, transmits the infraorbital nerve, artery, and vein. The lacrimal fossa, which contains the lacrimal gland in the superior temporal orbit. The supraorbital notch, located at the junction of the medial one third and temporal two thirds of the superior orbital rim, transmits the supraorbital nerve, artery, and vein. The supraorbital notch, the infraorbital foramen, and the lacri-

mal fossa are clinically palpable and function as major landmarks for administration of regional anesthesia.

The eye itself is actually one large sphere with part of a smaller sphere incorporated in the anterior surface, constituting a structure with two different radii of curvature. The coat of the eye is composed of three layers: sclera, uveal tract, and retina. The fibrous outer layer, or sclera, is protective, providing sufficient rigidity to maintain the shape of the eye. The anterior portion of the sclera, the cornea, is transparent, permitting light to pass into the internal ocular structures. The double-spherical shape of the eye exists because the corneal arc of curvature is steeper than the scleral arc of curvature. The focusing of rays of light to form a retinal image commences at the cornea.

The uveal tract, or middle layer of the globe, is vascular and in direct apposition to the sclera. A potential space, known as the suprachoroidal space, separates the sclera from the uveal tract. This potential space, however, may become filled with blood during an expulsive or suprachoroidal hemorrhage, often associated with surgical disaster. The iris, ciliary body, and choroid compose the uveal tract. The iris includes the pupil, which, by contractions of three sets of muscles, controls the amount of light entering the eye. The iris dilator is sympathetically innervated; the iris sphincter and the ciliary muscle have parasympathetic innervation. Posterior to the iris lies the ciliary body, which produces aqueous humor (see Formation and Drainage of Aqueous Humor). The ciliary muscles, situated in the ciliary body, adjust the shape of the lens to accommodate focusing at various distances. Large vessels and a network of small vessels and capillaries known as the choriocapillaris constitute the choroid, which supplies nutrition to the outer part of the retina.

The retina is a neurosensory membrane composed of 10 layers that convert light impulses into neural impulses. These neural impulses are then carried through the optic nerve to the brain. Located in the center of the globe is the vitreous cavity, filled with a gelatinous substance known as vitreous humor. This material is adherent to the most anterior 3 mm of the retina as well as to large blood vessels and the optic nerve. The vitreous humor may pull on the retina, causing retinal tears and retinal detachment.

The crystalline lens, located posterior to the pupil, refracts rays of light passing through the cornea and pupil to focus images on the retina. The ciliary muscle, whose contractile state causes tautness or relaxation of the lens zonules, regulates the thickness of the lens.

In addition, six extraocular muscles move the eye within the orbit to various positions. The bilobed lacrimal gland provides most of the tear film, which serves to maintain a moist anterior surface on the globe. The lacrimal drainage system, composed of the puncta, canaliculi, lacrimal sac, and lacrimal duct, drains into the nose below the inferior turbinate. Blockage of this system occurs not infrequently, necessitating procedures ranging from lacrimal duct probing to dacryocystorhinostomy, which involves anastomosis of the lacrimal sac to the nasal mucosa.

Covering the surface of the globe and lining the eyelids is a mucous membrane called the conjunctiva. Because drugs are absorbed across the membrane, it is a popular site for administration of ophthalmic drugs.

970 MANAGEMENT OF ANESTHESIA

Table 34-1. REQUIREMENTS OF OPHTHALMIC SURGERY

Safety
Akinesia
Profound analgesia
Minimal bleeding
Avoidance or obtundation of oculocardiac reflex
Control of intraocular pressure
Awareness of drug interactions
Smooth emergence

The eyelids consist of four layers: (1) the conjunctiva, (2) the cartilaginous tarsal plate, (3) a muscle layer composed mainly of the orbicularis and the levator palpebrae, and (4) the skin. The eyelids protect the eye from foreign objects; through blinking, the tear film produced by the lacrimal gland is spread across the surface of the eye, keeping the cornea moist.

Blood supply to the eye and orbit is by means of branches of both the internal and external carotid arteries. Venous drainage of the orbit is accomplished through the multiple anastomoses of the superior and inferior ophthalmic veins. Venous drainage of the eye is achieved mainly through the central retinal vein. All these veins empty directly into the cavernous sinus.

The sensory and motor innervations of the eye and its adnexa are very complex, with multiple cranial nerves supplying branches to various ocular structures. A branch of the oculomotor nerve supplies a motor root to the ciliary ganglion, which in turn supplies the sphincter of the pupil and the ciliary muscle. The trochlear nerve supplies the superior oblique muscle. The abducens nerve supplies the lateral rectus muscle. The trigeminal nerve constitutes the most complex ocular and adnexal innervation. In addition, the zygomatic branch of the facial nerve eventually divides into an upper branch, supplying the frontalis and the upper lid orbicularis, whereas the lower branch supplies the orbicularis of the lower lid.

OCULAR PHYSIOLOGY

Despite its relatively diminutive size, the eye is a complex organ, concerned with many intricate physiologic processes. The formation and drainage of aqueous humor and their influence on IOP in both normal and glaucomatous eyes are among the most important functions, especially from the anesthesiologist's perspective. An appreciation of the effects of various anesthetic manipulations on IOP requires an understanding of the fundamental principles of ocular physiology.

Formation and Drainage of Aqueous Humor

Two thirds of the aqueous humor is formed in the posterior chamber by the ciliary body in an active secretory process involving both the carbonic anhydrase and the cytochrome oxidase systems (Fig. 34-2). The remaining third is formed by passive filtration of aqueous humor from the vessels on the anterior surface of the iris.

At the ciliary epithelium, sodium is actively transported into the aqueous humor in the posterior chamber. Bicarbonate and chloride ions passively follow the sodium ions. This active mechanism results in the osmotic pressure of the aqueous being many times greater than that of plasma. It is this disparity in osmotic pressure that leads to an average rate of aqueous humor production of $2~\mu l \cdot min^{-1}$.

Aqueous humor flows from the posterior chamber through the pupillary aperture into the anterior chamber, where it mixes with the aqueous formed by the iris. During its journey into the anterior chamber, the aqueous humor bathes the avascular lens, providing essential metabolic materials and removing metabolic wastes. Once in the anterior chamber, the aqueous also bathes the corneal endothelium, maintaining healthy corneal metabolism. Then the aqueous flows into the peripheral segment of the anterior chamber and exits the eye through the trabecular network, Schlemm's canal, and the episcleral venous system. A network of connecting venous channels eventually leads to the superior vena cava and the right atrium. Thus, obstruction of venous return at any point from the eye to the right side of the heart impedes aqueous drainage, elevating IOP accordingly.

Maintenance of Intraocular Pressure

Intraocular pressure normally varies between 10 and 21.7 mm Hg and is considered abnormal above 22 mm Hg. This level varies 1–2 mm Hg with each cardiac contraction. Also, a diurnal

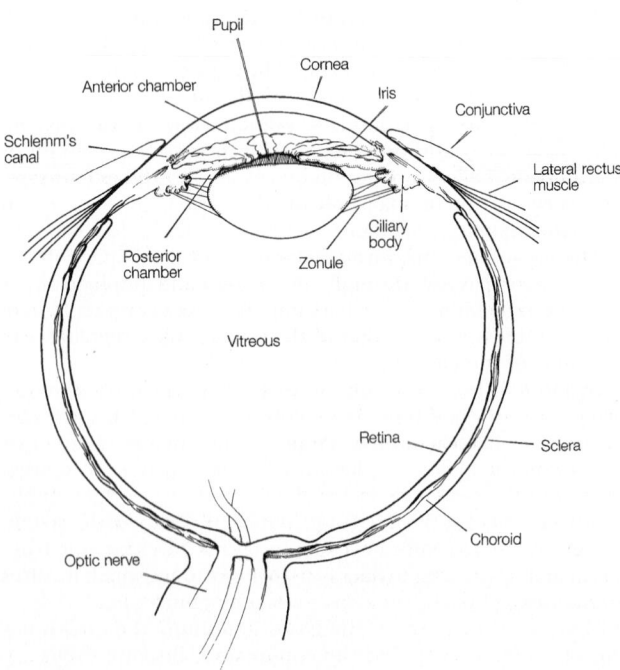

Figure 34-1. Diagram of ocular anatomy.

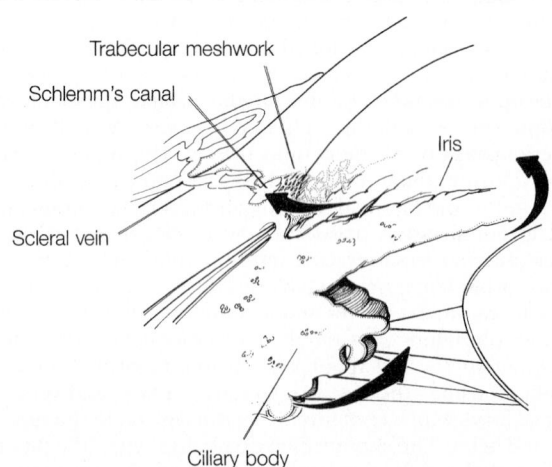

Figure 34-2. Ocular anatomy concerned with control of intraocular pressure.

variation of 2–5 mm Hg is observed, with a higher value noted on awakening. This higher awakening pressure has been ascribed to vascular congestion, pressure on the globe from closed lids, and mydriasis—all of which occur during sleep.

Intraocular pressure far exceeds not only tissue pressure (2–3 mm Hg) but intracranial pressure (7–8 mm Hg). Apparently the maintenance of such a relatively high pressure in the eye is demanded by the optical properties of refracting surfaces; the corneal surface should be kept at a constant curvature, and the stroma must be under constant high pressure to maintain a uniform refractive index.[3] However, an abnormally high pressure may result in opacities by interfering with normal corneal metabolism.

During anesthesia, a rise in IOP can produce permanent visual loss. If the IOP is already elevated, a further increase can trigger acute glaucoma. If penetration of the globe occurs when the IOP is excessively high, rupture of a blood vessel with subsequent hemorrhage may transpire. IOP becomes atmospheric once the eye cavity has been entered, and any sudden rise in pressure may lead to prolapse of the iris and lens, and loss of vitreous. Thus, proper control of IOP is critical.

Three main factors influence IOP: (1) external pressure on the eye by the contraction of the orbicularis oculi muscle and the tone of the extraocular muscles, venous congestion of orbital veins (as may occur with vomiting and coughing), and conditions such as orbital tumor; (2) scleral rigidity; and (3) changes in intraocular contents that are semisolid (lens, vitreous, or intraocular tumor) or fluid (blood and aqueous humor). Although all these factors are significant in affecting IOP, the major control of intraocular tension is exerted by the fluid content, especially the aqueous humor.

Sclerosis of the sclera, not uncommonly seen in the aged, may be associated with decreased scleral compliance and increased IOP. Other degenerative changes of the eye linked with aging can also influence IOP, the most significant being a hardening and enlargement of the crystalline lens. When these degenerative changes occur, they may lead to anterior displacement of the lens–iris diaphragm. A resultant shallowness of the anterior chamber angle may then occur, reducing access of the trabecular meshwork to aqueous. This process is usually gradual, but, if rapid lens engorgement occurs, angle-closure glaucoma may transpire.

Changes in the nature of the vitreous that affect the amount of unbound water also influence IOP. Myopia, trauma, and aging produce liquefaction of vitreous gel and a subsequent increase in unbound water, which may lower IOP by facilitating fluid removal. However, under different circumstances, the opposite may occur, that is, the hydration of more normal vitreous may be associated with elevation of IOP. Hence, it is often prudent to produce a slightly dehydrated state in the surgical patient with glaucoma.

Intraocular blood volume, determined primarily by vessel dilation or contraction in the spongy layers of the choroid, contributes significantly to IOP. Although changes in both arterial or venous pressure may secondarily affect IOP, excursions in arterial pressure have much less importance than do venous fluctuations. In chronic arterial hypertension, ocular pressure returns to normal levels after a period of adaptation brought about by compression of vessels in the choroid as a result of increased IOP. Thus, a feedback mechanism reduces the total volume of blood, keeping IOP relatively constant in patients with systemic hypertension.[4]

However, if venous return from the eye is disturbed at any point from Schlemm's canal to the right atrium, IOP increases substantially. This is caused both by increased intraocular blood volume and distention of orbital vessels, as well as by interference with aqueous drainage. Straining, vomiting, or coughing greatly increase venous pressure and raise IOP as much as 40 mm Hg or greater. The deleterious implications of these activities cannot be overemphasized. Laryngoscopy and tracheal intubation may also elevate IOP, even without any visible reaction to intubation, but especially when the patient coughs. Topical anesthetization of the larynx may attenuate the hypertensive response to laryngoscopy but does not reliably prevent associated increases in IOP.[5] Ordinarily, the pressure elevation from such increases in blood volume or venous pressure dissipates rapidly. However, if the coughing or straining occurs during ocular surgery when the eye is open, as in cataract extraction or in penetrating keratoplasty, the result may be a disastrous expulsive hemorrhage, at worst, or a disconcerting loss of vitreous, at best.

Despite the significant role of venous pressure, scleral rigidity, and vitreous composition, maintenance of IOP is determined primarily by the rate of aqueous formation and the rate of aqueous outflow. The most important influence on formation of aqueous humor is the difference in osmotic pressure between aqueous and plasma.[3] This fact is illustrated by the equation:

$$IOP = K[(OPaq - OPpl) + CP] \qquad (34\text{-}1)$$

where K = coefficient of outflow, OPaq = osmotic pressure of aqueous humor, OPpl = osmotic pressure of plasma, and CP = capillary pressure. The fact that a small change in solute concentration of plasma can markedly influence the formation of aqueous humor and hence IOP is the rationale for using hypertonic solutions, such as mannitol, to lower IOP.

Fluctuations in aqueous outflow may also produce a dramatic alteration in IOP. The most significant factor controlling aqueous humor outflow is the diameter of Fontana's spaces,[6] as illustrated by the equation:

$$A = \frac{r^4 \times (Piop - Pv)}{8\eta L} \qquad (34\text{-}2)$$

where A = volume of aqueous outflow per unit of time, r = radius of Fontana's spaces, Piop = IOP, Pv = venous pressure, η = viscosity, and L = length of Fontana's spaces. When the pupil dilates, Fontana's spaces narrow, resistance to outflow is increased, and IOP rises. Because mydriasis is undesirable in both closed- and open-angle glaucoma, miotics such as pilocarpine are applied conjunctivally in patients with glaucoma.

Glaucoma

Glaucoma is a condition characterized by elevated IOP, resulting in impairment of capillary blood flow to the optic nerve with eventual loss of optic nerve tissue and function. Two different anatomic types of glaucoma exist: open-angle or chronic simple glaucoma, and closed-angle or acute glaucoma. (Other variations of these processes occur but are not especially germane to anesthetic management.)

With open-angle glaucoma, the elevated IOP exists with an anatomically open anterior chamber angle. It is thought that sclerosis of trabecular tissue results in impaired aqueous filtration and drainage. Treatment consists of medication to produce miosis and trabecular stretching. Commonly used eyedrops are epinephrine, timolol, dipivefrin, and betaxolol. Closed-angle glaucoma is characterized by the peripheral iris moving into direct contact with the posterior corneal surface, mechanically obstructing aqueous outflow. People who have a narrow angle between the iris and posterior cornea are predisposed to this condition. In these patients, mydriasis can produce such increased thickening of the peripheral iris that corneal touch occurs and the angle is closed. Another mechanism producing acute, closed-angle glaucoma is swelling of the crystalline lens. In this case, pupillary block occurs, with the edematous lens blocking the flow of aqueous from the posterior to the anterior chamber. This situation can also develop if the lens is traumatically dislocated anteriorly, thus physically blocking the anterior chamber.

It was previously thought by some clinicians that patients with glaucoma should not be given atropine premedication. However, this claim is untenable. Atropine premedication in the dose range used clinically has no effect on IOP in either open- or closed-angle glaucoma. When 0.4 mg of atropine is given to a 70-kg person, approximately 0.0001 mg is absorbed by the eye.[7] Garde *et al*[8] reported, however, that scopolamine has a greater mydriatic effect than atropine and recommended not using scopolamine in patients with known or suspected closed-angle glaucoma.

Equation 34-2, describing the volume of aqueous outflow per unit of time, clearly demonstrates that outflow is exquisitely sensitive to fluctuations in venous pressure. Because a rise in venous pressure produces an increased volume of ocular blood as well as decreased aqueous outflow, it is obvious that considerable elevation of IOP occurs with any maneuver that increases venous pressure. Hence, in addition to preoperative instillation of miotics, other anesthetic goals for the patient with glaucoma include perioperative avoidance of venous congestion and of overhydration. Furthermore, hypotensive episodes are to be avoided because these patients are allegedly vulnerable to retinal vascular thrombosis.

Primary congenital glaucoma is classified according to age of onset, with the infantile type presenting any time after birth until 3 years of age. The juvenile type presents between the ages of 37 months and 30 years. Moreover, childhood glaucoma may also occur in conjunction with various eye diseases or developmental anomalies such as aniridia, mesodermal dysgenesis syndrome, and retinopathy of prematurity.[9]

Successful management of infantile glaucoma is crucially dependent on early diagnosis. Presenting symptoms include epiphora, photophobia, blepharospasm, and irritability. Ocular enlargement, termed *buphthalmos,* or "ox eye," and corneal haziness secondary to edema are common. Buphthalmos is rare, however, if glaucoma develops after 3 years of age because by then the eye is much less elastic.

Because infantile glaucoma is frequently associated with obstructed aqueous outflow, management of it often requires surgical creation, by goniotomy or trabeculotomy, of a route for aqueous humor to flow into Schlemm's canal. However, advanced disease may be unresponsive to even multiple goniotomies, and the more radical trabeculectomy or some other variety of filtering procedure may be necessary.

The juvenile form of glaucoma, in which the cornea and eye size are normal, is commonly associated with a family history of open-angle glaucoma and is treated similarly to primary open-angle glaucoma.

In cases of pediatric secondary glaucoma, goniotomy and filtering may be unsuccessful, whereas cyclocryotherapy may effect a reduction in IOP, pain, and corneal edema. The ciliary body is destroyed with a cryoprobe, cooled to $-70°C$, thus dramatically decreasing aqueous formation.

It is essential to appreciate that the high IOP frequently encountered in infantile glaucoma can be reduced by more than 15 mm Hg when surgical anesthesia is achieved. One study, however, demonstrated minimal effect of halothane on IOP when the concentration ranged narrowly between 0.5 and 1.0%.[10] Some clinicians maintain that ketamine is a useful drug to use for examination under anesthesia when infantile glaucoma is part of the differential diagnosis because ketamine does not appear to reduce IOP, giving a spuriously low reading. Moreover, even normal infants sporadically have pressures in the mid-20s. Hence, diagnosis is not based exclusively on the numerical pressure recorded under anesthesia. Other factors such as corneal edema and increased corneal diameter, tears in Descemet's membrane, and cupping of the optic nerve are considered in making the diagnosis. If these aberrations are noted, surgical intervention may be mandatory, even in the setting of a reputedly normal IOP.

EFFECTS OF ANESTHESIA AND ADJUVANT DRUGS ON INTRAOCULAR PRESSURE

Central Nervous System Depressants

Inhalation anesthetics purportedly cause dose-related decreases in IOP.[11] The exact mechanisms are unknown, but postulated etiologies include depression of a central nervous system (CNS) control center in the diencephalon,[4] reduction of aqueous humor production, enhancement of aqueous outflow, or relaxation of the extraocular muscles.[7] Moreover, virtually all CNS depressants, including barbiturates,[12] neuroleptics,[13] opioids, tranquilizers,[7] and hypnotics, such as etomidate[14] and propofol,[15] lower IOP in both normal and glaucomatous eyes. Etomidate, despite its proclivity to produce pain on intravenous (iv) injection and skeletal muscle movement, is associated with a significant reduction in IOP.[16] However, etomidate-induced myoclonus may be hazardous in the setting of a ruptured globe.

Controversy, however, surrounds the issue of ketamine's effect on IOP. Administered iv or intramuscularly (im), ketamine initially was thought to increase IOP significantly, as measured by indentation tonometry.[17] Corssen and Hoy[18] had also reported a slight but statistically significant increase in IOP that appeared unrelated to changes in blood pressure or depth of anesthesia. However, nystagmus made proper positioning of the tonometer difficult and may have resulted in less-than-accurate measurements.

Conflicting results arose from a study in which $2 \text{ mg} \cdot \text{kg}^{-1}$ of ketamine given iv to adults failed to have a significant effect on IOP.[19] Furthermore, a pediatric study reported no increase in IOP after an im ketamine dose of $8 \text{ mg} \cdot \text{kg}^{-1}$. Indeed, values obtained were similar to those reported with halothane and isoflurane.[20,21]

Some of the confusion may arise from differences in premedication practices and from the use of different instruments to measure IOP. More recent studies have used applanation tonometry rather than indentation tonometry. However, even if future studies should confirm that ketamine has minimal or no effect on IOP, ketamine's proclivity to cause nystagmus and blepharospasm makes it a less-than-optimal agent for many types of ophthalmic surgery.

Ventilation and Temperature

Hyperventilation decreases IOP, whereas asphyxia, administration of carbon dioxide, and hypoventilation have been shown to elevate IOP.[3,22]

Hypothermia lowers IOP. On initial consideration, hypothermia might be expected to raise IOP because of the associated increase in viscosity of aqueous humor. However, hypothermia is linked with decreased formation of aqueous humor and with vasoconstriction; hence, the net result is a reduction in IOP.

Adjuvant Drugs

Ganglionic Blockers, Hypertonic Solutions, and Acetazolamide

Ganglionic blockers such as tetraethylammonium[23] and pentamethonium effect a dramatic decrease in IOP. Trimethaphan also significantly lowers IOP in normal subjects, despite mydriasis.

Intravenous administration of hypertonic solutions such as dextran, urea, mannitol, and sorbitol elevates plasma osmotic pressure, thereby decreasing aqueous humor formation and reducing IOP.[24] As effective as urea is in reducing IOP, iv mannitol has the advantage of fewer side effects. Mannitol's onset, peak (30–45 minutes), and duration of action (5–6 hours) are similar to those of urea. Moreover, both drugs may produce acute intravascular volume overload. Sudden expansion of plasma volume secondary to efflux of intracellular water into the vascular compartment places a heavy workload on the kidneys and heart, often resulting in hypertension and dilution of plasma sodium. Furthermore, mannitol-associated diuresis, if protracted, may trigger hypotension in volume-depleted patients.

Glycerin has the advantage of being effective orally. However, the ocular hypotensive effect is said to be less predictable than that of mannitol. Onset usually occurs within 10 minutes of ingestion, and peak action is noted at 30 minutes. The duration of action is 5–6 hours. Unfortunately, glycerin may trigger nausea or vomiting, and gastric fluid trapping increases the risk of aspiration.

Intravenous administration of acetazolamide inactivates carbonic anhydrase and interferes with the sodium pump. The resultant decrease in aqueous humor formation lowers IOP. However, the action of acetazolamide is not limited to the eye, and systemic effects include loss of sodium, potassium, and water secondary to the drug's renal tubular effects. Such electrolyte imbalances may then be linked to cardiac dysrhythmias during general anesthesia.

An advantage of acetazolamide is its relative ease of administration. Whereas large volumes of hypertonic solutions must be infused to reduce IOP, acetazolamide is easily given as a typical adult dose of 500 mg dissolved in 10 ml of sterile water. Acetazolamide may also be given orally, and topical carbonic anhydrase inhibitors are commercially available.

Neuromuscular Blocking Drugs

Neuromuscular blocking drugs have both direct and indirect actions on IOP. Hence, a paralyzing dose of d-tubocurarine directly lowers IOP by relaxing the extraocular muscles.[25] The same is true of equipotent doses of the other nondepolarizing drugs, including pancuronium[26] (Fig. 34-3). However, if paralysis of the respiratory muscles is accompanied by alveolar hypoventilation, the latter secondary effect may supervene to increase IOP.

In contrast to nondepolarizing drugs, the depolarizing drug succinylcholine elevates IOP. Lincoff et al[27] reported extrusion of vitreous after succinylcholine administration to a patient with a surgically open eye. An average peak IOP increase of about 8 mm Hg is produced within 1–4 minutes of an iv dose. Within 7 minutes, return to baseline usually transpires.[28] The ocular hypertensive effect of succinylcholine has been attributed to several mechanisms, including tonic contraction of extraocular muscles,[7] choroidal vascular dilation, and relaxation of orbital smooth muscle.[29] One study speculates that the succinylcholine-induced increase in IOP is multifactorial but primarily the result of the cycloplegic action of succinylcholine producing a deepening of the anterior chamber and increased outflow resistance.[30] Because they studied eyes with the extraocular muscles detached and still observed an elevation in IOP, these investigators proposed that changes in extraocular muscle tone do not contribute significantly to the increase in IOP observed after succinylcholine administration.

A variety of methods have been advocated to prevent succinylcholine-induced elevations in IOP. In truth, although some attenuation of the increase results, none of these techniques consistently and completely blocks the ocular hypertensive response. Prior administration of such drugs as acetazolamide,[31] propranolol, and nondepolarizing neuromuscular blocking drugs has been suggested. The efficacy of pretreatment with nondepolarizing drugs is controversial.

In 1968, Miller et al,[32] using indentation tonometry, reported that pretreatment with small amounts of gallamine or d-tubocurarine prevented succinylcholine-associated increases in IOP. However, in 1978 Meyers et al,[33] using the more sensitive applanation tonometer, were unable consistently to circumvent the ocular hypertensive response after similar pretreatment therapy (Table 34-2). In addition, Verma[34] in 1979 had claimed that a "self-taming" dose of succinylcholine was protective, but Meyers et al[35] in 1980, in a controlled study using applanation tonometry, challenged this claim. Although iv pretreatment with lidocaine, 1–2 mg · kg⁻¹, may blunt the hemodynamic response to laryngoscopy,[5,36] such therapy does not reliably prevent the ocular hypertensive response associated with succinylcholine and intubation.[37] However, Grover and associates[38] claimed that pretreatment with lidocaine, 1.5 mg · kg⁻¹ iv, 1 minute before induction with thiopental and succinylcholine offered protection from IOP increases due to succinylcholine and may therefore be of value in rapid-sequence induction for open eye injuries.

Certainly, no one would disagree that succinylcholine—if unaccompanied by pretreatment with a nondepolarizing neuromuscular blocking drug—is contraindicated in patients with penetrating ocular wounds and should not be given for the first time after the eye has been opened. Nonetheless, it no longer is valid to recommend that succinylcholine be used only with extreme reluctance in ocular surgery. Clearly, any succinylcholine-induced increment in IOP is usually dissipated before surgery is started. Of concern, however, is Jampolsky's[39] warning that succinylcholine be avoided in patients undergoing repeat strabismus surgery because the forced duction test (FDT) does not return to baseline for approximately 30 minutes after administration of the drug. More recent and quantitatively sophisticated studies by France et al[40] have supported this caveat, although the latter investigators suggest waiting only 20 minutes after administration of succinylcholine before performing the FDT.

OCULOCARDIAC REFLEX

Bernard Aschner and Guiseppe Dagnini first described the oculocardiac reflex in 1908. This reflex is triggered by pressure on the globe and by traction on the extraocular muscles as well as on the conjunctiva or on the orbital structures. Moreover, the reflex may also be elicited by performance of a retrobulbar block,[41] by ocular trauma, and by direct pressure on tissue remaining in the orbital apex after enucleation.[42] The afferent limb is trigeminal and the efferent limb is vagal. Although the

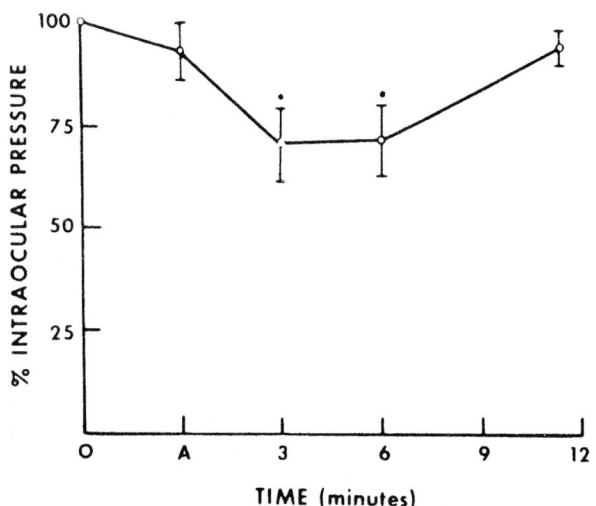

Figure 34-3. Mean intraocular pressure after administration of thiopental, 3–4 mg · kg⁻¹, and pancuronium, 0.08 mg · kg⁻¹ at 0. A = loss of lid reflux; *$p < 0.05$. (Reprinted with permission from Litwiller RW, DeFazio CA, Rushia EF: Pancuronium and intraocular pressure. Anesthesiology 42:750, 1975.)

Table 34-2. EFFECTS OF SUCCINYLCHOLINE ON INTRAOCULAR PRESSURE: DOUBLE-BLIND *d*-TUBOCURARINE OR GALLAMINE PRETREATMENT

Pretreatment*	Mean Age (yr)	Intraocular Pressure (mm Hg, mean ± SE)		
		Baseline	3 Minutes After Pretreatment	1 Minute After Succinylcholine[†]
d-Tubocurarine	13.4	13.0 ± 1.0	12.3 ± 1.2	24.0 ± 1.3
Gallamine	8.7	10.9 ± 1.1	10.6 ± 1.0	23.4 ± 2.3

* *d* Tubocurarine, 0.09 mg · kg^{-1}, or gallamine, 0.3 mg · kg^{-1}.
[†] 1 to 1.5 mg · kg^{-1} iv.
Reprinted with permission from Meyers EF, Krupin T, Johnson M *et al*: Failure of nondepolarizing neuromuscular blockers to inhibit succinylcholine-induced increased intraocular pressure: A controlled study. Anesthesiology 48:149, 1978.

most common manifestation of the oculocardiac reflex is sinus bradycardia, a wide spectrum of cardiac dysrhythmias may occur, including junctional rhythm, ectopic atrial rhythm, atrioventricular blockade, ventricular bigeminy, multifocal premature ventricular contractions, wandering pacemaker, idioventricular rhythm, asystole, and ventricular tachycardia.[43-45] This reflex may appear during either local or general anesthesia; however, hypercarbia and hypoxemia are thought to augment the incidence and severity of the problem, as may inappropriate anesthetic depth.

Reports on the alleged incidence of the oculocardiac reflex are remarkable in their striking variability. Berler's study[41] reported an incidence of 50%, but other sources quote rates ranging from 16 to 82%.[43,46] Commonly, those articles disclosing a higher incidence included children in the study population, and children tend to have more vagal tone.

A variety of maneuvers to abolish or obtund the oculocardiac reflex have been promulgated. None of these methods has been consistently effective, safe, and reliable. Inclusion of im anticholinergic drugs such as atropine or glycopyrrolate in the usual premedication regimen for oculocardiac reflex prophylaxis is ineffective.[47] Nearly complete vagolytic blockade in the adult mandates 2–3 mg of atropine or 0.03–0.05 mg · kg^{-1}.[48] Insofar as the peak action of im atropine occurs approximately 30 minutes after administration, it is not surprising that studies of the usual, routine, much smaller doses of atropine administered more than 1 hour before surgery have shown inconsistent protection against the oculocardiac reflex.

For the young child who is extremely apprehensive about "shots," giving oral atropine, 0.04 mg · kg^{-1}, with a small amount of water 60–90 minutes before surgery is an alternative.[49] However, the oral route has not enjoyed tremendous popularity with anesthesiologists because of its slower absorption and more erratic efficacy.

Atropine given iv within 30 minutes of surgery[46] is thought to effect a reduced incidence of the reflex. However, reports differ concerning dosage and timing. Moreover, some anesthesiologists claim that prior iv administration of atropine may yield more serious and refractory cardiac dysrhythmias[50] than the reflex itself. Clearly, atropine may be considered a potential myocardial irritant. A variety of cardiac dysrhythmias[51,52] and several conduction abnormalities,[53] including ventricular fibrillation, ventricular tachycardia, and left bundle-branch block, have been attributed to iv atropine.

Although administration of retrobulbar anesthesia may provide some cardiac antidysrhythmic value by blocking the afferent limb of the reflex arc, such a regional technique is not devoid of potential complications, which include, but are not limited to, optic nerve damage, retrobulbar hemorrhage, and stimulation of the oculocardiac reflex arc by the retrobulbar block itself.

It is generally believed that, in adults, the aforementioned

prophylactic measures, fraught with inherent hazards, are usually not indicated. If a cardiac dysrhythmia appears, initially the surgeon should be asked to cease operative manipulation. Next, the patient's anesthetic depth and ventilatory status are evaluated. Commonly, heart rate and rhythm return to baseline within 20 seconds after institution of these measures. Moreover, Moonie *et al*[54] noted that, with repeated manipulation, bradycardia is less likely to recur, probably secondary to fatigue of the reflex arc at the level of the cardioinhibitory center. However, if the initial cardiac dysrhythmia is especially serious or if the reflex tenaciously recurs, atropine should be administered iv, but only after the surgeon stops ocular manipulation.

During pediatric strabismus surgery, however, current popular practice favors administration of iv atropine, 0.02 mg · kg^{-1}, before commencing surgery.[55] Alternatively, glycopyrrolate, 0.01 mg · kg^{-1} administered iv, may be associated with less tachycardia than atropine in this setting.

Clearly, considerable controversy surrounds the issues of incidence and prophylaxis of the oculocardiac reflex. Nonetheless, there is consensus that continuous monitoring of the electrocardiogram (ECG) is important during all types of eye surgery to detect potentially dangerous cardiac rhythm disturbances.

ANESTHETIC RAMIFICATIONS OF OPHTHALMIC DRUGS

There is considerable potential for drug interactions during administration of anesthesia for ocular surgery. Topical ophthalmic drugs may produce undesirable systemic effects or may have deleterious anesthetic implications. Systemic absorption of topical ophthalmic drugs may occur from either the conjunctiva or the nasal mucosa after drainage through the nasolacrimal duct. In addition, some percutaneous absorption, from spillover, through the immature epidermis of the premature infant may transpire.[56] Occluding the nasolacrimal duct by pressing on the inner canthus of the eye for a few minutes after each instillation greatly decreases systemic absorption.

Some of the potentially worrisome topical ocular drugs include acetylcholine, anticholinesterases, cocaine, cyclopentolate, epinephrine, phenylephrine, and timolol. In addition, intraocular sulfur hexafluoride and other intraocular gases have important anesthetic ramifications. Furthermore, certain ophthalmic drugs given systemically may produce untoward sequelae germane to anesthetic management. Drugs in this category include glycerol, mannitol, and acetazolamide.

Acetylcholine

Acetylcholine is commonly used intraocularly after lens extraction to produce miosis. The local use of this drug may occasionally result in such systemic effects as bradycardia, increased salivation, and bronchial secretions, as well as bronchospasm. The side effects, including hypotension and bradycardia,[57] that may develop in patients given acetylcholine after cataract extraction may be rapidly reversed with iv atropine. Furthermore, vagotonic anesthetic agents such as halothane can accentuate the effects of acetylcholine.

Anticholinesterase Agents

Echothiophate is a long-acting anticholinesterase miotic that lowers IOP by decreasing resistance to the outflow of aqueous humor. Useful in the treatment of glaucoma, echothiophate is absorbed into the systemic circulation after instillation in the conjunctival sac. Any of the long-acting anticholinesterases may prolong the action of succinylcholine[58] because, after a month or more of therapy, plasma pseudocholinesterase activity may be less than 5% of normal.[59] It is said, moreover, that normal enzyme activity does not return until 4–6 weeks after discontinuation of the drug.[60] Hence, the anesthesiologist should anticipate prolonged apnea if these patients are given a usual dose of succinylcholine. In addition, a delay in metabolism of ester local anesthetics should be expected.

Cocaine

Cocaine, introduced to ophthalmology in 1884 by Koller, has limited topical ocular use because it can cause corneal pits and erosion. However, as the only local anesthetic that inherently produces vasoconstriction and shrinkage of mucous membranes, cocaine is commonly used in a nasal pack during dacryocystorhinostomy. The drug is so well absorbed from mucosal surfaces that plasma concentrations comparable to those after direct iv injection are achieved.[61] Because cocaine interferes with catecholamine uptake, it has a sympathetic nervous system potentiating effect.[61]

Historically, epinephrine had often been mixed with cocaine in hopes of augmenting the degree of vasoconstriction produced. This practice is both superfluous and deleterious because cocaine is a potent vasoconstrictor in its own right, and the combination of epinephrine with cocaine may trigger dangerous cardiac dysrhythmias. It has been shown that cocaine used alone, without topical epinephrine, to shrink the nasal mucosa in conjunction with halothane or enflurane does not sensitize the heart to endogenous epinephrine during halothane or enflurane anesthesia.[62] However, animal studies have shown that after pretreatment with exogenous epinephrine, cocaine facilitates the development of epinephrine-induced cardiac dysrhythmias during halothane anesthesia.[63]

The usual maximal dose of cocaine used in clinical practice is 200 mg for a 70-kg adult, or 3 mg · kg^{-1}. However, 1.5 mg · kg^{-1} is preferable, because this lower dose has been shown not to exert any clinically significant sympathomimetic effect in combination with halothane.[64] Although 1 g is considered to be the usual lethal dose for an adult, considerable variation occurs. Furthermore, systemic reactions may appear with as little as 20 mg.

Meyers[65] described two cases of cocaine toxicity during dacryocystorhinostomy, underscoring that cocaine is contraindicated in hypertensive patients or in patients receiving drugs such as tricyclic antidepressants or monoamine oxidase inhibitors. In addition, sympathomimetics such as epinephrine or phenylephrine should not be given with cocaine.

Obviously, before administering cocaine or another potent vasoconstrictor for dacryocystorhinostomy, the physician should carefully search out possible contraindications. To avoid toxic levels, doses of dilute solutions should be meticulously calculated and carefully administered. If serious cardiovascular effects occur, labetalol should be used to counteract them.[66] In the past, propranolol was widely used to control cocaine-induced hypertension,[67] but a lethal hypertensive exacerbation has been

ascribed to unopposed α-adrenergic stimulation.[68] Labetalol offers the advantage of combined α and β blockade.

Cyclopentolate

Despite the popularity of cyclopentolate as a mydriatic, it is not without side effects, which include CNS toxicity. Manifestations include dysarthria, disorientation, and frank psychotic reactions. Purportedly, CNS dysfunction is more likely to follow use of the 2% solution as opposed to the 1% solution.[69] Furthermore, cases of convulsions in children after ocular instillation of cyclopentolate have been reported.[70] Hence, for pediatric use, 0.5–1.0% solutions are recommended. At higher concentrations, cyclopentolate also causes cycloplegia.

Epinephrine

Although topical epinephrine has proved useful in some patients with open-angle glaucoma, the 2% solution has been associated with such systemic effects as nervousness, hypertension, angina pectoris, tachycardia, and other dysrhythmias.[71]

Some anesthesiologists have maintained that it is unwise to use epinephrine in patients being anesthetized with a halogenated hydrocarbon. However, Smith and colleagues[72] reported on the administration of epinephrine into the anterior chamber of patients undergoing cataract surgery by phacoemulsification and aspiration. They concluded it is safe to administer epinephrine into the anterior chamber in doses up to 68 μg · kg^{-1} under these circumstances. It was postulated that the iris, with its rich supply of adrenergic receptors, may be able to capture with extreme rapidity the epinephrine given into the eye. Apparently, there is not much systemic absorption from the globe.

Phenylephrine

Pupillary dilation and capillary decongestion are reliably produced by topical phenylephrine. Although systemic effects secondary to topical application of prudent doses are rare,[73] severe hypertension, headache, tachycardia, and tremulousness have been reported.[71]

In patients with coronary artery disease, severe myocardial ischemia, cardiac dysrhythmias, and even myocardial infarction may develop after topical 10% eyedrops. Those with cerebral aneurysms may be susceptible to cerebral hemorrhage after phenylephrine in this concentration. In general, a safe systemic level follows absorption from either the conjunctiva or the nasal mucosa after drainage by the tear ducts. However, phenylephrine should not be given in the eye after surgery has begun and venous channels are patent.

Children are especially vulnerable to overdose and may respond in a dramatic and adverse fashion to phenylephrine drops. Hence, the use of only 2.5%, rather than 10%, phenylephrine is recommended in infants and the elderly, and the frequency of application should be strictly limited in these patient populations.

Timolol and Betaxolol

Timolol, a nonselective β-adrenergic blocking drug, is a popular antiglaucoma drug. Because significant conjunctival absorption may occur, timolol should be administered with caution to patients with known obstructive airway disease, congestive heart failure, or greater than first-degree heart block. Life-threatening asthmatic crises have been reported after the administration of timolol drops to some patients with chronic, stable asthma.[74] Not unexpectedly, the development of severe sinus bradycardia in a patient with cardiac conduction defects (left anterior hemiblock, first-degree atrioventricular block, and incomplete right bundle-branch block) has been reported after timolol.[75] Moreover, timolol has been implicated in the exacerbation of myasthenia gravis[76] and in the production of postoperative apnea in neonates and young infants.[77,78]

In contrast to timolol, a newer antiglaucoma drug, betaxolol, a β_1 blocker, is said to be more oculospecific and have minimal systemic effects. However, patients receiving an oral β blocker and betaxolol should be observed for potential additive effect on known systemic effects of β blockade. Caution should be exercised in patients receiving catecholamine-depleting drugs. Although betaxolol has produced only minimal effects in patients with obstructive airways disease, caution should be exercised in the treatment of patients with excessive restriction of pulmonary function. Moreover, betaxolol is contraindicated in patients with sinus bradycardia, congestive heart failure, greater than first-degree heart block, cardiogenic shock, and overt myocardial failure.

Intraocular Sulfur Hexafluoride

For a patient with a retinal detachment, intraocular sulfur hexafluoride[79] or other gases such as certain perfluorocarbons may be injected into the vitreous to facilitate reattachment mechanically. These recommendations do not apply to open-eye procedures during which volume and pressure changes are readily compensated for by fluid and gas leak.

Stinson and Donlon[80] suggest terminating nitrous oxide 15 minutes before gas injection to prevent significant changes in the size of the intravitreous gas bubble. The patient is then given virtually 100% oxygen or a combination of oxygen and air (admixed with a small percentage of volatile agent) for the balance of the operation without adversely affecting intravitreous gas dynamics. Furthermore, if a patient requires reoperation and general anesthesia after intravitreous gas injection, nitrous oxide should be avoided for 5 days subsequent to air injection and for 10 days after sulfur hexafluoride injection[81] (Table 34-3).

Perfluoropropane and octafluorocyclobutane may also be used in vitreoretinal surgery to support the retina. Like sulfur hexafluoride, these gases are relatively insoluble and require discontinuance of nitrous oxide at least 15 minutes before injection. Should the patient require reoperation, it must be remembered that perfluoropropane lingers in the eye for longer than 30 days.[82]

Systemic Ophthalmic Drugs

In addition to topical and intraocular therapies, various ophthalmic drugs given systemically may result in complications of concern to the anesthesiologist. These systemic drugs include glycerol, mannitol, and acetazolamide. For example, oral glycerol may be associated with nausea, vomiting, and risk of aspiration. Hyperglycemia or glycosuria, disorientation, and seizure activity may occur after oral glycerol.

The recommended iv dose of mannitol is $1.5-2 \text{ g} \cdot \text{kg}^{-1}$ given over a 30- to 60-minute interval. However, serious systemic problems may result from rapid infusion of large doses of mannitol. These complications include renal failure, congestive heart failure, pulmonary congestion, electrolyte imbalance, hypotension or hypertension, myocardial ischemia, and, rarely, allergic reactions. Clearly, the patient's renal and cardiovascular status must be thoroughly evaluated before mannitol therapy.

Acetazolamide, a carbonic anhydrase inhibitor with renal tubular effects, should be considered contraindicated in patients with marked hepatic or renal dysfunction or in those with low sodium levels or abnormal potassium values. As is well known, severe electrolyte imbalances can trigger serious cardiac dysrhythmias during general anesthesia. Furthermore, people with chronic lung disease may be vulnerable to the development of severe acidosis with long-term acetazolamide therapy. Topically active carbonic anhydrase inhibitors have been developed[83] and are now commercially available. Such topical agents might well be expected to be relatively free of clinically significant systemic effects.

PREOPERATIVE EVALUATION

Establishing Rapport and Assessing Medical Condition

Preoperative preparation and evaluation of the patient begin with the establishment of rapport and communication among the anesthesiologist, the surgeon, and the patient. Most patients realize that surgery and anesthesia entail inherent risks, and they appreciate a candid explanation of potential complications, balanced with information concerning probability or frequency of permanent adverse sequelae. Such an approach also fulfills the medicolegal responsibilities of the physician to obtain informed consent.

A thorough history of the patient and physical examination are the *sine qua non* of safe patient care. A complete list of medications that the patient is currently taking, both systemic and topical, must be obtained so that potential drug interactions can be anticipated and essential medication will be administered during the hospital stay. Naturally, a history of any allergies to medicines, foods, or tape should be documented. Clearly, knowledge of any personal or family history of adverse reactions to anesthesia is mandatory. The requisite laboratory data vary depending on the age and physical status of the patient. An ECG is often obtained in men older than 40 years of age, in women older than 50 years of age, and in younger patients if their medical history suggests the possibility of cardiovascular disease.

The anesthesiologist must be aware of the anesthetic implications of congenital and metabolic diseases with ocular manifestations. Diabetics often present with ocular complications, and the anesthesiologist must be knowledgeable about the systemic disturbances of physiology that affect these patients. Indeed, the list of congenital and metabolic diseases associated with ocular pathologic effects that have significant anesthetic implications is lengthy. A partial summary includes such syndromes as Crouzon's, Apert's, Goldenhar's (oculoauriculovertebral dysplasia), Sturge-Weber, Marfan's, Lowe's (oculocerebrorenal syndrome), Down's (trisomy 21), Wagner-Stickler, and Riley-Day (familial dysautonomia). Other diseases in this category are homocystinuria, malignant hyperthermia, myotonia dystrophica, and sickle cell disease.[84]

Furthermore, eye patients are often at the extremes of age—ranging from premature babies to nonagenarians. Hence, special age-related considerations, such as altered pharmacokinetics and pharmacodynamics, apply. In addition, elderly patients not infrequently have thyroid dysfunction and cardiopulmonary and renal diseases.

Selection of Anesthesia

The requirements of ophthalmic surgery include safety, akinesia, profound analgesia, minimal bleeding, avoidance or obtundation of the oculocardiac reflex, prevention of intraocular hypertension, awareness of drug interactions, and a smooth

---

Table 34-3. DIFFERENTIAL SOLUBILITIES OF GASES

	Blood : Gas Partition Coefficients
Sulfur hexafluoride	0.004
Nitrogen	0.015
Nitrous oxide	0.468

emergence devoid of vomiting, coughing, or retching (see Table 34-1). Moreover, the exigencies of ophthalmic anesthesia mandate that the anesthesiologist be positioned remote from the patient's airway, and this necessity sometimes creates certain logistic problems.

Most ophthalmic procedures may be performed in adults under either local or general anesthesia. (In children, general anesthesia is almost always selected.) When local anesthesia is elected, the ophthalmologist usually administers the local or regional blockade, and the anesthesiologist is present to monitor the patient's ECG continuously, routinely check vital signs, and administer sedation appropriately. If a mature, cooperative patient and a gentle, communicative surgeon are involved, local anesthesia should provide satisfactory conditions for almost any ophthalmic operation of reasonable length. Local anesthesia is especially popular for anterior segment surgery of 2 hours' duration or less. Many retina operations of similar length, however, may also be done under local anesthesia.

The choice of anesthesia should be individualized according to the nature and duration of the procedure, the patient's coagulation status, the ability of the patient to communicate and cooperate, and the personal preference of the surgeon. Patients who are deaf or who speak a foreign language and those with claustrophobia or excessive anxiety are often poor candidates for local anesthesia. Other relative contraindications include tremors, chronic coughing, and inability to lie flat.

Retrobullar Block

Retrobulbar block is a practical means to achieve akinesis of the globe. Deep general anesthesia or nondepolarizing muscle relaxants also produce a motionless eye. Retrobulbar block entails injection of local anesthesia behind the eye into the muscle cone. In the past, patients were typically asked to gaze superonasally while the block was being performed. This maneuver theoretically freed the inferior oblique muscle from the course of the needle. More recently, however, Unsold et al[85] found that the eye was more vulnerable to optic nerve or ophthalmic artery injury in this position. Hence, they suggest performing the injection with the eye in neutral position or looking slightly downward and inward because these positions move the optic nerve sheath farther away from the path of the needle. A 25-gauge needle, no longer than 31 mm, is then introduced through the lower lid in the inferotemporal quadrant, at the junction of the lateral and middle thirds of the lower orbital rim. The needle is advanced along the inferotemporal wall of the orbit and is then directed upward and nasally toward the orbital apex. The plunger of the syringe is withdrawn to reveal an unwanted intravascular location, and 4 ml of local anesthetic is then injected. The retrobulbar injection should be followed by gentle massage of the globe to enhance dispersion of the local anesthetic.

Akinesia of the eyelids is then obtained by blocking the branches of the facial nerve supplying the orbicularis muscle. This is performed in conjunction with retrobulbar block to prevent squeezing of the eyelid that could result in extrusion of intraocular contents. Since first used for ophthalmic surgery by Van Lint in 1914,[86] numerous methods of facial nerve blockade have been described. All these techniques block the facial nerve after its exit point from the skull in the stylomastoid foramen. Moving distally to proximally to the foramen, the techniques include the Van Lint, Atkinson, O'Brien, and Nadbath-Rehman methods. Although each has advantages and disadvantages, the Nadbath-Rehman approach can potentially produce the most serious systemic consequences. With this approach, a 27-gauge, 12-mm needle is inserted between the mastoid process and the posterior border of the mandibular ramus. Owing to the proximity of the jugular foramen (10 mm medial to the stylomastoid foramen) to the injection site, ipsilateral paralysis of cranial nerves IX, X, and XI can occur, producing hoarseness, dysphagia, pooling of secretions, agita-

tion, respiratory distress, or laryngospasm. Moreover, because the Nadbath-Rehman block produces complete hemifacial akinesia that interferes with oral intake, this approach is not recommended for outpatients.

Available data have failed to demonstrate a significant difference in complications such as iris prolapse or vitreous loss between local and general anesthesia for cataract surgery,[87] and local anesthesia has proved safe for patients with certain types of cardiovascular disease such as a relatively recent myocardial infarction.[88] The clinician must not be lulled into a false sense of security, however, with local anesthesia, because this technique does not necessarily involve less physiologic trespass than general anesthesia. Complications associated with retrobulbar block may be local or systemic and may result in blindness and even death (Table 34-4). The most common complication is retrobulbar hemorrhage secondary to puncture of vessels in the retrobulbar space. This misadventure is characterized by the simultaneous appearance of an excellent motor block of the globe, closing of the upper lid, proptosis, and a palpable increase in IOP. If this develops, it is prudent to defer the proposed intraocular procedure and monitor the patient for several hours after the hemorrhage to follow central retinal artery pulsations to rule out retinal artery occlusion, and to watch for the possible appearance of the oculocardiac reflex as blood extravasates from the muscle cone. If external pressure on the globe is sufficient to produce retinal artery compression, then a deep lateral canthotomy should be performed to decompress the orbit rapidly. If this does not reestablish normal retinal blood flow, an anterior chamber paracentesis should be done to decompress the globe.

Other complications of retrobulbar block include direct intravascular injection; stimulation of the oculocardiac reflex; inadvertent intraocular injection; inadequate blockade of extraocular muscles with compression of the globe and extrusion of intraocular contents; puncture of the posterior segment of the globe, producing a posterior retinal tear resulting in retinal detachment and vitreous hemorrhage; and penetration of the optic nerve. Furthermore, retinal vascular occlusion, a potentially blinding situation, may result from direct trauma to the central retinal artery behind the globe or from the pharmacologic or compressive effects of the injected solution. Optic atrophy may follow direct injury to the nerve, injection into the nerve sheath with compressive ischemia, and intraneural sheath hemorrhage. An initially insidious but potentially lethal complication may also develop when accidental access to cerebrospinal fluid during performance of a retrobulbar nerve block occurs secondary to perforation of the meningeal sheaths that surround the optic nerve. One case report[89] described the gradual onset of unconsciousness and apnea over 7 minutes without any accompanying seizures or cardiovascular collapse. Hence, anesthesiologists and ophthalmologists should be exquisitely aware of the possibility of accidental brain stem anesthesia after retrobulbar block. In a series of 6000 retrobulbar blocks, Nicoll et al[90] reported 16 cases of apparent central spread of local anesthesia; respiratory arrest developed in 8 of the 16 patients. Clearly, there is a continuum of sequelae, depending on the

Table 34-4. COMPLICATIONS OF RETROBULBAR BLOCK

Stimulation of oculocardiac reflex arc
Retrobulbar hemorrhage
Puncture of posterior globe, resulting in retinal detachment and vitreous hemorrhage
Intra-arterial injection, producing immediate convulsions
Central retinal artery occlusion
Penetration of optic nerve
Inadvertent brain stem anesthesia
Inadvertent intraocular injection

amount of drug that gains entrance to the CNS and the specific area to which the drug spreads (Fig. 34-4). The protean CNS signs may include violent shivering; contralateral amaurosis; eventual loss of consciousness; apnea; and hemiplegia, paraplegia, quadriplegia, or hyper-reflexia. Blockade of cranial nerves VIII–XII results in deafness, vertigo, vagolysis, dysphagia, aphasia, and loss of neck muscle power. It is axiomatic that personnel skilled in airway maintenance and ventilatory and circulatory support should be immediately available whenever retrobulbar block is administered.

The issue of anticoagulant therapy in the setting of ocular regional anesthesia has been revisited in recent years. Discontinuing anticoagulant can have serious medical consequences, and several studies suggest that cataract surgery can be safely performed under regional anesthesia without discontinuing anticoagulants,[91–93] especially if the prothrombin time is approximately 1.5 times control.[94] Retinal surgery may be another matter, however.

Because the complications of retrobulbar block can be both vision threatening and life threatening, alternative approaches have been developed. Since the late 1980s, peribulbar block has become popular. The advantages of this technique include its safety and the fact that a lid block usually is superfluous because the relatively large volume of injected local anesthetic usually diffuses into the eyelids. Two injections are required; these are placed inferotemporally and then superonasally, between the supraorbital notch and trochlea. For both injections, the needle is held in a plane parallel to the orbit, careful aspiration is performed, and 4–5 ml of anesthetic solution is injected in each site. Onset is usually slower than with retrobulbar blockade and may be delayed for as long as 15–20 minutes. However, pH adjustment of a lidocaine–bupivacaine mixture or of plain bupivacaine with bicarbonate may accelerate the onset.[95] Another disadvantage includes increased forward pressure on the eyeball consequent to the larger volume of local anesthetic deposited in the orbit compared with retrobulbar block. However, no cases of either retrobulbar hemorrhage or brain stem anesthesia associated with peribulbar block have been documented to date. Indeed, Hamilton et al[96] reported 5714 peri-

bulbar blocks without a single case of brain stem anesthesia or respiratory arrest.

Ophthalmologists have also been returning to a technique that was popularized during the early 1900s—the use of topical anesthetic agents, particularly when the surgical incision is being made through clear cornea. Multiple advances in cataract surgery that have enabled faster operations, with greater control and less trauma, have allowed ophthalmologists to re-examine the use of topical anesthesia for this procedure. Phacoemulsification, with its small incisions, is clearly the procedure of choice in using topical anesthesia; however, planned extracapsular procedures can also be performed under topical anesthesia, thereby circumventing potential complications of peribulbar or retrobulbar block that can result in blindness or death. Potential disadvantages of topical anesthesia include eye movement during surgery, patient anxiety, and, rarely, allergic reactions. Patient selection is critical and should be restricted to individuals who are alert, able to follow instructions, and can control their eye movements. Patients who are demented, photophobic, or cannot communicate are inappropriate candidates, as are those with an inflamed eye. Similarly, patients with small pupils who may require significant iris manipulation or those who need large scleral incisions may be contraindicated for topical anesthesia.

A parabulbar method of sub-Tenon's infusion of anesthetic via a flexible, curved cannula also has been developed.[97] Because it does not involve the use of a sharp needle, it eliminates the risk of globe penetration, retrobulbar hemorrhage, and optic nerve trauma. Topical anesthetic is applied, and a buttonhole is made through the conjunctiva and Tenon's capsule in the inferior temporal or nasal quadrants. A flexible, curved cannula is passed through the buttonhole and slid 3–5 mm along the globe. Two milliliters of 4% lidocaine and 0.75% bupivacaine in a 50 : 50 mixture without hyaluronidase is infused. Immediate analgesia occurs; akinesia may require 5 minutes to develop.

Many advocate the administration of approximately 10–30 mg of methohexital iv immediately before performance of ocular regional anesthesia, provided that no contraindications to the use of this drug exist. Such a practice is usually quite satisfactory, affording considerable comfort and amnesia. Alternative approaches include 0.5–1 $\mu g \cdot kg^{-1}$ remifentanil, 0.3–0.5 $mg \cdot kg^{-1}$ of propofol iv,[98] or alfentanil 10–20 $\mu g \cdot kg^{-1}$ iv[99] just before placement of the retrobulbar or peribulbar block. What should be avoided at all costs, however, is the combination of local anesthesia with heavy sedation in the form of high doses of opioids, benzodiazepines, and hypnotics. This polypharmacology is highly unsatisfactory because of the pharmacologic vagaries in the geriatric population and the attendant risks of respiratory depression, airway obstruction, hypotension, CNS aberrations, and prolonged recovery time. This undesirable technique has all the disadvantages of a general anesthetic in the absence of a tracheal tube without the advantage of controllability that general anesthesia offers. The patient should be relaxed but awake to avoid head movement associated with snoring or sudden abrupt movement on awakening. Clearly, patients under conscious sedation must be capable of responding rationally to commands and must be able to maintain airway patency. Undersedation should likewise be avoided because tachycardia and hypertension may have deleterious effects, especially in patients with coronary artery disease. Moreover, patients with orthopedic deformities or arthritis must be meticulously positioned and given comfortable padding on the operating table. Adequate ventilation about the face is essential for all patients to avoid carbon dioxide accumulation, and each must be comfortably warm. (The hazards of shivering in patients with cardiac disease and, for that matter, in any patient having delicate eye surgery are well known.) Continuous ECG monitoring is vital, lest performance of the retrobulbar block, pressure on the orbit, or tugging on the extraocular muscles stimulate the oculocardiac reflex arc and produce dangerous cardiac dysrhythmias. Likewise, pulse oximetry is essential.

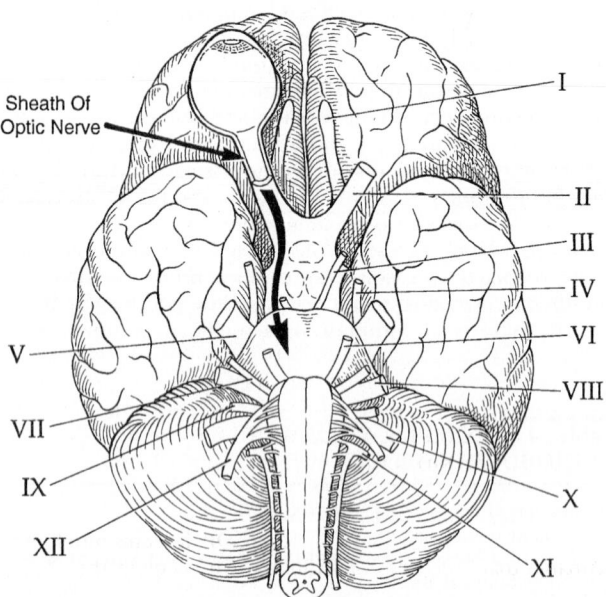

Figure 34-4. Base of the brain and the path that local anesthetic agents might follow if inadvertently injected into the subarachnoid space. This route includes the cranial nerves, pons, and midbrain. (Reprinted with permission from Javitt JC, Addiego R, Friedberg HL *et al:* Brain stem anesthesia after retrobulbar block. Ophthalmology 94:718, 1987.)

A question that is frequently asked is whether, for cardiac patients, epinephrine may be safely combined with local anesthetics to achieve vasoconstriction and increased anesthetic duration. Donlon and Moss[100] emphasize that release of endogenous catecholamines secondary to suboptimal analgesia may greatly exceed the relatively minute amount of injected exogenous catecholamine. Specifically, they mention that 0.06 mg epinephrine (12 ml of 1 : 200,000) produces some systemic uptake but no untoward clinical effects.[100] However, ocular perfusion may be reduced with epinephrine-containing solutions.

Given the economic pressures and fiscal constraints affecting our contemporary practice of medicine, it is critical to acknowledge that cataract surgery is the number one Medicare expenditure. With more than 1.3 million cataract operations performed annually in the United States, the economic impact of each aspect of cataract surgery, including preoperative preparation, intraoperative monitoring, and actual charges for surgery and supplies, can have a profound impact on the Health Care Finance Administration (HCFA) budget. Studies have confirmed that most cataract operations performed annually in the United States, are conducted with the patient under some form of local anesthesia (either retrobulbar, peribulbar, or parabulbar injection, or topical analgesia), with monitoring equipment used in 97% of cases and an anesthesiologist present in 78% of cases.[101] Indeed, many anesthesiologists have long wondered whether HCFA will decide not to reimburse for monitored anesthesia care for "routine" cataract cases.

An important study by Rosenfeld and colleagues[102] is the first to assess the need for monitored anesthesia care in cataract surgery. These investigators prospectively studied the incidence and the nature of interventions required by anesthesia personnel in 1006 consecutive cataract operations (both phacoemulsification and extracapsular techniques were included) performed under peribulbar block. They also analyzed the risk factors for intervention, including patient demographic data, medical history, and preoperative laboratory tests, for reliability in predicting those patients at greatest risk for intervention. They found that 37% of patients required some type of intervention and that, in general, the majority of those interventions could not have been predicted before surgery. The interventions ranged from minor forms, such as verbal reassurance and hand holding, to administering such iv medications as supplemental sedation or antihypertensive, pressor, or antiarrhythmic agents, or to providing respiratory assistance. Although hypertension, lung disease, renal disease, and a diagnosis of cancer were related to interventions, these four conditions combined accounted for only a small portion of the needed interventions. Moreover, although many of the interventions were relatively minor, several were more serious, and 30% of the interventions were considered (by the involved anesthesia personnel) to be critical to the success of the operation. The investigators concluded that monitored anesthesia care by qualified anesthesia personnel is reasonable and justified and contributes to the quality of patient care when cataract surgery is performed with local anesthesia. Although there were few, if any, injection-related problems, one wonders if the conclusion regarding need for anesthesia involvement would be different if the majority of cases had received topical analgesia.

ANESTHETIC MANAGEMENT IN SPECIFIC SITUATIONS
General Concepts and Objectives

Most patients undergoing eye surgery are either younger than 10 years of age or older than 55 years of age. In children, operations on the ocular adnexa, including lid surgery, repair of lacrimal apparatus, and adjustment of extraocular muscles, are common. However, surgery on the anterior segment, such as cataract removal, glaucoma procedures, and trauma repair, is

definitely not limited to the adult population. Nor are posterior segment operations such as scleral buckling and vitrectomy the exclusive domain of geriatrics.

Most ocular procedures demand profound analgesia but minimal skeletal muscle relaxation. The airway must be protected from obstruction, and the anesthesiologist must distance himself or herself—along with anesthetic apparatus—from the surgical field. Depending on whether the patient is a child or an adult and various other factors previously discussed, a decision is reached regarding selection of local or general anesthesia. Additional preparation must include, of course, identification of underlying diseases, such as asthma, diabetes mellitus, or nephropathy. The patient should also be prepared emotionally for the recovery period, when he or she will awaken with one or both eyes closed by bandages. This is important not only to spare him or her fear and anxiety but to prevent much of the thrashing about that fright might produce, to the detriment of the eye.

Preoperative sedation is chosen carefully. Except for strabismus correction, retinal detachment surgery, and cryosurgery, ophthalmic procedures usually are associated with little pain. Thus, the routine use of opioid premedication, replete with emetic potential, is ill advised. Rather, premedication should be prescribed with a view toward amnesia, sedation, and antiemesis. Reasonable selections would include a benzodiazepine, for sedative-hypnotic effect, or the phenothiazine derivative promethazine or the antihistaminic hydroxyzine for their sedative and antiemetic properties.

Analgesia and akinesis are then secured through either local or general anesthesia, with careful attention paid to proper control of IOP and to the possible appearance of the oculocardiac reflex. The anesthesiologist strives to provide a smooth intraoperative course and to prevent coughing, retching, and vomiting, lest harmful increases in IOP transpire that could hinder successful surgery. If general anesthesia is elected, extubation of the trachea should be accomplished before there is a tendency to cough. The administration of iv lidocaine, 1.5–2 $mg \cdot kg^{-1}$, before extubation of the trachea is helpful in attenuating coughing. Likewise, prophylactic iv droperidol is valuable in reducing the incidence and severity of nausea and vomiting.[103,104] Should droperidol be ineffective as a prophylactic agent, then the more expensive ondansetron or dolasetron may be administered as a "rescue" antiemetic.

"Open-Eye, Full-Stomach" Encounters

The anesthesiologist involved in caring for a patient with a penetrating eye injury and a full stomach confronts special challenges. He or she must weigh the risk of aspiration against the risk of blindness in the injured eye that could result from elevated IOP and extrusion of ocular contents.

As in all cases of trauma, attention should be given to the exclusion of other injuries, such as skull and orbital fractures, intracranial trauma associated with subdural hematoma formation, and the possibility of thoracic or abdominal bleeding.

Although regional anesthesia or an awake intubation are often valuable alternatives for the management of trauma patients who have recently eaten, such options are not available for patients with penetrating eye injuries. Retrobulbar blockade is ill advised in this setting because extrusion of intraocular contents may ensue. Moreover, although it is conceivable that a well conducted, extremely smooth awake intubation after topical anesthesia might not increase IOP, it seems much more probable that coughing or straining will occur in this setting, resulting in an increased IOP.

Preoperative prophylaxis against aspiration may involve administering H_2 receptor antagonists to elevate gastric fluid pH and to reduce gastric acid production. Metoclopramide may be given to induce peristalsis and enhance gastric emptying.

Not infrequently, a barbiturate, nondepolarizing neuromuscular blocking drug technique is described as the method of choice for the emergency repair of an open eye injury; the nondepolarizing drug pancuronium in a dose of 0.15 mg · kg^{-1} has been shown to lower IOP. However, this method has its disadvantages, including risk of aspiration and death during the relatively lengthy period—ranging from 75 to 150 seconds—that the airway is unprotected. Performance of the Sellick maneuver during this interval affords some protection. Furthermore, a premature attempt at intubation of the trachea produces coughing, straining, and a dramatic rise in IOP, emphasizing the need to confirm the onset of drug effect with a peripheral nerve stimulator while appreciating, nonetheless, that muscle groups vary in their response to muscle relaxants. Moreover, the cardiovascular side-effects of tachycardia and hypertension may prove worrisome in patients with coronary artery disease. Also, the long duration of action of intubating doses of pancuronium may mandate postoperative mechanical ventilation of the lungs. Intermediate-acting nondepolarizing drugs such as vecuronium have briefer durations of action, and less dramatic, if any, circulatory effects, but nevertheless have an onset of action similar to that of pancuronium.[105,106]

Several studies have explored the use of extremely large doses of nondepolarizing muscle relaxants to accelerate the onset of adequate relaxation for endotracheal intubation. Using vecuronium doses of 0.2 and 0.4 mg · kg^{-1}, Casson and Jones[107] found mean onset times of 95 and 87 seconds, respectively. Ginsberg et al[108] found comparable albeit slightly longer onset times. Ginsberg's group reported that the administration of high-dose (0.4 mg · kg^{-1}) vecuronium reduced the onset from 208 ± 41 seconds, as seen with the usual intubating dose of 0.1 mg · kg^{-1}, to 106 ± 35 seconds. However, the design of this study did not eliminate the possibility of bias being introduced by factors that could influence the quality of intubating conditions. For example, the doses of diazepam, fentanyl, and thiopental given before intubation of the trachea varied greatly among patients.

Succinylcholine offers the distinct advantages of swift onset, superb intubating conditions, and brief duration of action. If administered after careful pretreatment with a nondepolarizing drug and an induction dose of thiopental (4–6 mg · kg^{-1}), succinylcholine produces only small increases in IOP.[109,110] Although the advisability of this technique has been debated vociferously, there are no published reports of loss of intraocular contents from a pretreatment barbiturate–succinylcholine sequence when used in this setting.[111] On completion of surgery and return of spontaneous ventilation, an awake extubation of the trachea may be performed with the patient in a lateral, head-down position.

In managing certain pediatric patients in this situation, a reasonable approach might be to perform an inhalation induction with cricoid pressure and intubation of the trachea under deep halothane[112] or sevoflurane anesthesia. In these cases, attempting to start an iv infusion before induction of anesthesia can trigger struggling, sobbing, and screaming, and optimal visual outcome may be compromised. Moreover, it is important to keep in mind that much damage to the eye may already have occurred as a result of vomiting owing to pain or as a result of eye-rubbing and eye-squeezing by the child. The anesthesiologist cannot be held accountable for every insult to the eye.

What about the so-called priming principle?[113,114] This concept involves using approximately one tenth of an intubating dose of nondepolarizing drug, followed 4 minutes later by an intubating dose. Then, after waiting an additional 90 seconds, intubation of the trachea may be performed. However, studies in this area demonstrate wide variability and disconcerting scatter of data. Future investigations should use a randomized, double-blind design because studies of intubating conditions are notoriously difficult to interpret. Moreover, priming is not devoid of risk; a case of pulmonary aspiration after a priming dose of vecuronium has been reported.[115]

Rocuronium, with its purportedly rapid onset, may prove to be a useful drug in this setting provided adequate doses (1.2 mg · kg^{-1} iv) are administered. However, additional data are needed before rocuronium can be enthusiastically recommended in this challenging situation. Moreover, rocuronium has an intermediate duration of action that could be disadvantageous, compared with succinylcholine, in a patient with an unrecognized difficult airway. Perhaps rapacuronium (Org 9487) will emerge as a viable alternative to succinylcholine. However, considerably more data are needed in this context.

Perhaps the wisest approach to the management of open-eye, full-stomach situations is summarized by Baumgarten and Reynolds,[116] who wrote in 1985:

> It may be possible to devise a combination of intravenous anesthetics and nondepolarizing relaxants that totally prevents coughing after rapid intubation. Until this combination is devised and confirmed in a large, controlled double-blind series, clinicians should not apply the priming principle to the open eye-full stomach patient. Use of a blockade monitor to predict intubating conditions may be unreliable, since muscle groups vary in their response to nondepolarizing relaxants. At this time, succinylcholine with precurarization probably remains the most tenable compromise in the open eye-full stomach challenge.

Strabismus Surgery

Approximately 3% of the population has malalignment of the visual axes, which may be accompanied by diplopia, amblyopia, and loss of stereopsis (Table 34-5). Indeed, strabismus surgery is the most common pediatric ocular operation performed in the United States, and it entails a variety of techniques to weaken an extraocular muscle by moving its insertion on the globe (recession) or to strengthen an extraocular muscle by eliminating a short strip of the tendon or muscle (resection).

Infantile strabismus occurs within the first 6 months of life and is often observed in the neonatal period. Although most patients with strabismus are healthy, normal children, the incidence of strabismus is increased in those with CNS dysfunctions such as cerebral palsy and meningomyelocele with hydrocephalus. Moreover, strabismus may be acquired secondary to oculomotor nerve trauma or sensory abnormalities such as cataracts or refractive aberrations.

In addition to the well known propensity of strabismus surgery to trigger the oculocardiac reflex (previously discussed), there is also an increased incidence of malignant hyperthermia in patients with conditions such as strabismus or ptosis. This observation is consistent with the impression that people susceptible to malignant hyperthermia often have localized areas of skeletal

Table 34-5. CONCERNS WITH VARIOUS OCULAR PROCEDURES

Procedure	Concerns
Strabismus repair	Forced duction testing
	Oculocardiac reflex
	Oculogastric reflex
	Malignant hyperthermia
Intraocular surgery	Proper control of IOP
	Akinesia
	Drug interactions
	Associated systemic disease
Retinal detachment surgery	Oculocardiac reflex
	Proper control of IOP
	Nitrous oxide interaction with air, sulfur hexafluoride, or perfluorocarbons

IOP = intraocular pressure.

muscle weakness or other musculoskeletal abnormalities.[117-119] Other aspects of strabismus surgery of interest to anesthesiologists include succinylcholine-induced interference with the FDT and an increased incidence of postoperative nausea and vomiting.

In formulating a surgical treatment plan for incomitant strabismus, ophthalmologists often find the FDT to be exquisitely helpful in differentiating between a paretic muscle and a restrictive force preventing ocular motion. To perform the FDT, the surgeon grasps the sclera of the anesthetized eye with a forceps near the corneal limbus and moves the eye into each field of gaze, concomitantly assessing tissue and elastic properties. This simple test provides valuable clues to the presence and site of mechanical restrictions of the extraocular muscles and is most valuable in patients who have previously undergone strabismus surgery, in those who may have paralysis of one of the extraocular muscles, and in those who have sustained orbital trauma.

France et al[40] quantitated the magnitude and duration of change of the FDT after succinylcholine administration. They demonstrated that quantitation of the force necessary to rotate the globe remained significantly elevated over control for 15 minutes, even though the rise in IOP and the skeletal muscle paralysis lasted less than 5 minutes. Because succinylcholine interferes with FDT, its use is contraindicated less than 20 minutes before testing. Hence, France et al suggest performing the FDT on the anesthetized patient either while mask inhalation anesthesia is being administered, before intubation of the trachea; or after intubation, facilitated by nondepolarizing neuromuscular blocking drugs; or after intubation under moderately deep inhalation anesthesia, unaided by succinylcholine. However, when deep inhalational anesthesia is elected, atropine (0.02 mg·kg^{-1}, administered iv) should be given before or in the early stage of induction of anesthesia to prevent the fall in cardiac output that may accompany the significant dose-dependent depression of left ventricular function in children.[120] In addition, the use of iv atropine at this time affords some protection against elicitation of the oculocardiac reflex. For these reasons, many anesthesiologists administer iv atropine routinely to children scheduled for strabismus surgery.

Eye movement under general anesthesia is well documented, and in nonaligned eyes this tendency is augmented such that divergent squints diverge more and convergent squints converge less. A recent report discloses that surgeons at a regional eye teaching hospital in the United Kingdom who specialize in strabismus surgery are increasingly requesting that, if the FDT is being used, nondepolarizing neuromuscular blockade be incorporated into the anesthetic management so that muscle tone is minimal or absent during testing.[121]

Once intubation of the trachea has been accomplished, anesthesia is commonly maintained with halothane, desflurane, sevoflurane, or isoflurane, nitrous oxide, and oxygen. The patient is carefully monitored with a precordial stethoscope, ECG, blood pressure device, pulse oximeter, end-tidal carbon dioxide measurement, and temperature probe. If bradycardia occurs, the surgeon is asked to discontinue ocular manipulation and the patient's ventilatory status and anesthetic depth are quickly assessed. If additional iv atropine is deemed indicated, it is not given while the oculocardiac reflex is active lest even more dangerous cardiac dysrhythmias be triggered.

The laryngeal mask airway is gaining popularity for strabismus surgery in the United States, provided the patient is not at risk for aspiration. The laryngeal mask can be inserted without the use of muscle relaxants, causes significantly less hemodynamic perturbation, and is associated with less straining and coughing on removal.

Vomiting after eye muscle surgery is common, giving credibility to the existence of the oculogastric reflex. Abramowitz et al[103,104] reported that prophylactic iv administration of 0.075 mg·kg^{-1} of droperidol 30 minutes before termination of surgery was "highly effective" in reducing the frequency and severity of vomiting in pediatric patients undergoing repair of strabismus. (The incidence was decreased from 85 to 43%.) Fortunately, because strabismus surgery is commonly performed on an ambulatory basis, no significant prolongation of recovery time was observed with this protocol. More recently, the administration of droperidol, 0.075 mg·kg^{-1} at induction of anesthesia before manipulation of the eye, has been claimed to reduce the incidence of vomiting after strabismus surgery to a more clinically acceptable level of approximately 10%.[122] Moreover, a low dose of droperidol, 0.02 mg·kg^{-1} iv, administered immediately after anesthetic induction in patients with strabismus may decrease both the incidence and severity of nausea and vomiting.[123]

Although Warner and associates[124] reported an incidence of vomiting of approximately 16% when lidocaine, 2 mg·kg^{-1}, was given iv before tracheal intubation, others have not been able to document such favorable results after lidocaine prophylaxis.[125]

Prophylactic iv administration of metoclopramide[126] 0.25 mg·kg^{-1} or ondansetron[127] 0.15 mg·kg^{-1} also appears to be efficacious. More studies are needed to document the efficacy of some of the other serotonin receptor antagonists, such as dolasetron, granisetron, tropisetron, and ramosetron in this setting. Combination therapy consisting of a given antiemetic, plus a glucocorticoid such as dexamethasone is also gaining popularity in some venues. Moreover, a total iv technique with propofol has also been associated with a low incidence of emesis after strabismus surgery.[128] In addition, avoiding narcotics may be helpful. One study demonstrates that the nonopioid analgesic ketorolac, in a dose of 0.75 mg·kg^{-1} iv, provides analgesia comparable with that of morphine in pediatric patients with strabismus, but with a much lower incidence of nausea and vomiting in the first 24 hours.[129]

Intraocular Surgery

Advances in both anesthesia and in technology now permit a level of controlled intraocular manipulation not possible a quarter of a century ago (see Table 34-5).

Proper control of IOP is crucial for such intraocular procedures as glaucoma drainage surgery, open sky vitrectomy, penetrating keratoplasty (corneal transplantation), and traditional intracapsular cataract extraction. Before scleral incision (when IOP becomes equal to atmospheric pressure), a low-normal IOP is essential because abrupt decompression of a hypertensive eye could result in iris or lens prolapse, vitreous loss, or expulsive choroidal hemorrhage. Available data[87] have not demonstrated a major difference in the rate of complications such as vitreous loss and iris prolapse between local anesthesia and general anesthesia, and local anesthesia has proved to be a safe technique for eye patients with a recent myocardial infarction.[88]

Premedication is selected with a view toward antiemesis. Furthermore, atropine may be given safely, if desired, for antisialagogue properties. In the usual systemic premedicating dose, atropine is not harmful to patients with glaucoma.[130]

Many anesthetic techniques may be safely used for elective intraocular surgery. If general anesthesia is selected, virtually any of the inhalation drugs may be given after iv induction of anesthesia with a barbiturate or propofol and neuromuscular blocking drug and topical laryngeal lidocaine. Because complete akinesia is essential for delicate intraocular surgery, nondepolarizing drugs are administered, followed by neuromuscular function monitoring to ensure a 90-95% twitch suppression level during surgery. Because proper control of IOP is critical, controlled ventilation of the lungs is used, along with end-tidal carbon dioxide monitoring to ensure avoidance of hypercarbia.

Maximal pupillary dilation is important for many types of intraocular surgery and can be induced by continuous infusion of epinephrine 1:200,000 in a balanced salt solution, delivered through a small-gauge needle placed in the anterior chamber.

Almost simultaneous with its administration, the drug is removed by aspirating it from the anterior chamber. The iris usually dilates immediately on contact with the epinephrine infusion, and drug uptake is presumably limited by the associated intense vasoconstriction of the iris and ciliary body. However, epinephrine may also be potentially absorbed by drainage through Schlemm's canal into the venous system or by spillover of the infusion into the conjunctival vessels or drainage to the nasal mucosa.

Clearly, the extent of systemic absorption of epinephrine is of concern to the anesthesiologist, especially in view of the drug's cardiac dysrhythmogenic potential when given concomitantly with potent inhalation drugs. However, plasma catecholamine levels during epinephrine infusion into the anterior chamber have not been investigated extensively. Nonetheless, under halothane anesthesia, in both children and adults, Smith et al[72] were unable to show any increased incidence of cardiac dysrhythmias or signs of systemic effects after instillation of $1:1000$ epinephrine ($0.4-68\ \mu g \cdot kg^{-1}$) directly into the anterior chamber during cataract surgery. However, all patients were given lidocaine, $2\ mg \cdot kg^{-1}$, as topical laryngeal anesthesia. The authors postulated that the globe is not a fertile site for systemic absorption. Hence, general guidelines for subcutaneous injection may not be germane for intraocular injection.[72]

At the completion of surgery, any residual neuromuscular blockade is reversed. On resumption of spontaneous ventilation, the patient's trachea is extubated (often in the lateral position) still deeply anesthetized and after iv administration of lidocaine to prevent coughing. Atropine and neostigmine may be safely used to reverse neuromuscular blockade even in patients with glaucoma because this combination of drugs, in conventional doses, has minimal effects on pupil size and IOP.[131]

Retinal Detachment Surgery

Surgery to repair retinal detachments involves procedures affecting intraocular volume, frequently using a synthetic silicone band or sponge to produce a localized or encircling scleral indentation (see Table 34-5). Furthermore, internal tamponade of the retinal break may be accomplished by injecting an expandable gas such as sulfur hexafluoride into the vitreous. Owing to blood gas partition coefficient differences, the administration of nitrous oxide may enhance the internal tamponade effect of sulfur hexafluoride intraoperatively, only to be followed by a dramatic drop in IOP and volume on discontinuation of nitrous oxide. The injected sulfur hexafluoride bubble, in the presence of concomitant administration of nitrous oxide, can cause a rapid and dramatic rise in IOP, reaching a peak within 20 minutes[79-81] (see Intraocular Sulfur Hexafluoride). Because the resultant rise in IOP may compromise retinal circulation, Stinson and Donlon[80] recommend cessation of nitrous oxide administration 15 minutes before gas injection to prevent significant changes in the volume of the intravitreous gas bubble. Furthermore, Wolf et al[81] state that if a patient requires anesthesia after intravitreous gas injection, nitrous oxide should be omitted for 5 days after an air injection and for 10 days after sulfur hexafluoride injection. Perfluoropropane, moreover, remains in the eye longer than 30 days.

Alternatively, silicone oil, a vitreous substitute, may be injected to achieve internal tamponade of a retinal break.

Retinal detachment operations are basically extraocular but may briefly become intraocular if the surgeon elects to perforate and drain subretinal fluid. Furthermore, rotation of the globe with traction on the extraocular muscles may elicit the oculocardiac reflex, so the anesthesiologist must be vigilant about potential cardiac dysrhythmias. In addition, because it is desirable to have a soft eye while the sclera is being buckled, iv administration of acetazolamide or mannitol is common during retinal surgery to lower IOP.

These patients are usually managed in the same manner as those having intraocular surgery except that maintenance of intraoperative skeletal muscle paralysis is not as critical as during intraocular surgery. Hence, inhalational anesthetics need not be accompanied during surgery by nondepolarizing neuromuscular blocking drugs.

POSTOPERATIVE OCULAR COMPLICATIONS

The incidence of eye injuries associated with nonocular surgery is low. In a study by Roth and colleagues[132] of 60,965 patients undergoing nonocular surgery from 1988 to 1992, the incidence of eye injury was 0.056% (34 patients). Twenty-one of these 34 patients sustained corneal abrasion, although other injuries included conjunctivitis, blurry vision, red eye, chemical injury, direct ocular trauma, and blindness. Independent risk factors for greater relative risk of ocular injury were protracted surgical procedures, lateral intraoperative positioning, head or neck surgery, general anesthesia, and (for some unknown reason) surgery on a Monday. A specific mechanism of injury could be identified in only 21% of cases. In the ASA Closed Claims Study (which analyzed only cases involving litigation), eye injuries represented only 3% of all claims, but the serious nature of some of the injuries were reflected in large financial awards.[133] Similar to the findings of Roth et al, in the Closed Claims Study the specific mechanism of injury could be ascertained in only a minority of cases.

Although infrequent and often transient, eye injuries can result occasionally in blindness or more limited, but nonetheless permanent, visual impairment. Postoperative complications after nonocular surgery include corneal abrasion and minor visual disturbances, chemical injuries, thermal or photic injury, and serious visual disturbances, including blindness. Serious injury may result from such diverse conditions as acute corneal epithelial edema,[134] glycine toxicity and other visual disturbances associated with transurethral resection of the prostate, retinal ischemia, ischemic optic neuropathy, cortical blindness, and acute glaucoma. It appears that certain types of surgery, including complex spinal surgery in the prone position, operations involving extracorporeal circulation, and nasal or sinus surgery may increase the risk of serious postoperative visual complications.

Corneal Abrasion

Although the most common ocular complication of general anesthesia is corneal abrasion,[135] the incidence varies widely, depending on the perioperative circumstances. In a prospective study, Cucchiara et al[136] found a 0.17% incidence of corneal abrasion in 4652 neurosurgical patients whose eyes were protected, whereas Batra and Bali[135] one decade earlier reported a 44% incidence of corneal abrasion when eyes were left unprotected and partly open. A variety of mechanisms can result in corneal abrasion, including damage caused by the anesthetic mask, surgical drapes, and spillage of solutions. During intubation of the trachea, moreover, the end of plastic watch bands or hospital ID cards clipped to the laryngoscopist's vest pocket can injure the cornea. Ocular injury may also occur owing to loss of pain sensation, obtundation of protective corneal reflexes, and decreased tear production during anesthesia. Therefore, it may be prudent to tape the eyelids closed immediately after induction and during mask ventilation and laryngoscopy. In addition to taping the eyelids closed,[137] applying protective goggles, and instilling petroleum-based ointments (artificial tears) into the conjunctival sac may provide protection. Disadvantages of ointments include occasional allergic reactions; flammability, which may make their use undesirable during surgery around the face and contraindicated during laser surgery; and blurred vision in the early postoperative period.[137]

The blurring and foreign body sensation associated with ointments may actually increase the incidence of postoperative corneal abrasions if they trigger excessive rubbing of the eyes while the patient is still emerging from anesthesia. Moreover, halothane absorption into paraffin-based ointments can damage the cornea,[138] and even water-based (methylcellulose) ointments may be irritating and cause scleral erythema. It would seem prudent, therefore, to close the eyelids with tape during general anesthesia for procedures away from the head and neck. For certain procedures on the face, ocular occluders or tarsorrhaphy may be indicated. Special attention should also be devoted to frequent checking of the eyes during procedures on a prone patient.

Patients with corneal abrasion usually complain of a foreign body sensation, pain, tearing, and photophobia. The pain is typically exacerbated by blinking and ocular movement. It is wise to have an ophthalmologic consultation immediately. Treatment typically consists of the prophylactic application of antibiotic ointment and patching the injured eye shut. Although permanent sequelae are possible, healing usually occurs within 24 hours.

Chemical Injury

Spillage of solutions during skin preparation may result in chemical damage to the eye. The Food and Drug Administration reported serious corneal damage from eye contact with Hibiclens, a 4% chlorhexidine gluconate solution formulated with a detergent.[139] Again, with meticulous attention to detail, this misadventure is preventable. Treatment consists of liberal bathing of the eye with balanced salt solution to remove the offending agent. After surgery, it may be desirable to have an ophthalmologist examine the eye to document any residual injury or lack thereof.

Photic Injury

Direct or reflected light beams may permanently damage the eye. The potential for serious injury to the cornea or retina from certain laser beams requires that the patient's eyes be protected with moist gauze pads and metal shields and that operating room personnel wear protective glasses. These goggles must be appropriately tinted for the specific wavelength they are intended to block. Clear goggles may be worn when working with the carbon dioxide laser, whereas for work with the argon, Nd-YAG, or Nd-YAG-KTP laser, the goggles must be tinted orange, green, and orange-red, respectively.

Mild Visual Symptoms

After anesthesia, mild visual disturbances such as photophobia or diplopia are not uncommon. Blurred vision in the early postoperative period may reflect residual effects of petroleum-based ophthalmic ointments or ocular effects of anticholinergic drugs administered in the perioperative period (see Corneal Abrasion). Dhamee et al[140] reported a 7–14% incidence of benign, transient visual disturbances after gynecologic procedures.

By contrast, the complaint of postoperative visual loss is rare and is cause for alarm. Several of the following conditions may be associated with visual loss after anesthesia and surgery and should be included in the differential diagnosis: hemorrhagic retinopathy, retinal ischemia, retinal artery occlusion, ischemic optic neuropathy, cortical blindness, and acute glaucoma.

Hemorrhagic Retinopathy

Retinal hemorrhages that occur in otherwise healthy people secondary to hemodynamic changes associated with turbulent emergence from anesthesia or protracted vomiting are termed Valsalva retinopathy.[141] Fortunately, these venous hemorrhages are usually self-limiting and resolve completely in a few days to a few months.

Because no visual changes occur unless the macula is involved, most cases are asymptomatic. However, if bleeding into the optic nerve occurs, resulting in optic atrophy, or if the hemorrhage is massive, permanent visual impairment may ensue. In some instances of massive hemorrhage, vitrectomy may offer some improvement.

Retinal venous hemorrhage has been described also after injections of local anesthetics, steroids, or saline into the lumbar epidural space, and these cases have been summarized by Purdy and Ajimal.[142] The patients all received large injections (≥40 ml) into the epidural space and they subsequently developed blurry vision or headaches. On funduscopic examination, retinal hemorrhage was consistently observed. Eight of the nine patients described had complete recovery. It is thought that the hemorrhage is produced by rapid epidural injection, which causes a sudden increase in intracranial pressure. This increase in cerebrospinal fluid pressure causes an increase of retinal venous pressure, which may cause retinal hemorrhages. It is possible that obesity, hypertension, coagulopathies, pre-existing elevated cerebrospinal fluid pressure (as seen in pseudotumor cerebri), and such retinal vascular diseases as diabetic retinopathy may be risk factors. Caution is recommended when injecting drugs or fluid into the epidural space; a slow injection rate and using the minimal volume necessary to accomplish the desired objective are strongly recommended.

Retinal Ischemia

Retinal bleeding may also originate from the arterial circulation. This bleeding may be associated with extraocular trauma. Funduscopic examination shows cotton-wool exudates,[143] and this condition is known as Purtscher's retinopathy. Purtscher's retinopathy should be ruled out when a trauma patient complains of postanesthetic visual loss. This condition is associated with a poor prognosis, and most patients sustain permanent visual impairment.

Retinal ischemia or infarction may also result from direct ocular trauma secondary to external pressure exerted by an ill-fitting anesthetic mask, especially in a hypotensive setting, as well as from embolism during cardiac surgery[144] or from the intraocular injection of a large volume of sulfur hexafluoride in the presence of high concentrations of nitrous oxide. It may also result from increased ocular venous pressure associated with impaired venous drainage or elevated IOP.

The importance of carefully positioning patients and scrupulously monitoring external pressure on the eye cannot be overemphasized, especially when the patient is in the prone or jackknife positions. When the head is dependently positioned, venous pressure may be elevated. If external pressure is applied to the globe from improper head support, perfusion pressure to the eye is likely to be reduced. An episode of systemic hypotension in this setting could further decrease perfusion pressure and thereby decrease intraocular blood flow, resulting in possible retinal ischemia.

It is imperative that for procedures in the prone position a padded or foam headrest be used. The patient's eyes must be in the opening of this headrest and they must be checked at frequent intervals for pressure. If the patient's head is too large to fit properly into the headrest, then a pin head-holder should be used. During some spine procedures, a steep head-down position may be used to decrease venous bleeding and enhance surgical exposure. This position, in combination with deliberate hypotension and infusion of large quantities of crystalloid, may increase the risk of compromising the ocular circulation. It seems prudent to avoid combining these three risk factors to any significant degree.

Central retinal arterial occlusion and branch retinal arterial occlusion are important, and frequently preventable, causes of postoperative visual loss. Cases have occurred following spinal, nasal, sinus, or neck surgery as well as after coronary artery bypass graft (CABG) surgery. In addition to external pressure on the eye, causes can include emboli from carotid plaques or other sources, as well as vasospasm or thrombosis after radical neck surgery complicated by hemorrhage and hypotension, and after intranasal injection of α-adrenergic agonists. Several cases have followed intra-arterial injections of corticosteroids or local anesthetics in branches of the external carotid artery, with possible retrograde embolization to the ocular blood supply.[145] Mabry[146] has suggested that, in order to produce retrograde flow into the branches of the ophthalmic artery, the needle must be positioned intra-arterially and the perfusion pressure must be overcome during the injection. Therefore, when injecting in the nasal and sinus areas, topical vasoconstrictors should be applied to decrease the size of the vascular bed, and a small (25-gauge) needle on a low-volume syringe should be used to minimize injection pressure. Moreover, because some cases have followed injections of corticosteroids combined with other drugs, it is thought that this practice may predispose to formation of drug crystals and should therefore be discouraged.

In cases of central retinal arterial occlusion, funduscopic examination discloses a pale, edematous retina and a cherry-red spot. Platelet-fibrin, cholesterol, calcific, or crystalloid emboli may be found in narrowed retinal arterioles. Computed tomography (CT) and magnetic resonance imaging (MRI) studies are negative.

Prevention is much more successful than treatment. It may be possible to apply ocular massage (contraindicated if glaucoma is a possibility) to dislodge an embolus to more peripheral sites, and iv acetazolamide and 5% carbon dioxide inhalation have been used to increase retinal blood flow. The prognosis, however, is typically poor, and approximately 50% of patients with central retinal arterial occlusion eventually have optic atrophy.

Ischemic Optic Neuropathy

Ischemic optic neuropathy (ION) in the nonsurgical setting is the most common cause of sudden visual loss in patients older than 50 years, and it may be either arteritic or nonarteritic. Our discussion will be limited to postoperative ION and will contrast the similarities and differences between anterior ischemic optic neuropathy (AION) and posterior ischemic optic neuropathy (PION).

Anterior Ischemic Optic Neuropathy

Although the multifactorial pathophysiology of AION has not been completely established, it is thought to involve temporary hypoperfusion or nonperfusion of the vessels supplying the anterior portion of the optic nerve, although intra-axonal edema and disturbed autoregulation to the optic nerve head may also play a role.[145] Coexisting systemic disease, especially involving the cardiovascular system and (to a lesser extent) the endocrine system, is common in patients in whom AION develops. Male sex also strongly predominates. Other risk factors for postoperative AION include CABG and other thoracovascular operations, and spinal surgery. Although massive bleeding, anemia, and hypotension are commonly described intraoperative risk factors, a retrospective survey of surgeons who perform spinal fusion surgery disclosed that hypotension and anemia were equally prevalent in patients in whom ION developed and in those in whom it did not.[147] Other possible risk factors are increased IOP or orbital venous pressure. Although emboli may also play a role, AION is not usually caused by emboli because emboli preferentially lodge in the central retinal artery rather than in the short posterior ciliary arteries that supply the anterior optic nerve.

Increased IOP caused by extrinsic compression of the eye

decreases retinal blood flow that can produce both retinal and optic nerve injury. Moreover, increased IOP can result from large infusions of crystalloid when the head is steeply dependent, as during many spinal operations.[148] Increased orbital venous pressure results in a decreased perfusion pressure gradient to the optic nerve head. Interestingly, one patient who had ION despite perioperative normotension had marked facial edema after surgery of protracted duration.[148] Similarly, a study in cardiac surgery patients revealed that increases in IOP correlated with the degree of hemodilution and the use of crystalloid priming solution.[149] Patients with AION were more likely to have significant weight gain within 24 hours of open heart surgery, again suggesting the role of elevated ocular venous pressure in impeding blood flow to the optic nerve.

According to Roth and Gillesberg,[145] a complex interaction of factors such as ocular venous pressure, hemodilution, hypotension, release of endogenous vasoconstrictors, and individual risk factors such as atherosclerosis and aberrant optic nerve circulation may be implicated in the development of AION. Therefore, specific recommendations for preventative strategies are elusive. Clearly, however, external pressure on the eyes must be meticulously avoided. It also seems prudent to minimize time in the prone position when the head is notably dependent. In patients with pre-existing cardiovascular disease, significant hypertension, or glaucoma, it seems advisable to maintain systemic blood pressure as close to baseline as possible.[145] Recommendations about specific hematocrit levels are difficult to make at this time and should be individualized based on a constellation of circumstances, but it seems prudent to have a different "transfusion threshold" in high-risk patients.

Patients with AION typically have painless visual loss that may not be noted until the first postoperative day (or possibly later), an afferent pupillary defect, altitudinal field defects, and optic disc edema or pallor. MRI or CT initially show enlargement of the optic nerve. However, optic atrophy is detected by MRI later.

The prognosis for AION varies but is often grim. Although there is no recognized treatment for AION, Williams et al[150] have reviewed the various therapies that may be instituted. These include iv acetazolamide, furosemide, mannitol, and steroids. Maintaining the head-up position could be helpful if increased ocular venous pressure is operative. Surgical optic nerve sheath fenestration or decompression is not only ineffective, but may actually be harmful.[151]

Posterior Ischemic Optic Neuropathy

Posterior ischemic optic neuropathy is less common than AION despite the fact that the posterior optic nerve has a less luxuriant blood supply than the anterior optic nerve. In contrast to AION, relatively few cases have been reported after CABG, and PION appears to be less related to coexisting cardiovascular disease. As with AION, male patients outnumber female patient four to one. Many cases have been associated with surgery involving the neck, nose, sinuses, or spine. In approximately one third of cases reported, facial edema has been noted.[145]

Posterior ischemic optic neuropathy is produced by reduced oxygen delivery to the retrolaminar part of the optic nerve. Probably compression of the pial vessels (supplied by small collaterals from the ophthalmic artery) or embolic phenomena produce ischemia.[152] However, severe systemic hypotension, anemia, or venous stasis may also be contributory.[145]

A hypoxic insult in this region results in a slower development of ischemic damage, so a symptom-free period often precedes the loss of vision. In some patients, the onset of symptoms may be delayed several days. Typical findings include an afferent pupillary defect or nonreactive pupil. Disc edema is not a feature of PION owing to its retro-orbital position. CT scan in the early postoperative period may reveal enlargement of the intraorbital portion of the optic nerve. Bilateral blindness is more common with PION than AION, possibly indicating involvement of the optic chiasm. Concomitant disease of the eye or ocular blood supply may be related to PION.[145] Some cases may improve spontaneously, but usually no improvement is noted. Steroids may be considered for treatment. Preventative strategies are as outlined for AION.

Cortical Blindness

Brain injury rostral to the optic nerve may cause cortical blindness. The impairment is produced by damage to the visual path beyond the lateral geniculate nucleus or the visual cortex in the occipital lobe. Similar to AION, cortical blindness is a significant concern in patients undergoing CABG, and systemic disease is often present. Emboli and sustained, profound hypotension are common causes. Other events implicated in the pathophysiology include cardiac arrest, hypoxemia, intracranial hypertension, exsanguinating hemorrhage, vascular occlusion, thrombosis, and vasospasm.

Differential diagnostic features include a normal optic disc on fundoscopy and normal pupillary responses. There is, however, loss of optokinetic nystagmus with normal eye motility. CT and MRI are helpful to delineate the extent of brain infarction associated with cortical blindness. Occipital lesions are frequently bilateral and CT findings typically indicate posterior cerebral artery thrombosis, basilar artery occlusion, posterior cerebral artery branch occlusion, or watershed infarction. Lesions after CABG often include the parieto-occipital area.

Whereas most cases of ION do not improve significantly, visual recovery from cortical blindness in previously healthy patients may be considerable but prolonged. Preventive strategies include maintenance of adequate systemic perfusion pressure and, in cardiac surgery, minimizing manipulation of the aorta, meticulous removal of air and particulate matter during valvular procedures, and use of an arterial line filter in selected patients during bypass.

Visual Symptoms After Transurethral Resection of the Prostate

Visual disturbances associated with transurethral resection of the prostate (TURP) are transient and often the result of the TURP syndrome, wherein excessive absorption of irrigating fluid can produce cardiac failure, hyponatremia, serious dysrhythmias, seizures, and coma. Visual disturbances can extend the gamut from subtle changes, such as seeing halos or a bluish hue, to complete absence of light perception.

Liberal bladder irrigation is required during TURP to remove clots and other detritus to enhance visibility for the surgeon. Factors postulated to influence the volume of irrigant absorbed include the extent of opening of the prostatic venous sinuses, the hydrostatic pressure of the irrigation fluid, the venous pressure at the irrigant–blood interface, and, arguably, the duration of the resection.

Glycine 1.5%, although slightly hypo-osmolar, does not cause clinically significant hemolysis and is one of the most commonly used irrigating solutions. Glycine toxicity is probably the most important mechanism resulting in TURP-associated visual dysfunction, although the disturbance may be multifactorial. An inhibitory neurotransmitter in the CNS, glycine freely crosses the blood–brain barrier and depresses the spontaneous and evoked activity of retinal neurons.[153] Additionally, glycine is metabolized to serine and ammonia, both of which have been linked to CNS disturbances after TURP.[154] Serine is known to have inhibitory effects on the retina similar to those produced by glycine.[155]

Hyponatremia can occur independently of glycine toxicity and produce hypo-osmolality-induced CNS dysfunction. The degree of brain dysfunction is determined by the rapidity as well as the severity of the reduction in sodium concentration. Symptoms include hallucinations, psychosis, focal neurologic signs, seizures, and coma. It has been suggested that TURP-

associated hypo-osmolality produces occipital cortical edema, but this has not been definitively established.

Preventive strategy should focus on taking all possible measures to avoid excessive absorption of irrigating solution. Moreover, a high index of suspicion is necessary because significant amounts of irrigant may be absorbed even if the surgeon does not see any open venous sinuses. Thus, it is difficult, if not impossible, to estimate the degree of fluid absorption without confirmatory laboratory data.

Acute Glaucoma

Although topical application of such mydriatic drugs as atropine and scopolamine is contraindicated in patients with known, chronic glaucoma, the systemic use of anticholinergics in usual premedicating doses is safe for glaucomatous eyes.[130] The use of an atropine–neostigmine combination for reversal of neuromuscular blockade is also safe in patients with glaucoma.[131] Topical ophthalmic medications that are being administered to control glaucoma should be continued through the perioperative period.

Acute angle-closure glaucoma typically occurs spontaneously but has been reported rarely after spinal anesthesia as well as general anesthesia. Acute angle-closure glaucoma caused by pupillary block is a serious, multifactorial disease. Risk factors include genetic predisposition,[156] shallow anterior chamber depth,[157] increased lens thickness,[157] small corneal diameter,[157] female sex,[157] and advanced age.[156] One study[158] explored possible precipitating events in at-risk patients and found no evidence that the type of anesthetic agent, the duration of surgery, the volume of parenteral fluids, or the intraoperative blood pressure were related to the development of acute angle-closure glaucoma.

Despite its seriousness, acute angle-closure glaucoma may be difficult to recognize. However, physicians should be knowledgeable about this potential complication because diagnostic delay may detrimentally affect visual outcome and cause permanent optic nerve damage. Fazio et al[158] recommend that the preoperative evaluation include a thorough ocular history as well as a penlight examination to detect a shallow anterior chamber. Those patients considered at risk should then undergo a preoperative ophthalmic evaluation as well as perioperative miotic therapy. After surgery, these patients should be scrupulously watched for red eye or for complaints of pain and blurred vision. Acute glaucoma is a true emergency, and ophthalmologic consultation should be secured immediately to acutely decrease IOP with systemic and topical therapy. The intense periorbital pain typically described by these patients is an important aid in differential diagnosis.

Postcataract Ptosis

Ptosis after cataract surgery is not uncommon, and multiple factors have been implicated in its etiology.[159,160] These include the presence of a pre-existing ptosis, injection of anesthetic solution into the upper lid when performing facial nerve block, retrobulbar injection, injection of peribulbar anesthesia through the upper eyelid at the 12 o'clock position, ocular compression or massage, the eyelid speculum, placement of a superior rectus bridle suture with traction on the superior rectus–levator complex, creation of a large conjunctival flap, prolonged or tight patching in the postoperative period, and postoperative eyelid edema. Feibel and colleagues[159] believe that the development of postcataract ptosis is multifactorial, and no single aspect of cataract surgery is the sole contributor. Although local anesthetics clearly are myotoxic, that the local anesthetic injection cannot be isolated as the primary factor is underscored by the observation that postsurgical ptosis is seen in patients undergoing surgery with general anesthesia.

REFERENCES

1. Bruce RA: Ocular anatomy. In Bruce RA, McGoldrick KE, Oppenheimer P (eds): Anesthesia for Ophthalmology, p 3. Birmingham, Alabama, Aesculapius, 1982

2. Wolff E: Anatomy of the Eye and Orbit, 7th ed, p 1. Philadelphia, WB Saunders, 1976

3. Aboul-Eish E: Physiology of the eye pertinent to anesthesia. In Smith RB (ed): Anesthesia in Ophthalmology, p 1. Boston, Little, Brown, 1973

4. Adler FH: Physiology of the Eye: Clinical Application, 5th ed, p 249. St. Louis, CV Mosby, 1970

5. Stoelting RK: Circulatory changes during direct laryngoscopy and tracheal intubation: Influence of duration of laryngoscopy with or without prior lidocaine. Anesthesiology 47:381, 1977

6. Hill DW: Physics Applied to Anaesthesia. Norwalk, Connecticut, Appleton-Century-Crofts, 1968

7. Duncalf D, Foldes FF: Effect of anesthetic drugs and muscle relaxants on intraocular pressure. In Smith RB (ed): Anesthesia in Ophthalmology, p 21. Boston, Little, Brown, 1973

8. Garde JF, Aston R, Endler GC et al: Racial mydriatic response to belladonna preparations. Anesth Analg 57:572, 1978

9. Lee P: Congenital glaucoma. In Femann SS, Reinecke RD (eds): Handbook of Pediatric Ophthalmology. New York, Grune & Stratton, 1978

10. Watcha MF, Chu FC, Stevens JL, et al: Effects of halothane on intraocular pressure in anesthetized children. Anesth Analg 71:181, 1990

11. Al-Abrak MH, Samuel JR: Effects of general anesthesia on intraocular pressure in man: Comparison of tubocurarine and pancuronium in nitrous oxide and oxygen. Br J Ophthalmol 58:806, 1974

12. Joshi C, Bruce DL: Thiopental and succinylcholine: Action on intraocular pressure. Anesth Analg 54:471, 1975

13. Presbitero JV, Ruiz RS, Rigor BM et al: Intraocular pressure during enflurane and neuroleptic anesthesia in adult patients undergoing ophthalmic surgery. Anesth Analg 59:50, 1980

14. Famewo CE, Odugbesan CO, Osuntokun OO: Effect of etomidate on intraocular pressure. Canadian Anaesthetists Society Journal 24:712, 1977

15. Mirakhur RK, Shepherd WFI, Darrah WC: Propofol and thiopentone: Effects on intraocular pressure associated with induction of anaesthesia and tracheal intubation (facilitated with suxamethonium). Br J Anaesth 59:431, 1987

16. Thompson MF, Brock-Utne JG, Bean P et al: Anaesthesia and intraocular pressure: A comparison of total intravenous anaesthesia using etomidate with conventional inhalational anaesthesia. Anaesthesia 37:758, 1982

17. Yoshikawa K, Murai Y: Effect of ketamine on intraocular pressure in children. Anesth Analg 50:199, 1971

18. Corssen G, Hoy JE: A new parenteral anesthetic—CI581: Its effect on intraocular pressure. Journal of Pediatric Ophthalmology 4:20, 1967

19. Peuler M, Glass DD, Arens JF: Ketamine and intraocular pressure. Anesthesiology 43:575, 1975

20. Ausinsch B, Rayburn RL, Munson ES et al: Ketamine and intraocular pressure in children. Anesth Analg 55:773, 1976

21. Ausinsch B, Graves SA, Munson ES et al: Intraocular pressure in children during isoflurane and halothane anesthesia. Anesthesiology 42:167, 1975

22. Duncalf D, Weitzner SW: Ventilation and hypercapnia on intraocular pressure in children. Anesth Analg 43:232, 1963

23. Drucker AP, Sadove MS, Unna KR: Ocular manifestations of intravenous tetraethylammonium chloride in man. Am J Ophthalmol 33:1564, 1950

24. Galin MA, Aizawa F, McLean JM: Intravenous urea in the treatment of acute angle glaucoma. Am J Ophthalmol 50:379, 1960

25. Agarwal LP, Mathur SP: Curare in ocular surgery. Br J Ophthalmol 36:603, 1952

26. Litwiller RW, Difazio CA, Rushia EL: Pancuronium and intraocular pressure. Anesthesiology 42:750, 1975

27. Lincoff HA, Ellis CH, DeVoe AG et al: Effect of succinylcholine on intraocular pressure. Am J Ophthalmol 40:501, 1955

28. Pandey K, Badolas RP, Kumar S: Time course of intraocular hypertension produced by suxamethonium. Br J Anaesth 44:191, 1972

29. Bjork A, Hallidin M, Wahlin A: Enophthalmus elicited by succinylcholine. Acta Anaesthesiol Scand 1:41, 1957

30. Kelly RE, Dinner M, Turner LS et al: Succinylcholine increases intraocular pressure in the human eye with the extraocular muscles detached. Anesthesiology 79:948, 1993

31. Carballo AS: Succinylcholine and acetazolamide in anesthesia for ocular surgery. Canadian Anaesthetists Society Journal 12:486, 1965

32. Miller RD, Way WL, Hickey RF: Inhibition of succinylcholine-induced increased intraocular pressure by nondepolarizing muscle relaxants. Anesthesiology 29:123, 1968

33. Meyers EF, Krupin T, Johnson M et al: Failure of nondepolarizing neuromuscular blockers to inhibit succinylcholine-induced increased intraocular pressure: A controlled study. Anesthesiology 48:149, 1978

34. Verma RS: "Self-taming" of succinylcholine-induced fasciculations and intraocular pressure. Anesthesiology 50:245, 1979

35. Meyers EF, Singer P, Otto A: A controlled study of the effect of succinylcholine self-taming on IOP. Anesthesiology 53:72, 1980

36. Stoelting RK: Blood pressure and heart rate changes during short duration laryngoscopy for tracheal intubation: Influences of viscous or intravenous lidocaine. Anesth Analg 57:197, 1978

37. Smith RB, Babinski M, Leano N: Effect of lidocaine on succinylcholine-induced rise in IOP. Canadian Anaesthetists Society Journal 26:482, 1979

38. Grover VK, Lata K, Sharma S et al: Efficacy of lignocaine in the suppression of the intraocular pressure response to suxamethonium and tracheal intubation. Anaesthesia 44:22, 1989

39. Jampolsky A: Strabismus: Surgical overcorrections. Highlights in Ophthalmology 8:78, 1965

40. France NK, France TD, Woodburn JD et al: Succinylcholine alteration of the forced duction test. Ophthalmology 87:1282, 1980

41. Berler DK: Oculocardiac reflex. Am J Ophthalmol 12:56, 954, 1963

42. Kirsch RE, Samet P, Kugel V et al: Electrocardiographic changes during ocular surgery and their prevention by retrobulbar injection. Arch Ophthalmol 58:348, 1957

43. Bosomworth PP, Ziegler CH: The oculocardiac reflex in eye muscle surgery. Anesthesiology 19:7, 1958

44. Alexander JP: Reflex disturbances of cardiac rhythm during ophthalmic surgery. Br J Ophthalmol 59:518, 1975

45. Smith RB, Douglas H, Petruscak J: The oculocardiac reflex and sino-atrial arrest. Canadian Anaesthetists Society Journal 19:138, 1972

46. Taylor C, Wilson FM, Roesch R et al: Prevention of the oculocardiac reflex in children: Comparison of retrobulbar block and intravenous atropine. Anesthesiology 24:646, 1963

47. Mirakur RK, Clarke RSJ, Dundee JW et al: Anticholinergic drugs in anaesthesia: A survey of their present position. Anaesthesia 33:133, 1978

48. Gaviotaki A, Smith RM: Use of atropine in pediatric anesthesia. Int Anesthesiol Clin 1:97, 1962

49. Joseph MC, Vale RJ: Premedication with atropine by mouth. Lancet 2:1060, 1960

50. Katz RL, Bigger JT: Cardiac arrhythmias during anesthesia and operation. Anesthesiology 33:193, 1970

51. Massumi RA, Mason DT, Amsterdam EA et al: Ventricular fibrillation and tachycardia after intravenous atropine for treatment of bradycardias. N Engl J Med 287:336, 1972

52. Horgan J: Atropine and ventricular tachyarrhythmias. JAMA 223:693, 1973

53. McGoldrick KE: Transient left bundle branch block during local anesthesia. Anesthesiology Review 8(6):36, 1981

54. Moonie GT, Rees DI, Elton D: Oculocardiac reflex during strabismus surgery. Canadian Anaesthetists Society Journal 11:621, 1964

55. Steward DJ: Anticholinergic premedication for infants and children. Canadian Anaesthetists Society Journal 30:325, 1983

56. Nachman RL, Esterly NB: Increased skin permeability in preterm infants. J Pediatr 79:628, 1971

57. Rongey KA, Weisman H: Hypotension following acetylcholine. Anesthesiology 36:412, 1972

58. Humphreys JA, Holmes JH: Systemic effects produced by echothiophate iodide in treatment of glaucoma. Arch Ophthalmol 69:737, 1963

59. DeRoeth A, Detbarn W, Rosenberg P et al: Effect of phospholine iodide on blood cholinesterase levels of normal and glaucoma subjects. Am J Ophthalmol 59:586, 1965

60. Ellis EP, Esterdahl M: Echothiophate iodide therapy in children; effect upon blood cholinesterase levels. Arch Ophthalmol 77:598, 1967

61. Ritchie JM, Greene NM: Local anesthetics. In Gilman AG, Goodman LS, Rall TW et al (eds): The Pharmacological Basis of Therapeutics, 7th ed, p 302. New York, Macmillan, 1985

62. Chung B, Naraghi M, Adriani J: Sympathetic effects of cocaine and their influence on halothane and enflurane anesthesia. Anesthesiology Review 5:16, 1978

63. Koehntop DE, Liao J, Van Bergen FH: Effects of pharmacologic alterations of adrenergic mechanisms by cocaine, tropolone, aminophylline, and ketamine on epinephrine-induced arrhythmias during halothane–N₂O anesthesia. Anesthesiology 46:83, 1977

64. Barash PG, Kopriva CJ, Langou R et al: Is cocaine a sympathetic stimulant during general anesthesia? JAMA 243:1437, 1980

65. Meyers EF: Cocaine toxicity during dacryocystorhinostomy. Arch Ophthalmol 98:842, 1980

66. Gay GR, Loper KA: Control of cocaine-induced hypertension with labetalol (letter). Anesth Analg 67:92, 1988

67. Rappolt RT, Gay GR, Inaba DS: Propranolol: A specific antagonist to cocaine. Clin Toxicol 10:265, 1977

68. Ramoska E, Sacchetti AD: Propranolol-induced hypertension in treatment of cocaine intoxication. Ann Emerg Med 14:1112, 1985

69. Binkhorst RD, Weinstein GW, Baretz RM et al: Psychotic reaction induced by cyclopentolate: Results of pilot study and a double-blind study. Am J Ophthalmol 55:1243, 1963

70. Kennerdell JS, Wucher FP: Cyclopentolate associated with two cases of grand mal seizure. Arch Ophthalmol 87:634, 1972

71. Lansche RK: Systemic effects of topical epinephrine and phenylephrine. Am J Ophthalmol 49:95, 1966

72. Smith RB, Douglas H, Petruscak J et al: Safety of intraocular adrenaline with halothane anaesthesia. Br J Anaesth 44:1314, 1972

73. Brown MM, Brown GC, Spaeth GL: Lack of side effects from topically administered 10% phenylephrine eye drops: A controlled study. Arch Ophthalmol 98:487, 1980

74. Jones FL, Eckberg NL: Exacerbation of asthma by timolol. N Engl J Med 301:170, 1979

75. Kim JW, Smith PH: Timolol-induced bradycardia. Anesth Analg 59:301, 1980

76. Shavitz SA: Timolol and myasthenia gravis. JAMA 242:1612, 1979

77. Olson RJ, Bromberg BB, Zimmerman TJ: Apneic spells associated with timolol therapy in a neonate. Am J Ophthalmol 88:120, 1979

78. Bailey PL: Timolol and postoperative apnea in neonates and young infants. Anesthesiology 61:622, 1984

79. Fineberg E, Machemer R, Sullivan P et al: Sulfur hexafluoride in owl monkey vitreous cavity. Am J Ophthalmol 79:67, 1975

80. Stinson TW, Donlon JV: Interaction of SF6 and air with nitrous oxide. Anesthesiology 51:S16, 1979

81. Wolf GL, Capriano C, Hartung J: Effects of nitrous oxide on gas bubble volume in the anterior chamber. Arch Ophthalmol 103:418, 1985

82. Chang S, Lincoff HA, Coleman DJ et al: Perfluorocarbon gases in vitreous surgery. Ophthalmology 92:651, 1985

83. Lippa EA, Aasved H, Airaksinen PJ et al: Multiple-dose, dose-response relationship for the topical carbonic anhydrase inhibitor MK-927. Arch Ophthalmol 109:46, 1991

84. McGoldrick KE: Anesthetic implications of congenital and metabolic diseases. In Bruce RA, McGoldrick KE, Oppenheimer P (eds): Anesthesia for Ophthalmology, p 139. Birmingham, Alabama, Aesculapius, 1982

85. Unsold R, Stanley JA, DeGroot J: The CT-topography of retrobulbar anesthesia. Graefes Arch Clin Exp Ophthalmol 217:125, 1981

86. Van Lint A: Paralysie palperbrale temporaire provoquée dans l'operation de la cataracte. Ann Occul 151:420, 1914

87. Lynch S, Wolf GL, Berlin I: General anesthesia for cataract surgery: A comparative review of 2217 consecutive cases. Anesth Analg 53:909, 1974

88. Backer CL, Tinker JH, Robertson DM: Myocardial reinfarction following local anesthesia. Anesthesiology 51:S61, 1979

89. Chang J-L, Gonzalez-Abola E, Larson CE: Brain stem anesthesia following retrobulbar block. Anesthesiology 61:789, 1984

90. Nicoll JMV, Acharya PA, Ahlen K et al: Central nervous system complications after 6000 retrobulbar blocks. Anesth Analg 66:1298, 1987

91. McMahan LB: Anticoagulants and cataract surgery. J Cataract Refract Surg 14:569, 1988

92. Hall DL, Steen WH, Drummond JW et al: Anticoagulants and cataract surgery. Ophthalmic Surg 19:221, 1988

93. Robinson GA, Nylander A: Warfarin and cataract extraction. Br J Ophthalmol 73:702, 1989

94. Feitl ME, Krupin T: Retrobulbar anesthesia. Ophthalmol Clin North Am 3:83, 1990

95. Zahl K, Jordan A, McGroarty J et al: The use of pH-adjusted bupivacaine/hyaluronidase for peribulbar anesthesia. Anesthesiology 72:230, 1990

96. Hamilton RC, Gimbel HV, Strunin L: Regional anesthesia for 12,000 cataract extractions and intraocular lens implantation procedures. Can J Anaesth 35:615, 1988

97. Greenbaum S: Parabulbar anesthesia. Am J Ophthalmol 114:776, 1992

98. Ferrari LR, Donlon JV: A comparison of propofol, midazolam, and methohexital for sedation during retrobulbar and peribulbar block. J Clin Anesth 4:93, 1992

99. Yee JB, Schafer PG, Crandall AS et al: Comparison of methohexital and alfentanil on movement during placement of retrobulbar nerve block. Anesth Analg 79:320, 1994

100. Donlon JV, Moss J: Plasma catecholamine levels during local anesthesia for cataract operations. Anesthesiology 51:471, 1979

101. Norregaard JC, Schein OD, Bellan L et al: International variation in anesthesia care during cataract surgery: Results from the International Cataract Surgery Outcomes Study. Arch Ophthalmol 115:1304, 1997

102. Rosenfeld SI, Litinsky SM, Snyder DA et al: Effectiveness of monitored anesthesia care in cataract surgery. Ophthalmology 106:1256, 1999

103. Abramowitz MD, Epstein BS, Friendly DS et al: Effect of droperidol in reducing vomiting in pediatric strabismic outpatient surgery. Anesthesiology 55:A329, 1981

104. Abramowitz MD, Oh TH, Epstein BS: Antiemetic effect of droperidol following outpatient strabismus surgery in children. Anesthesiology 59:579, 1983

105. Savarese JJ: New neuromuscular blocking drugs are here. Anesthesiology 55:1, 1981

106. Basta SJ, Ali HH, Savarese JJ et al: Clinical pharmacology of atracurium besylate (BW33A): A new nondepolarizing muscle relaxant. Anesth Analg 61:723, 1982

107. Casson WR, Jones RM: Vecuronium induced neuromuscular blockade. Anaesthesia 41:354, 1986

108. Ginsberg B, Glass PS, Quill T et al: Onset and duration of neuromuscular blockade following high-dose vecuronium administration. Anesthesiology 71:201, 1989

109. Konchiergeri HN, Lee YE, Venugopal K: Effect of pancuronium on intraocular pressure changes induced by succinylcholine. Canadian Anaesthetists Society Journal 26:479, 1979

110. Smith RB, Leano N: Intraocular pressure following pancuronium. Canadian Anaesthetists Society Journal 20:742, 1973

111. Libonati MM, Leahy JJ, Ellison N: The use of succinylcholine in open eye surgery. Anesthesiology 62:637, 1985

112. McGoldrick KE: Pediatric anesthesia for ophthalmic surgery. In Bruce RA, McGoldrick KE, Oppenheimer P (eds): Anesthesia for Ophthalmology, p 75. Birmingham, Alabama, Aesculapius, 1982

113. Foldes FF: Rapid tracheal intubation with nondepolarizing neuromuscular blocking drugs: The priming principle. Br J Anaesth 56:663, 1984

114. Schwarz S, Ilias W, Lackner F et al: Rapid tracheal intubation with vecuronium: The priming principle. Anesthesiology 62:388, 1985

115. Musich J, Walts LF: Pulmonary aspiration after a priming dose of vecuronium. Anesthesiology 64:517, 1986

116. Baumgarten RK, Reynolds WJ: Priming principle and the open eye-full stomach. Anesthesiology 63:561, 1985

117. Beasley H: Hyperthermia associated with ophthalmic surgery. Am J Ophthalmol 77:76, 1974

118. Dodd MJ, Phattiyakul P, Silpasuvan S: Suspected malignant hyperthermia in a strabismus patient. Arch Ophthalmol 99:1247, 1981

119. Sessler DI: Malignant hyperthermia. J Pediatr 109:9, 1986

120. Barash PG, Glanz S, Katz D et al: Ventricular function in children during halothane anesthesia: An echocardiographic evaluation. Anesthesiology 49:79, 1978

121. Dell R, Williams B: Anesthesia for strabismus surgery: a regional review. Br J Anaesth 82:761, 1999

122. Lerman MD, Eustis S, Smith DR: Effect of droperidol pretreatment on postanesthetic vomiting in children undergoing strabismus surgery. Anesthesiology 65:322, 1986

123. Brown RE, James DG, Weaver RG et al: Low-dose droperidol versus standard-dose droperidol for prevention of postoperative vomiting after pediatric strabismus surgery. J Clin Anesth 3:306, 1991

124. Warner LO, Rogers GL, Marino JD et al: Intravenous lidocaine reduces the incidence of post-strabismus vomiting in children. Anesthesiology 68:618, 1988

125. Christensen S, Farrow-Gillespie A, Lerman J: Incidence of emesis and postanesthetic recovery after strabismus surgery in children: A comparison of droperidol and lidocaine. Anesthesiology 70:251, 1989

126. Lin DM, Furst SR, Rodarte A: A double-blinded comparison of metoclopramide and droperidol for prevention of emesis following strabismus surgery. Anesthesiology 76:357, 1992

127. Rose JB, Martin TM, Corddry DH et al: Ondansetron reduces the incidence and severity of poststrabismus repair vomiting in children. Anesth Analg 79:486, 1994

128. Watcha MF, Simeon RM, White PF et al: Effect of propofol on the incidence of postoperative vomiting after strabismus surgery in pediatric outpatients. Anesthesiology 75:204, 1991

129. Munro HM, Riegger LQ, Reynolds PI et al: Comparison of the analgesic and emetic properties of ketorolac and morphine for paediatric outpatient strabismus surgery. Br J Anaesth 72:624, 1994

130. Schwartz H, de Roeth A, Papper EM: Pre-anesthetic use of atropine in patients with glaucoma. JAMA 165:144, 1957

131. Rastron RE, Hutchinson BR: Pupillary and circulatory changes at the termination of relaxant anesthesia. Br J Anaesth 35:795, 1963

132. Roth S, Thisted RA, Erickson JP et al: Eye injuries after nonocular surgery: a study of 60,965 anesthetics from 1985-1992. Anesthesiology 85:1020, 1996

133. Gild WA, Posner KL, Caplan RA et al: Eye injuries associated with anesthesia. Anesthesiology 76:204, 1992

134. Richardson RB, McBride CM, Berkely RG et al: An unusual ocular complication after anesthesia. Anesthesiology 43:357, 1975

135. Batra YK, Bali M: Corneal abrasions during general anesthesia. Anesth Analg 56:363, 1977

136. Cucchiara R, Black S: Corneal abrasion during anesthesia and surgery. Anesthesiology 69:978, 1988

137. Siffring PA, Poulton TJ: Prevention of ophthalmic complications during general anesthesia. Anesthesiology 66:569, 1987

138. Boggild-Madsen N, Bundgard-Nielson P, Hammer U, Jakobsen B: Comparison of eye protection with methylcellulose and paraffin ointments during general anesthesia. Canadian Anaesthetists Society Journal 28:575, 1981

139. Tabor E, Bostwick DC, Evans CC: Corneal damage due to eye contact with chlorhexidine gluconate (letter). JAMA 261:557, 1989

140. Dhamee MS, Ghandi SK, Callen KM et al: Morbidity after outpatient anesthesia: A comparison of different endotracheal anesthetic techniques for laparoscopy. Anesthesiology 57:A375, 1982

141. DeVoe AG, Norton EWD, Kearns TP et al: Valsalva hemorrhagic retinopathy: Discussion. Trans Am Ophthalmol Soc 70:307, 1972

142. Purdy EP, Ajimal GS: Vision loss after lumbar epidural steroid injection. Anesth Analg 86:119, 1998

143. McLeod D: Reappraisal of the retinal cotton-wool spot. J R Soc Med 74:682, 1981

144. Gutman FA, Zegarra H: Ocular complications in cardiac surgery. Surg Clin North Am 51:1095, 1971

145. Roth S, Gillesberg I: Injuries to the visual system and other sense organs. In Benumof JL, Saidman LJ (eds): Anesthesia and Perioperative Complications, 2nd ed, p 377. St. Louis, Mosby, 1999.

146. Mabry RL: Visual loss after intranasal corticosteroid injection. Arch Otolaryngol 107:484, 1981

147. Myers MA, Hamilton SR, Bogosian AJ et al: Visual loss as a complication of spinal surgery. Spine 22:1325, 1997

148. Dilger JA, Tetzlaff JE, Bell GR et al: Ischemic optic neuropathy after spinal fusion. Can J Anaesth 45:63, 1998

149. Shapira OM, Kimmel WA, Lindsey PS et al: Anterior ischemic optic neuropathy after open heart operations. Ann Thorac Surg 61:660, 1996

150. Williams EL, Hart WM, Tempelhoff R: Postoperative ischemic optic neuropathy. Anesth Analg 80:1018, 1995

151. The Ischemic Optic Neuropathy Decompression Trial Research Group: Optic nerve decompression surgery is not effective and may be harmful. JAMA 273:625, 1995

152. Hayreh SS: Posterior ischemic optic neuropathy. Ophthalmologica 182:29, 1981

153. Gilbertson TA, Borges S, Wilson M: The effects of glycine and GABA on isolated horizontal cells from the salamander retina. J Neurophysiol 66:2002, 1991

154. Hoekstra PT, Kahnoski R, McCamish MA et al: Transurethral prostatic resection syndrome—a new perspective: Encephalopathy with associated hyperammonemia. J Urol 130:704, 1983

155. Slaughter MM, Miller RF: Characterization of serine inhibitory action on neurons in the mudpuppy retina. Neuroscience 41:817, 1991

156. Drance SM: Angle-closure glaucoma among Canadian Eskimos. Can J Ophthalmol 8:252, 1973

157. Alsbirk PH: Angle-closure glaucoma surveys in Greenland Eskimos. Can J Ophthalmol 8:260, 1973

158. Fazio DT, Bateman JB, Christensen RE: Acute angle-closure glaucoma associated with surgical anesthesia. Arch Ophthalmol 103:360, 1985

159. Feibel RM, Custer PL, Gordon MO: Postcataract ptosis: A randomized, double-masked comparison of peribulbar and retrobulbar anesthesia. Ophthalmology 100:660, 1993

160. Kaplan LJ, Jaffee NS, Clayman HM: Ptosis and cataract surgery. Ophthalmology 92:237, 1985

Clinical Anesthesia (4/e), edited by
Paul G. Barash, Bruce F. Cullen, and
Robert K. Stoelting. Lippincott Williams &
Wilkins, Philadelphia, © 2001.

CHAPTER 35

ANESTHESIA FOR OTOLARYNGOLOGIC SURGERY

ALEXANDER W. GOTTA, LYNNE R. FERRARI, AND
COLLEEN A. SULLIVAN

The anesthetic management of a patient undergoing surgery of the head, neck, ear, nose, and throat challenges the anesthesiologist to devise an anesthetic plan that will accommodates the needs of the surgeon, anesthesiologist, and patient. Among the problems that must be solved are the following:

1. Diagnosing alterations in a patient's airway created by infection, tumor, trauma, or congenital defect
2. Establishing and maintaining the airway in a patient whose anatomy has been distorted
3. Creating a shared operative field that enables the anesthesiologist to ventilate the patient's lungs and monitor the patient safely and the surgeon to perform his or her tasks
4. Selecting appropriate anesthetic drugs compatible with the surgical procedure
5. Defining the appropriate moment for extubating the trachea of the postoperative patient

EVALUATING THE AIRWAY

In the healthy human, air flow through the upper respiratory passages, and into the trachea, bronchi, bronchioles, and in and out of the alveoli occurs seemingly without either thought or effort, and the actual work of respiration in the unobstructed airway is minimal. However, airway obstruction due to tumor, infection, or trauma may significantly alter the clinical presentation and make gas exchange a laborious, energy-consuming process, leaving the patient exhausted, eventually incapable of maintaining adequate gas exchange, and finally succumbing to asphyxiation. Clinically evident upper airway obstruction is a late sign, whatever the causative process may be, and significant obstruction and anatomic distortion may be present in a patient with minimal evidence of disease. It is a most unwelcome experience for the anesthesiologist to discover a large, unexpected, and obstructing upper airway tumor at the time of attempted tracheal intubation.

In the presence of tumor or infection in the airway it may be useful to obtain radiologic evaluation of the airway via plain films of the tracheal and laryngeal air columns or computerized tomographic studies of the airway. Significant anatomic distortion is usually readily evident and may help the anesthesiologist to determine the most appropriate technique for securing the airway.

ANESTHESIA FOR PEDIATRIC EAR, NOSE, AND THROAT SURGERY

Particularly challenging to the anesthesiologist is the safe management of the pediatric patient undergoing surgery of the ear, nose, and throat (ENT). The restricted spaces in the airway of the child mandate an understanding and cooperative relationship between surgeon and anesthesiologist, and the use of specially adapted equipment suitable to these cramped areas. Tonsillectomy, adenoidectomy, myringotomy, and tube insertion (flexible and rigid bronchoscopy) are commonly performed on pediatric patients.

Tonsillectomy and Adenoidectomy

Untreated adenoidal hyperplasia may lead to nasopharyngeal obstruction, causing failure to thrive, speech disorders, obligate mouth breathing, sleep disturbances, orofacial abnormalities with a narrowing of the upper airway, and dental abnormalities. Surgical removal of the adenoids is usually accompanied by tonsillectomy; however, purulent adenitis, despite adequate medical therapy, and recurrent otitis media with effusion secondary to adenoidal hyperplasia are improved with adenoidectomy alone.

Tonsillectomy is one of the more commonly performed pediatric surgical procedures today.[1] Chronic or recurrent acute tonsillitis, peritonsillar abscess, and obstructive tonsillar hyperplasia are the major indications for surgery.[2,3] Patients with cardiac valvular disease are at risk for endocarditis from recurrent streptococcal bacteremia secondary to infected tonsils, and tonsillar hyperplasia may lead to chronic airway obstruction resulting in sleep apnea, CO_2 retention, cor pulmonale, failure to thrive, swallowing disorders, and speech abnormalities. These risks are eliminated with removal of the tonsils.

Obstruction of the oropharyngeal airway by hypertrophied tonsils leading to apnea during sleep is an important clinical syndrome referred to as *obstructive sleep apnea syndrome*. Despite only mild to moderate tonsillar enlargement on physical examination, these patients have upper airway obstruction while awake and apnea during sleep. The goals of treatment are to relieve airway obstruction and increase the cross-sectional area of the pharynx, which is successful in two thirds of cases. Some patients require the use of nasal constant positive airway pressure during sleep, whereas others may require a tracheostomy to bypass the chronic upper airway obstruction that is present. The two most frequent levels of obstruction during sleep are at the soft palate and the base of the tongue.[4] Most children will have tremendous improvement in their symptoms after tonsillectomy.

In children with long-standing hypoxemia and hypercarbia, increased airway resistance can lead to cor pulmonale (Fig. 35-1). Patients have electrocardiographic evidence of right ventricular hypertrophy and one third have chest radiographs consistent with cardiomegaly. Each apneic episode causes progressively increasing pulmonary artery pressure with significant systemic and pulmonary artery hypertension leading to ventricular dysfunction and cardiac dysrhythmias. Often, these patients have dysfunction in the medulla or hypothalamic areas of the central nervous system causing persistently elevated CO_2 despite relief of airway obstruction. This group of patients has a hyperreactive pulmonary vascular bed and the increased pulmonary vascular resistance and myocardial depression in response to hypoxia, hypercarbia, and acidosis are far greater than what is expected for that degree of physiologic alteration in the normal population. Cardiac enlargement is frequently reversible with digitalization and surgical removal of the tonsils and adenoids.

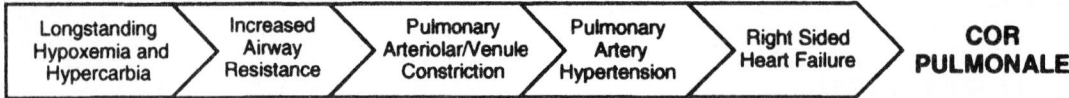

Figure 35-1. Events leading to cor pulmonale.

Preoperative Evaluation

A thorough history is the basis for the preoperative evaluation. Because patients requiring tonsillectomy and adenoidectomy have frequent infections, the parent should be questioned for current use of antibiotics, antihistamines, or other medicines. A history of sleep apnea should be sought. The physical examination should begin with observation of the patient. The presence of audible respirations, mouth breathing, nasal quality of the speech, and chest retractions should be noted. Mouth breathing may be the result of chronic nasopharyngeal obstruction. A longer face, retrognathic mandible, and a high-arched palate may be present.[5] The oropharynx should be inspected for evaluation of tonsillar size for determining the ease of mask ventilation and tracheal intubation (Fig. 35-2). The presence of wheezing or rales on auscultation of the chest may be a result of lower respiratory manifestation of pharyngitis or tonsillitis. The presence of inspiratory stridor or prolonged expiration may indicate partial airway obstruction from hypertrophied tonsils or adenoids.

Measurement of hematocrit and coagulation parameters may be suggested. Many nonprescription cold medications and antihistamines contain aspirin, which may affect platelet function, and this should be taken into consideration. Chest radiographs and electrocardiograms (ECG) are not required unless specific history of abnormalities in these areas is elicited, such as recent pneumonia, bronchitis, upper respiratory infection (URI), or history consistent with cor pulmonale. In those children with a history of cardiac abnormalities, an echocardiogram may be indicated.

Anesthetic Management

The goals of the anesthesia for tonsillectomy and adenoidectomy are to render the child unconscious in the most atraumatic manner possible, provide the surgeon with optimal operating conditions, establish intravenous (iv) access to provide a route for volume expansion and medications should they be necessary, and to provide rapid emergence so that the patient is awake and able to protect the recently manipulated airway. Premedication may be used as determined by the anesthesiologist during the preanesthetic visit. Sedative premedication may be avoided in children with obstructive sleep apnea, intermittent obstruction, or very large tonsils. An antisialagogue is often included to minimize secretions in the operative field.

Anesthesia is usually induced with a volatile drug, oxygen and nitrous oxide (N_2O) by mask. Parental presence in the operating room during mask induction is often helpful in the anxious unpremedicated child. Tracheal intubation is best accomplished under deep inhalation anesthesia or aided by a short-acting nondepolarizing muscle relaxant. The possibility exists for blood in the pharynx to enter the trachea during the surgical procedure. For this reason, the supraglottic area may be packed with petroleum gauze, or a cuffed endotracheal tube may be used provided an appropriate leak around the endotracheal tube is obtained. Monitoring consists of precordial stethoscope, ECG, automated blood pressure, pulse oximetry, and end-tidal CO_2.

Emergence from anesthesia should be rapid and the child should be alert before transfer to the recovery area. The child should be awake and able to clear blood or secretions in the oropharynx as efficiently as possible before removal of the endotracheal tube. Maintenance of airway and pharyngeal reflexes is of utmost importance in the prevention of aspiration, laryngospasm, and airway obstruction. Emergence airway complications have not been shown to be different in patients extubated deep or awake.[6]

The use of the laryngeal mask airway (LMA) for adenotonsil-

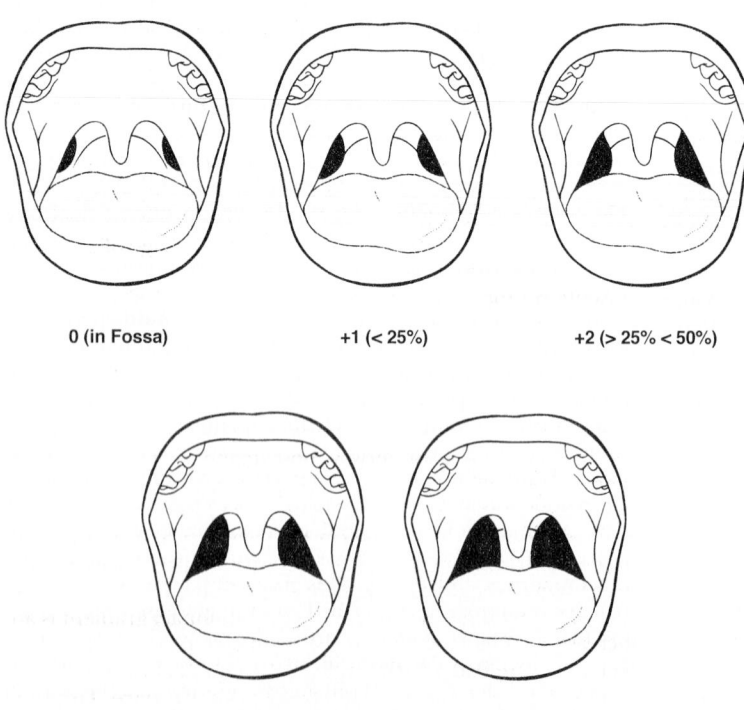

0 (in Fossa)   +1 (< 25%)   +2 (> 25% < 50%)

+3 (> 50% < 75%)   +4 (> 75%)

Figure 35-2. Classification of tonsil size, including percentage of oropharyngeal area occupied by hypertrophied tonsils.

lectomy was described in 1990; however, it was not until the widespread availability of a streamlined flexible model that it was widely used.[7,8] The wide, rigid tube of the original model did not fit under the mouth gag and was easily compressed or dislodged during full mouth opening. The newer, flexible model has a soft, reinforced shaft which easily fits under the mouth gag without becoming dislodged or compressed. Adequate surgical access can be achieved and the lower airway is protected from exposure to blood during the procedure.[9,10]

Insertion is possible after either the intravenous administration of 3.5 mg · kg^{-1} propofol or when sufficient depth of anesthesia is achieved using a volatile agent administered by mask. The same depth of anesthesia should be obtained during insertion of the LMA as would be required for performing laryngoscopy and endotracheal intubation. Positive-pressure ventilation should be avoided, although gentle assisted ventilation is both safe and effective if peak inspiratory pressure is kept below 20 cm H$_2$O.[11]

Tonsillar enlargement can make LMA insertion difficult, so care in placement is essential.[12] Maneuvers to overcome this difficulty include increased head extension, lateral insertion of the mask, anterior displacement of the tongue, pressure on the tip of the LMA using the index finger as it negotiates the pharyngeal curve, or use of the laryngoscope if all else fails. Dislodgement of the device does not occur during extreme head extension, assuming that good position and ventilation were obtained before to changes in head position.[13]

Advantages of the LMA over traditional endotracheal intubation are a decrease in the incidence of postoperative stridor and laryngospasm and an increase in immediate postoperative oxygen saturation. The LMA should be viewed as a useful adjunct to airway management, never a substitute for endotracheal intubation. If the child is breathing spontaneously at a regular rate and depth, the LMA may be removed before emergence from anesthesia. The oropharynx should be gently suctioned with a soft, flexible catheter, the LMA deflated and removed, an oral airway inserted, and the respirations assisted with 100% oxygen delivered by mask. It is often distressing for young children to awaken with the LMA still in place, and although the device is an appropriate substitute for oral airway in the adult population, the same is not so in children. If the practitioner wishes to remove the LMA when the child has emerged from anesthesia, it should be deflated and removed as soon as possible after the return to consciousness.

Complications

The incidence of emesis after tonsillectomy ranges from 30% to 65%.[14] Whether this is due to irritant blood in the stomach or interference with the gag reflex by inflammation and edema at the surgical site remains unclear. Central nervous system stimulation from the gastrointestinal tract, as may be seen with gastric distention from the introduction of swallowed or insufflated air, may trigger the emetic center.[15] Decompressing the stomach with an orogastric tube may be helpful in preventing this response. The nasal route of insertion should not be used because unremoved adenoidal tissue may become dislodged or bleeding may be induced at the surgical site if adenoidectomy has been performed. Postoperative administration of meperidine increases the probability of emesis, and other analgesic agents should be administered. Dehydration secondary to poor oral intake as a result of nausea, vomiting, or pain can occur after tonsillectomy.[16] Postoperative dehydration occurs at a frequency of 1.1%.[17] Vigorous iv hydration during surgery to restore intravascular volume can offset the physiologic effects of later decreases in fluid intake.

The most serious complication of tonsillectomy is postoperative hemorrhage, which occurs at a frequency of 0.1–8.1%.[17–19] Approximately 75% of postoperative tonsillar hemorrhage occurs within 6 hours of surgery. Most of the remaining 25% occurs within the first 24 hours of surgery, although bleeding may be noted until the sixth postoperative day.[20] Sixty-seven percent of postoperative bleeding originates from the tonsillar fossa, 27% in the nasopharynx, and 7% in both. Initial attempts to control bleeding may be made using pharyngeal packs and cautery. If this fails, patients must return to the OR for exploration and surgical hemostasis.

Unappreciated large volumes of blood originating from the tonsillar bed may be swallowed. These patients must be considered to have a full stomach, and anesthetic precautions addressing this situation must be taken. A rapid sequence induction accompanied by cricoid pressure and a styletted endotracheal tube are often recommended. Because the amount of blood swallowed can be considerable, blood pressure must be checked in both the erect and supine positions to look for orthostatic changes resulting from decreases in vascular volume. Intravenous access and hydration must be established before the induction of anesthesia. A variety of laryngoscope blades and endotracheal tubes as well as functioning suction apparatus should be prepared in duplicate because blood in the airway may impair visualization of the vocal cords and cause plugging of the endotracheal tube.

Pain after adenoidectomy is usually minimal but is severe after tonsillectomy. This contributes to poor fluid intake and overall discomfort of patients. An increase in postoperative pain medication requirements has been noted in patients having laser or electrocautery as part of the operative tonsillectomy compared with those having had sharp surgical dissection and ligation of blood vessels to achieve hemostasis.[21] Intraoperative administration of corticosteroids may decrease edema formation and subsequent patient discomfort.[22] Although infiltration of the peritonsillar space with local anesthetic and epinephrine has been shown to be effective in reducing intraoperative blood loss, it does not decrease postoperative pain.[23]

Peritonsillar abscess, or quinsy tonsil, is a condition that may require immediate surgical intervention to relieve potential or existing airway obstruction. An acutely infected tonsil may undergo abscess formation, producing a large mass in the lateral pharynx that can interfere with swallowing and breathing (Figs. 35-3 through 35-5). Fever, pain, and trismus are frequent symptoms. Treatment consists of surgical drainage of the abscess either with or without tonsillectomy and iv antibiotic therapy. Although the airway seems compromised, the peritonsillar abscess is usually in a fixed location in the lateral pharynx and does not interfere with ventilation of the patient by mask after induction of general anesthesia. Visualization of the vocal cords should not be impaired because the pathologic process is supraglottic and well above the laryngeal inlet. Laryngoscopy must be carefully performed, avoiding manipulation of the larynx and surrounding structures. Intubation should be gentle because the tonsillar area is tense and friable and inadvertent rupture of the abscess can occur, leading to spillage of purulent material into the trachea.

Acute postoperative pulmonary edema is an infrequent but potentially life-threatening complication encountered when airway obstruction is suddenly relieved. One proposed mechanism is that during inspiration before adenotonsillectomy, the negative intrapleural pressure that is generated causes an increase in venous return, enhancing pulmonary blood volume. In the healthy child without airway obstruction, pleural pressure ranges from −2.5 cm to −10.0 cm H$_2$O during inspiration. Intrapleural pressure generated in the child with airway obstruction can be as much as −30 cm H$_2$O which, when transmitted to the interstitial peribronchial and perivascular spaces, causes disruption of the capillary walls of the pulmonary microvasculature. Concurrent with a negative transpulmonary gradient is an increase in venous return to the right side of the heart, thus increasing preload, which, in the setting of "leaky capillaries," facilitates transudation of fluid into the alveolar space. To counterbalance this, positive intrapleural and alveolar pressure is generated during exhalation, which decreases pulmonary ve-

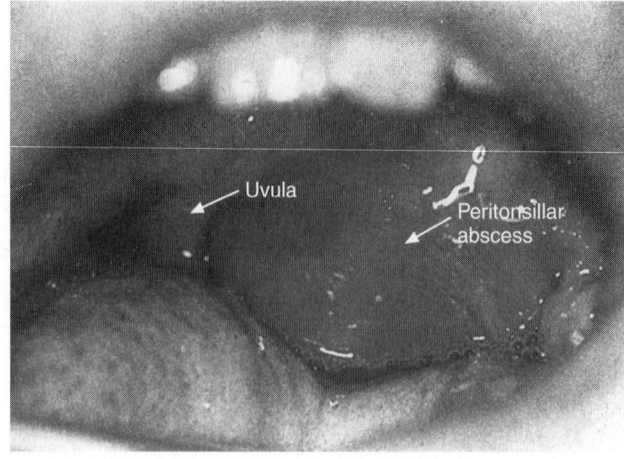

A

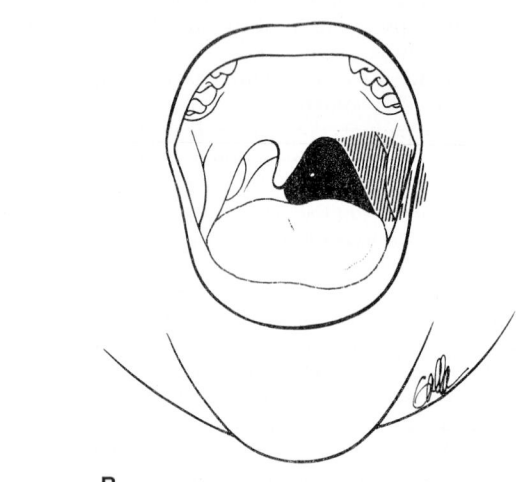

B

Figure 35-3. (*A*) Patient with a peritonsillar abscess on the left side. (*B*) Note the displacement of the uvula. (Courtesy of Michael Cunningham, M.D., Boston, Massachusetts.)

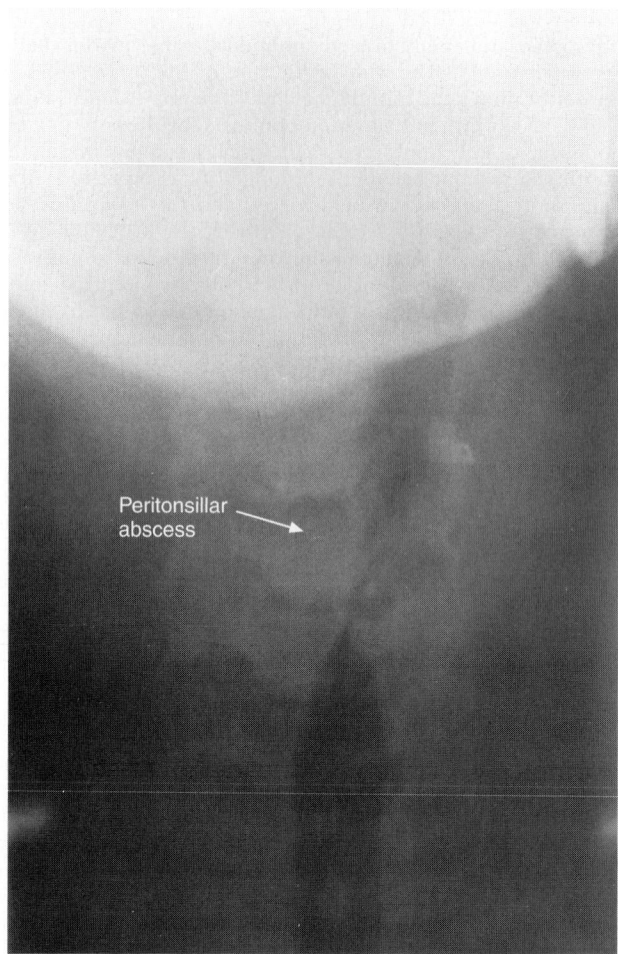

Figure 35-4. Neck radiograph of a patient with a peritonsillar abscess.

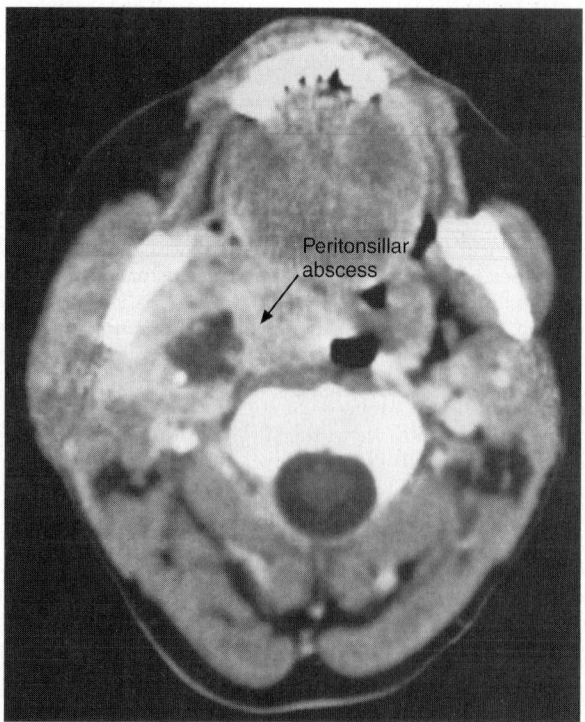

Figure 35-5. Computed tomography scan of a patient with a peritonsillar abscess.

nous return and blood volume. This is similar to an expiratory "grunt" mechanism in which the transpleural pressures generated are similar to those present during a Valsalva maneuver.

The rapid relief of airway obstruction results in decreased airway pressure, an increase in venous return, an increase in pulmonary hydrostatic pressure, hyperemia, and finally pulmonary edema. The all-important counterbalance of the expiratory "grunt" in limiting pulmonary venous return is lost when the obstruction is relieved. Contributing factors are the increased volume load on both ventricles as well as the inability of the pulmonary lymphatic system to remove acutely large amounts of fluid. The anesthesiologist may attempt to prevent this situation during induction of anesthesia by applying moderate amounts of continuous positive pressure to the airway, thus allowing time for circulatory adaptation to take place. This physiologic sequence is similar to that seen in patients with severe acute airway obstruction secondary to epiglottitis or laryngospasm.

Negative-pressure pulmonary edema is signaled by the appearance of frothy pink fluid in the endotracheal tube of an intubated patient or the presence of a decreased oxygen saturation, wheezing, dyspnea, and increased respiratory rate in the immediate postoperative period in a previously extubated patient. Mild cases may present with minimal symptoms. The differential diagnosis of negative-pressure pulmonary edema includes aspiration of gastric contents, adult respiratory distress syndrome, congestive heart failure, volume overload, and anaphylaxis. A chest radiograph illustrating diffuse, usually bilateral

Table 35-1. TONSILLECTOMY AND ADENOIDECTOMY INPATIENT GUIDELINES: RECOMMENDATION OF THE AMERICAN ACADEMY OF OTOLARYNGOLOGY–HEAD AND NECK SURGERY PEDIATRIC OTOLARYNGOLOGY COMMITTEE

Patients shall be admitted to the hospital after adenotonsillectomy if they meet any of the following criteria:

Age ≤3 y

Abnormal coagulation values with or without an identified bleeding disorder in the patient or family

Evidence of obstructive sleep disorder or apnea due to tonsillar or adenoidal hypertrophy

Systemic disorders that put the patient at increased preoperative cardiopulmonary, metabolic, or general medical risk

Child with craniofacial or other airway abnormalities including, but not limited to, syndromic disorders such as Treacher Collins syndrome, Crouzon's syndrome, Goldenhar syndrome, Pierre Robin anomalad, C.H.A.R.G.E. association, achondroplasia, and, most prominently, Down's syndrome, as well as isolated airway abnormalities such as choanal atresia and laryngotracheal stenosis

When the procedure is being done for acute peritonsillar abscess

When extended travel time, weather conditions, and home social conditions are not consistent with close observation, cooperation, and ability to return to the hospital quickly at the discretion of the attending physician

---

interstitial pulmonary infiltrates combined with an appropriate clinical history will confirm the diagnosis.[24]

Treatment is usually supportive, with maintenance of a patent airway, oxygen administration, and diuretic therapy in some cases. Endotracheal intubation and mechanical ventilation with positive end-expiratory pressure may be necessary in severe cases. Resolution is usually rapid and may occur within hours of surgery. Most cases resolve without treatment within 24 hours. There is currently no reliable method for predicting which children will experience this clinical syndrome after their airway obstruction has been resolved.[25]

Adenoidectomy patients may be safely discharged on the same day after recovering from anesthesia. Tonsillectomy has been a procedure that warranted postoperative admission of the patient to the hospital for observation, administration of analgesics, and hydration. Many centers are discharging tonsillectomy patients on the day of surgery without adverse outcome, and this trend will likely continue.[17,20,21,26] It is recommended that patients be observed for early hemorrhage for a minimum of 6 hours and be free from significant nausea, vomiting, and pain prior to discharge. Ability to take fluid by mouth is not a requirement for discharge home. However, iv hydration must be adequate to prevent dehydration. Excessive somnolence and severe vomiting are indications for hospital admission. There is a set of patients in whom early discharge is not advised, and those patients should be admitted to the hospital after tonsillectomy. The characteristics of such patients are listed in Table 35-1.[27]

Ear Surgery

The ear and its associated structures are target organs for many pathologic conditions. General anesthesia for surgery of the ear has its own set of unique considerations that must be addressed.

Myringotomy and Tube Insertion

Chronic serous otitis in children can lead to hearing loss, and drainage of accumulated fluid in the middle ear is effective treatment for this condition. Myringotomy, which creates an opening in the tympanic membrane for fluid drainage, may be performed alone. During healing, the drainage path may become occluded. Therefore, tube placement is usually included. The insertion of a small plastic tube in the tympanic membrane serves as a vent for the ostium and allows for continued drainage of the middle ear until the tubes are naturally extruded in 6 months to a year or surgically removed at an appropriate time (Fig. 35-6).

Myringotomy and tube insertion is a relatively short procedure and anesthesia may be effectively accomplished with a potent inhalation drug, oxygen, and N_2O administered by mask. Premedication is not recommended because most sedative drugs used for premedication will far outlast the duration of the surgical procedure. Patients with chronic otitis frequently have accompanying recurrent URIs. It is often the eradication of middle ear fluid that resolves the concomitant URI. Because tracheal intubation is not required for routine patients, the criteria for cancellation of surgery and anesthesia may be different for this procedure. No significant difference in perioperative morbidity between asymptomatic patients and those fulfilling URI criteria has been demonstrated.[28,29] It is recommended that patients with URI symptoms receive supplemental postoperative oxygen.[30]

Middle Ear and Mastoid

Tympanoplasty and mastoidectomy are two of the most common procedures performed on the middle ear and accessory structures. To gain access to the surgical site, the head is positioned on a head rest, which may be lower than the operative table, and extreme degrees of lateral rotation may be required. Extreme tension on the heads of the sternocleidomastoid muscles must be avoided. The laxity of the ligaments of the cervical spine as well as immaturity of odontoid process in children make them especially prone to C1–C2 subluxation. Up to 31% of patients with Down's syndrome and achondroplasia may have atlantoaxial instability.[31]

Ear surgery often involves surgical identification and preservation of the facial nerve, which requires isolation of the nerve by the surgeon and verification of its function by means of electrical stimulation (Figs. 35-7 and 35-8). This is accomplished by brainstem auditory evoked potential and electrocochleogram monitoring, and this is safest if profound skeletal muscle relaxation is avoided and a volatile drug is the primary anesthetic.[32] If an opioid-relaxant technique is chosen, however, at least 30% of the muscle response, as determined by a twitch monitor, should be preserved. There is evidence, however, that electri-

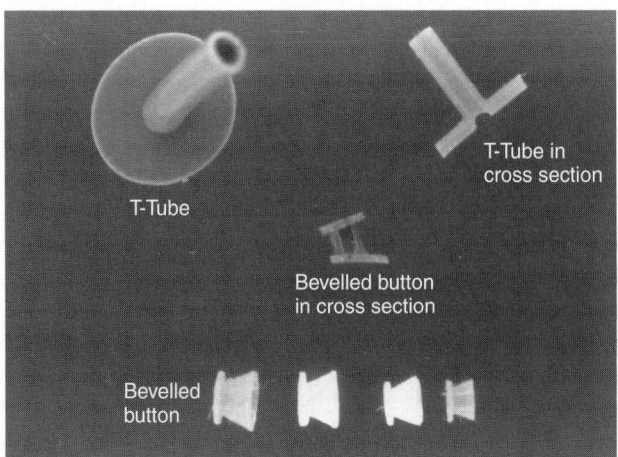

Figure 35-6. Two types of myringotomy tubes. Both are 2.5 mm in internal diameter. Both the ventilating T-tube and the beveled-button ventilating tube (large and small) are shown in full and cross-sectional views. (Courtesy of Michael Cunningham, M.D., Boston, Massachusetts.)

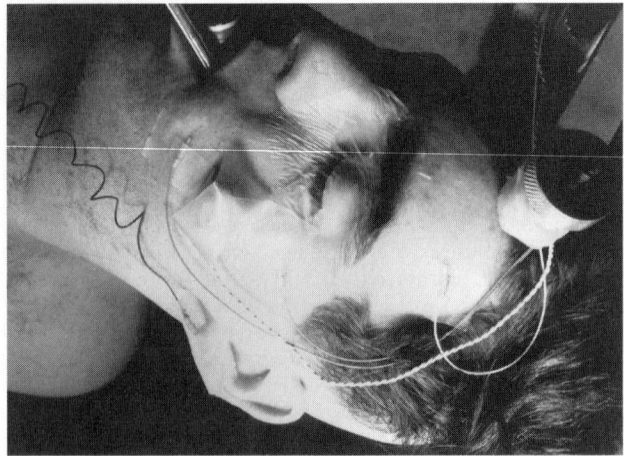

Figure 35-7. Anesthetized patient with facial nerve monitoring electrodes in place.

cally induced facial muscle activity persists and is easily visible even when neuromuscular blockade prevents a visible response to electrical stimulation of the thenar muscles.[33] This suggests that it is not mandatory to avoid skeletal muscle relaxants in the anesthetic management of patients undergoing surgical procedures when monitoring of facial nerve function is necessary.

Bleeding must be kept to a minimum during surgery of the small structures of the middle ear. Relative hypotension, keeping the mean arterial pressure 25% below baseline, is effective. Concentrated epinephrine solution, often 1:1000, can be injected in the area of the tympanic vessels to produce vasoconstriction. Close attention should be paid to the volume of injected epinephrine to avoid dysrhythmias and wide swings in blood pressure.

The middle ear and sinuses are air-filled, nondistendible cavities. An increase in the volume of gas in these structures results in an increase in pressure. N_2O diffuses along a concentration gradient into the air-filled middle ear spaces more rapidly than nitrogen moves out. Passive venting occurs at 20–30 cm H_2O pressure, and it has been shown that use of N_2O results in pressures that exceed the ability of the eustachian tube to vent the middle ear within 5 minutes, leading to pressure buildup.[34]

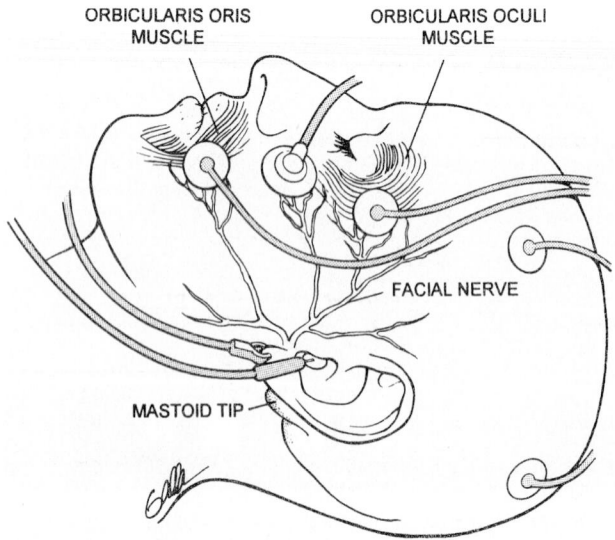

Figure 35-8. Illustration of facial nerve and monitoring electrodes. (Courtesy of Steve Ronner, Ph.D., Boston, Massachusetts.)

Intermittent venting of the middle ear leads to constant changes in middle ear pressure, which in turn cause movement of the tympanic membrane.[35] During procedures in which the ear drum is replaced or perforation is patched, N_2O should be discontinued or, if this is not possible, limited to a maximum of 50% the application of the tympanic membrane graft to avoid pressure-related displacement.

After N_2O is discontinued, it is quickly reabsorbed, creating a void in the middle ear with resulting negative pressure. This negative pressure may result in serous otitis, disarticulation of the ossicles in the middle ear, especially the stapes, and hearing impairment, which may last up to 6 weeks after surgery. The use of N_2O may cause a high incidence of postoperative nausea and vomiting, which is a direct result of negative middle ear pressure during recovery. The vestibular system is stimulated by traction placed on the round window by the negative pressure that is created. Although all patients have the potential for nausea and vomiting after surgery, children younger than 8 years of age seem to be most affected. If the use of N_2O cannot be avoided, vigorous use of antiemetics is warranted.

Special Considerations

Postoperative Nausea and Vomiting. Nausea and vomiting are among the most common postoperative problems. Although all are at risk, ENT procedures are associated with the highest incidence of postoperative emesis. Not only are patients uncomfortable after surgery, but delayed discharge from the postanesthesia care unit or unscheduled hospital admission is becoming an economic concern.

The act of vomiting is under the control of both the dorsal aspect of the lateral reticular formation and the chemoreceptor trigger zone in the area postrema of the floor of the fourth ventricle. Although the control of emesis is central in origin, the afferent stimuli originate primarily in the periphery from the gastrointestinal tract, the labyrinthine apparatus, or the oculomotor center. The anesthetic technique and drugs used can have an impact on the incidence of nausea and vomiting through effects on both central and peripheral structures. There are, however, some nonanesthetic factors that contribute to the incidence of nausea and vomiting, including a positive correlation with both obesity and prior history of motion sickness.

Both the conduct of the anesthetic and the use of specific drugs can help to prevent postoperative emesis, if not eliminate it completely. Decompressing the stomach after induction of general anesthesia empties the stomach of gas and fluid, thereby diminishing gastric distention. Limiting the use of opioids is helpful in those patients who fall into a high-risk category. The use of meperidine is known to cause emesis in children more frequently than adults, and other analgesics should be substituted. Ketamine, etomidate, and anticholinesterase inhibitors may promote emesis. Ketorolac is a nonsteroidal anti-inflammatory cyclo-oxygenase inhibitor analgesic that is effective as an adjuvant to volatile anesthetic drugs. It has been shown to provide excellent postoperative analgesia and less emesis compared with equipotent doses of morphine. Propofol has been widely used for both induction and maintenance of general anesthesia and has been associated with a dramatic decrease in postoperative nausea and vomiting. In one series of children undergoing strabismus repair, postoperative emesis occurred in only 24% of patients receiving propofol, compared with 71% receiving halothane. Butyrophenones such as droperidol are often given but are minimally effective and cause excessive somnolence. Metoclopramide, a benzamide that blocks central nervous system dopaminergic receptors, is a more effective prophylactic antiemetic that does not result in sedation and drowsiness, but in the recommended dose may cause extrapyramidal side effects. Postoperative pain, dizziness, and sudden changes in movement increase the frequency of nausea and vomiting and should be minimized in the postanesthesia care unit.

Table 35-2. CAUSES OF STRIDOR

Supraglottic Airway	Larynx	Subglottic Airway
Laryngomalacia	Laryngocele	Tracheomalacia
Vocal cord paralysis	Infection (tonsillitis, peritonsillar abscess)	Vascular ring
Subglottic stenosis	Foreign body	Foreign body
Hemangiomas	Choanal atresia	Infection (croup, epiglottitis)
Cysts	Cyst	
	Mass	
	Large tonsils	
	Large adenoids	
	Craniofacial abnormalities	

When postoperative emesis cannot be prevented, there are many effective treatments available. Metoclopramide is effective for treatment as well as prevention of nausea and vomiting. Ondansetron, a serotonin inhibitor, antagonizes central and peripheral 5-hydroxytryptamine type 3 receptors to prevent emesis. It is an effective antiemetic when administered iv. In children undergoing tonsillectomy, the iv administration of ondansetron $(0.15 \text{ mg} \cdot \text{kg}^{-1})$ after inhalational induction of anesthesia decreased but did not abolish the incidence of postoperative emesis.[36] In the same report, droperidol and metoclopramide had no significant effect on postoperative vomiting.

Airway Surgery

Stridor

Noisy breathing due to obstructed airflow is known as *stridor*. Inspiratory stridor results from upper airway obstruction; expiratory stridor results from lower airway obstruction; and biphasic stridor is present with midtracheal lesions. The evaluation of a patient with stridor begins with taking a thorough history. The age of onset suggests a cause because laryngotracheomalacia and vocal cord paralysis are usually present at or shortly after birth, whereas cysts or mass lesions develop later in life (Table 35-2). Information indicating positions that make the stridor better or worse should be obtained, and placing a patient in a position that allows gravity to aid in reducing obstruction can be of benefit during anesthetic induction.

Physical examination reveals the general condition of a patient as well as the degree of the airway compromise. Laboratory examination may include assessment of hemoglobin, a chest radiograph, and barium swallow, which can aid in identifying lesions that may be compressing the trachea. Computed tomography scan and tomograms may be indicated in isolated instances but are not routinely ordered. Specific note of the signs and symptoms listed in Table 35-3 should be made.

Laryngomalacia is the most common cause of stridor in infants. It is most often due to a long epiglottis that prolapses posteriorly, and prominent arytenoid cartilages with redundant aryepiglottic folds, that obstruct the glottic opening during inspiration.[37] The definitive diagnosis is obtained by direct laryngoscopy and rigid or flexible bronchoscopy. Preliminary examination is usually carried out in the surgeon's office. A small, flexible fiberoptic bronchoscope is inserted through the nares into the oropharynx, and the movement of the vocal cords is observed. Alternatively, it may be accomplished in the OR before anesthetic induction in an awake patient or in a lightly anesthetized patient during spontaneous respiration. Patients must be spontaneously breathing so that the vocal cords move freely. After deepening anesthesia, a rigid bronchoscope is inserted through the vocal cords and the subglottic area is inspected; the lower trachea and bronchi are evaluated with a rigid or flexible fiberoptic bronchoscope.

Bronchoscopy

Small infants may be brought into the operating room unpremedicated. Older children and adults may experience respiratory depression and worsening of airway obstruction if heavy premedication is administered, so light sedation is suggested. The airway must be protected from aspiration of gastric contents during prolonged airway manipulation; therefore, premedication with the full regimen of acid aspiration prophylaxis may be indicated.

The goals of anesthesia are analgesia, an unconscious patient, and a "quiet" surgical field.[38] Coughing, bucking, or straining during instrumentation with the rigid bronchoscope may cause difficulty for the surgeon and result in damage to the patient's airway. At the conclusion of the procedure, patients should be returned to consciousness quickly with airway reflexes intact. For most patients, a pulse oximeter, blood pressure cuff, ECG, and precordial stethoscope are applied before induction of anesthesia. Inhalation induction by mask is accompanied by oxygen and a volatile drug (usually halothane) administered in increasing concentrations in children, and iv drugs in adults. Patients should be placed in the position that produces the least adverse effect on airway symptoms (often the sitting position). An antisialagogue (atropine or glycopyrrolate) is often administered iv to decrease secretions that may obscure the view through the bronchoscope.

The size of a bronchoscope refers to the internal diameter. Because the external diameter may be significantly greater than in an endotracheal tube of similar size (Table 35-4), care must be taken to select a bronchoscope of proper external diameter to avoid damage to the laryngeal structures.

A rigid bronchoscope can be used for ventilation of the lungs during examination of the airway. It is inserted through the vocal cords and ventilation is accomplished through a side port, which can be attached to the anesthesia circuit. During ventilation with the viewing telescope in place, high resistance

Table 35-3. SIGNS AND SYMPTOMS SPECIFICALLY EXAMINED IN PATIENTS WITH STRIDOR

Respiratory rate
Heart rate
Wheezing
Cyanosis
Chest retractions
Nasal flaring
Level of consciousness

Table 35-4. COMPARISON OF EXTERNAL DIAMETER OF STANDARD ENDOTRACHEAL TUBES VERSUS RIGID BRONCHOSCOPE

Endotracheal Tube		Rigid Bronchoscope External Diameter (mm)
Internal Diameter (mm)	External Diameter (mm)	
2.5	3.5	4.2
3.0	4.3	5.0
3.5	4.9	5.7
4.0	5.5	6.7
5.0	6.8	7.8
6.0	8.2	8.2

Adapted with permission from Mallinckrodt Medical, Inc., St. Louis, Missouri.

may be encountered as a result of partial occlusion of the lumen. High fresh gas flow rates, large tidal volumes, and high inspired volatile anesthetic concentrations are often necessary to compensate for leaks around the ventilating bronchoscope and the high resistance encountered when the viewing telescope is in place. Manual ventilation at higher-than-normal rates is most effective in achieving adequate ventilation. Adequate time for exhalation must be provided for passive recoil of the chest.

An alternative method of ventilation is the Sander's jet ventilation technique. The principle of jet ventilation involves intermittent bursts of oxygen delivered under a pressure of 50 psi through a 16-gauge catheter attached to a rigid bronchoscope.[39] Intermittent flow is accomplished by depressing the lever of an on–off valve. The use of jet ventilation techniques is associated with the additional risks of pneumothorax or pneumomediastinum due to rupture of alveolar blebs or a bronchus.[40]

Because ventilation may be intermittent and at times suboptimal, it is recommended that oxygen be used as the carrier gas during bronchoscopic examination. Intravenous drugs that cause excessive respiratory depression should be avoided. It is wise to ask the surgeon if movement of the vocal cords will be observed at the conclusion of the procedure or if tracheal or bronchial dynamics will be evaluated during the procedure so that the anesthetic may be planned accordingly (i.e., spontaneous respirations preserved during light levels of anesthesia versus no respiratory efforts and the use of short-acting muscle relaxants).

Maintenance of anesthesia is usually accomplished with a volatile anesthetic. Intravenous anesthetics combined with muscle relaxation best maintain a constant level of anesthesia because the delivery of volatile anesthetics through the bronchoscope may be interrupted and anesthetic depth can vary. At the conclusion of rigid bronchoscopy, an endotracheal tube is usually placed in the trachea to control the airway during recovery of anesthesia; this tube is particularly important if muscle relaxants have been used because passive regurgitation of gastric contents may be more likely to occur in paralyzed patients. An additional advantage of placing an endotracheal tube is that if the surgeon should wish to examine the distal airways, a small, flexible fiberoptic bronchoscope can be passed through the endotracheal tube.

Pediatric Airway Emergencies

Upper airway emergencies may be life-threatening and demand immediate treatment. Rapid respiratory failure can occur in patients with from croup, epiglottitis, or foreign body aspiration, and few clinical situations are more challenging to the anesthesiologist.

Epiglottitis

Acute epiglottitis is one of the most feared infectious diseases in children and adults and is the result of *Haemophilus influenzae* type B. It can progress with extreme rapidity from sore throat to airway obstruction to respiratory failure and death if proper diagnosis and intervention are not rapidly effected. Patients are usually between 2 and 7 years of age, although epiglottitis has been reported in younger children and adults. Vaccination against *H. influenzae* type B polysaccharide is now recommended before 2 years of age to provide immunity before the greatest period of vulnerability in pediatric patients.

Characteristic signs and symptoms of acute epiglottitis include sudden onset of fever, dysphagia, drooling, thick, muffled voice, and preference for the sitting position with the head extended and leaning forward. Retractions, labored breathing, and cyanosis may be observed in cases where respiratory obstruction is present. However, in the early stages, the patient may be pale and toxic without respiratory distress. *Supraglottitis* may be a more appropriate designation because it is the tissues of the supraglot-

tic structures, from the vallecula to the arytenoids, that are involved in the infectious process. At no time (in the emergency room or radiography suite) should direct visualization of the epiglottis be attempted in the unanesthetized patient. The differential resulting from negative pressure inside and atmospheric pressure outside the extrathoracic airway results in slight narrowing during normal inspiration. The pressure differential on inspiration is exaggerated in the patient with airway obstruction. This dynamic collapse of the airway may become life-threatening in the struggling, agitated patient, and every attempt should be made in keeping him or her calm. Blood drawing, iv insertion, and excessive manipulation of the patient as well as sedation should be avoided before securing the airway to avoid the possibility of total obstruction.

If the clinical situation allows, oxygen should be administered by mask and lateral radiographs of the soft tissues in the neck may be obtained. Thickening of the aryepiglottic folds as well as swelling of the epiglottis may be noted. Radiologic examination should only be carried out if skilled personnel and adequate equipment accompany the patient at all times. The patient with severe airway compromise should proceed from the emergency department directly to the operating suite accompanied by the anesthesiologist and surgeon. Parental presence in this situation may calm an anxious and frightened child.

In all cases of epiglottitis, an artificial airway is established by means of tracheal intubation. In some centers where personnel experienced in the management of the compromised airway are not available, tracheostomy is a less favored alternative. In the OR, the child is kept in the sitting position while monitors are placed. A pulse oximeter and precordial stethoscope are essential. If it is thought to be helpful, one parent may accompany the child and remain in the OR during the induction of general anesthesia. The OR must be prepared with equipment and personnel for laryngoscopy, rigid bronchoscopy, and tracheostomy. Anesthetic induction is accomplished by inhalation of oxygen and increasing concentrations of halothane or sevoflurane. After loss of consciousness occurs, iv access should be secured and the child lowered into the supine position. Laryngoscopy followed by oral tracheal intubation is then accomplished without the use of muscle relaxants. The endotracheal tube chosen should be at least one size (0.5 mm) smaller than would normally be chosen, and a stylette is often useful. Once the surgeon has examined the larynx, noting the appearance of the epiglottis, aryepiglottic folds, and surrounding tissues, the endotracheal tube may be changed to a nasotracheal tube and secured. Tissue and blood cultures are taken and antibiotic therapy is initiated. The child is then transferred to the intensive care unit for continued observation and radiographic confirmation of tube placement. Sedation is appropriate at this time. Tracheal extubation is usually attempted 48–72 hours later in the OR, when a significant leak around the nasotracheal tube is present and visual inspection of the larynx by flexible fiberoptic bronchoscopy confirms reduction in swelling of the epiglottis and surrounding tissues.

Laryngotracheobronchitis

Laryngotracheobronchitis (LTB), or croup, occurs in children from 6 months to 6 years of age but is primarily seen in children less than 3 years of age. It is usually viral in etiology and its onset is more insidious than that of epiglottitis. The child presents with low-grade fever, inspiratory stridor, and a "barking" cough. Radiologic examination confirms the diagnosis, and subglottic narrowing of the airway column secondary to circumferential soft tissue edema produces the "steeple" sign characteristic of LTB. Approximately 6% of patients with LTB require admission to the hospital. Treatment includes cool, humidified mist and oxygen therapy, usually administered in a tent for mild to moderate cases. More severe cases of LTB are accompanied by tachypnea, tachycardia, and cyanosis. Racemic epinephrine administered by nebulizer is beneficial. The use of steroids has been surrounded by a great deal of controversy, but current opinion is that a short course of steroids may be beneficial. In rare circumstances, thick secretions are present in the airway and the child requires intubation to allow pulmonary toilet and suctioning to be carried out. Management in the intensive care unit and extubation are carried out in the same fashion as for epiglottitis.

Foreign Body Aspiration

A major cause of morbidity and mortality in children as well as adults is aspiration of a foreign body. Any history of coughing, choking, or cyanosis while eating (peanuts, popcorn, jelly beans, hot dogs) should suggest the possibility of foreign body aspiration. Any patient who presents to the emergency room with refractory wheezing should be suspected of this diagnosis. Physical findings include decreased breath sounds, tachypnea, stridor, wheezing, and fever. These signs indicate an obstructive–inflammatory process in the airway. Some foreign bodies are identifiable on radiologic examination; however, 90% are radiolucent and air trapping, infiltrate, and atelectasis are all that is noted. The most common site of foreign body aspiration is the mainstem bronchus, the right being more frequent than the left. Food particles comprise the majority of aspirated items; however, beads, pins, and small toys are not unusual. Each type of aspirated item has potential complications associated with it. Vegetable items expand with moisture encountered in the respiratory tract and can fragment into multiple pieces, thus creating a situation where the original foreign body is in one bronchus and with coughing a fragment is dislodged and transported to the other bronchus. Oil-containing objects, such as peanuts, cause a chemical inflammation and sharp objects cause bleeding in addition to the obstruction.

All aspirated foreign bodies in the airway should be removed in the OR and considered to be emergency situations. No sedation should be administered to patients before removal of the foreign body. If the patient has recently eaten, full stomach precautions must be taken and anesthesia should be induced iv (topical EMLA cream may be applied to the skin before iv insertion in small children) by rapid sequence and gentle cricoid pressure maintained during intubation of the trachea. If the child has not recently eaten, anesthesia may be induced by inhalation of halothane in oxygen by mask. Inhalation induction can be prolonged secondary to obstruction of the airway and N_2O should be avoided to reduce air trapping distal to the obstruction. After evacuation of the stomach by orogastric tube, the airway may be given over to the surgeon, who replaces the endotracheal tube with a rigid bronchoscope and removes the aspirated object.

Spontaneous ventilation should be preserved until the location and nature of the foreign body have been determined. Ventilation via the bronchoscope requires careful attention. Hypoxia and hypercarbia may occur because of inadequate ventilation caused by an excessively large leak around the bronchoscope or, more commonly, inability to provide adequate gas exchange through a narrow-lumen bronchoscope fitted with an internal telescope. These conditions are remedied by frequent removal of the telescope and withdrawal of the bronchoscope to the midtrachea, allowing effective ventilation. Bronchospasm may occur during examination of the respiratory tract and should be treated with increasing depths of anesthesia, nebulized albuterol, or iv bronchodilators. Although rare, pneumothorax should be suspected if acute deterioration occurs during the procedure.

Once the foreign body has been removed, examination of the entire tracheobronchial tree is carried out to detect any additional objects or fragments. Often, vigorous irrigation and suctioning distal to the obstruction are required to remove secretions and prevent the possibility of postobstructive pneumonia. Steroids are administered if inflammation of the airway mucosa is observed. Close postoperative observation of the patient is required so that early intervention may be instituted in the event of respiratory compromise secondary to airway edema or infection.

ANESTHESIA FOR PEDIATRIC AND ADULT SURGERY

Certain surgical procedures are commonly performed in both adults and children, including nasal surgery and laser surgery of the airway. Surgery for maxillofacial trauma and upper airway tumors or infection, as well as temporomandibular joint (TMJ) arthroscopy, are procedures done more commonly in adults.

Laser Surgery of the Airway

One of the greatest advances in airway surgery has been the use of the laser (*l*ight *a*mplification by *s*timulated *e*mission of *r*adiation). For use in the airway, the laser provides precision in targeting lesions, minimal bleeding and edema, preservation of surrounding structures, and rapid healing. The laser consists of a tube with reflective mirrors at either end and an amplifying medium between them to generate electron activity, resulting in the production of light.[41] The CO_2 laser is the most widely used in medical practice, having particular application in the treatment of laryngeal or vocal cord papillomas, laryngeal webs, resection of redundant subglottic tissue, and coagulation of hemangiomas. The laser is an especially useful modality for the surgeon because the invisible beam of light affords an unobstructed view of the lesion during resection. The energy emitted by a CO_2 laser is absorbed by water contained in blood and tissues. Human tissue is approximately 80% water, and laser energy absorbed by tissue water rapidly increases the temperature, denaturing protein and vaporizing the target tissue. The thermal energy of the laser beam cauterizes capillaries as it vaporizes tissues; thus, bleeding and postoperative edema are minimized.

The properties that give the laser a high degree of specificity also supply the route by which a misdirected laser beam may cause injury to a patient or to unprotected OR personnel.[42] The eyes are especially vulnerable, and all OR personnel should wear laser-specific eye goggles with side protectors to prevent injury. Due to the limited penetration (0.01 mm) of the CO_2 laser, it may cause injury only to the cornea. Other lasers, such as the neodymium–yttrium-aluminum-garnet (Nd-YAG), have deeper penetration and may cause retinal injury and scarring. The eyes of a patient undergoing laser treatment must be protected by taping them shut, followed by the application of wet gauze pads and a metal shield. Any stray laser beam is absorbed by the wet gauze, preventing penetration of the eyes. Laser radiation increases the temperature of absorbent material, and flammable objects such as surgical drapes must be kept away from the path of the laser beam. Wet towels should be applied to exposed skin of the face and neck when the laser is being used in the airway to avoid cutaneous burns from deflected beams. Laser smoke plumes may cause damage to the lungs, and interstitial pneumonia has been reported with long-term exposure. In addition, it has been postulated that, during laser application, cancer cells and virus particles, including human immunodeficiency virus, are vaporized and the resultant smoke plume, if inhaled, may be a vehicle for spread. The use of specially designed surgical masks for filtering laser smoke is recommended.

Most anesthetic techniques are suitable for laser surgery provided that patients are immobile and the laser beam can be directed at a target that is entirely still and in full view. Both N_2O and oxygen support combustion. The primary gas for anesthetic maintenance should consist of blended air and oxygen or helium and oxygen. A pulse oximeter should be used at all times.

Anesthesia during laser surgery may be administered with or without an endotracheal tube. The choice of endotracheal tube

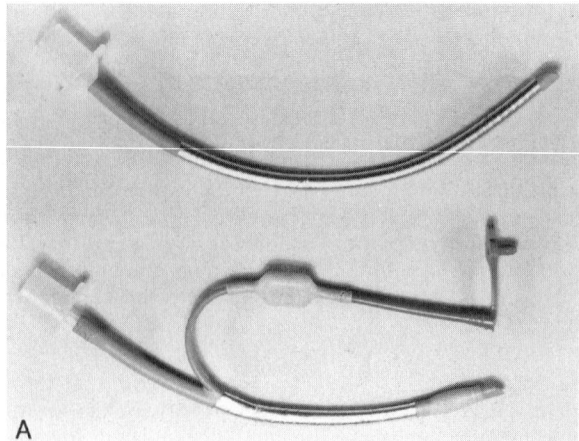

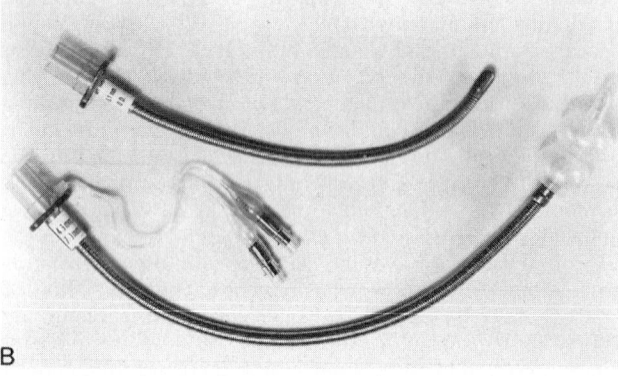

Figure 35-9. (*A*) Cuffed and uncuffed rubber endotracheal tubes wrapped with reflective metallic tape. (*B*) Cuffed and uncuffed flexible metal endotracheal tubes for use during laser surgery of the airway. (Reprinted with permission from Ferrari LR: Anesthesia for otorhinolaryngology procedures. In Cote C, Ryan J, Todres D, Goudsouzian N [eds]: A practice of Anesthesia for Infants and Children, 2nd ed., Chapter 18, Philadelphia, WB Saunders, 1993.)

used during laser surgery can affect the safety of the technique. All standard polyvinyl chloride (PVC) endotracheal tubes are flammable and can ignite and vaporize when in contact with the laser beam. Red rubber endotracheal tubes wrapped with reflective metallic tape do not vaporize but instead deflect the laser beam. The unwrapped cuff below the vocal cords is still vulnerable to laser injury. Cuffed endotracheal tubes should be inflated with sterile saline to which methylene blue has been added so that a cuff rupture from a misdirected laser spark is readily detected by the blue dye and extinguished by the saline.[43] Endotracheal tubes have been manufactured specifically for use during laser surgery. Some have a double cuff to ensure protection of the airway in the event of a cuff rupture, whereas others have a special matte finish that is effective in deflecting the laser beam throughout the entire length. Nonreflective flexible metal endotracheal tubes are also specifically manufactured for use during laser surgery. The outer diameter of each size of metal laser tube is considerably greater than the PVC counterpart, especially in the small sizes used for pediatric anesthesia (Figs. 35-9 and 35-10, Table 35-5).

An apneic technique is preferred by some surgeons, especially when working on the airway of small infants and children. The advantage of this technique is the absence of an endotracheal tube, which may obscure the surgical field. In this circumstance, a child is anesthetized and rendered immobile by use of a muscle relaxant or deep inhalation of a volatile anesthetic. The patient's trachea is not intubated and the airway is given over to the surgeon, who uses the laser for brief periods. Between laser applications, the patient's lungs are ventilated by mask. Because apnea is a component of this technique, it is prudent to ventilate the lungs with oxygen. Although this technique has been widely used with safety, there is a greater potential for debris and resected material to enter the trachea.

A modification of the apneic technique that does not require tracheal intubation but does provide for oxygenation during laser surgery uses a jet ventilator. The operating laryngoscope is fitted with a catheter through which oxygen is delivered under pressure through a variable reducing value (see Fig. 35-10). Additional room air is entrained and the patient's lungs are ventilated with this combination of gases. This technique produces a quiet surgical field because large chest excursions of the diaphragm are eliminated and ventilation of the patient is uninterrupted. In morbidly obese patients and those with severe small airway disease, effective ventilation is not accomplished with this technique, and an alternate technique should be used.

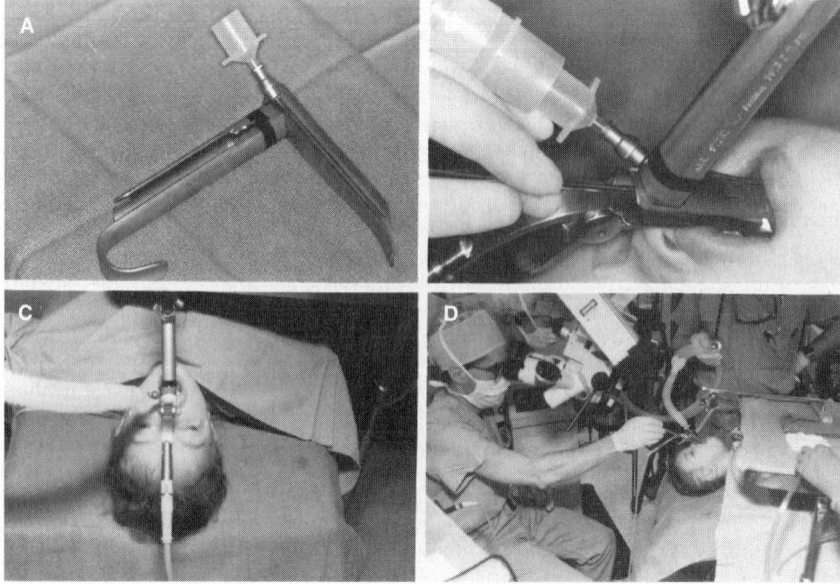

Figure 35-10. (*A*) The surgical laryngoscope fitted with an endotracheal tube connector. (*B*) The surgical laryngoscope positioned in the patient's pharynx and connected to the anesthesia circuit. (*C*) Surgical view of the anesthetized, spontaneously breathing patient. (*D*) Laser-aided resection of vocal cord lesion.

Table 35-5. COMPARISON OF STANDARD PLASTIC *VERSUS* METAL ENDOTRACHEAL TUBES

Internal Diameter (mm)	External Diameter (mm)	
	Plastic	*Metal*
3.0 (uncuffed)	4.3	5.2
3.5 (uncuffed)	4.9	5.7
4.0 (uncuffed)	5.5	6.1
4.5 (cuffed)	6.2	7.0
5.0 (cuffed)	6.8	7.5
5.5 (cuffed)	7.5	7.9
6.0 (cuffed)	8.2	8.5

The final technique that may be used without the aid of an endotracheal tube is spontaneous ventilation with the "oxiscope." In this technique, a surgical laryngoscope fitted with an oxygen insufflation port is inserted into the larynx. The volatile anesthetic gas is mixed with oxygen and administered through the side port. Anesthesia is maintained without muscle relaxant in the spontaneously breathing patient in this manner. Propofol may be infused to decrease the concentration of inhaled volatile anesthetic, and the vocal cords may be sprayed with 4% lidocaine to decrease reactivity. This technique is advantageous in that longer periods of uninterrupted laser application may be provided. Disadvantages include the absence of complete control of the airway, no protection from laryngospasm, no protection from debris entering the airway, motion of the vocal cords is present, and adequate scavenging is difficult.

Nasal Surgery

Nasal surgery may be successfully accomplished under either general anesthesia or conscious sedation. Whichever method is selected, profound vasoconstriction is required. Cocaine packs, local anesthetics, and epinephrine infiltration are often used simultaneously. All three of these agents can cause cardiac irritability, and both epinephrine and cocaine are known to produce varying degrees of hypertension. The simultaneous use of these medications causes cumulative and often dangerous side effects. Young, healthy patients may be able to tolerate these effects. The older patient or one who has known cardiovascular compromise may benefit from slow, sequential administration of these medications guided by heart rate, cardiac rhythm, and blood pressure. The potent inhalation anesthetics do have varying degrees of dysrhythmogenic potential and should be used with caution in the face of pharmacologically induced alterations in cardiac rhythm.

A moderate degree of controlled hypotension combined with head elevation decreases bleeding in the surgical site, but some blood may passively enter the stomach. The placement of an oropharyngeal pack or suctioning of the stomach at the conclusion of surgery may attenuate postoperative retching and vomiting.

Maxillofacial Trauma

Traumatic disruption of the bony, cartilaginous, and soft tissue components of the face and upper airway challenge the anesthesiologist to recognize the nature and extent of the injury and consequent anatomic alteration, create a plan for securing the airway safely, implement the plan without doing further damage, maintain the airway during the administration of an anesthetic, and determine when and how to extubate the patient's trachea, all the while creating an environment in which both surgeon and anesthesiologist can comfortably work together in the same cramped space.

Anatomy

It is conventional to divide the facial skeleton into thirds. The lower third consists of the mandible, with its subdivisions of midline symphysis, body, angle, ramus, condyle, and coronoid process. The middle third contains the zygomatic arch of the temporal bone, blending into the zygomaticomaxillary complex, the maxillae, nasal bones, and orbits. The superior third consists of the frontal bone. Actually, there are two skeletons, facial and cranial, each one in contiguity with the other. Great forces are generated within the facial skeleton during the normal physiologic process of mastication. To prevent injury of one skeleton against the other, there is a series of bony buttresses built into the relationship between the two skeletons. Horizontal posterior displacement of the facial skeleton is limited by the zygomatic process of the temporal bone, oblique posterior displacement by the pterygoid process of the sphenoid bone, and vertical posterior displacement by the greater wing of the sphenoid bone. Upward displacement is held in check by the zygomatic process of the frontal bone, the nasal part of the frontal bone, and the roof of the mandibular fossa.

In addition to the buttresses, there are two arches lending stability to the craniofacial skeleton. An arch extends from the mandibular condyle to the coronoid process, and another arch is created by the zygomatic arch of the temporal bone extending into the zygomaticomaxillary complex.

This combination of bony buttresses and arches creates a normal vector of force dispersion and distribution.[44] Thus, a blow to the mandible may be of sufficient magnitude to fracture the mandible at the point of impact, or elsewhere, but does not extend the fracture line into the base of the skull. However, a blow to the midface, especially from in front and above, does not follow a normal vector of force dispersion and redistribution and tends to create an abnormal shearing force, which may tear the facial skeleton from the cranial skeleton and extend the fracture into the base of the skull. In any patient with severe midfacial trauma, a fracture of the base of the skull must be considered.

The mandible is a tubular bone and, as such, derives its strength from the cortices and is least vulnerable to fracture where the cortex is thickest (*i.e.,* at the anteroinferior margin).[45] Moving posteriorly, the cortex thins and a greater incidence of fractures found at the angle of the mandible, the ramus, and the condyle.[46-49] Another common point of fracture is in the body of the mandible at the level of the first or second molar. These are laboratory observations, but clinical experience indicates that this distribution occurs after high-velocity, high-impact trauma, such as in an automobile accident. After personal trauma, such as inflicted by a fist, a blunt weapon, or a fall, there is a greater tendency for a fracture of the symphysis, parasymphysis, and body to occur. This may result from lesser versus greater energy impact and redistribution but also results from the person's tendency to turn the head away from an impending blow and thus take the force of impact on the side of the face and the body of the mandible rather than on the symphysis.[50]

The mandible has a unique, horseshoe shape that causes forces to gather at points of vulnerability, often distant from the point of impact.[48] If this phenomenon is unrecognized, it can create serious problems in diagnosis. It may be known, for example, that the patient was struck on the symphysis, but it must also be recognized that he may have a fracture of the condyle, perhaps with involvement of the TMJ and limitation of jaw mobility.

LeFort Classification of Fractures

In 1901 Rene LeFort of Lille, France, published the results of a series of rather bizarre experiments.[51] He attempted to determine if there is a reliable means of detecting facial fractures by examining the facial soft tissue injuries and using the nature and extent of these injuries as indicators of bony disruption. This relationship does not exist. Extensive soft tissue injury does not necessarily indicate bony trauma, and conversely, serious fractures may exist with relatively little soft tissue disruption. In the course of his studies LeFort determined the common lines of fracture of the midface, which are thus eponymous and called LeFort I, LeFort II, and LeFort III fractures.

The LeFort I fracture is a horizontal fracture of the maxilla, passing above the floor of the nose but involving the lower third of the septum, mobilizing the palate, maxillary alveolar process, and the lower third of the pterygoid plates and parts of the palatine bones. The fracture segment may be displaced posteriorly or laterally, rotated about a vertical axis, or any combination.

The LeFort II fracture is pyramidal, beginning at the junction of the thick upper part of the nasal bone and the thinner portion forming the upper margin of the anterior nasal aperture. The fracture crosses the medial wall of the orbit, including the lacrimal bone, beneath the zygomaticomaxillary suture, crosses the lateral wall of the antrum, and passes posteriorly through the pterygoid plates. The fracture segment may be displaced posteriorly or rotated about an axis.

In a LeFort III fracture, the line of fracture parallels the base of the skull, separating the midfacial skeleton from the base of the cranium. The line of fracture passes through the base of the nose and the ethmoid bone in its depth, and through the orbital plates. The cribriform plate of the ethmoid may or may not be fractured. The fracture line crosses the lesser wing of the sphenoid, then downward to the pterygomaxillary fissure and sphenopalatine fossa. From the base of the inferior orbital fissure, the fracture extends laterally and upward to the frontozygomatic suture and downward and backward to the root of the pterygoid plates. A LeFort III fracture results from massive force applied to the mid-face. The zygomata are displaced and rotational force applied to the zygomatic arches. The arches are usually fractured as a result.

With this fracture, the midface is mobilized and often distracted posteriorly. The normal convexity of the face may be replaced by a concavity, giving rise to the characteristic "dish face deformity" of a LeFort III fracture. Even if this facial concavity is not clinically evident, the presence of a LeFort III fracture should be suspected if the incisive edges of the maxillary and mandibular teeth are apposed, instead of the normal position in which the maxillary incisors shingle over the mandibular incisors. This apposition serves as a subtle clue to minimal posterior displacement of the midface.

Tumors

Neoplastic growths can occur anywhere within the upper airway and may achieve significant size with little evidence of airway obstruction. These tumors are often friable and bleed readily. Attempted tracheal intubation can induce significant hemorrhage and edema and cause severe compromise of the airway. Prior radiation therapy may cause extensive fibrosis, increased intraoperative bleeding, and ankylosis of the TMJ, making tracheal intubation under direct vision difficult or impossible. Consultation with a surgeon as to the nature and extent of the tumor its potential to bleed, together with review of appropriate radiographs and prior therapy, are important in determining techniques for airway management. Tumors of the head and neck are usually associated with abuse of both cigarettes and alcohol, with consequent abnormalities of both pulmonary and hepatic function.

Upper Airway Infection

Infectious processes in the upper airway may be of sufficient size to mimic neoplasms and present the same problems of airway distortion, compression, and compromise. The same precautions must be taken in dealing with airway abscesses as with tumors. An added problem is the ability of an abscess to leak spontaneously, dribbling pus into the lungs, contaminating and infecting them, and producing scattered areas of pneumonitis; or to rupture during tracheal intubation, flooding the lungs with purulent material.

Ludwig's Angina

Ludwig's angina is an overwhelming generalized septic cellulitis of the submandibular region.[52,53] It generally occurs after dental extraction, especially of the second or third mandibular molars, whose roots lie below the attachment of the mylohyoid muscle. The infection is bilateral and involves three fascial spaces: submandibular, submental, and sublingual.[54] Ludwig's angina is characterized by brawny induration of the upper neck, usually without obvious fluctuation, and the patient has a typical open-mouthed appearance. Involvement of the sublingual space pushes the tongue upward and backward, and it usually protrudes from the open mouth. Soft tissue swelling in the suprahyoid region, coupled with upward and posterior displacement of the tongue, and the frequent presence of laryngeal edema can close the airway and asphyxiate the patient.

Early signs and symptoms include chills, fever, drooling of saliva, inability to open the mouth, and difficulty in speaking. The cause is often hemolytic streptococci but may be a mixture of aerobic and anaerobic organisms, including gas-forming bacteria.[55] Although fluctuation is rarely appreciated, abscesses may be present but their presence hidden by the thick, indurated tissue of the neck. The infectious process may spread into the thorax, causing empyema, pericarditis, pericardial effusion, and pulmonary infiltrates.[56,57] Patients with Ludwig's angina often require incision and drainage of whatever purulent material is present, coupled with airway decompression. Airway management may be extremely difficult. While inhalation anesthesia and intubation have been advocated,[58] preliminary tracheostomy using local anesthesia in the awake patient is the safest course. The patient with Ludwig's angina is commonly septic and extremely ill, and often poorly hydrated.

Temporomandibular Joint Arthroscopy

Open surgery of the human TMJ was first described in 1887 in a discussion of operative repair of displaced interarticular cartilage of the joint.[59] Although open surgery of the joint is still sometimes considered necessary, the development of small-gauge arthroscopes and lasers has made arthroscopic surgery of the TMJ an increasingly popular technique, frequently performed on an ambulatory basis.[60,61] Common indications for arthroscopic correction of TMJ lesions include the following:[61] (1) internal joint derangement with closed lock, (2) internal joint derangement with painful clicking, (3) osteoarthritis, (4) hypermobility, (5) fibrous ankylosis, and (6) arthralgia. Other less common indicators include chondromalacia and synovitis.

Temporomandibular joint disease is usually caused by spasm of the muscles of mastication secondary to chronic tensing of these muscles as an involuntary mental tension–relieving mechanism.[62] The patient population is unique in that 86% of patients with chronic TMJ dysfunction have significant psychopathology, with major depression in 74% and somatoform disorder in 50%.[63] A total of 40% of the patients are preoccupied with facial pain yet have no physical findings accounting for the pain. Many of these patients habitually use mood-altering or tension-abating drugs such as benzodiazepines, phenothiazines, or lithium.

Nasotracheal intubation is usually preferred, allowing the surgeon the option of intraoral manipulation during surgery. Complications of TMJ arthroscopy are rare but include partial or total hearing loss, infection, hemorrhage requiring open arthrotomy, and temporary or permanent deficits of the fifth and eighth cranial nerves and temporary seventh nerve paresis.[61,64]

Of particular importance to the anesthesiologist is partial or even complete closure of the airway due to extracapsular extravasation of the fluid used to irrigate the joint during arthroscopy.[65] Significant amounts of fluid can leak into the soft tissues of the neck and compromise the airway. After TMJ arthroscopy, the patient's trachea should not be extubated until the oral cavity, especially on the affected side, and neck have been examined carefully and there is no evidence of unusual swelling that might indicate extravasated fluid.

Patient Evaluation

The patient who has sustained facial trauma or whose airway is clearly distorted by tumor or infection may present with an obvious pathologic process that can distract the physician from completing a total evaluation of the patient. In the patient with facial trauma, other injuries may not be as apparent but may represent a greater threat to the patient's well-being. In patients with maxillofacial injury due to low-velocity, low-impact blows (as from a fist), 4% had major (life-threatening) other injuries, and 10% had minor (non–life-threatening) injuries. With high-velocity, high-impact (motor vehicle) accidents, 32% had major and 31% minor other injuries.[66] Of great importance, cervical spine fractures occurred in 1.2% of high-velocity injuries. Other studies have reported a 5.5% incidence of cervical spine injury in patients with facial skeletal trauma.[67] Any level of the cervical spine may be involved, but injuries at C2 (31%) and C6–7 (50%) predominate. Cranial fractures and intracranial injury are also not uncommon.

SECURING THE AIRWAY

In most instances of anesthesia for head and neck surgery, tracheal intubation is effected without significant problems. Grave difficulties can arise in patients with tumor or infection or other facial trauma. If any of these processes has so altered the airway that attempted tracheal intubation risks airway compromise and an inability to ventilate the lungs, then awake tracheal intubation or preliminary tracheostomy is mandated. History, physical examination, appropriate radiographs, and surgical consultation are the foundation of airway evaluation and choice of intubating technique. The technique of an "awake look" before a decision to anesthetize and paralyze a patient is particularly hazardous and misleading. Muscle tone and labored respiration in the awake patient help to identify the rima glottis or some seemingly familiar anatomic structure but disappear once anesthesia and paralysis have been induced, and it may be impossible to identify the entrance to the airway and intubate the trachea.

For the anesthesiologist to be able to intubate the trachea of a patient under direct vision, the patient must be able, at a minimum, to open the mouth and extend the tongue beyond the incisors. After maxillofacial trauma, there may be serious limitation in mobility owing to one or more factors, including pain, trismus, edema, and mechanical dysfunction of the TMJ. Pain yields to an anesthetic and muscle relaxant and presents no problem.

Trismus is spasm of the masseter muscles, binding the jaw closed, secondary to trauma or infection. Trismus, too, succumbs to an anesthetic and muscle relaxant, but with an important caveat. If the trismus has been present for 2 weeks or if the jaw has been closed for some other reason for 2 weeks, the masseters acquire a degree of fibrosis that limits their response to an anesthetic and relaxant. A jaw closed for 2 weeks for whatever cause merits consideration for awake tracheal intubation. Edema varies in severity and consequences from mild

to extreme and may occasionally cause serious limitation in jaw mobility.

Mechanical dysfunction in the jaw arises from several causes. A fracture of the condyle in its articulation in the TMJ may create a situation in which the jaw is locked closed and unresponsive to an anesthetic and muscle relaxant. A fracture of the zygomatic arch of the temporal bone will always causes some decrease in jaw mobility. This bone is well protected, enveloped in the tough temporal fascia. Nonetheless, a severe blow to the side of the head may fracture the bone, pushing bony segments down onto the coronoid process of the mandible. There is a biphasic motion in the mandible, rotation about an axis passing through the condyles, and anterior motion (translation). This anterior motion is limited by the bony impingement on the coronoid process, and TMJ function is thus limited by the limitation in translation. Usually, the decrease in function is not severe enough to make tracheal intubation impossible, but it may be, and the decision whether to anesthetize and paralyze the patient or perform awake tracheal intubation may be difficult. The anesthesiologist in doubt is cautioned to err on the side of conservatism.

Patients with TMJ dysfunction undergoing arthroscopic surgery may present with either closed or open lock and be unsuitable for intubation of the trachea after induction of anesthesia. Patients with large cervical abscesses may require awake intubation or tracheostomy. If the abscess has caused anatomic distortion or respiratory difficulty, awake intubation or tracheostomy is usually mandatory. Early tracheostomy in Ludwig's angina is preferred, and no patient should ever be observed to the point of airway compromise.[68] In any instance in which awake intubation is elected in the infected patient provision must be available for immediate tracheostomy.

Awake Intubation

Passing an endotracheal tube through the mouth or nose and into the larynx and trachea of an awake patient is a formidable procedure that the patient resists fiercely, stimulated by the protestations of highly sensitive airway reflexes. To overcome these reflexes, the airway must be anesthetized using a combination of topical local anesthetic and superior laryngeal nerve block.

The *superior laryngeal nerve* is a branch of the vagus arising from the nodose ganglion and coursing with the main trunk of the vagus until it reaches the level of the larynx, where it springs forward and terminates in two branches, internal and external. The external branch of the superior laryngeal nerve penetrates and innervates the cricothyroid muscle, a tensor of the vocal cords. The internal branch penetrates the thyrohyoid membrane, ramifies, and provides sensory innervation from the base of the tongue to the vocal cords.[69] Once it has penetrated the thyrohyoid membrane, it lies in a closed space, bounded medially by the laryngeal mucosa, laterally by the thyrohyoid membrane, superiorly by the inferior border of the hyoid bone, and inferiorly by the superior surface of the thyroid cartilage. The anatomic landmarks for superior laryngeal nerve block are as follows:

1. The hyoid bone, a freely movable bone in the upper part of the neck, articulating with no other bone
2. The thyroid cartilage, the largest component of the larynx, usually easily identified
3. The thyrohyoid membrane binding the two together

With the patient lying supine, a 22-gauge needle attached to a syringe containing 2 ml of 2% lidocaine is aimed directly at the hyoid, traveling parallel to the operating table. When the needle strikes the hyoid, the operator can appreciate the characteristic gritty feeling of a needle on bone, similar to striking the rib while doing an intercostal block. The needle is then walked caudad until it just slips off the bone, penetrating the thyrohyoid membrane. After negative aspiration, lidocaine may be injected and the block repeated on the other side.[70,71]

Contraindications to a superior laryngeal nerve block are relative, not absolute, and include the following:

1. A full stomach, because of the possibility of vomiting and aspiration into an airway whose protective reflexes have been partially obtunded
2. Tumor at the site of block
3. Infection at the site of block

Tumor and infection are considered to be relative contraindications because of the possibility of dissemination of either tumor or infection secondary to the manipulation associated with the block. Risks must be weighed against benefit, and very often benefit wins. Protection against aspiration can be increased by the presence of knowledgeable help, an operating table that can swing quickly into the Trendelenburg position, and efficient suction apparatus.

Local anesthetic may be instilled into the nose for nasotracheal intubation and into the mouth and oropharynx for either nasal or oral intubation. A vasoconstrictor, such as 0.5% phenylephrine hydrochloride or 0.05% oxymetazoline, should also be instilled in the nose to shrink the nasal mucosa, decrease the risk of trauma, and create a larger passage for tracheal intubation. Topical anesthetic may be applied to the trachea below the level of the vocal cords by introducing a 22-gauge needle attached to a syringe containing 4 ml of 2% lidocaine and injecting the drug rapidly into the trachea at the end of the maximal expiration. The injection of the drug excites a vigorous cough reflex, spraying the local anesthetic along the tracheal side walls and inferior surface of the vocal cords. As a supplement to direct tracheal instillation of local anesthetic and bilateral superior laryngeal nerve block, local anesthetic (e.g., 2% lidocaine) may be nebulized in a hand-held nebulizer and inhaled by the patient. This is a tedious process, demanding long, slow breaths and inhalation of the nebulized anesthetic over the course of at least 20 minutes. The endotracheal tube may then be passed into the anesthetized airway using a guided, fiberoptic technique or blindly. Complications of superior laryngeal nerve block include intravascular injection of local anesthetic. The carotid sheath lies just posterior to the site of block and, if the needle is angled posteriorly, the sheath may be entered and the anesthetic injected directly into the carotid artery or internal jugular vein.

The role of the LMA in head and neck surgery awaits clarification. The LMA may be useful in temporarily securing a compromised airway. In any situation, however, where the airway is jeopardized by blood or pus, or the anatomy distorted by trauma, the airway must be secured with a cuffed endotracheal or tracheostomy tube. The intubating LMA may facilitate awake intubation.[72] The flexible LMA is unsafe in head and neck surgery in the presence of foreign material such as blood, bone fragments, or pus.[73]

LeFort III Fractures

A LeFort III fracture may involve the cribriform plate of the ethmoid bone, thus violating the separation of nasopharynx and base of the skull and allowing entrance into the intracranial subarachnoid space. Nasotracheal intubation risks the introduction of foreign material from the nasopharynx into the subarachnoid space and the consequent development of meningitis. More importantly, it risks the introduction of the endotracheal tube into the substance of the brain, with direct mechanical damage. Even positive-pressure bag and mask ventilation is contraindicated because the increase in volume and pressure within the nasopharynx can force foreign material[74] or air into the skull.[75]

The problems of securing the airway in a patient with a LeFort III fracture are ordinarily obviated by doing a preliminary tracheostomy using local anesthetic in an awake patient. This has the added advantage of separating surgeon and anesthesiologist and allowing each an adequate working space. Nasotracheal intubation can be performed in a patient with a LeFort III fracture provided three criteria are met: (1) absence of clinical signs of basal skull fracture, (2) absence of radiographic evidence of basal skull fracture, and (3) a compelling reason for doing so. Occasionally (rarely) these three criteria are fulfilled.

Anesthetic Management of the Traumatized Upper Airway

After tracheal intubation has been achieved or tracheostomy performed, general or iv anesthetics may be used. The use of ketamine as a sole anesthetic in an attempt to obviate the necessity of performing a difficult tracheal intubation is perilous and should be avoided. Ketamine is a potent respiratory depressant[76] in bolus doses, increases intracranial pressure[77] (ICP), and causes focal alterations in the cerebral metabolic rate.[78] Because there is a significant incidence of intracranial trauma associated with maxillofacial trauma, the brain must be protected and alterations in ICP avoided. Opioids have little effect on ICP and are useful in anesthetic management. However, the dose may be difficult to determine because of the high incidence of drug abuse associated with trauma. Inhalation anesthetics are safe and effective and ICP can be moderated by altering the Pa_{CO_2}. The halogenated ethers are particularly useful, but the halogenated alkane halothane should be avoided because of the high incidence of cardiac arrhythmias associated with its use.[79]

Extubation

When tracheostomy has been incorporated into the anesthetic-surgical plan, it is maintained at the termination of the procedure and the only decision facing the anesthesiologist is whether to allow spontaneous respiration or to create suitable conditions for continued mechanical ventilation by maintaining the patient anesthetized and paralyzed. This decision is contingent on such factors as the nature and duration of surgery, the patient's prior physical condition, and concurrent respiratory disease, a frequent concomitant of head and neck tumors.

After trauma, infection, or extensive oral resection for tumor, the endotracheal tube must not be removed until there is clearly subsidence of any edema that might compromise the unprotected airway. Particular attention must be given to the submandibular area, where extensive edema pushes the tongue upward and posteriorly and risk the airway. An edematous tongue protruding past the incisors is an ominous warning of dangerous edema. If substantial edema is present, a waiting period of 24–36 hours is usually indicated. Serious infection may require a longer period of time to resolve. An oral endotracheal tube may be removed over a tube changer. When removing a nasotracheal tube, a useful technique is to place a fiberoptic bronchoscope through the tube and into the airway and remove the tube over the bronchoscope, so that it can be replaced immediately if need demands.

REFERENCES

1. Brodsky L: Modern assessment of tonsils and adenoids. Pediatr Clin North Am 36:1551, 1989
2. Berkowitz RG, Zalzal GH: Tonsillectomy in children under 3 years of age. Arch Otolaryngol Head Neck Surg 116:685, 1990
3. Potsic WP, Pasquariello PS, Baranak CC et al: Relief of upper airway obstruction by adenotonsillectomy. Otolaryngol Head Neck Surg 94:476, 1986
4. Chaban R, Cole P, Hoffstein V: Site of upper airway obstruction in patients with idiopathic obstructive sleep apnea. Laryngoscope 98:641, 1988

5. Smith RM, Gonzallez C: The relationship between nasal obstruction and craniofacial growth. Pediatr Clin North Am 36:14423, 1989
6. Patel RI, Hannallah RS, Norden J et al: Emergence airway complications in children: A comparison of tracheal extubation in awake and deeply anesthetized patients. Anesth Analg 73:266, 1991
7. Alexander CA: A modified Intavent laryngeal mask for ENT and dental anaesthesia. Anaesthesia 45:892, 1990
8. Haynes SR, Morton NS: The laryngeal mask airway: A review of its uses in paediatric anaesthesia. Paediatr Anaesth 3:65, 1993
9. Nair I, Bailey PM: Review of uses of the laryngeal mask airway in ENT anaesthesia. Anaesthesia 50:898, 1995
10. Williams PJ, Bailey PM: Comparison of the reinforced laryngeal mask airway and tracheal intubation for adenotonsillectomy. Br J Anaesth 70:30, 1993
11. Devitt JH, Wenstone R, Noel AG, O'Donnell MP: The laryngeal mask airway and positive pressure ventilation. Anesthesiology 80:550, 1994
12. Manson DG, Bingham RM: The laryngeal mask airway in children. Anesthesia 45:760, 1990
13. Goudsouzian NG, Cleveland R: Stability of the laryngeal mask airway during marked extension of the head. Paediatr Anaesth 3:117, 1993
14. Ferrari LR, Donlon JV: Metoclopramide reduces the incidence of vomiting after tonsillectomy in children. Anesth Analg 75:351, 1992
15. Watcha MF, White PF: Postoperative nausea and vomiting. Anesthesiology 77:162, 1992
16. Broadman LM, Ceruzzi W, Patane PS et al: Metoclopramide reduces the incidence of vomiting following strabismus surgery in children. Anesthesiology 72:245, 1990
17. Conclasure JB, Graham SS: Complications of outpatient tonsillectomy and adenoidectomy: A review of 3340 cases. Ear Nose Throat J 69:155, 1990
18. Carithers JS, Gebhart DE, Williams JA: Postoperative risks of pediatric tonsilloadenoidectomy. Laryngoscope 97:422, 1987
19. Chiang TM, Sukis AE, Ross DE: Tonsillectomy performed on an outpatient basis: Report of a series of 40,000 cases performed without a death. Arch Otolaryngol 88:105, 1968
20. Crysdale WS, Russel D: Complications of tonsillectomy and adenoidectomy in 9409 children observed overnight. CMA J 135:1139, 1986
21. Linden BE, Gross CW, Long TE et al: Morbidity in pediatric tonsillectomy. Laryngoscope 100:120, 1990
22. Fairbanks DN: Uvulopalatopharyngoplasty complications and avoidance strategies. Otolaryngol Head Neck Surg 102:239, 1990
23. Broadman LM, Patel RI, Feldman BA et al: The effects of peritonsillar infiltration on the reduction of intraoperative blood loss and post-tonsillectomy pain in children. Laryngoscope 99:578, 1989
24. Galvis AG, Stool SE, Bluestone CD: Pulmonary edema following relief of acute upper airway obstruction. Ann Otol 89:124, 1980
25. Allen SJ: New concepts in the management of pulmonary edema. ASA Refresher Courses 22:11, 1994
26. Guida RA, Mattucci KF: Tonsillectomy and adenoidectomy: An inpatient or outpatient procedure? Laryngoscope 100:491, 1990
27. Brown OE, Cunningham MJ: Tonsillectomy and adenoidectomy inpatient guidelines. American Academy of Otololaryngology Head and Neck Surgery Bulletin 15(9):13, 1996
28. Tait AR, Knight PR: The effects of general anesthesia on upper respiratory tract infections in children. Anesthesiology 67:930, 1987
29. Pandit UA, Levy L, Randel GI et al: Perioperative respiratory complications in children with upper respiratory infections. Anesthesiology 71:A1011, 1989
30. DeSoto H, Patel R, Soliman I et al: Changes in oxygen saturation following general anesthesia in children with URI symptoms. Anesthesiology 65:A443, 1986
31. Williams JP, Sommerville GM, Miner ME et al: Alanto-axial subluxation and trisomy 21: Another perioperative complication. Anesthesiology 67:253, 1987
32. Levine RA, Ronner SF, Ojemann RG: Auditory evoked potential and other neurophysiologic monitoring techniques during tumor surgery in the cerebellopontine angle. In Loftus CM, Traynelis VC (eds): Intraoperative Monitoring Techniques in Neurosurgery, p 175. New York, McGraw-Hill, 1994
33. Paloheimo M, Edmonds HL, Wirtavuori K, Tammisto T: Assessment of anaesthetic adequacy with upper facial and abdominal wall EMG. Eur J Anaesthesiol 6:119, 1989
34. Casey WF, Drake-Lee AB: Nitrous oxide and middle ear pressure: A study of induction methods in children. Anaesthesia 37:896, 1982
35. Patterson ME, Bartlett PC: Hearing impairment caused by intratympanic pressure changes during general anesthesia. Laryngoscope 86:399, 1976
36. Furst SR, Rodarte A: Prophylactic antiemetic treatment with ondansetron in children undergoing tonsillectomy. Anesthesiology 81:799, 1994
37. Zalzal GH: Stridor and airway compromise. Pediatr Clin North Am 36:1389, 1989
38. Woods AM: Pediatric bronchoscopy, bronchography and laryngoscopy. In Berry FA (ed): Anesthetic Management of Difficult and Routine Pediatric Patients, p 189. New York, Churchill Livingstone, 1986
39. Sanders RD: Two ventilating attachments for bronchoscopes. Del Med J 39:170, 1967
40. Steward DJ: Percutaneous transtracheal ventilation for laser endoscopic procedures in infants and small children. Can J Anaesth 34:429, 1987
41. Hermens JM, Bennett MJ, Hirshman CA: Anesthesia for laser surgery. Anesth Analg 62:218, 1983
42. McLesky CH: Anesthetic management of patients undergoing endoscopic laser surgery. In IARS Review Course Lectures, p 135. Cleveland, International Anesthesia Research Society (IARS), 1988
43. Sosis MB, Dillon FX: Saline-filled cuffs help to prevent laser-induced polyvinylchloride endotracheal tube fires. Anesth Analg 72:187, 1991
44. Gotta AW: Maxillofacial trauma: Anesthetic considerations. ASA Refresher Courses 15:39, 1987
45. Haskell R: Applied surgical anatomy. In Rowe NL, Williams JL (eds): Maxillo Facial Injuries, p 3. Edinburgh, Churchill Livingstone, 1985
46. Huelke DF: Mechanics in the production of mandibular fractures: A study of the "stresscoat" technique. I. Symphyseal impacts. J Dent Res 40:1042, 1961
47. Huelke DF, Patrick LM: Mechanics in the production of mandibular fractures: Strain-gauge measurements of impacts to the chin. J Dent Res 43:437, 1964
48. Halazonetis JA: The "weak" regions of the mandible. Br J Oral Surg 6:37, 1968
49. Nahum AM: The biomechanics of facial bone fracture. Laryngoscope 85:140, 1975
50. Olson RA, Fonseca RJ, Zeitter DL, Osbon DB: Fractures of the mandible: A review of 580 cases. J Oral Maxillofac Surg 40:23, 1982
51. LeFort R: Etude experimentale sur les fractures de la machoire superieure. Rev Chir 23:208, 1901
52. Burke J: Angina Ludovici A translation, together with a biography of Wilhelm Frederick von Ludwig. Bull Hist Med. 7:1115, 1939
53. Ballenger JJ: Diseases of the Nose, Throat, Ear, Head and Neck, 14th ed, p 240. Philadelphia, Lea & Febiger, 1991
54. Moose SM, Marshall KJ: Acute infections of the oral cavity. In Kruger GO (ed): Oral and Maxillofacial Surgery, 6th ed, p 213. St. Louis, CV Mosby, 1984
55. Moreland LW, Corey J, McKenzie R: Ludwig's angina: Report of a case and review of the literature. Arch Intern Med 148:461, 1988
56. Strauss HR, Tilghma DM, Hankins J: Ludwig angina, empyema, pulmonary infiltration, and precarditis secondary to extraction of a tooth. J Oral Surg 38:223, 1980
57. Young JN, Samson PC: Extrapleural empyema thoracis as a direct extension of Ludwig's angina. Thorac Cardiovasc Surg 80:25, 1980
58. Loughnan TE, Allen DE: Ludwig's angina. The anesthetic management of nine cases. Anaesthesia 40:295, 1985
59. Annandale T: On displacement of the inter-articular cartilage of the lower jaw, and its treatment by operation. Lancet 1:411, 1887
60. Goss AN, Bosanquet AG: Temporomandibular arthroscopy. J Oral Maxillofac Surg 44:614, 1986
61. McCain JP, Sanders B, Koslin MG et al: Temporomandibular joint arthroscopy: A 6 year multicenter retrospective study of 4,831 joints. J Oral Maxillofac Surg 50:926, 1992
62. Laskin DM: Etiology of the pain-dysfunction syndrome. J Am Dent Assoc 79:147, 1969
63. Kinney RK, Gatchel RJ, Ellis E, Holt C: Major psychological disorders in chronic TMD patients. J Am Dent Assoc 123:49, 1992
64. Sanders B: Arthroscopic surgery of the temporomandibular joint: Treatment of internal derangement with persistent closed lock. Oral Surg Oral Med Oral Pathol 62:361, 1992
65. Hendler BH, Levin LM: Postobstructive pulmonary edema as a sequela of temporomandibular joint arthroscopy: A case report. J Oral Maxillofac Surg 51:315, 1993

66. Luce EA, Tubb TD, More AM: Review of 1,000 major facial fractures and associated injuries. Plast Reconstr Surg 63:26, 1979
67. Davidson JSD, Birdsell DC: Cervical spine injury in patients with facial skeletal trauma. J Trauma 29:1276, 1989
68. Har-El G, Aroesty JH, Shaha A, Lucente FE: Changing trends in deep neck abscess: A retrospective study of 110 patients. Oral Surg Oral Med Oral Pathol 77:446, 1994
69. Durham CF, Harrison TS: The surgical anatomy of the superior laryngeal nerve. Surgical Gynecology and Obstetrics 118:38, 1984
70. Gotta AW, Sullivan CA: Superior laryngeal nerve block: An aid to intubating the patient with fractured mandible. J Trauma 24:83, 1984
71. Gotta AW, Sullivan CA: Anaesthesia of the upper airway using topical anaesthetic and superior laryngeal nerve block. Br J Anaesth 53:1055, 1981
72. Ferson DZ, Brimacombe J, Brain AIJ, Verghese C: The intubating laryngeal mask airway. Intern Anesthesiol Clin 36:183, 1998
73. Bailey P, Brimacombe JR, Keller C: The flexible LMA: Literature considerations and practical guide. Intern Anesthsiol Clin 36:111, 1998
74. Kitahata LM, Collins WF: Meningitis as a complication of anesthesia in a patient with a basal skull fracture. Anesthesiology 32:282, 1970
75. DaCosta A, Billard J, Gery P et al: Posttraumatic intracerebral pneumatocele after ventilation with a mask: Case report. J Trauma 36:255, 1994
76. Zsigmand EK, Matsuki A, Kothafy SP: Arterial hypoxemia caused by intravenous ketamine. Anesth Analg 55:311, 1976
77. Gardner AE, Olson BE, Lichtiger M: Cerebrospinal-fluid pressure during dissociative anesthesia with ketamine. Anesthesiology 35:226, 1971
78. Takeshita H, Okuda Y, Sari A: The effects of ketamine on cerebral circulation and metabolism in man. Anesthesiology 36:69, 1972
79. Gotta AW, Sullivan CA, Pelkofski J et al: Aberrant conduction as a precursor to cardiac arrhythmias during anesthesia for oral surgery. J Oral Surg 34:421, 1976

Clinical Anesthesia (4/e), edited by
Paul G. Barash, Bruce F. Cullen, and
Robert K. Stoelting. Lippincott Williams &
Wilkins, Philadelphia, © 2001.

CHAPTER 36

THE RENAL SYSTEM AND ANESTHESIA FOR UROLOGIC SURGERY

TERRI G. MONK AND B. CRAIG WELDON

The kidney plays a central role in the implementation and control of a variety of homeostatic functions. Most important are the complementary tasks of excreting metabolic waste products in the form of urine and maintaining extracellular fluid volume and composition constant. Renal dysfunction may occur perioperatively as a direct result of surgical or medical disease, prolonged reduction in renal oxygen delivery, nephrotoxin insult, or, frequently, a combination of the three. Postoperative renal failure, although infrequent, is a serious complication that carries a high mortality rate. The first part of this chapter reviews renal physiology and pathophysiologic states as they relate to anesthetic practice, and then discusses strategies for recognizing and managing patients at risk for renal failure.

Since 1980, many exciting advances have occurred in urologic surgery. Lithotripsy and endoscopic surgery have replaced open surgical procedures for the treatment of urinary tract calculi. Laparoscopy is now used for numerous surgical procedures, and improved diagnostic tests for urologic cancers have dramatically increased the number of radical surgical procedures. These surgical advances have presented the anesthesiologist with enormous challenges. For example, minimally invasive surgical techniques have made it possible to treat patients who were once considered too sick to undergo open surgical procedures. The creation of a pneumoperitoneum during laparoscopic surgery produces unique physiologic alterations and increases the potential for complications. The second part of this chapter familiarizes the anesthesiologist with current surgical techniques in urology and their attendant anesthetic management issues.

RENAL ANATOMY AND PHYSIOLOGY

Anatomy and Innervation of the Genitourinary System

The kidneys are located in the retroperitoneal space, with their center at the L2 vertebral body. Renal pain sensation is conveyed back to spinal cord segments T10–L1 by sympathetic fibers. Sympathetic innervation is supplied by preganglionic fibers from T8–L1 whereas the vagus nerve provides parasympathetic innervation to the kidney (Fig. 36-1).

The ureters are also retroperitoneal structures and have sympathetic innervation and nociceptive projection to the spinal cord that is nearly identical to that of the kidneys. These spinal segments also provide somatic innervation to the lumbar area, flank, ilioinguinal area, and scrotum or labia. Accordingly, pain from the kidney and ureter is referred to those areas. Parasympathetic fibers from S2–4 spinal segments supply the ureters (Fig. 36-1).

The bladder is located in the retropubic space and receives its innervation from sympathetic nerves originating from T11–L2, which conduct pain, touch, and temperature sensations, whereas bladder stretch sensation is transmitted via parasympathetic fibers from segments S2–4. Parasympathetics also provide the bladder with most of its motor innervation (Fig. 36-2).

The prostate, penile urethra, and penis also receive sympathetic and parasympathetic fibers from the T11–L2 and S2–4 segments, respectively. The pudendal nerve provides pain sensation to the penis *via* the dorsal nerve of the penis. The sensory innervation of the scrotum is *via* cutaneous nerves, which project to lumbosacral segments, whereas testicular sensation is conducted to lower thoracic and upper lumbar segments (Fig. 36-2).

Anatomy of the Nephron

The *nephron* is the microscopic functional unit of the kidney and is elegantly designed to carry out its excretory and regulatory roles (Fig. 36-3). The *glomerulus* is a capillary network that serves as the basic filtering unit of the nephron and is situated in the outer cortex of the kidney. Blood to be filtered enters the glomerular tuft through the afferent arteriole and eventually exits the glomerulus through the efferent arteriole. The initial segment of the renal tubular system, called *Bowman's capsule*, envelops the glomerulus. The glomerular filtrate passes from Bowman's capsule into the proximal tubule and then into the descending loop of Henle, which dips deep into the medullary portion of the kidney. The ascending limb of the loop is made up of an initial thin segment, which gives rise to a thick-walled segment as it approaches the cortex. Once back in the cortex, the distal tubule comes in contact with both the afferent and efferent arterioles to form the juxtaglomerular apparatus. The distal tubule then proceeds through the cortex to join with other tubules to form cortical collecting ducts. These collecting ducts again plunge into the medulla, coalesce, and eventually empty urine into the renal pelvis, which is drained by the ureters. Blood supply to the entire tubular system comes from the glomerular efferent arteriole, which branches into an extensive capillary network. Some of these peritubular capillaries, the *vasa recta*, descend deep into the medulla to parallel the loops of Henle. The vasa recta then return in a cortical direction with the loops, join other peritubular capillaries, and empty into the cortical veins.

Renal Physiology

The kidney fulfills its dual roles of waste excretion and body fluid management by filtering large amounts of fluid and solutes from the blood, reabsorbing needed components of this filtrate, and secreting waste products into the tubular fluid.[1] Filtration and reabsorption are most susceptible to alterations by surgical illness and anesthesia and are the focus of discussion.

Glomerular Filtration

Urine production begins with the filtration of water and solutes from blood flowing through the afferent arteriole. The glomerular membrane serves as the filter, whereas Bowman's capsule acts as the initial receptacle for the filtrate. The kidneys receive ~20% of the systemic cardiac output and are able to filter 10%

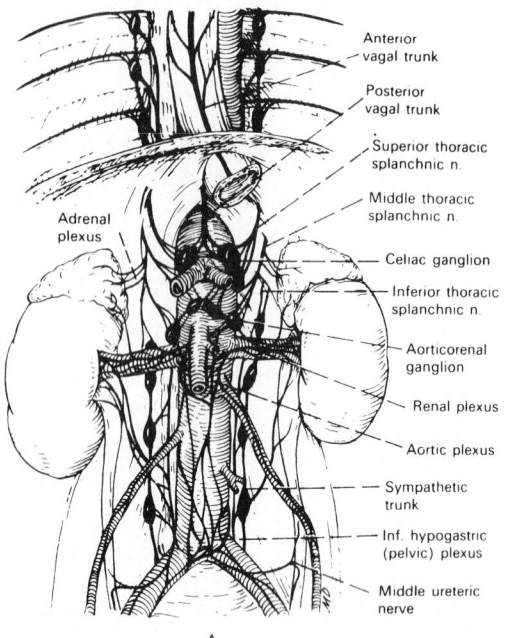

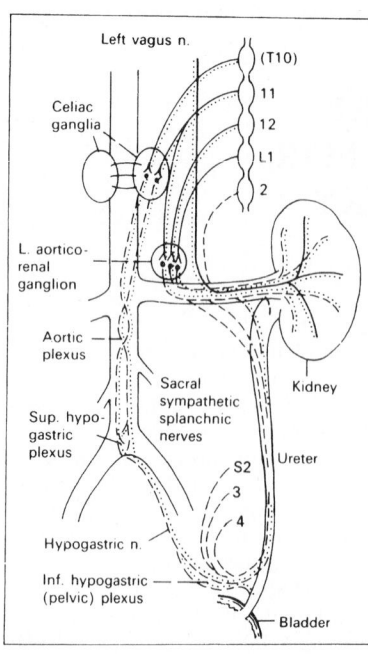

Figure 36-1. (*A*) Anatomy and innervation of the kidney and ureters. (*B*) Schematic illustration of the autonomic and sensory nerve pathways supplying the kidney and ureters. (Reprinted with permission from Ansell JS, Gee WF: Diseases of the kidney and ureter. In Bonica JJ [ed]: The Management of Pain, p 1233. Philadelphia, Lea & Febiger, 1990.)

of this volume to produce 180 l·day⁻¹ of glomerular filtrate. More than 99% of the filtered fluid is reabsorbed and returned to the circulation, resulting in 1–2 l of urine output per day in the healthy adult.

The *glomerular filtration rate* (GFR) is a measure of glomerular function expressed as milliliters of filtrate produced per minute. GFR can be thought of as the product of the tendency of the glomerular membrane to allow filtration to occur (*i.e.,* glomerular permeability and surface area) and the pressure inside the

glomerular capillary that forces fluid through the filter. Thus, the GFR can be expressed simply as:

$$GFR = Kf \text{ [Filtration pressure]}$$

where Kf is the ultrafiltration constant of the glomerulus. The glomerular filtration pressure is a complex value that can be calculated by subtracting oncotic forces from opposing hydrostatic forces:

$$\text{Filtration pressure} = (P_{GC} - P_{BC}) - (\pi_{GC} - \pi_{BC})$$

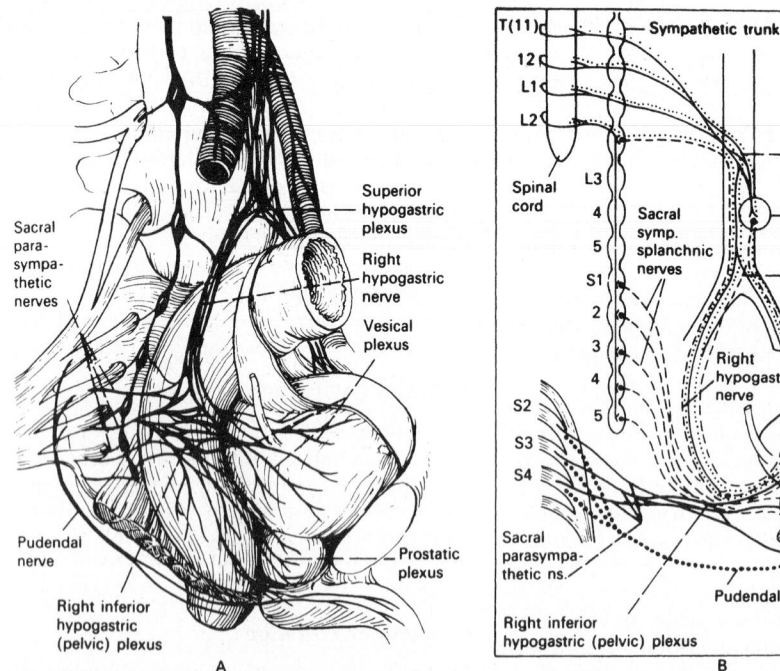

Figure 36-2. (*A*) Anatomy and innervation of the urinary bladder and prostate. (*B*) Schematic illustration of the innervation of the bladder, penis, and scrotum. *Solid lines* = preganglionic fibers; *dashed lines* = postganglionic fibers; *dotted lines* = sensory fibers. (Reprinted with permission from Gee WF, Ansell JS: Pelvic and peritoneal pain of urologic origin. In Bonica JJ [ed]: The Management of Pain, p 1369. Philadelphia, Lea & Febiger, 1990.)

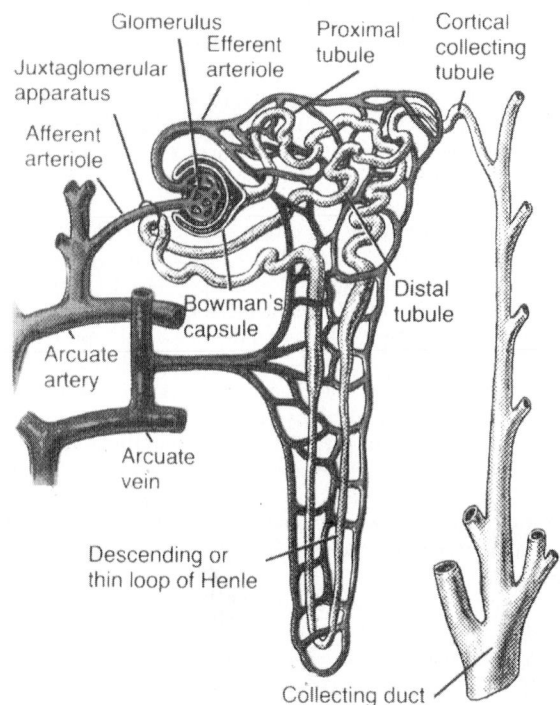

Figure 36-3. Anatomy of the nephron. (Reprinted with permission from Guyton AC: Formation of urine by the kidney: Renal blood flow, glomerular filtration, and their control. In Guyton AC [ed]: Textbook of Medical Physiology, 8th ed, p 287. Philadelphia, WB Saunders, 1991.)

where P_{GC} is the glomerular capillary pressure, P_{BC} is the pressure inside Bowman's capsule, π_{GC} is the glomerular capillary oncotic pressure (plasma oncotic pressure), and π_{BC} is Bowman's capsule oncotic pressure.

The *ultrafiltration constant* (Kf) is directly related to glomerular capillary permeability and glomerular surface area. Glomerular capillary permeability is relatively constant, but the glomerular surface area can be reduced by intense sympathetic or angiotensin II stimulation, which, in turn, decreases GFR.

Changes in glomerular filtration pressure exercise the greatest influence on GFR in both normal and pathologic states. The two major determinants of filtration pressure are glomerular capillary pressure (P_{GC}) and glomerular oncotic pressure (π_{GC}); changes in Bowman's capsule hydrostatic and oncotic pressures are of less importance. P_{GC} is directly related to the renal artery pressure but is heavily influenced by arteriolar tone at points upstream (afferent) and downstream (efferent) from the glomerulus. An increase in afferent arteriolar tone, as occurs with intense sympathetic or angiotensin II stimulation, causes filtration pressure and GFR to fall. Milder degrees of sympathetic or angiotensin activity cause a selective increase in efferent arteriolar tone, which tends to increase the filtration pressure and GFR. The π_{GC} is directly dependent on the plasma oncotic pressure but is also related to the rate of blood flow through the glomerulus. The capillary oncotic pressure tends to increase as fluid is filtered into Bowman's capsule, and this would inhibit further filtration but for fresh blood flowing through the glomerulus and diluting the "left-over" plasma proteins. Therefore, high renal (glomerular) blood flow keeps the π_{GC} lower, which promotes filtration. Afferent arteriolar dilation enhances GFR by increasing glomerular flow, which, in turn, elevates glomerular capillary pressure and keeps π_{GC} low. Efferent arteriolar constriction intense enough to slow glomerular blood flow produces opposing effects on the GFR. This occurs because any

increase in capillary pressure is partially offset by an increase in capillary oncotic pressure.

Autoregulation of Renal Blood Flow and Glomerular Filtration Rate

From the preceding discussion, it is apparent that renal blood flow (RBF) and perfusion pressure, in large part, determine GFR. To maintain relatively constant rates of RBF and glomerular filtration over a wide range of physiologic demands, the kidney must exercise some control over its own performance. Renal autoregulation of blood flow and filtration is accomplished by local feedback signals that modulate glomerular arteriolar tone.

Autoregulation of RBF is effective over a wide range of arterial pressure (Fig. 36-4). Two separate mechanisms for regulating blood flow to the glomerulus have been proposed, and both involve the modulation of afferent arteriolar tone. A myogenic reflex has been postulated in which an increase in arterial pressure causes the afferent arteriolar wall to stretch and then reflexly constrict, whereas a decrease in arterial pressure causes arteriolar dilation. The other mechanism of RBF autoregulation is a phenomenon called *tubuloglomerular feedback,* which is also responsible for the autoregulation of GFR.

Tubuloglomerular feedback control of RBF and GFR works by using the composition of distal tubular fluid to influence glomerular function through the *juxtaglomerular apparatus.* When RBF falls, the concomitant decrease in GFR results in less chloride ion delivery to the juxtaglomerular apparatus, which then signals the afferent arteriole to dilate. Glomerular flow and pressure then increase and the GFR returns to previous levels. Chloride ion also acts as the feedback signal for control of efferent arteriolar tone. When GFR falls, declining chloride ion delivery to the juxtaglomerular apparatus triggers release of *renin,* which causes the formation of *angiotensin* II. In response to angiotensin, efferent arteriolar constriction increases glomerular pressure, which increases glomerular filtration. Simultaneous afferent arteriolar dilation and efferent arteriolar constriction allow glomerular flow and filtration to increase.

Note from Figure 36-4 that autoregulation of urine flow does not occur and that there is a linear relationship between mean arterial pressure above 50 mm Hg and urine output.

Tubular Reabsorption of Sodium and Water

The renal tubular system is responsible for selectively reabsorbing the vast quantities of fluid and solutes filtered by the

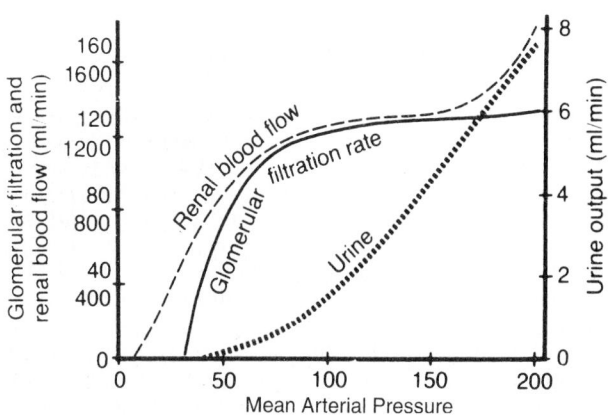

Figure 36-4. Autoregulation of glomerular filtration rate (GFR) and renal blood flow (RBF) over a wide range of arterial pressures. Note that urine output is not subject to autoregulation. (Reprinted with permission from Guyton AC: Formation of urine by the kidney: Renal blood flow, glomerular filtration, and their control. In Guyton AC [ed]: Textbook of Medical Physiology, 8th ed, p 293. Philadelphia, WB Saunders, 1991.)

glomeruli. Waste materials are thereby separated from essential solutes and excreted in the minimum volume of water possible. Sodium and water conservation by the kidney are closely related to the homeostatic mechanisms involved in the mammalian response to physiologic stress. The neurohumoral response to surgical stress and critical illness is primarily directed at maintaining blood pressure, circulating blood volume, and essential organ blood flow. Sodium and water reabsorption will be examined in the context of their roles as markers of the stress response.

The active, energy-dependent reabsorption of sodium begins almost immediately as filtrate enters the proximal tubule. Here, an adenosine triphosphatase pump drives the sodium into tubular cells while chloride ion passively follows. Glucose, amino acid, and other organic compound reabsorption is strongly coupled to sodium in the proximal tubule. Normally, the proximal tubule reabsorbs ~65% of the filtered sodium, but no active sodium transport occurs in the loop of Henle until the medullary thick ascending limb (mTAL) is reached. The cells of the mTAL are metabolically active in their role of reabsorbing sodium and chloride and have a high oxygen consumption compared with the thin portions of the descending and ascending limbs. Sodium pumps in the distal tubule and collecting duct are unique in that they are under the control of the adrenal hormone aldosterone.

The reabsorption of water is a passive, osmotically driven process that is tied to sodium and other solute reabsorption. Water reabsorption also depends on peritubular capillary pressure; high capillary pressure opposes water reabsorption in the proximal tubule and tends to increase urine output. The proximal tubule reabsorbs ~65% of filtered water in an isosmotic fashion with sodium and chloride. The descending limb of the loop of Henle allows water to follow osmotic gradients into the renal interstitium. However, the thin ascending limb and mTAL are relatively impermeable to water and play a key role in the production of concentrated urine. Only approximately 15% of filtered water is reabsorbed by the loop of Henle, and the remaining 20% of the filtrate volume flows into the distal tubule. There, and in the collecting duct, water reabsorption is controlled entirely by antidiuretic hormone (ADH) secreted by the pituitary gland.

The conservation of water and excretion of excess solute by the kidneys would become untenable without the ability to produce concentrated urine. This is accomplished by establishing a hyperosmotic medullary interstitium and regulating the water permeability of the distal tubule and collecting duct with ADH.

Medullary interstitial fluid hyperosmolarity is achieved primarily through the activity of nephrons whose glomeruli are located at the border of the cortex and medulla. These juxtamedullary nephrons send their loops of Henle very deep into the medulla and are able to produce an increasingly hyperosmolar interstitium by three mechanisms: (1) vigorous transport of ions by the mTAL into the interstitium while water is retained in the tubule, (2) active transport of ions into the medullary interstitium by the collecting ducts, and (3) passive diffusion of large quantities of urea from the collecting ducts into the interstitium. The medullary interstitium would eventually lose its hyperosmolarity by washout of solutes were it not for the unique role of the vasa recta. The vasa recta prevents medullary solute washout by providing for a countercurrent exchange of ions, which continually "recycles" solutes between its descending and ascending arms. The countercurrent exchange mechanism works because the vasa recta is extremely permeable to solutes and water, which allows for their rapid, passive movement between the two arms. The other important characteristic of the vasa recta is that its blood flow is sluggish (the inner medulla receives 2% of total RBF) and therefore, does not contribute to washout of solutes from the medulla. Low medullary blood flow is essential to renal concentrating ability but

may render the metabolically active mTAL vulnerable to ischemic injury during times of reduced RBF.[2]

All that is now necessary to produce a concentrated urine is to alter the water permeability of the distal tubule and collecting duct in response to bodily needs. ADH increases the water permeability of these structures and allows for passive diffusion of water (under considerable osmotic pressure) back into the circulation. The posterior pituitary releases ADH in response to an increase in either the extracellular sodium concentration or the extracellular osmolality. In addition, ADH release can be triggered by a perceived reduction in intravascular fluid volume. The arterial baroreceptors are activated when hypovolemia leads to a decrease in blood pressure, whereas atrial receptors are stimulated by a decline in atrial filling pressure. Both of these circulatory reflex systems stimulate release of ADH from the pituitary and cause retention of water by the kidney in an effort to return the intravascular volume toward normal. ADH also causes renal cortical vasoconstriction when it is released in large amounts, as during the physiologic stress response to trauma, surgery, or other critical illness. This induces a shift of RBF to the hypoxia-prone renal medulla.

The neurohumoral regulation of sodium reabsorption by the kidney is another important component of the physiologic response to stress. The hormonal messengers involved in sodium management also have potent vasoactive effects on both the renal and systemic vasculature.

Renin-Angiotensin-Aldosterone System. As discussed earlier, renin-angiotensin activity plays an important role in regulating RBF and GFR. Renin release by the renal afferent arteriole may be triggered by hypotension, increased tubular fluid chloride ion concentration, or sympathetic stimulation. Renin enhances angiotensin II production, which induces renal efferent arteriolar vasoconstriction. Angiotensin II also promotes ADH release from the posterior pituitary, sodium reabsorption by the proximal tubule, and aldosterone release by the adrenal medulla. Aldosterone, in turn, stimulates the distal tubule and collecting duct actively to reabsorb sodium (and water), resulting in intravascular volume expansion. Sympathetic nervous system stimulation may also directly cause the release of aldosterone. Thus, the response of the body to surgical stress uses existing mechanisms for sodium and water conservation. This results in renal cortical vasoconstriction, a shift in RBF to salt-and-water-conserving juxtamedullary nephrons, a decrease in GFR, and salt and water retention. Clinically, this tendency toward oliguria and edema formation may persist for several days into the postoperative period due to ongoing stress (pain, sepsis, hypovolemia).

Renal Vasodilator Mechanisms. Opposing the salt and water retention and vasoconstriction observed in stress states and mediated by the sympathetic nervous system, ADH, and the renin-angiotensin-aldosterone system are the actions of *atrial natriuretic peptide* (ANP), *nitric oxide*, and the renal *prostaglandin* system. ANP is released by the cardiac atria in response to increased stretch under conditions of relative hypervolemia. Both salt and water excretion increase as ANP blocks reabsorption of sodium in the distal tubule and collecting duct. ANP also increases GFR, causes systemic vasodilation, inhibits the release of renin, opposes the production and action of angiotensin II, and decreases aldosterone secretion.[3-5] Nitric oxide produced by the kidney opposes the renal vasoconstrictor effects of angiotensin II and the adrenergic nervous system, increases sodium and water excretion, and participates in the tubuloglomerular feedback system.[6]

Prostaglandins are produced by the kidney as part of a complex system that modulates RBF and opposes the actions of ADH, norepinephrine, and the renin-angiotensin-aldosterone system.[7] Stress states, renal ischemia, and hypotension stimulate the production of renal prostaglandins through the enzymes phospholipase A_2, and cyclo-oxygenase. The prostaglandins produced by cyclo-oxygenase activity cause dilation of renal arterioles (anti-angiotensin II), whereas their distal tubular effects result in an increase in sodium and water excretion (anti-ADH and aldosterone). The renal prostaglandin system is important in maintaining RBF and sodium and water excretion during times of high physiologic stress and poor renal perfusion.[7] This defensive role for the prostaglandins has been confirmed by experiments that demonstrate that cyclo-oxygenase inhibition has damaging effects in the ischemic kidney, but not in the unstressed state.[8] Conversely, the stimulation of prostaglandin synthesis or the administration of exogenous prostaglandin E_2 protects the kidney from hypoxic injury.[9]

RENAL DYSFUNCTION AND ANESTHESIA

Altered renal function can be represented as a clinical continuum that ranges from normal compensatory changes in renal function during stress to frank renal failure. Clinically, there is considerable overlap between compensated and decompensated renal dysfunctional states. For the anesthesiologist, there is little time or opportunity to make such a distinction in the operating room using laboratory tests. Nevertheless, it is worthwhile here to review the clinical spectrum of renal dysfunction-failure and comment on the implications for anesthesia practice.

The kidney under stress reacts in a predictable manner to help restore intravascular volume and maintain blood pressure. The sympathetic nervous system reacts to trauma, shock, or pain by releasing norepinephrine, which acts much like angiotensin II on the renal arterioles. Norepinephrine also activates the renin-angiotensin-aldosterone system and causes ADH release. The net result of modest activity of the stress response system is characterized by a shift of blood flow from the renal cortex to the medulla, avid sodium and water reabsorption, and decreased urine output. A more intense stress response may induce a decrease in RBF and GFR by causing afferent arteriolar constriction. If this extreme situation is not reversed, ischemic damage to the kidney may result and acute renal failure (ARF) may become clinically manifest. More often, some other insult contributes to renal failure in the "stressed" patient with co-existing renal vasoconstriction.[10]

With the exception of methoxyflurane and possibly enflurane, anesthetic agents do not directly cause renal dysfunction or interfere with normal compensatory mechanisms activated by the stress response. Nephrotoxicity of methoxyflurane appears to be due to its metabolism, which results in the release of fluoride ion thought to be responsible for the renal injury.[11] It has been suggested that renal, not hepatic, metabolism of methoxyflurane may be responsible for generating fluoride ions locally that contribute to nephrotoxicity.[12] Enflurane nephrotoxicity may occur,[13] but seems to be of minor clinical importance even in patients with pre-existing renal dysfunction.[14] Controversy over sevoflurane-induced nephrotoxicity appears to be waning and is discussed in Chapter 15. Anesthetic-induced reductions in RBF have been described for many agents but are clinically insignificant and reversible.[15,16] Likewise, anesthetic agents have not been shown to interfere with renal neurohumoral responses to physiologic stress.

Although direct anesthetic effects on the kidney are usually not harmful, indirect effects of anesthesia may combine with hypovolemia, shock, nephrotoxin exposure, or other renal vasoconstrictive states to produce renal dysfunction. If the chosen anesthetic technique causes a protracted reduction in cardiac output or sustained hypotension that coincides with a period of intense renal vasoconstriction, renal dysfunction or failure could result. This is true for either general or regional anesthesia. There are no comparative studies demonstrating superior renal protection or improved renal outcome with general versus regional anesthesia.

Acute Renal Failure

Acute renal failure is a sudden decrease in renal function resulting in the inability of the kidneys to excrete nitrogenous and other wastes. This is manifest by the accumulation of creatinine and urea in the blood (uremia) and is often accompanied by reduced urine production, although nonoliguric forms of postoperative ARF are common.[17] In surgical patients, (1) acute tubular necrosis (ATN) is the etiology for ARF in most patients; (2) ARF frequently occurs in the setting of critical surgical illness with multiple organ failure (MOF)/dysfunction—it is rarely an isolated event; and (3) the mortality rate is alarmingly high (up to 90%) and may be higher than for medical patients with renal failure.[18]

One explanation for the high death rate is that ARF is often part of an MOF–sepsis syndrome.[19,20] Major trauma, burns, and other critical events predispose surgical patients to sepsis, MOF, and ARF.[19] Nonseptic triggers of MOF have also been identified in seriously ill trauma patients.[21] The mortality rate in MOF is directly related to the number of organ systems involved.[22,23] To ascribe these deaths solely to failure of the kidneys overestimates the contribution that ARF makes to the overall syndrome, especially because isolated ARF carries a mortality rate of <10%.[23] A contributing factor to the poor outcome is the fact that extracorporeal renal support appears to have had little success in altering the course of ARF in critically ill surgical patients.[22,24] Even studies that advocate the use of extracorporeal technology report mortality rates of between 50% and 70%.[25-28]

Active renal failure can be classified as arising from *prerenal* factors causing renal hypoperfusion, numerous *intrinsic* renal etiologies, or *postrenal* causes (obstructive uropathy). There are many pathophysiologic similarities between the various causes of renal failure that ultimately lead to a common syndrome referred to as organic ARF (Fig. 36-5).

Prerenal Azotemia and Acute Tubular Necrosis

Prerenal azotemia is defined as the increase in blood urea nitrogen (BUN) associated with renal hypoperfusion or ischemia that has not caused renal parenchymal damage. As such, prerenal azotemia forms a continuum with ATN. As normal renal compensatory mechanisms are maximized to maintain RBF and GFR and conserve salt and water, increasing sympathetic activity and circulating blood levels of angiotensin II and ADH cause the afferent arteriole and mesangium to constrict and the efferent arteriole to paradoxically dilate. Global RBF decreases and the renal medulla is subjected to profound hypoxia. The metabolically active cells of the mTAL of Henle are especially vulnerable to hypoxic damage because of their relatively high oxygen consumption-to-delivery ratio.[2] The necrosis of tubular cells releases debris into the tubules, causing obstruction to flow, increased tubular pressure, and back leak of tubular fluid (Fig. 36-5). Often prerenal failure is precipitated in patients with pre-existing renal vasoconstriction (*e.g.*, volume depletion, congestive heart failure, sepsis), by nephrotoxin exposure, or a reduction in cardiac output.[29]

Intrinsic Acute Renal Failure

The term "intrinsic" implies a primary renal etiology of ARF but also includes ischemia and toxins as well as renal parenchymal diseases. ATN remains the most common ischemic lesion and represents an extension of prerenal azotemia, whereas cortical necrosis may follow a massive renovascular insult such as prolonged suprarenal aortic cross-clamping or renal artery embolism. Nephrotoxins often act in concert with hypoperfusion or underlying renal vasoconstrictive states to damage renal tubules or microvasculature. Several common nephrotoxins, some of which are difficult to avoid in a hospitalized patient population, are listed in Table 36-1. Renal parenchymal diseases may affect either the glomerulus or the interstitium and are frequently

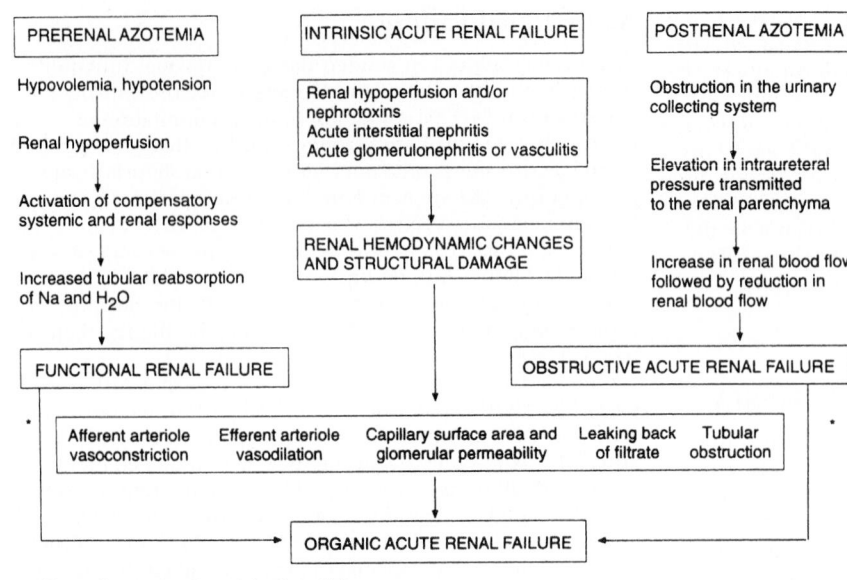

Figure 36-5. Mechanisms of acute renal failure. (Reprinted with permission from Pellanda MV, Fabris A, Ronco C: Etiology and pathophysiology of acute renal failure. In Pinsky MR, Dhainaut JFA [eds]: Pathophysiologic Foundations of Critical Care, p 575. Baltimore, Williams & Wilkins, 1993.)

immune mediated or part of a more systemic disorder that targets the kidney.

Postrenal Azotemia: Obstructive Uropathy

Downstream obstruction of the urinary collecting system is the least common pathway to organic ARF, accounting for <5% of cases.[29] The obstructing lesion may occur at any level of the collecting system, from the renal pelvis to the distal urethra. Intraluminal pressure then rises and is eventually transmitted back to the glomerulus, thereby reducing its filtration pressure. RBF transiently increases but soon falls as angiotensin II and thromboxane A_2 are generated and produce ischemic renal damage and ARF.

Intraoperative Oliguria: Prerenal Azotemia or Acute Tubular Necrosis

Several real-time RBF monitors are being developed for intraoperative and critical care use (see Perioperative Assessment of Renal Function). However, urine flow rate has traditionally been used as a measure of renal "well-being," a job for which it is ill suited.[30] Nevertheless, oliguria (a urine flow rate of <0.5 $ml \cdot kg^{-1} \cdot h^{-1}$) may be a useful sign of renal hypoperfusion when other objective signs of reduced systemic blood flow are present and the overall clinical scenario is appropriate. The presumption should be that intraoperative oliguria is a normal response to the stress of surgery and ongoing blood and fluid losses. If a fluid bolus improves the urine flow rate, or heart rate and blood pressure indicate hypovolemia, further fluid administration is indicated. Isolated hypovolemia can usually be corrected relatively quickly as long as ongoing loss of blood and intravascular fluid is also replaced. If oliguria persists and signs of congestive heart failure or volume overload appear, the patient's hemodynamic profile should be further assessed with a pulmonary artery catheter. The goal of pulmonary artery catheterization in this setting is to optimize cardiac output and systemic oxygen delivery and, in so doing, improve renal perfusion.

When sepsis is responsible for poor urine output, hypotension is a common finding and is usually secondary to systemic vasodilation, hypovolemia, and depressed myocardial contractility. Hypovolemia should be corrected with vigorous fluid resuscitation while combinations of inotropic–vasopressor agents, such as dopamine, norepinephrine, phenylephrine, and dobutamine, are used to increase cardiac output, systemic vascular resistance, and renal perfusion pressure.[31-33]

Chronic Renal Failure

Chronic renal failure (CRF) or *end-stage renal disease* (ESRD) are the terms used to describe a clinical syndrome that is characterized by multiple organ dysfunction that would prove fatal without dialysis. These patients have GFRs <25% of normal. Lesser degrees of renal dysfunction are categorized as renal insufficiency (25–40% of normal GFR) or decreased renal reserve (60–75% of normal GFR). Patients with decreased renal reserve are asymptomatic and frequently do not have abnormally elevated blood levels of creatinine or urea (Fig. 36-6). Renal insufficiency results in clearly abnormal creatinine and BUN values, but nocturia (due to decreased concentrating ability) may be the patient's only symptom.

The *uremic syndrome* represents the most extreme form of CRF that occurs as the surviving nephron population and GFR decrease below 10% of normal. The uremic syndrome results in the inability of the kidney to perform its two major duties: the regulation of the volume and composition of extracellular fluid and the excretion of waste products. The loss of homeostasis and the accumulation of cellular toxins cause the multiple organ system dysfunction seen in the uremic syndrome[34] (Table

Table 36-1. NEPHROTOXINS COMMONLY FOUND IN THE HOSPITAL SETTING

Exogenous	Endogenous
Antibiotics	Calcium (hypercalcemia)
Aminoglycosides, cephalosporins, amphotericin B, sulfonamide, tetracyclines, vancomycin	Uric acid (hyperuricemia and hyperuricosuria)
Anesthetic agents	Myoglobin (rhabdomyolysis)
Methoxyflurane, enflurane	Hemoglobin (hemolysis)
Nonsteroidal anti-inflammatory drugs (NSAIDs)	Bilirubin (obstructive jaundice)
Aspirin, ibuprofen, naproxen, indomethacin, ketorolac	Oxalate crystals
Chemotherapeutic–immunosuppressive agents	Paraproteins
Cisplatinum, cyclosporin A, methotrexate, mitomycin, nitrosoureas, tacrolimus	
Contrast media	

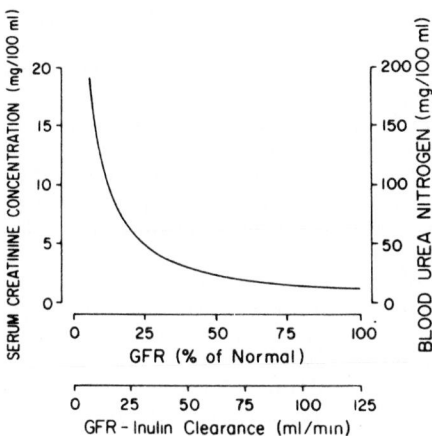

Figure 36-6. Relationship of serum creatinine concentration and blood urea nitrogen levels to glomerular filtration rate (GFR). (Reprinted with permission from Valtin H: Renal Dysfunction: Mechanisms Involved in Fluid and Solute Imbalance, p. 206, Boston, Little, Brown, 1979.)

36-2). Patients with the uremic syndrome usually require frequent or continuous dialysis. Dialytic therapy in the perioperative period is discussed in Chapter 52.

Water balance in ESRD becomes difficult to manage because the number of functioning nephrons is too small either to concentrate or fully dilute the urine. This results in the inability to conserve water as well as to excrete excess water. Eventually, as GFR continues to decline, the urine flow rate falls below a threshold that prevents water accumulation, and expansion of the extracellular fluid volume takes place. This has implications for sodium homeostasis, the cardiovascular system, and the respiratory system.

Electrolyte and acid-base disturbances associated with the uremic syndrome are listed in Table 36-2. Hyponatremia occurs, in part, because extracellular fluid expansion triggers natriuresis and results in an obligatory sodium loss that is characteristic of the end-stage kidney. Sodium restriction or overhydration of the patient with CRF may also precipitate hyponatremia. Potassium homeostasis is maintained in renal failure until the GFR is <10% of normal through increased distal tubule secretion, decreased reabsorption, and enhanced fecal potassium loss. Nevertheless, life-threatening hyperkalemia may occur in CRF because of slower potassium clearance than normal. Situations predisposing patients with renal failure to hyperkalemia are presented in Table 36-3. Derangements in calcium, magnesium, and phosphorus metabolism are also commonly seen in CRF (see Table 36-2).

Metabolic acidosis occurs in two forms in ESRD: a hyperchloremic, normal–anion-gap acidosis and a high-gap acidosis due to an inability to excrete titratable acids. Both render patients susceptible to an endogenous acid load as may occur in shock states, hypovolemia, or an increase in catabolism.

Cardiovascular complications of the uremic syndrome are primarily due to volume overload, high renin–angiotensin activity, autonomic nervous system hyperactivity, acidosis, and electrolyte disturbances. Hypertension due to extracellular fluid volume expansion, autonomic factors, and hyper-reninemia is an almost universal finding in ESRD. Together with volume overload, acidemia, anemia, and high-flow arteriovenous fistulae created for dialysis access, hypertension contributes to the development of myocardial dysfunction and congestive heart failure. Pericarditis may occur secondary to uremia or dialysis, with pericardial tamponade developing in 20% of the latter group.[35] Fatal dysrhythmias may result from acute elevation in serum potassium.[36]

The pulmonary problems associated with CRF are limited to changes in lung water and the control of ventilation. Pulmonary

Table 36-2. THE UREMIC SYNDROME

WATER HOMEOSTASIS
Extracellular fluid expansion

ELECTROLYTE AND ACID–BASE
Hyponatremia
Hyperkalemia
Hypercalcemia or hypocalcemia
Hyperphosphatemia
Hypermagnesemia
Metabolic acidosis

CARDIOVASCULAR
Congestive heart failure
Hypertension
Pericarditis
Myocardial dysfunction
Dysrhythmias

RESPIRATORY
Pulmonary edema
Central hyperventilation

GASTROINTESTINAL
Delayed gastric emptying, anorexia, nausea, vomiting, hiccups, upper gastrointestinal tract inflammation/hemorrhage

NEUROMUSCULAR
Encephalopathy, seizures
Sensory and motor polyneuropathy
Antonomic dysfunction

HEMATOLOGIC
Anemia
Platelet hemostatic defect

IMMUNOLOGIC
Cell-mediated and humoral immunity defects

ENDOCRINE–METABOLISM
Renal osteodystrophy
↓ Glucose intolerance
Hypertriglyceridemia, ↑ atherosclerosis

Table 36-3. FACTORS CONTRIBUTING TO HYPERKALEMIA IN CHRONIC RENAL FAILURE

POTASSIUM INTAKE
Increased dietary intake
Exogenous iv supplementation
Potassium salts of drugs
Sodium substitutes
Blood transfusion
Gastrointestinal hemorrhage

POTASSIUM RELEASE FROM INTRACELLULAR STORES
Increased catabolism, sepsis
Metabolic acidosis
β-Adrenergic blocking agents
Digitalis intoxication (Na-K-ATPase inhibition)
Insulin deficiency
Succinylcholine

POTASSIUM EXCRETION
Acute decrease in GFR
Constipation
Potassium-sparing diuretics
Angiotensin-converting enzyme inhibitors (decreased aldosterone secretion)
Heparin (decreased aldosterone effect)

Na-K-ATPase = Na-K-adenosine triphosphatase; GFR = glomerular filtration rate.

edema and restrictive pulmonary dysfunction are commonly seen in patients with renal failure and are responsive to dialysis. Hypervolemia, congestive heart failure, reduced serum oncotic pressure, and increased pulmonary capillary permeability are factors in the development of pulmonary edema. Chronic metabolic acidosis may be responsible, in part, for the hyperventilation seen in patients with ESRD, but increased lung water and poor pulmonary compliance also stimulate ventilation.

Gastrointestinal complaints, seen early in CRF, are almost universal in the uremic syndrome and consist of anorexia, nausea, vomiting, and hiccups. Delayed gastric emptying is of importance to the anesthesiologist and may improve with metoclopramide treatment or dialysis.

Uremic neuromuscular complications may take the form of central nervous system dysfunction, peripheral polyneuropathy, or autonomic dysfunction. The encephalopathy of uremia consists of alterations in the level of consciousness, tremors, myoclonus, and seizures. This picture can be mimicked or worsened by the accumulation of renally excreted, pharmacologically active metabolites of certain opioids and sedative-hypnotic drugs (see Anesthetic Agents in Renal Failure, later). Autonomic dysfunction may be manifest by sympathetic hyperactivity or hypoactivity, decreased baroreceptor responsiveness, or dialysis-associated hypotension.

The anemia of CRF is due to reduced levels of erythropoietin, red cell damage, ongoing gastrointestinal blood loss, and iron or vitamin deficiencies. Recombinant human erythropoietin has improved the management of anemia in ESRD.[37] Platelet dysfunction may aggravate blood loss but is responsive to dialysis, cryoprecipitate, and desmopressin (DDAVP). Acquired defects in both cellular and humoral immunity probably account for the high rate of serious infections (60%) and the high mortality rate due to sepsis in CRF (30%).

Anesthetic Agents in Renal Failure

Significant renal impairment may affect the disposition, metabolism, and excretion of commonly used anesthetic agents. The inhalational anesthetics are, of course, an exception to the rule that drugs with central nervous system activity (which generally are lipid soluble) must be converted to more hydrophilic compounds by the liver before being excreted by the kidney. Water-soluble metabolites of agents that are not inhaled may accumulate in renal failure and contribute to a prolongation of clinical effects if they possess even a small percentage of the pharmacologic activity of the parent drug. Drugs that are eliminated unchanged by the kidneys (e.g., certain nondepolarizing muscle relaxants, the cholinesterase inhibitors, many antibiotics, and digoxin) may have a prolonged elimination half-life when given to patients with renal failure. Many drugs used in the practice of anesthesia are highly protein bound and may demonstrate exaggerated clinical effects when protein binding is reduced by uremia. Renal failure may also increase the volume of distribution of certain agents, thereby prolonging their elimination half-life. There is a paucity of data concerning the effects of renal failure on anesthetic drug metabolism,[38,39] and suspected pharmacodynamic changes in patients with renal failure have proved difficult to document for most drugs.[40] Renal disease has a minimal effect on the pharmacokinetics of the inhaled anesthetics; therefore, the following discussion focuses on anesthetic agents that are not inhaled.

Induction Agents and Sedatives

Thiopental serves as an example of how reduced protein binding in CRF may affect the clinical use of an anesthetic agent. Burch and Stanski[41] have shown that the free fraction of a thiopental induction dose is nearly doubled in patients with renal failure. This accounts for the exaggerated clinical effects of thiopental in these patients and explains the need for a decreased induction dose in uremic patients compared with normal patients.

Ketamine is less extensively protein bound than thiopental, and renal failure appears to have minimal influence on its free fraction. Redistribution and hepatic metabolism are largely responsible for termination of the anesthetic effects, with <3% of the drug excreted unchanged in the urine. Norketamine, the major metabolite, has one third of the pharmacologic activity of the parent drug and is further metabolized before it is excreted by the kidney.[42] Poor renal function is not known to alter the pharmacokinetics or clinical profile of ketamine.[43] However, caution must be used when it is administered to patients with renal failure with hypertension because it may induce a dramatic increase in blood pressure.[44]

Etomidate, although only 75% protein bound in normal patients, has a larger free fraction in ESRD.[45] The decrease in protein binding does not seem to alter the clinical effects of an etomidate anesthetic induction in patients with renal failure. This may be due to its relative lack of cardiovascular-depressant effects.

Propofol undergoes extensive, rapid hepatic biotransformation to inactive metabolites that are renally excreted. Its pharmacokinetics appear to be unchanged in patients with renal failure,[46,47] and there are no reports of prolongation of its effects in ESRD. Use of the standard induction dose of propofol and a propofol infusion has been shown to be safe for patients with renal failure.[47,48]

The benzodiazepines, as a group, are extensively protein bound. CRF increases the free fraction of benzodiazepines in plasma, which may potentiate their clinical effect. Certain benzodiazepine metabolites are pharmacologically active and have the potential to accumulate with repeated administration of the parent drug to anephric patients. For example, 60–80% of midazolam is excreted as its (active) α-hydroxy metabolite,[49] which accumulates during long-term infusions in patients with renal failure.[50] ARF appears to slow the plasma clearance of midazolam itself,[50] while repeated diazepam or lorazepam administration in CRF may carry a risk of active metabolite-induced sedation.[39] Alprazolam is one of the few drugs related to anesthesia practice that has undergone pharmacodynamic studies in patients with CRF. Schmith et al[51] found that when decreased protein binding and increased free fraction of alprazolam are taken into account, patients with CRF are actually more sensitive to its sedative effects than normal people. It would seem that a single dose of benzodiazepine should be well tolerated but that the dose should be reduced because of the possibility of increased free fraction and increased patient sensitivity.

Opioids

Single-dose studies of morphine pharmacokinetics in renal failure do not demonstrate any alteration in its disposition. However, chronic administration results in the accumulation of its 6-glucuronide metabolite, which has potent analgesic and sedative effects.[52] There is also a decrease in protein binding of morphine in ESRD, which mandates a reduction in its initial dose. Meperidine is remarkable for its neurotoxic, renally excreted metabolite (normeperidine) and is not recommended for use in patients with poor renal function. Hydromorphone is metabolized to hydromorphone-3-glucuronide, which is excreted by the kidneys. This active metabolite accumulates in patients with renal failure and may cause cognitive dysfunction and myoclonus.[53] Oxycodone elimination was found to be prolonged in a single-dose study of patients with CRF.[54] Repeated dosing of oxycodone should result in prolonged opioid effects. Codeine also has the potential for causing prolonged narcosis in patients with renal failure and cannot be recommended for long-term use.[52]

Fentanyl appears to be an excellent opioid for use in ESRD because of its lack of active metabolites, unchanged free fraction, and short redistribution phase.[39] Small to moderate doses of fentanyl, titrated to effect, are well tolerated by uremic patients. However, a dose of 25 μg · kg^{-1} given to patients undergoing renal transplantation resulted in prolonged opioid effect that correlated with preoperative BUN.[55] Alfentanil has been shown to have reduced protein binding but no change in its elimination half-life or clearance in ESRD, and is extensively metabolized to inactive compounds.[56,57] Therefore, caution should be exercised in administering the loading dose of alfentanil, but the total dose and infusion dose should be similar to those for patients with normal renal function. The free fraction of sufentanil is unchanged in ESRD, but its pharmacokinetics are variable and it has been reported to cause prolonged narcosis.[58] Remifentanil is rapidly metabolized by blood and tissue esterases to a weakly active, renally excreted metabolite, GR90291. Renal failure has no effect on the clearance of remifentanil but GR90291 elimination is markedly reduced.[59] The long-term administration of remifentanil to anephric patients has not been studied to determine if accumulation of GR90291 has any clinical implications.

Muscle Relaxants

The muscle relaxants are the most likely group of drugs used in anesthetic practice to produce prolonged effects in ESRD because of their reliance on renal excretion (Table 36-4). (See also Chapter 16). Only succinylcholine, atracurium, cis-atracurium, and mivacurium appear to have minimal renal excretion of the unchanged parent compound. Most nondepolarizing muscle relaxants must either be hepatically excreted or metabolized to inactive forms to terminate their activity in the absence of renal function. Some muscle relaxants have renally excreted, active metabolites that may contribute to their prolonged duration of action in patients with ESRD. Although the following discussion focuses on the pharmacology of individual muscle relaxants, coexisting acidosis and electrolyte disturbances, as well as drug therapy (e.g., aminoglycosides, diuretics, immunosuppressants, and magnesium-containing antacids), may alter the pharmacodynamics of muscle relaxants in patients with renal failure.[60]

Succinylcholine has a long history of use in CRF that has been somewhat confused by conflicting reports of plasma cholinesterase activity in renal failure.[61-65] Its use can be justified as part of a rapid-sequence intubation because its duration of action in ESRD is not significantly prolonged. The use of a continuous infusion of succinylcholine, however, is more problematic because the major metabolite, succinylmonocholine, is weakly active and excreted by the kidney. Concern over the increase in serum potassium levels after succinylcholine administration (0.5 mEq · l^{-1} in normal subjects) dictates that a recent, normal potassium level be demonstrated in patients with renal failure. Recent dialysis (<24 hours before surgery) also lessens the risk of hyperkalemia in this population.[66,67]

The older nondepolarizing muscle relaxants (i.e., d-tubocurarine, metocurine, pancuronium, and gallamine) all have prolonged elimination half-lives in renal failure (see Table 36-4). A single small dose of these drugs should be well tolerated, but larger doses or repeated small doses may result in the accumulation of the parent drug and prolonged clinical effect. More recently introduced intermediate- and short-acting muscle relaxants are less likely to have a clinically significant prolongation of duration in ESRD.

The use of the long-acting muscle relaxants, doxacurium and pipecuronium, also might be questioned in patients with known renal insufficiency. In a single-dose study of doxacurium, Cook et al[68] demonstrated an increased elimination half-life, reduced plasma clearance, and prolonged duration of effect in patients with renal failure. These data support the observations of Cashman et al,[69] that renal failure nearly doubles the clinical duration of doxacurium. Similar findings have been reported for the pharmacokinetics of pipecuronium. Although the mean duration of action was not different between control subjects and patients with renal failure, the latter group had an unpredictable response to pipecuronium with a wide variability in duration of action of the drug.[70,71]

The intermediate-acting muscle relaxants (atracurium, cis-atracurium, vecuronium, and rocuronium) have a distinct advantage in ESRD precisely because of their shorter duration; the risk of a clinically significant, prolonged block is reduced. Atracurium and its derivative, cis-atracurium, undergo enzymatic ester hydrolysis and spontaneous nonenzymatic (Hoffman) degradation with minimal renal excretion of the parent compound. Their elimination half-life, clearance, and duration of action are not affected by renal failure,[72,73] nor have they been reported to cause prolonged clinical effect in ESRD. These characteristics strongly recommend atracurium and cis-atracurium for use in patients with renal disease. One potential concern is that an atracurium metabolite, laudanosine, causes seizures in experimental animals and may accumulate with repeated dosing or continuous infusion.[74] This concern, however, has not been realized in intensive care patients with renal failure receiving prolonged infusions of atracurium.[75] Consistent with its greater potency and lower dosing requirements, cis-atracurium metabolism results in lower laudanosine blood levels than atracurium in ESRD.[76]

The pharmacokinetics of vecuronium were initially reported as unchanged in renal failure,[77] but it was later demonstrated that its duration of action was prolonged as a result of reduced plasma clearance and increased elimination half-life.[78] In addition, the active metabolite, 3-desmethylvecuronium, was shown to accumulate in anephric patients receiving a continuous vecuronium infusion who subsequently had prolonged neuromuscular blockade.[79] Vecuronium is an acceptable muscle relaxant for patients with ESRD if it is not continuously infused for long periods and if maintenance doses are reduced and the dosing

Table 36-4. NONDEPOLARIZING MUSCLE RELAXANTS IN RENAL FAILURE[60, 64, 65, 68-71, 78, 80-84, 86, 87]

Drug	% Renal Excretion	Half-life (h) Normal/ESRD	Renally Excreted Active Metabolite	Use in ESRD
d-Tubocurarine	60	1.4–2.2	–	Avoid
Metocurine	45–60	6/11.4	–	Avoid
Pancuronium	30	2.3/4–8	+	Avoid
Gallamine	>85	2.5/6–20	–	Avoid
Pipecuronium	37	1.8–2.3/4.4	+	Avoid
Doxacurium	30	1.7/3.7	–	Avoid
Vecuronium	30	0.9/1.4	+	Normal single, smaller repeat doses; avoid prolonged CI
Rocuronium	30	1.2–1.6/1.6–1.7	–	Normal single, repeat doses, increased variability
Atracurium/cis-atracurium	<5	0.3/0.4	–	Normal single, repeat, CI doses
Mivacurium	<7	2 min/2 min	–	Duration 1.5 × normal, lower CI dose
Rapacuronium	<12	0.5/0.5	++	Normal single dose, much smaller repeat dose, avoid CI

CI = continuous infusion; ESRD = end-stage renal disease.

interval is increased. An intubating dose would be expected to last ~50% longer in patients with ESRD.[78]

Rocuronium, a rapid-onset muscle relaxant, has a pharmacokinetic profile in normal subjects that is similar to that of vecuronium.[80] Single-dose pharmacokinetic studies in patients with renal failure have reported conflicting findings. Szenhradszky et al[81] reported that renal failure increased the volume of distribution and elimination half-life of rocuronium, but had no effect on its clearance. Cooper et al[82] found that clearance was reduced and the duration of block widely variable in patients with renal failure, although the mean duration of clinical relaxation and spontaneous recovery was not statistically different from that in controls subject. Wide variation in the duration of neuromuscular block has been reported by others, who also found that repeated maintenance doses of rocuronium were well tolerated in patients with ESRD.[83]

The short-acting muscle relaxant mivacurium is enzymatically eliminated by plasma pseudocholinesterase at a somewhat slower rate than succinylcholine. Low pseudocholinesterase activity correlates with slower recovery from a bolus dose of mivacurium in anephric patients.[64,65,84] The maintenance infusion dose has been reported to be both lower[65] and similar[84] to that in normal control subjects. A single case report of neuromuscular blockade lasting 3 hours after an intubating dose of mivacurium implies that ESRD may significantly alter the clinical response to this drug.[85]

Rapacuronium is a rapid-onset, short-to-intermediate-acting muscle relaxant, that undergoes nonspecific hydrolysis to a very potent, renally excreted 3-hydroxy metabolite, Org9488.[86] The clearance of Org9488 is 85% slower in anephric patients compared with normal subjects.[87] Repeated dosing or continuous infusion of rapacuronium in this population should result in prolonged clinical effects.

The pharmacokinetics of the clinically available anticholinesterases (i.e., neostigmine, pyridostigmine, and edrophonium) are significantly affected by renal failure.[88–90] All three have a prolonged duration of action in ESRD due to their heavy reliance on renal excretion. The anticholinergic agents, atropine and glycopyrrolate, which are used in conjunction with the anticholinesterases, are similarly excreted by the kidney.[91] Therefore, no dosage alteration of the anticholinesterases is required when antagonizing neuromuscular blockade in patients with reduced renal function.

PRESERVATION OF RENAL FUNCTION

Prevention of renal failure in the surgical patient is preferable to treatment of established ARF based on the previous discussion of poor outcome of these patients. To prevent ARF, the clinician must first identify those patients who are particularly at risk for perioperative renal damage and then focus on preserving renal function in that group. Patients may be at risk for postoperative renal failure because of an underlying condition or pre-existing renal insufficiency. Several well known nephrotoxins may contribute to renal damage in hospitalized patients and must be identified so that their use can be avoided or limited in high-risk patients. Finally, certain surgical procedures are known to increase the chances of development of postoperative ARF. All three factors (patient status, nephrotoxin exposure, and surgical procedure) can be recognized before surgery, affording the anesthesiologist an opportunity to devise an anesthetic plan emphasizing renal preservation. Risk factors for postoperative ARF are listed in Table 36-5.

Patient-Based Risk Factors for Acute Renal Failure

Large, prospective studies of preoperative patient-based risk factors for ARF are lacking. Most often, retrospective reviews of ARF in surgical patients have revealed conflicting data that

Table 36-5. RISK FACTORS FOR POSTOPERATIVE RENAL FAILURE

PATIENT-BASED INDICATORS
  Preoperative renal dysfunction
  Perioperative cardiac dysfunction
  Sepsis
  Hepatic failure, obstructive jaundice, ascites
  Hypovolemia
  Advanced age?

NEPHROTOXIN EXPOSURE (SEE TABLE 36-1)

HIGH-RISK SURGICAL PROCEDURES
  Cardiac: cardiopulmonary bypass
  Aortic cross-clamping
  Trauma/burn (? emergency)
  Hepatic transplantation
  Renal transplantation

may be pertinent to a select patient population but cannot be generalized to a larger group of patients. Novis et al[92] published a review of the available prospective and retrospective studies examining patient-based risk factors for postoperative renal failure. Their report serves as the basis for the following discussion on preoperative risk factors, which can be easily identified with history, physical examination, and appropriate laboratory screening tests.

The single most reliable predictor of postoperative renal dysfunction is preoperative renal dysfunction.[92] Elevated BUN or creatinine levels, a history of renal dysfunction, or other evidence of pre-existing renal problems successfully predict postoperative ARF. It is likely that pre-existing renal disease predisposes patients to further renal insult, but it may also make further loss of function easier to recognize.[92] The presumption, of course, is that it is essential to preserve what renal function the patient has. The alternative (frank renal failure) is potentially catastrophic. Identifying patients with pre-existing renal dysfunction requires appropriate screening of BUN and creatinine in those who have other renal risk factors (history of renal problems, cardiac disease, sepsis) or are facing high-risk surgical procedures.

Preoperative cardiac dysfunction is another important predictor of postoperative ARF.[92] Shusterman et al[93] identified congestive heart failure as a risk factor in a mixed, surgical-medical population.[93] Specifically, evidence of left ventricular dysfunction or elevated pulmonary capillary wedge pressure (PCWP) has predictive value in identifying patients at risk for ARF. This is intuitively obvious when one considers that poor cardiac output reduces RBF and increases the potential for renal vasoconstriction and ischemic injury. Patients with a history and physical examination consistent with congestive heart failure should have a screening echocardiogram and chest radiograph. When the diagnosis of left ventricular dysfunction is confirmed, medical management should be optimized before surgery whenever possible. Intraoperative monitoring with a pulmonary artery catheter may be helpful in managing fluid administration, oliguria, respiratory dysfunction, or further deterioration in cardiac performance.

Sepsis poses a major threat to renal function in surgical patients.[19,20,93,94] The pathophysiology of ARF in sepsis involves systemic hemodynamic derangements,[95] inflammatory mediator-induced renal vasoconstriction,[96] and, frequently, nephrotoxin exposure in the form of aminoglycoside antibiotics.[97] The sepsis syndrome, once recognized, is managed by eradication of the septic focus with antibiotics and surgical excision (where feasible), fluid and blood component therapy, and manipulation of cardiovascular performance with vasopressors.

Volume depletion has been reported to be an ARF risk factor in both medical and surgical patients.[93] As with heart failure and sepsis, hypovolemia may induce renal vasoconstriction and render the kidney vulnerable to nephrotoxin exposure or a further reduction in oxygen delivery. Patients with diabetes mellitus (and microangiopathy) are particularly prone to development of ARF when they become volume depleted.[93]

Cholestatic jaundice has long been suspected to be a risk factor for postoperative ARF.[98,99] Patients with severe cirrhosis and ascites or hepatic failure are clearly predisposed to renal dysfunction as a result of portal vein sepsis. In up to 75% of patients with hepatic failure, associated renal dysfunction-failure (hepatorenal syndrome) develops.[100]

In patients presenting for liver transplantation surgery, 25% have some degree of renal dysfunction, and post-transplantation this percentage rises to almost 70%.[101] Preoperative serum creatinine levels can predict short-term survival of liver transplant recipients.[102]

Numerous investigators cite advanced age as a risk factor for postoperative ARF.[92] Elderly patients are frequently found to have reduced GFR, RBF, and renal reserve, making them less able to withstand a renal insult.[103] The aged also have a high incidence of cardiovascular disease and flow-limiting renal arterial atherosclerosis, which may account for their apparent increased risk of ARF. One study has convincingly demonstrated that advanced age increases the risk of ARF due to aminoglycoside toxicity.[93] However, age as an isolated risk factor has not been shown to predict postoperative ARF.[92]

Other risk factors for postoperative ARF were reviewed by Novis et al[92] but could not be conclusively shown to be of significance. These included aortic aneurysm, acute bacterial endocarditis, decreased serum albumin, malignancy, emergency surgery, and previous cardiac surgery.

Perioperative Assessment of Renal Function

Preoperative renal function appears to be the most reliable predictor of postoperative renal failure.[92] Although an accurate preoperative assessment of renal function is important in identifying the high-risk patient, it would be advantageous to be able to differentiate prerenal azotemia from early ATN and predict impending ARF. Kellen et al[30] examined the ability of commonly used measures of renal function to predict and diagnose early ARF in the critically ill patient. The findings of their meta-analysis of the specificity, sensitivity, and positive predictive value of renal function tests are summarized in Table 36-6.

Kellen et al[30] found that most of the standard renal function tests were unable to predict impending ATN and that many could not reliably differentiate between prerenal azotemia and early ATN. Urine flow rate, specific gravity, and osmolality are poor indicators of renal dysfunction because they are influenced by many nonrenal variables. Serum creatinine and BUN are good screening tools for preoperative renal dysfunction, but they are late warning signals of reduced GFR. A sizable loss of GFR may occur before serum creatinine and BUN values become abnormal (see Fig. 36-6). Unfortunately, creatinine and BUN are influenced by nonrenal variables such as catabolic rate and muscle mass, making isolated serum determinations unreliable in a rapidly changing scenario of critical illness. This is also true for tests based on creatinine and urea levels such as urine-to-plasma ratios of these compounds. Urine sodium excretion should increase when tubular injury results in a loss of reabsorptive ability, but isolated urine sodium (urine Na^+) values more accurately reflect the composition of resuscitative fluids than tubular function in the acute setting. The fractional excretion of sodium (percentage of filtered sodium that is excreted) can reliably distinguish prerenal azotemia from established ATN, but Kellen et al[30] found it unable to serve as an early indicator or predictor of ARF.[30] Free water clearance (C_{H_2O}) measures the diluting-concentrating ability of the kidney and should reflect tubular integrity. As a predictor of impending ARF, however, C_{H_2O} cannot be used by itself and should be combined with a creatinine clearance (Ccr) determination.[104] It would appear that the Ccr, as a sole indicator of imminent ARF, is the best test available to the clinician.[30]

The Ccr is a direct reflection of the GFR and may be either measured or calculated. The measured determination requires that urine and plasma creatinine (cr) levels be obtained and that the urine volume for 24 hours be collected and measured, such that:

$$Ccr = \frac{Urine\ cr \times Urine\ volume}{Plasma\ cr}$$

Traditionally, the need for a 24-hour urine collection has limited the usefulness of Ccr in the acute situation. However, a 2-hour Ccr correlates reasonably well with the standard 24-hour collection in critically ill surgical patients[105] and in nonoliguric intensive care patients.[106] Shin et al[104] used 1-hour Ccr determinations to predict the onset of renal dysfunction-failure in postoperative trauma patients. Despite normal blood pressure and urine flow rates in all patients studied, those with Ccr <25 $ml \cdot min^{-1}$ within the first 6 postoperative hours went on to have renal dysfunction or frank ARF.[104] A major advantage of the abbreviated Ccr determination is that it facilitates sequential monitoring of renal function during periods of rapidly changing patient status. Therapeutic interventions directed at improving renal function may be quickly assessed in this way.

Measured Ccr remains the most reliable predictor of renal dysfunction in critically ill surgical patients regardless of the urine collection duration. The ideal renal function monitor would provide real-time data using noninvasive, easily transportable, and interpretable technology. Real-time monitoring of renal function is under development using ultrasonography[107,108] and nuclear medicine[109-111] technology.

Table 36-6. CLINICAL USEFULNESS OF RENAL FUNCTION TESTS

Renal Function Test	Distinguish ATN *vs.* PRA	Predict Early ATN	Comments
Urine flow rate	Poor	Poor	
Urine specific gravity	Poor	Poor	Many nonrenal factors
Urine osmolality	Poor	Poor	Many nonrenal factors
Serum creatinine, BUN	Poor	Late findings	Rapid preoperative screen
Urine/plasma creatinine, BUN	Poor	Poor	
Urine Na^+	Poor	Poor	
Fractional excretion Na^+	Good in late ATN	Poor	
Free water clearance	—	Good with Ccr	Less sensitive than Ccr
Ccr	Good	Good	24-h collection?

ATN = acute tubular necrosis; PRA = prerenal azotemia; BUN = blood urea nitrogen; Ccr = creatinine clearance.

Nephrotoxins and Perioperative Acute Renal Failure

Nephrotoxin exposure is a common occurrence in hospitalized patients and frequently plays a role in the etiology of ARF in this population. Nephrotoxins may take the form of drugs, non-therapeutic chemicals, heavy metals, poisons, and endogenous compounds. A partial list is found in Table 36-1. The nephrotoxins most likely to contribute to renal dysfunction-failure in the perioperative period are certain antimicrobial and chemotherapeutic-immunosuppressive agents, radiocontrast media, nonsteroidal anti-inflammatory drugs (NSAIDs), and the endogenous heme pigments myoglobin and hemoglobin. These diverse groups of renal toxins share a common pathophysiologic characteristic: they disturb either renal oxygen delivery or oxygen utilization and thereby promote renal ischemia.

Antimicrobial and chemotherapeutic-immunosuppressive agents are effective for their designed purpose because they are cellular toxins. When these drugs are filtered, reabsorbed, secreted, and eventually excreted by the kidney, the potential for achieving toxic concentrations in renal cells can be realized.[112] The aminoglycoside antibiotics (neomycin, gentamicin, tobramycin, amikacin) and amphotericin B are particularly difficult to avoid because they are effective antimicrobials, with few available alternatives.[113] Cyclosporin A and tacrolimus are similarly indispensable agents but, in combination with other nephrotoxins and clinical factors, cause both acute and chronic renal injury in transplant recipients.[114]

Radiocontrast media pose a threat to the renal function of patients with diabetic nephropathy, pre-existing renal vasoconstriction (congestive heart failure, hypovolemia), or renal insufficiency.[115] Measures that can prevent ARF or lessen the severity of renal damage include prehydration, smaller contrast doses, and withholding other nephrotoxins, such as NSAIDs. Consideration should also be given to using an imaging technique that does not require contrast media. Future strategies to prevent radiocontrast-induced renal ischemia may include pretreatment with renal vasodilators such as fenoldopam, nifedipine, or ANP.

The NSAIDs produce reversible inhibition of prostaglandin synthesis and are well known nephrotoxins.[116] Except in cases of massive overdose, the NSAIDs produce renal dysfunction only in patients with coexisting renal hypoperfusion or vasoconstriction. Advanced age, hypovolemia, end-stage hepatic disease, congestive heart failure, sepsis, renal insufficiency, and major surgery are risk factors for the development of NSAID-induced ARF.[113] Of particular interest to anesthesiologists is *ketorolac*, a parenterally administered NSAID. Ketorolac may predispose the critically ill and elderly patient to ischemic ARF and acute, life-threatening hyperkalemia when given in the perioperative period.[113] Oliguric ARF has been observed after a single dose of ketorolac.[117] All NSAIDs must be used with caution in high-risk patients, and should be withheld before surgical procedures that carry a significant risk of renal dysfunction.

Myoglobin and hemoglobin are both capable of causing ARF in the context of critical surgical illness. Myoglobin seems to be a more potent nephrotoxin than hemoglobin because it is more readily filtered at the glomerulus and can be reabsorbed by the renal tubules, where it inhibits nitric oxide and induces medullary vasoconstriction and ischemia.[2,118] Hypovolemia and acidemia potentiate the toxicity of both pigments. Reduced intravascular volume causes a decrease in RBF and GFR, which results in a smaller volume of tubular fluid with a relatively higher concentration of pigment. Myoglobin and hemoglobin dissociate more easily to ferrihemate (a potent nephrotoxin) in acidic tubular fluid. There is also evidence to suggest that pigment precipitation inside the tubular lumen is enhanced under acidotic conditions and that tubular obstruction plays a role in the pathogenesis of ARF.[118,119]

Myoglobinuric renal failure occurs in the clinical scenario of massive rhabdomyolysis that may follow from a number of insults. The most common causes of massive rhabdomyolysis in surgical patients are major crush, thermal, or electrical injuries, acute muscle ischemia due to arterial occlusion or compartment syndrome, malignant hyperpyrexia, the extreme lithotomy position, and hyperlordotic position.[119–123] Potassium, phosphorus, and creatinine are released in large quantities from the necrotic muscle. The clinical picture of myoglobinuric ARF is one of oligo-anuria, rapidly rising creatinine, and life-threatening hyperkalemia. Unfortunately, the diagnosis of rhabdomyolysis is not straightforward and a high index of suspicion is necessary to identify patients at risk for ARF. A creatine phosphokinase level $>15,000$ units $\cdot l^{-1}$ is predictive of hyperkalemic ARF and a high risk of death.[124] A creatine phosphokinase level should be obtained and preventive treatment initiated in patients with suspected rhabdomyolysis.

Hemoglobinuric ARF is usually the result of massive hemolysis in association with renal hypoperfusion as is seen during exposure to extracorporeal circulation or cardiopulmonary bypass (CPB). Major transfusion reactions that occur in hypovolemic, acidemic, septic, or hemodynamically unstable patients may lead to renal injury, but rarely does isolated hemoglobinemia cause renal failure.[119]

Preventive treatment of pigmenturia-induced ARF is directed at increasing RBF and tubular (urine) flow while correcting any existing acidosis. These goals are accomplished by expanding the intravascular fluid volume with crystalloid infusion, stimulating an osmotic diuresis with mannitol, and increasing urine pH with alkali therapy.[125] Adequate systemic resuscitation from shock cannot be overemphasized as a prerequisite for prevention of ARF, especially in massive crush injuries and electrical burns. Forced mannitol-alkali diuresis is indicated as the second step in preventive treatment of myoglobinuric renal failure, with urine flow rates of up to 300 ml $\cdot$ hr^{-1} and urine pH 6.5 advocated for patients with massive crush injuries.[125] This treatment regimen is effective for moderate hyperkalemia, but life-threatening potassium levels may require urgent dialysis. Occasionally, acetazolamide therapy may be used to counteract excessive systemic alkalosis and promote a further increase in urine pH.[125]

High-Risk Surgical Procedures

Several common surgical procedures can place renal function at risk. These include surgery of the heart and aorta, trauma surgery, and hepatic transplantation. Renal transplantation poses other special problems for renal preservation and is discussed in more detail in Chapter 52.

Emergency surgery has been reported as a possible risk factor for ARF, with trauma surgery figuring as a prominent subgroup of emergency procedures.[92] ATN is the pre-eminent renal lesion associated with trauma and may be produced by any number of ischemic mechanisms. Most often, hypovolemic shock, pigmenturia, MOF, or exogenous nephrotoxins are responsible for sequential or simultaneous insults to the kidney.[126] ARF that develops in the trauma patient may be characterized by either an early, oliguric picture related to inadequate volume resuscitation or a later, often nonoliguric, syndrome associated with MOF, nephrotoxin exposure, or sepsis.[127] The outcomes of these two post-traumatic ARF scenarios are dramatically different. The early form is associated with up to 90% mortality rate, whereas only 20–30% of patients die with nonoliguric ARF.[94] Not surprisingly, trauma victims with pre-existing renal insufficiency have a higher mortality rate than previously healthy patients.[128]

Prevention of ARF in the patient presenting for emergency surgery begins with proper management of intravascular volume depletion and shock. The restoration of euvolemia and maintenance of cardiac output, systemic oxygen delivery, and RBF obviate renal vasoconstriction. Urine flow, once established, is maintained at ≥ 0.5 ml $\cdot$ kg^{-1} $\cdot$ hr^{-1}. Invasive hemodynamic monitoring may be required to guide the intraoperative management of ongoing cardiovascular instability due to surgical manipulation, blood loss, fluid shifts, and anesthetic effects. Nephrotoxin exposure should be kept to a minimum in the unstable trauma victim. Radiocontrast media, NSAIDs, and myoglobin pose the greatest threat in this patient group. There is no place for either furosemide or mannitol therapy in the early, resuscitative phase of trauma management except in the case of head injury with elevated intracranial pressure or when massive rhabdomyolysis is suspected. After surgery, 1 or 2-hour Ccr determinations can help identify those patients with impending ARF.[104] It is not yet clear whether renal function in these patients can be normalized with renal vasodilators, diuretics, supraphysiologic oxygen delivery, or other maneuvers.

Vascular surgery requiring cross-clamping of the aorta has deleterious effects on renal function regardless of the level of cross-clamp placement. Suprarenal cross-clamping results in an attenuated ATN-like lesion.[129] Infrarenal cross-clamping causes a smaller, short-lived reduction in GFR and is associated with a lower risk of ARF, whereas surgery involving the thoracic aorta has an incidence of renal failure of 25%.[130] It is hoped that the use of endoluminal aortic stents, which do not require aortic cross-clamping, will reduce the incidence of ischemic renal injury.[131,132] Two major predictors of ARF following aortic surgery appear to be pre-existing renal dysfunction and perioperative hemodynamic instability.[133] Olsen et al[24] reported that in a large series of patients undergoing abdominal aortic aneurysm repair, the overall incidence of ARF was 12%.[24] Those patients who had emergency surgery for ruptured aneurysm had a very high incidence of hemodynamic instability and ARF developed in 26%, whereas elective aortic surgery was associated with good hemodynamic control and a 4% incidence of renal failure.[24] Atheromatous renal artery emboli and prolonged cross-clamp time may contribute to the ischemic renal injury.

Efforts to improve renal outcome in aortic surgery should begin in the preoperative period by identifying patients with renal dysfunction. Ideally, these high-risk patients should not receive radiocontrast media or other nephrotoxins in the immediate preoperative period. The surgeon and anesthesiologist must also work together to provide as much hemodynamic stability as possible throughout the perioperative period.[134] Consideration should be given to using acute normovolemic hemodilution during infrarenal cross-clamping to improve systemic blood flow and RBF, thereby preserving renal function.[135]

Most efforts to preserve renal function in aortic surgery have centered on the use of diuretic and renal vasodilator therapy. Unfortunately, there are few data to support the use of either mannitol or low-dose dopamine to prevent the renal injury associated with aortic surgery. Indeed, a clinical infrarenal cross-clamp study found that combined mannitol and low-dose dopamine treatment was no more effective in preventing renal dysfunction than volume expansion with saline.[136] Pass et al[137] could demonstrate no benefit of mannitol, low-dose dopamine, or a combination of the two in a canine suprarenal cross-clamp model. Baldwin et al[138] compared low-dose dopamine with crystalloid volume loading and strict maintenance of euvolemia in patients undergoing infrarenal cross-clamping and found no difference in postoperative renal function between the two groups. Although other investigators have demonstrated an increase in urine flow rate with low-dose dopamine in sick postoperative patients,[139] evidence that low-dose dopamine preserves renal function during aortic surgery is lacking. Nifedipine prevented a postoperative decrease in GFR in a small, placebo-controlled study in aortic surgery patients.[140] Larger outcome trials are needed to confirm this preliminary finding. Insulin-

like growth factor-1 has been shown to speed healing in experimental ischemic ARF[141] and to improve renal function in patients with ESRD[142] and those undergoing aortic or renal artery surgery.[143] A synthetic form of ANP may be useful in the management of established oliguric ARF,[144] but it has not been used prophylactically in high-risk surgical patients. Fenoldopam, a selective dopamine-1 receptor agonist, shows great promise as a renal protective agent and should be the subject of future perioperative studies.[145]

Cardiac surgery requiring CPB can be expected to result in renal dysfunction or failure in up to 7% of patients.[146–150] Preoperative renal dysfunction is a major risk factor for postoperative ARF in this population,[146,149–151] yet patients with preoperative CRF appear to tolerate surgery and CPB well.[147] Renal hypoperfusion is considered the primary pathogenic mechanism involved in precipitating ARF. Preoperative left ventricular dysfunction[149,150,152] and the duration of CPB[146,149,150] are associated with post-CPB renal failure. The type of CPB (pulsatile versus nonpulsatile) and bypass pressure are less important factors in the pathogenesis of ARF than is protracted hemodynamic instability due to poor overall cardiovascular performance.[147–150,152,153]

Careful perioperative hemodynamic management is the basis of any strategy designed to promote renal perfusion in cardiac surgery. Early experience with non-CPB, "off pump", coronary revascularization suggests that it offers better renal preservation than the traditional, on-pump technique.[154] When CPB is used, mannitol can be used to protect against hemoglobin-induced ARF, promote urine flow, and reduce renal cell swelling.[155] Dopamine has been used as a renal vasodilator in cardiac surgery with mixed success. Costa et al[156] administered low-dose dopamine during CPB to patients with preoperative renal dysfunction and were able to induce a saluresis without affecting GFR or protecting the kidney from ischemic injury. When perioperative low-dose dopamine was used in patients undergoing elective coronary artery bypass surgery, it had no beneficial effect on urine output, Ccr, free water clearance, or the incidence of renal dysfunction compared with placebo.[157] Other investigators have warned that low-dose dopamine can increase dysrhythmias in postoperative cardiac surgery patients.[158] Dopexamine has been shown to improve Ccr and systemic oxygen delivery in cardiac surgery patients,[159] but studies examining the renal protective effects of fenoldopam, ANP, and insulin-like growth factor-1 in this population are not yet available.

As previously discussed, patients with hepatic failure or cholestatic jaundice are particularly susceptible to renal dysfunction. This probably accounts for the high likelihood of ARF after liver transplantation and biliary surgery.[98,99,160,161] Renal dysfunction-failure may occur in up to two thirds of liver transplant recipients.[101] Many transplantation candidates have overt hepatorenal syndrome, asymptomatic renal dysfunction, or underlying renal vasoconstriction. When such patients are exposed to intraoperative hemodynamic instability, massive transfusion, and nephrotoxins, ARF frequently follows.[160,161] Both preoperative and postoperative renal dysfunction contribute to early and long-term mortality.[102,160,162,163] Maintenance of adequate intravascular volume and aggressive management of hypoperfusion are basic tenets of anesthetic care of the liver transplant recipient, but investigators have sought a role for low-dose dopamine as well. In a retrospective study of liver transplant recipients who also received mannitol, low-dose dopamine administration during the perioperative period was thought to increase urine flow and Ccr and prevent postoperative renal dysfunction.[164] Swygert et al[165] attempted to confirm this observation with a randomized, prospective, double-blind study using low-dose dopamine in liver transplant recipients with normal preoperative renal function.[165] In this study, low-dose dopamine did not increase urine production or GFR compared with placebo, and the incidence of ARF was similar in both groups. Low-dose dopamine has been shown to be no better than preoperative hydration at preserving renal function in patients with obstructive jaundice.[166]

ANESTHESIA FOR ENDOUROLOGIC PROCEDURES

Since 1980, medical care has evolved toward nonoperative or minimally invasive surgical procedures. Incisional surgery in urology is being replaced by endoscopic procedures in which endoscopes are passed along natural pathways (*e.g.*, urethra, ureter) or through minimal incisions.[167] Economic considerations, patient convenience, and advances in instrumentation have all supported the trend toward endoscopy in urologic surgery. (Table 36-7)

Cystourethroscopy and Ureteral Procedures

Cystourethroscopy is commonly used to examine and treat lower urinary tract disease. This procedure provides direct visualization of the anterior and posterior urethra, bladder neck, and bladder. In the past, cystourethroscopy was performed with rigid endoscopes, and general or regional anesthesia was required for patient comfort. In 1973, the flexible endoscope was introduced, which can be gently passed over anatomic angles with less patient discomfort.[168] For brief cystoscopic procedures, 5–10 ml of lubricant anesthetic jelly (2% lidocaine hydrochloride jelly) can be instilled into the urethra prior to the procedure.[169] This local anesthetic technique provides adequate anesthesia for many patients undergoing simple cystoscopy. For longer or more extensive procedures, conscious sedation techniques utilizing a wide variety of sedative-hypnotic, anxiolytic, and analgesic drugs have been shown to combine excellent patient comfort and operating conditions with rapid patient recovery.[170,171] If general anesthesia is required for cystoscopy or urethral procedures, laryngeal mask airways are an attractive alternative to the traditional face mask.[172]

Numerous therapeutic procedures may also be performed using endoscopic techniques. Strictures of the bladder neck or urethra are treated with internal optical urethrotomy, which uses a "cold knife" to excise the scar. Ureteroscopy is an extension of cystoscopic techniques and provides access to the upper urinary tract and kidney for diagnostic endoscopy and biopsy, removal of ureteral and renal calculi, passage of a ureteral stent, dilation and incision of strictures, fulguration of tumors, and laser treatments.[167,173,174] Ureteroscopy usually requires dilation of the ureteral orifice and intramural ureter, often necessitating regional or general anesthesia.

Transurethral Resection of the Prostate

Benign prostatic hyperplasia (BPH), the most common benign tumor in men, refers to the regional nodular growth that occurs in the prostate gland of men as they age.[175] The prostate is a pear-shaped gland that surrounds the urethra at the base of

---

Table 36-7. COMMON ENDOUROLOGIC PROCEDURES

Cystourethroscopy
Internal optical urethrotomy
Ureteroscopy
Placement of ureteral stent
Distal stone manipulation/laser lithotripsy
Transurethral resection of prostate
Transurethral incision of the prostate
Balloon dilation of the prostate
Transurethral resection of bladder tumors
Extracorporeal shock wave lithotripsy
Percutaneous nephrostomy, nephroscopy, and nephrolithotomy

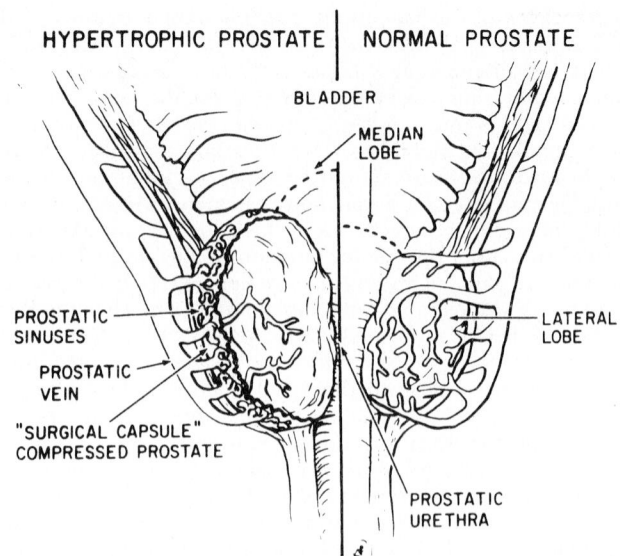

Figure 36-7. Anatomy of the normal and hypertrophic prostate gland. (Reprinted from Stoelting RK, Barash PG, Gallagher TJ: Advances in Anesthesia, p. 379, Chicago, Year Book Medical Publishers, 1986.)

the bladder (Fig. 36-7). Because of the anatomic position of the prostate gland, hypertrophy of this organ compresses the proximal urethra. Thus, BPH is responsible for the majority of the urinary symptoms in men over the age of 50 years of age and results in the need for prostatectomy in approximately one third of all men who live to 80 years of age.[176]

Transurethral resection of the prostate (TURP) is the primary treatment for symptomatic BPH. This procedure commences with an initial cystoscopy to rule out concomitant disease and to evaluate the size of the prostate gland.[177] The resectoscope, a specialized instrument with an electrode capable of both coagulating and cutting tissue, is then introduced through a modified cystoscope into the bladder, and the tissue protruding into the prostatic urethra is resected. Continuous irrigation of the bladder and the prostatic urethra is required to maintain visibility, distend the operative site, and remove dissected tissue and blood.[178]

The prostate gland contains a rich plexus of veins that can be opened during the surgical resection (see Fig. 36-7). If the pressure of the irrigating fluid during TURP procedures exceeds venous pressure, intravascular absorption of the fluid may occur via these open venous sinuses. The need for large volumes of irrigating fluid during the procedure and the potential for absorption of this fluid into the intravascular space may result in unique perioperative complications.

Irrigating Solutions for TURP

The ideal irrigating fluid for use during TURP would be isotonic and nonhemolytic if it were absorbed. In addition, it would be nonelectrolytic to disperse the electrical current, transparent to allow clear visibility for the operating surgeon, nonmetabolized, nontoxic, rapidly excreted, and inexpensive.[179] A variety of irrigating solutions are available for transurethral procedures (Table 36-8), but most of these solutions are hypo-osmolar (normal serum osmolality is 280–300 mOsm $\cdot$ l^{-1}) and acidic (pH of 4.5–6.5).[180]

Distilled water was the irrigating solution used by urologists in the past because it was nonconductive and interfered least with surgical visibility. However, because of its low tonicity, water absorbed into the circulation caused massive intravascular hemolysis, hemoglobinemia, and (rarely) renal failure.[181] Absorption of large amounts of distilled water also resulted in dilutional

Table 36-8. PROPERTIES OF COMMONLY USED IRRIGATING SOLUTIONS FOR TRANSURETHRAL RESECTION PROCEDURES

Solution	Osmolality (mOsm · l^{-1})	Advantages	Disadvantages
Distilled water	0	Improved visibility	Hemolysis Hemoglobinemia Hemoglobinuria Hyponatremia
Glycine (1.5%)	200	Less likelihood of transurethral resection syndrome	Transient postoperative visual impairment Hyperammonemia Hyperoxaluria
Sorbitol (3.3%)	165	Same as glycine	Hyperglycemia, possible lactic acidosis Osmotic diuresis
Mannitol (5%)	275	Isosmolar solution Not metabolized	Osmotic diuresis Possibility of acute intravascular volume expansion

Adapted with permission from Krongrad A, Droller MJ: Complications of transurethral resection of the prostate. In Marshall FF (ed): Urologic Complications: Medical and Surgical, Adult and Pediatric, 2nd ed, p 305. St. Louis, Mosby–Year Book, 1990.

hyponatremia. Emmett et al[182] demonstrated a 75% decrease in the hospital mortality rate after TURP when a nonhemolytic solution was substituted for distilled water. Although distilled water is still used for transurethral procedures that do not open venous sinuses and are not associated with absorption of irrigating fluid (i.e., cystoscopy), it is no longer used for TURP procedures.

Solutes such as sorbitol, mannitol, glycine, urea, and glucose have been added to water to make its osmolality closer to that of plasma[179,183] (see Table 36-8). It is essential that the anesthesiologist be aware of the type of irrigating solution being used during an endoscopic procedure because absorption of this fluid can be associated with numerous perioperative complications. Urea is no longer used because it freely passes into both the intracellular and extracellular spaces and results in elevated blood urea concentrations.[183] Electrolyte solutions such as Ringer's lactate or normal saline would not cause electrolyte imbalance if absorbed into the circulation, but cannot be used in conjunction with an electrocautery device because they are ionized and are able to conduct electrical currents. Sorbitol is metabolized to fructose and use of this solution can produce hyperglycemia. Sorbitol is also converted to lactate, which may cause systemic acidosis, or it may induce an osmotic diuresis leading to dehydration and a hyperosmolar state. Glucose solutions have many of the same complications as sorbitol; however, glucose solutions are rarely used because they are sticky and not easily handled in the urology suite.[183]

Glycine is a nonessential amino acid that is normally present in the circulation. It is metabolized in the liver by oxidative deamination into ammonia and glyoxylic acid.[184] Depressed mental status and coma secondary to hyperammonemia have been reported following TURP procedures in which glycine was used as the irrigating solution.[184,185] Blood ammonia levels as high as 834 μM · l^{-1} (normal 11–35 μM · l^{-1}) have been documented, although the central nervous system depression was transient in these patients and they recovered within 24–48 hours.[185] Other investigators have observed the development of hyperoxaluria in association with glycine irrigation.[186] Hyperoxaluria places the patient at risk for calcium oxalate deposition in the kidneys if fluid intake is not maintained in the postoperative period. Visual disturbances, including blurred vision and transient blindness, have been reported following TURP procedures with glycine-containing irrigation fluid.[187,188] Loss of vision after transurethral procedures was traditionally thought to be secondary to cerebral edema from the hypervolemia and hyponatremia that developed as irrigating fluid was absorbed. However, when a centrally acting mechanism, such as cerebral edema, is the cause of visual impairment, patients have normal pupillary light reflexes. A review of patients with blindness after TURP revealed that some patients had sluggish or nonreactive

pupils, suggesting an anterior pathway disturbance rather than cerebral edema.[188] Glycine acts as an inhibitory neurotransmitter in the brain, spinal cord, and retina. Elevated serum glycine levels could exert an inhibitory action on the retina and result in transient blindness consistent with the clinical picture seen in these patients.[188,189] It would appear that the visual disturbance after TURP may have more than one etiology.

Mannitol is an osmotic diuretic, occasionally used as an irrigating solution, which can cause dehydration and hyperosmolality if absorbed into the circulation in large quantities. In addition, marked intravascular volume expansion may occur when mannitol-containing irrigating fluid is absorbed.

Transurethral Resection Syndrome

The *transurethral resection (TUR) syndrome* (water intoxication syndrome) is a general term used to describe a wide range of neurologic and cardiopulmonary symptoms that occur when irrigating fluid is absorbed during TUR procedures, especially TURP. The principal components of this syndrome include respiratory distress secondary to volume expansion from rapid intravascular absorption of the irrigating fluid, dilution of electrolytes and proteins by the electrolyte-free irrigating fluid, and symptoms related to the type of irrigating solution used.[179,183,190–192] The average amount of irrigating fluid absorbed during TURP is ~20 ml · min^{-1} of resection time.[181,193] The volume of fluid absorbed during the procedure can be estimated with the following formula:[191]

$$\text{Volume absorbed} = \frac{\text{preoperative serum Na}^+}{\text{postoperative serum Na}^+ \times \text{ECF}} - \text{ECF}$$

where ECF = extracellular fluid volume.

The amount of irrigation fluid absorbed during the procedure is directly related to the number and size of venous sinuses opened, the duration of the resection, the hydrostatic pressure of the irrigating fluid, and the venous pressure at the irrigant–blood interface.[178] In an attempt to prevent excessive fluid absorption, it is recommended that resection time be limited to <1 hour and that the bag of irrigating fluid be suspended no more than 30 cm above the operating table at the beginning of the resection and 15 cm in the final stages of resection.[178,193] Investigations have demonstrated that ethanol-labeled irrigating fluid can be used to accurately assess the degree of fluid absorption during TUR procedures.[194,195] With this monitoring technique, a trace amount of ethanol is incorporated into the irrigating fluid so that the transfer of fluid to the patient can be detected by measuring the ethanol content of the patient's exhaled breath. The ethanol concentration in the expired breath is a reflection of the degree of uptake of irrigating fluid. When high

Table 36-9. SIGNS AND SYMPTOMS ASSOCIATED WITH ACUTE CHANGES IN SERUM NA⁺ LEVELS

Serum Na⁺	Central Nervous System Changes	Electrocardiogram Changes
120 mEq · l⁻¹	Confusion Restlessness	Possible widening of QRS complex
115 mEq · l⁻¹	Somnolence Nausea	Widened QRS complex Elevated ST segment
110 mEq · l⁻¹	Seizures Coma	Ventricular tachycardia or fibrillation

Adapted with permission from Jensen V: The TURP syndrome. Can J Anaesth 38:90, 1991.

concentrations of exhaled ethanol are detected, the surgeon is notified and the operation is terminated.[195]

Clinical manifestations of the TUR syndrome range from mild (restlessness, nausea, shortness of breath, or dizziness) to severe (seizures, coma, hypertension, bradycardia, or cardiovascular collapse). In the awake patient with a regional block, a classic triad of symptoms has been described that consists of an increase in both systolic and diastolic pressures associated with an increase in pulse pressure, bradycardia, and mental status changes.[179,180] During a general anesthetic, many of the more subtle signs of the TUR syndrome are obscured, making the early diagnosis of this problem more difficult. The initial hypertension and bradycardia are the result of acute volume overload, which may lead to left heart failure, pulmonary edema, and cardiovascular collapse.[190] With the continued absorption of electrolyte-free irrigation fluid, dilutional hyponatremia and cerebral edema develop. The acute decrease in serum sodium concentration is responsible for many of the signs and symptoms of the TUR syndrome[179] (Table 36-9). A serum sodium of 120 mEq · l⁻¹ is associated with the development of central nervous system symptoms due to neuronal edema and dysfunction. Restlessness and confusion progress to loss of consciousness and seizures as sodium concentrations decline further.[196] Hyponatremia can also disturb the electrophysiology of cardiac cells. Electrocardiographic changes are seen when serum sodium levels fall below 115 mEq · l⁻¹ followed by cardiac arrest at levels near 100 mEq · l⁻¹. Rapid changes in the serum sodium concentration are more deleterious than chronic hyponatremia.[197]

Symptoms related to absorption of a specific irrigating solution during the procedure may further complicate the TUR syndrome. For example, if excessive amounts of glycine are absorbed, the patient may become encephalopathic secondary to high blood ammonia concentrations.[184,185] Likewise, absorption of large volumes of sorbitol may produce hyperglycemia and coma, especially in diabetic patients.

Prompt intervention is necessary when the neurologic or cardiovascular complications of TUR procedures are recognized (Table 36-10). Oxygenation, ventilation and circulatory support of the patient must be ensured and other potentially treatable conditions such as diabetic coma, hypercarbia, or drug interactions should be considered.[179] The surgeon should be informed of the change in the patient's status so that the procedure can be terminated as quickly as possible. Rapid measurement of serum electrolytes, creatinine, glucose, and arterial blood gases, as well as recording of an electrocardiogram are indicated. The severity of symptoms dictates the treatment of hyponatremia. If the patient's symptoms are mild and the serum sodium concentration is >120 mEq · l⁻¹, fluid restriction and administration of a loop diuretic, usually furosemide, are all that is necessary to return the sodium level to normal. Treatment with hypertonic saline has been associated with the development of demyelinating central nervous system lesions due to rapid increases in plasma osmolality and should be reserved for patients with severe, life-threatening symptoms.[197,198] Three

percent sodium chloride solution should be infused at a rate no greater than 100 ml · h⁻¹ and discontinued as soon as the serum sodium is >120 mEq · l⁻¹. Once this goal is reached, treatment can continue with fluid restriction and diuretic therapy. The rate at which serum sodium is increased should not exceed 12 mEq · l⁻¹ in a 24-hour period.[198]

Other Complications of TURP

Bleeding associated with TURP comes from either open venous sinuses or unrecognized arterial bleeding sites. Estimation of blood loss during transurethral procedures is grossly inaccurate because the shed blood is mixed with copious amounts of irrigating fluid. Typically, blood loss ranges from 2 to 4 ml · min⁻¹ during the resection and total blood loss correlates with the weight of the resected prostate tissue.[178] Because blood loss is difficult to assess, serial hemoglobin or hematocrit levels, as well as the patient's vital signs should be evaluated to determine the need for transfusion.[180] The incidence of intraoperative blood transfusion is reported to be ~2.5%; therefore, a preoperative "type and screen" for blood is all that is indicated.[199]

Abnormal bleeding after TURP occurs in <1% of resections.[178] This situation occurs more commonly if a TURP procedure is performed in a patient with prostate cancer and may be caused by the release of thromboplastin, which is found in high concentrations in prostate cancer cells.[180] This thrombogenic stimulus produces disseminated intravascular coagulation in which an initial state of hypercoagulability is followed by a phase of secondary fibrinolysis. Continued fibrin formation and fibrinolysis cause hemorrhage from the depletion of coagulation factors and platelets. Treatment of this condition is supportive, including the administration of plasma and platelet transfusions to replace the deficient factors.[200] Another cause of postoperative bleeding after TURP is the release of tissue plasminogen activators from the prostate. These factors activate the coagulation system and convert plasminogen to plasmin, which, in turn, causes fibrinolysis. Despite the fact that excessive bleeding after TURP has never been directly correlated with

Table 36-10. TREATMENT OF THE TRANSURETHRAL RESECTION SYNDROME

Ensure oxygenation and circulatory support
Notify surgeon and terminate procedure as soon as possible
Consider insertion of invasive monitors if cardiovascular instability occurs
Send blood to laboratory for electrolytes, creatinine, glucose, and arterial blood gases
Obtain 12-lead electrocardiogram
Treat mild symptoms (with serum Na⁺ concentration >120 mEq · l⁻¹) with fluid restriction and loop diuretic (furosemide)
Treat severe symptoms (if serum Na⁺ <120 mEq · l⁻¹) with 3% sodium chloride iv at a rate <100 ml · h⁻¹
Discontinue 3% sodium chloride when serum Na⁺ >120 mEq · l⁻¹

the degree of fibrinolysis, suggested treatment includes ε-aminocaproic acid, an inhibitor of fibrinolysis.[201] The recommended dosage for ε-aminocaproic acid is 4–5 g infused intravenously (iv) over the first hour followed by a continuous infusion of 1 g·hr^{-1} for 8 hours or until the bleeding is controlled.

Perforation of the prostatic capsule occurs in ~1–2% of all patients undergoing TURP, usually resulting in extraperitoneal extravasation of fluid.[180,199] This complication occurs more commonly during transurethral resection of the bladder (TURB) and the management of this problem is discussed in that section of this chapter.

The development of a fever in the perioperative period suggests bacteremia secondary to spread of bacteria through open prostatic venous sinuses, which is fostered by the presence of an indwelling urethral catheter.[180] Most patients receive prophylactic antibiotics before the surgical procedure, which are continued until 2–3 days after the catheter is removed. This risk of sepsis is increased by the use of "high-pressure" irrigation during the procedure and can be significantly decreased if the irrigation pressure is maintained at ≤30 cm.[193]

If large volumes of room temperature irrigating fluids are used to remove blood from the operative site during TURP procedures, this may result in hypothermia in many patients, especially the elderly, who have a reduced thermoregulatory capacity. It has been shown that body temperature decreases ~1°C·h^{-1} of surgery and shivering occurs in 16% of patients who receive room-temperature irrigation fluids, whereas hypothermia does not develop if the irrigation solution is warmed to body temperature (95–100°F).[202,203]

Anesthetic Techniques for TURP

Regional anesthesia has long been considered the anesthetic technique of choice for TURP and is used in >70% of these procedures in the United States.[199,204] This anesthetic technique allows the patient to remain awake, which should facilitate the early diagnosis of TUR syndrome or the extravasation of irrigation fluid. Some studies have demonstrated decreased blood loss when TURP procedures are performed using regional anesthesia, whereas others have found no difference in blood loss between regional and general anesthesia.[205–208]

The use of longer-acting regional anesthesia, compared with general anesthesia, for patients undergoing TURP is associated with improved postoperative pain control and decreased postoperative pain medication requirements. Bowman et al[209] found that only 15% of patients receiving spinal anesthesia for TURP required any pain medication other than acetaminophen but that the need for analgesics was increased approximately fourfold after general anesthesia.

A prospective study comparing the effect of general versus spinal anesthesia on cognitive function after TURP found a significant decrease in mental status in both groups at 6 hours after surgery, but no differences in postoperative mental function at any time in the first 30 days after surgery.[210] Ghoneim et al[211] also found that the type of anesthesia (regional versus general) did not affect postoperative behavior in patients undergoing prostatectomy, hysterectomy, or joint replacement.

Perioperative morbidity and mortality among patients older than 90 years of age who underwent TURP do not depend on the type of anesthesia used.[212] A study of the occurrence of perioperative myocardial ischemia in patients undergoing transurethral surgery, assessed by Holter monitoring, determined that both the incidence and duration of myocardial ischemia increased following TUR surgery but that there was no difference between general or spinal anesthesia.[213] A second study confirmed these findings and concluded that the presence of short duration silent myocardial ischemia did not correlate with adverse outcome in elderly patients undergoing TURP procedures.[214] Thus, it appears that TURP can be performed safely with either type of anesthesia and the choice of anesthetic technique should be tailored to the individual patient.

If regional anesthesia is used for the procedure, a T10 dermatome anesthetic level is needed to block the pain from bladder distention by the irrigating fluid. However, an S3 level is reported to be adequate in ~25% of patients if the bladder is not allowed to overfill.[204] Spinal anesthesia is usually preferred over lumbar epidural anesthesia because sacral segments are sometimes inadequately blocked with lumbar epidural techniques.

Local anesthesia has also been used for TURP procedures in patients with small to moderately sized prostate glands.[215] This anesthetic technique involves infiltration of 1–3 ml of local anesthetic solution (0.25% bupivacaine, 1% lidocaine) into the bladder neck and lateral lobes of the prostate to block the inferior hypogastric plexus of nerves, along with transurethral injection of local anesthesia into the gland surrounding the prostatic urethra. With this type of anesthetic, the surgeon can remove small amounts of prostatic tissue with minimal patient discomfort. Although the authors reported that this technique was difficult to implement on a large scale, they speculated that it might prove useful in high-risk patients who cannot tolerate spinal or general anesthesia.[215]

Morbidity and Mortality After TURP

An American Urological Association (AUA) cooperative study evaluated postoperative complications in 3885 patients after TURP;[199] the average patient age was 69 years and most (>75%) patients had coexisting medical problems that involved many of the major organ systems. The complication rate for the intraoperative period was 6.9%, and the most common intraoperative problems were bleeding requiring transfusion in 2.5% of patients, the TUR syndrome in 2% of patients, cardiac dysrhythmias in 1% of patients, and extravasation of irrigating fluid in 0.9% of patients. No intraoperative deaths occurred. Immediate postoperative problems following TURP occurred in 18% of patients, with the most common problem during this period being failure to void. Other common postoperative problems were bleeding, clot retention, and infection. Patients at an increased risk for perioperative morbidity after TURP were identified as those patients with large prostate glands (>45 g), resection times longer than 90 minutes, acute urinary retention, or age >80 years.

Despite the high incidence of coexisting medical problems in patients undergoing TURP, the mortality rate in the first month after this procedure has declined over the years. In 1962, the mortality rate after TURP was 2.5%, whereas the AUA cooperative study evaluating these procedures during the years 1978–1987 found a mortality rate of 0.2%, even though patient age and the amount of prostate tissue resected had not changed from earlier surveys.[199]

The Future of TURP

Since 1980, TURP has been the most common operative procedure performed in urologic surgery.[216,217] In 1986, TURP accounted for >90% of prostatectomy procedures in the United States. However, since that time, the number of operations has fallen by nearly 20%.[217] Potential factors in the decline of TURP include the development of less invasive surgical alternative treatments, including balloon dilation, transurethral incision of the prostate (TUIP), laser prostatectomy, and prostate stents. In addition, drug therapy with α-blocking agents or 5α-reductase inhibitors is now available.[216]

Balloon dilation of the prostate has been used as an alternative to TURP since the 1980s.[193] With this technique, a balloon is inflated in the prostatic urethra and left in place for 10 minutes.[218] The advantages of this technique include lower cost and shorter hospital stay, as well as the fact that it can usually be performed under local anesthesia with supplemental iv sedation. However, the future of balloon dilation is in question because it has been shown to be no more effective than dilation with cystoscopy alone.[217]

Transurethral incision of the prostate is the alternative to TURP that comes closest to matching its effectiveness in relieving urinary symptoms.[219,220] The incision can be performed at a variety of locations around the bladder neck using laser or a cutting balloon.[220] This procedure can be performed on an outpatient basis and is associated with shorter surgical times and significantly less blood loss.[177] Although some patients need only local anesthesia with iv sedation for TUIP, most require a spinal or "light" general anesthetic.

The technique of laser prostatectomy has recently been approved by the U.S. Food and Drug Administration. A neodymium–yttrium-aluminum-garnet (Nd-YAG) laser can be used to coagulate the prostate tissue, and the coagulated tissue is sloughed for the next several months. This procedure is associated with minimal bleeding and a decreased risk of absorption of the irrigating fluid, thereby minimizing the risk of TUR syndrome.[221] Because of these advantages, laser prostatectomy is preferred over TURP in elderly patients with significant comorbidity.

Transurethral Resection of Bladder Tumors

Bladder cancer is the second most common urologic malignancy, with nearly 50,000 new cases diagnosed in the United States each year.[222,223] Bladder tumors occur with a male-to-female ratio of ~3:1. Although the etiology of this tumor is not known, numerous lifestyle and environmental factors have been associated with the development of bladder cancer, including cigarette smoking, coffee drinking, use of artificial sweeteners, pelvic irradiation, and exposure to industrial carcinogens.

Superficial transitional cell carcinoma accounts for ~90% of bladder cancers, and most patients undergo endoscopic procedures transurethral resection of the bladder for both the diagnosis and treatment of this disease.[222,223] This procedure can be performed with either regional or general anesthesia. If a regional anesthetic is employed, an anesthetic level to T10 is required to block the pain associated with bladder distention during the procedure. However, if the bladder tumor lies near the obturator nerve, general anesthesia with muscle relaxation is the preferred technique.

Complications During Transurethral Resection of the Bladder

Perforation of the bladder has been reported during transurethral surgery.[224,225] This complication can occur if the bladder is over distended in the later stages of the procedure, causing tears in bladder areas thinned by the resection. Perforation of the bladder results in intraperitoneal extravasation of the fluid that is being used to irrigate the bladder, causing an abnormal irrigating pattern in which fluid is instilled into the bladder but not recovered. The clinical diagnosis of bladder perforation is simplified if the procedure is performed under regional anesthesia. The conscious patient describes sudden, severe abdominal pain, often associated with referred pain to the shoulder.[181,224] Associated symptoms include pallor, sweating, abdominal rigidity, nausea, and vomiting. If extravasation is suspected, the operation should be terminated as quickly as possible. Small perforations with minimal intraperitoneal leakage rarely cause hemodynamic changes and can usually be managed with catheter drainage and diuretics. Open exploration with closure of the perforation is recommended for patients with respiratory embarrassment.[181,224]

The obturator nerve passes near the lateral bladder wall, bladder neck, and lateral prostatic urethra as it courses through the pelvis. Stimulation of the obturator nerve by an electrocautery device during transurethral surgery may cause the thigh muscles to contract violently, leading to inadvertent bladder perforation.[226,227] Spinal anesthesia, "deep" general anesthesia, nerve cooling, and changing either the electrocautery current frequency or site of the inactive electrode have all

been ineffective in blocking the muscle contraction.[226] However, this reflex may be eliminated either by use of a muscle relaxant during general anesthesia or local anesthetic infiltration of the obturator nerve as it passes through the obturator canal.[226–230]

Extracorporeal Shock Wave Lithotripsy

In the United States, the annual incidence of urolithiasis is 16.4 per 10,000 people, and it is estimated that 12% of all people will experience calculus disease in their lifetime.[231] This disease is three times more common in men than in women, with a peak age incidence in the third to fourth decade of life.[232] Small calculi of <4.0 mm usually pass spontaneously; however, 10–20% of stones cause enough symptoms to justify surgical treatment.[233] Several therapeutic modalities exist for the surgical treatment of urinary calculi. The final treatment decision is based on the size of the stone being treated, its location in the urinary tract, and its composition.[232,233]

The introduction of extracorporeal shock wave lithotripsy (SWL) in 1980 dramatically changed the management of urolithiasis. Before the development of this modality, open surgical removal was the most common technique for treatment of urethral and renal calculi.[234] Now only 5% of all urinary calculi require treatment with open surgical procedures. SWL has the advantages of being a minimally invasive technique that can be performed on an outpatient basis and is associated with minimal perioperative morbidity, which translates into a significant reduction in treatment costs.[235]

Technical Aspects of Shock Wave Lithotrips

All lithotriptors have four main components: an energy source, a focusing device, a coupling medium, and a stone localization system.[233] The original lithotriptor was the Dornier HM-3, in which the patient is placed in a hydraulically supported gantry chair and immersed in a water bath (Fig. 36-8). The Dornier HM-3 energy source is a spark-plug generator that creates an explosive impact and transmits very high pressures (shock waves) to the water when it discharges. An ellipsoidal reflector aims the shock waves at a focal point. Two fluoroscopes are oriented so that their beam paths intersect at the focal point above the ellipsoidal reflector, and the patient's position in the tub is adjusted so that the calculus is centered in these beam paths.[236] The water bath transmits the shock wave to the patient. It also serves as the coupling medium, allowing the shock wave to pass into the body without dissipation because the acoustic impedance of body tissue is close to that of water.[235]

During lithotripsy on the Dornier HM-3, the shock waves are delivered at an energy level of 18–20 kV, which corresponds to a pressure of ~900–1100 bar (1 bar = 14.7 psi) at the focal point on the calculus.[237] Initial SWL treatments were associated with ventricular ectopic beats and even ventricular tachycardia.[238] It was postulated that these dysrhythmias were caused by stimulation of the myocardium when shock waves were delivered during the repolarization phase of the heart. To avoid this problem, shock waves are now triggered off the electrocardiogram to occur 20 milliseconds after the R wave during the refractory period of the heart.[238] The average treatment on the Dornier HM-3 lithotriptor uses 1500–2000 shocks.[235]

Physiologic Effects of Immersion Lithotripsy

Placement of a patient into the water bath during lithotripsy produces a number of physiologic alterations in the cardiovascular system (Fig. 36-9). Immersion causes peripheral venous compression, resulting in an increase in central blood volume as well as central venous pressure (CVP) and PCWP.[239,240] The increases in CVP and PCWP are linearly related to the depth of immersion, with immersion to the clavicles increasing CVP by 10–14 cm H_2O.[241] Despite the increase in venous return during immersion, some patients experience hypotension as a result of vasodilatation from the warm water.[242,243] Other

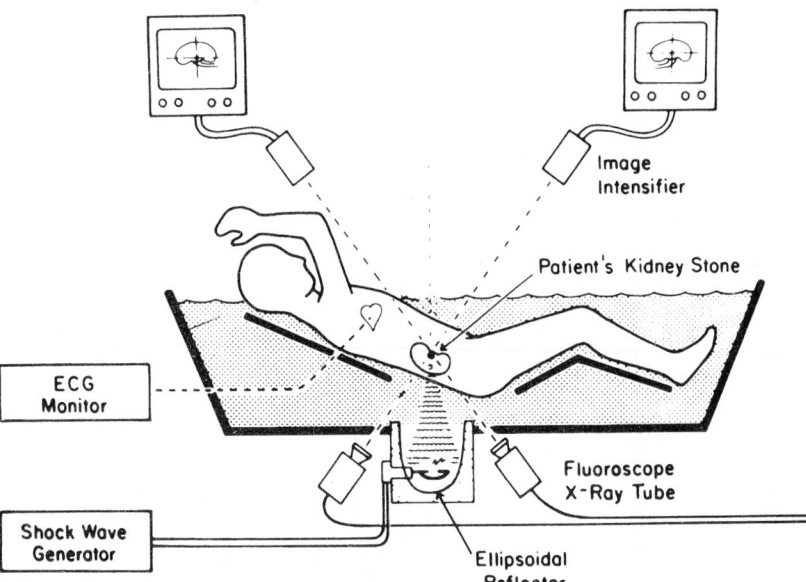

Figure 36-8. Schematic of patient positioned in the Dornier HM-3 lithotriptor. (Reprinted from Hunter PT II: The physics and geometry pertinent to ESWL. In Riehle RA Jr., Newman RC [eds]: Principles of Extracorporeal Shock Wave Lithotripsy, p 14. New York, Churchill Livingstone, 1987.)

investigators have reported an increase in blood pressure and a decrease in cardiac output secondary to increased systemic vascular resistance during these procedures.[244,245] The wide variety of cardiovascular changes that are possible during SWL procedures dictates the use of extreme caution when caring for patients with significant cardiac disease undergoing this procedure. For example, patients with congestive heart failure may decompensate as their central blood volume increases during immersion. Likewise, patients with coronary artery disease may experience myocardial ischemia if hypotension or large increases in cardiac work occur during the procedure. In patients at risk for cardiovascular problems, immersion should be achieved in a gradual fashion so that alterations in the cardiovascular system can be closely monitored and the process terminated, if necessary. The procedure can also be performed with minimal immersion so that only the entry site is covered with water, or a nonimmersion (second- or third-generation) lithotriptor may be used.

Immersion lithotripsy also affects the respiratory system. Placement of a patient in water to the level of the clavicles increases the work of breathing, and respirations often become shallow and rapid.[246,247] Other respiratory effects include a decrease in vital capacity and functional residual capacity secondary to extrinsic pressure on the upper abdomen and thorax. Bromage *et al*[247] demonstrated that the addition of iv sedation during SWL procedures resulted in a potentiation of the respiratory depressant effects of immersion. Continuous monitoring of respiratory gas exchange and oxygenation should be used in all patients undergoing SWL but are of paramount importance in patients with pre-existing respiratory disease.

Problems involving temperature regulation may occur during SWL, especially in elderly patients with impaired thermoregulatory systems. Water in the lithotriptor tub should be maintained in the temperature range of 35.8–37.5 °C.[237,248,249] Water temperature should be checked before immersion, temperature monitoring used in every patient, and temperature alarms installed in the tub to signal excessively high or low temperatures.[249]

Patient Selection for Lithotripsy Procedures

Lithotripsy was initially limited to the treatment of renal calculi, but the indications for SWL have been expanded to include most ureteral stones. The only absolute contraindications to this procedure are pregnancy, abnormal coagulation parameters, and the presence of an active urinary tract infection. Consequently, women of child-bearing potential should be carefully evaluated for pregnancy before lithotripsy to avoid possible fetal damage from exposure to shock waves or radiation. Other pretreatment testing should include coagulation tests (*i.e.*, prothrombin time, partial thromboplastin time, and platelet count), and a urine culture. The risk of subcapsular renal bleeding or perinephric hematoma mandates that all coagulation parameters be normalized before lithotripsy. Aspirin-containing medications and NSAIDs should be discontinued for a minimum of 10 days before surgery.[250] To minimize septic complications, all patients with active urinary tract infections should be treated with antibiotics before SWL.

Lithotripsy may be problematic in children or patients of small stature (height <48 inches) because positioning in the lithotriptor chair is more difficult and there is a higher risk of pulmonary contusion by shock waves.[250] The lungs of small patients can be shielded by foam padding during the treatment in an effort to prevent this complication.

It was initially thought that the presence of a cardiac pacemaker was a contraindication to SWL because of the possibility that electrical interference from the spark gap generating the shock wave might inhibit, reprogram, or damage the pacemaker.[235] However, a review of 142 SWL treatments in pacemaker-dependent patients found a low (<1%) incidence of major pacemaker complications in these patients with only one pacemaker deprogrammed during the treatment period.[251] Based on these findings, patients with pacemakers are considered acceptable candidates for lithotripsy provided that certain precautions are taken, including (1) preoperative determination of the type of pacemaker and its functional status, (2) availability of a magnet or programming device in the operating room along with a person skilled in its use, (3) availability of an alternative pacing device, and (4) positioning of the patient so that the pacemaker is not in the shock wave path.

Other relative contraindications to SWL include complete urinary tract obstruction distal to the stone, calcification or aneurysm of the renal artery or aorta, the presence of an orthopedic prosthesis, or renal insufficiency as indicated by serum creatinine level of ≥ 3 mg · dl^{-1}. Patients with small abdominal aortic aneurysms have been safely treated if they are carefully positioned; however, patients with aneurysms measuring >6 cm in diameter should not be treated because the risk of accidental rupture increases exponentially with size.[250]

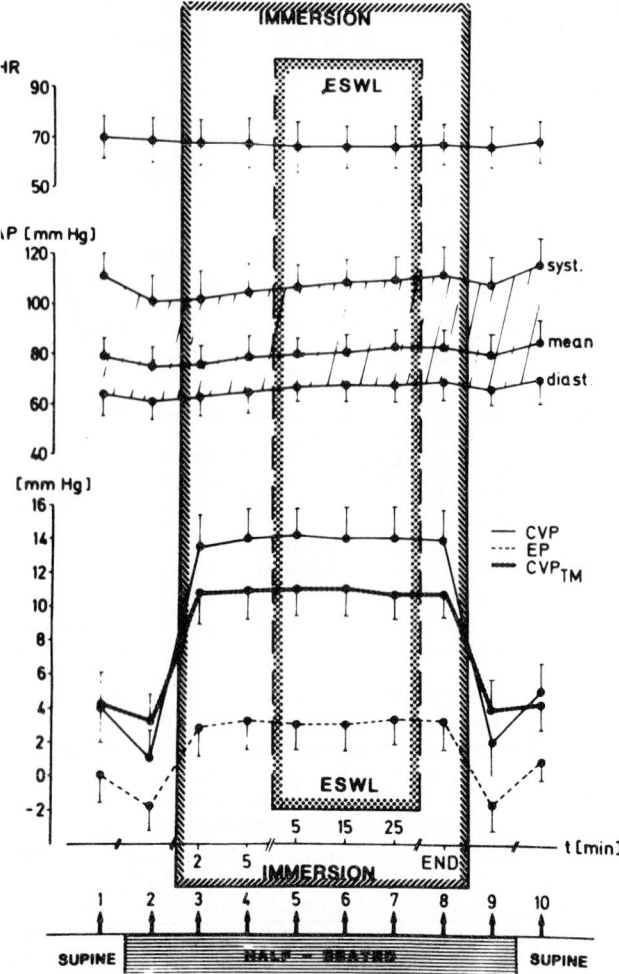

Figure 36-9. Effects of positioning, immersion, and immersion on heart rate (HR; beats · min⁻¹); systolic (syst.), mean and diastolic (diast.) arterial pressure (AP); and central venous (CVP) and esophageal (EP) pressures and transmural CVP (CVP$_{TM}$) in 25 patients during treatment with extracorporeal shock wave lithotripsy (ESWL). The numbers along the bottom refer to the number of measurements. Mean and standard deviations are shown. (Reprinted with permission from Weber W, Madler C, Keil B *et al*: Cardiovascular effects of ESWL. In Gravenstein JS, Peter K [eds]: Extracorporeal Shock-Wave Lithotripsy for Renal Stone Disease, p 105. Boston, Butterworths, 1986.)

Complications of Shock Wave Lithotripsy

Renal parenchymal damage is thought to be responsible for the hematuria that occurs in nearly all patients, while subcapsular hematoma is seen in only 0.5% of patients after lithotripsy.[234] These problems usually resolve spontaneously and bleeding that requires transfusion is rare.[252] Transient renal failure after SWL has been reported; however, there is no evidence that lithotripsy is associated with permanent renal dysfunction. Nevertheless, it seems prudent to avoid bilateral lithotripsy in a single procedure.[252]

After treatment, many patients complain of flank pain, which may be severe for several days.[252,253] Petechiae and soft tissue swelling are often seen at the entry site of the shock wave, especially in thin patients. These skin changes resolve quickly and appear to be of little clinical significance. Up to 10% of patients have significant urinary tract colic, occasionally requiring hospitalization and opioid analgesics. Broken stone fragments can also collect in the ureter and form a column of stone, which is commonly referred to as *steinstrasse* or "stone street." Although some patients have little pain associated with this

condition, others may experience severe postoperative pain. If *steinstrasse* results in total ureteral obstruction, rising creatinine levels, or severe pain, the patient may require an endoscopic procedure with ureteral stent placement to relieve the obstruction.[252]

Other potential complications following lithotripsy include damage to adjacent organs by the shock waves.[234] As previously mentioned, pulmonary contusions may occur if shock waves strike the lungs. Several cases of pancreatitis and transient gastrointestinal erosions have also been reported. Approximately 1% of patients have septic complications after SWL. Brachial plexus injuries have also occurred from improper positioning of patients in the lithotriptor chair. Despite the wide array of potential complications, the mortality rate after SWL was only 0.02% in a review of >62,000 patients.[234] It appears that with proper patient selection and cautious intraoperative management, most patients can safely undergo lithotripsy procedures.

Recent Advances in Lithotripsy

Modifications of the original Dornier HM-3 lithotriptor have produced second- and third-generation lithotriptors with several advantages.[233,234] First, newer lithotriptors generate shock waves within a "shock tube" that is coupled to the body surface with a water cushion, thus eliminating the water bath and all the problems associated with immersion of the patient. Second, recent modifications have focused on the development of pain-free lithotripsy by decreasing the power of the lithotriptor. Although newer lithotriptors cause less pain, they are not pain-free and most patients still require iv sedation during treatments. In addition, decreasing the power in these machines has reduced the efficiency of stone fragmentation and resulted in a higher retreatment rate compared with treatment on the HM-3 lithotriptor.[234] For this reason, many urologists prefer to use the HM-3, ensuring that anesthesiologists will continue to care for patients treated with immersion lithotripsy for some time to come.

Anesthetic Techniques for Shock Wave Lithotripsy

During lithotripsy shock waves release energy as they pass through the interface between substances of different acoustic density. It is the impact of the shock waves on the skin and viscera that is responsible for the pain experienced during the procedure.[254] The initial approach to anesthesia for lithotripsy on the Dornier HM-3 used either a regional or general technique. General anesthesia offers the advantages of control of patient ventilation and movement, as well as a rapid induction of anesthesia and a quicker recovery from anesthesia compared with epidural anesthesia.[255] However, patients have to be positioned in the lithotriptor chair while unconscious, increasing the risk of peripheral nerve injuries. With regional anesthesia, the patient is awake and cooperative during transport, simplifying patient positioning. In addition, the anesthetic can be used for additional operative procedures should they become necessary. Regional anesthetic techniques for this procedure require a sensory level of T6. Spinal anesthesia has a quicker onset and shorter preparation time compared with epidural anesthesia, but produces a more profound sympathetic blockade and is associated with a higher incidence of intraoperative hypotension.[256]

Conscious sedation techniques have been developed for use during lithotripsy.[253,257] A wide variety of sedative-hypnotic, anxiolytic, and analgesic drugs have been used, but the most successful regimens use agents with small volumes of distribution, rapid clearance rates, and short elimination half-lives. Monk *et al*[253] examined the use of propofol and fentanyl or midazolam and alfentanil for iv sedation during treatments on the Dornier HM-3 immersion lithotriptor. Both sedative-analgesic combinations provided good treatment conditions and were associated with a high degree of patient satisfaction. Compared with epidural anesthesia for the same procedures, anesthesia and recovery times were significantly shortened and hospital costs decreased by the use of iv sedation.[253] Local anesthetic infiltration of the flank alone or in combination with intercostal blocks and topical application of local anesthetic cream have also been used during lithotripsy on the Dornier HM-3 to decrease iv analgesic requirements for SWL.[254,258] Although both local anesthetic techniques produced cutaneous analgesia, iv analgesics were still required for intraoperative patient comfort. It is unclear whether the addition of local anesthesia decreases the overall need for iv medication. Currently, conscious sedation is the preferred anesthetic technique for most routine SWL procedures, particularly those performed using the newer-generation lithotriptors.[259,260]

Percutaneous Renal Procedures

Percutaneous nephrostomy (PCN) is commonly performed for the diagnosis and treatment of a wide variety of urologic problems, including relief of renal obstruction, stone removal, biopsy of tumors, and ureteral stent placement.[167] During a PCN procedure, a needle is passed into the renal collecting system under fluoroscopic guidance. After the needle is properly positioned, a guidewire is inserted through the needle and the needle is removed. A catheter is then placed over the guidewire, establishing access and drainage of the kidney. This procedure is performed with the patient prone, and local anesthesia with iv sedation is utilized for analgesia.[167] However, if the patient requires more than drainage catheter placement, the nephrostomy tract is dilated by the passage of graduated plastic dilators over the guidewire. Dilation of the nephrostomy tract is associated with considerable discomfort and requires either general or regional (spinal or epidural) anesthesia. PCN involves the passage of an endoscope through the nephrostomy tract. Percutaneous nephrolithotomy, a procedure to remove renal calculi too large to be treated with lithotripsy, is one of the most common endosurgical procedures requiring dilation of a nephrostomy tract.

Although percutaneous surgical techniques are considerably less invasive than open surgical procedures, a variety of complications may occur during these procedures.[261] During insertion of the nephrostomy tube, trauma to the spleen, liver, or kidney can result in acute blood loss necessitating an emergency open surgical procedure. Colon injury has been reported if a retrorenal colon overlies the lower pole of the kidney.[167] This problem is usually managed by the placement of a colostomy tube, but a colostomy may be indicated if the patient exhibits signs of peritonitis. Pleural injury may occur during nephrostomy tube placement when access is created above the 12th rib or the kidney lies in a more cephalad position than normal. Nephrostomy tract dilation causes bleeding in most patients, with the hemoglobin declining by an average of $1.2 \text{ g} \cdot \text{dl}^{-1}$. If excessive intraoperative bleeding occurs, it is wise to stop the procedure and insert a large-caliber nephrostomy tube or high-pressure balloon nephrostomy catheter to tamponade the bleeding.[261] In a study of 50 patients undergoing PCN for stone removal, the complication rate was 12%, with pleural effusion and hydropneumothorax the most common problems encountered.[262]

During nephroscopy procedures, continuous irrigation of fluid through the endoscope is necessary to prevent blood and debris from obscuring the surgeon's vision. Because extravasation of irrigation fluid into the retroperitoneal, intraperitoneal, intravascular, or pleural spaces is possible, it should be standard practice to compare the quantity of irrigating fluid used with the output of fluid into the suction and urinary catheters. If there is a discrepancy between the amount of fluid infused and the output from the patient, extravasation must be assumed to have occurred. If the discrepancy between intake and output exceeds 500 ml and the difference cannot be accounted for by spillage or other losses, consideration should be given to stopping the procedure.[261] Intravenous absorption of irrigation fluid during percutaneous renal procedures can create a situation similar to that seen with the TUR syndrome, in which electrolyte abnormalities and fluid overload can occur. Because electrocautery is rarely used during percutaneous renal procedures, the preferred irrigating solution is 0.9% sodium chloride.[263] If an electrocautery device is needed, the irrigation fluid is temporarily changed to sorbitol solution.

LASER SURGERY IN UROLOGY

Laser therapy has been shown to be effective in the treatment of a multitude of urologic problems, including condyloma acuminatum of the external genitalia and urethra, ureteral stricture or bladder neck contracture, interstitial cystitis, BPH, ureteral calculi, and superficial carcinoma of the penis, bladder, ureter, and renal pelvis.[264] The major advantages of laser surgery over traditional surgical approaches are minimal blood loss, decreased postoperative pain, and tissue denaturation, which reduces the risk of tumor implantation.

Because lasers are an integral part of urologic surgery, an understanding of the indications and limitations of each type of laser is essential.[265] The *carbon dioxide* (CO_2) *laser* produces intense heat with vaporization but has minimal tissue penetration and is unable to penetrate water. Thus, its use is limited to the treatment of cutaneous lesions of the external genitalia. The *argon laser* is poorly absorbed by water but is selectively absorbed by hemoglobin and melanin, making this laser useful for procedures in the bladder requiring coagulation of bleeding sites. The *pulsed dye laser* generates a pulsed output and is useful for destroying ureteral calculi. One of the most versatile and widely used lasers in urologic surgery is the *Nd-YAG laser*.[264] This laser produces deep tissue penetration *via* protein denaturation with minimal vaporization. It can be used in water or urine without loss of effectiveness and delivered with a fiberoptic laser delivery system for endourologic surgery. Excellent results have been reported after the treatment of lesions of the penis, urethra, bladder, ureters, and kidneys with the Nd-YAG laser. The *KTP-532 laser* is a frequency-doubled Nd-YAG laser that does not penetrate tissue as deeply as the Nd-YAG but has a better cutting effect.[265] It is extremely effective in the treatment of urethral strictures and bladder neck contractures.

Safety issues assume paramount importance during laser surgery. Damage to the eye is the potential injury that requires the greatest attention because both direct and reflected laser beams can cause eye injury.[266] The part of the eye that is damaged by the laser depends on the wavelength. CO_2 laser beams cause a corneal ulceration, but no energy is transmitted to the fundus. Argon, Nd-YAG, and *KTP-532* lasers pass through the anterior chamber of the eye with minimal absorption and can therefore damage the retina. Protective goggles with appropriate filtering lenses are available for each type of laser, and laser equipment should not be activated until all operating room personnel and the patient are wearing glasses. It is also desirable to limit access to the operating room during laser surgery. Although less critical than eye damage, inadvertent thermal injury to the skin may also occur during laser treatments. Thermal injuries are avoidable if the laser is placed in the "standby" mode when not in operation and the laser is activated only by the surgeon performing the procedure. During CO_2 laser therapy for condyloma acuminatum, the plume (smoke) from the vaporization of tissue contains active human papilloma virus particles.[267] To avoid inhalation of infectious agents, all operating room personnel involved in CO_2 laser procedures for genital lesions should wear protective laser masks that prevent small particles from being inhaled. In addition, the laser plume should be removed from the operating room with a smoke-evacuation system.

UROLOGIC LAPAROSCOPY

Urologic laparoscopy techniques are minimally invasive and have rapidly gained acceptance because they are associated with decreased postoperative pain, shorter hospital stays, and more rapid convalescence than open surgical procedures.[167] Laparoscopic procedures performed in urology include diagnostic procedures for the evaluation of undescended testis, orchiopexy, varicocelectomy, bladder suspension, pelvic lymphadenectomy, nephrectomy, nephroureterectomy, adrenalectomy, and cystectomy.

Unique cardiopulmonary changes may occur during laparoscopic surgery (see Chapter 38). Physiologic alterations during laparoscopy are often related to the surgical technique itself, in particular, the creation of the pneumoperitoneum and absorption of the insufflating gas.[268] A wide variety of intraoperative complications are also possible during laparoscopy (Table 36-11). Complication rates for large laparoscopy series are reported to range from 0.6% to 2.4%, with approximately one third of the complications being cardiopulmonary in nature.[269] These factors often make the intraoperative management of laparoscopic procedures more challenging for the anesthesiologist than open surgical procedures for the same indication.

Laparoscopic urologic procedures differ from conventional laparoscopy in several respects. Many structures in the genitourinary system are extraperitoneal (i.e., the pelvic lymph nodes, bladder, ureters, adrenal glands, and kidneys), and urologists often prefer extraperitoneal insufflation during laparoscopic surgery on these organs. Several studies have suggested that CO_2 absorption is greater with extraperitoneal compared with intraperitoneal insufflation. Mullet et al[270] reported that extraperitoneal laparoscopic pelvic lymphadenectomy caused a 76% increase in CO_2 elimination, whereas intraperitoneal diagnostic pelvic laparoscopy and laparoscopic cholecystectomy were associated with increases in CO_2 elimination of only 15% and 25%, respectively. A retrospective analysis of patients undergoing laparoscopic renal and pelvic surgery revealed that CO_2 elimination increased as much as 135% when the operation was approached with an extraperitoneal approach versus 61% when intraperitoneal insufflation was used.[271,272] The increased absorption of CO_2 during extraperitoneal laparoscopic techniques mandates that the anesthesiologist carefully monitor and adjust ventilation as needed to maintain normocarbia.

Some laparoscopic procedures in urology, namely, cystectomy and nephrectomy, tend to be lengthy. Prolonged insuffla-

---

Table 36-11. POTENTIAL INTRAOPERATIVE COMPLICATIONS DURING LAPAROSCOPIC SURGERY

PULMONARY
Pneumothorax
Pneumomediastinum
Hypoxemia
Hypercapnia
Aspiration

CARDIOVASCULAR
Dysrhythmias
Hypotension
Hypertension
Venous gas embolus
Venous thrombosis

MISCELLANEOUS
Vascular injury
Visceral perforation
Oliguria
Hypothermia
Peripheral nerve injury

---

tion times during these procedures increase the amount of CO_2 absorbed and also necessitate the use of general anesthesia to guarantee patient comfort. Oliguria has been associated with prolonged durations of pneumoperitoneum during laparoscopic nephrectomy surgery.[273] In a porcine laparoscopic model, McDougall et al[274] demonstrated that prolonged increases in intra-abdominal pressure of ≥15 mm Hg resulted in a significant decrease in urine output despite adequate circulating blood volume and cardiac output. The mechanism for the intraoperative renal dysfunction was considered to be decreased renal cortical blood flow and renal vein obstruction during insufflation. In this study, the intraoperative oliguria was transient and not associated with any permanent renal derangement in the postoperative period. A review of the first 10 patients undergoing laparoscopic nephrectomy found that transient congestive heart failure developed in two of the patients in the postoperative period.[275] The authors postulated that this problem occurred secondary to excessive fluid and blood administration to treat oliguria. Another possible mechanism for intraoperative oliguria during laparoscopic surgery is an increase in stress hormone levels, such as ADH.[276] Because intraoperative oliguria is often treated with fluid administration, it is important that the anesthesiologist be aware that oliguria during prolonged laparoscopic procedures may not reflect intravascular volume depletion.

RADICAL CANCER SURGERY

Most major, open surgical procedures in urology are performed to treat cancer of the prostate, bladder, or kidney. These procedures are often lengthy and require intraoperative patient positions that are associated with significant impact on cardiorespiratory function. Radical urologic surgery also carries a potential for hemorrhage and large intraoperative blood and fluid requirements. In addition, patients undergoing these procedures are often elderly with pre-existing medical conditions.

Radical Prostatectomy

Cancer of the prostate is the most commonly diagnosed cancer in men, as well as the second most common cause of prostate-related mortality in American men.[277] Localized prostate cancer (Stage A or B) is treated with either radical prostatectomy or radiation therapy. Considerable controversy exists over the best therapy for this disease because only one prospective, randomized trial to date has compared radical prostatectomy with radiation therapy in patients with organ-confined disease.[278] These investigators found that radical prostatectomy offered a "distinct survival advantage" for localized prostate cancer. In the United States, men with clinically localized prostate cancer whose life expectancy is 10 years or longer tend to undergo radical prostatectomy, whereas patients older than 70 years of age or with a life expectancy of less than 10 years usually opt for radiation therapy or observation.[279]

Radical prostatectomy has been the most commonly used curative procedure for the treatment of prostate cancer since its introduction into the United States in 1905. This procedure involves the en bloc surgical removal of the entire prostate gland, the seminal vesicles, the ejaculatory ducts, and a portion of the bladder neck. After these structures are removed, the remaining bladder neck is anastomosed to the membranous urethra over an indwelling urethral catheter. A limited pelvic lymphadenectomy is usually performed during the procedure to aid in cancer staging.[280] Radical prostatectomy can be performed with either a retropubic or perineal approach.

Radical retropubic prostatectomy is performed through a midline lower abdominal incision with the patient in the supine position. The operating room table is broken in the midline or the kidney rest is elevated to provide a slight hyperextension, which increases the distance from the symphysis pubis to the umbilicus. The table is then placed in the Trendelenburg position until the patient's legs are parallel to the floor.[280] Either general anesthesia or regional (epidural or spinal) anesthesia with sedation may be used for this procedure. If a regional anesthetic technique is utilized, a sensory block of T6–T8 is adequate.[204] Advocates of general anesthesia believe that it provides greater intraoperative patient comfort and improved airway control as well as a faster onset and more controllable duration of action. Other anesthesiologists suggest that regional anesthesia is preferable for this procedure because it is associated with decreased intraoperative blood loss, a lower incidence of thromboembolic complication, and less postoperative mortality. A prospective study evaluating the influence of anesthetic technique on postoperative morbidity after radical retropubic prostatectomy randomized patients to receive epidural, general, or combined epidural-general anesthesia for their prostatectomy procedure.[281] Epidural patient-controlled analgesia was maintained in all groups for 3–5 days after the procedure. There were no differences in postoperative morbidity among the three groups. None of the patients died or experienced a major pulmonary, cardiovascular, or neurologic complication in the initial 3 months after surgery. These authors concluded that the intraoperative anesthetic technique did not influence postoperative outcome in patients undergoing radical prostatectomy. A review of the surgical literature supports this finding.[282]

Proponents of radical perineal prostatectomy claim that the perineal approach is superior to the retropubic approach to the prostate because it is associated with less intraoperative blood loss, better exposure for the vesicourethral anastomosis, and shorter convalescence times.[283] During a radical perineal prostatectomy, the patient is placed in the exaggerated lithotomy position combined with slight flexion of the trunk and a Trendelenburg tilt. This position flexes the spine and results in the sacrum and the pelvis being tilted upward so that the perineum is horizontal and parallel to the floor.[204] The exaggerated lithotomy position places the abdominal contents upon the diaphragm, which may cause respiratory embarrassment (see Chapter 24). Rhabdomyolysis with secondary ARF has also been reported after perineal prostatectomy in the exaggerated lithotomy position.[120–122,284] These reports suggest that the muscle damage is probably secondary to ischemia of the muscles in the elevated legs or the lumbar and pelvic muscles that were compressed by the exaggerated position. Because of the positioning used for radical perineal prostatectomy, most anesthesiologists prefer either general or a combined epidural-general anesthetic for the procedure.[204]

The Trendelenburg position is used during both perineal and retropubic prostatectomy procedures. This position produces physiologic changes in the respiratory, circulatory, and cerebrovascular systems in proportion to the degree of head-down tilt.[285] The head-down position induces venous distention of the upper body and jugular venous distention, which can lead to edema of the airway, tongue, and face. Airway management can be difficult if intubation becomes necessary during a prostatectomy procedure using regional anesthesia. The increase in venous pressure during Trendelenburg positioning can also increase intracranial pressure and has the potential to decrease cerebral perfusion. Therefore, this position should be avoided in patients with pre-existing elevation of intracranial pressure or glaucoma.[286] Trendelenburg positioning during prostatectomy procedures places the operative site in the pelvis above the heart, creating a gravitational gradient between the prostatic fossa and the heart. An air embolism may occur if the prostatic venous network is opened while the patient is in this position.[287,288] Some authors recommend that patients be monitored with a precordial Doppler and have a multiorificed CVP line in place for air aspiration during radical prostatectomy.

The most common intraoperative problem during radical prostatectomy is hemorrhage.[280] Massive blood loss may occur if one of the branches of the hypogastric vein is inadvertently torn during pelvic lymphadenectomy or during transection of the dorsal venous complex. The potential for rapid blood loss is high and direct arterial blood pressure monitoring is recommended, especially in elderly or high-risk patients. Hemodynamic monitoring of volume status with a CVP catheter may be necessary because the bladder is opened during the procedure, making it impossible for the anesthesiologist to evaluate fluid status with urinary output. The potential for a venous air embolism during these procedures may also necessitate the use of a CVP catheter. In patients with severe pre-existing pulmonary or cardiovascular problems, a pulmonary artery catheter may be needed accurately to assess cardiac filling pressures and hemodynamic status.

Radical Cystectomy

The standard of care for the treatment of muscle-invasive bladder cancer is a radical cystectomy.[289] In men, this surgery involves the *en bloc* removal of the bladder, prostate, seminal vesicles, and proximal urethra. In women, it is necessary to remove the bladder, urethra, and anterior vaginal wall as well as to perform a total hysterectomy and bilateral salpingo-oophorectomy. At the completion of the procedure, a urinary diversion is performed, most commonly as an ileal conduit or a colon conduit.

Patient positioning and monitoring are similar to those used during radical retropubic prostatectomy procedures. Likewise, the same intraoperative problems may occur. However, this is an intraperitoneal procedure and fluid requirements are increased, similar to a major bowel procedure. The urinary diversion also prolongs the procedure, and most anesthesiologists find that the additional length and extent of surgery mandate a general or combined general-epidural anesthetic.[204] Patients with bladder cancer may have been treated with chemotherapy before their procedure. The most commonly chemotherapeutic agents used include methotrexate, vinblastine, cisplatinum, and doxorubicin. The anesthesiologist should be aware of the previous use of any chemotherapeutic agent so that any possible drug toxicity can be elucidated. In particular, doxorubicin has cardiotoxic effects, methotrexate may cause hepatic toxicity, and both cisplatinum and methotrexate are associated with neurotoxicity and renal injury.

Radical Nephrectomy

Renal cell carcinoma accounts for ~3% of all adult malignancies.[290] Surgery is the only effective method for treating renal cell carcinoma, with radical nephrectomy the treatment of choice. This surgical procedure involves the *en bloc* removal of the kidney and surrounding fascia, the ipsilateral adrenal gland, and the upper ureter. The tumor extends into the vena cava in ~5% of patients, and aggressive surgical therapy is warranted if there is no evidence of metastasis. On occasion, CPB and circulatory arrest have been used to treat extensive caval tumor invasion.

The kidney can be approached through a lumbar, transabdominal, or thoracoabdominal incision.[204] If a lumbar approach is used, the patient is placed in the flexed lateral decubitus position with the operative side up and the kidney rest elevated beneath the 12th rib. General anesthesia or combined epidural-general anesthesia is used for patients placed in the "kidney position" because the position is extremely uncomfortable. This position may predispose patients to nerve damage or cardiopulmonary alterations (see Chapter 24). During radical nephrectomy procedures, the anesthesiologist needs to be prepared for acute blood loss because of the proximity of the kidney to large blood vessels. The patient also needs to be adequately hydrated to optimize blood flow to the remaining kidney and to prevent hypotension from inferior vena caval compression during positioning. Pneumothorax may also occur during surgery if the chest is inadvertently entered. A chest radiograph should be obtained in the postanesthesia care unit if a pneumothorax is suspected. Venous air embolisms are also possible during nephrectomy procedures if the positioning places the operative site above the heart.

Radical Surgery for Testicular Cancer

Although testicular cancer accounts for only 1% of all cancers in men, it is the most common malignancy in men between 15 and 34 years of age.[291] All intratesticular masses are considered cancer until proven otherwise, and radical orchiectomy is performed for both definitive diagnosis and as the initial step of most treatment regimens. Either regional or general anesthesia can be used for this surgical procedure.

Subsequent treatment depends on the stage and histology of the testicular tumor. Potential treatment options include observation, radiation to the inguinal and retroperitoneal areas, chemotherapy, or retroperitoneal lymph node dissection. Because chemotherapy regimens change frequently, the National Cancer Institute's CancerNet Internet site (http://cancernet.nci.nih.gov) carries the current treatment protocols for each type and stage of testicular cancer. Prior to surgery, the anesthesiologist should identify the chemotherapeutic agents used and be aware of the side effects of these drugs. One commonly used chemotherapeutic agent, bleomycin, is an antitumor antibiotic used against germ cell tumors of the testis. Its use is associated with pulmonary toxicity and there are numerous reports of postoperative respiratory failure after retroperitoneal lymph node dissection in patients treated with bleomycin.[292-294] The onset of respiratory failure usually occurs 3–10 days after surgery. Risk factors for postoperative respiratory distress include preoperative evidence of pulmonary injury, recent exposure to bleomycin (within 1 to 2 months), a total dose of bleomycin >450 mg, or a Ccr of <35 ml · min^{-1}.[293] Although intraoperative exposure to hyperoxia (inspired oxygen concentrations >30%) has been linked to postoperative pulmonary toxicity, this relationship is controversial.[292,293] A retrospective study found that iv fluid management, including blood transfusion, was the most significant factor affecting postoperative pulmonary morbidity and clinical outcome.[292] These authors recommended that iv fluid administration should primarily consist of colloid administration and be limited to the minimum volume necessary to maintain hemodynamic stability and adequate renal output.

REFERENCES

1. Guyton AC: Formation of urine by the kidney: Renal blood flow, glomerular filtration, and their control. In Guyton AC (ed): Textbook of Medical Physiology, 8th ed, p 286. Philadelphia, WB Saunders, 1991
2. Brezis M, Rosen S: Hypoxia of the renal medulla: Its implications for disease. N Engl J Med 332:647, 1995
3. Awazu M, Ichikawa I: Biological significance of atrial natriuretic peptide in the kidney. Nephron 63:1, 1993
4. Espiner EA: Physiology of natriuretic peptides. J Intern Med 235:527, 1994
5. McIntyre RW, Schwin DA: Atrial natriuretic peptide. J Cardiothorac Anesth 3:91, 1989
6. Gabbai FB, Blantz RC: Role of nitric oxide in renal hemodynamics. Semin Nephrol 19:242, 1999
7. Mené P, Dunn MJ: Vascular, glomerular, and tubular effects of angiotensin II, kinins, and prostaglandins. In Seldin DW, Giesbisch G (eds): The Kidney: Physiology and Pathophysiology, 2nd ed, p 1205. New York, Raven Press, 1992
8. Satoh S, Zimmerman BG: Influence of the renin-angiotensin system on the effect of prostaglandin synthesis inhibitors in the renal vasculature. Circ Res 36(suppl 1):89, 1975
9. Silva P, Rosen S, Spokes K et al: Influence of endogenous prostaglandins on mTAL injury. J Am Soc Nephrol 1:808, 1990
10. Badr KF, Ichikawa I: Prerenal failure: A deleterious shift from renal compensation to decompensation. N Engl J Med 319: 623, 1988
11. Crandell WB, Pappas SG, MacDonald A: Nephrotoxicity associated with methoxyflurane anesthesia. Anesthesiology 27:591, 1966
12. Kharasch ED, Hankins DC, Thummel KE: Human kidney methoxyflurane and sevoflurane metabolism. Anesthesiology 82:689, 1995
13. Mazze RI, Calverley RK, Smith NT: Inorganic fluoride nephrotoxicity: Prolonged enflurane and halothane anesthesia in volunteers. Anesthesiology 46:265, 1977
14. Mazze RI, Sievenpiper TS, Stevenson J: Renal effects of enflurane and halothane in patients with abnormal renal function. Anesthesiology 60:161, 1984
15. Priano LL: The effects of anesthetic agents on renal function. In Barash PG (ed): ASA Refresher Courses in Anesthesiology, p 240. Philadelphia, JB Lippincott, 1985
16. Halperin BD, Feeley TW: The effect of anesthesia and surgery on renal function. Int Anesthesiol Clin 22:157, 1984
17. Anderson RJ, Linas SL, Berns AS et al: Nonoliguric acute renal failure. N Engl J Med 296:1134, 1977
18. Firmat J, Zucchini A, Martin R, Aguirre C: A study of 500 cases of acute renal failure (1978-1991). Ren Fail 16:91, 1994
19. Fry ED, Pearlstein L, Fulton RL, Polk HC: Multiple system organ failure. Arch Surg 115:136, 1980
20. Wardle EN: Acute renal failure and multiorgan failure. Nephron 66:380, 1994
21. Moore FA, Moore EE: Evolving concepts in the pathogenesis of postinjury multiple organ failure. Surg Clin North Am 75:257, 1995
22. Baudouin SV, Wiggins J, Koegh BF et al: Continuous veno-venous haemofiltration following cardio-pulmonary bypass. Intensive Care Med 19:290, 1993
23. Cameron JS: Acute renal failure in the intensive care unit today. Intensive Care Med 12:64, 1986
24. Olsen PS, Schroeder T, Perko M et al: Renal failure after operation for abdominal aortic aneurysm. Ann Vas Surg 4:580, 1990
25. Storck M, Hartl WH, Zimmerer E, Inthorn D: Comparison of pump-driven and spontaneous continuous haemofiltration in postoperative acute renal failure. Lancet 337:452, 1991
26. Gordon AC, Pryn S, Collin J et al: Outcome in patients who require renal support after surgery for ruptured abdominal aortic aneurysm. Br J Surg 81:836, 1994
27. Tominaga GT, Ingegno MD, Scannell G et al: Continuous arteriovenous hemodiafiltration in postoperative and traumatic renal failure. Am J Surg 166:612, 1993
28. Bellomo R, Farmer M, Boyce N: A prospective study of continuous venovenous hemodiafiltration in critically ill patients with acute renal failure. Journal of Intensive Care Medicine 10:187, 1995
29. Pellanda MV, Fabris A, Ronco C: Etiology and pathophysiology of acute renal failure. In Pinsky MR, Dhainaut JFA (eds): Pathophysiologic Foundations of Critical Care, p 571. Baltimore, Williams & Wilkins, 1993
30. Kellen M, Aronson S, Roizen MF et al: Predictive and diagnostic tests of renal failure: A review. Anesth Analg 78:134, 1994
31. Desjars P, Pinaud M, Bugnon D, Tasseau F: Norepinephrine therapy has no deleterious renal effects in human septic shock. Crit Care Med 17:426, 1989
32. Martin C, Papazian L, Perrin G et al: Norepinephrine or dopamine for the treatment of hyperdynamic septic shock? Chest 103:1826, 1993
33. Vincent JL, Preiser JC: Inotropic agents. New Horiz 1:137, 1993
34. Martinez-Maldonado M, Benabe JE, Cordova HR: Chronic clinical intrinsic renal failure. In Seldin DW, Giebisch (eds): The Kidney: Physiology and Pathophysiology, 2nd ed, p 3227. New York, Raven Press, 1992
35. Kuruvila KC, Schrier RW: Chronic renal failure. Int Anesthesiol Clin 22:101, 1984
36. Sieberth HG, Mann H, Kierdorf H: Acute complications in patients with chronic renal failure. In Pinsky MR, Dhainaut JFA (eds): Pathophysiologic Foundations of Critical Care, p 677. Baltimore, Williams & Wilkins, 1993
37. Eschbach JW: The anemia of chronic renal failure: Pathophysiology and the effects of recombinant erythropoietin. Kidney Int 35:134, 1989
38. Touchette MA, Slaughter RL: The effect of renal failure on hepatic drug clearance. Ann Pharmacother 25:1214, 1991
39. Sear JW: Kidney transplants: Induction and analgesic agents. Int Anesthesiol Clin 33:45, 1995

40. St. Peter WL, Halstenson CE: Pharmacologic approach in patients with renal failure. In Chernow B (ed): The Pharmacologic Approach to the Critically Ill Patient, 3rd ed, p 41. Baltimore, Williams & Wilkins, 1994

41. Burch PG, Stanski DR: Decreased protein binding and thiopental kinetics. Clin Pharmacol Ther 32:212, 1982

42. Trevor AJ: Biotransformation of ketamine. In Domino EF (ed): Status of Ketamine in Anesthesiology, p 93, Ann Arbor, Michigan, NPP Books, 1990

43. Reich DL, Silvay G: Ketamine: An update on the first twenty-five years of clinical experience. Can J Anaesth 36:186, 1989

44. White PF, Way WL, Trevor AJ: Ketamine: Its pharmacology and therapeutic uses. Anesthesiology 56:119, 1982

45. Carlos R, Calvo R, Erill S: Plasma protein binding of etomidate in patients with renal failure or hepatic cirrhosis. Clin Pharmacokinet 4:144, 1979

46. Morcos WE, Payne JP: The induction of anaesthesia with propofol (Diprivan) compared in normal and renal failure patients. Postgrad Med J 61(suppl 3):62, 1985

47. Kirvelä M, Olkkola KT, Rosenberg PH et al: Pharmacokinetics of propofol and haemodynamic changes during induction of anaesthesia in uraemic patients. Br J Anaesth 68:178, 1992

48. Ickx B, Cockshott ID, Barvais L et al: Propofol infusion for induction and maintenance of anaesthesia in patients with end-stage renal disease. Br J Anaesth 81:854, 1998

49. Vinik HR, Reves JG, Greenblatt DJ et al: The pharmacokinetics of midazolam in chronic renal failure patients. Anesthesiology 59:390, 1983

50. Driessen JJ, Vree TB, Guelen PJM: The effects of acute changes in renal function on the pharmacokinetics of midazolam during long-term infusion in ICU patients. Acta Anaesthesiol Belg 42:149, 1991

51. Schmith VD, Piraino B, Smith RB, Kroboth PD: Alprazolam in end-stage renal disease: II. Pharmacodynamics. Clin Pharmacol Ther 51:533, 1992

52. Chan GLC, Matzke GR: Effects of renal insufficiency on the pharmacokinetics and pharmacodynamics of opioid analgesics. Ann Pharmacother 21:773, 1987

53. Babul N, Darke AC, Hagen N: Hydromorphone metabolite accumulation in renal failure (letter). J Pain Symptom Manage 10:184, 1995

54. Kirvelä M, Lindgren L, Seppala T, Olkkola KT: The pharmacokinetics of oxycodone in uremic patients undergoing renal transplantation. J Clin Anesth 8:13, 1996

55. Koehntop DE, Rodman JH: Fentanyl pharmacokinetics in patients undergoing renal transplantation. Pharmacotherapy 17:746, 1997

56. Chauvin M, Lebrault C, Levron JC, Duvaldestin P: Pharmacokinetics of alfentanil in chronic renal failure. Anesth Analg 66:53, 1987

57. Davis PJ, Stiller RL, Cook DR et al: Effects of cholestatic hepatic disease and chronic renal failure on alfentanil pharmacokinetics in children. Anesth Analg 68:579, 1989

58. Wiggum DC, Cork RC, Weldon ST et al: Postoperative respiratory depression and elevated sufentanil levels in a patient with chronic renal failure. Anesthesiology 63:708, 1985

59. Hoke JF, Shlugman D, Dershwitz M et al: Pharmacokinetics of remifentanil in persons with renal failure compared with healthy volunteers. Anesthesiology 87:533, 1997

60. Smith CE, Hunter JM: Anesthesia for renal transplantation: Relaxants and volatiles. Int Anesthesiol Clin 33:69, 1995

61. Thomas JL, Holmes JH: Effect of hemodialysis on plasma cholinesterase. Anesth Analg 49:323, 1970

62. Wyant GM: The anaesthetist looks at tissue transplantation: Three years experience with kidney transplants. Can J Anaesth 14:255, 1967

63. Ryan DW: Preoperative serum cholinesterase concentration in chronic renal failure. Br J Anaesth 49:945, 1977

64. Cook DR, Freeman JA, Lai AA et al: Pharmacokinetics of mivacurium in normal patients and in those with hepatic or renal failure. Br J Anaesth 69:580, 1992

65. Phillips BJ, Hunter JM: Use of mivacurium chloride by constant infusion in the anephric patient. Br J Anaesth 68:492, 1992

66. Miller RD, Way WL, Hamilton WK et al: Succinylcholine induced hyperkalemia in patients with renal failure? Anesthesiology 36:138, 1972

67. Koide M, Waud BE: Serum potassium concentrations after succinylcholine in patients with renal failure. Anesthesiology 36:142, 1972

68. Cook DR, Freeman JA, Lai AA et al: Pharmacokinetics and pharmacodynamics of doxacurium in normal patients and in those with hepatic or renal failure. Anesth Analg 72:145, 1991

69. Cashman JN, Luke JJ, Jones RM: Neuromuscular block with doxacurium (BW A938U) in patients with normal or absent renal function. Br J Anaesth 64:186, 1990

70. Caldwell JE, Canfell PC, Castagnoli KP et al: The influence of renal failure on the pharmacokinetics and duration of action of pipecuronium bromide in patients anesthetized with halothane and nitrous oxide. Anesthesiology 70:7, 1989

71. Weirda JMKH, Szenohradszky J, Dewit APM et al: The pharmacokinetics, urinary and biliary excretion of pipecuronium bromide. Eur J Anaesthesiol 8:451, 1991

72. Boyd AH, Eastwood NB, Parker CJR, Hunter JM: Pharmacodynamics of the 1R cis-1′R cis isomer of atracurium (51W89) in health and chronic renal failure. Br J Anaesth 74:400, 1995

73. Fahey MR, Rupp SM, Fisher DM et al: The pharmacokinetics and pharmacodynamics of atracurium in patients with and without renal failure. Anesthesiology 61:699, 1984

74. Fahey MR, Rupp SM, Canfell C et al: Effect of renal failure on laudanosine excretion in man. Br J Anaesth 57:1049, 1985

75. Yate PM, Flynn PJ, Arnold RW et al: Clinical experience and plasma laudanosine concentration during the infusion of atracurium in the intensive therapy unit. Br J Anaesth 59:211, 1987

76. Eastwood NB, Boyd AH, Parker CJ, Hunter JM: Pharmacokinetics of 1R-cis 1′R-cis atracurium besylate (51W89) and plasma laudanosine concentrations in health and chronic renal failure. Br J Anaesth 75:431, 1995

77. Bencini AF, Scaf AHJ, Sohn YJ et al: Disposition and urinary excretion of vecuronium bromide in anesthetized patients with normal renal function or renal failure. Anesth Analg 65:245, 1986

78. Lynam DP, Cronnelly R, Castagnoli KP et al: The pharmacodynamics and pharmacokinetics of vecuronium in patients anesthetized with isoflurane with normal renal function or with renal failure. Anesthesiology 69:227, 1988

79. Segredo V, Caldwell JE, Matthay MA et al: Persistent paralysis in critically ill patients after long-term administration of vecuronium. N Engl J Med 327:524, 1992

80. Wierda JMKH, Kleef UW, Lambalk LM et al: The pharmacodynamics and pharmacokinetics of Org 9426, a new non-depolarizing neuromuscular blocking agent, in patients anaesthetized with nitrous oxide, halothane and fentanyl. Can J Anaesth 38:430, 1991

81. Szenohradszky J, Fisher DM, Segredo V et al: Pharmacokinetics of rocuronium bromide (ORG 9426) in patients with normal renal function or patients undergoing cadaver renal transplantation. Anesthesiology 77:899, 1992

82. Cooper RA, Maddineni VR, Mirakhur RK et al: Time course of neuromuscular effects and pharmacokinetics of rocuronium bromide (ORG 9426) during isoflurane anaesthesia in patients with and without renal failure. Br J Anaesth 71:222, 1993

83. Khuenl-Brady KS, Pomaroli A, Pühringer F et al: The use of rocuronium (ORG 9426) in patients with chronic renal failure. Anaesthesia 48:873, 1993

84. Blobner M, Jelen-Esselborn S, Schneider G et al: Effect of renal function on neuromuscular block induced by continuous infusion of mivacurium. Br J Anaesth 74:452, 1995

85. Mangar D, Kirchhoff GT, Rose PL, Castellano FC: Prolonged neuromuscular block with mivacurium in a patient with end-stage renal disease. Anesth Analg 76:866, 1993

86. Schiere S, Proost JH, Schuringa M, Wierda JM: Pharmacokinetics and pharmacokinetic-dynamic relationship between rapacuronium (Org 9487) and its 3-desacetyl metabolite (Org 9488). Anesth Analg 88:640, 1999

87. Szenohradszky J, Caldwell JE, Wright PM et al: Influence of renal failure on the pharmacokinetics and neuromuscular effects of a single dose of rapacuronium bromide. Anesthesiology 90:24, 1999

88. Cronnelly R, Stanski DR, Miller RD et al: Renal function and the pharmacokinetics of neostigmine in anesthetized man. Anesthesiology 51:222, 1979

89. Cronnelly R, Stanski DR, Miller RD, Sheiner LB: Pyridostigmine kinetics with and without renal function. Clin Pharmacol Ther 28:78, 1980

90. Morris RB, Cronnelly R, Miller RD et al: Pharmacokinetics of edrophonium in anephric and renal transplant patients. Br J Anaesth 53:1311, 1981

91. Ali-Melkkilä T, Kanto J, Iisalo E: Pharmacokinetics and related pharmacodynamics of anticholinergic drugs. Acta Anaesthesiol Scand 37:633, 1993

92. Novis BK, Roizen MF, Aronson S, Thisted RA: Association of preoperative risk factors with postoperative acute renal failure. Anesth Analg 78:143, 1994

93. Shusterman N, Strom BL, Murray TG et al: Risk factors and outcome of hospital-acquired acute renal failure. Am J Med 83:65, 1987

94. Stene JK: Renal failure in the trauma patient. Crit Care Clin 6: 111, 1990

95. Quezado ZMN, Natanson C: Systemic hemodynamic abnormalities and vasopressor therapy in sepsis and septic shock. Am J Kidney Dis 20:214, 1992

96. Badr KF: Sepsis-associated renal vasoconstriction: Potential targets for future therapy. Am J Kidney Dis 20:207, 1992

97. Zager RA: Endotoxemia, renal hypoperfusion, and fever: Interactive risk factors for aminoglycoside and sepsis-associated acute renal failure. Am J Kidney Dis 20:223, 1992

98. Dawson JL: The incidence of postoperative renal failure in obstructive jaundice. Br J Surg 52:663, 1965

99. Blamey SL, Fearon KCH, Gilmour WH et al: Prediction of risk in biliary surgery. Br J Surg 70:535, 1983

100. Ring-Larsen H: Associated renal failure. In Williams R (ed): Liver Failure, p 72. New York, Churchill Livingstone, 1986

101. Rimola A, Gavaler JS, Schade RR et al: Effects of renal impairment on liver transplantation. Gastroenterology 93:148, 1987

102. Cuervas-Mons V, Millan I, Gavaler JS et al: Prognostic value of preoperatively obtained clinical and laboratory data in predicting survival following orthotopic liver transplantation. Hepatology 6: 922, 1986

103. Lindeman RD: Overview: Renal physiology and pathophysiology of aging. Am J Kidney Dis 16:275, 1990

104. Shin B, Mackenzie CF, Helrich M: Creatinine clearance for early detection of posttraumatic renal dysfunction. Anesthesiology 64: 605, 1986

105. Wilson RF, Soullier G, Antonenko D: Creatinine clearance in critically ill surgical patients. Arch Surg 114:461, 1979

106. Sladen RN, Endo E, Harrison T: Two-hour versus 22-hour creatinine clearance in critically ill patients. Anesthesiology 67:1013, 1987

107. Aronson S, Thistlewaite RJ, Walker R et al: Safety and feasibility of renal blood flow determination during kidney transplant surgery with perfusion ultrasonography. Anesth Analg 80:353, 1995

108. Taylor GA, Barnewolt CE, Adler BH, Dunning PS: Renal cortical ischemia in rabbits revealed by contrast-enhanced power Doppler sonography. AJR 170:417, 1998

109. Rabito CA, Panico F, Rubin R et al: Noninvasive, real-time monitoring of renal function during critical care. J Am Soc Nephrol 4:1421, 1994

110. Haug CE, Lopez IA, Moore RH et al: Real-time monitoring of renal function during ischemic injury in the rhesus monkey. Ren Fail 17:489, 1995

111. Bauman LA, Watson NE Jr, Scuderi PE, Peters MA: Transcutaneous renal function monitor: precision during unsteady hemodynamics. J Clin Monit Comput 14:275, 1998

112. Walker RS, Duggin GG: Cellular mechanisms of drug nephrotoxicity. In Seldin DW, Giebisch G (eds): The Kidney: Physiology and Pathophysiology, 2nd ed, p 3571. New York, Raven Press, 1992

113. Hock R, Anderson RJ: Prevention of drug-induced nephrotoxicity in the intensive care unit. J Crit Care 10:33, 1995

114. Wilkinson AH, Cohen DJ: Renal failure in the recipients of nonrenal solid organ transplants. J Am Soc Nephrol 10:1136, 1999

115. Barrett BJ: Contrast nephrotoxicity. J Am Soc Nephrol 5:125, 1994

116. Garella S, Matarese RA: Renal effects of prostaglandins and clinical adverse effects of nonsteroidal anti-inflammatory agents. Medicine (Baltimore) 63:165, 1984

117. Quan DJ, Kayser SR: Ketorolac induced acute renal failure following a single dose. J Toxicol Clin Toxicol 32:305, 1994

118. Abassi ZA, Hoffman A, Better OS: Acute renal failure complicating muscle crush injury. Semin Nephrol 18:558, 1998

119. Dubrow A, Flamenbaum W: Acute renal failure associated with myoglobinuria and hemoglobinuria. In Brenner BM, Lazarus JM (eds): Acute Renal Failure, 2nd ed, p 279. New York, Churchill Livingstone, 1988

120. Ali H, Nieto JG, Rhamy RK et al: Acute renal failure due to rhabdomyolysis associated with the extreme lithotomy position. Am J Kidney Dis 22:865, 1993

121. Gabrielli A, Caruso L: Postoperative acute renal failure secondary to rhabdomyolysis from exaggerated lithotomy position. J Clin Anesth 11:257, 1999

122. Guzzi LM, Mills LM, Greenman P: Rhabdomyolysis, acute renal failure, and the exaggerated lithotomy position. Anesth Analg 77: 635, 1993

123. Uratsuji Y, Ijichi K, Irie J et al: Rhabdomyolysis after abdominal surgery in the hyperlordotic position enforced by pneumatic support. Anesthesiology 91:310, 1999

124. Veenstra J, Smit WM, Krediet RT, Arisz L: Relationship between elevated creatine phosphokinase and the clinical spectrum of rhabdomyolysis. Nephrol Dial Transplant 9:637, 1994

125. Better OS, Stein JH: Early management of shock and prophylaxis of acute renal failure in traumatic rhabdomyolysis. N Engl J Med 322:825, 1990

126. Sirinek KR, Hura CE: Renal failure. In Moore EE, Mattox KL, Feliciano DV (eds): Trauma, 2nd ed, p 927. Norwalk, Connecticut, Appleton & Lange, 1991

127. Baxter CR: Acute renal insufficiency complicating trauma and surgery. In Shires GT (ed): Principles of Trauma Care, 3rd ed, p 502. New York, McGraw-Hill, 1985

128. Cachecho R, Millham FH, Wedel SK: Management of the trauma patient with pre-existing renal disease. Crit Care Clin 10:523, 1994

129. Myers BD, Miller DC, Mehigan JT et al: Nature of the renal injury following total renal ischemia in man. J Clin Invest 73:329, 1984

130. Godet G, Fleron MH, Vicaut E et al: Risk factors for acute postoperative renal failure in thoracic or thoracoabdominal aortic surgery: a prospective study. Anesth Analg 85:1227, 1997

131. Baker AB, Lloyd G, Fraser TA et al: Retrospective review of 100 cases of endoluminal aortic stent-graft surgery from an anaesthetic perspective. Anaesth Intensive Care 25:378, 1997

132. Walker SR, Yusuf SW, Wenham PW, Hopkinson BR: Renal complications following endovascular repair of abdominal aortic aneurysms. J Endovasc Surg 5:318, 1998

133. Svensson LG, Coselli JS, Safi HJ et al: Appraisal of adjuncts to prevent acute renal failure after surgery on the thoracic or thoracoabdominal aorta. J Vasc Surg 10:230, 1989

134. Hollier LH, Moore WM: Avoidance of renal and neurologic complications following thoracoabdominal aortic aneurysm repair. Acta Chir Scand Suppl 555:129, 1990

135. Welch M, Knight DG, Carr HMH et al: The preservation of renal function by isovolemic hemodilution during aortic operations. J Vasc Surg 18:858, 1993

136. Paul MD, Mazer CD, Byrick RJ et al: Influence of mannitol and dopamine on renal function during elective infrarenal aortic clamping in man. Am J Nephrol 6:427, 1986

137. Pass LJ, Eberhart RC, Brown JC et al: The effect of mannitol and dopamine on the renal response to thoracic aortic cross-clamping. J Thorac Cardiovasc Surg 95:608, 1988

138. Baldwin L, Henderson A, Hickman P: Effect of postoperative low-dose dopamine on renal function after elective major vascular surgery. Ann Intern Med 120:744, 1994

139. Flancbaum L, Choban PS, Dasta JF: Quantitative effects of low-dose dopamine on urine output in oliguric surgical intensive care unit patients. Crit Care Med 22:61, 1994

140. Antonucci F, Calò L, Rizzolo M et al: Nifedipine can preserve renal function in patients undergoing aortic surgery with infrarenal cross-clamping. Nephron 74:668, 1996

141. Ding H, Kopple JD, Cohen A, Hirschberg R: Recombinant human insulin-like growth factor-I accelerates recovery and reduces catabolism in rats with ischemic acute renal failure. J Clin Invest 91: 2281, 1993

142. Vijayan A, Franklin SC, Behrend T et al: Insulin-like growth factor I improves renal function in patients with end-stage chronic renal failure. Am J Physiol 276:R929, 1999

143. Franklin SC, Moulton M, Sicard GA et al: Insulin-like growth factor I preserves renal function postoperatively. Am J Physiol 272:F257, 1997

144. Allgren RL, Marbury TC, Rahman SN et al: Anaritide in acute tubular necrosis: Auriculin Anaritide Acute Renal Failure Study Group. N Engl J Med 336:828, 1997

145. Singer I, Epstein M: Potential of dopamine A-1 agonists in the management of acute renal failure. Am J Kidney Dis 31:743, 1998

146. Abel RM, Buckley MJ, Austen WG et al: Etiology, incidence, and

prognosis of renal failure following cardiac operations. J Thorac Cardiovasc Surg 71:323, 1976

147. Anderson LG, Ekroth R, Bratteby LE et al: Acute renal failure after coronary surgery: A study of incidence and risk factors in 2009 consecutive patients. Thorac Cardiovasc Surg 41:237, 1993

148. Zanardo G, Michielon P, Paccagnella A et al: Acute renal failure in the patient undergoing cardiac operations: Prevalence, mortality rate and main risk factors. J Thorac Cardiovasc Surg 107:1489, 1994

149. Mangano CM, Diamondstone LS, Ramsay JG et al: Renal dysfunction after myocardial revascularization: Risk factors, adverse outcomes, and hospital resource utilization. The Multicenter Study of Perioperative Ischemia Research Group. Ann Intern Med 128:194, 1998

150. Conlon PJ, Stafford-Smith M, White WD et al: Acute renal failure following cardiac surgery. Nephrol Dial Transplant 14:1158, 1999

151. Anderson RJ, O'Brien M, MaWhinney S et al: Renal failure predisposes patients to adverse outcome after coronary artery bypass surgery. VA Cooperative Study #5. Kidney Int 55:1057, 1999

152. Hilberman M, Myers BD, Carrie BJ et al: Acute renal failure following cardiac surgery. J Thorac Cardiovasc Surg 77:880, 1979

153. Hilberman M, Derby GC, Spencer RJ, Stinson EB: Sequential pathophysiological changes characterizing the progression from renal dysfunction to acute renal failure following cardiac operation. J Thorac Cardiovasc Surg 79:838, 1980

154. Ascione R, Lloyd CT, Underwood MJ et al: On-pump versus off-pump coronary revascularization: evaluation of renal function. Ann Thorac Surg 68:493, 1999

155. Hilberman M: The kidneys: Function, failure, and protection in the perioperative period. In Ream AK, Fogdall RP (eds): Acute Cardiovascular Management Anesthesia and Intensive Care, p 806. Philadelphia, JB Lippincott, 1982

156. Costa P, Ottino GM, Matani A et al: Low-dose dopamine during cardiopulmonary bypass in patients with renal dysfunction. J Cardiothorac Anesth 4:469, 1990

157. Myles PS, Buckland MR, Schenk NJ et al: Effect of "renal-dose" dopamine on renal function following cardiac surgery. Anaesth Intensive Care 21:56, 1993

158. Chiolero R, Borgeat A, Fisher A: Postoperative arrhythmias and risk factors after open heart surgery. Thorac Cardiovasc Surg 39:81, 1991

159. Berendes E, Mullhoff T, Van Aken H et al: Effects of dopexamine on creatinine clearance, systemic inflammation, and splanchnic oxygenation in patients undergoing coronary artery bypass grafting. Anesth Analg 84:950, 1997

160. Pascual E, Gomez-Arnau J, Pensado A et al: Incidence and risk factors of early acute renal failure in liver transplant patients. Transplant Proc 25:1837, 1993

161. Haller M, Schönfelder R, Briegel J et al: Renal function in the postoperative period after orthotopic liver transplantation. Transplant Proc 24:2704, 1992

162. Brown RS Jr, Lombardero M, Lake JR: Outcome of patients with renal insufficiency undergoing liver or liver-kidney transplantation. Transplantation 27:1788, 1996

163. Fraley DS, Burr R, Bernardini J et al: Impact of acute renal failure on mortality in end-stage liver disease with or without transplantation. Kidney Int 54:518, 1998

164. Polson RJ, Park GR, Lindop MJ et al: The prevention of renal impairment in patients undergoing orthotopic liver grafting by infusion of low dose dopamine. Anaesthesia 42:15, 1987

165. Swygert TH, Roberts LC, Valek TR et al: Effect of intraoperative low-dose dopamine on renal function in liver transplant recipients. Anesthesiology 75:571, 1991

166. Parks RW, Diamond T, McCrory DC et al: Prospective study of postoperative renal function in obstructive jaundice and the effect of perioperative dopamine. Br J Surg 81:437, 1994

167. Clayman RV, Kavoussi LR: Endosurgical techniques for the diagnosis and treatment of noncalculous disease of the ureter and kidney. In Walsh PC, Retik AB, Stamey TA, Vaughan ED Jr. (eds): Campbell's Urology, 6th ed, p 2231. Philadelphia, WB Saunders, 1992

168. Kennedy TJ, Preminger GM: Flexible cystoscopy. Urol Clin North Am 15:525, 1988

169. Clayman RV: Diagnostic and therapeutic applications of outpatient cystourethroscopy. In Kaye KW (ed): Outpatient Urologic Surgery, p 111. Philadelphia, Lea & Febiger, 1985

170. Monk TG: Clinical applications of monitored anaesthesia care. Minimally Invasive Therapy 3(suppl 2):17, 1994

171. Schow DA, Jackson TL, Samson JM et al: Use of intravenous alfentanil-midazolam anesthesia for sedation during brief endourologic procedures. J Endourol 8:33, 1994

172. Jenstrup M, Fruergaard KO, Mortensen CR: Pollution with nitrous oxide using laryngeal mask or face mask. Acta Anaesthesiol Scand 43:663, 1999

173. Huffman JL: Ureteroscopy. In Walsh PC, Retik AB, Stamey TA, Vaughan ED Jr. (eds): Campbell's Urology, 6th ed, p 2195. Philadelphia, WB Saunders, 1992

174. Kahn RI: Outpatient endourologic procedures. Urol Clin North Am 14:77, 1987

175. Walsh PC: Benign prostatic hyperplasia. In Walsh PC, Retik AB, Stamey TA, Vaughan ED Jr. (eds): Campbell's Urology, 6th ed, p 1009. Philadelphia, WB Saunders, 1992

176. Riehmann M, Bruskewitz R: Evaluation of benign prostatic hyperplasia. In Bahnson RR (ed): Management of Urologic Disorders, p 1.2. London, Wolfe, 1994

177. Freiha FS, Deem S, Pearl RG: Urology: Transurethral resection of the prostate (TURP). In Jaffe RA, Samuels SI (eds): Anesthesiologist's Manual of Surgical Procedures, p 553. New York, Raven Press, 1994

178. Hatch PD: Surgical and anaesthetic considerations in transurethral resection of the prostate. Anaesth Intensive Care 15:203, 1987

179. Jensen V: The TURP syndrome. Can J Anaesth 38:90, 1991

180. Krongrad A, Droller MJ: Complications of transurethral resection of the prostate. In Marshall FF (ed): Urologic Complications: Medical and Surgical, Adult and Pediatric, 2nd ed, p 305. St. Louis, Mosby-Year Book, 1990

181. Marx GF, Orkin LR: Complications associated with transurethral surgery. Anesthesiology 23:802, 1962

182. Emmett JL, Gilbaugh JH Jr., McLean P: Fluid absorption during transurethral resection: Comparison of mortality and morbidity after irrigation with water and non-hemolytic solutions. J Urol 101:884, 1969

183. McDougal WS: Perioperative Care. In Gillenwater JY, Grayhack JT, Howards SS, Duckett JW (eds): Adult and Pediatric Urology, 2nd ed, p 445. St. Louis, Mosby Year Book, 1991

184. Roesch RP, Stoelting RK, Lingeman JE et al: Ammonia toxicity resulting from glycine absorption during a transurethral resection of the prostate. Anesthesiology 58:577, 1983

185. Hoekstra PT, Kahnoski R, McCamish MA et al: Transurethral prostatic resection syndrome-a new perspective: Encephalopathy with associated hyperammonemia. J Urol 130:704, 1983

186. Fitzpatrick JM, Kasidas GP, Rose GA: Hyperoxaluria following glycine irrigation for transurethral prostatectomy. Br J Urol 53:250, 1981

187. Ovassapian A, Joshi CW, Brunner EA: Visual disturbances: An unusual symptom of transurethral prostatic resection reaction. Anesthesiology 57:332, 1982

188. Barletta JP, Fanous MM, Hamed LM: Temporary blindness in the TUR syndrome. J Neuroophthalmol 14:6, 1994

189. Wang JM, Wong KC, Creel DJ et al: Effects of glycine on hemodynamic responses and visual evoked potentials in the dog. Anaesth Analg 64:1071, 1985

190. Hahn G: The transurethral resection syndrome. Acta Anaesthesiol Scand 35:557, 1991

191. Agin C: Anesthesia for transurethral prostate surgery. In Lebowitz PW (ed): Anesthesia for Urological Surgery, p 25. Boston, Little, Brown, 1993

192. Gravenstein D: Transurethral resection of the prostate (TURP) syndrome: a review of the pathophysiology and management. Anesth Analg 84:438, 1997

193. Rippa A: Transurethral resection of the prostate: aids and accessories. In Smith AD (ed): Smith's Textbook of Endourology, p 1190. St. Louis, Quality Medical, 1996

194. Hahn R, Mjöberg M: Immediate detection of irrigant absorption during transurethral prostatectomy: Case report. Can J Anaesth 36:86, 1989

195. Hahn RG, Larsson H, Ribbe T: Continuous monitoring of irrigating fluid absorption during transurethral surgery. Anaesthesia 50:327, 1995

196. Henderson DJ, Middleton RG: Coma from hyponatremia following transurethral resection of prostate. Urology 15:267, 1980

197. Narins RG: Therapy of hyponatremia: Does haste make waste? N Engl J Med 314:1573, 1986

198. Black RM: Disorders of plasma sodium and plasma potassium. In

Rippe JM, Irwin RS, Alpert JS, Fink MP (eds): Intensive Care Medicine, 2nd ed, p 794. Boston, Little, Brown, 1991

199. Mebust WK, Holtgrewe HL, Cockett ATK, Peters PC: Transurethral prostatectomy: Immediate and postoperative complications. A cooperative study of 13 participating institutions evaluating 3,885 patients. J Urol 141:243, 1989

200. Ansell JE: Acquired bleeding disorders. In Rippe JM, Irwin RS, Alpert JS, Fink MP (eds): Intensive Care Medicine, 2nd ed, p 1013. Boston, Little, Brown, 1991

201. Elliot JS, McDonald JK, Fowell AH: Blood loss and fibrinolysin levels during transurethral prostatic resection. J Urol 89:62, 1963

202. Allen TD: Body temperature changes during prostatic resection as related to the temperature of the irrigating solution. J Urol 110:443, 1973

203. Heathcote PS, Dyer PM: The effect of warm irrigation on blood loss during transurethral prostatectomy under spinal anaesthesia. Br J Urol 58:669, 1986

204. Raj PP, Gesund P, Phero J et al: Rationale and choice for surgical procedures. In Raj PP (ed): Clinical Practice of Regional Anesthesia, p 197. New York, Churchill Livingstone, 1991

205. Abrams PH, Shah PJR, Bryning K et al: Blood loss during transurethral resection of the prostate. Anaesthesia 37:71, 1982

206. Mackenzie AR: Influence of anaesthesia on blood loss in transurethral prostatectomy. Scot Med J 35:1, 1990

207. McGowan SW, Smith GFN: Anaesthesia for transurethral prostatectomy. Anaesthesia 35:847, 1980

208. Nielsen KK, Anderson K, Asbjfrn J et al: Blood loss in transurethral prostatectomy: Epidural versus general anaesthesia. Int Urol Nephrol 19:287, 1987

209. Bowman GW, Hoerth JW, McGlothlen JS et al: Anesthesia for transurethral resection of the prostate: Spinal or general? Journal of the American Association of Nurse Anesthetists 49:63, 1981

210. Chung FF, Chung A, Meier RH et al: Comparison of perioperative mental function after general anaesthesia and spinal anaesthesia with intravenous sedation. Can J Anaesth 36:382, 1989

211. Ghoneim MM, Hinrichs JV, O'Hara MW et al: Comparison of psychologic and cognitive functions after general or regional anesthesia. Anesthesiology 69:507, 1988

212. Hosking MP, Lobdell CM, Warner MA et al: Anaesthesia for patients over 90 years of age: Outcomes after regional and general anaesthetic techniques for two common surgical procedures. Anaesthesia 44:142, 1989

213. Edwards ND, Callaghan LC, White T, Reilly CS: Perioperative myocardial ischaemia in patients undergoing transurethral surgery: A pilot study comparing general with spinal anaesthesia. Br J Anaesth 74:368, 1995

214. Windsor A, French GWG, Sear JW et al: Silent myocardial ischaemia in patients undergoing transurethral prostatectomy. Anaesthesia 51:728, 1996

215. Sinha B, Haikel G, Lange PH et al: Transurethral resection of the prostate with local anesthesia in 100 patients. J Urol 135:719, 1986

216. Lu-Yao GL, Barry MJ, Chang CH et al: Transurethral resection of the prostate among Medicare beneficiaries in the United States: Time trends and outcomes. Urology 44:692, 1994

217. Kirby RS: Are the days of transurethral resection of prostate for benign prostatic hyperplasia numbered? Urologists must grasp the future. BMJ 309:716, 1994

218. Riehman M, Bruskewitz R: Treatment of benign prostatic hyperplasia. In Bahnson RR (ed): Management of Urologic Disorders, p 2.2. London, Wolfe, 1994

219. McCullough DL, Roth RA, Babayan RK et al: Transurethral ultrasound-guided laser-induced prostatectomy: National Human Cooperative Study results. J Urol 150:1607, 1993

220. Leach GE, Sirls L, Ganabathi K et al: Outpatient visual laser-assisted prostatectomy under local anesthesia. Urology 43:149, 1994

221. Watson G: Lasers. In Smith AD (ed): Smith's Textbook of Endourology, p 78. St. Louis, Quality Medical, 1996

222. Catalona WJ: Urothelial tumors of the urinary tract. In Walsh PC, Retik AB, Stamey TA, Vaughan ED Jr. (eds): Campbell's Urology, 6th ed, p 1094. Philadelphia, WB Saunders, 1992

223. Paola AS, Lamm DL: Bladder: Superficial transitional cell carcinoma. In Resnick MI, Kursh ED (eds): Current Therapy in Genitourinary Surgery, 2nd ed, p 68. St. Louis, Mosby–Year Book, 1992

224. Smith RB: Complications of transurethral surgery. In Smith RB, Ehrlich RM (eds): Complications of Urologic Surgery, 2nd ed, p 355. Philadelphia, WB Saunders, 1990

225. Kenyon HR: Perforations in transurethral operations. JAMA 142: 798, 1950

226. Hobika JH, Clarke BG: Use of neuromuscular blocking drugs to counteract thigh-adductor spasm induced by electrical shocks of obturator nerve during transurethral resection of bladder tumors. J Urol 85:295, 1961

227. Prentiss RJ, Harvey GW, Bethard WF et al: Massive adductor muscle contraction in transurethral surgery: Cause and prevention; development of new electrical circuitry. J Urol 93:263, 1965

228. Augspurger RR, Donohue RE: Prevention of obturator nerve stimulation during transurethral surgery. J Urol 123:170, 1980

229. Gasparich JP, Mason JT, Berger RE: Use of nerve stimulator for simple and accurate obturator nerve block before transurethral resection. J Urol 132:291, 1984

230. Fujita Y, Kimura K, Furukawa Y, Takaori M: Plasma concentrations of lignocaine after obturator nerve block combined with spinal anaesthesia in patients undergoing transurethral resection procedures. Br J Anaesth 68:596, 1992

231. Van Arsdalen KN, Levy JB: Urolithiasis. In Hanno PM, Wein AJ (eds): Clinical Manual of Urology, 2nd ed, p 229. New York, McGraw Hill, 1994

232. Drach GW: Urinary lithiasis: Etiology, diagnosis, and medical management. In Walsh PC, Retik AB, Stamey TA, Vaughan ED Jr. (eds): Campbell's Urology, 6th ed, p 2085. Philadelphia, WB Saunders, 1992

233. Preminger GM: Surgical management of calculus disease. In Bahnson RR (ed): Management of Urologic Disorders, p 14.2. London, Wolfe, 1994

234. McCullough DL: Extracorporeal shock wave lithotripsy. In Walsh PC, Retik AB, Stamey TA, Vaughan ED Jr. (eds): Campbell's Urology, 6th ed, p 2157. Philadelphia, WB Saunders, 1992

235. Eide TR: Anesthetic considerations for extracorporeal shock wave lithotripsy. In Lebowitz PW (ed): Anesthesia for Urological Surgery, p 47. Boston, Little, Brown, 1993

236. Hunter PT II: The physics and geometry pertinent to ESWL. In Riehle RA Jr, Newman RC (eds): Principles of Extracorporeal Shock Wave Lithotripsy, p 13. New York, Churchill Livingstone, 1987

237. Newman RC, Riehle RA Jr: Principles of treatment. In Riehle RA Jr, Newman RC (eds): Principles of Extracorporeal Shock Wave Lithotripsy, p 79. New York, Churchill Livingstone, 1987

238. Carlson CA, Gravenstein JS, Gravenstein N: Ventricular tachycardia during ESWL: Etiology, treatment, and prevention. In Gravenstein JS, Peter K (eds): Extracorporeal Shock-Wave Lithotripsy for Renal Stone Disease, p 119. Boston, Butterworths, 1986

239. Weber W, Chaussy C, Madler C et al: Cardiocirculatory changes during anesthesia for extracorporeal shock wave lithotripsy (ESWL). J Urol 4:246A, 1984

240. Farhi LE, Linnarsson D: Cardiopulmonary readjustments during graded immersion in water at 35 °C. Respir Physiol 30:35, 1977

241. Weber W, Madler C, Keil B et al: Cardiovascular effects of ESWL. In Gravenstein JS, Peter K (eds): Extracorporeal Shock-Wave Lithotripsy for Renal Stone Disease, p 101. Boston, Butterworths, 1986

242. Frank M, McAteer EJ, Cohen DG, Blair IJ: One hundred cases of anaesthesia for extracorporeal shock wave lithotripsy. Ann R Coll Surg Engl 67:341, 1985

243. Abbott MA, Samuel JR, Webb DR: Anaesthesia for extracorporeal shock wave lithotripsy. Anaesthesia 40:1065, 1985

244. Behnia R, Moss J, Graham JB et al: Hemodynamic and catecholamine responses associated with extracorporeal shock wave lithotripsy. J Clin Anesth 2:158, 1990

245. Behnia R, Shanks CA, Ovassapian A, Wilson LA: Hemodynamic responses associated with lithotripsy. Anesth Analg 66:354, 1987

246. Löllgen H, Nieding GV, Horres R: Respiratory and hemodynamic adjustment during head out of water immersion. Int J Sports Med 1:25, 1980

247. Bromage PR, Bonsu AK, El-Faqih SR, Husain I: Influence of Dornier HM3 system on respiration during extracorporeal shock-wave lithotripsy. Anesth Analg 68:363, 1989

248. Higgins TL, Miller EV, Roberts J: Accidental hyperthermia as a complication of extracorporeal shock-wave lithotripsy under general anesthesia. Anesthesiology 66:389, 1987

249. Malhotra V: Hyperthermia and hypothermia as complications of extracorporeal shock wave lithotripsy. Anesthesiology 67:448, 1987

250. Fuchs GJ, David RD, Fuchs AM, Chaussy CG: Complications of extracorporeal shock wave lithotripsy (ESWL). In Smith RB, Ehr-

lich RM (eds): Complications of Urologic Surgery, 2nd ed, p 181. Philadelphia, WB Saunders, 1990

251. Drach GW, Weber C, Donovan JM: Treatment of pacemaker patients with extracorporeal shock wave lithotripsy: Experience from 2 continents. J Urol 143:895, 1990

252. Segura JW: Complications of shock wave lithotripsy. In Marshall FF (ed): Urologic Complications: Medical and Surgical, Adult and Pediatric, 2nd ed, p 215. St. Louis, Mosby–Year Book, 1990

253. Monk TG, Bouré B, White PF et al: Comparison of intravenous sedative-analgesic techniques for outpatient immersion lithotripsy. Anesth Analg 72:616, 1991

254. Monk TG, Ding Y, White PF et al: Effect of topical eutectic mixture of local anesthetics on pain response and analgesic requirement during lithotripsy procedures. Anesth Analg 79:506, 1994

255. Richardson MG, Dooley JW: The effects of general versus epidural anesthesia for outpatient extracorporeal shock wave lithotripsy. Anesth Analg 86:1214, 1998

256. London RA, Kudlak T, Riehle RA: Immersion anesthesia for extracorporeal shock wave lithotripsy; review of two hundred twenty treatments. Urology 28:86, 1986

257. Monk TG, Rater JM, White PF: Comparison of alfentanil and ketamine infusions in combination with midazolam for outpatient lithotripsy. Anesthesiology 74:1023, 1991

258. Malhotra V, Long CW, Meister MJ: Intercostal blocks with local infiltration anesthesia for extracorporeal shock wave lithotripsy. Anesth Analg 66:85, 1987

259. Freilich JD, Brull SJ, Schiff S et al: Anesthesia for lithotripsy: Efficacy of monitored anesthesia care with alfentanil. Anesth Analg 70:S115, 1990

260. Baskin LS, Floth A, Stoller ML: Monitored anesthesia care with the standard Dornier HM3 lithotriptor. J Endourol 4:49, 1990

261. Segura JW: Complications of endourology. In Marshall FF (ed): Urologic Complications: Medical and Surgical, Adult and Pediatric, 2nd ed, p 200. St. Louis, Mosby–Year Book, 1990

262. Picus D, Weyman PJ, Clayman RV, McClennan BL: Intercostal-space nephrostomy for percutaneous stone removal. American Journal of Radiology 147:393, 1986

263. Schultz RE, Hanno PM, Wein AJ et al: Percutaneous ultrasonic lithotripsy: Choice of irrigant. J Urol 130:858, 1983

264. Smith JA Jr.: Urologic laser surgery. In Walsh PC, Retik AB, Stamey TA, Vaughan ED Jr. (eds): Campbell's Urology, 6th ed, p 2923. Philadelphia, WB Saunders, 1992

265. Malloy TR, Wein AJ: Complications of lasers in urology. In Marshall FF (ed): Urologic Complications: Medical and Surgical, Adult and Pediatric, 2nd ed, p 411. St. Louis, Mosby–Year Book, 1990

266. Smith JA Jr.: Complications of laser surgery. In Smith RB, Ehrlich RM (eds): Complications of Urologic Surgery, 2nd ed, p 629. Philadelphia, WB Saunders, 1990

267. Lundergan DK: Practical laser safety. In Smith JA Jr, Stein BS, Benson RC (eds): Lasers in Urologic Surgery, 2nd ed, p 165. Chicago, Year Book, 1989

268. Monk TG, Weldon BC: Anesthetic considerations for laparoscopic urology. In Das S, Crawford ED (eds): Urologic Laparoscopy, p 45. Philadelphia, WB Saunders, 1994

269. Wolf JS Jr., Monk TG: Anesthetic considerations. In Smith AD (ed): Smith's Textbook of Endourology, p 731. St. Louis, Quality Medical Publishing, 1996

270. Mullet CE, Viale JP, Sagnard PE et al: Pulmonary CO_2 elimination during surgical procedures using intra- or extraperitoneal CO_2 insufflation. Anesth Analg 76:622, 1993

271. Wolf JS Jr., Monk TG, McDougall EM et al: The extraperitoneal approach and subcutaneous emphysema are associated with greater absorption of carbon dioxide during laparoscopic renal surgery. J Urol 154:959, 1995

272. Wolf JS Jr., Clayman RV, Monk TG et al: Carbon dioxide absorption during laparoscopic pelvic operation. J Am Coll Surg 180:555, 1995

273. Kerbl K, Clayman RV, McDougall EM, Kavoussi LR: Laparoscopic nephrectomy: The Washington University experience. Br J Urol 73:231, 1994

274. McDougall EM, Monk TG, Hicks M et al: The effect of prolonged pneumoperitoneum on renal function in an animal model. J Am Coll Surg 182:317, 1996

275. Clayman RV, Kavoussi LR, Soper NJ et al: Laparoscopic nephrectomy: Review of the initial 10 cases. J Endourol 6:127, 1992

276. Oretga AE, Peters JH, Incarbone R et al: A prospective randomized comparison of the metabolic and stress hormonal responses of laparoscopic and open cholecystomy. J Am Coll Surg 183:249, 1996

277. Brawer MK: How to use prostate-specific antigen in the early detection or screening for prostatic carcinoma. Cancer J Clin 45:148, 1995

278. Paulson DF: Radiotherapy versus surgery for localized prostatic cancer. Urol Clin North Am 14:675, 1987

279. Walsh PC, Partin AW: Treatment of early stage prostate cancer: Radical prostatectomy. In DeVita VT, Heliman S, Rosenberg SA (eds): Important Advances in Oncology 1994, p 211. Philadelphia, JB Lippincott, 1994

280. Walsh PC: Radical retropubic prostatectomy. In Walsh PC, Retik AB, Stamey TA, Vaughan ED Jr. (eds): Campbell's Urology, 6th ed, p 2865. Philadelphia, W.B. Saunders, 1992

281. Shir Y, Frank SM, Brendler CB, Raja SN: Postoperative morbidity is similar in patients anesthetized with epidural and general anesthesia for radical prostatectomy. Urology 44:232, 1994

282. Monk TG: Cancer of the prostate and radical prostatectomy. In Malhotra V (ed): Renal Anesthesia for Renal and Genito-urologic Surgery, p 177. New York, McGraw-Hill, 1996

283. Frazier HA, Robertson JE, Paulson DF: Radical prostatectomy: The pros and cons of the perineal versus retropubic approach. J Urol 147:888, 1992

284. Bruce RG, Kim FH, McRoberts W: Rhabdomyolysis and acute renal failure following radical prostatectomy. Urology 47:427, 1996

285. Prentice JA, Martin JT: The Trendelenburg position: Anesthesiologic considerations. In Martin JT (ed): Positioning in Anesthesia and Surgery, 2nd ed, p 127. Philadelphia, WB Saunders, 1987

286. Wilcox S, Vandam LD: Alas, poor Trendelenburg and his position! A critique of its uses and effectiveness. Anesth Analg 67:574, 1988

287. Albin MS, Ritter RR, Reinhart R et al: Venous air embolism during radical retropubic prostatectomy. Anesth Analg 74:151, 1992

288. Razvi HA, Chin JL, Bhandari R: Fatal air embolism during radical retropubic prostatectomy. J Urol 151:433, 1994

289. Freiha FS: Open bladder surgery. In Walsh PC, Retik AB, Stamey TA, Vaughan ED Jr. (eds): Campbell's Urology, 6th ed, p 2750. Philadelphia, WB Saunders, 1992

290. deKernion JB, Belldegrun A: Renal tumors. In Walsh PC, Retik AB, Stamey TA, Vaughan ED Jr. (eds): Campbell's Urology, 6th ed, p 1053. Philadelphia, WB Saunders, 1992

291. Kinkade S: Testicular cancer. Am Fam Physician 59:2539, 1999

292. Donat SM, Levy DA: Bleomycin associated pulmonary toxicity: Is perioperative oxygen restriction necessary? J Urol 160:1347, 1998

293. Mathes DD: Bleomycin and hyperoxia exposure in the operating room. Anesth Analg 81:624, 1995

294. Ingrassia TS III, Ryu JH, Trastek VF, Rosenow EC III: Case report: Oxygen-exacerbated bleomycin pulmonary toxicity. Mayo Clin Proc 66:173, 1991

Clinical Anesthesia (4/e), edited by
Paul G. Barash, Bruce F. Cullen, and
Robert K. Stoelting. Lippincott Williams &
Wilkins, Philadelphia, © 2001.

CHAPTER 37

ANESTHESIA AND OBESITY AND GASTROINTESTINAL DISORDERS

F. PETER BUCKLEY AND KENNETH MARTAY

OBESITY

Obesity is usually defined relative to actuarially derived *ideal body weight* (IBW), or relative to height using indices such as the *body mass index* (BMI), defined as weight (kg) divided by height (m) squared (wt/ht²). For example, a 70-kg, 1.7-m patient has a BMI of 24. Patients who weigh 20% above IBW or have a BMI greater than 28 are regarded as obese. Approximately one third of the U.S. population meets these definitions of obesity,[1-3] and the prevalence of BMI greater than 28 has risen 8% since the early 1980s. The very obese, usually termed the *morbidly obese*, weigh more than 45 kg above IBW or have a BMI of greater than 35, and constitute some 3–5% of the U.S. population.[4]

Obesity is associated with a number of anatomic, physiologic, and biochemical deviations from normality that may affect all bodily systems. Even modest obesity (BMI = 28) is associated with increased risks for poor health and premature death[5] and, in the narrower anesthesiologic perspective, high risk for complications in the perioperative period.[3,6,7] Much of the information on the perioperative management of obese patients has come from studies of morbidly obese patients with no systemic clinical disease. Caution should be used when applying such information to the less obese, or to the morbidly obese population as a whole, which has a high prevalence of systemic clinical disease.

The physiologic and pathophysiologic consequences of obesity vary with the anatomic distribution of fat. Fat of primarily truncal distribution—android obesity—with a waist–hip circumference ratio of 0.9 in men and 0.8 in women, is associated with increased oxygen consumption ($\dot{V}O_2$) and an increased incidence of cardiovascular disease. Fat primarily of the buttocks and thighs—gynecoid obesity—is metabolically less active and less closely associated with cardiovascular disease.[8] Fat distributed intra-abdominally appears to be particularly associated with cardiovascular risk[9,10] and left ventricular (LV) dysfunction.[11]

Pathophysiology of Obesity

Respiratory System

Obese people have increased $\dot{V}O_2$ and carbon dioxide production ($\dot{V}CO_2$), but the basal metabolic rate, because it is related to body surface area, is usually normal.[12-14] Contributing to the increased $\dot{V}O_2$ are the metabolic activity of fat and an increase in energy expenditure for locomotion and breathing (to move the mass-loaded chest and abdomen, and to maintain a high minute volume in order to remain normocarbic with an increased $\dot{V}CO_2$). With exercise, $\dot{V}O_2$ and $\dot{V}CO_2$ rise more sharply than in people of normal body weight, as does the oxygen cost of respiration, implying respiratory muscle inefficiency.

Mass loading of the chest wall and abdomen by fat results in alterations in both the static and dynamic performance of the respiratory system. In the upright position, expiratory reserve volume and functional residual capacity (FRC) are reduced so that tidal ventilation may fall within the range of closing capacity, with ensuing ventilation–perfusion ($\dot{V}/\dot{Q}$) abnormalities,

or frank right-to-left shunt, with ensuing hypoxemia (Fig. 37-1). In the supine position, FRC often falls further within the range of closing capacity, with worsening hypoxemia (see Fig. 37-1). Fat mass loading of the chest and abdomen reduces chest wall compliance, with lung compliance remaining unaffected, and respiratory resistance increases.[15] Despite these changes in respiratory variables, the usual clinical tests of respiratory function (*e.g.*, forced vital capacity, forced expiratory volume in 1 second [FEV_1], and peak expiratory flow rate) are usually normal in the healthy obese patient.

Most obese patients maintain a sufficient minute volume of ventilation ($\dot{V}E$) to remain normocarbic and preserve a normal response to carbon dioxide challenge. However, with increasing obesity, intercurrent lung disease, and the changes wrought by pulmonary hypertension, their condition may deteriorate to the *obesity hypoventilation syndrome* (loss of hypercarbic drive, sleep apnea, hypersomnolence, and potential or overt airway difficulties) or to the worst end of the spectrum, the *pickwickian syndrome* (hypercarbia, hypoxemia, polycythemia, hypersomnolence, pulmonary hypertension, and biventricular failure).[16] The interactions of the respiratory and cardiovascular effects of obesity that lead to these conditions are shown schematically in Figure 37-2.

Cardiovascular System

In obese people, circulating blood volume, plasma volume, and cardiac output increase proportionately with rising weight and $\dot{V}O_2$. Cerebral and renal blood flows are similar to those in normal people, but splanchnic blood flow is 20% higher than in normal-weight people.[14,17-19] At rest, blood flow to fat is 2–3 ml · 100 g⁻¹ tissue; for a patient with a fat mass of 50 kg, blood flow to this fat mass accounts for an extra cardiac output of 1.5–2.0 l · min¹. The increase in cardiac output parallels the rise in $\dot{V}O_2$; thus, systemic arteriovenous oxygen difference remains normal or slightly above normal. The pulse rate in the obese person is usually within normal limits; thus, with an increased cardiac output, stroke volume is increased.

Arterial hypertension occurs frequently in the morbidly obese. It is severe in 5–10% of the obese population and moderate in 50%. The increase in cardiac output in response to exercise is more abrupt than in normal-weight people and may be accompanied by increases in LV end-diastolic pressure and pulmonary capillary wedge pressure.[18] Changes similar to those seen during exercise have been observed in the perioperative period.[19] Thus, patients with any degree of cardiovascular compromise are particularly at risk in the perioperative period.

The pathophysiologic effects of obesity on cardiac function are complex. In the setting of elevated circulating blood volume and cardiac output cardiomegaly is common, particularly in association with hypertension. Catheterization studies in the obese (IBW > 50%) without hypertension show increased filling pressures and increased chamber size but normal LV performance.[20] More severe obesity (BMI = 30) is associated with impairment of both diastolic and systolic function,[21-23] which are most severely affected in patients with congestive heart failure and may be improved by weight loss. Patients with sleep apnea appear to be particularly at risk for ventricular dysfunction.[24] Most morbidly obese patients can maintain a normal ejection fraction at rest but cannot produce a rise in ejection fraction in response to exercise.[25] Thus, in the more obese and older patients, and in those with demonstrable cardiac disease, a low threshold for performing detailed cardiac investigations is appropriate.

The pulmonary circulation is also vulnerable to the pathophysiologic changes produced by obesity. An increase in pulmonary blood volumes and flows predisposes obese patients to pulmonary hypertension, which may be accentuated or precipitated by hypoxic pulmonary vasoconstriction, which in turn occurs as a result of the static lung volume changes found in the morbidly obese (see Fig. 37-2).

Endocrine and Metabolic Systems

To maintain a stable weight, morbidly obese patients have to maintain a greater-than-normal caloric intake.[26] But, as with $\dot{V}O_2$, when this intake is related to body surface area, the values are similar to those of normal-weight people. Glucose tolerance is frequently impaired, with pancreatic islet cell hypertrophy and hyperinsulinemia, regardless of the state of carbohydrate tolerance, and is reflected in a high prevalence of diabetes mellitus in the morbidly obese. Abnormal serum lipid profiles are often found and may be associated with an increased prevalence of ischemic heart disease.

Gastrointestinal System

Morbidly obese patients have an increased prevalence of hiatal hernia and a linear increase in intra-abdominal pressure with increasing weight. At induction of anesthesia, 90% of fasted (>8 hours) morbidly obese patients presenting for elective surgery have a gastric fluid volume in excess of 25 ml and a gastric fluid pH of less than 2.5.[27] Such volume and pH figures are generally accepted as being indicative of a high risk for acid aspiration pneumonitis if the gastric fluid reaches the airway. The effects of more modern preoperative fasting regimens, which permit clear fluid intake up to a few hours before surgery, are unclear. Because both intra-abdominal pressure and the volume of gastric content increase during pregnancy, the pregnant morbidly obese woman is at particular risk for aspiration pneumonitis.

There is an increase in liver fat content in 90% of morbidly obese patients[26,28] that may not be evident with the usual clinical tests of hepatic function.[28] The increase appears to reflect the duration rather than the degree of obesity. The prevalence of hepatic dysfunction is particularly high in patients who have

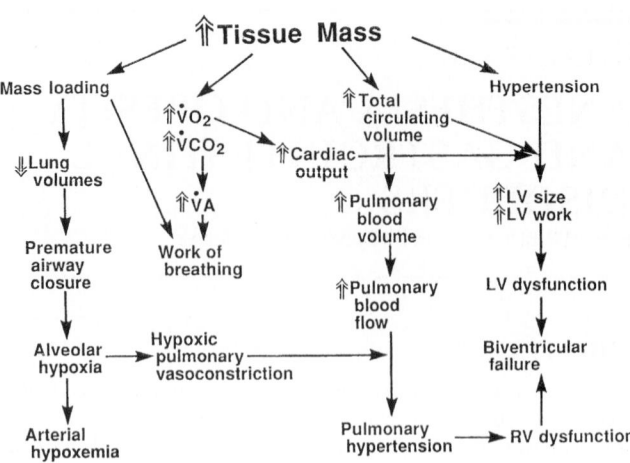

Figure 37-2. A schema interrelating the cardiovascular and respiratory abnormalities in morbidly obese patients to the pathophysiologic changes found in such patients. LV = left ventricular; RV= right ventricular.

undergone intestinal bypass operations.[29] The effect of gastric partitioning operations on hepatic function is uncertain.

Airway

Obesity produces a number of anatomic changes that can affect the airway. Flexion of the cervical spine and the atlantoaxial joint may be limited by numerous "chins" and by thoracic wall or breast fat. Extension of these joints may be limited by low cervical or upper thoracic fat pads. Mouth opening may be restricted by submental fat. Fleshy cheeks, a large tongue, and copious flaps of palatal, pharyngeal, and supralaryngeal soft tissue may narrow the airway. Moreover, the laryngeal aperture may occupy a "high and anterior" infantile position. The morbidly obese have a high prevalence of obstructive apnea syndrome (see Chapter 35).[30] Such patients often present particular airway difficulties when anesthetized.

Psychology of the Obese

In addition to its negative health consequences, obesity is associated with significant negative consequences in the educational, social, and economic spheres.[31] The attitudes of the public toward the obese and the purported stereotypic features of the obese are quite negative.[32] Neither medical students[33] nor physicians, who may characterize the obese as lazy, lacking in self-control, noncompliant with therapies, and difficult to manage,[34] are exempt from these negative attitudes. It is unclear whether the character traits attributed to the obese are attributed incorrectly or correctly. If correct, it is also unclear whether these features are inherent in their condition (the prevalence of psychopathology in the obese population as a whole is similar to that in the normal-weight population, but it may be somewhat higher in the morbidly obese[35]), or whether they result from the interactions of the obese with a population that holds them in negative regard, or is prejudiced against them. Whichever is the case, negative attitudes and behaviors from health care workers toward the obese will not change the characteristics or behavior of the obese, and should be avoided (see section on preoperative evaluation). In our experience with morbidly obese patients about to undergo gastric stapling operations, the patients were compliant with management regimens and conducted themselves normally throughout the perioperative period.[36] However, much time and effort were expended with this group, and the patients were obviously highly selected and motivated, having decided on a very dramatic course of action in an attempt to reduce their obesity.

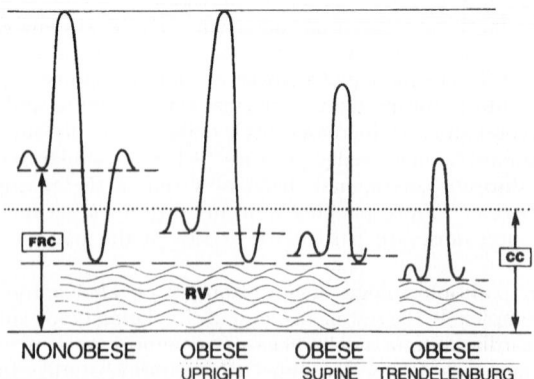

Figure 37-1. The effect of change in position on various lung volumes in nonobese and morbidly obese patients. FRC = functional residual capacity; RV = residual volume; CC = closing capacity. (Reprinted with permission from Vaughan RW: Pulmonary and cardiovascular derangements. In Brown BR [ed]: Anesthesia and the Obese Patient. Contemporary Anesthesia Practice Series, p 19. Philadelphia, FA Davis, 1982.)

Pharmacokinetics and Pharmacodynamics in the Obese

The many pathophysiologic deviations from normal that occur in the obese result in changes in drug pharmacokinetics and pharmacodynamics.[37,38] A summary of the deviations from normal and their consequences is given in Table 37-1.[38]

Physiologic changes in obesity that affect drug distribution include increased cardiac output, blood volume, lean body mass, organ size, and fat mass. In general, water-soluble compounds have smaller distribution volumes than lipophilic compounds and their distribution is less affected by obesity. Drugs with high affinity for fat show an increase in volume of distribution. Albumin binding of drugs is unchanged in the obese, although changes in levels of fatty acids, triglycerides, and α_1-acid glycoprotein may influence plasma protein binding.

Pathophysiologic changes in hepatic function in obesity may affect hepatically mediated drug clearance. Obesity is not associated with changes in Phase I metabolism (oxidation, reduction, hydrolysis), which affects drugs with low intrinsic clearance. Drugs eliminated through Phase II conjugation pathways (glucuronidation and sulfation) appear to be cleared faster in the obese.

Both renal glomerular filtration and tubular secretion are increased in the obese, and renally excreted drugs (e.g., aminoglycoside antibiotics, cimetidine) may need increased dosages.

Of specific drugs of interest to the anesthesiologist, lipophilic drugs such as the benzodiazepines[39] and thiopental[40] have an increased volume of distribution, more selective distribution to fat stores, and a longer elimination half-life in obese subjects than in normal-weight people, but clearance values are similar in both groups. For thiopental, the dosage suggestions are a larger absolute dose, but smaller dose per unit weight. An implication of the longer elimination half-life has been that fat-soluble volatile anesthetics may have a prolonged elimination time, with a consequent slow recovery. However, theoretical studies have shown that for prolonged recovery to occur, such agents would have to be administered for periods in excess of 24 hours.[41] Clinical studies of volatile agents administered to morbidly obese patients for commonly encountered operative times (2-4 hours) have shown normal recovery times.[42]

There are minimal data on the pharmacokinetics of propofol administered as a bolus. A dose based on IBW is advised. When used by infusion for maintenance of anesthesia, propofol volume of distribution and clearance rise in correlation with weight in the obese, but on average are similar to those in nonobese patients.[43] Moreover, speed of recovery, as judged by relatively crude methods, is similar in the obese and nonobese.[43]

Fentanyl, when administered to the obese patient on a $mg \cdot kg^{-1}$ body weight basis, has pharmacokinetic parameters similar to those in normal-weight subjects.[44] When administered on a $mg \cdot kg^{-1}$ body weight basis, sufentanil shows a large volume of distribution and a similar mean elimination half-life that is variable.[45] When administered on a $mg \cdot kg^{-1}$ lean body weight basis, alfentanil has a volume of distribution in obese patients similar to that in normal-weight patients, but a longer elimination half-life secondary to reduced clearance.[46] Remifentanil, when administered to obese patients on a $mg \cdot kg^{-1}$ body weight basis, produces higher peak blood levels of drug but shows pharmacokinetic parameters similar to those in the nonobese patient, but are most closely related to lean body mass of ideal weight, which should form the basis of dosage regimens.[47]

Hydrophilic drugs have similar volumes of distribution, elimi-

Table 37-1. FACTORS AFFECTING DRUG DISPOSITION AND RESPONSE IN OBESITY

Variable	Altered Physiology	Clinical Observations
Absorption	↔, ?	
Distribution		
Body composition	↑ Lean body mass ↑ Adipose tissue mass ↑ Organ size ↑ Blood volume ↑ Cardiac output	Lipid-soluble drugs tend to have ↑ volume of distribution
Protein binding	↔ Albumin and total protein ↑ α_1-Acid glycoprotein ↑ Triglycerides ↑ Cholesterol ↑ Free fatty acids	↔ Free fraction of acidic drugs ↑ Free fraction of basic drugs
Metabolism (hepatic)	↑ Splanchnic blood flow ↑ Number and size of parenchymal cells ↑ Parenchymal cell degeneration ↑ Fatty infiltration ↑ Bile pigment retention ↑ Periportal fibrous tissue ↑ Periportal cellular infiltration ↑ Focal necrosis	Studies have demonstrated ↓ clearance of high-extraction compounds
	↔, ↓, ? Phase 1 metabolism	Inconclusive studies on oxidation, reduction, and hydrolysis
	↑ Phase 2 metabolism ↔ Acetylation	Glucuronidated and sulfated drugs have ↑ clearance
Excretion (renal)	↑ Kidney size ↑ Glomerular filtration rate ↑ Tubular secretion	Drugs primarily filtered have ↑ renal clearance; compounds both filtered and secreted have demonstrated ↑ renal clearance values

↔ = no change; ? = effect unknown; ↑ = increased; ↓ = decreased.
Reprinted with permission from Blouin RA, Kolpek JH, Mann HJ: Influence of obesity on drug disposition. Clin Pharm 6:706, 1987.

nation half-lives, and clearance times in obese and nonobese patients. Morbidly obese patients have a higher pseudocholinesterase activity than nonobese subjects,[48] and dosages of 1.2–1.5 $mg \cdot kg^{-1}$ of succinylcholine are advised. When administered on a $mg \cdot kg^{-1}$ body weight basis, mivacurium has similar pharmacodynamics in normal-weight and morbidly obese patients.[49] To produce a given degree of neuromuscular blockade, a larger dose of pancuronium must be given to morbidly obese patients than to normal-weight patients. However, when this dose is related to body surface area, it is similar to the dose in normal-weight patients.[50] When vecuronium,[51] metocurine,[52] and rocuronium[53] are administered on a $mg \cdot kg^{-1}$ body weight basis, recovery in the morbidly obese is slower than in normal-weight subjects, probably as a consequence of relative overdose (higher blood levels).[51] In contrast, when atracurium is administered on a $mg \cdot kg^{-1}$ body weight basis, the speed of recovery is similar in both populations,[51,54] even though blood levels of atracurium at the time of recovery are higher in the morbidly obese patients.[54] Specific data on cisatracurium are lacking, but as its properties seem to be very similar to atracurium, and it is probably an acceptable drug to use in the obese. Specific data on rapacuronium use in the obese are lacking.

Preoperative Evaluation

Although obese people have a reputation for being difficult to manage, this difficulty can be minimized by a suitable preoperative evaluation and visit. The anesthesiologist should be aware of his or her feelings, attitudes, and prejudices toward obesity and avoid condescension. Obese patients should be evaluated in a thorough, nonjudgmental fashion, with particular emphasis on the difficulties obesity presents to the anesthesiologist. Time should be allowed for the patient to detail previous adverse experiences with anesthetics and operations, as well as any fears and anxieties about the upcoming experience. The various potential difficulties that the patient presents, and the specific anesthesia plan that is to be used to minimize or avoid such difficulties, should be discussed with the patient. The likely postoperative course should be discussed, and the patient should be allowed some degree of input and choice in the management plan.

Cardiovascular System

The evaluation should be directed toward the abnormalities detailed in the section on pathophysiology. Hypertension, signs of LV or right ventricular failure, and signs of pulmonary hypertension should be sought. Sites for venous access and, if needed, arterial cannulation should be identified. The electrocardiogram and chest radiograph should be scrutinized for evidence of ischemic heart disease, LV or right ventricular hypertrophy, and pulmonary congestion. The finding of any of these abnormalities should lead to appropriate investigations. For patients with the obesity hypoventilation syndrome or the pickwickian syndrome, a cardiologist's opinion should be sought, both to define the magnitude of the problem and for advice on how best to optimize the patient's condition before surgery.

Respiratory System

The clinical history should seek to identify symptoms indicative of severe degrees of respiratory disease (*e.g.*, orthopnea), obesity hypoventilation syndrome, or sleep apnea syndrome, and should elicit any history of upper airway obstruction, especially if associated with previous anesthesia and surgery. In young morbidly obese patients, the results of routine pulmonary function tests such as forced vital capacity, FEV_1, and peak expiratory flow rate are usually normal, but in older patients and those who smoke, the results may reveal unsuspected bronchospastic disease. Chest radiographs should be obtained, and blood gases should be measured with the patient seated and supine to rule out carbon dioxide retention and provide guidelines for perioperative oxygen administration.[55] More detailed pulmonary investigations should be reserved for those with severe disease. Because the degree of respiratory compromise in the postoperative period is often pronounced, it is imperative to optimize the patient's pulmonary status before embarking on anesthesia or surgery.

Endocrine, Metabolic, and Gastrointestinal Systems

Fasting blood glucose levels should be determined and the urine should be tested for ketones. If gross carbohydrate intolerance, diabetes, or ketosis is found, it should be corrected before either elective or emergency operations are begun. The patient should be closely questioned for symptoms of esophageal reflux and for a previous history of investigations or therapies that might be aimed at such a problem. Routine liver function tests should be performed.

Airway

A history of airway difficulties during previous anesthetics and operations should be obtained from the patient or previous anesthetic records. The patient should be questioned about symptoms suggestive of obstructive sleep apnea (excessive nocturnal snoring, with or without apneic episodes), which may suggest a potential for mechanical airway obstruction when the level of consciousness is decreased. Patients with such histories, and those presenting for operations designed to alleviate such conditions (tracheostomy, palatoplasty), should be scrutinized especially closely, because they may present formidable airway difficulties. Physical examination of the patient should include range-of-motion testing of the atlantoaxial joint and cervical spine, the degree to which the mouth can open, and the distance between the tip of the chin and the hyoid cartilage. The interior of the mouth and pharynx should be scrutinized for excessive folds of tissue. The Mallampati classification, based on an ability to visualize the uvula, may help identify those with potentially difficult laryngeal visualization. Lateral soft tissue radiographs of the neck in neutral and extended positions, computed tomographs of the pharynx, hypopharynx, and the larynx, or consultation with an otolaryngologist for a specialized work-up[56] may help delineate airway difficulties before surgery (see Chapter 23).

Pharmacologic Treatment of Obesity

A number of medications have been developed and used in attempts to assist the obese with weight loss. Perhaps the most notorious of these medications is the fenfluramine–phentermine combination that was withdrawn from the market because of concerns that the combination produced cardiac valve defects. More recently, sibutramine, a serotonin and norepinephrine uptake inhibitor, has been introduced. This drug appears to facilitate weight loss and is associated with modest hypertension and with the rare "serotonin syndrome."[57] There are no available data on interactions between sibutramine and anesthetic agents or techniques.

Perioperative Management

Premedication

Premedication, if any, should be given intravenously (iv) or orally. Attempts to give an intramuscular injection usually result in an intrafat injection, which leads to unpredictable absorption. In the morbidly obese patient, the effects of central nervous system–active drugs are not predictable and, because of the high prevalence of respiratory disease in this population, premedication should not be administered until the patient is in a safely monitored environment (*e.g.*, the holding area or the operating room). This is particularly true for any patient with a history of airway obstruction or cardiovascular or respiratory disease. Even when such drugs are administered in the operating room, the patient should be monitored diligently. If an awake intubation of the trachea is anticipated, anticholinergic drugs should be given in an attempt to reduce secretions.

Because the risk of gastric regurgitation is high in obese patients, specific measures should be taken to guard against it. If a large volume of gastric contents is suspected (*e.g.,* in an emergency situation), an attempt should be made to empty the stomach with a nasogastric tube. The tube should be removed before induction of anesthesia because of its potential for making a likely difficult tracheal intubation even more difficult. For elective cases, the preoperative administration of a clear antacid, metoclopramide, and histamine (H_2) blockers is advisable both to lower the volume and to increase the pH of gastric contents.[58-61] Suggested doses are metoclopramide, 10 mg iv; cimetidine, 300 mg; or ranitidine, 50 mg iv, given 1 hour before operation.

Operating Room Preparation

It is important to ensure that equipment such as gurneys, operating tables, and lithotomy stirrups are capable of bearing the load imposed by the obese patient. The heels, buttocks, and shoulders of obese people are at risk for development of decubitus ulcers. All vulnerable areas should be padded. The distribution of body fat may make the usual operating table positions hazardous to the obese. For example, excessive posterior extension of the shoulder with the potential for brachial plexus injury may occur when a patient with a large posterior thoracic fat pad is placed supine with arms abducted at 90 degrees to the body. Because the obese patient may have reduced respiratory compliance, increased respiratory resistance, and a need for a higher-than-normal minute volume, the use of ventilators more powerful than the usual operating room ventilators should be considered.

Monitoring

If cuff blood pressure monitoring is to be used, the cuff should be of an appropriate size (the bladder should enclose 70% of the arm). Cuff blood pressure monitoring may be both difficult and inaccurate in obese patients, and intra-arterial monitoring is advised for all but the shortest and simplest cases. Paradoxically, although it is often difficult to secure venous access in the obese, intra-arterial cannulation is usually no more difficult than in nonobese people. A V_5 or equivalent electrocardiogram lead should be used on all patients. Monitoring of patients with cardiovascular disease is dictated by their specific problem. Pulmonary artery catheterization and transesophageal echocardiography may be indicated in patients with LV compromise or pulmonary hypertension.[25]

Perioperative hypoxia is a constant threat in obese patients, and oxygenation should be monitored by pulse oximetry and by frequent arterial blood gas measurements. Capnography should be used to ensure adequacy of mechanical ventilation and to confirm correct endotracheal tube placement.

To ensure that any nondepolarizing neuromuscular blockade is adequate during surgery and fully reversed at the conclusion of the operation, such blockade must be monitored with a peripheral nerve stimulator. It may be difficult to achieve adequate peripheral nerve stimulation with skin electrodes because considerable amounts of tissue may separate skin electrodes from the relevant nerve. This problem may be circumvented by the use of percutaneous needle electrodes.

Because obese patients are no less likely than normal-weight patients to lose heat during surgery, body temperature should be monitored and maintained with forced air warming, which is effective in the obese.[62] It is best to avoid postoperative shivering in obese patients because this may result in further mixed

venous hypoxia and subsequent arterial hypoxia in patients who may be borderline normal in this regard.

Intraoperative Management

Airway Maintenance

Other than for the shortest general anesthetics in highly selected patients, general anesthesia should be delivered by an endotracheal tube. This is advocated because:

1. It may be difficult or impossible to maintain a gastight fit with a mask while maintaining an adequate airway and attending to the manual tasks necessary during anesthesia.
2. Obese patients are at high risk for aspiration of gastric contents.
3. Obese patients, if allowed to breathe spontaneously under general anesthesia, hypoventilate and become undesirably hypoxic or hypercarbic. Mechanical ventilation through an endotracheal tube is almost mandatory.

Difficulties with endotracheal intubation should be anticipated in all obese patients, and the person doing the intubation should thoroughly evaluate the patient and define all risks at the preoperative visit. All appropriate airway management equipment should be available, including a selection of oropharyngeal and nasopharyngeal airways, endotracheal tubes with introducers, a selection of laryngeal mask airways, intubation stylets, and laryngoscope blades of different patterns and sizes. If chest wall or breast fat is likely to obstruct the usual laryngoscope handles, a short-handled laryngoscope or a "polio blade" laryngoscope, which has a handle in the reverse of the usual direction, may be helpful. Fiberoptic intubation devices should also be available (see Chapter 23).

A carefully considered choice between awake and asleep tracheal intubation should be made in each case, bearing in mind the anticipated difficulties and the expertise of the anesthesiologist. An estimated 13% of morbidly obese patients pose difficulties for tracheal intubation using direct laryngoscopy.[36] Awake tracheal intubation has been recommended for all patients more than 75% above IBW,[63] but difficulties may also be encountered at weights below that cutoff point. Inability to visualize the patient's uvula with the mouth open may be helpful in identifying those patients in whom intubation is likely to be difficult.[55,64]

The "awake look" is a useful practice. The practitioner topically anesthetizes the mouth, pharynx, and supralaryngeal area with a local anesthetic and then gently introduces a standard laryngoscope and attempts to visualize the epiglottis and the larynx. If it is possible to see these structures, it is likely that intubation of the trachea after induction of anesthesia can be performed; if not, intubation of the trachea with the patient awake should be performed. If in doubt, the anesthesiologist should err on the side of caution and perform an awake intubation. Awake intubations should be accomplished with a fiberoptic instrument after suitable topical anesthesia. Any central nervous system depressant drug used to provide patient comfort should be kept to a minimum dosage and its effects monitored closely. Supplemental oxygen should be given during awake tracheal intubations.

Patients with a history suggestive of obstructive sleep apnea and those who are to undergo operations designed to alleviate such conditions almost invariably pose formidable endotracheal intubation difficulties. Endotracheal intubation attempted under general anesthesia in such patients frequently fails. Difficulty with bag-and-mask ventilation subsequent to a failed tracheal intubation, and the ensuing hypoxia, dictate that the trachea of many of these patients should be intubated while the patients are awake.

If tracheal intubation under general anesthesia is to be performed, it is a useful policy to have two people and two pairs of experienced hands available. If the initial attempt at intubation is not successful and it is necessary to resort to bag-and-mask ventilation, one person maintains a gastight mask fit and the airway, and the second person ventilates manually. A second pair of educated hands is also useful to cope with other difficulties.

Intubation under general anesthesia should be performed in a manner designed to avoid hypoxia and the aspiration of vomited or regurgitated gastric contents. Cricothyroid pressure (Sellick maneuver) is indicated in most cases. Thorough preoxygenation/denitrogenation by a conventional 3-minute period or a four-breath technique[65] is essential because intubation may take longer than usual, and obese patients have smaller-than-normal oxygen stores in their lungs (low FRC) and a high $\dot{V}o_2$ and therefore become hypoxic much faster than normal-weight patients.[65,66]

Regardless of the method used to place the endotracheal tube, correct tracheal placement should be confirmed with capnography because auscultation through chest wall fat may be difficult and inaccurate. Similarly, confirmation that the tip of the endotracheal tube is above the carina may necessitate fiberoptic bronchoscopy.

Choice of Anesthetic Technique

General Anesthesia. The doses of induction drugs used for the obese patient should be larger than for normal-weight patients (*e.g.*, thiopental, 7.5 mg · kg^{-1} IBW), but allowance should be made for any cardiovascular dysfunction. Nitrous oxide is a logical choice for maintenance of anesthesia because it is fat insoluble, has a rapid onset and decrement of action, and is subject to little metabolism. However, even in fit morbidly obese patients, it may be necessary to use an inspired oxygen concentration (Fio_2) in excess of 0.5 to maintain an adequate Pao_2;[67] thus, the usefulness of nitrous oxide is limited.

Obese patients metabolize volatile anesthetics to a greater extent than normal patients. The blood levels of fluoride after administration of methoxyflurane, halothane, and enflurane, and the blood levels of bromide after halothane are higher in the morbidly obese than in normal-weight patients.[68] Moreover, because the incidence of "halothane hepatitis" is allegedly higher in the obese, and because obese subjects metabolize some halothane by a potentially hepatotoxic reductive pathway,[68] this drug should be used with caution, if at all. However, simple tests of hepatic function are similarly marginally impaired after either halothane or enflurane anesthesia. Because morbidly obese patients metabolize isoflurane[69] and sevoflurane[70] to a minimal extent, and because desflurane appears strongly to resist biodegradation,[71] these are the volatile agents of choice in the obese patient.

The supposition that recovery from fat-soluble volatile anesthetics may be prolonged in the obese patient because such drugs may take a long time to leach out of fat stores has been elegantly disproved in theory[41] and in clinical studies of speed of awakening[42] (see Pharmacokinetics and Pharmacodynamics in the Obese).

When used in association with inhaled anesthetics at low dose, a propofol infusion at a rate of 6 mg · kg^{-1} · h^1 (where weight used for the calculation is IBW + [0.4 × excess weight]) appears to produce satisfactory anesthesia and rapid emergence (see Pharmacokinetics and Pharmacodynamics in the Obese).[43]

Great care should be exercised when giving opioids to obese patients. Unless the patient's trachea is to be left intubated and the patient provided with ventilator support in the immediate postoperative period, it is wise to keep the dose of opioid to a minimum. Maintenance of normal ventilation is already difficult for obese patients, and further respiratory depression with opioids could predispose to hypoxia or hypercarbia in the recovery room.

When administered on a mg · kg^{-1} body weight basis, the magnitude and duration of effect of succinylcholine are similar

in morbidly obese and normal-weight subjects.[48] Of the nondepolarizing neuromuscular blocking drugs, atracurium,[51,54] cisatracurium, vecuronium,[51] and rocuronium[53] are all reasonable choices.

Paramount among the changes in the physiology of obese patients produced by general anesthesia are respiratory abnormalities. With the induction of anesthesia, there is further disruption of the already altered FRC–closing capacity relationship, with a further deterioration in $\dot{V}/\dot{Q}$ relations or the development of a frank right-to-left shunt. The impairment of pulmonary hypoxic vasoconstriction by volatile agents contributes further to such changes. All obese patients should be considered at risk for hypoxia under general anesthesia. Obese patients should initially receive an Fio_2 of 1.0. Then, based on Spo_2 or Pao_2, the Fio_2 may be titrated downward, slowly. The application of positive end-expiratory pressure may improve Pao_2.[72,73]

Even in fit obese patients, intraoperative events that influence lung volumes may produce changes in oxygenation. The Trendelenburg or lithotomy position and the placement of subdiaphragmatic packs or retractors may lead to further decreases in Spo_2 and Pao_2.[14] Given these findings, it is important that particular attention be paid to oxygenation at the time of positional changes and various surgical maneuvers. The assumption of the prone position may improve some aspects of pulmonary function,[74] although this improvement may depend on the frame on which the patient is placed.[75] Morbidly obese patients may, however, be safely maintained by one-lung anesthesia performed through a double-lumen endobronchial tube during transthoracic operations.[76]

Because of the hypoventilation produced by general anesthesia, spontaneous respiration during general anesthesia is relatively contraindicated. Intermittent positive-pressure ventilation is best accomplished with large tidal volumes* at a rate of 8–10 breaths · min^{-1}. Hypocarbia with a $Paco_2$ of less than 30 mm Hg is best avoided because this may result in a rise in shunt fraction.[77]

At the conclusion of the operation, any neuromuscular blockade must be totally reversed, as judged by the response to peripheral nerve stimulation, and the parameters for extubation must be fulfilled. The trachea should not be extubated until the patient is fully awake and in control of the airway to avoid hazards of pulmonary aspiration or airway obstruction. Before extubating the patient, the anesthesiologist should ensure, either by pulse oximetry or arterial blood gas measurements, that hypoxia is not present.

Regional Anesthesia. Regional anesthesia would appear to be a useful alternative to general anesthesia but is accompanied by its own constellation of difficulties. The considerable body fat and the indistinct nature of bony landmarks make regional anesthesia technically difficult in the obese patient. For peripheral nerve blocks, these difficulties may be circumvented by the use of insulated needles and a peripheral nerve stimulator to ensure correct needle and drug placement.

Subarachnoid blockade may be more difficult to perform in obese patients than in normal-weight patients, but the difficulties are not insurmountable. The midline of the back in the lumbar region usually does not have as thick a layer of fat as do the more lateral portions, and subarachnoid puncture may be facilitated by having the patient sit up. Needles longer than

---

* By rearranging the BMI equation (BMI = weight [kg]/height² [m] to BMI × height² (m) = weight (kg), various body weights may be calculated for the person. Thus, a patient with a true body weight of 139 kg and a height of 1.77 m has a BMI of 139/1.77² = 44.4. At IBW, BMI = 25, and at low body weight (LBW), BMI = 30. Thus, for this patient, IBW = 25 × 1.77² = 78 kg and LBW = 30 × 1.77² = 94 kg. Intermittent positive-pressure ventilation at a rate of 12 ml · kg^{-1} at the LBW at a rate of 8–10 breaths · min^{-1} achieves a $Paco_2$ of approximately 30 mm Hg.[78]

usual often are needed. For a given age and height of a patient, the dose requirement for subarachnoid anesthesia in obese patients is approximately 75–80% that of normal,[79–81] and with more variability than in normal subjects.[81] However, the influence of body weight on dose requirements for spinal anesthesia is debatable (see Chapter 26). Evidence from case reports implies that the level of blockade produced by subarachnoid local anesthetics is not predictable and that the blockade is of slow onset and creeps insidiously higher over the first 30 minutes.[82] Anecdotal reports have implied that a high subarachnoid blockade tends to produce respiratory compromise, especially if patients are sedated.[82] However, in obese patients with a blockade at T5, both respiratory volume[83] and blood gases[84] show minimal change from baseline. If the blockade does extend higher in the thoracic area than T5, there is a distinct possibility of respiratory compromise, particularly in obese patients with respiratory disease. Moreover, the high extension of the blockade, with the variable extent of the autonomic blockade above the somatic blockade,[85] may lead to cardiovascular compromise, which can also be precipitated by panniculus retraction.[86] A strong case can be made for the use of a continuous subarachnoid block. This could provide all the benefits of regional anesthesia, allowing careful titration of the drug to the desired effect, thus circumventing the potential unpredictability of "single-shot" subarachnoid blocks. Moreover, the incidence of postdural puncture headache after large-bore needle dural puncture appears to be lower in the morbidly obese parturient than the nonobese parturient.[87]

Although technically more exacting than subarachnoid anesthesia, epidural anesthesia has been widely used and described in obese patients,[36,88,89] particularly for abdominal operations. The technique usually consists of a high lumbar or thoracic puncture, followed by the introduction of a catheter and induction of a segmental block. Catheter placement may be easier with fluoroscopic guidance.[89] The technique is usually used in combination with a light general anesthetic delivered by an endotracheal tube, with intermittent positive-pressure ventilation. Such a technique bypasses many of the problems of general anesthesia, reduces the volatile drug requirement, eliminates the need for neuromuscular blocking drugs, and permits rapid postoperative mobilization. As is true for subarachnoid anesthesia, the dose requirement for epidural anesthesia for operative procedures is approximately 75–80% that for normal-weight patients.[36,90] The use of epidural analgesia may confer some intraoperative and postoperative benefits on morbidly obese patients (decreased shunt fraction, LV work, A-VdO$_2$, and V̇o$_2$).[91] The catheter used to provide epidural anesthesia may be used again to provide postoperative analgesia either with local anesthesia[36,88] or with opioids,[92] which may be particularly beneficial in morbidly obese patients.[26,88] The epidural dose requirement for analgesia in obese patients appears to be similar to that in normal-weight patients for both local anesthetics[36,93] and opioids.[92]

Because it may be difficult to deal with respiratory or cardiovascular emergencies in the obese, any such potential hazards must be detected as early as possible and dealt with vigorously. The obese patient receiving a regional anesthetic should receive supplemental oxygen and minimal sedation or analgesia, and must be monitored in the same fashion as if he or she were receiving a general anesthetic. The anesthesiologist should not choose regional anesthesia for a patient unless prepared to convert to general anesthesia if the regional anesthesia is unsatisfactory for the surgical procedure or if respiratory difficulties develop in the patient.

Postoperative Care

Obese patients with a previous history of respiratory disease, those with obesity hypoventilation syndrome or pickwickian syndrome, and those who have undergone major abdominal and thoracic operations are likely to have a high incidence of postoperative respiratory complications. Thus, it may be wise to admit these patients electively to an intensive care unit. Their management in the intensive care unit depends on the individual patient but should include mechanical ventilation, if necessary, and aggressive prophylaxis against the development of respiratory complications. Obese patients are highly immobile after surgery; measures should be taken to assist them in moving by the provision of an adjustable bed, overhead trapeze, and sufficient nursing staff.

Respiratory Function

Even in healthy obese patients, postoperative hypoxemia is a universal hazard. Supplemental oxygen should be given during transport from the operating room to the recovery room. Respiratory monitoring should be particularly aggressive in the recovery room and should include pulse oximetry or arterial blood gas monitoring, or both. Patients should not be discharged to the ward until they have been shown capable of maintaining adequate oxygenation, and it may be appropriate to use long-term oxygen therapy on the ward. After intra-abdominal operations, arterial hypoxemia may last 4–6 days[94] and is of greater magnitude with vertical than with horizontal incisions. Postoperative hypoxemia can be minimized by having patients sit in bed. There is some evidence that the intraoperative and postoperative use of regional anesthesia techniques reduces the incidence of postoperative respiratory complications.[36,92]

Immobilization

Obese patients have a high incidence of postoperative deep vein thrombosis and pulmonary emboli. The use of low-dose heparin or intermittent leg compression prophylaxis may be appropriate. The use of regional anesthesia techniques may decrease the incidence of deep vein thrombosis and pulmonary emboli.[36]

Analgesia

Obese patients may have less need for postoperative analgesics than normal-weight patients.[95] For previously stated reasons, the use of opioid analgesics can be hazardous in obese patients. Moreover, the routine use of intramuscular injections may not result in predictable blood levels of the opioid. If opioids are used, they should be delivered directly into the intravascular compartment using devices such as patient-controlled analgesia (PCA) machines. An anecdotal report implies that PCA may be hazardous in patients with obstructive sleep apnea,[96] but PCA has been effectively and safely used in the morbidly obese.[97,98]

If an epidural catheter was placed for operative anesthesia, it may be used as the route for injecting either local anesthetic or opioid to provide postoperative analgesia. The use of local anesthesia[36] or opioids[92] is associated with faster postoperative recovery and a lower incidence of respiratory complications than the use of conventional opioid techniques. The doses of either local anesthetic or opioid necessary to provide postoperative epidural analgesia are similar to those in normal-weight patients. Epidural opioid analgesia may result in delayed respiratory depression, and, because of the difficulty of maintaining or securing the airway in obese patients, those receiving epidural opioids should probably be nursed in a closely monitored environment (*e.g.*, an intensive care unit) until the potential for such a complication has passed.

GASTROINTESTINAL DISORDERS
Functional Anatomy and Physiology

The mouth and pharyngeal musculature are under voluntary control as boluses of food and fluid are swallowed and delivered to the esophagus. Such boluses are lubricated by saliva, which amounts to approximately 1200 ml · day^{-1}.[99]

Esophagus

The esophageal musculature is under involuntary control and is innervated by the vagus nerve and a sympathetic component derived from segments T6–10. Waves of esophageal contraction pass boluses of food down to the gastroesophageal junction, which relaxes to allow them to enter the stomach.

At the gastroesophageal junction, reflux is prevented by a number of means, including the esophagus acting as a flap valve and the diaphragmatic crura pinching off the esophagus. The major barrier to gastroesophageal reflux is now believed to be the lower esophageal sphincter (LES). The LES is histologically similar to the rest of the esophagus but is functionally quite different. It may be identified by gastroesophageal manometry, in which a series of transducers is drawn from the stomach back through the gastroesophageal junction into the esophagus. The LES appears as an area of increased pressure (Fig. 37-3). It is usually 2–3 cm long and extends above and below the diaphragm. Peak pressure occurs just above the diaphragm and varies with respiration. The LES relaxes on swallowing, in contrast to the rest of the esophagus, which exhibits peristalsis.

The tendency for esophageal reflux is related to some degree to LES tone but more to the barrier pressure, that is, the difference between the LES pressure and the gastric pressure. Thus, if intragastric pressure is sufficiently high, it may surmount the LES to produce reflux. However, in health, the LES pressure usually rises in response to a rise in intragastric pressure. The LES tends to relax during pregnancy; thus, the tendency for reflux to occur is greater at that time. Patients with hiatal hernia may have a normal LES pressure, although in such patients the LES is nearly always above the diaphragm. Patients with gastroesophageal reflux tend to have lower barrier pressures, ranging from low to near normal, rather than exhibiting a distinct cutoff point. The LES is innervated by both vagal and sympathetic nerves, but the role of the innervation is uncertain; vagal denervation does not affect resting tone or active function. Clinical circumstances associated with reduced LES tone include pregnancy, obesity, and hiatal hernia. Patients with gastro-

Table 37-2. LOWER ESOPHAGEAL SPHINCTER EFFECT OF DRUGS USED IN ANESTHESIA

Increase	Decrease	No Change
Metoclopramide	Atropine	Propranolol
Domperidone	Glycopyrrolate	Oxprenolol
Prochlorperazine	Dopamine	Cimetidine
Cyclizine	Sodium nitroprusside	Ranitidine
Edrophonium	Ganglion blockers	Atracurium
Neostigmine	Thiopental	?Nitrous oxide
Histamine	Tricyclic antidepressants	
Suxamethonium	Halothane	
Pancuronium	Enflurane	
Metoprolol	Opioids	
Antacids	?Nitrous oxide	

esophageal reflux may also have reduced LES tone. A number of drugs may increase or decrease LES tone (Table 37-2).

Stomach

The stomach has various functions. As a distensible receptacle, it allows the storage of large amounts of food and fluids (it may accept 1–1.5 l of fluid with minimal rises in intragastric pressure). As a chamber, it is the site for mixing of ingested food and gastric secretions, and where digestion begins; as a system, it expels small and manageable amounts of gastric contents into the duodenum.[100]

The proximal part of the stomach is functionally a receptacle, exhibiting little mobility and in which little mixing occurs. Mixing occurs primarily in the distal stomach, with electrical activity originating from a "pacemaker," usually located near the midpoint of the greater curvature. The electrical activity and resulting mechanical activity spread circumferentially and longitudinally toward the pylorus. Pyloric relaxation occurs in response to the waves of gastric activity, permitting expulsion of small amounts of gastric contents into the duodenum. In health, gastric emptying occurs at a rate that closely approximates an exponential curve, although varying from this curve when the stomach is full or nearly empty.

The rate of gastric emptying can be influenced by physiologic factors such as the type of intake—liquids leave the stomach more quickly than solids—and by the volume, pH, and osmotic qualities of the gastric contents.[100] The customary 4-hour preoperative fast does not guarantee that the stomach is empty, and evidence is accumulating that modest feeding or intake of small amounts of fluid during the preoperative period may be associated with lower volumes of gastric contents and may shorten the usual NPO waiting period before elective surgery (see Chapter 21).[101] Certain groups of patients tend to have a high resting gastric content volume, including the pregnant, the obese, and the bedridden (Table 37-3). Pathologic states associated with high resting gastric content volume include pain, shock, and trauma. Laparotomy slows the rate of gastric emptying for approximately 24 hours, although this is probably the result of a combination of the mechanical effects of bowel handling and the postoperative use of opioids. A number of drugs may influence the rate of gastric emptying (see Table 37-3).

Gastric secretions are produced at a rate of nearly 2000 ml · day^{-1}. They have a pH of 1.0–3.5, are isotonic with extracellular fluid, and consist predominantly of hydrochloric acid, with a higher potassium content than extracellular fluid. The pH of gastric contents may be raised by the administration of antacids or H$_2$-blocking drugs.

Duodenum

In the duodenum, secretions of the pancreas and the biliary tract are mixed with the gastric contents. Secretions of the pancreas and biliary tract are predominantly alkaline, with pH

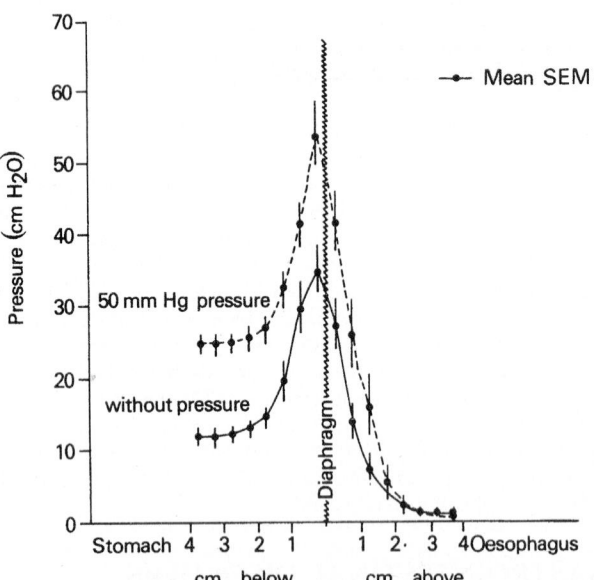

Figure 37-3. The pressures found by lower esophageal manometry, illustrating the relationship of the lower esophageal sphincter to the diaphragm. Note also the effect of increasing intra-abdominal pressure causing a concurrent rise in lower esophageal sphincter pressure. (Reprinted with permission from Colton BR, Smith G: The lower esophageal sphincter and anaesthesia. Br J Anaesth 56:37, 1984.)

Table 37-3. SOME FACTORS INFLUENCING GASTRIC EMPTYING RATE

	Accelerate	Delay
Physiologic	Gastric distention	Food
	Neuroticism	Acid
		High osmotic pressure
		Posture
		Pregnancy
Pathologic	Thyrotoxicosis	Shock
		Trauma and pain
		Myocardial infarction
		Pyloric stenosis
		Crohn's disease
		Celiac disease
		Diabetic autonomic neuropathy
Pharmacologic	Metoclopramide	Anticholinergics
	Neostigmine	Tricyclic antidepressants
	Propranolol	Aluminum hydroxide
	Sodium bicarbonate	Alcohol
	Cigaratte smoking	Isoprenaline
		Opioid analgesics

values in the region of 7.8–8.3 and daily volumes of 1200 and 700 ml, respectively. The pH of the resultant mix of gastric contents and duodenal secretions is a function of the respective volumes and pH of the gastric contents and the pancreatic and biliary tract secretions.

Small Intestine

At rest, the activity of the small intestine is governed by the migrating myoelectric complex. This complex has two components, electromyographic and manometric. Four phases may be seen: Phase I, the slow-wave electrical activity of the quiescent intestine; Phase II, characterized by slow-wave activity with some spikes, accompanied by periodic intestinal contractions; Phase III, characterized by intense spiking accompanied by electrical slow waves with vigorous mechanical contractions; and Phase IV, which reverts from Phase III to Phase I and is associated with rapid subsidence of contractions.

When food is taken, the migrating myoelectric complex is disrupted and there is contractile activity throughout the whole intestine. Postprandial intestinal activity can be divided into a cephalic phase, which may be abolished by vagotomy, a gastric phase, which is promoted by gastric distention, and an intestinal phase, which is provoked by perfusion of the intestine with nutrients.

The mode of control of small intestinal activity is not known with certainty. The parasympathetic system plays a role because parasympathetic stimulation results in increased activity, and suppression of the parasympathetic system results in decreased activity. The sympathetic nervous system also plays a role because sympathetic suppression causes an increase in activity and stimulation causes a decrease in activity, with the changes mediated by both catecholamines and dopaminergic receptors. However, with bowel denervation, there appears to be little change in activity, and it is likely that humoral secretions, especially pancreatic polypeptides and somatostatin, play a major role in mediating activity. Small intestinal activity is suppressed for 24–48 hours after laparotomy and may also be decreased by peritonitis and a reduction in serum potassium levels.

The small intestine secretes 2000 ml · day^{-1} of fluid with a pH of 7.0–8.0. The small intestine is the site of most of the absorption of fluid and nutrients in the gastrointestinal (GI) tract. It is presented with 5500 ml · day^{-1} of fluid (2000 ml from the stomach, 1500 ml from the pancreas and biliary tract, and 2000

ml from the small intestine), but passes on only 500 ml to the colon. Thus, the net turnover of fluid in the small intestine is of the order of approximately 5000 ml · day^{-1}. The absorptive abilities of the small intestine are impaired for approximately 36 hours after laparotomy.

Colon

Approximately 500–700 ml of bowel content is presented to the colon each day. The colon expels only 100–200 ml · day^{-1}; therefore, its function is predominantly absorptive. Colonic motility is controlled by a pacemaker located in the transverse colon. Three types of activity can be observed: (1) antiperistalsis from the transverse colon to the cecum, which permits maximal exposure of the feces for absorption of fluid; (2) peristalsis, which pushes feces forward to the distal parts of the colon; and (3) a powerful peristaltic movement that is responsible for the evacuation of fecal content; this movement proceeds anally in a series of large mass movements.

Parasympathetic neural control of the colon as far as the splenic flexure is furnished by the vagus nerve; beyond that point, it is furnished by the sacral parasympathetic outflow. The sympathetic supply is from segments T6–10. Parasympathetic stimulation increases motility, whereas sympathetic stimulation decreases activity. Administration of neostigmine increases both activity and tone, whereas morphine decreases them.[102]

Splanchnic Blood Flow

Splanchnic oxygenation can be influenced by changes in the blood oxygen-carrying capacity (such as anemia) and by changes in blood flow to the bowel. In normal circumstances of a normal cardiac output, splanchnic blood flow remains relatively stable, being regulated by the splanchnic vascular resistance through mechanisms similar to those regulating hepatic blood flow. Splanchnic vascular resistance is largely regulated by the sympathetic nervous system, with sympathectomy decreasing splanchnic vascular resistance, α-adrenergic stimulation promoting vasoconstriction, and β-adrenergic stimulation promoting vasodilation. Dopamine may act in the splanchnic vascular bed through two receptors, with α-adrenergic vasoconstriction predominating over the mild vasodilation produced by β-adrenergic stimulation. Parasympathetic stimulation results in an increase in blood flow and an increase in motor activity.

In stress states, a number of humoral agents may influence splanchnic blood flow, including catecholamines, vasopressin, and angiotensin II. With hemorrhage, splanchnic vascular resistance rises, presumably as a teleologic mechanism to permit the diversion of cardiac output to organs more vital to survival. A modest hemorrhage of 10–15% of circulating blood volume, which does not affect systemic arterial pressure, may markedly impair splanchnic blood flow. The restoration of circulating volume does not result in a rapid restoration of splanchnic blood flow, which may remain decreased for several hours. Although blood loss and hypotension are not particularly critical for the blood supply to the stomach and small bowel, which have a liberal vascular supply, such circumstances may be associated with an increased rate of colonic anastomotic dehiscence.

A number of perioperative factors may alter splanchnic blood flow. After trauma, there may be an increase in splanchnic blood flow, but laparotomy alone produces little change. Morphine decreases splanchnic vascular resistance and therefore increases splanchnic blood flow. There is an almost linear relationship between splanchnic blood flow and Pa_{CO_2}, with hypocapnia decreasing flow and hypercapnia increasing flow. Most inhaled anesthetics decrease splanchnic blood flow.[103] Regional anesthesia with high levels of sympathetic blockade results in an increase in splanchnic blood flow owing to a decrease in splanchnic vascular resistance, both as a consequence of the sympathectomy itself and of the fall in catecholamine levels associated with sympathetic blockade. However, if such a sympathectomy results in a fall in cardiac output, splanchnic blood flow may fall.

Sympathectomy does not influence the changes in splanchnic blood flow produced by changes in Pa_{CO_2}.[104] Neostigmine reduces mesenteric blood flow by 30–50% in association with the exaggerated motor activity of the intestine. Such decreases in blood flow may be somewhat ameliorated by the prior administration of atropine.

General Considerations for Anesthesia and the Gastrointestinal Tract

Regardless of the target of the surgery in the GI tract, a number of factors bearing on patient evaluation and management must be taken into consideration.

Airway Management and Protection

The oral, pharyngeal, and hypopharyngeal areas may be distorted by a number of pathologic processes, including tumor, infection, obstruction by an ingested foreign body, thermal or chemical damage, and nonmalignant variations on normal anatomy such as pharyngeal pouches. Thus, it is necessary to evaluate the patient carefully with respect to the site, type, and magnitude of the distortion and the pathologic process producing the airway abnormality. The choice of airway management and method of securing the airway should be based on clinical findings, supplemented as necessary by investigations such as direct or indirect laryngoscopy, soft tissue radiography, and computed tomography or magnetic resonance imaging of the abnormal area (see Chapter 23).

A major consideration in anesthesia for surgery on the GI tract is the prevention of inadvertent airway soiling by aspiration of GI contents during induction and maintenance of anesthesia. During routine anesthesia, the incidence of regurgitation of gastric contents is remarkably low; the incidence in adults and children is less than 1:1000.[105] Aspiration is most likely to occur during the induction of anesthesia, when the airway is not securely protected by an endotracheal tube and when active vomiting is most likely.

The consequences of regurgitation and subsequent aspiration of gastric contents into the airway depend on the character and volume of the aspirate. Solid matter produces an anatomic obstruction of the airway, and fluid of neutral pH produces the clinical picture of near drowning, whereas the aspiration of even small amounts of acidic fluid may be associated with the aspiration syndrome (Mendelson syndrome). The incidence of the latter is estimated at 0.05%.[105] It is generally accepted that a gastric content in excess of 25 ml with a pH of less than 2.5 implies a special risk for producing an aspiration syndrome if such fluid is aspirated. However, there is also opinion that acid aspiration syndromes can be produced by aspirates with a higher pH. Therefore, it is incumbent on anesthesiologists to attempt to reduce the volume and increase the pH of any gastric contents.

If the volume of gastric contents is suspected to be high, it may be reduced by emptying the stomach with a nasogastric tube or by inducing vomiting with apomorphine, although neither can guarantee complete gastric emptying. Gastric emptying can also be facilitated by using drugs to increase gastric motility. Several factors that influence gastric emptying are listed in Table 37-3. Application of any of these techniques does not absolve the anesthesiologist of the responsibility of taking other precautions to prevent regurgitation and possible aspiration of GI tract contents.

A major thrust in reducing the potential for acid aspiration syndrome has been to raise the pH of gastric contents. This may be done effectively with particulate antacids such as aluminum hydroxide or magnesium trisilicate. However, such drugs may cause lung damage if they are aspirated; thus, it is preferable to use nonparticulate antacids such as sodium citrate (0.3 mmol). Drugs that reduce acid secretion, such as the H_2 blockers (*e.g.*, ranitidine, famotidine), or proton pump inhibitors (*e.g.*, ome-

prazole, lansoprazole), effectively raise the pH.[50,51,106] Some anticholinergics, particularly glycopyrrolate, also reduce gastric acidity. Metoclopramide is of benefit because it increases gastric motility and increases LES tone.[106]

Studies of the acid aspiration syndrome have shown that a high proportion of patients who have this problem have an LES dysfunction. Thus, it is important to maintain LES function. Circumstances associated with a lowered LES tone are discussed in an earlier section; drugs that raise LES tone are listed in Table 37-2.

Before induction of anesthesia, the risk of regurgitation and pulmonary aspiration may be reduced by the following measures:

Avoiding airway instrumentation at inadequate levels of anesthesia

Reducing the volume of the stomach content

Using nasogastric tubes

Inducing vomiting

Accelerating gastric emptying with drugs such as metoclopramide

Raising the gastric content pH with clear antacids and H_2 blockers

Increasing LES tone with metoclopramide

Once the anesthesiologist has attempted to reduce the likelihood of regurgitation and aspiration, the airway should be secured coincident with the induction of anesthesia by the expeditious passage of an endotracheal tube. Although conventional wisdom holds that application of cricoid pressure (Sellick maneuver) should accompany induction of anesthesia in the patient with a "full stomach," in fact, application of cricoid pressure is associated with a relaxation of the gastroesophageal sphincter.[107]

Fluid and Electrolyte Balance

Patients with GI disease may be in fluid or electrolyte imbalance for a number of reasons, some of which are listed in the following (see Chapter 9).

1. *Inadequate intake.* Patients awaiting surgery are often kept NPO for varying periods before surgery. This is especially likely to be a problematic factor in children, small adults, and patients in a hot environment or with pyrexia, in whom insensible fluid losses may be high. In the chronically ill patient, there may be a long period of inadequate intake, or oral intake may be prevented by anorexia or GI tract obstruction.
2. *Sequestration of water and electrolytes into abdominal structures,* such as the bowel lumen, bowel wall, and peritoneum, in patients with inflammatory bowel disease or intestinal obstruction.
3. *Extracorporeal loss of fluid* such as from vomiting, diarrhea, loss through fistulae, nasogastric suction, or diuretics.

Frequently, the etiology of the fluid deficit is an amalgam of these three causes. The magnitude of the fluid and electrolyte deficit reflects the duration of the problem and the site of the fluid loss. Deficient intake and salivary loss, for example, in a patient with a pharyngeal tumor, is primarily water loss with minimal electrolyte loss.

Loss of fluid that is primarily gastric contents (which, in a patient with pyloric stenosis, may reach 2000 ml · day^{-1}) results in a hypochloremic alkalosis and hypokalemia. Not only is potassium lost in the gastric fluid, it is excreted by the kidney in response to the alkalosis.

If fluid is lost externally from the lower GI tract, the resulting deficit is predominantly a metabolic acidosis and hypochloremia. The loss may be up to 3000 ml · day^{-1}.

When small bowel obstruction occurs, a complex series of events takes place. The segment of bowel proximal to the obstruction dilates and contains gas (primarily swallowed gas) and fluids. The fluids result from bowel contents upstream and an increase in small bowel secretion with a decrease in fluid absorption. As bowel dilation increases, fluid is lost into the bowel wall and peritoneal cavity. Progressive dilation and edema of the bowel or of a volvulus may lead to impaired bowel blood supply, with potential bowel necrosis and perforation. In these circumstances, further rapid fluid loss occurs and the patient may contract bacterial toxemia or septicemia. The usually encountered abnormalities include hemoconcentration, a fall in circulating blood volume, and a fall in total body potassium.

Large bowel obstruction tends to occur more slowly and manifests less dramatically than small bowel obstruction. The effects of the obstruction depend on the competence of the ileocecal valve. If the valve is competent, the closed obstruction results in large bowel dilation, particularly of the right colon and cecum, with the potential for progression to impairment of colonic blood supply and necrosis and perforation. However, if the ileocecal valve is not competent, the bowel contents reflux into the small bowel, ultimately resulting in feculent vomiting. The speed of progression of symptoms in large bowel obstruction tends to be slower than in small bowel obstruction, but the fluid and electrolyte disturbances may be just as severe, with similar intravascular and extracellular fluid consequences.

Diarrhea may result from impaired intestinal absorption of water and electrolytes, from abnormal bowel motility, or from an increase in the osmotically active substances in the bowel lumen. The fluid and volume deficit reflects the hypotonic, potassium-containing nature of the stools and tends to produce a hypokalemic metabolic acidosis.

Preoperative evaluation of the patient's fluid and electrolyte deficit includes assessment of clinical parameters such as skin turgor, peripheral circulation, heart rate, blood pressure, and urine output. Useful laboratory studies include hematocrit, serum electrolytes, and blood urea nitrogen. If necessary, invasive monitoring such as central venous pressure and pulmonary artery pressure measurements should be used further to assess the patient's vascular volume. The speed with which resuscitation and rehydration should be accomplished depends on the urgency of the surgical procedure. Small bowel obstruction, which may rapidly progress to bowel ischemia and perforation, necessitates urgent operation. Therefore, resuscitation should be swift and aggressive and aimed at rendering the patient fit for operation in a brief time. Resuscitation for large bowel obstruction or for a more chronic fluid loss, from whatever source, may be accomplished in a somewhat more leisurely fashion. The type of fluid resuscitation depends on the volume of loss and the clinical and laboratory findings.

Malabsorption and Malnutrition

The GI tract is responsible for absorbing all nutrients; therefore, bowel abnormalities may be associated with malabsorption of nutrients and consequent malnutrition. The malabsorption may be of one element only, but more commonly it is of multiple elements and is usually associated with chronic rather than acute disease.

Gastric lesions and gastric resections are commonly associated with a poorly understood iron deficiency anemia and with megaloblastic vitamin B_{12} deficiency anemia owing to either lack of intrinsic factor or overgrowth of vitamin B_{12}-consuming bacteria in a blind loop. A deficiency of bile salt secretion impairs fat absorption, leading to steatorrhea and deficiencies of the fat-soluble vitamins A, D, and K and of calcium. Pancreatic insufficiency may lead to protein and fat malabsorption with steatorrhea and fat-soluble vitamin deficiency. Intestinal malabsorption may occur owing to motility disorders, a reduction in absorptive area, mucosal abnormalities, or bacterial overgrowth. The severity of the malabsorption and malnutrition is related to the magnitude, site, and duration of the disease and the magnitude of the decrease in absorptive surface. Malabsorption

is usually of protein, fats, and vitamins; carbohydrate absorption is relatively well preserved.

Malnutrition may also result from loss of bowel contents through fistulae or from intestinal loss of protein into the bowel lumen in diseases such as regional enteritis, ulcerative colitis, and allergic enteropathies.

Although the correction of malnutrition in the preoperative period is relatively unimportant for acute diseases, it may be extremely important in chronic disease states. Experience with preoperative elemental diets or hyperalimentation has shown that correction of malnutrition improves both wound healing and the overall outcome of surgical procedures for chronic bowel diseases. Adequate postoperative nutrition is also important to improve healing and to reduce the incidence of complications. After abdominal operations, most patients have increased needs for calories and protein, particularly patients with major abdominal infections (see Chapter 56).

Special Anesthesia Considerations for Bowel Surgery

Use of Nitrous Oxide

The solubility of nitrous oxide in blood is 34 times that of nitrogen. In consequence, nitrous oxide in the bloodstream enters gas-containing body cavities much faster than the nitrogen in those cavities can be removed by the circulation. If this occurs in the bowel, the gas-containing bowel distends.[108] The amount of distention depends on the following factors:

1. The amount of gas within the bowel. In health, the bowel contains approximately 100 ml of gas, most of which is swallowed; therefore, distention is relatively unimportant. However, with obstruction or aerophagy, the bowel may contain much larger amounts of gas, and the potential for expansion is much greater.
2. The duration of administration. During the initial administration of nitrous oxide, there is a linear increase in bowel gas cavity size. By approximately 100 minutes after the commencement of administration of nitrous oxide, bowel gas cavity size increases by 75–100%, and, at that time, the ratio of bowel nitrous oxide to end-tidal nitrous oxide is approximately 0.5.
3. The concentration of nitrous oxide. If the alveolar concentration is only 50%, the maximum possible increase in bowel gas is twofold. At 80%, the increase could potentially be fivefold.[108]

The distention of bowel by nitrous oxide may produce a number of problems. In a critical situation with an already distended bowel (*e.g.,* in bowel obstruction), the increases in size and intraluminal pressure may tip the balance toward bowel ischemia and necrosis. More commonly, the increase in size causes intraoperative difficulties for the surgeon, especially during abdominal closure. Therefore, although use of nitrous oxide for most abdominal procedures is appropriate, it is best to avoid nitrous oxide when the bowel contains significant quantities of gas. In such circumstances, it is probably safe to use nitrous oxide, limiting its concentration to 50% for a brief time (*e.g.,* 10–15 minutes), at the start of an operation to facilitate induction of anesthesia with a volatile drug. The nitrous oxide should be withdrawn thereafter and anesthesia should be maintained with oxygen and a volatile drug—a technique that leads to little or no increase in the size of gas-containing cavities.

Neostigmine

Parasympathetic activity results in increased bowel peristalsis. Thus, drugs that increase parasympathetic effects (*e.g.,* cholinesterase inhibitors such as neostigmine) also increase bowel activity. In normal bowel, neostigmine increases the frequency and magnitude of the pressure waves, particularly in the colon, and this effect is magnified in diseased bowel. Such effects may be reduced by the presence of anesthetic drugs or the previous administration of atropine or glycopyrrolate.[109] There is anecdotal evidence that the administration of neostigmine to patients with a large bowel anastomosis may lead to an increased incidence of anastomotic disruption, but this has never been verified experimentally.

Specific Disease States

Esophageal Perforation. Patients with this anomaly may be extremely ill, fluid depleted, and septic. They may have pneumomediastinum, pneumothorax, and pleural effusions. The patient's inability to swallow may complicate airway management.

Acute Pancreatitis. This entity is commonly associated with chronic alcohol ingestion; thus, the patient usually is compromised by the effects of alcoholism. The patient may be malnourished with impaired liver function and possibly an alcohol withdrawal syndrome. More acute problems include a fluid deficit, hypocalcemia, hyperglycemia, pleural effusions, and the adult respiratory distress syndrome.

Pancreatic Cysts and Pseudocysts. These cysts are usually a consequence of acute or chronic pancreatitis. Patients are usually malnourished and often septic.

Crohn's Disease. Patients with Crohn's disease are chronically ill, malnourished, and dehydrated owing to bowel obstruction, malabsorption, or loss of fluids and nutrients through fistulae. They are often very ill, taking large doses of steroids or immunosuppressive therapy.

Ulcerative Colitis. This chronic disease often results in electrolyte and fluid imbalance, vitamin B_{12} and folate deficiency, and extracolonic manifestations such as arthritis, iritis, and hepatitis. Operations in the quiescent phases are often undertaken for precancerous lesions. Acute problems that may necessitate urgent operation include hemorrhage, bowel perforation, bowel obstruction, and toxic megacolon. Patients undergoing operations in the acute phase are often very ill, taking large doses of steroids, and undergoing extensive operations (*e.g.*, total colectomy or total proctocolectomy). Careful resuscitation and intensive monitoring may be required.

Carcinoid Tumors. Although carcinoid tumors may occur at other anatomic sites, the GI tract is the source of most of them.[110-112] The tumors are usually small and frequently multiple. Most carcinoid tumors originate in the intestine, although approximately 20% can originate in the lung. Of those in the intestine, 50% occur in the appendix, 25% in the ileum (these are usually the source of metastatic tumors), and 20% in the rectum. The hormones secreted by nonmetastatic carcinoid tumors reach the liver by way of the portal vein and are usually inactivated there. However, once metastases to the liver have occurred, the hormones secreted by the hepatic metastases may have direct access to the systemic circulation, to produce the symptoms and signs of the *carcinoid syndrome*. Approximately 35% of patients with carcinoid tumors and metastases have symptoms of the carcinoid syndrome. The classic presentation of the carcinoid syndrome is not evident in all patients, and the presentation of the disease varies considerably between patients. Typical symptoms include cutaneous flushing, abdominal pain, vomiting, diarrhea, hypertension, hypotension, bronchospasm, and hyperglycemia.

Carcinoid tumors produce a variety of hormones, and the symptoms produced in each case probably depend on the hormone(s) secreted. A summary of the hormones secreted, their physiologic effects, and suggested treatments is given in Table 37-4.

The drug of choice for treatment of patients with carcinoid syndrome is the synthetic somatostatin analog octreotide.[112] Somatostatin suppresses release of serotonin and other vasoactive substances from the carcinoid tumor. Octreotide, with a half-life of approximately 160 minutes, has greatly improved preoperative and intraoperative management of carcinoid syndrome. Octreotide can be given subcutaneously in effect-titrated concentrations of 50–500 μg, 8-hourly, for prophylaxis, or 10–100 μg slowly iv 1 hour before surgery. During an intraoperative carcinoid crisis, it can be administered slowly iv in doses of 10–100 μg $\cdot$ h^{-1} or 100 μg $\cdot$ h^{-1} by iv drip, until symptoms cease. With the exception of steroids used for bronchospasm, other drugs used for carcinoid syndrome (*e.g.*, theophyllines for bronchospasm, aprotinin for flushing and hypotension, and cyproheptadine, methysergide, and ketanserin) are drugs of second choice and should be used only if octreotide has failed. Octreotide should be administered 100 μg subcutaneously, three times a day, for two weeks before surgery. If octreotide is discontinued after surgery, it should be weaned over a period of 1 week and not stopped abruptly.

Although carcinoid tumors are relatively rare, patients with carcinoid tumors who present for surgery are usually the worst affected and pose a number of problems. Carcinoid heart disease occurs in approximately one third of the patients, but its etiology is somewhat uncertain. The pathologic findings are predominantly right-sided fibrinous plaques deposited on the right ventricular wall and on the tricuspid valve, producing incompetence or, less frequently, stenosis or deposition on the pulmonary valve. Such plaques are rarely found on the left side of the heart. Invasive or noninvasive cardiologic evaluation is necessary to determine the magnitude and the effects of heart disease.

It is difficult to give blanket recommendations for the man-

Table 37-4. HORMONES RELEASED BY CARCINOID TUMORS AND THEIR MANAGEMENT

	Physiologic Effects	Treatment		
		Inhibiting Synthesis	*Hormone Depletion*	*Receptor Blockers*
Serotonin	Vasoconstriction Vasodilation Increased motility Tryptophan depletion	Parachlorophylalamine	Fenluranine	Methysergide Cyproheptadine Ketanserin
Kinins	Vasodilation Histamine release Bronchoconstriction	Steroids Aprotinin		
Histamine	Vasodilation H_1 = extravascular smooth muscle contraction H_2 = extravascular smooth muscle relaxation			H_2 antagonists Phenothiazines

agement of all patients with carcinoid syndrome because it is likely that the extent and proportion of hormonal secretion and the hormones' effects will vary from person to person. When anesthetizing a patient with a carcinoid syndrome, it may be possible to get clues to likely intraoperative events from the previous history, although this is not necessarily so (*e.g.,* 50% of the patients with intraoperative bronchospasm may have no previous history).

Choices of preoperative and intraoperative medication should be those that have low potential for provoking mediator release. Preoperative anxiety can trigger a carcinoid episode. Premedication with benzodiazepines, which do not release histamines, and antihistamines for any potential histamine release, is recommended. Perioperative factors that can trigger the release of carcinoid mediators (anxiety, hypothermia, hypercapnia, hypotension, hypertension) and drugs that can cause histamine release should be avoided. At induction of anesthesia, 100 μg of octreotide should be given iv. The induction of anesthesia should be smooth to avoid catecholamine release and is best performed with propofol or etomidate. Thiopental, with its potential for histamine release, is relatively contraindicated. Fentanyl and its derivatives, with their cardiovascular stability and non–histamine-releasing properties, are the opioids of choice. Morphine can cause histamine release and should be avoided. To facilitate tracheal intubation, nondepolarizing muscle relaxants are preferred because succinylcholine can cause histamine and peptide release from the liver. The use of succinylcholine should be limited to emergencies in which other agents are not considered suitable. Because of the potential for rapid and dramatic changes in systemic blood pressure, it may be wise to establish intra-arterial blood pressure monitoring before induction of anesthesia and to continue it after surgery. Central venous pressure and urinary output should be monitored because hypotension can be caused by both hypovolemia and mediator release from the carcinoid tumor. In patients with cardiac dysfunction, a pulmonary artery catheter or transesophageal echocardiographic monitor should be considered.

Anesthesia can be maintained with fentanyl or its derivatives, a nondepolarizing muscle relaxant, and an inhalation agent. Nitrous oxide, isoflurane, and sevoflurane are acceptable choices. Acceptable alternatives include continuous propofol infusion and spinal or epidural anesthesia. Regional anesthetic techniques require great care because sympathomimetic drugs, such as ephedrine, can trigger mediator release from carcinoid tumors.

Intraoperative hypotension is the most serious complication of the "carcinoid crisis" because it cannot be treated directly with sympathomimetics. The treatment of choice is fluid therapy and iv octreotide infused slowly. Hypertensive carcinoid crises can be treated by increasing the concentration of volatile anesthetic or with octreotide infusion. Bronchospastic carcinoid crises have been successfully treated with an iv bolus of octreotide (200 μg) and nebulized ipratropium bromide. Blood glucose levels should be closely monitored and hyperglycemia treated with an insulin infusion.

After surgery, the patient should be closely monitored for at least 24 hours because the effects of carcinoid mediators can continue after the tumor has been removed. Octreotide should be weaned slowly over a week.

REFERENCES

1. Flegal KM: The obesity epidemic in children and adults: Current evidence and research issues. Med Sci Sports Exerc 31(11 Suppl):S509, 1999
2. Van Itallie TB: Health implications of overweight and obesity in the United States. Ann Intern Med 103:983, 1985
3. Kuzmarski RJ, Flegal KM, Campbell SM, Johnson CL: Increasing prevalence of overweight amongst U.S. adults: The National Health and Nutrition Examination surveys 1960–1991. JAMA 272:205, 1994
4. Abraham S, Johnson CL: Prevalence of severe obesity in adults in the United States. Am J Clin Nutr 33:306, 1980
5. Willett WC, Dietz WH, Colditz GA: Guidelines for healthy weight. N Engl J Med 341:247, 1999
6. Fisher A, Waterhouse TD, Adams AP: Obesity: Its relation to anaesthesia. Anaesthesia 30:633, 1975
7. Shenkman Z, Shir Y, Brodsky JB: Perioperative management of the morbidly obese patient. Br J Anaesth 70:349, 1993
8. Bray GA, Gray DS: Obesity: Part 1. Pathogenesis. West J Med 149:429, 1988
9. Peiris AN, Sothmann MS, Hoffman RG et al: Adiposity, fat distribution and cardiovascular risk. Ann Intern Med 110:867, 1989
10. Rexrode KM, Carey VJ, Hennekens CH et al: Abdominal adiposity and coronary artery disease in women. JAMA 280:1843, 1998
11. Nakajima T, Fujioka S, Tokunaga K et al: Correlation of intraabdominal fat accumulation and left ventricular function in obesity. Am J Cardiol 64:369, 1989
12. Farebrother MJB: Respiratory function and cardiorespiratory response to exercise in obesity. Br J Dis Chest 73:211, 1979
13. Luce JM: Respiratory complications of obesity. Chest 78:626, 1980
14. Vaughan RW: Pulmonary and cardiovascular derangements in the obese patient. In Brown BR (ed): Anesthetics and the Obese Patient, p 19. Contemporary Anesthesia Practice Series. Philadelphia, FA Davis, 1982
15. Zerah F, Harf A, Perlmuter L et al: Effects of obesity on respiratory resistance. Chest 103:1470, 1993
16. Burwell CS, Robin ED, Whaley RD et al: External obesity associated with alveolar hypoventilation: A Pickwickian syndrome. Am Med 21:811, 1956
17. Reisin E, Frolich ED: Obesity: Cardiovascular and respiratory pathophysiological alterations. Arch Intern Med 141:431, 1981
18. Alexander JK: The cardiomyopathy of obesity. Prog Cardiovasc Dis 28:325, 1985
19. Paul DR, Hoyt IL, Boutros AR: Cardiovascular and respiratory changes in response to change of posture in the obese. Anesthesiology 45:73, 1976
20. Corrello BA, Gittens L: The cardiac mechanisms and function in obese normotensive persons with normal coronary arteries. Am J Cardiol 59:469, 1987
21. Bergalp B, Cesur V, Corapcioglu D et al: Obesity and left ventricular diastolic function. Int J Cardiol 52:23, 1995
22. Ferraro S, Pewrrone-Filiardi P, Desirderio A et al: Left ventricular systolic and diastolic function in severe obesity: a radionuclide study. Cardiology 87:347, 1996
23. Alpert MA, Terry BE, Mulekar M et al: Cardiac morphology and left ventricular function in normotensive morbidly obese patients with and without congestive heart failure and the effect of weight loss. Am J Cardiol 80:736, 1997
24. Noda A, Okada T, Yatsuma F et al: Cardiac hypertrophy in the obstructive sleep apnea syndrome. Chest 107:1538, 1995
25. Alpert MA, Singh A, Terry BE et al: Effect of exercise on left ventricular systolic function and reserve in morbid obesity. Am J Cardiol 63:1478, 1989
26. Vaughan RW: Biochemical and biotransformation alterations in obesity. In Brown BR (ed): Anesthesia and the Obese Patient, p 55. Contemporary Anesthesia Practice Series. Philadelphia, FA Davis, 1982
27. Vaughan RW, Bauer S, Wise L: Volume and pH of gastric juice in obese patients. Anesthesiology 43:686, 1975
28. Nomura F, Ohnishi K, Satomura Y et al: Liver function in moderate obesity: Study in 536 moderately obese subjects among 4613 male company employees. Int J Obes 10:349, 1986
29. Hocking MP, Davis GL, Franzini DA et al: Long term consequences after jejunoileal bypass for morbid obesity. Dig Dis Sci 43:2493, 1998
30. Wittels EH, Thompson S: Obstructive sleep apnea and obesity. Otolaryngol Clin North Am 23:751, 1990
31. Gortmaker SL, Must A, Perrin JM et al: Social and economic consequences of overweight in adolescence and young adulthood. N Engl J Med 329:1009, 1993
32. Time: January 16th, 1995, p 35
33. Blumberg P, Mellis LP: Medical students' attitudes towards the obese and the morbidly obese. Int J Eat Disord 4:169, 1985
34. Price JH, Desmond SM, Krol RA et al: Family practice physicians' attitudes and practices regarding obesity. Am J Prev Med 3:339, 1987

35. Wadden TA, Stunkard AJ: Social and psychological consequences of obesity. Ann Intern Med 103:1062, 1985

36. Buckley FP, Robinson NB, Simonowitz DA *et al:* Anesthesia in the morbidly obese: A comparison of anesthetic and analgesic regimens for upper abdominal surgery. Anaesthesia 38:840, 1983

37. Abernathy DR, Greenblatt DS: Pharmacokinetics of drugs in obesity. Clin Pharmacokinet 7:108, 1981

38. Blouin RA, Kolpek JH, Mann HJ: Influence of obesity on drug disposition. Clinical Pharmacy 6:706, 1987

39. Abernathy DR, Greenblatt DS, Divoll M *et al:* The influence of obesity on the pharmacokinetics of oral alprazolam and triazolam. Clin Pharmacokinet 9:177, 1984

40. Mayersohn M, Calkins JM, Perrier DG *et al:* Thiopental kinetics in obese patients. Anesthesiology 55:A178, 1981

41. Ladergaard-Pederson MJ: Recovery from general anesthesia in obese patients. Anesthesiology 55:720, 1981

42. Cork RC, Vaughan RW, Bentley JB: General anesthesia for morbidly obese patients: An examination of postoperative outcomes. Anesthesiology 54:310, 1981

43. Sevin F, Farinotti R, Haberer JP, Desmonts JM: Propofol infusion for maintenance of anesthesia in morbidly obese patients receiving nitrous oxide: A clinical and pharmacokinetic study. Anesthesiology 78:657, 1993

44. Bentley JB, Borel JD, Gillespie TS *et al:* Fentanyl pharmacokinetics in obese and nonobese patients. Anesthesiology 55:A177, 1981

45. Schwartz AE, Matteo RS, Ornstein E *et al:* Pharmacokinetics of sufentanil in obese patients. Anesth Analg 73:790, 1991

46. Bentley JB, Finley JM, Humphrey LR *et al:* Obesity and alfentanil pharmacokinetics. Anesth Analg 62:251, 1983

47. Egan TD, Huizinga B, Gupta SK *et al:* Remifentanil pharmacokinetics in obese versus lean patients. Anesthesiology 89:562, 1998

48. Bentley JB, Bond JB, Vaughan RW *et al:* Weight, pseudocholinesterase activity and succinylcholine requirements. Anesthesiology 57:48, 1982

49. Tuchy GK, Tuchy E, Bleyberg M *et al:* Pharmacodynamics of mivacurium in obese patients. Anesthesiology 81:A1069, 1994

50. Tseueda K, Warren JE, McCafferty LA: Pancuronium bromide requirement during anesthesia for the morbidly obese. Anesthesiology 48:483, 1978

51. Weinstein JE, Matteo RS, Ornstein E *et al:* Pharmacodynamics of vecuronium and atracurium in the obese surgical patient. Anesth Analg 65:684, 1986

52. Schwartz AE, Matteo RS, Ornstein E *et al:* Pharmacokinetics and dynamics of metocurine in the obese. Anesthesiology 65:A295, 1986

53. Puhringer FK, Keller C, Kleinsasser A *et al:* Pharmacokinetics of rocuronium bromide in obese female patients. Eur J Anesthesiol 16:507, 1999

54. Varin F, Ducharme J, Thoret Y *et al:* The influence of extreme obesity on body disposition and neuromuscular blocking effect of atracurium. Clin Pharmacol Ther 48:18, 1990

55. Herer B, Roche N, Carton M *et al:* Value of clinical, functional, and oximetric data for the prediction of obstructive sleep apnea in obese patients. Chest 116:1537, 1999

56. Norton ML, Brown ACD: Evaluating the patient with a difficult airway for anesthesia. Otolaryngol Clin North Am 23:771, 1990

57. McNeely W, Goa KL: Sibutramine: A review of its contribution to the management of obesity. Drugs 56:1093, 1998

58. Wilson SL, Manaltea NR, Malvesa JD: Effects of atropine, glycopyrrolate and cimetidine on gastric secretions in markedly obese patients. Anesth Analg 60:37, 1981

59. Goldberg ME, Rosenberg FL, Everts EA Jr *et al:* Metoclopramide and cimetidine pretreatment does not reduce the risk of acid aspiration in the morbidly obese patient. Anesthesiology 63:A279, 1985

60. Lam AM, Grace DM, Penny FJ *et al:* Prophylactic IV cimetidine reduces the risk of acid aspiration in morbidly obese patients. Anesthesiology 65:684, 1986

61. Manchikanti L, Roush JR, Colliver JR: Effect of preanesthetic ranitidine and metoclopramide on gastric contents of morbidly obese patients. Anesth Analg 65:195, 1986

62. Mason DS Sapaal JA, Wood MH *et al:* Influence of forced air warming on morbidly obese patients undergoing Roux-en-Y gastric bypass. Obesity Surgery 8:453, 1998

63. Lee JJ, Larson RM, Buckley JJ *et al:* Airway maintenance in the morbidly obese. Anesthesiol Rev 7:33, 1980

64. Mallampati SR, Gatt SP *et al:* A clinical sign to predict difficult tracheal intubation: A prospective study. Canadian Anaesthetists Society Journal 32:429, 1985

65. Moyer GA, Rein P: Preoxygenation in the morbidly obese patient. Anesth Analg 65:S106, 1986

66. Jense HG, Dubin SA, Silverstein PI *et al:* Effect of obesity on safe duration of apnoea in anesthetised humans. Anesth Analg 72:89, 1991

67. Vaughan RW, Wise L: Intraoperative hypoxemia in obese patients. Ann Surg 184:35, 1976

68. Bentley JB, Vaughan RW, Gandolfi J *et al:* Halothane biotransformation in obese and nonobese patients. Anesthesiology 57:94, 1982

69. Strube PJ, Hulands GM, Halsey MJ: Serum fluoride levels in morbidly obese patients: Enflurane compared with isoflurane. Anaesthesia 42:685, 1987

70. Frink EJ, Malan TP, Brown RA *et al:* Plasma inorganic fluoride levels with sevoflurane anesthesia in morbidly obese and non obese patients. Anesth Analg 76:1333, 1993

71. Sutton TS, Koblin DD, Gruenke LD *et al:* Fluoride metabolites after prolonged exposure of patients and volunteers to desflurane. Anesth Analg 73:180, 1991

72. Salem MR, Joseph N, Lim R *et al:* Respiratory and hemodynamic response to PEEP in grossly obese patients. Anesthesiology 61:A511, 1984

73. Pelosi P, Ravagnan I, Giurati G *et al:* Positive end expiratory pressure improves respiratory function in obese but not normal subjects during anesthesia and paralysis. Anesthesiology 91:1221, 1999

74. Pelosi P, Croci M, Callappi E *et al:* Prone positioning improves pulmonary function in obese patients during general anesthesia. Anesth Analg 83:578, 1996

75. Palmon SC, Kirsch JR, Depper JA *et al:* The effect of the prone position on pulmonary mechanics is frame dependent. Anesth Analg 87:1175, 1998

76. Brodsky JB, Wyner J, Ehrenwerth S *et al:* One lung ventilation anesthesia in morbidly obese patients. Anesthesiology 57:32, 1982

77. In-amani M, Kikuta Y, Nagai H *et al:* The increase in pulmonary venous admixture by hypocapnia is enhanced in obese patients. Anesthesiology 63:A520, 1985

78. Ferguson CL, Sivashankaran S, Dauchot PJ: Ventilator settings to mitigate hypocarbia in the obese patient. Anesth Analg 65:53, 1986

79. McCullough WJD, Littlewood DG: Influence of obesity on spinal analgesia with bupivacaine. Br J Anaesth 58:610, 1984

80. Pitkanen MJ: Body mass and the spread of spinal analgesia with bupivacaine. Anesth Analg 66:127, 1987

81. Taivainen T, Tuominen M, Rosenberg PM: Influence of obesity on the spread of spinal analgesia after injection of plain 0.5% bupivacaine at the L3–4 or L4–5 interspace. Br J Anaesth 64:542, 1990

82. Catennacci AJ, Anderson JD, Boersma D: Anesthetic hazards of obesity. JAMA 175:657, 1961

83. Catennacci AJ, Sampathakar DR: Ventilation studies in the obese patient during spinal anesthesia. Anesth Analg 48:48, 1969

84. Blass NM: Regional anesthesia in the morbidly obese. Regional Anesthesia 5(3):20, 1979

85. Chamberlain DD, Chamberlain BDL: Changes in skin temperature and their relationship to sympathetic blockade during spinal anesthesia. Anesthesiology 65:139, 1986

86. Hodgkinson R, Hussein FJ: Caesarian section associated with gross obesity. Br J Anaesth 52:919, 1980

87. Brown RS, Johnson MD, Zavisca F *et al:* Morbid obesity in the parturient reduces the risk of post dural puncture headache after large bore continuous spinal anesthesia. Anesthesiology 79:A1009, 1993

88. Fox GS, Whalley DG, Bevan DR: Anaesthesia for the morbidly obese: Experience with 110 patients. Br J Anaesth 53:811, 1981

89. Gelman S, Vitek JJ: Thoracic epidural catheter placement under fluoroscopic control in morbidly obese patients. Regional Anesthesia 4(4):19, 1980

90. Hodgkinson R, Hussein FJ: Obesity and the spread of analgesia following epidural administration of bupivacaine for caesarian section. Anesth Analg 59:89, 1980

91. Gelman S, Laws ML, Potzick J *et al:* Thoracic epidural vs. balanced anaesthesia in morbid obesity: An intraoperative and postoperative hemodynamic study. Anesth Analg 59:902, 1980

92. Rawal N, Sjostrand V, Christofferson E *et al:* Comparison of intramuscular and epidural morphine for postoperative analgesia in the grossly obese: Influence on postoperative ambulation and pulmonary function. Anesth Analg 63:583, 1986
93. Milligan KR, Cramp P, Schatz L *et al:* The effect of positioning and obesity on epidural analgesic spread. Anesth Analg 72:S185, 1991
94. Vaughan RW, Wise L: Intraoperative hypoxemia in obese patients. Ann Surg 180:872, 1974
95. Rand CSW, Kuldau JM, Yost RL: Obesity and postoperative pain. J Psychosom Res 29:43, 1985
96. Vandercar DH, Martinez AP, De Lisser EA: Sleep apnea syndromes: A potential contraindication for patient controlled analgesia. Anesthesiology 74:623, 1991
97. Graves DA, Batenhorst RL, Bennet RL *et al:* Morphine requirements using patient controlled analgesia: Influence of diurnal variation and morbid obesity. Clinical Pharmacy 2:49, 1982
98. Levin A, Klein SL, Brolin RE *et al:* Patient controlled analgesia for morbidly obese patients: An effective modality if used correctly. Anesthesiology 76:857, 1992
99. Scratcherd T, Grundy O: The physiology of intestinal motility and secretion. Br J Anaesth 56:3, 1984
100. Nimmo WS: Effect of anaesthesia on gastric motility and emptying. Br J Anaesth 56:29, 1984
101. Ferrari LR, Rooney FM, Rockoff MA: Preoperative fasting practices in pediatrics. Anesthesiology 90:978, 1999
102. Aitkenhead AR: Anaesthesia and bowel surgery. Br J Anaesth 56:95, 1984
103. Gelman S, Fowler KC, Smith LR: Regional blood flow during isoflurane and halothane anesthesia. Anesth Analg 63:557, 1986
104. Aitkenhead AR, Gilmour PS, Hothersall AP *et al:* Effects of subarachnoid nerve block and arterial PCO_2 on colon blood flow. Br J Anaesth 52:1071, 1980
105. Warner MA, Warner ME, Warner DO, *et al:* Perioperative pulmonary aspiration in infants and children. Anesthesiology 90:66, 1999
106. Manchikanti L, Colliver JA, Marrero T *et al:* Ranitidine and metoclopramide for prophylaxis of aspiration pneumonitis in elective surgery. Anesth Analg 63:903, 1984
107. Tournadre JP, Chassard D, Berrada KR *et al:* Cricoid cartilage pressure decreases lower esophageal sphincter tone. Anesthesiology 86:7, 1997
108. Eger EL III, Saidman LJ: Hazards of nitrous oxide in bowel obstruction and pneumothorax. Anesthesiology 26:61, 1965
109. Childes CS: Prevention of neostigmine induced colonic activity. Anaesthesia 39:1083, 1984
110. Longnecker M, Roizen MF: Patients with carcinoid syndrome. Anesthesiol Clin North Am 51:313, 1987
111. Vaughan DJ, Brunner MD: Anesthesia for patients with carcinoid syndrome. Int Anesthesiol Clin 35(4):129, 1997
112. Gray J, Jahr JS, Schneider P: Carcinoid syndrome and anesthetic use of octreotide: A review. Am J Anesth 26:377, 1999

Clinical Anesthesia (4/e), edited by
Paul G. Barash, Bruce F. Cullen, and
Robert K. Stoelting. Lippincott Williams &
Wilkins, Philadelphia, © 2001.

CHAPTER 38

ANESTHESIA FOR MINIMALLY INVASIVE PROCEDURES

ANTHONY J. CUNNINGHAM AND NOREEN DOWD

HISTORICAL PERSPECTIVES

The modern age of laparoscopic surgery was ushered in with the incorporation of a miniature video camera attached to the eyepiece of the laparoscope, allowing multiple assistants to view the operative field from the same vantage point.[1] Gynecologic laparoscopic surgery has been routinely performed since the 1970s. In 1987, Phillipe Mouret described the first laparoscopic cholecystectomy in France; the first series was reported by Peris-sat *et al*,[2] and the technique was introduced into the United States in 1988 by Reddick and Olsen.[3] Improved instrumentation allowed laparoscopic cholecystectomy to revolutionize upper abdominal surgery in the 1990s. Currently, laparoscopic gastroesophageal, hepatobiliary, colorectal, and solid-organ renal/splenic procedures, as well as herniorrhaphy, are routinely performed using minimal-access techniques.

Laparoscopic surgical techniques have been rapidly accepted by surgeons worldwide, with published reports describing the benefits of less postoperative pain, reduced hospital stay, and an earlier return to work.[4] Until the late 1980s, morbidity and mortality were accepted as unavoidable aspects of the therapeutic process. The current realization that less invasive methods of treatment may reduce the risks of death and morbidity has given rise to the concept of *minimally invasive therapy* with the general aim to "minimize the trauma of the interventional process whilst still achieving a satisfactory therapeutic result."[5] A United Kingdom report commissioned by the Department of Health[6] to assess the implications of minimally invasive therapy did not favor the term *minimally invasive surgery*, with its connotation of increased safety and minor procedures, preferring instead the term *minimal-access surgery*. The key feature of this technology-dependent surgery is that it produces significantly less trauma than does the conventional means of gaining access. The technology required is expensive, and its adoption has major implications for patient services, hospital design, operating room equipment, surgical specialty alignment, and training.[7]

Public perception that laparoscopic techniques are superior has led to the poorly controlled and audited introduction of laparoscopy-based surgical procedures. The percentage of cholecystectomies that are laparoscopic procedures has climbed from 0% in 1987 to 80% in 1992.[8] A State of New York Department of Health[9] memorandum reported 158 adverse incidents involving laparoscopic cholecystectomy between August 1990 and March 1992. Seventy-two percent of these incidents required remedial open surgical repair of the injury/complication. As the demand grew for laparoscopy-based procedures, the demand for training also increased. Approximately 15,000 general surgeons were trained in new laparoscopic techniques in the United States between 1990 and 1992.[8] The Society of American Gastrointestinal Endoscopy Surgeons suggested guidelines for the credentialing, training, and determination of competence in laparoscopy techniques for their members.[10]

For more than a century, surgeons have upheld the legacy of William Halsted, who believed that each surgical advance should be based on thoughtful observation, laboratory experimentation, and carefully planned clinical trials. The evolution of laparoscopic cholecystectomy, however, has represented a

departure from traditional surgical development. The National Laparoscopic Surgery Registry was established in the United States in 1990 with the support of independent educational grants to help evaluate the acquisition of technical skills, the outcome analysis of new laparoscopic procedures, and cost–benefit assessments. The initial mission of the Registry was to collect, organize, and disseminate clinical data relevant to laparoscopic cholecystectomy, but has been expanded to include all endocavity surgical procedures.[11]

The development and potential for advanced laparoscopic surgery, beyond laparoscopic cholecystectomy and diagnostic laparoscopy, were reviewed by Hunter.[12] Current limitations include a two-dimensional video image and the requirement for specialized surgical instrumentation. The laparoscopic port acts as a fulcrum that restricts the freedom of movement of the instruments.[1] The development of three-dimensional imaging and expected introduction of flexible laparoscopes and robotics in the future will herald a new age in interventional surgery.[1,13] The implications for anesthesia will be far reaching. The physiologic effects of prolonged CO_2 insufflation into an endocavity combined with variations in positioning have a major impact on cardiopulmonary function, particularly in American Society of Anesthesiologists (ASA) Class III or IV patients.[14] Introduction of "gasless laparoscopy" using an abdominal wall lifting device may obviate the requirement for pneumoperitoneum.[15]

CARDIAC AND THORACOSCOPIC PROCEDURES

Thoracoscopic Procedures

The history of thoracoscopic surgery has been reviewed.[16] Jacobaeus, in 1910, introduced therapeutic thoracoscopy by using the cystoscope in the pleural space to diagnose and treat patients with tuberculous effusions. Thoracoscopy is now commonly used in the diagnosis and treatment of pleuropulmonary disease.

The thoracoscopic management of pneumothorax and bullous lung disease was reviewed by Hazelrigg.[17] Thoracoscopy allows visualization of the causal lung lesion, its removal, and subsequent pleurodesis. Blebs may be resected using a ligature or linear stapler and thoracoscopic pleural abrasion or apical pleurectomy used to achieve pleurodesis. Open surgical procedures for idiopathic spontaneous pneumothorax are rapidly being replaced by analogous thoracoscopic procedures. Graeber and Jones[18] reviewed the application of thoracoscopic techniques in the management of traumatic thoracic injuries. After initial stabilization, they recommend thoracoscopic evaluation under general anesthesia through a double-lumen endobronchial tube in the operating room. Videothoracoscopy proved to be an accurate and safe procedure in the assessment of diaphragmatic injuries, control of continuing chest wall bleeding, and the early evacuation of clotted hemothorax.

Video-Assisted Thoracic Surgery

Video-assisted thoracic surgery (VATS) presents new challenges for the surgeon and anesthesiologist. Potential advantages include less postoperative pain, improved postoperative pulmonary function, shorter hospitalization, and earlier return to work. Applications of VATS (Table 38-1) include lobectomy, pneumonectomy, esophagectomy, and pericardial resection. More innovative applications include implantation of the implantable cardioverter–defibrillator,[19] excision of mediastinal masses, transthoracic endoscopic sympathectomy for the treatment of upper limb hyperhydrosis and painful causalgias,[20,21] and splanchnicectomy (celiac plexus block) for intractable pain from pancreatic cancer and pancreatitis.[22] VATS has been reported in the management of multiple diseases of the thoracic spine, including disc herniation, disc space abscesses, and spinal deformities.[23]

Early experience with video-assisted thoracoscopic lobectomy has been reported by Kirby *et al.*[24] A successful VATS lobectomy was accomplished *via* two thoracoscopy ports and a 6–8-cm ''access'' thoracotomy in 35 of 44 patients included in the study. Conversion to open thoracotomy was indicated in five patients because of dense pleural adhesions, difficulty dissecting the interlobar pulmonary artery, or a combination of these factors. The mean operative time for thoracoscopic lobectomy was 153 ± 26 minutes, and no major intraoperative complications were reported. The mean hospital stay was 5.7 ± 1.6 days. The authors concluded that VATS lobectomy was technically feasible and potentially safe. Walker *et al*[25] reported their experience with video-assisted thoracoscopic pneumonectomy and found that the lung was easily delivered through a small submammary incision. Adoption of VATS lobectomy and pneumonectomy has enabled curative surgery to be attempted as an alternative to compromise therapy in elderly patients.[26]

Anesthetic Implications

Anesthetic techniques for thoracoscopy were reviewed by Horswell.[27] Most VATS are performed under general anesthesia with one-lung ventilation (OLV) provided through a double-lumen endobronchial tube placed in the left mainstem bronchus and verified bronchoscopically (Fig. 38-1).

Anesthesia is maintained by a combination of intravenous (iv) and inhaled agents. A radial artery cannula is usually placed for continuous blood pressure measurement and blood gas analysis.[28] Continuous pulse oximetry and end-tidal carbon di-

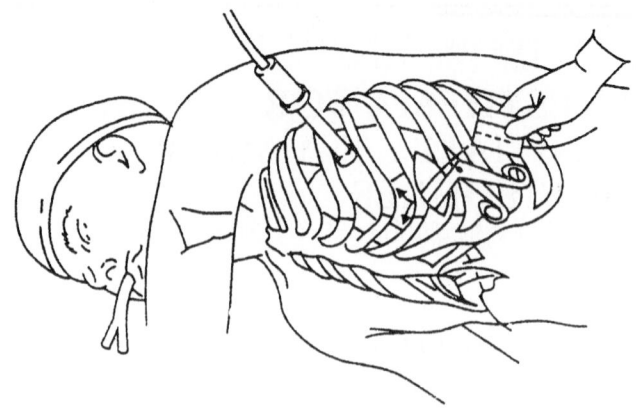

Figure 38-1. Thoracoscopic surgery.

oxide tension (PET_{CO_2}) are measured. Postoperative pain is managed by patient-controlled opioid analgesia, nonsteroidal anti-inflammatory drugs (NSAIDs), or regional techniques. VATS-assisted placement of paravertebral catheters during thoracoscopic procedures has been reported in the management of postoperative pain.[29]

The double-lumen endobronchial tube has evolved as the technique of choice for most cases of OLV, which creates an obligatory right-to-left transpulmonary shunt of blood flow through the nonventilated, nondependent lung. Consequently, OLV results in a much larger alveolar–arterial oxygen tension difference and a greater risk of intraoperative hypoxemia than two-lung ventilation.

The distribution of pulmonary blood flow and ventilation is influenced by the lateral decubitus position, and the anesthetized, paralyzed, closed/open chest conditions. Creation of an artificial pneumothorax by CO_2 insufflation has been advocated in an effort to provide complete nondependent lung collapse and optimal surgical conditions. Using an animal model, Jones *et al*[30] evaluated the hemodynamic response to varying insufflation pressures in eight mechanically ventilated pigs undergoing thoracoscopy. Significant hemodynamic compromise followed CO_2 insufflation. Cardiac index (CI), stroke volume, and left ventricular stroke work index (LVSWI) decreased 36%, 34%, and 49%, respectively, compared with baseline measurement at an insufflation pressure of 5 mm Hg. At an insufflation pressure of 15 mm Hg, mean arterial blood pressure (MABP) decreased 64%, CI decreased 81%, and LVSWI decreased 95% compared with baseline. The hemodynamic parameters returned to within 5% of baseline values when negative intrapleural pressure was restored by suction. The authors concluded that routine CO_2 insufflation during thoracoscopy could not be recommended because of significant hemodynamic compromise.

Patients with severe bilateral chronic lung disease who previously may not have been candidates for thoracotomy may be considered for VATS. Barker *et al*[31] described the anesthetic management of 22 such patients who underwent long periods of OLV during thoracoscopic laser ablation of emphysematous bullae. Thirteen patients in this series were receiving long-term supplemental oxygen and six patients were wheelchair bound. Despite this degree of respiratory impairment, OLV with 100% O_2 was instituted for a mean of 170 ± 53 minutes. Intraoperative hypoxemia was managed with differential lung ventilation and positive end-expiratory pressure as required. Only one patient failed to tolerate OLV. Elective postoperative ventilation was recommended.

Table 38-1. VIDEO-ASSISTED THORACIC SURGERY

Lungs
  Pneumonectomy
  Lobectomy
  Wedge, subsegmental, segmental resection
  Resection of pulmonary metastases
  Excision of blebs and bullae
Heart
  Pericardiocentesis
  Pericardiectomy
  Insertion of implantable cardioverter–difibrillator
Esophagus
  Esophagectomy
  Repair of esophageal perforation
  Fundoplication
Mediastinum
  Excision of tumors/cysts
Sympathetic nervous system
  Transthoracic endoscopic sympathectomy
Vagus
  Truncal vagotomy
Thoracic spine
  Disc herniation
  Deformity correction
  Abscess drainage

An overview of the emerging practice of thoracoscopy and VATS was provided by the Video Assisted Thoracic Surgery Study Group.[32] This group has collected data on 1820 patients from more than 40 institutions who have undergone a thoracoscopic procedure in an effort to define the role for this new technique. Lung nodules (47.5%) and pleural effusions (19.4%) represent the most frequent indication, and most commonly performed procedures were wedge resection (49%) and operation in the pleural space. Conversion to thoracotomy occurred in 24% of procedures. Half of these conversions were because of the need for more extensive resection, but other indications included inability to find the lesion, too large a lesion or difficult location, adhesions, equipment failure, and bleeding. Complications included prolonged air leak for more than 5 days (4.7%), atelectasis (1.9%), dysrhythmia (1.6%), bleeding requiring transfusion (2.0%), and pneumonia (1.9%). Rubin et al,[33] in an investigation of patients undergoing VATS or thoracotomy for limited diagnostic and therapeutic procedures, found that the VATS patients had significantly shorter hospitalizations (4.8 ± 2.7 versus 7.8 ± 4.6 days), fewer days of narcotic use for pain control (3.4 ± 2.1 versus 6.1 ± 3.6 days), and similar operating times compared with patients undergoing traditional thoracotomy.

Cardiac Procedures

Since the mid-1990s, minimally invasive cardiac surgery has evolved to avoid cardiopulmonary bypass (CPB; with its inherent risks), median sternotomy, or both. The media, patient preferences, and commercial developments (fiberoptic imaging technology) that made minimally invasive cardiac surgery possible have fueled this change.

Cardiovascular disease affects approximately one in four Americans, with approximately one million deaths per year.[34] The increasing numbers of elderly patients undergoing cardiac surgical procedures has major implications for health care costs.[35] To contain costs and minimize the major risks of conventional cardiac surgery, including median sternotomy (mediastinitis, sternal dehiscence, chest wall instability, wound pain) and deleterious effects of CPB (stroke, neuropsychological dysfunction, myocardial infarction, renal dysfunction and bleeding diatheses), less invasive direct procedures have been introduced[36] (Fig. 38-2).

Minimally invasive direct coronary artery bypass grafting (MIDCAB) is an alternative method of revascularization for certain categories of coronary artery disease.[37] The strategy is to use a small incision, thus avoiding median sternotomy, or to make an anastomosis on the beating heart without CPB, or both.[38] Port-access minimally invasive cardiac surgery uses a system of cannulae and catheters to provide CPB and myocardial protection without accessing the heart through a median sternotomy. In contrast, the strategy in valvular heart surgery is to avoid the median sternotomy. However, all valve procedures currently require CPB.

Benetti and colleagues[39] highlighted developments in minimally invasive cardiac surgery techniques between 1978 and 1990. In 1975, Ankeneny[40] reported a series of 143 patients undergoing coronary artery bypass graft surgery without CPB and the same year Trapp and Bisarya[41] reported a series of 63 patients. Buffolo et al[42] reported their series of 1274 patients in 1996 and concluded that the operation can be performed with an acceptable mortality rate of 2.5%. In addition, all types of arterial conduits can be used and the incidences of neurologic complications (1.1%) and dysrhythmias (5.5%) were lower than with conventional coronary artery bypass grafting with CPB (3.8% and 12.6%, respectively).[42] In contrast to MIDCAB, minimally invasive valve surgery is in its relative infancy, with the first such repair performed by Chitwood et al[43] in 1996. Cosgrove

and Sabik[44] at the Cleveland Clinic subsequently described and popularized a minimally invasive approach for aortic valve replacement.

The largest experience of minimally invasive cardiac surgery relates to coronary artery bypass surgery. The advantages of MIDCAB include early extubation, hospital discharge, and return to a functional level[45] (Table 38-2).

Diegeler and colleagues[46] reported an immediate and 6-month angiographic graft patency rate of at least 90% in a series of patients undergoing MIDCAB. The limited clinical experience of minimally invasive valve surgery prohibits firm conclusions about the utility and benefit of this technique. However, Weinschelbaum et al[47] reported that the minimally invasive approach was a useful technique in patients undergoing first-time valve surgery.

Surgical Techniques

Minimally invasive coronary artery bypass is particularly suitable for patients with isolated proximal left anterior descending coronary artery (LAD) disease or right coronary artery disease and minimal left ventricular impairment.[48] In addition, Del Rizzo et al[49] reported that high-risk patients (advanced age, urgent operation, impaired left ventricular function, redo operation) are also suitable candidates and have significantly lower mortality rates and intensive care unit (ICU) stays compared with predicted rates for similar patients undergoing conventional coronary artery bypass surgery. Relative contraindications include acute myocardial ischemia at the time of the procedure, a small LAD (lumenal diameter <1.5 mm), and cardiac arrhythmias (atrial fibrillation). An intramyocardial or calcified LAD represents an absolute contraindication.

Minimally invasive coronary artery bypass is performed using one of two types of approaches,[50] a series of small holes or "ports" in the chest (referred to as PACAB, PortCAB, or port-access coronary artery bypass) or a small incision directly over the coronary artery to be bypassed (i.e., MIDCAB). The latter may be used with a port access approach.

Port-Access Coronary Artery Bypass. Port-access coronary artery bypass currently uses CPB via the femoral vessels. Bypasses are performed using instruments passed through the ports during cardiac standstill. As with abdominal laparoscopic surgery, the cardiac surgeon typically views the operative field on a video monitor. More recently, a specially designed port-access system has been introduced by a group from Stanford in conjunction with Heartport (Redwood City, CA). Port-access coronary artery bypass surgery was initially attempted under thoracoscopic guidance, but small incisions are now used to allow direct anastomosis to the coronary arteries, similar to the MIDCAB procedure. This system is used for both minimally invasive coronary artery bypass and mitral valve surgery.

Minimally Invasive Direct Coronary Artery Bypass. MIDCAB uses a small incision directly over the coronary artery to be bypassed. The small incisions used most commonly for the left coronary circulation include a mini-anterior mediastinotomy, a minithoracotomy, and a mini- or partial sternotomy. Right coronary artery disease may also be treated by MIDCAB using a gastroepiploic artery graft, through a small subxiphoid incision. All of the approaches are suitable for off-pump coronary artery bypass grafting. Diegeler and colleagues[46] compared four techniques for minimally invasive coronary artery bypass surgery and found that MIDCAB using a minithoracotomy, without CPB, was the preferred technique for one-vessel graft procedure to the LAD or right coronary artery. The port-access system with CPB was reserved as a second option for young patients requiring multiple-vessel grafting to the left coronary circulation (LAD or circumflex arteries). For either the MIDCAB or port-access techniques, the procedure is converted to a standard median sternotomy and CPB in less than 5% of cases, when the artery lies inside the heart muscle and cannot be easily located.

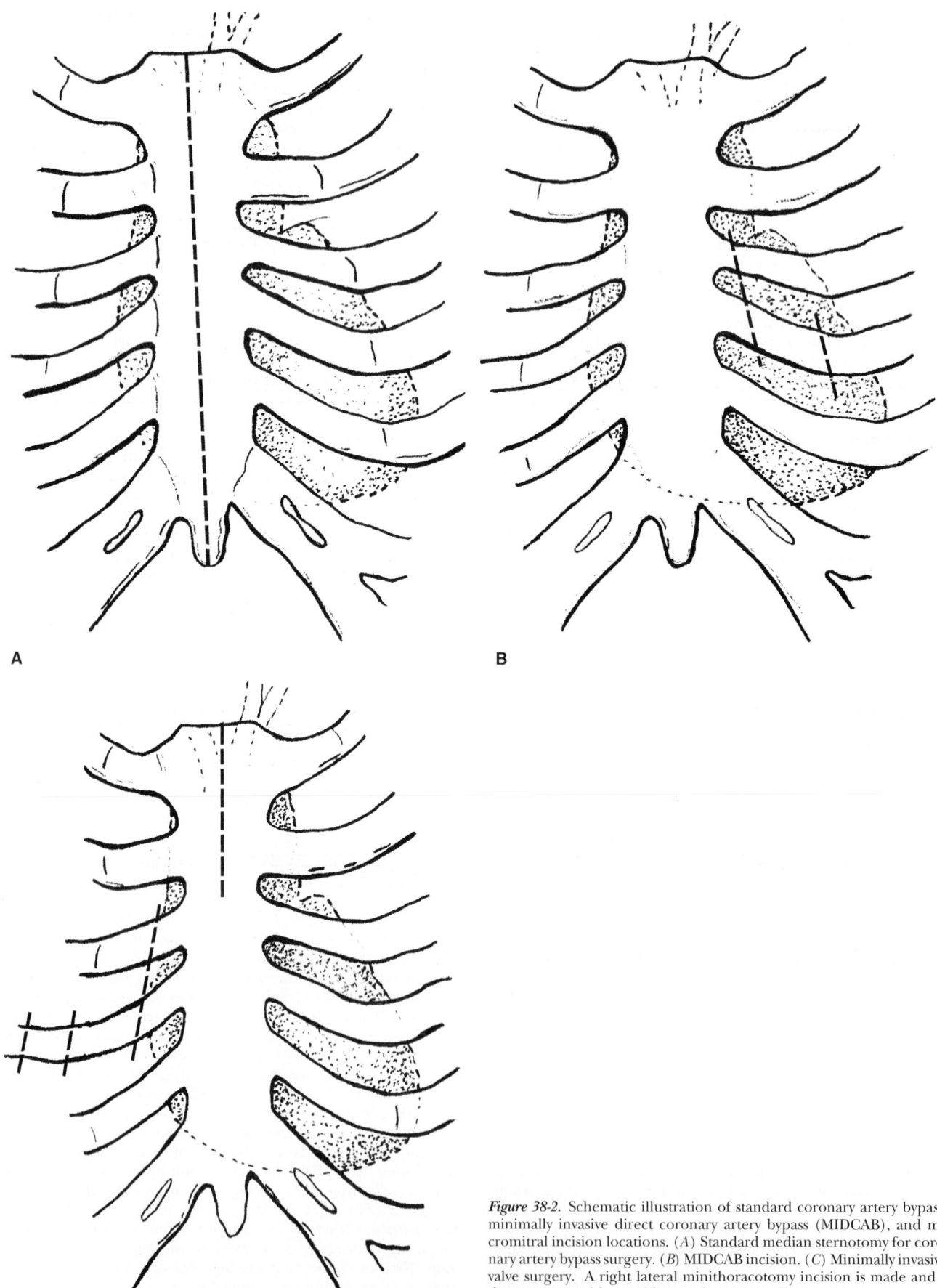

Figure 38-2. Schematic illustration of standard coronary artery bypass, minimally invasive direct coronary artery bypass (MIDCAB), and micromitral incision locations. (*A*) Standard median sternotomy for coronary artery bypass surgery. (*B*) MIDCAB incision. (*C*) Minimally invasive valve surgery. A right lateral minithoracotomy incision is made and a thoracoscope with or without other minimally invasive instruments is introduced to facilitate mitral valve repair. A partial sternal incision may be used to access either valve.

Table 38-2. ADVANTAGES OF MINIMALLY INVASIVE CARDIAC SURGERY

1. Suitable for internal mammary artery graft
2. Avoids complications of median sternotomy
   - Mediastinitis
   - Sternal dehiscence
   - Chest wall instability
   - Wound pain
3. Avoids complications of aortic cross-clamp and cardiopulmonary bypass
   - Stroke
   - Neuropsychological dysfunction
   - Myocardial infarction
   - Renal dysfunction
   - Bleeding diatheses
4. Reduces intubation time
5. Reduces intensive care unit length of stay
6. Reduces hospital length of stay
7. Promotes earlier return to functional capacity

Minimally invasive procedures for performing aortic/mitral valve repair or replacement involve small (~10 cm) parasternal or partial sternal access incisions. Patients are placed on CPB by cannulating either the common femoral artery and vein, or the right atrial appendage and the common femoral artery. Visualization of the mitral valve using this approach is described as superior to that obtained with the conventional median sternotomy, in contrast to the view obtained during aortic valve procedures, where the main advantage is avoidance of a full sternotomy.[51]

Anesthetic Considerations

Anesthetic techniques and monitoring strategies for minimally invasive cardiac surgery focus on detection and monitoring cardiac ischemia, maintaining perioperative hemodynamic stability, ensuring adequate pain relief, and facilitating early extubation.

Standard patient monitoring includes direct arterial and central venous or pulmonary artery pressure recordings and, in some cases, pulmonary artery catheterization for continuous cardiac output (CO) and mixed venous oxygen saturation ($S\bar{v}o_2$) measurements. Transesophageal echocardiography (TEE) is used in some institutions to detect regional myocardial ischemia or to facilitate placement of coronary sinus catheters for retrograde cardioplegia administration during port-access coronary artery bypass grafting. The operating room is set up as for a conventional coronary artery bypass procedure with the CPB machine and perfusion team on standby. The patient is placed in the supine position with external defibrillator pads in place. Conversion from MIDCAB to conventional coronary artery bypass surgery may be indicated if the symptomatic ischemia develops in the patient, if the arterial conduit is inadequate, or if the coronary artery target is inaccessible.

Early extubation, within 1–4 hours after surgery (in the operating room or in the cardiovascular ICU), is a major priority. Short-acting anesthetic and sedative agents facilitate this process. A benzodiazepine premedication is given 1 hour before surgery. Induction agents include low-dose fentanyl, midazolam, and thiopentone, whereas fentanyl and inhalational agents are used to maintain anesthesia. A double-lumen tube is used in some institutions when minithoracotomy is the surgical approach. Otherwise, standard single-lumen endotracheal tubes are inserted.

Coronary artery bypass without CPB requires local occlusion of the coronary artery to be grafted during anastomosis. Snares are placed to occlude both antegrade and retrograde flow and the anastomosis is performed on the beating heart. Commer-

cially available heart-stabilizing devices (Octopus) to facilitate the anastomosis of the graft to the coronary artery have made pharmacologic control of the heart rate, with β or calcium channel blockade, less of a management consideration. Variable periods of regional ischemia may occur during occlusion of the coronary arteries, and detection and treatment of this ischemia is an important component of anesthetic management. Ischemia may be manifested by hypotension, electrocardiogram ST segment elevation, elevated pulmonary capillary wedge pressure, reduced CO and $S\bar{v}o_2$, or TEE-detected new regional wall motion abnormalities. If such changes occur before grafting, the snares are released and the myocardium is reperfused and allowed to recover. Additional 5-minute occlusion periods have then been used to induce "ischemic preconditioning" with reperfusion for several minutes before reocclusion.[52] Other strategies to ameliorate regional ischemia during anastomosis include nitroglycerin infusion or β blockade. If ischemia persists and the patient becomes hemodynamically unstable, other options include instituting femorofemoral CPB or conversion to the conventional procedure with aortocaval CPB. Ventricular dysrhythmias may occur after reperfusion of the myocardium. Treatment options include prophylactic lidocaine before reperfusion or defibrillation using external defibrillator pads. Careful attention to electrolyte and acid-base balance is important in the prevention and management of these dysrhythmias.

The severity of pain reported after minimally invasive cardiac surgery is poorly quantified.[53] MIDCAB without a median sternotomy may be less painful. However, trauma to the costal cartilages (with or without rib segment removal) may be more painful than a median sternotomy. Ineffective treatment of pain from minithoracotomy or mini-anterior mediastinotomy incisions causes an increase in catecholamine release with consequent tachycardia, increased myocardial oxygen demand and myocardial ischemia, perioperative cardiac morbidity, and delayed hospital discharge.[53] In addition, lung volumes may be reduced with atelectasis and ventilation-perfusion ($\dot{V}/\dot{Q}$) mismatch.[54] Postoperative analgesic techniques include iv opioids, thoracic epidural analgesia, intercostal nerve block, and NSAIDs. Randomized, controlled trials are warranted to determine the optimal techniques and agents.

INTRA-ABDOMINAL LAPAROSCOPIC PROCEDURES

Cholecystectomy

Laparoscopic cholecystectomy involves changes in patient position from Trendelenburg to reverse Trendelenburg (rT), and intraperitoneal CO_2 insufflation (Fig. 38-3).

The laparoscopic approach combines the benefit of completely removing the gallbladder with the advantages of shorter hospital stays, more rapid return to normal activities, less pain associated with the small, limited incisions, and less postoperative ileus compared with the open laparotomy technique[55] (Table 38-3).

The Southern Surgeons Club,[56] in a prospective study of 1518 laparoscopic cholecystectomies performed by 59 surgeons in academic and private practice, defined a standard of care for the new procedure in 1991. Several other large series have also been reported from Europe[57] and North America.[58–60] Acute cholecystitis, obesity, and previous intra-abdominal surgery were initially considered to present difficult technical challenges. In late pregnancy, limited exposure was believed to compound the potential hazards of trocar insertion and the deleterious fetal effects of hypercarbia and pneumoperitoneum.

An impressive body of experience and literature has emerged in the 1990s confirming the safety and efficacy of laparoscopic cholecystectomy in the hands of experienced surgeons. Acute cholecystitis, despite concerns about technical difficulties with

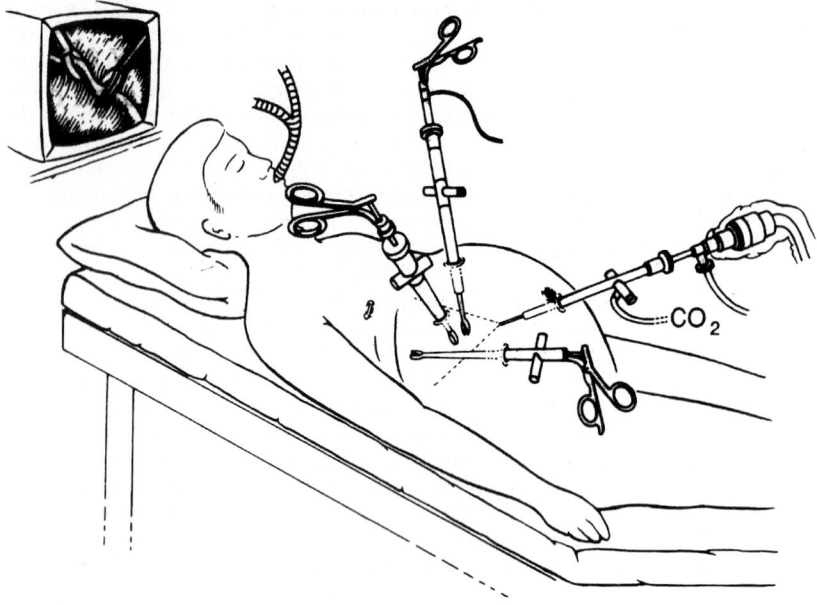

Figure 38-3. Laparoscopic cholecystectomy: patient positioning and equipment.

the associated edema, inflammation, and necrosis, is no longer considered a contraindication to laparoscopic cholecystectomy.[61] The conversion rate, however, is high, especially in patients older than 65 years of age with a history of biliary disease and an acute gangrenous gallbladder.[62] Although the incidence of symptomatic biliary disease in pregnancy is estimated at only 0.05%, the need for surgery in symptomatic patients is approximately 40%, and the risk of premature labor is inversely related to gestational age.[63] As with open cholecystectomy, conventional wisdom suggests delay until the postpartum period, if possible, when managing biliary colic in pregnancy. Case reports,[64] series,[65] studies,[66] and literature reviews[67] confirm that laparoscopic cholecystectomy can be safely performed in all trimesters of pregnancy, with acceptable maternal and fetal morbidity. The available data suggest that the safety and efficacy of laparoscopic cholecystectomy in pregnancy is increased by using the open Hasson technique for instrumentation; limiting intra-abdominal pressure (IAP) during the pneumoperitoneum; using appropriate maternal and fetal monitoring; ensuring adequate maternal oxygenation and normocapnia; preventing aortocaval compression by left tilt; and using active antithromboembolism measures, including calf compression.

Careful audit of large series has highlighted problems unique to or more commonly associated with the laparoscopic approach in North American and Australia/New Zealand practice.[68,69] Pre-existing umbilical and ventral hernia defects are major risk factors for postoperative trocar site hernia formation.

Table 38-3. POTENTIAL BENEFITS OF LAPAROSCOPIC CHOLECYSTECTOMY

Comparison with traditional open cholecystectomy
   Minimizes abdominal incision
   Preserves diaphragmatic function
Potential benefits
   Reduced adverse events
   Pulmonary function preserved
   Less postoperative ileus
   Early ambulation
   Economic benefits
      Shorter hospital stay
      Early return to work and normal activities

Critics of laparoscopic surgery cite the increased incidence of tumor recurrence at the trocar sites after laparoscopic cholecystectomy in patients incidentally found to have carcinoma of the gallbladder. There is considerable controversy regarding the appropriateness of laparoscopy in the treatment of known malignant disease. However, data suggest that gallbladder cancer is an aggressive malignancy and abdominal wall implantation is not increased with laparoscopic surgery, but is more likely a manifestation of the aggressive nature of the tumor.[70] Bile duct injuries are more common after laparoscopy compared with open cholecystectomy.[71] Furthermore, such injuries after laparoscopic cholecystectomy tend to be more extensive and higher in the duct system than those after open cholecystectomy, thus reducing the chance of a successful outcome from reconstruction. Roy et al[72] undertook a case series review of 21 patients who sustained bile duct injuries during laparoscopic cholecystectomy in two tertiary care centers over 2 years. Misidentification of the common duct, resulting in accidental division or resection, and obstruction by hemoclips were the most common injuries. Pain, jaundice, and bile collections were the typical presenting features of injuries that became evident after laparoscopic cholecystectomy. Twenty of the 21 patients required Roux-en-Y hepaticojejunostomy for definitive treatment.

Miscellaneous Intra-abdominal Procedures

The adoption of therapeutic endoscopy has triggered the single largest change in surgical practice for many decades. Proponents of the endoscopic approach claim that the minimally invasive aspect should decrease postoperative morbidity and allow the patient to return to normal activity and work earlier than after a conventional open procedure.

Mellinger and Ponsky[73] highlighted the minimally invasive surgery literature in 1996. The list of procedures now commonly performed endoscopically has grown rapidly with gastric, antireflux, colonic, and renal surgery following appendectomy and inguinal hernia repair (Table 38-4).

Raiser et al[74] reviewed the current status of minimally invasive antireflux surgery. They emphasized the importance of preoperative evaluation—endoscopy, biopsy, manometry, pH monitoring—in guiding patient selection for the most appropriate procedure, and in avoiding unnecessary or inappropriate operative misadventures. A laparoscopic Nissen fundoplication may prove a cost-effective technique for patients with gastroesophageal re-

Table 38-4. LAPAROSCOPIC INTRA-ABDOMINAL SURGICAL PROCEDURES

Cholecystectomy
Vagotomy
Hiatal hernia repair
Diaphragmatic hernia repair
Appendectomy
Colectomy
Inguinal hernia repair
Nephrectomy
Adrenalectomy

flux on long-term medical management, provided complication rates are comparable and surgical results are enduring. Interest in laparoscopic hernia repair continues, although conflicting reports have been published regarding its putative advantages over traditional surgical techniques. The laparoscopic surgical technique has evolved from external intraperitoneal onlay, to transabdominal preperitoneal, to totally extraperitoneal. The laparoscopic techniques involve the use of general anesthesia, and the associated higher operative costs and complication rates may not offset the potential benefits of less postoperative pain.[75] Laparoscopic approaches to solid abdominal organs, especially the spleen, kidney, and adrenal gland, continue to be described. A comparative study of laparoscopic and open splenectomy reported by a group from the University of California at San Francisco noted equivalent blood loss, complication rates, transfusion requirements, and hospital costs.[76] Longer operative times, earlier return to regular diet, and shorter hospital stay were features of the laparoscopic group. Goletti and Buccianti[77] reported a mean operative time of 109 minutes and a median postoperative stay of 3 days in their series of 25 patients undergoing laparoscopic adrenalectomies.

Despite the significant advances in surgery over the past century, the diagnosis of acute appendicitis continues to present problems for clinicians. In 20% of patients with appendicitis, the diagnosis was missed initially, and in 15–40% percent of those undergoing emergency operations for suspected appendicitis, the appendix was normal.[78] The laparoscopic appendectomy technique, in a prospective, randomized study, was associated with longer duration of surgery, shorter hospital stay, and no differences in terms of time to return to activity and work compared with conventional open surgery.[79] Case reports, with associated literature reviews and editorial comments, highlighted concerns about trocar site recurrence after laparoscopic colectomy for colorectal cancer.[80,81] Preliminary experimental data confirmed a significantly increased incidence of diffuse carcinomatosis, even when the procedure was performed for locally noninvasive tumors.[82]

PHYSIOLOGIC CHANGES AND COMPLICATIONS

Significant data have been accumulated on complications associated with laparoscopy.[83] The complications unique to laparoscopic cholecystectomy, reviewed by Strasberg and colleagues,[84] include bile duct injury and disruption of major blood vessels. Other problems relate to the cardiopulmonary effects of pneumoperitoneum, systemic CO_2 absorption, extraperitoneal gas insufflation, and venous gas embolism (Table 38-5).

Trocar Insertion

The establishment of a pneumoperitoneum during laparoscopy is essential for most laparoscopists before a trocar and laparoscope can be introduced into the peritoneal cavity. To achieve a pneumoperitoneum, a Veress needle is introduced into the peritoneal cavity and CO_2 gas is insufflated. Injuries have been reported to occur as the Veress needle or trocar is introduced blindly through the abdominal wall before insertion of the laparoscope (Fig. 38-4). Such injuries have included bleeding from abdominal wall vessels, gastrointestinal tract perforations, hepatic and splenic tears, major vascular trauma, avulsion of adhesions, omental disruption, and herniation at the trocar insertion site.[85] Near the level of the umbilicus, both the medial vessels (superficial and inferior epigastric) and lateral vessels (superficial and deep circumflex iliac) are at risk for injury.[86] To avoid injuries associated with blind Veress needle and trocar insertion, Hasson[87] has advocated a minilaparotomy technique for pneumoperitoneum creation. In this open technique, the first or primary trocar is inserted through a minilaparotomy incision, and the potential complications of blind Veress needle and trocar insertion are avoided.

Gees and Holden[88] retrospectively reviewed 2201 laparoscopic procedures performed in Columbus, Ohio between 1992 and 1995. There were three major vascular injuries—the left common iliac vein, the right common iliac artery, and the left internal iliac artery—for a combined incidence of 0.14%. Noga et al[89] highlighted the role of the anesthesiologists in the early diagnosis of retroperitoneal hematoma, a potentially fatal complication laparoscopic surgery.

Table 38-5. LAPAROSCOPIC SURGERY: SUMMARY OF POTENTIAL PHYSIOLOGIC CHANGES

TRENDELENBURG POSITION

Circulation
  Heart rate
  Stroke volume
Respiration
  Minute volume
  Work of breathing
  Lung volumes
  Gas exchange

PNEUMOPERITONEUM

Circulation
  Venous return (cardiac filling pressures)
  Contractility (neural/humoral)
  Afterload
Respiration
  Minute ventilation
  Airway pressure
  Lung volumes (functional residual capacity)
  Gas exchange (hypoxemia/hypercapnia)

EXOGENOUS CO_2

Circulation
  Dysrhythmias
  Contractility
  Venous gas embolization
Respiration
  Ventilation (dead space)
  CO_2 hemostasis

REVERSE TRENDELENBURG

Circulation
  Venous return
  Afterload
Respiration
  Lung volumes
  Work of breathing
  Minute ventilation
  Gas exchange

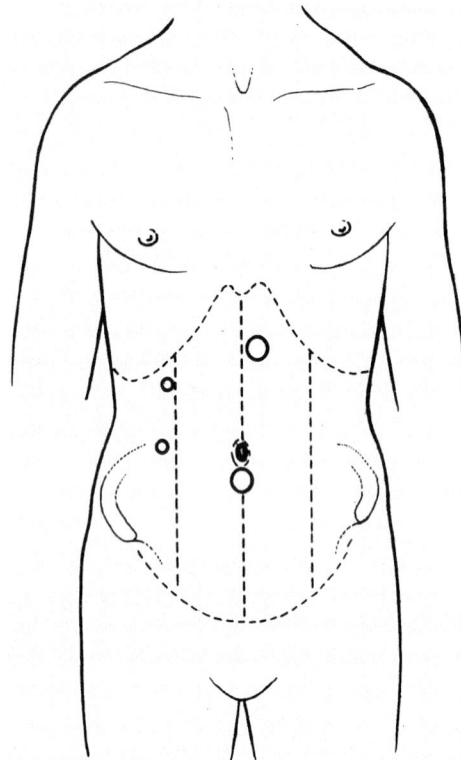

Figure 38-4. Laparoscopic cholecystectomy: surgical incision sites.

Patient Position

During laparoscopic surgery, the patient is positioned to produce gravitational displacement of the abdominal viscera away from the surgical site. Gravity has profound effects on the cardiovascular and pulmonary systems. The head-down tilt of 10–20 degrees commonly used both in gynecologic procedures and for the initial trocar insertion in laparoscopic cholecystectomy is accompanied by an increase in central blood volume[90] and a decrease in vital capacity and diaphragmatic excursion,[91] whereas the rT position favors improved pulmonary dynamics[92] but reduced venous return.[93,94] These changes associated with positioning may be influenced by the extent of the tilt,[95] the patient's age, intravascular volume status, and associated cardiac disease,[96,97] anesthetic drugs administered, and ventilation techniques. The potential for inadvertent right mainstem bronchial intubation and hypoxemia associated with Trendelenburg positioning was highlighted by Wilcox and Vandam.[98] A subsequent case report confirmed this possibility.[99] The proposed mechanism is that the endotracheal tube, firmly secured at its proximal end to the mandible, does not always move along with the trachea as the diaphragm causes cephalad displacement of the lung and carina.[100] In one report, prolonged laparoscopic surgery in the Trendelenburg position was complicated by brachial plexus injury.[101]

Creation of Pneumoperitoneum

Pneumoperitoneum creation involves the intraperitoneal insufflation of CO_2 through a Veress needle while the patient is in a 15–20-degree Trendelenburg position. The potential difficulties that may be encountered during creation of pneumoperitoneum are outlined in the following.

Technical Difficulties

Extraperitoneal insufflation of CO_2 is one of the most common complications of laparoscopy. The incidence of this complication has been reported to vary from 0.4 to 2%.[102] Such extraperitoneal insufflation may cause subcutaneous or retroperitoneal emphysema, prolonging surgery or causing its abandonment. Subcutaneous emphysema may occur if the tip of the Veress needle does not penetrate the peritoneal cavity before insufflation of gas. This may cause the insufflating gas to accumulate in the subcutaneous tissue or between the fascia and the peritoneum. Lew et al[103] reported extensive subcutaneous emphysema, which involved the neck, chest, and abdomen and extended to the groin, attributed to subcutaneous insufflation of CO_2 from a poorly stabilized Veress needle.

Extraperitoneal insufflation has been associated with higher levels of CO_2 absorption than intraperitoneal insufflation and may be the cause of a sudden rise in PET_{CO_2} during the procedure.[104]

Pneumomediastinum and Pneumothorax

Pneumothorax is a rare but potentially life-threatening complication of pneumoperitoneum. The history, pathogenesis, and management of such clinical situations were reviewed by Prystowsky and colleagues.[105] This complication occurs primarily on the right side. Insufflated gas may track around the aortic and esophageal hiatuses of the diaphragm into the mediastinum and then rupture into the pleural space. However, an anatomic basis for passage of gas into the thoracic cavity through a diaphragmatic defect is more likely. Commonly, these weak points or defects occur at the pleuroperitoneal hiatus or foramen of Bochdalek, the outer crus, or the esophageal hiatus. Pneumothoraces have been reported in association with subcutaneous emphysema and pneumomediastinum, whereas an isolated tension pneumothorax has been reported during laparoscopic cholecystectomy after trocar insertion and intraperitoneal CO_2 insufflation.[106] A congenital defect of the diaphragm (patent pleuroperitoneal canal) through which the insufflated gas passes into the thoracic cavity has been suggested as the underlying mechanism. Alternatively, a ruptured bleb or bulla could have produced the tension pneumothorax independent of the pneumoperitoneum.

Hasel et al[107] reported three cases in which extravasation of CO_2 during laparoscopic cholecystectomy resulted in subcutaneous emphysema associated with pneumomediastinum, pneumoscrotum, pneumothorax, and ocular emphysema. It was assumed that intraperitoneal CO_2 traversed into the mediastinum through a defect in the diaphragm, and to the scrotum along the spermatic cord through the inguinal canal. Excessively high IAPs during CO_2 insufflation may have contributed to these complications, which resolved uneventfully within 24 hours.

Undetected pneumothorax/pneumomediastinum can be life threatening. The diagnosis should be considered in the presence of increased airway pressure, hemodynamic compromise, oxygen desaturation, or unexpected hypoxemia-hypercarbia. Subcutaneous emphysema of the neck, chest wall, and face should alert the anesthesiologist to the possibility of such associated complications. As soon as this possibility is suspected, a chest radiograph should be obtained to rule out a pneumomediastinum or pneumothorax. If the hemodynamic status is stable and if there is clinical evidence of a tension pneumothorax, chest tube decompression and abdominal deflation are indicated before obtaining a chest radiograph. Once the chest drain is in a satisfactory position, the abdomen can be insufflated and the procedure continued if the patient remains stable. If the pneumothorax is recognized near the end of the operation and the patient is stable, the surgery can be completed without therapeutic intervention. Once the abdomen is deflated, the CO_2 in the pleural cavity is rapidly resorbed, obviating the necessity for a chest tube.

Cardiovascular Effects

The extent of cardiovascular changes associated with creation of the pneumoperitoneum depends on the interaction of factors that include positioning of the patient,[108] the IAPs obtained during insufflation,[109] and the neurohumoral effects of absorbed CO_2.[110] Preoperative cardiorespiratory status,[14] the intravascular volume,[111] and the anesthetic agents used may also be significant.

The physiologic changes associated with laparoscopy and pneumoperitoneum in gynecologic surgery have been well described.[112,113] This patient population in general comprises healthy women undergoing short procedures in the Trendelenburg position. In comparison, abdominal laparoscopic surgery has been recommended for elderly and infirm patients who may not tolerate conventional surgery,[114,115] although the technique requires complicated positioning and increased operating time.[6]

The hemodynamic effects of CO_2 insufflation and rT positioning were comprehensively reviewed by Wahba et al[116] in a meta-analysis of North American and United Kingdom literature. The dynamic physiologic changes that occur during laparoscopic abdominal surgery appear to have a phasic component. Joris et al[117] used flow-directed pulmonary artery catheters to assess the effects of CO_2 insufflation to an IAP of 14 mm Hg in healthy patients undergoing laparoscopic cholecystectomy. CI was reduced by 35–40% from baseline after induction of anesthesia and rT positioning, and further reduced to 50% of its preoperative value 5 minutes after the beginning of CO_2 insufflation. CI gradually improved after 10 minutes of CO_2 insufflation. Other studies support this phasic change in hemodynamic function.[118,119] However, some investigators have documented an unchanged CI during insufflation of CO_2.[120,121]

The filling pressures of the heart, central venous pressure, and pulmonary artery occlusion pressure (PAOP) initially are reduced after induction of anesthesia and venous pooling in the rT position. After CO_2 insufflation, the right- and left-sided filling pressures substantially increase.[14,117,122,123] The mechanical effects of insufflated CO_2 may explain some of these changes. Modern laparoscopic insufflators automatically terminate the gas flow when a preset IAP of 10–15 mm Hg is reached. The insufflated CO_2 compresses both the venous capacitance system and the arterial resistance vessels. The mechanical effect on the venous system involves transiently increased venous return followed by impedance.[124] However, the increase in IAP has been claimed to cause a proportionate increase in intrathoracic pressure, and this probably also contributes to the documented rise in central venous pressure and PAOP.[125,126]

The compressive effects on the arterial vasculature result in a dramatic increase in calculated systemic vascular resistance (SVR), particularly during the initial phase of CO_2 insufflation. MABP also rises substantially, reflecting the increased afterload with an associated deterioration in CI.[14,117,118] The magnitude of CI reduction is directly proportional to the insufflation pressure. Westerband et al,[118] using impedance cardiography, reported a 30% reduction in CI and a 79% increase in SVR immediately after peritoneal insufflation to 15 mm Hg. The safe upper limit of IAP insufflation was studied in an animal model investigating stepwise increases in IAP of 8, 12, and 16 mm Hg. The threshold pressure that had minimal effects on hemodynamic function was found at an IAP of ≤ 12 mm Hg. The authors recommend this pressure limit to avoid cardiovascular compromise during pneumoperitoneum.[109]

In a series of 13 otherwise healthy patients, Cunningham et al[108] found that left ventricular function, as determined by TEE, was preserved after CO_2 insufflation and patient position changes, despite variations in left ventricular loading conditions. However, CO_2 insufflation was associated with increases in left ventricular end-systolic wall stress, concomitant with increases in systemic arterial pressure. In addition, left ventricular

end-diastolic volume decreased after rT positioning, indicating reduced venous return. Left ventricular ejection fraction was maintained throughout the study period in this investigation of otherwise healthy patients. However, it might reasonably be speculated that the aforementioned changes in left ventricular loading conditions might have had deleterious consequences in a patient population with significant cardiovascular disease.

Safran et al[14] investigated ASA Class III–IV patients with severe heart disease. CO decreased and SVR and MABP increased after CO_2 insufflation. Significant reductions in $S\bar{v}O_2$ and oxygen delivery were noted in 50% of their patients. Feig and colleagues[127] documented significant increases in SVR, MABP, PAOP, and LVSWI occurring with insufflation pressures up to 15 mm Hg in 15 ASA Class III–IV patients. Persistent refractory acidemia and hypercarbia complicated four cases in the study. Two patients had significant cardiac arrhythmias requiring treatment during insufflation. Hypercarbia and respiratory acidosis may cause a decrease in myocardial contractility and a lowering of the arrhythmia threshold, particularly if the myocardium is already sensitized by the use of volatile anesthetic agents. Hypercarbia is reported to increase CO, MABP, heart rate, and plasma epinephrine and norepinephrine levels.[128] Because the direct effects of hypercarbia include arteriolar dilatation and myocardial depression, the overall change in cardiovascular function is thought to be mediated by the catecholamine release.

A number of case reports have described acute hypotension, hypoxemia, and cardiovascular collapse associated with laparoscopy.[129,130] Postulated causes included (1) hypercarbia, which may induce dysrhythmias; (2) reflex increases in vagal tone due to excessive stretching of the peritoneum; (3) compression of the inferior vena cava, leading to decreased CO; (4) hemorrhage; and (5) venous gas embolism. The clinical conditions associated with venous CO_2 embolism during laparoscopy have also been described.[131,132] Venous CO_2 embolism in these cases was associated with profound hypotension, cyanosis, and asystole after creation of pneumoperitoneum. Beck and McQuillan[131] noted a sudden decrease in $PETCO_2$ after 1 hour of surgery in a fatal case of embolism. The authors suggested that CO_2 could enter a tributary of the portal system during attempts at establishing the pneumoperitoneum. Rapid CO_2 exsufflation was reported to have precipitated acute hypotension, bradycardia, and hypoxemia.[133] Derouin and colleagues,[134] using TEE, observed CO_2 gas embolism in 11 of 16 patients studied (5 during peritoneal insufflation and 6 during gallbladder dissection). Cerebral arterial CO_2 embolism has been reported in a patient with an atrial septal defect.[135]

Renal and Hepatic Blood Flow

Intra-abdominal pressure, hypercarbia, and patient position may influence renal and hepatic blood flow. Head-up position and intraperitoneal pressure greater than 12 mm Hg compromised hepatic and renal blood flow in an experimental animal study.[136] The level and duration of IAP were responsible for elevations in serum bilirubin and hepatic aminotransferases during laparoscopic surgery.[137] Although no symptoms appeared in patients with normal hepatic function, patients with severe hepatic failure should probably not be subjected to prolonged laparoscopic procedures.

During pneumoperitoneum, the plasma concentrations of dopamine, vasopressin, epinephrine, norepinephrine, renin, and cortisol rise significantly.[138–141] Of particular importance is the time course of vasopressin and norepinephrine elevation. The plasma concentration–time course profile parallels that of the change in CI, MABP, and SVR,[138,140] suggesting a possible cause–effect relationship. It is probable that hypercarbia and pneumoperitoneum cause stimulation of the sympathetic nervous system and release of catecholamines.[141] The phasic restoration in CI may be a result of the direct arteriolar vasodilatory effects of CO_2 and the effects of anesthetic agents on the SVR. Overall, the hemodynamic effects of pneumoperitoneum are generally well tolerated by healthy people but require careful evaluation in compromised patients.

Respiratory Function

Carbon Dioxide Homeostasis

Peritoneal gas insufflation is essential to facilitate exposure, visualization, and manipulation of intra-abdominal contents. Although nitrous oxide has been used for diagnostic gynecologic procedures, it is flammable when electrocautery is used. Helium has not been accepted because of its insolubility in blood in the case of embolic phenomena.[142] CO_2 has evolved as the insufflation gas of choice for laparoscopic surgery because of its efficacy and safety during electrocautery and laser surgery and its capability for pulmonary excretion.[121]

Carbon dioxide insufflation into the peritoneal cavity increases arterial CO_2 tension, which is managed by increasing minute ventilation. The absorption of CO_2 from a closed cavity depends on its diffusibility and perfusion of the walls of that cavity, and not on the rate of insufflation of the gas into the cavity.[143] Mullet et al[144] hypothesized that the rate of CO_2 diffusion into the body depends on the duration and the site of CO_2 insufflation. They examined PET_{CO_2} and pulmonary CO_2 elimination during CO_2 insufflation under general anesthesia for gynecologic laparoscopy (intraperitoneal for 43 minutes), laparoscopic cholecystectomy (intraperitoneal for 125 minutes), and pelviscopy (extraperitoneal for 45 minutes). PET_{CO_2} and pulmonary CO_2 elimination increased in parallel from the 8th to the 10th minute after the start of CO_2 insufflation. A plateau was reached 10 minutes later in patients having intraperitoneal insufflation, whereas PET_{CO_2} and pulmonary CO_2 elimination continued to increase slowly throughout CO_2 insufflation during pelviscopy.

Wittgen et al[145] compared 20 healthy patients undergoing laparoscopic cholecystectomy with 10 ASA Class II-III patients. Compared with the healthy group, there were significant decreases in pH and increases in $PaCO_2$ during pneumoperitoneum in the ASA III group, and this group also had significantly higher minute ventilation and peak inspiratory pressures than baseline values. Increasing minute ventilation in most cases maintains $PaCO_2$ within normal limits but inevitably leads to some increase in airway pressure. However, in ASA Class III or IV patients, $PaCO_2$ may remain elevated despite adjusting minute ventilation to normalize PET_{CO_2}.[127] Preoperative evaluation with pulmonary function tests demonstrating forced expiratory volumes less than 70% of predicted values and diffusion defects less than 80% of predicted values can identify patients at risk for development of hypercarbia and respiratory acidosis after pneumoperitoneum. Hall et al[146] reported a case of acute profound hypercarbia occurring late in the procedure caused by CO_2 insufflation and first detected by capnography.

Intraoperative Changes

Respiratory function changes occurring during laparoscopic cholecystectomy may differ from those reported during gynecologic laparoscopic procedures, probably because of the intra-abdominal nature of the surgery and the prolonged insufflation times required. Functional residual capacity (FRC) and lung compliance decrease with assumption of the supine position and cephalad shift of the diaphragm and with induction of general anesthesia.[147] However, the insufflation of intraperitoneal CO_2 may exacerbate these changes. Lung and chest wall mechanical impedance increase with increasing IAP.[148] The increase depends on body configuration and is greater in a head-down position. These changes should be considered in patients for whom increases in impedance may be critical, such as obese patients and those with pulmonary disease.

Hypoxemia during laparoscopic abdominal surgery can have many causes, including a reduction in compliance, which may lead to diminished FRC relative to closing volume and $\dot{V}/\dot{Q}$ mismatch. Intraoperative hypoxemia is uncommon in healthy patients.[149,150] Joris et al[117] found no significant increased intrapulmonary shunt despite reductions in CO and oxygen delivery in 20 healthy patients during laparoscopic cholecystectomy. We reported a case of intraoperative hypoxemia complicating laparoscopy in an obese patient with sickle hemoglobinopathy.[151] Hypoxemia may be caused by regurgitation and aspiration of gastric contents. Duffy[152] reported gastric regurgitation in 2 of 93 fasted patients undergoing laparoscopic gynecologic surgery. Similarly, during laparoscopic cholecystectomy, there are several factors that predispose to regurgitation, including the initial steep head-down tilt, insufflation of intraperitoneal gas, and mechanical pressure exerted on the abdomen by the surgical team. The hazards of intraoperative pneumothorax are described earlier.

Postoperative Changes

There have been few prospective, randomized studies comparing laparoscopic and open cholecystectomy. Pulmonary dysfunction after open cholecystectomy is multifactorial and has been characterized as a restrictive pattern with a decrease in vital capacity and FRC. The common denominator is division of the abdominal musculature, which produces incisional pain, diaphragmatic dysfunction, and impairment of ventilatory mechanics. It has been suggested that laparoscopic surgery may reduce postoperative pulmonary complications by avoiding the restrictive pattern of breathing that usually follows upper abdominal surgery.

Schauer et al[153] observed that, compared with patients undergoing open cholecystectomy, the laparoscopic procedure was associated with 30–38% less impairment of pulmonary function, including FRC, forced expiratory volume in 1 second (FEV_1), maximum forced expiratory flow, and total lung capacity. Joris and colleagues[154] differentiated the influence of site of surgery, parietal trauma, intraoperative patient position, and pneumoperitoneum on pulmonary function and, by extension, clarified their roles in the pathophysiology of postoperative pulmonary dysfunction in women of normal body mass index and free of cardiopulmonary disease. Reductions in effort-dependent measures of pulmonary function—FEV_1, peak expiratory flow rate, and vital capacity—were less than those usually associated with "open" cholecystectomy, and return to normal function was more rapid. Although the incidence of surgical trauma to the gallbladder is almost identical with open and laparoscopic techniques, the advantage of the latter may relate to the minimal trauma to the abdominal wall.[155] Postoperative residual pneumoperitoneum per se may not explain the diaphragmatic dysfunction observed after laparoscopic cholecystectomy. Visceral afferents originating in the gallbladder area or somatic afferents arising from the abdominal wall, which exert an inhibitory action on phrenic discharge, may be the cause of this diaphragmatic dysfunction. Erice et al[156] concluded that the internal site of surgical intervention is the crucial variable determining diaphragmatic inhibition after they observed a decrease in maximum transdiaphragmatic pressure with laparoscopic cholecystectomy and not laparoscopic hernia repair.

ANESTHETIC MANAGEMENT

A number of reviews have highlighted the anesthetic considerations for laparoscopic cholecystectomy, including anesthetic technique, intraoperative opioid and nitrous oxide administration, and appropriate monitoring.[157,158] The choice of anesthetic technique for upper abdominal laparoscopic surgery is mostly limited to general anesthesia because of patient discomfort associated with creation of pneumoperitoneum and the extent of position changes associated with the procedure. Cuffed endotracheal tube placement minimizes the risk of acid aspiration if reflux occurs. Controlled ventilation is recommended because several factors may induce hypercarbia, including depression of ventilation by anesthetic agents, absorption of CO_2 from the peritoneal cavity, and mechanical impairment of ventilation by the pneumoperitoneum and the initial steep Trendelenburg position.

After induction of anesthesia, a urinary catheter and nasogastric tube are placed. Bladder catheterization is undertaken to decompress the bladder and thus avoid trauma to intraabdominal contents at the time of trocar insertion. Gastric decompression may also reduce the risk of visceral puncture, as well as improving laparoscopic visualization and facilitating retraction of the right upper quadrants.[159] Data reported by Goodale and colleagues[124] suggest that the increased IAP with pneumoperitoneum causes venous stasis. Measures to reduce stasis, such as pneumatic compressive stockings, may be indicated during these procedures. In general, local or regional anesthetic techniques have not been advocated for laparoscopic cholecystectomy or other upper abdominal laparoscopic procedures.

Anesthetic Agents

Limited data are available concerning the impact of anesthetic management on postoperative outcome after laparoscopic cholecystectomy. Rose et al[160] prospectively documented intraoperative critical observations and adverse outcomes in the recovery room for the first 101 patients undergoing laparoscopy at their institution. They compared the anesthetic management and outcome with patients undergoing open cholecystectomy. Intraoperative hypothermia (35°C nasal/oral) and hypotension (systolic blood pressure <80 mm Hg) were documented in 6.2% and 12.9%, respectively, of patients undergoing laparoscopic cholecystectomy, compared with 2.9% and 3.4% for open cholecystectomy. Of the laparoscopic cholecystectomy patients, 31.4% had skin temperature recordings of 35°C in the recovery room.

Most authors studying laparoscopic techniques have used balanced anesthetic techniques with oxygen, nitrous oxide, volatile anesthetic agents, relaxants, and opioids. Opioid or cholinergic agents have been reported to cause spasm of the sphincter of Oddi,[161] which can be antagonized by several drugs, including naloxone,[162] glucagon,[163] and nalbuphine.[164] The advent of parenteral perioperative NSAIDs and the tendency for less postoperative pain associated with the laparoscopic approach may obviate perioperative narcotic administration.

Pain after laparoscopic surgery may result from tissue injury, nociceptor sensitization, and activation of central pathways. Michaloliakou et al[165] used wound infiltration with local anesthesia and NSAIDs to attenuate peripheral pain and opioids for central pain modulation. This preoperative multimodal analgesic regime was associated with less postoperative pain, nausea, and vomiting and faster recovery and discharge.

Intraperitoneal administration of local anesthetics has been reported to reduce postoperative shoulder pain after minor gynecologic laparoscopic procedures. Experiences with intraperitoneal local anesthetic administration after laparoscopic cholecystectomy have ranged from significant reduction in postoperative pain during the first 48 hours with 10 ml of 0.5% bupivacaine,[166] to no effect in reducing postoperative pain, improving lung function, or attenuating metabolic endocrine responses with 20 ml 0.25% bupivacaine.[167] Joris and colleagues[168] investigated the time course of parietal (abdominal wall), visceral, and shoulder pain after laparoscopic cholecystectomy. Visceral pain accounted for most of the discomfort after laparoscopic cholecystectomy and was not attenuated by intraperitoneal administration of 80 ml 0.125% bupivacaine

Postoperative nausea and vomiting are among the most common and distressing symptoms after laparoscopic surgery.[169] Ondansetron, a highly potent and selective 5-hydroxytryptamine type 3 (5-HT3) receptor antagonist, has proved to be an effective oral and iv prophylaxis against postoperative emesis.[170]

Use of Nitrous Oxide

The use of nitrous oxide during laparoscopic surgery is controversial because of concerns over its ability to produce bowel distention during surgery and to increase postoperative nausea. The effects of nitrous oxide on bowel distention during surgery and bowel function after surgery were studied in 150 patients undergoing elective colonic surgery.[171] There was no difference between the air–oxygen group and the nitrous oxide–oxygen group in duration of anesthesia, distention of the bowel, and postoperative bowel function. The safety and efficacy of nitrous oxide specifically during laparoscopic cholecystectomy were investigated by Taylor et al.[172] There were no significant differences between the groups receiving air and nitrous oxide with respect to operating conditions or bowel distention. More important, there were no time-related changes in either variable during the course of surgery. Finally, the incidence of postoperative nausea and vomiting was similar in both treatment groups. However, a meta-analysis performed by Divatia and colleagues[173] noted that the omission of nitrous oxide reduced the risk of postoperative nausea and vomiting by 28%. In the subgroup analysis, the maximum effect of nitrous oxide omission was seen in female patients.

In summary, there is no conclusive evidence demonstrating a clinically significant effect of nitrous oxide on surgical conditions during laparoscopic cholecystectomy or on the incidence of postoperative emesis. With the caveats previously described, nitrous oxide therefore may still be a useful adjuvant during general anesthesia for this procedure.

Monitoring

Standard monitoring techniques are required for all patients undergoing laparoscopic surgery. PET_{CO_2} is most commonly used as a noninvasive substitute for Pa_{CO_2} in evaluating the adequacy of ventilation during laparoscopic cholecystectomy. Wahba and Mamazza[174] studied 28 otherwise healthy patients undergoing elective laparoscopic cholecystectomy to determine the increase in minute ventilation required to maintain the preinsufflation arterial CO_2 tension and whether PET_{CO_2} could safely be used as an index of Pa_{CO_2} and, therefore, of the adequacy of ventilation during pneumoperitoneum. Increasing minute ventilation by 12–16% maintained the Pa_{CO_2} close to the preinsufflation levels. PET_{CO_2} was not a satisfactory noninvasive index of Pa_{CO_2} if it exceeded 41 mm Hg and if large volumes of CO_2 were insufflated. Otherwise, PET_{CO_2} proved to be a reasonable approximation of Pa_{CO_2} in these patients free from cardiopulmonary disease. In contrast, patients with preoperative cardiopulmonary disease demonstrated significant increases in Pa_{CO_2} not reflected by comparable increases in PET_{CO_2} during insufflation.[145]

Pa_{CO_2} may be underestimated by PET_{CO_2} if there is a reduction in CO or an increase in $\dot{V}/\dot{Q}$ mismatch, and occasionally PET_{CO_2} may overestimate Pa_{CO_2}.[175] In patients with significant cardiopulmonary disease, it would seem prudent to monitor Pa_{CO_2} levels at times during the procedure to avoid problems with hypercarbia and acidosis. Preoperative pulmonary function test results with low forced expiratory and vital capacity volumes and high ASA grouping can predict those patients at risk for development of hypercarbia and acidosis during laparoscopic cholecystectomy, but patient age and duration of surgery do not seem to be influencing factors.[176]

Invasive hemodynamic monitoring may be required in ASA Class III–IV patients to monitor the cardiovascular response to insufflation and institute therapy. Because the CO is inversely proportional to the insufflation pressure in the abdomen, gradual insufflation should be monitored by the anesthesiologist and a limit of 8–12 mm Hg set as maximal inflationary pressure. Limiting the rT tilt may attenuate the reduction in CO during pneumoperitoneum.[177] Refractory persistent hypercarbia, acidosis, or a reduction in $S\overline{v}O_2$ may necessitate exsufflation of pneumoperitoneum or lowering of the insufflation pressure.[177] Finally, a decision to convert to an open procedure may be an important option in those patients with significant hemodynamic compromise.

SUMMARY

Minimally invasive therapy aims to minimize the trauma of any interventional process but still achieve a satisfactory therapeutic result. The development of "critical pathways," rapid mobilization, and early feeding have contributed to the goal of shorter hospital stay. This concept has been extended to include laparoscopic cholecystectomy and laparoscopic hernia repair.[178] Reports have been published confirming the safety of same-day discharge for most laparoscopic cholecystectomy patients.[179] The minimal-access nature of the surgical insult and the lack of opioid administration may minimize postoperative hypoxemia and sleep disturbance.[180] However, we caution against overenthusiastic ambulatory laparoscopic cholecystectomy based on the rational, but unproven, assumption that early discharge will lead to occasional delays in diagnosis and management of postoperative complications. A New South Wales group in Australia has reported a 1.37% incidence of ICU admissions after 725 general surgical procedures.[181] Surgical complications were associated with delayed diagnosis and longer ICU admissions.

Endoscopic-assisted intra-abdominal procedures recently introduced include appendectomy, herniorrhaphy, adhesiolysis, antireflux and acid-reducing procedures, and intestinal resections. Case reports of bile duct injuries after laparoscopic cholecystectomy and unusual modes of colorectal, renal, and gallbladder carcinoma recurrence after laparoscopic-assisted surgery confirm the need for rigorous prospective study of these new procedures.

Intraoperative complications of laparoscopic surgery are mostly due to traumatic injuries sustained during blind trocar insertion and physiologic changes associated with patient positioning and pneumoperitoneum creation. General anesthesia and controlled ventilation comprise the accepted anesthetic technique to reduce the increase in $Paco_2$. Investigators have documented the cardiorespiratory compromise associated with upper abdominal laparoscopic surgery, and particular emphasis is placed on careful perioperative monitoring of ASA Class III–IV patients during insufflation. Setting limits on the inflationary pressure is advised in these patients. Anesthesiologists must maintain a high index of suspicion for complications such as gas embolism, extraperitoneal insufflation and surgical emphysema, pneumothorax, and pneumomediastinum.

Postoperative nausea and vomiting are among the most common and distressing symptoms after laparoscopic surgery. A highly potent and selective 5-HT3 receptor antagonist, ondansetron, has proven to be an effective oral and iv prophylaxis against postoperative emesis in preliminary studies. Opioids remain an important component of the anesthesia technique, although the introduction of newer, more potent NSAIDs may diminish their use. A preoperative multimodal analgesic regimen involving skin infiltration with local anesthesia, NSAIDs to attenuate peripheral pain, and opioids for central pain may reduce postoperative discomfort and expedite patient recovery and discharge. There is no conclusive evidence to demonstrate clinically significant effects of nitrous oxide on surgical conditions during laparoscopic cholecystectomy or on the incidence of postoperative emesis. Laparoscopic cholecystectomy has proven to be a major advance in the treatment of patients with symptomatic gallbladder disease.

REFERENCES

1. Soper NJ, Brunt LM, Kerbl K: Laparoscopic general surgery (review article). N Engl J Med 330:409, 1994
2. Perissat J, Collet D, Belliard R: Gallstones: Laparoscopic treatment—cholecystectomy, cholecystotomy and lithotripsy—our own technique. Surg Endosc 4:1, 1990
3. Reddick EJ, Olsen DO: Laparoscopy laser cholecystectomy, a comparison with mini lap cholecystectomy. Surg Laparosc Endosc 1:2, 1990
4. Soper NJ, Barteau JA, Clayman RV et al: Comparison of early postoperative results for laparoscopic versus standard open cholecystectomy. Surgery, Gynecology and Obstetrics 174:114, 1992
5. Wickham JEA: Minimally invasive surgery: Future developments. BMJ 308:193, 1994
6. Working Group of Department of Health and the Scottish Department of Home Health: Minimal Access Surgery: Implications for the NHS. Edinburgh, Her Majesty's Stationery Office, 1994
7. Lawrence K: Minimal access surgery: Harnessing the revolution (editorial). Lancet 1:308, 1994
8. NIH Consensus Conference: Gallstones and laparoscopic cholecystectomy. JAMA 269:1018, 1993
9. State of New York Department of Health: Memorandum: Health Facilities Series H-18. New York, State of New York Department of Health, 1992
10. Society of American Gastrointestinal Endoscopic Surgeons (SAGES): Granting of privileges for laparoscopic general surgery. Am J Surg 161:324, 1991
11. White JV: Registry of laparoscopic cholecystectomy and new and evolving laparoscopic techniques. Am J Surg 165:536, 1993
12. Hunter JG: Advanced laparoscopic surgery. Am J Surg 173:14, 1997
13. Satava RM: 3-D vision technology applied to advanced minimally invasive surgery systems. Surg Endosc 7:429, 1993
14. Safran D, Sgambati S, Orlando R III: Laparoscopy in high risk cardiac patients. Surgery, Gynecology and Obstetrics 176:548, 1993
15. Smith RS, Fry WR, Tsoi EK et al: Gasless laparoscopy and conventional instruments. Arch Surg 128:1102, 1993
16. Braimbridge MV: The history of thoracoscopic surgery. Ann Thorac Surg 56:610, 1993
17. Hazelrigg SR: Thoracoscopic management of pulmonary blebs and bullae. Semin Thorac Cardiovasc Surg 5:327, 1993
18. Graeber GM, Jones DR: The role of thoracoscopy in thoracic trauma. Ann Thorac Surg 56:646, 1993
19. Ely SW, Kron IL: Thoracoscopic implantation of the implantable cardioverter defibrillator. Chest 103:271, 1993
20. Mack MJ: Thoracoscopy and its role in mediastinal disease and sympathectomy. Semin Thorac Cardiovasc Surg 5:332, 1993
21. Jedeikin R, Olsfanger D, Shachor D, Mansoor K: Anaesthesia for transthoracic endoscopic sympathectomy in the treatment of upper limb hyperhidrosis. Br J Anaesth 69:349, 1992
22. Cuschierei A, Shimi SM, Crosthwaite G, Joypaul V: Bilateral endoscopic splanchnicectomy through a posterior thoracoscopic approach. J R Coll Surg Edinb 39:44, 1994
23. Mack MJ, Regan JJ, Bobechkjo WP, Acuff TE: Application of thoracoscopy for diseases of the spine. Ann Thorac Surg 56:736, 1993
24. Kirby TJ, Mack MJ, Landreneau RJ, Rice TW: Initial experience with video-assisted thoracoscopic lobectomy. Ann Thorac Surg 56:1248, 1993
25. Walker WS, Carnochan FM, Mattar S: Video-assisted thoracoscopic pneumonectomy. Br J Surg 81:81, 1994
26. McKenna RJ Jr: Thoracoscopic lobectomy with mediastinal sampling in 80-year-old patients. Chest 106:1902, 1994.
27. Horswell JL: Anesthetic techniques for thoracoscopy. Ann Thorac Surg 56:624, 1993
28. Kaiser LR, Bavaria JE: Complications of thoracoscopy. Ann Thorac Surg 56:796, 1993
29. Soni AK, Conacher ID, Waller DA, Hilton CJ: Video-assisted thoracoscopic placement of paravertebral catheters: A technique for postoperative analgesia for bilateral thoracoscopic surgery. Br J Anaesth 72:462, 1994
30. Jones DR, Graeber GM, Tanguilig GG et al: Effects of insufflation on hemodynamics during thoracoscopy. Ann Thorac Surg 55:1379, 1993
31. Barker SJ, Clarke C, Trivedi N et al: Anesthesia for thoracoscopic laser ablation of bullous emphysema. Anesthesiology 78:44, 1993
32. Hazelrigg SR, Nunchuck SK, LoCicero J III et al: Video Assisted

Thoracic Surgery Study Group data. Ann Thorac Surg 56:1039, 1993

33. Rubin JW, Finney NR, Borders BM, Chauvin EJ: Intrathoracic biopsies, pulmonary wedge excision, and management of pleural disease: Is video-assisted closed chest surgery the approach of choice? Am Surg 60:860, 1994

34. Weinstein M, Coxson P, Williams L *et al:* Forecasting coronary heart disease incidence, mortality and cost: The coronary heart disease policy model. Am J Public Health 77:1417, 1987

35. Naylor CD, Phil D, Ugnat AM *et al:* Coronary artery bypass grafting in Canada: What is its rate of use? Which rate is right? CMAJ 146:851, 1992

36. Hensley FA Jr: Minimally invasive myocardial revascularisation surgery: Here to stay? J Cardiothorac Vasc Anesth 10:445, 1996

37. Subramanian VA, Guido S, Federico J *et al:* Minimally invasive coronary bypass surgery: A multi-centre report of preliminary experience. Circulation 92:645, 1995

38. Matsuda H, Sawa Y, Takahashi T *et al:* Minimally invasive cardiac surgery: Current status and perspective. Artif Organs 22:759, 1998

39. Benetti F, Naselli G, Wood M, Geffner L: Direct myocardial revascularization without extracorporeal circulation: Experience in 700 patients. Chest 100:312, 1991

40. Ankeney JL: Coronary vein graft without cardiopulmonary bypass: A surgical motion picture. Ann Thorac Surg 1:19, 1975

41. Trapp WS, Bisarya R: Placement of coronary artery bypass graft without pump oxygenator. Ann Thorac Surg 1:19, 1975

42. Buffolo E, de Andrade JCS, Branco JNR *et al:* Coronary artery bypass grafting without cardiopulmonary bypass. Ann Thorac Surg 61:63, 1996

43. Chitwood WR, Elbeery JR, Chapman WH *et al:* Video-assisted minimally invasive mitral valve surgery: The "micro mitral" operation. J Thorac Cardiovasc Surg 1997

44. Cosgrove DM III, Sabik JF: Minimally invasive approach for aortic valve operations. Ann Thorac Surg 62:596, 1996

45. Arom KV, Emery RW, Nicoloff DM: Minimally invasive coronary artery bypass surgery: Ministernotomy for CABG surgery. Ann Thorac Surg

46. Diegeler A, Falk V, Krahling M *et al:* Less-invasive coronary artery bypass grafting: Different techniques and approaches. Eur J Cardiothorac Surg 14(suppl 1):S13, 1998

47. Weinschelbaum E, Stuzbach P, Machain A *et al:* Valve operations through a minimally invasive approach. Ann Thorac Surg 66:1106, 1998

48. Gayes JM, Emery RW, Nissen MD: Anesthetic considerations for patients undergoing minimally invasive coronary artery bypass surgery: Mini-sternotomy and mini-thoracotomy approaches. J Cardiothorac Vasc Anesth 10:531, 1996

49. Del Rizzo DF, Boyd WD, Novek RJ: Safety and cost effectiveness of MIDCAB in high risk CABG patients. Ann Thorac Surg 66:1002, 1998

50. Hartz RS: Minimally invasive heart surgery. Circulation 94:2669, 1996

51. Elbeery JR, Chitwood WR: Minimally invasive cardiac surgery: Heart surgery for the 21st century. N C Med J 58:374, 1997

52. Greenspun HG, Adourian UA, Fonger JD *et al:* Minimally invasive direct coronary artery bypass grafting (MIDCAB): Surgical techniques and anaesthetic considerations. J Cardiothorac Vasc Anesth 10:507, 1996

53. Heres EK, Marquez J, Malkowski MJ *et al:* Minimally invasive direct coronary artery bypass (MIDCAB): Anesthetic, monitoring, and pain control considerations. J Cardiothorac Vasc Anesth 12:385, 1998

54. Gelfand RA, Matthews DE, Bier DM, Sherwin RS: Role of counterregulatory hormones in the catabolic response to stress. J Clin Invest 74:2238, 1984

55. Craig DB: Postoperative recovery of pulmonary function. Anesth Analg 60:46, 1981

56. Grace PA, Quereshi A, Coleman J *et al:* Reduced postoperative hospitalization after laparoscopic cholecystectomy. Br J Surg 78:160, 1991

57. Southern Surgeons Club: A prospective analysis of 1518 laparoscopic cholecystectomies. N Engl J Med 324:1073, 1991

58. Cuschieri A, Dubois F, Mouiel J *et al:* The European experience with laparoscopic cholecystectomy. Am J Surg 161:385, 1991

59. Litwin DEM, Girotti MJ, Poulin EC *et al:* Laparoscopic cholecystectomy: Trans-Canada experience with 2201 cases. Can J Surg 35:291, 1992

60. Stoker ME, Vose JO, Meara P, Maini BJ: Laparoscopic cholecystectomy: A clinical and financial analysis of 280 operations. Arch Surg 127:589, 1992

61. Lujan JA, Parrilla P, Robles R *et al:* Laparoscopic cholecystectomy vs open cholecystectomy in the treatment of acute cholecystitis: A prospective study. Arch Surg 133:173, 1998

62. Eldar S, Sabo E, Nash E, Abrahamson J, Matter I: Laparoscopic cholecystectomy for acute cholecystitis: Prospective trial. World J Surg 21:540, 1997

63. McKellar DP, Andersson CT, Bynton CJ: Cholecystectomy during pregnancy without fetal loss. Surgery, Gynecology and Obstetrics 174:292, 1992

64. Pucci RO, Seed RW: Case report of laparoscopic cholecystectomy in the third trimester of pregnancy. Am J Obstet Gynecol 165:401, 1991

65. Amos JD, Schorr SJ, Norman PF *et al:* Laparoscopic surgery during pregnancy. Am J Surg 171:435, 1996

66. Curet MJ, Allen D, Josloff RK *et al:* Laparoscopy during pregnancy. Arch Surg 131:546, 1996

67. Halpern NB: Laparoscopic cholecystectomy in pregnancy: A review of published experiences and clinical considerations. Seminars in Laparoscopic Surgery 5:129, 1998

68. Lee VS, Chari RS, Cucchiaro G, Meyers WC: Complications of laparoscopic cholecystectomy. Am J Surg 165:527, 1993

69. Deziel DJ, Millikan KW, Economou SG *et al:* Complications of laparoscopic cholecystectomy: A national survey of 4,292 hospitals and an analysis of 77,604 cases. Am J Surg 165:9, 1993

70. Ricardo AE, Feig BW, Ellis LM *et al:* Gallbladder cancer and trocar site recurrences. Am J Surg 174:619, 1997

71. Fletcher DR: Biliary injury at laparoscopic cholecystectomy: Recognition and prevention. Aust N Z J Surg 63:673, 1993

72. Roy AF, Passi RB, Lapointe RW *et al:* Bile duct injury during laparoscopic cholecystectomy. Can J Surg 36:509, 1993

73. Mellinger JD, Ponsky JL: Recent publications in laparoscopic surgery: An overview. Endoscopy 28:441, 1996

74. Raiser F, Hinder RA, McBride PJ: The technique of laparoscopic Nissen fundoplication. Chest Surg Clin North Am 5:437, 1995

75. Lawrence K, McWinnie D, Goodwin A: Randomized controlled trial of laparoscopic versus open repair of inguinal hernia. BMJ 311:981, 1995

76. Yee LF, Carvajal SH, de Lorimer AA: Laparoscopic splenectomy: The initial experience at the University of California. Arch Surg 130:874, 1995

77. Goletti O, Buccianti P: Laparoscopic adrenalectomy. Journal of Laparoendoscopic Surgery 5:221, 1995

78. Rao PM, Rhea TJ, Novelline RA *et al:* Effect of computed tomography of the appendix on treatment of patients and use of hospital resources. N Engl J Med 338:141, 1998

79. Martin LC, Puente I, Sosa JL: Open versus laparoscopic appendectomy: A prospective randomized comparison. Ann Surg 222:256, 1995

80. Jacquet P, Averbach AM, Stephens AD, Sugerbaker PH: Cancer recurrence following laparoscopic colectomy. Dis Colon Rectum 38:1110, 1995

81. Laparoscopic surgery for cure of colorectal cancer. Surg Endosc 11:797, 1997

82. Le Moine MC, Navarro F, Burgel JS *et al:* Experimental assessment of the risk of tumor recurrence after laparoscopic surgery. Surgery 123:427, 1998

83. Nord HJ: Complications of laparoscopy. Endoscopy 24:693, 1992

84. Strasberg SM, Sanabria JR, Clavien PA: Complications of laparoscopic cholecystectomy. Can J Surg 35:275, 1992

85. Ponsky JL: Complications of laparoscopic cholecystectomy. Am J Surg 161:393, 1991

86. Hurd WW, Pearl ML, DeLancey JO *et al:* Laparoscopic injury of abdominal wall blood vessels: A report of three cases. Obstet Gynecol 82:673, 1993

87. Hasson H: A modified instrument and method for laparoscopy. Am J Obstet Gynecol 70:886, 1971

88. Gees J, Holden C: Major vascular injury as a complication of laparoscopic surgery: A review of three cases and review of the literature. Am Surg 62:377, 1996

89. Noga J, Fredman B, Olsfanger D, Jedeikin R: Role of the anesthesiologist in the early diagnosis of life-threatening complications during laparoscopic surgery. Surg Laparosc Endosc 7:63, 1997

90. Miller AH: Surgical posture with symbols for its record on the anesthetists chart. Anesthesiology 1:241, 1940

91. Schiller WR: The Trendelenburg position: Surgical aspects. In Martin JT (ed): Positioning in Anesthesia and Surgery, 2nd ed, p 117. Philadelphia, WB Saunders, 1987

92. Don HF: The measurement of trapped gas in the lungs at functional residual capacity and the effects of posture. Anesthesiology 35:582, 1971

93. Sonkodi S, Agabiti-Rosei E, Fraser R: Response of the renin-angiotensin-aldosterone system to upright tilting and to intravenous furosemide: Effect of prior metoprolol and propranolol. Br J Clin Pharmacol 13:341, 1982

94. Williams GH, Cain JP, Dluly RG: Studies on the control of plasma aldosterone concentration in normal man: Response to posture, acute and chronic volume depletion and sodium loading. J Clin Invest 51:1731, 1972

95. Ward RJ, Danziger F, Bonica JJ: Cardiovascular effects of change of posture. Aerospace Med 37:257, 1966

96. Kubal K, Komatsu T, Sanchala V: Trendelenburg position used during venous cannulation increases myocardial oxygen demands. Anesth Analg 63:239, 1984

97. Pricolo VE, Burchard KW, Singh AK: Trendelenburg versus PASG application: Hemodynamic response in man. J Trauma 26:718, 1986

98. Wilcox S, Vandam LD: Alas, poor Trendelenburg and his position! A critique of its uses and effectiveness. Anesth Analg 67:574, 1988

99. Burton A, Steinbrook RA: Precipitous decrease in oxygen saturation during laparoscopic surgery. Anesth Analg 76:1177, 1993

100. Brimacombe JR, Orland H: Endobronchial intubation during upper abdominal laparoscopic surgery in the reverse Trendelenburg position. Anesth Analg 78:607, 1994

101. Gagnon J, Poulin EC: Beware of the Trendelenburg position during prolonged laparoscopic procedures. Can J Surg 36:505, 1993

102. Kabukoba JJ, Skillern LH: Coping with extraperitoneal insufflation during laparoscopy: A new technique. Obstet Gynecol 80:144, 1992

103. Lew JKL, Gin T, Oh TE: Anaesthetic problems during laparoscopic cholecystectomy. Anaesth Intensive Care 20:91, 1992

104. Kendall AP, Bhatt S, Oh TE: Pulmonary consequences of carbon dioxide insufflation for laparoscopic cholecystectomies. Anaesthesia 50:286, 1995

105. Prystowsky JB, Jerico BJ, Epstein HB: Spontaneous bilateral pneumothorax: Complication of laparoscopic cholecystectomy. Surgery 114:988, 1993

106. Seow LT, Khoo ST: Unilateral pneumothorax: An unexpected complication of laparoscopic cholecystectomy. Can J Anaesth 40:1000, 1993

107. Hasel R, Arora SK, Hickey DR: Intraoperative complications of laparoscopic cholecystectomy. Can J Anaesth 40:459, 1993

108. Cunningham AJ, Turner J, Rosenbaum S, Rafferty T: Transoesophageal echocardiographic assessment of haemodynamic function during laparoscopic cholecystectomy. Br J Anaesth 70:621, 1993

109. Ishizaki Y, Bandai Y, Shimomura K, Abe H: Safe intraabdominal pressure of CO_2 pneumoperitoneum during laparoscopic surgery. Surgery 114:549, 1993

110. Rasmussen JP, Dauchot PJ, De Palma RG: Cardiac function and hypercarbia. Arch Surg 113:1196, 1978

111. Ho HS, Saunders CJ, Corso FA, Wolfe BM: The effects of CO_2 pneumoperitoneum on haemodynamics in haemorrhaged animals. Surgery 114:381, 1993

112. Alexander GD, Noe FE, Brown EM: Anesthesia for pelvic laparoscopy. Anesth Analg 48:14, 1969

113. Calverly RK, Jenkins LC: The anaesthetic management of pelvic laparoscopy. Canadian Anaesthetists Society Journal 20:679, 1973

114. Fried GM, Clas D, Meakins JL: Minimally invasive surgery in the elderly patient. Surg Clin North Am 74:375, 1994

115. Carroll BJ, Chandra M, Phillips EH, Margulies DR: Laparoscopic cholecystectomy in critically ill cardiac patients. Am Surg 59:783, 1993

116. Wahba RWM, Beique F, Kleiman SJ: Cardiopulmonary function and laparoscopic cholecystectomy. Can J Anaesth 42:51, 1995

117. Joris JL, Noirot DP, Legrand MJ et al: Hemodynamic changes during laparoscopic cholecystectomy. Anesth Analg 76:1067, 1993

118. Westerband A, Van De Water JM, Amzallag M: Cardiovascular changes during laparoscopic cholecystectomy. Surgery, Gynecology and Obstetrics 175:535, 1992

119. Reid CW, Martineau RJ, Hull KA, Miller DR: Haemodynamic consequences of abdominal insufflation with CO_2 laparoscopic cholecystectomy. Can J Anaesth 39:A132, 1992

120. Morris JJ, Perkins SR, Hein HAT et al: Physiologic alterations during laparoscopic cholecystectomy in cardiac transplant patients. Anesth Analg 80:S329, 1995

121. Liu SY, Leighton T, Davis I: Prospective analysis of cardiopulmonary responses to laparoscopic cholecystectomy. Journal of Laparoendoscopic Surgery 1:241, 1991

122. Iwase K, Takenaka H, Yagura A et al: Hemodynamic changes during laparoscopic cholecystectomy in patients with heart disease. Endoscopy 24:771, 1992

123. Fox LG, Hein Hat, Gawey BJ et al: Physiological changes during laparoscopic cholecystectomy in ASA III & IV patients. Anesthesiology 79:A55, 1993

124. Goodale RL, Beebe DS, McNevin MP et al: Hemodynamic, respiratory and metabolic effects of laparoscopic cholecystectomy. Am J Surg 166:533, 1993

125. Smith I, Benzie RJ, Gordon NLM et al: Cardiovascular effects of peritoneal insufflation of carbon dioxide for laparoscopy. BMJ 3:410, 1971

126. Joris J, Honore P, Lamy M: Changes in oxygen transport and ventilation during laparoscopic cholecystectomy. Anesthesiology 77:A149, 1992

127. Feig BW, Berger DH, Dougherty TB et al: Pharmacological intervention can reestablish baseline hemodynamic parameters during laparoscopy. Surgery 116:733, 1994

128. Rasmussen JP, Dauchot PJ, DePalma RG et al: Cardiac function and hypercarbia. Arch Surg 113:1196, 1978

129. Shifren JL, Adelstein L, Finkler NJ: Asystolic cardiac arrest: A rare complication of laparoscopy. Obstet Gynecol 79:840, 1992

130. Beck DH, McQuillan PJ: Fatal carbon dioxide embolism and severe haemorrhage during laparoscopic salpingectomy. Br J Anaesth 72:243, 1994

131. Clarke CC, Weeks DB, Gusdon JP: Venous carbon dioxide embolism during laparoscopy. Anesth Analg 56:650, 1977

132. Root B, Levy MN, Pollack S et al: Gas embolism death after laparoscopy delayed by trapping in the portal circulation. Anesth Analg 57:232, 1978

133. Baraka A: Cardiovascular collapse after carbon dioxide exsufflation in a patient undergoing laparoscopic cholecystectomy (letter). Anesth Analg 78:603, 1994

134. Derouin M, Couture P, Boudreault D et al: Detection of gas embolism by transoesophageal echocardiography during laparoscopic cholecystectomy. Anesth Analg 82:119, 1996

135. Schindler E, Muller M, Kelm C: Cerebral carbon dioxide embolism during laparoscopic cholecystectomy. Anesth Analg 81:643, 1995

136. Junghans T, Bohm B, Grundel K et al: Does pneumoperitoneum with different gases, body positions, and intraperitoneal pressures influence renal and hepatic blood flow? Surgery 121:206, 1997

137. Morino M, Giraudo G, Festa V: Alterations in hepatic function during laparoscopic surgery. Surg Endosc 12:968, 1998

138. Aoki T, Tanii M, Takahashi K et al: Cardiovascular changes and plasma catecholamine levels during laparoscopic surgery. Anesth Analg 78:S8, 1994

139. Felber AR, Blobner M, Goegler S: Plasma vasopressin in laparoscopic cholecystectomy. Anesthesiology 79:A32, 1993

140. Joris J, Lamy M: Neuroendocrine changes during pneumoperitoneum for laparoscopic cholecystectomy. Br J Anaesth 70:A33, 1993

141. Mealy K, Gallagher H, Barry M et al: Physiological and metabolic responses to open and laparoscopic cholecystectomy. Br J Surg 79:1061, 1992

142. Wolf JS Jr, Carrier S, Stoller S: Gas embolism: Helium is more lethal than carbon dioxide. Journal of Laparoendoscopic Surgery 4:173, 1994

143. Piiper J: Physiological equilibria of gas cavities in the body. In Fenn WO, Rahn M (eds): Handbook of Physiology: 3. Respiration, p 1205. Washington, DC, American Physiology Society, 1965

144. Mullet CE, Viale JP, Sagard PE: Pulmonary CO_2 elimination during surgical procedures using intra- or extraperitoneal CO_2 insufflation. Anesth Analg 76:622, 1993

145. Wittgen CM, Andrus CH, Fitzgerald SD: Analysis of the hemodynamic and ventilatory effects of laparoscopic cholecystectomy. Arch Surg 126:997, 1991

146. Hall D, Goldstein A, Tynan E, Braunstein L: Profound hypercarbia late in the course of laparoscopic cholecystectomy: Detection by continuous capnometry. Anesthesiology 79:173, 1993

147. Wahba RWM: Perioperative functional residual capacity. Can J Anaesth 38:384, 1991

148. Fahy B, Barnas G, Flowers J et al: The effects of increased abdominal

pressure on lung and chest wall mechanics during laparoscopic surgery. Anesth Analg 81:744, 1995

149. Puri GD, Singh H: Ventilatory effects of laparoscopy under general anaesthesia. Br J Anaesth 68:211, 1992

150. Brown DR, Fishburne JI, Roberson VO: Ventilatory and blood gas changes during laparoscopy with local anaesthesia. Am J Obstet Gynecol 124:741, 1976

151. Cunningham AJ, Schlanger M: Intraoperative hypoxemia complicating laparoscopic cholecystectomy in a patient with sickle hemoglobinopathy. Anesth Analg 75:838, 1992

152. Duffy BL: Regurgitation during pelvic laparoscopy. Br J Anaesth 51:1089, 1979

153. Schauer PR, Luna J, Ghiatas AA *et al:* Pulmonary function after laparoscopic cholecystectomy. Surgery 114:389, 1993

154. Joris J, Kaba A, Lamy M: Postoperative spirometry after laparoscopy for lower abdominal or upper abdominal surgical procedures. Br J Anaesth 79:422, 1997

155. McKeague H, Cunningham AJ: Postoperative respiratory dysfunction: is the site of surgery crucial? Br J Anaesth 79:415, 1997

156. Erice F, Fox GS, Salib YM *et al:* Diaphragmatic function before and after laparoscopic cholecystectomy. Anesthesiology 79:966, 1993

157. Cunningham AJ, Brull SJ: Laparoscopic cholecystectomy: Anesthetic implications. Anesth Analg 76:1120, 1993

158. Chui PT, Oh TE: Anaesthesia for laparoscopic general surgery. Anaesth Intensive Care 21:163, 1993

159. Marco AP, Yeo CJ, Rock P: Anesthesia for a patient undergoing laparoscopic cholecystectomy. Anesthesiology 73:1268, 1990

160. Rose DK, Cohen MM, Soutter DI: Laparoscopic cholecystectomy: The anaesthetist's point of view. Can J Anaesth 39:809, 1992

161. Chesick KC, Black S, Hoye SJ: Spasm and operative cholangiography. Arch Surg 110:53, 1975

162. McCammon RL, Viegas OJ, Stoelting RK: Naloxone reversal of choledochoduodenal sphincter spasm associated with narcotic administration. Anesthesiology 48:437, 1978

163. Jones RM, Detmer M, Hill AB: Incidence of choledochoduodenal sphincter spasm during fentanyl-supplemented anesthesia. Anesth Analg 60:638, 1981

164. Humphrey HK, Fleming NW: Opioid induced spasm of the sphincter of Oddi apparently reversed by nalbuphine. Anesth Analg 74:308, 1992

165. Michaloliakou C, Chung F, Sharma S: Preoperative multimodal analgesia facilitates recovery after ambulatory laparoscopic cholecystectomy. Anesth Analg 82:44, 1996

166. Weber A, Munoz J, Garteiz D. *et al.* Use of subdiaphragmatic bupivacaine instillation to control postoperative pain after laparoscopic surgery. Surg Laparosc Endosc 7:6, 1997

167. Rademaker BMP, Kalkman CJ, Odoom J *et al:* Intraperitoneal local anaesthetics after laparoscopic cholecystectomy: Effects on postoperative pain, metabolic responses and lung function. Br J Anaesth 72:263, 1994

168. Joris J, Thiry E, Paris P *et al:* Pain after laparoscopic cholecystectomy: Characteristics and effect of intraperitoneal bupivacaine. Anesth Analg 81:379, 1995

169. Malins AF, Field JM, Nesling PM, Cooper GM: Nausea and vomiting after gynaecological laparoscopy: Comparison of premedication with oral ondansetron, metoclopramide and placebo. Br J Anaesth 72:231, 1994

170. Raphael JH, Norton AC: Antiemetic efficacy of prophylactic ondansetron in laparoscopic surgery: Randomized, double-blind comparison with metoclopramide. Br J Anaesth 71:845, 1993

171. Krogh B, Jensen PJ, Henneberg SW *et al:* Nitrous oxide does not influence operating conditions or postoperative course in colonic surgery. Br J Anaesth 72:55, 1994

172. Taylor E, Feinstein R, White PF, Sopor N: Anesthesia for laparoscopic cholecystectomy: Is nitrous oxide contraindicated? Anesthesiology 76:541, 1992

173. Divatia JV, Vaidya JS, Badwe RA, Hawaldar RW: Omission of nitrous oxide during anesthesia reduces the incidence of postoperative nausea and vomiting: A meta-analysis. Anesthesiology 85:1055, 1996

174. Wahba RWM, Mamazza J: Ventilatory requirements during laparoscopic cholecystectomy. Can J Anaesth 40:206, 1993

175. Bhavani-Shanker K, Moseley H, Kumar AY, Delph Y: Capnometry and anesthesia. Can J Anaesth 39:617, 1991

176. Wittgen CM, Naunhein KS, Andrus CH, Kaminski DL: Preoperative pulmonary evaluation for laparoscopic cholecystectomy. Arch Surg 128:880, 1993

177. Dhoste K, Karayan J, Lacoste L *et al:* Hemodynamic changes during laparoscopic cholecystectomy in the elderly. Br J Anaesth 72: A32, 1993

178. Stevenson ARL: Ambulatory laparoscopic surgery: The patient's perspective in an inpatient world. Aust N Z J Surg 68:753, 1998

179. Cuschieri A: Day-case (ambulatory) laparoscopic surgery: Let us sing from the same hymn sheet. Surg Endosc 11:1142, 1997

180. Rosenberg-Adamsen S, Skarbye M, Wildschiodtz G *et al:* Sleep after laparoscopic cholecystectomy. Br J Anaesth 77:572, 1996

181. Hayes C, Ambazidis S, Gani JS: Intensive care unit admissions following laparoscopic surgery: What lessons can be learned? Aust N Z J Surg 66:206, 1996

Clinical Anesthesia (4/e), edited by
Paul G. Barash, Bruce F. Cullen, and
Robert K. Stoelting. Lippincott Williams &
Wilkins, Philadelphia, © 2001.

CHAPTER 39

ANESTHESIA AND THE LIVER

PHILLIP S. MUSHLIN AND SIMON GELMAN

The liver occupies the epicenter of a diverse spectrum of vital physiologic functions and plays an essential role in maintaining perioperative homeostasis. For example, the liver moderates hypotensive responses to acute losses of blood via its reservoir function, and helps to prevent the development of coagulopathies though its synthesis of clotting factors and the degradation of fibrinolytic substances. Predictable termination of the pharmacologic effects of many anesthetic agents depends on hepatic clearance mechanisms. In addition, the liver nourishes the essential organs, helping to sustain them during the fasted state. Moreover, it defends the body against invading microorganisms, maintains immunologic surveillance, and modulates inflammatory processes. Such vital functions are often unappreciated when the liver is healthy.

The liver is a remarkably resilient organ, with an unparalleled regenerative capacity and substantial physiologic reserves. These reserves, however, enable insidious diseases, such as hepatitis C, to silently destroy a majority of the liver. Few, if any, symptoms develop and many patients remain unaware of their condition until irreversible hepatic damage has occurred. Identifying patients with marked limitations of hepatic reserve but no overt hepatic dysfunction is important and requires a careful preoperative history and physical examination. These patients are often at increased risk for perioperative complications and postoperative liver dysfunction, particularly when undergoing major operative procedures. Unfortunately, when the pathogenesis of postoperative hepatobiliary disorders is unclear, the anesthetic often gets the blame.

As therapies for stabilizing chronic hepatic diseases continue to improve, an increasing number of patients with moderate-to-severe liver disease will be presenting for surgery. Certain operative procedures (*e.g.*, laparotomy), when performed in patients with severe liver disease, have been associated with rates of morbidity and mortality that are stunning. For example, a British study documented a 30-day mortality rate after laparotomy of 31%, and reported that all patients with viral or alcoholic hepatitis died, as did most of those with ascites.[1] In a subsequent U.S. study, the 30-day mortality rate approached 83% in patients with severe hepatic disease and ascites, and reached 91% when their prothrombin time (PT) was prolonged by more than 2.5 seconds.[2] Because patients with hepatic dysfunction may be at extremely high risk for perioperative complications, anesthesiologists must understand the interactions between liver disease, surgical procedures, and anesthetic interventions, so that we can formulate and orchestrate therapeutic plans to optimize patient outcome.

HEPATIC ANATOMY

The liver is the largest gland in the human body, accounting for nearly 2% of the total body mass of an adult and about 5% of a newborn's mass.[3]

Lobes Versus Segments of the Liver

Physicians of prior eras viewed the liver as a bilobed organ, with right and left lobes separated by the falciform ligament (a peritoneal fold connecting the diaphragm and anterior abdominal wall). Contemporary anatomic classifications include lobar and segmental systems. The former system derives from topographic anatomy of the liver and specifies four distinct lobes (left, right, caudate and quadrate; Fig. 39-1), whereas the latter (French or Couinaud) relates to physiologic anatomy (Fig. 39-2). Couinaud partitions the liver into eight functionally independent segments, each with its own vascular inflow, vascular outflow, and biliary drainage. This system enables hepatic resections along segmental planes, which prevents major disruptions of hepatobiliary function and facilitates the preservation of vital tissue and extirpation of nonviable tissue.[4] By coupling segmental concepts with innovative imaging techniques, radiologists can construct precise, three-dimensional models of a patient's liver to pinpoint the proximity of lesion(s) to critical intrahepatic structures. Such information simplifies surgical decision making, enhances the resectability of a variety of lesions, and improves outcomes for patients undergoing hepatic operations for neoplasms or trauma.[5]

Vascular Supply of the Liver

The liver receives about 25% of the cardiac output, and therefore has an average blood flow of between 100 and 130 $ml \cdot min^{-1} \cdot 100 \ g^{-1}$. The hepatic artery delivers one-fourth of this flow but nearly one-half (45–50%) of the oxygen supply; the portal vein provides three-fourths of the hepatic flow and roughly one-half (50–55%) of the oxygen. Because portal venous blood has already perfused the preportal organs (stomach, intestines, spleen, and pancreas) (Fig. 39-3), it is partially deoxygenated and enriched with nutrients and other substances absorbed from the gastrointestinal tract.

The hepatic artery arises from the celiac axis (Fig. 39-3) and has abundant collateral circulation. The portal vein forms by the anastomosis of the superior mesenteric and splenic veins and has numerous tributaries (Fig. 39-1), which are normally of little importance. When patients develop portal hypertension, however, these normally rudimentary connections form large portosystemic shunts, permitting portal venous blood to return to the heart without traversing the liver. These shunts produce many of the pathologic findings and severe complications of portal hypertension (*e.g.*, esophageal varices).

Intrahepatic Circulation

As the hepatic artery and portal vein approach the porta hepatis, each bifurcates into left and right branches. These branches enter the liver, arborize in parallel, and diminish in caliber as they penetrate the hepatic parenchyma. At the end of their intrahepatic journeys, these vessels become terminal hepatic arterioles and terminal portal venules (Fig. 39-4).

Most terminal vessels drain directly into the hepatic sinusoids, delivering substrates to, and removing products from, the neighboring liver cells. Before emptying into the sinusoids, some hepatic arteriolar blood flows through the peribiliary capillary plexus, which plays a major role in bile secretion and absorption (Fig. 39-4).

A sinusoid is typically 7–15 μm wide, but its width may increase to 180 μm under certain physiologic conditions. The pressure within the sinusoids is normally 2–3 mm Hg above central venous pressure. Sinusoids have a large reservoir capacity, are highly compliant, and have an extremely low resistance.

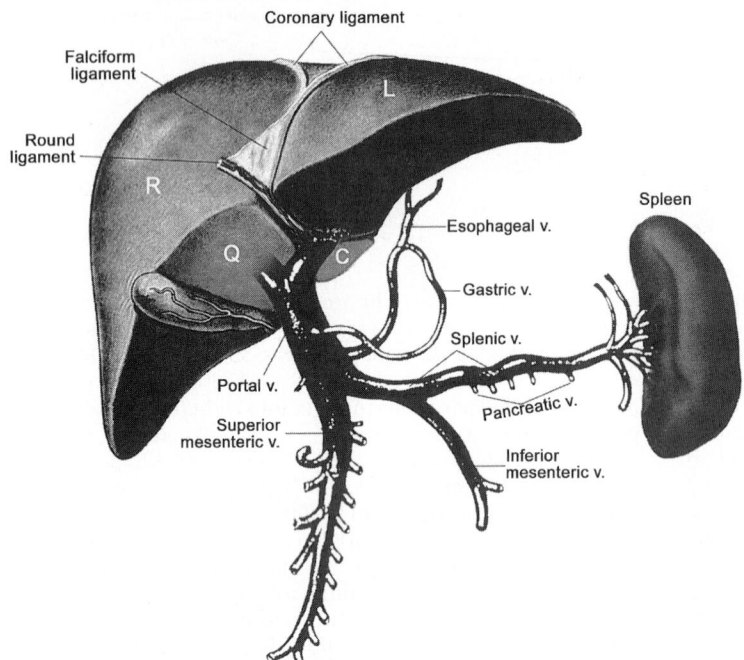

Figure 39-1. Schematic representation depicting the lobar classification of the liver and the extrahepatic portal venous circulation.

Blood egresses from the distal end of a sinusoid through a terminal hepatic venule, and immediately enters a central vein (Fig. 39-5). It then flows through sublobular veins to progressively larger tributaries that ultimately form one of the three major hepatic veins (right, middle, and left). A short extrahepatic segment joins each major vein to the inferior vena cava (IVC). If thrombosis of the major hepatic veins occurs (Budd-Chiari syndrome), the small posterior caudate veins become important for draining hepatic blood into the IVC.

Hepatic Microanatomy: Classic Liver Lobule Versus Acinar Lobule

The classic lobule is roughly a hexagonal prism of liver tissue. A central vein courses longitudinally through the prism's center and runs parallel to six vertically aligned portal canals that define the angles of the hexagonal structure (Fig. 39-5). Each canal contains connective tissue, lymphatics, nerves, and a portal triad (terminal branches of portal vein, hepatic artery, and bile duct). Viewed in transverse section, a lobule is an array of anastomosing cords of cuboidal hepatocytes, separated by vascular channels (lacunae) that radiate from the six portal areas and converge on a central vein at the middle of the hexagon. A lacunar labyrinth permeates the entire lobule, except for the most peripheral portion, where a limiting plate of hepatocytes forms a near continuous wall. This wall separates the interior of the lobule from the portal canals. Only tiny terminal branches of the hepatic artery, portal vein, and bile duct can penetrate the occasional fenestrae within the limiting plate.

Human livers, unlike those of several other species, lack well-defined interlobular connective tissue. Therefore, classic lobules are difficult to visualize in human livers. The quest to identify their boundaries led to the discovery of circumferential terminal hepatic arterioles, portal venules, and bile ductules. Reasoning that these encircling vessels supply segments of contiguous classic lobules that lie between two central veins (*i.e.,* terminal hepatic venules; Fig. 39-6), Rappaport developed the acinus lobule (acinus) concept.

The acinar concept partitions all liver cells supplied by a terminal branch of the portal vein and hepatic artery into three concentric circulatory zones, based on their proximity to the afferent vessels (Fig. 39-6). Blood enters the center of the acinus and flows centrifugally to the central veins. Zone 1 cells are closest to the portal axis and are therefore the first to receive blood. The oxygen content and nutritive value of the blood progressively decrease as blood flows from Zone 1 to Zone 3. Blood perfusing Zone 3 cells (acinar periphery) has already exchanged gases with, and collected waste products from, cells of Zones 1 and 2.

This unique microvascular arrangement allows for metabolic heterogeneity among the various zones. Cells of Zone 1 are amply equipped with mitochondria and contain the highest concentrations of Krebs cycle enzymes; they are ideally suited for oxidative metabolism and synthesis of glycogen. Zone 1 cells are of primary importance in the bile synthetic pathway that is dependent upon the plasma concentration of bile, being the first cells to encounter this readily absorbable detergent. On the other hand, cells of Zone 3 play the larger role in the bile salt–independent formation of bile.

Zone 3 cells are relatively anaerobic and well suited to regulate the rates of metabolic reactions that use molecular oxygen

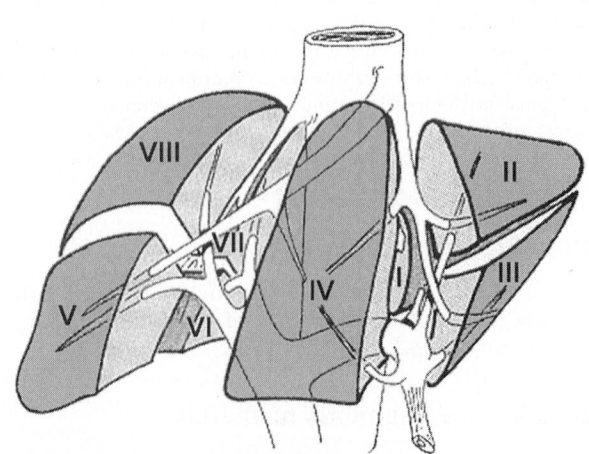

Figure 39-2. Segmental division of the liver according to Couinaud's nomenclature. (Reprinted with permission from Parks RW, Chrysos E, Diamond T: Br J Surg 86:1121, 1999.)

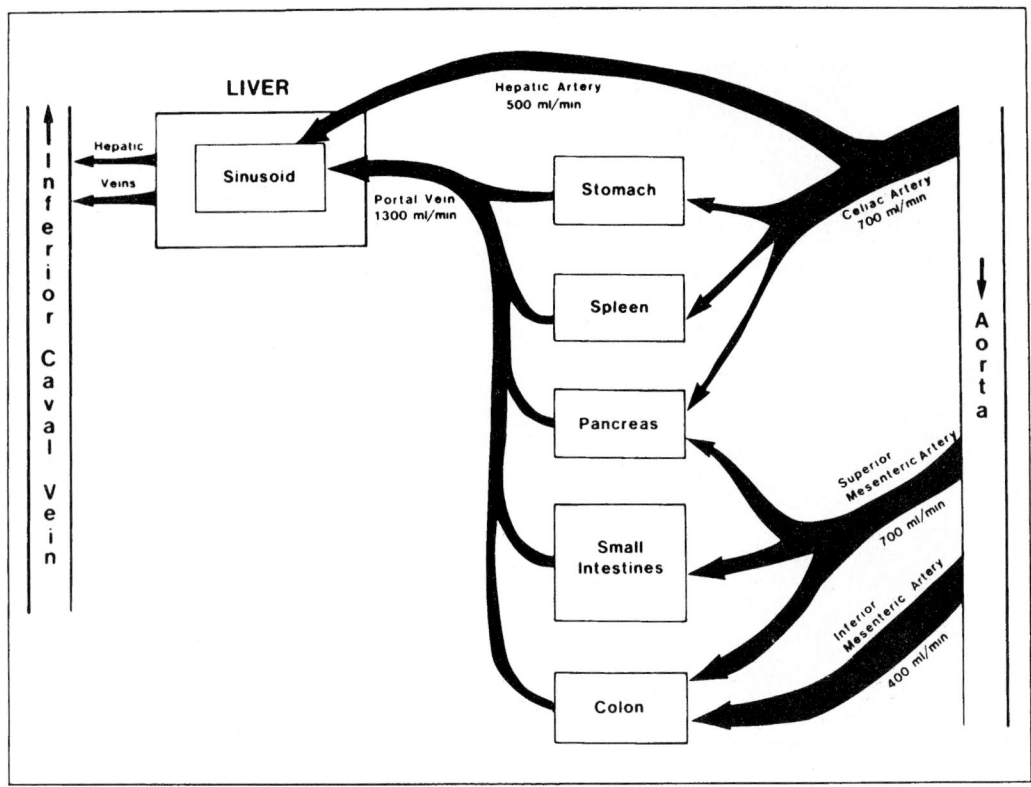

Figure 39-3. Schematic representation of splanchnic circulation. (Reprinted with permission from Gelman S: Effects of anesthetics on splanchnic circulation. In Altura BM, Halevy S [eds]: Cardiovascular Action of Anesthetics and Drugs Used in Anesthesia, p 127. Basel, Karger, 1986.)

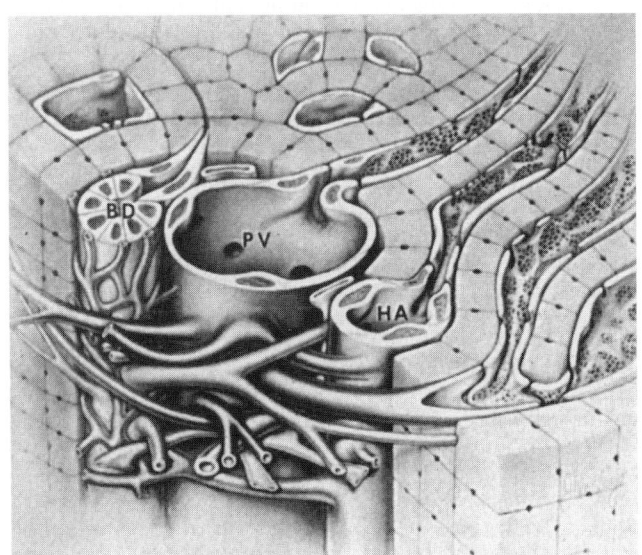

Figure 39-4. Relationship of branches of the portal vein (PV), hepatic artery (HA), and bile duct (BD). Notice the peribiliary capillary plexus that envelops the bile ducts. These three structures constitute a portal triad, which is a transverse section of a portal canal. (Reprinted with permission from Jones AL: Anatomy of the normal liver. In Zakim D, Boyer T (eds): Hepatology: A Textbook of Liver Disease, 3rd ed, p 3. Philadelphia, WB Saunders, 1996.)

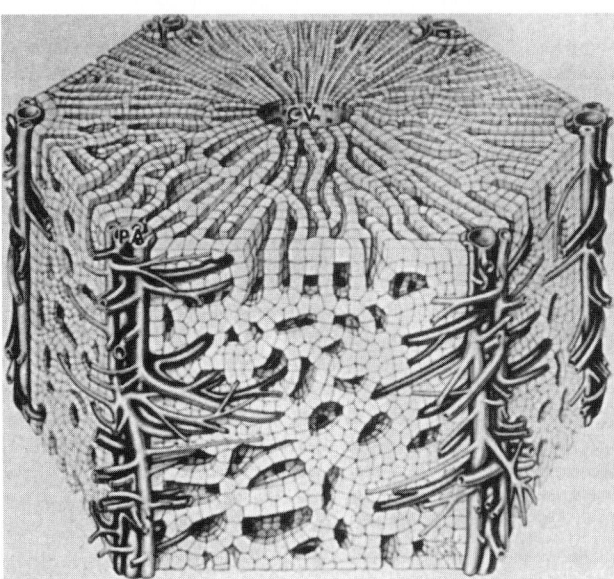

Figure 39-5. Schematic view of liver lobule: The central vein (CV) lies in the center of the figure surrounded by anastomosing cords of block-like hepatocytes. About the periphery of this schema are six portal areas (PA) consisting of branches of the portal vein, the hepatic artery, and the bile duct. (Reprinted with permission from Jones AL: Anatomy of the normal liver. In Zakim D, Boyer T (eds): Hepatology: A Textbook of Liver Disease, 3rd ed, p 3. Philadelphia, WB Saunders, 1996.)

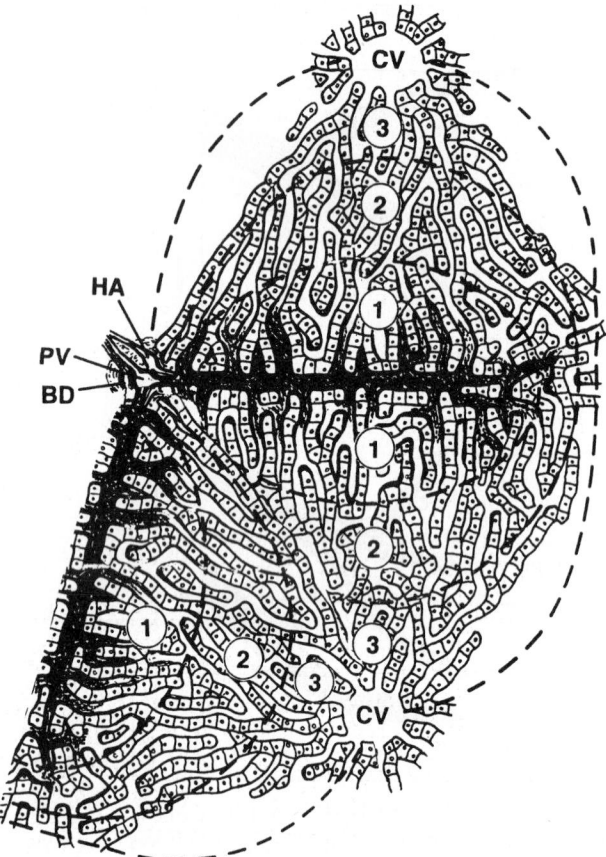

Figure 39-6. Blood supply of the simple liver acinus. The oxygen tension and the nutrient level of the blood in sinusoids decrease from Zone 1 through Zone 3. Note that the lower left side of the figure also depicts Zones 1, 2 and 3 in a portion of an adjacent acinar unit. BD = bile duct; HA = hepatic artery; PV = portal vein; CV = central vein. (Reprinted with permission from Jones AL: Anatomy of the normal liver. In Zakim D, Boyer T (eds): Hepatology: A Textbook of Liver Disease, 3rd ed, p 3. Philadelphia, WB Saunders, 1996.)

and produce reactive oxygen species. They have an abundance of smooth endoplasmic reticulum, reduced nicotinamide adenine dinucleotide phosphate (NADPH), and reduced cytochrome P-450, and play a major role in the metabolism of drugs, chemicals, and toxins. The anaerobic milieu of Zone 3, however, is also its Achilles' heel because these cells are exquisitely susceptible to injury from circulatory disturbances that cause ischemia or hypoxia (*e.g.*, hypotension, hypoxemia, severe anemia) and to toxic products of biotransformation. Thus, a decreased capacity of the liver to metabolize drugs and endogenous substances may be an early manifestation of hepatic dysfunction. Centrilobular necrosis is more likely to occur than periportal necrosis when pathophysiologic processes critically lower the oxygen supply-to-demand ratio in the liver by decreasing oxygen delivery or by increasing its extraction by cells of Zone 1 and Zone 2.

Innervation of the Liver

An anterior and a posterior plexus innervate the portal and pericapsular regions of the liver. The anterior plexus conveys postganglionic sympathetic nervous system (SNS) fibers from the celiac plexus (ganglia T7–T10), left-sided vagal fibers, and fibers from the right phrenic nerve. The anterior plexus communicates with the posterior plexus near the portal vein and bile ducts. SNS fibers innervate the hepatic arteries.

Disruption of neurotransmission through the anterior plexus can modify hepatobiliary physiology, producing alterations in the accumulation of hepatic fat and in the composition of secreted bile. Distension of the liver capsule or gallbladder causes referred pain, conveyed to the right shoulder or scapula via the third and fourth cervical nerves.

Hepatic Lymphatic System

The primary site of hepatic lymph formation is the perisinusoidal space of Disse (located between hepatocytes and the sinusoidal endothelium). This lymph travels through the periportal space of Mall (between the limiting plate and portal connective tissue), permeates the connective tissue, and drains into the lymphatic vessels of the portal canal. About 80% flows through progressively larger channels, ultimately reaching the collecting lymphatics, which exit the porta hepatis and empty into the thoracic duct at the cisterna chyli. The remaining 20% leaves the liver either via small lymphatic networks near the hepatic veins and IVC or in vessels that pierce the diaphragm and anastomose with retrosternal lymphatics. Hepatic lymph nodes are located in the porta hepatis, celiac region, and near the IVC. Small increases in hepatic venous pressure can drive an excess of intravascular fluid into the lymphatics, leading to its transudation through the hepatic capsule and into the peritoneal cavity (ascites).

REGULATION OF HEPATIC BLOOD FLOW

The hepatic circulation is regulated by mechanisms that are both intrinsic[6] and extrinsic to the liver. Intrinsic mechanisms help to provide a constant supply of blood and oxygen to the liver. In doing so, these mechanisms stabilize the hepatic clearances of many endogenous substances and drugs, and contribute to the maintenance of venous return and cardiac output.[6] Extrinsic mechanisms, which include a complex constellation of neural and humeral reflexes, moderate the hemodynamic consequences of major circulatory derangements. For example, when hypovolemia and hypotension occur, extrinsic reflexes are activated, resulting in the prompt deployment of the liver's blood reservoir and rapid diversion of its blood flow to essential, extrahepatic tissues, including the heart and brain.

Intrinsic Circulatory Regulation

Hepatic Arterial Buffer Response

Because the liver lacks the ability to directly regulate portal venous flow, intrinsic regulatory mechanisms operate almost exclusively by modulating hepatic arteriolar tone. The hepatic arterial buffer response—the most important of these mechanisms—causes hepatic arterial flow to vary reciprocally with changes in portal venous flow. The greatest reduction in arterial flow achievable by the buffer response occurs when portal venous flow doubles. Conversely, the buffer response produces an approximately twofold increase in arterial flow following severe reductions of portal venous flow, as occurs after placement of a portal–caval shunt or ligation of the superior mesenteric artery.[6] Thus, at least in theory, if portal venous flow were to decrease by more than 50%, the arterial buffer response would be unable to fully prevent a decrease in hepatic blood flow, although it could be expected to totally preserve hepatic oxygenation. (Because the hepatic artery supplies 25% of the liver's blood flow and 50% of its oxygen, a doubling of the arterial flow would yield 50% of the normal total blood flow and 100% of the normal oxygen supply.)

The hepatic buffer response appears to be mediated via adenosine. Presumably, this potent arteriolar dilator is synthesized at a constant rate (independent of oxygen supply or demand) and continuously secreted in the vicinity of the terminal hepatic arterioles and portal venules.[6] If flow through the portal vein decreases, less of the perivascular adenosine is "washed out," leading to its accumulation around hepatic arterioles. The result is a greater degree of arteriolar dilation and an increase in hepatic arterial flow. Conversely, an increase in portal venous flow would lower the peri-arteriolar concentration of adenosine, and thereby decrease hepatic arterial flow.

Hepatic Flow Autoregulation

The hepatic arterial system also undergoes flow autoregulation (constant pressure, variable flow) when the liver is very active metabolically (postprandial) but not during the fasted state. The metabolic state modifies the composition of portal venous and systemic blood, thereby influencing hepatic blood flow. Decreases in pH and O_2 content, or increases in Pco_2 of the portal blood promote increases of hepatic arterial flow.[7] Postprandial hyperosmolarity can increase both hepatic arterial and portal venous blood flow, but this effect would not be relevant in fasted patients. Thus, hepatic flow autoregulation is not an important mechanism during most anesthetics, given that they occur in fasted patients.

Extrinsic Circulatory Regulation

Extrinsic factors regulate blood flow through the portal vein by modulating the tone of arterioles in the preportal splanchnic organs (Fig. 39-3). Portal vein pressure (normally 7–10 mm Hg) therefore reflects both splanchnic arteriolar tone and intrahepatic resistance to portal flow. Portal venules (presinusoidal sphincters) affect the distribution of blood flow to the sinusoids; however, the hepatic venules (postsinusoidal sphincters) control venous resistance in the liver. Extrinsic mechanisms modulate this venular tone, with the sympathetic nervous system being the primary physiologic regulator. Stimulation of α_1-adrenergic receptors increases venular tone, leading to decreases in hepatic blood flow and a reduction of blood volume in the sinusoids.

Hepatic arteriolar tone is the main determinant of resistance in the hepatic arterial tree. Blood flow through the liver decreases with stimulation of certain arteriolar receptors (α_1-adrenergic or type 1 dopaminergic) and increases with activation of others (β_2-adrenergic receptors). As mentioned earlier, local and intrinsic mechanisms also modulate arteriolar tone, producing changes in arterial flow that are reciprocal to changes in portal flow (arterial buffer response). Thus, when the arterial buffer response is intact, changes in portal venous flow will induce compensatory alterations in hepatic arterial flow.

Humoral Regulators of Hepatic Blood Flow

Myriad humoral substances alter liver blood flow, including gastrin, glucagon, secretin, bile salts, angiotensin II, vasopressin, and catecholamines. Of the systemic hormones, epinephrine is most likely to attain concentrations that produce vasoactive effects. Both α- and β-adrenergic receptors exist in the hepatic arterial bed, whereas the portal vasculature has only α receptors. An injection of epinephrine directly into the hepatic artery causes vasoconstriction (α-adrenergic effect), followed by vasodilation (β_2-adrenergic effect). When injected into the portal bed, epinephrine produces only vasoconstriction. During activation of the sympathetic nervous system, the hepatic circulatory effects of epinephrine and norepinephrine would far exceed those of dopamine. Dopamine probably has little if any importance as a physiologic modulator of the hepatic circulation. Glucagon induces a graded, long-lasting dilation of hepatic arterioles; it also antagonizes arterial constrictor responses to a wide range of physiologic stimuli, including stress-induced sympathoadrenal outflow. Angiotensin II markedly constricts both hepatic arterial and portal beds, and significantly reduces mesenteric outflow; the result is a substantial decrease in total hepatic blood flow. Vasopressin also intensely constricts splanchnic vessels, markedly reducing flow into the portal vein. This action accounts for the efficacy of vasopressin to alleviate portal hypertension; of lesser importance is its ability to dilate intrahepatic portal vessels, which further lowers portal pressure.

MAJOR PHYSIOLOGIC FUNCTIONS OF THE LIVER

Blood Reservoir

The liver is a vital reservoir of whole blood in humans. It contains nearly 25–30 ml of blood per 100 g tissue, which represents 10–15% of a person's total blood volume. The autonomic innervation of the liver coupled with neurohumoral input from the systemic circulation allows for rapid, precise control of the reservoir volume. Intense sympathetic nervous system stimulation (e.g., pain, hypoxia, hypercarbia) abruptly decreases hepatic blood flow and blood volume; 80% of the hepatic blood volume (approximately 400–500 ml) can be expelled within a matter of seconds.

Anesthetics that suppress sympathetic nervous system outflow impair the reservoir function, and predispose to circulatory decompensation when significant decreases of intravascular volume occur without immediate replacement. Severe liver disease exacerbates hypotensive effects of hypovolemia by impairing vasoconstrictor responses to catecholamines. A total failure of vasoconstriction not only incapacitates the splanchnic reservoir, but also prevents the redirection of blood flow from skeletal muscle beds and splanchnic tissues to the heart and brain.

Regulator of Blood Coagulation

The liver helps maintain normal blood clotting function in numerous ways. It synthesizes all of the coagulation factors except VIII clotting factor, VIII vWF (endothelial), and IV (Ca). Through the synthesis of bile acids and the enterohepatic circulation, the liver ensures absorption of orally administered vitamin K; it uses this vitamin to bioactivate several clotting factors (II, VII, IX, and X). The liver also modulates platelet production through the synthesis of thrombopoietin, which stimulates bone marrow precursor cells to differentiate into platelet-generating megakaryocytes. Moreover, hepatic clearance of fibrinolysins and tissue plasminogen activators is necessary to prevent or control fibrinolytic states.

Endocrine Organ

The liver has important endocrine functions. It synthesizes and secretes essential hormones, including insulin-like growth factor-1 (IGF-1), angiotensinogen, and thrombopoietin. IGF-1, formerly called somatomedin, is the immediate stimulus for growth of the body. Thrombopoietin stimulates the bone marrow to produce platelets. Angiotensinogen, a precursor of angiotensin II, is intricately involved in the regulation of fluid and electrolyte balance in the body. The liver is also essential for the transport and metabolism of a variety of hormones including insulin, thyroxine, and estrogen.

Erythrocyte Breakdown and Bilirubin Excretion

Excretion of bilirubin, a breakdown product of heme, requires an intact biliary system. After reticuloendothelial cells phagocytize damaged erythrocytes and separate the protein portion of hemoglobin from the heme moiety, they convert heme to biliverdin and reduce this compound to bilirubin. Upon release into the blood, bilirubin binds tenaciously to albumin. Hepatocytes avidly extract bilirubin from albumin, conjugate it with glucuronic acid, and then actively excrete these conjugates into bile canaliculi; only a small portion of the conjugated bilirubin enters the plasma. Bacteria in the gut convert most of the conjugated bilirubin to urobilinogen. The intestinal mucosa reabsorbs some urobilinogen, which reaches the liver *via* the mesenteric blood. The liver efficiently extracts this molecule and returns it to the intestine (enterohepatic circulation); the kidneys excrete only about 5% of the urobilinogen produced. Exposure to air oxidizes urobilinogen to urobilin in the urine or to stercobilin in the feces.

The liver also scavenges free hemoglobin from blood, helping to conserve body iron. It synthesizes haptoglobin, which forms complexes with dimers of free intravascular hemoglobin. Receptors on hepatocytes remove these complexes from plasma and thereby prevent the loss of hemoglobin dimers in the urine. The decomposition of hemoglobin in plasma yields free oxidized heme (metheme). Hemopexin, another liver-derived protein, complexes with metheme; hepatocytes extract these hemopexin–metheme complexes from plasma and retain the iron.

Regulator of Intermediary Metabolism

The liver is the penultimate metabolic organ and is highly specialized to meet the energy requirements of the body. It expends nearly 20% of the energy and O_2 used by the body, while accounting for only about 2% of the total body mass. To feed itself, the liver prefers fatty acids to glucose.

Carbohydrate Metabolism

Normal hepatic function is important for maintaining euglycemia (glucose buffer function). Multiple metabolic pathways contribute to glucose homeostasis, including glycogen synthesis and degradation, conversion of galactose to glucose, and the *de novo* synthesis of glucose via gluconeogenesis. Important substrates for gluconeogenesis include lactate and amino acids. As prolonged fasting depletes hepatic and muscle stores of glycogen, the continued production of glucose requires muscle catabolism to provide the liver with amino acids (Cori cycle). Some amino acids, such as alanine, undergo oxidative deamination in the liver and are readily converted to glucose via gluconeogenesis. Others, including branched-chain amino acids (leucine, valine, and isoleucine), are not very useful in this capacity because they are relatively resistant to deamination or transamination by the liver.

Lipid Metabolism

During the fed state, with oxidative substrates in abundance, the liver transforms carbohydrates, proteins, and dietary lipids to fatty acids. It esterifies these acids with glycerol metabolites to yield triglycerides and phospholipids. Excess lipids attach to hepatically synthesized or reprocessed apoproteins to create lipoproteins, which are transported to adipocytes. The liver synthesizes a variety of important lipids including precursors and derivatives of cholesterol that provide the molecular framework of steroid hormones and bile acids. Bile salts form the micelles required to absorb essential lipids from the gut (*e.g.*, fat-soluble vitamins: D, E, and K). In the fasted state, the liver converts triglycerides and fatty acids to ketone bodies (*e.g.*, acetoacetate) via beta-oxidation. Rather than using these ketones for its own nourishment, the liver exports them to sustain other tissues (*e.g.*, brain, muscle, and kidney).

Amino Acid Metabolism

The liver synthesizes the nonessential amino acids either *de novo* or through a variety of pathways involving transamination or deamination reactions. Such reactions are essential in the catabolism of amino acids and are required for the elimination of nitrogenous waste products. Deamination of glutamine yields glutamic acid plus ammonia (NH_3). The urea cycle combines NH_3 with CO_2 to form urea, which the kidney excretes. Thus, a normal or low concentration of urea nitrogen in blood (BUN) provides no assurance that a patient has adequate renal function if the liver is failing. Decreased activities of urea cycle enzymes (secondary to zinc deficiency) may contribute to the development of hepatic encephalopathy.

Synthesis of Important Proteins

The liver produces a vast assortment of proteins with important extrahepatic functions. These proteins include blood clotting factors, hormones, acute phase proteins, and most of the plasma proteins, with a few notable exceptions (*e.g.*, immunoglobulins). Albumin accounts for nearly 10% of the protein synthesized by the liver. It constitutes about 60% (≥ 4 $g \cdot dl^{-1}$) of the total plasma protein pool and is the major determinant of the colloid oncotic pressure of plasma. Albumin also performs significant carrier functions: it transports unconjugated bilirubin to the liver for excretion; serves as a secondary carrier for thyroxine, cortisol, and heme; and is the only plasma protein that transports free fatty acids. Furthermore, albumin binds to, and therefore affects the responses to, a variety of pharmacologic agents.

Tissue injury and inflammation activate macrophages, which release cytokines (*e.g.*, tumor necrosis factor, interleukins) that can stimulate the hepatic synthesis of a variety of acute phase proteins while decreasing the production of albumin. (This may explain why plasma albumin levels generally decrease in all types of chronic diseases.) One of the acute phase proteins, ceruloplasmin, is an important transporter of copper, which also functions as an oxidase and perhaps as a free-radical scavenger. Estrogens stimulate ceruloplasmin synthesis via interactions with steroid receptors on hepatocytes, accounting for the substantial elevations of plasma ceruloplasmin that occur in pregnancy and in women taking estrogen-containing oral contraceptives.

Host Defender

Sinusoidal and perisinusoidal cells of the liver defend the body against microbial invaders, and modulate inflammatory and immune responses to foreign materials. Pit cells, sparsely located in the perisinusoidal space, possess natural killer and neuroendocrine activities. The ubiquitous Kupffer cells police the channels between the portal and systemic circulation, effectively clearing gut-derived toxins and antigens. These cells are aggressively involved in immune surveillance, participating in phagocytosis, cytolysis, antigen presentation to T cells, and perhaps regulation of T-cell proliferation. Kupffer cells produce a variety of inflammatory mediators and cytokines that initiate and modulate both local and systemic effects of hepatic injury. Impairment of Kupffer cell function may be an important harbinger of sepsis or multiorgan systems failure, particularly in the setting of severe gastrointestinal pathology or splanchnic ischemia.

Pharmacokinetics

The liver influences the plasma concentration and systemic availability of most orally and parentally administered substances. Through its synthesis of drug-binding proteins, the liver affects the partitioning of drugs into the various compartments of the body (apparent volume of distribution, V_d). Plasma proteins, especially albumin (preferentially binds acidic and neutral molecules) and α_1-acid glycoprotein (high affinity for alkaloids), act as sponges or sinks to decrease concentrations of free (unbound) drug. Consequently, changes in concentrations of plasma proteins often modify dose–response relationships of drugs. At times, hepatic diseases will be associated with simultaneous decreases of certain plasma proteins and increases of others, which may contribute to confusion about the impact of such diseases on pharmacokoinetics. A large decrease in albumin, for example, would be expected to enhance pharmacologic responses to drugs that are normally highly bound to albumin (*i.e.*, leftward shift of dose–response curve). Conversely, an elevation of other plasma proteins (*e.g.*, α_1-acid glycoprotein) may reduce the delivery of certain medications to the relevant receptors, thereby attenuating the pharmacologic response to any given dose of the drug (*i.e.*, rightward shift of dose–response curve).

Hepatic clearance is the sum of all processes by which the liver eliminates a drug from the body. The three major factors that determine a compound's hepatic clearance are its rate of delivery to the liver (liver blood flow), its intrinsic metabolic clearance (ratio of V_{max} to K_m), and its biliary excretion. Biliary excretion is a major mechanism for clearing peptides and proteins, whereas metabolic processes are primarily responsible for eliminating smaller molecules. Thus, the effects of liver disease on the hepatic clearance of a drug or endogenous substance depend both on the molecule's physicochemical properties and on the degree of impairment of hepatocellular and cholestatic function.[8]

Hepatic metabolic clearance occurs via phase 1 and phase 2 reactions. These reactions typically alter drugs in a manner that facilitates their elimination via renal or biliary mechanisms. In general, phase 1 reactions (oxidation, reduction, *N*-dealkylation) modify structural features of molecules to render them more hydrophilic, whereas phase 2 reactions increase hydrophilicity by conjugating compounds with endogenous molecules that are water-soluble. Products of phase 1 transformations often become substrates for phase 2 reactions. Phase 1 reactions, which involve a wide range of cytochrome P-450 isozymes, are much more susceptible to inhibition by advanced age or hepatic diseases than are phase 2 reactions.

The inherent ability of the liver to metabolize a drug is referred to as intrinsic metabolic clearance.[8] Intrinsic clearance, which reflects the fraction of the delivered drug load that is metabolized or extracted during a single pass through the liver, provides the basis for classifying drugs as high-, intermediate- or low-clearance compounds. High-clearance drugs (*e.g.*, lidocaine, diphenhydramine, or metoprolol) are so efficiently metabolized that their hepatic clearance approaches the rates at which they traverse the liver (*i.e.*, total hepatic blood flow; Fig. 39-7). In other words, hepatic blood flow determines the liver's ability to eliminate high-clearance drugs. Low-clearance drugs (*e.g.*, diazepam or antipyrine), however, are metabolized at rates that are usually far below their flow rates through the liver (Fig. 39-7); therefore, their hepatic clearances are relatively independent of liver blood flow. Factors that increase the free

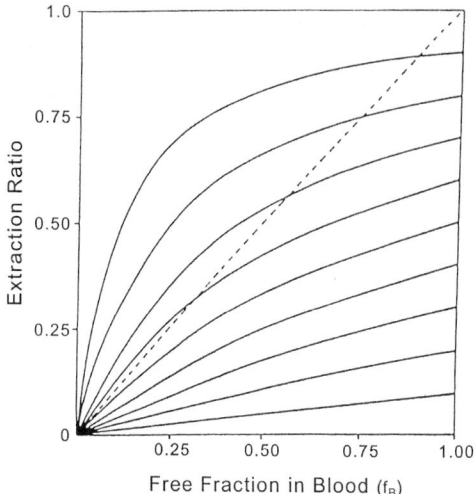

Figure 39-8. Relationship between hepatic extraction and fraction of unbound drug in blood: increasing free fraction (more unbound drug) usually produces increased extraction. This phenomenon is of greater importance for low-extraction drugs (with almost a direct linear change in extraction ratio with increasing free fraction) than for high-extraction drugs because the latter are almost completely cleared, regardless of extent of binding (nonrestrictive binding). The hepatic clearance (CL) reflects the changes in extraction ratio (E) if blood flow (Q) is constant (CL = Q · E). (Reprinted with permission from Wilkinson GR, Shand DG: A physiological approach to hepatic drug clearance. Clin Pharmacol Ther 18:377, 1975.)

fraction of drugs are much more consequential for low- than for high-extraction drugs. The clearance of low-extraction drugs increases almost linearly as the free fraction increases (Fig. 39-8). In contrast, a single pass through the liver metabolizes almost all of a high-clearance drug, irrespective of its extent of binding to plasma proteins (nonrestrictive binding).

Significant liver disease decreases the clearances and prolongs the terminal half-lives of most drugs eliminated by the liver. Nonetheless, the complex and poorly quantifiable effects of hepatic dysfunction on drug disposition may render pharmacokinetic, and even pharmacodynamic, predictions precarious. The rational selection of medications for patients with severe liver dysfunction mandates a careful risk–benefit analysis that integrates both pharmacodynamic and pharmacokinetic concerns. At times, cirrhotic patients with coexisting diseases will be better served by a hepatically cleared medication (superior efficacy, fewer untoward effects) than by one whose clearance is primarily extrahepatic. In such cases, careful titration of medications is imperative to achieve the desired pharmacologic responses with minimal adverse effects.

ASSESSMENT OF HEPATIC FUNCTION
Laboratory Evaluation of Hepatic Function

A broad array of laboratory and clinical tests are available to evaluate the hepatobiliary system (Table 39-1).[9] The majority of the so-called liver function tests (LFT) do not actually measure functions of the liver. Rather, they serve to detect hepatobiliary injury or suggest a general category of disease, such as hepatitis, biliary obstruction, or steatosis.

Increased serum activities of aspartate aminotransferase (AST, formerly SGOT [serum glutamic oxaloacetic transaminase]) and alanine aminotransferase (ALT, formerly SGPT [serum glutamic pyruvic transaminase]) reflect hepatocellular injury and occur in almost all types of hepatic disease. Small increases (less than 3-fold) are consistent with steatosis or chronic viral hepatitis. Larger increases (3 to 22-fold) suggest

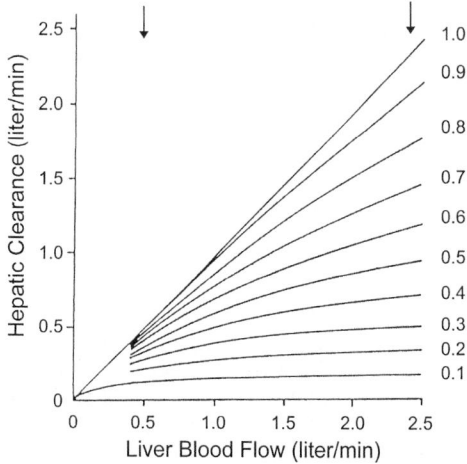

Figure 39-7. Relationship between hepatic clearance (*ordinate, on left*) and liver blood flow (*abscissa*) as determined by the extraction ratios (ER) of the drug (*ordinate, on right*). Hepatic clearances of compounds with low extraction ratios are nearly independent of liver blood flow whereas the clearances of compounds with high extraction ratios vary almost directly with changes in hepatic blood flow. The *arrows* indicate the normal physiologic range of liver blood flow. (Reprinted with permission from Wilkinson GR, Shand DG: A physiological approach to hepatic drug clearance. Clin Pharmacol Ther 18:377, 1975.)

Table 39-1. BLOOD TESTS AND THE DIFFERENTIAL DIAGNOSIS OF HEPATIC DYSFUNCTION

	Bilirubin Overload (Hemolysis)	Parenchymal Dysfunction	Cholestasis
Aminotransferases	Normal	Increased (may be normal or decreased in advanced stages)	Normal (may be increased in advanced stages)
Alkaline phosphatase	Normal	Normal	Increased
Bilirubin	Unconjugated	Conjugated	Conjugated
Serum proteins	Normal	Decreased	Normal (may be decreased in advanced stages)
Prothrombin time	Normal	Decreased (may be normal in early stages)	Normal (may be prolonged in advanced stages)
Blood urea nitrogen	Normal	Normal (may be decreased in advanced stages)	Normal
Sulfobromophthalein/indocyanine green	Normal	Retention	Normal or retention

From Gelman S: Anesthesia and the liver. In Barash P, Cullen B, Stoelting, R (eds): Clinical Anesthesia, 3rd ed, p 1011. Philadelphia, Lippincott-Raven, 1997.

acute hepatitis or exacerbations of chronic hepatitis (alcoholic hepatitis). The largest increases (greater than 20-fold) indicate massive hepatocellular necrosis and usually result from toxic reactions to drugs (including anesthetics) or other chemicals, circulatory shock, or severe viral hepatitis.

Changes in ALT or AST, however, do not necessarily reflect the severity or even the presence of hepatocellular injury. For example, decreases of ALT or AST in patients with severe hepatitis may indicate that the liver is either recovering from the disease or being destroyed by it, with few remaining hepatocytes to release these enzymes into the circulation. Moreover, AST or ALT may increase in the absence of liver disease, reflecting injuries to tissues such as heart or skeletal muscle. ALT resides primarily in the liver, and is therefore more specific than AST as a marker of hepatic injury; AST exists in a variety of organs including liver, heart, skeletal muscle, kidney, and brain.

Lactate dehydrogenase (LDH) activity serves as a test for hepatic injury. A marked increase of LDH may indicate hepatocellular necrosis, shock liver, or hemolysis combined with liver disease. However, LDH increases in many nonhepatic diseases and is therefore of little value as a diagnostic test for liver disease.

Glutathione S-transferase (GST) is a sensitive and specific test for detecting drug-induced hepatocellular damage.[10] Because of the rapid release of GST into the circulation following hepatic injury and its short plasma half-life (90 minutes), monitoring of plasma GST concentrations can provide detailed information about the time course of an injury, from onset to resolution. Unlike the aminotransferases, which are highly localized in the periportal region (Zone 1), GST is most abundant in centrilobular (Zone 3) hepatocytes.[11] This distinction is important because the centrilobular region contains the hepatocytes that are most susceptible to injuries from circulatory disturbances and toxic products of drug metabolism. Following such injuries, increases of GST may be disproportionately greater than increases of serum aminotransferases.

Alkaline phosphatase (AP) is a highly sensitive test for assessing the integrity of the biliary system. However, AP is not specific for hepatobiliary disease; alkaline phosphatase isozymes are present in bone, placenta, kidney, leukocytes, intestine, and liver. Routine laboratory testing reveals transient, mild increases of AP in up to one-third of patients in the absence of hepatobiliary disease. During pregnancy, AP can nearly double just from placental release of the enzyme. Nonetheless, the greatest increases in AP result from cholestatic disorders. In patients with fulminant hepatic failure, a low AP-to-serum bilirubin ratio portends a poor prognosis.

5'-Nucleotidase (5'NT) activity in blood is a highly specific test for hepatobiliary injury. (It has largely replaced GGT [serum glutamyl transpeptidase], which is a more sensitive indicator of biliary tract disease but relatively nonspecific.) Although 5'NT is present in numerous tissues (liver, brain, intestine, heart, blood vessels, and endocrine pancreas), only hepatobiliary tissue releases 5'NT into the circulation; the release may require the detergent action of bile salts on plasma membranes. 5'NT is an excellent test for assessing the hepatic origin of an increased AP because it closely correlates with AP in those patients with liver disease.

Measurement of serum bilirubin—unconjugated (indirect), conjugated (direct reacting), and total—is central to the evaluation of hepatobiliary disorders. Hyperbilirubinemia has a wide range of causes (Table 39-2). Serum concentrations of unconjugated bilirubin that are between 1 and 4 $mg \cdot dl^{-1}$ generally indicate a disorder of bilirubin metabolism, such as excessive production, impaired transport into hepatocytes, or defective

Table 39-2. CAUSES OF HYPERBILIRUBINEMIA

UNCONJUGATED (INDIRECT)

Excessive bilirubin production (hemolysis)
Immaturity of enzyme systems
   Physiologic jaundice of newborn
   Jaundice of prematurity
Inherited defects
   Gilbert's syndrome
   Crigler-Najjar syndrome
Drug effects

CONJUGATED (DIRECT)

Hepatocellular disease (hepatitis, cirrhosis, drugs)
Intrahepatic cholestasis (drugs, pregnancy)
Benign postoperative jaundice, sepsis
Congenital conjugated hyperbilirubinemia
   Dubin-Johnson syndrome
   Rotor's syndrome
Obstructive jaundice
   Extrahepatic (calculus, stricture, neoplasm)
   Intrahepatic (sclerosing cholangitis, neoplasm, primary biliary cirrhosis)

From Friedman L, Martin P, Munoz S: Liver function tests and the objective evaluation of the patient with liver disease. In Zakim D, Boyer T (eds). Hepatology: A Textbook of Liver Disease, 3rd ed, p 791. Philadelphia, WB Saunders, 1996, with permission.

conjugation by hepatocytes. The concentration of unconjugated bilirubin will rarely exceed 5 mg · dl^{-1} when hepatic function is normal, even if severe hemolysis occurs. Conjugated hyperbilirubinemia indicates the presence of intra- or extrahepatic cholestatic disease. If the biliary tract is completely obstructed, conjugated bilirubin levels may reach 35 mg · dl^{-1}; they rarely go higher because the kidney excretes conjugated bilirubin. A total bilirubin level that exceeds 35 mg · dl^{-1} suggests biliary obstruction combined with renal failure, or severe hepatocellular disease plus hemolysis.

Assays of coagulation function or serum albumin concentration are the most widely used methods for evaluating hepatic synthetic function. Proper interpretation of these tests requires an understanding of a patient's clinical status. For example, decreasing plasma albumin concentrations indicate a worsening of hepatic function in patients who have chronic liver disease but no other cause of hypoalbuminemia (poor nutritional status, hormonal imbalance, nephropathy, and derangements of osmotic pressure). Plasma albumin, however, is an insensitive and unreliable marker for acute hepatic dysfunction because of its long plasma half-life (nearly 20 days). In contrast to measurements of plasma albumin, coagulation tests (*e.g.,* prothrombin time [PT] or international normalized ratio [INR]; thromboelastography) are sensitive indicators of severe hepatic dysfunction whether patients have acute or chronic liver disease. Such tests, however, may not detect mild-to-moderate hepatic disease because the liver's capacity to synthesize clotting factors far exceeds the concentrations needed to maintain normal coagulation. Thus, a progressively increasing PT is usually ominous in liver-diseased patients, signaling the development of end-stage hepatic failure. Of course, a prolonged PT can be totally unrelated to liver disease, resulting instead from congenital deficiencies of coagulation factors or acquired conditions, such as consumptive coagulopathy, vitamin K deficiency, or ingestion of drugs that antagonize the prothrombin complex (coumarin).

Tests that measure hepatic blood flow and metabolic capacity can detect acute changes in hepatic circulation and function. The indocyanine green (ICG) method has been a standard technique for comparing effects of various anesthetics on hepatic blood flow. ICG is a nontoxic dye that binds avidly to plasma proteins. It is highly extracted by the liver following an intravenous injection; its extraction ratio (70–90%) exceeds that of bromsulfophthalein (BSP) (50–80%). Although the liver excretes ICG into the bile without metabolizing it, some extrahepatic clearance occurs, which limits the accuracy of the ICG method. Modifying the method by measuring ICG concentrations in hepatic veins circumvents this limitation; however, this modification also increases the invasiveness of the ICG method. Flow-dependent tests of hepatic metabolic function may offer some advantages over ICG for detecting rapid or abrupt changes in hepatic function. One test involves injecting lidocaine intravenously and monitoring its rate of conversion to monoethylglycinexylidide (MEGX). This test, which can help identify patients whose hepatic blood flow is inadequate to meet the liver's metabolic demands, may be more sensitive than ICG as an indicator of poor prognosis in critically ill patients.[12] Additional metabolic tests for assessing hepatic function include antipyrine clearance from plasma (C14 aminopyrine breath test), caffeine clearance, galactose elimination, and the maximum rate of urea synthesis. As a general rule, such tests employ highly extracted drugs (*e.g.,* lidocaine) to track changes in hepatic blood flow, and agents with low intrinsic clearance to assess the metabolic capacity of the liver, as their hepatic elimination depends mainly on the functional mass of the liver.

Several other laboratory tests are crucial for accurate diagnosis of liver disease but provide no specific information about hepatic function. Included in this category are serologic profiles for viral hepatitis and measurements of plasma immunoglobulins, which may reveal autoantibodies or antibodies to anesthetic-induced neoantigens (discussed later).

Liver Biopsy

Liver biopsy continues to play a central role in the evaluation of patients with suspected liver disease because it provides the only means of determining the precise nature of hepatic injury (necrosis, inflammation, steatosis or fibrosis). Postoperatively, liver biopsy can be invaluable. It often helps resolve diagnostic dilemmas by revealing the type and extent of various chronic hepatic disorders, the identity and location of intrahepatic viral antigens, and patterns of acute hepatic injury characteristic of hepatotoxic drugs. Liver biopsy is also useful for evaluating the efficacy of therapy for liver disease. The presence of coagulopathy (*e.g.,* PT that is 3 seconds greater than control, platelet count <60,000 mm^{-3}), however, contraindicates liver biopsy.

HEPATITIS CAUSED BY HALOGENATED VAPORS

The recognition that halothane can cause significant hepatotoxicity prompted a dramatic decrease in its use in adult patients in the United States. This paved the way for the newer agents: enflurane (1972), isoflurane (1981), desflurane (1993), and sevoflurane (1995). Several hundred cases of halothane hepatitis have been reported since the introduction of halothane into clinical practice in the 1950s.[13] This is many times more than the total number of cases attributed to all the other inhaled agents combined (Table 39-3). Thus far, enflurane has reportedly caused severe hepatic injury in approximately 50 cases,[13-15] and isoflurane may have been responsible for another 6 cases.[13,16] Three cases of hepatitis have been linked to sevoflurane use,[17-19] and only a single report implicates desflurane as a possible cause of hepatitis.[20]

Clinical Evidence That Halogenated Vapors Cause Hepatitis

Halothane

Several years elapsed between the clinical debut of halothane and the appearance of reports linking halothane anesthesia to severe liver damage. To determine the incidence of massive hepatic necrosis after halothane anesthesia, the Committee on Anesthesia of the National Academy of Sciences launched one of the largest epidemiologic studies ever completed: the National Halothane Study.[21] This retrospective review of 856,600 anesthetics performed over a 4-year period (from 1959 through 1962) reported an incidence of fulminant hepatic necrosis of about 1 per 35,000 anesthetics. It is important to recall that the National Halothane Study was not designed to determine the incidence of halothane hepatitis; it included only cases in which massive hepatic necrosis terminated in death and did not investigate lesser degrees of hepatic injury.[22] Based on more recent studies, the incidence of halothane hepatitis is probably somewhere between 1 in 3000 and 1 in 30,000.[23-26]

Halothane hepatitis characteristically develops after minor, uneventful procedures of brief duration (<30 minutes), and does not become clinically apparent for several days after the anesthetic. The classic presentation includes fever, anorexia, nausea, chills, myalgias, and a rash, followed by the appearance of jaundice 3–6 days later. Overt jaundice indicates severe disease and portends a mortality rate that may be as high as 40%. Other indicators of poor prognosis include a short latency between the anesthetic and onset of symptoms, certain demographic factors (age >40 years, obesity), and severe hepatic dysfunction (PT >20 seconds, bilirubin concentration >10 mg · dl^{-1}).[27]

The single most important risk factor for halothane hepatitis is prior exposure to halothane. Of the patients who develop jaundice after halothane, 71–95% have had at least one prior exposure to this agent.[22,25,28-32] Severe reactions occur

Table 39-3. RELATIONSHIP BETWEEN METABOLISM OF VOLATILE HALOGENATED AGENTS AND ANESTHETIC-INDUCED HEPATITIS

Agent	Year Introduced in United States	No. of Cases of Hepatitis	Percentage of Anesthetic Metabolized	Fluoroacetyl Metabolites
Halothane	1958	>500	20–46	Yes
Enflurane	1972	~50	2.5–8.5	Yes
Isoflurane	1981	6	0.2–2	Yes
Desflurane	1993	1	0.02	Yes
Sevoflurane	1995	3	2–5	No

From Mushlin PS, Gelman S: Liver dysfunction after anesthesia. In Benumof JL, Saidman LJ (eds): Anesthesia and Perioperative Complications, 2nd ed, p 440. St. Louis, Mosby, 1999, with permission.

nearly 10 times more often in patients who have had multiple halothane anesthetics than in those having their first-ever halothane anesthetic.[33] The shorter the interval between the two most recent exposures, the more rapid is the onset of jaundice and the more serious the disease.

Demographic factors also provide important information about the risk of halothane hepatitis. Obese women appear to be more likely than their nonobese counterparts to contract halothane hepatitis. The disease may have a genetic basis.[34] Some ethnic groups (Mexican-American) seem to be at greater risk,[35] and chromosomal differences have been noted between patients who recovered from halothane hepatitis and halothane-treated patients who never had the disease.[36] For reasons that are not yet clear, age is also a significant risk factor. Approximately 50% of the cases of halothane-associated fulminant hepatic failure occur in patients older than 50,[33] whereas children are highly resistant to the development of halothane hepatitis.[37–39] The rare cases documented in children have involved multiple exposures to halothane.[37] Notably, neither pre-existing liver disease nor concomitant administration of medication has been identified as a risk factor for halothane hepatitis.

Enflurane

About a decade after the clinical introduction of enflurane, Lewis et al[14] published a case-control study involving 24 cases of suspected enflurane hepatitis. The clinical, biochemical, and histopathologic profiles were similar to those seen in halothane hepatitis. Fever was the most common presenting feature (79%). Jaundice eventually occurred in 79% of the patients, with a latency of 8 days. A shorter latent period occurred in patients who had had prior anesthetics with either enflurane or halothane. Liver biopsy characteristically showed centrilobular necrosis, and 20% of the patients died from fulminant hepatic failure.

Eger et al[15] re-evaluated these data by creating a syndrome score for each patient, based on a composite of variables, including fever, chills, nausea, rash, eosinophilia, death, and hepatic histopathology. These investigators found no differences between the syndrome scores of patients identified in the prior study as having "probable postanesthetic enflurane hepatitis" and patients whose postoperative hepatitis was attributable to other causes (such as sepsis or shock). Consequently, they argued that there is still no proof that enflurane causes hepatitis. This conclusion notwithstanding, the many unexplained cases of massive or submassive necrosis that have followed enflurane anesthesia[40–42] provide presumptive evidence that the disorder exists. The risk factors for "enflurane hepatitis" appear to be the same as those for halothane hepatitis. According to Eger, even if all unexplained cases of hepatitis that have followed enflurane anesthetics were considered to be enflurane-induced, the incidence of enflurane hepatitis would be just 0.36 cases per million, about 1/200 that associated with halothane.

Isoflurane

It is plausible that isoflurane, on very rare occasions, can produce significant liver injury. Numerous reports describe severe, unexplained hepatic dysfunction following isoflurane anesthesia.[16,43–47] In many of the cases, the patients had had prior exposure to halogenated agents (e.g., halothane,[47] enflurane,[43] or isoflurane[48]). The Food and Drug Administration (FDA), having received notification of 47 cases of suspected isoflurane-induced hepatic injuries that occurred between 1981 and 1984, convened a committee to investigate the cases. In most instances, the committee identified likely causes other than isoflurane, such as sepsis, hypoxia, biliary obstruction, nutritional deficiency, circulatory shock, viral hepatitis (including herpes virus), and antibiotic therapy (erythromycin estolate). Nonetheless, the issue remains controversial. A brief review published in the *American Journal of Gastroenterology* in 1996 states that there is "direct evidence that isoflurane can induce liver injury and should therefore be considered as a potential cause of serum transaminase elevations in any patient who is exposed to this anesthetic."[46] This conclusion contrasts with that of the FDA committee, which found no compelling evidence of a causal relationship between isoflurane anesthesia and severe hepatic dysfunction.[44]

Sevoflurane

Although sevoflurane was first synthesized in the late 1960s, its commercial development was delayed because of concerns about the potential toxicity of its metabolites and breakdown products. Such concerns were mitigated by the apparent safety of sevoflurane in clinical trials, conducted initially in Japan and later throughout the world.[49] Sevoflurane was approved for clinical use in Japan in 1990. During the next few years, three case reports of sevoflurane-induced hepatitis appeared in the *Japanese Journal of Anesthesiology*[17–19]; two of those cases involved infants. By 1995, when sevoflurane became clinically available in the United States, more than 2 million Japanese patients had already received the anesthetic. Despite its extensive use in the American population and elsewhere in the world, there have been no additional reports of sevoflurane hepatitis.

Desflurane

To date, the literature provides only a single account of desflurane-induced hepatitis.[20] The case involved a healthy 65-year-old woman who developed pruritus, malaise, nausea, and polyarthralgia 12 days after a minor operation under desflurane anesthesia. Four days later she had a macular rash, dermal jaundice, epigastric pain, and laboratory evidence of significant hepatic dysfunction (serum ALT was 1886 IU, total bilirubin was 27 mg · dl^{-1}, and PT was 27 seconds, with negative serologies). She re-entered the hospital as a potential candidate for orthotopic liver transplantation (OLT); however, her condition gradually improved on conservative therapy. A blood sample collected on postoperative day 48 contained antibodies that reacted with trifluoroacylated (TF-acylated) liver microsomal proteins, providing circumstantial evidence for an immunologically mediated hepatitis.

Mechanisms of Anesthesia-Induced Hepatitis

Relationship Between Oxidative Metabolism and Immune Injury

The oxidative metabolism of the halogenated vapors relates to their potential to cause severe liver damage. Of the halothane taken up during anesthesia, 20–46% is metabolized,[50,51] compared to 2.5–8.5% for enflurane,[51,52] 2–5% for sevoflurane,[53,54] 0.2–2% for isoflurane,[51,55] and 0.02% for desflurane[56] (Table 39-3). Each of these anesthetics, with the exception of sevoflurane, is oxidized via cytochrome P-450 2El to yield highly reactive intermediates that bind covalently (acylation) to a variety of hepatocellular macromolecules (Fig. 39-9). Halothane anesthesia induces both neoantigens (arising via reaction of TF-acetyl chloride and hepatic proteins) and autoantigens (lacking TF-acetyl adducts).[57–61] Presumably, the TF-acetyl moiety acts as a hapten and enhances the immune recognition of the carrier protein. In susceptible people, these altered hepatic proteins may trigger an immunologic response that causes massive hepatic necrosis.[13]

Halothane hepatitis has many features of an immunologic disease. It is idiosyncratic, affecting only a tiny fraction of those anesthetized with halothane. Neither the incidence nor the severity of the hepatitis correlates with the halothane dose administered. The disease has a latency of days, unlike the hepatic injury produced by severe hypoxia or a potent cytotoxin, which typically appears within hours of the hepatic insult. Moreover, the disease is usually accompanied by clinical laboratory findings that are characteristic of an immunologically mediated disorder. Such findings include peripheral eosinophilia,[62] circulating immune complexes, organ nonspecific autoantibodies,[63] and antibodies that will bind to antigens isolated from halothane-treated animals (rabbits). Approximately 70% of the patients have antibodies that recognize neoantigens (TF-acetyl–modified epitopes), and 90% have antibodies that recognize autoantigens (non-TF-acetyl–modified epitopes). Therefore, preoperative testing for halothane antibodies might identify patients at risk for developing halothane hepatitis, whereas postoperative testing could help to determine if halothane anesthesia was the likely cause of unexplained postoperative hepatitis. Currently, however, no tests exist that are totally sensitive or specific for detecting the disease. The ELISA method of antibody detection has been reported to be approximately 75% sensitive and 88% specific.[59]

Metabolites of Halogenated Vapors Other Than Halothane

Enflurane metabolism produces acyl adducts (difluoromethoxydifluoroacetyl halide) that are similar, but not identical, to those derived from halothane (TF-acetyl halide). Nonetheless, antibodies isolated from patients with halothane hepatitis can bind to hepatic proteins that contain enflurane-induced adducts (neoantigens).[64]

Isoflurane metabolism also yields highly reactive intermediates (TF-acetyl chloride; acyl ester) that bind covalently to hepatic proteins (Fig. 39-9). The likelihood that isoflurane causes hepatitis via production of these intermediates appears to be extremely low, however, because just 0.2% of the isoflurane taken up into the body is actually metabolized. Only trace amounts of isoflurane-derived adducts are bound to hepatic proteins following isoflurane anesthesia.

Desflurane, which is similarly biotransformed to trifluoroacyl metabolites, appears even less likely than isoflurane to cause immune injury because only 0.02–0.2% of a desflurane dose is

metabolized (1/1000 that of halothane). Desflurane metabolites are usually undetectable in plasma, except after prolonged anesthetics with this agent. Furthermore, while antibodies from patients with halothane hepatitis clearly react with proteins isolated from halothane- or enflurane-treated rats, they do not appear to react with hepatic proteins from desflurane- or isoflurane-treated rats.[13]

Sevoflurane is metabolized more extensively than isoflurane or desflurane, slightly less than enflurane, and much less than halothane (see Table 39-3).[54,65] The metabolism of sevoflurane (primarily via cytochrome P-450 2E1)[53] is rapid (1.5–2 times faster than enflurane), and produces detectable plasma concentrations of fluoride and hexafluoroisopropanol (HFIP) within minutes of initiating the anesthetic. The liver conjugates most of the HFIP with glucuronic acid, and the kidney excretes the HFIP-glucuronide (Fig. 39-10). An important distinction between sevoflurane and the aforementioned vapors is that sevoflurane produces neither highly reactive metabolites nor fluoroacetylated liver proteins.[54] At present, there is no evidence that any sevoflurane metabolites cause severe hepatic injury.[66]

Immune Crossover

The concept of immune crossover might explain cases of hepatitis that have been associated with anesthetics other than halothane. According to the immune theory, exposure to an anesthetic that generates fluoroacyl-derived antigens (neoantigens or autoantigens) can predispose to hepatitis from subsequent anesthetics that stimulate the formation of the same or similar antigens. Indeed, many patients who develop unexplained hepatitis after anesthetics with halothane,[67] isoflurane,[43] or sevoflurane,[18] had prior enflurane anesthetics. Similarly, cases of unexplained hepatitis after isoflurane anesthesia have also occurred in patients with prior exposure to halogenated agents (e.g. halothane,[47] enflurane,[43] or isoflurane[48]). Furthermore, the only patient ever reported to have desflurane hepatitis[20] had had two prior halothane anesthetics more than a decade before she received desflurane. About 7 weeks after the desflurane anesthetic, her blood contained antibodies that reacted with TF-acylated liver microsomal proteins. Did her earlier exposures to halothane sensitize her to desflurane hepatitis? Or could this actually have been a case of halothane hepatitis, triggered by the release of trace amounts of halothane from an anesthesia machine that contained residual halothane from prior anesthetics? Whether desflurane by itself actually causes hepatitis is unclear. Moreover, it is still unclear whether the above-mentioned associations are merely coincidental or represent true immune crossover between the various halogenated agents.

Conclusions

At present, the preponderance of evidence supports the TF-acetyl–hapten (immune) theory of anesthesia-induced hepatitis. Nonetheless, it is conceivable that the antigen–antibody responses that accompany anesthesia-induced hepatitis are the result of the hepatic injury, rather than its cause. Proponents of the hapten theory must reconcile the facts that most (if not all) patients anesthetized with halothane form the same or a similar set of TF-acetylated liver proteins but few develop halothane hepatitis. Explanations for this disparity include the following possibilities: only a few of the TF-acetyl proteins are actually immunogenic; the triggering of an immune response requires a critical threshold of TF-acetylated proteins (antigenic threshold theory); and, only a tiny fraction of patients are genetically susceptible to the immunogenicity of these antigens.

HALOGENATED VAPORS CAUSE HEPATIC INJURIES OTHER THAN HEPATITIS

Mild hepatic injuries often occur after anesthetics with halogenated vapors. These injuries are typically asymptomatic and manifested only by minor abnormalities of LFTs.[10,33,68] The inci-

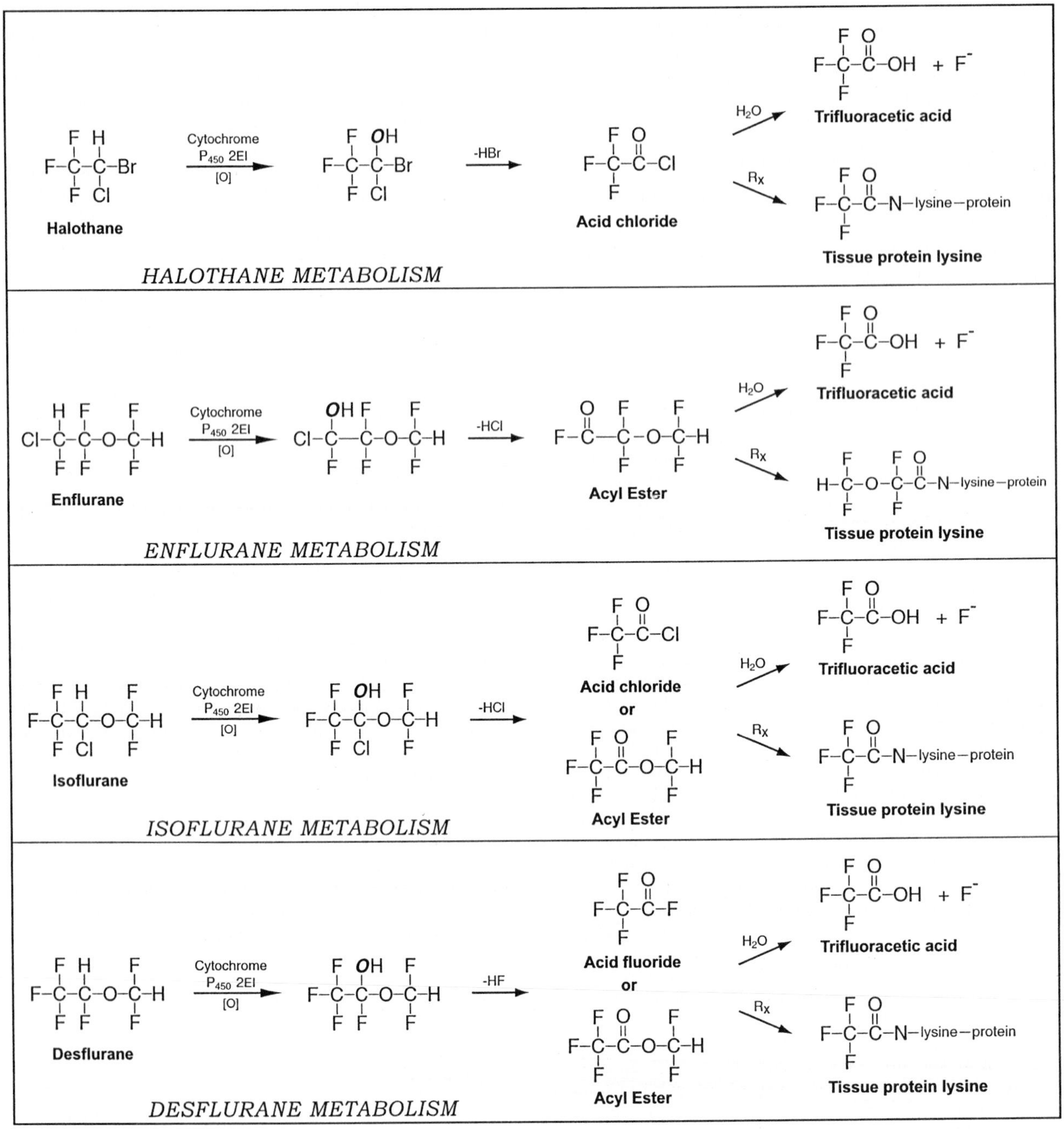

Figure 39-9. Proposed pathways of cytochrome P-450 2E1–catalyzed metabolism of halothane, enflurane, isoflurane, and desflurane that are involved in the production of highly reactive intermediates that acylate hepatic proteins. The acylated moieties of the liver proteins appear to function as haptens to elicit an immune response. Because there is no evidence that the metabolism of sevoflurane produces an acylating intermediate, sevoflurane metabolism is not included in this figure (see Fig. 39-10). (Reprinted with permission from Mushlin PS, Gelman S: Liver dysfunction after anesthesia. In Benumof JL, Saidman LJ (eds): Anesthesia and Perioperative Complications, 2nd ed, p 442. St Louis, Mosby, 1999; modified from Frink EJ Jr: Anesth Analg 81[suppl 6]:S46, 1995; Kenna JG, Jones RM: Anesth Analg 81[suppl 6]:S51, 1995.)

dence of these abnormalities appears to be related to the extent of an anesthetic's metabolism and the degree to which an anesthetic impairs hepatic perfusion and oxygenation. Whether such injuries predispose to halothane hepatitis is unclear.

Following halothane anesthetics, 20–50% of adult patients exhibit evidence of mild hepatic injury.[10,33,68–71] Serum aminotransferases (ALT or AST) increase in about 25% of halothane-treated patients,[33] and may remain elevated for nearly 2 weeks after the anesthetic.[69–72] GST, which is generally regarded as a more sensitive test than aminotransferases for detecting centrilobular injury,[10,68,73] increases in almost 50% of adults who re-

ceive halothane and in approximately 20% of those who have enflurane anesthetics for minor operative procedures. Isoflurane anesthesia is less likely than either agent to produce enzyme elevations.[10]

Halothane anesthesia can also produce hepatic enzyme elevations in children. A prospective study of 25 children who received at least 10 halothane anesthetics in a single year revealed minor increases of enzymes in 5–11% of the children.[74] Similar elevations occurred in 3% of children who had had repeated halothane anesthetics at intervals of less than 28 days. Such findings indicate that children are much less susceptible than

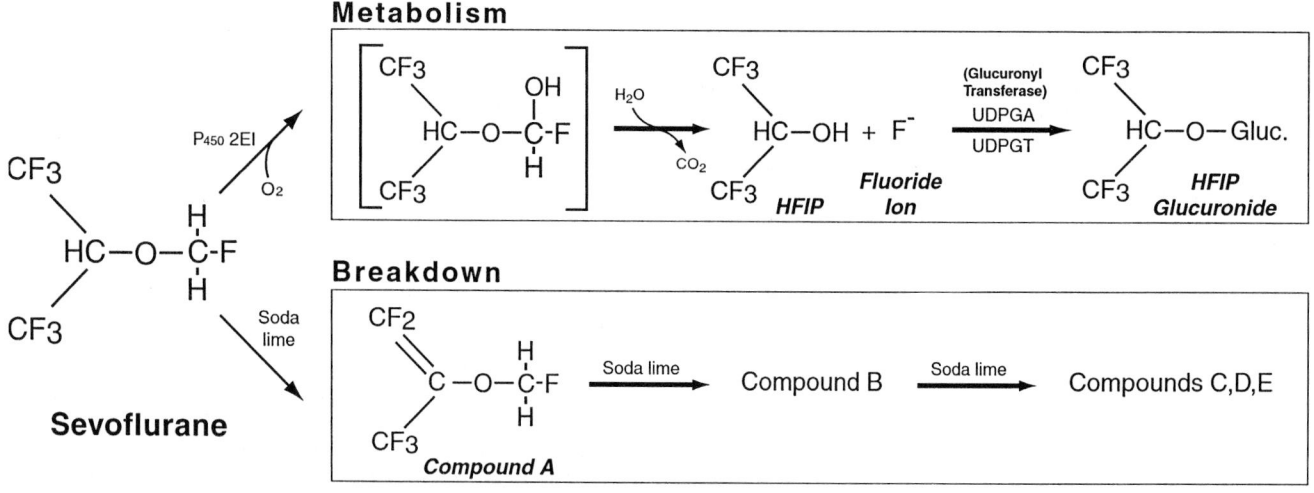

Figure 39-10. Cytochrome P-450 2E1-catalyzed biotransformation of sevoflurane produces inorganic fluoride and hexafluoroisopropanol (HFIP). The liver rapidly metabolizes HFIP to HFIP-glucuronide. Sevoflurane also undergoes breakdown in soda lime, yielding compound A, which is nephrotoxic but does not appear to be hepatotoxic. (Reprinted with permission from Mushlin PS, Gelman S: Liver dysfunction after anesthesia. In Benumof JL, Saidman LJ (eds): Anesthesia and Perioperative Complications, 2nd ed, p 442. St Louis, Mosby, 1999; modified from Frink EJ Jr: The hepatic effects of sevoflurane. Anesth Analg 81[suppl 6]:S46, 1995.)

adults to both subclinical hepatic injury and hepatitis from halothane anesthesia.

Effects of Halogenated Vapors on Hepatic Blood Flow and Oxygen Delivery

Hepatic injury occurs whenever the liver's supply of oxygen is insufficient to meet its metabolic needs. The severity of the injury relates directly to the degree of ischemia or hypoxia, regardless of the cause, be it hemorrhage, halothane, or isoflurane.[75] Conditions that decrease hepatic oxygen consumption, including hypothermia or inhibition of metabolism pathways (e.g., by cimetidine), can protect the liver from hypoxic injury.[76]

Halothane anesthesia significantly decreases hepatic blood flow and oxygen delivery in a variety of animal models, as well as in patients undergoing elective operations.[77] Studies in rats indicate that halothane anesthesia does not predictably cause dose-related hepatic injuries without employing special conditions, including those that stimulate the reductive metabolism of halothane (e.g., hypoxemic gas mixtures or phenobarbital pretreatment). However, such conditions also cause hepatic hypoxia, which creates confusion about the mechanism of the injury. Does it result primarily from the reductive metabolites of halothane or from halothane-induced decreases of oxygen delivery to a marginally hypoxic liver? Or does the injury stem from a combination of enhanced reductive metabolism and anesthesia-related decreases in hepatic oxygenation?

At least superficially, guinea pigs seem less complex than rats when it comes to studying halothane hepatotoxicity; halothane anesthesia by itself is sufficient to damage the guinea pig liver. This exquisite sensitivity to halothane presumably results from the unusually low hepatic arterial flow in guinea pigs (2–3% of the liver's total blood flow, versus 20–35% in other species). This low arterial flow renders guinea pigs unusually susceptible to hepatic injury from a variety of insults, including surgical stress and hemorrhage, as well as from anesthetic agents that are characteristically nontoxic (isoflurane, nitrous oxide). Both animal and human studies indicate that halothane is more likely than the other inhaled anesthetics to produce liver injury, probably because it causes the most cardiovascular and respiratory depression and the greatest reduction in hepatic arterial flow (see Fig. 39-11). Consequently, halothane is the most likely of the clinically used vapors to produce, or exacerbate, hepatic hypoxia when blood flow to the liver is critically limited and

the adequacy of the oxygen supply-to-demand balance is in question.

Excluding halothane, enflurane decreases hepatic blood flow and splanchnic perfusion more than any other halogenated vapor in clinical use. It induces dose-dependent decreases in portal venous blood flow[78,79] and either reduces[78] or does not change hepatic artery blood flow[79] (Fig. 39-11). Splanchnic perfusion decreases in parallel with decreases in mean arterial pressure (MAP) and cardiac output in patients anesthetized with enflurane.[80] Enflurane also increases splanchnic oxygen extraction and lowers both hepatic venous and mixed venous oxygen saturation.[80]

Desflurane anesthesia decreases hepatic blood flow in both experimental and clinical settings. Administration of 1 MAC desflurane to patients prior to skin incision reportedly decreases hepatic blood flow by 30% (measured by ICG), similar to the decreases associated with 1 MAC of halothane or iso-

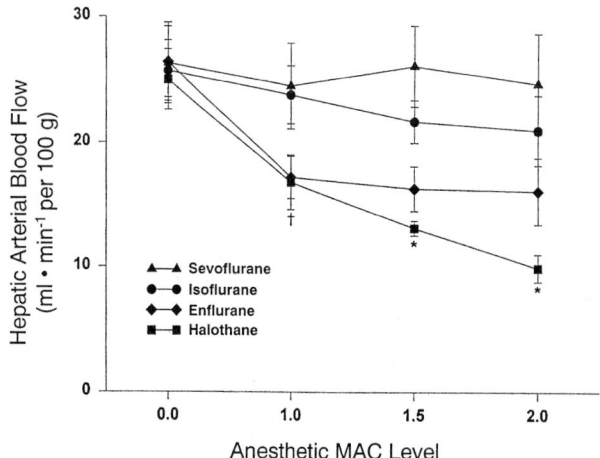

Figure 39-11. Dose-dependent effects of inhaled anesthetics on hepatic arterial flow in chronically instrumented dogs in the absence of a surgical stress. Sevoflurane and isoflurane preserve hepatic arterial flow even at the higher minimum alveolar anesthetic concentration (MAC) levels. *Differs from sevoflurane and isoflurane at same MAC values ($p < 0.05$). †Differs from sevoflurane at same MAC value ($p < 0.05$). (Reprinted with permission from Frink EJ Jr: The hepatic effects of sevoflurane. Anesth Analg 8[suppl 6]:S46, 1995.)

flurane.[81] Studies in domestic pigs indicate that desflurane anesthesia produces dose-dependent reductions of mean arterial blood pressure, cardiac output, and hepatic blood flow. At 0.5 MAC, it decreases blood flow through the portal vein and superior mesenteric artery, and at 1 MAC, it also decreases hepatic arterial flow.[82] Desflurane can markedly reduce oxygen delivery to the liver and small intestine without producing comparable reductions of hepatic oxygen uptake or hepatic and mesenteric metabolism. Therefore, desflurane anesthesia could decrease the oxygen reserve capacity of both the liver and small intestine.

Isoflurane is much less likely than halothane or enflurane to cause, or contribute to, hepatic injury. It undergoes minimal biodegradation,[51,55] and preserves hepatic blood flow[77] and oxygen delivery even during laparotomy.[83] It actually protects the liver from carbon tetrachloride (CCl$_4$) toxicity, probably by inhibiting the cytochrome P-450 isozyme that metabolizes CCl$_4$ and possibly by dismutating halo-peroxyl radicals.[84,85]

Sevoflurane anesthesia usually preserves blood flow and oxygen delivery to the liver, even in the presence of positive-pressure ventilation.[86] Patients having elective operations under sevoflurane anesthesia (1 or 2 MAC) experience significant reductions in mean arterial blood pressure, but maintain their hepatic blood flow (ICG clearance) at awake, preanesthetic levels. Experiments in chronically instrumented dogs indicate that sevoflurane produces dose-dependent increases of hepatic arterial flow that compensate for the dose-related decreases of portal venous flow.[87] At 2 MAC, sevoflurane produces a 33% decrease in portal flow and a 33% increase in hepatic arterial flow (mean arterial pressure and cardiac output decrease by 37% and 21%, respectively). By comparison, hepatic arterial flow decreases slightly with 2 MAC isoflurane,[87] moderately (approximately 30%) with 1 MAC of halothane or enflurane, and markedly with 1.5 MAC halothane. At 2 MAC, sevoflurane reduces portal flow more than isoflurane, but less than enflurane, and much less than halothane.[78] At 1.5 MAC, however, sevoflurane and isoflurane produce similar reductions of portal vein flow. Thus, sevoflurane appears to be the most effective of the inhaled anesthetics for maintaining both blood flow and oxygen delivery to the liver (Fig. 39-11).

Under a condition of marginal hepatic oxygen supply (hepatic artery ligation) in beagles, both sevoflurane and halothane decrease portal venous flow (electromagnetic flow meter) and hepatic oxygen supply more than isoflurane does. Hepatic oxygen uptake is reportedly higher with sevoflurane than halothane (3.7 vs. 2.7 ml · min^{-1} · 100 g^{-1} of liver), perhaps because halothane decreases hepatic metabolism and oxygen requirements more than sevoflurane does. Thus, the hepatic oxygen supply/uptake ratio may be lower with sevoflurane than with halothane anesthesia. Despite this, sevoflurane appears to better preserve hepatic function than halothane anesthesia (ICG clearance; 40 vs. 31 ml · min^{-1}),[88] even in the presence of hypoxia. The reason for this is unclear.

After minor operative procedures, sevoflurane anesthesia may produce slight elevations in blood concentrations of hepatic enzymes, which are comparable to those associated with isoflurane.[89] Sevoflurane anesthesia does not appear to cause significant postoperative hepatic dysfunction in patients undergoing major intra-abdominal operations.[90,91]

In animal studies (beagles), sevoflurane (1.8 MAC) produces minor, transient elevations of hepatic enzymes, similar to those that result from enflurane or halothane.[92] Multiple, prolonged sevoflurane anesthetics (up to 2 MAC, for 3 hours per day, 3 days per week) are well tolerated. Although aminotransferases and LDH increase within the first few weeks of sevoflurane administration, they subsequently return to normal. In an 8-week study in monkeys, sevoflurane anesthesia did not produce any gross pathologic, histopathologic, or ultrastructural abnormalities of the liver.[93]

Several breakdown products of sevoflurane, including compound A [CF$_2$=C(CF$_3$)OCH$_2$F and fluoromethyl-2,2-difluoro- L-(trifluoromethyl) vinyl ether], result from the extraction of hydrogen fluoride by CO$_2$ absorbents at low fresh gas flows (see Fig. 39-10). Compound A clearly causes renal injury in animals and could possibly be nephrotoxic in humans.[77] However, no significant hepatic abnormalities occurred during a 2-week study in dogs and rats, despite repeated administrations of sevoflurane (closed-circle, soda lime absorbent).[94] There are no laboratory or clinical reports indicating that compound A itself causes hepatotoxicity.

Conclusions About Halogenated Vapors and Liver Injury

Guidelines for the clinical use of halothane should take into consideration the following issues and concerns.[95] (1) In children, halothane hepatitis is extremely uncommon, even after repeated exposures to halothane. (2) In adults, the disease rarely occurs after a single exposure to halothane; repeated anesthetics, however, especially in obese, middle-aged women, over a brief period (<6 weeks) substantially increase the risk of the disease. (3) No totally reliable test exists for detecting halothane hepatitis or susceptibility to the disease. (4) Halothane can markedly decrease hepatic blood flow and oxygen supply and often causes mild, transient liver injury. (5) Halothane anesthetics have medicolegal implications, which may plague anesthesiologists whenever unexplained hepatic dysfunction develops in the postoperative period.

Why use halothane at all? The main advantage of halothane over other agents appears to be its low cost. However, when potential medicolegal costs are factored into the equation, the cost–benefit analysis might actually favor the elimination of halothane from anesthesia practice.[27]

Sevoflurane is less likely than either halothane or enflurane to induce liver injury, and no more toxic than either desflurane or isoflurane. Its metabolic products are less reactive, and therefore probably less injurious, than those resulting from halothane, enflurane, isoflurane, or even desflurane.[96] Sevoflurane better preserves hepatic blood flow and oxygen delivery than halothane, enflurane, or desflurane; its effects on hepatic perfusion and metabolic function are similar to those of isoflurane. It seems unlikely that sevoflurane will emerge as a clinically important cause of severe postoperative liver dysfunction.

Other than sevoflurane, desflurane is the least likely of the halogenated vapors to cause severe hepatic injury, based on the immune theory of anesthesia-induced hepatitis. Nonetheless, desflurane produces a greater reduction of hepatic blood flow and oxygen delivery than either isoflurane or sevoflurane. Hence, it may be more likely than the latter agents to cause liver injury in the setting of marginal hepatic oxygenation.

EFFECTS OF ANESTHETICS OTHER THAN HALOGENATED VAPORS ON HEPATIC FUNCTION

Nitrous Oxide

Cohen and co-workers[97] surveyed more than 60,000 dentists and chair-side assistants and found a higher prevalence of liver disease in professionals who were chronically exposed to nitrous oxide (N$_2$O); the prevalence was 1.7-fold higher in dentists and 1.6-fold higher in their assistants. The methodologic limitations of this study argue for cautious interpretation of the data. It is clear, however, that N$_2$O inhibits the enzyme methionine synthetase, which could produce toxic effects. Brief exposures to N$_2$O, at concentrations used clinically, are sufficient to produce time-related decreases in methionine synthetase activity in the livers of animals and humans.[98] Whether the resultant abnormalities in folate and methionine metabolism actually injure the liver is unclear.

Nitrous oxide by itself does not usually cause clinically significant changes in blood pressure and cardiac output. Hepatic circulation remains undisturbed when it is administered to conscious animals.[99] However, when used with a barbiturate to provide anesthesia during laparotomy, N_2O (30, 50 and 70%) induces dose-related decreases in both hepatic arterial flow and portal venous flow without altering hepatic oxygen consumption. In this setting, N_2O also increases mean arterial pressure, hepatic arterial resistance, and mesenteric vascular resistance. Taken together, these data suggest that N_2O can increase sympathetic nervous system activity, which decreases portal venous and hepatic arterial flows through stimulation of α-adrenergic receptors in the hepatic and mesenteric circulations.[100]

Hepatic injury may at times result from a N_2O-related decrease in hepatic oxygen tension. Nitrous oxide appears to increase selectively the potential of halothane to cause mild hepatic injury. For example, in a study of urologic patients, halothane anesthetics (100% O_2, or 70% N_2O + 30% O_2), but not isoflurane anesthesia with 70% N_2O (30% O_2), increased GST. The N_2O plus halothane group had a higher incidence than the halothane group of small, but significant, GST elevations 3–6 hours after anesthesia (35 *vs.* 24%, respectively).[68] The exact mechanisms of the GST increases are unknown, but the increases probably result from hepatic hypoxia caused by anesthesia-related decreases of hepatic blood flow and oxygen delivery. Another clinical investigation evaluated effects of inspired oxygen tension (including hyperbaric oxygenation) during halothane anesthesia on postoperative ALT levels; patients who received halothane at lower intraoperative oxygen tensions had the largest increases of ALT.[101] These results suggest that increases in oxygen tension may protect the liver from halothane-induced hypoxic injury.

The aforementioned studies suggest that N_2O-containing anesthetics do not cause liver injury in the absence of impaired hepatic oxygenation.[68,101] In another study, no hepatocellular injury resulted from up to 4 hours of anesthesia with 67% N_2O (in oxygen) and infusions of methohexital.[102] Moreover, no hepatic dysfunction developed when patients with mild alcoholic hepatitis received N_2O–opioid or N_2O–enflurane anesthetics for peripheral or superficial operations.[103] There is no convincing evidence that nitrous oxide *per se* causes hepatotoxicity[104] in the absence of a precarious oxygen supply/demand ratio in the liver.

Nonopioid Sedative–Hypnotic Agents

Intravenous anesthetic agents, such as propofol, etomidate, and midazolam, have not been shown to significantly alter hepatic function in patients undergoing minor operative procedures. Although very large doses of thiopental (>750 mg) may cause hepatic dysfunction, usual induction doses have little effect on the liver.[105] Ketamine induction may produce a moderate increase in serum concentrations of some liver enzymes.[75] Patients anesthetized with ketamine infusions plus oxygen show a dose-dependent increase in biochemical markers of hepatic injury.[106] It is unclear whether ketamine causes liver dysfunction by exerting direct hepatotoxic effects, altering hepatic metabolism, or by increasing serum catecholamines, which can decrease hepatic blood flow and oxygen delivery. However, none of the intravenous agents commonly used to induce anesthesia appears to produce serious hepatotoxicity.

Opioids

Opioids and intravenous anesthetics *per se* have little effect on hepatic function, provided that they do not impair hepatic blood flow and oxygen supply.

Opioids increase the tone of the common bile duct (Fig. 39-12) and sphincter of Oddi, leading to increases in biliary tract pressure and biliary spasm. Consequently, opioids may

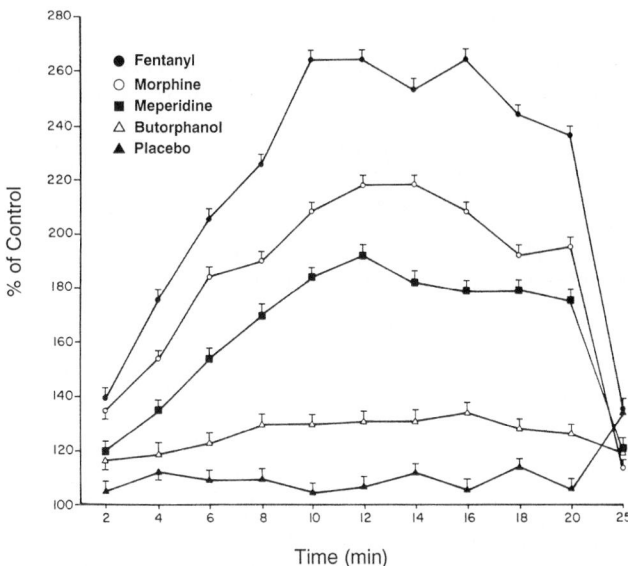

Figure 39-12. Effects of opioids and placebo on common bile duct pressure, expressed as a percentage of pretreatment values. (Reprinted with permission from Radnay PA, Duncalf D, Novakovic M, *et al:* Common bile duct pressure changes after fentanyl, morphine, meperidine, butorphanol, and naloxone. Anesth Analg 63:441, 1984.)

trigger severe epigastric or abdominal pain, and biliary spasms. This may occur in approximately 3% of patients receiving opioids and can cause false-positive results on intraoperative cholangiography.[107] Also, increases in serum lipase and amylase concentrations may occur, and persist for up to 24 hours after administration of a μ-agonist. At equianalgesic doses, fentanyl and morphine cause larger increases in biliary pressure than meperidine[108] or pentazocine.[109,110] Butorphanol[108] and nalbuphine[111] probably do not cause spasm of the sphincter of Oddi. Medications that can antagonize opioid-induced increases in biliary spasm include nitroglycerin, atropine, glucagon, and naloxone, as well as the volatile anesthetic agents.

Nonopioid Analgesics

Acetaminophen

Acetaminophen is widely prescribed for the treatment of postoperative pain, being used alone (Tylenol) or in combination with opioid analgesics, such as oxycodone (Percocet) and hydrocodone (Vicodin). Extremely large doses (suicide attempts) of acetaminophen are a well-known cause of fulminant hepatic failure, and it has recently become clear that analgesic doses can produce hepatotoxicity in susceptible individuals.[112] Daily doses in the range of 3–8 g may result in chronic liver injury.[113] In chronic alcoholics or patients with poor nutritional status, doses as low as 2 g per day may produce serious liver injury.[114] The American Liver Foundation has recommended that warning labels be placed on all acetaminophen-containing products to alert consumers of the potential for liver damage. Whenever acetaminophen hepatotoxicity seems probable, specific treatment (*N*-acetylcysteine) should be instituted without delay because it is highly effective with minimal risk to the patient.

Nonsteroidal Anti-inflammatory Drugs, Including Aspirin

Aspirin is a well-documented cause of a dose-related, reversible form of hepatotoxicity. This disorder may develop in days to weeks after initiation of high-dose aspirin therapy. Patients are usually asymptomatic, with mild-to-moderate increases of serum aminotransferase activities. Jaundice is uncommon, and severe clinical hepatitis is rare.

The FDA Arthritis Advising Committee concluded in 1992 that hepatotoxicity is a "class characteristic" of nonsteroidal anti-inflammatory drugs (NSAIDs). Major offenders in this regard have been diclofenac, sulindac, and phenylbutazone. Other offenders include piroxicam, ibuprofen, naproxen, and fenoprofen. The basis of hepatotoxicity from NSAIDs appears to be largely, but not entirely, idiosyncratic. Cross-sensitivity between different NSAID classes may occur.

NONPHARMACOLOGIC CAUSES OF PERIOPERATIVE LIVER DYSFUNCTION

Sepsis and Splanchnic Ischemia

The characteristic features of human sepsis occur in chronically instrumented, sedated sheep that receive a 24-hour infusion of *Escherichia coli* endotoxin. The earliest vascular abnormality is transient pulmonary arterial constriction, which is followed immediately by simultaneous, precipitous decreases in blood flow (to below 50% baseline values) through the celiac trunk, superior mesenteric artery, and portal vein. Hepatic arterial flow exhibits a biphasic response; an abrupt, transient decrease precedes a marked and sustained increase in flow. These early effects appear to be unrelated to systemic hemodynamics. The large increase in hepatic artery flow occurs independently of changes in portal venous flow, suggesting a dysregulation of the physiologic hepatic arterial buffer response. This phenomenon may be the result of an increase in hepatic oxygen demand, to support phagocytosis and digestion of the sudden overload of bacterial endotoxins.[115]

Endotoxin also ablates the hepatic arterial buffer response and autoregulation in anesthetized pigs.[116] Decreases in portal venous flow parallel and match decreases in cardiac output, without reciprocal increases in hepatic arterial flow. Selective inhibition of vascular endothelial function appears to mediate the impairment of the buffer response,[117] and nitric oxide may moderate this effect. During endotoxic shock, nitric oxide induces arterial hypotension, dilates hepatic arterioles, and attenuates the increases in both portal and pulmonary resistances.[116] The nitric oxide synthase inhibitor, $N(G)$-nitro-L-arginine methyl ester (L-NAME), markedly disrupts the hepatic circulation in experimental endotoxemia. This latter effect is rapidly and partially reversed by sodium nitroprusside.[117] Thus, inhibition of NO synthetase might worsen outcome in endotoxic shock by causing a loss of local control of liver blood flow and markedly increasing resistance to venous return across both the liver and lungs.

Splanchnic ischemia impairs hepatic function and appears to increase morbidity and mortality in critically ill patients. A prospective study, conducted in ICU patients with evidence of inadequate tissue perfusion, suggests that measurements of hepatic metabolic function and tonometric assessment of gastric intramucosal pH (pH_{im}) better predict patient outcome than standard liver blood tests.[12] The investigators noted that the survivors and nonsurvivors had similar values of bilirubin, AST, alkaline phosphatase, PT, and indocyanine green clearance (ICG). In contrast, hepatic metabolism of lidocaine to monoethylglycinexylidide (MEGX) differed markedly between survivors and nonsurvivors (MEGX levels of 16 ng·ml^{-1} and 2.4 ng·ml^{-1}, respectively). During the 3-day study period, MEGX levels in nonsurvivors had decreased from 20.6 to 2.4 ng·ml^{-1}. Such data suggest that critically ill patients can rapidly develop severe hepatic dysfunction. This rapid deterioration may result from an imbalance between hepatic metabolic demand and liver blood flow, and portends a poor prognosis.

Hepatic Injury Associated with Low Arterial Oxygen Content, Hypotension, and Shock

The liver is exquisitely sensitive to hypoxia. In one study, patients with chronic lung disease whose blood oxygen content fell below 9 ml·dl^{-1} all developed liver injury, without developing overt myocardial or cerebral damage.[118] Detrimental effects of oxygen deprivation on perioperative hepatic function can occur independent of anesthetic techniques.[119]

Passive congestion alone, no matter how severe or prolonged, seems to cause little if any damage to the liver,[120] even in patients with congestive heart failure. Hepatic dysfunction tends to be mild, and the prognosis primarily depends on the severity of the underlying cardiac or systemic illness. However, if moderate hypotension occurs, a hepatitis-like illness (ischemic hepatitis) may follow. Patients develop jaundice, systemic symptoms, and large increases of serum transaminases, which may persist for 3–11 days. Liver biopsy shows centrilobular necrosis with little or no inflammatory response.[121]

Patients with ischemic hepatitis typically have a history of inadequate systemic perfusion, along with marked increases of serum aminotransferases. The increases are usually of greater magnitude than those associated with viral hepatitis. Prolonged shock or sepsis can cause extreme liver injury; a hepatic lobe or the entire liver may become infarcted, even in the absence of portal venous or hepatic arterial occlusion.[120] The mechanism of ischemic hepatitis is unknown, but may involve free-radical production because hepatocytes contain very high concentrations of xanthine oxidase. (Ischemia and reperfusion increase xanthine oxidase activity; this enzyme catalyzes the oxidation of purines to uric acid and the associated reduction of O_2 to superoxide anion, which initiates toxic free-radical reactions.)

Surgery-Related Injury

Minor operations do not cause postoperative liver dysfunction in healthy patients. Even patients with marginal hepatic function usually tolerate peripheral procedures without hepatic complications, including those who receive halothane anesthesia.[122] A randomized study in patients with mild alcoholic hepatitis compared spinal *vs.* general anesthesia (enflurane plus N_2O or N_2O plus opioid) and found no anesthesia-related differences in values of LFTs following peripheral or superficial surgery.[103]

Major operations (especially laparotomy) are often associated with hepatic dysfunction or injury. The magnitude of the abnormality depends more on the type of operation than on a particular anesthetic technique.[122,123] Nonetheless, hepatic dysfunction subsequent to major surgery is rarely of concern in healthy patients. By contrast, patients with advanced hepatic disease (marginal hepatic function) who undergo major operations, such as laparotomy, have extremely high postoperative morbidity and mortality.[1,2,124,125] These patients are probably unable to tolerate the surgical stress, which contributes to decreased hepatic oxygen supply.

The surgical stress response includes the stimulation of the sympathetic nervous system, activation of the renin–angiotensin–aldosterone system, and the nonosmotic release of vasopressin; each of these neurohumoral responses can compromise the splanchnic circulation. These effects may persist for many hours or even days after surgery. Laboratory studies indicate that laparotomy induces marked mesenteric vasoconstriction and decreases gastrointestinal blood flow; acute hypophysectomy and administration of an angiotensin II antagonist can abolish these changes.[126] In addition to the surgical stress response, laparotomy by itself decreases blood flow through the intestine and the liver,[127] probably through traction and manipulation of the viscera.

Anesthetic agents might be expected to modify the effects of laparotomy on the liver because some of them (halothane or enflurane) cause much greater decreases of hepatic blood flow and oxygen supply than others (isoflurane or sevoflurane).[83,128–131] Support for this idea comes from experiments conducted in phenobarbital-pretreated rats (microsomal enzyme induction) that were anesthetized with either thiamylal, halothane, enflurane, or isoflurane for various operative interventions, including hepatic artery ligation.[131] Centrilobular necrosis occurred only in the rats anesthetized with halothane; the severity of the injury was related both to duration of anesthesia and to operative location. The hepatic damage that resulted from upper abdominal (sham for hepatic artery ligation) and lower abdominal operations was comparable, and exceeded that associated with peripheral surgery. Thus, the pathogenesis of laparotomy-induced hepatic injury appears to involve mesenteric vasoconstriction and reductions of hepatic and intestinal blood flow.

Laparoscopic Cholecystectomy

Acute cholecystitis occasionally develops in cirrhotic patients and requires surgical intervention. It is unclear whether a laparoscopic procedure is preferable to an open cholecystectomy because of the risk of intraoperative hemorrhage related to portal hypertension. A recent study compared complication rates and outcomes in cirrhotic patients ($n = 48$; Child-Pugh A or B severity) and noncirrhotic controls ($n = 187$) who underwent laparoscopic cholecystectomy for symptomatic cholelithiasis. No differences occurred in overall outcome, operation duration, or hospital stay. However, the group with cirrhosis required more transfusions and had a higher incidence of minor complications. Conversion to open cholecystectomy occurred in 8.3% of cirrhotic patients but in none of the controls (0/187). Thus, while laparoscopic cholecystectomy may appear safe in patients with mild-to-moderate cirrhosis and symptomatic gallstones, the overall complication rate is increased.[132]

Procedures Requiring Cardiopulmonary Bypass

Cardiac failure itself does not usually lead to significant hepatic dysfunction, but jaundice and hepatocellular necrosis may occur if severe hypotension develops.[133] Cardiopulmonary bypass with low-flow states and nonpulsatile perfusion can aggravate pre-existing hepatic dysfunction. Administration of catecholamines to improve cardiac performance, either before or after bypass, may decrease hepatic oxygen delivery. Hypothermia during cardiopulmonary bypass probably limits the hepatic injury created by the abnormal hemodynamics.

Hypotension and hemorrhage decrease portal blood flow, but the hepatic arterial buffer response and pressure-flow autoregulation tend to preserve hepatic arterial flow and oxygen delivery. Perfusion at $28°C$ increases portal flow and slightly decreases hepatic arterial flow. A pump flow rate of 2.4 $l \cdot min^{-1} \cdot m^{-1}$ better maintains total blood flow to the liver than a rate of $1.2 l \cdot min^{-1} \cdot m^{-1}$. Only at low pump rates does pulsatile flow appear to be more advantageous than nonpulsatile perfusion in terms of hepatic blood flow.[134]

Liver Transplantation

One to three hours after transplantation, mean cardiac output remains elevated ($9.5 l \cdot min^{-1}$) and hepatic blood flow represents 23% of cardiac output. The portal flow is disproportionately high, constituting 85% of total blood flow to the liver. Intentionally reducing the portal flow by 50% triggered a 30% increase in hepatic artery flow, indicating an intact hepatic arterial buffer response in the newly transplanted liver.[135]

Hemolysis and Transfusion

Reabsorption of large surgical hematomas and transfusions of red blood cells are major causes of postoperative jaundice in the absence of overt hepatocellular dysfunction. At least 10% of transfused erythrocytes hemolyze within the initial 24 hours following a blood transfusion (bilirubin load is about 250 mg per unit transfused). A normal liver readily clears the bilirubin load that results from mild hemolysis. With severe hemolysis, the excessive bilirubin loads lead to unconjugated hyperbilirubinemia, which persists until the liver conjugates and excretes the excess bilirubin.

Excessive bilirubin loads can also result from severe hemolytic disorders, including hemoglobinopathies (*e.g.*, sickle cell disease) or derangements of erythrocyte metabolism [glucose-6-phosphate dehydrogenase (G6PD) deficiency]. Thus unconjugated hyperbilirubinemia may be seen in the perioperative period as a result of exacerbations of sickle cell disease (via hypovolemia, hypoxia, hypothermia, stress) or G6PD deficiency (via sulfonamides, chloramphenicol, nitrofurantoin). Other causes of significant hemolysis include transfusion reactions and prosthetic cardiac valves.

HEPATIC AND HEPATOBILIARY DISEASES

Classification of Liver Diseases

For the purposes of the following discussion, liver diseases are divided into two large, heterogeneous groups: parenchymal diseases (*e.g.*, viral hepatitis, steatohepatitis, hepatic cirrhosis, and fulminant hepatic failure) and cholestatic diseases (*e.g.*, intrahepatic and extrahepatic biliary obstruction).

Prevalence of Hepatobiliary Disease

More than 100 distinct hepatic diseases have been described. Currently, nearly 10% of the American population (25 million) have some form of hepatobiliary disease. Hepatitis B or C viral infections afflict more than 5 million Americans. About 50% of those with hepatitis C may develop cirrhosis, which currently accounts for between 13,000 to 15,000 deaths each year. Alcoholic liver disease remains a problem, becoming severe in 10–15% of those who consume large amounts of alcohol over a prolonged period.

Viral Hepatitis

Viral hepatitides are important causes of perioperative hepatic dysfunction. They can elude preoperative detection, especially during the incubation period, when the disease is asymptomatic. Heterotropic viruses are the ones that most commonly cause hepatitis: hepatitis A (HAV), hepatitis B (HBV), hepatitis C (HCV), hepatitis D (HDV, delta), and hepatitis E (HEV). HDV is a defective but pathogenic agent that requires HBV for its replication.

Other important but much less common causes of viral hepatitis include cytomegalovirus (CMV), Epstein-Barr (EBV), herpes simplex, rubella, varicella zoster, measles, Coxsackie, and echoviruses. These viruses typically produce benign, anicteric disease, and often escape detection by surgical and anesthesia teams.[136,137] However, in rare circumstances, particularly in immunocompromised patients, they cause acute hepatitis, fulminant hepatic failure, and death.

The differential diagnosis of viral hepatitis and anesthesia-induced hepatitis can be quite difficult. The clinical presentations may be similar, laboratory findings may be inconclusive, and liver biopsy results may fail to provide a basis for etiologic differentiation. A diagnosis of viral hepatitis is based on a constellation of findings suggestive of viral infection coupled with hepatocellular necrosis.[138] The clinical presentation of viral hepatitis generally includes four phases: An *early prodromal phase*, resembling serum sickness, with fever, arthralgias, arthritis, rash, and angioneurotic edema; a *preicteric phase*, with nonspecific constitutional symptoms including malaise, unusual fatigue, myalgias, anorexia, nausea, vomiting, occasional midepigastric or right upper quadrant pain, and diarrhea; an *icteric phase*, marked by the onset of jaundice, a decrease in fever, and lessening of constitutional symptoms; a *convalescent phase*, in which jaundice begins to subside, constitutional symptoms disappear, and a sense of well-being returns to the patient.

HAV infection (infectious hepatitis) is not associated with blood transfusion. Viremia is short-lived, and the incubation period is only 3–4 weeks long. There are no chronic carriers, and chronic liver disease does not occur. Fulminant hepatic failure is rare (0.14–2%) in the absence of pre-existing liver disease. Patients with hepatitis B who acquire an HAV infection typically have an uncomplicated clinical course. However, approximately 41% of patients with chronic hepatitis C who acquire an HAV superinfection go on to develop fulminant hepatitis, which has a fatality rate of 35%. In these cases, propensity to develop liver failure is unrelated to the severity of pre-existing liver disease.[139] An HDV superinfection markedly increases the potential for HBV to cause fulminant hepatic failure.

HCV (previously called non-A, non-B hepatitis), which was discovered in 1989, was the major cause of transfusion-related hepatitis until the 1990s. Reports from earlier decades indicate that approximately 7 weeks elapsed between a transfusion and the onset of clinical hepatitis. It is now clear that the incubation period for HCV is 7 weeks, which is distinctly different from that of HAV (3–4 weeks) or HBV (12 weeks). HCV infections more often progress to chronic liver disease than do infections with the other viruses. Fortunately, serologic tests for HCV now exist. Because of their use in screening donated blood, the incidence of transfusion-related hepatitis from HCV has dropped precipitously. It continues to decline and is currently lower than that from HBV (about 1 case per 300,000 vs. 1 case per 60,000 units transfused).

Serologic tests have been the mainstay in the diagnosis of viral hepatitis. Serum immunoglobulin M (IgM) antibody to the HAV capsid or HAV RNA in stool documents an acute infection with HAV; recovery is associated with IgG anti-HAV. The diagnosis of HBV infection is made by identifying either HBsAg or antibody (IgM) to core antigen (HBV core), hepatitis Be antigen (HBeAg), antibody to HBeAg (anti-HBe), antibody to HBsAg (anti-HBs), or HBV DNA measured by polymerase chain reaction (PCR). IgM and total antibody to HDV document an infection with HDV, which requires a coexisting HBV infection. Anti-HCV or the presence of HCV RNA detects HCV. Assay for viral genome helps identify hepatitis G virus (HGV).

Autoantibodies often occur in both HBV and HCV infections, especially anti–smooth-muscle antibodies and antinuclear antibodies. The latter are associated with an HLA phenotype of Al,B8,DR3, which may be a marker for susceptibility to fulminant viral hepatitis. Anti-asialoglycoprotein receptor antibodies often appear in HAV infections, as well as in autoimmune hepatitis, but they are almost undetectable in HCV infections. HAV may trigger autoimmune mechanisms (partially primed by HCV) in susceptible patients, leading to massive hepatocellular necrosis.

Serologic tests used to diagnose viral hepatitis have their limitations; they are neither 100% sensitive nor 100% specific. Tests that screen for HBsAg are negative during the incubation period of HBV infections. Similarly, HDV infections generally suppress HBV replication; hence, patients with chronic liver disease caused by HBV, may have HDV but no detectable HbsAg in their blood. However, the identification of hepatitis B viral DNA in the blood of such patients indicates that the HbsAg assay may yield false-negative results in patients infected with HDV.[140] Acute HAV infections can cause previously detectable HBV DNA or HCV RNA to become undetectable until recovery from the HAV infection. Moreover, new hepatotoxic viruses continue to arise and may cause significant disease that eludes detection by present assays.

Fatty Liver Diseases

The most prevalent of the fatty liver diseases are alcoholic liver disease and nonalcoholic steatosis. These are the most common causes of cryptogenic cirrhosis. Morbid obesity or diabetes is present in about 70% of patients who develop cryptogenic cirrhosis. Increased fat appears to stress the hepatocyte and render it more susceptible to necrosis and apoptosis from other causes.

Nonalcoholic Steatohepatitis

Nonalcoholic steatohepatitis (NASH) is the most common cause of elevated liver blood tests in healthy blood donors. Up to 20% of these patients may have unsuspected fibrosis or cirrhosis. In this population, liver disease was the third most common cause of death, with a liver-related mortality of 11%.

Ethanol-Related Liver Diseases

Chronic alcoholism produces a wide spectrum of liver diseases, including steatosis (fatty liver), alcoholic hepatitis, and cirrhosis. Chronic alcoholism is notoriously difficult to detect by a brief patient history and physical examination. Laboratory values can be misleading, and the correlation between clinical presentation and hepatic histopathology is poor because compensatory mechanisms often mask extensive liver disease.[141] Alcohol abusers by definition consume more than 5 g of alcohol per day (≥5 drinks per day). Recent studies indicate alcohol abusers have a 2- to 3-fold increase in perioperative morbidity (Fig. 39-13).[142] The most frequent complications are bleeding, infections, and cardiopulmonary insufficiency. The pathogenic mechanisms include immune incompetence, subclinical cardiac insufficiency, hemostatic imbalance, and perhaps an exaggerated stress response to surgery or alcohol abstinence.

Hereditary Hemochromatosis

More than one million Americans absorb and store too much iron in their bodies. This condition, called hemochromatosis, is the most common inherited metabolic disease. Approximately 85–90% of patients with hemochromatosis are homozygous for a C282Y mutation on the short arm of chromosome 6. The highest prevalence is in people of western European, specifically Celtic, descent. Patients are usually diagnosed with the disease when they are between 40 to 60 years old; they complain of vague symptoms, including fatigue, abdominal pain, joint pain, and exhibit slightly elevated liver enzymes and bronze discoloration of the skin.

The pathophysiology of hereditary hemochromatosis (HHC) involves an up-regulation of iron absorption from the duodenal mucosa. Decreased mucosal ferritin concentrations are associated with increased transferrin receptor levels. The mucosa behaves as if the patient were iron-deficient, leading to deposition of increased quantities of iron in a variety of tissues including the liver, skin, heart, pancreas, and joints.

Hereditary hemochromatosis is associated with a 150- to 200-fold increase in the risk of developing hepatocellular carcinoma. Liver cancer occurs in about 30% of the advanced cases, leading to the need for transplantation. However, survival rates

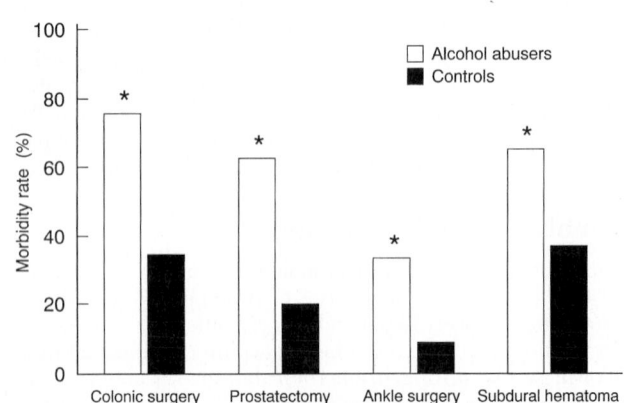

Figure 39-13. Prospective studies of postoperative morbidity in alcohol abusers and control subjects. *$p < 0.05$ vs. control subjects. (Reprinted with permission from Tonnesen H, Kehlet H: Preoperative alcoholism and postoperative morbidity. Br J Surg 86:869, 1999.)

after liver transplantation are much lower in hemochromatosis patients than in patients who undergo this procedure because of other liver diseases. This may relate to the devastating impact of untreated hemochromatosis on organs, such as the heart and pancreas.

Most of the clinical manifestations respond to phlebotomy. Once cirrhosis develops, however, phlebotomy will not reduce the risk of liver cancer. If HHC seems likely, it is important to obtain a liver biopsy and a quantitative iron determination because identification and treatment in the precirrhotic stage results in a normal long-term survival. The treatment of choice for these patients is quantitative phlebotomy performed on a weekly basis. Patients may have a total body iron content of 20–60 g. Since a unit of packed red blood cells contains 250 mg of iron, removal of excess iron stores may require 2–4 years. Thereafter, life-long phlebotomy treatments every 2–4 months will prevent accumulation of iron.

CIRRHOSIS: A PARADIGM FOR END-STAGE PARENCHYMAL LIVER DISEASE

For simplicity, this section discusses the pathophysiology of parenchymal liver disease with the example of hepatic cirrhosis as it relates to the practice of anesthesia. The most common clinical features of cirrhosis are an enlarged spleen and liver, ascites, mild to moderate jaundice, weakness, large esophageal varices, spider nevi, anorexia, nausea, vomiting, encephalopathy, and, sometimes, abdominal pain. Advanced parenchymal hepatic disease alters the function of nearly every organ and body system.

Cardiovascular Abnormalities

A hallmark of liver cirrhosis and portal hypertension is a hyperdynamic cardiovascular system, characterized by high cardiac output, low peripheral vascular resistance, and normal filling pressures, heart rate, and arterial pressure (Table 39-4). The earliest changes include arterial dilation and a decrease in peripheral vascular resistance. Stroke volume and cardiac index increases, which may even occur in patients with cardiomyopathy. The total blood volume tends to increase, but its maldistribution often leads to central hypovolemia and splanchnic hypervolemia. Peripheral blood flow markedly exceeds the metabolic oxygen requirements. Therefore, oxygen tension and saturation in the peripheral and mixed venous blood typically increase, and the arteriovenous difference in oxygen content narrows. The clinical and pathophysiologic syndrome is reminiscent of a peripheral arteriovenous fistula. This is not surprising, considering the extensive arteriovenous collateralization that occurs in many organs and tissues, including the splanchnic organs, lungs, skin, muscles, and probably others. The mechanism by which these collaterals develop is complex and not completely understood. Experimentally induced portal stenosis in rats increases arteriovenous shunting and blood flow in preportal tissues; 40% of this effect may be attributable to an increase in plasma glucagon.[143] The remaining 60% may be due to substances such as nitric oxide, ferritin, and vasoactive intestinal polypeptide (VIP), which can induce peripheral vasodilation, decrease vascular resistance, and increase arteriovenous shunting.

Cirrhosis reduces the responsiveness of the cardiovascular system to sympathetic discharge, as well as to endogenous and exogenous cardiovascular stimulants. These distorted responses probably relate to circulating vasodilating factors, but could also result from an impairment of baroreceptor reflexes. The mechanism of the decreased responsiveness to cardiovascular stimulation is not completely clear. Glucagon, whose concentration invariably increases in cirrhotic patients with portal hypertension, reduces the vascular responsiveness to infused catecholamines and other vasopressors in experimental settings.[144]

Does Nitric Oxide (NO) Mediate the Hyperdynamic Circulatory Changes?

Recent evidence indicates that nitric oxide (NO) may be an important mediator of the hyperdynamic changes, as well as the disorders of sodium and water excretion, that occur in cirrhosis and portal hypertension. NO-induced cyclic guanosine monophosphate (cGMP) production correlates with the degree of peripheral arterial dilation in experimental models of chronic portal hypertension (partial portal vein ligation and CCl_4-induced cirrhosis in rats). The CCl_4 model is characterized by significant decreases both in MAP (20 mm Hg) and in systemic vascular resistance (by 45%) and a marked increase (44%) in cardiac index (Fig. 39-14). Treatment with inhibitors of NO synthase returns these parameters to baseline values, as well as restoring the responsiveness of blood vessels to vasoconstrictor therapy. Moreover, inhibition of NO synthase restores plasma concentrations of aldosterone and arginine vasopressin to normal values, and corrects abnormalities of sodium and water excretion in experimental models of cirrhosis and portal hypertension (Fig. 39-15). Preliminary evidence in humans suggests that NO may mediate the hyperdynamic circulatory state that occurs clinically. Data from normal subjects and patients with cirrhosis reveal a positive correlation between the exhaled concentration of NO and cardiac index (Fig. 39-16). Based on such observations, it may be possible to develop a new class of therapeutic agents to treat the major causes of morbidity and mortality in cirrhosis.

Pulmonary Dysfunction

Patients with cirrhosis and portal hypertension will have some degree of pulmonary dysfunction; the severity is usually greatest in patients with the most advanced liver disease.[145] Hypoxemia commonly occurs for a variety of reasons (Table 39-5). Vasodilatory substances (*e.g.*, nitric oxide, glucagon, adenosine, or prostacyclin) may account for the impaired hypoxic pulmonary vasoconstriction associated with liver disease.[146] Erythrocyte concentrations of 2,3-diphosphoglycerate may increase, reducing the affinity of hemoglobin for oxygen and shifting the oxyhemoglobin dissociation curve to the right. Major intrapulmonary arteriovenous shunting of blood is present in some patients with advanced liver disease; these shunts are of great clinical concern and a characteristic feature of the hepatopulmonary syndrome. The development of severe ascites and pleural effusions leads to atelectasis, marked restrictions of lung volumes and capacities (including FRC and closing capacity) and causes major V/Q mismatching and severe hypoxemia.

Table 39-4. CARDIOVASCULAR FUNCTION IN HEPATIC CIRRHOSIS

Decreased vascular resistance (peripheral vasodilation, increased arteriovenous shunting)
Increased cardiac output
Maintained arterial blood pressure, filling pressures, and heart rate (deterioration is late)
Blood volume maintained or increased, but redistributed (splanchnic hypervolemia, central hypovolemia).
Possible cardiomyopathy
Increased O_2 content in mixed venous blood; decreased difference in the O_2 contents of arterial and venous blood
Diminished responsiveness to catecholamines
Increased blood flow in splanchnic (extrahepatic), pulmonary, muscular, and cutaneous tissues
Decreased total hepatic blood flow
   Maintained hepatic arterial blood flow
   Decreased portal venous blood flow
Maintained or decreased renal blood flow

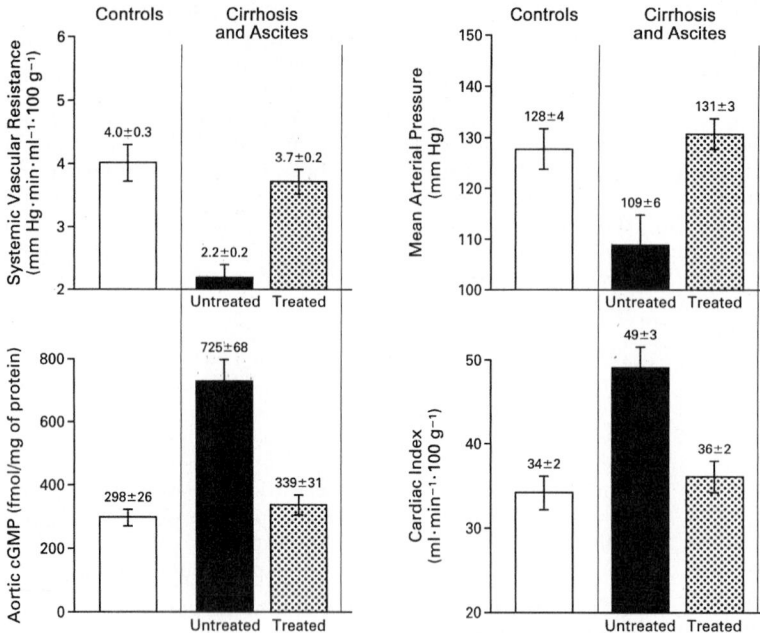

Figure 39-14. Effects of 7-day administration of L-NAME (N[G])-nitro-L-arginine methyl ester) on cyclic guanosine monophosphate (cGMP), mean arterial pressure, systemic vascular resistance, and cardiac index in cirrhotic rats with ascites. Rats were either untreated (*solid bars*) or treated (*stippled bars*) with L-NAME (0.5 mg · kg⁻¹ · day⁻¹). A group of normal untreated rats (*open bars*) served as controls. For each measurement, values in untreated cirrhotic rats with ascites differed significantly from those in the treatment and control groups ($p < 0.01$; $n = 8$ per group). Values for systemic vascular resistance and cardiac index are per 100 g of body weight. Values shown are means ± SE. (Reprinted with permission from Niederberger, M, Martin, PY, Gines, P *et al*: Normalization of nitric oxide production corrects arterial vasodilation and hyperdynamic circulation in cirrhotic rats. Gastroenterology 109:1624, 1995.)

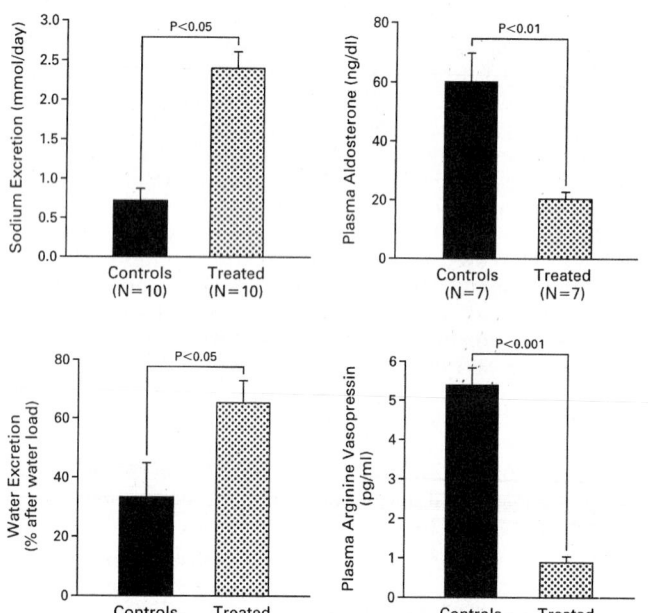

Figure 39-15. Effects of the inhibition of nitric oxide synthase with L-NAME (N[G]-nitro-L-arginine methyl ester) on mean urinary sodium excretion, plasma aldosterone concentrations, water excretion, and plasma vasopressin concentrations in rats with cirrhosis. (Reprinted with permission from Martin PY, Ohara M, Gines P *et al*: Nitric oxide synthase [NOS] inhibition for one week improves renal sodium and water excretion in cirrhotic rats with ascites [published erratum appears in J Clin Invest 102(3), 1998, inside back cover]. J Clin Invest 101: 235, 1998.)

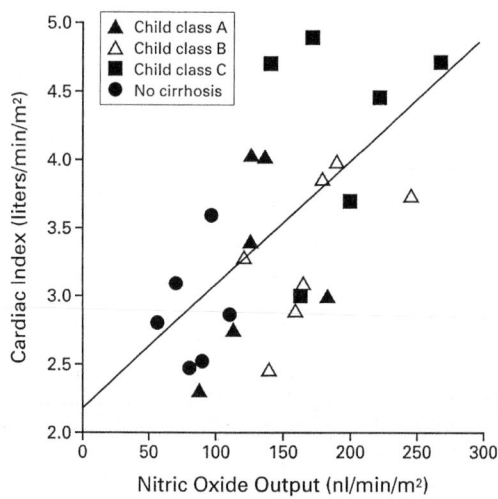

Figure 39-16. Relationship between nitric oxide in exhaled air and the cardiac index in 25 patients who had either normal hepatic function or cirrhosis with varying degrees hepatic dysfunction. (Severity of liver dysfunction increases progressively from Child class A to class C.) A positive correlation exists between nitric oxide output (expressed in nanoliters per minute per square meter of body surface area) and cardiac index (expressed in liters per minute per square meter). $r = 0.62$ and $p < 0.001$. (Reprinted with permission from Matsumoto, A, Ogura, K, Hirata, Y *et al*: Increased nitric oxide production in the exhaled air of patients with decompensated cirrhosis. Ann Intern Med 123:110, 1995.)

Table 39-5. HYPOXEMIA IN HEPATIC CIRRHOSIS

Rightward shift of the oxyhemoglobin dissociaton curve (increased 2, 3 = DPG)
Ventilation–perfusion abnormalities (impaired hypoxic pulmonary vasoconstriction)
Hypoventilation secondary to ascites
Decreases in pulmonary diffusing capacity secondary to increased extracellular fluid
Right-to-left pulmonary shunts caused by:
   Spider angiomas in the lungs
   Portopulmonary venous communications
   Humoral factors (*e.g.*, vasodilators, nitric oxide, glucagon)

Hepatic Hydrothorax

Hepatic hydrothorax occurs in 4–10% of cirrhotic patients. This disorder is characterized by pleural effusions in the absence of cardiopulmonary disease.[147] Most often, ascitic fluid fluxes from the peritoneal cavity into the pleural space through diaphragmatic defects. Initial treatment of hepatic hydrothorax consists of sodium restriction, diuretics, and thoracentesis; transjugular intrahepatic portosystemic stent shunts (TIPS) may be required in refractory cases. Because most of these patients have end-stage liver disease, liver transplantation becomes the preferred treatment if the above options fail.[147]

Pulmonary Pathophysiology in Patients with End-Stage Liver Disease

In a group of patients ($n = 362$) awaiting their first liver transplantation, 20% had mean pulmonary artery pressures that exceeded 25 mm Hg.[148] Only 4% of patients had pulmonary hypertension (defined as mean pulmonary artery pressure $\geq$25 mm Hg and pulmonary vascular resistance >120 dyn · s · cm^{-5}). Seven percent of patients had obstructive airways disease, 18% had restrictive disease, and 46% had low diffusion capacity on pulmonary function tests.

Ascites, Renal Dysfunction, and the Hepatorenal Syndrome

Portal hypertension alone does not impair renal circulation or cause obvious renal dysfunction. However, the combination of portal hypertension and cirrhosis leads to a spectrum of renal abnormalities. Derangements of sodium, potassium, and water metabolism and excretion occur commonly, as well as disorders of renal acidification. Glomerulopathy, acute renal failure, or hepatorenal syndrome often complicates severe liver disease.

Ascites and Edema

Nearly 50% of cirrhotic patients develop ascites within 10 years of being diagnosed with cirrhosis.[149] Ascites markedly worsens the prognosis of cirrhotic patients. Those with mild ascites retain sodium, but the problem usually corrects with diuretics. More severe forms, however, may be refractory to diuretic therapy (refractory ascites) and degenerate into hepatorenal failure. Of patients who have ascites, 18% develop hepatorenal syndrome at 1 year and 39% at 5 years.[150]

The most important treatments for patients with ascites are dietary sodium restriction and diuretic therapy, particularly spironolactone and furosemide. However, the overaggressive use of diuretics to increase urine output and decrease ascites often results in potentially serious complications, including hypovolemia, hyponatremia, hypokalemia, azotemia, and encephalopathy. Without proper fluid management, diuretics can severely diminish a patient's effective plasma volume, leading to azotemia or to the hepatorenal syndrome.

Pathogenesis of Ascites

The pathogenesis of ascites in cirrhosis is complex and not completely understood[149] (Fig. 39-17). Cardiovascular abnormalities (discussed previously) associated with advanced liver disease cause major alterations of renal function. The kidneys avidly retain sodium, which leads to the accumulation of extracellular fluid and the development of ascites and edema. It is thought that the sodium retention results from either a decrease in "effective" blood volume (traditional or arterial underfilling hypothesis[151]),[152] or from a renal tubular disorder (Fig. 39-17).

Schrier and Abraham[151] suggest that the concept of arterial underfilling provides the basis for a unifying hypothesis that explains the regulation of body-fluid volume in health and disease. The hypothesis states that "the integrity of the arterial circulation, as determined by cardiac output and peripheral arterial resistance, is the primary determinant of renal sodium and water excretion."[151] In other words, the body activates neurohumoral reflexes to retain sodium and water whenever it senses a decrease in the volume of the arterial system, whether the decrease results from a lowering of cardiac output or from an increased degree of arterial dilation. In cirrhotic patients, the effective (circulating) plasma volume decreases owing to the combined effects of arteriolar dilation (discussed earlier) and an imbalance of Starling forces in the hepatic sinusoids and splanchnic capillaries. This leads to excessive formation of lymph, which engorges the lymphatic system and transudes through Glisson's capsule, to accumulate in the peritoneal cavity as ascites. The total plasma volume remains normal or may even increase, but the effective plasma volume decreases. The neurohumoral response to the "ineffective" plasma volume triggers the kidney to retain sodium and water. Thus, the underfilling hypothesis explains renal sodium retention as a secondary rather than a primary phenomenon.

In contrast, the overflow hypothesis posits that abnormal sodium retention *per se* is the primary pathogenetic factor that

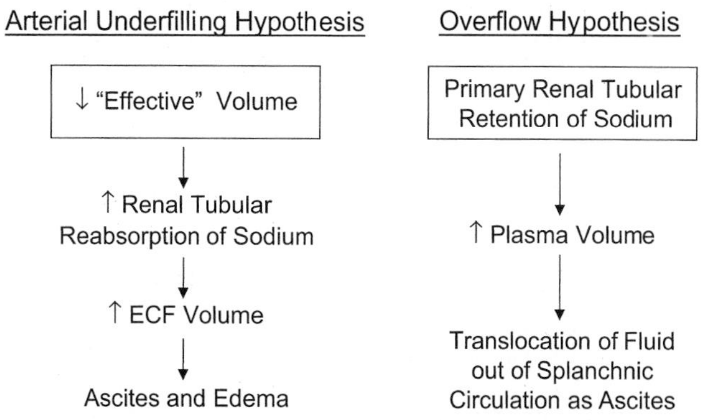

Figure 39-17. The presumed sequences of events that result in ascites formation according to the arterial underfilling hypothesis and the overflow hypothesis. The proposed primary disorders are shown in the boxes. According to the underfilling hypothesis, cirrhosis induces abnormal Starling forces in the portal venous circulation that cause an unfavorable distribution of the circulating blood volume (decreased effective blood volume). The diminished "effective" volume constitutes an afferent signal to the renal tubules to augment salt and water reabsorption. The attempt to replenish the diminished effective volume results in an expansion of the total blood volume to values far in excess of normal, with resultant ascites and edema formation. The overflow hypothesis holds that the primary disorder is retention of excessive sodium by the kidneys. In the setting of abnormal Starling forces in the portal venous bed, the expanded plasma volume is sequestered preferentially in the peritoneal sac. ECF = extracellular fluid. (Reprinted with permission from Epstein M: Renal functional abnormalities in cirrhosis: Pathophysiology and management. In Zakim D, Boyer TD [eds]: Hepatology: A Textbook of Liver Disease, p 448. Philadelphia, WB Saunders, 1982.)

increases plasma volume in cirrhotic patients. Accordingly, expansion of plasma volume causes portal hypertension (via increased hydrostatic pressure). This, in conjunction with a decrease in the colloid osmotic pressure of plasma, leads to ascites formation. Thus, the overflow hypothesis contends that renal sodium retention and plasma volume expansion, rather than plasma volume reduction are responsible for ascites formation.

Conceptually, these two hypotheses are not mutually exclusive; each may play a role in various stages of cirrhosis. Conceivably, in the early stages of cirrhosis, a primary defect in sodium excretion plays the more critical role, whereas with more advanced disease, a reduction in circulating plasma volume is more essential.[152]

Pathogenesis of Renal Dysfunction

A decrease in renal cortical blood flow is one of the earliest manifestations of impaired renal function in cirrhotic patients. Renal blood flow decreases because renal vascular resistance increases. This occurs despite a lowering of total peripheral vascular resistance and an elevation of cardiac output. Thus, the kidneys suffer from hypoperfusion while other tissues (preportal organs, skin, lungs, and muscles) tend to be hyperperfused. The increase in renal vascular resistance is greater in afferent than in efferent arterioles. Various neurohumoral substances as well as intrarenal factors mediate the increases in renal vascular resistance (Fig. 39-18).

Volume receptors detect decreases in effective plasma volume and activate the sympathetic nervous system. This causes the kidney to release renin, which leads to an increased production of angiotensin II (vasoconstrictor) and aldosterone. Both aldosterone and increased sympathetic nervous system outflow enhance tubular resorption of sodium. Norepinephrine concentrations are inversely related to renal blood flow, suggesting that the sympathetic nervous system plays an important role in sodium retention. Both norepinephrine and angiotensin II, through their vasoconstrictive actions, cause a redistribution of intrarenal blood flow, which further decreases sodium elimination. The kallikrein–kinin system also participates in modulating sodium retention. The concentration of endothelin, which is the most potent naturally occurring vasoconstrictor, is elevated in cirrhotic patients with ascites and probably contributes

to the renal dysfunction. Renal prostaglandin synthesis appears crucial to the preservation of renal function in patients with advanced liver disease because inhibitors of prostaglandin synthesis (*e.g.*, NSAIDs) markedly decrease renal plasma flow and glomerular filtration rate and can precipitate acute renal insufficiency. Cirrhotic patients without ascites do not seem to be susceptible to this untoward effect of NSAIDs. Thus, in cirrhotic patients with ascites, vasodilatory actions of prostaglandins synthesized in the kidney play an essential role in maintaining renal blood flow.

Hepatorenal Syndrome

The hepatorenal syndrome occurs primarily in hospitalized patients who have cirrhosis, portal hypertension, and moderate to severe ascites. The syndrome is typically associated with therapeutic interventions (or events) that can critically decrease plasma volume, including paracentesis, vigorous diuretic therapy, and gastrointestinal bleeding. Patients with hepatorenal syndrome continue to produce urine, although the rate of urine formation is somewhat decreased. Quite remarkably, this urine, even when concentrated, contains almost no sodium, similar to the urine of hypovolemic patients. Serum creatinine and blood urea nitrogen increase continuously as the syndrome progresses. When hepatorenal failure occurs, the kidneys are histologically intact and the renal damage is reversible; such kidneys, when transplanted, can function normally. Nonetheless, most patients with hepatorenal syndrome die. It is therefore imperative to prevent this syndrome by judicious management of diuretic therapy and volume status.

The pathogenesis of hepatorenal syndrome is complex and involves intense renal vasoconstriction and marked decreases in renal blood flow. The syndrome involves alterations of key vasoregulatory pathways, including the renin–angiotensin system, sympathetic nervous system, kallikrein–kinin system, prostaglandins synthesis, as well as the production and removal of endotoxin from blood. Endothelin-1 can produce intense renal vasoconstriction, which correlates with the severity of the renal dysfunction. Renal prostaglandins usually compensate for the intense vasoconstriction that occurs in patients with advanced liver disease. In hepatorenal syndrome, this compensatory mechanism fails to maintain renal perfusion. Concentrations

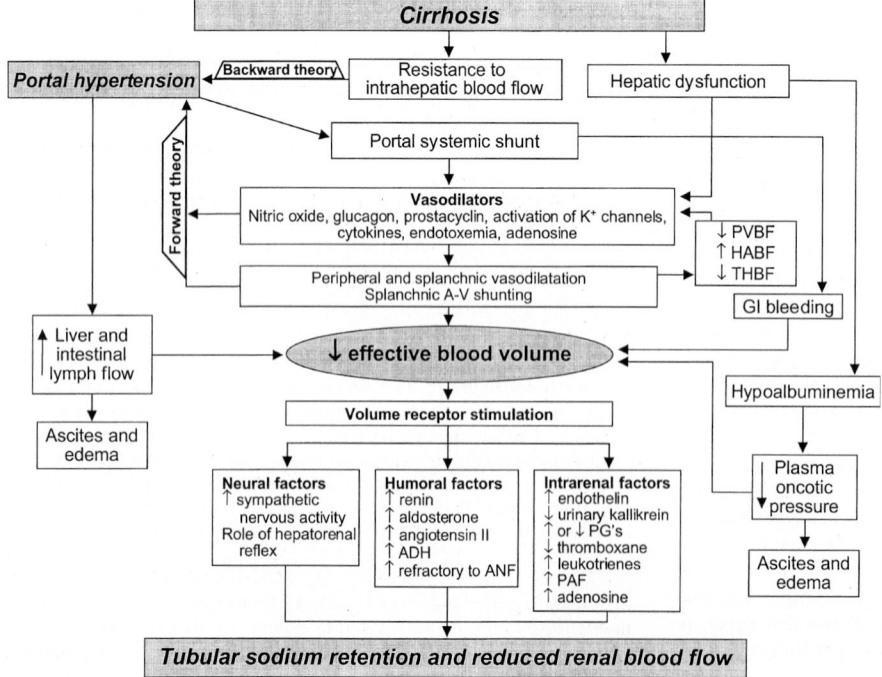

Figure 39-18. This schematic representation depicts the cirrhosis-induced development of portal hypertension, according to the forward theory and backward theory. Circulatory changes associated with cirrhosis and portal hypertension ultimately decrease the effective blood volume. This decrease stimulates volume receptors, which activate the neural, humoral, and intrarenal pathways that cause renal dysfunction (tubular sodium retention and decreased renal blood flow) in patients with hepatic cirrhosis. PVBF = portal vein blood flow; HABF = hepatic artery blood flow; THBF = total hepatic blood flow; A-V = arteriovenous; PG = prostaglandins; ADH = antidiuretic hormone; ANF = atrial natriuretic factor; PAF = platelet-activating factor.

Table 39-6. DIFFERENTIAL DIAGNOSIS OF ACUTE AZOTEMIA IN PATIENTS WITH LIVER DISEASE: IMPORTANT DIFFERENTIAL URINARY FINDINGS

	Prerenal Azotemia	Hepatorenal Syndrome	Acute Renal Failure (Acute Tubular Necrosis)
Urinary sodium concentration	<10 mEq$\cdot$l^{-1}	<10 mEq$\cdot$l^{-1}	>30 mEq$\cdot$l^{-1}
Urine-to-plasma creatinine ratio	$>30:1$	$>30:1$	$<20:1$
Urinary osmolality	Exceeds plasma osmolality by at least 100 mOsm	Exceeds plasma osmolality by at least 100 mOsm	Equal to plasma osmolality
Urinary sediment	Normal	Unremarkable	Casts, cellular debris

From Epstein M: Renal functional abnormalities in cirrhosis: Pathophysiology and management. In Zakim D, Boyer TD (eds): Hepatology: A Textbook of Liver Disease, p 460. Philadelphia, WB Saunders, 1982, with permission.

of atrial natriuretic factor, a powerful vasodilator, increase in cirrhotic patients, but the kidney is somewhat refractory to its vasodilatory effects.

Patients with hepatorenal syndrome usually have a decreased mean arterial pressure, which adds to the difficulty of successfully treating them. These patients have a rightward shift of their autoregulatory curve (renal blood flow and renal perfusion pressure); hence, small reductions in arterial pressure produce profound decreases in renal blood flow.

Acute Renal Failure and Acute Tubular Necrosis

Cirrhotic patients are also at risk for developing acute renal failure (ARF) and acute tubular necrosis (ATN), especially following infection or episodes of arterial hypotension. ATN appears to occur more often after operative interventions to relieve obstructive jaundice than following similar operations on nonjaundiced patients. Renal tubular injury may occur because patients with hepatic parenchymal disease and obstructive jaundice do not effectively mobilize blood from the splanchnic (including hepatic) vasculature to increase the central blood volume. Thus, even moderate hemorrhage may produce severe hypotension and cause ATN. In addition, conjugated bilirubin appears to be toxic to renal tubules and may contribute to the development of ATN in jaundiced patients.

The differential diagnosis of acute azotemia, shown in Table 39-6, indicates that the urinary characteristics of prerenal azotemia and hepatorenal syndrome are remarkably similar, but are clearly distinct from the urinary profile of ATN. Nonetheless, hepatorenal syndrome and ATN require similar therapeutic strategies. In both disorders, it is critically important to identify the underlying causes of renal insufficiency and to ensure an adequate circulating blood volume. To do this mandates prompt detection and treatment of bleeding and cautious use of diuretics.

Hepatic Circulatory Dysfunction

The pathogenesis of hepatic cirrhosis and portal hypertension is extremely complex and not well understood (see Fig. 39-18). Elevation of portal pressure stems from one or a combination of three factors: preportal blood flow, resistance to intrahepatic flow, and resistance to flow through the portacaval collaterals.

The classic "backward theory" posits that proliferation of fibrotic tissue, which gives rise to hepatic cirrhosis, increases the resistance to portal flow, thereby causing portal hypertension. However, many clinical and experimental observations do not fit the backward theory. For example, in experimental animals, restriction of transhepatic portal flow does not always produce portal hypertension comparable to that encountered clinically, nor does it produce bleeding from esophageal varices. In addi-

tion, when acute portal hypertension is produced by specifically narrowing the portal vein, splanchnic venous oxygen saturation decreases substantially, mesenteric arterial venous oxygen content difference increases, mesenteric vascular resistance increases, and mesenteric arterial flow decreases. Such changes are in diametric opposition to those observed in cirrhotic patients with portal hypertension.

To explain the clinical and physiologic features that are not well explained by the backward theory, a "forward theory" has been proposed.[153] This theory posits that certain mediators (nitric oxide, glucagon, prostacyclin, adenosine, and other compounds) cause vasodilation and formation of arteriovenous fistulae in the intestine and the spleen, thereby producing a hyperdynamic state with increased splanchnic blood flow and cardiac output. Portal blood flow to the liver decreases substantially, whereas hepatic arterial flow remains unchanged or increases. Thus, while total blood flow to the liver decreases, the hepatic oxygen supply is preserved. The decrease in total hepatic flow has pharmacokinetic implications: compounds, exogenous as well as endogenous, with high hepatic clearances are eliminated more slowly than in healthy people.

Hematologic and Coagulation Disorders

Anemia is common in cirrhotic patients for a variety of reasons. A dilutional anemia results from an increase in plasma volume, and is often exacerbated by erythrocyte loss from gastrointestinal bleeding. Malnutrition may lead to megaloblastic anemia because of deficiencies of vitamin B$_{12}$ and other vitamins, especially in alcoholics. There is an increased rate of hemolysis; the hemolytic activity is proportional to the size of the spleen but not to the degree of portal hypertension, and relates to reticulocytosis. Leukopenia and thrombocytopenia may also arise owing to hypersplenism or ethanol-induced depression of the bone marrow.

Most patients with liver cirrhosis have mild abnormalities of coagulation. Factor VII, owing to its relatively short half-life, decreases earlier and to lower levels than the other clotting factors produced by the liver. This is followed by a decrease in Factors V, X, and II (prothrombin); Factor I (fibrinogen) synthesis deteriorates last. The liver does not synthesize Factor VIII, which occasionally increases in cirrhotic patients. Usually, the concentration of fibrin degradation products is not increased, although severe disseminated intravascular coagulation develops in some settings, such as after LeVeen shunt surgery. When hepatic failure is severe, clotting factors synthesis decreases substantially, resulting in prolongation of the prothrombin (PT or INR) and partial thromboplastin times. Changes in the prothrombin time (PT or INR) usually provide an accurate reflection of the extent of liver dysfunction.

Endocrine Disorders

Cirrhotic patients often have abnormal glucose utilization. The mechanism of this phenomenon is rather complex and includes increased fatty acid concentrations in plasma, which antagonize the effects of insulin on glucose uptake by skeletal muscles. In addition, plasma concentrations of growth hormone and glucagon are often increased, and undoubtedly contribute to the glucose intolerance and other derangements of intermediary metabolism that occur in patients with hepatic dysfunction.

Abnormal metabolism of sex hormones causes gonadal dysfunction in both men and women. Men undergo feminization, often developing gynecomastia along with a decrease in the size of their testes and prostate gland. Testicular dystrophy is often apparent microscopically. The frequency of impotence increases and sperm counts typically decrease in those who still produce and ejaculate semen. In women with liver dysfunction, oligomenorrhea or amenorrhea commonly occurs.

Hepatic Encephalopathy

Hepatic encephalopathy is a complex neuropsychiatric syndrome with clinical manifestations ranging from subtle abnormalities, detectable only by psychometric testing, to confusion, obtundation, and deep coma. Some degree of encephalopathy occurs in 50–70% of patients with cirrhosis. Many of the encephalopathic changes are reversible with medical therapy. Even the most progressive, debilitating abnormalities, such as dementia, spastic paresis, cerebellar degeneration, and extrapyramidal movement disorders, may gradually improve after successful orthotopic liver transplantation. The encephalopathy may result from inadequate hepatocyte function, reduced hepatic blood flow, or diversion of portal flow through extrahepatic collateral vessels (*i.e.*, portacaval blood flow). These vessels include the portacaval collaterals that commonly develop in cirrhotic patients with portal hypertension (*e.g.*, esophageal, rectal) as well as surgically created portacaval shunts.

Patients with advanced hepatocellular dysfunction often have elevated ammonia levels in arterial blood, especially when significant portosystemic shunting is present. Ammonia levels, however, correlate poorly with the grade of hepatic encephalopathy and therefore are of little clinical value either for establishing a diagnosis of hepatic encephalopathy or for assessing prognosis. Of greater value are the physical examination and bedside psychometric tests (number-connection, trail-making tasks), which provide inexpensive, useful information about the progression and severity of the encephalopathy. The pathogenesis of hepatic encephalopathy is complex (Fig. 39-19). While ammonia seems to play the central role (inset; Fig. 39-19) a wide variety of pathologic changes probably contribute to the genesis of the encephalopathy. Putative mechanisms include neurotoxic effects of gut-derived molecules (*e.g.*, short-chain fatty acids, mercaptans, phenols, manganese), impairment of cerebral energy metabolism, disruption of the blood–brain barrier, and neuropathic changes that intensify neuroinhibition (*e.g.*, synthesis of endogenous ligands that activate central γ-aminobutyric acid–benzodiazepine receptors) or diminish neuroexcitation (*e.g.*, production of false neurotransmitters). For example, encephalopathic patients appear to form abnormal biogenic amines in the central nervous system that are released by neural stimulation along with, or instead of, normal neurotransmitters. Structurally, these amines are similar to norepinephrine or dopamine, but they are much less active in eliciting a response from the effector (*i.e.*, false neurotransmitters).

Despite recent insights into the etiology of hepatic encephalopathy, the ammonia hypothesis still provides the rationale for

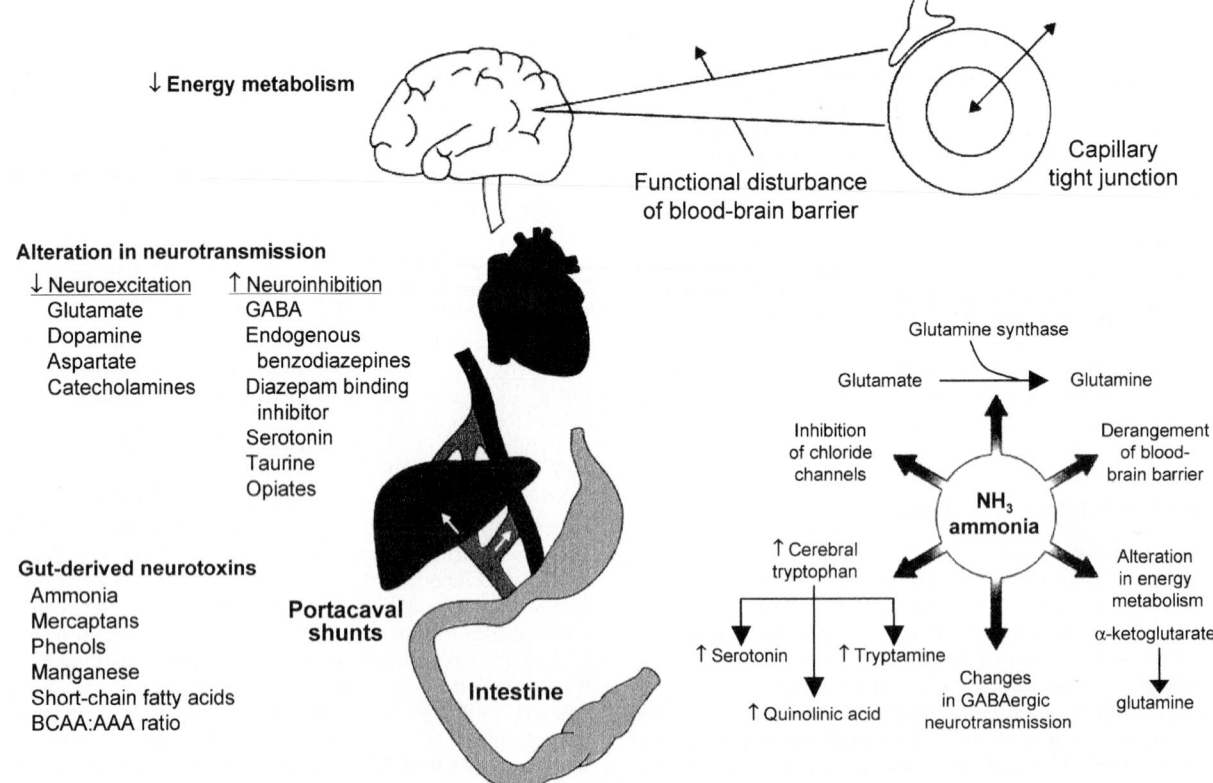

Figure 39-19. Schematic representation of pathogenesis of hepatic encephalopathy: *Inset:* proposed mechanisms of neurotoxicity of ammonia. AAA = aromatic amino acid; BCAA = branched-chain amino acid; GABA = γ-aminobutyric acid. (Reprinted with permission from Jalan R, Hayes PC: Hepatic encephalopathy and ascites. Lancet 350:1309, 1997.)

most therapies used to stabilize or reverse the encephalopathy. The diet should restrict the intake of nitrogen-containing food (protein) to minimize the synthesis of ammonia. Lactulose, which promotes ammonia excretion from the body by trapping it in the acidified fecal stream (ammonium), makes ammonia unavailable for absorption. It is especially important to prevent gastrointestinal bleeding, control infection (neomycin is usually the drug of choice), correct acid–base and electrolyte imbalances, and to titrate diuretic drugs and the fluid load. L-Dopa may facilitate renal excretion of ammonia. In addition, dopamine agonists and L-dopa may produce beneficial effects by promoting displacement of false neurotransmitters in the central nervous system.

It appears clear that encephalopathic changes are associated with clinically important alterations in pharmacodynamic and pharmacokinetics of various medications. For example, cerebral uptake of benzodiazepines increases substantially, which may reflect an increase in the density or affinity of benzodiazepine receptors or a leaky blood–brain barrier. Drugs administered to patients with advanced hepatic disease require careful titration against effect. The pathogenesis and management of hepatic encephalopathy are described in detail elsewhere.[149,152,154]

Effects on Responses to Pharmacologic Agents

Pharmacokinetic Alterations

Data concerning the pharmacokinetics of midazolam in patients with advanced liver disease are conflicting. One study[155] demonstrated a significant decrease in clearance and elimination half-life, whereas another study[156] demonstrated only slightly impaired disposition in cirrhotic patients. The pharmacokinetics of single doses of sufentanil[157] and propofol[158] were found to be similar in cirrhotic patients and those with normal hepatic function, although some differences in elimination time were observed. Such findings imply that administering infusions or multiple doses of certain intravenous drugs can result in prolonged pharmacologic effects because of impaired hepatic elimination in patients with advanced hepatic disease. The differences in the results of these studies are probably a consequence of certain differences in the binding proteins, as well as accumulation of endogenous binding inhibitors such as bilirubin. This might explain a smaller degree of midazolam protein binding in cirrhotic individuals, with a subsequent increase in the free fraction of the drug and enhancement of the pharmacologic effect in cirrhotic patients.

For thiopental, total plasma clearance and total apparent volume of distribution at the steady state are unchanged in cirrhotic patients. Therefore, the elimination half-life is not prolonged.[159] Thiopental has a low extraction ratio, so its clearance is independent of hepatic blood flow. Nonetheless, decreases in plasma protein binding, which are often unpredictable, may cause excessive pharmacologic responses to standard doses of the various agents used to induce anesthesia.

The plasma clearance of fentanyl is significantly lower in cirrhotic patients than in control subjects. The total apparent volume of distribution does not change, but the elimination half-life increases owing to decreased plasma clearance. With alfentanil, the free fraction also increases, and this agent exerts prolonged and pronounced effects in cirrhotic patients with advanced liver disease.[160]

The data regarding morphine pharmacokinetics in cirrhotic patients are contradictory. For example, Patwardhan *et al*[161] reported that the pharmacokinetics of morphine in cirrhotic patients and healthy people are similar. They suggested that "reported intolerance to the central effects of morphine cannot be explained by impaired drug elimination and increased availability of morphine to cerebral receptors."[161] Other investigators, however, reported that the clearances of free morphine and its metabolites are decreased and their half-lives prolonged in cirrhotic patients compared to healthy control subjects.[162]

Pharmacodynamic Alterations

Although hepatic disease often produces substantial pharmacokinetic changes, it also can lead to important pharmacodynamic alterations. Patients with cirrhosis, particularly those with hepatic encephalopathy, are much more sensitive to sedatives (*e.g.*, opioids and benzodiazepines) than are healthy people. For example, at equal plasma concentrations of diazepam, more pronounced encephalographic alterations occur in those with severe hepatic disease than in healthy people.[163] By contrast, pharmacologic responses to some medications decrease in patients with cirrhosis and portal hypertension as a result of the pathophysiologic changes associated with the disease. Increases in plasma concentrations of certain vasodilatory substance antagonize responses to catecholamines and other vasoconstrictors. Patients, as well as animals, with portal hypertension have elevations of plasma glucagon,[143] which substantially reduces the responses of a variety of blood vessels to catecholamines.[144] Thus, while patients with advanced liver disease often require reduced doses of central nervous system depressants (morphine, chlorpromazine, and benzodiazepines), they require increased doses of catecholamine or addition of a nonadrenergic vasoconstrictor (vasopressin) when such therapy is needed to support blood pressure.

Rational Drug Therapy

Rational drug selection mandates an understanding of the effects of hepatic disease on pharmacokinetics and pharmacodynamics, but it does not preclude the use of medications whose pharmacology is significantly altered by hepatic disease. Indeed, a drug's effects may be rendered less predictable by hepatic disease, but the drug may still be clinically preferable to an alternative agent whose pharmacology is unaffected by hepatic disease. As an illustration, cirrhotic patients require higher initial doses of *d*-tubocurarine than do healthy patients to achieve a similar degree of muscle relaxation.[164] This effect seems to be related purely to pharmacokinetic factors: cirrhotic patients have a larger volume of distribution for *d*-tubocurarine, primarily related to an increased γ-globulin fraction (greater binding of *d*-tubocurarine and a smaller free fraction). On the other hand, the presence of end-stage liver disease plus cholestasis (obstructive jaundice) results in an impairment of clearance and a potential for prolonged effects of all drugs excreted in bile, including muscle relaxants. To some clinicians, these observations might suggest the advisability of using gallamine or, particularly, atracurium, since these relaxants are not excreted with the bile.[165] However, pharmacokinetic data should not dictate therapeutic decisions, because pharmacodynamic factors, such as the undesirable effects of alternative medications, may be of greater clinical relevance. For example, severe liver disease may decrease vecuronium clearance and prolong its half-life, but it has no significant effect on gallamine clearance. This does not mean that vecuronium is contraindicated in cirrhotic patients. In fact, a cirrhotic patient with coronary artery disease may have a better outcome with cautious titration of vecuronium than with gallamine, which induces tachycardia. The lesson is clear. Owing to the pharmacodynamic and pharmacokinetic alterations that accompany hepatic disease, responses of cirrhotic patients to drugs are often unpredictable. Minimizing the adverse consequences of this unpredictability requires judicious drug selection and, perhaps more importantly, careful titration of the drug to the desirable effect.

CHOLESTATIC DISEASE

Cardiovascular Dysfunction

The presence of bile salts in circulating blood (cholemia) can impair myocardial contractility.[166] Cholemia also blunts the response to norepinephrine, angiotensin II, and isoproterenol,[167] probably by interfering with their binding to membrane receptors. Less severe hemodynamic perturbations occur in patients with biliary obstruction than in those with cirrhosis. However, the pattern of the pathophysiologic change is remarkably similar: peripheral vascular resistance decreases, cardiac output increases, portal venous pressure increases, and portal venous blood flow decreases.

Patients with hepatic disease, either parenchymal or cholestatic, have a reduced sensitivity to vasopressor drugs. The exact reasons for the decreased sensitivity is unclear. However, data from *in vitro* and *in vivo* experiments indicate that bile acids contribute to the vasodilation and hypotension that often occur in patients with biliary obstruction.[166] Conceivably, a decreased responsiveness to vasoactive substances (including catecholamines) is responsible for the interesting and clinically important observation that patients with biliary obstruction are often intolerant of even small blood losses. A moderate loss (10%) of blood volume in normal animals does not substantially decrease mean arterial pressure, but a 10% loss of blood volume in animals with experimentally induced biliary obstruction causes severe (~50%) arterial hypotension. Intact animals respond to such blood loss with an approximately 15% decrease in blood volumes in both the pulmonary and splanchnic vascular beds. Animals with biliary obstruction have only a 7% decrease of their pulmonary blood volume and no change in splanchnic blood volume.[167] If we can extrapolate these results to humans, patients with biliary obstruction would have an impaired hemodynamic response to blood loss. An impairment of the ability to translocate blood from pulmonary and splanchnic blood reservoirs to the systemic circulation would render patients highly susceptible to arterial hypotension from bleeding. Furthermore, the results would indicate the urgency of expeditiously replacing perioperative volume losses in this patient population. The anesthesiologist should be aware that biliary decompression may be accompanied by severe cardiovascular collapse.[168]

Coagulation Disorders

Patients with biliary obstruction are prone to certain coagulation disorders. During brief episodes of biliary obstruction, co-

agulopathy can result from a deficiency of coagulation factors whose activation depends on the presence of vitamin K. Absorption of vitamin K depends on the excretion of bile into the gastrointestinal tract. Long-lasting biliary obstruction can cause liver injury, with subsequent deterioration in the hepatic synthesis of proteins, including coagulation factors. Usually, the coagulation disorders are moderate, and parenteral vitamin K corrects the problem. If this treatment is not fully effective, one should suspect that the disease is not purely cholestatic, and that hepatic parenchymal injury exists. Should such patients need urgent surgery, the coagulopathy will require immediate treatment with fresh frozen plasma. The failure of parenteral vitamin K to correct a prolonged prothrombin time typically indicates the presence of severe hepatic parenchymal dysfunction and portends a poor prognosis.

CLINICAL APPROACH TO PATIENTS WITH ASYMPTOMATIC BIOCHEMICAL ABNORMALITIES OR OVERT LIVER DISEASE

A careful history and physical examination will usually suffice to detect patients with significant hepatic dysfunction. Unless liver disease is suspected, it is probably best not to order a panel of liver blood tests. This is because routine testing may yield false-positive results, engendering patient anxiety and prompting the performance of expensive, unnecessary, and potentially injurious invasive tests.

Perioperative physicians are presented with a dilemma when patients without clinically apparent hepatic disease have recently had liver blood tests with one or more abnormal results. The prudent course in patients with asymptomatic biochemical abnormalities may be to delay surgery and repeat the test(s) later (Fig. 39-20). This conservative approach helps to ensure that a patient is not in the early stages of a disease process that may abruptly worsen.

Assessing perioperative risks for patients with liver disease is an inexact science. Their risk of perioperative morbidity and mortality appears to depend on three major factors: (1) type

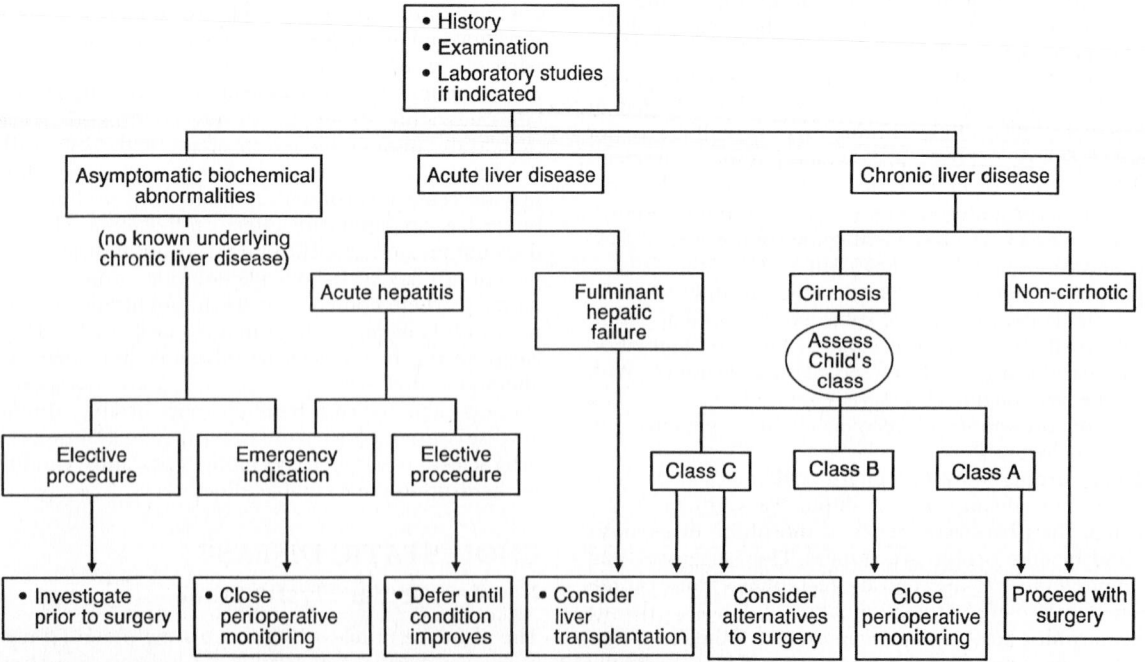

Figure 39-20. Preoperative approach to patient with known or suspected liver disease. (Modified with permission from Patel T: Surgery in the patient with liver disease. Mayo Clin Proc 74:593, 1999.)

of operation, (2) nature and severity of the underlying hepatic disease, and (3) extent of the hepatic dysfunction. Most of the data on perioperative risk derive from retrospective studies or clinical reports of cirrhotic patients undergoing abdominal surgeries rather than from large, prospective studies on the subject. Nonetheless, these data persuasively suggest that patients with severe hepatic dysfunction have a high risk for morbidity and mortality from major operative procedures. In addition, acute hepatitis (viral, alcoholic, ischemic, or drug-related) is associated with increase perioperative risk and mortality. These patients deserve supportive therapy; an improvement in their overall condition will diminish their perioperative risk. Therefore, in the presence of acute hepatic disease, elective surgery should be postponed (Fig. 39-20).

ANESTHESIA FOR PATIENTS WITH MODERATE-TO-SEVERE LIVER DISEASE (HEPATITIS, CIRRHOSIS)

Significant liver disease greatly increases the risk of postoperative hepatic complications, especially after emergency surgery.[169] These risks are greater for abdominal operations than for peripheral or superficial procedures. The severity of the hepatic dysfunction, as assessed by the Child-Pugh classification (Table 39-7), correlates with the incidence of both perioperative complications (liver failure, bleeding, infection, sepsis, renal failure, pulmonary failure, and ascites)[170,171] and mortality.[1]

Preoperative Evaluation

During the preoperative visit, the anesthesiologist should note current medications (including pharmaceutical and herbal preparations). The history should include mention of previous jaundice, blood product transfusions, gastrointestinal bleeding, prior surgeries and the anesthetic management techniques used. In addition to the routine examination of organs and systems, the physical examination should detail the patient's appearance, and document the degree of ascites and encephalopathy. The physical evaluation of a patient with chronic liver disease is particularly valuable, as the patient may feel unwell or look ill before there is evidence of hepatic dysfunction by liver blood tests.

Blood tests should include determinations of hemoglobin and hematocrit; platelet count; serum bilirubin; serum electrolytes; creatinine and blood urea nitrogen; arterial blood gases; serum proteins; prothrombin time; and several enzymes, including aminotransferases, alkaline phosphatase, lactate dehydrogenase, and hydroxybutyrate dehydrogenase (lactate dehydrogenase isoenzyme being more specific for liver function).

Preoperative Preparation

In nonemergent situations, surgical preparation of a patient with severe hepatic disease should focus on correcting clinical or laboratory abnormalities identified in the preoperative evaluation. A failure to correct coagulation abnormalities can predispose to major complications including hemorrhage, encephalopathy, or renal failure (hepatorenal syndrome). Significant coagulation abnormalities must be corrected before performance of spinal or epidural anesthesia to prevent the development of epidural hematomas. A patient with obstructive jaundice, who has a prolonged PT or an increased INR, can receive a trial of vitamin K (10 mg im 3 times a day for a few days) to correct the problem. If this therapy is unsuccessful, or if there is insufficient time for vitamin K to be effective, administration of fresh frozen plasma is indicated. Platelet transfusions should be considered for patients with evidence of platelet dysfunction or thrombocytopenia ($<100,000$ mm^{-3}). Each unit transfused into an average adult will increase the platelet count in blood by about 10,000 mm^{-3}.

The patient's fluid and electrolyte status should be optimized before elective surgery (to minimize the risk of hepatic, splanchnic, and renal ischemia). Urine output is generally considered adequate if it is at least 1 ml $\cdot$ kg$^{-1} \cdot$ hr^{-1}. If a patient has been aggressively diuresed, he or she may require proper fluid therapy to correct volume deficits and electrolyte abnormalities. A central venous catheter may suffice to guide fluid administration to patients with relatively normal myocardial and pulmonary function. For those with severe cardiorespiratory or renal dysfunction, however, pulmonary artery catheterization may be required. To tailor intravenous fluid therapy to meet the specific needs of each patient requires obtaining blood samples at appropriate intervals. Using this laboratory information, the appropriate fluids can be selected to normalize volume deficits, electrolyte imbalances (especially sodium, potassium, and ionized calcium), as well as abnormalities of blood glucose and hemoglobin. In patients with excessive intravascular fluid, diuretic therapy may include furosemide, mannitol, or both, and a low dose of dopamine (2–4 ml $\cdot$ kg$^{-1} \cdot$ min^{-1}), owing to its antialdosterone effect and ability to produce renal vasodilation. Perioperative administration of spironolactone may also be a diuretic of choice because of its strong antialdosterone activity.

Medications needed to control the myriad complications of severe liver disease should be continued throughout the periop-

Table 39-7. MODIFIED CHILD-PUGH SCORE

Presentation	Points*		
	1	2	3
Albumin (g $\cdot$ dl^{-1})	>3.5	2.8–3.5	<2.8
Prothrombin time			
Seconds prolonged	<4	4–6	>6
International normalized ratio	<1.7	1.7–2.3	>2.3
Bilirubin (mg $\cdot$ dl^{-1})†	<2	2–3	>3
Ascites	Absent	Slight–moderate	Tense
Encephalopathy	None	Grade I–II	Grade III–IV

* Class A = 5–6 points; B = 7–9 points; C = 10–15 points.
† Cholestatic diseases (*e.g.*, primary biliary cirrhosis) produce bilirubin elevations that are disproportionate to the hepatic dysfunction. Thus, the following adjustments should be made: assign 1 point for a bilirubin level of 4 mg $\cdot$ dl^{-1}; 2 points for bilirubin concentrations between 4 and 10 mg $\cdot$ dl^{-1}; and 3 points for bilirubin $>$ 10 mg $\cdot$ dl^{-1}.
From Kamath PS: Clinical approach to the patient with abnormal liver test results. Mayo Clin Pro 71:1089, 1996, with permission.

erative period. Preoperative sedatives, when indicated, should be used in lower doses because of the marked derangements in pharmacokinetics and pharmacodynamics associated with advanced liver disease. These patients may have a full stomach, even if they have not taken food or fluid for several hours, because of hiatal hernia, massive ascites, and decreased gastric and intestinal motility. Therefore, premedication may include an H_2 histamine receptor blocker (e.g., ranitidine), metoclopramide, as well as sodium citrate.

Monitoring

In addition to using the routine array of monitors required by the ASA, the need for invasive monitoring will be dictated by the severity of the liver disease and type of surgery. For severely ill patients or major operative procedures, cannulation of an artery is important for direct blood pressure monitoring, as well as for periodic determinations of blood gases, electrolytes, hematocrit, and other laboratory data as needed during surgery. Because patients with advanced liver disease require fluids to be titrated carefully, insertion of a pulmonary artery catheter, or at least a central venous catheter, is often necessary. It is always important to monitor the urine output of patients with advanced liver disease when they undergo operations lasting longer than an hour. Surgical procedures associated with extensive blood loss (e.g., liver transplantation) require monitoring of the blood coagulation status, including periodic determinations of prothrombin time, partial thromboplastin time, and platelet count. Thromboelastography may be helpful.[172] A transcutaneous nerve stimulator facilitates the titration of muscle relaxants, especially when treating cirrhotic patients in whom the effects of muscle relaxants are often unpredictable.

Selection of Anesthetic Technique

Regional anesthesia is generally the preferred anesthetic technique in patients without coagulation abnormalities who are undergoing peripheral surgery. However, it would be difficult to justify using regional anesthesia or analgesia for patients with overt coagulopathies who undergo major operations. Local anesthesia with sedation is usually the best approach for relatively minor procedures, such as sclerotherapy. A short-acting benzodiazepine, such as midazolam combined with remifentanil, or a low dose of fentanyl, will usually provide sedation, anxiolysis, and analgesia. As mentioned previously, patients with advanced hepatic disease have extensive pharmacodynamic and pharmacokinetic abnormalities, so each medication should be titrated carefully to achieve the desired effect.

Induction of General Anesthesia

Rapid-sequence induction (or awake intubation of the trachea) is indicated in patients perceived to be at risk for aspiration pneumonitis (full stomach). All widely used intravenous induction agents have been administered to patients with advanced hepatic disease. For patients who do not require rapid-sequence induction, careful titration of the anesthetic will minimize hemodynamic lability while achieving the desired anesthetic effect. Succinylcholine is a reasonable choice to facilitate endotracheal intubation. Although severe liver dysfunction can markedly decrease cholinesterase activity and may prolong the effect of succinylcholine somewhat, this rarely causes a clinical problem. When using nondepolarizing neuromuscular blocking agents to induce anesthesia, consider that the initial dose to achieve total relaxation may be higher than in healthy patients. This increased dose requirement results primarily from pharmacokinetic alterations and pertains to relaxants such as atracurium,[173] d-tubocurarine, and pancuronium,[174] but not to vecuronium.[175]

Maintenance of Anesthesia

Intraoperative liver injury can develop from oxygen deprivation, the stress response, drug toxicity, blood transfusion, and infection. An impairment of hepatic oxygen supply can occur at any step in the process of delivering oxygen to the liver. Hypoxic hypoxia may result from inadequate F_{IO_2} or hypoventilation. Anemic hypoxia may develop when the oxygen-carrying capacity of the blood (hematocrit) is inadequate. Circulatory hypoxia may result from systemic (hypovolemia, arterial hypotension, reduction in cardiac output) or regional (decrease in hepatic blood and oxygen supply) hemodynamic disorders. Delivery of blood and oxygen to the liver may decrease owing to systemic circulatory disturbances, surgical manipulation of the liver or adjacent structures, or from endogenous vasoconstrictors (e.g., renin–angiotensin, catecholamines, and antidiuretic hormone). Anesthetics or other medications that impair electron transport could also induce histotoxic hypoxia, but this mechanism does not appear to be clinically important.

In addition to assuring adequate oxygen supply, one must always consider the oxygen supply–demand relations in the liver. Experimental data indicate that severe surgical stress during fentanyl (moderate dose) anesthesia can produce a somewhat higher hepatic oxygen supply and uptake than an identical stress during isoflurane anesthesia; this results in similar values of hepatic oxygen supply–uptake ratio with the two anesthetics.[83] Taking this into consideration, the guiding principle is to maintain adequate pulmonary ventilation and cardiovascular function, including cardiac output, blood volume, and perfusion pressures. One should strive to prevent arterial hypotension by adequate blood and volume replacement and avoidance of relative overdoses of anesthetics or other blood pressure–lowering drugs. Vasodilation, a reduced perfusion pressure, and a decrease in blood velocity will inevitably increase oxygen extraction in all tissues, including those in the preportal area. A decreased blood velocity and an increased oxygen extraction will cause a decrease in venous oxygen content—in this case, decreased oxygen content in the portal venous blood. A reduction in portal blood oxygen content or flow usually leads to a compensatory increase in hepatic arterial flow. Thus, hepatic injury after moderate arterial hypotension is a relatively rare event. However, in the presence of severe liver dysfunction, the ability of autoregulatory mechanisms to increase hepatic arterial blood flow may be diminished or abolished.[176] Therefore, with severe hepatic disease, the hepatic arterial blood flow may not increase when portal blood flow or oxygen content decreases. This might lead to hepatic oxygen deprivation. Thus, the lesson is clear: take all precautions to avoid arterial hypotension as well as low cardiac output states.

When performing general anesthesia, it seems prudent to avoid halothane, and possibly enflurane, because they cause the most prominent decreases in hepatic blood and oxygen supply and are associated with the highest incidences of postoperative hepatic dysfunction. Isoflurane and probably sevoflurane appear to be the anesthetics of choice for inhalational anesthesia. Nitrous oxide does not appear to be associated with major hepatic complications in patients with advanced liver disease despite its abilities to produce sympathomimetic effects and to limit the maximum oxygen content of arterial blood. Opioids are reasonable to include in the anesthetics of patients with hepatic disease. Despite certain pharmacokinetic concerns (decreased clearance and prolonged half-life), fentanyl is probably the opioid of choice. Interestingly, fentanyl neither decreases the hepatic oxygen or blood supply nor prevents an increase in hepatic oxygen requirements when used in moderate doses. Therefore, the oxygen supply-demand relation in the liver is no better with a fentanyl-based anesthetic than during anesthesia with isoflurane.[83] It seems that anesthetic management using inhaled agents (especially isoflurane or sevoflurane) alone or in combination with small doses of fentanyl would be the method of choice, provided that adequate pulmonary ventilation, cardiac output, and arterial pressures are maintained. Many other agents also have favorable risk–benefit profiles for patients with advanced hepatic disease.

Because substantial alterations in pharmacokinetics occur in patients with advanced hepatic disease, dose requirements for a variety of medications can be unpredictable. For example, the hepatic clearance of lidocaine may be increased by more than 300%, and benzodiazepines by more than 100%. Drugs that bind to albumin (e.g., thiopental) usually have a decreased volume of distribution, so a lower initial dose will be required. The volume of distribution of other agents, such as muscle relaxants, may increase substantially for various reasons, including an increase in γ-globulin concentration or the presence of edema. This appears to account for the so-called resistance to such agents and explains why the initial dose requirements of these medications are increased in cirrhotic patients. However, subsequent dose requirements may be decreased, and drug effects prolonged, owing to decreases in hepatic blood flow, impaired hepatic clearance, and possible renal dysfunction (e.g., d-tubocurarine or pancuronium). Advanced hepatic disease does not appear to significantly affect the pharmacokinetics of vecuronium, although some dose-dependent pharmacokinetic alterations may occur.[175] This may be the result of a limited hepatic uptake capacity, which is usually exceeded at doses greater than 0.15 mg $\cdot$ kg^{-1}. At lower doses, hepatic dysfunction does not affect the pharmacokinetics or duration of action of vecuronium.[175]

Severe hepatic dysfunction per se does not contraindicate the use of any specific muscle relaxant. Atracurium has a theoretical advantage because its elimination occurs mainly by Hofmann decomposition, making its clearance relatively independent of renal or hepatic function. Thus, both the elimination half-life and clearance of atracurium are similar in healthy subjects and cirrhotic patients with impaired renal function. However, volumes of distribution are larger and, accordingly, the distribution half-life is shorter in patients with severe hepatorenal dysfunction compared with normal individuals.[173] The only situation that appears to prolong the elimination half-life of atracurium is marked metabolic acidosis, which may decrease the rate of Hofmann decomposition.[173] Rapacuronium, which has a more rapid onset and shorter duration of action than other currently used nondepolarizing agents, may have advantages in patients with cirrhosis. A recent study of cirrhotic patients (Child-Pugh score of 7; see Table 39-7) showed that the onset and recovery rate from a single bolus dose (1.5 mg $\cdot$ kg^{-1}) of rapacuronium is similar in cirrhotic patients and in patients with normal hepatic function.[177] The presence of cirrhosis did not affect the elimination half-life or plasma clearance of rapacuronium.

The pharmacokinetics of many muscle relaxants in conditions of cholestasis and obstructive jaundice may be altered: prolonged duration of action has been demonstrated.[178] However, when postoperative ventilation of the lungs is planned, vecuronium, atracurium, and pancuronium can be used successfully. Titration of any relaxant according to transcutaneous nerve stimulation monitoring is beneficial.

Although pharmacokinetic studies in patients with hepatic cirrhosis provide interesting results that are helpful in understanding the pathogenic aspects of chronic liver disease, the results do not have significant value for predicting the safety of a drug. The degree of hepatic dysfunction affects the degree of pharmacokinetic disorder; therefore, the best way to avoid complications when administering medications is to titrate to effect.

Renal function must be maintained by administering proper fluid therapy (volume and content), including diuretics, as needed. It can be extremely difficult to maintain the proper fluid balance without monitoring filling pressures. Therefore, insertion of a pulmonary artery catheter, or at least a central venous catheter, is often indicated. The contents of infused solutions should be initially selected and subsequently adjusted based upon periodic determinations of blood electrolyte concentrations. For example, when the serum sodium concentration is normal or elevated, a solution with a little or no sodium is indicated (5% glucose in water). A decrease in serum sodium below $130-135$ mEq $\cdot$ l^{-1} would favor the use of a sodium-containing solution such as Normosol. Furosemide and mannitol are often effective diuretics in these patients. Infusion of a low dose of dopamine ($2-4$ mg $\cdot$ kg^{-1} $\cdot$ min^{-1}) can also be beneficial owing to its many pharmacologic actions, including enhancement of renal perfusion and antagonism of the aldosterone effect.

The parameters of controlled ventilation should be carefully selected to avoid an unnecessary increase in intrathoracic pressure which may impede venous return, thereby decreasing cardiac output. Hypocarbia should probably be avoided because it can aggravate hepatic encephalopathy. As mentioned previously, opioids may induce spasm of the sphincter of Oddi (see Fig. 39-12) in nearly 3% of opioid-treated patients.[107] This spasm can be relieved by many agents, including antimuscarinic drugs such as atropine. The clinical disadvantage of this treatment is the accompanying tachycardia. Naloxone relaxes the sphincter of Oddi, but it also antagonizes the analgesic effects of the opioid, increasing the requirements for supplemental anesthetics. The potential of naloxone to produce cardiovascular complications should also be kept in mind. Glucagon effectively relaxes biliary smooth muscle; however, it might not be the drug of choice because it can cause many untoward effects, including hyperglycemia and a hyperdynamic cardiovascular state. Finally, nitroglycerin is effective in relieving opioid-induced spasm of the sphincter of Oddi. Volatile anesthetics similarly attenuate contractile responses of the sphincter to opioids.

Because coagulopathy can develop during surgery, perioperative monitoring of the coagulation state is important. Treatment may include administration of platelets, fresh frozen plasma, cryoprecipitate, and sometimes ε-aminocaproic acid. Interestingly, coagulopathies that develop during liver transplantation are occasionally caused by heparin, which had been sequestered in, and subsequently washed from, the graft. Protamine sulfate effectively reverses this effect of heparin. Although patients with advanced liver disease are at risk for fibrinolysis and disseminated intravascular coagulation, a note of caution is in order: overly aggressive treatment of a coagulopathy, especially in patients on anti-fibrinolytic therapy, may lead to a hypercoagulable state, thrombosis, and pulmonary embolism.

POSTOPERATIVE LIVER DYSFUNCTION: AN OVERVIEW

Postoperative liver dysfunction is common, but rarely severe. While it is usually asymptomatic, it may progress to overt liver failure on rare occasions.

Mild, transient increases in serum concentrations of hepatic enzymes are often detectable within hours of surgery but do not usually persist for more than 2 days. Such subclinical hepatocellular injury occurs in as many as 20% of patients who receive enflurane anesthesia and in nearly 50% of those receiving halothane.[122,179] Jaundice rarely occurs in healthy patients following minor operations but appears in up to 20% of patients after major surgical procedures.[179] Jaundice is typically the earliest sign of serious hepatic or hepatobiliary dysfunction and therefore requires prompt medical attention. Marked increases of serum aminotransferase activities are an ominous finding, reflecting extensive hepatocellular necrosis.

Severe Postoperative Liver Dysfunction

Some cases of severe postoperative liver dysfunction are apparent hours after surgery (e.g., with hypoxic injury), whereas other cases are delayed in onset for days to weeks (e.g., with anesthesia-induced hepatitis). With severe postoperative liver dysfunction, residual liver function may fall below a critical threshold, leading to the development of hepatic encephalopathy. If encephalopathy occurs within 2 weeks of the onset of jaundice or within 8 weeks of the initial manifestation of hepatic disease, the disorder is defined as fulminant hepatic failure. Fulminant hepatic failure has a variety of causes.[180] The mortality rate from fulminant hepatic failure correlates with the severity of encephalopathy. The shorter the interval between the appearance of jaundice and presentation of encephalopathy, the worse the prognosis.

Treatment of Fulminant Hepatic Failure

Successful treatment of patients with fulminant hepatic failure requires the clinician to make prompt and accurate predictions about the outcome of the disease. Proper recognition of reversible disease obviates unnecessary orthotopic liver transplantation (OLT). Irreversible cases of fulminant hepatic failure require immediate identification. Otherwise, the severe complications of fulminant hepatic failure that develop may render patients unacceptable candidates for OLT.

CAUSES OF POSTOPERATIVE LIVER DYSFUNCTION UNRELATED TO PERIOPERATIVE FACTORS

Asymptomatic Diseases

Although postoperative liver dysfunction can clearly result from anesthetic or surgical interventions, it is often unrelated to perioperative factors. For example, it can arise from pre-existing liver disease that has escaped preoperative detection. According to a study by Schemel[181] the prevalence of acute, asymptomatic liver disease in a healthy-appearing surgical population may approach 0.25%. During a 1-year period, Schemel and co-workers performed multiple laboratory screening tests in 7620 patients (ASA Physical Status 1) scheduled for elective surgical procedures. Eleven of these patients (approximately 1 per 700) were found to have abnormal increases of AST, ALT, and LDH, and the proposed surgeries were canceled. All 11 proved to have overt hepatic disorders (infectious mononucleosis, viral hepatitis, cirrhosis, or alcoholic hepatitis), and three later became clinically jaundiced (overall incidence of jaundice of 1:2540). Had any of these three patients actually received a halogenated anesthetic, with the subsequent development of overt hepatic disease between the 6th and 14th postoperative days, their diseases may well have been diagnosed erroneously as anesthesia-induced hepatitis. None of the 7609 patients who underwent anesthesia and surgery exhibited laboratory evidence of pre-existing hepatic disease, and none developed unexplained postsurgical jaundice. Another clinical study[182] has documented a prevalence of unsuspected preoperative hepatic dysfunction similar to that reported by Schemel. Thus, it appears that approximately 1 out of every 2500 healthy patients who undergo surgery and anesthesia may have clinically significant postoperative liver dysfunction that is totally unrelated to surgery or anesthesia.

Unrecognized Pre-existing Hepatic Injury Caused by Drugs or Medications

Because a pre-existing disease is more likely than an anesthetic agent to cause severe postoperative liver dysfunction, the preoperative evaluation should address the important risk factors for liver disease. These include use of potentially hepatotoxic medications or illicit drugs (cocaine), alcoholism, prior episodes of jaundice or history of viral hepatitis, congenital disorders (e.g., Gilbert's disease), and systemic diseases or conditions associated with hepatic pathology (e.g., pre-eclampsia). Exposure to environmental and occupational hepatotoxins should also be considered as possible causes of liver disease of unknown origin.[183] Hepatotoxins can produce a broad spectrum of liver disorders, including abnormal liver blood tests in asymptomatic patients, steatosis, acute or chronic hepatitis, fulminant hepatic necrosis, cirrhosis, veno-occlusive disease, and hepatic neoplasia.

Use of prescription and over-the-counter medications is ubiquitous. Polypharmacy is the rule rather than the exception, especially in elderly and debilitated patients who undergo major operations. Thus, the capacity of pharmacologic agents to injure the liver is an important perioperative concern. Some 500–1000 therapeutic agents have been implicated in a broad spectrum of liver diseases.[184] These diseases may be classified in accordance with whether the drug produces primarily direct cell toxicity (necrosis), cholestasis (cessation of bile flow), or steatosis (fatty liver). Most forms of drug-induced liver disease are benign and of little consequence (estrogen-induced cholestasis), producing only transient alterations of liver blood tests. Severe drug toxicities, which are typically dose-related (acetaminophen) or idiosyncratic (halothane), are responsible for 15–30% of the cases of fulminant hepatic failure and 20–50% of the cases of chronic hepatitis (nonviral). Moreover, when drug reactions produce hepatocellular necrosis, the estimated case fatality approaches 50%.

Drugs known to produce hepatocellular injury and centrilobular necrosis include acetaminophen, isoniazid, and methyldopa. Other cytotoxic drugs include oxyphenisatin, rifampin, papaverine, phenytoin,[185] indomethacin, monoamine oxidase inhibitors, and amitriptyline.[186] The use of dantrolene for treatment of muscle spastic disorders has been associated with the development of hepatic failure in patients receiving the drug for more than 60 days. Cholestatic reactions often result from drugs such as chlorpromazine, phenylbutazone, and androgenic and anabolic steroids. In at least one case, erythromycin (ethylsuccinate form) has caused hepatic failure that had initially been attributed to halothane administration.

A drug's potential to cause hepatotoxicity is influenced by various pharmacologic (other drugs) or pathophysiologic (hepatitis) factors. For example, the combination of trimethoprim sulfamethoxazole is nearly five times more frequently associated with hepatotoxicity than sulfamethoxazole alone. By inducing hepatic microsomal drug-metabolizing systems, some drugs can markedly increase the injurious potential of others by altering their metabolism to favor the production of toxic metabolites. For example, phenobarbital increases the hepatotoxicity of various drugs including chemotherapeutic agents (methotrexate) and antibiotics (tetracycline).[187]

Ethanol is obviously an important hepatotoxin. Although elective surgery is not contraindicated in patients with alcoholic steatosis, the mortality from acute alcoholic hepatitis, even without surgery, is significant. Animal studies indicate that alcohol ingestion increases the likelihood that centrilobular necrosis will develop after halothane anesthesia, which may relate to the ability of ethanol to increase hepatic hypoxia. Therefore, if alcoholic hepatitis is suspected, further examination of liver function is warranted before performing an elective operation.

Congenital Disorders

The most common cause of jaundice in the United States is a benign metabolic disorder known as Gilbert's syndrome (familial unconjugated hyperbilirubinemia). In this syndrome, bilirubin uptake by the liver is impaired and the activity of bilirubin glucuronyl transferase is decreased. Patients often do not manifest their disease until the second decade of life. Stress, fasting, fever, and infection can exacerbate this condition. Diagnosis is suggested by clinical (jaundice without dark urine) and laboratory (unconjugated hyperbilirubinemia) abnormalities.

A less common metabolic disorder, the Crigler-Najjar syndrome (type II), is also associated with unconjugated hyperbilirubinemia; surgical and anesthetic-related problems are apparently minimal. However, surgery can exacerbate the Dubin-Johnson syndrome.

Pregnancy-Related Disorders

Well known disorders of pregnancy that cause fulminant hepatic failure during the third trimester or in the immediate postpartum period include acute fatty liver of pregnancy (AFLP) and the HELLP syndrome (hemolysis, elevated liver enzymes, and low platelet count). In addition, parturients are unusually susceptible to morbidity and mortality from hepatitis E infection.[188] It is unclear how the natural courses of these diseases are affected by the analgesic or anesthetic techniques used for vaginal or abdominal deliveries.

Acute Fatty Liver of Pregnancy

A rare disease that occurs in the late stages of pregnancy, AFLP probably represents an abnormality of lipid metabolism. Jaundice, encephalopathy, hypoglycemia, and pre-eclampsia are common, but hypertension is rare (incidence of 1 in 13,000 births) with advanced liver failure. Liver biopsy shows infiltration of centrilobular hepatocytes with microvesicular fat, producing a histopathologic picture that is strikingly similar to that seen in disorders called hepatic microvesicular steatosis (including Reye's syndrome and injury produced by valproic acid or tetracycline). Serum aminotransferases typically do not exceed 1000 IU · l^{-1} because hepatocellular necrosis is not a major feature of this disease. When AFLP is diagnosed, delivery of the fetus is expedited, usually by induction of labor or, occasionally, cesarean section. Some patients continue to decline clinically after delivery, but most begin to recover by the third day postpartum. On rare occasions, liver transplantation has been necessary. Recurrence of AFLP with future pregnancy is uncommon.

Pre-eclampsia and HELLP

Defined by Louis Weinstein in 1982, the HELLP syndrome (Hemolysis Elevated Liver enzymes Low Platelets) is much more common and generally occurs earlier in pregnancy than AFLP. This syndrome, which appears to represent a severe manifestation of pre-eclampsia, affects about 10% of all pre-eclamptic women. In some cases, pregnancy-induced hypertension (in the absence of pre-eclampsia) adversely affects hepatic function. This presumably results from marginal hepatic perfusion, owing to profound peripheral vasoconstriction accompanied by hypovolemia and starvation.[189]

On liver biopsy, pre-eclampsia has three characteristic histopathologic features: diffuse fibrin deposition along the sinusoids; periportal and portal tract hemorrhage; and ischemic necrosis, which is usually focal but occasionally confluent. Because hepatocellular necrosis is present in all patients with HELLP, serum aminotransferases are almost invariably increased; mean values of AST and ALT are 434 and 239 IU · l^{-1}, respectively. At times, the degree to which laboratory abnormalities reflect hepatic dysfunction is difficult to assess. For example, hyperbilirubinemia, which occurs in approximately 40% of cases of HELLP, may be caused by a combination of hemolysis and liver dysfunction.

Hepatic hemorrhage or rupture probably results from confluent hepatocellular necrosis from pre-eclampsia. Abdominal computed tomography scans in women with few symptoms other than right upper quadrant abdominal pain suggest that hepatic hemorrhage may occur in up to 2% of women with

pre-eclampsia. The most important factors in ensuring maternal survival following hepatic rupture are prompt identification of this disorder before irreversible shock occurs, vigorous hemodynamic support, and emergency laparotomy if Glisson's capsule has ruptured.

CONCLUSION: PREVENTION AND TREATMENT OF POSTOPERATIVE LIVER DYSFUNCTION

Identifying patients at high risk for developing liver dysfunction or for having an exacerbation of pre-existing liver disease is of utmost importance for minimizing the morbidity and mortality in such patients. Thus, a careful preoperative evaluation is required to detect pre-existing liver disease and to identify important risk factors for anesthesia-induced hepatic injury. Perioperative physicians who are armed with an understanding of the interactions among liver disease, surgical procedures, and anesthetic interventions can formulate and orchestrate therapeutic plans to optimize patient outcome.

When liver abnormalities are recognized preoperatively, it is prudent to defer elective procedures until the course of the disease can be determined. For operations that cannot be deferred, clinically significant pathophysiologic changes associated with the liver disease (e.g., coagulopathy, fluid and electrolytes abnormalities) should be corrected as soon as practical.

Which anesthetic technique best preserves the function of the liver? The choice of anesthesia is usually an insignificant issue for peripheral or minor surgery (operations that do not affect splanchnic blood flow), even in patients with severe liver disease. Regional anesthetic techniques, when appropriate (e.g., absence of coagulopathy), are often preferred because they often minimize the cardiovascular and pulmonary perturbations associated with anesthesia. The selection of pharmacologic anesthetic agents may have important implications, especially in patients undergoing major operations. A rational approach to general anesthesia would include the use of agents that preserve cardiac output and do not adversely affect the oxygen supply–demand relationships of the liver (e.g., isoflurane, sevoflurane, fentanyl, remifentanil). Throughout the perioperative period, medications must be carefully titrated to achieve the desired pharmacologic effects while minimizing untoward effects; this can be challenging because pharmacokinetics and pharmacodynamics of many drugs are often unpredictable in patients with hepatobiliary dysfunction.

A primary goal during the maintenance of anesthesia is to ensure the adequacy of hepatic and renal perfusion, especially in patients with severe liver disease who undergo major abdominal operations. Although well tolerated in the absence of liver disease, hepatic hypoperfusion in patients recovering from infectious hepatitis or chronic alcoholics can have devastating consequences. These patients may be highly susceptible to hepatic ischemia because of critically compromised liver blood flow, impaired pressure-flow autoregulation, and a dysfunctional hepatic arterial buffer response. In such cases, invasive monitoring of the circulation is indicated, so that acute hypovolemia can be rapidly detected and expeditiously treated.

Although anesthesia-induced hepatitis rarely occurs, we must remain aware of the association between this disorder and the use of halogenated vapors. Halothane hepatitis produces high rates of morbidity and mortality, and survival of the most severely affected may necessitate liver transplantation. The disease affects primarily middle-aged people, particularly obese females. A history of fever or unexplained jaundice after a previous halothane anesthetic is a contraindication to another halothane anesthetic. A history of anesthesia-induced hepatitis may also be a reason to avoid general anesthesia with any inhaled vapor. This admonition, however, is predicated on remote possibilities: that immune crossover could occur with various halogenated vapors, or that the anesthesia apparatus could harbor residual amounts of the offending anesthetic, allowing trace amounts to enter the patient and trigger an allergic response. In the final analysis, avoiding the use of halothane is perhaps the single most effective way to decrease the frequency of anesthesia-induced hepatitis.

When postoperative hepatic injury occurs, the mainstay of therapy is supportive. A thorough search is required to identify any reversible cause of the injury. The hepatotoxic potentials of all medications merit consideration. Discontinue any medication that is suspect. Search for all sources of sepsis, as the presence of sepsis mandates rapid, aggressive therapy. Consider extrahepatic biliary obstruction in the differential diagnosis because this may require prompt surgical intervention. In some cases, identifying the pathogen or documenting the type of hepatic injury requires a percutaneous liver biopsy. Judicious use of biochemical tests and imaging studies, which can help delineate hepatocellular from cholestatic dysfunction, usually shortens the list of diagnostic possibilities and provides useful prognostic information.

REFERENCES

1. Powell-Jackson P, Greenway B, Williams R: Adverse effects of exploratory laparotomy in patients with unsuspected liver disease. Br J Surg 69:449, 1982
2. Aranha GV, Greenlee HB: Intra-abdominal surgery in patients with advanced cirrhosis. Arch Surg 121:275, 1986
3. Jones AL: Anatomy of the normal liver. In Zakim D, Boyer T (eds): Hepatology: A Textbook of Liver Disease, 3rd ed, p 3. Philadelphia, WB Saunders, 1996
4. Gazelle GS, Lee MJ, Mueller PR: Cholangiographic segmental anatomy of the liver. Radiographics 14:1005, 1994
5. Parks RW, Chrysos E, Diamond T: Management of liver trauma. [Review]. Br J Surg 86:1121, 1999
6. Lautt WW: The 1995 Ciba-Geigy Award Lecture: Intrinsic regulation of hepatic blood flow. Can J Physiol Pharmacol 74:223, 1996
7. Gelman S, Ernst EA: Role of pH, PCO_2, and O_2 content of portal blood in hepatic circulatory autoregulation. Am J Physiol 233:E255, 1977
8. Adedoyin A, Branch RA: Pharmacokinetics. In Zakim D, Boyer T (eds): Hepatology: A Textbook of Liver Disease, 3rd ed, p 307. Philadelphia, WB Saunders; 1996
9. Friedman L, Martin P, Munoz S: Liver function tests and the objective evaluation of the patient with liver disease. In Zakim D, Boyer T (eds): Hepatology: A Textbook of Liver Disease, 3rd ed, p 791. Philadelphia, WB Saunders; 1996
10. Hussey AJ, Aldridge LM, Paul D et al: Plasma glutathione S-transferase concentration as a measure of hepatocellular integrity following a single general anaesthetic with halothane, enflurane or isoflurane. Br J Anaesth 60:130, 1988
11. Redick JA, Jakoby WB, Baron J: Immunohistochemical localization of glutathione S-transferases in livers of untreated rats. J Biol Chem 257:15200, 1982
12. Maynard ND, Bihari DJ, Dalton RN et al: Liver function and splanchnic ischemia in critically ill patients. Chest 111:180, 1997
13. Njoku D, Laster MJ, Gong DH et al: Biotransformation of halothane, enflurane, isoflurane, and desflurane to trifluoroacetylated liver proteins: Association between protein acylation and hepatic injury. Anesth Analg 84:173, 1997
14. Lewis JH, Zimmerman HJ, Ishak KG, Mullick FG: Enflurane hepatotoxicity: A clinicopathologic study of 24 cases. Ann Intern Med 98:984, 1983
15. Eger EI, Smuckler EA, Ferrell LD et al: Is enflurane hepatotoxic? Anesth Analg 65:21, 1986
16. Carrigan TW, Straughen WJ: A report of hepatic necrosis and death following isoflurane anesthesia. Anesthesiology 67:581, 1987
17. Watanabe K, Hatakenaka S, Ikemune K et al: A case of suspected liver dysfunction induced by sevoflurane anesthesia [in Japanese]. Masui—Japanese Journal of Anesthesiology 42:902, 1993
18. Shichinohe Y, Masuda Y, Takahashi H et al: A case of postoperative hepatic injury after sevoflurane anesthesia [in Japanese]. Masui—Japanese Journal of Anesthesiology 41:1802, 1992
19. Ogawa M, Doi K, Mitsufuji T et al: Drug-induced hepatitis following

20. Martin JL, Plevak DJ, Flannery KD et al: Hepatotoxicity after desflurane anesthesia. Anesthesiology 83:1125, 1995
21. Anonymous: Summary of the National Halothane Study: Possible association between halothane anesthesia and postoperative hepatic necrosis. JAMA 197:775, 1966
22. Touloukian J, Kaplowitz N: Halothane-induced hepatic disease. Semin Liver Dis 1:134, 1981
23. Kenna JG, Jones RM: The organ toxicity of inhaled anesthetics. Anesth Analg 81(suppl 6):S51, 1995
24. Eger E: Anesthetic-induced hepatitis. In International Anesthesia Research Society Review Course Lectures, p 116. Cleveland, International Anesthesia Research Society, 1986
25. Inman WH, Mushin WW: Jaundice after repeated exposure to halothane: An analysis of reports to the Committee on Safety of Medicines. BMJ 1:5, 1974
26. Bottinger L, Dalen E, Hallen B: Halothane-induced liver damage: An analysis of the material reported to the Swedish Adverse Drug Reaction Committee 1966–1973. Acta Anaesthesiol Scand 20:40, 1976
27. Mushlin PS, Gelman S: Liver dysfunction after anesthesia. In Benumof JL, Saidman LJ (eds): Anesthesia and Perioperative Complications, 2nd ed, p 441. St. Louis, Mosby; 1999
28. Bottiger LE, Dalen E, Hallen B: Halothane-induced liver damage: an analysis of the material reported to the Swedish Adverse Drug Reaction Committee, 1966–1973. Acta Anaesthesiol Scand 20:40, 1976
29. Moult PJ, Sherlock S: Halothane-related hepatitis: A clinical study of twenty-six cases. QJM 44:99, 1975
30. Walton B, Simpson BR, Strunin L et al: Unexplained hepatitis following halothane. BMJ 1:1171, 1976
31. Peters RL, Edmondson HA, Reynolds TB et al: Hepatic necrosis associated with halothane anesthesia. Am J Med 47:748, 1969
32. Klion FM, Schaffner F, Popper H: Hepatitis after exposure to halothane. Ann Intern Med 71:467, 1969
33. Neuberger J, Williams R: Halothane anaesthesia and liver damage. BMJ 289:1136, 1984
34. Hoft R, et al: Halothane hepatitis in three pairs of closely related women. N Engl J Med 304:1023, 1981
35. Brown BJ, Gandolfi A: Adverse effects of volatile anaesthetics. Br J Anaesth 59:14, 1987
36. Otsuka S et al: HLA antigens in patients with unexplained hepatitis following halothane anesthesia. Acta Anaesthesiol Scand 29:497, 1985
37. Kenna J et al: Halothane hepatitis in children. BMJ 294:1209, 1987
38. Warner LO, Beach TP, Garvin JP, Warner EJ: Halothane and children: the first quarter century. Anesth Analg 63:838, 1984
39. Hassall E, Israel DM, Gunasekaran T, Steward D: Halothane hepatitis in children [see comments]. J Pediatr Gastroenterol Nutr 11:553, 1990
40. Schneider M: Fatal hepatic necrosis following cardiac surgery and enflurane anaesthesia [see comments]. Anaesth Intensive Care 23:225, 1995
41. Hausmann R, Schmidt B, Schellmann B, Betz P: Differential diagnosis of postoperative liver failure in a 12-year-old child. Int J Legal Med 109:210, 1996
42. Reeves M: Acute hepatitis following enflurane anaesthesia. Anaesth Intensive Care 25:80, 1997
43. Weitz J, Kienle P, Bohrer H et al: Fatal hepatic necrosis after isoflurane anaesthesia. Anaesthesia 52:892, 1997
44. Stoelting RK, Blitt CD, Cohen PJ, Merin RG: Hepatic dysfunction after isoflurane anesthesia. Anesth Analg 66:147, 1987
45. Shiraishi N, Saito H, Shiraishi H et al: A case of liver dysfunction after isoflurane anesthesia [in Japanese]. Masui—Japanese Journal of Anesthesiology 42:910, 1993
46. Sinha A, Clatch RJ, Stuck G et al: Isoflurane hepatotoxicity: A case report and review of the literature. Am J Gastroenterol 91:2406, 1996
47. Gunaratnam NT, Benson J, Gandolfi AJ, Chen M: Suspected isoflurane hepatitis in an obese patient with a history of halothane hepatitis. Anesthesiology 83:1361, 1995
48. Gelven PL, Cina SJ, Lee JD, Nichols CA: Massive hepatic necrosis and death following repeated isoflurane exposure: Case report and review of the literature. Am J Forensic Med Pathol 17:61, 1996
49. Brown B Jr: Sevoflurane: Introduction and overview. Anesth Analg 81:S1, 1995

sevoflurane anesthesia in a child [in Japanese]. Masui—Japanese Journal of Anesthesiology 40:1542, 1991

50. Cohen EN, Trudell JR, Edmunds HN, Watson E: Urinary metabolites of halothane in man. Anesthesiology 43:392, 1975
51. Carpenter RL, Eger EI, Johnson BH *et al:* The extent of metabolism of inhaled anesthetics in humans. Anesthesiology 65:201, 1986
52. Chase RE, Holaday DA, Fiserova-Bergerova V *et al:* The biotransformation of ethrane in man. Anesthesiology 35:262, 1971
53. Kharasch ED, Armstrong AS, Gunn K *et al:* Clinical sevoflurane metabolism and disposition: II. The role of cytochrome P450 2E1 in fluoride and hexafluoroisopropanol formation. Anesthesiology 82:1379, 1995
54. Kharasch ED: Biotransformation of sevoflurane. Anesth Analg 81:S27, 1995
55. Holaday DA, Fiserova-Bergerova V, Latto IP, Zumbiel MA: Resistance of isoflurane to biotransformation in man. Anesthesiology 43:325, 1975
56. Sutton TS, Koblin DD, Gruenke LD *et al:* Fluoride metabolites after prolonged exposure of volunteers and patients to desflurane. Anesth Analg 73:180, 1991
57. Callis AH, Brooks SD, Roth TP *et al:* Characterization of a halothane-induced humoral immune response in rabbits. Clin Exp Immunol 67:343, 1987
58. Hals J, Dodgson MS, Skulberg A, Kenna JG: Halothane-associated liver damage and renal failure in a young child. Acta Anaesthesiol Scand 30:651, 1986
59. Martin JL, Kenna JG, Pohl LR: Antibody assays for the detection of patients sensitized to halothane. Anesth Analg 70:154, 1990
60. Neuberger J *et al:* Specific serological markers in the diagnosis of fulminant hepatic failure associated with halothane anaesthesia. Br J Anaesth 55:15, 1983
61. Kenna JG, Neuberger J, Williams R: Specific antibodies to halothane-induced liver antigens in halothane-associated hepatitis. Br J Anaesth 59:1286, 1987
62. Fujiwara M, Watanabe A, Sato Y *et al:* Clinical significance of eosinophilia in the diagnosis of halothane-induced liver injury. Acta Med Okayama 38:35, 1984
63. Hubbard AK, Roth TP, Gandolfi AJ *et al:* Halothane hepatitis patients generate an antibody response toward a covalently bound metabolite of halothane. Anesthesiology 68:791, 1988
64. Christ DD, Kenna JG, Kammerer W *et al:* Enflurane metabolism produces covalently bound liver adducts recognized by antibodies from patients with halothane hepatitis. Anesthesiology 69:833, 1988
65. Shiraishi Y, Ikeda K: Uptake and biotransformation of sevoflurane in humans: A comparative study of sevoflurane with halothane, enflurane, and isoflurane [see comments]. J Clin Anesth 2:381, 1990
66. Kharasch ED: Metabolism and toxicity of the new anesthetic agents. Acta Anaesthiol Belg 47:7, 1996
67. Gogus FY, Toker K, Baykan N: Hepatitis following use of two different fluorinated anesthetic agents. Isr J Med Sci 27:156, 1991
68. Allan LG, Hussey AJ, Howie J *et al:* Hepatic glutathione S-transferase release after halothane anaesthesia: Open randomised comparison with isoflurane. Lancet 1:771, 1987
69. Trowell J, Peto R, Campton-Smith A: Controlled trial of repeated halothane hepatitis in patients of the uterine cervix treated with radium. Lancet 1:824, 1975
70. Fee JP, Black GW, Dundee JW *et al:* A prospective study of liver enzyme and other changes following repeat administration of halothane and enflurane. Br J Anaesth 51:1133, 1979
71. Wright R, Eade OE, Chisholm M *et al:* Controlled prospective study of the effect on liver function of multiple exposures to halothane. Lancet 1:817, 1975
72. Neuberger J: Halothane hepatitis. In Institute for Scientific Information Atlas of Science: Pharmacology, p 309. 1988
73. Hussey AJ, Howie J, Allan LG *et al:* Impaired hepatocellular integrity during general anaesthesia, as assessed by measurement of plasma glutathione S-transferase. Clin Chim Acta 161:19, 1986
74. Wark H, O'Halloran M, Overton J: Prospective study of liver function in children following multiple halothane anaesthetics at short intervals. Br J Anaesth 58:1224, 1986
75. Gelman S: General anesthesia and hepatic circulation. Can J Physiol Pharmacol 65:1762, 1987
76. Gelman S, Van Dyke R: Mechanism of halothane-induced hepatotoxicity: Another step on a long path. Anesthesiology 68:479, 1988
77. Kanaya N, Nakayama M, Fujita S, Namiki A: Comparison of the effects of sevoflurane, isoflurane and halothane on indocyanine green clearance. Br J Anaesth 74:164, 1995
78. Frink EJ Jr, Morgan SE, Coetzee A *et al:* The effects of sevoflurane, halothane, enflurane, and isoflurane on hepatic blood flow and oxygenation in chronically instrumented greyhound dogs. Anesthesiology 76:85, 1992
79. Bernard JM, Doursout MF, Wouters P *et al:* Effects of enflurane and isoflurane on hepatic and renal circulations in chronically instrumented dogs. Anesthesiology 74:298, 1991
80. Berendes E, Lippert G, Loick HM, Brussel T: Effects of enflurane and isoflurane on splanchnic oxygenation in humans. J Clin Anesth 8:456, 1996
81. Schindler E, Muller M, Zickmann B *et al:* Blood supply to the liver in the human after 1 MAC desflurane in comparison with isoflurane and halothane [in German]. Anasthesiol Intensivmed Notfallmed Schmerzther 31:344, 1996
82. Armbruster K, Noldge-Schomburg GF, Dressler IM *et al:* The effects of desflurane on splanchnic hemodynamics and oxygenation in the anesthetized pig. Anesth Analg 84:271, 1997
83. Gelman S, Dillard E, Bradley EL Jr: Hepatic circulation during surgical stress and anesthesia with halothane, isoflurane, or fentanyl. Anesth Analg 66:936, 1987
84. Gil F, Fiserova-Bergerova V, Altman NH: Hepatic protection from chemical injury by isoflurane. Anesth Analg 67:860, 1988
85. Baden JM: Hepatotoxicity and metabolism of isoflurane in rats with cirrhosis. Anesth Analg 68:214, 1989
86. Conzen PF, Vollmar B, Habazettl H *et al:* Systemic and regional hemodynamics of isoflurane and sevoflurane in rats. Anesth Analg 74:79, 1992
87. Bernard JM, Doursout MF, Wouters P *et al:* Effects of sevoflurane and isoflurane on hepatic circulation in the chronically instrumented dog. Anesthesiology 77:541, 1992
88. Fujita Y, Kimura K, Hamada H, Takaori M: Comparative effects of halothane, isoflurane, and sevoflurane on the liver with hepatic artery ligation in the beagle. Anesthesiology 75:313, 1991
89. Bito H, Ikeda K: Renal and hepatic function in surgical patients after low-flow sevoflurane or isoflurane anesthesia. Anesth Analg 82:173, 1996
90. Newman PJ, Quinn AC, Hall GM, Grounds RM: Circulating fluoride changes and hepatorenal function following sevoflurane anaesthesia. Anaesthesia 49:936, 1994
91. Quinn AC, Newman PJ, Hall GM, Grounds RM: Sevoflurane anaesthesia for major intra-abdominal surgery [see comments]. Anaesthesia 49:567, 1994
92. Nagata R, Sameshima H, Komaki T *et al:* The effect of inhalation of sevoflurane for an hour on the liver of beagles [in Japanese]. Masui—Japanese Journal of Anesthesiology 40:887, 1991
93. Soma LR, Tierney WJ, Hogan GK, Satoh N: The effects of multiple administrations of sevoflurane to cynomolgus monkeys: Clinical pathologic, hematologic, and pathologic study. Anesth Analg 81:347, 1995
94. Wallin RF, Regan BM, Napoli MD, Stern IJ: Sevoflurane: A new inhalational anesthetic agent. Anesth Analg 54:758, 1975
95. Stock JG, Strunin L: Unexplained hepatitis following halothane. Anesthesiology 63:424, 1985
96. Frink EJ Jr: The hepatic effects of sevoflurane. Anesth Analg 81(suppl 6):S46, 1995
97. Cohen EN, Gift HC, Brown BW *et al:* Occupational disease in dentistry and chronic exposure to trace anesthetic gases. J Am Dent Assoc 101:21, 1980
98. Koblin DD, Waskell L, Watson JE *et al:* Nitrous oxide inactivates methionine synthetase in human liver. Anesth Analg 61:75, 1982
99. Lundeen G, Manohar M, Parks C: Systemic distribution of blood flow in swine while awake and during 1.0 and 1.5 MAC isoflurane anesthesia with or without 50% nitrous oxide. Anesth Analg 62:499, 1983
100. Thomson IA, Hughes RL, Fitch W, Campbell D: Effects of nitrous oxide on liver haemodynamics and oxygen consumption in the greyhound. Anaesthesia 37:548, 1982
101. Pratilas V, Pratila MG, Bramis J, Smith H: The hepatoprotective effect of oxygen during halothane anesthesia. Anesth Analg 57:481, 1978
102. Prys-Roberts C, Sear JW, Low JM *et al:* Hemodynamic and hepatic effects of methohexital infusion during nitrous oxide anesthesia in humans. Anesth Analg 62:317, 1983
103. Zinn SE, Fairley HB, Glenn JD: Liver function in patients with mild alcoholic hepatitis, after enflurane, nitrous oxide-narcotic, and spinal anesthesia. Anesth Analg 64:487, 1985

104. Brodsky JB: Toxicity of nitrous oxide. In Eger EI (ed): Nitrous Oxide/N₂O, p 265. New York, Elsevier, 1985

105. Clarke R et al: Clinical studies of induction agents: XIII. Liver function after propanidid and thiopentone anaesthesia. Br J Anaesth 37:415, 1965

106. Dundee JW, Fee JP, Moore J et al: Changes in serum enzyme levels following ketamine infusions. Anaesthesia 35:12, 1980

107. Jones R, Detmar M, Hill A et al: Incidence of choledochoduodenal sphincter spasm during fenanyl-supplemented anesthesia. Anesth Analg 60:638, 1981

108. Radnay PA, Duncalf D, Novakovic M, Lesser ML: Common bile duct pressure changes after fentanyl, morphine, meperidine, butorphanol, and naloxone. Anesth Analg 63:441, 1984

109. Arguelles JE, Franatovic Y, Romo-Salas F, Aldrete JA: Intrabiliary pressure changes produced by narcotic drugs and inhalation anesthetics in guinea pigs. Anesth Analg 58:120, 1979

110. Economou G, Ward-McQuaid JN: A cross-over comparison of the effect of morphine, pethidine, pentazocine, and phenazocine on biliary pressure. Gut 12:218, 1971

111. Vatashsky E, Haskel Y: Effect of nalbuphine on intrabiliary pressure in the early postoperative period. Canadian Anaesthetists Society Journal 33:433, 1986

112. Bridger S, Henderson K, Glucksman E et al: Lesson of the week: Deaths from low dose paracetamol poisoning. BMJ 316:1724, 1998

113. Eriksson LS, Broome U, Kalin M, Lindholm M: Hepatotoxicity due to repeated intake of low doses of paracetamol. J Intern Med 231:567, 1992

114. Kaplowitz N: Drug metabolism and hepatotoxicity. In Kaplowitz N (ed): Liver and Biliary Diseases, p 112. Baltimore, Williams & Wilkins, 1996

115. Schiffer ER, Mentha G, Schwieger IM, Morel DR: Sequential changes in the splanchnic circulation during continuous endotoxin infusion in sedated sheep: Evidence for a selective increase of hepatic artery blood flow and loss of the hepatic arterial buffer response. Acta Physiol Scand 147:251, 1993

116. Ayuse T, Brienza N, Revelly JP et al: Role of nitric oxide in porcine liver circulation under normal and endotoxemic conditions. J Appl Physiol 78:1319, 1995

117. Gundersen Y, Saetre T, Scholz T et al: The NO donor sodium nitroprusside reverses the negative effects on hepatic arterial flow induced by endotoxin and the NO synthase inhibitor L-NAME. Eur Surg Res 28:323, 1996

118. Refsum H: Arterial hypoxaemia, serum activity of GO-T, GP-T and LDH, and central lobular liver cell necrosis in pulmonary insufficiency. Clin Sci 25:369, 1963

119. Sims J, Morris L, Orth O et al: The influence of oxygen and carbon dioxide levels during anesthesia upon postsurgical hepatic damage. J Lab Clin Med 38:388, 1951

120. Bynum TE, Boitnott JK, Maddrey WC: Ischemic hepatitis. Dig Dis Sci 24:129, 1979

121. Gibson PR, Dudley FJ: Ischemic hepatitis: Clinical features, diagnosis and prognosis. Aust N Z J Med 14:822, 1984

122. Clarke RS, Doggart JR, Lavery T: Changes in liver function after different types of surgery. Br J Anaesth 48:119, 1976

123. Viegas O, Stoelting RK: LDH5 changes after cholecystectomy or hysterectomy in patients receiving halothane, enflurane, or fentanyl. Anesthesiology 51:556, 1979

124. Garrison RN, Cryer HM, Howard DA, Polk HC Jr: Clarification of risk factors for abdominal operations in patients with hepatic cirrhosis. Ann Surg 199:648, 1984

125. Cryer HM, Howard DA, Garrison RN: Liver cirrhosis and biliary surgery: Assessment of risk. South Med J 78:138, 1985

126. McNeill JR, Pang CC: Effect of pentobarbital anesthesia and surgery on the control of arterial pressure and mesenteric resistance in cats: Role of vasopressin and angiotensin. Can J Physiol Pharmacol 60:363, 1982

127. Gelman SI: Disturbances in hepatic blood flow during anesthesia and surgery. Arch Surg 111:881, 1976

128. Gelman S, Rimerman V, Fowler KC et al: The effect of halothane, isoflurane, and blood loss on hepatotoxicity and hepatic oxygen availability in phenobarbital-pretreated hypoxic rats. Anesth Analg 63:965, 1984

129. Gelman S, Fowler KC, Smith LR: Regional blood flow during isoflurane and halothane anesthesia. Anesth Analg 63:557, 1984

130. Gelman S, Fowler KC, Smith LR: Liver circulation and function during isoflurane and halothane anesthesia. Anesthesiology 61: 726, 1984

131. Harper MH, Collins P, Johnson BH et al: Postanesthetic hepatic injury in rats: Influence of alterations in hepatic blood flow, surgery, and anesthesia time. Anesth Analg 61:79, 1982

132. Fernandes NF, Hilsenbeck SG, Gross GW: Laparoscopic cholecystectomy in cirrhotic patients. Am J Gastroenterol 94:2656, 1999

133. Maze M, Baden J: Anesthesia for patients with liver disease. In Miller R (ed): Anesthesia. New York, Churchill Livingstone, 1986

134. Mathie RT: Hepatic blood flow during cardiopulmonary bypass. Crit Care Med 21:S72, 1993

135. Henderson JM, Gilmore GT, Mackay GJ et al: Hemodynamics during liver transplantation: The interactions between cardiac output and portal venous and hepatic arterial flows. Hepatology 16:715, 1992

136. Douglas HJ, Eger EI, Biava CG, Renzi C: Hepatic necrosis associated with viral infection after enflurane anesthesia. N Engl J Med 296:553, 1977

137. Scully R et al: Case records of the Massachusetts General Hospital. N Engl J Med 322:318, 1990

138. Seeff L: Diagnosis, therapy, and prognosis of viral hepatitis. In Zakim D, Boyer T (eds): Hepatology: A Textbook of Liver Disease, 3rd ed, p 1067. Philadelphia, WB Saunders, 1996

139. Vento S, Garofano T, Renzini C et al: Fulminant hepatitis associated with hepatitis A virus superinfection in patients with chronic hepatitis C. N Engl J Med 338:286, 1998

140. Brechot C et al: Hepatitis B virus DNA in patients with chronic liver disease and negative tests for hepatitis B surface antigen. N Engl J Med 312:270, 1985

141. Maddrey W: Alcoholic hepatitis. In Williams R, Maddrey W (eds): Liver. London, Butterworth, 1984

142. Tonnesen H, Kehlet H: Preoperative alcoholism and postoperative morbidity. Br J Surg 86:869, 1999

143. Benoit JN, Granger DN: Splanchnic hemodynamics in chronic portal hypertension. Semin Liver Dis 6:287, 1986

144. Bomzon A, Blendis L: Vascular reactivity in experimental portal hypertension. Am J Physiol 252:G158, 1987

145. Rakela J, Krowka M: Cardiovascular and pulmonary complications of liver disease. In Zakim D, Boyer T (eds): Hepatology: A Textbook of Liver Disease, 3rd ed, p 675. Philadelphia, WB Saunders, 1996

146. Daoud FS, Reeves JT, Schaefer JW: Failure of hypoxic pulmonary vasoconstriction in patients with liver cirrhosis. J Clin Invest 51: 1076, 1972

147. Lazaridis KN, Frank JW, Krowka MJ, Kamath PS: Hepatic hydrothorax: Pathogenesis, diagnosis, and management. Am J Med 107: 262, 1999

148. Castro M, Krowka MJ, Schroeder DR et al: Frequency and clinical implications of increased pulmonary artery pressures in liver transplant patients. Mayo Clin Proc 71:543, 1996

149. Jalan R, Hayes PC: Hepatic encephalopathy and ascites [see comments]. Lancet 350:1309, 1997

150. Gines A, Escorsell A, Gines P et al: Incidence, predictive factors, and prognosis of the hepatorenal syndrome in cirrhosis with ascites [see comments]. Gastroenterology 105:229, 1993

151. Schrier RW, Abraham WT: Hormones and hemodynamics in heart failure. N Engl J Med 341:577, 1999

152. Epstein M: Renal functional abnormalities in cirrhosis: Pathophysiology and management. In Zakim D, Boyer T (eds): Hepatology: A Textbook of Liver Disease, p 446. Philadelphia, WB Saunders, 1982

153. Witte CL, Witte MH: Splanchnic circulatory and tissue fluid dynamics in portal hypertension. Fed Proc 42:1685, 1983

154. Riordan SM, Williams R: Treatment of hepatic encephalopathy [see comments]. N Engl J Med 337:473, 1997

155. MacGilchrist AJ, Birnie GG, Cook A et al: Pharmacokinetics and pharmacodynamics of intravenous midazolam in patients with severe alcoholic cirrhosis. Gut 27:190, 1986

156. Trouvin JH, Farinotti R, Haberer JP et al: Pharmacokinetics of midazolam in anaesthetized cirrhotic patients. Br J Anaesth 60:762, 1988

157. Chauvin M, Ferrier C, Haberer JP et al: Sufentanil pharmacokinetics in patients with cirrhosis. Anesth Analg 68:1, 1989

158. Servin F, Desmonts JM, Haberer JP et al: Pharmacokinetics and protein binding of propofol in patients with cirrhosis. Anesthesiology 69:887, 1988

159. Pandele G, Chaux F, Salvadori C et al: Thiopental pharmacokinetics in patients with cirrhosis. Anesthesiology 59:123, 1983

160. Ferrier C, Marty J, Bouffard Y et al: Alfentanil pharmacokinetics in patients with cirrhosis. Anesthesiology 62:480, 1985

161. Patwardhan RV, Johnson RF, Hoyumpa A Jr *et al:* Normal metabolism of morphine in cirrhosis. Gastroenterology 81:1006, 1981
162. Mazoit JX, Sandouk P, Zetlaoui P, Scherrmann JM: Pharmacokinetics of unchanged morphine in normal and cirrhotic subjects. Anesth Analg 66:293, 1987
163. Branch R, Morgan M, James J *et al:* Intravenous administration of diazepam in patients with chronic liver disease. Gut 17:975, 1976
164. Baraka A, Gabali F: Correlation between tubocurarine requirements and plasma protein pattern. Br J Anaesth 40:89, 1968
165. Parker C, Hunter J: Pharmacokinetics of atracurium and laudanosine in patients with hepatic cirrhosis. Br J Anaesth 62:177, 1989
166. Better OS: Renal and cardiovascular dysfunction in liver disease [clinical conference]. Kidney Int 29:598, 1986
167. Bomzon A, Monies-Chass I, Kamenetz L, Blendis L: Anesthesia and pressor responsiveness in chronic bile-duct-ligated dogs. Hepatology 11:551, 1990
168. Tamakuma S, Wada N, Ishiyama M *et al:* Relationship between hepatic hemodynamics and biliary pressure in dogs: Its significance in clinical shock following biliary decompression. Japanese Journal of Surgery 5:255, 1975
169. Friedman L, Maddrey W: Surgery in the patient with liver disease. Med Clin North Am 71:454, 1987
170. Bloch RS, Allaben RD, Walt AJ: Cholecystectomy in patients with cirrhosis: A surgical challenge. Arch Surg 120:669, 1985
171. Brown MW, Burk RF: Development of intractable ascites following upper abdominal surgery in patients with cirrhosis. Am J Med 80:879, 1986
172. Kang Y, Gelman S: Liver transplantation. In Gelman S (ed): Anesthesia and Organ Transplantation, p 139. Philadelphia, WB Saunders, 1987
173. Ward S, Neill E: Pharmacokinetics of atracurium in acute hepatic failure (with acute renal failure). Survey of Anesthesia 28:364, 1984
174. Duvaldestin P, Agoston S, Henzel D *et al:* Pancuronium pharmacokinetics in patients with liver cirrhosis. Br J Anaesth 50:1131, 1978
175. Arden J, Cannon J, Lynam D *et al:* Vecuronium pharmacokinetics and pharmacodynamics in hepatocellular disease. Anesth Analg 66:S3, 1987
176. Gelman S, Ernst E: Hepatic circulation during sodium nitroprusside infusion in the carbon tetrachloride-treated dog. Alabama Journal of Medical Science 19:371, 1982
177. Duvaldestin P, Slavov V, Rebufat Y: Pharmacokinetics and pharmacodynamics of rapacuronium in patients with cirrhosis. Anesthesiology 91:1305, 1999
178. Westra P, Houwertjes C, DeLange A *et al:* Effect of experimental cholestasis on neuromuscular blocking drugs in cats. Br J Anaesth 52:747, 1980
179. Evans C, Evans M, Pollock AV: The incidence and causes of postoperative jaundice: A prospective study. Br J Anaesth 46:520, 1974
180. Sussman N: Fulminant hepatic failure. In Zakim D, Boyer T (eds): Hepatology: A Textbook of Liver Disease, 3rd ed, p 618. Philadelphia, WB Saunders, 1996
181. Schemel WH: Unexpected hepatic dysfunction found by multiple laboratory screening. Anesth Analg 55:810, 1976
182. Wataneeyawech M, Kelly K: Hepatic diseases: Unsuspected before surgery. New York State Journal of Medicine 75:1278, 1975
183. Gitlin N: Clinical aspects of liver disease caused by industrial and environmental toxins. In Zakim D, Boyer T (eds): Hepatology: A Textbook of Liver Disease, 3rd ed, p 1018. Philadelphia, WB Saunders, 1996
184. Bass N, Ockner R: Drug-induced liver disease. In Zakim D, Boyer T (eds): Hepatology: A Textbook of Liver Disease, 3rd ed, p 962. Philadelphia, WB Saunders, 1996
185. Dossing M, Andreasen PB: Drug-induced liver disease in Denmark: An analysis of 572 cases of hepatotoxicity reported to the Danish Board of Adverse Reactions to Drugs. Scand J Gastroenterol 17:205, 1982
186. Brown B: Anesthesia in Hepatic and Biliary Tract Disease. Philadelphia, FA Davis, 1988
187. Gilman A: The Pharmacological Basis of Therapeutics. In Gilman A, *et al* (eds): 7th ed. New York, MacMillan, 1985
188. Van Dyke R: The liver in pregnancy. In Zakim D, Boyer T (eds): Hepatology: A Textbook of Liver Disease, 3rd ed, p 1734. Philadelphia, WB Saunders, 1996
189. James F, Wheeler A, Dewan D: Obstetric Anesthesia: The Complicated Patient. Philadelphia, FA Davis, 1988

Clinical Anesthesia (4/e), edited by
Paul G. Barash, Bruce F. Cullen, and
Robert K. Stoelting. Lippincott Williams &
Wilkins, Philadelphia, © 2001.

CHAPTER 40

ANESTHESIA FOR ORTHOPAEDIC SURGERY

TERESE T. HORLOCKER AND DENISE J. WEDEL

Orthopaedic anesthesia is a logical outgrowth of the subspecialization that has taken place in the field of anesthesiology. Several factors bind this diverse patient group together. Although patients vary in age from very young to very old, the surgical procedures involving bone, muscle, and related soft tissues require similar monitoring and anesthetic techniques. For example, many orthopaedic surgical procedures lend themselves to the use of regional anesthesia. Regional anesthetic techniques allow intraoperative surgical anesthesia as well as postoperative pain relief, and create a further subspecialty within orthopaedic anesthesia. Another seemingly trivial but vitally important part of orthopaedic anesthesia is patient positioning. Unusual patient positioning is a common feature in orthopaedic cases. Experience and specific knowledge are required to produce optimal surgical conditions and avoid potential injuries. Orthopaedic procedures are frequently associated with major blood loss and its related risks. The orthopaedic anesthesia care provider must be experienced in techniques that decrease these risks, must be able to use intraoperative hypotension and blood salvage techniques, and must be able to manage transfusion-related complications. The orthopaedic surgical patient is also at risk for deep venous thrombosis and pulmonary embolus. Knowledge of the current pharmacologic and mechanical methods of thromboprophylaxis is required to prevent the occurrence of these thromboembolic complications. Likewise, potential interactions between anticoagulants and anesthetic drugs or regional anesthetic techniques must be thoroughly understood to reduce the risk of perioperative bleeding.

Knowledge of specific orthopaedic surgical techniques, including duration, extent, predicted blood loss, and associated complications, is invaluable to the anesthesia care provider working in a team to provide the best possible patient care. Orthopaedic surgical patients usually require early mobilization and rehabilitation, both of which can be expedited by appropriate selection of anesthetic techniques and management of postoperative analgesia. In this chapter, we discuss the various aspects of orthopaedic anesthesia, emphasizing the anesthetic techniques and patient management issues unique to this practice.

PREOPERATIVE ASSESSMENT

The anesthesiologist's preoperative assessment is crucial to the formulation and execution of the anesthetic plan. The patient must be evaluated for pre-existing medical problems, previous anesthetic complications, potential airway difficulties, and considerations relating to intraoperative positioning. This evaluation, coupled with an appreciation of the surgeon's needs, is used to formulate the anesthetic plan.

Pre-existing medical conditions may have a profound impact on anesthetic choice and perioperative management. Optimal patient management balances the pathophysiology of concurrent medical conditions, the cause and significance of physiologic changes to regional block or general anesthesia, and the results of outcome studies. *Advancing age* is often accompanied by decreases in physiologic function that can progress to significant illness. *Hypertension* is the most prevalent medical problem seen in elderly patients undergoing orthopaedic surgery. Hypertensive patients experience wider fluctuations in intraoperative

blood pressure than normotensive patients. Noxious stimuli lead to exaggerated hypertensive responses. Conversely, because hypertensive patients tend to be intravascularly depleted, once general or neuraxial anesthesia is induced, hypotension may occur. Intraoperative blood loss exacerbates this response. In general, hypertensive patients should continue their antihypertensive medications during the perioperative period.

Patients with *coronary artery disease* pose unique problems to the anesthesiologist. For the patient who has experienced a myocardial infarction, elective surgery should typically be delayed by 6 months to avoid significant cardiac morbidity and mortality. Patients with unstable angina require a cardiac evaluation before elective surgery to determine the extent of disease and plan appropriate interventions. However, it is often difficult to assess exercise tolerance or a recent progression of cardiac symptoms because of the limitations in mobility induced by the underlying orthopaedic condition. Antianginal medications should be continued during the perioperative period. During surgery, patients may require intravenous nitrates to improve coronary blood flow and β blocking agents to control heart rate.

Many patients undergoing orthopaedic surgery have *rheumatoid arthritis*. Systemic manifestations of this disease include pulmonary, cardiac, and musculoskeletal involvement. Particularly significant to the anesthesiologist is involvement of the cervical spine, temporomandibular joint, and larynx. Rheumatoid involvement of the cervical spine may result in limited neck range of motion, which interferes with airway management. Atlantoaxial instability, with subluxation of the odontoid process, can lead to spinal cord injury during neck extension. Patients with rheumatoid arthritis are often on chronic steroid therapy and require perioperative steroid replacement.

Management of orthopaedic *trauma* patients involves unique preoperative considerations. Trauma patients requiring emergency surgical intervention are assumed to have full stomachs because of delayed gastric emptying secondary to the traumatic event, and because of opioid administration. Patients who have sustained cervical spine trauma require careful and controlled airway management to avoid further injury. Associated injuries and blood loss may further complicate management of otherwise routine orthopaedic surgery in the trauma patient.

The *past medical history*, including the *past anesthetic history* of the patient and his or her family, should be reviewed. A history of coagulation disorders associated with easy bruising or bleeding in the patient or family may make regional anesthesia inadvisable. Other familial traits, such as sickle cell disease or porphyria, affect surgical and anesthetic management. Some hereditary diseases, such as plasma cholinesterase deficiency or malignant hyperthermia, may not be diagnosed until the patient or a member of his or her family is anesthetized.

Preoperative evaluation should include a focused *physical examination*. Patients should be assessed for limitation in mouth opening or neck extension, adequacy of thyromental distance (measured from the lower border of the mandible to the thyroid notch), and state of dentition. The heart and lungs should be auscultated. In addition, the site of proposed injection for regional anesthesia should be assessed for evidence of infection and anatomic abnormalities or limitations. At this time, the patient should also be evaluated for any potential positioning difficulties related to arthritic involvement of other joints or body habitus.

CHOICE OF ANESTHETIC TECHNIQUE

Orthopaedic surgery can often be completed under either regional or general anesthesia. The risks and benefits of each are discussed in the following sections. Any patient who has an absolute contraindication to regional anesthesia (patient refusal, infection at the site of needle placement, systemic anticoagulation) is a candidate for general anesthesia. General anesthesia provides the patient with amnesia, analgesia, and muscle relaxation.

Many orthopaedic surgical procedures, because of their localized peripheral site, lend themselves to regional anesthetic techniques. Neural structures may be blocked at the peripheral nerve, plexus, or neuraxial level. A regional anesthetic provides the patient with surgical analgesia and muscle relaxation; intravenous sedatives can be used to provide mild sedation and amnesia during the operative procedure. The regional technique and local anesthetic solution used depend on a variety of factors, including duration of surgery, length of desired postoperative analgesia, and indication for postoperative sympathectomy.

Regional anesthetics offer several advantages over general anesthetics in patients undergoing orthopaedic procedures, including improved postoperative analgesia, decreased incidence of nausea and vomiting, less respiratory and cardiac depression, improved perfusion *via* sympathetic block, reduced blood loss, and decreased risk of thromboembolism. It is important to explain these benefits and encourage regional anesthesia where appropriate.

SURGERY TO THE UPPER EXTREMITIES

Orthopaedic surgical procedures to the upper extremity are well suited to regional anesthetic techniques. Surgery to the elbow, forearm, and hand may be accomplished with regional blockade alone, whereas surgery to the shoulder and upper arm can be performed under regional blockade alone or a combination of regional and general anesthesia. In addition to intraoperative anesthesia, brachial plexus and peripheral nerve blocks may be used in the treatment and prevention of reflex sympathetic dystrophy. Continuous catheter techniques provide postoperative analgesia and allow early limb mobilization. However, although the benefits of regional anesthesia in this patient population are well established, orthopaedic surgical procedures often involve peripheral nerves with pre-existing deficits, such as ulnar nerve transposition and carpal tunnel release. In addition, the operative site may be adjacent to neural structures, as with total shoulder arthroplasty or fractures of the proximal humerus. Improper surgical positioning and the use of a tourniquet or constrictive casts or dressings may also result in perioperative neurologic ischemia. The use of regional techniques in the patient at increased risk for perioperative nerve injury remains controversial. Therefore, the patient should be examined before surgery to document pre-existing neurologic deficits. Meticulous regional anesthetic technique with appropriate use of local anesthetic solutions and vasoconstrictors, careful patient positioning, and serial postoperative neurologic examinations reduce the incidence of neurologic dysfunction.

Local anesthetic selection should be based on the duration and degree of sensory or motor block required. Although prolonged blockade of the lower extremities interfere with ambulation and therefore delay outpatient discharge, persistent upper extremity block is not a contraindication to hospital dismissal. However, during the postoperative visit, the patient should be informed of the anticipated duration of analgesia and instructed to protect the blocked extremity until block resolution.

Surgery to the Shoulder and Upper Arm

Reconstructive shoulder surgery, including total shoulder arthroplasty and rotator cuff repair, presents unique management and positioning considerations to the anesthesiologist. These surgical procedures are typically performed with the patient in the ''beach chair'' position. The patient is flexed at the hips and knees and placed in a 10–20-degree reverse Trendelenburg position to promote venous return. The patient is shifted laterally to the edge of the operating table to allow unrestricted surgical access to the upper extremity. The patient's head, neck, and hips must be secured to prevent additional lateral movement. The head and neck must remain firmly supported by the operating table and secured in a neutral position; excessive rotation or flexion of the head away from the operative side results in stretch injury to the brachial plexus. Care also must be taken to avoid pressure on the eyes and ears. All airway connections should be tightened and possibly reinforced with tape because after surgical draping, access to the patient's face and airway is limited. Hypotension can be minimized by gradual assumption of the beach chair position and by delaying head elevation until the time of surgical incision. A tourniquet cannot be used during proximal upper extremity surgical procedures, and significant blood loss may occur. Therefore, arterial cannulation may be helpful for direct blood pressure measurement and monitoring of intraoperative hemoglobin concentrations during total shoulder arthroplasty and reduction of humeral fractures. In theory, venous air embolism (VAE) may occur during surgical procedures to the shoulder because the operative site is higher than the heart. However, this complication has not been reported in the literature. Patients with a documented right-to-left shunt may be monitored with a precordial Doppler to allow prompt diagnosis and treatment of VAE.

Surgery to the shoulder and humerus may be performed under regional or general anesthesia.[1] With careful positioning and appropriate sedation, interscalene or supraclavicular blockade alone can provide excellent surgical anesthesia. However, general anesthesia or a combination of regional and general anesthesia is often chosen because of limited access to the patient's airway during these surgical procedures. Interscalene brachial plexus block may be performed before surgical incision or after postoperative upper extremity neurologic function has been determined. Although preoperative interscalene block reduces the intraoperative requirement of volatile anesthetic and opioids, and in theory provides pre-emptive analgesia, postoperative evaluation of neurologic function will not be possible until block resolution.

Nerve injury often occurs in association with upper extremity trauma. Radial nerve palsy is identified in up to 18% of patients with humeral shaft fractures, whereas injury to the axillary nerve and brachial plexus is associated with proximal humerus fractures. In addition, 4% of patients undergoing total shoulder arthroplasty have a documented postoperative neurologic deficit, including 3% of patients with injury to the brachial plexus. The level of injury is at the level of the nerve trunks, which is the level at which an interscalene block is performed, making it impossible to determine the etiology of the nerve injury (surgical *vs.* anesthetic). Most of these nerve injuries represent a neurapraxia; 90% resolve in 3–4 months.[2] However, the significant incidence of neurologic deficits demonstrates the importance of clinical examination before regional anesthetic techniques in these patients. Interscalene block should be performed with caution in patients with a pre-existing brachial plexopathy because of the risk of perioperative exacerbation of neurologic deficits. The ipsilateral diaphragmatic paresis and 25% loss of pulmonary function produced by interscalene block also contraindicates this block in patients with severe pulmonary disease.[3] The reduction in pulmonary function is present for the duration of the interscalene block and is present even with concentrations of bupivacaine as low as 0.125%.

Surgery to the Elbow

Surgical procedures to the distal humerus, elbow, and forearm are commonly performed under regional anesthetic techniques. Infraclavicular and supraclavicular approaches to the brachial plexus are the most reliable and provide consistent anesthesia to the four major nerves of the brachial plexus: median, ulnar, radial, and musculocutaneous. However, the small but definite risk of pneumothorax associated with supraclavicular and infraclavicular blocks makes this approach unsuitable for outpatient procedures. Typically, the pneumothorax occurs 6–12 hours after hospital discharge; therefore, a postoperative chest radiograph is not helpful. Although chest tube placement is advised for pneumothorax greater than 20% of lung volume, the lung may also be re-expanded with a small Teflon catheter under fluoroscopic guidance, eliminating the need for hospital admission. The axillary approach to the brachial plexus eliminates the risk of pneumothorax and reliably provides adequate anesthesia for surgery near the elbow.[4] Injection of greater volumes of local anesthetic solution into the axillary sheath or supplemental musculocutaneous nerve block at the level of the axilla, in the coracobrachialis muscle, increases the probability of successful block of the brachial plexus and the surgical field.

Surgery to the Wrist and Hand

Surgery to the distal forearm, wrist, and hand may be performed under general or regional anesthesia. Brachial plexus block provides comprehensive and consistent regional anesthesia for the distal upper extremity.[5] Although the brachial plexus may be successfully blocked at several sites, the interscalene approach is seldom used for wrist and hand procedures because incomplete anesthesia of the ulnar nerve is produced in 15–30% of patients. In addition, although the supraclavicular approach results in blockade of all four major nerves, the risk of pneumothorax reduces its suitability for outpatient procedures. Therefore, the axillary approach is most commonly used for surgical procedures to the forearm, wrist, and hand.

Minor hand procedures such as carpal tunnel release, reduction of phalanx fractures, and superficial wound débridements may require only local infiltration or peripheral blockade at the mid-humeral, elbow, or wrist level. Inflation of an upper arm tourniquet in these patients causes significant discomfort in 45–60 minutes, and limits the duration of the surgical procedure. Intravenous regional anesthesia (Bier block) using a double tourniquet permits more extensive surgery and longer tourniquet times. However, the Bier block has several disadvantages, including the potential for high blood levels of local anesthetic solutions, a maximum anesthetic duration of 90–120 minutes, and rapid termination of anesthesia (and analgesia) on tourniquet deflation.

Continuous Brachial Plexus Anesthesia

Indwelling brachial plexus catheters allow prolonged upper extremity anesthesia and postoperative analgesia. A continuous infusion of local anesthetic solution, such as bupivacaine 0.125%, prevents vasospasm and increases circulation after limb replantation or vascular repair. More concentrated solutions of bupivacaine result in complete sensory block and allow early joint mobilization after painful surgical procedures to the elbow. Brachial plexus catheters may be inserted using interscalene, infraclavicular, and axillary approaches. However, the axillary approach is most common. The catheter is inserted 5–10 cm through a medium-gauge needle after elicitation of a paresthesia (or motor response if the nerve stimulator technique is used), and 45–50 ml of local anesthetic is injected. Although *analgesia* is produced in all nerve distributions, the block may not provide satisfactory surgical *anesthesia*, even with administra-

tion of more potent local anesthetic solutions. Therefore, for surgical procedures, the continuous brachial plexus block is often supplemented with a general anesthetic. After surgery, the catheters may be left indwelling for 4–7 days without adverse effects.

SURGERY TO THE LOWER EXTREMITIES

Although orthopaedic procedures to the lower extremity may be performed under both general and regional anesthesia, the ability to provide superior postoperative analgesia, rapid postoperative rehabilitation, and reduced cost of medical care may result from thoughtfully implemented regional anesthetic and analgesic techniques.

Multiple studies demonstrate significantly reduced intraoperative blood loss during total hip arthroplasty (THA) completed under central neuraxial blockade compared with general anesthesia.[6] The reasons for this reduction are unproved but may be influenced by the decrease in mean arterial pressure, blood flow redistribution to larger-caliber vessels, and locally reduced venous pressure. Decreased postoperative blood loss can be demonstrated when the epidural local anesthetic is continued for analgesia.

Postoperative pulmonary thromboembolism (PTE) from deep venous thrombosis (DVT) is an important cause of morbidity and mortality in orthopaedic surgical patients. A variety of authors have identified decreased incidence of DVT and PTE in patients whose surgery was conducted under regional anesthesia.[7–9] However, these patients did not receive anticoagulants. The potential benefit of regional anesthesia in reducing thromboembolic complications is discussed later in this chapter.

Surgery to the Hip

In 1990, more than 120,000 total hip replacements were performed in North America. Patients undergoing surgical procedures to the hip for arthritic conditions typically are elderly and often have pre-existing medical conditions that may affect perioperative outcome. In addition, because hospital costs appear to be directly related to the length of hospital stay, anesthetic techniques associated with improved recovery and reduced complications may decrease the total hospital costs among these patients.

Positioning

The lateral decubitus position is frequently used to facilitate surgical exposure for THA, whereas the fracture table is often used for repair of femur fractures. In transferring the patient from the supine to lateral decubitus position, care must be taken to maintain the head and shoulders in a neutral position. Ideally, a separate person is responsible for moving the legs, the torso, the shoulders, and the head. The patient is supported while the position is secured with hip rests or other mechanical devices. The dependent arm is abducted and placed on a padded arm rest; a rolled towel or wrapped intravenous fluid bag is placed in the axilla to avoid compression of the brachial plexus and vascular structures. The upper arm is placed on a padded over-arm board.

Positioning on the fracture table (Fig. 40-1) also requires adequate personnel to move the patient, with one person assigned to apply traction to the fractured limb. The fracture table affords two advantages: maintenance of traction on the fractured extremity, allowing manipulation for closed reduction and fixation; and access to the fracture site for radiography in several planes. The patient must be carefully monitored for hemodynamic changes during positioning, whether under regional or general anesthesia. Care must be taken to pad the perineal post before positioning the patient's pelvis. Usually the arm ipsilateral to the fractured hip is placed on an arm board or in a sling to keep it from obstructing the fluoroscopic view.

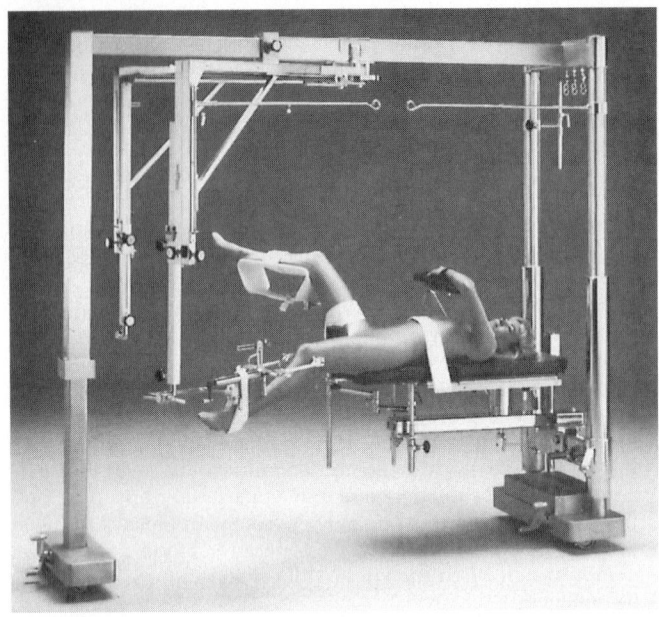

Figure 40-1. The fracture table. The patient must be moved carefully with continuous traction on the fractured limb. The ipsilateral arm is positioned on an arm board or sling without stretching the brachial plexus. (Courtesy of Midmark Corporation, Versailles, OH.)

Anesthetic Technique

Regional anesthetic techniques are well suited to procedures involving the hip. Central neuraxial blockade, including spinal and epidural blockade, is commonly used. Regional anesthesia may be instituted with the patient sitting or in the lateral decubitus position. Both hypobaric and isobaric spinal anesthetic solutions are effective. After establishment of spinal anesthesia, a dense sensory and motor block progresses quickly. Adequate intravenous hydration before placing the spinal block protects against a precipitous drop in blood pressure that can occur secondary to sympathetic blockade and peripheral vasodilation. In any patient, there is a risk of postdural puncture headache, but this risk diminishes with increasing age and decreasing needle gauge. Epidural blockade also provides excellent surgical anesthesia. Placement of a catheter allows the anesthesiologist to provide prolonged anesthesia as well as postoperative analgesia.

Regional anesthetic techniques reduce blood loss in patients undergoing hip surgery. Deliberate hypotension can also be used with general anesthesia as a means of reducing surgical blood loss and has been recommended when the benefits can be expected to outweigh the risks. In a comparative study, average blood loss during induced nitroprusside hypotension with nitrous oxide–halothane anesthesia for hip arthroplasty was 1.3 l, whereas neuroleptanalgesia or nitrous oxide–halothane without hypotension yielded blood losses of 2.6 and 2 l, respectively.[10] Diltiazem, nitroprusside with and without captopril, β blockers, and nitroglycerin have also been used to induce hypotension.

Surgery to the Knee

The most common surgical procedures to the knee are arthroscopy, anterior cruciate ligament repair, and total knee arthroplasty. Oral opioids and other adjuvant analgesics relieve postoperative pain after ambulatory knee surgery. However, open knee procedures are extremely painful. Therefore, continuous regional anesthetic techniques are helpful in facilitating rehabilitation and maintaining adequate joint range of motion.

Regional anesthetic techniques that can be used for surgical procedures about the knee include neuraxial as well as peripheral leg blocks. Spinal anesthesia can be accomplished with hyperbaric or isobaric solutions, although the latter are favored by most orthopaedic anesthesiologists. Injection of hyperbaric solutions often results in a higher level of sensory and motor blockade than needed for the surgical procedure, with subsequent earlier offset of anesthesia. Epidural blockade offers the advantage of a continuous catheter technique that can be continued into the postoperative period. These procedures are often associated with significant postoperative pain, particularly when continuous-motion machines are applied to the affected joint. The patient undergoing amputation of a lower limb often benefits from the use of regional anesthesia, although adequate sedation is imperative.

Peripheral nerve blocks of the lower extremity are not as popular as upper extremity blocks. Whereas the brachial plexus is a compact and conveniently located grouping of nerves that may be blocked at a single injection site, there is no anatomic correlate in the lower extremity. To provide surgical anesthesia of the lower extremity using peripheral nerve blocks, each major nerve is blocked individually at separate locations. These blocks do offer the advantage of limiting sympathectomy to the extremity blocked. Also, depending on the local anesthetic agent used, significant postoperative analgesia can be provided.

Surgical anesthesia for operative procedures on the knee in which a tourniquet will be used requires blockade of all four nerves (femoral, lateral femoral cutaneous, obturator, and sciatic nerves) innervating the leg. Although it is possible to perform major knee surgery under peripheral nerve blocks, more often a femoral three-in-one or lumbar plexus (psoas) block is combined with a spinal or general anesthetic. This is less difficult technically, reduces the amount of local anesthetic (and associated systemic toxicity), and provides postoperative analgesia for 12–24 hours. Continuous lumbar plexus and sciatic techniques allow for prolonged postoperative analgesia.

Minor knee procedures with limited tourniquet inflation times, such as knee arthroscopy, may be performed solely under femoral or lumbar plexus block. Thus peripheral lower extremity blocks provide adequate surgical anesthesia and also allow for rapid recovery and early hospital dismissal for ambulatory patients.

The supine position optimizes surgical exposure during knee arthroscopy or arthroplasty, lower extremity amputations, and procedures to the tibia and fibula. Care must be taken to cushion the extremities and bony prominences.

Surgery to the Ankle and Foot

Innervation of the foot is provided by the femoral nerve (*via* the saphenous nerve) and by the sciatic nerve (*via* the posterior tibial, sural, and deep and superficial peroneal nerves). Therefore, central neuraxial blockade and peripheral nerve blocks at the upper leg, knee, or ankle are appropriate regional anesthetic techniques for foot surgery. The selection of the regional technique is based on the surgical site, use of a calf or thigh tourniquet, degree of weight bearing/ambulation, and the need for postoperative analgesia. For example, inflation of a thigh tourniquet for longer than 15–20 minutes necessitates a general or neuraxial anesthetic, regardless of surgical site. Common surgical procedures and considerations regarding the choice of regional technique are discussed in Table 40-1.[11]

The distal surgical site and the ability to block the pain pathways at multiple sites give regional anesthesia an advantage over general anesthesia for surgery to the ankle and foot. Peripheral blockade avoids the cardiovascular and respiratory side effects and the urinary retention associated with neuraxial and general anesthesia. Often patients undergoing lower extremity peripheral techniques may be discharged directly from the operating room to the outpatient nursing station, reducing recovery time and charges. The use of long-acting local anesthetics and the addition of epinephrine or clonidine allow prolongation of postoperative analgesia. However, additional onset time is required with bupivacaine and ropivacaine. Mepivacaine and lidocaine may be more appropriate in the ambulatory setting, where fast-onset and reliable surgical anesthesia are essential. The main disadvantage of peripheral blocks is the technical expertise required for consistent success; neuraxial techniques are a suitable alternative. The additional time that is often required for induction of regional anesthesia, as opposed to general anesthesia, can also be problematic in an era promoting increased surgical through-put and health care cost reduction.

Postoperative Analgesia

Systemic opioids remain a popular postoperative regimen for major orthopaedic surgery because they are relatively simple to administer, safe, and cost effective. Delivery of opioids using patient-controlled analgesia (PCA) devices results in improved analgesia, decreased total opioid consumption, and increased patient and nurse satisfaction. However, the pain after total joint replacement, particularly total knee arthroplasty, is severe. Adequate analgesia achieved with systemic opioids is frequently associated with side effects, including sedation, nausea, and pruritus. Anti-inflammatory medications and acetaminophen are valuable adjuvants to systemic opioids. The addition of non-opioid analgesics reduces opioid use, improves analgesia, and decreases opioid-related side effects.

Studies have demonstrated that epidural analgesia or peripheral nerve blocks provide better pain relief and faster postoperative rehabilitation than intravenous PCA with morphine after total joint replacement. For example, after total knee arthroplasty, patients receiving epidural analgesia or continuous femoral three-in-one block reported lower pain scores, better knee flexion, faster ambulation, and shorter hospital stays compared with patients who received intravenous PCA morphine.[12,13] In addition, the patients with continuous femoral three-in-one blocks had the fewest side effects. These studies support the movement toward peripheral nerve blocks as a valuable technique for providing postoperative analgesia after major joint replacement. However, additional studies are needed further to define their use, duration, and application.

MICROVASCULAR SURGERY

Microvascular surgery includes both replantation, the reattachment of a completely severed body part, and revascularization, the re-establishment of blood flow through a severed body part. Most replantation surgery involves the upper extremity. Anesthetic management in microvascular surgery includes maintenance of blood flow through microvascular anastomoses, positioning considerations associated with a long surgical procedure during which the patient must lie completely still, and replacement of blood and fluid losses, which may be extensive.

Maintenance of blood flow through microvascular anastomoses is paramount to limb or graft viability. Blood flow may be improved by increasing the perfusion pressure, preventing hypothermia, and using vasodilators and sympathetic blockade. Microvascular perfusion pressure depends on both adequate intravascular volume and oncotic pressure. Blood loss during microvascular surgery is typically continual and insidious. Unrecognized bleeding and migration of intravascular fluid into the third space reduce microvascular perfusion pressure, and must be corrected. However, overzealous use of crystalloid results in generalized edema, including the replanted body part, whereas excessive transfusion of blood products increases blood viscosity and therefore decreases flow. Evidence suggests that use of phenylephrine to support blood pressure does not jeopardize blood flow to the tissue being replanted.[14] Rheologically, the oxygen-carrying capacity of blood is optimized with a hematocrit of 30%. Normovolemic hemodilution may be used to

Table 40-1. ANESTHETIC TECHNIQUES FOR COMMON FOOT AND ANKLE OPERATIONS

	Surgical Procedure	Regional Technique	Comments
Forefoot*	Hallux valgus	Metatarsal, ankle, popliteal blockade	Sural nerve block not necessary for surgery
	Amputations	Ankle, popliteal blockade	Popliteal blockade is the technique of choice in the presence of infection or swelling
Midfoot*	Transmetatarsal amputations	Popliteal, ankle blockade	
Hindfoot*	Ankle arthroscopy	Spinal, epidural, or general anesthesia	Operation typically requires good muscle relaxation for manipulation; thigh tourniquet
	Achilles tendon repair	Spinal, epidural, or popliteal blockade	Spinal or epidural anesthesia whenever thigh tourniquet is required
	Ankle fractures	Spinal, epidural, or popliteal blockade	Epidural block requires blockade of L5–S1
	Triple arthrodesis	Spinal or epidural	Neuraxial technique preferred for bone graft harvesting; popliteal blockade for postoperative analgesia

* Femoral or saphenous block required if the incision extends to the medial aspect of the foot or ankle.
From Hadzic A, Vloka JD: Anesthesia for ankle and foot surgery. Techniques in Regional Anesthesia and Pain Management 3:113, 1999, with permission.

improve tissue blood flow and decrease transfusion requirements in patients without significant cardiovascular, cerebrovascular, and renal disease.[15] Preoperative autologous blood donation and intraoperative use of a cell saver also significantly reduce the number of transfused homologous units. Arterial cannulation allows frequent assessment of hemoglobin levels and acid–base status, as well as direct blood pressure measurement.

Body temperature is also a determinant of blood flow. Hypothermia not only results in peripheral vasoconstriction, but causes sympathetic activation, shivering, increased oxygen demand, a leftward shift of the oxygen–hemoglobin dissociation curve, and altered coagulation. Therefore, hypothermia must be prevented in microvascular surgical patients. The operating room temperature should be increased to 21°C, intravenous solutions should be warmed,[16] and the patient covered with a forced-air warming blanket.

The use of vasodilators has also been studied in the treatment of perioperative vasospasm. Local anesthetics and papaverine, applied *topically,* may be used to provide relaxation of vascular smooth muscle in the intraoperative setting.[17] All of the volatile anesthetics are potent vasodilators, and can increase tissue blood flow 200–300%, even at typical expired anesthetic concentrations. Direct-acting vasodilating agents, such as sodium nitroprusside, trimethaphan, and hydralazine, produce vasodilation but do not prevent vasospasm due to direct surgical stimulation. Nitroprusside has been shown to reduce perfusion in a microvascular free flap.[14] In addition, the volatile anesthetics and intravenous agents also may result in hypotension and decreased microvascular perfusion pressure. Regional anesthetic techniques provide sympathectomy and vasodilation to the proximal (innervated) segment of an extremity, but have no effect on vasospasm in the replanted (denervated) tissue. Currently, antithrombotics (heparin), fibrinolytics (streptokinase, urokinase, low–molecular-weight dextran), and smooth muscle relaxants (papaverine, local anesthetics) are used to preserve blood flow in microvascular anastomoses.

Microvascular surgery may be performed under regional or general anesthesia. Regional anesthesia has several advantages over general anesthesia. The sympathectomy associated with local anesthetic blockade results in vasodilation and increased blood flow. A "single-shot" regional anesthetic technique may be of insufficient duration for many microvascular procedures. However, placement of an indwelling catheter (intrathecal, epidural, or axillary) provides extended intraoperative anesthesia and continuous postoperative analgesia. General anesthesia is more reliable, ensures airway access, and reduces the possibility of patient movement during critical surgical events. A combination of general and continuous regional anesthesia allows prolonged intraoperative anesthesia and postoperative analgesia, reduces the amount of inhalational agent, and increases the patient's acceptance of lengthy surgical procedures. However, regardless of anesthetic technique, conditions that stimulate vasospasm or vasoconstriction, such as pain, hypotension, and hypovolemia, must be avoided. Whether administration of a vasopressor with vasoconstrictive qualities, or addition of epinephrine to local anesthetic solutions may decrease anastomotic blood flow is controversial.[14]

PEDIATRIC ORTHOPAEDIC SURGERY

Pediatric patients present with a variety of orthopaedic conditions, including congenital deformities, traumatic injuries, infections, and malignancies. Anesthetic management of the pediatric orthopaedic patient involves not only the usual pediatric patient considerations, such as airway management, fluid replacement, and maintenance of body temperature, but the unique concerns associated with orthopaedic surgery. Coexisting neuromuscular conditions, such as arthrogryposis or myelo-

meningocele, may predispose pediatric orthopaedic patients to latex allergy and malignant hyperthermia. In addition, patient positioning and the use of regional techniques for intraoperative anesthesia and postoperative analgesia must be considered.

Regional techniques are readily adaptable to the pediatric orthopaedic patient. Often, regional anesthetic procedures are technically easier to perform on children because the relative lack of subcutaneous tissue facilitates identification of bony and vascular landmarks as well as spread of local anesthetic solutions. The advantages of regional anesthesia in children are similar to those in adults and include earlier ambulation and hospital discharge, decreased incidence of nausea and vomiting, and prolonged postoperative analgesia. However, pediatric patients often are not considered candidates for regional techniques. The preoperative visit is essential in building a patient–parent–physician relationship and establishing an anesthetic plan. The use of preoperative and preblock sedation (oral and intranasal midazolam, intramuscular ketamine, and rectal methohexital) decreases anxiety and increases acceptance of regional anesthesia in the pediatric patient.

Orthopaedic procedures may be performed under regional, general, or a combination of anesthetic techniques. The patient's age, operative site and positioning, and surgical duration are important factors in selection of an anesthetic. Children older than 7 years of age may tolerate a primary regional anesthetic technique, whereas younger children may benefit from a general or combination regional/general anesthesia. Neural blockade may be initiated after induction of general anesthesia and before surgical incision, to provide possible pre-emptive analgesia, or on completion of the surgical procedure to extend the duration of postoperative analgesia.

Surgical procedures to the lower extremity may be safely and successfully performed under caudal, epidural, and spinal anesthesia.[18] However, the anatomic differences between the pediatric and adult spine and spinal cord must be appreciated.[19] In addition, femoral, lateral femoral cutaneous, and sciatic nerve blocks allow prolonged anesthesia and analgesia to the blocked extremity, but often require additional intraoperative supplementation with intravenous or inhalational agents.[20]

Upper extremity procedures may be performed with any of the anesthetic techniques previously described for adults. The superficial location of the brachial plexus, decreased neural diameter, and rapid diffusion of local anesthetics contribute to the high success rate, which approaches 100%, even with a variety of techniques.[21] Blockade of the brachial plexus is usually accomplished with perivascular, sheath, or nerve stimulator techniques in children younger than 7 years of age because elicitation of paresthesias is regarded as uncomfortable (and therefore unacceptable) by the younger pediatric patients. Intravenous regional (Bier) block is particularly useful in the pediatric population for limited procedures such as closed reduction of forearm fractures. The use of local anesthetic eutectic creams minimizes patient discomfort during intravenous catheter placement. Once intravenous access has been established, and the patient sedated, placement of a second venous cannula in the operative extremity is well tolerated. The small size of the upper arm often precludes the use of a double tourniquet in pediatric patients, limiting the duration of the surgical procedure to 45–60 minutes.

SURGERY TO THE SPINE
Spinal Cord Injuries

Spinal injury occurs at a rate of 11,000 cases per year. Approximately one half of these are at the cervical level. The examination of a person with a suspected spinal cord injury begins with a prompt neurologic examination and a rapid assessment for possible injury to other systems. Cervical injuries are frequently associated with head injury, thoracic fractures with pulmonary and cardiovascular injury, and lumbar fractures with abdominal and long bone injuries. The patient should be examined immediately for signs of respiratory insufficiency, airway obstruction, rib fractures, and chest wall or facial trauma.

Serial neurologic examination is necessary to assess function of the spinal cord above the level of the fracture. The fifth cervical segment is perhaps the most important in providing clinical evidence of cervical spinal injury. This segment controls motor function of the deltoid, biceps, brachialis, and brachioradialis muscles. If these muscles are flaccid, the fifth cervical nerve is involved and there will be partial diaphragmatic paralysis. A complete lesion at the fourth cervical segment is not compatible with survival unless artificial respiration is initiated.

Tracheal Intubation

Airway management is critical in patients with cervical spinal cord injury. The most common cause of death with acute cervical spinal cord injury is respiratory failure. All patients with severe trauma or head injuries should be assumed to have an unstable cervical fracture until proven otherwise radiographically. During transport, the patient should be moved on a spine board with the neck immobilized to prevent further injury. Fiberoptic intubation of an awake patient may be necessary. Blind nasotracheal intubation can be used when there is no evidence of facial or basal skull fractures. In a truly emergent situation, oral intubation with direct laryngoscopy is the usual approach. The trachea should be intubated with minimum flexion or extension of the neck.

Surgical Management

Surgical treatment of spinal cord injuries is based on the presence or absence of neurologic function and the radiographic evaluation of vertebral displacement and instability. Patients with unstable spines who are not quadriplegic or paraplegic may become so during positioning for surgery. The period of greatest risk is associated with turning the patient prone. Safe positioning for posterior cervical and thoracolumbar procedures may be performed by using a Foster frame, Jackson table, or other rotating bed. When appropriate, line placement, intubation, and positioning can be performed while the patient is awake with general anesthesia induced only after voluntary upper and lower extremity movement is confirmed. Cervical spine fractures are most often surgically treated by anterior open reduction and fusion. The surgical incision approximates the anterior border of the sternocleidomastoid muscle, and is therefore near critical anatomic structures. Lateral retraction of the carotid artery may endanger blood flow to the brain, particularly in the elderly patient.[22] Retraction of the esophagus and trachea medially may cause pharyngeal laceration, laryngeal edema, and recurrent laryngeal nerve paralysis. Cerebrospinal fluid leaks and trauma to the vertebral artery have also been reported. Thoracolumbar dislocations are typically posterior.

Maintaining Spinal Cord Integrity

Spinal shock occurs acutely and results in complete cessation of spinal cord functions below the level of the lesion. This results in flaccid paralysis, loss of visceral and somatic sensation, and paralytic ileus. Vasopressor reflexes are also lost. Spinal shock may persist from a few days to 3 months.

All patients with spinal cord trauma should be considered to have compromised spinal cords, and an important component of anesthetic management is the preservation of spinal cord blood flow. Blood pressure and intravascular volume should be maintained within normal levels to ensure adequate spinal cord perfusion pressure. Sustained hypotension may worsen neurologic deficits. Hyperventilation should be avoided because hypocarbia decreases spinal cord blood flow. Neurophysiologic monitoring, such as the use of somatosensory evoked potentials (SSEPs), motor evoked potentials (MEPs), or electromyography, assists in prompt diagnosis of neurologic changes and early intervention in situations of potential neurologic ischemia. The wake-up test may also be used to confirm neurologic dysfunction in the presence of changes in MEP or SSEP waveforms.

Respiratory Considerations

Ventilatory impairment increases with the higher level of spinal injury. A high cervical lesion that includes the diaphragmatic segments (C4–5) results in respiratory failure, and death occurs unless artificial pulmonary ventilation is used. Lesions between C5 and T7 cause significant alterations in respiratory function owing to the loss of abdominal and intercostal support. The indrawing of flaccid thoracic muscles during inspiration produces paradoxical respirations, resulting in a vital capacity reduction of 60%. Inability to cough and effectively clear secretions results in atelectasis and infection.

Cardiovascular Considerations

During spinal shock, there is loss of sympathetic vascular tone below the injury. If the cardioaccelerator fibers (T1–4) are damaged, bradycardia results. Therefore, hemorrhagic shock may not produce a compensatory tachycardia in these patients; the rate may remain at $40–60$ beats $\cdot$ min^{-1}. Monitoring of central venous or pulmonary artery pressures may be necessary as an aid to fluid management in a patient with a high cervical lesion. Autonomic instability should be treated with vasoconstrictors, vasodilators, and positive chronotropic drugs as needed.

Succinylcholine-Induced Hyperkalemia

In patients with motor deficits from spinal cord injuries, hyperkalemia may develop after administration of succinylcholine. The amount of potassium released depends on the degree of paralysis. It is usually safe to administer succinylcholine for the first 48 hours. After that time, there is a proliferation of acetylcholine receptors in muscle and they become supersensitive to depolarizing muscle relaxants.[23] The increases in serum potassium are maximal between 4 weeks and 5 months after spinal injury. Serum potassium levels may increase from normal to as high as 14 mEq $\cdot$ l^{-1}, causing ventricular fibrillation or cardiac arrest. Therefore, succinylcholine should be avoided in all spinal cord-injured patients after 48 hours. There are no contraindications to the nondepolarizing agents.

Temperature Control

Disruption of the sympathetic pathways carrying temperature sensation and subsequent loss of vasoconstriction below the level of injury cause spinal cord-injured patients to be poikilothermic. Maintenance of normal temperature can be achieved by applying exogenous heat to the skin, increasing ambient air temperature, warming intravenous fluids, and humidifying gases.

Autonomic Hyper-reflexia

After recovery from spinal shock, 85% of patients exhibit autonomic hyper-reflexia when there has been complete cord transection above T5. The syndrome can also occur with injuries at lower levels and is characterized by severe paroxysmal hypertension with bradycardia, arrhythmias, and cutaneous vasoconstriction below and vasodilation above the level of the injury. The episode is typically precipitated by distention of a viscus (bladder or rectum), but can be induced by any noxious stimulus. The lack of supraspinal inhibition allows the sympathetic outflow below the lesion to react to the stimulus unopposed. If untreated, the hypertensive crisis may progress to seizures, intracranial hemorrhage, or myocardial infarction. If autonomic hyper-reflexia occurs, it should be treated by removal of the stimulus, deepening anesthesia, and administration of direct-acting vasodilators.

Scoliosis

Scoliosis is a deformity of the spine resulting in lateral curvature and rotation of the vertebrae as well as deformity of the rib cage (Fig. 40-2). The incidence of scoliosis predominantly reflects the incidence of idiopathic scoliosis, which represents 75–90% of cases. The remaining 10–25% of cases are associated with neuromuscular diseases, congenital abnormalities including congenital heart disease, trauma, and mesenchymal disorders. A diagno-

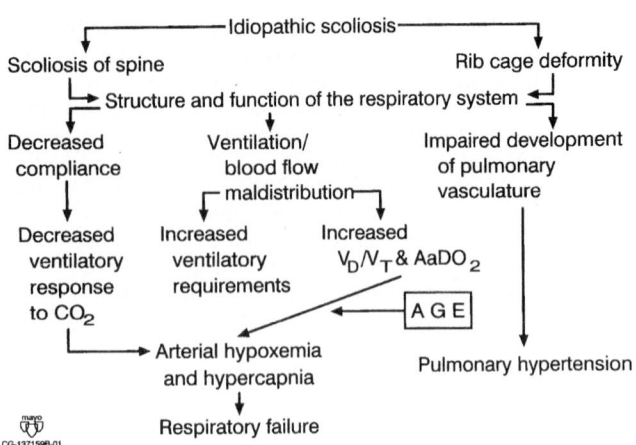

Figure 40-3. The factors in idiopathic scoliosis that contribute to respiratory function abnormalities and failure. (Reprinted with permission from Kafer ER: Respiratory and cardiovascular functions in scoliosis. Bull Eur Physiopathol Respir 13:299, 1977.)

sis of scoliosis in a patient should therefore include a family history and physical examination with particular attention to the respiratory, cardiac, and neuromuscular systems.

Respiratory Function

Scoliosis has profound effects on the respiratory and cardiovascular systems (Fig. 40-3). In patients with untreated scoliosis, respiratory failure and death usually occur by 45 years of age. Vital capacity appears to be a reliable prognostic indicator of perioperative respiratory reserve. Postoperative ventilation will most likely be required for patients with a vital capacity less than 40% of predicted. Although the long-term effect of scoliosis repair is to halt the decline in respiratory function, pulmonary function acutely deteriorates for 7–10 days after surgery.

The primary abnormality in gas exchange is ventilation–perfusion maldistribution, which contributes to hypoxemia. However, hypercapnia develops with increasing age as compensatory mechanisms fail. Prolonged hypoxia, hypercapnia, and pulmonary vascular constriction may result in irreversible pulmonary vascular changes and pulmonary hypertension. In general, the prognosis of scoliosis associated with neuromuscular disease is worse than that of idiopathic scoliosis. These patients frequently need postoperative ventilatory support.

Cardiovascular Function

Cardiovascular function is also affected in patients with scoliosis. At autopsy, these patients exhibit right ventricular hypertrophy and hypertensive pulmonary vascular changes. Prolonged alveolar hypoxia due to hypoventilation and ventilation–perfusion mismatch eventually causes irreversible vasoconstriction and pulmonary hypertension. Scoliosis is also associated with congenital heart conditions, including mitral valve prolapse, coarctation, and cyanotic heart disease, suggesting a common embryonic insult or collagen defect.

Preoperative Assessment

The primary aim of preoperative evaluation of patients with scoliosis is to detect the presence and extent of cardiac or pulmonary compromise. Respiratory reserve is assessed by exercise tolerance, vital capacity, and arterial blood gases. Cardiac studies are performed as indicated to optimize preoperative cardiovascular status. A brief neurologic examination is also performed at the time of the preoperative evaluation to document pre-existing neurologic deficits. Finally, cervical mobility and upper airway anatomy are assessed to discover any potential airway or positioning difficulties and the need for fiberoptic intubation. Patients should also be encouraged to participate

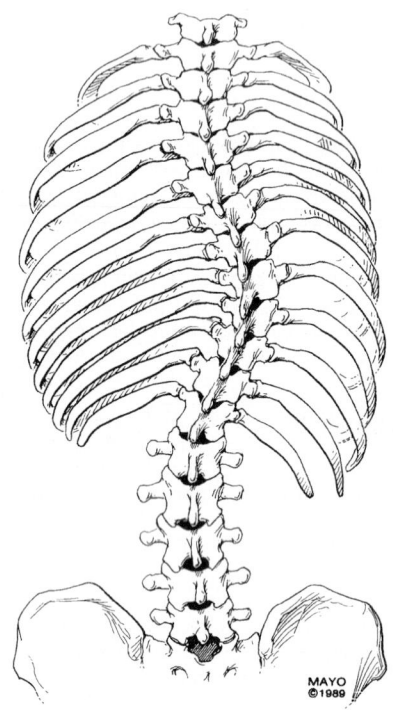

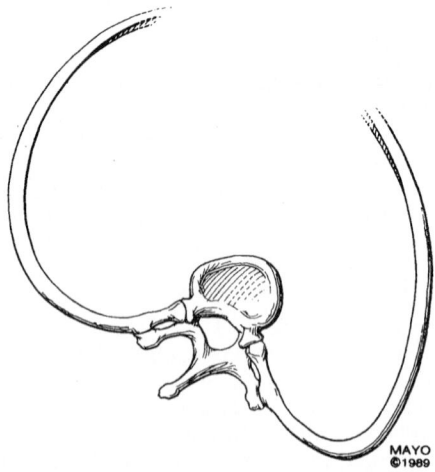

Figure 40-2. Deformity of the vertebrae and rib cage in scoliosis. Primary curvature occurs most frequently in the thoracic and lumbar regions. The vertebral bodies are wedge shaped and the posterior angles of the ribs are shallow on the side of concavity. On the convex side, the rib angles are more acute. (Reprinted with permission from Horlocker TT, Cucchiara RF, Ebersold MJ: Vertebral column and spinal cord surgery. In Cucchiara RF, Michenfelder JD [eds]: Clinical Neuroanesthesia, p 325. New York, Churchill Livingstone, 1990.)

in preoperative autologous blood donation. Usually 4 or more units of blood can be collected in the month before surgery.

Anesthetic Management

Anesthetic considerations in orthopaedic surgery for scoliosis include management of a patient in the prone position, hypothermia secondary to a long procedure with an extensive exposed area, and replacement of blood and fluid losses, which may be extensive.[24] Recently, attention has been focused on the maintenance of spinal cord integrity, the prevention and treatment of VAE, and reduction of blood loss through hypotensive anesthetic techniques.

Adequate monitoring and venous access are essential in management of patients undergoing spinal fusion and instrumentation. The radial artery is cannulated for direct blood pressure measurement and assessment of blood gases. A central venous catheter is helpful in evaluating blood and fluid management and can be used to aspirate air should VAE occur. Patients with evidence of pulmonary hypertension or severe coexistent cardiovascular or pulmonary disease may require a pulmonary artery catheter.

After anesthetic induction and establishment of vascular access are completed, the patient is positioned for surgery. The prone position is used for the posterior approach. Pressure points should be carefully padded. An orthopaedic frame, such as the Jackson table or Wilson frame, can be used to free the chest and abdomen. In correct prone positioning for thoracolumbar spine surgery, the head is turned, the neck is slightly flexed, and the arms are anteriorly flexed and abducted to reduce tension on the brachial plexus (Fig. 40-4). If only one arm is abducted, the head should be laterally rotated toward the ipsilateral arm to prevent stretch injury to the brachial plexus. Because rotation of the neck in patients with cervical spondylosis may alter cerebrovertebral circulation and compromise the spinal cord, patients should be evaluated for neck pain or neurologic symptoms with neck rotation before surgery. The chest and iliac crest are supported by chest rolls or other supports to leave the abdomen free. Breasts should be positioned medially to avoid traumatic injury. The dependent ear and eye should be checked frequently during surgery to avoid injury and ischemia. Pressure on the globe can result in retinal damage, especially in patients with glaucoma. Unilateral and bilateral blindness have been reported after spinal surgery, and have been attributed to multiple causes, including anemia, hypotension, and improper positioning.[25,26] Eyes should be taped closed to avoid corneal abrasion, which occurs in the dependent eye with a frequency of 0.17%. Necrosis of the dependent ear cartilage may occur if the pinna is doubled back on itself.

A nitrous oxide–narcotic–relaxant technique supplemented as necessary by volatile anesthetics is most commonly used for maintenance of anesthesia. The use of low concentrations of inhalational anesthetics helps maintain normotension, reduces

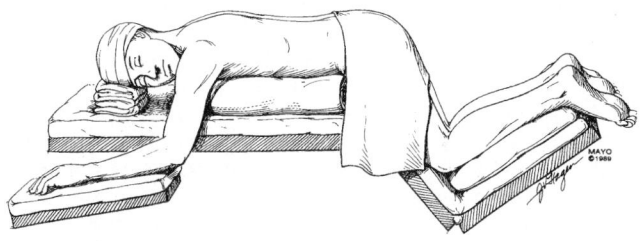

Figure 40-4. Prone position. The head is turned with the dependent ear and eye protected from pressure. Chest rolls are in place, the arms are brought forward without hyperextension, and the knees are flexed. (Reprinted with permission from Horlocker TT, Cucchiara RF, Ebersold MJ: Vertebral column and spinal cord surgery. In Cucchiara RF, Michenfelder JD [eds]: Clinical Neuroanesthesia, p 325. New York, Churchill Livingstone, 1990.)

total narcotic requirements, and still allows satisfactory interpretation of SSEPs. Narcotics may be administered by either bolus or continuous infusion. However, continuous infusion may reduce total narcotic requirement by over 50% and results in a smoother and more rapidly achievable wake-up test.[27]

Blood Loss

Most of the blood loss in spinal instrumentation and fusion occurs with decortication and is proportional to the number of vertebral levels decorticated. Blood loss and transfusion requirements may be reduced through proper positioning and the use of intraoperative blood salvage, induced hypotension, and intraoperative hemodilution, although reported results are inconsistent.[28–31]

Patient positioning should minimize epidural venous engorgement by freeing the abdomen. Preoperative donation of autologous blood or infusion of a large volume of crystalloid before surgical incision to reduce the hematocrit to 25–28% decreases blood viscosity and enhances organ blood flow. Normovolemic hemodilution combined with induced hypotension and autotransfusion can decrease or eliminate the need for homologous transfusion.[30]

Moderate induced hypotension (reduction of systolic pressure 20 mm Hg from baseline or lowering mean arterial pressure to 65 mm Hg in the normotensive patient) has been shown to decrease blood loss, reduce transfusion requirements by 50%, and shorten operating times.[30] However, induced hypotension is not without risk and has been reported to cause cord ischemia and neurologic deficit, including blindness.[25,32] Factors associated with increased risk of spinal cord injury include preoperative hypertension, hypocapnia, intraoperative mean arterial pressure less than 60 mm Hg, rapid decrease in blood pressure, and anemia.

The various agents used to induce hypotension in scoliosis surgery include trimethaphan, nitroglycerin, sodium nitroprusside, volatile anesthetics, calcium channel blockers, and α and β antagonists.[33] The volatile agents provide anesthesia as well as hypotension. However, all volatile anesthetics produce a dose-dependent deterioration of evoked potential waveforms. Therefore, a combination of intravenous hypotensive agents and volatile anesthetics is frequently used.

Venous Air Embolus

Several catastrophic events may occur during spine surgery. The large amount of exposed bone and the elevated location of the surgical incision relative to the heart predispose to VAE. The actual incidence of VAE in scoliosis surgery is unknown; however, six cases have been reported in the literature, four of which were fatal.[34–37] The presenting sign in all cases was unexplained hypotension and an increase in the end-tidal nitrogen concentration. The anesthesiologist, therefore, should be aware of the possibilities of VAE because prompt diagnosis and treatment increase patient survival. Should VAE be suspected, the wound should be irrigated with saline, nitrous oxide discontinued, and vasopressors administered. Massive embolism may necessitate turning the patient supine and initiating cardiopulmonary resuscitation.

Another rare complication during spine surgery is trauma to the aorta, vena cava, or iliac vessels. Unexplained hypotension or signs of hypovolemia without obvious blood loss should alert the anesthesiologist to this possibility.

Anterior–Posterior Spinal Surgery

Combined anterior and posterior spinal procedures yield higher union rates and greater correction in patients undergoing scoliosis correction. It remains unclear whether these two major procedures should be performed on the same day or whether the posterior fusion should be delayed to allow the patient to recover from the anterior (first) procedure. Furthermore, the actual timing of the second procedure remains controversial. Although the degree of correction and the arthrodesis rates are similar for one- or two-stage procedures, the morbidity and number of complications, such as increased blood loss and transfusion requirements, decreased nutritional parameters, and longer hospital stays, may be increased for staged procedures.[38] However, these results are not consistent.[39] Because the risk of significant complications is present with either same-day or staged anterior–posterior fusion, prospective studies are needed to clarify this issue.

Degenerative Vertebral Column Disease

Spinal stenosis, spondylosis, and spondylolisthesis are all forms of degenerative vertebral column disease. It is not unusual for more than one of these degenerative changes in the spine to occur concomitantly, leading to a more rapid progression of neurologic symptoms and the need for surgical intervention.

Positioning

Cervical laminectomy is performed in the prone, lateral, or sitting position, whereas thoracolumbar laminectomy is usually performed prone. Considerations for positioning a prone patient have been previously discussed. Patients undergoing cervical laminectomy should be assessed before surgery for cervical range of motion and the presence of neurologic symptoms during flexion, extension, or rotation. Awake fiberoptic intubation may be necessary in patients with severely limited cervical movement.

The use of the sitting position for cervical laminectomy has become increasingly popular. Blood flows away from the site of operation, producing a clear operative field and better surgical exposure. In this position, the patient sits with head, arms, and chest supported. The patient must be carefully positioned and dependent areas padded to prevent compression injuries to nerves and skin. Extreme cervical flexion may obstruct the airway. Hypotension can be minimized by gradual attainment of the sitting position.

A disadvantage of the sitting position is the increased occurrence of VAE. Although the incidence of VAE in sitting posterior fossa cases is 40%, the incidence is only 5–25% in sitting cervical spine procedures. This decreased incidence may alter the need for a central venous pressure catheter. The use of capnography, mass spectrometry, and precordial Doppler should be routine for such cases because they are noninvasive yet effective in detecting VAE. VAE can occur in all positions associated with laminectomies because the wound is above the cardiac level. Incidences of VAE (defined by aspiration of air through a central venous catheter) in patients undergoing neurosurgical procedures in the sitting, supine, prone, and lateral positions are 25, 18, 10, and 8%, respectively.[40]

Anesthetic Management

Both general and regional anesthesia can be safely administered for lower thoracic and lumbar surgery. Some anesthesiologists and surgeons prefer the use of spinal anesthesia; typically, a hypobaric solution is used. Advocates of regional anesthesia maintain that this type of anesthesia reduces blood loss and improves operating conditions by shrinking epidural veins. If a regional technique is used, a local anesthetic of sufficient duration must be selected. Should surgery last longer than the regional block, conversion to general anesthesia is difficult. Most spine surgery, however, is performed under general endotracheal anesthesia. General anesthesia is preferred for essentially all thoracic and cervical procedures because of the high spinal level that would be required with a regional technique. In addition, general anesthesia ensures airway access, is associated with greater patient acceptance, and can be used for lengthy operations. Succinylcholine should be avoided if there are progressive neurologic deficits because of the possible hyperkalemic response.

Spinal Cord Monitoring

Paraplegia is one of the most feared complications of spinal surgery. The incidence of neurologic injuries associated with scoliosis correction is 1.2%, with partial or complete paraplegia occurring in one half of cases. When patients awaken paraplegic, neurologic recovery is unlikely, although immediate removal of instrumentation improves the prognosis. It is therefore essential that any intraoperative compromise of spinal cord function be detected as early as possible and reversed immediately. The two methods developed to accomplish this are the wake-up test and neurophysiologic monitoring.

The *wake-up test*, first described by Vauzelle *et al*,[41] consists of the intraoperative awakening of patients after completion of spinal instrumentation. Surgical anesthesia is typically provided with a balanced technique of nitrous oxide, a volatile drug, and opioids, although use of opioids and a short-acting volatile anesthetic (such as sevoflurane) alone is also possible. The opioids are important to provide analgesia while the patient is awake and to permit the patient to tolerate the endotracheal tube. During the 30–45 minutes before intraoperative wake-up, the volatile anesthetic is discontinued and the patient is allowed gradually to awaken. Muscle relaxants should be allowed to wear off, or be reversed. Awakening is accomplished by withdrawing the nitrous oxide. The patient is addressed by name and asked to move both hands, and after a positive response, both feet. Patients usually respond within 5 minutes. If there is satisfactory movement of the hands, but not the feet, the distraction on the rod is released one notch, and the wake-up test repeated. Increasing the blood pressure and blood volume may be attempted to increase spinal cord perfusion. Although recall of the event occurs in only 0–20% of patients and is rarely viewed as unpleasant,[27] it is important to describe what will transpire to the patient before surgery so that anxiety will be minimized should the patient be fully aware.

The wake-up test is associated with few false-negative results. That is, it is extremely rare for a patient who was neurologically intact when awakened during surgery to have a neurologic deficit on completion of the procedure. However, certain hazards of the wake-up test do exist and include recall, pain, air embolism, dislocation of spinal instrumentation, and accidental tracheal extubation or removal of intravenous and arterial lines. In addition, the wake-up test requires patient cooperation and may be difficult to perform on young children or mentally deficient patients.

An adjunct or alternative to the wake-up test is neurophysiologic monitoring. Neurophysiologic monitoring, including SSEPs, MEPs, and electromyography, is also discussed in Chapter 25. Although the use of MEPs remains limited, SSEP monitoring is widely accepted. However, somatosensory stimulation follows the dorsal column pathways of proprioception and vibration, pathways supplied by the posterior spinal artery. The motor pathway, which is supplied by the anterior spinal artery, is not monitored. MEPs, on the other hand, monitor motor pathways but are technically more difficult to use. Muscle relaxants cannot be used in patients having MEP monitoring. It is of critical importance to note that postoperative paraplegia has occurred in at least one patient with preserved intraoperative SSEPs.[42]

A number of variables are known to alter SSEP waveforms.[43,44] In addition to neural injury, SSEPs are altered by hypercarbia, hypoxia, hypotension, and hypothermia. All the volatile anesthetics produce a dose-related decrease in the amplitude and an increase in the latency of SSEPs.

Acute alterations in SSEP amplitude or latency signify spinal cord compromise and may be the result of direct trauma, ischemia, compression, or hematoma. Should changes occur, it is recommended that surgery be discontinued, blood pressure be returned to normal or 20% above normal, and volatile agents decreased or discontinued. Arterial blood gases may be drawn to rule out a metabolic derangement. If the waveform does not return to normal, the surgeon should release distraction on the cord. A wake-up test is often performed at this time definitely to exclude neurologic deficits.

Postoperative Care

Most patients undergoing posterior spinal fusion can be extubated immediately after the operation if the procedure was relatively uneventful and preoperative vital capacity values were acceptable. Residual opioid or muscle relaxant may lead to hypoventilation or apnea, especially in patients with an associated neuromuscular disease. Some patients who have experienced considerable blood loss and who have received large amounts of intravenous fluids, particularly if they were prone, may have severe facial edema that renders immediate tracheal extubation unwise. Aggressive postoperative pulmonary care, including incentive spirometry, is necessary to avoid atelectasis and pneumonia. Continued hemorrhage in the postoperative period is another concern. Careful monitoring of systemic and central venous pressures, urine output, and wound drainage is essential. Neurologic status must also be monitored closely for deterioration.

Epidural and Spinal Anesthesia After Major Spine Surgery

Previous spinal surgery has been considered to represent a relative contraindication to the use of regional anesthesia. Many of these patients experience chronic back pain and are reluctant to undergo epidural or spinal anesthesia, fearing exacerbation of their pre-existing back complaints. Several postoperative anatomic changes make needle or catheter placement more difficult and complicated after major spinal surgery. Degenerative changes such as spondylolisthesis occur in the spine below the level of fusion, increasing the potential for spinal cord ischemia and neurologic complications with regional anesthesia.[45] The ligamentum flavum may be injured during surgery, resulting in adhesions within or obliteration of the epidural space. Spread of epidural local anesthetic may be affected by adhesions, producing an incomplete or "patchy" block. Obliteration of the epidural space may increase the incidence of dural puncture and make subsequent epidural blood patch placement impossible. Finally, needle placement in an area of the spine that has undergone bone grafting and fusion may not be possible with either midline or lateral approaches; needle insertion can be accomplished only at unfused segments.

Several retrospective studies have demonstrated that epidural anesthesia may be successfully performed in patients with previous spinal surgery; however, successful catheter placement was possible on the first attempt in only 50% of patients, even with an experienced anesthesiologist. In addition, although adequate epidural anesthesia was eventually produced in 40–95% of patients, there appeared to be a higher incidence of traumatic needle placement, inadvertent dural puncture, and unsuccessful epidural needle or catheter placement, especially if spinal fusion extended to L5–S1.[46–48]

Spinal anesthesia may produce a more reliable block and cause less trauma than epidural anesthesia, although this has not been studied. However, it is reasonable to believe that although needle placement may be more difficult or traumatic in these patients, the spread of local anesthetic in the subarachnoid space and quality of block would not be affected. A spinal anesthetic may be more desirable after spinal surgery because the technique does not depend on a subjective loss of resistance, but instead has a definite end point—the presence of cerebrospinal fluid. In addition, the presence of postoperative spinal stenosis or other degenerative changes in the spine or pre-existing neurologic symptoms may preclude the use of regional anesthesia in these patients.

OTHER CONSIDERATIONS

Anesthesia for Nonsurgical Orthopaedic Procedures

Many orthopaedic procedures requiring anesthesia are carried out in areas other than the operating room. These include cast and dressing changes in pediatric patients, pin removal, hip and shoulder relocation, closed reduction of fractures, and joint manipulations. Although some of the minor procedures require only light sedation, those procedures involving bone and joint manipulation usually require a full anesthetic intervention. It is critically important that patients undergoing these procedures be managed with the same careful attention afforded those scheduled for a standard operating room. The orthopaedic surgeon is usually eager to proceed with these surgically straightforward procedures, often without the same preoperative consideration given to a patient undergoing a more extensive surgery.

Regional anesthesia, usually with a short-acting local anesthetic, can be a good choice for these procedures, especially when the patient wishes to leave the hospital on the same day with minimal residual anesthetic effects.

Regional Anesthesia in the Outpatient

The use of regional anesthesia in the outpatient population is associated with several theoretic benefits for the patient. Studies have demonstrated decreased nausea and vomiting, less drowsiness, improved pain control, and shorter stays in the outpatient unit.[5,20,21] However, management of the outpatient regional anesthetic presents a number of unique problems as well. In many cases, residual blockade at the time of discharge is not desirable. This is particularly true when central neural blockade is used. In such cases, a local anesthetic should be chosen to provide a short duration of blockade, and the patient should be fully recovered by the time of discharge. Full recovery implies return of all motor and sensory function along with evidence that the sympathetic blockade has also dissipated. This can best be evaluated by performing orthostatic blood pressure checks, as well as a nursing assessment of the patient's ability to stand upright and ambulate without assistance. It is also prudent to require that the patient be able to urinate before discharge to prevent overdistention of the bladder, and to demonstrate return of autonomic and somatic nerve function.

Return of full neurologic function may be less important immediately after peripheral nerve blocks. Persisting neural blockade provides excellent pain relief and increased blood flow to the surgical site, both of which may be desirable side effects. However, the risk of accidental nerve trauma in a blocked extremity is theoretically higher outside of the hospital environment. The patient should be informed of the risks and instructed in appropriate care of the extremity. Patients who are unable or unwilling to comply with recommended medical care may not be good candidates for regional anesthesia techniques, and should be fully recovered before discharge.

In all cases, a follow-up telephone call on the first postoperative day should include questions concerning residual areas of neural blockade or altered neural function, such as paresthesias. Any patient concerns regarding the anesthetic or surgery should also be discussed. In the case of outpatient spinal anesthesia or accidental dural puncture during epidural anesthesia, the patient should be informed of the risk of postspinal headache and given a contact person in the anesthesia department to call if problems arise. Postdural puncture headache should be managed conservatively for 24–72 hours with bed rest and rehydration. If it persists, epidural blood patch may be considered.

Tourniquets

Peripheral orthopaedic procedures involving removal of tumors, muscle, and bone may be quite bloody. Tourniquets are often used to minimize blood loss. The cuff should be applied over limited padding or none at all. Padding can cause irritation owing to wrinkling or folds, or by absorbing iodophor. During skin preparation, the cuff and padding may be protected with a plastic drape placed just distal to the cuff. The cuff should be large enough comfortably to circle the limb to ensure circumferentially uniform pressure. The point of overlap should be placed 180 degrees from the neurovascular bundle because there is some area of decreased compression at the overlap point. The width of the inflated cuff should be more than half the limb diameter. Pressure is usually maintained by compressed gas (air or oxygen) and must be monitored continually while the tourniquet is in use. Before tourniquet inflation, the limb should be elevated for approximately 1 minute and tightly wrapped with an elastic bandage distally to proximally. Limb tourniquets are relatively contraindicated when there is infection or tumor.

Opinions differ as to the pressure required in tourniquets to prevent bleeding. Some gauges are marked with average arm and leg pressures, but varying patient sizes render such averages irrational. Leg tourniquets are often pressurized more than arm tourniquets, on the theory that larger limbs require more pressure than smaller limbs. In general, a cuff pressure 100 mm Hg above a patient's measured systolic pressure is adequate for the thigh, and 50 mm Hg above systolic pressure is adequate for the arm, with the understanding that if hypertensive episodes occur, the cuff pressure should be increased. Bleeding from the surgical site after cuff inflation may rarely be due to inadequate occlusion of the major arterial inflow, which is corrected by cuff reapplication and use of the proper degree of inflation. Oozing is more commonly due to intramedullary blood flow in the long bones, particularly in the skeletally immature, and to small arterial vessels between the two bones of distal extremities. Overinflation of the tourniquet does not resolve these problems.

The duration of safe tourniquet inflation is unknown. Recommendations range from 30 minutes to 4 hours. Five minutes of intermittent perfusion between 1- and 2-hour inflations, followed by repeated exsanguination through elevation and compression, may allow more extended use.[49] Local hypothermia has been shown to protect muscle from ischemia,[50,51] and decreased muscle activity after neural block may also be protective.

Damage to underlying vessels, nerves, and skeletal muscles has been reported.[52] Injury is a function of both inflation pressure and duration of inflation.[53,54] Direct pressure from the cuff is more damaging than the ischemia distally.[53,55] Arterial spasm, venous thrombosis, and nerve injury are all demonstrable after several hours, depending on the technique used to search for injury. Clinical examination, electromyography, and effluent blood analysis all show completely reversible changes for inflations of 1 to 2 hours, which is the basis for the recommendation of this period as the safe duration for tourniquet use.[56]

Transient systemic metabolic acidosis and increased arterial carbon dioxide levels have been demonstrated after tourniquet deflation, and do not cause deleterious effects in healthy patients.[57,58] Measurable changes include a 10–15% increase in heart rate, a 5–10% increase in serum potassium, and a rise of 1–8 mm Hg in carbon dioxide tension in blood. Prolonged inflation or the simultaneous release of two tourniquets may produce clinically significant acidosis, particularly in patients with an underlying acidosis due to other causes. Tourniquet release has also been associated with cerebral embolic phenomena.[59]

When a pneumatic tourniquet is used with regional anesthetic techniques, some patients complain of dull, aching pain or become restless, even though seemingly adequate analgesia exists for the operation itself. Patient discomfort usually appears approximately 45 minutes after the tourniquet is inflated and becomes more intense with time. No satisfactory explanation for its genesis has been found. Current explanations involve pain transmission through both A delta and C fibers, and its modulation in the dorsal horn synapses. The C (slow pain) fibers recover faster as the block wanes. Analogous phenomena may be observed at the same time point during general anesthesia. Evidence of lightening anesthesia (increase in blood pressure and pulse rate) may appear even though the same concentrations of anesthetic are being delivered.[60,61] The definitive treatment for tourniquet pain is release of the tourniquet. Relief of pain is prompt and complete. During surgery, however, opioids and hypnotics are usually effective.

Fat Embolus Syndrome

Fat embolus syndrome (FES) is associated with multiple traumatic injuries and surgery involving long bone fractures.[62] Risk factors include male sex, age (20–30 years), hypovolemic shock, intramedullary instrumentation, rheumatoid arthritis, THA using the technique of cementing femoral stems designed for press-fit application, and bilateral total knee surgery. The incidence of FES in isolated long bone fractures is 3–4%, and the mortality rate associated with this condition is significant, ranging from 10 to 20%.

Clinical and laboratory signs of FES have been classified by Gurd[63] as major or minor (Table 40-2), with a diagnosis requiring at least one major and four minor criteria as well as the exclusion of other post-traumatic causes of hypoxemia. Major signs of the syndrome include the presence of axillary or subconjunctival petechiae, significant hypoxemia, central nervous system depression in excess of that expected due to the level of hypoxemia, and pulmonary edema. Classified as minor signs are tachycardia, hyperthermia, retinal fat emboli on funduscopic examination, urinary fat globules, an unexplained decrease in hematocrit or platelets, an increased erythrocyte sedimentation rate, and fat globules in the sputum. Symptoms usually occur 12–40 hours after the injury and can range from mild dyspnea to frank coma. Decreased arterial oxygen tension is the most consistent abnormal laboratory value.[62] Fulminant episodes can occur within hours of the traumatic injury, causing severe hypoxemia, respiratory failure, and severe neurologic impairment. Disseminated intravascular coagulation can also occur in conjunction with FES. Not all trauma patients who have demonstrated evidence of fat emboli fit the criteria for diagnosis of

---

Table 40-2. CRITERIA FOR DIAGNOSIS OF FAT EMBOLUS SYNDROME

MAJOR

Axillary/subconjunctival petechiae
Hypoxemia ($Pao_2 < 60$ mm Hg; $Fio_2 < 0.4$)
Central nervous system depression (disproportionate to hypoxemia)
Pulmonary edema

MINOR

Tachycardia (>110 beats·min^{-1})
Hyperthermia
Retinal fat emboli
Urinary fat globules
Decreased platelets/hematocrit (unexplained)
Increased erythrocyte sedimentation rate
Fat globules in sputum

Diagnosis of fat embolus syndrome requires at least one sign from the major and four signs from the minor criteria categories.
From Gurd AR: Fat embolism: An aid to diagnosis. J Bone Joint Surg Br 52:732, 1970, with permission.

FES. Two theories are hypothesized to explain the mechanism of this syndrome: the mechanical theory and the biochemical theory. The mechanical theory proposes that long bone trauma results in release of fat droplets that enter the vascular system through torn veins. These droplets are transported to the pulmonary vascular bed where they act as microemboli. The biochemical theory can be divided into two mechanisms, toxic and obstructive. The toxic mechanism proposes that free fatty acids released at the time of trauma directly affect pneumocytes in the lung and cause adult respiratory distress syndrome. This effect would be enhanced by the trauma-induced release of catecholamines, which would result in further mobilization of free fatty acids. The obstructive theory hypothesizes that an unspecified chemical event at the site of the fracture releases mediators that affect lipid solubility, resulting in coalescence of lipids and consequent embolization. Some or all of these theories may play a role in development of FES. Other predisposing or aggravating factors such as shock, hypovolemia, sepsis, or disseminated intravascular coagulation may be required to trigger the conversion of fat emboli to FES.

Appropriate treatment of FES requires early recognition of the syndrome, reversal of possible aggravating factors such as hypovolemia, early surgical stabilization of fracture sites, and aggressive respiratory support. Corticosteroid therapy is controversial, but may be beneficial. Other pharmacologic interventions, including heparin and dextran, have not been shown to be effective in treating FES.

Deep Venous Thrombosis and Pulmonary Embolus

Orthopaedic surgical procedures are associated with a variety of complications due to embolic phenomena. Reported emboli occurring during and after surgery include fat, cement, air, and thrombus. These may be caused by multiple factors such as positioning, fracture of long bones, injection of cement under pressure, and predisposing medical conditions. VAE can occur in orthopaedic surgical patients undergoing spine surgery in the prone position and shoulder surgery in the sitting position, and is discussed earlier in this chapter.

Incidence of Thromboembolic Complications

Venous thromboembolism is a major cause of death after surgery or trauma to the lower extremities. Without prophylaxis, venous thrombosis develops in 40–80% of orthopaedic patients, and 1–24% show clinical or laboratory evidence of pulmonary embolism. Fatal pulmonary embolism occurs in 0.2–13% of patients[64] (Table 40-3). The incidence of fatal pulmonary embolism is highest in patients who have undergone surgery for hip fracture. Although fatal pulmonary embolism may be the most common preventable cause of hospital death, many physicians fail to use prophylaxis appropriately because of concern about bleeding complications from anticoagulation. Effective throm-

boprophylaxis requires knowledge of clinical risk factors in individual patients such as advanced age, prolonged immobility or bed rest, prior history of thromboembolism, cancer, pre-existing hypercoagulable state, and major surgery. In many patients, multiple risk factors may be present, and the risks are cumulative. After identification of the risk of thromboembolism, an assessment may be made regarding the risks and benefits of physical or pharmacologic techniques used to prevent thromboembolic complications.

Thromboembolic Prophylaxis

Patients undergoing major orthopaedic surgery are at increased risk for thromboembolism. Although it is recommended that some form of prophylaxis be used in all patients, the method and duration of prophylaxis remain controversial (Table 40–4). Nonpharmacologic measures include graded elastic compression stockings, intermittent pneumatic compression, and early ambulation.

Multiple thromboprophylaxis regimens for patients undergoing total hip replacement have been studied. Although aspirin and subcutaneous unfractionated heparin are more efficacious than placebo, the risk of thromboembolism remains significant, and a higher level of anticoagulation is required. In addition, although adjusted-dose administration of unfractionated heparin (to attain an activated partial thromboplastin time in the upper normal range) is effective, most orthopaedic surgeons consider adjusted-dose heparin prophylaxis impractical. The most popular method of thromboprophylaxis after total hip replacement is oral anticoagulation with warfarin, with the first dose administered the evening before surgery and a target international normalized ratio (INR) of 2.0–3.0. Low–molecular-weight heparin (LMWH) has also been demonstrated to be equally efficacious and cost effective.[64]

Thromboembolic complications occur after total knee replacement despite aggressive measures. Intermittent pneumatic compression devices may be effective, but must be applied during surgery and worn continuously after surgery except during ambulation. Patient intolerance limits their use, however. Subcutaneous heparin and aspirin are also ineffective. Therefore, the two most common anticoagulant-based methods of thromboprophylaxis after total knee replacement are warfarin and LMWH. Current data suggest that LMWH is slightly more effective than warfarin in this patient population.

The optimal duration of anticoagulation after either total hip or knee replacement is unknown. Although available information implies that a minimum of 7–10 days of prophylaxis is required, significant risk for thromboembolism may persist for 1–2 months after surgery. Discontinuation of LMWH or warfarin therapy on hospital discharge (approximately 5 days after surgery) may be inadequate.

Prophylaxis in patients sustaining a hip fracture remains a challenge. Although these patients are at significant risk of thromboembolism, their overall medical condition may also

---

Table 40-3. VENOUS THROMBOEMBOLISM PREVALENCE AFTER ORTHOPEDIC SURGERY

Procedure	Deep Venous Thrombosis*		Pulmonary Embolism	
	Total (%)	Proximal (%)	Total (%)	Fatal (%)
Total hip replacement	45–57%	23–36%	0.7–30%	0.34–6%
Total knee replacement	40–84%	9–20%	1.8–7%	0.2–0.7%
Hip fracture surgery	36–60%	17–36%	4.3–24%	3.6–12.9%

* Total or proximal deep venous thrombosis prevalence among placebo or control groups in clinical trials requiring mandatory postoperative venography.
From Dalen JE, Hirsh J: The fifth ACCP Consensus Conference on Antithrombotic Therapy. Chest 114:531S, 1998, with permission.

Table 40-4. ANTITHROMBOTIC REGIMENS TO PREVENT THROMBOEMBOLISM IN ORTHOPEDIC SURGICAL PATIENTS

ADJUSTED-DOSE SUBCUTANEOUS HEPARIN

3500 U heparin q8h with dose adjustments to maintain aPTT at high-normal values

LOW–MOLECULAR-WEIGHT HEPARIN AND HEPARINOIDS*

Ardeparin 50 U · kg^{-1} twice daily starting 12–24 h after surgery
Dalteparin 5000 U 8–12 h before surgery and once daily starting 12 h after surgery
Danaparoid 750 U 1–2 h before surgery and once daily after surgery
Enoxaparin 3000 U twice daily starting 12–24 h after surgery or 4000 U once daily starting 10–12 h before surgery
Nadroparin 40 U · kg^{-1} starting 2 h before surgery and once daily after surgery for 3 days. The dose is then increased to 60 U · kg^{-1} once daily.
Tinzaparin 50 U · kg^{-1} 2 h before surgery and once daily after surgery, or 75 U · kg^{-1} once daily starting 12–24 h after surgery

ADJUSTED-DOSE PERIOPERATIVE WARFARIN

Start daily warfarin dose 5 mg the day of surgery or the day after surgery; adjust dose for INR 2–3 by day 5

* Dosage expressed as anti–factor Xa units. Use with caution in patients receiving neuraxial anesthesia/analgesia. Ardeparin, enoxaparin, dalteparin, and danaparoid are approved by the Food and Drug Administration.
aPTT = activated partial thromboplastin time; INR = international normalized ratio.
From Dalen JE, Hirsh J: The fifth ACCP Consensus Conference on Antithrombotic Therapy. Chest 114:531S, 1998, with permission.

place them at risk for bleeding complications. In addition, no data are available to assess the efficacy of nonpharmacologic methods such as intermittent pneumatic compression. Although prophylaxis with either LMWH or warfarin therapy is preferable, administration of standard subcutaneous heparin or aspirin may be acceptable in some patients.[64]

Neuraxial Anesthesia and Analgesia in the Orthopaedic Patient Receiving Thromboprophylaxis

Several studies show a decrease in the incidence of both DVT and PTE in patients undergoing hip surgery under epidural[7-9] and spinal[65-67] anesthesia. Similar findings have been reported for knee surgery performed under epidural anesthesia.[68,69] Proposed mechanisms for this effect include (1) rheologic changes resulting in hyperkinetic lower extremity blood flow, reducing venous stasis and preventing thrombus formation; (2) beneficial circulatory effects from epinephrine added to the local anesthetic solutions; (3) altered coagulation and fibrinolytic responses to surgery under central neural blockade, resulting in a decreased tendency for blood to clot and better fibrinolytic function;[70] (4) the absence of positive-pressure ventilation and its concomitant effects on circulation; and (5) direct local anesthetic effects such as decreased platelet aggregation. Although the improved lower extremity rheology associated with spinal and epidural anesthesia seems self-evident, other cited mechanisms are difficult to prove. Interpretation of studies that examine these factors must take into consideration variations in surgical techniques, fluid management, patient positioning, and other parameters. Finally, most of the studies examining the value of epidural and spinal anesthesia in preventing DVT and PTE involved patients who were not receiving currently recommended pharmacologic prophylaxis. The role of regional anesthesia needs to be re-evaluated in this population to determine the extent of protection as well as the risk of performing neural blockade in partially anticoagulated patients so that a reasonable risk–benefit ratio can be determined.

Despite the advantages of neuraxial techniques, patients receiving perioperative anticoagulants and antiplatelet medications are often not considered candidates for spinal or epidural anesthesia/analgesia because of the risk of neurologic compromise from expanding spinal hematoma. The actual incidence of neurologic dysfunction resulting from hemorrhagic complications associated with neuraxial blockade is unknown; however, the incidence cited in the literature is estimated to be less than 1 in 150,000 epidural and less than 1 in 220,000 spinal anesthetics.[71] The frequency of spinal hematoma is increased in patients who receive perioperative anticoagulation.[72] The clinician must be aware of the pharmacologic properties of

thromboprophylactic medications to evaluate patients for neuraxial block as well as determine the timing of catheter removal.

Extensive clinical testing and use of LMWH in Europe in the 1990s suggested that there was not an increased risk of spinal hematoma in patients undergoing neuraxial anesthesia while receiving perioperative LMWH thromboprophylaxis.[72] However, 5 years after the release of LMWH for general use in the United States in May 1993, over 40 cases of spinal hematoma associated with neuraxial anesthesia administered in the presence of perioperative LMWH prophylaxis had been reported to the manufacturer.[73] Many of these events occurred when LMWH was administered during or soon after surgery to patients undergoing continuous epidural anesthesia and analgesia. Concomitant antiplatelet therapy was administered in several cases. The apparent difference in incidence in Europe compared with the United States may be a result of a difference in dose and dosage schedule. For example, in Europe the recommended dose of enoxaparin is 40 mg once daily (with LMWH therapy initiated 12 hours before surgery), rather than 30 mg every 12 hours. However, timing of catheter removal may also have an impact. It is likely that the lack of a trough in anticoagulant activity associated with twice-daily dosing resulted in catheter removal during significant anticoagulant activity. The incidence of spinal hematoma in patients undergoing neuraxial block in combination with LMWH has been estimated at 1 in 40,800 spinal anesthetics and 1 in 3100 continuous epidural anesthetics.[74] Although patients with postoperative initiation of LMWH thromboprophylaxis may safely undergo single-dose and continuous catheter techniques, the first dose of LMWH should be administered no earlier than 24 hours after surgery. In addition, it is recommended that indwelling catheters be removed before initiation of LMWH thromboprophylaxis. The decision to implement LMWH thromboprophylaxis in the presence of an indwelling catheter must be made with care.[73] Since anti–factor Xa activity is not predictive of the risk of bleeding, monitoring of the anti–factor Xa level is not recommended. Concomitant administration of medications affecting hemostasis, such as antiplatelet drugs, standard heparin, or dextran, should be avoided in patients receiving LMWH to reduce the risk of surgical or anesthetic-related bleeding complications.

Anesthetic management of patients receiving perioperative anticoagulation with warfarin depends on dosage and timing of initiation of therapy. Patients receiving warfarin therapy during epidural analgesia should have their prothrombin time and INR monitored on a daily basis, and checked before catheter removal if the initial dose of warfarin was more than 36 hours beforehand. There is no definitive recommendation for removal of neuraxial catheters in patients with therapeutic levels of anticoagulation; the trauma associated with catheter removal must be compared with the ongoing trauma produced by an indwelling catheter in an anticoagulated patient, as well as the degree and duration of anticoagulation.[75]

Many orthopaedic patients receive perioperative antiplatelet agents such as aspirin or ibuprofen. Antiplatelet drugs, by themselves, appear to represent no added significant risk for the development of spinal hematoma in patients having epidural or spinal anesthesia. It is not necessary to discontinue antiplatelet medications or assess platelet function before neuraxial anesthesia. However, careful preoperative assessment of the patient to identify alterations of health that might contribute to bleeding is crucial.[76] The relative risk of other antiplatelet agents such as ticlopidine and clopidogrel remains undetermined.

In summary, the decision to perform spinal or epidural anesthesia/analgesia and the timing of catheter removal in the orthopaedic patient receiving thromboprophylaxis should be made on an individual basis; alternative anesthetic and analgesic techniques exist for patients considered to be at an unacceptable risk. The patient's coagulation status should be optimized at the time of spinal or epidural needle/catheter placement, and the level of anticoagulation must be carefully monitored during the period of epidural catheterization. Patients respond with variable sensitivities to anticoagulant medications. Indwelling catheters should not be removed in the presence of therapeutic anticoagulation because this appears to significantly increase the risk of spinal hematoma.[72,73] In addition, communication between clinicians involved in the perioperative management of patients receiving anticoagulants for thromboprophylaxis is essential to decrease the risk of serious hemorrhagic complications.

The patient should be closely monitored in the perioperative period for signs of cord ischemia. If spinal hematoma is suspected, the treatment of choice is immediate decompressive laminectomy. Recovery is unlikely if surgery is postponed for more than 10–12 hours; less than 40% of the patients in a series reported by Vandermeulen et al[72] had partial or good recovery of neurologic function.

Methyl Methacrylate

Methyl methacrylate is an acrylic bone cement used during arthroplastic procedures. Insertion of this cement is associated with sudden onset of hypotension in some patients. This hypotension has been attributed to absorption of the volatile monomer of methyl methacrylate, embolization of air and bone marrow during femoral reaming, lysis of blood cells and marrow induced by the exothermic reaction, and conversion of methyl methacrylate to methacrylate acid. Adequate hydration and maximizing inspired oxygen concentration minimize the hypotension and hypoxemia that can accompany cementing of the prosthesis. Because air can be entrained during this procedure, nitrous oxide should be discontinued several minutes before this point.

Intra-articular Injections

Peripheral opioid receptors may be increased in the presence of chronic inflammation. Intra-articular injection of local anesthetics can be used during arthroscopic procedures along with local infiltration to provide surgical anesthesia. These agents can be injected into the articular space before the start of surgery or added to the irrigation solution. Longer-acting local anesthetic agents alone, or combined with opioids or nonsteroidal agents, can provide postoperative pain relief when injected at the end of the procedure.

Intra-articular injections of local anesthetics, opioids, or combinations have become routine for perioperative pain management after arthroscopic knee surgery. A number of reports enthusiastically recommend the use of this technique; however,

the results remain conflicting.[77,78] Comparison of reports is difficult because of variability in underlying anesthetic techniques, different dosages and concentrations of local anesthetic, and lack of control groups. The safety of injecting large volumes of intra-articular bupivacaine has been ascertained,[79] and side effects are rare after intra-articular doses of morphine. Because these techniques are simple and low risk and seem to afford pain relief under some conditions, they will likely be continued. Carefully controlled studies are necessary to determine which techniques are efficacious and under what clinical circumstances they should be applied.

REFERENCES

1. Conn RA, Cofield RH, Byer DE, Linstromberg JW: Interscalene block anesthesia for shoulder surgery. Clin Orthop 216:94, 1987
2. Lynch NM, Cofield RH, Silbert PL, Hermann RC: Neurologic complications after total shoulder arthroplasty. J Shoulder Elbow Surg 5:53, 1996
3. Urmey WF, Talts KH, Sharrock NE: One hundred percent incidence of hemidiaphragmatic paresis associated with interscalene brachial plexus anesthesia as diagnosed by ultrasonography. Anesth Analg 72:498, 1991
4. Schroeder LE, Horlocker TT, Schroeder DR: The efficacy of axillary block for surgical procedures about the elbow. Anesth Analg 83:747, 1996
5. Davis WJ, Lennon RL, Wedel DJ: Brachial plexus anesthesia for outpatient surgical procedures on an upper extremity. Mayo Clin Proc 66:470, 1991
6. Sculco TP: Global blood management in orthopaedic surgery. Clin Orthop 357:43, 1998
7. Modig J, Borg T, Karlstrom G et al: Thromboembolism after total hip replacement: Role of epidural and general anesthesia. Anesth Analg 62:174, 1983
8. Modig J, Hjelmsted A, Sahlstedt B, Maripuu E: Comparative influences of epidural and general anaesthesia on deep venous thrombosis and pulmonary embolism after total hip replacement. Acta Chir Scand 147:125, 1981
9. Modig J, Borg T, Bagge L, Saldeen T: Role of extradural and of general anaesthesia in fibrinolysis and coagulation after total hip replacement. Br J Anaesth 55:625, 1983
10. Rosberg B, Fredin H, Gustafson C: Anesthetic techniques and surgical blood loss in total hip arthroplasty. Acta Anaesthesiol Scand 26:189, 1982
11. Hadzic A, Vloka JD: Anesthesia for ankle and foot surgery. Techniques in Regional Anesthesia and Pain Management 3:113, 1999
12. Singelyn FJ, Deyaert M, Joris D et al: Effects of intravenous patient-controlled analgesia with morphine, continuous epidural analgesia, and continuous three-in-one block on postoperative pain and knee rehabilitation after unilateral total knee arthroplasty. Anesth Analg 87:88, 1998
13. Capdevila X, Barthelet Y, Biboulet P et al: Effects of perioperative analgesic technique on the surgical outcome and duration of rehabilitation after major knee surgery. Anesthesiology 91:8, 1999
14. Banic A, Krejci V, Erni D et al: Effects of sodium nitroprusside and phenylephrine on blood flow in free musculocutaneous flaps during general anesthesia. Anesthesiology 90:147, 1999
15. MacDonald DJF: Anaesthesia for microvascular surgery. A physiological approach. Br J Anaesth 57:904, 1985
16. Bird TM, Strunin L: Anaesthetic considerations for microsurgical repair of limbs. Canadian Anaesthetists Society Journal 31:51, 1984
17. Geter RK, Winters RRW, Puckett CL: Resolution of experimental microvascular spasm and improvement in anastomotic patency by direct topical agent application. Plast Reconstr Surg 66:690, 1980.
18. Yaster M, Maxwell LG: Pediatric regional anesthesia. Anesthesiology 70:324, 1989
19. Dalens B: Regional anesthesia in children. Anesth Analg 68:654, 1989
20. Wedel DJ: Femoral and lateral femoral cutaneous nerve block for muscle biopsies in children. Regional Anesthesia 14:63, 1989
21. Wedel DJ, Krohn JS, Hall J: Brachial plexus anesthesia in pediatric patients. Mayo Clin Proc 66:583, 1991
22. Sloan TB, Ronai AK, Koht A: Reversible loss of somatosensory evoked potentials during anterior cervical spinal fusion. Anesth Analg 65:96, 1986
23. Martyn JA, White DA, Gronert GA et al: Up-and-down regulation of

skeletal muscle acetylcholine receptors: Effects on neuromuscular blockers. Anesthesiology 76:822, 1992

24. Winkler M, Marker E, Hetz H: The peri-operative management of major orthopaedic procedures. Anaesthesia 53(suppl 2):37, 1998

25. Dilger JA, Tetzlaff JE, Bell GR et al: Ischaemic optic neuropathy after spinal fusion. Can J Anaesth 45:63, 1998

26. Wolfe SW, Lospinuso MF, Burke SW: Unilateral blindness as a complication of patient positioning for spinal surgery. Spine 17:600, 1992

27. Pathak KS, Brown RH, Nash CL, Cascorbi HF: Continuous opioid infusion for scoliosis fusion surgery. Anesth Analg 62:841, 1983

28. Copley LA, Richards BS, Safavi FZ, Newton PO: Hemodilution as a method to reduce transfusion requirements in adolescent spine fusion surgery [see discussion]. Spine 24:219, 1999

29. Murray DJ, Forbes RB, Titone MB, Weinstein SL: Transfusion management in pediatric and adolescent scoliosis surgery: efficacy of autologous blood. Spine 22:2735, 1997

30. Mandel RJ, Brown MD, McCollough NC et al: Hypotensive anesthesia and autotransfusion in spinal surgery. Clin Orthop 154:27, 1981

31. Brodsky JW, Dickson JH, Erwin WD, Rossi CD: Hypotensive anesthesia for scoliosis surgery in Jehovah's Witnesses. Spine 16:304, 1991

32. Grundy BL, Nash CL, Brown RH: Deliberate hypotension for spinal fusion: prospective randomized study with evoked potential monitoring. Canadian Anaesthetists Society Journal 29:452, 1982

33. Patel NJ, Patel BS, Paskin S, Laufer S: Induced moderate hypotensive anesthesia for spinal fusion and Harrington-rod instrumentation. J Bone Joint Surg Am 67:1384, 1985

34. Lang SA, Duncan PG, Dupius PR: Fatal air embolism in an adolescent with Duchenne muscular dystrophy during Harrington instrumentation. Anesth Analg 69:132, 1989

35. Frankel AS, Holzman RS: Air embolism during posterior spinal fusion. Can J Anaesth 35:511, 1988

36. McCarthy RE, Lonstein JE, Mertz JD, Kuslich SD: Air embolism in spinal surgery. J Spinal Disord 3:1, 1990

37. Horlocker TT, Wedel DJ, Cucchiara RF: Venous air embolism during spinal instrumentation and fusion in the prone position (Letter). Anesth Analg 75:152, 1992

38. Ferguson RL, Hansen MM, Nicholas DA, Allen BL: Same-day versus staged anterior-posterior spinal surgery in a neuromuscular scoliosis population: The evaluation of medical complications. J Pediatr Orthop 16:293, 1996

39. McDonnell MF, Glassman SD, Dimar JR et al: Perioperative complications of anterior procedures on the spine. J Bone Joint Surg Am 78:839, 1996

40. Albin MS, Chang JL, Babinski M et al: Intracardiac catheters in neurosurgical anesthesia. Anesthesiology 50:67, 1979

41. Vauzelle C, Stagnara P, Jouvinroux P: Functional monitoring of spinal cord activity during spinal surgery. Clin Orthop 93:173, 1973

42. Ginsburg HH, Shetter AG, Raudzens PA: Postoperative paraplegia with preserved intraoperative somatosensory evoked potentials. J Neurosurg 63:296, 1985

43. Burke D, Hicks RG: Surgical monitoring of motor pathways. J Clin Neurophysiol 15:194, 1998

44. Pathak KS, Ammadio M, Kalamchi A et al: Effects of halothane, enflurane, and isoflurane on somatosensory evoked potentials during nitrous oxide anesthesia. Anesthesiology 66:753, 1987

45. Laasonen EM, Soini J: Low-back pain after lumbar fusion: Surgical and computed tomographic analysis. Spine 14:210, 1989

46. Daley MD, Morningstar BA, Rolbin SH et al: Epidural anesthesia for obstetrics after spinal surgery. Regional Anesthesia 15:280, 1990

47. Crosby ET, Halpern SH: Obstetric epidural anaesthesia in patients with Harrington instrumentation. Can J Anaesth 36:693, 1989

48. Hubbert CH: Epidural anesthesia in patients with spinal fusion. Anesth Analg 64:843, 1985

49. Sapega A, Heppenstall RB, Chance B et al: Optimizing tourniquet application and release times in extremity surgery. J Bone Joint Surg Am 67:303, 1985

50. Irving GA, Noakes TD: The protective role of local hypothermia in tourniquet-induced ischaemia of muscle. J Bone Joint Surg Br 67:297, 1985

51. Ikemoto Y, Kobayashi H, Usui M, Ishii S: Changes in serum myoglobin levels caused by tourniquet ischemia under normothermic and hypothermic conditions. Clin Orthop 234:296, 1988

52. Hamilton WK, Sokoll MD: Tourniquet paralysis. JAMA 199:37, 1967

53. Patterson S, Klenerman L: The effect of pneumatic tourniquets on ultrastructure of skeletal muscle. J Bone Joint Surg Br 61:178, 1979

54. Hurst LN, Weinglein O, Brown WF, Campbell GJ: The pneumatic tourniquet: A biomechanical and electrophysiologic study. Plast Reconstr Surg 67:648, 1981

55. Miller SH, Price G, Buck D et al: Effects of tourniquet ischemia and postischemic edema on muscle metabolism. J Hand Surg 4:547, 1979

56. Heppenstall RB, Balderston R, Goodwin C: Pathophysiologic effects distal to a tourniquet in the dog. J Trauma 19:234, 1979

57. Kadoi Y, Ide M, Saito S et al: Hyperventilation after tourniquet deflation prevents an increase in cerebral blood flow velocity. Can J Anaesth 46:259, 1999

58. Bourke DL, Silberberg MS, Ortega R, Willock MM: Respiratory responses associated with release of intraoperative tourniquets. Anesth Analg 69:541, 1989

59. Della Valle CJ, Jazrawi LM, Di Cesare PE, Steiger DJ: Paradoxical cerebral embolism complicating a major orthopaedic operation: A report of two cases. J Bone Joint Surg Am 81:108, 1999

60. Valli H, Rosenberg PH: Effects of three anaesthetic methods on haemodynamic responses connected with the use of thigh tourniquets in orthopaedic patients. Acta Anaesthesiol Scand 29:142, 1985

61. Hagenouw RPM, Bridenbaugh PO, van Egmond J, Stuebing R: Tourniquet pain: A volunteer study. Anesth Analg 65:1175, 1986

62. Carr JB: Fulminant fat embolism. Orthopedics 13:258, 1990

63. Gurd AR: Fat embolism: An aid to diagnosis. J Bone Joint Surg Br 52:732, 1970

64. Dalen JE, Hirsh J: The fifth ACCP Consensus Conference on Antithrombotic Therapy. Chest 114:531S, 1998

65. Thorburn J, Louden JR, Vallance R: Spinal and general anaesthesia in total hip replacement: Frequency of deep vein thrombosis. Br J Anaesth 52:1117, 1980

66. Donadoni R, Baele G, Devulder J, Rolly G: Coagulation and fibrinolytic parameters in patients undergoing total hip replacement: Influence of the anaesthesia technique. Acta Anaesthesiol Scand 33:588, 1989

67. Davis FM, Laurenson VG, Gillespie WJ et al: Deep vein thrombosis after total hip replacement: A comparison between spinal and general anaesthesia. J Bone Joint Surg 71:181, 1989

68. Sharrock NE, Haas SB, Hargett MJ et al: Effects of epidural anesthesia on the incidence of deep-vein thrombosis after total knee arthroplasty. J Bone Joint Surg 73:502, 1991

69. Nielsen PT, Jorgensen LN, Albrecht-Beste E et al: Lower thrombosis risk with epidural blockade in knee arthroplasty. Acta Orthop Scand 61:29, 1990

70. Simpson PJ, Radford SG, Forster SJ et al: The fibrinolytic effects of anaesthesia. Anaesthesia 37:3, 1982

71. Tryba M: Epidural regional anesthesia and low molecular heparin: Pro (in German). Anasthesiol Intensivmed Notfallmed Schmerzther 28:179, 1993

72. Vandermeulen EP, Van Aken H, Vermylen J: Anticoagulants and spinal-epidural anesthesia. Anesth Analg 79:1165, 1994

73. Horlocker TT, Wedel DJ: Neuraxial block and low molecular weight heparin: Balancing perioperative analgesia and thromboprophylaxis. Reg Anesth Pain Med 23:164, 1998

74. Schroeder DR: Statistics: Detecting a rare adverse drug reaction using spontaneous reports. Reg Anesth Pain Med 23:183, 1998

75. Enneking KF, Benzon HT: Oral anticoagulants and regional anesthesia: A perspective. Reg Anesth Pain Med 23:140, 1998

76. Urmey WF, Rowlingson JC: Do antiplatelet agents contribute to the development of perioperative spinal hematoma? Reg Anesth Pain Med 23:146, 1998

77. Stein C, Comisel K, Haimeri E et al: Analgesic effect of intraarticular morphine after arthroscopic knee surgery. N Engl J Med 325:1123, 1991

78. Hughes DG: Intra-articular bupivacaine for pain relief in arthroscopic surgery. Anaesthesia 40:84, 1985

79. Katz JA, Kaeding CS, Hill JR, Henthorn TK: The pharmacokinetics of bupivacaine when injected intra-articularly after knee arthroscopy. Anesth Analg 67:872, 1988

Clinical Anesthesia (4/e), edited by
Paul G. Barash, Bruce F. Cullen, and
Robert K. Stoelting. Lippincott Williams &
Wilkins, Philadelphia, © 2001.

CHAPTER 41

ANESTHESIA AND THE ENDOCRINE SYSTEM

JEFFREY J. SCHWARTZ, STANLEY H. ROSENBAUM, AND
GEORGE J. GRAF

THYROID GLAND

The thyroid gland secretes thyroid hormones, thyroxine (T_4) and 3,5,3'-1-tri-iodothyronine (T_3), which are the major regulators of cellular metabolic activity. Thyroid hormones influence a variety of proteolytic reactions by regulating the synthesis and activity of various proteins. They are necessary for proper cardiac, pulmonary, and neurologic function during both health and illness.

Thyroid Metabolism and Function

The production of thyroid hormone is initiated by the active uptake and concentration of iodide in the thyroid gland (Fig. 41-1). Dietary iodine is reduced to iodide in the gastrointestinal (GI) tract. Circulating iodide is taken up by the thyroid gland where it is then bound to tyrosine residues to form various iodotyrosines. After organification, monoiodotyrosine or diiodotyrosine is coupled enzymatically by thyroid peroxidase to form either T_3 or T_4. These hormones are attached to the thyroglobulin protein and stored as colloid in the gland. The release of T_3 and T_4 from the gland is accomplished through proteolysis from the thyroglobulin and diffusion into the circulation. Thyrotropin (thyroid-stimulating hormone; TSH) is produced in the anterior pituitary gland, and its secretion is regulated by thyrotropin-releasing hormone, produced in the hypothalamus. TSH is responsible for maintaining the uptake of iodide and proteolytic release of thyroid hormone. Excess iodine inhibits the synthesis and secretion of thyroid hormone. Circulating thyroid hormone inhibits thyroid-releasing hormone and TSH secretion in a negative feedback loop. The thyroid gland is solely responsible for the daily secretion of T_4 (80–100 $\mu g \cdot day^{-1}$). The half-life of T_4 in the circulation is 6–7 days.

Approximately 80% of T_3 is produced by the extrathyroidal deiodination of T_4 and 20% by direct thyroid secretion. The half-life of T_3 is 24–30 hours. Most of the effects of thyroid hormones are mediated by the more potent and less protein bound T_3. The degree to which these hormones are protein bound in the circulation is the major factor influencing their activity and degradation. T_4 is metabolized by monodeiodination to either T_3 or reverse T_3 (rT_3). T_3 is biologically active, whereas rT_3 is inactive. The major fraction of circulating hormone is bound to thyroid-binding globulin (TBG), with a smaller fraction bound to albumin and thyroid-binding prealbumin. Less than 0.1% is present as free, unbound hormone. Changes in serum binding protein concentrations have a major effect on total T_3 and T_4 serum concentrations. The plasma normally contains 5–12 $\mu g \cdot dl^{-1}$ of T_4 and 80–220 $ng \cdot dl^{-1}$ of T_3. Many drugs can affect thyroid function, including amiodarone and dopamine.[1]

Although the thyroid hormone is important to many aspects of growth and function, the anesthesiologist is most often concerned with the cardiovascular manifestations of thyroid disease. Thyroid hormones affect tissue responses to sympathetic stimuli and increase the intrinsic contractile state of cardiac muscle. β-adrenergic receptors are increased in number and cardiac α-adrenergic receptors are decreased by thyroid hormone.[2]

Tests of Thyroid Function

Serum Thyroxine

The serum T_4 assay is the standard screening test for evaluation of thyroid gland function (Table 41-1). The total T_4 is elevated in approximately 90% of patients with hyperthyroidism, and it is low in 85% of those who are hypothyroid. The concentration of T_4 is measured by radioimmunoassay (RIA). The serum T_4 concentration is influenced by thyroid hormone protein-binding capacity. An increase or decrease in TBG levels or in protein binding may therefore alter the total T_4 but not the concentration of the free T_4. Because of the effect of TBG on circulating total T_4, T_4 levels should never be used alone to evaluate thyroid disease. Elevations in the TBG concentration are the most common cause of hyperthyroxinemia in euthyroid patients. Increases in TBG due to acute liver disease, pregnancy, or drugs (oral contraceptives, exogenous estrogens, clofibrate, opioids) may be responsible. Because a total T_4 can be misleadingly high in euthyroidism or normal in hypothyroidism, some measure of free thyroid hormone activity (free T_4) must also be used.

Serum Triiodothyronine

The serum T_3 is also measured by RIA. Serum T_3 levels are often determined to detect disease in patients with clinical evidence of hyperthyroidism in the absence of elevations of T_4. T_3 may be the only thyroid hormone produced in excess. T_3 concentrations may be depressed by factors that impair the peripheral conversion of T_4 to T_3 (sick euthyroid syndrome). In 50% of hypothyroid patients, the serum T_3 concentration is low; in the remaining 50% it is normal.

Tests for Assessing Thyroid Hormone Binding

It is necessary to find some measure of thyroid binding proteins, mostly TBG, to interpret correctly total thyroxine levels. The "T uptake" test measures the ability of the patient's serum to bind exogenously introduced T_4 and reflects the amount of TBG and the extent of T_4 saturation on TBG. The T uptake is inversely related to the degree of unsaturation of TBG. The T uptake can be used to calculate the T_4-binding capacity, which is directly related to the degree of unsaturation of TBG. The T uptake or T_4-binding capacity can be used to calculate the estimated free T_4 or free T_4 index, which reflect the free T_4 concentration in the blood independent of binding proteins.

Thyroid-Stimulating Hormone

The RIA for this hormone has proved most useful in detecting patients who are hypothyroid. It is often higher than 20 $\mu IU \cdot ml^{-1}$ in primary hypothyroidism (normal, 8 $\mu IU \cdot ml^{-1}$). In the past, the TSH assay was not sensitive enough to discriminate between the normal levels associated with euthyroid states and the suppressed levels associated with hyperthyroidism, but current assays have made the measurement of TSH a valuable adjunct in the diagnosis of hyperthyroidism. A condition characterized by elevated TSH and normal T_4 may represent subclinical hypothyroidism. A low TSH level in a clinically hy-

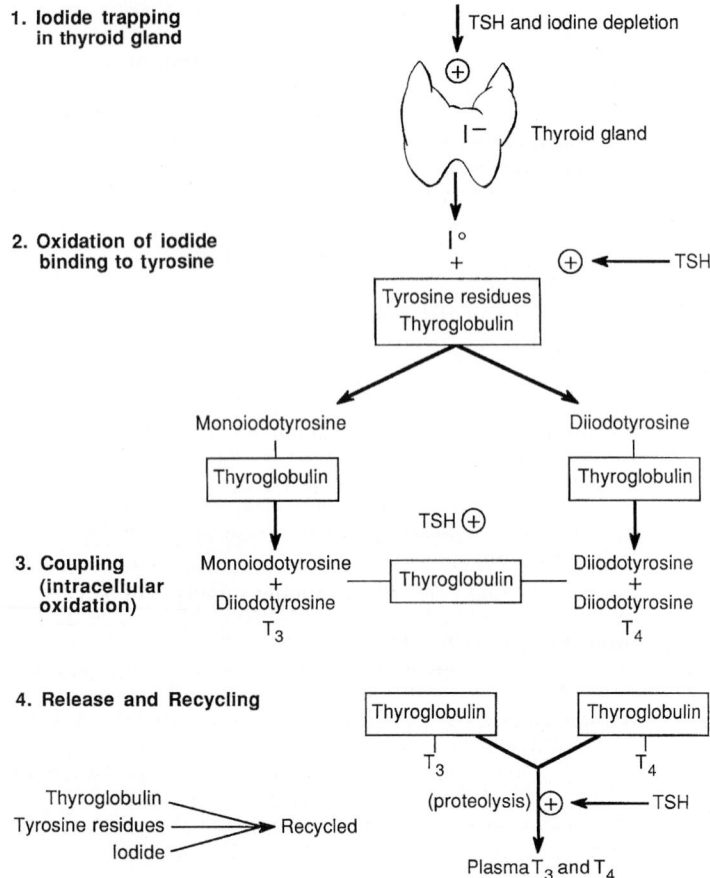

1. Iodide trapping in thyroid gland

TSH and iodine depletion

Thyroid gland

2. Oxidation of iodide binding to tyrosine

I°
+
TSH

Tyrosine residues
Thyroglobulin

Monoiodotyrosine   Diiodotyrosine

Thyroglobulin   Thyroglobulin

TSH ⊕

3. Coupling (intracellular oxidation)

Monoiodotyrosine
+
Diiodotyrosine
T_3

Thyroglobulin

Diiodotyrosine
+
Diiodotyrosine
T_4

4. Release and Recycling

Thyroglobulin   Thyroglobulin
T_3 T_4

Thyroglobulin
Tyrosine residues ——→ Recycled
Iodide

(proteolysis) ⊕ ← TSH

Plasma T_3 and T_4

Figure 41-1. Thyroid hormone biosynthesis consists of four stages: (1) organification, (2) binding, (3) coupling, and (4) release. TSH = thyroid-stimulating hormone; T_3 = triiodothyronine; T_4 = thyroxine.

pothyroid patient indicates disease at the pituitary or hypothalamic level. The goal of thyroid replacement therapy is to normalize TSH levels.[3] Starvation, fever, stress, corticosteroids, and T_3 or T_4 can all depress TSH levels.

Radioactive Iodine Uptake

The thyroid gland has the ability to concentrate large amounts of inorganic iodide. The oral administration of radioactive iodine (^{131}I) can be used to indicate thyroid gland activity. Thyroid uptake is elevated in hyperthyroidism unless the hyperthyroidism is caused by thyroiditis, in which case the uptake is low or absent. Because of overlap in values, it is difficult to distinguish euthyroid from hypothyroid people. Radioactive iodide uptake may be increased by a variety of factors, including dietary iodine deficiency, renal failure, and congestive heart failure. Because uptake is under TSH control, elevated free T_4 levels and corticosteroids decrease radioactive iodide uptake. Functioning ("hot") thyroid tissue is rarely malignant. Nonfunctioning ("cold") tissue may be malignant or benign.

Hyperthyroidism

Hyperthyroidism results from the exposure of tissues to excessive amounts of thyroid hormone (Table 41-2). The most common etiology is the multinodular diffuse goiter of Graves' disease. This typically occurs between the ages of 20 and 40 years and is predominant in women. Most of these patients demonstrate a syndrome characterized by diffuse glandular enlargement, ophthalmopathy, dermopathy, and clubbing of the fingers. A thyroid-stimulating autoantibody may be present. Thyroid adenoma is the second most common cause. Another cause of increased thyroid hormone synthesis is thyroiditis. Subacute thyroiditis frequently follows a respiratory illness and is characterized by a viral-like illness with a firm, painful gland. This type of thyroiditis is frequently treated with anti-inflammatory agents alone. Rarely, subacute thyroiditis may occur in a patient with a normal-sized, painless gland. Hashimoto's thyroiditis is a chronic autoimmune disease that usually produces hypothyroidism but may occasionally produce hyperthyroidism.

Table 41-1. TESTS OF THYROID GLAND FUNCTION

	T_4	THBR	T_3	TSH
Hyperthyroidism	Elevated	Elevated	Elevated	Normal or low
Primary hypothyroidism	Low	Low	Low or normal	Elevated
Secondary hypothyroidism	Low	Low	Low	Low
Sick euthyroidism (decreased peripheral conversion of T_4 to T_3)	Normal	Normal	Low	Normal
Pregnancy	Elevated	Low	Normal	Normal

T_4 = total serum thyroxine; T_3 = serum triiodothyronine; TSH = thyroid-stimulating hormone; THBR = thyroid hormone binding rate.

Table 41-2. CAUSES OF HYPERTHYROIDISM

Intrinsic Thyroid Disease
Hyperfunctioning thyroid adenoma
Toxic multinodular goiter

Abnormal TSH Stimulator
Graves' disease
Trophoblastic tumor

Disorders of Hormone Storage or Release
Thyroiditis

Excess Production of TSH
Pituitary thyrotropin (rare)

Extrathyroidal Source of Hormone
Struma ovarii
Functioning follicular carcinoma

Exogenous Thyroid
Iatrogenic
Iodine-induced

TSH = thyroid-stimulating hormone.

Hyperthyroidism may also be associated with pregnancy, ^{131}I therapy, thyroid carcinoma, trophoblastic tumors, or TSH-secreting pituitary adenomas. Iatrogenic hyperthyroidism may follow thyroid hormone replacement or may occur after iodide exposure (angiographic contrast) in patients with chronically low iodide intake (Jodbasedow phenomenon). The antiarrhythmic agent amiodarone is iodine rich and is another cause of iodine-induced thyrotoxicosis.[4]

The major manifestations of hyperthyroidism are weight loss, diarrhea, skeletal muscle weakness and stiffness, warm, moist skin, heat intolerance, and nervousness. Cardiovascular manifestations include increased left ventricular contractility and ejection fraction, tachycardia, elevated systolic blood pressure, and decreased diastolic blood pressure. Hypercalcemia, thrombocytopenia, and a mild anemia may be present. Elderly patients may present with heart failure owing to papillary muscle dysfunction, atrial fibrillation, or other cardiac dysrhythmias without other systemic signs or symptoms of hyperthyroidism (apathetic hyperthyroidism).

Treatment and Anesthetic Considerations

The most important goal in managing the hyperthyroid patient is to make the patient euthyroid before any surgery, if possible. The drugs propylthiouracil and methimazole are thiourea derivatives that inhibit the synthesis of thyroid hormone.[5] Propylthiouracil also decreases the peripheral conversion of T_4 to T_3. Normal thyroid glands usually contain a store of hormone that is large enough to maintain a euthyroid state for several months, even if all synthesis is abolished. Therefore, hyperthyroid patients are unlikely to be regulated to a euthyroid state with antithyroid drugs alone in less than 6–8 weeks. Toxic reactions from these drugs are uncommon but include skin rash, nausea, fever, agranulocytosis, hepatitis, and a lupus-like syndrome.

Inorganic iodide inhibits iodide organification and thyroid hormone release. Iodide is also effective in reducing the size of the hyperplastic gland and has a role in the preparation of the patient for emergency thyroid surgery.

β-Adrenergic antagonists are effective in attenuating the manifestations of excessive sympathetic activity.[6] For example, propranolol given over 12–24 hours decreases tachycardia, heat intolerance, anxiety, and tremor. β-adrenergic blockade alone does not inhibit hormone synthesis, but it does impair the peripheral conversion of T_4 to T_3 over 1–2 weeks. The combination of propranolol (in doses titrated to effect) plus potassium iodide (two to five drops every 8 hours) is frequently used before surgery to ameliorate cardiovascular symptoms and reduce circulating concentrations of T_4 and T_3. Preoperative preparation usually requires 7–14 days. β-adrenergic antagonists should not be used routinely in patients with symptoms of congestive heart failure or bronchospasm. Heart failure secondary to poorly controlled paroxysmal atrial fibrillation may improve with slowing of the ventricular rate, but abnormalities of left ventricular function secondary to hyperthyroidism may not be corrected with the use of β antagonists. If a hyperthyroid patient with clinically apparent disease requires emergency surgery, β-adrenergic blockade should be administered to achieve a heart rate less than 90 beats · min^{-1}. Glucocorticoids such as dexamethasone (8–12 mg · day^{-1}) are used in the management of severe thyrotoxicosis because they reduce thyroid hormone secretion and reduce the peripheral conversion of T_4 to T_3.

Radioactive iodine therapy is an effective treatment for some patients with thyrotoxicosis.[7] It should not, however, be administered to pregnant patients because it crosses the placenta and may destroy the fetal thyroid. A side effect of RAI therapy is hypothyroidism; 10–60% of cases occur in the first year of therapy, and an additional 2% occur per year thereafter.

A variety of anesthetic techniques and drugs have been used for hyperthyroid patients undergoing surgery. The key to the management of these patients is delaying the stress of surgery until the patient has been brought to a euthyroid state. All antithyroid medications are continued through the morning of surgery. The goal of intraoperative management in the hyperthyroid patient is to achieve a depth of anesthesia that prevents an exaggerated sympathetic response to surgical stimulation while avoiding the administration of medication that stimulates the sympathetic nervous system. It is best to avoid using ketamine even when a patient is clinically euthyroid.[8] Hypotension that occurs during surgery is best treated with direct-acting vasopressors rather than a medication that provokes the release of catecholamines. The appropriate selection of neuromuscular blocking drug deserves mention. Pancuronium has the ability to increase the heart rate and should be avoided; muscle relaxants that provide greater cardiovascular stability (vecuronium, atracurium) should be used. The incidence of myasthenia gravis is increased in hyperthyroid patients; thus, the initial dose of muscle relaxant should be reduced and a twitch monitor should be used to guide all subsequent administration of neuromuscular blocking agents. Regional anesthesia is an excellent alternative when appropriate; however, epinephrine-containing solutions should be avoided.

Thyroid storm is a life-threatening exacerbation of hyperthyroidism that may occur during or immediately after surgery. Operating on an acutely hyperthyroid patient may provoke thyroid storm, although this is probably not due to mechanical release of hormone.[9] Thyroid storm may develop in the undiagnosed hyperthyroid patient because of the stress of surgery and nonthyroid illness.[10] Its manifestations include hyperthermia, tachycardia, dysrhythmias, congestive heart failure, agitation, and confusion. It must be distinguished from, or considered with, pheochromocytoma, malignant hyperthermia, and light anesthesia. Although free T_4 levels are often markedly elevated, no laboratory test is diagnostic. Treatment is with large doses of propylthiouracil and supportive measures to control fever and restore intravascular volume. Hemodynamic monitoring (pulmonary artery catheter, arterial catheter) is especially useful in guiding the treatment of patients with significant left ventricular dysfunction (Table 41-3). Again, it is essential to remove or treat the precipitating event.

Complications of surgery in hyperthyroid patients occur more frequently when preoperative preparation has been inadequate. Airway obstruction is a potential problem in the patient with a large substernal goiter, although rarely a problem with goiters exclusively in the neck. Preoperative computed tomography of the neck provides valuable information about airway anatomy.[11]

Table 41-3. MANAGEMENT OF THYROID STORM

Administer iv fluids.

Administer sodium iodide, 250 mg po or iv q6h.

Administer propylthiouracil, 200–400 mg po or pNGT q6h.

Administer hydrocortisone, 50–100 mg iv q6h.

Administer propanolol 10–40 mg po q4–6h or esmolol infusion to treat hyperadrenergic signs.

Cooling blankets and acetaminophen and meperidine (25–50 mg) iv q4–6h may be used to prevent shivering.

Using digoxin for heart failure especially in the presence of atrial fibrillation with rapid ventricular response.

iv = intravenous; po = oral; NGT = nasogastric tube.

Anesthesia for Thyroid Surgery

Subtotal thyroidectomy as an alternative to prolonged medical therapy is used less frequently today than in the past. It is usually performed under general endotracheal anesthesia, although the use of the laryngeal mask airway is increasing. Use of a laryngeal mask airway allows real-time visualization of vocal cord function because the patient is allowed to breath spontaneously. The complications after subtotal thyroidectomy include recurrent laryngeal nerve damage, tracheal compression secondary to hematoma or tracheomalacia, and hypoparathyroidism.[12] Hypoparathyroidism secondary to the inadvertent surgical removal of parathyroid glands is most frequently seen after total thyroidectomy. The symptoms of hypocalcemia develop within the first 24–96 hours after surgery.[13] Laryngeal stridor progressing to laryngospasm may be one of the first indications of hypocalcemic tetany. The intravenous (iv) administration of calcium chloride or calcium gluconate is warranted in this situation. Magnesium levels should also be monitored and corrected if low. Bilateral recurrent laryngeal nerve injury is an extremely rare injury and necessitates reintubation. Unilateral nerve injury is more common and is often transient.[14] Unilateral damage to the recurrent laryngeal nerve is characterized by hoarseness and a paralyzed vocal cord, whereas bilateral injury causes aphonia. It is wise to evaluate vocal cord function before and after surgery by laryngoscopy or by asking the patient to phonate by saying the letter ''e''. Routine postoperative visualization of the vocal cords is not warranted.[15] Postoperative extubation of the trachea should be performed under optimal conditions. Intraoperative laryngeal nerve injury or collapse of the tracheal rings from previous weakening may mandate emergency reintubation.

Hypothyroidism

Hypothyroidism is a relatively common disease (0.5–0.8% of the adult population) that results from inadequate circulating levels of T_4 or T_3, or both.[16] The development of hypothyroidism is often slow and progressive, making the clinical diagnosis difficult, especially in the more subtle cases. Hypofunctioning of the thyroid gland has many causes (Table 41-4). Primary failure of the thyroid gland refers to decreased production of thyroid hormone despite adequate TSH production and accounts for 95% of all cases of thyroid dysfunction. The remainder are caused by either hypothalamic or pituitary disease (secondary hypothyroidism) and are associated with other pituitary deficiencies.

A lack of thyroid hormone produces a variety of signs and symptoms. These early findings are often nonspecific and difficult to recognize. A history of RAI therapy, external neck irradiation, or the presence of a goiter are all helpful in making a diagnosis. There is a generalized reduction in metabolic activity, resulting in lethargy, slow mental functioning, cold intolerance, and slow movements. The cardiovascular manifestations of hy-

pothyroidism reflect the importance of thyroid hormone for myocardial contractility and catecholamine function. These patients exhibit bradycardia and depressed myocardial contractility. The accumulation of a cholesterol-rich pericardial fluid produces low voltage on the electrocardiogram (ECG). Impaired myocardial contractility generally correlates with the severity of hypothyroidism, although myxedema rarely produces congestive heart failure in the absence of coexisting heart disease. Angina pectoris itself is unusual in hypothyroidism and usually appears when thyroid hormone treatment is initiated (catecholamine hypersensitivity). Ventilatory responsiveness to hypoxia and hypercapnia is depressed in hypothyroid patients. This depression is potentiated by sedatives, opioids, and general anesthesia. Postoperative ventilatory failure requiring prolonged ventilation is rarely seen in hypothyroid patients in the absence of coexisting lung disease, obesity, or myxedema coma. Other abnormalities found in hypothyroidism include anemia, hypothermia, sleep apnea, and impaired renal free water clearance with hyponatremia. Basal plasma levels of cortisol are usually normal in hypothyroidism; however, in long-standing or severe disease, the stress response may be blunted and adrenal depression may occur.

Treatment and Anesthetic Considerations

Treatment of symptomatic hypothyroidism is with hormone replacement therapy.[17] Controversy remains regarding the preoperative anesthetic management of the hypothyroid patient. Although it seems logical to recommend that all hypothyroid surgical candidates be restored to a euthyroid state before surgery, such a recommendation is, in general, based on individual case reports. There have been few controlled studies to support the position that most hypothyroid patients are unusually sensitive to anesthetic drugs, have prolonged recovery times, or have a higher incidence of cardiovascular instability or collapse.

No increase in serious complications in patients with mild or moderate hypothyroidism undergoing general anesthesia has been noted. One study[18] noted a higher incidence of intraoperative hypotension and postoperative GI and neuropsychiatric complications in mild and moderately hypothyroid patients undergoing noncardiac surgery but still noted there were no compelling clinical reasons to postpone surgery in these patients. Surgery in severely hypothyroid patients should be postponed when possible until these patients are at least partially treated.

The management of hypothyroid patients with symptomatic coronary artery disease has been a subject of particular controversy.[19] The need for thyroid hormone replacement therapy must be weighed against the risk of precipitating myocardial ischemia. Several studies and a literature review[20] found no differences in the frequency of intraoperative or postoperative

Table 41-4. CAUSES OF HYPOTHYROIDISM

Primary Hypothyroidism

Autoimmune

Irradiation to the neck

Previous ^{131}I therapy

Surgical removal

Thyroiditis (Hashimoto's)

Severe iodine depletion

Medications (iodines, propylthiouracil, methimazole)

Hereditary defects in biosynthesis

Congenital defects in gland development

Secondary or Tertiary Hypothyroidism

Pituitary

Hypothalamic

Reproduced with permission from Petersdorf RG (ed): Harrison's Principles of Internal Medicine, 10th ed. New York, McGraw-Hill, 1983.

Table 41-5. MANAGEMENT OF MYXEDEMA

Tracheal intubation and controlled ventilation as needed
Levothyroxine 200–300 μg iv over 5–10 min initially, and 100 μg iv q24h
Hydrocortisone, 100 mg iv, then 25 mg iv q6h
Fluid and electrolyte therapy as indicated by serum electrolytes
Cover to conserve body heat; no warming blankets

iv = intravenous.

complications when mild or moderately hypothyroid patients underwent cardiac surgery. In symptomatic patients or unstable patients with cardiac ischemia, thyroid replacement should probably be delayed until after coronary revascularization.

There appears to be little reason to postpone elective surgery in patients who have mild or moderate hypothyroidism. Thyroid replacement therapy is, however, indicated for patients with severe hypothyroidism or myxedema coma and for pregnant patients who are hypothyroid. Untreated hypothyroidism in pregnant patients is associated with an increased incidence of spontaneous abortion and mental and physical abnormalities in the offspring.

A number of anesthetic medications have been used without difficulty in hypothyroid patients. Although ketamine has been proposed as the ideal induction agent, thiopental has also been used in the hypothyroid patient. The maintenance of anesthesia may be safely achieved with either iv or inhaled anesthetics. There appears to be little if any decrease in the minimum alveolar concentration for volatile agents.[21] Regional anesthesia is a good choice in the hypothyroid patient provided that the intravascular volume is well maintained. Monitoring is directed toward the early recognition of hypotension, congestive heart failure, and hypothermia. Scrupulous attention should be paid to maintaining normal body temperature.

Myxedema coma represents a severe form of hypothyroidism characterized by stupor or coma, hypoventilation, hypothermia, hypotension, and hyponatremia. This is a medical emergency with a high mortality rate (50%) and as such requires aggressive therapy (Table 41-5). Only life-saving surgery should proceed in the face of myxedema coma. Intravenous thyroid replacement is initiated as soon as the clinical diagnosis is made. An iv loading dose of T_4 (sodium levothyroxine, 200–300 μg) is given initially and followed by a maintenance dose of T_4, 50–200 mg · day^{-1} iv.[22] Alternatively, T_3 may be used because it has a more rapid onset. Improvements in heart rate, blood pressure, and body temperature may occur within 24 hours. Replacement therapy with either form of thyroid hormone may precipitate myocardial ischemia, however. There is also an increased likelihood of acute primary adrenal insufficiency in these patients, and they should receive stress doses of hydrocortisone. Steroid replacement continues until normal adrenal function can be confirmed.

PARATHYROID GLANDS
Calcium Physiology

The normal adult body contains approximately 1–2 kg of calcium (Ca^{2+}), of which 99% is in the skeleton. Plasma calcium is present in three forms: (1) a protein-bound fraction (40%); (2) an ionized fraction (50%); and (3) a diffusible but nonionized fraction (10%) that is complexed with phosphate, bicarbonate, and citrate. This division is of interest because it is the ionized fraction that is physiologically active and homeostatically regulated. The normal total serum calcium concentration is 8.8–10.4 mg · dl^{-1}. Albumin binds approximately 90% of the protein-bound fraction of calcium, and total serum Ca^{2+} conse-

quently depends on albumin levels. In general, an increase or decrease in albumin of 1 g · dl^{-1} is associated with a parallel change in total serum Ca^{2+} of 0.8 mg · dl^{-1}. The serum ionized Ca^{2+} concentration is affected by temperature and blood pH through alterations in Ca^{2+} protein binding to albumin. Acidosis decreases protein binding (increases ionized Ca^{2+}), and alkalosis increases protein binding (decreases ionized Ca^{2+}). The concentration of free Ca^{2+} ion is of critical importance in regulating skeletal muscle contraction, coagulation, neurotransmitter release, endocrine secretion, and a variety of other cellular functions. As a consequence, the maintenance of serum Ca^{2+} concentration is subject to exquisite hormonal control by parathyroid hormone (PTH) and vitamin D (Fig. 41-2).

Parathyroid hormone acts to maintain the extracellular fluid Ca^{2+} concentration through direct effects on bone resorption and renal Ca^{2+} resorption at the distal tubule, and indirectly through its effects on the synthesis of 1,25-dihydroxyvitamin D. The renal effects of PTH include phosphaturia and bicarbonaturia, in addition to enhanced Ca^{2+} and magnesium resorption. Most evidence suggests that rapid changes in blood Ca^{2+} levels are due primarily to hormonal effects on bone and to a lesser extent to renal Ca^{2+} clearance, whereas maintenance of Ca^{2+} balance depends more on the indirect effects of the hormone on intestinal calcium absorption. The effects of PTH are mediated by specific hormone-target cell membrane interaction. Hormone receptor activation of adenylate cyclase leads to increased intracellular cyclic adenosine monophosphate (cAMP). Presumably, the rapid rise in cAMP promotes an increase in protein kinase, leading to a phosphorylation of key effector

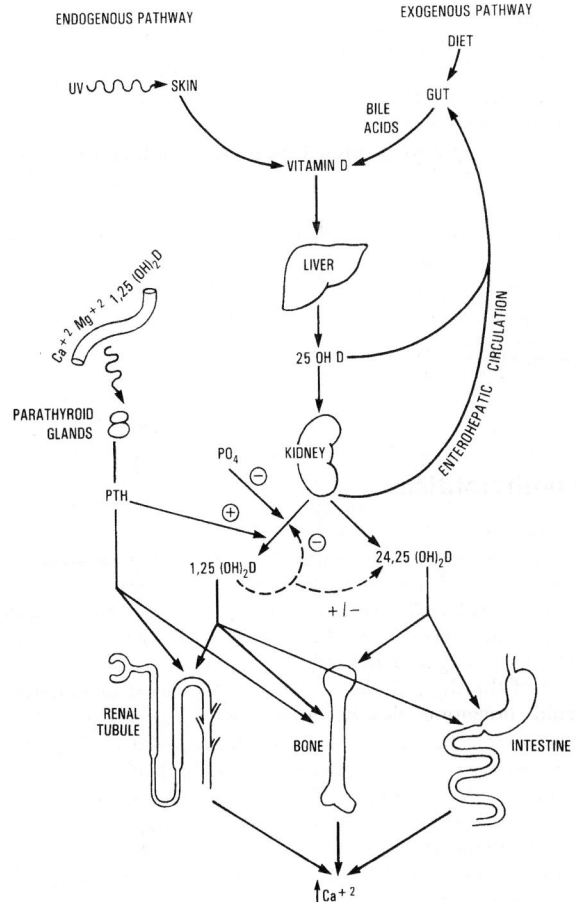

Figure 41-2. Parathyroid hormone and vitamin D metabolism and action. PTH = parathyroid hormone; UV = ultraviolet. (Reproduced with permission from Geelhoed GW, Chernow B [eds]: Endocrine Aspects of Acute Illness. New York, Churchill Livingstone, 1985.)

proteins that initiate the hormonal effect. After the administration of PTH, there is a rise in urinary cAMP. This cAMP leaks from renal tubular cells and provides an index of the biologic activity of PTH.

Parathyroid hormone secretion is primarily regulated by the serum ionized Ca^{2+} concentration. This negative feedback mechanism is exquisitely sensitive in maintaining calcium levels in a normal range. Release of PTH is also influenced by phosphate, magnesium, and catecholamine levels. Acute hypomagnesemia directly stimulates PTH release, whereas chronic magnesium depletion appears to inhibit proper functioning of the parathyroid gland. The plasma phosphate concentration has an indirect influence on PTH secretion by causing reciprocal changes in the serum ionized Ca^{2+} concentration.

Vitamin D Metabolism

Vitamin D is absorbed from the GI tract and can be produced enzymatically by ultraviolet irradiation of the skin. Vitamin D (cholecalciferol) is made from cholesterol metabolites and is inactive. Calciferol is hydroxylated in the liver to 25-hydroxycholecalciferol (25-OHD) and in the kidney is further hydroxylated to 1,25-dihydroxycholecalciferol [1,25 $(OH)_2D$] or 24,25-dihydroxycholecalciferol [24,25$(OH)_2D$]. 25-OHD is the major circulating form of vitamin D. The synthesis of this hormone is not regulated by a hormone or by Ca^{2+} or phosphate levels. 1,25$(OH)_2D$ and 24,25$(OH)_2D$ are the major active metabolites of vitamin D, and their production is reciprocally regulated at the kidney. Hypocalcemia and hypophosphatemia cause an increased production of 1,25$(OH)_2D$ and a decreased production of 24,25$(OH)_2D$. 1,25$(OH)_2D$ stimulates bone, kidney, and intestinal absorption of calcium and phosphate. Vitamin D deficiency can lead to decreased intestinal absorption of Ca^{2+} and secondary hyperparathyroidism.

Hyperparathyroidism

Primary hyperparathyroidism is most commonly due to a benign parathyroid adenoma (90% of cases) or hyperplasia (9%) and very rarely to a parathyroid carcinoma. Primary hyperparathyroidism may also exist as part of a multiple endocrine neoplastic (MEN) syndrome. Hyperplasia usually involves all four glands. Although most patients with primary hyperparathyroidism are hypercalcemic, most are asymptomatic at the time of diagnosis. When symptoms occur, they usually result from the hypercalcemia that accompanies the disease. Primary hyperparathyroidism occurring during pregnancy is associated with a high maternal and fetal morbidity rate (50%). The placenta allows the fetus to concentrate calcium, promoting fetal hypercalcemia and leading to hypoparathyroidism in the newborn. Pregnant women with primary hyperparathyroidism should be treated with surgery.

Hypercalcemia is responsible for a broad spectrum of signs and symptoms. Nephrolithiasis is the most common manifestation, occurring in 60–70% of patients. Polyuria and polydipsia are also common complaints. An increase in bone turnover may lead to generalized demineralization and subperiosteal bone resorption; however, only a small group of patients (10–15%) have clinically significant bone disease. Patients may experience generalized skeletal muscle weakness and fatigability, epigastric discomfort, peptic ulceration, and constipation. Psychiatric manifestations include depression, memory loss, confusion, or psychosis. Between 20 and 50% of patients are hypertensive, but this usually resolves with successful treatment of the disease. Cardiac function is enhanced in the early stages of hypercalcemia. Calcium flux into the cells is reflected in the plateau phase of the action potential (Phase 2). As extracellular calcium increases, the inward flux is more rapid, and Phase 2 is shortened. The corresponding ECG change is a shorter QT interval. Cardiac contractility may increase until a level between

15 and 20 mg $\cdot$ dl^{-1} is reached. At this point, there is a prolongation of the PR segment and QRS complex that can result in heart block or bundle-branch block. Bradycardia also occurs.

An elevated serum Ca^{2+} concentration is a valuable diagnostic indicator of primary hyperparathyroidism. The serum phosphate concentration is nonspecific, with many patients having normal or near-normal levels. The reported incidence of hyperchloremic acidosis varies widely in primary hyperparathyroidism, but most patients usually have a serum chloride concentration in excess of 102 mEq $\cdot$ l^{-1}. Rarely does a patient with hypercalcemia secondary to ectopic PTH production (malignancy) present with hyperchloremic acidosis. The definitive diagnosis of primary hyperparathyroidism is made by RIA demonstration of an elevation in PTH levels in the presence of hypercalcemia. An elevated nephrogenous cAMP is noted in more than 90% of patients with primary hyperparathyroidism.

Hypercalcemia may also result from the ectopic production of PTH or PTH-like substances from lung, genitourinary, breast, GI, and lymphoproliferative malignancies. Tumors may also produce hypercalcemia through direct bone resorption or the production of osteoclast-activating factor. In the absence of a clinically obvious neoplasm, there may be difficulty in differentiating between PTH-producing malignancies and primary hyperparathyroidism. PTH fragments from malignant tissue differ from native PTH and aid in distinguishing between ectopic PTH production and primary hyperparathyroidism.

Secondary hyperparathyroidism represents an increase in parathyroid function as a result of conditions that produce hypocalcemia or hyperphosphatemia. Chronic renal disease is a common cause of hyperphosphatemia (due to decreased phosphate excretion) and decreased vitamin D metabolism. The hypocalcemia that results leads to an increased production of PTH. GI disorders accompanied by malabsorption may also lead to a secondary increase in parathyroid activity. Tertiary hyperparathyroidism refers to the development of hypercalcemia in a patient who has had prolonged secondary hyperparathyroidism that has caused adenomatous changes in the parathyroid gland and PTH production to become autonomous.

Treatment and Anesthetic Considerations

Surgery is the treatment of choice for the patient with symptomatic disease. Considerable controversy, however, surrounds the choice of treatment in the asymptomatic patient. It is not clear that mild primary hyperparathyroidism decreases longevity. Surgery is often chosen over medical therapy because it offers definitive treatment and is generally safe.

Preoperative preparation focuses on the correction of intravascular volume and electrolyte irregularities. It is particularly important to evaluate the patient with chronic hypercalcemia for abnormalities of the renal, cardiac, or central nervous systems. Emergency treatment of hypercalcemia is undertaken before surgery when the serum Ca^{2+} concentration exceeds 15 mg $\cdot$ dl^{-1} (7.5 mEq $\cdot$ l^{-1}). Lowering of the serum Ca^{2+} concentration is initially accomplished by expanding the intravascular volume and establishing a sodium diuresis. This is achieved with the iv administration of normal saline and furosemide. Rehydration alone is capable of lowering the serum Ca^{2+} level by ≥ 2 mg $\cdot$ dl^{-1}. Hydration dilutes the serum Ca^{2+}, and a sodium diuresis promotes Ca^{2+} excretion through an inhibition of sodium and Ca^{2+} resorption in the proximal tubule. Hypokalemia and hypomagnesemia may result. Another element in the treatment of hypercalcemia is the correction of hypophosphatemia. Hypophosphatemia increases GI absorption of Ca^{2+}, stimulates the breakdown of bone, and impairs the uptake of Ca^{2+} by bone. Low serum phosphate levels impair cardiac contractility and may contribute to congestive heart failure. Hypophosphatemia also causes skeletal muscle weakness, hemolysis, and platelet dysfunction.

Other medications that have a role in lowering the serum Ca^{2+} include bisphosphonates, mithramycin, calcitonin, and glucocorticoids. Bisphosphonates are pyrophosphate analogues that inhibit osteoclast action. They are the drugs of choice for severe hypercalcemia. Toxic effects include fever and hypophosphatemia. Mithramycin, a cytotoxic agent, inhibits PTH-induced osteoclast activity and can lower the serum Ca^{2+} levels by ≥ 2 mg·dl^{-1} in 24–48 hours. Toxic effects include azotemia, hepatotoxicity, and thrombocytopenia. Calcitonin is useful in transiently lowering the serum Ca^{2+} level 2–4 mg·dl^{-1} through direct inhibition of osteoclastic bone resorption. The advantages of calcitonin are that side effects are mild (urticaria, nausea) and the onset of activity is rapid. Calcitonin resistance usually develops within 24–48 hours. Glucocorticoids are effective in lowering the serum Ca^{2+} concentration in several conditions (sarcoidosis, some malignancies, hyperthyroidism, vitamin D intoxication) through their actions on osteoclast bone resorption, GI absorption of calcium, and the urinary excretion of calcium. Glucocorticoids are usually of no benefit in the treatment of primary hypercalcemia. Finally, hemodialysis or peritoneal dialysis can be used to lower the serum Ca^{2+} level when alternative regimens are ineffective or contraindicated.

There is no evidence that a specific anesthetic drug or technique has advantages over another. A thorough knowledge of the clinical manifestations attributable to hypercalcemia is of the greatest value in choosing an anesthetic technique. Special monitoring is usually not required. Because of the unpredictable response to neuromuscular blocking drugs in the hypercalcemic patient, a conservative approach to muscle paralysis makes sense. There is an increased requirement for vecuronium, and probably all nondepolarizing muscle relaxants, during onset of neuromuscular blockade.[23] Careful positioning of the osteopenic patient is necessary to avoid pathologic bone fractures.

Anesthesia for Parathyroid Surgery

General anesthesia is most commonly used, but cervical plexus block and local anesthesia with hypnosedation have been used successfully.[24] Postoperative complications include recurrent laryngeal nerve injury, bleeding, and transient or complete hypoparathyroidism. Unilateral recurrent laryngeal nerve injury is characterized by hoarseness and usually requires no intervention. Bilateral recurrent laryngeal nerve injury is a rare complication, producing aphonia and requiring immediate tracheal intubation. After successful parathyroidectomy, a decrease in the serum Ca^{2+} level should be observed within 24 hours. Patients with significant preoperative bone disease may have hypocalcemia after removal of the PTH-secreting glands. This "hungry bone" syndrome comes as a result of the rapid remineralization of bone.[25] Thus, serum Ca^{2+}, magnesium, and phosphorus levels should be closely monitored until stable. The serum Ca^{2+} nadir usually occurs within 3–7 days.

Hypoparathyroidism

An underproduction of PTH or resistance of the end-organ tissues to PTH results in hypocalcemia (<8 mg·dl^{-1}). The normal physiologic response to hypocalcemia is an increase in PTH secretion and $1,25(OH)_2D$ synthesis with an increase in Ca^{2+} mobilization from bone, GI absorption, and renal tubule reclamation. The most common cause of acquired PTH deficiency is inadvertent removal of the parathyroid glands during thyroid or parathyroid surgery. Other causes of acquired hypoparathyroidism include ^{131}I therapy for thyroid disease, neck trauma, granulomatous disease, or an infiltrating process (malignancy or amyloidosis). Idiopathic hypoparathyroidism is rare and may occur as an isolated disease or as part of an autoimmune polyglandular process (hypothyroidism, adrenal insufficiency). Pseudohypoparathyroidism is an inherited disorder in which parathyroid gland function is normal but the end-organ response to the PTH is deficient. Affected patients have hypocalcemia and hyperphosphatemia. They are characterized by mental retardation, a short stature, obesity, and shortened metacarpals. Pseudopseudohypoparathyroid patients are characterized by the same physical findings but have normal serum calcium and phosphate levels. Severe hypomagnesemia (<0.8 mEq·l^{-1}) from any cause can produce hypocalcemia by suppressing PTH secretion. Renal insufficiency leads to phosphorus retention and impaired $1,25(OH)_2D$ synthesis, and this results in hypocalcemia. These patients are commonly treated with vitamin D, which increases intestinal calcium absorption and suppresses secondary increases in PTH secretion. Hypocalcemia due to pancreatitis and burns results from the suppression of PTH and from the sequestration of calcium.

Clinical Features and Treatment

The clinical features of hypoparathyroidism are a manifestation of hypocalcemia. Neuronal irritability and skeletal muscle spasms, tetany, or seizures reflect a reduced threshold of excitation. Latent tetany may be demonstrated by eliciting Chvostek's or Trousseau's sign. Chvostek's sign is a contracture of the facial muscle produced by tapping the facial nerve as it passes through the parotid gland. Trousseau's sign is contraction of the fingers and wrist after application of a blood pressure cuff inflated above the systolic blood pressure for approximately 3 minutes. Other common complaints of hypocalcemia include fatigue, depression, paresthesias, and skeletal muscle cramps. The acute onset of hypocalcemia after thyroid or parathyroid surgery may manifest as stridor and apnea. Cardiovascular manifestations of hypocalcemia include congestive heart failure, hypotension, and a relative insensitivity to the effects of β-adrenergic agonists. Delayed ventricular repolarization results in a prolonged QT interval on the ECG. Although prolongation of the QT interval may be a reliable sign of hypocalcemia in an individual patient, the ECG is relatively insensitive for the detection of hypocalcemia.

The treatment of hypoparathyroidism consists of electrolyte replacement. The objective is to have the patient's clinical symptoms under control before anesthesia and surgery. Hypocalcemia caused by magnesium depletion is treated by correcting the magnesium deficit. Serum phosphate excess is corrected by the removal of phosphate from the diet and the oral administration of phosphate-binding resins (aluminum hydroxide). The urinary excretion of phosphate can be increased with a saline volume infusion. Ca^{2+} deficiencies are corrected with Ca^{2+} supplements or vitamin D analogues. Patients with severe symptomatic hypocalcemia are treated with iv calcium gluconate (10–20 ml of 10% solution) given over several minutes and followed by a continuous infusion (1–2 mg·kg^{-1}·h^{-1}) of elemental Ca^{2+}. The correction of serum Ca^{2+} levels should be monitored by measuring serum Ca^{2+} concentrations and following clinical symptoms. When oral or iv calcium is inadequate to maintain a normal serum ionized calcium level, vitamin D is added to the regimen.

ADRENAL CORTEX

The adrenal cortex functions to synthesize and secrete three types of hormones. Endogenous and dietary cholesterol is used in the adrenal biosynthesis of glucocorticoids (cortisol), mineralocorticoids (aldosterone and 11-deoxycorticosterone), and androgens (dehydroepiandrosterone). Cortisol and aldosterone are the two essential hormones, whereas adrenal androgens are of relatively minor physiologic significance in adults. The major biologic effects of adrenal cortical hyperfunction or hypofunction occur as a result of cortisol or aldosterone excess or deficiency. Abnormal function of the adrenal cortex may render a patient unable to respond appropriately during a period of surgical stress or critical illness.

Glucocorticoid Physiology

Cortisol (hydrocortisone) is the most potent glucocorticoid and is produced by the inner portions of the adrenal cortex. Cortisone is a glucocorticoid produced in small amounts. Cortisol is produced under the control of adrenocorticotropic hormone (ACTH; corticotropin), a polypeptide synthesized and released by the anterior pituitary gland. Glucocorticoids exert their biologic effects by diffusing into the cytoplasm of target cells and combining with specific high-affinity receptor proteins.

The daily production of endogenous cortisol is approximately 20 mg. The maximal output is 150–300 mg · day^{-1}. Most of the circulating hormone is bound to the α-globulin transcortin (cortisol-binding globulin). It is the relatively small amount of free hormone that exerts the biologic effects. Glucocorticoids such as cortisol are inactivated primarily by the liver and are excreted in the urine as 17-hydroxycorticosteroids. Cortisol is also filtered at the glomerulus and may be excreted unchanged in the urine. Although the rate of cortisol secretion is decreased by approximately 30% in the elderly patient, plasma cortisol levels remain in a normal range because of a corresponding decrease in hepatic and renal clearance.

Cortisol secretion is directly controlled by ACTH, which in turn is regulated by the corticotropin-releasing factor (CRF) from the hypothalamus. ACTH is synthesized in the pituitary gland from a precursor molecule that also produces β-lipotropin and β-endorphin. The secretion of ACTH and CRF is governed chiefly by glucocorticoids, the sleep-wake cycle, and stress. Cortisol is the most potent regulator of ACTH secretion, acting by a negative feedback mechanism to maintain cortisol levels in a physiologic range. ACTH release follows a diurnal pattern, with maximal activity occurring soon after awakening. This diurnal pattern of activity occurs in normal subjects as well as in those with adrenal insufficiency. Psychological or physical stress (trauma, surgery, intense exercise) also promotes ACTH release regardless of the level of circulating cortisol or the time of day.[26]

Cortisol has multiple effects on intermediate carbohydrate, protein, and fatty acid metabolism. Glucocorticoids enhance gluconeogenesis, elevate blood glucose, and promote hepatic glycogen synthesis.[27,28] The catabolic effect of glucocorticoids is partially blocked by insulin. The net effect on protein metabolism is enhanced degradation of muscle tissue and negative nitrogen balance. In supraphysiologic amounts, glucocorticoids suppress growth hormone secretion and impair somatic growth. The anti-inflammatory actions of cortisol relate to its effect in stabilizing lysosomes and promoting capillary integrity. Cortisol also antagonizes leukocyte migration inhibition factor, thus reducing white cell adherence to vascular endothelium and diminishing leukocyte response to local inflammation. Phagocytic activity does not decrease, although the killing potential of macrophages and monocytes is diminished. Other diverse actions include the facilitation of free water clearance, maintenance of blood pressure, a weak mineralocorticoid effect, promotion of appetite, stimulation of hematopoiesis, and induction of liver enzymes.

Mineralocorticoid Physiology

Aldosterone is the most potent mineralocorticoid produced by the adrenal gland. This hormone binds to receptors in sweat glands, the alimentary tract, and the distal convoluted tubule of the kidney. Aldosterone is a major regulator of extracellular volume and potassium homeostasis through the resorption of sodium and the secretion of potassium by these tissues. The major regulators of aldosterone release are the renin–angiotensin system and serum potassium (Fig. 41-3). The juxtaglomerular apparatus that surrounds the renal afferent arterioles produces renin in response to decreased perfusion pressures and sympathetic stimulation. Renin splits the hepatic precursor angiotensinogen to form the decapeptide, angiotensin I, which is then altered enzymatically by converting enzyme (primarily in the lung) to form the octapeptide angiotensin II. Angiotensin II is the most potent vasopressor produced in the body. It directly stimulates the adrenal cortex to produce aldosterone. The renin–angiotensin system is the body's most important protector of volume status. Other stimuli that increase the production of aldosterone include hyperkalemia and, to a limited degree, hyponatremia, prostaglandin E, and ACTH.

Glucocorticoid Excess (Cushing's Syndrome)

Cushing's syndrome, caused either by the overproduction of cortisol by the adrenal cortex or exogenous glucocorticoid therapy, results in a syndrome characterized by truncal obesity, hypertension, hyperglycemia, increased intravascular fluid volume, hypokalemia, fatigability, abdominal striae, osteoporosis, and muscle weakness. Most cases of Cushing's syndrome that occur spontaneously are due to bilateral adrenal hyperplasia secondary to ACTH produced by an anterior pituitary microadenoma or nonendocrine tumor (e.g., of the lung, kidney, or pancreas). The primary overproduction of cortisol and other adrenal steroids is caused by an adrenal neoplasm in approximately 20–25% of patients with Cushing's syndrome. These tumors are usually unilateral, and approximately half are malignant. When Cushing's syndrome occurs in patients older than 60 years of age, the most likely cause is an adrenal carcinoma or ectopic ACTH produced from a nonendocrine tumor. Finally, an increasingly common cause of Cushing's syndrome is the prolonged administration of exogenous glucocorticoids to treat a variety of illnesses.

The signs and symptoms of Cushing's syndrome follow from the known actions of glucocorticoids. Truncal obesity and thin

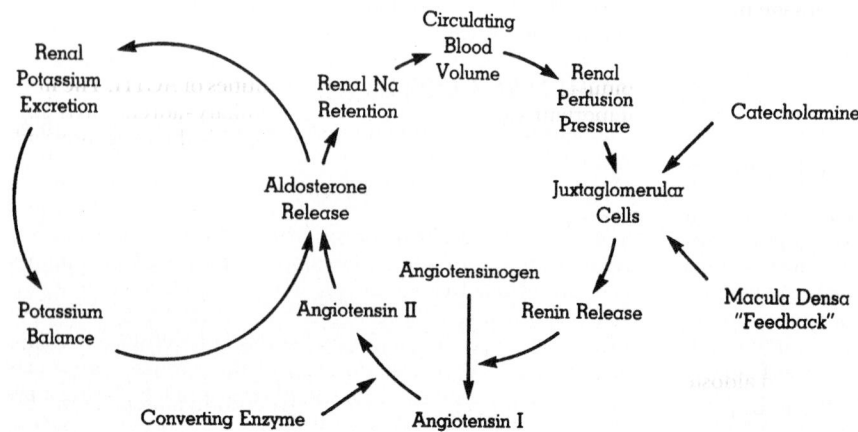

Figure 41-3. The inter-relationship of the volume and potassium feedback loops on aldosterone secretion. (Reproduced with permission from Petersdorf RG [ed]: Harrison's Principles of Internal Medicine, 10th ed. New York, McGraw-Hill, 1983.)

extremities reflect increased muscle wasting and a redistribution of fat in facial, cervical, and truncal areas. Impaired calcium absorption and a decrease in bone formation may result in osteopenia. Sixty percent of patients have hyperglycemia, but overt diabetes mellitus occurs in less than 20%. Hypertension and fluid retention are seen in most patients. Profound emotional changes ranging from emotional lability to frank psychosis may be present. An increased susceptibility to infection reflects the immunosuppressive effects of corticosteroids. Hypokalemic alkalosis without distinctive physical findings is common when adrenal hyperplasia is caused by ectopic ACTH production from a nonendocrine tumor.

The biochemical diagnosis of hyperadrenocorticism is based on a variable elevation in plasma and urinary cortisol levels, urinary 17-hydroxycorticosteroids, and plasma ACTH. The diagnosis can be established by failure normally to suppress endogenous cortisol secretion after the exogenous administration of dexamethasone. Patients with pituitary adenomas frequently show depression in cortisol and 17-hydroxycorticosteroid levels when a high dose of dexamethasone is administered because the tumor retains some negative feedback control. The ectopic production of ACTH by a nonendocrine tumor usually shows no suppression with low- or high-dose dexamethasone.

Anesthetic Management

General considerations for the preoperative preparation of the patient include regulating hypertension and diabetes and normalizing intravascular fluid volume and electrolyte concentrations. Diuresis with the aldosterone antagonist spironolactone helps to mobilize fluid and normalize the potassium concentration. Careful positioning of the osteopenic patient is important to avoid fractures. Intraoperative monitoring is planned after evaluation of the patient's cardiac reserve and consideration of the site and extent of the proposed surgery. When unilateral or bilateral adrenalectomy is planned, glucocorticoid replacement therapy is initiated at a dose equal to full replacement of adrenal output during periods of extreme stress (see Steroid Replacement During the Perioperative Period). The total dosage is reduced by approximately 50% per day until a daily maintenance dose of steroids is achieved ($20-30$ mg · day^{-1}). Hydrocortisone given in doses of this magnitude exerts significant mineralocorticoid activity, and additional exogenous mineralocorticoid usually is not necessary during the perioperative period. The oral administration of mineralocorticoid is usually started on day 5. After bilateral adrenalectomy, most patients require $0.05-0.1$ mg · day^{-1} of fludrocortisone (9-α-fluorohydrocortisone). Slightly higher doses may be needed if prednisone is used for glucocorticoid maintenance (little intrinsic mineralocorticoid activity). The fludrocortisone dose is reduced if congestive heart failure, hypokalemia, or hypertension develops. For the patient with a solitary adrenal adenoma, unilateral adrenalectomy may be followed by normalization of function in the contralateral gland over time. Treatment plans should therefore be individualized, and adjustments in dosage may be necessary. The production of glucocorticoids or ACTH by a neoplasm may not be eliminated if the tumor is unresectable. These patients often need continuous medical therapy with steroid inhibitors such as metyrapone to control their symptoms.

There are no specific recommendations regarding the use of a particular anesthetic technique or medication in patients with hyperadrenocorticism. When significant skeletal muscle weakness is present, a conservative approach to the use of muscle relaxants is warranted.

Mineralocorticoid Excess

Hypersecretion of the major adrenal mineralocorticoid aldosterone increases the renal tubular exchange of sodium for potassium and hydrogen ions. This leads to potassium depletion, skeletal muscle weakness, fatigue, and hypokalemic alkalosis. Possibly as much as 1% of unselected hypertensive patients have primary hyperaldosteronism. The increase in renal sodium reabsorption and extracellular volume expansion is in part responsible for the high incidence of diastolic hypertension in these patients. Patients with primary hyperaldosteronism (Conn's syndrome) characteristically do not have edema. Secondary aldosteronism results from an elevation in renin production. The diagnosis of primary or secondary hyperaldosteronism should be entertained in the nonedematous hypertensive patient with persistent hypokalemia who is not receiving potassium-wasting diuretics. Hyposecretion of renin that fails to increase appropriately during volume depletion is an important finding in primary aldosteronism. The measurement of plasma renin levels is useful in distinguishing these two from one another; however, it is of limited value in differentiating patients with primary aldosteronism from those with other causes of hypertension because renin activity is also suppressed in approximately 25% of patients with essential hypertension.

Anesthetic Considerations

Preoperative preparation for the patient with primary aldosteronism is directed toward restoring the intravascular volume and the electrolyte concentrations to normal. Hypertension and hypokalemia may be controlled by restricting sodium intake and administration of the aldosterone antagonist spironolactone. This diuretic works slowly to produce an increase in potassium levels, with dosages in the range of $25-100$ mg every 8 hours. Total body potassium deficits are difficult to estimate and may be in excess of 300 mEq. Whenever possible, potassium should be replaced slowly to allow equilibration between intracellular and extracellular potassium stores. The usual complications of chronic hypertension need to be assessed.

Adrenal Insufficiency

The undersecretion of adrenal steroid hormones may develop as the result of a primary inability of the adrenal gland to elaborate sufficient quantities of hormone or as the result of a deficiency in the production of ACTH.

Clinically, primary adrenal insufficiency is usually not apparent until at least 90% of the adrenal cortex has been destroyed. The predominant cause of primary adrenal insufficiency during the early part of the century was tuberculosis; however, today, the most frequent cause of Addison's disease is idiopathic adrenal insufficiency secondary to autoimmune destruction of the gland. Autoimmune destruction of the adrenal cortex causes both a glucocorticoid and a mineralocorticoid deficiency. A variety of other conditions presumed to have an autoimmune pathogenesis may also occur concomitantly with idiopathic Addison's disease. Hashimoto's thyroiditis in association with autoimmune adrenal insufficiency is termed *Schmidt's syndrome*. Other possible causes of adrenal gland destruction include certain bacterial or fungal infections, metastatic cancer, sepsis and hemorrhage.

Secondary adrenal insufficiency occurs when the anterior pituitary fails to secrete sufficient quantities of ACTH. The most important cause of hypothalamic–pituitary–adrenal axis suppression confronting the anesthesiologist is the exogenous administration of glucocorticoids. Pituitary failure may also result from tumor, infection, surgical ablation, or radiation therapy.

Clinical Presentation

Several important differences exist between primary adrenal insufficiency and hypopituitarism. The cardinal symptoms of idiopathic Addison's disease include asthenia, weight loss, anorexia, abdominal pain, nausea, vomiting, diarrhea, and constipation. Hypotension is almost always encountered in the disease process. Diffuse hyperpigmentation occurs in most patients with primary adrenal insufficiency and is secondary to the compensatory increase in ACTH and β-lipotropin. These hormones stimulate an increase in melanocyte production. Mineralocorticoid deficiency is characteristically present in primary adrenal disease, and, as a result, there is a reduction in urine sodium conservation and a decreased pressure response to circulating catecholamines. Hyperkalemia may be a cause of life-threatening cardiac dysrhythmias. Female patients may exhibit decreased axillary and pubic hair growth owing to the loss of adrenal androgen secretion. Adrenal insufficiency secondary to pituitary suppression is not associated with cutaneous hyperpigmentation or mineralocorticoid deficiency. Salt and water balance is usually maintained unless severe fluid and electrolyte losses overwhelm the subnormal aldosterone secretory capacity. Organic lesions of pituitary origin require a diligent search for coexisting hormone deficiencies.

It is important to recognize the patient with adrenal insufficiency secondary to exogenous steroid therapy because it is possible for acute adrenal crisis to occur if high-dose glucocorticoids are abruptly withdrawn or if deficient patients are subjected to surgical stress.[29] Because patients who have received exogenous glucocorticoids may exhibit pituitary–adrenal suppression for up to 12 months after cessation of therapy, these patients receive supplemental glucocorticoid coverage during periods of increased stress (e.g., trauma, surgery, infection). Patients receiving inhaled or topical steroids may also exhibit pituitary–adrenal suppression for up to 9 months after the cessation of therapy.

Diagnosis

The patient's pituitary-adrenal responsiveness should be determined when the diagnosis of primary or secondary adrenal insufficiency is first suspected. Biochemical evidence of impaired adrenal or pituitary secretory reserve unequivocally confirms the diagnosis. Patients who are clinically stable may undergo testing before treatment is initiated. Those thought to have acute adrenal insufficiency should receive immediate therapy.

Plasma cortisol levels are measured before and 30 and 60 minutes after the iv administration of 250 μg of synthetic ACTH. In patients with adequate adrenal reserve, plasma cortisol rises at least 7 mg · dl^{-1} (or to a total of 18 mg · dl^{-1}) 60 minutes after the injection of the synthetic ACTH.[30] Patients with adrenal insufficiency usually demonstrate little or no adrenal response.

Treatment and Anesthetic Considerations

Normal adults secrete 20 mg of cortisol (hydrocortisone) and 0.1 mg of aldosterone per day. Glucocorticoid therapy is usually given twice daily in sufficient dosage to meet physiologic requirements. A typical regimen may consist of prednisone, 5 mg in the morning and 2.5 mg in the evening, or hydrocortisone, 20 mg in the morning and 10 mg in the evening. The daily glucocorticoid dosage is typically 50% higher than basal adrenal output to cover the patient for mild stress. Replacement dosages are adjusted in response to the patient's clinical symptoms or the occurrence of intercurrent illnesses. Patients with Addison's disease should be instructed to increase glucocorticoid medication to three or four times their usual daily dosage during periods of increased stress. Mineralocorticoid replacement is also administered on a daily basis; most patients require 0.05–0.1 mg · day^{-1} of fludrocortisone. The mineralocorticoid dose may be reduced if severe hypokalemia, hypertension, or congestive heart failure develops, or it may be increased if postural hypotension is demonstrated. Children with Addison's disease receive lesser daily amounts of steroids. Twelve milligrams of cortisol per square meter of body surface area is usually sufficient.

Secondary adrenal insufficiency often occurs in the presence of multiple hormone deficiencies. A decrease in ACTH production results in the decreased secretion of cortisol and adrenal androgens, but aldosterone control by more dominant mechanisms remains intact. A liberal salt diet is encouraged. Glucocorticoid substitution follows the same guidelines previously outlined for primary adrenal insufficiency.

Perioperatively, patients with adrenal insufficiency require additional corticosteroids to mimic the increased output of the normal adrenal gland during stress (see Steroid Replacement During the Perioperative Period). Acute adrenal insufficiency is usually precipitated by sepsis, trauma, or surgical stress in the setting of hypovolemic shock and severe electrolyte imbalance in a patient with inadequate adrenal reserves. Immediate therapy is mandatory regardless of the etiology and consists of fluid and electrolyte resuscitation and steroid replacement (Table 41-6).

In critically ill patients, adrenal insufficiency may not present with classic symptoms. The clinical picture may resemble that of sepsis without a source of infection.[31] A high degree of suspicion must be maintained if the patient has cardiovascular instability without a defined cause.[32,33]

Initial therapy of acute adrenal insufficiency begins with the rapid iv administration of an isotonic crystalloid solution (D$_5$NS); 100 mg of hydrocortisone is administered as an iv bolus over several minutes. Steroid replacement is continued during the first 24 hours with 100 mg iv hydrocortisone given every 6 hours. If the patient is stable, the steroid dose is reduced starting on the second day. After adequate fluid resuscitation, if the patient continues to be hemodynamically unstable, inotropic support may be necessary. Invasive monitoring is extremely valuable as a guide to both diagnosis and therapy.

Mineralocorticoid Insufficiency

Isolated mineralocorticoid insufficiency has been reported as a congenital biosynthetic defect, after unilateral adrenalectomy for removal of an aldosterone-secreting adenoma, during protracted heparin therapy, and in patients with a deficiency in renin production. This syndrome is commonly seen in patients with mild renal failure and long-standing diabetes mellitus. A feature common to all patients with hypoaldosteronism is a failure to increase aldosterone production in response to salt restriction or volume contraction.

Most patients present with hypotension, hyperkalemia that may be life threatening, and a metabolic acidosis that is out of proportion to the degree of coexisting renal impairment. Patients with low renin secretion, hypoaldosteronism, and renal dysfunction respond to ACTH stimulation. Nonsteroidal anti-inflammatory drugs, which inhibit prostaglandin synthesis, may further inhibit renin release and exacerbate the condition. Patients with isolated hypoaldosteronism are given fludrocortisone orally in a dose of 0.05–0.1 mg · day^{-1}. Patients with low renin secretion usually require higher doses to correct the electrolyte abnormalities. Caution should be observed in patients with hypertension or congestive heart failure. An alternative approach in these patients is the administration of furosemide alone or in combination with mineralocorticoid.

Exogenous Glucocorticoid Therapy

The therapeutic use of supraphysiologic doses of glucocorticoids has expanded, and, as a consequence, the clinical implications of such therapy are important. The relative glucocorticoid

---

Table 41-6. MANAGEMENT OF ACUTE ADRENAL INSUFFICIENCY

Hydrocortisone 100 mg intravenous bolus followed by hydrocortisone 100 mg q6h for 24 h

Fluid and electrolyte replacement as indicated by vital signs, serum electrolytes, and serum glucose

Table 41-7. GLUCOCORTICOID PREPARATIONS

Generic Name	Trade Name	Relative Potency* Anti-inflammatory	Relative Potency* Mineralocorticoid	Approximate Equivalent Dose (mg)
Short-Acting				
Hydrocortisone (cortisol)	Cortef	1.0	1.0	20.0
Cortisone	Cortigen	0.8	0.8	25.0
Prednisone	Deltasone	4.0	0.25	5.0
Prednisolone	Hydeltrasol	4.0	0.25	5.0
Methylprednisolone	Medrol	5.0	±	4.0
Intermediate-Acting				
Triamcinolone	Aristocort	5.0	±	4.0
Long-Acting				
Dexamethasone	Decadron	30.0	±	0.75

* Relative milligram comparisons with cortisol. The glucocorticoid and mineralocorticoid properties of cortisol are set as 1.0.

and mineralocorticoid properties of the various preparations are listed in Table 41-7. Dexamethasone, methylprednisolone, and prednisone have less mineralocorticoid effect than do cortisone and hydrocortisone. The anti-inflammatory activity of a glucocorticoid depends on the hydroxyl group at the carbon 11 position. Therefore, glucocorticoids such as cortisone and prednisone must undergo hepatic conversion from 11-keto compounds to 11-β-hydroxyl compounds before anti-inflammatory activity can occur. Consequently, prednisone and cortisone should probably be avoided in the presence of severe liver disease. Because most side effects from steroids are related to the dose and duration of administration, the smallest effective dose is used for the shortest time.

Patients at particular risk for development of complications related to steroid therapy include those with diabetes mellitus, pre-existing infection, hypertension, or congestive heart failure. Aseptic necrosis of the bones, subcapsular cataracts, pancreatitis, benign intracranial hypertension, and glaucoma are complications associated with exogenous steroid administration. Although the overall prevalence of steroid-associated peptic ulceration is small (2%), patients receiving exogenous steroids have approximately twice the risk for development of peptic ulceration or GI hemorrhage as do control subjects.

Steroid Replacement During the Perioperative Period

The normal adrenal gland can secrete up to 200 mg of cortisol per day or more during the perioperative period. During periods of extreme stress, the adrenal gland may be exogenously stimulated to secrete between 200 and 500 mg·day^{-1} of cortisol.[34] The pituitary–adrenal axis is usually considered to be intact if a plasma cortisol level of greater than 22 mg·dl^{-1} is measured during acute stress. The degree of adrenal responsiveness has been correlated with the duration of surgery and the extent of surgical trauma. The mean maximal plasma cortisol level measured during major surgery (colectomy, hip osteotomy) was 47 mg·dl^{-1}. Minor surgical procedures (herniorrhaphy) resulted in mean maximal plasma cortisol levels of 28 mg·dl^{-1}. Adrenal activity may also be affected by the anesthetic technique used. Regional anesthesia is effective in postponing the elevation in cortisol levels during surgery of the lower abdomen and extremities.[35] Deep general anesthesia may also suppress the elevation of stress hormones such as ACTH and cortisol during the surgical procedure.[36-38]

Although symptoms indicative of clinically significant adrenal insufficiency have been reported during the perioperative period, these clinical findings have rarely been documented in direct association with glucocorticoid deficiency.[39] There is evidence in adrenally suppressed primates that subphysiologic steroid replacement causes perioperative hemodynamic instability and increased mortality. Because acute adrenal crisis is life threatening, and because there is relatively little risk in providing steroid coverage for isolated periods of stress, most clinicians empirically administer supplemental steroids to all patients who have received daily steroid replacement for at least 1–2 weeks in the 6–12 months before surgery. Provocative testing with ACTH stimulation to identify patients at risk is too costly to justify compared with the risk of brief steroid supplementation.

The question is how much steroid to give. There is no proven optimal regimen for perioperative steroid replacement (Table 41-8). A "low-dose" cortisol replacement program using an iv infusion of 25 mg of cortisol before the induction of anesthesia, followed by a continuous infusion of cortisol (100 mg) in the next 24 hours has been advocated[40] (Fig. 41-4). This low-dose cortisol replacement program was used in patients with proven adrenal insufficiency and resulted in plasma cortisol levels as high as those seen in healthy control subjects subjected to a similar operative stress. One study with a limited number of patients found no problems with cardiovascular instability if patients received their usual dose of steroids.[41] Although the low-dose approach appears logical, many clinicians are unwilling to adopt this regimen until further trials have been undertaken in patients receiving physiologic steroid replacement. A popular regimen calls for the administration of 200–300 mg of hydrocortisone per 70 kg body weight in divided doses on the day of surgery. The lower dose is adjusted upward for longer and more extensive surgical procedures. Patients who are using steroids at the time of surgery receive their usual dose on the morning of surgery and are supplemented at a level that is at least equivalent to the usual daily replacement. Glucocorticoid coverage is reduced to the patient's normal maintenance dosage during the postoperative period. Although there is no conclusive evidence supporting an increased incidence of infection or abnormal wound healing when supraphysiologic doses of supplemental steroids are used acutely, the goal of therapy is to use the minimal drug dosage necessary adequately to protect the patient.

Table 41-8. MANAGEMENT OPTIONS FOR STEROID REPLACEMENT IN THE PERIOPERATIVE PERIOD

Hydrocortisone 25 mg iv at time of induction followed by hydrocortisone infusion 100 mg over 24 h
Hydrocortisone 100 mg iv before, during, and after surgery

iv = intravenous.

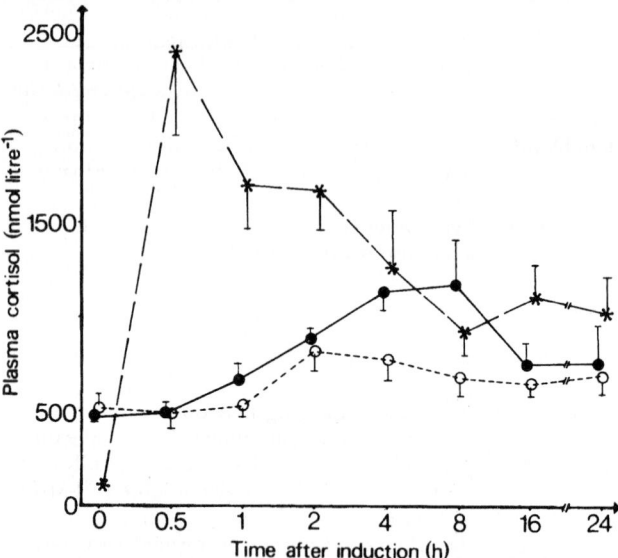

Figure 41-4. Plasma cortisol concentrations (mean ± SEM) were measured in three groups of patients undergoing elective surgery. Group I control patients, $n = 8$ (*closed circles*), had never received corticosteroids. Group II patients, $n = 8$ (*open circles*), received preoperative corticosteroids with a normal response to preoperative adrenocorticotropic hormone (ACTH; corticotropin) stimulation testing. These patients and control patients received no corticosteroid substitution during the perioperative period. Group III, $n = 6$ (*asterisks*), consisted of patients receiving long-term corticosteroid therapy with an abnormal response to ACTH stimulation testing during the perioperative period. These patients (Group III) received intravenous (iv) cortisol, 25 mg, after the induction of anesthesia plus a continuous iv infusion of cortisol, 100 mg, during the next 24 hours. Plasma cortisol levels in Group III were significantly lower than in the other two groups before the induction of anesthesia. After iv administration of cortisol to Group III patients, plasma concentrations were significantly higher than in Groups I and II for the next 2 hours ($p < 0.01$). Thereafter, the mean plasma concentrations were similar for all groups. There were no clinical signs of circulatory insufficiency in any group. (Reproduced with permission from Symreng T, Karlberg BE, Kagedol B, Schildt B: Physiological cortisol substitution of long-term steroid-treated patients undergoing major surgery. Br J Anaesth 53:949, 1981.)

ADRENAL MEDULLA

The adrenal medulla is derived embryologically from neuroectodermal cells. As a specialized part of the sympathetic nervous system, the adrenal medulla synthesizes and secretes the catecholamines epinephrine (80%) and norepinephrine (20%). Preganglionic fibers of the sympathetic nervous system bypass the paravertebral ganglia and pass directly from the spinal cord to the adrenal medulla. The adrenal medulla is analogous to a postganglionic neuron, although the catecholamines secreted by the medulla function as hormones, not as neurotransmitters.

The synthesis of norepinephrine begins with hydroxylation of tyrosine to dopa (Fig. 41-5). This rate-limiting step in catecholamine biosynthesis is regulated so that synthesis is coupled to release. In the adrenal medulla and in those rare central neurons using epinephrine as a neurotransmitter, most of the norepinephrine is converted to epinephrine by the enzyme phenylethanolamine-N-methyltransferase. It is likely that the capacity of the adrenal medulla to synthesize epinephrine is influenced by the flow of glucocorticoid-rich blood from the adrenal cortex through the intra-adrenal portal system because it is known that high concentrations of glucocorticoid are able to induce the enzyme phenylethanolamine-N-methyltransferase.

In the adrenal medulla, catecholamines are stored in chro-

maffin granules complexed with adenosine triphosphate and Ca^{2+}. The normal adrenal releases epinephrine and norepinephrine by exocytosis in response to stimulation by preganglionic sympathetic neurons. The circulatory half-life (10–30 seconds) of these catechols is considerably longer than the brief receptor activity of norepinephrine released as a neurotransmitter from postganglionic sympathetic nerve endings. Biotransformation of circulating norepinephrine and epinephrine is accomplished chiefly by the enzyme catechol-O-methyltransferase, located in the liver and kidney. Monoamine oxidase is of less importance in the metabolism of circulating catechols. Metanephrines and vanillylmandelic acid (VMA) are the major end products of catecholamine metabolism. These metabolites and a small amount of unchanged catecholamine (1%) appear in the urine.

The outflow of postganglionic sympathetic neurotransmitters and circulating catecholamine from the adrenal medulla is coordinated by higher cortical centers connected to the brain stem. The intrinsic activity of the brain stem sympathetic areas is modulated by higher cortical functions, emotional reactions (anger, fear), and various physiologic stimuli, including changes in the physical and chemical properties of the extracellular fluid (hypoglycemia, hypotension). The adrenal medulla and sympathetic nervous system are often stimulated together in a generalized fashion, although many physiologic conditions exist in which they act independently.

Pheochromocytoma

The only important disease process associated with the adrenal medulla is pheochromocytoma. These tumors produce, store, and secrete catecholamines. Most pheochromocytomas secrete both epinephrine and norepinephrine, with the percentage of secreted norepinephrine being greater than that secreted by the normal gland. Although pheochromocytomas occur in fewer than 0.1% of hypertensive patients, it is important aggressively to evaluate the patient with clinically suspect symptoms because surgical extirpation is curative in more than 90% of patients and complications are often lethal in undiagnosed cases. Postmortem series have reported high perioperative mortality rates in undiagnosed patients undergoing relatively minor

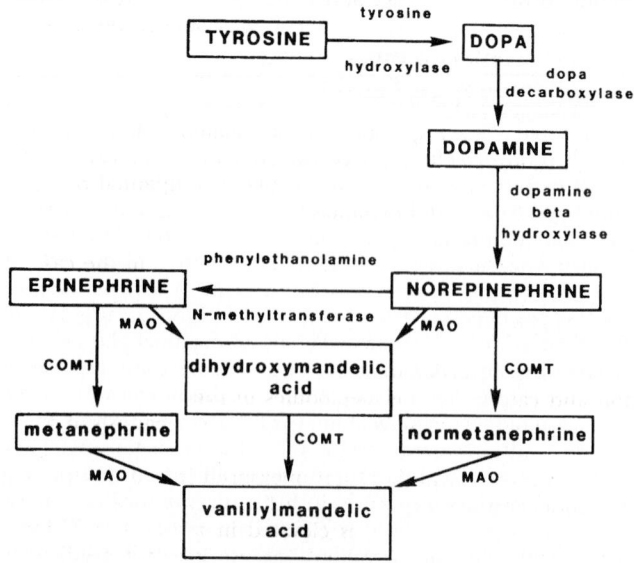

Figure 41-5. The synthesis and metabolism of endogenous catecholamines. COMT = catechol-O-methyltransferase; MAO = monoamine oxidase. (Reproduced with permission from Stoelting RK, Dierdorf SF [eds]: Anesthesia and co-existing disease. New York, Churchill-Livingstone, 1983.)

surgical procedures. Most deaths are from cardiovascular causes. Of particular importance to the anesthesiologist is that anesthetic drugs, in particular, halothane and histamine-releasing drugs, can exacerbate the life-threatening cardiovascular effects of the catecholamines secreted by these tumors.

Most (85–90%) pheochromocytomas are solitary tumors localized to a single adrenal gland, usually the right. Approximately 10% of adults and 25% of children have bilateral tumors. The tumor may originate in extra-adrenal sites (10%) anywhere along the paravertebral sympathetic chain; however, 95% are located in the abdomen, and a small percentage are located in the thorax, urinary bladder, or neck. Malignant spread of these highly vascular tumors occurs in approximately 10% of cases.

In approximately 5% of cases, this tumor is inherited as a familial autosomal dominant trait. It may be part of the polyglandular syndrome referred to as MEN Type IIA or IIB. Type IIA includes medullary carcinoma of the thyroid, parathyroid hyperplasia, and pheochromocytoma; Type IIB consists of medullary carcinoma of the thyroid, pheochromocytoma, and neuromas of the oral mucosa. Pheochromocytomas may also arise in association with von Recklinghausen's neurofibromatosis or von Hippel-Lindau disease (retinal and cerebellar angiomatosis). The pheochromocytoma of the familial syndromes is rarely extra-adrenal or malignant. Bilateral tumors occur in approximately 75% of cases. When these patients present with a single adrenal pheochromocytoma, the chances of subsequent development of a second adrenal pheochromocytoma are sufficiently high that bilateral adrenalectomy should be considered. Every member of a MEN family should be considered at risk for pheochromocytoma.

Clinical Presentation

Pheochromocytoma may occur at any age, but it is most common in young to mid-adult life. The clinical manifestations are mainly due to the pharmacologic effects of the catecholamines released from the tumor. These tumors are not innervated, and catecholamine release is independent of neurogenic control. Although most patients (90%) are hypertensive, the blood pressure profile is labile in half of these cases. Forty percent have only paroxysmal hypertension. When true paroxysms occur, the blood pressure may rise to alarmingly high levels, placing the patient at risk for cerebrovascular hemorrhage, heart failure, dysrhythmias, or myocardial infarction. Headache, palpitations, tremor, profuse sweating, and either pallor or flushing may accompany an attack. There are reports of pheochromocytoma manifesting as malignant hyperthermia.[42] Physical examination of the patient with pheochromocytoma may be unrevealing during the period between attacks unless the patient presents with symptoms and signs of sequelae related to long-standing hypertension. A well described catecholamine-induced cardiomyopathy may manifest as myocarditis accompanied by heart failure and cardiac dysrhythmias. Paroxysms commonly are not associated with clearly defined events but may be precipitated by displacement of the abdominal contents or, in the case of a bladder tumor, by micturition.

Diagnosis

Biochemical determination of free catecholamine concentration and catecholamine metabolites in the urine is the most common screening test used to establish the diagnosis of pheochromocytoma.[43] Urinary VMA and unconjugated norepinephrine and epinephrine levels are measured in a 24-hour urine collection and are expressed as a function of the creatinine clearance. The VMA level is elevated in most cases. Urinary metanephrine is not quantified because it is not predictably elevated in pheochromocytoma. Free catecholamines represent less than 1% of the originally released hormone, and urinary levels are not always elevated to a significant degree. Hence, differentiation from normal subjects may be difficult. A change in the ratio of unconjugated epinephrine to norepinephrine may be the only biochemical finding. Certain drugs interfere with urinary assays, and some patients with paroxysmal hypertension have normal values between attacks.

Although routine laboratory data are unlikely to provide specific diagnostic insight, the ECG, chest radiograph, and complete blood cell count can provide valuable information to the clinician who entertains the diagnosis. Left ventricular hypertrophy and nonspecific T-wave changes are two of the more common ECG findings. Evidence of acute myocardial infarction or tachyarrhythmia has also been reported. The chest radiograph may reveal cardiomegaly, and the blood count often shows an elevated hematocrit consistent with a reduced intravascular volume and hemoconcentration. Standardized imaging methods such as computed tomography and magnetic resonance imaging (MRI) are used in the noninvasive localization of these tumors.[44] Improvements in imaging may obviate the need for abdominal exploration or venous sampling to localize the tumor in selected patients.[45] Ultrasound and MRI are especially useful in pregnant patients. ^{131}I-Metaiodobenzylguanidine (^{131}I-MIBG) scintigraphy is also effective in localizing recurrent or extra-adrenal masses. Arteriography must be performed with extreme care in these patients because a hypertensive crisis can be precipitated.

Anesthetic Considerations

Preoperative Preparation. The reduction in perioperative mortality rates from a high of 45% to between zero and 3% with the excision of pheochromocytoma followed the introduction of α-antagonists for preoperative therapy. Perioperative blood pressure fluctuations, myocardial infarction, congestive heart failure, cardiac dysrhythmias, and cerebral hemorrhage all appear to be reduced in frequency when the patient has been treated before surgery with α blockers and the intravascular fluid compartment has been re-expanded. Extended treatment with α antagonists is also effective in treating the clinical manifestations of catecholamine myocarditis. However, α blocker therapy has never been studied in a controlled way and there are some groups that question its necessity.[46] A list of drugs frequently used in the management of pheochromocytoma is given in Table 41-9.

α-Adrenergic blockade is initiated once the diagnosis of pheochromocytoma is established. The patient receives phenoxybenzamine, a long-acting (24–48 hours), noncompetitive presynaptic (α_2) and postsynaptic (α_1) blocker, at doses of 10 mg every 8 hours. Increments are added until the blood pressure is controlled and paroxysms disappear. Most patients need between 80 and 200 mg $\cdot$ day^{-1}. The absorption after oral administration is variable, and side effects are common. Certain cardiovascular reflexes, such as the baroreceptor reflex, are blunted, and postural hypotension is common. α-adrenergic blockade also causes nasal stuffiness and impairs ejaculation. Prazosin, a competitive postsynaptic (α_1) blocking agent with a shorter half-life than phenoxybenzamine, has also been used effectively. Because postural hypotension can be pronounced with the commencement of therapy, the initial 1-mg dose is given at bedtime. Postural changes are also seen with maintenance therapy (6–10 mg $\cdot$ day^{-1}). A comparison of patients with pheochromocytoma receiving phenoxybenzamine and prazosin has shown both drugs to be equally effective in controlling the blood pressure. A case report of severe hypertension in a prazosin-treated patient after the initiation of β blocker therapy suggested that a less selective blockade of both α_1 and α_2 receptors (phenoxybenzamine) might be preferable in patients with severe hypertension.[47] Although the optimal period of preoperative treatment has not been established, most clinicians recommend beginning α blockade therapy at least 10–14 days before the proposed surgery; however, periods as short as 3–5 days have been used.[48] During this time, the contracted intravascular volume and hematocrit return toward normal and the blood pressure is stabilized. Despite the real possibility of hypotension after vascular

Table 41-9. DRUGS USED IN THE MANAGEMENT OF PHEOCHROMOCYTOMA

Drug	Action	Pressor Crisis	Preoperative Blood Pressure Control	Comment
Phentolamine	α Blocker	iv 2–5 mg	—	Rapid onset, short-acting; give bolus every 5 min or infuse initially 1 mg·min^{-1}
Phenoxybenzamine	α Blocker	—	Oral 30 mg·day^{-1}, increasing daily dosage by 30 mg	Long half-life; may accumulate; give twice or three times daily
Prazosin	α Blocker	—	Oral 1.0 mg single dose, increasing to tid regimen	First-dose phenomenon; may cause syncope, so start with low dose before bedtime
Propanolol	β Blocker	iv 1.0 mg bolus to total of 10 mg	Oral 40 mg bid; increase to 480 mg·day^{-1}	Should never be given without first creating α blockade
Atenolol	β Blocker	—	Oral 50 mg·day^{-1} initially; may increase to 100 mg·day^{-1}	Long-acting, selective β_1 antagonist eliminated unchanged by kidney
Esmolol	β Blocker	iv 500 μg·kg^{-1}·min^{-1} loading followed by maintenance infusion	—	Ultrashort-acting selective β_1 antagonist; may be used during anesthesia
Labetalol	α and β Blocker	iv 10 mg bolus to 150 mg	Oral 200 mg tid	A much weaker α-blocker than β blocker; may cause pressor response in pheochromocytoma
Nitroprusside	Vasodilator	iv infusion initially 0.5–1.5 μg·kg^{-1}·min^{-1}	—	Powerful vasodilator; short-acting; may be used during anesthesia
Magnesium sulfate	Vasodilator	iv 40–60 mg·kg^{-1} bolus followed by 2 g·h^{-1} and additional 20 mg·kg^{-1} boluses as needed	—	May potentiate neuromuscular blockade
Diltiazem	Calcium channel blocker	iv 3–10 μg·kg^{-1}·min^{-1}	—	May also directly block release of catecholamines
Nicardipine	Calcium channel blocker	iv 2–6 μg·kg^{-1}·min^{-1}	—	Better vasodilator than diltiazem
α-Methyl-tyrosine	Inhibitor of biosynthesis of cathecholamines	—	Oral 1–4 g·day^{-1}	Suitable for patients not amenable to surgery; may be nephrotoxic

iv = intravenous.

isolation of the tumor, most clinicians continue α blockers up until the morning of surgery.

β-Adrenergic blockade is often added after α blockade has been established. This addition is considered in patients with persistent tachycardia or cardiac dysrhythmias that may be exacerbated by α blockade. β Blockers should not be given until adequate α blockade is ensured to avoid the possibility of unopposed α-mediated vasoconstriction. There is no clear preoperative advantage of one β antagonist over another, although the short half-life of esmolol may allow better control of heart rate and arrhythmias in the perioperative setting. Labetalol, a β-adrenergic antagonist with α-blocking activity, is effective as a second-line medication, but there are reports of increases in blood pressure when this drug is used alone.[49]

Acute hypertensive crises are treated with iv infusions of nitroprusside or phentolamine. Phentolamine is a short-acting α-adrenergic antagonist that may be given as an iv bolus (2–5 mg) or by continuous infusion. Tachydysrhythmias are controlled with iv boluses of propranolol (1-mg increments) or by a continuous infusion of the ultrashort-acting selective β_1-adrenergic antagonist esmolol. The disadvantage of long-acting β blockers may be persistence of bradycardia and hypotension after the tumor is removed. Even esmolol may be problematic because there are cases of cardiac arrest after clamping of the venous drainage in patients on large doses of esmolol.

α-Methyl tyrosine is an agent that inhibits the enzyme tyrosine hydroxylase, the rate-limiting step in catecholamine biosynthesis. This medication is currently reserved for patients with meta-static disease or for situations in which surgery is contraindicated and long-term medical therapy is required. When α-methyl tyrosine is used in combination with α-adrenergic-blocking agents, there is a significant reduction in catecholamine biosynthesis.

Unrecognized pheochromocytoma during pregnancy may be life threatening to the mother and fetus. Although the safety of adrenergic-blocking agents during pregnancy has not been established, these agents probably improve fetal survival in pregnant patients with pheochromocytoma. The trend is to perform surgery during the first trimester or at the time of cesarean delivery. There is no reason to terminate an early pregnancy, but the patient should be aware of the risk of spontaneous abortion resulting from abdominal surgery to remove the tumor.[50]

Perioperative Anesthetic Management. Symptomatic patients continue to receive medical therapy until tachycardia, cardiac dysrhythmias, and paroxysmal elevations in blood pressure are well controlled. Occasionally, a patient with pheochromocytoma unaccompanied by hypertension is referred for consultation before surgery. These patients are difficult to manage with α blockade therapy on an outpatient basis because of the fear of clinically significant orthostatic hypotension. These patients are admitted to the hospital at least 24 hours before surgery to institute bed rest, "prophylactic" α-adrenergic blockade (prazosin), and fluid therapy. Central venous and peripheral artery pressure monitoring is routinely used to guide preoperative intervention. Because of the unpredictable and potentially lethal nature of the patient response to the stress of anesthesia and surgery, all patients presenting for pheochromocytoma surgery should receive a preoperative anesthesiology consultation. Experience suggests that pretreated patients have fewer cardiac dysrhythmias and less fluctuation in blood pressure and heart rate during the induction of anesthesia than other, "normotensive" patients who do not receive preoperative α blockade therapy. If it is not possible to initiate α-blocking therapy before surgery, or if the patient has received less than 48 hours of intensive treatment, it is frequently necessary to infuse nitroprusside during the induction of anesthesia. A low-dose infusion is often initiated in anticipation of the marked blood pressure elevations that can occur with laryngoscopy and surgical stimulation.

Until recently, a transperitoneal approach was necessary to allow the surgeon to assess for multiple or bilateral disease. Improvements in imaging now allow selected patients with solitary tumors less than 5 cm to undergo a retroperitoneal or laparoscopic approach. During laparoscopic surgery, creation of the pneumoperitoneum may cause release of catecholamines and large changes in hemodynamics that can be controlled with a vasodilator.[51]

Although there is no clear advantage to one anesthetic technique over another, drugs that are known to liberate histamine are avoided. Because of the potential for ventricular irritability, halothane is not administered. A potent sedative–hypnotic in combination with an opioid analgesic is used for induction. It is extremely important to achieve an adequate depth of anesthesia before proceeding with laryngoscopy to minimize the sympathetic nervous system response to this maneuver. Maintenance is provided with an opioid analgesic and a potent inhalation agent. Manipulation of the tumor may produce marked elevations in blood pressure, which are controlled with nitroprusside and, if necessary, phentolamine. Tachydysrhythmias are treated with iv β blockers. Many adjuvant drugs have been tried and recommended to control arterial pressure often seen during surgery. Magnesium sulfate given as an infusion with intermittent boluses has successfully controlled blood pressure.[52] Nicardipine, nitroglycerin, diltiazem, and prostaglandin E₁ have all been used anecdotally. The reduction in blood pressure that may occur after ligation of the tumor's venous supply should be anticipated through close communication with the surgical team. Restitution of any intravascular fluid deficit is the initial therapy in this situation. After replenishment of the intravascular volume, if the patient remains hypotensive, phenylephrine is administered. After surgery, catecholamine levels return to normal over several days. Approximately 75% of patients become normotensive within 10 days.[53]

DIABETES MELLITUS

Diabetes mellitus is the most commonly occurring endocrine disease found in surgical patients.[54] It has a broad spectrum of severity, and its manifestations can be altered in reaction to the patient's metabolic stress. Although the most serious complications of diabetes mellitus are related to its character as a chronic disease, it can cause difficulties in the short-term management of acute illness. Occasionally, diabetes remains clinically inapparent until exacerbated by the stress of trauma or surgery.

The principles of the treatment of diabetes will be easier to understand if we review the physiology of glucose metabolism and the stress response and then consider some of the specific pathologic entities that make up the clinical picture of diabetes mellitus.

Classification

Diabetes mellitus is primarily a disease of carbohydrate metabolism; however, it has numerous manifestations and interactions with a large range of hormonal and endocrinologic functions. Despite a variety of etiologic factors, its hallmark is a deficiency, either absolute or relative, in the amount of insulin available to the tissues.

Diabetes is often divided into two broad types. Type I, or insulin-dependent diabetes mellitus (IDDM), is distinguished from Type II, or non–insulin-dependent diabetes mellitus (NIDDM). The patient with IDDM typically experiences the onset of disease early in life.[55] Consequently, this form is also referred to as juvenile-onset diabetes. In general, the patient with IDDM is not obese, had an abrupt onset of the disease, and has very low levels of circulating insulin. Disease in these patients cannot be controlled with diet or oral hypoglycemic agents and mandates treatment with insulin. Patients in this group are often difficult to maintain in good glucose balance, are more likely to become ketotic, and are likely to sustain the end-organ complications of diabetes if they live long enough.

Patients with NIDDM, also called maturity-onset diabetes, typically experience a gradual onset of the disease later in life. They are often obese and have some degree of resistance to the effects of insulin. They may have normal or even elevated levels of insulin. In milder forms, this version of diabetes can often be treated with diet or oral hypoglycemic agents. Because these patients are relatively resistant to ketosis, their disease may be clinically inapparent until exacerbated by the stress of surgery or intercurrent illness.

This classification of diabetes mellitus is only a generalization. The milder, NIDDM form occasionally occurs in young people, and many older adults acquire a severe and brittle form of IDDM. Diabetes can also be a secondary result of a disease that damages the pancreas and thus impairs insulin secretion. Pancreatic surgery, chronic pancreatitis, cystic fibrosis, and hemochromatosis can damage the pancreas and thus impair insulin secretion sufficiently to produce clinical diabetes. Diabetes can result from one of the endocrine diseases that produces a hormone that opposes the action of insulin. Hence, a patient with a glucagonoma, pheochromocytoma, or acromegaly may be diabetic. An increased effect of glucocorticoids, either from Cushing's disease or steroid therapy, may also oppose the effect of insulin enough to elicit clinical diabetes and would certainly complicate the management of pre-existing diabetes. Patients with circulating anti-insulin receptor antibodies in association with other autoimmune processes are also diabetic. Finally, there is a clinical triad of severe insulin resistance in young, hirsute women with polycystic ovaries who have decreased insulin receptors.

Physiology

Insulin has multiple and complex interactions with lipid, protein, and glucose metabolism.[56] For our purposes, it is easiest to regard the effects of insulin on glucose metabolism as primary and to view its effects on other metabolic functions only as they relate to glucose.

Insulin is a small protein produced by the β cells of the islets of Langerhans in the pancreas. Normal production in the adult human is approximately 40–50 units·day⁻¹. Insulin acts through receptor sites on cells. The half-life of insulin in the circulation is only a few minutes. However, it may clinically appear to have a longer duration of action, owing to delays in binding and release from the cellular receptors. These facts lead us to the important principle that once a high level of insulin saturates all the binding sites, insulin will not have a more potent effect, just a more long-lasting effect. This is crucial to understanding insulin therapy, which is discussed in the following paragraphs.

Insulin is metabolized in the liver and kidney. In patients with hepatic dysfunction, the loss of gluconeogenesis as well as a prolongation of insulin effect increases the risk of hypoglycemia. Renal disease is another risk factor for hypoglycemia and is an important consideration in managing the use of exogenous insulin in diabetic patients.

Insulin release is related to a number of events. First is the direct effect of glucose (and amino acids) to stimulate insulin release. The mechanism involves interaction with hormones from the GI tract released during enteral feeding. The autonomic nervous system, also through vagal stimulation, increases insulin release, as does β-adrenergic stimulation and α-adrenergic blockade.

The most fundamental action of insulin is to stimulate increased cellular uptake of glucose. This is particularly important in skeletal muscle cells, where muscle activity also increases glucose uptake and is an important variable in the management of the physically active diabetic patient. (The brain and liver are exceptional areas where insulin does not affect glucose transport.) Hence, the diabetic patient has hyperglycemia because of inadequate cellular uptake of glucose. Along with glucose, potassium enters the cells under the influence of insulin, so the diabetic patient is also likely to have an imbalance of potassium concentrations across cell membranes.

Other important metabolic functions of insulin include the stimulation of glycogen formation and the suppression of gluconeogenesis and lipolysis. The patient with insulin deficiency has low glycogen stores and active gluconeogenesis. This implies that in the diabetic patient, owing to an absence of glycogen, protein must be broken down to make glucose. Insulin also increases the uptake of amino acids into muscle cells. Hence, an insulin deficiency leads to catabolism and negative nitrogen balance.

Fat metabolism is also abnormal in the diabetic state, with acceleration of lipid catabolism and increased formation of ketone bodies. A deficiency of insulin leads to increased fatty acid liberation from adipose tissue. These fatty acids have multiple metabolic effects, including interference with carbohydrate phosphorylation in muscle, which leads to further hyperglycemia. Low concentrations of insulin, which may be inadequate to prevent hyperglycemia, are often sufficient to block lipolysis. This effect explains the common clinical situation in which a patient is hyperglycemic without being ketotic.

Glucagon is a polypeptide released from the α cells of the pancreas and acts both to stimulate the release of insulin and oppose some of the effects of insulin. Hence, it has both a direct and an indirect ability to increase circulating glucose levels. In some patients, after total pancreatic resection, glucose balance is not as poor as might be expected because of the concomitant absence of glucagon. Glucagon release is stimulated by hypoglycemia as well as by epinephrine and cortisol, and is suppressed by glucose ingestion.

The metabolic effects of stress are intricately involved with the same pathways as those involved in diabetes mellitus. During stress, elevations in the circulating levels of cortisol, glucagon, catecholamines, and growth hormones all act to cause hyperglycemia. In addition, glucagon and epinephrine exert a suppressive effect on insulin release. Mild hyperglycemia may occur in the stressed patient who does not have diabetes mellitus. In the diabetic patient, stress makes the diabetes more difficult to control. In a patient with minimal or subclinical diabetes before the stressful episode, the glucose balance may become difficult to manage during the stress-related event.

Treatment

Patients with Type I diabetes require insulin to survive. Further, the risk of microvascular complications can be decreased if tight glycemic control maintains near-normal levels of blood glucose. Patients may be on a range of doses of both short- and intermediate-acting insulin, with doses given one to six times a day depending on the desire for tight control.

Patients with Type II diabetes may initially be treated with diet control and exercise. If this fails to control glucose levels, or if the diabetes worsens, therapy with an oral agent is indicated.[57] Sulfonylureas enhance β-cell insulin secretion. Metformin is a biguanide that enhances the sensitivity of both hepatic and peripheral tissues to insulin.[58] Rosiglitazone (Avandia) and pioglitazone (Actos) are thiazolidinediones that also increase insulin sensitivity. If oral agents cannot maintain acceptable glucose levels, insulin is used.

Anesthetic Management

Successful management of the diabetic patient depends as much, if not more, on the proper management of the chronic complications of the disease as on acute glycemic management.

Preoperative

A thorough preoperative search must be done for end-organ complications of diabetes. In addition to a thorough history and physical, a recent ECG, blood urea nitrogen, potassium, creatinine, glucose, and urinalysis are essential.

Atherosclerosis develops earlier and is more widespread in diabetic patients compared with nondiabetic people. Manifestations include coronary artery disease, peripheral vascular disease, cerebrovascular disease, and renovascular disease. The incidence of postoperative myocardial infarction is increased in diabetic patients.[59] Silent myocardial ischemia and infarction occur more commonly in diabetic patients, perhaps because of sensory neuropathy of the visceral afferents to the heart. Diabetes may be associated with a cardiomyopathy in the face of angiographically normal coronary arteries, possibly with diffuse disease in arteries too small to be visualized.

Laryngoscopy in up to 40% of juvenile patients with diabetes presenting for renal transplantation can be difficult.[60] This may be due to diabetic stiff joint syndrome, a frequent complication of IDDM, leading to decreased mobility of the atlanto-occipital joint. The "prayer sign," an inability to approximate the palmar surfaces of the interphalangeal joints, is associated with stiff joint syndrome and may predict difficult laryngoscopy.

Diabetic nephropathy eventually occurs in up to 40–50% of patients with IDDM. Albuminuria usually precedes a steady decline in renal function.

Diabetic patients with autonomic neuropathy are at increased risk for intraoperative hypotension requiring vasopressor support, and perioperative cardiorespiratory arrest.[61-64] There may be an exaggerated pressor response to tracheal intubation.[65] Autonomic function may be tested by measuring the beat-to-beat variation in heart rate during breathing, heart rate response to a Valsalva maneuver, and orthostatic changes in diastolic blood pressure and heart rate.

Diabetic patients may have delayed gastric emptying as a result of diabetic autonomic neuropathy, and therefore be at increased risk of aspiration. Autonomic function tests can predict the presence of solid food particles in gastric contents but not increased gastric volume or acidity.[66] Metoclopramide may be useful in emptying the stomach of solid food.

It is axiomatic that the patient should attain the best possible preoperative metabolic control. If the patient's glucose level has been unstable, especially with episodes of hypoglycemia, adjustment of insulin therapy is required. Traditionally, oral hypoglycemics have been held before surgery because of fear of hypoglycemia in the fasted patient. With today's shorter-acting agents, this may be unnecessary because the risk is much reduced. Metformin should be discontinued preoperatively because it has been associated with severe lactic acidosis during episodes of hypotension, poor perfusion, or hypoxia. Unless the patient has a surgical emergency, patients with diabetic ketoacidosis or hyperosmolar coma should receive intensive medical management before coming to the operating room (see Emergencies).

Intraoperative

The details of the anesthetic plan depend intimately on the end-organ complications. Invasive monitoring may be indicated for the patient with heart disease; awake intubation may be necessary if a difficult intubation is predicted; fluid management and drug choices may depend on renal function; and aspiration must be considered if there is gastroparesis.

Blood glucose levels should be measured before and after surgery. The need for additional measurements is determined by the duration and magnitude of surgery and the brittleness of the diabetes. Hourly measurements are reasonable in high-risk patients.

On the basis of a preoperative osmotic diuresis, the diabetic patient may reach the operating room with clinically significant dehydration. In addition to the usual principles of perioperative fluid management, it is important to note the amount of glucose administered iv to avoid a massive overdose of glucose. The standard glucose dosage for an adult patient is $5-10 \text{ g} \cdot \text{h}^{-1}$ (100–200 ml of 5% dextrose solution hourly). It is best to monitor and record the dextrose administered separately from the fluids given. It would be wrong to give large amounts of dextrose (contained in the iv solutions) just because that patient needed vigorous fluid replacement. If this happens, the patient is likely to be very hyperglycemic in the postanesthesia care unit. It is difficult to determine the proper dose of insulin to correct this iatrogenic hyperglycemia, and prolonged observation and therapy may be required.

Monitoring of the patient who arrives in the operating room with significant metabolic impairment, such as diabetic ketoacidosis, is similar to management in the medical intensive care unit, including hourly determinations of blood glucose, arterial pH, electrolytes, and fluid balance. Frequent reassessments with medical consultation as necessary guide the use of fluids, electrolytes (especially potassium), insulin, phosphate, and glucose.[67]

Another area of patient monitoring that is extremely important in the diabetic patient is positioning on the operating table. Injuries to the limbs or nerves are more likely in the patient who arrives in the operating room already compromised by diabetic peripheral vascular disease or neuropathy. The peripheral nerves may already be partly ischemic and therefore particularly vulnerable to pressure or stretch injuries.[68]

Management Regimens

There is no consensus about the optimal way to manage perioperative metabolic changes in diabetic patients; many options are available. Factors to consider in selecting a plan include whether the patient is insulin dependent, whether the surgery is minor and in an ambulatory unit, whether the surgery is elective or an emergency, the desire to maintain "tight" perioperative control of glucose levels, and the ability of hospital resources safely to administer a complex plan. The goal of any regimen should be to minimize metabolic derangements and, most obviously, to avoid hypoglycemia. Because hypoglycemia may develop insidiously and be difficult to detect quickly, insulin and glucose therapy is usually administered to bring about a mild, transient hyperglycemia that can gradually be corrected in the postoperative period. Mild hyperglycemia is not an acute problem, and there is no need for it to be corrected rapidly. It is never simple to determine the precise dose of insulin needed to correct hyperglycemia. Excessively rapid correction may lead to glucose instability and fluctuations that can persist for hours to days. There are clinical situations in which lower glucose levels may be desirable. Hyperglycemia may exacerbate neuronal ischemic damage. Patients undergoing surgical procedures associated with cerebral ischemia such as intracranial surgery, carotid endarterectomy, and cardiopulmonary bypass may benefit from maintenance of glucose levels less than 200 $\text{mg} \cdot \text{dl}^{-1}$.[69,70] Wound strength, wound healing, and phagocyte activity may all be impaired by hyperglycemia.

For some diabetic patients, the best method of diabetic management is to give no insulin. For short procedures in unstressed patients, especially if they are not chronically receiving insulin, there may be enough endogenous production of insulin to maintain reasonable glucose balance in the unfed state. Glucose should still be given during surgery as protection against the delayed effects of prior oral hypoglycemic agents or long-acting insulin and to prevent the occurrence of mild ketosis.

Patients receiving short-acting oral hypoglycemic agents should omit them the morning of surgery. Long-acting agents should be converted to short-acting agents several days before surgery.

Another common method of management is to administer a fraction of the patient's usual morning NPH insulin dose the morning of the day of surgery. Often, half the usual NPH dose suffices to maintain the patient through the day. It is critical for the patient who is NPO and receiving insulin also to receive an iv infusion of a dextrose solution. If $5-10 \text{ g} \cdot \text{h}^{-1}$ of dextrose (100–200 ml $\cdot \text{h}^{-1}$ of 5% dextrose solution) is administered to the adult, the risk of hypoglycemia is small. Nevertheless, the patient's usual dosage depends on caloric intake and physical activity, which are different in the hospital setting.

The "sliding scale" regimen for insulin administration is popular and easy to use. Varying doses of regular insulin are administered on a 4- to 6-hour schedule, depending on the blood or urine glucose levels and the patient's prior responses to insulin. This method of management guarantees that the glucose levels are checked frequently. Large fluctuations in blood glucose can occur if insulin is administered in the presence of high glucose levels and no insulin is given for normal or intermediate levels. This can be avoided if some insulin is always present. Small doses of insulin can be prescribed for all but the lowest levels of blood glucose, or the sliding scale can be combined with a small morning dose of long-acting NPH insulin.

A continuous, carefully titrated variable-rate infusion of insulin has been advocated as the ideal method for perioperative diabetic management.[71] Except in the patient with renal failure, in whom insulin effects are difficult to predict, the continuous-infusion method has the advantage of allowing rapid adjustment of the insulin effect by changing the rate of infusion. Also, alterations in cutaneous blood flow need not result in unpredictable serum insulin concentrations. In the adult with normal renal function, 7–10 units of regular insulin in 1 liter of 5% dextrose, infused at a rate of 75–100 ml $\cdot \text{h}^{-1}$, provides 0.5–1 unit $\cdot \text{h}^1$ of insulin. This tends to be a low dose, and many patients need more insulin, which can be given either as an increased insulin concentration in the infusion or as a sliding scale subcutaneous regimen. Alternatively, 50 units of regular insulin can be mixed in 500 ml of normal saline and administered at 10 ml $\cdot \text{h}^{-1}$. Sufficient glucose can be administered by a separate iv infusion. Glucose–insulin–potassium infusions have been used. The advantage of a combination solution is that any accidental variation in the infusion rate affects all components equally. The disadvantage is that a new bag must be prepared if the nominal concentrations do not achieve good control. In all iv regimens, a small amount of iv insulin is lost by adherence to the wall of the tubing and containers, but this loss is not clinically significant and should not be a deterrent to this route of administration.

Emergencies

Patients may present with metabolic instability, or it may develop perioperatively. Stress, trauma, and infection may all lead to increased insulin requirements and insulin resistance.

Hyperosmolar Nonketotic Coma

An occasional elderly patient with minimal or mild diabetes may present with remarkably high blood glucose levels and profound dehydration. Such patients usually have enough endogenous insulin activity to prevent ketosis; even with blood sugar concentrations of 1000 mg $\cdot \text{dl}^{-1}$, they are not in ketoacidosis. Presumably, it is the combination of an impaired thirst response and mild renal insufficiency that allows the hyperglycemia to develop. The marked hyperosmolarity may lead to coma and seizures, with the increased plasma viscosity producing a tendency to intravascular thrombosis. It is characteristic of this syndrome that the metabolic disturbance responds quickly to rehydration and small doses of insulin. One to 2 liters of normal saline, or equivalent, should be infused over 1–2 hours if there are no cardiovascular contraindications. Insulin, by bolus or infusion, should be administered. With rapid correction of the hyperosmolarity, cerebral edema is a risk, and recovery of mental acuity may be delayed after the blood glucose level and circulating volume have been normalized.

Diabetic Ketoacidosis

If the diabetic patient has insufficient insulin effect to block the mobilization and metabolism of free fatty acids, the metabolic by-products acetoacetate and β-hydroxybutyrate accumulate.[72] These ketone bodies are organic acids and cause a metabolic acidosis with an increased unmeasured anion gap. Clinically, the patient often presents because of intercurrent illness, trauma, or the untoward cessation of insulin therapy. Although hyperglycemia is almost always present, the degree of hyperglycemia does not correlate with the severity of the acidosis. Blood sugar levels are often in the 300–500 mg $\cdot$ dl^{-1} range. The patient is always dehydrated because of the combination of the hyperglycemia-induced osmotic diuresis and the nausea and vomiting typical of this syndrome. Because leukocytosis, abdominal pain, GI ileus, and mildly elevated amylase levels are all common in ketoacidosis, an occasional patient is misdiagnosed as having an intra-abdominal surgical problem.

Treatment of diabetic ketoacidosis includes insulin administration and fluid and electrolyte replacement (Table 41-10). An iv bolus of 10–20 units of insulin achieves rapid maximal effect. Further insulin can be administered by iv infusion or intermittent bolus every 30–60 minutes. When blood glucose levels decrease below 250 mg $\cdot$ dl^{-1}, glucose should be added to the iv fluid while insulin therapy continues. Fluid requirements can be marked; 1–2 liters of normal saline, or equivalent, should be given over 1–2 hours. Further deficits can be replaced more gradually. Potassium replacement is a key concern in patients with diabetic ketoacidosis. Because of the diuresis, the total body potassium stores are reduced. However, acidosis by itself causes a shift of potassium ions out of the cell. Thus, the serum potassium concentration may be normal or even slightly elevated while the patient is acidotic. As soon as the metabolic acidosis is corrected, the potassium ions shift back into the cells. Consequently, the serum potassium concentration can decline acutely. Therefore, early and vigorous potassium replacement is required in these patients, with the exception of those patients in renal failure. Hypophosphatemia also occurs with the correction of the acidosis and, if severe, may cause impairment of ventilation resulting from skeletal muscle weakness in the vulnerable patient. Instead of diabetic ketoacidosis, the diabetic

---

Table 41-10. MANAGEMENT OF DIABETIC KETOACIDOSIS

Regular insulin 10 units iv bolus followed by an insulin infusion nominally at (blood glucose/150) units $\cdot$ h^{-1}

Isotonic iv fluids as guided by vital signs and urine output; anticipate 4–10 l deficit

When urine output is >0.5 ml $\cdot$ kg^{-1} $\cdot$ h^{-1}, give potassium chloride 10–40 mEq $\cdot$ h^{-1} (with continuous ECG monitoring when the rate is greater than 10 mEq $\cdot$ h^{-1})

When serum glucose decreased to 250 mg $\cdot$ dl^{-1}, add dextrose 5% at 100 ml $\cdot$ h^{-1}

Consider sodium bicarbonate to correct pH <7.1

---

iv = intravenous.

---

patient with a metabolic acidosis may have lactic acidosis, which results from poor tissue perfusion or sepsis. It is diagnosed by the presence of an increased serum lactate concentration without an elevated ketone concentration.

Diabetic ketoacidosis must also be distinguished from the syndrome of alcoholic ketoacidosis. This typically occurs in the poorly nourished alcoholic patient after acute intoxication. Except for the presence of chemical ketoacidosis, alcoholic ketoacidosis is not clinically related in any way to diabetes mellitus. The alcoholic patient may be hypoglycemic or mildly hyperglycemic. The predominant ketone in this syndrome is β-hydroxybutyrate, which tends to react less sensitively in the standard laboratory nitroprusside reaction measurement of ketones. Hence, the diagnosis may be obscured. Administration of dextrose and parenteral fluids is the specific treatment for alcoholic ketoacidosis; insulin is not indicated (except in the rare circumstance in which the patient also has clear-cut diabetes mellitus).

Hypoglycemia

Hypoglycemia is the clinical occurrence most feared in the management of diabetic patients.[73] The precise level at which symptomatic hypoglycemia occurs is variable. The normal, fasted patient may have blood sugar levels lower than 50 mg $\cdot$ dl^{-1} without symptoms. However, the diabetic patient who has a chronically elevated blood sugar level may be symptomatic at levels significantly above this glucose concentration. Hypoglycemia is almost impossible to diagnose clinically in the unconscious patient.

In the awake patient, hypoglycemia often produces central nervous system changes ranging from light-headedness to coma with seizures. Often the patient recognizes the symptoms and can tell that the blood sugar is low before any overt clinical signs develop. With hypoglycemia, there is a reflex catecholamine release that produces overt sympathetic hyperactivity causing tachycardia, lacrimation, diaphoresis, and hypertension. In the anesthetized patient, these signs of sympathetic hyperactivity can easily be misinterpreted as inadequate or "light" anesthesia. In the anesthetized, sedated, or seriously ill patient, the mental changes of hypoglycemia are also unrecognizable. Furthermore, in patients being treated with β-adrenergic blocking agents or in patients with advanced diabetic autonomic neuropathy, the sympathetic hyperactivity of hypoglycemia may be obscured. Thus, the clinical diagnosis of hypoglycemia in the surgical patient may be difficult to make, and only a high degree of suspicion and frequent blood glucose checks can prevent this complication.

Hypoglycemia is more likely to occur in the diabetic surgical patient under certain circumstances. With renal insufficiency, the action of insulin and oral hypoglycemic agents is prolonged. This is a common problem owing to the prevalence of renal disease in the diabetic. Because some of the oral agents, especially chlorpropamide, can have long-lasting effects, an accurate medical history with attention to medications taken in the past day or two is essential. A frequent and totally avoidable cause of inadvertent hypoglycemia is the administration of insulin to a patient who is not receiving sufficient oral or iv caloric input. For the purpose of preventing hypoglycemia, transfused blood has a low glucose concentration (even with citrate–phosphate–dextrose added, it contains only ~2 g of glucose per unit); lactated Ringer's solution is also inadequate (the lactate is metabolized to produce ~9 kcal $\cdot$ l^{-1}).

The anesthesiologist must recognize that hypoglycemia in the critically ill or anesthetized patient is a serious hazard that may be difficult to diagnose. It is therefore reasonable to aim for mild hyperglycemia as the goal in diabetes management in these patients. There is considerable discussion by endocrinologists over how close to normal the blood sugar level should be maintained (chronic management) in long-standing diabetes to avoid the end-organ damage that diabetes can produce in the eyes, kidneys, nerves, and blood vessels. In the perioperative period, it is unlikely that such chronic damage is exacerbated by mild hyperglycemia.

PITUITARY GLAND

The pituitary gland is located below the base of the brain in a bony structure, the sella turcica. The pituitary gland and the hypothalamus together form a central unit that regulates the release of various hormones. The pituitary gland is divided into two components. The anterior pituitary (adenohypophysis) secretes prolactin, growth hormone, gonadotropins (luteinizing hormone and follicle-stimulating hormone), TSH, and ACTH. The posterior pituitary (neurohypophysis) secretes the hormones vasopressin and oxytocin. Hormone release from the anterior and posterior pituitary is regulated by the hypothalamus. Regulatory peptides or preformed hormones from the hypothalamus are transported to the pituitary gland through vascular or tissue connections.

Anterior Pituitary

Hyposecretion of anterior pituitary hormones is usually due to compression of the gland by tumor. This may begin as an isolated deficiency, but it usually develops into multiglandular dysfunction. Male impotence or secondary amenorrhea in the woman is an early manifestation of panhypopituitarism. Panhypopituitarism after postpartum hemorrhagic shock (Sheehan's syndrome) is due to necrosis of the anterior pituitary gland. Radiation therapy delivered to the sella turcica or nearby structures and surgical hypophysectomy are other causes of panhypopituitarism. Panhypopituitarism is treated with specific hormone replacement therapy, which should be continued in the perioperative period. Stress doses of corticosteroids are necessary for patients receiving steroid replacement due to inadequate ACTH.

The hypersecretion of various anterior pituitary hormones is usually caused by an adenoma. Excess prolactin secretion with galactorrhea is a common hormonal abnormality associated with pituitary adenoma. Cushing's disease may occur secondary to excess ACTH production, and gigantism or acromegaly may occur as a consequence of excess growth hormone production in the child or adult, respectively. Excessive secretion of TSH is rare.

Acromegaly in the adult patient may pose several problems for the anesthesiologist.[74] Excess hypertrophy occurs in skeletal, connective, and soft tissues.[75] The tongue and epiglottis are enlarged, making the patient susceptible to upper airway obstruction. Hoarseness may reflect thickening of the vocal cords or paralysis of a recurrent laryngeal nerve due to stretching. Dyspnea or stridor is associated with subglottic narrowing. Peripheral nerve or artery entrapment, hypertension, and diabetes mellitus are other common findings. The anesthetic management of these patients is complicated by distortion of the facial anatomy and upper airway. Induction of general anesthesia may put the patient at increased risk if mask fit or vocal cord visualization is impaired. When the preoperative history suggests upper airway or vocal cord involvement, it is prudent to consider intubation of the trachea while the patient is awake.

Posterior Pituitary

The posterior pituitary, or neurohypophysis, is composed of terminal nerve endings that extend from the ventral hypothalamus. Vasopressin (antidiuretic hormone [ADH]) and oxytocin are the two principal hormones secreted by the posterior pituitary. Both hormones are synthesized in the supraoptic and paraventricular nuclei of the hypothalamus. They are bound to inactive carrier proteins, neurophysins, and transported by axons to membrane-bound storage vesicles located in the posterior pituitary. ADH is a nonapeptide that circulates as a free peptide after its release. The primary functions of ADH are the maintenance of extracellular fluid volume and regulation of plasma osmolality. Oxytocin elicits contraction of the uterus and promotes milk secretion and ejection by the mammary glands.

Vasopressin

Antidiuretic hormone promotes resorption of solute-free water by increasing cell membrane permeability to water alone. The target sites for ADH are the collecting tubules of the kidneys. A decrease in free water clearance causes a decrease in serum osmolality and a corresponding increase in circulating blood volume. Under normal conditions, the primary stimulus for the release of ADH is an increase in serum osmolality.

Osmoreceptors located in the hypothalamus are sensitive to changes in the normal serum osmolality of as little as 1% (normal osmolality is approximately 285 mOsm · l⁻¹). Stretch receptors in the left atrium and perhaps pulmonary veins, which are sensitive to moderate reductions in the blood volume, are also capable of stimulating ADH secretion. The need to restore plasma volume may at times override osmotic inhibition of ADH release. Various physiologic and pharmacologic stimuli also influence the secretion of ADH. Positive pressure ventilation of the lungs, stress, anxiety, hyperthermia, β-adrenergic stimulation, and any histamine-releasing stimulus can promote the release of ADH.

Antidiuretic hormone also has other actions. ADH can increase blood pressure by constricting vascular smooth muscle. This activity is most significant in the splanchnic, renal, and coronary vascular beds and provides the rationale for administering exogenous vasopressin in the management of hemorrhage due to esophageal varices. Caution must be taken when this drug is used in patients with coronary artery disease. ADH (even in small doses) can precipitate myocardial ischemia through vasoconstriction of the coronary arteries. It is unclear whether selective arterial infusion is safer than systemic administration with regard to cardiac and vascular side effects.

Antidiuretic hormone also promotes hemostasis through an increase in the level of circulating von Willebrand factor and factor VIII. Desmopressin (DDAVP), an analogue of ADH, administered to patients after cardiopulmonary bypass in a dose of 0.3 μg · kg⁻¹ significantly decreased blood loss and reduced transfusion requirements compared with a group of patients who did not receive the drug. DDAVP is also frequently used to reverse the coagulopathy of renal failure.

Diabetes Insipidus

This disorder results from inadequate secretion of ADH or resistance on the part of the renal tubules to ADH (nephrogenic diabetes insipidus). Failure to secrete adequate amounts of ADH results in polydipsia, hypernatremia, and a high output of poorly concentrated urine. Hypovolemia and hypernatremia may become so severe as to be life threatening. This disorder usually occurs after destruction of the pituitary gland by intracranial trauma, infiltrating lesions, or surgery. Patients in whom diabetes insipidus develops secondary to severe head trauma or subarachnoid hemorrhage often have impending brain death.[76] The treatment of diabetes insipidus depends on the extent of the hormonal deficiency. During surgery, the patient with complete diabetes insipidus receives an iv infusion of aqueous ADH (100–200 mU · h⁻¹) combined with administration of an isotonic crystalloid solution. The serum sodium and plasma osmolality are measured on a regular basis, and therapeutic changes are made accordingly. ADH also may be given intramuscularly (as vasopressin tannate in oil). DDAVP administered intranasally has prolonged antidiuretic activity (12–24 hours) and is associated with a low incidence of pressor effects. As a consequence of the large outpouring of ADH in response to surgical stress, patients with a residually functioning gland usually do not need parenteral ADH during the perioperative period unless the plasma osmolality rises above 290 mOsm · l⁻¹.

Nonhormonal agents that have efficacy in the treatment of incomplete diabetes insipidus include the oral hypoglycemic chlorpropamide (200–500 mg · day^{-1}). This drug stimulates the release of ADH and sensitizes the renal tubules to the hormone. Hypoglycemia is a serious side effect that limits the usefulness of the drug. Clofibrate, a hypolipidemic agent, is also capable of stimulating ADH release and has been used in the outpatient setting. None of these medications is effective in the patient with nephrogenic diabetes insipidus. Paradoxically, the thiazide diuretics exert an antidiuretic action in patients with this disorder.

Inappropriate Secretion of Antidiuretic Hormone

The inappropriate and excessive secretion of ADH may occur in association with a number of diverse pathologic processes, including head injuries, intracranial tumors, pulmonary infections, small cell carcinoma of the lung, and hypothyroidism. The clinical manifestations occur as a result of a dilutional hyponatremia, decreased serum osmolality, and a reduced urine output with a high osmolality. Weight gain, skeletal muscle weakness, and mental confusion or convulsions are presenting symptoms. Peripheral edema and hypertension are rare. The diagnosis of the syndrome of inappropriate ADH (SIADH) secretion is one of exclusion, and other causes of hyponatremia must first be ruled out. The prognosis is related to the underlying cause of the syndrome.

The treatment of patients with mild or moderate water intoxication is restriction of fluid intake to 800 ml · day^{-1}. Patients with severe water intoxication associated with hyponatremia and mental confusion may require more aggressive therapy, with the iv administration of a hypertonic saline solution. This may be administered in conjunction with furosemide. Caution must be observed in patients with poor left ventricular function. Isotonic saline is substituted for hypertonic solutions once the serum sodium is brought into a safe range. Too-rapid correction of hyponatremia may induce central pontine myelinolysis and cause permanent brain damage. Serum sodium should not be raised by more than 12 mEq · l^{-1} in 24 hours. Other drugs that may be used in the patient with SIADH are demeclocycline and lithium. Demeclocycline interferes with the ability of the renal tubules to concentrate urine and is frequently used in outpatients. Lithium usually is not used because of the high incidence of toxicity.

ENDOCRINE RESPONSE TO SURGICAL STRESS

Anesthesia, surgery, and trauma elicit a generalized endocrine metabolic response characterized by an increase in the plasma levels of cortisol, ADH, renin, catecholamines, and endorphins and by metabolic changes such as hyperglycemia and a negative nitrogen balance.[77,78] Various neural and humoral factors (*e.g.*, pain, anxiety, acidosis, local tissue factors, hypoxia) play a role in activating this stress response.

The induction of anesthesia increases the levels of circulating catecholamines and is a form of metabolic stress. Regional anesthesia may block part of the metabolic stress response during surgery, probably by blockade of the neural communications from the surgical area. It is theorized that the persistently high levels of circulating catecholamines in trauma and critical illness lead to stress hyperglycemia through a direct inhibition of insulin release. Bypass of the gut hormonal actions in patients receiving iv glucose feedings, especially if given in large amounts, contributes to the impairment of insulin release during illness and can create a particularly difficult management problem for diabetic patients.

Endorphins are a group of endogenous peptides with opioid activity that have been isolated from the central nervous system. It is well documented that β-endorphin is released from the anterior pituitary, where it is contained as part of β-lipoprotein,

a 91-chain amino acid, which is a cleavage product of the precursor peptide for ACTH. Large increases in the central nervous system and plasma concentrations of endorphins in response to emotional or surgical stimuli suggest that these substances play a role in the body's response to stress. These substances modulate painful stimuli by binding to opiate receptors located throughout the brain and spinal cord.

Numerous experiments have focused on the stress response and its relationship to the depth of anesthesia. Regional anesthesia and general anesthesia appear to blunt the release of various stress hormones during the period of surgical stimulation in a dose-dependent fashion. Historically, anesthesiologists have relied on the indirect measurement of hemodynamic variables such as blood pressure and heart rate to evaluate the level of autonomic activity in response to anesthesia and surgery. It is assumed that the physiologic manifestations of stress are potentially harmful, especially in patients with limited functional reserve. As such, our anesthetic techniques and pain management strategies are designed to limit this neurohormonal response, in the hope of providing the patient with some benefit. Further investigations are needed to assess the impact of these efforts on perioperative morbidity and mortality.

REFERENCES

1. Surks MI, Sievert R: Drugs and thyroid function. N Engl J Med 333:1688, 1995
2. Bilezikian J, Loeb JN: The influence of hyperthyroidism and hypothyroidism on alpha and beta adrenergic receptor systems and adrenergic responsiveness. Endocr Rev 4:378, 1983
3. Mandel SJ, Brent GA, Larsen PR: Levothyroxine therapy in patients with thyroid disease. Ann Intern Med 119:492, 1993
4. Mulligan DC, McHenry CR, Kinney W, Esselstyn CB Jr: Amiodarone-induced thyrotoxicosis: Clinical presentation and expanded indications for thyroidectomy. Surgery 114:1114, 1993
5. Gittoes NJL, Franklyn JA: Hyperthyroidism: Current treatment guidelines. Drugs 55:543, 1998
6. Geffner DL, Hershman JM: Beta-adrenergic blockade for the treatment of hyperthyroidism. Am J Med 93:61, 1992
7. Franklyn JA: The management of hyperthyroidism. N Engl J Med 330:1731, 1994
8. Kaplan JA, Cooperman LH: Alarming reactions to ketamine in patients taking thyroid medication treatment with propranolol. Anesthesiology 35:229, 1971
9. Hermann M, Richter B, Roka R, Freissmuth M: Thyroid surgery in untreated severe hyperthyroidism: Perioperative kinetics of free thyroid hormones in the glandular venous effluent and peripheral blood. Surgery 115:240, 1994
10. Smallridge RC: Metabolic and anatomic thyroid emergencies: A review. Crit Care Med 20:276, 1992
11. Wade JSH: Respiratory obstruction in thyroid surgery. Annals of the College of Surgeons of England 62:15, 1980
12. Kahky MP, Weber RS: Complications of surgery of the thyroid and parathyroid glands. Surg Clin North Am 73:307, 1993
13. Szubin L, Kacker A, Kakani R et al: The management of postthyroidectomy hypocalcemia. Ear Nose Throat J 75:612, 1996
14. Wagner HE, Seiler C: Recurrent laryngeal nerve palsy after thyroid gland surgery. Br J Surg 81:226, 1994
15. Jarhult J, Lindestad PA, Nordenstrom J, Perbeck L: Routine examination of the vocal cords before and after thyroid and parathyroid surgery. Br J Surg 78:1116, 1991
16. Lindsay RS, Toft AD: Hypothyroidism. Lancet 349:413, 1997
17. Toft AD: Thyroxine therapy. N Engl J Med 331:174, 1994
18. Ladenson PW, Levin AA, Ridgway EC, Daniels GH: Complications of surgery in hypothyroid patients. Am J Med 77:261, 1984
19. Whitten CW, Latson TW, Klein KW et al: Anesthetic management of a hypothyroid cardiac surgical patient. J Cardiothorac Vasc Anesth 5:156, 1991
20. Drucker DJ, Burrow GN: Cardiovascular surgery in the hypothyroid patient. Arch Intern Med 145:1585, 1985
21. Babad AA, Eger EI: The effects of hyperthyroidism and hypothyroidism on halothane and oxygen requirements in dogs. Anesthesiology 29:1087, 1968
22. Weinberg AD, Ehrenwerth J: Anesthetic considerations and periop-

erative management of patients with hypothyroidism. Advances in Anesthesia 4:185, 1987

23. Roland EJ, Wierda JM, Eurin BG, Roupie E: Pharmacodynamic behaviour of vecuronium in primary hyperparathyroidism. Can J Anaesth 41:694, 1994

24. Meuriaaw M, Hamoir E, Defechereux T et al: Bilateral neck exploration under hypnosedation. Ann Surg 229:401, 1999

25. Al-Zahrani, Levine MA: Primary hyperparathyroidism. Lancet 349:1233, 1997

26. Sainsberg JRC, Stoddard JC, Watson MJ: Plasma cortisol levels: A comparison between sick patients and volunteers given intravenous cortisol. Anaesthesia 36:16, 1981

27. Munck A, Guyre PM: Glucocorticoid physiology, pharmacology and stress. Adv Exp Med Biol 196:81, 1986

28. Fischer JE, Hasselgren PO: Cytokines and glucocorticoids in the regulation of the "hepato-skeletal muscle axis" in sepsis. Am J Surg 161:266, 1991

29. Knudsen L, Christiansen LA, Lorentzen JE: Hypotension during and after operation in glucocorticoid-treated patients. Br J Anaesth 53:295, 1981

30. Oelkers W: Adrenal insufficiency. N Engl J Med 335:1206, 1996

31. Lamberts SWJ, Bruining HA, DeJong FH: Corticosteroid therapy in severe illness. N Engl J Med 337:1285, 1997

32. Bennett N, Gabrielli A: Hypotension and adrenal insufficiency. J Clin Anesth 11:425, 1999

33. Sutherland FWH, Naik SK: Acute adrenal insufficiency after coronary artery bypass grafting. Ann Thorac Surg 62:1516, 1996

34. Chin R: Adrenal crisis. Crit Care Clin 7:23, 1991

35. Engquist A, Brandt MR, Fernandes A, Kehlet H: The blocking effect of epidural analgesia on the adrenocortical and hyperglycemic responses to surgery. Acta Anaesthesiol Scand 21:330, 1977

36. Lehtinen AM, Fyhrquist F, Kivalo I: The effect of fentanyl on arginine, vasopressin and cortisol secretion during anesthesia. Anesth Analg 63:25, 1984

37. Namba Y, Smith JB, Fox GS, Challis: Plasma cortisol concentrations during cesarean section during anesthesia. Br J Anaesth 52:1027, 1980

38. Oyama T, Taniguchi K, Jin T et al: Effects of anesthesia and surgery on plasma aldosterone concentration and renin activity in man. Br J Anaesth 51:747, 1979

39. Salem M, Tainsh RE Jr, Bromberg J et al: Perioperative glucocorticoid coverage: A reassessment 41 years after emergence of a problem. Ann Surg 219:416, 1994

40. Symreng T, Karlberg BE, Kagedal B, Schildt B: Physiological cortisol substitution of long-term steroid-treated patients undergoing major surgery. Br J Anaesth 53:949, 1981

41. Glowniak JV, Loriaux DL: A double-blind study of perioperative steroid requirements in secondary adrenal insufficiency. Surgery 121:123, 1997

42. Allen GC, Rosenberg H: Pheochromocytoma presenting as acute malignant hyperthermia, a diagnostic challenge. Can J Anaesth 37:593, 1990

43. Giffird RW Jr, Manger WM, Bravo EL: Pheochromocytoma. Endocrinol Metab Clin North Am 23:387, 1994

44. Samaan NA, Hickey RC, Shutts PE: Diagnosis, localization and management of pheochromocytoma. Cancer 62:2451, 1988

45. Geoghegan JG, Emberton M, Bloom R, Lynn JA: Changing trends in the management of phaeochromocytoma. Br J Surg 85:117, 1998

46. Ulchaker JC, Goldfarb DA, Bravo EL, Novick AC: Successful outcomes in pheochromocytoma surgery in the modern era. J Urol 161:764, 1999

47. Knapp HR, Fitzgerald GA: Hypertensive crisis in prazosin-treated pheochromocytoma. South Med J 77:535, 1984

48. Russell WJ, Metecalfe IR, Tonkin AL, Frewin DB: The preoperative management of phaeochromocytoma. Anaesth Intensive Care 26:196, 1998

49. Briggs RSJ, Birtwell AJ, Pohl JEF: Hypertensive response to labetalol in pheochromocytoma. Lancet 1:1045, 1978

50. Hamilton A, Sirrs S, Schmidt N, Onrot J: Anaesthesia for phaeochromocytoma in pregnancy. Can J Anaesth 44:654, 1997

51. Joris JL, Hamoir EE, Hartstein GM et al: Hemodynamic changes and catecholamine release during laparoscopic adrenalectomy for pheochromocytoma. Anesth Analg 88:16, 1999

52. Drolet P, Girard M: The use of magnesium sulfate during surgery of pheochromocytoma: Apropos of 2 cases. Can J Anaesth 40:521, 1993

53. Jovenich JJ: Anesthesia in adrenal surgery. Urol Clin North Am 16:583, 1989

54. Gusberg RJ, Moley J: Diabetes and abdominal surgery. Yale J Biol Med 56:285, 1983

55. Atkinson MA, Maclaren NK: The pathogenesis of insulin-dependent diabetes mellitus. N Engl J Med 331:1428, 1994

56. Stevens A, Roizen MF: Patients with diabetes mellitus and disorders of glucose metabolism. Anesthesiol Clin North Am 5:339, 1987

57. DeFronzo RA: Pharmacologic therapy for type 2 diabetes mellitus. Ann Intern Med 131:281, 1999

58. Bailey CJ, Turner RC: Metformin. N Engl J Med 334:574, 1996

59. Treiman GS, Treiman RL, Foran RF et al: The influence of diabetes mellitus on the risk of abdominal aortic surgery. Am Surg 60:436, 1994

60. Hogan K, Rusy D, Springman SR: Difficult laryngoscopy and diabetes mellitus. Anesth Analg 67:1162, 1988

61. Charlson ME, MacKenzie CR, Gold JP: Preoperative autonomic function abnormalities in patients with diabetes mellitus and patients with hypertension. J Am Coll Surg 179:1, 1994

62. Burgos LG, Ebert TJ, Asiddao C et al: Increased intraoperative cardiovascular morbidity in diabetics with autonomic neuropathy. Anesthesiology 70:591, 1989

63. Latson TW, Ashmore TH, Reinhart DJ et al: Autonomic reflex dysfunction in patients presenting for elective surgery is associated with hypotension after anesthesia induction. Anesthesiology 80:326, 1994

64. Page MM, Watkins PJ: Cardiorespiratory arrest and diabetic autonomic neuropathy. Lancet 1:14, 1978

65. Vohra A, Kumar S, Charlton AJ et al: Effect of diabetes mellitus on the cardiovascular responses to induction of anesthesia and tracheal intubation. Br J Anaesth 71:258, 1993

66. Ishihara H, Singh H, Giesecke AH: Relationship between diabetic autonomic neuropathy and gastric contents. Anesth Analg 78:943, 1994

67. Cefalu WT: Diabetic ketoacidosis. Crit Care Clin 7:89, 1991

68. Harati Y: Diabetic peripheral neuropathies. Ann Intern Med 107:546, 1987

69. Lanier WL: Glucose management during cardiopulmonary bypass: Cardiovascular and neurologic implications. Anesth Analg 72:423, 1991

70. Sieber FE: The neurologic implications of diabetic hyperglycemia during surgical procedures at increased risk for brain ischemia. J Clin Anesth 9:334, 1997

71. Hirsch IB, McGill JB, Cryer PE, White PF: Perioperative management of surgical patients with diabetes mellitus. Anesthesiology 74:346, 1991

72. Foster DW, McGarry JD: The metabolic derangements and treatment of diabetic ketoacidosis. N Engl J Med 309:159, 1983

73. Fischer KF, Lees JA, Newman JM: Hypoglycemia in hospitalized patients. N Engl J Med 315:1245, 1986

74. Melmed S: Acromegaly. N Engl J Med 322:966, 1990

75. Kitahata LM: Airway difficulties associated with anaesthesia in acromegaly. Br J Anaesth 43:1187, 1971

76. Wong MF, Chin NM, Lew TW: Diabetes insipidus in neurosurgical patients. Ann Acad Med Singapore 27:340, 1998

77. Weissman C: The metabolic response to stress: An overview and update. Anesthesiology 73:308, 1990

78. Woolf PD: Hormonal responses to trauma. Crit Care Med 20:216, 1992

Clinical Anesthesia (4/e), edited by
Paul G. Barash, Bruce F. Cullen, and
Robert K. Stoelting. Lippincott Williams &
Wilkins, Philadelphia, © 2001.

CHAPTER 42

OBSTETRIC ANESTHESIA

ALAN C. SANTOS, DAVID A. O'GORMAN, AND
MIECZYSLAW FINSTER

PHYSIOLOGIC CHANGES OF PREGNANCY

During pregnancy, there are major alterations in nearly every maternal organ system. These changes are initiated by hormones secreted by the corpus luteum and placenta. The mechanical effects of the enlarging uterus and compression of surrounding structures play an increasing role in the second and third trimesters. This altered physiologic state has relevant implications for the anesthesiologist caring for the pregnant patient. The most relevant changes, involving hematologic, cardiovascular, ventilatory, metabolic, and gastrointestinal functions, are considered here (Table 42-1).

Hematologic Alterations

Increased mineralocorticoid activity during pregnancy produces sodium retention and increased body water content.[1] Thus, plasma volume and total blood volume begin to increase in early gestation, resulting in a final increase of 40–50% and 25–40% respectively, at term. The relatively smaller increase in red blood cell volume (20%) accounts for a reduction in hemoglobin (to 11–12 g · dl^{-1}) and hematocrit (to 35%).[1] The leukocyte count ranges from 8000–10,000 per mm^3 throughout pregnancy, whereas the platelet count remains unchanged. Plasma fibrinogen concentrations increase during normal pregnancy by approximately 50%, whereas clotting factor activity is variable.[2] Serum cholinesterase activity declines to a level of 20% below normal by term, and reaches a nadir in the puerperium. However, it is doubtful that moderate succinylcholine doses lead to prolonged apnea in otherwise normal circumstances.[3] Total plasma protein concentration declines to less than 6 g · dl^{-1} at term, whereas the total amount in the circulation increases.[4] The albumin–globulin ratio declines because of the relatively greater reduction in albumin concentration. A decrease in serum protein concentration may be clinically significant, in that the free fractions of protein-bound drugs can be expected to increase.

Cardiovascular Changes

As oxygen consumption increases during pregnancy, the maternal cardiovascular system adapts to meet the metabolic demands of a growing fetus. Decreased vascular resistance due to estrogens, progesterone, and prostacyclin may be the initiating factor.[5] Lowered resistance is found in the uterine, renal, and other vascular beds; at term, there is an increase in heart rate (15–25%), and cardiac output (up to 50%) above that of the nonpregnant state. Arterial blood pressure decreases slightly because the decrease in peripheral resistance exceeds the increase in cardiac output. Additional increases in cardiac output occur during labor (when cardiac output may reach 12–14 · min^{-1}) and also in the immediate postpartum period owing to added blood volume from the contracted uterus.

From the second trimester, aortocaval compression by the enlarged uterus becomes progressively more important, reaching its maximum at 36–38 weeks, after which it may decrease as the fetal head descends into the pelvis.[6] Studies of cardiac output, measured with the patient in the supine position during the last weeks of pregnancy, have indicated a decrease to nonpregnant levels; however, this decrease was not observed when patients were in the lateral decubitus position.[6] Supine hypotensive syndrome, which occurs in 10% of pregnant women because of venous occlusion, results in maternal tachycardia, arterial hypotension, faintness, and pallor.[7] Compression of the lower aorta in this position may further decrease uteroplacental perfusion and result in fetal asphyxia. Therefore, uterine displacement or lateral pelvic tilt should be applied routinely during the second and third trimesters of pregnancy.

Changes in the electrocardiogram may also occur. Left axis deviation results from the upward displacement of the heart by the gravid uterus, and there is also a tendency toward premature atrial contractions, sinus tachycardia, and paroxysmal supraventricular tachycardia.

Ventilatory Changes

Increased extracellular fluid and vascular engorgement may not only lead to edema of the extremities but may compromise the upper airway. Many pregnant women complain of difficulty with nasal breathing, and the friable nature of the mucous membranes during pregnancy can cause severe bleeding, especially on insertion of nasopharyngeal airways or nasogastric and endotracheal tubes. Airway edema may be particularly severe in women with pre-eclampsia, in patients placed in the Trendelenburg position for prolonged periods, or with concurrent use of tocolytic agents. It may also be difficult to perform laryngoscopy in obese, short-necked parturients with enlarged breasts. Use of a short-handled laryngoscope has proved helpful.

The level of the diaphragm rises as the uterus increases in size, and is accompanied by an increase in the anteroposterior and transverse diameters of the thoracic cage. From the fifth month, the expiratory reserve volume, residual volume, and functional residual capacity (FRC) decrease, the latter to 20% less than in the nonpregnant state.[8] Concomitantly, there is an increase in inspiratory reserve volume, so that total lung capacity remains unchanged. In most pregnant women, a decreased FRC does not cause problems, but those with pre-existing alterations in closing volume as a result of smoking, obesity, or scoliosis may experience early airway closure with advancing pregnancy, leading to hypoxemia. The Trendelenburg and supine positions also exacerbate the abnormal relationship between closing volume and FRC. The residual volume and functional residual capacity return to normal shortly after delivery.

Progesterone-induced relaxation of bronchiolar smooth muscle decreases airway resistance, whereas lung compliance remains unchanged. Minute ventilation increases from the beginning of pregnancy to a maximum of 50% above normal at term.[8] This is accomplished by a 40% increase in tidal volume and a 15% increase in respiratory rate. Dead space does not change significantly, and thus alveolar ventilation is increased by 70% at term. After delivery, as blood progesterone levels decline, ventilation returns to normal within 1–3 weeks.[9]

Metabolism

Basal oxygen consumption increases during early pregnancy, with an overall increase of 20% by term.[8] However, increased alveolar ventilation leads to a reduction in the partial pressure of carbon dioxide in arterial blood ($Paco_2$) to 32 mm Hg and an increase in the partial pressure of oxygen in arterial blood

Table 42-1. SUMMARY OF PHYSIOLOGIC CHANGES OF PREGNANCY AT TERM

Variable	Change	Amount
Total blood volume	Increase	25–40%
Plasma volume	Increase	40–50%
Fibrinogen	Increase	50%
Serum cholinesterase activity	Decrease	20–30%
Cardiac output	Increase	30–50%
Minute ventilation	Increase	50%
Alveolar ventilation	Increase	70%
Functional residual capacity	Decrease	20%
Oxygen consumption	Increase	20%
Arterial carbon dioxide tension	Decrease	10 mm Hg
Arterial oxygen tension	Increase	10 mm Hg
Minimum alveolar concentration	Decrease	32–40%

(Pa_{O_2}) to 106 mm Hg. The plasma buffer base decreases from 47 to 42 $mEq \cdot l^{-1}$, and therefore the pH remains practically unchanged. The maternal uptake and elimination of inhalational anesthetics is enhanced because of the increased alveolar ventilation and decreased FRC.[9] However, the decreased FRC and increased metabolic rate predispose the mother to development of hypoxemia during periods of apnea/hypoventilation, such as may occur during airway obstruction or prolonged attempts at tracheal intubation.[10]

Human placental lactogen and cortisol increase the tendency toward hyperglycemia and ketosis, which may exacerbate preexisting diabetes mellitus. The patient's ability to handle a glucose load is decreased, and the transplacental passage of glucose may stimulate fetal secretion of insulin, leading in turn to neonatal hypoglycemia in the immediate postpartum period.[11]

Gastrointestinal Changes

Enhanced progesterone production causes decreased gastrointestinal motility and slower absorption of food. Gastric secretions are more acidic and lower esophageal sphincter (LES) tone is decreased. A delay in gastric emptying can already be demonstrated by the end of the first trimester.[12] Uterine growth leads to upward displacement and rotation of the stomach, with increased pressure and a further delay in gastric emptying. By the 34th week, evacuation of a watery meal may be prolonged by 60%.[13] Pain, anxiety, and administration of opioids (systemic or neuraxial) and belladonna alkaloids may further exacerbate this delay.

The risk of regurgitation on induction of general anesthesia depends, in part, on the gradient between the LES and intragastric pressures. In most patients, the gradient increases after succinylcholine administration because the increase in LES pressure exceeds the increase in intragastric pressure. However, in parturients with "heartburn," the LES tone is greatly reduced.[14] The efficacy of prophylactic nonparticulate antacids is diminished by inadequate mixing with gastric contents, improper timing of administration, and the tendency for antacids to increase gastric volume. Administration of histamine (H_2) receptor antagonists, such as cimetidine and ranitidine, requires careful timing. A good case can be made for the administration of intravenous (iv) metoclopramide before elective cesarean section. This dopamine antagonist hastens gastric emptying and increases resting LES tone in both nonpregnant and pregnant women.[15] However, conflicting reports have appeared on its efficacy and on the frequency of side effects such as extrapyramidal reactions and transient neurologic dysfunction.[16,17] Although no routine prophylactic regimen can be recommended with certainty, it is the authors' preference to administer at least a nonparticulate antacid before cesarean section and to use regional anesthesia whenever possible. A rapid-sequence induc-

tion of anesthesia, application of cricoid pressure, and intubation with a cuffed endotracheal tube are required for all pregnant women receiving general anesthesia from the 12th week of gestation.[12] These recommendations also pertain to women in the immediate postpartum period because there is uncertainty as to when gastric volume returns to normal.

Altered Drug Responses

The minimum alveolar concentration (MAC) for inhalational agents is decreased by 8–12 weeks of gestation and may be related to an increase in progesterone levels.[18] In addition, lower doses of local anesthetic are needed per dermatomal segment of epidural or spinal block. This has been attributed to an increased spread of local anesthetic in the epidural and subarachnoid spaces, which occurs as a result of epidural venous engorgement. An increased neural sensitivity to local anesthetics also has been suggested, which may be mediated by progesterone.[19]

FETAL EXPOSURE TO DRUGS USED IN OBSTETRIC ANESTHESIA

It is generally accepted that most drugs, including anesthetic agents, readily cross the placenta. The development of highly sensitive and specific techniques for drug analysis and a better understanding of the fetal circulation have improved our comprehension of fetal drug exposure.

Placental Transfer

Several factors influence the placental transfer of drugs, including the physicochemical characteristics of the drug itself, maternal drug concentrations in the plasma, properties of the placenta, and hemodynamic events within the fetomaternal unit.

Drugs cross biologic membranes by simple diffusion, the rate of which is determined by the Fick principle, which states that:

$$Q/t = KA(C_m - C_f)/D$$

where Q/t = rate of diffusion, K = diffusion constant, A = surface area available for exchange, C_m = concentration of free drug in maternal blood, C_f = concentration of free drug in fetal blood, and D = thickness of diffusion barrier.

The diffusion constant (K) of the drug depends on physicochemical characteristics such as molecular size, lipid solubility, and degree of ionization. Compounds with a molecular weight of less than 500 daltons are unimpeded in crossing the placenta, whereas those with molecular weights of 500–1000 daltons are more restricted. Most drugs commonly used by the anesthesiologist have molecular weights that permit easy transfer.

If blood flow to the fetal side of the placenta can be measured, as in some animal models, calculating the placental clearance may be a more appropriate way of expressing drug transfer to the fetus.[20]

Drugs that are highly lipid soluble cross biologic membranes more readily, and the degree of ionization is important because the nonionized moiety of a drug is more lipophilic than the ionized one. Local anesthetics and opioids are weak bases, with a relatively low degree of ionization and considerable lipid solubility. In contrast, muscle relaxants are less lipophilic and more ionized, and their rate of placental transfer is therefore more limited. The relative concentrations of drug existing in the nonionized and ionized forms can be predicted from the Henderson-Hasselbalch equation:

$$pH = pKa + \log(base)/(cation)$$

The ratio of base to cation becomes particularly important with local anesthetics because the nonionized form penetrates tissue barriers, whereas the ionized form is pharmacologically active in blocking nerve conduction. The pKa is the pH at which the concentrations of free base and cation are equal. For the amide local anesthetics, the pKa values (7.7–8.1) are sufficiently close to physiologic pH that changes in maternal or fetal biochemical status may significantly alter the proportion of ionized and nonionized drug present (Fig. 42-1). At equilibrium, the concentrations of nonionized drug in the fetal and maternal plasma are equal. In the case of the acidotic fetus, a greater tendency for drug to exist in the ionized form, which cannot diffuse back across the placenta into the maternal plasma, causes a larger total amount of drug to accumulate in the fetal plasma and tissues. This is the mechanism for the phenomenon termed *ion trapping*.[21]

The effects of maternal plasma protein binding on the rate and amount of drug transferred to the fetus are not so well understood. Animal studies have shown that the transfer rate is slower for drugs that are extensively bound to maternal plasma proteins, such as bupivacaine.[22] In sheep, the low fetomaternal ratio of bupivacaine plasma concentrations has been attributed to the difference between fetal and maternal plasma protein binding, rather than to extensive fetal tissue uptake.[23] However, if enough time is allowed for fetomaternal equilibrium to be approached, substantial accumulation of highly protein-bound drugs, such as bupivacaine, can occur in the fetus.[24]

As already stated, the driving force for placental drug transfer is the concentration gradient of free drug between the maternal and fetal blood. On the maternal side, the following factors interact: the dose administered, the mode and site of administration, and, in the case of local anesthetics, the use of vasoconstrictors. The rates of distribution, metabolism, and excretion of the drug, which may vary at different stages of pregnancy, are equally important. In general, higher doses result in higher maternal blood concentrations. The absorption rate varies with the site of drug injection. Compared with other forms of administration, an iv bolus results in the highest blood concentrations. It was believed that intrathecal administration of local anesthetics resulted in negligible plasma concentrations because of the small doses used and the relatively poor vascularity of this area. However, spinal anesthesia induced with lidocaine 75 mg has resulted in maternal plasma concentrations of drug that were similar to those reported by others after epidural anesthesia.[25] Furthermore, significant levels of the drug were found in the umbilical vein at birth.

Increased maternal blood concentrations after repeated administration of a drug greatly depend on the dose and frequency of reinjection, in addition to the kinetic characteristics of the drug. The elimination half-life of amide local anesthetic agents is relatively long, so that repeated injection may lead to accumulation in the maternal plasma[26] (Fig. 42-2). In contrast, 2-chloroprocaine, an ester local anesthetic, undergoes rapid enzymatic hydrolysis in the presence of pseudocholinesterase. After epidural injection, the mean half-life in the mother was shown to be approximately 3 minutes; after reinjection, 2-chloroprocaine could be detected in the maternal plasma for only 5–10 minutes, and no accumulation of this drug was evident[27] (Fig. 42-3).

Pregnancy is associated with physiologic changes that may influence maternal pharmacokinetics and the action of anesthetic drugs. These changes may be progressive during the course of gestation and are often difficult to predict. Kinetic studies after thiopental injection for induction of anesthesia showed a longer elimination half-life and a larger volume of distribution than were noted in a group of nonpregnant women.[28] In contrast, the elimination half-life of bupivacaine after epidural injection was similar in pregnant and nonpregnant women.[29] Alterations in ventilation and lung volumes have a significant effect on the rate of uptake and excretion of inhalation agents. Of most concern to the anesthesiologist is a 20% reduction in FRC.[8] As a result, the equilibration time between the alveolar and inspired concentrations of inhalation agents is shortened.

Placenta

Maturation of the placenta can affect the rate of drug transfer to the fetus, as the thickness of the trophoblastic epithelium decreases from 25 to 2 mm at term. In pregnant mice, diazepam and its metabolites are transferred more rapidly in late than in early pregnancy.[30]

Uptake and biotransformation of anesthetic drugs by the placenta would decrease the amount transferred to the fetus. However, placental drug uptake is limited, and there is no evidence to suggest that this organ metabolizes any of the agents commonly used in obstetric anesthesia.

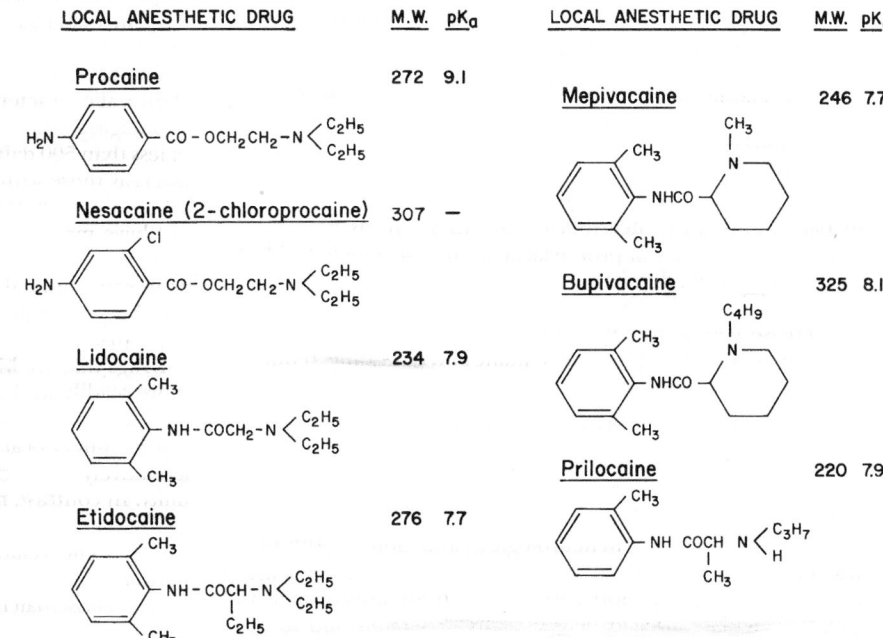

Figure 42-1. Chemical structures, pKa, and molecular weights of commonly used local anesthetics. (Reprinted with permission from Finster M, Pedersen H: Placental transfer and fetal uptake of local anesthetics. Clin Obstet Gynecol 18:556, 1975.)

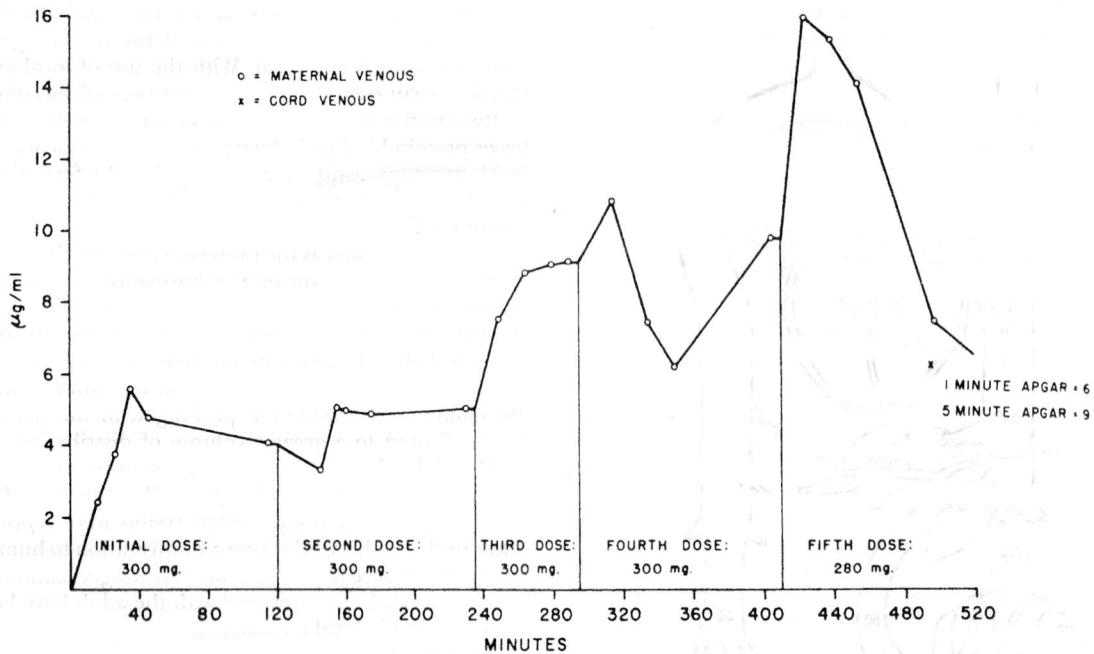

Figure 42-2. Increased levels of mepivacaine with each reinforcing dose in a patient receiving continuous caudal anesthesia during parturition. (Reprinted with permission from Moore DC, Bridenbaugh LD, Bagdi PA *et al:* Accumulation of mepivacaine hydrochloride during caudal block. Anesthesiology 29:585, 1968.)

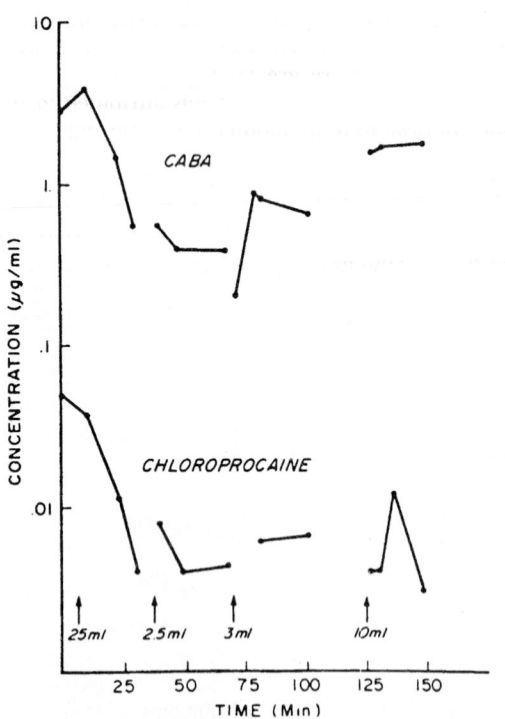

Figure 42-3. Plasma concentrations of chloroprocaine and chloroaminobenzoic acid (CABA) in a typical patient after epidural anesthesia (multiple injections) for vaginal delivery. (Reprinted with permission from Kuhnert BR, Kuhnert PM, Prochaska AL *et al:* Plasma levels of 2-chloroprocaine in obstetric patients and their neonates after epidural anesthesia. Anesthesiology 53:21, 1980.)

Hemodynamic Factors

Any factor decreasing placental blood flow, such as aortocaval compression, hypotension resulting from sympathetic blockade, or hemorrhage, can decrease drug delivery to the fetus. During labor, uterine contractions intermittently reduce perfusion of the placenta. If a uterine contraction coincides with a rapid decline in plasma drug concentration after an iv bolus injection, by the time perfusion has returned to normal, the concentration gradient across the placenta has been greatly reduced. When women were given an iv injection of diazepam, administered at the onset of contraction in one group and during uterine diastole in the other, less drug was found in infants born to mothers in the former group.[31]

Several characteristics of the fetal circulation delay equilibration between the umbilical arterial and venous blood, and thus delay the depressant effects of anesthetic drugs (Fig. 42-4). The liver is the first fetal organ perfused by umbilical vein blood, which carries drug to the fetus. Substantial uptake by this organ has been demonstrated for a variety of drugs, including thiopental, lidocaine, and halothane. During its transit to the arterial side of the fetal circulation, the drug is progressively diluted as blood in the umbilical vein becomes admixed with fetal venous blood from the gastrointestinal tract, the lower extremities, the head and upper extremities, and, finally, the lungs. Because of this unique pattern of fetal circulation, continuous administration of anesthetic concentrations of nitrous oxide or cyclopropane during elective cesarean sections caused newborn depression only if the induction-to-delivery interval exceeded 5–10 minutes. Because of the rapid decline in maternal plasma drug concentrations, administration of thiopental or thiamylal as a single bolus injection not exceeding 4 mg · kg⁻¹ was followed by fetal arterial concentrations of barbiturate below a level that would result in neonatal depression[32] (Fig. 42-5).

Fetal regional blood flow changes can also affect the amount of drug taken up by individual organs. For example, during asphyxia and acidosis, a greater proportion of the fetal cardiac output perfuses the fetal brain, heart, and placenta. Infusion

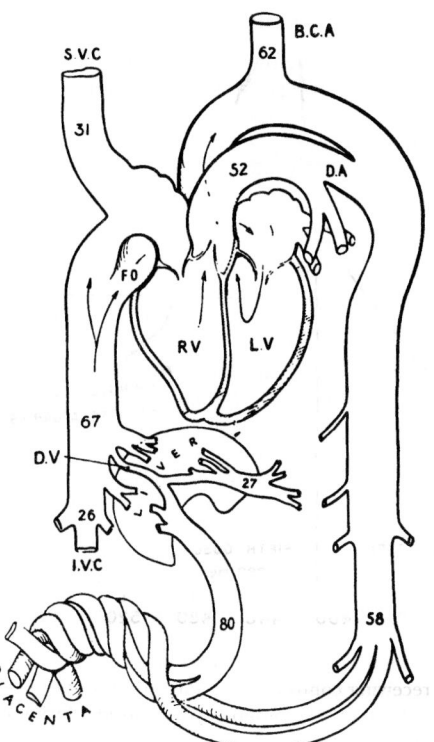

Figure 42-4. Diagram of the circulation in the mature fetal lamb. The numerals indicate the mean oxygen saturation (%) in the great vessels of six lambs: right ventricle (RV); left ventricle (LV); superior vena cava (SVC); inferior vena cava (IVC); brachiocephalic artery (BCA); foramen ovale (FO); ductus arteriosus (DA); ductus venosus (DV). (Reprinted with permission from Born GVR, Dawes GS, Mott JC *et al:* Changes in the heart and lungs at birth. Cold Spring Harbor Symp Quant Biol 19:103, 1954.)

of lidocaine resulted in increased drug uptake in the heart, brain, and liver of asphyxiated baboon fetuses compared with nonasphyxiated control fetuses.[33]

Fetus and Newborn

Any drug that reaches the fetus undergoes metabolism and excretion. In this respect, the fetus has an advantage over the newborn in that it can excrete the drug back to the mother once the concentration gradient of the free drug across the placenta has been reversed. With the use of local anesthetics, this may occur even though the total plasma drug concentration in the mother may exceed that in the fetus, because there is lower protein binding in fetal plasma.[23] There is only one drug, 2-chloroprocaine, that is metabolized in the fetal blood so rapidly that even in acidosis, substantial accumulation in the fetus is avoided.[27]

In the term as well as the preterm newborn, the liver contains enzymes essential for the biotransformation of amide local anesthetics. A study comparing the pharmacokinetics of lidocaine among adult ewes and lambs (fetal and neonatal) showed that the metabolic clearance in the newborn was similar to, and renal clearance greater than, that in the adult.[34] Nonetheless, the elimination half-life was prolonged in the newborn. This was attributed to a greater volume of distribution and tissue uptake of the drug, so that at any given time the neonate's liver and kidneys were exposed to a smaller fraction of lidocaine accumulated in the body. Similar results were reported in another study involving lidocaine administration to human infants in a neonatal intensive care unit.[35] Prolonged elimination half-lives in the newborn compared with the adult have been noted for other amide local anesthetics.

The question remains whether the fetus and newborn are more sensitive than adults to the depressant and toxic effects of drugs. Laboratory investigations have shown that the newborn is, in fact, more sensitive to the depressant effects of opioids. With local anesthetics, neonatal depression occurred at blood concentrations of mepivacaine or lidocaine that were approximately 50% less than those producing toxic manifestations in the adult. However, infants accidentally injected *in utero* with mepivacaine, intended for maternal caudal anesthesia, stopped convulsing when the drug concentration decreased below the threshold level for convulsions in the adult.[36] The relative central nervous and cardiorespiratory toxicity of several local anesthetics has been studied in adult ewes and lambs (fetal and neonatal).[37] The doses required to produce toxicity in the fetus and newborn were greater than those required in the adult. In the fetus, this difference was attributed to placental clearance of drug into the mother and better maintenance of blood gas tensions during convulsions, whereas in the newborn, a larger volume of distribution is probably responsible for the higher doses needed to induce toxic effects.

Bupivacaine has been implicated as a possible cause of neonatal jaundice because its high affinity for fetal erythrocyte mem-

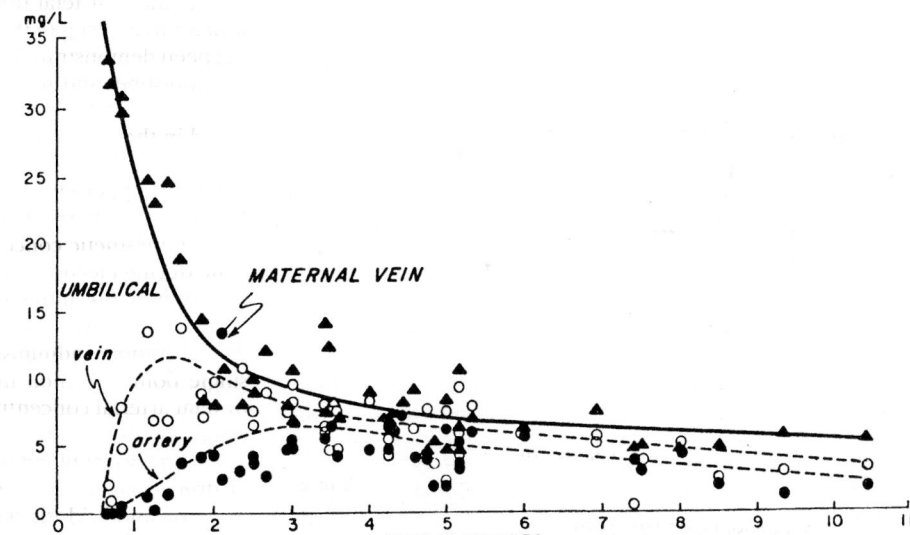

Figure 42-5. Cesarean section. Thiamylal concentrations in maternal vein (▲—▲), umbilical vein (○—○) and umbilical artery (●—●). Curves drawn by inspection. (Reprinted with permission from Kosaka Y, Takahashi T, Mark LS: Intravenous thiobarbiturate anesthesia for cesarean section. Anesthesiology 31:489, 1969.)

branes may lead to a decrease in filterability and deformability, rendering them more prone to hemolysis. However, a more recent study has failed to show increased bilirubin production in newborns whose mothers received bupivacaine for epidural anesthesia during labor and delivery.[38] Finally, neurobehavioral studies have revealed subtle changes in newborn neurologic and adaptive function. In the case of most anesthetic agents, these changes are minor and transient, lasting for only 24–48 hours.[39]

ANESTHESIA FOR LABOR AND VAGINAL DELIVERY

Most women experience moderate to severe pain during parturition. In the first stage of labor, pain is caused by uterine contractions, associated with dilation of the cervix and stretching of the lower uterine segment. Pain impulses are carried in visceral afferent type C fibers accompanying the sympathetic nerves. In early labor, only the lower thoracic dermatomes (T11–12) are affected, but with progressing cervical dilation in the transition phase, adjacent dermatomes may be involved and pain referred from T10 to L1. In the second stage, additional pain impulses due to distention of the vaginal vault and perineum are carried by the pudendal nerves, composed of lower sacral fibers (S2–4).

Well conducted obstetric analgesia, in addition to relieving pain and anxiety, may benefit the mother. For instance, in animal studies, pain has been shown to result in maternal hypertension and reduced uterine blood flow.[40] During the first and second stages of labor, epidural analgesia blunts the increases in maternal cardiac output, heart rate, and blood pressure that occur with painful uterine contractions and "bearing-down" efforts.[41] In reducing maternal secretion of catecholamines, epidural analgesia may convert a previously dysfunctional labor pattern to normal.[42] Maternal analgesia may also benefit the fetus by eliminating maternal hyperventilation, which often leads to a reduced fetal arterial oxygen tension because of a leftward shift of the maternal oxygen–hemoglobin dissociation curve.[43]

The most frequently chosen methods for relieving the pain of parturition are psychoprophylaxis, systemic medication, and regional analgesia. Inhalational analgesia, conventional spinal analgesia, and paracervical blockade are less commonly used. General anesthesia is rarely necessary but may be indicated for uterine relaxation in some complicated deliveries.

Psychoprophylaxis

The philosophy of prepared childbirth maintains that lack of knowledge, misinformation, fear, and anxiety can heighten a patient's response to pain and consequently increase the need for analgesics. Although there is no question that an informed patient is better equipped for the stresses of parturition, few women are able to withstand labor without some pharmacologic analgesia.[44] The most popular method of prepared childbirth is that introduced by Lamaze. It provides an educational program on the physiology of parturition and attempts to diminish cortical pain perception by encouraging responses such as specific patterns of breathing and focused attention on a fixed object.[45] However, labors do vary in length and intensity; thus, it is realistic to encourage the mother in the Lamaze method while recognizing individual variations in pain tolerance and need for pain relief. Of course, medication should not be withheld if required. Neonatal outcome appears to be similar for women who deliver infants solely with the Lamaze technique and for women who receive appropriate supplementary analgesia.

Systemic Medication

The advantages of systemic analgesics include ease of administration and patient acceptability. However, the drug, dose, time, and method of administration must be chosen carefully to avoid maternal or neonatal depression. Drugs used for systemic analgesia are opioids, tranquilizers, and occasionally ketamine.

Opioids

Meperidine is the most commonly used systemic analgesic and is reasonably effective in ameliorating pain during the first stage of labor. It can be administered by iv injection (effective analgesia in 5–10 minutes) or intramuscularly im (im; peak effect in 40–50 minutes). The major side effects are a high incidence of nausea and vomiting, dose-related depression of ventilation, orthostatic hypotension, and the potential for neonatal depression. Meperidine may cause transient alterations of the fetal heart rate, such as decreased beat-to-beat variability and tachycardia. Among other factors, the risk of neonatal depression is related to the interval from the last drug injection to delivery.[46] The placental transfer of an active metabolite, normeperidine, which has a long elimination half-life in the neonate (62 hours), has also been implicated in contributing to neonatal depression and subtle neonatal neurobehavioral dysfunction.[46]

Experience with the newer synthetic opioids, such as fentanyl and alfentanil, has been limited. Although they are potent, their use during labor is restricted by their short duration of action. For example, a single iv injection of fentanyl, up to $1 \ \mu g \cdot kg^{-1}$, results in prompt pain relief without severe neonatal depression.[47] These drugs offer an advantage when analgesia of rapid onset but short duration is necessary (e.g., with forceps application). For more prolonged analgesia, fentanyl can be administered with patient-controlled delivery devices.[48] Remifentanil is a new opioid that is rapidly metabolized by serum and tissue cholinesterases, and consequently, has a short (3-minute), context-sensitive half-time.[49] In one study, Apgar and neurobehavioral scores were good in neonates whose mothers were given an intravenous infusion of remifentanil, $0.1 \ \mu g \cdot kg^{-1} \cdot min^{-1}$, during cesarean delivery under epidural anesthesia.[50] Unfortunately, there are no studies of the use of remifentanil for labor analgesia. Opioid agonists–antagonists, such as butorphanol and nalbuphine, have also been used for obstetric analgesia. These drugs have the proposed benefits of a lower incidence of nausea, vomiting, and dysphoria, as well as a "ceiling effect" on depression of ventilation. However, studies for the most part have not demonstrated a clear advantage over meperidine during parturition.[51] Butorphanol is probably most popular; unlike meperidine, it is biotransformed into inactive metabolites and has a ceiling effect on depression of ventilation in doses exceeding 2 mg. A potential disadvantage is a high incidence of maternal sedation. The recommended dose is 1–2 mg by iv or im injection. Nalbuphine, 10 mg iv or im, is an alternative to butorphanol.

Naloxone, a pure opioid antagonist, should not be administered to the mother shortly before delivery to prevent neonatal ventilatory depression because it reverses maternal analgesia at a time when it is most needed and, in some instances, has caused maternal pulmonary edema and even cardiac arrest. If necessary, the drug should be given directly to the newborn im $(0.1 \ mg \cdot kg^{-1})$.

Ketamine

Ketamine is a potent analgesic. However, it may also induce unacceptable amnesia that may interfere with the mother's recollection of the birth. Nonetheless, ketamine is a useful adjunct to incomplete regional analgesia during vaginal delivery or for obstetric manipulations. In low doses $(0.2–0.4 \ mg \cdot kg^{-1})$, ketamine provides adequate analgesia without causing neonatal depression.

Regional Analgesia

Regional techniques provide excellent analgesia with minimal depressant effects in mother and fetus. The regional techniques most commonly used in obstetric anesthesia include central neuraxial blocks (spinal, epidural, and combined spinal–epidural), paracervical and pudendal blocks, and, less frequently, lumbar sympathetic blocks (LSB). Hypotension resulting from sympathectomy is the most frequent complication that occurs with central neuraxial blockade. Therefore, maternal blood pressure must be monitored at regular intervals, typically every 2–5 minutes for approximately 15–20 minutes after the initiation of the block and at routine intervals thereafter. The use of regional analgesia may be contraindicated in the presence of severe coagulopathy, acute hypovolemia, or infection at the site of needle insertion. Chorioamnionitis itself, without frank sepsis, is not a contraindication to central neuraxial blockade in obstetrics.

Epidural Analgesia

Epidural analgesia may be used for pain relief during labor, vaginal delivery, and for anesthesia during cesarean delivery, if required. Effective analgesia during the first stage of labor may be achieved by blocking the T10–L1 dermatomes with low concentrations of local anesthetic. For the second stage of labor and delivery, because of pain due to vaginal distention and perineal pressure, the block should be extended to include the S2–4 segments.

Because of ethical considerations and methodologic difficulties, it is difficult to design clinical studies to examine the effects of epidural analgesia on the progress of labor and mode of delivery. In general, the first stage of labor is not prolonged by epidural analgesia, provided aortocaval compression is avoided.[52–56] There has been concern that early initiation of epidural analgesia during the latent phase of labor (2–4 cm cervical dilation) in nulliparous women may result in a higher incidence of dystocia and cesarean delivery.[54–57] However, this has largely been dispelled by several large, randomized, prospective studies. Chestnut et al[52,53] demonstrated that there was no significant difference in the incidence of cesarean delivery between nulliparous women having epidural analgesia initiated during the latent phase (<4 cm dilation) compared with control group whose analgesia was initiated during the active phase. Similarly, other investigators have demonstrated that epidural analgesia was not associated with an increased incidence of cesarean delivery compared with patient-controlled iv analgesia in nulliparous women.[55,56] However, a prolongation of the second stage of labor has been reported in nulliparous women, possibly owing to a decrease in expulsive forces or malposition of the vertex.[52–57] Thus, with use of epidural analgesia, the American College of Obstetricians and Gynecologists have redefined an abnormally prolonged second stage of labor as greater than 3 hours in nulliparous and 2 hours in multiparous women.[58] Prolongation of the second stage may be minimized by the use of an ultradilute local anesthetic solution in combination with opioid.[59] Long-acting amides such as bupivacaine, ropivacaine, or levobupivacaine are most frequently used because they produce excellent sensory analgesia while sparing motor function, particularly at the low concentrations used for epidural analgesia. Analgesia for the first stage of labor may be achieved with 5–10 ml of bupivacaine, ropivacaine, or levobupivacaine (0.125–0.25%), followed by a continuous infusion (8–12 ml · h^{-1}) of 0.0625% bupivacaine or levobupivacaine, or 0.1% ropivacaine. Addition of fentanyl 1–2 μg · ml^{-1} or sufentanil 0.3–0.5 μg · ml^{-1} is often required. During the delivery, the sacral dermatomes may be blocked with 10 ml of 0.5% bupivacaine, 1% lidocaine, or, if a rapid effect is required, 2% chloroprocaine, in the semirecumbent position.

There is controversy regarding the need for a test dose when using an ultradilute solution of local anesthetic.[60,61] Because catheter aspiration is not always diagnostic, some authors believe that a test dose should be administered to improve detection of an intrathecally or intravascularly placed catheter (see Lumbar Epidural Anesthesia for cesarean section).

Patient-controlled epidural analgesia (PCEA) is a safe and effective alternative to conventional bolus or infusion techniques.[62] Maternal satisfaction is excellent and demands on anesthesia manpower reduced. Analgesia is initially achieved with bolus doses of local anesthetic. Once the mother is comfortable, PCEA may then be started with a maintenance infusion (4–8 ml · h^{-1}) of local anesthetic (bupivacaine, levobupivacaine, ropivacaine, 0.0625–0.125%), with or without opioid (fentanyl 1–2 μg · ml^{-1}, sufentanil 0.3–0.5 μg · ml^{-1}). The patient-controlled analgesia pump may be programmed to deliver an epidural bolus of 4 ml with a lockout period of 10 minutes between doses.[62]

The caudal approach may result in a faster onset of perineal analgesia and therefore, when an imminent vaginal delivery is anticipated, may be preferable to the lumbar epidural approach. However, caudal analgesia is no longer popular because of occasionally painful needle placement, a high failure rate, potential contamination at the injection site, and risks of accidental fetal injection. Before caudal injection, a digital rectal examination must be performed to exclude needle placement in the fetal presenting part.[36] Low spinal "saddle block" has virtually eliminated the need for caudal anesthesia in modern practice.

Spinal Analgesia

A single subarachnoid injection for labor analgesia has the advantages of a reliable and rapid onset of neural blockade. However, repeated intrathecal injections may be required for a long labor, thus increasing the risk of postdural puncture headache (PDPH). In addition, the motor block may be uncomfortable for some parturients and may prolong the second stage of labor. Spinal anesthesia is a safe and effective alternative to general anesthesia for instrumental delivery.

Microcatheters were introduced for continuous spinal anesthesia in the 1980s. They were subsequently withdrawn when found to be associated with neurologic deficits, possibly related to maldistribution of local anesthetic in the cauda equina region.[63] Fortunately, in a recent multi-institutional study, there were no cases of neurologic complaints after the use of 28-gauge microcatheters for continuous spinal analgesia in laboring women.[64]

Combined Spinal–Epidural Analgesia

Combined spinal–epidural analgesia (CSE) is an ideal analgesic technique for use during labor. CSE combines the rapid, reliable onset of profound analgesia resulting from spinal injection with the flexibility and longer duration of epidural techniques. After identification of the epidural space using a conventional (or specialized) needle, a longer (127-mm), pencil-point spinal needle is advanced into the subarachnoid space through the epidural needle. After intrathecal injection, the spinal needle is removed and an epidural catheter is inserted. Intrathecal injection of fentanyl 10–25 μg or sufentanil 5–10 μg, alone or more commonly in combination with 1 ml of isobaric bupivacaine 0.25%, produces profound analgesia lasting for 90–120 minutes with minimal motor block.[65] Although opioid alone may suffice for the early latent phase, addition of bupivacaine is usually necessary for satisfactory analgesia during advanced labor. An epidural infusion of bupivacaine 0.03–0.0625% with added opioid may be started within 10 minutes of spinal injection. Alternatively, the epidural component may be activated when necessary. Women with hemodynamic stability and preserved motor function who do not require continuous fetal monitoring may ambulate with assistance.[66,67] Before ambulation, women should be observed for 30 minutes after intrathecal or epidural drug administration to assess maternal and fetal well-being.

The most common side effects of intrathecal opioids are pruritus, nausea, vomiting, and urinary retention. Rostral spread resulting in delayed respiratory depression is rare with fentanyl and sufentanil, and usually occurs within 30 minutes of injection.[68] Transient nonreassuring fetal heart rate patterns may occur because of uterine hyperstimulation, presumably as a result of a rapid decrease in maternal catecholamines, or because of hypotension after sympatholysis.[69] A preliminary study by O'Gorman et al[70] suggests that fetal bradycardia may occur in the absence of uterine hyperstimulation or hypotension and is unrelated to uteroplacental insufficiency. The incidence of fetal heart rate abnormalities may be greater in multiparous women with rapidly progressing, painful labors.[71] Most studies have demonstrated that the incidence of emergency cesarean delivery is no greater after CSE than after conventional epidural analgesia.[72,73]

Postdural puncture headache is always a risk after intrathecal injection. However, it has been demonstrated that the incidence of cephalalgia is no greater with CSE compared with standard epidural analgesia.[74]

Unintentional intrathecal catheter placement through the dural puncture site is also extremely rare after use of a 26-gauge spinal needle for CSE.[74] The potential exists for epidurally administered drug to leak into the subarachnoid space after dural puncture, particularly if large volumes of drug are rapidly injected. Indeed, epidural drug requirements are approximately 30% less with CSE than with standard lumbar epidural techniques.[75]

Paracervical Block

Although paracervical block effectively relieves pain during the first stage of labor, the technique has fallen out of favor because it was associated with a high incidence of fetal asphyxia and poor neonatal outcome, particularly with the use of bupivacaine. This may be related to uterine artery constriction or increased uterine tone.[76] The technique is basically simple and involves a submucosal injection of local anesthetic at the vaginal fornix, near the neural fibers innervating the uterus.

Paravertebral Lumbar Sympathetic Block

Paravertebral LSB is a reasonable alternative when contraindications exist to central neuraxial techniques. LSB interrupts the painful transmission of cervical and uterine impulses during the first stage of labor.[77] Although there is less risk of fetal bradycardia with LSB compared with paracervical blockade, technical difficulties associated with the performance of the block and risks of intravascular injection have decreased its use in standard practice.

Pudendal Nerve Block

The pudendal nerves, derived from the lower sacral nerve roots (S2–4), supply the vaginal vault, perineum, rectum, and parts of the bladder. The nerves are easily anesthetized transvaginally where they loop around the ischial spines. Ten milliliters of local anesthetic deposited behind each sacrospinous ligament can provide adequate anesthesia for outlet forceps delivery and episiotomy repair.

Inhalation Analgesia

Inhalation analgesia is easily administered and although it does not relieve pain completely, it may make uterine contractions more tolerable. During delivery, a combination of inhalation analgesia with a pudendal block or infiltration of the perineum with a local anesthetic may be satisfactory. A particular advantage of inhalation analgesia is that the desired level of analgesia can be easily and rapidly titrated. However, a major disadvantage of inhalational analgesia is the need for a waste gas scavenging system.

Inhalation anesthetic agents can be self-administered by the patient under supervision. A nitrous oxide inhaler is commercially available for self-administration. The system must be able to deliver a precise concentration of agent over a wide range of inspiratory flow rates. The parturient is instructed to breathe deeply from the inhaler when she detects the onset of uterine contraction, so that analgesia is established at its peak. Nitrous oxide, 50% by volume, is the most commonly used inhalation agent for analgesia during labor. However, the analgesia provided by intermittently self-administered 50% nitrous oxide alone has been shown to be equivalent to that of a placebo.[78]

General Anesthesia

General anesthesia is rarely used for vaginal delivery, and precautions against gastric aspiration must always be observed. It may be required when time constraints prevent induction of regional anesthesia. Potent inhalation drugs (1.5–2.0 MAC for short periods) can provide uterine relaxation for obstetric maneuvers such as second twin delivery, breech presentation, or postpartum manual removal of a retained placenta. In all cases, preoxygenation and rapid iv induction of anesthesia with the use of cricoid pressure and placement of a cuffed endotracheal tube are required. High inspiratory flows ensure quick delivery of the drug. The depth of anesthesia must be monitored to avoid maternal hemodynamic instability. Immediately after the obstetric manipulation is completed, the potent inhalational agent should be discontinued or reduced to prevent uterine atony and hemorrhage. An intravenous infusion of oxytocin 10–20 units should be commenced to promote uterine contraction. The endotracheal tube should not be removed until the woman is awake and airway reflexes have returned. In current practice, intravenous nitroglycerin (50–500 μg) has replaced the need for general anesthesia for uterine relaxation.[79,80]

ANESTHESIA FOR CESAREAN SECTION

Despite efforts to promote vaginal birth after previous cesarean delivery, the frequency of cesarean section has remained elevated. The most common indications include failure to progress, nonreassuring fetal status, cephalopelvic disproportion, malpresentation, prematurity, and prior uterine surgery involving the corpus. The choice of anesthesia should depend on the urgency of the procedure, in addition to the condition of the mother and fetus. After a comprehensive discussion of the risks and benefits of all anesthesia options, the mother's wishes should be considered.

Regional Anesthesia

A 1992 survey of obstetric anesthesia practices in the United States revealed that most patients undergoing cesarean section do so under spinal or epidural anesthesia.[81] Regional techniques have several advantages: they lessen the risk of gastric aspiration, avoid the use of depressant anesthetic drugs, and allow the mother to remain awake during delivery. It has also been suggested that operative blood loss is less with regional than with general anesthesia. In elective cesarean sections, the duration of antepartum anesthesia does not affect neonatal outcome provided that there is no protracted aortocaval compression or hypotension.[82] The risk of hypotension is greater than during vaginal delivery because the block must extend to at least the T4 dermatome. In this regard, epidural anesthesia is advantageous because of its slower onset and controllability. Proper positioning and prehydration with at least 10–20 ml·kg^{-1} of a crystalloid solution is recommended.[83] If hypotension occurs despite these measures, left uterine displacement should be increased, the rate of iv infusion augmented, and iv ephedrine 10–15 mg administered incrementally.

Spinal Anesthesia

Subarachnoid block is probably the most commonly administered regional anesthetic for cesarean delivery because of its speed of onset and reliability. It has become an alternative to general anesthesia for emergency cesarean section.[84] Hyperbaric solutions of lidocaine 5%, tetracaine 1.0%, or bupivacaine 0.75% are available for spinal use. The dosages and duration of action of these local anesthetics are listed in Table 42-2. Using 0.75% hyperbaric bupivacaine, Norris[85] has shown that it is not necessary to adjust the dose of drug based on the patient's height. Hemodynamic monitoring during cesarean section should be similar to that used for other surgical procedures. Before delivery, oxygen should be routinely administered to optimize fetal oxygenation.

Despite an adequate dermatomal level for surgery, women may experience varying degrees of visceral discomfort, particularly during exteriorization of the uterus and traction on abdominal viscera. Improved perioperative analgesia can be provided by the addition of fentanyl 6.25 μg or 0.1 mg of preservative-free morphine to the local anesthetic solution.[86] Nausea and vomiting may be alleviated by the administration of droperidol or metoclopramide. Maternal sedation should be avoided if possible.

Lumbar Epidural Anesthesia

In contrast to spinal anesthesia, epidural anesthesia is associated with a slower onset of action and a larger drug requirement to establish an adequate sensory block. The advantages are a reduced risk of PDPH and the ability to titrate the local anesthetic through the epidural catheter. To avoid inadvertent intrathecal or intravascular injection, correct placement of the epidural catheter is essential. This is especially a concern when administering the large doses of local anesthetic required for cesarean delivery.

Aspiration of the epidural catheter for blood or cerebrospinal fluid is not reliable for detection of catheter misplacement. Thus, administration of a test dose has become popular. A small dose of local anesthetic, lidocaine 45 mg or bupivacaine 5 mg, produces a readily identifiable sensory and motor block if injected intrathecally. Addition of epinephrine (15 μg) with careful hemodynamic monitoring may signal intravascular injection when followed by a transient increase in heart rate and blood pressure. However, the use of an epinephrine test dose is controversial because false-positive results do occur in the presence of uterine contractions. In addition, epinephrine may reduce uteroplacental perfusion. Electrocardiography and application of a peak-to-peak heart rate criterion may improve detection.[87] Use of isoproterenol may be preferable to epinephrine because in the event of intravascular injection, tachycardia is reliably achieved without affecting uteroplacental blood flow,[88] but, before its use in clinical practice, safety and efficacy studies must be performed. Rapid injection of 1 ml of air with simultaneous precordial Doppler monitoring appears to be a reliable indicator of intravascular catheter placement.[89] A negative test, although reassuring, does not eliminate the need for fractional administration of local anesthetic.

The most commonly used agents are 2-chloroprocaine 3%, bupivacaine 0.5%, and lidocaine 2% with epinephrine 1:200,000. Adequate anesthesia is usually achieved with 15–25 ml of the solution, given in divided doses. The patient should be monitored as with spinal anesthesia. Because of its extremely high rate of metabolism in maternal and fetal plasma, 2-chloroprocaine provides a rapid-onset, reliable block with minimal risk of systemic toxicity.[26] It is the local anesthetic of choice in the presence of fetal acidosis and when a pre-existing epidural block is to be rapidly extended for an urgent cesarean section.[84] Transient neurologic deficits after massive inadvertent intrathecal administration of the drug have occurred with the formulation containing a relatively high concentration of sodium bisulfite, at a low pH.[90] In a new formulation of 2-chloroprocaine (Nesacaine-MPF), ethylene diaminetetra-acetic acid (EDTA) has been substituted for sodium bisulfite and, to date, no new cases of neurologic deficit have been reported. However, severe spasmodic back pain has been described after epidural injection of large volumes of Nesacaine-MPF in surgical patients, but not in parturients.[91] This complication has been attributed to EDTA-induced leaching of calcium from paravertebral muscles. The most recent formulation of 2-chloroprocaine contains no additives and is packaged in an amber vial to prevent oxidation. Bupivacaine 0.5% provides profound anesthesia for cesarean section of slower onset but longer duration of action. Considerable attention has been focused on the drug since it was reported that unintentional intravascular injection could result not only in convulsions but in almost simultaneous cardiac arrest, with patients often refractory to resuscitation.[92] The greater cardiotoxicity of bupivacaine (and etidocaine) compared with other amide local anesthetics has been well established.[93] Lidocaine has an onset and duration intermediate to those of 2-chloroprocaine and bupivacaine. The need to include epinephrine in the local anesthetic solution to ensure adequate lumbosacral anesthesia limits the use of lidocaine in the setting of maternal hypertension and uteroplacental insufficiency.

Prolonged postoperative pain relief can be provided by epidural administration of an opioid, such as morphine 4 mg. PCEA is another option. Delayed respiratory depression may occur, particularly with the use of morphine, and hence the

Table 42-2. LOCAL ANESTHETICS COMMONLY USED FOR CESAREAN SECTION WITH SUBARACHNOID BLOCK

	Lidocaine 5% in 7.5% Dextrose	Tetracaine 1% in Equal Volume of 10% Dextrose	Bupivacaine 0.75% in 8.25% Dextrose
Dosage (mg) according to height (cm)			
150–160	65	8	8
160–182	70	9	10
182 and taller	75	10	12
Onset of action (min)	1–3	3–5	2–4
Duration of action (min)	45–75	120–180	120–180

patient must be monitored carefully in the postoperative period.

General Anesthesia

General anesthesia may be necessary when contraindications exist to regional anesthesia or when time precludes central neuraxial blockade. General anesthesia with a potent halogenated agent may also be useful in situations where uterine relaxation will facilitate delivery, as with breech presentation, transverse lie, or in women with multiple gestation, who often do not tolerate regional blocks owing to dyspnea and supine hypotension syndrome. General anesthesia should be used cautiously in women with asthma, upper respiratory tract infection, obesity, or a history of difficult tracheal intubation. Preoperative airway evaluation is particularly important in pregnant women because inability to intubate the trachea and provide effective ventilation is the leading cause of maternal death related to anesthesia.[81] If airway difficulties are anticipated, a regional anesthetic technique should be considered, or an awake tracheal intubation performed. Premedication is usually not necessary, except for administration of 15–30 ml of a nonparticulate antacid within 30 minutes of induction of anesthesia. The patient should be positioned with a wedge in place to prevent aortocaval compression. Routine monitoring should be the same as with regional anesthetic techniques, and comply with national standards.

To minimize the risk of hypoxemia during induction, denitrogenation for 3–5 minutes with a tight-fitting mask is essential. In an emergency, four deep breaths with 100% oxygen suffices. A "defasciculating" dose of a nondepolarizing muscle relaxant is not necessary. Rapid-sequence induction is performed with thiopental (4 mg·kg^{-1}), ketamine (up to 1 mg·kg^{-1}), or a combination of thiopental (2–3 mg·kg^{-1}) and ketamine (0.5 mg·kg^{-1}), followed by succinylcholine (1–1.5 mg·kg^{-1}) to facilitate intubation. Cricoid pressure is applied by a trained assistant until the airway is properly secured with a cuffed endotracheal tube. If there is difficulty in securing the airway, cricoid pressure should be maintained throughout and the mother ventilated with 100% oxygen before a subsequent attempt at tracheal intubation is made. It is safer to permit the mother to awaken and to reassess the method of induction than to persist with traumatic efforts at tracheal intubation, which may result in loss of the airway because of edema and bleeding (Fig. 42-6). Once placement of the endotracheal tube is confirmed, with capnography and auscultation, the obstetrician may proceed with incision. In the predelivery interval, anesthesia is maintained with a 50:50 mixture of nitrous oxide in oxygen and 0.5 MAC of a potent agent. Severe maternal hyperventilation should be avoided because it may reduce uterine blood flow. A few minutes before delivery is anticipated, the concentration of the potent agent may be increased temporarily to 2 MAC, when uterine relaxation is desired to facilitate delivery.

The newborn's condition after cesarean section with general anesthesia is comparable with that seen with regional techniques.[94] The uterine incision-to-delivery interval seems to be more important to neonatal outcome than the induction of anesthesia-to-delivery interval. Lower Apgar scores at 1 minute and acidosis were reported in cases in which the uterine incision-to-delivery time interval exceeded 180 seconds, whereas anesthesia for up to 30 minutes before delivery appears to have no adverse effects on the infant.[95] In contrast, with use of nitrous oxide 70–75% in oxygen, neonatal depression has been reported to occur within approximately 10 minutes of anesthesia. Increasing the Fio$_2$ to 50% has the additional benefit of increasing the fetal Pao$_2$.[96]

After delivery of the infant, 20 units of oxytocin should be added to the infusion and anesthesia is deepened with an opioid or benzodiazepine, as necessary. At the end of the procedure, the mother's trachea is extubated once she is awake and extubation criteria have been met. The usual blood loss at a cesarean section is 750–1000 ml, and transfusion is rarely necessary.

ANESTHETIC COMPLICATIONS
Maternal Mortality

A study of anesthesia-related deaths in the United States between 1979 and 1990 revealed that the case fatality rate with general anesthesia was 16.7 times greater than that with regional anesthesia. Most anesthesia-related deaths were a result of cardiac arrest due to hypoxemia when difficulties securing the airway were encountered.[81] Pregnancy-induced anatomic and physiologic changes, such as reduced FRC, increased oxygen consumption, and oropharyngeal edema, may expose the patient to serious risks of desaturation during periods of apnea and hypoventilation (see Physiologic Changes of Pregnancy).

Pulmonary Aspiration

The risk of inhalation of gastric contents is increased in pregnant women, as discussed previously, particularly if difficulty is encountered establishing the airway. Measures to decrease the risks of aspiration include comprehensive airway evaluation, prophylactic administration of nonparticulate antacids, and preferred use of regional anesthesia. Occasionally, general anesthesia may be unavoidable in obstetric anesthesia practice, and therefore awake intubation may be indicated in women in whom airway difficulties are anticipated.

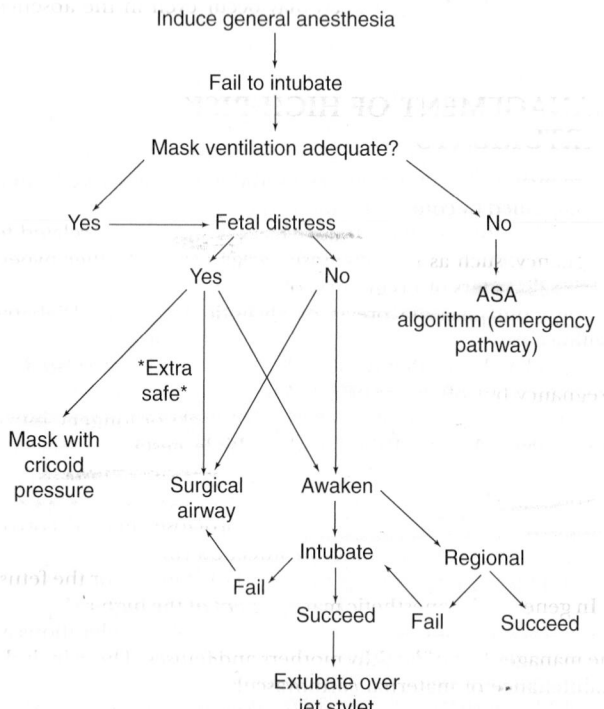

Figure 42-6. Management of the difficult airway in pregnancy with special reference to the presence or absence of fetal distress. When mask ventilation is not possible, the clinician is referred to the American Society of Anesthesiologists (ASA) algorithm for the emergency airway management found in Chapter 23. (Adapted with permission from Reisner LS, Benumof JL, Cooper SD. The difficult airway: Risk, prophylaxis, and management. p 607. In Chestnut DH (ed): Obstetric Anesthesia: Principles and Practice, p 607. St. Louis, Mosby, 1999.)

Hypotension

Regional anesthesia is commonly associated with hypotension, which is related to the degree and rapidity of local anesthetic-induced sympatholysis. Thus, more hemodynamic stability is usually observed with epidural anesthesia, where careful titration of local anesthetic may be performed.

In addition, the risk of hypotension is lower in women who are in labor compared with nonlaboring women.[97] Maternal prehydration with 10–20 ml · kg^{-1} of lactated Ringer's solution before initiation of regional anesthesia, and avoidance of aortocaval compression after induction, may decrease the incidence of hypotension. It has been demonstrated that for effective prevention of hypotension, the blood volume increase from preloading must be sufficient to result in a significant increase in cardiac output.[98] This was possible only with the administration of hetastarch, 0.5–1 liter.[98] Nonetheless, controversy exists regarding the efficacy of volume loading in the prevention of hypotension.[99,100] If hypotension does occur despite prehydration, therapeutic measures include increased displacement of the uterus, rapid infusion of iv fluids, titration of iv ephedrine (5–10 mg), oxygen administration, and placement of the patient in the Trendelenburg position. In the presence of maternal tachycardia, phenylephrine 25–50 μg may be substituted for ephedrine, in women with normal uteroplacental function. Continued vigilance and active management of hypotension can prevent serious sequelae in both mother or neonate.[97,101]

Total Spinal Anesthesia

High or total spinal anesthesia is a rare complication of intrathecal injection, and occurs after excessive cephalad spread of local anesthetic in the subarachnoid space. Unintentional intrathecal administration of epidural medication as a result of dural puncture or catheter migration may also result in this complication. Left uterine displacement, placement in the Trendelenburg position, and continued fluid and vasopressor administration may be necessary to achieve hemodynamic stability. Rapid control of the airway is essential and endotracheal intubation may be necessary to ensure oxygenation without aspiration.

Local Anesthetic–Induced Seizures

Unintended intravascular injection or drug accumulation after repeated epidural injection can result in high serum levels of local anesthetic. Rapid absorption of local anesthetic from highly vascular sites of injection may also occur after paracervical and pudendal blocks.

Resuscitation equipment should always be available when any major nerve block is undertaken. Intravenous access, airway equipment, emergency drugs, and suction equipment should be immediately accessible. To avoid systemic toxicity of local anesthetic agents, strict adherence to recommended dosages and avoidance of unintentional intravascular injection are essential.

Despite these precautions, life-threatening convulsions and, more rarely, cardiovascular collapse may occur. Seizure activity should be treated with iv thiopental 50–100 mg or diazepam 5–10 mg; larger doses may enhance local anesthetic-induced myocardial depression. The maternal airway should be secured and oxygenation maintained. If cardiovascular collapse does occur, cesarean delivery may be required to relieve aortocaval compression and to ensure the efficiency of cardiac massage.[102]

Postdural Puncture Headache

By virtue of age and sex, pregnant women are at a higher risk for developing PDPH. In addition, after delivery, the reduced epidural pressure increases the risk of cerebrospinal fluid leakage through the dural opening.

The frequency of PDPH development is related to the diameter of the dural puncture, ranging from in excess of 70% after use of 16-gauge needles to less than 1% with the smaller 25- or 26-gauge spinal needles. The incidence of cephalalgia is reduced with the use of atraumatic pencil-point needles (Whitacre or Sprotte), which are thought to separate the dural fibers, compared with the diamond-shaped (Quincke) cutting needles. Conservative treatment is indicated in the presence of mild to moderate discomfort, and includes bed rest, hydration, and simple analgesics. Caffeine (500 mg iv or 300 mg orally) and theophylline have also been used in treatment of PDPH.[103–105] Severe headache that does not respond to conservative measures is best treated with autologous blood patch. Using an aseptic technique, 10–15 ml of the patient's blood is injected into the epidural space close to the site of dural puncture. This procedure may be repeated as necessary and is associated with excellent success rates. If an epidural catheter is in place after delivery, 15–20 ml of autologous blood may be injected through the catheter before removal. This may decrease the risk of a headache developing.[106]

Nerve Injury

Neurologic sequelae of central neuraxial blockade, although rare, have been reported. Pressure exerted by a needle or catheter on spinal nerve roots produces immediate pain and necessitates repositioning. Infections such as epidural abscess or meningitis are very rare and may be a manifestation of systemic sepsis. Epidural hematoma can also occur, usually in association with coagulation defects. Nerve root irritation may have a protracted recovery, lasting weeks or months. Peripheral nerve injury as a result of instrumentation, lithotomy position, or compression by the fetal head may occur even in the absence of neuraxial technique.

MANAGEMENT OF HIGH-RISK PARTURIENTS

Pregnancy and parturition are considered "high risk" when accompanied by conditions unfavorable to the well-being of the mother or fetus, or both. Maternal problems may be related to pregnancy, such as pre-eclampsia–eclampsia and other hypertensive disorders of pregnancy, or antepartum hemorrhage resulting from placenta previa or abruptio placentae. Diabetes mellitus; cardiac, chronic renal, neurologic, or sickle cell disease; and asthma, obesity, and drug abuse are not related to pregnancy but often are affected by it. Prematurity (gestation of less than 37 weeks), postmaturity (42 weeks or longer), intrauterine growth retardation, and multiple gestation are fetal conditions associated with risk. During labor and delivery, fetal malpresentation (breech, transverse lie), placental abruption, compression of the umbilical cord (prolapse, nuchal cord), precipitous labor, or intrauterine infection (prolonged rupture of membranes) may increase the risk to the mother or the fetus.

In general, the anesthetic management of the high-risk parturient is based on the same maternal and fetal considerations as the management of healthy mothers and fetuses. These include maintenance of maternal cardiovascular function and oxygenation, maintenance and possibly improvement of uteroplacental blood flow, and creation of optimal conditions for a painless, atraumatic delivery of an infant without significant drug effects. However, there is less room for error because many of these functions may be compromised before the induction of anesthesia. For example, significant acidosis is prone to develop in fetuses of diabetic mothers when delivered by cesarean section with spinal anesthesia complicated by even brief maternal hypotension.[11] Because the high-risk parturient may have received a variety of drugs, anesthesiologists must be familiar with potential interactions between these drugs and the anesthetic drugs they plan to administer.

Pre-eclampsia–Eclampsia

Hypertensive disorders, which occur in approximately 7% of all late pregnancies, are among the major causes of maternal mortality, accounting for approximately one-fifth of maternal deaths, and have been estimated to result in 30,000 neonatal deaths and stillbirths per year in the United States alone. Pre-eclampsia is diagnosed on the basis of development of hypertension with proteinuria or edema, or both. The added appearance of convulsions makes for the diagnosis of eclampsia. Pre-eclampsia–eclampsia is a disease unique to human pregnancy, occurring predominantly in young nulliparas. Symptoms usually appear after the 20th week of gestation, occasionally earlier than that if in association with a hydatidiform mole. Thus, the condition requires the presence of a trophoblast but not a fetus.

The origin of pre-eclampsia–eclampsia is unknown. One theory invokes immunologic rejection of fetal tissues by the mother, which causes a placental vasculitis and ischemia. This theory explains why the disease is more common among nulliparas (no previous exposure to a trophoblast) and in conditions associated with an abnormally large mass of trophoblastic tissues, as in hydatidiform mole, multiple pregnancy, diabetes, and Rh incompatibility. Various studies have demonstrated an abnormal maternal immune responsiveness in pre-eclampsia. Placental ischemia results in a release of uterine renin and an increase in angiotensin activity (Fig. 42-7). This would lead to a widespread arteriolar vasoconstriction, causing hypertension, tissue hypoxia, and endothelial damage. Adherence of platelets at sites of endothelial damage would result in coagulopathies, occasionally in disseminated intravascular coagulation. Enhanced angiotensin-mediated aldosterone secretion would lead to an increased sodium reabsorption and edema. Proteinuria, another symptom of pre-eclampsia, may also be attributed to placental ischemia, which would lead to local tissue degeneration and a release of thromboplastin with subsequent deposition

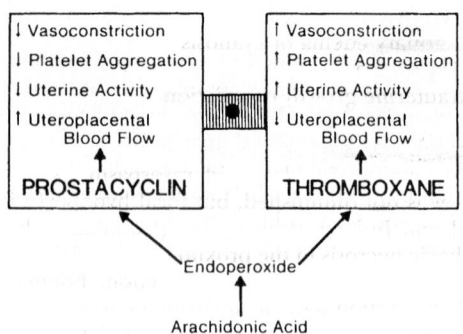

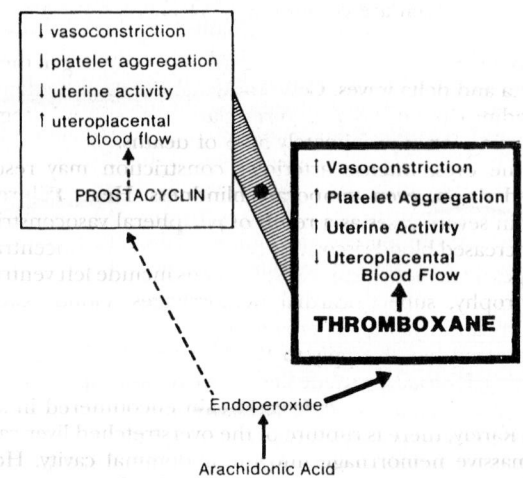

PREECLAMPSIA

Figure 42-8. Comparison of the balance in the biologic actions of prostacyclin and thromboxane in normal pregnancy with the imbalance of increased thromboxane and decreased prostacyclin in pre-eclamptic pregnancy. (Reprinted with permission from Walsh SW: Preeclampsia: An imbalance in placental prostacyclin and thromboxane production. Am J Obstet Gynecol 152:335, 1985.)

of fibrin in constricted glomerular vessels and increased permeability to albumin and other plasma proteins. Furthermore, there is thought to be a decreased production of prostaglandin E, a potent vasodilator secreted in the trophoblast, which normally would balance the hypertensive effects of the renin–angiotensin system.

Many of the symptoms associated with pre-eclampsia, including placental ischemia, systemic vasoconstriction, and increased platelet aggregation, may result from an imbalance between the placental production of prostacyclin and thromboxane (Fig. 42-8). During normal pregnancy the placenta produces equivalent quantities of these prostaglandins, whereas in pre-eclamptic pregnancy, there is seven times more thromboxane than prostacyclin.[107] According to the latest theory, endothelial cell injury is central to the development of pre-eclampsia.[108] This injury occurs as a result of reduced placental perfusion leading to a production and release of substances (possibly lipid peroxidases) causing endothelial cell injury. Abnormal endothelial cell function contributes to an increase in peripheral resistance and other abnormalities noted in pre-eclampsia through a release of fibronectin, endothelin, and other substances.

Pre-eclampsia is classified as severe if it is associated with any of the following:

1. Systolic blood pressure of 160 mm Hg
2. Diastolic blood pressure of 110 mm Hg
3. Proteinuria of 5 g · 24 h^{-1}
4. Oliguria (400 ml · 24 h^{-1})

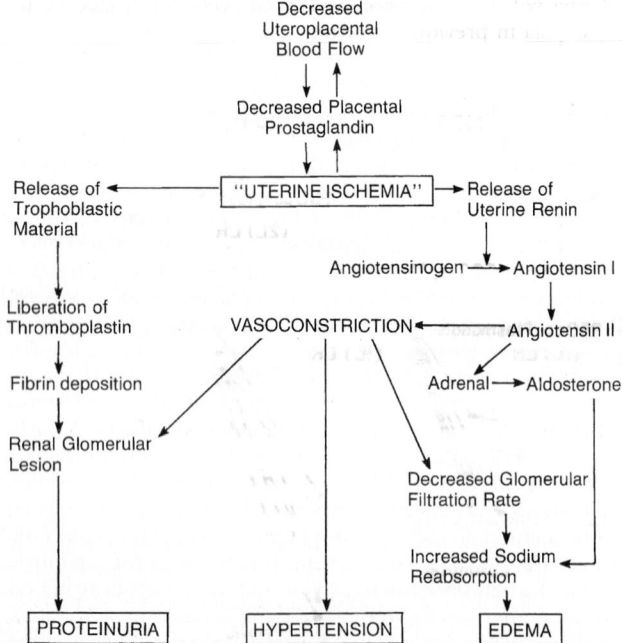

Figure 42-7. Proposed scheme of pathophysiologic changes in toxemia of pregnancy. (Reprinted with permission from Speroff L: Toxemia of pregnancy: Mechanism and therapeutic management. Am J Cardiol 32:582, 1973.)

the recovery room or intensive care setting. In patients with blood clotting abnormalities, the risk of inadvertent puncture of the carotid artery associated with internal jugular cannulation may be averted by inserting the line in the basilic or external jugular vein.

Antihypertensive therapy in pre-eclampsia is used to lessen the risk of cerebral hemorrhage in the mother while maintaining, even improving, tissue perfusion. Plasma volume expansion combined with vasodilation fulfills these goals.[110] Hydralazine is the most commonly used vasodilator in pre-eclampsia because it increases uteroplacental and renal blood flows. It can be administered orally, im, or iv. Nitroprusside, a potent vasodilator of resistance and capacitance vessels, with an immediate but evanescent action, is useful in preventing dangerous elevations in systemic and pulmonary artery blood pressure during laryngoscopy and intubation and is ideal for treatment of hypertensive emergencies. Its infusion can be decreased gradually in the interim as a longer-acting agent, such as hydralazine, begins to take effect. Infusion rates of nitroprusside less than $5-10$ mg $\cdot$ kg^{-1} $\cdot$ min^{-1}, depending on the length of administration, can be maintained without undue risk of cyanide toxicity to the mother and fetus. Trimethaphan, a ganglionic blocking agent, is particularly useful in hypertensive emergencies when cerebral edema and increased intracranial pressure are of particular concern because it does not cause vasodilation in the brain. Other agents used to control maternal blood pressure in pre-eclampsia include α-methyldopa and nitroglycerin. Labetalol, a nonselective β blocker with some α_1-blocking effects, is now frequently used.[111,112]

Consumption coagulopathy may require corrective measures such as infusion of fresh whole blood, platelet concentrates, fresh frozen plasma, and cryoprecipitate. The administration of conduction anesthesia is contraindicated in patients with severe coagulopathy because of the increased risk of an epidural hematoma, leading to permanent neurologic damage.

Anesthetic Management

Epidural anesthesia (or CSE) for labor and delivery should no longer be considered contraindicated, provided there is no severe clotting abnormality or plasma volume deficit.[113] In volume-repleted patients positioned with left uterine displacement, epidural anesthesia does not cause an unacceptable reduction in blood pressure and leads to a significant improvement in placental perfusion.[114] With the use of radioactive xenon, it was shown that the intervillous blood flow increased by approximately 75% after the induction of epidural analgesia (10 ml of bupivacaine 0.25%).[115] The total maternal body clearance of amide local anesthetics is prolonged in pre-eclampsia, and repeated administration of these drugs can lead to higher blood concentrations than in normotensive patients.[116]

For cesarean section, the sensory level of regional anesthesia must extend to T3–4, making adequate fluid therapy and left uterine displacement even more vital. Epidural anesthesia has been preferred to spinal anesthesia in pre-eclamptic women because of its slower onset of action and controllability. The rapid onset of spinal anesthesia may be associated with hypotension, particularly in a volume-depleted patient. However, in two recent studies, the incidence of hypotension, perioperative fluid and ephedrine administration, and neonatal conditions were found to be similar in pre-eclamptic women who received either epidural or spinal anesthesia for cesarean delivery.[117,118] There is an increased sensitivity to vasopressors in pre-eclampsia; therefore, lower doses of ephedrine are usually required to correct hypotension.

General anesthesia in pre-eclamptic patients has its particular hazards. Rapid-sequence induction of anesthesia and intubation of the trachea necessary to avoid aspiration are occasionally difficult because a swollen tongue, epiglottis, or pharynx distorts the anatomy. In patients with impaired coagulation, laryngoscopy and intubation of the trachea may provoke profuse bleeding. Marked systemic and pulmonary hypertension occurring at intubation and extubation enhance the risk of cerebral hemorrhage and pulmonary edema (Fig. 42-10). However, these hemodynamic changes can be minimized with appropriate antihypertensive therapy, such as administration of a trimethaphan or nitroprusside infusion. The use of ketamine and ergot alkaloids should be avoided. As already mentioned, magnesium sulfate may prolong the effects of all muscle relaxants through its actions on the myoneural junction. Therefore, relaxants should be administered with caution (using a nerve stimulator) to avoid overdosage. General anesthesia may be necessary in acute emergencies, such as abruptio placentae, and in patients who do not meet the criteria for epidural anesthesia.

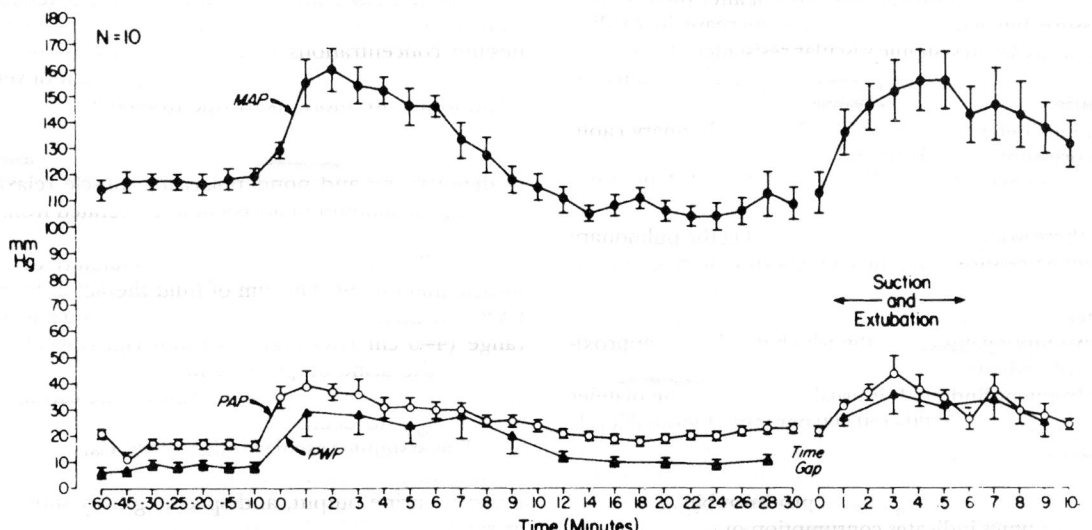

Figure 42-10. Mean and SE of mean arterial pressure (MAP), mean pulmonary artery pressure (PAP), and pulmonary wedge pressure (PWP) in patients with severe pre-eclampsia receiving thiopental and nitrous oxide (40%) with 0.5% halothane anesthesia for cesarean section. (Reprinted with permission from Hodgkinson R, Husain FJ, Hayashi RH: Systemic and pulmonary blood pressure during cesarean section in parturients with gestational hypertension. Canadian Anaesthetists Society Journal 27:389, 1980.)

Antepartum Hemorrhage

Antepartum hemorrhage occurs most commonly in association with placenta previa (abnormal implantation on the lower uterine segment, and partial to total occlusion of the internal cervical os) and abruptio placentae. Placenta previa occurs in 0.1–1.0% of all pregnancies, resulting in up to a 0.9% incidence of maternal and a 17–26% incidence of perinatal mortality. It may be associated with abnormal fetal presentation, such as transverse lie or breech. Placenta previa should be suspected whenever a patient presents with painless, bright red vaginal bleeding, usually after the seventh month of pregnancy. The diagnosis is confirmed by ultrasonography. If the bleeding is not profuse and the fetus is immature, obstetric management is conservative to prolong pregnancy. In severe cases, or if the fetus is mature at the onset of symptoms, prompt delivery is indicated, usually by cesarean section. An emergency hysterectomy may be required because of severe hemorrhage, even after delivery of the placenta, because of uterine atony. The risk of severe hemorrhage after attempted removal of a placenta previa is greatly increased in patients who have undergone prior uterine surgery, including cesarean section. This is due to a higher incidence of placenta accreta, which results from the penetration of myometrium by placental villi. After one previous cesarean delivery, placenta accreta was reported to occur in 20–25% of patients with placenta previa, and after four or more prior cesarean sections, the incidence is greater than 67%.[119]

Abruptio placentae occurs in 0.2–2.4% of pregnant women, usually in the final 10 weeks of gestation and in association with hypertensive diseases. Complications include Couvelaire uterus (when extravasated blood dissects between the myometrial fibers), renal failure, disseminated intravascular coagulation, and anterior pituitary necrosis (Sheehan's syndrome). The maternal mortality rate is high (1.8–11.0%), and the perinatal mortality rate is even higher, in excess of 50%. The diagnosis of abruptio placentae is based on the presence of uterine tenderness and hypertonus and vaginal bleeding of dark, clotted blood. Bleeding may be concealed if the placental margins have remained attached to the uterine wall. If the blood loss is severe (>2l), there may be changes in the maternal blood pressure and pulse rate indicative of hypovolemia. Fetal movements may increase during acute hypoxia or decrease if hypoxia is gradual. Fetal bradycardia and death may ensue. Management of milder cases of abruption includes artificial rupture of amniotic membranes and oxytocin augmentation of labor, if required. In the presence of fetal distress, an emergency cesarean section should be performed.

The anesthesiologist is involved in maternal resuscitation and provision of anesthesia. This may include the establishment of invasive monitoring (an arterial and a central venous catheter are usually adequate) and blood volume replacement, preferably through 14- or 16-gauge cannulae. To correct clotting abnormalities, blood components such as fresh frozen plasma, cryoprecipitate, and platelet concentrates may be required. The anesthesiologist also performs the traditional role of providing appropriate anesthesia for a cesarean section or, occasionally, a hysterectomy. Epidural anesthesia should be considered, but general anesthesia is indicated in the presence of uncontrolled hemorrhage and coagulation abnormalities.[120] As usual, it should be preceded by adequate denitrogenation. In hypovolemic patients, induction may be accomplished with ketamine iv, 0.5–1.0 mg · kg⁻¹. In all obstetric patients, proper precautions should be taken to prevent aspiration of gastric contents. These include the administration of a clear antacid and rapid-sequence induction of anesthesia with application of cricoid pressure until tracheal intubation.

Heart Disease

Heart disease during pregnancy occurs in 0.4–4.1% of patients and is the leading nonobstetric cause of maternal mortality, with a mortality rate ranging from 0.4% among patients in Class I or II of the New York Heart Association's functional classification to 6.8% among those in Classes III and IV. The following lesions pose the greatest risk for the mother: pulmonary hypertension, particularly with Eisenmenger's syndrome; mitral stenosis with atrial fibrillation; tetralogy of Fallot; Marfan's syndrome; and coarctation of the aorta. Cardiac decompensation and death occur most commonly at the time of maximum hemodynamic stress, that is, in the third trimester of pregnancy, during labor and delivery, and particularly during the immediate postpartum period. During labor, cardiac output increases above antepartum levels. Between contractions this increase is approximately 15% in the early first stage, approximately 30% during the late first stage, approximately 45% during the second stage, and, after delivery, 30–50%.[41] With each uterine contraction, approximately 200 ml of blood is squeezed out of the uterus into the central circulation. Consequently, stroke volume, cardiac output, and left ventricular work increase, and each contraction consistently increases cardiac output by 10–25% above that of uterine diastole. The greatest change occurs immediately after delivery of the placenta, when cardiac output increases to an average of 80% above prepartum values, and in some patients it may increase by as much as 150%. These changes in cardiac output can be reduced by administration of regional anesthesia. In patients managed with continuous caudal anesthesia, cardiac output increased only 24% above prepartum control values during the second stage and 59% immediately postpartum.[41]

Until 1960, rheumatic fever was responsible for almost 90% of the heart disease encountered in pregnant women. Since that time, with improved medical care and surgical techniques, more patients with congenital disease survive to reach childbearing age. Simultaneously, better living conditions and antibiotic treatment have reduced the incidence of rheumatic heart disease, and the ratio of rheumatic to congenital heart disease among parturients has declined to 3:1.

Rheumatic Heart Disease

Mitral stenosis is the sole or predominant valvular lesion in most parturients with rheumatic heart disease. The primary defect is obstruction to diastolic blood flow from the left atrium to the left ventricle. This becomes hemodynamically significant when the valve orifice is diminished or the rate of blood flow through the constricted orifice is increased sufficiently to raise left atrial pressure and, consequently, pressure in the pulmonary veins and capillaries.

The physiologic changes of pregnancy usually aggravate the problems of mitral stenosis. An increased pulse rate necessitates a higher diastolic flow rate across the mitral orifice to maintain cardiac output. The flow rate is also augmented by the increased cardiac output that pregnancy requires. In the presence of significant mitral stenosis, these increases in flow rate can be accomplished only by an increase in left atrial and pulmonary venous pressure. The increased blood volume in the lungs that occurs during pregnancy may also contribute to the distention of pulmonary capillaries. Atrial fibrillation may occur in the presence of an enlarged left atrium, leading to pulmonary edema with an associated maternal mortality rate as high as 17%. Cardioversion should be undertaken if drug therapy does not decrease ventricular rate. Mitral commissurotomy may be necessary because of symptoms of congestive heart failure or, less frequently, because of hemoptysis or emboli. When performed in the second or early third trimester, closed as well as open commissurotomies have been well tolerated by the mother and were accompanied by fetal survival rates in excess of 80%. Fortunately, 90% of pregnant women with mitral stenosis are in functional Classes I and II. These patients usually tolerate childbearing well. The relatively small number in functional Classes III and IV account for most maternal cardiac deaths.

Other valvular diseases, namely mitral regurgitation, aortic stenosis, or regurgitation, are much less frequent in pregnant cardiac patients. Together they account for 10–35% of all cases. Pure mitral regurgitation is rarely a problem. Properly managed patients can have repeated pregnancies without serious complications. Similarly, pure aortic insufficiency rarely causes disability in the absence of bacterial endocarditis. Aortic stenosis is frequently associated with aortic insufficiency and mitral stenosis. Myocardial failure secondary to pure aortic stenosis is rare in patients of childbearing age because symptoms develop in most patients when they are in their fifth or sixth decades. Left ventricular hypertrophy and a relatively fixed stroke volume develop in those with significant aortic stenosis. These changes reduce their tolerance to decreases in systemic vascular resistance, bradycardia, and decreased venous return (and left ventricular filling).

Continuous epidural block offers particular advantages to the pregnant cardiac patient. It not only eliminates pain and tachycardia throughout labor and delivery but prevents the progressive increase in cardiac output and stroke volume that normally occurs in parturition.[41] It also abolishes the bearing-down reflex. CSE may be expected to produce the same salutary effects. In view of these advantages, continuous lumbar epidural and CSE techniques are recommended for most pregnant women with rheumatic valvular diseases, whether they are to have vaginal or cesarean section deliveries, with the exception of those with severe symptomatic aortic stenosis. In patients with this condition, even transient episodes of hypotension may cause serious coronary hypoperfusion, arrhythmias, and even cardiac arrest. However, use of a pulmonary artery catheter, careful titration of anesthetic dose, and the use of phenylephrine for changes in blood pressure may permit the use of regional anesthesia in selected patients. Intrathecal opioids have been used in an attempt to provide adequate obstetric analgesia during labor without the risk of hypotension. Morphine, 0.5–1.0 mg, or fentanyl, 10–20 μg, alone or in combination, relieves the pain of uterine contractions. Pudendal block is needed for delivery. Should general anesthesia be deemed necessary for cesarean section, the standard thiopental–nitrous oxide–halogenated anesthetic–muscle relaxant technique is recommended. In cases of severe mitral stenosis, etomidate, 0.2–0.3 mg · kg^{-1}, or a slower induction with halothane or iv fentanyl is preferred. The benefit of high-dose narcotic induction should be weighed against the risk of transient neonatal depression. In patients with severe aortic stenosis and evidence of left ventricular compromise, halogenated agents should be avoided.

Congenital Heart Diseases

Patent ductus arteriosus, atrial septal defect, and ventricular septal defect are the more common congenital cardiovascular abnormalities. In all these conditions, anomalous communicating channels exist between the cardiac chambers or the great vessels. Normally, pressures on the left side of the circulation are higher than those on the right and there is a left-to-right shunt. Late in the natural history of these diseases, pulmonary hypertension may develop, causing a reversal of the shunt (Eisenmenger's syndrome). Patients with Eisenmenger's syndrome rarely live beyond the age of 40 years. Pregnancy is poorly tolerated because the gestational decrease in systemic vascular resistance in the presence of fixed pulmonary vascular resistance results in a significant increase in the right-to-left shunt. Changes in systemic and pulmonary pressures are also likely to occur with the aortocaval compression near the end of pregnancy, hypotension caused by epidural or spinal anesthesia, and bearing-down efforts of parturition. Severe shunt disturbances induced by these changes may lead to further cyanosis, even death.

Tetralogy of Fallot is the most common cyanotic congenital heart defect. It consists of an interventricular septal defect, pulmonary stenosis, displacement of the aortic orifice so that it overlies the ventricular septal defect, and right ventricular hypertrophy. The pulmonary stenosis leads to increases in right ventricular systolic pressure with dilation and hypertrophy of that chamber. Blood from the right ventricle is shunted through the septal defect, and the overriding aorta receives venous blood from this source and oxygenated blood from the left ventricle. Reduced arterial oxygenation leads to cyanosis, polycythemia, and clubbing. Symptoms develop in patients during the first few months of life, with their severity related to the degree of the pulmonic stenosis. However, the introduction of cardiac surgery has increased the number of patients surviving to childbearing age.

Anesthesia for parturients with cyanotic heart disease should provide effective pain relief while avoiding hypotension, struggling, or coughing, and eliminating bearing-down efforts, all of which could increase the right-to-left shunt. For labor, intrathecal opioids rather than conventional epidural anesthesia can be administered. Light planes of general anesthesia are usually well tolerated for cesarean section.

PRETERM DELIVERY

Preterm labor and delivery present a significant challenge to the anesthesiologist because the mother and the infant may be at risk. The definition of prematurity was altered to distinguish between the preterm infant, born before the 37th week of gestation is completed, and the small-for-gestational-age infant, who may be born at term but whose weight is more than 2 standard deviations below the mean. Although preterm deliveries occur in 8–10% of all births, they account for approximately 80% of early neonatal deaths. In general, the mortality and morbidity rates are higher among preterm infants than among small-for-gestational-age infants of comparable weight. Severe problems, including respiratory distress syndrome, intracranial hemorrhage, hypoglycemia, hypocalcemia, and hyperbilirubinemia, are prone to develop in preterm infants. Fortunately, with improved neonatal intensive care, severe, lasting impairment, such as cerebral palsy, mental retardation, or chronic lung disease, has become infrequent among the survivors.

Obstetricians frequently try to inhibit preterm labor to enhance fetal lung maturity. Delaying delivery by even 24–48 hours may be beneficial if glucocorticoids are administered to the mother. Various agents have been used to suppress uterine activity (tocolysis), including ethanol, magnesium sulfate, prostaglandin inhibitors, β-sympathomimetics, and calcium channel blockers. β-Adrenergic drugs, such as ritodrine and terbutaline, are the most commonly used tocolytics. These agents are initially administered by an iv infusion at the rate of 0.05–0.1 mg · min^{-1} for ritodrine and 0.01 mg · min^{-1} for terbutaline. Their predominant effect is β_2 receptor stimulation, resulting in myometrial inhibition, vasodilation, and bronchodilation. Numerous maternal complications have been reported: hypotension, hypokalemia, hyperglycemia, myocardial ischemia, pulmonary edema, and death.[121] Complications also may occur because of interactions with anesthetic drugs and techniques. With the use of regional anesthesia, peripheral vasodilation caused by β-adrenergic stimulation increases the risk of hypotension. Acute prehydration must be managed carefully to avoid pulmonary edema. General anesthesia may be associated with increased risks of hemodynamic instability in the presence of pre-existing tachycardia, hypotension, and hypokalemia. Caution should be exercised with use of halothane (cardiac dysrhythmias), atropine, and pancuronium (tachycardia). In nonemergent situations, delay of anesthesia by at least 3 hours from the cessation of tocolysis allows β-mimetic effects to dissipate. Potassium supplementation is usually not necessary because the intracellular potassium concentration is normal despite a reduction in serum concentrations.

It has become axiomatic that the premature infant is more vulnerable than the term newborn to the effects of drugs used in obstetric analgesia and anesthesia. However, there have been few systematic studies to determine the maternal and fetal pharmacokinetics and dynamics of drugs throughout gestation. There are several postulated causes of enhanced drug sensitivity in the preterm newborn: less protein available for drug binding; higher levels of bilirubin, which may compete with the drug for protein binding; greater drug access to the central nervous system because of a poorly developed blood–brain barrier; greater total body water and lower fat content; and a decreased ability to metabolize and excrete drugs. However, these deficiencies of the preterm infant should not be as serious as we have been led to believe. Although the serum albumin and α_1-acid glycoprotein concentrations are lower in the preterm fetus, this would primarily affect drugs that are highly bound to these proteins. However, most drugs used in anesthesia exhibit only low to moderate degrees of binding in the fetal serum: approximately 50% for etidocaine and bupivacaine, 25% for lidocaine, 52% for meperidine, and 75% for thiopental.

The placenta efficiently eliminates fetal bilirubin. Thus, the hyperbilirubinemia of prematurity normally occurs in the postpartum period. With the exception of diazepam, bilirubin does not compete with anesthetic drugs because most are bound to other serum proteins (*e.g.*, meperidine and local anesthetics to α_1-acid glycoproteins). It seems likely that the human blood–brain barrier develops substantially in early gestation. Thus, factors such as tissue affinity changes may account for differences between immature and mature animals in brain uptake of highly lipid-soluble drugs.

Greater total body water in the preterm fetus results in a greater volume of distribution for drugs. Thus, to achieve equal blood concentrations, the immature fetus must receive a greater amount of drug transplacentally than the mature fetus. A study of age-related toxicity of lidocaine in sheep showed that the greater the volume of distribution, the greater the dose required to achieve toxic blood concentrations of the drug.[37] Decreased ability to metabolize or excrete drugs, associated with prematurity, is certainly not a universal phenomenon. In a study comparing the pharmacokinetics of lidocaine in preterm newborns and adults, plasma clearance was similar in both groups.[35] Neonates excreted much more unchanged lidocaine than did adults. Similarly, although meperidine metabolism is more limited in the neonate than in the adult, urinary excretion of the unchanged drug is greater in the neonate.

Another factor is gestational changes in maternal serum albumin and α_1-acid glycoprotein concentrations, which tend to decrease. Serial determinations of protein binding of diazepam, phenytoin, and valproic acid in maternal serum, performed in early (8–16 weeks), middle (17–32 weeks), and late pregnancy, showed a progressive increase in the unbound fraction of these drugs.[122] This increases drug availability for placental transfer. Placental permeability itself increases as pregnancy progresses because of the increased area and decreased thickness of tissue barriers.[30]

In a largely ignored, prospective study of more than 1000 premature labors, during which mothers received meperidine alone or with scopolamine, medication had no effect on the perinatal death rate, the incidence of respiratory distress syndrome, Apgar scores, the need for resuscitation, and the incidence of severe neurologic defects within 1 year.[123]

Therefore, it appears that in selection of the anesthetic drugs and techniques for delivery of a preterm infant, concerns regarding drug effects on the newborn are far less important than prevention of asphyxia and trauma to the fetus. For labor and vaginal delivery, well conducted epidural anesthesia is advantageous in providing good perineal relaxation. The anesthesiologist should ascertain that the fetus is neither hypoxic nor acidotic before induction of epidural blockade. Asphyxia results in a redistribution of fetal cardiac output, which increases oxygen delivery to vital organs such as the brain, heart, and adrenals. These changes in the preterm fetus may be better preserved with bupivacaine or chloroprocaine than with lidocaine.[124,125]

Preterm infants with breech presentation are usually delivered by cesarean section. General anesthesia with uterine relaxation, provided by a halogenated drug, facilitates delivery of the aftercoming head. If regional anesthesia is used, nitroglycerin should be available for uterine relaxation.

FETAL AND MATERNAL MONITORING

The development of biophysical and biochemical monitoring of the fetus during labor and delivery has had a tremendous impact on obstetric practice since the early 1970s. Monitoring procedures are now performed routinely, and it is important that the anesthesiologist understand the basic principles of the technology, as well as the interpretation of results, because they relate to both mother and fetus.

During the same period, there has been an explosion in monitoring technology in the fields of anesthesiology and intensive care. The mother with serious medical problems requiring intensive care or the one whose infant is delivered in an operating room under an anesthesiologist's care is subject to the same standards of monitoring as any other surgical patient. It is generally agreed that the use of intensive peripartum monitoring is appropriate in a high-risk pregnancy. In contrast, patients with routine labor are frequently observed in the same way that patients were many generations ago (*i.e.*, with intermittent blood pressure readings). With the growing sophistication of electronic devices, and specifically the science of telemetry, we can look forward to better surveillance of both mother and fetus without the loss of maternal freedom and activity that monitoring currently entails.

Biophysical Monitoring

A fetal monitor is a two-channel recorder of fetal heart rate and uterine activity. In the direct system, the fetal ECG is obtained from an electrode attached to the presenting part. Intrauterine pressure is measured continuously with a transducer connected to a saline-filled catheter that is inserted transcervically. Direct monitoring is quantitative but requires rupture of the membranes and a cervical dilation of at least 1.5 cm. In addition, the presenting part must dip into the true pelvis. Indirect fetal monitoring uses data obtained from transducers secured to the mother's abdomen with adjustable straps. Ultrasound cardiography is the most commonly used indirect method of obtaining fetal heart rate signals. Uterine activity is monitored with a tocodynamometer triggered by the changing shape of the uterus during the contraction. Indirect monitoring is mostly qualitative. Its advantage is that it can be applied without rupture of membranes, even before the onset of labor.

The following variables are considered when fetal well-being is determined: baseline heart rate, beat-to-beat variability, periodic patterns, and uterine activity. The baseline fetal heart rate is measured between contractions and ranges between 120–160 beats $\cdot$ min^{-1} in the normal fetus. An acceleration of fetal heart rate in response to fetal stimulation, such as during vaginal examination or fetal capillary blood sampling, is a reassuring sign that the fetus is not acidotic. Persistently elevated rates may be associated with chronic fetal distress, maternal fever, or administration of drugs such as ephedrine and atropine. Abnormally low rates may be encountered in fetuses with congenital heart block or as a late occurrence during the course of fetal hypoxia and acidosis.

The baseline fetal heart rate variability, which is normally present, reflects the beat-to-beat adjustments of the parasympathetic and sympathetic nervous systems to a variety of internal and external stimuli. Fetal central nervous system depression by asphyxia may decrease baseline variability. Therefore, a smooth fetal heart rate tracing may be an ominous finding. Studies comparing beat-to-beat variability with fetal acid–base analysis indicate a good correlation between the two parameters.[126] However, drugs can also decrease fetal heart rate variability by depressing mechanisms in the central nervous system that integrate cardiac control (tranquilizers, opioids, barbiturates, anesthetics) or by blocking the transmission of control impulses to the cardiac pacemaker (atropine). In contrast, ephedrine administration may increase beat-to-beat variability.[127]

Periodic fetal heart rate patterns consist of decelerations or accelerations of relatively brief duration in association with uterine contractions (Fig. 42-11). There are three major forms of fetal heart rate deceleration: early, late, and variable. Early decelerations are U-shaped, with the heart rate usually not decreasing to less than 100 beats·min⁻¹. The fetal heart begins to slow with the onset of the contraction, the low point coincides with the peak of the contraction, and the rate usually returns to the baseline as the uterus relaxes. This type of deceleration has been attributed to fetal head compression, leading to increased vagal tone. It is not ameliorated by increasing fetal oxygenation but is blocked by atropine administration. Early decelerations are transitory and well tolerated by the fetus because there is no systemic hypoxemia or acidosis.[128]

Late decelerations are also U-shaped. They begin 20–30 seconds or more after the onset of uterine contraction, and the low point of the deceleration occurs well after the peak of the contraction. Myocardial ischemia resulting from uteroplacental insufficiency is believed to cause this pattern. The pattern of late deceleration can be corrected by improving fetal oxygenation, which may be accomplished with oxygen administration to the mother, correction of maternal hypotension, or aortocaval compression, or by taking measures that decrease uterine activity. If this pattern is repetitive, continuous, and progressive in severity, there is a significant correlation with fetal acidosis, and delivery may be required.[128]

Variable decelerations, which result from umbilical cord compression, are the most common periodic patterns observed in the intrapartum period. They are variable in shape and onset, with the rate usually decreasing to less than 100 beats·min⁻¹. Although the initial fetal heart rate changes are of reflex origin, if the cord compressions are frequent or prolonged, fetal asphyxia may result in direct myocardial depression.[128]

Cervical dilation and descent of the presenting part during the first stage of labor result primarily from uterine contractions. During the active phase, contractions should occur every 2–3 minutes, with peak intrauterine pressures of 50–80 mm Hg and resting pressures of 5–20 mm Hg. Uterine activity may be abnormally elevated in association with abruptio placentae or the injudicious use of oxytocics. Tetanic uterine contractions have been reported after the use of methoxamine, a pure α-adrenergic agonist. In the first and second trimesters of pregnancy, increased uterine tone may be induced with ketamine in doses greater than 1.1 mg·kg⁻¹. At term, ketamine does not appear to have this effect.[129]

Poor uterine contractility may result from overdistention (polyhydramnios, multiple pregnancy) or maintenance of the supine position. During early labor, administration of opioids, sedatives, or regional anesthesia may delay the onset of the active phase by diminishing uterine activity. However, regional anesthesia instituted during the active phase has no untoward effects on uterine activity as long as hypotension and the supine position are avoided. The addition of epinephrine to a local anesthetic solution may have a dose-related inhibitory effect on uterine activity.

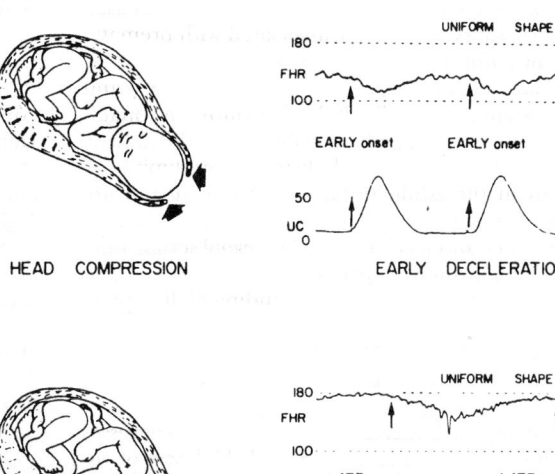

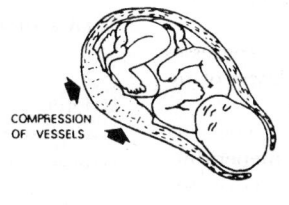

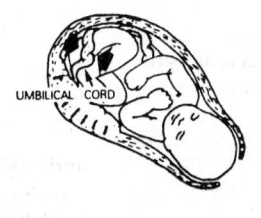

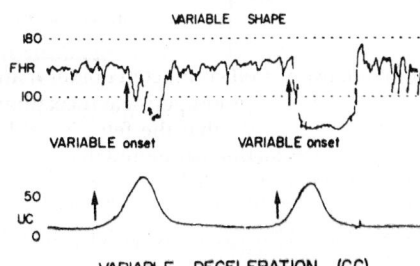

Figure 42-11. Classification and mechanism of fetal heart rate patterns. (Reprinted with permission from Hon EH: An Introduction to Fetal Heart Rate Monitoring, p 29. New Haven, Connecticut, Harty Press, 1969.)

Biochemical Monitoring

Before labor, the normal fetus is neither hypoxic nor acidotic. During labor, many events, including uterine contractions, cord compression, aortocaval compression, and maternal hypotension from any cause, may decrease uteroplacental blood flow sufficiently to produce fetal hypoxia and acidosis. Acidosis associated with short-term placental hypoperfusion primarily results from carbon dioxide accumulation (respiratory acidosis). In prolonged asphyxia, hypercarbia is accompanied by metabolic acidosis resulting from anaerobic metabolism. Thus, fetal acid–base indices, such as Pco_2 and base deficit, usually reflect the degree and duration of asphyxia.

Assessment of acid–base status of the fetus became possible in the early 1960s, with the development of a fetal capillary blood-sampling technique. Blood is usually obtained from the scalp but may also be sampled from the breech. It is collected into a heparinized glass capillary tube, and pH, Pco_2, Po_2, and base deficit are determined immediately with an appropriate electrode system adapted to the small sample size.

This technique has been validated in animal and clinical studies. It has been shown in fetal monkeys that the blood values obtained from the scalp are closely correlated with those in simultaneously obtained samples from the carotid artery and jugular vein.[130] A fetal capillary blood pH of 7.25 is the lowest limit of normal. A pH below 7.20 indicates fetal acidosis, and values between 7.20 and 7.24 are considered preacidotic. The last predelivery fetal pH correlated with the Apgar score at 1 or 2 minutes after birth.[131,132] Ninety-two percent of infants scored 7 or better when the pH was above 7.25. With the pH below 7.16, 80% of infants scored 6 or less.[131] In general, when the pH is normal immediately before delivery, it can be assumed that the infant will be in good condition. However, there is a small incidence of false-positive and false-negative results. In one study, normal pH was associated with low Apgar scores (false-positive results) in approximately 10% of cases[132] (Fig. 42-12). In approximately 8% of cases (false-negative results), a vigorous infant was born despite a low capillary scalp pH. The major factors contributing to false-positive outcomes are administration of sedative drugs or anesthetics, infection, airway obstruction, and congenital anomalies. False-negative outcomes are usually associated with maternal acidosis, which may occur after prolonged labor, excessive muscular activity, or inadequate fluid and caloric intakes. Obtaining a maternal sample (arterial or free-flowing venous blood) for the evaluation of the acid–base status helps identify this group. If fetal acidosis is of maternal origin, the mother's blood shows a large base deficit value, and the difference between the fetal and maternal base deficit values (DBD) is small. In contrast, fetal acidosis resulting from prolonged asphyxia is reflected in a large fetal but a normal maternal base deficit value; consequently, the difference in base deficit values is large. Fetal acidosis of maternal origin can be treated by correcting the maternal acid–base imbalance.

Complications

There are data correlating direct fetal monitoring with maternal infection.[133] However, conclusions from these reports are tenuous because most of the affected patients had prolonged rupture of membranes. A less frequent complication of internal monitoring is uterine perforation. The firm plastic cannula used to introduce the intra-amniotic pressure catheter has been implicated. Fetal complications related to scalp electrodes are ecchymoses, lacerations, leakage of cerebrospinal fluid, osteomyelitis of the skull, sepsis, scalp abscesses, and a case of meningitis with ventriculitis and hydrocephalus. The overall incidence of these complications is unknown. Scalp abscess is the most commonly reported.

Scalp capillary blood sampling can also lead to fetal complications. The two major ones are hemorrhage and abscess formation. Bleeding from the sampling site is usually self-limited, but massive hemorrhage resulting in severe anemia and, rarely, neonatal death has been reported. Prenatal and postnatal bleeding from a sampling incision may be the first manifestation of a severe fetal coagulation disorder.

The costs and benefits of fetal monitoring are still being questioned. There is a conflict between the desire for a "natural" childbirth experience and the physician's concern for maternal and fetal safety. It is generally agreed that the use of intensive intrapartum monitoring is appropriate in high-risk pregnancies. Debate continues concerning the benefits of these methods to low-risk fetuses. A large, randomized, controlled trial comparing continuous electronic fetal monitoring with traditional intermittent auscultation of the fetal heart (with an option to measure fetal scalp capillary blood pH) showed that neonatal seizures and abnormal neurologic signs occurred twice as frequently in the group with intermittent auscultation. In addition, the study showed no difference in the cesarean section rate between the two groups.[134]

NEWBORN RESUSCITATION IN THE DELIVERY ROOM

Of the approximately 3.5 million infants born in the United States each year, 6% require resuscitation in the delivery room. Among those weighing 1500 g or less, the incidence is approximately 80%. The following factors may contribute to depression of the newborn: drugs used in labor or during delivery, including anesthetic agents; trauma of precipitate labor and operative obstetrics; and birth asphyxia (i.e., hypoxia and hypercapnia with acidosis).

Fetal Asphyxia

Fetal asphyxia, the best-studied cause of neonatal depression, usually develops as a result of interference with maternal or fetal perfusion of the placenta. As stated previously, the normal fetus is neither hypoxic nor acidotic before labor. Experimental data have revealed that transplacental gradients for pH and Pco_2 are approximately 0.05 pH units and 5 mm Hg, respectively. Although oxygen tension is low, oxygen saturation is relatively high (80–85%) by virtue of the shift to the left of the fetal oxyhemoglobin dissociation curve.

During labor, uterine contractions decrease the blood flow

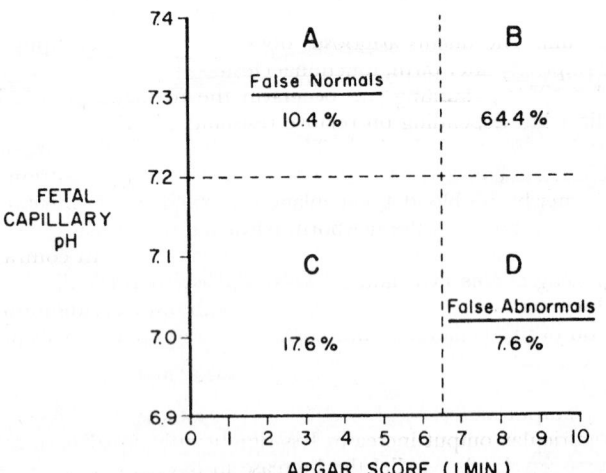

Figure 42-12. Fetal pH as an index of infant's condition at birth in 355 patients during labor. Segment A: depressed infants with normal pH; segment B: vigorous infants with normal pH; segment C: depressed infants with low pH; segment D: vigorous infants with low pH. (Reprinted with permission from Bowe ET, Beard RW, Finster M *et al*: Reliability of fetal blood sampling. Am J Obstet Gynecol 107:279, 1970.)

through the intervillous space of the placenta or may stop it completely. On the fetal side, cord compression occurs during the final stages of approximately one third of vaginal deliveries. Thus, mild degrees of hypoxia and acidosis occur even during normal labor and delivery, and play an important role in initiation of ventilation. On average, healthy, vigorous infants (at birth) have an oxygen saturation of 21%, a pH of 7.24, and a Pco_2 of 56 mm Hg.

Severe fetal asphyxia occasionally develops as a result of fetal and maternal complications such as a tight nuchal cord, prolapsed cord, premature separation of the placenta, uterine hyperactivity, or maternal hypotension. During asphyxia, changes in blood gases and hydrogen ion concentration are rapid. The decrease in pH results from accumulation of carbon dioxide and end products of anaerobic glycolysis. After oxygen stores are exhausted, the ability of fetal brain and myocardium to derive energy from anaerobic metabolism is essential for survival. However, anaerobic glycolysis is pH dependent, and its rate is greatly diminished when the pH decreases below 7.0. Other untoward effects of severe hypoxia and acidosis include depression of the myocardium resulting from a decrease in its responsiveness to catecholamines; a shift to the right of the fetal oxyhemoglobin dissociation curve, resulting in reduced oxygen-carrying capacity; and an increase in pulmonary vascular resistance, which plays an important role during circulatory readjustment after birth.

Ventilatory and cardiovascular responses to controlled experimental asphyxia have been investigated extensively in newborn monkeys (Fig. 42-13). During the initial phase of asphyxia, the unanesthetized animal exhibits respiratory efforts that increase in depth and frequency for up to 3 minutes. This period, called

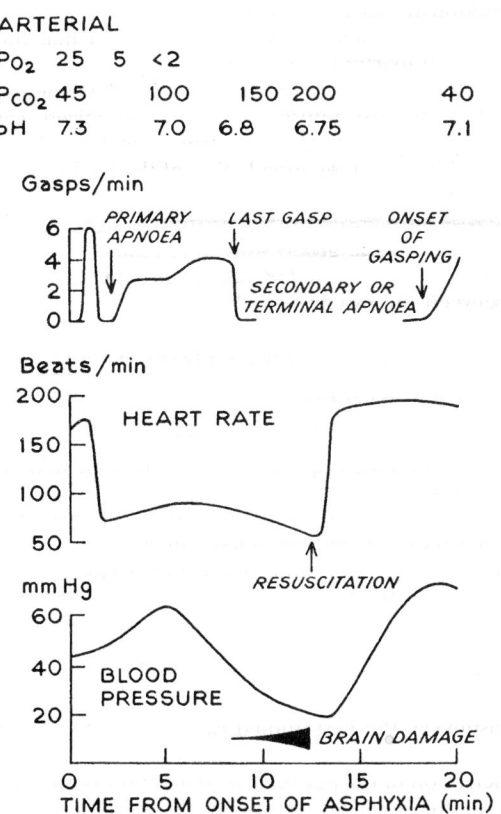

Figure 42-13. Schematic diagram of changes in rhesus monkeys during asphyxia and with resuscitation by positive-pressure ventilation. Brain damage was assessed by histologic examination some weeks or months later. (Reprinted with permission from Dawes GS: Foetal and Neonatal Physiology: A Comparative Study of the Changes at Birth, p 149. Chicago, Year Book Medical Publishers, 1968.)

primary hyperpnea, is followed by primary apnea, which lasts for approximately 1 minute. Rhythmic gasping then begins and is maintained at a fairly constant rate of approximately 6 gasps · min^{-1} for 4–5 minutes. Thereafter, the gasps become weaker and slower. Their cessation at approximately 8.5 minutes after the onset of asphyxia marks the beginning of secondary apnea. Administration of opioids and systemic anesthetic agents to the mother can abolish the period of primary hyperpnea and prolong primary apnea.

There is a linear relationship between the duration of asphyxia and the onset of gasping and rhythmic spontaneous breathing. In the newborn monkey, for each minute of asphyxia beyond the last gasp, 2 additional minutes of artificial ventilation is required before gasping begins again and 4 minutes before rhythmic breathing is established.[135] This indicates that the longer artificial ventilation of the lungs is delayed during secondary apnea, the longer it will take to resuscitate the infant. Furthermore, in the newborn monkey, prolongation of asphyxia for 4 minutes beyond the last gasp is accompanied by extensive damage to brain stem nuclei, whereas animals resuscitated before the last gasp show little or no brain damage. Thus, a relatively short delay in resuscitation can have serious sequelae.

Neonatal Adaptations at Birth

During this period, and through the early hours and days of life, many morphologic and functional changes take place, with the cardiovascular and ventilatory systems undergoing the most dramatic alterations. In the normal newborn, two events occur almost simultaneously, and within seconds of delivery: the arrest of umbilical circulation through the placenta and expansion of the lungs. These events change the fetal circulation toward the adult type. Survival of the neonate depends primarily on prompt expansion of the lungs and establishment of effective ventilation.

The onset of ventilation and expansion of the lungs opens up the pulmonary vascular bed, resulting in decreased resistance and a significant increase in pulmonary blood flow. Pulmonary vascular resistance decreases as oxygen tension increases and carbon dioxide levels decrease. As soon as pulmonary perfusion increases, the foramen ovale, which constitutes a communication between the inferior vena cava and the left atrium, undergoes functional closure because of pressure changes across the valve of the foramen (see Fig. 42-4). Cessation of the umbilical circulation reduces pressure in the inferior vena cava and right atrium, whereas the increase in pulmonary blood flow increases venous return and pressure in the left atrium. The ductus arteriosus does not constrict abruptly or completely after birth; functional closure may take hours, even days. Thus, shunting still occurs in the neonatal period, its direction depending on relative resistances in the pulmonary and systemic vascular beds. The smooth muscle of the ductus arteriosus constricts in response to increased oxygen tension in the newborn's blood. Catecholamines, which exist in increased concentrations in the newborn, particularly during the first 3 hours of life, also constrict the ductus arteriosus. In contrast, prostaglandins PGI_2 and PGE_2, produced by the wall of the ductus arteriosus, relax the ductal smooth muscle. Administration of prostaglandin synthesis inhibitors to fetal animals promotes constriction of the ductus arteriosus.

Cardiac output and its distribution also increase; left ventricular output increases ~150–400 ml · kg^{-1} · min^{-1}, whereas right ventricular output increases less significantly. Cardiac output changes closely parallel the increase in oxygen consumption. The redistribution of cardiac output also leads to increases in myocardial, renal, and gastrointestinal blood flow and decreases in cerebral, adrenal, and carotid flow.

During fetal life, respiratory gas exchange takes place through the placenta. Delivery of the infant's trunk relieves the thoracic compression that occurs as the infant passes through the birth

Table 42-4. RESUSCITATION EQUIPMENT IN THE DELIVERY ROOM

Radiant warmer
Suction with manometer and suction trap
Suction catheters
Wall oxygen with flow meter
Resuscitation bag ($\leq$750 ml)
Infant face masks
Infant oropharyngeal airways
Endotracheal tubes, 2.5, 3.0, 3.5, and 4.0 mm
Endotracheal tube stylets
Laryngoscope(s) and blade(s)
Sterile umbilical artery catheterization tray
Needles, syringes, three-way stopcocks
Medications and solutions
  1:10,000 epinephrine
  Naloxone hydrochloride
  Sodium bicarbonate
  Volume expanders

canal, and the thorax and the lungs expand. Most infants initiate respiratory efforts a few seconds after birth. After the first inspiration, a cry usually results as the infant exhales against a partially closed glottis, thus increasing intrathoracic pressure significantly. Negative pressures in excess of 40 cm H_2O bring about the initial entry of air into fluid-filled alveoli. In the mature, normal neonate, the lungs expand almost completely after the first few breaths, and the pressure–volume changes achieved with each respiration resemble those of the adult. After lung expansion, the FRC approximates 70 ml in the term newborn and changes little over the first 6 days of life. The tidal volume varies between 10 and 30 ml, the breathing frequency ranges from 30–60 breaths $\cdot$ min^{-1}, and minute ventilation exceeds 500 ml. After delivery and prompt lung expansion, reoxygenation is rapid, but it takes 2 or 3 hours to achieve a relatively normal acid–base balance, primarily by pulmonary excretion of carbon dioxide. By 24 hours, the healthy neonate has reached the same acid–base state as that of the mother before labor.

Resuscitation

The delivery room must be prepared for adequate and prompt treatment of severe neonatal depression at birth. All members of the delivery room team should be trained in resuscitation methods because both mother and infant may encounter difficulty simultaneously. Every piece of apparatus necessary for emergency resuscitation should be checked carefully before delivery (Table 42-4). An overview of resuscitation in the delivery room is provided in Figure 42-14.

Initial Treatment and Evaluation of All Infants

Immediately after delivery, the infant should be held head down while the cord is clamped and cut. The infant should then be placed supine under a radiant heat source, with the head kept low with a slight lateral tilt, and the skin should be dried

promptly. A nurse or assistant should listen to the heart beat immediately, indicating the rate by finger movement. If help is not available, the rate can be detected from pulsation of the umbilical cord. At the same time, the resuscitator should aspirate the mouth, pharynx, and nose with a catheter. This suction should be brief, not exceeding 30 seconds. Slapping the infant's soles lightly or rubbing its back frequently aids in initiating a deep breath or cry. The initial appraisal of the newborn should start from the moment of birth, with particular attention paid to the first few breaths and the evenness and ease of respiration. Most infants are vigorous and cough or cry within seconds of delivery. Their heart rate is above 100 beats $\cdot$ min^{-1}. The administration of free-flowing oxygen rapidly improves their oxygenation and decreases pulmonary vascular resistance. Mildly to moderately depressed infants constitute the largest group requiring some form of resuscitation at birth. These infants are pale or cyanotic, have not established sustained respiration even at 1 minute after delivery, and may be nearly flaccid. However, their heart rate is usually above 100 beats $\cdot$ min^{-1}. The severely depressed infant is flaccid, unresponsive, and pale, and may often have a heart rate below 100 beats $\cdot$ min^{-1}. The scoring system introduced by Apgar is a useful method of clinically evaluating the infant, particularly at 1 and 5 minutes after delivery (Table 42-5).

Treatment of Moderately Depressed Infants

If initial resuscitative methods, including rubbing the back or slapping the feet once or twice, have produced no response, that is, the infant is apneic or its heart rate remains below 100 beats $\cdot$ min^{-1}, positive-pressure ventilation by bag and mask should be instituted at a rate of 40 breaths $\cdot$ min^{-1}. The initial breath may require pressures of 30–40 cm H_2O. Subsequently, the inflation pressures should be reduced to 15–20 cm H_2O in an infant with normal lungs. A small plastic oropharyngeal airway may be needed to maintain patency of the upper airway. If after 15–30 seconds of ventilation the heart rate is below 60 beats $\cdot$ min^{-1}, or maintained between 60 and 80 beats $\cdot$ min^{-1}, chest compressions should be initiated.

Treatment of Severely Depressed Infants

Ventilation should be established without delay. The glottis should be inspected immediately with the laryngoscope. If meconium or thick meconium-stained mucus has been aspirated into the trachea, it must be suctioned out at once through an endotracheal tube before the lungs are inflated. It is usually possible to accomplish this within 1–2 minutes of delivery. Severely depressed infants may require 3–8 minutes of artificial ventilation before a spontaneous gasp is taken. The endotracheal tube can be removed as soon as quiet and sustained respiration is established.

Use of Cardiac Massage

If the blood pressure or heart rate is unduly low at the beginning of resuscitation, positive-pressure ventilation is unlikely to be successful unless cardiac massage is used. The technique preferred by the authors consists of intermittent compression of the lower third of the sternum 120 times per minute with the index and middle fingers. During chest compressions, positive-

Table 42-5. APGAR SCORES

Sign	0	1	2
Heart rate	Absent	<100 beats $\cdot$ min^{-1}	>100 beats $\cdot$ min^{-1}
Respiratory effort	Absent	Slow, irregular	Good, crying
Muscle tone	Limp	Some flexion of extremities	Active motion
Reflex irritability	No repsonse	Grimace	Cough, sneeze, or cry
Color	Pale, blue	Body pink, extremities blue	Completely pink

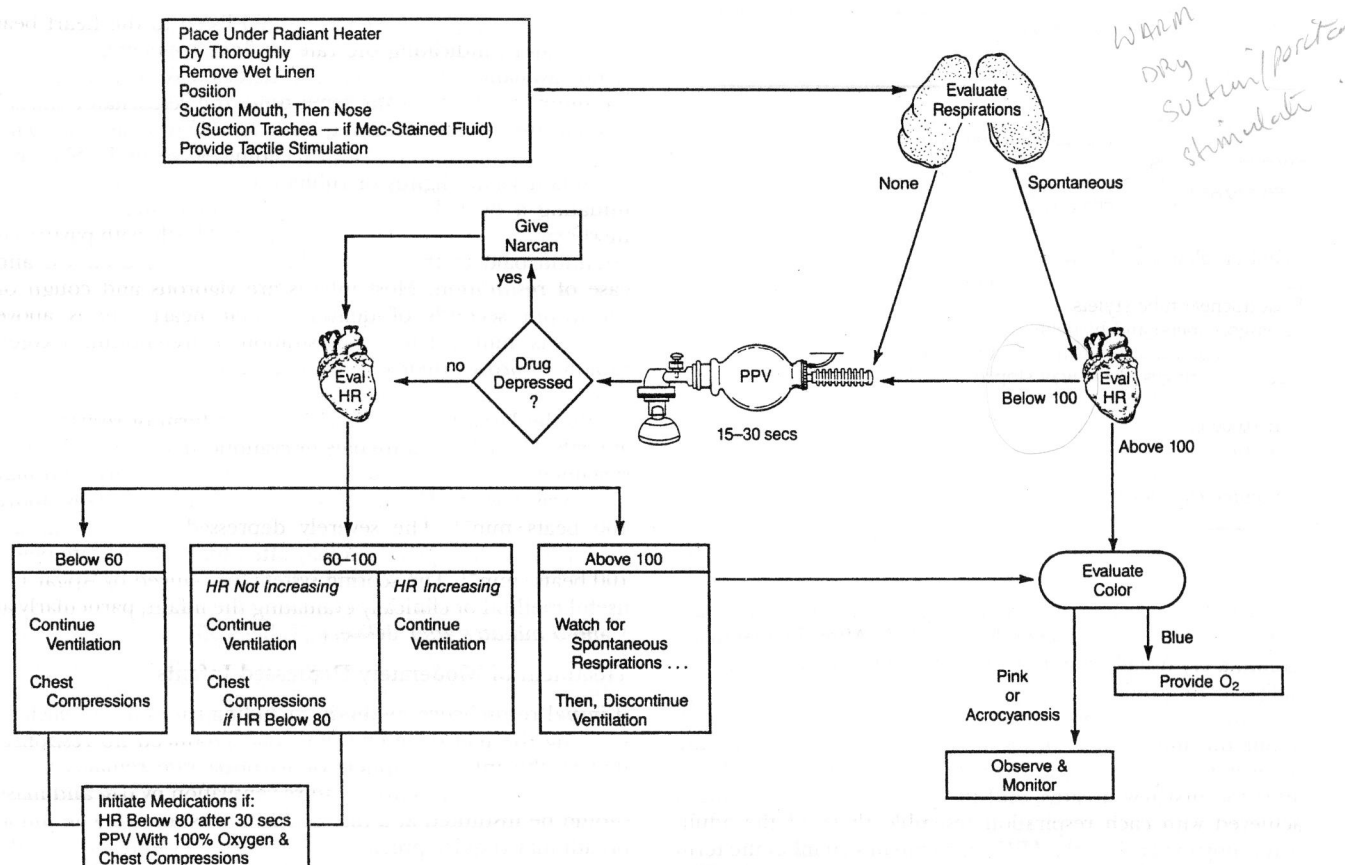

Figure 42-14. Overview of resuscitation in the delivery room. HR = heart rate; PPV = positive-pressure ventilation. (Reprinted with permission from Bloom RS, Copley C: Textbook of Neonatal Resuscitation. Elk Grove Village, Illinois, American Heart Association/American Academy of Pediatrics, 1990.)

pressure ventilation with 100% oxygen should be performed at a rate of 40–60 per minute. Cardiac massage and ventilation should be maintained until the heart rate exceeds 100 beats · min^{-1}.

Rapid Correction of Acidosis

In clinical practice, severe acidosis (pH <7.0 or a base deficit >15 mEq · l^{-1}) should be corrected promptly to improve pulmonary perfusion and oxygenation. For that purpose, a 3.5- or 5.0-French catheter should be inserted, under sterile conditions, into the umbilical vein and advanced until the tip of the catheter is just below the skin level. A solution of sodium bicarbonate, 0.5 mEq · ml^{-1} (4.2%), is then infused over at least 2 minutes, up to a total dose of 2 mEq · ml^{-1} (Fig. 42-15). Adequate pulmonary ventilation should be ensured during the infusion.

Other Drugs and Fluids

If it is believed that persistent depression has resulted from maternal opioid medication, naloxone should be given after adequate ventilation has been established (Table 42-6). The recommended dose of 0.1 mg · kg^{-1} may be injected iv, im, subcutaneously, or by endotracheal tube. The initial dose may be repeated as needed. Naloxone should be avoided in infants born to opioid-addicted mothers so as not to precipitate acute withdrawal. A severely asphyxiated newborn might require cardiotonic drugs during early resuscitation. Epinephrine should be used to treat asystole or persistent bradycardia despite adequate ventilation and external cardiac massage. A dose of 0.1–0.3 ml · kg^{-1} of a 1:10,000 solution should be injected iv

or by endotracheal tube, and repeated every 5 minutes if necessary.

Hypovolemia frequently follows severe birth asphyxia because a greater than normal portion of fetal blood remains in the placenta. The infant appears pale and has low arterial pressure, tachycardia, and tachypnea. Acute blood volume expansion may be accomplished with the iv administration of the following solutions over 5–10 minutes: O negative blood, cross-matched with the mother's blood, 10 ml · kg^{-1}; 5% albumin, 10 ml · kg^{-1}; and normal saline or lactated Ringer's solution, 10 ml · kg^{-1}.

Diagnostic Procedures

After the neonate is successfully resuscitated and stabilized, several diagnostic procedures are indicated. To rule out choanal atresia, each nostril should be obstructed. Because newborns must breathe through their noses, occlusion of the nostril on the patent side causes respiratory obstruction. To rule out esophageal atresia, a suction catheter is inserted into the stomach. Gastric contents are aspirated; volume in excess of 12 ml after vaginal delivery and 20 ml after cesarean section may result from an abnormality of the upper gastrointestinal tract.

ANESTHESIA FOR NONOBSTETRIC SURGERY IN THE PREGNANT WOMAN

Approximately 1.6–2.2% of pregnant women undergo surgery for reasons unrelated to parturition.[136,137] Apart from trauma, the most common emergencies are abdominal, involving torsion or rupture of an ovarian cyst and acute appendicitis, but breast

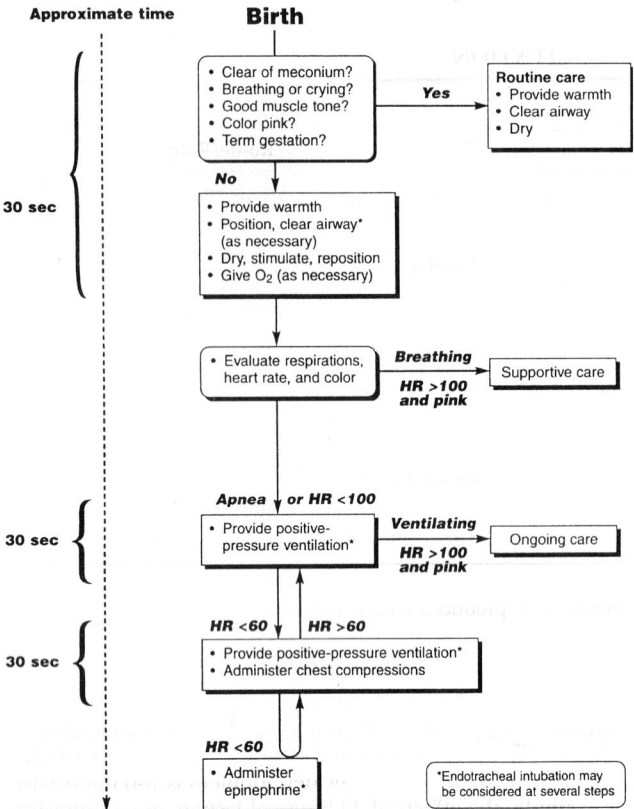

Approximate time

Birth

- Clear of meconium?
- Breathing or crying?
- Good muscle tone?
- Color pink?
- Term gestation?

Yes →

Routine care
- Provide warmth
- Clear airway
- Dry

No ↓

- Provide warmth
- Position, clear airway* (as necessary)
- Dry, stimulate, reposition
- Give O₂ (as necessary)

30 sec

- Evaluate respirations, heart rate, and color

Breathing → Supportive care
HR >100 and pink

Apnea or **HR <100**

- Provide positive-pressure ventilation*

Ventilating → Ongoing care
HR >100 and pink

30 sec

HR <60 ↓ **HR >60**

- Provide positive-pressure ventilation*
- Administer chest compressions

30 sec

HR <60 ↓

- Administer epinephrine*

*Endotracheal intubation may be considered at several steps

Figure 42-15. Algorithm for resuscitation of the newly born heart.

tumors are not uncommon, as are serious conditions such as intracranial aneurysms, cardiac valvular disease, and pheochromocytoma. Surgery to correct an incompetent cervix with Shirodkar or McDonald sutures is more related to the pregnancy itself.

When the necessity for surgery arises, anesthetic considerations are related to the alterations in maternal physiologic condition with advancing pregnancy, the teratogenicity of anesthetic drugs, the indirect effects of anesthesia on uteroplacental blood flow, and the potential for abortion or premature delivery. The risks must be balanced to provide the most favorable outcome for mother and child.

Four major studies have attempted to relate surgery and anesthesia during human pregnancy to fetal outcome as determined by anomalies, premature labor, or intrauterine death.[136–140] Although they failed to correlate surgery and anesthetic exposure with congenital anomalies, all of them demonstrated an increased incidence of fetal death, particularly after operations during the first trimester. No particular anesthetic agent or technique was implicated, and it seemed that the condition that necessitated surgery was the most relevant factor, with fetal mortality greatest after pelvic surgery or procedures performed for obstetric indications (*i.e.,* cervical incompetence).

Two studies deserve mention. A review was taken of the entire population of the province of Manitoba, Canada, between the years 1971 and 1978.[139] State health insurance records were used to identify approximately 2500 pregnant women who had undergone surgery during this period. Each patient was matched with a woman of similar age, living in the same area, with a pregnancy-related condition but no surgical intervention.

As in earlier studies, there was no increase in the incidence of congenital anomalies in the offspring of mothers who had had surgery. However, there was an increased risk of spontaneous abortion in women who had received general anesthesia during the first or second trimesters, which was most evident after gynecologic operations. Few of the surgical group had had procedures to treat cervical incompetence, suggesting that factors other than the obstetric condition itself might be important. The results also might have been influenced by the fact that a small number of gynecologic procedures were performed with anesthesia other than general, so that the effect of the surgical site alone could not be distinguished. The authors emphasized a multiplicity of factors other than choice of anesthetic agent (*e.g.,* diagnostic radiologic procedures, antibiotics, analgesics, infection, decreased uterine perfusion, and stress) that might have been responsible for the increased risk of abortion.

The largest study to date regarding reproductive outcome after surgery during pregnancy is a Swedish registry review covering the years 1973–1981.[140] During this period, there were a total of 720,000 births, 5405 of them after anesthesia and surgery during pregnancy. The results of this study are reassuring in that there was no increased incidence of congenital anomalies or stillbirths among infants exposed *in utero* to maternal surgery and anesthesia. However, in this group there was an increased frequency of very low and low birth weights, and of deaths within 168 hours after delivery. The reasons for this are unclear and are not related to any specific type of operation. The authors postulated that the maternal illness itself may have been a major contributor to adverse neonatal outcome.

Studies of the effects of chronic exposure to subanesthetic concentrations of inhalation agents on pregnancy offer a different approach to the question of outcome. Evidence originates from animal studies and from epidemiologic surveys performed on operating room personnel and their offspring. A nationwide survey conducted by the American Society of Anesthesiologists found a higher incidence of cancer among female anesthesia personnel as well as increased rates of abortion and congenital abnormalities in their infants.[141] Furthermore, the last of these misfortunes also applied, although to a lesser degree, to unexposed wives of male operating room personnel. The results of these studies have been disputed because of possible statistical inaccuracies and inappropriate choices of control groups. Another survey conducted among dentists and their female assistants compared the incidence of spontaneous abortions and congenital abnormalities among those exposed to inhalation anesthetics and those using only local anesthetics in their daily practices.[142] A significant increase in these complications occurred among assistants and wives of dentists exposed to inhalation drugs. Because of the controversy surrounding this issue, the American Society of Anesthesiologists commissioned an independent review by a team of epidemiologists.[143] This group found the data from most of the surveys to be flawed for a variety of reasons. These included responder bias, inappropriate control groups, failure to document exposure levels or verify medical data, and inability to ascertain which of the many environmental factors present in operating rooms might be blamed. The group concluded that, although exposed women appeared to have an increased risk of abortion (and, to a much lesser extent, congenital anomalies), the increase was small enough to be accounted for by bias and uncontrolled variables. Some of these problems are absent in two subsequent studies in which questionnaire information was matched with information obtained from medical records or registries of abortions, births, and congenital malformations.[144,145] Neither of these studies found significant deviations from expected rates of threatened abortion in exposed women. In addition, no differences in birth weight distribution, perinatal mortality, or congenital malformations in the infants of exposed and nonexposed women were

Table 42-6. THERAPEUTIC GUIDELINES FOR NEONATAL RESUSCITATION

Drug or Volume Expander	Concentration to Administer	Preparation (Based on Recommended Concentration)	Dosage	Route/Rate
Epinephrine	1:10,000	1 ml in a syringe Can dilute 1:1 with normal saline if given IT	0.1–0.3 ml · kg^{-1}	iv or IT Give rapidly
Volume expanders	Whole blood 5% albumin/saline solution Normal saline Lactated Ringer's	40 ml to be given by syringe or iv drip	10 ml · kg^{-1}	Give over 5–10 min
Sodium bicarbonate	0.5 mEq · ml^{-1} (4.2% solution)	20 ml in a syringe or two 10-ml prefilled syringes	2 mEq · kg^{-1}	iv Give slowly over at least 2 min (1 mEq · kg^{-1} · min^{-1})
Naloxone hydrochloride	Narcan Neonatal 0.02 mg · ml^{-1}	2 ml in a syringe	0.5 ml · kg^{-1}	iv, im, sc, or IT Give rapidly

im = intramuscular; iv = intravenous; IT = intratracheal; sc = subcutaneous.
Adapted from Bloom RS, Cropley C, Drew CR: Textbook of Neonatal Resuscitation. Reproduced with permission of the American Heart Association, American Academy of Pediatrics, Dallas, 1987.

detected.[145] The authors point out that their results do not indicate that there is no reproductive hazard relating to working in operating rooms; effects that might have been missed include very early abortions not requiring hospitalization, congenital abnormalities not apparent at birth, and infertility.

Direct Effects of Anesthetic Agents on Embryo and Fetus

The idea that surgical anesthesia, although deemed necessary for the patient, might have detrimental effects on the growth and development of the human fetus has led to a great deal of investigation, both *in vitro* and in experimental animals. These studies present difficulties in interpretation because the concentrations of anesthetic and the duration of exposure are frequently far in excess of what is clinically used and because most of the studies were performed in lower animals.

Animals exposed to toxic substances and anesthetics show a dose-related response, the first change being decreased fertility and increased fetal death. With increasing dose, the number of surviving fetuses with anomalies begins to increase, with the peak incidence occurring at a dose that causes a 50% incidence of fetal death.[146] The teratogenic effects between species and also within the same species vary significantly. The developmental stage is crucial, with dramatic sensitivity to exposure at certain times and little or no effect at a later time.[146] The period of organogenesis is most critical. In humans, it corresponds to the 15th–56th days of gestation.

Many congenital malfunctions show a pattern of multifactorial inheritance. In this mode, maldevelopment may result from a combination of factors in one person, such as hereditary predisposition, sensitivity to a given drug, and exposure at a vulnerable time in development. There are numerous other factors contributing to the potential teratogenicity of anesthesia. The cytotoxicity of anesthetic agents is closely associated with biodegradation, which, in turn, is influenced by oxygenation and hepatic blood flow. Thus, the complications associated with anesthesia, such as maternal hypoxia, hypotension, administration of vasopressors, hypercarbia, hypocarbia, and electrolyte disturbances, may possibly be a greater cause for concern as regards teratogenesis than the use of the agents

themselves.[147] Hypoxia is certainly a well documented teratogen in the incubating chick embryo.[148] The role of maternal carbohydrate metabolism on embryonic development is also important. For example, the effects of 48 hours of fasting and administration of insulin to pregnant rats have included a large number of skeletal deformities.[149]

Experimental evidence on exposure to specific drugs and agents is highlighted briefly, with the consideration that it is difficult to extrapolate laboratory data to the clinical situation in humans. Very large numbers of patients must be exposed to a suspected teratogen before its safety can be ascertained. Complicating factors include the frequency of maternal exposure to a multiplicity of drugs; the difficulty in separating the effects of the underlying disease process and surgical treatment from those of the drug administered; differing degrees of risk with stage of gestation; and the variety, rather than the consistency, of anomalies that appear in association with one agent. Of the premedicants, anticholinergics have not been found to be teratogenic, whereas tranquilizers and sedatives such as phenothiazines and barbiturates produce anomalies in some species.[150] Several reports have described a specific relationship between diazepam and oral clefts, but another study has not confirmed this.[151,152] Intravenous agents such as thiopental, methohexital, and ketamine in doses normally used in the operating room have not been associated with birth defects. Only one study has shown musculoskeletal deformities involving the joints after infusion of a muscle relaxant (*d*-tubocurarine) in the chick embryo between the 7th and 15th day of incubation.[153] Local anesthetics have not been shown to be teratogenic in animals or humans.[147] Halogenated inhalation drugs have produced conflicting results. Pregnant rats exposed to halothane 0.8% for 12 hours at various times during gestation have increased incidences of anomalous skeletal development and fetal death.[154] Other investigators have failed to show teratogenic effects of halothane in rats, rabbits, and mice exposed to subanesthetic concentrations for brief periods. Subanesthetic concentrations of enflurane do not appear to be teratogenic. However, mice exposed to 1% enflurane for 4 h · day^{-1} on days 6–15 of gestation showed an increased incidence of cleft palates and minor skeletal and visceral abnormalities.[155] In a subsequent study by the same authors, teratogenic changes after exposure to 0.6% isoflurane in mice were similar to those found with enflurane, but the incidence of cleft palate was six times more frequent (12 vs. 1.9%).[156] Cleft palate readily develops in mice, and its occurrence as an isolated finding suggests that this might be a species-specific response. To clarify the results from earlier studies, rats were exposed to 0.75 MAC halothane, isoflurane, or enflurane; 0.55 MAC nitrous oxide; or a known teratogen, retinoic acid, for two 6-hour periods at three different stages of pregnancy.[157] No major morphologic abnormalities occurred in any of the anesthetic-exposed groups.

Nitrous oxide has been the most extensively investigated agent since the 1955 observation that leukopenia developed in patients with tetanus after they inhaled nitrous oxide for several days. Numerous studies have demonstrated significant effects on fetal growth, skeletal development, and death rate in both pregnant rats and incubating chicks exposed to concentrations of between 50 and 80%, for periods ranging from hours to days.[158] The question arises whether adverse effects at such high doses resulted from the anesthetic itself or from the accompanying physiologic derangements.

Although the mechanism of the teratogenic effect of nitrous oxide has not been determined, it may be related to the inhibitory effect of the agent on methionine synthetase activity and vitamin B_{12}. A dose-dependent decrease in both maternal and fetal methionine synthetase activity occurred in pregnant rats receiving 10 or 50% nitrous oxide for periods ranging from 60–240 minutes.[159] It is possible that failure of this enzyme to convert homocysteine to the essential amino acid methionine may lead to abnormalities of myelination of nerve fibers (Fig. 42-16). Furthermore, inhibition of methionine synthesis results in decreased thymidine production, which in turn can lead to decreased DNA synthesis and inhibition of cell division. Because there is evidence that nitrous oxide adversely affects methionine synthetase activity, it has been recommended that it not be administered to pregnant women in the first two trimesters.[160,161] However, a more recent human study demonstrated no significant changes in plasma methionine concentrations after anesthesia with 60–70% nitrous oxide for up to 4 hours.[162] Two other reviews of exposure to this agent, this time for cervical cerclage procedures, showed no effects on fetal outcome.[163,164] Further, in the already mentioned Swedish birth registry study, nitrous oxide was administered to almost all of 2929 patients receiving general anesthesia without adverse fetal consequences.[140] In rats, the teratogenic effects of nitrous oxide could be prevented by the concomitant administration of isoflurane or halothane.[165] It is controversial whether pretreatment with folinic acid, the concentration of which is reduced when methionine synthetase is inhibited, affords protection against the effects of nitrous oxide.[165] Because a single exposure to anesthetic agents seems unlikely to result in fetal abnormality, the selection of agent should be based on specific surgical requirements.

Indirect Effects of Agents and Techniques

The adequacy of the uteroplacental circulation, so vital to the well-being of the fetus, is easily affected by drugs and anesthetic procedures. As discussed previously, perfusion of the intervillous space of the placenta may be diminished consequent on maternal systemic hypotension, which in turn may result from the use of epidural or spinal anesthesia, from aortocaval compression with the patient in the supine position, or from hemorrhage. Similarly, increased uterine activity may result in reduced placental perfusion. Thus, the use of α-adrenergic drugs to correct maternal hypotension and anesthetics such as ketamine (in doses above $1 \text{ mg} \cdot \text{kg}^{-1}$) may produce increased uterine tone sufficient to endanger the fetus. Severe hyperventilation of the mother may also reduce uterine blood flow. Finally, it has been shown in experimental animals that epinephrine or norepinephrine infusion results in decreased uterine blood flow and deterioration of fetal condition. Maternal pain and apprehension may similarly affect the fetus.[166]

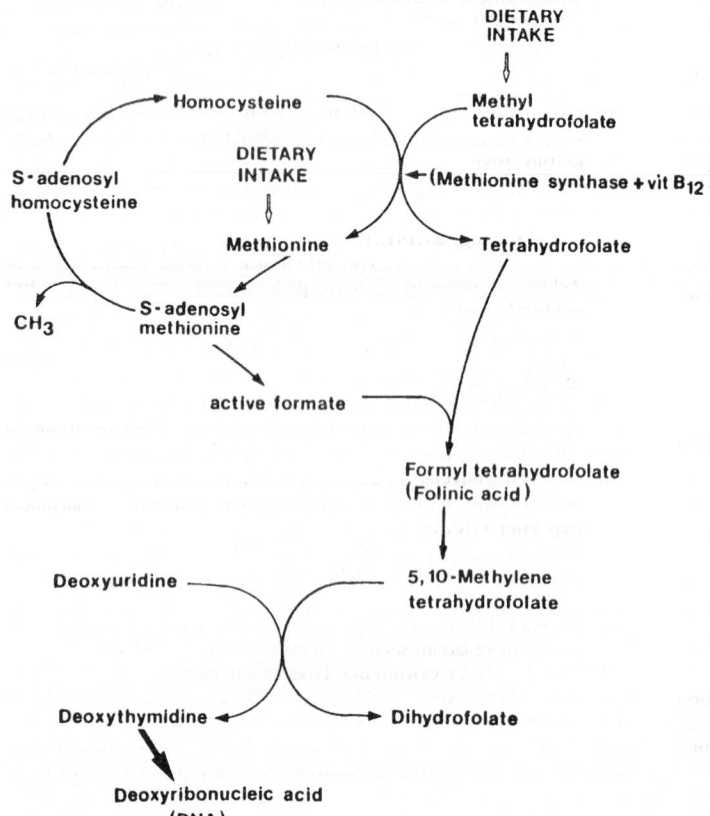

Figure 42-16. Abridged metabolic map showing the relationship between methionine and deoxythymidine syntheses. (Reprinted with permission from Nunn JF: Interaction of nitrous oxide and vitamin B_{12}. Trends Pharmacol Sci 5:225, 1984.)

Practical Suggestions

It is generally agreed that only emergency surgery should be performed during pregnancy, particularly in the first trimester. The possibility of pregnancy should be considered in all female surgical patients of reproductive age. Based on the maternal and fetal hazards already described, the following approach to anesthesia seems indicated:

1. The patient's apprehension should be allayed as much as possible by personal reassurance during the preanesthetic visit and by adequate sedation and premedication.
2. Pain should be relieved whenever present.
3. An antacid, 15–30 ml, should be administered within half an hour before induction of anesthesia. Ranitidine and metoclopramide may be useful.
4. Beginning in the second trimester, uterine displacement must be maintained at all times.
5. Hypotension related to spinal or epidural anesthesia should be prevented as much as possible by rapid iv infusion of crystalloid solution before induction. If the mother becomes hypotensive, ephedrine should be promptly administered iv.
6. General anesthesia should be preceded by careful denitrogenation.
7. The risk of aspiration should be minimized by application of cricoid pressure and rapid tracheal intubation with a cuffed tube.
8. To reduce fetal hazard, particularly during the first trimester, it appears preferable to choose drugs with a long history of safety; these drugs include thiopental, morphine, meperidine, muscle relaxants, and low concentrations of nitrous oxide.
9. Avoid maternal hyperventilation and monitor end-expiratory $Paco_2$ or arterial blood gases.
10. Fetal heart rate should be monitored continuously throughout surgery and anesthesia, provided that placement of the transducer does not encroach on the surgical field[167] (this becomes technically feasible from the 16th week of pregnancy). Uterine tone may also be monitored with an external tocodynamometer if the uterus reaches the umbilicus or above.
11. Monitoring of uterine activity should be continued after operation, and tocolytic agents may be required.
12. Special procedures such as hypothermia and induced hypotension might be necessary to facilitate surgery, despite the potential fetal hazard. It is reassuring to know that there was successful fetal outcome after both procedures for intracranial operations.[168,169] There are numerous reports of cardiopulmonary bypass being performed during pregnancy, with generally good maternal and fetal results.[170,171]

REFERENCES

1. Lund CJ, Donovan JC: Blood volume during pregnancy. Am J Obstet Gynecol 98:393, 1967
2. Maternal adaptation to pregnancy. In Pritchard JA, Macdonald PC (eds): Williams Obstetrics, p 236. New York, Appleton-Century-Crofts, 1980
3. Wildsmith JAW: Serum pseudocholinesterase, pregnancy and suxamethonium. Anaesthesia 27:90, 1972
4. Coryell MN, Beach EF, Robinson AR et al: Metabolism of women during the reproductive cycle: XVII. Changes in electrophoretic patterns of plasma proteins throughout the cycle and following delivery. J Clin Invest 29:1559, 1950
5. Goodman RP, Killom AP, Brash AR et al: Prostacyclin production during pregnancy: Comparison of production during normal pregnancy and pregnancy complicated by hypertension. Am J Obstet Gynecol 142:817, 1982
6. Kerr MG, Scott DB, Samuel E: Studies of the inferior vena cava in late pregnancy. BMJ 1:532, 1964
7. Howard BK, Goodson JH, Mengert WF: Supine hypotensive syndrome in late pregnancy. Obstet Gynecol 1:371, 1953
8. Prowse CM, Gaensler EA: Respiratory and acid-base changes during pregnancy. Anesthesiology 26:381, 1965
9. Moya F, Smith BE: Uptake, distribution and placental transport of drugs and anesthetics. Anesthesiology 26:465, 1965
10. Archer GW, Marx GF: Arterial oxygenation during apnoea in parturient women. Br J Anaesth 46:358, 1974
11. Datta S, Kitzmiller JL, Naulty JS et al: Acid-base status of diabetic mothers and their infants following spinal anesthesia for cesarean section. Anesth Analg 61:662, 1982
12. Simpson KH, Stakes AF, Miller M: Pregnancy delays paracetamol absorption and gastric emptying in patients undergoing surgery. Br J Anaesth 60:24, 1988
13. Davison JS, Davison MC, Hay DM: Gastric emptying time in late pregnancy and labour. Journal of Obstetrics and Gynaecology of the British Commonwealth 77:37, 1970
14. Brock-Utne JG, Dow TGB, Dimopoulos GE et al: Gastric and lower oesophageal sphincter (LOS) pressures in early pregnancy. Br J Anaesth 53:381, 1981
15. Wyner J, Cohen SE: Gastric volume in early pregnancy: Effect of metoclopramide. Anesthesiology 57:209, 1982
16. Cohen SE, Woods WA, Wyner J: Antiemetic efficacy of droperidol and metoclopramide. Anesthesiology 60:67, 1984
17. Scheller MS, Sears KL: Post-operative neurologic dysfunction associated with preoperative administration of metoclopramide. Anesth Analg 66:274, 1987
18. Gin T, Chan MTV: Decreased minimum alveolar concentration of isoflurane in pregnant humans. Anesthesiology 81:829, 1994
19. Datta S, Lambert DH, Gregus J et al: Differential sensitivities of mammalian nerve fibers during pregnancy. Anesth Analg 62:1070, 1983
20. Reynold F, Knott C: Pharmacokinetics in pregnancy and placental drug transfer. In Milligan SR (ed): Oxford Reviews of Reproduction Biology, Vol II, p 389. New York, Oxford University Press, 1989
21. Brown WU, Bell GC, Alper MH: Acidosis, local anesthetics and the newborn. Obstet Gynecol 48:27, 1976
22. Hamshaw-Thomas A, Rogerson N, Reynolds F: Transfer of bupivacaine, lignocaine and pethidine across the rabbit placenta: Influence of maternal protein binding and fetal flow. Placenta 5:61, 1984
23. Kennedy RL, Miller RP, Bell JU et al: Uptake and distribution of bupivacaine in fetal lambs. Anesthesiology 65:247, 1986
24. Kuhnert PM, Kuhnert BR, Stitts BS et al: The use of a selected ion monitoring technique to study the disposition of bupivacaine in mother, fetus and neonate following epidural anesthesia for cesarean section. Anesthesiology 55:611, 1981
25. Kuhnert BR, Philipson EH, Pimental R et al: Lidocaine disposition in mother, fetus, and neonate after spinal anesthesia. Anesth Analg 65:139, 1986
26. Morishima HO, Daniel SS, Finster M et al: Transmission of mepivacaine hydrochloride (Carbocaine) across the human placenta. Anesthesiology 27:147, 1966
27. Kuhnert BR, Kuhnert PM, Prochaska AL et al: Plasma levels of 2-chloroprocaine in obstetric patients and their neonates after epidural anesthesia. Anesthesiology 53:21, 1980
28. Morgan DJ, Blackman GL, Paul JD et al: Pharmacokinetics and plasma binding of thiopental: II. Studies at cesarean section. Anesthesiology 54:474, 1981
29. Pihlajamäki K, Kanto J, Lindberg R et al: Extradural administration of bupivacaine: Pharmacokinetics and metabolism in pregnant and non-pregnant women. Br J Anaesth 64:556, 1990
30. Idanpaan-Heikkila JE, Taska RJ, Allen HA et al: Placental transfer of diazepam:14C in mice, hamsters and monkeys. J Pharmacol Exp Ther 176:752, 1971
31. Haram K, Bakke OM, Johannessen KH et al: Transplacental passage of diazepam during labor: Influence of uterine contractions. Clin Pharmacol Ther 24:590, 1978
32. Kosaka Y, Takahashi T, Mark LC: Intravenous thiobarbiturate anesthesia for cesarean section. Anesthesiology 31:489, 1969
33. Morishima HO, Covino BG: Toxicity and distribution of lidocaine in nonasphyxiated and asphyxiated baboon fetuses. Anesthesiology 54:182, 1981
34. Morishima HO, Finster M, Pedersen H et al: Pharmacokinetics of lidocaine in fetal and neonatal lambs and adult sheep. Anesthesiology 50:431, 1979
35. Mihaly GW, Moore RG, Thomas J et al: The pharmacokinetics and

metabolism of the anilide local anaesthetics in neonates. Eur J Clin Pharmacol 13:143, 1978

36. Finster M, Poppers PJ, Sinclair JC et al: Accidental intoxication of the fetus with local anesthetic drug during caudal anesthesia. Am J Obstet Gynecol 92:922, 1965

37. Morishima HO, Pedersen H, Finster M et al: Toxicity of lidocaine in adult, newborn and fetal sheep. Anesthesiology 55:57, 1981

38. Gale R, Ferguson JE II, Stevenson D: Effect of epidural analgesia with bupivacaine hydrochloride on neonatal bilirubin production. Obstet Gynecol 70:692, 1987

39. Brockhurst NJ, Littleford JA, Halpern SH: The neurological and adaptive capacity score: A systematic review of its use in obstetric anesthesia research. Anesthesiology 92: 237, 2000

40. Morishima HO, Yeh M-N, James LS: Reduced uterine blood flow and fetal hypoxemia with acute maternal stress: Experimental observation in the pregnant baboon. Am J Obstet Gynecol 134:270, 1979

41. Ueland K, Hansen JM: Maternal cardiovascular dynamics: III. Labor and delivery under local and caudal analgesia. Am J Obstet Gynecol 103:8, 1969

42. Moir DD, Willocks J: Management of incoordinate uterine action under continuous epidural analgesia. BMJ 2:396, 1967

43. Miller FC, Petrie RH, Arce JJ et al: Hyperventilation during labor. Am J Obstet Gynecol 120:489, 1974

44. Melzack R, Taenzer P, Feldman P et al: Labour is still painful after prepared childbirth training. CMAJ 125:357, 1981

45. Scott JR, Rose NB: Effect of psychoprophylaxis (Lamaze preparation) on labor and delivery in primiparas. N Engl J Med 294:1205, 1976

46. Kuhnert BR, Linn PL, Kennard MJ et al: Effect of low doses of meperidine on neonatal behavior. Anesth Analg 64:335, 1985

47. Eisele JH, Wright R, Rogge P: Newborn and maternal fentanyl levels at cesarean section. Anesth Analg 61:179, 1982

48. Muir HA, Breen T, Campbell DC et al: Is intravenous PCA fentanyl an effective method for providing labor analgesia? Anesthesiology (suppl):A28, 1999

49. Kapila A, Glass PS, Jacobs JR et al: Measured cortex and sensitive half times of remifentanil and alfentanil. Anesthesiology 83:968, 1995

50. Kan RE, Hughes SC, Rosen M et al: Intravenous remifentanil: placental transfer, maternal and neonatal effects. Anesthesiology 88:1467, 1998

51. Maduska AL, Hajghassemali M: A double blind comparison of butorphanol and meperidine in labor: Maternal pain relief and effect on newborn. Can Anaesth Soc J 25:398, 1978

52. Chestnut DH, Vincent RD, McGrath JM et al: Does early administration of epidural analgesia affect obstetric outcome in nulliparous women who are receiving intravenous oxytocin? Anesthesiology 80:1193, 1994

53. Chestnut DH, McGrath JM, Vincent RD et al: Does early administration of epidural analgesia affect obstetric outcome in nulliparous women who are in spontaneous labor? Anesthesiology 80:1201, 1994

54. Thorp JA, Hu DH, Albin RM et al: The effect of intrapartum epidural analgesia on nulliparous labor: A randomized, controlled, prospective trial. Am J Obstet Gynecol 169:851, 1993

55. Sharma SK, Sidawi JE, Ramin SM et al: Cesarean delivery: A randomized trial of epidural versus patient controlled meperidine analgesia during labor. Anesthesiology 87:487, 1997

56. Halpern SH, Leighton BL, Ohlsson A et al: Effect of epidural vs parenteral opioid analgesia in the progress of labor: A meta-analysis. JAMA 280:2105, 1998

57. Ramin SM, Gambling DR, Lucas MJ et al: Randomized trial of epidural versus intravenous analgesia in labor. Obstet Gynecol 86:783, 1995

58. American College of Obstetrics and Gynecology: Obstetric forceps. ACOG Committee on Obstetrics, Maternal and Fetal Medicine, Committee Opinion No. 71, 1989

59. Chestnut DH, Laszewski LJ, Pollack RL et al: Continuous epidural infusion of 0.0625% bupivacaine-0.0002% fentanyl during the second stage of labor. Anesthesiology 72:613, 1990

60. Birnbach DJ, Chestnut DH: The epidural test dose in obstetric practice: Has it outlived its usefulness? Anesth Analg 88:971, 1999

61. Norris MC, Ferrenbach D, Dalman H et al: Does epinephrine improve the diagnostic accuracy of aspiration during labor epidural analgesia? Anesth Analg 88:1073, 1999

62. Viscomi C, Eisenach JC: Patient-controlled epidural analgesia during labor. Obstet Gynecol 77:348, 1991

63. Rigler ML, Drasner K, Krejcie TC et al: Cauda equina syndrome after continuous spinal anesthesia. Anesth Analg 72:275, 1991

64. Arkoosh VA, Palmer CM, Van Maren GA et al: Continuous intrathecal labor analgesia: Safety and efficacy. Anesthesiology (suppl):A8, 1998

65. Campbell DC, Camann WR, Datta S: The addition of bupivacaine to intrathecal sufentanil for labor analgesia. Anesth Analg 81:305, 1995

66. Collis RE, Davies DWL, Aveling W: Randomized comparison of combined spinal epidural and standard epidural analgesia in labour. Lancet 345:1413, 1995

67. McLeod A, Fernando R, Page F et al: An assessment of maternal balance and gait using computerized posturograph. Anesthesiology (suppl):A8, 1999

68. Cohen SE, Cherry CM, Holbrook RH et al: Intrathecal sufentanil for labor analgesia: Sensory changes, side-effects and fetal heart rate changes. Anesth Analg 77:1155, 1993

69. Clarke VT, Smiley RM, Finster M: Uterine hyperactivity after intrathecal injection of fentanyl for analgesia during labor: A cause of fetal bradycardia? Anesthesiology 81:1083, 1994

70. O'Gorman DA, Birnbach DJ, Kuczkowski KM et al: Use of umbilical flow velocimetry in the assessment of the pathogenesis of fetal bradycardia following combined spinal epidural analgesia in parturients. Anesthesiology (suppl):A2, 2000

71. Riley ET, Vogel TM, El-Sayed YY et al: Patient selection bias contributes to an increased incidence of fetal bradycardia after combined spinal epidural analgesia for labor. Anesthesiology 91:A1054, 1999

72. Nielson PE, Erickson R, Abouleish E et al: Fetal heart rate changes after intrathecal sufentanil or epidural bupivacaine for labor analgesia: incidence and clinical significance. Anesth Analg 83:742, 1996

73. Albright GA, Forester RM: Does combined epidural analgesia with subarachnoid sufentanil increase the incidence of emergency cesarean section? Regional Anesthesia 22:400, 1997

74. Norris MC, Grieco WM, Borkowski M et al: Complications of labor analgesia: Epidural versus combined spinal epidural techniques. Anesth Analg 79:529, 1995

75. Leighton BL, Arkoosh VA, Haffnagle S et al: The dermatomal spread of epidural bupivacaine with and without prior intrathecal sufentanil. Anesth Analg 83:526, 1996

76. Baxi LV, Petrie RH, James LS: Human fetal oxygenation following paracervical block. Am J Obstet Gynecol 135:1109, 1979

77. Leighton BL, Halpern SH, Wilson DB: Lumbar sympathetic blocks speed early and second stage induced labor in nulliparous women. Anesthesiology 90:1039, 1999

78. Carstoniu J, Levytam S, Norman P et al: Nitrous oxide in early labor: Safety and analgesic efficacy assessed by a double-blind, placebo controlled study. Anesthesiology 80:30, 1994

79. Peng ATC, Gorman RS, Shulman SM et al: Intravenous nitroglycerin for uterine relaxation in the postpartum patient with retained placenta. Anesthesiology 71:172, 1989

80. DeSimone CA, Norris MC, Leighton BL: Intravenous nitroglycerin aids manual extraction of a retained placenta. Anesthesiology 73:787, 1990

81. Hawkins JL, Gibbs CP, Orleans M et al: Obstetric anesthesia workforce survey: 1992 vs 1981. Anesthesiology 81:A1128, 1994

82. Shnider SM, Levinson G: Anesthesia for cesarean section. In Shnider SM, Levinson G (eds): Anesthesia for Obstetrics, 2nd ed, p 159. Baltimore, Williams & Wilkins, 1987

83. Rout CC, Rocke DA, Levin J et al: A reevaluation of the role of crystalloid preload in the prevention of hypotension associated with spinal anesthesia for elective cesarean section. Anesthesiology 79:262, 1993

84. Marx GF, Luykx WM, Cohen S: Fetal-neonatal status following cesarean section for fetal distress. Br J Anaesth 56:1009, 1984

85. Norris MC: Height, weight and the spread of subarachnoid hyperbaric bupivacaine in the term parturient. Anesth Analg 67:555, 1988

86. Hunt CO, Naulty S, Bader AM et al: Perioperative analgesia with subarachnoid fentanyl-bupivacaine for cesarean delivery. Anesthesiology 71:535, 1989

87. Leighton BL, Norris MC, Sosis M et al: Limitations of epinephrine as a marker of intravascular injection in laboring women. Anesthesiology 66:688, 1987

88. Leighton BL, DeSimone CA, Norris MC et al: Isoproterenol is an

effective marker for intravenous injection in laboring women. Anesthesiology 71:206, 1989

89. Leighton BL, Norris MC, DeSimone CA *et al:* The air test as a clinically useful indicator of intravenously placed epidural catheters. Anesthesiology 73:610, 1990

90. Gissen AJ, Datta S, Lambert D: The chloroprocaine controversy: Is chloroprocaine neurotoxic? Regional Anaesthesia 9:135, 1984

91. Hynson JM, Sessler DI, Glosten B: Back pain in volunteers after epidural anesthesia with chloroprocaine. Anesth Analg 72:253, 1991

92. Albright GA: Cardiac arrest following regional anesthesia with etidocaine or bupivacaine. Anesthesiology 51:285, 1979

93. Tanz RD, Heskett T, Loehning RW *et al:* Comparative cardiotoxicity of bupivacaine and lidocaine in the isolated perfused mammalian heart. Anesth Analg 63:549, 1984

94. James FM III, Crawford JS, Hopkinson R *et al:* A comparison of general anesthesia and lumbar epidural analgesia for elective cesarean section. Anesth Analg 56:228, 1977

95. Datta S, Ostheimer GW, Weiss JB *et al:* Neonatal effect of prolonged anesthetic induction for cesarean section. Obstet Gynecol 58:331, 1981

96. Marx GF, Mateo CV: Effects of different oxygen concentrations during general anaesthesia for elective caesarean section. Canadian Anaesthetists Society Journal 18:587, 1971

97. Brizgys RV, Dailey PA, Shnider SM *et al:* The incidence and neonatal effects of maternal hypotension during epidural anesthesia for cesarean section. Anesthesiology 67:782, 1987

98. Ueyama H, He YL, Tanigami H, *et al:* Effects of crystalloid and colloid preload or blood volume in the parturient undergoing spinal anesthesia for elective cesarean section. Anesthesiology 91:1571, 1999

99. Rout CC, Roche DA, Levin J *et al:* A reevaluation of the role of crystalloid preload in the prevention of hypertension associated with spinal anesthesia for elective cesarean section. Anesthesiology 79:262, 1993

100. Rout CC, Roche DA: Spinal hypotension associated with cesarean section: Will preload ever work? Anesthesiology 91:1565, 1999

101. Ramanathan S, Grant GJ: Vasopressor therapy for hypotension due to epidural anaesthesia. Acta Anaesthesiol Scand 32:559, 1988

102. Kasten GW, Martin ST: Resuscitation from bupivacaine-induced cardiovascular toxicity during partial inferior vena cava occlusion. Anesth Analg 65:341, 1986

103. Jarvis AP, Greenwalt JW, Fagraeus L: Intravenous caffeine for postdural puncture headache. Anesth Analg 65:313, 1986

104. Camann WR, Murray RS, Mushlin PS *et al:* Effects of oral caffeine on postdural puncture headache: A double-blind, placebo-controlled trial. Anesth Analg 70:181, 1990

105. Schwalbe SS, Schiffmiller MW, Marx GF: Theophylline for postdural puncture headache (abstract). Anesthesiology 75:A1082, 1991

106. Brownridge P: The management of headache following accidental dural puncture in obstetric patients. Anaesth Intensive Care 11:4, 1983

107. Walsh SW: Preeclampsia: An imbalance in placental prostacyclin and thromboxane production. Am J Obstet Gynecol 152:335, 1985

108. Roberts JM, Taylor RN, Musci TJ *et al:* Preeclampsia: An endothelial cell disorder. Am J Obstet Gynecol 161:1200, 1989

109. Chesley LC: Plasma and red cell volumes during pregnancy. Am J Obstet Gynecol 112:440, 1972

110. Groenendijk R, Trimbos MJ, Wallenburg HCS: Hemodynamic measurements in preeclampsia: Preliminary observations. Am J Obstet Gynecol 150:232, 1984

111. Cotton DB, Gonik B, Dorman K *et al:* Cardiovascular alterations in severe pregnancy-induced hypertension: Relationship of central venous pressure to pulmonary capillary wedge pressure. Am J Obstet Gynecol 151:762, 1985

112. Rodgers RPC, Levin J: A critical reappraisal of the bleeding time. Semin Thromb Hemost 161:1, 1990

113. Hogg B, Hauth JC, Caritis SN *et al:* Safety of labor epidural anesthesia for women with severe hypertensive disease. Am J Obstet Gynecol 181:1099, 1999

114. Newsome LR, Bramwell RS, Curling PE: Severe preeclampsia: Hemodynamic effects of lumbar epidural anesthesia. Anesth Analg 65:31, 1986

115. Jouppila P, Jouppila R, Hollmen A *et al:* Lumbar epidural analgesia to improve intervillous blood flow during labor in severe preeclampsia. Obstet Gynecol 59:158, 1982

116. Ramanathan J, Botorff M, Jeter JN *et al:* The pharmacokinetics and maternal and neonatal effects of epidural lidocaine in preeclampsia. Anesth Analg 65:120, 1986

117. Wallace DH, Leveno KJ, Cunningham FG *et al:* Randomized comparison of general and regional anesthesia for cesarean delivery in pregnancies complicated by severe preeclampsia. Obstet Gynecol 86:193, 1995

118. Hood DD, Curry R: Spinal versus epidural anesthesia for cesarean section in severely preeclamptic patients: a retrospective survey. Anesthesiology 90:1276, 1999

119. Clark SL, Koonings PP, Phelan JP: Placenta previa/accreta and prior cesarean section. Obstet Gynecol 66:89, 1985

120. Chestnut DH, Dewan DM, Redick LF *et al:* Anesthetic management for obstetric hysterectomy: A multi-institutional study. Anesthesiology 70:607, 1989

121. Benedetti TJ: Maternal complications of parenteral beta-sympathomimetic therapy for premature labor. Am J Obstet Gynecol 145:1, 1983

122. Krauer B, Krauer F, Hytten F: Drug prescribing in pregnancy. Current Reviews in Obstetrics and Gynaecology, Vol 7, p 44. Edinburgh, Churchill Livingstone, 1984

123. Kaltreider DF: Premature labor and meperidine analgesia. Am J Obstet Gynecol 99:989, 1967

124. Santos AC, Yun EM, Bobby PD *et al:* The effects of bupivacaine, L nitro-L-arginine-methyl-ester and phenylephrine on cardiovascular adaptations to asphyxia in the preterm fetal lamb. Anesth Analg 84:1299, 1997

125. Morishima HO, Pedersen H, Santos AC *et al:* Adverse effects of maternally administered lidocaine on the asphyxiated preterm fetal lamb. Anesthesiology 71:110, 1989

126. Martin CB, Gingerich B: Factors affecting the fetal heart rate: Genesis of FHR patterns. Journal of Obstetric and Gynecologic Nursing 5(suppl):30S, 1976

127. Wright RG, Shnider SM, Levinson G *et al:* The effect of maternal administration of ephedrine on fetal heart rate and variability. Obstet Gynecol 57:734, 1981

128. Finster M, Petrie RH: Monitoring of the fetus. Anesthesiology 45:198, 1976

129. Oats JN, Vasey DP, Waldron BA: Effects of ketamine on the pregnant uterus. Br J Anaesth 51:1163, 1979

130. Adamsons K, Beard RW, Cosmi EV *et al:* The validity of capillary blood in the assessment of the acid-base state of the fetus. In Adamsons K (ed): Diagnosis and Treatment of Fetal Disorders, p 175. New York, Springer-Verlag, 1968

131. Beard RW: Fetal blood sampling. Br J Hosp Med 3:523, 1970

132. Bowe ET, Beard RW, Finster M *et al:* Reliability of fetal blood sampling. Am J Obstet Gynecol 107:279, 1970

133. Gibbs RS, Listwa HM, Read JA: The effect of internal monitoring on maternal infection following cesarean section. Obstet Gynecol 48:653, 1976

134. MacDonald D, Grant A, Sheridan-Pereira M *et al:* The Dublin randomized controlled trial of intrapartum fetal heart rate monitoring. Am J Obstet Gynecol 152:524, 1985

135. Adamsons K, Behrman R, Dawes GS *et al:* Resuscitation by positive pressure ventilation and Tris-hydroxymethylaminomethane of rhesus monkeys asphyxiated at birth. J Pediatr 65:807, 1964

136. Shnider SM, Webster GM: Maternal and fetal hazards of surgery during pregnancy. Am J Obstet Gynecol 92:891, 1965

137. Brodsky JB, Cohen EN, Brown BW Jr *et al:* Surgery during pregnancy and fetal outcome. Am J Obstet Gynecol 138:1165, 1980

138. Smith BE: Fetal prognosis after anesthesia during gestation. Anesth Analg 42:521, 1963

139. Duncan PG, Pope WDB, Cohen MM *et al:* Fetal risk of anesthesia and surgery during pregnancy. Anesthesiology 64:790, 1986

140. Mazze RI, Källén B: Reproductive outcome after anesthesia and operation during pregnancy: A registry study of 5405 cases. Am J Obstet Gynecol 161:1178, 1989

141. Ad Hoc Committee on the Effect of Trace Anesthetics on the Health of Operating Room Personnel, American Society of Anesthesiologists: Occupational disease among operating room personnel: A national study. Anesthesiology 41:321, 1974

142. Cohen EN, Brown BW, Wu M: Anesthetic health hazards in the dental operatory. Anesthesiology 51:S256, 1976

143. Buring JE, Hennekens CH, Mayrent SL: Health experiences of operating room personnel. Anesthesiology 62:325, 1985

144. Axelsson G, Rylander R: Exposure to anesthetic gases and sponta-

neous abortion: Response bias in postal questionnaire study. Int J Epidemiol 11:250, 1982

145. Ericson HA, Källén AJB: Hospitalization for miscarriage and delivery outcome among Swedish nurses working in operating rooms, 1973–1978. Anesth Analg 64:981, 1985

146. Smith BE: Teratogenicity of inhalation anesthetics. In: Progress in Anesthesiology, p 589. London, Excerpta Medica, 1970

147. Heinonen OP, Slone O, Shapiro S: Birth Defects and Drugs in Pregnancy, p 516. Littleton, Massachusetts, Publishing Sciences Group, 1977

148. Grabowski CT, Paar JA: The teratogenic effects of graded doses of hypoxia on the chick embryo. Am J Anat 103:313, 1958

149. Hannah RS, Moore KL: Effects of fasting and insulin on skeletal development in rats. Teratology 4:135, 1971

150. Hartz SC, Heinonen OP, Shapiro S et al: Antenatal exposure to meprobamate and chlordiazepoxide in relation to malformations, mental development and childhood mortality. N Engl J Med 292:726, 1975

151. Sáxen I, Sáxen L: Association between maternal intake of diazepam and oral clefts. Lancet 2:498, 1975

152. Safra MJ, Oakley GP: Association between cleft lip with or without cleft palate and prenatal exposure to diazepam. Lancet 2:478, 1975

153. Drachman DB, Coulombre AJ: Experimental clubfoot and arthrogryposis multiplex congenita. Lancet 2:523, 1962

154. Basford AB, Fink BR: The teratogenicity of halothane in the rat. Anesthesiology 29:1167, 1968

155. Wharton RS, Mazze RI, Wilson AI: Reproduction and fetal development in mice chronically exposed to enflurane. Anesthesiology 54:505, 1981

156. Mazze RI, Wilson AI, Rice SA et al: Effects of isoflurane on reproduction and fetal development in mice. Anesth Analg 63:249, 1984

157. Mazze RI, Fujinaga M, Rice SA et al: Reproductive and teratogenic effects of nitrous oxide, halothane, isoflurane and enflurane in Sprague-Dawley rats. Anesthesiology 64:339, 1986

158. Smith BE, Gaub MI, Moya F: Teratogenic effects of anesthetic agents: Nitrous oxide. Anesth Analg 44:726, 1965

159. Baden JM, Serra M, Mazze RI: Inhibition of fetal methionine synthase by nitrous oxide. Br J Anaesth 56:523, 1984

160. Nunn JF, Chanarin I: Nitrous oxide inactivates methionine synthetase. In Eger EI II (ed): Nitrous Oxide/N₂O, p 221. New York, Elsevier-Dutton, 1985

161. Eger EI II: Should we not use nitrous oxide? In Eger EI II (ed): Nitrous Oxide/N₂O, p 339. New York, Elsevier-Dutton, 1985

162. Nunn JF, Sharer NM, Battiglieri T et al: Effect of short-term administration of nitrous oxide on plasma concentration of methionine, tryptophan, phenylalanine, and S-adenosyl methionine in man. Br J Anaesth 58:1, 1986

163. Crawford JS, Lewis M: Nitrous oxide in early human pregnancy. Anaesthesia 41:900, 1986

164. Aldridge LM, Tunstall ME: Nitrous oxide and the fetus: A review and the results of a retrospective study of 175 cases of anaesthesia for insertion of Shirodkar suture. Br J Anaesth 58:1348, 1986

165. Fujinaga M, Baden JM, Yhap EO et al: Halothane and isoflurane prevent the teratogenic effects of nitrous oxide in rats, folinic acid does not. Anesthesiology 67:A456, 1987

166. Adamsons K, Mueller-Heubach E, Myers RE: Production of fetal asphyxia in the rhesus monkey by administration of catecholamines to the mother. Am J Obstet Gynecol 109:148, 1971

167. Katz JD, Hook R, Barash PG: Fetal heart rate monitoring in the pregnant patient under surgery. Am J Obstet Gynecol 125:267, 1976

168. Hehre RW: Hypothermia for operations during pregnancy. Anesth Analg 44:424, 1965

169. Kofke WA, Wuest HP, McGinnis LA: Cesarean section following ruptured cerebral aneurysm and neuroresuscitation. Anesthesiology 60:242, 1984

170. Estafanous FG, Buckley S: Management of anesthesia for open heart surgery during pregnancy. Cleve Clin Q 43:121, 1976

171. Trimakas AP, Maxwell KD, Berkay S et al: Fetal monitoring during cardiac pulmonary bypass for removal of a left atrial myxoma during pregnancy. Johns Hopkins Med J 144:156, 1979

After this book went into production, new CPR guidelines were published. Here is the full reference for these algorithms: American Heart Association: Guidelines 2000 for Cardiopulmonary Resuscitation and Emergency Cardiovasciular Care: International Concensus on Science. Circulation 102(8), 2000.

Clinical Anesthesia (4/e), edited by
Paul G. Barash, Bruce F. Cullen, and
Robert K. Stoelting. Lippincott Williams &
Wilkins, Philadelphia, © 2001.

CHAPTER 43

NEONATAL ANESTHESIA

FREDERIC A. BERRY AND BARBARA A. CASTRO

PHYSIOLOGY OF THE INFANT AND THE TRANSITION PERIOD

The first year of life is characterized by an almost miraculous growth in size and maturity. The body weight alone changes by a factor of 3, and there is no other period in extrauterine life when changes occur so rapidly. Before birth, fetal growth and development depend on the genetic composition of the fetus, the mother's placental function, and potential exposure to chemicals or infectious agents that can affect mother, fetus, or both. The journey down the birth canal (or through the abdominal wall)—called the most dangerous trip in a person's life—ends the fetal period, and the newborn must adapt to extrauterine life. This change from fetal to extrauterine life is called the period of transition or adaptation.

The newborn infant is an infant in the first 24 hours of life. This chapter focuses on the neonatal period, which is defined as the first 30 days of extrauterine life and includes the newborn period.

The most significant part of transition occurs in the first 24–72 hours after birth. All systems of the body change during transition, but the most important to the anesthesiologist are the circulatory, pulmonary, hepatic, and renal systems. The circulatory and pulmonary systems are so interdependent that they are discussed together.

Transition of the Cardiopulmonary System

Fetal Circulation

Fetal circulation is characterized by the presence of three main shunts (Fig. 43-1*A*). These shunts are the placenta, foramen ovale, and ductus arteriosus. The relatively low pressure in the left atrium and the high pressure in the right atrium result in the foramen ovale being open. The pulmonary vascular bed has a high vascular resistance because the alveoli are relatively closed and filled with fluid and the blood vessels are compressed. In addition, the low partial pressure of oxygen in arterial blood (Pao_2) and *p*H increase pulmonary vascular resistance. However, the ductus arteriosus represents a low-resistance system because it is dilated secondary to a low Pao_2. Therefore, the blood that leaves the right ventricle by the pulmonary artery is shunted preferentially (90%) through the ductus arteriosus and down the descending aorta, whereas only 10% of the output of the right ventricle flows through the pulmonary artery into the pulmonary vascular bed. The pulmonary vascular bed requires only enough blood flow to ensure growth and development of the pulmonary tissue, including surfactant production.

The placenta oxygenates the blood, which then courses up the inferior vena cava into the right atrium. The right atrium is divided by a structure called the crista dividens, so that this relatively well oxygenated blood is shunted from the right atrium through the foramen ovale into the left atrium, thereby bypassing the right ventricle and the pulmonary vascular bed. This blood, the best oxygenated in the fetus, progresses from the left atrium to the left ventricle and out the ascending aorta to provide oxygenation for the brain and upper extremities. Blood returns from the upper body to the right heart by the superior vena cava, where it is directed by the crista dividens into the right ventricle, from which it is then pumped out the pulmonary artery.

Clamping of the umbilical cord and initiation of ventilation produce enormous circulatory changes in the newborn (Fig. 43-1*B*). The transition of the alveoli from a fluid-filled to an air-filled state results in a reduced compression of the pulmonary alveolar capillaries with a reduction in pulmonary vascular resistance; there is a rapid reduction in the first several hours of life. However, it takes 3–4 days for the pulmonary vascular resistance to decrease to the eventual level that it will achieve during the neonatal period. Nitric oxide is an integral part of the reduction in pulmonary vascular resistance; its clinical use is discussed later in the chapter. The initial moderate decrease in pulmonary vascular resistance is accompanied by constriction of the ductus arteriosus secondary to oxygenation. This results in an increase in pulmonary blood flow and an increase in left atrial pressure, so that the foramen ovale functionally closes. Closure of these two neonatal shunts (*i.e.*, the ductus arteriosus and the foramen ovale) is initially only a functional closure. Both shunts usually close permanently in the first several months of life. However, an autopsy study of normal hearts has demonstrated a 30% incidence of patent foramen ovale during the first 30 years of life and a 20% incidence for people 30 years of age and older.[1]

Incidence of Patent Ductus Arteriosus in the Premature Infant

A study by Reller *et al*[2] demonstrated that a patent ductus arteriosus (PDA) on or beyond the fourth day of life is abnormal regardless of gestational age. Prematurity, unless complicated by acute asphyxia or the respiratory distress syndrome, is not a risk factor for persistent PDA. In their study, 95% of premature infants, regardless of gestational age, had closure of the ductus by day 4. The incidence of a PDA in premature infants with the respiratory distress syndrome without a history of birth asphyxia was 11%, a percentage that is somewhat less than is commonly assumed.

Persistent Pulmonary Hypertension

The major transition of the circulatory system occurs over the first 24 hours of life. Figure 43-2 illustrates the correlation of the mean pulmonary artery pressure with age during the first 3 days of life. The pulmonary circulation is extremely sensitive to oxygen, *p*H, and nitric oxide. Hypoxia and acidosis, along with inflammatory mediators, may cause pulmonary artery pressure either to persist at a high level, or, after initially decreasing, to increase to pathologic levels. The result is termed *persistent pulmonary hypertension* (PPH). The pathophysiologic characteristics of pulmonary hypertension comprise a spectrum, ranging from normal pulmonary vasculature to abnormal pulmonary vasculature that is characterized by extension of smooth muscle into the distal respiratory units (Fig. 43-3). There are all degrees in between. Vasoconstriction of the muscle in the blood vessels of the pulmonary vascular bed results in pulmonary hypertension with a right-to-left shunt through the foramen ovale or the ductus arteriosus (Fig. 43-4).

Persistent pulmonary hypertension is a syndrome that may be primary with no recognized etiology, or it may be secondary to meconium aspiration, sepsis, pneumonia, respiratory distress, and congenital diaphragmatic hernia (CDH). Currently, the basic treatment depends on the degree of respiratory failure and the response to therapy. The goals of therapy are to achieve

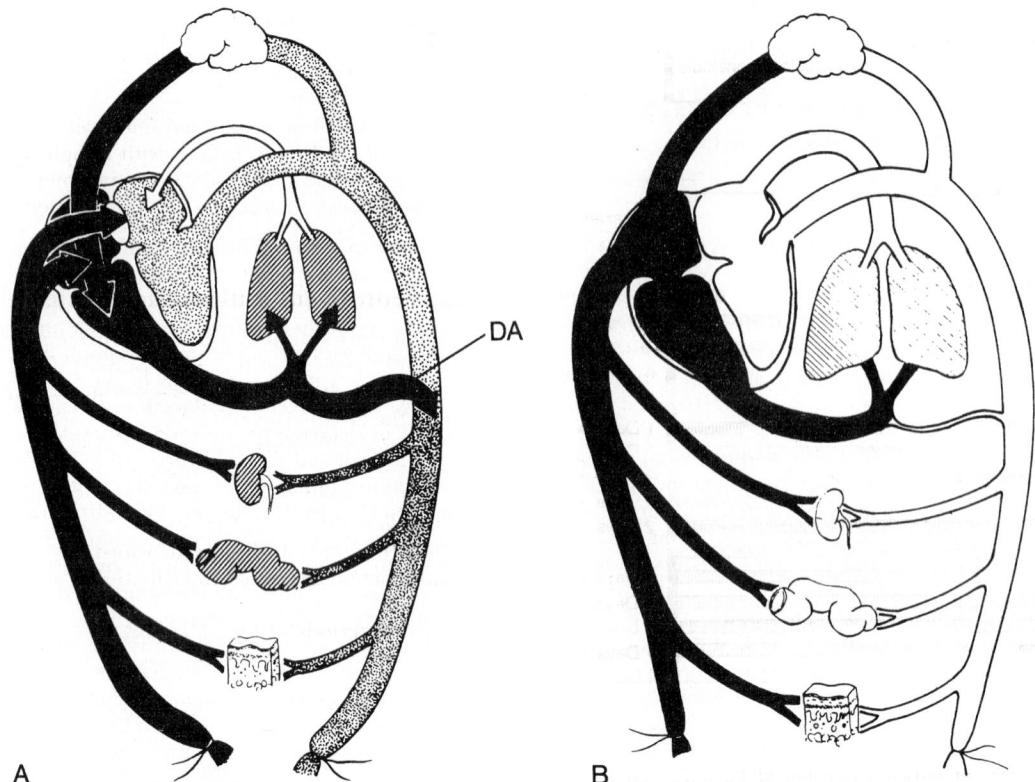

Figure 43-1. (*A*) Schematic representation of the fetal circulation. Oxygenated blood leaves the placenta in the umbilical vein (*vessel without stippling*). Umbilical vein blood joins blood from the viscera (represented here by the kidney, gut, and skin) in the inferior vena cava. Approximately half of the inferior vena cava flow passes through the foramen ovale to the left atrium, where it mixes with a small amount of pulmonary venous blood, and this relatively well oxygenated blood (*light stippling*) supplies the heart and brain by way of the ascending aorta. The other half of the inferior vena cava stream mixes with superior vena cava blood and enters the right ventricle (blood in the right atrium and ventricle has little oxygen, which is denoted by *heavy stippling*). Because the pulmonary arterioles are constricted, most of the blood in the main pulmonary artery flows through the ductus arteriosus (DA), so that the descending aorta's blood has less oxygen (*heavy stippling*) than does blood in the ascending aorta (*light stippling*). (*B*) Schematic representation of the circulation in the normal newborn. After expansion of the lungs and ligation of the umbilical cord, pulmonary blood flow and left atrial and systemic arterial pressures increase. When left atrial pressure exceeds right atrial pressure, the foramen ovale closes so that all the inferior and superior vena cava blood leaves the right atrium, enters the right ventricle, and is pumped through the pulmonary artery toward the lung. With the increase in systemic arterial pressure and decrease in pulmonary artery pressure, flow through the ductus arteriosus becomes left-to-right and the ductus constricts and closes. The course of circulation is the same as in the adult. (Reprinted with permission from Phibbs R: Delivery room management of the newborn. In Avery GB [ed]: Neonatology, Pathophysiology and Management of the Newborn, p 184. Philadelphia, JB Lippincott, 1981.)

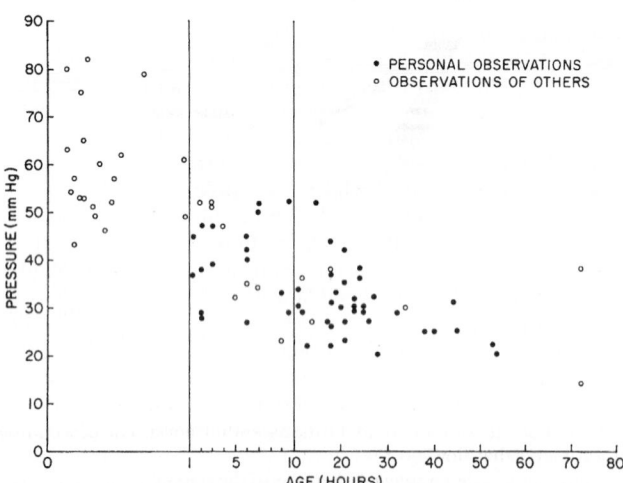

Figure 43-2. Correlation of mean pulmonary arterial pressure with age in 85 normal-term infants studied during the first 3 days of life. (Reprinted with permission from Emmanouilides GC, Moss AJ, Duffie ER, Adams FH: Pulmonary arterial pressure changes in human newborn infants from birth to 3 days of age. J Pediatr 65:327, 1964.)

a PaO_2 between 50 and 70 and a $PaCO_2$ between 40 and 60 cm H_2O. Problems of PPH or hypoxemic respiratory failure involve not only preterm but term infants. There have been major changes in therapy in the 1990s with the introduction of surfactant, high-frequency ventilation, inhaled nitric oxide, and extracorporeal membrane oxygenation (ECMO). The technique and degree of intervention depend on the response to supportive care. Surfactant and various ventilatory techniques are used as the first-line treatment. These techniques include intermittent mandatory ventilation, assist control ventilation, and proportional assist ventilation.[3–5] Studies with proportional assist ventilation demonstrate that gas exchange can be maintained with smaller transpulmonary pressure changes, which may reduce the incidence of chronic lung disease in low–birth-weight infants.[5]

A number of reports have discussed the use of ECMO.[4,6,7] The therapy is aimed at resting the infant's lungs while providing adequate oxygenation for survival and lung repair. It is hoped that the rested lung can recover its function by repairing the pulmonary parenchyma and restructuring the pulmonary vascular bed. The lung is ventilated with low pressures, namely, 20 cm H_2O pressure with 5 cm H_2O of positive end-expiratory pressure (PEEP) and an FIO_2 of 0.21 to 0.3. As the infant's pulmonary function improves, evidenced by increasing PaO_2 levels, the ECMO is reduced accordingly. This is an extremely expensive and high-

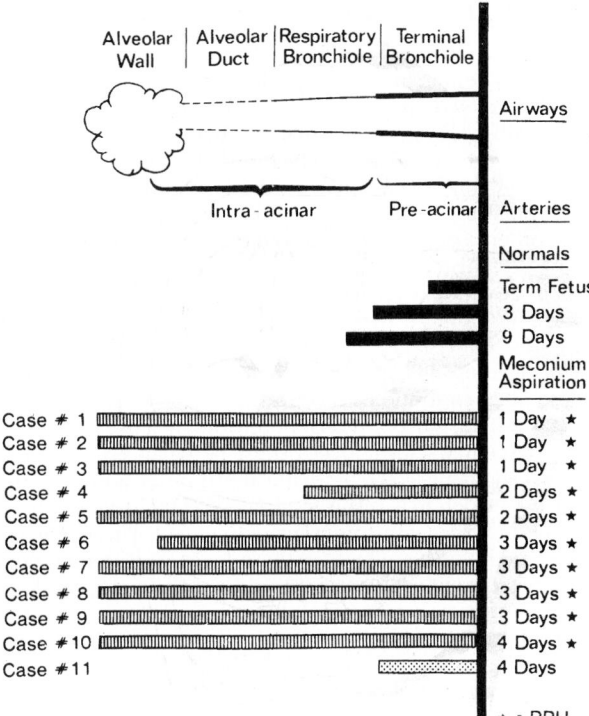

Figure 43-3. Diagram of muscle extension along pulmonary arterial branches (*shaded bars*). In the normal newborn, virtually no intra-acinar artery is muscular. In 9 of 10 infants with meconium aspiration and persistent pulmonary hypertension (PPH), muscle extended into the most peripheral arteries; the infant with meconium aspiration without PPH (case 11) had normal intra-acinar arteries. (Reprinted with permission from Murphy JD, Vawter GF, Reid LM: Pulmonary vascular disease in fetal meconium aspiration. J Pediatr 104:758, 1984.)

risk technique that requires an experienced and talented team. The vascular shunt is performed through either a venovenous or a venoarterial circuit. Heparin must be administered to the infants, and this may increase the chance of intracranial bleeding. The use of ECMO therapy has increased tremendously in the past several years; however, there is a definite associated morbidity and mortality rate.[8,9] Many infants with respiratory failure who are candidates for ECMO have been successfully treated with nitric oxide, and ECMO has been avoided.

Meconium Aspiration

Interference with the normal maternal placental circulation in the third trimester may cause chronic fetal hypoxia. Fetal hypoxia can result in an increase in the amount of muscle in the blood vessels of the distal respiratory units.[10] Figure 43-3 illustrates the muscle increase found in blood vessels of a series of 11 infants who died of PPH.[11] Chronic fetal hypoxia leads to the passage of meconium *in utero*. The fetus breathes *in utero* so that the meconium enters the pulmonary system. It is thought that the meconium *per se* does not cause the extension of the muscle of the pulmonary vascular system but that such muscle extension along pulmonary arterial branches is due to fetal hypoxia. Meconium aspiration can be a marker of chronic fetal hypoxia in the third trimester. This condition is different from the meconium aspiration that occurs during delivery. This meconium at birth is thick and tenacious and mechanically obstructs the tracheobronchial system. Meconium aspiration syndrome leads to varying degrees of respiratory failure, which can be fatal in spite of all treatment modalities.

Until relatively recently, tracheal intubation and suctioning were recommended for all infants with frank meconium aspiration or meconium staining (approximately 10% of newborns).

Now a more conservative approach should be used because routine intubation may cause unnecessary respiratory complications.[8,9,12] Routine oropharyngeal suctioning is recommended immediately at the time of delivery, but tracheal intubation and suctioning should be performed selectively, depending on the condition of the infant. Infants with a high Apgar score (*i.e.*, 7–9) need no additional airway management. Infants with a low Apgar score or who are clinically obstructed with meconium should have the appropriate resuscitative measures taken.

Transition of the Pulmonary System

The pulmonary system transition occurs more quickly than the circulatory system transition. The primary event of the pulmonary system transition is the initiation of ventilation, which changes the alveoli from a fluid-filled to an air-filled state. During the first 5–10 minutes of extrauterine life, normal ventilatory volumes develop and a normal tidal ventilation is established. The initial negative intrathoracic pressures that the newborn generates are often in the range of 40–60 cm H_2O. By 10–20 minutes of life, the newborn has achieved its near-normal functional residual capacity (FRC) and the blood gases are well stabilized. Table 43-1 lists the normal blood gases for the various periods of life. A recent study in preterm infants

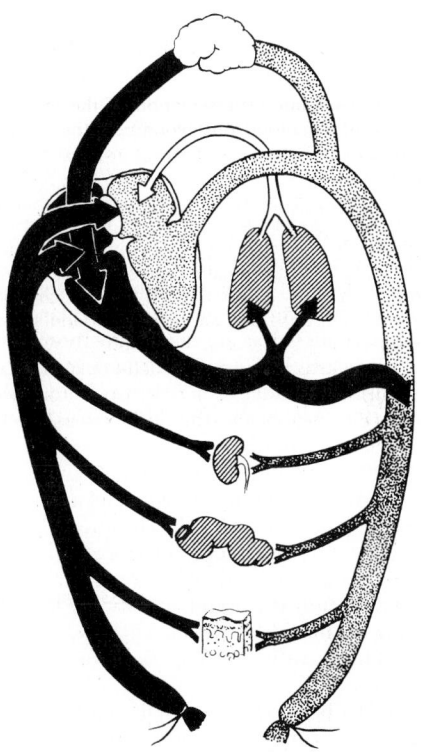

Figure 43-4. Schematic representation of the circulation in an asphyxiated newborn with incomplete expansion of the lungs. Pulmonary vascular resistance is high, pulmonary blood flow is low (note the small caliber of the pulmonary vein), and flow through the ductus arteriosus is high. With little pulmonary venous flow, left atrial pressure decreases below right atrial pressure, the foramen ovale opens, and vena cava blood flows through the foramen into the left atrium. This partially venous blood flows to the brain by the ascending aorta. The descending aorta blood that flows to the viscera has less oxygen than that of the ascending aorta (*heavy stippling*) because of the right-to-left flow through the ductus arteriosus. The circulation is the same in the fetus except that there is no oxygenated blood in the inferior vena cava from the umbilical vein. (Reprinted with permission from Phibbs R: Delivery room management of the newborn. In Avery GB [ed]: Neonatology, Pathophysiology and Management of the Newborn, p 184. Philadelphia, JB Lippincott, 1981.)

Table 43-1. NORMAL BLOOD GAS VALUES IN THE NEWBORN

Subject	Age	Po_2 (mm Hg)	Pco_2 (mm Hg)	pH
Fetus (term)	Before labor	25	40	7.37
Fetus (term)	End of labor	10–20	55	7.25
Newborn (term)	10 min	50	48	7.20
Newborn (term)	1 hr	70	35	7.35
Newborn (term)	1 wk	75	35	7.40
Newborn (preterm, 1500 g)	1 wk	60	38	7.37

older than 26 weeks' gestational age demonstrated that a single dose of dexamethasone given within 2 hours of delivery resulted in lower ventilator settings and a higher mean blood pressure during the first week of life.[13] In addition, fewer infants in this group received indomethacin to treat a PDA.

Transition and Maturation of the Renal System

The fetal kidneys and the fetal lungs have certain similarities. During the fetal period, both have a relatively low blood flow compared with that during the newborn and neonatal periods because both organs need only enough blood flow for growth and development. The maternal placenta removes fetal waste material. The major function of the fetal kidneys is the production of urine, which contributes to the formation of amniotic fluid, which is important for the normal development of the fetal lung and acts as a shock absorber for the fetus. The fetal kidney is characterized by a low renal blood flow (RBF) and glomerular filtration rate (GFR).[14] There are four major reasons for the low RBF and GFR: low systemic arterial pressure, high renal vascular resistance, low permeability of the glomerular capillaries, and the small size and number of glomeruli. The low systemic arterial pressure and high vascular resistance are the two characteristics that are similar to those found in the fetal lung. This results in a low RBF, which in turn results in a low GFR. Transition changes the first two factors: the systemic arterial pressure increases and the renal vascular resistance decreases. Again, this is similar to what occurs in the lung. The other two factors are changed through maturation. The limited ability of the newborn's kidney to concentrate or dilute urine results from the low GFR at birth. However, during the first 3–4 days, the circulatory changes increase RBF and GFR and improve the neonate's ability to concentrate and dilute the urine. The maturation continues, and by the time the normal full-term infant is 1 month of age, the kidneys are approximately 70% mature. This is sufficient renal function to handle almost any contingency.

The neonatal kidney does have certain limitations. The renin–angiotensin–aldosterone system is the primary compensatory system for the reabsorption of sodium and water to compensate for the loss of plasma, blood, gastrointestinal tract fluid, and third-space fluid. Although the neonate has a normal renin–angiotensin–aldosterone system, the neonatal kidney cannot completely conserve sodium, even with a severe sodium deficit. Aldosterone facilitates the reabsorption of sodium in the distal tubule. The immature tubular cells cannot completely reabsorb sodium under the stimulus of aldosterone, so that the neonate continues to excrete sodium in the urine even in the presence of a severe sodium defect. For this reason, the neonate is considered an "obligate sodium loser." In the mature state, the distal tubule can reabsorb essentially all of the sodium, so that the urine has less than 5–10 mEq of sodium per liter of urine. In the neonate, this number may be as high as 20–25 mEq of sodium per liter of urine.

Fluid and Electrolyte Therapy in the Neonate

The inability of the neonatal distal tubule to respond fully to aldosterone results in the obligatory sodium loss in the urine. Therefore, intravenous (iv) fluids in the neonate must contain sodium. Most operations on neonates involve loss of blood and extracellular fluid, which must be replaced with a fluid of similar electrolyte content (i.e., a balanced salt solution: lactated Ringer's, Plasmalyte).

The other problems of the neonate are those of appropriate glucose administration. Infants of diabetic mothers and those small for gestational age have particular problems with hypoglycemia. These infants need to have their blood glucose values monitored until stable. Neonates scheduled for surgery who have been receiving hyperalimentation fluids or supplementary glucose must continue to receive that fluid during surgery or must have their glucose levels monitored because of concerns of hypoglycemia. This concern must be balanced against the potential augmentation of ischemic injury by the administration of glucose, which may result in glycemia. One issue of glucose metabolism is what constitutes hypoglycemia.[15] There is no consensus on this issue. The anesthesiologist and neonatologist have very different problems in this area. For the neonatologist, the issue is not one or two episodes of hypoglycemia, but the recurrent problem of hypoglycemia over a period of days, which has been demonstrated to result in brain damage. The anesthesiologist is faced with a different picture, in which the issues are whether the glucose-containing solution may be interrupted or, conversely, if a bolus of the solution should be administered along with various medications that may be required during the anesthetic. For this reason, the balanced salt solution used for replacement therapy during surgery should either be administered through a separate iv line or as close to the iv port as possible. If there is any question about the glucose level, it should be checked during surgery.

Premature infants and neonates must receive full-strength balanced salt solution for the replacement of third-space and blood losses during the perioperative period.[10] There is a misconception that these infants cannot tolerate the salt load; therefore, they are often given hypotonic fluids. It is not unusual to see premature infants with postoperative sodium values of $125–130$ mEq $\cdot$ l^{-1}. Alone, these levels may not be a major problem, but when added to the residual effects of muscle relaxants and antibiotics in a sick infant, they may result in depression of neuromuscular function.

Atrial Natriuretic Factor

There has been interest in the role of atrial natriuretic factor (ANF, a peptide) in sodium homeostasis of the infant. ANF is released from the atria and reduces sodium overload in the body. ANF affects renal function by altering renal hemodynamics and increasing urinary sodium and water excretion; it also increases the GFR, which results in a significant natriuresis without an alteration in total RBF. In addition, ANF opposes the renin system. The renin–angiotensin–aldosterone system is a tightly controlled system that immediately activates when there is a challenge to arterial blood pressure as well as a deficit of sodium. Sometimes this system overshoots and the patient acquires an excessive sodium load.

ANATOMIC AND MATURATIONAL FACTORS OF NEONATES AND THEIR CLINICAL SIGNIFICANCE

The anatomic and maturational factors unique to the neonate have far-reaching clinical implications (Fig. 43-5). Neonates are obligate nose breathers; therefore, anything that obstructs the nares compromises the neonate's ability to breathe. For this

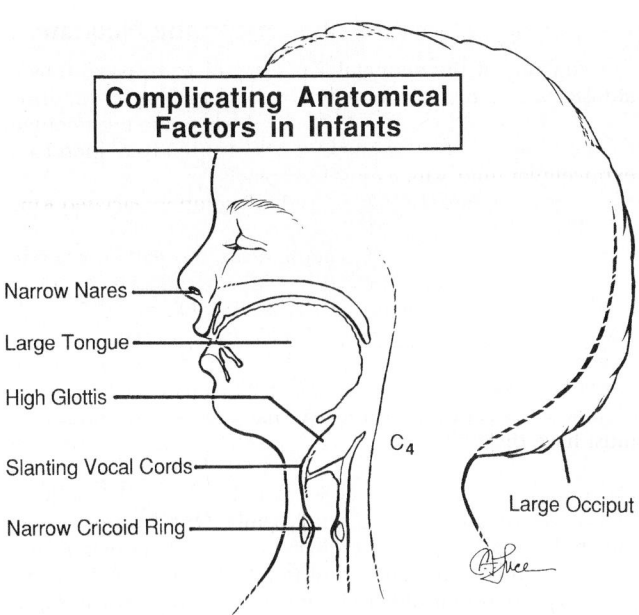

Complicating Anatomical Factors in Infants

Narrow Nares
Large Tongue
High Glottis
Slanting Vocal Cords
Narrow Cricoid Ring

C₄

Large Occiput

Figure 43-5. Complicating anatomic factors in infants. (Modified with permission from Smith RM: Anesthesia for Infants and Children, 4th ed. St. Louis, CV Mosby, 1980.)

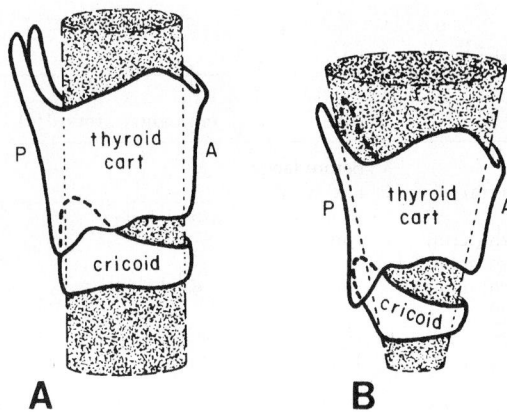

thyroid cart
cricoid

thyroid cart
cricoid

A **B**

Figure 43-7. Configuration of the adult (*A*) versus the infant larynx (*B*). The adult larynx has a cylindric shape. The infant larynx is funnel shaped because of the narrow, undeveloped cricoid cartilage. (Reprinted with permission from The pediatric airway. In Ryan JF, Todres ID, Cote CJ *et al* [eds]: A Practice of Anesthesia for Infants and Children, 2nd ed., p 61. Orlando, Florida, Grune & Stratton, 1992.)

reason, choanal atresia is a life-threatening surgical problem for the infant. The large tongue occupies relatively more space in the infant's airway and makes it difficult to conduct a laryngoscopic examination and intubate the infant's trachea. In the normal adult, the glottis is at the level of C5. In the full-term infant, the glottis is at the level of C4, and in the premature infant it is at the level of C3. The combination of a large tongue and a relatively high glottis means that on laryngoscopic examination it is more difficult to establish a line of vision between the mouth and larynx: there is relatively more tissue in less distance. Therefore, the infant's larynx appears to be anterior. When combined with the anterior-slanting vocal cords, the result is a more difficult laryngoscopic examination and intubation. Application of cricoid pressure by the anesthesiologist or an assistant improves visualization of the neonate's larynx. If the anesthesiologist's hand is large enough, cricoid pressure can be applied with the little finger (Fig. 43-6). This is more effective than having an assistant apply pressure because

the anesthesiologist can determine the best position for intubation.

A narrow cricoid ring is significant because it means that the narrowest portion of the neonate's airway is not the vocal cords but the cricoid ring. In the mature state, the airway from the vocal cords down the trachea is of equal dimensions (Fig. 43-7), and if the endotracheal tube passes comfortably through the vocal cords, it will not be tight within the cricoid cartilage. However, the neonate's laryngeal structures resemble a funnel; even though the endotracheal tube may pass through the vocal cords, which are at the midpoint of the funnel, the endotracheal tube may be tight within the cricoid ring. This tight fit may cause temporary or permanent damage to the cricoid cartilage, resulting in short- or long-term airway difficulties. The infant has a large occiput so that the head flexes forward onto the chest when the infant is lying supine with its head in the midline (Fig. 43-8A). Extreme extension can also obstruct the airway, so that a mid-position of the head with slight extension is preferred for airway maintenance. This is accomplished by placing a small roll at the base of the neck and shoulders (see Fig. 43-8B).

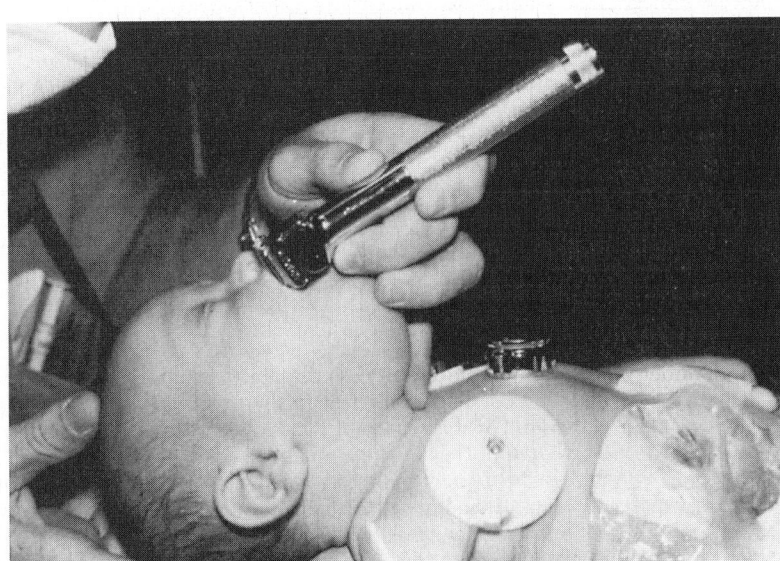

Figure 43-6. Cricoid pressure applied with little finger. (Reprinted with permission from Physiology and surgery of the infant. In Berry FA [ed]: Anesthetic Management of Difficult and Routine Pediatric Patients, p 129. New York, Churchill Livingstone, 1990.)

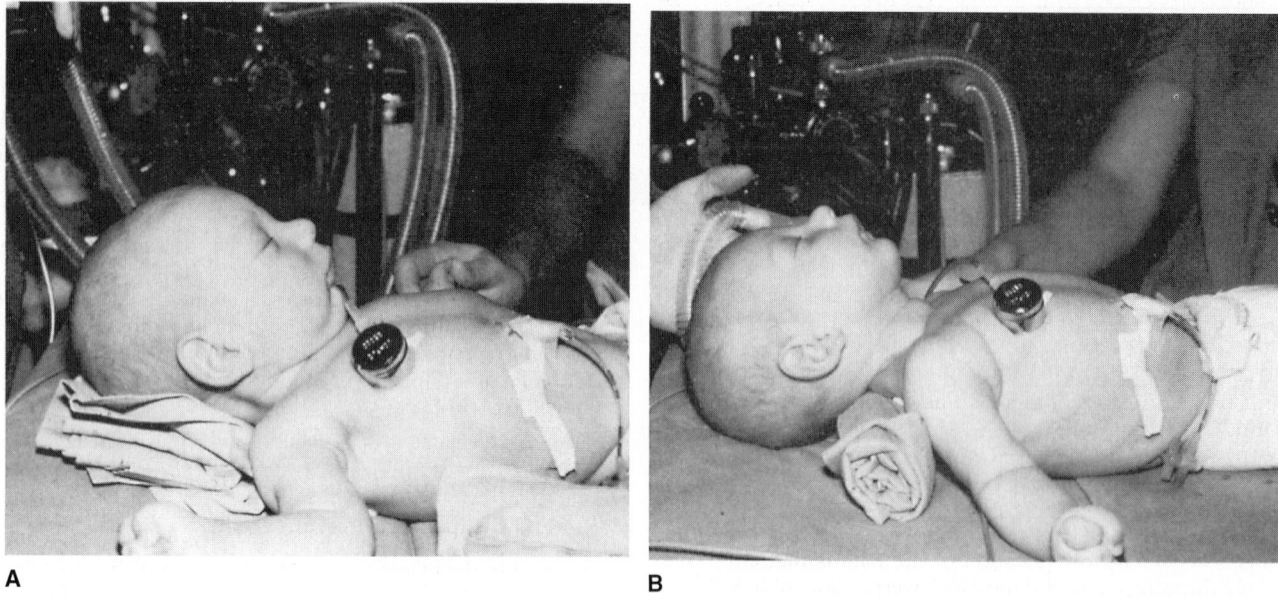

A   **B**

Figure 43-8. (A) Pad placed under occiput in an attempt to achieve a "sniffing" position obstructs the infant's airway. (B) Pad is placed under infant's neck to improve the airway patency and for laryngoscopic examination.

Anatomic and Physiologic Factors of the Pulmonary System

Anatomically and physiologically, the neonate's pulmonary system differs in at least four respects from that of the adult: a high oxygen consumption, high closing volumes, a high ratio of minute ventilation to FRC, and pliable ribs. The oxygen consumption of the infant is $7–9 \; ml \cdot kg^{-1} \cdot min^{-1}$, whereas in the adult it is $3 \; ml \cdot kg^{-1} \cdot min^{-1}$. Therefore, varying degrees of airway obstruction have more impact on oxygen delivery and reserve in the neonate, infant, and child than in adults.

The high closing volumes of the neonate's lungs are within the lower range of the normal tidal volume (Fig. 43-9). Closing volumes are the lung volumes at which alveoli close, resulting

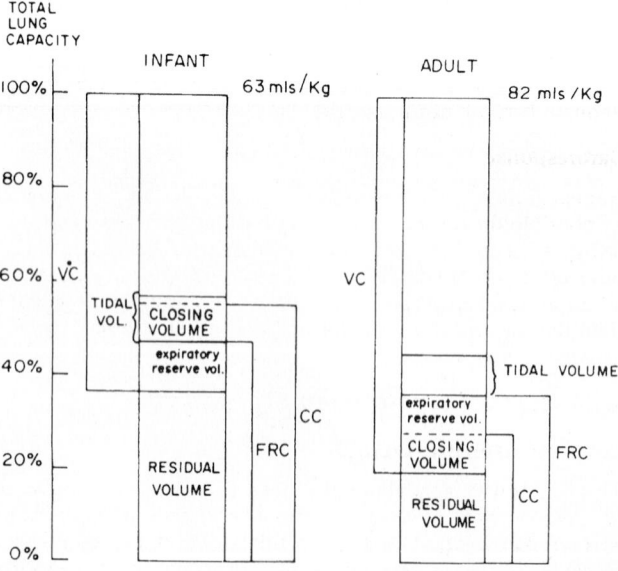

Figure 43-9. Static lung volumes of infants and adults. (Reprinted with permission from Smith CA, Nelson NM: Physiology of the Newborn Infant, 4th ed. Springfield, Illinois, Charles C Thomas, 1976.)

in the shunting of blood by a closed alveolus. If an infant experiences mild laryngospasm and a reduction in lung volume, the high closing volume contributes to shunting of blood and rapid desaturation. When a high oxygen consumption is combined with a high closing volume in the presence of laryngospasm, the rapidity with which desaturation occurs is breathtaking not only for the infant but also for the anesthesiologist. When coughing and breath-holding occur with an endotracheal tube in place, the situation is not much different because there is an inability to ventilate the alveoli. Positive pressure ventilates the large airways, but there is no oxygen delivery to the closed alveoli. Therefore, even though an endotracheal tube may be in the appropriate anatomic location, severe desaturation can occur in infants who are lightly anesthetized and are coughing on the endotracheal tube. At times, because of inability to oxygenate the infant, it might be incorrectly believed that the endotracheal tube has come out of the trachea. The high intrathoracic pressure along with hypoxia, which increases pulmonary vascular resistance, may well cause right-to-left shunting either through the ductus arteriosus or through the foramen ovale. Management of the patient in this situation entails deepening the anesthesia or paralysis. This can be done with either small iv doses of succinylcholine, $0.5 \; mg \cdot kg^{-1}$, or iv lidocaine, $1.5 \; mg \cdot kg^{-1}$. Caution must be taken not to exceed this dose of lidocaine in the neonate.

The third unique pulmonary feature of the neonate is the high ratio of minute ventilation to FRC, which is similar to that of the term pregnant woman but occurs for different reasons. The pregnant woman has a reduction in FRC because of elevation of the diaphragm by the uterus. The neonate has an increased alveolar ventilation because of the need to increase oxygen delivery secondary to the high oxygen consumption. Table 43-2 compares the normal respiratory values for newborns and adults.

The tidal ventilation for an infant is the same, in milliliters per kilogram, as for the adult; therefore, with an oxygen consumption that is three times greater, the respiratory rate must be three times greater, which results in an alveolar ventilation that is three times greater. Consequently, the ratio of minute ventilation to FRC is 5:1 in the neonate, whereas in adults it is 1.5:1. The clinical implication of the high ratio of minute

Table 43-2. COMPARISON OF NORMAL RESPIRATORY VALUES IN INFANTS AND ADULTS

Parameter	Infant	Adult
Respiratory frequency	30–50	12–16
Tidal volume (ml·kg^{-1})	7	7
Dead space (ml·kg^{-1})	2–2.5	2.2
Alveolar ventilation (ml·kg^{-1}·min^{-1})	100–150	60
Functional residual capacity (ml·kg^{-1})	27–30	30
Oxygen consumption (ml·kg^{-1}·min^{-1})	7–9	3

ventilation to FRC is that there is a much more rapid induction of inhalational anesthesia, as well as more rapid awakening. The more rapid induction of anesthesia also results from a higher percentage of the neonate's body weight consisting of vessel-rich tissues. Figure 43-10 compares the predicted versus observed ratio of end-tidal to inspired halothane in infants and adults. The practical implication of the data is that clinicians who use the adult curve and the usual overpressure of halothane for induction will find the neonate more rapidly induced and perhaps at risk for an overdose of anesthetic (see Uptake and Distribution of Anesthetic Agents).

The fourth anatomic difference of the neonate is a pliable rib cage. When increased minute ventilation is needed, which requires an increase in respiratory frequency or tidal volume, the pliable ribs of the neonate are a disadvantage. The neonate's diaphragm is the major ventilatory muscle. To increase oxygen delivery by either an increase in frequency or excursion, the contraction of the diaphragm results in greater negative intrathoracic pressures. In mature people with a fixed rib cage, this results in an increase in air movement. However, with a pliable rib cage, the resulting increase in negative intrathoracic pressure results in retractions of ribs as well as retraction in the subcostal and supraclavicular area. This results in less efficient ventilation and a high energy price for the effort involved. This is one of the reasons why neonates are susceptible to fatigue with airway obstruction, pneumonia, and any other condition that results in interference with pulmonary function; another reason is the immaturity of the muscles.

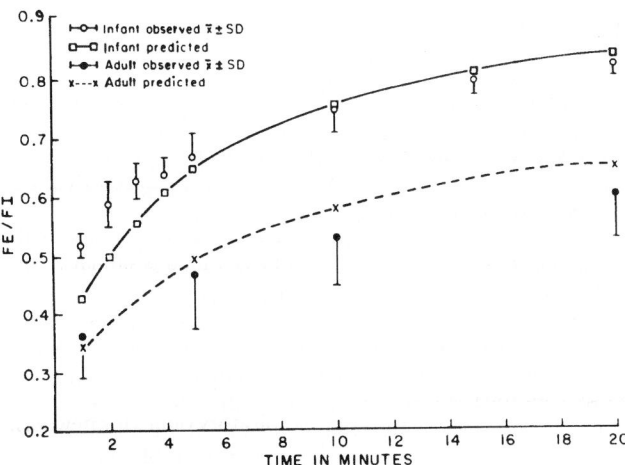

Figure 43-10. Predicted versus observed ratio of end-tidal to inspired halothane (FE/FI) in infants and adults. Predicted FE/FI values are those generated by a computer program of anesthetic uptake and distribution. In infants, the minute ventilation averaged 1.9 l; in adults, 6.9 l. The inspired fraction of halothane was 0.5% in both cases. (Reprinted with permission from Brandom BW, Brandom RB, Cook DR: Uptake of halothane in infants. Anesth Analg 62:404, 1983.)

Maturation of Respiratory Muscles

There are two types of muscles: Type 1, slow-twitch, high-oxidative muscles, which are necessary for sustained muscle activity; and Type 2, fast-twitch, low-oxidative muscles, which have an immediate but short activity.[16] The development of Type 1 muscles is necessary for sustained ventilatory activity. The premature infant has 10% Type 1 and the newborn 25% Type 1 muscles in the diaphragm, which is the primary muscle for ventilation. The infant's diaphragm achieves maturity of Type 1 muscles at approximately 8 months of age. At that point, he or she has approximately 55% Type 1 muscles. The intercostal muscles are the other ventilatory muscles. The premature infant has 20% Type 1 intercostal muscles and the newborn, 46%. The age of maturity for these muscles is 2 months, when Type 1 muscles comprise 65% of the total.

Maturation of the Cardiovascular System

Heart and Sympathetic Nervous System

The ability of the neonate's immature cardiovascular system to respond to stress is limited by the relatively low contractile mass per gram of cardiac tissue, which results in a limited ability to increase myocardial contractility as well as a reduction in ventricular compliance.[17] The clinical implication of this limited stretchability or compliance of the ventricle means that, although there may be some ability to increase stroke volume, it is extremely limited. Therefore, any increase in cardiac output must be accomplished by an increase in heart rate. For this reason, the infant is said to be rate dependent for its cardiac output. Thus, any slowing of the heart rate is reflected in a reduction in cardiac output. This is why bradycardia has such serious consequences for the infant. Hypoxia is a major cause of bradycardia in the neonate. Even in the absence of stress, the neonatal heart has limited ability to increase cardiac output compared with the mature heart (Fig. 43-11). The resting cardiac output of the immature heart is very close to the maximal cardiac output, so there is a limited reserve. The mature heart can increase cardiac output by 300%, whereas the immature heart can only increase cardiac output by 30–40%.

In summary, the neonatal heart has some significant limitations. The resting cardiac output is much higher relative to body weight than in the adult. The neonatal heart is less able to handle a volume or pressure change. Stimulation of the myocardium produces a limited increase in contractility and cardiac output. The sympathetic nervous system, which usually provides the important chronotropic and inotropic support to the mature circulation during stress, is severely limited in the neonate because of immaturity.

Baroresponse

Neonates have immature baroreceptors. The baroreceptor is responsible for the reflex tachycardia that occurs in response to hypotension. Therefore, the immaturity of this reflex would limit the neonate's ability to compensate for hypotension. In addition, the baroresponse of the neonate is more depressed than that of the adult at the same level of anesthesia.

ANESTHESIA FOR THE NEONATE

Anticholinergic Drugs

There is controversy about the need for premedication with anticholinergics. However, two special concerns in the neonate and immature infant distinguish them from the more mature infant and child: an active vagal reflex and secretions. Because of these concerns, many anesthesiologists routinely administer anticholinergics either before or during surgery to infants younger than 6 months of age. We administer anticholinergics

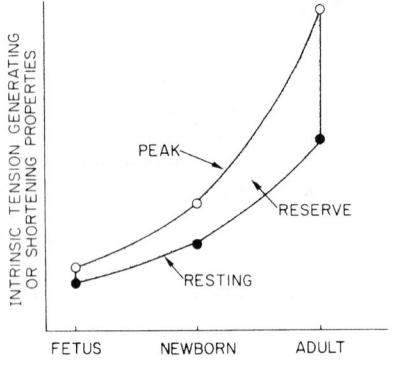

A

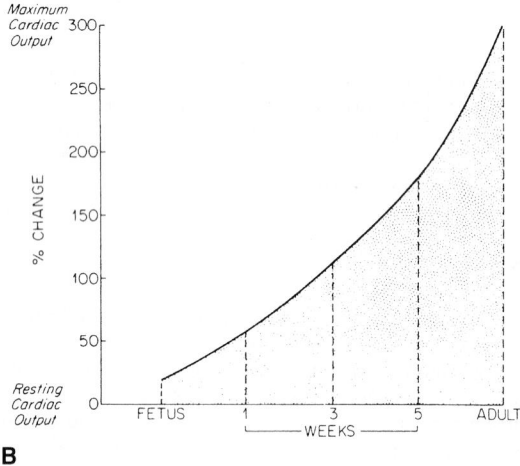

B

Figure 43-11. Schema of reduced cardiac reserve in fetal and newborn animal hearts compared with adult hearts. (*A*) In the newborn infant, resting cardiac muscle performance is close to a peak of ventricular function because of limitations in diastolic, systolic, and heart rate reserve. (*B*) Similarly, pump reserve early in life is limited by these factors as well as by much higher resting cardiac output relative to body weight, compared with that in adults. (Reprinted with permission from Friedman WF, George BL: Treatment of congestive heart failure by altering loading conditions of the heart. J Pediatr 106:700, 1985.)

only for specific indications (*i.e.,* reactive airway disease or excessive secretions).

One of the major indications for anticholinergics is to reduce secretions. The management of the combination of a difficult infant airway and excessive secretions can be simplified by reducing secretions. The dose of atropine in the neonate is 0.02 mg · kg⁻¹; for glycopyrrolate it is 0.01 mg · kg⁻¹.

Tracheal Intubation

One of the frequently asked questions about the anesthetic management of neonates is whether tracheal intubation is routinely needed or if the airway and ventilation can be managed with the laryngeal mask airway. The answer to this question depends on the skill of the anesthesiologist and the surgical procedure, but in most clinical situations, the neonate should be intubated because of various anatomic and physiologic considerations. If the anesthesiologist is skilled and the surgery is short, intubation may not be necessary and a laryngeal mask airway can be used. This is a clinical judgment that must be determined individually by each anesthesiologist and in each situation. Another question is whether to control the ventilation of all neonates. If the overall condition of the neonate is healthy and the procedure is short, then spontaneous ventilation is certainly acceptable. However, if the neonate is debilitated, has

had a relatively long-standing illness, has circulatory instability, and requires muscle relaxation for the surgery, then intraoperative controlled ventilation of the lungs is certainly indicated.

Opinion on whether to perform awake tracheal intubation in the neonate has changed in the last several years. There is concern that awake tracheal intubation causes hypertension and that the hypertension can rupture the fragile intracerebral vessels, particularly in premature infants. There are times when awake tracheal intubation would seem to be the technique of choice, such as in neonates who are critically ill and need resuscitation. Neonates who are persistently vomiting should have an awake tracheal intubation if at all possible. An awake tracheal intubation can be accomplished with topical anesthesia of the oropharynx and lidocaine, 1.5 mg · kg⁻¹ iv, to blunt the response to the intubation. If problems of a full stomach and the resulting concern for aspiration are not present, the current trend is to perform tracheal intubation after the induction of anesthesia (see Anesthetic Management of the Neonate).

The question of extubation of the trachea is considerably easier to answer. The awake state is associated with control of the airway reflexes. Partially anesthetized infants are susceptible to laryngospasm and its associated apnea. Laryngospasm, apnea, and a high oxygen consumption are a devastating combination. Therefore, the trachea should be extubated when the neonate is awake. An awake neonate opens his or her eyes, grasps the endotracheal tube, and cries. Crying cannot be heard because of the endotracheal tube but can be readily visualized. Any of these findings indicates that the infant is ready for extubation. If there is any doubt, however, the neonate should remain intubated until the clinician feels comfortable that the neonate can be extubated.

Does the Neonate Need Anesthesia?

There was some question in past years about whether the premature infant needed anesthesia for surgery. However, the neonate and premature infant should be considered as any other patient who needs anesthesia.[18] The selection of anesthetic techniques for the neonate is based on the same criteria as for any patient, while recognizing the pharmacokinetic and pharmacodynamic differences.

Impact of Surgical Requirements on Anesthetic Technique

Blood loss and muscle relaxation are two areas of concern for the surgeon and anesthesiologist. Parents and health care workers also are concerned about the transmission of acquired immunodeficiency syndrome and hepatitis through transfusion of blood and blood products. The use of blood and blood products should be minimized whenever possible. One way to minimize blood replacement is to minimize blood loss. This can be achieved through the control of blood pressure by the various anesthetics and muscle relaxants. The anesthetic techniques used can be directed toward preventing hypertension, which often occurs with the use of nitrous oxide or an opioid plus muscle relaxant, by inducing controlled normovolemic hypotension. Therefore, it is extremely important for the anesthesiologist and surgeon to discuss the impact of blood pressure on the surgical procedure, as well as the potential for loss of blood. Blood replacement is indicated if the neonate has demonstrated circulatory instability and considerable blood loss is anticipated. However, if the neonate is basically healthy, and the anticipated blood loss is 25–30% of the blood volume, and the final hemoglobin is in the range of 8–9 g · dl⁻¹, then blood transfusion probably can be avoided. The anesthesiologist can tailor the anesthetic to control the blood pressure and thereby reduce blood loss. This requires an appreciation of the cardiovascular effects of anesthetics and muscle relaxants.

Cardiovascular Effects of Muscle Relaxants

Although *d*-tubocurarine does trigger a dose-related histamine release that causes peripheral vasodilation, the incremental administration of *d*-tubocurarine minimizes, if not eliminates, any effect on the blood pressure. Pancuronium has vagolytic and sympathomimetic actions that cause tachycardia and an increase in blood pressure[19] (Table 43-3). If a neonate is moribund or in shock or there is concern about the volume status, then pancuronium may well be the muscle relaxant of choice. However, in a relatively normal neonate with a normal blood pressure and normal blood volume, the use of pancuronium may result in hypertension, which has the potential to increase blood loss. In such an infant, cisatracurium or rocuronium would be a more logical choice of muscle relaxant. Atracurium and rocuronium have certain advantages over vecuronium in the infant younger than 1 year of age because vecuronium is metabolized by the liver. The duration of action of vecuronium is approximately twice that observed in older children because of liver immaturity, and it would be similar to pancuronium in its length of action. If a long-acting nondepolarizing muscle relaxant were desired, vecuronium would have advantages in a child with a normal blood pressure, blood volume, and cardiovascular system.[20] The length of action of cisatracurium and rocuronium in the neonate is similar to that in the older infant or child. The infant's neuromuscular junction is more sensitive to muscle relaxants, and the infant has a larger volume of distribution because of a large extracellular fluid volume. These two effects tend to balance each other, so that, roughly speaking, the dose of a nondepolarizing muscle relaxant for an infant is similar to that for a child on a milligram per kilogram basis. The major difference in neonates is the great variability in response to the nondepolarizing muscle relaxants, so that dose–response effects must be carefully observed to avoid either overdose or underdose. A neuromuscular stimulator is a very useful monitor in infants as well as in older children and adults.

There is some increase in succinylcholine requirement in the infant compared with the older child.[21] The intramuscular dose of succinylcholine is $4 \text{ mg} \cdot \text{kg}^{-1}$ in the infant. The iv dose of succinylcholine in the infant and child is $2 \text{ mg} \cdot \text{kg}^{-1}$. The recent succinylcholine controversy has called into question the use of succinylcholine in male children younger than 8 years of age.[22] The reports of hyperkalemia with cardiac arrest in such children with unrecognized muscular dystrophy has led some clinicians to take the position that succinylcholine should not be used routinely for this group of patients. The occurrence of this problem is somewhere in the range of 1 in 250,000 anesthetics, with a mortality rate of 50%. However, succinylcholine is still recommended in rapid-sequence situations, a potentially difficult airway, or if there are airway emergencies with a developing desaturation. The anesthesiologist must know how to recognize and treat hyperkalemia;[23] hyperkalemia can be recognized by peaked T waves. However, the clinician may not see this particular electrocardiographic change because it occurs 2–3 minutes after drug administration, when the anesthesiologist is attending to the airway. The hyperkalemia interferes with conduction, leading to a bradycardia and, if severe enough, cardiac arrest. If the heart rate slows, then the drug of first choice is calcium $10–15 \text{ mg} \cdot \text{kg}^{-1}$ in a diluted solution. However, if the circulation is unstable with severe bradycardia and hypotension or cardiac arrest, the drug of first choice is epinephrine $5–10 \text{ } \mu\text{g} \cdot \text{kg}^{-1}$. One of the actions of epinephrine is to stimulate the sodium–potassium pump and cause the potassium to re-enter the cell, thereby reducing the serum level. If there is no response at this dose level, it should be increased incrementally until there is a response. Magnesium has been described as a treatment for hyperkalemia because it also antagonizes the effects of hyperkalemia, as does calcium.[24] The use of sodium bicarbonate to treat any metabolic acidosis that may occur with arrest is also thought to be useful because alkalosis decreases hyperkalemia. At the same time, the patient should be hyperventilated to reduce the CO_2, thereby encouraging a respiratory alkalosis.

In the emergency airway situation, the clinician should not wait to use succinylcholine until the patient becomes severely desaturated and bradycardic. When it is evident that a neonate is obstructed by laryngospasm or any other reason and no progress is made in ventilation, then either intramuscular succinylcholine ($4–5 \text{ mg} \cdot \text{kg}^{-1}$) if there is no iv, or an iv dose of $1–2 \text{ mg} \cdot \text{kg}^{-1}$ is given. When succinylcholine is used on an elective basis for a rapid-sequence induction or for any other reason, then curare in a dose of $0.05 \text{ mg} \cdot \text{kg}^{-1}$ should be administered 2–3 minutes before the administration of succinylcholine. The curare reduces the degree and length of the hyperkalemia that is associated with up-regulation of the neuromuscular junction.

Cisatracurium and rocuronium appear to be the drugs of choice among the intermediate-acting, nondepolarizing muscle relaxants. The dose of rocuronium is $0.3–0.4 \text{ mg} \cdot \text{kg}^{-1}$. If a larger dose of rocuronium is used to avoid using succinylcholine, then these doses cause rocuronium to be a relatively long-acting muscle relaxant, and this needs to be kept in mind. Cisatracurium does not have a prolonged effect in the neonate. Its metabolism is by Hofmann elimination, ester hydrolysis, and the liver and kidney. The recommended dose is $0.4–0.6 \text{ mg} \cdot \text{kg}^{-1}$. The use of nondepolarizing muscle relaxants should be guided by monitoring of neuromuscular function with a nerve stimulator. There is some controversy about the routine reversal of nondepolarizing muscle relaxants if a nerve stimulator indicates only a 75–80% return of function. One opinion is that if the usual time for the spontaneous reversal of neuromuscular function has been exceeded by a factor of two, and if neuromuscular function is determined to be normal as judged clinically and by the nerve stimulator, there is no need for reversal. The other opinion is that, regardless of time, there is relatively little risk in administering neuromuscular reversal drugs. We do not favor routine reversal of muscle relaxants.

Table 43-3. CARDIOVASCULAR EFFECTS OF MUSCLE RELAXANTS

Drug	Mechanism of Action on Circulation	Circulatory Changes
Curare	Histamine release	Slow administration—minimal Rapid administration—20–30% decrease in blood pressure
Atracurium	Histamine release	Rapid administration, high dose—20% decrease in blood pressure
Metocurine	None	Minimal change
Vecuronium	None	No change
Pancuronium	Vagal blockade, indirect adrenergic stimulation	Increased pulse and blood pressure

Reversal of Nondepolarizing Neuromuscular Blocking Agents

Edrophonium in a dose of 1 mg · kg^{-1} achieves a 90% reversal of a neuromuscular block in 2 minutes, whereas neostigmine in a dose of 0.06 mg · kg^{-1} requires 10 minutes for a 90% reversal of neuromuscular block. This difference in time to peak effect allows the anesthesiologist to decide which agent is needed. A word of caution: when edrophonium is used to reverse neuromuscular blockade, the effect is so rapid that atropine should be administered before the edrophonium; and there some believe that atropine is superior to glycopyrrolate for this reversal. The dose of atropine is 0.01–0.02 mg · kg^{-1}. Neostigmine is a suitable alternative for reversal of nondepolarizing muscle relaxants in neonates. The muscarinic effects of neostigmine can be blocked with atropine or glycopyrrolate (0.01 mg · kg^{-1}), and the drugs can be given concurrently. The two advantages of edrophonium over neostigmine are a more rapid reversal and fewer muscarinic side effects.

Cardiovascular Effects of the Anesthetic Drugs

Opioids are mild vasodilators but have little direct effect on cardiac function. Cholinergic side effects may decrease the heart rate. If the neonate is hypovolemic, the administration of opioids may decrease blood pressure. However, if the infant is adequately volume resuscitated, the administration of opioids should have little effect on the blood pressure.[25,26] Ketamine has unique cardiovascular effects.[27] Its action is centrally mediated through the sympathetic nervous system, and it can cause a release of norepinephrine. Ketamine *in vitro* has negative inotropic effects. However, on balance, ketamine can override the depressant effects on the myocardium and overall results in support of the cardiovascular system. Therefore, ketamine is a useful agent for the infant who has an unstable cardiovascular system or in whom there is some question about volume repletion. The iv induction dose of ketamine is 1–2 mg · kg^{-1} in titrated doses, followed by 0.5–1 mg · kg^{-1} every 15–30 minutes.

Nitrous oxide usually is considered a reasonably benign anesthetic drug from the standpoint of the cardiovascular system. However, in adult patients, when nitrous oxide is combined with opioids, the cardiac index and arterial pressure decrease because of myocardial depression.[27] Nitrous oxide has mild depressant effects on systemic hemodynamics in sedated infants, similar to those reported in adults, but does not produce the elevations in pulmonary artery pressure and pulmonary vascular resistance that are seen in adults. Therefore, it appears that nitrous oxide is a reasonable drug in neonates if there is no concern for expanding gas pockets within the body (*i.e.,* pneumoencephalos, intestinal obstruction, pneumothorax) and no need for a high FIo$_2$ to maintain saturation.

All of the volatile anesthetics affect the cardiovascular system. Halothane has little effect on peripheral vascular resistance; therefore, the decrease in blood pressure that accompanies the administration of halothane results from myocardial depression. However, isoflurane, desflurane, and sevoflurane decrease systemic vascular resistance so that the major effect on blood pressure is a decrease in peripheral vascular resistance.[28]

Anesthetic Dose Requirements of Neonates

Neonates and premature infants have lower anesthetic requirements than older infants and children.[29] The minimum alveolar concentration (MAC) of halothane for the premature infant is 0.6%; it is 0.89% for full-term neonates and 1.12% for 2- to 4-month-old infants.[29,30] Isoflurane has the same differences in MAC requirement as does halothane. The easiest way to remember the MAC values is that the MAC value in the mature state (*i.e.,* late teenager or adult) is the same as for a full-term infant. By 6 months of age, the MAC value has increased by 50%. In the premature infant, the MAC value decreases by 20–30%. The reasons for the lower MAC requirements are thought to be an immature nervous system, progesterone from the mother, and elevated blood levels of endorphins, coupled with an immature blood–brain barrier. The neonate has an immature central nervous system with attenuated responses to nociceptive cutaneous stimuli. These responses rapidly mature in the first several months of an infant's life, along with an increase in the MAC. Progesterone has been shown to reduce the MAC of the pregnant mother. The newborn infant has elevated progesterone levels, similar to those of the mother. In a study in lambs, Gregory et al[31] showed that the MAC increased progressively over the first 12 hours of life, with a concomitant decrease in progesterone levels. Elevated levels of β-endorphin and β-lipotropin have been demonstrated in infants in the first few days of postnatal life. The levels returned to mature concentrations by the time the infants were 24 days of age. Endorphins do not cross the blood–brain barrier in adults; however, it is thought that the neonate's blood–brain barrier is more permeable and that endorphins might well pass into the central nervous system, thus elevating the pain threshold and reducing the MAC requirement.

ANESTHETIC MANAGEMENT OF THE NEONATE

The anesthesiologist has a host of anesthetic techniques from which to choose and can tailor the anesthetic to the requirements of the surgery and the condition of the neonate. The neonate who is moribund or who has a severely compromised cardiovascular status needs resuscitation. If muscle relaxants are needed, pancuronium is the relaxant of choice. As the neonate's status improves, anesthetic drugs may be titrated in. The neonate with a questionable cardiovascular and volume status needs anesthetic drugs such as ketamine or an opioid. However, in neonates who have a stable cardiovascular state, the choice of drugs depends on the type of surgery and on whether the neonate will be extubated at the end of surgery.

The three major factors to consider in selecting an anesthetic technique are (1) whether it is anticipated that the neonate will be extubated at the end of surgery or shortly thereafter, (2) the need to control blood pressure, and (3) the need for postoperative pain relief. The drugs and techniques available to achieve these goals are many and include inhalational anesthetics, regional techniques, muscle relaxants, opioids, and ketamine. If extubation is anticipated at the end of surgery or shortly thereafter, the anesthetic must be tailored so that there are minimal residual effects from inhalational agents and muscle relaxants, thereby allowing the infant to be awake and in control of its airway reflexes, which promotes early extubation. The muscle relaxant of choice in this situation is atracurium because of its moderate duration of action (30–45 minutes), which is the same in the neonate as in the older child and adult. Vecuronium, by contrast, is metabolized by the liver and in the neonate is a long-acting muscle relaxant. The use of a regional anesthesia technique, such as a caudal technique, reduces the need for inhalational agents, opioids, and muscle relaxants. There are great advantages to using a combined general and regional technique when early extubation is anticipated. Yet, if the management plan is to leave the infant intubated and ventilated for a longer time, then the choice of anesthetic technique and muscle relaxant depends on other factors, such as the need to control blood pressure and the length of postoperative ventilation.

Nitrous oxide can be added provided oxygenation is closely monitored and expansion of any gas pocket in the body is considered. In the case of intestinal obstruction, the use of air along with appropriate concentrations of oxygen and a volatile drug is indicated. The normal full-term neonate has a systolic blood pressure between 60 and 70 mm Hg. For purposes of controlled hypotension, a blood pressure of 45–50 mm Hg is desired. The use of ketamine or opioids and a muscle relaxant can be advantageous when caring for the hemodynamically unstable infant. A study of the dose–response relationship of fentanyl in neonates undergoing surgery demonstrated that, in doses of $10–12.5$ mg $\cdot$ kg^{-1}, fentanyl produced a stable hemodynamic state and reliable anesthesia as determined by the heart rate and blood pressure.[26] The doses were given in increments of 2.5 mg $\cdot$ kg^{-1}. In all infants in the study, heart rate and systolic blood pressure decreased with the administration of fentanyl. One of the concerns with the administration of opioids in neonates is the altered pharmacokinetics and pharmacodynamics.[32,33] In one study, $25–50$ mg $\cdot$ kg^{-1} of fentanyl resulted in unpredictable respiratory effects and, in some neonates, postoperative respiratory depression. Four of 14 neonates studied, none of whom had any respiratory impairment secondary to surgery or disease, needed ventilatory support for 11–40 hours after operation. All infants had a rebound of fentanyl blood levels. There was a prolonged metabolism of the fentanyl, particularly in those with increased intra-abdominal pressure. This was thought to be due to a reduction in liver blood flow and hence metabolism of fentanyl—evidence of altered pharmacokinetics. In addition, it also appeared that newborns were more sensitive at the same plasma level to the respiratory depressant effects of fentanyl—evidence of altered pharmacodynamics.

Regional Anesthesia

There has been a tremendous increase in the use of regional anesthesia in children. In general, the regional techniques are combined with general anesthesia to permit early extubation and provide postoperative pain relief. Early extubation is possible because the use of regional anesthetic techniques eliminates the need for intraoperative narcotics in neonates, reduces or eliminates the need for muscle relaxants, and reduces the concentration of volatile agents needed for relaxation. Spinal anesthesia has been reported to be effective when used as the sole anesthetic technique in premature and high-risk infants, but this technique requires excellent cooperation between the anesthesiologist and an experienced surgeon. Even at a dose of 0.5 mg $\cdot$ kg^{-1}, the effects of tetracaine last only approximately 90 minutes in the neonate. Total spinal anesthesia, produced either with a primary spinal technique or secondary to an attempted epidural puncture, presents as respiratory insufficiency rather than as hypotension because of the lack of sympathetic tone in infants.[34] The exact mechanism for the lack of cardiovascular change with spinal anesthesia in infants and young children is not clear. Initially it was thought that there was a relative lack of development of the sympathetic nervous system. A more recent study, however, suggests that the sympatholysis that results from high thoracic spinal anesthesia and is expected to cause a decrease in heart rate and blood pressure is offset by a decrease in parasympathetic activity resulting in the withdrawal of cardiac vagal activity. The overall effect is no change in heart rate and blood pressure.[35] The first indication of trouble is a falling oxygen saturation rather than a falling blood pressure. Sedation can be added to regional anesthesia but may cause problems of apnea in ex-premature infants.

The techniques of caudal, spinal, brachial plexus, and other blocks should be considered in all neonates. Caudal epidural block is frequently used for abdominal and thoracic surgery in neonates. There are several different techniques described for performing a caudal. We prefer the 22-gauge short-bevel needle; the caudal space is identified both by the loss of resistance and the ease of administering the anesthetic. Once the sacrococcygeal membrane is penetrated and there is a loss of resistance, gentle aspiration is applied to the needle to determine if there is blood or cerebrospinal fluid (CSF). Injection of the anesthetic is then attempted. If there is difficulty in injecting the solution, the tip of the needle is not in the caudal space and it needs to be repositioned. If the anesthetic can be injected easily, this confirms placement in the epidural space. The needle is not advanced up the caudal canal after proper placement in the caudal space has been accomplished. In one study that uses Longwell catheters for the caudal epidural, the catheter is advanced up the caudal canal.[36] They report an iv injection incidence of approximately 6% with this technique. Evidence of an intravascular injection includes (1) peaked T-waves (which may be of relatively short duration, *e.g.*, 30 seconds), and (2) an increase in heart rate. Epinephrine is added to local anesthetic solutions for the purposes of determining if there is an intravascular injection of the anesthetic. The other technique to minimize the potential difficulties of an intravascular injection is to fractionate the dose by dividing the dose into three aliquots and waiting approximately 20–30 seconds between each aliquot before continuing the injection. A recent survey details the epidemiology and morbidity of regional anesthesia in children.[37]

Caudal anesthesia is particularly effective at reducing the concentrations of volatile anesthetics needed as well as relaxants and opioids. In addition, a single-injection caudal anesthetic can provide analgesia for 6–8 hours. The two local anesthetics currently in use are 0.25% bupivacaine or 0.2% ropivacaine. Epinephrine is added to local anesthetics to assist in determining if there has been an iv injection. The amount of epinephrine added should result in a 1:200,000 dilution of epinephrine (5 μg $\cdot$ ml^{-1}). Although ropivacaine has not been approved for use in infants, it does have several theoretical advantages. Because it is used in a concentration of 0.2%, compared with 0.25% for bupivacaine, there is less drug being administered per milliliter of injectate. In addition, ropivacaine has been reported to be less cardiodepressant than equipotent doses of bupivacaine. If a caudal catheter is placed, an infusion of bupivacaine can be administered and provide analgesia for several days. Close attention must be paid to the dosing of bupivacaine for postoperative infusions. Several studies have reported cardiovascular and central nervous system toxicity. Current recommendations for infusions in neonates and young infants are for an initial loading dose of 0.2–0.25 mg $\cdot$ kg^{-1}; after 1–2 hours, an infusion can be begun in a dose of 0.2 mg $\cdot$ kg$^{-1} \cdot$ h^{-1}. For older infants, toddlers, and children, the dosage range is 0.4–0.5 mg $\cdot$ kg$^{-1} \cdot$ h^{-1}.

Another block that has become popular is a simple ring block of the penis for circumcision. Bupivacaine 0.25% is injected subcutaneously in a ring about the base of the penis. This way, there is no danger of causing a hematoma, which occasionally occurs with a penile block.

Postoperative Ventilation

The choice of an anesthetic drug should also be determined by the need for postoperative management of ventilation and by the drug's effects on the circulation. If the surgical procedure or the neonate's condition is such that postoperative ventilation is likely, the prolonged respiratory effects of opioids or any other drug are of little concern. However, if the surgical procedure is relatively short and by itself does not require postoperative ventilation, the clinician should carefully select drugs and doses of anesthetic drugs and relaxants that will not necessitate prolonged postoperative ventilation or intubation. Postoperative ventilation places the neonate at added risk because of the problems associated with mechanical ventilation, the trauma to the subglottic area, and the potential development of postoperative subglottic stenosis or edema. However, if there is any question about the neonate's ability to maintain protective airway reflexes or normal ventilation after anesthesia, the neonate should be returned to the recovery room or newborn intensive care unit with the trachea intubated, and either ventilated or treated with a small amount of PEEP (2–4 cm H_2O).

Postoperative Pain Management

The concepts of postoperative pain management are well known to most anesthesiologists. The use of intraoperative epidural anesthesia followed by postoperative epidural local anesthetics or opioids has been popular in older children and adults, and these techniques are being applied to neonates. In addition, most neonatologists are experienced with the iv administration of opioids for patient comfort. Each technique has its own risks and benefits.

Uptake and Distribution of Anesthetics in Neonates

Rapid induction of anesthesia with volatile drugs can cause a greater degree of hypotension in young infants than in older infants and children.[38] However, no adverse effects from this fall in blood pressure were reported in these studies. There are several possible reasons for this observation. Young infants achieve a higher end-tidal halothane or isoflurane concentration more rapidly than older children and adults because the uptake of anesthetic drugs is more rapid in infants than in adults. Brandom et al[39] reported a study of both computer-simulated and measured halothane concentrations in infants (see Fig. 43-10). Whereas in the adult it takes 15–20 minutes to arrive at approximately a 50–60% equilibration of the end-tidal to the inspired halothane concentration, the infant is 70–80% equilibrated in the same period. The computer simulation similarly showed a higher concentration of halothane in the hearts of infants (Fig. 43-12). The same anesthetic concentration would also be present in the brain.

Various reasons for the faster uptake of anesthetics in infants have been proposed: (1) the ratio of alveolar ventilation to FRC is 5:1 in the infant and 1.5:1 in the adult; (2) in the neonate, more of the cardiac output goes to the vessel-rich group of organs, which includes the heart and brain; (3) the neonate has a greater cardiac output per kilogram of body mass; and (4) the infant has a lower blood gas partition coefficient for volatile anesthetics. An appreciation of the lower MAC in neonates, along with recognition of the more rapid uptake, suggests that care must be taken not to "overpressure" the concentration of the volatile drugs to as great a degree or for as long before intubation as would be done with an older infant or adult. The use of end-tidal gas measurements to determine both inspired and end-tidal anesthetic concentrations of the various volatile drugs can be helpful. Another not well-recognized factor that may result in higher concentrations of volatile anesthetics being administered to infants has to do with the use of nonrebreathing systems such as the Bain or a Mapleson "D" circuit. When an adult circle system is used with infant tubes and bag, the clinician experienced with this equipment is used to reading the inspired and end-tidal as well as the dialed concentration. In the circle system, the inspired concentration is a result of the combination of the end-tidal concentration that is rebreathed through the soda lime absorber and the dialed concentration. The inspired concentration is always lower than the dialed concentration, unless the flow rates are so high that a nonrebreathing system has been created. In the nonrebreathing system, the dialed concentration is the inspired concentration. Clinicians who use one system or the other are accustomed to these subtle differences. However, if the clinician switches back and forth between the circle system and a nonrebreathing circuit, but does so infrequently, there is a danger of not recognizing the possibility of excessive overpressure of volatile anesthetics with the nonrebreathing systems.

SURGICAL PROCEDURES IN NEONATES

For the purposes of discussion, surgical procedures in neonates are arbitrarily divided into two periods: those performed in the first week and those performed in the first month. Except for gastroschisis, which should be attended to within 12–24 hours, there are really no acute emergency operations in the neonate. This means that a period of 2–3 days can be allowed for stabilization or transport to an appropriate pediatric center for treatment. There is more to neonatal emergency surgery than just the immediate anesthetic and surgical procedure. Many of these infants require the support services of specialized nursing units, pediatric radiologists, pediatric intensive care physicians, and so forth. Managed care considerations should never take precedence over the appropriate care of infants and children.

Surgical Procedures in the First Week of Life

The five most frequent major surgical procedures performed in the first week of life are for congenital diaphragmatic hernia (CDH), omphalocele and gastroschisis, tracheoesophageal fistula (TEF), intestinal obstruction, and meningomyelocele. Some of these conditions, such as CDH, omphalocele and gastroschisis, and meningomyelocele, are obvious at birth. It may take hours or days for a TEF or intestinal obstruction to become manifest.

Two confounding factors in neonatal surgery are prematurity and associated congenital anomalies. The presence of one congenital anomaly increases the likelihood of another congenital anomaly. In conditions such as TEF, the mortality rate from the associated congenital heart defect is far higher than that from the surgical correction of the TEF. Prematurity, particularly when associated with the respiratory distress syndrome, may adversely affect surgical outcome. The use of surfactant in the treatment of the respiratory distress syndrome has greatly increased the number of survivors and has decreased the complexity of the issues of the infant with a combination of TEF and the respiratory distress syndrome. A neonatologist should be consulted in the case of any neonate with a congenital defect who is considered for surgery. The most serious associated congenital lesion is that of the cardiovascular system. Approximately 25–30% of infants with CDH have a cardiac anomaly.[40] Approximately 15–25% of infants with TEF have an associated congenital cardiac anomaly.[41]

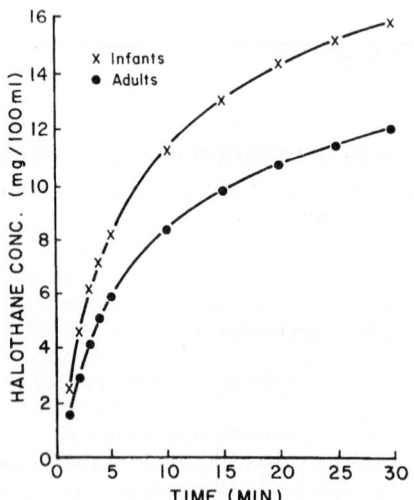

Figure 43-12. Predicted concentration of halothane in the heart. The values were derived from a computerized model of anesthetic uptake and distribution. The model infant weighed 4 kg; the model adult weighed 70 kg. In both cases, normal ventilation and a constant inspired fraction of 0.5% halothane were used. Tissue levels are given in milligrams per 100 ml of tissue. (Reprinted with permission from Brandom BW, Brandom RB, Cook DR: Uptake of halothane in infants. Anesth Analg 62:404, 1983.)

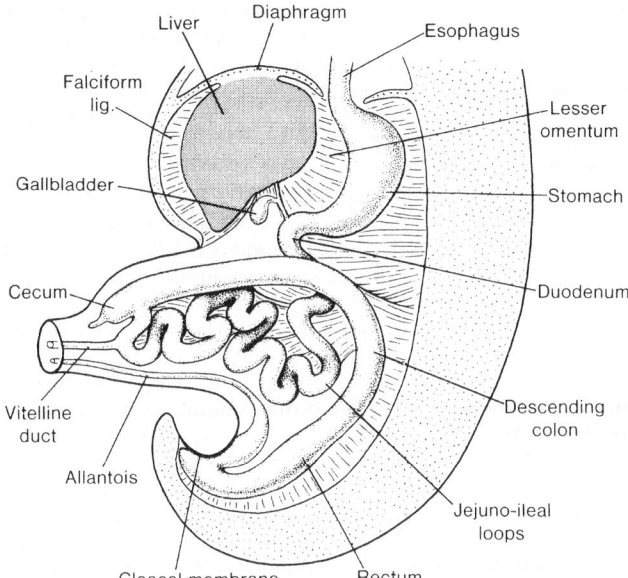

Figure 43-13. Umbilical herniation of the intestinal loops in an embryo of approximately 8 weeks' gestation (crown-rump length, 35 mm). Coiling of the small intestinal loops and formation of the cecum occur during the herniation. (Reprinted with permission from Body cavities and serous membranes. In Sadler TW: Langman's Medical Embryology, 5th ed., p 150. Baltimore, Williams & Wilkins, 1985.)

Maternal Cocaine Use During Pregnancy

Maternal cocaine use during pregnancy leads to a host of problems for the fetus and neonate. Cocaine results in a reduced catecholamine reuptake, which may result in the accumulation of catecholamines. This has circulatory effects on the uterus, the umbilical blood vessels, and the fetal cardiovascular system. The three major problems affecting the infant are premature birth, intrauterine growth retardation, and cardiovascular abnormalities.[42] One report documented a low cardiac output in infants of mothers who abused cocaine.[43] The cardiac output and stroke volume were reduced on the first day of life but had returned to normal by the second day. The clinical implication of this finding is that in infants of mothers who have abused cocaine, it may be advantageous to postpone any surgery until the second or third day of life. Cardiovascular abnormalities also were found in these infants. There was an increase in structural cardiovascular malformations and electrocardiographic abnormalities. The most frequent lesions were peripheral pulmonic stenosis, right ventricular conduction delay, right ventricular hypertrophy, and ST segment and T-wave changes.

Congenital Diaphragmatic Hernia

Congenital diaphragmatic hernia occurs with an incidence of approximately 1 in 4000 live births. Despite intensive, often heroic postoperative measures, the mortality rate from CDH remains in the range of 40–50% because of severe underdevelopment of the lung. A brief discussion of the embryologic characteristics of CDH will help the clinician understand the potentially enormous postoperative problems that may be encountered. It will become evident that the defect is more than a hernia of the diaphragm.

Early in fetal development, the pleuroperitoneal cavity is a single compartment. The gut is herniated or extruded to the extraembryonic coelom during the 5th to 10th weeks of fetal life (Fig. 43-13). During this period, the diaphragm develops to separate the thoracic and abdominal cavities (Fig. 43-14). The development of the diaphragm is usually completed by the seventh fetal week. In the 9th to 10th weeks, the developing gut returns to the peritoneal cavity. If there is delay or incomplete closure of the diaphragm, or if the gut returns early and prevents normal closure of the diaphragm, a diaphragmatic hernia will develop, producing varying degrees of herniation of the intestinal contents into the chest. The left side of the diaphragm closes later than the right side, which results in the higher incidence of left-sided diaphragmatic hernias (foramen of Bochdalek). Approximately 90% of hernias detected in the first week of life are on the left side.

The clinical presentation and the outcome from a diaphragmatic hernia are varied. At one end of the spectrum, the diaphragmatic hernia may develop early in fetal life so that the abdominal contents compress the developing lung bud, resulting in an extremely small, hypoplastic lung. Bilateral hypoplastic lungs may be found, with no chance for survival. At the other end of the spectrum, a moderately small diaphragmatic hernia may develop later in fetal life, so that the lung is normal but compressed by the abdominal viscera. In between is a large range of possibilities. At the mild end of the scale the infant might have a relatively normal pulmonary vascular bed with varying degrees of PPH that may revert to normal. At the more serious end of the spectrum are severe pulmonary hypoplasia and abnormal pulmonary vasculature with a very low chance for survival. There is an irreducible mortality rate with CDH.

After closure of the pleuroperitoneal membrane, muscular development of the diaphragm occurs. Incomplete muscularization of the diaphragm results in the development of a hernia sac because of intra-abdominal pressure. The condition is known as eventration of the diaphragm, and the diaphragm may extend well up into the thoracic cavity. The other possibility is that the innervation of the diaphragm is incomplete and the muscle atonic. Eventration of the diaphragm usually is not symptomatic in the first week of life.

Figure 43-14. Schematic drawings illustrating the development of the diaphragm. (*A*) The pleuroperitoneal folds appear at the beginning of the sixth week. (*B*) The pleuroperitoneal folds have fused with the septum transversum and the mesentery of the esophagus in the seventh week, thus separating the thoracic cavity from the abdominal cavity. (*C*) In a transverse section at the fourth month of development, an additional rim derived from the body wall forms the most peripheral part of the diaphragm. (Reprinted with permission from Body cavities and serous membranes. In Sadler TW: Langman's Medical Embryology, 5th ed., p 147. Baltimore, Williams & Wilkins, 1985.)

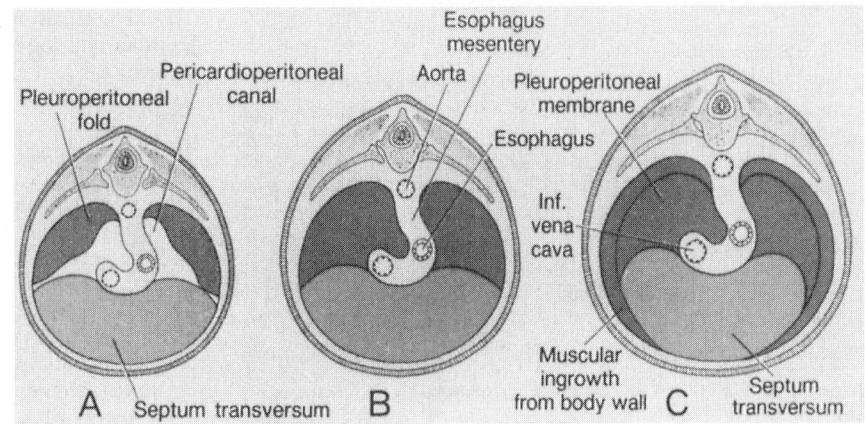

Clinical Presentation

Because the infant's status immediately at birth is determined primarily by the oxygenation of the placenta, the 1-minute Apgar score may well be normal. The occurrence of symptoms depends on the degree of herniation and interference with pulmonary function. At times, the degree of interference is so great that the neonate's clinical condition begins to deteriorate immediately, whereas in other situations it may be several hours before the infant's condition is fully appreciated. In the severely involved newborn, the initial clinical findings are usually classic and readily discerned. The infant has a scaphoid abdomen secondary to the absence of intra-abdominal contents, which have herniated into the chest (Fig. 43-15). Breath sounds on the affected side are reduced or absent. The diagnosis can be confirmed with an immediate radiograph. Immediate supportive care entails tracheal intubation and control of the airway, along with decompression of the stomach. Excessive airway pressure carries a high risk for pneumothorax and worsening of a bad situation.

Antenatal Diagnosis

The diagnosis of CDH can be made prenatally by fetal ultrasonography or ultrafast fetal magnetic resonance imaging. Antenatal diagnosis has led to the identification of a "hidden mortality" in CDH, fetuses who did not survive gestation and neonates who died before diagnosis. One of the hopes of prenatal diagnosis is to identify predictors of poor postnatal outcome. Various factors have been proposed, including early gestation diagnosis, severe mediastinal shift, polyhydramnios, a small lung-to-thorax transverse area ratio, and the herniation of liver or stomach. The single most predictive factor is the right lung area-to-head circumference ratio, defined as the lung area measured at the level of the four-chamber view divided by the head circumference to account for fetal size. New techniques in fetal surgery, such as temporary fetal tracheal occlusion, may prove beneficial to fetuses with CDH who are identified to be at risk for not surviving to term.[44,45] The other obvious advantage of prenatal diagnosis is that plans can be made for maternal or neonatal transport to a center with advanced neonatal critical care.

Preoperative Care

Congenital diaphragmatic hernia was traditionally treated as a surgical emergency. The infants were taken immediately to surgery for decompression and repair. The thought was that removing the abdominal viscera from the thorax would allow for re-expansion of the lung and improved oxygenation. However, as the pathophysiology of CDH was more clearly defined—

irreversible pulmonary hypoplasia associated with a hyper-reactive pulmonary vasculature—a strategy of preoperative stabilization with delayed surgical repair was adopted. Frenckner et al[46] have used this strategy of prolonged preoperative stabilization since 1990 and report survival rates of 90%, significantly better than the frequently quoted rates of 40–60%.

The stabilization of an infant with CDH may require multiple treatment modalities. The use of aggressive ventilation strategies to induce hyperventilation alkalosis has been abandoned secondary to the high incidence of iatrogenic lung injury. Conventional ventilation with permissive hypercapnia is now favored. The goal is to maintain preductal arterial saturation above 90% using peak inspiratory pressures below 35 cm H_2O and allowing the P_{CO_2} to rise to 60–65 mm Hg. High-frequency oscillatory ventilation has been used in place of conventional ventilation in an attempt to reduce barotrauma, but has not been shown to improve survival.[47] The Neonatal Inhaled Nitric Oxide Study Group (NINOS) was unable to demonstrate a beneficial effect for inhaled nitric oxide in infants with CDH and hypoxic respiratory failure unresponsive to aggressive conventional therapy, although it may have some benefit post-ECMO.[48] Neonates born with CDH may also have a component of surfactant deficiency, and studies have shown improvement in oxygenation in those infants given surfactant prophylactically.[47] Partial liquid ventilation with oxygenated perfluorocarbon is also being studied in infants with CDH.[47]

The use of ECMO in infants with CDH was initiated in the mid-1980s. Since then, over 2000 infants with CDH have been placed on ECMO. Despite extensive literature on the subject, there remains an ongoing debate as to whether ECMO improves survival in neonates with CDH. It is difficult to compare studies between institutions because of the different selection criteria used to initiate ECMO therapy. Some institutions use an oxygenation index (OI = [MAP × F_{IO_2} × 100]/Pa_{O_2}) of >40, whereas others use pH, preductal or postductal Pa_{O_2}, alveolar–arterial gradients, or ventilatory index (mean airway pressure × respiratory rate). The Congenital Diaphragmatic Hernia Study Group analyzed data from the multicenter CDH Registry and determined that ECMO improves the survival rate in CDH neonates with a predicted high risk of mortality (≥80%) based on birth weight and 5-minute Apgar score.[49]

Perioperative Care

Because delayed surgical repair of CDH is now the norm, neonates with CDH frequently present to the operating room already intubated and on some form of ventilatory support. Despite a period of preoperative stabilization, some infants still have a component of reactive pulmonary hypertension. The goals of ventilatory management are to ensure adequate oxygenation and avoid barotrauma. Any sudden deterioration in oxygen saturation with or without associated hypotension should raise suspicion of pneumothorax. It is important to avoid hypothermia because this increases the oxygen requirement and could precipitate pulmonary hypertension. Blood loss and fluid shifts are usually not a problem, although maintenance of intravascular volume is essential to avoid acidosis, which could also precipitate pulmonary hypertension.

The anesthetic technique chosen depends on the size of the defect and the anticipated postoperative respiratory status. In those infants who will remain intubated after surgery, inhalational agents and narcotics may be used as tolerated. In those infants with a small defect who present to the operating room with little or no respiratory distress, it may be beneficial to avoid intraoperative narcotics and provide regional analgesia in anticipation of extubation. The use of nitrous oxide should be avoided, particularly in those situations in which abdominal closure could be difficult. Muscle relaxation is often needed to facilitate abdominal closure.

Some centers are performing repairs of CDH while the neonate is on ECMO. This may be performed in the operating room

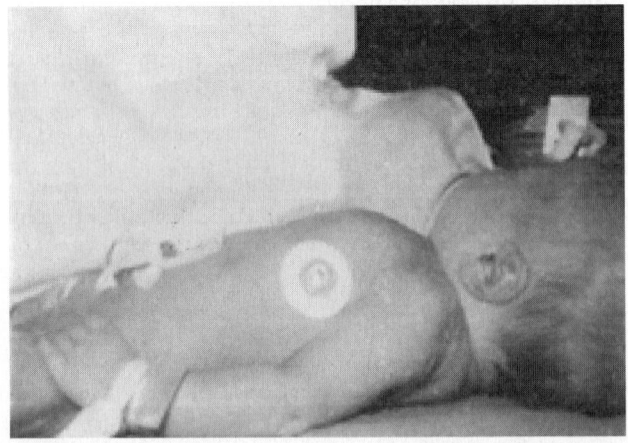

Figure 43-15. Infant with congenital diaphragmatic hernia. Note scaphoid abdomen.

or in the neonatal intensive care unit (NICU). The anesthetic technique usually consists of narcotics with muscle relaxation. Surgical repair while on ECMO can be associated with significant bleeding, making fluid management more challenging and increasing the mortality rate. The use of antifibrinolytic therapy has been associated with decreased hemorrhage and improved outcome.[46]

Postoperative Care

Most infants with CDH require intensive postoperative care. Recovery depends on the degree of pulmonary hypertension and pulmonary hypoplasia. It was previously believed that pulmonary hypoplasia was responsible for most deaths; however, it is now thought that potentially reversible pulmonary hypertension may be responsible for as much as 25% of reported deaths.[50]

Most infants require some form of ventilatory support in the postoperative period. Occasionally infants who were stabilized on conventional ventilation in the preoperative period require ECMO or inhaled nitrous oxide in the postoperative period. Some infants have long-term persistence of pulmonary hypertension. A study by Iocono et al[50] identified two parameters that were predictive of identifying patients with postnatal PPH at discharge with 100% sensitivity: an echocardiographic examination at 2 months of age demonstrating pulmonary hypertension; or requirement for respiratory support, either mechanical ventilation or supplemental oxygen, at 3 months of age.

There is evidence to suggest that cardiac development is impaired in infants with CDH. Relative left ventricular hypoplasia with an attenuated muscle mass and cavity size have been described. Many studies have confirmed that a calculated left ventricular mass less than $2 \ g \cdot kg^{-1}$ on pre-ECMO echocardiography was predictive of subsequent death.[51]

Omphalocele and Gastroschisis

Although omphalocele and gastroschisis sometimes appear similar and may be confused, they have entirely different origins and associated congenital anomalies.[52] During the 5th to 10th weeks of fetal life, the abdominal contents are extruded into the extraembryonic coelom, and the gut returns to the abdominal cavity at approximately the 10th week (see Fig. 43-13). Failure of part or all of the intestinal contents to return to the abdominal cavity results in an omphalocele that is covered with a membrane called the amnion. The amnion protects the abdominal contents from infection and the loss of extracellular fluid. The umbilical cord is found at approximately the apex of the sac (Fig. 43-16). Gastroschisis, by contrast, develops later in fetal

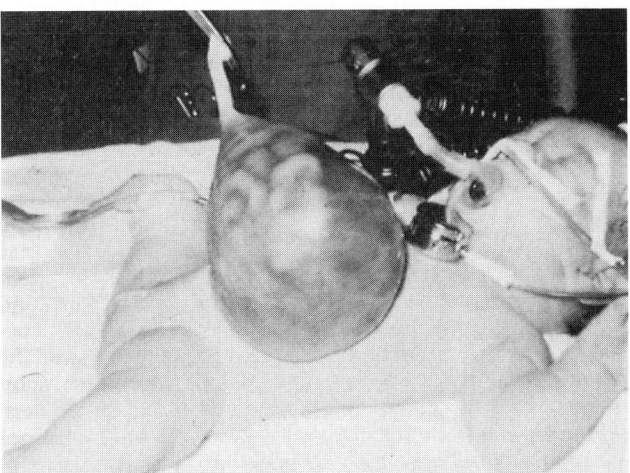

Figure 43-16. Omphalocele. (Reprinted with permission from Physiology and surgery of the infant. In Berry FA [ed]: Anesthetic Management of Difficult and Routine Pediatric Patients, p 152. New York, Churchill Livingstone, 1990.)

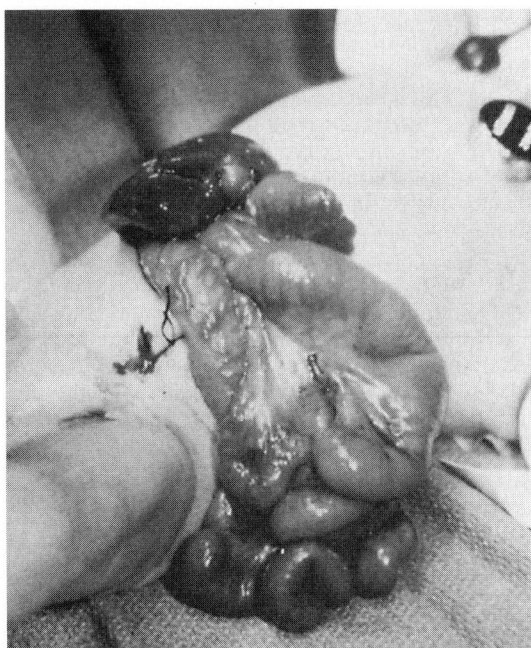

Figure 43-17. Gastroschisis.

life, after the intestinal contents have returned to the abdominal cavity. It results from interruption of the omphalomesenteric artery, which results in ischemia and atrophy of the various layers of the abdominal wall at the base of the umbilical cord. The gut then herniates through this tissue defect (Fig. 43-17). The degree of herniation may be slight, or major amounts of the abdominal viscera may be found outside the peritoneal cavity. The umbilical cord is found to one side of the intestinal contents. The intestines and viscera are not covered by any membrane and therefore are highly susceptible to infection and loss of extracellular fluid. There is a high incidence of associated congenital anomalies with omphalocele, but not with gastroschisis. The Beckwith-Wiedemann syndrome consists of mental retardation, hypoglycemia, congenital heart disease, a large tongue, and an omphalocele. Congenital heart lesions are found in approximately 20% of infants with omphalocele. Other associated congenital defects are found with gastroschisis and omphalocele; most involve the gastrointestinal tract and consist primarily of intestinal atresia or stenosis and malrotation.

Antenatal Diagnosis

α-Fetoprotein (AFP) is a normal closure protein present in fetal tissues during fetal development. Closure of the abdominal wall and the neural tube (see Meningomyelocele) prevents release of large quantities of this protein into the amniotic fluid. High levels of AFP in the amniotic fluid can cross the placenta and be detected in maternal blood. Thus, abnormal levels of AFP in the mother raise concerns over the possibility of either an abdominal wall defect or a neural tube defect in the fetus, as do high levels of AFP in fluid obtained during amniocentesis. Ultrasonography is reliable in helping to diagnose either condition.

Preoperative Care

There is controversy over the appropriate mode of delivery, vaginal or cesarean section, in parturients in whom the antenatal diagnosis has been made. Advocates of operative delivery maintain that it is necessary to prevent trauma to the exposed bowel and that it allows better coordination of the various medical specialties needed for immediate surgical management of the defect. Advocates of vaginal delivery point out that most infants with abdominal wall defects are born without injury to the bowel. The aspect of delivery room care unique to an infant with gastroschisis is the need to protect the exposed bowel and minimize fluid and temperature loss. This is best achieved by "bagging" the neonate, that is, placing its lower body in a sterile, clear plastic bag. The bag is then filled with warm saline and a drawstring is used to tighten the bag against the infant's body. This fluid must be maintained at body temperature to prevent hypothermia. Use of a fluid-filled bag helps protect against infection and the massive fluid loss that can occur with exposed bowel. This procedure is not necessary with omphalocele because the bowel is still enclosed by amnion.

Preoperative stabilization of the neonate with an abdominal wall defect includes management of respiratory insufficiency, establishment of adequate iv access, and an assessment for associated congenital anomalies. Respiratory failure at birth in infants with omphalocele is a significant predictor of mortality.[53] Lung hypoplasia and abnormal thoracic development may be significant in infants with large omphaloceles. Fluid losses can be excessive, particularly in neonates with gastroschisis. Central venous access may be necessary to provide adequate fluid resuscitation. Serum electrolytes and glucose should be obtained before to going to the operating room. In addition, the infant with an omphalocele should be assessed for any associated congenital anomalies prior to going to the operating room. Congenital heart disease is found in approximately 20% of patients. A difficult airway can be anticipated in the patient with Beckwith-Wiedemann syndrome. Infants with gastroschisis are at high risk for infection because of exposed bowel; therefore, the initial stabilization includes antibiotic therapy.

Traditionally, neonates with gastroschisis have been taken to the operating room urgently, within the first 12–24 hours, for reduction of closure. A recent British study describes a technique of "minimal intervention management" for gastroschisis. After a short period of stabilization in the NICU, midgut reduction was performed in the conscious neonate without anesthesia. The reduction was performed through the umbilical cord while monitoring respiratory status and lower extremity circulation. The reported advantages of such a technique include the avoidance of ventilation, a shorter time until full enteral feedings are established, and a scarless abdomen with an aesthetically normal umbilicus.[54]

Surgery is not urgent in the neonate with an omphalocele, and can be delayed for several days until the infant is assessed and stabilized. In those infants with severe respiratory distress or congenital heart disease who are too unstable for surgery, nonsurgical treatment with topical antiseptics and delayed closure is an option.

Perioperative Care

The two major perioperative concerns are fluid loss and ventilation. The fluid volume management of the infant often entails administration of large amounts of full-strength balanced salt solution. The adequacy of the peripheral circulation and urine output is an indicator of the adequacy of the volume resuscitation. Both conditions may present an intraoperative challenge to the anesthesiologist because with an omphalocele, after the amniotic membrane is removed, large volumes of fluid may transudate or exudate from the exposed abdominal viscera. The fluid that is lost is extracellular fluid, which should be replaced with full-strength balanced salt solution. An arterial line is often used for blood pressure monitoring and frequent blood gas monitoring to assess acid–base status.

If the defect in the abdominal wall is small, a primary repair of the deficit can be accomplished. However, with a large defect, it may be difficult to return the abdominal viscera to the peritoneal cavity because the muscle and peritoneum are underdeveloped. Because of concern for the increase in the volume of gas in the intestine, nitrous oxide should not be used. Excellent skeletal muscle relaxation is necessary to allow closure of the abdomen. With moderate-sized abdominal wall defects, it may not be possible to close the peritoneum, but there may be sufficient skin to close the defect. With large defects, the peritoneal cavity may be too small to contain the viscera, and attempted closure can impair circulation to the bowel, kidneys, and lower extremities as well as compromise respiration. A pulse oximeter probe on the foot can be helpful in monitoring circulation to the lower extremities during abdominal wall closure.

Attempts have been made to find objective criteria by which to determine whether the infant will tolerate primary closure of the defect and to avoid or minimize the circulatory and ventilatory problems. One study that measured intragastric pressure in infants who underwent primary closure found that if the intragastric pressure was 20 mm Hg or more, the infant needed reoperation and placement of a Dacron silo (Fig. 43-18) within 24 hours of the primary closure.[55] If the intragastric pressure was less than 20 mm Hg, the defect was successfully closed primarily. Intragastric pressure is measured by placing a nasogastric tube in the stomach and using a column of saline to measure the pressure. A value of 20 mm Hg is approximately 27 cm H_2O. Studies in dogs revealed a close correlation between

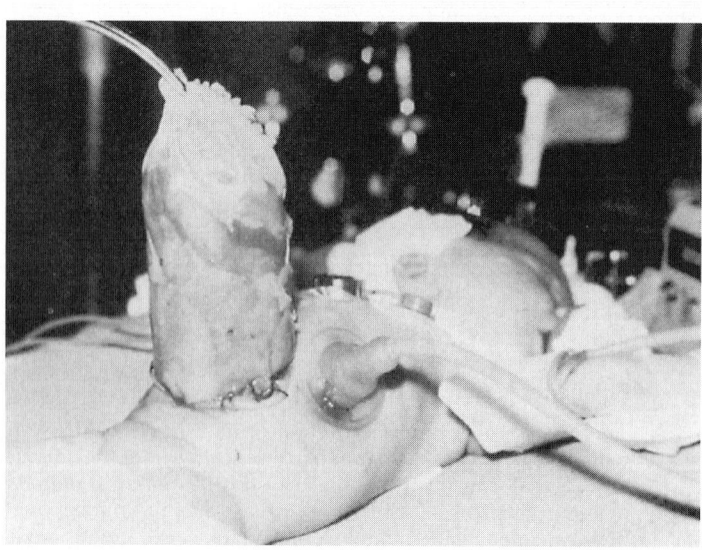

Figure 43-18. Dacron silo for extruded viscera. (Reprinted with permission from Physiology and surgery of the infant. In Berry FA [ed]: Anesthetic Management of Difficult and Routine Pediatric Patients, p 154. New York, Churchill Livingstone, 1990)

bladder pressure and intra-abdominal pressure; thus, bladder pressure can be used as an alternative measurement of intra-abdominal pressure.[56]

If primary closure is impossible, a silo is incorporated into the abdominal wall to contain and cover the abdominal viscera. The repair is then staged from this point onward. Every 2 or 3 days, the size of the silo is reduced, in much the same fashion that a tube of toothpaste is squeezed. The infant may feel some degree of discomfort as the peritoneum and skin are stretched. Small doses of ketamine, $0.5–1.0 \text{ mg} \cdot \text{kg}^{-1}$, are titrated as the silo is reduced. The infant is allowed to breathe spontaneously and without intubation. Oxygen saturation should be monitored with a pulse oximeter, and the infant's pulse and blood pressure are also monitored. These measurements help the surgeon and anesthesiologist determine the appropriate silo reduction that allows adequate ventilation and circulation. This is a situation that requires clinical judgment. After several stages of silo reduction, the final operation is complete closure of the abdominal wall defect under full anesthesia with complete muscle relaxation.

Postoperative Care

The postoperative care of infants with omphalocele or gastroschisis is critical. Some need tracheal intubation and assisted ventilation of the lungs for as long as 3–7 days. Additional complications include postoperative hypertension and edema of the extremities. The increased abdominal pressure can reduce the circulation to the kidneys, which results in a release of renin. Renin activates the renin–angiotensin–aldosterone system, which is thought to cause the hypertension. Obstruction of the venous circulation of the lower body may cause a large amount of edema of the legs. These infants need large amounts of extracellular fluid resuscitation.

Tracheoesophageal Fistula

The treatment of esophageal atresia and TEF can be both challenging and satisfying for the anesthesiologist. Death in the perioperative period typically results from prematurity or from an associated congenital heart defect. TEF occurs in approximately 1 in 3000 live births. Approximately 85% consist of a fistula from the distal trachea to the esophagus and a blind proximal esophageal pouch. In 10% of cases, there is a blind proximal esophageal pouch with no TEF (Fig. 43-19). The embryologic defect results from imperfect division of the foregut into the anteriorly positioned larynx and trachea and the posteriorly positioned esophagus; the division should occur between the fourth and fifth weeks of intrauterine life. Fifty percent of affected infants have associated congenital anomalies, of which approximately 15–25% involve the cardiovascular system.

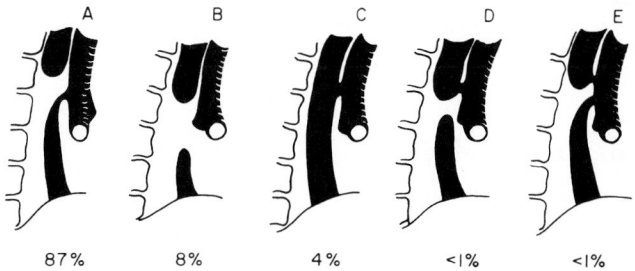

Figure 43-19. Diagrams of the five most commonly encountered forms of esophageal atresia and tracheoesophageal fistula, shown in order of frequency. (Reprinted with permission from Herbst JJ: Gastrointestinal tract. In Behrman RE, Kleigman RM, Nelson WE, Vaughan III WC [eds]: Nelson Textbook of Pediatrics, 14th ed, p 942. Philadelphia, WB Saunders, 1992.)

Clinical Presentation

Atresia of the esophagus leads to inability of the fetus to swallow amniotic fluid and the subsequent development of polyhydramnios. Ultrasound may well raise the possibility of a congenital anomaly. For that reason, if polyhydramnios is present, attempts should be made to pass a nasogastric tube shortly after delivery. Passing a nasogastric tube is not routine in the delivery room; therefore, the diagnosis may not become apparent until the infant is fed. Cyanosis and choking with oral feedings should raise suspicion.

There are two major complications of esophageal atresia with a distal tracheal fistula: aspiration pneumonia and dehydration. The presence of a distal TEF increases the likelihood of reflux of gastric juice up the esophagus and into the pulmonary system. Dehydration results from the fact that the proximal esophagus does not communicate with the stomach. Therefore, preoperative preparation of these infants is aimed at evaluation and treatment of the pulmonary system and ensuring adequate hydration and electrolyte balance. At times, the degree of reflux and pneumonia is so great that a gastrostomy must be performed to protect the pulmonary system, and a period of several days is needed to improve the general condition of the infant. However, if the infant is in good condition, primary repair can be performed at 24–48 hours. This consists of ligation of the fistula and a primary repair with approximation of the two ends of the esophagus.

Anesthetic Considerations

The presence of a gastrostomy reduces the potential for reflux of gastric juice during the surgical procedure. If a gastrostomy is present, the gastrostomy tube should be open to air and left at the head of the table under the anesthesiologist's observation to avoid kinking and obstruction. Not all patients need a gastrostomy, however. There is some difference of opinion concerning the technique for intubation of the trachea. Some clinicians prefer an awake intubation, and others prefer intubation after induction of anesthesia. The important issue is to avoid excessive positive pressure ventilation, which distends the stomach, thereby increasing the risk for reflux and ventilatory compromise. If an awake tracheal intubation is done, it can be facilitated by the topical administration of lidocaine and with the use of $1 \text{ mg} \cdot \text{kg}^{-1}$ of lidocaine iv 1–2 minutes before laryngoscopic examination. Most clinicians prefer the technique described in the following paragraph.

There are two approaches to tracheal intubation after induction of anesthesia. One is to use an inhalation induction, followed by topical application of lidocaine and intubation while the infant is breathing spontaneously. The other technique is to use an iv or inhalation induction and intubate the trachea after muscle paralysis. This technique may lead to distention of the fistula and stomach with excessive positive-pressure ventilation. With either technique, topical anesthesia of the larynx may be achieved with $4–5 \text{ mg} \cdot \text{kg}^{-1}$ of 2% lidocaine sprayed on the larynx and vocal cords. Lidocaine 2% is preferred to higher concentrations in these small infants because it is easier to control the dose. When controlled ventilation of the lungs is used, attempts must be made to minimize the distention of the stomach and the potential for reflux. If a gastrostomy tube is in place, the point is moot. Alternatively, because the fistula is usually located just above the carina on the posterior wall of the membranous trachea, the endotracheal tube can be placed just distal to the TEF. To do this, the endotracheal tube is inserted until it enters one or the other mainstem bronchi. This is judged by unilateral expansion of the chest and unilateral breath sounds. The endotracheal tube is then slowly withdrawn until bilateral chest movement and breath sounds are confirmed.

The endotracheal tube might inadvertently enter the fistula either during the initial tracheal intubation of the infant, when the infant is turned, or during surgical manipulation. The clinical indications for this are increased difficulty in ventilation of the lungs and decreased oxygen saturation and end-tidal CO_2. Because these findings may also be present when the lung is packed away to perform the surgery, and because there are other explanations for these findings, intubation of the fistula should always be included in the differential diagnosis. Any time ventilation is difficult and desaturation is occurring, the surgeon must stop the procedure and the lungs should be ventilated. The surgeon will be able to palpate the tip of the tube in the fistula if this is the problem.

The localization and isolation of H-type fistulas can be difficult. In this situation, bronchoscopy is performed by the surgeon, the fistula is identified, and a guide wire is fed through the fistula tract into the esophagus. The infant is then intubated, with care taken not to dislodge the guide wire. Once intubated esophagoscopy is performed, the guide wire is visualized and brought out through the mouth. In this way the surgeon can use fluoroscopy to determine the level of the fistula and decide whether a cervical or thoracic approach is necessary. During surgery, the anesthesiologist can apply traction to the wire loop to facilitate the localization of the fistula by the surgeon.[57]

Other techniques for obliterating H-type fistulas, such as electrocauterization and neodymium–ytrrium-aluminum-garnet laser, have been attempted with varying success.[58]

Postoperative Care

Although there have been great advances in the treatment of TEF and esophageal atresia, postoperative care can be complicated by associated congenital heart disease, respiratory distress syndrome, and a need for continued postoperative ventilation. The compression of the lung for several hours, along with pre-existing aspiration pneumonia in some of these infants, suggests the need in the more difficult cases for a short period of postoperative ventilation or at least intubation with PEEP, as the most conservative technique for postoperative airway management. Some infants are in excellent condition at the time of surgery with no complicating factors, and therefore should be considered for extubation immediately at the end of surgery or shortly thereafter. If extubation of the trachea is planned for the end of surgery, the anesthetic technique must be tailored accordingly. Caudal anesthesia as part of the technique is useful in these situations, reducing the concentration of maintenance volatile anesthetics, the amount of muscle relaxants, and the need for intraoperative narcotics.

A high percentage of infants with esophageal atresia have residual difficulties of the tracheobronchial tree and esophagus for many years. These include tracheomalacia, gastroesophageal reflux, esophageal stricture, and recurrent fistulas.

Intestinal Obstruction

For purposes of discussion, obstruction of the gastrointestinal system can be arbitrarily divided into obstruction of the upper gastrointestinal tract (*i.e.*, duodenum) and obstruction of the lower gastrointestinal tract (*i.e.*, terminal ileum, colon, imperforate anus). Obstruction of the upper gastrointestinal tract usually is evident within the first 24 hours of life, when the institution of feedings leads to vomiting, whereas obstruction of the lower gastrointestinal tract becomes evident somewhere between 2 and 7 days of age, as the infant becomes progressively distended, little or no stool is passed, and there is vomiting.

Upper Gastrointestinal Tract Obstruction

If there has been persistent vomiting, this usually means that a deficit of fluids or electrolytes will develop in the infant. The stomach contains approximately 100–130 mEq·l^{-1} of sodium and 5–10 mEq·l^{-1} of potassium. The greatest deficit is for sodium. Another major concern in the infant with upper gastrointestinal tract obstruction is aspiration of gastric contents.

Therefore, awake tracheal intubation may be indicated. Techniques for this are discussed in an earlier section.

The anesthetic management of these patients is directed toward ensuring adequate relaxation for abdominal exploration, repair of the congenital defect, and closure of the abdomen. Nitrous oxide can be used in high intestinal obstruction because there is essentially no gas in the gastrointestinal tract. The next concern is whether the infant's trachea should be extubated at the end of surgery. If the infant is robust, extubation of the trachea at the end of surgery can be anticipated. The preferred technique is for general anesthesia combined with caudal epidural anesthesia. This allows very light levels of volatile agent and minimal muscle relaxant use, resulting in an early extubation. Opioids are not administered until the postoperative period. However, if the infant is moderately debilitated or if the surgical incision is extensive, a period of postoperative intubation with PEEP may well be indicated, particularly if moderate doses of opioids have been used. These infants are also candidates for regional techniques.

Lower Gastrointestinal Tract Obstruction

The problems associated with lower gastrointestinal tract obstruction usually develop within 2–7 days after birth. It may take this long for the lesion to become evident because it is low in the gastrointestinal tract. An imperforate anus should be recognizable shortly after birth. Some of these infants may have vomiting secondary to the obstruction, which poses a problem for fluid and electrolyte management. An enormous amount of fluid can be sequestered within the intestinal tract. This fluid is essentially extracellular fluid and has a high sodium content. Therefore, these infants should be prepared carefully for surgery and have a serum sodium level of at least 130 mEq·l^{-1} and a urine volume of 1–2 ml·kg^{-1}·h^{-1}.

If the infant has had minimal or no vomiting, rapid-sequence induction of anesthesia and tracheal intubation can be done. Rapid-sequence induction in an infant is the same as in an adult, with iv barbiturate or propofol, muscle relaxant, cricoid pressure, and oxygenation. If the infant is experiencing vomiting in the immediate preoperative period, the most conservative approach is an awake tracheal intubation after gastric decompression. Although a nasogastric tube may be in place, there is no guarantee that the stomach is empty. Nitrous oxide should not be used in any infant who has gaseous distention of the intestine, which is easily determined from the preoperative radiograph. Providing adequate muscle relaxation for surgery can be accomplished with various anesthetic techniques such as volatile anesthesia, muscle relaxants, and caudal epidural block.

The criteria for tracheal extubation at the end of surgery are the same as those described for upper gastrointestinal tract obstruction. When in doubt, leave the tracheal tube in place with PEEP. This is not to suggest that prolonged tracheal intubation is benign; it is not. There is a small but significant risk for the development of subglottic stenosis, but this is a situation in which the risk of subglottic stenosis and other airway trauma must be weighed against the risk of too early tracheal extubation with vomiting, aspiration, and airway obstruction.

Meningomyelocele

Clinical Presentation

Myelomeningocele is the most common congenital primary neural tube defect, occurring in approximately 1 of every 1000 live births. It results from failure of neural tube closure during the fourth week of gestation. Neural tube defects can be identified on prenatal ultrasound. Elevated maternal serum AFP detects 50–90% of open neural tube defects but has a false-positive rate of 5%. Amniotic fluid AFP is more reliable. Evidence also supports a relation between folic acid deficiency and the development of neural tube defects.

By definition, the lesion involves both the meninges and neural components, as compared with a meningocele, which does not contain neural elements. The infant is born with a cystic mass on the back comprising a neural placode, arachnoid, dura, nerve tissue and roots, and CSF. The lesion most commonly occurs in the lumbosacral or sacral region. The bony canal is also malformed, leading to multiple orthopedic problems as the child matures. Urologic complications correlate with the level of the spinal lesion.

Most infants born with myelomeningocele have an associated anomaly of the brain stem known as the Arnold-Chiari II (Chiari II) malformation. The Chiari II malformation is characterized by caudal displacement of the cerebellar vermis through the foramen magnum, caudal displacement of the medulla oblongata and the cervical spine, kinking of the medulla, and obliteration of the cisterna magna. Hydrocephalus requiring shunting develops in approximately 90% of infants with myelomeningocele. On the other hand, only 20% of patients have symptoms of brain stem dysfunction as a result of the Chiari II malformation, but the mortality rate among those symptomatic patients is high. Symptoms of brain stem dysfunction include stridor, apnea and bradycardia, aspiration pneumonia, sleep-disordered breathing patterns, vocal cord paralysis, incoordination, and spasticity. If the symptoms are not improved by shunting, posterior fossa decompression is necessary.[59–61]

The infant with a myelomeningocele is usually operated on within the first 72 hours of life. This reduces the risk for development of ventriculitis or progressive neurologic deficits. Most centers close the defect and place a shunt at the same time. However, some centers may delay placement of a shunt until the infant shows symptoms of hydrocephalus. There is some evidence that intrauterine repair of myelomeningocele may decrease the morbidity associated with the Chiari II malformation and brain stem dysfunction.[62]

Preoperative Care

The safest route of delivery of an infant with a myelomeningocele remains controversial. Some question whether labor and vaginal delivery can adversely affect neurologic outcome. However, there are studies suggesting no difference in neurologic deficits between infants delivered vaginally or by cesarean section.

The preoperative stabilization period focuses on the prevention of infection, maintenance of extracellular fluid volume, and assessment for other congenital anomalies. The exposed neural placode is susceptible to trauma, leakage, and infection. The infant is usually placed in the prone position and the placode is covered with saline-soaked gauze to prevent desiccation. Because of the high risk of infection, antibiotic therapy is initiated in the preoperative period. Rupture of the cyst on the back can lead to ongoing CSF leakage. This fluid is replaced with full-strength balanced salt solution. The infant is also assessed for any potentially life-threatening congenital anomalies.

Perioperative Care

The high prevalence of clinical latex allergy and latex sensitization in children with myelomeningocele has drawn much attention. Studies show that the prevalence increases with increasing age. It is believed that an early, intense exposure to the allergen, as occurs with frequent surgery and bladder catheterization, contributes to this high prevalence. As a result, these infants are now labeled as latex sensitive and cared for in a latex-free environment.[63]

Positioning is critical in the infant with myelomeningocele. For induction of anesthesia, the infant may be placed supine with the defect resting in a "donut" to minimize trauma. Alternatively, the induction can be performed with the infant in the lateral position, although this makes intubation more challenging. The infant is turned prone for surgery. Rolls are positioned to ensure that the abdomen and chest are free, avoiding pressure on the epidural venous plexus to minimize bleeding and allowing for adequate ventilation.

In most instances, the infant has an iv line placed before surgery and an iv induction is performed. Succinylcholine may be used to facilitate intubation without risking hyperkalemia.[64] Because increased intracranial pressure is rarely present before closure of the defect, inhalational induction is an alternative in the infant with difficult iv access. Identification of neural tissue may require nerve stimulation, and therefore muscle relaxants are avoided. Narcotics are used with caution in these infants because of the abnormal response to hypoxia and hypercarbia, predisposing to apnea and bradycardia. Careful monitoring of temperature is necessary because prolonged exposure during repair can lead to hypothermia. These infants must remain intubated until they are fully awake. The effects of general anesthesia in association with the abnormalities of respiratory control may warrant a prolonged period of respiratory support in some infants with myelomeningocele.

Regional anesthesia has been reported as a safe alternative to general anesthesia in the neonate with myelomeningocele. Viscomi et al[65] successfully administered tetracaine spinals to 14 infants undergoing repair of myelomeningocele. In this small series, there was no evidence of anesthetic-induced neurologic damage. Two of the 14 infants had a postoperative respiratory event (1 transient apnea/bradycardia and 1 brief desaturation with bradycardia). Both of these infants had received intraoperative midazolam for sedation.

Postoperative Care

These infants must be monitored closely in the postoperative period. Respiratory complications, including stridor, apnea and bradycardia, cyanosis, and respiratory arrest may develop after surgery in these infants with known brain stem abnormalities and potential disorders of central respiratory control. In addition, those infants who were not shunted during repair may show signs of hydrocephalus, including lethargy, vomiting, seizures, apnea and bradycardia, or cardiovascular instability. These infants need to return to the operating room for insertion of a shunt.

Hydrocephalus

Hydrocephalus may occur after closure of a meningomyelocele because of the Arnold-Chiari malformation. The cranial sutures in the neonate are open, so that intracranial pressure increases are blunted or minimized. However, infants with hydrocephalus eventually have an increase in head size and sometimes in intracranial pressure, resulting in lethargy, vomiting, and cardiorespiratory problems. The anesthetic approach and the technique for tracheal intubation depend on the infant's condition. The major concern is protection of the airway and control of intracranial pressure. Awake tracheal intubation, crying, struggling, and straining can increase intracranial pressure. A rapid-sequence induction of anesthesia to control the airway and intracranial pressure is preferred. Pretreatment before a rapid-sequence induction consists of the administration of iv curare or atracurium in a dose of $0.05 \text{ mg} \cdot \text{kg}^{-1}$. A rapid-sequence induction with $3–4 \text{ mg} \cdot \text{kg}^{-1}$ of thiopental or $2–3 \text{ mg} \cdot \text{kg}^{-1}$ of propofol, $2 \text{ mg} \cdot \text{kg}^{-1}$ of succinylcholine, and cricoid pressure can lead to rapid control of the airway. Hyperventilation, along with the administration of barbiturate, rapidly controls intracranial pressure. Volatile drugs, nitrous oxide, and opioids are all reasonable choices for maintenance of anesthesia. Noninvasive intracranial pressure measurements in neurologically normal preterm neonates have shown a decrease in intracranial pressure with all drugs, including ketamine, fentanyl, isoflurane, and halothane. The failure of volatile anesthetics and ketamine to increase intracranial pressure as in adults is attributed to the compliance of the neonate's open-sutured cranium. After surgery, the trachea of these infants should remain intubated and they should receive PEEP if they were experiencing periods of apnea or bradycardia before surgery because of the intracranial abnormalities. If not, the trachea can be extubated as soon as the protective reflexes have recovered.

Surgical Procedures in the First Month of Life

Surgical procedures in the first month also are considered emergent, or at least urgent, surgery. The six most frequent surgical procedures in the first month are exploratory laparotomy for necrotizing enterocolitis (NEC), inguinal hernia repair, correction of pyloric stenosis, PDA ligation, a shunt procedure for hydrocephalus, and placement of a central venous catheter.

Necrotizing Enterocolitis

Necrotizing enterocolitis is a disease that primarily affects premature infants who have survived the first days of life. One of the theories about NEC is that earlier, more rapid feeding places infants at greater risk for development of NEC. A study by Kliegman et al[66] supports this theory. They found that delayed feeding was related to a delayed onset of NEC. Another factor in the feeding issue is that the larger the feeding, the higher the incidence of NEC. It primarily affects the very–low-birth-weight infant, but it may also affect the larger premature and occasionally full-term neonates. The incidence of NEC among very–low-birth-weight infants varies between 5 and 15%.[67] It has been postulated that because the use of surfactant increases the survival of very small premature infants with respiratory distress syndrome, it may also increase the incidence of NEC.[67]

The exact pathophysiology of NEC has yet to be determined. Kosloske proposed the hypothesis that NEC occurs by the coincidence of two of three pathologic events: intestinal ischemia, colonization by pathogenic bacteria, and excess protein substrate in the intestinal lumen.[68] NEC is more likely to appear after quantitative extremes (i.e., severe ischemia, highly pathogenic flora, or significant excess of substrate). NEC develops only if a threshold of injury sufficient to initiate intestinal necrosis is exceeded. The condition is characterized by a cascade of pathologic events, beginning with an immature intestine that has a decreased ability to absorb substrate, leading to stasis. Stasis encourages bacterial proliferation, which leads to local infection. The picture is complicated by further pooling of fluid. The ischemia and infection may lead to necrosis of the intestinal mucosa, followed by perforation. The perforation leads to gangrene, fluid loss, peritonitis, septicemia, and disseminated intravascular coagulation. The first signs that NEC may be developing are abdominal distention, irritability, and the development of metabolic acidosis. NEC is primarily a medical disease and is treated by cessation of oral intake and administration of antibiotics and supportive care, particularly fluid and electrolyte therapy. In nonresponsive cases, the infant becomes more septic with severe peritonitis, and the only solution is to perform an exploratory laparotomy to remove the gangrenous bowel and create an ileostomy.

The preoperative problems are an acute abdomen with severe peritonitis, necrosis and gangrene of the intestine, septicemia, metabolic acidosis, and hypovolemia. These neonates may also have a coagulopathy. Preparation of the patient is directed toward these problems. Often the septicemia, coupled with the distended abdomen and the overall clinical deterioration of the infant, also necessitates the use of intubation and ventilation in the NICU. The anesthetic requirements are continuation of resuscitation, provision of abdominal relaxation for the surgery, and careful titration of anesthetic drugs. These infants are often so critically ill that they tolerate minimal anesthesia. One choice is to start with small doses of ketamine, 0.5–1 mg·kg⁻¹. This can be administered every 20–30 minutes. If the condition improves, fentanyl, 2–3 mg·kg⁻¹, can be administered, up to a total dose of 10–12 mg·kg⁻¹. If the infant's condition improves

dramatically, small doses of volatile drug can be added as well. The use of nitrous oxide should be avoided because of the gas pockets in the abdomen.

These infants are among the most challenging cases in all of pediatric anesthesia. Monitoring of intra-arterial pressure and arterial blood gases has usually been started in the NICU. The fluid loss can be enormous. They need full-strength balanced salt solution for maintenance of blood pressure and urine output. If the hematocrit is below 30–35%, blood should be administered. These infants are returned to the NICU and their postoperative care coordinated carefully with the surgeon, neonatologist, or pediatrician.

Inguinal Hernia Repair in the Neonate

The development of a hernia in the premature infant or neonate is a different clinical problem from the development of a hernia in an infant older than 1 year of age.[69,70] In one study of 100 infants younger than 2 months of age who needed inguinal hernia repair, 30% were premature, 42% had a history of respiratory distress syndrome, 16% had been ventilated, and 19% had congenital heart disease.[69] Furthermore, 31% of the infants had incarcerated hernias, 9% had an intestinal obstruction, and 2% had gonadal infarction. These data preclude waiting until a premature infant or neonate is 6 months or 1 year of age before performing "elective" surgery. The potential for emergent or urgent intervention is so great that surgical repair should be accomplished within a reasonable amount of time after an inguinal hernia is discovered. The "reasonable" time depends on the infant's condition. If the infant is normal and has no other life-threatening medical problems, repair can be done within several days or weeks. If the infant has another problem, the waiting period should be sufficient to stabilize the infant's condition.

Perioperative complications are frequent in these infants. In the 100 patients reported by Rescorla and Grosfeld,[69] 2 had apnea and bradycardia, 4 needed postoperative ventilatory support, 1 had a cardiac arrest resulting from digoxin toxicity, and 1 acquired Klebsiella sepsis. It has long been recognized that premature infants undergoing elective surgery have a higher rate of complications than full-term infants undergoing the same type of surgery.

Postoperative Apnea

A major concern with surgery in neonates is the development of apnea in the postoperative period. The infants at highest risk are those born prematurely, those with multiple congenital anomalies, those with a history of apnea and bradycardia, and those with chronic lung disease. The etiology of this apnea is multifactorial. Decreased ventilatory control and hyporesponsiveness to hypoxia and hypercarbia may be potentiated by anesthetic agents. Respiratory muscle fatigue may also play a role because neonates have a smaller percentage of Type I fibers in their diaphragm and intercostal muscles. Hypothermia and anemia may also contribute to the development of postoperative apnea.[71–74] The treatment of postoperative apnea may be as simple as tactile stimulation with "blow by" oxygen. However, some infants require prolonged intubation in ventilatory support. Infants with life-threatening apnea and bradycardia before surgery may be on central nervous system stimulants. Caffeine or theophylline both act by increasing central respiratory drive and lowering the threshold of response to hypercarbia as well as stimulating contractility in the diaphragm. Administering supplemental intraoperative doses to those infants to ensure adequate serum levels of drugs may prevent the need for prolonged periods of postoperative ventilatory support.[75,76]

Those infants at high risk for development of postoperative apnea may benefit from the use of a regional anesthetic as opposed to general anesthesia. Multiple studies have shown that spinal anesthesia without supplemental sedation decreases the incidence of postoperative apnea and bradycardia in high-risk infants. Once supplemental sedation is used, inhalation or ketamine, this advantage is lost.[77,78] The question remains as to which infant should be monitored after surgery, and for how long. The most conservative approach is to monitor all infants younger than 60 weeks postconceptual age for 24 hours after surgery.[71] Many reports show that the incidence of significant apnea and bradycardia is highest in the first 4–6 hours after surgery, but they have been reported up to 12 hours after surgery. In addition, the incidence of apnea directly correlates to postconceptual age. Therefore, the most widely accepted guideline is to monitor all infants younger than 50 weeks postconceptual age for at least 12 hours after surgery, even infants who have had a spinal as their sole anesthetic.[72,73]

Anesthetic Techniques for Hernia Repair

Surgical procedures below the umbilicus can be performed with either general or regional anesthesia. There is no consensus about which is preferred. The choice of whether to do general or regional depends on the preference of the surgeon or the anesthesiologist. Regional anesthesia can be used entirely for the surgery or as an adjunct to reduce general anesthetic requirements and produce postoperative analgesia. There has been some concern that general anesthesia is associated with a slightly higher incidence of postoperative apnea, although there have been no bad outcomes reported from the apnea. These episodes have not been increased when pure regional anesthesia is used, but if sedatives are added to regional anesthesia, then the same incidence of postoperative apnea occurs as with general anesthesia. Other methods of providing intraoperative anesthesia and postoperative analgesia include the ilioinguinal–iliohypogastric nerve block or local infiltration. Ilioinguinal-iliohypogastric nerve block with 0.25% bupivacaine or 0.2% ropivacaine, with epinephrine, can be administered shortly after the induction of general anesthesia; it affords excellent postoperative analgesia without the need for opioids.

Pyloric Stenosis

Pyloric stenosis is a relatively frequent surgical disease of the neonate and infant. It can appear as early as the second week of life. The pathologic characteristics include hypertrophy of the pyloric smooth muscle with edema of the pyloric mucosa and submucosa. This process, which develops over a period of days to weeks, leads to progressive obstruction of the pyloric valve, causing persistent vomiting. The vomiting leads to varying losses of fluids and electrolytes. Pediatricians are now adept at the early diagnosis of pyloric stenosis with ultrasound, so it is rare to find an infant with severe fluid and electrolyte derangements. However, an infant is occasionally seen whose problem has developed slowly over a period of weeks, resulting in severe fluid and electrolyte derangements. The stomach contents contain sodium, potassium, chloride, hydrogen ions, and water. The classic electrolyte pattern in infants with severe vomiting is a hyponatremic, hypokalemic, hypochloremic metabolic alkalosis with a compensatory respiratory acidosis. The anesthesiologist, pediatrician, and surgeon are all responsible for preparing these infants for surgery. Pyloric stenosis is a medical emergency and should not be converted into an anesthetic nightmare by premature surgical repair before adequate fluid and electrolyte homeostasis has been achieved. The infant should have normal skin turgor, and the correction of the electrolyte imbalance should produce a sodium level that is greater than 130 mEq $\cdot$ l^{-1}, a potassium level that is at least 3 mEq $\cdot$ l^{-1}, a chloride level that is greater than 85 mEq $\cdot$ l^{-1} and increasing, and a urine output of at least 1–2 ml $\cdot$ kg^{-1} $\cdot$ h^{-1}. These patients need a resuscitation fluid of full-strength balanced salt solution, and, after the infant begins to urinate, the addition of potassium chloride.

Anesthetic Management

One of the concerns in the anesthetic management of patients with pyloric stenosis is the aspiration of gastric contents. Affected infants are usually older and stronger than those in whom an intestinal obstruction appears in the first day or so of life. For this reason, a slightly different approach is used. A large orogastric tube is passed and the stomach contents aspirated.[79] This procedure greatly reduces the quantity of gastric fluid. Intubation of the trachea can be done while the patient is awake or after induction of anesthesia, which is preferred by most clinicians. If an iv line is not in place and cannot be placed with reasonable ease, then after the stomach-emptying regimen is followed, an inhalation induction of anesthesia is done with nitrous oxide and sevoflurane or halothane. Sevoflurane has proved to be an excellent volatile agent for the induction of anesthesia and establishment of endotracheal intubation. There is very little irritation of the respiratory tract and it has a very rapid onset. Use of nitrous oxide should be discontinued as soon as the infant loses the lid reflex. If a vein becomes evident, an iv line is placed and rapid intubation of the trachea accomplished with the use of succinylcholine or a nondepolarizing muscle relaxant and cricoid pressure. If an iv line still cannot be placed easily, two options exist: the anesthesiologist should either deepen inhalation anesthesia with halothane or sevoflurane, insert the laryngoscope, topically anesthetize the vocal cords with 4 mg $\cdot$ kg^{-1} of lidocaine, and intubate the trachea; or administer 4 mg $\cdot$ kg^{-1} of succinylcholine intramuscularly before intubation. If iv access has already been obtained, a rapid-sequence tracheal intubation technique is preferred. The infant is preoxygenated with high-flow oxygen; curare 0.05 mg $\cdot$ kg^{-1} is given, followed by thiopental 3–4 mg $\cdot$ kg^{-1} or 3 mg $\cdot$ kg^{-1} propofol, and succinylcholine 2 mg $\cdot$ kg^{-1}. If a nondepolarizing muscle relaxant is chosen, the dose is cisatracurium 0.4–0.6 mg $\cdot$ kg^{-1} or rocuronium 0.4 mg $\cdot$ kg^{-1}. Cricoid pressure is applied as soon as tolerated and the infant's trachea is intubated. Anesthesia can be maintained by almost any technique the clinician prefers. The point to remember is that surgeons need muscle relaxation twice: when they deliver the pylorus at the beginning of surgery and when they replace the pylorus into the abdomen at the end of surgery, shortly before closing the peritoneum. Administration of a caudal anesthetic (1.25 ml $\cdot$ kg-1 of 0.25% bupivacaine with epinephrine) after the induction of general anesthesia with tracheal intubation is recommended. Caudal anesthesia provides intraoperative relaxation, reduces the anesthetic requirement, and provides postoperative analgesia. Controlled ventilation with sevoflurane reduces or eliminates the need for muscle relaxants for this surgery. The infant's trachea should remain intubated until he or she is awake with eyes opened and is reaching for the endotracheal tube, or is crying. There has been some concern about the risk of postoperative apnea in these infants. With the use of regional anesthesia and avoidance of narcotics, these infants do not appear to be at increased risk.[80]

Ligation of a Patent Ductus Arteriosus

As the number of small premature infants who survive has increased, so also has the number of infants who have PDA with heart failure and respiratory failure. Prostaglandins relax the smooth muscle of the ductus so that it cannot constrict. Indomethacin, a prostaglandin synthetase inhibitor, is administered to encourage closure of the ductus. However, indomethacin is often unsuccessful in the small premature infant because of the lack of muscle within the ductus. Infants with a PDA and heart failure need maximal medical management with fluid restriction and diuretics. These infants are at special risk because of the reduced blood volume and precarious cardiopulmonary system. Fentanyl with pancuronium is a frequent choice for anesthesia. The clinician must be prepared to augment volume rapidly with $10-15$ ml $\cdot$ kg^{-1} of lactated Ringer's solution. If the lactated Ringer's solution accompanies the administration of $20-25$ mg $\cdot$ kg^{-1} of fentanyl and pancuronium, the pressure changes are minimal and the infant will be appropriately anesthetized. The tracheas of these infants usually remain intubated and the lungs ventilated in the postoperative period, so concern about the length of action of muscle relaxants and opioids is minimized.

A new technique for closing the PDA in low–birth-weight infants has been developed, called video-assisted ligation of the PDA.[81] Under general anesthesia, four small thoracotomy incisions are made that allow the insertion of an endoscope and various other instruments to ligate the PDA. The operation is accomplished without either spreading the ribs or cutting muscles, thereby offering a minimally traumatic and safe technique for the surgery. This operation has been accomplished both in the operating room as well as in the NICU; where the surgery is performed is more of a "turf" issue than a technical one.

Placement of a Central Venous Catheter

The use of a central venous catheter for monitoring serum electrolytes for hyperalimentation and for administering medications is increasing. It can be placed either as part of the surgical procedure or at some other time as a separate procedure. The three major concerns in central venous catheter placement are airway management, pneumothorax, and bleeding. The airway should be secured by an endotracheal tube in small infants because of the difficulty in sharing the head, neck, and upper chest with the surgeon and as an adjunct for treating complications such as pneumothorax and bleeding. The anesthetic technique depends on the infant's condition. A pneumothorax may occur with attempts at subclavian vein puncture. The first indication of trouble may be a decreasing oxygen saturation, hypotension, or difficulty with ventilation of the lungs. Because a fluoroscope is often used for central venous catheter placement, it can be used rapidly to diagnose a pneumothorax. If not, the chest should be rapidly aspirated for both diagnostic and therapeutic reasons. Bleeding is an unusual but serious complication of central venous catheter placement. It usually becomes manifest in the perioperative period as a hemothorax or as hypovolemia with a decreasing hematocrit or blood pressure. The question of whether an infant needs an iv catheter placed before proceeding with a central line has never been answered. The reason for the central line is usually that the infant has no veins and the clinician is left with a tradeoff between prolonged attempts at starting an iv versus proceeding without an iv line to obtain central venous line placement. The subclavian approach has a higher incidence of problems than an external or internal jugular approach. An iv catheter should be started when possible if it can be done within a reasonable time (i.e., 15–20 minutes). If not, then central catheter placement continues as described previously, without an iv catheter, after discussion and agreement with the surgeon.

Respiratory Distress Syndrome

Because of the enormous technical ability of the neonatologist and the resources of NICUs, many very small infants survive who need surgery. One of the frequent problems of these infants is the occurrence of the respiratory distress syndrome secondary to a deficiency of surfactant. Respiratory distress syndrome is not an all-or-none disease; there are varying degrees of the disease and various treatments for it. Exogenous surfactant has been widely used in premature infants of low birth weight either to prevent or to treat respiratory distress syndrome.[82] As a result, fewer infants now die of this entity, and the incidence of bronchopulmonary dysplasia in survivors has fallen. However, the use of exogenous surfactant appears to have had little impact on other complications of prematurity such as PDA, NEC, or intraventricular hemorrhage.

Retinopathy of Prematurity

Advances in neonatal medicine have led to the survival of extremely premature infants (i.e., infants weighing <1000 g and infants <28 weeks' gestation). These infants are at high risk for development of retinopathy of prematurity (ROP).[83] ROP is a common cause of blindness in these extremely premature infants. Although the exact etiology is unknown, variations in arterial oxygenation (hypoxia or hyperoxia) and prolonged exposure to bright light are believed to play a significant role. Hyperoxic vasoconstriction of retinal vessels, induction of vascular endothelial growth factor, and damage to spindle cells by oxygen free radicals are some of the currently supported hypotheses in the pathogenesis of ROP.[84]

Advances in the treatment of ROP have followed the advances in neonatal care that led to the increased incidence of ROP. ROP is staged as follows:

Stage 1: Presence of a demarcation line between vascularized and avascularized retina

Stage 2: Presence of a demarcation line that has height, width, and volume (ridge)

Stage 3: Presence of a ridge with extraretinal fibrovascular proliferation

Stage 4: Partial retinal detachment

Stage 5: Total retinal detachment

The early stages are treated with cryotherapy or laser. These treatments may be performed with sedation in the NICU or under general anesthesia in the operating room. The later stages require retinal surgery (scleral buckle or vitrectomy) to be performed under general anesthesia.[85] In addition, the anesthesiologist may be called on to anesthetize an infant with ROP for an unrelated surgery, such as hernia repair or ventriculoperitoneal shunt or central line placement.

The question the anesthesiologist faces is what inspired oxygen concentration is safe under general anesthesia. There are no studies that document some threshold Pao$_2$ above which ROP develops. In addition, there are no studies that document the length of time that the Pao$_2$ has to remain above some threshold number. A study by Flynn et al[86] suggested that the longer the time the premature infant had a documented Tco$_2$ (transcutaneous oxygen) above 80 mm Hg, the higher the incidence of ROP. The guidelines for the administration of oxygen in premature infants is a goal of $50-80$ mm Hg.[87] An oxygen saturation of $90-95\%$ represents a Pao$_2$ of somewhere between 60 and 80 mm Hg. Therefore, it seems reasonable to try to maintain an oxygen saturation of 95% with minimal inspired oxygen while these premature infants are under general anesthesia. If the infant is experiencing episodes of hypotension or problems with ventilation, then attempts to micromanage the oxygen saturation should be secondary to the management of the primary problems. However, if an infant is stable, it might be appropriate to dilute the inspired oxygen with room air, nitrogen, or nitrous oxide until the saturation is in the neighborhood of 95%.

Sudden Infant Death Syndrome

Sudden infant death syndrome (SIDS) is defined as the sudden death of an infant younger than 1 year of age that remains unexplained after complete autopsy, death scene investigation, and review of family history. SIDS is the most frequent cause of death in infants between the ages of 1 month and 1 year. Death from SIDS is relatively rare in the first month of life, with the peak occurring at the third to fourth months of life. Premature infants are known to be at increased risk to die of SIDS. However, studies have failed to prove a relationship between apnea of prematurity and SIDS.[88] Epidemiologic studies suggest that the risk factors for SIDS include low birth weight, maternal smoking, maternal cocaine use, young maternal age, low socioeconomic status, and African-American race.[89] There is currently no evidence that general anesthesia triggers SIDS.[90]

The relationship between infant sleep position and SIDS was evaluated in the early 1990s. It was noted that there was a 50% reduction of SIDS rates in those countries where there was a decline in prone positioning of infants. As a result, the American Academy of Pediatrics recommended that all well infants at term with no other problems be placed either on their side or back when sleeping.[91,92]

Sudden infant death syndrome remains a mystery in many ways. Multiple theories have been proposed over the years, including the "infant apnea syndrome." The more current theories focus on abnormalities of cardiorespiratory control during sleep states. Recent evidence suggests an abnormality in the maturational process of brain stem nuclei, particularly the arcuate nucleus. As a result, it is believed that these infants lack the normal homeostatic mechanisms necessary to respond to exogenous stressors during sleep.[93] A separate theory focuses on abnormalities in autonomic control during obstructive sleep events in infants at risk.[94]

REFERENCES

1. Hagen PT, Scholz DG, Edwards WD: Incidence and size of patent foramen ovale during the first 10 decades of life: An autopsy study of 965 normal hearts. Mayo Clin Proc 59:17, 1984
2. Reller MD, Rice MJ, McDonald RW: Review of studies evaluating ductal patency in the premature infant. J Pediatr 122:S59, 1993
3. Sahni R, Wung J-T, James LS: Controversies in management of persistent pulmonary hypertension of the newborn. Pediatrics 94:307, 1994
4. UK Collaborative ECMO Trial Group: UK collaborative randomised trial of neonatal extracorporeal membrane oxygenation. Lancet 348:75, 1996
5. Schulze A, Gerhardt T, Musante G et al: Proportional assist ventilation in low birth weight infants with acute respiratory disease: A comparison to assist/control and conventional mechanical ventilation. J Pediatr 135:339, 1999
6. Kanto WP: A decade of experience with neonatal extracorporeal membrane oxygenation. J Pediatr 124:335, 1994
7. Walsh-Sukys M, Stork EK, Martin RJ: Neonatal ECMO: Iron lung of the 1990s? J Pediatr 124:427, 1994
8. Katz VL, Bowes WA: Meconium aspiration syndrome: Reflections on a murky subject. Am J Obstet Gynecol 166:171, 1992
9. Wiswell TE, Henley MA: Intratracheal suctioning, systemic infection, and the meconium aspiration syndrome. Pediatrics 89:203, 1992
10. Berry FA: Practical aspects of fluid and electrolyte therapy. In Berry FA (ed): Anesthetic Management of Difficult and Routine Pediatric Patients, p 89. New York, Churchill Livingstone, 1990
11. Murphy JD, Vawter GF, Reid LM: Pulmonary vascular disease in fatal meconium aspiration. J Pediatr 104:758, 1984
12. Wiswell TE, Tuggle JM, Turner BS: Meconium aspiration syndrome: Have we made a difference? Pediatrics 85:715, 1990
13. Kopelman AE, Moise AA, Holbert D, Hegemier SE: A single very early dexamethasone dose improves respiratory and cardiovascular adaptation in preterm infants. J Pediatr 135:345, 1999
14. Berry FA, Castro BC: Anesthesia for genitourinary anesthesia. In Gregory GA (ed): Pediatric Anesthesia, 4th ed. New York, Churchill Livingstone, 1999
15. Cornblath M, Schwartz R, Aynsley-Green A et al: Hypoglycemia in infancy: The need for a rational definition. Pediatrics 85:834, 1990
16. Keens TG, Bryan AC, Levison H et al: Developmental pattern of muscle fiber types in human ventilatory muscles. J Appl Physiol 44:909, 1978
17. Friedman WF, George BL: Treatment of congestive heart failure by altering loading conditions of the heart. J Pediatr 106:697, 1985
18. Berry FA, Gregory GA: Do premature infants require anesthesia for surgery? Anesthesiology 67:291, 1987
19. Cabal LA, Siassi B, Artal R et al: Cardiovascular and catecholamine changes after administration of pancuronium in distressed neonates. Pediatrics 75:284, 1985
20. Miller RD, Rupp SM, Fisher DM et al: Clinical pharmacology of vecuronium and atracurium. Anesthesiology 61:444, 1984
21. Meakin G, McKiernan EP, Morris P, Baker RD: Dose-response curves for suxamethonium in neonates, infants and children. Br J Anaesth 62:655, 1989
22. Morell RC, Berman JM, Royster RI et al: Revised label regarding use of succinylcholine in children and adolescents (letter). Anesthesiology 80:242, 1994
23. Parker SF, Bailey A, Drake AF: Infant hyperkalemic arrest after succinylcholine. Anesth Analg 80:206, 1995
24. Kraft LF, Katholi RE, Woods WT, James TN: Attenuation by magnesium of the electrophysiologic effects of hyperkalemia on human and canine heart cells. Am J Cardiol 45:1189, 1980
25. Hickey PR, Hansen DD, Wessel DL et al: Pulmonary and systemic hemodynamic responses to fentanyl in infants. Anesth Analg 64:483, 1985
26. Yaster M: The dose response of fentanyl in neonatal anesthesia. Anesthesiology 66:433, 1987
27. Friesen RH, Morrison JE Jr: The role of ketamine in the current practice of paediatric anaesthesia. Paediatr Anaesth 4:79, 1994
28. Mannion D, Doherty P: Desflurane in paediatric anaesthesia. Paediatr Anaesth 4:301, 1994
29. LeDez KM, Lerman J: The minimum alveolar concentration (MAC) of isoflurane in preterm neonates. Anesthesiology 67:301, 1987
30. Lerman J, Robinson S, Willis MM et al: Anesthetic requirements for halothane in young children 0–1 month and 1–6 months of age. Anesthesiology 59:421, 1983
31. Gregory GA, Wade JG, Beihl DR et al: Fetal anesthetic requirement (MAC) for halothane. Anesth Analg 62:9, 1983
32. Koehntop DE, Rodman JH, Brundage DM et al: Pharmacokinetics of fentanyl in neonates. Anesth Analg 65:227, 1986
33. Gauntlett IS, Fisher DM, Hertzka RE et al: Pharmacokinetics of fentanyl in neonatal humans and lambs: Effects of age. Anesthesiology 69:683, 1988
34. Bailey A, Valley R, Bigler R: High spinal anesthesia in an infant. Anesthesiology 70:560, 1989
35. Oberlander TF, Berde CB, Lam KH et al: Infants tolerate spinal anesthesia with minimal overall autonomic changes: Analysis of heart rate variability in former premature infants undergoing hernia repair. Anesth Analg 80:20, 1995
36. Fisher QA, Shaffner DH, Yaster M: Detection of intravascular injection of regional anaesthetics in children. Can J Anaesth 44:592, 1997
37. Giaufre E, Dalens B, Gombert A: Epidemiology and morbidity of regional anesthesia in children: A one-hear prospective survey of the French-language society of pediatric anesthesiologists. Paediatr Anesth 83:904, 1996
38. Friesen RH, Lichtor JL: Cardiovascular effects of inhalation induction with isoflurane in infants. Anesth Analg 62:411, 1983
39. Brandom BW, Brandom RB, Cook DR: Uptake of halothane in infants. Anesth Analg 62:404, 1983
40. Greenwood RD, Rosenthal A, Nadas AS: Cardiac anomalies associated with congenital diaphragmatic hernia. Pediatrics 57:92, 1976
41. Greenwood RD, Rosenthal A: Cardiovascular malformations associated with tracheoesophageal fistula and esophageal atresia. Pediatrics 57:87, 1976
42. Lipshultz SE, Frassica JJ, Orav EJ: Cardiovascular abnormalities in infants prenatally exposed to cocaine. J Pediatr 118:44, 1991
43. van de Bor M, Walther FJ, Ebrahimi M: Decreased cardiac output in infants of mothers who abused cocaine. Pediatrics 85:30, 1990
44. Kitano Y, Adzick NS: New developments in fetal lung surgery. Curr Opin Pediatr 11:193, 1999
45. Skarsgard ED, Meuli M, Vanderwall KJ et al: Fetal endoscopic tracheal occlusion ("Fetendo-PLUG") for congenital diaphragmatic hernia. J Pediatr Surg 31:1335, 1996
46. Frenckner B, Ehren H, Granholm T et al: Improved results in patients who have congenital diaphragmatic hernia using preoperative stabilization, extracorporeal membrane oxygenation, and delayed surgery. J Pediatr Surg 32:1185, 1997
47. Katz AL, Wiswell TE, Baumgart S: Contemporary controversies in the management of congenital diaphragmatic hernia. Clin Perinatol 25:219, 1998
48. The Neonatal Inhaled Nitric Oxide Study Group (NINOS): Inhaled nitric oxide and hypoxic respiratory failure in infants with congenital diaphragmatic hernia. Pediatrics 99:838, 1997
49. The Congenital Diaphragmatic Hernia Study Group: Does extracorporeal membrane oxygenation improve survival in neonates with congenital diaphragmatic hernia? J Pediatr Surg 34:720, 1999

50. Iocono JA, Cilley RE, Mauger DT *et al:* Postnatal pulmonary hypertension after repair of congenital diaphragmatic hernia: Predicting risk and outcome. J Pediatr Surg 34:349, 1999

51. Schwartz SM, Vermillion RP, Hirschl RB: Evaluation of left ventricular mass in children with left-side congenital diaphragmatic hernia. J Pediatr 125:447, 1994

52. Grosfeld JL, Weber TR: Congenital abdominal wall defects: Gastroschisis and omphalocele. Curr Probl Surg 19:158, 1982

53. Tsakayannis DE, Zurakowski D, Lillehei CW: Respiratory insufficiency at birth: A predictor of mortality for infants with omphalocele. J Pediatr Surg 31:1088, 1996

54. Bianchi A, Dickson AP: Elective delayed reduction and no anesthesia: "Minimal intervention management" for gastroschisis. J Pediatr Surg 33:1338, 1998

55. Yaster, Buck JR, Dudgeon DL *et al:* Hemodynamic effects of primary closure of omphalocele/gastroschisis in human newborns. Anesthesiology 69:84, 1988

56. Iberti TJ, Lieber CE, Benjamin E: Determination of intra-abdominal pressure using a transurethral bladder catheter: Clinical validation of the technique. Anesthesiology 70:47, 1989

57. Garcia NM, Thompson JW, Shaul DB: Definitive localization of isolated tracheoesophageal fistula using bronchoscopy and esophagoscopy for guide wire placement. J Pediatr Surg 33:1645, 1998

58. Bhatnagar V, Lal R, Sriniwas M *et al:* Endoscopic treatment of tracheoesophageal fistula using electrocautery and the Nd:YAG laser. J Pediatr Surg 34:464, 1999

59. McLone DG: Care of the neonate with a myelomeningocele. Neurosurg Clin North Am 1:111, 1998

60. Dias MS, Li V: Pediatric neurosurgical disease. Pediatr Clin North Am 45:1539, 1998

61. Rowe MI, O'Neill JA, Grosfeld JL, Fonkalsrud EW, Coran AG: Neurosurgical disorders. In Essentials of Pediatric Surgery, p 831. St. Louis, Mosby, 1995

62. Tulipan N, Hernanz-Schulman M, Bruner JP: Reduced hindbrain herniation after intrauterine myelomeningocele repair: A report of four cases. Pediatr Neurosurg 29:274, 1998

63. Shah S, Cawley M, Gleeson R *et al:* Latex allergy and latex sensitization in children and adolescents with meningomyelocele. J Allergy Clin Immunol 101:741, 1998

64. Dierdorf SF, McNiece WL, Rao CC *et al:* Failure of succinylcholine to alter plasma potassium in children with myelomeningocele. Anesthesiology 64:272, 1986

65. Viscomi CM, Abajian JC, Wald SL *et al:* Spinal anesthesia for repair of meningomyelocele in neonates. Anesth Analg 81:492, 1995

66. Kliegman RM: Neonatal necrotizing enterocolitis: Bridging the basic science with the clinical disease. J Pediatr 117:833, 1990

67. Fujiwara T, Konishi M, Chida S: Surfactant replacement therapy with a single postventilatory dose of a reconstituted bovine surfactant in preterm neonates with respiratory distress syndrome: Final analysis of a multicenter, double-blind, randomized trial and comparison with similar trials. Pediatrics 86:753, 1990

68. Kosloske AM: Pathogenesis and prevention of necrotizing enterocolitis: A hypothesis based on personal observation and a review of the literature. Pediatrics 74:1086, 1984

69. Rescorla FJ, Grosfeld JL: Inguinal hernia repair in the perinatal period and early infancy: Clinical considerations. J Pediatr Surg 19:832, 1984

70. Peevy KJ, Speed FA, Hoff CJ: Epidemiology of inguinal hernia in preterm neonates. Pediatrics 77:246, 1986

71. Steward DJ: Preterm infants are more prone to complications following minor surgery than are term infants. Anesthesiology 1982; 56:304, 1982

72. Liu LMP, Coté CJ, Goudsouzian NG *et al:* Life-threatening apnea in infants recovering from anesthesia. Anesthesiology 59:506, 1983

73. Kurth CD, Spitzer AR, Broennle AM, Downes JJ: Postoperative apnea in preterm infants. Anesthesiology 66:483, 1987

74. Kurth CD, LeBard SE: Association of postoperative apnea, airway obstruction, and hypoxemia in former premature infants. Anesthesiology 75:22, 1991

75. Welborn LG, Hannallah RS, Fink R *et al:* High-dose caffeine suppresses postoperative apnea in former preterm infants. Anesthesiology 71:347, 1989

76. Lee TC, Charles B, Steer P *et al:* Population pharmacokinetics of intravenous caffeine in neonates with apnea of prematurity. Clin Pharmacol Ther 61:628, 1997

77. Welborn LG, Rice LJ, Hannallah RS *et al:* Postoperative apnea in former preterm infants: Prospective comparison of spinal and general anesthesia. Anesthesiology 72:838, 1990

78. Krane EJ, Haberkern CM, Jacobson LE: Postoperative apnea, bradycardia, and oxygen desaturation in formerly premature infants: Prospective comparison of spinal and general anesthesia. Anesth Analg 80:7, 1995

79. Cook-Sather SD, Tulloch HV, Liacouras CA, Schreiner MS: Gastric fluid volume in infants for pyloromyotomy. Can J Anaesth 44:278, 1997

80. Chipps BE, Moynihan R, Schieble T *et al:* Infants undergoing pyloromyotomy are not at risk for postoperative apnea. Pediatr Pulmonol 27:278, 1999

81. Burke RP, Jacobs JP, Cheng W *et al:* Video-assisted thoracoscopic surgery for patent ductus arteriosus in low birth weight neonates and infants. Pediatrics 104:227, 1999

82. Willson DF: Surfactant in pediatric respiratory failure. Reviews, overviews, and updates. Respiratory Care 43:1070, 1998

83. Hussain N, Clive J, Bhandari V: Current incidence of retinopathy of prematurity. Pediatrics 104:552, 1999

84. Spaeth JP, O'Hara IB, Kurth CD: Anesthesia for the micropremie. Semin Perinatol 22:390, 1998

85. Andrews AP, Hartnett ME, Hirose T: Surgical advances in retinopathy of prematurity. In Surgical Advances in Retinopathy of Prematurity, p 275

86. Flynn JT, Bancalari E, Snyder ES, *et al:* A cohort study of transcutaneous oxygen tension and the incidence and severity of retinopathy of prematurity. N Engl J Med 326:1050, 1992

87. Phelps DL: Retinopathy of prematurity. N Engl J Med 326:1078, 1992

88. Metzl K: Telephone advice: to charge or not to charge, that is the question. Pediatrics 102:969, 1998

89. Gibson E, Cullen JA, Spinner S: Infant sleep position following new AAP guidelines. Pediatrics 96:69, 1995

90. Steward DJ: Is there a risk of general anesthesia triggering SIDS? Possibly not! Anesthesiology 63:326, 1985

91. Kattwinkel J, Brooks J, Myerberg D: Positioning and SIDS: AAP Task Force on Infant Positioning and SIDS. Pediatrics 89:1120, 1992

92. Willinger M, Hoffman HJ, Hartford RB: Infant sleep position and risk for sudden infant death syndrome: Report of meeting held January 13 and 14, 1994, National Institutes of Health, Bethesda, MD. Pediatrics 93:814, 1994

93. Gaultier C: Early disturbances in cardiorespiratory control. Pediatr Pulmonol 16:225, 1997

94. Franco P, Szliwowski H, Dramaix M, Kahn A: Decreased autonomic responses to obstructive sleep events in future victims of sudden infant death syndrome. Pediatr Res 46:33, 1999

Clinical Anesthesia (4/e), edited by
Paul G. Barash, Bruce F. Cullen, and
Robert K. Stoelting. Lippincott Williams &
Wilkins, Philadelphia, © 2001.

CHAPTER 44

PEDIATRIC ANESTHESIA

JOSEPH P. CRAVERO AND LINDA JO RICE

The provision of safe anesthesia for the pediatric patient requires a clear understanding of the psychological, physiologic, and pharmacologic differences between a premature infant and an adolescent, as well as between a newborn and a toddler. A thorough understanding of these differences must be applied to each pediatric patient presenting for surgery. This chapter presents an overview of the important issues in pediatric anesthesia. There are many specialized pediatric anesthesia texts that expand on topics introduced here.[1-6] In addition, neonatal anesthesia, pediatric pharmacology, equipment, and other general topics are covered elsewhere in this text.

During the first several months of life, an infant experiences rapid growth, organ maturation, and neurologic development. In the first 3 months of life, circulatory and ventilatory adaptation are completed and thermoregulation is altered to a more adult state. The sizes of body fluid compartments approach adult values. Skeletal muscle mass and hepatic enzyme systems are developing and renal function is maturing (Table 44-1). Over the next 18 months, the infant is physically transformed to a miniature adult. Psychological maturation (which continues through adolescence) is a much more gradual process[7] (Table 44-2).

PREANESTHETIC EVALUATION AND PREPARATION

The preoperative visit and preparation of the child for surgery is more important than the choice of premedication. During this brief period, the anesthesiologist evaluates the medical condition of the child, integrating this information with the planned surgical procedures. The history should begin with a review of the perinatal period and seek information regarding history of a recent or intercurrent upper respiratory infection.[8] The pediatric anesthesiologist should be aware of the increasing prevalence of reactive airway disease in pediatric patients; routine or "as-needed" use of nebulized bronchodilators occurs in up to 10% of pediatric patients, especially during high-risk times of the year. The possibility of loose teeth should be evaluated in school-age children. The anesthesiologist should recall that congenital anomalies frequently present in combination rather than as single entities. Other medical problems should be assessed and pediatric caregivers consulted as appropriate to ascertain that the child is in the best possible physiologic state before surgery.[9-11]

In addition, the anesthesiologist must assess the psychological makeup of the child and family. He or she should establish rapport with the child and reassure the parents. In addition, the anesthesiologist must realize that the entire family is undergoing the psychological stress of the child's surgery, in addition to the feelings of guilt, helplessness, and inconvenience that even outpatient surgery may cause. Parental anxieties concerning both the anesthesia and surgical procedure are transmitted to even very young children. Both realistic concerns and misconceptions ("How do they put the eye back in its socket after they fix the muscles?") can be addressed during the preoperative interview.

Anesthesia and surgery represent an enormous time of stress for the child. The reasons for the stress are many, but include primarily (1) separation from parents, (2) strange surroundings, (3) painful procedures, (4) frightening procedures, and (5) survival. Coping with this stress and pain requires honest and consistent communication between the child and his or her parents, all physicians involved in the anesthesia and surgery, and all other staff involved in the child's care. The more information the parents and child have, the more easily they will cope with the period leading up to surgery and hospitalization. Presurgical programs, including written literature, videotapes, or hospital tours, have been shown to decrease preoperative anxiety in both the patient and the family.[12] Unfortunately, the stress caused by mask induction of anesthesia and postoperative care is not necessarily ameliorated by these interventions.

Many institutions have adopted policies that allow parents to participate actively in the anesthetic induction.[13-15] Very young children benefit most from parental reassurance and a hypnotic voice, whereas older children and adolescents benefit from choices and ability to maintain some control over their environment.[16] Although many parents prefer to be with their child during the stressful and somewhat frightening time of anesthesia induction, not all parents and not all children benefit from this opportunity. In fact, one prospective, randomized study found that only certain personality types of children and parents had improvement in anxiety levels at the time of induction when parents were allowed to be present.[17] Parents can become quite emotional if their child continues to struggle even in their presence, and again when the child lies quietly, not moving, at the end of induction. Parents who have been questioned after such an experience express the need for a great deal of education about what to expect and how they can help their child. In addition, institutions that have such a program emphasize the need for an escort to provide support (and be certain that the parent leaves the operating room or induction room). A consistent policy for age and medical status of children who are eligible to have parental accompaniment is also important, as is the recognition that the final decision always rests in the hands of the anesthesiologist responsible for the safe care of that child during that anesthetic. Other children, even preschoolers, may benefit from the opportunity to exhibit independence and bravery.

Preoperative sedation has been studied carefully with respect to effect on stress and postoperative behaviors. The most complete and recent information suggests that adequate preoperative sedation (midazolam $0.5 \text{ mg} \cdot \text{kg}^{-1}$ orally) decreases anxiety for parents and children in the immediate presurgical time frame and at the time of mask induction. Preoperative sedation has been found to be superior to parental presence for decreasing anxiety during induction of anesthesia and increasing cooperation with inhalation induction.[18] In addition, children who are sedated before coming to the operating room may have fewer stress-related behavioral changes in the immediate postoperative time compared with groups of patients who receive no sedation. Almost all of these behaviors extinguish by 2 weeks after the operation, however, and much of this work was performed on first-time surgical patients. Further studies are needed to clarify the role of sedation with respect to postoperative behavior changes.[19]

Minimal Laboratory Evaluation

As with adults, preoperative laboratory evaluation is guided by the medical history.[20] Most children require no laboratory evaluation, and can be spared the psychological and physical pain of venipuncture. Determination of electrolytes or other

Table 44-1. BODY COMPOSITION DURING GROWTH

Body Compartment	Percentage of Body Weight	
	Infant	Adult
Total body water	73	60
Extracellular fluid	44	15–20
Blood volume	8–10	7
Intracellular water	33	40
Muscle mass	20	50
Fat	12	18

chemistries should be limited to those children who have a clinical history consistent with a significant probability of abnormalities. Many institutions still require preoperative hematocrits for infants younger than 2 months of age, largely because the frequency of postoperative apnea and bradycardia in newborns has been shown to increase with anemia. Outside of this subgroup, there is little evidence that testing for hematocrit levels is helpful in the management of routine pediatric outpatients.[21]

There is controversy as to what constitutes the minimal acceptable hemoglobin value for elective pediatric surgery. The arbitrary value of 10 g · dl^{-1} (the nadir of hemoglobin in a healthy term infant) has been cited for infants older than 3 months, with higher values for the younger infants, depending on gestational age and general health status. Children whose hemoglobin values are less than this arbitrary standard should have the cause of their anemia investigated and corrected. A decision to proceed with anesthesia and surgery should include an assessment of the surgical procedure and the possibility of blood loss. Elective major surgery in which blood loss is anticipated, but transfusion is not usually required, should be postponed until the anemia is corrected. A decision to proceed with major surgery in which blood transfusion is planned, as well as brief minor surgery with little anticipated blood loss, might be appropriate in a child with iron-deficiency anemia.

Transfusion to raise a hemoglobin value to an arbitrary number to perform elective surgery is rarely justified. Even in premature infants, where apnea is correlated with anemia, appropriate supervision in the postoperative period and perioperative caffeine to treat apnea is preferred over the risks of transfusion.

Patients with sickle cell anemia or other hemoglobinopathies

Table 44-2. SPECIFIC ANXIETIES OF PEDIATRIC PATIENTS

0–6 mo:	Maximum stress for parents, minimum for child because he or she is not old enough to be frightened of strangers or to remember unpleasant events.
6 mo–4 yr:	Fear of separation at maximum, able to remember but not to understand previous hospital experiences.
	Hospitalization is followed by the most severe emotional upset and behavioral regression.
4–6 yr:	Almost able to understand explanations. Accepts separation more easily. Concerned about integrity of body and may have wild misconceptions of surgical mutilation.
6 yr–adolescence:	Tolerates separation well. Better able to understand explanations. May communicate fear of waking during surgery or "not waking up."
Teenagers:	"Physiologic schizophrenia." Developing sexuality. Need for conformity. Need for dignity. Fear of losing control, narcosis. Need for information.

require special preoperative preparation. Debate continues as to the exact need for preoperative transfusion to a target hemoglobin level, or to a given percentage of hemoglobin A.[22] This is reviewed in the standard texts mentioned previously.[1–6]

Preoperative Fasting Period

Evidence is accumulating that children allowed clear fluids until 2 hours before surgery have similar gastric contents as those fasted for more than 4 hours.[23,24] In fact, Coté et al[25] have demonstrated that up to 76% of children have sufficient volume of acid gastric contents at time of induction to cause chemical pneumonitis regardless of their fasting status. In spite of this, the best estimates of aspiration in pediatric patients place the incidence at a relatively rare 1 in 5000–10,000.[26]

The exact length of time that a child must not eat or drink various foods and liquids before surgery has not been completely settled. A survey of pediatric anesthesia fellowship programs found significant variation in recommendations for restriction of breast feeding, formula feeding, and solids.[27] Various experts recommend 2- or 4-hour restriction of breast feeding, 4- or 6-hour restriction of formula feeding, and 6-hour or "after midnight" restrictions on solids. In spite of the lack of complete agreement among pediatric anesthesiologists, an American Academy of Pediatrics/American Society of Anesthesiologists task force has set recommendations that advise restriction of clear fluids for 2 hours, breast milk for 4 hours, formula or light meals for 6 hours, and fatty solid meals for 8 hours.

When counseling parents, recommendations need to be unambiguous. Clear liquids should be specifically listed and the time that they should stop should be noted. Many pediatric institutions have chosen to make the absolutely nothing by mouth (NPO) time 4 hours before scheduled surgery, although it is recognized that 2 hours is sufficient for gastric emptying of clear fluids. The longer fasting times allow for flexibility in patient scheduling; should an earlier surgical case be canceled, the next child can be safely moved up. Of course, gastric emptying after trauma is delayed in children as well as adults, and even a prolonged fast may not result in significant gastric emptying.

If these details of feeding and fasting are not clearly defined with stated hours, infants and children are likely to go without fluids for protracted times.[28,29] Because young children do not understand the need for fasting, they should still be scheduled early in the day, or at least at a specified time to minimize their discomfort and that of the parents, who must keep them away from the water fountain. Anesthesiologists should be alert to delays and make sure that the child's fluid restriction is modified if a long delay is anticipated.

Preanesthetic Medications

Preanesthetic sedation is usually used to decrease apprehensiveness and stress for pediatric surgical patients and their families. Preoperative anxiolytics may also greatly improve cooperation with mask induction of anesthesia. The large number of studies in this area have produced approximately the same results: all sedatives are effective in a large percentage of patients if administered in a timely fashion. Other preanesthetic medications may be administered to prevent vagal reflexes or dry oral secretions in a child with an anticipated difficult airway. In some cases, premedications can serve to reduce gastric volume and acidity in a child with increased risk of vomiting.

Because of children's exaggerated psychological response to needles, other routes of administration are almost always preferable. Some children simply refuse to cooperate at all with preanesthetic medication, and for them the only sure method of administration is intramuscular or intravenous. Although it is desirable to provide anxiolysis for the child who is to undergo anesthesia and surgery, the respiratory "cost" of this state may sometimes be excessive, particularly in patients who have predisposing factors that increase the respiratory effects of sedation. An example of such a patient would be an obese 3-year-old with sleep apnea coming for a tonsillectomy. In addition, although a heavily sedated and unresponsive child will have no memory of the surgery, he or she may also undergo prolonged emergence from anesthesia and experience postoperative respiratory depression, especially after short surgical procedures.

Oral

By far the most popular oral premedication at this time is midazolam, in a dose of 0.5–0.75 mg · kg^{-1}. Midazolam is first and foremost an anxiolytic; the child's eyes are usually open and he is aware of the environment, but nothing seems to disturb him. The effects of this medication peak approximately 30 minutes after administration, and last approximately 30 minutes.[30,31] An oral syrup preparation is now available in a concentration of 2 mg · ml^{-1} that is palatable to all but the most uncooperative of patients.

Serious side effects after oral midazolam are uncommon. However, loss of balance and head control occurs in as many as 20% of children receiving oral midazolam. Consequently, strict adult supervision is necessary in children who receive this drug. Dysphoria has also been noted—in these patients, the drug has the opposite effect to that desired. The crying and disorientation that ensue usually abate with the drug effect.

As mentioned in the Preoperative Preparation section of this chapter, midazolam has been shown in one study to be superior to parental presence in decreasing perioperative stress for patients and families. It has been shown to increase cooperation with induction of anesthesia and has also been suggested to decrease the incidence of adverse behavioral changes that may occur in the 2 weeks after a surgical intervention.[18] Further studies are required to confirm these findings.

Oral ketamine has also been used as a sedation medication. One study evaluated doses of 5–6 mg · kg^{-1} for children 1–6 years of age.[32] Maximal sedation occurred within 20 minutes. Nystagmus occurred in 60% of children, and increased oral secretions in 33%, but there were no emergence phenomena in any child at these doses. Nausea and vomiting rates were slightly increased in children who received oral ketamine. Discharge from the day surgery unit was slightly delayed compared with children sedated with midazolam. Although effective, this drug is probably best reserved for patients who would benefit from the tachycardia and increased blood pressure that usually accompany its administration.

Oral transmucosal fentanyl represents the first commercial attempt to deliver medication to children by the transmucosal oral route.[33] It is available in 200-, 300-, and 400-μg strengths; onset is 10–20 minutes, with a duration of action of 30 minutes. The current dosage recommendation is 10–15 μg · kg^{-1}. Intense supervision is required to ensure the medication is absorbed by the transmucosal route and not chewed and swallowed. In addition, difficulties with perioperative emesis and arterial oxygen desaturation have been reported.[34] One advantage of oral transmucosal fentanyl is its postoperative analgesic properties. The dose indicated previously offers similar pain control as that provided by 2 μg · kg^{-1} given iv. However, safe use of this medication does require more intensive nursing care than do the other oral sedatives commonly in use.

Nasal

Although this route of administration also bypasses the dreaded "shot," any parent who has administered nose drops to a child recognizes that lack of cooperation may also defeat this mode of administration. Most clinicians have found this mode of drug administration no better than intramuscular injection, and consequently its use has never been widespread. Rapid absorption as well as avoidance of first-pass hepatic metabolism of medications are advantages of this route of administration. This route

should be reserved for the rare patient who refuses oral medication and has a contraindication to intramuscular injection.

When required, midazolam (for intravenous use) can be administered undiluted (5 mg · ml^{-1}) by dropper or syringe to the nose in a dose of 0.2 mg · kg^{-1}. Clinical effects of midazolam are evident in 10 minutes, and these children are conscious but glassy-eyed, just as with oral administration.[35] Drawbacks of this form of administration are the intense stinging of nose drops on the nasal mucosa and the undisguised bitterness of the medication that reaches the oral cavity.

The use of sufentanil and other sedatives intranasally has largely been abandoned because of untoward side effects.

Rectal

Both methohexital and thiopental have been used in rectal formulations in a dose of 25 mg · kg^{-1}. Onset of sedation requires approximately 10 minutes. Respiratory depression and oxygen desaturation may occur because of variable absorption of the medication in the rectum. Care must be taken that the medication is not expelled immediately on placement. In spite of these drawbacks, there are a number of institutions that report a high success rate in infants and toddlers with this type of preoperative sedative.

Intramuscular

Parenteral administration of sedation may be the only alternative in a child who refuses to cooperate with other modalities. Injection should be accomplished with a very small gauge needle or a CO_2-powered needleless injection system. When done quickly, intramuscular injection can be less upsetting than the other modes of delivery mentioned previously.

Intramuscular midazolam in a dose of 0.3 mg · kg^{-1} provides anxiolysis in 5–10 minutes and dissipates in 25–30 minutes.

Ketamine in an intramuscular dose of 3–4 mg · kg^{-1} provides a quiet, breathing, yet minimally responsive patient in approximately 5 minutes. Analgesia for intravenous placement is more than adequate. Previous studies have shown that smaller doses of 2–3 mg · kg^{-1} provide sedation without prolonging hospital stay even after brief procedures.[36]

A combination of intramuscular morphine 0.05–0.1 mg · kg^{-1}, atropine 0.02 mg · kg^{-1}, and pentobarbital 4 mg · kg^{-1} is still used in children presenting for repair of congenital heart disease in some institutions. Although mixtures such as this are effective in experienced hands, they also markedly increase the chance of medication errors and respiratory depression. The use of these combinations is no longer widespread.

ANESTHETIC AGENTS

The choices of anesthetic drugs for infants and children are not strikingly different from those for adults. There are few specific contraindications to any of the commonly used drugs on the basis of age alone. Selection of drugs and techniques should be based on the anesthesiologist's experiences, preferences, and skill. Nitrous oxide in combination with potent inhalation agents or intravenous drugs is frequently used to induce and maintain anesthesia in pediatric patients; muscle relaxants and local anesthetics are also common adjuncts to anesthesia.

Potent Inhalation Agents

Mask induction of general anesthesia is the most common induction technique in the United States. Although in general very safe, it can be complicated by breath-holding, laryngospasm, dysrhythmias, and distention of the stomach by anesthetic gases (both from crying and from difficulty in ventilation). Difficulty in maintaining a mask fit may also occur, particularly in a struggling infant.

Although very young infants may interpret the mask as a nipple and attempt to suck as they breathe, increasing the concentrations of anesthetic agents, toddlers and preschool children usually fight the claustrophobic feeling of a tight mask fit. Older children may be persuaded to assist in holding the mask if they have chosen this induction over a "shot." Halothane and sevoflurane are the only agents available for reliable and safe inhaled induction of anesthesia. The incidence of bradycardia, hypotension, and cardiac arrest during inhalation induction of anesthesia is higher in infants younger than 1 year of age than in older children and adults.[37] This greater propensity for untoward events from potent inhalational agents may be attributed to age-related differences in uptake, anesthetic requirements, and sensitivity of the cardiovascular system.[38] Uptake of inhalational anesthetics is faster in infants and small children than in adults because of the much greater ratio of alveolar ventilation to functional residual capacity and the altered distribution of cardiac output. The high inspired concentrations (overpressure) used early in induction can lead to very high tissue concentrations of anesthetic early in induction and result in severe cardiac depression.[39] The incidence of severe myocardial depression is similar with equipotent concentrations of both halothane and sevoflurane.[40,41] Mask anesthesia induction in this age group must be accompanied by vigilant monitoring of blood pressure and pulse. Early administration of muscle relaxants to facilitate intubation in young infants may be more prudent than attempting endotracheal intubation under deep volatile anesthesia alone.

Although intracardiac shunts can, in theory, alter the uptake of anesthetic agents and affect the speed of induction, this is rarely clinically evident. A right-to-left shunt slows the induction of anesthesia because anesthetic concentration in the arterial blood increases more slowly. A left-to-right shunt should have the opposite effect; volatile agent induction is speeded up because the rate of anesthetic transfer from the lungs to the arterial blood is increased. In practice, decreased delivery of anesthetic to the target tissues largely negates the increased uptake.

The minimum alveolar concentration (MAC) of anesthetic required in pediatric patients differs with age, usually in an inverse relationship (Fig. 44-1). Two- to 3-month-old infants actually have the highest anesthetic requirements.

Halothane has a long history of efficacy as an inhaled agent for pediatric anesthesia. It has the least noxious smell of the

older agents and is very well accepted by most patients. In terms of emergence characteristics (in spite of a higher blood–gas partition coefficient), studies of time to awakening have shown little clinical difference between halothane and isoflurane.[42] Although there has been some concern regarding sensitization of the myocardium to catecholamines, there is little problem in the absence of hypercarbia or light anesthesia.[43] Up to 10 $\mu g \cdot kg^{-1}$ of epinephrine may be used with minimal risk of cardiac dysrhythmia in normocarbic pediatric patients.

Halothane can cause myocardial depression. This effect is exaggerated in young children, and in those who are relatively hypovolemic. Addition of muscle relaxants to a lighter halothane anesthetic (in conjunction with regional anesthetic techniques or opioids) can ameliorate this effect.

Isoflurane has a long track record as a safe and efficacious agent for maintenance of anesthesia in infants and children. Like halothane, it decreases blood pressure in pediatric patients. Although the myocardial depression in children may be less than that caused by halothane in equipotent doses, isoflurane reduces peripheral vascular resistance, whereas halothane does not. (In neonates, equal myocardial depression has been demonstrated with both drugs.[44]) The major disadvantage of isoflurane is its pungent odor and high incidence of laryngospasm when this agent is used for inhaled induction of anesthesia. It should not be used for inhaled induction of anesthesia.

Desflurane has also been used as a maintenance anesthetic in pediatric patients of all ages. Unfortunately, an unacceptable incidence of coughing, increased secretions, and laryngospasm preclude its use as a mask induction agent.[45] Although desflurane appears to be associated with faster initial awakening when used as a maintenance anesthetic agent in pediatric patients, studies have shown no difference between halothane and desflurane in time to discharge after ambulatory surgery.[46]

Sevoflurane is now well established as an excellent choice for inhaled induction of anesthesia of anesthesia in pediatric patients. Its low blood-gas solubility allows rapid induction and emergence from anesthesia. There appears to be a relatively low level of myocardial depression even when given at maximum vaporizer output for induction of anesthesia. Numerous studies have documented a decreased incidence of dysrhythmias compared with halothane. However, some confusion is apparent in studies citing sevoflurane's superiority over other potent inhalational agents; in many studies, higher MACs of halothane are compared with lower MACs of sevoflurane.[40,41]

The nonpungent smell of sevoflurane allows smooth mask induction.[47,48] Its safety and efficacy have been well established in hundreds of studies from around the world. In spite of its excellent clinical track record, concerns about the possible accumulation of toxic metabolites in a rebreathing circuit at low fresh gas flows remain to be worked out; at this time, flows of $2 \; l \cdot min^{-1}$ or greater are recommended. Sevoflurane is also relatively expensive compared with the other inhalation agents. In addition, the one advantage of any agent with low solubility (*i.e.*, rapid awakening) is accompanied by a high rate of postoperative excitement.[49,50] Close attention to postoperative analgesia is imperative when either desflurane or sevoflurane is used.

Intravenous Agents

Sedative–Hypnotics

Sedative–hypnotic medications are often used after intravenous placement in pediatric patients (after mask induction) to facilitate deepening of anesthesia. Older children frequently undergo intravenous induction rather than mask inhalational anesthesia induction. Application of EMLA (eutectic mixture of local anesthetics) cream or iontophoresis of lidocaine can increase cooperation and patient comfort during venous cannulation, particularly in children who must undergo frequent needle procedures.[51,52] Propofol, thiopental, methohexital, and keta-

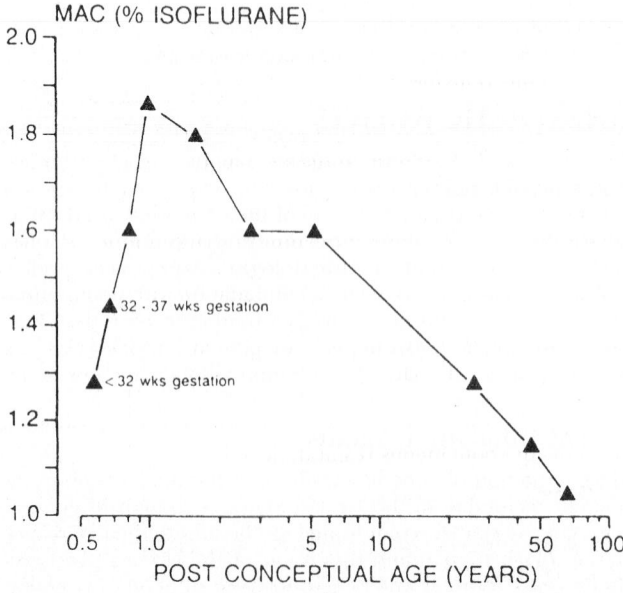

Figure 44-1. The minimum alveolar concentration (MAC) of isoflurane and postconceptual age. (Data from Le Dez KM, Lerman J: The minimum alveolar concentration [MAC] of isoflurane in preterm neonates. Anesthesiology 67:301, 1987.)

mine have been used extensively for anesthetic induction in pediatric patients; there is much less experience with etomidate. Children usually require larger doses of these drugs (on a per kilogram basis) to achieve obtundation than adults. Pediatric patients receiving antiseizure medications require even larger doses than their nonmedicated counterparts to achieve the same effect.

Propofol's chemistry and pharmacokinetics are reviewed elsewhere in this text. Induction doses of 2.5–3 mg·kg^{-1} are required in children younger than 2 years of age, whereas older children need doses of 2.0–2.5 mg·kg^{-1}.[53] The major drawback with use of this drug (aside from the requirement for intravenous access) is pain on administration. This pain is enhanced if the drug is injected into a small vein. The injection of intravenous lidocaine 0.2–1 mg·kg^{-1} immediately before propofol injection can reduce this pain, as can administration through a small-gauge (22–27) catheter in a large antecubital vein. As in adults, a modest reduction in systolic blood pressure usually accompanies bolus administration. Propofol may be used for induction or maintenance of anesthesia. When used for maintenance of anesthesia (150–200 µg·kg^{-1}·min^{-1}), propofol is associated with decreased postoperative vomiting.[53] In addition, propofol infusions can be very useful for sedation during magnetic resonance imaging as well as other minimally invasive procedures where patient cooperation is essential.[54]

Opioids

Fentanyl 1–3 µg·kg^{-1} or morphine 0.05–0.1 mg·kg^{-1} are often used as adjuncts to nitrous oxide–volatile agent anesthetics. Sufentanil 1–2 µg·kg^{-1} or alfentanil 50–100 µg·kg^{-1} have also been successfully used in pediatric patients. In addition to blunting hemodynamic responses to intubation and decreasing required MAC for inhaled agents, these doses of fentanyl and morphine also provide postoperative analgesia. The ultra–short-acting opioid remifentanil has been successfully used in children for both general anesthesia and sedation.[55] No postoperative analgesia is provided, and further experience is required to prove its cost effectiveness and safety.

The issue of sensitivity to the respiratory depressant effects of opioids and at what age it decreases has yet to be resolved. It is apparent that altered pharmacokinetics and immaturity of the blood–brain barrier may alter disposition of these drugs in very young children. Morphine is the least lipophilic of the opioid class; a greater proportion of any blood concentration may be able to cross the immature blood–brain barrier of the neonate or young infant compared with adults. Therefore, this medication should be administered with caution in infants younger than 6 months of age.

Bradycardia and chest wall rigidity are two other potential difficulties associated with opioid anesthesia. Early administration of a vagolytic agent or muscle relaxant should be considered in all infants when using these medications.

Muscle Relaxants

Succinylcholine has a long history of use in children. Since 1990, the drug has received much attention because of the severity of its possible complications.[56] Reports of rhabdomyolysis, hyperkalemia, masseter spasm, and malignant hyperthermia have caused the U.S. Food and Drug Administration to label this drug relatively contraindicated in pediatric patients.

The hydrophilic nature of succinylcholine and its rapid redistribution into the extracellular fluid volume mandate higher doses in infants (2 mg·kg^{-1}) than in older patients. Optimal intubating conditions are achieved within 1 minute when administered iv. Reliable muscle relaxation is also achieved within 1–2 minutes after intramuscular administration of 4–5 mg·kg^{-1}; this route may be life saving if laryngospasm occurs before establishment of intravenous access.

Atropine is frequently administered before or with succinylcholine to prevent potential associated dysrhythmias such as marked bradycardia or sinus arrest, especially with repeat dosing. Although both of these cardiac dysrhythmias may occur at any age, they are more frequent in young pediatric patients.

Succinylcholine administration has also been associated with spasm of the masseter muscles. There is an association of masseter spasm with malignant hyperthermia, and some debate remains as to the appropriate action when masseter spasm occurs.[57] At the very least, extreme vigilance for signs of malignant hyperthermia is warranted whenever masseter spasm occurs. Malignant hyperthermia is evidenced by high end-tidal carbon dioxide along with tachycardia and hypertension. Treatment with cooling measures and dantrolene must be initiated immediately to avoid serious morbidity and mortality.

Although malignant hyperthermia remains the most dreaded consequence of succinylcholine administration, another life-threatening complication has been reported.[58] Succinylcholine-induced hyperkalemic cardiac arrest has been reported in children with previously undiagnosed myopathies. Hyperkalemic cardiac arrest is heralded by tall, peaked T waves on the electrocardiogram, proceeding swiftly to bizarre, wide-complex tachydysrhythmias, ventricular tachycardia, and possible ventricular fibrillation. In addition to immediate cardiopulmonary resuscitation efforts, calcium and bicarbonate administration can be life saving in this situation.

In spite of the aforementioned catastrophes, airway-related complications are a far more frequent cause of serious morbidity in pediatric patients undergoing anesthesia. Although use of succinylcholine should probably be limited to patients with a full stomach or laryngospasm, it remains the drug of choice when rapid onset of muscle relaxation is essential.

All of the nondepolarizing muscle relaxants used in adults are effective for pediatric patients as well. Neonates have a significantly larger volume of distribution for these drugs than older children and adults.[59] In addition, infants appear relatively sensitive to nondepolarizing muscle relaxants. The recommended effective doses for nondepolarizing muscle relaxants (reviewed elsewhere in this text) are similar in children and adults, but the duration of action tends to be slightly longer in pediatric patients. Selection of muscle relaxant should be done with an understanding of side effects and desired duration of effect. Rocuronium has the fastest onset of action in this class (60–90 seconds for a 1 mg·kg^{-1} dose); however, the variability of onset time in pediatric patients has left its use as a reliable rapid-sequence drug uncertain. Although intramuscular administration of rocuronium provides rapid onset of muscle relaxation, intubating conditions are inadequate.[60] Thus, succinylcholine remains the only reliable intramuscular muscle relaxant.

The new, rapid-onset agent rapacuronium is being evaluated in children. Early reports indicate that the same profiles of hemodynamic stability and rapid onset noted in adults are evident in pediatric patients. Higher doses administered intramuscularly provided optimum intubating conditions much less rapidly than succinylcholine, although faster than rocuronium.[61]

Antagonism of neuromuscular blockade should be carefully considered in all neonates and small infants, even if they have recovered clinically. Any increase in the work of breathing may cause fatigue and respiratory failure, particularly if concomitant opioid administration occurs. In general, if an infant or child can vigorously flex at the hips, adequate muscle strength is present for spontaneous respiration.

Antinausea Medications

Nausea and vomiting are among the most frequent causes for unanticipated hospital admission in pediatric ambulatory surgery patients. This is a particular problem in children undergoing tonsillectomy, strabismus surgery, or orchiopexy.

The same medications have been shown to be effective in children as in adults. Droperidol in doses of 20–70 µg·kg^{-1} has been successfully used; however, some studies report a delay in discharge at higher doses.[62] Metoclopramide has also been used in doses of 0.15 mg · kg^{-1}, whereas ondansetron at doses of 0.05–0.15 mg · kg^{-1} has also proven useful.[63] Use of propofol as a *primary* anesthetic decreases nausea and vomiting after surgeries associated with a high rate of nausea; use of propofol solely as an induction agent does not decrease nausea and vomiting.[64] Many studies have demonstrated that the use of high doses of dexamethasone decreases nausea and vomiting after tonsillectomy and other procedures.[65,66]

What is lacking in pediatric, as in adult patients, is a clear cost–benefit analysis showing a hierarchy of use of these various medications as either prophylactic or rescue medications.[67] It is clear, however, that in addition to pharmacologic intervention, the simple policy of not requiring children to drink fluids before discharge itself decreases vomiting.[68] It is also clear that administration of even a single dose of opioid increases nausea and vomiting. Optimal use of nonsteroidal anti-inflammatory drugs (NSAIDs), acetaminophen, and regional analgesia techniques can help avoid this annoying complication.[69]

AIRWAY MANAGEMENT

Attention to appropriate management of the airway in pediatric patients remains the single most important aspect of pediatric anesthesia. Many pediatric anesthetics in older infants and children are conducted by face mask or (more often) laryngeal mask airway (LMA). Most pediatric anesthesiologists still believe that endotracheal intubation is particularly valuable in young infants and neonates. Mask ventilation is technically more difficult in young infants, and sizing/securing an LMA can be uncertain. In addition, these infants are more sensitive to the myocardial depressant effects of volatile anesthetics and often benefit from the use of muscle relaxants as part of the anesthetic technique.

Laryngeal mask airways are available in sizes for all patients, including newborns.[70] Their use has become ubiquitous in outpatient pediatric anesthesia. The LMA is now a standard airway for lower extremity and genito-urinary surgery. More recently, it has been incorporated into tonsillectomy and adenoidectomy procedures as well as eye muscle surgery.[71,72] In addition, the LMA has proven useful in assisting airway management in infants and children with difficult airways, particularly those for whom conventional mask ventilation may be difficult.[73] As in older patients, the use of LMAs is not without problems; oxygen desaturation and difficulty in placement as well as aspiration around the device can occur.

Tracheal intubation in infants and children is not more difficult than in the adult, but the anesthesiologist must be familiar with the anatomic differences of the pediatric airway as well as the specialized equipment required. Trauma can be minimized by gentle airway manipulation at a sufficiently deep plane of anesthesia or after adequate muscle relaxation. The most common morbidity associated with endotracheal intubation (postextubation croup) has been associated with tight endotracheal tube fit. An air leak at 20–25 cm H_2O pressure or lower has been shown to decrease the risk of postextubation croup; use of a cuffed endotracheal tube usually requires a half-size decrease in tube diameter to provide the same leak as an uncuffed tube, but its use is by no means contraindicated.

Several formulas have been used for endotracheal tube selection; for children older than 1 year of age, (age/4) + 4.5, or French size + 18/4 are two of the more popular formulas. Appropriate size has also been correlated with the tip of the child's fifth finger. It is important to have endotracheal tube sizes above and below the estimated size, and to begin with the smaller tube if an estimated size falls between available tubes. If an air leak is present at too low a pressure, replacement of a smaller tube with one a half-size larger causes less trauma than the reverse.

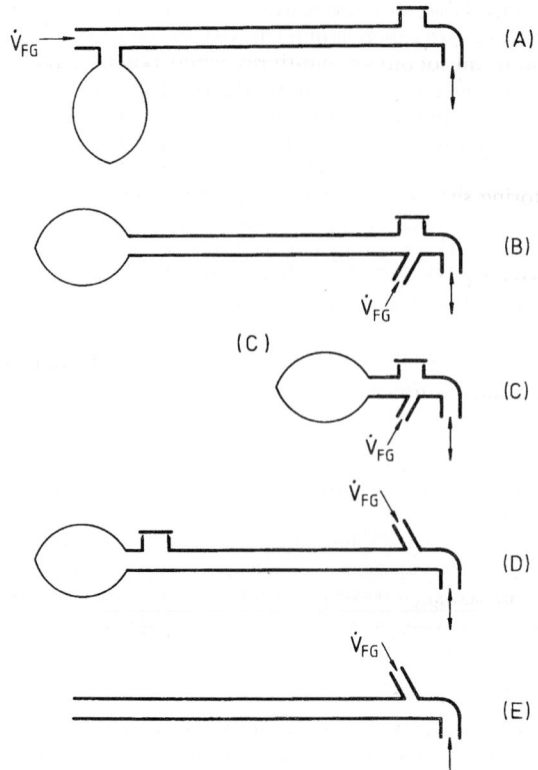

Figure 44-2. Mapleson classification (A–E) of some rebreathing systems. $\dot{V}_{FG}$ is the fresh gas flow. (From Mushin WW, Jones PL: Physics for the Anaesthetist, 4th ed, p 375. Boston, Blackwell Scientific, 1987.)

PEDIATRIC BREATHING CIRCUITS

Much has been written about the advantages and disadvantages of various anesthesia circuits for use in pediatric patients (see Chapter 22). Pediatric circuit design has been directed to the physiology of the neonate and ways of reducing the work of breathing while preventing rebreathing. Nonrebreathing circuits minimize the work of breathing because they have no valves to be opened by the patient's respiratory effort. In addition, because the total volume of the circuit is less, the partial pressure of inhaled agent increases faster. Compression and compliance volumes are also decreased compared with a standard breathing circuit.

A number of combinations of the simple T-piece tubing, reservoir bag, and sites of fresh gas entry and overflow are possible. Mapleson classified the various combinations into five types (Fig. 44-2). The Jackson Rees modification is functionally identical to the Mapleson D, as are coaxial systems. Carbon dioxide is removed most effectively in the D configuration when controlled ventilation is used, whereas spontaneous ventilation is most effective in the A system.

Circle breathing systems can also be used very effectively in infants and children. Newer anesthesia machines use valves with much less resistance than older models. In addition, most neonates and small infants (for whom resistance would be the biggest problem) are ventilated mechanically during surgery, making work of breathing a nonissue. Dead space in these systems is no more than that of the Mapleson circuits.[74,75]

MONITORING

Monitoring decisions for pediatric patients are similar to those in adults. The pediatric patient should be monitored continuously with precordial or esophageal stethoscope. This simple device allows the anesthesiologist to detect changes in the rate, quality, and intensity of the heart sounds, which is helpful in evaluating the depth of anesthesia when potent inhalational agents are used. Pulse oximetry, capnometry, blood pressure (measured noninvasively with appropriately sized cuffs), temperature, and electrocardiogram should also be monitored routinely in children as in adults. More invasive or sophisticated monitoring should be used in appropriate circumstances.

INTRAVENOUS FLUID THERAPY

Fluid therapy is divided into three portions: deficit, maintenance, and third-space/blood replacement. Fortunately, modern fasting guidelines have greatly reduced the fluid deficit that pediatric surgical patients must replace. It is, however, important to elicit when the child last took fluid, and an estimate of how much the child drank.

An understanding of intravenous fluid management in the pediatric patient must consider the high metabolic demands and the high ratio of body surface area to weight that children have.[76] The basis for calculating maintenance fluid need derives from the fact that daily fluid requirements depend directly on metabolic demand; 100 ml of water is required for each 100 calories of expended energy. Relating this to weight produces the hourly fluid requirements, as seen in Table 44-3.

There is a trend to provide maintenance fluids, as well as deficit fluids with a balanced salt solution, with or without glucose. The optimum fluid to avoid hypoglycemia and hyperglycemia is dextrose 2.5% in lactated Ringer's solution; however, this fluid is not commercially available.[28] Even though symptomatic hypoglycemia is very rare in children beyond the infant age, it is important to monitor blood glucose if it is not included in the intravenous therapy for infants. Another approach might be to provide 5% dextrose in 0.45% normal saline (D_5 0.45 NS) for maintenance, piggybacked into a balanced salt solution for the deficit and third-space fluid. This double-iv fluid system may be quite costly because it does require a second intravenous administration setup.

The fluid deficit incurred during fasting should be replaced during anesthesia. Vasodilation from anesthetic agents may cause hypotension, even in patients who are not significantly hypovolemic. Aggressive intravenous hydration improves patient well-being. As mentioned earlier, aggressive hydration in the perioperative period combined with no requirement for oral intake before discharge decreases both postoperative nausea and vomiting and time to discharge home in pediatric outpatients.[77]

Assuming a healthy infant is in water and electrolyte balance at the time oral feeding stopped, the fluid deficit at the start of anesthesia can be calculated by multiplying the infant's hourly maintenance fluid requirement by the number of hours since the last oral intake. This deficit may be replaced by giving half of the calculated volume during the first hour of anesthesia, and the other half over the next 2 hours in addition to intraoperative maintenance fluids. An alternative formula for short surgical cases is to administer 20 mg · kg⁻¹ of deficit fluid, plus 5 mg · kg⁻¹ of maintenance fluid in the first hour, followed by maintenance

fluid for the rest of the brief procedure. It is important not to give large amounts of hypotonic solutions or dextrose in water (D_5W) because these hypotonic solutions can result in hyponatremia.[78]

Replacement of third-space intraoperative losses and blood is administered in a fashion similar to that in adult patients. The magnitude of third-space loss varies with the surgical procedure, and is highest in infants undergoing intestinal surgery. Evaporative losses are also highest in these procedures. Estimated third-space loss during intra-abdominal surgery varies from 6 to 15 ml · kg⁻¹ · h⁻¹, whereas in intrathoracic surgery it is less (4–7 ml · kg⁻¹ · h⁻¹). Lactated Ringer's solution is frequently used to replace these third-space losses. In cases of massive volume replacement, some advocate the use of 5% albumin. The end point of fluid therapy is sustained adequate blood pressure, tissue perfusion, and urine volume (0.5–1 ml · kg⁻¹ · h⁻¹). Because baroreceptor reflexes are blunted by volatile anesthetic agents, pulse rate often is not an accurate reflection of decreased intravascular volume.

All blood loss should be replaced in some way. Accurate measurement and calculation of acceptable blood loss in the infant are vital to any replacement plan. The concept of the maximum allowable blood loss (MABL) takes into account the effects of patient age, weight, and starting hematocrit on blood volume. In general, blood volume is approximately 100–120 ml · kg⁻¹ for the preterm infant, 90 ml · kg⁻¹ for the term infant, 80 mg · kg⁻¹ for the child 3–12 months of age, and 70 mg · kg⁻¹ for the patient older than 1 year. These estimates of blood volume can be used in calculating the individual patient's blood volume by multiplying the child's weight by the estimated blood volume (EBV) per kilogram:

$$MABL = \frac{EBV \times (\text{starting hematocrit} - \text{target hematocrit})}{\text{Starting hematocrit}}$$

Therefore, if an infant weighs 6 kg and has a starting hematocrit of 32%, and if clinical judgment estimates the desired postoperative hematocrit to be 25%, the calculation would be:

$$MABL = \frac{(6 \times 90) \times (32 - 25)}{32} = \frac{540 \times 7}{32} = 118 \text{ ml}$$

This MABL would be replaced with 3 ml of lactated Ringer's per milliliter of blood loss (118 × 3 = 354 ml). If blood loss remains less than MABL, no further blood loss is anticipated in the perioperative period, and hemodynamics remain stable, there is no need for blood transfusion. If significant perioperative blood loss occurs or is anticipated, discussion of potential transfusion needs with the surgeon is important.

As mentioned earlier, the incidence of apnea is higher in neonates and premature infants with hematocrits below 30%. A discussion with the surgeon and neonatologist may be helpful regarding transfusion management for surgical procedures for which significant perioperative blood loss is anticipated in these tiny patients.

Packed red blood cells have a hematocrit between 55 and 65%. On the average, 1 ml · kg⁻¹ of packed red blood cells increases the hematocrit by 1.5%. Units of blood can be subdivided into pediatric packs of 50–100 ml; thus, the remainder of a single unit is not wasted.

Rapid administration of citrated blood products can result in hypocalcemia as well as hypothermia. Fresh frozen plasma contains the greatest amount of citrate per unit volume of any blood product; rapid administration of fresh frozen plasma causes the greatest decrease in ionized calcium. Although under most circumstances, mobilization of calcium and hepatic metabolism of citrate are sufficiently rapid to prevent precipitous decreases in ionized calcium, infants have smaller stores of calcium. Infusion of fresh frozen plasma at a rate of 1–2.5 ml · kg⁻¹ · min⁻¹ may be associated with transient decreases in ionized calcium and decreased arterial blood pressure.

Table 44-3. MAINTENANCE FLUID REQUIREMENTS FOR PEDIATRIC PATIENTS (LEAN BODY MASS)

Weight (kg)	Hourly Fluid (ml)	24-hr Fluid (ml)
<10	4 ml · kg⁻¹	100 ml · kg⁻¹
11–20	40 ml + 2 ml · kg⁻¹ > 10 kg	1000 ml + 50 ml · kg⁻¹ > 10
>20	60 ml + 1 ml · kg⁻¹ > 20 kg	1500 ml + 20 ml · kg⁻¹ > 20

POSTANESTHETIC CARE
Monitoring

Continued monitoring of vital signs is important in infants and children, just as in adults. Pulse oximetry, pulse rate, and noninvasive blood pressure measurement should continue in the postanesthesia care unit, just as in older patients. Administration of supplemental oxygen may be guided by pulse oximetry.

Analgesia

It is the responsibility of the adult to provide analgesia, not the responsibility of the child to request pain relief. Pain assessment in pediatric patients is complicated by children's changing but relatively limited cognitive ability to understand measurement instructions or to articulate descriptions of their pain.[79] Children's responses are also affected by their developing behavioral repertoire and their constantly changing psychology.

Children older than 4–6 years of age can self-report pain. Younger children are usually assessed using a behavioral or physiologic–behavioral scale. Pain in children is much more difficult to assess than in adults because discrimination between pain and distress may be very challenging, particularly in the younger pediatric patient. Selecting a consistent means of pain assessment, performing that assessment at regular intervals, intervening, and reassessing are probably more important than which tool is selected. The prevailing philosophy among pediatric anesthesiologists is as follows: if I were having the procedure/surgery that this child is undergoing, would I require pain medication? If the answer is yes, the child is assessed, pain medication is administered, and a reassessment is made. If the reassessment shows a decrease of pain behaviors, pain management is considered successful, and continued evaluations are planned. If pain behaviors persist, the child receives additional pain treatment.

In addition, it is recognized that the emotional component of pain is very strong in children. Nonpharmacologic methods of pain management are also important. Although the most important of these is minimal separation from parents, other methods such as reassurance, cuddling, stroking, and distraction should also be used.

Nonopioid analgesics, usually acetaminophen or an NSAID, act at peripheral sites of injury by inhibiting prostaglandin synthesis and decreasing activation of primary afferent nerve injuries. These analgesics are useful for the treatment of mild to moderate discomfort (such as in many ambulatory procedures). When given in appropriate doses, all of these medications reduce the need for opioids in more severe pain conditions by approximately 30%.

The most common oral analgesic used in pediatric patients continues to be acetaminophen. This medication has been shown to be safe and efficacious in neonates as well as older children, with similar pharmacodynamics and pharmacokinetics in all but the youngest age groups.[80] Doses of 15 mg · kg^{-1} orally every 4 hours or 30–40 mg · kg^{-1} rectally as a loading dose followed by 15–20 mg · kg^{-1} every 6 hours, with a maximum dose of 90 mg · 24 h^{-1}, produce therapeutic plasma levels with good analgesia.[81] Acetaminophen should be administered only for a few consecutive days to reduce the risk of hepatic toxicity. Although rectal administration is less convenient and absorption more erratic than oral doses, acetaminophen suppositories can be inserted after induction of anesthesia to achieve effective blood levels in approximately 90 minutes.

Ketorolac has been shown to be an effective and safe analgesic for pediatric patients.[82] Because a child often denies pain rather than submit to an intramuscular injection, intravenous administration of ketorolac has become very popular—in spite of the fact that it is an off-label use of the drug. Intramuscular doses of 0.75 mg · kg^{-1} provide highly effective postoperative analge-

sia, as does an intravenous dose of 1 mg · kg^{-1} as a loading dose, with 0.5 mg · kg^{-1} administered every 6 hours thereafter.

As with other NSAIDs, ketorolac should be avoided in patients with pre-existing nephropathy or bleeding diathesis. Attention to fluid balance is also important; acute renal failure can occur with the use of NSAIDs in dehydrated patients after even one dose. Gastritis does not appear to be a problem. Although the bleeding time is not increased after administration of this drug, there is an increasing tendency to avoid its administration in surgical procedures that place a large stress on platelet and clotting mechanisms, such as tonsillectomy and adenoidectomy.

Ibuprofen is the most popular NSAID given orally to children. It comes in several palatable preparations. When given in the recommended oral dose of 10 mg · kg^{-1} it has similar analgesic effects as acetaminophen or ketorolac. Gastrointestinal side effects are uncommon.

Codeine can be administered orally or parenterally, and provides effective control of mild to moderate postoperative pain. The bioavailability of codeine after oral administration is approximately 60%. Orally administered codeine (0.5–1 mg · kg^{-1}) is often combined with acetaminophen (10 mg · kg^{-1}). This combination reduces the overall codeine requirement, thus limiting dose-dependent side effects. Although available, this medication is rarely used in its intravenous form because it has no advantage over morphine, and may be associated with a higher incidence of nausea and vomiting. Oxycodone (0.2 mg · kg^{-1}) is available only as a tablet, and is also often combined with acetaminophen or an NSAID. This agent appears to cause less nausea than codeine at equipotent doses.

As mentioned in the Opioids section of this chapter, all of the intravenous opioids used in adult patients can be successfully used in the pain management of children. Doses need to be reduced for neonates and infants younger than 4–6 months of age. Patient-controlled analgesia with opioids is used very effectively in children. The developmental level of the child must be considered, but most 5-year-olds and almost all 6-year-olds can be taught to use patient-controlled analgesia for postoperative pain control.

Regional anesthetic techniques have been shown to be particularly useful in pediatric ambulatory surgery procedures. They are most often used as adjuncts to general anesthesia, decreasing volatile agent requirement and providing postoperative analgesia. Simple techniques such as ilioinguinal–iliohypogastric nerve block, ring block of the penis, or caudal block can be very useful for common pediatric surgical procedures.[83-85] Direct local infiltration of surgical wounds can also be very helpful. Strict attention must be paid to the dose of local anesthetic, the dose of epinephrine (if used), and the technique of administration. More sophisticated techniques such as continuous caudal or epidural analgesia using combinations of opioids and local anesthetics are useful for inpatients after thoracic, abdominal, or lower extremity procedures. These regional techniques usually are used in combination with general anesthesia (catheters are placed after the child is induced) and the regional block is maintained for postoperative pain control.[86] Meticulous attention to technique and close monitoring of the child must take place when these continuous infusions are used.

Subglottic Edema (Postextubation Croup)

Subglottic edema after extubation usually manifests itself by arrival in the postanesthesia care unit, and if not, within 2 to 4 hours. In most cases, a "barky" cough and stertorous respirations are observed. With severe croup, there may be suprasternal retractions, tachypnea, labored respirations, and arterial oxygen desaturation.[87]

Mild cases require little therapy other than high concentrations of humidified oxygen. Racemic epinephrine (0.5 ml of a 2% solution diluted to a volume of 2–4 ml) administered by nebulizer is the next step. If this treatment is used, the child should be observed for 4 hours before discharge so that an evaluation of respiratory status postepinephrine effect can be made. If a second treatment is required, the child should be admitted for overnight observation and treatment.

Even if racemic epinephrine is not used, if there is any doubt as to the child's fitness for discharge, admission is the prudent course. Although their efficacy is unproven, systemic steroids are often administered in severe cases of postextubation croup.

CONCLUSION

"Children are not just little adults." However, most principles of adult anesthesia are also applicable in pediatric patients. A thorough understanding of the differences is crucial to the skilled administration of anesthesia to this challenging group of patients. The smaller the child, the less margin of reserve is present. The smile on the face of a child who is comfortable in her mother's arms in the postanesthesia care unit is one of the greatest rewards any practitioner can receive.

REFERENCES

1. The Virtual Anaesthetic Textbook (online). Available: http://www.usyd.edu.au/su/anaes/VAT/VAT.html (website coordinator, Dr. Chris Thompson)
2. Motoyama EK, Davis PJ (eds): Smith's Anesthesia for Infants and Children, 6th ed. St. Louis, Mosby, 1995
3. Gregory GA (ed): Pediatric Anesthesia, 3rd ed. New York, Churchill Livingstone, 1994
4. Katz J, Steward D (eds): Anesthesia and Uncommon Pediatric Diseases, 2nd ed. Philadelphia, WB Saunders, 1993
5. Badgwell JM (ed): Clinical Pediatric Anesthesia. Philadelphia, Lippincott-Raven, 1997
6. Berry FA (ed): Anesthetic Management of Difficult and Routine Pediatric Patients, 2nd ed. New York, Churchill Livingstone, 1990
7. Steward DJ: Psychological preparation and premedication. In Gregory GA (ed): Pediatric Anesthesia, 3rd ed, p 179. New York, Churchill Livingstone, 1994
8. Martin LD: Anesthetic implications of an upper respiratory infection in children. Pediatr Clin North Am 41:121, 1994
9. Mulroy JJ, Lynn AM: The medical evaluation of pediatric patients. Seminars in Anesthesiology 11:200, 1992
10. Berry FA, Steward DJ: Pediatrics for the Anesthesiologist. New York, Churchill Livingstone, 1993
11. Maxwell LG, Deshpande JK, Wetzel RC: Preoperative evaluation of children. Pediatr Clin North Am 41:93, 1994
12. Kain ZN, Caramico LA, Mayes LC et al: Preoperative preparation programs in children: A comparative examination. Anesth Analg 87:1249–55, 1998
13. McGraw T: Preparing children for the operating room: psychological issues. Can J Anaesth 41:1094, 1994
14. Bevan JC, Johnston C, Haig MJ et al: Preoperative parental anxiety predicts behavioral and emotional responses to induction of anaesthesia in children. Can J Anaesth 37:177, 1990
15. Kain ZN: Parental presence and induction of anesthesia. Paediatr Anaesth 5:209, 1995
16. Vetter TR: The epidemiology and selective identification of children at risk for preoperative anxiety reactions. Anesth Analg 77:96, 1993
17. Kain ZN, Mayes LC, Caramico LA et al: Parental presence during induction of anesthesia: A randomized controlled trial. Anesthesiology 84:1060, 1996
18. Kain ZN, Mayes LC, Wang SM et al: Parental presence during induction of anesthesia versus sedative premedication: Which intervention is more effective? Anesthesiology 89:1147, 1998
19. Kotiniemi LH, Ryhänen PT, Moilanen IK: Behavioral changes following routine ENT operations in two-to-ten-year-old children. Paediatr Anaesth 6:45, 1996
20. Steward DJ: Screening test before surgery in children. Can J Anaesth 38:693, 1991
21. Hackman T, Steward DJ, Sheps SB: Anemia in pediatric day-surgery patients: Prevalence detection. Anesthesiology 75:27, 1991
22. McClain BC, Redd SA, Turner EA: Sickle cell disease: A 90's perspective on an old disease. Advances in Anesthesia 16:129, 1999

23. Schreiner MS, Nicolson SC: Pediatric ambulatory anesthesia: NPO—before or after surgery? J Clin Anesth 7:589, 1995
24. Splinter WM, Schaeffer JD: Unlimited clear fluid ingestion two hours before surgery in children does not affect volume or pH of stomach contents. Anaesth Intensive Care 18:522, 1990
25. Coté CJ, Goudsouzian NG, Liu LMP et al: Assessment of risk factors related to the acid aspiration syndrome in pediatric patients: Gastric pH and residual volume. Anesthesiology 56:70, 1982
26. Borland LM, Sereika MS, Woelfel SR: Pulmonary aspiration in pediatric patients during general anesthesia: incidence and outcome. J Clin Anesth 10:95, 1998
27. Ferrari LR, Rooney FM, Rockoff MA: Preoperative fasting practices in pediatrics. Anesthesiology 90:978, 1999
28. Welborn LG, McGill WA, Hannallah RS et al: Perioperative blood glucose concentrations in pediatric outpatients. Anesthesiology 65:543, 1986
29. Veall GRQ, Dorman T: Prolonged starvation in paediatric surgery. Anaesthesia 50:458, 1995
30. Jones RDM, Visram AR, Kornberg JP et al: Premedication with oral midazolam in children an assessment of psychomotor function, anxiolysis, sedation and pharmacokinetics. Anaesth Intensive Care 22:539, 1994
31. Weldon BC, Watcha MF, White PF: Oral midazolam in children: effect of time and adjunctive therapy. Anesth Analg 75:51, 1992
32. Alderson PJ, Lerman J. Oral premedication for paediatric ambulatory anaesthesia: A comparison of midazolam and ketamine. Can J Anaesth 41:221, 1994
33. Ashburn MA, Streisand JB, Tarver SD et al: Oral transmucosal fentanyl citrate for premedication in paediatric outpatients. Can J Anaesth 37:857, 1990
34. Epstein RH, Mendel HG, Witkowski TA et al: The safety and efficacy of oral transmucosal fentanyl citrate for preoperative sedation in young children. Anesth Analg 83:1200, 1996
35. Davis PJ, Tome JA, McGowan FX et al: Preanesthetic medication with intranasal midazolam for brief pediatric surgical procedures. Anesthesiology 82:2, 1995
36. Hannallah RS, Patel RI: Low-dose intramuscular ketamine for anesthesia pre-induction in young children undergoing brief outpatient procedures. Anesthesiology 70:598, 1989
37. Keenan RL, Shapiro JH, Dawson K: Frequency of anesthetic cardiac arrests in infants: Effect of pediatric anesthesiologists. J Clin Anesth 3:433, 1991
38. Friesen RH, Lichtor JL: Cardiovascular depression during halothane anesthesia in infants: A study of three anesthetic techniques. Anesth Analg 61:42, 1982
39. Lerman J: Pharmacology of inhalational anaesthetics in infants and children. Paediatr Anaesth 2:191, 1992
40. Holzki J, Kretz FJ: Changing aspects of sevoflurane in paediatric anaesthesia: 1975–99. Paediatr Anaesth 8:283, 1999
41. Kern C, Erb T, Frei FJ: Hemodynamic responses to sevoflurane compared with halothane during inhalational induction in children. Paediatr Anaesth 7:439, 1997
42. Fisher DM, Robinson S, Brett CM et al: Comparison of enflurane, halothane, and isoflurane for diagnostic and therapeutic procedures in children with malignancies. Anesthesiology 63:647, 1985
43. Rolf N, Coté CJ: Persistent cardiac arrhythmias in pediatric patients: Effects of age, expired carbon dioxide values depth of anesthesia, and airway management. Anesth Analg 73:720, 1991
44. Friesen RH, Henry DB: Cardiovascular changes in preterm neonates receiving isoflurane, halothane, fentanyl, and ketamine. Anesthesiology 64:238, 1986
45. Welborn LG, Hannallah RS, McGill WA et al: Induction and recovery characteristics of desflurane and halothane anaesthesia in paediatric outpatients. Paediatr Anaesth 4:359, 1994
46. Welborn LG, Hannallah RS, Norden JM: Comparison of emergence and recovery characteristics of sevoflurane, desflurane, and halothane in pediatric ambulatory patients. Anesth Analg 83:917, 1996
47. Naito Y, Tamai S, Shingu K et al: Comparison between sevoflurane and halothane for paediatric ambulatory anaesthesia. Br J Anaesth 67:387, 1991
48. Epstein RH, Mendel HG, Suarnieri KM et al: Sevoflurane versus halothane for general anesthesia in pediatric patients: A comparative study of vital signs, induction, and emergence. J Clin Anesth 7:237, 1995
49. Lapin SL, Auden SM, Goldsmith LJ, Reynolds A-M: Effects of sevoflurane anaesthesia on recovery in children: A comparison with halothane. Paediatr Anaesth 9:299, 1999

50. Wells LT, Rasch DK: Emergence "delirium" after sevoflurane anesthesia: A paranoid delusion? Anesth Analg 98:1308, 1999

51. Gajraj NM, Pennant JH, Watcha MF: Eutectic mixture of local anesthetics (EMLA) cream. Anesth Analg 78:574, 1994

52. Zempsky WT, Anand KJS, Sullivan KM et al: Lidocaine iontophoresis for topical anesthesia before intravenous line placement in children. J Pediatr 132:1061, 1998

53. Hannallah RS, Britton JT, Schafer PG et al: Propofol anaesthesia in paediatric ambulatory patients: A comparison with thiopentone and halothane. Can J Anaesth 41:12, 1994

54. Kain ZN, Gaal DJ, Kain TS et al: A first-pass cost analysis of propofol versus barbiturates for children undergoing magnetic resonance imaging. Anesth Analg 79:1102, 1994

55. Davis PJ, Lerman J, Suresh S et al: A randomized multicenter study of remifentanil compared with alfentanil, isoflurane, or propofol in anesthetized pediatric patients undergoing elective strabismus surgery. Anesth Analg 84:982, 1997

56. Blanc VF: Atropine and succinylcholine: Beliefs and controversies in paediatric anaesthesia. Can J Anaesth 42:1, 1995

57. O'Flynn RP, Schutack JG, Rosenberg H, Fletcher JE: Masseter muscle rigidity and malignant hyperthermia susceptibility in pediatric patients. Anesthesiology 80:1228, 1994

58. Sullivan M, Thompson WK, Hill GD: Succinylcholine-induced cardiac arrest in children with undiagnosed myopathy. Can J Anaesth 41:497, 1994

59. Gronert BJ, Brandom BW: Neuromuscular blocking drugs in infants and children. Pediatr Clin North Am 41:73, 1994

60. Kaplan RF, Uejima T, Lobel TG et al: Intramuscular rocuronium in infants and children. Anesthesiology 91:633, 1999

61. Kaplan RF, Fletcher JE, Hannallah RS et al: The potency (ED_{50}) and cardiovascular effects of rapacuronium (Org 9487) during narcotic–nitrous oxide–propofol anesthesia in neonates, infants and children. Anesth Analg 89:1172, 1999

62. Litman RS, Wu CL, Lee A, Griswold JD et al: Prevention of emesis after strabismus repair in children: A prospective, double-blinded, randomized comparison of droperidol versus ondansetron. J Clin Anesth 7:58, 1995

63. Watcha MF, Bras PJ, Cieslak GD, Pennant JH: The dose–response relationship of ondansetron in preventing postoperative emesis in pediatric patients undergoing ambulatory surgery. Anesthesiology 82:47, 1995

64. Watcha MF, Simeon RM, White PF: Effect of propofol on the incidence of postoperative vomiting after strabismus surgery in pediatric outpatients. Anesthesiology 75:204, 1991

65. Henzi I, Walder B, Tramèr MR: Dexamethasone for the prevention of postoperative nausea and vomiting: A qualitative systematic review. Anesth Analg 90:186, 2000

66. Pappas LS, Sukhani R, Hotaling AJ: The effect of preoperative dexamethasone on the immediate and delayed postoperative morbidity in children undergoing adenotonsillectomy. Anesth Analg 87:57, 1998

67. Lerman J: Are antiemetics cost-effective for children? Can J Anaesth 42:263, 1995

68. Schreiner MS, Nicolson SC, Martin T, Whitney L: Should children drink before discharge from day surgery? Anesthesiology 76:528, 1992

69. Weinstein MS, Nicolson SC, Schreiner MS: A single dose of morphine sulfate increases the incidence of vomiting after outpatient inguinal surgery in children. Anesthesiology 81, 572, 1994

70. McGinn G, Haynes SR, Morton NS: An evaluation of the laryngeal mask airway during routine paediatric anaesthesia. Paediatr Anaesth 3:23, 1993

71. Hatcher IS, Stack CG: Postal survey of the anaesthetic techniques used for paediatric tonsillectomy surgery. Paediatr Anaesth 9:311, 1999

72. Ruby RR, Webster AC, Morley-Rorster PK, Dain S: Laryngeal mask airway in paediatric otolaryngologic surgery. J Otolaryngol 24:288, 1995

73. Markakis DA, Sayson SC, Schreiner MS: Insertion of the laryngeal mask airway in awake infants with the Robin sequence. Anesth Analg 75:822, 1992

74. Fisher D: Anesthesia equipment for pediatrics. In Gregory GA (ed): Pediatric Anesthesia, 3rd ed, p 197. New York, Churchill Livingstone, 1994

75. Conterato JP, Lindahl SGE, Meyer DM, Bires JA: Assessment of spontaneous ventilation in anesthetized children with use of a pediatric circle or a Jackson-Reese system. Anesth Analg 69:484, 1989

76. Keyes MA: Perioperative fluid therapy for the pediatric patient. Seminars in Anesthesiology 11:252, 1992

77. Kearney R, Mack C, Entwistle L: Withholding oral fluids from children undergoing day surgery reduces vomiting. Paediatr Anaesth 8:331, 1998

78. Arieff AL. Postoperative hyponatraemic encephalopathy following elective surgery in children. Paediatr Anaesth 8:1, 1998

79. Houck CS, Berde CB, Anand KJS: Pediatric pain management. In Gregory GA (ed): Pediatric Anesthesia, 3rd ed, p 743. New York, Churchill Livingstone, 1994

80. Lesko SM, Mitchell AA: The safety of acetaminophen and ibuprofen among children younger than two years old (online). Available: http://:www.pediatrics.org/cgi/content/full/104/4/e39

81. Birmingham PK, Tobin MJ, Henthorn TK et al: Twenty-four-hour pharmacokinetics of rectal acetaminophen in children: an old drug with new recommendations. Anesthesiology 87:244, 1997

82. Splinter WM, Reid CW, Roberts DJ, Bass J: Reducing pain after inguinal hernia repair in children: Caudal anesthesia versus ketorolac tromethamine. Anesthesiology 87:542, 1997

83. Rice LJ: Regional anesthesia. In Motoyama ES, Davis PD (eds): Smith's Anesthesia for Infants and Children, 6th ed., p 403. St. Louis, Mosby, 1995

84. Broadman LM, Rice LJ: Neural blockade for pediatric surgery. In Cousins MJ, Bridenbaugh PO (eds): Neural Blockade in Clinical Anesthesia and Management of Pain, 3rd ed, p 615. Philadelphia, JB Lippincott, 1996

85. Dalens BJ: Regional anesthesia in children. In Cocchiara RF, Miller ED, Reves JG, et al (eds): Anesthesia, 5th ed. New York, Churchill Livingstone, 1999

86. Dalens BJ: Lumbar epidural anesthesia. In Dalens BJ (ed): Regional Anesthesia in Infants, Children, and Adolescents, p 207. London, Williams & Wilkins, 1995

87. Patel R, Rice LJ: Special considerations in recovery of children from anesthesia. Int Anesthesiol Clin 29:55, 1991

Clinical Anesthesia (4/e), edited by
Paul G. Barash, Bruce F. Cullen, and
Robert K. Stoelting. Lippincott Williams &
Wilkins, Philadelphia, © 2001.

CHAPTER 45

ANESTHESIA FOR THE GERIATRIC PATIENT

STANLEY MURAVCHICK

Advances in nutrition, public health, education, and social services have produced major changes in human longevity in industrialized societies. Life expectancy for adult males has increased by more than 30 years since the introduction of the term "geriatrics" at the beginning of the twentieth century.[1] Elderly patients account for 48% of all hospital care days in the United States. Currently, at least one of every four surgical patients is 65 years of age or older, and an even larger fraction is anticipated in the next two decades Therefore, unless intentionally limited to pediatrics or obstetric patients, every anesthesiologist in contemporary practice must acquire expertise in geriatric medicine. The sections that follow define the current concepts of aging that are relevant to anesthetic practice. They discuss the distinction between aging and age-related disease and present strategies useful for perioperative assessment of the elderly patient, and they summarize practical aspects of anesthetic management and anticipating perioperative outcome in geriatric surgical patients.

CONCEPTS OF AGING AND GERIATRICS

Extreme variability of signs, symptoms, and physical presentation among older patients has long been recognized as an important characteristic of geriatric medicine. As they age, adults exhibit an increasingly varied array of physical responses to concurrent disease states which, in turn, reflect life-long exposure to environmental and socioeconomic conditions and to the accumulated stigmata of prior traumatic injuries and medical therapies. Prolonged longevity also enables complete expression of intrinsic genetic qualities in all their subtle physiologic manifestations. Discrete "biologic markers of aging" such as visual acuity or the racemization of structural amino acids in connective tissue have been of some value for highly specialized nonclinical applications such as the evaluation of "anti-aging" therapies administered to laboratory animals. Currently, however, there is no consensus as to when the "geriatric" era begins in human subjects or whether any single physiologic marker can identify a physiologically "elderly" patient. Therefore, establishing a rigid and finite chronological definition of the term "geriatric" has little medical value other than for administrative, actuarial, or epidemiologic applications. For clarity and consistency, however, the terms "elderly" and "geriatric" will be used synonymously within this chapter to describe human subjects who, by arbitrary convention, are about 65 years of age or older. Because clinical experience and large-scale outcome studies suggest that there may be some predictive value in subdividing elderly patients into chronological subgroups, the term "aged" will be used to describe individuals older than 80 years.

"Life-span" is an idealized, species-specific, relatively fixed biologic parameter that quantitates maximum attainable individual age under optimal conditions. Historical anecdote and contemporary demographic data suggest that human life span has, indeed, remained constant at about 110–115 years for the past 20 centuries.[2] In contrast, "life-expectancy" describes typical longevity under prevailing conditions in society. This has changed dramatically during different periods in history. Recently, advances in medical science and health care have improved life expectancy and have increased the relative "aged-

ness" of voting populations in democratic societies to the point that the economics and politics of healthcare for the elderly have, for the first time, assumed roles of major importance.

Most studies of human aging are cross-sectional studies that measure physiologic parameters simultaneously in young and elderly subjects. Although straightforward in design and in execution, even a comprehensive cross-sectional approach may not identify patients with subtle preclinical manifestations of disease. In addition, cross-sectional experimental design cannot be controlled for cohort-specific factors such as nutritional and environmental history, for genetic background, or for prior exposure to infectious agents. Therefore, many changes now known to be due to age-related disease have been attributed erroneously to aging. The "young" and "old" patient groups being compared in cross-sectional studies often differ not only in age but also in terms of their overall physiologic, anatomic, and biochemical characteristics. Therefore, data from cross-sectional studies rarely permit unambiguous conclusions regarding the effect of age itself on a measured parameter.

Longitudinal studies of aging, in contrast, require that the investigator obtain repeated measurements in each individual subject over several decades. Each subject therefore generates his own "young adult" control value for comparison with subsequent measurements. If any of the subjects in a longitudinal study eventually manifest signs of age-related disease, their data points can be excluded from the study, thereby leaving behind a smaller but more homogeneous group of healthy elderly subjects. Although difficult and expensive to organize and maintain, long-term longitudinal studies have produced substantial amounts of extremely valuable data related to human aging.

Despite considerable efforts by many scientists, however, the mechanisms that control the aging process remain unknown. The impressive consistency of observed life span may not, as was once believed, necessarily imply a genetically or centrally coordinated, hypothalamic "biological clock" for each species. Instead, age-related decline in organ and tissue function may simply be the inevitable accumulation of nonspecific, degenerative phenomena such as ionizing radiation.[3] Currently, there is also great interest in the role of declining mitochondrial bioenergetics as the underlying mechanism for deterioration of organ function. Throughout adulthood, increasing levels of oxygen-derived free radicals within the mitochondria appear to disrupt the structural and enzymatic machinery of oxidative phosphorylation.[4] As the ability to scavenge these byproducts of aerobic metabolism declines, it creates a "vicious cycle of aging" within the mitochondria (Fig. 45-1). Viewed from this perspective, the unique life span demonstrated by each species could be explained as a stochastic interaction between genetically determined biochemical and physiologic attributes for each species and the destructive environmental factors that disorder biologic systems.

AGING AND ORGAN FUNCTION

For these reasons, contemporary definitions of aging are conceptual rather than quantitative. Aging is a universal and progressive physiologic phenomenon characterized by degenerative changes in both the structure and the function of organs

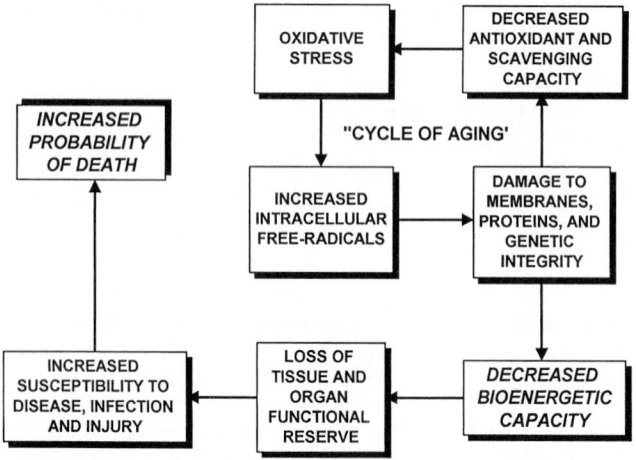

Figure 45-1. At a cellular level, there may be a self-sustaining "cycle of aging" within mitochondria in which oxidative stress damages the metabolic machinery needed to provide adequate bioenergetic capacity for full organ system functional reserve.

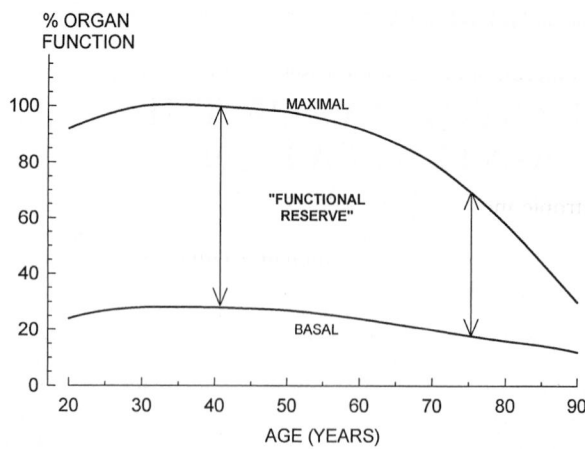

Figure 45-3. For any organ system "functional reserve" represents the difference between basal (minimal) and maximal organ system function. The age-related decline in functional reserve may not be clinically apparent until demands made upon the organ system are increased by stress, disease, polypharmacy, or surgical intervention.

and tissues. At one time, global age-related physiologic degeneration was depicted as linear decline of maximal function beginning in young adulthood and continuing inexorably downward thereafter. However, a more contemporary analysis describes nonlinear change in maximal organ function that first becomes apparent following the years that represent the peak of somatic maturation, in the fourth decade of human life (Fig. 45-2). Additional decrements of function during the middle adult years appear to be relatively subtle but subsequently become progressively more dramatic during the traditional years of geriatric senescence, the seventh decade of life and beyond. Elderly patients who maintain greater than average functional capacities are considered "physiologically young." When organ function declines at an earlier age than usual, or at a more rapid rate, elderly patients appear to be "physiologically old."

Nevertheless, the competence of integrated organ system function varies greatly from one elderly patient to the next, even in the absence of disease, and is significantly altered by activity level, social habits, diet, and genetic background. In healthy geriatric patients, however, maximum organ system function at all ages is greater than basal demand. The difference between maximal organ system capacity and basal function rep-

resents organ system functional reserve (Fig. 45-3). Organ system functional reserve is the "safety margin" of organ capacity available to meet, for example, the additional demands for cardiac output, carbon dioxide excretion, or protein synthesis imposed upon the patient by trauma or disease, or by surgery and convalescence. Cardiopulmonary functional reserve can be assessed clinically and quantified using various exercise or aerobic stress tests. It is generally assumed that the functional reserve of all organ systems is progressively and significantly reduced in elderly patients, although there are at present no techniques for assessment of hepatic, immune, or nervous system functional reserve. In fact, many gerontologists consider the increased susceptibility of elderly patients to stress- and disease-induced organ system decompensation to be a defining characteristic of physiologic aging. Consequently, preoperative testing in the elderly patient is most effective when it provides the anesthesiologist with a quantifiable assessment of organ system reserve and it is clinically directed according to symptoms and complaints referable to age-related disease and the erosion of physiologic homeostasis.

CARDIOPULMONARY FUNCTION

Classic studies suggested that aging inevitably produces a progressive depression of cardiac output. This conclusion, however, is contradicted by more recent studies of fit and active elderly subjects in whom demand for cardiopulmonary function is maintained through daily exercise or even enhanced by aerobic training.[5] In young and elderly adults alike, resting cardiac output appears to be determined largely by the metabolic demands of lean tissue mass, and maximal cardiac output responds to vigorous physical activity. Consequently, the modest decrease in resting cardiac index observed in most healthy elderly subjects is not evidence of degenerative cardiovascular change. Rather, it represents an appropriate integrated response to the reduced requirements for perfusion and metabolism that occur with age-related atrophy of skeletal muscle and the loss of tissue mass in major organs with high intrinsic metabolic rates.[6] From the perspective of integrated cardiovascular function, exercise, and aerobic capacity, aging simply produces a progressively smaller "machine."

Under conditions of submaximal demand, myocardial contractility as assessed by rates of myocardial shortening and ventricular pressure generation or ejection fraction appears to remain uncompromised by increasing age, at least until the eighth decade.[7] Similarly, there is little evidence of significant change

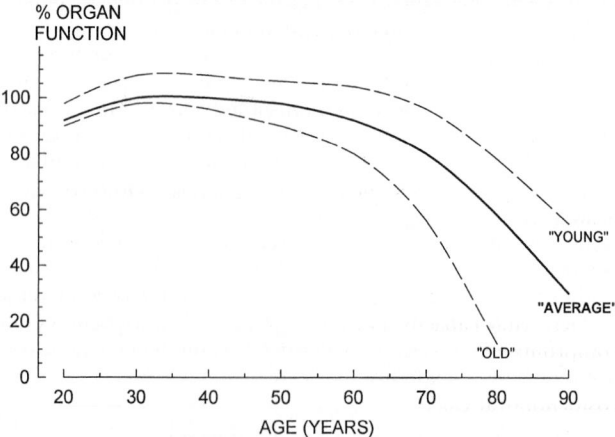

Figure 45-2. Differences in the rate at which maximal organ system functions decline with increasing age, and, to a lesser extent, differences in initial functional levels explain the inevitable variability seen in geriatric patients commonly described as physiologically "younger" or "older" than average.

at a cellular level in the contractile proteins or in the enzymatic substrate required for energy production within the myocardial sarcomeres. Short-term increases in cardiac output are accomplished in the elderly patient at first by modest increases in heart rate, and then by increased left ventricular end-diastolic volumes and pressures that produce progressively larger stroke volumes (Fig. 45-4). However, because aging reduces both the inotropic and chronotropic responses to adrenergic stimulation and to β-agonists, maximal heart rate is age-limited, and unlike young adults, older adults exhibit little enhancement of ejection fraction under these conditions.

The heart, unlike other major organs, does not atrophy significantly with age. Both heart size and myocardial tissue mass are increased in older adults. However, the aging left ventricle is thicker and less elastic than its younger counterpart, exhibiting symmetric hypertrophy and an increase in collagen cross-linking in the myocardial cytoskeleton to which the myocytes are attached.[8] The stiffer, less compliant ventricular and atrial myocardium of the aging heart therefore undergoes complete myocardial relaxation relatively late in diastole, and the contribution of passive ventricular filling, which occurs during the early phase of diastole, is significantly reduced (Fig. 45-5). The hemodynamic importance of diastolic dysfunction has been recognized only recently, but it is now clear that age-related diastolic dysfunction makes the elderly subject significantly more dependent upon the synchronous atrial contraction of sinus rhythm for complete ventricular filling at end-diastole.[9] Therefore, relatively small decreases in venous return such as those produced by positive-pressure ventilation, surgical hemorrhage, or venodilator drugs may significantly compromise stroke volume, especially when cardiac dysrhythmias are present.

Virtually all longitudinal studies of aging confirm the universal nature of progressive systolic arterial hypertension, a phenomenon due to fibrotic replacement of elastic tissues within the cardiovascular system. Age reduces the ability of the aorta and large arteries to store hydraulic energy, increasing vascular impedance to cardiac ejection and raising ventricular wall tensions and cardiac workload. These forces appear to explain the development of symmetric ventricular hypertrophy described above. Because vascular impedance is a frequency-dependent form of hydraulic resistance, increases in impedance to ejection of stroke volume can occur even when systemic vascular resistance (SVR) is unchanged.[10] Increased vascular stiffness and

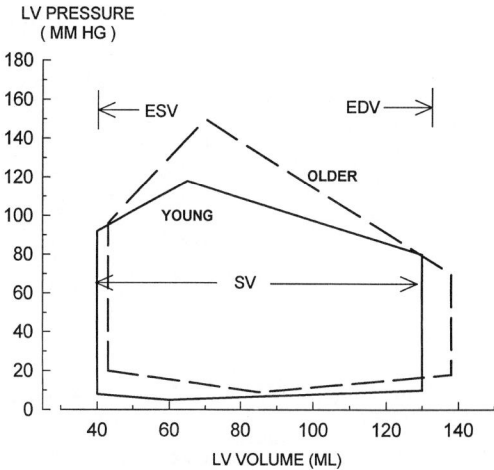

Figure 45-5. Left ventricular (LV) cardiac pressure–volume loops for fit young (*solid line*) and elderly (*broken line*) subjects. Older subjects have a slightly higher end-diastolic ventricular volume (EDV) and larger stroke volume (SV) as well as slightly elevated intracavitary pressures throughout the cardiac cycle because of increased myocardial stiffness and delayed active relaxation during diastole.

loss of arterial cross-sectional area increase the reflection of arterial pressure waves within the arterial tree, producing the familiar "overshoot" characteristics of radial artery waveform tracings in geriatric patients as well as generating large discrepancies between blood pressure values obtained by invasive techniques and those measured by more traditional occlusive cuff techniques. In the absence of disease, however, neither intrinsic myocardial contractility nor integrated cardiovascular function actually limits cardiac output at rest or during moderate exercise. The heart increases its output to meet imposed metabolic demands as needed within the limits of its maximal capacity. Even sedentary geriatric subjects benefit dramatically from programmed increases in aerobic activity, and many aged individuals participate in strenuous athletic events such as marathon running events.

Age-related loss of tissue elasticity is ubiquitous. It occurs in the lung as well as in the cardiovascular system. In fact, loss of lung elastic recoil is a primary anatomic mechanism by which aging exerts deleterious effects on pulmonary gas exchange.[11] With increasing age, there is an increase in fibrous connective tissue within the lung parenchyma and progressive degeneration and cross-linking of lung elastin fibers. It remains unclear whether there is an actual decline in lung elastin content, however. Whatever the mechanism, elderly individuals experience virtually inevitable emphysema-like increases in lung compliance because lung elastic recoil declines. The patency of small airways, normally maintained by elastic recoil, may be compromised, moving closing capacity (CC) above functional residual capacity (FRC), the volume of the lung at rest.[12] However, calcification and stiffening of the costochondral joints of the thorax actually reduce chest wall compliance, so net pulmonary compliance is almost unchanged.[13]

Although aging produces only a minor progressive increase in FRC, vital capacity (VC) is significantly and progressively compromised[14] as residual volume increases at the expense of inspiratory and expiratory reserve volumes (Fig. 45-6). The costochondral calcification that makes the thorax more rigid and decreases the compliance of the chest wall also increases the work of breathing in elderly subjects. Increased airway resistance associated with partial obstruction of small airways also produces a modest increase in the total work of breathing of elderly subjects. Although the strength and endurance of muscles of ventilation remain adequate for moderate demands,[15] compro-

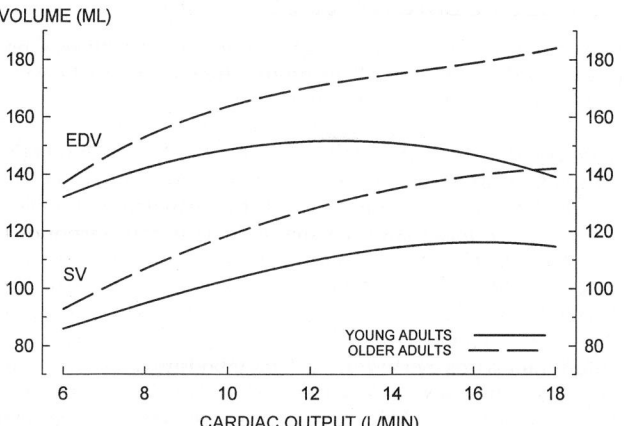

Figure 45-4. In healthy elderly subjects (*broken lines*), demand for increased cardiac output is met by significant increases in stroke volume (SV) and left ventricular end-diastolic volume (LVEDV) that compensate for reduced maximal heart rate. In contrast, high levels of cardiac output are achieved in younger subjects (*solid lines*) through large increases in heart rate and only modest enhancement of SV, the latter achieved through β-adrenoceptor-mediated inotropy that increases ejection fraction but actually reduces LVEDV.

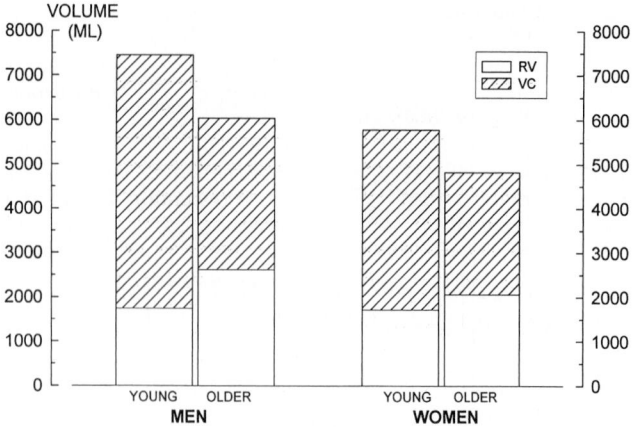

Figure 45-6. Total lung capacity, the sum of vital capacity (VC) and residual volume (RV), is reduced only modestly in older adults of either gender. VC, however, is markedly compromised by age-related increases in thoracic rigidity and loss of ventilatory muscle power. RV increases because intrinsic lung elastic recoil is progressively reduced.

mised ability to meet heavy ventilatory workloads predisposes the elderly patient to acute postoperative ventilatory failure.[16]

These changes in the physical composition of the lung parenchyma also reduce the efficiency of gas exchange within the aging lung. Although, as in every organ system, variability is great, age-related decline in perioperative arterial oxygenation is significant and progressive. Breakdown of alveolar septae reduces total alveolar surface area, increasing both anatomic and alveolar dead space. Because these changes in the physical properties of the lungs are nonuniform, they severely disrupt the normal matching of ventilation and perfusion, increasing both physiologic shunting and dead space.[17] Therefore, pulmonary dysfunction in older adults during general anesthesia is best described as diffuse ventilation–perfusion mismatch (Fig. 45-7) due to deterioration of alveolar architecture and anesthetic-induced depression of active hypoxic pulmonary vasoconstriction. Consequently, virtually all surgical patients 70 years of age or older should receive supplemental oxygen perioperatively because they are at increased risk of hypoxemia following sedation, diagnostic procedures, or surgical intervention.

In contrast, the moment-to-moment control of ventilation by neural structures and the ventilatory responses to changes in

pH and respiratory gases appear to be essentially unchanged in healthy elderly subjects. However, the cardiovascular and the ventilatory stimulation normally mediated by homeostatic reflex mechanisms in response to imposed hypoxia or hypercarbia are delayed in onset, and of considerably smaller magnitude, in geriatric patients.[18] For reasons not completely understood, elderly subjects also experience a higher incidence of transient apnea and episodic respiration when given narcotics, and may be more sensitive to the respiratory depression produced by non-narcotic central nervous system depressant drugs such as the benzodiazepines.

Opioid-induced rigidity of the chest wall also occurs more frequently in older than in younger adults, although this may be a manifestation of opiate-induced nervous system toxicity. Like virtually all forms of sensory input in elderly subjects, the threshold stimulus magnitude needed for vocal cord closure is markedly elevated,[19] increasing the risk of pulmonary injury due to aspiration of gastric contents in older patients, especially if level of consciousness is depressed. Consequently, geriatric surgical patients are clearly at greater risk of unrecognized respiratory failure in the typical postoperative setting of residual anesthetic depression and the use of opioids for pain management.

HEPATORENAL AND IMMUNE FUNCTION

In general, age is associated with loss of hepatic tissue mass and splanchnic blood flow and not a qualitative impairment of hepatocellular function. Hepatic enzyme activities are similar to those of young adults,[20] and "normal" values for plasma concentrations of transaminases and other hepatocyte-derived enzymes are unchanged in the elderly adults,[21] although the bromsulphthalein (BSP) retention approaches the upper limit of the "normal" range by the seventh decade of life even in individuals who demonstrate no other evidence of hepatic dysfunction. Nevertheless, the overall functional capacity of the liver is largely determined by its size and blood flow, and age-related changes in hepatic and splanchnic anatomy are dramatic. Age-related loss of hepatic tissue mass is generally thought to be the primary explanation for the delayed biotransformation and prolonged clinical effects of narcotics and many other xenobiotics in geriatric subjects.[22] Liver tissue mass declines about 40% by the age of 80 years, and hepatic blood flow is reduced proportionally.[23]

Some clinical studies suggest that this organ system may undergo subtle physiologic changes that are both age- and gender-specific. For example, elderly women metabolize benzodiazepines at rates close to that of their younger counterparts, yet elderly men do not. Elderly men, but not women, frequently have significant reductions in the activity of the hepatically synthesized enzyme plasma cholinesterase.[24] Hepatic metabolism and drug biotransformation may also be unpredictably altered in this patient subpopulation because they are also likely to have sustained exposure to the polypharmacy of age-related chronic disease. For example, cimetidine, widely used in geriatric patients to relieve gastritis that occurs because of age-impaired secretion of protective gastric mucus, significantly depresses the hepatic biotransformation of benzodiazepines. Although liver blood flow remains relatively constant as a percentage of cardiac output and therefore provides adequate function to meet basal metabolic needs, the hepatic synthetic reserve needed for wound healing or response to sepsis may be inadequate, especially if associated with arterial hypotension, low cardiac output, hypothermia, or any form of direct hepatic injury.

Age-related tissue atrophy is also evident in anatomic and postmortem observations of the kidneys,[25] with 30% of renal tissue mass lost by the eighth decade. Total renal blood flow decreases almost 50%, a decline of about 10% per decade begin-

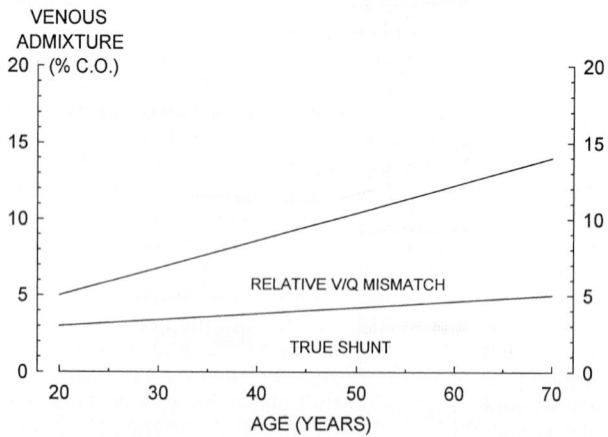

Figure 45-7. During general anesthesia, the efficiency of oxygenation decreases with age. Venous admixture, expressed as the percentage of cardiac output, rises significantly as both intrapulmonary shunting and relative ventilation/perfusion ($\dot{V}/\dot{Q}$) mismatch become more prevalent. (Data courtesy of Dr. G. Hedenstierna.)

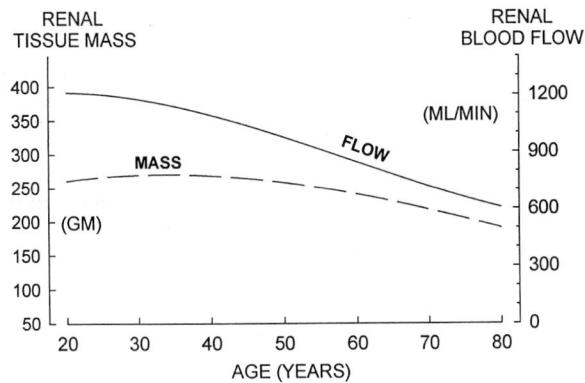

Figure 45-8. Renal blood flow (*solid line*) declines more rapidly than does renal tissue mass (*broken line*) with increasing age. Glomerular filtration rate (not shown) falls somewhat more slowly than plasma flow because filtration fraction actually increases in some elderly individuals.

ning in early adulthood (Fig. 45-8). Cellular attrition is especially marked in the renal cortex, although the extent of parenchymal loss is grossly masked by a reciprocal increase in renal fat and by a diffuse and generalized process of interstitial fibrosis. The effects of aging on the renal microarchitecture is dramatic. More than one-third of the glomeruli and their associated nephron tubular structures disappear in the elderly.[26] In 10–20% of those glomeruli that remain, sclerosis impairs effective filtration by producing tubular diverticuli and dysfunctional continuity between afferent and efferent glomerular arterioles.[27]

The renal cortex appears to be particularly sensitive to progressive reduction of tissue vascularity, with relative sparing of the renal medulla. Shifting of renal perfusion from cortex to medulla appears to produce a slight compensatory increase in filtration fraction in elderly subjects. Therefore, although both renal plasma flow and glomerular filtration rate (GFR) decline more rapidly than would be expected from the loss of renal tissue mass alone,[28] GFR decreases less rapidly than expected. Despite compromise of renal functional reserve, serum creatinine concentration usually remains within the normal range in elderly patients because their declining skeletal muscle mass generates a progressively smaller creatinine load. A lower level of basal renal function is therefore adequate to maintain metabolic equilibrium, and GFR is sufficient to avoid uremia and to maintain normal plasma osmolarity and electrolyte concentrations.[29]

Elderly patients release large concentrations of antidiuretic hormone (ADH) in response to a hypertonic saline load, but water retention is still less efficient than that of young adults. The elderly also demonstrate a decreased maximal reabsorption rate for glucose as well as significant impairment of the response to aldosterone and the extent to which they conserve sodium. Excretion of a free water load is also markedly delayed. Diminished thirst, poor diet, and the use of diuretic agents to decrease age-related hypertension also predispose elderly surgical patients to intravascular and intracellular dehydration.[30] Geriatric surgical patients do not appear to require a unique fluid replacement protocol, but their renal functional reserve is usually inadequate to withstand gross disruptions of water and electrolyte balance. They may not respond promptly or appropriately to imposed contractions or expansions of intravascular volume, and they therefore require meticulous monitoring and management of fluid and electrolyte balance.

Even fit elderly subjects exhibit some general characteristics of decreased immune responsiveness. The quantitative age-related change in thymic mass and progressive alteration of thymic cellular composition both play a central role in senescence of the immune system. Lymphocyte numbers remain

within the range established as normal for young adults, yet older adults have decreased B- and T-cell lymphocyte activity and depressed serum titers of immunoglobulin E, depressed skin response to allergens, and compromise of delayed hypersensitivity.[31] Aging appears to have little effect upon macrophage and other phagocytic activity, yet older adults are particularly predisposed to streptococcal pneumonia, meningitis, and septicemia.[32] In fact, sepsis is second only to respiratory failure as a cause of morbidity and mortality in elderly trauma patients.[33]

METABOLISM, BODY COMPOSITION, AND PHARMACOKINETICS

Aging, particularly in men, produces a progressive and generalized loss of skeletal muscle mass as well as atrophy of metabolically active areas in brain, liver, and kidney.[34] Reciprocal increases in the lipid fraction of total body mass are typical during the middle adult years but are extremely variable in magnitude. In general, changes in body composition reduce the basal metabolic requirements of aging patients by 10–15% compared with their young adult counterparts.[35] Reduction in body heat production and impairment of autonomically mediated thermoregulatory vasoconstriction[36] put the elderly surgical patient at increased risk for inadvertent intraoperative hypothermia. Intraoperative core temperature decreases at a rate twice as great as that observed in young adults under comparable conditions.[37] The time needed for spontaneous rewarming postoperatively also appears to increase in direct proportion to the patient's age.[38] Because skeletal muscle and liver normally provide storage for carbohydrates, aging is also associated with progressive impairment of the ability to handle a glucose challenge. However, because both the timing and the magnitude of insulin release itself appear to remain normal, age-related glucose intolerance may also reflect, at least in part, a progressive impairment of insulin function[39] or subtle antagonism of its effect on these target tissues.[40] In any case, iv fluid replacement using glucose-containing solutions should be limited to environments that permit frequent measurement of blood sugar levels in elderly patients.

From young adulthood on, most men initially gain about 12 kg of adipose tissue and lose about 8 kg of skeletal muscle mass, changes that may eventually result in the loss of 10–15% of their total body water (Fig. 45-9). The change in total body

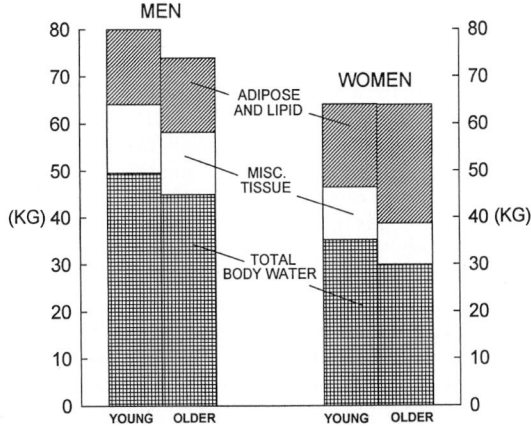

Figure 45-9. Age-related changes in body composition are gender-specific. In women, total body mass remains constant because increases in body fat (*upper shaded segment*) offset bone loss (*middle segment*) and intracellular dehydration (*lower shaded segment*). In men, body mass declines despite maintenace of body lipid and skeletal tissue elements because accelerating loss of skeletal muscle and other components of lean tissue mass produces marked contraction of intracellular water (*lower shaded segment*).

weight seen during and following the young adult years is bipha-sic, characterized by the middle-adult–year increases in adipose fraction and total body weight commonly described as "middle-aged spread." However, in aged men, continuing loss of muscle and central organ atrophy eventually produce a significant de-cline in total body weight, often to levels less than those of young adulthood.[41] In women, however, dehydration and bone loss due to osteoporosis are largely offset by increasing body fat, and total body weight usually returns to, but rarely below, young adult body weight. Virtually all of the age-related changes in body water remain limited to intracellular compartments, with decrease in circulating blood volume usually restricted to the deconditioned elderly subject or to those with essential hypertension.[42] Plasma volume, red cell mass, and extracellular fluid volumes are normally well maintained in nonhypertensive elderly individuals who maintain their habits of daily physical ac-tivity.

These age-related changes in body composition are universal, progressive, and relatively irreversible, although the rate at which skeletal muscle mass is lost may be minimized by vigorous exercise, and the progressive increase in adipose tempered by changes in diet or by maintenance of high caloric expenditure. Nevertheless, many of these physiologic and anatomic changes reflect the unavoidable consequences of genetic predisposition and reduced testosterone, thyroid hormone, or other endoge-nous modulators of tissue metabolism at least as much as they reflect individual lifestyle and the social environment. There-fore, as aging increases the lipid fraction of body mass relative to the proportion of aqueous, well-perfused body tissues, it also enlarges the distribution volumes available to function as reservoirs for inhalational anesthetics, benzodiazepines, barbi-turates, and other drug molecules that are preferentially soluble in lipid.[43] If iv drugs are administered in dosage determined by total body weight, the increased lipid fraction of total body weight seen in elderly subjects may delay elimination to a degree greater than would be expected solely from reduced rates of hepatic and renal drug clearance. Consequently, age-related changes in body composition have a significant impact on the elimination or beta-phase pharmacokinetic processes that occur after anesthesia,[44] although immediate recovery from anesthetic effects is predominantly determined by redistribution or alpha-phase parameters.

CENTRAL NERVOUS SYSTEM

Many age-related changes within the human brain and spinal cord are well described, yet their functional significance remains unclear. As in other organ systems, it is often difficult to distin-guish between aging and age-related disease. Many aspects of "senile" neurologic dysfunction, in particular those with a neu-rohumoral basis, may eventually be recategorized as age-related diseases and no longer seen simply as the inevitable deteriora-tion of an aging nervous system. Nevertheless, there are some unequivocal hallmarks of aging within this organ system. Aging reduces brain size. Average adult brain mass is about 20% less by the age of 80 years than respective values measured postmor-tem in young adults.[45] The fraction of intracranial volume occu-pied by brain tissue falls from 92% to 82% over the same time period, with the most rapid reduction in gray matter tissue mass and the greatest rate of compensatory increase in cerebrospinal fluid occurring after the sixth decade. Aging, in effect, produces a form of low-pressure hydrocephalus.[46] Most of this loss of nervous system tissue reflects attrition of neurons, particularly in the gray matter because there appears to be little atrophy of the supportive, non-neuronal glial cells that normally constitute almost half of total brain mass. Estimates of the average rate of neuronal cell death, 50,000 per day from an initial pool of about 10 billion, are a misleading generalization because neuronal loss is highly selective according to type and region, and the rate

of neuronal loss also varies greatly at different ages and under different circumstances.[47]

In general, the most metabolically active, highly specialized neuronal subpopulations, particularly those that synthesize neu-rotransmitters, appear to suffer the most severe degree of loss. Fully 30–50% of the neuronal population of the cerebral and cerebellar cortices, thalamus, locus ceruleus, and basal ganglia disappear in the aged subject. The residual neuropil also dem-onstrates a markedly simplified pattern of synaptic interconnec-tion.[48] There are reduced intraneuronal stores of dopamine, noradrenaline, tyrosine, and serotonin, and a simultaneous in-crease in the activity of enzymes essential to the destruction of the neurotransmitters such as monoamine oxidase and cate-chol-O-methyltransferase.[49] The up-regulation or increase in number of neurotransmitter receptor sites that appear in young neural tissues in response to a reduction of neurotransmitter activity appears to be slow and incomplete in the aging brain.[50]

In the healthy elderly individual, decreased cerebral blood flow (CBF) is a consequence, not a cause, of brain tissue atrophy. Total CBF falls in proportion to reduced brain tissue mass. Specific CBF in the gray matter, expressed per 100 g of brain tissue, declines 20–30% from the maximal values seen in the young adult, a rate that parallels the age-related decline in the neuronal density of cortical tissues. Nevertheless, the intrinsic mechanisms that couple regional cortical and subcortical perfu-sion to local variation of metabolic demands is maintained in older adults,[51] and the blood–brain barrier is functionally intact. Age does not impair autoregulation of cerebrovascular resis-tance (CVR) in response to changes in arterial blood pressure, and the cerebral vasoconstrictor response to hyperventilation remains intact in the healthy geriatric patient.[52] Therefore, the use of controlled hyperventilation to produce deliberate cere-bral vasoconstriction should be appropriate for use in elderly neurosurgical patients, at least in those individuals without ex-tensive cerebrovascular disease.

Despite the long-established bias that aging inevitably pro-duces deterioration of mental function, most recent studies suggest that the most complex aspects of "crystallized intelli-gence" such as language skills, esthetics, and personality do not decline with increasing age. Even in aged individuals, general knowledge base, comprehension, and long-term memory are well maintained in active and fit older adults,[53] although there may be some unavoidable decline in short-term memory, visual and auditory reaction time, and other aspects of "fluid intelli-gence."[54] It remains unclear whether those intellectual func-tions that require immediate processing or rapid retrieval of information suffer intrinsic deterioration or whether they are incidentally compromised by an age-related limitation of atten-tion span. In general, however, across the entire range of adult life span, complex nervous system functions persist at levels sufficiently close to those seen in young adults that they are more dependent upon individual capabilities than upon age itself. Anatomic and functional redundancy within the central nervous system appear to compensate adequately for the attri-tion of cellular elements, reduction of neurotransmitter concen-trations, and the simplification of neuronal interconnections within the neuropil that occur in the aging brain.

Some elderly patients with impaired cognition of uncertain etiology may have hypothalamic–pituitary–adrenal (HPA) dys-regulation and elevated cortisol levels. Aging within the central nervous system leads to selective hippocampal cell loss. Neu-ronal attrition in the hippocampus produces symptoms of im-paired cognition as well as activation of the HPA axis due to removal of chronic hippocampal suppression of HPA activity. The resulting long-term increase in plasma cortisol further ac-celerates hippocampal cell loss and perpetuates the stress/in-jury cycle (Fig. 45-10). In fact, increases in serum cortisol levels over time may predict the development of cognitive deficits in an otherwise healthy elderly individual.[55] Acute stress-related glucocorticoid responses to tissue injury, pain, or the psychoso-

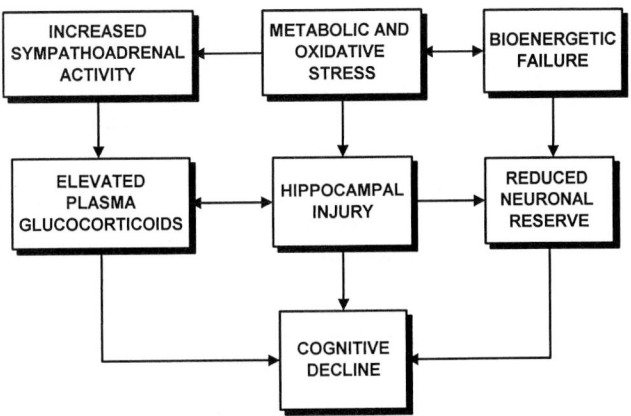

Figure 45-10. Perioperative cognitive decline in elderly adults may reflect the complex interaction of neuroendocrine stress, decreased neuronal reserve due to neuron and transmitter loss, and bioenergetic decline from mitochondrial injury.

cial consequences of disability are also now thought to produce or accelerate cognitive decline in aged adults in whom nervous system tissue and neurotransmitter reserve is most severely reduced.[56]

PERIPHERAL NERVOUS SYSTEM

Within the geriatric era, the threshold intensities of stimuli needed to initiate all forms of perception, including vision, hearing, touch, joint position sense, smell, peripheral pain, and temperature are all markedly elevated (Fig. 45-11). This process of progressive age-related deafferentation is due, at least in part, to degenerative changes within specialized sense organs such as the pain-generating Meissner's corpuscles in skin. However, there are also age-related changes at central sites of pain processing such as the thalamus and throughout peripheral pathways for conduction of pain impulses. In addition, attrition of the individual nerve fibers within afferent conduction pathways in both the peripheral nervous system and spinal cord reduce the velocity and amplitude of both evoked sensory potentials.

Similarly, peripheral motor nerve conduction velocity decreases by about $0.15\,\mathrm{m}\cdot\mathrm{sec}^{-1}\cdot\mathrm{yr}^{-1}$,[57] and impairment of efferent corticospinal transmission increases the time needed between intention and onset of voluntary motor activity. Isometric muscle strength appears to be well maintained, but failing proximodistal protoplasmic transport in aging motor neurons re-

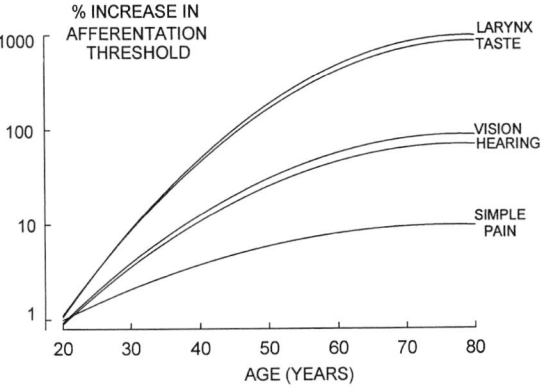

Figure 45-11. Age-related processes of deafferentation produce logarithmic increases in the thresholds for the various sensory modalities and increase the risk of hypoxia by raising the threshold for activation of protective laryngeal reflexes.

duces the myotrophic support normally provided to skeletal muscle. Although mitochondrial volume within skeletal muscle cells is reduced, there appear to be no significant changes in skeletal muscle metabolism or intrinsic contractile function.[58] Nevertheless, this process of neurogenic skeletal muscle atrophy[59] causes the dynamic strength, control, and ability to maintain steadiness of the skeletal muscles in the extremities to decline 20–50% by the age of 80 years and produces disseminated neurogenic atrophy at the neuromuscular junction.[60] The postjunctional muscle membrane thickens and spreads and new, atypical ''extrajunctional'' cholinoceptors appear on the skeletal muscle surface.[61] The increase in the total number of cholinoceptors at each endplate and in the surrounding areas of the muscle cell surface appears to mask the age-related decline in the number and the density of motor neuron/endplate units.

AUTONOMIC NERVOUS SYSTEM

As in all of the peripheral nervous system, neurons in sympathoadrenal pathways are subject to significant cellular attrition. Adrenal tissue mass atrophies and cortisol secretion declines at least 15% by the age of 80. Nevertheless, plasma concentrations of norepinephrine are 2- to 4-fold higher in elderly subjects than in younger adults during sleep, at rest, and even in response to exercise-induced physical stress.[62] Plasma epinephrine levels are far less predictable. High plasma levels of catecholamines are rarely apparent clinically in elderly patients, however, because aging markedly and progressively depresses autonomic endorgan responsiveness.[63] There is a significant impairment of the ability of β agonists such as isoproterenol to enhance the velocity and force of cardiac contraction and a general decline in maximal chronotropic response.[64] In effect, aging produces ''endogenous β blockade.'' There appears to be little change in α-adrenoceptor or muscarinic cholinoceptor activity in older adults and no intrinsic changes in the basic contractile properties of peripheral vascular smooth muscle.[65]

The complex integrated autonomic reflex responses that maintain cardiovascular and metabolic homeostasis precisely in young adults are nevertheless progressively impaired in elderly individuals.[66] This may explain the increased incidence and severity of arterial hypotension seen in older patients following anesthetic induction.[67] Baroreflex responsiveness, the vasoconstrictor response to cold stress, and beat-to-beat heart rate responses following postural change in elderly subjects become progressively less rapid in onset, smaller in magnitude, and less effective in stabilizing blood pressure under a variety of circumstances.[68] The autonomic nervous system in the elderly patient is ''underdamped,'' permitting wider variation from homeostatic set points and delayed restabilization during hemodynamic stress.[69] Therefore, anesthetic agents that disrupt endorgan function or reduce plasma catecholamines, or techniques associated with a pharmacologic sympathectomy such as spinal or epidural anesthesia produce arterial hypotension that is more severe in elderly than in young patients.[70]

ANALGESIC AND ANESTHETIC REQUIREMENTS

The age-related structural and functional changes within the nervous system described above are measurable and consistent, but their net effect on pain-related neurologic function remains controversial. The study of amplification, modulation, and selectivity of afferent input within the spinal cord, thalamus, and other locations within the aging nervous system does not yet permit broad generalizations regarding aging and perception of pain.[71] Some clinical evidence suggests that elderly patients have slightly elevated thresholds for discrete and superficial discomfort.[72] However, severe visceral or postoperative pain is

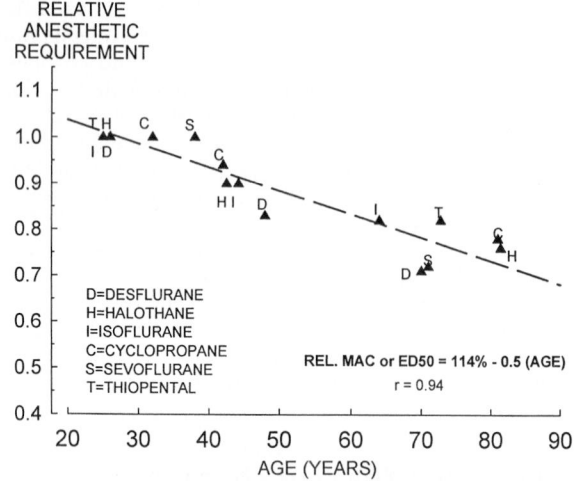

Figure 45-12. The age-related decline in relative anesthetic requirement (MAC or ED₅₀) in unsedated human subjects is a consistent characteristic reported for a wide variety of inhaled and injected anesthetic agents.

a diffuse, emotionally enhanced phenomenon. Therefore, perceived intensity of pain perioperatively is extremely unpredictable[73] and appears to be far more dependent upon anxiety, personality, and the prospect of long-term debility than upon age itself.[74]

Nevertheless, systemic morphine requirements have also long been known to be inversely related to patient age and essentially independent of body weight.[75] When a fixed drug dose and volume of local anesthetics protocol is used, slightly higher levels of sensory blockade occur in elderly patients undergoing spinal anesthesia.[76] Segmental dose requirements for epidural analgesia are also reduced,[77] suggesting a modest reduction in afferent peripheral pain traffic or increased susceptibility to neural blockade. Some recent data[78] suggest that these clinical observations may be due largely to pharmacokinetic, not pharmacodynamic, phenomena, and in any case the age-dependent aspects of major conduction anesthesia become clinically insignificant after middle age.[79]

The effect of nervous system aging on requirements for general anesthesia is less controversial. Between young adulthood and the geriatric era, relative minimum alveolar concentration (MAC) values for the newer inhalational agents decline progressively by as much as 30%,[80,81] the same decrement seen with older anesthetics (Fig. 45-12). The mechanisms producing age-related increases in sensitivity to anesthetic agents remain unknown, but the consistency of this phenomenon for anesthetic agents with markedly different chemical characteristics[82] suggests that it is the result of a fundamental neurophysiologic process such as loss of neuronal mass or cerebral blood flow. The decline in anesthetic requirements also parallels the reduction in brain neurotransmitter activity that occurs with increasing age, however, and a direct relationship between brain catecholamine levels and MAC is well established for patients treated with drugs that deplete or to enhance these neurotransmitters.[83] Whatever the mechanism of age-related increase in anesthetic potency, changes in anesthetic requirement may be a clinically relevant indicator of nervous system functional reserve.

The data for the effect of aging on the pharmacodynamics, or dose requirements, for opioids, barbiturates, and benzodiazepines are less consistent than those for inhalational anesthetics. There is considerable controversy as to whether the clinically apparent age-related increase in the potency of these drugs is truly a pharmacodynamic phenomenon or whether it simply reflects age-related changes in "alpha" or early-phase redistribution pharmacokinetics because plasma drug concentrations

immediately after intravenous injection are often higher in elderly subjects than in young adults.[84] This may reflect delayed intercompartmental transfer of drug rather than a decreased initial volume of distribution.[85] In any case, the concentrations of short-acting iv agents in plasma change so rapidly, and in such a complex manner, that the traditional two-compartment pharmacokinetic model may be of little value for studying the early- or alpha-phase behavior of these drugs and their subsequent redistribution in elderly subjects.[86]

Interpretation of data from clinical studies of iv agents is further complicated by difficulty in defining the anesthetic endpoint in a process, that, in contrast to the conditions under which MAC is determined, does not represent pharmacokinetic equilibrium. Therefore, both onset and duration of clinical effects can be influenced by pharmacodynamic (drug sensitivity) or by pharmacokinetic (molecular drug disposition) processes. Clinical experience suggests that there are significant age-related reductions in the dose requirements for thiopental[87] as well as virtually all other agents that depress consciousness. Most studies also suggest that aging increases brain sensitivity to narcotics,[88,89] but there are only insignificant pharmacodynamic changes for barbiturates or etomidate.[90] Overall, it appears that there is a complex interaction in older patients between subtle changes in pharmacodynamics and altered alpha-phase redistribution pharmacokinetics due to age-related hemodynamic factors[91] that must be characterized for each drug in order to predict the implications of aging for clinical drug action and drug dosage.[92]

Despite the inevitable loss of skeletal muscle mass in elderly subjects, the median effective doses (ED₅₀) and steady-state plasma concentrations required for half-maximal neuromuscular blocking effect (EC₅₀) remain virtually unchanged or may actually increase slightly in the elderly patient.[93] However, maximal relaxant effect may be delayed in onset relative to that produced in young adults.[94,95] Duration of neuromuscular blockade is markedly prolonged (Fig. 45-13) for those relaxants requiring hepatic or renal elimination because plasma clearance declines dramatically with increasing age.[96,97] However, as in younger adults, the intensity of neuromuscular blockade at time of antagonism or "reversal" by neostigmine or edrophonium

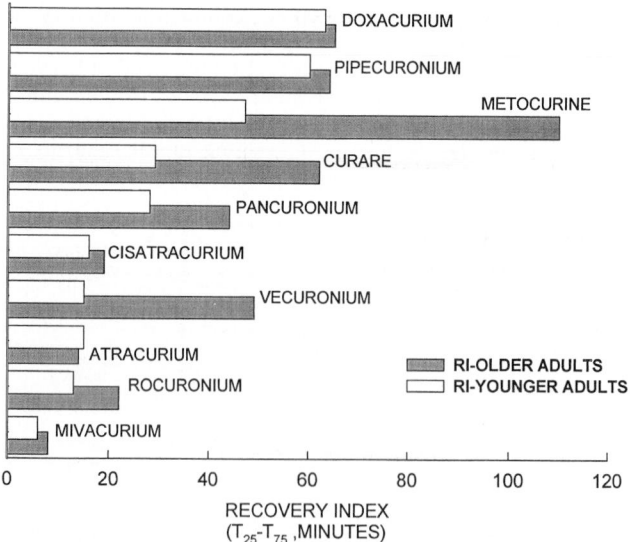

Figure 45-13. The time needed for clinical recovery from neuromuscular blockade (RI = recovery index—the time required for spontaneous recovery from 25% to 75% of the control evoked neuromuscular response) is significantly increased in older adults (*shaded bars*) for nondepolarizing relaxants that requires organ-based clearance from plasma but is little different for atracurium, cisatracurium, or mivacurium because they are hydrolyzed in plasma.

and the choice and dosage of reversal agent, not patient age itself, determine the speed and the completeness of recovery of neuromuscular transmission.

PERIOPERATIVE MANAGEMENT AND OUTCOME

Overall, perioperative mortality and major morbidity increase with advancing age after young adulthood. However, age-related disease, not aging itself, largely determines the morbidity and mortality that characterizes an elderly surgical population,[98–101] although advanced age itself may have additional negative prognostic significance if associated with severe multiple organ system dysfunction. Morbidity and mortality rates, therefore, are higher in elderly surgical patients largely because this surgical patient subpopulation has a greater incidence and severity of concurrent disease, and greater exposure to invasive medical interventions, than do younger adults (Fig. 45-14). The high prevalence of polypharmacy associated with chronic disease and its treatment also produces an age-related increase in adverse drug reactions that complicate perioperative management. Therefore, there are probably no healthy patients "too old" for anesthesia, even for ambulatory surgical procedures.[102]

The probability of a serious pulmonary or hemodynamic complication after surgery is determined both by the site of operation and by the patient's physical status. When they occur in geriatric surgical patients, adverse outcomes show a relative predominance of disorders of cardiac rate or rhythm, myocardial ischemia, or general hemodynamic instability. Pulmonary complications, infections and sepsis, and renal failure also contribute significantly to their morbidity. Many members of the geriatric surgical population summarily "cleared" for major surgery by medical consultants on empirical clinical grounds may nevertheless have mild to severe cardiopulmonary functional deficits. Consequently, adequate time for diagnosis, treatment, and preparation of the anesthetic plan is essential if the rate and severity of complications are to be reduced.[103]

Although many clinical studies have shown that some perioperative complications are associated more frequently with one form of anesthesia than another,[104–108] it may not be possible to determine whether there is a single "best" anesthetic for elderly patients.[109] All anesthetic techniques are appropriate and in widespread use for geriatric patients in general, and none appears to have universal advantage for the elderly surgical patient

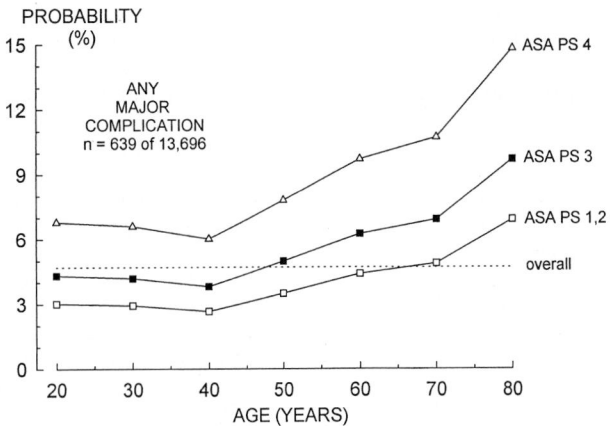

Figure 45-15. The probability of adverse postoperative outcome increases only gradually with age across middle adulthood. Analyzed prospectively from a large series of randomized patients,[99] pre-existing cardiovascular or pulmonary disease and physical status (*solid lines*) were found to be the primary determinants of perioperative morbidity, although the widening of the separation between physical status lines shown here suggests that age itself may further amplify the negative prognostic value of impaired physical status in surgical patients who are well into the geriatric era.

with regard to survival. From the perspective of major adverse surgical outcome and eventual mortality, a brief intraoperative period of exposure to anesthesia is often only an insignificant component of a prolonged, difficult, and complex hospital course. In effect, neither regional anesthesia nor general anesthesia has clearly demonstrable superiority of outcome in elderly patients, although one or the other may be preferred for use in specific procedures or certain patients for other medical reasons.[110] The use of newer intravenous agents such as remifentanil[111,112] and cisatracurium[113] minimizes dependence upon organ system functional reserve for drug elimination. New inhalation agents such as desflurane and sevoflurane provide rapid recovery of consciousness even in the aged adult. Therefore, well-conducted general anesthesia is a safe and appropriate anesthetic plan for older adults, even for those having same-day surgery in which rapid recovery and prompt ambulation are essential.[114]

Prompt and complete postoperative recovery of mental function is particularly important in elderly patients if mentation is already compromised by age-related disease or drug therapy. Recent large-scale prospective studies of outpatients suggest that there is less nausea and vomiting in older adults[115] after general anesthesia but a greater likelihood of prolonged postoperative confusion.[116] The most common cause of failure to emerge promptly from anesthesia is simply the use of too much anesthesia or too many anesthetic agents.[117] Local anesthesia or regional techniques, if they can be comfortably performed without heavy intravenous sedation, may significantly improve postoperative mental function immediately after surgery, although there is no evidence of any long-term benefits to this approach.[118,119] In addition, nerve palsies, residual paresthesias, and other neuropraxias due to regional anesthesia may occur more often in older than in young adults.[120–122]

Even when anesthetic management of the older patient is appropriate and surgical convalescence uncomplicated, full return of cognitive function to preoperative levels may require 5–10 days after a prolonged general anesthetic. Perioperative environmental factors such as chronic medication and drug interaction,[123] disorientation due to sensory deprivation, or the disruption of normal routine needed to maintain "implicit" memory[124] may also explain the high incidence of "delirium"

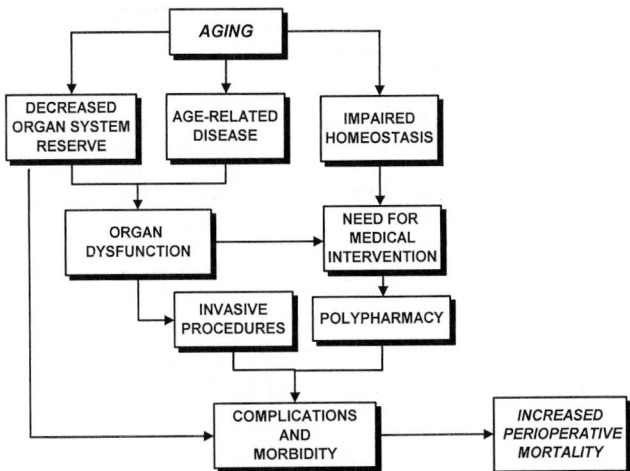

Figure 45-14. Increased rates of perioperative morbidity and mortality in elderly surgical patients can be attributed primarily to interactions between age-related decreases in organ system reserve, a high prevalence of disease in the elderly, and the inherent risk associated with therapy and surgical intervention.

in older surgical patients.[125] However, the neurophysiologic or pharmacologic explanation for prolonged disruption of nervous system function remains unknown. Psychometrically defined postoperative cognitive dysfunction can be demonstrated 3 months after otherwise uncomplicated surgery in 10–15% of patients 60 years of age or older who have had major procedures and a hospital stay of 4 or more days.[126] This suggests that, at least in older adults with reduced central nervous system functional reserve, either the process of general anesthesia itself or the drugs used to produce it may have effects upon the metabolic and neurotransmitter functions of neuronal tissue that can actually produce residual neurologic injury.

The physical management of elderly patients in the operating room and afterward also requires specific precautions. Aged skin and bones are fragile, joints are stiff, and their range of motion is limited, especially if compromised by age-related arthritic processes. The elderly surgical patient therefore requires gentle and expert routine care if traumatic injuries from improper positioning, bandaging, or enforced bed rest are to be avoided. Avoiding hypothermia is important, but active heating devices in contact with poorly perfused skin or connective tissue pressure points can quickly produce ischemic lesions requiring surgical treatment. In all elderly patients, postoperative bleeding diatheses or hypercoagulable states and bacterial infection are more frequent than in younger adults.[127] Because of diastolic dysfunction and increased ventricular stiffness, rates of iv fluid administration that would be modest for young adults may, in the geriatric patient, produce increases in atrial and pulmonary artery pressures large enough to disrupt the fragile balance of forces that control lung water, precipitating congestive heart failure and pulmonary edema.

Whatever anesthetic approach is selected, major surgery and the resultant tissue injury produce extensive neuroendocrine and sympathoadrenal stress. Suppression of excessive sympathetic activity appears to promote rewarming and healing, reduce cardiovascular and pulmonary demands, and eliminate the long periods of emotional stress due to the inadequate analgesia sometimes imposed upon geriatric patients owing to exaggerated fears of opioid side-effects. To some extent, "ageism" may influence caregivers to withhold diagnostic or therapeutic measures that would be offered routinely to a younger adult.[128] Untreated pain and related emotional stress itself may significantly impair immune responsiveness in older adults and increase the risk of perioperative infection.[129] Therefore, an anesthetic plan that includes postoperative epidural sympathectomy and analgesia[130] or a parenteral sympathetic modulator such as dexmedetomidine[131] may be of special value in the elderly surgical patient. Overall, elderly and aged patients do not require a "special" kind of anesthetic. Rather, if complications are to be minimized, their perioperative care simply requires the highest standards of preparation and diagnosis and control of pre-existing disease, vigilance, and meticulous execution of all details of anesthetic and postoperative management.

REFERENCES

1. Nascher IL: Geriatrics. NY Med J 90:358, 1909
2. Schneider EL, Reed JD Jr: Life extension. N Engl J Med 312:1159, 1985
3. Hayflick L: Biologic and theoretical perspectives of human aging. In Katlic MR (ed): Geriatric Surgery: Comprehensive Care of the Elderly Patient, p 3. Baltimore, Urban and Schwarzenberg, 1990
4. Ozawa T: Genetic and functional changes in mitochondria associated with aging. Physiol Rev 77:425, 1997
5. Rodeheffer RJ, Gerstenblith G, Becker LC et al: Exercise cardiac output is maintained with advancing age in healthy human subjects: Cardiac dilatation and increased stroke volume compensate for diminished heart rate. Circulation 69:203, 1984
6. Tzankoff SP, Norris AH: Effect of muscle mass decrease on age-related BMR changes. J Appl Physiol 43:1001, 1977
7. Aronow WS, Stein PD, Sabbah HN, Koenigsberg M: Resting left ventricular ejection fraction in elderly patients without evidence of heart disease. Am J Cardiol 63:368, 1989
8. Folkow B, Svanborg A: Physiology of cardiovascular aging. Physiol Rev 73:725, 1993
9. Pagel PS, Grossman W, Haering JM, Warltier DC: Left ventricular diastolic function in the normal and diseased heart. Perspectives for the anesthesiologist. Anesthesiology 79:836, 1104, 1993
10. Nichols WW, O'Rourke MF, Avolio AP et al: Ventricular/vascular interaction in patients with mild systemic hypertension and normal peripheral resistance. Circulation 74:455, 1986
11. Cohn JE, Donoso HD: Mechanical properties of lung in normal men over 60 years old. J Clin Invest 42:1406, 1963
12. Allen SJ: Respiratory considerations in the elderly surgical patient. Clin Anaesthesiol 4:899, 1986
13. Dauchot PJ, Graber RG: The aging respiratory system. Prob Anesth 9:498, 1997
14. Wahba WM: Influence of aging on lung function—clinical significance of changes from age twenty. Anesth Analg 62:764, 1983
15. Tolep K, Kelsen SG: Effect of aging on respiratory skeletal muscles. Clin Chest Med 14:363, 1993
16. Rose DK, Cohen MM, Wigglesworth DF, DeBoer DP: Critical respiratory events in the postanesthesia care unit. Anesthesiology 81:410, 1994
17. Holland J, Milic-Emili J, Macklem PT, Bates DV: Regional distribution of pulmonary ventilation and perfusion in elderly subjects. J Clin Invest 47:81, 1968
18. Peterson DD, Pack AI, Silage DA, Fishman AP: Effects of aging on ventilatory and occlusion pressure responses to hypoxia and hypercapnia. Am Rev Resp Dis 124:387, 1981
19. Pontoppidan H, Beecher HK: Progressive loss of protective reflexes in the airway with the advance of age. JAMA 174:2209, 1960
20. Hunt CM, Westerkam WR, Stave GM: Effect of age and gender on the activity of human hepatic CYP3A. Biochem Pharmacol 44:275, 1992
21. Schemel WH: Unexpected hepatic dysfunction found by multiple laboratory screening. Anesth Analg 55:810, 1976
22. Swift CG, Homeida M, Halliwell M, Roberts CJ: Antipyrine disposition and liver size in the elderly. Eur J Clin Pharmacol 14:149, 1978
23. Zoli M, Iervese T, Abbati S et al: Portal blood velocity and flow in aging man. Gerontology 35:61, 1989
24. Shanor SP, Van Hees GR, Baart N et al: The influence of age and sex on human plasma and red cell cholinesterase. Am J Med Sci 242:357, 1961
25. McLachlan MSF: The ageing kidney. Lancet 2:143, 1978
26. Rowe JW: Renal function and aging. In Reff ME, Schneider EL (eds): Biological Markers of Aging, p 228. NIH Publication No. 82–2221, 1982
27. Lindeman RD: Renal physiology and pathophysiology of aging. Contrib Nephrol 105:1, 1993
28. Hollenberg NK, Adams DF, Solomon HS et al: Senescence and the renal vasculature in normal man. Circulation Res 34:309, 1974
29. Lubran MM: Renal function in the elderly. Ann Clin Lab Sci 25:122, 1995
30. Phillips PA, Johnston CI, Gray L: Disturbed fluid and electrolyte homeostasis following dehydration in elderly people. Age Ageing 22:S26, 1993
31. Stoy PJ, Roitman-Johnson B, Walsh G et al: Aging and serum immunoglobin E levels, immediate skin tests, and RAST. J Allergy Clin Immunol 68:421, 1981
32. Miller RA: The aging immune system: Primer and prospectus. Science 273:70, 1996
33. Tornetta P 3rd, Mostafavi H, Riina J et al: Morbidity and mortality in elderly trauma patients. J Trauma-Injury Infect Crit Care 46:702, 1999
34. Forbes GB: The adult decline in lean body mass. Human Biology 48:161, 1976
35. Tzankoff SP, Norris AH: Effect of muscle mass decrease on age-related BMR changes. J Appl Physiol 43:1001, 1977
36. Kurz A, Plattner O, Sessler DI et al: The threshold for thermoregulatory vasoconstriction during nitrous oxide/isoflurane anesthesia

is lower in elderly than in young patients. Anesthesiology 79: 465, 1993

37. Frank SM, Beattie C, Christopherson R et al: Epidural versus general anesthesia; ambient operating room temperature, and patient age as predictors of inadvertent hypothermia. Anesthesiology 77: 252, 1992

38. Carli F, Gabrielczyk M, Clark MM, Aber VR: An investigation of factors affecting postoperative rewarming of adult patients. Anaesthesia 41:363, 1986

39. Cefalu WT, Wang ZQ, Werbel S et al: Contribution of visceral fat mass to the insulin resistance of aging. Metab Clin Exper 44: 954, 1995

40. Davidson MB: The effect of aging on carbohydrate metabolism: A review of the English literature and a practical approach to the diagnosis of diabetes in the elderly. Metab 28:688, 1979

41. Hornick TR: Effects of advanced age on body composition and metabolism. Prob Anesth 9:461, 1997

42. Fulop T Jr, Worum I, Csongor J et al: Body composition in elderly people. Gerontol 31:6, 1985

43. Richey DP, Bender AD: Pharmacokinetic consequences of aging. Ann Rev Pharmacol Tox 17:49, 1977

44. Hoppel CL, Lina AA: Pharmacology and pharmacokinetics of aging. Prob Anesth 9:471, 1997

45. Terry RD, DeTeresa R, Hansen LA: Neocortical cell counts in normal human aging. Ann Neurol 21:530, 1987

46. Creasey H, Rapoport SI: The aging human brain. Ann Neurol 17:2, 1985

47. Schjeide OA: Relation of development and aging: Pre- and postnatal differentiation of the brain as related to aging. Adv Behav Biol 16:37, 1975

48. Feldman ML: Aging changes in the morphology of cortical dendrites. In Terry RD, Gershon S (eds): Neurobiology of Aging, p 11. New York, Raven Press, 1976

49. McGeer EG, McGeer PL: Age changes in the human for some enzymes associated with metabolism of catecholamines, GABA, and acetylcholine. Adv Behav Biol 16:287, 1975

50. Greenberg LH: Regulation of brain adrenergic receptors during aging. Fed Proc 45:55, 1986

51. Duara R, London ED, Rapoport SI: Changes in structure and energy metabolism of the aging brain. In Finch CE, Schneider EL (eds): Handbook of the Biology of Aging, 2nd ed, p 595. New York, Van Nostrand Reinhold, 1985

52. Meyer JS, Terayama Y, Takashima S: Cerebral circulation in the elderly. Cerebrovasc Brain Metab Rev 5:122, 1993

53. Rogers RL, Meyer JS, Mortel KF: After reaching retirement age physical activity sustains cerebral perfusion in normal aging. J Am Geriatric Soc 38:123, 1990

54. van Boxtel MP, Langerak K, Houx PJ, Jolles J: Self-reported physical activity, subjective health, and cognitive performance in older adults. Exp Aging Res 22:363, 1996

55. Meaney MJ, O'Donnell D, Rowe W et al: Individual differences in hypothalamic-pituitary-adrenal activity in later life and hippocampal aging. Exper Gerontol 30:229, 1995

56. O'Brien JT: The 'glucocorticoid cascade' hypothesis in man: Prolonged stress may cause permanent brain damage. Br J Psychiat 170:199, 1997

57. Dorfman LJ, Bosley TM: Age-related changes in peripheral and central nerve conduction in man. Neurol 29:38, 1979

58. Taylor DJ, Crowe M, Bore PJ et al: Examination of the energetics of aging skeletal muscle using nuclear magnetic resonance. Gerontol 30:2, 1984

59. Swash M, Fox KP: The effect of age on human skeletal muscle: Studies of the morphology and innervation of muscle spindles. J Neurol Sci 16:417, 1972

60. Gutmann E, Hanzlikova V, Jaboubek B: Changes in the neuromuscular system during old age. Exp Gerontol 3:141, 1968

61. Martyn JAJ, White DA, Gronert GA et al: Up- and down-regulation of skeletal muscle acetylcholine receptors: Effects on neuromuscular blockers. Anesthesiology 76:822, 1992

62. Ziegler MG, Lake CR, Kopin IJ: Plasma noradrenaline increases with age. Nature 261:333, 1976

63. Vestal RE, Wood AJJ, Shand DG: Reduced adrenoceptor sensitivity in the elderly. Clin Pharmacol Ther 26:181, 1979

64. Seals DR, Taylor JA, Ng AV, Esler MD: Exercise and aging: Autonomic control of the circulation. Med Sci Sports Exer 26(5): 568, 1994

65. Docherty JR: Effect of age on the response of target organs to autonomic neurotransmitters. In Amenta F (ed): Aging of the Autonomic Nervous System, p 109. Boca Raton, FL, CRC Press, 1993

66. Rooke GA, Robinson BJ: Cardiovascular and autonomic nervous system aging. Prob Anesth 9:482, 1997

67. Latson TW, Ashmore TH, Reinhart DJ et al: Autonomic reflex dysfunction in patients presenting for elective surgery is associated with hypotension after anesthesia induction. Anesthesiology 80: 326, 1994

68. Pfeifer MA, Weinberg CR, Cook D et al: Differential changes of autonomic nervous system function with age in man. Am J Med 75:249, 1983

69. Shannon RP, Maher KA, Santinga JT et al: Comparison of differences in the hemodynamic response to passive postural stress in healthy subjects greater than 70 years and less than 30 years of age. Am J Cardiol 67:1110, 1991

70. Carpenter RL, Caplan RA, Brown DL et al: Incidence and risk factors for side effects of spinal anesthesia. Anesthesiology 76: 906, 1992

71. Melding PS: Is there such a thing as geriatric pain? (editorial). Pain 46:119, 1991

72. Harkins SW, Chapman CR: Detection and decision factors in pain perception in young and elderly men. Pain 2:253, 1976

73. Tobias MD, Muravchick S: New approaches to the management of postoperative pain. Adv Urol 8:325, 1995

74. Hapidou EG, DeCatanzaro D: Responsiveness to laboratory pain in women as a function of age and childbirth pain experience. Pain 48:177, 1992

75. Bellville JW, Forrest WH, Miller E, Brown BW: Influence of age on pain relief from analgesics: A study of postoperative patients. JAMA 217:1835, 1971

76. Cameron AE, Arnold RW, Ghoris MW, Jamieson V: Spinal analgesia using bupivacaine 0.5% plain: Variation in the extent of block with patient age. Anaesthesia 36:318, 1981

77. Sharrock NE: Epidural dose responses in patients 20 to 80 years old. Anesthesiology 49:425, 1978

78. Veering BT, Burm AGL, Vletter AA et al: The effect of age on systemic absorption and systemic disposition of bupivacaine after subarachnoid administration. Anesthesiology 74:250, 1991

79. Curatolo M, Orlando A, Zbinden AM et al: A multifactorial analysis of the spread of epidural analgesia. Acta Anaesthesiol Scand 38: 646, 1994

80. Gold MI, Abello D, Herrington C: Minimum alveolar concentration of desflurane in patients older than 65 years. Anesthesiology 79:710, 1993

81. Nakajima R, Nakajima Y, Ikeda K: Minimum alveolar concentration of sevoflurane in elderly patients. Br J Anaesth 70:273, 1993

82. Munson ES, Hoffman JC, Eger EI II: Use of cyclopropane to test generality of anesthetic requirement in the elderly. Anesth Analg 63:998, 1984

83. Miller RD, Way WL, Eger EI II: The effects of alpha-methyl dopa, reserpine, guanethidine, and iproniazid on minimum alveolar anesthetic requirement (MAC). Anesthesiology 29:1153, 1968

84. Singleton MA, Rosen JI, Fisher DM: Pharmacokinetics of fentanyl in the elderly. Br J Anaesth 60:619, 1988

85. Avram MJ, Krejcie TC, Henthorn TK: The relationship of age to the pharmacokinetics of early drug distribution: The concurrent disposition of thiopental and indocyanine green. Anesthesiology 72:403, 1990

86. Hull CJ: How far can we go with compartmental models? (editorial). Anesthesiology 72:399, 1990

87. Muravchick S: Effect of age and premedication on thiopental sleep dose. Anesthesiology 61:333, 1984

88. Scott JC, Stanski DR: Decreased fentanyl and alfentanil dose requirements with increasing age. A simultaneous pharmacokinetic and pharmacodynamic evaluation. J Pharmacol Exp Ther 240: 159, 1987

89. Minto CF, Schnider TW, Egan TD et al: Influence of age and gender on the pharmacokinetics and pharmacodynamics of remifentanil. Anesthesiology 86:10, 1997

90. Arden JR, Holley FO, Stanski DR: Increased sensitivity to etomidate in the elderly: Initial distribution versus altered brain response. Anesthesiology 65:19, 1986

91. Bjorkman S, Wada DR, Stanski DR: Application of physiologic

models to predict the influence of changes in body composition and blood flows on the pharmacokinetics of fentanyl and alfentanil in patients. Anesthesiology 88:657, 1998

92. Shafer SL, Varvel JR: Pharmacokinetics, pharmacodynamics, and rational opioid selection. Anesthesiology 74:53, 1991
93. Shanks CA: Pharmacokinetics of the nondepolarizing neuromuscular relaxants applied to calculation of bolus and infusion dosage regimens. Anesthesiology 64:72, 1986
94. Koscielniak-Nielsen ZJ, Bevan JC, Popovic V et al: Onset of maximum neuromuscular blockade following succinylcholine or vecuronium in four age groups. Anesthesiology 79:229, 1993
95. Sarooshian SS, Stafford MA, Eastwood NB et al: Pharmacokinetics and pharmacodynamics of cisatracurium in young and elderly adult patients. Anesthesiology 84:1083, 1996
96. Lien CA, Matteo RS, Ornstein E et al: Distribution, elimination, and action of vecuronium in the elderly. Anesth Analg 73:39, 1991
97. Matteo RS, Ornstein E, Schwartz AE et al: Pharmacokinetics and pharmacodynamics of rocuronium (Org 9426) in elderly surgical patients. Anesth Analg 77:1193, 1993
98. Lewin I, Lerner AG, Green SH et al: Physical class and physiologic status in the prediction of operative mortality in the aged sick. Ann Surg 174:217, 1971
99. Forrest JB, Rehder K, Cahalan MK, Goldsmith CH: Multicenter study of general anesthesia. III: Predictors of severe perioperative adverse outcomes. Anesthesiology 76:3, 1992
100. Arvidsson S, Ouchterlony J, Nilsson S et al: The Gothenburg study of perioperative risk. I: Preoperative findings, postoperative complications. Acta Anaesthesiol Scand 38:679, 1994
101. Pedersen T: Complications and death following anaesthesia: A prospective study with special reference to the influence of patient-, anaesthesia-, and surgery-related risk factors. Danish Med Bull 41:319, 1994
102. Kortilla K: Aging, medical disease, and outcome of ambulatory surgery. Curr Opin Anaesthesiol 6:546, 1993
103. Kennedy RH, al Mufti RA, Brewster SF et al: The acute surgical admission: Is mortality predictable in the elderly? Ann Roy Coll Surg Eng 76:342, 1994
104. Hole A, Terjesen T, Breivik H: Epidural versus general anaesthesia for total hip arthroplasty in elderly patients. Acta Anaesthesiol Scand 24:279, 1980
105. Wickstrom I, Holmberg I, Stefansson T: Survival of female geriatric patients after hip fracture surgery: A comparison of 5 anaesthetic methods. Acta Anaesthesiol Scand 26:607, 1982
106. Valentin N, Lomholt B, Jensen JS et al: Spinal or general anaesthesia for surgery of the fractured hip? Br J Anaesth 58:284, 1986
107. Davis FM, Woolner DF, Frampton C et al: Prospective, multi-centre trial of mortality following general or spinal anaesthesia for hip fracture surgery in the elderly. Br J Anaesth 59:1080, 1987
108. Sutcliffe AJ, Parker M: Mortality after spinal and general anaesthesia for surgical fixation of hip fractures. Anaesthesia 49:237, 1994
109. Go AS, Browner WS: Cardiac outcomes after regional or general anesthesia: Do we have the answer? (editorial). Anesthesiology 84:1, 1996
110. Christopherson R, Beattie C, Frank SM et al: Perioperative morbidity in patients randomized to epidural or general anesthesia for lower extremity vascular surgery. Anesthesiology 79:422, 1993
111. Westmoreland CL, Hoke JF, Sebel PS et al: Pharmacokinetics of remifentanil (GI87084B) and its major metabolite (GI90291) in

patients undergoing elective inpatient surgery. Anesthesiology 79: 893, 1993
112. Minto CF, Schnider TW, Egan TD et al: Influence of age and gender on the pharmacokinetics and pharmacodynamics of remifentanil. Anesthesiology 86:10, 1997
113. Wright PMC, Ornstein E: Pharmacokinetics, pharmacodynamics and safety of cisatracurium in elderly patients. Curr Opin Anaesth 9(suppl 1):S30, 1996
114. Nathanson MH, Fredman B, Smith I, White PF: Sevoflurane versus desflurane for outpatient anesthesia: A comparison of maintenance and recovery profiles. Anesth Analg 81:1186, 1995
115. Sinclair DR, Chung F, Mezel G: Can postoperative nausea and vomiting be predicted? Anesthesiology 91:109, 1999
116. Tzabar Y, Asbury AJ, Millar K: Cognitive failures after general anaesthesia for day-case surgery. Br J Anaesth 76:194, 1996
117. Muravchick S: Immediate and long-term nervous system effects of anesthesia in elderly patients. Clin Anaesthesiol 4:1035, 1986
118. Chung F, Meier R, Lautenschlager E et al: General or spinal anesthesia: Which is better in the elderly? Anesthesiology 67:422, 1987
119. Chung FF, Chung A, Meier RH et al: Comparison of perioperative mental function after general anaesthesia and spinal anaesthesia with intravenous sedation. Can J Anaesth 36:382, 1989
120. Warner MA, Martin JT, Schroeder DR et al: Lower-extremity motor neuropathy associated with surgery performed on patients in a lithotomy position. Anesthesiology 81:6, 1994
121. Hampl KF, Heinzmann-Wiedmer S, Luginbuehl I et al: Transient neurologic symptoms after spinal anesthesia. Anesthesiology 88: 629, 1998
122. Martinez-Bourio R, Arzuaza M, Quintana JM et al: Incidence of transient neurologic symptoms after hyperbaric subarachnoid anesthesia with 5% lidocaine and 5% prilocaine. Anesthesiology 88:624, 1998
123. Jolles J, Verhey FR, Riedel WJ, Houx PJ: Cognitive impairment in elderly people: Predisposing factors and implications for experimental drug studies. Drugs Aging 7:459, 1995
124. Inouye SK, Bogardus ST, Charpentier PA et al: A multicomponent intervention to prevent delirium in hospitalized older patients. N Engl J Med 340:669, 1999
125. O'Keefe ST, Ni Conchubhair A: Postoperative delirium in the elderly. Br J Anaesth 73:673, 1994
126. Moller JT, ISOPCD investigators: Long-term postoperative cognitive dysfunction in the elderly; ISPOCD1 study. Lancet 351:857, 1998
127. Yardumian A, Machin SJ: Hypercoagulable states. Int Anesthesiol Clin 23(2):141, 1985
128. Giugliano RP, Camargo CA Jr, Lloyd-Jones DM et al: Elderly patients receive less aggressive medical and invasive management of unstable angina: Potential impact of practice guidelines. Arch Int Med 158:1113, 1998
129. Esterling BA, Kiecolt-Glaser JK, Glaser R: Psychosocial modulation of cytokine-induced natural killer cell activity in older adults. Psychosom Med 58:264, 1996
130. Yeager MP, Glass DD, Neff RK, Brinck-Johnsen T: Epidural anesthesia and analgesia in high-risk surgical patients. Anesthesiology 66:729, 1987
131. Talke P, Richardson CA, Scheinin M, Fisher DM: Postoperative pharmacokinetics and sympatholytic effects of dexmedetomidine. Anesth Analg 85:1136, 1997

Clinical Anesthesia (4/e), edited by
Paul G. Barash, Bruce F. Cullen, and
Robert K. Stoelting. Lippincott Williams &
Wilkins, Philadelphia, © 2001.

CHAPTER 46

ANESTHESIA FOR AMBULATORY SURGERY

J. LANCE LICHTOR

The first ether anesthetic was given for ambulatory surgery. The patient, James M. Venable, had a small cystic tumor removed from the back of his neck by Dr. Crawford W. Long on the evening of March 30, 1842, after school was dismissed. The patient described the procedure in this way: "I commenced inhaling the ether before the operation was commenced and continued it until the operation was over. I did not feel the slightest pain from the operation and could not believe the tumor was removed until it was shown to me."[1] The modern concept of an independent surgical center for outpatients was popularized in the early 1970s by Wallace Reed. Since then, ambulatory surgery has been so well accepted that the majority of patients currently return home within 24 hours of an operative procedure. Because of this fact, anesthesiologists have had to refine the method of performing anesthesia so that the anesthetic is not responsible for hindering a patient from returning to normal activities.

Cost-savings partially prompted the original ambulatory centers. In the late 1960s, an uninsured barber's two children needed myringotomies, which in those days meant 2 days of hospitalization before the procedure. The surgeons, astounded by how many haircuts they would receive instead of payment, began the cost-reducing measure of ambulatory surgery. Patient selection today is based on the desire to reduce cost while at the same time maintaining quality of care, so that morbidity from the procedure or pre-existing disease is no greater than if the patient were hospitalized. The length and complexity of operations performed in an ambulatory setting have increased, especially with the arrival of many new procedures. In the past, only patients with physical status evaluated as American Society of Anesthesiologists (ASA) Class I or II were candidates for ambulatory surgery. Today, patients classified as ASA III or IV whose systemic disease is medically stable are considered for procedures as outpatients. Preoperative screening, preferably in a clinic or by telephone, is essential both for reduction of patient anxiety and to ensure that medical management is appropriate. Specific laboratory tests before these operations are discussed elsewhere (see Chapter 18). In this chapter, we review the patients and procedures suitable for ambulatory surgery and how to manage anesthesia for outpatients. An excellent review of the history of ambulatory surgery is provided by Vandam.[2]

PLACE, PROCEDURES, AND PATIENT SELECTION

Ambulatory surgery occurs in a variety of settings. Some centers are within a hospital or in a freestanding satellite facility that is either part or independent of a hospital. Physicians' offices may also serve for procedures. In fact, by 2005, 20% of all surgical procedures will be performed in doctors' offices.[3] The independent facilities are often for-profit and not located in rural or inner city areas. Although freestanding, independent facilities continue to grow, some consumers prefer care in units affiliated with hospitals.

Procedures appropriate for ambulatory surgery are those associated with postoperative care that is easily managed at home, and with low rates of postoperative complications that require

intensive physician or nursing management. The definition of a low rate of postoperative complication depends on the relative aggressiveness of the facility, surgeon, patient, and payer. For example, procedures such as cholecystectomy, vaginal hysterectomy, reduction mammoplasty, open arthrotomy with ligament repair, and thyroidectomy are performed in some ambulatory surgery centers, whereas in other settings, these procedures are limited to inpatients. Lists of ambulatory procedures quickly become outdated simply because they exclude certain procedures which in a short time may become routine in ambulatory settings. In 1986, a patient would have been hospitalized for cholecystectomy but not for cataract extraction. When laparoscopic cholecystectomy was first introduced, a much higher percentage of patients required open cholecystectomy afterward, hence inpatient admission. Now some ambulatory surgery centers perform cholecystectomy on selected outpatients (generally healthy ones who live nearby) when an uneventful operative procedure is anticipated. Patients undergoing breast surgery have, in the past, been hospitalized for 1–7 days afterward. Yet in one series of 118 patients undergoing various types of breast surgery, including modified radical mastectomies and axillary node dissection, only three patients required hospital admission for relatively minor complications.[4] For modified radical mastectomy performed as ambulatory surgery, compared to the same surgery with a three-day hospital stay, hospital costs were reduced by 75%. Some have argued that ambulatory tonsillectomy is not advisable because of the risk of hemorrhage as much as 24 hours after the procedure. Tonsillectomies, however, are performed safely in outpatients unless they are suffering from allergic episodes during the pollen season; have bleeding abnormalities or sickle cell anemia; are within 5 weeks of an acute attack of tonsillitis; have heart disease, sleep apnea, or congenital malformations; or experience bleeding within 8 hours of the procedure.[5] It is suggested also that tonsillectomies for outpatients be performed in the morning. In another series, preoperative apnea, age less than 12 months, and the presence of accompanying medical conditions were associated with a higher incidence of postoperative airway complications.[6] The investigators recommended that tonsillectomy in patients younger than 36 months be planned as an inpatient procedure.

Length of surgery is not a criterion for ambulatory procedures because there is little relationship between length of anesthesia and recovery (Fig. 46-1).[7] Patients undergoing longer procedures, though, should have their operations earlier in the day. In a study of unplanned admission of patients undergoing ambulatory ophthalmic surgery, the variable most highly correlated with admission was the completion of surgery later in the day.[8] The need for transfusion also is not a contraindication for ambulatory procedures. Some patients undergoing liposuction as outpatients, for example, are given autologous blood. Some surgeons, however, are uneasy about performing transfusion-requiring operations in an ambulatory setting because blood loss is a factor in unexpected hospital admission after surgery.[9,10]

Preterm infants (gestation age 37 weeks) who are younger than 50 weeks postconceptual age should not be discharged from an ambulatory surgery center for at least 23 hours after a procedure because they are at risk of developing apnea even without a history of apnea. In one study using pneumography, 37% of infants as old as 55 postconceptual weeks had prolonged

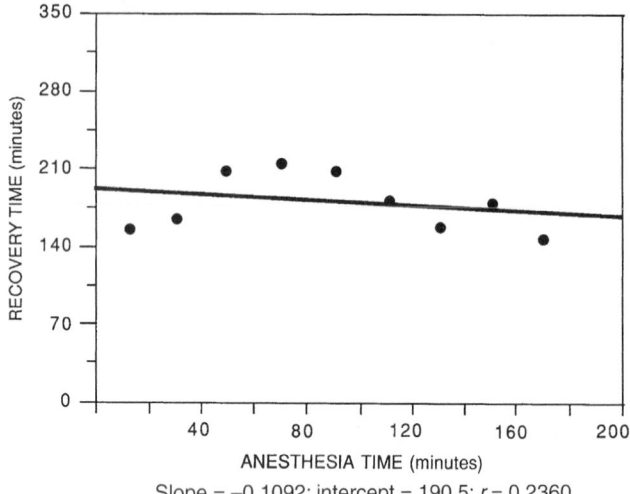

Slope = −0.1092; intercept = 190.5; r = 0.2360.

Figure 46-1. Length of anesthesia has little correlation with recovery time. (Reprinted with permission from Meridy HW: Criteria for selection of ambulatory surgical patients and guidelines for anesthetic management: A retrospective study of 1553 cases. Anesth Analg 61:921, 1982.)

apnea up to 12 hours after operation.[11] This study prompted the suggestion that the upper age limit for infants admitted for overnight stays should be extended to 60 postconceptual weeks. Some of the infants in the study underwent typical outpatient procedures like herniorrhaphy; others underwent laparotomy. In a similar study of infants who underwent inguinal herniorrhaphy only, 64% with a conceptual age of less than 44 weeks had periodic breathing afterward, two as late as 5 hours postoperatively.[12] No infant who was 44 conceptual weeks or older had periodic breathing postoperatively (conceptual age = gestational age plus postnatal age). Anemia (hematocrit < 30%) is also associated with an increased incidence of apnea in preterm infants less than 60 postconceptual weeks old at the time of operation.[13]

Some techniques have been tried to eliminate postoperative apnea in infants to allow them to go home on the same day of a procedure. When caffeine 10 mg·kg^{-1} was administered immediately after induction of anesthesia, no preterm infants ≤44 conceptual weeks old developed postoperative apnea.[14] Spinal anesthesia, without the use of other drugs intraoperatively or postoperatively, also was not associated with apnea (Fig. 46-2).[15] Although preterm infants who have received caffeine or an unsupplemented spinal anesthetic may be discharged on the day of the procedure, they should probably be observed overnight in a hospital until more data confirm the safety of this practice.

At the other extreme of life, advanced age alone is not a reason to disallow surgery in an ambulatory setting. Age, however, does affect the pharmacokinetics of drugs. Even short-acting drugs such as midazolam and propofol have decreased clearance in older individuals. In a study of outcome after 6000

procedures, some for patients older than 90 years, longer recovery time was not correlated with older age.[16] Transurethral resection of the prostate is performed in the ambulatory setting. In two studies, increased age was correlated with unexpected hospital admissions.[17,18] In a third study of more than 6,000 patients undergoing ambulatory surgery, age was not a predictor of return; however, patients <40 years who returned after ambulatory procedures were more likely to be treated in the emergency room, whereas patients >65 years were more likely to be hospitalized.[19] Admission, by itself, is not necessarily bad if it results in a better quality of care or uncovers the need for more extensive surgery. With proper patient selection for ambulatory procedures, which are usually elective, the incidence of readmission should be very low. Most medical problems that older individuals may experience after ambulatory procedures are not caused by age, but by specific organ dysfunction. For that reason, all individuals, whether young or old, deserve a careful preoperative history and physical examination.

Whatever their age, ambulatory surgery is no longer restricted to patients of ASA physical status I or II. Patients of ASA physical status III or IV are appropriate candidates, providing their systemic diseases are medically stable. In one study of 6000 ambulatory surgery procedures in a public teaching hospital, perioperative complications related to surgery (1:105) were more frequent than those related to pre-existing medical problems (1:500).[16] Nonetheless, pre-existing medical illness is a factor in both intraoperative difficulties and postoperative complications that require unexpected patient admission.

Patients who undergo ambulatory surgery should have someone to take them home and stay with them afterward to provide care. Before the procedure, the patient should receive information about the procedure itself, where it will be performed, laboratory studies that will be ordered, and dietary restrictions. The patient must understand that he or she will be going home on the day of surgery. The patient, or some responsible person, must be able to see that all instructions are carried out. Once at home, the patient must be able to tolerate the pain from the procedure, assuming adequate pain therapy is provided. The majority of patients are satisfied with early discharge, although a few prefer a longer stay in the hospital. Patients for certain procedures such as laparoscopic cholecystectomy or transurethral resection of the prostate should live close to the ambulatory facility because postoperative complications may require their prompt return. "Reasonable" distance and time for the patient to get care if problems arise are not easily defined. This issue must be addressed by each facility and by each patient and depends on the type of surgery to be performed. In one series, one-half of the deaths in patients within 30 days of ambulatory surgery were due to traffic accidents.[20]

PREOPERATIVE EVALUATION AND REDUCTION OF PATIENT ANXIETY

Each outpatient facility should develop its own method of preoperative screening to be conducted before the day of surgery. The patient may visit the facility, or staff members may telephone to

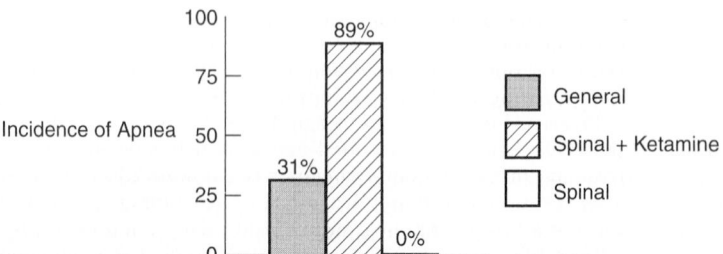

Figure 46-2. Postoperative apnea in premature infants with and without a history of apnea is significantly less if only spinal anesthesia is used. (Reprinted with permission from Welborn LG, Rice LJ, Hannallah RS *et al*: Postoperative apnea in former preterm infants: Prospective comparison of spinal and general anesthesia. Anesthesiology 72:838, 1990.)

obtain necessary information about the patient, including a complete medical history of the patient and family, the medications the patient is taking, and the problems the patient or the patient's family may have had with previous anesthetics. In a study of the usefulness of a preoperative screening telephone call, patients were less likely to cancel surgery if they had been screened beforehand.[21] Unscreened patients were more likely to be hospitalized after surgery. Overall, cancellation rates did not differ between patients evaluated within 24 hours of surgery or days or weeks before surgery. The screening may uncover the need for transportation to the facility or the need for child care. The process also provides the staff with an opportunity to remind patients of arrival time, suitable attire, and dietary restrictions (*e.g.*, nothing to eat or drink after midnight, no jewelry or makeup). Staff members can determine whether a responsible person is available to escort the patient to and from the facility and care for the patient at home after surgery. The screening is the ideal time for the anesthesiologist to talk with the patient, but if that is not possible, the anesthesiologist may review the screening record to determine whether additional evaluation by other consultants is necessary and if laboratory tests must be obtained.

Automated history-taking may also prove beneficial during the screening of a patient. Computerized questionnaires or checklists with plastic overlays automate the taking of patient histories, flag problem areas, and suggest laboratory tests to be ordered. Such devices can also be used in a surgeon's office, both to guide the surgeon in the selection of laboratory tests and to serve as a medical summary for the anesthesiologist. Such devices are particularly useful to control the cost of preoperative testing. They enable test ordering based on information obtained from a patient's responses to health questions, thus eliminating requests for tests that are not warranted by history or physical examination.

Another important reason for preoperative screening is to help alleviate a patient's anxiety. In a classic study, Egbert *et al*[22] found that a preoperative visit by an anesthesiologist was more effective in decreasing anxiety than administration of a barbiturate. Other authors also have confirmed the value of a preoperative visit. Preoperative reassurance from nonanesthesia staff and the use of booklets also reduce preoperative anxiety. Patients given maximally informative booklets to prepare them for surgery have less anxiety than those given minimally informative booklets or only routine care.[23] However, use of such booklets is less effective than a preoperative visit by the anesthesiologist. Audiovisual instructions also reduce preoperative anxiety. Certain relaxation techniques for reducing anxiety are best taught before the surgery. In one study, for example, relaxation training was given to ambulatory patients scheduled for excision of a skin cancer without general anesthesia.[24] The relaxation response was elicited for 20 min · day^{-1} until the day of surgery; the control group spent 20 min · day^{-1} reading. Patients who were taught the relaxation response said their anxiety was highest before entering the study; control patients said their anxiety was greatest during surgery and when facing the results of biopsy. However, anxiety levels (as assessed by the State-Trait Anxiety Inventory) were the same immediately before and after surgery for both the control and study groups. In another study of outpatients, in which a tape-recorded procedure guided relaxation, the treatment significantly reduced preoperative anxiety, the time required for the induction of anesthesia, and the amount of anesthetic agent (isoflurane) needed to maintain anesthesia.[25] Patients receiving the relaxation treatment also had more favorable perceptions of their treatment than did a control group.

For children, information-modeling and coping-based programs have been shown to reduce anxiety and enhance coping, particularly during the preoperative period. Behavior during induction, in the PACU, or postoperatively does not seem to be affected by this effort. A child's anxiety seems

to be maximally reduced if the effort to reduce it is made before surgery.

Chronic Medications Before Ambulatory Surgery

As the severity of illness increases in patients who present for ambulatory surgery, the number of potent drugs that they may be taking to treat disease also increases. Drugs that may significantly affect anesthetic management may be proscribed before a procedure. What follows is a partial list of some long-term medications and how they interact with drugs commonly used for ambulatory anesthesia.

Antihypertensive Agents

Withdrawal of antihypertensive therapy can exacerbate intraoperative hypertension. Most antihypertensive agents affect storage, uptake, metabolism, or release of neurotransmitters and thus may interact with drugs used intraoperatively. In addition, they can produce adverse effects such as depression, nightmares, and drowsiness. Clonidine, an α_2-adrenergic agonist that centrally inhibits release of catecholamines, has been used as a premedicant to control intraoperative hypertension. Calcium channel–blocking drugs inhibit the transmembrane flux of calcium ions into cardiac and vascular smooth muscle. The effects of inhalation agents with calcium channel–blocking drugs may be additive, causing a decrease in blood pressure and contractility. Calcium channel–blocking drugs may also protect against myocardial ischemia or dysfunction during anesthesia, reduce anesthetic requirement, and potentiate both depolarizing and nondepolarizing muscle relaxants. Withdrawal of β-adrenergic receptor blocking drugs, such as propranolol, is associated with an increase in sympathetic stimulation. Antihypertensive agents, except for diuretics, should be continued on the day of surgery.

Mood-Altering Drugs

Mood-altering drugs, such as fluoxetine (Prozac), the monoamine oxidase inhibitors, lithium, and tricyclic antidepressants, are among the most common chronic medications. Fluoxetine, a selective inhibitor of the neuronal uptake of 5-hydroxytryptamine (5-HT), is probably the most frequently prescribed antidepressant. No interactions have been described between anesthetics and fluoxetine or ondansetron, a 5-HT$_3$ antagonist. Fever may result when fluoxetine is combined with drugs with antidopaminergic properties that control nausea.

The tricyclic antidepressants inhibit, to a varying degree, the neuronal uptake of norepinephrine, 5-HT, and dopamine; and they act as antagonists at muscarinic, cholinergic, α_1-adrenergic, and H$_1$ and H$_2$ receptors. These actions may produce dry mouth, tachycardia, delirium, and urinary retention. Because these drugs block the reuptake of norepinephrine, injections of epinephrine (with local anesthetics) or indirectly acting sympathomimetics, such as ephedrine, can result in severe hypertension. Cardiac dysrhythmias and sinus tachycardia are more prevalent when imipramine pretreatment is followed by halothane and pancuronium. Anesthetic requirement may be greater because of increased central levels of norepinephrine.

Lithium is used to treat manic depression and, in particular, the manic portion of this illness. It can replace sodium during an action potential, prolong neuromuscular blockade with either depolarizing or nondepolarizing muscle relaxants, and prolong the time for reversal by neostigmine. Because lithium blocks brainstem release of epinephrine or norepinephrine, anesthetic requirements may be decreased.

Monoamine oxidase (MAO) inhibitors block the enzyme MAO from breaking down catecholamines. They are used to treat depression when tricyclic or other antidepressants, or even electroconvulsive therapy, cannot be used. Their interactions with drugs and foods containing amines produce serious effects including severe hypertension, intracranial bleeding, and death. Five patients who had taken the MAO inhibitor dextromethorphan died after receiving meperidine for analgesia.[26] With phenelzine, pseudocholinesterase levels may be reduced, so that the action of succinylcholine could be prolonged. With reversible inhibitors of MAO-A alone, rather than the nonspecific blockers of both A and B enzyme activity, the potential for fatal reaction is probably reduced.

Aspirin

Many people in the United States take aspirin or other nonsteroidal anti-inflammatory agents. These drugs can alter platelet function within a few hours of ingestion and prolong bleeding times for at least 7 days. Studies of patients undergoing hip arthroplasty or coronary bypass surgery showed that blood loss was greater in patients who took aspirin or nonsteroidal anti-inflammatory drugs before surgery. If bleeding times are normal, though, blood loss may not be increased. Although no large study in patients undergoing ambulatory surgery has been performed to show that it makes any clinical difference if patients do or do not stop taking aspirin, there is no reason to discontinue aspirin when the risk of bleeding during surgery is small.

Upper Respiratory Tract Infection (URI)

A patient might be seen several days before surgery without any contraindication to the upcoming procedure. On the day of surgery, the patient may have a URI. Some retrospective studies have noted an increased incidence of laryngospasm or bronchospasm in such patients. Other studies have failed to show an effect of URI. In one study of patients who developed laryngospasm, they were more than twice as likely to have a URI compared to control patients.[27] Once the decision is made to perform surgery in spite of URI, there is no difference in incidence of laryngospasm if a laryngeal mask airway or endotracheal tube is used.[28] Generally, if a patient with a URI has a normal appetite, does not have a fever or an elevated respiratory rate, and does not appear toxic, it is probably safe to proceed with the planned procedure.

Restriction of Food and Liquids Before Ambulatory Surgery

To decrease the risk of aspiration of gastric contents, patients are routinely asked not to eat or drink anything (*non per os* [NPO], "nothing by mouth") for at least 6–8 hours before surgery. Gastric volumes are actually less when patients are allowed to drink some fluids before surgery. One study comparing patients given diazepam orally with 50 ml of water and a similar group given diazepam im found that gastric volume was smaller (median volume 1.5 vs. 20 ml) and pH was higher (median pH 2.4 vs. 1.8) for patients given diazepam and water.[29] When 100 ml of water was ingested 2 hours before surgery without a pill but in conjunction with an im premedicant (meperidine and promethazine), gastric volume and pH were not affected by ingestion of water.[30] In one study, patients either drank orange juice or coffee 2–3 hours before surgery or fasted overnight.[31] The incidence of gastric volume exceeding 25 ml and of gastric $pH < 2.5$ did not differ between the groups.

Similar findings are reported in children. For example, when $3 \text{ ml} \cdot \text{kg}^{-1}$ of apple juice was given 2.6 ± 0.4 hours preoperatively to healthy children 5–10 years of age, gastric volume was less and gastric pH was no different than if they had fasted.[32] In addition, patients who drank fluids beforehand were less irritable, less thirsty, less hungry, and better able to tolerate the preoperative waiting period. Similar results were found in a study of children who were allowed to drink clear liquids *ad libitum* until 2 hours before surgery, with the last intake before

surgery limited to 240 ml.[33] In a national survey of preoperative fasting practices conducted in 1992 and published in 1996, the majority of respondents abided by the traditional NPO policy (NPO after midnight); 24% allowed liquids up to 4 hr before surgery; 68% allowed liquids for children (Table 46-1).[34] One advantage of allowing coffee drinkers their morning coffee is that the incidence of headaches after surgery is reduced.[35]

MANAGING THE ANESTHETIC: PREMEDICATION

The outpatient is not that different from the inpatient undergoing surgery. In both, premedication is useful to control anxiety, postoperative pain, nausea, and vomiting and to reduce the risk of aspiration during induction of anesthesia. Because the outpatient is going home on the day of surgery, the drugs given before anesthesia should not hinder recovery afterward. Most premedicants do not prolong recovery when given in appropriate doses for appropriate indications. For example, when patients who received $1 \text{ } \mu\text{g} \cdot \text{kg}^{-1}$ fentanyl and $0.04 \text{ mg} \cdot \text{kg}^{-1}$ midazolam before induction were compared with patients who received no premedication, maintenance requirements (desflurane), airway irritability, and blood pressure increases during induction were reduced for the former and discharge times were unaffected.[36]

Controlling Anxiety

Patients scheduled to undergo surgery tend to be anxious long before they come to the outpatient area. In one study, the level of anxiety was measured daily from 4 days before hospital admission to several days after surgery.[37] Anxiety was high before admission, between admission and surgery, and 2 days after surgery (Fig. 46-3). Some patients, however, are not anxious. A study to examine the efficacy of drugs for relief of anxiety in outpatients undergoing gynecologic surgery was unsuccessful simply because of the low levels of preoperative anxiety present.[38] Some operations certainly can generate more anxiety than others. Increased anxiety has been noted in females, in those accompanied by a friend or relative to the preoperative holding area, in patients undergoing mutilating surgery or surgery for malignancy, in those undergoing surgery for the first time, in young patients, and in those with a previous bad anesthetic experience. The need to remove dentures is also associated with increased preoperative stress. Some patients worry more about their family than themselves immediately before surgery. If in doubt about patient anxiety, ask: predictive accuracy in determining whether patients are anxious increases when they are asked.[39]

Like adults, children should have some idea of what to expect during a procedure. But much of a child's anxiety before surgery concerns separation from parent(s). A child is more likely to demonstrate problematic behavior from the time of separation from parents to induction of anesthesia if a procedure has not been explained preoperatively. Similarly, extreme anxiety during the induction of anesthesia is associated with increased occurrence of postoperative negative behavioral changes, such as bad dreams/waking up crying, disobeying parents, separation anxiety, and temper tantrums.[40] Both parents and children need to be involved in preoperative discussions so that the anxiety of the parents is not transmitted to the child. The transmission of anxiety is at least as problematic as is the separation itself (*e.g.*, experiences of children being left with baby-sitters). If the parents are calm and can effectively manage the physical transfer to a warm and playful anesthesiologist or nurse, premedication is not necessary. Semisedation may be awkward and recovery after premedication may be prolonged. Nonetheless, at least in one study, both parental and child anxiety around

Table 46-1. CURRENT NPO GUIDELINES FOR CLEAR LIQUIDS FROM A NATIONAL SURVEY OF AMBULATORY SURGERY CENTERS AND UNIVERSITY ANESTHESIOLOGY PROGRAMS, CONDUCTED IN 1992

	Freestanding		University Affiliates		All Respondents	
	Adults n (%)	Children n (%)	Adults n (%)	Children n (%)	Adults n (%)	Children n (%)
NPO after midnight or 6–8 hr	63 (59.4)	40 (39.2)	48 (57.8)	16 (20.8)	111 (58.7)	56 (31.3)
NPO policy: 2 hr preoperatively	3 (2.8)	8 (7.8)	6 (7.2)	6 (7.8)	9 (4.8)	14 (7.8)
3 hr preoperatively	16 (15.1)	38 (37.3)	13 (15.7)	39 (50.6)	29 (15.3)	77 (43.0)
4 hr preoperatively	3 (2.8)	9 (8.8)	4 (4.8)	11 (14.3)	7 (3.7)	20 (11.2)
Flexible NPO policy	21 (19.8)	7 (6.9)	12 (14.5)	5 (4.8)	33 (17.5)	12 (6.7)
Total	106	102	83	77	189	179

the time of induction was better managed with oral midazolam rather than by having the parents present.[41]

Although historically many classes of drugs (*e.g.,* barbiturates and antihistamines) have been used to reduce anxiety and to induce sedation, benzodiazepines are at present the drugs most commonly used. Oral transmucosal fentanyl may be useful for reducing anxiety in children. Propofol also has some anxiety-reduction properties.

Benzodiazepines

Midazolam is the benzodiazepine most commonly used preoperatively. It is water-soluble with an initial distribution half-life of 7.2 minutes and an elimination half-life of 2.5 hours (range 2.1–3.4 hr), which increases to 5.6 hours in the elderly and to 8.4 hours in obese patients.[42] Fifty percent of an orally administered dose undergoes first-pass metabolism in the liver, and extrahepatic metabolism may also occur. The metabolites of midazolam have negligible soporific effects. Although midazolam does not produce thrombosis or thrombophlebitis, it may cause nausea occasionally. The drug's dose should be decreased with increasing age (Fig. 46-4).[43] A dose of midazolam of 0.1 mg · kg^{-1} iv in a 60-year-old patient would be equivalent to a dose of 0.03 mg · kg^{-1} iv in a 90-year-old patient and a dose of 0.15 mg · kg^{-1} in a 20-year-old patient. Midazolam 0.07 mg · kg^{-1} iv given to 40 elderly patients for sedation before endoscopy of the esophagus, stomach, and duodenum was effective based on time to achieve

sedation, adequacy of sedation, and absence of gagging during the procedure.[44] In a 20-year-old, effective sedation for 20–40 minutes is usually provided at doses of 0.07–0.15 mg · kg^{-1}. Cardiovascular, respiratory, and psychomotor depression are adverse effects of midazolam.

Oral midazolam is a useful premedicant for children. The U.S. Food and Drug Administration (FDA) approved an oral formulation of midazolam in October 1998. Oral midazolam in a dose of 0.5 mg · kg^{-1} produces effective sedation and reduces anxiety. With this dose, children can be effectively separated from their parents after 10 minutes.[45] When midazolam is given before procedures lasting about 30 minutes with a halothane anesthetic, recovery is not prolonged (Fig. 46-5).[46] Initial recovery after shorter acting anesthetics, *e.g.,* sevoflurane or desflurane, may be prolonged; discharge time, however, is not affected. With the antifungal agents itraconazole or ketoconazole, serum concentrations of midazolam are increased, thereby increasing the potential for intense and prolonged sedation as well as respiratory depression.

Diazepam is recommended for oral use by patients who are identified as anxious before coming for ambulatory surgery. Orally administered diazepam is well absorbed from the intestine. Plasma levels peak 60 minutes after ingestion, when anxiolytic effects are measurable. The drug is effective for several hours. Dose requirements decrease approximately 10% per decade of patient age. We prescribe diazepam in a dose of 2–5

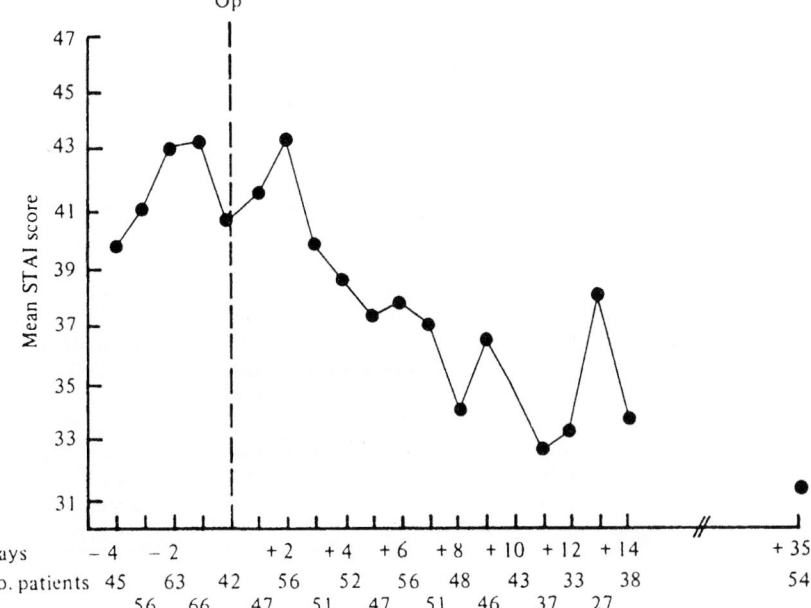

Figure 46-3. Mean scores for the State-Trait Anxiety Inventory (STAI), which were obtained daily beginning 4 days before surgery, at home, at the time of admission to the hospital, and up to 35 days after surgery (at this time, most patients had been discharged). "Op" indicates day of surgery. The level of anxiety was high not only before surgery but also at 2 days after surgery. (Reprinted with permission from Johnston M: Anxiety in surgical patients. Psychol Med 10:145, 1980.)

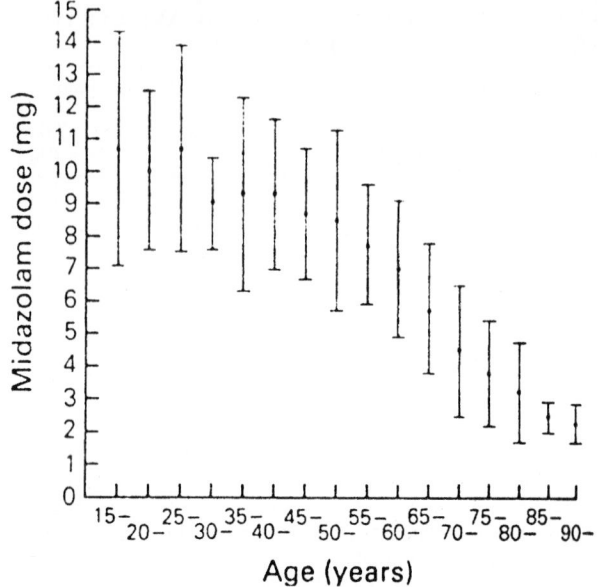

Figure 46-4. The mean dose (±SD) of iv midazolam required to produce adequate sedation before upper gastrointestinal endoscopy decreases with age. (Reprinted with permission from Bell GD, Spickett GP, Reeve PA *et al:* Intravenous midazolam for upper gastrointestinal endoscopy: A study of 800 consecutive cases relating dose to age and sex of patient. Br J Clin Pharmacol 23:241, 1987.)

mg · 70 kg⁻¹ adult. Its metabolite, desmethyldiazepam, has pharmacologic properties similar to those of the parent drug; concentrations can be detected after 2 hours and decrease only after 36 hours. The elimination half-life of diazepam and desmethyldiazepam is longer in older subjects than in young ones. The activity of this drug, however, does not depend on plasma concentration alone. When younger and older patients with equal plasma levels of diazepam are compared, the central nervous system of elderly patients is more sensitive to the depressant effects.

At proper doses, midazolam places patients at no additional risk for cardiovascular and respiratory depression than does diazepam. Decrease in blood pressure in healthy individuals with the benzodiazepines is trivial (10%); but in older patients, particularly those with heart disease, decreases may range from 20% to 35% and may be associated with apnea.[47] A decrease in blood pressure is greater when other drugs, such as fentanyl, propofol, or thiopental, are coadministered. Decreased oxygen saturation has also been reported after injection of midazolam.

In 100 patients undergoing endoscopy, average baseline oxygen saturation of 95% decreased to 92% after iv administration of midazolam and to 89% during endoscopy (Fig. 46-6).[48] Oxygen saturation was below 80% in 7% of patients. Routine administration of supplemental oxygen with or without continuous monitoring of arterial oxygenation is recommended whenever benzodiazepines are given intravenously. This precaution is important not only when midazolam is given as a premedicant, but also when it is used alone or with other drugs for conscious sedation.

Fatigue associated with the effects of anxiolytics may delay or prevent the discharge of patients on the day of surgery, although more frequently patients are not discharged because of the effects of the operation. With regard to anesthesia effects, patients normally stay in the hospital not because they are too sleepy but because they are nauseous.

The potential for amnesia after premedication is another concern, especially for patients undergoing ambulatory surgery. Anterograde amnesia occurs, yet no controlled studies have shown that retrograde amnesia has occurred in patients given midazolam or diazepam. In one study, 42% of patients given a placebo, but only 2.8% of patients given midazolam (0.1 mg · kg⁻¹ im), could remember induction of anesthesia for cervical dilation and uterine curettage (*p* < 0.0001).[49] It is noteworthy, however, that so many patients given placebo could not remember induction.

Opioids and Nonsteroidal Analgesics

Opioids can be administered preoperatively to sedate patients, to control hypertension during tracheal intubation, and to decrease pain before surgery. Meperidine (but not morphine or fentanyl) is sometimes helpful in controlling shivering in the operating room or postanesthesia care unit (PACU), although treatment is usually instituted at the time of shivering and not in anticipation of the event. The effectiveness of opioids in relieving anxiety is controversial and probably nonexistent, particularly in adults. In children, a lozenge form of fentanyl (oral transmucosal fentanyl citrate) reduced anxiety, increased sedation, and improved quality of induction.[50] Like all opioids, fentanyl in this form can decrease respiratory rate and oxygen saturation.[51] This effect usually can be reversed by having the child breathe deeply or take a big breath. Oxygen saturation should be monitored, particularly when the drug is used in this form. Pruritus, nausea, and vomiting can also be problematic. Droperidol, 50 μg · kg⁻¹, given to 2- to 8-year-olds, did not reduce the incidence of vomiting.[51] With fentanyl, PACU stay is not prolonged and postoperative analgesia requirements are less, although if children are required to drink fluids before they can be discharged, vomiting may delay their release. In adults, as in children, postoperative analgesia requirements are

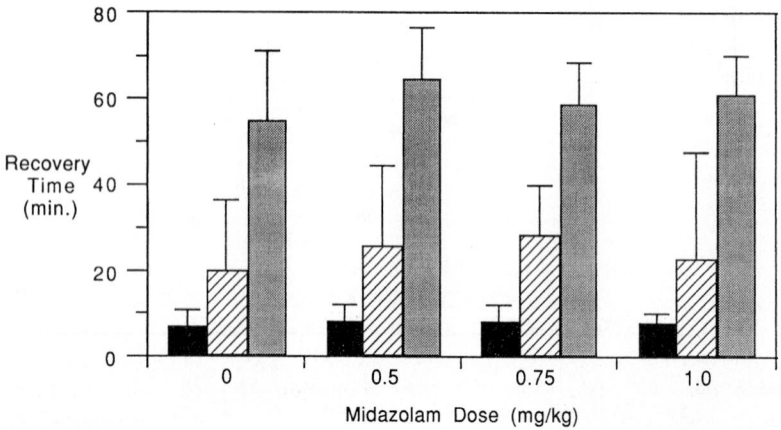

Figure 46-5. Recovery is not affected by the preoperative use of midazolam (*black* = surgery to PACU; *stippled* = PACU to eye opening; *gray* = PACU to discharge). (Reprinted with permission from McMillan CO, Spahr-Schopfer IA, Sikich N *et al:* Premedication of children with oral midazolam. Can J Anaesth 39:545, 1992.)

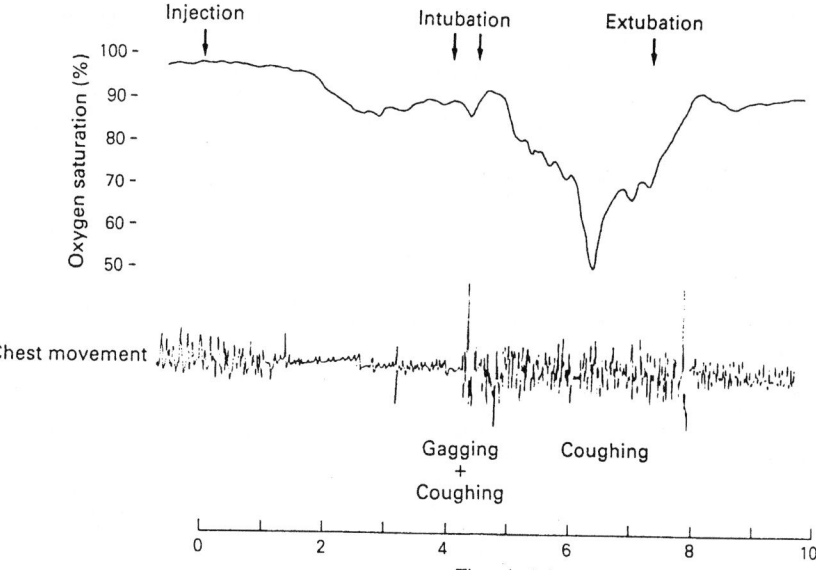

Figure 46-6. Oxygen saturation and chest wall movements decreased in a patient after injection of midazolam during gastroscopy. After introduction of the gastroscope, the patient coughed and oxygen saturation decreased even more. (Reprinted with permission from Bell GD, Reeve PA, Moshiri M *et al:* Intravenous midazolam: A study of the degree of oxygen desaturation occurring during upper gastrointestinal endoscopy. Br J Clin Pharmacol 23:703, 1987.)

decreased, but the nausea that may accompany opioids can be problematic.

Opioids are useful in controlling hypertension during tracheal intubation. Opioid premedication prevents increases in systolic pressure in a dose-dependent fashion. After tracheal intubation, however, systolic, diastolic, and mean arterial blood pressures sometimes decrease below baseline values.

Preoperative administration of opioids or nonsteroidal anti-inflammatory drugs is also useful for controlling pain in the early postoperative period. Patients undergoing laparoscopy received ketorolac 60 mg, dezocine 6 mg, or fentanyl 100 μg before the start of operation.[52] In the PACU 61% of patients who received fentanyl needed supplemental analgesia compared with 34% who received ketorolac and 25% who received dezocine; the amount of narcotic required was also less in the ketorolac and dezocine groups. Nausea was greatest after dezocine. In other studies, preoperative administration of diclofenac or naproxen to patients who underwent laparoscopy significantly reduced postoperative pain as well as the need for supplemental analgesia. Ibuprofen, an anti-inflammatory drug with analgesic action, can be given rectally to children preoperatively.

Propofol

Propofol is used for sedation, induction, and maintenance of anesthesia; the drug is discussed more completely in the section on General Anesthesia. However, propofol has other properties, such as anxiety reduction. When patients could administer propofol in 0.7-mg $\cdot$ kg^{-1} boluses to themselves during different ambulatory surgical procedures, they described a feeling of well-being and relaxation.[53] Anxiety reduction and sedation were similar when propofol was compared with midazolam and methohexital for sedation for retrobulbar and peribulbar ocular block.[54] Of patients who received either propofol or thiopental for induction and then enflurane, nitrous oxide, and oxygen for maintenance of anesthesia, anxiety increased postoperatively only in the thiopental group.[55]

Preoperative sedation is not needed for every patient. The following is our practice when patients require drugs to relieve anxiety. For the patient who has been seen at least 24 hours before a scheduled procedure and expresses a desire for medication to relieve anxiety or has anxiety that cannot be relieved with comforting, oral diazepam, 2–5 mg $\cdot$ 70 kg^{-1} body weight, is prescribed for the night before and at 6:00 A.M. on the day

of surgery (even if surgery is scheduled for 1:00 P.M. or later). For patients seen for the first time in the preoperative holding area who seem to need medication, midazolam, 0.03 mg $\cdot$ kg^{-1}, is administered iv, or the patient is brought into the operating room and propofol, 0.7 mg $\cdot$ kg^{-1}, is injected iv. For children, when necessary, oral midazolam, 0.5 mg $\cdot$ kg^{-1} is administered in the preoperative holding area.

Controlling the Risk of Aspiration

Patients who undergo ambulatory surgery may be at some small risk for aspiration of gastric contents, although this risk is no greater than for inpatients. At greater risk for aspiration are pregnant or morbidly obese patients or patients with hiatal hernia. Preoperative anxiety probably has no effect on gastric acidity for individuals without a history of duodenal ulcer.

H$_2$ Receptor Antagonists

Cimetidine and ranitidine antagonize the action of histamine on H$_2$ receptors, causing a reduction in concentration of hydrogen ions; they also decrease gastric volume. The effect of cimetidine begins 60–90 minutes after administration and lasts for at least 3 hours. Ranitidine is 4–6 times as potent as cimetidine, yet the elimination half-lives are similar (2–3 hours).[56] Famotidine and nizatidine, two new H$_2$ receptor antagonists, are similar to cimetidine and ranitidine. On an equimolar basis, famotidine is ~7.5 times more potent than ranitidine and 20 times more potent than cimetidine. Cimetidine inhibits metabolism of drugs dependent on biotransformation by cytochrome P-450. Cimetidine also decreases blood flow in the liver by 25% if administered acutely to a fasting patient and by 33% if administered chronically. Thus, drugs such as propranolol, which depend on blood flow in the liver for hepatic elimination, are eliminated from the body more slowly when given in conjunction with cimetidine. Cimetidine sometimes causes mental confusion, particularly in elderly patients,[57] and usually within 48 hours of the first dose. This syndrome is associated with trough concentrations of 2.0 mg $\cdot$ ml^{-1}.

Omeprazole

Omeprazole is a substituted benzimidazole that inhibits the gastric enzyme, hydrogen-potassium-adenosine-triphosphatase (ATPase), which mediates the production of hydrochloric acid in the gastric parietal cell. The half-life of omeprazole ranges from 0.3 to 2.5 hours.[58] Its metabolite is also active and binds irreversibly to gastric hydrogen-potassium-ATPase. Like cimetidine, omeprazole inhibits cytochrome P-450, and therefore reduces the metabolism of drugs depending on cytochrome P-450 systems. When omeprazole, 80 mg, was given to ambulatory patients the night before surgery, gastric volume was unchanged and gastric pH was increased.[59]

Sodium Citrate

Soluble antacids such as sodium citrate or Bicitra are useful because if aspirated, they produce less severe hypoxia and lung abnormalities than do nonabsorbable antacids, such as Mylanta. Customary doses (30 ml) of soluble antacids raise gastric pH but can also increase gastric volume. Very small doses of sodium bicarbonate (1.6 ml) can increase gastric pH without affecting gastric volume.[60]

Metoclopramide

Metoclopramide is a dopamine antagonist that increases the pressure of the lower esophageal sphincter, speeds gastric emptying, and prevents or alleviates nausea and vomiting. To reduce gastric volume even more, metoclopramide is combined with other drugs. For example, the combination of cimetidine and metoclopramide given to ambulatory patients during the preinduction phase was better than either drug alone for increasing gastric pH and decreasing gastric volume.[61] Metoclopramide is also an effective antiemetic. Patients given metoclopramide before surgery may experience less nausea and vomiting not only during, but also after surgery. However, the duration of action of metoclopramide is relatively brief, and its antiemetic effectiveness may be negligible with doses that are too low. Oral doses of $0.15-0.3$ mg $\cdot$ kg^{-1}, typical for patients undergoing anesthesia, were not effective in preventing emesis induced by cisplatin, an antineoplastic drug given to cancer patients, whereas iv doses of 2 mg $\cdot$ kg^{-1} were effective.[62] These higher doses, however, have not been used perioperatively.

In our practice, sodium citrate and metoclopramide or an H$_2$ receptor antagonist is routinely administered to patients at risk for acid aspiration, particularly those with hiatal hernia, the morbidly obese, parturients, and those with a history of duodenal ulcer.

Controlling Postoperative Nausea Preoperatively

Nausea, with or without vomiting, is probably the most important factor contributing to a delay in discharge of patients and an increase in unanticipated admissions of both children and adults after ambulatory surgery (Fig. 46-7).[63] Women, especially those who are pregnant, have a higher incidence of postoperative nausea and vomiting. Other risk factors include a previous history of motion sickness or postanesthetic emesis; surgery within 1–7 days of the menstrual cycle; and procedures such as laparoscopy; lithotripsy; and ear, nose, or throat surgery. Narcotics given for premedication may exacerbate the problem of postoperative nausea and vomiting. Other drugs such as metoclopramide may help alleviate this condition.

Droperidol

Droperidol has been variably successful as an antiemetic in patients undergoing surgery. Lower doses (0.25–0.5 mg) seem to be more effective than higher doses and recovery after anesthesia is not delayed.[64,65] The use of doses as low as 1.25 mg can produce untoward effects in the postoperative period (e.g., restlessness).[66] In children, $50-75$ μg $\cdot$ kg^{-1} is useful to control postoperative nausea, although this dose is also associated with

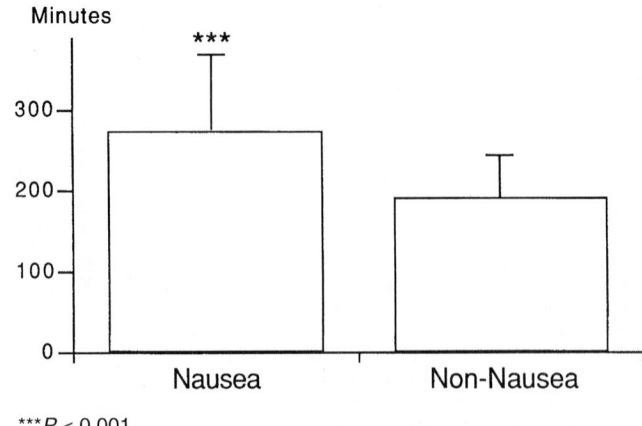

Figure 46-7. Time to home-readiness (mean $\pm$ SD) in nauseated versus non-nauseated patients. Home-readiness is significantly delayed ($p < 0.001$) if a patient is nauseous. (Reprinted with permission from Green G, Jonsson L: Nausea: The most important factor determining length of stay after ambulatory anaesthesia. A comparative study of isoflurane and/or propofol techniques. Acta Anaesthesiol Scand 37:742, 1993.)

a delay in discharge. When propofol and droperidol were compared, postoperative nausea in patients was similar, but droperidol patients were fit for discharge 1 hour later.[67]

Promethazine

Promethazine is the most common phenothiazine derivative used in children to control postoperative nausea and vomiting. The usual dose is $0.5-1.0$ mg $\cdot$ kg^{-1}. In patients undergoing strabismus surgery, promethazine, 0.5 mg $\cdot$ kg^{-1} iv and im, was significantly more effective than droperidol in controlling overall postoperative vomiting, particularly vomiting that occurred after the children left the hospital.[68]

Serotonin Antagonists

Ondansetron is the most studied drug in this class. It has a half-life that is approximately 3.5 hours in adults but shorter in children and longer in the elderly (mean 7.9 hr).[69] The primary adverse effect it produces is headache, although patients may also have diarrhea, constipation, sedation, and transient minor elevations in liver function tests. The drug is not associated with extrapyramidal reactions. Studies of patients undergoing anesthesia showed that doses of 4–8 mg were very effective antiemetics, although 4 mg was not less effective than 8 mg (Fig. 46-8).[70] Ondansetron, 4 mg, was superior to metoclopramide for control of postoperative nausea or vomiting.[71] An 8-mg dose was superior to droperidol, 1.25 mg, and metoclopramide, 10 mg.[72] In children, ondansetron, 100 μg, was more effective than droperidol, 75 μg $\cdot$ kg^{-1}, or placebo.[73] In another study that compared ondansetron to placebo followed by a "rescue" antiemetic of 20 mg of iv metoclopramide and 25 mg of iv hydroxyzine, reduction of postoperative nausea in patients was similar.[74] Overall, though, ondansetron is most effective when given at the end of surgery.[75]

Acupressure

Acupressure may also decrease postoperative nausea and vomiting. Acupressure bands that were placed preoperatively and removed 6 hr postoperatively reduced nausea and vomiting by 50% (Fig. 46-9).[76] The pressure bands cost just $8.00 and are reusable.

The routine use of antiemetics is controversial, given that a large percentage of patients do not experience postoperative nausea and vomiting. We use propofol for induction (see below), and then metoclopramide and a low dose of droperidol

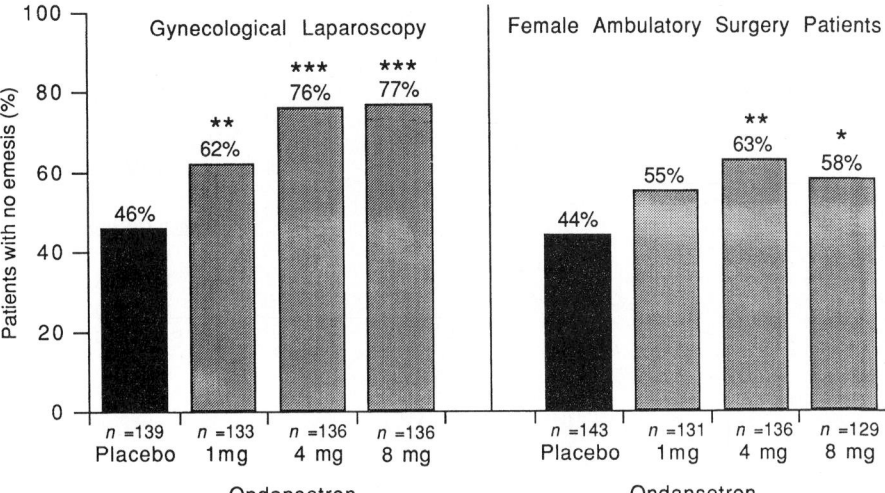

Figure 46-8. Nausea and vomiting were significantly less in ambulatory surgery patients with 4 or 8 mg ondansetron given before induction of anesthesia compared with placebo or 1 mg ondansetron. (Reprinted with permission from Pearman MH: Single dose intravenous ondansetron in the prevention of postoperative nausea and vomiting. Anaesthesia 49[suppl]:11, 1994.)

early in the case. If, despite this regimen, patients are nauseous or vomiting in the PACU, we use ondansetron. For children at risk for emesis, after an inhalation induction, we convert to an infusion of propofol.

Fluid Administration Before Surgery

Generally, before they are brought to the operating room, all patients have an intravenous catheter inserted with fluids infusing. Exceptions are children or adults afraid of needles or those who do not have a vein that can be easily accessed. Once the intravenous catheter has been inserted, we give an initial fluid bolus of 10 ml · kg^{-1}. Patients who received 10 ml · kg^{-1} of fluid in an initial bolus preoperatively were less thirsty, drowsy, and dizzy postoperatively than patients who were given 2 ml · kg^{-1} of fluid.[77]

INTRAOPERATIVE MANAGEMENT: CHOICE OF ANESTHETIC METHOD

There are several choices among anesthetic methods: general anesthesia or regional or local anesthesia with or without sedation. Except for obstetric cases for which regional anesthesia

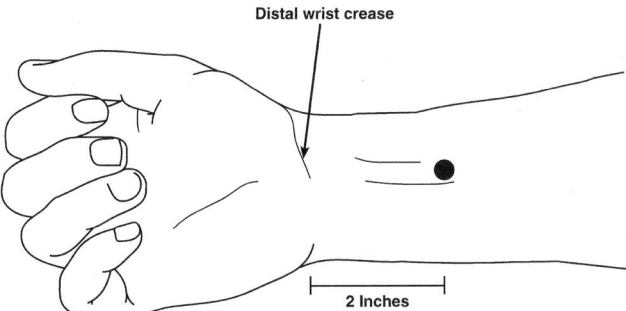

Figure 46-9. The treatment point P.6 is located on the anterior surface of the forearm, 2 inches proximal to the distal wrist crease between the tendons of musculus flexor carpi radialis and musculus palmaris longus. The forearm of the patient from the transverse crease of the wrist to the cubital crease is measured as 12 inches, or one-sixth of the forearm. (Reprinted with permission from Fan C, Tanhui E, Joshi S *et al*: Acupressure treatment for prevention of postoperative nausea and vomiting. Anesth Analg 84:821, 1997.)

may be safer than general anesthesia, both are otherwise equally safe. However, even for experienced anesthesiologists, there is a failure rate associated with regional anesthesia. Certainly, some procedures are possible only with a general anesthetic. For others the preference of patients, surgeons, or anesthesiologists may determine selection. Cost may be a factor: the cost of sedation is usually less than the cost of a general anesthetic. Time to recovery may also influence the choice of anesthetic method. Of 1180 ambulatory surgery patients, two-thirds of whom had general anesthesia for their procedures while the remainder had a local anesthetic supplemented by iv sedation, the three patients who required admission on the day of surgery had undergone general anesthesia.[78] The incidence of postoperative nausea and vomiting in the recovery room after local anesthesia and sedation was 6% compared with 14% after general anesthesia. Recovery times were also shorter after local anesthesia and sedation. In a study comparing regional anesthesia and sedation with general anesthesia for abortion, patients' blood pressures and pulse rates tended to be higher with the former (Fig. 46-10).[79] In that study, during local block with sedation, patients had more perioperative complaints, although few recalled any discomfort, presumably because of amnesia caused by benzodiazepines. Also, time spent in the operating room was longer with regional anesthesia because more time was needed to institute the block than the general anesthetic; however, time in the PACU was shorter because patients were more alert and in less pain. In a similar study of 136 patients undergoing arthroscopy, intra-articular bleeding and onset time were less, and the success rate was much higher after general anesthesia than local anesthesia: for 16 of 66 patients who received local anesthesia it was either partially successful or unsatisfactory, whereas general anesthesia was successful for all procedures.[80] Another study of patients undergoing minor gynecologic procedures showed an advantage of general anesthesia. Oxygen saturation was normal in all the patients who received general anesthesia, whereas sedated patients had significant oxygen desaturation.[81] Some of the sedated patients made movements that interfered with surgery, and 6% of sedated patients were switched to a general anesthetic.

One adverse effect associated with spinal anesthesia is headache, but headaches are also experienced by patients after general anesthesia. Especially when smaller spinal needles are used, the incidence of headache after either technique may be similar. In one study, after either method of anesthesia, incidence of headache ranged between 11% and 15%.[82] In that study, backache was higher (26%) after spinal anesthesia than general anesthesia (4%). However, incidence of sore throat (24%) and

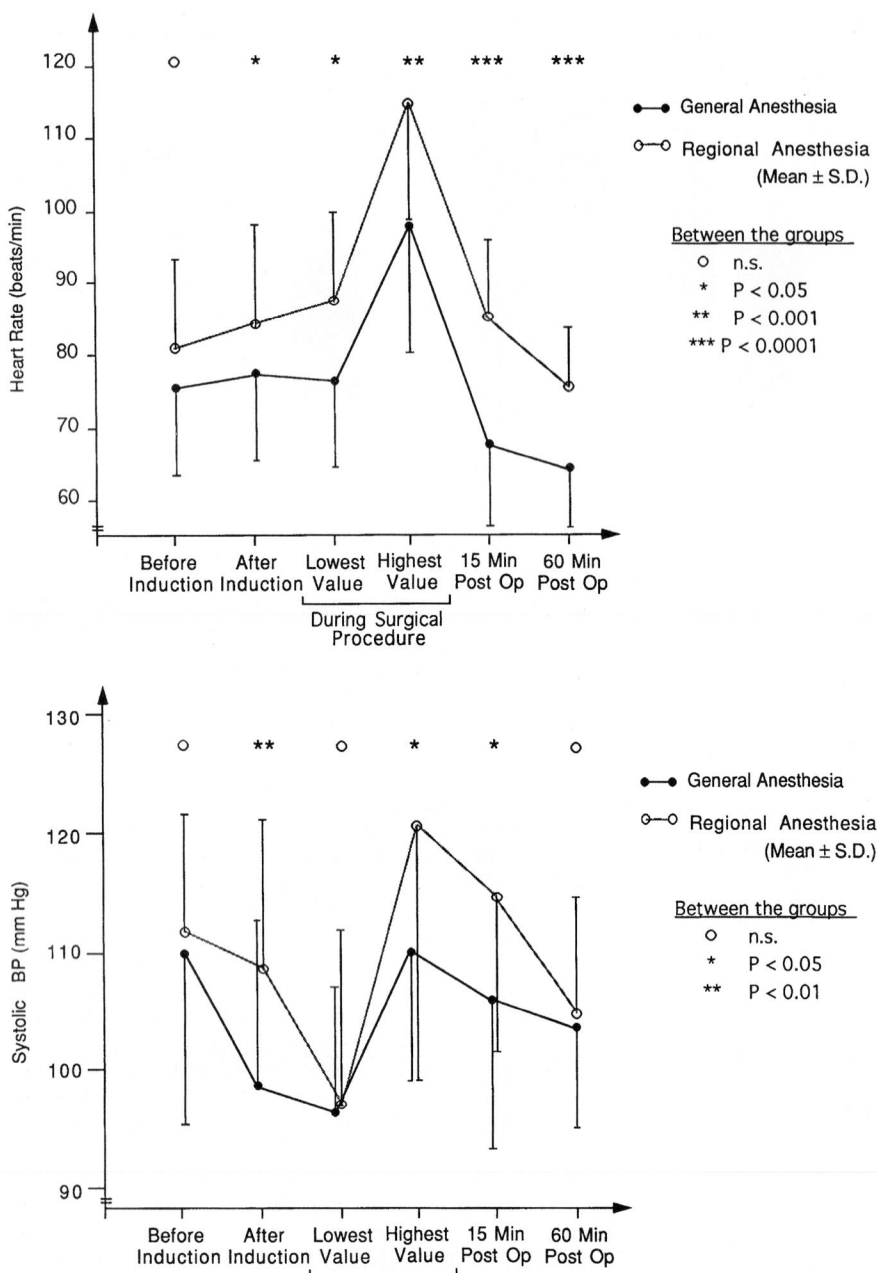

Figure 46-10. Heart rate and blood pressure were higher with regional anesthesia and sedation than with general anesthesia. (Reprinted with permission from Raeder JC: Propofol anaesthesia versus paracervical blockade with alfentanil and midazolam sedation for outpatient abortion. Acta Anaesthesiol Scand 36:31, 1992.)

nausea (22%) was higher after general anesthesia than spinal anesthesia (6% for both). For some procedures (*e.g.,* immersion lithotripsy), iv sedation techniques may reduce preparation and recovery time and the need for invasive monitors (*e.g.,* Foley catheter) when compared with regional techniques.[83] More large studies of patients undergoing ambulatory surgery are needed, particularly with some of the newer drugs used for both sedation and general anesthesia (*e.g.,* propofol, desflurane, and mivacurium) and some newer techniques (*e.g.,* spinal anesthesia with Sprotte needles), to show that regional anesthesia is better than general anesthesia or that general anesthesia is better than conscious sedation.

Regional Techniques

Local anesthesia and regional anesthesia have long been used for ambulatory surgery. As early as 1963, for example, 56% of ambulatory procedures were performed with the use of these

techniques.[84] Regional techniques commonly used for ambulatory surgery, in addition to spinal and epidural anesthesia, include local infiltration, brachial plexus and other peripheral nerve blocks, and iv regional anesthesia. General anesthesia can also be supplemented with regional nerve blocks. Performing a block takes longer than inducing general anesthesia and the incidence of failure is higher. Unnecessary delays can be obviated by performing the block beforehand in a preoperative holding area. Because the duration of effect of the newer general anesthesics and muscle relaxants is very short, recovery after a regional technique may take longer than after a general anesthetic. An occasional patient may experience syncope when the needle for the regional block is inserted. In the experience of oral and maxillofacial surgeons in Massachusetts in the late 1980s, 1 of 228 patients fainted when local anesthesia was injected.[85] The incidence was reduced by a factor 2 when parenteral sedation was also provided (see monitored anesthesia care below). Patients usually experience less pain when local or regional anesthesia has been used. Patients might still have a numb extremity (*e.g.*, after a brachial plexus block) but otherwise might meet all criteria for discharge. In such instances, the extremity must be well protected with a sling and patients must be cautioned to protect against injury because they are without normal sensations that would warn them of vulnerability. Reassurance that sensation will return should be provided.

Spinal Anesthesia

Spinal anesthesia is useful for ambulatory procedures in children who were born prematurely. The procedure is best performed with the child in the sitting position, head supported and somewhat extended, to prevent occlusion of the airway. Tetracaine, 0.8 mg · kg^{-1}, mixed with an equal volume of 10% dextrose, is injected into the L4–5 interspace with a 22-gauge Quincke needle 3.75 cm long. Since a leg raised may drive the spinal higher, the child must be kept flat when, for example, the Bovie pad is placed on the back. Hypotension is less common after spinal anesthesia in infants than adults, although it occurs when the spinal is very high. An iv line can be started in a lower extremity after the spinal is in place, the extremity is anesthetized, and vasodilatation is present.

The use of spinal needles with pencil-point noncutting tips has prompted a resurgence of spinal anesthesia for ambulatory surgery in adults. Epidural or spinal anesthesia is suitable for pelvic, lower abdominal, and lower extremity surgery but not for laparoscopic procedures because most people have difficulty breathing in the head-down position with the abdomen distended with air. Motor block of the legs with either technique may delay a patient's ability to walk; however, the use of a short-acting local anesthetic through an epidural catheter, for example, will minimize this problem while allowing the duration of anesthesia to match the sometimes unpredictable duration of surgery. Nausea is much less frequent after epidural or spinal anesthesia than after general anesthesia.

Different drugs and drug concentrations have been used for spinal anesthesia. Lidocaine and mepivacaine are ideal for ambulatory surgery because of their short duration of action, although lidocaine use has been problematic because of transient neurologic symptoms. In one study comparing patients who underwent knee arthroscopy with either 45 mg 1.5% mepivacaine or 60 mg 2% lidocaine, 22% of patients who received lidocaine had transient neurologic symptoms (back pain or dysesthesia). The symptoms were treated by NSAIDs and resolved within 5 days; no patients who received mepivacaine developed transient neurologic symptoms.[86]

For spinal anesthesia, needle size and shape are important to reduce the incidence of postdural puncture headache. The Sprotte and Whitacre needles are less traumatic to the lumbar dura mater than are Quincke needles. Incidence of postdural puncture headache with pencil-point Sprotte and Whitacre needles was 1–4% in one study,[87] but failure of anesthesia was higher when a Sprotte needle was used. In that study, spinal anesthetic required supplementation with additional parenteral drugs for 17% of patients with use of the Sprotte needle and for only 3% with the Whitacre needle. The position of the needle tip and the need to insert the Sprotte needle a little farther once cerebral spinal fluid is identified may have been factors. Rates of failed block have been shown to be higher with smaller gauge needles and are similar with Quincke and Whitacre needles. In some studies, incidence of postdural puncture headache after use of needles with a cutting tip, such as the Quincke 25–27 gauge, was higher than with the Sprotte needle. When same size Whitacre and Quincke needles were compared, the incidence of postdural puncture headache was higher with the Quincke (8.5%) than with the Whitacre needle (3%).[88] Another study reported incidence of headache with 25-gauge Quincke needles at 15% and with 22-gauge Whitacre needles at 6%.[89]

Smaller gauge needles result in a lower incidence of postdural puncture headache. With 25-gauge needles, the incidence of postdural puncture headache reported was four times that with 26-gauge needles; with 26-gauge needles, it was 9.6%; and with 27-gauge needles, it was 1.5%.[90,91] Needles of 27 gauge are associated with increasingly difficult insertion, a higher rate of failed block, and the risk of a spinal anesthetic with the use of the introducer. The incidence of postspinal headache is higher in younger individuals, particularly in women.[92] Backaches can be problematic after spinal anesthesia, especially when more than two attempts have been made to insert a spinal needle.[93] Women also tend to have more complaints of backache than do men.[94]

For those patients who do receive spinal anesthesia, it is incumbent upon the anesthesiologist and the facility to have follow-up with telephone calls to ensure that no disabling symptoms of headache have developed. If the headache does not respond to bed rest, analgesics, and oral hydration, the patient must return to the hospital for a course of caffeine iv therapy or an immediate epidural blood patch.

Spinal anesthesia should not be avoided in ambulatory surgery patients simply because they may be more active postoperatively than inpatients. Bed rest does not reduce the frequency of headache.[95] Early ambulation may decrease the incidence.[96] Further study is needed to assess the relative risk–benefit ratio of spinal anesthesia as a technique for the ambulatory surgery patient.

Epidural and Caudal Anesthesia

Epidural anesthesia takes longer to perform than spinal anesthesia. Onset with spinal anesthesia is more rapid, although recovery may be the same with either technique. Some studies suggest that bicarbonate can be added to solutions for faster onset of epidural anesthesia. An advantage of the epidural block is that it can be performed outside the operating room, and after the surgical procedure is completed, the problem of postdural puncture headache is usually avoided. In one study of 682 patients, 90% were discharged within 5 hours of the operation.[97] Two patients in that series required a blood patch, and the overall incidence of backache was 9.3%.

Caudal anesthesia is a form of epidural anesthesia commonly used in children before surgery below the umbilicus as a supplement to general anesthesia and to control postoperative pain. Bupivacaine, 0.175–0.25%, in a volume of 0.5–1.0 ml · kg^{-1} may be used. The block may be more difficult in children, particularly those who weigh more than 10 kg and are obese, if landmarks for the block are difficult to locate. The block is usually administered while the child is anesthetized. After injection, the depth of general anesthesia can be reduced. Because of better pain control after a caudal block, children can usually ambulate earlier and be discharged sooner than without a caudal block. In one study, patients who received a dose of 0.175% bupivacaine for caudal block went home more than 1 hour before patients who received higher or lower concentrations of drug.[98] Pain control and discharge times were no different whether the caudal block had been placed before surgery or after it was completed.[99]

Nerve Blocks

Among the different nerve blocks, the axillary nerve block is popular for hand surgery, particularly useful in an ambulatory setting because postoperative nausea, vomiting, and pain are less. An interscalene block is useful for shoulder surgery. To decrease pain after inguinal hernia repair in children or adults, an ilio-inguinal-hypogastric nerve block is often successful. A femoral nerve block with genitofemoral nerve infiltration is useful for procedures that require saphenous vein stripping. In one study that compared femoral nerve block to spinal anesthesia for vein stripping surgery, femoral nerve block resulted in a shorter hospital stay and less postoperative pain (both in the

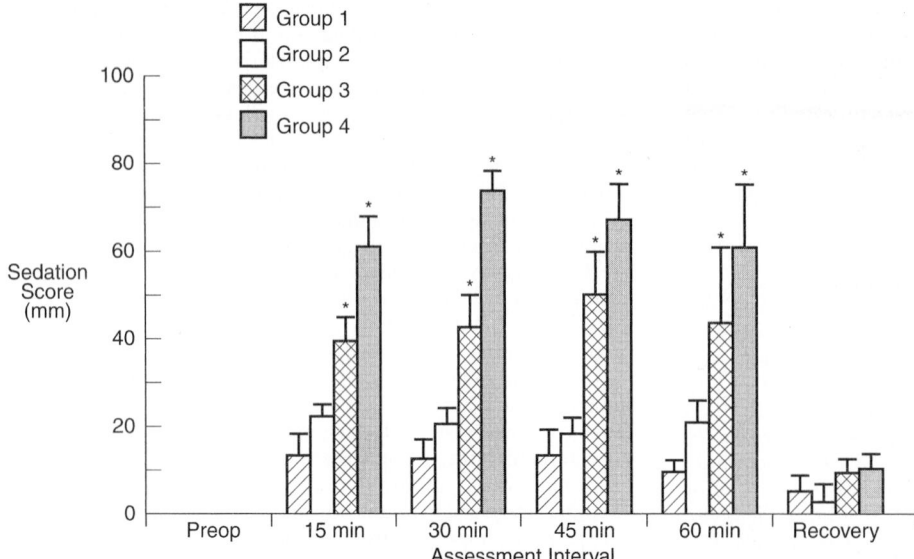

Figure 46-11. Sedation produced by increasing propofol dose in patients with spinal anesthesia. Group 1 = propofol 0.2 mg · kg^{-1} bolus and 0.5 mg · kg^{-1} · hr^{-1}; Group 2 = propofol 0.4 mg · kg^{-1} bolus and 1 mg · kg^{-1} · hr^{-1}; Group 3 = propofol 0.5 mg · kg^{-1} bolus and 2 mg · kg^{-1} · hr^{-1}; Group 4 = propofol 0.7 mg · kg^{-1} bolus and 4 mg · kg^{-1} · hr^{-1}. Mean values ± SEM; *p < 0.05 from lowest dose group. (Reprinted with permission from Smith I, Monk TG, White PF, Ding Y: Propofol infusion during regional anesthesia: Sedative, amnestic and anxiolytic properties. Anesth Analg 79:313, 1994.)

PACU and at home), backache, and headache; furthermore, patient satisfaction was greater with the nerve block.[100]

Sedation and Analgesia

Many patients who undergo surgery with local or regional anesthesia prefer to be sedated and to have no recollection of the procedure. Sedation is important, in part, because injection with local anesthetics can be painful, and lying on a hard operating room table for any time can be uncomfortable. Levels of sedation vary from light, during which a patient's consciousness is minimally depressed, to very deep, in which protective reflexes are partially blocked and response to physical stimulation or verbal command may not be appropriate. When patients are unsuitable for outpatient general anesthesia, surgery can often be performed if local or regional anesthesia is supplemented with conscious sedation. In such cases, however, patients may be at much greater risk for complications after conscious sedation. In one study of approximately 100,000 anesthetics, monitored anesthesia care was associated with the highest rate of mortality (209 deaths per 10,000 anesthetic episodes).[101] Children who have surgery usually will not remain immobile unless they are deeply sedated or receive general anesthesia.

During conscious sedation, medication is administered to provide amnesia and sedation, to reduce anxiety, and to control pain. Agents commonly used in adults for sedation include benzodiazepines for anxiety reduction and amnesia, opioids to control pain, and low doses of iv or inhalation anesthetics to provide sedation. Benzodiazepines, such as midazolam, or the iv anesthetic propofol may be used alone because both reduce anxiety and cause amnesia. For more painful procedures, or when a block does not seem to be working well, opioids (*e.g.,* fentanyl, 25–50 µg · 70 kg^{-1}) are usually added. Nonsteroidal analgesics such as ketorolac are also useful.

For adults, the iv route of administration is the most popular. Drugs are often titrated to effect, although bolus dosing may produce a faster effect. The challenge lies in selecting appropriate drugs and titrating their doses. Usually, drugs from the sedative-hypnotic and analgesic classes are administered. Propofol is particularly useful because during low-dose infusions, degree of sedation can be adjusted precisely. Infusion rates between 25 and 100 mg · hr^{-1} produce dose-dependent levels of sedation (Fig. 46-11).[102] Fentanyl with or without an NSAID is often used for analgesia.

In children multiple drug combinations are used to achieve sedation. One combination often given is im meperidine (2 mg · kg^{-1}), promethazine (1 mg · kg^{-1}), and chlorpromazine (1 mg · kg^{-1}). With this combination, sedation is long-lasting for painful procedures. In one study of 63 patients, the onset time for sedation was 27 minutes, and the children were sitting upright after the procedure in ~100 minutes.[103] Rectal thiopental is also used for sedation; however, children particularly dislike shots or rectal injections. Chloral hydrate, not as useful for painful procedures, is given in a dose of 20–100 mg · kg^{-1} orally or rectally and onset time occurs after ~1 hour. Other popular drugs for sedation include oral midazolam, pentobarbital (5–7 mg · kg^{-1}), and a combination of oral meperidine (2 mg · kg^{-1}) and promethazine (0.5 mg · kg^{-1}). Unfortunately, chloral hydrate is bitter. Oral transmucosal fentanyl citrate (described above) may be a more readily accepted alternative. Ketamine, which provides analgesia, amnesia, and sedation, can be given intravenously, orally, rectally, or intramuscularly. It is commonly used in the operating room to sedate children who have become uncontrollable and refuse to inhale anything after an attempt at induction with an inhalation anesthetic has failed. A dose of 2 mg · kg^{-1} im is usually adequate.[104] For oral doses, 5 mg · kg^{-1} resulted in onset of action after 20 minutes, similar to that with oral midazolam, although patients who received midazolam were discharged from the hospital sooner.[105] Nitrous oxide can also be used, but achieving sedation may be difficult when nitrous oxide is not supplemented with other agents.

In one survey of 89 pediatric residency programs, the most popular method for sedating children for medical procedures was use of chloral hydrate; a combination of parenteral meperidine, promethazine, and chlorpromazine was second; and pentobarbital was third.[106] Those sedation regimens were associated with few serious adverse effects, except for two deaths reported in infants with congenital heart disease who were sedated with a combination of meperidine, promethazine, and chlorpromazine.

For adults, the proper dose might be selected by having the patient control dosage, as has been successful with postoperative analgesia. When anesthetist versus patient control of sedation with midazolam was compared during bilateral extraction of third molar teeth, the total dose of midazolam administered was similar, 5.0–5.3 mg, but 67% of patients reported that they could sedate themselves better than the anesthetist could.[107] Equal numbers preferred either one or the other technique and overall satisfaction with both techniques was high. In a similar study in which patient-controlled sedation with propofol was compared with anesthetist-administered midazolam and

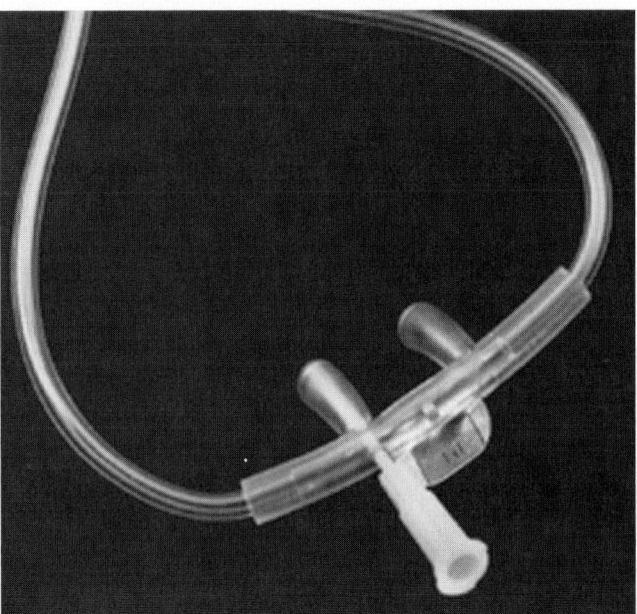

Figure 46-12. Modification of a nasal cannula to measure end-tidal CO_2. (Reprinted with permission from Prstojevich SJ, Sabol SR, Goldwasser MS, Johnson C: Utility of capnography in predicting venous carbon dioxide partial pressure in sedated patients during outpatient oral surgery. J Oral Maxillofac Surg 50:37, 1992.)

fentanyl for third molar tooth extraction, satisfaction was higher with patient-controlled sedation for both subjective intraoperative feelings and willingness to have the procedure again.[108] When using such techniques, though, it is important to adjust dose for patient variables, such as patient age. In a study of 30 patients, aged 26–72 years, who received a fixed propofol dose of 0.7 mg·kg^{-1} when they pressed a button, older age was significantly correlated with a deeper maximum level of sedation.[53] When a drug is administered by an anesthetist or anesthesiologist for sedation, the amount needed may be unclear. Eye signs and verbal responses from the patient are important monitors. To determine an adequate amount of midazolam, good patient markers are ptosis, with the eyelid halfway across the pupil, or a loss of interest in maintaining conversation with a tendency toward monosyllabic replies. The latter marker is associated with a shorter duration of amnesia after a procedure; the former, with more intense amnesia during the procedure.[109] During patient-controlled administration of propofol, sedation no deeper than full eyelid closure with prompt response to verbal command was reported.[53] In summary, patient-controlled sedation may or may not be associated with equal or less drug administered. The patient, though, has some control over medication, which produces a positive psychological response.

As with any other instance in which the potential exists for complete loss of consciousness, appropriate monitoring and availability of resuscitation equipment are essential. The monitoring standards for general anesthesia also apply for monitored sedation. A member of the anesthesia care team must be continuously present and an anesthesiologist must be immediately available. Cardiac and respiratory monitoring is required. Pulse oximetry is essential and oxygen, if necessary, should be provided. Capnography is also invaluable, even when a nasal cannula is used to administer oxygen (Fig. 46-12).[110] All drugs used during conscious sedation can cause hypoxia, and oxygen should be routinely used (see Fig. 46-6). Monitoring patient awareness or level of consciousness by speaking to the patient frequently is also an important component of this type of anesthetic. The patient must be reassured, particularly during times of distress or discomfort, and, if necessary, given additional

medication. The patient must also be warned of stimulating events about to take place (*e.g.,* injection of local anesthetic, laparoscope insertion, tourniquet inflation). An expected event is less stimulating than an unanticipated one. Conversation is also important because some drugs, *e.g.,* the benzodiazepines, which normally reduce anxiety, may, in some individuals, increase it. A patient may appear sleepy but not calm or, conversely, calm but not sleepy. Conversation with the patient may better determine how the patient is really feeling. An excellent review of this topic is provided by Sá Rêgo *et al.*[111]

General Anesthesia

The drugs selected for general anesthesia determine how long patients stay in the postanesthesia recovery unit after surgery, and for some patients, whether or not they can be discharged to go home. Some of the pertinent issues, *i.e.,* problems with nausea and vomiting and drowsiness, have already been discussed in the premedication section (Managing the Anesthetic: Premedication).

Induction

Since its introduction, propofol has almost become the induction agent of choice for patients undergoing ambulatory surgery. This fact in part relates to its half-life: the elimination half-life of propofol is 1–3 hours, shorter than that of methohexital (6–8 hr) or thiopental (10–12 hr). Although the effect of drugs given for induction seems to be transient, these drugs can depress psychomotor performance for several hours. When induction doses of propofol and thiopental were compared, psychomotor impairment in patients was evident for up to 5 hours after thiopental, but only for 1 hour after propofol (Fig. 46-13).[112] When a volatile anesthetic is used after induction with propofol, recovery is much more rapid than after induction with thiopental, methohexital, or etomidate. For arthroscopic surgery lasting 30–40 minutes, patients who received isoflurane for maintenance of anesthesia recovered 1 hour sooner with propofol induction than with thiopental.[113] The differences in recovery are also apparent in children. In a study of children who received propofol, halothane, or thiopental for induction, recovery was associated with less nausea and discharge home was much more rapid after propofol.[114] Postoperatively patients have much less nausea and vomiting after an induction with propofol; such a reduction is even more apparent when propofol is also used for maintenance of anesthesia.

Pain on injection can be a problem with propofol. Pain is more likely on injection into dorsal hand veins and is minimized if forearm or larger antecubital veins are used. Some individuals, though, experience pain if the drug is injected into proximal larger veins. Nonetheless, thrombophlebitis does not appear to be a problem after iv administration of this agent. The addition of 1 ml lidocaine (1%) to 19 ml propofol significantly reduced the incidence and severity of pain on injection (Fig. 46-14).[115] Lidocaine injected immediately before propofol only partially reduced the incidence.

Most children and some adults prefer not to have an intravenous catheter inserted before the start of anesthesia. Sevoflurane has a relatively low blood-gas partition coefficient and the speed of induction is similar to, albeit somewhat slower than, that of propofol. In one study of 146 adults, when sevoflurane with nitrous oxide and fentanyl for induction was compared with propofol, fentanyl, and nitrous oxide, induction with sevoflurane was approximately 60 sec longer than with propofol; sevoflurane for induction and maintenance was associated with a higher incidence of postoperative emetic sequelae compared with propofol.[116] Yet, when a vital capacity inhaled induction with sevoflurane was compared with an iv induction with propofol for ambulatory surgery in adults, sevoflurane resulted in a faster loss of consciousness (30 sec). Adverse effects, recovery times, and patient satisfaction were similar to those after a

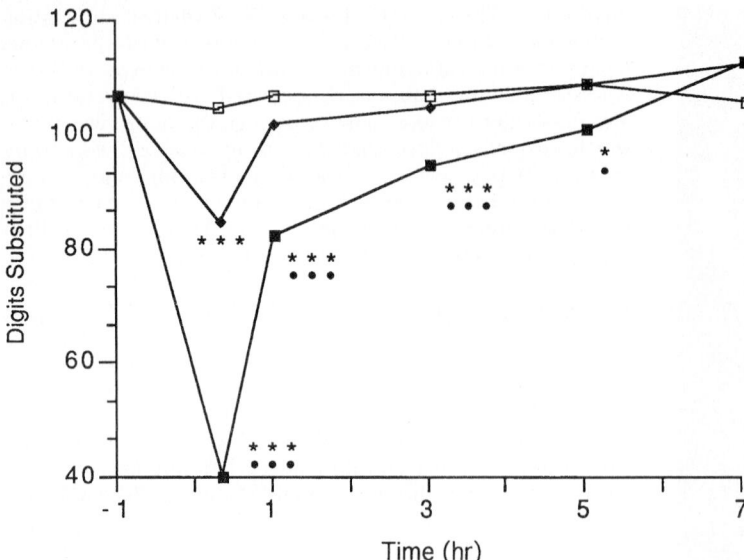

Figure 46-13. Performance on the digit symbol substitution test after either propofol 2.5 mg·kg^{-1}, then 1 mg·kg^{-1} (*diamonds*); thiopental 5 mg·kg^{-1}, then 2.0 mg·kg^{-1} (*filled squares*); or control (*open squares*) in 12 healthy volunteers (*$p < 0.05$, ***$p < 0.001$ vs. control; •$p < 0.05$, •••$p < 0.001$ vs. propofol). (Reprinted with permission from Korttila K, Nuotto EJ, Lichtor L *et al:* Clinical recovery and psychomotor function after brief anesthesia with propofol or thiopental. Anesthesiology 76:676, 1992.)

propofol induction.[117] When sevoflurane was compared to halothane for induction of anesthesia in children, induction times were not clinically different.

Parental presence is becoming more accepted during induction of anesthesia in children, even though scientific evidence of its advantages is not conclusive. Some studies show that children are less upset and have fewer behavioral changes after surgery if a parent is present during induction. Others have suggested that parents can become upset when they see their anesthetized child, who appears to be dead, albeit breathing and with a beating heart. Separation anxiety on the part of the parents is probably no different if the child is awake or asleep.

For short procedures, some patients may not require neuromuscular blocking drugs; others may need an ultra–short-acting agent to facilitate tracheal intubation or a muscle relaxant during the procedure. Succinylcholine, a depolarizing relaxant, is used to facilitate tracheal intubation and to provide a short period of profound relaxation. Skeletal muscle aches and pains can be problematic with the drug. Myalgia may occur up to the fourth postoperative day and be more painful than the surgery itself. The incidence of myalgia was significantly higher in patients who walked shortly after surgery (66%) than in inpatients who remained resting in bed (13.9%); the pain can persist for 2–3 days.[118] Pretreatment with a variety of drugs (*d*-tubocurarine, 0.05 mg·kg^{-1}; diazepam, 0.05 mg·kg^{-1}; calcium gluconate, 1000 mg; succinylcholine, 10 mg) has been reported to lessen and even eliminate the myalgia that occurs after administration of succinylcholine. Succinylcholine should be used with caution in children because of the possibility of cardiac arrest related to malignant hyperthermia or unsuspected muscular dystrophy, particularly Duchenne's disease.

Nondepolarizing drugs such as rapacuronium or rocuronium have rapid onset times that are similar to those with succinylcholine. Rapacuronium's duration of action is similar to duration with succinylcholine. In one study, onset time was 67 sec for succinylcholine vs. 83 sec for rapacuronium, and conditions for endotracheal intubation were similar.[119] Times until clinically sufficient recovery from neuromuscular block induced after succinylcholine (time until $T_1 = 90\%$) was 10.6 min and after rapacuronium was 11.6 min with reversal by neostigmine. Not all anesthesiologists have found that intubating conditions are as good after rapacuronium as after succinylcholine. Rapid recovery from block is a desired characteristic if, for example, tracheal intubation is not possible. In one study, when 0.07 mg neostigmine was given 2 minutes after rapacuronium administration, the time to 25% T_1 twitch recovery decreased from 16 minutes in control patients to 8–10 minutes.[120] When rocuronium and succinylcholine were compared, 1 mg·kg^{-1} of succinylcholine had an onset time (as measured by suppression of twitch tension to 5% of control value) of 0.8 minutes, and 0.6 mg·kg^{-1} rocuronium had an onset time of 1.2 minutes.[121] The time to recovery of twitch was of the same order of magnitude as time with vecuronium. The nondepolarizing drugs are useful because they are not associated with postoperative muscle pain. Postoperative nausea may be less, in particular with rapacuronium, because reversal of the drug (after single injection) with neostigmine may not be necessary. Priming doses can also accelerate onset time. A priming dose of mivacurium, for example, can reduce the time for onset of action of the drug. When mivacurium was given in a bolus dose of 0.15 mg·kg^{-1}, onset time was 3.5 minutes; onset time was reduced to 2 minutes when a priming dose was used, longer by 1.5 minutes compared

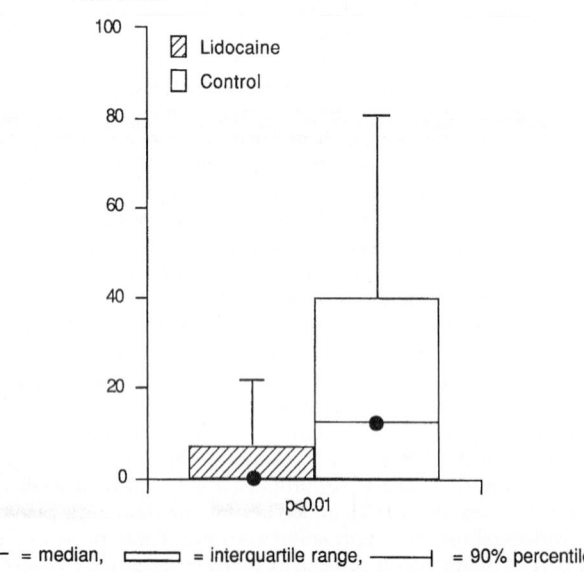

Figure 46-14. Pain on injection of propofol with and without lidocaine. Median, interquartile range and 90th percentile are illustrated. (Reprinted with permission from Helbo-Hansen S, Westergaard V, Krogh BL, Svendsen HP: The reduction of pain on injection of propofol. The effect of lignocaine. Acta Anesthesiol Scand 32:502, 1988.)

with onset time of succinylcholine.[122] If a higher dose of nondepolarizing drugs is used, onset time should be shorter, particularly when a priming dose is also used. Certainly, other longer-acting, nondepolarizing drugs can also be used for tracheal intubation of ambulatory surgical patients. Tracheal intubation can also be performed without the use of muscle paralytics. Combinations of alfentanil and propofol have been described. Nonetheless, succinylcholine provides the most rapid onset of paralysis, which is particularly useful when there is a risk of aspiration or hypoxia.

Maintenance

Although many factors affect the choice of agents for maintenance of anesthesia, one primary consideration for ambulatory anesthesia is speed of wake-up. Time to recovery may be measured by various criteria; however, for an ambulatory center, a patient may be considered awake when able to leave the center. Actual discharge from an ambulatory center, though, may depend on administrative issues, such as a written order from a surgeon or anesthesiologist. The time necessary before a patient can be taken from the operating room after completion of surgery, or a patient's ability to skip the post-anesthesia care unit and go directly to a step-down unit may be directly related to the anesthetic and result in cost savings for an institution. Does choice of maintenance agent affect recovery after anesthesia? The relatively new drugs, propofol, desflurane, and sevoflurane, have characteristics that make them ideal for maintenance of anesthesia for ambulatory surgery. Propofol has a short half-life, and when used as a maintenance agent, results in rapid recovery and few side effects. Desflurane and sevoflurane, halogenated ether anesthetics with low blood–gas partition coefficients, seem to be ideal for general anesthesia for ambulatory surgery. Sevoflurane, unlike desflurane, facilitates a smooth inhalation induction of anesthesia, the preferred technique to ensure rapid recovery of children in ambulatory surgery centers. For children who receive either sevoflurane or halothane, or halothane and then desflurane for induction and maintenance of anesthesia, recovery times are significantly shorter after sevoflurane or desflurane. Studies with desflurane and sevoflurane have shown that recovery afterward, even by comparison with that after propofol for maintenance, is rapid. In one study of laparoscopic surgery, patients emerged from anesthesia with desflurane and nitrous oxide significantly faster than after propofol or sevoflurane and nitrous oxide, although the ability to sit up, stand, and tolerate fluids and the time to fitness for discharge were no different (Fig. 46-15).[123] On arrival in the PACU, a significantly higher percentage of patients who had

received desflurane or sevoflurane were eligible to skip the PACU for recovery. Nausea was greater, albeit not significantly, when desflurane was used for maintenance. Other studies have shown relatively equal times to discharge with propofol, desflurane, and enflurane; propofol for maintenance of anesthesia resulted in less nausea and vomiting than did the two inhalation anesthetics. When propofol was used for induction, and maintenance was with halothane, enflurane, isoflurane, or propofol, no differences were readily apparent among the four agents 4 hours after the end of anesthesia when the patient was discharged.[124] Children who received desflurane or halothane to maintain anesthesia for ambulatory surgery (induction was with halothane after premedication with midazolam), awakened more rapidly after desflurane (10 min vs. 21 min).[125] The desflurane group was in the PACU 8 fewer minutes, although discharge times were unaffected. Desflurane is not recommended for induction in children because it causes a high incidence of coughing and laryngospasm. In one study, halothane was used first, and then children received desflurane, after which no airway irritability was reported.[125]

Desflurane can be problematic in individuals with hypertension when the concentration of the drug is increased rapidly. Rapid changes in concentration of isoflurane or desflurane were associated with sympathetic and renin–angiotensin system activity and with transient increases in arterial blood pressure and heart rate.[126] Increases were greater in patients who received desflurane. These patients also had a transient increase in plasma vasopressin concentration. This response can be avoided if the concentration is increased more slowly or if other drugs that attenuate the sympathetic response, such as opioids, are also administered.

The use of nitrous oxide for ambulatory anesthesia is an issue because the incidence of emesis may be greater after nitrous oxide than after other inhalation agents. Yet many studies have shown that nitrous oxide can be used successfully for ambulatory anesthesia. A meta-analysis, designed to determine if nitrous oxide significantly reduced the odds of postoperative nausea and vomiting (PONV) included 26 trials from 24 studies.[127] Overall, the use of nitrous oxide increased the risk of PONV by 28% (Fig. 46-16). The maximal benefit of nitrous oxide avoidance was seen in females (46%).

Propofol is better than some other agents for ambulatory anesthesia because it is associated with less nausea. When patients undergoing laparoscopy or arthroscopy received either propofol or isoflurane for maintenance, initial recovery was faster after isoflurane, although nausea was much less in the group who received propofol.[63] After outpatient restorative den-

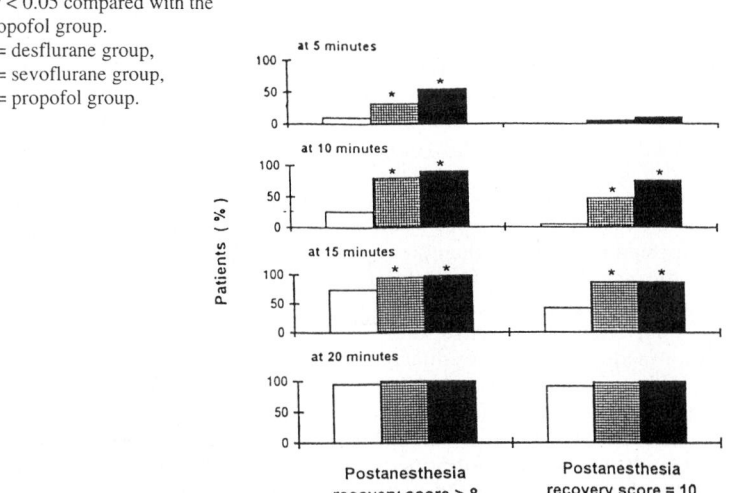

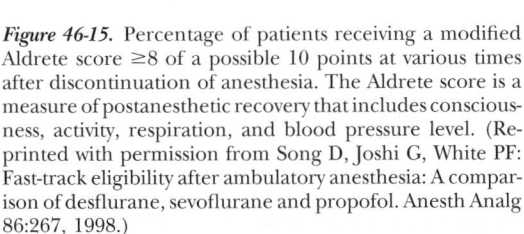

Figure 46-15. Percentage of patients receiving a modified Aldrete score ≥8 of a possible 10 points at various times after discontinuation of anesthesia. The Aldrete score is a measure of postanesthetic recovery that includes consciousness, activity, respiration, and blood pressure level. (Reprinted with permission from Song D, Joshi G, White PF: Fast-track eligibility after ambulatory anesthesia: A comparison of desflurane, sevoflurane and propofol. Anesth Analg 86:267, 1998.)

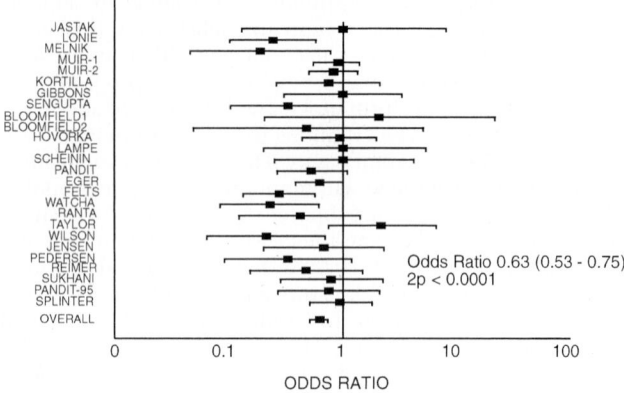

Figure 46-16. Meta-analysis of randomized trials comparing incidence of PONV with or without the use of nitrous oxide.[127] The odds ratios (OR) are plotted on the *x*-axis using a logarithmic scale. The position of each solid square represents the OR of each trial. The horizontal line indicates the 95% confidence interval. In each trial, squares to the left of unity (OR = 1) imply that omission of nitrous oxide reduced the incidence of nausea and vomiting; conversely, squares to the right of unity signify the omission of nitrous oxide increased the likelihood of nausea and vomiting. (Reprinted with permission from Divatia JV, Vaidya JS, Badwe RA, Hawaldar RW: Omission of nitrous oxide during anesthesia reduced the incidence of postoperative nausea and vomiting: A meta-analysis. Anesthesiology 85:1055, 1996.)

tal surgery lasting 2–4 hours, patients who received propofol went home sooner than those who received isoflurane, primarily because of less nausea.[128] Less postoperative nausea after propofol has been reported when it was compared with enflurane, isoflurane, or desflurane. Despite the greater initial cost of propofol, overall costs may be less because treatment for nausea and vomiting is eliminated. In one study of patients undergoing office-based surgical procedures, patients received either propofol or sevoflurane for induction and maintenance.[129] Costs of drugs used for anesthesia were the same; yet, when wasted propofol was also considered, propofol costs were greater by approximately $5.00. Overall, though, average cost per patient was lowest when propofol was used for both induction and maintenance, primarily because of the costs of treating nausea and vomiting ($46 propofol induction and maintenance; $63 propofol induction and sevoflurane maintenance; $72 sevoflurane induction and maintenance).

Muscle relaxation for ambulatory anesthesia extends beyond the time of relaxation for intubation, particularly when nondepolarizing drugs have been used. The clinical effect of the nondepolarizing agent mivacurium, given as a bolus injection to 25% recovery, lasts 12–18 minutes, the shortest duration of effect for the neuromuscular blockers. The duration of action of rocuronium, vecuronium, rapacuronium, and atracurium ranges from 25 to 40 minutes. Because mivacurium is dependent on plasma cholinesterase for metabolism, recovery can be prolonged in the presence of atypical plasma cholinesterase. In patients with normal plasma cholinesterase levels, postoperative vomiting might be reduced if mivacurium does not have to be reversed. Reversal agents must be used unless there is no doubt that muscle relaxation has been fully reversed. When an ambulatory surgery case is expected to last more than 30 minutes, mivacurium may not be indicated. Particularly for children, in whom muscle relaxants generally have decreased potency, thereby enabling more rapid recovery, longer-acting drugs, such as pancuronium, may be used without sequelae. When residual muscle paralysis was examined in children undergoing ambulatory surgery who had received pancuronium, atracurium, or vecuronium, no postoperative weakness could be observed in the PACU.[130]

Opioids, when given intraoperatively, are useful to supplement both intraoperative and postoperative analgesia. Fentanyl

is probably the most popular drug, although all other available narcotics have been tried. All narcotics can cause nausea, sedation and dizziness, which can delay a patient's discharge. Nonsteroidal analgesics are not effective as supplements during general anesthesia, although they are useful in controlling postoperative pain, particularly when given before skin incision. For example, in a study of patients undergoing breast biopsy, patients received intravenous tenoxicam (20 mg) either 30 min before surgery (37 patients) or after incision (40 patients); tenoxicam given before surgery resulted in lower postoperative pain scores, a longer time before additional postoperative analgesia was needed, and lesser amounts of postoperative pain medications than tenoxicam administered after incision.[131] Nerve blocks can also be used in conjuction with general anesthesia, both to decrease intraoperative anesthesia requirement and to effectively reduce postoperative pain.

Certain devices or equipment are commonly used during anesthesia for inpatients. The usefulness of forced-air warmers for the ambulatory surgery patient has been questioned. Patients undergoing general anesthesia for arthroscopic surgery were warmed either with blankets or with a forced-air warmer. Those warmed with forced air were initially 0.4°C warmer in the PACU and 0.6°C warmer after 1 hour, but shivering rates were not different (about 35%) and discharge rates were the same.[132] Routine aspiration of gastric contents to decrease postoperative nausea and vomiting is probably unwarranted, except for laparoscopic surgery. Despite what is commonly stated, insertion of an orogastric tube was associated with an increased incidence of nausea and vomiting (incidence for both was doubled) in ambulatory surgery patients.[133] Bispectral index (BIS) monitors are thought to decrease anesthesia requirement without sacrificing amnesia during general anesthesia. One group found that for ambulatory patients, inhalation anesthetic requirement was reduced with the BIS monitor. However, paralytic use increased to prevent coughing or bucking, and discharge times were no different with or without the use of the BIS monitor.[134]

Using a laryngeal mask airway (LMA) provides several advantages for allowing a patient to return to baseline status quickly. Muscle relaxants required for intubation can be avoided. Coughing is less than with tracheal intubation. Anesthetic requirements are reduced. Hoarseness and sore throat are also reduced. Overall, cost savings result with the use of LMAs. Because of gastric insufflation, though, nausea and vomiting may be greater. The use of the LMA has been described for laparoscopic procedures, although the potential for aspiration exists because of an inflated abdomen during laparoscopy.

MANAGEMENT OF POSTANESTHESIA CARE

Many recovery issues are part of patient selection and perioperative management and must be considered before the patient enters the PACU. Managing common problems in the PACU quickly and effectively is as important as appropriate patient selection and choice of anesthetic technique if the patient is to return home on the day of surgery. The three most common reasons for delay in patient discharge from the PACU are drowsiness, nausea and vomiting, and pain. All three are a function of intraoperative management; but nausea, vomiting, and pain also can be treated in the PACU.

Reversal of Drug Effects

Reversal of muscle relaxants is not unique to the ambulatory surgery patient and will not be discussed here. Reversal of opioids may sometimes be necessary. However, to prevent pain postoperatively, longer-acting drugs, such as morphine, may be used. Flumazenil, a benzodiazepine receptor antagonist, has primarily been used to reverse the effects of sedation after

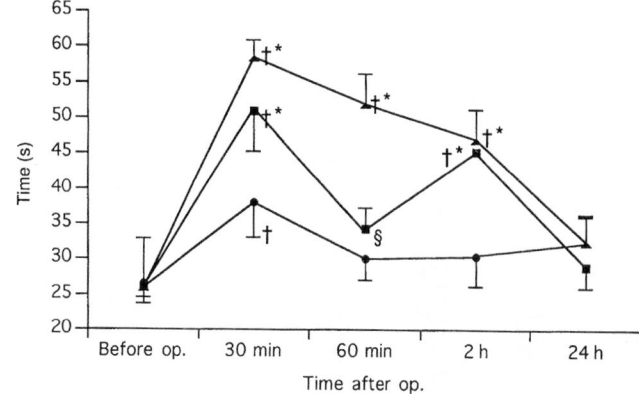

Figure 46-17. Time to perform the serial 7s test (reverse counting aloud from 100 to 44 in steps of 7) after midazolam alone, midazolam and then flumazenil given 60 min after the operation, or propofol. Performance initially improved after flumazenil, but 2 hr after the operation, performance in the two midazolam groups was similarly impaired compared to performance after propofol. (Reprinted with permission from Kestin IG, Harvey PB, Nixon C: Psychomotor recovery after three methods of sedation during spinal anaesthesia. Br J Anaesth 64:675, 1990.)

Midazolam-saline (MS)(●), midazolam-flumazenil (MF)(■) and propofol (P)(▲) groups. $P < 0.05$ compared with: *group P; § group MS; † preoperative baseline.

endoscopy and spinal anesthesia. Reversal of psychomotor impairment with flumazenil is not complete, and the subjective experience of sedation is not necessarily attenuated.[135,136] After 1 hour there was usually no difference in psychomotor performance from control (Fig. 46-17).[136] Even patients who appeared awake still suffered some psychomotor impairment.[135] Reversal of amnesia with flumazenil is only partial, and the duration of the reversal effect may not be long enough to be clinically significant. Flumazenil should not be used routinely as a benzodiazepine antagonist, but only when sedation appears to be excessive. In addition, reversal of benzodiazepine-induced sedation by flumazenil should not replace appropriate ventilatory assistance and, if necessary, placement of an endotracheal tube.

Nausea and Vomiting

Nausea and vomiting are the most common reasons both children and adults have protracted stays in the PACU or unexpected hospital admission. Nausea and vomiting are also the most common adverse effect in patients in the PACU.[137] Much research has been undertaken to study prophylactic treatment of this problem before surgery and the practice techniques in the operating room that can minimize nausea and vomiting in the PACU. The treatment of this problem, once it occurs in the PACU, has not received as much study. Drugs that are useful for this problem include metoclopramide 20 mg, hydroxyzine 25 mg, or droperidol 0.625–1.25 mg. Metoclopramide, 0.15 mg · kg^{-1}, is useful for children.[138] Ondansetron and propofol have also been shown to be effective. In a study of the treatment of nausea and vomiting after ambulatory surgery in more than 500 patients at 10 medical centers, ondansetron doses of 1, 4, and 8 mg were found to be equally effective.[139] Ondansetron 8 mg was similarly effective against nausea or vomiting after laparoscopy.[73] Propofol, 10 mg, prevented nausea with an 81% success rate (vs. 35% with placebo) in the PACU.[140] A dose of 0.5 mg · kg^{-1}, given at the end of an inhalation anesthetic, prolonged awakening time but reduced emesis, request for antiemetic rescue, and time to home readiness by at least 30 minutes.[141] Propofol also can be infused at low doses (8–12 µg after a loading dose of 10 mg) for 2 hr.[142] Because anxiety may be associated with persistent nausea and vomiting, midazolam also has been used for treatment.[143] Because pain may be associated with nausea, treatment of pain frequently decreases nausea.

Pain

Postsurgical pain must be treated quickly and effectively. It is important for the practitioner to differentiate postsurgical pain from the discomfort of hypoxemia, hypercapnia, or a full bladder. Factors that correlate with greater postoperative pain are younger age of patient, less serious illness, greater body mass index; operative site, and duration of surgery.[144] Medications for pain control should be given in small iv doses (e.g., 1–3 mg · 70 kg^{-1} morphine or 10–25 µg · 70^{-1} kg fentanyl). Intramuscular injection of opioid for pain control in the PACU is probably not necessary. Onset of action of drugs is faster after intravenous than after oral administration. Control of postoperative pain may include administration of opioid analgesics or nonsteroidal anti-inflammatory agents, which are not associated with respiratory depression, nausea, or vomiting. Fentanyl is the narcotic frequently used to control postoperative pain, although the effects of morphine last longer. Patients who received fentanyl for pain control required additional injections and went home no sooner compared to patients who received morphine.[145] Patients given ketorolac both iv in the PACU and then orally for up to 6 days postoperatively had less somnolence and earlier return of bowel function than those who received fentanyl in the PACU and codeine with aspirin afterward.[146] In another study, ibuprofen controlled postoperative pain, gave pain relief for a longer period than fentanyl, and was associated with less nausea and vomiting (Fig. 46-18).[147] The effects of iv ketorolac lasted longer than the effects of oral ibuprofen or aspirin.[148] Nonsteroidal anti-inflammatory drugs (NSAIDs) can increase bleeding, although there is no evidence at this time of such a danger for most ambulatory surgery procedures. When swelling and pain are problematic postoperatively, e.g., tooth extraction, NSAIDs can be more effective than opioids in relieving both.[149] Particularly for operations associated with moderate pain, butorphanol, in a nasal spray for delivery, may afford satisfactory relief. Onset of action is rapid (2–3 minutes), and the effects last for 4–5 hours. Because the spray can be taken home for pain treatment, this method of delivery seems ideal for patients undergoing ambulatory surgery. This method is also ideal for children, particularly when no iv is used for (painful) surgery, e.g., myringotomy. Butorphanol is lipophilic, quickly absorbed, and has no vasoactive effects.

We manage pain in both adults and children initially either with a short-acting opioid analgesic, e.g., fentanyl (25 µg · 70 kg^{-1}), or with an injection of ketorolac 60 mg · 70^{-1} kg im or iv. Fentanyl is repeated at 5-minute intervals until pain is controlled. For children, we also use an elixir of acetaminophen containing codeine (120 mg acetaminophen, 12 mg codeine, in each 5 ml of solution). Five milliliters is administered to children between the ages of 3 and 6, and 10 ml to children between the ages of 7 and 12. Children are returned to parental care as soon as they are awake. We find frequently that infants younger than 6 months of age usually need to be reunited with their mothers for nursing (or bottle feeding) after a procedure not associated with severe pain. For older infants and young children in the PACU, acetaminophen, 60 mg per year of age

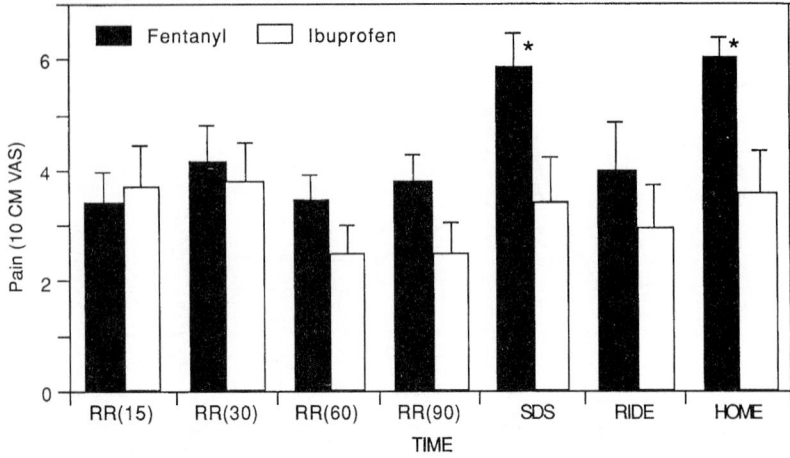

* P < 0.05

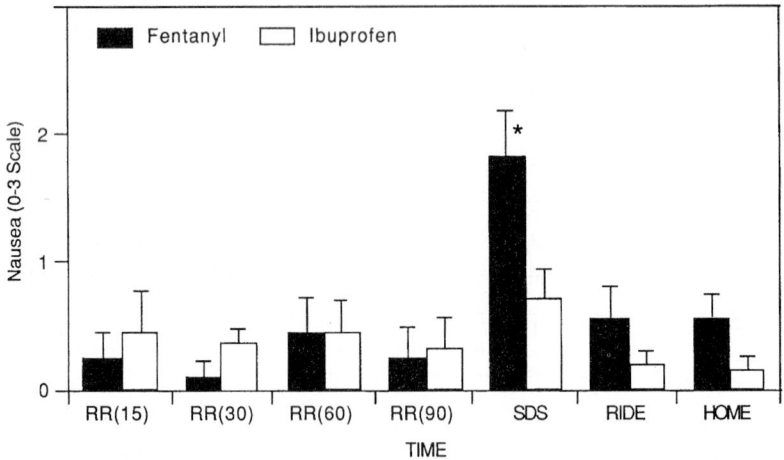

Figure 46-18. Pain and nausea were much less in the same-day surgery stepdown unit, during the ride home, and after arrival home with ibuprofen when either ibuprofen or fentanyl was given preoperatively to patients undergoing laparoscopic surgery. (Reprinted with permission from Rosenblum M, Weller RS, Conard PL *et al:* Ibuprofen provides longer lasting analgesia than fentanyl after laparoscopic surgery. Anesth Analg 73: 255, 1991.)

(given orally or rectally), is commonly used to relieve mild pain. Intravenous fentanyl (up to a dose of 2 μg $\cdot$ kg^{-1} is preferred for more severe pain). Meperidine (0.5 mg $\cdot$ kg^{-1}) and codeine (1–1.5 mg $\cdot$ kg^{-1}) can be given im if an iv route has not been established.

Preparation for Discharging the Patient

In addition to the PACU, many ambulatory surgery centers in the United States have another area, often known as a Phase II recovery room, where patients may stay until they are able to tolerate liquids, walk, and/or void. With the anesthetics that are typically used in ambulatory surgery ORs, patients who are awakened in the OR and are evaluated as 9 or 10 according to the modified Aldrete scoring system may be transferred directly to Phase II recovery from the OR. Some criteria for discharge from the Phase II recovery, however, have been created without scientific basis. One criterion is the ability to tolerate liquids before being discharged. When this criterion was applied to patients 1–18 years of age, incidence of postoperative nausea was greater and hospital stay was 20 minutes longer than in the control groups (Fig. 46-19).[150] Patients who were not required to drink were not readmitted because of dehydration. Similar results have been found in adults.[151] Even though it is warranted after spinal or epidural anesthesia, some data suggest that requiring low-risk patients to void before discharge may be unduly conservative if patients are willing to return to a medical facility if they are unable to void.[152] Perhaps some patients do not need to go to the PACU before going to the Phase II recovery area. We frequently transfer all patients who have had sedation and

some patients who have had a general anesthetic directly to the Phase II recovery area if they can tolerate sitting in a chair in the operating room and can breathe comfortably. Practical criteria for patient discharge from the operating room, from the PACU, and from the Phase II recovery area are needed that in no way compromise patient safety. The value of psychomotor tests to measure different phases of recovery (except for research purposes) is questionable.

Scoring systems have been developed to guide transfer from the PACU to the Phase II recovery room and from Phase II recovery to home (Table 46-2).[153] These criteria do little to test higher levels of function, such as the ability to use one's hands, to drive a car, or to remain alert for long enough to drive. Patients may feel fine after they leave the hospital, but they should be advised against driving for at least 24 hours after a procedure. Patients and responsible parties should be reminded that the patient should not operate power tools or be involved in major business decisions for up to 24 hours. Once the patient leaves the medical facility, supervision may not be as good as it was in the hospital. Therefore, before a patient is discharged, dressings should be checked. It is wise to include the responsible person in all discharge instructions, which are best made available on printed forms.

Patients should also be informed that they may experience pain, headache, nausea, vomiting, or dizziness and, if succinylcholine was used, muscle aches and pains apart from the incision for at least 24 hours. A patient will be less stressed if the described symptoms are expected in the course of a normal recovery. Written instructions are important. In 100 consecutive outpatients who were given no written instructions at discharge,

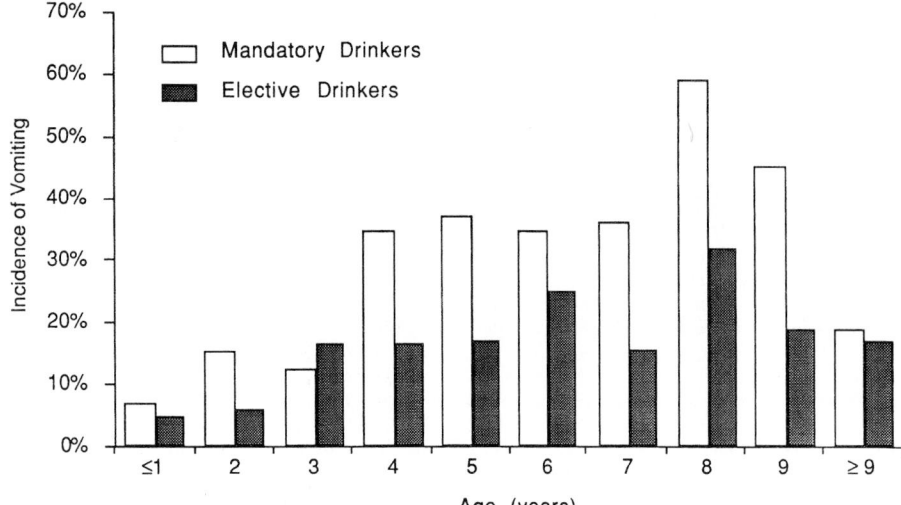

Figure 46-19. The incidence of vomiting in the day surgery unit was significantly less in those individuals who were allowed to drink electively compared with those who were required to drink prior to discharge. (Reprinted with permission from Schreiner MS, Triebwasser A, Keon TP: Ingestion of liquids compared with preoperative fasting in pediatric outpatients. Anesthesiology 72:593, 1990.)

despite oral instructions to the contrary, 31% of patients went home unaccompanied by a responsible adult; 73% of car owners drove within 24 hours of surgery (30% within 12 hours); 9% of patients drove themselves home; and a bus driver returned to work on the same day, to drive a busload of passengers a distance of 95 miles.[154] The addition of written and oral education techniques at discharge has a significant impact on improving compliance.

For patients with a language barrier (*e.g.,* in a population with a high percentage of immigrants), consent forms, procedural explanation, and discharge information may have to be written in languages other than English and the services of an interpreter may be necessary. Nursing staff should assess the adult who will take the patient home to determine whether he or she is in fact a responsible person. A responsible person is someone who is physically and intellectually able to take care of the patient at home. Facilities should develop a method of follow-up after the patient has been discharged. At some facilities staff members telephone the patient the next day to determine the progress of recovery; others use follow-up postcards.

Table 46-2. POSTANESTHETIC DISCHARGE SCORING SYSTEM*

Vital signs
   2 = within 20% of preoperative value
   1 = 20–40% of preoperative value
   0 = 40% of preoperative value
Ambulation and mental status
   2 = oriented × 3 and has a steady gait
   1 = oriented × 3 or has a steady gait
   0 = neither
Pain or nausea
   2 = minimal
   1 = moderate
   0 = severe
Surgical bleeding
   2 = minimal
   1 = moderate
   0 = severe
Intake and output
   2 = has had po fluids and has voided
   1 = has had po fluids or has voided
   0 = neither

* The total score is 10; if the patient's score is 9, then the patient is fit for discharge. Reprinted with permission from Chung F: Are discharge criteria changing? J Clin Anesth 5:64S, 1993.

Whenever we become innovative in the management of our outpatients, we must assess how a cost-effective "no frills" approach to care affects patient safety. We must determine what we can do for the patient who lives alone, the patient whose responsible person is unable to manage his or her needs, the patient without means of transportation, and the patient with limited insurance coverage. Hospital beds can be set aside for patients who require observation. Patients in these beds after an ambulatory surgical procedure are still considered outpatients. They are charged for the hours spent in the observation area. Some hospitals have joined with management firms to build a hospital hotel or medical motel close to the hospital itself. The hotel, usually a nonmedical facility, offers the outpatient a comfortable, inexpensive, and convenient place to recuperate while being cared for by family or nurses. Home health care nursing may be appropriate after surgical procedures such as reduction mammoplasty, abdominoplasty, vaginal hysterectomy, and major open ligament repairs of the knee. The various services for outpatient observation and home health care stand today where outpatient surgery stood in the health care delivery system 20 years ago. Prospective studies are needed to assess the quality of care and the effect these innovative approaches have on patient safety.

Patient, procedure, availability and quality of aftercare, and anesthetic technique must be individually and collectively assessed to determine acceptability for ambulatory surgery. A delicate balance must be maintained between the physical status of patient, the proposed surgical procedure, and the appropriate anesthetic technique, to which must be added the expertise level of the anesthesiologist caring for a patient.

Anesthesia for ambulatory surgery is a rapidly evolving specialty. Patients once thought unsuitable for ambulatory surgery are now considered to be appropriate candidates. Operations once thought unsuitable for outpatients are now routinely performed in the morning so that the patient can be discharged in the afternoon or evening. The appropriate anesthetic management before these patients come to the operating room, during their operation, and then afterwards is the key to success. The availability of both shorter-acting anesthetics and longer-acting analgesics and antiemetics enables us to care for patients in ambulatory centers effectively.

REFERENCES

1. Packard FR: History of Medicine in the United States. New York, Paul B Hoeber, 1931
2. Vandam LD: A history of ambulatory anesthesia. Anesthesiol Clin North Am 5:1, 1987

3. Zuger A: Surgeons leaving the O.R. for the office. New York Times May 18, 1999, Section F, page 1

4. McManus SA, Topp DA, Hopkins C: Advantages of outpatient breast surgery. Am Surg 60:967, 1994

5. Yardley MPJ: Tonsillectomy, adenoidectomy and adenotonsillectomy: Are they safe day case procedures? J Laryngol Otol 106:299, 1992

6. Tom LWC, DeDio RM, Cohen DE *et al:* Is outpatient tonsillectomy appropriate for young children? Laryngoscope 102:277, 1992

7. Meridy HW: Criteria for selection of ambulatory surgical patients and guidelines for anesthetic management: A retrospective study of 1553 cases. Anesth Analg 61:921, 1982

8. Freeman LN, Schachat AP, Manolio TA, Enger C: Multivariate analysis of factors associated with unplanned admission in "outpatient" ophthalmic surgery. Ophthalmic Surg 19:719, 1988

9. Lammers PK, Palmer PN: Surgeons discuss ambulatory surgery, legislative concerns, dangers of transfusions, surgical advances. AORN J 53:16, 1991

10. Meeks GR, Waller GA, Meydrech EF, Flautt FH Jr: Unscheduled hospital admission following ambulatory gynecologic surgery. Obstet Gynecol 80:446, 1992

11. Kurth CD, Spitzer AR, Broennle AM, Downes JJ: Postoperative apnea in preterm infants. Anesthesiology 66:483, 1987

12. Welborn LG, Ramirez N, Oh TH *et al:* Postanesthetic apnea and periodic breathing in infants. Anesthesiology 65:658, 1986

13. Welborn LG, Hannallah RS, Luban NLC *et al:* Anemia and postoperative apnea in former preterm infants. Anesthesiology 74:1003, 1991

14. Welborn LG, Hannallah RS, Fink R *et al:* High-dose caffeine suppresses postoperative apnea in former preterm infants. Anesthesiology 71:347, 1989

15. Welborn LG, Rice LJ, Hannallah RS *et al:* Postoperative apnea in former preterm infants: Prospective comparison of spinal and general anesthesia. Anesthesiology 72:838, 1990

16. Osborne GA, Rudkin GE: Outcome after day-care surgery in a major teaching hospital. Anaesth Intensive Care 21:822, 1993

17. Biswas TK, Leary C: Postoperative hospital admission from a day surgery unit: A seven-year retrospective survey. Anaesth Intensive Care 20:147, 1992

18. Levin P, Stanziola A, Hand R: Postoperative hospital retention following ambulatory surgery in a hospital-based program. Qual Assur Util Rev 5:90, 1990

19. Twersky R, Fishman D, Homel P: What happens after discharge? Return hospital visits after ambulatory surgery. Anesth Analg 84:319, 1997

20. Warner MA, Shields SE, Chute CG: Major morbidity and mortality within 1 month of ambulatory surgery and anesthesia. JAMA 270:1437, 1993

21. Patel RI, Hannallah RS: Preoperative screening for pediatric ambulatory surgery: Evaluation of a telephone questionnaire method. Anesth Analg 75:258, 1992

22. Egbert LD, Battit GE, Turndorf H, Beecher HK: The value of the preoperative visit by an anesthetist. JAMA 185:553, 1963

23. Wallace LM: Psychological preparation as a method of reducing the stress of surgery. J Human Stress 10:62, 1984

24. Domar AD, Noe JM, Benson H: The preoperative use of the relaxation response with ambulatory surgery patients. J Human Stress 13:101, 1987

25. Markland D, Hardy L: Anxiety, relaxation and anaesthesia for day-case surgery. Br J Clin Psychol 32:493, 1993

26. Hill S, Yau K, Whitwam J: MAOIs to RIMAs in anaesthesia: A literature review. Psychopharmacology 106:S43, 1992

27. Schreiner MS, O'Hara I, Markakis DA, Politis GD: Do children who experience laryngospasm have an increased risk of upper respiratory tract infection? Anesthesiology 85:474, 1996.

28. Tait AR, Pandit UA, Voepel-Lewis T *et al:* Use of the laryngeal mask airway in children with upper respiratory tract infections: A comparison with endotracheal intubation. Anesth Analg 86:706, 1998

29. Hjortsø E, Mondorf T: Does oral premedication increase the risk of gastric aspiration? A study to compare the effect of diazepam given orally and intramuscularly on the volume and acidity of gastric aspirate. Acta Anaesthesiol Scand 26:505, 1982

30. McGrady EM, Macdonald AG: Effect of the preoperative administration of water on gastric volume and pH. Br J Anaesth 60:803, 1988

31. Hutchinson A, Maltby JR, Reid CRG: Gastric fluid volume and pH in elective inpatients: Part I: Coffee or orange juice versus overnight fast. Can J Anaesth 35:12, 1988

32. Splinter WM, Stewart JA, Muir JG: The effect of preoperative apple juice on gastric contents, thirst, and hunger in children. Can J Anaesth 36:55, 1989

33. Schreiner MS, Triebwasser A, Keon TP: Ingestion of liquids compared with preoperative fasting in pediatric outpatients. Anesthesiology 72:593, 1990

34. Green CR, Pandit SK, Schork MA: Preoperative fasting time: Is the traditional policy changing? Results of a national survey. Anesth Analg 83:123, 1996

35. Fennelly M, Galletly DC, Purdie GI: Is caffeine withdrawal the mechanism of postoperative headache? Anesth Analg 72:449, 1991

36. Kelly RE, Hartman GS, Embree PB *et al:* Inhaled induction and emergence from desflurane anesthesia in the ambulatory surgical patient: The effect of premedication. Anesth Analg 77:540, 1993

37. Johnston M: Anxiety in surgical patients. Psychol Med 10:145, 1980

38. Aantaa R, Jaakola M-L, Kallio A *et al:* A comparison of dexmedetomidine, an α_2-adrenoceptor agonist, and midazolam as i.m. premedication for minor gynaecological surgery. Br J Anaesth 67:402, 1991

39. Badner NH, Nielson WR, Munk S *et al:* Preoperative anxiety: Detection and contributing factors. Can J Anaesth 37:444, 1990

40. Kain ZN, Wang SM, Mayes LC *et al:* Distress during the induction of anesthesia and postoperative behavioral outcomes. Anesth Analg 88:1042, 1999

41. Kain ZN, Mayes LC, Wang SM *et al:* Parental presence during induction of anesthesia versus sedative premedication: Which intervention is more effective? Anesthesiology 89:1147, 1998

42. Greenblatt DJ, Abernethy DR, Locniskar A *et al:* Effect of age, gender, and obesity on midazolam kinetics. Anesthesiology 61:27, 1984

43. Bell GD, Spickett GP, Reeve PA *et al:* Intravenous midazolam for upper gastrointestinal endoscopy: A study of 800 consecutive cases relating dose to age and sex of patient. Br J Clin Pharmacol 23:241, 1987

44. Brophy T, Dundee JW, Heazelwood V *et al:* Midazolam, a water-soluble benzodiazepine, for gastroscopy. Anaesth Intensive Care 10:344, 1982

45. Levine MF, Spahr-Schopfer IA, Hartley E *et al:* Oral midazolam premedication in children: The minimum time interval for separation from parents. Can J Anaesth 40:726, 1993

46. McMillan CO, Spahr-Schopfer IA, Sikich N *et al:* Premedication of children with oral midazolam. Can J Anaesth 39:545, 1992

47. Samuelson PN, Reves JG, Kouchoukos NT *et al:* Hemodynamic responses to anesthetic induction with midazolam or diazepam in patients with ischemic heart disease. Anesth Analg 60:802, 1981

48. Bell GD, Reeve PA, Moshiri M *et al:* Intravenous midazolam: A study of the degree of oxygen desaturation occurring during upper gastrointestinal endoscopy. Br J Clin Pharmacol 23:703, 1987

49. Raeder JC, Breivik H: Premedication with midazolam in out-patient general anaesthesia. A comparison with morphine-scopolamine and placebo. Acta Anaesthesiol Scand 31:509, 1987

50. Feld LH, Champeau MW, van Steennis CA, Scott JC: Preanesthetic medication in children: A comparison of oral transmucosal fentanyl citrate versus placebo. Anesthesiology 71:374, 1989

51. Friesen RH, Lockhart CH: Oral transmucosal fentanyl citrate for preanesthetic medication of pediatric day surgery patients with and without droperidol as a prophylactic anti-emetic. Anesthesiology 76:46, 1992

52. Ding Y, White PF: Comparative effects of ketorolac, dezocine, and fentanyl as adjuvants during outpatient anesthesia. Anesth Analg 75:566, 1992

53. Grattidge P: Patient-controlled sedation using propofol in day surgery. Anaesthesia 47:683, 1992

54. Ferrari LR, Donlon JV: A comparison of propofol, midazolam, and methohexital for sedation during retrobulbar and peribulbar block. J Clin Anesth 4:93, 1992

55. Winwood MA, Jago RH: Anxiety levels following anaesthesia for day-case surgery: A comparison of state anxiety levels following induction of anaesthesia with propofol or thiopentone. Anaesthesia 48:581, 1993

56. Douglass WW: Histamine and 5-hydroxytryptamine (serotonin) and their antagonists. In Gilman AG, Goodman LS, Rall TW, Murad F (eds): Goodman and Gilman's The Pharmacological Basis of Therapeutics, 7th ed, p 624. New York, Macmillan, 1985

57. Schentag JJ, Cerra FB, Calleri G *et al:* Pharmacokinetic and clinical

studies in patients with cimetidine-associated mental confusion. Lancet 1:177, 1979

58. Cederberg C, Andersson T, Skanberg I: Omeprazole: Pharmacokinetics and metabolism in man. Scand J Gastroenterol 24 (suppl):33, 1989

59. Haskins DA, Jahr JS, Texidor M, Ramadhyani U: Single-dose oral omeprazole for reduction of gastric residual acidity in adults for outpatient surgery. Acta Anaesthesiol Scand 36:513, 1992

60. Faure EA, Lim HS, Block BS et al: Sodium bicarbonate buffers gastric acid during surgery in obstetric and gynecologic patients. Anesthesiology 67:274, 1987

61. Dimich I, Katende R, Singh PP et al: The effects of intravenous cimetidine and metoclopramide on gastric pH and volume in outpatients. J Clin Anesth 3:40, 1991

62. Gralla RJ: Metoclopramide: A review of antiemetic trials. Drugs 25(suppl):63, 1983

63. Green G, Jonsson L: Nausea: The most important factor determining length of stay after ambulatory anaesthesia. A comparative study of isoflurane and/or propofol techniques. Acta Anaesthesiol Scand 37:742, 1993

64. Millar JM, Hall PJ: Nausea and vomiting after prostaglandins in day case termination of pregnancy: The efficacy of low dose droperidol. Anaesthesia 42:613, 1987

65. O'Donovan N, Shaw J: Nausea and vomiting in day-case dental anaesthesia: The use of low-dose droperidol. Anaesthesia 39:1172, 1984

66. Melnick B, Sawyer R, Karambelkar D et al: Delayed side effects of droperidol after ambulatory general anesthesia. Anesth Analg 69:748, 1989

67. Watcha MF, Simeon RM, White PF, Stevens JL: Effect of propofol on the incidence of postoperative vomiting after strabismus surgery in pediatric outpatients. Anesthesiology 75:204, 1991

68. Blanc VF, Ruest P, Milot J et al: Antiemetic prophylaxis with promethazine or droperidol in paediatric outpatient strabismus surgery. Can J Anaesth 38:54, 1991

69. Chaffee BJ, Tankanow RM: Ondansetron—the first of a new class of antiemetic agents. Clin Pharm 10:430, 1991

70. Pearman MH: Single dose intravenous ondansetron in the prevention of postoperative nausea and vomiting. Anaesthesia 49 (suppl):11, 1994

71. Malins AF, Field JM, Nesling PM, Cooper GM: Nausea and vomiting after gynaecological laparoscopy: Comparison of premedication with oral ondansetron, metoclopramide and placebo. Br J Anaesth 72:231, 1994

72. Alon E, Himmelseher S: Ondansetron in the treatment of postoperative vomiting: A randomized, double-blind comparison with droperidol and metoclopramide. Anesth Analg 75:561, 1992

73. Davis PJ, McGowan FX Jr, Landsman I et al: Effect of antiemetic therapy on recovery and hospital discharge time. A double-blind assessment of ondansetron, droperidol, and placebo in pediatric patients undergoing ambulatory surgery. Anesthesiology 83:956, 1995

74. Bodner M, White PF: Antiemetic efficacy of ondansetron after outpatient laparoscopy. Anesth Analg 73:250, 1991

75. Tang J, Wang B, White PF et al: The effect of timing of ondansetron administration on its efficacy, cost-effectiveness, and cost–benefit as a prophylactic antiemetic in the ambulatory setting. Anesth Analg 86:274, 1998

76. Fan CF, Tanhui E, Joshi S et al: Acupressure treatment for prevention of postoperative nausea and vomiting. Anesth Analg 84:821, 1997

77. Yogendran S, Asokumar B, Cheng DCH, Chung F: A prospective randomized double-blinded study of the effect of intravenous fluid therapy on adverse outcomes on outpatient surgery. Anesth Analg 80:682, 1995

78. Chye EP, Young IG, Osborne GA, Rudkin GE: Outcomes after same-day oral surgery: A review of 1180 cases at a major teaching hospital. J Oral Maxillofac Surg 51:846, 1993

79. Raeder JC: Propofol anaesthesia versus paracervical blockade with alfentanil and midazolam sedation for outpatient abortion. Acta Anaesthesiol Scand 36:31, 1992

80. Fairclough JA, Graham GP, Pemberton D: Local or general anaesthetic in day case arthroscopy? Ann R Coll Surg Engl 72:104, 1990

81. Yeo SW, Tay D, Chong JL, Tan TK: General anaesthesia vs sedation for minor gynaecological procedures—a comparative study. Singapore Med J 34:395, 1993

82. Dahl JB, Schultz P, Anker-Møller E et al: Spinal anaesthesia in

young patients using a 29-gauge needle: Technical considerations and an evaluation of postoperative complaints compared with general anaesthesia. Br J Anaesth 64:178, 1990

83. Monk TG, Bouré B, White PF et al: Comparison of intravenous sedative-analgesic techniques for outpatient immersion lithotripsy. Anesth Analg 72:616, 1991

84. Cohen DD, Dillon JB: Anesthesia for outpatient surgery. JAMA 196:1114, 1966

85. D'Eramo EM: Morbidity and mortality with outpatient anesthesia: The Massachusetts experience. J Oral Maxillofac Surg 50:700, 1992

86. Liguori GA, Zayas VM, Chisholm MF: Transient neurologic symptoms after spinal anesthesia with mepivacaine and lidocaine. Anesthesiology 88:619, 1998

87. Campbell DC, Douglas MJ, Pavy TJG et al: Comparison of the 25-gauge Whitacre with the 24-gauge Sprotte spinal needle for elective caesarean section: Cost implications. Can J Anaesth 40:1131, 1993

88. Buettner J, Wresch KP, Klose R: Postdural puncture headache: Comparison of 25-gauge Whitacre and Quincke needles. Reg Anaesth 18:166, 1993

89. Lynch J, Arhelger S, Krings-Ernst I et al: Whitacre 22-gauge pencil-point needle for spinal anaesthesia: A controlled trial in 300 young orthopaedic patients. Anaesth Intensive Care 20:322, 1992

90. Kang SB, Goodnough DE, Lee YK et al: Comparison of 26- and 27-G needles for spinal anesthesia for ambulatory surgery patients. Anesthesiology 76:734, 1992

91. Sarma VJ, Boström U: Intrathecal anaesthesia for day-care surgery: A retrospective study of 160 cases using 25- and 26-gauge spinal needles. Anaesthesia 45:769, 1990

92. Despond O, Meuret P, Hemmings G: Postdural puncture headache after spinal anaesthesia in young orthopaedic outpatients using 27-g needles. Can J Anaesth 45:1106, 1998

93. Shutt LE, Valentine SJ, Wee MYK et al: Spinal anaesthesia for caesarean section: Comparison of 22-gauge and 25-gauge Whitacre needles with 26-gauge Quincke needles. Br J Anaesth 69:589, 1992

94. Brattebo G, Wisborg T, Rodt SA, Bjerkan B: Intrathecal anaesthesia in patients under 45 years: Incidence of postdural puncture symptoms after spinal anaesthesia with 27G needles. Acta Anaesthesiol Scand 37:545, 1993

95. Carbaat PAT, van Crevel H: Lumbar puncture headache: Controlled study on the preventive effect of 24 hours' bed rest. Lancet: 2:1133, 1981

96. Thornberry EA, Thomas TA: Posture and post-spinal headache: A controlled trial in 80 obstetric patients. Br J Anaesth 60:195, 1988

97. Sarma VJ, Lundström J: Epidural anaesthesia for day care surgery: A retrospective study. Anaesthesia 44:683, 1989

98. Gunter JB, Dunn CM, Bennie JB et al: Optimum concentration of bupivacaine for combined caudal–general anesthesia in children. Anesthesiology 75:57, 1991

99. Rice IJ, Pudimat MA, Hannallah RS: Timing of caudal block placement in relation to surgery does not affect duration of postoperative analgesia in paediatric ambulatory patients. Can J Anaesth 37:429, 1990

100. Vloka JD, Hadzic A, Mulcare R et al: Femoral and genitofemoral nerve blocks versus spinal anesthesia for outpatients undergoing long saphenous vein stripping surgery. Anesth Analg 84:749, 1997

101. Cohen MM, Duncan PG, Tate RB: Does anesthesia contribute to operative mortality? JAMA 260:2859, 1988

102. Smith I, Monk TG, White PF, Ding Y: Propofol infusion during regional anesthesia: Sedative, amnestic and anxiolytic properties. Anesth Analg 79:313, 1994

103. Terndrup TE, Dire DJ, Madden CM et al: A prospective analysis of intramuscular meperidine, promethazine, and chlorpromazine in pediatric emergency department patients. Ann Emerg Med 20:31, 1991

104. Hannallah RS, Patel RI: Low-dose intramuscular ketamine for anesthesia pre-induction in young children undergoing brief outpatient procedures. Anesthesiology 70:598, 1989

105. Alderson PJ, Lerman J: Oral premedication for paediatric ambulatory anaesthesia: A comparison of midazolam and ketamine. Can J Anaesth 41:221, 1994

106. Cook BA, Bass JW, Nomizu S, Alexander ME: Sedation of children for technical procedures: Current standard of practice. Clin Pediatr 31:137, 1992

107. Rodrigo MRC, Tong CKA: A comparison of patient and anaesthe-

tist controlled midazolam sedation for dental surgery. Anaesthesia 49:241, 1994

108. Osborne GA, Rudkin GE, Curtis NJ *et al:* Intra-operative patient-controlled sedation: Comparison of patient-controlled propofol with anaesthetist-administered midazolam and fentanyl. Anaesthesia 46:553, 1991

109. Church JA, Pollock JSS, Still DM, Parbrook GD: Comparison of two techniques for sedation in dental surgery. Anaesthesia 46:780, 1991

110. Prstojevich SJ, Sabol SR, Goldwasser MS, Johnson C: Utility of capnography in predicting venous carbon dioxide partial pressure in sedated patients during outpatient oral surgery. J Oral Maxillofac Surg 50:37, 1992

111. Sá Rêgo MM, Watcha MF, White PF: The changing role of monitored anesthesia care in the ambulatory setting. Anesth Analg 85:1020, 1997

112. Korttila K, Nuotto EJ, Lichtor JL *et al:* Clinical recovery and psychomotor function after brief anesthesia with propofol or thiopental. Anesthesiology 76:676, 1992

113. Gupta A, Larsen LE, Sjöberg F *et al:* Thiopentone or propofol for induction of isoflurane-based anaesthesia for ambulatory surgery? Acta Anaesthesiol Scand 36:670, 1992

114. Hannallah RS, Britton JT, Schafer PG *et al:* Propofol anaesthesia in paediatric ambulatory patients: A comparison with thiopentone and halothane. Can J Anaesth 41:12, 1994

115. Helbo-Hansen S, Westergaard V, Krogh BL, Svendsen HP: The reduction of pain on injection of propofol: The effect of addition of lignocaine. Acta Anaesthesiol Scand 32:502, 1988

116. Fredman B, Nathanson MH, Smith I *et al:* Sevoflurane for outpatient anesthesia: A comparison with propofol. Anesth Analg 81:823, 1995

117. Philip BK, Lombard LL, Roaf ER *et al:* Comparison of vital capacity induction with sevoflurane to intravenous induction with propofol for adult ambulatory anesthesia. Anesth Analg 89:623, 1999

118. Churchill-Davidson HC: Suxamethonium (succinylcholine) chloride and muscle pains. Br Med J 1:74, 1954

119. Wierda JM, van den Broek L, Proost JH *et al:* Time course of action and endotracheal intubating conditions of ORG 9487, a new short-acting steroidal muscle relaxant; a comparison with succinylcholine. Anesth Analg 77:579, 1993

120. Purdy R, Bevan DR, Donati F, Lichtor JL: Early reversal of rapacuronium with neostigmine. Anesthesiology 91:51, 1999

121. Pühringer FK, Khuenl-Brady KS, Koller J, Mitterschiffthaler G: Evaluation of the endotracheal intubating conditions of rocuronium (ORG 9426) and succinylcholine in outpatient surgery. Anesth Analg 75:37, 1992

122. Hwang KH, Kim SC, Kim SY *et al:* Neuromuscular and hemodynamic effects of mivacurium and succinylcholine in adult patients during nitrous oxide-propofol-fentanyl anesthesia. J Korean Med Sci 8:374, 1993

123. Song D, Joshi G, White PF: Fast-track eligibility after ambulatory anesthesia: A comparison of desflurane, sevoflurane, and propofol. Anesth Analg 86:267, 1998

124. Pollard BJ, Bryan A, Bennett D *et al:* Recovery after oral surgery with halothane, enflurane, isoflurane or propofol anaesthesia. Br J Anaesth 72:559, 1994

125. Davis PJ, Cohen IT, McGowan FX Jr, Latta K: Recovery characteristics of desflurane versus halothane for maintenance of anesthesia in pediatric ambulatory patients. Anesthesiology 80:298, 1994

126. Weiskopf RB, Moore MA, Eger EI II *et al:* Rapid increase in desflurane concentration is associated with greater transient cardiovascular stimulation than with rapid increase in isoflurane concentration in humans. Anesthesiology 80:1035, 1994

127. Divatia JV, Vaidya JS, Badwe RA, Hawaldar RW: Omission of nitrous oxide during anesthesia reduces the incidence of postoperative nausea and vomiting: A meta-analysis. Anesthesiology 85:1055, 1996

128. Valanne J: Recovery and discharge of patients after long propofol infusion vs isoflurane anaesthesia for ambulatory surgery. Acta Anaesthesiol Scand 36:530, 1992

129. Tang J, Chen L, White PF *et al:* Recovery profile, costs, and patient satisfaction with propofol and sevoflurane for fast-track office-based anesthesia. Anesthesiology 91:253, 1999.

130. Baxter MR, Bevan JC, Samuel J *et al:* Postoperative neuromuscular function in pediatric day-care patients. Anesth Analg 72:504, 1991

131. Colbert ST, O'Hanlon DM, McDonnell C *et al:* Analgesia in day case breast biopsy—the value of pre-emptive tenoxicam. Can J Anaesth 45:217, 1998

132. Smith I, Newson CD, White PF: Use of forced-air warming during and after outpatient arthroscopic surgery. Anesth Analg 78:836, 1994

133. Trepanier CA, Isabel L: Perioperative gastric aspiration increases postoperative nausea and vomiting in outpatients. Can J Anaesth 40:325, 1993

134. Song D, Joshi GP, White PF: Titration of volatile anesthetics using bispectral index facilitates recovery after ambulatory anesthesia. Anesthesiology 87:842, 1997

135. Sanders LD, Piggott SE, Isaac PA *et al:* Reversal of benzodiazepine sedation with the antagonist flumazenil. Br J Anaesth 66:445, 1991

136. Kestin IG, Harvey PB, Nixon C: Psychomotor recovery after three methods of sedation during spinal anaesthesia. Br J Anaesth 64:675, 1990

137. Duncan PG, Cohen MM, Tweed WA *et al:* The Canadian four-centre study of anaesthetic outcomes: III. Are anaesthetic complications predictable in day surgical practice? Can J Anaesth 39:440, 1992

138. Ferrari LR, Donlon JV: Metoclopramide reduces the incidence of vomiting after tonsillectomy in children. Anesth Analg 75:351, 1992

139. Scuderi P, Wetchler B, Sung YF *et al:* Treatment of postoperative nausea and vomiting after outpatient surgery with the 5-HT$_3$ antagonist ondansetron. Anesthesiology 78:15, 1993

140. Borgeat A, Wilder-Smith OH, Saiah M, Rifat K: Subhypnotic doses of propofol possess direct antiemetic properties. Anesth Analg 74:539, 1992

141. Song D, Whitten CW, White PF *et al:* Antiemetic activity of propofol after sevoflurane and desflurane anesthesia for outpatient laparoscopic cholecystectomy. Anesthesiology 89:838, 1998

142. Gan TJ, Glass PSA, Howell ST *et al:* Determination of plasma concentrations of propofol associated with 50% reduction in postoperative nausea. Anesthesiology 87:779, 1997

143. Di Florio T: The use of midazolam for persistent postoperative nausea and vomiting. Anaesth Intensive Care 20:383, 1992

144. Chung F, Ritchie E, Su J: Postoperative pain in ambulatory surgery. Anesth Analg 85:808, 1997

145. Claxton AR, McGuire G, Chung F, Cruise C: Evaluation of morphine versus fentanyl for postoperative analgesia after ambulatory surgical procedures. Anesth Analg 84:509, 1997

146. Wong HY, Carpenter RL, Kopacz DJ *et al:* A randomized, double-blind evaluation of ketorolac tromethamine for postoperative analgesia in ambulatory surgery patients. Anesthesiology 78:6, 1993

147. Rosenblum M, Weller RS, Conard PL *et al:* Ibuprofen provides longer lasting analgesia than fentanyl after laparoscopic surgery. Anesth Analg 73:255, 1991

148. Morrison NA, Repka MX: Ketorolac versus acetaminophen or ibuprofen in controlling postoperative pain in patients with strabismus. Ophthalmology 101:915, 1994

149. Lysell L, Anzen B: Pain control after third molar surgery—a comparative study of ibuprofen (Ibumetin) and a paracetamol/codeine combination (Citodon). Swed Dent J 16:151, 1992

150. Schreiner MS, Nicolson SC, Martin T, Whitney L: Should children drink before discharge from day surgery? Anesthesiology 76:528, 1992

151. Jin F, Norris A, Chung F, Ganeshram T: Should adult patients drink fluids before discharge from ambulatory surgery? Anesth Analg 87:306, 1998

152. Pavlin DJ, Pavlin EG, Gunn HC, *et al:* Voiding in patients managed with or without ultrasound monitoring of bladder volume after outpatient surgery. Anesth Analg 89:90, 1999

153. Chung F: Are discharge criteria changing? J Clin Anesth 5(suppl 1):64S, 1993

154. Ogg TW: An assessment of postoperative outpatient cases. Br Med J 4:573, 1972

Clinical Anesthesia (4/e), edited by
Paul G. Barash, Bruce F. Cullen, and
Robert K. Stoelting. Lippincott Williams &
Wilkins, Philadelphia, © 2001.

CHAPTER 47

MONITORED ANESTHESIA CARE

SIMON C. HILLIER

Monitored anesthesia care is usually provided to patients undergoing therapeutic or diagnostic procedures that would otherwise be unacceptably uncomfortable or unsafe without the continuous attention of an anesthesiologist who is solely dedicated to optimizing the patient's comfort and safety. Monitored anesthesia care commonly, but not necessarily, involves the administration of drugs with anxiolytic, hypnotic, analgesic, and amnestic properties, either alone or as a supplement to a local or regional technique.

TERMINOLOGY

It is important to distinguish between "monitored anesthesia care" and "sedation/analgesia." *Sedation/analgesia,* which has replaced the previously used term "conscious sedation," is the term currently used by the American Society of Anesthesiologists (ASA) in their recently published Practice Guidelines for Sedation and Analgesia by Non-anesthesiologists.[1] *Conscious sedation,* a term first introduced by the American Dental Association (ADA), described the level of sedation provided to patients during dental procedures.[2] The ADA defined conscious sedation as "a depressed level of consciousness that allows the patient the ability to independently and continuously maintain an airway and respond appropriately to physical stimulation and verbal command." The current ASA definition of sedation/analgesia is "a state which allows patients to tolerate unpleasant procedures while maintaining adequate cardiorespiratory function and the ability to respond purposefully to verbal command or tactile stimulation." Thus, conscious sedation or sedation/analgesia is intended to be a lighter level of sedation than may be encountered during monitored anesthesia care. The term sedation/analgesia is used most frequently in the context of care provided by nonanesthesiologists, and implies a level of vigilance that is less than that required for general anesthesia.[3] The ASA specifically states that those patients whose only response is reflex withdrawal from a painful stimulus are sedated to greater degree than encompassed by the term sedation/analgesia. Significant inter-patient variability in dose response will cause some patients intended to receive sedation/analgesia to be rapidly sedated to a level much deeper than intended. Indeed, some patients may have no movement in response to painful stimulus (general anesthesia). This situation compromises patient safety and may increase morbidity and mortality. Education of nonanesthesiologist providers as described by the ASA practice guidelines is intended to reduce the likelihood of such outcomes. *Monitored anesthesia care* implies the potential for a deeper level of sedation than that provided by sedation/analgesia and is always administered by an anesthesiologist provider. The standards for preoperative evaluation, intraoperative monitoring, continuous presence of a member of the anesthesia care team, etc. are no different from those for general or regional anesthesia.[4]

Conceptually, monitored anesthesia care is attractive because it should invoke less physiologic disturbance and allow a more rapid recovery than general anesthesia. It is instructive to review the ASA position statement approved by the House of Delegates in 1986 and last amended in 1998.[4] The ASA definition of monitored anesthesia care is as follows:

Monitored anesthesia care is a specific anesthesia service in which an anesthesiologist has been requested to participate in the care of a patient undergoing a diagnostic or therapeutic procedure.

Monitored anesthesia care includes all aspects of anesthesia care—a preprocedure visit, intraoperative care and postprocedure anesthesia management.

During monitored anesthesia care, the anesthesiologist or a member of the anesthesia care team provides a number of specific services, including but not limited to:

Monitoring of vital signs, maintenance of the patient's airway and continual evaluation of vital functions

Diagnosis and treatment of clinical problems which occur during the procedure

Administration of sedatives, analgesics, hypnotics, anesthetic agents or other medications as necessary to ensure patient safety and comfort

Provision of other medical services as needed to accomplish the safe completion of the procedure

Monitored anesthesia care often includes the administration of doses of medications for which the loss of normal protective reflexes or loss of consciousness is likely. Monitored anesthesia care refers to those clinical situations in which the patient remains able to protect the airway for the majority of the procedure. If, for an extended period of time, the patient is rendered unconscious and/or loses normal protective reflexes, then anesthesia care shall be considered a general anesthetic.

Because monitored anesthesia care is a physician service provided to an individual patient and is based on medical necessity, it should be subject to the same level of reimbursement as general or regional anesthesia. Accordingly, the ASA Relative Value Guide provides for the use of proper basic procedural units, time units and age and risk modifier units as the basis for determining reimbursement.

The ASA also states that monitored anesthesia care should be requested by the attending physician and be made known to the patient, in accordance with accepted procedures of the institution. In addition, the ASA states that the service must include the following:

1. Performance of a preanesthetic examination and evaluation.
2. Prescription of anesthetic care.
3. Personal participation in, or medical direction of, the entire plan of care.
4. Continuous physical presence of the anesthesiologist or, in the case of medical direction, of the resident or nurse anesthetist being medically directed.
5. Proximate presence, or in the case of medical direction, availability of the anesthesiologist for diagnosis and treatment of emergencies.

Furthermore, the ASA states that all institutional regulations pertaining to anesthesia services shall be observed, and all the usual services performed by the anesthesiologist shall be furnished, including but not limited to:

1. Usual noninvasive cardiocirculatory and respiratory monitoring.

2. Oxygen administration, when indicated.
3. Administration of sedatives, tranquilizers, antiemetics, narcotics, other analgesics, beta-blockers, vasopressors, bronchodilators, antihypertensives, or other pharmacologic therapy as may be required in the judgment of the anesthesiologist.

From the statements above it is apparent that monitored anesthesia care always involves preoperative assessment and evaluation and intraoperative monitoring but does not necessarily involve the administration of sedative drugs. It should be self-evident that whenever monitored anesthesia care is planned, the facilities and expertise to secure the airway and provide general anesthesia should be immediately available.

PREOPERATIVE ASSESSMENT

The preoperative evaluation is an essential prerequisite to monitored anesthesia care and should be as comprehensive as that performed prior to any general or regional anesthetic (see Chapter 18). However, in addition to the usual evaluation for the patient who is planned to undergo general anesthesia, there are additional considerations unique to monitored anesthesia care that may ultimately determine the success or failure of the procedure. Because the patient will be conscious during monitored anesthesia care, it is important to evaluate the patient's ability to remain motionless and, if necessary, actively cooperate throughout the procedure. Thus, it is important to evaluate the patient's psychological preparation for the planned procedure. It is also important to elicit the presence of coexisting sensorineural or cognitive deficits. These factors or the inability to communicate with the patient may on occasion make general anesthesia a more appropriate alternative. Verbal communication between physician and patient is very important for three reasons: (1) as a monitor of the level of sedation and cardiorespiratory function, (2) as a means of explanation and reassurance for the patient, and (3) as a mechanism of communication when the patient is required to actively cooperate. Although cardiorespiratory disease is often an indication to perform a procedure using monitored anesthesia care rather than general anesthesia, there are occasions when cardiorespiratory disease may reduce the utility of monitored anesthesia care. For example, the presence of a persistent cough may make it very difficult for the patient to remain immobile, which can be particularly dangerous during ophthalmologic or awake neurosurgical procedures. Attempts to attenuate coughing with sedation techniques are likely to be unsuccessful and potentially harmful, as a significant level of anesthesia is required to abolish the cough reflex. Similarly, some patients with significant cardiovascular disease may experience orthopnea and be unable to lie flat for an extended period.

SEDATION TECHNIQUES FOR MONITORED ANESTHESIA CARE

Sedative hypnotics are commonly administered intravenously during monitored anesthesia care. The desired endpoint is to provide patient comfort, maintain cardiorespiratory stability, improve operating conditions, and to prevent recall of unpleasant perioperative events. It is helpful to delineate and individualize the goals of the sedation technique in each patient in order to formulate an appropriate regimen. The ideal sedation technique involves the administration of either individual or combinations of analgesic, amnestic, and hypnotic drugs. There should be a minimal incidence of side-effects, such as cardiorespiratory depression, nausea and vomiting, delayed emergence, and dysphoria. There should be a rapid and complete recovery after completion of the procedure. Ideally, the sedation technique will allow the patient to be able to communicate during the procedure. Experience shows that this level of sedation is optimal for the patient's comfort and safety. If the level of sedation is deepened to the extent that verbal communication is lost, most of the advantages of sedation/analgesia are lost and the risks of the technique approximate those of general anesthesia with an unprotected and uncontrolled airway (Table 47-1). Monitored anesthesia care may or may not involve the provision of sedation. However, because monitored anesthesia care is provided by anesthesiologists, the range of sedation can safely be expanded to include significantly deeper sedation techniques than those provided by nonanesthesiologists during sedation/analgesia.

The word "sedation" is derived from the Latin *sedatus*, meaning composed or calm. However, in current anesthetic practice "sedation" is often used loosely to describe analgesia, anxiolysis, and hypnosis, either individually or in combination.[5,6] Ideally, any sedation technique should strive to identify specific causes of and provide specific therapy for pain, anxiety, and agitation. Pain may be treated by local or regional analgesia, systemic analgesics, or removal of the painful stimulus. Anxiety may be reduced by the use of an anxiolytic such as a benzodiazepine and reassurance by the anesthesiologist. Patient agitation may be a result of pain or anxiety, but it is also vitally important to eliminate life-threatening factors such as hypoxia, hypercarbia, impending local anesthetic toxicity, and cerebral hypoperfusion. Other, less ominous, but often overlooked, causes of discomfort and agitation include a distended bladder, hypothermia, hyperthermia, pruritus, nausea, positional discomfort, uncomfortable oxygen masks and nasal cannulae, iv cannulation site infiltration, a member of the surgical team leaning on the patient, and prolonged pneumatic tourniquet inflation.

Pharmacologic Basis of Conscious Sedation Techniques—Optimizing Drug Administration

During conscious sedation, drugs are administered in the expectation that the desired therapeutic effects will result. Ideally, the therapeutic effects are as predicted. Occasionally, however, the result can depart significantly from expected, leading to an adverse effect upon patient comfort and safety. The ability to predict the effects of the drugs in our armamentarium demands an understanding of their pharmacokinetic and pharmacodynamic properties. This understanding is a fundamental prerequisite for the design of an effective sedation regimen and greatly increases the probability of producing the desired therapeutic effect. Context-sensitive half-time, effect–site equilibration time, and quantification of anesthetic/sedative drug interactions are all recently introduced concepts that are particularly useful in the context of conscious sedation and will be discussed in some detail.

The ultimate objective of any dosing regimen is to deliver a therapeutic concentration of drug to its site of action. The concentration of drug that is achieved as a result of a drug administration regimen is determined by the unique pharmacokinetic properties of that drug in that particular patient. The therapeutic response to a particular drug concentration is described by the pharmacodynamics of that particular patient–drug combination. There is a large degree of pharmacokinetic and pharmacodynamic variability, producing a significant variability in the dose–response relationship in clinical practice. Variability in drug response is an especially important consideration during MAC because these patients have unprotected airways. Excessive sedation may result in cardiac or respiratory depression. Inadequate sedation may result in patient discomfort and potential morbidity due to lack of cooperation. As a general principle, to avoid excessive levels of sedation, drugs should be titrated in small increments or by adjustable infusions rather than administered in larger doses according to predeter-

Table 47-1. COMPARISON OF THE IMPORTANT FEATURES OF A SEDATION/ ANALGESIA TECHNIQUE AND A DEEP SEDATION TECHNIQUE

Sedation/Analgesia	Deep Sedation or General Anesthesia with an Unprotected Airway
Verbal communication possible	Verbal communication impossible
Patient cooperation possible	Patient cooperation impossible
Patient reassurance possible	Patient reassurance impossible
Airway reflexes intact	Airway reflexes attenuated
Aspiration unlikely	Aspiration possible
Airway dilator muscles functional	Airway dilator muscles dysfunctional
Obstruction unlikely	Obstruction likely
Work of breathing normal	Work of breathing increased
Respiratory control intact	Respiratory control impaired
Hypoventilation unlikely	Hypoventilation likely
Airway intervention unlikely	Airway intervention likely
Unplanned intubation unlikely	Unplanned intubation likely
Respiratory complications unlikely	Respiratory complications likely
	Aspiration
	Obstruction
	Post-obstructive edema
	Hypoxia/hypercarbia
	Hypoxic neurologic injury

mined notions of efficacy. In an ideal dosing regimen, an effective concentration of drug is achieved and then adjusted according to the magnitude of the noxious stimulus. If the noxious stimulus is increased or decreased, the concentration is increased or decreased accordingly. By the end of the procedure, the drug concentration should have decreased to a level compatible with rapid recovery. This approach requires the use of drugs that are easily titratable, such as propofol. When using drugs such as propofol, adjustable-rate continuous infusions are the most logical method of maintaining a desired therapeutic concentration. When the traditional method of intermittent bolus administration is used, significant fluctuations in drug concentration occur. Under these circumstances, the plasma concentrations are either above or below the desired therapeutic range for a significant proportion of the procedure (Fig. 47-1). Continuous infusions are superior to intermittent bolus dosing because they produce less fluctuation in drug concentration, thus reducing the number of episodes of inadequate or excessive sedation. Administration of drugs by continuous infusion rather than by intermittent dosing also reduces the total amount of drug administered and facilitates a more prompt recovery.[7]

Distribution, Elimination, Accumulation, and Duration of Action

Following the administration of iv anesthetic drugs, the immediate distribution phase causes a brisk decrease in plasma levels as the drug is transported to the rapidly equilibrating vessel-rich group of tissues. There is a simultaneously occurring distribution of drug to the less well perfused tissues such as muscle and skin. Over time, the drug is also distributed to the poorly perfused tissues such as bone and fat. Although the latter compartments are poorly perfused, they may accumulate significant amounts of lipophilic drugs over the course of prolonged drug administration. This peripheral depot of drug may contribute to a delayed recovery when it is eventually released back into the central compartment after its administration is discontinued. These redistributive factors are extremely important determinants of drug effect and may increase or decrease the plasma concentration of a drug in a time-dependent fashion.

The Elimination Half-Life

Until recently, the elimination half-time was the predominant pharmacokinetic parameter utilized as the predictor of an anesthetic drug's duration of action. In everyday clinical practice, however, this parameter has not greatly enhanced our ability to predict anesthetic drug disposition. Only in single-compartment models does the elimination half-time actually represent the time required for a drug to reach half of its initial concentration after administration. This is because in a single-compartment model elimination is the only process that can alter drug concentration. Intercompartmental distribution cannot occur because there are no other compartments for the drug to be distributed to and from. Most drugs in the anesthesiologist's armamentarium are lipophilic and are therefore more suited to multicompartmental modeling than single-compartment modeling. Similarly, other pharmacokinetic parameters, such as distribution half-time, distribution volume, intercompartmental rate constants, and so forth, do not provide us with a practical means of predicting drug disposition. In multicompartmental models, the metabolism and excretion of some iv anesthetic drugs may have only a minor contribution to changes in plasma concentration when compared with the effects of intercompartmental distribution.

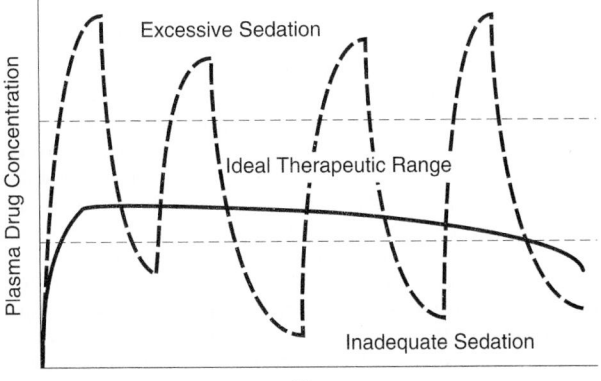

Figure 47-1. The changes in drug concentration during differing administration techniques. The heavy line represents a continuous infusion of a drug. In this situation the drug is maintained within the therapeutic range for most of the procedure. The lighter line represents the drug concentration resulting from intermittent bolus administration. The drug concentration is significantly above or below the desired therapeutic level for most of the procedure.

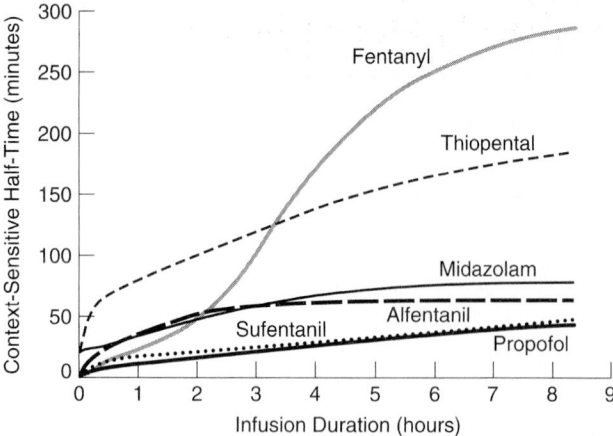

Figure 47-2. Context-sensitive half-times as a function of infusion duration. These data were generated from the computer model of Hughes *et al.*[8] It can be seen that the context-sensitive half-time of propofol demonstrates a minimal increase as the duration of the infusion increases. Also note that for infusions of short duration sufentanil has a shorter half-time than alfentanil. (Reproduced with permission from Hughes MA, Glass PSA, Jacobs JR: Context-sensitive half-time in multicompartment pharmacokinetic models for intravenous anesthetic drugs. Anesthesiology 76:334, 1992.)

Context-Sensitive Half-Time

In order to improve the description and understanding of anesthetic drug disposition, the concept of context-sensitive half-time has been developed.[8] This concept has greatly improved our understanding of anesthetic drug disposition and is clinically applicable. The effect of distribution upon plasma drug concentration varies in magnitude and direction over time and is dependent upon the drug concentration gradients that exist between the various compartments. For example, during the early part of an infusion of a lipophilic drug, distributive factors will tend to decrease plasma concentrations as the drug is transported to the unsaturated peripheral tissues. Later, after the infusion is discontinued, drug will return from the peripheral tissues and re-enter the central circulation. The relative effect on plasma concentrations of distributive processes versus elimination varies over time and from drug to drug. The context-sensitive half-time describes the time required for the plasma drug concentration to decline by 50% after terminating an infusion of a particular duration. This parameter is calculated by utilizing computer simulation of multicompartmental models of drug disposition (Fig. 47-2). The context-sensitive half-time reflects the combined effects of distribution and metabolism on drug disposition. There are several interesting aspects of these data. First, the data confirm the clinical impression that as the infusion duration increases, the context-sensitive half-time of all the drugs increases; this phenomenon is not described in any way by the elimination half-life. The increase in context-sensitive half-time is particularly marked with fentanyl and thiopental. In the case of fentanyl, drug that is irreversibly eliminated from the plasma by hepatic clearance is immediately replaced by drug returning from the peripheral compartments. Thus, although fentanyl has a shorter elimination half-life than that of sufentanil (462 vs. 577 min), its context-sensitive half-time is much greater than that of sufentanil after an infusion of duration longer than 2 hours. The storage and later release of fentanyl from peripheral binding sites delays the decline in plasma concentration that would otherwise occur. The context-sensitive half-times of all the drugs bear no constant relationship to their elimination half-times. Note also that that the context-sensitive half-time of propofol is short compared with that of thiopental. Although the context-sensitive half-times of propofol and thiopental are comparable following a brief

infusion, the context-sensitive half-time of thiopental increases rapidly following all but the shortest infusions. This finding confirms the clinical impression that thiopental is not an ideal drug for continuous infusion during ambulatory procedures. The context-sensitive half-time of propofol is prolonged to a minimal extent as the infusion duration increases. After an infusion of propofol, the drug that returns to the plasma from the peripheral compartments is rapidly cleared by metabolic processes and is therefore not available to retard the decay in plasma levels. This difference between thiopental and propofol is attributable to (1) the high metabolic clearance of propofol compared to thiopental and (2) the relatively slow rate at which propofol returns to the plasma from peripheral compartments.

Alfentanil is the opioid that has, until recently, been most frequently studied, described, and promoted in the context of ambulatory techniques. This is because alfentanil has a very short elimination half-time, one-fifth that of sufentanil (111 vs. 577 min). However, despite sufentanil's short elimination half-time, its context-sensitive half-time is actually less than that of alfentanil for infusions up to 8 hours in duration. This phenomenon is explained in part by the huge distribution volume of sufentanil. After termination of a sufentanil infusion, the decay in plasma drug concentrations is accelerated not only by elimination but also by the continued redistribution of sufentanil into peripheral compartments. On the other hand, the small distribution volume of alfentanil equilibrates rapidly; therefore, peripheral distribution of drug away from the plasma is not a significant contributor to the decay in plasma concentration after an infusion. The data derived from computer simulation by Hughes *et al*[8] show that the plasma decay of alfentanil is slower than that of sufentanil following infusions of similar duration to those used during conscious sedation. Thus, despite its short elimination half-time, alfentanil may not necessarily be superior to sufentanil for ambulatory sedation techniques.

How Does the Context-Sensitive Half-Time Relate to the Time to Recovery? Although the context-sensitive half-time represents a significant advance in our ability to describe drug disposition, this parameter does not directly describe how long it will take the patient to recover from conscious sedation. The context-sensitive half-time merely describes how long it will take for the plasma concentration of the drug to decrease by 50%. The time to recovery is dependent upon other additional factors. The difference between the plasma concentration at the end of the infusion and the plasma concentration below which awakening can be expected is an obvious factor in determining time to recovery. For example, if the drug concentration is maintained at a level just above that required for awakening, the time to recovery will be more rapid than after an infusion during which the drug concentration is much greater than that required for awakening (Fig. 47-3). Furthermore, although context-sensitive half-time is a reflection of plasma drug decay, awakening from anesthesia is actually a function of effect–site (*i.e.*, brain) concentration decay. Changes in effect–site concentration demonstrate a variable time lag behind changes in plasma drug concentration. Effect–site equilibration is a concept that is particularly relevant to iv sedation. When a drug is administered iv by bolus or infused rapidly, there is a delay before the onset of clinical effect. This delay occurs because the plasma is not usually the site of action but is merely the route by which the drug reaches its effect site. If some parameter of drug effect can be measured (*e.g.*, power spectrum electroencephalographic [EEG] analysis in the case of opioids), the half-time of equilibration between drug concentration in the blood and the drug effect can then be determined.[9] This parameter is abbreviated $t_{1/2}k_{e0}$. Drugs with a short $t_{1/2}k_{e0}$ will equilibrate rapidly with the brain and have a shorter delay in onset than drugs that have a longer $t_{1/2}k_{e0}$. Thiopental, propofol, and alfentanil have short $t_{1/2}k_{e0}$ values compared with midazolam, sufentanil, and fentanyl. The $t_{1/2}k_{e0}$ allows predictions to be made of the time course of equilibration of the drug between the blood and the brain. A distinct time

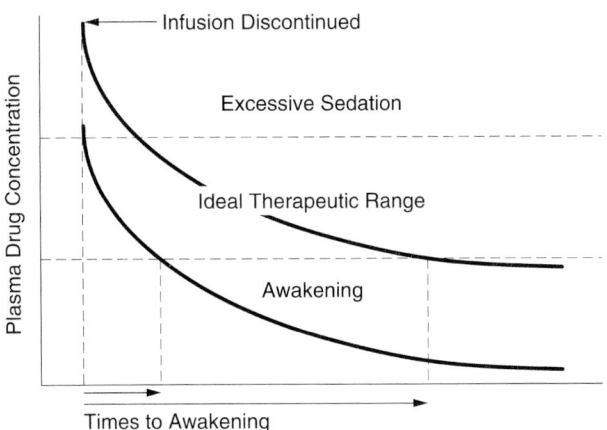

Figure 47-3. The context-sensitive half-time is not the sole determinant of the time it takes for the patient to awaken. This parameter merely reflects the time taken for the plasma concentration of a drug to decrease by 50%. The time to awakening is determined in addition by the difference in concentration at the end of the procedure and the concentration below which awakening will occur.

lag between the peak serum fentanyl concentration and the peak EEG slowing can be seen. In contrast, following alfentanil administration, the EEG changes closely parallel serum concentrations. The $t_{1/2}k_{e0}$ for fentanyl is 6.4 minutes compared with a $t_{1/2}k_{e0}$ of 1.1 minutes for alfentanil. If an opioid is required to blunt the response to a single brief stimulus, alfentanil might represent a logical choice over fentanyl. The $t_{1/2}k_{e0}$ is an important determinant of bolus spacing when titrating drugs to clinical effect. In the case of drugs like midazolam, which have a relatively long equilibration time (midazolam $t_{1/2}k_{e0} = 0.97–5.6$ min), boluses of drug should be spaced far enough apart to allow the full peak effect to be clinically appreciated before further drug administration in order to avoid inadvertent overdosing.[10,11] For example, even if the shortest quoted equilibration half-time for midazolam (0.9 min) is used, it will take 2.7 minutes for effect–site concentrations to be 87.5% equilibrated. Other factors are also important determinants of bolus size and spacing. For example, a low cardiac output will markedly delay drug arrival at the site of action. If sufficient time is not given for the drug to take effect before giving additional drug increments, significant cardiorespiratory compromise may occur. Furthermore, the effects of initial doses of most drugs in anesthetic practice are terminated by redistribution, which is dependent upon blood flow to redistribution sites. If there is reduced blood flow to redistribution sites because of pre-existing and iatrogenic decreases in cardiac output, the dangerous adverse effects of these drugs are likely to be markedly prolonged. An example of the above scenario is the patient with a hemodynamically compromising cardiac tachydysrhythmia that requires sedation for cardioversion. Careful, well-spaced, small boluses of drug should be given to induce the appropriate level of sedation, bearing in mind that it may take several minutes for the full effect of a small bolus dose to become apparent.

DRUG INTERACTIONS IN CONSCIOUS SEDATION

At the present time, no one inhaled or iv drug can provide all the components of conscious sedation (i.e., analgesia, anxiolysis, and hypnosis) with an acceptable margin of safety or ease of titratability. Therefore, patient comfort is usually maintained with a combination of drugs. Combinations of drugs should theoretically enable reductions in the dose requirements of individual drugs, thereby resulting in a reduction in adverse drug effects. For example, during general anesthesia, the combi-

nation of propofol and fentanyl by infusion has been shown to produce a more rapid recovery and better stress response abolition than the use of propofol alone.[12] Under most circumstances, the hypnotic effect of combinations of barbiturates or propofol with either opioids or benzodiazepines is synergistic. However, the decision whether to use a particular drug combination depends upon to what extent the synergistic interaction also extends to the undesirable nonhypnotic interactions of the drugs such as cardiorespiratory depression.

Drug interactions may have both a pharmacodynamic and a pharmacokinetic basis and may vary depending on the combination of drugs being coadministered, the dose range over which these drugs are administered, and the specific clinical effect that is measured. For example, because fentanyl is primarily an analgesic rather than a hypnotic, it reduces propofol requirements for suppression of response to skin incision to a much greater degree than it reduces propofol requirements for induction of anesthesia.[13] On the other hand, because midazolam has significant hypnotic properties, it displays significant synergism with propofol or thiopental when used to induce hypnosis.[14,15]

The plasma concentration of a drug at steady state that is required to abolish purposeful movement at skin incision in 50% of patients ($Cp_{ss}50$) is a measure of potency that is analogous to the familiar parameter of minimum alveolar concentration (MAC) of the volatile inhaled anesthetics. Intravenous anesthetic interactions may be evaluated by their effect upon the $Cp_{ss}50$ in a manner analogous to the expression of the effects of opioids on volatile anesthetic requirements in terms of MAC reduction. For example, during general anesthesia, opioid requirements to suppress the responses to noxious stimuli are 10-fold higher when used as the sole agent compared to when they are used in conjunction with a nitrous oxide/potent inhaled vapor technique. This interaction is likely to persist at the lighter levels of anesthesia encountered during conscious sedation. Therefore, in an ambulatory conscious sedation setting, it is likely that a rapid recovery would be facilitated by using opioids in combination with other agents (e.g., propofol/midazolam) rather than as the sole drug.

Drug interactions are dose-dependent. For example, when fentanyl is combined with isoflurane, the greatest reduction in isoflurane MAC occurs within the analgesic concentration range of fentanyl, i.e., 1–2 ng·ml^{-1}. At a fentanyl concentration of 1.7 ng·ml^{-1} the minimum alveolar concentration of isoflurane is reduced by 50%.[16] Once the fentanyl concentration is increased beyond 3 ng·ml^{-1}, there appears to be minimal further reduction with a maximum MAC reduction of 80%. Likewise, the MAC of desflurane is reduced by approximately 50% 25 minutes after a 3-μg·kg^{-1} iv bolus of fentanyl.[17] However, when the fentanyl bolus is increased to 6 μg·kg^{-1}, there is no significant further decrease in the MAC of desflurane. The interactions between propofol and opioids are important because these agents are frequently used during conscious sedation. When analgesic concentrations of fentanyl (0.6 ng·ml^{-1}) are used in combination with propofol for anesthesia, the $Cp_{ss}50$ of propofol is reduced by 50% compared with when propofol is used as the sole agent.[15] However, when the dose of fentanyl is increased, there is no significant further reduction of the $Cp_{ss}50$ for propofol beyond a fentanyl concentration of 3 ng·ml^{-1}.

Although the data presented above pertain to patients under general anesthesia, these findings have important implications for monitored anesthesia care. These studies demonstrate that the potentiating effects of opioids upon coadministered sedatives are pronounced within the dose range commonly used during conscious sedation. Furthermore, the data suggest that the dose–response curve is likely to be steep within this dose range, thus supporting the clinical impression that significant increases in depth of sedation can occur with only modest increments in opioid or hypnotic/sedative dosage. The following clinical recommendations can be made: During conscious sedation, the maximum benefit of opioid supplementation, in terms of potentiation of other administered sedatives, will accrue when the opioid is used in the analgesic dose range. Within this dose range there is great potential for adverse cardiorespiratory interaction.

Opioid and benzodiazepine combinations are frequently used to achieve the components of hypnosis, amnesia, and analgesia. The opioid–benzodiazepine combination displays marked synergism in producing hypnosis. Approximately 25% of the ED_{50} for each individual drug is required in combination to induce hypnosis in 50% of patients.[18] If the combination were simply additive, hypnosis would be induced in only approximately 25% of patients. Even subanalgesic doses of alfentanil ($3 \ \mu g \cdot kg^{-1}$) produce a profound reduction in midazolam requirements for hypnosis.[19] This synergism also extends to the unwanted effects of these drugs, producing the life-threatening complications of respiratory and cardiac depression.[20] Several fatalities have been reported after the use of midazolam, the majority of these being related to adverse respiratory events. In many of these cases, midazolam was used in combination with an opioid. The effects of midazolam and fentanyl upon respiratory function in healthy volunteers have been examined by Bailey et al.[21] Whereas midazolam produced no significant respiratory effects alone, and fentanyl alone produced hypoxemia (oxyhemoglobin saturation 95%) in half of the subjects, the combination of midazolam $0.05 \ mg \cdot kg^{-1}$ and fentanyl $2.0 \ \mu g \cdot kg^{-1}$ resulted in hypoxemia in 11 of 12 subjects and apnea (no spontaneous respiratory effort for 15 seconds) in 6 of 12 subjects. The combination of midazolam and fentanyl places patients at high risk for developing hypoxemia and apnea. The respiratory depressant effects of this drug combination are likely to be even more significant in the patient with coexisting respiratory or CNS disease or at the extremes of age. In clinical practice, the clinical advantages of the synergy between opioids and benzodiazepines for the maintenance of patient comfort should be carefully weighed against the disadvantages of the potentially adverse effect of this drug combination on the cardiovascular and respiratory systems.

SPECIFIC DRUGS USED FOR CONSCIOUS SEDATION

Propofol

Propofol has many of the ideal properties of a sedative-hypnotic for use in conscious sedation. Its pharmacokinetic profile, i.e., a context-sensitive half-time that remains short even after infusions of prolonged duration and a short effect–site equilibration time, makes it an easily titratable drug with an excellent recovery profile. The quality of recovery and the low incidence of nausea and vomiting make propofol particularly well suited to ambulatory conscious sedation procedures. A significant body of experience with the use of propofol for conscious sedation has emerged. Propofol has significant advantages compared with benzodiazepines when used as the hypnotic component of a conscious sedation technique. Although midazolam has a relatively short elimination half-time, its context-sensitive half-time is approximately twice that of propofol. Whereas propofol is noted for the rapid return to clearheadedness, midazolam is often associated with prolonged postoperative sedation and psychomotor impairment, particularly in the elderly. Propofol in typical conscious sedation doses ($25–75 \ \mu g \cdot kg^{-1} \cdot min^{-1}$) has minimal analgesic properties. However, the unique advantages of propofol can be exploited to the maximum when propofol is used to provide sedation when the analgesic component is provided by a local or regional analgesic technique. The use of propofol ($50–70 \ \mu g \cdot kg^{-1} \cdot min^{-1}$) to provide sedation (defined as sleep with preservation of the eyelash reflex and purposeful reaction to verbal or mild physical stimulation) as an adjunct to spinal anesthesia for lower limb surgery has been examined.[22] After

termination of infusions of approximately 100 minutes in duration, patients regained consciousness in approximately 4 minutes. The authors also noted the ease with which general anesthesia could be induced if necessary by increasing the propofol infusion. The same group also compared propofol (60.5 $\mu g \cdot kg^{-1} \cdot min^{-1}$) to midazolam (4.3 $\mu g \cdot kg^{-1} \cdot min^{-1}$) as an adjunct to spinal anesthesia. The propofol group had faster immediate recovery than the midazolam group (2.3 vs. 9.2 min to spontaneous eye opening). Furthermore, psychomotor function was comparable to baseline values following propofol sedation but did not return to baseline until 2 hours after midazolam administration. White and Negus also compared propofol and midazolam sedation for local and regional anesthesia.[23] These investigators examined several recovery parameters and demonstrated that propofol produced less postoperative sedation, drowsiness, confusion, and clumsiness than midazolam but that discharge times were similar. It should be noted that most investigators have shown that propofol does not reliably produce amnesia in subhypnotic doses.[24] Although recall of intraoperative events is generally thought to be undesirable, propofol's lack of amnestic properties may be preferable when patients are required to remember important instructions they are given in the postoperative period. Theoretically, a combination of propofol and midazolam could produce reliable amnesia for intraoperative events yet allow a rapid recovery of psychomotor function at the end of the procedure.

The use of propofol for conscious sedation has been examined in several diverse clinical settings, including propofol alone for upper gastrointestinal endoscopy[25] and magnetic resonance imaging in children,[26] with fentanyl for extracorporeal shock wave lithotripsy,[27] and with alfentanil for transvaginal oocyte retrieval.[28] The provision of conscious sedation during dental care to the mentally and physically handicapped is a significant anesthetic challenge. Propofol has been used successfully in the mentally and physically handicapped undergoing dental surgery.[29] However, the authors of that study expressed concern about the purported proconvulsive properties of propofol, particularly when used in the handicapped population, which has a high prevalence of epilepsy. However, a follow-up study by the same group examined the EEG effects of propofol sedation on epileptic patients undergoing dental surgery and found no increase in EEG or clinical epileptoid activity during propofol sedation.[30]

There is a general clinical impression that patients recovering from propofol not only recover rapidly but often experience an increased sense of well-being. However, a study specifically addressing the issue of the subjective effects of low-dose propofol in volunteers could find no evidence for a euphoric effect of propofol.[31] The authors postulate that the sense of well-being arises from the feeling of relief that the procedure is over. This feeling of relief may be inhibited by the prolonged psychomotor impairment that often follows other anesthetic techniques.

General anesthesia with propofol is generally associated with less nausea and vomiting than most other anesthetic techniques. There is now evidence that even subhypnotic doses of propofol (a single 10-mg dose in an adult) also possess direct antiemetic properties.[32] Thus, it is likely that the beneficial effects of propofol upon nausea and vomiting will be a feature of conscious sedation techniques using this drug. On the other hand, even during low-dose infusions used for conscious sedation, pain during injection of propofol may be troublesome in 33–50% of patients.[33,34] Several strategies for reducing the pain of propofol administration are described in Table 47-2.[35]

Benzodiazepines

Benzodiazepines are commonly utilized during conscious sedation for their anxiolytic, amnestic, and hypnotic properties. In the past, diazepam enjoyed great popularity as a major component of conscious sedation techniques. However, midazolam

Table 47-2. PUBLISHED STRATEGIES FOR REDUCING THE PAIN ON IV INJECTION OF PROPOFOL

Using larger veins in antecubital fossa
Decreasing the speed of injection
Injection into a fast-running iv
Diluting with 5% glucose or 10% intralipid
Adding lidocaine to propofol
Pretreating with lidocaine and venous occlusion
Pretreatment with opioid
Pretreatment with pentothal
Cooling to 4°C prior to injection
Injecting cooled saline (4°C) prior to injection
Discontinuing iv fluid administration during injection

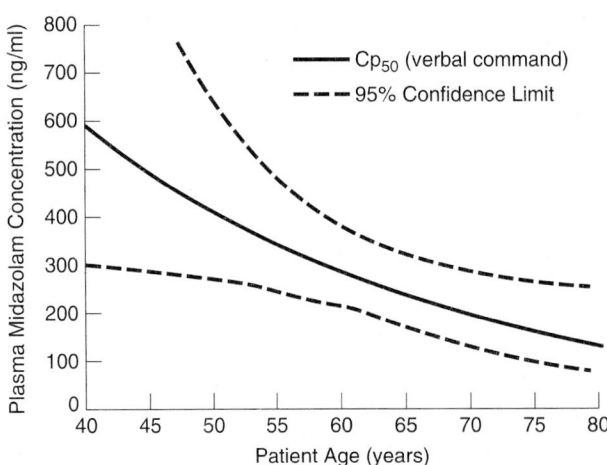

Figure 47-4. Midazolam Cp50 (the concentration at which 50% of subjects will fail to respond to a verbal command) as a function of age. There is a marked decrease in midazolam requirements as patient age increases. (Reproduced with permission from Jacobs JR, Reves JG, Marty J *et al*: Aging increases pharmacodynamic sensitivity to the hypnotic effects of midazolam. Anesth Analg 80:143,1995.)

has many advantages and has now displaced diazepam as the most commonly utilized benzodiazepine for conscious sedation. The important differences between midazolam and diazepam are listed in Table 47-3.[36] Although midazolam has a short elimination half-time, there is often significant and prolonged psychomotor impairment following conscious sedation techniques using midazolam as a significant component. With the recent availability of propofol, midazolam may be better utilized in a modified role by using lower doses prior to the start of a propofol infusion to provide the specific amnestic and perhaps anxiolytic component of a "balanced" sedation technique rather than as the major hypnotic component.[37] This allows the more evanescent and titratable propofol to provide the desired level of conscious sedation in an adjustable manner according to the specific stimulus. The analgesic component, if required, of a balanced conscious sedation technique could be provided by regional/local techniques or opioids. However, when using opioids with benzodiazepines, the potential for significant respiratory impairment should be considered.

Clinical experience suggests that the dose of a particular benzodiazepine required to reach a desired clinical endpoint is reduced in the elderly compared with younger patients. This difference in dosing requirements in the elderly is due mainly to pharmacodynamic factors, as evidenced by the 3-fold decrease in steady-state plasma concentration of midazolam at which 50% of patients would be expected not to respond to verbal command (Cp50) in the 80-year-old compared to the 40-year-old (Fig. 47-4).[38]

Although benzodiazepines are valuable components of conscious sedation techniques because they enhance patient comfort, improve operating conditions, and provide amnesia, recovery of psychomotor and cognitive function may be significantly prolonged following benzodiazepine sedation, especially when compared with sedative–hypnotic techniques utilizing propofol as the major component.[39] The recent introduction of a specific benzodiazepine antagonist flumazenil provides the potential to improve the recovery profile of benzodiazepines by permitting the active termination of their sedative and amnestic effects. Several studies have demonstrated that flumazenil facilitates

early recovery from benzodiazepine sedation without invoking adverse side-effects. However, the potential for resedation remains an obstacle to the routine use of benzodiazepine reversal, particularly in patients undergoing ambulatory procedures. Flumazenil has a very short elimination half-life of only 60 minutes, which is shorter than that of most clinically used benzodiazepines.[40] Although the more clinically relevant context-sensitive half-times have not been published for flumazenil, it is likely that the plasma concentration of flumazenil following a bolus will decrease by 50% in less than 12 minutes, or in less than 20 minutes in the case of an infusion lasting up to 2 hours (Dr. Steven L. Shafer, Stanford University Department of Anesthesia, personal communication, 1994). By contrast, the plasma concentration of midazolam will decrease by 50% in approximately 40 minutes following a 2-hour infusion.[8] The effective duration of a dose of flumazenil will depend upon the dose and elimination half-life of the benzodiazepine, the dose of flumazenil, and the time elapsed between benzodiazepine and flumazenil administration.[41] The effects of midazolam may recur up to 90 minutes following the administration of flumazenil.[42] Thus, it is possible that patients could be discharged prematurely to a less well-monitored area, or even out of the hospital in the case of ambulatory surgery, and later experience recurrence of benzodiazepine effects. An important additional issue is that of cost. The routine use of flumazenil-antagonized benzodiazepine sedation has a significant cost disadvantage. Ghouri *et al*[42] demonstrated that flumazenil-antagonized midazolam sedation was more expensive than propofol sedation ($68.67 vs. $27.80). Typical dose requirements are listed in Table 47-4.

Table 47-3. COMPARISON OF THE IMPORTANT PROPERTIES OF MIDAZOLAM AND DIAZEPAM

Midazolam	Diazepam
Water-soluble, does not require propylene glycol for solubilizing	Lipid-soluble, requires propylene glycol for solubilizing
Nonvenoirritant, usually painless	Venoirritant, pain on injection
Thrombophlebitis rare	Thrombophlebitis common
Short elimination half-time (1–4 hours)	Long elimination half-time (>20 hours)
Clearance unaffected by H_2 antagonists	Clearance reduced by H_2 antagonists
Inactive metabolites (1-hydroxy-midazolam)	Active metabolites (desmethyl-diazepam, oxazepam)
Resedation unlikely	Resedation more likely

Table 47-4. RECOMMENDED REGIMEN FOR THE USE OF FLUMAZENIL TO ANTAGONIZE BENZODIAZEPINE EFFECTS

Initial recommended dose of 0.2 mg

If desired level of consciousness is not achieved in 45 seconds, repeat 0.2-mg dose
0.2-mg doses may need to be repeated every 60 seconds until a maximum of 1 mg is administered
Be aware of the potential for resedation

Opioids

Opioids are most logically used in the context of conscious sedation to provide the specific analgesic component of a "balanced conscious sedation" technique. With the availability of drugs with specific and potent hypnotic and amnestic properties, such as propofol and midazolam, opioids are no longer required to play a significant role as the sole or major component of a sedation technique. Before the introduction of remifentanil, the available opioids did not reliably produce a controllable degree of sedation without a significant risk of respiratory depression. Furthermore, the significant increase in the incidence of nausea and vomiting associated with opioid use increased morbidity in ambulatory patients. Opioid analgesics are indicated when regional or local anesthetic techniques are inappropriate or ineffective. Opioids may also play an important role during the initial injection of local anesthetic solution or during other periods of intense patient discomfort. Pain relief may be required for factors other than the procedure itself, such as uncomfortable positioning, propofol injection, pneumatic tourniquet pain, or other pain not relieved by the local anesthetic technique.

A situation in which the patient must cooperate and remain motionless for a brief period is during the placement of a retrobulbar block prior to ophthalmic procedures. Patient movement during block placement may increase the incidence of complications such as brain stem anesthesia and cardiac arrest. Retrobulbar block placement affords an excellent opportunity to study the effects of drugs on the response to a standardized ethically acceptable brief painful stimulus. The ideal drug for block placement would provide a brief period of intense analgesia yet allow the patient to be awake and cooperative without causing cardiorespiratory depression, cause minimal nausea and vomiting, and not significantly prolong recovery.[43] Alfentanil (20 μg · kg^{-1}) has a rapid onset and offset of intense analgesia and was compared with methohexital (0.5 mg · kg^{-1}) for retrobulbar block placement.[43] Patients receiving methohexital were unresponsive to verbal command at the time of block placement and demonstrated more movement upon injection than those receiving alfentanil, who were mostly (87%) awake and cooperative at the time of injection. The authors note that one elderly patient out of the 15 who received alfentanil became apneic for 30 seconds, and suggested that the dose of opioids be reduced in the elderly. They also noted that the personnel performing the block were accustomed to the patient being "asleep" during methohexital sedation, but took some time to become at ease with the awake yet comfortable and cooperative patient who had received alfentanil.

The well-described phenomenon of patient awareness and subsequent recall of intraoperative events following high-dose opioid anesthesia is taken as evidence that opioids lack significant amnestic properties. However, when the effects of low-dose fentanyl upon memory were specifically examined in volunteers, it was found that although the subjects appeared to be awake during the fentanyl infusion, there was significant memory impairment.[44] However, the degree of stimulation was

probably less than that experienced by a patient undergoing a painful surgical procedure. Recall for a painful stimulus may not be impaired to the same degree as recall for the less noxious stimuli that the subjects of this study experienced.

Alfentanil appears to have a pharmacokinetic advantage for the treatment of discrete stimuli because of its short effect–site equilibration time, which allows rapid access of the drug to the brain and facilitates titration. However, sufentanil may have a more favorable recovery profile when used over a longer period of time because of its shorter context-sensitive half-time. In clinical practice, however, there is a marked interpatient variability in opioid pharamacokinetics and dynamics. This interpatient variability may be more significant than the interdrug differences, making it difficult to predict with any precision the effects of a given drug dose in an individual patient.

Remifentanil

In the context of monitored anesthesia care, the analgesic properties of opioids are extremely valuable. However, their adverse effects, including respiratory depression, muscle rigidity, and emesis, are undesirable in the spontaneously breathing patient with an unprotected airway and significantly limit our ability to consistently provide effective analgesic doses. A further complicating issue is that our ability to predict the effect of a given dose of opioid in a particular patient is limited by significant interpatient pharmacokinetic and pharmacodynamic variability. This problem is usually overcome in practice by the cautious incremental administration of small, carefully spaced boluses or by titrating infusions to the desired effect.

Remifentanil, a recently introduced μ-opioid receptor agonist, has pharmacodynamic properties similar to those of other potent μ-opioid receptor agonists such as fentanyl and alfentanil. However, unlike previously available opioids, remifentanil is predominantly metabolized by nonspecific esterases generating an extremely rapid clearance and offset of effect.[45] The context-sensitive half-time of remifentanil is consistently short, 3–5 minutes, increasing to a minimal degree with the duration of the infusion. Furthermore, remifentanil has a comparatively short effect–site equilibration time ($t_{1/2}k_{e0}$) of 1.0–1.5 minutes. This $t_{1/2}k_{e0}$ is slightly longer than that of alfentanil (0.6–1.2 min) but shorter than that of fentanyl (4–5 min) and much shorter than that of morphine (~20 min), and makes the onset of effect after drug administration very rapid. The rapid onset and offset of remifentanil greatly facilitate titration of effect during MAC.

In clinical practice, remifentanil has been used successfully as the analgesic component of sedation techniques for regional and local anesthesia. Its unique pharmacokinetic profile makes it well suited for ambulatory sedation/analgesia techniques. Published experience with the use of remifentanil suggests that it is possible to titrate remifentanil administration to provide effective analgesia with minimal respiratory depression. The published data can be used to generate some practical clinical guidelines,[46] which are discussed below.

1. As with other potent opioids used during sedation techniques, the most logical therapeutic endpoint for remifentanil administration is effective analgesia and patient comfort rather than sedation. When opioids are titrated to preconceived levels of sedation rather than patient comfort, an unacceptable degree of respiratory depression may occur. Drugs such as propofol or midazolam can be used in combination with remifentanil to provide the hypnotic–amnestic component of the sedation technique, remembering that the concomitant administration of midazolam decreases remifentanil dose requirements by up to 50%.[47]

2. Published data suggest that bolus administration of remifentanil is associated with an increased incidence of respiratory depression and chest wall rigidity. Because these

side-effects are likely to be related to high peak concentrations of drugs, it is recommended that remifentanil boluses be administered slowly (over 30–90 sec) or avoided completely by utilizing a pure infusion technique. Furthermore, the administration of remifentanil boluses during the concomitant administration of remifentanil infusions is also associated with an increased incidence of respiratory depression, the most likely mechanism again being excessive peak drug concentrations. These episodes of respiratory depression are of significant concern, particularly in the spontaneously breathing patient with an unprotected airway. However, once they were recognized and the remifentanil administration was reduced or discontinued, they resolved with a median time of 3 minutes. Thus, despite the pharmacokinetic advantages of remifentanil, the level of vigilance required for its administration should be no different from that for any other potent opioid. Although the offset time of remifentanil is rapid, it still requires the recognition of respiratory depression to trigger a downward adjustment in dosage. On the other hand, the short $t_{1/2}k_{e0}$ of remifentanil suggests that sudden respiratory depression may occur in response to upward adjustments in dosage. Despite the potential for respiratory depression, the efficacy of remifentanil boluses during MAC has been investigated by several groups. The most logical scenario in which a bolus dose could be utilized is immediately prior to a brief but very painful stimulus, such as placement of a retrobulbar block.[48] A bolus of 1 $\mu g \cdot kg^{-1}$ over 30 seconds was administered 90 seconds prior to block placement. More than three-quarters of patients receiving remifentanil did not report any pain during subsequent block placement. However, 15% of the patients given a single bolus alone had significant respiratory depression (respiratory rates <8 breaths per minute), and 19% of those given a bolus followed by an infusion had significant respiratory depression.

3. The effects of coadministration of benzodiazepines and opioids are well documented. The addition of midazolam to provide the anxiolytic–sedative and amnestic components of a sedation technique has been shown to increase patient satisfaction and significantly reduce remifentanil dose requirements. The combination of remifentanil with midazolam significantly reduces patient anxiety when compared to the use of the opioid alone.[49] Even relatively low-dose midazolam (2 mg iv) produces significant reductions in remifentanil requirements and patient anxiety. During breast or lymph node biopsy, remifentanil infusion requirements were 0.065 $\mu g \cdot kg^{-1} \cdot min^{-1}$ when preceded by midazolam compared to 0.123 $\mu g \cdot kg^{-1} \cdot min^{-1}$ when used alone. The advantages of coadministration of small doses of midazolam include increased patient satisfaction, increased amnesia, decreased nausea and vomiting, and decreased anxiety. The disadvantages include a tendency toward increased respiratory depression, apnea, and excessive sedation.

4. Because most painful stimuli are of unpredictable duration and because the risk of adverse respiratory events is increased following bolus administration, the most logical method for the administration of remifentanil during MAC is by an adjustable infusion. This should ideally be preceded by a small bolus of midazolam. Most investigators have used infusion rates that start at 0.1 $\mu g \cdot kg^{-1} \cdot min^{-1}$ approximately 5 minutes prior to the first painful stimulus. This initial "loading" infusion is then weaned to approximately 0.05 $\mu g \cdot kg^{-1} \cdot min^{-1}$ to maintain patient comfort. The maintenance infusion is adjusted upward in response to pain or hemodynamic response or downward in response to excessive sedation, respiratory depression, or apnea. A typical incremental change in infusion rate is 0.025 $\mu g \cdot kg^{-1} \cdot min^{-1}$. The use of remifentanil infusions

Table 47-5. TYPICAL DOSE RANGES OF SEDATIVE, HYPNOTIC AND ANALGESIC DRUGS

Drug	Typical Adult iv Dose Range (titrated to effect in small increments)
Benzodiazepines	
Midazolam	1–2 mg prior to propofol or remifentanil infusion
Diazepam	2–8 mg as major component
	2.5–10 mg
Opioid analgesics	
Alfentanil	5–20-$\mu g \cdot kg^{-1}$ bolus 2 min prior to stimulus
Fentanyl	0.5–2.0-$\mu g \cdot kg^{-1}$ bolus 2–4 min prior to stimulus
Remifentanil	Infusion 0.1 $\mu g \cdot kg^{-1} \cdot min^{-1}$ 5 min prior to stimulus
	Wean to 0.05 $\mu g \cdot kg^{-1} \cdot min^{-1}$ as tolerated
	Adjust up or down in increments of 0.025 $\mu g \cdot kg^{-1} \cdot min^{-1}$
	Reduce dose accordingly when coadministered with midazolam or propofol
	Avoid boluses
Hypnotics	
Propofol	250–500-$\mu g \cdot kg^{-1}$ boluses
	25–75 $\mu g \cdot kg^{-1} \cdot min^{-1}$ infusion

of 0.2 $\mu g \cdot kg^{-1} \cdot min^{-1}$ is associated with an increased incidence of respiratory depression that is not necessarily associated with superior analgesia. As in the case of propofol administration, inadvertent interruption of remifentanil administration will result in abrupt offset of effect, which may result in patient discomfort, hemodynamic instability, and even morbidity due to patient movement. It is therefore very important to ensure that the drug delivery system is monitored carefully during the procedure. Remifentanil is supplied as a powder that must be reconstituted prior to use. It is particularly important when administering this drug to patients with an unsecured airway to ensure that there are no errors in drug dilution that would result in inadvertent dosing errors.

Typical adult dose recommendations for opioids and other drugs discussed in the text are listed in Table 47-5.

Patient-Controlled Sedation and Analgesia

There is increasing interest in techniques that allow the patient some direct control of the level of sedation. Patient participation in the perioperative process may positively affect patient satisfaction.[50] The degree of sedation desired by the patient varies significantly and the individual response to drugs is variable. Patient-controlled sedation (PCS) appears to be an attractive solution to this problem. One approach to PCS has been to use a conventional patient-controlled analgesia (PCA) delivery system set to deliver 0.7-mg $\cdot kg^{-1}$ boluses of propofol with a 3-minute lockout period.[51] Other approaches include fixed-dose combinations of 0.5 mg midazolam and 25 μg fentanyl with a 5-minute lockout interval between doses.[52] This technique was as safe and effective as anesthesiologist-controlled drug delivery. However, some workers have noted greater post-procedure sedation following self-administration compared to physician-controlled sedation.[53] The pharmacokinetic profile of alfentanil is ideal for the treatment of short, discrete episodes of pain. These properties have been exploited during vaginal ovum retrieval procedures, when ultrasonically guided needles are passed through the vaginal wall under monitored anesthesia care. Zelcer et al utilized a PCA delivery system to allow self-administration of alfentanil during this procedure.[54] After midazolam premedication and a loading dose of alfentanil, patients received 5-$\mu g \cdot kg^{-1}$ boluses of alfentanil via the PCA pump with a mandatory 3-minute lockout period. Patient acceptability, alfentanil dosage, respiratory variables, and pain scores were similar to those obtained with physician-controlled analgesia. From the limited data that are available, intraoperative PCA during monitored anesthesia care appears to be an effective alternative to physician-administered analgesia.

RESPIRATORY FUNCTION AND SEDATIVE–HYPNOTICS

During monitored anesthesia care there is significant potential for respiratory compromise mediated *via* several important mechanisms. These include adverse effects on respiratory drive, either directly as a result of sedative–hypnotic or opioid administration or indirectly as a consequence of brain stem hypoperfusion resulting from hypotension, such as that occurring during spinal or epidural anesthesia. There may also be a marked increase in the work of breathing due to increased resistance to gas flow in the upper airway.[55] During sedation it is likely that protective airway reflexes will be attenuated. On the other hand, sedative doses of benzodiazepines appear to have variable effects upon respiratory system mechanics, decreasing, increasing, or having no effect upon functional residual capacity.[56-58]

Sedation and Upper Airway Patency

The upper airway is located outside the thorax. During normal inspiration, the pressure within the upper airway is subatmospheric; thus, there is a tendency for the upper airway to collapse under the influence of the surrounding atmospheric pressure. However, in the normal subject this tendency for airway collapse is opposed by upper airway dilator muscle tone. These muscles probably both increase the diameter and reduce the compliance of the upper airway. An increase in upper airway dilator muscle tone occurs during inspiration, commencing just prior to diaphragmatic contraction.[59] Several studies have confirmed the importance of coordinated activation of the diaphragmatic and upper airway respiratory muscles in maintaining airway patency. Upper airway dilator muscle control appears to be extremely sensitive to sedative–hypnotic drug administration.[60] For example, sedative doses of midazolam have been reported to increase inspiratory subglottic airway resistance by 3- to 4-fold.[61] Sedative doses of diazepam selectively suppress genioglossal muscle activity to a greater degree than diaphragmatic activity; furthermore, this effect is exaggerated in the elderly.[62] In all these examples the increased upper airway resistance markedly increased the work of breathing. The response to this obstruction is a significant increase in intercostal and accessory muscle activity. However, this response is only partially effective because the increase in inspiratory force will further decrease intraluminal upper airway pressure, predisposing to further airway collapse. It is likely that these effects will be of greatest significance in patients with pre-existing respiratory compromise, such as the elderly or those with chronic obstructive pulmonary disease. These patients often have limited respiratory reserve and are unable to increase their respiratory muscle activity in response to the increased work of breathing induced by sedation and may become hypercarbic, acidotic, and hypoxic.

Sedation and Protective Airway Reflexes

Competent laryngeal and upper airway reflexes are required to protect the lower airway from aspiration. It is well documented that protective laryngeal and pharyngeal reflexes are depressed by anesthesia and sedation. Furthermore, it is also well documented that protective airway reflexes are compromised by advanced age and debilitation. Therefore, it is likely that significant depression of airway reflexes could occur during sedation in the elderly or debilitated patient. Aspiration of gas-

tric contents could occur either in the operating room or during recovery, particularly if oral intake is allowed before the return of adequate upper airway protective reflexes. The time required for the return of protective reflexes varies considerably. Complete recovery of the swallowing reflex occurs approximately 15 minutes after the return of consciousness following propofol anesthesia.[63] However, the iv administration of 15 mg of diazepam has been shown to depress the swallowing reflex for up to 4 hours.[64] The swallowing reflex is significantly depressed for up to 2 hours following the administration of midazolam despite the return to a normal state of consciousness.[65] In otherwise healthy adult male volunteers the inhalation of 50% nitrous oxide was associated with marked depression of the swallowing reflex.[66]

It is apparent from the sources quoted above that the protective airway reflexes alone cannot be relied upon to protect the lower airway from aspiration during sedation. Thus, patients who are deemed to be at risk from aspiration of gastric contents should be maintained at the lightest level of sedation possible. Ideally, the patient should be awake enough to recognize the regurgitation of gastric contents and be able to protect his or her own airway. If the ability of the patient to protect his or her own airway cannot be reliably guaranteed and regurgitation/aspiration is thought to be a significant risk, placement of a cuffed endotracheal tube under general or local anesthesia should be seriously considered.

Sedation and Respiratory Control

Clinical experience would lead most anesthesiologists to predict that the administration of sedative–hypnotic drugs is associated with the depression of respiratory drive. However, the findings of scientific studies in this area are often conflicting and confusing, on occasion finding minimal, if any, effects of sedative drugs upon ventilatory responsiveness. However, it is important to note that in many cases the methods used to measure respiratory drive may affect the outcome of the study by stimulating the subject, thus attenuating the negative effect of the drug upon respiratory drive. In clinical practice it is likely that during regional anesthesia there is a degree of deafferentation that will potentiate the respiratory depressant effects of sedative–hypnotic drugs.[67] Most studies have demonstrated that opioids depress the ventilatory response to hypercapnia and hypoxia.[68] Reports of the effects of sedative doses of benzodiazepines upon carbon dioxide responsiveness have shown variable results, including no significant effect[69] and clinically significant depression.[70] However, when opioids and benzodiazepines are used in combination, there appears to a marked negative effect upon respiratory responsiveness.[21] However, initial clinical investigation examining the combination of propofol and opioids has shown little potentiation of the adverse effects of opioids by sedative doses of propofol.[28]

SUPPLEMENTAL OXYGEN ADMINISTRATION

Hypoxia as a result of alveolar hypoventilation is a relatively common occurrence following the administration of sedatives, analgesics, and hypnotics. In the absence of significant lung disease, the administration of only modest concentrations of supplemental oxygen is frequently effective in restoring the patient's oxygen saturation to an acceptable level. This concept is well illustrated by reference to the familiar alveolar gas equation. An extreme example illustrates the point: an otherwise healthy adult male breathing room air receives a dose of an opioid that causes marked alveolar hypoventilation such that his alveolar P_{CO_2} is increased to 80 mm Hg. The alveolar gas equation predicts that his arterial P_{O_2} will fall to approximately 40 mm Hg as shown below:

$$P_{AO_2} = P_{IO_2} - P_{ACO_2}/R$$

$$P_{IO_2} = F_{IO_2} \times (P_B - P_{H_2O})$$

$$P_{IO_2} = 0.21 \times (760 - 47) = 150 \text{ mm Hg}$$

$$P_{AO_2} = 150 - 80/0.8$$

$$P_{AO_2} = 50 \text{ mm Hg}$$

Assuming a normal A–a gradient, his P_{aO_2} will be 40 mm Hg, corresponding to an arterial oxygen saturation of 75%. If while initiating definitive therapy for hypoventilation this patient were to receive only a modest increase in inspired oxygen, a marked improvement in arterial saturation would be achieved:

$$F_{IO_2} \text{ increased to } 28\%$$

$$P_{IO_2} = 0.28 \times (760 - 47) = 200 \text{ mm Hg}$$

$$P_{AO_2} = 200 - 80/0.8$$

$$P_{AO_2} = 100 \text{ mm Hg}$$

This theoretical example serves to highlight several points. First, in isolated hypoventilation modest increases in inspired oxygen are remarkably effective at restoring oxygen saturation to acceptable levels. However, a patient who is receiving minimal supplemental oxygen and has an acceptable oxygen saturation may have significant undetected alveolar hypoventilation. Therefore, before making the decision to discharge patients to a less well monitored environment without supplemental oxygen, it is useful to measure their oxygen saturation while breathing room air.

MONITORING DURING MONITORED ANESTHESIA CARE

ASA Standards

The ASA standards for basic anesthetic monitoring are applicable to all levels of anesthesia care, including monitored anesthesia care. It is useful to review the components of the ASA standards that are pertinent to monitored anesthesia care as approved by the house of delegates on October 21, 1986 and subsequently amended on October 21, 1998.[71] (See Chapter 2, Table 2-1, for the current ASA standards.)

Communication and Observation

A conscientious and well-trained anesthesia caregiver is the single most vital monitor in the operating room. However, his or her effectiveness will be markedly enhanced by the use of the basic quantitative and qualitative monitoring devices, which should be readily available in all operating rooms. It is important that the anesthesiologist continually evaluate the patient's response to verbal stimulation to effectively titrate the level of sedation and to allow the earlier detection of neurologic or cardiorespiratory dysfunction. Continuous visual, tactile, and auditory assessment of physiologic function should include observation of the rate, depth, and pattern of respiration; palpation of the arterial pulse; and assessment of peripheral perfusion by extremity temperature and capillary refill. In addition, the patient should be continually observed for diaphoresis, pallor, shivering, cyanosis, and acute changes in neurologic status.

Auscultation

Auscultation of heart and breath sounds has long been a vital component of monitoring during anesthesia. Placement of a precordial stethoscope near the sternal notch of a nonintubated patient provides important information concerning upper airway patency as well as a continuous monitor of heart sounds and ventilation. Continuous precordial auscultation is an inexpensive, effective, and essentially risk-free process that serves

an additional important purpose by bringing the anesthesia care provider closer to the patient. If access to the patient is limited during the procedure, FM wireless or infrared remote transmission systems are now commercially available.

Pulse Oximetry

No monitor of oxygen transport has had a greater impact on the practice of anesthesiology than the pulse oximeter.[72] Despite occasional mechanical interference due to limb movement, this technology is readily applied and is positively indicated in the context of monitored anesthesia care. Pulse oximetry is noninvasive, safe, and comfortable to the awake patient; it is also technically simple to apply and interpret, and allows continuous real-time monitoring of arterial oxygenation. The use of a quantitative measure of oxygenation is specifically mandated by the ASA standards for intraoperative monitoring. The important mechanisms whereby respiratory function may be compromised during monitored anesthesia care include the effects of sedatives and opioids upon respiratory drive, upper airway patency, and protective airway reflexes. Additional important risk factors for arterial desaturation include obesity, pre-existing upper airway obstruction and respiratory disease, the extremes of age, and the lithotomy position.[73] The fundamental importance of monitoring oxygenation during monitored anesthesia care can be appreciated from the closed-claim study of Caplan et al,[67] who examined 14 cases of sudden cardiac arrest in otherwise healthy patients who received spinal anesthesia. These major anesthetic mishaps occurred before the routine adoption of pulse oximetry. One of the major findings of this study was that cyanosis frequently heralded the onset of cardiac arrest, suggesting that unappreciated respiratory insufficiency may have played an important role. Further support for the use of pulse oximetry comes from the ASA Committee on Professional Liability analysis of closed anesthesia claims. Examination of the data from the closed-claims project reveals that respiratory events constitute the single largest source of adverse outcome. Furthermore, review of these cases suggests that pulse oximetry in combination with capnometry would have prevented the adverse outcome in the vast majority of cases. During monitored anesthesia care, patient movement can occasionally interfere with effective pulse oximetry. One solution to this problem has been developed by Nellcor Inc. (Hayward, CA). This company has developed a system whereby the pulse oximeter compares the pulsatile absorbance signal with the simultaneous electrocardiogram (ECG) waveform.[72] Absorbance pulsations that are not synchronous with an ECG complex are rejected. This system (C-Lock®, Nellcor Inc.) is generally effective but requires a clean ECG signal, which can also be adversely affected by patient movement. On the other hand, pulse oximeter artifacts due to shivering have proved to be a difficult problem to overcome, further emphasizing the need to monitor and maintain body temperature during monitored anesthesia care.[74]

Capnography

Although capnography is most effective in the intubated patient, some useful information may be obtained from a spontaneously breathing, nonintubated patient. Sidestream capnographs have been adapted for use with facemasks, nasal airways, and nasal cannulae and have been used successfully during monitored anesthesia care.[75–78] Nasal cannulae for oxygen delivery have been modified to provide an integral port for respiratory gas sampling and are available commercially. Alternatively, capnograph sampling lines can be attached to shortened iv catheters and inserted inside nasal oxygen probes.

Cardiovascular System

At a minimum, the ECG must be continually displayed and the blood pressure measured and recorded at least every 5 minutes during monitored anesthesia care. The pulse should be monitored by palpation, oximetry, or auscultation. The selection of additional hemodynamic monitoring is usually determined more by the cardiovascular status of the patient than the magnitude of the procedure. Most procedures performed under monitored anesthesia care do not involve major hemorrhage, fluid shifts, or major physiologic trespass. Decisions concerning choice of monitoring for myocardial ischemia and other adverse hemodynamic events will need to be individualized on a case-by-case basis. Monitoring modalities that may be considered include automated ECG ischemia detection, invasive arterial pressure monitoring, central venous and pulmonary artery catheters, urinary catheterization, and transesophageal echocardiography (very uncomfortable in the awake patient).

Temperature Monitoring and Management During Monitored Anesthesia Care

The value of temperature monitoring is well established during general anesthesia, the perioperative period being frequently complicated by hypothermia and hyperthermia. Although sedation techniques used during monitored anesthesia care do not generally trigger malignant hyperthermia, there is potential for significant inadvertent hypothermia, particularly during neuraxial anesthesia. Even monitored anesthesia care techniques unaccompanied by regional anesthesia are associated with hypothermia at the extremes of age, both the old and very young having impaired thermoregulatory mechanisms. The elderly also have markedly reduced muscle mass and therefore basal heat production. Although the anesthesiologist may be able to exert some control over the ambient temperature in the operating room, he or she may be unable to influence the temperature at remote anesthetizing locations. Radiology suites are often maintained at lower temperatures to accommodate the computer systems that are used to reconstruct images. Radiant heating lamps, forced-air heaters, fluid warmers, or warming blankets, all common items in operating rooms, may be unavailable and unsuitable for use at remote locations. Forced-air heating has been shown to be an effective means of maintaining normothermia, and can be combined with iv fluid warming.[79] Even mild perioperative hypothermia (i.e., 1–2°C) accompanying general anesthesia is associated with adverse myocardial outcomes, increased bleeding tendency and transfusion requirements, wound infections, and delayed wound healing and hospital discharge.[80] There is no evidence suggesting that the morbidity associated with perioperative hypothermia is any less during monitored anesthesia care than during general anesthesia. The morbidity associated with perioperative hypothermia is well described in high-risk patients; this is a group of patients that are very likely to undergo procedures under monitored anesthesia care. When hypothermia is significant, shivering may interfere with the planned procedure and markedly increase oxygen requirements and predispose susceptible patients to myocardial ischemia or respiratory insufficiency. The major thermoregulatory defenses against hypothermia include vasoconstriction, shivering, and behavior. Vasoconstriction and shivering are impaired during major conduction anesthesia. Behavioral thermoregulation is impaired even in the conscious patient. The patient undergoing a procedure is immobile, unable to move to a warmer environment, or put on warmer clothes. Furthermore, neuraxial or regional techniques and the presence of impaired consciousness will impair the patients' ability to perceive that they are hypothermic. Regional anesthesia has major effects on thermoregulation.[81] Lower extremity vasodilatation causes central cooling via a redistribution of heat from the core to the periphery. Afferent input to the hypothalamus from the warm peripheral compartment counteracts conflicting input from the cooling central compartment, thus delaying the initiation of compensatory thermoregulation. In the absence of reliable temperature monitoring it is possible that the first indication

of hypothermia would be the onset of shivering, by which time considerable central cooling may have occurred.

Frank and co-workers have examined the issue of temperature monitoring and management during neuraxial anesthesia and found that temperature monitoring is significantly underutilized, only one-third of patients being monitored.[82] Furthermore, the method that was most frequently used to monitor temperature may not accurately reflect core temperature, the most important determinant of thermoregulatory response and perioperative morbidity. Forehead skin surface was the most commonly monitored site followed by the axilla. Forehead skin surface monitoring usually utilizes liquid crystal thermometry. This site is chosen for convenience, accessibility, minimal forehead subcutaneous insulation, and because the site has few arteriovenous shunts. However, forehead skin surface temperature is significantly dependant upon vasomotor tone and the ambient temperature. The commercially available liquid crystal devices supplied for this purpose usually incorporate a 2–3°C offset to account for the difference between skin and core temperature under normal conditions. The accuracy of these devices for perioperative temperature monitoring remains controversial; they do not reliably detect malignant hyperthermia and are not sufficiently accurate for fever screening purposes in children.[83] Sessler recommends the use of a properly positioned axillary probe or intermittent oral temperature monitoring during neuraxial anesthetics.[81]

Some of the more accurate methods of measuring core temperature—pulmonary artery, distal esophagus, and nasopharynx—are clearly not well tolerated in the awake patient. However, other sites such as tympanic membrane, urinary bladder (with neuraxial techniques), and rectum can provide accurate indications of core temperature. Sessler notes the important distinction between properly positioned tympanic membrane thermocouples and infrared aural canal thermocouples, the accuracy and precision of the latter being clearly inferior.[81]

Patients will frequently complain of feeling too warm when covered by heavy drapes. Although malignant hyperthermia is rare during monitored anesthesia care because the common triggering agents are rarely used, hyperthermia is still possible as a result of thyroid storm or malignant neuroleptic syndrome. The subjective sensation of hyperthermia may also be the first indicator of important adverse events in evolution such as hypoxia, hypercarbia, cerebral ischemia, local anesthetic toxicity, and myocardial ischemia.

Bispectral Index Monitoring During Monitored Anesthesia Care

The bispectral index (BIS) is a processed EEG parameter that was developed specifically to evaluate patient response during drug-induced anesthesia and sedation. Sedation monitoring is attractive because of the potential to titrate drugs more accurately, avoiding the adverse effects of both over- and under-dosing. BIS monitoring has some potential advantages over conventional intermittent techniques of patient assessment. Conventional assessment involves patient stimulation at frequent intervals to determine the level of consciousness, requires patient cooperation, and is subject to testing fatigue. An example of a conventional assessment tool is the Observer's Assessment of Alertness/Sedation Scale (OAA/S; see Table 47-6).[84] The bispectral index has been shown to be a useful monitor of drug-induced sedation and recall in volunteers and has been shown to correlate with OAA/S scores during propofol-induced sedation in patients undergoing surgery with regional anesthesia.[85] An increasing depth of sedation was associated with a predictable decrease in the BIS index. Absence of recall was associated with BIS values below 80. These findings correspond with those of Kearse et al, who found no intraoperative recall at BIS values below 79 during midazolam-, isoflurane-, and pro-

Table 47-6. OBSERVER'S ASSESSMENT OF ALERTNESS/SEDATION SCALE[84,85]

Responsiveness	Speech	Facial Expression	Eyes	Composite Score
Responds readily to name spoken in normal tone	Normal	Normal	Clear, no ptosis	5 (alert)
Lethargic response to name spoken in normal tone	Mild slowing or thickening	Mild relaxation	Glazed or mild ptosis (less than half the eye)	4
Responds only after name is called loudly or repeatedly	Slurring or prominent slowing	Marked relaxation (slack jaw)	Glazed and marked ptosis (half the eye or more)	3
Responds only after mild prodding or shaking	Few recognizable words			2
Does not respond to mild prodding or shaking				1 (asleep)

pofol-induced sedation.[86] However, the inability to recall a non-noxious stimulus such as a picture, as used in the above studies, may not necessarily correspond to amnesia to noxious events such as surgical stimulation. Despite this caveat, Liu and co-workers suggest that using a combination of propofol and midazolam to achieve a BIS value below 80 will minimize the possibility of intraoperative recall.[85] Although the use of BIS to monitor sedation is appealing, conventional assessment of sedation is an important mechanism whereby continuous patient contact is maintained. Ideally, BIS monitoring will be employed in the future as an adjunct to clinical evaluation rather than as the primary monitor of consciousness.

Preparedness to Recognize and Treat Local Anesthetic Toxicity

Monitored anesthesia care is often provided in the context of regional or local anesthetic techniques. It is vitally important that the anesthesiologist responsible for the patient have a high index of suspicion and be fully prepared to recognize and treat local anesthetic toxicity immediately (see Chapter 17). This point deserves special emphasis, particularly in view of the fact that monitored anesthesia care is often provided to the elderly or debilitated patient who has been deemed "unfit" for general anesthesia; these are the patients most likely to suffer adverse reactions to local anesthetic drugs. Even if the anesthesiologist does not perform the block personally, he or she is in a unique position to fulfill an important "preventive" role by advising the surgeon about the most appropriate volume, concentration, and type of local anesthetic drug or technique to be used.

Systemic local anesthetic toxicity occurs when plasma concentrations of drug are excessively high. Plasma concentrations will increase when the rate of entry of drug into the circulation exceeds the rate of drug clearance from the circulation. The clinically recognizable effects of local anesthetics on the central nervous system are concentration-dependent. At low concentrations, sedation and numbness of the tongue and circumoral tissues and a metallic taste are prominent features. As concentrations increase, restlessness, vertigo, tinnitus, and difficulty of focusing may occur. Higher concentrations result in slurred speech and skeletal muscle twitching, which often herald the onset of tonic–clonic seizures.

The conduct of monitored anesthesia care may modify the individual's response to the potentially toxic effects of local anesthetic administration and adversely affect the margin of safety of a regional or local technique. For example, a patient with compromised cardiovascular function may experience a further decline in cardiac output during sedation. The resultant reduction in hepatic blood flow will reduce the clearance of local anesthetics that are metabolized by the liver and have a high hepatic extraction ratio, thereby increasing the likelihood of achieving toxic plasma concentrations. A patient receiving sedation may experience respiratory depression and a subsequent increase in arterial carbon dioxide concentration. Hypercarbia adversely affects the margin of safety in several ways. By increasing cerebral blood flow, hypercarbia will increase the amount of local anesthetic that is delivered to the brain, thereby increasing the potential for neurotoxicity. By reducing neuronal axoplasmic pH, hypercarbia increases the intracellular concentration of the charged, active form of local anesthetic, thus also increasing its toxicity. In addition, hypercarbia, acidosis, and hypoxia all markedly potentiate the cardiovascular toxicity of local anesthetics. Furthermore, the administration of sedative–hypnotic drugs may interfere with the patient's ability to communicate the symptoms of impending neurotoxicity. However, the anticonvulsant properties of benzodiazepines and barbiturates may attenuate the seizures associated with neurotoxicity. In both of the above circumstances, it is possible that the symptoms of cardiotoxicity will be the first evidence that an adverse reaction has occurred. Thus, appropriate treatment is delayed or inadvertent intravascular injection is continued because of the absence of any clinical evidence of neurotoxicity. Cardiovascular toxicity usually occurs at a higher plasma concentration than neurotoxicity, but when it does occur, it is usually much more difficult to manage than neurotoxicity. Although cardiotoxicity is usually preceded by neurotoxicity, it may occur *de novo* when bupivacaine is being used.

Regional anesthetic techniques may have adverse effects upon respiratory function. The effects of clinically relevant concentrations of local anesthetics on respiratory control have been examined in two studies. In one of these studies, lidocaine was found to depress the ventilatory response to hypoxia.[87] The authors postulate that patients with carbon dioxide retention whose resting ventilation depends upon hypoxic drive may be at risk for ventilatory failure when lidocaine is administered (such as for arrhythmia control or regional anesthesia). However, lidocaine and bupivacaine have both been shown to increase the ventilatory response to carbon dioxide.[88,89] There appear to be few data concerning the combined effects of local anesthetics and sedative–hypnotics on respiratory control.

Sedation and Analgesia by Nonanesthesiologists

Although anesthesiologists have specific training and expertise to provide sedation and analgesia, in clinical practice these services are frequently provided by nonanesthesiologists. The specific reasons for nonanesthesiologist involvement differ from institution to institution and from case to case. Putative causes include: convenience, availability, and scheduling issues; perceived lack of anesthesiologist enthusiasm; perceived cost issues;

and a perceived lack of benefit concerning patient satisfaction and safety when sedation/analgesia is provided by anesthesiologists. Despite our frequent noninvolvement in these cases, anesthesiologists can be indirectly involved in the care of these patients by participating in the development of institutional policies and procedures for analgesia and sedation. To assist anesthesiologists in this process, an ASA task force has developed practice guidelines for sedation and analgesia by nonanesthesiologists.[1] Practice guidelines are recommendations that can be adopted, modified, exceeded, or rejected according to local institutional demands and resources.

The ASA practice guidelines define specifically the desired level of sedation that should be achieved by nonanesthesiologist providers. The term "sedation and analgesia" is used in preference to "conscious sedation": "Sedation and analgesia describes a state that allows patients to tolerate unpleasant procedures while maintaining adequate cardiorespiratory function and the ability to respond purposefully to verbal command and/or tactile stimulation." The practice guidelines specifically state that the patient whose only response is reflex withdrawal is sedated to a greater degree than defined by the term "sedation and analgesia." Excessive sedation may result in cardiorespiratory compromise. If cardiorespiratory compromise is not immediately diagnosed and treated appropriately, hypoxic brain damage or death may occur.

The guidelines emphasize the importance of preprocedure patient evaluation, patient preparation, and appropriate fasting periods. The importance of continuous patient monitoring is discussed: in particular, the response of the patient to commands as a guide to the level of consciousness. The appropriate monitoring of pulmonary ventilation, oxygenation, and hemodynamics is also discussed and recommendations are made for the contemporaneous recording of these parameters. The task force strongly suggests that an individual other than the person performing the procedure be available to monitor the patient's comfort and physiologic status. Education and training of providers is recommended. Specific educational objectives include: the potentiation of sedative-induced respiratory depression by concomitantly administered opioids, adequate time intervals between doses of sedative/analgesics to avoid cumulative overdosage, and familiarity with sedative/analgesic antagonists. The routine administration of supplemental oxygen is recommended. At least one person with advanced life support skills should be present during the procedure. This individual should have the ability to recognize airway obstruction, establish an airway, and maintain oxygenation and ventilation. The practice guidelines recommend that appropriate patient size emergency equipment be readily available, specifically including equipment for establishing an airway and delivering positive pressure ventilation with supplemental oxygen, emergency resuscitation drugs, and a working defibrillator. As discussed earlier in this chapter, the use of drug combinations may be more effective than using single agents to achieve adequate sedation/analgesia. However, in the context of nonanesthesiologist-provided sedation/analgesia it is important that the potential adverse effects on ventilatory function of drug combinations be well understood. When using combinations of drugs, the importance of careful individual drug titration rather than the use of fixed-dose combinations is emphasized. The presence of reliable intravenous access until the patient is no longer at risk for cardiorespiratory depression will improve safety. Adequate post-procedure recovery care with appropriate monitoring must be provided until discharge. Certain high-risk patient groups (e.g., uncooperative patients, extremes of age, severe cardiac, pulmonary, hepatic, renal, or central nervous system disease, morbid obesity, sleep apnea, pregnancy, drug or alcohol abuse) will be encountered. The guidelines recommend that preprocedure consultation with cardiologists, pulmonologists, and so forth be performed *before* administration of analgesia/sedation by nonanesthesiologists.

CONCLUSION

Through the use of monitored anesthesia care and conscious sedation, an often terrifying and painful procedure can be made safe and comfortable for the patient. Monitored anesthesia care presents an opportunity for our patients to observe us at work. For the anesthesiologist, monitored anesthesia care presents an opportunity to provide a more prolonged and intimate level of care and reassurance to our patients that is in contrast to the more limited exposure that occurs during and after general anesthesia. Our airway management skills and our daily practice of applied pharmacology make us uniquely qualified to provide this service. Monitored anesthesia care presents us with an opportunity to display these skills and increase our recognition in areas outside the operating room. The availability of drugs with a more favorable pharmacologic profile allows us to tailor our techniques to provide the specific components of analgesia, sedation, anxiolysis, and amnesia with minimal morbidity and to facilitate a prompt recovery. As the population ages, increasing numbers of patients will become candidates for monitored anesthesia care. Significant advances in nonsurgical fields, *e.g.,* interventional radiology, will increase the number of procedures that are ideally performed under monitored anesthesia care. It is our responsibility to clearly demonstrate to our nonanesthesia colleagues that anesthesiologist-provided monitored anesthesia care contributes to the best outcome for our patients. If anesthesiologists are not willing or able to provide these services, others, who are less well qualified, are prepared to assume that role.

REFERENCES

1. American Society of Anesthesiologists Task Force on Sedation and Analgesia by Non-anesthesiologists: Practice guidelines for sedation and analgesia by non-anesthesiologists. Anesthesiology 84:459, 1996
2. McCarthy FM, Solomon AL, Jastak JT *et al:* Conscious sedation: Benefits and risks. J Am Dental Assoc 109:546, 1984
3. Sa Rego MM, Watcha MF, White PF: The changing role of monitored anesthesia care in the ambulatory setting. Anesth Analg 85:1020, 1997
4. American Society of Anesthesiologists (ASA): Position on monitored anesthesia care. In ASA Directory of Members, p 481. Park Ridge, IL, American Society of Anesthesiologists, 1999
5. Wansbrough SR, White PF: Sedation scales: Measures of calmness or somnolence? Anesth Analg 76:219, 1993
6. Villieneuve A: Clinical differences between anxiolytics and sedatives. Mod Prob Pharmacopsychiatry 14:1, 1979
7. Ausems ME, Vuyk J, Hug CC Jr, Stanski DR: Comparison of a computer-assisted infusion versus intermittent bolus administration of alfentanil as a supplement to nitrous oxide for lower abdominal surgery. Anesthesiology 68:851, 1988
8. Hughes MA, Glass PSA, Jacobs JR: Context-sensitive half-time in multicompartment pharmacokinetic models for intravenous anesthetic drugs. Anesthesiology 76:334, 1992
9. Scott JC, Ponganis KV, Stanski DR: EEG quantitation of narcotic effect: The comparative pharmacodynamics of fentanyl and alfentanil. Anesthesiology 62:234, 1985
10. Mandema JW, Tuk B, van Stveninck AL *et al:* Pharmacokinetic-pharmacodynamic modeling of the central nervous system effects of midazolam and its main metabolite α-hydroxy-midazolam in healthy volunteers. Clin Pharmacol Ther 51:715, 1992
11. Buhrer M, Maitre PO, Crevoisier C, Stanski DR: Electroencephalographic effects of benzodiazepines. II. Pharmacodynamic modeling of the effects of midazolam and diazepam. Clin Pharmacol Ther 48:555, 1990
12. Glass P, Dyar O, Jhaveri R *et al:* TIVA-propofol and combinations of propofol with fentanyl [abstract]. Anesthesiology 75:A44, 1991
13. Smith C, McEwan AI, Jhaveri R *et al:* Reduction of propofol Cp50 by fentanyl [abstract]. Anesthesiology 77:A340, 1992
14. Short TG, Chui PT: Propofol and midazolam act synergistically in combination. Br J Anaesth 67:539, 1991
15. Short TG, Plummer JL, Chui PT: Hypnotic and anesthetic interactions between midazolam, propofol and alfentanil. Br J Anaesth 69:162, 1992
16. McEwan A, Smith C, Dyar O *et al:* MAC reduction of isoflurane by fentanyl [abstract]. Anesthesiology 75:A43, 1991

17. Sebel PS, Glass PSA, Fletcher JE *et al:* Reduction of the MAC of desflurane with fentanyl. Anesthesiology 76:52, 1992
18. Vinik HR, Bradley EL, Kissin I: Midazolam–alfentanil synergism for anesthetic induction in patients. Anesth Analg 69:213, 1989
19. Kissin I, Vinik HR, Castillo R, Bradley EL: Alfentanil potentiates midazolam-induced unconsciousness in subanalgesic doses. Anesth Analg 71:65, 1990
20. Federal Food and Drug Administration: Warning reemphasized in midazolam labeling. FDA Drug Bulletin 5, 1987
21. Bailey PL, Pace NL, Ashburn MA *et al:* Frequent hypoxemia and apnea after sedation with midazolam and fentanyl. Anesthesiology 73:826, 1990
22. Mackenzie N, Grant IS: Propofol for intravenous sedation. Anaesthesia 42:3, 1987
23. White PF, Negus JB: Sedative infusions during local and regional anesthesia: A comparison of midazolam and propofol. J Clin Anesth 3:32, 1991
24. Smith I, Monk T, White PF, Ding Y: Propofol infusion during regional anesthesia: Sedative, hypnotic and amnestic properties. Anesth Analg 79:313, 1994
25. Dubois A, Balatoni E, Peeters JP, Baudoux M: Use of propofol for sedation during gastrointestinal endoscopies. Anaesthesia 43(suppl):75, 1988
26. Kain ZN, Gaal D, Jaeger DD, Rimar S: Sedation for MRI in children: Propofol vs. barbiturates [abstract]. Anesthesiology 79:A1158, 1993
27. Monk TG, Boure B, White PF *et al:* Comparison of intravenous sedative-hypnotic techniques for outpatient immersion lithotripsy. Anesth Analg 72:616, 1991
28. Sherry E: Admixture of propofol and alfentanil: Use for intravenous sedation and analgesia during transvaginal oocyte retrieval. Anaesthesia 47:477, 1992
29. Oei-Lim LB, Vermeulen-Cranch DME, Bouvry-Berends ECM: Conscious sedation with propofol in dentistry. Br Dent J 170:340, 1991
30. Oei-Lim VLB, Kalkman CJ, Bouvry-Berends ECM *et al:* A comparison of the effects of propofol and nitrous oxide on the electroencephalogram in epileptic patients during conscious sedation for dental procedures. Anesth Analg 75:708, 1992
31. Whitehead C, Sanders LD, Oldroyd G *et al:* The subjective effects of low dose propofol. Anaesthesia 49:490, 1994
32. Borgeat A, Wilder-Smith OHG, Saiah M, Rifat K: Subhypnotic doses of propofol possess direct antiemetic properties. Anesth Analg 74:539, 1992
33. White PF, Negus JB: Sedative infusions during local and regional anesthesia: A comparison of midazolam and propofol. J Clin Anesth 3:32, 1991
34. Ghouri AF, Ramirez Ruiz MA, White PF: Effect of flumazenil on recovery after midazolam and propofol sedation. Anesthesiology 81:333, 1994
35. Smith I, White PF, Nathanson M, Gouldson R: Propofol: An update on its clinical use. Anesthesiology 81:1005, 1994
36. Stoelting RK: Benzodiazepines. In Pharmacology and Physiology in Anesthetic Practice, 2nd ed, p 118. Philadelphia, JB Lippincott, 1991
37. Taylor E, Ghouri AF, White PF: Midazolam in combination with propofol for sedation during local anesthesia. J Clin Anesth 4:213, 1992
38. Jacobs JR, Reves JG, Marty J *et al:* Aging increases pharmacodynamic sensitivity to the hypnotic effects of midazolam. Anesth Analg 80:143, 1995
39. Pratila MG, Fischer ME, Alagesan R *et al:* Propofol vs. midazolam for monitored sedation: A comparison of intraoperative and recovery parameters. J Clin Anesth 5:268, 1993
40. Klotz U, Kanto J: Pharmacokinetics and clinical uses of flumazenil. Clin Pharmacokinet 14:1, 1988
41. Gellar E, Halpern P: Benzodiazepines and their antagonists in anesthesia (IARS review course lecture). Anesth Analg 76:136, 1993
42. Ghouri AF, Ramirez Ruiz MA, White PF: Effect of flumazenil on recovery after midazolam and propofol sedation. Anesthesiology 81:333, 1994
43. Yee JB, Schafer PG, Crandall AS, Pace NL: Comparison of methohexital and alfentanil on movement during placement of retrobulbar nerve block. Anesth Analg 79:320, 1994
44. Veselis RA, Reinsel RA, Feshchenko VA *et al:* Impaired memory and behavioural performance with fentanyl at low plasma concentrations. Anesth Analg 79:952, 1994
45. Glass PSA, Gan TJ, Howell S: A review of the pharmacokinetics and pharmacodynamics of remifentanil. Anesth Analg 89(suppl):S7, 1999
46. Servin F, Desmonts JM, Watkins WD: Remifentanil as an analgesic adjunct in local/regional anesthesia and monitored anesthesia care. Anesth Analg 89(suppl):S28, 1999
47. Avramov MN, Smith I, White PF: Interactions between midazolam and remifentanil during monitored anesthesia care. Anesthesiology 85:1283, 1996
48. Ahmad S, Leavell M, Fragen RJ *et al:* Remifentanil versus alfentanil as analgesic adjuncts during placement of ophthalmologic nerve blocks. Reg Analg Pain Med. 24:331, 1999
49. Gold MI, Watkins WD, Sung YF *et al:* Remifentanil versus remifentanil/midazolam for ambulatory surgery during monitored anesthesia care. Anesthesiology 87:51, 1997
50. Perry F, Parker RK, White PF *et al:* Role of psychological factors in postoperative pain control and recovery with patient-controlled analgesia. Clin J Pain 10:57, 1994
51. Rudkin GE, Osborne GA, Curtis NJ: Intraoperative patient controlled sedation. Anaesthesia 46:90, 1991
52. Park WY, Watkins PA: Patient-controlled sedation during epidural anesthesia. Anesth Analg 72:304, 1991
53. Cork R, Guillory E, Viswanathan S: Effect of patient-controlled sedation on recovery from ambulatory monitored anesthesia care [abstract]. Anesthesiology 81:A31, 1994
54. Zelcer J, White PF, Chester S *et al:* Intraoperative patient-controlled analgesia: An alternative to physician administration during outpatient monitored anesthesia care. Anesth Analg 75:41, 1992
55. Montravers P, Duriel B, Molliex S, Desmonts JM: Effects of intravenous midazolam on the work of breathing. Anesth Analg 79:558, 1994
56. Gelb A, Southorn P, Redher K, Didier E: Sedation and respiratory mechanics in man. Br J Anaesth 57:1104, 1983
57. Morel DR, Forster A, Bachmann M, Suter PM: Effect of intravenous midazolam on breathing pattern and chest wall mechanics in humans. J Appl Physiol 55:419, 1983
58. Prato FS, Knill RL: Diazepam sedation reduces functional residual capacity and alters the distribution of ventilation in man. Anesth Analg 61:209, 1982
59. Cohen MI: Phrenic and recurrent laryngeal discharge patterns and the Hering-Breuer reflex. Am J Physiol 228:1489, 1975
60. Gottfried SR, Strohl KP, Van de Graaff W *et al:* Effects of phrenic stimulation on upper airway resistance in anesthetized dogs. J Appl Physiol 55:419, 1983
61. Montravers P, Dureuil B, Desmonts JM: Effects of i.v. midazolam on upper airway resistance. Br J Anaesth 68:27, 1992
62. Leiter JC, Knuth SL, Krol ZRC, Bartlett D: The effects of diazepam on genioglossal muscle activity in normal subjects. Am Rev Respir Dis 132:216, 1985
63. Rimaniol JM, D'Honneur G, Duvaldestin P: Recovery of the swallowing reflex after propofol anesthesia. Anesth Analg 79:856, 1994
64. Groves ND, Rees JL: Effects of benzodiazepines on laryngeal reflexes. Anaesthesia 42:808, 1987
65. Lambert Y, D'Honneur G, Abhay K, Gall O: Depression of swallowing reflex two hours after midazolam [abstract]. Anesthesiology 75:A891, 1991
66. Nishino T, Takizawa K, Yokokawa N, Hiraga K: Depression of the swallowing reflex during sedation and/or relative analgesia produced by inhalation of 50% nitrous oxide in oxygen. Anesthesiology 67:995, 1987
67. Caplan RA, Ward RJ, Posner K, Cheney FW: Unexpected cardiac arrest during spinal anesthesia: A closed claims analysis of predisposing factors. Anesthesiology 68:5, 1988
68. Weil JV, McCullocugh RE, Kline JS, Sodal IE: Diminished ventilatory response to hypoxia and hypercapnia after morphine in normal man. N Engl J Med 292:1103, 1975
69. Power SJ, Morgan M, Chakrabarti MK: Carbon dioxide response curves following midazolam and diazepam. Br J Anaesth 55:837, 1983
70. Jordan C, Lehane JR, Jones JG: Respiratory depression following diazepam: Reversal with high dose naloxone. Anesthesiology 53:293, 1980
71. American Society of Anesthesiologists: Standards for Basic Intraoperative Monitoring. 1999 Directory of Members, p 462. Park Ridge, IL, American Society of Anesthesiologists, 1999
72. Barker SJ, Tremper KK: Pulse oximetry. In Ehrenworth J, Eisenkraft J (eds): Anesthetic Equipment: Principles and Applications, p 249. St Louis, CV Mosby, 1993

73. Raemer DB, Warren DL, Morris R *et al:* Hypoxemia during ambulatory gynecologic surgery as evaluated by the pulse oximeter. J Clin Monit 3:244, 1987

74. Wukitsch MW, Tobler D, Pologe J *et al:* Pulse oximetry: An analysis of theory, technology, and practice. J Clin Monit 4:290, 1988

75. Pressman MA: A simple method for measuring end-tidal CO_2 during MAC and major regional anesthesia. Anesth Analg 67:900, 1988

76. Norman EA, Zeig NJ, Ahmad I: Better designs for mass spectrometer monitoring of the awake patient (letter). Anesthesiology 64:664, 1986

77. Bowe EA, Boysen PG, Brome JA *et al:* Accurate determination of end-tidal CO_2 through nasal cannulae. J Clin Monit 5:105, 1989

78. Goldmann JM: A simple and inexpensive method for monitoring end-tidal CO_2 through nasal cannulae (letter). Anesthesiology 67:606, 1987

79. Kurz A, Kurz M, Poeschl G *et al:* Forced-air warming maintains intraoperative normothermia better than circulating-water mattresses. Anesth Analg 77:89, 1993

80. Frank SM, Fleisher LA, Breslow MJ *et al:* Perioperative maintenance of normothermia reduces the incidence of morbid cardiac events: a randomized trial. JAMA 277:1127, 1997

81. Sessler DI: Temperature monitoring and management during neuraxial anesthesia. Anesth Analg 88:243, 1999

82. Frank SM, Nguyen JM, Garcia CM *et al:* Temperature monitoring practices during regional anesthesia. Anesth Analg 88:373, 1999

83. Scholefield JH, Gerber MA, Dwyer P. Liquid crystal forehead temperature strips. Am J Dis Child 136:198, 1982

84. Chernik DA, Gillings D, Laine H *et al:* Validity and reliability of the observer's assessment of alertness/sedation scale: Study with intravenous midazolam. J Clin Psychopharmacol 10:244, 1990

85. Liu J, Singh HS, White PF: Electroencephalographic bispectral index correlates with intraoperative recall and depth of propofol induced sedation. Anesth Analg 84:185, 1997

86. Kearse LA, Manberg P, Chamoun N *et al:* Bispectral analysis of the electroencephalogram correlates with patient movement to skin incision during propofol/nitrous oxide anesthesia. Anesthesiology 81:1365, 1994.

87. Gross JB, Caldwell CB, Shaw LM, Apfelbaum JL: The effect of lidocaine infusion on the ventilatory response to hypoxia. Anesthesiology 61:662, 1984

88. Negre I, Labaille T, Samii K, Noviant Y: Ventilatory response to CO_2 following axillary blockade with bupivacaine. Anesthesiology 63:401, 1985

89. Labaille T, Clergue F, Samii K *et al:* Dual effects of lidocaine on the ventilatory response to CO_2 [abstract]. Anesthesiology 61: A227, 1984

Clinical Anesthesia (4/e), edited by
Paul G. Barash, Bruce F. Cullen, and
Robert K. Stoelting. Lippincott Williams &
Wilkins, Philadelphia, © 2001.

CHAPTER 48

TRAUMA AND BURNS

LEVON M. CAPAN AND SANFORD M. MILLER

Injuries are the most common cause of death in Americans between the ages of 1 and 45 years; more than 50% of all deaths in people between 5 and 34 years of age result from trauma.[1] Although the proportionate mortality rate from trauma (6.3%) is far less than those of heart disease (31.5%) and cancer (23.3%), these are most often diseases of older people.[1] Thus, injuries remain the largest contributor (34%) to the 13.6 million years of productive life lost annually in the population younger than 75 years of age. As of 1996, years of productive life lost from trauma were 4.6 million; malignancy, 4.4 million; heart disease, 3.5 million; and human immunodeficiency virus infection, 1.1 million.[1]

In the United States, deaths from unintentional injuries are most often the result of motor vehicle accidents, falls, poisoning, fires, or drowning.[1] In the last few years, although the number of deaths from unintentional injuries has been stable at approximately 92,000 per year, the per capita mortality rate has been decreasing because the population has been increasing.[1] However, this improvement has been thwarted by an alarming increase in violent injuries, especially in inner cities, mostly caused by firearms, and usually affecting young men of minority groups.[2,3] In 1996, the death toll from homicide was 20,971 and from suicide 30,903, a total intentional injury mortality of approximately 52,000.

Although the time of death after trauma may be influenced by the type and severity of injury and the effectiveness of prehospital and hospital care, existing data suggest that between 34 and 76% of trauma deaths occur immediately at the scene of the accident or during transport to the hospital.[4-6] Central nervous system (CNS) injuries, exsanguination, or both are responsible for 90% of these deaths;[6] hypoxia as a result of airway obstruction, aspiration of gastric contents, or pneumothorax may also contribute. Any improvement in prehospital care is unlikely to better the outcome of these unsalvageable patients.

Approximately 75% of the hospital mortality from trauma occurs within 48 hours after admission,[4,6,7] most commonly from thoracic, abdominal or retroperitoneal, vascular, or CNS injuries.[6,7] Hypoxia, systemic air embolism, and cardiac failure may also be direct or contributing factors.[6] Approximately one third of these patients die within the first 4 hours after admission, representing most of operating room trauma deaths.[4,5] Of the remaining 25% of hospital deaths, 5–10% occur between the third and seventh day of admission, usually from CNS injuries,[4,5,7] and the rest in subsequent weeks, most commonly as a result of multiorgan failure.[6] Pulmonary thromboembolism and infectious complications may also contribute to mortality during this phase.[6,7] The quality of life may also be affected; approximately 80% of survivors of major trauma have significant functional limitation at 12 and 18 months after injury.[8]

TRAUMA CENTERS

The American College of Surgeons (ACS) has published guidelines for the organization of centers structured to care for injuries of various grades of severity.[9] A Level I trauma center must manage at least 1200 patients annually, 20% of whom should have injury severity scores of 15 or greater.[9] Other requirements include around-the-clock coverage in a fully staffed emergency department by a physician experienced in management of injuries, with continuous availability of a surgeon, a neurosurgeon,

and other consultants who can be present within a short time. There should always be an operating room prepared and staffed, along with available anesthesia personnel, an intensive care unit (ICU), a fully equipped laboratory and blood bank, and a radiology facility that can perform portable chest radiographs, computed tomography (CT), angiography, and ultrasound studies. Level I and II trauma centers must have anesthesia services available in-house 24 hours a day.[9] Preferably, anesthesia care in a Level I or II trauma center should be controlled by an anesthesiologist interested and experienced in the care of the injured.[9] In Level I and II trauma centers, senior anesthesia residents (chief residents as described in the ACS manual) or certified registered nurse anesthetists (CRNA) experienced in trauma care can initiate emergency care, including surgical anesthesia, as long as an attending physician is notified and can arrive promptly.[9] In Level III trauma centers, a CRNA may provide initial care, as long as an anesthesiologist is immediately available, or in the worst circumstances, the CRNA is supervised by a physician skilled in airway management.[9] Approximately 12% of injured patients require Level I care.[10]

Unfortunately, the changing demographics of trauma victims has put severe financial pressure on designated trauma centers. As discussed previously, in some areas the previously predominant population of blunt trauma victims, more than 70% of whom are insured and, proportional to their injury severity, generate significant profit to the institution,[11] is being replaced by an increasing number of people injured by firearms, who are mostly underinsured or uninsured, and whose medical expenses are either covered by public funds or written off as bad debt. In a population-based study in California, annual medical charges for 9193 hospitalized firearm injuries were $164 million. Seventy-five percent of these patients were either uninsured or had publicly financed health insurance.[12] This is part of the reason that 66 of 600 designated trauma centers closed between 1983 and 1992.[13] This trend has been reversed since 1992 by the passage of the Trauma Care Systems Planning and Development Act of 1990 (Public Law 101-590). Under this law, in 1993 development grants were given to 19 states for initiation of trauma systems, while an additional 16 states received funds to improve their existing programs.[14]

The economic impact of trauma on society is enormous. In 1998, the estimated total cost of unintentional injuries alone exceeded $500 billion, including wage and productivity losses of $246 billion and medical expenses of $76 billion, in addition to other costs.[1]

INITIAL EVALUATION AND RESUSCITATION

The Advanced Trauma Life Support (ATLS) Course developed by the Committee on Trauma of the ACS provides the trauma team with a common base of clinical knowledge and skills that facilitates coordination and clear, rapid, and accurate communication during the initial phase of treatment.[15] The main emphasis in the ATLS Course is on the recognition of clinical priorities that proceed in a stepwise fashion to assess and treat injuries in order from the most to the least life threatening. Although this vertical or sequential care design is safe and frequently practiced in centers with limited manpower, in hospitals where personnel from various clinical disciplines can readily form a multidisciplinary team, a horizontal or simultaneous approach is used. In this manner, each group of physicians carries out its role in resuscitation, coordinated by a team leader who applies the same priority-oriented care principles.[9] As part of the team, the anesthesiologist, aside from managing the airway, contributes to evaluation and resuscitation while gathering information needed for possible future anesthetic management.

The clinical strategy of initial management can be defined as a continuous, priority-driven process of patient assessment, resuscitation, and reassessment. The general approach to evaluation of the acute trauma victim has three sequential components: rapid overview, primary survey, and secondary survey[15] (Fig. 48-1). Resuscitation is initiated, if needed, at any time during this continuum. *Rapid overview* takes only a few seconds and is used to determine whether the patient is stable, unstable, dead, or dying. The *primary survey* involves rapid evaluation of functions that are crucial to survival. The "ABCs" of airway patency, breathing, and circulation are assessed. Then a brief neurologic examination is performed and the patient is examined for injuries that might have been overlooked.

The *secondary survey* involves a more elaborate systematic examination of the entire body to identify additional injuries. Radiographic and other diagnostic procedures may also be performed if the stability of the patient permits. Within this general framework, the anesthesiologist identifies injuries, pre-existing conditions, and any resulting functional abnormalities that require either immediate treatment or provision for resuscitative and anesthetic management.

RAPID OVERVIEW

(Differentiation between stable, unstable and dead or dying patient)

PRIMARY SURVEY

(Evaluation and Concurrent Resuscitation)

1) Airway
2) Breathing
3) Circulation
4) Neurologic Function
5) Examination of undressed patient

(Essential Laboratory and Radiologic Examination)

SECONDARY SURVEY

(Detailed and Systematic Evaluation of Injury to each Anatomic Region and Resuscitation at any time, if necessary)

Operating Room for Emergency Surgery

Radiology Suite For Special X-rays (CT Scan, arteriogram, esophagram)

Observation in ER Or ICU

Operating Room

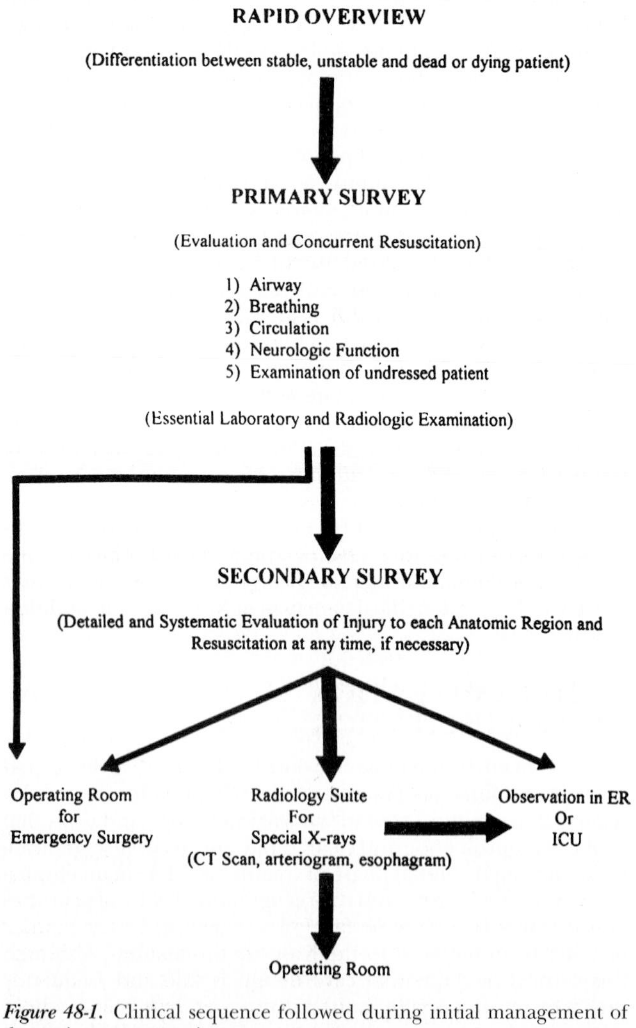

Figure 48-1. Clinical sequence followed during initial management of the major trauma patient.

An important issue should be emphasized at this time. Many trauma victims are carriers of hepatitis B, hepatitis C, tuberculosis, or human immunodeficiency virus.[16–18] Universal infection control precautions are the standard and must be used during every stage of management of these patients.

It is possible that injuries may be missed during initial evaluation and even during emergency surgery. An Australian study demonstrated that many clinically significant injuries were undiagnosed, resulting in significant pain, complications, residual disability, delay of treatment, or death.[19] Examples of missed diagnoses included cervical spine, thoracoabdominal, pelvic, nerve, and external soft tissue injuries, and extremity fractures. Some of these injuries may present during anesthesia, such as spinal cord damage during airway management in a patient with unrecognized cervical spine injury, massive intraoperative bleeding from an unrecognized thoracoabdominal injury during extremity surgery, or sudden intraoperative hypoxemia in a patient with unrecognized pneumothorax. A *tertiary survey* within the first 24 hours after admission (that may include a period of anesthesia), which involves repeating the primary and secondary examinations and reviewing the radiologic and laboratory results, has been shown to diagnose 90% of clinically significant injuries missed during initial evaluation.[19]

Airway Evaluation and Intervention

Airway evaluation (see also Chapter 23) involves the diagnosis of any trauma to the airway or surrounding tissues, recognition and anticipation of the respiratory consequences of these injuries, and prediction of the potential for exacerbation of these or other injuries by any contemplated airway management maneuvers. Although nontraumatic causes of airway difficulty, such as pre-existing factors, may be present, only the management of trauma-related problems is discussed in this section.

Asphyxia or Hypoxia

Airway obstruction, hypopnea or apnea, thoracic trauma, inhalation injury, and pulmonary embolism (PE; air, fat, or thrombus) are the most frequent causes of this complication. Rapid intervention is required to restore airway patency, administer oxygen, establish ventilation, and ultimately secure the airway. Hypoxia may be difficult to recognize in the severely injured patient; its symptoms may be masked or attributed to other causes. For example, cyanosis may be undetectable in the presence of coexisting anemia, a low-flow state, or dark skin pigmentation. Apprehension and restlessness may be attributed to fear and anxiety rather than to hypoxia. If the patient can talk, serious airway obstruction is unlikely, although inability to respond verbally may also be caused by respiratory or CNS dysfunction.

Airway obstruction is probably the most frequent cause of asphyxia, and may result from posteriorly displaced or lacerated pharyngeal soft tissues, hematoma, bleeding, secretions, foreign bodies, or displaced bone or cartilage fragments. Bleeding into the cervical region may produce airway obstruction not only because of direct airway occlusion by the hematoma but from venous congestion and upper airway edema as a result of compression of neck veins.[20] Signs of upper and lower airway obstruction include dyspnea, hoarseness, stridor, dysphonia, subcutaneous emphysema, and hemoptysis. Cervical deformity, edema, crepitation, tracheal deviation, or jugular venous distention may be present before appearance of these symptoms and may help to indicate that specialized airway management techniques are required.

The initial steps in airway management are chin lift, jaw thrust, clearing of the oropharyngeal cavity, placement of an oropharyngeal or nasopharyngeal airway, and in inadequately breathing patients, ventilation with a self-inflating bag. These measures should follow immobilization of the cervical spine and should include administration of oxygen. Blind passage of a nasopharyngeal airway on a nasogastric or nasotracheal tube should be avoided if a basilar skull fracture is suspected; it may enter the anterior cranial fossa.[21] A cuffed oropharyngeal airway (COPA) with a standard connector may permit ventilation by a self-inflating bag, although it provides no protection against aspiration of gastric contents. If these measures do not provide adequate ventilation, the trachea must be intubated immediately using either direct laryngoscopy or a cricothyroidotomy, depending on the results of airway assessment. Whenever possible, the airway should be secured only after adequate ventilation and oxygenation are provided by mask. Maxillofacial, neck, and chest injuries and cervicofacial burns are the most common trauma-related causes of difficult tracheal intubation. Appropriate personnel and equipment must be ready to establish an emergency surgical airway in case attempts at direct laryngoscopy fail. Airway assessment should therefore include a rapid examination of the anterior neck for the feasibility of access to the cricothyroid membrane. Tracheostomy is not desirable during initial management because it takes longer to perform than a cricothyroidotomy and requires neck extension, which may cause or exacerbate cord trauma in cervical spine–injured patients. Conversion to a tracheostomy should be considered to prevent laryngeal damage if a cricothyroidotomy will be in place for more than 2–3 days. Possible contraindications to cricothyroidotomy include age younger than 12 years and suspected laryngeal trauma; laryngeal damage may result in the former and uncorrectable airway obstruction may occur in the latter situation.

A high rate of success in prehospital airway management by paramedics is possible using the laryngeal mask airway (LMA), esophageal–tracheal combitube, tracheal intubation under direct laryngoscopy with or without rapid-sequence induction, and surgical cricothyroidotomy.[22–24] Proper placement of these devices should be confirmed, preferably with capnography, as soon as possible. Esophageal lacerations presenting as subcutaneous emphysema, pneumomediastinum, or pneumoperitoneum have been described secondary to esophageal–tracheal combitube use.[25,26]

Full Stomach

A full stomach is a background condition in acute trauma; the urgency of securing the airway most often does not permit adequate time for pharmacologic measures to reduce gastric volume and acidity. Thus, rather than relying on these agents, the emphasis should be placed on selection of a safe technique for securing the airway when necessary: rapid-sequence induction with cricoid pressure for those patients without serious airway problems, and awake intubation with sedation and topical anesthesia, if possible, for those patients who may present with serious airway difficulties. Excessive cricoid pressure is unnecessary and may increase the likelihood of a reduction in expired tidal volume, an increase in peak airway pressure, and even complete airway obstruction.[27] Posterior displacement of a vertebral bone fragment, with potential damage to the spinal cord, may also occur when cricoid pressure and manual inline stabilization (MIS) are applied to cervical spine–injured patients.[28] Modifying this technique by supporting the back of the neck with another hand may alleviate this problem.[27]

The probability of a full stomach precludes the use of an LMA or any other device that does not protect the trachea as a definitive airway in trauma patients. However, there are some potential benefits to using this device. It can serve as a bridge for a brief period to re-establish airway patency or to facilitate intubation aided by a flexible fiberoptic bronchoscope. In patients with maxillofacial injuries, aspiration of pharyngeal blood or secretions is more likely than aspiration of gastric contents.[29] If it can be inserted in these circumstances, an LMA may protect the lungs. Positive-pressure ventilation may be used with the LMA provided that peak airway pressures do not exceed 25 cm H_2O.[27] However, trauma patients with pulmonary contusion,

edema, or aspiration may be difficult to ventilate with this device. Difficulty may also be encountered when inserting an LMA in the presence of cricoid pressure and MIS of the cervical spine.[27,30] These problems may be somewhat circumvented with the intubating laryngeal mask (ILM); adequate ventilation is more likely, blind tracheal intubation is more successful, and an endotracheal tube up to 8 mm can be placed by ILM, as opposed to the maximum of 6 mm that can be passed through an LMA.[31,32] An important disadvantage of the ILM is that its metal part may exert considerable pressure against cervical vertebrae, potentially exacerbating an unstable injury in this region.[33]

The selection of an airway management technique in the trauma patient is affected by his or her hemodynamic condition. The presence of uncorrectable hypotension from hemorrhage, hypovolemia, or pericardial tamponade may necessitate omitting intravenous (iv) anesthetics from the rapid-sequence technique. Muscle relaxants alone may be sufficient. If only a mild to moderate degree of hypovolemia is present, reduced doses (30–50%) of iv anesthetics should be administered.[34] Although there is no evidence that the choice of iv agent affects outcome, ketamine and etomidate may confer advantages over thiopental and propofol. In equipotent doses, in normovolemic patients, they have less cardiovascular depressant effects. The resulting better muscle perfusion promotes increased drug delivery to the neuromuscular junction, accelerating the onset time of muscle relaxants.[35] Although succinylcholine, with its short onset time and duration, is still the muscle relaxant of choice for rapid-sequence induction, the nondepolarizing relaxants rocuronium (0.9–1.2 $mg \cdot kg^{-1}$) and rapacuronium[36] (1.5–2.5 $mg \cdot kg^{-1}$) have onset times almost comparable with that of succinylcholine and do not have the undesirable side effects associated with succinylcholine (*e.g.*, increased intragastric, intraocular, and intracranial pressure, and potassium release in patients with burns and neurologic diseases).[37,38] Bradycardia, dysrhythmias, and cardiac arrest have been described after succinylcholine in the presence of hypoxia and hypercarbia; however, these complications may also follow apparently uneventful intubation performed without succinylcholine.

There is no consensus about the extent of the airway that can be safely anesthetized with topical agents to facilitate awake tracheal intubation in the trauma patient. Anesthesia of the entire pharynx, larynx, and trachea clearly provides the most optimal conditions. Avoiding transtracheal and superior laryngeal nerve blockade helps to preserve glottic and cough reflexes, although tracheal intubation is technically more difficult. Another approach is to block the superior laryngeal nerves in addition to topically anesthetizing the mouth and pharynx, using the rationale that even in the absence of glottic closure, an intact cough reflex will cause the expulsion of aspirated material. To our knowledge, there are no data to verify which method is superior.

Agitated and uncooperative patients present a difficult situation. Topical anesthesia of the airway may be impossible, whereas administration of sedative agents may result in apnea or airway obstruction, with an increased risk of aspiration of gastric contents and inadequate conditions for tracheal intubation. After locating the cricothyroid membrane and denitrogenating the lungs, a rapid-sequence induction may be used to permit securing the airway with direct laryngoscopy or, if necessary, with immediate cricothyroidotomy. Personnel and material necessary to perform translaryngeal ventilation or cricothyroidotomy must be secured before induction of general anesthesia.[39]

Head, Open Eye, and Contained Major Vessel Injuries

The principles of tracheal intubation are similar for all of these injuries. Apart from the need to ensure adequate oxygenation and ventilation, these patients require deep anesthesia and profound muscle relaxation before airway manipulation. This helps to prevent hypertension, coughing, and bucking, and thereby minimizes intracranial, intraocular, or intravascular pressure elevation, which can result in herniation of the brain, extrusion of eye contents, or dislodgment of a hemostatic clot from an injured vessel, respectively. The preferred anesthetic sequence to achieve this goal includes preoxygenation and opioid loading followed by relatively large doses of an iv anesthetic and muscle relaxant. Because of its rapid onset and short duration, remifentanil has been considered for opioid loading; a $1 \ \mu g \cdot kg^{-1}$ bolus with or without a $0.5 \ \mu g \cdot kg^{-1}$ infusion can attenuate the pressor response to laryngoscopy and intubation.[40,41] In one study, however, almost one half of the patients had hypotension and bradycardia unless glycopyrrolate was also given.[41] Hemodynamic responses to the opioid should be carefully monitored and promptly corrected. Systemic hypotension, intracranial pressure (ICP) elevation, and decreased cerebral perfusion pressure (CPP) may occur whether cerebral autoregulation is present or absent, and if untreated can produce secondary ischemic insults.[42] Ketamine is probably contraindicated in patients with head and vascular injuries because it may increase both intracranial[43,44] and systemic vascular pressures; however, no significant increase in intraocular pressure (IOP) has been documented.[45] Any muscle relaxant, including succinylcholine, may be used as long as the fasciculations produced by this agent are inhibited by prior administration of an adequate dose of a nondepolarizing muscle relaxant.[46] Alternatively, rocuronium can be administered; intubating conditions may be achieved within 60 seconds with a dose of $1.6–2.0 \ mg \cdot kg^{-1}$, although the neuromuscular blockade produced by this dose lasts approximately 2 hours.[47] Intravenous lidocaine may be used although its attenuating effect on the pressor response to airway instrumentation is mild and unpredictable. Of course, neither muscle relaxants nor iv anesthetics are indicated when initial assessment suggests a difficult airway. If the patient is hypotensive, the same precautions used during intubation in any other trauma victim apply: little or no iv anesthetic is administered.

Cervical Spine Injury

Cervical spine injury may be present in any trauma patient, but it is more likely in those sustaining high-velocity blunt injuries, especially above the clavicle. Evidence of a serious new spinal cord injury or accentuation of existing neurologic abnormalities has been documented after intubation of patients with unsuspected cervical spine injuries.[48,49] Immobilization of the neck in a neutral position is indicated in all unconscious patients, in conscious patients with cervical pain or tenderness, and whenever the pain of other injuries is likely to mask neck pain.[50] The combined use of a semirigid collar, sandbags placed on both sides of the head and neck, bindings, and a backboard provides the most reliable immobilization.[50] For airway management purposes, however, MIS, with assistants holding the head and torso of the patient, is a practical and safe method if the neck is not otherwise reliably stabilized.[50] A semirigid neck collar alone does not provide reliable protection. Of course, the airway must be evaluated before administration of any anesthetics or muscle relaxants. The anterior part of the cervical collar can be removed for this purpose. Protection of the neck should be maintained after tracheal intubation until a cervical spine injury has been ruled out.

Nasotracheal intubation carries the risks of epistaxis, failure of intubation, and the possibility of entry of the endotracheal tube into the cranial vault or the orbit if there is damage to the cranial base or the maxillofacial complex. Absence of the usual signs of cranial base fracture (Battle sign, raccoon eyes, or bleeding from the ear or the nose) cannot be relied on to exclude the possibility of its occurrence because with rapid prehospital transport, these signs may not be immediately apparent. Thus, nasotracheal intubation cannot be routinely recommended for the early phase of trauma management. Orotracheal intubation with direct laryngoscopy is more desirable, although stabilization of the neck, which limits head extension, may make glottic visualization difficult. The incidence of inadequate exposure of the larynx increases from less than 3% in the general population to approximately 10% with immobilization of the neck.[51,52]

A variety of devices and techniques, including the McCoy laryngoscope, rigid fiberoptic laryngoscopes (Bullard or WuScope), flexible fiberoptic endoscope, light-wand, translaryngeal (retrograde) intubation, and cricothyroidotomy, can be used to secure the airway in patients requiring cervical spine immobilization.[27] In most instances, successful, safe, and rapid tracheal intubation can be achieved with a conventional laryngoscope in spite of limited visualization of the larynx.[53] The McCoy laryngoscope with its flexible tip is able to lift the epiglottis and improve the laryngeal view without adding to the time and complexity of the procedure.[27] A gum-elastic bougie passed through the endotracheal tube, or a satin-sheathed stylet placed through its Murphy aperture may also be helpful because they can be inserted through the larynx more easily than the tube itself; their small diameter does not block the view of the glottis during direct laryngoscopy.[54] Other specialized techniques require operator experience and a longer preparation and performance time; thus, they should probably be used in cervical spine–stabilized patients only when tracheal intubation is suspected or proven to be impossible. Of these, the WuScope provides a consistently good laryngeal view with a high success rate of intubation and minimal neck movement.[55] The Bullard scope is also considered useful, although there have been no studies comparing it with the WuScope.[51]

Although flexible fiberoptic laryngoscopy and translaryngeal guided intubation (see Maxillofacial Injuries) cause almost no neck movement, the presence of blood or secretions in the airway, a long preparation time, and difficulty in their use in comatose, uncooperative, or anesthetized patients reduce their utility during initial management.

Direct Airway Injuries

Direct airway damage can occur anywhere between the nasopharynx and the bronchi; sometimes more than one site may be involved, resulting in persistent airway dysfunction after one of the problems is corrected.[56] The clinical presentation and management of airway compromise resulting from direct trauma are determined by the type of injury and its location.

Maxillofacial Injuries. In addition to soft tissue edema of the pharynx and peripharyngeal hematoma, blood or debris in the oropharyngeal cavity may be responsible for partial or complete airway obstruction in the acute stage of these injuries. Occasionally teeth or foreign bodies in the pharynx may be aspirated into the airway, causing some degree of obstruction, which may occur or be recognized only during attempts at tracheal intubation. Another problem is the dynamic nature of soft tissue injuries in this region. A hematoma or edema in the head or neck may expand during the 6–12 hours after injury and ultimately occlude the airway.[57] Serious airway compromise may develop within a few hours in up to 50% of patients with major penetrating facial injuries or multiple trauma as a result of progressive inflammation or edema resulting from liberal administration of fluids.[58,59] Prophylactic intubation of the trachea or very close and repeated examination of the upper airway may help detect the potential for airway compromise before its occurrence.

Certain facial fractures may also produce airway compromise. In bilateral parasymphyseal fractures of the mandible, a posteriorly shifted bone fragment may encroach on the pharynx and the larynx; traction on this fragment with the hand or a clamp can relieve the airway obstruction. Bilateral, but not unilateral, mandibular condyle fractures may prevent adequate mouth opening, thus causing problems with laryngoscopy. In the midface, trimalar fractures can cause the free fragment of the zygoma to descend in front of the coronoid process of the mandible and interfere with mouth opening. These mechanical problems should be differentiated from the limitation of jaw movement produced by pain and trismus. Fentanyl in titrated doses of up to 2–4 $\mu g \cdot kg^{-1}$ over a period of 10–20 minutes may produce an improvement in the patient's ability to open the mouth in the latter case.

LeFort fractures of the midface are the most severe types of facial trauma. Of these, LeFort 1 involves the maxilla and the maxillary sinus. Airway management is easy in these patients because the fracture mobilizes the upper jaw, leaving more maneuvering room for the laryngoscope. Both LeFort 2 and LeFort 3 fractures involve the thick portion of the nasal bone; LeFort 2 extends to the medial side of the orbit, whereas the LeFort 3 involves the orbit laterally and extends toward the temporal bone. From the airway management standpoint, the degree of posterior extension of these fractures is important. The pterygoid plate, an inferior process of the sphenoid bone, is the only buttress that prevents the midface from shifting posteriorly. In LeFort 2 and 3 fractures, the pterygoid plate is fractured at its base, often in combination with the cranial base, including the cribriform plate. With disruption of the posterior buttress, the entire midface of the patient with one of these fractures moves backward and may encroach on the pharynx[60] (Fig. 48-2).

The selection of an airway management technique in the presence of a maxillofacial fracture is based on the presenting condition. Most patients with isolated facial injury do not require emergency tracheal intubation. Surgery for facial injuries may be delayed for approximately a week without adverse effect on the repair. Patients who present with airway compromise may be intubated using direct laryngoscopy; the use of anesthetics and muscle relaxants is based on the results of airway evaluation. When there is bleeding into the oropharynx, a flexible fiberoptic laryngoscope may be useless because of obstruction of the view. A retrograde technique, using a wire or epidural catheter passed through a 14-gauge catheter introduced into the trachea through the cricothyroid membrane, may be used if the patient can open his or her mouth. A surgical airway is indicated when there is airway compromise, when direct laryngoscopy has failed or is considered impossible, when the jaws will be wired, or when a tracheostomy tube will be placed anyway after definitive repair of the fracture. Nasogastric or nasotracheal intubation should be avoided when basilar skull or maxillary fracture is suspected because of the possibility that the tube may enter the cranium or the orbital fossa. Cranial and cervical spine injuries are commonly associated with midface fractures; the airway management must be tailored accordingly.[61] The likelihood of cranial injury increases in midface fractures involving the frontal sinus and the orbitozygomatic and orbitoethmoid complexes.[62]

Cervical Airway Injuries. Injury to the cervical air passages can result from blunt or penetrating trauma. In the latter category, stab wounds are usually easier to manage than gunshot wounds. Clinical signs such as escape of air, hemoptysis, and coughing are present in almost all patients with penetrating injuries, facilitating the diagnosis. In contrast, major blunt laryngotracheal damage may be missed, either because the patient is asymptomatic or unresponsive, or because suggestive signs and symptoms are missed in the initial evaluation.[56] The typical presentation includes hoarseness, muffled voice, dyspnea, stridor, dysphagia, odynophagia, cervical pain and tenderness, ecchymosis, subcutaneous emphysema, and flattening of the thyroid cartilage protuberance (Adam's apple).[63] Whether the trauma is blunt or penetrating, attempts at blind tracheal intubation may produce further trauma to the larynx and complete airway obstruction if the endotracheal tube enters a false passage or disrupts the continuity of an already tenuous airway.[64,65] Thus, whenever possible, intubation of the trachea should be performed using a flexible fiberoptic bronchoscope, or an airway should be established surgically. A CT scan of the neck provides valuable information and should be performed before any airway intervention in all stable patients without respiratory and hemodynamic compromise.

The strategy for tracheal intubation depends on the clinical presentation.[64] The tracheas of some patients with penetrating airway injuries, especially stab wounds, may be intubated through the airway defect without the need for anesthetics or optical equipment.[51] Patients with a normal airway on endoscopy can be intubated orotracheally under general anesthesia. The presence of cartilaginous fractures or mucosal abnormalities necessitates awake intubation with a fiberoptic bronchoscope or awake tracheostomy. Laryngeal damage precludes cricothyroidotomy. Tracheostomy should be performed with extreme caution because up to 70% of patients with blunt laryngeal injuries may have an associated cervical spine injury.[64] Uncooperative or confused patients may not tolerate awake airway manipulation. It may be best to transport these patients to the operating room, induce anesthesia with inhalational agents, and intubate the trachea without muscle relaxants.[64] Episodes of airway obstruction during spontaneous breathing under an inhalational anesthetic can be managed by positioning the patient upright in addition to usual maneuvers. In extreme situations such as near-complete transection of the larynx and trachea, femorofemoral bypass or percutaneous cardiopulmonary support should be considered.[66]

Thoracic Airway Injuries. Whereas penetrating trauma can cause damage to any segment of the intrathoracic airway, blunt injury usually involves the posterior membranous portion of the trachea and the mainstem bronchi, usually within approximately 3 cm from the carina. Pneumothorax, pneumomediastinum, pneumopericardium, subcutaneous emphysema, and a continuous air leak from the chest tube are the usual signs of this injury; they occur frequently, but are not specific for thoracic airway damage. When tracheal intubation is performed without the suspicion of an underlying tracheal injury, difficulty in obtaining a seal around the endotracheal tube, or the presence on a chest radiograph of a large radiolucent area in the trachea corresponding to the cuff, suggests a perforated airway.[67] Other radiographic findings include a radiolucent line along the prevertebral fascia due to air tracking up from the mediastinum, peribronchial air or sudden obstruction along

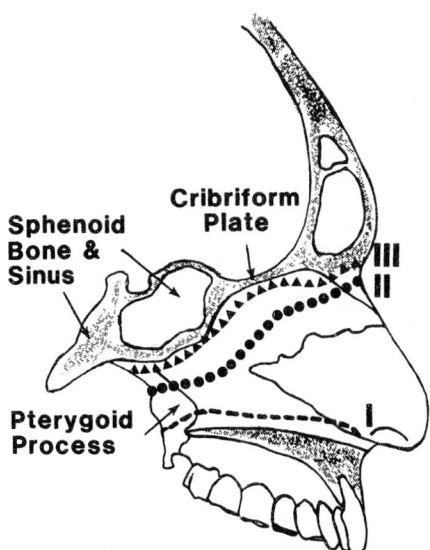

Sphenoid Bone & Sinus

Cribriform Plate

Pterygoid Process

III

II

I

Figure 48-2. Anteroposterior fracture lines of LeFort 1 (I), LeFort 2 (II) and LeFort 3 (III) injuries. Note that in LeFort 3 fracture the pterygoid process, the only facial buttress posteriorly, is injured from its base, allowing the entire midface to shift posteriorly. In this injury, the cribriform plate may also be fractured. (Reprinted by permission from Capan LM, Miller, SM, Glickmann R: Management of facial injuries. In Capan LM, Miller SM, Turndorf H [eds]: Trauma: Anesthesia and Intensive Care, p 383. Philadelphia, JB Lippincott, 1991.)

an air-filled bronchus, and the "dropped lung" sign. The latter occurs when complete intrapleural bronchial transection causes the apex of the collapsed lung to descend to the level of the hilum.[68]

The principles of airway management are similar to those of cervical airway injury. Although in both cervical and thoracic airway injuries, administration of anesthetics and especially muscle relaxants may result in irreversible airway obstruction, presumably because of relaxation of structures that maintain the airway patent in the awake state, airway loss may also occur during attempts at awake intubation.[69] Certain manipulations may also lead to sudden airway obstruction. For example, cricoid pressure during a rapid-sequence induction in a patient with injury to this cartilage may completely occlude the trachea.[56] Thus, the cricothyroid membrane should be located before administration of any anesthetic induction agents to permit securing the airway surgically if there are serious problems with direct laryngoscopy.[69]

After intubation of the trachea, the adequacy of the airway intervention is evaluated by clinical examination, capnography, and pulse oximetry. Pulmonary contusion, atelectasis, diaphragmatic rupture with thoracic migration of the abdominal contents, and pneumothorax may complicate the interpretation of chest auscultation. Likewise, CO_2 elimination may be decreased or absent in shock and cardiac arrest.

Management of Breathing Abnormalities

Of the several causes that may alter respiration after trauma, tension pneumothorax, flail chest, and open pneumothorax are immediate threats to the patient's life and therefore require rapid diagnosis and treatment. Hemothorax; closed pneumothorax; pulmonary contusion; diaphragmatic rupture with herniation of abdominal contents; and atelectasis from a mucus plug, aspiration, or chest wall splinting can also interfere with breathing and pulmonary gas exchange and deteriorate into life-threatening complications. Nevertheless, they do not usually carry the same gravity of risk as the first three conditions.

Although cyanosis, tachypnea, hypotension, neck vein distention, tracheal deviation, and diminished breath sounds on the affected side are the classic signs of tension pneumothorax, neck vein distention may be absent in hypovolemic patients and tracheal deviation may be difficult to appreciate. The definitive diagnosis is established by chest radiograph; however, in hypoxemic and hypotensive patients, immediate insertion of a 14-gauge angiocatheter through the fourth intercostal space in the midaxillary line or, at times, through the second intercostal space at the midclavicular line, is essential. There is no time for radiologic confirmation in this setting.

A flail chest results from comminuted fractures of at least three adjacent ribs or rib fractures with associated costochondral separation or sternal fracture.[70] Respiratory insufficiency or failure in this situation results from coexisting hemopneumothorax, lung contusion, paradoxical chest wall movement, or splinting because of intense pain. Because of splinting, not all trauma victims with flail chest manifest respiratory paradox during initial assessment. The diagnosis, which is primarily based on physical findings, may be delayed in approximately 15% of patients.[71] Repeated evaluation by physical examination, chest radiograph, and arterial blood gas (ABG) determinations is essential for early recognition of flail chest and a possible underlying pulmonary contusion, the clinical manifestations of which may also be delayed.[72] Patients in whom respiratory insufficiency or failure develop despite analgesic treatment require tracheal intubation and mechanical ventilation[70–72] (Table 48-1).

Without significant gas exchange abnormalities, chest wall instability alone is not an indication for respiratory support. There is evidence that liberal use of mechanical ventilation in the presence of a flail chest or pulmonary contusion increases

Table 48-1. INDICATIONS FOR MECHANICAL VENTILATION IN PATIENTS WITH FLAIL CHEST

Respiratory failure manifested by one or more of the following criteria:
  Clinical signs of progressive fatigue or deterioration.
  Respiratory rate >35 breaths · min^{-1} or <8 breaths · min^{-1}
  Pao_2 <60 mm Hg at Fio_2 ≥0.5
  $Paco_2$ >55 mm Hg
  Pao_2 / Fio_2 ratio ≤200
  Vital capacity <15 ml · kg^{-1}
  Forced expiratory volume in 1 s (FEV_1) ≤10 ml · kg^{-1}
  Inspiratory force ≥−25 cm H_2O
  Alveolar–arterial oxygen gradient (A–a $\dot{D}o_2$ in mm Hg at Fio_2 of 1.0) >450
  Shunt fraction (Qs/Qt) >0.2
  Dead space/tidal volume ratio (Vd/Vt) >0.6
Clinical evidence of severe shock
Associated severe head injury with absent airway control or need to hyperventilate
Severe associated injury requiring surgery
Airway obstruction
Significant pre-existing chronic pulmonary disease.

Reprinted with permission from Cogbill TH, Landercasper J: Injury to the chest wall. In Moore EE, Mattox KL and Feliciano DV (eds): Trauma, 2nd ed, p 338. Norwalk, Connecticut, Appleton and Lange, 1991.

the rate of pulmonary complications and mortality and prolongs the hospital stay.[71,72] Effective pain relief by itself can improve respiratory function and often avoid the need for mechanical ventilation. For this purpose, continuous epidural analgesia with local anesthetics and opioids, preferably directed to thoracic segments, provides better pain relief and ventilatory function than parenteral opioids, reducing morbidity and mortality in elderly patients with chest wall trauma.[73,74] Coagulopathy, spine injury, and suspected abdominal injury, however, can be contraindications to epidural analgesia. Other therapeutic measures in patients with chest wall injury include supplemental oxygen, airway humidification, chest physiotherapy, incentive spirometry, bronchodilators, airway suctioning using fiberoptic bronchoscopy if necessary, and nutritional support.[70] Fluid therapy should also be adjusted carefully. Overzealous infusion of fluids may result in deterioration of oxygenation by worsening underlying pulmonary injury.[72]

The life-threatening hypoxia and hypercarbia that may complicate an open pneumothorax result from atmospheric air following the path of least resistance and entering the pleural cavity through the chest wall instead of the normal air passages. Immediate management in spontaneously breathing patients involves covering the defect with a dressing taped on three sides, so that a one-way valve is created that prevents air entry into the pleural cavity and allows egress of air during expiration. Another effective maneuver is to apply an occlusive dressing and insert a chest tube at a site distant from the wound. For very large defects, positive-pressure ventilation with pleural decompression is the wisest choice.

Another rare but life-threatening complication that requires special attention during the early phase of trauma is systemic air embolism.[75] It occurs mainly after penetrating lung trauma and blast injuries, and rarely after blunt thoracic trauma that produces lacerations of both distal air passages and pulmonary veins. The normal response to these injuries is bleeding into the respiratory tree. However, positive-pressure ventilation after tracheal intubation may lead to entrance of air into the systemic circulation through the pulmonary veins. Hemoptysis and circulatory and CNS dysfunction immediately after artificial ventilation and detection of air in the retinal vessels establish the diagnosis. Air bubbles in the coronary arteries may be seen during thoracotomy. Definitive management involves immediate thoracotomy and clamping the hilum of the lacerated lung. Respiratory maneuvers that minimize or eliminate air entry into the systemic circulation have been described:[75] isolating and collapsing the lacerated lung by means of a double-lumen tube used as a bronchial blocker, and ventilating with low tidal volumes or high frequency. If available, transesophageal echocardiography (TEE) may permit visualization of air bubbles in the left heart and their disappearance with therapeutic maneuvers.

Management of Shock

Hypotension occurring shortly after a traumatic event may have many causes, but hemorrhage is the most common etiology of this complication. Among the other causes of traumatic shock are abnormal pump function (myocardial contusion, pericardial tamponade, pre-existing cardiac disease, or coronary artery or cardiac valve injury), pneumothorax or hemothorax, spinal cord injury, and, rarely, anaphylaxis or sepsis (Table 48-2).

Evaluation of the severity of hemorrhagic shock in the initial phase is based on a few relatively insensitive and nonspecific clinical signs. For example, the heart rate, which is traditionally used as an index of hypovolemia, may go up or down depending on the amount and rapidity of bleeding, on drugs or alcohol the victim may have taken before the injury, or on the effects of the patient's injuries on different systems. A prolonged decrease in blood volume may cause an increase in vagal activity, thereby restoring the pulse to normal, or even subnormal, levels.[76] Patients with a history of chronic cocaine use may also exhibit bradycardia with severe hypovolemia, particularly under general anesthesia;[76,77] acute cocaine intoxication causes tachycardia and hypertension.[78] The overall incidence of paradoxical or relative bradycardia in severely injured patients is between 2 and 3%; however, up to 30% of hypotensive trauma patients may exhibit paradoxical bradycardia.[78]

In contrast, tissue injury and associated pain may exacerbate the tachycardia induced by hypovolemia without necessarily increasing the cardiac index or tissue oxygen delivery.[79] In fact, in this setting an increase in intestinal vascular resistance and a decrease in intestinal blood flow may occur, increasing the likelihood of subsequent sepsis and organ failure.[80] Thus, although tachycardia is one of the earliest signs of hemorrhagic shock, the heart rate does not necessarily correlate with the blood loss. Furthermore, the systemic blood pressure may be sustained by compensatory mechanisms if hypovolemia is not sudden and severe. Equating a normal systemic blood pressure with normovolemia during initial resuscitation may lead to loss of valuable time for treating an underlying occult hypovolemia or hypoperfusion. Nevertheless, heart rate, systemic blood pres-

Table 48-2. GUIDELINES FOR MANAGEMENT OF TRAUMATIC SHOCK

	Etiology					
	Hemorrhage or Extensive Tissue Injury	Cardiac Tamponade	Myocardial Contusion	Pneumothorax or Hemothorax	Spinal Cord Injury	Sepsis
PRIMARY MECHANISMS	Hypovolemia	Ventricular inflow restriction	Diminished ventricular performance and elevated pulmonary vascular resistance	Lung collapse Mediastinal shift, causing inflow and outflow obstruction of the heart	Vasodilatation and relative hypovolemia caused by loss of sympathetic tone	Intestinal perforation causing peritoneal contamination
TYPICAL SIGNS AND SYMPTOMS	Tachycardia Narrow pulse pressure Cold, clammy skin from vasoconstriction	Tachycardia Hypotension Dilated and engorged neck veins Muffled heart sounds Diminished BP response to fluid challenge	Dysrhythmia Tachycardia Hypotension	Tachycardia Hypotension Dilated and engorged neck veins Absent breath sounds Hyper-resonance to percussion Tracheal shift Dyspnea Subcutaneous emphysema	Hypotension without tachycardia, cutaneous vasoconstriction, or narrow pulse pressure	Develops mainly a few hours after colon injury In hypovolemic patients, signs and symptoms indistinguishable from hypovolemic shock In normovolemic patients, fever, modest tachycardia, warm, pink skin, near normal BP, wide pulse pressure Hypotension may develop
TREATMENT CONTINUUM, FROM LEAST TO MOST INTENSE	Crystalloids initially Transfusion if 2000 ml of crystalloid in 15 min does not restore BP	Pericardiocentesis Pericardial window Emergency room thoracotomy	Fluids Fluids and vasodilators Fluids and inotropes	Release of air with 14-gauge catheter Chest tube	Fluids Fluids and vasopressors Fluids, vasopressors, and inotropes, if myocardial damage is present	Fluids and antibiotics Fluids, anibiotics, and inotropes for hypotension

BP = blood pressure.

sure, pulse pressure, respiratory rate, urine output, and mental status remain the best available early indicators of the severity of hemorrhagic shock[81] (Table 48-3).

The response of the pulse and blood pressure to initial fluid therapy also aids in assessment of the degree of hypovolemia.[81] In hypotensive and tachycardic patients, administration of lactated Ringer's (LR) solution, 2000 ml over 15 minutes in adults, or 20 ml · kg^{-1} in children, should normalize the vital signs if hemorrhage is mild (10–20%). A transient improvement after fluid infusion suggests a 20–40% decrease in circulating volume or continuing blood loss. More crystalloids and possibly blood transfusion are required in these patients. If the vital signs do not respond to initial fluid resuscitation, there has probably been severe (>40%) hemorrhage, which must be replaced by rapid infusion of crystalloids, colloids, and blood.

If the blood loss has been moderate, the 45 minutes needed for blood typing and cross-matching is acceptable. In more severe hemorrhage, type-specific blood can be available in approximately 15 min. If the situation dictates immediate transfusion, type O, Rh(+) blood is satisfactory in most situations: O, Rh(−) blood should be given to women of childbearing age. However, because of the scarcity of Rh(−) blood, some women require an Rh(+) transfusion. The immunogenicity of the D antigen can be neutralized by administration of Rh immune globulin (anti-Rh antibody).

Invasive hemodynamic monitoring is rarely indicated during initial resuscitation because it slows treatment and thus may be counterproductive. However, if time permits, placement of an arterial catheter during this phase of therapy, and drawing of blood for serial measurements of hemoglobin or hematocrit, can be of great help in determining the need for transfusion. During fluid infusion, a reasonable transfusion threshold is a hematocrit below 25% for young, healthy patients and below 30% for older patients or those with coronary or cerebrovascular disease.[82] This may not apply to the trauma patient whose underlying medical diseases often are unknown, and the extent of stress-induced by injuries may require a safety buffer. Control of active bleeding has a higher priority than restoration of blood volume in the initial resuscitation of hemorrhage. It has even been suggested that fluid should be withheld until the patient is in the operating room. Fluid administration in the field or in the emergency department after penetrating trauma may accelerate blood loss.[83]

Parenthetically, after normalization of these parameters within the first hour, recognition of occult hypoperfusion with hemodynamic and oxygenation monitoring, and prompt treatment within the first 24 hours of injury decreases the incidence of post-traumatic multisystem organ failure and improves outcome.[84] Although a variety of methods have been proposed to monitor organ perfusion and oxygenation, currently the serum lactate level, base deficit, or gastric mucosal pH have been accepted as reliable end points for resuscitation in trauma patients.[85] Preferably, all three of these values should be within normal limits: lactate <2 mmol · l^{-1}, base deficit less than 3, and gastric intramucosal pH >7.33.[85]

Rapid establishment of venous access with large-bore cannulae placed in peripheral veins that drain both above and below the diaphragm is essential for adequate fluid resuscitation in the severely injured patient. When vascular collapse and extremity injury impair access to arm or leg vessels, percutaneous cannulation of the internal jugular, subclavian, or femoral veins, or a cutdown to a saphenous or arm vein can be rapidly performed in older children and adults. In children younger than 5 years of age, intraosseous cannulation has a high success rate and a low incidence of complications. Infusion rates comparable with those obtained with iv lines are possible in small children, although a pressure infusion device may be necessary to achieve adequate flow.[86] A special screw-type needle or the needle of a 16- or 18-gauge angiocatheter is introduced into the bone marrow of the distal femur or proximal tibia at the level of its tuberosity. Care should be taken not to injure the epiphyseal plate during puncture. Proper placement is indicated by loss of resistance to fluid injection or aspiration of marrow.

A few words of caution are necessary: internal jugular and subclavian vein catheterization carries the danger of infusing large volumes of fluids into the pleural cavity in patients with hemothorax; aspiration of blood or a "central venous pressure" fluctuation does not necessarily indicate that the cannula is in a blood vessel.[87] The common femoral vein may be accessed 1 cm medial to the artery just below the ilioinguinal ligament. If the femoral artery pulsation is not palpable, the vein may be located at a point one third of the distance from the pubic tubercle to the anterior superior iliac spine, below the ilioinguinal ligament.[88]

Although little, if any, survival benefit has been demonstrated for patients transported within urban areas from the prehospital use of military antishock trousers (MAST), the device is probably useful in rural regions, in combat, and in patients with extensive pelvic fractures.[89,90] It may help maintain hemodynamic stability during a relatively long prehospital transport, and reduces bleeding from pelvic vessels by stabilizing the fractures.[89,90] It should not be applied to patients with head and penetrating chest injuries and to those already in respiratory distress. In the emergency department, deflation of this device may be associated with significant hypotension; it should be deflated one segment at a time starting with the abdominal compartment, and a pump should always be available for reinflation of the MAST if the blood pressure falls.

Table 48-3. ADVANCED TRAUMA LIFE SUPPORT CLASSIFICATION OF HEMORRHAGIC SHOCK*

	Class I	Class II	Class III	Class IV
Blood loss (ml)	≤750	750–1500	1500–2000	≥2000
Blood loss (% blood volume)	≤15	15–30	30–40	≥40
Pulse rate (per min)	<100	>100	>120	≥140
Blood pressure	Normal	Normal	Decreased	Decreased
Pulse pressure	Normal or increased	Decreased	Decreased	Decreased
Respiratory rate (breaths · min^{-1})	14–20	20–30	30–40	<35
Urine output (ml · hr^{-1})	≥30	20–30	5–15	Negligible
Mental status	Slightly anxious	Mildly anxious	Anxious and confused	Confused, lethargic
Fluid replacement (3:1 rule)†	Crystalloid	Crystalloid	Crystalloid + blood	Crystalloid + blood

* For a 70-kg male patient; based on initial presentation.
† 3:1 rule is based on empiric observation that most patients require 300 ml balanced electrolyte solution for each 100 ml blood loss. Without other clinical and monitoring parameters, this guideline may result in excessive or inadequate fluid resuscitation.
Adapted with permission from American College of Surgeons Committee on Trauma: Shock. In American College of Surgeons (ed): Advanced Trauma Life Support Course for Physicians, p 108. Chicago, American College of Surgeons, 1997.

Emergency Room Thoracotomy

Patients who arrive in the emergency department in cardiac arrest require advanced cardiac life support. However, the success rate of external cardiac massage in hypovolemic trauma victims is likely to be low.[91] Emergency department thoracotomy not only permits performance of open cardiac massage but aids resuscitation efforts by allowing drainage of pericardial blood, control of cardiac and great vessel bleeding, application of a cross-clamp to the aorta, and rapid administration of fluids through a small Foley catheter introduced into the right atrium, or in desperate situations, through a large-bore catheter or introducer into the descending aorta. This procedure is not indicated in blunt torso trauma; the mortality rate is similar regardless of whether it is attempted.[92] In penetrating injuries, success depends on the presence of a blood pressure, spontaneous respiration, and a resuscitatable cardiac rhythm (sinus, ventricular tachycardia, or fibrillation), and on the duration of resuscitation before the thoracotomy is performed. Patients in asystole or idioventricular rhythm, and those who have required cardiopulmonary resuscitation for more than 5 minutes before the performance of the thoracotomy, are unlikely to survive.[92,93] Tracheal intubation and ventilation with oxygen seem to increase the time limit to 10 minutes and increase the success rate of the procedure.[92] Unfortunately, there is a major discrepancy between the rates of initial successful resuscitation and of survival without neurologic complications to hospital discharge. Although the initial survival rate of emergency department thoracotomy may be as high as 70%, only 10% of these patients are discharged from the hospital.[92,93] Serious questions, therefore, have been raised about the indications for and the appropriateness of the procedure.[94]

EARLY MANAGEMENT OF SPECIFIC INJURIES

Head Injury

Approximately 40% of deaths from trauma are caused by head injury, and indeed, even moderate brain injury may increase the mortality rate of patients with other injuries.[95] In the United States each year, approximately 56,000 head-injured patients die and 90,000 are left with long-term disabilities.[96] In 65% of nonsurvivors, progression of the damaged area beyond the directly injured region (secondary brain injury) can be demonstrated at autopsy.[97] The major factor in secondary injury is tissue hypoxia, which results in lactic acidosis, free radical generation, lipid peroxidation, prostaglandin synthesis, release of excitatory amino acids (primarily glutamate), breakdown of cell membranes, and entry of large quantities of sodium and calcium into the cells.[97] Of all the possible insults to the injured brain, hypotension and hypoxia have the greatest detrimental impact[98,99] (Table 48-4).

The vulnerability of the brain to decreases in blood pressure and oxygen supply is not surprising. It consumes 3.5 ml of $O_2 \cdot min^{-1} \cdot 100 \ g^{-1}$ (~50 ml of $O_2 \cdot min^{-1}$), requiring a high blood flow (700 $ml \cdot min^{-1}$) and high O_2 extraction ratio (~0.35). Brain injury by itself does not cause hypotension in adults except as a preterminal event. However, more than half of patients with severe head trauma have other injuries that render approximately 15% of them hypotensive; approximately 30% are hypoxic on admission as a result of central respiratory depression or associated chest injuries.[100] Furthermore, exposure to these insults is likely to occur during any phase of the continuum of hospital care: in the radiology unit, the operating room, the recovery room, the ICU, and so forth. The most common early complications of head trauma are intracranial hypertension, brain herniation, seizures, neurogenic pulmonary edema, cardiac dysrhythmias, bradycardia, systemic hypertension, and coagulopathy.

Table 48-4. EFFECTS ON OUTCOME OF SECONDARY INSULTS OCCURRING FROM TIME OF INJURY THROUGH RESUSCITATION*

Secondary Insults	No. of Patients	% of Total Patients	6-Month Outcome (%)		
			Good/ Moderate	Severe/ Vegetative	Dead
Total cases	717	100	43.0	20.2	36.8
Neither	308	43.0	63.9	10.2	26.9
Hypoxia	161	22.4	50.3	21.7	28.0
Hypotension	62	11.4	32.9	17.1	50.0
Both	166	23.2	20.5	22.3	57.2

* Data from hospital emergency departments enrolled in Traumatic Coma Data Bank.
Reprinted with permission from Prough DS, Lang J: Therapy of patients with head injuries: Key parameters for management. J Trauma 42 (suppl): 10S, 1997, with permission.

Diagnosis

Because the injured brain is acutely sensitive to hypotension and hypoxia, every effort should be made to support the blood pressure and ensure adequate oxygenation before the unconscious patient is evaluated.[101] Indeed, intubating the trachea of the unconscious patient in the field may significantly increase his or her chances of survival.[102] A baseline neurologic examination should be performed after initial resuscitation, but before any sedative or muscle relaxant agents are administered, and should be repeated at frequent intervals because the patient's condition may change rapidly. A brief initial evaluation includes assessment of consciousness, pupillary response, and motor activity of the extremities. Consciousness can be assessed within a few seconds using the AVPU system[103] (alert; responds to verbal stimuli; responds to painful stimuli; unresponsive; Table 48-5). More precise information is provided by the Glasgow

Table 48-5. TWO-LEVEL INITIAL EVALUATION OF CONSCIOUSNESS

LEVEL 1. AVPU SYSTEM

A = Alert
V = Responds to verbal stimuli
P = Responds to painful stimuli
U = Unresponsive

LEVEL 2. GLASGOW COMA SCALE (GCS)

Eye-opening (E)	
Spontaneous, already open and blinking	4
To speech	3
To pain	2
None	1
Verbal response (V)	
Oriented	5
Answers but confused	4
Inappropriate but recognizable words	3
Incomprehensible sounds	2
None	1
Best motor response (M)	
Obeys verbal commands	6
Localizes painful stimulus	5
Withdraws from painful stimulus	4
Decorticate posturing (upper extremity flexion)	3
Decerebrate posturing (upper extremity extension)	2
No movement	1

GCS ≤8 = deep coma, severe head trauma, poor outcome.
GCS 9–12 = concious patient with moderate injury.
GCS >12 = mild injury.

Coma Scale[103] (GCS; see Table 48-5). In this test, the sum of the scores obtained for eye opening, verbal response, and motor activity correlates with the state of consciousness, the severity of the head injury, and the prognosis.[104,105] Anesthetic and adjunct drugs render an adequate neurologic examination impossible; thus, long-acting muscle relaxants, opioids, sedatives, or hypnotics should be given selectively.[101]

Mental impairment after trauma may have any of several etiologies. However, the possibility of hypoxia and shock must always be considered first. If consciousness remains depressed despite ventilation and fluid replacement, a head injury is assumed to be present and the patient is managed accordingly. Only after all of these causes are excluded should the possibility of toxic or metabolic etiologies be considered. Dilatation and sluggish response of the pupil is a sign of compression of the oculomotor nerve by the medial portion of the temporal lobe (uncus). A maximally dilated and unresponsive "blown" pupil suggests uncal herniation under the falx cerebri. The presence of similar findings in ocular injuries makes interpretation of pupillary findings difficult when eye and head injuries coexist. However, the pupillary reaction to light is usually more sluggish in the head-injured patient. Assessment of motor function should be performed on the extremity that responds best. The limb affected by neurologic injury is examined, but the result is not considered in the GCS.

Computed tomography scanning is used for the diagnosis of most acute head injuries. Magnetic resonance imaging offers additional advantages: it can demonstrate nonhemorrhagic brain contusion (ischemia), indicate the severity of diffuse axonal injury, and may predict the development of a delayed intracerebral hematoma.[106] However, because of its impracticality in the injured patient, it is rarely used. Positive CT findings after acute head injury include midline shift, distortion of the ventricles and cisterns, effacement of the sulci in the uninjured hemisphere, and the presence of a hematoma at any location in the cranial vault. Subdural hematomas usually have a concave border, whereas epidural hematomas present with a convex outline classically termed a *lenticular* configuration. Patients in coma (GCS <8) have a 40% likelihood of an intracranial hematoma.[107] Those with a higher GCS score are less likely to have intracranial bleeding, although it is now evident that the significant incidence of this complication even in these patients necessitates a CT study, preferably with contrast enhancement.[108] Other benefits of CT scanning include detection of intracranial air and depressed skull fractures.

Management

The primary objective in the early management of brain trauma is to prevent or alleviate the secondary injury process that may follow any complication that decreases the oxygen supply to the brain, including systemic hypotension, hypoxemia, anemia, raised ICP, acidosis, and possibly hyperglycemia (serum glucose >200 mg · dl^{-1}).[109] These insults cause exacerbation of trauma-induced cerebral ischemia and metabolic derangements, worsening the outcome.[98,109]

The most important therapeutic maneuvers in these patients are aimed at maintaining CPP and oxygen delivery. Although there are wide variations among the various trauma centers in the specific details of managing the head-injured patient, certain aspects of treatment are virtually universal.[101,110–113] They include normalization of systemic blood pressure (mean blood pressure >80) and arterial oxygenation (Sao$_2$ >95), sedation and paralysis if necessary, mannitol and possibly a loop diuretic to shrink the brain and decrease the ICP, drainage of cerebrospinal fluid through a ventriculostomy catheter, and mechanical hyperventilation if the ICP does not respond to other measures.

Antidysrhythmics and fresh frozen plasma (FFP) are required in those patients with cardiac or hemostatic abnormalities. If the ICP still does not respond, pentobarbital (3–10 mg · kg^{-1} given over 0.5–2.5 hours, followed by a maintenance infusion of 0.5–3.0 mg · kg^{-1} · hr^{-1}, aimed at a serum concentration between 2.5 and 4.0 mg · dl^{-1}) may be required.[114] High-dose barbiturates, however, are of no value in the routine therapy of head injury, and should be used only for refractory ICP elevation. Of course, immediate surgical decompression, especially of epidural hematomas, is an important factor in reducing morbidity and mortality. Whether active normalization of an elevated serum glucose (a common occurrence in the head-injured patient) has any salutary effect on outcome is not known.

Measurement of the jugular bulb O$_2$ saturation (Sjvo$_2$) is used in many centers as a guide to therapy of the head-injured patient.[115] A catheter is passed retrograde into the jugular bulb. The O$_2$ saturation may be measured with a co-oximeter or continuously by means of a fiberoptic sensor. An Sjvo$_2$ of <50% is considered critical desaturation. The value of this technique depends on the fact that the difference between the arterial and jugular venous O$_2$ content can be used as a measure of the amount of oxygen used by the brain.

The arteriovenous O$_2$ difference

$$AVDo_2 = 1.34 \cdot Hgb \cdot (Sao_2 - Sjvo_2)$$

is an indicator of the relationship between the demand of the brain for O$_2$ and its supply by the blood. The normal AVDo$_2$ is approximately 6. An increase in this value is a sign of insufficient blood flow, whereas a subnormal level indicates hyperemia. Unfortunately, several shortcomings of the technique have hindered its universal acceptance. Because all of the cerebral veins drain into the torcula and from there into the jugular bulbs, AVDo$_2$ measures only global O$_2$ consumption, which may well be different from regional areas within the brain or the situation in the injured region. Patient or catheter movement may also alter the measured Pjvo$_2$. Thus, there may be a high proportion of inaccurate values—as high as nearly two thirds in one study[116]—although recent advances in the technique have probably reduced these errors. Cruz[117] has suggested that jugular venous monitoring should be used only in sedated, paralyzed patients.

Several therapeutic maneuvers deserve further comment. Hyperventilation to a Paco$_2$ level of 25–30 mm Hg was used routinely until the mid-1990s in the initial management of the severely head-injured patient to decrease ICP and correct cerebral acidosis (Table 48-6). Available data suggest that brain ischemia, which is probably the most threatening consequence of head injury, is likely to occur during the first 6 hours after trauma.[118–120] This decrease in blood flow may be present even when the CPP (the difference between the mean arterial pressure and the ICP) is maintained above the generally recommended 60–70 mm Hg.[121] Thus, the initial hypoperfusion seems to be caused largely by increased cerebral vascular resistance, which may be enhanced by hyperventilation. Ward et al[122] showed that patients ventilated to a Paco$_2$ of 24 mm Hg had a significantly worse outcome than did those maintained at a Paco$_2$ of 35 mm Hg. In an attempt to correct cerebral acidosis

---

Table 48-6. CLASSIC AND CONTEMPORARY TREATMENT OF SEVERE HEAD INJURY

Old Treatment	New Treatment
Hyperventilation	Normal ventilation; hyperventilation only when needed
Fluid restriction	Normovolemia
Steroids?	No steroids
Mannitol	Mannitol or hypertonic saline
CPP >70 mm Hg	CPP ≥60 mm Hg (50 mm Hg in Lund protocol)
Normotension/mild hypertension	Lund protocol—clonidine, metoprolol, ergotamine
	Sjvo$_2$?

CPP = cerebral perfusion pressure.

induced by the head injury and hyperventilation, they also administered tris(hydroxymethyl)aminomethane (THAM), an amine buffer, to one of their study groups. There was no difference in outcome between the patients treated with hyperventilation alone and those who also received THAM. However, subsequent studies have demonstrated that THAM may produce an immediate decrease in ICP, limit wide fluctuations of ICP during hyperventilation, and reduce the need for mannitol.[123,124] Although the role of THAM is not yet clear, some degree of hyperventilation may be necessary in patients who have severe injuries and elevated ICP that does not respond to normal ventilation and diuretics.[120] Its use after the initial phase should be based on monitoring of the ICP and, if available, the $SjvO_2$ and $AVDO_2$. A reduction in ICP with elevation of CPP during treatment is reflected by a rise in $SjvO_2$ and a narrowing of the $AVDO_2$, presumably reflecting an improvement in the circulation to the brain.[120,125]

Effective reduction in ICP can be provided, or at least aided, by administration of mannitol ($0.25–0.5\ g \cdot kg^{-1}$). In addition to its osmotic diuretic effect, this agent may improve cerebral blood flow (CBF) and O_2 delivery by reducing blood viscosity.[126] There is a risk of hypovolemia and thus of hypotension when therapeutic doses of mannitol are used. The aim in administration of this agent is a normal volume of mildly hypertonic ($\sim$295 $mOsm \cdot l^{-1}$) plasma. If the ICP elevation persists, additional doses of mannitol should be given with great care. Acute mannitol toxicity, manifested by hyponatremia, high serum osmolality, and a gap between calculated and measured serum osmolality $>10\ mOsm \cdot l^{-1}$, may result when the drug is given in large doses ($2–3\ g \cdot kg^{-1}$) or to patients with renal failure.[127] Hyponatremia in these patients results from intravascular volume expansion rather than sodium loss; thus, treatment with saline solutions is not appropriate. Because of a synergistic action between mannitol and loop diuretics in improving the ICP, addition of furosemide may be a safer and more effective treatment than increasing the dose of mannitol when intracranial hypertension persists.[114]

Both intracranial hematomas and hemorrhage in other regions have a high surgical priority. In the multiple trauma victim, prioritization between the two is based on the severity of each injury. Because there is no time to obtain a CT scan of the head in patients with both profuse hemorrhage and brain herniation, the patient is brought directly to the operating room for simultaneous control of the bleeding site and evacuation of the intracranial hematoma. The site of the craniotomy can be determined by a ventriculogram or an ultrasound examination with a pencil-tip probe; both tests may be performed under local anesthesia through a frontal bur hole. If the patient is hemodynamically stable, a CT scan is performed; the strictest attention should be paid to ensuring adequate oxygenation, ventilation, blood pressure, and ICP control during the procedure. If the patient is hemodynamically unstable or requires emergency surgery for associated injuries, and has a history suggesting a head injury even though a significant intracranial hematoma is unlikely on clinical grounds, intraoperative ICP monitoring is indicated to permit rapid detection of ICP elevation.

Excessive fluid resuscitation of the multiple trauma patient with a head injury poses the problem of augmentation of brain edema. Rapid and adequate restoration of the intravascular volume with isotonic crystalloid and, if necessary, with colloid solutions should be aimed at maintaining the CPP while attempting to minimize further brain swelling. LR solution, which is slightly hypotonic ($Na^+ = 130\ mEq \cdot l^{-1}$ and osmolality $\sim$255 $mOsm \cdot l^{-1}$), may promote edema in noninjured areas of the brain if it is given in large quantities; edema tends to occur in injured brain regions regardless of the type of solution administered because of increased permeability of the blood–brain barrier. To minimize edema formation, it is wise to monitor serum osmolality and to replace LR solution with truly isotonic normal saline. If serum osmolality cannot be measured, this change can be made empirically after 3 l of LR solution.

There are data suggesting that the addition of relatively small volumes of hypertonic saline in concentrations between 3% ($6–8\ ml \cdot kg^{-1}$) and 7.5% ($4\ ml \cdot kg^{-1}$) followed by infusion of LR may be beneficial in multiple trauma patients with head injury.[128,129] In head-injured children, administration of 3% saline was associated with an average 4 mm Hg decline in ICP, compared with a 0.7 mm Hg decline after normal saline.[130] Hypertonic saline draws fluid from the intracellular space and, thus, in addition to restoring the blood volume, it reduces brain edema and prevents elevation of the ICP as effectively as 20% mannitol.[130–132] The intravascular volume expansion produced by hypertonic saline is transient; it can be prolonged by addition of 6% dextran-70 or hetastarch to the solution.[133] The effects of this combination on coagulation are minimal.[134] However, administration of hypertonic saline cannot be maintained for long periods. It may cause hypernatremia, hyperosmolality, or hyperchloremic acidosis; the latter probably results from renal bicarbonate loss secondary to the increased levels of Cl^-. Serum concentrations of Na^+ and Cl^- and the patient's acid–base status should be followed, and the administration of hypertonic saline should be discontinued if plasma Na^+ reaches 160 $mEq \cdot l^{-1}$. Resuscitation with colloid solutions (hetastarch, pentastarch, pentafraction, human albumin 5% and 25%, or dextran) provides a sustained improvement in vital signs, but the increase in colloid osmotic pressure produced by these solutions may not have an important role in reducing brain edema.[135]

Two recently reviewed therapeutic approaches suggest that it may be possible to improve the long-term survival of severely head-injured patients significantly[110,136–139] (Table 48-7). In 1998, Cruz[137] described the use of continuous fiberoptic $SjvO_2$ monitoring in 178 comatose patients (GCS <8) with diffuse brain swelling. The major principles of this approach are not only to maintain an adequate CPP, but to keep ICP below 25 mm Hg and the cerebral extraction of O_2 ($CEO_2 = SaO_2 - SjvO_2$) within the normal range of 24–42%. All of the patients in the study group were mechanically ventilated, and otherwise treated according to a standard protocol similar to that described previously. In addition, the CEO_2 was monitored. When ICP >20 mm Hg was associated with a normal to low CEO_2, ventilation was increased until both parameters normalized. On the other hand, when elevated ICP was associated with normal to increased CEO_2, mannitol boluses were administered, again aiming at normalization of ICP and CEO_2. Thus, in addition to treating decreased cerebral perfusion, this protocol aims to reverse the effects of hyperperfusion as well.

The Lund Treatment is based on an attempt to control increased ICP by reducing the formation of cerebral edema.[136] There are several components to the protocol. Normovolemia is maintained by colloids and blood products. Sympathetic outflow and catecholamine levels are decreased by the α_2-agonist clonidine, which helps to maintain CBF because catecholamines produce intracerebral vasoconstriction. An additional antihypertensive effect is produced by the β_1-adrenergic antagonist, metoprolol, which seems to improve cerebral microcirculation despite a reduction in mean arterial blood pressure.[140] Precapillary vasoconstriction is provided by low-dose thiopental ($0.5–3\ mg \cdot kg^{-1} \cdot h^{-1}$) and dihydroergotamine. The latter agent also constricts the large cerebral veins, further reducing the ICP. A CPP of approximately 60 mm Hg is the usual end point, although in some circumstances 50 mm Hg is accepted in adults, and 40 mm Hg in children. More recently, the Lund group has added prostacyclin infusion to the treatment[141] to improve the microcirculation, prevent blood cell aggregation, and reduce capillary permeability. The results of this protocol have been very impressive in the 53 patients in their series (see Table 48-7); however, a larger, controlled study is clearly necessary to prove its value.

Table 48-7. SIX-MONTH OUTCOMES FOR BRAIN-INJURED PATIENTS IN VARIOUS STUDIES

Study	No. of Patients	Year	6-Month Outcome (%)			Comments
			Good/ Moderate	*Severe/ Vegetative*	*Dead*	
3-Country (Jennett et al[138])	700	1977	38	11	51	Various treatments; some untreated
Miller et al[139]	158	1981	47	12	40	Ventilation, surgery, intracranial pressure monitoring and treatment
Traumatic Coma Data Bank[110]	717	1997	43	20	37	Total patients, standard therapy
Traumatic Coma Data Bank[110]	308	1997	54	19	27	Same therapy; patients without hypotension or hypoxia
Eker et al[136]	53	1998	79	13	8	Lund protocol
Cruz[137]	132	1998	74	17	9	CEO_2 group

CEO_2 = Cerebral extraction of O_2.

The common factor in these newer protocols appears to be reduction in brain swelling. Cruz[137] seems to accomplish this by hyperventilation—and thus arteriolar constriction—of patients with cerebral hyperperfusion, whereas the Lund group uses a carefully controlled pharmacologic approach. It may be that future improvements in the survival of the head-injured patient will be provided not only by maintaining oxygenation, arterial blood pressure, and CPP, but by limiting the formation of cerebral edema. In any case, the outlook for the head-injured patient has improved significantly since the mid-1990s.[113]

Spine and Spinal Cord Injury

Initial Evaluation

The incidence of cervical spine injury in trauma center admissions is 4.3%; 3% of injured patients have bony fractures without spinal cord injury, and 0.7% have a cord injury without a fracture.[142] Delayed diagnosis occurs in 0.01% of trauma admissions.[142]

The objective in the evaluation of spinal trauma is to diagnose instability of the spine and the extent of neurologic involvement. Often the urgency of associated injuries precludes a definitive assessment, necessitating spine protection until a satisfactory diagnosis is established. In the conscious patient, the diagnosis is relatively easy: a history of a motor vehicle, industrial, or athletic accident or a fall; penetrating trauma resulting in a neurologic deficit below a specific spinal level; or pain and tenderness over the involved vertebrae strongly suggests a spine injury. Obviously, these symptoms are difficult to elicit in the comatose patient. In these circumstances, flaccid areflexia, loss of rectal sphincter tone, diaphragmatic breathing, and bradycardia in a hypovolemic patient suggest the diagnosis. In cervical spine trauma, an ability to flex but not to extend the elbow and response to painful stimuli above but not below the clavicle also indicate neurologic injury. Current guidelines consider absence of neck pain or paresthesia and a negative physical examination—lack of tenderness with palpation and during voluntary flexion and extension of the neck—in a neurologically intact, conscious patient as adequate indications for ruling out a cervical spine injury without further radiologic studies.[143,144] Alcohol intoxication and distracting associated injuries do not seem to alter these guidelines as long as the patient is alert, conscious, and able to concentrate.[145]

Depending on the degree of deficit, spinal cord injuries are categorized as *complete* or *incomplete*. Intact sensory perception over the sacral distribution and voluntary contraction of the anus (sacral sparing) are present in incomplete, but not in complete, injuries. There is practically no possibility of neurologic recovery in complete injury, whereas functional restoration may occur in up to 50% of patients after incomplete injuries.[146] In some patients the development of *spinal shock,* which is manifested by absolute flaccidity and loss of reflexes, precludes distinguishing between complete and incomplete injuries during the initial phase of injury. Therefore, even in the absence of sacral sparing, the possibility of neurologic recovery dictates that all possible efforts be made in the early stages of the injury to prevent further damage and to preserve cord function. A similar principle applies to the evaluation of the level of injury. After the first few days, spinal cord edema subsides and the final level is commonly a few segments lower than on initial presentation. Thus, early therapeutic efforts should not be abandoned even in the patient with a high-level injury, which carries a grim functional prognosis.

Spinal shock is probably caused by direct trauma to the spinal cord, and usually subsides within days to weeks.[147] The term is frequently used as a misnomer for *neurogenic shock,* which is defined as hypotension and bradycardia caused by the loss of vasomotor tone and sympathetic innervation of the heart as a result of functional depression of the descending sympathetic pathways of the spinal cord. It is usually present after high thoracic and cervical spine injuries and improves within 3–5 days.

Radiologic Evaluation

In patients with neck pain and those who are unable to describe their symptoms, the diagnosis of spine injury is made radiologically. Some clinicians believe that radiologic evaluation is necessary to eliminate cervical spine injury in all blunt trauma victims, even those with normal clinical findings, and request lateral cervical spine films. However, the cross-table lateral view is capable of detecting only 35–65% of fracture–dislocations in this region.[145] The sixth and seventh cervical and the first thoracic vertebrae must be visualized clearly because 30–35% of all cervical spine injuries occur at these levels.[146] Higher injuries may also be missed if the radiologic examination is limited to a single lateral view. Other views (anteroposterior, open-mouth, and oblique) may be necessary for definitive diagnosis. The CT scan is the most reliable diagnostic technique for cervical spine fracture detection, but not for ligamentous injuries. Woodring and Lee[148] found that CT scans detected 90% of the fractures, but only 54% of the subluxation–dislocations, whereas plain films identified only 58% of the fractures but 93% of the subluxation–dislocations. Thus, plain films and CT scans are complementary and together increase the likelihood of accurate diagnosis. A recent strategy is to obtain a three- or five-view series of radiographs and to examine suspect or suboptimally visualized areas with limited, focused CT scans. Examination of the entire cervical spine with CT scanning necessitates obtaining narrowly spaced images, which may require as much as 1 hour with a conventional scanner. Berne *et al*[149] suggested that a complete examination of the cervical spine with the new spiral CT scanner had a sensitivity of 90%, specificity of 100%, positive predictive value of 100%, and negative predictive value of 95%. The expense of this technique, however, is higher than that of plain radiographic or focused CT evaluation.[149] Of course, when associated injuries dictate immediate management, radiographic diagnosis may have to be postponed for several hours or days as long as proper immobilization of the spine is maintained. On the other hand, patients, especially when they are paralyzed, should not be left on a rigid spine board for longer than 1 hour because of the risk of decubitus ulcers. Radiologic evaluation of the thoracolumbar vertebrae requires a minimum of two views: lateral and anteroposterior.

It is important that any radiologic examination be performed with the patient in supine position until a spine injury is ruled out, so that the risk of displacement of the fracture is minimized. A systematic evaluation of spine radiographs involves examination of the vertebrae, the vertebral alignment, and the adjacent soft tissue.[150] Bony parts are assessed by examining the height of the vertebral bodies and the integrity of the spinous and transverse processes, laminae, facets, and pedicles. Vertebral alignment is determined on the lateral cervical radiograph by evaluating four longitudinal curves: the anterior and posterior borders of the vertebral bodies (the latter representing the anterior border of the spinal canal), the posterior border of the spinal canal, and the tips of the spinous processes[150] (Fig. 48-3). Vertebral dislocation should be suspected if there is >3 mm of malalignment in any of these curves. The prevertebral space measures 10 mm at the level of the anterior arch of the atlas, 4 mm between C2 and C4, and 15 mm below C4[150] (see Fig. 48-3). An increase in these measurements by >5 mm suggests a hematoma, presumably caused by a body fracture. Irregularity of the prevertebral fat also suggests a fracture at that level. Enlargement of the prevertebral space in the neck may incidentally also be due to a retropharyngeal hematoma, which may cause tracheal deviation and tenderness and complicate airway management. Radiologic interpretation of thoracolumbar fractures is based on principles similar to those applied to cervical injuries.

Despite cervical pain and tenderness, cervical spine radiographs may at times be normal. A high index of suspicion of an unstable injury should appropriately lead to obtaining a flexion–extension series, which may demonstrate a fracture or dislocation that has been missed by the standard views.

Initial Management

The spinal cord is a microcosm of the brain. Thus, it is also vulnerable to a secondary injury process that may be a product of hypotension, hypoxia, and probably other physiologic complications.[151] Therefore, prompt recognition and treatment of these insults, which usually result from associated injuries, may minimize exacerbation of spinal cord lesions and significantly improve the long-term outlook of patients with spinal cord injuries.[105,152]

Steroids

For several years, high-dose methylprednisolone has been used in many centers in an attempt to improve the outcome from spinal cord injuries. The drug is usually given as a bolus of 30 mg · kg^{-1} within 8 hours of injury followed in 1 hour by an infusion of 5.4 mg · kg^{-1} · hr^{-1} for the next 23–47 hours. The National Acute Spinal Cord Injury Studies (NASCIS-2 and NASCIS-3)[153-155] demonstrated some improvement in motor function in treated patients who had partial sensory and motor loss. The results were best in patients who received 24 hours of therapy starting within 3 hours of injury, and those receiving 48 hours of treatment starting within 3–8 hours of injury. There

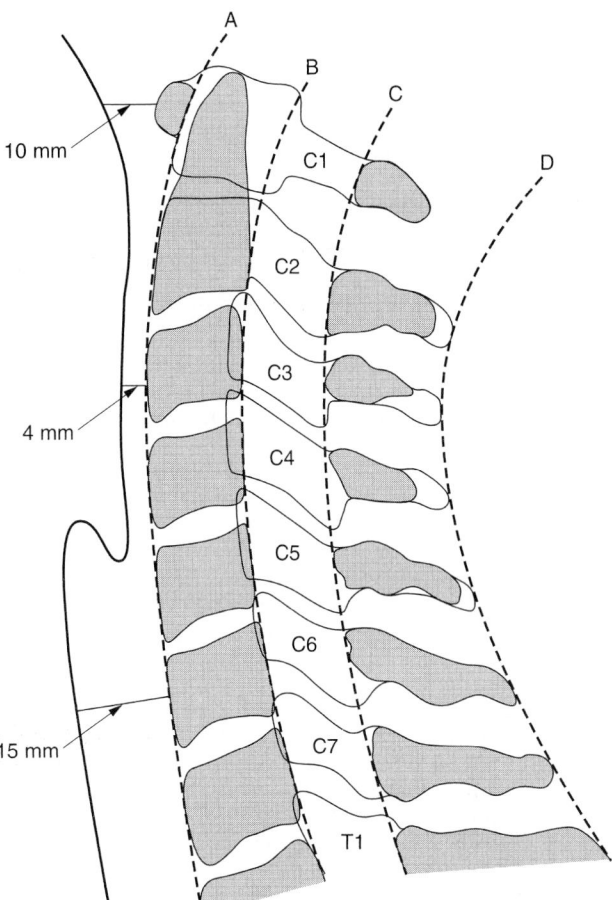

Figure 48-3. Normal cervical spine alignment and soft tissue measurement. Measurements denote normal width of soft tissues. (*A*) Anterior vertebral line; (*B*) posterior vertebral line; (*C*) spinolaminar line; (*D*) spinous process line. (Reprinted with permission from Bernstein RL, Rosenberg AD: Trauma. In Bernstein RL, Rosenberg AD [eds]: Manual of Orthopedic Anesthesia and Related Pain Syndromes, p 66. New York, Churchill Livingstone, 1993.)

was no improvement in sensory scores in any of the groups. There was little or no difference from untreated patients in groups with more severe injuries or in those who were treated after 8 hours. Furthermore, although some improvement could be demonstrated by neurologic examination, the change in the functional status of most of the patients was at best minimal.

Unfortunately, there are many problems with the design and analysis of the NASCIS trials.[156] Serious questions have been raised about the randomization of the patients, the analysis of the results, the clinical end points used, the definitions of motor levels, and the reliability of data collection. Furthermore, the results of these studies have not been duplicated in any other prospective or retrospective trials.[157-159]

The most definite finding of NASCIS-2 was that such large doses of methylprednisolone over a 24-hour period were not associated with an increased rate of complications. Unfortunately, NASCIS-3 patients who were treated for 48 hours had a higher incidence of both severe sepsis and severe pneumonia. In another study,[160] even patients who had been treated for only 24 hours had a 2.6-fold increase in the incidence of pneumonia and an increase in ventilated and intensive care days, although there was some decrease in the period of rehabilitation. Given these results, the best that can be said about the use of methylprednisolone in the spinal cord–injured patient is that there is a small chance that it may help some patients, but certainly its usefulness in the treatment of spinal cord injury remains to be clarified.

Immobilization

Maintenance of immobilization of the injured spine is of paramount importance. All changes in the patient's position must be performed carefully. If a cervical spine fracture is suspected, immobilization or MIS of the neck is necessary before the patient is moved. If the patient has a thoracic or lumbar injury, a careful log-rolling maneuver should be used.

Respiratory Complications

Respiratory complications are common in all phases of the care of spinal cord–injured patients. During the initial period, respiratory dysfunction caused by paralysis of the accessory muscles may be augmented by associated brain, neck, chest, or abdominal injury, alcohol intoxication, or the effects of self-administered or iatrogenic drugs. Accessory respiratory muscle paresis may cause a significant loss of expiratory reserve even when the injury involves the lower spinal segments.[161] The need for ventilatory assistance depends on the level of the spinal cord involved. Injuries at C5 or lower are usually associated with normal tidal volumes because the function of the diaphragm is intact, whereas patients with levels at C4 or above require ventilatory assistance.

Pulmonary edema is another significant cause of respiratory dysfunction. A severe catecholamine surge follows acute trauma to the spinal cord.[162] Although the resultant hypertension lasts for only a few minutes, its effects persist; it may produce both pulmonary capillary damage, as a result of shifting of a large portion of the blood volume into the pulmonary circulation, and left ventricular dysfunction. Overzealous fluid therapy to treat the patient's initial hypotension may lead to acute pulmonary edema when the sympathetic activity returns approximately 3–5 days after the injury.

Paradoxical respiration in the quadriplegic patient results from partial chest wall collapse during inspiration; it may produce limitation of the tidal volume and an increased risk of hypoventilation. The situation is aggravated when the patient is in an upright position. The diaphragm cannot maintain its normal domed shape, the only way it can contract efficiently, because the weight of the thoracic contents is not opposed by the normal tone of the abdominal muscles. Thus, in contrast to other diseases that produce respiratory insufficiency, the supine position improves respiration in persons with quadriplegia.

Other causes of inadequate respiration in the early phase of spinal cord injury are aspiration of gastric contents, atelectasis, and bronchoconstriction. Management includes careful observation of the patient's breathing and preparation to intubate the trachea and ventilate the lungs at the first sign of respiratory depression.

Severe bradycardia or dysrhythmias may result from unopposed vagal activity during tracheal intubation or suctioning: the patient must be preoxygenated and atropine (0.4–0.6 mg) should be given before any instrumentation. If bradycardia develops during airway management, treatment includes additional atropine, glycopyrrolate, isoproterenol, or, if necessary, cardiac pacing.

Hemodynamic Management

Hemodynamic management of patients with quadriplegia includes a complete assessment, if necessary, with a pulmonary artery catheter, as early as possible after injury. In as many as 25% of patients with cervical spinal cord injuries, left ventricular dysfunction may contribute to the hypotension.[163] Decreased preload can be treated with fluid infusion using cardiac function curves as a guide. In general, volume may be safely replaced to a pulmonary capillary wedge pressure (PCWP) of 18 mm Hg.[163] This avoids, or at least limits, the severity of the pulmonary edema described previously. Hypotension despite adequate fluid infusion, acidosis, or low mixed venous Po_2 requires treatment with inotropes such as dopamine.

Anesthetic Considerations

Any anesthetic technique compatible with the patient's general condition is satisfactory for the spinal cord–injured patient. Hypotension is very common during anesthesia in quadriplegic patients. Placement of a central venous or pulmonary artery catheter may facilitate management of the patient's volume and blood pressure status.

The danger of administering succinylcholine to spine-injured patients is well known.[164] Succinylcholine produces massive and simultaneous depolarization of all the involved muscles; within 3 minutes a sudden, severe increase in serum K^+ occurs. Levels as high as $14\ mEq \cdot l^{-1}$ may be reached: the result may be irreversible ventricular dysrhythmias and cardiac arrest. Although succinylcholine is probably safe during the first week after injury, it is probably best to avoid it altogether in the paraplegic patient and use rapid-onset nondepolarizing agents such as rocuronium or rapacuronium when a rapid-sequence induction is required.

Neck Injury

In addition to the cervical spine, penetrating and blunt trauma may injure the other major structures in the neck: vessels, respiratory and digestive tracts, and nervous system. Devastating complications, including hemorrhage, asphyxia, mediastinitis, paralysis, stroke, or death, may result from these injuries if they are not promptly recognized and treated. Successful anesthetic and airway management also depends on timely diagnosis of these injuries. A chart designed by Demetriades et al[165] provides a systematic tool for assessing penetrating neck trauma and minimizing the rate of missed injuries (Fig. 48-4). With minor modifications it may also be used for evaluation of blunt cervical trauma.

Physical signs and symptoms are often sufficient for evaluating penetrating neck injuries; they usually present with obvious clinical manifestations. Blunt cervical trauma may be more subtle. Airway compromise or obstruction, brisk bleeding from the wound site, an expanding pulsatile hematoma, and shock with or without external bleeding are obvious signs of cervical vascular injuries and dictate immediate airway management and vascular control. Decreased or absent upper extremity or distal carotid pulses, and carotid bruit or thrill are pathognomonic for cervical arterial injury; however, these often do not require immediate surgery. Hemothorax, pneumothorax, and signs of air embolism are also suggestive. Respiratory distress, cyanosis, or stridor are obvious signs of airway injury and require immediate tracheal intubation. Other signs that strongly suggest airway injury are dysphonia, hoarseness, cough, hemoptysis, air bubbling from the wound, subcutaneous crepitus, laryngeal tenderness, pneumothorax, and hemothorax. Because of their dynamic nature, cervical airway injuries may rapidly progress to obstruction; the patient therefore should be observed carefully and the trachea intubated at the first sign of problems.

Esophageal injuries, whether in the neck or the chest, are insidious and difficult to diagnose. Dysphagia, odynophagia, hematemesis, subcutaneous crepitus, prevertebral air on a lateral cervical radiograph, and major concomitant injuries to other cervical structures suggest an esophageal injury and call for confirmation with an esophagram.

The neurologic manifestations of a penetrating neck injury vary depending on the injured structure. Partial spinal cord transection produces the Brown-Sequard syndrome with ipsilateral motor and contralateral sensory deficit below the injury. Complete spinal cord transection, depending on the level of injury, produces paraplegia or quadriplegia, usually with neurogenic shock. Occasionally luminal occlusion of the carotid and vertebral arteries may lead to hemispheric cerebrovascular acci-

A. Site of Injury:

    ☐ Anterior neck triangle (anterior to SMS muscle)
    ☐ Posterior neck triangle (posterior to SMS muscle)
    ☐ Zone I (between clavicles and cricoid)
    ☐ Zone II (between cricoid and angle of mandible of skull)
    ☐ Zone III (between angle of mandible and base of skull)

Wound Tract:

    ☐ Towards midline
    ☐ Towards clavicle
    ☐ Away from midline or
    ☐ Can't assess

B. Vascular Structures

    1. Active bleeding: ☐ None, ☐ Minor, ☐ Moderate, ☐ Severe
    2. Hypovolemia: ☐ BP >100, ☐ BP 60–90, ☐ BP <60
    3. Hematoma: ☐ None, ☐ Small, ☐ Moderate, ☐ Large, ☐ Expanding, ☐ Pulsatile
    4. Peripheral pulses (compare with contralateral):
        Distal carotid: ☐ normal, ☐ diminished, ☐ absent
        Superficial temporal: ☐ normal, ☐ diminished, ☐ absent
        Brachial or radial: ☐ normal, ☐ diminished, ☐ absent
    5. Bruit: ☐ No. ☐ Yes. (If so where_____)

C. Larynx/trachea, esophagus

    1. Hemoptysis (ask patient to cough) ☐ yes, ☐ no
    2. Air bubbling through wound? ☐ yes, ☐ no (ask patient to cough)
    3. Subcutaneous emphysema: ☐ yes, ☐ no
    4. Hoarseness: ☐ yes, ☐ no
    5. Pain on swallowing sputum: ☐ yes, ☐ no
    6. Hematemesis: ☐ yes, ☐ no

D. Nervous system

    1. GCS: ☐ eye response, ☐ verbal response, ☐ motor response
       Total GCS_____
    2. Localizing signs:
        Pupils:
        Limbs:
        Cranial nerves:
            Facial n.: ☐ normal, ☐ abnormal
            Glossopharyngeal n.: (check midline portion of soft palate) ☐ normal, ☐ abnormal
            Recurrent laryngeal n. (hoarseness, effective cough): ☐ normal, ☐ abnormal
            Accessory n. (lift the shoulder): ☐ normal, ☐ abnormal
            Hypoglossal n. (check midline position of tongue): ☐ normal, ☐ abnormal
            Spinal cord: ☐ normal, ☐ abnormal (specify)
            Horners syndrome (myosis, ptosis): ☐ yes, ☐ no
            Brachial plexus: median n. (fist): ☐ normal, ☐ abnormal
                              radial n. (wrist extension): ☐ normal, ☐ abnormal
                              ulnar n. (abduction/adduction of fingers): ☐ normal, ☐ abnormal
                              musculocutaneous n. (flexion of forearm): ☐ normal, ☐ abnormal
                              axillary n. (abduction of arm): ☐ normal, ☐ abnormal

Figure 48-4. Comprehensive evaluation chart used for penetrating neck trauma in Los Angeles County/University of Southern California Medical Center. (Reprinted with permission from Demetriades D, Asensio JA, Velmahos G, Thal E: Complex problems in penetrating neck trauma. Surg Clin North Am 76:661, 1996.)

dent; associated hypotension increases the likelihood of this event.

Patients with severe active bleeding, persistent hypotension, and air bubbling through the wound require immediate surgery without further diagnostic studies.[165] Controversy exists over the indications for surgical management of stable penetrating neck injuries. Mandatory exploration is associated with negative findings in approximately 70% of patients.[165] Thus, in many centers patients are evaluated with an angiogram, an esophagram, or a color flow Doppler, and undergo surgery only when there are positive findings.[165]

Blunt cervical vascular injuries usually present with a hematoma that may displace the airway and produce pharyngeal and laryngeal congestion. Injury to an artery may produce an intimal tear, pseudoaneurysm, fistula, or thrombosis.[166] If a carotid or vertebral artery is involved, cerebral ischemia may occur. Often thrombosis develops gradually over minutes to a few hours; therefore, the appearance of neurologic symptoms may be delayed in approximately 40% of patients.[166]

Blunt carotid injury, a rare entity before 1980, is now being diagnosed more frequently, probably because of increasing awareness and the increased use of shoulder belts that may compress the neck during automobile collisions. Although there are no reliable means to suspect this injury before neurologic abnormalities develop, knowledge of associated injuries should arouse suspicion in asymptomatic patients.[167] Carotid injury can occur with a history of severe hyperextension or flexion and rotation of the neck during an accident; concomitant cervical spine and displaced facial fractures; a basilar skull fracture involving the sphenoid, mastoid, or petrous bones, or the foramen lacerum; and significant soft tissue injury of the anterior part of the neck. Symptomatic patients may present with a cervical bruit, altered mental status, or lateralizing neurologic deficits including hemiparesis, transient ischemic attacks, amaurosis fugax, or Horner's syndrome. The mortality rate associated with blunt carotid injury varies between 15 and 28%, and 15–50% of survivors have neurologic deficits.[166,167] Identification of a blunt carotid injury in an asymptomatic patient using CT, magnetic resonance angiography, or four-vessel arteriography not only allows early institution of antiplatelet therapy, systemic anticoagulation, endovascular intervention, or surgical repair,[166,167] but occasionally it may prevent the neurologic deficits that may follow surgery for associated injuries in an unprotected patient.

Airway injuries after blunt trauma are rare, occurring in approximately 1/137,000 patients, with an overall mortality rate of 2%.[168] Their severity varies from a simple mucosal tear or hematoma to a comminuted laryngeal cartilage fracture or complete cricotracheal separation. They frequently require primary laryngeal repair or tracheostomy. Anesthetic management is not only complicated by relatively complex airway management problems[64-66] (discussed in the section on Airway Evaluation and Intervention), but with associated skull base, intracranial, open neck, cervical spine, esophageal, or pharyngeal injuries.[168]

Chest Injury

Trauma to almost any structure in the chest may produce serious and often life-threatening complications that require prompt diagnosis and intervention. Although a high percentage of these injuries can be treated conservatively, patients who need surgery may have major intraoperative physiologic disturbances.

Chest Wall Injury

The type and severity of trauma to the chest wall (ribs, sternum, and scapula) can, to a certain extent, predict the likelihood and severity of internal injuries. As is well known, rib fractures may produce pneumothorax or hemothorax, but both the frequency and severity of visceral injuries also increase as the number of fractured ribs increases. Patients with three or more

fractured ribs have a greater likelihood of hepatic and splenic injury, a higher mortality rate, a higher injury severity score, and longer ICU and hospital stays than those with fewer rib fractures.[169] Patients with lower rib fractures may have underlying spleen or liver injury. Because of the large amount of energy required to fracture the first rib in its protected location, injury to this bone indicates severe underlying trauma, commonly to the aorta, the subclavian vessels, the heart, or the abdominal viscera, but also to the maxillofacial complex, the brain, or the spinal cord.[170,171] Of the remaining components of the chest wall, scapular fractures suggest severe injuries in other locations, especially the heart and lungs.[172] Sternal fractures are mainly encountered in elderly female motor vehicle occupants wearing seat belts; they are usually not associated with serious trauma to the thoracic or abdominal viscera.[173,174]

The management principles for chest wall injuries are similar to those previously described for flail chest. Of course, the need for mechanical ventilation is less likely in single rib fractures than in a flail chest. Effective pain relief, preferably with continuous thoracic epidural anesthetics or opioids, is central to management.[73,74]

Pleural Injury

Two life-threatening chest injuries, tension and open pneumothorax, have already been discussed. Uncomplicated closed pneumothorax most commonly develops as a result of lung puncture by a displaced rib fracture after blunt trauma, or by missile injuries or stab wounds. The presence of subcutaneous emphysema suggests coexisting pneumothorax, although this finding alone is not an indication for chest tube placement; a tracheobronchial or esophageal perforation, interstitial lung injury, chronic pleural adhesions from pre-existing disease, facial injury with tracking of air through the fascial planes of the neck, and retroperitoneal air escape through the esophageal hiatus may also produce this finding. Tension pneumothorax involving >50% of a hemithorax presents with dyspnea, tachycardia, cyanosis, agitation, diaphoresis, neck vein distention, tracheal deviation, and displacement of the maximal cardiac impulse to the contralateral side.

The definitive diagnosis of this and other chest injuries is made by plain chest radiograph, a routine film obtained during initial evaluation of all trauma victims. Although an upright film provides the best opportunity for detection of pleural air, this position may be impossible or contraindicated in patients who are experiencing major hemorrhage or those with suspected spine or severe head injury. The supine chest radiograph can detect most pneumothoraces large enough to require immediate thoracostomy. Intrapleural free air in supine patients tends to move to the highest portion of the chest, which corresponds to the cardiophrenic or anteromedial and subpulmonic spaces.[175] Air in these regions is most likely to be detected with a lateral radiograph. Nevertheless, a small pneumothorax can easily be missed under these conditions. CT of the chest is more reliable than plain radiography for diagnosis of these so-called "occult pneumothoraces," which occur in approximately 6% of patients with blunt abdominal trauma.[176] There is a recent suggestion that a small closed pneumothorax can be safely managed by observation alone, without a chest tube, even in those patients who require positive-pressure ventilation, as long as continuing vigilance is maintained.[176] However, based on an earlier study[177] and our own experience, we strongly believe that once diagnosed, a traumatic pneumothorax, no matter how small, should be treated with thoracostomy drainage before tracheal intubation and positive-pressure ventilation.

Bleeding intercostal vessels are responsible for most hemothoraces. Severe airway deviation may be produced by a hemothorax, although it is not as common as it is after a pneumothorax. Treatment consists of drainage with a 30–40 French chest tube (26–32 French is used for pneumothorax). Initial drainage of 1000 ml of blood, or collection of >200 ml·hr^{-1} is an indication for thoracotomy. Additional indications for thoracotomy are a "white lung" appearance on the anteroposterior chest radiograph, a continuous major air leak from the chest tube, which may result from a direct airway injury or major lung laceration, and evidence of pericardial tamponade. Hemodynamically stable patients with persistent bleeding of <150 ml · hr^{-1} are managed with video-assisted thoracoscopic surgery (VATS) to control bleeding.[178] This procedure requires placement of a double-lumen tube to collapse the lung on the involved side; it can also be useful in diagnosis of suspected diaphragmatic, cardiac, or mediastinal injuries; evaluation of some bronchopleural fistulas; and evacuation of clotted blood or an empyema that does not drain with a chest tube.[178] Use of VATS decreases the need for open thoracotomy and the number of negative explorations in trauma patients.[179] Parenthetically, blood drained from the pleural space does not coagulate. This defibrinated blood can be collected into citrate-phosphate-dextrose–containing bags and returned to the patient.

Pulmonary Contusion

Pathologically, pulmonary contusion can be described as intra-alveolar hemorrhage and edema, with atelectasis, parenchymal disruption, and lung consolidation resulting from a sudden increase in intra-alveolar pressure and rupture of the alveolar–capillary interface. There is evidence to suggest that prostanoids are also involved in the development and progression of pulmonary abnormalities on the injured side as well as in the contralateral lung.[180] The presence of a pulmonary contusion cannot be predicted from rib fractures; severe chest wall injuries may be associated with no lung damage and vice versa. Pulmonary contusion may not be apparent on admission, although physiologic, clinical, and radiologic manifestations usually begin to appear within 4 hours after injury. In all patients with suspected blunt chest trauma, ABGs and a chest radiograph should be obtained on admission and several times during the first day. Even a small contusion may enlarge to involve most of a lung volume within a few hours.[181] Patients with involvement of >60% of a lung at any time within the first 24 hours after admission, or a Pao$_2$/Fio$_2$ ratio of <300 are very likely to need positive-pressure ventilation and are at increased risk of death.[181]

Initial management of pulmonary contusion is supportive, and includes tracheal intubation; mechanical ventilation, preferably with positive end-expiratory pressure (PEEP), judicious fluid resuscitation, and frequent tracheobronchial suctioning. Clearing of airway secretions is important; many trauma patients smoke and have copious secretions that may cause bronchial plugging and atelectasis in the acute stage and pneumonia later if they are not cleared; the presence of rib fractures probably increases the likelihood of these complications.

Experimental studies suggest that, probably because of pulmonary vascular changes, a pulmonary contusion may interfere with the accuracy of the PCWP as an estimate of left ventricular end-diastolic pressue. The central venous pressure (CVP) may be a better measure of cardiac preload than the PCWP in this situation.[182] Furthermore, significant myocardial depression, probably due to circulating arachidonic acid metabolites, has been seen after isolated pulmonary contusion. Thus even without direct cardiac injury, pulmonary contusion may contribute to the development of congestive heart failure.[182]

Penetrating Cardiac Injury

Pericardial tamponade, cardiac chamber perforation, and fistula formation between the cardiac chambers and the great vessels are the consequences of this type of trauma. Any penetrating wound of the chest, especially one within the "cardiac window" (midclavicular lines laterally, clavicles superiorly, and costal margins inferiorly), can cause this injury. Pneumopericardium visible on a plain chest radiograph after penetrating chest trauma should increase the suspicion, although it is not seen in all patients. Unstable patients require immediate sternotomy

or left thoracotomy; transthoracic two-dimensional echocardiography (TTE) can be used for screening stable patients.[183] Transthoracic two-dimensional echocardiography may be inconclusive in obese patients and in those with pneumothorax; TEE may provide an accurate diagnosis in these patients.[184] Alternative diagnostic measures are more problematic. The CVP is not always accurate, and a subxiphoid pericardial window is invasive, must be performed in the operating room under general anesthesia, takes longer, and cannot detect an intracardiac shunt.

Pericardial Tamponade

The classic findings of pericardial tamponade—tachycardia, hypotension, distant heart sounds, distended neck veins, pulsus paradoxus, or pulsus alternans—are difficult to appreciate or may be absent in a hypovolemic trauma patient. Transthoracic echocardiography or TEE can demonstrate blood in the pericardial sac and the presence of ventricular "diastolic collapse," which indicates at least a 20% reduction in cardiac output. Initial management consists of intravenous fluids and, if necessary, careful selection and titration of anesthetic agents. Ketamine and etomidate, which produce little myocardial depression, are the agents of choice. Evacuation of the pericardial blood by pericardiocentesis or surgery should be performed as soon as possible.

Myocardial Contusion

This injury is probably present in a large proportion of blunt chest trauma victims, but it usually is not recognized because its symptoms are absent, vague, or nonspecific. The prominent clinical findings are angina-like pain, which may or may not respond to nitrates, dysrhythmias of any type, and right- or left-sided congestive heart failure. Initial management includes identification of those patients in whom dysrhythmias or pump dysfunction may develop. Echocardiography, creatine phosphokinase MB (CPK-MB) isoenzyme determination, and electrocardiography (ECG) seem to be most helpful for this purpose. Of these, two-dimensional echocardiography appears to be the most reliable test,[185,186] especially when it is combined with a color Doppler study. Findings that suggest the presence of this injury are segmental wall motion abnormalities, increased end-diastolic wall thickness, right ventricular (RV) dilatation, septal shift, myocardial hematoma, and an intracavitary filling defect produced by the hematoma in the myocardium. Valvular dysfunction and pericardial fluid may also be seen. CPK-MB isoenzyme elevation usually occurs within the first day after the injury. The usual ECG abnormalities are ST segment and T-wave changes, axis shift, bundle-branch block, and dysrhythmias; they may be detectable for a few days.[187] Diagnosis can be made on the basis of clinical data and positive results of all three of the screening tests,[185] which indicate a clinically significant myocardial contusion; cardiac failure is unlikely if only one or two tests are positive.[188] Patients with a normal admission ECG are unlikely to have a significant cardiac abnormality, and further diagnostic studies are not indicated.[143]

Thoracic Aortic Injury

A history of high-impact trauma, especially to the chest, should raise the suspicion of thoracic aortic injury. It occurs most frequently in the proximal portion of the descending aorta; injury to the ascending aorta and the arch is much less likely. Clinical findings are not always detectable in the emergency department (Table 48-8). A widened mediastinum on the chest radiograph should prompt a search for this injury. This sign is a reflection of mediastinal hemorrhage due to aortic injury in only 20% of cases; at other times, it is a result of bleeding from other thoracic or cervical vessels.[189] Although biplanar aortography is the definitive diagnostic test, it has major drawbacks: a prolonged procedure time and the risks of vascular catheterization, dye injection, and transport of a potentially

Table 48-8. COMMON CLINICAL, RADIOGRAPHIC, AND ULTRASOUND FEATURES OF THORACIC AORTIC INJURIES

Clinical	Radiographic	Spiral Computed Tomography	Ultrasound
Increased arterial pressure and pulse amplitude in upper extremities	Widened mediastinum	Mediastinal hematoma	Intimal flap
Decreased arterial pressure and pulse amplitude in lower extremities	Blurring of the aortic contours	Aortic wall irregularity	Turbulent flow
Absent or weak left radial artery pulse	Widened paraspinal interfaces	Intimal flap	
Osler's sign: discrepancy between left and right arm blood pressure	Opacified pulmonary window		
Retrosternal or interscapular pain	Broadened paratracheal stripe		
Hoarseness	Displacement of the left mainstem bronchus		
Systolic flow murmur over the precordium or medial to the left scapula	Rightward deviation of the esophagus and trachea		
Neurologic deficits in the lower extremities	Left hemothorax		
	Sternal or upper rib fractures		

unstable patient to the radiology suite. Less invasive diagnostic tests have, therefore, been attempted. A thoracic CT scan may be problematic. The procedure time may be prolonged; in some cases, the scan is incapable of adequately visualizing parts of the aorta and its branches; and it may be difficult to demonstrate an intimal flap or aortic wall irregularities. Diagnosis is made by identifying the mediastinal hemorrhage and demonstrating its proximity to the aorta or other great vessels. With the spiral CT, power-injected contrast studies have a high degree of accuracy. Although this technique is reliable for the diagnosis of aortic injuries, there has been little experience with trauma around the aortic arch.[189] TEE is a relatively simple, minimally invasive diagnostic test.[190] An intimal flap and turbulent flow (detected by the Doppler technique) are the characteristic signs of aortic injury on TEE. It can be used during surgery for patients with unstable injuries that preclude preoperative examination of the aorta. Nevertheless, neither the CT scan nor the TEE are absolutely reliable diagnostic tests[190]; aortography is still indicated whenever there is uncertainty about the results of these studies, or when there are contraindications to their use.

Thoracic aortic rupture rarely presents without an associated injury. Surgical prioritization depends on the hemodynamic and neurologic status of the patient. Although the aorta should be repaired as early as possible, control of active hemorrhage from other sites and surgery for intracranial hematomas have a higher surgical priority, unless the aorta is leaking.[191] In most instances, a blood clot between the aorta and the mediastinal pleura occludes the vessel. Any disturbance of the vessel in the tamponaded region may reinitiate bleeding. A rapid flow of blood in a large artery tends to pull its endothelium with it and thus may rupture an injured vessel that is sealed with a clot or a hematoma. Such an increase in the aortic blood flow is usually caused by increased myocardial contractility. Thus, during management of patients with aortic injury, every effort should be made to prevent hypertension.

Diaphragmatic Injury

In addition to interfering with the competence of the esophagogastric junction, a diaphragmatic injury may permit migration of abdominal contents into the chest where they may compress the lung, producing abnormalities of gas exchange, or the heart, resulting in dysrhythmias. Even when the abdominal contents do not migrate, there may be breathing abnormalities because of diaphragmatic dysfunction. Patients usually present with shortness of breath and, less frequently, with symptoms of gastrointestinal obstruction. Other injuries often accompany diaphragmatic trauma. Because the defect produced by blunt trauma is larger than that resulting from a penetrating injury, migration of abdominal contents, which requires a defect of at least 6 cm in diameter, is also more common after blunt

trauma.[192] The liver protects the right side of the diaphragm, thus traumatic herniation is more common on the left side.[192] The abdominal contents may rarely herniate into the mediastinum and cause persistent tachycardia, which may be attributed to other factors.

With the exception of laparoscopy, all of the available methods of abdominal diagnosis have their limitations. Nevertheless, noting that the end of a nasogastric tube is above the diaphragm on the chest radiograph is a certain sign that the stomach is displaced into the chest. Failure to retrieve the instilled fluid during diagnostic peritoneal lavage (DPL) also suggests this injury.[193] If a thoracostomy tube is in place, drainage of DPL fluid from the chest is another indication of a ruptured diaphragm.[193] A chest radiograph with or without a contrast study of the gastrointestinal tract that shows intestinal markings and lung compression is diagnostic in patients with intestinal contents in the chest.[193] A contrast-enhanced abdominal CT scan that includes the lower third of the thorax can also provide important information.[193] As mentioned previously, laparoscopic examination or VATS provides a definitive intraoperative diagnosis.

Abdominal and Pelvic Injuries

The management of acute abdominal injuries has changed significantly in the 1990s, and the current trend suggests that there will be additional modifications in the future. Thus, preferences in management of abdominal trauma vary widely among centers. Table 48-9 summarizes the strengths and weaknesses of the currently available diagnostic tools used for abdominal injuries.[194] Because of the unpredictable course of bullets in the body, exploratory laparotomy or, in selected cases, laparoscopy is required after any gunshot wound of the abdomen. Stab wounds may be managed with tractotomy to determine whether the peritoneum is involved, and then a DPL may be performed if necessary. A positive DPL is an indication for laparotomy. In some hemodynamically stable patients, abdominal and flank gunshot wounds may be managed safely with an initial CT scan.[195] Patients with a negative study are observed, whereas those with positive findings undergo exploratory surgery. Equivocal CT results are followed by a laparoscopy and, if this is positive, by laparotomy.

Blunt abdominal trauma requires a diagnostic workup before a laparotomy is performed, unless the patient is hemodynamically unstable and there are overt abdominal signs such as tenderness, guarding, and gross distention. Absence of abdominal distention, however, does not rule out intra-abdominal bleeding; at least 1 liter of blood can accumulate before the smallest change in girth is apparent, and the diaphragm can also move

Table 48-9. DIAGNOSTIC TOOLS IN ABDOMINAL TRAUMA: STRENGTHS AND WEAKNESSES

Diagnostic Tool	Strength	Weakness
Physical examination	Expeditious, safe, and inexpensive; potential for serial examination	Diagnosis of specific injury (*e.g.,* diaphragm)
Diagnostic peritoneal lavage	Expeditious, safe, and inexpensive	Diagnosis of diaphragmatic injury, hollow viscus injury, retroperitoneal injury; can be oversensitive and nonspecific
Computed tomography	Evaluation of peritoneum and retroperitoneum Staging of solid organ injury	Diagnosis of diaphragmatic injury, hollow viscus injury Expensive; controversial need for contrast
Ultrasonography	Expeditious, safe, and inexpensive; accurate for free peritoneal fluid Potential for serial examinations	Diagnosis of diphragmatic injury, hollow viscus injury Less accurate in the presence of large retroperitoneal hematomas
Laparoscopy	Diagnosis of peritoneal penetration, diaphragmatic injury Evaluation of bleeding or solid organ injury Potential for therapy	Diagnosis of hollow viscus injury, retroperitoneal injury Expensive (especially in OR); difficult to perform in busy emergency department
Video-assisted thoracic surgery	Evaluation of lung, diaphragm, mediastinum, chest wall and pericardium; potential for treatment	Requires OR; expensive

OR = operating room.
Reprinted with permission from Villavicencio RT, Aucar JA: Analysis of laparoscopy in trauma. J Am Coll Surg 189:11, 1999.

cephalad, allowing further significant blood loss without any change in abdominal circumference.

In hemodynamically stable patients, there are two major diagnostic algorithms: focused approach with sonography for trauma (FAST; Fig. 48-5) and the conventional approach, without ultrasonography (Fig. 48-6). The diagnostic accuracy of these algorithms is similar, but FAST requires one-third of the time and is 3.5 times less expensive than the conventional approach.[196] Screening with abdominal ultrasonography is performed by placing the probe (3.0–5.0 MHz) on four distinct areas of the abdomen: subxiphoid, to detect pericardial blood; right upper quadrant, for blood in the hepatorenal pouch; left upper quadrant, to detect perisplenic blood; and just above the pubic symphysis, for blood in the rectovesical pouch. FAST

provides rapid, cost-effective results, and may be implemented by the physician responsible for initial evaluation in the emergency department. It is accurate for detection of hemoperitoneum,[196,197] and can also identify solid organ injuries, although experience with these is limited. It cannot reliably detect trauma to the intestines unless they are associated with bleeding.[197] Fortunately, isolated intestinal injuries are uncommon after blunt trauma. Depending on the results of FAST, patients are managed with observation, repeat FAST, DPL, abdominal CT, laparoscopy, or laparotomy[196] (see Fig. 48-5). Patients managed with the conventional algorithm are evaluated by CT if they are stable, and DPL if they are hemodynamically or neurologically unstable; depending on the results of these studies, they are observed or undergo surgery[196] (see Fig. 48-6).

Diagnostic peritoneal lavage is considered positive if (1) >10 ml of gross blood is obtained, or (2) the erythrocyte count is >100,000 per mm^3, the leukocyte count is >500 per mm^3, the

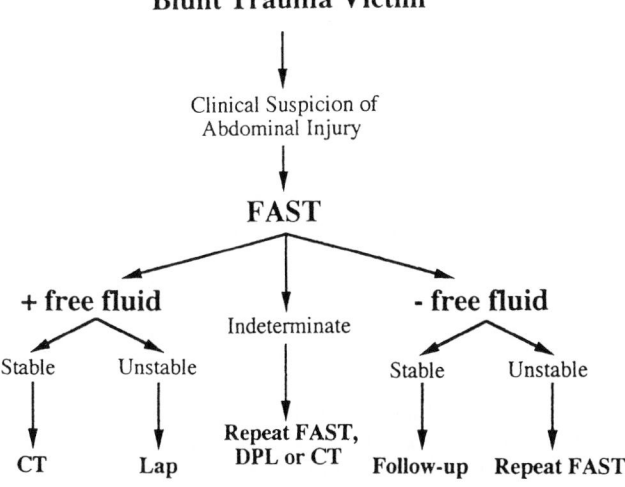

Figure 48-5. Algorithm using focused assessment with sonography for trauma for evaluation of blunt abdominal injury. CT = computed tomography; DPL = diagnostic peritoneal lavage; FAST = focused approach with sonography for trauma; Lap = laparotomy. (Reprinted with permission from Boulanger BR, McLennan BA, Brennemann FD *et al:* Prospective evidence of the superiority of a sonography-based algorithm in the assessment of blunt abdominal injury. J Trauma 47:632, 1999.)

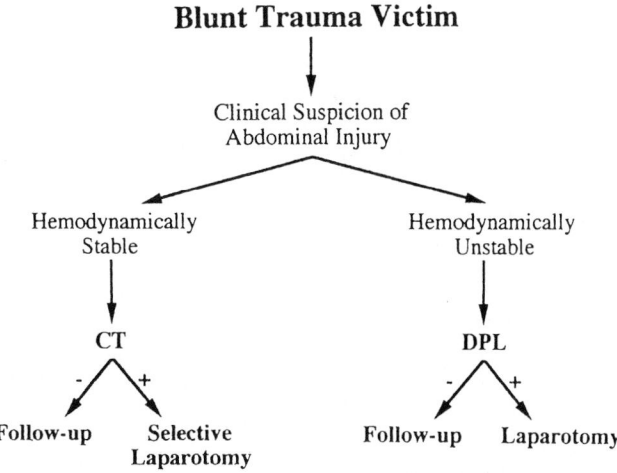

Figure 48-6. Conventionally used algorithm for evaluation of blunt abdominal injury. CT = computed tomography; DPL = diagnostic peritoneal lavage. (Reprinted with permission from Boulanger BR, McLennan BA, Brennemann FD *et al:* Prospective evidence of the superiority of a sonography-based algorithm in the assessment of blunt abdominal injury. J Trauma 47:632, 1999.)

amylase level is above 200 U · l⁻¹, and there are bacteria in the drainage fluid. Using these criteria, the overall sensitivity of DPL is 91%, specificity 94%, accuracy 93%, positive predictive value 80%, and negative predictive value 98%.[198] Nevertheless, intestinal injuries may be missed with these criteria.[199]

Problems with DPL include its lack of organ specificity, inability to evaluate the retroperitoneal region, and potential to perforate an organ in patients with abdominal adhesions. Abdominal CT scanning presents none of these difficulties. It is an excellent diagnostic technique in flank injuries, which usually involve retroperitoneal structures. More important, it permits the use of an organ injury scaling system, which has decreased the rate of diagnostic laparotomy. In this system, the injury to each organ is classified according to its severity; patients with lower scores are treated conservatively. The overall sensitivity of the CT scan is approximately 74%, the specificity 99.5%, and the accuracy 92%.[200] If there is leukocytosis combined with free fluid on abdominal CT, this should raise the suspicion of a hollow viscus injury.[201]

Laparoscopy is an excellent screening tool in trauma patients. An analysis showed that it avoided laparotomy in 63% of patients and missed only 1% of the injuries.[194] However, it is not an accurate tool for identifying injuries to specific organs; the missed injury rate per patient was 44–77%.[194] Although the therapeutic advantages of laparoscopy have not been demonstrated in trauma patients, it is possible that diaphragm, bladder, and solid organ injuries may be repaired with this technique. The complication rate of laparoscopy in trauma is approximately 1%, including pneumothorax, small bowel injury, intraabdominal vascular injury, and extraperitoneal CO_2 insufflation.[194]

Fractures of the Pelvis

Pelvic fractures result in major hemorrhage in 25% and exsanguination in 1% of patients.[202] Although there is no reliable way to predict the extent of bleeding in a given patient, as a simple guide, all patients with "open book" fractures (disruption of the pubic symphysis) and those with >0.5 cm displacement on an anteroposterior pelvic film can be considered candidates for administration of between 4 and 10 units of blood within 48 hours after the injury.[203] In most trauma victims with pelvic fractures, bleeding results from disruption of veins by the bone fragments. Pelvic retroperitoneal bleeding is self-limited in most patients with venous injuries, except those with open fractures, in whom the tamponading effect does not occur. Approximately 18–20% of patients have arterial bleeding, which does not stop. The retroperitoneal space in these patients may serve as a distensible container, expanding superiorly and anteriorly toward the abdominal wall and totally obliterating the lower part of the abdominal cavity. Thus, DPL, as in pregnant trauma patients, should be performed above the umbilicus. Large retroperitoneal hematomas may also cause respiratory difficulty because of pressure on the diaphragm. Application of MAST to prevent friction of fracture fragments and thus bleeding can worsen the respiratory difficulty in these patients.

Angiography after external pelvic fixation provides information about the type and location of bleeding. Arterial bleeding is treated with embolization; the angiography suite should be prepared in advance not only for anesthesia but for invasive monitoring and resuscitation. Pelvic fractures may also injure the bladder and the urethra. Thus, a urethrogram should be performed before insertion of a urinary catheter.

Extremity Injuries

Surgical repair of extremity fractures, whether they are open or closed, should be performed as soon as possible. Delayed fracture repair is associated with increased risk of deep vein thrombosis (DVT), pneumonia, sepsis, and the pulmonary and cerebral complications of fat embolism.[204] Thus, contrary to the old understanding that considered skeletal injuries a low surgical priority, the current belief is that long bone fractures must be reduced and pelvic fractures immobilized with external fixators during the initial surgery, simultaneously with or shortly after the repair of thoracoabdominal and brain injuries. In open fractures, an additional important concern is infection. Wounds left unrepaired for more than 6 hours are likely to become septic. Other factors that influence the incidence of extremity infection include the extent of soft tissue damage, the location of the injury (upper extremities are less likely to become infected than lower extremities), the mechanism of trauma, the use of prophylactic antibiotics, the type of fixation, and the amount of blood transfused.[205]

Associated vascular trauma must be recognized early. Most vascular injuries exhibit at least some part of the classic syndrome of pain, pulselessness, pallor, paresthesias, and paresis. The definitive diagnosis is made with arteriography; in selected patients a duplex ultrasound study may be used as a screening test. *Compartment syndrome*, which is characterized by severe pain in the affected extremity or calf pain on dorsiflexion of the foot, should be recognized early so that emergency fasciotomy can be effective in preventing irreversible muscle and nerve damage. In unconscious patients, swelling and tenseness of the extremity indicate the presence of this complication. The definitive diagnosis is made by measuring compartment pressures, using a transducer attached to a fluid-filled extension tube and a needle inserted into the various compartments of the extremity. A pressure exceeding 40 cm H_2O is an indication for immediate surgery. Caution must be exercised when using epidural or nerve block analgesia for perioperative pain relief in the presence of extremity fractures. Absence of pain could delay diagnosis of a compartment syndrome.

Burns

Determination of the size and depth of the burn sets the guidelines for resuscitation as well as the indications for surgical intervention.[206] A partial-thickness burn is red, blanches to touch, and is sensitive to painful stimuli and heat. Superficial partial-thickness (first-degree) burns involve the epidermis and upper dermis and heal spontaneously. Deep partial-thickness (second-degree) burns involve the deep dermis and require excision and grafting to ensure rapid return of function. A full-thickness (third-degree) burn does not blanch even with deep pressure and is insensate. Complete destruction of the dermis requires wound excision and grafting. Some limitation of function due to scar formation results. Fourth-degree burns involve muscle, fascia, and bone, necessitating complete excision and leaving the patient with limited function. The size of the burned area as a fraction of the total body surface area (TBSA) is estimated by the "rule of nines." In an adult, the head contributes to 9%, the upper extremities, 18%, the trunk, 36%, and the lower extremities, 36% of the TBSA. These proportions are somewhat different in children.

Information about the mechanism of injury facilitates the diagnosis of associated clinical abnormalities. For example, thermal trauma caused by flames in a closed space is likely to be associated with airway damage. Burns resulting from motor vehicle, airplane, or industrial accidents may be complicated by other traumatic injuries. Finally, burns caused by electrocution may show little external evidence but may be associated with severe fractures, hematomas, visceral injury, and skeletal and cardiac muscle injury resulting in pain, myoglobinuria, and dysrhythmias or other ECG abnormalities.

Full-thickness burns involving >10% of the TBSA; partial-thickness burns covering >25% of TBSA in adults and over 20% at the extremes of age; burns involving the face, hands, feet, or perineum; inhalation, chemical, and electrical burns; and burns in patients with severe pre-existing medical disorders are considered to be *major burns*.[206] A severe burn is a systemic disease that stimulates the release of mediators locally—producing wound edema—and into the circulation, that cause immune suppression, hypermetabolism, protein catabolism, sepsis, and multisystem organ failure.[206]

Airway Complications

Respiratory distress in the initial phase of a burn is usually caused by airway injury involving the pharynx or the trachea. Singed facial hair, facial burns, dysphonia or hoarseness, cough, soot in the mouth or nose, and swallowing difficulties in patients without respiratory distress should increase the suspicion of upper (frequent) and lower (occasional) airway injury. In the upper airway, particles with high heat capacity, such as plastics and absorbed chemicals, cause glottic and periglottic edema and copious, thick secretions, resulting in obstruction and possibly interfering with laryngeal protection of the lower airway. Fluid resuscitation probably contributes greatly to upper airway obstruction even in the absence of significant inhalation injury.[207] The trachea and bronchi may be damaged by toxic gases. Decreased surfactant and mucociliary function, mucosal necrosis and ulceration, edema, tissue sloughing, and secretions produce bronchial obstruction, air trapping, and bronchopneumonia. The development of parenchymal lung injury takes approximately 1–5 days and presents with the clinical picture of adult respiratory distress syndrome. Pneumonia and PE are late complications that occur 5 or more days after burns. The presence of respiratory difficulty markedly increases the mortality rate from thermal injuries.[208]

Administration of the highest possible concentration of O_2 by face mask is the first priority in moderately to severely burned patients with a patent airway. In patients with massive burns, stridor, respiratory distress, hypoxemia, hypercarbia, loss of consciousness, or altered mentation, immediate tracheal intubation is indicated.[209] The intubation technique selected depends on the operator's experience, the age of the patient, and the extent of airway compromise. In adults, awake fiberoptic intubation under adequate topical anesthesia is probably the safest approach. In most pediatric patients, awake intubation is not possible. An inhalation induction with O_2 and halothane or sevoflurane, followed by intubation using a fiberoptic bronchoscope or conventional laryngoscope is appropriate.[206] Personnel and equipment should be available for a possible needle or formal cricothyroidotomy or tracheostomy. It is generally believed that a surgical airway entails a significant risk of pulmonary sepsis, late upper airway sequelae, and death in burned patients; it should be reserved for those whose airway management cannot be handled in any other way.[206,210] Immediately after securing the airway, ventilation with low levels of PEEP may prevent the pulmonary edema that may develop secondary to loss of laryngeal auto-PEEP in patients with significant airway obstruction before intubation.[211] Airway humidification, bronchial toilet, and bronchodilators if needed for bronchospasm, are also indicated.

Decisions about airway management can be difficult. Some patients may not have overt signs and symptoms initially, but may later develop airway compromise with progressive supraglottic edema or pulmonary abnormalities. The pediatric airway is particularly challenging because it may be occluded by minimal amounts of swelling owing to its small diameter. Prophylactic intubation may therefore be required in children who are suspected of having an inhalation injury even though they are not yet in respiratory distress. Prophylactic tracheal intubation may also be indicated in adults when the resources for careful follow-up are insufficient.[211] However, this approach may subject some patients to unnecessary risks of laryngeal sequelae such as granuloma formation, bleeding, or vocal cord paralysis. Information obtained from radiologic, ABG, and endoscopic examinations and pulmonary function testing may be useful to predict which patient will need tracheal intubation.[209]

Fiberoptic laryngoscopy is easy to perform and can provide direct information about the glottic and periglottic structures. It may avoid tracheal intubation in patients who would otherwise be considered candidates for this procedure.[209] Fiberoptic bronchoscopy has the additional advantage of providing information about the lower airway, although it is more uncomfortable for the patient and requires topical anesthesia of the tracheobronchial tree.[212] These studies should be performed every 3–4 hours for the first 12 hours after injury. In cooperative patients, pulmonary function testing may aid in the evaluation of airway obstruction. A sawtoothed or flattened inspiratory flow and an extrathoracic obstruction pattern on the flow/volume loop suggest upper airway obstruction. Decreased peak expiratory flow, forced vital capacity, and pulmonary compliance, and increased airway resistance suggest lower airway injury.

The initial chest radiograph is usually negative even in patients with pulmonary complications. However, a baseline film should be obtained for later comparison. Perivascular fuzziness and peribronchial cuffing within the first 24 hours of a burn suggest inhalation injury. Grading the severity of chest radiograph findings within the first 5 days after a thermal injury has been shown to correlate with the increase in lung water and pulmonary shunting, and the decrease in lung compliance.[213] As expected, the more extensive the pulmonary edema, the more severe are the functional abnormalities of the lung. The treatment of smoke inhalation in burns involves ventilatory management, intensive care, and treatment of carbon monoxide (CO) and cyanide (CN^-) toxicity.

Carbon Monoxide Toxicity

The patient's inspired oxygen should be maintained at the highest possible concentration, even when there is no evidence of significant smoke-induced lung injury, until CO toxicity is ruled out by measurement of blood carboxyhemoglobin (COHb). A high F_{IO_2} not only improves oxygenation but promotes elimination of CO; an F_{IO_2} of 1.0 decreases the blood half-life of COHb from the 4 hours seen in room air to <1 hour.[206] A normal oxygen saturation on a pulse oximeter does not exclude the possibility of CO toxicity, although low arterial O_2 saturation measured by a co-oximeter should raise the suspicion.[214] Similarly, the mixed venous oximeter catheters that are used for continuous in vivo measurement of $S\bar{v}O_2$ overestimate oxyhemoglobin concentration in the presence of CO.[215] If CO toxicity is not accompanied by a lung injury and thus by decreased PaO_2, tachypnea is absent; the carotid bodies are sensitive to the arterial O_2 tension and not to the O_2 content. The classic cherry-red color of the blood is also absent in most patients because it occurs only at COHb concentrations above 40%, and it may also be obscured by coexistent hypoxia and cyanosis.

Although CO may interfere with mitochondrial cytochrome function, it produces tissue hypoxia primarily by its 200-fold greater affinity for hemoglobin than oxygen and by its ability to shift the hemoglobin dissociation curve to the left. Thus, it reduces the oxyhemoglobin concentration and blood oxygen content and oxygen-carrying capacity, and impairs the release of oxygen to tissues.[216,217] The greater the blood concentration of COHb, the more severe are the presenting symptoms (Table 48-10). Delayed neuropsychiatric disorders have been described in patients exposed to toxic levels of CO, and there is evidence to suggest that early hyperbaric O_2 treatment may prevent these symptoms.[206] The decision to institute this treatment should be based on comparing the risks of transport, decreased patient access, and delay in emergency treatment against the possible neurologic sequelae. MacLennan et al[206] recommend hyperbaric O_2 for patients with COHB >30% at admission if the treatment of life-threatening problems will not be compromised.

Cyanide Toxicity

Another cause of tissue hypoxia in burned patients is CN^- toxicity. Cyanide or hydrocyanic acid is produced by incomplete

Table 48-10. SYMPTOMS OF CO TOXICITY AS A FUNCTION OF THE BLOOD CARBOXYHEMOGLOBIN (COHb) LEVEL

Blood COHb Level (%)	Symptoms
<15–20	Headache, dizziness, and occasional confusion
20–40	Nausea, vomiting, disorientation, and visual impairment
40–60	Agitation, combativeness, hallucinations, coma, and shock
>60	Death

combustion of synthetic materials, and may be inhaled or absorbed through mucous membranes. As in CO toxicity, the usual clinical presentation is unexplained metabolic acidosis. Nonspecific neurologic symptoms such as agitation, confusion, or coma are also common findings. Elevated plasma lactate levels in severe burns may result from hypovolemia, CO toxicity, or CN^- toxicity. However, lactic acidosis after smoke inhalation in a patient without a major burn suggests CN^- toxicity.[218] The definitive diagnosis can be made only by determination of the blood cyanide level, which is toxic above $0.2 \text{ mg} \cdot l^{-1}$ and lethal at levels beyond $1 \text{ mg} \cdot l^{-1}$.[219] A spectrophotometric assay using methemoglobin as a colorimetric indicator provides a timely and reliable determination of blood CN^-.[220] Increased CN^- in the blood can cause generalized cardiovascular depression and cardiac rhythm disturbances, especially in patients with lactic acidosis. Fortunately, the half-life of CN^- is short (approximately 1 hour),[218] and rapid improvement of hemodynamics should be expected after rescue of the victim from the toxic environment. Immediate administration of O_2, which is required for all burn victims, may be life saving for this complication. Although there are specific therapies for CN^- toxicity (e.g., amyl nitrate, sodium nitrite, thiosulfate), given the short half-life of the ion, it is not clear whether these measures offer significant help to the patient whose blood CN^- usually decreases to low levels during transport from the field to the hospital.[221] Of course, hyperbaric O_2 treatment can be used for all of the complications of thermal injury: CO and CN^- poisoning, smoke-induced lung damage, and cutaneous burns.[222] However, as mentioned, placement of a critically ill patient who may have other injuries in a hyperbaric chamber is technically difficult and fraught with complications.

Fluid Replacement

Immediately after a burn, microvascular permeability increases for 3–5 days in the injured tissues, and for less than a day in normal tissues, causing a loss of a substantial amount of protein-rich fluid.[206] This fluid flux is enhanced by increased intravascular hydrostatic and interstitial osmotic pressures and a decrease in interstitial hydrostatic pressure. In addition, cardiac contractility decreases because of circulating mediators, a diminished response to catecholamines, decreased coronary blood flow, and increased systemic vascular resistance.[206] This may result in shock, whose origin is primarily hypovolemic and to a small extent cardiogenic. If the hypotension is treated appropriately with fluids, the hemodynamic picture is replaced within 24 to 48 hours by one resembling sepsis or septic shock, with increased cardiac output and diminished systemic vascular resistance caused by the release of inflammatory mediators.[206]

Fluid resuscitation is essential in the early care of the burned patient, but restoration of intravascular volume should be done with utmost care to prevent excessive edema formation in both damaged and intact tissues resulting from the generalized increase in capillary permeability caused by the injury. Edema from overaggressive resuscitation has many deleterious and po-

tentially life-threatening effects. Mention has already been made of the facilitation of upper airway edema after rapid fluid infusion in large cutaneous burns with or without smoke inhalation.[207] Likewise, chest wall edema may develop after administration of large quantities of fluid, causing respiratory difficulties and necessitating excision of burned tissue from the anterior axillary line to improve breathing. Abdominal edema may also occur and occasionally increase intra-abdominal pressure and impede venous return. Edema formation may also increase the tissue pressure in the burned area, resulting in reduction of blood flow to distal sites. This, together with decreased tissue oxygen tension, may produce necrosis of damaged but viable cells, increasing the extent of injury and the risk of infection.

Both crystalloid and colloid solutions are effective in restoring tissue perfusion. However, colloids do not seem to offer any advantage over crystalloids in most instances, and are more expensive. The ACS Committee on Trauma recommends the use of crystalloids for this reason.[206] Nevertheless, crystalloid resuscitation, especially in children, may cause a rapid decline in plasma protein concentration and necessitate colloid administration.[223] Normal saline is isotonic and inexpensive, and can be used in most burn patients during initial resuscitation. Because of its slight hypotonicity, large quantities of LR solution may cause edema in intact tissues. However, it is used frequently in thermal injuries because it contains electrolytes in addition to Na^+ and Cl^-. Patients with inhalation injury require a larger volume of fluids than those without it, and thus are prone to edema formation with isotonic solutions.[224] Hypertonic salt solutions draw intracellular water into the bloodstream and thus decrease the fluid volume needed to maintain perfusion. Patients with burns occupying >50% of the TBSA, circumferential extremity burns, or inhalational injury may benefit from these solutions, which both maintain extracellular volume and limit the severity of edema.[206] Unfortunately, hypertonic solutions cause hypernatremia and intracellular water depletion; patients receiving these fluids for burn therapy had an unacceptably high incidence of renal failure and death compared with those receiving LR.[225]

Various burn centers have developed guidelines for fluid resuscitation[216] (Table 48-11). Of these, the Evans and Brooke formulas suggest the combined use of colloid, crystalloid, and 5% dextrose solutions. However, the early glucose intolerance seen in burn patients, especially in children, should probably preclude sugar-containing fluids in the first 24 hours after injury. These formulas are guidelines only, and none can be expected to provide adequate restoration of intravascular volume in all burn victims, especially small children and patients with inhalation injuries.[216] Therefore, administration of fluids during the initial phase should be titrated to specific goals such as a urine output of approximately $0.5 \text{ ml} \cdot kg^{-1} \text{ hr}^{-1}$; a heart rate of 110–120 beats min^{-1}; a minimal base deficit; a normal blood lactate level; and, if a pulmonary artery catheter is placed, acceptable filling pressures and a mixed venous oxygen tension ($P\bar{v}o_2$) of 35–40 mm Hg. Careful monitoring of the hematocrit may also guide fluid management. An increase in hematocrit during the first day suggests inadequate fluid resuscitation because hemolysis and sequestration are actually expected to cause a decrease in this parameter. Acute anemia, as may occur during excision and grafting of burns, is usually well tolerated. Blood replacement is usually not initiated until the hematocrit is below 15–20% in healthy patients requiring limited operations, approximately 25% in those who are healthy but need extensive procedures, and 30% or more when there is a history of preexisting cardiovascular disease.[226]

Pulmonary artery catheters should not be used indiscriminately because they are associated with a high rate of complications, including septic emboli, in these patients.[216] On the other hand, in severe burns urine output and vital signs alone may not provide reliable information about the hemodynamic status of the patient.[227,228] In major burns, invasive central monitoring

Table 48-11. INITIAL FLUID RESUSCITATION AFTER THERMAL INJURY

EVANS FORMULA*

1.0 ml crystalloid/kg/% burn/24 hr
1.0 ml colloid/kg/% burn/24 hr
2000 ml 5% dextrose in water/24 hr

BROOKE FORMULA*

1.5 ml crystalloid/kg/% burn/24 hr
0.5 ml colloid/kg/% burn/24 hr
2000 ml 5% dextrose in water/24 hr

MODIFIED BROOKE FORMULA*

2.0 ml lactated Ringer's/kg/% burn/24 hr

PARKLAND FORMULA*

4.0 ml crystalloid/kg/% burn/24 hr

HYPERTONIC LACTATED SALINE†

Volume adjusted to promote a urine flow of 30 ml · hr^{-1} with a solution containing 300 mEq · l^{-1} sodium, 200 m Eq · l^{-1} lactate, and 100 mEq · l^{-1} chloride (usually amounts to 2 ml · kg^{-1}/% burn/24 hr)

DEXTRAN-CRYSTALLOID-PROTEIN‡

Dextran 40 or dextran 70 ≥ 2 ml · kg^{-1}/hr^{-1} to maintain plasma dextran levels at or in excess of 2 g · dl^{-1} and crystalloid as needed (1.0 ml · kg^{-1}/% burn/8 hr) during the first 8 hr after injury (followed by plasma protein 0.5–1.0 ml · kg^{-1}/% burn/16 hr with necessary additional crystalloid infusion).

---

* Fifty percent of calculated volume is given during the first 8 hr, 25% is given during the second 8 hr, and the remaining 25% is given during the third 8 hr.
† Hypertonic saline is usually administered during the first 8 hr. Elevation of serum Na$^+$ concentration above 160 mEq · l^{-1} dictates replacement of hypertonic solution with isotonic saline or lactated Ringer's.
‡ Used in patients admitted in shock to restore adequate volume and perfusion rapidly.
Reprinted with permission from Welch GW: Care of the patient with thermal injury. In Capan LM, Miller SM, Turndorf H (eds): Trauma Anesthesia and Intensive Care, p 632. Philadelphia, JB Lippincott, 1991.

and inotropic agents are often indicated. Rarely, initial fluid resuscitation may fail in patients with large, deep burns, inhalational injury, or pre-existing disease, and those at the extremes of age. Plasma exchange may be useful in these patients.[206]

OPERATIVE MANAGEMENT

Pre-existing Diseases

Pre-existing medical conditions have an overall prevalence of at least 19% in the population of trauma patients, increasing to >30% in those older than 55 years of age.[229] Coexisting cirrhosis, cardiovascular, pulmonary, and renal diseases, coagulation disorders, and diabetes increase trauma-related morbidity and mortality.[229] Alcohol intoxication or substance abuse is very common in injured patients, especially in those sustaining intentional injury. Surveys have shown that nearly 50% of trauma patients test positive for alcohol or drugs.[230,231] Table 48-12 summarizes the clinical implications and management of some of these conditions in trauma patients.[232]

Premedication

Premedication is not indicated in most trauma patients, particularly those who are hypovolemic, head injured, or intoxicated. If deemed necessary, it can be given intravenously to patients with adequate circulating volume and unimpaired mental sta-

tus. Small doses of opioid (morphine, 1–2 mg; fentanyl, 25–50 μg) or sedative (diazepam, 2.5 mg; midazolam, 0.5–1 mg) are administered with close monitoring of vital signs, and repeated as required to obtain the desired degree of analgesia and sedation. Regional techniques may also provide analgesia for some patients with skeletal injuries awaiting surgery. Femoral nerve block, for example, provides excellent analgesia for fractures of the femur.

Preinduction Phase

The operating room must be ready to receive critically injured patients on a moment's notice. This requires not only advance preparation of anesthetic equipment, supplies, and drugs but rapid coordination of adequate help from other departments such as nursing, blood bank, radiology, and the laboratory. All equipment necessary for anesthetic management of the trauma patient must be prepared in advance; consideration should be given to timely provision of those items that are essential but not routinely used (Table 48-13). Stocking and periodic checking of a dedicated "trauma anesthesia cart" are essential. In addition, availability of sophisticated equipment such as TEE, a rapid infusion system, and an autotransfusion (cell saver) device is highly desirable.

Transport of the trauma victim to the operating room should take place with close monitoring of blood pressure, heart rate, O$_2$ saturation, and, in intubated patients, end-expired CO$_2$. In intubated patients, correct position and patency of the endotracheal tube must be confirmed, and oxygen must be administered to all patients immediately on arrival in the operating room. Severe hypoxemia is likely to develop in the operating room after chest trauma despite acceptable blood gases in the emergency department. This may be secondary to progressive inflammatory response to injury with pulmonary contusion and aspiration pneumonitis, development of heart failure and pulmonary edema, respiratory insufficiency or failure in those with rib fractures, or lung collapse in patients with diaphragmatic rupture and hernia, hemothorax, or pneumothorax. Auscultation of breath sounds, examination of the chest film, and measurement of ABGs provide a baseline with which subsequent intraoperative changes can be compared. Rapid clinical determination of the patient's fluid volume status is difficult. Gross estimation of intravascular volume can be made by observing blood pressure, pulse rate, external bleeding, chest tube drainage, and the rate and amount of fluid infusion. Performance of a "tilt test" for orthostatic hypotension[232] is unreliable and delays necessary management of the patient.[233]

Continued assessment of the patient for missed injuries is important before and during surgery. Information is obtained from the surgeon, evaluation of the patient, and review of radiographs and laboratory results. Injuries that if missed in initial evaluation can lead to major perioperative complications include those of the head and cervical spine, eye, airway, diaphragm, liver, and spleen, and conditions such as hemothorax, pneumothorax, pulmonary and cardiac contusion, hemopericardium, and injury to major thoracic and abdominal vessels. In addition, if time permits, appropriate resuscitative measures should be ensured before induction. The anesthesiologist should check venous lines for proper and unimpeded flow, monitor arterial pressure and CVP and waveforms on the oscilloscope, observe the amount and color of the urine, and monitor the ECG for heart rate, dysrhythmias, and ST segment and T-wave abnormalities. In patients presenting with impalement injuries, the impaling object, which may have injured a large internal vessel, should not be manipulated until the patient is anesthetized, and then only by the surgeon.

Monitoring

Table 48-14 lists monitoring techniques currently used in the operating room and indicates their relative importance in the

Table 48-12. IMPLICATIONS OF PRE-EXISTING CONDITIONS FOR INTRAOPERATIVE MANAGEMENT OF THE TRAUMA PATIENT

Pre-existing Condition	Implications	Management
Substance Abuse		
Alcohol	Decreased gastric motility increasing the risk of vomiting, regurgitation, and aspiration during airway management	Rapid control of the airway
	Alcohol-induced vasodilation, myocardial depression, and diuresis enhancing the severity of hypotension	Careful titration of anesthetics; use of vasopressors and inotropes if necessary
	Dysrhythmias and enhancement of cardiac, brain, and probably other organ damage in acute alcohol intoxication; underlying cardiomyopathy in chronic alcoholics	Use of antiarrhythmics and inotropes
	Potentiation of trauma induced hypothermia by alcohol-induced skin vasodilation	Use of forced-air warming (Bair Hugger), warm inspired gases, warm intravenous fluids
	Hemostatic defects in chronic alcoholics with liver disease complicating trauma and massive transfusion-induced coagulopathy	Consideration of FFP and/or DDAVP
	Difficulty in differentiating trauma-induced metabolic acidosis from alcoholic ketoacidosis and lactic acidosis	Interpretation of hemodynamic data, plasma lactate, urinary ketone levels, and blood sugar
	Alteration in drug pharmacokinetics due to increased volume of distribution, decreased plasma albumin concentration, increased globulin fraction, and decreased pseudocholinesterase	
	Postoperative alcohol withdrawal (within 6 to 8 hr)	Use of benzodiazepines, thiamine, and multivitamins
Cocaine	Unpredictable hemodynamic response to hemorrhage, resuscitation, and anesthetics	Use of sympathetic blockers to treat hypertension and tachycardia caused by cocaine can lead to severe hypotension in hypovolemic patients
	Occasional sudden arrhythmias or unexplained cardiac decompensation	Use of direct-acting vasopressors in chronic cocaine users; careful titration of these agents in acute cocaine use; reduction of epinephrine dose
Opioids	Delayed gastric emptying	Rapid airway control
	Peripheral vasodilation potentially causing profound hypotension and hypothermia	Careful monitoring, prevention, and treatment of hypothermia
	Difficulty in placing intravenous lines	
	Consequences of the adverse effects of diluting agents (talc, quinine, or starch)	
	Conduction delays, dysrhythmias, hypotension from quinine	
	Enhancement of the pulmonary insult from hypovolemic shock	
	Unexplained hypotension, tachycardia, increased airway pressure, and pulmonary edema intraoperatively from opiate withdrawal	Administration of opioids
	Opiate withdrawal symptoms	
Hypertension	Decreased tolerance to hypovolemia	Maintenance of normal BP using appropriate monitoring, adequate volume loading, and vosoactive drugs (esmolol, nitroglycerin, nitroprusside, dobutamine)
	Exaggerated hypertensive response to pain	
	Increased likelihood of myocardial ischemia and dysrhythmias	
Ischemic heart disease	Increased likelihood of myocardial ischemia due to trauma induced hypovolemia:	Maintenance of hematocrit between 25 and 35%
	Increased myocardial O_2 demand	Maintenance of adequate diastolic BP
	Elevated systemic vascular resistance and heart rate	Avoidance of hypoxia, hypertension, and tachycardia
	Decreased left ventricular filling pressure	Routine monitoring of SpO_2, $ETCO_2$, electrocardiogram (lead II and V_5), arterial line, and possibly central venous pressure
Anemia	Difficulty in diagnosis of chronic anemia in acute trauma	History of disease or treatment that may cause anemia
	Decreased tissue O_2 delivery in shock when compensatory physiologic changes would maintain tissue oxygenation in normal patients	Close hemodynamic and oxygen monitoring
Sickle cell disease	Sickle cell trait is asymptomatic, but in extreme hypoxia and acidosis it can cause sickling	Avoid triggering factors such as hypoxia, hypothermia, and acidosis
Coagulation disorders	Hemophilia A and von Willibrand's disease are the most likely coagulation disorders	
	Marginally adequate levels of hemostatic factors (factor VIII:c or VIII:von Willebrand's factor) may be diluted with fluid resuscitation	Bleeding into body regions where there is no evidence of significant injury or more hemorrhage than expected in injured areas may suggest diathesis
		Consultation should be obtained from the hematology service if time permits
		Factor VIII concentrate for hemophilia if available; cryoprecipitate and DDAVP (0.4 $\mu g \cdot kg^{-1}$) for von Willebrand's disease and hemophilia A (if factor VIII concentrate is not available).
		FFP may be used, but large volumes are needed

(continued)

Table 48-12. IMPLICATIONS OF PRE-EXISTING CONDITIONS FOR INTRAOPERATIVE MANAGEMENT OF THE TRAUMA PATIENT (continued)

Pre-existing Condition	Implications	Management
Diabetes mellitus	Delay in gastric emptying	Airway control may be difficult because of obesity and decreased motility of atlanto-occiptal and temporomandibular joints
	Decreased response to resuscitative measures in patients with autonomic neuropathy	
	Increased likelihood of coronary artery disease, possibly increasing mortality from trauma	Treatment of hyperglycemia (serum glucose >250 mg·dl^{-1}) with regular insulin (5–10-unit bolus followed by 1–10 unit·hr^{-1} infusion)
	Augmentation of trauma-induced hyperglycemia; may be detrimental in patients with head injury or hypovolemia (diuresis)	Measurement of filling pressures, lactate level, urinary ketone bodies, and serum glucose
	Difficulty in differentiating the cause of metabolic acidosis in trauma patients	Monitoring of plasma electrolytes and treatment of hypopotassemia and hypophosphatemia
	Electrolyte abnormalities	
Asthma	Trauma-induced events such as pain, anxiety, smoke inhalation, burns, stress, and pulmonary contusion can induce an asthma attack, although catecholamine surge from trauma may counteract bronchospasm	Preanesthetic administration of bronchodilator (β_2 agonist) and anti-inflammatory agent (inhaled steroids)
		Avoidance of anesthetic and adjunct drugs that have the potential to release histamine
		Airway manipulation only after adequate general or topical anesthesia; consideration of induction with ketamine

FFP = fresh frozen plasma; DDAVP = desmopressin; BP = blood pressure.

Table 48-13. EQUIPMENT, SUPPLIES, AND DRUGS THAT MAY BE NEEDED IN ADDITION TO THOSE USED FOR ROUTINE ANESTHETIC CARE DURING INTRAOPERATIVE MANAGEMENT OF TRAUMA

EQUIPMENT
Fiberoptic bronchoscope with light source
Critical care ventilator*
Jet ventilator system
Positive end-expiratory pressure valves
Blood and fluid bag pressurizing devices
Level 1 countercurrent fluid infusion and warming system
Rapid infusion system (Haemonetics)
Autotransfusion device
Forced dry air warming device (Bair Hugger)
Heated humidifier to warm inspired gases
Calibrated infusion pumps
Transesophageal or transthoracic echocardiograph
Pneumatic tourniquet
Cardiopulmonary bypass pump†
Defibrillator

SUPPLIES
Equipment for special airway management (jet ventilation, retrograde intubation, cricothyroidotomy, tracheostomy, lung isolation)
Equipment for placement of arterial and pulmonary artery lines

DRUGS
Vasopressors and inotropes (ephedrine, phenylephrine, dopamine, dobutamine, amrinone, milrinone, epinephrine)
Calcium chloride or gluconate
THAM (possibly sodium bicarbonate)
Topical anesthetics

THAM = tris(hydroxymethyl)aminomethane.
* For ventilation of patients with severely decreased lung compliance (e.g., pulmonary contusion, aspiration).
† For management of patients with penetrating cardiac injury involving a major coronary artery.

intraoperative care of the trauma patient.[234] Clearly, valuable time can be lost if the placement of invasive monitors takes precedence over resuscitation.

Hemodynamic Monitoring

There is no effective substitute for direct intra-arterial pressure monitoring, which permits beat-to-beat data acquisition and sampling for measurement of blood gases. Every effort must be made to place this line before surgery, even if it requires surgical cut-down. A relatively stable patient may rapidly become unstable when the abdomen or chest is opened. The radial artery is most commonly used because it is accessible, easy to cannulate, and relatively free from serious complications. It is the artery of choice in abdominal or chest trauma in which the aorta may be cross-clamped, making a femoral or dorsalis pedis cannula nonfunctional. The right radial artery is preferred in cases of chest trauma in which cross-clamping of the descending aorta might result in occlusion of the left subclavian artery. In mechanically ventilated patients, the magnitude of systolic pressure variation (the difference between the maximum and minimum systolic pressure over the respiratory cycle) and its Δdown component (the difference between systolic pressure at end-expiration and the lowest value during the respiratory cycle) can provide reliable information about the intravascular volume status (Fig. 48-7). A systolic pressure variation >5 mm Hg and a Δdown >2 mm Hg suggest hypovolemia.[235] Most trauma patients are young, with a healthy heart. Consequently, delaying emergent surgery to place a central venous line is rarely indicated unless a large-bore catheter is needed for volume resuscitation. Reasonable assessment of the patient's volume status can be made by repeated observation of blood pressure, urine output, hematocrit, and ABG. However, if the patient is elderly, there is a likelihood of myocardial damage, or there is multiple organ damage with requirement for prolonged surgery and massive fluid replacement, early placement of a CVP or pulmonary artery catheter is indicated before the development of coagulopathy renders it hazardous.

Both CVP and PCWP assess preload indirectly from pressure measurements that are subject to error in the presence of altered ventricular compliance or, in the case of PCWP, significant pulmonary abnormality such as contusion. Volumetric assess-

Table 48-14. TECHNIQUES TO MONITOR PHYSIOLOGIC PARAMETERS AND THEIR IMPORTANCE IN INTRAOPERATIVE MANAGEMENT OF THE TRAUMA PATIENT

Physiological Parameter	Degree of Importance	Monitoring Equipment	Specific Intraoperative Uses in the Trauma Patient
Cardiac rate, rhythm, and myocardial ischemia	Essential	Five-lead electrocardiograph system with oscilloscope, digital display, recorder, and printer (three-lead system can be used)	Routine
Arterial blood pressure	Essential	Indirect Blood pressure cuff Doppler system Programmable oscillometric system Direct Pressure transducer with calibrated oscilloscope and recorder	Routine
Central venous pressure	Useful	Pressure transducer with calibrated oscilloscope and recorder	Hypovolemia Pericardial tamponade, myocardial contusion Air embolism Pulmonary contusion
Pulmonary artery pressures	Essential in multiple trauma	Pressure transducer with calibrated oscilloscope and recorder	Blunt chest injury (pericardial tamponade, myocardial contusion) Adult respiratory distress syndrome Differentiation of low- and high-pressure pulmonary edema Traumatic (cardiac contusion) or pre-existing heart failure
Cardiac output	Useful in some patients	Thermodilution cardiac output computer with recorder and printer	Same as pulmonary artery pressure measurement
Cardiac wall motion abnormalities, myocardial ischemia, flow through valves or septal defects	Useful in some patients	Transesophageal echocardiograph	Cardic contusion Coronary artery injuries? Septal injuries Air embolism Thoracic aortic rupture Shock
Ventilation	Essential	End-tidal CO_2 monitor with waveform display and recording	Routine Head injury Air embolism
Arterial oxygenation	Essential	Airway pressure Pulse oximeter Arterial blood gases (intermittent or continuous)	Routine
Tissue oxygenation	Useful	Pulmonary artery catheter ($P\overline{v}O_2$ Arterial/venous lactate analyzer Base deficit	Low perfusion states
Renal function	Essential	Foley catheter and graduated container	In all major trauma patients
Temperature	Essential	Esophageal or rectal probe	Routine
Neuromuscular function	Essential	Peripheral nerve stimulator Electromyograph	Head injury Open globe Sealed major vessel injury
Neurologic function	Useful	Intracranial pressure measurement with bolt, catheter, or fiberoptic sensor Jugular bulb O_2 saturation Bispectral Index (BIS) monitor	Head injury Intraoperative awareness
Blood coagulation	Useful	Prothrombin time/partial thromboplastin time/platelet count/fibrinogen, tube test, thrombelastograph	Shock Massive transfusion Pre-existing coagulation abnormalities

Modified by permission from Capan LM, Gottlieb G, Rosenberg A: General principles of anesthesia for major acute trauma. In Capan LM, Miller SM, Turndorf H (eds): Trauma Anesthesia and Intensive Care, p 259. Philadelphia, JB Lippincott, 1991.

ment of preload appears to correlate better with cardiac index than the CVP or PCWP.[236,237] A pulmonary artery catheter equipped with a rapid-response thermistor and intracardiac electrodes is capable of measuring RV cardiac output and ejection fraction, and calculating RV end-diastolic volume index. The latter appears to correlate with cardiac output better than CVP and PCWP in trauma patients. An RV end-diastolic volume index >130 ml·m^{-2} is considered optimal for organ perfusion.[236,237]

Transesophageal echocardiography provides valuable diagnostic information in myocardial contusion, cardiac septal or valvular damage, coronary artery injury, pericardial tamponade, and aortic rupture.[184] Intraoperative TEE can permit assessment of cardiac function, including right and left ventricular volume, ejection fraction, wall motion abnormalities, pulmonary hypertension, and cardiac output, and detects acute ischemia more accurately than either ECG or pulmonary artery pressure monitoring.[238] Monitoring left ventricular volume alone can provide

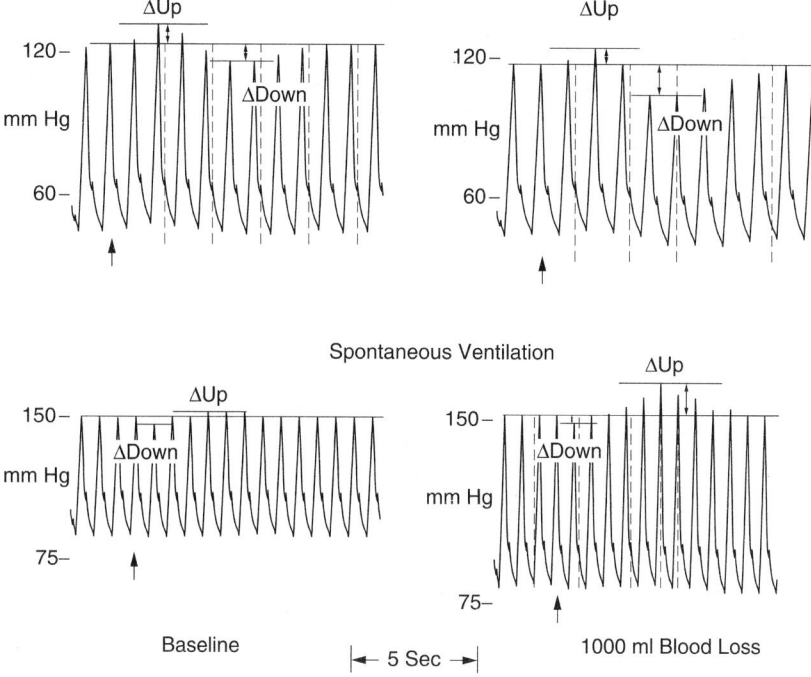

Figure 48-7. Arterial pressure records of a mechanically ventilated patient before (*left*) and after (*right*) 1000 ml blood loss. Note the increase in systolic pressure variation and Δdown component following blood loss. Decrease in blood pressure occurs during exhalation with mechanical ventilation, and inspiration in spontaneously breathing subjects (*upgoing arrow* defines inhalation). ΔUp is the difference between the end-expiratory systolic pressure and the maximum systolic pressure over a respiratory cycle. See text for definition of systolic pressure variation and Δdown component. (Reprinted with permission from Rooke GA, Schwid HA, Shapira Y: The effect of graded hemorrhage and intravascular volume replacement on systolic pressure variation in humans during mechanical and spontaneous ventilation. Anesth Analg 80:925, 1995.)

information about the adequacy of the intravascular volume. This technique also allows visualization of fat and air entry into the right heart, or the left heart through a patent foramen ovale, during internal fixation of lower extremity fractures.[239] The complication rate from insertion of TEE probe is small (0.18%); esophageal perforation and bleeding from esophageal varices are the most frequent problems.[240] In the trauma setting, it is possible that the TEE probe may be introduced into an unrecognized esophageal tear because the insidious nature of esophageal injury makes diagnosis difficult during the first 24 hours after trauma.

In most hypovolemic trauma patients, almost all available methods of determining cardiac preload correlate poorly with circulating blood volume.[241] Preload remains stable up to a critical level of volume reduction because of a compensatory increase in sympathetic tone. Therefore, a direct measurement of circulating blood volume may be advantageous in this setting. Japanese investigators using a pulsed dye densitometer, a technique that relies on indocyanine green distribution and elimination, were able to measure blood volume at 20-minute intervals.[242]

Urine Output

Urine output is routinely monitored as an indicator of organ perfusion, hemolysis, skeletal muscle destruction, and urinary tract integrity after trauma. As a rough guideline, urine output should be maintained at $>0.5 \ \text{ml} \cdot \text{kg}^{-1} \cdot \text{hr}^{-1}$. Caution should be exercised in interpretation of urine output as an indicator of intravascular volume and kidney perfusion. After prolonged shock, renal failure (low or high output) may already be present at the time of the patient's arrival in the operating room. Osmotic diuresis produced by preoperative radiopaque dye or mannitol also reduces the reliability of urine output as an index of renal perfusion. Dark, cola-colored urine in the trauma patient suggests either hemoglobinuria resulting from incompatible blood transfusion, or myoglobinuria caused by massive skeletal muscle destruction after blunt or electrical trauma. Rapid differential diagnosis can be made by centrifugation of a blood specimen. Pink-stained serum suggests hemoglobinuria, whereas unstained serum indicates myoglobinuria. Both of these conditions may result in acute renal failure. Prevention involves mannitol diuresis and, in myoglobinuria, alkalinization of the urine with sodium bicarbonate to pH levels above 5.6. Red-colored urine usually is caused by hematuria, which, in the traumatized patient, suggests urinary tract injury. It should be investigated with iv pyelography, if possible. Intravenous injection of methylene blue (5–10 ml) or indigo carmine may be useful in helping the surgeon to locate the site of urinary tract injury during laparotomy.

Organ Perfusion and Oxygen Utilization

Mention has already been made about the importance of occult hypoperfusion that may not be detected by traditional hemodynamic monitoring such as blood pressure, heart rate, and urine output.[84,85] Unrecognized or untreated, this condition may lead to organ failure and death. The intestinal mucosa lacks autoregulatory control in splanchnic ischemia and is particularly vulnerable to occult hypoperfusion. Ischemia and resulting acidosis in the intestinal wall then permits the passage of luminal microorganisms into the circulation and release of inflammatory mediators, causing sepsis and multiorgan failure.[84] Thus, efforts have been made to find a monitoring technique that can promptly and reliably detect organ hypoperfusion in the *apparently* resuscitated patient and set the optimal end points of resuscitation.

Oxygen transport variables, blood lactate level, base deficit, and gastric intramucosal pH (pHi) are considered as acceptable markers of organ perfusion and O_2 utilization.[85] Currently, only the blood lactate level and base deficit and, in some instances, O_2 transport variables are used during surgery. However, with improved technology, alimentary tract pHi or Pco_2 may also be used in this setting.

Oxygen delivery ($\dot{D}o_2$), O_2 consumption ($\dot{V}o_2$), and O_2 extraction ratio are the three monitored O_2 transport variables:

$$\dot{D}o_2 = \text{Cardiac output (Qt)} \cdot Cao_2$$
$$\dot{V}o_2 = Qt \cdot (Cao_2 - Cvo_2)$$
$$O_2 \text{ extraction ratio} = \dot{V}o_2 / \dot{D}o_2$$

Shock induces an oxygen debt, which is defined as the amount of O_2 that cells are deprived of as a result of the imbalance between $\dot{D}o_2$ and $\dot{V}o_2$. Correction of this debt is one of the end points of resuscitation. Achieving supernormal values of cardiac index ($4.5 \ l \cdot min^{-1} \cdot m^{-2}$), $\dot{D}o_2$ index ($600 \ ml \cdot min^{-1} \cdot m^{-2}$), and $\dot{V}o_2$ index ($170 \ ml \cdot min^{-1} \cdot m^{-2}$) by fluid infusion and inotropes is a possible way to repay this debt and salvage tissues.[85] Although some clinicians believe in this concept, others have found that this approach actually may increase mortality.[85] Resuscitation with fluids and inotropes in patients who cannot increase their $\dot{V}o_2$ because of the damage sustained from shock may be deleterious. Nevertheless, monitoring these parameters with a pulmonary artery catheter may provide useful information.

Determination of plasma lactate is a more direct way to evaluate hypoperfusion-induced metabolic dysfunction. Normal plasma lactate concentration is $0.5-1.5 \ mmol \cdot l^{-1}$; higher levels, especially above $5 \ mmol \cdot l^{-1}$, suggest lactic acidosis.[243] Because the half-life of lactic acid is approximately 3 hours, improvement in blood lactate levels occurs rather gradually after the cause of the problem is corrected.[243] Failure to clear lactate within 24 to 48 hours after hypovolemic shock is a predictor of increased mortality.[244]

The base deficit, which is the amount of base required to titrate 1 liter of whole blood to a normal pH at normal Pao_2, $Paco_2$, and temperature, has been shown to be a good indicator of metabolic dysfunction during hypovolemic shock.[245] Base deficit reliably reflects the severity of shock, oxygen debt, changes in oxygen delivery, the adequacy of fluid resuscitation, and the likelihood of survival.[246,247] A base deficit between 2 and $5 \ mmol \cdot l^{-1}$ suggests mild hypovolemia, $6-14 \ mmol \cdot l^{-1}$ indicates moderate hypovolemia, and $>14 \ mmol \cdot l^{-1}$ is a sign of severe hypovolemia. Normalization of the base deficit is usually considered the end point of resuscitation.

Carbon dioxide accumulates in gastric mucosal cells as a result of ischemia. pHi is calculated from intracellular CO_2, which diffuses freely across the gastric mucosa and equilibrates with saline contained in a silicone balloon attached to the distal end of a nasogastric tube.[248] It takes 30–60 minutes for gastric luminal CO_2 to equilibrate, after which the saline is recovered and its Pco_2 measured. After applying a correction factor for gastric luminal Pco_2, pHi is calculated using the Hasselbach-Henderson equation. Patients are given histamine (H_2) blockers to prevent errors caused by gastric acid. The normal Pco_2 value is approximately 50 mm Hg and the lower limit for pHi is 7.33, approximately 0.06 lower than the blood pH.[248] An intramucosal pH of <7.32 is considered a sign of splanchnic ischemia. A pHi of <7.25 and a gradient between mucosal and arterial Pco_2 >18 mm Hg is predictive of multiple organ failure and death,[248] as is a delay in normalization of pHi of >24 hours.[85] Resuscitation is therefore aimed at obtaining a $pHi >7.32$. Obviously, this technique is cumbersome and cannot be used in the operating room. A recently designed fiberoptic Pco_2 probe obviates this problem and measures luminal Pco_2 directly.[249] It can easily be introduced into the stomach through a standard nasogastric tube. It has significant advantages over tonometry: it is continuous, easy to use, and noninvasive, and provides real-time data. A more promising variant of this technology, sublingual capnometry, has been introduced by Weil et al.[250] A CO_2 sensor is applied sublingually and mucosal Pco_2 is measured directly. The normal value for sublingual Pco_2 is approximately 45–50 mm Hg. They noted a significant elevation (81 ± 24 mm Hg) in patients with circulatory shock and a blood lactate level >2.5. Patients who were not in circulatory shock had values of 53 ± 8 mm Hg. Values over 70 mm Hg correlated with shock, and those under 70 mm Hg were predictive of survival. Combined measurement of O_2 transport variables, base deficit, lactate, and pHi or intramucosal Pco_2 is likely to be a more accurate indicator of the patient's condition than any of these values alone.

Coagulation

Conventional blood coagulation monitoring includes a baseline and subsequent serial measurements of prothrombin time (PT),

activated partial thromboplastin time (aPTT), platelet count, blood fibrinogen level, and fibrin degradation products (FDP). Although not always possible, a trauma center laboratory should provide results of the standard coagulation tests in <1 hour. A blood sample should be sent to the laboratory to determine, at least retrospectively, the etiology of any coagulation abnormality. The "tube test," which involves obtaining a tube of blood with no anticoagulant and observing coagulation, clot retraction, and clot lysis, is a practical intraoperative method of coagulation monitoring. If a good-quality clot does not form, or does so only after 10–20 minutes, clotting factor deficiency is the most likely cause. Failure of clot retraction within 1 hour after blood sampling suggests platelet depletion or dysfunction. Clot lysis earlier than 6 hours indicates fibrinolysis, which is infrequent in trauma patients.[251] However, disseminated intravascular coagulation (DIC) occurs frequently after trauma and is associated with absence of spontaneous clotting in the tube test. In addition to causing bleeding, it may prevent typing and cross-matching of blood.[252]

Thromboelastography (TEG) is similar in principle to the tube test but provides a quantitative, graphic evaluation of clotting function.[253] TEG determines the time necessary for initial fibrin formation, the rapidity of fibrin deposition, clot consistency, the rate of clot formation, and the times required for clot retraction and lysis[253] (Fig. 48-8). Basically, the R and K values are indices of formation, buildup, and cross-linking of fibrin and depend on the function of coagulation factors. The maximum amplitude (MA) corresponds to the widest portion of the curve and indicates the absolute strength of the fibrin clot. It represents the function of platelets. The α angle is the slope of the external divergence of the tracing from the R value point, indicating the speed of clot formation and fibrin cross-linking. The value of this index is determined by both coagulation factors and platelets. Hypothermia causes coagulopathy by interfering with both platelet and coagulation factor functions.[254–256] When the blood of a cold and coagulopathic patient is placed in the TEG cuvette, which is normally heated to 37°C, a near-normal trace may be obtained.[256] Newer TEG devices are temperature adjustable; thus, the temperature in the cuvette can be adjusted to that of the patient.

Coagulation test (PT, aPTT) results are often abnormal in major trauma patients. However, these findings do not necessarily indicate that factor and platelet therapy should be initiated, unless there is a clinical indication to do so.[257] The administration of FFP is generally recommended when PT and aPTT

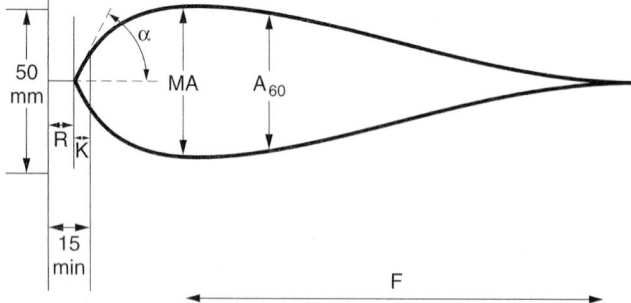

Figure 48-8. Thrombolastogram. R = time interval from blood deposition in the cuvette to an amplitude of 1 mm on the thromboelastogram; K = time interval between the end of R and a point with an amplitude of 20 mm on the thromboelastogram; MA = maximum amplitude of thromboelastogram; α angle = slope of the external divergence of the tracing from the R value point; A_{60} = amplitude of thromboelastogram 60 minutes after maximum amplitude; F = time from MA to return to 0 amplitude (normal >300 minutes). (Reprinted with permission from Capan LM, Gottlieb G, Rosenberg A: General principles of anesthesia for major acute trauma. In Capan LM, Miller SM, Turndorf H [eds]: Trauma: Anesthesia and Intensive Care, p 259. Philadelphia, JB Lippincott, 1991.)

exceed 1.5 times control,[258] but treatment is based primarily on clinical bleeding (oozing from puncture sites and wound), the amount of blood lost, and the quantity transfused. The likelihood of bleeding, for example, after one blood volume is replaced, increases to 60%, so that platelet and factor replacement becomes almost unavoidable once replacement exceeds this volume.[259,260] The results of coagulation tests have little primary impact on treatment. Nevertheless, they should be performed to determine the direction and extent of coagulation dysfunction over time.

Anesthetic and Adjunct Drugs

Apart from regional anesthesia techniques, which are used in patients with minor extremity injuries and stable hemodynamics, anesthetic and adjunct drugs for general anesthesia need to be tailored to five major clinical conditions. The varying contribution of these conditions to the clinical picture of a given patient necessitates priority-oriented planning.

Airway Compromise

The primary issue in these patients is whether to manage the airway with or without the use of anesthetics and muscle relaxants. The principles are discussed in the section on initial management. In general, these agents should be avoided if there is significant airway obstruction or if there is doubt as to whether the patient's trachea can be intubated because of anatomic limitations. If time permits, lateral neck radiographs, CT scanning, and endoscopy can be used to define the problem better. Topical anesthesia with mild sedation can be used with or without a flexible fiberoptic scope, Bullard blade, WuScope, or other aids, and with surgical standby for cricothyroidotomy should intubation attempts be unsuccessful.[57]

Hypovolemia

Hypovolemic patients are sensitive to the cardiovascular depressant action of iv and inhalational anesthetics. These not only have direct effects, but they inhibit hemodynamic compensatory mechanisms such as central catecholamine output and baroreflex (neuroregulatory) mechanisms, which maintain systemic pressure in hypovolemia. Among iv agents, etomidate has the least[261] and thiopental, propofol, and midazolam the greatest direct cardiovascular depressant activity;[262,263] ketamine has stimulatory effects when the autonomic nervous system is intact.[264] Among the inhalational agents, isoflurane depresses the myocardium least but it produces a decrease in mean arterial pressure comparable with that of halothane and enflurane, and offers no distinct advantage over the other agents.[265] Nitrous oxide has a direct depressant action on the myocardium, but *in vivo* it increases sympathetic activity, resulting in a negligible overall change in systemic blood pressure.[266]

There are also differences among anesthetics in the direction and extent of their effects on compensatory mechanisms. For example, the baroreceptor depression produced by iv agents is usually milder than that of inhalational agents. Data from animal and human studies have demonstrated that thiopental, propofol, and ketamine depress the baroreflex mechanism most and for approximately 10 minutes, whereas etomidate has little effect; the effects of midazolam, diazepam, and droperidol are intermediate.[267-269] Among inhalational agents, isoflurane has less of an inhibitory effect on the baroreflex mechanism than halothane or enflurane.[270] Opioid agents have little direct cardiovascular or baroreflex depressant effect. However, these agents can cause hypotension by inhibiting central sympathetic activity, especially in the hypovolemic trauma patient whose apparent hemodynamic stability is maintained by hyperactive sympathetic tone.[271] In addition, experimental data suggest a significant alteration in fentanyl pharmacokinetics, resulting in elevated plasma concentrations due to decreased volume of distribution and clearance.[272]

Two important principles in the use of anesthetic agents are accurate estimation of the degree of hypovolemia and reduction of the dose accordingly. The presence of hypotension suggests uncompensated hypovolemia, in which case anesthetics almost invariably produce further deterioration of systemic blood pressure and sometimes cardiac standstill. Intravascular volume, to the extent possible, must be restored before their use. When time constraints or continuing hemorrhage prevent restoration of blood volume, the airway must be secured without the benefit of anesthesia (perhaps using only rapidly acting muscle relaxants and very small doses of opioids, etomidate, or ketamine), even though this approach may result in recall of induction and intraoperative events. In a study by Bogetz and Katz,[273] only 11% of patients to whom ketamine and low-dose inhalational anesthetics were administered had recall. When hypovolemia precluded the use of anesthesia for 20 minutes, the incidence of recall increased to 43%. Studies of memory performance during general anesthesia in acute trauma patients with varying injury severity indicated that hypnotic depth plays an important role in reducing the occurrence of memory.[274] The memory detected in these patients is implicit rather than explicit, and is not associated with postoperative recall. Use of the Bispectral Index (BIS) monitor in these patients showed that significant implicit memory persisted even at BIS values between 40 and 60, which correspond to an acceptable level of surgical anesthesia.[274] Nevertheless, these patients did not recall auditory events after surgery. It is possible they would have had recall if anesthetics were titrated to higher BIS values. Although as yet unproved, intraoperative use of the BIS monitor and, whenever possible, titrating anesthetics to levels <60 may prevent recall in trauma patients. Hypothermia, alcohol intoxication, drug use before anesthesia, and metabolic disturbances in the acute trauma patient cannot reliably prevent recall. Scopolamine, 0.6 mg, given before airway management may decrease the likelihood of this complication, however.

Hypotension is also likely after administration of anesthesia in normotensive but hypovolemic patients. In these patients, restoration of volume as well as selection of an agent with the least cardiovascular depressant effect appears logical. Ketamine, because of its stimulatory action on the circulation,[264] and etomidate, because of its lack of histamine release and relatively mild cardiovascular depressant effect, are the preferred induction agents.[262,267,269,275] At low doses, however, other iv anesthetics are also unlikely to produce hypotension. Therefore, although ketamine and etomidate confer some hemodynamic advantages over other iv agents in acutely hypovolemic trauma patients, the use of any of these drugs in reduced doses is probably more important than the particular agent chosen.[276,277] Usually, reducing the dose of the anesthetic does not result in inadequate anesthesia because the dose needed for induction is also decreased in the hypovolemic patient secondary to a variety of effects, such as decreased volume of distribution, preferential distribution of the cardiac output to the brain and the heart, brain hypoxia, dilutional hypoproteinemia, acidosis, and increased sensitivity of the brain to anesthetics.[34] If there is concern that inadequate anesthesia will result from reducing the dose of anesthetic, patients may be pretreated with small doses of opioids. These principles may become especially important for the anesthesiologist if the concept of delayed fluid resuscitation, with hypovolemia prolonged until hemorrhage is controlled surgically, becomes widely accepted.[83]

The maintenance of anesthesia in the hypovolemic trauma patient raises concerns similar to those pertaining to induction of anesthesia. Although normally nitrous oxide's myocardial depressant effect is somewhat counterbalanced by its ability to increase sympathetic outflow, in acute hemorrhage there is already a dramatic increase in sympathetic activity and stimulation of baroreceptors. Under these circumstances, patients are unlikely to respond to the sympathetic effect of N_2O, and the cardiovascular depressant properties of the gas are unmasked.

Weiskopf and Bogetz[278] have demonstrated that in swine with 30% blood volume loss, hemodynamic and oxygenation indices produced by N_2O were the same as those caused by equipotent doses of halothane. In addition, N_2O, by reducing FIO_2, incurs a risk of hypoxemia in patients with reduced cardiac output or pulmonary compromise. Isoflurane, despite causing little impairment of reflex tachycardia and having a vasodilatory action that preserves organ blood flow in normovolemic patients, can impair cardiac output and organ blood flow in hypovolemia—that is, it can cause cardiovascular depression. Desflurane and sevoflurane are not significantly better than isoflurane in this regard. Because of their low solubility in blood, severe hemodynamic depression produced by these agents can be rapidly reversed, preventing suboptimal perfusion for a significant time.[279] In summary, in the hypovolemic patient, all inhalational agents may reduce both global and regional blood flows, and therefore should be used only in small concentrations (<1 minimum alveolar concentration [MAC]). Opioid supplementation is usually well tolerated and often indicated.

Head and Open Eye Injuries

The importance of deep anesthesia and adequate muscle relaxation during airway management of patients with head or open eye injuries has already been discussed. Anesthetic agents selected for management of brain injury should produce the least increase in ICP, the least decrease in mean arterial pressure, and the greatest reduction in cerebral metabolic rate ($CMRO_2$). As demonstrated by intraoperative $SjvO_2$ measurements in acutely head-injured patients, the most important factor in causing cerebral ischemia is increased ICP from intracranial hematoma.[280] Prompt decompression is the most crucial means of ensuring cerebral well-being. Hypotension caused by anesthetics or other factors contributes to the development or progression of cerebral ischemia. Utmost attention should be paid during anesthesia to avoidance of hypotension (mean arterial pressure <80 mm Hg) and, more important, if reliable $SjvO_2$ monitoring is in place, to avoid values <55–60%. Perhaps with the exception of ketamine,[44] all iv anesthetics cause comparable degrees of cerebrovascular constriction.[281-284] Thiopental, midazolam, propofol, and etomidate therefore also produce a dose-dependent reduction in cerebrospinal fluid formation.[285] Again with the exception of ketamine, $CMRO_2$ is also reduced by all of the available iv anesthetics.[44,281-284] An important drawback to these agents is that their cardiovascular depressant effects may reduce CPP.[281,282,284] This problem can be ameliorated by administering pretreatment doses of opioids (fentanyl, 2–3 $mg \cdot kg^{-1}$), which permit reduction of the anesthetic dose. This may also prevent the myoclonic movements associated with etomidate and occasionally with propofol, and thus reduce the risks of ICP and IOP increase. Nevertheless, myoclonus is best prevented by careful timing of the dose of muscle relaxants.[286] Another measure to preserve CPP during anesthesia is to administer vasopressors, while taking care not to mask hypovolemia by their use.

Ordinarily, administration of succinylcholine should follow pretreatment doses of nondepolarizing agents to prevent fasciculation-induced elevation of ICP and IOP.[46,287] The results of clinical trials in search of an induction technique to avoid IOP rise without precurarization are inconsistent. However, the combination of propofol, 2 $mg \cdot kg^{-1}$ and alfentanil, 40 $\mu g \cdot kg^{-1}$ prevented IOP elevation caused by succinylcholine, laryngoscopy, and intubation in all but one patient, without producing hemodynamic depression.[288] Avoiding succinylcholine usually does not alleviate the problem because laryngoscopy and tracheal intubation themselves produce a greater and longer-lasting increase in IOP and ICP.[288] However, rocuronium, at a dose of 0.9–1.2 $mg \cdot kg^{-1}$ has an onset time comparable with that of succinylcholine.[289] Mivacurium has a longer onset time than rocuronium and, unlike rocuronium, can cause vasodilatation and hypotension.[290] Finally, rapacuronium 1.5–2.5 $mg \cdot kg^{-1}$ most closely resembles to succinylcholine in onset of action and

duration and may be an appropriate agent for head- or eye-injured patients.[38] None of the nondepolarizing muscle relaxants causes elevation of ICP or IOP in the absence of associated endotracheal intubation.

All inhalation anesthetics may increase cerebral blood flow (CBF), cerebral blood volume (CBV), and thus the ICP.[281] Cerebral autoregulation, CO_2 responsiveness, and $CMRO_2$ are reduced. Unlike most iv anesthetics, which decrease both CBF and $CMRO_2$ in parallel, inhalational anesthetics decrease $CMRO_2$ while increasing the CBF. The extent of this uncoupling varies with the agent and the dose. Halothane has the greatest vasodilatory effect, whereas isoflurane has the least; enflurane is intermediate. $CMRO_2$ is reduced least by halothane and most by isoflurane.[291] Because it produces the most pronounced CBF–$CMRO_2$ uncoupling, halothane is not a desirable agent in brain injury. Enflurane produces a better CBF–$CMRO_2$ relationship, but its convulsive potential, which is increased by the hyperventilation frequently used in brain injury, makes it an undesirable agent as well. Isoflurane is the most widely used inhalation anesthetic, although desflurane and sevoflurane have similar effects on the cerebral circulation.[292] In hyperventilated patients with cerebral tumors or mild edema, isoflurane does not raise the ICP if it is administered at an inspired concentration of <1 MAC.[293] In the presence of severe head injury, when cerebral autoregulation and CO_2 responsiveness are impaired, isoflurane has the potential to increase CBF and ICP even if it is given at levels below 1 MAC and with hyperventilation.[293] Therefore, it may be prudent not to use this agent at high concentrations in the presence of elevated ICP, at least until the skull is opened and the ICP is controlled. In these patients, anesthesia can be maintained initially with opioids plus thiopental, propofol, midazolam, or etomidate. There is also some evidence to suggest that increasing PaO_2 to levels above 250–300 mm Hg by elevation of FIO_2 can partly compensate for the possible increase in cerebral ischemia caused by hyperventilation.[294] Thus, if hyperventilation is used to compensate for isoflurane-induced cerebral vasodilation, it should be accompanied by high levels of FIO_2.

Nitrous oxide may increase CBF, CBV, and ICP when administered with inhalation anesthetics if the $PaCO_2$ is normal or increased.[295] This effect may be eliminated when this agent is administered with adequate doses of barbiturates or hyperventilation. The effect on $CMRO_2$ is variable: both an increase and decrease have been observed. Thus, N_2O probably is not deleterious in head-injured patients with minimal ICP elevation, in hypocapnic patients, and if it is used after a bolus dose or during infusion of iv anesthetics.

Opioids are frequently used during induction and maintenance of anesthesia in neurotrauma. In a spontaneously breathing patient, they may produce hypoventilation with an associated increase in CBF and ICP; they should, therefore, be used only in mechanically ventilated head trauma patients. Some reports suggest that opioids and, to a smaller extent, opiates may interfere with CPP by increasing ICP, decreasing mean arterial pressure, or both.[42,296] Fentanyl and sufentanil are most implicated, and it appears that this phenomenon occurs when the head injury is severe.[297,298] As mentioned before, ICP increased in patients with both preserved and altered cerebral autoregulation.[42] It also appears that mechanisms other than cerebral vasodilation are responsible for these changes. The clinical significance of these findings is not yet clear. However, it is prudent to administer fentanyl or its analogues slowly, when the arterial pressure is normal or slightly elevated, possibly after establishing mild hypocarbia, and ensuring preservation of systemic blood pressure with vasoactive agents, if necessary.

Cardiac Injury

If there is pericardial tamponade, preload and myocardial contractility should be maintained. Any decrease in these parameters may exacerbate an already existing RV inflow occlusion. A decrease in heart rate should also be treated promptly to maintain adequate cardiac output. Because all of the available anesthetics can depress myocardial contractility and cause vasodilation, it is preferable to administer these agents after evacuation of pericardial blood under local anesthesia. If this is not possible, an agent that best preserves sympathetic tone should be selected. In chronic pericardial effusion, ketamine supports the cardiac index better than diazepam.[299] In acute pericardial tamponade, even minor insults can bring cardiac activity to a halt. Ketamine thus remains the agent of choice. It should be given in small doses after adequate fluid infusion. Similar principles apply to the use of maintenance agents, which should be given in the smallest possible doses until the heart is decompressed. If general anesthesia is required to relieve the tamponade, induction should be delayed until the patient is prepared and draped. Both anesthetics and controlled ventilation impair cardiac output. Deep anesthesia and high airway pressures should be avoided before evacuation of the hemopericardium.

In patients with myocardial contusion, the objective is not only to maintain cardiac contractility but to lower the elevated pulmonary vascular resistance that may result from concomitant pulmonary contusion or aspiration. All anesthetics should preferably be administered after restoration of intravascular volume and titrated to maintain adequate systemic blood pressure and cardiac output. If necessary, inotropes, preferably amrinone or milrinone, which produce some pulmonary vasodilation, may be used. Anesthetic maintenance by infusion of iv anesthetics and opioids to avoid the myocardial depression produced by inhalational agents should also be considered.

Burns

Anesthesia may be required during all three phases of burn injury: during the resuscitation phase (first 24–48 hours), during convalescence (a few weeks) for escharotomies, and during reconstruction (6 months). Extensive and repeated escharotomies may be required during the initial phase of convalescence, usually between the second day and the second week after injury, often necessitating massive transfusion, temperature control, and management of fluid, electrolyte, and coagulation abnormalities. A hypermetabolic state characterized by tachycardia, tachypnea, catecholamine surge, increased O_2 consumption, and augmented catabolism follows the initial few hours of a burn injury and continues into the convalescent phase, necessitating increased oxygen, ventilation, and nutrition.[206]

Anesthetic management of escharotomies presents several difficulties. Burned tissue may prevent access for ECG, pulse oximeter, neuromuscular function, and noninvasive blood pressure monitoring; needle electrodes or surgical staples, a reflectance pulse oximeter, and an arterial catheter may be necessary. Large-bore iv catheters are essential. Hyperthermia occurs, but hypothermia is more likely in the operating room and is to be avoided. Exposure and evaporative fluid loss necessitate maintenance of the operating room temperature between 28° and 32°C, use of countercurrent fluid and blood warming devices, surface heating with forced dry, warm air, and humidified inspired gases. Blood loss can be controlled by restricting the escharotomy to 15–20% of TBSA, use of extremity tourniquets, applying dilute epinephrine solution topically (1:10,000) or by injection (0.5 mg per 1000 ml), and using compression bandages. Epinephrine doses of up to 6.7 mg topically or 0.8 mg by injection into the surgical area are well tolerated[300]; the affinity of β-adrenergic receptors to ligands is decreased after burns. The administration of a large amount of blood and blood products subjects the patient to complications of transfusion such as coagulopathy. Although citrate-induced hypocalcemia is a relatively rare complication of transfusion,[301] monitoring of Ca^{2+} and administration of calcium chloride (2.5–5.0 mg · kg^{-1}) or gluconate (7.5–10.0 mg · kg^{-1}) should be considered when blood products are administered rapidly. A preliminary report demonstrated that reconstituted whole blood minimizes coagulation abnormalities and septic and pulmonary complications in pediatric burn patients.[302] Transfusion-related coagulopathy is less common now than formerly because of the measures we have described to reduce blood loss and because lower hematocrit levels are now accepted.[206]

The multiple pathophysiologic changes that occur with burns, such as shock, hyperdynamic circulation, decreased serum albumin concentration, increased α_1-acid glycoprotein concentration, and altered receptor sensitivity, alter the response to various drugs during the resuscitative and convalescent phases.[206,216] As in hypovolemic trauma patients, the doses of iv anesthetics should be reduced during the resuscitation phase to prevent excessive hemodynamic depression. Anesthesia should be maintained with opioid or inhalational agents as the hemodynamic status of the patient permits. However, burn patients have excruciating pain and exceedingly high opioid requirements. A proven anesthetic regimen for excision and grafting of burns is isoflurane plus large doses of opioid. The response to depolarizing and nondepolarizing muscle relaxants remains unaltered during the first 24 hours after burn injury. However, after the first day, succinylcholine should be avoided for at least 1 year because it can result in a potentially lethal increase of serum K$^+$ when the burn size exceeds 10% of TBSA. Resistance develops to all nondepolarizing muscle relaxants in patients with burns of >30% TBSA starting approximately 1 week and peaking 5–6 weeks after injury. Pharmacodynamic causes, such as an increased number of acetylcholine receptors in the neuromuscular junction, may be responsible, but the exact mechanism is not known.[206,216]

Ketamine is a commonly used anesthetic for serial wound débridements during the convalescent phase. It allows adequate spontaneous ventilation at a surgical plane of anesthesia, does not depress hemodynamics, and produces excellent analgesia. However, patients often experience dysphoric reactions with ketamine. Participation of an anesthesiologist using more common drugs and techniques is a safe and effective alternative.[206]

Management of Intraoperative Complications

Persistent Hypotension

Persistent hypotension is usally the result of one of four mechanisms in the trauma setting: bleeding, tension pneumothorax, neurogenic shock, and cardiac injury. Although many other causes, such as citrate intoxication (hypocalcemia), hypothermia, coronary artery disease, allergic reactions, or incompatible transfusion, can be responsible for this complication, they occur less frequently.

Hypotension due to bleeding is most likely. The source may be obvious, such as external bleeding from the skull or an open vessel in the extremities, or occult. The thoracic and abdominal cavities and the pelvic retroperitoneal space are the most common sites of occult hemorrhage that results in hypotension. Management includes early diagnosis and control of the bleeding site plus effective fluid resuscitation. The latter can best be accomplished using an infusion system with large-diameter tubing (5 mm) and a countercurrent heat exchanger, such as the Level 1 system (Level 1 Technologies, Inc., Marshfield, MA). Up to 1000 ml · min^{-1} of crystalloid solution or 600 ml · min^{-1} of packed cells can be given if a box-type pressure pump and a large-bore iv cannula are used.[303] The system should be connected to 14-gauge or larger cannulae, preferably inserted into veins both above and below the diaphragm. If a pulmonary artery catheter introducer is used, the tubing should be connected directly to the hub because the flow rate from its side port is equal to that of a 16-gauge catheter. The rapid infusor system (Haemonetics, Braintree, MA), which consists of a reservoir, countercurrent heating system, and roller pump, is capable of delivering up to 1600 ml · min^{-1} of warm fluids once the rate of infusion is programmed. Although a more powerful system than the Level 1, it is more costly, difficult to assemble, and infrequently necessary in the trauma patient.

Lactated Ringer's solution is the crystalloid of choice in most centers. However, it is slightly hypotonic (273 mOsm·l⁻¹), acidic (pH 5.1), and contains a small amount of Ca^{2+}, which may counteract the citrate anticoagulant in packed red blood cells (PRBC). Normal saline does not cause this problem, but, as mentioned, its infusion in large quantities may result in hyperchloremic acidosis. Both Plasma-lyte A and Normosol-R have the advantages of a pH of 7.4, no Ca^{2+}, and a normal osmolarity (295 mOsm). Because of their prolonged intravascular retention and decreased tendency to produce edema, colloid solutions may be used in selected trauma patients such as those with head injury and those in whom edema develops due to inflammatory reactions or prior administration of large amounts of crystalloids. However, consistent evidence for the benefit of colloids over crystalloids is lacking.[304] Human serum albumin (5 and 25%) and hydroxyethyl starch are the most commonly used solutions. Hydroxyethyl starch may produce coagulation abnormalities primarily by reducing the levels of fibrinogen, factor VIII, and von Willebrand's factor, and by reducing platelet function. This is especially important in head-injured patients in whom fatal intracranial hemorrhage may develop.[305] The recommended safe dose of this agent as a component of therapy for surgical blood loss is 20 ml·kg⁻¹, although a review suggests that there is little support for this recommendation.[305]

Ideally, transfusion of hemorrhaging trauma patients should be done with whole blood so that depletion of the patient's coagulation factors can be prevented. Even labile factors (V and VIII) rarely decrease below a critical 20–30% level as long as whole blood is administered.[258] However, of the 8 million units of blood administered annually in the United States, only 3% are provided as whole blood. Practically speaking, therefore, PRBC is the only preparation that is available for trauma resuscitation in this country (see also Chapter 10).

Inconvenience, safety, and cost factors associated with transfusion therapy prompted the development of artificial oxygen-carrying solutions. Various hemoglobin solutions and new-generation perfluorochemicals are in the advanced stage of human research. In a preliminary study, modified human polymerized hemoglobin was administered to 44 trauma patients and judged safe and effective as an oxygen-carrying solution.[306] Despite a reduction in red cell mass, tissue oxygenation was maintained by the plasma hemoglobin. Nevertheless, systemic hypertension, as a result of endothelial nitric oxide binding, and pancreatitis may occur after administration of hemoglobin solutions.

Hypotension due to tension pneumothorax continues and frequently leads to fatality unless this complication is diagnosed and treated rapidly.

Neurogenic shock must always be considered as a cause of hypotension. Spinal cord injury may be missed during initial evaluation, especially in unconscious patients. Intraoperative hemodynamic management of these patients is primarily by judicious administration of fluids and, if needed, vasopressors and inotropes. However, differentiation of neurogenic shock from hemorrhagic shock is important[307]; often patients are bradycardic and respond to catecholamine infusion readily. Misdiagnosing neurogenic for hemorrhagic shock may lead to excessive fluid infusion and pulmonary edema. The reverse error may also occur: depriving patients with hemorrhagic shock of fluids because of misdiagnosis of neurogenic shock.[307] Invasive central hemodynamic monitoring may be indicated in these patients.[163] In some patients, of course, hemorrhagic and neurogenic shock may coexist.

Cardiac causes of persistent hypotension include myocardial contusion, pericardial tamponade, valvular injury, and septal perforation. Intraoperative TEE can be useful in the differential diagnosis. In myocardial contusion, the RV is most commonly

injured. If there is a concomitant increase in pulmonary vascular resistance (e.g., from an associated pulmonary contusion), the RV pressure increases while its output decreases, resulting in an increased CVP. The raised RV pressure causes the interventricular septum to shift toward the left, decreasing left ventricular compliance and increasing its diastolic pressure. The net effect is a decreased cardiac output. In addition to demonstrating wall motion abnormalities, TEE can display the septal shift and altered left ventricular dynamics, information that can be useful during interpretation of elevated cardiac filling pressures.[308]

In the absence of TEE, a pulmonary artery catheter may be helpful. Equalization of pressures across the cardiac chambers during diastole suggests pericardial tamponade. A similar picture may also be seen in severe myocardial contusion, causing difficulty in differential diagnosis. This effect is rare and usually associated with severe hemodynamic instability. Differential diagnosis in these instances can be established by pericardiocentesis. Septal encroachment into the left ventricle from RV contusion results in an increase in pulmonary artery wedge pressure. Decreasing the rate of fluid infusion in these patients results in a further decrease in cardiac output. Treatment includes fluid infusion, pulmonary vasodilators if the systemic blood pressure is normal, and inotropic support if the systemic blood pressure is low. Absence of response to this treatment is an indication for placement of an intra-aortic balloon pump. Pulmonary artery catheterization is also helpful in demonstrating an oxygen step-up from septal injury. During thoracotomy, a distended RV should also raise the suspicion of a septal defect.

Hypothermia

Shock, alcohol intoxication, exposure to cold, fluid resuscitation, and abnormalities in thermoregulatory mechanisms render the major trauma patient hypothermic during the initial phase of injury. The mortality rate after trauma increases with decreasing temperature. Severe hypothermia, which in the trauma patient is defined as core temperature below 32°C, was associated with a 100% mortality rate in one study.[309] The intraoperative risk of hypothermia is also higher for the trauma victim than for electively operated patients. Heat loss increases in patients with spinal cord, extensive soft tissue, and burn injuries, and in those who consumed ethanol before surgery.

The impact of hypothermia on already compromised vital functions may be devastating. There may be reduced cardiac output, cardiac conduction abnormalities, diminished cerebral and renal blood flows, decreased oxygen release from red cells caused by the leftward shift of the O_2 dissociation curve, altered platelet and clotting enzyme function, and abnormalities of K^+ and Ca^{2+} homeostasis.[255] These effects may further compromise poor organ perfusion, oxygenation, blood coagulation, and metabolism.

Aggressive therapy and correction of body temperature to normal within a short time appear to decrease mortality rate, blood loss, fluid requirement, organ failure, and length of ICU stay.[310] Convective warming with forced dry air at 43°C can prevent a temperature drop in most trauma patients but cannot effectively treat severe hypothermia; because of its low specific heat, air has little heat content to give to the cold trauma patient.[310] Airway rewarming can reduce heat loss caused by latent heat of vaporization, but this technique also transfers very little heat.[310] Administration of warm iv fluids is the most effective way to prevent and treat hypothermia in the trauma patient, provided that fluids are being administered at a relatively rapid rate. For each liter of fluid given at 40°C to a patient with a body temperature of 33°C, 7 kcal of heat energy is gained. Countercurrent heat exchanging systems (Level 1 Technologies) are more effective than dry heat or still-water bath warmers. They warm the fluid to 40°C, and the delivered fluid temperature is not affected by rapid rates of administration.[303] The most effective method, however, is continuous arteriovenous rewarming, which can be achieved using a modified Level 1 countercurrent system (Fig. 48-9). The blood exits the body from a percutaneously placed femoral arterial catheter at the patient's own pressure, is warmed in the infusion system, and returned to the body through a venous cannula. Because the circuit tubing is heparin bonded, there is no need for heparinization. Experience with this technique in the ICU has been encouraging.[310,311]

Coagulation Abnormalities

During elective surgery, coagulation abnormalities result primarily from dilution of platelets and coagulation factors (see also Chapter 10). In trauma, other factors may also be responsible for this complication. These include hypothermia, acidosis, tissue hypoxia, and tissue thromboplastin release. Hypothermia and diminished tissue perfusion aggravate existing coagulation abnormalities,[312] and hypothermia by itself can cause clotting deficiencies in the absence of platelet or factor deficiency.[255] Hypothermia affects platelet morphology, function, and sequestration and retards enzyme activity, slowing the initiation and propagation of both platelet plug and fibrin clot.[313] Decreased body temperature may also enhance fibrinolytic activity.[313]

Perioperative diagnosis of coagulopathy is often made by observing bleeding from wounds or puncture sites, rather than by interpretation of laboratory tests. However, differential diagnosis between consumptive and dilutional coagulopathy requires laboratory testing, although the results of these tests are usually delayed. Usually, the inability to determine the type of coagulopathy does not present a problem because the initial treatment is similar for both conditions. Nevertheless, the diagnosis of DIC has prognostic significance because its treatment involves elimination of its causes. A blood sample without heparin should be sent for measurement of circulating fibrin degradation products (FDP/fdp). An FDP/fdp level >10 mg $\cdot$ ml^{-1} is suggestive of DIC, whereas a value >40 mg $\cdot$ ml^{-1} is diagnostic.

In patients who have not received blood products, simultaneous determination of fibrinogen level, platelet count, and PT may be helpful in diagnosis of the DIC. A fibrinogen level <150 mg $\cdot$ dl^{-1}, platelet count $<150,000$, and PT >15 seconds is highly suggestive. If only two of the three are abnormal, FDP/fdp should be measured.

Prompt platelet administration should always be considered once abnormal bleeding is noted. Each unit of platelet concentrate contains 55 billion platelets, which normally increase the platelet count by 5,000–10,000 per microliter (μl). If there is ongoing surgical bleeding, administration of platelets should perhaps be delayed until it is controlled; otherwise the platelets will be wasted. On the other hand, severe thrombocytopenia may contribute to the bleeding. Indications for FFP and cryoprecipitate are not clear. However, it has been shown that transfusion of PRBC in elective surgery results in depletion of coagulation factors earlier than of platelets.[258,314] Thus, it is not unreasonable to administer FFP or cryoprecipitate simultaneously with platelets in emergency trauma surgery. The minimum dose of FFP for adults is 2 units ($\sim$600 ml) and is given within less than 1 hour. Fibrinogen concentration <80 mg $\cdot$ dl^{-1} is an indication for cryoprecipitate administration. Ten units increase plasma fibrinogen concentration by approximately 100 mg $\cdot$ dl^{-1}.[260]

In the absence of abnormal bleeding, prophylactic administration of platelets, FFP, or cryoprecipitate is unwarranted even if coagulation tests indicate platelet and factor depletion.[315] However, once transfusion of factor-deficient PRBC and fluids exceeds one blood volume, clinical coagulopathy is likely even in the absence of shock, hypothermia, or other aggravating factors.[259,260] Thus, in trauma patients who receive between one and two blood volume replacements, platelet or factor administration is almost always indicated. In hypothermic patients with clinical coagulopathy, the critical treatment is rewarming rather than platelet and coagulation factor administration, although circumstances may require both.[256,316]

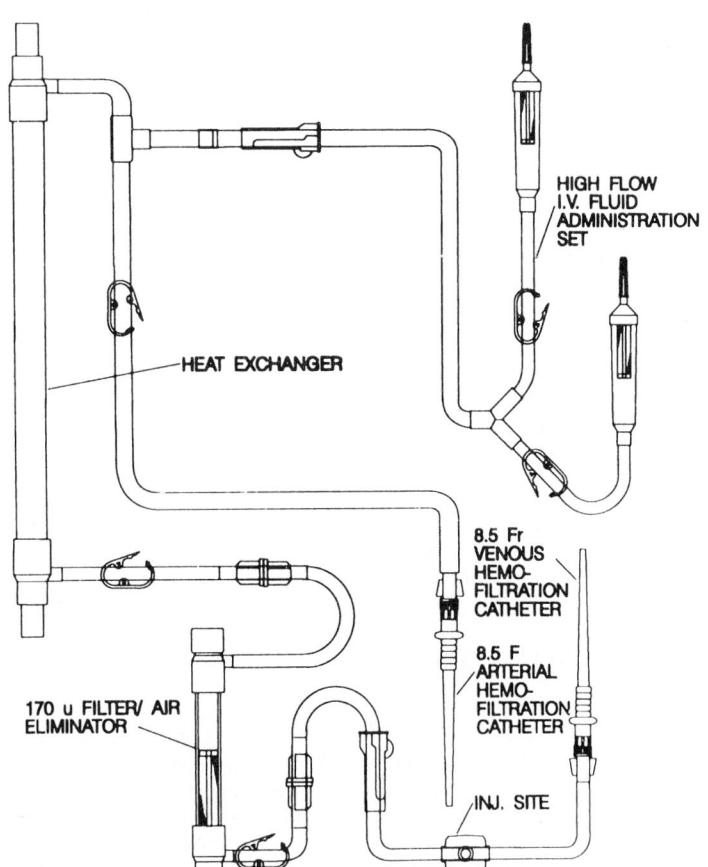

HIGH FLOW I.V. FLUID ADMINISTRATION SET

HEAT EXCHANGER

8.5 Fr VENOUS HEMO-FILTRATION CATHETER

8.5 F ARTERIAL HEMO-FILTRATION CATHETER

170 u FILTER/ AIR ELIMINATOR

INJ. SITE

Figure 48-9. Schematic drawing of the system used for continuous arteriovenous rewarming. (Reprinted with permission from Gentilello LM, Cobean R, Offner PJ *et al:* Continuous arteriovenous rewarming: rapid reversal of hypothermia in critically ill patients. J Trauma 32:316, 1992.)

Electrolyte and Acid–Base Disturbances

Intraoperative hyperpotassemia may develop as a result of three mechanisms. First, in patients with irreversible shock, cell membrane permeability is altered so that massive K^+ efflux results in severe hyperpotassemia; in this situation, the patient will not survive. Second, after repair of a major vessel, subsequent reperfusion of the ischemic tissues results in a sudden release of K^+. Third, transfusion at a rate faster than 1 unit every 4 minutes to an acidotic and hypovolemic patient may cause an increase in plasma K^+ levels.[317] Massive transfusion of a patient whose aorta is temporarily clamped below the diaphragm to prevent hemorrhage from the abdominal or pelvic vessels can also cause hyperpotassemia; the K^+ load is distributed into a small volume of blood in this instance. Frequent monitoring of serum K^+, gradual and intermittent unclamping of vascular shunts, and avoiding transfusion at higher rates than needed help reduce the rate of K^+ increase. If a rise in K^+ is detected, treatment with regular insulin, 10 units iv, with 50% dextrose, 50 ml; and sodium bicarbonate, 8.4%, 50 ml is indicated. If there is a dysrhythmia, $CaCl_2$, 500 mg should also be administered.[318] Insulin and dextrose can be repeated two or three times at 30–45 minute intervals if necessary. Hemodialysis may be indicated in desperate situations.

Metabolic acidosis is caused by shock in most trauma patients. Other causes of metabolic acidosis in this population are alcoholic lactic acidosis, alcoholic ketoacidosis, diabetic ketoacidosis, and CO or CN^- poisoning after inhalation injuries. Alcoholic lactic acidosis occurs in patients who become hypoperfused while intoxicated. Under normal circumstances, the liver can clear moderate amounts of lactic acid. In intoxicated patients, however, preferential metabolism of alcohol by the liver interferes with the utilization of lactate by this organ. Alcoholic ketoacidosis may also occur in those who are both starved and deprived of alcohol. Starvation usually results in lipolysis, which in turn produces free fatty acids. Alcohol ingestion prevents the conversion of free fatty acids to ketones. When a starved alcoholic is also deprived of alcohol, free fatty acids easily convert to ketones and produce alcoholic ketoacidosis. The differential diagnosis between hypovolemic, diabetic, and alcoholic acidosis, all of which have anion gaps, requires measurement of blood lactate, urinary ketone bodies, blood sugar, and invasive monitoring to assess intravascular volume. Alcoholic ketoacidosis is treated with iv dextrose, whereas diabetic ketoacidosis is managed with insulin. No specific treatment except iv normal saline exists for alcoholic lactic acidosis.

Treatment of metabolic acidosis involves correction of the underlying cause. This may involve management of hypoxemia, restoration of intravascular volume, optimization of cardiac function, or treatment of CO or CN^- toxicity. Symptomatic treatment with sodium bicarbonate has serious disadvantages, including leftward shift of the oxyhemoglobin dissociation curve causing decreased O_2 unloading, a hyperosmolar state secondary to the excessive sodium load, hypokalemia, further hemodynamic depression, overshoot alkalosis a few hours after giving the drug, and intracellular acidosis if adequate ventilation or pulmonary blood flow cannot be provided.[319] Development of intracellular acidosis is especially likely in patients who are being resuscitated from cardiac arrest. Nevertheless, because of the belief that severe acidosis itself can cause dysrhythmias, myocardial depression, hypotension, and resistance to exogenous catecholamines, to "buy time" some clinicians administer bicarbonate if the pH is <7.2.

Intraoperative Death

Death is a much greater threat during emergency trauma surgery than it is in any other operative procedure. Approximately 0.7% of patients admitted for trauma die in the operating room, accounting for approximately 8% of postinjury deaths.[320] Uncontrollable bleeding is the cause of approximately 80% of intraoperative mortality; brain herniation and air embolism are

Table 48-15. CLINICAL FEATURES ASSOCIATED WITH INTRAOPERATIVE MORTALITY

Category	Clinical Features
Mechanism of injury	Gunshot wound
	Pedestrian injuries
Injury severity	Mean Injury Severity Score (ISS) >41
	Mean Revised Trauma Score (RTS) >3.0
Preoperative physiologic profile	Mean BP in the field <50 mm Hg
	Mean BP on arrival to ED <60 mm Hg
	Best systolic BP in the ED <90 mm Hg
	Circulatory shock time >10 min
	Best mean pH <7.18
	Mean preoperative crystalloid resuscitation >3850 ml
	Mean red cell transfusion >834 ml
Type of injury	Significant head, chest, abdominal, and pelvic injuries individually or in combination after blunt trauma
	Significant chest and abdominal injuries individually or in combination after penetrating trauma
Organ injury	Brain
	Liver
	Aorta or other major vascular injury
	Cardiac injury
Operating room resuscitation and physiologic status	Systolic BP <90 mm Hg during first hour
	Systolic BP <90 mm Hg for >30 min
	Deterioration of mean pH from 7.19 to 7.01
	Mean intraoperative blood loss 5172 ml
	Mean blood replacement 4541 ml
	Mean platelet transfusion 784 ml
	Mean fresh frozen plasma 1418 ml
	Mean intraoperative temperature 32.2°C
	Intraoperative cardiac arrest

ED = emergency department; BP = blood pressure.
Data from Hoyt DB, Bulger EM, Knudson MM *et al*: Death in the operating room: An analysis of a multi-center experience. J. Trauma 37:426, 1994.

the most common causes of death in the remaining patients.[320] A multicenter, retrospective study has defined certain features that increase the likelihood of operating room death[320] (Table 48-15). Rapid transport to the operating room, concentrating efforts on life-threatening injuries while deferring definitive surgery, simultaneous thoracotomy and laparotomy for thoracoabdominal injuries, appropriate management of retroperitoneal hematoma, early correction of hypothermia and shock, and early packing of severe liver injuries may reduce intraoperative mortality rates.[320]

EARLY POSTOPERATIVE CONSIDERATIONS

The concerns in the early postoperative period are similar to those of the intraoperative phase. Re-evaluation and optimization of the circulation, oxygenation, temperature, CNS function, coagulation, electrolyte and acid–base status, and renal function are the hallmarks of postoperative management.

Sedation and Analgesia

Pain control in this group of patients may have more than a humanitarian purpose; it can improve pulmonary function, ventilation, and oxygenation in patients with chest injury or a long abdominal incision (see Chapter 54). For sedation in mechanically ventilated patients, both propofol and midazolam infusions alone or in combination are equally effective and safe, although wake-up time in patients receiving midazolam is longer (660 ± 400 minutes) than in those receiving propofol alone (110 ± 50 minutes) or both agents combined (190 ± 200 minutes).[321] Head-injured patients tolerate all three regimens well because the ICP, CPP, and Sjvo$_2$ remain unchanged.[321] The dose should be titrated to effect, but the usual infusion rates are as follows: midazolam, $0.1-0.2$ mg $\cdot$ kg^{-1} $\cdot$ hr^{-1}; propofol, $1.5-6$ mg $\cdot$ kg^{-1} $\cdot$ hr^{-1}, and the combination, midazolam, $0.1-0.2$ mg $\cdot$ kg^{-1} $\cdot$ hr^{-1} and propofol, $50-150$ mg $\cdot$ kg^{-1} $\cdot$ hr^{-1}. Larger doses may result in hemodynamic depression. Morphine $0.02-0.04$ mg $\cdot$ kg^{-1} $\cdot$ hr^{-1} or fentanyl $1-3$ μg $\cdot$ kg^{-1} $\cdot$ hr^{-1} may be added for analgesia. Small boluses of midazolam (3–5 mg), propofol (50 mg), morphine (2–3 mg), or fentanyl (25–50 μg) may also be given as required.[321]

Acute Renal Failure

Acute renal failure is a possibility if prolonged shock occurred during early management. In patients who have not received an osmotic load (radiopaque material, mannitol) or diuretic, postoperative determination of 2- or 6-hour creatinine and free water clearances may help predict the development of post-traumatic renal dysfunction.[322] Creatinine clearance <25 ml $\cdot$ min^{-1} and free water clearance ≥ -15 ml $\cdot$ hr^{-1} suggest the likelihood of acute renal failure. Decreased urine flow rate is not a good predictor, and the blood urea nitrogen does not rise until at least 24 hours after surgery or trauma.[322]

Abdominal Compartment Syndrome

An abdominal compartment syndrome as a result of intra-abdominal hypertension is a recently appreciated phenomenon that occurs after major abdominal trauma and surgery, although some patients may have the syndrome without surgery.[323] This complication results from massive edema of intra-abdominal organs produced by shock-induced inflammatory mediators, fluid resuscitation, and surgical manipulation. The significant impairment of cardiac, pulmonary, renal, gastrointestinal, hepatic, and CNS function caused by this syndrome results in a high mortality rate[323] (Fig. 48-10). Clinically, a tense, distended

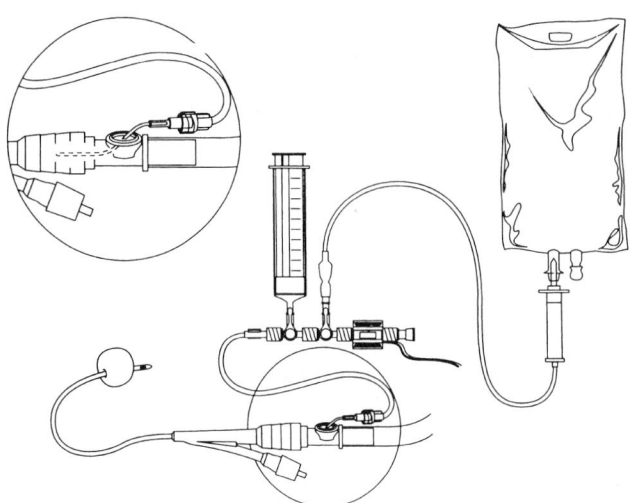

Figure 48-11. System used to measure intravesicular pressure in abdominal compartment syndrome. (Reprinted with permission from Cheatham ML: Intra-abdominal hypertension and abdominal compartment syndrome. New Horiz 7:96, 1999.)

abdomen should direct the clinician to measure the intravesical pressure, which reflects the intra-abdominal pressure. The system used for intravesical pressure measurement is shown in Figure 48-11.[323] Values >20–25 mm Hg indicate inadequate organ perfusion and necessitate abdominal decompression, which, if delayed, results in progression to multiorgan failure and death. After decompression, the abdominal pressure may remain high for a few days before decreasing to the normal range (3–10 mm Hg). Use of a volumetric pulmonary artery catheter for assessment of preload by left ventricular end-diastolic volume index determination may be more accurate than measuring CVP or PCWP in these patients.[323]

Thromboembolism

Trauma patients are prone to development of thromboembolic complications. The overall incidence of DVT in the proximal femoral veins, the major source of PE, is approximately 18% in trauma patients.[324] However, DVT occurs in 24% of lower extremity injuries, 27% of spine injuries, 20% of major head injuries, and 15% of serious injuries of the face, chest, or abdomen.[324] When injuries involve more than one of these high-risk regions, the likelihood of DVT is even higher. For example, up to 77% of patients with combined head and lower extremity injuries may have both distal and proximal DVT.[324] Fortunately, only a relatively small fraction (approximately 0.3–2%) of severely injured patients have PE.[324, 325] Apart from the type and severity of injury, older age, blood transfusion, and surgery appear to facilitate the development of this complication.[324] Almost half of all cases of PE occur within the first week, suggesting that DVT develops shortly after trauma.[325] In most instances, DVT is asymptomatic, and in many of those in whom leg swelling develops, concurrent lower extremity injuries may be implicated. The diagnosis of proximal DVT in symptomatic patients can be made by duplex ultrasonography, but this method has low sensitivity in the absence of symptoms.[326] Venography, which is the gold standard, can be performed in equivocal cases, although it is associated with complications and inherent logistical problems. Hypoxemia, especially when sudden and associated with dyspnea and hemodynamic abnormalities, is highly suggestive of PE. The definitive diagnosis is established by spiral CT and pulmonary angiography, pulmonary ventilation–perfusion scans are infrequently performed. In hemodynamically unstable patients, resuscitation takes precedence over ra-

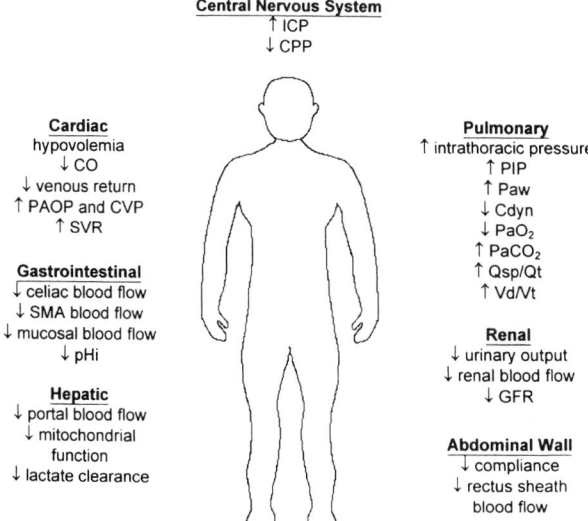

Figure 48-10. Physiologic effects of abdominal compartment syndrome. ICP = intracranial pressure; CPP = cerebral perfusion pressure; CO = cardiac output; PAOP = pulmonary artery occlusion pressure; CVP = central venous pressure; SVR = systemic vascular resistance; PIP = peak inspiratory pressure; Paw = mean airway pressure; Cdyn = dynamic pulmonary compliance; Qsp/Qt = intrapulmonary shunt; Vd/Vt = dead space ventilation; SMA = superior mesenteric artery; pHi = intramucosal pH; GFR = glomerular filtration rate. (Reprinted with permission from Cheatham ML: Intra-abdominal hypertension and abdominal compartment syndrome. New Horiz 7:96, 1999.)

diologic diagnosis. Management is symptomatic, and includes tracheal intubation, positive pressure ventilation with F_{IO_2} of 1.0, administration of fluids and inotropes (amrinone or milrinone), and continuous arterial and CVP or pulmonary artery monitoring. TEE is helpful because it may demonstrate RV performance, tricuspid regurgitation, or, in some cases, the thrombus within the pulmonary artery, the right heart chambers, or in transit through a patent foramen ovale to the left atrium.

In patients with relatively minor injuries, PE is treated with anticoagulants. Low-molecular-weight heparin may be used if bleeding is unlikely to exacerbate the injury. Consideration should be given to placement of a vena cava filter if the risk of bleeding is unacceptably high. Other indications for vena cava filter placement are recurrent PE despite full anticoagulation; proximal DVT with contraindications to, or major bleeding during, full anticoagulation; and progression of an iliofemoral clot despite full anticoagulation. Although widely performed in the past, placement of a vena cava filter before development of DVT in high-risk injuries such as pelvic fractures has decreased because of the severity of associated complications and the apparent ineffectiveness of this procedure. The current recommendation for prophylaxis in most trauma patients is low-molecular-weight heparin.[326] Low-dose unfractionated heparin appears to be ineffective in trauma patients.[327] Mechanical devices such as sequential compression devices and foot pumps should be applied as early as possible after injury.

REFERENCES

1. National Safety Council. Injury Facts: Chicago, National Safety Council, 1999
2. Violence Prevention Task Force of the Eastern Association for the Surgery of Trauma: Violence in America: A public health crisis—The role of firearms. J Trauma 38:163, 1995
3. Eachempati SR, Reed RL II, St. Louis JE, Fischer RP: "The demographics of trauma in 1995" revisited: An assesment of the accuracy and utility of trauma predictions. J Trauma 45:208, 1998
4. Trunkey DD, Blaisdell FW: Epidemiology of trauma. Sci Am 4:1, 1988
5. Wyatt J, Beard D, Gray A et al: The time of death after trauma. BMJ 310:1502, 1995
6. Sauaia A, Moore FA, Moore EE et al: Epidemiology of trauma deaths: A reassessment. J Trauma 38:185, 1995
7. Acosta JA, Yang JC, Winchell RJ et al: Lethal injuries and time of death in a level 1 trauma center. J Am Coll Surg 186:528, 1998
8. Holbrook TL, Anderson JP, Sieber WJ et al: Outcome after major trauma: 12-month and 18-month follow-up results from the trauma recovery project. J Trauma 46:765, 1999
9. American College of Surgeons Committee on Trauma: Trauma center descriptions and their role in trauma system. In American College of Surgeons (ed): Resources for Optimal Care of the Injured Patient, p 9. Chicago, American College of Surgeons, 1999
10. MacKenzie EJ, Morris JA, Smith GS, Fahey M: Acute hospital costs of trauma in the United States: Implications for regionalized systems of care. J Trauma 30:1096, 1990
11. Taheri PA, Butz DA, Watts CM et al: Trauma services: a profit center? J Am Coll Surg 188:349, 1999
12. Vassar MJ, Kizer KW: Hospitalizations for firearm-related injuries: A population based study of 9562 patients. JAMA 275:1734, 1996
13. Cornwell EE, Berne TV, Belzberg H et al: Health care crisis from a trauma center perspective. JAMA 276:940, 1996
14. Bazzoli GJ, Madura KJ, Cooper GF et al: Progress in the development of trauma systems in the United States. JAMA 273:395, 1995
15. American College of Surgeons Committee on Trauma: Initial assessment and management. In American College of Surgeons (ed): Advanced Trauma Life Support Course Instructor Manual, p 21. Chicago, American College of Surgeons, 1997
16. Janssen RS, St. Louis ME, Satten GA et al: HIV infection among patients in U.S. acute care hospitals: Strategies for counseling and testing of hospital patients. N Engl J Med 331:1153, 1994
17. Selwyn PA, Sckell BM, Aleales P et al: High risk of active tuberculosis in HIV-infected drug users with cutaneous anergy. JAMA 268:504, 1992
18. Kelen GD, Green GB, Purcell RH et al: Hepatitis B and hepatitis C in emergency department patients. N Engl J Med 326:1399, 1992
19. Janjua KJ, Sugrue M, Deane SA. Prospective evaluation of early missed injuries and the role of tertiary trauma survey. J Trauma 44:1000, 1998
20. O'Sullivan JC, Wells DG, Wells GR. Difficult airway management with neck swelling after carotid endarterectomy. Anaesth Intensive Care 14:460, 1986
21. Muzzi DA, Losasso TJ, Cucchiara RF: Complication from a nasopharyngeal airway in a patient with a basilar skull fracture. Anesthesiology 74:366, 1991
22. Jacobson LE, Gomez G, Sobieray RJ et al: Surgical cricothyroidotomy in trauma patients: Analysis of its use by paramedics in the field. J Trauma 41:15, 1996
23. Martin SE, Ochsner MG, Jarman RH et al: Use of laryngeal mask airway in air transport when intubation fails. J Trauma 47:352, 1999
24. Calkins MD, Robinson TD: Combat trauma airway management: Endotracheal intubation versus laryngeal mask airway versus combitube use by navy SEAL and reconnaissance combat corpsman. J Trauma 46:927, 1999
25. Vezina D, Lessard MR, Bussières J et al: Complications associated with the use of the esophageal-tracheal combitube. Can J Anaesth 45:76, 1998
26. Klein H, Williamson M, Sue-Ling HM et al: Esophageal rupture associated with the use of the combitube. Anesth Analg 85:937, 1997
27. Gabbott DA, Baskett PJF: Management of the airway and ventilation during resuscitation. Br J Anaesth 79:159, 1997
28. Gabbott DA: The effect of single handed cricoid pressure on neck movement after application of manual in line neck stabilization. Anaesthesia 52:586, 1997
29. McNicholl BP: The golden hour and prehospital care. Injury 25:251, 1994
30. Asai T, Neil J, Stacey M: Ease of placement of the laryngeal mask during manual inline neck stabilization. Br J Anaesth 80:617, 1998
31. Choyce A, Avidan MS, Patel C et al: Comparison of laryngeal mask and intubating laryngeal mask insertion by the naive intubator. Br J Anaesth 84:103, 2000
32. Fukutome T, Amaha K, Nakazawa K et al: Tracheal intubation through the intubating laryngeal mask airway (LMA-Fastrach) in patients with difficult airways. Anaesth Intensive Care 26:387, 1998
33. Brimacombe J, Keller C: Cervical spine instability and the intubating laryngeal mask-a caution (letter). Anaesth Intensive Care 26:708, 1998
34. Weiskopf RB, Bogetz MS: Haemorrhage decreases the anesthetic requirement for ketamine and thiopentone in the pig. Br J Anaesth 57:1022, 1985
35. Fuchs-Buder T, Sparr HJ, Ziegenfust T: Thiopental or etomidate for rapid sequence induction with rocuronium? Br J Anaesth 80:504, 1998
36. Levy JH, Pitts M, Thanopoulous A et al: The effects of rapacuronium on histamine release and hemodynamics in adult patients undergoing general anesthesia. Anesth Analg 89:290, 1999
37. Leiman BC, Katz J, Butler BD: Mechanism of succinylcholine induced arrhythmias in hypoxic or hypoxic hypercarbic dogs. Anesth Analg 66:1292, 1987
38. Schwab TM, Greaves TH: Cardiac arrest as a possible sequela of critical airway management and intubation. Am J Emerg Med 16:609, 1998
39. Ibarra P, Capan LM, Wahlander S, Sutin KM: Difficult airway management in a patient with traumatic asphyxia. Anesth Analg 85:216, 1997
40. McAtamney D, O'Hare R, Hughes D et al: Evaluation of remifentanil for control of hemodynamic response to tracheal intubation. Anaesthesia 53:1209, 1998
41. Thompson JP, Hall AP, Russell J et al: Effect of remifentanil on the haemodynamic response to orotracheal intubation. Br J Anaesth 80:467, 1998
42. de Nadal M, Munar F, Poca MA et al: Cerebral hemodynamic effects of morphine and fentanyl in patients with severe head injury: Absence of correlation to cerebral autoregulation. Anesthesiology 92:11, 2000
43. Gardner AE, Dannemiller FJ, Dean D: Intracranial cerebrospinal fluid pressure in man during ketamine anesthesia. Anesth Analg 51:741, 1972
44. Shapiro HM, Wyte SR, Harris AB: Ketamine anesthesia in patients with intracranial pathology. Br J Anaesth 44:1200, 1972

45. Badrinath SK, Vazeery A, McCarthy RJ, Ivankovich AD: The effect of different methods of inducing anesthesia on intraocular pressure. Anesthesiology 65:431, 1986

46. Stirt JA, Grosslight KR, Bedford RF, Vollmer D: ''Defasciculation'' with metocurine prevents succinylcholine-induced increases in intracranial pressure. Anesthesiology 67:50, 1987

47. Heier T, Caldwell JE: Rapid tracheal intubation with large-dose rocuronium: A probability based approach. Anesth Analg 90:175, 2000

48. Hastings RH, Kelley SD: Neurologic deterioration associated with airway management in a cervical spine-injured patient. Anesthesiology 78:580, 1993

49. Muckart DJJ, Bhagwanjee S, van der Merwe R: Spinal cord injury as a result of endotracheal intubation in patients with undiagnosed cervical spine fractures. Anesthesiology 87:418, 1997

50. Hastings RH, Marks JD: Airway management for trauma patients with potential cervical spine injuries. Anesth Analg 73:471, 1991

51. Hastings RH, Vigil AC, Hanna R et al: Cervical spine movement during laryngoscopy with the Bullard, Macintosh and Miller laryngoscopes. Anesthesiology 82:859, 1995

52. Hastings RH, Wood PR: Head extension and laryngeal view during laryngoscopy with cervical spine stabilization maneuvers. Anesthesiology 80:825, 1994

53. Smith CE, Pinchak AB, Sidhu TS et al: Evaluation of tracheal intubation difficulty in patients with cervical spine immobilization: Fiberoptic (Wu Scope) versus conventional laryngoscopy. Anesthesiology 91:1253, 1999

54. Nolan JP, Wilson ME: Orotracheal intubation in patients with potential cervical spine injuries. Anaesthesia 48:630, 1993

55. Sandhu NS, Schaffer S, Capan LM, Turndorf H: Comparison of the WuScope and Macintosh #3 blade in normal and cervical spine stabilized patients. Anesthesiology 91:A480, 1999

56. Cicala RS, Kudsk KA, Butts A et al: Initial evaluation and management of upper airway injuries in trauma patients. J Clin Anesth 3:91, 1991

57. Capan LM: Airway management. In Capan LM, Miller SM, Turndorf H (eds): Trauma: Anesthesia and Intensive Care, p 43. Philadelphia, JB Lippincott, 1991

58. Dolin J, Scalea T, Mannor L et al: The management of gunshot wounds to the face. J Trauma 33:508, 1992

59. Kihtir T, Ivatury RR, Simon RJ et al: Early management of civilian gunshot wounds to the face. J Trauma 35:569, 1993

60. Capan LM, Miller SM, Glickman R: Management of facial injuries. In Capan LM, Miller SM, Turndorf H (eds): Trauma: Anesthesia and Intensive Care, p 383. Philadelphia, JB Lippincott, 1991

61. Davidson JSD, Bindsell DC: Cervical spine injury in patients with facial skeletal trauma. J Trauma 29:1276, 1989

62. Brandt KE, Burruss GL, Hickerson WL et al: The management of mid-face fractures with intracranial injury. J Trauma 31:15, 1991

63. Capan LM, Miller SM, Turndorf H: Management of neck injuries. In Capan LM, Miller SM, Turndorf H (eds): Trauma: Anesthesia and Intensive Care, p 409. Philadelphia, JB Lippincott, 1991

64. O'Connor PJ, Russell JD, Moriarty DC: Anesthetic implications of laryngeal trauma. Anesth Analg 87:1283, 1998

65. Deshpande S: Laryngotracheal separation after attempted hanging. Br J Anaesth 81:612, 1998

66. Yamazaki M, Sasaki R, Masuda A, Ito Y: Anesthetic management of complete tracheal disruption using percutaneous cardiopulmonary support system. Anesth Analg 86:998, 1998

67. Rollins RJ, Tocino I: Early radiographic signs of tracheal rupture. AJR Am J Roentgenol 148:695, 1987

68. Klumpe DH, Sang OHK, Wayman SA: A characteristic finding in unilateral complete bronchial transection. AJR Am J Roentgenol 110:704, 1970

69. Shearer VE, Giesecke AH: Airway management for patients with penetrating neck trauma: A retrospective study. Anesth Analg 77:1135, 1993

70. Cogbill TH, Landercasper J: Injury to the chest wall. In Moore EE, Mattox KL, Feliciano DV (eds): Trauma, 2nd ed, p 327. Norwalk, CT, Appleton and Lange, 1991

71. Shackford SR, Virgilio RW, Peters RM: Selective use of ventilator therapy in flail chest injury. J Thorac Cardiovasc Surg 81:194, 1981

72. Richardson JD, Adams L, Flint LM: Selective management of flail chest and pulmonary contusion. Ann Surg 196:481, 1982

73. Wisner DH: A stepwise logistic regression analysis of factors affecting morbidity and mortality after trauma: Effect of epidural analgesia. J Trauma 30:799, 1990

74. Wu CL, Jani ND, Perkins FM, Barquist E: Thoracic epidural analgesia versus intravenous patient-controlled analgesia for the treatment of rib fracture pain after motor vehicle crash. J Trauma 47:564, 1999

75. Ho AM-H, Ling E: Systemic air embolism after lung trauma. Anesthesiology 90:564, 1999

76. Little RA: Heart rate changes after haemorrhage and injury. J Trauma 29:903, 1988

77. Bernards CM, Cullen BF, Powers KM, Kern C: Effect of chronic cocaine administration on the hemodynamic response to acute hemorrhage in awake sheep. J Trauma 42:42, 1997

78. Demetriades D, Chan LS, Bhasin P et al: Relative bradycardia in patients with traumatic hypotension. J Trauma 45:534, 1998

79. Rady MY: Possible mechanisms for the interaction of peripheral somatic nerve stimulation, tissue injury, and hemorrhage in the pathophysiology of traumatic shock. Anesth Analg 78:761, 1994

80. Mackway-Jones K, Foex BA, Kirkman E, Little RA: Modification of the cardiovascular response to hemorrhage by somatic afferent nerve stimulation with special reference to gut and skeletal muscle blood flow. J Trauma 47:481, 1999

81. American College of Surgeons Committee on Trauma: Shock. In American College of Surgeons (ed): Advanced Trauma Life Support Instructor Manual, p 97. Chicago, American College of Surgeons, 1997

82. Nacht A: The use of blood products in shock: Crit Care Clin 8:255, 1992

83. Bickell WH, Wall MJ, Pepe PE et al: Immediate versus delayed fluid resuscitation for hypotensive patients with penetrating torso injuries. N Engl J Med 331:1105, 1994

84. Blow O, Magliore L, Claridge JA et al: The golden hour and the silver day: Detection and correction of occult hypoperfusion within 24 hours improves outcome from major trauma. J Trauma 47:964, 1999

85. Porter JM, Ivatury RR: In search of the optimal end points of resuscitation in trauma patients: A review. J Trauma 44:908, 1998

86. Neufeld JDG, Marx JA, Moore EE, Light AI: Comparison of intraosseous, central, and peripheral routes of crystalloid infusion for resuscitation of hemorrhagic shock in a swine model. J Trauma 34:422, 1993

87. Pina J, Morujao N, Castro-Tavares J: Internal jugular catheterization: Blood reflux is not a reliable sign in patients with thoracic trauma. Anaesthesia 47:1275, 1992

88. Getzen LC, Pollack EW: Short-term femoral vein catheterization: A safe alternative for venous access. Am J Surg 138:875, 1979

89. Wiedman JE, Rignault DP: Civilian versus military trauma dogma: Who do you trust? Milit Med 164:256, 1999

90. Mucha PJ, Welch TJ: Hemorrhage in major pelvic fractures. Surg Clin North Am 68:757, 1988

91. Luna GK, Pavlin EG, Kirkman T et al: Hemodynamic effects of external cardiac massage in trauma shock. J Trauma 29:1430, 1989

92. Durham LA, Richardson RJ, Wall MJ et al: Emergency center thoracotomy: Impact of prehospital resuscitation. J Trauma 32:775, 1992

93. Millham FH, Gridlinger GA: Survival determinants in patients undergoing emergency room thoracotomy for penetrating chest injury. J Trauma 34:332, 1993

94. Esposito TS, Jurkovich GJ, Rice CL et al: Reappraisal of emergency room thoracotomy in a changing environment. J Trauma 31:881, 1991

95. McMahon CG, Yates DW, Campbell FM et al: Unexpected contribution of moderate traumatic brain injury to death after major trauma. J Trauma 47:891, 1999

96. Kraus JF, McArthur DL: Neuroepidemiology: Epidemiologic aspects of brain injury. Neurol Clin 14:435, 1996

97. Shackford SR, Mackersie RC, Davis JW et al: Epidemiology and pathology of traumatic deaths occurring at a level I trauma center in a regionalized system: The importance of secondary brain injury. J Trauma 29:1392, 1989

98. Chesnut RM, Marshall LF, Klauber MR et al: The role of secondary brain injury in determining outcome from severe head injury. J Trauma 34:216, 1993

99. Chesnut RM: Avoidance of hypotension: Conditio sine qua non of successful head injury management. J Trauma 42(suppl):4S, 1997

100. Miller JD, Becker DP: Secondary insults to the injured brain. J R Coll Surg Edinb 27:292, 1982

101. American College of Surgeons Committee on Trauma: Trauma center descriptions and their role in trauma system. In American

College of Surgeons (ed): Resources for Optimal Care of the Injured, Appendix B, p 105. Chicago, American College of Surgeons, 1999

102. Winchell RJ, Hoyt DB: Endotracheal intubation in the field improves survival in patients with severe head injury. Arch Surg 132:592, 1997

103. Teasdale G, Jennett B: Assessment of coma and impaired consciousness: A practical scale. Lancet 2:81, 1974

104. American College of Surgeons Committee on Trauma: Head trauma. In American College of Surgeons (ed): Advanced Trauma Life Support Instructor Manual, p 228. Chicago, American College of Surgeons, 1999

105. Miller SM: Management of central nervous system injuries. In Capan LM, Miller SM, Turndorf H (eds): Trauma: Anesthesia and Intensive Care, p 321. Philadelphia, JB Lippincott, 1991

106. Yokota H, Kurokawa A, Otsuka T et al: Significance of magnetic resonance imaging in acute head injury. J Trauma 31:351, 1991

107. Miller JD: Assessing patients with head injury. Br J Surg 77:241, 1990

108. Shackford SR, Wold SL, Ross SE et al: The clinical utility of computed tomographic scanning and neurologic examination in the management of patients with minor injuries. J Trauma 33:385, 1992

109. Lam AM, Winn HR, Cullen BF, Sundling N: Hyperglycemia and neurological outcome in patients with head injury. J Neurosurg 75:545, 1991

110. Chesnut RM: The management of severe traumatic brain injury. Emerg Med Clin North Am 15:581, 1997

111. Stocchetti N, Rossi S, Buzzi F et al: Intracranial hypertension in head injury: Management and results. Intensive Care Med 25:371, 1999

112. Prough DS, Lang J: Therapy of patients with head injuries: Key parameters for management. J Trauma 42(suppl): 10S, 1997

113. Unterberg A: Severe head injury: Improvement of outcome. Intensive Care Med 25:348, 1999

114. Wald SL: Advances in the early management of patients with head injury. Surg Clin North Am 75:225, 1995

115. Feldman Z, Robertson CS: Monitoring of cerebral hemodynamics with jugular bulb catheters. Crit Care Clin 13:51, 1997

116. Scheinberg M, Kanter MJ, Robertson CS et al: Continuous monitoring of jugular venous oxygen saturation in head-injured patients. J Neurosurg 76:212, 1992

117. Cruz J: Jugular venous oxygen saturation monitoring. J Neurosurg 77:162, 1992

118. Marion DW, Darby J, Yonas H: Acute regional cerebral blood flow changes caused by severe injuries. J Neurosurg 74:407, 1991

119. Bouma GJ, Muizelaar P, Choi SC et al: Cerebral circulation and metabolism after severe traumatic brain injury: The elusive role of ischemia. J Neurosurg 75:685, 1991

120. Yundt KD, Diringer MN: The use of hyperventilation and its impact on cerebral ischemia in the treatment of traumatic brain injury. Crit Care Clin 13:163, 1997

121. Zhuang J, Schmoker JD, Shackford SR, Pietropaol JA: Focal brain injury results in severe cerebral ischemia despite maintenance of cerebral perfusion pressure. J Trauma 33:83, 1992

122. Ward JD, Choi S, Marmarou A et al: Effect of prophylactic hyperventilation on outcome in patients with severe head injury. In Hoff JT, Betz AL (eds): Intracranial Pressure, Vol II, p 630. Berlin, Springer-Verlag, 1989

123. Muizelaar JP, Marmarou A, Ward JD et al: Adverse effect of prolonged hyperventilation in patients with severe head injury: A randomized clinical trial. J Neurosurg 75:731, 1991

124. Wolf AL, Levi L, Marmarou A et al: Effect of THAM upon outcome in severe head injury: A randomized prospective clinical trial. J Neurosurg 78:54, 1993

125. Chan K-H, Dearden NM, Miller JD et al: Multimodality monitoring as a guide to treatment of intracranial hypertension after severe brain injury. Neurosurgery 32:547, 1993

126. Paczynski RP: Osmotherapy: Basic concepts and controversies. Crit Care Clin 13:105, 1997

127. Huff JS: Acute mannitol intoxication in a patient with normal renal function. Am J Emerg Med 8:338, 1990

128. Ducey JP, Mozingo DW, Lamiell JM et al: A comparison of the cerebral and cardiovascular effects of complete resuscitation with isotonic and hypertonic saline, hetastarch, and whole blood following hemorrhage. J Trauma 29:1510, 1989

129. Gunnar W, Jonasson O, Merlotti G et al: Head injury and hemorrhagic shock: Studies of the blood brain barrier and intracranial pressure after resuscitation with normal saline solution, 3% saline solution, and dextran-40. Surgery 103:398, 1988

130. Fisher B, Thomas D, Peterson B: Hypertonic saline lowers raised intracranial pressure in children after trauma. J Neurosurg Anesthesiol 4:4, 1992

131. Freshman SP, Battistella FD, Mateucci M, Wisner DH: Hypertonic saline (7.5%) versus mannitol: A comparison for treatment of acute head injuries. J Trauma 35:344, 1993

132. Gemma M, Cozzi S, Tommassino C et al: 7.5% hypertonic saline versus 20% mannitol during elective neurosurgical supratentorial procedures. J Neurosurg Anesthesiol 9:329, 1997

133. Hartl R, Ghajar J, Hochleuthner H et al: Hypertonic/hyperoncotic saline reliably reduces ICP in severely head-injured patients with intracranial hypertension. Acta Neurochir Suppl (Wien) 70:126, 1997

134. Hess JR, Dubick MA, Summary JJ et al: The effects of 7.5% NaCL/ 6% dextran 70 on coagulation and platelet aggregation in humans. J Trauma 32:40, 1992

135. Kaieda R, Todd MM, Cook LN, Warner DS: Acute effects of changing plasma osmolality and colloid oncotic pressure on the formation of brain edema after cryogenic injury. Neurosurgery 24:671, 1989

136. Eker C, Asgeirsson B, Gründe P-O et al: Improved outcome after severe head injury with a new therapy based on principles for brain volume regulation and preserved microcirculation. Crit Care Med 26:1881, 1998

137. Cruz J: The first decade of continuous monitoring of jugular bulb oxyhemoglobin saturation: Management strategies and clinical outcome. Crit Care Med 26:344, 1998

138. Jennett B, Teasdale G, Galbraith S: Severe head injuries in three countries. J Neurol Neurosurg Psychiatry 40:291, 1977

139. Miller JD, Butterworth JF, Gudeman SK et al: Further experience in the management of severe head injury. J Neurosurg 54:289, 1981

140. Asgeirsson B, Gründe P-O, Nordsröm C-H et al: Effects of hypotensive treatment with α_2-agonist and β_1-antagonist on cerebral haemodynamics in severely head injured patients. Acta Anaesthesiol Scand 39:347, 1995

141. Jahr J, Ekelund U, Gründe P-O: In vivo effects of prostacyclin on segmental vascular resistances, on myogenic activity, and on capillary fluid exchange in cat skeletal muscle. Crit Care Med 23:523, 1995

142. Grossman MD, Eilly PM, Gillett T, Gillett D: National survey of the incidence of cervical spine injury and approach to cervical spinal clearance in U.S. trauma centers. J Trauma 47:684, 1999

143. Pasquale M, Fabian T, EAST Ad Hoc Committee on Practice Management Guideline Development: Practice management guidelines for trauma from the Eastern Association for the Surgery of Trauma. J Trauma 44:941, 1998

144. American College of Surgeons Committee on Trauma: Spine and spinal cord trauma. In American College of Surgeons (ed): Advanced Trauma Life Support Course Instructor Manual, p 263. Chicago, American College of Surgeons, 1997

145. Gonzalez RP, Fried PO, Bukhalo M et al: Role of clinical examination in screening for blunt cervical spine injury. J Am Coll Surg 189:152, 1999

146. Sommer RM, Bauer RD, Errico TJ: Cervical spine injuries. In Capan LM, Miller SM, Turndorf H (eds): Trauma, Anesthesia and Intensive Care, p 447. Philadelphia, JB Lippincott, 1991

147. Atkinson PP, Atkinson JL: Spinal shock. Mayo Clin Proc 71:384, 1996

148. Woodring JH, Lee C: Limitations of cervical radiography in the evaluation of acute cervical trauma. J Trauma 34:32, 1993

149. Berne JD, Velmahos GC, El-Tawil Q et al: Value of complete cervical helical computed tomographic scanning in identifying cervical spine injury in the unevaluable blunt trauma patient with multiple injuries: A prospective study. J Trauma 47:896, 1999

150. Bernstein RL, Rosenberg AD: Trauma. In Bernstein RL, Rosenberg AD (eds): Manual of Orthopedic Anesthesia and Related Pain Syndromes, p 66. New York, Churchill Livingstone, 1993

151. Amar AP, Levy ML: Pathogenesis and pharmacological strategies for mitigating secondary damage in acute spinal cord injury. Neurosurgery 44:1027, 1999

152. Vale FL, Burns J, Jackson AB, Hadley MN: Combined medical and surgical treatment after acute spinal cord injury: Results of a pilot study to assess the merits of aggressive medical resuscitation and blood pressure management. J Neurosurg 87:239, 1997

153. Bracken MB, Shepard MJ, Collins WFJ et al: Methylprednisolone or naloxone treatment after acute spinal cord injury: Results of the Second National Acute Spinal Cord Injury Study. J Neurosurg 76:23, 1992

154. Bracken MB, Shepard MJ, Collins WF et al: A randomized, controlled trial of methylprednisolone or naloxone in the treatment of acute spinal cord injury: Results of Second National Spinal Cord Injury Study. N Engl J Med 322:1405, 1990

155. Bracken MB, Shepard MJ, Holford TR et al: Methylprednisolone or tirilazad mesylate after acute spinal cord injury: Results of the third National Acute Spinal Cord Injury randomized controlled trial. J Neurosurg 89:699, 1998

156. Nesathurai S: Revisiting the NASCIS 2 and NASCIS 3 trials. J Trauma 45:1088, 1998

157. Poynton AR, O'Farrell DA, Shannon F et al: An evaluation of the factors affecting neurological recovery following spinal cord injury. Injury 28:545, 1997

158. Levy ML, Gans W, Wijesenghe HS et al: Use of methylprednisolone as an adjunct in the management of patients with penetrating spinal cord injury: Outcome analysis. Neurosurgery 39:1141, 1996

159. Petitjean ME, Pointillart V, Dixmerias F et al: Traitement medicamenteux de la lesion medullaire traumatique au stade aigu. Ann Fr Anesth Reanim 17:114, 1998

160. Gerndt SJ, Rodriguez JL, Pawlik JW et al: Consequences of high-dose steroid therapy for acute spinal cord injury. J Trauma 42:279, 1997

161. Roth EJ, Lu A, Primack S et al: Ventilatory function in cervical and high thoracic spinal cord injury: Relationship to level of injury and tone. Am J Phys Med Rehabil 76:262, 1997

162. Theodore J, Robin ED: Pathogenesis of neurogenic pulmonary edema. Lancet 2:749, 1975

163. Mackenzie CF, Shin B, Krishnaprasad D et al: Assessment of cardiac and respiratory function during surgery on patients with acute quadriplegia. J Neurosurg 62:843, 1985

164. Gronert GA, Theye RA: Pathophysiology of hyperkalemia induced by succinylcholine. Anesthesiology 43:89, 1975

165. Demetriades D, Asensio JA, Velmahos G, Thal E: Complex problems in penetrating neck trauma. Surg Clin North Am 76:661, 1996

166. Fabian TC, Patton JH, Croce MA et al: Blunt carotid injury: Importance of early diagnosis and anticoagulant therapy. Ann Surg 223:513, 1996

167. Biffl WL, Moore EE, Ryu RK et al: The unrecognized epidemic of blunt carotid arterial injuries: Early diagnosis improves neurologic outcome. Ann Surg 228:462, 1998

168. Jewett BS, Shockley WW, Rutledge R: External laryngeal trauma: analysis of 392 patients. Arch Otolaryngol Head Neck Surg 125:877, 1999

169. Lee RB, Bass SM, Morris JA, Mackenzie EJ: Three or more rib fractures as an indicator for transfer to a level I trauma center. J Trauma 30:689, 1990

170. Philips EH, Rogers WF, Gaspar MR: First rib fracture: Incidence of vascular injury and indications for angiography. Surgery 89:42, 1981

171. Kirsh MM: Acute thoracic injuries. In Siegel J (ed): Trauma, Emergency Surgery and Critical Care, p 863. New York, Churchill-Livingstone, 1987

172. McGinnis M, Denton JR: Fractures of the scapula: A retrospective study of 40 fractured scapulae. J Trauma 29:1488, 1989

173. Hills MW, Delfrado AM, Deane SA: Sternal fractures: Associated injuries and management. J Trauma 35:55, 1993

174. Brookes JG, Dunn RJ, Rogers IR: Sternal fractures: A retrospective analysis of 272 cases. J Trauma 35:46, 1993

175. Tocino IM, Miller MH, Fairfax WR: Distribution of pneumothorax in the supine and semirecumbent critically ill adult. AJR Am J Roentgenol 144:901, 1985

176. Brasel KJ, Stafford RE, Weigelt JA et al: Treatment of occult pneumothoraces from blunt trauma. J Trauma 46:987, 1999

177. Enderson BL, Abdalla R, Frame SB et al: Tube thoracostomy for occult pneumothorax: A prospective randomized study of its use. J Trauma 35:726, 1993

178. Carrillo EH, Heniford BT, Etoch SW et al: Video assisted thoracic surgery in trauma patients. J Am Coll Surg 184:316, 1997

179. Mineo TC, Ambrogi V, Cristino B et al: Changing indications for thoracotomy in blunt chest trauma after the advent of videothoracoscopy. J Trauma 47:1088, 1999

180. Davis KA, Fabian TC, Croce MA, Proctor KG: Prostanoids: Early mediators in the secondary injury that develops after unilateral pulmonary contusion. J Trauma 46:824, 1999

181. Tyburski JG, Collinge JD, Wilson RF, Eachempati SR: Pulmonary contusions: Quantifying the lesions on chest x-ray films and the factors affecting prognosis. J Trauma 46:833, 1999

182. Moomey CB, Fabian TC, Croce MA et al: Determinants of myocardial performance after blunt chest trauma. J Trauma 45:988, 1998

183. Rozycki GS, Feliciano DV, Ochsner G et al: The role of ultrasound in patients with possible penetrating cardiac wounds: A prospective multicenter study. J Trauma 46:543, 1999

184. Porembka DT, Johnson DJ, Hoyt BD et al: Penetrating cardiac trauma: A perioperative role for transesophageal echocardiography. Anesth Analg 77:1275, 1993

185. Helling TS, Duke P, Beggs CW, Crouse LJ: A prospective evaluation of 68 patients suffering blunt chest trauma for evidence of cardiac injury. J Trauma 29:961, 1989

186. Reif J, Prager RL: Selective monitoring of patients with suspected blunt cardiac injury. Ann Thorac Surg 50:530, 1990

187. Fabian TC, Cicala RS, Croce MA et al: A prospective evaluation of myocardial contusion: correlation of significant arrhythmias and cardiac output with CPK-MB measurements. J Trauma 31:653, 1991

188. Lampl L, Bock KH: Myocardial contusion in multisystem trauma: Diagnostic delimitation. Br J Anaesth 74:A418, 1995

189. Mirvis SE, Shanmuganathan K, Buell J, Rodriguez A: Use of spiral computed tomography for the assessment of blunt trauma patients with potential aortic injury. J Trauma 45:922, 1998

190. Patel NH, Stephens KE, Mirvis SE et al: Imaging of acute thoracic aortic injury due to blunt trauma. Radiology 209:335, 1998

191. Wahl WL, Michaels AJ, Wang SC et al: Blunt thoracic aortic injury. J Trauma 47:254, 1999

192. Symbas PN, Vlasis SE, Hatcher CRJ: Blunt and penetrating diaphragmatic injuries with or without herniation of organs into the chest. Ann Thorac Surg 42:158, 1986

193. Kearney PA, Vahey T, Burney RE et al: Computed tomography and diagnostic peritoneal lavage in blunt abdominal trauma. Arch Surg 124:344, 1989

194. Villavicencio RT, Aucar JA: Analysis of laparoscopy in trauma. J Am Coll Surg 189:11, 1999

195. Ginzburg E, Carillo EH, Kopelman T et al: The role of computed tomography in selective management of gunshot wounds to the abdomen and flank. J Trauma 45:1005, 1998

196. Boulanger BR, McLellan BA, Brenneman FD et al: Prospective evidence of the superiority of a sonography based algorithm in the assessment of blunt abdominal injury. J Trauma 47:632, 1999

197. FAST Consensus Conference Committee: Focused assessment with sonography for trauma (FAST): Results from an international consensus conference. J Trauma 46:466, 1999

198. Hanneman PL, Marx JA, Moore EE et al: Diagnostic peritoneal lavage: Accuracy in predicting necessary laparotomy following blunt and penetrating trauma. J Trauma 30:1345, 1995

199. McAnena OJ, Marx JA, Moore EE: Peritoneal lavage enzyme determinations following blunt and penetrating abdominal trauma. J Trauma 31:1161, 1991

200. Meyer DM, Thal ER, Weigelt JA, Redman HC: Evaluation of computed tomography and diagnostic peritoneal lavage in blunt abdominal trauma. J Trauma 29:1168, 1989

201. Harris HW, Morabito DJ, Mackersie RC et al: Leukocytosis and free fluid are important indicators of isolated intestinal injury after blunt trauma. J Trauma 46:656, 1999

202. Patel KP, Capan LM, Grant GJ, Miller SM: Musculoskeletal injuries. In Capan LM, Miller SM, Turndorf H (eds): Trauma: Anesthesia and Intensive Care, p 511. Philadelphia, JB Lippincott, 1991

203. Cryer HM, Miller FB, Evers BM et al: Pelvic fracture classification: Correlation with hemorrhage. J Trauma 28:973, 1988

204. Seibel R, La Duca J, Hassett JM et al: Blunt multiple trauma (ISS 36), femur traction, and the pulmonary failure-septic state. Ann Surg 202:283, 1985

205. Dellinger EP, Miller SD, Wertz MJ et al: Risk of infection after open fracture of the arm or leg. Arch Surg 123:1320, 1988

206. MacLennan N, Heimbach DM, Cullen BF: Anesthesia for major thermal injury. Anesthesiology 89:749, 1998

207. Haponik EF, Meyers DA, Munster AM et al: Acute upper airway injury in burn patients: Serial changes of flow volume curves and nasopharyngoscopy. American Review of Respiratory Disease 135:360, 1987

208. Smith DL, Cairns BA, Ramadan F et al: Effect of inhalation injury,

burn size and age on mortality: A study of 1447 consecutive burn patients. J Trauma 37:655, 1994

209. Muehlberger T, Kunar D, Munster A, Couch M: Efficacy of fiberoptic laryngoscopy in the diagnosis of inhalation injuries. Arch Otolaryngol Head Neck Surg 124:1003, 1998

210. Jones WG, Madden M, Finkelstein J et al: Tracheostomies in burn patients. Ann Surg 209:471, 1989

211. Venus B, Matsuda C, Copozio JB et al: Prophylactic intubation and continuous positive airway pressure in the management of inhalation injury in burn patients. Crit Care Med 9:519, 1981

212. Masanes MJ, Legendre C, Lioret N et al: Fiberoptic bronchoscopy for the early diagnosis of subglottic inhalation injury: Comparative value in the assessment of prognosis. J Trauma 36:59, 1994

213. Peitzman AB, Shires GT, Teixidor HS et al: Smoke inhalation injury: Evaluation of radiographic manifestations and pulmonary dysfunction. J Trauma 29:1232, 1989

214. Vegfors M, Lennmarken C: Carboxyhemoglobinaemia and pulse oximetry. Br J Anaesth 66:625, 1991

215. Haney M, Tait AR, Tremper KK: Effect of carboxyhemoglobin on the accuracy of mixed venous oximetry monitors in dogs. Crit Care Med 22:1181, 1994

216. Welch GW: Care of the patient with thermal injury. In Capan LM, Miller SM, Turndorf H (eds): Trauma: Anesthesia and Intensive Care, p 629. Philadelphia, JB Lippincott, 1991

217. Van Hoesen KB, Camporesi EM, Moon RE et al: Should hyperbaric oxygen be used to treat the pregnant patient for acute carbon monoxide poisoning? A case report and literature review. JAMA 261:1039, 1989

218. Baud FJ, Barriot P, Toffis V et al: Elevated blood cyanide concentrations in victims of smoke inhalation. N Engl J Med 325:1761, 1991

219. Silverman SH, Purdue GF, Hunt JL, Bost RO: Cyanide toxicity in burned patients. J Trauma 28:171, 1988

220. Tung A, Lynch J, McDade WA: A new biological assay for measuring cyanide in blood. Anesth Analg 85:1045, 1997

221. Breen PH, Isserles SA, Westley J et al: Combined carbon monoxide and cyanide poisoning: A place for treatment? Anesth Analg 80:671, 1995

222. Kulig K: Cyanide antidotes and fire toxicology (editorial). N Engl J Med 325:1801, 1991

223. Warden GD: Burn shock resuscitation. World J Surg 16:16, 1992

224. Lalonde C, Picard L, Youn YK et al: Increased early post burn fluid requirements and oxygen demands are predictive of the degree of airways injury by smoke inhalation. J Trauma 38:175, 1995

225. Huang PP, Stucky FS, Dimick AR et al: Hypertonic sodium resuscitation is associated with renal failure and death. Ann Surg 221:543, 1995

226. Mann R, Heimbach DM, Engrav LH, Foy H: Changes in transfusion practices in burn patients. J Trauma 37:220, 1994

227. Dries DJ, Waxman K: Adequate resuscitation of burn patients may not be measured by urine output and vital signs. Crit Care Med 19:327, 1991

228. Bernard F, Guegniaud PY, Bouchard C et al: Hemodynamic parameters in the severely burnt patient during the first 72 hours. Ann Fr Anesth Reanim 11:623, 1992

229. Morris JR, MacKenzie EJ, Edelstein SL: The effect of preexisting conditions on mortality in trauma patients. JAMA 263:1942, 1990

230. Madan AK, Yu K, Beech DJ: Alcohol and drug use in victims of life threatening trauma. J Trauma 47:568, 1999

231. Soderstrom C, Smith GS, Dischinger PC et al: Psychoactive substance use disorders among seriously injured trauma patients. JAMA 277:1769, 1997

232. Knopp R, Claypool R, Leonardi D: Use of the tilt test in measuring acute blood loss. Ann Emerg Med 9:72, 1980

233. McGee S, Abernethy WB, Simel DL: Is this patient hypovolemic? JAMA 281:1022, 1999

234. Capan LM, Gottlieb G, Rosenberg A: General principles of anesthesia for major acute trauma. In Capan LM, Miller SM, Turndorf H (eds): Trauma: Anesthesia and Intensive Care, p 259. Philadelphia, JB Lippincott, 1991

235. Rooke GA, Schwid HA, Shapira Y: The effect of graded hemorrhage and intravascular volume replacement on systolic pressure variation in humans during mechanical and spontaneous ventilation. Anesth Analg 80:925, 1995

236. Chang MC, Blinman TA, Rutherford EJ et al: Preload assessment in trauma patients during large-volume shock resuscitation. Arch Surg 131:728, 1996

237. Cheatham ML, Safcsak K, Block EF et al: Preload assessment in patients with an open abdomen. J Trauma 46:16, 1999

238. Cahalan MK, Litt L, Botvinick EH et al: Advances in noninvasive cardiovascular imaging: Implications for the anesthesiologist. Anesthesiology 66:356, 1987

239. Capan LM, Miller SM, Patel KP: Fat embolism. Anesthesiol Clin North Am 11:25, 1993

240. Daniel WG, Erbel R, Kasper W et al: Safety of transesophageal echocardiography: A multicenter survey of 10,419 examinations. Circulation 83:817, 1991

241. Shippy CR, Appel PL, Shoemaker WC: Reliability of clinical monitoring to assess blood volume in critically ill patients. Crit Care Med 12:107, 1984

242. Haruna M, Kumon K, Yahagi N et al: Blood volume measurement at the bedside using ICG pulse spectrophotometry. Anesthesiology 89:1322, 1998

243. Mizock BA, Falk JL: Lactic acidosis in critical illness. Crit Care Med 20:80, 1992

244. Abramson D, Scalea TM, Hitchcock R et al: Lactate clearance and survival following injury. J Trauma 35:584, 1993

245. Kincaid EH, Miller PR, Meredith JW et al: Elevated arterial base deficit in trauma patients: A marker of impaired oxygen utilization. J Am Coll Surg 187:384, 1998

246. Davis JW, Shackford SR, Mackersie RC, Hoyt DB: Base deficit as a guide to volume resuscitation. J Trauma 28:1464, 1988

247. Rutherford EJ, Morris JA, Reed GW, Hall KS: Base deficit stratifies mortality and determines therapy. J Trauma 33:417, 1992

248. Kolkman JJ, Otte JA, Groenveld ABJ: Gastrointestinal luminal PCO_2 tonometry: An update on physiology, methodology and clinical applications. Br J Anaesth 84:74, 2000

249. Knichwitz G, Rötker J, Brüssel T et al: A new method for continuous intramucosal PCO_2 measurement in the gastrointestinal tract. Anesth Analg 83:6, 1996

250. Weil MH, Nakagawa Y, Tang W et al: Sublingual capnometry: A new noninvasive measurement for diagnosis and quantitation of severity of circulatory shock. Crit Care Med 27:1225, 1999

251. Harrigan C, Lucas CE, Ledgerwood AM: The effect of hemorrhagic shock on the clotting cascade in injured patients. J Trauma 29:1416, 1989

252. Ordog GJ, Wasserberger J, Balasubramanian S: Coagulation abnormalities in traumatic shock. Ann Emerg Med 14:650, 1985

253. Mallett SV, Cox JA: Thromboelastography. Br J Anaesth 69:307, 1992

254. Johnston TD, Chen Y, Reed RL: Functional equivalence of hypothermia to specific clotting factor deficiencies. J Trauma 37:413, 1994

255. Gubler KD, Gentilello LM, Hassantash SA, Maier RV: The impact of hypothermia on dilutional coagulopathy. J Trauma 36:847, 1994

256. Douning L, Bierig P, Fang X et al: Temperature effect on thromboelastograph: A comparative study. Anesth Analg 80:S107, 1995

257. Ciavarella D, Reed RL, Counts RB et al: Clotting factor levels and the risk of diffuse microvascular bleeding in the massively transfused patient. Br J Haematol 67:365, 1987

258. Miller RD: Coagulation and packed red blood cell transfusions (editorial). Anesth Analg 80:215, 1995

259. Murray DJ, Olsen J, Strauss R, Tinker JH: Coagulation changes during packed red cell replacement of major blood loss. Anesthesiology 69:839, 1988

260. Murphy WG, Davies MJ, Eduardo A: The haemostatic response to surgery and trauma. Br J Anaesth 70:205, 1993

261. Wauquier A, Hermans C, Van den Broeck W et al: Resuscitative drug effects in hypovolemic hypotensive animals. Part 1: Comparative cardiovascular effects of an infusion of saline, etomidate, thiopental, or pentobarbital in hypovolemic dogs. Janssen Research Products, 1981

262. Gauss A, Heinrich H, Wilder-Smith OHG: Echocardiographic assessment of the haemodynamic effects of propofol: A comparison with etomidate and thiopentone. Anaesthesia 46:99, 1991

263. Adams P, Gelman S, Reves JG et al: Midazolam pharmacodynamics and pharmacokinetics during acute hypovolemia. Anesthesiology 63:140, 1985

264. Lippmann M, Appel PL, Mok MS et al: Sequential cardiorespiratory patterns of anesthetic induction with ketamine in critically ill patients. Crit Care Med 11:730, 1983

265. Theye RA, Perry LB, Brzica SM: Influence of anesthetic agent on response to hemorrhagic hypotension. Anesthesiology 40:32, 1974

266. Ebert TJ, Kampine JP: Nitrous oxide augments sympathetic out-

flow: Direct evidence from human peroneal nerve recordings. Anesth Analg 69:444, 1989

267. Priano LL, Bernards C, Marrone B: Effect of anesthetic induction agents on cardiovascular neuroregulation in dogs. Anesth Analg 68:344, 1989

268. Ebert TJ, Kanitz DD, Kampine JP: Inhibition of sympathetic neural outflow during thiopental anesthesia in humans. Anesth Analg 71:319, 1990

269. Ebert TJ, Muzi M, Berens R et al: Sympathetic responses to induction of anesthesia in humans with propofol or etomidate. Anesthesiology 76:725, 1992

270. Takeshima R, Dohi S: Comparison of arterial baroreflex function in humans anesthetized with enflurane or isoflurane. Anesth Analg 69:284, 1989

271. Flacke JW, Davis LJ, Flacke WE et al: Effects of fentanyl and diazepam in dogs deprived of autonomic tone. Anesth Analg 64:1053, 1985

272. Egar TD, Kuramkote S, Gong G et al: Fentanyl pharmacokinetics in hemorrhagic shock: A porcine model. Anesthesiology 91:156, 1999

273. Bogetz MS, Katz JA: Recall of surgery for major trauma. Anesthesiology 61:6, 1984

274. Lubke GH, Kerssens C, Phaf H et al: Dependence of explicit and implicit memory on hypnotic state in trauma patients. Anesthesiology 90:670, 1999

275. Doenicke A, Lorenz W, Bregl et al: Histamine release after intravenous application of short acting hypnotics: A comparison of etomidate, althesin, and propanidid. Br J Anaesth 45:1097, 1973

276. Brown DL: Anesthetic agents in trauma surgery: Are there differences? Int Anesthesiol Clin 25:75, 1987

277. Weiskopf RB, Bogetz MS, Roizen MF, Reid IA: Cardiovascular and metabolic sequelae of inducing anesthesia with ketamine or thiopental in hypovolemic swine. Anesthesiology 60:214, 1984

278. Weiskopf RB, Bogetz MS: Cardiovascular actions of nitrous oxide or halothane in hypovolemic swine. Anesthesiology 63:509, 1985

279. Warltier DC, Pagel PS: Cardiovascular and respiratory actions of desflurane: Is desflurane different from isoflurane? Anesth Analg 75:S17, 1992

280. Gopinath SP, Cormio M, Ziegler J et al: Intraoperative jugular desaturation during surgery for traumatic intracranial hematomas. Anesth Analg 83:1014, 1996

281. Shapiro HM: Intracranial hypertension: Therapeutic and anesthetic considerations. Anesthesiology 43:445, 1975

282. Reves JG, Fragen RJ, Vinik R, Greenblatt DJ: Midazolam: Pharmacology and uses. Anesthesiology 62:310, 1985

283. Modica PA, Tempelhoff R: Intracranial pressure during induction of anesthesia and tracheal intubation with etomidate-induced EEG burst suppression. Can J Anaesth 39:236, 1992

284. Smith I, White PF, Nathanson M, Gouldson R: Propofol: An update on its clinical use. Anesthesiology 81:1005, 1994

285. Artru AA: Dose-related changes in the rate of cerebrospinal fluid formation and resistance to reabsorption of cerebrospinal fluid following administration of thiopental, midazolam and etomidate in dogs. Anesthesiology 69:541, 1988

286. Berry JM, Merin RG: Etomidate myoclonus and the open globe. Anesth Analg 69:256, 1989

287. Libonati MM, Leahy MJ, Ellison N: The use of succinylcholine in open eye surgery. Anesthesiology 62:637, 1985

288. Zimmerman AA, Funk K, Tidwell JL: Propofol and alfentanil prevent the increase in intraocular pressure caused by succinylcholine and endotracheal intubation during a rapid sequence induction of anesthesia. Anesth Analg 83:814, 1996

289. Magorian T, Flannery KB, Miller RD: Comparison of rocuronium, succinylcholine, and vecuronium for rapid-sequence induction of anesthesia in adult patients. Anesthesiology 79:913, 1993

290. Savarese JJ, Ali HH, Basta SJ et al: The clinical neuromuscular pharmacology of mivacurium chloride (BW B 1090 U). Anesthesiology 68:723, 1988

291. Newberg LA, Milde JH, Michenfelder JD: The cerebral metabolic effects of isoflurane at and above concentrations that suppress cortical electrical activity. Anesthesiology 59:23, 1983

292. Eger EI II: New inhaled anesthetics. Anesthesiology 80:906, 1994

293. Grosslight K, Coleman A, Bedford RF: Isoflurane anesthesia: Risk factors for increase in intracranial pressure. Anesthesiology 63:533, 1985

294. Thiagarajan A, Goverdhan P, Chari P, Somasunderam K: The effect of hyperventilation and hyperoxia on cerebral venous oxygen saturation in patients with traumatic brain injury. Anesth Analg 87:850, 1998

295. Field LM, Dorrance DE, Krzeminska EK, Barsoum LZ: Effect of nitrous oxide on cerebral blood flow in normal humans. Br J Anaesth 70:154, 1993

296. Moss E: Alfentanil increases intracranial pressure when intracranial compliance is low. Anaesthesia 47:134, 1992

297. Albanese J, Durbec O, Viviand X et al: Sufentanil increases intracranial pressure in patients with head trauma. Anesthesiology 79:493, 1993

298. Sperry RJ, Bailey PL, Reichman MV et al: Fentanyl and sufentanil increase intracranial pressure in head trauma patients. Anesthesiology 77:416, 1992

299. Kingston HGG, Bretherton KW, Halloway AM, Downing JW: A comparison between ketamine and diazepam as induction agents for pericardiectomy. Anaesth Intensive Care 6:66, 1978

300. Missavage AE, Bush RL, Kien ND, Reilly DA: The effect of clysed and topical epinephrine on intraoperative catecholamine levels. J Trauma 45:1074, 1998

301. Coté CJ, Drop LJ, Hoaglin DC et al: Ionized hypocalcemia after fresh frozen plasma administration to thermally injured children: Effects of infusion rate, duration, and treatment with calcium chloride. Anesth Analg 67:152, 1988

302. Barret JP, Desai MH, Herndon DN: Massive transfusion of reconstituted whole blood is well tolerated in pediatric burn surgery. J Trauma 47:526, 1999

303. Uhl L, Pacini D, Kruskail MS: A comparative study of blood warmer performance. Anesthesiology 77:1022, 1992

304. Schierhout G, Roberts I: Fluid resuscitation with colloid or crystalloid solutions in critically ill patients: A systematic review of randomised trials. BMJ 1998;316:961

305. Warren BB, Durieux ME: Hydroxyethyl starch: Safe or not? Anesth Analg 84:206, 1997

306. Gould SA, Moore EE, Hoyt DB et al: The first randomized trial of human polymerized hemoglobin as a blood substitute in acute trauma and emergent surgery. J Am Coll Surg 187:113, 1998

307. Zipnick RI, Scalea TM, Trooskin SZ et al: Hemodynamic responses to penetrating spinal cord injuries. J Trauma 35:578, 1993

308. Johnson SB, Kearney PA, Smith MD: Echocardiography in the evaluation of thoracic trauma. Surg Clin North Am 75:193, 1995

309. Jurkovich GJ, Greiser WB, Luterman A et al: Hypothermia in trauma victims: An ominous predictor of survival. J Trauma 27:1019, 1987

310. Gentilello LM: Advances in the management of hypothermia. Surg Clin North Am 75:243, 1995

311. Gentilello LM, Cobean R, Offner PJ et al: Continuous arteriovenous rewarming: Rapid reversal of hypothermia in critically ill patients. J Trauma 32:316, 1992

312. Ferrara A, Mac Arthur JD, Wright HK et al: Hypothermia and acidosis worsen coagulopathy in the patient requiring massive transfusion. Am J Surg 160:515, 1990

313. Patt A, McCroskey BL, Moore EE: Hypothermia induced coagulopathies in trauma. Surg Clin North Am 68:775, 1988

314. Murray DJ, Pennell BJ, Weinstein SL, Olson JD: Packed red cells in acute blood loss: Dilutional coagulopathy as a cause of surgical bleeding. Anesth Analg 80:336, 1995

315. Reed RL, Ciavarella D, Heimbach DM et al: Prophylactic platelet administration during massive transfusion: A prospective, randomized, double-blind clinical study. Ann Surg 203:40, 1986

316. Reed RL II, Johnston TD, Hudson JD, Fisher RP: The disparity between hypothermic coagulopathy and clotting studies. J Trauma 33:465, 1992

317. Linko K, Tigerstedt I: Hyperpotassemia during massive blood transfusions. Acta Anaesthesiol Scand 28:220, 1984

318. Erdmann E, Reuschel-Janetschek E: Calcium for resuscitation? Br J Anaesth 67:178, 1991

319. Arieff AI: Indications for use of bicarbonate in patients with metabolic acidosis. Br J Anaesth 67:165, 1991

320. Hoyt DB, Bulger EM, Knudson MM et al: Death in the operating room: An analysis of a multi-center experience. J Trauma 37:426, 1994

321. Sanchez-Izquierdo-Riera JA, Caballero-Cubedo RE, Perez-Vela JL et al: Propofol versus midazolam: Safety and efficacy for sedating the severe trauma patient. Anesth Analg 86:1219, 1998

322. Shin B, Mackenzie CF, Helrich M: Creatinine clearance for early detection of posttraumatic renal dysfunction. Anesthesiology 64:605, 1986

323. Cheatham ML: Intra-abdominal hypertension and abdominal compartment syndrome. New Horiz 7:96, 1999

324. Geerts WH, Code KI, Jay RM *et al:* A prospective study of venous thromboembolism after major trauma. N Engl J Med 331:1601, 1994

325. Owings JT, Kraut E, Battistella F *et al:* Timing of the occurrence of pulmonary embolism in trauma patients. Arch Surg 132:862, 1997

326. Jongbloets LM, Lensing AW, Koopman MM *et al:* Limitations of compression ultrasound for the detection of symptomless postoperative deep vein thrombosis. Lancet 343:1142, 1994

327. Geerts WH, Jay RM, Code KI *et al:* A comparison of low-dose heparin with low-molecular-weight heparin as prophylaxis against venous thromboembolism after major trauma. N Engl J Med 335:701, 1996

Clinical Anesthesia (4/e), edited by
Paul G. Barash, Bruce F. Cullen, and
Robert K. Stoelting. Lippincott Williams &
Wilkins, Philadelphia, © 2001.

CHAPTER 49

THE ALLERGIC RESPONSE

JERROLD H. LEVY

Allergic reactions during anesthesia represent an important cause of perioperative complications. Anesthesiologists routinely manage patients during their perioperative medical care where they are exposed to a range of foreign substances, including drugs (*i.e.,* antibiotics, anesthetic agents, neuromuscular blocking agents, sedative hypnotics), polypeptides (protamine, aprotinin), blood products, and environmental antigens (*i.e.,* latex). Anesthesiologists must be able to rapidly recognize and treat anaphylaxis, the most life-threatening form of an allergic reaction.[1] Latex represents an important and potentially overlooked environmental antigen.[1]

The allergic response represents just one limb of the pathologic response the immune system can mount again foreign substances. As part of normal host surveillance mechanisms, a series of cellular and humoral elements monitors foreign structures called *antigens* to provide host defense. These foreign substances (antigens) consist of molecular configurations located on cells, bacteria, viruses, proteins, or complex macromolecules.[1-4] Immunologic mechanisms have the following characteristics: they (1) involve antigen interaction with antibodies or specific effector cells, (2) are reproducible, and (3) are specific and adaptive, capable of distinguishing foreign substances and amplifying reactivity through a series of inflammatory cells and proteins. The immune system serves to protect the body against external microorganisms and toxins and internal threats from neoplastic cells; however, it can respond inappropriately to cause hypersensitive (allergic) reactions. Life-threatening allergic reactions to drugs and other foreign substances observed perioperatively may represent different manifestations of the immune response.[1,2]

BASIC IMMUNOLOGIC PRINCIPLES

Host defense systems can be divided into cellular and humoral elements.[1-4] The humoral system includes antibodies, complement, cytokines, and other circulating proteins, whereas cellular immunity is mediated by specific lymphocytes of the T-cell series. Lymphocytes have receptors that distinguish between antigens of host and foreign origin. When lymphocytes react with foreign antigens, they respond to orchestrate immunosurveillance, regulate immunospecific antibody synthesis, and destroy foreign invaders. Individual aspects of the immune response and their importance are considered separately.

Antigens

Molecules capable of stimulating an immune response (antibody production or lymphocyte stimulation) are called *antigens.*[4] Only a few drugs used by anesthesiologists, such as polypeptides (protamine) and other large macromolecules (dextrans), are complete antigens (Table 49-1). Most commonly used drugs are simple organic compounds of low molecular weight (approximately 1000 daltons). For such a small molecule to become immunogenic, it must form a stable bond with circulating proteins or tissue micromolecules to result in a complete antigen (hapten–macromolecular complex). Small–molecular-weight substances such as drugs or drug metabolites that bind to host proteins or cell membranes to sensitize patients are called *haptens.* Haptens are not antigenic by themselves. Often, a reactive drug metabolite (*i.e.,* penicilloyl derivative of penicil-

lin) is thought to bind with macromolecules to become antigens, but for most drugs this has not been proved.

Thymus-Derived (T-Cell) and Bursa-Derived (B-Cell) Lymphocytes

The thymus of the fetus differentiates immature lymphocytes into thymus-derived cells (T cells). T cells have receptors that are activated by binding with foreign antigens and secrete mediators that regulate the immune response. The subpopulations of T cells that exist in humans include helper, suppressor, cytotoxic, and killer cells.[5] The two types of regulatory T cells are helper cells (OKT4) and suppressor cells (OKT8). Helper cells are important for key effector cell responses, whereas suppressor cells inhibit immune function. Infection of helper T cells with a retrovirus, the human immunodeficiency virus, produces a specific increase in the number of suppressor cells. Cytotoxic T cells destroy mycobacteria, fungi, and viruses. Other lymphocytes, called natural killer cells, do not require specific antigen stimulation to initiate their function. Both the cytotoxic T cells and natural killer cells participate in defense against tumor cells and in transplant rejection. T cells produce a spectrum of mediators that influence the response of other cell types involved in the recognition and destruction of foreign substances.

B cells represent a specific lymphocyte cell line that can differentiate into specific plasma cells that synthesize antibodies, a step controlled by both helper and suppressor T-cell lymphocytes.[5] B cells are also called bursa-derived cells because in birds, the bursa of Fabricius is important in producing cells responsible for antibody synthesis.

Antibodies

Antibodies are specific proteins called *immunoglobulins* (Ig) that can recognize and bind to a specific antigen.[6] The basic structure of the antibody molecule is illustrated in Figure 49-1. Each antibody has at least two heavy chains and two light chains that are bound together by disulfide bonds. The Fab fragment has the ability to bind antigen, and the Fc, or crystallizable, fragment is responsible for the unique biologic properties of the different classes of immunoglobulins (cell binding and complement activation). Antibodies function as specific receptor molecules for immune cells and proteins. When antigen binds covalently to the Fab fragments, the antibody undergoes conformational changes to activate the Fc receptor. The results of antigen–antibody binding depend on the cell type, which causes a specific type of activation (*i.e.,* lymphocyte proliferation and differentiation into antibody-secreting cells, mast cell degranulation, and complement activation).

Five major classes of antibodies occur in humans: IgG, IgA, IgM, IgD, and IgE. The heavy chain determines the structure and the function of each molecule. The basic properties of each antibody are listed in Table 49-2.

Effector Cells and Proteins of the Immune Response

Cells

Monocytes, neutrophils (polymorphonuclear leukocytes [PMNs]), and eosinophils represent important effector cells

Table 49-1. AGENTS ADMINISTERED DURING ANESTHESIA THAT ACT AS ANTIGENS

Haptens	Macromolecules
Penicillin and its derivatives	Blood products
Anesthetic drugs(?)	Chymopapain
	Colloid volume expanders
	Muscle relaxants
	Protamine
	Latex

that migrate into areas of inflammation in response to specific chemotactic factors, including lymphokines, cytokines, and complement-derived mediators. The deposition of antibody or complement fragments on the surface of foreign cells is called *opsonization*, a process that facilitates the killing of foreign cells by effector cells. In addition, lymphokines and cytokines produce chemotaxis of other inflammatory cells in a manner described in the following sections.

Monocytes and Macrophages. Macrophages regulate immune responses by processing and presenting antigens to effect inflammatory, tumoricidal, and microbicidal functions. Macrophages arise from circulating monocytes or may be confined to specific organs such as the lung. They are recruited and activated in response to microorganisms or tissue injury. Macrophages ingest antigens before they interact with receptors on the lymphocyte surface to regulate their action. Macrophages synthesize mediators to facilitate both B- and T-lymphocyte responses.

Polymorphonuclear Leukocytes (Neutrophils). The first cells to appear in acute inflammatory reaction are neutrophils that contain acid hydrolases, neutral proteases, and lysosomes. Once activated, they produce hydroxyl radicals, superoxide, and hydrogen peroxide, which aid in microbial killing.

Eosinophils. The exact function of the eosinophil in host defense is unclear; however, inflammatory cells recruit eosinophils to accumulate at sites of parasitic infections, tumors, and allergic reactions.[1]

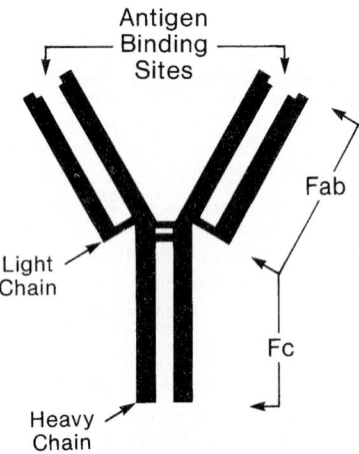

Figure 49-1. Basic structural configuration of the antibody molecule representing human immunoglobulin G (IgG). Immunoglobulins are composed of two heavy chains and two light chains bound by disulfide linkages (represented by *crossbars*). Papain cleaves the molecule into two Fab fragments and one Fc fragment. Antigen binding occurs on the Fab fragments, whereas the Fc segment is responsible for membrane binding or complement activation. (Reproduced with permission from Levy JH: Anaphylactic Reactions in Anesthesia and Intensive Care, 2nd ed. Boston, Butterworth-Heinemann, 1992.)

Basophils. Basophils comprise 0.5–1% of circulating granulocytes in the blood.[1] On the surface of basophils are IgE receptors, which function similarly to those on mast cells.

Mast Cells. Mast cells are important cells for immediate hypersensitivity responses. They are tissue fixed and located in the perivascular spaces of the skin, lung, and intestine.[1] On the surface of mast cells are IgE receptors, which bind to specific antigens. Once activated, these cells release a spectrum of physiologically active mediators important to immediate hypersensitivity responses (see IgE-Mediated Pathophysiology in section on Anaphylactic Reactions). Mast cells can be activated by a series of both immune and nonimmune stimuli.

Proteins

Cytokines/Interleukins. Cytokines are inflammatory cell activators that are synthesized by macrophages to act as secondary messengers and activate endothelial cells and white cells.[7] Interleukin-1 and tumor necrosis factor are examples of cytokines considered to be important mediators of the biologic responses to infection and other inflammatory reactions. Liberation of interleukin-1 and tumor necrosis factor produces fever, neuropeptide release, endothelial cell activation, increased adhesion molecule expression, neutrophil priming, hypotension, myocardial suppression, and a catabolic state.[7] The term *interleukin* was coined for a group of cytokines that facilitates communication between and among ("inter") leukocytes ("leukin"). Interleukins are a group of different regulatory proteins that act to control many aspects of the immune and inflammatory responses. The interleukins are polypeptides synthesized in response to cellular activation and produce their inflammatory effects by activating specific receptors on inflammatory cells and vasculature. T-cell lymphocytes influence the activity of other immunologic and nonimmunologic cells by the production of an array of interleukins that they secrete. A spectrum of different interleukins of this class have been isolated and characterized; they function as short-range or intracellular soluble mediators of the immune and inflammatory responses. The interleukin family of cytokines has been rapidly growing in number because of advances in gene cloning.

Complement. The primary humoral response to antigen and antibody binding is activation of the complement system.[8] The complement system consists of approximately 20 different proteins that bind to activated antibodies, other complement proteins, and cell membranes. The complement system is an important effector system of inflammation. Complement activation can be initiated by IgG or IgM binding to antigen, by plasmin through the classic pathway, by endotoxin, or by drugs through the alternate (properdin) pathway[8] (Fig. 49-2). Specific fragments released during complement activation include C3a, C4a, and C5a, which have important humoral and chemotactic properties (see Non–IgE-Mediated Reactions). The major function of the complement system is to recognize bacteria both directly and indirectly by the attraction of phagocytes (chemotaxis), as well as the increased adherence of phagocytes to antigens (opsonization), and cell lysis by activation of the complete cascade.

A series of inhibitors regulates activation to ensure regulation of the complement system. Hereditary (autosomal dominant) or acquired (associated with lymphoma, lymphosarcoma, chronic lymphatic leukemia, macroglobulinemia) angioneurotic edema is an example of a deficiency in an inhibitor of the C1 complement system (C1 esterase deficiency). This syndrome is characterized by recurrent increased vascular permeability of specific subcutaneous and serosal tissues (angioedema), which produces laryngeal obstruction and respiratory and cardiovascular abnormalities after tissue trauma and surgery, or even without any obvious precipitating factor.[9] One of the important pathologic manifestations of complement activation is acute pulmonary vasoconstriction associated with protamine administration.[1]

Table 49-2. BIOLOGIC CHARACTERISTICS OF IMMUNOGLOBULINS

	IgG	IgM	IgA	IgE	IgD
Heavy chain	γ	μ	α	ϵ	δ
Molecular weight	160,000	900,000	170,000	188,000	184,000
Subclasses	1,2,3,4	1,2	1,2		
Serum concentration, mg · dl⁻¹	6–14	0.5–1.5	1–3	$< -0.5 \times 10^3$	<0.1
Complement activation	All but IgG₄	+	–	–	–
Placental transfer	+	–	–	–	–
Serum half-life (days)	23	5	6	1–5	2–8
Cell binding	Mast cells (IgG₄)	Lymphocytes		Mast cells	Neutrophils
	Neutrophils			Basophils	Lymphocytes
	Lymphocytes			Lymphocytes	
	Mononuclear cells				
	Platelets				

Modified with permission from Levy JH: Anaphylactic Reactions in Anesthesia and Intensive Care, 2nd ed. Boston, Butterworth-Heinemann, 1992.

Effects of Anesthesia on Immune Function

Anesthesia and surgery depress a spectrum of nonspecific host resistance mechanisms, including lymphocyte activation and phagocytosis.[6] Immune competence during surgery can be affected by direct and hormonal effects of anesthetic drugs, by immunologic consequences of other drugs used, by the type of surgery, by coincident infections, and by transfused blood products. Blood represents a complex spectrum of humoral and cellular elements that may alter immunomodulation to a variety of antigens. Although multiple studies demonstrate *in vitro* alterations of immune function, no studies have ever demonstrated their actual importance.[6] Furthermore, such alterations are likely of minor importance compared with the hormonal aspects of stress responses.

HYPERSENSITIVITY RESPONSES (ALLERGY)

Gell and Coombs[3] first described a scheme for classifying immune responses to understand specific diseases mediated by immunologic processes. The immune pathway functions as a protective mechanism, but can also react inappropriately to produce a hypersensitivity or allergic response. They defined four basic types of hypersensitivity, Types I–IV. It is useful first to review all four mechanisms to understand the different immune reactions that occur in humans.

Type I Reactions

Type I reactions are anaphylactic or immediate-type hypersensitivity reactions (Fig. 49-3). Physiologically active mediators are released from mast cells and basophils after antigen binding to IgE antibodies on the membranes of these cells. Type I

hypersensitivity reactions include anaphylaxis, extrinsic asthma, and allergic rhinitis.

Type II Reactions

Type II reactions are also known as antibody-dependent cell-mediated cytotoxic hypersensitivity or cytotoxic reactions (antibody-dependent cell-mediated cytotoxic) (Fig. 49-4). These reactions are mediated by either IgG or IgM antibodies directed against antigens on the surface of foreign cells. These antigens may be either integral cell membrane components (A or B blood group antigens in ABO incompatibility reactions) or haptens that absorb to the surface of a cell, stimulating the production of anti-hapten antibodies (autoimmune hemolytic anemia). The cell damage in Type II reactions is produced by (1) direct cell lysis after complete complement cascade activation, (2) increased phagocytosis by macrophages, or (3) killer T-cell lymphocytes producing antibody-dependent cell-mediated cytotoxic effects. Examples of Type II reactions in humans are ABO-incompatible transfusion reactions, drug-induced immune hemolytic anemia, and heparin-induced thrombocytopenia.

Type III Reactions (Immune Complex Reactions)

Type III reactions result from circulating soluble antigens and antibodies that bind to form insoluble complexes that deposit in the microvasculature (Fig. 49-5). Complement is activated and neutrophils are localized to the site of complement deposition to produce tissue damage. Type III reactions include classic serum sickness observed after snake antisera or antithymocyte globulin, and immune complex vascular injury, and may occur through mechanisms of protamine-mediated pulmonary vasoconstriction.[1]

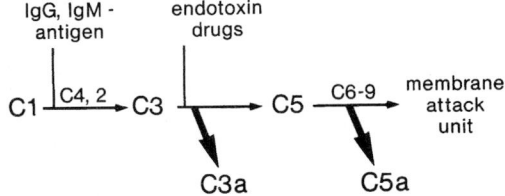

Figure 49-2. Diagram of complement activation. Complement system can be activated by either the classic pathway (IgG, IgM–antigen interaction) or the alternate pathway (endotoxin, drug interaction). Small peptide fragments of C3 and C5 called anaphylatoxins (C3a, C5a) that are released during activation are potent vasoactive mediators. Formation of the complete complement cascade produces a membrane attack unit that lyses cell walls and membranes. An inhibitor of the complement cascade, the C1 esterase inhibitor, ensures that the complement system is turned off most of the time.

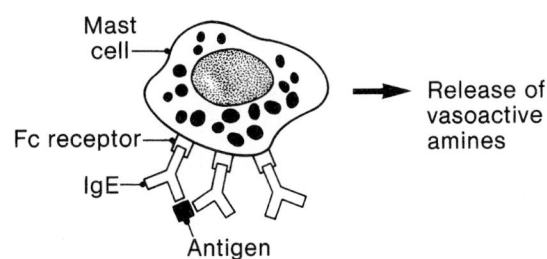

Figure 49-3. Type I immediate hypersensitivity reactions (anaphylaxis) involve IgE antibodies binding to mast cells or basophils by way of their Fc receptors. On encountering immunospecific antigens, the IgE becomes cross-linked, inducing degranulation, intracellular activation, and release of mediators. This reaction is independent of complement.

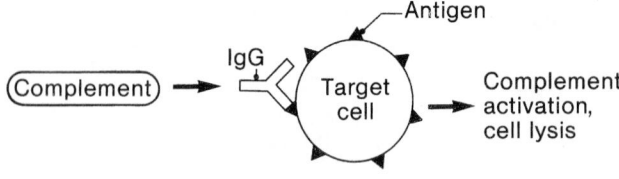

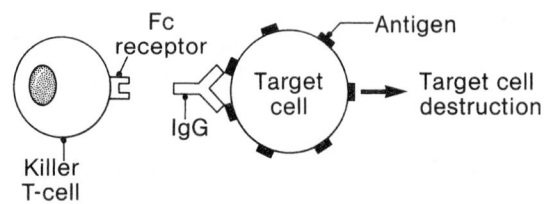

Figure 49-4. Type II or cytotoxic reactions. Antibody of an IgG or IgM class is directed against antigens on an individual's own cells (target cell). The antigens may be integral membrane components or foreign molecules that have been absorbed. This may lead to complement activation, including cell lysis (*upper figure*) or to cytotoxic action by killer T-cell lymphocytes (*lower figure*).

Type IV Reactions (Delayed Hypersensitivity Reactions)

Type IV reactions result from the interactions of sensitized lymphocytes with specific antigens (Fig. 49-6). Delayed hypersensitivity reactions are predominantly mononuclear, manifest in 18–24 hours, peak at 40–80 hours, and disappear in 72–96 hours. Antigen-lymphocyte binding produces lymphokine synthesis, lymphocyte proliferation, generation of cytotoxic T cells, and the attraction of macrophages and other inflammatory cells. Cytotoxic T cells are generated specifically to kill target cells that bear antigens identical to those that triggered the reaction. This form of immunity is important in tissue rejection, graft-versus-host reactions, contact dermatitis (*e.g.*, poison ivy), and tuberculin immunity.

Intraoperative Allergic Reactions

Intraoperative allergic reactions occur once in every 5000–25,000 anesthetics, with a 3.4% mortality rate.[10,11] More than

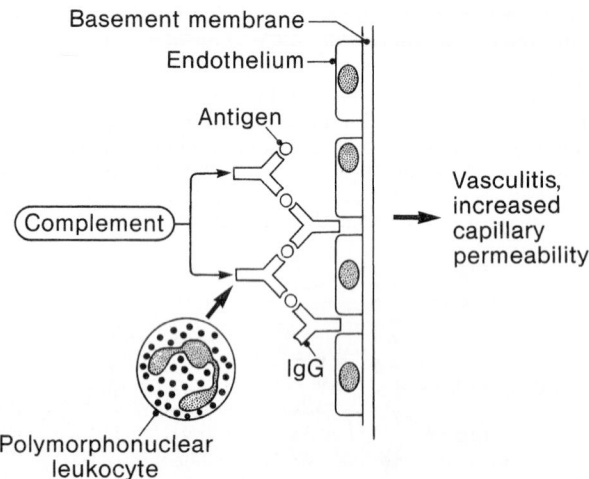

Figure 49-5. Type III immune complex reactions. Antibodies of an IgG or IgM type bind to the antigen in the soluble base and subsequently are deposited in the microvasculature. Complement is activated, resulting in chemotaxis and activation of polymorphonuclear leukocytes at the site of antigen–antibody complexes and subsequent tissue injury.

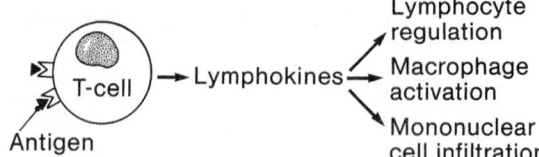

Figure 49-6. Type IV immune complex reactions (delayed hypersensitivity or cell-mediated immunity). Antigen binds to sensitized T-cell lymphocytes to release lymphokines after a second contact with the same antigen. This reaction is independent of circulating antibody or complement activation. Lymphokines induce inflammatory reactions and activate as well as attract macrophages and other mononuclear cells to produce delayed tissue injury.

90% of the allergic reactions evoked by intravenous (iv) drugs occur within 5 minutes of administration. In the anesthetized patient, the most common life-threatening manifestation of an allergic reaction is circulatory collapse, reflecting vasodilation with resulting decreased venous return (Table 49-3). The only manifestation of an allergic reaction may be refractory hypotension.[12] Portier and Richet first used the word *anaphylaxis* (from *ana*, "against," and *prophylaxis*, "protection") to describe the profound shock and subsequent death that sometimes occurred in dogs immediately after a second challenge with a foreign antigen.[13] When life-threatening allergic reactions mediated by antibodies occur, they are defined as anaphylactic. When antibodies are not responsible for the reaction or when antibody involvement in the reaction cannot be proven, the reaction is called *anaphylactoid*.[14] Anaphylactic and anaphylactoid reactions cannot be distinguished from one another on the basis of clinical observation.

ANAPHYLACTIC REACTIONS
IgE-Mediated Pathophysiology

Antigen binding to IgE antibodies initiates anaphylaxis (Fig. 49-7). Prior exposure to the antigen or to a substance of similar

Table 49-3. RECOGNITION OF ANAPHYLAXIS DURING REGIONAL AND GENERAL ANESTHESIA

Systems	Symptoms	Signs
Respiratory	Dyspnea	Coughing
	Chest discomfort	Wheezing
		Sneezing
		Laryngeal edema
		Decreased pulmonary compliance
		Fulminant pulmonary edema
		Acute respiratory failure
Cardiovascular	Dizziness	Disorientation
	Malaise	Diaphoresis
	Retrosternal oppression	Loss of consciousness
		Hypotension
		Tachycardia
		Dysrhythmias
		Decreased systemic vascular resistance
		Cardiac arrest
		Pulmonary hypertension
Cutaneous	Itching	Urticaria (hives)
	Burning	Flushing
	Tingling	Periorbital edema
		Perioral edema

Reproduced with permission from Levy JH: Anaphylactic Reactions in Anesthesia and Intensive Care, 2nd ed. Boston, Butterworth-Heinemann, 1992.

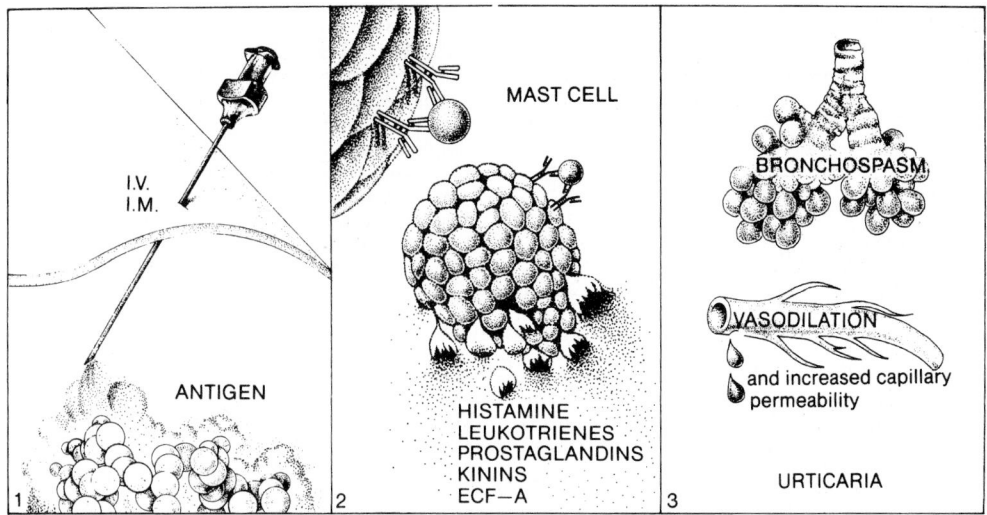

Figure 49-7. During anaphylaxis (Type I immediate hypersensitivity reaction), (1) antigen enters a patient during anesthesia through a parenteral route. (2) It bridges two IgE antibodies on the surface of mast cells or basophils. In a calcium- and energy-dependent process, cells release various substances—histamine, eosinophilic chemotactic factor or anaphylaxis, leukotrienes, prostaglandins, and kinins. (3) These released mediators produce the characteristic effects in the pulmonary, cardiovascular, and cutaneous systems. The most severe and life-threatening effects of the vasoactive mediators occur in the respiratory and cardiovascular systems. (Reproduced with permission from Levy JH: Identification and Treatment of Anaphylaxis: Mechanisms of Action and Strategies for Treatment Under General Anesthesia. Chicago, Smith Laboratories, 1983.)

structure is required to produce sensitization, although an allergic history may be unknown to the patient. On re-exposure, binding of the antigen to bridge two immunospecific IgE antibodies located on the surfaces of mast cells and basophils liberates stored mediators, including histamine, tryptase, and chemotactic factors.[15-17] Arachidonic acid metabolites (leukotrienes and prostaglandins), kinins, and cytokines are subsequently synthesized and released in response to cellular activation.[18] The liberated mediators produce a symptom complex of bronchospasm and upper airway edema in the respiratory system, vasodilation and increased capillary permeability in the cardiovascular system, and urticaria in the cutaneous system. Different mediators are released from mast cells and basophils after activation.

Chemical Mediators of Anaphylaxis

Histamine stimulates H_1, H_2, and H_3 receptors. H_1 receptor activation releases endothelium-derived relaxing factor (nitric oxide) from vascular endothelium, increases capillary permeability, and contracts airway and vascular smooth muscle.[1,19,20] H_2 receptor activation causes gastric secretion, inhibits mast cell activation, and contributes to vasodilation.[19] When injected into skin, histamine produces the classic wheal (increased capillary permeability producing tissue edema) and flare (cutaneous vasodilation) response in humans.[21] Histamine undergoes rapid metabolism in humans by the enzymes histamine *N*-methyltransferase and diamine oxidase located in endothelial cells.[1]

Peptide Mediators of Anaphylaxis

Factors are released from mast cells and basophils that cause granulocyte migration (chemotaxis) and collection at the site of the inflammatory stimulus.[18] Eosinophilic chemotactic factor of anaphylaxis (ECF-A) is a small–molecular-weight peptide chemotactic for eosinophils.[22] Although the exact role of ECF-A or the eosinophil in acute allergic response is unclear, eosinophils release enzymes that can inactivate histamine and leukotrienes.[18] In addition, a neutrophilic chemotactic factor is released that causes chemotaxis and activation.[18,23] Neutrophil activation may be responsible for recurrent manifestations of anaphylaxis.

Arachidonic Acid Metabolites

Leukotrienes and prostaglandins are both synthesized after mast cell activation from arachidonic acid metabolism of phospholipid cell membranes through either lipoxygenase or cyclooxygenase pathways.[24,25] The classic slow-reacting substance of anaphylaxis is a combination of leukotrienes C_4, D_4, and E_4.[25] Leukotrienes produce bronchoconstriction (more intense than that produced by histamine), increased capillary permeability, vasodilation, coronary vasoconstriction, and myocardial depression.[25] Prostaglandins are potent mast cell mediators that produce vasodilation, bronchospasm, pulmonary hypertension, and increased capillary permeability.[18,25] Prostaglandin D_2, the major metabolite of mast cells, produces bronchospasm and vasodilation.[25] Elevated plasma levels of thromboxane B_2 (the metabolite of thromboxane A_2), also a prostaglandin synthesized by mast cells as well as by PMNs, have been demonstrated after protamine reactions associated with pulmonary hypertension.[26,27]

Kinins

Small peptides called *kinins* are synthesized in mast cells and basophils to produce vasodilation, increased capillary permeability, and bronchoconstriction.[18,28] Kinins can stimulate vascular endothelium to release vasoactive factors, including prostacylin, and endothelial-derived relaxing factors like nitric oxide.[1]

Platelet-Activating Factor

Platelet-activating factor (PAF), an unstored lipid synthesized in activated human mast cells, is an extremely potent biologic material, producing physiologic effects at concentrations as low as 10^{-10} M.[18] PAF aggregates and activates human platelets, and perhaps leukocytes, to release inflammatory products. PAF causes a profound wheal-and-flare response, smooth muscle contraction, and increased capillary permeability.[18]

Recognition of Anaphylaxis

The onset and severity of the reaction relate to the mediator's specific end-organ effects. Antigenic challenge in a sensitized individual usually produces immediate clinical manifestations of anaphylaxis, but the onset may be delayed 2–20 minutes.[29,30]

Table 49-4. BIOLOGIC EFFECTS OF ANAPHYLATOXINS

Biologic Effects	C3a	C5a
Histamine release	+	+
Smooth muscle contraction	+	+
Increased vascular permeability	+	+
Chemotaxis		+
Leukocyte and platelet aggregation		+
Interleukin release	+	+

Table 49-5. DRUGS CAPABLE OF NONIMMUNOLOGIC HISTAMINE RELEASE

Antibiotics (vancomycin, pentamidine)
Basic compounds
Hyperosmotic agents
Muscle relaxants (d-tubocurarine, metocurine, atracurium, mivacurium, doxacurium)
Opioids (morphine, meperidine, codeine)
Thiobarbiturates

The reaction may include some or all of the symptoms and signs listed in Table 49-3. Individuals vary greatly in their manifestations and course of anaphylaxis.[31,32] A spectrum of reactions exists, ranging from minor clinical changes to the full-blown syndrome leading to death.[31,33] The enigma of anaphylaxis lies in the unpredictability of occurrence, the severity of the attack, and the lack of a prior allergic history.

Non–IgE-Mediated Reactions

Other immunologic and nonimmunologic mechanisms liberate many of the mediators previously discussed independent of IgE, creating a clinical syndrome identical to anaphylaxis. Specific pathways important in producing the same spectrum of clinical manifestations are considered later.

Complement Activation

Complement activation follows both immunologic (antibody-mediated, i.e., classic pathway) or nonimmunologic (alternative) pathways to include a series of multimolecular, self-assembling proteins that liberate biologically active complement fragments of C3 and C5.[10,34] C3a and C5a are called anaphylatoxins because they release histamine from mast cells and basophils, contract smooth muscle, increase capillary permeability, and cause interleukin synthesis (Table 49-4). C5a interacts with specific high-affinity receptors on PMNs and platelets, initiating leukocyte chemotaxis, aggregation, and activation.[35] Aggregated leukocytes embolize to various organs, producing microvascular occlusion and liberation of inflammatory products such as arachidonic acid metabolites, oxygen free radicals, and lysosomal enzymes (Fig. 49-8). Antibodies of the IgG class directed against antigenic determinants or granulocyte surfaces can also produce leukocyte aggregation.[36] These antibodies are called leukoagglutinins. Investigators have implicated complement activation and PMN aggregation in producing the clinical manifestation of transfusion reactions,[36,37] pulmonary vasoconstriction after protamine reactions,[27] adult respiratory distress syndrome,[36] and septic shock.[38]

Nonimmunologic Release of Histamine

Many diverse molecules administered during the perioperative period release histamine in a dose-dependent, nonimmunologic fashion[39-43] (Table 49-5, Fig. 49-9). The mechanisms involved in nonimmunologic histamine release are not well understood, but appear to represent selective mast cell but not basophil activation.[43,44] (Fig. 49-10). Human cutaneous mast cells are the only cell population that releases histamine in response to both drugs and endogenous stimuli (neuropeptides).[1] Nonimmunologic histamine release may involve mast cell activation through specific cell-signaling activation[40] (Fig. 49-11). Different molecular structures release histamine in humans, which suggests that different mechanisms are involved. Histamine release is not dependent on the μ receptor because fentanyl and sufentanil, the most potent μ receptor agonists clinically available, do not release histamine in human skin.[39] Although the newer muscle relaxants may be more potent at the neuromuscular junction, drugs that are mast cell degranulators are equally capable of releasing histamine.[39,40] On an equimolar basis, atracurium is as potent as d-tubocurarine or metocurine in its ability to degranulate mast cells.[40] Newer aminosteroidal agents like rocuronium and rapacuronium at clinically recommended doses have minimal effects on histamine release.[44,45]

Antihistamine pretreatment before administration of drugs that are known to release histamine in humans does not inhibit histamine release; rather, the antihistamines compete with histamine at the receptor and may attenuate decreases in systemic vascular resistance.[1] However, the effect of any drug on systemic vascular resistance may depend on other factors in addition to histamine release.[46,47]

Treatment Plan

A plan for the treatment of anaphylactic or anaphylactoid reactions must be established before the event. Airway maintenance, 100% oxygen administration, intravascular volume expansion, and epinephrine are essential to treat the hypotension and hypoxia that result from vasodilation, increased capillary permeability, and bronchospasm.[1] Table 49-6 lists a protocol for the management of anaphylaxis during general anesthesia, with representative doses for a 70-kg adult. The treatment plan is the same for life-threatening anaphylactic or anaphylactoid reactions. Therapy must be titrated to desired effects with careful monitoring.[1] Severe reactions require aggressive therapy and may be protracted, with persistent hypotension, pulmonary hypertension, lower respiratory obstruction, or laryngeal obstruction that may persist 5–32 hours despite vigorous therapy.[48] All patients who have experienced an anaphylactic reaction should be admitted to an intensive care unit for 24 hours of monitoring because manifestations may recur after successful treatment.

Initial Therapy

Although it may not be possible to stop the administration of antigen, limiting antigen administration may prevent further mast cell and basophil activation.

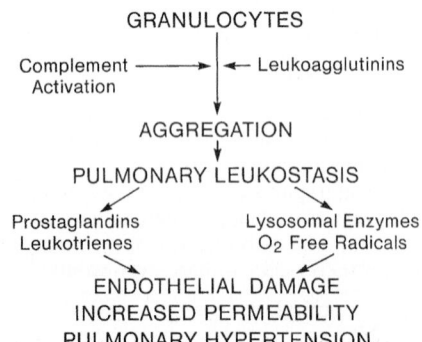

GRANULOCYTES

Complement Activation ⟶ ← Leukoagglutinins

AGGREGATION

PULMONARY LEUKOSTASIS

Prostaglandins Leukotrienes   Lysosomal Enzymes O₂ Free Radicals

ENDOTHELIAL DAMAGE
INCREASED PERMEABILITY
PULMONARY HYPERTENSION

Figure 49-8. Sequence of events producing granulocyte aggregation, pulmonary leukostasis, and cardiopulmonary dysfunction. (Reproduced from Levy JH: Anaphylactic Reactions in Anesthesia and Intensive Care, 2nd ed. Boston, Butterworth-Heinemann, 1992.)

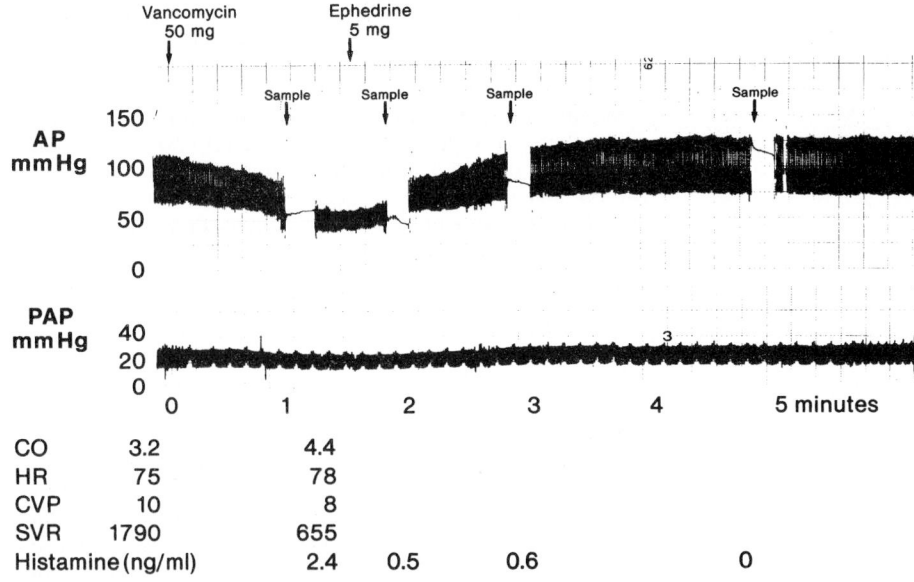

Figure 49-9. Example of an anaphylactic reaction after rapid vancomycin administration in a patient. Hypotension is associated with an increased cardiac output and decreased calculated systemic vascular resistance. Plasma histamine levels 1 minute after the vancomycin administration were 2.4 ng · ml^{-1} and subsequently decreased to zero. The patient was given ephedrine, 5 mg, and blood pressure returned to baseline values. (Reproduced from Levy JH, Kettlekamp N, Goertz P *et al:* Histamine release by vancomycin: A mechanism for hypotension in man. Anesthesiology 67:122, 1987.)

Maintain Airway and Administer 100% Oxygen. Profound ventilation–perfusion abnormalities producing hypoxemia can occur with anaphylactic reactions.[49] Always administer 100% oxygen along with ventilatory support as needed. Arterial blood gas values may be useful to follow during resuscitation.

Discontinue All Anesthetic Drugs. Inhalational anesthetic drugs are not the bronchodilators of choice in treating bronchospasm after anaphylaxis, especially during hypotension. These drugs interfere with the body's compensatory response to cardiovascular collapse, and halothane sensitizes the myocardium to epinephrine.

Provide Volume Expansion. Hypovolemia rapidly ensues during anaphylactic shock.[50] Fisher[50] has reported up to 40% loss of intravascular fluid into the interstitial space during reactions. Therefore, volume expansion is extremely important in conjunction with epinephrine in correcting the acute hypotension. Initially, 2–4 l of lactated Ringer's solution, or colloid or normal saline should be administered, keeping in mind that an additional 25–50 ml · kg^{-1} may be necessary if hypotension persists. Refractory hypotension after volume and epinephrine administration requires additional hemodynamic monitoring. The use

of transesophageal echocardiography for rapid assessment of intraventricular volume and ventricular function and to determine other occult causes of acute cardiovascular dysfunction can be important for accurate assessment of intravascular volume and guidance of rational therapeutic interventions. Fulminant noncardiogenic pulmonary edema with loss of intravascular volume can occur after anaphylaxis. This condition requires intravascular volume repletion with careful hemodynamic monitoring until the capillary defect improves. Colloid volume expansion has not proved to be more effective than crystalloid volume expansion for treating anaphylactic shock.

Administer Epinephrine. Epinephrine is the drug of choice when resuscitating patients during anaphylactic shock. α-Adrenergic effects vasoconstrict to reverse hypotension; β_2 receptor stimulation bronchodilates and inhibits mediator release by increasing cyclic adenosine monophosphate (cAMP) in mast cells and basophils.[32] The route of epinephrine administration and the dose depend on the patient's condition. Rapid and timely intervention is important when treating anaphylaxis. Furthermore, patients under general anesthesia may have altered sympathoadrenergic responses to acute anaphylactic shock,

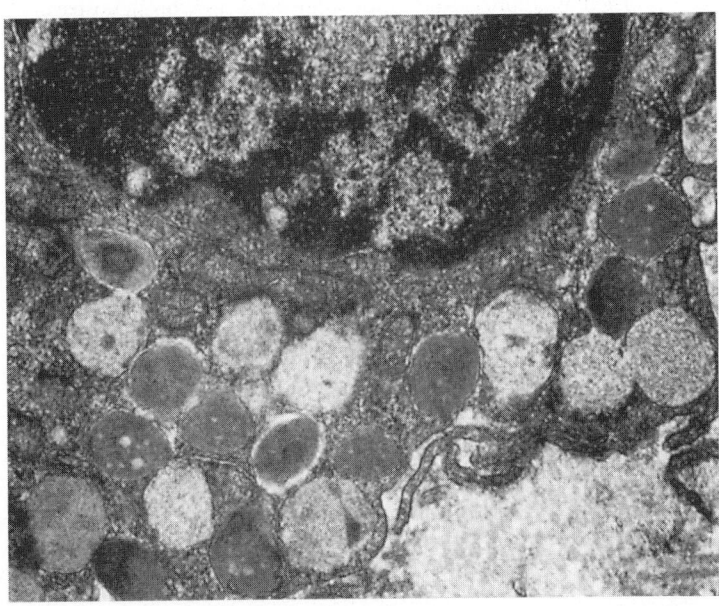

Figure 49-10. Electron micrograph of human cutaneous mast cell after injection of dynorphin, a κ opioid agonist. The cell outline is rounded and most of the cytoplasmic granules are swollen, exhibiting varying degrees of decreased electron density and flocculence consistent with ongoing degranulation. The perigranular membranes of the adjacent granules at the periphery of the cell are fused to each other and to plasma membrane. Original magnification × 72,000. (Reproduced from Casale TB, Bowman S, Kaliner M: Induction of human cutaneous mast cell degranulation by opiates and endogenous opioid peptides: Evidence for opiate and nonopiate receptor participation. J Allergy Clin Immunol 73:778, 1984.)

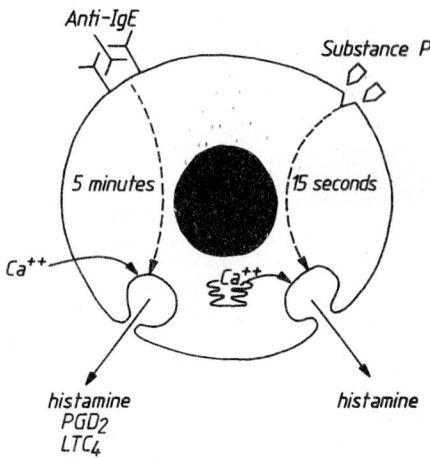

Figure 49-11. Different mechanisms of mediator release from human cutaneous mast cells stimulated immunologically by anti-IgE and by nonimmunologic stimuli with substance P. Anti-IgE stimulation, like antigen stimulation, initiates the release of histamine, prostaglandin D_2 (PGD_2), or leukotriene C_4 (LTC_4) by a mechanism that takes 5 minutes to reach completion and requires the influx of intracellular calcium. Nonimmunologic activation with drugs or substance P releases histamine but not PGD_2 or LTC_4 by a mechanism that is complete within 15 seconds and uses calcium mobilized from intracellular sources. (Reproduced from Caulfield JP, El-Lati S, Thomas G, Church MK: Dissociated human foreskin mast cells degranulate in response to anti-IgE and substance P. Lab Invest 63:502, 1990.)

whereas the patient under spinal or epidural anesthesia may be partially sympathectomized and may need even larger doses of catecholamines.[51]

In hypotensive patients, 5–10-μg boluses of epinephrine should be administered iv and incrementally titrated to restore blood pressure.* Additional volume and incrementally in-

---

Table 49-6. MANAGEMENT OF ANAPHYLAXIS DURING GENERAL ANESTHESIA

Initial Therapy

1. Stop administration of antigen
2. Maintain airway and administer 100% O_2
3. Discontinue all anesthetic agents
4. Start intravascular volume expansion (2–4 l of crystalloid/colloid with hypotension)
5. Give epinephrine (5–10 μg iv bolus with hypotension, titrate as needed; 0.1–1.0 mg iv with cardiovascular collapse)

Secondary Treatment

1. Antihistamines (0.5–1 mg · kg^{-1} diphenhydramine)
2. Catecholamine infusions (starting doses: epinephrine, 4–8 μg · min^{-1}; norepinephrine, 4–8 μg · min^{-1}; or isoproterenol, 0.5–1 μg · min^{-1} as a drip; titrated to desired effects)
3. Aminophylline (5–6 mg · kg^{-1} over 20 min with persistent bronchospasm)
4. Corticosteroids (0.25–1 g hydrocortisone; alternatively, 1–2 g methylprednisolone)*
5. Sodium bicarbonate (0.5–1 mEq · kg^{-1} with persistent hypotension or acidosis)
6. Airway evaluation (before extubation)

---

* Methylprednisolone may be the drug of choice if the reaction is suspected to be mediated by complement.
Reproduced with permission from Levy JH: Anaphylactic Reactions in Anesthesia and Intensive Care, 2nd ed, p 162. Boston, Butterworth-Heinemann, 1992.

---

* This dose of epinephrine can be obtained with 0.05–0.1 ml of a 1:10,000 dilution (100 μg · ml^{-1}) or by mixing 2 mg epinephrine with 250 ml of fluid to yield an 8 μg · ml^{-1} solution.

---

creased doses of epinephrine should be administered until hypotension is corrected. Although infusion is an ideal method of administering epinephrine, it is usually impossible to infuse the drug through peripheral iv access lines during acute volume resuscitation. With cardiovascular collapse, full iv cardiopulmonary resuscitative doses of epinephrine, 0.1–1.0 mg, should be administered and repeated until hemodynamic stability resumes. Patients with laryngeal edema without hypotension should receive subcutaneous epinephrine. Epinephrine should not be administered iv to patients with normal blood pressures.[52]

Secondary Treatment

Antihistamines. Because H_1 receptors mediate many of the adverse effects of histamine, the iv administration of 0.5–1 mg · kg^{-1} of an H_1 antagonist such as diphenhydramine may be useful in treating acute anaphylaxis. Antihistamines do not inhibit anaphylactic reactions or histamine release, but compete with histamine at receptor sites. H_1 antagonists are indicated in all forms of anaphylaxis. The H_1 antagonists available for parenteral administration may have antidopaminergic effects and should be given slowly to prevent precipitous hypotension in potentially hypovolemic patients.[1] The indications for administering an H_2 antagonist once anaphylaxis has occurred remain unclear.

Catecholamines. Epinephrine infusions may be useful in patients with persistent hypotension or bronchospasm after initial resuscitation.[1] Epinephrine infusions should be started at 0.05–0.1 μg · kg^{-1} · min^{-1} (5–10 μg · min^{-1}) and titrated to correct hypotension. Norepinephrine infusions may be needed in patients with refractory hypotension due to decreased systemic vascular resistance. It may be started at 0.05–0.1 μg · kg^{-1} · min^{-1} (5–10 μg · min^{-1}) and adjusted to correct hypotension.

Aminophylline. Aminophylline, a nonspecific phosphodiesterase inhibitor, bronchodilates and decreases histamine release from mast cells or basophils in part by increasing intracellular cAMP. In addition, it increases right and left ventricular contractility and decreases pulmonary vascular resistance. Aminophylline should be considered in patients with persistent bronchospasm and hemodynamic stability, although β_2-adrenergic drugs are the first-line drugs of choice. An iv loading dose of 5–6 mg · kg^{-1} of aminophylline given over 20 minutes should be followed by an infusion of 0.5–0.9 mg · kg^{-1} · hr^{-1}.[1]

Corticosteroids. Corticosteroids have a series of anti-inflammatory effects mediated by multiple mechanisms, including altering the activation and migration of other inflammatory cells (*i.e.*, PMNs) after an acute reaction.[53, 54] Corticosteroids may require 12–24 hours to work and, despite their unproven usefulness in treating acute reactions, they are often administered as adjuncts to therapy when refractory bronchospasm or refractory shock occurs after resuscitative therapy.[55] Although the exact corticosteroid dose and preparation are unclear, investigators have recommended 0.25–1 g iv of hydrocortisone in IgE-mediated reactions. Alternately, 1–2 g of methylprednisolone (30–35 mg · kg^{-1}) iv may be useful in reactions thought to be complement mediated, such as catastrophic pulmonary vasoconstriction after protamine transfusion reactions.[56] Administering corticosteroids after an anaphylactic reaction may also be important in attenuating the late-phase reactions reported to occur 12–24 hours after anaphylaxis.[48]

Bicarbonate. Acidosis develops rapidly in patients with persistent hypotension. This diminishes the effect of epinephrine on the heart and systemic vasculature. Therefore, with refractory hypotension or acidemia, sodium bicarbonate, 0.5–1 mEq · kg^{-1}, may be given and repeated every 5 minutes or as dictated by arterial blood gas valves.

Airway Evaluation. Because profound laryngeal edema can occur, the airway should be evaluated before extubation of the trachea.[29] Persistent facial edema suggests airway edema. The trachea of these patients should remain intubated until the edema subsides. The development of a significant air leak after endotracheal tube cuff deflation and before extubation of the trachea is useful in assessing airway patency. If there is any question of airway edema, direct laryngoscopy should be performed before the trachea is extubated.

PERIOPERATIVE MANAGEMENT OF THE PATIENT WITH ALLERGIES

Allergic drug reactions account for 6–10% of all adverse reactions.[57] DeSwarte[58] suggests that the risk of an allergic drug reaction occurring is approximately 1–3% for most drugs, and that approximately 5% of adults in the United States may be allergic to one or more drugs. Unfortunately, patients often refer to adverse drug effects as being allergic in nature. For example, opioid administration can produce nausea, vomiting, or even local release of histamine along the vein of administration. Patients will say they are ''allergic'' to a specific drug when in fact their adverse reaction is independent of allergy. Approximately 15% of adults in the United States believe they are allergic to specific medication(s) and therefore may be denied treatment with an indicated drug. To understand allergic reactions, the spectrum of adverse reactions to drugs needs to be considered.

Predictable adverse drug reactions account for approximately 80% of adverse drug effects. They are often dose dependent, related to known pharmacologic actions of the drug, and typically occur in normal patients. Most serious, predictable adverse drug reactions are toxic and are directly related to the amount of drug in the body (overdosage) or to an inadvertent route of administration (e.g., lidocaine-induced seizures or cardiovascular collapse). Side effects are the most common adverse drug reactions and are undesirable pharmacologic actions of the drugs occurring at usual prescribed dosages. Most anesthetic drugs exhibit multiple side effects that can produce precipitous hypotension. For example, morphine dilates the venous capacitance bed, thereby decreasing preload; releases histamine from cutaneous mast cells, thereby producing arterial and venous dilation; slows the heart rate; and decreases sympathetic tone. However, the net effects of morphine on blood pressure and myocardial function depend on the patient's blood volume, sympathetic tone, and ventricular function. Hypotension rapidly develops in a volume-depleted trauma patient in pain who is given morphine. Drug interactions also represent important predictable adverse drug reactions. Intravenous fentanyl or sufentanil administration to a patient who has just received iv benzodiazepines or other sedative–hypnotic drugs may produce precipitous hypotension that results from decreased sympathetic tone.[59] This represents a dose-dependent, predictable adverse drug reaction that is independent of allergy.

Unpredictable adverse drug reactions are usually dose independent and usually not related to the drugs' pharmacologic actions, but are often related to the immunologic response (allergy) of the individual. On occasion, adverse reactions can be related to genetic differences (i.e., idiosyncratic) in a susceptible individual who has an isolated genetic enzyme deficiency. In most allergic drug reactions, an immunologic mechanism is present or, more often, presumed. Providing that the initiating event involves a reaction between the drug or drug metabolites with drug-specific antibodies or sensitized T lymphocytes is often impractical. In the absence of direct immunologic evidence, criteria that may be helpful in distinguishing an allergic reaction from other adverse reactions include the following: Allergic reactions occur in only a small percentage of patients receiving the drug, and the clinical manifestations do not resemble known pharmacologic actions. In the absence of prior drug exposure, allergic symptoms rarely appear after less than 1 week of continuous treatment. After sensitization, the reaction develops rapidly on re-exposure to the drug. In general, drugs that have been administered without complications for several months or longer are rarely responsible for producing drug allergy.

The time span between exposure to the drug and noticed manifestations is often the most vital information in determining which drugs administered were the cause of a suspected allergic reaction.

Although the reaction may produce a life-threatening response in the cardiopulmonary system (anaphylaxis), a variety of cutaneous manifestations, fever, and pulmonary reactions have been attributed to drug hypersensitivity. Usually the reaction may be reproduced by very small doses of the suspected drug or other agents possessing similar or cross-reacting chemical structures. On occasion, drug-specific antibodies or lymphocytes have been identified that react with the suspected drug, although the relationship is seldom diagnostically useful in practice. Even when an immune response to a drug is demonstrated, it may not be associated with a clinical allergic reaction. As with adverse drug reactions in general, the reaction usually subsides within several days of discontinuation of the drug.

Immunologic Mechanisms of Drug Allergy

Different immunologic responses to any antigen can occur. Drugs have been associated with all of the immunologic mechanisms proposed by Gell and Coombs.[3] Although more than one mechanism may contribute to a particular reaction, any one can occur. Penicillin may produce different reactions in different patients or a spectrum of reactions in the same patient. In one patient, penicillin can produce anaphylaxis (Type I reaction), hemolytic anemia (Type II reaction), serum sickness (Type III reaction), and contact dermatitis (Type IV reaction).[58] Therefore, any one antigen has the ability to produce a diffuse spectrum of allergic responses in humans. Why some patients have localized rashes or angioneurotic edema in response to penicillin while others sustain complete cardiopulmonary collapse is unknown. Most anesthetic drugs and agents administered perioperatively have been reported to produce anaphylactic/anaphylactoid reactions[31,39-45,60-81] (Table 49-7). Muscle relaxants are the most common drugs responsible for evoking intraoperative allergic reactions.[67] In this regard, there is cross-sensitivity between succinylcholine and the nondepolarizing muscle relaxants. Unexplained intraoperative cardiovascular collapse has been attributed to anaphylaxis triggered by latex (natural rubber), and certain patients, including those with a history of spina bifida, are at a greater risk for reactions.[1,68] Even vascular graft material has been reported as a cause of intraoperative allergic reactions.[69]

Life-threatening allergic reactions are more likely to occur in patients with a history of allergy, atopy, or asthma. Nevertheless, because the incidence is low, the history is not a reliable predictor that an allergic reaction will occur and does not mandate that such patients should be investigated or pretreated, or that specific drugs be selected or avoided.[60] Although different mechanisms have been proposed, no one hypothesis has been proved.[1] The drugs and foreign substance listed in Table 49-7 may have both immunologic and nonimmunologic mechanisms for adverse drug reactions in humans.

Evaluation of Patients With Allergic Reactions

Identifying the drug responsible for a suspected allergic reaction still depends on circumstantial evidence indicating the temporal sequence of drug administration. Conventional in vivo and in vitro methods of diagnosing allergic reactions to most anesthetic drugs are unavailable or not applicable. The most important factor in diagnosis is the awareness of the physician that an untoward event may be related to a drug that the patient received. The physician must always be aware of the ability of any drug to produce an allergic reaction. The history is extremely important when evaluating whether an adverse drug reaction is allergic and whether the drug can be readministered. Although a prior allergic reaction to the drug in question is

Table 49-7. AGENTS IMPLICATED IN ALLERGIC REACTIONS DURING ANESTHESIA

Anesthetic Agents

Induction agents (cremophor-solubilized drugs, barbiturates, etomidate, propofol)
Local anesthetics (para-aminobenzoic ester agents)
Muscle relaxants (succinylcholine, gallamine, pancuronium, d-tubocurarine, metocurine, atracurium, vecuronium, mivacurium, doxacurium)
Opioids (meperidine, morphine, fentanyl)

Other Agents

Antibiotics (cephalosporins, penicillin, sulfonamides, vancomycin)
Aprotinin
Blood products (whole blood, packed cells, fresh frozen plasma, platelets, cryoprecipitate, fibrinin glue, gamma globulin)
Bone cement
Chymopapain
Corticosteriods
Cyclosporin
Drug additives (preservatives)
Furosemide
Insulin
Mannitol
Methylmethacrylate
Nonsteroidal anti-inflammatory drugs
Protamine
Radiocontrast dye
Latex (natural rubber)
Streptokinase
Vascular graft material
Vitamin K
Colloid volume expanders (dextrans, protein fractions, albumin, hydroxyethyl starch)

Reproduced with permission from Levy JH: Anaphylactic Reactions in Anesthesia and Intensive Care, 2nd ed. Boston, Butterworth-Heinemann, 1992.

important, this is rarely the case. Direct challenge of a patient with a test dose of drug is the only way to establish reaction, but this is potentially hazardous and not recommended. Although the anesthesiologist commonly administers small test doses of anesthetic drugs, these are pharmacologic test doses and have nothing to do with immunologic dosages. The demonstration of drug-specific IgE antibodies is generally accepted as evidence that the patient may be at risk for anaphylaxis if the drug is administered.[58] Different clinical tests are available to confirm or diagnose drug allergy; several are considered in the following section.

Testing for Allergy

After an anaphylactoid reaction, it is important to identify the causative agent to prevent readministration. When one particular drug has been administered and there is a clear correlation between the time of administration and the occurrence of a reaction, testing may be unnecessary, and general avoidance of the drug should be instituted. However, when patients have simultaneously received multiple drugs (e.g., an opioid, muscle relaxant, hypnotic, and antibiotic), it is often difficult to establish which particular drug caused the reaction. Furthermore, the reaction might have been caused by the vehicle or by one of the preservatives. For patients who want to know which drug was responsible and for patients scheduled for subsequent procedures, some degree of allergy evaluation should be undertaken to evaluate the drug at risk. Unfortunately, very few in vitro tests exist for anesthetic drugs; therefore, the available allergy tests are discussed.

Leukocyte Histamine Release. Leukocyte histamine is performed by incubating the patient's leukocytes with the of-

fending drug and measuring histamine release as a marker for basophil activation, although false-positive results can occur.[31] This test is not easy to perform, although modifications allow the use of whole blood instead of isolated PMNs.[76,82]

Radioallergosorbent Test. The radioallergosorbent test (RAST) allows *in vitro* detection of specific IgE directed toward particular antigens.[83] In this test, antigens are linked to insoluble material to make an immunoabsorbent.[83,84] When incubated with the serum in question, antibodies of different classes directed toward the antigen bind to it. After washing, the antigen–antibody complex on the immunoabsorbent is incubated with radiolabeled antibodies directed against human IgE, and counted in a scintillation counter. The concentration of specific IgE in the patient's serum directed toward the allergen is measured. The RAST is more quantitative than skin tests and avoids the potential of re-exposure.[84] RAST testing has been used to detect the presence of antibodies to meperidine,[49] succinylcholine,[85] and thiopental.[86] Two major limitations to this test include the commercial availability of the drug prepared as an antigen and false-positive test results in patients with elevated IgE levels.[87]

Enzyme-Linked Immunosorbent Assay. The enzyme-linked immunosorbent assay (ELISA) measures antigen-specific antibodies. The basis of the ELISA is similar to that of the RAST; however, immunospecific IgE directed against the antigen in question is determined by the addition of an anti-IgE coupled to an enzyme such as peroxidase that acts as a chromogen.[5] A colorless substrate is acted on by peroxidase to produce a colored by-product. The ELISA has been used to demonstrate IgE antibodies to chymopapain and protamine and has been developed to screen for other antibodies to diverse agents.

Intradermal Testing (Skin Testing). Skin testing is the method most often used in patients after anaphylactic reaction to anesthetic drugs after the history has suggested the relevant antigens for testing.[88,89] Within minutes after antigen introduction, histamine released from cutaneous mast cells causes vasodilation (flare) and localized edema from increased vascular permeability (wheal). Fisher[67,88] suggests that this is a simple, safe, and useful method in establishing a diagnosis in most cases of anaphylactoid reactions occurring in the perioperative period. If the strict protocols established by Fisher[88] are used, intradermal reactions are helpful. Intradermal testing is of no value in reactions to contrast media or colloid volume expanders. Cross-sensitivity between drugs of similar structures can often be evaluated on the basis of skin testing. Skin testing to local anesthetics is considered a direct challenge or provocative dose testing.[90] Local anesthetic drugs are injected in increasing quantities under controlled circumstances. This testing determines if the person can safely receive amide derivatives (e.g., lidocaine) and can also be used to determine if the person is sensitive to the para-aminobenzoic ester agents (e.g., procaine, tetracaine).

Agents Implicated in Allergic Reactions

Multiple agents, including antibiotics, induction agents, muscle relaxants, nonsteroidal anti-inflammatory drugs, protamine, colloid volume expanders, and blood products, are the etiologic agents often responsible for anaphylaxis in surgical patients.[1] However, any agent the patient receives as an injection, infusion, or environmental antigen has the potential to produce an allergic reaction.[1] Almost everything has been reported to produce an allergic reaction at some time, but usually from a case report or small series. The agents most often implicated include antibiotics, blood products, colloid volume expanders, latex, polypeptides, and neuromuscular blocking agents. If patients are truly allergic to a muscle relaxant, there is a potential for cross-reactivity because of the similarity of the active site, a quaternary ammonium molecule, among the different types of relaxants, and alternatives cannot be chosen without some degree of immunologic testing. Because of the ubiquity of latex as a perioperative environmental antigen, latex allergy is considered separately.

Latex Allergy

For the anesthesiologist, latex represents an environmental agent often implicated as an important cause of perioperative anaphylaxis[91–99] (see Chapter 4). Latex is the milky sap derived from the tree *Hevea brasiliensis* to which multiple agents, including preservatives, accelerators, and antioxidants are added to make the final rubber product. Latex is present in a variety of different products. In March, 1991, the U.S. Food and Drug Administration alerted health care professionals about the potential of severe allergic reactions to medical devices made of latex. The first case of an allergic reaction due to latex was reported in 1979 and was manifested by contact urticaria. In 1989, the first reports of intraoperative anaphylaxis due to latex were reported.

Health care workers and children with spina bifida, urogenital abnormalities, or certain food allergies have also been recognized as people at increased risk for anaphylaxis to latex.[91–99] Brown et al[95] reported a 24% incidence of irritant or contact dermatitis and a 12.5% incidence of latex-specific IgE positivity in anesthesiologists. Of this group, 10% were clinically asymptomatic although IgE positive. A history of atopy was also a significant risk factor for latex sensitization. Brown et al[95] suggest these people are in their early stages of sensitization and perhaps, by avoiding latex exposure, their progression to symptomatic disease can be prevented. Patients allergic to bananas, avocados, and kiwis have also been reported to have antibodies that cross-react with latex.[96,97] Multiple attempts are being made to reduce latex exposure to both health care workers and patients. If latex allergy occurs, then strict avoidance of latex from gloves and other sources needs to be considered, following recommendations as reported by Holzman.[91] Because latex is such a ubiquitous environmental antigen, this represents a daunting task.

More important, anesthesiologists must be prepared to treat the life-threatening cardiopulmonary collapse that occurs after anaphylaxis, as previously discussed. The most important preventive therapy is to avoid antigen exposure; although clinicians have used pretreatment with antihistamine (diphenhydramine and cimetidine) and corticosteroids, there are no data in the literature to suggest that pretreatment actually prevents anaphylaxis or decreases its severity.[1] Two patients in a series reported by Gold et al[93] were pretreated yet still had life-threatening reactions to latex. Patients in whom latex allergy is suspected should be referred to an allergist for appropriate evaluation and potential *in vitro* testing (RAST) for definitive diagnosis. When this is not possible, patients should be treated as if they were latex allergic, and antigen avoided. Patients with a documented history of latex allergy should wear Medic Alert bracelets.

SUMMARY

Although the immune system functions to provide host defense, it can respond inappropriately to produce hypersensitivity or allergic reactions. A spectrum of life-threatening allergic reactions to any drug or agent can occur in the perioperative period. The enigma of these reactions lies in their unpredictable nature. However, a high index of suspicion, prompt recognition, and appropriate and aggressive therapy can help to avoid a disastrous outcome.

REFERENCES

1. Levy J: Anaphylactic Reactions in Anesthesia and Intensive Care, 2nd ed. Boston, Butterworth-Heinemann, 1992
2. deShazo RD, Kemp SF: Allergic reactions to drugs and biologic agents. JAMA 278:1895, 1997
3. Gell PGH, Coombs RRA, Lachmann PJ (eds): Clinical Aspects of Immunology, 3rd ed. Oxford, Blackwell Scientific Publications, 1975
4. Butler VP Jr, Beiser SM: Antibodies to small molecules: Biologic and clinical applications. Adv Immunol 17:255, 1973
5. Holgate ST, Church MK (eds): Allergy. London, Gower Medical Publishing, 1993
6. Stevenson GW, Hall SC, Rudnick S et al: The effects of anesthetic agents on the human immune response. Anesthesiology 72:144, 1990
7. Pober JS, Cotran RS: Cytokines and endothelial cell biology. Physiol Rev 70:427, 1990
8. Frank MM: Complement: A brief review. J Allergy Clin Immunol 84:411, 1988
9. Wall RT, Frank M, Hahn M: A review of 25 patients with hereditary angioedema requiring surgery. Anesthesiology 71:309, 1989
10. Fisher MMD, More DG: The epidemiology and clinical features of anaphylactic reactions in anaesthesia. Anaesth Intensive Care 9:226, 1981
11. Weiss ME, Adkinson NF, Hirshman CA: Evaluation of allergic reactions in the perioperative period. Anesthesiology 71:438, 1989
12. Laxenaire MC, Moneret-Vautrin DA, Boileau S, Moeller R: Adverse reactions to intravenous agents in anaesthesia in France. Klin Wochenschr 60:1006, 1982
13. Portier MM, Richet C: De l'action anaphylactique de certains venins. C R Seances Soc Biol Fil 54:170, 1902
14. Watkins J: Anaphylactoid reactions to I. V. substances. Br J Anaesth 51:51, 1979
15. Costa JJ, Weller PF, Galli SJ: The cells of the allergic response: Mast cells, basophils, and eosinophils. JAMA 278:1815, 1997
16. Kazimierczak W, Diamant B: Mechanisms of histamine release in anaphylactic and anaphylactoid reactions. Prog Allergy 4:295, 1978
17. Winslow CM, Austen KF: Enzymatic regulation of mast cell activation and secretion by adenylate cyclase and cyclic AMP-dependent protein kinases. Fed Proc 41:22, 1982
18. Wasserman SI: Mediators of immediate hypersensitivity. J Allergy Clin Immunol 72:101, 1983
19. Reinhardt D, Borchard V: H1 receptor antagonists: Comparative pharmacology and clinical use. Klin Wochenschr 60:983, 1982
20. Ginsburg R, Bristow MR, Stinson EB et al: Histamine receptors in the human heart. Life Sci 26:2245, 1980
21. Majno G, Palade GE: Studies on inflammation: I. The effect of histamine and serotonin on vascular permeability. An electron microscopic study. Journal of Biophysical and Biochemical Cytology 11:571, 1961
22. Wasserman SI, Goetzl EJ, Austen KF: Preformed eosinophil chemotactic factor of anaphylaxis (ECF-A). J Immunol 112:351, 1974
23. Mathe AA, Hedqvist P, Strandberg K et al: Aspects of prostaglandin function in the lung. N Engl J Med 296:850, 910, 1977
24. Holgate ST, Bradding P, Sampson AP: Leukotriene antagonists and synthesis inhibitors: New directions in asthma therapy. J Allergy Clin Immunol. 98:1, 1996
25. Lazarus SC: Inflammation, inflammatory mediators, and mediator antagonists in asthma. J Clin Pharmacol 38:577, 1998
26. Schulman ES, Newball HH, Demers LM et al: Anaphylactic release of thromboxane A2, prostaglandin D2, and prostacyclin from human lung parenchyma. American Review of Respiratory Disease 124:402, 1981
27. Morel DR, Zapol WM, Thomas SJ et al: C5a and thromboxane generation associated with pulmonary vaso- and bronchoconstriction during protamine reversal of heparin. Anesthesiology 66:597, 1987
28. Meier HL, Kaplan AP, Lichtenstein LM et al: Anaphylactic release of a prekallikrein activator from human lung in vitro. J Clin Invest 72:574, 1983
29. Delage C, Irey NS: Anaphylactic deaths: A clinicopathologic study of 43 cases. J Forensic Sci 17:525, 1972
30. Smith Laboratories: Chymodiactin Post Marketing Surveillance Report. Chicago, Smith Laboratories, 1984
31. Laxenaire MC, Moneret-Vautrin DA, Vervloet D et al: Accidents anaphylactoides graves peranesthesiques. Ann Fr Anesth Reanim 4:30, 1985
32. Bochner BS, Lichtenstein LM: Anaphylaxis. N Engl J Med 324:1785, 1991
33. Pavek K, Wegmann A, Nordström L et al: Cardiovascular and respiratory mechanisms in anaphylactic and anaphylactoid shock reactions. Klin Wochenschr 60:941, 1982

34. Atkinson JP, Frank MM: Role of complement in the pathophysiology of hematologic disease. Prog Hematol 10:211, 1977

35. Jacobs HS, Craddock PR, Hammerschmidt DE et al: Complement-induced granulocyte aggregation: An unsuspected mechanism of disease. N Engl J Med 302:789, 1980

36. Dubois M, Lotze MT, Diamond WI et al: Pulmonary shunting during leukoagglutinin-induced noncardiogenic pulmonary edema. JAMA 244:2186, 1980

37. Teissner B, Brandslund I, Grunnet N et al: Acute complement activation during an anaphylactoid reaction to blood transfusion and the disappearance rate of C3c and C3d from the circulation. J Clin Lab Immunol 12:63, 1983

38. Hammerschmidt DE, Weaver LJ, Hudson LD et al: Association of complement activation and elevated plasma-C5a with adult respiratory distress syndrome. Lancet 1:947, 1980

39. Levy JH, Brister NW, Shearin A et al: Wheal and flare responses to opioids in humans. Anesthesiology 70:756, 1989

40. Levy JH, Adelson DM, Walker BF: Wheal and flare responses to muscle relaxants in humans. Agents Actions 34:302, 1991

41. Veien M, Holdin J, Szlam F et al: Mechanisms of non-immunological histamine and tryptase release from human cutaneous mast cells. Anesthesiology 92:1074, 2000

42. Levy JH, Kettlekamp N, Goertz P et al: Histamine release by vancomycin: A mechanism for hypotension in man. Anesthesiology 67:122, 1987

43. Caulfield JP, El-Lati S, Thomas G, Church MK: Dissociated human foreskin mast cells degranulate in response to anti-IgE and substance P. Lab Invest 63:502, 1990

44. Casale TB, Bowman S, Kaliner M: Induction of human cutaneous mast cell degranulation by opiates and endogenous opioid peptides: Evidence for opiate and nonopiate receptor participation. J Allergy Clin Immunol 73:775, 1984

45. Levy JH, Davis GK, Duggan J, Szlam F: Determination of the hemodynamics and histamine release of rocuronium (Org 9426) when administered in increased doses under N_2O/O_2-sufentanil anesthesia. Anesth Analg 78:318, 1994

46. Levy JH, Pitts M, Thanopoulos A et al: The effects of rapacuronium on histamine release and hemodynamics in adult patients undergoing general anesthesia. Anesth Analg 89:290, 1999

47. Hirshman CA, Downes H, Butler J: Relevance of plasma histamine levels to hypotension. Anesthesiology 57:424, 1982

48. Stark BJ, Sullivan TJ: Biphasic and protracted anaphylaxis. J Allergy Clin Immunol 78:76, 1986

49. Levy JH, Rockoff MR: Anaphylaxis to meperidine. Anesth Analg 61:301, 1982

50. Fisher MM: Blood volume replacement in acute anaphylactic cardiovascular collapse related to anaesthesia. Br J Anaesth 49:1023, 1977

51. Barnett A, Hirshman CA: Anaphylactic reaction to cephapirin during spinal anesthesia. Anesth Analg 58:337, 1979

52. Levy JH: Anaphylactic-anaphylactoid reactions during cardiac surgery. J Clin Anesthesiol 1:426, 1989

53. Austen KF: Tissue mast cells in immediate hypersensitivity. Hosp Pract 17:98, 1981

54. Hammerschmidt DE, White JG, Craddock PR et al: Corticosteroids inhibit complement-induced granulocyte aggregation: A possible mechanism for their efficacy in shock states. J Clin Invest 63:798, 1979

55. Halevy S, Altura BM: Pathophysiological basis for the use of steroids in the treatment of shock and trauma. Klin Wochenschr 60:1021, 1982

56. Sheagren JN: Septic shock and corticosteroids (editorial). N Engl J Med 305:456, 1981

57. Borda IT, Slone D, Jick H: Assessment of adverse reactions within a drug surveillance program. JAMA 205:645, 1968

58. DeSwarte RD: Drug allergy: Problems and strategies. J Allergy Clin Immunol 74:209, 1984

59. Tomicheck RC, Rosow CG, Philbin DM et al: Diazepam-fentanyl interaction: Hemodynamic and hormonal effect in coronary artery surgery. Anesth Analg 62:881, 1983

60. Fisher MM, Outhred A, Bowey CJ: Can clinical anaphylaxis to anaesthetic drugs be predicted from allergic history? Br J Anaesth 59:690, 1987

61. Christman D: Immune reaction to propanidid. Anaesthesia 39:470, 1984

62. Watkins J, Clarke SJ: Report of a symposium: Adverse responses to intravenous agents. Br J Anaesth 50:1159, 1978

63. Driggs RL, O'Day RA: Acute allergic reaction associated with methohexital anaesthesia: Report of six cases. J Oral Surg 30:906, 1972

64. Watkins J, Salo M: Incidence of immediate adverse response to intravenous anaesthetic drugs. In Trauma, Stress and Immunity in Anaesthesia and Surgery, p 272. London, Butterworth & Co, 1982

65. Schwartz HJ, Sher TH: Bisulfite sensitivity manifesting as allergy to local dental anaesthesia. J Allergy Clin Immunol 75:525, 1985

66. Brown DT, Beamins D, Wildsmith JAW: Allergic reaction to an amide local anesthetic. Br J Anaesth 53:435, 1981

67. Fisher MM, Munro I: Life-threatening anaphylactoid reactions to muscle relaxants. Anesth Analg 62:559, 1983

68. Swartz J, Braude BM, Gilmour RF et al: Intraoperative anaphylaxis to latex. Can J Anaesth 37:589, 1990

69. Roizen MF, Rodgers GM, Valone FH et al: Anaphylactoid reactions to vascular graft material presenting with vasodilation and subsequent disseminated intravascular coagulation. Anesthesiology 71:331, 1989

70. Laxenaire MC, Moneret-Vautrin DA, Watkins J: Diagnosis of the causes of anaphylactoid anaesthetic reactions. Anaesthesia 38:147, 1983

71. Vervloet D, Nizankowska E, Arnaud A et al: Adverse reactions to suxamethonium and other muscle relaxants under general anesthesia. J Allergy Clin Immunol 71:552, 1983

72. Harle DG, Baldo BA, Fisher MM: Detection of IgE antibodies to suxamethonium after anaphylactoid reactions during anaesthesia. Lancet 1:930, 1984

73. Zucker-Pinchoff B, Ramanathan S: Anaphylactic reaction to epidural fentanyl. Anesthesiology 71:599, 1989

74. Hilgard P: Immunological reactions to blood and blood products. Br J Anaesth 51:45, 1979

75. Sheffer AL, Pennoyer DS: Management of adverse drug reactions. J Allergy Clin Immunol 74:580, 1984

76. Levy JH, Zaidan JR, Faraj B: Prospective evaluation of risk of protamine reactions in NPH insulin-dependent diabetics. Anesth Analg 65:739, 1986

77. Levy JH, Schwieger IM, Zaidan JR et al: Evaluation of patients at risk for protamine reactions. J Thorac Cardiovasc Surg 98:200, 1989

78. Goldberg M: Systemic reactions to intravascular contrast media: A guide for the anesthesiologist. Anesthesiology 60:46, 1984

79. Isbister JP, Fisher MM: Adverse effects of plasma volume expanders. Anaesth Intensive Care 8:145, 1980

80. Colman WR: Paradoxical hypotension after volume expansion with plasma protein fraction. N Engl J Med 299:97, 1978

81. Ring K, Messmer K: Incidence and severity of anaphylactoid reactions to colloid volume substitutes. Lancet 1:466, 1977

82. Grant JA, Cooper JR, Arens JF et al: Anaphylactic reactions to protamine in insulin-dependent diabetics during cardiovascular surgery. Anesthesiology 59:A74, 1983

83. Berg TLO, Johansson SGO: Allergy diagnosis with the radioallergosorbent test: A comparison with the results of skin and provocation tests in an unselected group of children with asthma and hay fever. J Allergy Clin Immunol 54:209, 1974

84. Johansson SGO: In vitro diagnosis of reagin-mediated allergic diseases. Allergy 33:292, 1978

85. Baldo BA, Fisher MM: Detection of serum IgE antibodies that react with alcuronium and tubocurarine after life-threatening reactions to muscle relaxants. Anaesth Intensive Care 11:194, 1983

86. Harle DG, Baldo BA, Smal MA et al: Detection of thiopentone-reactive IgE antibodies following anaphylactoid reactions during anesthesia. Clin Allergy 16:493, 1986

87. Dueck R, O'Connor RD: Thiopental: False positive RAST in patient with elevated serum IgE. Anesthesiology 61:337, 1984

88. Fisher MM: Intradermal testing after anaphylactoid reaction to anaesthetic drugs: Practical aspects of performance and interpretation. Anaesth Intensive Care 12:115, 1984

89. Sage D: Intradermal drug testing following anaphylactoid reactions during anesthesia. Anaesth Intensive Care 9:381, 1981

90. Shatz M: Skin testing and incremental challenge in the evaluation of adverse reactions to local anesthetics. J Allergy Clin Immunol 74:606, 1984

91. Holzman RB: Clinical management of latex-allergic children. Anesth Analg 85:529, 1997

92. Kibby T, Akl M: Prevalence of latex sensitization in a hospital employee population. Ann Allergy Asthma Immunol 78:41, 1997

93. Gold M, Swartz JS, Braude BM et al: Intraoperative anaphylaxis: An

association with latex sensitivity. J Allergy Clin Immunol 87:662, 1991

94. Holzman RS: Latex allergy: An emerging operating room problem. Anesth Analg 76:635, 1993

95. Brown RH, Schauble JF, Hamilton RG: Prevalence of latex allergy among anesthesiologists: Identification of sensitized but asymptomatic individuals. Anesthesiology 89:292, 1998

96. Lavaud F, Prevost A, Cossart C *et al:* Allergy to latex, avocado, pear,

and banana: Evidence for a 30 kd antigen in immunoblotting. J Allergy Clin Immunol 95:557, 1995

97. Blanco C, Carrillo T, Castillo R *et al:* Latex allergy: Clinical features and cross-reactivity with fruits. Ann Allergy 73:309, 1994

98. Lebenbom-Mansour MH, Oesterle JR, Ownsby DR *et al:* The incidence of latex sensitivity in ambulatory surgical patients: A correlation of historical factors with positive serum immunoglobin E levels. Anesth Analg 85:44, 1997

Clinical Anesthesia (4/e), edited by
Paul G. Barash, Bruce F. Cullen, and
Robert K. Stoelting. Lippincott Williams &
Wilkins, Philadelphia, © 2001.

CHAPTER 50

DRUG INTERACTIONS

CARL ROSOW

Modern drug regimens for medical ailments like hypertension, angina, bronchospasm, or malignancy nearly always involve the use of multiple agents in combination. This strategy is frequently successful because many medical conditions are responsive to groups of drugs that act by different mechanisms and have different dose-limiting toxicities. The goal in each case is to produce increased therapeutic effect (or decreased toxicity) compared with treatment with individual agents. Unfortunately, the mixing of drugs is not without risk, and hundreds of research papers on the benefits and drawbacks of drug interactions appear every year. A sizable industry has now evolved to provide clinicians with reference books and computer databases on the subject.

Anesthesiologists face the same dilemma as all other physicians: drug combinations are a useful and necessary part of practice, but they are occasionally a source of morbidity. This chapter reviews the reasons that drugs are combined and the ways in which the combinations can alter either pharmacokinetics or pharmacodynamics. This is *not* a comprehensive list of anesthetic drug interactions—entire books are devoted to the subject.[1] The examples included have been chosen largely on the basis of proven or likely clinical relevance and the strength of their documentation. When possible, prototypic interactions are illustrated with examples that have direct relevance to anesthesia, although in some cases no such examples are available. The emphasis throughout is on mechanism, but it will quickly be apparent that our understanding of mechanism is incomplete for many pharmacodynamic interactions. Finally, it is important to know how to read the literature, and a short section is devoted to some of the common ways interactions can be studied.

HISTORICAL PERSPECTIVE

Historically, anesthesiologists were trained to regard drug interactions as a danger and something to be avoided. The generations of clinicians who administered open-drop diethyl ether probably had good reason to limit the number of anesthetic drugs administered: ether, by itself, could produce hypnosis, reasonable levels of analgesia, and muscle relaxation. Ventilation and blood pressure were usually well maintained because ether has respiratory stimulant and sympathomimetic properties. Clinicians could adjust the dose of this single agent fairly accurately using Guedel's criteria for pupil size, respiratory pattern, muscle tone, and so forth. All of this meant that a patient requiring even major abdominal surgery could be anesthetized using nothing more than a can of ether and a simple mask.

Before the Second World War, endotracheal intubation and controlled ventilation were usually not options, and muscle relaxants had not been introduced. Clinicians in this era were well served to keep things simple: if an anesthesiologist chose to add morphine to an ether anesthetic, the pupil and respiratory signs would no longer be reliable, muscle relaxation would probably decrease, and ventilatory depression (if it occurred) could not be treated easily.

The introduction of muscle relaxants, opioid-based anesthesia, and modern intravenous (iv) and inhaled anesthetics completely changed these considerations. The signs and stages of ether are no longer applicable, and controlled or assisted ventilation is often necessary because most of these drugs are profound respiratory depressants. Most important, clinicians now realize that anesthetics are highly specific drugs, and no single agent can produce all of the "desirable" components of anesthesia by itself. There is good evidence that even the potent volatile anesthetics are not sufficient to produce optimal anesthetic conditions when given alone. Zbinden *et al*[2] have shown that even moderately high concentrations of isoflurane in oxygen cannot suppress many cardiovascular responses to surgical stimuli. This finding is reflected in common clinical practice because isoflurane is routinely supplemented with opioids and other drugs to control blood pressure and heart rate.

Our views of what is desirable in anesthesia have also changed markedly. For example, most patients now expect and prefer an iv hypnotic rather than a mask for anesthetic induction. Similarly, the long emergence after ether is no longer expected or acceptable. A smooth recovery, free of pain or delirium is now considered routine within minutes after major surgical interventions. These goals are difficult to accomplish without using multiple drugs.

PROBLEMS CREATED BY DRUG–DRUG INTERACTION

There are almost no data on the true incidence of perioperative drug interaction, although there are data on general inpatient populations. We know that the probability of a drug–drug interaction increases with the number of drugs administered. Hospitalized patients are commonly given 10 or more drugs, and those in intensive care units may be receiving 15–20. In a frequently cited 1966 study, Smith *et al*[3] examined the frequency of drug "reactions" in hospitalized patients. The data showed that a linear increase in the number of drugs led to an exponential increase in the number of reactions (Table 50-1). The authors attributed the excess morbidity to drug interaction and concluded that there is a 24% chance of an "adverse interaction" when 10–15 drugs are administered concurrently.

Most anesthesiologists probably believe that this overstates the magnitude of the problem, at least as it applies to the intraoperative situation. Many patients are routinely taking 3 or 4 antihypertensives, antidepressants, or gastrointestinal drugs in the preoperative period, and most of them receive 5–10 drugs during general anesthesia, yet we do not normally hear about significant complications attributable to drug interaction. There are a number of possible explanations for this.

1. Interactions may occur, but they usually do not present a problem. In a sense, the practice of anesthesia is the diagnosis and treatment of drug "toxicity." Anesthesia practitioners are always prepared to titrate drugs and deal with the possibility of significant respiratory, central nervous system (CNS), or cardiovascular depression. Toxicity from a drug interaction is likely to become a source of morbidity primarily when it occurs in a setting where it is not rapidly recognized and treated. This happened when opioid–midazolam combinations were first used by nonanesthesia personnel for endoscopic and radiologic procedures. The unexpectedly large sedative and ventilatory effects led to numerous deaths.[4]

Table 50-1. ADVERSE DRUG REACTIONS: EFFECT OF TOTAL NUMBER OF DRUGS ADMINISTERED

No. Drugs	No. Patients	No. Reactions	Rate (%)
0–5	335	14	4.2
6–10	378	28	7.4
11–15	132	32	24.2
16–20	35	14	40.0
21+	20	9	45.0
Total	900	97	10.8

From Smith JW, Seidl LG, Cluff LG: Studies on the epidemiology of adverse drug reactions: V. Clinical factors influencing susceptibility. Ann Intern Med 65:629, 1966, with permission.

2. Variability in response to anesthetic drugs is the rule: the data on iv opioids[5] and hypnotics,[6] for example, show that different patients may have a three- to fivefold difference in the therapeutic and toxic effects of a given dose—even when the drug is given alone. We can assume that this variability is due to a large number of genetic and environmental factors, so the variability introduced by adding a second or third drug is usually only one more source of clinical "noise."

3. The qualitative nature of most anesthetic interactions is predictable even though the magnitude of the responses might not be known with certainty. It is no secret to an anesthesiologist that two cardiovascular depressants almost always produce more hypotension. Similarly, combinations of CNS depressants produce more, not less, depression. Drugs that interact to produce a totally unexpected or dangerous effect stand out because of their rarity. A notorious example of such an idiosyncratic interaction is the CNS excitation that may occur when meperidine is administered to patients taking monoamine oxidase (MAO) inhibitors (discussed later).

4. Many iv anesthetic drugs (diazepam, meperidine) have large safety margins—especially when respiration is supported—so small changes in drug concentration are not terribly important. The mere fact that a measurable interaction exists does not mean it will cause a difference in outcome or the need for intervention. Clinically meaningful interactions most often involve drugs like warfarin, digoxin, and theophylline, agents with only small differences between therapeutic and toxic concentrations.

5. Finally, it is likely that many instances of anesthetic drug interaction go unrecognized (a clinician must consider the possibility to make the diagnosis). Excessive drug effects are often attributed to some ill-defined patient "sensitivity." When a drug *fails* to produce an effect, it is because the patient is "tolerant" or "resistant." It is almost never considered a drug reaction or interaction.

WHY COMBINE DRUGS?

The goal of combining drugs is to decrease toxicity while maintaining or increasing efficacy. It is interesting to see how this principle has been applied in other areas of medicine.

1. Combination therapy is relatively straightforward in the treatment of hypertension. For example, a β-adrenergic antagonist and a vasodilator have at least additive effects on blood pressure, but their side effects are different and (presumably) nonadditive. Lower doses of each drug may be used in combination, so dose-related side effects are decreased.

2. The goals are different in combination chemotherapy for malignancy. To produce the maximum decrease in tumor burden, each chemotherapeutic drug is given at its maximally tolerated dose, an end point determined by its toxic effects on some normal cell population. Drugs such as alkylating agents and vinca alkaloids are combined because they have different dose-limiting organ toxicities (bone marrow and nerve, respectively), so each drug can be given at a full tumor-suppressing dose.

3. Finally, multiple-drug therapy is not usually the first choice for epilepsy. The mainstay drugs for prophylaxis of grand mal seizures (phenytoin, carbamazepine) have similar dose-limiting side effects such as ataxia and drowsiness. There is little to be gained by combining these drugs, so monotherapy tends to be the preferred mode of treatment.

PHARMACEUTICAL INTERACTIONS

A *pharmaceutical* interaction is a chemical or physical interaction that occurs before a drug is administered or absorbed systemically. The most obvious pharmaceutical interactions are the incompatibilities that can occur between iv drugs in solution:

- Precipitation of barbiturate may occur when thiopental or ketamine is injected together with succinylcholine into the iv line.
- Bicarbonate can decrease the solubility of bupivacaine and cause it to precipitate out of solution.
- Catecholamine solutions (norepinephrine, epinephrine) can be inactivated if they are alkalinized by the addition of sodium bicarbonate, a circumstance that could occur during cardiopulmonary resuscitation.

The number of these incompatibilities is very large, and the anesthesiologist is well advised to avoid mixing drugs unless they are known to be compatible. Information on specific iv drug incompatibilities is readily available from most hospital pharmacists.

Occasionally two drugs may interact chemically to form a toxic compound.

- The halogenated anesthetics, desflurane, enflurane, and isoflurane have been shown to interact with dry soda lime or baralyme to produce carbon monoxide.[7] Desiccation of soda lime is most likely to occur when oxygen has been left flowing through the canister overnight. Older anesthesiologists recall that trichloroethylene interacted with soda lime to produce the neurotoxin, dichloroacetylene.
- Nitric oxide (NO) is a selective pulmonary vasodilator that has been approved in the United States for treatment of primary pulmonary hypertension in the newborn.[8] If NO is allowed more than fleeting contact with oxygen, it forms nitrogen dioxide (NO_2). The latter compound can be quite toxic, and concentrations >10 ppm can produce pulmonary edema and alveolar hemorrhage. The problem is circumvented by allowing oxygen and NO to mix in the breathing circuit just before administration.

PHARMACOKINETIC INTERACTIONS

A *pharmacokinetic* interaction occurs when one drug alters the absorption, distribution, metabolism, or elimination of another. Many of the basic pharmacokinetic principles underlying these interactions are reviewed in Chapter 11.

Absorption

Alteration of absorption may occur because of direct chemical or physical interaction between drugs in the body or because one drug alters the physiologic mechanisms governing absorption of the second:

- Orally administered tetracycline can be inactivated by chelation if it is given together with antacids containing polyvalent cations like Mg^{2+}, Ca^{2+}, or Al^{3+}.

- Oral antidiarrheal drugs like kaolin and pectin can physically adsorb digoxin and prevent it from being absorbed.
- The bile acid–binding resin, cholestyramine, can bind to warfarin and prevent its absorption. On the other hand, it can also reduce the absorption of vitamin K and other fat-soluble compounds.

Another interaction of significance to anesthesiologists is the delay of gastric emptying produced by a variety of medications like opioids and anticholinergics.

Opioids produce hypertonus of smooth muscle, reduction of peristalsis, and contraction of sphincters throughout the gastrointestinal tract, and it appears that both central and peripheral mechanisms play a role in this effect. There are two important implications of delayed gastric emptying:

1. Opioid-premedicated patients are at increased risk for having a "full stomach" at the time of anesthesia induction.
   - Murphy et al[9] showed that when volunteers were given 500 ml of distilled water to drink, 0.09 mg · kg^{-1} of morphine increased the half-time for gastric emptying from 5.5 to 21 minutes.
2. The overall absorption of other drugs may also be reduced because the primary site for absorption of most orally administered drugs is the small intestine, and gastric emptying is rate-limiting.
   - Asai et al[10] have demonstrated in patients that morphine significantly reduces the absorption of oral acetaminophen.

Changes in regional blood flow (vasodilators, vasoconstrictors) can affect the absorption of parenterally administered drugs. Shock or congestive heart failure decrease perfusion of peripheral tissues like skin and muscle, so the onset and intensity of effect may become unpredictable for drugs given by intramuscular or subcutaneous injection.

- Local administration of epinephrine and other vasoconstrictors retards absorption of local anesthetics and therefore prolongs their effects.
- Numerous drugs can affect the pulmonary uptake of other drugs. Opioids and other drugs that decrease effective pulmonary ventilation have the potential to alter uptake of volatile anesthetics. Drugs that increase minute ventilation, reduce intrapulmonary shunting, or relieve bronchospasm can increase the uptake of volatile anesthetics, even though the inspired concentration remains constant.
- The rapid uptake of nitrous oxide can increase the alveolar concentration of concomitantly administered volatile anesthetics (the "second-gas effect").

Distribution

Many drug–drug interactions occur when one drug alters the distribution of a second. This may occur due to alterations in hemodynamics, drug ionization, or binding to plasma and tissue proteins. Much has been written about the involvement of these mechanisms in drug interactions (particularly the last two), but there are few examples of proven relevance to anesthesia.

There is little question that drug-induced hemodynamic compromise affects pharmacokinetics. Drugs like β blockers, calcium channel blockers, and vasodilators can decrease cardiac output by a variety of mechanisms (dysrhythmia, depression of contractility, decreased preload) and can produce significant changes in drug distribution. For a given rate of drug administration, a decrease in cardiac output increases the arterial drug concentration in highly perfused tissues like brain and myocardium.[11]

- In a patient with borderline cardiac function, normal doses of intravenous anesthetics like propofol and thiopental can produce substantial myocardial depression and hypotension. This is due to both pharmacodynamic and pharmacokinetic factors: the failing heart is often more sensitive to

Table 50-2. IONIZATION CONSTANTS (pK$_a$) OF SOME COMMON DRUGS*

Weak Acids		Weak Bases	
Acetaminophen	9.5	Albuterol	9.3
Aspirin	3.5	Alfentanil	6.5
Chlorothiazide	6.8, 9.4	Amiodarone	6.5
Furosemide	3.9	Amphetamine	9.8
Ibuprofen	4.4, 5.2	Atropine	9.7
Levodopa	2.3	Bupivacaine	8.1
Methyldopa	2.2, 9.2	Chlorpromazine	9.3
Pentobarbital	8.1	Clonidine	8.3
Phenobarbital	7.4	Cocaine	8.5
Phenytoin	8.3	Codeine	8.2
Theophylline	8.8	Desipramine	10.2
Thiopental	7.6	Diazepam	3.3
Tolbutamide	5.3	Diphenhydramine	9.0
Warfarin	5.0	Ephedrine	9.6
		Epinephrin	8.7
		Fentanyl	8.4
		Hydralazine	7.1
		Isoproterenol	8.6
		Kanamycin	7.2
		Lidocaine	7.9
		Methadone	8.4
		Metoprolol	9.8
		Morphine	7.9
		Norepinephrine	8.6
		Pentazocine	9.7
		Phenylephrine	9.8
		Physostigmine	7.9, 1.8
		Procainamide	9.2
		Procaine	9.0
		Propranolol	9.4
		Quinidine	8.5, 4.4
		Scopolamine	8.1
		Terbutaline	10.1

* The pK$_a$ is the pH at which 50% of drug is ionized. Some drugs have more than one ionizable group.

depressant medications, and the drugs attain higher tissue concentrations. There are animal data to suggest that brain sensitivity can be increased as well: dogs[12] or rats[13] with acute hemorrhagic hypovolemia have increased CNS sensitivity to the depressant effects of benzodiazepines.

- A patient with a low cardiac output state also has increased end-tidal concentrations of the potent volatile anesthetics and increased CNS effects.

Drug-induced changes in pH in a particular body region or fluid compartment can alter the distribution of other drugs by so-called "ion-trapping." Most of our therapeutic agents are weak acids or bases that are partially ionized at normal body pH (Table 50-2). It is only the nonionized fraction that can cross lipid membranes and come to equilibrium. The amount ionized can be determined for acids or bases from the general form of the Henderson-Hasselbalch equation:

$$\frac{[\text{Protonated}]}{[\text{Unprotonated}]} = 10^{(p\text{K}_a - p\text{H})}$$

Recall that an unprotonated acid is ionized, whereas an unprotonated base is nonionized. It is apparent from this relationship that a weak base (fentanyl, lidocaine) will be progressively ionized as the pH decreases, whereas a weak acid (aspirin, phenobarbital) will be more nonionized.

For certain membrane barriers, such as those in the stomach, placenta, or renal tubule, the pH on either side is different, and this creates the necessary conditions for ion trapping. Consider the case of a weak acid (ionization constant [pK$_a$] = 3.4) that is distributing between stomach and blood. In stomach acid (pH 2.4),

$$\frac{[\text{Nonionized}]}{[\text{Ionized}]} = 10^{(3.4-2.4)} = 10$$

In blood (*p*H 7.4),

$$\frac{[\text{Nonionized}]}{[\text{Ionized}]} = 10^{(3.4-7.4)} = 0.0001$$

At equilibrium, the concentrations of nonionized drug must be the same on either side of the gastric membrane barrier. This means that a 10,000-fold concentration gradient is established for total drug (nonionized + ionized):

STOMACH (*p*H 2.4)		BLOOD (*p*H 7.4)	
Nonionized	1 ⇌	1	Nonionized
	⇅	⇅	
Ionized	0.1	10,000	Ionized
Total	1.1	10,001	Total

It is easy to see why weak acids like aspirin are well absorbed from the stomach. The potential for drug interaction is great. Even moderate changes in *p*H can have large effects on this equilibrium: raising intragastric *p*H to 5.4 decreases the concentration gradient by 100-fold.

- Administration of antacid, histamine type 2 receptor antagonist, or omeprazole can reduce the gastric absorption of some acidic drugs. Alteration of *p*H has been shown to change the bioavailability of ketoconazole[14] and midazolam.[15]
- Lipid-soluble basic drugs like fentanyl and meperidine can be secreted *into* the stomach from the bloodstream. They become ionized and trapped in gastric acid only to be reabsorbed when they enter the more alkaline environment of the proximal jejunum. This gastric "recycling" is thought to be the basis for secondary increases in plasma concentrations of these opioids.[16]
- Alteration of urine *p*H can markedly alter the renal clearance of certain drugs (described in the section on Drug Elimination, later).

Much has been written about the role of plasma protein binding in drug–drug interaction. The fraction of the drug dose that is not distributed outside of the vascular space is either free or bound to circulating proteins. Acidic drugs bind to a greater or lesser degree to circulating proteins such as albumin and various globulin fractions. Many basic drugs like meperidine, lidocaine, bupivacaine, and propranolol bind to α_1-acid glycoprotein. Various pathophysiologic conditions can alter protein binding. α_1-Acid glycoprotein is an acute-phase reactant, so concentrations of this protein increase after surgery and in certain other conditions like burns, myocardial infarction, trauma, and malignancies. Conversely, hepatic cirrhosis and the nephrotic syndrome are often accompanied by hypoproteinemia and decreases in both albumin and globulin fractions.

The extent to which drug is bound versus free is important because it is only the unbound fraction that is available for crossing membranes, entering tissues, and binding to receptors to produce the pharmacologic effect. Protein-bound drug is not filtered by a normal glomerulus and (for some drugs) is not acted on by drug-metabolizing enzymes. A drug that is highly bound to plasma protein effectively exists in a "depot," not unlike a drug given by deep intramuscular injection. The potential therefore exists that one drug could alter the disposition, clearance, or biologic effect of another by altering its binding.

- The classic example of such an interaction is drug displacement of bilirubin in infants. Premature infants have immature glucuronyl transferase and are unable to conjugate bilirubin formed by destruction of erythrocytes. Much of the load of unconjugated bilirubin is bound to albumin and thus prevented from entering tissues. Sulfonamides and other drugs can compete for albumin binding sites, and the bilirubin they displace can enter tissues. Excessive levels of bilirubin in the brain can lead to kernicterus, a potentially fatal problem. This effect was discovered accidentally in 1956 during a clinical drug trial. When premature infants were given a penicillin–sulfonamide mixture, the mortality rate increased, and many were found to have kernicterus at autopsy.[17]
- The same mechanism has been described for numerous drug–drug interactions. Highly bound, potentially toxic drugs like warfarin and phenytoin may be displaced by other highly bound drugs. Warfarin is >98% bound to albumin, meaning that only 1–2% of the circulating drug accounts for the entire biologic effect. Phenylbutazone is a nonsteroidal anti-inflammatory drug (NSAID) that competes effectively for the same binding sites. If phenylbutazone displaces only 2% of warfarin, this theoretically doubles the free (active) fraction and greatly increases the anticoagulant effect.

The displacement interaction has been dogma for years, but the true clinical relevance of this type of interaction is actually not clear.[18] The argument has been made that, for many drugs, altered plasma protein binding causes only small or temporary changes in effect. The reasoning is as follows:

1. Most drugs are widely distributed in the body, and most of the administered dose is found outside of the vascular space. In the case of warfarin, over two thirds of the total is *extravascular*. Even a large change in plasma unbound fraction (*e.g.*, 10%) will therefore release only 3–4% of total warfarin in the body.
2. The body acts as a sink or buffer against large changes in unbound fraction (any unbound drug ultimately is distributed into peripheral tissues).

Some caution is still warranted for anesthesiologists and other clinicians who use iv drug regimens with doses often in the toxic range (*e.g.*, high doses of opioids, hypnotics, and muscle relaxants). In these circumstances, it is possible that even a temporary change in drug concentration can have clinical consequences.

Metabolism

There are numerous examples in anesthesia of drugs that increase or decrease the metabolism of others. Interactions may occur in extrahepatic or hepatic sites of metabolism.

Many drugs—especially those with ester linkages—undergo hydrolysis by specific or nonspecific esterases found in blood and peripheral tissues.

- Drugs given to inhibit acetylcholinesterase at the motor end plate usually inhibit butyrylcholinesterase (pseudocholinesterase) in plasma. Thus, administration of neostigmine or pyridostigmine intensifies and prolongs the effects of succinylcholine and could theoretically affect ester local anesthetics (procaine, chloroprocaine, tetracaine, cocaine) as well. Enzyme inhibition probably needs to be substantial (<20% of normal activity remaining) before the clinical effects of these local anesthetics become prolonged.[19,20] The prolongation of effect depends on the specific inhibitor. Neostigmine, for example, can prolong the effect of succinylcholine by several hours. The organophosphate, echothiophate, is a powerful miotic used topically for refractory glaucoma. This compound irreversibly inhibits pseudocholinesterase.[19,21] The effect persists for weeks, so the risk for interaction is prolonged.
- Drugs like esmolol and remifentanil are hydrolyzed by so-called "nonspecific" esterases in blood and peripheral tissues.[22] These drugs are not good substrates for cholinesterases, so they are not subject to this interaction.[23] The nonspecific esterases constitute a large group of isozymes with extremely high capacity and low substrate specificity. This enzyme system is not likely to be involved in drug–drug

interactions because inhibition of any one isozyme usually does not affect overall drug clearance.

Monamide Oxidase Interactions

The enzyme, MAO, is found in tissues throughout the body, with the largest amounts found in liver, kidney, and brain. MAO is located on the outer surface of mitochondria in the presynaptic terminals of noradrenergic, dopaminergic, and serotonergic neurons in the CNS and periphery. It acts to regulate the presynaptic pool of norepinephrine, dopamine, epinephrine, and serotonin available for synaptic transmission (see Chapter 12). MAO exists in two isoforms: MAO-A preferentially metabolizes serotonin, dopamine, and norepinephrine, whereas MAO-B preferentially metabolizes phenylethylamine and tyramine.

The MAO inhibitors (MAOI) are used mainly for the treatment of refractory endogenous depression and certain other mood disorders. They have gained some notoriety in medicine because they are the cause of more clinically important drug–drug interactions than almost any other class of drugs. Many of the purported interactions are poorly documented, although they cannot be discounted completely.

There are currently only three MAOI marketed in the United States. Phenelzine (Nardil) is an older, nonselective MAOI derived from hydrazine. It irreversibly inhibits the enzyme, and synthesis of new enzyme can take 10–14 days. Tranylcypromine (Parnate) is a slightly shorter-acting MAOI derived from amphetamine. The newest member of this class is selegiline (deprenyl, Eldepryl), a selective MAO-B inhibitor used as an adjunct in the treatment of Parkinson's disease. The antibiotic furazolidone and the chemotherapeutic drug procarbazine also cause substantial inhibition of MAO and can potentially cause many of the same interactions. The herbal supplement St. John's Wort has been used for depression and was originally thought to have some MAOI effects. This has not been borne out in subsequent studies.

Reported MAOI interactions are broadly of two types: the first group involves drugs that affect sympathetic neurotransmission:

- The well-known interaction with indirect-acting sympathomimetic drugs (ephedrine, amphetamine, metaraminol) occurs because MAOI treatment increases the amount of presynaptic transmitter that can be released by these drugs. Normal doses of ephedrine can produce exaggerated sympathetic responses, including severe hypertensive crises. Deaths have been attributed to severe hyperpyrexia and cerebral hemorrhage.
- The "wine and cheese" reaction is essentially the same interaction. Many foods like aged cheese contain tyramine, a phenylethylamine that has ephedrine-like actions at sympathetic nerve endings. Normally, exogenous tyramine is degraded by MAO in the gut wall and liver, but patients on an MAOI may achieve high systemic concentrations and consequently have hypertensive crises.
- Paradoxically, a patient who has been taking an MAOI for some time may actually have *decreased* adrenergic responsiveness (some of the older MAOIs were marketed as treatments for hypertension). Even with good dietary compliance, these patients absorb some tyramine. Chronic exposure to low levels of tyramine allows this compound to be taken up by adrenergic terminals (in place of tyrosine), where it is metabolized to octopamine (rather than norepinephrine). Octopamine is a "false transmitter" with little activity, so sympathetic nerve function may eventually be impaired.
- Because MAO plays only a small role in the metabolism of compounds in the synaptic cleft, the response to sympathomimetics that act directly on postsynaptic receptor sites (phenylephrine, norepinephrine, epinephrine) should be affected less by such interactions. In a small study of four

healthy volunteers (two receiving tranylcypromine and two receiving phenelzine), there was a moderate (twofold) increase in the response to phenylephrine, but the responses to norepinephrine and epinephrine were not exaggerated.[24] This is reassuring, but any sympathomimetic drug should still be administered with caution to patients on an MAOI.

- Adverse interactions have been described with older MAOIs and levodopa,[25] possibly because both drugs increase dopamine concentrations. Nevertheless, there is a small beneficial effect in patients with Parkinson's disease receiving levodopa and selegiline (the MAOI is given in this case to prevent free radical formation thought to be involved in neuronal degeneration).[26]
- Inhibition of norepinephrine reuptake by tricyclic antidepressants (TCAs) increases the amount of neurotransmitter in the synaptic cleft. This would seem to be a recipe for adverse interaction with MAOIs, but with careful monitoring, this combination has been used successfully for therapy.

The second group of MAOI interactions involves CNS depressants. As stated previously, many of these are poorly documented, and the mechanisms are unknown.

- The most important interaction is unquestionably with meperidine. When meperidine is given to a patient on an MAOI, a life-threatening reaction may occur, accompanied by excitation, hyperpyrexia, hypertension, profuse sweating, and rigidity.[27] This may progress to seizures, coma, and death. The reaction does not occur in every instance. It has also been described with selegiline,[28] but not yet with experimental inhibitors selective for MAO-A. There are one or two case reports suggesting that a toxic interaction may occur with the antitussive, dextromethorphan.[29] Other than some poorly documented case reports, the evidence suggests that other opioids like morphine and fentanyl do not produce this interaction.[30] The mechanism of meperidine–MAOI interaction is unknown, but animal models suggest that it involves elevations in brain concentrations of serotonin.[31]
- Anecdotal reports have appeared regarding adverse MAOI interactions with other psychotropic drugs, including alcohol, phenothiazines, benzodiazepines, and barbiturates,[32,33] but the evidence is weak. Some wines, like Chianti, could be dangerous because they contain tyramine. It is possible (but probably not advisable) to use ketamine for induction of anesthesia in such patients.[34]

Should MAOIs be discontinued before elective surgery? The issue is still a matter of debate,[35] although drug package inserts usually advise an extremely conservative position (*i.e.*, waiting 2 weeks for the enzyme to regenerate). Current clinical opinion probably favors continuing MAOI therapy up to the time of surgery, and our own anecdotal experience supports this view. Most patients are receiving these drugs for moderate to severe psychiatric disorders that have not responded to other treatments. It is unpleasant and possibly risky for a patient with refractory depression to endure 2–3 weeks without effective therapy. If a general anesthetic is planned, it seems prudent to use the fewest possible drugs. Avoiding drugs with substantial sympathetic effects (*e.g.*, pancuronium, cocaine, ketamine) probably makes sense.

There is little doubt that patients taking MAOIs have the potential for perioperative hemodynamic instability, yet β blockers, direct vasodilators, and direct-acting pressors appear to be safe and effective treatments in most circumstances. Roizen[36] has concluded, "The major problem with continuing MAO inhibitors preoperatively is not the hemodynamic fluctuations that might occur . . . but rather the rare instance of hyperpyrexic coma following narcotic administration. . . ." Because opioids like fentanyl appear safe, and there are no major interactions with local anesthetics or NSAIDs, providing analgesia without meperidine should not be a hardship.

Hepatic Biotransformation

Many anesthetic drugs undergo oxidative metabolism by one of the isoforms of cytochrome P-450 found in liver microsomes. The P-450 isoforms have low substrate specificity, which means that drugs of diverse structures, such as general inhalation anesthetics, meperidine, barbiturates, and benzodiazepines, can be biotransformed by a single group of enzymes. It is not surprising that inhibitors or inducers of these enzymes can also affect the clearance of broad groups of drugs.

The removal of drug from the blood by hepatic biotransformation (hepatic clearance) is a function of two independent variables, the hepatic blood flow and the intrinsic clearance (the maximal ability of the liver to metabolize that drug). The intrinsic clearance is often expressed as the *extraction ratio* (ER)—the fraction of drug that can be metabolized in a single pass through the liver (see Chapter 11)

$$ER = \frac{C_a - C_v}{C_a}$$

where C_a is the drug concentration coming to the liver (mixed portal vein + hepatic artery) and C_v is the drug concentration leaving (hepatic vein). So,

Hepatic clearance = ER × hepatic blood flow

Drugs may be classed broadly as "high extraction" and "low extraction," a distinction with important implications for drug interaction:

A high-extraction drug (*e.g.,* lidocaine, propranolol) may have an ER of 0.7–0.8 or more (70–80% is cleared in one pass through the liver). For these drugs, hepatic blood flow is the rate-limiting factor in overall hepatic clearance, that is, the delivery of drug to the liver determines the amount cleared. Clearance is decreased by drugs or maneuvers that lower hepatic blood flow, such as β blockade, cimetidine, halothane, hypotension, and upper abdominal surgery. The clearance of these rapidly metabolized drugs is much less sensitive to changes in enzyme activity. Nor does plasma protein binding have a large effect: the enzymes are so active that a drug like lidocaine is simply stripped off its binding proteins as it traverses the liver.

- Decreases in hepatic blood flow secondary to decreased cardiac output elevate lidocaine concentrations in humans.[37]
- Pressor administration can also accomplish the same thing. This effect was elegantly demonstrated by Benowitz *et al*[38] in rhesus monkeys (Fig. 50-1). Steady-state infusions of lidocaine were established, and then hepatic blood flow was increased or decreased by infusions of isoproterenol or norepinephrine, respectively. During isoproterenol infusion, the concentration of lidocaine decreased, indicating increased clearance. During norepinephrine infusion, lidocaine concentrations increased.
- Lidocaine clearance is decreased and toxicity is increased when patients are treated chronically with cimetidine.[39] It is not clear whether single-dose premedication with cimetidine produces the same effect.
- Other high-extraction drugs, such as morphine and sufentanil, are affected the same way. The clearance of morphine may be very slow in a patient with congestive heart failure and hepatic congestion.

Low-extraction drugs like diazepam, alfentanil, or mepivacaine have ERs of 0.3 or less. These drugs behave quite differently because hepatic enzyme activity is rate limiting (hepatic clearance is limited by intrinsic clearance). Stimulation or inhibition of enzyme activity can have a large effect on overall pharmacokinetics. Protein binding is also more likely to affect clearance because the bound forms of these drugs are protected from hepatic metabolism.

The most common reason for increased intrinsic clearance is enzyme induction. Many drugs of importance in anesthesiology are metabolized by the cytochrome P-450 enzymes (so-called microsomal or CYP enzymes). Several families and numerous subfamilies of these enzymes have been identified based on the homology of their amino acid sequences. The most important subfamily appears to be CYP3A, which is found in greatest abundance in human liver and is responsible for the metabolism of a huge number of drugs. Other subfamilies play important roles in drug metabolism, such as CYP2C19 (diazepam) or CYP2E1 (defluorination of volatile anesthetics). There are hundreds of drugs and environmental toxins that can stimulate or "induce" microsomal enzymes. Typically, a single inducer can affect the products of several gene families. For example, phenobarbital can increase the amount of the P-450 enzymes CYP2B, 2C, 2E, 3A, and 4B.[40] The increase in the quantity of enzyme protein can therefore increase the clearance of many drugs simultaneously. Not all inducers affect the same enzymes, however.

Treatment with an enzyme inducer (Table 50-3) can make an otherwise stable drug regimen ineffective or inconsistently effective.

- A classic example is the interaction between phenobarbital and coumarin-type anticoagulants (Fig. 50-2).

Increased metabolism may also result in the production of an active or toxic metabolite.

- In rat microsomal preparations, the liberation of inorganic fluoride by isoflurane, methoxyflurane, and enflurane can be increased by pretreatment with barbiturates,[41] but this interaction appears to be clinically important only for methoxyflurane.[42] In humans, phenobarbital does not induce the defluorination of enflurane.
- Reductive pathways also involve P-450 enzymes, and the production of toxic reduced intermediates has been postulated as a mechanism for halothane hepatitis. In animal models, administration of halothane after enzyme inducers can lead to centrilobular necrosis.[43] The clinical relevance of this finding is unknown.

There are many examples of drugs that inhibit the hepatic biotransformation of other drugs.

- When two drugs are substrates for the same P-450 enzymes, they can interact competitively and reduce the clearance of both. For example, it has been demonstrated that midazolam and fentanyl are competitive inhibitors *in vitro* of metabolism by CYP3A4.[44] This pharmacokinetic interaction is probably far less important than the pharmacodynamic interaction between these drugs (described later).
- Another study concluded that propofol competitively inhibits CYP3A4, and it can reduce the clearance of midazolam by 37%.[45] Propofol itself appears to be metabolized by a different isoform, CYP1A2.[46]
- Alfentanil and erythromycin are both metabolized by CYP3A4, and the antibiotic has been greatly shown to prolong the effect of the opioid.[47] Sufentanil and fentanyl are also metabolized by CYP3A4,[48] but the clearance of sufentanil is not changed by erythromycin.[49] Perhaps this is because these are higher-clearance opioids.
- Cimetidine has an imidazole group that binds to the heme iron of cytochrome P-450 and forms an inactive complex. Cimetidine inhibits the metabolism of many drugs, including warfarin, diazepam, phenytoin, and morphine. Several studies have demonstrated that coadministration of cimetidine and diazepam causes clinically significant elevations in the concentration of both diazepam and its active metabolite.[50] As stated previously, cimetidine can decrease hepatic blood flow, so it can also decrease the clearance of high-extraction drugs.[39]
- Protease inhibitors like saquinavir[51] and ritonavir[52] can inhibit the metabolism of midazolam and fentanyl, respectively, by inhibiting CYP3A4.

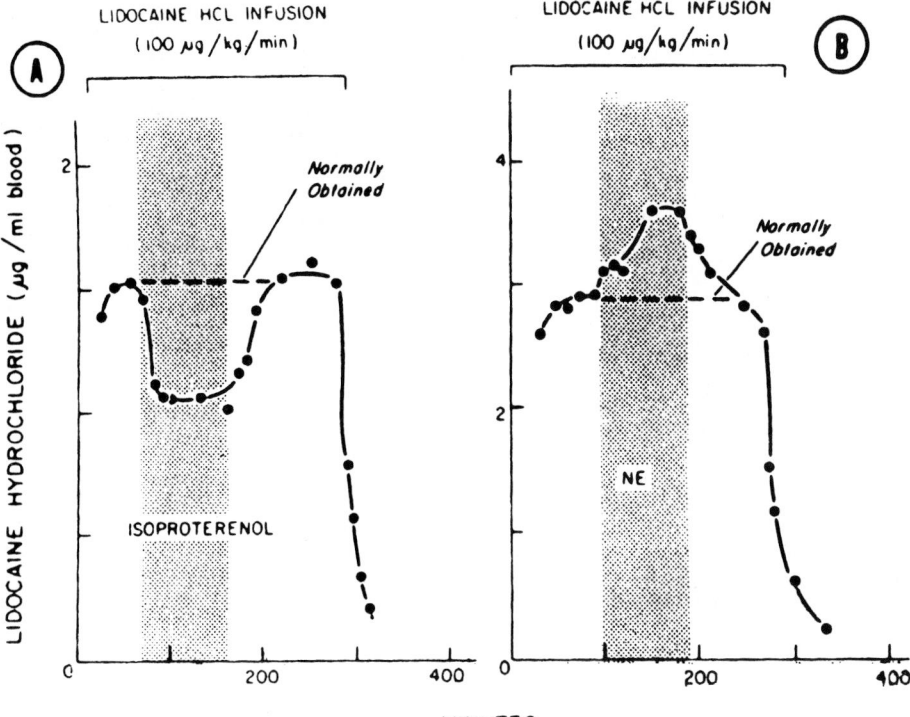

Figure 50-1. The effects of increasing or decreasing hepatic blood flow with isoproterenol (*A*) and norepinephrine (NE) (*B*) on steady-state arterial lidocaine concentrations in the rhesus monkey. The pressors were administered during the period indicated by the *shaded bar*. The *dashed lines* show the steady-state concentration expected in the absence of pressors. (From Benowitz N *et al:* Lidocaine disposition kinetics in monkey and man: II. Effects of hemorrhage and sympathomimetic drug administration. Clin Pharmacol Ther 16:99, 1974, with permission.)

- Other imidazole drugs like the antihistamine, astemizole, and the antifungals, ketoconazole and itraconazole, can inhibit a wide variety of microsomal enzymes. The antifungals, in particular, have been shown to decrease the clearance (and increase the toxicity) of glyburide, terfenadine, digoxin, midazolam, theophylline, and warfarin.
- The related benzimidazole, etomidate, blocks the synthesis of cortisol and aldosterone by inhibiting the P-450–dependent mitochondrial enzymes, 17α- and 11β-hydroxylase.[53] Etomidate can inhibit the metabolism of other drugs, but the effects do not appear to be clinically important.

Drug Elimination

The final category of pharmacokinetic interaction is through alteration in drug elimination. These interactions usually involve altered renal clearance, but they may also involve changes in pulmonary excretion.

The mechanism for ion-trapping was discussed earlier. Ion trapping can be the basis for large changes in renal drug excretion when the pK_a of the drug is close to the normal range of urine pH.

- A weak acid like phenobarbital (pK_a = 7.4) is largely nonionized when the urine pH is 6.0. This means that much of the filtered drug is in a relatively lipid-soluble form and available for tubular reabsorption. If the urine pH is raised

to 8 or 9 with sodium bicarbonate, most of the phenobarbital becomes ionized, reabsorption decreases, and clearance increases. For a weak base, the reverse situation is true—excretion can be promoted when the urine is acidified. This type of interaction is used therapeutically in certain cases of drug overdose.

Organic anions and cations are actively secreted by separate transporters in the renal tubule. The cation system handles the elimination of atropine, isoproterenol, neostigmine, and meperidine. The anion system is involved in the excretion of salicylate, penicillins, cephalosporins, and most of the potent diuretics. The various anions and cations can compete for their respective transport sites.

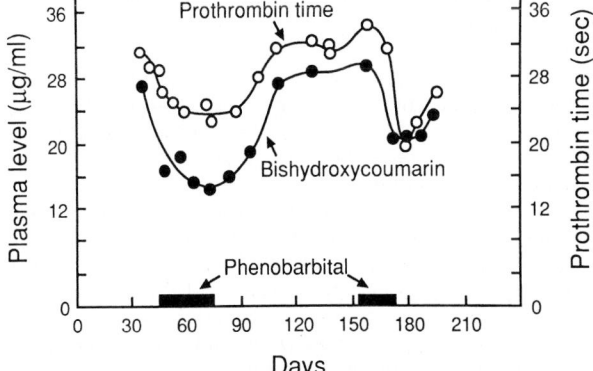

Figure 50-2. Effect of phenobarbital on plasma levels of bishydroxycoumarin. The anticoagulant was given at a dose of 75 mg · day^{-1}. Phenobarbital, 65 mg · day^{-1}, was given during the periods indicated on the x-axis. Induction of hepatic enzymes decreased anticoagulant concentrations and reduced the effect. (From Cucinell SA, Conney AH, Sansur M *et al:* Drug interactions in man: I. Lowering effect of phenobarbital on plasma levels of bishydroxy coumarin [dicumarol] and diphenylhydantoin [Dilantin]. Clin Pharmacol Ther 6:420, 1965, with permission.)

Table 50-3. DRUGS THAT INDUCE OR INHIBIT HEPATIC DRUG METABOLISM IN HUMANS

Inducers	Inhibitors
Phenobarbital	Cimetidine
Phenytoin	Ketoconazole
Rifampicin	Erythromycin
Carbamazepine	Disulfiram
Ethanol	Ritonavir

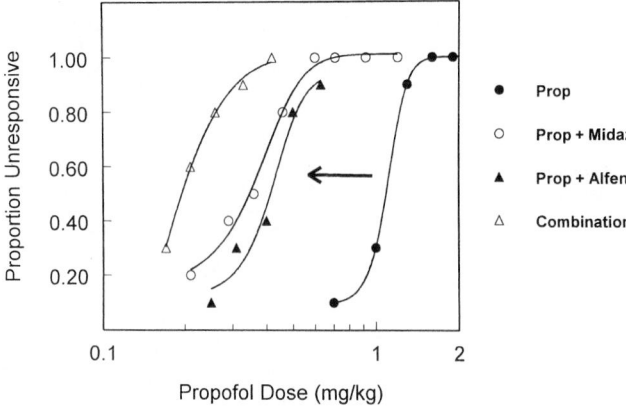

Figure 50-3. Dose–response curves for loss of consciousness after an intravenous bolus dose of propofol (Prop) alone, propofol plus midazolam (Midaz), propofol plus alfentanil (Alfent), or all three drugs. Drug combinations were given as constant ratios, based on the measured ED₅₀s of the individual drugs. Both the benzodiazepine and the opioid shifted the dose–response curve for propofol significantly to the left. (From Short TG, Plummer JL, Chui PT: Hypnotic and anaesthetic interactions between midazolam, propofol and alfentanil. Br J Anaesth 69:162, 1992, with permission.)

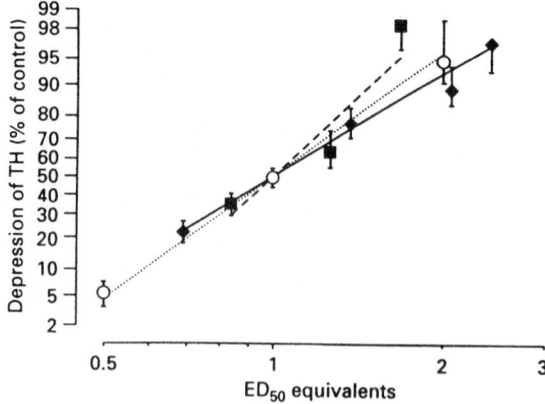

Figure 50-4. The interaction of rocuronium and vecuronium is additive in man. Log dose-probit graph plots twitch height (TH) as percentage of control value. Dose is given in terms of ED₅₀ multiples. *Dark diamonds, dark squares,* and *open circles* represent rocuronium, vecuronium, and the combination, respectively. The dose–response curve for the combination cannot be distinguished from those of the individual drugs. (From Naguib M, Samarkandi AH, Bakhamees HS *et al:* Comparative potency of steroidal neuromuscular blocking drugs and isobolographic analysis of the interaction. Br J Anaesth 75:37, 1995, with permission.)

- Probenecid inhibits the secretion of penicillin, increasing plasma concentrations and prolonging the duration of action.
- Quinidine has been shown to decrease both the volume of distribution and the renal clearance of digoxin, and plasma digoxin concentrations may increase by 2–5 fold.[54] The renal effect is thought to be due to a reduction in tubular secretion of digoxin.

PHARMACODYNAMIC INTERACTIONS

Up to this point, we have been discussing pharmacokinetic interactions that change the amount of active drug reaching receptor sites. A *pharmacodynamic* interaction occurs when one drug alters the sensitivity of a target receptor or tissue to the effects of a second drug. This means that the dose–response or concentration–response curve for one drug is shifted by another (Fig. 50-3). It is often difficult to assign a specific mechanism to these interactions. We commonly classify them by their direction and intensity, that is, additive, antagonistic, or supra-additive (synergistic).

Additive interactions are most likely to occur when drugs with identical mechanisms are combined. The clinician normally expects additivity when combining two benzodiazepines, two fentanyl analogues, or two volatile anesthetics. Most additive interactions tend not to be particularly surprising, although some are clinically useful.

- The administration of two aminosteroid nondepolarizing muscle relaxants like rocuronium and vecuronium gives an additive effect[55] (Fig. 50-4). Notably, the interactions between nondepolarizing relaxants of different chemical classes is often synergistic (see later).
- The interaction of two volatile anesthetics or nitrous oxide with volatile anesthetics is additive.[56–58]
- In animals, mixtures of lidocaine–tetracaine or lidocaine–etidocaine produce approximately additive CNS toxicity when given iv.[59]

The most common *antagonistic drug interactions* in anesthesia are those involving deliberate reversal with competitive antagonists such as neostigmine, naloxone, or flumazenil. Pharmacodynamic antagonism that is *unintended* is a much less common event.

- There is an antagonistic interaction between succinylcholine and the nondepolarizing relaxants.[60]
- When epidural morphine or fentanyl is administered after establishing a block with 2-chloroprocaine, both the duration and the intensity of opioid analgesia are decreased.[61] The mechanism for this interaction is unclear.
- Several years ago, we studied the memory effects of the drugs butorphanol and midazolam, both alone and in combination.[62] As expected, the anterograde amnestic effects of midazolam were profound, whereas the opioid agonist–antagonist produced much less amnesia (Fig. 50-5). When butorphanol was combined with midazolam, the mixture had less amnestic effect than midazolam alone. In this instance, the opioid may simply have been diluting the effects of the benzodiazepine.

The most interesting and clinically important interactions tend to be the *synergistic interactions,* in which small doses of

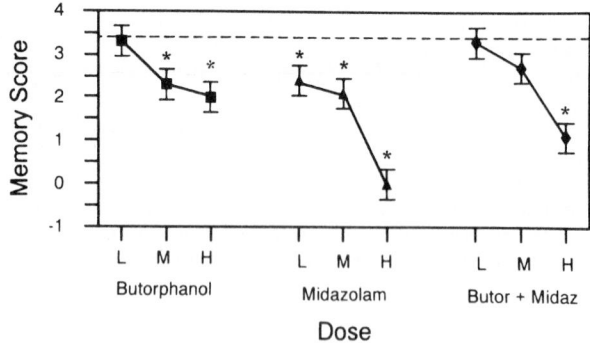

Figure 50-5. Memory scores of patients 5 minutes after receiving butorphanol, midazolam, or the combination. L, M, and H signify low, medium, and high doses (7.1, 22.5, and 71.4 μg · kg⁻¹ butorphanol; 4.3, 13.6, and 42.9 μg · kg⁻¹ midazolam; or 3.6 + 2.2, 11.3 + 6.8, and 35.7 + 21.5 μg · kg⁻¹ butorphanol and midazolam in combination). The *dashed line* indicates mean pretreatment value. Midazolam, but not butorphanol, produced a profound anterograde amnestic effect. Giving one-half the dose of each drug in combination produced an effect that was less than that after midazolam alone. (From Dershwitz M, Rosow CE, DiBiase PM *et al:* A comparison of the sedative effects of butorphanol and midazolam. Anesthesiology 74:717, 1991, with permission.)

two or more drugs can sometimes produce very large effects. Synergy is most likely to occur when drugs of different classes, or even those with slightly different mechanisms, are used to produce the same effects.

- The potentiation of opioids by NSAIDs is a classic and useful interaction between analgesic drugs with completely different mechanisms.[63–66]
- The potentiation of nondepolarizing relaxants by the various volatile anesthetics is a useful interaction on a daily basis. The exact mechanism is unknown, but several theories have been proposed, including increased blood flow to muscle, depression of centrally mediated muscle tone, decreased neurotransmitter release, and decreased sensitivity of postjunctional or muscle membranes.
- A much subtler supra-additive interaction occurs between aminosteroid and benzylisoquinoline relaxants. Pancuronium and *d*-tubocurarine were shown to produce a synergistic relaxant effect in combination,[67] and this is also seen with similar combinations across these two chemical classes (atracurium and vecuronium, *d*-tubocurarine and vecuronium, mivacurium and rocuronium[55]). Various mechanisms have been proposed, including multiple binding sites[68] (presynaptic for aminosteroids versus postsynaptic for benzylisoquinolines) and allosteric interactions between separate agonist and antagonist binding sites.[69]
- Another clinically important synergistic interaction occurs between barbiturates and benzodiazepines (discussed later), hypnotics with related mechanisms of action. Both drugs act on the γ-aminobutyric acid-A (GABA_A)–chloride ionophore complex, and both ultimately cause CNS depression by increasing neuronal chloride conductance. However, the mechanisms of action are slightly different: benzodiazepines act indirectly by facilitation of GABA action; barbiturates bind to a separate site and affect the chloride channel more directly.

STUDYING DRUG INTERACTIONS

As already discussed, a study that demonstrates that a drug–drug interaction exists does not necessarily establish its mechanism, its magnitude, or its clinical relevance. What information do we need to conclude that an interaction is pharmacodynamic rather than pharmacokinetic? How do we know it is really synergistic? Let us consider four possible ways to study the benzodiazepine–barbiturate interaction mentioned earlier.

1. In the simplest study design, two groups of patients are randomly assigned to receive midazolam–thiopental or placebo–thiopental. The percentage that becomes unresponsive in each group is assessed at a standard time after thiopental administration. The data show that midazolam increases the percentage unresponsive.
   Such a study is severely limited: it tells us that an interaction has occurred, but the results cannot be generalized beyond the conditions examined (a single dose of midazolam, a single dose of thiopental). Nothing may be inferred about mechanism.
2. A more complex (but more useful) experiment would be to study a series of thiopental doses (a dose–response curve) in the presence and absence of midazolam. This would show that the dose of thiopental required to produce hypnosis in half the patients (ED50) is decreased by midazolam.
   These results allow us to conclude that the interaction occurs over a range of thiopental doses relevant to clinical practice. The data still apply only to a single dose of midazolam, and they tell us nothing about the mechanism of the interaction.
3. A further useful modification of this experiment is to administer the thiopental by a constant-rate infusion and measure its concentration at the point response is lost.

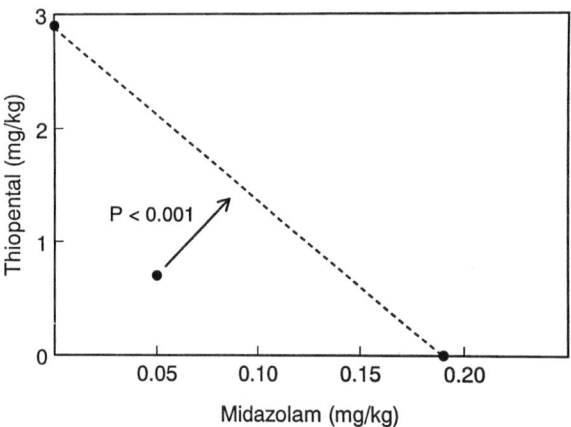

Figure 50-6. Isobolographic analysis of the interaction between midazolam and thiopental in humans (see text for details). The ED_50 of the combination was significantly less than predicted by the dotted ''line of additivity.'' (Redrawn from data of Tverskoy M, Fleyshman G, Bradley EL Jr, Kissin I: Midazolam-thiopental anesthetic interaction in patients. Anesth Analg 67:342, 1988, with permission.)

The data show that similar concentrations of thiopental are achieved in both groups, but the concentration needed to produce hypnosis in half the patients (the EC_50) is decreased.
This tells us that midazolam has not changed the pharmacokinetics of thiopental, so the interaction must have a pharmacodynamic mechanism.

4. Finally, how can we determine that this pharmacodynamic interaction is truly synergistic, that is, more than expected from simple addition? There are a number of experimental designs for quantitatively assessing the effects of drug combinations, and these have been reviewed in the clinical literature.[70] Two of the most common techniques used by experimental pharmacologists are algebraic (fractional)[71] and isobolographic[72,73] analysis, and clinical anesthesia studies using this method are increasingly more common. The interaction of thiopental and midazolam was studied with an isobolographic technique, and the results are shown in Figure 50-6.[74] In general, this analysis requires a minimum of *three* dose–response experiments, one with each drug alone and one with the drugs in combination. The drug combination can be studied as a fixed ratio, or one of the drugs can be given at a fixed dose and the dose of the second drug varied. From these experiments, three estimates of ED_50 are made, and an isobologram is constructed as shown in Figure 50-6. The ED_50s for thiopental and midazolam alone are graphed on the two axes, and these points are connected by the theoretic ''line of additivity.'' If the two drugs are simply additive when combined, we would expect the ED_50 of the mixture to fall somewhere along this line. Because the actual ED_50 of the mixture is significantly less than predicted by this line, the interaction is synergistic (an ED_50 greater than predicted would have signified antagonism).

SPECIFIC INTERACTIONS AFFECTING HEMODYNAMICS

The treatment of hypertension, angina, dysrhythmias, and congestive heart failure involves the use of drugs with powerful effects on autonomic function and cardiovascular homeostasis. Until the 1970s, the teaching was generally that cardiovascular depressant or stimulant medications should be discontinued before surgery because they interfered with protective responses

Table 50-4. EFFECTS OF ANTIHYPERTENSIVE DRUGS DURING ANESTHESIA

Class	Drugs	Effects
α Blockers	Phenoxybenzamine Phentolamine Prazosin	Hypotension/vasodilation Reflex tachycardia
β Blockers	Propranolol Metoprolol Atenolol	Hypotension Decreased contractility Bradycardia AV Block
Mixed α/β blocker	Labetalol	Hypotension/vasodilation Bradycardia AV Block
Calcium channel blockers	Verapamil Diltiazem Nifedipine Nicardipine	Hypotension/vasodilation Decreased contractility Bradycardia AV Block
Direct vasodilators	Nitroglycerin Isosorbide Hydralazine	Hypotension/vasodilation Reflex tachycardia
Angiotensin-converting enzyme inhibitors	Captopril Enalapril Lisinopril	Hypotension/vasodilation Hyperkalemia
Angiotensin II blocker	Losartan Valsartan	Hypotension/vasodilation Hyperkalemia
Diuretics	Thiazides Furosemide Bumetanide	Hypovolemia Hypokalemia Possible vasodilation

AV = atrioventricular.

to the trauma of anesthesia and surgery. There is now a substantial body of evidence showing that most cardiovascular medications need not and should not be stopped before surgery. Hypertensive patients who remain well controlled are less likely to have wide swings in pressure during surgery. Even small doses of β blockers given before surgery can reduce the incidence of myocardial ischemia and improve outcome.[75,76] One week of perioperative treatment with atenolol can produce long-term benefits.[77,78] Conversely, the abrupt discontinuation of vasoactive medications can actually increase cardiovascular instability, and in the case of β blockers and clonidine, the rebound hypertension and dysrhythmias may be dangerous.

Given the foregoing observations, it is fortunate that most cardiovascular drug–drug interactions are simply extensions of the known pharmacology of the agents (Table 50-4). In short, the hypotensive effects of general or regional anesthesia may be increased by all antihypertensive medications. Using similar logic, the antidysrhythmic drugs like amiodarone or bretylium increase the possibility of bradycardia, hypotension, and decreased cardiac output.

With few exceptions, there is little reason to withhold most vasoactive medications before surgery. It may be prudent to stop diuretic treatment before procedures with large anticipated fluid requirements or significant use of nephrotoxic antibiotics. Some studies suggest that continuation of the angiotensin-converting enzyme inhibitors (ACEI) leads to a very high incidence of severe hypotension during induction of general anesthesia.[79,80] In hypertensive patients, ACEI-induced hypotension is due to left ventricular diastolic dysfunction coupled with anesthetic-induced reduction in preload. There is by no means complete agreement that ACEIs should always be withheld before surgery, and some have found them to be beneficial during surgery.[81] The adverse effects are most likely to be problematic in patients with moderate to severe pre-existing cardiovascular dysfunction, and there seems to be no reliable way to predict the magnitude of hypotension. These considerations may or may not apply to patients receiving ACEIs for chronic congestive heart failure. ACEIs are given to these patients for afterload reduction; they improve baroreceptor sensitivity, reduce ventric-

ular remodeling, and decrease the mortality rate. Use of ACEIs in this population may not increase the already high incidence of hypotension during induction.[82]

Most perioperative hemodynamic interactions involve the use of cardiovascular depressants. It is also useful to consider several groups of patients who are treated (or "self-treat") before surgery with cardiovascular *stimulants*.

1. Patients with bronchospasm may require treatment with rapid-acting β_2 agonists (albuterol, terbutaline) or phosphodiesterase inhibitors (theophylline). These patients are at increased risk for tachydysrhythmias and ectopic rhythms. Similar considerations apply to the patient receiving the intravenous β_2 agonist, ritodrine, for premature labor.

2. Patients who receive TCAs like imipramine, desipramine, amitriptyline, and nortriptyline present several possible scenarios for adverse drug interaction. The drugs work by blocking presynaptic reuptake of norepinephrine or serotonin, so they can theoretically increase the effects of direct- or indirect-acting agonists at these synapses. Most TCAs have prominent anticholinergic effects as well. In therapeutic doses and in overdose situations, TCAs can create a range of cardiovascular toxicity that includes sinus tachycardia, prolonged PR, QRS, QT intervals, ST segment and T-wave changes, bundle-branch block, dysrhythmias, second- and third-degree atrioventricular block, postural hypotension, decreased myocardial contractility, congestive heart failure, myocardial infarction, and sudden death.[83] In spite of this, hypotension and tachydysrhythmias are not common intraoperative problems with TCAs. This may reflect the fact that during chronic administration, TCAs act to *down-regulate* central adrenergic and serotonergic receptors. In patients taking these older antidepressants, it seems reasonable to avoid pancuronium, halothane, and other agents with the potential to increase the incidence of dysrhythmias. Should TCA-induced hypotension occur, there is disagreement about the best way to treat it.[83] One case report[84] describes a patient on chronic

nifedipine and nortriptyline therapy who had hypotension that was resistant to ephedrine, phenylephrine, and dopamine (norepinephrine was eventually successful).

3. Finally, all of us must be prepared to treat patients who are acutely or chronically intoxicated with cocaine. In addition to its local anesthetic properties, cocaine decreases norepinephrine reuptake, like TCAs. Acute intoxication presents a particular challenge. Young, otherwise healthy people may present with fulminant hypertension, tachycardia, and myocardial ischemia (the latter may be severe because cocaine can induce a thrombotic diathesis). From the standpoint of drug interaction, acute cocaine intoxication resembles pheochromocytoma: these patients need both vasodilators and β blockers. Administration of a β blocker alone may allow unopposed α-adrenergic stimulation and a huge increase in systemic vascular resistance. Patients with chronic cocaine intoxication are less of a problem, but they are still at risk for dysrhythmias (avoiding halothane, pancuronium, atropine, and sympathomimetics still seems like a good idea). Chronic cocaine exposure increases halothane minimum alveolar concentration (MAC) in dogs[85] and isoflurane MAC in sheep,[86] and it may increase the sedative effects of benzodiazepines in humans.[87] This is an interesting contrast to chronic treatment with amphetamine, which appears to decrease MAC in dogs.[88] It might be thought that the adrenergic overactivity induced by cocaine would produce receptor down-regulation over time, but several animal studies suggest that chronic cocaine treatment does not decrease brain catecholamine content or sympathetic responsiveness over time.[89,90] The relevance of these data to human cardiovascular responses remains to be proven.

SPECIFIC INTERACTIONS AFFECTING ANALGESIA OR HYPNOSIS

As stated previously, combinations of CNS depressants almost always produce additive or synergistic increases in CNS effect. These interactions are usually useful and predictable. All of the common iv and inhaled anesthetic agents have been tested in combination in humans. The following sections highlight some of the most important interactions.

Opioid–Hypnotic

This is arguably the most commonly used synergistic combination in iv anesthesia.

- Fentanyl and alfentanil have been shown to reduce the requirement for thiobarbiturates, and there is some evidence that the interaction is a beneficial one. Reducing the total dose of thiopental[91] or thiamylal[92] during short procedures decreases the time to awakening and orientation.
- Opioids also potentiate propofol, but it has been much more difficult to show that the combination improves recovery compared with propofol alone. Short et al[93] found that a small dose of alfentanil can reduce the hypnotic ED_{50} of propofol by 50% (see Fig. 50-3). A typical premedication dose of fentanyl (100 μg) has been shown to decrease induction time and reduce the propofol requirement, but in extremely short outpatient cases it did not significantly improve recovery time or the subjective assessment of the quality of anesthesia.[94]
- During total iv anesthesia, infusions of remifentanil or alfentanil tremendously reduce the infusion rate of propofol needed to suppress responses to surgical stimuli[95,96] (Table 50-5). Target effect-site concentrations of only 1–2 μg · ml^{-1} of propofol produce adequate anesthesia in many cases.

Table 50-5. REMIFENTANIL INFUSION RATES (μg · kg^{-1} · min^{-1}) IN COMBINATION WITH PROPOFOL, WHICH PREVENTED RESPONSES TO INTUBATION AND INCISION IN MOST PATIENTS*

	Target Effect Site Concentration of Propofol (μg · ml^{-1})		
	1	2	4
Intubation	0.6	0.3	0.2
Incision	0.4	0.3	0.2

* Propofol was administered by computer-controlled infusion to target three specific effect-site concentrations.
From Fragen RJ, Randel GI, Librojo ES et al: The interaction of remifentanil and propofol to prevent response to tracheal intubation and the start of surgery for outpatient knee arthroscopy. Anesthesiology 81:A376, 1994, with permission.

There are concentrations routinely achieved with propofol doses used for conscious sedation (25–50 μg · kg^{-1} · min^{-1}).

Opioid–Benzodiazepine

This important interaction was alluded to earlier, and it illustrates why opioids are so commonly used in combination with diazepam or midazolam. Opioids are highly selective CNS depressants; they can produce sedation, but they are relatively weak hypnotics. Even huge doses of fentanyl and its congeners do not dependably produce sleep by themselves.[97] We have demonstrated, for example, that alfentanil doses as high as 100–200 μg · kg^{-1} cannot always induce unconsciousness in unpremedicated patients.[98] Such opioid doses uniformly produce apnea, rigidity, and profound analgesia.

Kissin and coworkers[99] found, however, that a tiny dose of alfentanil (3 μg · kg^{-1}) is sufficient to reduce the hypnotic ED_{50} of midazolam by 50%. This dose is subanalgesic and subhypnotic when given alone.

This means that a small dose of opioid (50 μg fentanyl, 500 μg alfentanil) may have almost no hypnotic effect by itself, but can still be an extremely effective potentiator of other hypnotics. It also means that when fentanyl and midazolam are combined for conscious sedation, the opioid is producing sleep as well as analgesia.

Benzodiazepine–Hypnotic

The theoretic basis for the interaction between barbiturates and benzodiazepines was discussed earlier, and the thiopental–midazolam interaction is shown in Figure 50-6.

- Thiopental–midazolam interaction has been studied in humans, and the combination was found to have 1.8 times the expected potency of the individual agents.[74,100] Similar results have been described with the combination of midazolam and methohexital.[101]
- Propofol also acts by modulation of GABA neurotransmission, and its hypnotic effects are potentiated when it is combined with midazolam.[93]

The clinical benefits of benzodiazepine premedication are most obvious during the preoperative period. Intraoperative benefits (i.e., increased efficacy or reduced toxicity) of benzodiazepine–hypnotic combinations have not been demonstrated. The patient premedicated with midazolam needs less thiopental or propofol for induction (or maintenance), but it is not known whether this results in a smoother anesthetic or more rapid awakening.

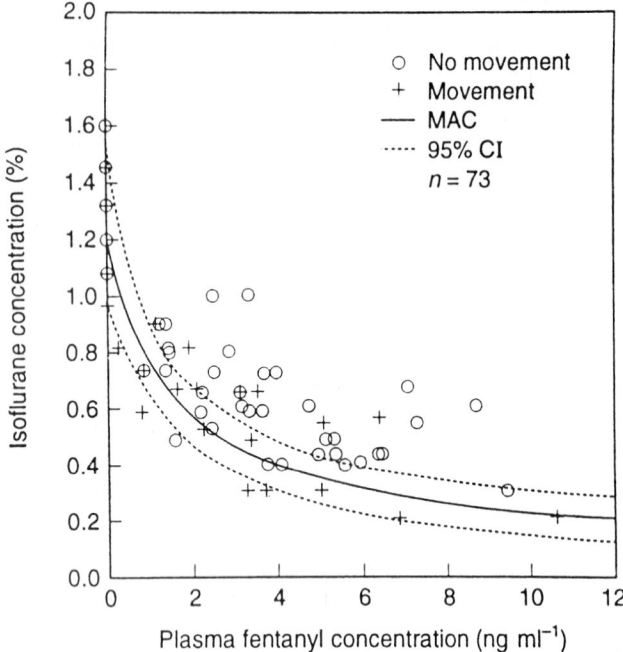

Figure 50-7. The interaction between fentanyl and isoflurane. The *solid line* represents the concentration of the two drugs that prevents movement in 50% of patients. MAC = minimum alveolar concentration; CI = confidence interval. (From McEwan AI, Smith C, Dyar O *et al:* Isoflurane minimum alveolar concentration reduction by fentanyl. Anesthesiology 78:864, 1993, with permission.)

Volatile Anesthetic–Opioid

Opioids produce dose- and concentration-dependent decreases in MAC for all of the inhalation anesthetics.

- A steady-state plasma fentanyl concentration of 1.67 ng · ml^{-1} decreases human isoflurane MAC by 50%[102] (Fig. 50-7).
- Opioid partial agonists like nalbuphine and butorphanol produce smaller reductions in MAC.[103]
- Animal data consistently show that an approximately 70% reduction in MAC is the maximum effect obtainable with a full agonist like fentanyl.[104] The mechanism for this interaction is unknown, but Licina *et al*[105] showed that administration of lumbar intrathecal morphine (15 μg · kg^{-1}) does not alter halothane MAC in humans. This suggests that the effect may be due to supraspinal opioid actions. These findings are particularly interesting in view of the work by Rampil *et al*,[106] who showed that MAC in the rat is not altered when the cerebral cortex and all other precollicular brain structures are removed. MAC therefore appears to reflect an action of the volatile anesthetics on the spinal cord, whereas MAC reduction by opioids is most likely to be mediated by structures in the brain stem or higher. One possible site for interaction is the locus ceruleus (LC; see later).

Opioids and volatile agents are often combined to smooth the intraoperative and postoperative course. In some patients, the combination of opioid and volatile agent is hemodynamically better tolerated than the volatile agent alone. Addition of an opioid may also reduce the incidence of emergence delirium.

Is there any evidence that the combination speeds awakening? Reduction of MAC clearly leads to lower end-tidal concentrations at the end of surgery. Faster emergence occurs only if the concentration of inhaled agent that produces hypnosis (*e.g.,* "MAC-awake," the concentration at which 50% of subjects respond to voice) is not reduced by a comparable amount. A few data indicate that MAC-awake is not decreased by opioids,

suggesting that the combination improves recovery.[107] There have been no studies specifically designed to test this hypothesis.

Other iv agents such as lidocaine,[108] midazolam,[109] and α$_2$ agonists (see later) have been shown to decrease MAC in experimental animals. For lidocaine and midazolam, the plasma concentrations required to produce a meaningful decrease in MAC are so high that the interaction is unlikely to have clinical utility. There is some evidence that the simultaneous use of volatile anesthetics and benzodiazepines causes increased cortical binding of the latter.[110]

α$_2$ Agonist Interactions

It has long been known that drugs that depress central sympathetic nervous system function can produce sedation and potentiate anesthesia. Older antihypertensives like reserpine and α-methyldopa can produce drowsiness and reduce halothane MAC.[111] The newer autonomic modulators—α$_2$ agonists like clonidine or dexmedetomidine—are powerful sedatives and analgesics in humans.

- In animals, dexmedetomidine produces marked potentiation of opioid analgesia and benzodiazepine-induced hypnosis.[112]
- Dexmedetomidine also lowers halothane MAC by nearly 100% through a specific postsynaptic α$_2$ mechanism.[113]

What is the neural basis for this effect? Dexmedetomidine interacts with both presynaptic and postsynaptic α$_2$-adrenergic receptors to decrease central sympathetic tone. Its hypnotic effect is due largely to depression of function in the LC, the main adrenergic nucleus in the brain.[114] There is evidence to suggest that the LC is an important site for control of sleep, attention, memory, analgesia, and autonomic function.[115] The LC contains receptors for glutamate, GABA, acetylcholine, opioids, and benzodiazepines, and experimental evidence suggests that it may be the site for some important anesthetic drug effects and interactions:

1. The LC is the rostral portion of an important descending inhibitory pathway, which plays a part in the production of opioid analgesia.[116]
2. In the rat, destroying the LC produces a state of narcolepsy and decreases halothane MAC by 30–40%.[117]
3. Agonists at GABA, opioid, and α$_2$ receptors are all inhibitory when injected into the LC. These drugs all have sedative-hypnotic properties, and all of them lower the requirement for volatile anesthetics.
4. Acetylcholine and glutamate receptor agonists are excitatory in the LC, and antagonists at these receptors (*e.g.,* scopolamine, ketamine) are hypnotics. Some glutamate effects are mediated by NO, and inhibitors of neuronal NO synthase can decrease the requirement for halothane[118] and isoflurane.[119]

Three-Way Interactions

In clinical practice, it is common to combine more than two drugs with sedative–hypnotic effects. We have relatively little information on what happens when a third drug is added to two that already have synergistic effects.

- Short *et al*[93] performed a clinical study of hypnotic interactions among propofol, midazolam, and alfentanil (see Fig. 50-3). Propofol requirement was reduced by 82% with the three-way combination, but it produced less potentiation than would have been predicted by adding the effects of the two-way combinations.
- Vinik *et al*[120] studied the same combination and also found profound hypnotic synergism: the dose of propofol could be decreased by 86% in the presence of alfentanil and midazolam. The data also suggested that the interaction between midazolam and alfentanil was a marked potentia-

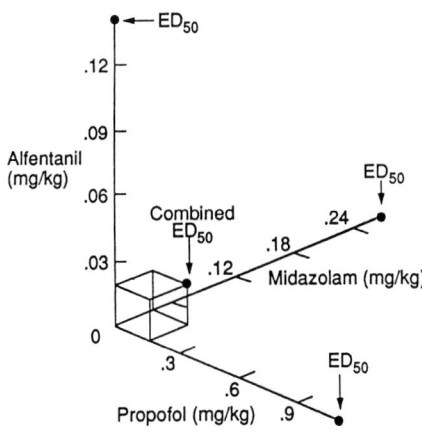

Figure 50-8. ED_{50} isobolograms for the three-way hypnotic interactions among midazolam, alfentanil, and propofol. The viewer can imagine a triangular "plane of additivity" with its corners at the individual ED_{50} values. The ED_{50} for the triple combination was significantly lower than predicted by additivity. (From Vinik HR, Bradley EL Jr, Kissin I: Triple anesthetic combination: Propofol-midazolam-alfentanil. Anesth Analg 78:354,1994, with permission.)

tion, but the addition of propofol did not produce significant additional change. Figure 50-8 shows the data from this experiment analyzed with a three-way isobologram.[120]

• A three-way interaction involving enflurane, dexmedetomidine, and fentanyl was investigated in dogs. Salmenpera et al[121] found that each of the two iv agents lowered enflurane MAC, and combining the three drugs produced a MAC reduction that was probably greater than predicted by simple additivity. In this case, the three-way combination produced more bradycardia than enflurane alone.

MODELS FOR THE FUTURE: DRUG INTERACTION DURING TOTAL INTRAVENOUS ANESTHESIA

Anesthesia must always be titrated to effect, but the clinician usually begins dosing each drug with some notion of a "normal" dose range and a reasonable incremental dose. As additional drugs are added to the anesthetic, these doses need to be modified. Are there any reliable data to guide the administration of anesthetic drugs in combination? The answer for most routine balanced anesthetics is probably "no." As we have seen, almost all anesthetic drugs interact in a nonlinear, synergistic fashion, and the magnitude of the interaction depends on the specific doses of each agent. If the drugs are given by bolus injection or variable-rate infusion, the interaction changes constantly with time. Predicting anesthetic interaction, then, is like aiming at a moving target. Even a relatively simple anesthetic seems to require the analysis of an impossibly large number of potential variables.

In spite of the obstacles, there have been some attempts to apply quantitative models to total iv anesthesia (TIVA). The TIVA technique offers several advantages in this regard:

1. Anesthesia is often induced and maintained with only two drugs, a rapid-acting hypnotic (*e.g.,* propofol) and a rapid-acting opioid (*e.g.,* alfentanil, remifentanil). The pharmacokinetics and pharmacodynamics of these drugs are exceptionally well studied.
2. The drugs have pharmacokinetics well suited to administration by continuous infusion with microprocessor-driven pumps. During anesthesia, plasma concentrations of the drugs may be held relatively constant, so blood and brain attain pseudoequilibrium. The researcher may vary the

infusion of each drug independently and relate stable plasma concentrations to clinical effects.

In a frequently cited study, Vuyk and colleagues[96] gave computer-controlled infusions of propofol and alfentanil to women undergoing lower abdominal surgery. First, the target concentration of alfentanil was held constant and propofol was varied; then, the reverse experiment was done. The onset of sleep and the time to awakening were measured, as was presence or absence of somatic and hemodynamic responses to laryngoscopy, intubation, incision, and opening of peritoneum. Arterial blood samples were collected, and the EC_{50} of alfentanil for each clinical end point was related to blood propofol concentration. As expected, the data showed that propofol potentiated the analgesic effects of alfentanil, and alfentanil potentiated the hypnotic effects of propofol. More important, the authors were able to relate various concentrations of each agent to a given end point.

The interest in these data lies in the way they can be used to simulate drug interactions.[122] In Figure 50-9, Vuyk et al have simulated the time to regain consciousness at different ratios of propofol and alfentanil. The graph is a somewhat complex, but it is worth considering for a few moments. Vuyk and colleagues assume that a 180-minute anesthetic has been given with propofol and alfentanil targeted at various combinations. Each combination is sufficient to prevent response to intraabdominal surgery in 50% of patients. The three-axis graph relates the concentrations of each drug to the time after discontinuation of the infusions. At time 0 (the floor of the graph), we see the steady-state concentrations just when the infusions are stopped. The disappearance of drug differs depending on how much of the mixture is propofol and how much is alfentanil, and the family of plasma decay curves is depicted on the graph surface. The curved line that crosses the time versus concentration surface identifies the time at which a patient has a 50% probability of awakening. The fastest emergence (10 minutes)

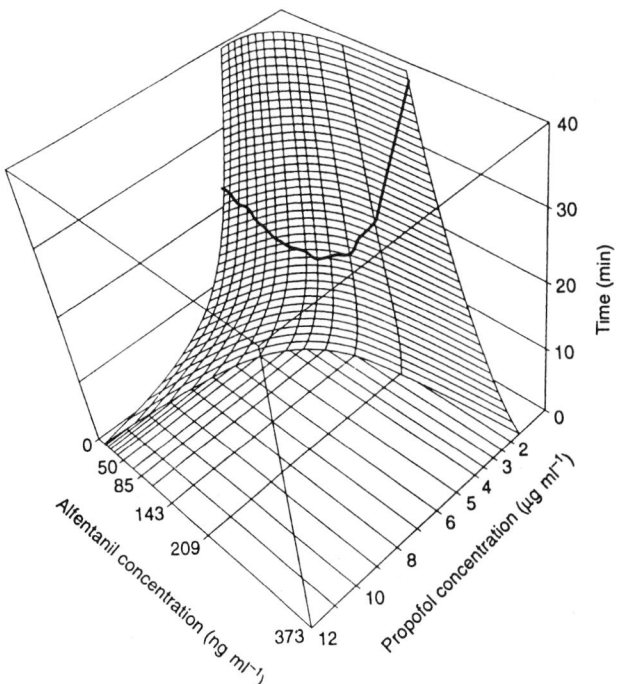

Figure 50-9. Computer simulation of the decay in blood propofol and plasma alfentanil concentrations during the first 40 minutes after the termination of a computer-controlled infusion (see text for details). (From Vuyk J, Lim T, Engbers FHM et al: The pharmacodynamic interaction of propofol and alfentanil during lower abdominal surgery in women. Anesthesiology 83:8, 1995, with permission.)

occurs when propofol and alfentanil are targeted at concentrations of 3.5 $\mu g \cdot ml^{-1}$ and 85 $ng \cdot ml^{-1}$, respectively. Emergence will be significantly longer if the anesthetic is mostly propofol or mostly alfentanil.

How will these data help anyone give an anesthetic? What if the infusion is much shorter or longer than 180 minutes? What if the patients are old and sick? What if the anesthesiologist does not have a computer or an infusion pump? The answer could be another set of questions: "What is the value of knowing that the MAC of halothane is 0.74 vol%, the induction dose of propofol is 2.5 $mg \cdot kg^{-1}$ or the analgesic dose of morphine is 0.1 $mg \cdot kg^{-1}$?" We all understand that the value of such numbers is to give us a frame of reference for titrating the agents. The value of Vuyk and colleagues' model is not as a "recipe" for a good iv anesthetic—it is a way to think about dosing guidelines for two or more drugs simultaneously. This was a difficult study to perform and analyze, but it is likely to be repeated with other drugs and other populations. It is not far-fetched to imagine that the U.S. Food and Drug Administration will some day require information on "optimal combinations" for each new pharmacologic agent.

REFERENCES

1. Smith NT, Corbascio AN (eds): Drug Interactions in Anesthesia, 2nd ed. Philadelphia, Lea and Febiger, 1986
2. Zbinden AM, Petersen-Felix S, Thomson DA: Anesthetic depth defined using multiple noxious stimuli during isoflurane/oxygen anesthesia: II. Hemodynamic responses. Anesthesiology 80:261, 1994
3. Smith JW, Seidl LG, Cluff LG: Studies on the epidemiology of adverse drug reactions: V. Clinical factors influencing susceptibility. Ann Intern Med 65:629, 1966
4. Bailey PL, Pace NL, Ashburn MA et al: Frequent hypoxemia and apnea after sedation with midazolam and fentanyl. Anesthesiology 73:826, 1990
5. Ausems ME, Hug CC Jr, Stanski DR et al: Plasma concentrations of alfentanil required to supplement nitrous oxide anesthesia for general surgery. Anesthesiology 65:362, 1986
6. Dundee JW, Robinson FP, McCullum JS et al: Sensitivity to propofol in the elderly. Anaesthesia 41:482, 1986
7. Baxter PJ, Garton K, Kharasch ED: Mechanistic aspects of carbon monoxide formation from volatile anesthetics. Anesthesiology 89:929, 1998
8. Steudel W, Hurford WE, Zapol WM: Inhaled nitric oxide: Basic biology and clinical applications. Anesthesiology 91:1090, 1999
9. Murphy DB, Sutton JA, Prescott LF et al: Opioid-induced delay in gastric emptying: A peripheral mechanism in humans. Anesthesiology 87:765, 1997
10. Asai T, McBeth C, Stewart JIM et al: Effect of clonidine on gastric emptying of liquids. Br J Anaesth 78:28, 1997
11. Johnson KB, Kern SE, Hamber EA et al: The influence of hemorrhagic shock on remifentanil: A pharmacokinetic analysis (abstract). Anesthesiology 89:A524, 1998
12. Adams P, Gelman S, Reves JG et al: Midazolam pharmacodynamics and pharmacokinetics during acute hypovolemia. Anesthesiology 63:140, 1985
13. Klockowski PM, Levy G: Kinetics of drug action in disease states: XXV. Effect of experimental hypovolemia on the pharmacodynamics and pharmacokinetics of desmethyldiazepam. J Pharmacol Exp Ther 245:508, 1988
14. van der Meer JWM, Keuning JJ et al: The influence of gastric acidity on the bioavailability of ketoconazole. J Antimicrob Chemother 6:552, 1980
15. Elwood RJ, Hildebrand PJ et al: Influence of ranitidine on uptake of oral midazolam. Br J Anaesth 55:241, 1983
16. Trudnowski RJ, Gessner T: Gastric excretion of intravenously administered meperidine in surgical patients. Anesth Analg 58:88, 1979
17. Silverman WA, Andersen DH, Blanc WA et al: A difference in mortality rate and incidence of kernicterus among premature infants allotted to two prophylactic antibacterial regimens. Pediatrics 18:614, 1956
18. Holford NHG, Benet LZ: Pharmacokinetics and pharmacodynamics: Dose selection and the time course of drug action. In Katzung
19. BG (ed): Basic and Clinical Pharmacology, p 48. Stamford, Connecticut, Appleton and Lange, 1998
19. Brodsky JB, Campos FA: Chloroprocaine analgesia in a patient receiving echothiophate eye drops. Anesthesiology 48:288, 1978
20. Kuhnert BR et al: A prolonged chloroprocaine epidural block in a postpartum patient with abnormal pseudocholinesterase. Anesthesiology 56:477, 1982
21. Lanks WK, Sklar GS: Pseudocholinesterase levels and rates of chloroprocaine hydrolysis in patients receiving adequate doses of phospholine iodide. Anesthesiology 52:434, 1980
22. Selinger K, Nation RL, Smith GA: Enzymatic and chemical hydrolysis of remifentanil (abstract). Anesthesiology 83:A385, 1995
23. Stiller RL, Davis PJ, McGowan FX et al: In vitro metabolism of remifentanil: The effects of pseudocholinesterase deficiency (abstract). Anesthesiology 83:A381, 1995
24. Boakes AJ et al: Interactions between sympathomimetic amines and antidepressant agents in man. BMJ 1:311, 1973
25. Friend DG et al: The action of L-dihydroxyphenylalanine in patients receiving nialamide. Clin Pharmacol Ther 6:362, 1965
26. Parkinson's Study Group: Effects of tocopherol and deprenyl on the progression of disability in early Parkinson's disease. N Engl J Med 328:176, 1993
27. Evans-Prosser CDG: The use of pethidine and morphine in the presence of monoamine oxidase inhibitors. Br J Anaesth 40:279, 1968
28. Zornberg G et al: Severe interaction between pethidine and selegiline. Lancet 337:246, 1991
29. Rivers N, Horner B: Possible lethal reaction between nardil and dextromethorphan (letter). CMAJ 103:85, 1970
30. Michaels I, Serrins M, Shier NQ et al: Anesthesia for cardiac surgery in patients receiving monoamine oxidase inhibitors. Anesth Analg 63:1041, 1984
31. Fahim I, Ismail M, Osman OH: The role of serotonin and norepinephrine in the hyperthermic reaction induced by pethidine in rabbits pretreated with pargyline. J Pharmacol 46:416, 1972
32. Domino EF et al: Barbiturate intoxication in a patient treated with a MAO inhibitor. Am J Psychiatr 118:941, 1962
33. Sjoqvist F: Psychotropic drugs (2): Interaction between monoamine oxidase (MAO) inhibitors and other substances. Proc R Soc Med 58:967, 1965
34. Doyle DJ: Ketamine induction and monoamine oxidase inhibitors. J Clin Anesth 2:324, 1990
35. El-Ganzouri AR, Ivankovich AD, Braverman B et al: Monoamine oxidase inhibitors: Should they be discontinued preoperatively? Anesth Analg 64:592, 1985
36. Roizen MF: Monoamine oxidase inhibitors: Are we condemned to relive history or is history no longer relevant? J Clin Anesth 2:293, 1990
37. Stenson RE, Constantino RT, Harrison DC: Interrelationship of hepatic blood flow, cardiac output and blood levels of lidocaine in man. Circulation 18:205, 1971
38. Benowitz N et al: Lidocaine disposition kinetics in monkey and man: II. Effects of hemorrhage and sympathomimetic drug administration. Clin Pharmacol Ther 16:99, 1974
39. Feely J et al: Increased toxicity and reduced clearance of lidocaine by cimetidine. Ann Intern Med 96:592, 1982
40. Tukey RH, Johnson EF: Molecular aspects of regulation and structure of the drug-metabolizing enzymes. In Pratt WB, Taylor P (eds): Principles of Drug Action: The Basis of Pharmacology, 3rd ed, p 435. New York, Churchill Livingstone, 1990
41. Greenstein LR, Hitt BA, Mazze RI: Metabolism in vitro of enflurane, isoflurane, and methoxyflurane. Anesthesiology 42:420, 1975
42. Mazze RI, Trudell JR, Cousins MJ: Methoxyflurane metabolism and renal dysfunction: Clinical correlation in man. Anesthesiology 35:247, 1971
43. Sipes JG, Brown BR Jr: An animal model of hepatotoxicity associated with halothane anesthesia. Anesthesiology 45:622, 1976
44. Oda Y, Hase I, Mizutani K: Metabolism of fentanyl is competitively inhibited by midazolam (abstract). Anesthesiology 89:A510, 1998
45. Hamaoka N, Oda Y, Hase I et al: Propofol decreases the clearance of midazolam by inhibiting CYP3A4: In vivo and in-vitro study (abstract). Anesthesiology 91:A451, 1999
46. Yutaka O, Hamaoka N, Hase I et al: Involvement of human liver CYP1A2 in the metabolism of propofol (abstract). Anesthesiology 91:A450, 1999
47. Bartkowski RR, Goldberg ME, Larijani GE et al: Inhibition of

alfentanil metabolism by erythromycin. Clin Pharmacol Ther 46:99 1989

48. Tateishi T, Krivoruk Y, Ueng Y et al: Identification of human liver cytochrome P-450 3A4 as the enzyme responsible for fentanyl and sufentanil N-dealkylation. Anesth Analg 82:167, 1996

49. Bartkowski RR, Goldberg ME, Huffnagle S et al: Sufentanil disposition. Anesthesiology 78:260, 1993

50. Klotz U, Reimann I: Delayed clearance of diazepam due to cimetidine. N Engl J Med 302:1012, 1980

51. Palkama VJ, Ahonen J, Neuvonen J et al: Effect of saquinavir on the pharmacokinetics and dynamics of oral and intravenous midazolam (abstract). Anesthesiology 91:A442, 1999

52. Olkkola KT, Palkama VJ, Neuvonen PJ: Ritonavir's role in reducing fentanyl clearance and prolonging its half life (abstract). Anesthesiology 91:A449, 1999

53. Wagner RL, White PF, Kan PB et al: Inhibition of adrenal steroidogenesis by the anesthetic etomidate. N Engl J Med 310:1415, 1984

54. Leahey EB et al. Interaction between quinidine and digoxin. JAMA 240:533, 1978

55. Naguib M, Samarkandi AH, Bakhamees HS et al: Comparative potency of steroidal neuromuscular blocking drugs and isobolographic analysis of the interaction. Br J Anaesth 75:37, 1995

56. Quasha AL, Eger EI II, Tinker JH: Determination and applications of MAC. Anesthesiology 53:315, 1980

57. Murray DJ, Mehta MP, Forbes RB et al: Additive contribution of nitrous oxide to halothane MAC in infants and children. Anesth Analg 71:120, 1990

58. Eger EI II. Does 1 + 1 = 2? Anesth Analg 41:482, 1989

59. Munson ES, Paul WL, Embro WJ: Central nervous system toxicity of local anesthetic mixtures in monkeys. Anesthesiology 46:179, 1977

60. Kim KS, Na DJ, Chon SU: Interactions between suxamethonium and mivacurium or atracurium. Br J Anaesth 77:612, 1996

61. Eisenach JC et al: Effect of prior anesthetic solution on epidural morphine analgesia. Anesth Analg 73:119, 1991

62. Dershwitz M, Rosow CE, DiBiase PM et al: A comparison of the sedative effects of butorphanol and midazolam. Anesthesiology 74:717, 1991

63. Maves TJ, Pechman PS, Meller ST et al: Ketorolac potentiates morphine antinociception during visceral nociception in the rat. Anesthesiology 80:1094, 1994

64. Laitinen J, Nuutinen L: Intravenous diclofenac coupled with PCA fentanyl for pain relief after total hip replacement. Anesthesiology 76:194, 1992

65. Gillies GWA, Kenny GNC, Bullingham RES et al: The morphine sparing effect of ketorolac tromethamine. Anaesthesia 42:727, 1987

66. Ready LB, Brown CR, Stahlgren LH et al: Evaluation of intravenous ketorolac administered by bolus or infusion for treatment of postoperative pain: A double-blind, placebo-controlled, multicenter study. Anesthesiology 80:1277, 1994

67. Lebowitz PW, Ramsey FM, Savarese JJ et al: Potentiation of neuromuscular blockade in man produced by combinations of pancuronium and metocurine or pancuronium and d-tubocurarine. Anesth Analg 59:604, 1980

68. Bowman WC, Prior C, Marshall IG: Presynaptic receptors in the neuromuscular junction. Ann NY Acad Sci 604:69, 1990

69. Standaert FG: Basic chemistry of acetylcholine receptors. Anesth Clin North Am 11:205, 1993

70. Tallarida RJ: Statistical analysis of drug combinations for synergism. Pain 49:93, 1992

71. Berenbaum MC: Synergy, additivism and antagonism in immunosuppression. J Clin Exp Immunol 28:1, 1989

72. Berenbaum MC: What is synergy? Pharm Rev 41:93, 1989

73. Tallarida RJ, Porreca F, Cowan A: Statistical analysis of drug-drug and site-site interactions with isobolograms. Life Sci 45:947, 1989

74. Tverskoy M, Fleyshman G, Bradley EL Jr, Kissin I: Midazolam-thiopental anesthetic interaction in patients. Anesth Analg 67:342, 1988

75. Stone JG, Foex P, Sear JW: Myocardial ischemia in untreated hypertensive patients: Effect of a single small oral dose of a beta-adrenergic blocking agent. Anesthesiology 68:495, 1988

76. Pasternack PF, Grossi EA, Baumann FG et al: Beta blockade to decrease silent myocardial ischemia during peripheral vascular surgery. Am J Surg 158:113, 1989

77. Wallace A, Layug B, Tateo I et al: Prophylactic atenolol reduces postoperative myocardial ischemia. Anesthesiology 88:7, 1998

78. Warltier DC: β-Adrenergic-blocking drugs: Incredibly useful, incredibly underutilized. Anesthesiology 88:2, 1998

79. Colson P, Saussine M, Séguin JR et al: Hemodynamic effects of anesthesia in patients chronically treated with angiotensin-converting enzyme inhibitors. Anesth Analg 74:805, 1992

80. Coriat P, Richer C, Douraki T et al: Influence of chronic angiotensin-converting enzyme inhibition on anesthetic induction. Anesthesiology 81:299, 1994

81. Licker M, Bednarkiewicz M, Neidhart P et al: Preoperative inhibition of angiotensin-converting enzyme improves systemic and renal haemodynamic changes during aortic abdominal surgery. Br J Anaesth 76:632, 1996

82. Ryckwaert F, Colson P: Hemodynamic effects of anesthesia in patients with ischemic heart failure chronically treated with angiotensin-converting enzyme inhibitors. Anesth Analg 84:945, 1997

83. Rosenthal JA: American Heart Association recommendations for treating tricyclic antidepressant-induced hypotension (letter). Anesthesiology 87:1259, 1997

84. Sprung J, Schoenwald P, Levy P et al: Treating intraoperative hypotension in a patient on long-term tricyclic antidepressants: A case of aborted aortic surgery. Anesthesiology 86:990, 1997

85. Stoelting RK, Creasser CW, Martz RC: Effect of cocaine administration on halothane MAC in dogs. Anesth Analg 54:422, 1975

86. Bernards C, Kern C, Cullen BF: Chronic cocaine administration reversibly increases isoflurane minimum alveolar concentration in sheep. Anesthesiology 85:91, 1996

87. Bernards C, Teijeiro A: Illicit cocaine ingestion during anesthesia. Anesthesiology 84:218, 1995

88. Johnston R, Way W, Miller R: Alteration of anesthetic requirement by amphetamine. Anesthesiology 36:357, 1972

89. Seidler F, Slotkin T: Fetal cocaine exposure causes persistent noradrenergic hyperactivity in rat brain regions: Effects on neurotransmitter turnover and receptors. J Pharmacol Exp Ther 263:413, 1992

90. Kelley K, Han D, Fellingham G et al: Cocaine and exercise: Physiological responses of cocaine-conditioned rats. Med Sci Sports Exerc 27:65, 1995

91. Epstein B, Levy M-L, Thein M et al: Evaluation of fentanyl as an adjunct to thiopental-nitrous oxide-oxygen anesthesia for short procedures. Anesthesia Reviews 2:24, 1985

92. Rosow CE, Latta WB, Keegan CR et al: Alfentanil for use in short surgical procedures. In Estafanous FG (ed): Opioids in Anesthesia, p 93. Boston, Butterworth, 1984

93. Short TG, Plummer JL, Chui PT: Hypnotic and anaesthetic interactions between midazolam, propofol and alfentanil. Br J Anaesth 69:162, 1992

94. Thomas VL, Sutton DN, Saunders DA: The effect of fentanyl on propofol requirements for day case anaesthesia. Anaesthesia 43(suppl):73, 1988

95. Fragen RJ, Randel GI, Librojo ES et al: The interaction of remifentanil and propofol to prevent response to tracheal intubation and the start of surgery for outpatient knee arthroscopy. Anesthesiology 81:A376, 1994

96. Vuyk J, Lim T, Engbers FHM et al: The pharmacodynamic interaction of propofol and alfentanil during lower abdominal surgery in women. Anesthesiology 83:8, 1995

97. Bailey PL, Wilbrink J, Zwanikken P et al: Anesthetic induction with fentanyl. Anesth Analg 64:48, 1985

98. Silbert BS, Rosow CE, Keegan CR et al: The effect of diazepam on induction of anesthesia with alfentanil. Anesth Analg 65:71, 1986

99. Kissin I, Vinik HR, Castillo R et al: Alfentanil potentiates midazolam-induced unconsciousness in subanalgesic doses. Anesth Analg 71:65, 1990

100. Short TG, Galletly DC, Plummer JL: Hypnotic and anesthetic action of thiopentone and midazolam alone and in combination. Br J Anaesth 66:13, 1991

101. Tverskoy M, Ben-Shlomo I, Finger EJ et al: Midazolam acts synergistically with methohexitone for induction of anaesthesia. Br J Anaesth 63:109, 1989

102. McEwan AI, Smith C, Dyar O et al: Isoflurane minimum alveolar concentration reduction by fentanyl. Anesthesiology 78:864, 1993

103. Murphy MR, Hug CC Jr: The enflurane sparing effect of morphine, butorphanol and nalbuphine. Anesthesiology 57:489, 1982

104. Murphy RM, Hug CC Jr: The anesthetic potency of fentanyl in terms of its reduction of enflurane MAC. Anesthesiology 57:485, 1982

105. Licina MG, Schubert A, Tobin JE et al: Intrathecal morphine

does not reduce minimum alveolar concentration of halothane in humans: Results of a double-blind study. Anesthesiology 74:660, 1991

106. Rampil IJ, Mason P, Singh H: Anesthetic potency (MAC) is independent of forebrain structures in the rat. Anesthesiology 78:707, 1993

107. Gross JB, Alexander CM: Awakening concentrations of isoflurane are not affected by analgesic doses of morphine. Anesth Analg 67:27, 1988

108. Himes RS, DiFazio CA, Burney RG: Effects of lidocaine on the anesthetic requirements for nitrous oxide and halothane. Anesthesiology 47:437, 1977

109. Hall RI, Schwieger IM, Hug CC: The anesthetic efficacy of midazolam in the enflurane-anesthetized dog. Anesthesiology 68:862, 1988

110. Hansen TD, Warner DS, Todd MM et al: The influence of inhalational anesthetics on in vivo and in vitro benzodiazepine receptor binding in the rat cerebral cortex. Anesthesiology 74:97, 1991

111. Miller RD, Way WL, Eger EI II: The effects of alpha-methyldopa, reserpine, guanethidine and iproniazide on minimum alveolar anesthetic concentration (MAC). Anesthesiology 29:1156, 1968

112. Salonen M, Reid K, Maze M: Synergistic interaction between α-2-adrenergic agonists and benzodiazepines in rats. Anesthesiology 76:1004, 1992

113. Segal IS, Vickery RG, Walton JK et al: Dexmedetomidine diminishes halothane anesthetic requirements in rats through a postsynaptic α-2-adrenergic receptor. Anesthesiology 69:818, 1988

114. Correa-Sales C, Rabin BC, Maze M: A hypnotic response to dexmedetomidine, an α-2- agonist, is mediated in the locus coeruleus in rats. Anesthesiology 76:948, 1992

115. Scheinin M, Schwinn DA: The locus coeruleus: Site of hypnotic actions of α-2-adrenoceptor agonists? (editorial). Anesthesiology 76:873, 1992

116. Advokat C: The role of descending inhibition in morphine-induced analgesia. Trends Pharmacol Sci 9:330, 1988

117. Roizen MF, White PF, Eger EI II et al: Effects of ablation of serotonin or norepinephrine brain-stem areas on halothane and cyclopropane MACs in rats. Anesthesiology 49:252, 1978

118. Johns RA, Moscicki JC, DiFazio CA: Nitric oxide synthase inhibitor dose-dependently and reversibly reduces the threshold for halothane anesthesia: A role for nitric oxide in mediating consciousness? Anesthesiology 77:779, 1992

119. Pajewski TN, DiFazio CA, Moscicki JC et al: Nitric oxide synthase inhibitors, 7-nitro-indazole and nitroG-L-arginine-methyl ester, dose-dependently reduce the threshold for isoflurane anesthesia. Anesthesiology 85:1111, 1996

120. Vinik HR, Bradley EL Jr, Kissin I: Triple anesthetic combination: Propofol-midazolam-alfentanil. Anesth Analg 78:354,1994

121. Salmenpera M, Szlam F, Hug CC Jr: Anesthetic and hemodynamic interactions of dexmedetomidine and fentanyl in dogs. Anesthesiology 75:A307, 1991

122. Stanski DR, Shafer SL: Quantifying anesthetic drug interaction. Implications for drug dosing (editorial). Anesthesiology 83:1, 1995

Clinical Anesthesia (4/e), edited by
Paul G. Barash, Bruce F. Cullen, and
Robert K. Stoelting. Lippincott Williams &
Wilkins, Philadelphia, © 2001.

CHAPTER 51

ANESTHESIA PROVIDED AT ALTERNATIVE SITES

CHARLES E. LAURITO

Not all anesthesia is given within a hospital operating room. Advances in medical technology, improved monitoring devices, the development of newer anesthetic agents, and economic pressures have changed the landscape of contemporary surgery. Anesthesiologists work at sites far removed from the conventional operating rooms where they received the bulk of their training. Anesthesia is provided in ambulatory care centers, both in hospitals or freestanding, and in remote areas such as surgeons' and dentists' offices. Additionally, anesthesia is provided for procedures performed in other departments throughout the hospital by radiologists, urologists, gastroenterologists, and cardiologists.

The role of the anesthesia provider in these different settings is to give thoughtful care, ensure the comfort and safety of the patient, and facilitate performance of the procedure. Doing this in remote sites presents additional challenges. The risks and benefits of providing anesthesia away from a hospital operating room have to be weighed carefully. Discussions with surgeons, dentists, and others performing interventional procedures have to include contingencies for adverse outcomes. Additional plans and agreements have to be developed and put into place to optimize patient safety.

GENERAL PRINCIPLES

It is important to have a single standard of patient care. This continually evolves with medical advances and is based on scientific principles and documented clinical outcomes. The standards are to apply regardless of the site at which medical care is delivered. Monitors and anesthesia equipment at alternative sites should be comparable to those within conventional operating rooms. The American Society of Anesthesiologists (ASA) established guidelines for nonoperating room anesthetizing locations[1] which state that uniformity of anesthesia equipment enhances safety and that regularly scheduled maintenance of the equipment is essential. Providers need to be particularly vigilant in their care for patients because the remote location may preclude obtaining immediate help from other qualified personnel. Thorough preoperative and preprocedural preparation is important. The provider must become familiar with all of the anesthesia equipment and the physical layout of the site, and must have a clear understanding of whom to call should an adverse outcome occur. The guidelines emphasize the importance of a reliable source of suction, oxygen supplies, and equipment to perform cardiopulmonary resuscitation.

Several problems are specific to the alternative site. Many of these facilities were not designed with an eye toward fulfilling the ASA guidelines or meeting the needs of anesthetic care for the patient. It is important that the areas be large enough to house routine anesthesia equipment, including self-inflating bags to deliver positive-pressure ventilation, oxygen cylinders, emergency resuscitation drugs, and a defibrillator. A reliable source of suction, appropriate lighting, a sufficient number of electrical outlets, and adequate space for anesthesia personnel to work are essential. Two-way communication systems between the provider and support staff should be established and tested so that backup personnel can be immediately called if help is needed.[1] Unless safeguards are taken and energies are directed toward careful planning, alternative sites for anesthesia care

may be more dangerous for patients than conventional hospital operating rooms.

The standards for monitoring in remote sites should be the same as those in the operating room. This applies whether the patient is receiving monitored anesthesia care, regional anesthesia, or a general anesthetic. Blood pressure and heart rate should be obtained frequently and documented at least every 5 minutes. An electrocardiogram (ECG) should be continuously displayed, as well as the SpO_2 from a pulse oximeter. If the patient undergoes a general anesthetic, the provider should continuously monitor ventilation with qualitative or quantitative end-tidal carbon dioxide measurements. The off-site facility should be as carefully maintained as the operating room and have modern anesthesia equipment available.[1] If general anesthesia is provided with volatile agents, the anesthesia machine must be equipped for the scavenging of waste anesthetic gases.[1] The oxygen concentration delivered to the patient should be monitored by an oxygen analyzer equipped with a low-concentration alarm. Although not mandatory, it is preferable to have a central oxygen supply instead of relying on tanks. Finally, all sites should have state-of-the-art patient physiologic monitors. This is particularly evident in radiology suites where the anesthesiologist must often leave the patient's side during treatment.

At the conclusion of a procedure in alternative locations, provision for recovery of the patient should be comparable to that for those treated in an operating room. Areas should be designated for patient recovery and assessment criteria should be established for discharge home. In areas remote from the hospital, patient transport and recovery within a post-anesthesia care unit (PACU) can maximize safety for the patient and convenience for the staff. Appropriate monitoring equipment, oxygen, power supplies, medications, and resuscitation equipment should be available in all recovery areas.

ANESTHESIA CARE

Anesthesia care spans a continuum (Fig. 51-1). *Light sedation* is the least invasive form in which medication is administered *via* oral (po), rectal (pr), intramuscular (im), or intravenous (iv) routes. The medications are provided primarily for the patient's comfort. Several procedures in the radiology suites are painless but require the patient to lie absolutely still during imaging. Patients are usually anxious about the potential findings, and the procedures can be highly stressful. Additionally, they occur with noisy equipment in cramped quarters. After obtaining iv access and administering oxygen by nasal cannulae, light sedation can be achieved with fentanyl, $2-4\ \mu g \cdot kg^{-1}$, midazolam 2–5 mg, and/or droperidol 2–4 mg. The goal should be to titrate the medications to patient comfort. Ideally, the patient will be completely still and less acutely aware of the surroundings, yet able to breathe normally, respond to verbal commands, and protect the airway.

Although the terms are not well differentiated because of overlap, the aim is to achieve a level of "conscious sedation" as opposed to "deep sedation." *Conscious sedation* is a state in which the patient is calm and relaxed, yet able to respond to verbal or physical stimulation. The patient is able to maintain a patent airway and protective airway reflexes during this minimally depressed level of consciousness.[2] *Deep sedation* is more

Sedation and Analgesia for Procedures Is a Continuum:

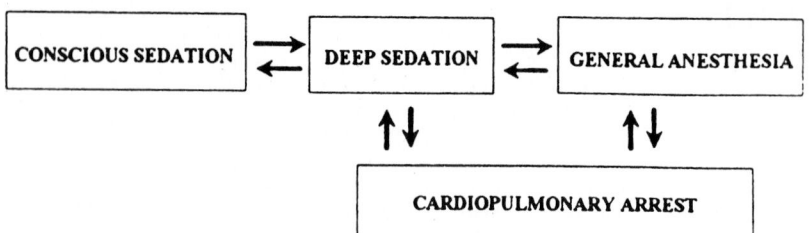

Figure 51-1. Anesthesia care spans a continuum. (Reprinted with permission from Kaplan RF: 1996 Annual Refresher Course Lectures. ASA Annual Meeting, October, 1996, No. 531, p 1. American Society of Anesthesiologists, Park Ridge, Illinois, 1996.)

hazardous. In this state, there is a controlled, depressed level of consciousness. There may be a loss of protective airway reflexes and a loss in the patient's ability to independently maintain his or her airway. The patient may be difficult to arouse immediately; and adverse physiologic changes including hypotension, respiratory depression, and apnea may occur.[3] In many situations these levels of sedation are inadequate for the procedure. For example, the patient may move too much during conscious sedation for an accurate image to be obtained. If additional sedation is provided, the patient may become too sedated, such that the airway becomes unprotected and jeopardized. In these situations, a general anesthetic must be administered.

Dentists and doctors from a variety of specialties administer sedatives and analgesics to their patients to provide conscious sedation. Their interventions are performed at sites far removed from operating rooms with no availability of anesthesiologists for backup help. Several specialty organizations have developed guidelines to maximize the safe use of sedatives and analgesics. These include standards for monitoring as well as working definitions of the level of sedation that is desired.[2,4,5] The Joint Commission on Accreditation of Healthcare Organizations (JCAHO) defined anesthesia care as the administration of iv, im, or inhalational agents that may result in the loss of the patient's protective reflexes. JCAHO standards require that the anesthesia service of a hospital participate with nonanesthesiology departments in setting up a uniform quality of care.[6,7] The expectation is that nonanesthesiology practitioners will administer conscious sedation with appropriate training and with the use and understanding of monitoring. Personnel from the anesthesiology department should be involved in patient care if deep sedation or general anesthesia is required within a JCAHO-approved facility. The ASA Standards for Basic Anesthetic Monitoring should apply in all cases involving anesthesiology personnel.[8]

Guidelines for the establishment of nonoperating room anesthetizing locations have been established.[1] In the office environment, however, little regulatory oversight is in place at the present time. Relatively few of these sites have sought approval from regulatory bodies. As the economics and politics of medicine continue to change, the sites and individual practitioners working at remote sites will begin to seek credentialing from the various regulatory bodies.

Monitored anesthesia care (MAC), regional, and general anesthesia can be provided at nonoperating room locations both within and outside of the hospital. Experience has shown that safe and efficient care can be provided at areas that are far removed from the operating room. The choice of technique should be dictated by the requests of the patient, the specific medical condition, the requirements for the particular procedure, and the expertise of the practitioner. No single drug or drug dosage is optimal in all situations. A sedative or amnestic may be appropriate and sufficient for some patients; others may require the additional use of an opioid. With some agents, such as the benzodiazepines, variability in response from patient to

patient is large. Substitute medications may be indicated. The practitioner's familiarity with the procedure and the patient's response to drug titration should guide drug administration. These principles apply regardless of the anesthetic, analgesic, or sedative chosen.

RADIOLOGY AND RADIATION THERAPY

A common alternative site where anesthesia services are required is within the radiology department. Diagnostic and therapeutic procedures performed by radiologists include angiography, magnetic resonance imaging (MRI), and computed tomography (CT). In more recent years, interventional radiology has become more aggressive in treating patients with advanced disease states. Procedures undertaken include angiographic embolization of arteriovenous malformations and aneurysms, removal of vascular occlusions, creation of vascular shunts, placement of stents, external beam radiation, and intraoperative radiation therapy. Most of these procedures are relatively painless. But the patient must remain motionless if the intervention is to be made successfully. An exception is the use of sclerotherapy to obliterate the vessels leading to an arterovenous malformation. This is quite painful. Also, patients experience brief periods of pain during angiography with cannulation of the vessel and subsequent injection of the contrast dye. Dye injections are described as episodes of burning. Finally, owing to a variety of factors, some patients are unable to lie still for prolonged procedures.

Most adult patients who have received adequate teaching and reassurance before and during the procedures are able to tolerate interventions without sedation. The more invasive procedures are difficult to tolerate without at least some degree of sedation. For some procedures, such as those done by neuroradiologists, the anesthesia care requires greater skill and finesse. Brief periods of intense sedation and analgesia are required for arterial catheterization (usually femoral) and can be accomplished with the use of short-acting agents. Then, a lesser level of sedation is required for the remainder of the procedure, when patient cooperation is necessary. Transfemoral access is obtained with the placement of a large introducer sheath. Through this sheath a coaxial catheter is positioned, with fluoroscopy, to the general region of interest. Finally, a much smaller, superselective catheter is introduced for the injection of embolic agents, sclerosing agents, or filaments (Fig. 51-2).

Patients with intracranial hypertension, trauma, decreased levels of consciousness, or a compromised airway can be particularly challenging. Similarly, when patients are confused and either unwilling or unable to remain motionless, an additional level of anesthesia skill will be required. Many of these patients suffer from claustrophobia, movement disorders, or simply cannot tolerate the radiologic procedures. Pediatric patients have additional needs that must be addressed. It is difficult to perform these procedures on children without the use of general anesthesia. Most children cannot tolerate the interventions owing to separation anxiety and fear of the medi-

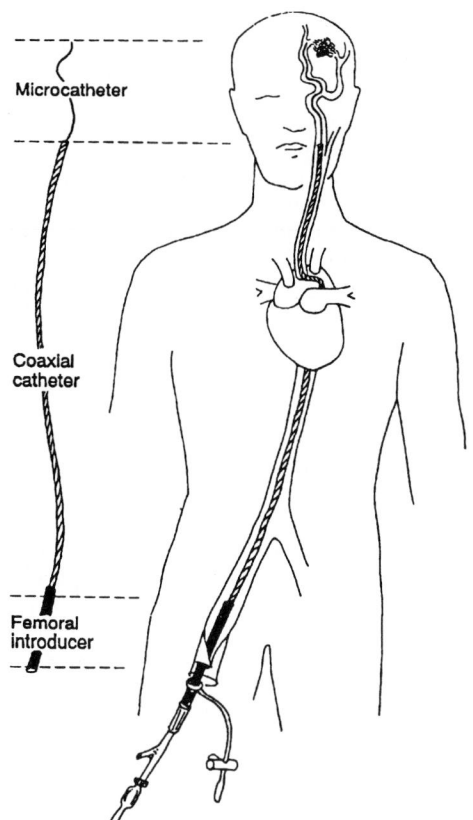

Figure 51-2. Representation of a superselective catheter. (Reprinted with permission from Young WL, Pile-Spellman J: Anesthetic considerations for interventional neuroradiology. Anesthesiology 80:427, 1994.)

cal staff and equipment. If arterial catheterization or other painful procedures are to be performed, general anesthesia is usually required.

Contrast Agents and Adverse Reactions

Contrast agents are required for many radiologic procedures. The newer agents have a low osmolality and are nonionic. Adverse reactions to the intravascular injection of these contrast dyes are diminished; fatal reactions occur in approximately 1 of 100,000 procedures.[9-11] Many factors contribute to the development of adverse reactions: the method of injection (either slow infusion or bolus), the type of dye employed, and the total dose administered. The specific technique performed and the site studied also influence the degree and severity of adverse reactions. Coronary artery and cerebral angiography are associated with a high risk of reactions.[9] Patients with a history of atopy or allergy to shellfish or seafood are more prone to contrast-related adverse reactions.[9,12] Adverse reactions are classified as mild, moderate, or severe (Table 51-1).

Table 51-1. ADVERSE REACTIONS TO CONTRAST MEDIA

Mild	Moderate	Severe
Urticaria	Tissue edema	Prolonged hypotension
Chills	Bronchospasm	Cyanosis
Fever	Hypotension	Anoxia
Facial flushing	Seizures	Pulmonary edema
Nausea		Angina
Vomiting		Dysrhythmias

Adapted from Goldberg M: Systemic reactions to intravascular contrast media. Anesthesiology 60:45, 1984.

Nausea and vomiting are mild reactions to dye injection. These, however, occur as prodromal symptoms in as many as 20% of all anaphylactoid reactions.[9] Hypotension, urticaria, and bronchospasm are also common side-effects. Hypotension frequently occurs with dye reactions. It may be preceded by a brief period of systemic hypertension. This elevation in blood pressure is a function of the high osmolarity of the injectate. Older contrast dyes consist of iodine-containing anions ionically linked to one of several cations, such as magnesium, calcium, and methylglucamine. The dyes are hyperosmolar when compared with blood plasma. Their osmolarities can be as high as $2100 \ mOsmol \cdot l^{-1}$. Newer agents are nonionic and have osmolarities in the $600-700 \ mOsmol \cdot l^{-1}$ range. Patients receiving contrast usually diurese large volumes of urine because of the osmotic load of the dye. Adequate hydration of these patients should be assured to prevent worsening of pre-existing hypovolemia or azotemia. Patients with renal dysfunction need extra care.[13] Many centers advocate the use of a Foley catheter in procedures lasting longer than 1 hour when dye loads are administered.

If patients have a history of a reaction to dyes or if a dye reaction is anticipated, prophylactic treatment with diphenhydramine, 25–50 mg iv, and/or steroids (methylprednisolone, 100–1000 mg iv, or prednisone, 50 mg po given in two doses prior to the procedure) is beneficial.[14,16] The medical treatment of adverse reactions following dye injection should be tailored to the severity of the reaction. Supportive care may be all that is necessary. Establishing intravenous access, administering fluids, airway management, and frequent monitoring of the patient's hemodynamic and respiratory functions are essential. In addition, there should be immediate access to oxygen and emergency drugs, including epinephrine, atropine, diphenhydramine, steroids, benzodiazepines, and methylxanthines (such as aminophylline).

Protection from Ionizing Radiation

Patients, physicians, and other health care workers are frequently exposed to ionizing radiation, usually in the form of X-rays. Exposure to gamma radiation or, rarely, alpha or beta radiation from radioactive isotopes may also occur during implantation or removal procedures. Ionizing radiation exposure may occur directly from the source, as leakage from the ionizing device, or as scatter from the equipment. Direct exposure must be avoided. High radiation exposure occurs with fluoroscopy or digital subtraction angiography. The dose delivered to the patient's skin during these procedures may be greater than 8000 mrem. During fluoroscopy for cardiac angiography, the total delivered dose may be greater than 75,000 mrem.[17,18]

Radiation exposure during fluoroscopy is often from scatter. A single CT scan exposes the patient to ~1–3 cGy.[17] Fortunately, the exposure of health-care workers to the radiation emitted from a CT scanner is relatively low. The beam of radiation is highly focused. Radiation intensity and exposure decrease with the inverse square of the distance from its source.[16] A minimum distance of 3–6 feet is recommended. With the routine use of a lead apron, protective goggles, and thyroid shield, exposure to radiation can be kept to a low level by maximizing the distance from the energy source. Radiation dosages and terminology are listed in Table 51-2.

SPECIFIC RADIOLOGIC PROCEDURES
Angiography

Simple angiographic studies are usually straightforward and do not require the participation of anesthesia personnel. Many radiologists are adept in the use of local anesthesia and are safely able to provide a light level of conscious sedation for their patients. Complex interventional radiologic procedures

Table 51-2. RADIATION TERMINOLOGY AND DOSAGE

Term	Definition
Radiation absorbed dose	A measure of an absorbed dose equal to 100 erg $\cdot$ g^{-1} of any absorber (SI units Gray [Gy]: 1 Gy = 100 rad)
Roentgen	Total dosage of either X-rays or gamma rays; 1 roentgen = 86.9 erg $\cdot$ g^{-1} of dry air
Roentgen-equivalent-man (rem)	Dose of ionizing radiation with the same biologic tissue effect as 1 rad of X-rays

Maximum Dose Recommended by the National Council of Radiation Protection

Exposure	<100 mrem $\cdot$ wk^{-1} <5000 mrem $\cdot$ yr^{-1}

Adapted from Davies D: Subspecialty monitoring techniques—miscellaneous. In Gravenstein N (ed): Problems in Anesthesia Monitoring, p 138. Philadelphia, JB Lippincott, 1987.

take longer periods of time and usually require concurrent care from an anesthesiologist. The techniques and medications chosen for use are dictated by the needs of the radiologist and the patient's underlying medical condition. The required level of anesthesia may range from monitored anesthesia care, with or without sedation, to general anesthesia with placement of an endotracheal tube. Attention to hydration is essential since patients will have fasted prior to the procedure and an osmotic diuresis will occur after contrast dye has been given.

The patient must be positioned comfortably and in a position suitable for the procedure, yet with an eye to providing necessary access for the anesthesiologist. A preformed headrest is helpful in minimizing unwanted movement; a support under the patient's knees provides flexion and reduces back discomfort during long cases. This does not interfere with catheter placement within the femoral veins or arteries. Arms should be padded and tucked at the sides of the body or comfortably restrained on arm boards. Monitors and iv lines often require additional extensions since the anesthesiologist is usually several feet away from the patient during the intervention. This arrangement minimizes radiation exposure and allows for movement of the imaging machinery. For therapeutic procedures, a larger-bore iv may be necessary. If the patient is not anesthetized, oxygen should be delivered by nasal cannula or face mask. An end-tidal CO_2 monitoring port allows for the documentation of exhaled air and confirms respiration.

When administered by appropriately trained personnel, propofol is particularly useful as a sedative during angiographic procedures. It can be initiated at small doses (20 μg $\cdot$ kg^{-1} $\cdot$ min^{-1}), then rapidly titrated up or down as needed; and, when discontinued, it allows a rapid return to consciousness at the conclusion of the procedure. The goal is to provide sedation while allowing the patient to maintain the airway. Peripheral body temperature should be monitored, and all attempts made to maintain normothermia. Shivering results in patient movement and, aside from exposing the patient to discomfort and additional risks, will obscure details of the image. When femoral artery cannulation is performed, the pulse oximeter probe can be placed on a toe of the leg that is cannulated. In addition to permitting measurement of SpO_2, placement at this site will allow early detection of femoral artery obstruction or distal thromboembolism. Locating the device on the toe is also useful once the catheter is removed and pressure applied to the vessel. Overly vigorous pressure can completely compress the vessel and stop blood flow to the foot. This will be detected by a corresponding fall in SpO_2.[16]

Specific angiographic procedures deserve special attention. In many of these procedures, "roadmapping" is employed in which a bolus of contrast agent is injected into the circulation to outline the vascular anatomy. Once this is obtained, the image is superimposed on live fluoroscopic imaging. The radiologist can correlate the progress of the microcatheter as it is advanced to a specific site. Although deep sedation has been used, this procedure usually requires general anesthesia with dense muscle relaxation and occasional periods of apnea. Movement during these procedures will slow the procedure. Time must then be spent for a repeat injection of dye to make another roadmap consistent with the patient's different position.[16]

Cerebral Angiography

Cerebral angiography is indicated for a variety of disorders including cerebrovascular disease, brain tumors, arteriovenous malformations, and cerebral aneurysms.[15] Medical conditions that increase the risk of complications during and following angiography include a history of cerebrovascular disease, stroke, diabetes, seizures, and transient ischemic attacks. Determining the patient's medical history from a reliable source is vital. Continuous arterial blood pressure monitoring is often necessary in addition to standard ASA monitors. This is particularly true whenever the systemic pressure will be modified with the use of vasoactive drugs. Radiologists may request changes in blood pressure to help with the placement of the catheters and to determine that blood flow to watershed areas will be adequate when the normal blood pressure is lowered somewhat, as occurs during sleep.

General anesthesia is required in patients who are unable to cooperate or who require airway protection. For patients presenting for cerebral angiography who are at risk for intracranial hypertension, control of arterial blood pressure and carbon dioxide partial pressure levels is mandatory.[15,16,19] Proper positioning of the patient (head up, head in the midline position, no compression of neck veins) will help to minimize increases in intracranial pressure (ICP). Tracheal intubation is challenging in these patients. Special care must be used to provide an adequate depth of anesthesia before the stimulus of laryngoscopy and intubation, since these maneuvers may increase blood pressure and the ICP. Once tracheal intubation is accomplished, mild hyperventilation will improve the quality of the angiographic study by inducing cerebral vasoconstriction, slowing the cerebral circulation, reducing dye washout, and increasing dye concentration within the brain. This allows for a more detailed image.[16]

Hypotension and bradycardia are occasionally seen during cerebral angiography once contrast dye is injected. These changes usually respond to administration of iv fluid and small doses of atropine.[19] Because contrast material may cross the blood–brain barrier, some of the dye can enter the brain and cause seizures. Whether this is a result of direct toxicity of the dye or activation of the chemoreceptor trigger zone is unclear.[9,19,20] Other complications of the procedure include embolization of plaques, bleeding, thrombosis, and hematoma at the arterial puncture site.[20] The overall incidence of complications from cerebral angiography ranges from 8 to 14%.[16,20,21] A standard management plan needs to be in place should the patient develop a neurologic catastrophe such as hemorrhage or stroke. Members of the care team must know the course of action to be taken as soon as the complication is recognized (Fig. 51-3).[15,16]

Coagulation

Careful management of coagulation is required during and after angiography and other invasive cardiovascular procedures. The goal is to prevent thromboemboli. Anticoagulation guidelines are controversial for the individual procedures; most agree that higher levels are indicated whenever test or permanent occlusions are performed. Intravenous heparinization is performed routinely during superselective catheterizations because

Initial resuscitation
    Communicate with radiologists
    Call for assistance
    Secure the airway and hyperventilate with 100% O₂
    Determine if problem is hemorrhagic or occlusive
        Hemorrhagic: immediate heparin reversal (1 mg protamine for
            each 100 units heparin given) and low normal pressure
        Occlusive: deliberate hypertension, titrated to neurologic
            examination, angiography, or physiologic imaging studies
            (*e.g.*, TCD, CBF)
Further resuscitation
    Head up 15° in neutral position
    Titrate ventilation to a Paco₂ of 26–28 mm Hg
    0.5 g/kg mannitol, rapid intravenous infusion
    Anticonvulsants: dilantin (give slowly, 50 mg/min) and
        phenobarbitol
    Titrate thiopental infusion to electroencephalogram burst
        suppression
    Allow body temperature to fall as quickly as possible to 33–34°C
    Consider dexamethasone 10 mg*

Figure 51-3. Acute management of neurologic catastrophes. (Reprinted with permission from Young WL, Pile-Spellman J: Anesthetic considerations for interventional neuroradiology. Anesthesiology 80:427, 1994.)

so much endothelial damage is created by the physical passage of the catheter itself. After placement of the femoral introducer catheter, a baseline activated clotting time (ACT) is measured, heparin $5000 \ U \cdot 70 \ kg^{-1}$ is given and another ACT obtained. Usually, the target measurement for ACT is 2.5 times the baseline level. Repeat ACTs should be measured hourly throughout the procedure to confirm adequate anticoagulation. The risks from excessive anticoagulation are small in comparison to thrombus formation. A heparin–ACT plot can be generated during long procedures to anticipate the need for subsequent doses. This makes it easier to follow trends. In many centers, heparin is continued throughout the first night of the case. The effects of the heparin are then allowed to dissipate. Only at this point is the introducer catheter sheath removed from the groin and pressure applied.[16]

Superselective Functional Examination

Superselective testing is performed following meticulous catheter placement within a segment of the brain (see Fig. 51-2). The procedure allows for the assessment of specific neurologic function or dysfunction at a particular site. The technique is used immediately prior to therapeutic embolization in patients who suffer from arteriovenous malformations. It is also used to isolate the seizure focus in patients with intractable epilepsy. Patients are given sedation and analgesia for the catheter placement through the skin, but they must then be awake and able to respond. A directed and detailed neurologic assessment is performed immediately prior to the procedure. Sedation is then stopped such that the patient is awake and able to respond to questioning. It may be necessary to use naloxone or flumazenil to antagonize opioids and/or benzodiazepine sedatives. Once catheter placement is confirmed, a small dose of sodium amobarbital (30 mg) or lidocaine (30 mg) mixed with contrast agent is injected through the catheter. The doses and volumes are tailored to fit the clinical situation and information that is to be obtained. Amobarbital is used to investigate areas of gray matter; lidocaine is used to evaluate white matter tracts. Immediately after the barbiturate is administered, a repeat neurologic examination is performed. Attention is directed toward "quiet areas" that would be missed if only a sensory or motor examination were performed. Patients are awake for these procedures and asked to answer specific questions. This indicates that parts of the brain involved in the use of language are intact. The changes that are seen following this "anesthesia" of a selected

site in the brain are used to predict the changes that will be associated with embolization or resection at that site.

Embolization Procedures

Angiographic embolizations are performed to treat cerebral vascular malformations, aneurysms, cavernous sinus fistulas, and brain tumors. A successful arterial embolization offers a relatively safe, nonsurgical cure provided in the radiology suite. If an open procedure is subsequently required, the embolization can minimize bleeding that will occur during the craniotomy. Anesthetic management for embolization is similar to that for standard angiographic procedures. Choice of sedation and use of either regional or general anesthesia depend on patient preference and the clinical indications. Awake but sedated patients may help with detection and avoidance of neurologic complications during intracranial embolization, but embolizations can be painful and lengthy procedures. Some interventional radiologists insist on general anesthesia with dense neuromuscular blockade.

Once the patient is positioned for the procedure, sophisticated imaging techniques, including digital subtraction, allow the catheter to be placed immediately before treatment. Deliberate hypotension is induced to slow the flow of blood in an arteriovenous malformation. This occurs directly before the injection of glue or foreign bodies to occlude the lesion. Since many of the patients are young and otherwise healthy, large amounts of medications are sometimes required. Esmolol, administered as a $1\text{-}mg \cdot kg^{-1}$ bolus with a starting infusion of $0.5 \ mg \cdot kg^{-1} \cdot min^{-1}$, can be used to reduce blood pressure to targeted levels. Labetolol, nitroprusside, and nitroglycerine can also be utilized to achieve hypotension. One must be aware of the potential danger of "overshooting" and causing episodes of profound hypotension. If the blood pressure is to be elevated, phenylephrine, administered as a $1\text{-}\mu g \cdot kg^{-1}$ bolus or as an infusion, is effective. Increasing the blood pressure is required if neurologic deficits are noted with planned or inadvertent vascular occlusions. The increase in blood pressure will increase blood flow through the collateral circulation to the areas of ischemia and can serve as an important temporizing measure.[15,16]

Embolizations are performed by selectively thrombosing an arteriovenous malformation. This is done by the careful introduction of small foreign bodies (pieces of polymeric plastics, detachable balloons, or threads of various materials) at the site of the pathology. Balloons can be inflated to a large diameter such that aneurysms or feeder vessels are occluded through small percutaneous arteriotomies. Sclerosing agents, such as N-butyl cyanoacrylate or ethyl alcohol, can also be employed to close the vascular malformation. Patients must be examined during and following the procedure because disruption of a vessel's integrity will allow for flow of these solids and sclerosing liquids into adjacent vascular beds within the brain. The procedures are highly invasive. If complications arise, contingency plans should be in place for emergent patient transport to the operating room for a craniotomy.

The cumulative dose of contrast dye used during these procedures is quite high because the angiographic catheter positioning must be tested repeatedly. All of the dyes act as osmotic diuretics; in addition, the use of diuretics such as furosemide or mannitol may be indicated for the procedure. Adequate hydration is necessary and a Foley catheter desirable. Nausea and vomiting are common complications. Metoclopramide, ranitidine, droperidol, and ondansetron are all useful adjuvant drugs.

Computed Tomography

Computed tomography (CT) scanning is noninvasive and painless. It is frequently used for intracranial, thoracic, and abdominal imaging. Interventional CT scanning is essential for needle placement for nerve blockade, biopsy, and needle aspiration of masses.[22] The early CT scanners generated a cross-sectional image of the patient and took several minutes. It was essential that the patient be motionless during this time.[19] Modern scanners obtain a cross-sectional image in just a few seconds, and state-of-the-art spiral scanners can image a slice of the body in less than 1 second. Thus, the problems with motion artifacts are greatly minimized. The majority of adult patients will tolerate CT scanning without anesthesia if given verbal assurances. Sedation or general anesthesia is usually required only during procedures for children or for adults who have difficulty remaining still. Patients requiring a more intensive level of care (e.g., following trauma) usually need the continuous presence of an anesthesiologist.

Children experience fear and separation anxiety when inside the scanning room. It is usually wiser to induce pediatric patients away from the scanner and position them once they are anesthetized. Temperature monitoring and attention to patient warming is necessary since the CT suites are cool, and hypothermia will develop rapidly in an anesthetized child. For patients undergoing general anesthesia or deep sedation, the primary concerns are related to airway management and adequate oxygenation. Positioning and movement of the gantry during various procedures may cause kinking of the endotracheal tube or disconnection of the anesthesia circuit. These problems must be anticipated. Also, patients undergoing emergency procedures and those who receive oral contrast agents are considered to have full stomachs and must be treated appropriately for airway protection.[23]

Stereotactic-guided needle placement and surgery is performed using CT scanning. Most of these procedures involve biopsies or aspirations, often of intracranial masses. The stereotactic approach minimizes injury to adjacent structures. It involves placement of a radiolucent frame around the head. The frame is held in place by pins inserted directly into the skull. This aspect of the procedure is painful. Transient deep sedation or general anesthesia may occasionally be necessary in combination with the injection of local anesthetic at the insertion sites. Sedation must be used with caution in patients with suspected intracranial hypertension. If the sedation causes hypoventilation, the arterial CO_2 will rise and the cerebral blood vessels will dilate, further increasing ICP. Once the frame is affixed to the skull, the patient can be positioned on the gantry and a motionless field is assured.

Magnetic Resonance Imaging

Magnetic resonance imaging (MRI) provides more detail of intracranial, spinal, and soft tissue lesions than does CT. MRI is noninvasive and produces no ionizing radiation. There are no reports of harm from tissue contact with the magnetic field itself. The device has gained universal popularity, and is one of the most important advances in imaging during the past decades. The patient is placed in a cylindrical tunnel surrounded by a high-intensity magnetic field coil. A high-quality image takes from 30 minutes to an hour to obtain. During this time the patient must remain motionless inside the magnetic bore, or the image will be degraded by artifact.[24,25]

Several days of energy input are required to establish the MRI's intense magnetic field. The field is constantly present, even in the absence of a patient to study. It is rarely allowed to fade away; this is done only in an emergency.[24,25] The way in which the device works is straightforward. Atoms with an odd numbers of protons in their nuclei, most notably, hydrogen, are aligned in one direction by the magnetic field.[22] Once this alignment occurs, the atoms comprising the tissues are subjected to intense radiofrequency pulses that temporarily change the protons' orientations. As the radiofrequency pulses are discontinued, the protons return to their original alignment (i.e., they "relax") within the original magnetic field. In conforming

to this orientation, they give off energy. It is this release of energy over a variable time span that is measured and used to generate the MRI image. The time it takes for the energy to dissipate as realignment is achieved is termed the relaxation time. These times are specific for given tissues.[22,26] The hydrogen atom is particularly useful in imaging. It is present in all tissues both as mobile water and as immobile triglycerides. Since the chemical environments surrounding these atoms differ from site to site, their relaxation rates differ, and body structures are differentiated by the images created.

High energy levels are used to generate the magnetic fields of the MRI. Ferromagnetic equipment cannot be safely used near the scanner.[24,25] Standard monitoring equipment must be modified to allow for proper function of the devices and to prevent distortion of the image. There are several types of physiologic monitors, oxygen-powered ventilators, laryngoscopy equipment, and anesthesia machines that can be used within the MRI suite.[24,25] Most of the equipment differs in that it is made of aluminum or other nonferromagnetic material. Absolute and relative contraindications for MRI scanning include patients with cardiac pacemakers near the site for scanning, aneurysm clips, or intravascular wires.[22,27–30] It has been suggested that MRI be avoided in women in the first trimester of pregnancy, although no strong data support such avoidance.[31] Large metal implants in patients may heat up when subjected to torque from the magnet's force. These sites should be monitored for temperature changes when the patient is within the magnetic field.

Anesthetic management of patients during MRI is similar to that for CT scanning. The environment for the MRI, however, is significantly different in that it is very confining. With a closed MRI, the patient is positioned on a long, thin table. This table is then advanced into the magnetic bore. The incidence of claustrophobia or anxiety-related problems for awake patients within the gantry ranges from 7–30%.[32] Procedures that require a long duration are uncomfortable for even the most cooperative patient. The equipment is noisy. Continual reassurances by the staff are helpful for the patient. When sedation or general anesthesia is required, the provider must pay particular attention to the patient's position and the placement of the anesthesia circuitry. Propofol (1–2-mg $\cdot$ kg^{-1} bolus followed by an infusion of 100 μg $\cdot$ kg^{-1} $\cdot$ min^{-1}, titrated to effect) is commonly used in spontaneously breathing patients. This tends to avoid some of the issues regarding incompatible anesthesia equipment close to the magnetic field. Direct access to the patient during the procedure is difficult. Although the anesthesiologist can remain in attendance in the scanning room, most people prefer to stay outside due to the excessive noise. Open MRI scanners have been developed over the last few years. The patient is still positioned on a narrow table, but the gantry is larger and there are fewer complaints of patients' feeling confined. As the technology continues to improve, the images from these newer models will rival those from the conventional devices.

Monitoring of MRI patients receiving sedation and regional or general anesthesia should include continuous ECG, automated blood pressure cuff, and pulse oximetry. ECG telemetry and capnography systems minimize distortion of the MRI signal while permitting accurate patient assessments.[28] When general anesthesia is required, induction is usually performed in a room adjacent to the MRI. Laryngoscopy is difficult within the MRI suite because the magnetic field affects conventional laryngoscope batteries. Anesthesia machines and ventilators constructed specifically for use in MRI are commercially available but are expensive. If the anesthesia machine is kept outside of the MRI, extra breathing tubing will be required to reach the patient. Mapleson and Bain circuits are used with MRI and may provide additional visual and tactile monitoring of the patient's breathing and airway.[24] As always, vigilance is required in caring for the patient during this procedure. Unusual complications must be anticipated and measures taken to prevent them. For example, a tissue burn from the heating of a pulse oximetry probe placed within the MRI magnetic field has been reported.[33]

Radiation Therapy

Two different types of radiation therapy commonly require anesthesia care—external beam radiation treatments (usually for children with malignancies) and intraoperative radiation to tumor masses that cannot be completely resected. Four general groups of radiation-sensitive malignancies occur in children: (1) central nervous system leukemias, (2) radiosensitive ocular tumors, (3) intracranial tumors, and (4) a variety of intra-abdominal tumors. These patients should be examined before each treatment for signs or symptoms of sepsis or increased ICP. Table 51-3 lists several radiosensitive tumors for which external beam radiation has proved useful.

Patients are typically scheduled for a series of treatments over several weeks. Radiation doses are in the range of 180–250 cGy. Since the dose is so high, all medical personnel must leave the room during the actual treatment. Direct observation of the patient is not possible. Closed-circuit television and telemetric microphones are used. Standard monitoring is interfaced with the remote location. Television cameras are mounted so that anesthesiologists may observe the patient and anesthesia equipment in one scene. In the event of a problem with the patient or a circuit disconnect, shutdown of the radiation beam and immediate access to the patient are crucial (within 20–30 seconds).[34]

The need for patient immobility is a primary reason anesthesia is required for these procedures. It is difficult for children to keep completely still with the use of sedation only. If it is attempted, airway management problems increase, and the recovery period is greatly prolonged. General anesthesia offers several advantages to conscious sedation. The treatments proceed with efficiency and precision, while patient and parent satisfaction is high. Use of a general anesthetic is especially important when a radiation therapy site treats 20–30 patients each day. General anesthesia may be tailored to the procedures with the use of agents and techniques that are of short duration. Most of the children in this subset of patients have indwelling catheters that facilitate iv induction. Airway management will vary with the individual patient and clinical situation. Since there is no surgical stimulation, patients can be maintained at light levels of anesthesia. Emergence and recovery are rapid. Changes in treatment plans or modification in anesthetic regimen may be necessary as the patients' conditions change.

Extremely high radiation levels are used as palliation for a variety of tumors. Intraoperative radiation therapy treatments are provided after the masses are exposed to view. Patients with pancreatic, colon and rectal cancers, radiation-sensitive sarcomas, and specific types of ovarian cancers receive this form of treatment.[34] Doses of 5000–6000 cGy may be used during a single, intraoperative treatment. These patients typically suffer from advanced cancers. They will have the attendant nutritional deficiency, dehydration, electrolyte imbalances, and coagulopathies that often complicate anesthetic management.

Table 51-3. COMMON RADIATION-SENSITIVE TUMORS

Neuroblastoma
Retinoblastoma
Medulloblastoma
Wilms' tumor
Rhabdomyosarcoma
Leukemia

Some newer hospitals are equipped with combination radiation therapy/operating room suites; however, most centers require that surgical exploration be performed in the traditional operating room. The anesthetized patient is subsequently transported to the radiology suite. Often, this can be a considerable distance. Portable monitors and methods for delivery of oxygen and agents to maintain general anesthesia during transport are all required. Intravenous anesthetics tend to be more efficacious than inhaled agents.[34] The standards for monitoring are the same as for procedures performed exclusively within the operating room.

Requirements for patient monitoring for intraoperative radiation are comparable to those described for external beam radiation. Personnel must leave the room during the actual treatment. Equipment interfaced to an external control desk allows careful monitoring with observation of the patient and anesthesia equipment with closed-circuit television. After treatment, patients must be transported back to the operating room for surgical closure. Occasionally, closure can be performed in radiology and the patient taken directly to the PACU.

Cardiac Catheterization

Anesthetic care is needed for patients who cannot keep still during imaging procedures or who require an increased level of care due to the severity of their underlying disease. Anesthesia is usually needed when a patient undergoes a cardiac catheterization, angioplasty, atherectomy, or a valvuloplasty.

Catheterization of children is most commonly performed to diagnose suspected congenital heart disease (CHD).[35] Presenting signs and symptoms include cyanosis, dyspnea, failure to thrive, and congestive heart failure. Adequate premedication and sedation are important to alleviate anxiety and fear. Anxiety, with its corresponding increases in heart rate and blood pressure, will exacerbate several cardiopulmonary abnormalities. The changes are particularly dangerous for patients with intracardiac shunts. Rapid changes follow myocardial depression from dye loads or anesthetic induction agents that produce abrupt falls in preload or afterload. They are also seen with excessive sympathetic stimulation. Normocarbia should be maintained. When patients are dependent on blood flow through a patent ductus arteriosis (e.g., coarctation of the aorta), high oxygen tensions should be avoided since elevations in oxygen partial pressures can lead to ductal closures. In these patients, prostaglandin E_1 infusions can be used to maintain the patency of the ductus. Polycythemia is commonly seen in cardiac patients with cyanotic CHD. The elevated hematocrit increases the blood viscosity and the risk of deep vein thrombosis. Lowering the hematocrit, however, can be detrimental in that it lowers the oxygen delivery to the peripheral tissues. The depth of analgesia, sedation, or general anesthesia must be titrated to prevent tachycardia, hypertension, and changes in cardiac function. The pharmacokinetics of anesthetic agents are affected by left-to-right and right-to-left cardiovascular shunts. Some of these patients have morbidity from dysrhythmias. Atropine premedication, especially for those children with cyanotic disease, is important. During cardiac catheterization in children, the information obtained from standard monitoring with an ECG, pulse oximeter, and blood pressure cuff is augmented with catheterization data and arterial blood gas analyses.

Adults rarely require more than conscious sedation for catheter insertion and performance of the procedure. Some studies have shown benefit from general anesthesia during angioplasty procedures for acute myocardial infarction, but the main benefit seems to be enhanced patient satisfaction during the procedure itself.[36] Patients undergoing atherectomy will experience discomfort during the excision of the atheroma. A need for increased analgesia should be anticipated and provided at the appropriate time. Monitoring should focus on the detection and management of ischemic episodes and cardiac dysrhythmias.

Additionally, catheter insertion may stimulate a conduction block, although these acute changes are usually transient and have minimal hemodynamic significance. Episodes of ischemia, ventricular tachycardia, and fibrillation can occur subsequent to the administration of contrast media. Immediate access to oxygen, nitroglycerin, vasopressors, inotropes, resuscitative agents, and a defibrillator is required. If acute decompensation occurs during catheterization, cardiopulmonary resuscitation (CPR) is indicated. Direct access to the patient may be difficult because the fluoroscopic equipment is in the way. A plan must be formulated, agreed upon, and in place to obtain immediate access to the patient in the event of this complication.

CARDIOVERSION

Most cardioversions are scheduled in advance. There is adequate time for optimal preparation of the patient and the equipment. Patients scheduled for elective cardioversion need sedation and airway management for a very short period of time. Occasionally, anesthesia is needed for emergency cardioversion. This is almost always a result of an acute change causing severe hemodynamic instability. In this situation, adherence to basic ACLS protocols will provide a satisfactory plan of action. The algorithms indicate what medications and procedures are to be employed.

Elective cardioversions are often performed in areas near the operating room, usually in the PACU. They are typically performed early in the morning before these sites fill with patients following surgery. Additional anesthesia personnel are available should help be needed, and the site is well stocked with additional drugs, airway management equipment, and anesthetic agents. Atrial fibrillation and atrial flutter are the most common dysrhythmias treated with elective cardioversion. These will occur spontaneously or subsequent to valvular heart disease or recent coronary artery bypass grafting. Supraventricular tachycardias, which are refractory to medical management, are also treated with cardioversions.

Although the procedure is brief, a detailed history and physical examination should be performed for each patient. The current health status, use of concurrent medications, particularly heparin or coumadin, and history of prior gastroesophageal reflux are important considerations. Patients should be kept NPO in preparation for the procedure. A high level of anticoagulation is often required before cardioversion is performed. This will decrease the chance that thrombotic emboli will be showered into the pulmonary or systemic vascular systems. Any history of previous thromboembolization should be noted, and a brief neurologic assessment performed immediately prior to the procedure. This will allow assessment of acute post-procedure CNS dysfunction. Many of these patients will have coexisting cardiovascular disease and myocardial dysfunction.

Standard monitoring is routinely employed. Invasive monitoring is rarely required for cardioversion. The patient's physical status and general medical condition will dictate special monitoring needs. Intubating equipment, medications, supplemental oxygen, and a method to provide positive-pressure ventilation, suction, and resuscitation equipment should be readily available. A variety of iv agents have been used successfully, including the benzodiazepines, thiopental, methohexital, etomidate, and propofol.[37-42] Although midazolam is associated with longer recovery times, reversal with flumazenil is effective and causes a more rapid awakening.[37,41-43] Etomidate provides more hemodynamic stability than many of the other agents; however, the myoclonus, which it induces in 40% of patients, may interfere with ECG interpretation. In some centers, this side-effect precludes its use. Propofol produces hypotension when given as a bolus because it is a direct myocardial depressant. A slow induction with a low-dose infusion can attenuate this drop in systemic blood pressure.[38,41]

Adequate preoxygenation is performed before the induction of anesthesia. The onset of unconsciousness is often delayed in these patients because the dysrhythmia decreases the cardiac output and prolongs the circulation time. Once the patient is assessed and the level of anesthesia is found to be adequate, a synchronized countershock is administered. The airway is maintained and ventilation supported until the patient regains consciousness. The patient must be closely monitored following cardioversion for recurrence of the dysrhythmia or a different rhythm disturbance. Once the patient is awake and alert, outpatient discharge or admission to a monitored bed is individualized.

Some centers are routinely performing transesophageal echocardiographic examinations immediately prior to cardioversion in order to evaluate for the present of thrombus in the atria.[44] This complicates the anesthetic management since the patient must be sufficiently obtunded to tolerate esophageal placement of the probe, yet control of the airway is not readily achieved. One approach is to topically anesthetize the patient's airway prior to the procedure so that deep levels of sedation can be avoided.

ELECTROCONVULSIVE THERAPY

In the 1930s, mental health clinicians observed that patients who suffered from both schizophrenia and occasional seizure activity experienced improvements in their schizophrenic states following a seizure. This observation led to the development of pharmacologically induced seizures as a treatment for mental illnesses.[45] For a time, hypoglycemic states were deliberately caused by insulin injections to elicit grand mal seizures. Glucose was subsequently administered for rescue. Electroconvulsive therapy (ECT) was introduced in the late 1930s as an alternative mechanism for seizure induction, and it continues to be used today for the treatment of a number of major affective disorders.[45,46] Its use has been studied extensively, and it is found to be a relatively safe procedure with a mortality rate of 2–4 per 100,000 treatments. The most common use of ECT today is for the treatment of severe depression. ECT is also used as the initial treatment for the acutely ill patient for whom a rapid clinical response is essential, for example, severe catatonia in previously healthy young people. The therapy is also used after unsuccessful trials of antidepressant medications in patients with recurrent episodes of depression. The cellular and physiologic mechanisms for the beneficial effects are unknown, but various theories have been suggested.[45-50] Empirically, the treatment seems to work, and it has strong supporters.

Depression is a psychological and biologic disorder.[47,48] Patients are afflicted with persistent feelings of worthlessness, anorexia/hyperphagia, insomnia/hypersomnia, and unhappiness. Signs of poor nutritional status and dehydration are often present. Patients are often noncompliant with medication regimens. Depression may occur as a primary illness or appear as a secondary manifestation of another disease. For instance, patients afflicted with Parkinson's disease, acquired immune deficiency disease, or cerebrovascular accidents commonly suffer from depression.[48] Firstline treatments for depression are pharmacotherapeutic agents such as tricyclic antidepressants, monoamine oxidase (MAO) inhibitors, and selective serotonin-reuptake inhibitors (SSRI). Patients presenting for ECT may also take a variety of other psychotropic and mood-enhancing agents. In addition, since depression tends to affect an older population with pre-existing illnesses, patients may commonly take medications for their concurrent medical problems. The likelihood of drug interactions during anesthesia is high.[51]

Tricyclic antidepressants are structurally related to the phenothiazines. They block the reuptake of catecholamines at the presynaptic nerve terminals. They increase circulatory catecholamine levels and increase the patient's resting vascular tone. Administration of sympathomimetic drugs, such as ephedrine, may generate an exaggerated pressor response. Most of these agents also have anticholinergic properties. MAO inhibitors block the enzyme monoamine oxidase. As a result of this inhibition, additional neurotransmitter accumulates within the nerve terminals. Indirect-acting sympathomimetics can precipitate hypertensive crises because of the release of these additional neurotransmitters. Sympathomimetic drugs should be avoided or used in greatly reduced doses for these patients. MAO inhibitors also exaggerate the effects of direct-acting sympathomimetics like phenylephrine, but to a lesser extent. There is a controversy as to the concurrent use of MAO inhibitors in patients scheduled for ECT. For a time it was thought that these medications should be discontinued several weeks prior to the therapy,[45] but clinical experience has shown that problems during ECT are rarely encountered.[51] Many depressed patients need the medication up to and following the ECT. The use of meperidine is specifically contraindicated in patients who receive MAO inhibitors. Although the mechanism is not understood, in combination, the two agents interact to cause a hypermetabolic syndrome that can be fatal. Fluoxetine blocks the neuronal uptake of serotonin but has not been shown to have adverse interaction with anesthetic agents or with ECT. Lithium is used to treat manic-depressive illness as well as recurrent depression. It acts by interrupting action of the sodium–potassium pump at the cell membrane. This, in turn, alters the transmembrane potential and interferes with the production of cyclic adenosine monophosphate. Elevated lithium levels can prolong the time until awakening from general anesthesia; they can produce ECG changes and prolong the action of some neuromuscular blocking agents.[45,46,51]

The therapeutic effect produced by ECT is caused by the grand mal seizure, not by the electrical stimulus.[52,53] The smallest electrical stimulus that will evoke the seizure is used. This is characteristically a short, square-pulse wave. It is effective at producing the seizure while minimizing the side-effects of memory loss and confusion.[45,54] The duration of the seizure is also of clinical importance. Seizures lasting less than 30 seconds are often not as therapeutic. Electrical stimulation usually results in production of a grand mal seizure lasting up to several minutes and consisting of a short, 10–15-second tonic phase followed by a more prolonged clonic phase, which lasts 30–60 seconds. The cumulative seizure duration for effective therapy is thought to be 210–1000 seconds.[55] As a result, most patients receive 10–20 treatments over several weeks.

The seizure itself causes physiologic changes (Table 51-4). The initial stimulation produces a transient period of increased vagal tone. Bradycardia and some degree of hypotension are measured. This is followed by a period of increased sympathetic output, which corresponds to the clonic phase of the seizure. The patient becomes tachycardic and hypertensive. This phase can be a major physiologic stress, resulting in myocardial ischemia or infarction. To anticipate and prevent these stresses, a number of treatment regimens have been suggested. These include the use of beta-blockers, opioids, and short-acting vasodilators. The agents need to be tailored to the situation since pronounced bradycardia and asystole have occasionally been reported following their use.[56]

Anesthetic Considerations

As always, a history and physical examination are performed on all patients. Any interval change is documented since different personnel may be involved in the care of the patient over several weeks of treatment. A review of the record from prior ECT treatments is particularly helpful to note the doses used and the responses to the agents. Patients with pre-existing cardiac or cardiovascular disease, including recent myocardial infarction, congestive heart failure, valvular heart disease, or thoracic aneurysm, require additional planning and monitoring. The benefits of successful treatment have to be weighed against the risks

Table 51-4. PHYSIOLOGIC EFFECTS OF ELECTROCONVULSIVE THERAPY

Cardiovascular Effects

Initial Phase
Bradycardia
Hypotension

Later Phase
Tachycardia
Dysrhythmia
Hypertension
Increased systemic and myocardial oxygen consumption

Cerebral Effects

Increased cerebral blood flow
Elevated intercranial pressure
Increased oxygen consumption

Other Effects

Elevated intraocular pressure
Elevated intragastric pressure

Adapted from Gaines GY III, Rees DI: Anesthetic considerations for electroconvulsive therapy. South Med J 85:469, 1992.

of the acute physiologic changes. For particularly ill patients, invasive cardiovascular monitoring may be indicated, as well as continued close monitoring throughout the recovery period.[52,57] ECT should rarely be performed on patients with intracranial mass lesions because of the risk of elevated ICP and possible brain herniation. In patients with recent cerebrovascular accidents, ECT should be performed only after resolution of the acute insult has been achieved. This usually entails a waiting period of approximately 3 months.[45,52] Patients with retinal detachment are at increased risk because of the concomitant rise in intraocular pressure. Other relative contraindications to ECT include pregnancy, presence of long bone fractures, thrombophlebitis, and acute or severe pulmonary disease.[45,46,52] If a pregnant patient is treated, close monitoring of the fetus should be performed. Esophageal reflux and hiatal hernia are common findings in patients receiving ECT.[45,52] Pretreatment with sodium citrate, histamine antagonists, or metoclopramide may be indicated.

The anesthetic focus for ECT includes amnesia, airway management, prevention of bodily injury from the seizure, control of hemodynamic changes, and a smooth, rapid emergence.[45,46,52] Preoxygenation is routinely administered before each treatment. Barbiturates are most commonly employed (methohexital $0.5–1$ mg $\cdot$ kg^{-1} or thiopental $1.5–3$ mg $\cdot$ kg^{-1}). Methohexital causes a lower incidence of dysrhythmias when compared with other induction agents.[58] Etomidate is associated with seizures of longer duration. Propofol is effective for ECT, and its effect on outcome is similar to that of barbiturate use.[59,60] Several investigators have noted that it tends to result in seizures of shorter duration, however. Muscle relaxants are needed to prevent injury to the patient during the grand mal seizure. Succinylcholine is most commonly used because of its rapid onset and short duration. Doses range from $0.5–1.0$ mg $\cdot$ kg^{-1}.

ANESTHESIA FOR DENTAL SURGERY

Most dental procedures are performed in the office with no sedation and only local anesthesia injected at the site. Anesthesia may be required during more complicated or prolonged cases and when patients are uncooperative, phobic, or mentally challenged.

Providing anesthesia for mentally challenged and pediatric patients can present unique difficulties. Mentally challenged children can have a number of associated problems. Cardiac disease, including conduction abnormalities and structural defects, are associated with trisomy 21. Macroglossia, hypoplastic maxilla, palatal abnormalities, or mandibular protrusion are airway anomalies often seen in these patients.[61] If the patient is in the head-up position in the dental chair, vasodilating and myocardial depressant effects of anesthetics can be pronounced, especially in patients with cardiovascular diseases. Patients with neuromuscular diseases may have a history of aspiration and episodes of chronic recurrent pneumonitis that must be addressed before therapy.

When providing dental anesthesia, standard monitoring devices should be employed. Availability of temperature monitoring is important for children who may be susceptible to malignant hyperthermia. Both the anesthesiologist and the dentist should assure that the airway is protected. Blood, saliva, and dental debris will enter the trachea if precautions are not taken. Airway obstruction is always a concern if throat packs are used to prevent the swallowing of blood.

The range of anesthetic techniques depends on the condition of the patient. Different strategies have been suggested to facilitate induction and maintenance.[62–65] For the mentally challenged patient, or children, ketamine is commonly recommended for use as a primary anesthetic agent or to facilitate induction. It has the advantage of administration through oral, intramuscular, or intravenous routes. In addition, preservation of laryngeal and oropharyngeal reflexes makes it well suited for dental surgery. If intravenous access is difficult to achieve prior to induction in uncooperative patients, an im dose of ketamine, e.g., 2 mg·kg^{-1}, can provide a sufficient depth of anesthesia for iv placement within a few minutes.[63] In more cooperative, anxious patients, oral ketamine (0.5–8 mg·kg^{-1}) premedication smooths induction. Oral midazolam is also popular. A dose of 0.5 mg·kg^{-1} is dissolved in a small amount of liquid. Oral premedication, which obtunds the patient prior to needle sticks and masks, causes less anxiety for the patient and the parent.

Ketamine stimulates the sympathetic nervous system and acts to increase the heart rate and blood pressure. It also causes additional salivation. Glycopyrrolate, scopolamine, and atropine are often used. If iv access is available, barbiturates (methohexital, thiopental, and thiamylal) and propofol are well suited for induction.[65] Anesthesia can be maintained with intravenous infusions or inhalation agents. The use of inhalational agents requires that scavenging systems be in place so that waste gases do not contaminate the office.[66] Concerns about the possibility of triggering malignant hyperthermia need to be addressed and dantrolene must be immediately available. A continuous remifentanil or alfentanil infusion can be a useful iv technique for oral restorations in children. In conjunction with amnestic agents, it provides stable maintenance and permits a more rapid emergence. A disadvantage is that postoperative nausea and vomiting can be a problem and keep the patient in the facility for a long period of time.[64] After induction, nasal–tracheal intubations are most commonly used for dental procedures. The dentist or oral surgeon will have easier access for the work to be performed. Because of bleeding and the use of oropharyngeal packing, patients need close observation during emergence and recovery. Emergence excitation, shivering, residual sedation, pain, episodes of nausea, and respiratory obstruction need to be addressed as the patient returns to his or her baseline of mental functioning and is readied for discharge home.

TRANSPORT OF PATIENTS

Patients who receive anesthesia or sedation within the hospital but at sites removed from the operating room often require transport to the PACU after the procedure is completed. This transport entails moving a sedated or recovering patient significant distances, often by way of elevators. The ASA standards state that these patients should be accompanied by a member of the anesthesia team and that evaluation, monitoring, treatment, and support appropriate to the patient's medical condition be maintained.[8] Vigilance is especially important because hypoxemia following the use of sedation or general anesthesia is particularly dangerous with the additional distractions associated with patient transport.[67–69] While in transit, the lighting is less intense and the visual recognition of hypoxemia becomes more difficult. Supplemental oxygen is usually indicated for both children and adults.[70,71] Monitoring, in addition to auditory and tactile awareness, should include a noninvasive blood pressure device, ECG, and pulse oximetry. For critically ill patients who are transported to ICUs, more sophisticated monitors that permit continuous displays of vital signs may be required. Small, lightweight monitors have been designed specifically for patient transport. Many are equipped with modules such that the transducers used at the remote location can plug directly into their bases.

When critically ill patients are transported within the hospital, the personnel need to have additional supplies available. These include emergency medications, vasopressor agents, drugs for resuscitation, and, at times, a portable defibrillator. Patients who need ventilatory support should be transported with a self-inflating bag and the equipment needed to maintain an airway and reintubate the trachea should the endotracheal tube become dislodged. Oxygen-powered portable ventilators are available should the patient be difficult to ventilate manually. The stretcher needs to be equipped with a pole that can hold infusion pumps, transducers, and display screens. Tanks must contain an adequate supply of oxygen. Battery power and access to wall power should be assessed before transport is begun. The battery-powered supplies and quantity of oxygen must exceed the anticipated need in case unplanned delays occur during the transport back to the ICU.

OFFICE-BASED ANESTHESIA

Office-based anesthesia is an old endeavor that has regained popularity. Anesthetics that were once administered exclusively in the hospital or ambulatory surgery center are again being routinely provided directly within a surgeon's office. Medical advances have decreased the morbidity and mortality. Minimally invasive surgical techniques and short-acting agents now allow invasive procedures to be performed at sites far removed from the hospital.

Twenty-eight million people undergo a surgical procedure of some type each year.[72] Most of them require some form of concurrent anesthesia. All estimates indicate that the number of cases performed annually will increase as the U.S. population ages. For example, the number of patients over the age of 65 who will undergo noncardiac surgery is predicted to double from 7 to 14 million during the next three decades.[73] The total number of surgical procedures performed at that time will also increase from 28 to just under 40 million cases annually.

As this demand for surgical procedures has increased, a trend away from conventional sites of care has emerged.[74] The number of elective surgical procedures performed in hospital operating rooms has markedly declined. Initially, the move was from operating rooms to other sites within the hospital and to freestanding surgical centers. Now, a greater number of cases are performed directly within the surgeon's office.[75] This rate of rise has been dramatic. In the early 1980s, 80% of surgical procedures were performed in operating rooms for hospital inpatients, 18% for outpatients, and just 2% in freestanding clinics and offices. By 1994, approximately 35% of operations were performed for hospital inpatients and 57% for hospital outpatients, i.e., those presenting to freestanding clinics and outpatient surgery centers. The number of elective procedures performed directly within the physician's office had climbed to 8% (Fig. 51-4). This trend should continue. Estimates indicate that 14–20% of all elective surgery will be performed in the surgeon's

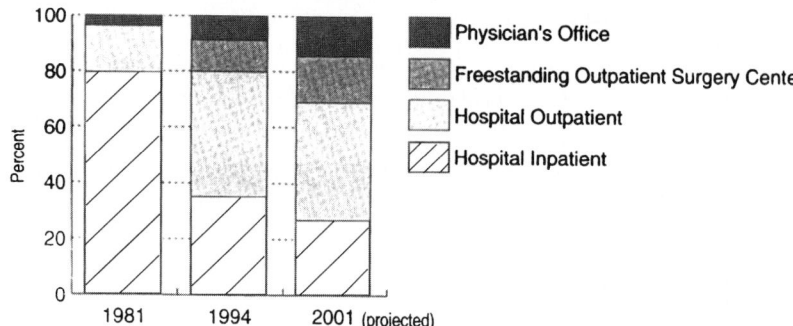

Figure 51-4. Location of anesthesia procedures. (Reprinted with permission from ASA Newsletter 60:11, 1996.)

office by the year 2001.[74,75] The total volume of surgical procedures will continue to increase following changes in the marketplace: an older, sicker population and an increased demand for services.

Operations performed in the office tend to be less invasive than those in the hospital operating room, and they do not require prolonged recovery. Thus, patients often infer that the procedure will be flawless, and that no delays or complications can arise. Consequently, even minor discomforts and inconveniences can result in exaggerated patient complaints. Patients need to be specifically prepared for an operation in an office. They have to understand that anesthetics are potent medicines and that side-effects do, indeed, occur. Since it is impossible to consistently perform flawless work, it is mandatory that all of the care providers plan ahead to anticipate complications and problems. What, specifically, will occur if the escort does not arrive on time? Or what if the patient is nauseated when it's time for the office to close? How will the practitioners maintain identical standards of patient care in an office, given that most standards were formulated with a hospital operating room in mind? Unusual outcomes are always just around the corner. The criteria for preoperative screening, intraoperative monitoring, oral intake restrictions, discharge criteria, and the need for an escort must be met for every patient, regardless of the planned anesthetic.

More invasive procedures are being performed in offices on a daily basis. This move is led by the plastic surgeons who offer cosmetic procedures to cash-paying patients, in which case prior approval for payment from the insurance company need not be sought. Other cases that are also leaving the hospital and surgical center at a rapid rate include ophthalmologic procedures and those involving assisted fertilization.[74-76]

Although economic factors cannot be ignored, medical advances are the most significant factors allowing a shift to performing surgery in less intensive settings. Examples of developments include new minimally invasive technology (*e.g.,* laparoscopic and arthroscopic),[79-81] better trained anesthesia providers, improved monitoring devices, short-acting anesthetics, and improved medications for postoperative pain and nausea.[72,74,75,77,78]

Progress in Anesthetic Devices and Monitors

New devices permit improved monitoring and anesthetic care of patients in an office setting. Pulse oximetry noninvasively measures oxygenation and the heart rate.[82-84] It is relatively inexpensive and allows for continuous monitoring. The laryngeal mask airway (LMA) provides a less invasive method for tracheal intubation for airway management.[85,86] Its use has increased over the past few years, in large part because it eliminates the need for laryngoscopy and tracheal intubation. A shortcoming with the LMA is that it cannot reliably protect against the risk of aspiration.[86] Therefore, it is not commonly used in obese patients, patients with pulmonary disease, pregnant patients, or those with a history of symptomatic hiatal hernia. With appropriate patient selection and a well-placed device, positive-pressure ventilation can be used for some surgical procedures. Most practitioners agree that LMAs are most appropriate in spontaneously breathing patients, or with controlled ventilation when the inflating pressures are under 20 cm H_2O. The device has also proved useful when unexpectedly difficult airways are discovered after induction.

Financial incentives for health care providers have completely changed under managed care organization. Under contracts with capped reimbursements, physicians must perform procedures economically in order to remain viable. Often this translates into performing cases in offices, far removed from hospitals and freestanding surgical centers. The availability of sophisticated computer programs and data entry systems has allowed third-party payers to look more closely at surgical outcomes in an attempt to justify the moneys paid to providers. HMO Blue in New Jersey, for example, offers a 15% bonus on certain procedures if they are performed directly within offices instead of hospitals or surgical centers.[76] The financial pressures that surround contemporary health care mandate this shift. The overall emphasis on cost-effectiveness with lower total reimbursements speeds the change.

Many surgeons prefer to work in their own offices because of the lower cost, increased convenience, and improved profit margin. Few would argue with the observation that the physician is better able to perform a simple procedure at minimal cost in his own office. This is particularly true for gynecologic, ophthalmologic, dental, plastic, and urologic procedures. Yet, in the past few years, other more invasive procedures have moved to the offices, including appendectomy, laparoscopic herniorrhaphy, and laparoscopic cholecystectomy. Specific cost comparisons are difficult to perform. The developing science of cost analysis in medicine is able to differentiate direct, indirect, and intangible costs. Attempts are being made to distinguish cost savings from cost shiftings. Several studies have compared the cost savings realized in performing cases in offices as opposed to hospitals and ASCs. One in particular compared the "office costs" with "hospital charges" for identical surgical procedures. For inguinal herniorrhaphy performed conventionally, the comparison is roughly $900 versus $2200. When the same procedure is performed laparoscopically, the comparisons are $1500 to $5500. The cost of an "in-office" laparoscopic cholecystectomy is $1900 versus the hospital charges of $6400. The potential savings to the patient and insurer, as well as increased profits for the surgeon, are large.[87]

Preparation for In-Office Anesthetic Care

Safe care for a patient in an office requires planning. The anesthesiologist is in the best position to understand nuances of office set-up, equipment requirements, and criteria for satisfactory recovery. The anesthesiologist can assume the role of perioperative manager. Anesthesia spans a continuum from minimally to maximally invasive control of consciousness and life-sustaining reflexes (see Fig. 51-1). Appropriate care in some settings allows the patient to breathe room air with no airway manipulation and no depression of reflexes; other cases require major nerve block or general anesthesia with endotracheal intubation. With this range of intervention in mind, several basic issues must be addressed before any anesthetic care is rendered.

Foremost is a clear plan should a medical disaster occur. The surgeon and anesthesiologist must have a plan that allows for an efficient interface between the office and a nearby emergency room. Few situations could cause more harm to the patient, or reflect more poorly on the office, than to have a patient develop a serious complication for which the practitioners have no recourse but to dial 911 and hope for a rapid response. Specific issues of how the patient will be carried from the site of care to the ambulance must be assessed. Will the stretcher fit into the elevator, and can it be negotiated around corners in the hallway? The response time for the local emergency medical service and ambulance should be determined, and the time for transport from the office to the emergency room clocked. Often these communications have political overtones, since work performed within an office reflects the decrease in hospital use. The hospital administration may not want its facility to serve as a safety net for procedures performed outside its walls. Discussions are best focused on the advantages to the particular hospital of providing medical care in an emergency situation. Although the potential for political problems in contract negotiations is daunting, this safety net should be established before the practitioner offers care.[88]

The office must be properly equipped. Even if the plan of intervention calls only for mild sedation for podiatric services under local blockade, certain devices must be present and readily available.[88–92] These include a reliable source of oxygen, motor-driven suction, capabilities for providing positive-pressure ventilation, and emergency airway management equipment—oral and nasal airways, a laryngoscope, and endotracheal tubes. Basic medications include sedatives, hypnotics, and opioids, as well as medications required to initiate and continue cardiac life support. Portable defibrillators are now readily available and reasonably priced. These devices and medications will be life-saving while waiting for an emergency response from the community should a medical disaster occur. Essential monitoring equipment for the least invasive cases includes a blood pressure device, pulse oximetry, and an electrocardiograph. The facility should have a backup power supply should a power failure occur during a procedure.

Patient selection is clearly an important factor for surgery performed in the office. It is always tempting to care for additional patients—patients who almost, but not quite, meet the criteria. This mirrors the evolution in care provided in ambulatory surgery centers in the 1980s. Surgical practices that initially accepted only ASA I and II patients began to care for the occasional ASA III patient. This occurred gradually as the staff became more familiar with the routines. Few data are available to assess outcomes in individual offices. Practitioners and organizations are just now looking at the care delivered. Answers to basic questions concerning quality of care in the office, as opposed to the hospital or surgical center, will be forthcoming as data are gathered and analyzed. This information will eventually determine the most desirable and cost-efficient site. For the present, most providers do not offer office anesthesia to patients whose coexisting medical conditions are likely to cause problems. No one needs the personal stress (patient, physicians), medical liability, or scheduling disruptions that follow a delay or a bad outcome. Frequent types of patients who are poor candidates for office surgery are those who have had recent cardiovascular events, are obese, or suffer medical conditions that would interfere with a rapid recovery.

Preoperative Testing

The first step in any anesthetic is the preoperative assessment. Its goal is to reduce the morbidity of surgery. When the assessment is performed in a preoperative screening clinic by an anesthesiologist, as opposed to a surgeon, requests for medical consultations are reduced by 75%.[92,93] Cancellations of procedures because of unresolved medical problems are reduced by 80%, and the cost of laboratory tests are reduced by 55%, or approximately $110 per patient. The advantages arise from having the anesthesiologist obtain the history and make decisions for further evaluation of the particular patient. This contrasts with the older practice of ordering batteries of blood tests for multiphasic screening.[92,93] The process seemed logical at the time because of the ease and relatively low cost of performing the tests. However, it is now known that routine screening tests are unnecessary and very costly. Most patients, unless they have significant comorbidity, do not require any laboratory tests prior to office surgery. A history and physical examination are the most efficient ways to determine if a patient has a disease that places them at increased risk for anesthesia.[94] Tests should be performed only if called for by the patient's medical condition.[92,93,95]

Anesthesia in the Office

The gradations in anesthesia care from conscious sedation to general anesthesia have been described above. The definitions are fluid because the depth of sedation and anesthesia changes over time depending on the degree of stimulation. Loosely defined, "conscious" sedation is a state of medically induced and controlled depression of consciousness in which the patient is able to maintain a patent airway and make appropriate responses to verbal commands. "Deep" sedation begins when the patient may not be able to maintain the airway independently and is unable to respond appropriately to physical stimulation or a verbal command.[91] Any drug used for conscious sedation can also cause deep sedation when given in excess or the level of stimulation falls. This change can, in turn, lead to hypoventilation, hypoxia, and cardiopulmonary collapse.

Routine Workloads

Unlike the work performed in hospitals and surgical centers, many of the procedures done in offices are highly routine. It is quite common for the same kind of anesthesia for the same surgical intervention to be performed over and over again. This is particularly true at office sites staffed by a few surgeons who work in one field only. For example, in an ophthalmology practice routine cataract extractions are performed sequentially. There is little or no variation in the practice from case to case. All health care professionals who work in the office know the routines of each of the other practitioners. The goal is to work quickly, efficiently, and safely. All efforts are focused on getting the patient in and out with no complication. If the nursing personnel who clean the instruments are delayed, the physicians may help clean and prepare the room. The offices encourage a team approach. Practitioners who work exclusively with ophthalmologists providing monitored anesthesia care (MAC) for eye operations develop techniques to maximize efficiency, cost savings, and patient safety. These attitudes permit the efficient use of newer medications that would otherwise be too expensive to allow for profitability.

The following, for example, is a cost-effective technique to provide sedation for cataract patients. A 1-mg vial of remifentanil is diluted in a 100-ml bag of saline. Ten different 10-ml syringes of the diluted remifentanil are drawn up at a concentration of $10 \ \mu g \cdot ml^{-1}$. Each cataract patient has a dose calculated at 0.5, 0.75, or $1.0 \ \mu g \cdot kg^{-1}$: the very elderly and frail receive $0.5 \ \mu g \cdot kg^{-1}$, the typical patient receives $0.75 \ \mu g \cdot kg^{-1}$, and the younger, healthier patient receives a full $1.0 \ \mu g \cdot kg^{-1}$. Nasal cannula are applied and the flow is set to 10 l $O_2 \cdot min^{-1}$ for 1 minute prior to a retrobulbar block. The injection of remifentanil is given over 15 seconds; then 90 seconds elapse before the surgeon performs the block. Patients have excellent anesthesia and amnesia for the block.[96]

The first two patients for the day are seen in a recovery area adjacent to the operating room, and the first two remifentanil injections and eye blocks are performed sequentially. When the first patient is taken to the recovery area at the conclusion of the first operation, the remifentanil injection and eye block are then administered to the third patient. This sequence continues throughout the workday. Occasionally, there is a transient decrease in the oxygen saturation, but it is rare. Within a few moments, the patient responds to verbal commands and takes deep breaths. Since only one vial is used for 10 cases each day, the cost for the agent is very low. Since patients recover from the effects of remifentanil before the surgery is completed, they are discharged home almost immediately after the procedure.[96]

Costs of Anesthesia Equipment and Supplies

It is possible to deliver a quality anesthetic to a patient in an office setting at a reasonable cost. There is a large range of fees charged in the office, and a savvy practitioner with an eye toward the bottom line can safely economize on many costs.[96,97] The following supplies are typically consumed for an office anesthetic: alcohol wipes, cloth tape, intravenous catheter, tubing, stopcock, a bag of crystalloid, midazolam, propofol, and a short-acting opioid (remifentanil or alfentanil). Rough costs when dealing with a discount supplier can be less than $50. If the oxygen and/or other gases for the office must be provided, these costs must be included. If the patient is at high risk for postoperative nausea (previous experience, history of motion sickness, or in the higher-risk phase of the menstrual cycle), a preemptive antiemetic may be given, further increasing costs.

In an office limited exclusively to performing cosmetic procedures, the estimated costs can be even further reduced.[97,98] Propofol and ketamine mixtures can be effectively infused and bolused during cosmetic surgery. The procedures performed may reflect the whole spectrum of cosmetic surgery, including face and brow lifts, blepharoplasty, rhinoplasty, otoplasty, facial resurfacing, fat transfer, breast augmentation, abdominoplasty, and liposuction. Despite the variety of surgical procedures, the anesthesia can be limited to the administration of midazolam, propofol, ketamine, and glycopyrrolate . . . exclusively.[98-100] Patients are sedated but awake enough to breathe room air spontaneously. No supplemental oxygen is provided. The approach is to infuse propofol continuously and then bolus ketamine to produce a dissociative state immediately prior to the injection of local anesthetic by the surgeon. The propofol/ketamine technique is a form of monitored anesthesia care (MAC) that is most properly called dissociative anesthesia, not total intravenous anesthesia (TIVA).

As the demand for office anesthesia grows, ketamine is enjoying a resurgence.[99,100] Ketamine differs from opioids in that it permits spontaneous ventilation. The agent enhances laryngeal reflexes (as opposed to the depression seen with opioids), making aspiration unlikely. It is not associated with postoperative nausea and vomiting. Ketamine hallucinations, as administered by the above protocol, are rarely seen.[99,100] A possible reason is that the ketamine is given only after midazolam is administered, and all doses of ketamine are nested within the propofol infusion. Patients are awake, with a mild euphoria. In a series of 1200 cases, only two instances of intraoperative emesis occurred, neither with aspiration. SpO_2 levels remained above 90% throughout all cases.[99,100] Patients emerged without harm, and there were no hospital admissions for nausea or pain. The majority of patients were discharged by the end of the first postoperative hour. Although some patients underwent 9-hour procedures and required 2 hours of observation before discharge, none required supplemental oxygen or support of the airway to maintain $SpO_2 > 95\%$.[99] In a 5-year review of 1264 cases at this site, the costs of the supplies and medications were approximately $40 per hour of MAC.[97] The anesthetic technique provides an appropriate depth of sedation, yet it allows the patient to breathe air spontaneously. The monitoring equipment in the office is compact, portable, and battery-operated. Resuscitative equipment and medication are stored in the surgeon's office and maintained by the staff.

Regulations for Office-Based Procedures

There is a large body of information regarding ambulatory surgery centers; however, not very much of this can be directly applied to patient care in an office. The problem is the inherent differences between the sites. Surgery centers have several different surgeons performing disparate operations. The center must be accredited by a variety of agencies, not the least of which is the state that issues a Certificate of Need for the construction and use of the facility. Because of the strict regulations concerning usage, all centers are relatively similar in their organization and physical structure.[101] Offices, on the other hand, run the gamut. A single site of anesthesia care within an office is currently unregulated in 47 states—all but California, Florida, and New Jersey. The range of facilities is quite broad; some are well equipped suites that mirror the operating rooms in hospitals. Others are small areas off to the side of an examining room. More importantly, the scope of the practice in an office is usually quite limited: one or two practitioners doing the same kinds of procedures repetitively. Consequently, not much of the data collected by those who work in the surgery centers can be extrapolated to the office.

There are, of course, some similarities between centers and offices; several of the basic concerns and issues overlap. Both require that a patient arrive at a site of surgical care, receive treatment, then leave to return home. Both have benefited from the advances in the fields of surgery and anesthesia. And both provide a continuum of anesthesia care to different patients. Newer induction agents, inhalational anesthetics, muscle relaxants, and opioids have allowed for specific tailoring of the anesthetic to the desired results.[72,77] The medications allow for a more rapid onset and offset of action, such that less time is required for clearance of the drug and dissipation of the effect.

The Scope of Care Provided in the Office

MAC

Monitored anesthesia care (MAC) has evolved over the past several years as new drugs have become available, older drugs are used in a more tailored fashion, and patient acceptance has increased.[102] A common practice is to combine a regional or local block with the intravenous infusion of medications to alleviate anxiety and prevent pain from the needle insertion. The combination of local anesthetics with MAC is particularly well suited for the office; many surgical procedures are performed this way. To some, the term MAC implies that the degree of vigilance is lower because fewer changes are produced by the medications than during a general anesthetic. This is not true. A patient can quickly move from a minimally depressed state of consciousness to deep sedation and general anesthesia when significant doses of depressant drugs have been administered and/or the degree of surgical stimulation is decreased. All patients who receive MAC should be monitored by a designated individual who is primarily responsible for the administration of the sedative and analgesic drugs, as well as monitoring of the patient's vital signs. The same standards of anesthetic care should be provided during MAC as are required for general or regional anesthesia.

A wide range of agents has been recommended for MAC, most with iv administration. Nitrous oxide has been used in the past, and many argue that low-dose sevoflurane may provide similar advantages in this setting. An activated charcoal filter is available to scavenge inhalation agents and minimize contamination of the office. Useful iv agents include benzodiazepines, ketamine, barbiturates, propofol, and opioids. Midazolam is particularly well suited for the office because it has an amnestic effect, and a short duration of action with a half-life of approximately 100 minutes. It is associated with less pain on injection than is diazepam, it is easy to administer, and its effects can be reversed with flumazenil $0.1 \text{ mg} \cdot \text{kg}^{-1}$. Sedation causes mild depression of the hypoxic ventilatory response, and severe respiratory depression can occur if the agent is combined with opioids. When contrasted with comparable doses of diazepam, midazolam provides more profound amnesia, sedation, and anxiolysis.[102,103]

Fentanyl is a synthetic opioid that is approximately 100 times stronger than morphine.[104] It has a rapid onset and a duration of action of only 30–45 minutes. This combination makes it ideal for short or painful procedures. Unfortunately, its respiratory depressant effect is longer than its analgesic effect. Doses of $0.5–1 \ \mu g \cdot \text{kg}^{-1}$ are slowly titrated to effect. Respiratory depression is more pronounced when the agent is combined with a sedative. For procedures performed under regional anesthesia, a stable level of sedation can be attained by the use of a small dose of midazolam (1–2 mg) followed by an infusion of propofol $25–100 \ \mu g \cdot \text{kg}^{-1} \cdot \text{min}^{-1}$. This can generally be supplemented with boluses of fentanyl (25 μg) or ketamine (5 mg) as needed. Careful titration of the agents is key to avoid respiratory depression or loss of airway reflexes.[102]

Local Anesthetics and Regional Techniques

When applicable, the use of local or regional anesthesia in an office is almost always preferable to the use of a general anesthetic.[105,106] Issues of airway trauma, bronchospasm, aspiration, prolonged sedation, paralysis, malignant hyperthermia, nausea, and vomiting are either bypassed or greatly reduced. Regional anesthesia offers fewer chances for drug interactions, cardiac or respiratory depression, or airway problems. It results in shorter time intervals to the intake of fluids, the ability to void, and to ambulate. At the end of the case, regional techniques allow for a reduced intensity of postoperative care, fewer side-effects, and, in some circumstances, a decreased recovery time. Often, they also provide excellent short-term pain control.

Regional anesthesia is the standard of care in an office devoted exclusively to patients for orthopedic procedures. In this setting, the techniques are particularly appropriate for the facility, surgeon, and patients. Those who provide the blocks are secure that the techniques will be successful a high percentage of the time. Performing a regional anesthetic can be a stress for the provider. A less than perfect block can be a public embarrassment that is evident to the surgeon, patient, and nurses. Because of this potential, it is important that the anesthesiologist maximize chances for success. It must be remembered that blocks take time to perform properly. Regional anesthesia is almost always most successful when it is the norm for the facility. Those involved with the care of the patient know that the time spent at the beginning of the case avoids delays in discharge that can follow general anesthesia. When all works well, regional techniques can allow the patient to bypass the first phase of recovery entirely, thereby decreasing the time to discharge. This is particularly evident when using intravenous regional, popliteal, brachial plexus, and retrobulbar blocks.[106] Central neuraxial blocks, such as spinal or epidural, tend to be long-acting and are generally not useful for rapid-turnover office procedures.

Skillfully managed regional techniques are valuable because they allow more patients to be discharged home uneventfully. Data collected from surgery centers indicate that persistent nausea, vomiting, or pain caused approximately 40% of the unanticipated hospital admissions. The rate following general anesthesia was 2.9%; after regional, the rate was less than half

that number, at 1.2%.[107] Although the local anesthetics have a good record of clinical safety, 5% lidocaine in a hyperbaric dextrose solution has been implicated as causing a painful radicular sensation lasting for one or two days. The phenomenon has been labeled *transient radicular irritation*s (TRI).[108,109] TRI has not been associated with intrathecal bupivacaine. Surgical positioning, especially use of dorsolithotomy, is thought to contribute to the radicular pain. It is not clear why these complaints are appearing now after decades of intrathecal lidocaine use.

Lower extremity procedures can be easily performed with spinal or epidural blockade. In general, a spinal is easier to perform, has a more definite endpoint, and provides a faster onset with a denser block. Additionally, a smaller dose of anesthetic is used, and patients report fewer backaches (11% vs. 30%).[106,110] The problem with the routine use of spinal blockade is the possibility for post–dural puncture headache, especially in younger patients. The risk can be lowered with the use of small-gauge needles (*e.g.,* 25 gauge) with pencil-point tips or attention to the orientation of the bevel on insertion.

Cost Savings with Regional Techniques. Data from nonhospital surgery centers indicate that regional anesthesia may offer savings when compared to general anesthesia.[105–107] Appropriately selected and managed regional anesthesia is usually associated with a reduced intraoperative time, a decreased need for intense postoperative care, fewer side-effects, shorter recovery times, and diminished postoperative pain. The use of regional techniques allows for persistence of postoperative analgesia and diminished needs for narcotics.[111]

Are there potential disadvantages to the use of regional techniques? Yes. Some of them include systemic toxicity from the local anesthetic, PDPH, allergy to the anesthetic, pneumothorax, low back pain, nerve injury, and hematoma formation. However, the techniques are region-specific and economical. General anesthesia must always be available as a backup to a regional technique.

General Anesthesia

Propofol is widely used for induction and maintenance of general anesthesia in the office setting.[112,113] Before propofol's introduction, thiopental was the drug of choice for induction. Thiopental, noted for its ease of administration and rapid onset, has a reasonably short period of hypnotic activity, but accumulates with repeated doses and is not appropriate for continuous infusions. It is associated with prolonged drowsiness and an increased incidence of nausea and vomiting upon emergence. Propofol, on the other hand, produces unconsciousness for a very short duration, does not accumulate, and is suitable for continuous infusions. Experience has shown that at infusion rates of $2.5–5.5 \text{ mg} \cdot \text{kg}^{-1} \cdot \text{hr}^{-1}$, patients undergoing leg surgery under spinal anesthesia were sedated/asleep but arousable with verbal commands.[102] These patients were completely awake a few minutes after the propofol infusion was stopped. A low-dose infusion of propofol allows patient comfort for the performance of a nerve block or regional anesthetic, and the infusion allows sedation throughout the procedure. Propofol sedation will control restlessness and anxiety during noninvasive procedures such as MRI and radiation therapy. Its antiemetic properties and short recovery times are additional benefits. Because it is supplied in a lipid vehicle that supports microbial growth, the contents of an ampule must be used within 6 hours of opening, and syringes or infusions of propofol must be for single-patient use only.

Nitrous oxide is used in hospitals and surgery centers to supplement more potent volatile agents. Its use in office settings is less common because of the expense of delivering tanks to the facility, its low potency, and its tendency to cause nausea and vomiting.[114] Isoflurane is the most commonly used inhalation agent in adults,[72] but it is relatively long-acting compared to the newer inhaled anesthetics. Desflurane, an anesthetic with low blood solubility and short action, has not gained general acceptance because it is expensive, it requires a special vaporizer for administration, and it is pungent. The odor makes it difficult to use for inhalational inductions.

Sevoflurane, a newer fluorinated anesthetic with minimal apparent toxicity,[72] is particularly well suited to office use because of its pleasant odor and rapid action. A theoretical concern is the development of vinyl ether, or compound A, when the agent is in prolonged contact with soda lime. Compound A has been implicated as causing renal tubular necrosis in laboratory animals given large doses. The potential for harm has generated dozens of papers and talks, yet no damage has been reported in patients despite extensive use of the agent in over 45 countries. The metabolism of sevoflurane results in measurable blood levels of free fluoride. Isosthenuric renal failure is another theoretical concern that has never been reported. Because sevoflurane has a pleasant odor and is easily inhaled, it is an excellent alternative to halothane for both children and adults. Patients rapidly emerge when the agent is discontinued. Effective methods for scavenging this agent in an office setting are being developed and refined.

Muscle relaxants are essential for certain types of operations. They abolish motor reflexes, ease the control of ventilation, and provide for immediate airway management. Both depolarizing drugs (succinylcholine) and nondepolarizing relaxants (mivacurium, vecuronium, atracurium, cisatracurium) are used in offices. Succinylcholine reliably and reproducibly causes complete muscle relaxation, but complications from routine use include myalgias and transient increases in intragastric and intraocular pressures. The most useful nondepolarizing relaxants are those with a short, predictable duration of action. Mivacurium has a favorable overall profile and is rapidly hydrolyzed by plasma cholinesterase. A typical intubating dose will provide onset within 2–3 minutes and 20 minutes of relaxation. Histamine release mandates a slow injection of the drug. For longer procedures, vecuronium and cisatracurium are logical choices, although they are more expensive than traditional nondepolarizing relaxants such as pancuronium. Succinylcholine, as well as all of the volatile inhalational agents, can trigger malignant hyperthermia (MH). Office-based physicians should have dantrolene immediately available. Should MH develop, treatment with dantrolene should be initiated before the patient is transported to an emergency room.

Potent, synthetic opioids have been developed that are many times stronger than morphine. These agents can be used to blunt the sympathetic response to laryngoscopy and intubation, and they can provide intense analgesia in the perioperative period. Opioids must be titrated because of their ability to cause profound hypoventilation and skeletal muscle rigidity. They can be used as the exclusive supplement to local anesthetics; however, they do not reliably cause sedation unless given in doses that can cause respiratory depression.[102] Alfentanil has a very low pK_a, which allows for more bioavailability at physiologic pH. The onset of action is rapid, and the duration is brief. Sufentanil is more lipid-soluble and tends to produce more depression of the sensorium than do the other synthetic opioids. Fentanyl has continued to be widely used. Doses of 50–100 μg iv have an onset time of 3–5 minutes and a duration of effect of 45–60 minutes. Even very small doses can cause respiratory depression when combined with a sedative. The latest synthetic opioid, remifentanil, is so short-acting that it has minimal application as an adjunct for general anesthesia. Patients have little postoperative analgesia. On the other hand, remifentanil can be effective when profound analgesia is required for a very brief period, such as during injection of local anesthetic.

Postoperative Analgesia

A major criterion for the performance of a procedure in an office setting is the ability to control the postoperative pain. Severe pain is a common reason for delayed discharge and for unanticipated hospital admission after ambulatory surgery.[78,115]

A large study examined consecutive ambulatory surgical patients. Nerve blocks and nonsteroidal anti-inflammatory agents (NSAIDs) were not routinely used as a part of the technique. Most patients received either general anesthesia or MAC. The patients were assessed for pain in the PACU, ambulatory surgical unit, and 24 hours postoperatively. Younger male adults and patients with a higher body mass index (BMI) had a higher incidence of severe pain. Those patients undergoing orthopedic procedures on the shoulder experienced the greatest incidence of severe postoperative pain. The group with severe pain had a longer stay in the PACU and in the surgical facility than did those in the group without severe pain.[78]

NSAIDs have become popular for perioperative analgesia. They avoid many of the side-effects caused by opioids, particularly respiratory depression. Ketorolac is a parenterally active NSAID that can be used as the sole analgesic supplement to local anesthetic, or as an adjunct to a propofol infusion. Use of iv ketorolac as compared to fentanyl is associated with a decreased incidence of nausea, vomiting, and pruritis. Ketorolac provides dense analgesia even following invasive procedures such as arthroscopy and laparoscopy. Ketoralac, like other NSAIDs, inhibits platelet function and, in large or repeated doses, has the potential to cause renal dysfunction or gastric bleeding.[102]

Postoperative Nausea

Although data on office-based outcomes are not yet available, experience in freestanding surgery centers indicate that postoperative nausea and vomiting (PONV) accounts for the majority of unanticipated admissions to the hospital. The incidence of these complications is highest with fentanyl-based anesthetics. The incidence is lower when propofol is used in place of thiopental. Several agents are available to prevent or decrease the incidence of PONV. These include promethazine, atropine, and droperidol. Ondansetron and granisetron are very effective in controlling postoperative nausea, although they are relatively costly. The additional cost is, however, easily justified if it prevents an unplanned hospital admission.

Discharge Criteria

There is now a move toward "criteria-based" recovery standards. These criteria will eliminate any mandatory time patients must spend in a recovery area. An essential aspect of care in the office is the timing for discharge home. At discharge, the patient should be clinically stable, ready to ambulate, and able to tolerate oral intake. Discharge from the facility should be to the care of a responsible adult. A post-anesthetic discharge scoring system (PADSS) has been developed that is based on five criteria: vital signs, activity and mental status, pain and nausea, surgical bleeding, and intake and output. Each of the items is graded from 0 to 2 such that a summed score of 9 or 10 indicates fitness for discharge from the office (Table 51-5). A major advantage to the use of the PADSS, as opposed to conventional criteria, is that it replaces the subjective clinical impressions with objective indicators. It indicates fitness for discharge home.[116]

Comparisons of Outcomes

Few data on specific practices and outcomes exist for office-based anesthesia. The practitioners have been too scattered and the field too ill-defined for information to have been collected. The establishment of standards is desirable for the patient, payer, and the provider. If standards are agreed upon and met, a bad clinical outcome is more likely to be seen as a complication of care as opposed to malpractice. Several guidelines already exist for the provision of anesthesia in settings outside of the traditional operating room. They address the use of sedation by nonanesthesiologists and discuss the necessary skills, supplies, and monitors that must be available. Recommendations

Table 51-5. A POST-ANESTHESIA DISCHARGE SCORING SYSTEM

Post-Anesthesia Discharge Scoring System (PADSS)	Clinical Discharge Criteria (CDC)

1. Vital signs
  2 = within 20% of preoperative value
  1 = 20–40% of preoperative value
  0 = >40% of preoperative value
2. Activity and mental status
  2 = oriented ×3 AND has a steady gait
  1 = oriented ×3 OR has a steady gait
  0 = neither
3. Pain, nausea, and/or vomiting
  2 = minimal
  1 = moderate, having required treatment
  0 = severe, requiring treatment
4. Surgical bleeding
  2 = minimal
  1 = moderate
  0 = severe
5. Intake and output
  2 = has had po fluids AND has voided
  1 = has had po fluids OR has voided
  0 = neither
	1. Stable vital signs
	2. Patient is alert and oriented
	3. Patient is free of nausea and/or vomiting
	4. Steady of gait
	5. Patient has no significant bleeding

From Chung F, Chan V, Ong D: A post-anesthetic discharge scoring system for home readiness after ambulatory surgery. J Clin Anesth 7:501, 1995.

have been published by the American Society of Anesthesiologists (1996), American Dental Society, American College of Surgeons (1994), American Academy of Pediatrics (1992), Sedation Guidelines–Pediatric Dentistry (1993), and others.[1,2,4–6,89]

If we examine these guidelines, we see a pattern. They match the level of care and sophistication of monitoring to the intensity of anesthesia intervention that is needed. This continuum ranges from conscious sedation through major nerve blockade to general anesthesia. Many states have introduced legislation to regulate the anesthesia care that is provided in an office. These laws aim to address wide variations in care that are found from site to site. Specific concerns include licensing issues, transfer agreements, medical record keeping, quality assurance and quality improvement, peer review of the medical practice, credentialing of practitioners, and documentation of outcomes.[117] The focus is on certification of the facility, not the practitioners. Some office settings "may be operating in a manner which is injurious to the public health, welfare, and safety," even though the professionals delivering health care services in those settings are licensed and qualified.[117] In California, the intent of the law was to create regulations that impact safety; it was not intended to require standards in excess of those requirements or to require physical modification of facilities unless the modifications or standards directly affect safety and are cost-effective.[117] Undoubtedly, new laws affecting office-based surgery will continue to evolve.[118]

The office-based surgery arena is dynamic, evolving as the country adapts to a new model of medical care delivery. Radically different trends will emerge to enhance cost-effective and safe care of patients in new and different settings. The guidelines presented by the American College of Surgeons in 1994 and reflected by Florida state legislation may emerge as universal standards. They focus on quality of care as a primary goal and follow the model of classifying surgical procedures according to the intensity of anesthesia care required. In brief, all surgical procedures are stratified into three classes according to the intensity of anesthesia care that is required.[89,119]

Class A office surgery permits topical or local agents or both, but no drug-induced alterations of consciousness other than minimal preoperative tranquilization of the patient. No assistance from any personnel other than the operator is required. Basic life support (BLS) certification is recommended but not mandatory. Required equipment and supplies include oxygen,

a positive-pressure ventilation device, epinephrine, corticosteroids, antihistamines, and atropine.

Class B office surgery encompasses those cases in which perioperative medication and sedation are required. Examples include herniorrhaphy, hemorrhoidectomy, breast biopsy, and colonoscopy. A transfer agreement between the operating physician and a local hospital is mandatory if the physician does not have privileges to perform the same procedure in the hospital. The hospital must be within a "reasonable distance" from the office, although the number of miles is not specified. Anesthetic care is limited to local injection or peripheral nerve block, including intravenous regional anesthesia (Bier block). Intravenous or intramuscular sedation is permitted. Vital reflexes are to be monitored and maintained at all times during and immediately after the procedure. The surgeon must have at least one assistant and both must be certified in BLS. It is recommended that at least one have advanced cardiac life support (ACLS) certification. In some specific situations, additional assistance may be required. Equipment and supplies include a full and current "crash cart," a defibrillator, and resuscitative medications.

Class C office surgery permits the use of preoperative sedation and general anesthesia or major nerve block. The physician must have staff privileges to perform the same procedures as are performed in the office setting at a licensed hospital within reasonable proximity. The surgeon and at least one assistant must be certified in BLS. It is recommended that at least one member of the team be certified in ACLS as well. Emergency procedures to be performed in response to serious complications should be formulated, written, periodically reviewed, practiced, updated, and posted in conspicuous locations. Equipment, medication, and post-anesthesia recovery must be available, with qualified nursing personnel. The facility, in terms of general preparation, equipment and supplies, must be comparable to a freestanding ambulatory surgical center. Equipment for patient monitoring, an operating table capable of rotation to the Trendelenburg position, and proper record keeping are also specifically mentioned.

Future Trends

Bolder use of the office setting is inevitable. Patient demand and obvious economic incentives will move more cases to this site. More invasive and prolonged procedures will be performed. Surgeons and anesthesia providers have already tested the limits by undertaking extensive and prolonged cosmetic procedures. A 1997 U.S. Supreme Court case, *Abbott v. Bradgon*,[120] concerned an HIV-positive patient who sued a dentist who refuses to treat her in the office, despite a lack of symptoms or signs of AIDS. The dentist was concerned about the appropriateness of care and insisted that the patient check into, and pay for, a hospital stay. The advantages of an office setting, as opposed to a hospital, were developed as a part of the arguments heard. Inherent to the case is the cost savings and convenience of care in a less intensive arena. This was tested as a right.

SUMMARY

Anesthesia provided at alternative sites is economical, safe, and popular. Proper attention must be paid to the physical site, the abilities of the provider, and the patient before any case is undertaken. Backup plans have to be in place to anticipate a misadventure. For the anesthetic itself, overall experiences indicate that the least amount of anesthetic that can be used is the best dose. Local and monitored anesthesia care are preferable to regional techniques. Regional techniques are preferable to general anesthesia. The number of anesthetics provided outside of conventional operating rooms is growing rapidly. More anesthesiologists are working in these settings. Advances in surgical techniques and the development of newer anesthetic agents have made the provision of care in an office both possible and practical. The cost savings of bypassing the hospitals and dedicated surgery centers are large. Operative care in the individual office is more convenient for the patient and economically advantageous for all involved. Patients will increasingly want the services a well-trained anesthesiologist who is adept at providing care at sites far removed from hospital operating rooms.

REFERENCES

1. American Society of Anesthesiologists: Guidelines for nonoperating room anesthetizing locations. ASA Directory of Members, p 476. Park Ridge, Illinois, 1999
2. Committee on Drugs, Section on Anesthesiology: Guidelines for the elective use of conscious sedation, deep sedation, and general anesthesia in pediatric patients. Pediatrics 76:317, 1985
3. Greenberg DJ, Romanoff ME: Anesthesia outside the operating room. In Romanoff ME, Miranda JV (eds): Problems in Anesthesia: Anesthesia in Remote Locations, Part 1, p 299. Philadelphia, JB Lippincott, 1992
4. Rosenberg MB, Campbell RL: Guidelines for intraoperative monitoring of dental patients undergoing conscious sedation, deep sedation and general anesthesia. Oral Surg Oral Med Oral Pathol 71:2, 1991
5. American Society for Gastrointestinal Endoscopy: Monitoring the patients undergoing gastrointestinal endoscopic procedures. Gastrointest Endosc 37:120, 1991
6. Joint Commission on Accreditation of Healthcare Organizations: Accreditation Manual for Hospitals, p 269. Oakbrook Terrace, Illinois, 1991
7. Gross JB, Epstein BS: ASA task force on analgesia and sedation by non-anesthesiologists. American Society of Anesthesiologists Newsletter 58:22, 1994
8. American Society of Anesthesiologists: Standards for basic anesthesia monitoring. ASA Directory of Members, p 462. Park Ridge, Illinois, 1999
9. Goldberg M: Systemic reactions to intravascular contrast media. Anesthesiology 60:45, 1984
10. Caro JJ, Trindale E, McGregor M: The risks of death and of severe non-fatal reactions with high versus low osmolality contrast media. Am J Radiol 159:869, 1991
11. Steinberg EP, Moore RD, Powe NR et al: Safety and cost effectiveness of high osmolality as compared to low osmolality contrast material in patients undergoing cardiac angiography. N Engl J Med 326:425, 1992
12. Shehadi W: Adverse reactions to intravascularly administered contrast media. Am J Radiol 124:145, 1975
13. Anto H, Chon S, Porush J et al: Infusion intravenous pyelography and renal function: Effects of hypertonic mannitol in patients with chronic renal insufficiency. Arch Intern Med 141:1652, 1981
14. Greenberger P, Patterson R, Kelly J et al: Administration of radiographic contrast media in high risk patients. Invest Radiol 15:540, 1980
15. Young WL, Pile-Spellman J: Interventional neuroradiology. In Albin MS (ed): Textbook of Neuroanesthesia, p 807. McGraw-Hill, 1997
16. Young WL, Pile-Spellman J: Anesthetic considerations for interventional neuroradiology. Anesthesiology 80:427, 1994
17. Davies D: Subspecialty monitoring techniques—miscellaneous. In Gravenstein N (ed): Problems in Anesthesia Monitoring, p 138. Philadelphia, JB Lippincott, 1987
18. Carmichael J, Henshaw E: Radiation hazards of diagnostic radiology. In Ansell GE, Wilkins RA (eds): Complications in Diagnostic Imaging, p 457. Oxford, Blackwell Scientific Publications, 1987
19. Wolfson B, Hetrick W: Anesthesia for neuroradiologic procedures. In Cottrell JE, Turndorf H (eds): Anesthesia and Neurosurgery, p 104. St Louis, CV Mosby, 1986
20. Earnest F, Forbes G, Samdok D et al: Complications of cerebral angiography. Am J Radiol 142:247, 1984
21. Dion J, Gates P, Fox A et al: Clinical events following neuroangiography. Stroke 18:997, 1987
22. Weston G, Strunin L, Amundson G: Imagery for anesthetists: A review of the methods and anaesthetic implications of diagnostic imagery techniques. Can Anaesth Soc J 32:552, 1985
23. Forestner J: Anesthesia for radiologic procedures. In Murphy C, Murphy M (eds): Radiology for Anesthesia and Critical Care, p 239. New York, Churchill Livingstone, 1987
24. Patteson SK, Chesney JT: Anesthetic management for magnetic resonance imaging: Problems and solutions. Anesth Analg 74:121, 1992
25. Jorgensen NH, Messick JM Jr, Gray J et al: ASA monitoring standards and magnetic resonance imaging. Anesth Analg 79:1141, 1994
26. Bydder GM: Magnetic resonance imagery of the brain. Radiol Clin North Am 22:779, 1984
27. Davis P, Crooks L, Arakawa M et al: Potential hazard in NMR. Am J Radiol 137:857, 1981
28. Roth J, Nugent M, Gray J et al: Patient monitoring during magnetic resonance imaging. Anesthesiology 62:80, 1985
29. Pavlicek W, Geisiuiger M, Castle L et al: The effects of nuclear magnetic resonance on patients with cardiac pacemakers. Radiology 147:149, 1983
30. Fetter J, Aram G, Holmes D et al: Nuclear magnetic resonance imagery of external and implantable cardiac pacemakers. Chest 84:345, 1983
31. Osbakken M, Griffith J, Taczanowsky P: A gross morphologic, histologic, and blood chemistry study of adult and neonatal mice chronically exposed to high magnetic fields. Magn Reson Med 3:502, 1986
32. Melendez JC, McCrank E: Anxiety-related reactions associated with magnetic resonance imaging examinations. JAMA 270:745, 1993
33. Shellock FG, Slimp GL: Severe burn of the finger caused by using a pulse oximeter during MR imaging. Am J Radiol 153:1105, 1989
34. Bashein G, Russell A, Momil S: Anesthesia and remote monitoring for intraoperative radiation therapy. Anesthesiology 64:805, 1986
35. Steward D: Cardiac surgery and cardiologic procedures. In Steward D (ed): Manual of Pediatric Anesthesia, 2nd ed, p 213. New York, Churchill Livingstone, 1985
36. DeBruijn N, Hlatky M, Jacobs JR et al: General anesthesia during percutaneous transluminary coronary angioplasty for acute myocardial infarction. Anesth Analg 68:201, 1989
37. Gale DW, Grissom TE, Mirenda JV: Titration of intravenous anesthetics for cardioversion: A comparison of propofol, methohexital, and midazolam. Crit Care Med 21:1509, 1993
38. Hullander RM, Leivers D, Wingler K: A comparison of propofol and etomidate for cardioversion. Anesth Analg 77:690, 1993
39. Sternlo JE, Hagerdal M: Anaesthesia for cardioversion: Clinical experiences with propofol and thiopentone. Acta Anaesthesiol Scand 35:606, 1991
40. Ford SR, Maze M, Gaba DM: A comparison of etomidate and thiopental anesthesia for cardioversion. J Cardiothorac Vasc Anesth 5:563, 1991
41. Canessa R, Lema G, Urz'ua J et al: Anesthesia for elective cardiover-

sion: A comparison of four anesthetic agents. J Cardiothorac Vasc Anesth 5:566, 1991

42. Gupta A, Lennmarken C, Vegfors M et al: Anaesthesia for cardioversion: A comparison between propofol, thiopentone and midazolam. Anaesthesia 45:872, 1990

43. Fennelly ME, Powell H, Galletly DC et al: Midazolam sedation reversed with flumazenil for cardioversion. Br J Anaesth 68:303, 1992

44. Irani WN, Grayburn PA, Afridi I: Prevalence of thrombus, spontaneous echo contrast, and atrial stunning in patients undergoing cardioversion of atrial flutter. A prospective study using transesophageal echocardiography. Circulation 95(4):962, 1997

45. Gaines GY III, Rees DI: Anesthetic considerations for electroconvulsive therapy. South Med J 85:469, 1992

46. Ellis JS: Anesthesia for electroconvulsive therapy. In Romanoff ME, Mirenda JV (eds): Problems in Anesthesia: Anesthesia for Remote Locations, Part 1, p 381. Philadelphia, JB Lippincott, 1992

47. American Psychiatric Association: Diagnostic and Statistical Manual of Mental Disorders: DSMIII-R, 3rd ed. Washington, DC, American Psychiatric Association, 1987

48. Gold P, Goodwin F, Chronsos G: Clinical and biochemical manifestations of depression: I. Relation to the neurobiology of stress. N Engl J Med 319:348, 1988

49. Sackeim HA: The anticonvulsant hypothesis of the mechanisms of action of ECT: Current status. J Electroconvulsive Ther 15(1):5, 1999

50. Mathe AA: Neuropeptides and electroconvulsive treatment. J Electroconvulsive Ther 15(1):60, 1999

51. Cullen BF: Drug interactions for the anesthesiologist. Fiftieth Annual Refresher Course Lectures and Clinical Update Program, No. 431, p 1. Park Ridge, Illinois, American Society of Anesthesiologists, 1999

52. Selvin BL: Electroconvulsive therapy. Anesthesiology 67:367, 1987

53. Fink M, Johnson L: Monitoring the duration of electroconvulsive therapy seizures: Cuff and EEG methods compared. Arch Gen Psychiatry 39:1189, 1982

54. Fling J, Moulton CH: Electrical design considerations for ECT apparatus. Convulsive Therapy Bulletin with Tardive Dyskinesia Notes 1:37, 1976

55. Maletzky B: Seizure duration and clinical effect in electroconvulsive therapy. Compr Psychiatry 19:541, 1978

56. Wulfson HD, Askanazi J, Finck AD: Propranolol prior to ECT associated with asystole. Anesthesiology 60:255, 1984

57. McPherson R, Lipsey J: Electroconvulsive therapy. In Rodgers M (ed): Current Practice in Anesthesiology, p 212. Philadelphia, BC Decker, 1988

58. Mokriski BK, Nagle SE, Papuchis GC et al: Electroconvulsive therapy induced cardiac arrhythmias during anesthesia with methohexital, thiamylal, or thiopental sodium. J Clin Anesth 4:208, 1992

59. Fredman B, d'Etienne J, Smith I et al: Anesthesia for electroconvulsive therapy: Effects of propofol and methohexital on seizure activity and recovery. Anesth Analg 79:75, 1994

60. Martenson B, Bartfai A, Hall'en B et al: A comparison of propofol and methohexital as anesthetic agents for ECT: Effects on seizure duration, therapeutic outcome, and memory. Biol Psychiatry 35:179, 1994

61. Gullikson J: Oral findings in children with Down's syndrome. J Dent Child 40:293, 1973

62. Bragg C, Miller B: Oral ketamine facilitates induction in a combative mentally retarded patient. J Clin Anesth 3:121, 1990

63. Carrel R: Ketamine: A general anesthetic for manageable ambulatory patients. J Dent Child 40:288, 1973

64. Davis P, Chopyk JB, Mazif M: Continuous alfentanil infusion in pediatric patients undergoing general anesthesia for complete oral restoration. J Clin Anesth 3:125, 1991

65. Oei-Lim LB, Vermeulen-Cranch DM, Bouvy-Berends EC: Conscious sedation with propofol in dentistry. Br Dent J 170:340, 1991

66. White P: Anesthesia for ambulatory surgery. In Stoelting RK (ed): Advances in Anesthesia, vol 2, p 1. Chicago, Year Book, 1985

67. Motoyama E, Glazener C: Hypoxemia after general anesthesia in children. Anesth Analg 65:267, 1986

68. Bailey P, Pace N, Ashbury M et al: Frequent hypoxemia and apnea after sedation with midazolam and fentanyl. Anesthesiology 73:826, 1990

69. Moller J, Wittrap M, Johansen S: Hypoxemia in the postanesthesia care unit: An observer study. Anesthesiology 73:890, 1990

70. Murray R, Raemer D, Morris R: Supplemental oxygen after ambulatory surgical procedures. Anesth Analg 67:967, 1988

71. Chripko D, Bevan J, Archer D et al: Decreases in arterial oxygen saturation in pediatric outpatients during transfer to the postanesthesia recovery room. Anesthesiology 65:180, 1986

72. Wiklund RA, Rosenbaum SH: Anesthesiology: Medical progress, Part I. N Engl J Med 337:1132, 1997

73. Mangano DT: Preoperative risk assessment. Many studies, few solutions: Is a cardiac risk assessment paradigm possible? Anesthesiology 83:897, 1995

74. American Hospital Association: Hospital statistics, Chicago, 1995

75. Forecast of surgical volume in hospital/ambulatory settings: 1994–2001. Chicago, SMG Marketing Group, 1996

76. Moss E: MD-office safety regs stalled in New Jersey. Anesthesia proposal follows office death. Anesthesia Patient Safety Foundation (APSF) Newsletter 11(4):37, 1996–7

77. Wiklund RA, Rosenbaum SH: Anesthesiology: Medical progress, Part II. N Engl J Med 337:1215, 1997

78. Chung F, Ritchie E, Su J: Postoperative pain in ambulatory surgery. Anesth Analg 85:808, 1997

79. Johnson A: Laparoscopic surgery. Lancet 349:631, 1997

80. Cuschieri A: Whither minimal access surgery: Tribulations and expectations. Am J Surg 169:9, 1995

81. Rutkow IM: Laparoscopic hernia repair: The socio-economic tyranny of surgical technology. Am J Surg 127:1271, 1992

82. Moller JT, Pedersen T, Rasmussen LS et al: Randomized evaluation of pulse oximetry in 20,802 patients. I. Design, demography, pulse oximetry failure rate, and overall complication rate. Anesthesiology 78:436, 1993

83. Moller JT, Pedersen T, Rasmussen LS et al: Randomized evaluation of pulse oximetry in 20,802 patients. II. Perioperative events and post-operative complications. Anesthesiology 78:445, 1993

84. Eichhorn JH: Pulse oximetry as a standard of practice in anesthesia. Anesthesiology 78:423, 1993

85. Brain AIJ: The laryngeal mask—a new concept in airway management. Br J Anaesth 55:801, 1983

86. Pennant JH, White PF: The laryngeal mask airway: Its uses in anesthesiology. Anesthesiology 79:144, 1993

87. Schultz LS: Cost analysis of office surgery clinic with comparison to hospital outpatient facilities for laparoscopic procedures. Int Surg 79:273, 1994

88. Koch ME: Anesthesiologists must take active role in regulating office-based surgery. Anesthesiology News 23(8), 1997

89. American College of Surgeons: Guidelines for optimal office-based surgery. Board of Governors' committee on ambulatory surgical care, Oct, 1994

90. Guidelines on sedation and analgesia by nonanesthesiologists. Park Ridge, Illinois, American Society of Anesthesiologist, 1995

91. Kaplan RF: Sedation and analgesia in pediatric patients for procedures outside the operating room. ASA refresher course lectures, No 531, p 1. Park Ridge, Illinois, 1996

92. Cohn S: Preoperative evaluation for elective surgery: What laboratory tests are really needed. Society of Office Based Anesthesia (SOBA) Newsletter 2(4):3, 1997

93. Roizen MF, Kaplan EB, Schreider BD et al: The relative roles of the history and physical examination, and laboratory testing in preoperative evaluation for outpatient surgery: The "Starling" curve of preoperative laboratory testing. Anesthesiol Clin North Am 5(1):15, 1987

94. Delahunt B, Turnbull PR: How cost effective are routine preoperative investigations? NZ Med J 92:431, 1980

95. Narr BJ, Hansen TR, Warner MA: Preoperative laboratory screening in healthy Mayo patients: Cost-effective elimination of tests and unchanged outcomes. Mayo Clinic Proc 66:155, 1991

96. Balaklaw LA: Sedation for cataract patients. Society of Office Based Anesthesia (SOBA) Newsletter 2(4):2 (letter), 1997

97. Friedberg B: www.soba.org. Clinical Forum. Costs of Office Based Anesthesia 12/97

98. Friedberg BL: Hypnotic doses of propofol block ketamine induced hallucinations. Plast Reconstr Surg 91(1):196, 1993

99. Friedberg BL: Propofol-ketamine technique. Anesth Plast Surg 17:297, 1993

100. Vinnik CA: An intravenous dissociation technique for outpatient plastic surgery: Tranquility in the office surgical facility. Plast Reconstr Surg 67(6):199, 1981

101. Joint Commission on Accreditation of Healthcare Organizations: Comprehensive Accreditation Manual, Oakbrook Terrace, Illinois, JCAHO 1996
102. Rego MM, Watcha MF, White PF: The changing role of monitored anesthesia care in the ambulatory setting. Anesth Analg 85:1020, 1997
103. Magni VC, Frost RA, Leung JW *et al:* A randomized comparison of midazolam and diazepam for sedation in upper gastrointestinal endoscopy. Br J Anaesth 55:1095, 1983
104. Bowdle TA, Rooke GA: Postoperative myoclonus and rigidity after anesthesia with opioids. Anesth Analg 78:783, 1994
105. Johnstone RE, Martinec CL: Costs of anesthesia. Anesth Analg 76:840, 1993
106. Greenberg CP: Practical, cost-effective regional anesthesia for ambulatory surgery. J Clin Anesth 7:614, 1995
107. Meridy HW: Criteria for selection of ambulatory surgery patients and guidelines for anesthetic management: A retrospective study of 1553 cases. Anesth Analg 61:921, 1982
108. Rigler ML, Drasner K, Krejcie TC *et al:* Cauda equina syndrome after continuous spinal anesthesia. Anesth Analg 72:275, 1991
109. Pollock JE, Neal JM, Stephenson CA *et al:* Prospective study of the incidence of transient radicular irritation in patients undergoing spinal anesthesia. Anesthesiology 84:1361, 1996
110. Seeberger MD, Lang ML, Drewe J *et al:* Comparison of spinal and epidural anesthesia for patients younger than 50 years of age. Anesth Analg 78:667, 1994
111. Mulroy MF: Regional anesthesia for the adult outpatient. ASA refresher course lectures, No 142, p 1. Park Ridge, Illinois, 1994
112. Sebel PS, Lowdon JD: Propofol: A new intravenous anesthetic. Anesthesiology 71:260, 1989
113. Smith I, White PF, Nathanson M *et al:* Propofol: An update on its clinical use. Anesthesiology 81:1005, 1994
114. Hartung J: Twenty-four of twenty-seven studies show a greater incidence of emesis associated with nitrous oxide than with alternative anesthetics. Anesth Analg 83:114, 1996
115. Twersky R, Fishman D, Homel P: What happens after discharge? Return hospital visits after ambulatory surgery. Anesth Analg 84:319, 1997
116. Chung F, Chan VWS, Ong D: A post-anesthetic discharge scoring system for home readiness after ambulatory surgery. J Clin Anesth 7:500, 1995
117. Assembly Bill 595, Medical Board of California, Division of Licensing, Affiliated healing arts program. Sacramento, California, 1996
118. Assembly Bill 745, Medical Board of California, Division of Licensing, Affiliated healing arts program. Sacramento, California, 1997
119. Standards of Care for Office Surgery. The Board of Medicine. 59F-9.009 Florida State Statutes. 1997
120. Abbott v Bragdon, 107F.3d 934; 1997 U.S. App Lexis 32203 (1st Cir 1997)

Clinical Anesthesia (4/e), edited by Paul G. Barash, Bruce F. Cullen, and Robert K. Stoelting. Lippincott Williams & Wilkins, Philadelphia, © 2001.

CHAPTER 52

ANESTHESIA FOR ORGAN TRANSPLANTATION

LEONARD L. FIRESTONE AND SUSAN FIRESTONE

Transplantation of a variety of tissues is now routine in clinical practice. Bone, tendon, cartilage, and fascia readily provide a partially inert framework for the ingrowth of healthy native cells. Cornea, blood vessels, heart valves, and certain endocrine tissues such as parathyroid are also, to some extent, immunologically privileged and have been successfully transplanted. Bone marrow can be used to replace the entire hematopoietic and lymphopoietic systems. More recently, transplantation of vital organs with distinct vasculature, including the kidneys, liver, heart, and lungs, has achieved the status of preferred therapeutic option for end-stage visceral disease. Technical and biologic factors have thus far prevented widespread introduction of pancreas and small bowel transplantation, but the intensity of current research suggests that important advances will be forthcoming.

The role of anesthesiologists in transplantation may involve caring for organ donors, prospective recipients, or patients who have already received transplants but require further surgery. To do so, specialized knowledge is required in a multitude of disciplines as diverse as organ preservation, biomedical ethics, transplantation immunology, and the physiology of brain death.

ANESTHESIA CARE OF ORGAN DONORS

In the United States, most viscera for transplantation are derived from brain-dead organ donors through voluntary programs established by state and federal law. To supplement these programs, many states have also enacted "required request" legislation, obliging hospital personnel to ask the family of a brain-dead patient to grant permission for organ donation. Organs are distributed through a nationwide organ and transplantation network developed, under federal contract, by the United Network for Organ Sharing (UNOS). UNOS is also responsible for collecting data, reporting statistics, and educating the public about organ donation and transplantation.[1]

Brain death is usually a consequence of catastrophic neurologic injury after blunt head trauma (most often from motor vehicle accidents), penetrating head injury (from gunshot wounds), or intracranial hemorrhage (cerebrovascular accidents). In general, suitable donors will not have sustained prolonged periods of circulatory compromise or septicemia. Donors are screened for serologic evidence of hepatitis B or human immunodeficiency virus infection, as well as active toxoplasmosis, herpes, or tuberculosis. All of these infectious processes disqualify organ donation. In contrast, most transplant centers use organs obtained from donors with prior cytomegalovirus (CMV) infection for recipients with previous CMV exposure. Autoimmune disease in general has not been a criterion for disqualification of donors, despite the report that idiopathic thrombocytopenic purpura can be transmitted by liver transplantation.[2] Cardiac donors are usually younger than 50 years of age and without pre-existing myocardial or coronary artery disease. Myocardial contractility must be adequate as judged by echocardiography, and there should be no history of use of intracardiac injections or high doses of inotropes. Hepatic function tests are useful to screen potential liver donors who may have abused drugs or alcohol. Urinalysis and cultures, blood urea nitrogen, and creatinine levels are standard tests for potential kidney donors. However, given that there are currently 62,000 people waiting for an organ,[3] and some 4000 will die while waiting this year, more compromised donor organs may make their way into patient care.

Viscera for transplantation are also obtained from living donors. Almost all viscera derived from living donors are kidneys, although partial liver and lung resections have been performed to create reduced-size allografts for relatively few recipients. Living donors must be closely related to recipients if there is to be any benefit. The strategy underlying living-related kidney transplantation is that human leukocyte antigen (HLA) identity between donor and recipient results in significantly greater graft survival than even a partially matched organ.[4] Discussion of the perioperative care of living donors is continued in the section on Kidney Transplantation.

Diagnosis of Brain Death

The need for a uniform definition of brain death arose with the advent of heart transplantation in the late 1960s. Before that time, retrieval of kidneys, which are tolerant of a short period of warm ischemia, was performed after cessation of the donor's heartbeat. After several legislative efforts to address the issue, a special panel of medical consultants to the President's Commission for the Study of Ethical Problems in Medicine and Biomedical and Behavior Research issued a report that defined brain death as "irreversible cessation of all function of the entire brain, including the cortex and brain stem, determined in accordance with accepted medical standards."[5] The concept of brain death is now widely recognized in Western societies, although the medical standards of its determination have been the subject of much debate.[6,7]

Cerebral cortical function is deemed absent when no spontaneous movement or response to noxious external stimuli can be elicited by an experienced physician (Table 52-1). However, studies supporting these physical findings are often obtained in accordance with local "medical standards," which may include electroencephalography or cortical blood flow determinations. An electrically silent (flat) electroencephalogram is consistent with the diagnosis of brain death, although residual activity may still be found after cessation of cerebral blood flow.[8] Four-vessel cerebral angiography has been used to establish brain death,[9] but less invasive methods, such as transcranial Doppler[10] and xenon-enhanced computed tomography,[11] are gaining popularity.

Brain stem infarction is indicated by loss of reflexes mediated by bulbar cranial nerve and respiratory nuclei. These include the direct pupillary light reflex (absent when bright light fails to constrict the homolateral pupil); the oculocephalic reflex (absent when ocular position is fixed during rotation of the head ["doll's eyes"]); the corneal reflex (absent when lightly touching the cornea fails to elicit a blink); and the oculovestibular reflex (absent when irrigation of the external auditory canal with ice water fails to produce nystagmus ["cold caloric test"]). Respiratory reflexes are assessed by the apnea test.[12] In most protocols, after a period of mechanical ventilation on 100% oxygen, the ventilator is disconnected (although oxygen is still supplied) and respiratory effort is judged by serial determinations of Pa_{CO_2}. By this means, an accurate assessment of respiratory brain stem function can be obtained in 10 minutes of

Table 52-1. CRITERIA FOR THE DIAGNOSIS OF BRAIN DEATH

LOSS OF CEREBRAL CORTICAL FUNCTION
No spontaneous movement
Unresponsive to external stimuli

LOSS OF BRAIN STEM FUNCTION
Absent respiratory reflex (apnea test)
Absent cranial nerve reflexes
   Pupillary light reflex
   Corneal reflex
   Oculocephalic reflex
   Oculovestibular reflex
   Atropine resistance

SUPPORTING STUDIES
Electroencephalography
Cerebral flow studies
   Angiography
   Transcranial Doppler examination
   Xenon computed tomography scan

observation if the patient remains otherwise physiologically stable.[13]

Irreversibility is implicit in the diagnosis of brain death and is established by the lack of improvement in the neurologic examination for 12–24 hours. Factors that may confound this diagnosis include generalized seizures, centrally active drug effects, hypothermia, and cardiovascular or metabolic instability because all may reversibly depress brain function. Therefore, it is also important that the cause of brain death is known and sufficient to account for this diagnosis. In young children, the potential for recovery from neurologic insults may be less predictable than in adults, so it has been recommended that an experienced pediatric neurologist be consulted to evaluate these young brain-injured patients.[14]

Physiologic Derangements With Brain Death

Brain death is frequently accompanied by marked physiologic instability, and treatment is often necessary to maintain the viability of donor organs (Table 52-2). Hypotension, hypoxemia, or arrhythmias may be part of the pathogenesis of brain death or else a consequence of brain stem infarction. Hypotension results from the loss of descending vasomotor control and is exacerbated by hemorrhage, massive diuresis from diabetes in-

Table 52-2. COMMON PHYSIOLOGIC DERANGEMENTS AFTER BRAIN DEATH

Condition	Cause
Hypotension	Hypovolemia (diabetes insipidus; hemorrhage)
	Neurogenic shock
Hypoxemia	Neurogenic pulmonary edema
	Pulmonary contusion
	Pneumonia
	Gastric aspiration
	Fluid overload
Hypothermia	Hypothalamic infarction
	Exposure
Dysrhythmia (especially bradycardia)	Intracranial injury or herniation
	Hypothermia
	Hypoxia
	Electrolyte abnormality
	Myocardial contusion, ischemia

sipidus or radiographic dyes, or dehydration therapy for cerebral edema. Treatment consists of restoration of intravascular volume with colloid and crystalloid solutions, and, if necessary, vasopressin administration (Pitressin $0.5–15 \text{ U} \cdot \text{h}^{-1}$) or vasoactive drug infusion. Because phenylephrine may diminish splanchnic perfusion and thereby jeopardize abdominal donor organs, dopamine ($2–5 \text{ mg} \cdot \text{kg}^{-1} \cdot \text{min}^{-1}$) is recommended for blood pressure support in this setting. Hypoxemia may follow from overzealous fluid administration during resuscitation attempts, atelectasis, aspiration, pneumothorax, pulmonary contusion, or pneumonia. The F_{IO_2}, minute volume of ventilation, and positive end-expiratory pressure (PEEP) are usually adjusted to maintain systemic arterial saturation in excess of 95%. Atrial and ventricular arrhythmias, as well as varying degrees of conduction blockade, have been noted after brain death.[15] Etiologies include intracranial hypertension, vagal nucleus infarction, myocardial ischemia or contusion, hypothermia, and abnormal pH or serum electrolytes. Bradycardia is resistant to atropine[16] but responds to direct-acting chronotropic agents (*e.g.*, dopamine, isoproterenol).

Numerous endocrine responses have been associated with brain death, including diabetes insipidus. This diagnosis is confirmed when polyuria is accompanied by relative hyposmolarity of the urine ($300 \text{ mOsm} \cdot \text{l}^{-1}$) despite serum hyperosmolarity ($310 \text{ mOsm} \cdot \text{l}^{-1}$) and hypernatremia (serum sodium $150 \text{ mEq} \cdot \text{l}^{-1}$). Treatment consists of replacement of free water losses while restoring normal serum electrolyte and osmolarity values, and infusion of aqueous vasopressin (Pitressin, $0.5–15 \text{ U} \cdot \text{h}^{-1}$ intravenously [iv]). Infrequently, catecholamine and cortisol levels are markedly elevated, and thyroid hormone (T_3) or insulin activity reduced after brain death. However, there is no consistent pattern; therefore, replacement therapies are not routinely used.

Donor Operation

Anesthesia care for multiple organ retrieval should continue the focus on maintenance of donor organ perfusion and oxygenation begun in the intensive care unit. Although cortical and brain stem function is absent, both visceral and somatic reflexes that can lead to physiologic responses during the procedure may be present.[17] For example, reflex pressor responses may accompany surgical stimuli and can jeopardize the renal microvasculature. Vasodilator infusion is sufficient treatment because general anesthetics are unnecessary under these circumstances. Reflex neuromuscular activity mediated by spinal somatic reflexes is suppressed with relaxants.

After surgical preparation in the supine position, a midline incision is made from the suprasternal notch to the pubic symphysis, followed by sternotomy. Once exposed, the liver is freed of its ligamentous attachments to the diaphragm. To minimize warm ischemic time and surgical trauma to the harvested viscera, the typical donor operation involves regional cooling and preservation of organs *in situ*, followed by *en bloc* removal.[18] Thus, after the abdominal aorta is encircled with a ligature above the celiac artery, either the splenic or inferior mesenteric vein is cannulated and the liver is flushed through the portal system with cold preservative solution. The donor is then systemically heparinized and the abdominal aorta is cannulated, cross-clamped, and perfused with cold preservative. This cools the donor's kidneys and liver, and once the ureters are dissected and divided, *en bloc* graft nephrectomy can be accomplished by transecting the aorta and inferior vena cava (IVC) above and below the renal pedicles. The hepatic artery and common bile duct are then divided and the donor liver can now be removed. Donor cardiectomy begins once *in situ* preservation of the abdominal viscera is begun; further details about the cardiac donor procedure are found in Heart Transplantation. After all donor organs are removed, ventilatory and circulatory support is discontinued and the anesthesiologist's involvement ends.

Death is always certified before the donor procedure and is not considered to have occurred in the operating room.

ORGAN PRESERVATION

Organ transplantation depends on the temporary separation of a donor organ from blood supply and protection from ischemia while *ex vivo*. Organ-sharing networks are based on distant procurement, which may extend the period of ischemia to the biologically tolerable limit. The protection strategy combines hypothermia to decrease metabolism with preservative solutions of specific electrolyte composition to maintain cellular integrity. These solutions may also contain chemical additives that are cryoprotective and prevent cellular swelling, vasospasm, and buildup of toxic metabolites and provide a source of energy.

Preservation strategies are based on the control of the adverse cellular events that follow ischemia and reperfusion. Preventing these chain reactions is the rationale for using free radical scavengers (*e.g.,* mannitol, superoxide dismutase) and synthesis blockers (allopurinol) as additives to preservative solutions.

Preservation Solutions

Collins *et al*[19] first developed a series of isotonic flushing solutions for renal preservation. Their compositions usually resembled that of intracellular fluid (*i.e.,* low sodium and high potassium), which was shown to diminish renal cortical respiration. Other additives included heparin, phenoxybenzamine, and procaine, all meant to prevent agonal vasospasm and thrombosis in cadaver kidneys. Today, among the most widely used kidney flushing solutions in the United States and Europe is a modified Collins solution, termed Euro-Collins (Table 52-3). Euro-Collins solution is modestly hyperosmotic, does not contain additives, and supports kidney viability *ex vivo* for more than 48 hours.[20]

The high metabolic rate of the liver makes it relatively vulnerable to ischemia, and its large bulk prevents rapid, uniform cooling during procurement. As a consequence, the most common cause of postoperative hepatic graft dysfunction is ischemic injury. UW (University of Wisconsin) solution[21] was shown to extend hypothermic preservation of donor livers for at least 24 hours *ex vivo*, and possibly longer.[21,22] The key additives in UW solution (see Table 52-3) include lactobionate and raffinose, which are used as impermeants to suppress hypothermia-induced cellular swelling.

Protection of the heart is based on cellular metabolic arrest and uniform cooling, both of which prevent the generation of cytotoxic free radicals.[23] Techniques that provide myocardial protection, particularly cardioplegia, developed in parallel with heart transplantation and greatly facilitated distal procurement.[24] Compared with other preservative regimens, cardioplegia solutions (see Table 52-3) were shown to reduce the need for inotropic support after implantation[24] and are now generally used for *ex vivo* myocardial preservation. Under laboratory conditions, cardioplegia is able to preserve cardiac function for up to 24 hours. However, in humans, the practical limit of ischemic time is 4–6 hours.[24,25]

TRANSPLANTATION IMMUNOLOGY

Tissue derived from a (nontwin) donor of the same species for transplantation is termed an *allograft*. When an immunocompetent recipient is confronted with foreign antigens present on the cell surfaces of an allograft, an immune response occurs. All elements of a recipient's immune system contribute to the response provoked by transplanted tissue; these include humoral factors (immunoglobulins secreted by B lymphocytes as well as complement proteins) and cellular elements (T cells, other leukocytes, and macrophages). T lymphocytes play a primary role in the immune response by initial antigen recognition and ultimate allograft destruction. On the basis of their specific

Table 52-3. COMMON ORGAN PRESERVATION SOLUTIONS

Solution	Amount per Liter
EURO-COLLINS SOLUTION*	
Potassium	115 mEq
Sodium	10 mEq
Chloride	15 mEq
Bicarbonate	10 mEq
Dihydrogen phosphate	15 mEq
Monohydrogen phosphate	85 mEq
Measured osmolality	375 mOsm
pH (4°C)	7.25
UNIVERSITY OF WISCONSIN (UW) OR BELZER'S SOLUTION†	
K+ Lactobionate	100 mmol
KH$_2$PO$_4$	25 mmol
Adenosine	5 mmol
MgSO$_4$	5 mmol
Glutathione	3 mmol
Raffinose	30 mmol
Allopurinol	1 mmol
Insulin	100 units
Penicillin	40 units
Dexamethasone	8 mg
Hydroxyethyl starch	50 g
Osmolality	320–330 mOsm
pH (4°C)	7.4
CRYSTALLOID CARDIOPLEGIA‡	
Potassium	30 mEq
Sodium	25 mEq
Chloride	30 mEq
Bicarbonate	25 mEq
Dextrose	50 g
Mannitol	12.5 g
Osmolality	440 mOsm
pH (4°C)	8.1–8.4

* "Modified" Euro-Collins contains 5 ml · l^{-1} of 50% glucose and 1 g · l^{-1} of magnesium sulfate. Adapted with permission from Collins GM, Bravo-Schuarman M, Teraskai PI: Kidney preservation for transplantation: Initial perfusion and 30 hours ice storage. Lancet 2:1219, 1969.

† Adapted with permission from Belzer FO, Southard JH: Principles of solid organ preservation by cold storage. Transplantation 45:673, 1988.

‡ Adapted with permission from Hardesty RL, Griffith BP, Deep GM et al: Improved cardiac function using cardioplegia during procurement and transplantation. Transplant Proc 15:1253, 1983.

reactivity to certain monoclonal antibodies or their cell surface antigens, T lymphocytes can be subdivided into at least four subpopulations:[26] cytotoxic T cells, helper T cells, delayed hypersensitivity T cells, and suppressor T cells. All are important participants in the reaction to foreign tissue.

The cell surface glycoproteins that establish the immunologic identity of donor tissues are termed the *major histocompatibility complex* (MHC) antigens. Class I MHC antigens, also called HLA-A, -B, and -C, are found on all nucleated cells. These are the classic transplantation antigens as well as the primary targets for cytotoxic cells.[27] Class II MHC antigens, also termed HLA-DR, -DQ, and -DP, are located on activated T cells, B cells, dendritic cells, and macrophages, and are the primary targets for helper T cells.[28] There is an enormous diversity of alleles at the chromosomal loci encoding for the HLA antigens, and this accounts for the varying degrees of HLA matching observed. Finally, the major blood group antigens (ABO) are particularly potent transplantation antigens, such that organs transplanted into patients with known preformed isohemagglutinins against the donor blood type can be expected to provoke the most

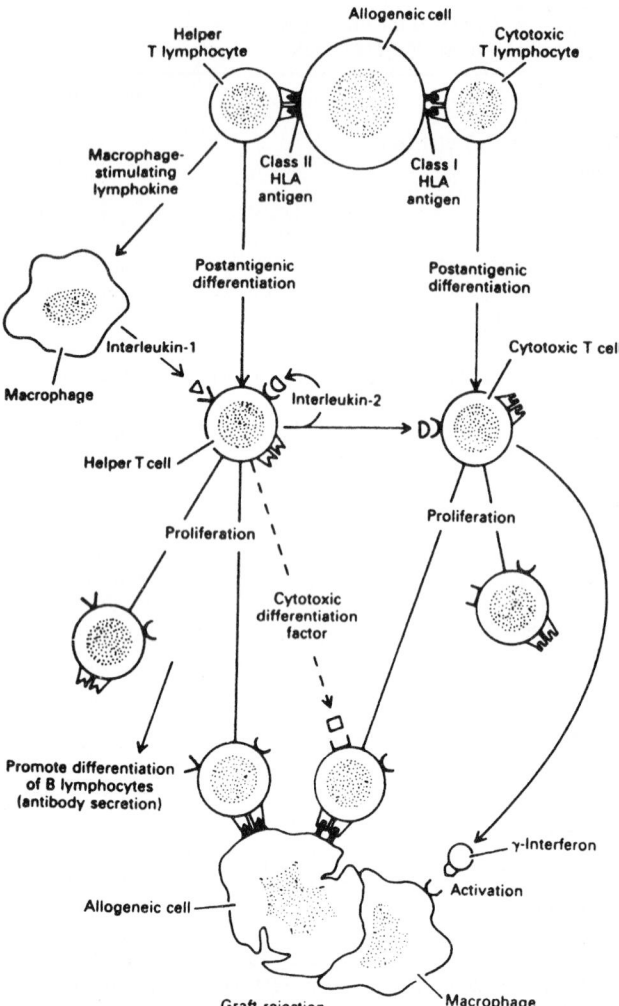

Figure 52-1. Immune response to allogenic tissue. The cellular and humoral events that comprise the immune cascade are illustrated, starting with recognition of an allogenic (foreign) cell by T lymphocytes at the top of the figure. See text for details. HLA = human leukocyte antigen. (Reprinted with permission from Strom TB: Immunosuppressive agents in renal transplantation. Kidney Int 26:353, 1984.)

rapid form of rejection (hyperacute rejection) because of thrombosis in the microvasculature.

Mechanisms of Allograft Rejection

Unless suppressed, the immune response to transplanted tissue begins with the recognition of the donor antigens as foreign or "nonself," proceeds with proliferation of immunocompetent cells, and culminates in an effector phase. Briefly, recognition involves a binding reaction between an immunogenic histocompatibility antigen present on the surface of the allogeneic (donor) cell and a receptor on the surface of a helper or cytotoxic T cell (Fig. 52-1). After T cells are bound, accessory macrophages secrete "monokines," notably interleukin-1 (IL-1), to further enhance T cell activation. IL-2 and other lymphokines are secreted by helper T cells, promoting lymphocyte proliferation and differentiation. Differentiated lymphocytes, in turn, secrete effector molecules including γ-interferon, which activate and enlist macrophages and leukocytes to cooperate in the process of graft rejection.

Clinical Immunology of Organ Transplantation

Hyperacute rejection of renal allografts, characterized by microvascular thrombosis rapidly followed by graft necrosis, occurs

in the presence of major blood group (ABO) incompatibilities.[29] However, like blood transfusion, kidneys from type O donors can be transplanted into compatible, nonidentical (A, B, or AB) recipients. In some centers, ABO-incompatible, living-related donor kidney transplants are performed with good results, but only under special immunosuppression protocols that include splenectomy, plasmapheresis, donor-specific platelet transfusion, and cyclosporine administration. The importance of HLA histocompatibility matching in kidney transplantation is controversial; HLA-incompatible, living-related donor transplantation yields excellent results, but survival rates of HLA-matched cadaver allografts are superior. The presence of preformed cytotoxic antibodies to the donor's T lymphocytes (anti-lymphocyte antibodies) increases the risk of hyperacute rejection and usually precludes kidney transplantation.[30] One other immunologic parameter that may affect renal allograft survival is the panel-reactive antibody (PRA). In this test, cross-match testing is done between patient sera and donor cells to detect the presence of preformed antibodies. It has been reported that patients with lymphocytotoxic antibodies that react against more than 50% of the random test panel have a greater rate of rejection.[31]

Donor-specific ABO isoagglutinins may induce hyperacute reactions of cardiac allografts;[32] thus, ABO matching is considered to be essential. The role of HLA matching in heart transplantation is more controversial. Some studies indicate that HLA mismatching does not correlate with the number of cardiac rejection episodes or survival,[33] whereas others find that HLA mismatching has clinically important consequences.[34] However, until the tolerable donor heart ischemic time is extended beyond the present 4–6 hours, full prospective histocompatibility matching and PRA screening will remain impractical and limit their application.

In contrast to the heart and kidneys, hyperacute rejection has not been reported to occur in liver allografts,[35] supporting the assertion that the liver is resistant to such antibody-mediated injury.[36] Consequently, liver transplantation is often performed despite major ABO incompatibility, although the risk of subsequent rejection is elevated.[29,37] When ABO matching is done, short-term survival is better with ABO-identical than with ABO-compatible, nonidentical allografts,[29] and the longer-term trend is similar.[38] There does not seem to be any relation between either HLA matching or T-cell crossmatch and allograft survival.

In summary, the distribution of renal allografts depends mostly on immunologic factors such as ABO match, HLA histocompatibility, T-cell crossmatch, and PRA profile. In contrast, except for ABO matching, the distribution of donor livers and hearts depends more on factors such as size compatibility and medical urgency than on immunologic criteria.

Mechanisms of Immunosuppression

In clinical practice, the immune response must be controlled to avoid allograft rejection. Immunosuppressant drugs have been developed for this purpose, but their use is accompanied by significant morbidity. Because of side effects and toxicities (as discussed in Evaluation of Patients With a Prior Organ Transplant), immunosuppression is warranted only for grafts essential for life. For example, a thyroid allograft would be inappropriate because it is easily substituted by a medication.

Ideally, immunosuppressants should inhibit only that lymphocyte subset directed against donor-specific alloantigens, but the drugs in current use are immunologically nonspecific. Antirejection regimens usually combine low doses of several agents to provide superior immunosuppression and to minimize side effects.

Glucocorticoids

Glucocorticoids (Table 52-4) are potent anti-inflammatory agents and have been a mainstay in almost all immunosuppressive regimens. These agents decrease macrophage production

Table 52-4. MECHANISMS OF IMMUNOSUPPRESSANT ACTION

Agent	Main Effect(s)
Glucocorticoids	Decrease IL-1 production from macrophages (reducing effectiveness of T-helper cells)
	Decrease IL-2 production from T cells (reducing clonal expansion of T-helper and cytotoxic cells)
Azathioprine	Inhibits DNA and RNA synthesis (reducing lymphocyte proliferation)
Cyclosporine	Prevents T-helper cell activation by antigen
	Inhibits elaboration of T-cell–derived factors, particularly IL-2
Tacrolimus (FK 506)	Inhibits T-cell production of IL-2
	Inhibits production of IL-2 receptors on T cells
	Prevents B-cell activation
Antilymphocyte globulin	Diminishes populations of both T and B lymphocytes
OKT3	Inactivates T cells and prevents reactivation

IL = interleukin.

of IL-1, a critical factor in helper T-cell development.[39] In addition, T-cell secretion of IL-2 is also diminished, preventing clonal expansion of helper and cytotoxic T cells.[40]

Azathioprine

Azathioprine is an imidazole derivative of 6-mercaptopurine, an analogue of the purine hypoxanthine. Thioinosinic acid, a metabolite of azathioprine, competes with inosinic acid for conversion to xanthylic acid, an essential substrate for *de novo* purine synthesis required for production of both DNA and RNA. As a result, protein synthesis and both T- and B-lymphocyte proliferation are inhibited.[41]

Cyclosporine, Tacrolimus, Mycophenolate, and Rapamycin

Cyclosporine is a lipophilic undecapeptide antibiotic isolated from a soil fungus that virtually revolutionized viscera transplantation by making it feasible routinely to achieve results comparable with those obtained in transplants between identical twins. Its major target is the T cell, which is inhibited from elaborating key lymphokines such as IL-2.[42] Cyclosporine also prevents activation of helper T cells by foreign antigens and inhibits the production of IL-1 by macrophages.

Tacrolimus (FK 506) and rapamycin are newer macrolide antibiotic immunosuppressants currently undergoing clinical trials. Both are highly potent and may have somewhat more immunospecificity and less toxicity than cyclosporine. These agents diminish activation and proliferation of T cells as well as lymphokine production, but do so through distinct intracellular signaling pathways.

Mycophenolate mofetil has shown promise in early clinical trials. It is hydrolyzed to mycophenolic acid, which inhibits the enzyme inosine monophosphate dehydrogenase. In turn, this disrupts guanosine nucleotide synthesis in T and B lymphocytes, reducing their ability to proliferate during an immune response.[43] Whether its immunospecificity and toxicity profiles are better than those of the aforementioned compounds remains to be seen.

Antilymphocyte Globulin and OKT3

Antilymphocyte globulin (ALG) is a polyclonal antibody produced by immunizing animals with human lymphoid cells and isolating the IgG fraction from resulting antisera. ALG seems rapidly to diminish the availability of activated T lymphocytes, interrupting the chain of events leading to rejection. ALG may also have a sustained effect on T-cell proliferation, perhaps by promoting formation of nonspecific suppressor T cells.[44] Similarly, the OKT series of murine monoclonal antibodies directed against T-cell surface antigens are added to some immunosuppression regimens to treat rejection. OKT3 is specifically directed against the T3 (CD3) complex on the surface of mature T lymphocytes. The T3 complex is located adjacent to the T-cell receptor involved in recognition of foreign antigens; binding of OKT3 blocks the recognition of MHC antigens and, consequently, the immune response cascade.[45] Administration of OKT3 also results in removal of opsonized T cells by the reticuloendothelial system.

GENERAL PREANESTHETIC EVALUATION OF TRANSPLANT CANDIDATES

The general indication for organ transplantation is failure of medical or other surgical management to enhance the quality of life for patients with end-stage organ disease or significantly to improve their chances for long-term survival. Because major organ transplantation procedures are now associated with reasonably low perioperative mortality rates, this option is considered in virtually all such cases.

The major contraindications to organ transplantation are incurable malignancy; the presence of another systemic disease; active, poorly controlled infection; and physical or social factors that would either impede recovery or lead to recurrent disease (Table 52-5). Rather than being considered absolute, these criteria are under continuous evolution in light of new information. For example, diabetes mellitus was formerly considered to contraindicate organ transplantation, but many diabetic patients have now undergone renal transplantation and 1-year allograft survival is the same as for nondiabetic patients. Patients with diabetic nephropathy now comprise the largest segment of adults who undergo renal transplantation. Similarly, many elderly patients have undergone heart transplantation with results that are comparable with those for younger subpopulations.

Candidates for organ transplantation often manifest physical findings or laboratory abnormalities indicative of secondary organ involvement (*e.g.*, hepatomegaly consequent to right ventricular failure). It is important to verify that such findings do not represent a coexistent primary disease process (which might disqualify potential recipients) and to bear in mind that compromised organs may be especially vulnerable to acute insults. Because recipients will be immunosuppressed, occult infection (*e.g.*, tuberculosis) should assiduously be ruled out. For the same reason, it is standard to order CMV-negative blood for transfusion unless recipients are seropositive. On occasion, technical feasibility may become the overwhelming source of concern (*e.g.*, with atypical vascular anatomy or body habitus, or multiple previous surgeries).

Because of the shortage of suitable donor organs, patients may remain on a waiting list for many months while their conditions continue to deteriorate. Interval changes, as well as corre-

Table 52-5. GENERAL CONTRAINDICATIONS TO VISCERA TRANSPLANTATION

Incurable malignancy
Other major systemic illness
Old ("physiologic") age
Active systemic or incurable infection
Significant obesity
Current alcohol, drug, or tobacco abuse
Evidence of emotional instability or lack of supportive social milieu

Table 52-6. ETIOLOGY OF END-STAGE RENAL DISEASE IN RENAL TRANSPLANT RECIPIENTS*

Etiology	Total Cases (%)
Diabetic glomerulonephropathy	43.6
Other glomerulonephritides	23.2
Polycystic kidney disease	5.8
Chronic pyelonephritis	5.4
Obstructive uropathy	3.4
Alport's syndrome	2.1
Lupus nephritis	1.6
Miscellaneous, including unknown	14.9

* Data derived from 2591 cases at the University of Minnesota performed between 1963 and 1990.
Adapted with permission from Belani KG, Palahniuk RJ: Kidney transplantation. In Firestone LL (ed): Anesthesia and Organ Transplantation, p 17. Boston, Little, Brown, 1991.

sponding alterations in their medical regimens, should be ascertained. The urgency of surgery may, by necessity, influence the acceptability of an available donor organ.

With organs for which the safe ischemic time is less than 24 hours, transplantation procedures are usually performed under emergency circumstances. The patient to receive the organ may have eaten recently and arrives in the operating room without the benefit of premedication. The remaining management considerations are specific to the particular type of transplantation procedure, as discussed in the following sections.

KIDNEY TRANSPLANTATION

Approximately 10,000 renal transplantations are performed each year in the United States. This comprises 5–10% of patients with end-stage renal disease who are otherwise dependent on dialysis. Dialysis is clearly effective in prolonging life, but considerable morbidity and mortality are associated with its use. For example, in 1988 the 1-year mortality rate after renal transplantation was 5%; in some studies the yearly mortality rate of patients on chronic dialysis is at least twice as high.[46]

Renal transplantation is a highly successful procedure. According to data from the national organ procurement and transplantation network UNOS, cadaveric renal allografts have a 1-year survival rate of 81%, whereas the same statistic for living-related donor organs is 91%.[47] Studies from large centers indicate that longer-term graft survival is also comparably favorable, as are other measures of outcome. In adults with end-stage renal disease, kidney transplantation improves the quality of life[48] while remaining cost-effective,[49] and for children, transplantation provides superior growth and development.[50] For these reasons, renal transplantation has become the treatment of choice for end-stage renal disease,[51] with its growth limited only by the supply of available donor organs.

Pathophysiology of End-Stage Renal Disease

End-stage renal disease can result from numerous causes (Table 52-6), all of which ultimately lead to the uremic syndrome. In uremia, patients are unable to regulate the volume and composition of their body fluids, resulting in fluid overload, acidemia, and imbalance of electrolytes such as potassium, phosphorus, magnesium, and calcium. In addition, there is usually evidence of secondary dysfunction in other organ systems (Table 52-7). Even patients maintained by dialysis may have peripheral neuropathy, pericardial or pleural effusions, renal osteodystrophy, and gastrointestinal (GI) as well as immunologic dysfunction.

Specific Indications and Contraindications

A large proportion of adults with end-stage renal disease are candidates for kidney transplantation. Aside from the general contraindications to viscera transplantation (see Table 52-5), relative contraindications specific to renal transplantation are disease processes likely to recur in the transplanted kidney. Hemolytic–uremic syndrome, membranoproliferative glomerulonephritis, and metabolic derangements that produce toxic deposits in the kidney (e.g., gout, oxalosis, cytinosis) fall into this group. In practice, however, patients with such disorders may derive years of benefit from transplantation, and thus at many centers are still considered eligible. Similarly, diabetic nephropathy can also recur in allografts, but diabetes mellitus is no longer considered a contraindication to renal transplantation.

Preanesthetic Considerations

Because the tolerable ischemic time for kidneys is at least 48 hours,[20] cadaver allografts may be transplanted semielectively. With living-related donation, renal transplantation is an elective procedure. In either case, sufficient time is available for ABO matching, cross-matching of the recipient's serum with donor lymphocytes, and, at some institutions, HLA tissue typing. Likewise, dialysis may precede transplantation to correct serious electrolyte and volume derangements. After dialysis, it is important to ascertain the net volume status of patients; the final hematocrit, electrolyte, and bicarbonate levels; and whether there is any residual heparin effect. The serum potassium should be normal, and the serum calcium supplemented if <7 mg · dl^{-1} to prevent tetanus. Most uremic patients, even those on dialysis, have hemoglobin levels in the 6–8 g · dl^{-1} range. However, in chronically anemic patients, compensatory changes promote tissue oxygen unloading, and, on this basis alone, preoperative

Table 52-7. COMMON PATHOPHYSIOLOGIC CONSEQUENCES OF END-STAGE RENAL DISEASE

Organ System	Consequence
Nervous system	Peripheral neuropathy
	Lethargy → coma
Hematologic	Anemia
	Diminished erythrocyte survival
	Platelet dysfunction
	Shift in P_{50} of oxyhemoglobin dissociation curve
Cardiovascular	Congestive heart failure
	Pericarditis
	Hypertension
	Dysrhythmias (abnormal electrolytes)
	Capillary fragility
Pulmonary	Pleural effusions
	Pulmonary edema
Musculoskeletal	Generalized muscle weakness
	Renal osteodystrophy
	Metastatic calcification
	Gout, pseudogout
Gastrointestinal	Nausea, vomiting
	Ileus
	Peptic and colonic ulceration
Endocrine	Pancreatitis
	Glucose intolerance
Integument	Pruritus
	Hyperpigmentation
Immunologic	Impaired cellular immunity

Adapted with permission from Belani KG, Palahniuk RJ: Kidney transplantation. In Firestone LL (ed): Anesthesia and Organ Transplantation, p 17. Boston, Little, Brown, 1991.

transfusion is not mandatory. But transfusion may enhance allograft survival; thus, it has become a standard part of the preoperative regimen at some centers. On occasion, pleural or pericardial effusions may require treatment if there is functional impairment; in patients on chronic steroids, preoperative administration of full replacement doses of glucocorticoids should be considered.

Because many adult recipients are diabetic, the possibility of coexistent ischemic heart disease is usually evaluated by exercise stress testing and, if indicated, coronary angiography.[52] Diffuse coronary disease has not been considered a contraindication to renal transplantation, provided that ventricular function is not seriously diminished and the patient is willing to assume the added risk. In such patients, appropriate invasive monitoring (arterial and pulmonary artery catheters) is warranted; in all others, a central venous pressure catheter is sufficient to monitor intravascular volume for optimal renal perfusion. Finally, transplanted kidneys, particularly those derived from cadaver donors, may not be functional immediately, so it is vital to protect existing arteriovenous fistulas or other routes for postoperative hemodialysis or peritoneal dialysis.

Donor Procedure and Related Considerations

The procedure used for harvesting abdominal viscera from cadaver donors is reviewed in Anesthesia Care of Organ Donors. If the cadaver is brain dead but the circulation is intact, harvesting may proceed at leisure through the transperitoneal route. If the circulation fails, however, the kidneys must be rapidly removed and flushed with preservative solution to minimize warm ischemic time.

Living donors are the source of 20% of the kidneys transplanted in the United States and 60% of those in Europe. Because results with unrelated living donors are no better than those achieved with cadaver donors, living donors are virtually always close relatives. Most are healthy adults, because any significant systemic disease increases the risk of general anesthesia and surgery, giving rise to ethical conflicts. For similar reasons, donors who are 45 (male) or 50 years (female) of age usually undergo noninvasive studies to detect occult coronary ischemia. The use of living-related donors has gained widespread acceptance because the overall incidence of serious perioperative morbidity in this population is small (≤2%), and deaths are extremely rare.[53] Furthermore, long-term follow-up studies indicate that donors have no greater risk of renal failure or hypertension.[54]

Before surgery, donors undergo renal arteriography and iv pyelography and are screened for ABO blood group compatibility and CMV titer. Then, 2–4 weeks before the procedure, several units of blood are donated for autologous transfusion. During the night preceding harvesting, donors are hydrated with crystalloid solutions to promote an active diuresis, and at the time of nephrectomy, a minimum urine output of 1 ml · min^{-1} is achieved by means of mannitol and furosemide. The timing of the donor and recipient procedures is coordinated so that the kidney's ischemic interval is minimized. Heparin is administered systemically before removal of the organ from the donor, which is then flushed free of blood with a cold crystalloid solution and transplanted immediately.

Anesthesia Induction for Recipients

Diabetic patients can have delayed gastric emptying;[55] therefore, rapid induction may be warranted. Provided the serum potassium is normal after recent dialysis, there is no contraindication to the use of succinylcholine. Drugs that are highly protein bound (e.g., thiopental) should be administered in reduced dosages. Further discussion of the kinetics and dynamics of drugs in renal failure patients is found in Chapter 36.

Central venous catheters are useful for the reasons discussed earlier but are usually inserted after induction. Many renal transplant recipients are moderately hypertensive and maintained on combinations of appropriate medications. Most have recently been dialyzed and are volume depleted. Thus, the possibility of synergistic interactions between strongly vasodilating anesthetics (e.g., isoflurane, fentanyl), antihypertensives (e.g., hydralazine, diltiazem, captopril), and hypovolemia should be considered.

Anesthesia and Surgical Procedures

Although regional anesthetic techniques have been advocated by some,[56] the use of general anesthesia is more common.[57] With general anesthesia, there is superior control of ventilation, which becomes particularly important when surgical retraction is close to the diaphragm. In addition, the duration of renal transplant procedures in most centers makes regional techniques impractical. Enflurane is seldom chosen because its biotransformation results in inorganic fluoride that is nephrotoxic. Nitrous oxide is often omitted to avoid distention of the bowel, particularly in children, so either opioids and benzodiazepines are used in combination, or a potent inhaled agent is used alone. Atracurium and vecuronium are the preferred muscle relaxants because they are least dependent on renal metabolism, although laudanosine, a metabolite of atracurium, may accumulate in patients with end-stage renal disease.[58] Laudanosine increases the minimum alveolar concentration of halothane in laboratory animals but does not seem to cause an analogous clinical effect in humans.[59] The response to vecuronium may be variable in renal failure,[60] and because it is not clear precisely when renal metabolic function is restored after transplantation, neuromuscular monitoring is highly recommended.

In adults, the kidney is implanted retroperitoneally in the upper pelvis using a paramedian lower-abdominal approach; in children weighing <20 kg, abdominal implantation is the rule. Revascularization of the allograft in adults involves anastomoses of the renal vessels to an iliac vein and artery. This necessitates clamping the common iliac vessels, resulting in lower extremity ischemia, usually for less than 60 minutes. After the anastomoses are complete, the circulation is restored to the allograft and lower extremities. To promote renal perfusion, a high-normal blood pressure is achieved by reducing the depth of anesthesia, bolus administration of crystalloid, or temporary dopamine infusion. When the vascular clamps are released, renal preservative solution and the venous drainage from the legs are also released into the circulation. These effluents are relatively rich in potassium and acid metabolites, but in adults, have little systemic effect. The final stage of the procedure involves ureteral implantation for urinary drainage.

Postoperative Management

Varying periods of oliguria or anuria due to acute tubular necrosis are associated with cadaveric renal transplantation in approximately one third of cases;[61] thus, fluids must be administered judiciously to reduce the risk of postoperative pulmonary edema. In contrast, the ischemic time for organs derived from living-related donors is minimal and urine flow is usually immediate. Emergence is often accompanied by both pain and hypertension, which are particularly hazardous in diabetic patients with coexistent ischemic heart disease. In such cases, preparations should be made to administer potent analgesics (e.g., by epidural catheter) and antihypertensives in the recovery room, if myocardial ischemia is to be avoided. Other early postoperative complications include atelectasis, bleeding and thrombosis of vascular anastomoses, urinary obstruction or leak, and, rarely, gastric aspiration. Hyperacute rejection may also occur and lead to anuria; definitive diagnosis requires a renal biopsy. This complication has become rare because both ABO matching

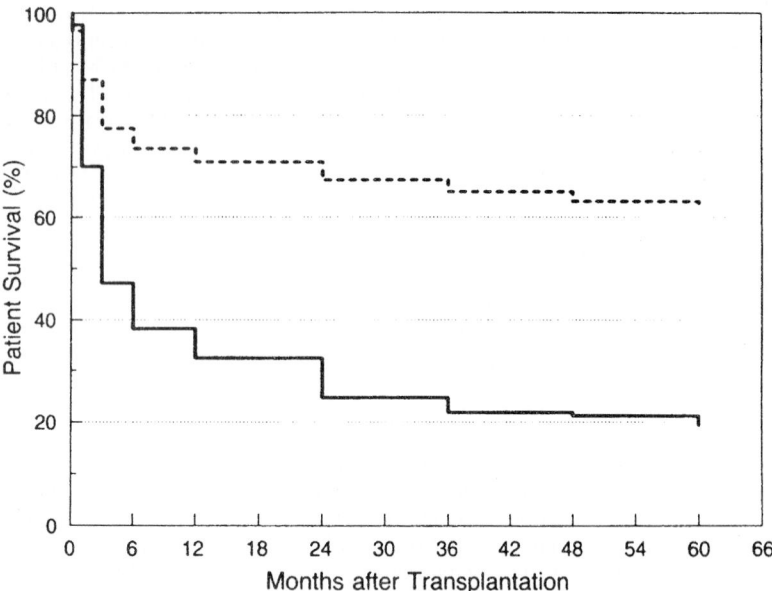

Figure 52-2. Survival of liver transplant recipients treated before and after the availability of cyclosporine. Data are derived from 170 "before" (*solid line*) and 1258 "after" (*dashed line*) recipients. Survival is calculated using the life-table method. (Reprinted with permission from Starzl TE, Demetris AJ, van Thiel DH: Liver transplantation. N Engl J Med 321:1014, 1092, 1989.)

and crossmatching of the recipient's serum to donor lymphocytes are routinely performed.

Immunosuppression with "triple therapy" (cyclosporine, azathioprine, prednisone) is usually begun before transplantation of living-related donor organs or after transplantation of cadaveric kidneys. Long-term complications of renal transplantation related to immunosuppression are discussed in Evaluation of Patients With a Prior Organ Transplant.

LIVER TRANSPLANTATION

Medical treatment for chronic end-stage liver disease is supportive but does little to prolong or improve the quality of life, particularly after serious complications (*e.g.,* GI bleeding, coma, uremia) develop. In acute hepatic failure, the salvage rate with medical treatment is between 5 and 20%.[62] In contrast, in the cyclosporine era, the overall 1-year survival rate of orthotopic liver recipients is 76%, with an allograft survival rate of 69%.[47] Longer-term survival is also comparatively high (Fig. 52-2). Moreover, the quality of life for a high proportion of transplantation survivors is markedly improved.[63]

The yearly rate of liver transplantations in the United States has reached approximately 2500, although it has been argued that more than twice that number are needed.[63] The overwhelming majority of these procedures are orthotopic, involving native hepatectomy and implantation of the donor organ in anatomic position in the right upper quadrant. Heterotopic (also called auxiliary) transplantation, where the donor liver is implanted adjacent to the native liver, which is left *in situ,* has been used on rare occasion for reversible hepatic failure and in patients too frail for the orthotopic procedure.[64]

Pathophysiology of End-Stage Liver Disease

The liver has numerous synthetic and metabolic functions (see Chapter 39); thus, end-stage liver disease has ramifications that extend to virtually every other organ system (Table 52-8). In disease processes that destroy the normal hepatic architecture, portal hypertension results and extensive venous collaterals develop in the abdominal wall, mesentery, retroperitoneum, and GI tract. Aside from the significant morbidity associated with hemorrhage from esophageal varices, the extensive network of arteriovenous communications results in low systemic vascular resistance and high cardiac output. Intrapulmonary shunting is also seen frequently in patients with end-stage liver disease,[65]

leading to hypoxemia that is exacerbated by pleural effusions and bibasilar atelectasis from abdominal distention. Renal function may be impaired from hepatorenal syndrome or prerenal azotemia. Ascites develops as a result of venous hypertension, decreased albumin synthesis, and sodium and water retention from a relative excess of aldosterone and antidiuretic hormone. Treatment often consists of diuretics, which in turn may cause electrolyte and acid–base derangements and intravascular volume depletion. Blood coagulation is abnormal because synthesis of the hepatically derived clotting factors (I [fibrinogen], II [prothrombin], V, VII, IX, X) and clearance of fibrinolytic factors are compromised. Hypersplenism may also markedly

Table 52-8. COMMON PATHOPHYSIOLOGIC CONSEQUENCES OF END-STAGE LIVER DISEASE

Organ System	Consequence
Central nervous system	Encephalopathy (mild confusion → coma)
	Brain edema (fulminant hepatitis)
Cardiovascular	Hyperdynamic circulation
	Reduced systemic resistance
	Increased plasma volume
	Pericardial effusion
Pulmonary	Pleural effusion
	Interstitial edema (hypoalbuminemia)
	Atelectasis
	Ventilation–perfusion mismatch and shunting
Gastrointestinal	Esophageal varices
	Ascites
	Portal hypertension
	Delayed gastric emptying
Hematologic	Reduced clotting factor levels
	Anemia
	Thrombocytopenia (hypersplenism)
	Reduced clearance of fibrinolytic substances and tissue plasminogen activators
Endocrine	Glucose intolerance
	Diminished glycogen stores
Renal	Oliguria (hepatorenal syndrome, prerenal azotemia)
	Hyponatremia (diuretics, increased antidiuretic hormone activity)
	Hypokalemia (poor nutrition, diuretics, gastrointestinal losses)

Table 52-9. PREOPERATIVE PATHOLOGIC DIAGNOSES IN LIVER TRANSPLANT RECIPIENTS*

Disease	No. of Cases
PARENCHYMAL	
Postnecrotic cirrhosis	348
Alcoholic cirrhosis	76
Acute liver failure	54
Budd-Chiari syndrome	18
Congenital hepatic fibrosis	9
Cystic fibrosis	6
Neonatal hepatitis	8
Hepatic trauma	3
CHOLESTATIC	
Biliary atresia	217
Primary biliary cirrhosis	186
Sclerosing cholangitis	100
Secondary biliary cirrhosis	25
Familial cholestasis	16
INBORN ERRORS OF METABOLISM	114
TUMORS	
Benign	10
Primary malignant	60
Metastatic	8

* Data derived from 400 pediatric and 858 adult recipients of liver transplants at the University of Pittsburgh, 1981–1988.
Adapted with permission from Starzl TE, Demetris AJ, van Thiel DH: Liver transplantation. N Engl J Med 321:1014, 1092, 1989.

diminish the platelet count. Eventually, even the central nervous system is affected, resulting in a progressive toxic encephalopathy and cerebral edema, which presage death.

Specific Indications and Contraindications

The decision to transplant is difficult to base on objective liver function test results because these values vary considerably according to the specific pathologic process. Instead, the degrees of medical, social, and psychological impairment are considered in combination, then balanced against the mortality associated with conservative management.[63] Ideally, liver transplantation is undertaken before the degree of organ failure becomes severe and the patient incapacitated,[62] to reduce perioperative morbidity.

There is little debate that liver transplantation is indicated for nonmalignant end-stage liver disease that will not recur in the hepatic graft. Most often, this procedure is used to treat benign parenchymal diseases, including postnecrotic cirrhosis and any of the causes of acute liver failure or cholestatic processes (*e.g.*, primary biliary cirrhosis or biliary atresia in children; Table 52-9). In all, more than 60 disease entities have now been successfully treated by liver transplantation.[63] Transplanting in the presence of a disease when recurrence is a possibility is somewhat more controversial, considering the limited supply of donor organs. Alcoholic cirrhosis was once considered an absolute contraindication to transplantation, but multidisciplinary care and careful selection have led to results with Laennec's cirrhosis that are comparable with those with other liver diseases.[66] Similarly, transplantation for cirrhosis from hepatitis B virus infection has proved to be beneficial for many patients[63] despite the inability to prevent infection in the donor liver. Advanced age was also once a contraindication, but recipients older than 50 years have been shown to have a 5-year survival rate after transplantation comparable with that of younger adults.[67]

Treatment of hepatic cancers by transplantation is being studied at several centers and is the subject of considerable debate.

Patients with primary liver and bile duct cancers, as well as hepatic metastases from GI and endocrine tumors, have undergone liver transplantation with varying duration of remission.[68,69] But recurrence of tumor is the rule, so transplantation is usually reserved for selected cases with isolated tumors and deteriorating liver function. If hepatic function remains preserved in the presence of a liver tumor, major hepatic resection is the recommended alternative.

Other possible contraindications relate to specific surgical obstacles, including thromboses of major abdominal veins and scarring from multiple abdominal procedures. However, the successful use of vein grafts and accumulation of practical experience with the transplantation procedure have rendered even these contraindications obsolete.

Preanesthetic Considerations

Candidates for liver transplantation present a broad clinical spectrum, ranging from chronic fatigue with mild jaundice to coma with multiorgan failure. Hepatic encephalopathy may be reversible; thus, the timing of liver transplantation can be critical to outcome. Emergency transplantation for fulminant hepatic failure can have a salvage rate of 55–75%[70] provided that symptoms have not progressed to Grade 4 encephalopathy.[63] Without transplantation, most causes of fulminant hepatic failure are associated with much poorer prognoses.

Certain uncommon diseases treated by liver transplantation have additional implications for anesthesiologists. For example, after transplantation for the Budd-Chiari syndrome, which typically is associated with extensive hepatic venous thrombosis, patients may require anticoagulation.[71] In children with an even rarer disorder, Crigler-Najjar syndrome (bilirubin uridine diphosphate–glucuronyl transferase deficiency), drugs that interfere with bilirubin binding to albumin (*e.g.*, barbiturates) should be avoided.[72]

Many of the physiologic derangements associated with end-stage liver disease are not correctable until after transplantation. Therefore, the major emphasis in the preanesthetic evaluation should be on identifying the most important areas of physiologic compromise and treating only those that threaten the safe induction of anesthesia. For example, pleural effusions may be responsible for profound hypoxemia, and despite clotting abnormalities, preoperative thoracentesis may be a necessity. However, defects in coagulation are usually not corrected at this point unless there is active hemorrhage. If blood product administration is essential, but limited by oliguric hypervolemia, hemofiltration has been used in parallel to the venovenous bypass circuit.[73]

Preparation of fluid-warming units, gas circuit humidifiers, warming blankets, and nonconductive wraps for the head and extremities is essential before induction; otherwise, hypothermia will rapidly result from transfusion, convective and evaporative losses from exposure of abdominal organs, diminished hepatic energy production, and implantation of a cold donor organ of large thermal mass. A thromboelastograph is also prepared at many centers as a relatively rapid means to elucidate a need for specific blood product replacement under conditions of massive transfusion.[74]

Finally, as a result of the primary disease process or subsequent multiple transfusions, recipient serologies may be positive for hepatitis A, B, or C. The health care team should be aware of the potential for infectious contamination and take appropriate precautions.

Anesthesia Induction

Liver transplantation involves transection and reanastomosis of several major venous structures (portal vein and IVC), and the ability to transfuse rapidly is vital to successful outcome.[75] At the University of Pittsburgh, at least two large-bore peripheral

Table 52-10. OVERVIEW OF THE ORTHOTOPIC LIVER TRANSPLANTATION PROCEDURE

Phase	Surgical Procedures	Physiologic Changes
Preanhepatic	Dissection of porta hepatis	Third space losses (ascites)
	Release of hepatic attachments	Hemorrhage (venous collaterals)
Anhepatic	Clamp hepatic aorta, portal vein	Obstruction of venous return
	Venovenous bypass (adults)	Oliguria (venous congestion)
	Clamp IVC	
	Retraction on diaphragm	Atelectasis, decreased compliance
Neohepatic	Anastomosis of IVC	Hemorrhage (coagulopathy)
	Flush hepatic allograft	
	Anastomosis of portal vein, hepatic artery	Citrate intoxication
		Hyperkalemia
	Biliary drainage procedure	Hypothermia
		Metabolic acidosis

IVC = inferior vena cava.

venous cannulae are inserted, one of which is 8.5 French units to facilitate the use of a rapid transfusion device. Because major shifts in intravascular volume are common and reperfusion of the donor liver has been associated with hypotension,[76] invasive monitoring with arterial and pulmonary artery catheters is standard. Both radial and femoral artery catheters are often placed because distal arterial flow may be compromised by aortic clamps during hepatic artery anastomoses. The balance of the monitoring array is similar to that used for any critically ill patient undergoing a major general surgical procedure.

Patients with end-stage liver disease have numerous reasons for delayed gastric emptying, such as ascites or active upper GI bleeding. Therefore, aspiration precautions are mandatory and induction of general anesthesia should proceed by either a rapid-sequence technique or, in patients with hemodynamic instability or significant hypovolemia, awake intubation.

Anesthesia and Surgical Procedures

Anesthesia is maintained by agents that preserve splanchnic flow (*e.g.,* opioids or isoflurane) combined with muscle relaxants, except in cases of fulminant hepatic failure in which the possibility of intracranial hypertension contraindicates potent inhaled agents. Nitrous oxide is not contraindicated but is usually avoided because of its ability to distend the bowel and increase the size of gas bubbles entrained in the circulation. Pharmacokinetic alterations associated with end-stage liver disease are complex and are described in Chapter 39 and reviewed by Howrie and Burckart.[77] The net effect of these factors for nondepolarizing muscle relaxants is to increase the loading dose requirements and prolong the durations of action. In contrast, fentanyl kinetics are not markedly changed.[78] Although well preserved liver allografts can rapidly begin to metabolize drugs,[79] many of the pharmacokinetic changes (*e.g.,* diminished serum albumin, enlarged volumes of distribution) persist beyond the transplantation procedure.

The orthotopic procedure involves replacing the diseased native liver with a cadaveric organ in the most anatomic position possible. It consists of three stages: the preanhepatic, anhepatic, and neohepatic stages[80] (Table 52-10).

The preanhepatic stage involves dissection of the structures of the porta hepatis and mobilization of the native liver. Cardiovascular instability is common during this phase because of hypovolemia from acute third-space losses (ascites) and hemorrhage from venous collaterals in the body wall and mesentery.

Citrate-induced hypocalcemia,[81] hyperkalemia from rapid transfusion and hemolysis, embarrassment of venous return from retraction, or precipitous drops in intra-abdominal pressure and consequent venous pooling also contribute to hemodynamic instability. During sudden volume shifts, previously asymptomatic pericardial effusions may reduce cardiac output, so they are often drained under direct vision. Hemorrhage may be exacerbated by clotting factor deficiencies or hemodilution, and fibrinolysis.[82] These defects should be treated as specifically as is feasible using either conventional studies (prothrombin time, partial thromboplastin time, bleeding time, fibrinogen, fibrin split product levels, and platelet count) or thromboelastography. At the University of Pittsburgh, a rapid infusion system designed to deliver prewarmed fluids or blood products at a rate of up to $1.5 \, l \cdot min^{-1}$ is routinely used (Fig. 52-3). Line pressure monitors, filters, air detectors, and fluid-level sensors are built into the device to minimize trauma to the blood and to prevent transfusion of air. Blood salvaging ("autotransfusion") systems, which collect and wash extravasated blood, are also used, provided that there is no active infection or malignancy.

Metabolic acidosis may accompany hypotension and persist in the absence of hepatic metabolic function. Sodium bicarbonate is used for treatment, although if acidosis is severe, THAM (tromethamine [tris(hydroxymethyl)aminomethane]) is an alternative that avoids hyperosmolar hypernatremia.[75] Oliguria is also common in this phase, and once prerenal causes are ruled out, aggressive treatment with osmotic or potent loop diuretics, as well as renal-dose dopamine ($2.5 \, mg \cdot kg^{-1} \cdot min^{-1}$), is begun.

The anhepatic stage begins when the native diseased liver is removed after transection of its blood supply (hepatic artery and portal vein) as well as occlusion of the suprahepatic and infrahepatic portions of the IVC. If large esophageal varices seem at high risk for rupturing during IVC clamping, a Sengstaken-Blakemore tube may be placed temporarily. To avoid drastic decreases in venous return and cardiac output, as well as venous congestion in the lower body, bowel, and kidneys, many centers use a venovenous bypass system.[83] The venovenous circuit drains blood from the portal and femoral veins and routes it extracorporeally to the axillary vein. A centrifugal pump propels blood through the circuit at a flow rate 20–50% of usual total systemic flow. The circuit makes use of heparin-bonded tubing, which at the flow rates typically used obviates the need for systemic heparinization. Although venous bypass may help to preserve renal function,[83] it may not improve overall morbidity and mortality[84] and can lead to venous air embolism[85] and thrombosis. The use of venous bypass can also prolong the procedure and contribute to heat loss.[86] Moreover, support of cardiac output with positive inotropes may still be required.

Removal of the native liver and implantation of the allograft usually require vigorous retraction near the diaphragm, decreasing respiratory compliance and causing atelectasis and hypoventilation. Adding PEEP and raising inspiratory pressures may help minimize these effects. Because of the lack of liver metabolic function during the anhepatic phase, citrate intoxication from rapid transfusion is a more likely possibility, and calcium must be infused to maintain the ionized calcium level above $1.0 \, mmol \cdot l^{-1}$. Calcium chloride is often chosen, but even in the absence of hepatic function, calcium gluconate has effectively treated ionized hypocalcemia.[87] Progressive hyperkalemia may be treated with an insulin infusion, despite the absence of liver, but metabolic acids, including lactate, remain largely uncleared during the anhepatic period.

The neohepatic or postreperfusion stage begins with reanastomoses of the major vascular structures. Before removal of all clamps, the allograft is flushed of air, debris, and preservative solution with blood released from the portal vein. Despite this, subsequent final unclamping can cause release of a large load of potassium and metabolic acids into the circulation.[88] Dysrhythmias, hypotension, and cardiac arrest may ensue, and the anesthesiologist should be prepared to treat the underlying

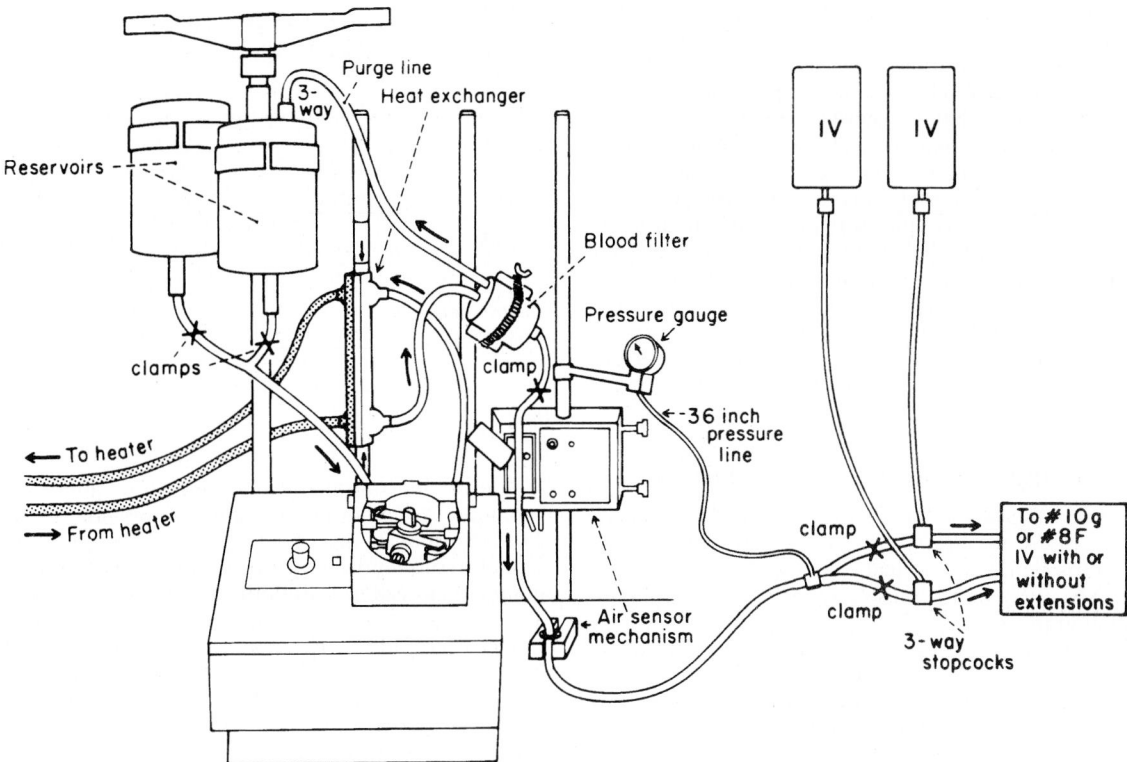

Figure 52-3. Rapid infusion system used during liver transplantation at the University of Pittsburgh. (Reprinted with permission from Kang YG, Martin DJ, Marquez J *et al:* Intraoperative changes in blood coagulation and thromboelastographic monitoring in liver transplantation. Anesth Analg 64:888, 1985.)

metabolic causes specifically. Inotropic support may be needed to treat hypotension stemming from myocardial depression by putative vasoactive mediators,[76] or right heart failure from venous air embolism.[89,90] Appearance of significant end-tidal nitrogen from venous air embolism by mass spectroscopy is useful to differentiate between these alternatives. Pulmonary thromboembolism has also been reported to be a cause of cardiovascular collapse during reperfusion.[90,91]

Once the allograft begins to function, hemodynamic and metabolic stability is gradually restored.[80] The need for inotropic support usually diminishes, and urine output improves even in patients with prior hepatorenal syndrome.[92] Clotting parameters can usually be normalized with specific replacement therapy, and fibrinolysis controlled with, ε-aminocaproate (Amicar). The procedure ends with some form of biliary reconstruction, either direct bile duct anastomosis or a Roux-en-Y choledochojejunostomy (Fig. 52-4).

Postoperative Management

In a well-functioning allograft, metabolic acids, including lactate, continue to be metabolized and systemic alkalosis may result. Meticulous postoperative pulmonary toilet is vital and may be complicated by injury to the diaphragm, nosocomial pneumonia, adult respiratory distress syndrome from massive transfusion, and weakness from nutritional deficiencies. Primary nonfunction of the allograft is now a rare complication of liver transplantation, perhaps because of the widespread use of UW solution for preservation. Recovery from primary nonfunction has occurred, but most often retransplantation has been necessary.

The full immunosuppression regimen of cyclosporine or tacrolimus, azathioprine, and prednisone is begun in the early postoperative period, yet rejection episodes are still common and may be treated with the monoclonal antibody OKT3. Other

complications include biliary or vascular anastomotic leaks, abdominal abscesses, and thrombosis of the hepatic artery or portal vein. As in other patients on long-term immunosuppression with cyclosporine, recipients are also at risk for development of lymphoproliferative malignancies and opportunistic infections (see Evaluation of Patients With a Prior Organ Transplant). Cases of transplantation for hepatitis B or neoplasms may also be complicated by recurrence of the original disease.[93]

HEART TRANSPLANTATION

It is estimated that as many as 14,000 patients per year in the United States alone could benefit from heart transplantation.[94]

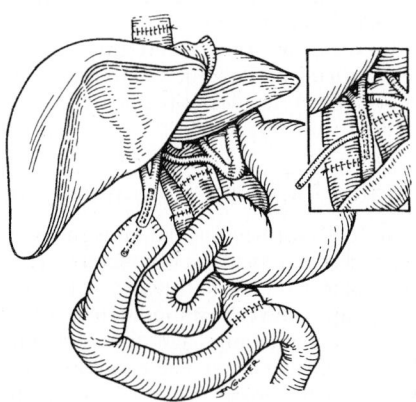

Figure 52-4. Biliary reconstruction after orthotopic liver transplantation. Biliary drainage can be accomplished via a Roux-en-Y (choledochojejunostomy) or "duct-to-duct" anastomosis (*inset*). (Reprinted with permission from Starzl TE, Demetris AJ, van Thiel DH: Liver transplantation. N Engl J Med 321:1014, 1092, 1989.)

However, after rapid growth in the mid-1980s, the number of heart transplantations per year has now reached a plateau of approximately 3000 cases worldwide because of the limited availability of donor organs. The orthotopic procedure has accounted for the overwhelming majority of cases.[95]

Growth in heart transplantation has been encouraged by dramatic increases in survival. Before the introduction of cyclosporine, the 1-year survival rate was approximately 40%. In the 1990s, cyclosporine, coupled with intensive immunologic surveillance by endomyocardial biopsy and aggressive antirejection treatment with lymphocyte-specific monoclonal antibodies, has boosted overall survival rates of orthotopic transplant recipients worldwide to >80% at 1 year, and >70% at 5 years.[95] Individual centers have reported survival rates to be as high as 90% at 4 years.[96] Other outcome variables, such as patients' quality of life, are favorable as well.

Pathophysiology of End-Stage Heart Disease

End-stage heart disease may result from either congenital or acquired diseases of the heart or vascular system. The leading causes include ischemic and valvular disease and primary cardiomyopathy. Depending on the cause, a varying period of physiologic adaptation precedes the onset of decompensation, which is usually manifested by congestive heart failure. Once this symptom is present, the overall 5-year survival rate is less than 50%, although patients with rapidly progressive symptoms seem even less likely to survive.[97] Dysrhythmias and laboratory evidence of pump failure (e.g., low ejection fraction) are also associated with a relatively poorer prognosis.

As the left ventricle fails, the main compensatory mechanism is an increase in left ventricular end diastolic volume, which enhances resting myocardial fiber length and promotes more effective fiber shortening. Such changes restore stroke volume, at the cost of increasing left atrial pressure and producing pulmonary venous congestion. Other compensations include elevation in catecholamines and increased renin production, resulting in salt and water retention.

Progression of the underlying pathophysiologic process eventually reduces ejection fraction and results in severe congestive heart failure refractory to conventional drug therapy. At this point, some patients may still be ambulatory but have little functional reserve; others are not ambulatory because of dyspnea or dependence on iv inotropes, mechanical circulatory support, or mechanical ventilation. Protracted periods of low cardiac output compromise other vital organ functions (e.g., passive congestion of the liver and prerenal azotemia) and may culminate in inadequate perfusion to the heart itself, initiating a final, irreversible downward spiral. Patients may enter a transplant program during any of these stages, or even after mechanical circulatory support with an intra-aortic balloon or ventricular assist device becomes necessary. Interestingly, survival rates remain relatively high in patients requiring mechanical circulatory support as a bridge to transplantation,[98] even in those receiving a temporary artificial heart.[99]

Specific Indications and Contraindications

The indication for heart transplantation is fulfilled when New York Heart Association Class IV status (severely compromised) and prognosis (guarded despite therapy) persist despite maximal medical therapy. The typical candidate is a 40–60-year-old man with a pretransplantation diagnosis of ischemic cardiomyopathy and left ventricular ejection fraction of <20%. The other common diagnoses are idiopathic cardiomyopathy and viral cardiomyopathy, and end-stage congenital heart disease accounts for the remainder. In the latter group, the congenital defect is often associated with a cardiomyopathy secondary to long-standing cyanosis or myocardial hypertrophy, making further palliation impossible.[100]

Table 52-11. PATHOPHYSIOLOGIC CONSEQUENCES OF DILATED CARDIOMYOPATHY

Organ System	Consequence
Pulmonary	Pulmonary venous congestion
	Interstitial edema
Renal	Prerenal azotemia
	Oliguria
Hepatic	Chronic passive congestion
	Hepatomegaly
	Ascites
Central nervous	Confusion (low cardiac output)
Endocrine	Elevated serum catecholamines
	Elevated renin levels

The list of contraindications has undergone considerable evolution in the last decade and will probably continue to do so. For example, the upper age limit was formerly 50 years. However, substantial numbers of older patients have now undergone this procedure without disproportionate morbidity, and, as a consequence, "physiologic" rather than chronologic age is now emphasized when deciding on candidacy. Diabetes mellitus had also been an absolute contraindication; however, it now seems that even insulin-dependent diabetic patients can be successfully immunosuppressed without the aid of steroids, and short-term results seem favorable. A history of cancer was once an absolute contraindication as well, but strict exclusion on this basis became obsolete as true long-term cures for certain malignancies (e.g., Hodgkin's lymphoma) were demonstrated. The presence of certain systemic diseases may also contraindicate heart transplantation; for example, the cardiomyopathy accompanying sarcoidosis could respond to medical therapy, and amyloidosis might recur in the donor organ.

Severe, irreversible pulmonary hypertension remains one of the few absolute contraindications to orthotopic heart transplantation because the right ventricle of a normal donor heart is unable acutely to cope with a markedly elevated, fixed pulmonary vascular resistance and rapidly decompensates.[101] The precise level of pulmonary hypertension deemed unacceptable is still a matter of debate: the traditional values are 6–8 Wood units (6–8 mm Hg [$1 \cdot min^{-1}$], or in metric resistance units, 480–640 dyne $\cdot s^{-1} \cdot cm^{-5}$), or a transpulmonary gradient (mean pulmonary artery pressure—mean pulmonary capillary wedge pressure) of 10–15 mm Hg. If irreversible pulmonary hypertension is present, heterotopic heart transplantation is one option, although more recently, as long as suitable organs are available, heart–lung transplantation is preferred.

Preanesthetic Considerations

Given the candidacy criteria, the recipient's other vital organs are usually not seriously impaired. However, low cardiac output may lead to chronic passive liver congestion and oliguria, and there may be corresponding physical signs and abnormal laboratory values (Table 52-11).

Candidates for heart transplantation are usually maintained on oral or iv inotropes (e.g., digoxin, amrinone), vasodilators (captopril, amrinone), and diuretics, and, when appropriate, antidysrhythmics. Patients with large, dilated hearts and low cardiac output are prone to form intracardiac thrombi and therefore are anticoagulated with warfarin. In such cases, fresh-frozen plasma is required after cardiopulmonary bypass, and appropriate arrangements should be made before induction. Blood products should be CMV free for patients without antibody evidence of prior exposure, considering the likelihood and morbidity of CMV sepsis in immunosuppressed recipients.[102] Bacterial pneumonia is relatively common early after heart transplantation,[103] so preparation of the anesthesia machine with a fresh, sterile breathing circuit and bacterial filter seems prudent. It has not been found necessary to sterilize tracheal intubation equipment, although at most institutions, factory-sterilized disposable endotracheal tubes are standard.

Some transplantation candidates have previously undergone coronary bypass or other thoracic or mediastinal procedures. If so, they are likely to require more than the usual time for insertion of vascular catheters and cannulation for cardiopulmonary bypass. To avoid unnecessary prolongation of donor organ ischemic times, the surgical and anesthesia teams must factor in these potential sources of delay.

Donor Procedure and Related Considerations

Cardiac harvesting is best done simultaneously with the harvesting of abdominal viscera. This approach, which involves local perfusion with preservative solutions after cross-clamping the abdominal and thoracic aortae, avoids inadvertent cardiac arrest before cardiectomy and damage to the allograft. Donor cardiectomy begins with pericardiotomy; after which the epicardial coronary arteries are grossly palpated for plaques. The aorta and both venae cavae are dissected, and after systemic heparinization, the superior vena cava is ligated and the IVC and a pulmonary vein are transected. The heart is then exsanguinated, and cardioplegia is administered through the aortic root. After cardiac arrest the aorta is cross-clamped, the heart is topically cooled, and the remaining pulmonary veins are individually transected. Finally, the great arteries are divided, and the heart is rinsed and examined for a patent foramen ovale or valvular lesions and then placed in a sterile plastic bag containing cold saline, which, in turn, is placed inside an insulated cooler. In laboratory studies, hearts have been preserved for as long as 24 hours with excellent subsequent graft function. Currently, however, the generally accepted limit on human donor heart ischemic time (measured from the time the cross-clamp is applied, to the time of cross-clamp removal after implantation) is 4–6 hours.[25,104] In view of this limited duration, the only immunologic matching performed prospectively is ABO compatibility.

Cardiac trauma, cardiac arrest, hypoxemia, and excessive requirement for exogenous catecholamines may render a potential donor's heart unacceptable for transplantation. However, as long as there is echocardiographic evidence of good contractility, such criteria do not necessarily mandate exclusion.[105] In most transplantation centers, there is no absolute age limit for eligibility as a heart donor, but in donors older than 40 years, careful physical examination at the time of harvest is essential to avoid transplanting organs with significant coronary lesions.

Anesthesia Induction

Candidates are often on the transplant list for extended periods and build up considerable apprehension. Despite this, preoperative sedation must be used judiciously because residual cardiac performance depends on elevated endogenous catecholamines. The monitoring regimen used by most heart transplantation centers includes intra-arterial and pulmonary artery pressure monitoring. Although avoidance of sepsis is important, conventional aseptic techniques for catheter insertions have proved to be sufficient.[106] At the University of Pittsburgh, pulmonary artery catheterization is routinely performed through the right internal jugular vein and does not seem to jeopardize access for future endomyocardial biopsies. Correct pulmonary artery catheter positioning is often more difficult in this population owing to severe orthopnea (necessitating a semisitting position), cardiac dilatation (promoting intraventricular coiling), tricuspid regurgitation, atrial fibrillation or other arrhythmias, or congenital vascular anomaly. Once the catheter is placed, a long, sterile

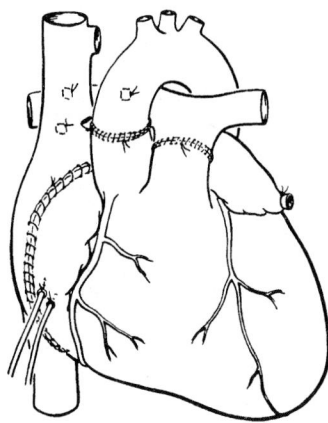

Figure 52-5. Sites of anastomoses after the mid-atrial excision orthotopic cardiac transplantation procedure. (Reprinted with permission from Reitz BA, Fowles RE, Ream AK: Cardiac transplantation. In Ream AK, Fogdall RP [eds]: Acute Cardiovascular Management, p 549. Philadelphia, JB Lippincott, 1982.)

sheath is always used because this catheter is pulled back to "central venous pressure position" before caval cannulation.

Whether already in the hospital or newly admitted through the emergency department, most of these patients have recently eaten and thus require rapid inductions. There have been numerous descriptions of anesthetic techniques under these circumstances,[107–109] all based on agents compatible with the pathophysiology of end-stage heart disease. In one study of induction regimens, a combination of etomidate 0.3 mg · kg^{-1}, fentanyl 10 μg · kg^{-1}, and succinylcholine 1.5 mg · kg^{-1} iv was shown rapidly to produce adequate intubating conditions without significant cardiovascular depression.[110] Anesthesia can then be maintained using a regimen compatible with extremely poor ventricular function (*e.g.*, O$_2$–fentanyl 35–75 μg · kg^{-1} iv [total] + scopolamine 0.3 mg iv).

After induction, tracheal intubation is accomplished without specially sterilized laryngoscopy equipment, and broad-spectrum prophylactic antibiotics and the immunosuppressant azathioprine are infused. Patients with end-stage heart disease are often exquisitely sensitive to changes in preload or afterload; thus, hypotension may stem from relatively small degrees of hypovolemia or alterations in systemic vascular resistance. Because one or both ventricles are usually extremely noncompliant, filling pressures may not accurately reflect intracavitary volumes, so transesophageal echocardiography can be especially helpful in maintaining cardiovascular stability.

Surgery and Cardiopulmonary Bypass

In the prepump phase of the orthotopic procedure, manipulation of the heart is minimized to avoid dislodging any intracardiac thrombi. After individual cannulation of the venae cavae as well as the aorta, cardiopulmonary bypass is initiated and patients are cooled as for conventional cardiac procedures (26–30°C). During cooling the diseased heart is excised, leaving an atrial cuff containing the caval and pulmonary venous orifices and long remnants of the aorta and pulmonary artery. The donor heart's back wall (atrium) is trimmed appropriately, then anastomosed with the recipient's atrial remnant. Special care must be taken to keep the anterior wall of the donor heart cold even during posterior wall anastomosis because warming may contribute to poor right ventricular function later. The heart is then filled with cold saline to displace most of the air, the aorta is anastomosed, and after de-airing once again, the cross-clamp is removed (ending the ischemic time). Often electromechanical activity resumes spontaneously and, finally, the pulmonary artery anastomosis is completed (Fig. 52-5). A more

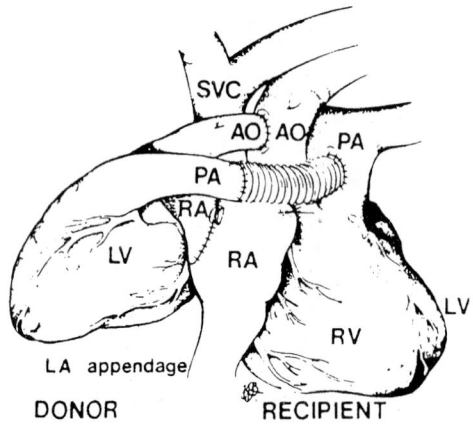

Figure 52-6. Heterotopic transplantation of a donor heart. Abbreviations are standard. (Reprinted with permission from Cooper DKC, Lanza LP: Heart Transplantation: The Present Status of Orthotopic and Heterotopic Heart Transplantation. Lancaster, United Kingdom MTP Press, 1984.)

recently introduced variation, the complete atrioventricular heart transplantation operation, involves bicaval anastomoses with preservation of the entire donor atria. The principal advantage seems to be a lower prevalence of tricuspid regurgitation.[111]

For the heterotopic procedure (Fig. 52-6), after sternotomy, a right pleuropericardial flap is created. When cardiopulmonary bypass is initiated, the native heart undergoes cardioplegic arrest for myocardial protection, and the donor heart is placed in the right thorax anterior to the compressed lung. The donor and recipient superior venae cavae and right atria are incised and sutured together, and the donor's aorta is sutured end-to-side to the recipient's ascending aorta. The donor's pulmonary artery is then connected to the recipient's main pulmonary artery by means of a Dacron graft.

Because many patients with end-stage heart disease are maintained on diuretics, mannitol or furosemide may be necessary to maintain a urine flow. In some cases, these patients may have markedly expanded blood volumes and benefit from hemoconcentration on bypass. At many centers, just before release of the aortic cross-clamp, to reduce the possibility of hyperacute immune response, methylprednisolone 500–1000 mg iv is administered. Immediately after release of the aortic cross-clamp, slow junctional rhythms or arteriovenous nodal dysfunction is relatively common. An infusion of either isoproterenol or another catecholamine with positive chronotropic effects is often begun temporarily to support heart rate. Most of these dysrhythmias resolve, but a small percentage do persist after surgery, even in the absence of rejection. Ultimately, approximately 5% of recipients require implantation of a permanent pacemaker, although the balance of survivors do not seem particularly prone to other serious dysrhythmias.

Immediately before weaning from cardiopulmonary bypass, the posterior anastomosis is rechecked because leaks in this area are difficult to repair later. After final de-airing, the superior vena caval cannula is removed, the pulmonary artery catheter advanced and repositioned, and the serum ionized calcium restored to normal. If heart rate is less than 60–70 beats · min[-1], epicardial electrodes are placed and pacing is begun.

Cardiac performance is often mildly compromised immediately after heart transplantation, and many transplantation centers routinely use inotropic infusions to wean patients from cardiopulmonary bypass. Although there have been reports of exaggerated effects, in practice, responses to catecholamine infusions seem qualitatively similar to those in other cardiac surgical patients.[112] Further discussion of the physiology and pharmacology of cardiac denervation is found in Evaluation of the Patient With a Prior Organ Transplant.

Markedly elevated pulmonary vascular resistance is a contraindication to orthotopic transplantation, but transient pulmonary vasospasm can occur during weaning, even in patients with previously normal pulmonary artery pressures, producing life-threatening right heart failure. Prostaglandin E_1 (PGE_1), at infusion rates of between 0.025 and 0.2 mg · kg[-1] · min[-1], has been shown effectively to unload the right heart,[113] although simultaneous norepinephrine or phenylephrine infusion may be required to support systemic vascular resistance. Elevated pulmonary vascular resistance often falls within hours of the procedure,[114] allowing PGE_1 infusions to be discontinued, but as a last resort, mechanical right ventricular assist has been used for varying periods with success.[115]

Postoperative Management

The short-term management goals in the intensive care unit include cardiovascular support and prevention of rejection and infection.[103] Most patients receive triple immunosuppression (cyclosporine–azathioprine–prednisone)[95] and, at some centers, OKT3. The sources of fever or pulmonary infiltrates are sought aggressively. Early in the postoperative period, bacterial pneumonias with typical nosocomial organisms are encountered. Later, opportunistic infection with CMV, *Pneumocystis*, or *Legionella*[116] may occur, and transbronchoscopic brushing may be necessary to establish the etiology. There may be bradydysrhythmias or atrioventricular block in this period, with temporary pacing required. Persistently low cardiac output may result from rejection or from reperfusion injury, and endomyocardial biopsy may be the only means to establish the diagnosis.

Excessive mediastinal bleeding and coagulopathy may be encountered in patients who had previously undergone a cardiac surgical procedure, and are treated in the conventional fashion. If hemodynamic stability is maintained, evidence of mild organ compromise present before transplantation will gradually disappear. If, however, the transplanted heart functions poorly, organs with preoperative impairment may rapidly decompensate.

HEART–LUNG TRANSPLANTATION

Heart–lung transplantation is the procedure of choice for patients with end-stage lung disease complicated by irreversible right ventricular failure, or end-stage congenital heart disease with secondary pulmonary vascular involvement (Eisenmenger's syndrome). Specific pathologic diagnoses in recipients have included primary pulmonary hypertension, emphysema, multiple pulmonary emboli, cystic fibrosis, and granulomatous and fibrotic diseases of the lung. Suitable donor blocs are in extremely short supply because both the lungs and heart must fulfill the criteria for acceptability (see Other Viscera Transplantation Procedures). Such blocs consist of the entire heart and lungs, including a tracheal segment long enough to facilitate anastomosis. Distal procurement is made feasible by flushing the harvested bloc with modified Euro-Collins or UW solution, to which PGE_1 or other pulmonary vasodilators may be added.

Considerations for monitoring and induction of anesthesia are in general similar to those for heart transplantation, but air trapping during ventilation and pulmonary hypertension are additional factors that may lead to hemodynamic instability. Difficulty with the airway during induction can result in hypercarbia or hypoxia and further elevate pulmonary vascular resistance. Patients with congenital heart disease may have bidirectional intracardiac shunts, which can become predominantly right-to-left and lead to profound hypoxemia. Such shunts may also lead to paradoxical air emboli, so bubbles in iv tubing should be scrupulously avoided. Chronically cyanotic patients are often severely polycythemic (hematocrit >60%) and manifest clotting derangements. Under these circumstances, phlebotomy and hemodilution are beneficial. In all recipients, large-sized endotracheal tubes are preferred to facilitate therapeutic bronchoscopies.

In the prebypass phase, surgical dissections may be complicated by extensive pleural adhesions; however, once on bypass, *en bloc* implantation is relatively straightforward and accomplished by sequential tracheal (or bibronchial), right atrial, and aortic anastomoses. The phrenic, vagus, and recurrent laryngeal nerves may be damaged by both dissection and topical cooling, and must be protected. The tracheal anastomosis usually involves some technique to prevent dehiscence, such as a "telescope" anastomosis or wrapping the suture line with vascularized omentum. Re-expansion of transplanted lungs may require bronchoscopy to relieve mechanical obstruction by secretions; occasionally, bronchodilators are useful to treat bronchospasm. Because of the extensive mediastinal and pleural dissection, the early postbypass period may be complicated by hemorrhage leading to coagulopathy. Pulmonary compliance and gas exchange may deteriorate during this time because of pulmonary hemorrhage or inadequate preservation, and the use of PEEP is often required.

After surgery, rejection episodes are relatively common and are characterized by infiltrates, fever, and deteriorating gas exchange. Pulmonary allografts may be rejected without significant abnormalities in endomyocardial specimens,[117] so low cardiac output is not necessarily a symptom of rejection. Recipients are also highly susceptible to bacterial pneumonia, which presents with the same clinical picture as rejection; bronchoalveolar lavage or transbronchial biopsy may be necessary for definitive diagnosis. A dreaded problem soon after heart–lung transplantation is dehiscence of the tracheal or bronchial suture lines, which can lead to fatal mediastinitis. Later, bronchiolitis obliterans develops in a significant proportion of survivors. The etiology is unknown, but this condition is associated with a progressive decline in exercise tolerance. Bronchiolitis obliterans and the physiology of transplanted lungs are discussed further in Other Viscera Transplantation Procedures.

In the future, heart–lung transplantation will probably have even fewer indications, as experience with isolated lung transplantation accumulates. The latter operation will then be used in patients with end-stage lung disease before right ventricular failure becomes irreversible and necessitates the combined heart–lung procedure.

LUNG TRANSPLANTATION

End-stage lung disease from destruction of the pulmonary parenchyma or vasculature is a leading cause of disability and death among adults. Several lung transplantation operations have been developed to treat end-stage lung disease, each having certain conceptual and practical advantages. These include the heart–lung, *en bloc* double-lung, single-lung, and bilateral sequential single-lung procedures. In the setting of chronically elevated pulmonary vascular resistance with right ventricular failure, heart–lung transplantation usually is chosen. However, when cardiac performance is preserved, isolated lung transplantation has been shown to be of benefit to carefully selected patients with end-stage lung disease[118] (Table 52-12).

End-stage pulmonary parenchymal diseases are either restrictive, obstructive, or infectious. Briefly, restrictive lung diseases are characterized by interstitial fibrosis with a loss of lung elasticity and compliance. Most fibrotic diseases are idiopathic, but they may also be caused by an inhalation injury or immune process. Interstitial lung disease may affect the blood vessels as well, so pulmonary hypertension is often found. Functionally, diseases in this category are associated with diminished lung volumes and diffusion capacity, but preserved air flow rates. Respiratory muscle strength is usually excellent because the work of breathing is chronically elevated. The most common cause of end-stage obstructive lung disease is smoking-induced emphysema, but other causes include asthma and several com-

Table 52-12. PATHOLOGIC DIAGNOSES IN LUNG TRANSPLANT RECIPIENTS*

Diagnosis	No.
Chronic obstructive pulmonary disease	20
α_1-Antitrypsin deficiency	19
Cystic fibrosis	8
Pulmonary hypertension	8
Pulmonary fibrosis	7
Bronchiectasis	2
Eosinophilic granuloma	1
Lymphangiomyomatosis	1

* Data derived from 66 consecutive patients who underwent lung transplantation at Barnes Hospital, St Louis, between July 1988 and January 1991.
Adapted with permission from Trulock EP, Cooper JD, Kaiser LR *et al:* The Washington University–Barnes Hospital experience with lung transplantation. JAMA 266:1943, 1991.

paratively rare congenital disorders. Among these, α_1-antitrypsin deficiency is associated with severe bullous emphysema in the fourth or fifth decade of life. With obstructive diseases, airway resistance is elevated, expiratory flow rates are diminished, air trapping may be prominent, and ventilation–perfusion mismatching severe. The common infectious etiologies of end-stage lung disease include cystic fibrosis and bronchiectasis. Cystic fibrosis, which occurs in 1 of every 2000 live births in the United States, produces mucus plugging of peripheral airways, chronic bronchitis, and bronchiectasis. Smoking and environmental exposures may also lead to bronchiectasis. End-stage pulmonary vascular disease may be a consequence of primary pulmonary hypertension, which is a relatively rare disease of unknown etiology characterized by marked elevation of pulmonary vascular resistance from hyperplasia of the muscular pulmonary arteries and fibrosis of smaller arterioles. Congenital heart disease with Eisenmenger's syndrome, and diffuse arteriovenous malformations, are other causes of destruction of the pulmonary arterial bed.

The general indications for transplantation with any of the end-stage lung diseases are progressive exercise intolerance, increasing oxygen requirements, and carbon dioxide retention. Other factors favoring the transplantation option are recurrent need for phlebotomy and increasing physical and social debilitation. The timing of surgery depends on the rate of functional deterioration and ability of the right ventricle to tolerate the progression of pulmonary hypertension. Considering the limited supply of donor organs, specific contraindications to lung transplantation include severe debilitation, neuromuscular disease, or mechanical ventilator dependence (because respiratory muscle strength is crucial to recovery); severe chest deformity or pleural disease (complicating surgical procedures and postoperative ventilation); advanced right ventricular failure; or glucocorticoid dependence (because healing of airway anastomoses is impeded by steroids).

The choice of lung transplantation procedure is based largely on the consequences of leaving the native lung *in situ*. For example, single-lung transplantation is not an option if infection or severe bullous emphysema is present in the contralateral lung. Infection would cross-contaminate the healthy transplanted lung, and severe bullous disease in the native lung could lead to gross ventilation–perfusion mismatching and shifting of the mediastinum. Instead, double-lung transplantation would be chosen for such cases. Similarly, double-lung transplantation may also lead to better functional outcomes in the treatment of end-stage pulmonary hypertension.[118,119] The other major factor influencing the choice of procedure is the relative rate of perioperative complications. For example, single-lung transplantation is feasible without cardiopulmonary bypass and is seldom complicated by bleeding diatheses. In contrast, *en bloc* double-lung transplantation mandates cardiopulmonary bypass with full systemic heparinization and extensive mediastinal dissection—both risk factors for development of postoperative coagulation defects. Another advantage of single-lung transplantation is that it makes use of bronchial anastomoses, which heal with significantly fewer complications than the tracheal repairs typical of the *en bloc* double-lung procedure. Bilateral sequential lung transplantation, an alternative to *en bloc* double-lung transplantation, combines advantages by using bibronchial anastomoses and avoiding cardiopulmonary bypass.

Donor Lungs

Donor lungs may be jeopardized by massive fluid resuscitation, aspiration, contusion, and exposure to nonphysiologic oxygen tensions because most organ donors are trauma victims. Ideally, the donor's history should indicate early tracheal intubation with no evidence of aspiration, minimal fluid administration in the course of resuscitation, and absence of chest tubes, pleural diseases, or tracheostomy at any time. Suitable donors should have a minimal alveolar–arterial O_2 gradient (*i.e.*, a Pao_2 of >400 mm Hg while breathing 100% O_2, or 100 mm Hg on 40% $O_2/5$ cm H_2O PEEP), as well as a clear chest radiograph and sputum examination within 2 hours of harvesting.[120] If bronchoscopy fails to elucidate any pathologic process, iv glucocorticoids and antibiotics are administered and the lungs harvested. Because both the heart and lungs may be harvested from the same donor, a method has been developed for cardiectomy without jeopardizing the use of the lungs.[121] First, the heart is removed, but a cuff of left atrium is left attached to the donor lungs. The trachea is then stapled and divided at its midpoint, and the lungs removed *en bloc* and immersed in cold preservative solution. In some centers, before removal, the donor is treated with a pulmonary vasodilator (*e.g.*, PGE_1) to improve the distribution of a large volume of either a blood-based or intracellular-type cold crystalloid preservative solution, infused through the pulmonary artery. Finally, the lungs may be inflated before immersion in preservative solution and stored for transportation.

Preanesthetic Considerations

Preanesthetic considerations for lung recipients have been described.[122-125] Briefly, size matching is achieved by comparing the vertical and transverse radiologic chest dimensions of the donor and recipient. Organs are also matched on the basis of ABO compatibility, but because the need for histocompatibility is still unknown and the tolerable ischemic time for the lung is relatively short (approximately 4 hours), HLA matching is done only in retrospect. Preoperative pulmonary function and right heart catheterization studies, ventilation–perfusion scans, and arterial blood gas values are helpful to predict the difficulties likely to be encountered during and after induction. For example, diminished expiratory flow rates and air trapping may exacerbate hypoxemia and hypercapnia and lead to hemodynamic instability during mask ventilation and after tracheal intubation. Elevated pulmonary artery pressures may indicate a likelihood that cardiopulmonary bypass will be necessary because right ventricular failure can suddenly result when one-lung ventilation or ligation of a pulmonary artery is begun. Even in the absence of pulmonary hypertension, many centers recommend "pump standby" for these cases because gas exchange is so precarious. Clearly, both systemic and pulmonary arterial pressure monitoring are vital during lung transplantation procedures, although profound dyspnea may make internal jugular cannulation difficult before induction. Pulmonary artery catheters should be inserted through a sterile sleeve to allow withdrawal during the anastomosis and subsequent repositioning. Finally, candidates may have recently undergone weaning from glucocorticoids, but "stress doses" are avoided in the perioperative period to protect from systemic sepsis or suture line dehiscence.

Single-Lung Transplantation

The single-lung transplantation procedure involves pneumonectomy and implantation of a new lung, sometimes preceded by mobilization of omentum with its vascular pedicle for bronchial wrapping. If the native lungs are equally impaired and no pleural scarring is present, the left lung is often chosen for transplantation for technical reasons: the native right pulmonary veins are less accessible than those on the left, the recipient's left bronchus is longer, and the left hemithorax can more easily accommodate a somewhat oversized donor lung. Most surgeons prefer that the lung to be removed is collapsed during dissection; both bronchial blockers and double-lumen endobronchial tubes have been used for this purpose. Because the right upper lobe bronchial orifice is relatively close to the origin of the mainstem bronchus, left-sided endobronchial double-lumen tubes have been recommended for both right and left single-lung transplants as well as for the bilateral sequential operation.

For the induction of anesthesia by the rapid-sequence technique, drugs that do not release histamine or depress the myocardium are usually preferred (*e.g.*, etomidate, vecuronium). Nitrous oxide is avoided in patients with bullae or elevated pulmonary vascular resistance and when 100% oxygen is needed to maintain acceptable arterial saturation. Both high-dose opioids and potent inhaled agents, supplemented with long-acting relaxants, have been used successfully for the maintenance of anesthesia. With the onset of one-lung ventilation, acute deterioration in gas exchange or hemodynamics is the rule. Strategies for improving oxygenation under these circumstances, discussed in detail in Chapter 30, include the use of PEEP in the dependent lung, continuous positive airway pressure or high-frequency ventilation in the nondependent lung, or ligation of the (nondependent) pulmonary artery. If pulmonary artery pressures rise sharply at this point, right ventricular failure may ensue. Vasodilators or inotropes may diminish right heart strain; if not, one-lung ventilation should be abandoned. Similarly, if hemodynamics or systemic arterial saturations deteriorate when the pulmonary artery is clamped in anticipation of pneumonectomy, cardiopulmonary bypass may be necessary.

Immediately before implantation, the donor lung is trimmed to match the size of the recipient bronchus, branch pulmonary artery, and atrial cuff containing the orifices of the pulmonary veins. While attempting to keep the allograft cold, the atrial, pulmonary artery, and bronchial anastomoses are completed in sequence. The circulation is then restored to the donor lung, ending the ischemic interval, but until ventilation to the allograft is restarted, systemic arterial saturation suffers. Flexible bronchoscopy is prudent at this stage to visualize the anastomosis directly or reinflate the allograft by removing secretions or blood from the airway. Once the anastomosis is secure, a pedicle of omentum with its blood supply intact may be brought into the chest and wrapped around the bronchial anastomosis. Finally, after the chest is closed, the supine position can be restored and the endobronchial tube exchanged for a standard endotracheal type (except if "split" ventilation is planned).

Double-Lung Transplantation

Double-lung transplantation is most often used in patients with primary pulmonary hypertension or cystic fibrosis. The *en bloc* operation is performed in the supine position, and because both lungs are replaced at once, cardiopulmonary bypass is mandatory. Cardioplegic arrest is used to accomplish anastomosis of the left atrial cuff containing all four pulmonary venous orifices. The airway is typically interrupted at the level of the

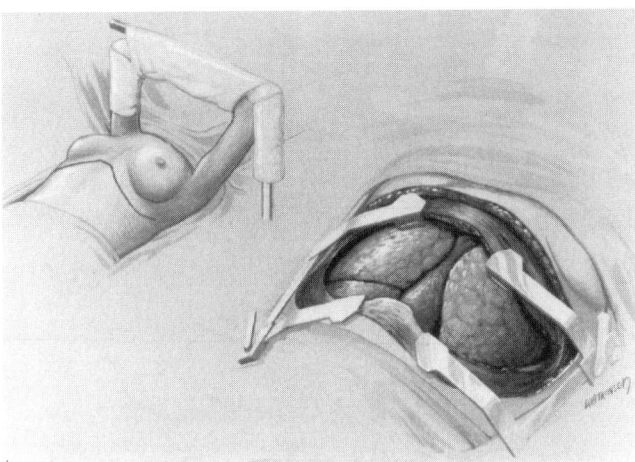

Figure 52-7. Positioning and surgical approach for bilateral sequential lung transplantation. The incision consists of bilateral anterior thoracotomies with a transverse sternotomy. After insertion of vascular catheters, the patient's arms are wrapped and suspended from the ether screen. (Reprinted with permission from Cooper JD, Patterson GA: Isolated lung transplantation. In Kapoor AS, Laks H, Schroeder JS et al [eds]: Cardiomyopathies and Heart–Lung Transplantation, p 429. New York, McGraw-Hill, 1991.)

trachea, so a standard endotracheal tube is suitable. Because systemic arterial supply to the trachea is permanently interrupted, an omental wrap may be added. The extensive retrocardiac dissection required often leads to cardiac denervation and postoperative bleeding that is difficult to control.[126]

Bilateral sequential single-lung transplantation was introduced to treat the same spectrum of patients as the *en bloc* procedure but obviates the need for cardiopulmonary bypass and tracheal anastomosis. Access to the hilar structures is gained in the supine position through a rather extensive incision that includes a transverse sternotomy ("clamshell" incision; Fig. 52-7). Another relative disadvantage is that serial implantation results in a longer ischemic time for the second allograft.

Postoperative Management

Postoperative management of patients after isolated lung transplantation involves intensive respiratory support and differentiating between lung infection and rejection using transbronchial biopsies obtained by flexible bronchoscopy.[127] Early respiratory insufficiency may be due to pulmonary venous (anastomotic) obstruction or reperfusion injury, which is characterized by large alveolar–arterial oxygen gradients, poor pulmonary compliance, and parenchymal infiltrates despite low cardiac filling pressures. Mechanical ventilation with PEEP is essential, but in consideration of new airway anastomoses, inflation pressures are kept to a minimum. FIO_2 values are also maintained at the lowest levels compatible with acceptable oxygen saturation. After single-lung transplantation for an obstructive disease, the endobronchial tube may be left in place for several days, and special respiratory support in the form of split (individual lung) ventilation used to avoid overinflation of the native lung, gross ventilation–perfusion mismatching, and shifting of the mediastinum.[128]

The lung is unique among transplanted viscera because it is exposed to the external environment. Lymphatic disruption, poor mucociliary function, and the presence of suture lines across the airway are other factors increasing the susceptibility of transplanted lungs to infection. In the first postoperative month, bacteria are the most frequent cause of pneumonia; nosocomial gram-negative organisms comprise the bulk of isolates.[129] After this period, CMV pneumonitis becomes more common, particularly if lungs from a CMV-seropositive donor are used in a seronegative recipient.[120] There is a high rate of acute rejection episodes after lung transplantation, which on clinical grounds alone are often difficult to distinguish from infection. This distinction is vital, however, because steroid boluses used to treat rejection may worsen pneumonia or promote systemic sepsis. Bronchoalveolar lavage fluid or sputum specimens obtained by fiberoptic bronchoscopy may be helpful in diagnosing an infectious etiology; transbronchial or, occasionally, open lung biopsy is needed to establish the diagnosis of rejection.[127]

Hemorrhage is a complication that most frequently occurs after *en bloc* double-lung transplantation, particularly in patients with pleural disease or Eisenmenger's syndrome with extensive mediastinal vascular collaterals. The recurrent laryngeal, phrenic, and vagal nerves are jeopardized during lung transplantation, and injury complicates the process of weaning from mechanical ventilation. Primary healing occurs with most bronchial anastomoses; rarely, bronchial fistulae lead to stenoses that can be successfully treated by silicone stents and dilatation. In contrast, tracheal anastomotic leaks often lead to fatal mediastinitis. Long-term complications include lung infections with opportunistic organisms, such as *Pneumocystis carinii* and *Candida albicans*. Bronchiolitis obliterans, a pathologic condition characterized by luminal destruction of small respiratory bronchioles, has been noted after heart–lung transplantation,[130] but so far seems less common after single-lung transplantation.

Outcome results of lung transplantation series from specialized centers are promising. The Washington University Lung Transplantation Group[118] has reported on a series of 69 procedures and found the actuarial survival at 1 year to be 90% after single-lung transplantation and 82% after the bilateral sequential operation. Pulmonary function tests, pulmonary arterial pressure and resistance, arterial blood gases, and exercise capacities all improved significantly after operation. In an earlier analogous series from Toronto, there were no ventilatory limitations noted in lung transplantation survivors or significant desaturation during exercise testing.[119]

OTHER VISCERA TRANSPLANTATION PROCEDURES

There is considerable interest in transplantation of the pancreas and small intestine, particularly in view of the sizable patient populations that stand to benefit. These are relatively fragile viscera, and optimal preservation regimens and implantation procedures have yet to be defined.

Pancreas Transplantation

There are as many as 20,000 new cases of Type 1 (juvenile-onset, insulin-dependent) diabetes mellitus in the United States each year.[131] This disease destroys the insulin-producing pancreatic β cells by an inflammatory process. The microangiopathy that results from diabetes is among the leading causes of blindness and renal failure.

Pancreatic transplantation by surgical means was first attempted in the mid-1960s, and by 1989 the annual rate of such cases reported to the International Pancreas Transplantation Registry was 554.[132] At specialized centers, the operative mortality rate was low ($\leq$1%), the 1-year survival rate was at least 90%, and normoglycemia and insulin independence was achieved in 50–70% of cases at 1 year.[133] In many of these cases, patients received both kidney and pancreas allografts, which seemed to prevent the recurrence of diabetic nephropathy in the transplanted kidney[134] as well as some of the other microvascular complications.

Pancreatic transplantation is usually reserved for diabetic patients with the most severe and rapidly progressive complications in view of the considerable side effects of immunosuppression. Preoperative screening consists of thorough evaluation of the organ systems most affected by diabetes; metabolic studies, including a glucose tolerance test; and urine and serum C-peptide levels ("connecting" peptide is cleaved from proinsulin before secretion into the circulation); glycosylated hemoglobin levels (an index of glycemic control during preceding months); and insulin and islet cell antibodies. Ultrasonography of the gallbladder is conducted to rule out cholelithiasis. In addition to tight preoperative plasma glucose control, mechanical and antibiotic bowel preparation is usually undertaken.

Most pancreatic transplantations are accomplished using the bladder drainage technique. This involves extraperitoneal pancreatic placement and exocrine drainage by duodenocystostomy. After surgery, patients seldom require intensive care, although assiduous control of plasma glucose using an insulin infusion is recommended. Once oral feeding is resumed, insulin is unnecessary unless allograft function is lost. A major advantage of the bladder drainage technique is the ability to monitor allograft exocrine function, which deteriorates during episodes of rejection. Urinary *p*H may fall, reflecting a decrease in pancreatic bicarbonate secretion, and urinary amylase may diminish. Other postoperative complications include graft thrombosis and intra-abdominal infection.

Pancreatic islet transplantation, in which only the required cell type is introduced, has undergone numerous clinical trials.[135] In this procedure, which does not require surgical intervention, just the islets are isolated by cell separation techniques then infused into the portal vein. In some cases, islet cells may become fully functional over several weeks and restore insulin independence;[135] in others, insulin requirement has been reduced but not eliminated.

Multiviscera Transplantation

Simultaneous replacement of multiple digestive organs, known as the *cluster operation*, has been introduced to treat two diseases: short gut syndrome and locally confined GI tumors.[136] With short gut syndrome from any cause, parenteral feeding may lead to liver failure, and *en bloc* transplantation of the liver combined with the pancreas, stomach, duodenum, and jejunum (Fig. 52-8) has met with some success.[137] In children, multiviscera transplantation is performed primarily for short gut syndrome resulting from necrotizing enterocolitis or midgut volvulus.

Tumors such as hepatomas and cholangiocarcinomas, as well as carcinomas of the proximal GI tract or pancreas, have also been treated by cluster operation after upper abdominal exenteration. Without surgery, the prognosis for these cancers is uniformly dismal, and even partial resections combined with chemotherapy or radiation offer little improvement in overall survival. In contrast, although experience is still limited, multiviscera transplantation is associated with 1-year survival rates of 70% (with sarcomas or GI-derived neuroendocrine tumors) or 44% (primary liver cancers).[138]

Anesthetic management of cluster surgery has been reviewed in detail.[139] Briefly, the types and doses of previous chemotherapy should be ascertained during the preoperative visit because some agents have long-lasting toxic effects on the heart or kidneys. Hormone-secreting tumors, producing carcinoid crisis, can be suppressed with octreotide acetate, a somatostatin analogue; with ketanserin, a serotonin antagonist; or by arterial embolization. During surgery, the management issues are similar to those for liver transplantation alone, namely, massive transfusion, coagulopathies, hypothermia, electrolyte abnormalities, and the use of venovenous bypass for systemic venous return. Postoperative complications include a high incidence of rejection, particularly of the small bowel, sepsis from loss of the intestinal barrier, and graft-versus-host disease. The likelihood of graft-versus-host disease is proportional to the length of intestine transplanted, presumably reflecting the quantity of lymphoid tissue contained in the wall of this organ.

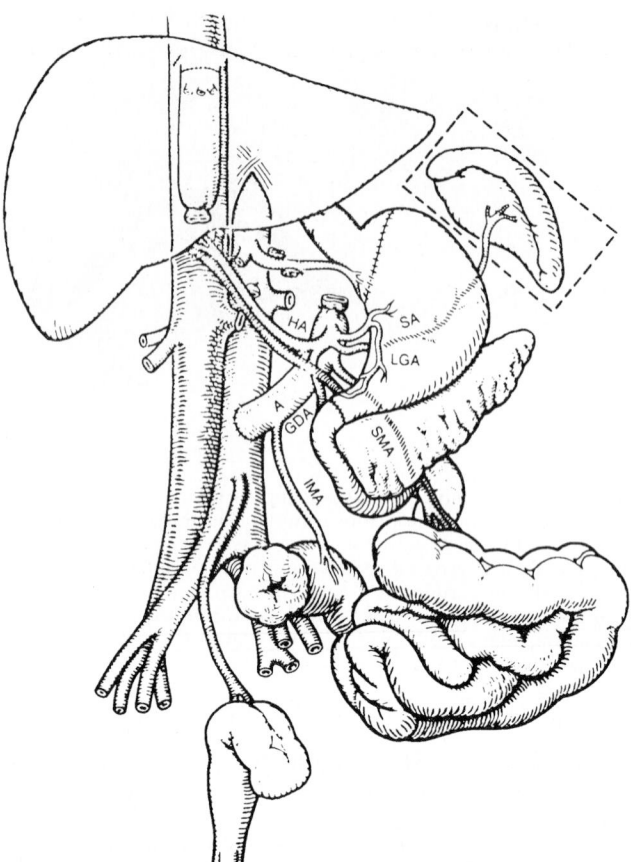

Figure 52-8. Schematic representation of the recipient procedure for multiviscera transplantation. (A = donor aorta; HA = hepatic artery; SA = splenic artery, LGA = left gastric artery; SMA = superior mesenteric artery; IMA = inferior mesenteric artery; GDA = gastroduodenal artery.) (Reprinted with permission from Starzl TE, Rowe MI, Todo S *et al:* Transplantation of multiple abdominal viscera. JAMA 261:1449, 1989.)

VISCERA TRANSPLANTATION IN CHILDREN

The clinical manifestations of end-stage organ disease in children are in general similar to those in adults; however, the pathologic processes leading to organ failure often differ. For example, the etiology of end-stage renal disease noted in the pediatric population (Table 52-13) differs markedly from that for the general population (see Table 52-6). During childhood, developmental anomalies and genetic defects, anatomic or functional (*i.e.*, inborn errors of metabolism), may lead to end-

Table 52-13. ETIOLOGY OF END-STAGE RENAL DISEASE IN CHILDREN

	Total Cases (%)
Urinary tract malformations	29
Chronic glomerulonephritis	24
Renal dysplasia/hypoplasia	23
Hereditary nephropathies	14
Miscellaneous	10

Adapted with permission from Turcotte JG, Campbell DA, Dafoe DC *et al:* Pediatric renal transplantation. In Cerilli GJ (ed): Organ Transplantation and Replacement, p 349. Philadelphia, JB Lippincott, 1988.

stage organ disease. Congenital anomalies may be confined to a single organ system (*e.g.*, reflux nephropathy) or be part of a constellation of abnormalities. For example, in Alagille's syndrome, end-stage liver disease is accompanied by congenital heart disease, hypercholesterolemia, and renal dysfunction. Clearly, awareness of such syndromes is necessary to anticipate coexistent pathologic processes in other organ systems.

Ethical Considerations

The ethics of transplantation are also somewhat different in the pediatric age group. The legally adopted criteria for brain death are not universally accepted as applicable in the immediate neonatal period,[140] so organ donation from this population is controversial. Size considerations place additional constraints on the organ-matching process in children, exacerbating the shortages. To remedy this, procedures for living-related donation have been developed for kidney transplantation, and, more recently, liver[141] and lung[142] transplantation. Although living-related renal transplantation has gained acceptance because of its particular benefits for children, the liver and lung procedures are more controversial owing to higher morbidity and mortality in the donors. Other ethical dilemmas, such as whether transplantation can provide truly long-term survival, and whether transplanted organs grow and develop normally in children, remain unresolved. In addition, long-term immunosuppression with cyclosporine increases the risk for development of a lymphoproliferative malignancy, perhaps related to Epstein-Barr virus infection or reactivation. Although the overall incidence is reasonably low, the shift to earlier presentation of aggressive malignancies raises new concerns.[143]

Renal Transplantation

Although pharmacologic agents combined with dialysis can be used to treat end-stage renal disease in children, medical management has an overall high morbidity rate and adversely affects growth and development.[144] Children treated medically during their maximum growth years show a marked decrease in eventual height and weight,[145] as well as cognitive development,[146] compared with control subjects. Early transplantation seems to reduce the severity of these problems,[147,148] justifying the current recommendation "expectantly" to transplant children with progressive renal insufficiency, sometimes even before dialysis is required.

The most common diseases leading to renal transplantation in children are related to congenital anomalies; acquired nephropathies and a group of miscellaneous diseases account for the remainder (Table 52-14). Living-related renal transplantation is most often done in children and confers significant advantages: both short- and long-term mortality rates are improved, and graft survival is superior,[149] perhaps because the risk of minor antigenic mismatch is reduced. Organ survival in children receiving a living-related donor kidney approaches 100% at 1 year and 70% at 10 years.[149] Because perioperative mortality and renal rejection are greater in infants, current practice is to avoid transplantation until later in childhood.

In contrast to adults, pediatric renal transplantation relies on intra-abdominal placement of the organ. This allows adult-sized kidneys to be transplanted into very small children and increases the size of the donor pool. During surgery, however, placement of the allograft can acutely cause hypothermia and sequester relatively large proportions of the child's blood volume. As a consequence, hypotension can occur when adequate perfusion is critical. To prevent this, fluid boluses and vasoactive infusions are used to maintain systemic blood pressure in the high-normal range. As in adults, living-related donor kidneys usually function at once, whereas cadaver kidneys may take hours to resume urine production. Fluid management must take this into account. In either case, adult kidneys initially

produce adult-sized volumes of urine, so maintenance fluids must be adjusted accordingly.

Liver Transplantation

Approximately 20% of the orthotopic liver transplantations performed worldwide are in children, and most recipients are younger than 5 years of age.[150] Biliary atresia is by far the most common cause of liver failure in this population (Table 52-15), followed by inborn errors of metabolism, which include disorders such as α_1-antitrypsin deficiency, glycogen storage diseases, Wilson's disease, and tyrosinemia. The latter three conditions primarily involve biochemical defects in hepatocytes and are therefore considered cured by liver transplantation.

Several aspects of the orthotopic liver transplantation procedure are unique to children. For example, patients with biliary atresia have usually undergone prior decompression with a Kasai (choledochojejunostomy) procedure, and this may complicate abdominal dissection during the preanhepatic phase of liver transplantation, as well as later biliary reconstruction. Venovenous bypass is not feasible in patients weighing <20 kg, so the lower body venous congestion that accompanies portal vein and IVC occlusion often leads to oliguria and intestinal complications in this group. An oversized allograft may sequester a substantial proportion of the blood volume, increase the risk of excessive potassium release after reperfusion, and lead to severe hypothermia. In children whose temperature falls below

Table 52-14. PATHOLOGIC DIAGNOSES IN PEDIATRIC RENAL TRANSPLANT RECIPIENTS AT THE UNIVERSITY OF MINNESOTA*

	Total Cases (%)
Obstructive uropathy	16.8
Renal hypoplasia	15.3
Glomerulonephritis	15.3
Congenital nephrotic syndrome	8.5
Steroid-resistant nephrotic syndrome	7.2
Medullary cystic disease	4.5
Pyelonephritis	4.1
Hemolytic–uremic syndrome	4.0
Alport's syndrome	2.6
Oxalosis	2.3
Miscellaneous, including unknown	19.4

* Data derived from a total of 531 cases performed betwen 1963 and 1990.
Adapted with permission from Belani K, Palahniuk R: Kidney transplantation. In Firestone L (ed): Anesthesia and Organ Transplantation, p 17. Boston, Little, Brown, 1991.

Table 52-15. PATHOLOGIC DIAGNOSES IN PEDIATRIC ORTHOTOPIC LIVER TRANSPLANT RECIPIENTS*

	Total Cases (%)
Biliary atresia	44
α_1-Antitrypsin deficiency	20
Other inborn errors of metabolism	10
Other obstructive disease (*e.g.*, Alagille's and Byler's syndromes)	12
Miscellaneous	14

* Data derived from 50 pediatric orthotopic liver transplant recipients at Children's Hospital of Pittsburgh between 1981 and 1983. Adapted with permission from Borland LM, Roule M, Cook DR: Anesthesia for pediatric orthotopic liver transplantation. Anesth Analg 64:117, 1985.

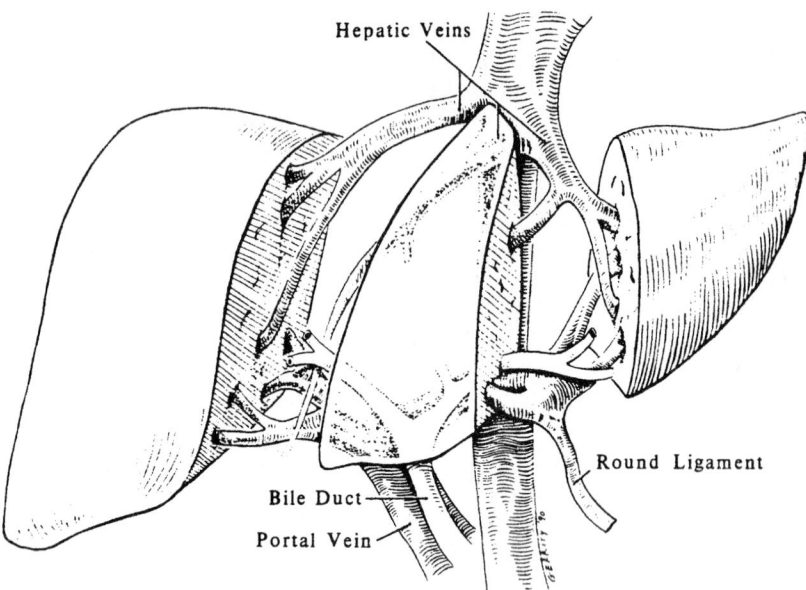

Figure 52-9. A schematic for *ex vivo* dissection of an adult liver to create reduced-size liver allografts with vascular supplies and biliary orifices. Donor iliac arteries or veins are used as needed to extend the vessels. (Adapted and reprinted with permission from Broelsch CE, Edmond JC, Whitington PF *et al:* Application of reduced-size liver transplants as split grafts, auxiliary orthotopic grafts, and living related segmental transplants. Ann Surg 212:368, 1990.)

34°C, lavage of the peritoneal cavity with warm saline is effective in raising core temperature.

The limited availability of suitably sized organs for small patients has prompted the development of techniques for transplanting part of a liver. Figure 52-9 illustrates the technique that is used to create a reduced-size ("split") liver and enable one donor liver to be used for multiple patients. There is a significantly higher complication rate with this method, including greater blood loss,[151] risk of organ necrosis, and diminished patient survival,[151,152] so it is usually reserved for patients who are rapidly deteriorating. Living-related (partial) liver donation has also been promoted by the contention that up to one half of pediatric liver transplantation candidates die while awaiting a suitable organ. However, in view of the potential for donor morbidity and the relatively reduced survival of recipients of reduced-size livers, few centers offer this option.

The overall 1-year survival rate in children after orthotopic liver transplantation is 70–75%, but results for younger (<3 years) and smaller (<12 kg) patients are not as good (45–50% 1-year survival rate).[150,152] This discrepancy probably stems from two factors: the greater incidence of hepatic artery thrombosis in small children, which in turn is related to arterial size, and the use of reduced-size livers.[141,153]

Heart Transplantation

Cardiac transplantation for congenital heart disease is the major indication for this procedure in children younger than 5 years of age.[154] In older children, dilated cardiomyopathy remains most common. However, mortality rates for the young children remain higher than for older children and adults (25% *vs.* 10% 30-day mortality, respectively),[154] which results in lower overall survival. Cardiac-related complications are responsible for most early deaths, stemming from the presence of complex vascular anatomy, previous cardiac surgery, and elevation of pulmonary vascular resistance. The latter factor is a well recognized contraindication to heart transplantation in adults, but it is often difficult accurately to quantify the "fixed" component of pulmonary vascular resistance in infants. If pulmonary vascular resistance is fixed at a high level, the normal allograft's right ventricle cannot acutely adjust to the afterload, and refractory right-heart failure ensues. Long-term survival may be limited by an accelerated form of coronary atherosclerosis,[155] as is seen in adults.

Generally accepted indications for heart transplantation in

newborns include aortic atresia and hypoplastic left heart syndrome. If reconstruction of the aortic arch is required, profound hypothermia and circulatory arrest are usually necessary. Positional or size discrepancies of the great vessels and abnormal arrangements of systemic or pulmonary venous return can complicate these procedures, and have so far limited overall survival rates for neonates to 66% at 1 year.[156]

A scientifically provocative aspect of transplantation unique to neonates is that the immature immune system seems relatively tolerant of foreign antigens.[157] By several criteria, the neonatal immune response to allograft tissue is attenuated, although the response to infective organisms and active immunization is comparatively intact. The mechanisms responsible are unclear but may involve neonatal suppressor cells or maternal cells that enter the circulation during gestation.

Other Viscera Transplantation Procedures

Rarely, heart–lung transplantation is indicated before early adulthood for cystic fibrosis, Eisenmenger's syndrome, or primary pulmonary hypertension.[158] Isolated lung transplantation may offer the only chance of survival to children with severe developmental anomalies of the lung, including cystadenomatous malformations and congenital diaphragmatic hernia with pulmonary hypoplasia or, in older children, cystic fibrosis. The scarcity of suitable donor organs has led to instances of living-related lung donation,[142] but the merits of this approach have yet to be fully evaluated.

Multiviscera transplantation, which combines liver and small bowel transplantation, has been tried in children with short gut syndrome (as a result of necrotizing enterocolitis or midgut volvulus) further complicated by hepatic failure after long-term hyperalimentation. So far, intra-abdominal infection and repeated episodes of bowel rejection have limited survival, and thus the approach is still considered experimental.

EVALUATION OF PATIENTS WITH A PRIOR ORGAN TRANSPLANT

Transplant recipients may return for a staged repair (*e.g.,* bile duct reconstruction after liver transplantation) or for entirely unrelated surgery. They may also present with a surgical illness superimposed on organ rejection, where the usual signs and symptoms are masked.

Immunosuppression increases the risk of opportunistic infec-

Table 52-16. IMMUNOSUPPRESSANT SIDE EFFECTS AND TOXICITIES

Agent	Side Effect/Toxicity
Glucocorticoids	Adrenal suppression
	Glucose intolerance
	Cushingoid appearance
	Integument fragility
	Aseptic necrosis
	Peptic ulceration
Azathioprine	Anemia
	Thrombocytopenia
	Leukopenia
	Pancreatitis
	Hepatitis
	Decrease nondepolarizing relaxant requirement
Cyclosporine, tacrolimus	Glomerulosclerosis (elevation of blood urea nitrogen, creatinine)
	Hypertension
	Hepatotoxicity
	Neurotoxicity
	Enhanced renal sensitivity to insults
Antilymphocyte globulin	Leukopenia
	Thrombocytopenia
	Systemic symptoms
OKT3	Systemic symptoms
	Increased susceptibility to cytomegalovirus infections

tion, so many recipients are maintained on a fixed-dose combination of trimethoprim–sulfamethoxazole, which is effective in preventing such illnesses.[159] Postoperative bacterial infections are also more common in this group, so an attempt should be made to minimize exposure to nosocomial sources, such as urinary and intravascular catheters, and mechanical ventilators. Immunosuppressants also have numerous other adverse effects that can influence perioperative management.

Immunosuppressant Side Effects and Toxicities

Although immunosuppressants are usually administered in combination to diminish the risk of dose-related toxicity from any single agent, significant morbidity is still associated with their use (Table 52-16).

Glucocorticoids

Glucocorticoids produce glucose intolerance, cushingoid habitus, fragility of the integument, aseptic necrosis, and exacerbation of peptic ulcer disease. Yet attempts to eliminate them from immunosuppression regimens usually have not met with success, with the possible exception of neonatal heart transplant recipients. Chronic glucocorticoid use is also associated with adrenal suppression. Although some authors advocate administration of preoperative stress doses of glucocorticoids, this was shown to be unnecessary in at least one large series of patients who underwent a surgical procedure after renal transplantation.[160]

Azathioprine

Azathioprine is a myelosuppressant, producing anemia, thrombocytopenia, and occasionally marrow aplasia. It has also been associated with hepatitis, alopecia, and GI upset, and through an allergic mechanism, pancreatitis. Azathioprine has been reported to increase the requirement for nondepolarizing relaxants to a modest degree, probably by presynaptic inhibition of phosphodiesterase in the motor nerve terminal.[161]

Cyclosporine and Tacrolimus

Cyclosporine is both acutely and chronically nephrotoxic, producing interstitial renal fibrosis and tubular atrophy. Chronic toxicity is common, leading to elevations in blood urea nitrogen and creatinine levels, as well as systolic and diastolic hypertension.[162] Management with conventional antihypertensives is usually successful, but the kidneys of such patients may be more vulnerable to acute insults, such as radiographic dye- or hypotension-induced nephropathy. Cyclosporine may be hepatotoxic, producing hyperuricemia, gingival hypertrophy, or seizures and neurotoxicity at high serum levels. The toxicity profile of tacrolimus seems to be qualitatively similar.

Antilymphocyte Globulin and OKT3

Antilymphocyte globulin is a polyclonal antibody, and as such is "contaminated" with antibodies other than those directed against lymphocytes. These may give rise to marked leukopenia and thrombocytopenia, and systemic symptoms such as fever, chills, pruritus, GI upset, and even frank serum sickness. The first dose of OKT3 is frequently followed by systemic symptoms such as fever, dyspnea, and nausea, unless patients are pretreated with hydrocortisone, acetaminophen, and diphenhydramine. Subsequent reactions are less pronounced. OKT3 has also been associated with episodes of pulmonary edema, aseptic meningitis, and an unusually high incidence of CMV infection.

Early after transplantation, bacterial infections related to wound infection, urinary catheters, and pneumonia are most common (e.g., with *Staphylococcus aureus*, *Escherichia coli*, and *Streptococcus pneumoniae*, respectively). After 1 month, immunosuppressed patients become vulnerable to opportunistic infections (*P. carinii* pneumonia, herpes zoster infections, and CMV sepsis).[102] These episodes need not be fatal and can be overcome if diagnosis is rapid and treatment specific. The most common viral infection is CMV, which can occur as a primary infection from contaminated blood or allograft tissue in seronegative recipients, or as reactivated infection in seropositive patients.[163]

Immunosuppressed patients are also more likely to have one of several histologically distinct types of lymphoproliferative malignancy. For example, the incidence of B-cell lymphoma in patients with renal allografts is approximately 350-fold higher than that seen in the normal age-matched population, and the same is probably true for cardiac recipients. Some studies have documented a causal role for Epstein-Barr virus,[164] and it is speculated that cyclosporine may diminish the cytotoxic response of suppressor T cells to autologous Epstein-Barr virus–infected B cells. Unfortunately, the mortality rate associated with these malignancies is relatively high; in one series, the 5-year mortality rate was 37%.[165]

Other Preanesthetic Considerations

Transplant recipients depend on immunosuppressants to avoid rejection, and these regimens must be restarted soon after surgery. If oral intake is expected to be delayed, appropriate parenteral formulations should be used. Certain drugs used in the perioperative period may inhibit the cytochrome P-450 system and interfere with metabolism of cyclosporine (e.g., cimetidine), whereas others may induce the P-450 enzymes and decrease cyclosporine levels (e.g., phenobarbital and phenytoin). Cyclosporine increases the hypnotic duration of pentobarbital in laboratory animals,[166] but because it does not increase the requirement for inhaled agents,[167] such an effect may be pharmacokinetic in origin. Cyclosporine has also been reported to prolong the action of pancuronium,[168] but controlled data are lacking.

The transplant population is also particularly prone to bacterial pneumonia and CMV sepsis,[102] so early extubation of the trachea is an important goal after any surgical procedure, and the use of CMV-negative blood is mandatory. In addition, intra-

Table 52-17. GENERAL SURGICAL DIAGNOSES IN PATIENTS AFTER HEART TRANSPLANTATION

Diagnosis	Time After Transplantation
Perforated sigmoid diverticulum	8 mo; 29 mo; 39 mo
Small bowel perforation	4 mo; 5 mo
Free intraperitoneal air	3 days; 5 wk
Cholecystitis	2 wk; 21 mo
Vagus nerve injury	3 mo
Ventral hernia	26 mo
Inguinal hernia	7 mo
Perirectal abscess	20 mo
Pancreatitis	18 mo; 1 mo; 2 mo
Diverticulitis	18 mo

Adapted with permission from Steed DL, Brown B, Reilly JJ et al: General surgical complications in heart and heart–lung transplantation. Surgery 98:739, 1985.

vascular catheterization is used only when specifically indicated, although standard aseptic cannulation techniques seem sufficient.

Anesthesia After Kidney Transplantation

Although renal transplantation is usually highly successful, some recipients still require dialysis. Thus, it is important to ascertain the degree of residual renal impairment and treat such patients accordingly. If the allograft is functional, renal excretion of drugs may be expected to be comparable with that through native kidneys.

Many of these patients are diabetic and return to the operating room for ophthalmologic or peripheral vascular procedures. Perioperative complications leading to loss of the renal allograft are uncommon,[160,169] but sepsis is a major cause of morbidity. Management of blood glucose may be complicated by steroid immunosuppressants and fever; in such cases, insulin infusions are often necessary.

Because kidney recipients are maintained on cyclosporine, other agents with nephrotoxic potential (e.g., enflurane) are usually avoided. Cyclosporine may render allografts particularly sensitive to insults, so maintaining a brisk urine flow during anesthesia is recommended. During long procedures, this may justify the use of central venous pressure and urinary catheters.

Anesthesia After Liver Transplantation

In a well functioning liver allograft, common biochemical pathways for drug metabolism are unimpaired.[170] Provided that the metabolic and synthetic functions of the transplanted liver are also intact, the anesthetic care of these patients differs little from that of any other visceral transplant recipient. Within the first 2 months after liver transplantation, the most common surgical procedures are exploratory laparotomy for biliary leak or abscess drainage, or open liver biopsy. Regional anesthesia is avoided unless the coagulation profile has returned to normal, and the likelihood of ileus or elevated intra-abdominal pressure indicates the use of rapid-sequence induction. Later, patients may require biliary reconstruction procedures.

Anesthesia After Heart Transplantation

Heart transplant recipients return to the operating room for noncardiac surgery with some regularity. Such procedures do not always follow the transplantation immediately, instead occurring months or even years later. Overall, 25–30% of these patients require a general surgical procedure (Table 52-17) within 2 years of transplantation.[171,172] Infectious causes for sur-

gery (e.g., drainage of abscesses) can clearly be attributed to immunocompromise, but a relatively high incidence of cholecystitis is unexplained. In addition to these common general surgical problems, orthopedic procedures are frequently required secondary to joint complications arising from chronic steroid use. Despite numerous case reports of cardiac recipients undergoing noncardiac surgery,[173,174] there are no prospective data addressing the risks of anesthesia in this physiologically unique population.

During orthotopic heart transplantation, the aorta and the main pulmonary artery are transected (see Fig. 52-6). As a result, the cardiac plexus is divided, resulting in autonomic afferent and efferent denervation. Myocardial tissue obtained from hearts transplanted for as long as 12 years fails to reveal evidence of abundant reinnervation.[175] Some of the nerve cells present in such specimens probably represent postganglionic parasympathetics because significant amounts of acetylcholine do remain.[176] Although early canine studies indicated that implanted hearts underwent efferent reinnervation and thus regained autonomic control,[177] in humans, with rare exception,[178,179] studies of transplanted heart rate responses to exercise and respiratory stimuli[176,180–182] indicate that autonomic efferent denervation is permanent. Afferent reinnervation may occur in some cases, as suggested by clinical and biochemical criteria.[183]

In the absence of rejection or significant pulmonary hypertension, long-term follow-up studies after heart transplantation have demonstrated that despite denervation, the resting stroke volume and indices of myocardial contractility are often normal[184] or only subtly reduced.[185] However, with demands for increased cardiac output (e.g., during exercise), the response of the denervated heart is demonstrably different (Fig. 52-10). In the normally innervated heart, immediate increases in cardiac output are mediated by elevation in heart rate with little

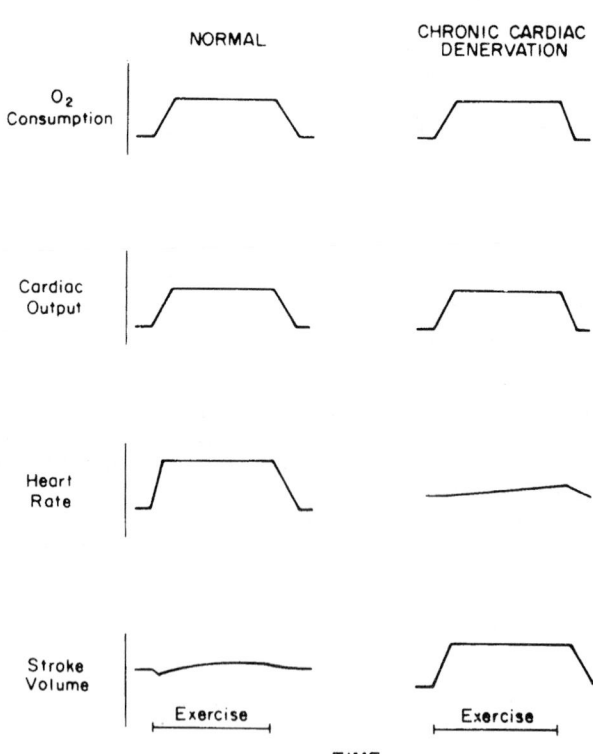

Figure 52-10. Schematic representation of the cardiac physiologic responses to moderate supine exercise in humans. Responses of normal subjects are represented on the left; those following cardiac denervation are on the right. (Reprinted with permission from Kent KIM, Cooper T: The denervated heart: A model for studying autonomic control of the heart. N Engl J Med 291:1017, 1974.)

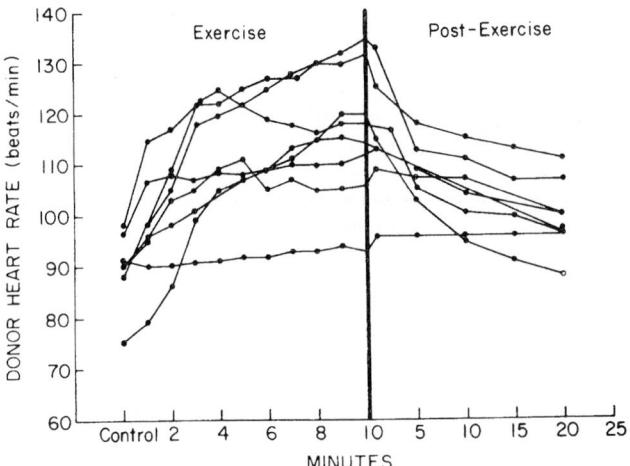

Figure 52-11. Donor heart rates during supine bicycle exercise by eight patients 1 year after heart transplantation. The rates of achieving a maximal pulse are slower than in patients with innervated hearts. "Control" refers to measurements made at the start of exercise. The postexercise scale is compressed. (Reprinted with permission from Stinson EB, Griepp RB, Schroeder JS et al: Hemodynamic observations one and two years after cardiac transplantation in man. Circulation 45:1183, 1972.)

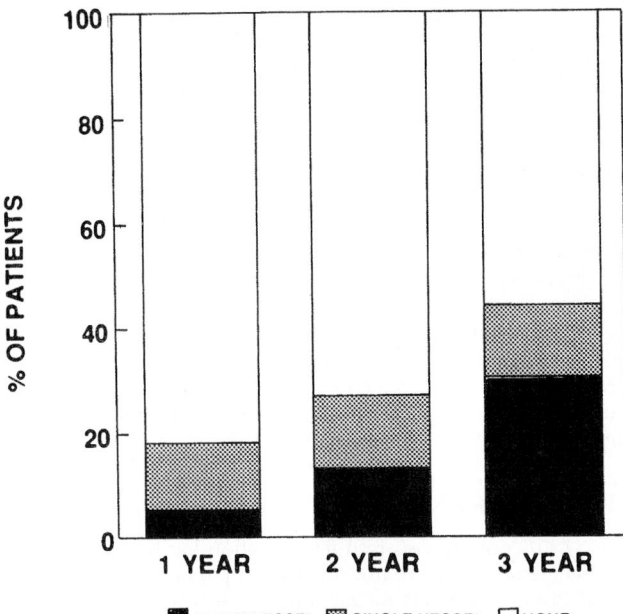

MULTI-VESSEL   SINGLE VESSEL   NONE

Figure 52-12. Life-table analysis showing the risk, in humans, for development of coronary artery disease over the first 3 years after cardiac transplantation. (Reprinted with permission of the authors and the American Heart Association. From Uretsky BF, Murali S, Reddy PS et al: Development of coronary artery disease in cardiac transplant patients receiving immunosuppressive therapy with cyclosporine and prednisone. Circulation 76:827, 1987.)

change in stroke volume. In contrast, the denervated heart responds to such demands by increases in stroke volume rather than in heart rate. Cardiac recipients are thus preload dependent and must have adequate central volume to meet the demands of stress or anesthetic techniques that redistribute vascular volume to the periphery.

The denervated heart eventually can manifest increases in heart rate, albeit with some delay (Fig. 52-11). In cardiac transplant recipients, the maximal achievable pulse rate during exercise develops more slowly than in control subjects, and the return of heart rate to baseline is slower. The delay in achieving a maximal heart rate corresponds to the time required for secretion and circulation of adrenal catecholamines, and the slow return is probably related to the absence of vagal input.

As a consequence of the mid-atrial orthotopic surgical technique, the transplant recipient retains remnants of the native atria, and the electrocardiogram may contain both donor and native P waves. Because the sinus node is normally under the continual influence of autonomic (vagal) nerves, the rate of the transplanted atria usually exceeds that of the native atria.[186] With parasympathetic activation (*e.g.*, by visceral traction, including laryngoscopy or drug effects), the native atrial rate may diminish but the transplanted heart rate remains unchanged because vagal input is absent. In contrast, sympathetic stimulation (whether from hypoxemia, hypercapnia, hypotension, or pain) can still increase the donor heart's sinus rate, although, importantly, such responses are delayed. In contrast to effects on the sinoatrial node, denervation usually does not alter the arteriovenous conduction time or affect ventricular conduction.[187]

By 3 years, approximately 30% of survivors have multivessel coronary stenoses[188] (Fig. 52-12). These lesions are diffuse, concentric narrowings of the coronary lumen, and are thought to arise from areas of immune-mediated endothelial damage. In some cases, lesions are amenable to angioplasty or surgical bypass, but often, myocardial ischemia and infarction limit the useful life of the allograft. Although the ability of these patients to perceive angina pectoris has been documented,[183] afferent innervation seems to be lacking in most, rendering episodes of myocardial ischemia silent. Thus, diagnostic electrocardiographic monitoring is essential throughout the perioperative period, and paroxysmal dyspnea, which may be the only indication of ischemia, should be regarded as an ominous symptom.

Clearly, drugs that act indirectly on the heart fail to produce their typical effects after denervation; for example, administration of atropine or pancuronium does not elevate heart rate (Table 52-18), although neostigmine can cause bradycardia in this population.[189] In contrast, agents that act directly on myocardium or cardiac conduction tissues manifest their usual effects; for example, isoproterenol increases contractility and heart rate, whereas propranolol has the opposite effects. Digoxin, which has mixed direct–indirect actions,[190] acts only directly after transplantation. An iv bolus of digoxin fails to alter either the functional or effective refractory periods of the atrioventricular node,[190] whereas it significantly increases the refractory period in normal patients. This suggests that digoxin's acute, chronotropic effects are vagotonic, dependent on intact autonomic innervation. When treated chronically with digoxin, cardiac transplant recipients demonstrate an inotropic response from a direct effect independent of autonomic innervation. Norepinephrine is another cardioactive drug with somewhat atypical effects in this population. Infusions at conventional

Table 52-18. ALTERED RESPONSES TO COMMON CARDIOVASCULAR DRUGS AFTER CARDIAC DENERVATION

Drug	Response
Atropine	No vagolytic effect
Pancuronium	No vagolytic effect
Edrophonium	No vagotonic effect
Ephedrine	Less cardiostimulatory effect
Nifedipine	No depression of nodal conduction
Digoxin	No acute vagotonic effect
Norepinephrine	Enhanced β-stimulatory effect
Phenylephrine	Diminished vasoconstrictive effects with long-standing heart failure

doses may be accompanied by more pronounced chronotropic effects than usual, through a direct β-adrenergic receptor–mediated effect on the sinus node that is normally masked by vagal reflexes. Cardiac transplant recipients with previous long-standing heart failure may also have a persistently blunted response to α-adrenergic agonists.[191] This probably results from adjustment of the peripheral vasculature or the baroreceptors to chronically elevated catecholamine levels. Finally, there is electrophysiologic evidence of moderate supersensitivity to adenosine after transplantation.[192]

Cardiac rejection may be superimposed on the surgical illness and may be the cause of low cardiac output and dysrythmias. Rejection can thus impair responses to the stress of surgery and anesthesia. Endomyocardial biopsy may be necessary for definitive diagnosis of rejection, and aggressive immunotherapy with high-dose steroids or antilymphocyte globulin may be started in the perioperative period.

FUTURE TRENDS

Since its inception, viscera transplantation has been limited by a shortage of suitable donor organs. For patients with end-stage renal disease, this has meant longer periods on dialysis with greater costs and morbidity, but for prospective heart and liver recipients, there is a 10–40% mortality rate while awaiting transplantation.[193] One remedy lies in further improvements in organ preservation because prolonging tolerable organ ischemic time increases the potential donor pool. The size of this pool will also increase as the criteria for donor acceptability expand (*e.g.,* to include older donors, donors with certain systemic diseases, and terminally ill and fetal donors).[3] Other approaches to deal with the limited supply of organs include cellular transplantation, where healthy allograft cells derived from one organ may be infused into multiple recipients, and xenotransplantation from genetically "humanized" animals.[194]

Optimizing use of the available donor organs will also be important. For example, early application of isolated lung transplantation could make the heart–lung procedure obsolete and allow each heart–lung bloc to serve several patients. Accelerated atherosclerosis is a major factor limiting the useful life span of donor hearts; development of an effective therapy would represent a major breakthrough.

For the foreseeable future, immunosuppressant drugs will continue to be necessary to prevent the response to foreign tissue antigens. Development of agents with greater immunoselectivity and reduced toxicity is of the highest priority. Noninvasive methods to diagnose organ rejection would also substantially improve the quality of life for transplantation survivors. Longer-term approaches to the problem of rejection currently under investigation include induction of tolerance to foreign antigens by promoting cell migration and "chimerism;"[195] definition of the most critical elements for histocompatibility; and development of better "rescue" drugs once rejection has begun.

REFERENCES

1. United Network for Organ Sharing (UNOS): UNOS receives federal contract to develop OPTN. UNOS Update 2:1(Oct), 1986
2. Friend PJ, McCarthy LJ, Filo RS *et al:* Transmission of idiopathic (autoimmune) thrombocytopenic purpura by liver. Ann Thorac Surg 41:520, 1986
3. United Network for Organ Sharing (UNOS) web site: http://www.unos.org, 1999
4. Simmons RL, Canafax DM, Fryd DS *et al:* New immunosuppressive drug combinations for mismatched and cadaveric renal transplantation. Transplant Proc 18(suppl 1):76, 1986
5. Guidelines for the Determination of Death: Report of the medical consultants on the diagnosis of death to the President's Commission for the Study of Ethical Problems in Medicine and Biomedical and Behavioral Research. JAMA 246:2184, 1981
6. Black PM: Brain death. N Engl J Med 299:338, 1978
7. Van Norman GE: A matter of life and death (review). Anesthesiology 91:275, 1999
8. Grigg MM, Kelly MA, Celesia GG *et al:* Electroencephalographic activity after brain death. Arch Neurol 44:948, 1987
9. Lynn J: Diagnosis of brain death. JAMA 250:612, 1983
10. Ropper AH, Kehne SM, Wechsler L: Transcranial Doppler in brain death. Neurology 37:1733, 1987
11. Ashwal S, Schneider S, Thompson J: Xenon computed tomography measuring cerebral blood flow in the determination of brain death in children. Ann Neurol 25:539, 1989
12. Earnest MP, Beresford HR, McIntyre HB: Testing for apnea in suspected brain death: Methods used by 129 clinicians. Neurology 36:542, 1986
13. Belsh JM, Blatt R, Schiffman PL: Apnea testing in brain death. Arch Intern Med 146:2385, 1986
14. Report of special task force: Guidelines for determination of brain death in children. Pediatrics 80:298, 1988
15. Logigian EL, Ropper AH: Terminal electrocardiographic changes in brain-dead patients. Neurology 35:915, 1985
16. Vaghadia H: Atropine resistance in brain dead organ donors. Anesthesiology 65:711, 1986
17. Conci F, Procaccio F, Arosio M *et al:* Viscero-somatic and viscero-visceral reflexes in brain death. J Neurol Neurosurg Psychiatry 9:695, 1986
18. Starzl TE, Miller C, Broznick B *et al:* An improved technique for multiple organ harvesting. Surgery, Gynecology and Obstetrics 165:343, 1987
19. Collins GM, Bravo-Shuarman M, Teraskai PI: Kidney preservation for transplantation: Initial perfusion and 30 hours ice storage. Lancet 2:1219, 1969
20. Baron P, Heil J, Condie R *et al:* 96-Hour renal preservation with silica gel precipitated plasma cold storage versus pulsatile perfusion. Transplant Proc 22:464, 1990
21. Belzer FO, Southard JH: Principles of solid organ preservation by cold storage. Transplantation 45:673, 1988
22. Todo S, Nery J, Yanaga K *et al:* Extended preservation of human liver grafts with UW solution. JAMA 261:711, 1989
23. Downey JM: Free radicals and their involvement during long-term myocardial ischemia and reperfusion. Annu Rev Physiol 52:487, 1990
24. Hardesty RL, Griffith BP, Deep GM *et al:* Improved cardiac function using cardioplegia during procurement and transplantation. Transplant Proc 15:1253, 1983
25. Watson DC, Reitz BA, Baumgartner WA *et al:* Distant heart procurement for transplantation. Surgery 86:56, 1979
26. Reinherz EL, Sclossman SF: The differentiation and function of human T-lymphocytes. Cell 19:821, 1980
27. Harris HW, Gill TJ III: Expression of class I transplantation antigens. Transplantation 42:109, 1986
28. Bach FH, Sach DH: Current concepts: Transplantation immunology. N Engl J Med 317:489, 1987
29. Iwaki Y, Ashizaqa T, Cook D *et al:* ABO matching in liver transplantation. Transplant Proc 20(suppl 1):564, 1988
30. Patel R, Terasaki PI: Significance of the positive cross-match test in kidney transplantation. N Engl J Med 14:735, 1969
31. Opelz G: Effect of HLA matching, blood transfusions, and presensitization in cyclosporine-treated kidney transplant recipients. Transplant Proc 17:2179, 1985
32. Weil R, Clarke DR, Iwaki Y *et al:* Hyperacute rejection of a transplanted human heart. Transplantation 32:71, 1981
33. Stinson EB, Payne R, Griepp RB *et al:* Correlation of histocompatibility matching with graft rejection and survival after cardiac transplantation in man. Lancet 2:459, 1971
34. Zerbe T, Arena V, Kormos R *et al:* Role of major histocompatibility complex (HLA) matching in cardiac allograft rejection. Transplant Proc 20(suppl 1):74, 1988
35. Starzl TE, Tzakis A, Makowka L *et al:* The definition of ABO factors in transplantation: Relation to other humoral antibody states. Transplant Proc 19:4492, 1987
36. Gordon RD, Iwatsuki S, Esquivel CO *et al:* Liver transplantation across ABO blood groups. Surgery 100:342, 1986
37. Demetris AJ, Jaffe R, Tzakis A *et al:* Antibody-mediated rejection of human orthotopic liver allografts: A study of liver transplantation across ABO blood group barriers. Am J Pathol 132:489, 1988
38. Gordon RD, Fung JJ, Markus B *et al:* The antibody crossmatch in liver transplantation. Surgery 100:705, 1986

39. Snyder DS, Unanue ER: Corticosteroids inhibit immune macrophage's Ia expression and interleukin-1 production. J Immunol 129:1803, 1982

40. Dupont E, Wybran J, Toussant C: Glucocorticosteroids and organ transplantation. Transplantation 37:331, 1984

41. Keown PA, Stiller CR: Kidney transplantation. Surg Clin North Am 66:517, 1986

42. Kahane BD: Cyclosporine. N Engl J Med 321:1725, 1989

43. Sollinger HW: Update on preclinical and clinical experience with mycophenolate mofetil. Transplant Proc 28:24, 1996

44. Maki T, Simpson M, Monaco MP: Development of suppressor T cells by antilymphocyte serum treatment in mice. Transplantation 34:376, 1982

45. Acuto O, Reinherz EL: The human T cell receptor: Structure and function. N Engl J Med 312:1100, 1985

46. Hull AR, Parker TF: Proceedings from the Morbidity, Mortality and Prescription of Dialysis Symposium, Dallas, Texas, Sept. 15–17, 1989. Am J Kidney Dis 15:375, 1990

47. United Network for Organ Sharing: United Network for Organ Sharing Newsletter, January 21, 1991

48. Evans RW, Manninen DL, Garrison LP et al: The quality of life of patients with end-stage renal disease. N Engl J Med 312:553, 1985

49. Eggers PW: Effect of transplantation on the Medicare end-stage renal disease program. N Engl J Med 318:223, 1988

50. Inglefinger J, Grupe W, Harmon W et al: Growth acceleration following renal transplantation in children less than 7 years of age. Pediatrics 68:255, 1981

51. Flechner SM: Current status of renal transplantation. Urol Clin North Am 21:265, 1994

52. Velez RL, Vergne-Marini P: Pretransplantation evaluation. In Toledo-Pereyra LH (ed): Kidney Transplantation, p 50. Philadelphia, FA Davis, 1988

53. Bay WH, Herbert LA: The living donor in kidney transplantation. Ann Intern Med 106:719, 1987

54. Spital A, Spital M, Spital R: The living kidney donor: Alive and well. Arch Intern Med 146:1993, 1986

55. Minami H, McCallum RW: The physiology and pathophysiology of gastric emptying in humans. Gastroenterology 86:1592, 1984

56. Lincke CL, Merin RG: A regional anesthetic approach for renal transplantation. Anesth Analg 55:69, 1976

57. Graybar GB: Choice of anesthesia. In Graybar GB, Bready LL (eds): Anesthesia for Renal Transplantation, p 139. Boston, Martinus Nijhoff, 1987

58. Fahey MR, Rupp SM, Canfell C et al: Effect of renal failure on laudanosine excretion in man. Br J Anaesth 57:1049, 1985

59. Belani KG, Palahniuk RJ: Kidney transplantation. In Firestone LL (ed): Anesthesia and Organ Transplantation, p 17. Boston, Little, Brown, 1991

60. Fahey MR, Morris RB, Miller RD et al: Pharmacokinetics of ORG NC45 (Norcuron) in patients with and without renal failure. Br J Anaesth 53:1049, 1981

61. Chapman JR, Allen RD: Dialysis and transplantation. In Morris PJ (ed): Kidney Transplantation: Principles and Practice, p 37. Philadelphia, WB Saunders, 1988

62. Bernuau J, Rueff B, Benhamou JP: Fulminant and subfulminant liver failure: Definition and causes. Semin Liver Dis 6:97, 1986

63. Starzl TE, Demetris AJ, van Thiel DH: Liver transplantation. N Engl J Med 321:1014, 1092, 1989

64. Terpstra OT, Schalm SW, Weimar W et al: Auxiliary partial liver transplantation for end-stage chronic liver disease. N Engl J Med 319:1507, 1988

65. Krowka MJ, Cortese DA: Pulmonary aspects of chronic liver disease and liver transplantation. Mayo Clin Proc 60:407, 1985

66. Starzl TE, van Thiel DH, Tzakis AG et al: Orthotopic liver transplantation for alcoholic cirrhosis. JAMA 260:2542, 1988

67. Starzl TE, Todo S, Gordon R et al: Liver transplantation in older patients. N Engl J Med 316:484, 1987

68. Starzl TE, Todo S, Tzakis A et al: Abdominal organ cluster transplantation for the treatment of upper abdominal malignancies. Ann Surg 210:374, 1989

69. Makowka L, Tzakis AG, Massaferro V et al: Transplantation of the liver for metastatic endocrine tumors of the intestine and pancreas. Surgery, Gynecology and Obstetrics 168:107, 1989

70. Bismuth H, Samuel D, Gugenheim J et al: Emergency liver transplantation for fulminant hepatitis. Ann Intern Med 107:337, 1987

71. Campbell DA, Rolles K, Jamieson N et al: Hepatic transplantation and long-term anticoagulation as treatment for Budd-Chiari syndrome. Surgery, Gynecology and Obstetrics 166:511, 1988

72. Pett S, Mowat AP: Crigler-Najjar syndrome types I and II: Clinical experience—King's College Hospital 1972–1978. Phenobarbitone, phototherapy, and liver transplantation. Mol Aspects Med 9:473, 1987

73. Tobias MD, Jobes CS, Aukburg SJ: Hemofiltration in parallel to the venovenous bypass circuit for oliguric hypervolemia during liver transplantation. Anesthesiology 90:909, 1999

74. Kang YG, Martin DJ, Marquez J et al: Intraoperative changes in blood coagulation and thromboelastographic monitoring in liver transplantation. Anesth Analg 64:888, 1985

75. Kang Y: Liver transplantation. In Firestone LL (ed): Anesthesia and Organ Transplantation, p 59. Boston, Little, Brown, 1991

76. Aggarwal S, Kang Y, Freeman JA et al: Postreperfusion syndrome: Cardiovascular collapse following hepatic reperfusion during liver transplantation. Transplant Proc 19(suppl 3):54, 1987

77. Howrie DL, Burckart GJ: Drug disposition in organ transplantation. In Cook DR, Davis PJ (eds): Anesthetic Principles for Organ Transplantation, p 55. New York, Raven Press, 1994

78. Haberer JP, Schoeffler P, Coudere E et al: Fentanyl pharmacokinetics in anaesthetized patients with cirrhosis. Br J Anaesth 54:1267, 1982

79. Rosenberg PH, Oikkonen MP, Orko RH et al: A transplanted liver rapidly begins to metabolize enflurane in humans. Anesth Analg 63:1131, 1984

80. Carton EG, Plevak DJ, Kranner PW et al: Perioperative care of the liver transplant patient: Part II. Anesth Analg 78:382, 1994

81. Marquez J, Martin D, Virji MA et al: Cardiovascular depression secondary to citrate intoxication during hepatic transplantation in man. Anesthesiology 65:457, 1986

82. Lewis JH, Bontempo FA, Awad SA et al: Liver transplantation: Intraoperative changes in coagulation factors in 100 first transplants. Hepatology 9:710, 1989

83. Shaw BW, Martin DJ, Marquez JM et al: Venous bypass in clinical liver transplantation. Ann Surg 200:524, 1984

84. Wall WJ, Grant DR, Duff JH et al: Blood transfusion requirement and renal function in patients undergoing liver transplantation without venous bypass. Transplant Proc 19(suppl 3):17, 1987

85. Khoury GF, Mann ME, Porot MJ et al: Air embolism associated with veno-venous bypass during orthotopic liver transplantation. Anesthesiology 67:848, 1987

86. Paulsen AW, Whitten CW, Ramsay MAE et al: Considerations for anesthetic management during veno-venous bypass in adult hepatic transplantation. Anesth Analg 68:489, 1989

87. Martin TJ, Kang Y, Marquez JM et al: Ionization and hemodynamic effects of calcium chloride and calcium gluconate in the absence of hepatic function. Anesthesiology 73:62, 1990

88. Martin DJ, Marquez JM, Kang YG et al: Liver transplantation: Hemodynamic and electrolyte changes seen immediately following revascularization (abstract). Anesth Analg 63:246, 1984

89. Prager MC, Gregory GA, Ascher NL et al: Massive venous air embolism during orthotopic liver transplantation. Anesthesiology 72:198, 1990

90. Ellis JE, Lichtor JL, Feinstein SB et al: Right heart dysfunction, pulmonary embolism and paradoxical embolization during liver transplantation. Anesth Analg 68:777, 1989

91. Navalgund AA, Kang Y, Sarner JB et al: Massive pulmonary thromboembolism during liver transplantation. Anesth Analg 67:400, 1988

92. Iwatsuki S, Popovtzer MM, Corman JL et al: Recovery from "hepatorenal syndrome" after orthotopic liver transplantation. N Engl J Med 289:1155, 1973

93. Starzl TE, Demetris AJ (eds): Candidacy, original disease, and outcome. In: Liver Transplantation, p 119. Chicago, Yearbook Publishers, 1990

94. Evans RW, Manninen DL, Overcast TD et al: The National Heart Transplantation Study: Final Report. Seattle, Battelle Human Affairs Research Centers, Health Care Financing Administration (HCFA) Publications, 1984

95. Hosenpud JD, Bennett LE, Keck BM et al: The Registry of the International Society for Heart and Lung Transplantation: Sixteenth official report—1999. J Heart Lung Transplant 18:611, 1999

96. Clark NJ, Martin RD: Anesthetic considerations for patients undergoing cardiac transplantation. Journal of Cardiothoracic Anesthesia 2:519, 1988

97. Massie BM, Conway M: Survival of patients with congestive heart failure: Past, present, future prospects. Circulation 75:11, 1987

98. Hardesty RL, Griffith BP, Trento A et al: Mortally ill patients and excellent survival following cardiac transplantation. Ann Thorac Surg 41:126, 1986

99. Griffith BP, Hardesty RL, Kormos RL et al: Temporary use of the Jarvik-7 total artificial heart before transplantation. N Engl J Med 316:130, 1987

100. Menkis AH, McKenzie FN, Novick RJ et al: Special considerations for heart transplantation in congenital heart disease. Journal of Heart Transplantation 9:602, 1990

101. Addonizio LJ, Gersony WM, Robbins RC et al: Elevated pulmonary vascular resistance and cardiac transplantation. Circulation 76(suppl 5):52, 1987

102. Dummer JS: Infectious complications of transplantation. In Thompson ME (ed): Cardiac Transplantation, p 163. Philadelphia, FA Davis, 1990

103. Stein KL, Darby JM, Grenvik A: Intensive care of the cardiac transplant recipient. Journal of Cardiothoracic Anesthesia 2:543, 1988

104. Watson DC, Reitz BA, Baumgartner WA et al: Distant heart procurement for transplantation. Surgery 86:56, 1979

105. Gilbert EM, Krueger SK, Murray JL et al: Echocardiographic evaluation of potential cardiac transplant donors. J Thorac Cardiovasc Surg 95:1003, 1988

106. Walsh TR, Syttendorf J, Dummer S et al: The value of protective isolation procedure in cardiac allograft recipients. Ann Thorac Surg 47:539, 1989

107. Keats AS, Strong JM, Girigis KZ et al: Observations during anesthesia for cardiac homotransplantation in ten patients. Anesthesiology 30:192, 1969

108. Fernando NA, Keenan RL, Boyan CP: Anesthetic experience with cardiac transplantation. J Thorac Cardiovasc Surg 75:531, 1978

109. Demas K, Wyner J, Mihm FG et al: Anaesthesia for heart transplantation. Br J Anaesth 58:1357, 1986

110. Waterman PM, Bjerke R: Rapid-sequence induction technique in patients with severe ventricular dysfunction. Journal of Cardiothoracic Anesthesia 2:602, 1988

111. Bainbridge AD, Cave M, Roberts M: A prospective randomized trial of complete atrioventricular transplantation versus ventricular transplantation with atrioplasty. J Heart Lung Transplant 18:407, 1999.

112. Cannon DS, Rider AK, Stinson EB et al: Electrophysiological studies in the denervated transplanted human heart: II. Response to norepinephrine, isoproterenol, and propranolol. Am J Cardiol 36:859, 1975

113. Armitage JM, Hardesty RL, Griffith BP: Prostaglandin E1: An effective treatment of right heart failure after orthotopic heart transplantation. Journal of Heart Transplantation 6:348, 1987

114. Bhatia SJS, Kirshenbaum M, Shemin RJ et al: Time course of resolution of pulmonary hypertension and right ventricular remodeling after orthotopic cardiac transplantation. Circulation 76:819, 1987

115. Fonger JD, Borkon AM, Baumgartner WA et al: Acute right heart failure following heart transplantation: Improvement with PGE1 and right ventricular assist. Journal of Heart Transplantation 5:317, 1986

116. Renlund DG, Bristow MR, Lee HR et al: Medical aspects of cardiac transplantation. Journal of Cardiothoracic Anesthesia 2:500, 1988

117. Griffith BP, Hardesty RL, Trento A et al: Asynchronous rejection of heart and lungs following cardiopulmonary transplantation. Ann Surg 40:488, 1985

118. Arcasoy SM, Kotloff RM: Lung transplantation (review). N Engl J Med 340:1081, 1999

119. Miyoshi S, Trulock EP, Schaefers HJ et al: Cardiopulmonary exercise testing after single and double lung transplantation. Chest 97:1130, 1990

120. Griffith BP, Zenati M: The pulmonary donor. Clin Chest Med 11:217, 1990

121. Todd TR, Goldberg M, Koshal A et al: Separate extraction of cardiac and pulmonary grafts from a single organ donor. Ann Thorac Surg 46:356, 1988

122. Conacher ID: Isolated lung transplantation: A review of problems and guide to anaesthesia. Br J Anaesth 61:468, 1988

123. Conacher ID, McNally B, Choudhry AK et al: Anaesthesia for isolated lung transplantation. Br J Anaesth 60:588, 1988

124. Gayes JM, Giron L, Nissen MD et al: Anesthetic considerations for patients undergoing double-lung transplantation. Journal of Cardiothoracic Anesthesia 4:486, 1990

125. Thomas BJ, Siegel LC: Anesthetic and postoperative management of single-lung transplantation. J Cardiothorac Vasc Anesth 5:266, 1991

126. Schaefers H-J, Waxman MB, Patterson GA et al: Cardiac innervation after double lung transplantation. J Thorac Cardiovasc Surg 99:22, 1990

127. Bierman MI, Stein KL, Stuart RS et al: Critical care management of lung transplant recipients. Journal of Intensive Care Medicine 6:135, 1991

128. Smiley RM, Navedo AT, Kirby T et al: Postoperative independent lung ventilation in a single-lung transplant recipient. Anesthesiology 74:1144, 1991

129. Dauber JH, Paradis IL, Dummer JS: Infectious complications in pulmonary allograft recipients. Clin Chest Med 11:291, 1990

130. Burke CM, Theodore J, Dawkins KD et al: Post-transplant obliterative bronchiolitis and other late lung sequelae in human heart-lung transplantation. Chest 86:824, 1984

131. National Diabetes Data Group: Diabetes in America. NIH publication no. 85–1467. Washington, DC, U.S. Department of Health and Human Services, August 1985

132. Sutherland DER, Gillingham K, Moudry-Munns KC: Registry report on clinical pancreas transplantation. Transplant Proc 23:55, 1991

133. Sutherland DER, Dunn DL, Goetz FC et al: A 10-year experience with 290 pancreas transplants at a single institution. Ann Surg 210:274, 1989

134. Bilous RW, Mauer SM, Sutherland DER et al: The effects of pancreas transplantation on the glomerular structure of renal allografts in patients with insulin-dependent diabetes. N Engl J Med 321:80, 1989

135. Tzakis AG, Ricordi C, Alejandro R et al: Pancreatic islet transplantation after upper abdominal exenteration and liver replacement. Lancet 336:402, 1990

136. Starzl TE, Rowe MI, Todo S et al: Transplantation of multiple abdominal viscera. JAMA 261:1449, 1989

137. Grant D: Intestinal transplantation: Current status. Transplant Proc 21:2869, 1989

138. Tzakis AG, Todo S, Madariaga J et al: Upper abdominal exenteration in transplantation for extensive malignancies of the upper abdomen: An update. Transplantation 51:727, 1991

139. DeWolf A: Multiviscera and pancreas transplantation. In Firestone LL (ed): Anesthesia and Organ Transplantation, p 111. Boston, Little, Brown, 1991

140. Report of Special Task Force: Guidelines for the determination of brain death in children. Pediatrics 80:298, 1988

141. Broelsch CE, Emond JC, Thistlethwaite JR et al: Liver transplantation, including the concept of reduced-size liver transplants in children. Ann Surg 208:410, 1988

142. Starnes VA, Barr ML, Cohen MG: Lobar transplantation: Indications, technique, and outcome. J Thorac Cardiovasc Surg 108:403, 1994

143. Penn I: The changing pattern of posttransplant malignancies. Transplant Proc 23:1101, 1991

144. Turcotte JG, Campbell DA, Dafoe DC et al: Pediatric renal transplantation. In Cerelli GJ (ed): Organ Transplantation and Replacement, p 349. Philadelphia, JB Lippincott, 1988

145. Warady B, Kriley M, Farrell S et al: Growth and development of infants with end-stage renal disease receiving long-term peritoneal dialysis. J Pediatr 112:714, 1988

146. McGraw ME, Haka-Ikse K: Neurologic developmental sequelae of chronic renal failure in infancy. J Pediatr 106:579, 1985

147. Ingelfinger J, Grupe W, Harmon W et al: Growth acceleration following renal transplantation in children less than 7 years of age. Pediatrics 68:255, 1981

148. Fennell K, Rasbury W, Fennell E et al: Effects of kidney transplantation on cognitive performance in a pediatric population. Pediatrics 74:273, 1984

149. Van Meurs IP, Terasaki PI, Cecka JM et al: A report from the UNOS scientific renal transplant registry. Transplant Proc 23:53, 1991

150. Gordon RD, Bismuth H: Liver transplant registry report. Transplant Proc 23:58, 1991

151. Lichtor JL, Emond J, Chung MR et al: Pediatric orthotopic liver transplantation: Multifactorial predictions of blood loss. Anesthesiology 68:607, 1988

152. Salt A, Barnes AP, Mowat R *et al:* Five years' experience of liver transplantation in children. Transplant Proc 22:1514, 1991

153. Bismuth H, Houssin D: Reduced-size orthotopic liver graft in hepatic transplantation in children. Surgery 95:367, 1984

154. Kriett JM, Kaye MP: The registry of the International Society for Heart Transplantation: Seventh official report, 1990. Journal of Heart Transplantation 9:323, 1990

155. Pahl E, Fricker FJ, Armitage J *et al:* Coronary arteriosclerosis in pediatric heart transplant survivors: Limitation of long term survival. J Pediatr 116:177, 1990

156. Starnes V, Oyer P, Bernstein D *et al:* Heart and heart-lung transplantation in the first year of life. J Heart Lung Transplant 10:162, 1991

157. Bailey L, Kahan B, Nehlsen-Cannarella S: The neonatal immune system: Window of opportunity? J Heart Lung Transplant 10:828, 1991

158. Smyth RL, Scott JP, Whitehead G *et al:* Heart-lung transplantation in children. Transplant Proc 22:1470, 1990

159. Gryzan S, Paradis IL, Zeevi A *et al:* Unexpectedly high incidence of *Pneumocystis carinii* infection after lung-heart transplantation: Implications for lung defense and allograft survival. American Review of Respiratory Disease 137:1268, 1988

160. Leapman SB, Vidne BA, Butt KM *et al:* Elective and emergency surgery in renal transplant patients. Ann Surg 183:262, 1976

161. Dretchen KL, Morgenroth VH, Standaert FG *et al:* Azathioprine: Effects on neuromuscular transmission. Anesthesiology 45:604, 1986

162. Hunt SA, Gamberg P, Stinson EB *et al:* The Stanford experience: Survival and renal function in the pre-Sandimmune era compared to the Sandimmune era. Transplant Proc 22(suppl 1):1, 1990

163. Weir MR, Irwin BC, Maters AW *et al:* Incidence of cytomegalovirus disease in cyclosporine-treated renal transplant recipients based on donor/recipient pretransplant immunity. Transplantation 43:187, 1987

164. Hanto DW, Simmons RL, Najarian JS: Epstein-Barr virus-induced lymphoproliferative diseases in renal allograft recipients. Journal of Heart Transplantation 3:121, 1984

165. Nalesnik MA, Locker J, Jaffe R *et al:* Clonal characteristics of posttransplant lymphoproliferative disorders. Transplant Proc 20:280, 1988

166. Cirella VN, Pantuck CB, Lee YJ *et al:* Effects of cyclosporine on anesthetic action. Anesth Analg 66:703, 1987

167. Firestone LL, Martin T, Liu P *et al:* The effect of cyclosporine on the potencies of general anesthetics. Anesth Analg 70:S105, 1990

168. Crosby E, Robblee JA: Cyclosporine-pancuronium interaction in a patient with a renal allograft. Can J Anaesth 35:300, 1988

169. Bakkaloglu M, Hamilton DNH, MacPherson SG *et al:* Morbidity and mortality in renal transplant patients after incidental surgery. Br J Surg 65:228, 1978

170. Mehta MU, Venkataramanan R, Burckart GJ *et al:* Antipyrine kinetics in liver disease and liver transplantation. Clin Pharmacol Ther 39:372, 1986

171. Steed DL, Brown B, Reilly JJ *et al:* General surgical complications in heart and heart-lung transplantation. Surgery 98:739, 1985

172. Colon R, Frazier OH, Kahan BD *et al:* Complications in cardiac transplant patients requiring general surgery. Surgery 103:32, 1988

173. Camann WR, Goldman GA, Johnson MD *et al:* Cesarean delivery in a patient with a transplanted heart. Anesthesiology 71:618, 1989

174. Kanter SF, Samuels SI: Anesthesia for major operations on patients who have transplanted hearts: A review of 29 cases. Anesthesiology 46:65, 1977

175. Rowan RA, Billingham ME: Myocardial innervation in long-term heart transplant survivors: A quantitative ultrastructural survey. Journal of Heart Transplantation 7:448, 1988

176. Kaye MP: Denervation and reinnervation of the heart. In Randall WC (ed): Nervous Control of Cardiovascular Function, p 278. New York, Oxford University Press, 1984

177. Dong E, Hurley EJ, Lower RR *et al:* Performance of the heart two years after autotransplantation. Surgery 56:270, 1964

178. Johnson TH, Kubo SH, McGinn AL *et al:* Physiologic importance of sympathetic reinnervation after cardiac transplantation (abstract). Journal of Heart Transplantation 10:178, 1991

179. Wilson RF, Christensen BV, Olivari MT *et al:* Evidence for structural sympathetic reinnervation after orthotopic cardiac transplantation in humans. Circulation 83:1210, 1991

180. Pope SE, Stinson EB, Daughters GT *et al:* Exercise response of the denervated heart in long-term cardiac transplant recipients. Am J Cardiol 46:213, 1980

181. Mason JW, Harrison DC: Electrophysiology and electropharmacology of the transplanted human heart. In Narula OS (ed): Cardiac Arrhythmias: Electrophysiology, Diagnosis and Management, p 66. Baltimore, Williams & Wilkins, 1979

182. Kavanagh T, Yacoub MH, Mertens DJ *et al:* Cardiorespiratory responses to exercise training after orthotopic cardiac transplantation. Circulation 77:162, 1988

183. Stark RP, McGinn AL, Wilson RF: Chest pain in cardiac-transplant recipients. N Engl J Med 324:1791, 1991

184. Stinson EB, Griepp RB, Clark DA *et al:* Cardiac transplantation in man: VIII. Survival and function. J Thorac Cardiovasc Surg 60:303, 1970

185. Verani MS, George SE, Leon CA *et al:* Systolic and diastolic ventricular performance at rest and during exercise in heart transplant recipients. Journal of Heart Transplantation 7:145, 1988

186. Cannom DS, Graham AF, Harrison DC: Electrophysiologic studies in the denervated transplanted human heart: Response to atrial pacing and atropine. Circ Res 32:268, 1973

187. Firestone LL: Autonomic influence on cardiac performance: Lessons from the transplanted (denervated) heart. Int Anesthesiol Clin 27:283, 1988

188. Uretsky BF: Physiology of the transplanted heart. In Thompson ME (ed): Cardiac Transplantation, p 21. Philadelphia, FA Davis, 1990

189. Beebe DS, Shumway SJ, Maddock R: Sinus arrest after intravenous neostigmine in two heart transplant recipients. Anesth Analg 78:779, 1994

190. Goodman DJ, Rossen RM, Cannom DS *et al:* Effect of digoxin on A-V conduction: Studies in patients with and without autonomic innervation. Circulation 51:251, 1975

191. Borow KM, Neumann A, Arensman FW *et al:* Cardiac and peripheral vascular responses to adrenoceptor stimulation and blockade after cardiac transplantation. J Am Coll Cardiol 14:1229, 1989

192. Ellenbogen KA, Thames MD, DiMarco JP *et al:* Electrophysiological effects of adenosine in the transplanted human heart. Circulation 81:821, 1990

193. Baumgartner WA, Augustine S, Borkon AM *et al:* Present expectations in cardiac transplantation. Ann Thorac Surg 43:585, 1987

194. Lu CY, Khaair-El-Din TA, Davidson IA *et al:* Xenotransplantation (review). FASEB J 8:1122, 1994.

195. Ascher NL: Microchimerism in organ transplantation (review). Liver Transpl Surg 1:43, 1995

SIX

POST ANESTHESIA AND CONSULTANT PRACTICE

Clinical Anesthesia (4/e), edited by
Paul G. Barash, Bruce F. Cullen, and
Robert K. Stoelting. Lippincott Williams &
Wilkins, Philadelphia, © 2001.

CHAPTER 53

POSTOPERATIVE RECOVERY

ROGER S. MECCA

An individualized, problem-oriented approach to the assessment of surgical patients is essential to ensure appropriate postoperative recovery with minimum risk and expense. Facility design, equipment, and staffing requirements for a state-of-the-art postanesthesia care unit (PACU) are reviewed elsewhere.[1]

VALUE OF POSTANESTHESIA CARE UNIT CARE

Indicators of PACU quality include not only clinical results but the "value" of care, defined as the improvement in clinical outcome per dollar spent on a PACU admission. The impact of PACU care on clinical outcomes in a surgical population varies with incidence and severity of underlying illness, the frequency, urgency, and type of surgical procedures, and the blend of surgical and anesthetic techniques used. Training, skill, and preferences of surgeons, anesthesia providers, and PACU nurses also affect how important a PACU admission might be to a patient. The effectiveness of PACU staff at recognizing complications, the quality of diagnostic and consultative services, and the efficiency with which physicians institute therapy are also important. The patient's impressions during the PACU stay have a major impact on perception of the entire surgical episode. Friendliness and empathy from the PACU staff is an important element of patient satisfaction that contributes to a pleasant working environment.

Actual cost of PACU care incorporates space, staff, and hardware. Triage, admission, and discharge policies affect how many admissions occur and what resources each admission consumes. The greatest PACU cost is for staffing. Mix of nursing staff (*e.g.,* amount of training and experience; salaries and benefit levels), the staffing ratios (*e.g.,* number of patients per caregiver, number of support staff), and the duration of PACU stay determine an overall personnel cost per admission. Level of monitoring provided affects capital expenditure for equipment and operating expenditure for disposable items. Patient mix also determines expenditures for staffing and for equipment such as intravenous (iv) pumps, and ventilators. The type of physician coverage (*e.g.,* dedicated versus on-demand coverage, response times) affects the efficiency of care. Routine postoperative diagnostic testing increases costs for securing and processing tests, and for professional interpretation. Finally, use of routine therapies (*e.g.,* oxygen, antiemetics, respiratory therapy) increases the expenditure per patient for drugs and disposable items, and can add to the staffing resources required per patient.

Cost comparisons between institutions are difficult because factors affecting impact and cost are facility specific and vary among institutions and over time. Regulatory requirements, standards of care, and medicolegal climates also vary among regions or between facilities in the same locale. Attempts to establish national benchmarks of "cost-effectiveness" of PACU care are fraught with inaccuracy. Despite this complexity, emphasis on containment of health care expenditures forces each surgical facility to evaluate the value of its PACU care to an individual patient.

Postanesthesia care unit directors are challenged to optimize clinical results while minimizing expenditure. Innovative PACU practices can guarantee safe care, minimize cost, and fulfill regulatory requirements. Medical leaders must identify those interventions that have actual yield versus those that are "wasteful." The actual impact of many PACU interventions on clinical

outcome is not substantiated by controlled scientific analysis. Useless testing, unnecessary or unjustifiably expensive therapy, and inappropriate PACU admission should be eliminated. However, using a more expensive therapy can sometimes generate real savings by decreasing admissions or length of stay. Finally, integration of the PACU service with other elements of the surgical continuum is essential. The most important interface is between the PACU and the intraoperative anesthesiology service. In one study, 22.1% of 37,000 patients had a minor anesthesia-related event or complication that prolonged PACU stay and consumed PACU resources.[2] Consumption of PACU resources is definitely linked to anesthetic duration and technique,[3] so close coordination between services should reduce the frequency and impact of such events.

It is important to distinguish between potential and actual cost savings. Improvements in care might create an opportunity to shorten length of stay in the PACU and discharge unit, but the actual impact is frequently reduced by transportation delays, persistence of pain or nausea, waiting for space, or surgeon discharge delays.[4,5] Also, administrators should beware of cost-saving measures in other areas that increase the cost of PACU care. For example, use of a cheaper, longer-acting muscle relaxant might trim cost in anesthesiology but increase length of stay, complication rates, and cost in the PACU.[6] Also, savings are illusory unless an operational change yields an actual decrease in expenditures for staff, supplies, or equipment. Nurse staffing is the largest variable direct cost in the PACU.[7] Innovative scheduling of operating room cases, shortening PACU length of stay, and bypassing the PACU create an opportunity for savings that is realized only if the number of paid nursing hours is reduced or if a larger number of patients is serviced with the same hours. If excess hours are consumed by ineffective scheduling, by using nurses for low-yield clerical or maintenance tasks, or by staff subterfuge, then no savings are realized. Finally, trimming costs sometimes entails an increase in risk, no matter how small. Differentiating between cost-effective postanesthetic care and unsafe clinical practice must remain a matter of professional judgment.

LEVELS OF POSTOPERATIVE CARE

For both ambulatory and inpatient surgery, the level of postoperative care a patient requires is determined by the degree of underlying illness, the duration and complexity of anesthesia and surgery, and the risk postoperative complications. As less invasive surgical techniques and shorter-duration anesthetic regimens become more prevalent, many patients exhibit minimal cardiovascular or respiratory depression after surgery. Using a less intensive postanesthesia setting for selected patients can reduce cost for a surgical procedure and allow the facility to divert scarce PACU resources to patients with greater needs. Alert patients are more satisfied when spared the unnecessary assessments and interventions and the upsetting environment of PACU care. Amenities such as recliners, reading material, television, music, and food improve perceptions without affecting quality or safety. Earlier reunion with family in lower-intensity recovery settings is desirable. This of course assumes that postoperative care is safe and appropriate.

Creation of separate PACUs for inpatients and ambulatory patients is one possible way to streamline PACU care for straightforward cases. If separation is not feasible, then linking the level of monitoring and coverage to the degree of postoperative impairment achieves similar results in one PACU. However, full-intensity PACU care must always be available, given the incidence of complications after anesthesia and surgery.[8] As the aging population generates an increase in the complexity of surgical care in the face of dwindling resources,[9] maintaining appropriate PACU capacity will be increasingly important.

Requirements of state and national agencies sometimes impede the implementation of innovative PACU care policies. Codes and regulations might be outdated, poorly substantiated, or interpreted by regulators with clinical experience from a different era. Flexibility and logic need to be incorporated into regulation for complete evolution of postanesthesia care to occur.

POSTOPERATIVE TRIAGE

Patients must be carefully evaluated to determine which level of postoperative care is most appropriate. Triage should be based on clinical condition and the potential for complications that require intervention. Alternatives to PACU care must be used in a nondiscriminatory fashion. Artificial triage categories based on age, American Society of Anesthesiologists classification, ambulatory versus inpatient status, or type of insurance should not be used. A wide margin of safety must be preserved, and applicable PACU standards observed when appropriate[10] (see Table 2-3). If doubt exists about a patient's safety in a lower-intensity setting, the patient should be admitted to a "full-service" PACU. The clinician always errs for patient safety, regardless of cost.

After superficial procedures using local infiltration or minor blocks and sedation, patients can almost always recover with less intensive monitoring and coverage. Healthy patients undergoing more extensive procedures (e.g., hernia repairs, arthroscopic procedures, minor joint procedures) under local or plexus blockade might also bypass the PACU. Selected patients who meet the PACU discharge criteria at the end of general anesthesia can bypass the PACU and be transferred from the operating room directly to a discharge area.[11] Innovative anesthetic techniques and use of bispectral index monitoring help facilitate this "fast-track" postoperative care, although inadequate control of pain and postoperative nausea and vomiting (PONV) often reduces the impact of PACU bypass on resource expenditure.[12]

SAFETY IN THE PACU

The PACU medical director must ensure that the PACU environment is as safe as possible. Beyond usual policies ensuring safe clinical care, staffing levels and training must ensure that appropriate coverage and skill mix are available to deal with unforeseen crises. Ideally, all staff should have PACU certification, and staffing ratios should never fall below accepted standards.[10] Each medical director must guarantee that less skilled staff are appropriately supervised and that a sufficient number of certified personnel is available to handle worst case scenarios.

The PACU staff protects patients who are temporarily incompetent. They safeguard the patient's right to informed consent for additional procedures and to observance of advanced directives. The staff is obligated to preserve each patient's privacy and dignity, and to minimize the psychological impact of unpleasant or frightening events. Medical directors must address the potential for personal assault of patients during recovery. Access to the PACU should be strictly controlled, and unobserved coverage of a PACU patient by one staff member for prolonged periods avoided, especially if there is a gender difference.

The PACU environment must also be safe for professionals. Air handling in the PACU should guarantee that personnel are not exposed to unacceptable levels of trace anesthetic gases, although trace gas monitoring is not necessary.[13] Staff must receive appropriate vaccinations, including that for hepatitis B. All practitioners must adhere to policies for radiation safety, infection control, disposal of sharps, universal precautions for bloodborne diseases, and safeguarding against exposure to pathogens like methicillin-resistant *Staphylococcus* or tuberculosis. Masks, gloves, eye protection, and appropriate personal respiratory equipment must always be available. Staff should never risk personal injury while lifting and positioning patients or while dealing with emergence reactions because sufficient help is not available. Compulsive documentation and clear lines of clinical responsibility protect staff against unnecessary medicolegal exposure.

ADMISSION CRITERIA

Every patient admitted to a PACU should have heart rate and rhythm, systemic blood pressure, and ventilatory rate and character recorded. Assessment every 5 minutes for the first 15 minutes and every 15 minutes thereafter is a prudent minimum, with contemporaneous recording of results. Temperature should be documented at least on admission and discharge, along with level of consciousness, airway patency, and skin color. Order diagnostic tests only for specific indications.

Every patient should be monitored with a pulse oximeter and a single-lead, continuous electrocardiogram (ECG). Capnography is necessary only for patients receiving mechanical ventilation or those at risk for compromised ventilatory function. The output from invasive monitors such as central venous, systemic, or pulmonary arterial catheters must be transduced, and results from monitors recorded and timed on the record.

Anesthesiology personnel should manage the patient until PACU staff secure admission vital signs and attach appropriate monitors. A succinct but thorough report that includes sufficient information to allow rapid evaluation and intervention for postoperative complications must be legibly recorded (Table 53-1). A standardized format printed on the PACU record is useful. Document the time, amount, and route of administration of all neuromuscular relaxants, respiratory depressant medications, and reversal agents, and clearly outline orders, specific therapeutic end points, and how to contact the responsible anesthesiologist. Responsibility should never be turned over to PACU personnel until the patient's airway status, ventilation, and hemodynamics are appropriate. The anesthesiologist checks the function of indwelling cannulae, iv catheters, and monitors just before leaving.

POSTOPERATIVE PAIN MANAGEMENT

Relief of surgical pain with minimal side effects is a primary goal of PACU care and a very high priority for both anesthesiologists and patients[14] (see also Chapter 54). Inadequate postoperative analgesia is a major source of preoperative fear and postoperative dissatisfaction for surgical patients. In addition to improving patient comfort, relief of pain reduces sympathetic nervous system (SNS) response and helps avoid hypertension, tachycardia, and dysrhythmias. In hypovolemic patients who rely on SNS activity for cardiovascular homeostasis, analgesics can precipitate hypotension, especially if direct or histamine-induced vasodilation occurs. A tachycardic patient with low or normal blood pressure who complains of severe pain must be carefully assessed before analgesics are given. Eliminating pain also precipitates hypoventilation by accentuating the depressant effects of previously administered opioids or residual anesthetics.

The actual degree of postoperative pain can be difficult to establish. Severity of pain varies among different surgical proce-

Table 53-1. COMPONENTS OF A POSTANESTHESIA CARE UNIT ADMISSION REPORT

PREOPERATIVE HISTORY

Medication allergies or reactions
Pertinent earlier surgical procedures
Underlying medical illness
Chronic medications
Acute problems (ischemia, acid–base status, dehydration)
Premedications
NPO status

INTRAOPERATIVE FACTORS

Surgical procedure
Type of anesthetic
Relaxant/reversal status
Time and amount of opioids administered
Type and amount of intravenous fluids administered
Estimated blood loss
Urine output
Unexpected surgical or anesthetic events
Intraoperative vital sign ranges
Intraoperative laboratory findings
Drugs given (*e.g.,* steroids, diuretics, antibiotics, vasoactive medications)

ASSESSMENT AND REPORT OF CURRENT STATUS

Airway patency
Ventilatory adequacy
Level of consciousness
Heart rate and heart rhythm
Endotracheal tube position
Systemic pressure
Intravascular volume status
Function of invasive monitors
Size and location of intravenous catheters
Anesthetic equipment (*e.g.,* epidural catheters)
Overall impression

POSTOPERATIVE INSTRUCTIONS

Expected airway and ventilatory status
Acceptable vital sign ranges
Acceptable urine output and blood loss
Surgical instructions (positioning, wound care)
Anticipated cardiovascular problems
Orders for therapeutic interventions
Diagnostic tests to be secured
Therapeutic goals and end points before discharge
Location of responsible physician

dures and anesthetic techniques. Staff are relatively ineffective at quantifying a patient's discomfort. Inexperienced nurses overestimate a patient's pain, whereas more experienced nurses tend to underestimate.[15] Either error leads to inappropriate treatment. A wide divergence can exist between cognitive perception of pain and SNS response, related to psychological, cultural, and cardiovascular differences among individuals. Some perceive severe pain with minimal SNS activity, whereas others have hypertension, tachycardia, and dysrhythmias with minimal complaint of discomfort. The best barometer of adequate analgesia is usually the patient's own perception. Careful planning of analgesic requirements and medication transitions is necessary to provide seamless pain control beyond the PACU.[16] In a study of postoperative pain in 10,008 ambulatory patients, 5.3% related severe pain in the PACU but only 1.7% in the discharge area. Surprisingly, 5.3% related severe pain again 24 hours after surgery[17] (Fig. 53-1).

To avoid masking signs of an unrelated condition or a surgical complication, ascertain that the nature and intensity of pain are appropriate for the surgical procedure before analgesics or sedatives are administered. The central nervous system (CNS) signs of hypoxemia, acidemia, or cerebral hypoperfusion often mimic those of pain, especially during emergence. Evaluating orientation, the level of arousal, and cardiovascular or pulmonary status usually identifies such patients. Administration of parenteral analgesics or sedatives can acutely worsen hypoventilation, airway obstruction, or hypotension, causing sudden deterioration and arrest.

Incisional pain can be effectively treated with iv opioids.[18] Opioid administration in the PACU should be part of a planned analgesic continuum that begins with the induction of surgical anesthesia and continues throughout the postoperative course. During iv titration, analgesia is achieved while incremental respiratory or cardiovascular depression is assessed. Sufficient analgesia is the end point, even if large doses of opioids are necessary in tolerant patients. Short-acting iv opioids are useful to expedite discharge and minimize nausea in ambulatory settings,[19] although short duration of analgesia can be a problem.[20] Disadvantages of the intramuscular route include larger dose requirements, delayed onset, and unpredictable uptake in hypothermic patients. Oral and transdermal analgesics have a limited role in the PACU but are helpful for ambulatory patients. Rectal

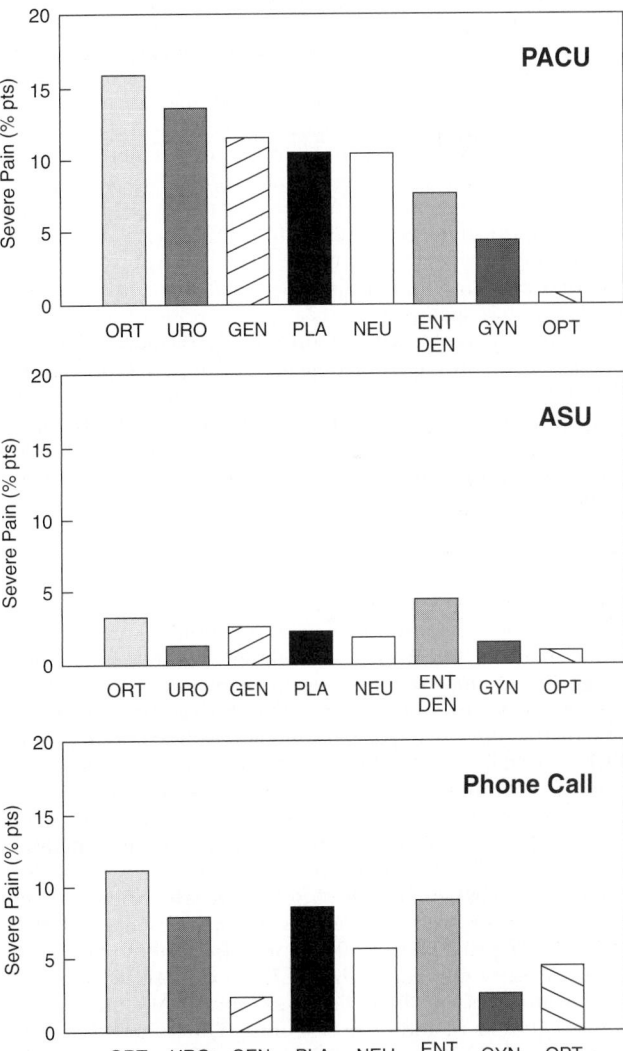

Figure 53-1. Percentage of patients experiencing severe pain in the postanesthesia care unit (PACU), the ambulatory surgery unit (ASU), and during a postanesthesia phone call at 24 hours. (From Chung F, Ritchie E, Su J: Postoperative pain in ambulatory surgery. Anesth Analg 85:808, 1997.)

analgesics are useful in children. Agonist–antagonist analgesics offer little advantage.

Ketorolac is an effective analgesic and anti-inflammatory that lowers opioid requirements, although possibility of hemorrhage due to its antiplatelet properties limits its use. Ketorolac might also decrease ischemic events in patients with coronary artery disease through analgesic and antiplatelet actions.[21] Oral acetaminophen or ibuprofen is effective, especially when administered before surgery.[22,23] Use of clonidine to supplement analgesic is effective but can cause hypotension.[24] N-methyl-D-aspartate antagonists such as dextromethorphan are claimed beneficial for inflammatory components of pain.[25]

Fear, anxiety, and confusion often accentuate postoperative pain, especially after general anesthesia. Titration of an iv sedative such as diazepam or midazolam attenuates this psychogenic component, although analgesic requirements may increase because of effects of benzodiazepines on γ-aminobutyric acid receptors. It is important to separate requirements for analgesia and for sedation. Opioids are poor sedatives, whereas benzodiazepines are poor analgesics. Interventions such as repositioning, reassurance, or extubation can also help minimize discomfort.

Other analgesic modalities provide pain relief beyond the PACU. Intravenous opioid loading in the PACU is important for smooth transition to patient-controlled analgesia. Injection of opioids into the epidural or subarachnoid space during anesthesia or in the PACU yields prolonged postoperative analgesia in selected patients.[26,27] Epidural opioid analgesia is effective after thoracic and upper abdominal procedures and helps wean patients with obesity or chronic obstructive pulmonary disease (COPD) from mechanical ventilation. Immediate and delayed ventilatory depression can occur, related to vascular uptake and cephalad spread in cerebrospinal fluid.[28,29] Nausea and pruritus are troubling side effects. Nausea resolves with antiemetics, whereas pruritus often responds to naloxone infusion. Ondansetron has been proposed as treatment for pruritus as well as opiate-induced nausea.[30] Epidural analgesia may also improve surgical outcomes after orthopedic and urologic procedures. Addition of local anesthetic or clonidine enhances analgesia and decreases the risk of side effects from epidural opioids,[24] although local anesthetics add risk of hypotension or motor blockade. Addition of other potentiating agents such as neostigmine is not yet widely used.

Placement of long-acting regional analgesic blocks reduces pain, controls SNS activity, and often improves ventilation. Percutaneous intercostal blocks reduce analgesic requirements after thoracic or high abdominal incision, although beneficial effects on postoperative pulmonary function are questionable. After shoulder and upper extremity procedures, interscalene block yields almost complete pain relief with only moderate inconvenience from motor impairment. Paralysis of the ipsilateral diaphragm can impair postoperative ventilation in patients with marginal reserve, although the impact is small in most.[31] Use of more dilute anesthetic solutions might decrease the incidence of this problem.[32] Suprascapular nerve block might be an alternative to avoid this very common and potentially serious side effect.[33] Caudal analgesia is effective in children after inguinal or genital procedures, whereas infiltration of local anesthetic into joints, soft tissues, or incisions decreases the intensity of pain. Instillation of opioids or neostigmine into joints is also somewhat analgesic. Input of positive suggestion during anesthesia probably has no significant influence on analgesic requirement and recovery course. Other modalities, such as transcutaneous nerve stimulation, "white noise," acupuncture, or hypnosis have limited utility for surgical pain.

Use of patient-controlled analgesia, spinal opioids, or neural blockade mandates anticipation of risk beyond the PACU. Again, the anesthesiologist must plan for extended postoperative analgesia before induction of surgical anesthesia and orient the anesthetic and PACU care toward that plan. If one analgesic modality proves inadequate, particular care must be taken implementing a second, innovative technique.

DISCHARGE CRITERIA

When possible before discharge, each patient should be sufficiently oriented to assess his or her physical condition and to summon assistance. Airway reflexes and motor function must be adequate to prevent aspiration of vomitus or secretions. Assure that ventilation and oxygenation are acceptable, with sufficient reserve to cover minor deterioration in unmonitored settings. Blood pressure, heart rate, and indices of peripheral perfusion should be relatively constant for at least 15 minutes. Achieving normal body temperature is not an absolute requirement, but resolution of shivering is. Acceptable analgesia must be achieved and vomiting appropriately controlled. Patients should be observed for at least 15 minutes after the last iv opioid or sedative is administered to assess peak effects and side effects. After reinforcement of regional anesthetics, longer observation could be appropriate. Oxygen saturation should be monitored for 15 minutes after discontinuation of supplemental oxygen to detect hypoxemia. Assess likely surgical complications (e.g., bleeding, vascular compromise, pneumothorax) or complications of underlying conditions (e.g., coronary artery disease, diabetes, hypertension, asthma). The results of postoperative diagnostic tests should be reviewed. If these generic criteria cannot be met, postponement of discharge or transfer to a specialized unit is advisable.

Fixed PACU discharge criteria must be used with caution because variability among patients is tremendous. Scoring systems that quantify physical status or establish thresholds for vital signs are useful for assessment but cannot replace individual evaluation.[34,35] Ideally, each patient should be evaluated for discharge by an anesthesiologist using a consistent set of criteria (Table 53-2), considering the severity of underlying disease, the anesthetic and recovery course, and the level of care at the destination, especially for ambulatory patients (see Chapter 46).

CARDIOVASCULAR COMPLICATIONS
Postoperative Hypotension

Systemic hypotension, a common postoperative complication, can cause hypoperfusion of vital organ systems. Consequent tissue hypoxia promotes inefficient anaerobic metabolism and accumulation of lactic acid, leading to unexplained metabolic acidemia. During hypotension, the SNS diverts blood flow to preserve the brain, heart, and kidneys. Symptoms of hypotension referable to these organs (e.g., disorientation, nausea, loss of consciousness, angina, reduced urine output) indicate that compensatory mechanisms have been exhausted. Complications of hypotension include ischemia or infarction of the myocardium, cerebrum, renal tubules, spinal cord, or bowel. Reduced venous flow rate increases risk of deep vein thrombosis and pulmonary embolism. Decreased hepatic oxygen delivery might change metabolic pathways for drugs, causing hepatic damage by toxic metabolites. The degree of hypotension at which risk of complications increases varies with the preoperative blood pressure, and is higher in patients with arteriosclerotic disease, stenotic vascular lesions, chronic hypertension, increased intracranial pressure, or renal failure.

Spurious Hypotension

Identifying spurious hypotension avoids unnecessary treatment and iatrogenic hypertension. A blood pressure cuff that is too large yields falsely low values. Cuff width should approximate two thirds of arm circumference. A transducer system that is improperly zeroed or excessively damped by air bubbles or catheter obstruction yields artificially low readings from an arterial catheter. Arterial constriction caused by hypothermia or

Table 53-2. GUIDELINES FOR DISCHARGE EVALUATION FROM POSTANESTHESIA CARE UNIT

General condition	Oriented to time, place, and surgical procedure
	Responds to verbal input and follows simple instructions
	Acceptable color without cyanosis, splotchiness, or paleness
	Adequate muscular strength and mobility for minimal self-care
	Absence or control of specific acute surgical complications (*e.g.*, bleeding, edema, neurologic weakness, diminished pulse)
	Suitable control of nausea and emesis
	Destination unit appropriate for patient's status
System blood pressure	Within ±20% of resting preoperative value
Heart rate and rhythm	Relatively constant for at least 30 min
	Resolution of any new dysrhythmia
	Acceptable intravascular volume status
	Any suspicion of myocardial ischemia rectified
Ventilation and oxygenation	Ventilatory rate >10, <30 breaths $\cdot$ min^{-1}
	Forced vital capacity approximately twice tidal volume
	Adequate ability to cough and clear secretions
	Qualitatively acceptable work of breathing
Airway maintainance	Protective reflexes (swallow, gag) intact
	Absence of stridor, retraction, or partial obstruction
	No further need for artificial airway support
Control of pain	Ability to localize and identify intensity of surgical pain
	Adequate analgesia, at least 15 min since last opioid
	Safe, appropriate orders for postdischarge analgesics
Renal function	Urine output >30 ml $\cdot$ h^{-1} (catheterized patients)
	Appropriate color and appearance of urine, evaluation of hematuria
	Follow-up orders *in re* output if spontaneous voiding has not occurred
Metabolic/laboratory	Acceptable hematocrit level in view of hydration, blood loss, and potential for future losses
	Suitable control of blood glucose
	Appropriate electrolyte homeostasis
	Evaluation of chest radiograph, electrocardiogram, and other tests as appropriate
Ambulatory patients	Ability to ambulate without dizziness, hypotension, or support
	Suitable control of nausea and vomiting after ambulation

Not all criteria will be satisfied by every patient, especially if discharge is to a critical care unit. Clinical judgment must always supersede established guidelines if the patient's condition is less than optimal in a given area. Whenever doubt exists about diagnosis or patient safety, discharge should be delayed.

α-adrenergic agonist drugs can reduce radial or brachial blood pressure below aortic pressure.

Hypovolemia

A reduction in circulating intravascular volume ("absolute" hypovolemia) decreases ventricular filling and cardiac output. SNS-mediated tachycardia, increased systemic vascular resistance (SVR), and venoconstriction might compensate for a 15–20% loss of intravascular volume. Greater deficits cause hypotension.

Failure to replace preoperative fluid deficit and fluid or blood lost during surgery frequently causes absolute hypovolemia. In the PACU, ongoing hemorrhage, sweating, and exudation of fluid into tissues (third-space losses) exacerbate hypovolemia. Blood loss is often occult, as with retroperitoneal bleeding, diffuse oozing related to coagulopathy, or hemorrhage into muscle after trauma or orthopedic procedures. Third-space losses can continue for up to 48 hours after surgery and can be massive during high-permeability pulmonary edema or accumulation of ascites. In a hypothermic, venoconstricted patient, a low intravascular volume might maintain cardiac output on PACU admission but cause hypotension when venous capacity increases during rewarming.

Sometimes, a "normal" intravascular volume is inadequate to maintain blood pressure (relative hypovolemia). Sudden decreases in endogenous SNS activity caused by relief of pain or vasovagal responses can acutely increase venous capacity, as can medications that mimic α-adrenergic receptor blockade (droperidol, chlorpromazine), release histamine (morphine), or directly dilate veins (nitrates, furosemide). Spinal or epidural anesthesia interferes with SNS regulation of venous tone, increasing venous capacitance and preventing constriction of veins in response to hemorrhage or positional changes. Compression of thoracic veins from positive intrathoracic pressure during mechanical ventilation impedes venous return, as does inferior vena caval compression from a gravid uterus or increased intra-abdominal pressure. Pericardial tamponade or air embolism also impedes ventricular filling.

On the patient's admission to the PACU, his or her intravascular volume is estimated, considering preoperative status, type and duration of surgery, estimated blood loss, fluid replacement, and hemostasis. Monitoring urine output as an index of intravascular volume can be misleading. Surgery and anesthesia impair renal tubular concentrating ability and glycosuria causes osmotic diuresis, each falsely indicating that intravascular volume is adequate. The variation of systolic blood pressure seen on an arterial catheter or pulse oximeter trace during positive-pressure ventilation provides a qualitative warning of reduced intravascular volume.[36] Central venous or pulmonary arterial pressure or transesophageal ultrasound monitoring helps clarify volume status.

Ventricular Dysfunction

Postoperative hypotension caused by ventricular dysfunction usually indicates that baseline ventricular contractility is reduced. Such patients often need high left ventricular end-diastolic pressure and elevated SNS activity to maintain cardiac output. Excessive fluid administration causes ventricular dilation, decreased cardiac output, and hypotension, often complicated by hydrostatic pulmonary edema. Overhydration may not be evident. If sympathetic blockade during spinal or epidural anesthesia is treated with excessive fluids, ventricular filling pressures can be normal during early recovery despite hypervolemia. When SNS blockade resolves, a characteristically high level of SNS outflow mobilizes large fluid volumes to the central circulation, precipitating ventricular failure. Depression from residual inhalational anesthetics and opiates contributes to decreased SNS outflow and reduced ventricular contractility. Although β-adrenergic receptor–blocking drugs reduce myocardial contractility, hypotension usually occurs only in patients who rely on maximal SNS activity for cardiovascular stability. Profound metabolic or respiratory acidemia reduces ventricular performance by interfering with catecholamine–receptor interaction and by depressing central SNS outflow. Low ionized calcium levels caused by dilution, chelation, or acute alkalemia also reduce ventricular contractility. Right ventricular dysfunction caused by pulmonary thromboembolism often presents with systemic hypotension.

Myocardial Ischemia

Postoperative myocardial ischemia is often initiated in high-risk patients by tachycardia or hypotension. Among patients with coronary disease, risk is higher for those with a history of congestive heart failure, smoking, and hypertension, and those having emergency surgery.[37] Patients are at significant risk of ischemia after both general and regional anesthetics.[38] In the PACU, tachycardia caused by pain, hypotension, acidemia, anxiety, or medications decreases diastolic filling time and generates ischemia. Inadequate diastolic blood pressure also causes ischemia. Increased ventricular wall tension secondary to overhydration, hypertension, or increased SNS activity increases myocardial oxygen consumption and initiates ischemia even when diastolic pressure is adequate. Severe hypoxemia, anemia, or carbon monoxide (CO) poisoning generates ischemia independent of coronary perfusion. The lowest tolerable hematocrit is highly individualized to each patient, but usually higher in patients with vascular disease.[39] Most postoperative angina is truly silent, and risk of early morbidity is high.[21,40] Postoperative anginal chest pain might be overshadowed by pain from surgical incisions and gastric distention, or masked by analgesia from residual anesthetics or opioids. The incidence of ischemic dysrhythmias is difficult to determine, given the high incidence of benign postoperative dysrhythmias. Hypotension caused by ischemic ventricular dysfunction can quickly cause irreversible infarction. Close evaluation of the hemodynamic responses to fluid challenge, the ST segment and T-wave morphology on the ECG, and the pulmonary artery (PA) pressures can sometimes uncover ischemia before hypotension occurs (Fig. 53-2). However, the predictive value of these indices is controversial. In high-risk patients, control of precipitating factors and timely therapy with analgesia, nitrates, and especially β-adrenergic blocking agents helps decrease morbidity from postoperative myocardial ischemia.[41,42]

Cardiac Dysrhythmia

Pre-existing myocardial disease or rhythm disturbances increase the risk of postoperative hypotension caused by a cardiac dysrhythmia. Sinus or nodal bradycardia with ventricular rates below 40 beats $\cdot$ min^{-1} decreases cardiac output and blood pressure, as do slow ventricular rhythms associated with complete heart block. A tachydysrhythmia that generates ventricular rates of 140–150 beats $\cdot$ min^{-1} can decrease cardiac output because ventricular filling time is compromised. Ventricular fibrillation, asystole, or electromechanical dissociation causes life-threatening reductions of output. Swings in autonomic nervous system activity place patients with valvular abnormalities at particular risk of hypotension from rhythm changes. An increased heart rate in patients with aortic stenosis reduces systolic ejection time, whereas tachycardia in patients with mitral stenosis impedes ventricular filling. Both decrease cardiac output and cause hypotension.

Decreased Systemic Vascular Resistance

Hypotension associated with regional anesthesia, α-adrenergic receptor–blocking drugs, blood components, or warming is caused by decreased SVR as well as by reduced venous return. Severe systemic acidemia decreases SVR by directly dilating vessels and by interfering catecholamine–α receptor interaction. Antihypertensive medications like hydralazine and nitroprusside reduce blood pressure in hypovolemic patients by interfering with arteriolar constriction. Sepsis interferes with arteriolar constriction, generating a high-output, low-resistance hypotension.

Postoperative hypotension is occasionally caused by the effects of anesthesia or surgery on baroreceptor function or by intracranial disease. Rarely, hypotension reflects steroid deficiency in patients whose adrenal axis is suppressed by exogenous steroid use. Hypotension secondary to steroid deficiency is often preceded by lethargy, fever, or nausea and by hyponatremia, hyperkalemia, and hypoglycemia.

Treatment of Postoperative Hypotension

In general, symptoms of vital organ hypoperfusion or a 20–30% reduction in systolic pressure from preoperative levels is an indication to treat. If risk for complication from hypotension is high, acceptable limits for pressure and heart rate should be defined during PACU admission.

A low blood pressure determination should be quickly validated. Auscultation of heart sounds and palpation of carotid or femoral pulses are useful qualitative indicators of central blood pressure. Supplemental oxygen should be administered and the iv infusion rate increased to maximum because hypovolemia is the most common etiology. If hypotension is spurious or caused by a reduced SVR or ischemia, the amount of fluid infused while these diagnoses are established is usually inconsequential. Check breath sounds and the cardiac rate and rhythm. Recent drug administration should be evaluated, and infusions that might cause vasodilation stopped. A 12-lead ECG, arterial blood gas determination, and chest radiography might be indicated.

Therapy is directed at the etiology of reduced systemic blood pressure, and the diagnosis reconfirmed. Simple maneuvers such as reducing airway pressure, placing pregnant patients in a lateral tilt position, or placing patients with orthostatic changes in a supine position should be used when appropriate. Tension pneumothorax must be evacuated. Infusion of crystalloid solutions is usually sufficient, although plasma expanders or blood facilitate more rapid volume expansion. Sympathomimetic α-adrenergic pressors such as phenylephrine that increase SVR and venous return temporarily maintain systemic pressure until sufficient volume can be infused. Ephedrine is less desirable because increased heart rate and contractility are usually unnecessary.

If fluid administration (300–500 ml) does not improve hypotension, myocardial dysfunction should be considered. For dysfunction not related to ischemia, drugs that augment contractility, perhaps in conjunction with systemic vasodilators, restore

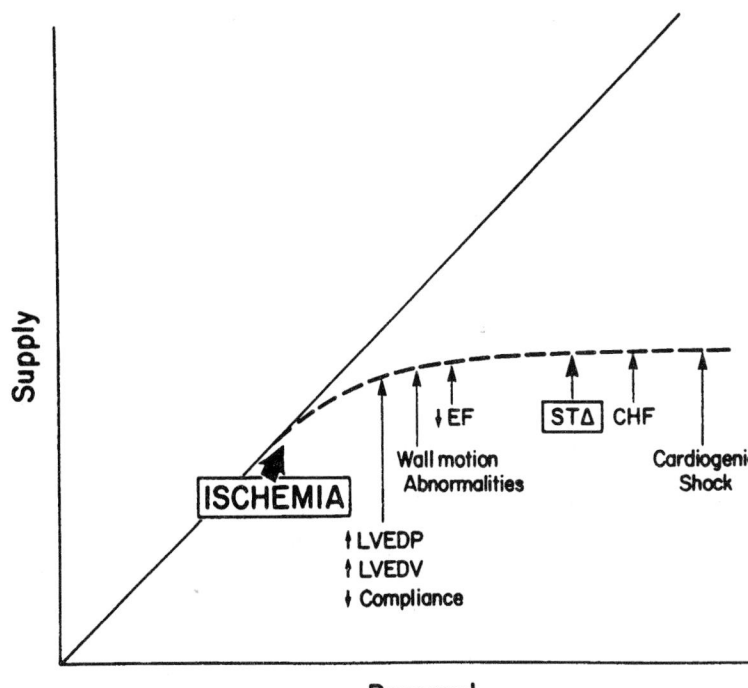

Figure 53-2. Physiologic consequences of myocardial ischemia. Note that changes in ventricular pressure and compliance may precede electrocardiographic changes (ST segment). LVEDP = left ventricular end-diastolic pressure; LVEDV = left ventricular end-diastolic volume; EF = ejection fraction; STD = ST segment change; CHF = congestive heart failure. (Reproduced with permission from Barash PG: Monitoring myocardial oxygen balance: Physiologic basis and clinical application. In Barash PG, Deutsch S, Tinker J [eds]: Refresher Courses in Anesthesiology, vol 13, p 21. Philadelphia, JB Lippincott, 1985.)

cardiac output and systemic pressure. If hypotension is caused by ischemia, resolution of the ischemia usually restores baseline cardiac function. Support of aortic diastolic pressure with an α receptor agonist and reduction of left ventricular end-diastolic pressure with nitroglycerin help maximize the coronary artery pressure gradient. Heart rate control with analgesics, sedatives, and especially β receptor blockers is important. Accurate diagnosis of ischemia is critical because therapy for ischemia can worsen hypotension caused by hypovolemia or other causes. PA catheterization or transesophageal echocardiography might be useful to estimate left ventricular filling and cardiac output, although the actual predictive value of PA readings is questionable.

If hypotension is caused by metabolic acidemia, iv bicarbonate or another alkalinizing agent helps restore pH while the underlying cause is remedied. Severe hypoxemia or respiratory acidemia mandates tracheal intubation and mechanical ventilation with supplemental oxygen. Sinus bradycardia unrelated to hypoxemia usually responds to iv atropine, glycopyrrolate, or ephedrine. Refractory bradycardia caused by sinus node disease or complete heart block is managed with iv epinephrine or isoproterenol, or with cardiac pacing. Digitalization or calcium channel blockade reduces the ventricular rate from acute-onset atrial fibrillation, whereas re-entrant paroxysmal atrial tachycardia often disappears with maneuvers or drugs that change cardiac conduction rates. If hypotension from a tachydysrhythmia is severe, immediate low-energy direct-current cardioversion (50 J) is indicated.

Hypotension caused by a low SVR is treated with an α-adrenergic agent. Sympathectomy from regional anesthesia responds to low levels of α stimulation. During advanced sepsis or catecholamine depletion, norepinephrine infusions may be required. If decreased SVR is caused by acidemia, correction of pH is necessary before pressor therapy will be effective.

Postoperative Hypertension

A moderate elevation in systemic blood pressure is common and acceptable in well-hydrated postoperative patients.[8,43] However, excessively high blood pressure can cause hemorrhage and third-space losses from arterial and venous sources, and might

disrupt vascular suture lines. High ventricular intracavitary pressure might lead to dilation, myocardial fiber stretch, and increased wall tension, precipitating ischemia or dysrhythmias. Elevated intraocular or intracranial pressure, cerebral edema, and intracranial hemorrhage also potentially increase morbidity.

A blood pressure cuff that is too small yields erroneously high readings, especially in obese or very muscular patients. A transducing system that is improperly zeroed or exhibits excessive resonance overestimates systolic pressure. Overshoot does not significantly change the accuracy of diastolic readings.

Patients with pre-existing hypertension exhibit exaggerated blood pressure responses because they have noncompliant vasculature, elevated peripheral vascular tone, and high levels of baseline endogenous SNS activity. Baroreceptor control of heart rate is impaired,[44] especially after anticholinergic administration during reversal of neuromuscular relaxation. After carotid endarterectomy, abnormal baroreceptor function can also generate hypertension.

Enhanced SNS activity frequently causes hypertension in the PACU. Peripheral arteriolar and venous constriction mediated by α-adrenergic stimulation increases SVR and venous return, whereas increased β_1 receptor stimulation increases ventricular contractility and heart rate. Intravascular volume expansion also increases cardiac output, especially when hypothermia leads to systemic vasoconstriction. SNS outflow most often reflects an appropriate response to noxious stimuli or adverse physiologic conditions (Table 53-3). SNS activity might also be a manifestation of exogenous sympathomimetics, monoamine oxidase inhibition, or pheochromocytoma. Cerebral vascular accidents, hypoxic encephalopathy, increased intracranial pressure, or severe osmotic changes interfere with central SNS regulation, causing autonomic dysfunction and severe hypertension.

Indications for treatment include a systolic or diastolic pressure 20–30% above baseline, signs or symptoms of complications (*e.g.,* headache, bleeding, ocular changes, angina, ST segment depression), or an unusual risk of morbidity (*e.g.,* increased intracranial pressure, mitral regurgitation, open eye injury). In patients with chronic hypertension, achieving a "normal" systemic pressure could promote vital organ hypoperfusion, so blood pressure should be reduced toward preoperative

Table 53-3. FACTORS THAT INCREASE POSTOPERATIVE CARDIAC SYMPATHETIC INFLUENCE

FACTORS INCREASING SYMPATHETIC ACTIVITY

Noxious stimuli
    Pain, anxiety, cranial stimulation, full bladder, tracheal intubation
Adverse physiologic conditions
    Hypercarbia/acidosis, hypoxemia, hypotension, hypoglycemia, congestive heart failure, increased intracranial pressure, myocardial ischemia
Medications
    β-Mimetic pressors, ephedrine, isoproterenol, epinephrine
    Dopamine, dobutamine
    Bronchodilators
        Terbutaline, aminophylline
    Anesthetics
        Ketamine, isoflurane
    Antihypertensives
        Hydralazine, nitroprusside

FACTORS DECREASING PARASYMPATHETIC ACTIVITY

Medications
    Parasympatholytics
        Atropine, glycopyrrolate
    Relaxants
        Pancuronium

levels. Therapy should be oriented toward causes of increased SNS activity. Administering analgesics or sedatives, correcting acidemia or hypoxemia, and ensuring ability to void are helpful. If hypertension persists, iv antihypertensive medications such as hydralazine with propranolol, labetalol, esmolol, or nicardipine yield temporary control. Incorporation of clonidine into the overall regimen is useful for both augmenting analgesia and for blood pressure control.[44] Clonidine may also blunt the postoperative SNS response to stimuli.[45] Potent vasodilators (nitroprusside, nitroglycerin) are reserved for refractory or profound hypertension.

Cardiac Dysrhythmias in the Postoperative Period

Asymptomatic Electrocardiographic Abnormalities

General anesthesia causes ECG changes in axis, intraventricular conduction, P- and T-wave morphology, and ST segments that are not related to cardiac abnormality (see Appendix). These changes reflect electrophysiologic effects of hypothermia, inhalation anesthetics, autonomic nervous system imbalance, and mild electrolyte abnormalities, and usually resolve within 3–6 hours. If persistent ECG changes indicate ischemia in a patient at risk, myocardial oxygen supply and demand should be optimized and serial ECG and enzyme determinations followed. Prolonged monitoring may be appropriate.

Bradycardia

In the PACU, increased parasympathetic nervous system (PNS) activity or decreased SNS influence promotes sinus bradycardia[46] (Table 53-4). Sick sinus syndrome, sinoatrial nodal ischemia, or severe hypoxemia also reduce sinus rate. Sinus bradycardia is benign unless it causes hypotension, usually when the rate falls below 40–45 beats · min⁻¹. Therapy involves restoring SNS/PNS balance to normal. Bradycardia caused by excess PNS activity usually responds to muscarinic-blocking drugs such as atropine or glycopyrrolate. Decreased SNS activity usually responds to a β-mimetic drug like ephedrine.

Emergence of a nodal pacemaker in the lower atrioventricular (AV) node or the bundle of His is also usually caused by autonomic imbalance. Increased PNS activity seems to suppress

a dominant sinoatrial pacemaker more than other pacemaker cells, allowing a slower focus to emerge. Factors that stop sinus impulses from reaching the ventricle also promote nodal rhythms. Nodal rhythms are benign unless a low ventricular rate or lack of coordinated atrial contraction reduces cardiac output and blood pressure. If hypotension occurs, atropine or β-mimetic medications can restore a sinus rhythm. These measures sometimes only increase nodal rate, necessitating support of blood pressure until spontaneous resolution occurs.

Risk of complete heart block in patients with bifascicular block or left bundle-branch block is small but real.[47] Idioventricular bradycardia seldom generates adequate cardiac output, and usually indicates life-threatening heart block, hypoxemia, acidemia, or myocardial ischemia. Atropine might improve AV nodal conduction enough to allow supraventricular impulses to reach the ventricles with acute third-degree AV nodal block. Atropine does not increase rate of ventricular pacemaker cells because they lack PNS innervation. Epinephrine, isoproterenol, or cardiac pacing accelerate the ventricular rate.

Tachycardia

Postoperative sinus tachycardia is nearly always associated with a physiologic increase in SNS influence (see Table 53-3). Tachycardia is usually harmless, but it can precipitate acute myocardial ischemia in patients with coronary artery disease. Sinus tachycardia seldom interferes with ventricular filling, but compromises cardiac output in patients with stenotic valvular lesions. Tachycardia exacerbates hypertension and might herald acidemia, hypoxemia, or malignant hyperthermia. Sinus tachycardia is treated by controlling its underlying cause. Giving analgesics for pain, iv fluids for hypovolemia, or sedatives to calm anxiety is usually sufficient. Decompressing a full bladder is helpful. Tachycardia caused by sympathomimetic drugs resolves as drug levels fall. If SNS activity is beyond control or tachycardia presents a threat, β blockade helps control rate. Digoxin is ineffective unless ventricular failure is the underlying cause.

Sudden-onset atrial fibrillation sometimes generates ventricular rates greater than 150 beats · min⁻¹ and might appear as a fast, nearly regular supraventricular tachycardia on the ECG. Patients recovering from thoracic surgical procedures or those with mitral valvular disease or pulmonary emboli have a higher incidence.[48] Fast ventricular rate might cause hypotension or myocardial ischemia. Digoxin or calcium channel blockers de-

Table 53-4. FACTORS THAT INCREASE POSTOPERATIVE PARASYMPATHETIC INFLUENCE

FACTORS INCREASING PARASYMPATHETIC ACTIVITY

Vagal reflexes
    Carotid sinus massage, Valsalva maneuver, gagging, rectal examination, increased ocular pressure, bladder distention, pharyngeal stimulation
Parasympathomimetic medications
    Acetylcholinesterase inhibitors
        Neostigmine, edrophonium
    α-Adrenergic drugs
        Neosynephrine, norepinephrine
    Opioids
        Morphine, fentanyl
    Succinylcholine

FACTORS DECREASING SYMPATHETIC ACTIVITY

High spinal or epidural anesthesia
Withdrawal of stimulus, extubation, emptying bladder
Severe acidemia/hypoxemia
Sympatholytic medications
    β Receptor blockers (propranolol)
    Opioids/sedatives/general anesthetics
    Ganglionic blockers
    Local anesthetics

crease the number of impulses that traverse the AV node per minute. For serious hypotension, direct-current cardioversion can convert fibrillation to sinus rhythm.

Atrial flutter is rare in postoperative patients. Treatment decreases the ventricular rate and regularizes atrial electrical activity. Paroxysmal atrial tachycardia usually reflects circus re-entry in a loop of conduction tissue, although 10–15% of cases are caused by discrete, rapidly firing atrial cells. Fast rates can interfere with ventricular filling and compromise cardiac output. Treatment involves slowing conduction velocities to interrupt re-entrant synchrony by increasing PNS influence (see Table 53-4). Digoxin or calcium channel blockers are also useful. Paroxysmal atrial tachycardia caused by a rapidly firing atrial pacemaker slows with β blockade.

Postoperative ventricular tachycardia or fibrillation almost always reflects severe myocardial ischemia, systemic acidemia, or hypoxemia, although re-entrant ventricular tachycardia does occur. Cardiopulmonary resuscitation, β-mimetic pressors, cardioversion, and control of ventilation, oxygenation, and serum pH help restore a synchronized rhythm.

Premature Contractions

An aberrant impulse arising in the atrium, AV node, or upper bundle of His generates an atrial premature contraction (APC), causing an early but otherwise normal QRS complex that often is not preceded by a P wave. In postoperative patients, APCs usually appear with increased SNS activity and seldom cause hemodynamic compromise. Control of stimuli causing increased SNS activity often eliminates APCs (see Table 53-3).

Ventricular ectopy present before surgery usually reappears in the PACU, with somewhat decreased frequency. Ectopy does not usually predict postoperative outcome.[49] In postoperative patients, abnormal ventricular complexes are almost always benign and seldom require treatment. Relatively few high-amplitude, wide, bizarre QRS complexes represent abnormal impulses that originate in ventricular conducting tissue. Most represent aberrantly conducted APCs or re-entrant rhythms. Most actual premature ventricular contractions (PVCs) are caused by nonthreatening conditions.

Actual PVCs usually occur at varying intervals from a previous normal QRS and often exhibit a full compensatory pause. In postoperative patients, benign PVCs frequently accompany excessive PNS or SNS activity. Increased PNS influence allows emergence of ventricular escape beats. Increased SNS activity accelerates ventricular automatic cells, promoting depolarization between supraventricular impulses, and fosters emergence of parasystolic foci. PVCs resolve when autonomic nervous system balance is restored. Benign postoperative PVCs can also be generated by stretch of myocardial fibers from hypertension and mechanical stimulation from central vascular catheters. PVCs that reflect digitalis toxicity, myocardial ischemia, or electrolyte disturbances are much rarer but more serious. Antidysrhythmics such as lidocaine, procainamide, and bretylium control automaticity in ischemic ventricular tissues.

An early supraventricular impulse that enters the ventricular conduction system before all pathways have recovered excitability generates asynchronous ventricular depolarization and a wide, high-amplitude ECG complex. This aberrantly conducted APC is sometimes preceded by an abnormal P wave, often exhibits a noncompensatory pause, and often resembles normal complexes in general shape. Delayed recovery of excitability after general anesthesia favors aberrant conduction.

If a sinus impulse is delayed in a ventricular conduction pathway long enough to encounter tissue that has recovered excitability, the impulse depolarizes this tissue a second time and spreads through the entire heart. This "re-entrant" depolarization generates a wide, high-amplitude QRS similar to a true PVC. Re-entrant complexes are uniform in configuration, manifest full compensatory pauses, follow the preceding normal complex by a constant interval (fixed coupling), and often

appear in a bigeminal pattern. Re-entry is often seen with increased SNS activity in patients recovering from halothane anesthesia.

If ectopic beats are so frequent that cardiac output is compromised, control of autonomic nervous system imbalance usually restores a regular rhythm. Antidysrhythmics are seldom necessary, although β receptor blockade might be useful. Treatment of re-entrant impulses is based on elimination of factors that cause conduction delay or nonuniform recovery of excitability, and on control of SNS activity.

POSTOPERATIVE PULMONARY DYSFUNCTION

Mechanical, hemodynamic, and pharmacologic factors related to surgery and anesthesia impair ventilation, oxygenation, and airway maintenance.[50] Heavy smoking, obesity, sleep apnea, severe asthma, and COPD increase the risk of postoperative ventilatory events.[43,51] Preoperative pulmonary function testing has limited predictive value for postoperative complications,[52,53] perhaps with the exception of postoperative bronchospasm in smokers.[54]

Inadequate Postoperative Ventilation

In the PACU, elevated Pa_{CO_2} does not necessarily indicate inadequate postoperative ventilation. Inadequate ventilation should be suspected when (1) respiratory acidemia occurs coincident with tachypnea, anxiety, dyspnea, labored ventilation, or increased SNS activity; (2) hypercarbia reduces the arterial pH below 7.25; or (3) Pa_{CO_2} progressively increases with a progressive decrease in arterial pH.

Inadequate Respiratory Drive

In PACU patients, mild respiratory acidemia is expected. Residual effects of iv or inhalational anesthetics blunt the ventilatory responses to both hypercarbia and hypoxemia.[55] Residual neuromuscular relaxants might also depress cholinergic portions of the hypoxic drive neural arc.[56] Sedatives augment depression from opioids and anesthetics, ablate the conscious will to ventilate (sometimes a significant component of ventilatory drive), and might directly depress ventilation.[57]

Serious hypoventilation and hypercarbia often evolve insidiously during transfer to the PACU. Effects of intraoperative medications are usually waning, but the peak depressant effect of iv opioid given just before transfer occurs in the PACU. Parallel depression of medullary centers that regulate the SNS blunts signs of acidemia or hypoxemia such as hypertension, tachycardia, and agitation, concealing hypoventilation. Patients might communicate lucidly and even complain of severe pain while experiencing significant opioid-induced hypoventilation.[58] A balance must be struck between an acceptable level of postoperative ventilatory depression and a tolerable level of pain or agitation.[59] If hypoventilation from opioids is excessive, titration of iv naloxone reverses respiratory depression without affecting analgesia. Flumazenil directly reverses depressant effects of benzodiazepines on ventilatory drive.[60]

The abrupt diminution of a noxious stimulus (e.g., tracheal extubation, regional analgesic block) may promote airway obstruction or hypoventilation by altering the balance between depression from medication and arousal from discomfort. Intracranial hemorrhage or edema sometimes presents with apnea, especially after posterior fossa craniotomy. Bilateral carotid body injury after endarterectomy can ablate peripheral hypoxic drive. Chronic respiratory acidemia from COPD alters CNS sensitivity to pH and makes hypoxic drive dominant, but hypoventilation from supplemental oxygen rarely occurs in the PACU. Patients with abnormal CO_2/pH responses from morbid obesity, chronic airway obstruction, or sleep apnea are more sensitive to respiratory depressants.[61] Risk for apnea after anesthesia in preterm infants depends on type of anesthetic, postconceptual age, and preoperative anemia.[62] Preterm infants should be monitored for at least 12 hours after surgery (see Chapter 43).

Increased Airway Resistance

High resistance to gas flow through airways increases work of breathing and CO_2 production. If inspiratory muscles cannot generate sufficient pressure gradients to overcome resistance, alveolar ventilation falls and progressive respiratory acidemia occurs.

In the PACU, high upper airway resistance is caused by obstruction in the pharynx (posterior tongue displacement, change in anteroposterior and lateral dimensions from soft tissue collapse), in the larynx (laryngospasm, laryngeal edema), or in the large airways (extrinsic compression from hematoma or tumor, tracheal stenosis).[63,64] Weakness from residual neuromuscular relaxation[65] or myasthenia gravis[66] is often contributory, but seldom is the primary etiology of airway compromise. If the airway is clear of vomitus or foreign bodies, simple maneuvers such as lateral positioning, chin lift, mandible elevation, or placement of an oropharyngeal or nasopharyngeal airway usually relieve obstruction. A nasopharyngeal airway is better tolerated with functional gag reflexes. Improving the level of consciousness is useful.

During emergence, stimulation of the pharynx or vocal cords by secretions, foreign matter, or extubation generates laryngospasm.[67] Laryngeal constrictor muscles tightly occlude the tracheal inlet and severely reduce air flow. Children with upper respiratory infections,[68] smokers,[50] children chronically exposed to secondhand smoke,[69] patients with irritable airway conditions, and patients recovering from upper airway surgery are at highest risk. Laryngospasm can usually be overcome with gentle positive pressure in the oropharynx with 100% oxygen. Prolonged laryngospasm is relieved with a small dose of succinylcholine (*e.g.*, 0.1 mg · kg^{-1}). An intubating dosage of succinylcholine should never be used to break postoperative laryngospasm, especially if the alveolar partial pressure of oxygen (P_{AO_2}) has been decreased by a period of apnea. The rate of P_{AO_2} decline invariably causes serious hypoxemia before restoration of spontaneous ventilation unless assisted ventilation is given[70] (Fig. 53-3). If obesity or surgical factors have reduced the func-

tional residual capacity (FRC), the decreased volume of O_2 available in the lungs accelerates the development of hypoxemia.

Acute extrinsic upper airway compression, as seen with an expanding neck hematoma, must be relieved. Soft tissue edema worsens airway obstruction, especially in children and in adults recovering from carotid endarterectomy, thyroid surgery, or other procedures on the neck.[71] Nebulized vasoconstrictors help somewhat, but systemic steroids have little effect.[72] Patients with C1 esterase inhibitor deficiency can have severe, refractory angioneurotic edema after even slight surgical trauma to the upper airway.[73] If airway obstruction is fixed (*e.g.*, epiglottitis, retropharyngeal abscess, encroaching tumors), emergency tracheal intubation might be necessary. Airway manipulation is dangerous because minor trauma from intubation attempts can convert a marginal airway into a total obstruction. Use of sedatives or muscle relaxants to facilitate intubation can worsen obstruction by compromising the patient's volitional efforts to maintain the airway and by eliminating spontaneous ventilation. Equipment and personnel necessary for emergency cricothyroidotomy or tracheostomy should be available. Cricothyroidotomy using a 14-gauge iv catheter permits oxygenation and marginal ventilation until the airway can be secured (Fig. 53-4), especially if jet ventilation with 100% oxygen is used.

Reduction of cross-sectional area in small airways increases overall airway resistance because resistance varies inversely with the fourth power of radius during laminar flow and with the fifth power during turbulent flow. In the PACU, pharyngeal or tracheal stimulation from secretions, suctioning, aspiration, or tracheal intubation can trigger a reflex constriction of bronchial smooth muscle in patients with reactive airways. Histamine release precipitated by medication or allergic reactions also increases airway smooth muscle tone. Decreased radial traction on small airways reduces cross-sectional area in patients with COPD or with decreased lung volume secondary to obesity, surgical manipulation, excessive lung water, or splinting.[74] If ventilatory requirements are increased by warming, hyperthermia, or elevated work of breathing, high flow rates convert laminar flow to higher-resistance turbulent flow.

Smokers and patients with bronchospastic conditions are at highest risk for bronchospasm after surgery.[75] Preoperative spirometric evidence of increased airway resistance predicts an increased risk of postoperative bronchospasm.[54] In postoperative patients, prolonged expiratory time or wheezing during

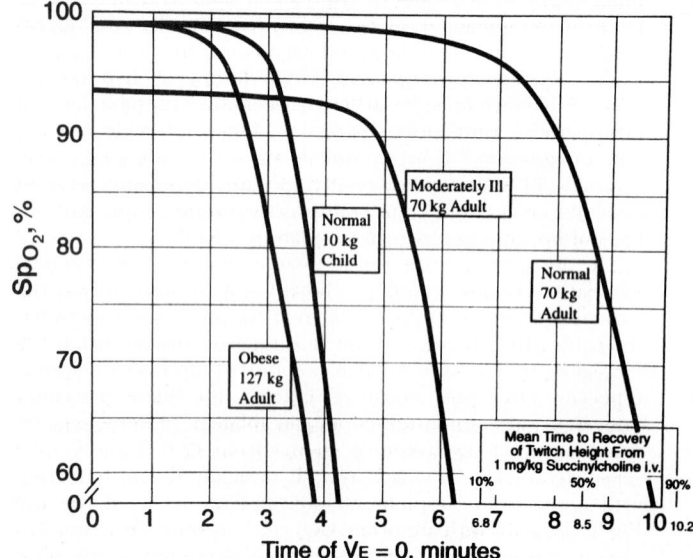

TIME TO HEMOGLOBIN DESATURATION WITH INITIAL F$_{AO_2}$ = 0.87

Figure 53-3. Rate of Sp_{O_2} decline after onset of apnea. (From Benumof JL, Dagg R, Benumof R: Critical hemoglobin desaturation will occur before return to an unparalyzed state following 1 mg/kg intravenous succinylcholine. Anesthesiology 87:979, 1997.)

a forced vital capacity expiration often unmasks high airway resistance. (Resistance is higher during expiration because intermediate-diameter airways are compressed by positive intrathoracic pressure.) High airway resistance does not always cause audible turbulent air flow (wheezing) because flow might be so impeded that no sound is produced. Signs of increased resistance mimic those of decreased pulmonary compliance. Spontaneously breathing patients exhibit accessory muscle recruitment, labored ventilation, and increased work of breathing with either condition. Mechanically ventilated patients exhibit high peak inspiratory pressure for a given tidal volume.

The treatment of small airway resistance is directed at an underlying etiology. Laryngeal or airway stimulation should be eliminated. Patients often respond well to their existing regimen of albuterol, pirbuterol, or salmeterol inhalers. Isoetharine or metaproterenol nebulized in oxygen resolves postoperative bronchospasm with minimal tachycardia. Intramuscular or sublingual terbutaline can be added. If ventilation is still compromised or unduly labored, an aminophylline loading dose and maintenance infusion might be administered. Bronchospasm resistant to β_2-sympathomimetic medication may improve with an anticholinergic medication such as atropine or ipratropium. If bronchospasm is life-threatening, an iv epinephrine infusion usually yields profound bronchodilation.

Increased small airway resistance caused by mechanical factors (*e.g.*, loss of lung volume, retained secretions, pulmonary edema) usually does not resolve with bronchodilators. Restoration of lung volume with incentive spirometry or deep tidal ventilation increases radial traction on small airways. Reducing left ventricular filling pressures might relieve airway resistance caused by increased lung water, although resistance can persist because interstitial fluid accumulation requires time to resolve. After prolonged bronchospasm, a patient might seem resistant to bronchodilators. Extended contraction of airway smooth muscle obstructs venous and lymphatic flow, leading to airway wall edema that resolves slowly.

Decreased Compliance

Extrinsic factors that reduce pulmonary compliance accentuate the work of breathing. In the extreme, low compliance causes progressive respiratory muscle fatigue, hypoventilation, and respiratory acidemia. Gas in the stomach or bowel and tight chest or abdominal dressings also reduce pulmonary compli-

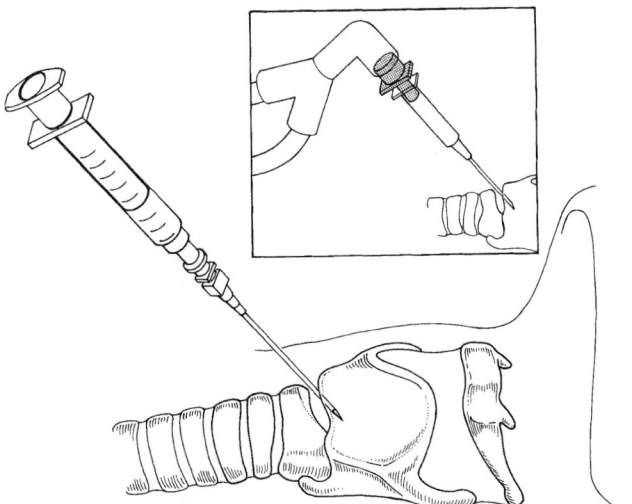

Figure 53-4. Cricothyroidotomy using a large-bore (14-gauge) intravenous catheter attached to syringe. After entry into the trachea, the needle is directed toward the carina.

ance. Obesity affects compliance, especially when adipose tissue compresses the thoracic cage or increases intra-abdominal pressure in supine or lateral positions. An intra-abdominal tumor, hemorrhage, ascites, bowel obstruction, or pregnancy also impairs diaphragmatic excursion and reduces compliance.

Parenchymal changes affect compliance. Reduction of FRC leads to small airway closure and distal lung collapse, requiring greater energy expenditure to re-expand the lung. Pulmonary edema increases the lung's weight and inertia, making expansion more difficult. Fluid in air spaces also elevates surface tension by interfering with surfactant activity. Pulmonary contusion or hemorrhage interferes with lung expansion, as do restrictive lung diseases, skeletal abnormalities, intrathoracic lesions, hemothorax, pneumothorax, or cardiomegaly.

In the PACU, the work of breathing is improved by resolving problems that reduce compliance. Allowing patients to recover in a semisitting position (rather than supine or full sitting position) reduces work of breathing. Incentive spirometry and chest physiotherapy restore lung volume, as does positive end-expiratory pressure (PEEP) or continuous positive airway pressure (CPAP). In patients with COPD and highly compliant lungs, positive airway pressure might force the rib cage and diaphragms toward their excursion limits, accentuating muscular effort required during inspiration.

Neuromuscular and Skeletal Problems

Postoperative airway obstruction and hypoventilation are sometimes caused by incomplete reversal of neuromuscular relaxation. Residual paralysis compromises cough, airway patency, ability to overcome airway resistance, and airway protection.[76] Intraoperative use of shorter-acting relaxants might decrease the incidence of residual paralysis, but does not eliminate the problem.[77] Marginal reversal can be more dangerous than near-total paralysis because an agitated patient exhibiting uncoordinated movements and airway obstruction is more easily identified. A somnolent patient exhibiting mild stridor and shallow ventilation from marginal neuromuscular function might be overlooked. Insidious hypoventilation with respiratory acidemia or regurgitation with aspiration then occur later into recovery.

Patients with neuromuscular abnormalities such as myasthenia gravis, Eaton-Lambert syndrome, periodic paralysis, or muscular dystrophies exhibit exaggerated or prolonged responses to muscular relaxants. Even without relaxant administration, they can exhibit postoperative ventilatory insufficiency from inadequate neuromuscular reserve. Medications potentiate neuromuscular relaxation (*e.g.*, antibiotics, furosemide, propranolol, phenytoin), as does hypocalcemia or hypermagnesemia.

Diaphragmatic contraction is compromised in some postoperative patients, forcing more reliance on intercostal muscles and reducing the ability to deal with decreased compliance or increased ventilatory demands.[78] Impairment of phrenic nerve function from interscalene block, trauma, or thoracic and neck operations "paralyzes" one or rarely both diaphragms.[31] Adequate ventilation can normally be maintained with only one diaphragm and marginal ventilation by external intercostal muscles alone. However, with high work of breathing, muscle weakness, or increased ventilatory demands, a nonfunctional diaphragm impairs ventilation. Thoracic spinal or epidural blockade interferes with intercostal muscle function and reduces ventilatory reserve, especially in patients with COPD. Abnormal motor neuron function (*e.g.*, Guillain-Barré syndrome, cervical spinal cord trauma), flail chest, or severe kyphosis or scoliosis can cause postoperative ventilatory insufficiency.

Simple bedside tests help assess mechanical ability to ventilate. Forced vital capacity of 10–12 ml · kg^{-1} and inspiratory pressure more negative than −25 cm H$_2$O imply that strength of ventilatory muscles is adequate to sustain ventilation. The ability to sustain head elevation in a supine position is a rough index of muscular recovery. Tactile train-of-four assessment accurately assesses ability to ventilate. However, none of these clinical end points reliably predicts recovery of airway protective reflexes.[79,80] Hand grip, pedal flexion, and other maneuvers are less reliable indicators. Failure on these tests does not necessarily indicate the need for assisted ventilation.

Occasionally, a clinical picture suggesting ventilatory insufficiency appears when ventilation is adequate. Voluntary limitation of chest expansion to avoid pain causes labored, rapid, shallow breathing characteristic of inadequate ventilation. This pattern seldom causes actual hypoventilation and usually regularizes with repositioning and analgesia. Ventilation with small tidal volumes due to thoracic restriction or reduced compliance generates afferent input from pulmonary stretch receptors, leading to dyspnea, labored breathing, and accessory muscle recruitment in spite of appropriate minute ventilation. (This also occurs during mechanical ventilation with low volumes.) Occasional large, "satisfying" lung expansions often relieve these symptoms. Finally, spontaneous hyperventilation to compensate for a metabolic acidemia might generate tachypnea or labored breathing, which is mistaken for ventilatory insufficiency.

Increased Dead Space

Ventilation of poorly perfused alveoli with high ventilation/perfusion ($\dot{V}/\dot{Q}$) ratios or of unperfused dead space is less effective in removing CO_2. Expansion of dead space volume or reduction of tidal volume increases the fraction of each breath wasted in dead space ($\dot{V}D/\dot{V}T$) and the amount of CO_2 from the previous exhalation that is rebreathed. A proportionally larger increase in total minute ventilation is also required to meet any increase in CO_2 production. Patients with high $\dot{V}D/\dot{V}T$ are at greater risk for postoperative ventilatory failure.

In an occasional postoperative patient, an acute increase in dead space contributes to postoperative respiratory acidemia. Although upper airway dead space is reduced after tracheal intubation and nearly eliminated by tracheostomy, excessive tubing volume or valve reversal in breathing circuits promotes rebreathing of CO_2. PEEP or CPAP elevates anatomic dead space, especially in patients with high pulmonary compliance. Pulmonary embolization with air, thrombus, or cellular debris increases physiologic dead space, although impact on CO_2 excretion is often masked by accelerated minute ventilation from hypoxic drive or reflex responses. Pulmonary hypotension can transiently increase $\dot{V}D/\dot{V}T$ by decreasing perfusion to well ventilated, nondependent lung. Irreversible increases in dead space occur if adult respiratory distress syndrome (ARDS) related to sepsis, massive transfusion, or hypoxia destroys pulmonary microvasculature.

Dead space may appear high if an inhalation interrupts the previous exhalation and a portion of spent alveolar gas is rebreathed. This "gas trapping" occurs when high airway resistance lengthens the time required to exhale completely, or if improper inspiration/expiration ratios or excessive ventilatory rates are used during mechanical ventilation.

Increased Carbon Dioxide Production

Carbon dioxide production varies directly with metabolic rate, body temperature, and substrate availability. During anesthesia, CO_2 production falls to approximately 60% of the normal 2–3 $ml \cdot kg^{-1} \cdot min^{-1}$ as hypothermia lowers metabolic activity and neuromuscular relaxation reduces tonic muscle contraction. In the PACU, metabolic rate and CO_2 production can increase by 40% as they return toward normal. Shivering, high work of breathing, infection, SNS activity, or rapid carbohydrate metabolism during iv hyperalimentation also accelerate CO_2 production. Malignant hyperthermia generates CO_2 production many

times greater than normal, which rapidly exceeds ventilatory reserve and causes severe respiratory acidemia.

Even mild increases of CO_2 production can precipitate respiratory acidemia if compliance, airway resistance, or neuromuscular paralysis interferes with ventilation. With the exception of adjusting hyperalimentation or treating malignant hyperthermia, there is little yield from adjusting CO_2 production in the PACU. Rarely, when increased dead space precludes delivery of adequate mechanical ventilation, deliberate hypothermia and paralysis are instituted to reduce CO_2 production in the hope that increased $\dot{V}D/\dot{V}T$ is reversible.

Inadequate Postoperative Oxygenation

Systemic arterial partial pressure of oxygen (PaO_2) is the best indicator of pulmonary oxygen transfer from alveolar gas to pulmonary capillary blood. Arterial hemoglobin saturation monitored by pulse oximetry yields less information on alveolar–arterial gradients and is not helpful to assess impact of hemoglobin dissociation curve shifts or carboxyhemoglobin.[81] Evaluation of metabolic acidemia or mixed venous oxygen content yields better insight into peripheral oxygen delivery and utilization. Adequate arterial oxygenation does not mean that cardiac output, arterial perfusion pressure, or distribution of blood flow will maintain tissue oxygenation. Sepsis, hypotension, anemia, hemoglobin dissociation abnormalities, or CO poisoning generate tissue ischemia in spite of adequate oxygenation.

In the PACU, the acceptable lower limit for PaO_2 varies with individual patient characteristics. A PaO_2 below 65–70 mm Hg causes significant hemoglobin desaturation, although tissue oxygen delivery might be maintained at lower levels. Maintaining PaO_2 between 80 and 100 mm Hg (saturation 93–97%) ensures adequate peripheral oxygen availability. Little benefit is derived from elevating PaO_2 above 110 mm Hg because hemoglobin is saturated and the amount of additional oxygen dissolved in plasma is negligible. During postoperative mechanical ventilation, a PaO_2 above 80 mm Hg with 0.4 FiO_2 and 5 cm H_2O PEEP or CPAP usually sustains peripheral oxygenation after tracheal extubation.

Distribution of Ventilation

Loss of dependent lung volume commonly causes $\dot{V}/\dot{Q}$ mismatching and hypoxemia. A reduction in FRC decreases radial traction on small airways, leading to collapse and distal atelectasis that can worsen for 36 hours after surgery.[82] Reduced ventilation in dependent lung is particularly damaging because gravity directs pulmonary blood flow to dependent areas. Certain patients are at increased risk. Obese patients sustain large decreases in FRC during surgery.[74] Older patients normally exhibit airway closure at end-expiration (Fig. 53-5). Those with COPD have more severe closure that is exacerbated by small reductions in FRC. Retraction, packing, manipulation, or peritoneal insufflation during upper abdominal surgery reduces FRC, as does compression from leaning surgical assistants.[83] Prone, lithotomy, or Trendelenburg positions are disadvantageous, especially in obese patients. Right upper lobe collapse secondary to partial right mainstem intubation is a frequently overlooked cause. During thoracic surgery, the weight of unsupported mediastinal contents, pressure from abdominal contents on the dependent diaphragm, and lung compression all reduce dependent lung volume. Gravity and lymphatic obstruction also promote interstitial fluid accumulation, which accentuates $\dot{V}/\dot{Q}$ mismatching. This "down lung syndrome" may appear as unilateral pulmonary edema on the chest film.

In the PACU, acute pulmonary edema from overhydration, ventricular dysfunction, or increased capillary permeability leads to hypoxemia by interfering with both $\dot{V}/\dot{Q}$ matching and diffusion of oxygen. Strong inspiratory efforts against an obstructed airway decrease FRC and promote negative-pressure pulmonary edema. Small airway occlusion from extrinsic compression, retained secretions, aspirate, or mainstem intubation leads to distal hypoventilation and hypoxemia. Pneumothorax, hemothorax, pulmonary contusion, or pulmonary hemorrhage also reduce lung volume.

Conservative measures that restore lung volume often improve oxygenation. If possible, obese patients should recover in a semisitting position to reduce the pressure of abdominal contents on the diaphragms. Deep ventilation, vigorous cough, chest physiotherapy, and incentive spirometry help expand FRC, mobilize secretions, and accustom a patient to incisional discomfort. Pain with ventilation encourages rapid, shallow breathing that provides adequate ventilation but does not promote expansion. Analgesia helps maintain FRC, especially with upper abdominal or chest wall incisions.

For serious postoperative reduction of lung volume, positive pressure is effective for restoring FRC. CPAP (5–7 cm H_2O) can be delivered by face mask for several hours until factors promoting loss of lung volume resolve. If hypoxemia is severe or patient acceptance of mask CPAP is poor, tracheal intubation is usually required. Intubation for delivery of CPAP does not mandate positive-pressure ventilation. Ventilatory requirements should be assessed independently, considering $PaCO_2$, arterial pH, and work of breathing. Usually, 5–10 cm H_2O of CPAP or PEEP restores lung volume and PaO_2 without risking hypotension, increased intracranial pressure, or barotrauma. If PaO_2 does not improve, the etiology must be re-evaluated. During routine postoperative care, airway pressure >10 cm H_2O is transmitted more to thoracic veins and is associated with higher incidence of barotrauma. An occasional patient with ARDS or severe pulmonary contusion might exhibit improvement in oxygenation and compliance with higher pressures.

Tracheal intubation eliminates expiratory resistance and the "physiologic PEEP" (2–5 cm H_2O) that might help maintain lung volume during spontaneous ventilation. Exposing an intubated trachea to ambient airway pressure may cause a gradual, progressive reduction in FRC. It may be helpful to allow intubated patients to exhale against a slight degree of CPAP.

Healthy, slender patients left intubated without positive pressure for short periods can usually restore reduced FRC after extubation.

Distribution of Perfusion

Poor distribution of pulmonary perfusion also interferes with $\dot{V}/\dot{Q}$ matching and oxygenation. The distribution of pulmonary blood flow is primarily determined by hydrodynamic factors (pulmonary arterial and venous pressures, arteriolar and capillary resistance), which in turn are affected by gravity, airway pressure, lung volume, and cardiovascular dynamics. Distribution of blood flow is modulated by hypoxic pulmonary vasoconstriction (HPV), which diverts flow away from air spaces that exhibit low PaO_2.

After surgery, SNS activity increases cardiac output and pulmonary vascular resistance, elevating PA pressure. High PA pressure increases blood flow to less dependent lung and through the bronchial circulation, interfering with $\dot{V}/\dot{Q}$ matching. Reduction in PA pressure might compromise perfusion to well ventilated midlung parenchyma. If low compliance in dependent lung simultaneously redistributes fresh ventilation to upper lung, regional $\dot{V}/\dot{Q}$ mismatch results. Also, the effectiveness of HPV varies with PA pressure in a bimodal fashion.

Position changes affect oxygenation if gravity forces blood flow to areas with reduced ventilation. Placing a poorly ventilated lung in a dependent position can seriously reduce PaO_2, but placing the unventilated parenchyma in a nondependent position could improve $\dot{V}/\dot{Q}$ matching. Care should be taken when positioning a diseased lung in the "up" position to avoid draining purulent material to the unaffected lung.

Distribution of blood flow is affected by changes in airway pressure and lung volume. Positive-pressure lung inflation might increase resistance in intra-alveolar and extra-alveolar vessels, whereas negative-pressure expansion probably decreases extra-alveolar resistance. Reduced lung volume has complex effects on microvascular resistance.

Other factors affect $\dot{V}/\dot{Q}$ matching in PACU patients. Residual inhalational anesthetics, vasodilators, and sympathomimetics alter PA pressure and directly affect vascular tone and HPV,

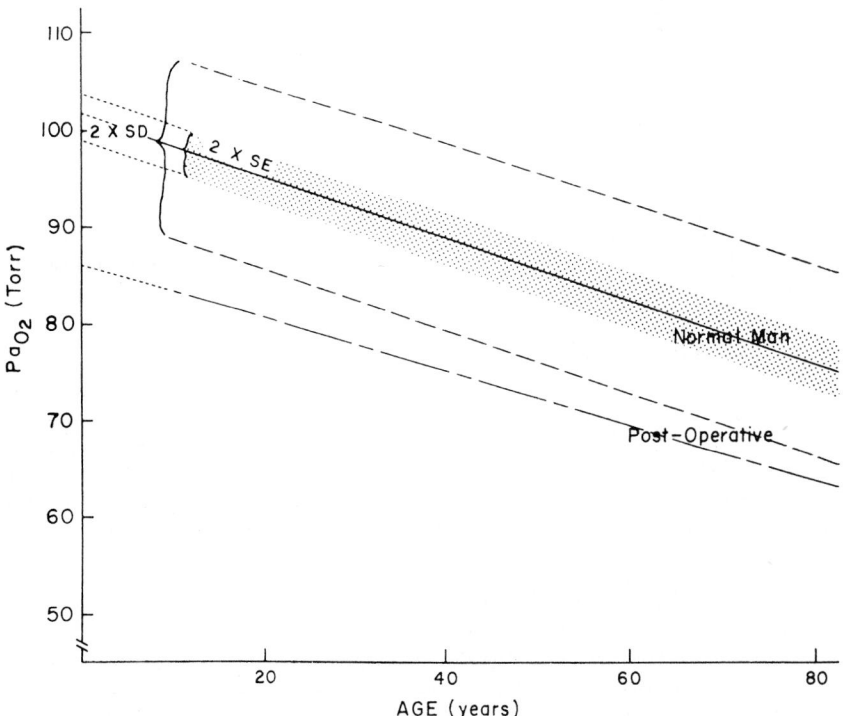

Figure 53-5. The influence of age on PaO_2. For any given age, the PaO_2 is lower in the postoperative period. The *dashed line* indicates range of normal individual values; the *shaded area* indicates the range of normal mean values. (Reproduced with permission from Marshall BE, Wyche MQ Jr: Hypoxemia during and after anesthesia. Anesthesiology 37:178, 1972.)

partially explaining larger alveolar–arterial oxygen gradients after general anesthesia. (Changes in lung volume and distribution of ventilation also contribute.) Patients with cirrhosis of the liver exhibit poor $\dot{V}/\dot{Q}$ matching caused by circulating humoral substances related to abnormal hepatic metabolism. Circulating endotoxin impairs HPV, contributing to hypoxemia in septic patients.

In the PACU, few interventions are useful to improve $\dot{V}/\dot{Q}$ matching by changing pulmonary blood flow. Postoperative $\dot{V}/\dot{Q}$ abnormalities are more effectively resolved by improving the distribution of ventilation. PA pressure should be maintained within an acceptable range and, when possible, placing severely diseased lung tissue in a dependent position should be avoided. Eliminating β-mimetic or vasodilatory medications may improve Pa_{O_2}, but benefits from the medication usually outweigh drawbacks of impaired HPV.

Inadequate Alveolar P_{AO_2}

Postoperative hypoxemia is occasionally caused by a global reduction of P_{AO_2}, usually from inadequate ventilation. If oxygen uptake from alveoli exceeds delivery by ventilation, P_{AO_2} decreases. Hypoxemia might occur if opioids or residual anesthetic levels depress ventilatory drives, or during periodic apnea. Hypoventilation must be severe to cause hypoxemia based on a reduction in oxygen delivery to alveoli. Complete apnea or airway obstruction by foreign bodies, soft tissue edema, or laryngospasm leads to rapid depletion of alveolar oxygen, as does very high small airway resistance, which precludes effective ventilation. If cessation of ventilation does occur, the rate of P_{AO_2} decline varies with age, body habitus, degree of underlying illness, and initial P_{AO_2}[70] (see Fig. 53-3).

Partial airway obstruction does not usually reduce P_{AO_2}, especially when patients are receiving supplemental oxygen. Increasing the oxygen content of the FRC safeguards against hypoxemia from hypoventilation or airway obstruction. Occasionally, excessive concentrations of other gases reduce P_{AO_2}. At the end of general anesthesia, rapid outpouring of nitrous oxide from PA blood displaces alveolar gas and can lower P_{AO_2} to dangerous levels if a patient is hypoventilating or breathing ambient air. This "diffusion hypoxia" usually occurs before PACU admission unless a patient is severely hypoventilating. Volume displacement of oxygen could also occur during severe hypercarbia in a patient breathing ambient air, although respiratory acidemia is often a greater problem than hypoxemia.

Reduced Mixed Venous P_{O_2}

Systemic venous partial pressure of oxygen ($P\bar{v}_{O_2}$) is affected by arterial oxygen content, cardiac output, distribution of peripheral blood flow, and tissue oxygen extraction. If arterial oxygen content decreases or tissue extraction increases, $P\bar{v}_{O_2}$ falls. The lower the $P\bar{v}_{O_2}$ in blood that is shunted or flows through low $\dot{V}/\dot{Q}$ units, the greater the reduction of Pa_{O_2}. Blood with a low $P\bar{v}_{O_2}$ also extracts larger volumes of oxygen from alveolar gas, amplifying the effect of hypoventilation or airway obstruction on P_{AO_2}. Very low $P\bar{v}_{O_2}$ increases the risk of resorption atelectasis in poorly ventilated alveoli. In PACU patients, shivering, infection, and hypermetabolism lower $P\bar{v}_{O_2}$ by increasing peripheral oxygen extraction. Low cardiac output or hypotension also lower $P\bar{v}_{O_2}$ by decreasing tissue oxygen delivery. Supplemental oxygen minimizes the impact of low $P\bar{v}_{O_2}$ on alveolar oxygen extraction and on arterial oxygenation.

Carbon Monoxide Poisoning

Carbon monoxide reversibly binds to hemoglobin with 200 times the affinity of oxygen, creating carboxyhemoglobin, which impedes both the binding of oxygen and the dissociation of oxygen from oxyhemoglobin. During general anesthesia, patients can be exposed to CO generated by a reaction between inhalation anesthetics and dry CO_2-absorbing agents. Overall risk of exposure is estimated as 0.26%, but risk increases to 0.46% for first cases of the day, and to 2.9% for first cases performed in peripheral anesthetizing locations.[84]

Because CO poisoning is difficult to recognize, a PACU patient can be severely hypoxic but appear well oxygenated by routine indices. Symptoms of moderate CO exposure such as headache, nausea, vomiting, irritability, and altered visual or motor skills are nonspecific and common during recovery. CO seldom causes cyanosis. A pulse oximeter interprets carboxyhemoglobin as oxyhemoglobin, so Sp_{O_2} reads falsely high. (A co-oximeter differentiates between carboxyhemoglobin and oxyhemoglobin.) The Pa_{O_2} is often high, although Sp_{O_2} is low and metabolic acidemia is significant.

Anemia

Preoperative hematocrit and intraoperative hemorrhage determine a patient's red cell mass and oxygen-carrying capacity after surgery. Reduction of hematocrit caused by dilution has less impact on oxygen-carrying capacity than reduction by hemorrhage. The hematocrit at which oxygen delivery becomes insufficient to match tissue needs varies with cardiac reserve, oxygen consumption, hemoglobin dissociation, Pa_{O_2}, blood flow distribution, and other factors. Each patient has a minimum hematocrit below which tissues use inefficient anaerobic metabolism, generating a lactic acidemia. Patients with vascular disease are at increased risk of vital organ ischemia as hematocrit falls.

Supplemental Oxygen

The incidence of hypoxemia in postoperative patients is high. In one study of PACU patients placed on room air, 30% of patients younger than 1 year of age, 20% aged 1–3 years, 14% aged 3–14 years, and 7.8% of adults had hemoglobin saturations fall below 90%, with many falling below 85%[85] (Fig. 53-6). Clinical observation and assessment of cognitive function do not accurately screen for hypoxemia, so monitoring with oximetry is essential throughout the PACU admission.[81] Predicting which patients will become hypoxemic in the PACU or when hypoxemia will occur is difficult. Patients with lung disease or obesity, those recovering from thoracic or upper abdominal procedures, and those with preoperative hypoxemia are probably at increased risk.[86] Perioperative hypoxemia occurs in children, especially those with respiratory infections or chronic adenotonsillar hypertrophy.[87] Hypoxemia occurs frequently after regional anesthesia.[27,28]

Supplemental oxygen could be administered only to patients at high risk of hypoxemia or with low Sp_{O_2} readings.[88,89] However, if a patient requires PACU admission (especially given evolving PACU bypass criteria), he or she should probably receive supplemental oxygen during initial recovery and perhaps during transport to the PACU.

Supplemental oxygen improves Pa_{O_2}, although the effect is variable. The inspired concentration delivered by face masks or nasal prongs is unpredictable because ambient gas is entrained during inspiration. Use of oxygen neither consistently prevents hypoxemia nor addresses underlying causes.[90] Oxygen has a negligible effect on hypoxemia caused by shunting because shunted blood is not exposed to increased F_{IO_2}, whereas blood passing ventilated alveoli is already saturated. If hypoxemia is caused by low $\dot{V}/\dot{Q}$, increasing oxygen content in marginally ventilated air spaces improves arterial saturation. Increased oxygen content in the FRC delays the onset of serious hypoxemia during airway obstruction or hypoventilation. If CO poisoning reduces oxygen-carrying capacity, 100% oxygen displaces CO from hemoglobin and markedly accelerates the CO elimination. Hyperbaric oxygen therapy may be indicated for severe cases.

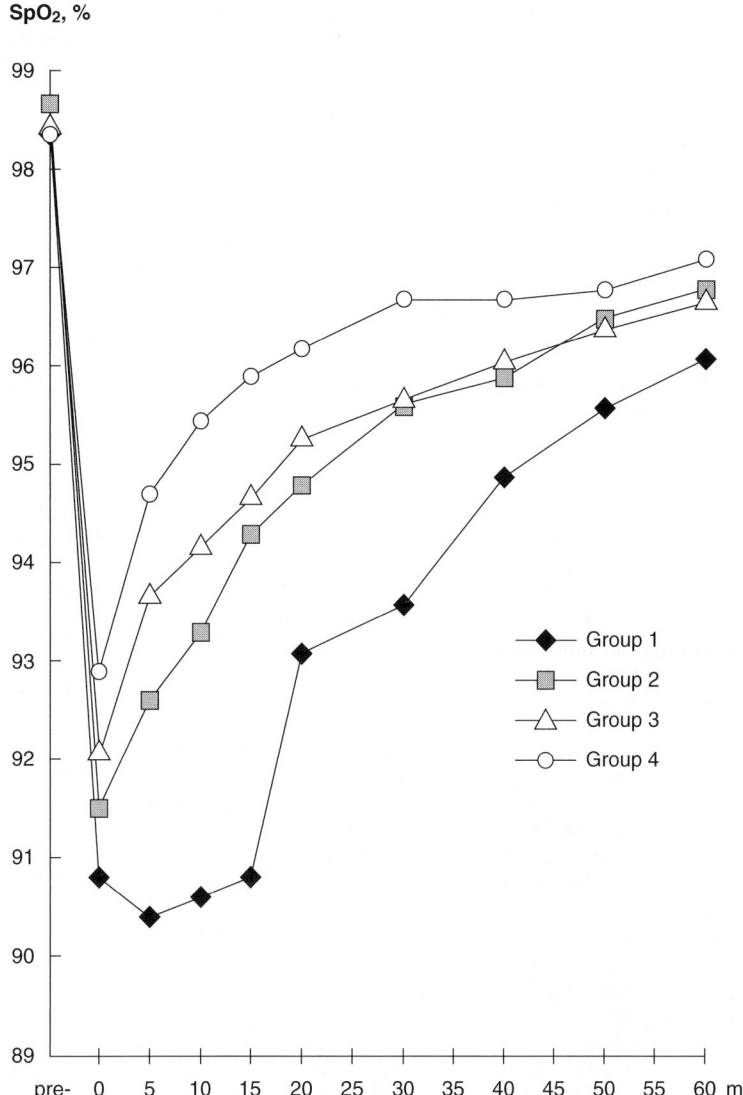

SpO₂, %

Figure 53-6. Spo₂ versus postanesthesia care unit (PACU) time in patients spontaneously ventilating on room air after general anesthesia (Group 1 = 0–1 year of age; Group 2 = 1–3 years; Group 3 = 3–14 years; Group 4 = 14–58 years). (From Xue FS, Huang YG, Tong SY *et al:* A comparative study of early postoperative hypoxemia in infants, children, and adults undergoing elective plastic surgery. Anesth Analg 83:709, 1996.)

Cost of supplemental oxygen is minimal, inconvenience to patients is minor, and risk is small. An $FIO_2 > 0.8$ promotes resorption atelectasis as inert nitrogen is replaced with oxygen in poorly ventilated alveoli. Inspiration of 100% oxygen for 24–36 hours generates early signs of pulmonary oxygen toxicity. Toxicity is accelerated in patients receiving hyperbaric oxygen therapy. If arterial oxygen saturation is adequate, PaO_2 should be maintained below 150 mm Hg. Risk of oxygen toxicity is not increased after bleomycin therapy. Although oxygen might cause minor mucosal drying, routine humidification is of little benefit unless intubation bypasses natural humidification. Oxygen apparatus might cause corneal abrasion during emergence.

Perioperative Aspiration

During anesthesia, airway reflexes are frequently ineffective, placing patients at risk for pulmonary aspiration. Pulmonary morbidity from perioperative aspiration varies with the type and volume of the aspirate. Although aspiration of gastric contents is most widely feared, surgical patients also experience other aspiration syndromes.

Aspiration of clear oral secretions during induction, face mask ventilation, or emergence is common and usually insig-

nificant. Cough, mild tracheal irritation, or transient laryngospasm are usual sequelae, although large-volume aspiration might predispose to infection, small airway obstruction, or pulmonary edema. Aspiration of blood secondary to trauma, epistaxis, or surgery in the oropharynx or large airways generates marked changes on the chest radiograph that are out of proportion with clinical signs. Aspirated "sterile" blood causes minor airway obstruction but is rapidly cleared by mucociliary transport, resorption, and phagocytosis. Massive blood aspiration interferes with gas exchange and leads to fibrinous changes in air spaces and to pulmonary hemochromatosis from iron accumulation in phagocytic cells. Secondary infection is a threat, especially if tissue or purulent matter is also aspirated.

Aspiration of food, small objects, pieces of teeth, or dental appliances causes persistent cough, diffuse reflex bronchospasm, airway obstruction with distal atelectasis, or pneumonia. Complications are often localized and treated with antibiotics and supportive care once the foreign matter is expelled or removed by bronchoscopy. Secondary thermal, chemical, or traumatic airway injury from aspirated objects may require later surgical intervention. Of course, complete upper airway or tracheal obstruction by an aspirated object is a life-threatening emergency.

Aspiration of acidic gastric contents during vomiting or regurgitation causes chemical pneumonitis characterized initially by diffuse bronchospasm, hypoxemia, and atelectasis. In serious cases, airway epithelial degeneration, interstitial and alveolar edema, and hemorrhage into air spaces rapidly progresses to ARDS with high-permeability pulmonary edema. Destruction of pneumocytes, decreased surfactant activity, hyaline membrane formation, and atelectasis or emphysematous changes can all occur, leading to $\dot{V}/\dot{Q}$ mismatching and reductions in compliance. Destruction of pulmonary microvasculature increases pulmonary vascular resistance and $\dot{V}_D/\dot{V}_T$. The morbidity increases directly with volume of acid aspirate and inversely with the pH of the aspirate. Classically, aspirates above 0.4–1.0 ml · kg^{-1} and with pH below 2.0–2.5 are most serious. Aspiration of partially digested food worsens and prolongs pneumonitis, especially if vegetable matter is present. Food particles mechanically obstruct airways and are a nidus for secondary bacterial infection.

The risk of aspiration is still high in PACU patients, although the incidence is relatively low.[91] Frequency of vomiting remains high, especially if gas has accumulated in the stomach. Hypotension, hypoxemia, or acidemia cause both emesis and obtundation, increasing aspiration risk. Protective airway reflexes such as cough, swallowing, and laryngospasm are suppressed by depressant medications such as inhalation anesthetics, barbiturates, and opiates, so patients with decreased levels of consciousness in the PACU must be observed carefully. Persisting effects of laryngeal nerve blocks or topical local anesthetics used to reduce airway irritability decrease postoperative airway protection, as does residual sedation. Reflexes are also impaired by residual neuromuscular paralysis.[79] Ability to sustain airway patency and spontaneous ventilation does not indicate that neuromuscular recovery is sufficient to maintain airway protection. Patients can pass a head lift test, have a tactile train-of-four T4/T1 ratio greater than 0.7, exhibit full recovery of ventilation, and still have impaired airway reflexes from to residual paralysis.[80] The T4/T1 ratio might need to exceed 0.9 before reflexes are completely competent.[92] Risk of aspiration also increases if reversal is omitted after paralysis with short-acting relaxants.[93]

Preventing aspiration is critical because effective therapy is limited. Evolution of guidelines for preoperative fasting and analysis of outcomes have demonstrated the safety of shorter fasting periods for clear liquids in all patients and for feedings in young children.[94,95] For patients at high risk, preoperative administration of nonparticulate antacids such as sodium citrate increase the pH of gastric fluid without excessively increasing volume. Particulate antacids must be avoided. Histamine type 2 receptor blockers like cimetidine or ranitidine reduce the volume and increase the pH of gastric secretions. Metoclopramide increases gastroesophageal sphincter tone and accelerates gastric emptying. Inserting a nasogastric tube is often ineffective to remove particulate matter and interferes with gastroesophageal sphincter integrity.

In the PACU, vigilance for regurgitation and aspiration is important. Trendelenburg position might promote regurgitation, but aids in airway clearance if regurgitation or vomiting occurs. Head elevation in unconscious patients should be avoided because it creates a gravitational gradient from pharynx to lung. High-risk patients should not have the trachea extubated until airway reflexes are fully restored. Aspiration of acidic fluid can still occur around an inflated tracheal tube cuff. Cuff deflation should be avoided because the rigid tube impairs laryngospasm and increases. The pharynx should be completely suctioned before extubation, and extubation done at end-inspiration with positive airway pressure to promote expulsion of material trapped below the cords but above the inflated cuff. Careful observation is essential after extubation because airway reflexes might be temporarily impaired.

Postoperative anatomic distortion from mandibular fractures or airway soft tissue trauma interferes with airway protection.

Mandibular fixation makes expulsion of vomitus, blood, or secretions difficult, so equipment for release of fixation must be available. Patients recovering with mandibular fixation must demonstrate cognitive and physical ability to clear the airway before the trachea is extubated.

Discovery of gastric secretions in the pharynx mandates immediate lateral head positioning (assuming cervical spine integrity) and suction of the airway. If airway reflexes are compromised, tracheal intubation is often appropriate. After intubation, the trachea is suctioned through the tracheal tube before positive-pressure ventilation; this avoids widely disseminating aspirated material into distal airways. Instillation of saline or alkalotic solutions is not recommended. Assessing the pH of tracheal aspirate is useless because buffering is immediate. Checking pharyngeal aspirate pH is more reliable but of little practical value.

Suspicion that aspiration has occurred mandates 24–48 hours of monitoring for development of aspiration pneumonitis. If likelihood of aspiration is high, the patient should be admitted to the hospital. Observation includes serial temperature checks, white blood cell counts with differential, and blood gas determination or pulmonary function testing if appropriate. Fluffy infiltrates may appear on the chest radiograph any time within 24 hours. Hypoxemia might develop quickly or evolve insidiously as lung injury progresses, so continuous pulse oximetry monitoring is important. Chest physiotherapy, incentive spirometry, and reinstitution of medications for pre-existing pulmonary conditions minimize the loss of lung volume, $\dot{V}/\dot{Q}$ mismatching, and infection. If the likelihood of aspiration is small, follow-up can be done on an outpatient basis, assuming hypoxemia, cough, wheezing, or radiographic abnormalities do not appear within 4–6 hours. Give the patient explicit instructions to contact a medical facility at the first appearance of malaise, fever, cough, chest pain, or other symptoms of pneumonitis.

If hypoxemia, increased airway resistance, consolidation, or pulmonary edema evolves, the patient is supported with supplemental oxygen, PEEP, or CPAP. Mechanical ventilation is often necessary. Therapy is similar to that for ARDS. Pulmonary edema usually reflects increased capillary permeability and should not be treated with diuretics unless high filling pressures or hypervolemia exist. Hypovolemia from fluid losses into the lung can necessitate aggressive fluid management. Steroids yield little real improvement of long-term outcome. Bacterial infection does not always follow aspiration, so prophylactic antibiotics merely promote colonization by resistant organisms. If evidence of bacterial infection appears, antibiotic therapy should be instituted based on Gram stain and culture of sputum. If culture results are equivocal, broad-spectrum antibiotics should be used with coverage for gram-negative rods and anaerobes, including *Bacteroides fragilis*.

POSTOPERATIVE RENAL COMPLICATIONS

Monitoring kidney function during recovery reduces morbidity in patients with marginal cardiovascular or renal status.

Ability to Void

The ability to void should be assessed because autonomic effects of regional anesthetics or opioids interfere with sphincter relaxation and promote urine retention.[96] Urinary retention is common after urologic, inguinal, and genital surgery, and frequently delays discharge.[97] It is reasonable to discharge inpatients to a surgical floor and selected ambulatory surgical patients from the facility before they void.[98] However, it is important to ensure that urine output is monitored after discharge from the PACU to avoid urinary retention. Give ambulatory patients who are discharged without voiding a specific time interval in which to void (*i.e.,* 10–12 hours after discharge). If retention persists, the patient is instructed to contact a health care facility. Higher-than-average return rates after urologic procedures are partially related to urinary retention.[99] An ultrasonic bladder scan is helpful to assess bladder volume before discharge, avoiding the archaic practice of "straight catheterization." Neither the patient nor staff can estimate the need to void through sensation or palpation, respectively.[100] Patients with indwelling urinary catheters should have output recorded hourly. Use of urinary output to gauge intravascular volume status or renal viability can be misleading given the prevalence of osmotic diuresis and impaired renal regulatory mechanisms in recovering patients.

Renal Tubular Function

Analysis of urine yields information about postoperative renal tubular function. Urine color is not useful for assessing tubular function such as concentrating ability, but color can signal hematuria, hemoglobinuria, or pyuria. Urine osmolarity (reflecting the number of particles in solution) is a more reliable index of tubular function than is specific gravity, which is affected by molecular weight. An osmolarity of 450 mOsm $\cdot$ l^{-1} indicates intact tubular concentrating ability. A urine sodium concentration far below or a potassium concentration above serum concentrations also indicates renal tubular viability. Acidification or alkalinization of urine requires intact tubular function, so urinary pH evaluation is useful. Osmolarity, electrolyte, and pH values close to those in serum may indicate poor tubular function and acute tubular necrosis.

Inorganic fluoride released during metabolism of inhalation anesthetics causes a transient reduction of maximum tubular concentrating ability after long anesthetics. Higher fluoride levels cause nephrotoxicity and renal tubular necrosis. Interaction between sevoflurane and carbon dioxide absorbents generates compound A, a vinyl ether. The amount of compound A generated varies directly with absorbent dryness and sevoflurane concentration, and inversely with flow rate. Cytochrome P-450 degrades compound A, increasing free inorganic fluoride in serum. In rats, compound A is lethal in high concentrations and nephrotoxic in lower concentrations. Although transient increases in protein excretion and decreases in concentrating ability may occur, prolonged use of sevoflurane does not have a serious impact on renal function.[101] Given the relationship between compound A and dry CO_2 absorbents, the anesthesiologist must be aware that polyuria or proteinuria in patients who received sevoflurane during first cases or cases performed in peripheral anesthetizing locations might be related to compound A exposure.

Oliguria

Oliguria ($\leq$0.5 ml $\cdot$ kg^{-1} $\cdot$ h^{-1}) occurs frequently during recovery and usually reflects an appropriate renal response to hypovolemia or systemic hypotension. However, a decreased urine output might indicate abnormal renal function. The acceptable degree and duration of oliguria vary with underlying renal status, the surgical procedure, and the anticipated postoperative course. If intraoperative manipulations or events could jeopardize renal function (possible ureteral ligature, aortic cross-clamping, severe hypotension, massive transfusion), oliguria must be aggressively evaluated. In patients without catheters, bladder volume and interval since last voiding should be checked to help differentiate between oliguria and inability to void. Urinary catheters should be checked for kinking and for obstruction by blood clots or debris. Patient position might also hold the catheter tip above the urinary level in the bladder.

Systemic pressure must be adequate for renal perfusion (based on preoperative pressures). A 300–500-ml iv crystalloid bolus given after urine sent for electrolyte and osmolarity determinations helps assess whether oliguria represents a renal response to hypovolemia. If output does not improve, a larger bolus or a diagnostic trial of furosemide, 5 mg iv, should be considered. Furosemide interferes with tubular resorption and increases urine output if oliguria reflects retention of fluid by the kidneys. Also, some patients on chronic diuretic therapy might require a diuretic effect to maintain brisk postoperative urine output.

Persistence of oliguria despite hydration, adequate perfusion pressure, and a furosemide challenge increases the likelihood of acute tubular necrosis, ureteral obstruction, renal artery or vein occlusion, or inappropriate antidiuretic hormone secretion. Administration of desmopressin for hematologic purposes seldom affects postoperative urinary output. Cystoscopy, iv pyelography, angiography, or radionuclide scanning may help clarify renal status. Osmotic or loop diuretics and low-dose dopamine or dobutamine are probably useful to attenuate renal damage, but consultation with a nephrologist is prudent.

Polyuria

Profuse postoperative urine output usually reflects generous intraoperative fluid administration. Osmotic diuresis caused by hyperglycemia and glycosuria is another cause, particularly if glucose-containing crystalloid solutions are infusing. Polyuria might also reflect intraoperative diuretic administration. However, sustained polyuria (4–5 ml $\cdot$ kg^{-1} $\cdot$ h^{-1}) can indicate abnormal regulation of water clearance, especially if urinary losses compromise intravascular volume and systemic blood pressure. Polyuria related to diabetes insipidus occurs secondary to intracranial surgery, pituitary ablation, head trauma, increased intracranial pressure, or inadvertent omission of preoperative vasopressin. The diagnosis is made by comparing urine and serum electrolytes and osmolarity. Diagnostic or therapeutic administration of vasopressin is useful. High-output renal failure also should be considered as a cause.

METABOLIC COMPLICATIONS
Postoperative Acid–Base Disorders

Categorization of postoperative acid–base abnormalities into discrete primary and compensatory disorders is difficult because a rapidly changing pathophysiologic process often generates two or more primary disorders.

Respiratory Acidemia

Respiratory acidemia is frequently encountered in PACU patients because anesthetics, opioids, and sedatives promote hypoventilation by depressing CNS sensitivity to pH and CO_2. In awake, spontaneously breathing PACU patients receiving adequate analgesia, hypercarbia and acidemia are usually mild (Paco$_2$ 45–50 mm Hg, pH 7.36–7.32). Anesthetized or deeply sedated patients exhibit more profound acidemia unless supplemental ventilation is used. Some postoperative patients cannot sustain adequate ventilation despite an appropriate CNS drive. Residual neuromuscular paralysis, increased airway resistance, or decreased pulmonary compliance might impede ventilation and lead to progressive respiratory acidemia, especially if dead space is increased. Elevated CO_2 production caused by shivering, hyperalimentation, fever, or malignant hyperthermia amplifies the problem. The kidneys require many hours to generate a compensatory metabolic alkalosis, so compensation for acute respiratory acidemia is limited.

Symptoms of respiratory acidemia include agitation, confusion, ventilatory dissatisfaction, and tachypnea. SNS responses to low pH cause hypertension, tachycardia, and dysrhythmias which increase the risk of myocardial ischemia, bleeding, or cerebrovascular accident. Respiratory acidemia caused by CNS depression often produces less intense signs of SNS activity because autonomic responses are also depressed. At very low pH, catecholamines cannot interact with adrenergic receptors, so heart rate and blood pressure decrease precipitously. Respiratory acidemia increases cerebral blood flow and potentially increases intracranial pressure in patients with head injury, intracranial tumors, or cerebral edema.

Treatment consists of correcting the imbalance between CO_2 production and alveolar ventilation. Reversal of opioids or neuromuscular relaxants and raising the level of consciousness improves ventilatory drive. Relieving airway obstruction, reducing airway resistance, or improving ventilatory mechanics is useful. If spontaneous ventilation cannot maintain CO_2 excretion, tracheal intubation and mechanical ventilation are necessary. Reducing CO_2 production by eliminating high glucose loads or controlling fever, shivering, and the work of breathing may be helpful. Extreme measures such as core cooling or paralysis are seldom useful in the PACU.

Metabolic Acidemia

Evaluation of acute postoperative metabolic acidemia is relatively straightforward. Patients with renal failure, renal tubular acidosis, or small bowel drainage usually exhibit a preoperative metabolic acidemia. Excessive saline infusion during surgery can generate a mild hyperchloremic metabolic acidemia in the PACU.[102] Substituting lactated Ringer's solution helps resolve this problem. Postoperative metabolic acidemia is occasionally caused by ketoacidosis in patients with severe diabetes mellitus. Serum glucose levels are elevated, and ketones are detectable in blood or urine. Rarely, a patient manifests acidemia from toxic ingestion of phenformin, aspirin, or methanol.

Once these unusual causes are excluded, postoperative metabolic acidemia almost always represents lactic acid accumulation secondary to insufficient delivery or utilization of oxygen in peripheral tissues. Hypotension leading to peripheral hypoperfusion is often caused by low cardiac output (hypovolemia, cardiac failure, dysrhythmia) or decreased SVR (sepsis, catecholamine depletion, sympathectomy). Arteriolar constriction from hypothermia or inappropriate pressor administration reduces tissue perfusion, as does poor distribution of blood flow. Hypoxemia, severe anemia, impaired hemoglobin dissociation (alkalemia, hypothermia), and inability to utilize oxygen in the mitochondria (cyanide or arsenic poisoning) also generate lactic acidemia. When evaluating lactic acidemia after general anesthesia, the real possibility of CO poisoning must be considered, especially in early cases from peripheral locations.

A spontaneously breathing patient with intact ventilatory drive quickly generates a respiratory alkalosis to compensate for postoperative metabolic acidemia. However, anesthetics and analgesics interfere with this ventilatory response. The sympathetic response to acute metabolic acidemia is often milder than the response to respiratory acidemia because hydrogen and bicarbonate ions cross the blood–brain barrier with more difficulty than CO_2.

Treatment consists of resolving the condition causing accumulation of metabolic acid. Ketoacidosis is treated with iv potassium, insulin, and glucose. If lactic acidemia is mild and conditions causing lactate accumulation are improved, acidemia resolves through metabolism and renal excretion of hydrogen ions. Improving cardiac output or systemic blood pressure can reduce lactic acid production, as can rewarming. If acidemia is severe or progressive, iv bicarbonate or a substitute helps restore pH toward normal.

Respiratory Alkalemia

Excessive pain or anxiety during emergence causes hyperventilation and acute respiratory alkalosis. Excessive mechanical ventilation also generates respiratory alkalemia, especially if hypothermia or paralysis has decreased CO_2 production. Pathologic causes of "central" hyperventilation include sepsis, cerebrovascular accident, or paradoxical CNS acidosis (an imbalance of bicarbonate concentration across the blood–brain barrier caused by prolonged mechanical hyperventilation).

Acute respiratory alkalemia generates confusion or dizziness, atrial dysrhythmias, or mild cardiac conduction abnormalities. If the alkalemia is severe, reduced serum ionized calcium concentration precipitates muscle fasciculation or hypocalcemic tetany. Alkalemia decreases cerebral blood flow, causing hypoperfusion and even stroke in patients with cerebrovascular disease. Very high pH levels depress cardiovascular, CNS, and catecholamine receptor functions. Metabolic compensation for acute respiratory alkalemia is limited, again because renal time constants for bicarbonate excretion are large. Correction of respiratory alkalemia necessitates reducing alveolar ventilation, usually by administering analgesics and sedatives for pain and anxiety. Rebreathing of CO_2 has little application in the PACU.

Metabolic Alkalemia

Metabolic alkalemia is rare in PACU patients unless vomiting, gastric suctioning, dehydration, alkaline ingestion, or potassium-wasting diuretics caused an alkalemia that existed before surgery. Excessive intraoperative bicarbonate administration causes postoperative metabolic alkalemia, but alkalemia from metabolism of lactate or citrate usually does not appear within the first 24 hours. Respiratory compensation through retention of CO_2 is rapid but limited because hypoventilation eventually causes hypoxemia. Hydration and correction of hypochloremia and hypokalemia allow the kidney to excrete excess bicarbonate. An iv hydrochloric acid infusion is seldom necessary but can be used through a central venous catheter to treat life-threatening alkalemia.

Glucose Disorders

Serum glucose determination is superior to urine glucose measurement for managing blood sugar abnormalities. However, urine glucose concentration helps assess osmotic diuresis and estimate renal transport by comparison with serum levels.

Hyperglycemia

Glucose infusions and stress responses commonly elevate serum glucose levels after surgery. In diabetic patients, hyperglycemia may indicate insulin deficiency and potential for ketoacidosis. Moderate hyperglycemia ($200–300$ mg $\cdot$ dl^{-1}) usually resolves spontaneously and probably has little effect on wound healing. Higher glucose levels cause glycosuria with osmotic diuresis and interfere with serum electrolyte determinations. Severe hyperglycemia increases serum osmolality to a point that cerebral disequilibrium and hyperosmolar coma occur. Titration of iv regular insulin by incremental doses or by continuous infusion allows adjustment of blood glucose without the uptake delay of subcutaneous, longer-acting insulin. Potassium replacement and serial blood glucose determinations are essential.

Hypoglycemia

Hypoglycemia in the PACU can be caused by endogenous insulin secretion or by excessive or inadvertent insulin administration. Serious postoperative hypoglycemia is rare and easily treated with iv 50% dextrose followed by glucose infusion. Both sedation and excessive SNS activity mask signs and symptoms of hypoglycemia during recovery.

Electrolyte Disorders

Hyponatremia

Postoperative hyponatremia occurs if free water is infused intravenously during surgery or if sodium-free irrigating solution is absorbed during transurethral prostatic resection or hysteroscopy. Accumulation of serum glycine or its metabolite, ammonia, might exacerbate symptoms. Free water retention is also caused by inappropriate antidiuretic hormone secretion, prolonged induction of labor with oxytocin, or respiratory uptake of nebulized droplets. Excessive intraoperative administration of isotonic saline expands extracellular volume, leading to excretion of hypertonic urine and iatrogenic hyponatremia through desalination.[103] Symptoms of moderate hyponatremia include agitation, disorientation, visual disturbances, and nausea, whereas severe hyponatremia causes unconsciousness, impaired airway reflexes, and CNS irritability that progresses to grand mal seizures. Therapy includes gradual administration of iv saline and iv furosemide to promote renal wasting of free water in excess of sodium. Infusion of hypertonic saline may be necessary for severe hyponatremia. Monitoring of sodium concentration and osmolarity is essential.

Hypokalemia

Although usually inconsequential, postoperative hypokalemia might generate serious dysrhythmias, especially in patients taking digoxin. A potassium deficit from chronic diuretic therapy, nasogastric suctioning, or vomiting often underlies hypokalemia. Urinary and hemorrhagic losses, dilution, and insulin therapy generate more acute hypokalemia that worsens during respiratory alkalemia. Excess SNS activity or infusion of calcium, insulin, or β-mimetic medications exacerbates effects of hypokalemia. Addition of potassium to peripheral iv fluids usually restores serum concentration, but infusion of concentrated solutions through a central catheter may be necessary.

Hyperkalemia

Serious postoperative hyperkalemia occurs after excessive potassium administration or in patients with chronic renal failure or malignant hyperthermia. Acute acidemia exacerbates hyperkalemia. Administration of succinylcholine in the PACU could increase serum potassium to dangerous levels in patients with burns, severe trauma, or chronic neurologic injuries. Treatment with iv insulin and glucose acutely lowers serum potassium, whereas iv calcium counters myocardial effects. β-Mimetic medications might also have a role. An inexplicably high serum potassium raises the suspicion of spurious hyperkalemia from a hemolyzed specimen or from sampling near an iv containing potassium or banked blood.

Calcium and Magnesium

Although underlying parathyroid disease or massive fluid replacement reduces total-body and ionized calcium, symptomatic postoperative hypocalcemia seldom occurs in the PACU. A rare patient might exhibit hypocalcemia and upper airway obstruction after parathyroid excision. Further reduction of the ionized fraction by alkalemia may cause myocardial conduction and contractility abnormalities, decreased vascular tone, or tetany. Administration of calcium chloride or calcium gluconate to hypocalcemic patients improves cardiovascular dynamics and the response to iv fluid administration. Transfusion of blood containing chelating agents (e.g., citrate) rarely causes symptomatic hypocalcemia unless the rate of blood infusion exceeds $500 \ ml \cdot min^{-1}$.

Magnesium plays a key role in restoration of neuromuscular function after surgery and in maintenance of cardiac rhythm and conduction.

MISCELLANEOUS COMPLICATIONS
Nausea and Vomiting

Avoiding postoperative nausea and vomiting (PONV) is a high priority for physicians and patients.[14] PONV remains a significant problem. Aside from unpleasantness for the patient and staff, PONV poses medical risks. Increased intra-abdominal pressure jeopardizes abdominal or inguinal suture lines, whereas elevated central venous pressure increases morbidity after ocular, tympanic, or intracranial procedures. Risk of aspirating gastric contents increases, especially if airway reflexes or ability to expel secretions are impaired. SNS response to emesis elevates heart rate and systemic blood pressure, increasing the risk of myocardial ischemia or dysrhythmias. Movement during PONV worsens postoperative pain and accentuates autonomic responses. Gagging and retching might also elicit parasympathetic responses with bradycardia and hypotension. Finally, PONV delays discharge or necessitates admission of ambulatory patients, reducing patient satisfaction and the efficiency of services.

The incidence of PONV varies with many factors.[8,104] Reported incidence is lower in the PACU than over 24 to 48 hours because emesis often appears after PACU discharge. Delayed emesis may reflect timing of oral intake, waning effects of antiemetics, or greater post-discharge pain. A prospective study of 17,638 ambulatory patients revealed increased risk in younger patients.[104] Likelihood of PONV decreased 13% per decade of age. Women had a 3-fold higher incidence than men. Ear–nose–throat and dental procedures had a high incidence (14.3%), followed by orthopedic shoulder procedures and cosmetic surgery. The risk of PONV is very high after procedures involving extraocular muscle traction,[105] middle ear manipulation, peritoneal or intestinal irritation, or testicular traction. A history of postoperative emesis or motion sickness predicts PONV. Smokers have a significantly lower risk of PONV than nonsmokers.[104,106] Undergoing a general anesthetic near menses increases the incidence in women, perhaps related to circulating E_2 estrogen levels.[107,108]

Perioperative factors contribute to emergence of PONV. Starvation, autonomic imbalance, pain, and effects of anesthetics on the chemotactic center probably increase the incidence. Conditions that affect the gastroesophageal junction (obesity, hiatal hernia) increase the likelihood of emesis in the PACU. Swallowed blood or secretions promotes PONV, as does gas in the stomach from face mask ventilation, nitrous oxide diffusion, or esophageal intubation. Incidence of PONV is lower after regional than general anesthesia, although this difference narrows once parenteral opioids are needed to control postoperative pain. Meta-analyses reveal that exclusion of nitrous oxide from an anesthetic appears to reduce the incidence of PONV.[109] The incidence of nausea does not differ greatly among inhalation anesthetics, although desflurane and sevoflurane might generate slightly higher rates. Barbiturate induction seems less offensive than etomidate or ketamine, whereas propofol offers a still lower risk. Administration of opioid analgesics increases the incidence PONV when compared with "pure" inhalational techniques, especially after ambulatory surgery. Using small doses of shorter-acting opioids might decrease incidence, but short duration of analgesia offsets this advantage. Supplementation of opioids with nonopioid analgesics such as ketorolac, acetaminophen, or ibuprofen might reduce the frequency of emesis. It is unclear whether administration of neostigmine to reverse neuromuscular relaxation or physostigmine to counteract sedation also increases the incidence of PONV. The choice of anticholinergic during reversal of paralysis might also affect incidence.

Several interventions have been evaluated to prevent PONV. Evacuation of stomach contents with an orogastric tube to avoid gastric distention is of questionable value. Hydration appears to reduce the incidence of PONV,[110] but postoperative drinking is often a triggering event. Children or high-risk patients can be appropriately discharged before they take oral fluids.[111] Whether this decreases incidence of PONV or merely delays onset is unclear. Limiting postoperative vestibular stimulation by minimizing brisk head motion is helpful.

Studies of medications for prophylaxis and treatment of PONV reveal that droperidol and ondansetron are probably equal in efficacy, cost effectiveness, and patient satisfaction,[105,112] whereas metoclopramide holds a weak third place.[113] These antiemetics have different sites of action, so combination therapy might generate better results by simultaneously treating two or more precipitating factors.[114]

Ondansetron, a serotonin receptor blocker, is a very useful antiemetic for PONV. Optimum iv dosage in adults seems to be 4 mg administered near the end of surgery or on PACU admission.[115] Ondansetron appears to be particularly useful for PONV related to stimulation of gastric enterochromaffin cells by blood.[116] Ondansetron has few side effects. Bothersome headache occurs after iv administration,[113] and transient liver enzyme elevation is seen in a small percentage of patients.[117] Ondansetron is cost effective if its use shortens PACU length of stay, avoids admission, and improves patient satisfaction. Granisetron, tropisetron, dolasetron, and the newer ramosetron all are effective antiemetics, but none appears to surpass ondansetron for efficacy.

Droperidol decreases the incidence and severity of PONV, although efficacy varies among procedures and patients. A total iv dose of $1-2$ $\mu g \cdot kg^{-1}$ ($0.625-1.25$ mg in adults) seems optimal.[113,114] Although mild sedation might delay discharge slightly, delay from untreated PONV is usually greater. Transient restlessness and rare extrapyramidal side effects are usually inconsequential.[113] Droperidol treats breakthrough nausea in patients who have received prophylaxis. α-Adrenergic blocking properties can precipitate hypotension in hypovolemic patients.

Other agents exhibit antiemetic properties. Propofol does not compare with droperidol or ondansetron as a first-line antiemetic.[105] Propofol has short-term antiemetic properties and is useful for anesthesia in patients at high risk for PONV.[118] Dexamethasone has an antiemetic effect when used during upper airway procedures such as adenotonsillectomy, perhaps secondary to its anti-inflammatory properties.[119,120] Although cimetidine decrease gastric acidity and ranitidine improves gastric emptying, neither is useful to treat PONV. Dimenhydrinate or thiethylperazine are also relatively ineffective. Intravenous scopolamine causes unacceptable psychogenic reactions, whereas transdermal scopolamine is ineffective and causes postoperative visual disturbances. Efficacy of ephedrine for treating PONV related to ambulation or motion is unclear. The antiemetic effect of midazolam in children is likely related to the relationship between vomiting and crying or agitation. Acupuncture and acupressure might reduce the incidence of PONV.[121] These modalities are unlikely to gain wide acceptance unless they prove clearly superior to antiemetic medications.

Before treating PONV, more serious causes of nausea and emesis should be considered, such as hypotension, hypoxemia, hypoglycemia, intracranial pressure, or gastric bleeding.

Incidental Trauma

Ocular Injuries

Anesthetized patients sustain incidental trauma from positioning, equipment, and manipulation. Corneal abrasion caused by drying or inadvertent eye contact during face mask ventilation or intubation is a common eye injury encountered in the PACU. Corneal abrasion occurs more frequently in elderly patients, after long cases, with lateral positioning, and after head or neck surgery.[122] Corneal injury also occurs in the PACU if a rigid oxygen face mask rides up on the eye or if the eye is rubbed with a digital pulse oximeter probe. Abrasion causes tearing, decreased visual acuity, pain, and photophobia. Fluorescein staining is useful for diagnosis. Abrasion usually heals spontaneously within 72 hours without scarring, but severe injury can cause cataract formation and impair vision. Symptomatic treatment includes artificial tears and eye closure.

Visual acuity is often impaired after anesthesia. Autonomic side effects of medications impair accommodation, and residual ocular lubricant clouds vision. Impairment of retinal perfusion by ocular compression generates postoperative visual disturbances ranging from loss of acuity to permanent blindness.[123] Ischemic optic atrophy also occurs in the absence of external compression.[124] Risk is higher after long procedures in the prone position, and in patients with vascular disease and anemia. The anesthesiologist must be alert for visual impairment and perform a cursory check of acuity when assessing patients at higher risk for ischemic optic atrophy.

Oral, Pharyngeal, and Laryngeal Injuries

Laryngoscopy, rigid airways, and dentition all can cause trauma of oral soft tissues. Lip, tongue, or gum abrasions heal quickly and are treated with an ice pack and analgesia. Penetrating injuries caused by tissue entrapment between teeth and a laryngoscope blade or airway may require topical antibiotics. After a traumatic tracheal intubation, hematoma or edema might cause partial airway obstruction. Nebulized racemic epinephrine often improves stridor. If damaged teeth or dental appliances are noted, it is necessary to obtain a dental consultation and observe for signs of foreign body aspiration.[125] Dental damage can also occur during emergence if a patient bites on a rigid oral airway or forcefully clenches his or her teeth.

Sore throat and hoarseness after tracheal intubation occur in 20–50% of patients, depending on the degree of trauma during laryngoscopy and oropharyngeal suctioning, the duration of intubation, and the type of tube (see also Chapter 23). Mucosal irritation often presents as an unquenchable dryness in mouth and throat. The use of local anesthetic ointments to lubricate endotracheal tubes does not help and may cause additional mucosal irritation. During surgery, impact of cuff expansion with nitrous oxide is avoided by inflating the cuff with a sample of the anesthetic mixture. Topical viscous lidocaine attenuates irritation from nasogastric tubes during recovery but may increases risk of aspiration. In children, the severity of postextubation laryngeal edema or tracheitis depends on age, intubation trauma, duration of intubation, and tube movement. Most children recover with cool mist therapy, but nebulized racemic epinephrine is also effective. Dexamethasone might also decrease edema. Laryngoscopy and intubation can also cause hypoglossal, lingual, or recurrent laryngeal nerve damage, vocal cord evulsion, desquamation of laryngeal or tracheal mucosa, airway wall edema or ulceration, and tracheal perforation. Sore throat can also occur without intubation, related to drying from unhumidified gases or trauma from airways and suctioning.

Nerve Injuries

Injuries caused by improper positioning during anesthesia generate serious long-term complications (see Chapter 24). Spinal cord injury can be caused by positioning for intubation or by hematoma accumulation after placement of regional anesthetics. Peripheral nerve compression during general or regional anesthesia sometimes causes permanent sensory and motor deficits, as do stretch injuries from hyperextension of an extremity.[126] Any bruising or skin breakdown should prompt evaluation for underlying nerve damage. Many postoperative neuropathies occur without an identifiable cause. This is particularly true for ulnar neuropathy, which may be related to subtle positioning problems,[127] pre-existing impairment,[128] or unusual sensitivity of the nerve to ischemia. Every complaint of pain, numbness, or weakness from a postoperative patient should be evaluated.

In spite of improvements in spinal needle design, postdural puncture headache often first emerges in the PACU. Positional headache is more frequent after difficult subarachnoid anesthetics with multiple attempts[129] and after dural puncture during attempted epidural placement. Subarachnoid air bubbles from loss-of-resistance testing may contribute. In the PACU, treatment is supportive with hydration, analgesics, and positioning. In severe cases, an early epidural blood patch might be considered.

Mechanical nerve injury secondary to puncture, laceration, or intraneuronal injection during placement of regional anesthesia is rare but does occur.[126,130] In the PACU, patients complain of pain, focal numbness, residual paresthesia, or dysesthesia. Symptoms are usually transient. In one study, 6.3% of 4767 patients experienced paresthesia during placement of spinal anesthesia, but only 0.126% had persisting symptoms.[131] Analgesia should be administered, and the patient reassured and closely observed to ensure that neurologic symptoms do not indicate a more serious complication.

During recovery from spinal anesthesia, some patients exhibit lower extremity discomfort, buttock pain, and other signs of sacral neurologic irritation. This problem is more common in obese patients, after procedures in lithotomy position, and after spinal anesthesia with 5% lidocaine.[132] Symptoms are transient and treated supportively. Rarely, a patient exhibits headache and meningeal signs caused by chemical meningitis after injection of a spinal drug that is contaminated or outside the acceptable pH range.

Soft Tissue and Joint Injuries

If pressure points are improperly padded during long procedures, soft tissue ischemia and necrosis occur, especially with lateral or prone positioning. Prolonged scalp pressure causes localized alopecia, whereas entrapment of ears, breasts, genitalia, or skin folds causes inflammation or necrosis. Regional ischemia from major arterial compression is rare. Thermal, electrical, or chemical burns from cautery equipment, preparatory solutions, or adhesives also appear. Extravasation of iv medications can cause sloughing or localized chemical neuropathy; extravasation of fluid or blood can cause a compartment syndrome. Excessive joint or muscle extension leads to postoperative backache, joint pain or stiffness, and even joint instability.

Each patient admitted to the PACU should be carefully evaluated for traumatic complications. Discovery or suspicion of a complication necessitates careful documentation, notification of physicians responsible for extended postoperative care, consultation with specialists, and follow-up.

Skeletal Muscle Pain

Postoperative muscle pain is caused by many intraoperative factors. Prolonged lack of motion or unusual muscle stretch during positioning often contributes to muscle stiffness and aching in the PACU. Fasciculation during depolarizing blockade has implicated succinylcholine as a cause of postoperative myalgias. A small dose of nondepolarizing relaxant may reduce the incidence or severity, but pretreatment with a "self-taming" dose of succinylcholine does not appear to be protective. Acute myalgia also occurs after administration of other relaxants and in patients receiving no relaxant. Delayed-onset muscle fatigue can appear days after surgery and resolve spontaneously.

Hypothermia and Shivering

Although intraoperative temperature maintenance is a standard, patients still exhibit hypothermia after surgery. Heat is lost by evaporation during skin preparation, by humidification of dry gases in the airway, and by radiation and convection from the skin and wound. Core temperature reduction is accelerated by cold iv fluids and low ambient temperatures. Thermoregulatory vasoconstriction decreases heat loss but is less effective under anesthesia. Rate of heat loss is approximately the same during general or regional anesthetics, but patients rewarm more slowly after regional anesthetics because residual vasodilation and paralysis impede heat generation and retention. Cachectic, traumatized, or burned patients experience more serious temperature reduction. Infants are at increased risk given their low ratio of body mass to surface area. Humans actively regulate body temperature once it falls below the thermoregulatory threshold temperature, which is decreased by approximately 2.5°C during general anesthesia.[133] Ability to maintain body temperature is compromised because paralysis and anesthesia impair shivering, and because nonshivering thermogenesis is relatively ineffective in adults.

Postoperative hypothermia increases SNS activity, elevates peripheral vascular resistance, and decreases venous capacitance.[134] Risk of myocardial ischemia is increased.[135] Severe hypothermia interferes with cardiac rhythm generation and impulse conduction, lengthens PR, QRS, or QT intervals, and generates J waves on the ECG. Risk of dysrhythmia from mechanical myocardial stimulation is increased. Spontaneous ventricular fibrillation occurs at temperatures <28°C. Hypoperfusion promotes tissue hypoxia and metabolic acidemia and jeopardizes marginal tissue grafts. The alveolar–arterial gradient for oxygen is increased even after temperature correction, and increased avidity of hemoglobin for oxygen compromises oxygenation in hypothermic tissues. Platelet sequestration, decreased platelet function, and reduced clotting factor activity contribute to coagulopathy. Moderately hyperglycemia occurs, cellular immune responses are compromised, and postoperative infection rates increase.[136] A decrease in the minimal alveolar concentration of inhalation anesthetics of 5–7% per 1°C reduction in core temperature accentuates sedation from residual inhalation anesthetics. Reduced perfusion and impaired biotransformation might increase the duration of neuromuscular relaxants and sedatives.

Hypothermia complicates care in the PACU. Vasoconstriction interferes with the reliability of pulse oximetry, intra-arterial pressure monitoring, and peripheral nerve stimulation. Duration of PACU stay averages 90 minutes longer for hypothermic patients, and 40 minutes longer if rewarming is not used as a discharge criteria.[137] To increase endogenous heat production, hypothalamic regulation accelerates metabolic activity and generates shivering during emergence.[138] Shivering increases the risk of incidental trauma or disruption of medical devices, interferes with accuracy of ECG and pulse oximetry monitoring, and makes bedside interventions more difficult. Oxygen consumption and CO_2 production increase by up to 800% during shivering. Associated increases in minute ventilation and cardiac output can precipitate ventilatory failure in patients with limited reserve, or myocardial ischemia in patients with coronary artery disease.[135] Shivering is accentuated by tremors related to emergence from inhalation anesthesia. Tremors exhibit both clonic and tonic components and likely reflect decreased cortical influence on spinal cord reflexes.

For most patients, shivering during warming from mild to moderate hypothermia is uncomfortable but self-limited, and needs no treatment other than warmth and reassurance. Many medications have been shown to suppress shivering, including meperidine, morphine, sufentanil, droperidol, physostigmine, clonidine, propofol, nalbuphine, chlorpromazine, and magnesium.[139] Withholding reversal of relaxants in ventilated, sedated patients attenuates shivering but increases rewarming time. Administration of additional relaxant to avoid shivering is seldom indicated in the PACU.

Hyperthermia

Hyperthermia is relatively uncommon in the PACU. Occasionally, a patient exhibits self-limited hyperthermia from close draping or aggressive intraoperative heat preservation. Postoperative fever sometimes reflects an existing infection exacerbated by the surgical procedure (e.g., resection of infected tonsils or appendix, abscess drainage, urinary tract manipulation) or by a previously asymptomatic condition (e.g., sinusitis, upper respiratory or urinary tract infection). Atelectasis secondary to loss of lung volume, retained secretions, or aspiration is another cause, although fever often appears after PACU discharge. Elevated temperature might indicate a drug or transfusion reaction. Muscarinic blocking agents like atropine interfere with a patient's ability to cool and might contribute to fever, but are seldom the cause. High fever occurs with malignant hyperthermia, but signs such as muscle rigidity, dysrhythmia, hyperventilation, and acidemia establish the diagnosis first. Other hypermetabolic states like thyroid storm must be considered.

Ambient cooling, chest physiotherapy, incentive spirometry, and antipyretics are usually sufficient to treat postoperative fever. Offending medications or blood products should be withheld if a drug or transfusion reaction is suspected. The physician responsible for extended care must be notified to ensure evaluation is continued beyond the PACU. Therapy for malignant hyperthermia or thyroid storm is well described elsewhere.

Persistent Sedation

The evaluation of prolonged unconsciousness after anesthesia requires an organized analysis. Because 90% of patients regain consciousness within 15 minutes of admission, unconsciousness persisting for a greater period is considered prolonged.[140] Even a highly susceptible patient should respond to a stimulus within 30–45 minutes after a reasonably conducted general anesthetic.

The level of preoperative responsiveness should be researched to uncover intoxication with drugs and alcohol or pre-existing mental dysfunction. The time and amount of all preoperative and intraoperative sedative medications are noted, and any unusual intraoperative events reviewed. Physical assessment should include a firm tactile stimulus such as a light skin pinch. Tactile stimulation elicits more arousal than verbal stimulation, perhaps because sensory input is amplified through the reticular activating system. The rate and character of spontaneous ventilation helps judge residual anesthesia depth, whereas the heart rate, rhythm, and systemic blood pressure qualitatively indicate adequacy of cerebral perfusion. Diagnostic value of pupillary size and response is low.

Residual sedation from inhalation anesthetics is a frequent cause of prolonged unconsciousness, especially after long procedures, in obese patients, or when high inspired concentrations are continued through the end of surgery. Sedation from intraoperative opioid or sedative administration is dose related. Long-acting sedatives used for premedication (*e.g.*, pentobarbital, hydroxyzine, promethazine, droperidol, lorazepam, scopolamine) contribute to postoperative somnolence. To assess degree of sedation from opioids, low-dose iv naloxone is administered (0.04-mg increments every 2 minutes, up to 0.2 mg). With careful titration, respiratory depression and sedation are reversed without precipitating dangerous reversal of analgesia. If unconsciousness is related to residual opioid effects, ventilatory rate and arousal increase with 0.2 mg or less of iv naloxone unless a patient has received a massive opioid overdose. Flumazenil (0.2 mg iv per min to a total of 1.0 mg), a competitive benzodiazepine antagonist, reverses sedation from midazolam and diazepam, although duration of action is short. Administration of iv physostigmine (1.25 mg) counteracts but does not reverse sedation caused by inhalation anesthetics and other sedatives. If administration of naloxone, flumazenil, or physostigmine does not elicit a response, unconsciousness is most likely not related to residual anesthetic medications. However, it is still possible that an unrecognized, preoperative overdose with depressant oral drugs is responsible.

Profound residual neuromuscular paralysis might rarely mimic unconsciousness by precluding any motor response to stimuli. This might occur after gross overdosage, if reversal agents are omitted, in patients with unrecognized neuromuscular disease, or in patients with Phase II blockade caused by excessive succinylcholine administration or pseudocholinesterase deficiency. Observation of any purposeful motion, spontaneous ventilation, or reflex activity eliminates residual paralysis as an explanation.

Children who were exhausted before surgery are often difficult to arouse after anesthesia, especially if sleep patterns are disrupted by emergency surgery at night. Hypothermia below 33°C impairs consciousness and increases the depressant effect of medications. Core temperatures below 30°C cause fixed pupillary dilation, areflexia, and coma. A serum glucose level should be evaluated to eliminate severe hypoglycemia or hyperglycemic, hyperosmolar coma as causes. Suspicion that unresponsiveness is caused by hypoglycemia indicates an immediate empiric trial of iv 50% dextrose. Hyposmolar states (<260 mOsm · l^{-1}) such as acute hyponatremia (Na < 125 mEq · l^{-1}) are ruled out by serum electrolyte and osmolarity determination. Arterial blood gas analysis reveals CO_2 narcosis (PaCO_2 > 200–250 mm Hg). A patient may also be feigning unresponsiveness or having a hysterical reaction that presents as unconsciousness.[141]

If a diagnosis remains elusive, a neurologist should perform a neurologic evaluation. CNS depression secondary to iv local anesthetic toxicity or inadvertent subarachnoid injection can mimic postoperative coma. Occasionally unresponsiveness reflects subclinical grand mal seizures secondary to delirium tremens or an underlying seizure disorder. Cerebral anoxia from intraoperative hypotension, dysrhythmias, or hypoxemia must be considered as a potential cause. Neither adequate PaO_2 from a blood gas nor hemoglobin saturation from a pulse oximeter rules out cerebral hypoxia from CO poisoning. Laboratory co-oximetry detects carboxyhemoglobinemia. The possibility of unrecognized head trauma, intracerebral hemorrhage, or increased intracranial pressure from bleeding or edema must be considered in injured patients or those recovering from intracranial surgery. Patients sometimes awaken very slowly after long intracranial procedures.[142] Paradoxical air or fat embolism through a right-to-left intracardiac shunt should be considered. Cerebral thromboembolism is another possibility after cardiac, proximal major vascular, or invasive neck surgery, or in patients who have undergone internal jugular or subclavian cannulation. Patients with atrial fibrillation, carotid bruits, or hypercoagulable states are also at increased risk of thromboembolism. Postoperative cerebrovascular accidents in other patients are very rare and usually occur after the PACU.

Altered Mental Status

Recovering patients often exhibit inappropriate mental reactions, ranging from lethargy and confusion to physical combativeness and extreme disorientation. Aside from the disturbance to staff and other patients, there are serious medical consequences. The risk of incidental trauma increases, including contusion or fracture from contact with equipment or side rails, corneal abrasion from dislodged oxygen apparatus, and sprains from violent struggling against restraints. Forceful, thrashing movements jeopardize suture lines, orthopedic fixations, vascular grafts, drains, tracheal tubes, and indwelling vascular catheters. Agitated patients manifest high levels of SNS tone. Resulting tachycardia and hypertension can cause serious medical complications. Least appreciated is the risk of injury to PACU staff struggling to protect a combative patient.

Adverse psychological responses during awakening from general anesthesia are the most frequent cause of emergence reactions. For a short period after regaining consciousness, some patients appear unable to process sensory input appropriately. Many exhibit somnolence, slight disorientation, and sluggish mental reactions that gradually clear. Others experience wide emotional swings such as uncontrollable weeping or escalating resistance to positioning and restraint.

Predicting which patients will have emergence reactions is difficult. Recovery of cognitive functions is slower in the elderly.[143,144] Emergence reactions are more prevalent in children and young adults, especially after anesthesia with sevoflurane and desflurane.[145] In young children, anxiety is heightened by parental separation. Patients with mental retardation, psychiatric disorders, organic brain dysfunction, or hostile preoperative interactions manifest those problems after surgery. Inability to speak secondary to oral fixation or tracheal intubation generates frustration or fear, which exaggerates emergence reactions. Ethnic, cultural, and psychological characteristics play some role. A language barrier accentuates an emergence reaction because reassuring input from PACU staff might not be understood. The incidence of stormy emergence is probably higher after procedures that are charged with anxiety or emotional significance such as breast or testicular biopsies. Recall of intraoperative events can generate severe panic and anxiety during emergence.[146]

Disorientation or clouded sensorium might reflect chronic use of psychogenic drugs or premedication with long-acting sedatives. Intoxication or withdrawal elicits bizarre emergence behavior in patients who abuse alcohol, opioids, cocaine, or other illicit drugs.[147] Disorientation, paranoia, and combativeness occur after administration of parenteral scopolamine as a premedication or antiemetic. This can be treated with iv physostigmine. Patients receiving atropine premedication or chronic meperidine therapy might exhibit anticholinergic-induced delirium. Ketamine may cause dysphoria and hallucination, although acute reactions are rare. The use of etomidate for induction contributes to restlessness.

Surgical pain amplifies agitation, confusion, and aggressive behavior during emergence.[148] Ensure adequate postoperative analgesia early in the PACU course. Urinary urgency or gastric distention from trapped gas generates discomfort and agitation, as do tight dressings, painful phlebotomy, and poor positioning. Pain from endotracheal or nasogastric tubes, urinary catheters, or infiltrated vascular catheters is equally discomforting. Unrecognized sources of pain such as corneal abrasion, entrapment of sensitive body parts, or small devices left beneath a patient should be checked.

Nausea and dizziness are very distressing during emergence, as is severe pruritus. Some patients struggle vigorously to move from a supine into a more comfortable semisitting position. This is common in patients with gastroesophageal reflux, pulmonary congestion, or obesity. Patients often resist physical restraint until the restraint is relaxed. Residual paralysis elicits severe agitation and violent, uncoordinated motions that make a patient appear disoriented and combative, even when ventilation is adequate. Weakness, a peculiar flapping nature of voluntary motion, and electrical nerve stimulation are helpful in the diagnosis. However, patients can appear fully recovered by train-of-four monitoring, head lift, and other bedside indices but still perceive significant impairment of swallowing, visual acuity, and overall sense of strength.[79]

Combativeness, confusion, or delirium might also reflect serious respiratory dysfunction. Moderate hypoxemia often presents with clouded mentation, disorientation, and agitation resembling that caused by pain. Respiratory acidemia caused by airway obstruction or poor ventilatory mechanics elicits profound agitation. (Hypercarbia caused by ventilatory center depression generates less agitation because higher CNS functions are also depressed.) Hypercarbia without acidemia is usually asymptomatic. Limitation of inspiratory volume by chest dressings, gastric distention, or splinting evolves a vague dissatisfaction with lung inflation similar to air hunger. This also occurs during mechanical ventilation with low delivered volumes, and is probably mediated by stretch receptors in the lung. Inability to generate a forceful cough or clear secretions causes distress, as does high work of breathing. Early interstitial pulmonary edema elicits symptoms of chest fullness and air hunger before airway flooding occurs. Agitation can be profound even though ventilation and oxygenation are adequate.

Metabolic abnormalities interfere with lucidity. Lactic acidemia causes anxiety and mild disorientation, whereas acute hyponatremia clouds the sensorium. Cerebral fluid shifts also occur in patients on dialysis and after repletion of severe dehydration. Hyperosmolarity from hyperglycemia or hypernatremia clouds consciousness, whereas severe hypoglycemia

causes first agitation and then diminished responsiveness. Cerebral hypoperfusion produces lethargy, disorientation, agitation, and combativeness. This is a medical emergency that requires aggressive resolution. Administration of sedative or analgesic medications for a mistaken diagnosis of anxiety or pain generates a catastrophic cardiopulmonary collapse in such a patient.

Once reversible causes of delirium or agitation are eliminated, a primary neurologic problem must be considered. Cerebral embolism, hemorrhage, or infarct may initially manifest with disorientation, inability to vocalize, or a reduced level of consciousness. Seizure activity might mimic agitation and combativeness, or disorientation and somnolence during the postictal phase. Seizures should be suspected in patients with epilepsy, head trauma, chronic alcohol intoxication, or cocaine abuse.

There are few interventions that prevent emergence reactions. Use of preoperative sedatives in children does not decrease the incidence of emergence delirium,[149] and preoperative suggestion or reassurance seems ineffective. Altered mental status is treated supportively because most emergence reactions disappear within 10–15 minutes as residual anesthesia dissipates. Verbal reassurances that surgery is completed and the patient is doing well are invaluable. The patient's and the surgeon's name should be used frequently, and the time and location stressed. When practical, patients can be allowed to choose their own positions. Adequate analgesia must be provided. In selected cases, light parenteral sedation relieves fear or anxiety and smooths emergence. Identifying whether a patient is reacting to pain or to anxiety is important. Benzodiazepines and barbiturates are ineffective analgesics, whereas opioids are poor sedatives. Physical restraint is used only when a patient's physical safety is jeopardized. Sedative or analgesic medications should not be administered if altered mental status reflects a physiologic abnormality (e.g., hypoxemia, hypoglycemia, hypotension, acidemia); instead, the abnormality should be resolved.

REFERENCES

1. DeFranco M: Planning the physical structure of the PACU. In Frost EAM (ed): Post Anesthesia Care Unit, p 187. St. Louis, CV Mosby, 1990
2. Bothner U, Georgieff M, Schwilk B: The impact of minor perioperative anesthesia related incidents, events and complications on postanesthetic care unit utilization. Anesth Analg 89:506, 1999
3. Waddle JP, Evers AS, Piccirillo JF: Postanesthesia care unit length of stay: Quantifying and assessing dependent factors. Anesth Analg 87:628, 1998
4. Chung F: Recovery pattern and home readiness after ambulatory surgery. Anesth Analg 80:896, 1995
5. Pavlin DJ, Rapp SE, Polissar NL et al: Factors affecting discharge time in adult outpatients. Anesth Analg 87:816, 1998
6. Ballantyne JC, Chang Y: The impact of choice of muscle relaxant on postoperative recovery time: A retrospective study. Anesth Analg, 85:476, 1997
7. Dexter F, Tinker JH: Analysis of strategies to decrease post anesthesia care unit costs. Anesthesiology, 82:94, 1995
8. Hines R, Barash PG, Watrous G et al: Complications occurring in the postanesthesia care unit: A survey. Anesth Analg 74:503, 1992
9. Kolpfenstein CE, Herrmann FR, Michel JP et al: The influence of an aging surgical population on the anesthesia workload: A ten year survey. Anesth Analg 86:1165, 1998
10. Sullivan E, Mamaril M, Bauer J et al: Standard of Peri-Anesthesia Nursing Practice. Thorofare, New Jersey, American Society of Post Anesthesia Nursing, 1998
11. Gan TJ, Glass TS, Windsor A et al: Bispectral index monitoring allows faster emergence and improved recovery from propofol, alfentanil, and nitrous oxide anesthesia. Anesthesiology 87:808, 1997
12. Song D, Joshi G, White PF: Fast track eligibility after ambulatory anesthesia: A comparison of desflurane, sevoflurane, and propofol. Anesth Analg 86:267, 1998

13. McGregor DG, Senjem DH, Mazze RI: Trace nitrous oxide levels in the postanesthesia care unit. Anesth Analg 89:472, 1999
14. Macario A, Weinger M, Truong P et al: Which clinical anesthesia outcomes are both common and important to avoid? The perspective of a panel of expert anesthesiologists. Anesth Analg 88:1085, 1999
15. Rundshagen I, Schnabel K, Standl T et al: Patients' vs. nurses' assessments of postoperative pain and anxiety during patient or nurse controlled analgesia. Br J Anaesth 82:374, 1999
16. Lynch EP, Lazor MA, Gellis J et al: Patient experience of pain after elective non cardiac surgery. Anesth Analg 85:117, 1997
17. Chung F, Ritchie E, Su J: Postoperative pain in ambulatory surgery. Anesth Analg 85:808, 1997
18. Sear JW: Recent advances and developments in the clinical use of IV opioids during the perioperative period. Br J Anaesth 81:38, 1998
19. Peng PWH, Sandler AN et al: A review of the use of fentanyl analgesia in the management of acute pain in adults. Anesthesiology 90:576, 1999
20. Claxton AR, McGuire G, Chung F et al: Evaluation of morphine versus fentanyl for postoperative analgesia after ambulatory surgical procedures. Anesth Analg 84:509, 1997
21. Beattie WS, Warriner CB, Etches R et al: The addition of continuous intravenous infusion of ketorolac to a patient controlled analgesic morphine regime reduced postoperative myocardial ischemia in patients undergoing elective total hip or knee arthroplasty. Anesth Analg 84:715, 1997
22. Plummer JL, Owen H, Ilsley AH et al: Sustained release ibuprofen as an adjunct to morphine patient controlled analgesia. Anesth Analg 83:92, 1996
23. Korpela R, Korvenoja P, Meretoja OA: Morphine sparing effect of acetaminophen in pediatric day case surgery. Anesthesiology 91:442, 1999
24. De Kock M, Crochet B, Morimont C et al: Intravenous or epidural clonidine for intra- and postoperative analgesia. Anesthesiology 79:525, 1993
25. Henderson DJ, Withington BS, Wilson JA et al: Perioperative dextromethorphan reduces postoperative pain after hysterectomy. Anesth Analg 89:399, 1999
26. Gwirtz KH, Young JV, Byers RS et al: The safety and efficacy of intrathecal opioid analgesia for acute postoperative pain: Seven years experience with 5969 surgical patients at Indiana university hospital. Anesth Analg 88:599, 1999
27. DeLeon-Casasola OA: Postoperative epidural opioid analgesia. Anesth Analg 83:867, 1996
28. Boylan JF, Katz J, Kavanagh BP et al: Epidural bupivacaine-morphine analgesia versus patient controlled analgesia following abdominal aortic surgery. Anesthesiology 89:585, 1998
29. Motamed C, Spencer A, Farhat F et al: Postoperative hypoxaemia: Continuous extradural infusion of bupivacaine and morphine vs patient controlled analgesia with intravenous morphine. Br J Anaesth 80:742, 1998
30. Borgeat A, Stirnemann HR: Ondansetron is effective to treat spinal or epidural morphine-induced pruritus. Anesthesiology 90:432, 1999
31. Casati A, Fanelli G, Cedrati V et al: Pulmonary function changes after interscalene brachial plexus anesthesia with 0.5% and 0.75% ropivacaine: A double blind comparison with 2% mepivacaine. Anesth Analg 88:587, 1999
32. Al-Kaisy AA, Chan VWS, Perlas A: Respiratory effects of low dose bupivacaine interscalene block. Br J Anaesth 82:217, 1999
33. Ritchie ED, Tong D, Chung F et al: Suprascapular nerve block for postoperative pain relief in arthroscopic shoulder surgery: a new modality. Anesth Analg 84:1306, 1997
34. Aldrete JA: The post-anesthesia recovery score revisited. J Clin Anesth 7:89, 1995
35. White PF, Song D: New criteria for fast tracking after outpatient anesthesia: A comparison with the Modified Aldrete's scoring system. Anesth Analg 88:1069, 1999
36. Rooke GA, Schwid HA, Shapira Y: The effect of graded hemorrhage and intravascular volume replacement on systolic pressure variation in humans during mechanical and spontaneous ventilation. Anesth Analg 78:46; 1995
37. Howell SJ, Sear JW, Sear YM et al: Risk factors for cardiovascular death within 30 days after anaesthesia and urgent or emergency surgery: A nested, case controlled study. Br J Anaesth 82:679, 1999
38. Bois S, Couture P, Boudreault D et al: Epidural analgesia and intravenous patient controlled analgesia result in similar rates of postoperative myocardial ischemia after aortic surgery. Anesth Analg 85:1233, 1997
39. Wahr JR: Myocardial ischaemia in anaemic patients. Br J Anaesth 81(suppl 1):10, 1998
40. Badner NH, Knill RL, Brown JE et al: Myocardial infarction after noncardiac surgery. Anesthesiology 88:572, 1998
41. Mangano DT, Layug EL, Wallace A et al, for the Multicenter Study of Perioperative Ischemia Research Group: Effect of atenolol on mortality and cardiovascular morbidity after non cardiac surgery. N Engl J Med 335:1713, 1996
42. Raby KE, Brull SK, Timimi F et al: The effect of heart rate control on myocardial ischemia among high risk patients after vascular surgery. Anesth Analg 88:477, 1999
43. Chung F, Mezei G, Tong D: Pre-existing medical conditions as predictors of adverse events in day case surgery. Br J Anaesth 83:262, 1999
44. Parlow JL, Begou G, Sagnard P et al: Cardiac baroreflex during the postoperative period in patients with hypertension: The effect of clonidine. Anesthesiology 90:681, 1999
45. Dorman T, Clarkson K, Rosenfeld BA et al: Effects of clonidine on prolonged postoperative sympathetic response. Crit Care Med 25:1147, 1997
46. Atlee JL, Bosnjak ZJ: Mechanisms for cardiac dysrhythmias during anesthesia. Anesthesiology 72:347, 1990
47. Gauss A, Hubner C, Radermacher P et al: Perioperative risk of bradyarrhythmias in patients with asymptomatic chronic bifascicular block or left bundle branch block: Does an additional first degree atrioventricular block make any difference? Anesthesiology 88:679, 1998
48. Amar D, Roistacher N, Burt M et al: Clinical and echocardiographic correlates of symptomatic tachydysrhythmias after non cardiac thoracic surgery. Chest 108:349, 1995
49. Mahla E, Rotman B, Rehak P et al: Perioperative ventricular dysrhythmias in patients with structural heart disease undergoing noncardiac surgery. Anesth Analg 86:16, 1998
50. Rose DK, Cohen MM, Wigglesworth DF et al: Critical respiratory events in the postanesthesia care unit: patient, surgical and anesthetic factors. Anesthesiology 81:410, 1994
51. Schwilk B, Bothner U, Schraag S et al: Perioperative respiratory events in smokers and nonsmokers undergoing general anesthesia. Acta Anaesthesiol Scand 41:348, 1997
52. Lawrence VA, Dhanda R, Hilsenbeck SG et al: Risk of pulmonary complications after elective abdominal surgery. Chest 110:774, 1996
53. Ballantyne JC, Carr DB, DeFerranti S et al: The comparative effects of postoperative analgesic therapies on pulmonary outcome: Cumulative meta-analyses of randomized, controlled trials. Anesth Analg 86:598, 1998
54. Warner DO, Warner MA, Offord KP et al: Airway obstruction and perioperative complications in smokers undergoing abdominal surgery. Anesthesiology 90:372, 1999
55. Dahan A, Sarton E, Teppema I et al: Sex related differences in the influence of morphine on ventilatory control in humans. Anesthesiology 88:903, 1998
56. Erikson LI: The effects of residual neuromuscular blockade and volatile anesthetics on the control of ventilation. Anesth Analg 89:243, 1999
57. Etches RC: Respiratory depression associated with patient controlled analgesia: A review of eight cases. Can J Anaesth 41:125, 1994
58. Wheatley RG, Shephard D. Jackson IJB et al: Hypoxaemia and pain relief after upper abdominal surgery: Comparison of IM and patient controlled analgesia in the postoperative patient. Br J Anaesth 69:558, 1992
59. Borgbjerg FM, Nielsen K, Franks J: Experimental pain stimulates respiration and attenuates morphine induced respiratory depression: A controlled study in human volunteers. Pain 64:123, 1996
60. Gross JB, Blouin RT, Zandsberg S et al: Effect of flumazenil on ventilatory drive during sedation with midazolam and alfentanil. Anesthesiology 85:713, 1996
61. Strauss SG, Lynn AM, Bratton SL et al: Ventilatory response to CO_2 in children with obstructive sleep apnea from adenotonsillar hypertrophy. Anesth Analg 89:328, 1999
62. Welborn LG, Hannallah RS, Luban NL et al: Anemia and postoperative apnea in former preterm infants. Anesthesiology 74:1003, 1991

63. Drummond GB: Comparison of sedation with midazolam and ketamine: Effects on airway muscle activity. Br J Anaesth 76:663, 1996

64. Mathru M, Esch O, Lang J et al: Magnetic resonance imaging of the upper airway. Anesthesiology 84:273, 1996

65. D'Honneur G, Lofaso F, Drummond GB et al: Susceptibility to upper airway obstruction during partial neuromuscular block. Anesthesiology 88:371, 1998

66. Putnam MT, Wise RA: Myasthenia gravis and upper airway obstruction. Chest 109:400, 1996

67. Asai T, Koga K, Vaughan RS: Respiratory complications associated with tracheal intubation and extubation. Br J Anaesth 80:767, 1998

68. Schreiner MS, O'Hara I, Markakis DA et al: Do children who experience laryngospasm have an increased risk of upper respiratory tract infection? Anesthesiology 85:475, 1996

69. Skolnick ET, Vomvolakis MA, Buck KA et al: Exposure to environmental tobacco smoke and the risk of adverse respiratory events in children receiving general anesthesia. Anesthesiology 88:1144, 1998

70. Benumof JL, Dagg R, Benumof R: Critical hemoglobin desaturation will occur before return to an unparalyzed state following 1 mg/kg intravenous succinylcholine. Anesthesiology 87:979, 1997

71. Carmichael FJ, Mcguire GP, Wong DT et al: Computed tomographic analysis of airway dimensions after carotid endarterectomy. Anesth Analg 83:12, 1996

72. Ho LI, Harn HJ, Lien TC et al: Postextubation laryngeal edema in adults: Risk factor evaluation and prevention by hydrocortisone. Intensive Care Med 22:933, 1996

73. Jansen NF, Weiler JM: C1 esterase inhibitor deficiency, airway compromise, and anesthesia. Anesth Analg 87:480, 1998

74. Pelosi P, Croci M, Ravagnan I et al: The effects of body mass on lung volumes, respiratory mechanics, and gas exchange during general anesthesia. Anesth Analg 87:654, 1998

75. Warner DO, Warner MA, Barnes RD et al: Perioperative respiratory complications in patients with asthma. Anesthesiology 85:460; 1996

76. Berg H, Viby-Mogensen J, Roed J et al: Residual neuromuscular block is a risk factor for postoperative pulmonary complications: A prospective, randomized, and blinded study of postoperative pulmonary complications after atracurium, vecuronium, and pancuronium. Acta Anaesthesiol Scand 41:1095, 1997

77. Bevan DR, Kahwaji R, Arsermino JM et al: Residual block after mivacurium with or without edrophonium reversal in adults and children. Anesthesiology 84:362, 1996

78. Sharma RR, Axelsson H, Oberg A et al: Diaphragmatic activity after laparoscopic cholecystectomy. Anesthesiology 91:406, 1999

79. Kopman AF, Yee PS, Neuman GG: Relationship of the train-of-four fade ratio to clinical signs and symptoms of residual paralysis in awake volunteers. Anesthesiology 86:765, 1997

80. Kopman AF, Ng J, Zank LM et al: Residual postoperative paralysis: Pancuronium versus mivicurium, does it matter? Anesthesiology 85:1253, 1996

81. Moller JT, Johannessen NW, Espersen K et al: Randomized evaluation of pulse oximetry in 20,802 patients: Perioperative events and postoperative complications. Anesthesiology 78:445, 1993

82. Rothen HU, Sporre B, Engberg G et al: Airway closure, atelectasis and gas exchange during anaesthesia. Br J Anaesth 81:68, 1998

83. Karayiannakis AJ, Makki GG, Mantzioka A et al: Postoperative pulmonary function after laparoscopic and open cholecystectomy. Br J Anaesth 77:448, 1996

84. Baxter PJ, Garton K, Kharasch ED: Mechanistic aspects of carbon monoxide formation from volatile anesthetics. Anesthesiology 89:929, 1998

85. Xue FS, Huang YG, Tong SY et al: A comparative study of early postoperative hypoxemia in infants, children, and adults undergoing elective plastic surgery. Anesth Analg 83:709, 1996

86. Xue FS, Li BW, Zhang GS et al: The influence of surgical sites on early postoperative hypoxemia in adults undergoing elective surgery. Anesth Analg 88:213, 1999

87. Levy L, Pandit UA, Randel GI et al: Upper respiratory tract infections and general anaesthesia in children: Perioperative complications and oxygen saturation. Anaesthesia 47:678, 1992

88. DeBenedeto RJ, Craves SA, Gravenstein N et al: Pulse oximetry monitoring can change routine oxygen supplementation practices in the postanesthesia care unit. Anesth Analg 78:365, 1994

89. Gift AG, Stanik J, Karpenick J et al: Oxygen saturation in postoperative patients at low risk for hypoxemia: Is oxygen therapy needed? Anesth Analg 80:368, 1995

90. Moller JT, Wittrup M, Johansen SH: Hypoxemia in the postanesthesia care unit: An observer study. Anesthesiology 73:890, 1990

91. Warner MA, Warner ME, Warner DO et al: Perioperative pulmonary aspiration in infants and children. Anesthesiology 90:66, 1999

92. Eriksson LI, Sundman E, Olsson R et al: Functional assessment of the pharynx at rest and during swallowing in partially paralyzed humans: Simultaneous videomanometry and mechanomyography of awake human volunteers. Anesthesiology 78:1035, 1997

93. Tramer MR, Fuchs-Buder T: Omitting antagonism of neuromuscular block: Effect on postoperative nausea and vomiting and risk of residual paralysis. A systematic review. Br J Anaesth 82:379, 1999

94. American Society of Anesthesiologists Task Force on Preoperative Fasting: Practice guidelines for preoperative fasting and the use of pharmacologic agents to reduce the risk of pulmonary aspiration: Application to healthy patients undergoing elective procedures. Anesthesiology 90:896, 1999

95. Splinter WM, Schreiner MS: Preoperative fasting in children. Anesth Analg 89:80, 1999

96. Kamphius ET, Ionescu TI, Kuipers PWG et al: Recovery of storage and emptying functions of the urinary bladder after spinal anesthesia with lidocaine and with bupivacaine in men. Anesthesiology 88:310, 1998

97. Pavlin DJ, Rapp SE, Polissar NL et al: Factors affecting discharge time in adult outpatients. Anesth Analg 87:816, 1998

98. Marshall SI, Chung F: Discharge criteria and complications after ambulatory surgery. Anesth Analg 88:508, 1999

99. Twersky R, Fishman D, Homel P: What happens after discharge? Return hospital visits after ambulatory surgery. Anesth Analg 84:319, 1997

100. Pavlin DJ, Pavlin EG, Gunn HC et al: Voiding in patients managed with or without ultrasound monitoring of bladder volume after outpatient surgery. Anesth Analg 89:90, 1999

101. Higuchi H, Sumita S, Wada H et al: Effects of sevoflurane and isoflurane on renal function and on possible markers of nephrotoxicity. Anesthesiology 89:307, 1999

102. Scheingraber S, Rehm M, Sehmisch C et al: Rapid saline infusion produces hyperchloremic acidosis in patients undergoing gynecologic surgery. Anesthesiology 90:1265, 1999

103. Steele A, Gowrishankar M, Abrahamson S et al: Postoperative hyponatremia despite near-isotonic saline infusion: A phenomenon of desalination. Ann Intern Med 126:20, 1997

104. Sinclair DR, Chung F, Mezei G: Can postoperative nausea and vomiting be predicted? Anesthesiology 91:109, 1999

105. Tramer M, Moore A, McQuay H: Prevention of vomiting after paediatric strabismus surgery: A systematic review using the numbers needed to treat method. Br J Anaesth 75:556, 1995

106. Duncan PG, Cohen MM, Tweed WA et al: The Canadian Four Centre Study of Anaesthetic Outcomes: III. Are anaesthetic complications predictable in day surgical practice? Can J Anaesth 39:440, 1992

107. Haigh CG, Kaplan LA, Durham FM et al: Nausea and vomiting after gynaecological surgery: A meta-analysis of factors affecting their incidence. Br J Anaesth 71:517, 1993

108. Beattie WS, Lindblad T, Buckley DN et al: Menstruation increases the risk of nausea and vomiting after laparoscopy: A prospective, randomized study. Anesthesiology 78:272, 1993

109. Hartung J: Twenty four of twenty seven studies show a greater incidence of emesis associated with nitrous oxide than with alternative anesthetics. Anesth Analg 83:114, 1996

110. Yogendran S, Kumar B, Cheng D et al: A prospective, randomized double blinded study of the effect of intravenous fluid therapy on adverse outcomes from outpatient surgery. Anesth Analg 80:682, 1995

111. Fengling J, Norris A, Chung F et al: Should adult patients drink fluids before discharge from ambulatory surgery? Anesth Analg 87:306, 1998

112. Tramer MR, Walder B: Efficacy and adverse effects of prophylactic antiemetics during patient controlled analgesia therapy: A quantitative systematic review. Anesth Analg 88:1354, 1999

113. Domino KB, Anderson EA, Polissar NL et al: Comparative efficacy and safety of ondansetron, droperidol, and metoclopramide for preventing postoperative nausea and vomiting: A meta analysis. Anesth Analg 88:1370, 1999

114. McKenzie R, Lim NT, Riley TJ et al: Droperidol/ondansetron

combination controls nausea and vomiting after tubal banding. Anesth Analg 83:1218, 1996

115. Tang J, Wang B, White P *et al:* The effect of timing of ondansetron administration on its efficacy, cost effectiveness, and cost benefit as a prophylactic antiemetic in the ambulatory setting. Anesth Analg 86:274, 1998

116. Hamid SK, Selby IR, Sikich N *et al:* Vomiting after adenotonsillectomy in children: A comparison of ondansetron, dimenhydrinate, and placebo. Anesth Analg 86:496, 1999

117. Tramer MR, Reynolds JM, Moore A *et al:* Efficacy dose response, and safety of ondansetron in prevention of postoperative nausea and vomiting: A quantitative, systematic review of randomized, placebo controlled trials. Anesthesiology 87:1277, 1997

118. Gan TJ, Glass PSA, Howell ST *et al:* Determination of plasma concentrations of propofol associated with 50% reduction in postoperative nausea. Anesthesiology 87:779, 1997

119. Pappas ALS, Sukhani R, Hotaling AJ *et al:* The effect of preoperative dexamethasone on the immediate and delayed postoperative morbidity in children undergoing adenotonsillectomy. Anesth Analg 87:57, 1998

120. Wang JJ, Shung TH, Lee SC *et al:* The prophylactic effect of dexamethasone on postoperative nausea and vomiting in women undergoing thyroidectomy: A comparison of droperidol with saline. Anesth Analg 89:200, 1999

121. Lee A, Done ML: The use of non-pharmacologic techniques to prevent postoperative nausea and vomiting: A meta analysis. Anesth Analg 88:1362, 1999

122. Roth SR, Thisted RA, Erickson JP *et al:* Eye injuries after nonocular surgery: A study of 60,965 anesthetics from 1988–1992. Anesthesiology 85:1020, 1996

123. Myers MA, Hamilton SR, Bogosian AJ: Visual loss as a complication of spine surgery: A review of 37 cases. Spine 22:1325, 1997

124. Williams EL, Hart WM, Templehoff R: Postoperative ischemic optic neuropathy. Anesth Analg 80:1018, 1995

125. Warner ME, Benenfeld SM, Warner MA *et al:* Peri-anesthetic dental injuries: Frequency, outcomes and risk factors. Anesthesiology 90:1302, 1999

126. Cheney FW, Domino KB, Caplan RA *et al:* Nerve injury associated with anesthesia: A closed claims analysis. Anesthesiology 90:1062, 1999

127. Prielipp RC, Morell RC, Walker FO *et al:* Ulnar nerve pressure: Influence of arm position and relationship to somatosensory evoked potentials. Anesthesiology 91:345, 1999

128. Warner MA, Warner DO, Matsumoto JY *et al:* Ulnar neuropathy in surgical patients. Anesthesiology 90:54, 1999

129. Seeberger MD, Kaufmann M, Staender S *et al:* Repeated dural punctures increase the incidence of post dural puncture headache. Anesth Analg 82:302, 1996

130. Auroy Y, Narchi P, Messiah A *et al:* Serious complications related to regional anesthesia: Results of a prospective survey in France. Anesthesiology 87:479, 1997

131. Horlocker TT, McGregor DG, Matsushige DK *et al:* A retrospective review of 4767 consecutive spinal anesthetics: Central nervous system complications. Anesth Analg 84:578, 1997

132. Hodgson PS, Neal JM, Pollock JE *et al:* The neurotoxicity of drugs given intrathecally (spinal). Anesth Analg 88:797, 1999

133. Sessler DI: Perioperative hypothermia. N Engl J Med 336:1730, 1997

134. Frank SM, Higgins MS, Fleisher LA *et al:* The adrenergic respiratory, and cardiovascular effects of core cooling in humans. Am J Physiol 272:R557, 1997

135. Frank SM, Fleisher LA, Breslow MJ *et al:* Perioperative maintenance of normothermia reduces the incidence of morbid cardiac events: A randomized clinical trial. JAMA 277:1127, 1997

136. Kurz A, Sessler DI, Lenhardt R *et al:* Perioperative normothermia to reduce the incidence of the surgical would infection and shorten hospitalization. N Engl J Med 334:1209, 1996

137. Lenhardt R, Marker E, Goll V *et al:* Mild intraoperative hypothermia prolongs post anesthetic recovery. Anesthesiology 87:1318, 1997

138. Horn EP, Sessler DI, Standl T *et al:* Non-thermoregulatory shivering in patients recovering from isoflurane or desflurane anesthesia. Anesthesiology 89:878, 1998

139. Horn EP, Standl T, Sessler DI *et al:* Physostigmine prevents postanesthetic shivering as does meperidine or clonidine. Anesthesiology 88:108, 1998

140. Zelcer J, Wells DG: Anaesthetic-related recovery room complications. Anaesth Intensive Care 15:168, 1996

141. Adams AP, Goroszeniuk T: Hysteria: A cause of failure to recover after anaesthesia. Anaesthesia 46:932, 1991

142. Schubert A, Mascha EJ, Bloomfield EL *et al:* Effect of cranial surgery and brain tumor size on emergence from anesthesia. Anesthesiology 85:513, 1996

143. Dodds C, Allison J: Postoperative cognitive deficit in the elderly surgical patient. Br J Anaesth 81:449, 1998

144. O'Keefe ST, Ni Chonchubhair A: Postoperative delirium in the elderly. Br J Anaesth 73:673, 1994

145. Welborn LG, Hannallah RS, Norden JM *et al:* Comparison of emergence and recovery characteristics of sevoflurane, desflurane, and halothane in pediatric ambulatory patients. Anesth Analg 83:917, 1996

146. Schwender D, Kunze-Kronawitter H, Dietrich P *et al:* Conscious awareness during general anaesthesia: Patients' perceptions, emotions, cognition and reactions. Br J Anaesth 80:133, 1998

147. Spies CD, Rommelspacher H: Alcohol withdrawal in the surgical patient: prevention and treatment. Anesth Analg 88:946, 1999

148. Lynch EP, Lazor MA, Gellis JE *et al:* The impact of postoperative pain on the development of postoperative delirium. Anesth Analg 86:781, 1998

149. Kain ZN, Mayes LC, Wang SM *et al:* Postoperative behavioral outcomes in children: Effects of sedative premedication. Anesthesiology 90:758, 1999

Clinical Anesthesia (4/e), edited by
Paul G. Barash, Bruce F. Cullen, and
Robert K. Stoelting. Lippincott Williams &
Wilkins, Philadelphia, © 2001.

CHAPTER 54

MANAGEMENT OF ACUTE POSTOPERATIVE PAIN

TIMOTHY R. LUBENOW, ANTHONY D. IVANKOVICH, AND
ROBERT J. MCCARTHY

Acute postoperative pain is a complex physiologic reaction to tissue injury, visceral distention, or disease. It is a manifestation of autonomic, psychological, and behavioral responses that result in an unpleasant, unwanted sensory and emotional experience. Patients often perceive postoperative pain as one of the more ominous aspects of undergoing surgery. In the past, the treatment of postoperative pain was given a low priority by both surgeons and anesthesiologists, and pain was considered a requisite part of the postoperative experience.

With the development of an expanding awareness of the epidemiology and pathophysiology of pain, more attention has been focused on the management of pain in an effort to improve quality of care and patient outcome. The natural progression of this focus was the formation of the postoperative analgesia service or acute pain service, involving a group of individuals who specialize in pain management and who apply an ever-increasing number of modalities to control postoperative pain. This chapter reviews the pathophysiology of pain, examines some pharmacologic considerations, and compares the use of oral, parenteral, and central neuraxial analgesics. Peripheral nerve blocks that have application for postoperative pain relief are highlighted, as are some nonpharmacologic therapies. Incorporation of this knowledge into clinical practice is the basis and the rationale for the effective management of acute postoperative pain.

FUNDAMENTAL CONCEPTS

Nociception

Nociception refers to the detection, transduction, and transmission of noxious stimuli. Stimuli generated from thermal, mechanical, or chemical tissue damage may activate nociceptors, which are free nerve endings. Nociceptors can be further classified into exteroceptors, which receive stimuli from skin surfaces, and interoceptors, which are located in the walls of viscera or deeper body structures. Although nociceptors are free nerve terminals, they are adjacent to small blood vessels and mast cells, with which they operate as a functional unit.[1] In addition to nociceptors, the skin is richly innervated by specialized somatosensory receptors that are sensitive to other forms of stimulation (Table 54-1). Each sensory unit includes an end-organ receptor, accompanying axon, dorsal root ganglion, and axon terminals in the spinal cord. In contrast to other special somatosensory receptors, nociceptors exhibit high response thresholds and persistent discharge to suprathreshold stimuli without rapid adaptation and are associated with small receptive fields and small afferent nerve fiber endings.

Peripheral Nerve Afferent Fibers

Nerve fibers were first described according to their type of covering and the presence or absence of myelination. Neural fibers may be covered with neurolemma or myelin, or both. Speed of conduction is determined by fiber size and the presence or absence of myelination. Small, unmyelinated fibers transmit at slower speed than larger myelinated afferent fibers.

With the invention of the oscilloscope, Erlanger and Gasser[2] were able to describe a more functional classification of peripheral nerve fibers. Nerve fibers were categorized into three groups (A, B, and C), depending on size, degree of myelination, rapidity of conduction, and distribution of fibers. A refinement of this classification is the functional subdivision of the Class A fibers into the subtypes of alpha, beta, gamma, and delta.[3]

Class A. These neurons, composed of large myelinated fibers, exhibit a low threshold for activation, conduct impulses at a speed of $5-100$ m · sec^{-1}, and measure $1-20$ μm in diameter. Class A delta fibers mediate pain sensation, whereas Class A alpha fibers transmit motor and proprioceptive impulses. Class A beta and gamma fibers are responsible for cutaneous touch and pressure as well as regulation of muscle spindle reflexes.

Class B. These neurons constitute the medium-sized myelinated fibers with a conduction velocity ranging from 3 to 14 m · sec^{-1} and a diameter less than 3 μm. They have a higher threshold (lower excitability) than Class A fibers but a lower threshold than Class C fibers. The postganglionic sympathetic and visceral afferents belong to this group.

Class C. These fibers are unmyelinated or thinly myelinated and have conduction velocities in the range of $0.5-2$ m · sec^{-1}. This class is composed of preganglionic autonomic fibers and pain fibers. Approximately $50-80\%$ of C fibers modulate nociceptive stimuli.

An additional classification of afferent muscle nerve fibers used by neurophysiologists divides the large myelinated fibers into three functional groups (Ia, Ib, II), placing the thinly myelinated (III) and unmyelinated fibers (IV) into separate groups. The muscle afferents of Erlanger and Gasser's Class A alpha fibers are subdivided into two groups, Ia and Ib. Fibers from the annulospiral endings of the muscle spindles compose the Ia Group, whereas Group Ib fibers emanate from the Golgi tendon organs. Group II consists of the tactile and proprioceptive fibers of Classes A beta and gamma, respectively, whereas the primary nociceptive nerve fibers of Classes A delta and C are equivalent to Groups III and IV, respectively, within this classification.[4]

Spinal Cord and Brain Pathways

The peripheral afferent neuron, termed the *first-order neuron*, has its cell body located in the dorsal root ganglion and sends axonal projections into the dorsal horn and other areas of the spinal cord. At this point, a synapse occurs with a second-order afferent neuron, which can be categorized, depending on the afferent input it receives, as a nociceptive-specific or wide–dynamic-range neuron. Nociceptive-specific neurons process afferent impulses only from nociceptive afferent fibers, whereas A beta, A delta, and C fibers communicate with wide–dynamic-range neurons. In the dorsal horn, further synaptic connections occur between first-order neurons and regulatory internuncial neurons. First-order neurons also communicate with the cell bodies of the sympathetic nervous system and ventral motor nuclei, either directly or through the internuncial neurons.[5] The cell body of the second-order neuron lies in the dorsal horn, and axonal projections of this neuron cross to the contralateral hemisphere of the spinal cord (Fig. 54-1). This second-order afferent neuron ascends from that level in the lateral spinothalamic tract to synapse in the thalamus. Along the way, this neuron divides and sends axonal branches that synapse in the

Table 54-1. SOMATOSENSORY RECEPTORS

Receptor	Sensation Perceived
Nerve fibers on hair follicles	Touch
Merkel's disks	Touch
Meissner's corpuscles	Touch
Free nerve endings (nociceptors)	Pain
Krause's end bulbs	Cold
Ruffini's endings	Heat
Pacinian corpuscles	Pressure
Golgi-Mazzoni endings	Pressure

regions of the reticular formation, nucleus raphe magnus, peri-aqueductal gray, and other areas in the brain stem. In the thalamus, the second-order neuron synapses with a third-order afferent neuron, which sends axonal projections into the sensory cortex.

Modulation of Nociception

Even though nociceptors and the afferent sensory neural pathways detect and transmit noxious stimuli reliably, modulation occurs at several levels in the pathway before perception of the signal at the cortical levels. Modulation can occur either in the periphery or at any point where synaptic transmission occurs.

Peripheral Modulation

Peripheral modulation occurs either by the liberation or elimination of allogeneic substances in the vicinity of the nociceptor.

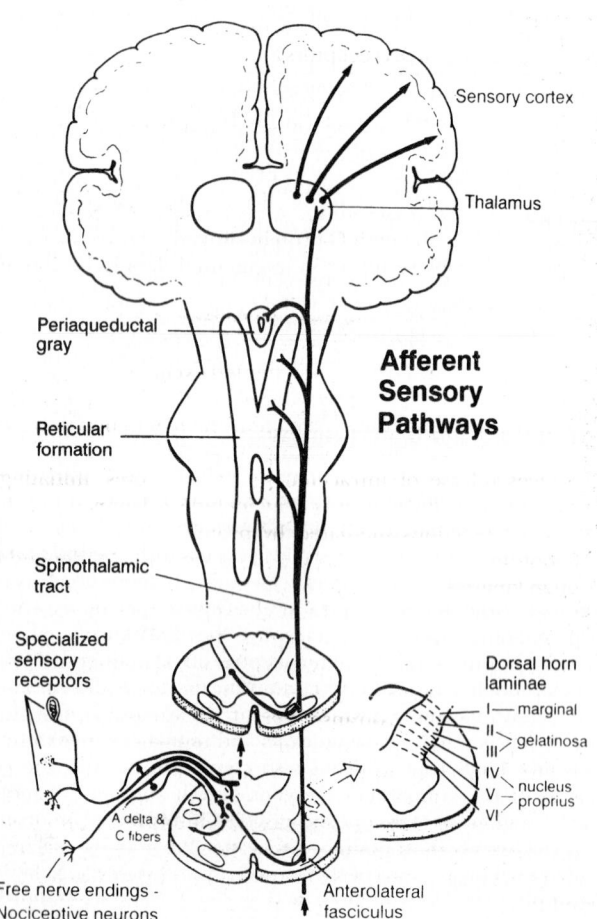

Afferent Sensory Pathways

- Sensory cortex
- Thalamus
- Periaqueductal gray
- Reticular formation
- Spinothalamic tract
- Specialized sensory receptors
- A delta & C fibers
- Free nerve endings - Nociceptive neurons
- Anterolateral fasciculus
- Dorsal horn laminae
  - I — marginal
  - II — gelatinosa
  - III
  - IV
  - V — nucleus
  - VI — proprius

Figure 54-1. Afferent sensory pathways for detection and transmission of nociceptive impulses.

Tissue injury activates nociceptors in the periphery by causing the release of neurotransmitters such as substance P and glutamate, which directly activate nociceptors. Other allogenic mediators—such as potassium and hydrogen ions, lactic acid, serotonin, bradykinin, histamine, and the prostaglandins—further sensitize and excite nociceptors and act as mediators of inflammation. The sources of these substances include ischemic damaged cells and mast cells in the area of the injury, as well as plasma and platelets in the microcirculation surrounding the nociceptors.[1] Aspirin, nonsteroidal anti-inflammatory drugs (NSAIDs), and specific cyclo-oxygenase-2 (COX-2) inhibitors exert an analgesic effect by inhibiting prostaglandin synthesis and reducing prostaglandin E_1- and E_2-mediated sensitization of peripheral nociceptors.

Spinal Modulation

Modulation in the spinal cord results from the action of neurotransmitter substances in the dorsal horn or from spinal reflexes, which convey efferent impulses back to the peripheral nociceptive field. The excitatory amino acid transmitters L-glutamate and aspartate, and several neuropeptides, including vasoactive intestinal peptide, calcitonin gene-related peptide, and neuropeptide Y, are found in central terminals of the first-order neurons and have been shown to modulate transmission of nociceptive afferent signals.[6] Substance P, which is found in the synaptic vesicle of unmyelinated C fibers, is also an important neuromodulator that can enhance or aggravate pain.[7] Prostaglandins produced in response to inflammation play a role in inflammation-evoked central sensitization of spinal cord neurons.[8]

Inhibitory substances involved in the regulation of afferent impulses in the dorsal horn include the enkephalins, β-endorphins, norepinephrine, dopamine, and adenosine.[6] Somatostatin, a neuropeptide found in cells that do not contain substance P, may represent another inhibitory neuropeptide involved in afferent modulation. Acetylcholine is also involved in afferent signal processing. Muscarinic receptors of the M_1 and M_2 subtypes have been identified on the nerve terminals of the first-order neurons in laminae II and III of the spinal cord.[9] Cell bodies staining for choline acetyltransferase have been found in laminae III, IV, and V,[10] with dendritic projections into laminae I, II, and III, sites that are primarily involved in processing of nociceptive impulses.[11] Cholinergic agonists have been demonstrated to produce analgesia,[12] as has neostigmine, which inhibits the breakdown of the endogenous neurotransmitter acetylcholine.[13] Acetylcholine acts at muscarinic (M_1 or M_3) receptors that appear to mediate spinal antinociception.[14] The analgesic efficacy of modulating the cholinergic system depends on the tonic release of acetylcholine at muscarinic receptors involved in afferent signal processing, because acetylcholine has actions at other spinal sites (inhibition of motor neuron activity, excitation of sympathetic outflow) that produce unwanted side effects.[13]

Afferent modulating mechanisms at the spinal level may also involve spinal reflexes in which afferent signals directly evoke somatic or sympathetic efferent impulses. These impulses discharge in the area of the efferent nociceptive signal. For example, skeletal muscle spasm in an injured area is part of a somatic efferent reflex that is induced as a result of nociceptive afferent signals. Increased skeletal muscle tone initiates more nociceptive signals in a positive feedback loop system from the muscles (Fig. 54-2). In addition, spinal reflexes may involve the discharge of efferent sympathetic signals evoked from the nociceptive impulse (see Fig. 54-2). Efferent sympathetic signals emanate from cell bodies located in the intermediolateral column of the spinal cord. These cell bodies receive internuncial projections from the dorsal horn of the gray matter. This sympathetic reflex produces smooth muscle spasm, vasoconstriction, and liberation of norepinephrine in the vicinity of the wound, thereby generating more

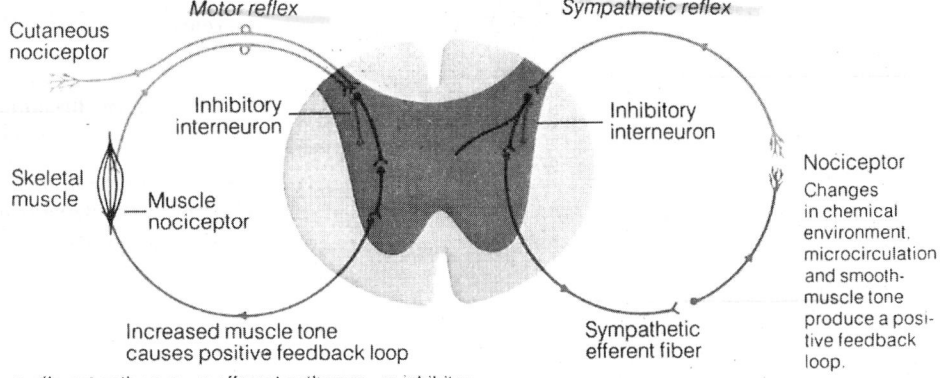

Figure 54-2. Schematic representation of spinal reflexes involved in pain modulation. (Reprinted with permission from Bonica JJ, Liebeskind JC, Albe-Fessard DG [eds]: Advances in Pain Research and Therapy, p 3. New York, Raven Press, 1979.)

pain. Release of norepinephrine has been shown to produce or augment pain after injury.

Neuroplasticity: The Dynamic Modulation of Neural Impulses. The preceding description of the neurophysiology of afferent signal transmission and processing is based on the concept that neural connections involve isolated, unaltered transmission of a single impulse or group of impulses between neurons. Using this model, modulation of noxious efferent signals could be described by gating mechanisms, which have formed the basis for therapeutic analgesic interventions. More recently, however, the description of neural activity–dependent plasticity has enhanced our understanding of the dynamic nature of the nociceptive response to injury. As peripheral nociceptors are sensitized by local tissue mediators of injury (potassium, prostaglandins, and bradykinins), the excitability and frequency of neural discharge increase. This primary hyperalgesia permits previously subnoxious stimuli to generate action potentials and be transduced orthodromically in the spinal cord (Fig. 54-3). The facilitation of impulse transduction in the first-order neuron is partially mediated by noxious substances released from damaged tissues. In addition, axonal reflexes exaggerate this response by releasing substance P, which produces vasodilation and mast cell degranulation, liberating histamine and serotonin and effectively enlarging the peripheral receptive field to include adjacent noninjured tissue, resulting in secondary hyperalgesia.[15]

The increased frequency of impulse transmission to the dorsal horn reduces the gradient between the resting and the critical threshold potential of second-order neurons in the spinal cord. As peripheral nerve firing increases, other changes also occur in the excitability of spinal cord neurons, altering their response to afferent impulses. This central sensitization to afferent impulses results from a functional change in spinal cord processing, termed *neuroplasticity* (see Fig. 54-3). The temporal summation of the number and duration of action potentials elicited per stimulus that occurs in dorsal horn neurons (or in the motor neurons of the ventral horn) has been referred to as the *"windup" phenomenon.*[16] In general, the windup phenomenon requires a minimum stimulus frequency of 0.5 Hz, arising from C fibers. Once the stimulus frequency reaches a critical threshold, the postsynaptic depolarizing responses of these second-order afferent neurons summate to produce bursts of action potential discharges instead of a single action potential. The windup phenomenon results in a persistence of action potentials for up to 60 seconds after the discontinuance of the stimulus, and results in a change in spinal cord processing that can last for 1–3 hours.[17] As this process repeats, more permanent changes in these second-order neurons occur and have been termed *long-term potentiation.*

The cellular mechanisms of spinal cord sensitization involve the relatively slow-onset and long-duration synaptic potentials elicited by A delta and C fibers in dorsal horn neurons.[16] These potentials persist up to 20 seconds (approximately 2000 times longer than the fast potentials of A beta fibers). These slow potentials are mediated through release by the afferent axon of the excitatory neurotransmitter glutamate and the neuropeptides substance P and neurokinin A[16,18] (see Fig. 54-3). As peripheral afferent nerve activity increases, progressively more and longer-lasting second-order neuron depolarizations occur because of the accumulation of these excitatory neurotransmitters and summation of these slow potentials. The net result is that a few seconds of C-fiber activity can result in several minutes of postsynaptic depolarization.

Spinal cord synaptic plasticity involves the binding of glutamate to the *N*-methyl-D-aspartate (NMDA) receptor as well as binding of substance P and neurokinins to tachykinin receptors.[16,19] High-frequency presynaptic activity causes release of glutamate and tachykinins from presynaptic vesicles. Binding of glutamate to NMDA receptors alters a magnesium-dependent block of ion channels, subsequently increasing cellular permeability to all cations, especially calcium and sodium. Glutamate also activates the α-amino-3 hydroxy-5-methyl-4-isoxazole propionic acid (AMPA) and metabotropic receptors on the postsynaptic cell. AMPA receptors control depolarization primarily through modulation of sodium influx into the cell. Neurokinins and substance P, through G-protein–linked receptors, increase enzymatic activity, resulting in augmented depolarization and increases in stores of secondary neurotransmitters. In aggregate, stimulation of these three receptor groups enhances the excitability of the second-order neuron (see Fig. 54-3).

In addition to modulating augmented excitability, these transmitter and cellular mechanisms mediate changes in the postsynaptic cell, leading to more permanent changes in nerve conduction, or long-term potentiation.[17] Extracellular calcium influx enhances release of intracellular calcium stores, initiating a series of intracellular events that include calcium-dependent enzymatic reactions mediated by protein kinase C, calcium-calmodulin, and cyclic adenosine monophosphate–dependent protein kinase A. These enzymes phosphorylate membrane proteins, namely receptors and ion channels on the postsynaptic cell, which further increases excitability. AMPA receptors become more numerous on the postsynaptic cell membrane, and a retrograde factor is released that diffuses back to the presynaptic cell, augmenting neurotransmitter release in response to a given presynaptic action potential. Finally, changes in second messengers also activate immediate early gene products, transcription factors that can alter the expression of particular genes, which in turn can result in more persistent changes in neural processing.

Although much of the preceding discussion of altered spinal cord processing in response to nociceptive input has been derived from the study of chronic pain, similar changes in spinal cord processing occur even after a minor surgical incision.[20] These changes result in an increase in primary hyperalgesic response to noxious stimulus that persists for many days in the

Spinal Cord

Peripheral Nerves

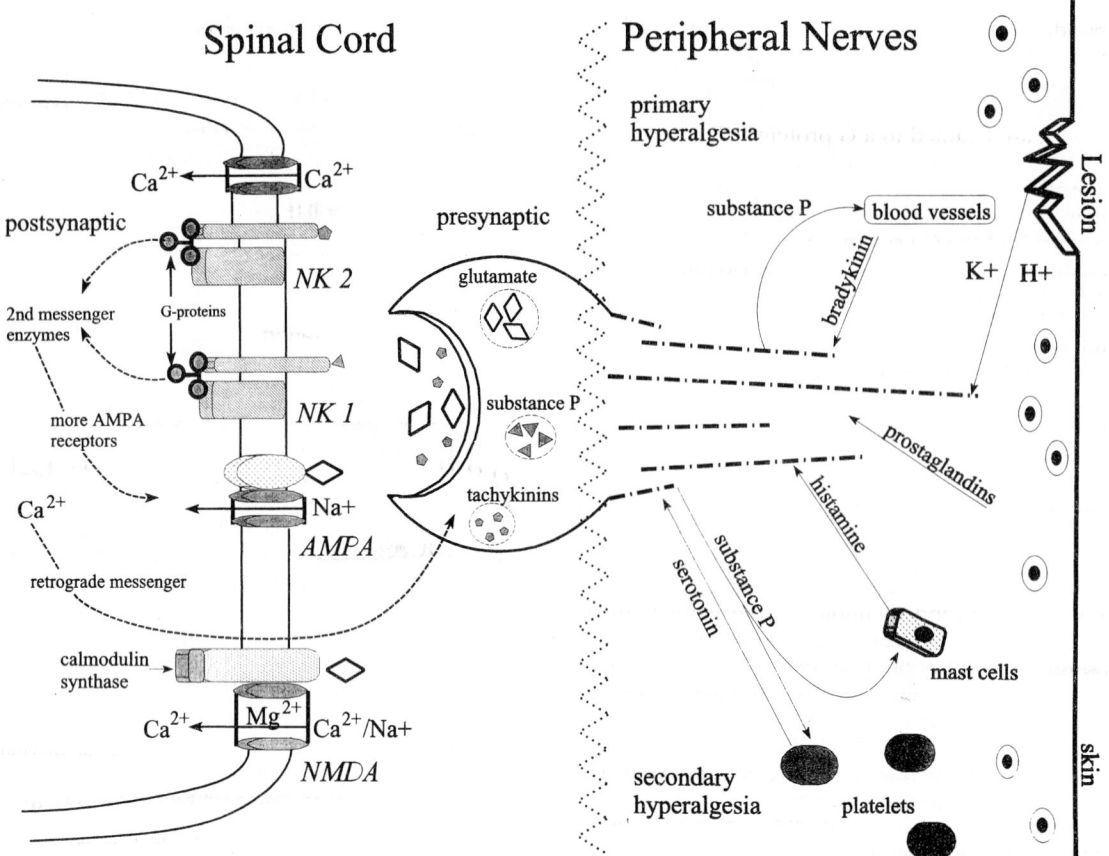

Figure 54-3. Schematic representation of peripheral and spinal mechanism involved in neuroplasticity. Primary hyperalgesia results from tissue release of toxic substances, which spread to adjacent tissues, prolonging the hyperalgesic state (secondary hyperalgesia). As C-fiber terminals increase in frequency of release of neurotransmitters such as glutamate, substance P, and tachykinins, the effects of these neurotransmitters are summated, resulting in prolonged depolarizations of second-order neurons ("windup"). Function changes at the second order neuron occur as a result of neurotransmitter binding to postsynaptic receptors, which results in activity-dependent plasticity of the spinal cord. See text for details. AMPA = α-amino-3 hydroxy-5-methyl-4-isoxazole propionic acid; NK = neurokinin; NMDA = N-methyl-D-aspartate.

area of the incision as well as secondary hyperalgesia of shorter duration in surrounding tissues.[21]

Supraspinal Modulation

Brain Stem. Descending inhibitory tracts at the brain stem level originate from cell bodies located in the region of the periaqueductal gray, reticular formation, and nucleus raphe magnus. These inhibitory tracts descend into the dorsolateral fasciculus and synapse in the dorsal horn. Neurotransmitters act presynaptically on the first-order neuron and postsynaptically on the second-order neuron of the spinothalamic tract or on the internuncial neuron pool. Internuncial neurons can be inhibitory and can regulate synaptic transmission between primary and secondary afferent neurons in the dorsal horn. At least two groups of nerve fibers have been identified as participants in this inhibitory modulation. One group of fibers involves the opioid system and contains the neurotransmitters β-endorphin and the enkephalins, as well as other neuropeptides. Analgesia is produced during electrical stimulation of the periaqueductal gray, and this effect is blocked by naloxone.[22] These opioid projections from the nucleus raphe magnus and reticular formation interface presynaptically with the first-order afferent neurons. Neurotransmitters released from these projections hyperpolarize Class A delta and C fibers, which serves to negate or shunt out the depolarizing current that approaches the terminal end plate, thereby diminishing the release of neurotransmitters such as substance P[23] (Fig. 54-4). In addition to this presynaptic modulation, exogenously applied opioids

inhibit L-glutamate–evoked discharge of dorsal horn neurons, suggesting that opioids exert a direct postsynaptic effect.[24] In summary, opioids modulate transmission of afferent impulses in the dorsal horn presynaptically at the level of the first-order neuron. The enkephalinergic transmitter that is released from the descending inhibitory pathways hyperpolarizes the afferent terminals to block neurotransmitter release. Opioids also exert a direct inhibitory effect on the postsynaptic membrane potential (see Fig. 54-4).

In addition to the opioid descending inhibitory pathway, a monoamine pathway has been identified that also originates from locations in the periaqueductal gray and reticular formation. Stimulation of these pathways inhibits synaptic transmission in the dorsal horn in a manner similar to the inhibiton produced by the opioid system. Electrical stimulation of these pathways and intracerebral injections of α_2-adrenergic agonists can inhibit spinal nociceptive reflexes, and this effect can be antagonized by intrathecally administered α_2-adrenergic antagonists.[25] Further evidence of a monoamine pathway stems from the observation that the intrathecal administration of α_2-adrenergic agonists produces analgesia, implying that α_2 adrenoreceptors are responsible for this antinociceptive effect.[26] These fibers descend into the dorsolateral fasciculus, in a manner similar to that of the opioid fibers, and synapse in the substantia gelatinosa region of the dorsal horn. Norepinephrine is released from these nerve terminals and produces hyperpolarization of the first-order neurons, internuncial neurons, and wide–dynamic-range neurons in the spinothalamic tract. In addition, there are some α_2-adrenoreceptor projections into the ventral gray matter area of the motor nuclei.

The opioid and the α_2 receptors share a common mechanism of action. At the cellular level, these receptors belong to a family of receptors that are coupled to a G protein[27] (Fig. 54-5). The G protein exerts its membrane function through a secondary messenger protein capable of converting guanosine triphosphate to guanosine diphosphate. When the receptor is occupied, the α subunit of the G protein releases from the β and γ subunits and modulates cellular functions such as ion exchange, adenyl cyclase, and phospholipase C activity. Hyperpolarization of the nerve results in decreased transmission of the action potential and decreased release of stored neurotransmitter. Hyperpolarization of the nerve most likely occurs because of the opening of potassium channels and the inhibition of calcium movement.[27,28]

Higher Central Nervous System. A basic review of the dimensions of perceptual psychology is required to understand the role of higher cortical function. Perception is the phenomenon by which noxious stimuli reach consciousness. Input from the cerebral cortex is necessary to provide interpretation and to give meaning to the stimuli. Perception can be subdivided into two categories: cognition and attention. Cognitive functions are those abilities that recognize, discriminate, memorize, or judge afferent information that stems from external stimuli. Therefore, cognitive modulation of pain involves the patient's ability to relate a painful experience to another event. For example, pain experienced in a pleasant environment elicits a less intense response than pain experienced in a setting of depression. The other area of perception is attention. Attention operates on the premise that only a fixed number of afferent stimuli can reach cortical centers. If a patient in pain concentrates on a separate

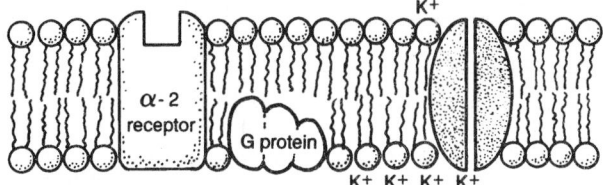

Nociceptive nerve membrane without alpha-2 activation

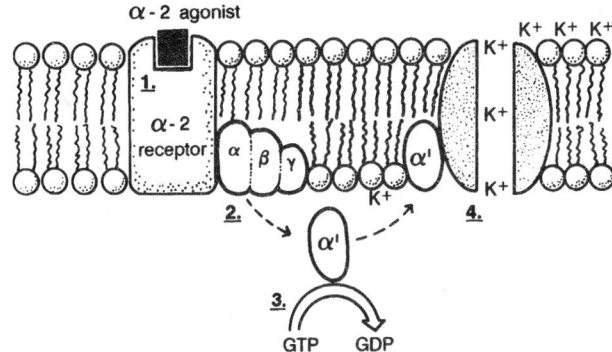

with alpha-2 activation

Figure 54-5. Schematic representation of cellular mechanisms of G-protein–linked receptor, depicted as an α_2-adrenergic receptor. Binding of agonist at receptor causes conformational change in G protein, allowing for cleavage of α subunit. Activation of α subunit occurs by hydrolysis of GTP to active state α', which is capable of increasing K^+ movement and resulting in membrane hyperpolarization. GTP = guanosine triphosphate; GDP = guanosine diphosphate. (Adapted with permission from Maze M: Alpha-2 adrenoreceptor agonists: Defining the role in clinical anesthesia. Anesthesiology 74:581, 1991.)

and unrelated image, it is possible to reduce the effect of a painful sensation. This is achieved because the patient is focused on something else. The positive impact on pain from biofeedback or hypnosis operates on this principle.

PATHOPHYSIOLOGY OF PAIN

Components of the Surgical Stress Response

It has been well established that surgical patients receiving routine, intermittent on-demand opioid analgesics remain in moderate to severe pain. Provision of effective postoperative analgesia is important not only for humanitrian reasons but because of the deleterious effects of postoperative pain on specific organ systems and the negative impact on postoperative recovery (Table 54-2).

Neuroendocrine

Surgical stress and pain elicit a consistent and well defined metabolic response, involving release of neuroendocrine hormones and cytokines, that leads to a myriad of detrimental effects.[29] In addition to the rise in catabolically active hormones such as catecholamines, cortisol, angiotensin II, and antidiuretic hormone, stress causes an increase in adrenocorticotropic hormone, growth hormone, and glucagon.[30] The stress response results in lower levels of anabolic hormones, such as testosterone and insulin. Epinephrine, cortisol, and glucagon produce hyperglycemia by promoting insulin resistance and increases in gluconeogenesis. They induce protein catabolism and lipolysis to provide substrates for gluconeogenesis. The stress response causes a negative postoperative nitrogen balance. Aldosterone, cortisol, and antidiuretic hormone influence water and electro-

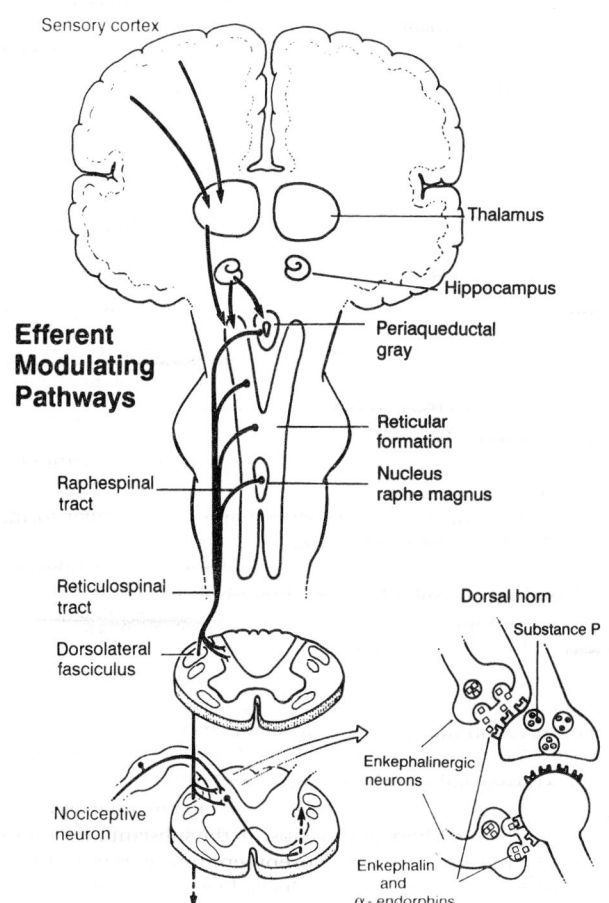

Figure 54-4. Efferent pathways involved in nociceptive regulation.

Table 54-2. ADVERSE PHYSIOLOGIC SEQUELAE OF PAIN

Organ System	Clinical Effect
RESPIRATORY	
Increased skeletal muscle tension	Hypoxemia
Decreased total lung compliance	Hypercapnia
	Ventilation–perfusion abnormality
	Atelectasis
	Pneumonitis
ENDOCRINE	
Increased adrenocorticotropic hormone	Protein catabolism
Increased cortisol	Lipolysis
Increased glucagon	Hyperglycemia
Increased epinephrine	
Decreased insulin	
Decreased testosterone	Decreased protein anabolism
Decreased insulin	
Increased aldosterone	Salt and water retention
Increased antidiuretic hormone	
Increased cortisol	Congestive heart failure
Increased catecholamines	Vasoconstriction
Increased angiotensin II	Increased myocardial contractility
	Increased heart rate
CARDIOVASCULAR	
Increased myocardial work (mediated by catecholamines, angiotensin II)	Dysrhythmias
	Angina
	Myocardial infarction
	Congestive heart failure
IMMUNOLOGIC	
Lymphopenia	Decreased immune function
Depression of reticuloendothelial system	
Leukocytosis	
Reduced killer T-cell cytotoxicty	
COAGULATION EFFECTS	
Increased platelet adhesiveness	Increased incidence of thromboembolic phenomena
Diminished fibrinolysis	
Activation of coagulation cascade	
GASTROINTESTINAL	
Increased sphincter tone	Ileus
Decreased smooth muscle tone	
GENITOURINARY	
Increased sphincter tone	Urinary retention
Decreased smooth muscle tone	

lyte reabsorption by promoting Na$^+$ and water retention while expending potassium. This contributes to increases in the extravascular fluid compartment both peripherally and within the pulmonary parenchymal tissue. Local release of cytokines such as interleukin-2, interleukin-6, and tumor necrosis factor may contribute to abnormal physiologic responses such as alterations in heart rate, temperature, blood pressure, and ventilation.[31] Finally, catecholamines sensitize peripheral nociceptive endings, which serve to propagate more intense pain and may contribute to a vicious pain–catecholamine release–pain cycle.[32] The magnitude of these neuroendocrine and cytokine responses is related to the severity of tissue injury and correlates with outcome after injury.[33,34]

Cardiovascular

The cardiovascular effects of pain are initiated by the release of catecholamines from sympathetic nerve endings and the adrenal medulla, of aldosterone and cortisol from the adrenal cortex, and of antidiuretic hormone from the hypothalamus, and by activation of the renin–angiotensin system. These hormones have direct effects on the myocardium and vasculature, and they augment salt and water retention, which places a greater burden on the cardiovascular system.

Angiotensin II causes generalized vasoconstriction, whereas catecholamines increase heart rate, myocardial contractility, and systemic vascular resistance. The sympathoadrenal release of catecholamines and the effects of angiotensin II may result in hypertension, tachycardia, and dysrhythmias and may lead to myocardial ischemia in susceptible patients as a consequence of increased oxygen demand. In addition, a significant proportion of perioperative myocardial ischemia is related to reductions in myocardial supply without hemodynamic aberrations. Activation of the sympathetic nervous system may trigger coronary vasoconstriction, which may result in myocardial ischemia in the presence of atherosclerotic coronary artery disease. This may occur through direct activation of cardiac sympathetic nerves[35] as well as through circulating catecholamines, which may contribute to hypercoagulability, a known mediator of adverse outcome in patients with ischemic heart disease. Salt and water retention secondary to aldosterone, cortisol, and antidiuretic hormone, in combination with the previously described effects of catecholamines and angiotensin II, can also precipitate congestive heart failure in patients with limited cardiac reserve.

Respiratory

Increases in extracellular lung water may contribute to ventilation-perfusion abnormalities. For surgical procedures performed on the thorax and abdomen, pain-induced reflex increases in skeletal muscle tension may lead to decreased total lung compliance, splinting, and hypoventilation. These changes then promote atelectasis, contribute to further ventilation-perfusion abnormalities, and result in hypoxemia. In major surgical procedures or in high-risk patients, these respiratory effects of pain may lead to a significant reduction in functional residual capacity ranging from 25–50% of preoperative values.[36] Hypoxemia stimulates increases in minute ventilation. Although tachypnea and hypocapnia are common initially, prolonged increases in the work of breathing may result in hypercapnic respiratory failure. Pulmonary consolidation and pneumonitis may occur because of hypoventilation and further aggravate the clinical scenario. These sequelae are especially significant in patients with pre-existing pulmonary disease, upper abdominal and thoracic incisions,[37] advanced age, or obesity.[36]

Gastrointestinal

Pain-induced sympathetic hyperactivity may cause reflex inhibition of gastrointestinal function.[38] This promotes postoperative ileus, which contributes to postoperative nausea, vomiting, and discomfort and delays resumption of an enteral diet. Failure to resume early enteral feeding may be associated with postoperative morbidity, including septic complications and abnormal wound healing.[39]

Genitourinary

An increase in sympathetic activity responses to pain causes reflex inhibition of most visceral smooth muscle, including urinary bladder tone. This can result in urinary retention with subsequent urinary tract infections and related complications.

Immunologic

The pain-related stress response suppresses both cellular and humoral immune function[40,41] and results in lymphopenia, leukocytosis, and depression of the reticuloendothelial system. In addition, some anesthetic agents reduce chemotaxis of neutrophils and may be one factor involved in the reduction of monocyte activity. Many known mediators of the stress response are potent immunosuppressants, and both cortisol and epinephrine infusions decrease neutrophil chemotaxis.[42] These effects can lower resistance to pathogens and may be key factors in the development of perioperative infectious complications.[43] In patients with neoplasms in whom surgical manipulation of the tumor causes release of tumor cells, the postoperative stress response may reduce the cytotoxicity of killer T cells. Increases in catecholamines, glucocorticoids, and prostaglandins in response to stress may impair immunologic responses important for patients with neoplasms.[44]

Coagulation

Stress-related alterations in blood viscosity, platelet function, fibrinolysis, and coagulation pathways have been described.[45-48] These stress-mediated effects include increased platelet adhesiveness, diminished fibrinolysis, and promotion of a hypercoagulable state. When these effects are coupled with the microcirculatory effects of catecholamines as well as immobilization of the patient in the postoperative period, thromboembolic events are more likely to occur.

General Well-Being

Pain increases skeletal muscle tone in the area of the surgical field. This postoperative impairment of muscle function may lead to physical immobility and a delayed return to normal function. Poorly controlled pain also contributes to insomnia, anxiety, and a feeling of helplessness. These psychological factors, coupled with the immobilization that occurs because of the increased skeletal muscle tone, create a postoperative scenario feared by many patients.

Attenuation of Central Sensitization and the Stress Response

As discussed earlier, acute tissue injury results in peripheral as well as central neural sensitization. It is also evident that acute nociceptive stimulation can result in neuroplastic responses that compound the intensity of pain perception in concert with other deleterious systemic effects, including those modulated as part of the stress response. Because most of these events are not manifest until after surgery, most efforts to attenuate the cascade of events precipitated by intraoperative trauma have focused on the postoperative period. These efforts are well founded because of the need to interrupt and limit central sensitization propagated by ongoing tissue injury. However, perioperative anesthetic and analgesic strategies must also consider the temporal relation of nociceptive stimulation to the initiation of central sensitization. The ideal perioperative intervention should focus on preventive, rather than primarily therapeutic measures to control the adverse sequelae of central sensitization and the stress response. Our current understanding of the pathophysiologic consequences of tissue injury has therefore prompted the application of preoperative and intraoperative techniques that prevent or minimize this postinjury hypersensitivity, and has fostered the concept of preemptive analgesia.

The relative importance of preemptive analgesia in preventing adverse sequelae depends on several factors, including preoperative patient status and the magnitude and site of the surgical intervention. It is widely believed that preemptive analgesia has a greater impact in patients with impaired physiologic reserve than in healthier patients who can better tolerate the perturbations induced by surgery. Minor, peripheral surgical procedures performed with the use of local anesthesia usually produce minimal systemic or central neuraxial changes. The more extensive the surgical procedure, the greater the magnitude of the neuroendocrine stress response. Procedures associated with greater degrees of surgical trauma may also contribute to greater central sensitization than less invasive procedures.

From the previous discussion, it is apparent that the postoperative physiologic changes are not homeostatic mechanisms but are reproducible adverse responses to tissue injury that result in a myriad of adverse physiologic events that likely modulate perioperative outcome. Research efforts have therefore been focused on the effectiveness of various anesthetic and analgesic strategies targeted to modify the adverse neural and systemic derangements commonly observed after surgery.

Influence of Anesthesia on the Surgical Stress Response and Outcome

General Anesthesia

It has been demonstrated that general anesthesia, either with intravenous (iv) or inhalational anesthetics, does not effectively attenuate the neuroendocrine stress response.[49] One exception to this assertion is the administration of high-dose opioid anesthesia. Extremely high doses of certain opioids can inhibit some aspects of the stress response, but lower doses of opioids usually are unable to hinder the neuroendocrine effects of stress.[50,51] The effect of opioids on immune function is controversial because both immune-suppressing and immune-enhancing effects have been described.[52] High doses of inhalational agents (1.5 of minimum alveolar concentration) may suppress the intraoperative catecholamine response but do not diminish the catecholamine response that develops after surgery.

Regional Anesthesia and Analgesia

Mitigation of nociception at the peripheral and central level may be accomplished through a variety of techniques. A regional anesthetic or analgesic modality is ideally suited to produce this desired effect because it diminishes the intensity of afferent impulses reaching the spinal cord. Regional anesthesia and analgesia have been shown to reduce catecholamine and other stress hormone responses during the perioperative period for certain surgical procedures.[30,47,53] The finding that regional anesthesia and analgesia can ablate the neuroendocrine stress responses is not universal. Some studies have demonstrated that central neuraxial techniques have no significant influence on cortisol release. The differing results may be related to the level of the afferent neural blockade. Another confounding variable is the region of the body where the surgical procedure was performed. In studies where regional anesthesia did not have an influence on the cortisol response, surgery was performed in the upper abdomen, whereas in most studies that demonstrate inhibition, surgery was performed on a lower extremity or the lower abdomen. Sensory blocks below L1 usually have no effect on cortisol response. To prevent a cortisol response to surgery, all afferent pathways from the surgical site must be blocked.[54]

Besides reducing the neuroendocrine stress response, regional anesthesia can reduce myocardial work and oxygen consumption by reducing heart rate, arterial pressure, and left ventricular contractility. Left ventricular ejection fraction is not significantly affected by epidural anesthesia in normal patients, whereas patients with chronic stable angina experience a modest but significant improvement in left ventricular ejection fraction and left ventricular wall motion, provided that volume loading is limited.[55] In patients with unstable angina that is refractory to treatment with nitrates, β blockers, and Ca^{2+} antagonists, thoracic epidural analgesia alleviates chest pain without changing coronary perfusion pressure, cardiac output, or systemic vascular resistance.[56] Studies evaluating regional myocardial blood flow distribution in intact animals indicate that epidurally administered local anesthetics can improve endocardial-to-epicardial blood flow ratios, shifting blood flow to the area of myocardium at greatest risk of ischemia and infarction.[57] A reduction in infarct size in experimental models of acute coronary occlusion has also been demostrated.[57]

Administration of epidural local anesthetics or opioids in the postoperative period can reduce the incidence of myocardial ischemia and dysrhythmias compared with systemic opioids.[58,59] Beneficial effects of epidural anesthesia and analgesia on cardiac outcomes have been demonstrated only in high-risk populations undergoing major operations, perhaps because such patients experience a high incidence of complications, allowing differences to be detected in relatively small samples. Epidural anesthesia and analgesia was associated with both statistically and clinically significant reductions in serious cardiovascular morbidity compared with general anesthesia with on-demand opioid analgesia alone in a population of patients undergoing major intrathoracic, intra-abdominal, or vascular surgery,[60] as well as in a series of patients undergoing major peripheral vascular surgery (approximately 45% of operations involving the abdominal aorta).[45] Another study in abdominal aortic reconstructive surgery comparing general anesthesia with combined epidural anesthesia and general anesthesia found no differences in cardiovascular or other outcomes, although postoperative analgesia techniques were not controlled or randomized.[61] In aggregate, these findings are consistent with the hypothesis that outcome improvement requires that intraoperative initiation of central neuraxial blockade be accompanied by postoperative continuation of this modality. Other studies investigating lower-risk patient populations[62] or less invasive surgical procedures (infrainguinal revascularizations)[63] with a lesser magnitude of surgical insult had lower incidences of cardiac morbidity and could not demonstrate significant effects on cardiac morbidity despite other beneficial effects of epidural anesthesia and analgesia. Therefore, the benefits of epidural analgesia on cardiac morbidity remain controversial, and formation of definitive conclusions has been hindered by the absence of studies with sufficient numbers of patients and the multifactorial causation of cardiac morbidity, which mandates a tightly controlled study design. Most studies with negative results have not consistently continued the intraoperative epidural technique for postoperative analgesia.

The beneficial effects of epidural anesthesia and analgesia on some aspects of cardiovascular outcome may be intimately related to modulation of the hypercoagulable state that occurs and persists after major surgical trauma, especially in patients with atherosclerotic vascular disease and others with a predisposition to hypercoagulability.[64] General anesthesia with parenteral opioid analgesia has little effect on postoperative hypercoagulability.[45,46,63,65] Epidural anesthesia using local anesthetics with or without opioids enhances fibrinolytic activity,[46,66] hastens the return of antithrombin III from elevated to normal levels, and attenuates postoperative increases in platelet activity. These effects probably occur through multiple mechanisms, including block of sympathetic efferent nerves, reduced levels of circulating catecholamines and anticoagulant properties of even low levels of systemically absorbed local anesthetics. These reductions in postoperative hypercoagulability appear to reduce the incidence of thromboses of vascular grafts in patients undergoing lower extremity revascularization,[45,63] and also reduce the incidence of deep venous thromboses and risk of pulmonary thromboembolism in patients undergoing total hip replacements. The reduced incidence of thrombotic phenomena in these settings may be related to an inhibitory effect on platelet aggregation as well as to improvements in lower limb blood flow.[67] Similar reductions in thromboembolic complications have been reported with the use of epidural anesthesia and analgesia (with local anesthetics) after other procedures, including knee arthroplasty[68] and open prostatectomy.[69] The differences in coagulability associated with epidural anesthesia and analgesia have been observed only in patients inherently at high risk for vaso-occlusive events.

Epidural analgesia is associated with improved pulmonary function after surgery compared with intramuscular (im) and iv opioid.[36,70-73] Diaphragmatic function is commonly impaired after abdominal or thoracic surgery, probably as a result of reflex inhibition of phrenic nerve activity.[74,75] Although analgesia provided by parenterally or epidurally administered opioids alone does not significantly improve this dysfunction,[76] thoracic epidural analgesia with local anesthetic may improve postoperative diaphragmatic function by neural blockade of the inhibitory reflex[74,75] as well as by changing chest wall compliance.

Although epidural and parenteral opioids are associated with similar frequencies of episodic postoperative hypoxemia,[77] epidural analgesia with local anesthetics reduces the frequency and severity of early postoperative hypoxemia. It is likely that reductions in the work of breathing and other beneficial effects of improved analgesia such as enhanced ability to cough and facilitation of chest physiotherapy also play an important role in preventing postoperative respiratory complications. The former effects may be related to improved analgesia during activity, particularly when epidural local anesthetics and opioid are combined.[78]

Several studies have demonstrated reductions in the incidence of postoperative pneumonia and respiratory failure in high-risk patients undergoing thoracic or abdominal operations.[36,45] Similar differences in pulmonary morbidity between parenteral postoperative opioids and epidural analgesia have not been observed in healthy patients undergoing low-risk operations or when postoperative analgesia was not managed using well defined protocols.[55,79-81]

In summary, epidural anesthesia and analgesia can reduce the frequency and severity of postsurgical stress–induced physiologic perturbations. The effect of epidural anesthesia and postoperative analgesia on mediators of the stress response appears to have the greatest impact on perioperative outcome in patients at high risk of complications. The relative importance of preemptive intraoperative initiation compared with postoperative application of epidural local anesthetics (versus opioid alone or in combination), as well as the cost effectiveness of these analgesic techniques compared with other modalities for management of postoperative pain, depends on the patient's preoperative status and the specific operative procedure.

PHARMACOLOGY OF POSTOPERATIVE PAIN MANAGEMENT

Drugs administered orally for postoperative pain management can be grouped by their mechanism of effect as nonopioid or opioid analgesics.

Nonopioid Analgesics

Mechanisms of Analgesic Effects

Aspirin, acetaminophen, the NSAIDs, and the selective COX-2 inhibitors are the principal nonopioid analgesics used to treat minor or moderate acute postoperative pain (Table 54-3). Although these compounds represent diverse chemical entities, their common mechanism of action is inhibition of prostaglandin-mediated amplification of chemical and mechanical irritants on the sensory pathways. Although sensitization or intensification of painful stimuli is mediated by the prostaglandins and lowers the threshold for further activation of the nociceptors, the prostaglandins directly evoke little painful response.

Most of these agents modulate prostaglandin synthesis through inhibition of the action of the enzyme prostaglandin endoperoxide synthase (COX), which is one of the first steps in the conversion of arachidonic acid into prostaglandins, thromboxanes, and prostacyclin. By reducing prostaglandin synthesis, COX inhibitors block the nociceptive response to endogenous mediators of inflammation such as bradykinin, acetylcho-

Table 54-3. PHARMACOKINETIC PARAMETERS/MAXIMUM DOSAGE RECOMMENDATIONS OF NON-NARCOTIC ANALGESICS

	Route	Time to Peak Levels (h)	Half-Life (h)	Analgesic Actions (h) Onset	Analgesic Actions (h) Duration	Maximum Recommended Daily Dose (mg)
SALICYLATES						
Aspirin/sodium salicylate	po	0.5–2	2–3*	0.5–1	2–4	3600
Diflunisal	po	2–3	8–12	1–2	8–12	2000
PROPIONIC ACIDS						
Fenoprofen	po	1–2	2–3	1	4–6	3200
Fluriboprofen	po	1.5	5.7	—		300
Ibuprofen	po	1–2	1.8–2.5	0.5	4–6	3200
Ketoprofen	po	0.5–2	2.4	—	4–6	300
Naproxen	po	2–4	12–15	1	4–7	1500
Naproxen sodium	po	1–2	12–13	1	4–7	1375
ACETIC ACIDS						
Etodolac	po	1–2	7.3	0.5	4–12	200
Indomethacin	po	1–2	4.5	0.5	4–6	200
Indomethacin	po	2–4	4.5–6	0.5	4–6	150
Ketorolac	im	1	2.4–6†	0.5–1	4–6	120‡
	po		5–9§			40‖
Nabumetone	po	2.4–4	22.5–30#	1	4–12	2000
Sulindac	po	2–4	7.8 (16.4)#	—	—	400
Tolmecin	po	0.5–1	1–1.5	—	—	2000
FENAMATES (ANTHRANILIC ACIDS)						
Meclofenamate	po	0.5–1	2 (3.3)¶	0.5–1	4–6	400
Mefanamic Acid	po	2.4	2–4	1	4–6	1000
OXICAMS						
Piroxicam	po	3–5	30–86	1	48–72	20
PHENYLACETIC ACIDS						
Diclofenac sodium	po	2–3	2	1	4–6	200
p-AMINOPHENOLS						
Acetaminophen	po	0.5–1	1–4	0.5	2–4	4000
SELECTIVE CYCLO-OXYGENASE-2 INHIBITORS						
Celecoxib	po	2–3	11–13	1	8–12	400**
Rofecoxib	po	2–3	17	0.45–1	12–24	50

Po = oral; im = intramuscular.
* Half-life of aspirin is dose–dependent.
† Half-life in healthy adults.
‡ Daily recommended dose for first day of therapy 150 mg.
§ Half-life in renal failure.
‖ Daily recommended dose for oral dosing.
Half-life of active metabolite.
¶ Half-life with multiple dosing.
** Daily recommended doses for pain not defined.

line, and serotonin. Although the exact mechanism for the participation of endogenous substances such as prostaglandins in the generation and transduction of nociceptive stimuli is unknown, the effect is greatest in tissues that have been subjected to trauma and inflammation.[82] The prostaglandins represent a diverse group of compounds that mediate many cellular and subcellular functions. The order of the sensitizing or hyperalgesic effect that is usually observed with this group is $PGE_1 > PGE_2 > PGF_{2a}$, whereas PGA_1, PGB_2, and PGI_2 exhibit little sensitizing effect.

Although mediation of the peripheral inflammatory response is an important component of pain modulation by this group of drugs, inhibition of central mechanisms of hyperalgesia is

likely.[83,84] Acetaminophen and ketorolac are COX inhibitors that are equipotent to aspirin in inhibiting prostaglandin synthesis in the central nervous system but much less potent in inhibiting prostaglandin synthesis at peripheral sites. The site of activity of these agents may be a result of pharmacokinetic factors such as drug distribution, but more likely it reflects differences in these enzyme systems throughout the body. Studies in mammalian cells indicate that COX exists as two unique isoenzymes, COX-1 and COX-2.[85] Major differences between these isoenzymes involve dissimilar regulation and expression, with COX-1 found in most tissues, especially platelets, vascular endothelial cells, and collecting tubules. Unlike COX-1, under basal conditions COX-2 usually is undetectable in most tissues except the brain and renal cortex.[86] The COX-1 isoform primarily produces prostaglandins that regulate renal, gastric, and vascular homeostasis. In the presence of inflammation or tissue injury, inflammatory cytokines induce the expression of the COX-2 enzyme, which generates the prostaglandins involved in pain. Both isoforms of the enzyme are membrane associated and have a long, narrow tunnel into which arachidonic acid is drawn for conversion to a prostaglandin. NSAIDs block the tunnel at approximately its midpoint. Although the enzymes are not selective for substrate, a valine amino acid substitution (for isoleucine) in the COX-2 isoform allows for the synthesis of isoform-specific inhibitors. The smaller valine amino acid exposes an area in the tunnel into which larger side-chain substitutions of the enzyme inhibitor can fit. Because of these bulkier side groups, these same drugs have much less COX-1 activity, resulting in analgesic/anti-inflammatory properties with diminished effects on platelet, gastric mucosal, and renal functions.[87]

Because not all NSAIDs block COX to the same degree, membrane stabilization has also been attributed to these drugs.[88] Membrane stabilization may account for decreased prostaglandin release seen at drug concentrations that are lower than those needed for effective COX inhibition. This theory is supported by the correlation of analgesic potency with the octanol/water partition coefficient in this group.[88] Corticosteroids, which are membrane stabilizers, are known selectively to inhibit the expression of COX-2 during inflammation. NSAIDs, tricyclic antidepressants, and local anesthetics may also function through this mechanism of action, which explains some of their beneficial effects when they are used for acute pain management.

Absorption/Biotransformation/Elimination

After oral administration, nonopioid analgesics are rapidly and completely absorbed. Food usually delays absorption but does not affect absolute bioavailability. Intramuscular absorption of ketorolac is complete and occurs within 50 minutes of administration.[89] With the exception of acetaminophen, protein binding for this group exceeds 80%. Displacement of other highly protein-bound drugs, such as warfarin, may occur when these agents are administered concurrently. Biotransformation by liver enzyme systems and renal excretion of conjugated metabolites are the primary modes of elimination of these agents. Caution must be exercised in patients with renal and liver dysfunction.

Adverse Effects

Gastrointestinal discomfort and central nervous system disturbances are the most common adverse effects of short-term therapy with nonopioid analgesics. Nausea, vomiting, dyspepsia, heartburn, and epigastric discomfort occur in 5–25% of patients receiving aspirin and in 3–9% of patients receiving other NSAIDs. Selective COX-2 inhibitors have a similar incidence of prototypical NSAID gastrointestinal side effects; however, the incidence of endoscopically confirmed gastrointestinal ulceration is reduced with these drugs. Dizziness, headache, and drowsiness occur in approximately 1–9% of patients receiving NSAIDs. Prolonged bleeding is a result of the action of these drugs on COX-1 in platelets. This effect is usually reversible with the NSAIDs 24–48 hours after discontinuing therapy. It is more prolonged after discontinuation of aspirin because of the irreversible acetylation of the platelet surface. Although this effect of aspirin persists for the life of the platelet, clinical prolongation of bleeding time is thought to be reversed in approximately 1 week. More severe adverse effects include an exacerbation of bronchospasm and rhinitis induced by aspirin or other NSAIDs in patients with a history of nasal polyps, asthma, and rhinitis. Ulceration and bleeding of the gastrointestinal mucosa can occur because of direct irritation by the drug. This effect, coupled with the inhibition of prostaglandin-mediated bicarbonate and mucus secretion, allows for further erosion of the tissue. Patients with diabetes or gastric or peptic ulcers are at higher risk for gastrointestinal bleeding, ulceration, and even perforation. Misoprostol, a synthetic PGE_2, can be used to increase bicarbonate and mucus production in high-risk patients. An acute renal insufficiency syndrome—hyperkalemia and peripheral edema—can be precipitated in elderly patients, those with congestive heart failure or renal or hepatic dysfunction, or patients on diuretic therapy. This is a result of the blockade of prostaglandin-mediated effects on renal blood flow. Proteinuria, interstitial nephritis, and papillary necrosis have been reported, but the mechanism of their association with prostaglandin inhibition is less clear. Despite its usefulness as an injectable NSAID, ketorolac should be restricted to short-term postoperative administration to limit the risk of renal dysfunction. In general, acetaminophen is free of adverse effects in dosages used for acute pain management.

Clinical Uses

Unlike the opioid analgesics, the mechanisms of analgesia with the nonopioid analgesics are not specifically involved in interrupting the transmission of the nociceptive stimulus. The effectiveness of these agents depends on the central and peripheral inflammatory responses to tissue injury, although they have little or no inhibitory effect on classic catabolic stress hormones, acute-phase protein, and other immunologic responses.[52] The reduction in prostaglandin-mediated inflammatory response can serve to enhance the analgesic effect when these agents are combined with opioids, such as the use of acetaminophen with codeine and its congeners. Based on their pharmacologic mechanisms, it is predictable that the analgesic effect of nonopioid drugs is confined to somewhat narrow therapeutic ranges above which there is little increase in analgesia but a considerable increase in toxicity. To reduce the postoperative amplification of the nociceptive response to tissue injury, the most efficacious use of these agents is before surgery. This is because the effect of PGE_2 can last for many hours and the sensitizing effects of circulating prostaglandins are not reversed by COX inhibitors. These agents also appear to be more effective in procedures involving musculoskeletal, post-traumatic, and inflammatory pain and in conditions such as dysmenorrhea, renal colic, and biliary obstruction, in which prostaglandins are known to be involved in the pathogenesis of the pain.

Opioid Analgesics

Mechanism of Analgesic Effects

Morphine and related compounds act as agonists, producing their biologic effects by interacting with stereoselective and saturable membrane-bound receptors that are nonuniformly distributed throughout the central nervous system. The major sites of opioid activity in the central nervous system include the periaqueductal and periventricular gray, nucleus reticularis gigantocellularis, medial thalamus, mesencephalic reticular formation, lateral hypothalamus, raphe nuclei, and spinal cord. The endogenous neuromodulating peptides of the enkephalin and β-endorphin classes also bind to this family of receptors, which are collectively referred to as the *opioid receptors*. The unique properties of the individual drugs of this group are a result of their specific receptor activity and affinity. Currently, five distinct classes of opioid receptors have been identified (mu [μ], kappa [κ], delta [δ], sigma [σ]; and epsilon [ε]), as well as subtypes of the μ, κ, and σ receptors. The cellular mechanisms of these interactions have been discussed previously in this chapter. A peripheral effect of opioids that results in "local analgesia" is more pronounced in chronically inflamed tissues,[90,91] where opioid receptors that are synthesized in the dorsal root ganglia have been transported and activated on primary afferent neurons in response to inflammation.[92] The

Table 54-4. PHARMACOLOGY OF OPIOID RECEPTORS

	Mu (μ)		Delta (δ)	Kappa (κ)	Sigma (σ)
	μ$_1$	μ$_2$			
EFFECT					
Analgesia	Supraspinal	Sedation	Spinal	Spinal	
Affect	Euphoria	Sedation		Sedation	Dysphoria/hallucinations
Pupil	Miosis			Miosis	Mydriasis
Respiratory		Depression	Depression		Tachypnea
Gastrointestinal	Nausea/vomiting	Constipation	Nausea/vomiting		
Genitourinary	Urinary retention		Urinary retention	Diuresis	
Temperature	Increase				
Other	Pruritus		Pruritus		
Physical dependence/ tolerance	Yes		Yes	Little	
Cross-tolerance	δ		μ	No	

BINDING PROPERTIES	Affinity	Activity	Affinity	Activity	Affinity	Activity	Affinity	Activity
Agonists								
Morphine	+++	+++	++	++	+	+		
Meperidine	++	++	++	++	+	+		
Fentanyl	++++	++++	+	+				
Agonist–antagonists								
Pentazocine	++	0			+++	+++	+++	+++
Nalbuphine	++	0			+++	+++	++	+
Butorphanol	++	0			+++	++	++	++
Buprenorphine	+++	+			++			
Dezocine	+++	+	++	+	+	+		

Affinity: ++++ = very high; +++ = high; ++ = moderate; + = low.
Activity: 0 = no activity; + = low activity; ++ = moderate activity; +++ = high activity; ++++ = very high activity.
Adapted from Benedetti C, Butler SH: Systemic analgesics. In Bonica JJ (ed): The Management of Pain, vol II, 2nd ed, p 1640. Philadelphia, Lea & Febiger, 1990.

local analgesic effects of opioids such as morphine have been clinically useful after surgery. Application of morphine at the nerve terminal (e.g., intra-articular injections after orthopedic procedures) often produces effective, long-lasting analgesia of similar potency to conventional local anesthetics.[93–98] Peripherally acting μ-receptor agonists that do not cross the blood-brain barrier are being investigated.[99]

Affinity and activity at four of the opioid receptor classes (μ, δ, κ, and σ) are responsible for the pharmacologic effects of the opiates (Table 54-4). The enkephalins and opiates have affinity and activity at the μ$_1$ receptor, which mediates supraspinal analgesia, prolactin release, and euphoria. Opiate-selective μ$_2$ receptors appear to mediate respiratory depression and physical dependence. The δ and κ receptors are at least partially responsible for spinal analgesia. Miosis and sedation are a result of κ receptor activity, whereas σ activity can produce dysphoria and hallucinations. Pure opioid agonists (Table 54-5) have affinity and exhibit at least moderate activity at the μ$_1$, μ$_2$, δ, and κ receptors, which explains their central and spinal analgesic effect as well as their dose-related side effects and addictive potential. The differences in potency and side effects among drugs in this class are a result of receptor selectivity, affinity, and lipophilicity of the drug.

Tramadol, a synthetic 4-phenyl-piperidine analogue of codeine, is a centrally acting analgesic that possesses weak affinity for the μ opioid receptor and modifies transmission of nociceptive impulses through inhibition of monoamine (norepinephrine and serotonin) reuptake but not production. Receptor-blocking studies have demonstrated that these mechanisms work synergistically to produce the therapeutic analgesic effects of tramadol.[100–102] Intravenous and im tramadol has been found to be approximately 1/10 as potent an analgesic as morphine in treating moderate (but not severe) pain. At similar analgesic doses, tramadol has less effect on the respiratory center than morphine and has not been associated with a high abuse potential.[103]

The pharmacologic properties of the mixed agonist–antagonist analgesics are also a result of their affinity for the opioid receptors. Unlike pure agonists, however, not all of these agents produce an agonist effect when they interact with the receptor. There are two distinct groupings of the agonist–antagonist drugs based on their receptor affinity and activity. The first of these groups is characterized by high μ receptor affinity with activity less than or similar to that of morphine. Agents in this category include buprenorphine and dezocine. The second group of agonist–antagonist analgesics includes pentazocine, butorphanol, and nalbuphine. This group possesses only moderate affinity without activity at the μ receptor, high affinity with at least moderate activity at the κ receptor, and at least moderate affinity and some activity at the σ receptor, which accounts for the highly sedative effects and potential for psychomimetic reactions seen with these drugs. In addition, because of the affinity of both of these classes for the μ receptor, with activity less than that of the pure agonists, all of these drugs have the potential for reversing the effect of an agonist, including precipitation of withdrawal symptoms.

Absorption/Biotransformation/Elimination

Although opioid analgesics are well absorbed from the gastrointestinal tract, differences in analgesic equivalence between oral and parenteral doses result from significant first-pass metabolism by the liver. Codeine, oxycodone, and hydrocodone do not undergo extensive first-pass metabolism owing to the methoxy substitution of the phenolic component of the phenanthrene ring, and they have greater oral-to-parenteral equivalency than morphine. Parenteral administration results in a more rapid onset of effect compared with oral and rectal administration. Distribution depends on the lipophilicity of the drug; smaller amounts of the more hydrophobic morphine equilibrate in the brain as opposed to more lipophilic agents such as methadone, meperidine, and codeine. Biotransformation followed by renal elimination of conjugated metabolites is the primary mode of

Table 54-5. PHARMACOKINETIC PARAMETERS AND MAXIMUM DOSAGE RECOMMENDATIONS OF ORAL AND PARENTERAL OPIOID ANALGESICS

	Dosage		Half-Life (hr)	Analgesic Action (hr)			Equivalency Ratio	Comment
	Route	mg		Onset	Peak	Duration		
AGONISTS								
Naturally Occurring Alkaloids								
Morphine	iv	15–25	2–3.5		0.125			Rapid onset, peak respiratory depression 10 min
	im	10–15		0.3	0.5–1.5	3–4	1	
	po	30–60		0.5–1	1.2	4	6	Equivalency to im decreases with repeated dosing
Codeine	im	15–60	3	0.25–5	1–5	4–6	12	Intramuscular has little advantage compared with morphine
	po	15–60	2–3.5	0.25–1	1.5–2	3–4	20	Oral potency due to low first-pass effect
Partially Synthetic Derivatives of Morphine								
Hydromorphone	im	1–4	2–3	0.3–5	1	2–3	0.2	Potent analgesic, short duration limits usefulness
	po	1–4		0.5–1	1	3–4	0.6	Well absorbed from gastrointestinal tract
Oxymorphone	im	0–1.5	2–3	0.5	1	2–3	0.1	
Hydrocodone	po	5–7.5	3.3–4.5	0.25–0.5	1–2	3–8	3	Similar but more potent than codeine, preparations contain acetaminophen
Oxycodone	po	5	2–3	0.5	1–2	3–6	3	Short-acting, preparations contain acetaminophen
Synthetic Compounds								
Morphans								
Levorphanol	im	2–3	12–16	1	2	4–6	0.2	Drug accumulation precludes usefulness
	po	2–4		1.5	2	4–6	0.4	Well absorbed after oral administration
Phenylheptylamines								
Methadone	im	2.5–10	15–30	0.25	0.5–1	4–6	1	Used more widely in Europe
	po	2.5–10		0.5–1	1.5–2	4–8	1	
Propoxphene HCl	po	32–65	3–4	0.25–1	1–2	3–6	30	Weak narcotic, optical enantiomorph of methadone
Propoxphene Napsylate	po	50–100					100	Delayed absorption compared with hydrochloride salt
Phenylpiperidines								
Meperidine	im	50–100	3–4	0.12–5	1	2–4	10	Short duration of effect One-tenth as potent as morphine
	po	50–100	14–20	0.5–1	1–2	2–3	20	Active metabolite normeperidine accumulation in renal failure
MIXED AGONIST–ANTAGONISTS								
Buprenorphine	im	0.3–0.6	2–3	0.12	1	6–8	0.04	High mu affinity, may precipitate withdrawal
	iv	0.03–0.2*						Decreased onset and duration compared with im
Butorphanol	im	2–4	2.5–3.5	0.1–0.2	0.5–1	3–4	0.2	May precipitate withdrawal
Dezocine	im	5–20	2.5	0.25–0.5	0.5–1.5	2.4	1	Potency similar to morphine
	iv	5–10		0.25				
Nalbuphine	im	10–20	5	0.25	1	3–6	1	May precipitate withdrawal
	iv	1–5						Onset 2–3 min
Pentazocine	im	30–60	2–3	0.12–0.5	1–3	3–6	6	Used primarily for cancer pain
	po	50				4–7	18	

im = intramuscular; iv = intravenous; po = oral.
* Intravenous route usually used for antagonist properties.
Adapted from Intrurrsi CE, Foley KM: Narcotic analgesics in the management of pain. In Kuhar M, Pasternak G (eds): Analgesics: Neurochemical, Behavioral, and Clinical Perspectives, pp 257–258. New York, Raven Press, 1984.

elimination. Active metabolites of morphine (morphine-6-glucuronide), codeine (morphine), meperidine (normeperidine), and propoxyphene (norpropoxyphene) add to the primary pharmacologic effect as well as to the toxicity of these drugs. Metabolism of tramadol, including production of its primary metabolite O-demethyl tramadol and its conjugates, is influenced by debrisoquine polymorphism.[104] This metabolite has a greater affinity for opioid receptors than the parent drug; however, the elimination half-life of this metabolite is not significantly greater than that of tramadol itself.[105] Renal elimination of the opioids and their metabolites is primarily by glomerular filtration, with small fractions of drug and metabolites excreted in the feces.

Adverse Effects

With short-term, moderate-dose therapy, central nervous system and gastrointestinal side effects predominate. Sedation, dizziness, lightheadedness, miosis, nausea, vomiting, and constipation are extensions of the pharmacologic actions of these drugs and occur in dose-dependent fashion. Tolerance to the sedative and other central nervous system effects develops rapidly over the first few days of therapy or after an increase in dosage. Constipation is a result of decreased peristalsis of the bowel and decreased secretory actions of the stomach, biliary tract, and pancreas. Spasm of the sphincter of Oddi can increase pressure in the common bile duct and contribute to epigastric distress. This effect can persist for up to 24 hours after a single therapeutic dose of an opioid. Low doses of naloxone and vasodilating agents have been used to relieve this discomfort. Biliary colic tends to occur more often in patients after morphine administration than after meperidine administration, despite the similar rise in biliary pressure seen with both these agents. The agonist–antagonists tend to produce less of a rise in biliary pressure than pure agonists. Stool softeners and laxatives are warranted in patients with severe constipation. Urinary retention may also result from the increase in sphincter tone. Physical dependence and analgesic tolerance usually are not problems in short-term use but may occur after chronic opioid therapy. Unlike the NSAIDs, opioid analgesics do not interfere with healing processes or inhibit platelet function. Ventilatory depression, apnea, cardiac arrest, circulatory collapse, coma, and death can occur after large iv doses.

Clinical Uses

Opioids remain the primary pharmacologic therapy for moderate to severe postoperative pain. Analgesia is achieved by blunting the central response to noxious stimuli without loss of consciousness or affecting tactile, visual, or auditory sensation. Dose-limiting side effects such as nausea, vomiting, constipation, urinary retention, and ventilatory depression can be overcome by proper selection of the agent and route of administration. Sedation and euphoria may be desired in the immediate postoperative period. Analgesic potency is not necessarily an advantage because at equianalgesic doses there are parallel increases in side effects. Agonist–antagonists can be effective analgesics in the postoperative period and have a ceiling effect for ventilatory depression. Unfortunately, dose escalations with these agents may also produce a ceiling for their analgesic effects while increasing their sedative and dysphoric properties.

Therapeutic approaches using on-demand administration have been replaced with continuous or regularly scheduled dosing methods. As postoperative analgesic requirements diminish, the transition from parenteral to oral opioid analgesia usually involves replacing the opioid with an opioid-NSAID combination such as acetaminophen with codeine. Codeine, hydrocodone, and oxycodone are limited in their analgesic potency because of their high incidence of side effects at equianalgesic doses compared with morphine or meperidine, and are best used for minor to moderate pain.

METHODS OF ANALGESIA

Pain relief may involve administration of analgesic drugs by various routes or nonpharmacologic application of mechanical, electrical, or psychological techniques. In any patient, the optimal combinations of these techniques depend on the type and degree of pain, the patient's perception of the pain, and the underlying medical, social, and environmental conditions in which the pain is managed.

Routes of Analgesic Delivery

Oral

Oral analgesics are usually considered less than optimal for moderate to severe acute postoperative pain management because of their lack of titratability and prolonged time to peak effect, and because they require a functional gastrointestinal system. In general, hospitalized patients receive systemically administered opioids and then are converted to oral analgesics when the need for rapid adjustments in the level of analgesia has diminished. However, with the focus on more rapid hospital discharge, early use of longer-acting, potent oral opioids facilitates transition of patients from parenteral opioids to oral therapy. Both nonopioid and opioid analgesic agents are available for oral administration, alone or in combination.

Transepithelial

With the increased number and complexity of surgical procedures being performed in the outpatient setting, there is a growing need for efficacious analgesic regimens for moderate to severe acute postoperative pain in this subset of patients. Methods of drug delivery such as transdermal[106] or transmucosal[107] administration have been evaluated as alternatives to oral analgesics. These techniques permit delivery of potent analgesics that would be less effective when administered orally because of significant first-pass metabolism. Pharmacokinetic characteristics, primarily in absorption, confer important clinical differences to these routes of administration. For example, to achieve optimal analgesic efficacy, transdermal fentanyl must be applied several hours before emergence from anesthesia, whereas transmucosal fentanyl is more rapidly absorbed. As with the oral route, titratability can be problematic and there may be unpredictability of drug absorption. Although transdermal fentanyl combined with patient-controlled analgesia (PCA) using morphine can reduce the number of demand doses, total opioid requirements as well as side effects are not decreased.[108]

Parenteral

Parenteral administration of opioid analgesics remains the primary pharmacologic route for the treatment of moderate to severe postoperative pain. The use of computerized, patient-controlled delivery systems has played an important role in refining this method of delivery and reducing side effects of parenterally administered drugs.

Intramuscular. Intramuscular administration of postoperative analgesics produces a more rapid onset and time to peak effect than oral administration. It is also simple to administer analgesics by this route because no special infusion device is needed. However, pain at the injection site, patient apprehensiveness of needle sticks, the potential for delayed ventilatory depression, and wide variability in drug serum concentrations limit the viability of this route. Absorption from im sites depends on the lipophilicity of the agent and blood flow in the area of the injection. After im injections of morphine or meperidine, plasma concentrations may vary as much as 3-fold to 5-fold, and time to peak concentration may vary from 4 to 108 minutes among patients.[109] On the other hand, there is much less variability in the minimum analgesic plasma concentration for any patient.[110] Small changes in plasma concentrations (10–20%)

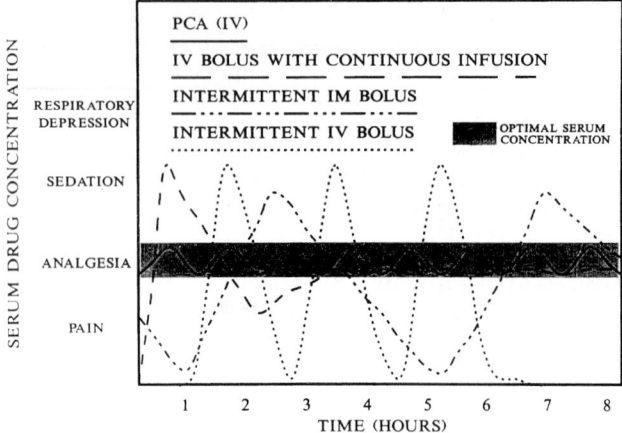

Figure 54-6. Relationship between serum drug concentration, pharmacologic effect, and method of administration. (Reprinted with permission from Tuman KJ, McCarthy RJ, Ivankovich AD: Pain control in the postoperative cardiac surgery patient. Hospital Formulary 23:580, 1988.)

for a patient may represent a spectrum of effects from inadequate analgesia to complete pain relief.[111]

The relationship between plasma concentrations, effect, and time is depicted in Figure 54-6. Plasma concentrations after im administration of high doses of an opioid analgesic such as morphine at long dosing intervals establish a cyclic pattern of sedation, analgesia, and finally inadequate analgesia. When morphine is administered by this route on a 3- or 4-hour basis, plasma concentrations exceed or meet analgesic requirements for only approximately 35% of the dosing interval because of the delayed absorption and narrow therapeutic window. This situation is exacerbated by the dynamic nature of analgesic requirements. PCA and continuous epidural infusions circumvent many of the problems of im administration and may provide more effective analgesia with fewer side effects by maintaining tighter control of plasma levels.

Most opioids can be administered by the im route; however, only one NSAID, ketorolac, is available for parenteral injection to manage postoperative pain. Ketorolac has efficacy equal to that of moderate doses of opioids for treatment of moderate to severe pain after general, gynecologic, or orthopedic surgeries.

Intravenous.   Intermittent iv bolus infusions of opioids can be administered in situations when close continuous monitoring of the patient is feasible. With a small iv bolus, the delay until analgesic effect and the variability in plasma concentrations seen with im administration can be reduced. Rapid redistribution of the drug shortens the duration of effect after a single iv administration compared with im injections. The numerous personnel needed to supervise frequent administration of boluses and monitoring of the fluctuations seen in plasma concentrations has led to the use of continuous iv infusions.

Continuous iv infusions offer the advantages of maintaining nearly constant plasma drug concentrations and reducing the peak-and-valley effect inherent in intermittent injections. Without the use of an initial bolus loading injection, continuous infusion techniques are inadequate because of the long time required for the drug to reach steady state (four to five half-lives). Initiating therapy with a loading dose eliminates this problem but still does not allow for rapid dosage adjustments as analgesic requirements change.

Patient-Controlled Analgesia.   By combining the advantages of a continuous infusion with the flexibility of interposing low bolus doses as analgesic requirements vary, PCA appears to be the answer for many patients' analgesic needs. This method has evolved as advances in computer technology have met the needs for improved drug delivery. Early PCA devices permitted

a patient to titrate analgesic needs by delivering a small bolus dose of an opioid such as morphine sulfate when he or she activated a switch. Limits could be placed on the number of activations per unit time the patient was allowed and the minimum time that would have to elapse between activations (lockout interval). Refinements of this system permit administration of a continuous background infusion superimposed on patient-controlled boluses. Background infusion concomitant with intermittent PCA boluses is advantageous in maintaining serum drug levels within the analgesic range and further attenuates fluctuations in levels, resulting in improved analgesia and patient satisfaction without producing additional unwanted side effects.[112] In addition to combining infusion and bolus dosing, current devices record a profile of the drug administration, including number and time of bolus delivery, number of activations that did not result in drug delivery, and total amounts of the agent that were administered per unit time.

Compared with traditional methods of on-demand analgesic delivery, PCA has been shown to provide superior analgesia, with less total drug use, less sedation, fewer nocturnal sleep disturbances, and a more rapid return to physical activity.[113] Most patients tend to titrate PCA to a level of pain at which they feel comfortable and taper their dosage requirements as they convalesce.[114] In addition, patient acceptance of PCA is high because patients feel that they have significant control over their therapy.[115]

One limitation to PCA therapy is the selection of agents available for use in the PCA devices (Table 54-6). Ideally, a drug administered by PCA should be highly efficacious, have a rapid onset of action and a moderate duration of effect, should not accumulate or change pharmacokinetic properties with repeated administration, and should have a large therapeutic window. Morphine and meperidine, the drugs most widely prescribed by this route, are far from ideal, and limitations imposed by the pharmacology of the agonist–antagonist group have made their use in these devices disappointing. Despite theoretic advantages, the use of fentanyl for PCA has not been shown to be clearly superior to morphine,[116] although it may improve the initial PCA demand-to-delivery ratio.[117]

Other problems encountered with PCA therapy are primarily a result of operator or mechanical errors.[118] Because patients titrate their own therapy, they must be capable of understanding the concepts of the device, be able to activate the trigger, and be willing to participate. This often makes the use of PCA devices more difficult in pediatric and in older and debilitated patients.

Optimum results from PCA therapy are obtained only when the patient's analgesic needs can be met within the prescribed parameters set on the device. The patient's age, surgical procedure, need for a continuous background infusion, number and amount of boluses allowed, and total analgesic requirements are considered. Anesthesiologists must incorporate some flexibility into protocols for ordering PCA therapy to account for the variability introduced by these factors.

Central Neuraxial Analgesia

The technique of spinal analgesia was described by Bier and Tuffler in 1898, and that of sacral epidural analgesia by Sicard and Cathelin in 1901. In 1949, a major advance in the application of central neuraxial analgesia was the description by Cleland[119] of the use of a continuous catheter epidural infusion for postoperative analgesia. Analgesia was maintained for 1–5 days after surgery by administering intermittent bolus doses of a local anesthetic. Although effective analgesia was obtained, a significant sympathetic block accompanied the analgesia, and all patients required at least one dose of a vasopressor. Additional shortcomings of this technique, as with any intermittent dosing regimen, were the fluctuating levels of analgesia that occur as the effect of the bolus dissipates, and the medical staff required to reinject the patient every several hours.

Because of the shortcomings of intermittent dosing, the con-

Table 54-6. GUIDELINES REGARDING THE BOLUS DOSAGES, LOCKOUT INTERVALS, AND CONTINUOUS INFUSIONS FOR VARIOUS PARENTERAL ANALGESICS WHEN USING A PATIENT-CONTROLLED ANALGESIA SYSTEM

Drug	Loading Dose (mg)	Intermittent Bolus Dose (mg)	Lockout Interval (min)	Continuous Infusion (mg · h⁻¹)	4-Hour Limit (mg)
AGONISTS					
Fentanyl citrate	0.025–0.075	0.015–0.05	3–10	0.02–0.1	0.2–0.4
Hydromorphone hydrochloride	0.25–0.5	0.10–0.5	5–10	0.2–0.5	
Meperidine hydrochloride	50–100	5–30	10–20	5–40	200–300
Methadone hydrochloride		0.5–3	10–20		
Morphine sulfate*	5–10	0.5–3	5–12	1–10	20–30
Sufentanil citrate	0.002–0.005	0.002–0.01	2–10		
AGONISTS–ANTAGONISTS					
Nalbuphine hydrochloride	2–5	1–5	5–15	1–8	20–30

* For pediatric dosing, see text.

tinuous infusion of local anesthetics along the central neuraxis was subsequently recommended as an alternative to the intermittent bolus technique. The continuous infusion of local anesthetics simplifies maintenance of analgesia, but the use of local anesthetics in concentrations sufficient to produce pain relief usually results in sensory and occasional motor blockade. These are unwanted effects in the postoperative period because sensory and motor blockade prohibit ambulation, an important factor in postoperative convalescence.

Although it has long been recognized that application of local anesthetic agents along the spinal canal could provide effective analgesia, the demonstration that opioids could produce analgesia by this route has been responsible for the widespread application of the practice of central neuraxial analgesia. The enthusiasm for this route of administration has also been a direct result of the shortcomings of im and iv therapies. By interrupting pain pathways at the level of communication between the first- and second-order neurons, a method for providing effective analgesia without the associated central nervous system depression and cyclical nature of pain associated with other parenteral routes of administration is achieved.

Intrathecal. The intrathecal administration of opioids has the advantage of providing long-lasting analgesia after a single injection. The onset of analgesic effect after the intrathecal administration of an opioid is directly proportional to the lipid solubility of the agent, whereas the duration of the effect is longer with more hydrophilic compounds. Morphine, for example, has been shown to produce peak analgesic effects in 20–60 minutes that last for 2–12 hours when doses ranging from 0.25 to 4 mg were administered intrathecally to adults.[120,121] In routine clinical practice, 0.25–1 mg morphine can be expected to provide effective analgesia, whereas doses in the range of 0.25–0.5 mg generally maintain analgesic efficacy while minimizing the potential for ventilatory depression.[120]

Intrathecal bolus injections share many of the problems of other intermittent techniques, including lack of titratability and extensive time requirements for monitoring and reinjection. In addition, the potential for infection, a greater risk of ventilatory depression owing to rostral spread of the drug, and a higher incidence of side effects make this technique less desirable than epidural administration (Table 54-7). Widespread clinical experience has shown that continuous epidural infusions may be preferable to intrathecal techniques for central neuraxial analgesia. The practical aspects of maintaining a catheter in the intrathecal space for a prolonged period and reports of cauda equina syndrome after continuous spinal anesthesia also may favor the continuous epidural technique.[122] Although intrathecal analgesic techniques are infrequently used outside the setting of labor analgesia, the use of a combined spinal anesthesia followed by continuous epidural analgesia has gained

increasing popularity because it provides the advantages of spinal anesthesia (rapid onset, dense neural blockade) while facilitating the transition to an effective and titratable postoperative analgesia method after major surgery.[123]

Epidural. Epidural administration of opioids and local anesthetics has evolved in parallel with intrathecal techniques. As noted, the advantages of epidural administration of drugs such as opioids and local anesthetics include the reduced incidence of side effects and a diminished propensity for opioid-induced ventilatory depression compared with the intrathecal route. When a drug is placed in the epidural space, it must first cross the dura before it can reach the spinal cord. Besides the physical barrier presented by the dura, the epidural space is highly vascularized, and a significant redistribution of drug to the systemic circulation occurs. The epidural space also contains fat, connective tissues, a lymphatic network, and the dorsal and ventral roots of the spinal nerves, all of which can serve as a repository for lipophilic agents.[124]

The influence of these factors can be demonstrated by an examination of the pharmacokinetics of epidurally administered hydrophilic (morphine) and lipophilic (fentanyl) opioids. Ten milligrams of morphine, given either iv or epidurally, produce peak serum levels and decay curves that are nearly identical (Fig. 54-7). Whereas the duration of pain relief from iv administration is short-lived (1–2 hours), epidural morphine can provide 12 or more hours of analgesia. This indicates that although

Table 54-7. COMPLICATIONS OF NEURAXIAL OPIOIDS

Complication	Reported Incidence (%)*		Treatment
	Spinal	*Epidural*	
Respiratory depression	5–7	0.1–2	Support ventilation; naloxone
Pruritus	60	1–100	Antihistamine; naloxone
Nausea and vomiting	20–30	20–30	Antiemetic; transdermal scopolamine; naloxone
Urinary retention	50	15–25	Catheterize; naloxone

* Reported incidences vary widely, appear to be related to dose, and are higher with spinal than with epidural administration.

Reprinted with permission from Ready LB: Regional analgesia with intraspinal opioids. In Bonica JJ (ed): The Management of Pain, vol II, 2nd ed, p 1976. Philadelphia, Lea & Febiger, 1990

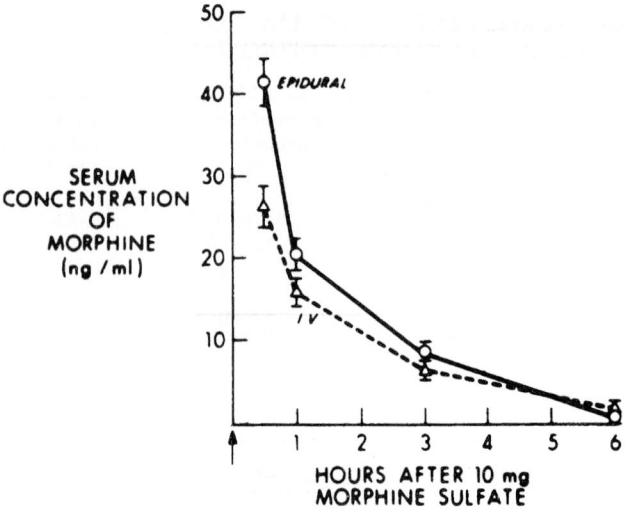

Figure 54-7. Serum concentration of morphine (mean ± SEM) after intravenous and lumbar epidural administration of 10 mg of morphine sulfate in 10 subjects; triangles = intravenous; circles = epidural. (Reprinted with permission from Bromage PR, Camporesi EM, Durant PAC, Nielsen CH: Nonrespiratory side effects of epidural morphine. Anesth Analg 61:490, 1982.)

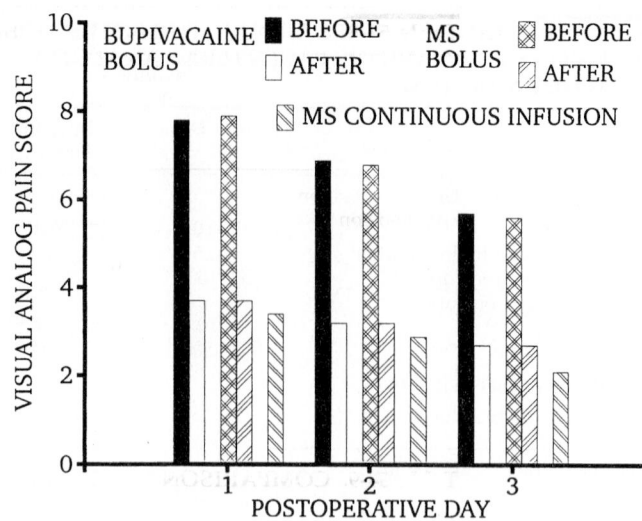

Figure 54-8. Analgesic effectiveness of continuous morphine epidural infusion compared with epidural bolus doses of morphine sulfate (MS) or bupivacaine. See text for details. (Adapted from El-Baz NI, Faber LP, Jensik RJ: Continuous epidural infusion of morphine for treatment of pain after thoracic surgery: A new technique. Anesth Analg 63:757, 1984.)

much of an epidural dose is absorbed into the systemic circulation, a small fraction of the morphine dose (~2–10%) diffuses across the dura to bind spinal opiate receptors and produce analgesia. In contrast, when epidural fentanyl 200 µg is given in a similar manner, peak serum levels are only approximately 50% of those after a similar im injection. However, serum levels of fentanyl 24 hours after a continuous rate infusion are similar to those obtained from a similar iv infusion.[125] This implies that with the initial bolus of fentanyl, there is redistribution of the drug to lipophilic tissues, which become saturated after continuous administration. Therefore, only a small fraction of a typically administered epidural dose is necessary to produce spinally mediated analgesia.

Because the diffusion of drugs across the dura is both concentration and time dependent, it is necessary to administer significantly larger amounts of drugs than those that effectively saturate spinal opiate receptors. These higher doses are more likely to produce unwanted side effects from systemic and rostral distribution of the drug, but fewer than those associated with equianalgesic intrathecal doses. When these factors are considered, the margin of therapeutic safety and the decrease in side effects with epidural administration make this route preferred for postoperative analgesia.

Intermittent epidural bolus doses of morphine sulfate (≤15 mg over 24 hours) have been used for postsurgical analgesia.[72] Although this method of administration provides excellent analgesia for up to 12 hours, side effects associated with these bolus doses limits the widespread application of this technique. An intermittent bolus technique also has the disadvantage of limiting the number of usable opioids to the longer-acting drugs (*e.g.*, morphine and hydromorphone).

In an effort to mitigate the frequency and severity of opioid-induced side effects associated with bolus techniques, El-Baz *et al*[126] described the use of a continuous epidural morphine infusion (100 µg·h⁻¹) and found equivalent analgesia and fewer side effects than after epidural boluses of either bupivacaine (0.5%) or morphine (5 mg; Fig. 54-8 and Table 54-8). It is now well accepted that continuous epidural infusions of opioids provide effective analgesia while reducing the side effects associated with bolus administration.[127–129]

Because the laws of mass action apply to diffusion of drugs out of the epidural space to their sites of action, several hours

are often required to achieve adequate analgesia when using continuous infusions alone. Effective analgesia with epidural infusions administered at a continuous rate may take as long as 3–4 hours to achieve. Delay in onset of effective analgesia can be reduced by adjusting the infusion rate to provide the equivalent of a small (5–10 ml) bolus of the epidural solution over 5–15 minutes before beginning the maintenance infusion. This allows an adequate concentration of the analgesic drug(s) to be present at their site(s) of action in a shorter time.

In addition to a reduction in adverse effects, another advantage of a continuous epidural infusion over an epidural bolus injection is the ability to titrate the amount of analgesia (Table 54-9). Although morphine usually provides 12 hours of pain relief after a single epidural injection, wide variability has been reported in the duration of effective analgesia (4–24 hours) depending on the site and extent of surgical trauma and age of the patient. Because of this variability, it becomes difficult to titrate uniform levels of analgesia. A continuous infusion provides easier analgesic titration, particularly when shorter-acting opioids such as fentanyl are used. Fentanyl has an onset of action within 4–5 minutes and a peak effect within 20 minutes.[130,131] Because of the rapid onset, it becomes much easier to adjust dosage, observe the desired effect, and titrate to an optimal intensity of analgesia. Morphine, on the other hand, has an onset time of 30 minutes with a time to peak effect ranging from 60 to 90 minutes.

Mirroring the evolution of PCA, a refinement in delivery of analgesics by the epidural route is the use of superimposed patient-controlled bolus doses with a continuous basal infusion. Early application of this technique for delivery of epidural analgesia used relatively large intermittent demand doses alone or combined with a low-rate continuous infusion, and the intermittent demand doses provided the preponderance of analgesia. This dosing paradigm has reduced efficacy because of fluctuations in analgesia occurring as a consequence of large intermittent bolus dosing. Using higher basal infusion rates and smaller patient-activated bolus doses, the continuous infusion maintains a more constant intensity of analgesia, whereas the bolus doses provide supplemental analgesia for transient increases in analgesic requirements[132] (Table 54-10). Patient-controlled epidural analgesia is particularly useful to manage dynamic changes in pain related to patient activity (*e.g.*, coughing, chest physiother-

Table 54-8. SIDE EFFECTS WITH POSTOPERATIVE EPIDURAL ANALGESIA

Side Effect	Group A (Bupivacaine 25 mg · 5 ml⁻¹, 0.5% Epidural Bolus)	Group B (Morphine 5 mg Epidural Bolus)	Group C (Morphine 100 μg · h⁻¹ Epidural Infusion)
Urinary retention	30 (100%)	30 (100%)	2 (7%)
Hypotension	7 (23%)	0	0
Weakness of hands	12 (40%)	0	0
Pruritus	0	12 (40%)	1 (3%)
Depressed consciousness	0	8 (27%)	0

Adapted from El-Baz MI, Faber LP, Jensik RJ: Continuous epidural infusion of morphine for treatment of pain after thoracic surgery: A new technique. Anesth Analg 63:757, 1984.

Table 54-9. COMPARISON OF EPIDURAL ADMINISTRATION TECHNIQUES

Advantages	Disadvantages
CONTINUOUS EPIDURAL INFUSIONS	
1. Less rostral spread so side effects are minimized	1. Need for sophisticated infusion device
2. Provides continuous analgesia avoiding the peaks and nadir seen with intermittent bolus	
3. Allows for concomitant use of dilute local anesthetic solutions	
4. Allows the use of shorter-acting opiates such as fentanyl or sufentanil	
5. Less potential risk of contamination for injection because the catheter system has fewer breaks in sterile technique	
6. Simple and easy maintenance; removes the need for anesthesia personnel to inject patients periodically	
INTERMITTENT EPIDURAL BOLUS	
1. Simple (providing resident or nursing staff accepts the responsibility of epidural catheter injections)	1. Limited number of suitable opioids
2. No need for infusion devices	2. Higher incidence of side effects
	3. Extra effort to inject catheter every 8–12 hr
	4. Excludes the use of local anesthetics
	5. More difficult to titrate dose

Table 54-10. EPIDURAL OPIOIDS: LATENCY AND DURATION OF POSTOPERATIVE ANALGESIA

Agent	Bolus Dose	Analgesic Effect Onset (min)	Analgesic Effect Peak (min)	Duration (hr)	Continuous Infusion Rate Range (ml · hr⁻¹)	Continuous Infusion Rate Base (ml · hr⁻¹)	Patient Assisted Bolus	Interval (min)
Meperidine	30–100 mg	5–10	12–30	4–6				
Meperidine 0.1–0.25% + bupivacaine 0.1%					2–10	5	1	12
Morphine	5 mg	23.5 ± 6	30–60	12–24				
Morphine 0.01%						1–6		
Morphine 0.01–0.1% + bupivacaine 0.1%					3–6	3	1	20
Methadone	5 mg	12.5 ± 2	17 ± 3	7.2 ± 4.6				
Hydromorphone	1 mg	13 ± 4	23 ± 8	11.4 ± 5.5				
Hydromorphone 0.05%					1–8			
Fentanyl	100 μg	4–10	20	2.6 ± 5.7				
Fentanyl 0.001%					4–12			
Fentanyl 0.001% + bupivacaine 0.1%					4–10	5	1	12
Diamorphine	5 mg	5	9–15	12.4 ± 6.5				
Sufentanil	10–60 μg	7.3 ± 5.6	26.5 ± 8.1	3.9–6.9				
Sufentanil 0.0001%					5–10			
Alfentanil	15 μg · kg⁻¹	15		1–2				

Adapted from Cousins MJ, Mather LE: Intrathecal and epidural administration of opioids. Anesthesiology 61:276, 1984.

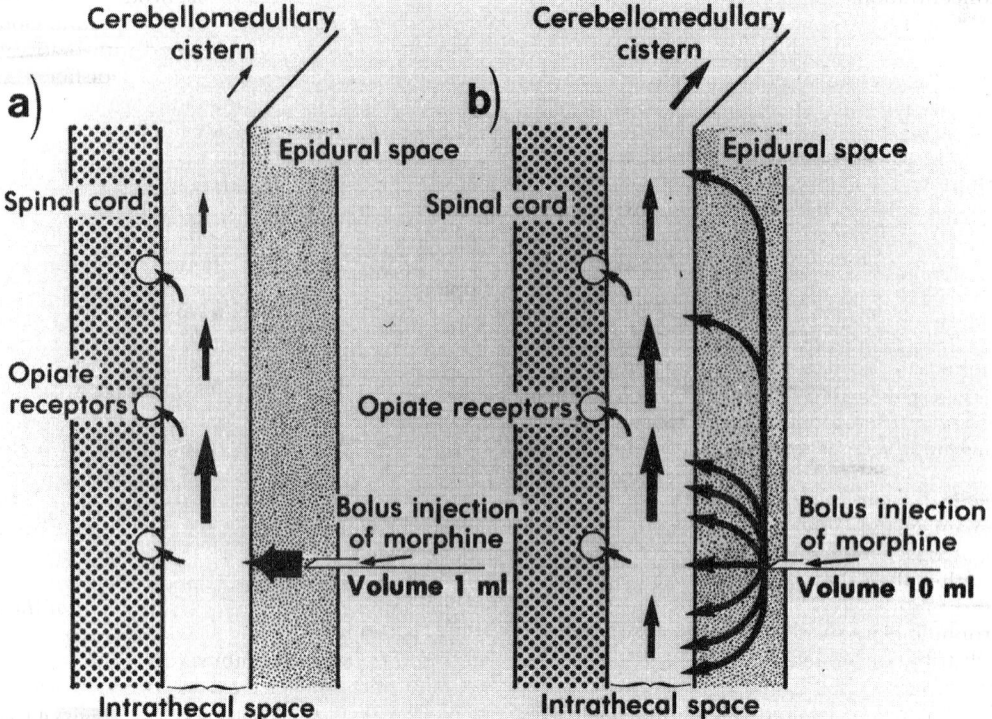

Figure 54-9. Rostral spread of central neuraxial morphine. (*a*) Spread in small injection volumes of 1 ml after dura penetration into the intrathecal space. (*b*) Spread in high injection volumes of 10 ml in the intrathecal and epidural space. (Reprinted with permission from Chrubasik J: Investigations on respiratory repression. In Chrubasik J [ed]: Spinal Infusions of Opiates and Somatostatin, p 19. Obersul, Germany, Verlag Hygeineplan, 1985.)

apy).[133] The development of new infusion devices has allowed such combined modes of administration of epidural analgesia to be readily delivered (see Appendix 54-1).

INITIATION AND MAINTENANCE OF THERAPY   Based on the preceding considerations, achievement of optimal results with a continuous epidural analgesia technique requires appropriate perioperative planning and assessment. This strategy includes identifying patients who may benefit from epidural analgesia and scheduling the epidural catheter placement as part of the anesthetic plan. At the authors' institution, epidural catheters are commonly placed while the patient is in the holding area before being taken to the operating room. This practice allows the anesthesiologist to administer a test dose of local anesthetic while the patient is still awake. The application of bolus administration followed by a continuous infusion mandates that the test dose be administered to an awake patient. This facilitates diagnosis of intrathecal, intravascular, or subdural catheter placement and allows confirmation of segmental epidural analgesia when the test dose of local anesthetic is administered. This practice also allows the continuous epidural infusion to be started during surgery. Solutions of morphine (0.1 mg · ml^{-1}) with bupivacaine (1 mg · ml^{-1}), or fentanyl (10 μg · ml^{-1}) with bupivacaine (1 mg · ml^{-1}), are most commonly used. Concentrations of opioid are reduced for patients with increased risk of serious opioid-induced side effects (see later). The infusion is begun during surgery at a rate of 4–6 ml · h^{-1}, augmenting the general anesthetic and providing sufficient time to achieve good analgesia and smooth emergence. If the surgical procedure is relatively short (1–2 hours), a 5- to 10-ml bolus of the epidural solution may be given as a rapid infusion as described earlier, to hasten the onset of analgesia. As an alternative, the patient may be given an epidural bolus of 0.5% bupivacaine combined with either fentanyl (50–100 μg) or morphine (2–5 mg). If the surgical procedure is expected to exceed 3–4 hours, bolus dosing may not be needed because sufficient time is allowed

for continuous epidural infusion alone to achieve analgesia on the patient's awakening.

PLACEMENT OF EPIDURAL CATHETER   Hydrophilic compounds such as morphine, when injected epidurally, result in cerebrospinal fluid concentrations of the drug that allow it to follow the rostral spread of the cerebrospinal fluid[134] (Fig. 54-9). Because of this property, epidural morphine may be infused at a lower lumbar level and still provide analgesia for surgical procedures performed on the upper abdomen and thorax. Lipophilic drugs such as fentanyl tend to provide more of a segmental analgesic effect.[135] This may in part be the result of the lipophilic compounds partitioning into lipid compartments in the spinal canal, such as epidural fat and the spinal cord. This segmental nature of analgesia mandates the need to place an epidural catheter in a location to cover the dermatomes included in the surgical field. A general guideline for the catheter locations in various types of surgery is as follows: thoracic surgery—upper to lower thoracic; upper abdominal and renal surgery—low thoracic to high lumbar; orthopedic procedures of the lower extremities and lower abdominal and gynecologic surgery—lumbar region. Alternatively, catheter placement should be approximately at the dermatomal level that corresponds to a point intersecting the upper one third and lower two thirds of the surgical incision. In general, placement of the epidural catheter at a level lower than that described previously necessitates increased epidural drug dosing to achieve effective analgesia, especially when lipophilic opioids are used, and this may lead to an increase in side effects.

SELECTION OF ANALGESICS   The differences among the opioids used for epidural analgesia relate to their duration of action and propensity to produce side effects. Patient factors such as advanced age, small body habitus, morbid obesity, history of sleep apnea, and general debilitation should be considered when initiating epidural analgesia because these conditions are associated with a greater propensity for respiratory complications. Reduced concentrations of opioids should be used when initiating epidural analgesia in such patients (see Appendices 54-1–54-3).

Pain relief lasts longer with hydrophilic agents such as morphine than with the more lipid-soluble hydromorphone or fentanyl (see Table 54-10). The relatively long duration of action of epidural or intrathecal morphine allows it to be used effectively as an intermittent bolus given every 12 hours, whereas because of a shorter duration of analgesia, fentanyl is better suited for continuous epidural infusions. Morphine can be used as a continuous epidural infusion and has been associated with reduced side effects compared with epidural bolus injections.[126] Hydromorphone, which has a lipid solubility between that of morphine and fentanyl, is 7–10 times as potent as morphine. Intermittent epidural bolus administration of hydromorphone provides effective analgesia for 7–12 hours with a reduced incidence of pruritus and nausea compared with morphine.[136]

Lipophilic compounds such as fentanyl and sufentanil and, to a lesser extent, hydromorphone partition into the spinal cord and lipid structures in the epidural space more than hydrophilic agents, which remain in the cerebrospinal fluid to a greater extent. Therefore, it may be preferable to use lipophilic opioids such as fentanyl rather than the more hydrophilic morphine to produce a more segmental level of analgesia. Although the tendency of hydrophilic drugs for rostral ascension facilitates the dermatomal distribution of analgesia, it also can result in a higher incidence of some side effects.[134]

Epidural coadministration of opioids with local anesthetics takes advantage of the desirable properties of each drug. The desired result of these combinations is achievement of potentiated analgesia at lower opioid doses with a concentration of a local anesthetic that does not produce significant motor blockade. This potentiation may be a result of antinociception at different sites in the spinal cord.[137] Opioids produce analgesia by binding to opiate receptors in the substantia gelatinosa, whereas local anesthetics block transmission of afferent impulses at the nerve roots and dorsal root ganglia.[138] Another advantage of the combination using reduced doses is the concomitant decrease in the incidence and severity of side effects. Despite wide acceptance, not all studies have demonstrated analgesic potentiation when bupivacaine and fentanyl have been used in combination.[139]

Receptors of the α_2 class modulate nociceptive impulses in the dorsal horn of the spinal cord as well as throughout the central nervous system. Agonists of these receptors produce antinociception with minimal ventilatory depression compared with opioids.[140] Clonidine has been the most widely used α_2 agonist for epidural analgesia, producing dose-dependent analgesia when given as a bolus.[141,142] Epidural clonidine has been associated with hypotension and with bradycardia because of inhibition of preganglionic sympathetic fibers. This is most prevalent at lower doses, whereas increased doses normalize blood pressure because of systemic vasoconstriction that overrides the central hypotensive effect. Although epidural clonidine has been used as a single agent to provide postoperative analgesia,[143] it has more frequently been used in combination with local anesthetics[144] or opioids[145,146] to potentiate analgesia and minimize side effects. Optimal ratios for combining α_2 agonists with opioid or local anesthetics are yet to be defined[147] because these drugs exhibit nonlinear synergism.[148] Other α_2 agonists that may be introduced into clinical pain management include dexmetotomidine and tizanidine.[149] Dexmetotomidine is an α_2 agonist with a very high α_2-to-α_1 selectivity (1600) compared with clonidine (ratio of 200).[150] Tizanidine, an analogue of clonidine, produces analgesia in a manner similar to clonidine but has fewer cardiovascular effects.[149,151]

MANAGEMENT OF INADEQUATE ANALGESIA Although epidural analgesia is usually effective, patients may occasionally experience inadequate pain relief. A systematic approach is necessary to evaluate and manage inadequate epidural analgesia. The initial step in this process is verification of the integrity of the catheter system, followed by a bolus (5–7 ml) of the epidural solution (typically a combination of dilute local anesthetic with opioid), with analgesic assessment after a short interval (15–30 minutes). If analgesia remains inadequate, a test dose of a local anesthetic solution, such as 2% lidocaine with 1:200,000 epinephrine, can be given further to evaluate epidural catheter location (Fig. 54-10). The test dose usually yields one of three results. If bilateral sensory block occurs in a few segmental dermatomes, epidural catheter location is confirmed. In this case, volume of the infusion was likely insufficient for adequate dermatomal coverage, resulting in inadequate analgesia, and increasing the rate of infusion may produce effective analgesia. A unilateral sensory block after administration of a test dose of local anesthetic is suggestive of the catheter tip residing laterally in or near a neuroforamen. Withdrawal of the catheter 1–2 cm is usually associated with a bilateral sensory block after a subsequent test dose. Once bilateral sensory blockade has been documented, adequate analgesia can be maintained with bolus administration of the epidural solution, followed by adjustments of the continuous epidural infusion or patient-controlled epidural infusion parameters.

Finally, a lack of sensory blockade after test dose administration indicates that the epidural catheter does not reside in the

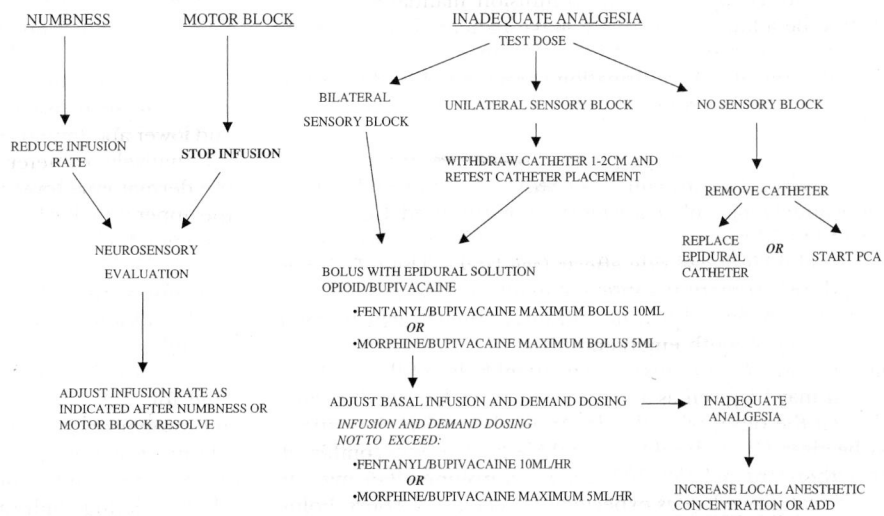

Figure 54-10. Postoperative epidural management algorithm. The test dose, given by anesthesia personnel, is two percent lidocaine with epinephrine 1:200,000 (5 ml for lumbar catheters; 3 ml for thoracic catheters).

epidural space. In this situation, the catheter is removed and the patient is given the option of having another epidural catheter placed or switching to PCA therapy.

SAFETY CONSIDERATIONS   Serious complications that can occur with a continuous epidural technique include accidental intrathecal administration of drug, infection-related problems, epidural hematoma, and ventilatory depression. To decrease the incidence of these complications, the authors propose the following guidelines:

1. A low concentration of local anesthetic (*e.g.*, 0.1% bupivacaine) in combination with an opioid analgesic allows subarachnoid catheter migration to be identified earlier by the onset of progressive sensory blockade. Low concentrations of local anesthetics do not interfere with neurologic assessments because they do not usually produce significant sensory or motor block when administered epidurally. If sensory or motor deficits are present, discontinuation of the infusion should allow for regression of these anesthetic effects within 2–4 hours. Persistent impairment of sensory or motor function should prompt appropriate evaluation to identify potentially serious causes of neurologic dysfunction, especially in anticoagulated patients (Fig. 54-10).

2. Catheter sites should be examined daily, temperature curves monitored, and the patient periodically evaluated for signs of meningism. Symptoms of epidural abscess include neurologic deficits, elevated body temperature, and back pain, although meningitis is uncommon.[152] If any findings consistent with infection are present, the catheter is removed and cultures performed. In the authors' experience of more than 23,000 cases of postoperative epidural analgesia, only a single case of epidural abscess has been encountered, and this patient was successfully treated without neurologic compromise. In a small number of patients, infections limited to the cutaneous structures have developed and resolved with conservative therapy.

3. Epidural catheters should be placed at least 1 hour before iv heparinization in patients without preoperative coagulation defects but requiring intraoperative anticoagulation with unfractionated heparin. At least one published series has shown that if epidural catheters are placed at least 1 hour before heparinization, the incidence of clinically significant epidural hemorrhage does not appear to increase.[153]

4. The risk of epidural hematoma formation related to epidural catheter placement in patients receiving certain forms of perioperative anticoagulation is controversial. Historically, concern for epidural hematoma formation with epidural catheterization has been generated primarily in the setting of intraoperative anticoagulation with unfractionated heparin. With the introduction of low–molecular-weight heparins (LMWH), increased risk of epidural hematoma formation related to epidural catheterization has been attributed to the perioperative use of such fractionated heparin compounds. Similar to unfractionated heparin, LMWH binds to antithrombin III; however, the resulting complex also diminishes thrombin generation by inhibiting factor Xa. In contrast to unfractionated heparin, the anticoagulating effects of LMWH are of longer duration and not effectively monitored with the activated clotting time or activated partial thromboplastin time.[154] Based on consensus opinion, after assessing the risks and benefits of epidural anesthesia/analgesia on an individual patient basis, it has been recommended that epidural catheterization (as well as removal of epidural catheters) be performed at least 10–12 hours after a dose of LMWH.[155] In addition, dosing of LMWH should not occur for at least 2 hours after removal of an epidural catheter to avoid manipulation during the peak anticoagulant effect.[155] Although some clinicians remove epidural catheters before postoperative initiation of LMWH, others continue postoperative epidural analgesia for longer than 24 hours in some patients. In such instances, LMWH administration may be delayed or alternative methods of thromboprophylaxis selected. The risks of spinal hematoma are incrementally increased when LMWH is used concomitantly with other drugs that affect hemostasis, including antiplatelet drugs, standard heparin, and dextran. The entire patient care team must be cognizant of this whenever postoperative epidural analgesia is used, and the postoperative analgesia service should interface with other managing clinicians to determine the optimal management of patients with these considerations. Whenever perioperative anticoagulation is used in patients managed with epidural analgesia, monitoring of anticoagulation and neurologic status is imperative.

5. With appropriate monitoring of coagulation status, epidural catheters may be inserted safely in patients who receive perioperative warfarin.[156] In patients with international normalized ratio values exceeding 1.5, neurologic checks should be continued for at least 24 hours after epidural catheter removal.[157]

6. Respiratory rates and level of sedation should be monitored every hour for the first 24 hours of the epidural infusion and every 4 hours thereafter. Apnea monitors can be used to supplement, but cannot replace, direct patient observation. Patients at increased risk for respiratory compromise include the elderly and those with sleep apnea or any debilitating disease. In the authors' institution, an apnea monitor is usually used for the first 24 hours when epidural bolus doses of morphine 2 mg or greater are given as loading doses.

In summary, a continuous infusion technique alone or in combination with patient-controlled epidural boluses simplifies maintenance of epidural analgesia and allows greater analgesic titratability than intermittent epidural bolus dosing. Proper patient selection, catheter placement, and methods to identify and treat inadequate analgesia are important aspects of postoperative pain management. Patient safety is paramount and guidelines should be established within each facility for prevention, early diagnosis, and treatment of complications.

Caudal.   Caudal nerve blocks play a minor role in acute postoperative pain management in adults. Because they are technically more difficult to perform in adults than other efficacious forms of lumbar epidural blocks, they are used less frequently in adults than in the pediatric population. Continuous caudal analgesia for postoperative pain has a limited utility because of the difficulty of securing a catheter, but it may have a role in select patients such as those who have had extensive lumbar or thoracic spine surgery. In those unusual situations where continuous caudal analgesia is used, the standard solutions for lumbar epidural analgesia may be used, although infusion rates may need to be higher than those with a lumbar epidural infusion.

Pediatric ("kiddie") caudals have become popular for intraoperative supplementation and postoperative pain relief. Palpation of the sacral hiatus is much easier in the pediatric population, and a distinct "pop" can be heard as the needle pierces the sacrococcygeal membrane. A short, 22- or 23- gauge needle should be used; the block is usually performed with the child in the lateral position. After needle insertion, needle aspiration should be performed to avoid inadvertent injection into the intrathecal or vascular space. Volumes of local anesthetic ranging from 0.75 to 1 ml·kg⁻¹ body weight of 0.25% bupivacaine should provide analgesia to the T10 level, which is sufficient for procedures in the groin and lower extremities. Although bupivacaine usually provides 4–6 hours of effective pain relief, children receiving caudal nerve blocks at the time of surgery exhibit better pain relief and use significantly fewer supplemental opioids during the first 12 postoperative hours.

As with other combined regional and general techniques, a relatively lighter plane of general anesthesia is required to maintain adequate surgical anesthesia when this block is instituted before the surgical incision, and this may represent an advantage over the use of a caudal block placed at the conclusion of the procedure. Blocks placed before surgical incisions also allow the patient to awaken more quickly and to benefit from a smoother emergence from general anesthesia.

Peripheral Nerve Blocks

General Considerations.   Peripheral application of local anesthetics to block nociceptive neural transmission can be a useful adjunct in the treatment of acute postoperative pain. Although peripheral neural blocks are simple to perform and have a hisorical record of safety, the relatively short duration of analgesia and the selective nature of these blocks preclude their general application to all patient populations. With proper selection of the patient and the local anesthetic, the pain relief afforded by regional nerve blocks may be superior to that achievable with systemic opioids.

MECHANISM OF ACTION OF LOCAL ANESTHETICS   The electrophysiology of local anesthetics is described in detail elsewhere in this textbook (see Chapter 17). Local anesthetics produce their neuronal blocking effect by diffusing across the nerve membrane and inhibiting sodium channels, thereby preventing the normal influx of sodium ions necessary for depolarization and nerve transmission. Thus, the membrane is left in its normal polarized state, and neither local miniature endplate potentials nor action potentials are generated.

Local Infiltration.   Local infiltration, the instillation of local anesthetics in the vicinity of the surgical incision, is a simple technique for providing postoperative analgesia for the first several hours after a minor surgical procedure. Needle aspiration before injection should be performed to avoid intravascular injection or perforation of deep vascular structures. Even when blood has not been aspirated before injection, it is still possible for local anesthetic to be delivered intravascularly during a local infiltration. In addition to intravascular injection, exceeding recommended total volume and dosages of local anesthetic is another factor that can be responsible for untoward reactions.

The primary advantages of the local infiltration technique are simplicity and the ability to block afferent nerve activity in the area of the incision without affecting the general sensorium. A major disadvantage is the limited duration of analgesia, which usually lasts only several hours. The most commonly used local anesthetics for this procedure are bupivacaine and ropivacaine because of their long duration of effect compared with most other local anesthetics.

A special type of local infiltration is the intra-articular injection of local anesthetics after arthroscopic procedures. This technique decreases postoperative discomfort and facilitates postsurgical recuperation.[158] Bupivacaine is the most commonly used local anesthetic, with doses of 100 mg providing effective analgesia while maintaining serum concentrations below toxic levels.[158,159]

Intercostal.   Intercostal blocks are useful for providing analgesia after operations of the thorax and upper abdomen. A 22- or 25-gauge needle is advanced at the midaxillary or postaxillary line until a rib is contacted. The needle is then walked off the inferior border and advanced 1 mm. When performing intercostal blocks for large thoracic incisions, it is important to identify the sensory dermatomes supplying the surgical incision so that each can be blocked. Dermatomes that supply the area where thoracostomy drainage tubes may be inserted should also be blocked. When abdominal incisions are large and lie in or extend across the midline, a large volume of local anesthetic is needed for optimal pain relief. Providing adequate analgesia for these types of incisions usually requires multiple bilateral intercostal blocks. In general, postoperative pain management for abdominal surgery is better conducted with continuous epidural infusion of opioids or with opioid and local anesthetic solutions. An additional problem with intercostal blocks is the potential for pneumothorax and respiratory compromise. Bupivacaine or bupivacaine with epinephrine is recommended for postsurgical pain relief with an intercostal nerve block. Intercostal blocks should be performed in the midaxillary or posterior axillary line. The site of the injection must be proximal or more posterior to the area of incision. This may occasionally present technical difficulties because the ribs tend to project more anteriorly as they approach the posterior midline. Adequate analgesia for a surgical incision usually requires application of local anesthetic to a minimum of two intercostal segments, and optimal analgesia usually requires that a minimum of three segments be blocked.

An alternative to the injection of local anesthetic on the intercostal nerve is the use of a cryoprobe, which is designed to produce local intercostal nerve freezing (cryoanalgesia).[160] This technique has been reported to produce reversible nerve disruption while preserving intraneural and peridural connective tissues. For optimal results, the cryoprobe should be applied on the intercostal nerve from within the chest by piercing the parietal pleura, and two to three levels above and below the incision should be blocked. Two to three weeks after cryoanalgesia, nerve function and structure begin to recover, with complete recovery occurring within 1–3 months. Advantages reported with this technique include a low incidence of neuritis or neuroma formation. Because of the extended period of postoperative analgesia, this technique is advantageous when prolonged effective postoperative analgesia is desirable, such as in the patient with chest trauma or significantly limited respiratory function.[161]

Ilioinguinal.   An ilioinguinal nerve block is useful for pain relief after inguinal or femoral herniorrhaphy, appendectomy, or procedures involving the scrotum. A simple technique to perform ilioinguinal nerve block involves palpation of the anterior superior iliac spine.[162] Next, a position is located two fingerbreadths medial and two fingerbreadths superior until an imaginary line drawn from the anterosuperior iliac spine to the umbilicus is reached. At this point, a 22-gauge, 8.75-cm spinal needle is advanced perpendicular to the skin. The needle is advanced slowly and bounced every several millimeters until a paresthesia is elicited. This is indicative of needle contact with the fascia immediately outside the external oblique muscle pierced by the ilioinguinal nerve on its path to more superficial structures. Once the needle is in this location, 10–15 ml of local anesthetic is injected after aspiration. The needle is then withdrawn by several centimeters and redirected laterally until the tip reaches the medial edge of the anterior superior iliac spine. An additional 10–15 ml of local anesthetic solution is them injected. Complications of ilioinguinal nerve blocks include hemorrhage and hematoma at the injection site. Occasionally, numbness in the distribution of the lateral femoral cutaneous nerve can be demonstrated. Ilioinguinal nerve blocks are useful for acute postoperative analgesia after outpatient procedures such as inguinal herniorrhaphy.

Penile.   A penile nerve block performed with 0.25% bupivacaine can provide effective analgesia after circumcision or orchiopexy. Two techniques are described for performing this block. One involves injecting half of the volume of local anesthetic at the 10 o'clock position at the base of the penis, with the remainder at the 2 o'clock position. An alternative involves placing the local anesthetic in a ring of the subcutaneous tissue 360 degrees around the base of the penis. Epinephrine-containing local anesthetic should not be used for penile blocks because of the risk of vasoconstriction and ischemic necrosis of the skin.

Brachial Plexus.   Continuous postoperative brachial plexus analgesia can be achieved using catheters placed by the infraclavicular, supraclavicular, axillary, or interscalene approach. A catheter-over-needle technique using an 18-gauge, 5-cm Teflon-coated iv catheter threaded over a 22-gauge, 8.75-cm spinal needle is one method. A nerve stimulator is essential to elicit paresthesias and identify when the neurovascular bundle is contacted. Another method for catheter placement uses the Seldinger technique. With this technique, the needle is positioned with the aid of a nerve stimulator, and after paresthesias are elicited, a guidewire is passed through the needle. Sterile alligator clips connected to the nerve stimulator can then be placed on the guidewire after the needle has been removed to confirm that the guidewire is still contacting the brachial plexus. A 20-gauge catheter is passed over the guidewire, which is then removed. For rapid sequential confirmation of correct catheter placement, the guidewire can be reinserted through the catheter at any time and a nerve stimulator used to determine if paresthesia can be elicited.

Postoperative brachial plexus analgesia has been described using bupivacaine 0.25% at rates ranging from 6 to 10 ml · h^{-1}. When infusion rates are maintained in this range, toxic serum levels are unlikely to occur. Application of this regimen does not preclude the use of any commonly used doses and volumes of local anesthetics currently recommended for surgical anesthesia with brachial plexus blockade. Patient-controlled interscalene brachial plexus analgesia has also been used in patients after shoulder surgery.[163] One disadvantage to this technique is postoperative catheter migration, and the infraclavicular and interscalene approaches may be better suited to continuous postoperative analgesia of the upper extremity because there tends to be less catheter migration than with the axillary approach.

Intrapleural. Intrapleural regional analgesia involves the percutaneous placement of a catheter in the thoracic cage between the visceral and parietal pleurae. The procedure is usually performed with the patient in the lateral decubitus position. An intercostal space between the fifth and tenth ribs is usually chosen, and a 17-gauge Touhy needle is inserted in the posterior axillary line over the superior aspect of the rib. A saline-lubricated glass syringe filled with 3–4 ml of air is attached to the needle, and the syringe and needle unit is advanced with the needle bevel directed in a cephalad direction. Once the pleural space is entered, the negative interpleural pressure draws the syringe plunger down in a manner analogous to the hanging drop technique of Gutierrez used for locating the epidural space. An epidural catheter may then be advanced 6 cm into the pleural space, rapidly to prevent the development of a clinically significant pneumothorax. If patients are mechanically ventilated, positive-pressure ventilation should be interrupted while the needle and catheter are being inserted to prevent injury to the pulmonary parenchyma. When patients are breathing spontaneously, the needle and catheter procedure should be performed during end exhalation.

Local anesthetics placed in the pleural cavity diffuse across the parietal pleura to the intercostal neurovascular bundle, producing a unilateral intercostal nerve block at multiple levels. To achieve a more extensive block, two catheters may have to be placed in the interpleural space. Interpleural analgesia using intermittent boluses of local anesthetic may be used to provide postoperative analgesia after upper abdominal surgical procedures, such as open cholecystectomy with subcostal incision as well as laparoscopic cholecystectomy. Effective postoperative pain relief requires intermittent intrapleural injections every 6 hours with approximately 20 ml of 0.25–0.5% bupivacaine. As in other intermittent bolus techniques, peaks and valleys in intrapleural analgesia occur when sequential doses are separated by hours.

Intrapleural analgesia may be less effective for post-thoracotomy pain than after other procedures in which the pleura is intact and there are no pleural drainage tubes to divert the local anesthetic from its site of action. Certain intercostal incisions, particularly those used for anterior thoracotomies, require that pleural drainage tubes be clamped for a short time after each intermittent local anesthetic injection to allow the local anesthetic to cross the parietal pleura and provide effective analgesia.

Intermittent clamping of the pleural drainage tube after injection of the local anesthetic may not be tolerated in patients with a moderate or large air leak from the pulmonary parenchyma after thoracotomy. The risk of pneumothorax and the problems of fluctuating levels of analgesia with intermittent dosing of intrapleural catheters suggest that other techniques, such as continuous thoracic epidural analgesia, may be preferable after thoracotomy when there is an anterior intercostal incision.

Other Modalities

Transcutaneous and Percutaneous Electrical Nerve Stimulation

Although transcutaneous electrical nerve stimulation (TENS) was initially prescribed for relief of chronic pain, its use has been extended to postoperative pain. TENS is a simple, conservative technique that uses electrical stimulation of the skin to provide pain relief. Two or four electropads are placed on the skin adjacent to the skin incision. These pads are then connected to a battery-operated pulse generator with varying modes, frequencies, and strengths of stimulation. Current strength can be varied from 100 to 200 mA, with mixed low 2-Hz and high 100-Hz frequencies providing a greater opioid-sparing effect than either low or high frequencies alone.[164] The mechanism by which TENS produces pain relief is thought to involve the release of endogenous endorphins by the electrical stimulation of afferent cutaneous nerves. The endogenous endorphin release has an inhibitory effect on the dorsal horn and augments the descending inhibitory modulating pathways. Partial reversal by naloxone of the analgesia produced by TENS supports this hypothesis. The degree of pain relief that patients experience is highly variable. Percutaneous electrical nerve stimulation is a modification of TENS in which needle electrodes are used instead of electropads. This method may reduce the interpatient variability in responses by avoiding the high resistance of the skin.

Psychological Interventions for Postoperative Analgesia

The use of various analgesic techniques involving nerve blocks and of opioids applied to the central neuraxis as well as administered by iv infusions has produced dramatic changes in the management of pain. Nevertheless, it is sometimes necessary to augment these techniques with various psychological interventions. Psychological interventions are used widely in the treatment of chronic pain, and the benefit of these behavioral strategies for the management of acute pain is now recognized. This often involves approaching the treatment of pain on a cognitive basis and using interventions such as distraction or imagery that attempt to focus attention away from the painful event. Other, simpler methods consist of educating patients about their surroundings, disease state, treatment plans, and the hospital environment in an effort to reduce fear and anxiety about unknown events or situations in the perioperative period. Despite the banality of this approach, it is a frequently overlooked element when dealing with patients who often are unfamiliar with the hospital environment. Other psychological interventions that may be effective are relaxation techniques such as deep breathing exercises or muscle relaxation training, which can reduce anxiety and muscle tension.

ORGANIZATION OF A POSTOPERATIVE ANALGESIA SERVICE

With the increasing number and complexity of modalities for treating postoperative pain, it is logical that an organized, systematic approach involving all members of the health care team has evolved in the form of the postoperative analgesia service. The anesthesiologist is uniquely qualified to lead this team because of his or her knowledge of the neurophysiology, pathophysiology, pharmacology, and anatomic pathways involved in the modulation of acute pain. Furthermore, with the postoperative analgesia service under the direction of the anesthesiologist, continuity of pain care management is enhanced because the anesthesiologist is routinely involved in the preoperative assessment, intraoperative management, and postoperative follow-up of surgical patients. Because anesthesiologists are the logical choice for managing the postoperative analgesia service, it is desirable that each department of anesthesiology assume responsibility for organizing and maintaining efficient operation of the service.

When initiating a postoperative analgesia service, it is essential that the department of anesthesiology have one or more members who will assume the position of director or co-director. This ensures that at least one person will be responsible for communication with the pharmacy, nursing, and surgical departments, development of policy and procedural protocols, and departmental representation when issues concerning postoperative pain management arise.

The delivery of central neuraxial opioid analgesia requires cooperation among the anesthesiology, nursing, surgery, and pharmacy staffs. Success of such an interdisciplinary program for postoperative analgesia often requires significant flexibility to satisfy the needs of all the parties concerned. Each institution must identify the approach that is practical and most beneficial for its patients after considering available resources. With these considerations, protocols that reflect individual practice patterns can be effectively developed. These protocols should include written policy and procedure manuals for nursing staff (see Appendices 54-2 and 54-4) as well as preprinted epidural analgesia orders (see Appendix 54-3). Postoperative pain relief has generated intense interest and fostered the introduction of several new analgesic modalities. Although these techniques have been shown to provide better pain relief than conventional im administration of opioids, the complexity of these modalities requires the use of an organized approach to maximize efficacy while minimizing potentially adverse effects. The transition phase from the operating room to the recovery area and then to the patient ward is a crucial period for intervention by the postoperative analgesia service. Optimization of analgesia (while the effects of anesthesia are dissipating) and potential reduction in the incidence or severity of side effects requires proactive evaluation and management in the recovery area by personnel trained and dedicated to these aspects of patient care.

When formulating the strategy for development and initiation of an epidural analgesia service, consideration must be given to the choice of continuous infusion techniques, intermittent bolus regimens, or combinations of these methods. In addition, with the use of PCA devices, similar protocols outlining the initial parameters for starting therapy should be established to facilitate effective use when these devices are prescribed (see Table 54-6).

The basic goals of the postoperative analgesia service are (1) administering and monitoring postoperative analgesia, and (2) identifying and managing complications or side effects of postoperative analgesic techniques. Implicit in these goals is the inclusion of an active quality assurance program directed at maintaining high-quality patient care while minimizing complications. When the postoperative analgesia service is managed by anesthesiologists, quality assurance monitoring can be applied to the heterogeneous surgical population so that the goals of pain management can be refined for the individual patient. This is much more difficult to achieve when particular surgical services are charged with the management of postoperative pain. Nonetheless, successful implementation of these principles requires the cooperation and involvement of health care providers outside of the department of anesthesiology, such as surgeons, nurses, and pharmacy personnel.

The foundation of an effective postoperative analgesia service is based on education of all members of the interdisciplinary health care team. This educational process must begin within the department of anesthesiology and be directed by those physicians with special qualifications in pain management and regional anesthesia. A corollary of this educational process is the use of a standardized approach to the initiation of pain management, which may include choices among fixed medication protocols, algorithms to identify and treat inadequate analgesia, and preprinted postoperative orders. The use of such methods increases efficiency, serves as a guideline for health care providers involved with the postoperative analgesia service, and gives the postoperative analgesia service team the flexibility to individualize therapy. This approach also facilitates the education of ancillary personnel, such as nursing staff, necessary to the functioning of the service.

Ideally, all members of each anesthesia department should become well versed in the basic principles necessary for the day-to-day operation of the postoperative analgesia service. Although its management usually is the responsibility of a limited number of anesthesia personnel, education of all members of the department ensures the smooth operation of the service when those key individuals are not available after hours or on weekends. Although patients receiving postoperative analgesia should be seen on a regular basis by the anesthesiologist, it may be necessary for nurse clinicians or anesthesiology residents to assist in performing these functions if the service is very large. It is the responsibility of the anesthesiologist to educate these people in the principles of pain management. Nurse clinicians often have excellent rapport with other nursing staff and can act as effective liaisons. In addition, nurse clinicians can facilitate the operation of the postoperative analgesia service by performing tasks such as charting daily progress notes, inspecting epidural catheter sites, removing epidural catheters when therapy is discontinued, notifying the anesthesiologist of any problems pertaining to pain management, and collecting patient data to facilitate quality assurance. The participation of anesthesiology residents in the postoperative analgesia service allows them to gain knowledge and expertise in this area of perioperative care. Depending on the size of the surgical population and the scope of the service, additional support may be required from clinical pharmacologists, nurse anesthetists, or other physicians. Developing this solid foundation is an important consideration when establishing a postoperative analgesia service.

In addition to 24-hour-a-day support from the anesthesia department, a successful postoperative analgesia service requires the cooperation and education of nursing staff so that they are responsive to the needs of the patients. In-service training of hospital nurses requires instruction in the principles of analgesic techniques, including appropriate aspects of neuroanatomy, neuropharmacology, side effects and their treatment, monitoring skills, analgesia assessment, and the technical aspects of the operation of PCA and epidural infusion devices. This instruction should be conducted under the supervision of the anesthesiologist in charge of the postoperative analgesia service but may also involve a clinical nurse specialist trained by the anesthesiology department, who may assist in solving nursing problems related to the operation of the service. To minimize dosing and medication errors and to improve patient comfort by early treatment of inadequate analgesia and complications such as pruritus, nurses must understand the use of the standardized protocols.

One additional benefit of such a model is the ability to transition patients from epidural or PCA techniques to oral or other analgesia delivery systems, facilitating postoperative discharge. This can usually be accomplished for most surgical patients by converting from the parenteral techniques to an orally administered acetaminophen–hydrocodone or acetaminophen–codeine preparation. However, some patients experience difficulty with transition from parenteral therapy and require more potent opioids and other nonopioid adjuvants. Such patients have typically received opioids chronically for pain, and have higher analgesic requirements to achieve satisfactory postoperative pain control.[165] Because of their experience with the principles and use of the more potent, longer-acting oral opioid preparations (in the setting of chronic pain management), anesthesiologists can facilitate the management of this complicated set of patients. For example, combining sustained-release forms of long-duration drugs such as oxycodone or morphine sulfate every 6–12 hours can be effective in the transition from parenteral analgesic therapy. Using such an approach, this transition may be accomplished more efficiently and potentially hastens postsurgical discharge in patients who have received opioids chronically for pain.

Another key aspect to the initiation of a postoperative analgesia service is the identification of patient populations that are most likely to benefit from improved postoperative pain management. Patients undergoing thoracic and upper abdominal procedures, major orthopedic operations such as hip surgery, and high-risk vascular surgical procedures are examples of groups in whom effective postoperative pain management produces the most rewarding results. It is often useful to consider a pilot program using PCA or epidural analgesia when surgeons are doubtful or hesitant about the efficacy of these methods. After the utility of the postoperative analgesia service has been demonstrated to surgeons, referring physicians, and others, the service can expand logically to patient populations in which improved analgesia will be obvious but in which the effects on outcome may be more subtle. Initiation of the service in any subset of patients also requires the education of surgical staff regarding (1) the advantages to their practice of being able to offer patients surgery with less postoperative discomfort, and (2) the potential differences in outcome when using certain methods of postoperative analgesia. Despite the lack of large-scale, randomized studies to demonstrate that improved postoperative analgesia (especially the use of epidural analgesia in high-risk patients) is definitively associated with improved outcomes (such as shorter, less expensive hospital stays, with fewer major complications), there is more than enough evidence currently in the literature to support the important role of epidural anesthesia and analgesia in clinical practice. Surgeons must understand that their patients will receive attentive care and that an essential element of the postoperative analgesia service is the maintenance of a cooperative spirit among disciplines.

Once the appropriate subsets of patients have been identified and educated, the physicians in charge of initiating the postoperative analgesia service must make plans for the provision of the capital resources necessary to operate the service. Plans must be made regarding types of equipment needed for continuous or patient-controlled iv or epidural analgesia, whether such devices are to be rented or purchased, types of monitoring equipment deemed necessary, any pharmacy-related factors necessary to prepare solutions of drugs for administration, and the printing of standard orders for the postoperative management of pain and treatment of complications. Decisions regarding funding sources for these capital expenses often must involve discussions with hospital administrators. In the present medical–economic climate, hospital administrators may be opposed to the purchase of new equipment if old methods appear to be functional. It is important to educate administrators who are reluctant to support the concept of a postoperative analgesia service about the potential benefits to some patients in terms of shorter, less complicated, less expensive hospital stays. Not only can the service be cost effective, but sometimes it can be used by hospital administrators as a marketing tool to attract surgical patients. Preprinted order forms usually require approval from the hospital's medical records/forms department. Job descriptions and resources are necessary to define and fund support staff such as nurse clinicians, psychologists, or clinical pharmacologists. Thus, a significant degree of planning, effort, and commitment is necessary to initiate a properly functioning postoperative analgesia service. When such efforts are expended, the establishment of such a service allows the anesthesi-

ologist to play an important role in the postoperative period and to provide a valuable service to patients.

SPECIAL CONSIDERATIONS IN PEDIATRIC ACUTE PAIN MANAGEMENT

Acute pain management in the pediatric patient poses a unique challenge to the anesthesiologist. It is often more difficult to evaluate pain intensity in children because the expression of pain is manifested over a broad emotional spectrum. For instance, some children withdraw and become nonverbal with the onset of pain, whereas others become emotionally labile, with crying, screaming, and violent behavior. Psychological distress is often compounded in children by separation from their parents and inadequate understanding of their disease and its treatment. Furthermore, depending on age, lack of cognitive development makes it more difficult to communicate relevant concepts to children. In view of these difficulties, a useful monitor of analgesic efficacy in children is behavior observation. Some behavior such as crying can be easily understood, but social withdrawal and the inability to be distracted often indicate that a young patient has distressing pain.

The selection and dosing of analgesic agents also requires special attention in the pediatric patient (Table 54-11). Neonates and infants, because of immature hepatic function and reduced plasma proteins and plasma protein-binding capacity, exhibit a higher fraction of free drug in the central compartment. This effect is offset to some degree by the higher total body water and extracellular fluid, and larger blood volume in this group compared with adults. Increased susceptibility to the respiratory depressant component of opioids may be a result of the increased fraction of cardiac output to the developing brain, or reduced metabolic pathways leading to accumulation of opioids and their metabolites. Morphine exhibits an increase in half-life and respiratory depressant effect in infants younger than 1 month of age owing to immature glucuronidation pathways. The half-lives of meperidine and fentanyl are similarly increased during the first 3 months of life. The pharmacokinetics of local anesthetics exhibit a similar pattern of development in neonates and infants. Free fractions of local anesthetics approach those seen in adults by 6 months of age (Table 54-12).

Oral Analgesics

Nonopioid

Nonsteroidal anti-inflammatory drugs are useful oral drugs for acute postoperative pain management in the pediatric population. Ibuprofen can be administered at 6- to 8-hour intervals in doses of 8 mg · kg^{-1}. Contraindications to the use of NSAIDs in the pediatric population are similar to those in adults. The most frequently encountered adverse effects are gastrointestinal. Platelet function alteration can occur, but this is usually not a significant clinical problem after short-term administration in the postoperative period. Acetaminophen has fewer side effects than ibuprofen and can be administered in doses of 5–15 mg · kg^{-1} orally or 20 mg · kg^{-1} rectally every 4–6 hours. Ketorolac in doses of 0.4–1.0 mg · kg^{-1} is also useful for mild to moderate postoperative pain in children when parenteral administration is desirable, but may be associated with a greater incidence of vomiting than morphine.[166,167]

Opioid

Codeine in combination with acetaminophen is a commonly used oral preparation for moderate postoperative pain in the pediatric population. The recommended oral dosage range is 0.5–1 mg · kg^{-1} every 4–6 hours.

Patient-Controlled Analgesia

Patient-controlled analgesia is an opioid delivery system that has been used with increasing frequency to treat acute postoperative

Table 54-11. PHARMACOLOGIC CONSIDERATIONS FOR PEDIATRIC PATIENTS

Drug	Dose (Age >6 mo)*	Interval (hr)	Route	Comments
NONOPIOID				
Acetaminophen	$5–15\ mg \cdot kg^{-1}$	4–6	po	Overdose may cause hepatotoxicity
	$20\ mg \cdot kg^{-1}$	4–6	Rectal	
Ibuprofen	$8\ mg \cdot kg^{-1}$	6	po	
Naproxen	$5\ mg \cdot kg^{-1}$	8–12	po	
Ketorolac	$0.4–1\ mg \cdot kg^{-1}$	6	iv/im	Vomiting may be greater than with morphine
	$0.25\ mg \cdot kg^{-1}$	6	po	Maximum dose $1\ mg \cdot kg^{-1} \cdot d^{-1}$
OPIOID				
Codeine	$0.5–1\ mg \cdot kg^{-1}$	4–6	po	Most commonly combined with acetaminophen
Oxycodone	$.005–0.15\ mg \cdot kg^{-1}$	4–6	po	Similar to codeine
Meperidine	$1–1.5\ mg \cdot kg^{-1}$	3–4	im	May cause less constipation, ileus, and urinary
	$0.8–1\ mg \cdot kg^{-1}$	2–3	iv	retention than morphine
Morphine	$0.1–0.15\ mg \cdot kg^{-1}$	3–4	im	
	$0.08–0.1\ mg \cdot kg^{-1}$	2	iv	
	$0.05–0.06\ mg \cdot kg^{-1} \cdot hr^{-1}$		iv	Continuous infusion
	$50\ \mu g \cdot kg^{-1}$	12–24	epi	Abdominal surgery
	$120–150\ \mu g \cdot kg^{-1}$	12–24	epi	Thoracic surgery
	$50–100\ \mu g \cdot kg^{-1}$	12–24	Caudal	Diluted in equal volume of normal saline
Fentanyl	$1–1.5\ \mu g \cdot kg^{-1}$	1–2	iv	Minimum age 1 yr
	$2–4\ \mu g \cdot kg^{-1} \cdot hr^{-1}$		iv	Continuous infusion

Epi = epidural (L3–L5); caudal = (S4–S5); im = intramuscular; iv = intravenous; po = oral.
* Fractionation of dose is recommended for age <6 mo.

pain in children. Morphine sulfate given as a loading dose of $0.1–0.2\ mg \cdot kg^{-1}$ and administered as small incremental boluses of $0.01–0.03\ mg \cdot kg^{-1}$ can be used to initiate PCA therapy. After this, maintenance doses of morphine sulfate, $0.01–0.015\ mg \cdot kg^{-1}$, given every 6–10 minutes with a 4-hour limit of $0.25\ mg \cdot kg^{-1}$, are appropriate. Incorporation of a continuous infusion of $0.01–0.015\ mg \cdot kg^{-1} \cdot h^{-1}$ into the regimen may be beneficial.[168] Lower doses of morphine may be used if ketorolac is used in conjunction with PCA.[169] Meperidine in maintenance doses of $0.15–0.20\ mg \cdot kg^{-1}$ with a 4-hour limit of $2–3\ mg \cdot kg^{-1}$ has been used and may be associated with fewer side effects than morphine.

Epidural Opioids

Like other methods of pain control, the use of epidural opioids has not been extensively studied in the pediatric population. Lumbar epidural analgesia has been used for young patients undergoing abdominal, urologic, or orthopedic procedures. Because lumbar epidural catheters may be more difficult to place in the pediatric patient than in adults, an alternative is to perform a "kiddie caudal" with a mixture of local anesthetic and opioid for postoperative analgesia. Morphine is the preferable drug for single-injection techniques and can be adminis-

tered as a $0.05\ mg \cdot kg^{-1}$ bolus, in volumes appropriate for the age and weight of the child.[170] Additional information on caudal analgesia is reported in earlier sections of this chapter.

RELATIONSHIP BETWEEN ACUTE AND CHRONIC PAIN

For an individual patient, the development of a chronic pain syndrome may simply be the extension of inadequately treated acute pain after trauma or surgery. Differentiation between acute and chronic pain is important in clinical practice because therapy usually is vastly different. It is generally agreed that pain persisting longer than 6 months can be viewed as chronic pain. Acute pain management techniques usually are not effective and may add to the problems when applied to chronic pain. For instance, systemic opioids for long-term use are often associated with the development of tolerance and, occasionally, drug dependency. Chronic pain is not simply the extension of acute pain as an isolated entity but involves multiple other factors such as altered mechanisms of nociceptive modulation and amplification of neural responses that account for the differences in clinical presentation and, more important, in choice of therapeutic modality.

SUMMARY

This chapter has reviewed the physiology of nociception and the production of acute postoperative pain as well as compared and contrasted various methods for analgesia. In addition, the rationale behind the development of a team of health care personnel aimed at managing postoperative pain has been addressed. Postoperative pain management requires continued study to refine, explore, and open new avenues for further improvement of current techniques.

Table 54-12. MAXIMUM LOCAL ANESTHETIC DOSES IN INFANTS AND CHILDREN

Drug	Infant Dose ($mg \cdot kg^{-1}$): Age	Child Dose ($mg \cdot kg^{-1}$)
Lidocaine (plain)	5: from birth on	5
Lidocaine (epinephrine)	7: from birth on	7
Mepivacaine	4: <6 mo	5
Bupivacaine (plain)	2: <3 mo	3
Bupivacaine (epinephrine)	2: <3 mo	4
Chloroprocaine (plain)	4: <6 mo	8
Chloroprocaine (epinephrine)	5: <6 mo	10

Reprinted with permission from Vetter TR: Acute pediatric pain management. Advances in Anesthesia 8:29, 1991.

REFERENCES

1. Sorkin L, Wallace MS. Acute pain mechanisms. Surg Clin North Am 79:213, 1999
2. Erlanger J, Gasser HS: The compound nature of the action current of nerve as disclosed by cathode ray oscillograph. Am J Physiol 70:624, 1924

3. de Jong RH: Function and diameter of nerve fiber. In de Jong RH (ed): Physiology and Pharmacology of Local Anesthesia, p 97. Springfield, Illinois, Charles C Thomas, 1970

4. Guyton AC: Sensory receptors; neuronal circuits for processing information. In Guyton AC (ed): Textbook of Physiology, 8th ed, p 495. Philadelphia, WB Saunders, 1991

5. Kerr FWL: The structured basis of pain: Circulatory and pathway. In Ng LWY, Bonica JJ (eds): Pain, Discomfort and Humanitarian Care, p 49. New York, Elsevier, 1980

6. Dougherty PM, Staats PS: Intrathecal drug therapy for chronic pain. Anesthesiology 91:1891, 1999

7. Henry JL: Effects of substance P on functionally identified units in cat spinal cord. Brain Res 114:439, 1976

8. Ebersberger A, Grubb BD, Willingale HL et al: The intraspinal release of prostaglandin E₂ in a model of acute arthritis is accompanied by an up-regulation of cyclo-oxygenase-2 in the spinal cord. Neuroscience 93:775, 1999

9. Gilbert PG, Askmark H: Changes in cholinergic and opioid receptors in the rat spinal cord, dorsal root and sciatic nerve after ventral and dorsal root lesion. J Neural Transm 85:31, 1991

10. Barber RP, Phelps PE, Houser CR et al: The morphology and distribution of neurons containing choline acetyltransferase in the adult rat spinal cord: An immunocytochemical study. J Comp Neurol 229:329, 1984

11. Ribeiro-Da-Silva A, Cuello AC: Choline acetyltransferase-immunoreactive profiles are presynaptic to primary sensory fibers in the rat superficial dorsal horn. J Comp Neurol 295:370, 1990

12. Iwamoto ET, Marion L: Characterization of the antinociception produced by intrathecally administered muscarinic agonists in rats. J Pharmacol Exp Ther 266:329, 1993

13. Hood DD, Eisenach JC, Tuttle R: Phase I safety assessment of intrathecal neostigmine methylsulfate in humans. Anesthesiology 82:331, 1995

14. Naguib M, Yaksh TL: Characterization of muscarinic receptor subtypes that mediate antinociception in the rat spinal cord. Anesth Analg 85:847, 1997

15. Treede R-D, Meyer RA, Raja SN, Cambell JN: Peripheral and central mechanisms of cutaneous hyperalgesia. Prog Neurobiol 38:397, 1992

16. Thompson SWN, King AE, Woolf CJ: Activity-dependent changes in rat ventral horn neurons in vitro, summation of prolonged afferent evoked depolarizations produce a D-2-amino-5-phosphonovaleric acid sensitive windup. Eur J Neurosci 2:638, 1990

17. Pockett S: Spinal cord plasticity and chronic pain. Anesth Analg 80:173, 1995

18. Urban L, Randic M: Slow excitatory transmission in rat dorsal horn: Possible mediation by peptides. Brain Res 290:336, 1992

19. Nagy J, Maggi CA, Dray A et al: The role of neurokinin and N-methyl-s-aspartate receptors in synaptic transmission from capsaicin sensitive primary afferents in the rat spinal cord in vitro. Neuroscience 52:1029, 1993

20. Zahn PK, Brennan TJ: Incisional-induced changes in receptive field properties of rat dorsal horn neurons. Anesthesiology 91:772, 1999

21. Zahn PK, Brennan TJ: Primary and secondary hyperalgesia in a rat model for human postoperative pain. Anesthesiology 91:863, 1999

22. Hosobuchi Y, Adams JE, Linchitz R: Pain relief by electrical stimulation of central grey matter in humans and its reversal by naloxone. Science 197:183, 1977

23. Yaksh TL: Multiple opioid receptor systems in brain and spinal cord: Part 2. Eur J Anesthesiol 1:201, 1984

24. Zieglgansberger W, Tulloch IF: The effects of methionine and leucine-enkephalin on spinal neurones of the cat. Brain Res 167:53, 1979

25. Camarata PJ, Yaksh TL: Characterization of the spinal adrenergic receptors mediating the spinal effects produced by microinjection of morphine into the periaqueductal gray. Brain Res 336:133, 1985

26. Reddy SV, Maderdrut JL, Yaksh TL: Spinal cord pharmacology of adrenergic agonist mediated antinociception. J Pharmacol Exp Ther 213:525, 1980

27. Maze M, Tranquilli W: Alpha-2 adrenoreceptor agonists: Defining the role in clinical anesthesia. Anesthesiology 74:581, 1991

28. Sabbe MB, Yaksh TL: Pharmacology of spinal opioids. J Pain Symptom Manage 5:191, 1990

29. Weissman C: The metabolic response to stress: An overview and update. Anesthesiology 73:308, 1990

30. Hagen C, Brandt MR, Kehlet H: Prolactin, LH, FSH, GH and cortisol response to surgery and the effect of epidural analgesia. Acta Endocrinologica 94:151, 1980

31. Michie HR, Wilmore DW: Sepsis, signals, and surgical sequelae (a hypothesis). Arch Surg 125:531, 1990

32. Levin JD, Coderne JS, Basbaum AI: The peripheral nervous system and the inflammatory process. In Dubner R, Gebhart GF, Bond MR (eds): Proceedings of the Vth World Congress on Pain, p 33. Amsterdam, Elsevier Science Publishers, 1988

33. Marano MA, Fong Y, Moldawer LL et al: Serum cachectin/tumor necrosis factor in critically ill patients with burns correlates with infection and mortality. Surgery, Gynecology and Obstetrics 170:32, 1990

34. Chernow B, Alexander HR, Smallridge RC et al: Hormonal responses to graded surgical stress. Arch Intern Med 147:1273, 1987

35. Lee DD, Kimura S, DeQuattro V: Noradenergic activity and silent ischemia in hypertensive patients with stable angina: Effect of metoprolol. Lancet 1:403, 1989

36. Rawal N, Sjostrand U, Christoffersson E et al: Comparison of intramuscular and epidural morphine for postoperative analgesia in the grossly obese: Influence on postoperative ambulation and pulmonary function. Anesth Analg 63:583, 1984

37. Rademaker BM, Ringers J, Oddom JA et al: Pulmonary function and stress response after laparoscopic cholecystectomy: Comparison with subcostal incision ans influence of thoracic epidural analgesia. Anesth Analg 75:381, 1992

38. Livingston E, Passaro E: Postoperative ileus. Dig Dis Sci 35:121, 1990

39. Moore FA, Feliciano DV, Andeassy RJ et al: Early enteral feeding, compared with parenteral, reduces postoperative septic complications. Ann Surg 216:172, 1992

40. Saol M: Effects of anesthesia and surgery on the immune response. Acta Anaesthesiol Scand 36:201, 1992

41. Toft P, Svendsen P, Tonnesen E et al: Redistribution of lymphocytes after major surgical stress. Acta Anaesthesiol Scand 37:245, 1993

42. Davis JM, Albert JD, Tracy KJ et al: Increased neutrophil mobilization and decreased chemotaxis during cortisol and epinephrine infusion. J Trauma 31:725, 1991

43. Akca O, Melischek M, Scheck T: Postoperative pain and subcutaneous oxygen tension [letter]. Lancet 354:41, 1999

44. Pollock RE, Lotzoua E, Stanford SD: Mechanism of surgical stress impairment of human perioperative natural killer cell cytotoxicity. Arch Surg 126:338, 1991

45. Tuman KJ, McCarthy RJ, March RJ et al: Effects of epidural anesthesia and analgesia on coagulation and outcome after major vascular surgery. Anesth Analg 73:696, 1991

46. Rosenfeld BA, Beattie C, Christopherson R et al: The effects of different anesthetic regimens on fibrinolysis and the development of postoperative arterial thrombosis. Anesthesiology 79:435, 1993

47. Breslow MJ, Parker SD, Frank SM et al: Determinants of catecholamine and cortisol responses to lower-extremity revascularization. Anesthesiology 79:1202, 1993

48. Rosenfeld BA, Faraday N, Campbell D et al: Hemostatic effects of stress hormone infusion. Anesthesiology 81:1116, 1994

49. Oyama T: Influence of anesthesia on the endocrine system. In Stoeckel H, Oyama T (eds): Endocrinology in Anaesthesia and Surgery, p 39. New York, Springer-Verlag, 1980

50. Roizen MF, Horrigan RW, Frazer BM: Anesthetic doses blocking adrenergic (stress) and cardiovascular response to incision: MAC BAR. Anesthesiology 54:390, 1981

51. Kehlet H: Modification of response to surgery by neural blockade: Clinical implications. In Cousins MJ, Bridenbaugh PO (eds): Neural Blockade in Clinical Anesthesia and Management of Pain, p 129. Philadelphia, Lippincott-Raven, 1998

52. Kehlet H: Acute pain control and accelerated postoperative recovery. Surg Clin North Am 79:431, 1999

53. Moeller IW, Rem J, Brandt MR, Kehlet H: Effect of posttraumatic epidural analgesia on the cortisol and hyperglycemic response to surgery. Acta Anaesthesiol Scand 26:56, 1980

54. Cosgrove DO, Jenkins JS: The effect of epidural anaesthesia on the pituitary-adrenal response to surgery. Clin Sci Mol Med 46:403, 1974

55. Baron JF, Coriat P, Mundler O et al: Left ventricular global and regional function during lumbar epidural anesthesia in patients with and without angina pectoris: Influence of volume loading. Anesthesiology 66:621, 1987

56. Blomberg S, Curelaru I, Emanuelsson H et al: Thoracic epidural

anaesthesia in patients with unstable angina pectoris. Eur Heart J 10:437, 1989

57. Davis R, DeBoer LWV, Maroko PR: Thoracic epidural analgesia reduces myocardial infarct size after coronary artery occlusion in dogs. Anesth Analg 65:711, 1986

58. Kataja J: Thoracolumbar anesthesia and isoflurane to prevent hypertension and tachycardia in patients undergoing abdominal aortic surgery. Eur J Anaesthesiol 8:427, 1991

59. Breslow MJ, Jordan DA, Christopherson R et al: Epidural morphine decreases postoperative hypertension by attenuating sympathetic nervous system hyperactivity. JAMA 261:3577, 1989

60. Yeager MP, Glass DD, Neff RK, Brinck-Johnsen T: Epidural anesthesia and analgesia in high-risk surgical patients. Anesthesiology 66:729, 1987

61. Baron JF, Bertrand M, Barre E et al: Combined epidural and general anesthesia *versus* general anesthesia for abdominal aortic surgery. Anesthesiology 75:611, 1991

62. Hjortso NC, Neumann P, Frosig F et al: A controlled study on the effect of epidural analgesia with local anaesthetics and morphine on morbidity after abdominal surgery. Acta Anaesthesiol Scand 29:705, 1985

63. Christopherson R, Beattie C, Frank SM et al: Perioperative morbidity in patients randomized to epidural or general anesthesia for lower-extremity vascular surgery. Anesthesiology 79, 422, 1993

64. McDaniel MD, Pearce WH, Yao JS et al: Sequential changes in coagulation and platelet function following femorotibial bypass. J Vasc Surg 1:261, 1984

65. Lichtenfeld K, Schiffer D, Helrich M: Platelet aggregation during and after general anesthesia and surgery. Anesth Analg 58:293, 1979

66. Modig J, Borg T, Bagge L, Saldeen T: Role of extradural and of general anesthesia in fibrinolysis and coagulation after total hip replacement. Br J Anaesth 55:625, 1983

67. Modig J, Malberg P, Karlstrom G: Effect of epidural versus general anesthesia on calf blood flow. Acta Anaesthesiol Scand 24:305, 1980

68. Jorgensen L, Rasmussen L, Nielsen P et al: Antithrombotic efficacy of continuous extradural analgesia after knee replacement. Br J Anaesth 66:8, 1991

69. Hendolin H, Mattila MAK, Poikolainen E: The effect of lumbar epidural analgesia on the development of deep vein thrombosis of the legs after open prostatectomy. Acta Chirurgica Scandinavica 147:425, 1981

70. Cuschieri RJ, Morran CG, Howie JC, McArdle CS: Postoperative pain and pulmonary complications: Comparison of three analgesic regimens. Br J Surg 72:495, 1985

71. Hedolin H, Lahtinen J, Länsimies E et al: The effect of thoracic epidural analgesia on respiratory function after cholecystectomy. Acta Anaesthesiol Scand 31:645, 1983

72. Bromage PR, Camporessi E, Chestnut D: Epidural narcotics for postoperative analgesia. Anesth Analg 59:473, 1980

73. Shulman M, Sandler AN, Bradley JW et al: Postthoracotomy pain and pulmonary function following epidural and systemic morphine. Anesthesiology 61:569, 1984

74. Pansard J-L, Mankikian B, Bertrand M et al: Effects of thoracic extradural block on diaphragmatic electrical activity and contractility after upper abdominal surgery. Anesthesiology 78:63, 1993

75. Mankikian B, Cantineau JP, Bertrand M et al: Improvement of diaphragmatic function by a thoracic extradural block after upper abdominal surgery. Anesthesiology 68:379, 1988

76. Simonneau G, Vivien A, Saberne R et al: Diaphragm dysfunction induced by upper abdominal surgery: Role of postoperative pain. American Review of Respiratory Disease 128:899, 1983

77. Wheatley R, Somerville I, Sapsford D, Jones J: Postoperative hypoxaemia: Comparison of extradural, I.M., and patient-controlled analgesia. Br J Anaesth 64:267, 1990

78. Kehlet H, Dahl JB: The value of multi-modal or balanced analgesia in postoperative pain relief. Anesth Analg 77:1048, 1993

79. Schulze S, Roikjaer O, Hasselstrøm L et al: Epidural bupivacaine and morphine plus systemic indomethacin eliminates pain but not systemic response and convalescence after choleystectomy. Surgery 103:321, 1988

80. Jayr C, Thomas H, Rey A et al: Postoperative pulmonary complications: Epidural analgesia using bupivacaine and opioids versus parenteral opioids. Anesthesiology 78:666, 1993

81. Jayr C, Mollie A, Bourgain JL et al: General anesthesia with postop-

erative parenteral morphine compared with epidural analgesia. Surgery 104:57, 1987

82. Ferreira SH: Prostaglandins hyperalgesia and the control of inflammatory pain. In Bonta IL, Bray MA, Parnham MJ (eds): Handbook of Inflammation, vol 5: The Pharmacology of Inflammation, p 108. New York, Elsevier, 1985

83. Malberg AB, Yaksh TL: Hyperalgesia mediated by spinal glutamate substance P receptor blocked by spinal cyclooxygenase inhibition. Science 257:28, 1992

84. Ferreira SH: Prostaglandins: Peripheral and central analgesia. Advances in Pain Research and Therapy 5:627, 1983

85. Hawkey CJ: COX-2 inhibitors. Lancet 353:307, 1999

86. Ehrich EW, Dallob A, DeLepeleire I et al: Characterization of rofecoxib as a cyclooxygenase-2 isoform inhibitor and demonstration of analgesia in the dental pain model. Clin Pharmacol Ther 65:336, 1999

87. Blanco FJ, Guitan R, Moreno J et al: Effect of anti-inflammatory drugs on COX-1 and COX-2 activity in human articular chondrocytes. J Rheumatol 26:1366, 1999

88. Lee VC: Non-narcotic modalities for the management of acute pain. Anesthesiology Clinics of North America 7:101, 1989

89. Jung D, Mroszczak E, Bynum L: Pharmacokinetics of ketorolac tromethamine in humans after intravenous, intramuscular and oral administration. Eur J Clin Pharmacol 35:423, 1988

90. Antonijevic I, Mousa SA, Schäfer M, Stein C: Perineurial defect and peripheral opioid analgesia in inflammation. J Neurosci 15:165, 1995

91. Stein C: Peripheral mechanisms of opioid analgesia. Anesth Analg 76:182, 1993

92. Zhou L, Zhang Q, Stein C, Schafer M: Contribution of opioid receptors on primary afferent versus sympathetic neurons to peripheral opioid analgesia. J Pharmacol Exp Ther 286:1000, 1998

93. Stein C, Comisel K, Haimeri E et al: Analgesic effect of intraarticular morphine after arthroscopic knee surgery. N Engl J Med 325:1123, 1991

94. Khoury GF, Chen ACN, Garland DF, Stein C: Intraarticular morphine, bupivacaine, and morphine/bupivacaine for pain control after knee videoarthroscopy. Anesthesiology 77:263, 1992

95. Joshi GP, McCarroll SM, O'Brien TM, Lenane P: Intraarticular analgesia following knee arthroscopy. Anesth Analg 76:333, 1993

96. DeAndres J, Bellver J, Barrera L et al: A comparative study of analgesia after knee surgery with intraarticular bupivacaine, intraarticular morphine and lumbar plexus block. Anesth Analg 77:727, 1993

97. Dalsgaard J, Felsby S, Juelsgaard P, Froekjaer J: Low-dose intraarticular morphine analgesia in day case knee arthroscopy: A randomized double-blinded study. Pain 56:151, 1994

98. Heine MF, Tillet ED, Tsueda K et al: Intra-articular morphine after arthroscopic knee operation. Br J Anaesth 73:413, 1994

99. Nozaki-Taguchi N, Yaksh TL: Characterization of the antihyperalgesic action of a novel peripheral mu-opioid receptor agonist-loperamide. Anesthesiology 90:225, 1999

100. Raffa RB, Friderichs E, Reimann W et al: Opioid and nonopioid components independently contribute to the mechanism of action of tramadol, an "atypical" opioid analgesic. J Pharmacol Exp Ther 260:275, 1992

101. Kayser V, Besson JM, Guilbaud G: Effects of the analgesic agent tramadol in normal and arthritic rats: comparison with the effects of different opioids, including tolerance and cross-tolerance to morphine. Eur J Pharmacol 195:37, 1991

102. Kayser V, Besson JM, Guilbaud G: Evidence for nonadrenergic component in the antinociceptive effect of the analgesic agent tramadol in an animal model of clinical pain. Eur J Pharmacol 224:83, 1992

103. Lehman KA: Tramadol for management of acute pain. Drugs 47:19, 1994

104. Collart L, Luthy C, Dayer P: Multimodal analgesic effect of tramadol. Annual Meeting of the American Society of Clinical Pharmacology and Therapeutics, Honolulu, March 1993. Clin Pharmacol Ther 53:233, 1993

105. Lee CR, McTavish D, Sorkin EM: Tramadol: A preliminary review of its pharmacodynamic and pharmacokinetic properties, and therapeutic potential in acute and chronic pain states. Drugs 46:313, 1993

106. Lehmann LJ, DeSio JM, Radvany T, Bikhazi GB: Transdermal fentanyl in postoperative pain. Regional Anesthesia 22:24, 1997

107. Lichtor JL, Sevarino FB, Joshi GP et al: The relative potency of

oral transmucosal fentanyl citrate compared with intravenous morphine in the treatment of moderate to severe postoperative pain. Anesth Analg 89:732, 1999

108. Sevarino FB, Paige D, Sinatra RS, Silverman DG: Postoperative analgesia with parenteral opioids: Does continuous delivery utilizing a transdermal opioid preparation affect analgesic efficacy or patient safety? J Clin Anesth 9:173, 1997

109. Rigg JR, Browne RA, Davis C et al: Variation in the disposition of morphine after administration in surgical patients. Br J Anaesth 5:1125, 1978

110. Gourlay GK, Kowalski SR, Plummer JL et al: Fentanyl blood concentration-analgesic response relationship in the treatment of postoperative pain. Anesth Analg 67:329, 1988

111. Edwards DJ, Svensson CK, Visco JP, Lalka D: Clinical pharmacokinetics of pethidine: 1982. Clin Pharmacokinet 7:421, 1982

112. Berde CB, Lehn BM, Yee JD et al: Patient controlled analgesia in children and adolescents: A randomized, prospective comparison with intramuscular administration of morphine for postoperative pain. J Pediatr 118:460, 1991

113. Egbert AM, Parks LH, Short LM, Burnett ML: Randomized trial of postoperative patient-controlled analgesia vs intramuscular narcotics in frail elderly men. Arch Intern Med 150:1897, 1990

114. Sidebotham D, Dijkhuizen MR, Schug SA: The safety and utilization of patient-controlled analgesia. J Pain Symptom Manage 24:202, 1997

115. Egan KJ, Ready LB: Patient satisfaction with intravenous PCA or epidural morphine. Can J Anaesth 41:6, 1994

116. Woodhouse A, Ward ME, Mather LE: Intra-subject variability in postoperative patient-controlled analgesia: Is the patient satisfied with morphine, pethidine and fentanyl? Pain 80:545, 1999

117. Ginsberg B, Gil KM, Muir M et al: The influence of lockout intervals and drug selection on patient-controlled analgesia following gynecological surgery. Pain 62:95, 1995

118. White PF: Mishaps with patient-controlled analgesia. Anesthesiology 66:81, 1987

119. Cleland JG: Continuous peridural caudal analgesia in surgery and early ambulation. NW Med J 48:26, 1949

120. Abboud TK, Dror A, Mosaad P et al: Mini-dose intrathecal morphine for the relief of post-cesarean section pain: Safety, efficacy and ventilatory responses to carbon dioxide. Anesth Analg 67:137, 1988

121. Aun C, Thomas D, St. John-Jones L et al: Intrathecal morphine in cardiac surgery. Eur J Anaesthesiol 2:419, 1985

122. Rigler ML, Drasner K, Krejcie TC et al: Cauda equina syndrome after spinal anesthesia. Anesth Analg 72:275, 1991

123. Eisenach JC: Combined spinal-epidural analgesia in obstetrics. Anesthesiology 1:299, 1999

124. van Lersberghe C, Camu F, de Keersmaecker E, Sacré S: Continuous administration of fentanyl for postoperative pain: A comparison of the epidural, intravenous, and transdermal routes. J Clin Anesth 6:308, 1984

125. Loper KA, Ready LB, Downey M et al: Epidural and intravenous fentanyl infusions are clinically equivalent after knee surgery. Anesth Analg 70:72, 1990

126. El-Baz NM, Faber LP, Jensik RJ: Continuous epidural infusion of morphine for treatment of pain after thoracic surgery: A new technique. Anesth Analg 63:757, 1984

127. Chestnut DH, Owen CL, Bates JN et al: Continuous infusion epidural analgesia during labor: A randomized double-blind comparison of 0.0625% bupivacaine/0.0002% fentanyl versus 0.125% bupivacaine. Anesthesiology 68:754, 1988

128. Cullen ML, Staren ED, el-Ganzouri A et al: Continuous thoracic epidural analgesia after major abdominal operations: A randomized prospective double-blind study. Surgery 98:718, 1985

129. Logas WG, el-Baz N, el-Ganzouri A et al: Continuous thoracic epidural analgesia for prospective pain relief following thoracotomy: A randomized prospective study. Anesthesiology 67:787, 1987

130. Cousins MJ, Mather LE: Intrathecal and epidural administration of opioids. Anesthesiology 61:276, 1984

131. Rutter DV, Skewes DG, Morgan M: Extradural opioids for postoperative analgesia: A double blind comparison of pethidine, fentanyl and morphine. Br J Anaesth 53:915, 1981

132. Lubenow TR, Tanck EN, Hopkins EM et al: Comparison of patient-assisted epidural analgesia with continuous-infusion epidural analgesia for postoperative patients. Regional Anesthesia 19:206, 1994

133. Paech MJ, Moore JS, Evans SF: Meperidine for patient-controlled analgesia after cesarean section. Anesthesiology 80:1268, 1994

134. Angst MS, Ramaswamy B, Riley ET, Stanski DR: Lumbar epidural morphine in humans and supraspinal analgesia to experimental heat pain. Anesthesiology 92:312, 2000

135. Hansdottir V, Woestenborghs R, Nordberg G: The cerebrospinal fluid and plasma pharmacokinetics of sufentanil by the lumbar versus thoracic route after thoracotomy. Anesth Analg 78:215, 1994

136. Shulman MS, Wakerlin G, Yamaguchi L, Brodsky JB: Experience with epidural hydromorphone for post-thoracotomy pain relief. Anesth Analg 66:1331, 1987

137. Akerman B, Arwenstrom E, Post C: Local anesthetic potentiates spinal morphine antinociception. Anesth Analg 67:943, 1988

138. Solomon RE, Gebhart GF: Synergistic antinociceptive interaction among drugs administered to the spinal cord. Anesth Analg 78:1164, 1994

139. Badner NH, Reimer EJ, Komar WE, Moote CA: Low-dose bupivacaine does not improve postoperative epidural fentanyl analgesia in orthopedic patients. Anesth Analg 72:237, 1991

140. Eisenach J, Detweiler D, Hood D: Hemodynamic and analgesic actions of epidurally administered clonidine. Anesthesiology 78:277, 1993

141. Eisenach JC, Lysaks Z, Viscomi CM: Epidural clonidine following surgery: Phase I. Anesthesiology 71:640, 1989

142. Eisenach JL, Rauch RL, Buzzanell C, Lysak SZ: Epidural clonidine for intractable cancer pain: Phase I. Anesthesiology 71:647, 1989

143. DeKock M, Gautier P, Pavlopoulou A et al: Epidural clonidine or bupivacaine as the sole analgesic agent during and after abdominal surgery. Anesthesiology 90:1354, 1999

144. Klimscha W, Chiari A, Krafft P et al: Hemodynamic and analgesic effects of clonidine added repetitively to continuous epidural and spinal blocks. Anesth Analg 80:322, 1995

145. DeKock M, Crochet B, Morimont C, Scholtes JL: Intravenous or epidural clonidine for intra- and postoperative analgesia. Anesthesiology 79:525, 1993

146. Motsch J, Graber E, Ludwig K: Addition of clonidine enhances postoperative analgesia from epidural morphine: A double-blind study. Anesthesiology 73:1067, 1990

147. Curatolo M, Schnider TW, Petersen-Felix S et al: A direct search procedure to optimize combinations of epidural bupivacaine, fentanyl, and clonidine for postoperative pain. Anesthesiology 92:325, 2000

148. Tallarida RJ, Stone DJ Jr, McCary JD, Raffa RB: Response surface analysis of synergism between morphine and clonidine. J Pharmacol Exp Ther 289:8, 1999

149. Asano T, Dohi S, Ohta S et al: Antinociception by epidural and systemic α2-adrenoceptor agonists and their binding affinity in rat spinal cord and brain. Anesth Analg 90:400, 2000

150. Nagasaka H, Yaksh TL: Pharmacology of intrathecal adrenergic agonists: Cardiovascular and nociceptive reflexes in halothane-anesthetized rats. Anesthesiology 73:1198, 1990

151. McCarthy RJ, Kroin JS, Lubenow TR et al: Effect of intrathecal tizanidine on antinociception and blood pressure in the rat. Pain 40:333, 1990

152. Wang LP, Hauerberg J, Schmidt JF: Incidence of spinal epidural abscess after epidural analgesia. Anesthesiology 91:1928, 1999

153. Rao TL, El-Etr AA: Anticoagulation following placement of epidural and subarachnoid catheters: An evaluation of neurologic sequelae. Anesthesiology 56:618, 1981

154. Vandermeulen EP, Van Aken M, Vermylen J: Anticoagulants and spinal epidural anesthesia. Anesth Analg 79:1165, 1994

155. Horlocker TT, Wedel DJ: Neuraxial block and low molecular weight heparin: balancing perioperative analgesia and thromboprophylaxis. Reg Anesth Pain Med 23(6 Suppl 2):129;1998

156. Horlocker TT, Wedel DJ, Schlichting JL: Postoperative epidural analgesia and oral anticoagulant therapy. Anesth Analg 79:89, 1994.

157. Enneking FK, Benzon HT. Oral anticoagulants and regional anesthesia: a perspective. Reg Anesth Pain Med 23(6 Suppl 2):140; 1998

158. Katz JA, Kaeding CS, Hill JR, Henthorn TK: The pharmacokinetics of bupivacaine when injected intraarticularly after knee arthroscopy. Anesth Analg 67:872, 1988

159. Kaeding CC, Hill JA, Katz J, Benson L: Bupivacaine use after knee arthroscopy: Pharmacokinetics and pain control study. Arthroscopy 6:33, 1990

160. Katz J, Nelson W, Forest R et al: Cryoanalgesia for postthoracotomy pain. Lancet 1:512, 1980

161. Benumof JL: Management of postoperative pain. In Benumof JL

(ed): Anesthesia for Thoracic Surgery, p 467. Philadelphia, WB Saunders, 1987

162. Moore DC: Regional block. In Moore DC (ed): A Handbook for Use in the Clinical Practice of Medicine and Surgery, p 169. Springfield, Illinois, Charles C Thomas, 1981

163. Singelyn FJ, Seguy S, Gouverneur JM: Interscalene brachial plexus analgesia after open shoulder surgery: Continuous versus patient controlled infusion. Anesth Analg 89:1216, 1999

164. Hamza MA, White PF, Ahmed HE, Ghoname EA: Effect of frequency of transcutaneous electrical nerve stimulation on the postoperative opioid analgesic requirements and recovery profile. Anesthesiology 5:1232, 1999

165. Rapp SE, Ready LB, Nessly ML: Acute pain management in patients with prior opioid consumption: A case-controlled retrospective review. Pain 61:195, 1995

166. Forrest JB, Heitlinger EL, Revell S: Ketorolac for postoperative pain management in children. Drug Saf 16:309, 1997

167. Lieh-Lai MW, Kauffman RE, Uy HG *et al*: A randomized comparison of ketorolac tromethamine and morphine for postoperative analgesia in critically ill children. Crit Care Med 27:2786, 1999

168. Lubenow TR, Ivankovich AD: Patient-controlled analgesia for postoperative pain. Crit Care Nurs Clin North Am 3:35, 1991

169. Sutters KA, Shaw BA, Gerardi JA, Herbert D: Comparison of morphine patient controlled analgesia with and without ketorolac for postoperative analgesia in pediatric orthopedic surgery. Am J Orthop 28:351, 1999

170. Tyler D, Krane E: Postoperative pain management in children. Anesthesiology Clinics of North America 7:155, 1989

APPENDIX 54-1
Solutions and Rates of Patient-Controlled Epidural Analgesia
Standard Solutions

Fentanyl 3000 μg with bupivacaine 300 mg in 300 ml normal saline (NS)—adults <70 yr, >50 kg

Fentanyl 1500 μg with bupivacaine 300 mg in 300 ml NS—adults ≥70 yr, ≤50 kg, history of sleep apnea

Maximum continuous rate 10 ml · hr^{-1} for lumbar epidural catheters (total infusion rate ≤40 ml · 4 hr^{-1})

Examples of continuous and demand dosing combinations:
- 4 ml · hr^{-1} continuous, demand mode 1 ml q10min, 40 ml · 4 hr^{-1} lockout
- 4 ml · hr^{-1} continuous, demand mode 2 ml q20min, 40 ml · 4 hr^{-1} lockout
- 5 ml · hr^{-1} continuous, demand mode 1 ml q12min, 40 ml · 4 hr^{-1} lockout
- 6 ml · hr^{-1} continuous, demand mode 1 ml q15min, 40 ml · 4 hr^{-1} lockout
- 6 ml · hr^{-1} continuous, demand mode 2 ml q30min, 40 ml · 4 hr^{-1} lockout
- 7 ml · hr^{-1} continuous, demand mode 1 ml q20min, 40 ml · 4 hr^{-1} lockout
- 8 ml · hr^{-1} continuous, demand mode 1 ml q30min, 40 ml · 4 hr^{-1} lockout
- 8 ml · hr^{-1} continuous, demand mode 2 ml q60min, 40 ml · 4 hr^{-1} lockout
- 9 ml · hr^{-1} continuous, demand mode 1 ml q60min, 40 ml · 4 hr^{-1} lockout
- 10 ml · hr^{-1}, no demand mode

Morphine 30 mg with bupivacaine 300 mg in 300 ml NS—adults <70 yr, >50 kg

Morphine 15 mg with bupivacaine 300 mg in 150 ml NS—adults ≥70 yr, ≤50 kg, history of sleep apnea

Maximum continuous rate 6 ml · hr^{-1} for lumbar or thoracic epidural catheters (total infusion rate ≤24 ml · 4 hr^{-1})

Examples of continuous and demand dosing combinations:
- 3 ml · hr^{-1} continuous, demand mode 1 ml q20min, 24 ml · 4 hr^{-1} lockout
- 4 ml · hr^{-1} continuous, demand mode 1 ml q30min, 24 ml · 4 hr^{-1} lockout
- 5 ml · hr^{-1} continuous, demand mode 1 ml q60min, 24 ml · 4 hr^{-1} lockout
- 6 ml · hr^{-1} continuous, no demand mode

APPENDIX 54-2
Policy and Procedures for Initiation and Nursing Care of Patients with Postoperative Epidural Analgesia

I. Purpose
- A. To list guidelines for the initiating and monitoring of patients receiving postoperative epidural analgesia and to provide quality assurance and patient safety.

II. Candidates
- A. Postsurgical patients who have no previous history of allergy to the ordered analgesics.
- B. Patients must not have any contraindications to the placement of an epidural catheter (*e.g.,* sepsis, severe coagulopathy abnormality, hypovolemia, head injury).

III. Equipment
- A. Epidural infusion pump
- B. Cassette tubing
- C. Epidural catheter tray
- D. Micropore tape
- E. Tegaderm dressing
- F. Apnea monitor (if required—see below)
- G. Naloxone 0.4 mg · ml^{-1}—two ampules
- H. 3-ml syringes with needles
- I. Alcohol wipes
- J. Epidural solution
  1. Fentanyl 0.001%/bupivacaine 0.1%—300 ml (age <70 yr)
  2. Fentanyl 0.0005%/bupivacaine 0.1%—300 ml (age >70 yr, ≤50 kg, history of sleep apnea)
  3. Morphine 0.01%/bupivacaine 0.1%—300 ml (age <70 yr)
  4. Morphine 0.005%/bupivacaine 0.1%—300 ml (age >70 yr, ≤50 kg, history of sleep apnea)

IV. Treatment initiation and guidelines
- A. Placement of epidural catheter is performed by the anesthesiologist.
- B. Epidural order sheet must be completed by the anesthesiologist.
  1. Anesthesiologist's written order for epidural solution to include the name and amount of fluid, rate of infusion, name and dosage of any medications added, and supplemental intravenous/intramuscular pain medications as required.
- C. Epidural solution must be administered by designated infusion pump.
- D. Baseline blood pressure and respiratory rate must be documented before initiating epidural infusion.
- E. Blood pressure, heart rate, level of consciousness, and temperature are to be monitored every 4 hours for the first 24 hours of the epidural infusion.
- F. Respiratory monitoring
  1. An apnea monitor is required for patients who received epidural narcotic bolus of MSO$_4$ ≥2 mg. Patients may receive an epidural bolus of fentanyl 50–150 μg without the routine use of an apnea monitor.

2. Respiratory rate to be monitored every hour for the first 24 hours of the epidural infusion.
   a. Naloxone, syringe, and needle are to be readily available at all times.
G. The epidural solution bag and volumetric pump cassette are not changed unless otherwise ordered.

V. Nursing responsibilities
A. Record vital signs (blood pressure, level of consciousness, ambulation, temperature) every 4 hours for first 24 hours of epidural infusion, then as ordered.
B. Record respiratory rates every 1 hour for the first 24 hours of the epidural infusion and every 4 hours thereafter.
   1. If the respiratory rate falls below 8 per minute, notify the postoperative analgesia service (PAS) and administer naloxone as ordered.
C. Record all analgesic medications administered on the medication record.
D. Using the Visual Analog Scale, record patient's subjective level of pain with vital signs on flow sheet.
   1. Scale for pain: 0–10, with 0 = no pain and 10 = worst pain ever.
E. Assess epidural catheter integrity and check dressing for wetness every shift and as needed.
   1. Reinforce with dry 4 × 4 gauze if dressing is wet.
   2. Cover with clear plastic tape.
   3. Notify PAS if excessive wetness or integrity of catheter is in question.
      a. If epidural catheter becomes dislodged or disconnected.
         i. Notify PAS.
         ii. If catheter is disconnected, cover end of catheter with 4 × 4 gauze (do not reconnect).
         iii. If catheter becomes dislodged, keep for inspection by anesthesiologist.
F. Assess and document signs and symptoms of side effects.
   1. Pruritus with and without rash
   2. Nausea or vomiting
   3. Paresthesia, numbness, motor weakness
   4. Headache
   5. Backache
   6. Signs of infection around catheter site
   7. Urinary retention
G. Assess and document the following if patient is on anticoagulation medication:
   1. Notify PAS if patient receiving warfarin has an international normalized ratio (INR) >1.8.
   2. Notify PAS if a second anticoagulant is ordered.
H. Record any prescribed treatment administered for side effects or supplemental analgesics on patient care record.

VI. Postoperative analgesia service responsibilities
A. Team members will see patients daily and chart progress notes documenting adequacy of pain relief and the occurrence of side effects or problems associated with epidural use. Will adjust therapy or institute test dose algorithm if current protocol is associated with inadequate analgesia, side effects or complications. Will collect and maintain data for review by anesthesiologist on a weekly basis.
B. Organize and conduct inservice training of hospital nursing staff.
C. Review epidural medication record to ensure adequate documentation of use and disposal of medications.
D. Evaluate and make recommendations regarding new equipment for epidural analgesia.
E. Analyze data, identify problems, propose changes if any, and evaluate changes for quality assurance purposes.
F. Review anticoagulation medication taken along with coagulation status before epidural catheter removal.
   1. The epidural catheter should not be removed for at least 4 hours after the previous dose of subcutaneous standard heparin or discontinuation of intravenous heparin infusion. The next subcutaneous dose or the resumption of the intravenous infusion should be at least 2 hours after catheter removal.
   2. The epidural catheter should not be removed for at least 10 hours after the previous dose of a low-molecular-weight heparin. The next dose should be held for at least 2 hours after catheter removal.
   3. Patients receiving warfarin should not should have the epidural catheter removed until INR <1.8 and platelet count >80,000 per mm³. After epidural catheter removal in patients with INR >1.5, order neurosensory assessments to be made every 4 hours for the next 24 hours.

VII. Pharmacy responsibilities
A. Daily log of all patients receiving epidural analgesia with type of solution and amount dispensed.
B. Computer printout of all patients started on epidural analgesia in the last 24 hours. Printout should be available in pharmacy at 8 A.M. Monday through Saturday mornings. Patients started on epidural analgesia on Saturday or Sunday will be on the Monday morning printout. This list will be picked up by the PAS personnel to aid in identifying those patients started on epidural analgesia.
C. Collaborate with PAS personnel in quality assurance matters.

VIII. Termination
A. Epidural infusions ordinarily will be terminated by the PAS in conjunction with the primary surgical service using guidelines established for the type of surgical procedure and patients' analgesic requirements.

IX. Questions/problems
A. Any questions or problems regarding epidural drip or catheter are referred to the PAS between 8:00 A.M. and 4:30 P.M., or to the anesthesiologist on call after 4:00 P.M. and weekends.

APPENDIX 54-3
Postoperative Epidural Analgesia Order Sheet

(PLEASE CIRCLE ORDERS TO BE IMPLEMENTED AND COMPLETE BLANKS WHERE APPROPRIATE)
(DATE AND TIME FOR EACH PROCEDURE IS TO BE NOTED)

1. Admit to PAR or SIT, routine PAR or SIT VS.
2. Discharge from PAR per anesthesia care team.
3. On floor (circle):
   a. Monitoring
      1. Apnea monitor
      2. Telemetry
      3. Pulse oximetry
   b. VS q4h, respiratory rate q1h for the first 24 hours.
   c. Tape two ampules of naloxone with syringe and needle at bedside.
   d. If respiratory rate <8 per minute, give 0.4 mg naloxone iv stat and call anesthesia.
4. Epidural solution (circle one):
   a. MSO_4 15 mg with bupivacaine 300 mg in 300 ml NS, rate _____ ml·hr⁻¹ (age ≥70 yr, ≤50 kg, history of sleep apnea)

b. MSO$_4$ 30 mg with bupivacaine 300 mg in 300 ml NS, rate _____ ml·hr^{-1}

c. Fentanyl 1500 μg with bupivacaine 300 mg in 300 ml NS, rate _____ ml·hr^{-1} (age ≥70 y, ≤50 kg, history of sleep apnea)

d. Fentanyl 3000 μg with bupivacaine 300 mg in 300 ml NS, rate _____ ml·hr^{-1}

e. PATIENT-ASSISTED EPIDURAL MODE _____ ml q _____ min, with _____ ml·4 hr^{-1} lockout

5. Supplemental medications (circle):
   a. MSO$_4$ 2 mg iv, im, or sq q2–4h prn for pain
   b. Metoclopramide 10 mg im q4–6h prn for nausea
   c. Nalbuphine 10 mg im or sq q4–6h prn for pruritus
   d. Ketorolac 30 mg im q6h × 48 h prn for pain; if patient >65 y or <65 kg, give 15 mg im q6h × 48 h prn for pain

6. Nursing staff on floor call postoperative analgesia service × 24 hours a day if any problems arise or if catheter needs to be discontinued.

7. All other preoperative orders, medications, and diet per service with the exception of opioids and sedatives.

Signed _____, M.D.   Date _____

PAR = postanesthesia recovery; VS = vital signs; SIT = surgical intensive therapy unit; iv = intravenously; im = intramuscularly; sq = subcutaneously; NS = normal saline.

APPENDIX 54-4
Patient-Controlled Analgesia (PCA) Service Protocol for Postsurgical Pain Relief

I. Purpose
   A. To list guidelines to follow when PCA is ordered and to provide quality assurance and patient safety.

II. Candidates
   A. Postsurgical patients who have no previous history of allergy to the ordered analgesics.
   B. Patients must be mentally alert, understand basic instructions, and be physically capable of operating the PCA infusion device.

III. Treatment initiation
   A. Treatment may be initiated by any surgical service as well as by anesthesia personnel. PCA treatment initiated by surgical services must conform to the guidelines listed below.

IV. Postoperative PCA guidelines
   A. The physician's order for PCA must include the following:
      1. Drug (only morphine and meperidine are available for routine use for postsurgical pain. Fentanyl and other drugs may be used only with the approval of the postoperative analgesia service [PAS] physician or anesthesiologist on call when the PAS service is not available)
      2. Loading dose (if patient has pain when PCA is ordered)
      3. Maintenance infusion (if desired)
      4. Incremental or maintenance dose
      5. Lockout interval
      6. Four-hour limit
      7. Mode of operation—PCA
   B. Recommended starting parameters
      1. Loading dose, morphine 1–4 mg, meperidine 10–40 mg
      2. Maintenance dose, morphine 1 mg, meperidine 10 mg
      3. Lockout interval, 6–10 minutes
      4. Four-hour limit, morphine 20 mg, meperidine 200 mg
      5. Mode of operation—PCA

V. Surgical staff
   A. Initiate preprinted order sheet.
   B. Evaluate adequacy of therapy.
   C. Contact PAS personnel if inadequate pain relief or patient has requirements for more complex PCA dosing.
   D. Monitor for complications.

VI. Nursing responsibilities
   A. Obtain and assure prompt delivery of PCA morphine/meperidine vials from pharmacy to nursing units.
   B. Verify proper and patent intravenous line.
   C. Monitor and record vital signs per orders.
   D. Reinforce patient teaching on use of PCA, if needed.
   E. Assess pain level and effectiveness of PCA.
   F. Change PCA tubing every 48 hours.
   G. Document accurate dosage of narcotic used or wasted in separate PCA medication sheets (two signatures needed for drug wasted).
   H. Verify that PCA is programmed to deliver dosage as ordered.
   I. At the change of shift, the incoming and outgoing nurses will check the PCA flow sheet, the pump readout, and the labeled syringe. The amount of drug administered in the previous 8 hours will be recorded on the PCA medication sheet.
   J. Notify PAS personnel and primary surgical service if the patient experiences side effects, complications, or inadequate analgesia.
   K. Assess and document signs and symptoms of side effects.
      1. Pruritus with and without rash
      2. Nausea or vomiting.
      3. Sedation/decreased mentation
      4. Decreased respiration
      5. Ileus/constipation
      6. Signs of infection or infiltration around catheter site
      7. Urinary retention
   L. Record any prescribed treatment administered for side effects or supplemental analgesics on patient care record.

VII. Postoperative analgesia service responsibilities
   A. Instruct patients on the use of PCA when ordered by anesthesia and provide additional teaching if PCA is ordered by surgical service.
   B. Team members will see patients daily and chart progress notes documenting adequacy of pain relief and the occurrence of side effects or problems associated with PCA use. Will adjust therapy or substitute with a new protocol if current therapy is associated with inadequate analgesia, side effects or complications. Will collect and maintain data for review by anesthesiologist on a weekly basis.
   C. Organize and conduct inservice training of hospital nursing staff.
   D. Review epidural medication record to ensure adequate documentation of use and disposal of medications.
   E. Evaluate and make recommendations regarding new equipment of epidural analgesia.
   F. Analyze data, identify problems, propose changes, if any, and evaluate changes for quality assurance purposes.

VIII. Pharmacy responsibilities
   A. Daily log of all patients receiving PCA with type of solution and amount dispensed.

B. Computer printout of all patients started on epidural analgesia in the last 24 hours. Printout should be available in pharmacy at 8 A.M. Monday through Saturday mornings. Patients started on PCA on Saturday or Sunday will be on the Monday morning printout. This list will be picked up by the PAS personnel to aid in identifying those patients started on epidural analgesia.

C. Collaborate with PAS personnel in quality assurance matters.

IX. Termination
   A. Epidural infusions ordinarily will be terminated by the PAS in conjuction with the primary surgical service using guidelines established for the type of surgical procedure and patients analgesic requirements.

X. Questions/problems
   A. Any questions or problems regarding epidural drip or catheter are referred to the postoperative analgesia service between 8:00 A.M. and 4:30 P.M. or to the anesthesiologist on call after 4:00 P.M. and weekends.

Clinical Anesthesia (4/e), edited by
Paul G. Barash, Bruce F. Cullen, and
Robert K. Stoelting. Lippincott Williams &
Wilkins, Philadelphia, © 2001.

CHAPTER 55

CHRONIC PAIN MANAGEMENT

STEPHEN E. ABRAM AND CHRISTIAN R. SCHLICHT

A generation ago, when confronted by patients who failed to respond to reasonable therapeutic measures, we had few explanations for our failures. The gate control theory helped to direct our thinking away from the concept of a hardwired, straight-through pain transmission system. We have made enormous progress in delineating the peripheral and central mechanisms of pain perception, and we have developed some novel methods for managing intractable pain. However, we are still frustrated by a substantial number of patients for whom we cannot provide effective pain control. Part of our failure to manage some patients effectively is the fact that pain complaints are related to factors independent of either nociception or aberrant neuronal activity within the pain projection system. Patients with somatization disorders, dysfunctional learned behaviors, secondary-gain issues, and substance abuse problems are likely to fail physiologically directed treatment regimens. Even when psychosocial issues are adequately addressed, the pathophysiologic processes leading to the perception of pain may not be successfully managed by treatment options that are currently available. Patients with pain following spinal cord injury or stroke are notoriously resistant to treatment. Although the number of treatment options is expanding, the complexity and cost of care are increasing as well, and the resources available to pay for these therapies are shrinking.

In order to successfully manage a wide range of chronic pain problems, one must have a good understanding of the physiology and anatomy of pain perception. One must understand the endogenous mechanisms that serve to heighten or suppress the neural activity associated with pain perception. In addition, an understanding of the pathophysiology of the more common painful disorders is essential, as is an understanding of the pharmacology of a wide range of medications, many of which are not analgesic *per se*. Other required skills include physical examination and psychological assessment techniques, regional anesthesia skills, and familiarity with an increasingly complex range of interventional management techniques. The management of difficult chronic pain patients is being done increasingly by physicians with subspecialty training in this field.

PAIN PATHWAYS AND MECHANISMS

Pain is most often experienced as a result of injury. Its survival value to an organism is based on the fact that it is initiated by tissue injury or by stimuli that threaten damage and that it produces sufficient arousal and distress that it is unlikely to be ignored. It is tempting to envision pain as a straightforward receptive system, with transducers that respond to intense, tissue-threatening stimuli, and neurons that project to areas of the brain capable of processing pain information. Unfortunately, such a view of pain perception fails to explain the tremendous variation in pain sensitivity between individuals or the dramatic shifts in sensitivity that can occur in a single individual. It also fails to explain chronic pain that is experienced without any noxious stimulation. Oversimplified anatomic concepts also predispose to simplistic therapeutic interventions, such as neurectomy or rhizotomy, that may intensify pain or create new and often more distressing pain.

In reality, the nociceptive system is highly complex and highly adaptable. Sensitivity of most of its components can be reset by a variety of physiologic and pathologic conditions. Injury to neural elements may result in loss of ability to perceive pain or may cause spontaneous pain or heightened pain sensitivity.

The ability to understand acute pain requires a knowledge of the physiology of receptors that respond to tissue-threatening stimuli, the anatomy of peripheral and central nervous system (CNS) pathways that are activated, and the mechanisms by which various components of the pain projection system can be sensitized or suppressed. Mechanisms of chronic pain are even more complex. Chronic injury may lead to irreversible alterations in nociceptor sensitivity, to spontaneous firing of peripheral or central pain projection fibers, and to dramatic changes in the reaction of the CNS to sensory inputs. This section provides an overview of the anatomic pathways, the physiologic modulating mechanisms, and the pathologic alterations that are important to the perception of pain.

ANATOMIC PATHWAYS

Nociceptors

Receptors that respond exclusively to intense, potentially tissue-damaging stimuli are well characterized. Cutaneous nociceptors have been extensively studied. Considerably less is known about receptors responsive to intense stimuli found in deep somatic structures. Still less is known about the physiology of visceral pain.

Cutaneous Nociceptors

Most cutaneous nociceptors respond to both intense mechanical stimulation and to high temperatures and are termed mechano-heat nociceptors.[1] They do not respond to low-threshold mechanical stimulation (light touch, pressure) or to warm temperatures below the noxious range. C-fiber mechano-heat (CMH) nociceptors respond to temperatures above 43°C. Firing frequency increases in a roughly linear fashion as skin temperature is increased within the noxious range (Fig. 55-1). Repeated or prolonged exposure to suprathreshold stimuli may lead to a reduction in response, or habituation. However, under certain circumstances, previous exposure to a noxious stimulus may lead to an enhanced response (sensitization).

There are two types of A-fiber mechano-heat nociceptors (AMHs). Type I AMHs have a very high threshold to thermal stimuli (53°C or greater) and are considered by some investigators to be mechanical nociceptors, or high-threshold mechanoreceptors. These nociceptors are found principally in glabrous skin. While most have afferent fibers with conduction velocities in the A-delta range ($\sim$30 m·sec^{-1}), some have conduction velocities as high as 55 m·sec^{-1}, and would be considered A-b fibers. Type II AMHs are activated by temperatures below activation thresholds of type I AMHs and conduct at about 15 m·sec^{-1}. These nociceptors also have a much shorter delay between stimulus onset and receptor activation. They are generally found in hairy skin and on the face.

The receptive fields for mechanical and thermal nociception are essentially identical for both CMHs and AMHs. However, there may be differences in the transducer mechanisms for mechanical versus thermal nociception. For instance, application of capsaicin to the skin produces analgesia to noxious

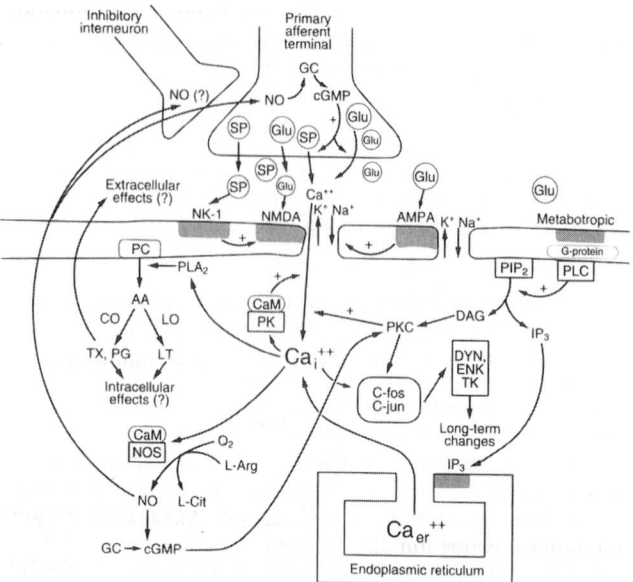

Figure 55-1. Sequence of events leading to sensitization of dorsal horn neurons following injury and intense nociceptive stimulation. Intense activation of primary afferent neuron stimulates release of glutamate (Glu) and substance P (SP). The NMDA receptor, at physiologic Mg^{2+} levels, is initially unresponsive to Glu; but following depolarization of the AMPA receptor by Glu on the metabotropic receptor it stimulates G-protein–mediated activation of phospholipase C (PLC), which catalyzes hydrolysis of phosphatidylinositol 4,5-biphosphate (PIP_2) to produce inositol triphosphate (IP_3) and diacylglycerol (DAG). DAG stimulates production of protein kinase C (PKC), which is activated in the presence of high levels of intracellular Ca^{2+} (Ca^{2+}). IP_3 stimulates release of intracellular Ca^{2+} from intracellular stores within the endoplasmic reticulum (Ca_{er}^{2+}). Increased PKC induces a sustained increase in membrane permeability and, in conjunction with increased intracellular Ca^{2+}, leads to increased expression of proto-oncogenes such as *c-fos* and *c-jun*. The proteins produced by these proto-oncogenes encode a number of neuropeptides such as enkephalins (ENK), dynorphin (DYN), and tachykinins (TK). Increased Ca_i^{2+} also leads to activation of phospholipase A_2 (PLA_2) and to activation of nitric oxide synthase (NOS) through a calcium/calmodulin mechanism. PLA_2 catalyzes the conversion of phosphatidyl choline (PC) to prostaglandins (PG) and thromboxanes (TX) and by lipoxygenase (LO) to produce leukotrienes (LT). NOS catalyzes the production of protein kinases, such as PKC, and alterations in gene expression. NO diffuses out of the cell to the primary afferent terminal, where, through a GC/cGMP mechanism, it increases the release of glutamate. It is speculated that NO may interfere with release of inhibitory neurotransmitters from inhibitory neurons. (From Hogan QH, Abram SE: Diagnostic and prognostic neural blockade. In Cousins MJ, Bridenbaugh PO [eds]: Neural Blockade in Clinical Anesthesia and Management of Pain, p 837. Philadelphia, Lippincott-Raven, 1998.)

thermal, but not mechanical stimulation. Cutaneous AMHs and CMHs are poorly responsive to cooling stimuli, and there is some evidence that afferent fibers from vascular structures are capable of signaling cold pain.[2]

Some cutaneous nociceptors are insensitive to noxious mechanical stimuli, and are termed mechanically insensitive afferents. Some of these may be chemically responsive, while others are responsive only to intense heat or cold. Some of these receptors develop mechanosensitivity following the development of inflammation.

A number of chemical mediators that are released following injury are capable of either acitvating or sensitizing both CMHs and AMHs. These substances include bradykinin, serotonin, prostaglandins, leukotrienes, histamine, and substance P. Bradykinin, which is released locally following tissue injury, is capable of evoking pain on intradermal injection, and has been shown to activate both CMHs and AMHs when administered within a nerve's receptive field. In addition, bradykinin pro-

duces hyperalgesia to heat stimuli through receptor sensitization. Serotonin can activate nociceptors and potentiates bradykinin-induced pain. Low *p*H is also capable of producing pain, both by nociceptor activation and by sensitization to mechanical stimuli.[1]

Nociceptors in Other Somatic Structures

A large number of A-delta and C fibers found in muscle, fascia, and tendons are poorly responsive to normal stretching or contraction and are probably nociceptive in function. Many of the C fibers are responsive to chemical irritants, heat, and strong pressure.[3] A few respond to strong contraction and to ischemia, whereas others fire in response to muscle stretching. Some A-delta fibers in muscle have relatively low sensitivity to mechanical stimuli, responding best to chemicals, such as bradykinin. Others, which tend to be arranged near muscle–tendon junctions, respond to local pressure, stretch, and contractions.[3]

Nociceptors in joints are located in the joint capsule, ligaments, periosteum, and articular fat pads, but probably not in cartilage. Small myelinated and unmyelinated fibers terminate in free nerve endings in joints, and A-delta fibers form a widespread plexus in capsules, fat pads, and ligaments.[4] Some of the A-delta axons respond to noxious stimuli. Intracapsular bradykinin in animals produces generalized nociceptive responses that are enhanced by prostaglandins.

Corneal sensitivity serves a primarily protective function, and most stimuli to corneal epithelium are sensed as pain. Innervation is mainly from A-delta fibers, with fine terminals devoid of Schwann cell covering.[3] These fibers have activation thresholds similar to low-threshold mechanoreceptors in skin,[5] but low-intensity stimulation is capable of evoking pain. Tooth pulp afferents respond to a variety of chemical stimuli, strong heating, cooling, and pressure. Electrical stimulation produces almost exclusively painful sensations.[3]

Visceral Pain Receptors

Because of the infrequency with which visceral structures are exposed to potentially damaging events, it would not seem efficient to provide these structures with receptors designed solely to detect intense stimuli in the environment. Although severe pain of visceral origin is a common clinical phenomenon, there is little evidence that specialized pain receptors exist in visceral structures. Many damaging stimuli, such as cutting, burning, or clamping, produce no pain when applied to visceral structures. On the other hand, inflammation, ischemia, mesenteric stretching, or dilation or spasm of hollow viscera may produce severe pain. These stimuli are usually associated with pathologic processes, and the pain they induce may serve a survival function by promoting immobility.

For almost all intrathoracic, intra-abdominal, and pelvic viscera, pain perception is a function of visceral afferent (sometimes termed sympathetic afferent) nerve activity.[3] These neurons accompany sympathetic efferent axons in the sympathetic chain and intra-abdominal and intrathoracic plexuses; but most, like other afferent fibers, have their cell bodies in the dorsal root ganglia and synapse with dorsal horn neurons.

Pain Perception in the Gut

It has been widely accepted that nociceptive-specific fibers do not exist in the gut. Pain is thought to result from intense activation of afferent fibers that serve other functions, such as stretch receptors. High-frequency activation of these visceral afferents in turn activates dorsal horn pain projection neurons, producing pain perceived within cutaneous referral sites. This referred pain is probably the result of viscerosomatic convergence, the phenomenon of a single spinothalamic tract (STT) neuron that can be activated by either visceral or somatic stimuli. Another type of convergence, reported by Bahr *et al*,[6] is based on the existence of afferent neurons with two sensory branches, one visceral (sympathetic afferent) and one somatic. It is not possible to locate the site of a painful stimulus to the gut with any accuracy because stimulation of widely distant sites can give rise to the same referred sensations.

Cardiac Pain

Cardiac afferent fibers, conducting in the C and A-delta range, have been shown to fire at high rates in response to coronary occlusion or to intracoronary bradykinin.[7] However, to designate these nerves as nociceptors, they should respond only to noxious stimuli and should exhibit no background discharge. Malliani[7] has shown that these putative nociceptors are tonically active, demonstrate mechanosensitivity, and respond to normal hemodynamic events. It is likely that cardiac afferents that are responsive to tissue-threatening stimuli have physiologic functions under normal circumstances, but give rise to volleys of activity that can cause poorly localized pain referred to somatic structures. Viscerosomatic convergence probably occurs with these fibers.

Other Visceral Structures

Pain associated with gallbladder disease is similar in character and location to angina pectoris.[8] Mechanical stimulation of the gallbladder or the application of chemical stimuli can affect the electrical activity and contractility of the heart.[9] Stretching of the bile ducts and gallbladder activates two populations of afferent fibers, one responding to small changes in pressure and the other responding only to high pressures (>25 mm Hg).[10] The high-threshold stretch receptors may have a nociceptive function. Gallbladder distension activates spinothalamic cells in the T1–5 portion of the cord, cells that are also activated by cardiac afferents and somatic afferents from the medial aspect of the arm and the chest wall.

Pain from the upper portions of the esophagus is most likely caused by activation of vagal afferents.[3] Heartburn pain may be a vagally mediated phenomenon, but little study of the activation of pain by acids in the esophagus has been carried out.

Distension of the renal pelvis or ureters is known to produce pain, but few studies have characterized afferent responses from the urinary tract. Pain of urethral origin is probably transmitted via sacral nerve roots rather than through sympathetic afferents. Urinary bladder distension is capable of producing cardiovascular responses, but, unlike gallbladder distension, is associated with reduced heart rate and contractility.

Dorsal Horn Mechanisms

The spinal dorsal horn and its analog in the medulla are exceedingly complex sensory processing areas. They contain the central terminals of peripheral afferent fibers, projection neurons of spinothalamic and other ascending tracts, local neurons that activate or inhibit projection neurons, and axon terminals of descending brain stem fibers.

As nerve roots approach the dorsal horn, segregation of fibers according to size takes place, with large myelinated afferents becoming arranged medially and small unmyelinated and thinly myelinated fibers arranged laterally. Most large myelinated fibers enter the cord medial to the dorsal horn. Many of these axons bifurcate, sending one branch rostrally in the dorsal columns. The other branch enters deeper layers of the dorsal horn, sending terminals into laminae IV and V and extensive arborizations into the substantia gelatinosa (laminae II and III).

Most unmyelinated or thinly myelinated afferents pass directly through the outer layer of lamina I, where they synapse with marginal layer cells and send a few branches into the underlying substantia gelatinosa. Some axons pass ventrally through these outer layers to terminate in laminae V and X.[11]

There are two groups of cells in the dorsal horn that respond to noxious stimulation in the periphery. One group, located mainly in lamina I, responds exclusively to noxious stimulation. Most of these cells, termed nociceptive-specific, have relatively limited receptive fields, confined to some fraction of a dermatome. The second group of cells, termed wide dynamic range neurons, can be activated by either tactile or noxious stimuli. Most of these cells are located in lamina V. They have large, complex receptive fields that often have a central area of responsiveness to either noxious or tactile stimulation, surrounded by an area of responsiveness only to noxious stimulation. Stimulation just outside the entire receptive field may produce inhibition. It is generally accepted that wide dynamic range neurons contribute to pain perception and that their selective activation is sufficient to cause pain. It is likely that many of the neurons in laminae I and V that respond to noxious stimuli are STT neurons.

Activation of the Dorsal Horn Projection System

There is considerable evidence that excitatory amino acids (EAAs) such as glutamate and aspartate are the principal neurotransmitters responsible for activation of dorsal horn neurons following noxious stimulation. Evidence for this conclusion is based on localization of these substances in nerve terminals in the dorsal horn, detection of release of EAAs following noxious stimulation, and behavioral evidence of hyperalgesia following intrathecal (IT) administration of EAAs in animals.[12]

Several types of EAA receptors are involved in the initiation of neuronal excitation that leads to the transmission of pain information. The AMPA receptor responds briefly (tens of milliseconds) and unconditionally to the release of glutamate.[13] Activation of the NMDA receptor results in postsynaptic potentials that may last much longer, on the order of seconds to minutes. The NMDA receptor is normally unresponsive to EAAs because of a voltage-dependent block that occurs at normal resting membrane potentials and physiologic concentrations of Mg^{2+}. Following a period of depolarization of the AMPA receptor or activation of neurokinin (NK-1) receptors by substance P (which is released from nociceptive afferent terminals following intense activation), the NMDA receptor becomes responsive to EAAs and produces a relatively prolonged postsynaptic response (see Fig. 55-1). In such a way, the brief response to a short-lived stimulus is converted to a prolonged response, one likely to be perceived as pain, following prolonged repetitive stimulation. The phenomenon of "windup,"[14] the progressive increase in response to repetitive, brief C-fiber intensity stimulation, appears to be NMDA receptor–mediated, and can be blocked by pretreatment with NMDA receptor antagonists. It has been proposed that the NMDA receptor is principally activated by aspartate released from excitatory interneurons in the dorsal horn, while the AMPA receptor is usually activated by glutamate released directly from afferent nerve terminals.

There is evidence for still more prolonged increases in sensitivity of spinal cord neurons to sensory inputs occurring in response to ongoing nociceptor activation. Changes in dorsal horn neural function known as long-term potentiation (LTP) can occur in the spinal cord and may last hours to days. A similar phenomenon is seen in the hippocampus, and is associated with learning and memory function. As with the spinal cord phenomenon of augmented transmission of nociceptive transmission (allodynia, hyperalgesia), LTP in the hippocampus is NMDA receptor–mediated. It has been shown that prolonged excitation and release of EAAs in certain areas of the CNS can lead to damage or loss of neurons, and that such neurotoxicity is mediated at least in part by the NMDA receptor.[15] Following some types of peripheral nerve lesions in animals, the appearance of small darkly staining neurons in the substantia gelatinosa occurs coincidentally with the development of thermal hyperalgesia.[16] It has been proposed that these cells represent degenerating inhibitory interneurons damaged by the large amounts of EAAs released by barrages of neural discharge from the injured nerve segment.[13]

Several neuropeptides that are released in the dorsal horn in response to noxious stimulation, including SP, neurokinin A, somatostatin, CGRP, and galanin, are thought to play a role in modulating the neural responses of dorsal horn cells sensory inputs.[16] The role of SP is perhaps best understood. It activates a postsynaptic NK-1 receptor resulting in reduction of K^+ efflux (μ-opioids and α_2-adrenergic agonists enhance K^+ efflux), thereby increasing neuronal excitability. Its activity is limited by rapid enzymatic degradation. Neurokinin A also acts as an NK-1 receptor agonist but is more slowly broken down and may actively enhance dorsal horn transmission for a period of many minutes to a few hours following injury.[17]

Intense or prolonged noxious stimulation produces sustained depolarization of dorsal horn neurons leading to a series of intracellular events that alter cellular responsiveness to subsequent sensory input. Ca^{2+} influx into dorsal horn cells is generated by both membrane depolarization and NMDA receptor activation. Ca^{2+} influx then results in a series of intracellular events. These include the activation of phospholipase A_2 (PLA_2) and increased production of intracellular arachidonic acid and the products of the prostaglandin cascade. The resultant spinal cord accumulation of prostaglandins augments the hyperalgesic state through mechanisms not yet identified. Evidence for this proposal is provided by the fact that intrathecal prostaglandins are indeed capable of inducing a hyperalgesic state,[12] and that hyperalgesia induced by IT NMDA is inhibited by IT administration of NSAIDs.[19]

Another mechanism by which Ca^{2+} influx enhances responsiveness to noxious stimulation is through an increase in the production of intracellular nitric oxide (NO). Intracellular Ca^{2+} activates the enzyme nitric oxide synthase (NOS) through a calcium–calmodulin mechanism. NO is produced by the action of the enzyme on L-arginine. NO, which is rapidly diffusible both within and outside the cell, activates protein kinases through a cyclic GMP mechanism, leading to enhanced release of neurotransmitters from primary afferent terminals and enhanced responsiveness of the NMDA receptor in postsynaptic neurons. IT administration of substances that block the synthesis NO has been shown to inhibit nociceptor-induced spinal sensitization.[20]

Still other intracellular events, triggered by the action of EAAs and neuropeptides on metabotropic receptors, may lead to enhanced sensory processing. The activation of intracellular phospholipase C (PLC) stimulates the formation of inositol triphosphate (IP_3) and diacylglycerol (DAG). IP_3 stimulates release of intracellular Ca^{2+} stores, while DAG leads to increased production of protein kinase C (PKC). PKC further enhances NMDA receptor excitation and increases the expression of proto-oncogenes such as *c-fos* and *c-jun*, which control transcription of genes encoding a variety of neuropeptides that modulate responses to noxious stimuli.[16] Agents that inhibit production of PLC (*e.g.*, neomycin) or PKC (*e.g.*, H-7) reduce the delayed hyperalgesic response to subcutaneous formalin injection in rats (see Fig. 55-1).[21]

PKC is involved in the development of opioid tolerance.[22] Following prolonged occupation of opioid receptors on postjunctional dorsal horn neurons, there is translocation and activation of PKC, which in turn may uncouple the G protein that activates the potassium channel from the opioid receptor, producing tolerance. Thus activated, PKC may also enhance calcium influx through the NMDA receptor, producing sensitization of the cell as described above. In addition, PKC activated by the activity of EAAs on the NMDA receptor is capable of uncoupling the opiate receptor mechanism, reducing opioid responsiveness (see Fig. 55-2). Thus, prolonged opioid administration can lead to spinal sensitization, and prolonged EAA release, as occurs with neuropathic pain states, can reduce responsiveness to opioids.[22]

There are several systems capable of suppressing activity in STT neurons. There is substantial evidence that both descending and segmental neuronal inputs can inhibit activa-

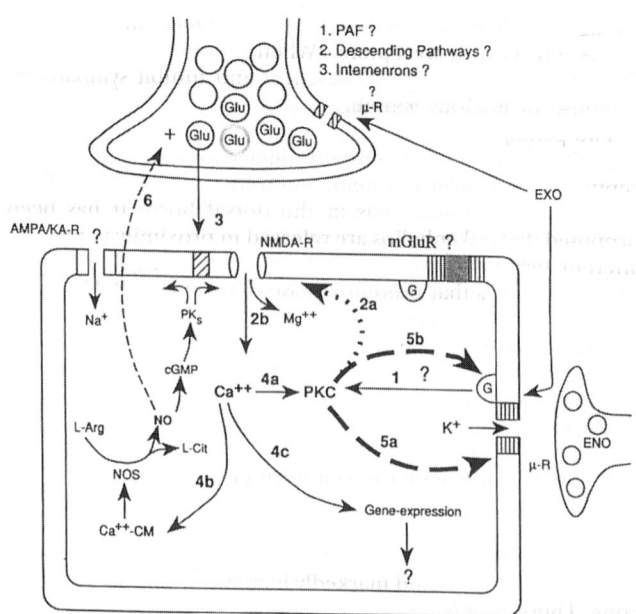

Figure 55-2. A spinal cord model of morphine tolerance. Postsynaptic opioid (μ) receptor occupation by an exogenous ligand such as morphine may initiate GTP binding protein-mediated kinase C (PKC) translocation and activation (*step 1*). PKC translocation/activation (*step 2a*) causes a removal of the Mg^{2+} blockade of the NMDA receptor (*step 2b*). With this blockade removed, even small amounts of EAA ligands, which could be released from presynaptic terminals of primary afferent fibers, supraspinal descending pathways, and/or spinal dorsal horn interneurons, could activate the NMDA receptor (*step 3*) and allow localized Ca^{2+} channel opening. An elevation of the intracellular Ca^{2+} level leads to activation of additional PKC (*step 4a*), production of NO via Ca^{2+}–calmodulin mediated activation of NO synthase (*step 4b*), as well as regulation of relevant gene expression (*step 4c*). PKC may then modulate μ-opioid activated, G-protein-coupled K^+ channels (*5a*) or uncouple the G-protein with the μ-opioid receptor (*5b*). In addition, NO may activate various protein kinases via cGMP and thus participates in the modulation of the μ-opioid activated, G-protein-coupled K^+ channels within the same cell. Perhaps more importantly, NO may diffuse out of the neuron enhancing presynaptic release of endogenous EAAs, resulting in a positive feedback (*step 6*). In this way, exogenous opiates may increase the basal level of presynaptic EAA release via the NO mechanism initiated by postsynaptic opioid action. This model suggests that morphine-induced presynaptic EAA release, postsynaptic NMDA receptor activation, and intracellular biochemical consequences are critical, and these factors operate in concert to result in the development of morphine tolerance. The role of presynaptic μ-opioid receptors in the development of morphine tolerance remains to be determined (see the text for a detailed discussion). Since many of the intracellular steps following the activation of the NMDA receptor in this proposed model of morphine tolerance are similar to those that occur following injury-induced hyperalgesia (see Fig. 55-1), it is conceivable that NMDA receptor–mediated intracellular changes initiated by exogenous opiate administration may also lead to the development of hyperalgesic states by means of increasing efficacy of the NMDA receptor–activated Na^+ channels and/or metabotropic EAA receptors. It is also likely that hyperalgesic states following the development of tolerance may contribute to signs of physical dependence in the process of opiate abstinence. Abbreviations not appearing in Fig. 55-1: μ-R = μ-opioid receptor; EXO = exogenous opiates; ENO, endogenous opioids. (From Mao J, Price DD, Mayer D: Mechanisms of hyperalgesia and morphine tolerance: A current view of their possible interactions. Pain 62:259, 1995.)

tion of nociceptive-specific and wide dynamic range neurons. The amino acids glycine and γ-aminobutyric acid (GABA) are known to be inhibitors of synaptic transmission, and there is some speculation that they are important mediators of segmental inhibition of nociception. There are two known GABA recognition sites: $GABA_A$, for which muscimol and isoguvacine are agonists, and $GABA_B$, for which baclofen is an agonist. Benzodiazepines act to enhance the effect of GABA on GABA$_A$ receptors. When administered spinally, they produce a mild analgesic effect and inhibit sympathetic response to noxious stimuli.

Two pentapeptides, leucine enkephalin and methionine enkephalin, appear to be important spinal cord inhibitors of nociception. STT neurons in laminae I and V receive input from enkephalin-containing cells in the dorsal horn. It has been proposed that enkephalins are released in proximity to primary afferent terminals in the dorsal horn, activating presynaptic opiate receptors that prevent release of substance P. However, the presence of direct synaptic contact between enkephalin-containing cells and STT neurons suggests that their inhibitory mechanism is, at least in part, postsynaptic. Enkephalins are found in highest concentrations in laminae I and II but are also present in deeper laminae. Most dorsal horn enkephalins originate from intrinsic neurons.

It is not clear whether dorsal horn enkephalins function in a tonic fashion or whether their activity is stimulated for the most part by descending or peripheral segmental activity. If there is significant tonic inhibition by enkephalins, administration of naloxone should markedly increase activity in STT neurons. There is only equivocal evidence for such disinhibition. Release of enkephalins in response to descending neural activity has not been well documented. There is, however, evidence of enkephalin release in response to segmental activity.[23]

Serotonin, or 5-hydroxytryptamine (5-HT) produces analgesia when injected intrathecally, and its antagonist methysergide attenuates the analgesia produced by certain pharmacologic interventions. It is likely that this neurotransmitter is involved in descending control mechanisms that originate in the midbrain and medulla. It has been speculated that the analgesic effect of some of the tricyclic antidepressants may be related to an increase in serotonin availability in the CNS. However, the class of antidepressants known as serotonin-specific reuptake inhibitors (SSRIs) appears to have little or no beneficial effect on those conditions that typically respond to tricyclics.

Norepinephrine is also an important neurotransmitter in descending inhibitory pathways. Spinally administered adrenergic agonists, such as epinephrine, have been shown to have analgesic effects in animals. This analgesic effect is mediated by α_2-adrenergic receptors. Evidence for this is provided by the fact that α_2 agonists such as clonidine and dexmedetomidine produce analgesia when injected spinally and that α_2 antagonists such as yohimbine and idazoxan block their analgesic effects. IT clonidine is now in use for the treatment of intractable cancer pain. It appears to be helpful in some opioid-tolerant patients.

Adenosine receptors appear to play a role in the modulation of nociceptive transmission in the dorsal horn. There are two receptor subtypes: A$_1$, which inhibits adenylcyclase activity, and A$_2$, which stimulates it.[24] Adenosine receptors may play a role in the analgesia provided by transcutaneous electrical stimulation, as it has been demonstrated that dorsal horn inhibition induced by high-frequency stimulation is blocked by methylxanthines, which antagonize adenosine receptor activity.[25] The adenosine receptor may also play a role in the mediation of analgesia induced by spinally administered opiates. Adenosine agonists have been shown to reduce the tactile hyperesthesia induced by low-dose spinal strychnine, a glycine receptor antagonist, and may prove to be effective in certain hyperalgesic states.

In summary, the dorsal horn functions as a relay center for nociceptive and other sensory activity. The degree of activation of ascending pain projection systems depends on the degree of activation of segmental and descending inhibitory neurons in the dorsal horn, the pre-existing concentration of excitatory neurotransmitters, the level of activation of inhibitory neurotransmitters, the intensity of the noxious stimulus, and the degree of sensitization of nociceptors in the periphery.

Ascending Pathways

The STT has been considered for many years to be the most important pathway transmitting nociceptive stimuli to the brain. Although it is important to normal perception of pain, it is by no means the only pathway with that function. The ability of patients to perceive pain following spinothalamic tractotomy provides evidence that other pathways are involved.

Many of the neurons in laminae I and V that respond to noxious stimulation are probably cells of origin of the STT. The majority of STT fibers cross near their level of origin. There are thought to be two functionally distinct divisions of the STT: the neospinothalamic tract, whose fibers tend to be more lateral, and the paleospinothalamic tract, located in the medial portion of the pathway. The phylogenetically newer neospinothalamic tract projects to posterior nuclei of the thalamus, such as the ventral posterolateral nucleus, and is thought to be involved with discriminative functions, *e.g.,* location, intensity, and duration of noxious stimulation.[26] The paleospinothalamic tract projects to medial thalamic nuclei, and its activation is probably associated with autonomic and unpleasant emotional aspects of pain. This older portion of the STT is likely to be important in pain associated with denervation dysesthesia. Stimulation of the thalamic projections of the paleospinothalamic tract in patients with denervation dysesthesia reproduces the burning pain these patients experience spontaneously.[27]

The spinoreticular tract is likely to play a role in pain perception. Its cells of origin are unknown. It is thought to produce arousal associated with pain perception and probably contributes to neural activity underlying motivational, affective, and autonomic responses to pain.[28] The spinomesencephalic tract projects to the midbrain reticular formation. It probably evokes nondiscriminative painful sensations and may be important in the activation of descending antinociceptive pathways.[28]

Following bilateral spinothalamic tractotomy, it is still possible for patients to perceive pain from peripheral stimulation. There must necessarily be pathways in the dorsal portions of the spinal cord that are capable of producing pain perception. The spinocervical tract is a likely candidate for such a function. It is located in the dorsolateral funiculus. Its fibers ascend uncrossed to the lateral cervical nucleus, which serves as a relay, sending fibers to the contralateral thalamus.[28] There is also evidence that some fibers in the dorsal columns are responsive to noxious stimuli.

Descending Control

In the early 1970s several reports showed that electrical stimulation of the periaqueductal gray (PAG) area of the midbrain could produce widespread analgesia in animals and humans. The PAG was later found to have high concentrations of endogenous opiates and to be rich in opiate receptors. Microinjection of small quantities of morphine into that area produces generalized analgesia. Anatomic connections from the PAG area to the nucleus raphe magnus and to the medullary reticular formation were subsequently described. From the nucleus raphe magnus, serotoninergic fibers descend via the dorsolateral funiculus to spinal cord dorsal horn cells. It is not clear whether serotoninergic fibers produce a direct, postsynaptic inhibition of STT neurons or whether they act by activation of inhibitory neurons that release enkephalins or GABA.

There are also adrenergic fibers that descend in the dorsolateral funiculus that are thought to be inhibitors of pain. The cells of origin of these descending adrenergic pathways are believed to lie in the locus ceruleus and parabrachial regions of the medulla. Stimulation of spinal α_2-adrenergic receptors produces analgesia through G-protein–mediated K$^+$ channel activation.

Multiple environmental factors appear to activate descending pain control mechanisms. Nociceptive inputs and various types of stress can produce generalized increases in pain threshold. Anxiety, depression, and emotional distress can reduce pain threshold. The descending control mechanisms described may respond to such factors. Under normal circumstances, inhibitory and pronociceptive neurons located in the midbrain periaqeductal gray rostral ventromedial medulla (RVM) play an important role in integrating and coordinating behavioral and autonomic responses to noxious stimuli.[29] Following a brief noxious stimulus, certain cells, known as "off-cells," in the RVM abruptly cease firing. It is thought that these cells produce tonic inhibition of nociceptive reflexes, and their cessation is associated with loss of such inhibition. Other cells, known as "on-cells," show a sudden burst of activity just before a behavioral response to a noxious stimulus. Their activation appears to produce a facilitatory influence on nociceptive transmission. At least some on-cells are GABAergic and exert an inhibitory influence on descending inhibitory neurons, including off-cells. On-cell activity is inhibited by local application of opioids, which block their inhibitory effect on pain-inhibitory pathways.

Pain and Nerve Injury

Spontaneous discharge of injured peripheral nerves was demonstrated by Wall and Gutnick,[30] who reported spontaneous neural activity originating from experimentally induced neuromas. It was later demonstrated that sympathetic stimulation or norepinephrine infusion could increase such abnormal firing.[31] There is now considerable evidence that changes in ion channel configuration and distribution are responsible for functional changes in the behavior of injured axons. Following nerve injury, there is an increase in the occurrence of large intramembranous particles, which represent surface proteins such as receptors and channel proteins. In addition, the membrane properties of a regenerating nerve tip differ from those of intact nerves. There is disappearance of the sodium-dependent action potential and an increase in in conductance to Na^+, K^+, and Ca^{2+}.[32]

In addition to impulse generation originating from the site of injury, there is considerable evidence that impulse generation occurs at points of membrane instability proximal to the injury. Wall and Devor[33] reported spontaneous discharge originating from dorsal root ganglia in sciatic nerve–sectioned rats. They proposed that the dorsal root ganglia impulses could contribute to pain after peripheral nerve injury.

Another possible mechanism for chronic pain following peripheral nerve lesions involves the short-circuiting of action potentials (ephaptic transmission, cross-talk) across demyelinated segments. Several possible types of interaction might exist. Demyelination of large afferent fibers could cause activation of nociceptors at the site of injury in response to stimulation of mechanoreceptors by non-noxious stimuli. Injury of motor fibers could cause nociceptor activation in response to motoneuron activation. Loss of Schwann cell protection of postganglionic sympathetics could produce nociceptor firing in response to sympathetic discharge.

Intact peripheral nerve pathways are essential for normal function of pain projection neurons and inhibitory interneurons in the dorsal horn. Following loss of peripheral nerve activity, there may be an increase in sensitivity or onset of spontaneous activity in STT neurons. It has been postulated that disruption of large afferents, which send extensive arborizations into the substantia gelatinosa, decreases the activity of inhibitory neurons in those areas.

Spontaneous activity or heightened sensitivity of neurons is thought to occur at more central locations within the pain projection system as well. Thalamic cells may undergo such changes following cord injury or some cerebrovascular accidents. Sensitization of central neurons may also occur some time after peripheral nerve injuries.

Sympathetically Maintained Pain

There are several mechanisms by which the sympathetic nervous system influences the perception of pain. Interactions between sympathetic outflow and spontaneous depolarization of injured nerve segments have already been discussed. Following trauma, surgery, and certain illnesses, a syndrome of pain, hyperalgesia, autonomic dysfunction, and dystrophy, known as complex regional pain syndrome (CRPS), can occur. A common explanation is that there is interference with the normal regulatory function of the sympathetics to the affected area induced by pain or injury, hence the former name of the syndrome, reflex sympathetic dystrophy (RSD). Periods of heightened sympathetic activity are thought to result in vasoconstriction, ischemia, changes in interstitial environment, and, perhaps, release of prostaglandins, bradykinin, and other pain-sensitizing substances. This explanation is highly simplistic and is contradicted by several clinical findings: (1) early in the course of the syndrome the affected limb is usually warm and erythematous, (2) microneurographic recording studies have failed to demonstrate alterations in sympathetic outflow in the affected limb, and (3) venous catecholamine levels in the affected limb are not elevated. There may be central dysregulation of autonomic function in these patients, however. Experimental evidence for interference with sympathetic regulatory function following injury was provided by Blumberg and Janig,[34] who demonstrated loss of the normal reciprocity between skin and muscle vasoconstrictors in animals with peripheral nerve lesions. Skin vasoconstrictors are normally under the influence of hypothalamic centers. They are important in thermoregulation and tend to be inhibited by stimuli that activate muscle vasoconstrictors, which are under medullary control. Following peroneal nerve lesions, skin vasoconstrictors begin to respond like muscle vasoconstrictors and appear to be under medullary control.[34]

Another possible interaction between sympathetic activity and pain perception involves ephaptic transmission, or "cross-talk," between different fiber types at injured nerve segments. Segmental loss of myelin or protective Schwann cell sheaths could lead to depolarization of nociceptor fibers by efferent sympathetic transmission. Although such segmental demyelination has been demonstrated anatomically, physiologic evidence for the phenomenon is scant.

Another proposal is the direct sensitization of nociceptor nerve endings by sympathetic nerve terminals. Again, there is little evidence that such nociceptor sensitization occurs. There is, however, considerable evidence that sympathetic fibers are in direct contact with mechanoreceptors and that sympathetic activity can sensitize mechanosensitive afferents. Roberts[35] has proposed that a combination of sensitization of mechanoreceptors plus disinhibition of wide dynamic range neurons could occur in certain post-traumatic states. Such a situation would lead to high-frequency firing of STT neurons and pain perception in response to non-noxious mechanical stimulation.

Several studies have demonstrated sprouting of sympathetic neurons following nerve injury. These neurons, which are not normally present in the dorsal root ganglion, invade this structure to form elaborate arborizations, known as baskets, surrounding neuronal cell bodies.[36] It is not known as yet whether there is synaptic contact between the sympathetic fibers and the cell bodies, nor have the types of afferents whose somata are invaded by sympathetic sprouts been characterized. Nerve growth factor (NGF) and the cytokines leukemia inhibitor factor (LIF) and interleukin 6 (IL-6) appear to contribute to the initiation of sympathetic sprouting. There is considerable speculation, though so far no proof, that the interactions between sympathetic sprouts and DRG cell bodies is responsible in part for sympathetically maintained pain in some clinical states.

PSYCHOLOGICAL MECHANISMS

No discussion of chronic pain is complete without some consideration of the psychological factors that are related to pain. In 1986, the International Association for the Study of Pain published a taxonomy of pain-related terms to promote uniformity of usage and to enhance accurate reporting of clinical and experimental phenomena.[37] Pain was defined as "an unpleasant sensory and emotional experience associated with actual or potential tissue damage, or described in terms of such damage." The salient features of that definition are that (1) pain is unpleasant, which is no surprise to most; (2) it may have a sensory component, also not surprising; (3) it has an emotional component, which distinguishes it from other sensory experiences such as touch, pressure, and vibration; and, most importantly, (4) it is an experience and, as such, is subjective, personal, private, and verifiable only by report of the individual suspected of suffering from pain. This last point cannot be overemphasized. While much of what a physician does when dealing with pain patients is objectively verifiable by monitors, touch, or direct vision, these clinical tools only allow us to make inferences about another's suffering. The gold standard for determining if a patient is in pain is to ask the patient if he or she hurts. Other observations may aid in formulating a diagnostic impression, but only the patient can tell you if he or she has pain.

Psychological mechanisms can contribute to the pain experience in two general ways. A direct influence is exemplified by a situation in which psychological factors are entirely the cause of a report of pain. An example of this is psychogenic pain, which is considered to be rare. The psychological construct that is invoked to explain this involves the production of a perception of pain as a result of purely psychological factors, such as the need to suffer, as a means of assuaging guilt, or as a way to resolve some other intrapsychic conflict. This type of condition does exist but is frequently overdiagnosed. In fact, the likelihood of diagnosing psychogenic pain is inversely proportional to the skill and expertise of the physician examining the patient. The histories of these patients present no clear patterns or similarities, making a neat diagnostic algorithm impossible. Dramatic presentations or, conversely, apparent indifference, are not pathognomonic.[38]

Other direct psychological influences are found in the somatization disorders. These are a group of psychiatric disorders that are typified by a preoccupation with bodily function or symptoms.[39] Hypochondriasis is a condition in which the individual is preoccupied with the notion that he or she is sick, despite continual reassurance from physicians. The exact psychological mechanism is not well understood, but this condition should be treated by a psychologist or psychiatrist. In suspecting this diagnosis, it is wise to remember that the term arose from patients describing pain below the right costal margin (hypochondriac) at a time when cholecystitis was not recognized as a bona fide medical entity. Patients with fears or convictions that they are ill do, on occasion, turn out to be right,[40] so a careful history and physical examination coupled with performance of clearly indicated tests is advisable.

Somatization disorder is characterized by an onset of physical symptoms before the age of 30 years and includes at least 12 (for men) or 14 (for women) of 37 symptoms involving various organ systems. These symptoms are of sufficient severity to cause the individual to seek medical attention, to take medicines, or to otherwise alter his or her lifestyle. These patients typically have undergone extensive investigations, usually from multiple physicians, all of which have yielded negative, equivocal, or conflicting results. Frequent surgeries, usually of an exploratory nature, are a common historical feature. These features are superimposed on any genuine somatic diseases suffered by the person, presenting a complex clinical picture. The mechanism

for this disorder is not proved, but it is suspected that these persons come from families in which little credence or attention is given to display of emotion, yet care and attention are provided in response to physical symptoms. Thus, the theory goes, the patient learns that the exhibition of a physical symptom results in attention to the patient's needs. This modus operandi becomes ingrained on a subconscious level and then becomes part of the person's psychic constitution. This condition is not nearly so rare as psychogenic pain and, therefore, is likely to be seen with some frequency by a physician treating patients presenting with pain.

Factitious disorders (Munchausen's syndrome) present with reporting of symptoms and the intentional creation of signs that are intended to lead a physician to suspect a medical or surgical disorder. Patients have been known to instrument their urethra to cause hematuria and complain of flank pain or to use tourniquets to induce edema of the limb. The motivation for this behavior appears to be to occupy the role of a patient. The reasons for this goal are poorly understood.

Another similar condition is malingering, which is differentiated only by motivation. In this case, the motivation to assume the role of a patient is driven by the wish to avoid some other alternative that the individual feels is distasteful, such as military service or apprehension by the police, or to achieve financial gain. Fortunately, these charades are usually transparent to the astute physician. The incidence of this disorder in pain clinics is probably low.

Indirect psychological effects that influence the pain experience are common in chronic pain syndromes. At its most basic level, the presence of an ongoing nociceptive process that is not well relieved and produces continual suffering is bound to have some psychological sequelae that will color the whole pain experience. Such secondary effects as sleep deprivation, fatigue, irritability, and anger are commonly observed.[41]

The issue of depression and pain has been discussed by several authors.[38,42,43] It is not surprising that most patients with chronic pain are likely to show signs of depression. It is difficult at times, however, to clarify the distinction between a set of depressive features that are reactive to having chronic pain and an episode of major depression because there can be so much overlap in symptoms.[43] The Diagnostic and Statistical Manual of Mental Diseases[39] includes many somatic and related symptoms in its criteria for diagnosing major depression. Most chronic pain patients will have several of these, but the genesis of the symptom (e.g., insomnia) may be due to the pain itself rather than depression. It is clear, however, that a negative affective state such as depression serves to enhance the suffering of a person with chronic pain.

Another indirect influence is that of pain behavior. Pilowsky et al[44] have described the concept of illness behavior as it applies to pain patients. Simply stated, an illness is the individual's reaction or response to a disease. Illness behaviors arise from the patient's underlying physical condition and may consist of active behaviors, such as taking pills and visiting physicians, or passive behaviors, such as not working and lying down or sitting much of the day. In many chronic pain patients the illness behaviors must become a focus of treatment.

Behaviors of any type are subject to influence by operant factors.[45] Operant conditioning states that the likelihood of a behavior being expressed in a given situation can be altered by the consequences of the behavior. In chronic pain, for example, pain behavior (moaning) may be unwittingly reinforced by a spouse (showing attention), resulting in an increased frequency of the behavioral expression in the presence of the spouse. This is an example of positive reinforcement. By rewarding the behavior, its frequency is increased. The term secondary gain is often used to describe the type of paradigm wherein the individual, despite suffering with pain, does receive some benefit from it. Negative reinforcement increases the frequency of the behavior by removing a noxious condition from the environment in response to the behavior. Avoiding taking the garbage out by complaining of back pain is an example. Punishment, or the provision of undesirable consequences in response to a behavior, and extinction, the provision of no consequences, lead to decreased frequency of a behavior.

Cognitive factors also influence a pain experience. The belief that a person has about the meaning of his or her pain can substantially alter the actual perception of the pain. An important issue in this regard is the perceived degree of control over the pain. Using this fact, it is common practice for dentists to tell patients to raise their finger if anything hurts during the procedure. This granting of control allows patients to tolerate procedures with greater comfort. Contrast this with a patient suffering from poorly controlled cancer. Here, every time a pain is experienced, it reminds the patient of the cancer and the likelihood of an imminent and probably painful death.

MANAGEMENT OF COMMON CHRONIC PAIN SYNDROMES

It is beyond the scope of this chapter to consider the entire spectrum of long-term pain problems. Instead, the medical management of several painful conditions that are likely to respond to regional analgesic techniques or other modalities that anesthesiologists are likely to use are discussed. In addition, this section presents, in general terms, the use of some pharmacologic agents that are helpful in certain pain syndromes and gives a brief overview of the psychological principles that are important in managing chronic pain.

Low Back Pain

Several low back structures are innervated by nociceptors and act as sources of pain under certain pathologic conditions. The outer third of the annulus of the intervertebral disk has sensory innervation. Pain associated with annular tears is generally thought of as occurring only in the back; but during discography, distension of the annulus commonly produces pain in the thigh and lower leg.[46] There is also evidence that, in the presence of chronic degenerative or inflammatory conditions, the vertebral bodies and vertebral endplates may become sources of pain.[47] Facet joints receive sensory innervation and, particularly if there are inflammatory changes in the joint, mechanical stimulation or injection of the joint may result in pain which may be localized to the back or may radiate to the buttock, thigh, and lower leg. A study using saline-controlled diagnostic local anesthetic injections of the facet joint indicated that in 40% of patients the facet joint was a source of low back pain.[48] Similarly, the sacroiliac joint is a source of pain in some patients, and injection of the joint reproduces back and lower extremity pain in some patients who have evidence of SI joint pathology. Using a rigorous paradigm requiring pain relief after two separate joint injections, Maigne et al[49] concluded that only 20% of patients with clinical symptoms compatible with sacroiliac arthropathy had pain of sacroiliac joint origin. Mechanical compression or traction on a normal nerve root produces painless paresthesias. However, similar stimulation of a chronically injured or inflamed nerve root produces sciatica, or pain in the normal sensory distribution of that nerve root.[50]

Lumbosacral Radiculopathy

Mechanical nerve root compression was originally presumed to be the cause of pain in discogenic radiculopathy. The lack of uniform success with surgical decompression and the fact that many asymptomatic patients demonstrate substantial disk protrusion on myelography or on subsequent postmortem examination suggests that other mechanisms must be operative as well. Following a period of mechanical nerve root compression, an acute inflammatory process may ensue, leading to intraneural accumulation of serum proteins and fluid, raised intraneural

pressure, ischemia, and axonal degeneration.[51] There is considerable evidence that the contents of the intervertebral disk can produce severe inflammation in the spinal canal. Gertzbein et al[52] found that patients with lumbar disk disease in which sequestration of nucleus pulposus occurred were highly likely to exhibit cellular immune responses to homogenates of lumbar disk material, whereas patients who did not show sequestration were less likely to show such a response. These findings led the authors to propose an inflammatory autoimmune mechanism for the radicular pain associated with disk rupture. Marshall and Trethwie[53] were able to demonstrate the production of antibodies to glycoproteins from nucleus pulposus among patients who suffered from acute lumbar disk disease. They also demonstrated severe inflammatory reaction to nuclear glycroproteins following pulmonary arterial injection in a guinea pig heart–lung preparation.

A different line of evidence for the development of inflammation in response to disk rupture was presented by Saal et al.[54] They collected human disk samples removed at surgery from patients with symptomatic radiculopathy and analyzed the material for PLA_2 activity. They found extremely high levels in this material, 20- to 100-fold higher than activity from human inflammatory synovial effusion. They conclude that the high PLA_2 activity leads to inflammation at the site of disk herniation by action of the enzyme to liberate arachidonic acid from cell membranes.

Cytokines, including interleukins, nerve growth factor (NGF), interferons, and tumor necrosis factor (TNF-α), are thought to play an important role in the pathophysiology of radiculopathic pain. Intrathecal administration of the interleukin IL-6 can produce touch-evoked allodynia in rats, and substances that block the effects of TNF-α are capable of blocking the hyperalgesic effect of experimental mononeuropathy or endotoxin.[55]

It has been proposed that epidural or subarachnoid injection of corticosteroids provides beneficial effects by reducing the inflammation initiated by either mechanical or chemical insult to the nerve root.[57] The earliest use of epidural steroids was published by Lievre et al[56] in 1957, who reported good to excellent results in 50% of patients following injection of cortisone acetate plus radiographic dye. Most subsequent series of epidural steroid injections used a combination of local anesthetic and suspensions of insoluble steroids. To determine whether local anesthetic alone provided benefit for patients with sciatica, Coomes[58] compared patients receiving bed rest plus epidural injections of procaine with patients treated with bed rest alone. He found that patients treated with procaine became ambulatory in 11 days, while it took the noninjected patients an average of 31 days to regain ambulation. Swerdlow and Sayle-Creer,[59] in a nonrandomized study, found consistently better results among chronic pain patients treated with epidural lidocaine and methylprednisolone than for patients treated with epidural saline or lidocaine injections. There was no difference in success rates among the three treatment groups for patients with acute or recurrent sciatica. Winnie et al[60] compared patients treated with epidural methylprednisolone with patients treated with local anesthetic combined with the steroid. Success was close to 100% in both groups, suggesting that the steroid, rather than the local anesthetic, was providing the benefit.

Reports on more than 7000 patients appear in the English language literature attesting to the beneficial effects of epidural steroid injections for the treatment of sciatica. However, while there have been anecdotal reports or noncontrolled case series attesting to the beneficial effect of epidural steroids in several thousand patients, only thirteen controlled, randomized studies of the use of caudal or lumbar epidural steroid injections have been published. Koes et al[61] found that more than half of these controlled studies had substantial methodologic flaws. Of four studies that had reasonable methodologies, two reported positive (beneficial) results and two reported negative results. Watts and Silagy[62] performed a meta-analysis of nearly the same group of studies (11 randomized studies with 907 patients). In assessing the rate of treatment success, defined as >75% improvement for up to 60 days, they found the odds ratio for success in the steroid treatment group to be 2.61 (95% CI 1.90–3.77). For long-term (>12 months) treatment success, the odds ratio for the steroid treatment group was 1.87 (95% CI 1.31–2.68). There was no significant difference in outcomes between the caudal and lumbar route of injection. A more recent controlled study, not included in either of the above reviews, compared epidural methylprednisolone acetate to epidural saline.[63] The steroid-treated group experienced more improvement in sensory function and flexibility, but only at the three-week assessment.

Few studies have evaluated the long-term effects of epidural steroids. Abram and Hopwood[64] compared the long-term responses of patients who initially experienced a favorable response to epidural steroid injections to those of patients who were considered treatment failures. After 6 months, patients in the initial success group were significantly more likely to rate their pain level lower, had significantly less sleep disruption, and were significantly less likely to be unemployed as a result of their pain when compared with initial failure patients.

The L5 and S1 nerve roots are most commonly affected by disk disease. Those roots pass through a narrow lateral bony recess as they exit the spinal canal, a circumstance that increases the likelihood of root compression.[65] Symptoms of lumbosacral radiculopathy consist of varying degrees of low back pain, pain radiating a varying distance into the lower extremity, and, in more severe cases, motor and sensory loss consistent with damage to the affected root. Typical signs and symptoms are listed in Table 55-1. As noted above, the pain typically associated with nerve root pathology is often in the same distribution as pain associated with lumbosacral or facet arthropathy or with annular tears without nerve root pathology. The presence of sciatic stretch signs (positive straight leg raising, Lasegue's sign) or single segment sensory, motor, or reflex changes increase the likelihood that the pain is related to radiculopathy.

If bowel and bladder dysfunction are present, indicative of a large midline disk, prompt surgical intervention may be indicated. Otherwise, initial treatment of acute discogenic radiculopathy consists of short periods (a few days) of immobilization and mild analgesics followed by gradual resumption in physical activity. Prolonged immobilization has been shown to be counterproductive. If severe pain persists after reasonable trials of conservative management, epidural steroids may be used.

Triamcinolone diacetate or methylprednisolone acetate are the most commonly used preparations. Injections are generally performed as close to the affected nerve root as possible. Addition of a small volume (3–4 ml) of local anesthetic will produce considerable analgesia if it reaches the affected nerve root,

confirming proper drug placement. In occasional patients, particularly those with S1 pathology, the drug will not spread adequately to the affected root. In that situation, caudal injection may result in better drug access to the injured nerve. Likewise, caudal introduction of a radioopaque catheter, advanced under fluoroscopic control to the appropriate neural foramen, may provide a better result. Reassessment should be carried out 1–2 weeks after the initial treatment. If the patient has little or no pain at the time of the return visit, repeating the injection is relatively unlikely to be of benefit. However, if it was felt that the drug may not have reached the affected root at the time of the initial injection, a repeat procedure is a reasonable option. If symptoms are improved at the time of the follow-up visit, but some pain is still present, it is likely that a repeat injection will produce further improvement. A third block can be performed 1–2 weeks later if some symptoms persist. An algorithm for epidural steroid treatment is shown in Figure 55-3.

There appears to be extremely little risk of serious complications associated with the use of epidural steroid injections. Animal studies tend to confirm the safety of neuraxial administration of depo steroids.[66,67] Allegations that the 3% polyethylene glycol vehicle of methylprednisolone acetate (MPA) and triamcinolone diacetate (TD) is capable of producing neurologic damage[68] are based on studies of high concentrations of propylene glycol (80–100%) and appear to be unfounded. The doses of corticosteroids commonly used for the treatment of sciatica are capable of producing adrenal suppression for up to several weeks, and there are occasional reports of cushingoid side-effects, sometimes lasting for weeks or longer. For example, a single injection of triamcinolone into the epidural space for the treatment of low back pain in adult patients has been shown to acutely suppress the hypothalamic–pituitary–adrenal (HPA) axis as reflected by decreased plasma cortisol and adrenocorticotrophic hormone levels in response to a provocative stimulus.[69] When three epidural triamcinolone injections were administered at 7-day intervals, the median suppression of the HPA axis was less than 1 month following the last injection and all patients had recovered by 3 months. Sedation with midazolam in conjunction with the epidural steroid injection accentuates the suppression of the HPA axis.[69] These observations suggest the possible need for exogenous steroid coverage in patients undergoing major stress during the period that the HPA axis may be suppressed by epidural steroids. Epidural steroid injections should be used with caution in diabetic patients, who may be at added risk for epidural infections, and whose glucose control may be compromised. Because of the immunosuppression associated with the steroid, aseptic technique should be meticulous.

Most of the literature documenting the safety of epidural steroids comes from reports on the use of a small number of injections, usually one to three, and with modest doses, usually 40–80 mg MPA or 50 mg TD. There are few data to support

Table 55-1. PAIN DISTRIBUTION AND PHYSICAL SIGNS ASSOCIATED WITH ACUTE DISK HERNIATION

Level of Herniation	Pain Distribution	Numbness	Weakness	Reflex Changes
L3–4 disk (L4 root)	Low back, buttock, lateral thigh, anterior calf, ankle, and occasionally big toe	Lower anterior thigh and patella	Mid (quadriceps)	Diminished (knee jerk)
L4–5 disk (L5 root)	Low back, buttock, lateral thigh, calf, ankle, big toe	Lateral calf, web space of first and second toe	Foot (dorsiflexion)	None
L5–S1 disk (S1 root)	Low back, buttock, posterior thigh, and calf	Posterior calf, lateral heel, and foot	Foot (plantar flexion)	Diminished or absent (ankle jerk)

Reprinted with permission from Abram SE: Management of pain. In Cottrell JE, Turndorf H (eds): Anesthesia and Neurosurgery, p 496. St Louis, CV Mosby, 1986.

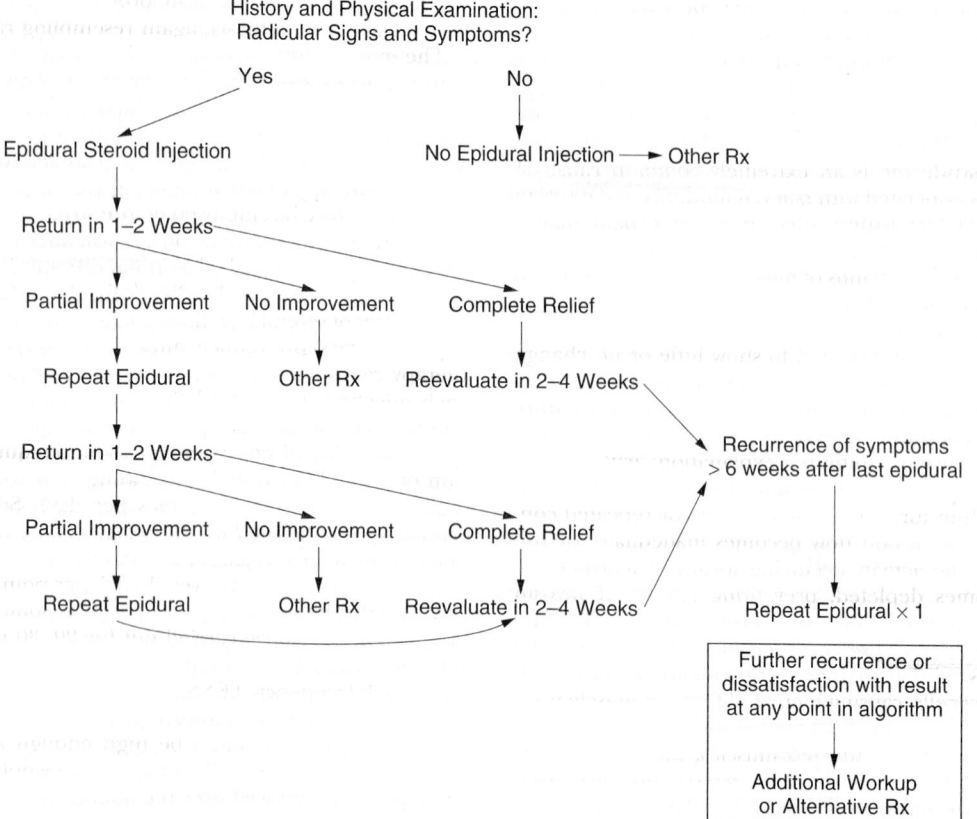

Figure 55-3. Algorithm for treatment of sciatica with epidural steroid injections.

the safety of this treatment when higher doses are used or when treatment is extended beyond 3 or 4 injections over a period of several weeks.

There is some evidence that complications can occur following IT steroid injections. Aseptic meningitis[70] and bacterial meningitis[71] appear to be uncommon but real risks. Arachnoiditis[72] and cauda equina syndrome[73] have been reported, but these cases are rare and have occurred after multiple injections over a prolonged time interval. Nevertheless, some physicians are using a test dose of local anesthetic prior to injection of steroid in order to rule out intrathecal placement of the needle.

Patients with chronic radicular low back pain are much less likely to benefit from epidural steroid injections than are patients with more acute symptoms. Abram and Anderson[74] reported in a retrospective study that patients with long-standing symptoms were much less likely to experience even transient relief from epidural steroid injections. Similar findings were seen in a subsequent prospective study.[64] Patients who had undergone previous back surgery also had a much lower success rate. Several mechanisms may lead to chronic radicular pain that is unresponsive to steroid injections. Spontaneous activity or ephaptic transmission may occur from the injured, demyelinated root. Scarring of the root, with replacement of neural elements with fibrous tissue, causes inelasticity of the nerve. The nerve root can no longer stretch with leg motion, and chronic mechanical irritation ensues.[51] Loss of large afferent fibers may lead to disruption of dorsal horn gating mechanisms and disinhibition of spinothalamic projection cells. Loss of disk height following herniation can lead to narrowing of intervertebral foramina, with subsequent root irritation laterally, or may cause redundancy and buckling of the posterior longitudinal ligament, which can effectively narrow the spinal canal. Loss of disk height can lead to facet joint subluxation and degeneration, producing pain from the joint itself and to osteophyte formation, which can narrow foramina or the central canal. Injury

to the vertebral plate, the cartilaginous portion of the vertebral body adjacent to the disk, often accompanies disk disease and may lead to osteophytic growth into the central canal.

Lumbosacral Arthropathies

Degeneration and inflammation of the lumbar facet joints and sacroiliac joints can produce low back pain that is often difficult to distinguish from radicular pain. Both conditions may cause pain that radiates to the lower extremities. Computed tomographic scanning is a fairly reliable method of demonstrating pathology in these joints.[75,76] Bone scans, particularly single-photon emission computed tomography (SPECT) scanning, may also be useful diagnostically.

When facet arthropathy is the suspected cause of low back pain, the diagnosis can be confirmed by injection of local anesthetic into the facet joint. The procedure can be done easily under fluoroscopic control. The patient is placed prone and the affected side is tilted upward until the joint space is visualized (Fig. 55-4). Proper needle placement can be confirmed by injection of 0.5–1 ml of nonionic contrast. The injection should transiently reproduce the patient's pain, and the dye will outline the extent of the capsule. Injection of 1 ml of local anesthetic should produce dramatic relief of arthropathic pain. Injection of a small volume of insoluble corticosteroid into an affected joint has been reported to produce analgesia lasting 6 months or longer in about one third of patients who experience relief from the local anesthetic. Nonsteroidal anti-inflammatory drugs may be of some benefit.

When sacroiliac pathology is demonstrated, injection of the joint with local anesthetic will help confirm the diagnosis. In an uncontrolled study, we found that 25 of 35 patients with suspected sacroiliac disease experienced pain relief from local anesthetic injection of the joint. After injection of triamcinolone diacetate, 7 of 20 patients who were followed long-term experienced at least 6 months of moderate to complete pain relief

(Abram SE, unpublished data). As noted previously, a more rigorous local anesthetic treatment paradigm showed only a 20% response to local anesthetic injection.[49]

Myofascial Pain

The myofascial syndrome is an extremely common cause of somatic pain. It is associated with marked tenderness of discrete points (trigger points) within affected muscles, pain that is referred to areas some distance from the trigger point, and the appearance of tight, ropy bands of muscle. Autonomic changes, such as vasoconstriction and skin conductivity changes, may occur some distance from the affected muscle.[77] Biopsies of trigger points have been reported to show little or no change or to show degenerative changes, the severity of which corresponds to the intensity of the symptoms.[77] Although the pathophysiology of the condition has not been clearly defined, Travell and Simons[77] propose the following explanation: acute muscle strain causes disruption of sarcoplasmic reticulum and release of calcium, which in turn produces sustained or repeated contraction and fatigue. Blood flow becomes inadequate for the degree of metabolic activity occurring locally. Adenosine triphosphate becomes depleted, preventing release of myosin from actin, causing sarcomeres to become rigid and affected muscles to become taut. Nociceptor-sensitizing substances, such as prostaglandins, bradykinin, and serotonin, are released from platelets and mast cells, causing increased firing of muscle nociceptors.

Many of the commonly affected muscles, the sites of their trigger points, and their zones of referred pain have been mapped out.[78] The scapulocostal syndrome, one of the most common patterns of myofascial pain, is characterized by a trigger point located just medial and superior to the upper portion of the scapula and pain that can radiate to the occipital region, shoulder, medial aspect of the arm, or anterior chest wall.[79] Myofascial pain involving gluteal muscles produces pain referred into the posterior thigh and calf, mimicking S1 radiculopathy. Myofascial pain involving the piriformis muscle, which overlies the sciatic nerve, can produce sciatic irritation and, occasionally, hypoesthesia, again resembling radiculopathy.

The most important aspect of treatment for myofascial pain is to regain muscle length and elasticity. This is best done by maneuvers that gently stretch affected muscles. Because of the sensitization of muscle afferents, appropriate physical therapeutic maneuvers are often painful and may reinitiate muscle contraction. Therapy aimed at reducing muscle pain and sensitivity should therefore be employed before stretching exercises. Trigger point injection, infiltration of local anesthetic directly into the trigger point, is a valuable initial therapy. Pain relief following injection confirms the diagnosis of myofascial syndrome, and a series of several injections performed daily or every several days can markedly reduce muscle sensitivity. Fairly vigorous therapy can be carried out during the analgesic period after each injection. Ultrasound therapy applied over the affected muscle may also produce periods of analgesia.

Trigger point injections and ultrasound require the participation of trained personnel, precluding their use on a frequent regular basis (*e.g.*, several times per day). Several treatment modalities can be used by the patient alone or with the help of family members. Transcutaneous electrical nerve stimulation (TENS), applied directly over the trigger points, may produce analgesia during stimulation and often for some time afterward. Stimulation should be carried out for 20–30 minutes prior to stretching exercises. Some patients who do not respond to the usual high-frequency TENS may benefit from a brief period (about 5–10 minutes) of low-frequency (2–4 Hz) high-intensity TENS. The current should be high enough to cause muscle contraction and mild discomfort. Vapocoolant spray (*e.g.*, fluorimethane) sprayed over the affected muscle may produce transient analgesia sufficient to facilitate physical therapy. Massage of the affected muscle with ice may also be of some benefit.

Injection of myofascial trigger points with botulinum toxin, which produces a long-lasting block of acetylcholine release from peripheral nerves, has been shown to provide lasting pain relief in myofascial syndrome.[80] Pain relief begins within one to several days after injection and generally lasts several weeks. The principal side-effect is weakness in the injected and adjacent muscles.

Myofascial pain often develops in patients whose response to stress is an increase in muscle tone. This mechanism frequently contributes to the pathophysiology of tension headache. Surface measurement of electromyography in such patients will often demonstrate extremely high activity at rest. Electromyographic biofeedback is a useful added therapy for such patients and appears to be helpful in preventing future painful episodes for patients with recurrent problems.

Complex Regional Pain Syndromes

The term *reflex sympathetic dystrophy* (RSD) has been widely used to describe a group of conditions associated with burning pain in an extremity, dystrophic changes in skin, hair, nails and joints, allodynia, and signs of autonomic dysfunction, including skin temperature changes and alterations of sweat gland activity. The term *causalgia* has been used to describe a syndrome with similar clinical features following injury to a major nerve trunk. The term *sympathetically maintained pain* (SMP) has been used synonymously with both of these syndromes, implying that the autonomic nervous system is somehow involved in the pathophysiology of these conditions. While autonomic dysfunction is clearly evident in some cases of causalgia and RSD, it is not a prominent feature in some cases, and many patients with these conditions fail to respond to blockade or ablation of sympathetic fibers. Therefore, the term *complex regional pain syndrome* (CRPS) has become widely accepted.[81] Complex regional pain syndrome type I (CRPS-I) is the term that has replaced the term RSD, and CRPS-II is now used in place of the term causalgia. The term *sympathetically maintained pain* describes

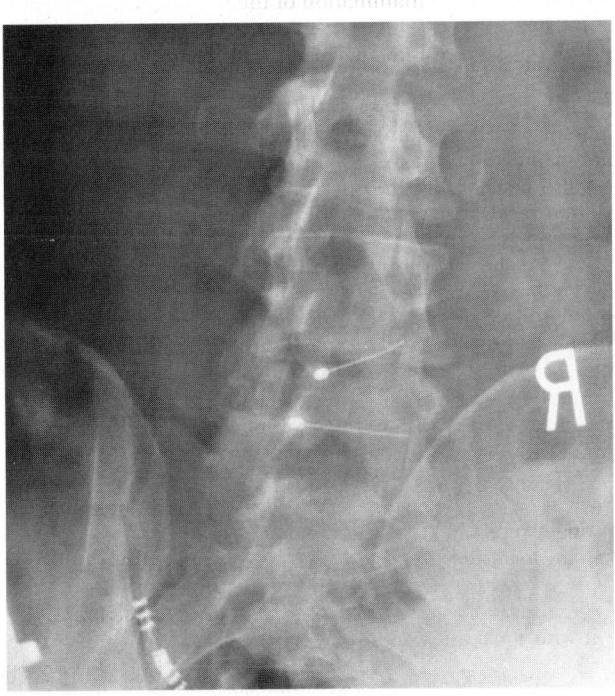

Figure 55-4. Right L4–5 and L5–S1 facet injections. Note the slight bending of needle at the L4–5 level, which is typical when the needle lies within the joint space.

that component of pain that is initiated or maintained by activity in the sympathetic nervous system, including both efferent sympathetic nervous system activity and circulating catecholamines. Painful conditions that are not typical of CRPS may have a sympathetically mediated component. Patients with certain types of neuropathic pain do not exhibit the typical clinical features of CRPS and yet experience significant pain relief following sympathetic blockade. Likewise, some patients with typical features of CRPS experience no relief from sympathetic denervation. Pain that does not appear to be sympathetically mediated is termed *sympathetically independent pain* (SIP).

CRPS-I

Common antecedents to the development of this syndrome include crush injuries, lacerations, fractures, sprains, and burns. Many postoperative cases occur after surgery involving the median nerve distribution, such as carpal tunnel release or palmar fasciectomy. The syndrome occasionally occurs after cerebrovascular accident or myocardial infarction. The pain is usually burning in quality and is often accompanied by diffuse tenderness and pain on light touch. The hand or foot are commonly the major sites of pain. The pain and hypersensitivity often spread beyond the original sites of pain.

Autonomic dysfunction is manifested as changes in skin temperature, cyanosis, edema, and hyperhydrosis. Early in the course of the disease, the skin may be warm and erythematous, with occasional to frequent bouts of intense vasoconstriction. As the process becomes more chronic, the involved extremity is usually cool and pale or cyanotic. The vascular phase of bone scanning often demonstrates differences in flow between the normal and the affected extremity. Thermography or local measurement of skin temperature using surface thermistors is also useful in documenting differences in regional blood flow.

Dystrophic changes become increasingly evident with time if the condition is untreated. Skin of the affected area becomes smooth and glossy. Bone demineralization takes place to a much greater extent than would be expected on the basis of reduced activity. Joints in the affected extremity become stiff and painful as a result of synovial edema, hyperplasia, fibrosis, and perivascular inflammation.

Local anesthetic blockade of the sympathetic chain is useful diagnostically, particularly when only a portion of the spectrum of possible symptoms is present. Cervicothoracic sympathetic block is usually carried out by injection of local anesthetic on the anterior tubercle of C6 (Fig. 55-5) or on the medial portion of the transverse process of C7. Unfortunately, a moderate number of patients experience a Horner's syndrome but fail to demonstrate evidence of sympathetic denervation of the upper extremity. Using MRI scans, Hogan *et al*[82] demonstrated that solutions injected paratracheally at the C6 or C7 anterior tubercle often fail to spread to the stellate ganglion. Subsequently, he and his colleagues described a CT-guided technique for direct injection of the stellate ganglion just anterior to the head of the first rib.[83] Using this technique, evidence of sympathetic denervation of the extremity is often seen after injection of as little as 1 ml of local anesthetic. Lumbar sympathetic block is performed by injecting local anesthetic at the anterolateral aspect of the lumbar spine (Fig. 55-6). Placement of the needle at the lower border of the L2 vertebral body minimizes needle contact with the nerve root and places the needle tip in plane of the sympathetic chain.

Pain relief following sympathetic blockade does not guarantee that there is a sympathetically mediated component to the patient's pain. Pain relief may be the result of a placebo effect, spread of anesthetic to somatic afferent fibers, blockade of afferent fibers located in the sympathetic chain, or the systemic effect of absorbed local anesthetic.[84] Similarly, failure to achieve pain relief following sympathetic block does not guarantee that the pain is not sympathetically mediated. There may be sympathetic efferent fibers to the limb that do not travel with that portion of the sympathetic chain that has been interrupted.[84]

Once it has been established that there is a sympathetically mediated component to the patient's pain, treatment consists of a series of local anesthetic sympathetic blocks. For patients with lower extremity pain, if lumbar sympathetic block is technically difficult or is particularly painful to the patient, repeated or continuous lumbar epidural blockade can be used instead. Injections are generally continued until symptoms are minimal. Three to seven blocks are usually sufficient, but the series may occasionally be longer. Physical therapy, consisting of desensitizing techniques and active or active-assisted range of motion, is usually indicated and should be carried out immediately after each sympathetic block. Vigorous passive range of motion and heavy weights should be avoided, as they may retrigger symptoms. Patients whose condition is diagnosed and treated early are more likely to respond to sympathetic blocks. Success rates of 90% or more have been reported.[85] Unfortunately, few if any controlled studies documenting the long-term effects of sympathetic blockade exist, and the high success rates associated with early intervention may simply reflect the natural history of the process.

Hannington-Kiff[86] described an alternative technique for producing temporary sympathetic blockade using iv regional injection of guanethidine. The technique has been shown to be as

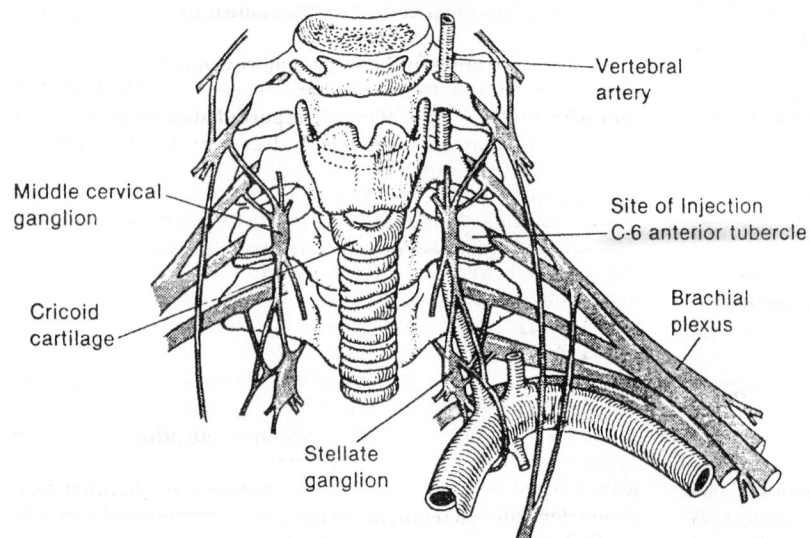

Figure 55-5. Site of injection for the C6 paratracheal approach to the cervicothoracic sympathetic chain. (From Abram SE, Boas RA: Sympathetic and visceral nerve blocks. In Benumof JL [ed]: Clinical Procedures in Anesthesia and Intensive Care, p 787. Philadelphia, JB Lippincott, 1992.)

Vertebral artery

Middle cervical ganglion

Cricoid cartilage

Site of Injection C-6 anterior tubercle

Brachial plexus

Stellate ganglion

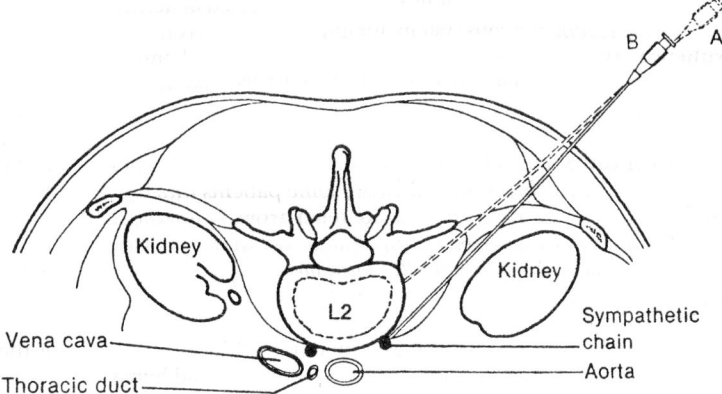

Figure 55-6. Initial needle position (*A*) and final needle position (*B*) for lumbar sympathetic block. Contact should be made at the lower portion of the L2 vertebral body, just cephalad to the L2–3 disk. (Reprinted with permission from Stanton-Hicks M, Abram SE, Nolte H: Sympathetic blocks. In Raj PP [ed]: Practical Management of Pain, p 674. Chicago, Year Book, 1986.)

effective as local anesthetic blockade[87] and has the advantage of being safer in anticoagulated patients. No reports have yet shown the technique to be superior to local anesthetic blocks. Unfortunately, injectable guanethidine is not available in some countries. Intravenous regional bretyllium has been used in a similar fashion, but there are no well-controlled studies documenting lasting benefit.

The use of systemic sympathetic blocking drugs is occasionally useful clinically. Prazosin and phenoxybenzamine, both α-adrenergic blocking agents, provide partial symptomatic relief in some patients, particularly those patients exhibiting signs of vasoconstriction. Intravenous phentolamine, given in small incremental doses up to 30 mg maximum, is helpful in predicting response to oral α-adrenergic blockers. Oral and transdermal clonidine are also occasionally useful. Other systemic medications that have been used with variable success include calcium channel blockers, tricyclic antidepressants, and anticonvulsants. Gabapentin has been used with some success, and is better tolerated than most of the older anticonvulsants.

Kozin *et al*[88] reported substantial benefit from treatment of RSD with a brief course of high-dose corticosteroids. Their success rate was 82%, which is particularly impressive in that many of their patients had experienced long-term symptoms. However, it is not clear whether improvement was permanent in these patients. In addition, their criteria for diagnosing RSD were somewhat vague and did not include response to sympathetic block, allodynia, hyperpathia, or burning pain. Side-effects from high-dose systemic steroids are often troublesome. An alternative treatment is the intravenous regional injection of soluble steroids in the affected limb.[89] TENS can be a useful adjunctive treatment for RSD. Increased skin temperature during stimulation has been documented in patients who experience pain relief following treatment,[90] and TENS has been reported to provide substantial clinical benefit when used as the sole therapy for RSD.[91]

Patients with long-standing symptoms of RSD, who develop dystrophic changes and, frequently, the behavioral and psychological profiles typical of chronic pain patients, are extremely resistant to the types of intervention described previously. Surgical or neurolytic sympathectomy has been suggested as a treatment for RSD patients who respond only transiently to sympathetic blocks. It is the authors' experience, however, that most patients with chronic RSD get no relief or only a few days to weeks of benefit from sympathetic ablation. Therapy instead should be directed toward extinguishing pain behavior, increasing strength and mobility, and developing coping strategies.

CRPS-II

The term *causalgia,* which has been used to indicate a specific syndrome of burning pain and autonomic dysfunction associated with major nerve trunk injury,[85] has been replaced by the term *complex regional pain syndrome type II,* or CRPS-II.

Most cases of CRPS-II are caused by gunshot wounds. Rapid, violent deformation of the nerve seems to play a major pathophysiologic role. Most cases involve partial injury to the brachial plexus, median nerve, or tibial division of the sciatic nerve proximal to the elbow or knee. Pain often begins immediately after injury and may spread to involve previously unaffected areas. There is usually severe burning pain, allodynia, and hyperpathia, often accompanied by deep shooting, crushing, or stabbing pains. The pain is aggravated by movement or any physical stimulation, such as light touch or pressure. Stimuli that increase sympathetic activity, such as a loud noise, a flash of light, or anxiety, often increase the severity of the pain. Pain may persist for many years in inadequately treated patients. There is usually evidence of reduced sympathetic activity in the affected extremity, which is generally warm, dry, and venodilated. Vasoconstriction, hyperhydrosis, cyanosis, and edema are occasionally seen. Dystrophic changes of skin, bone, and joints, similar to those encountered in CRPS-I patients, often begin early.

Reports on the therapy of causalgia from the early 1900s described surgical destruction of peripheral nerves, which was uniformly unsuccessful. Opioid analgesics were likewise ineffective. In 1930, Spurling[92] published encouraging results of treatment with sympathetic ganglionectomy. Since then, numerous reports have documented the efficacy of such treatment. Mayfield[93] reported complete relief of symptoms in 91% of 105 causalgia victims treated with surgical sympathectomy. Bonica,[85] in a review of 500 cases, found that 80% of patients responded to sympathectomy.

More recently, less invasive therapy has been undertaken in the management of CRPS-II. Neurolytic lumbar sympathetic block has been proposed as an alternative to surgical lumbar sympathectomy and has been shown to produce long-term sympathetic denervation in the large majority of patients.[94] Aggressive treatment with local anesthetic sympathetic blockade has met with some success. Bonica[85] reported success in 10 of 17 causalgia patients managed with frequent local anesthetic blocks. The authors have treated three patients with early, severe causalgia who responded dramatically to continuous-infusion lumbar epidural blockade or continuous-infusion brachial plexus block that was maintained for 5–7 days (unreported findings).

Herpes Zoster

Herpes zoster is caused by the varicella zoster virus, which, following a chicken pox infection, lies dormant in dorsal root ganglia. As immunity to the virus declines with advancing age or immunosuppression, the virus becomes active again. In patients with normal immune systems, the infection is confined to a single dermatomal segment. In immunocompromised patients, multiple segments may be involved.

Herpes zoster most commonly involves the thoracic and trigeminal dermatomes, with the ophthalmic division of the trigeminal nerve being second most common.[95] Autopsy studies have shown evidence of viral DNA in trigeminal ganglia in 87% of patients and in thoracic dorsal root ganglia in 53% of patients.

The incidence of herpes zoster in the general population is 1–2/1000 per year. It is higher among older patients, whose incidence is 5–10/1000 per year. Postherpetic neuralgia has been defined as pain persisting well beyond healing of the skin rash (4 weeks to 6 months). Overall incidence among patients with herpes zoster infection has been reported to range from 9 to 34%.[96] Incidence is considerably higher in older patients (16% in patients under 60, 47% in patients over 60).[97] Patients with severe pain during the acute phase of the disease are more likely to develop postherpetic neuralgia.

As the latent virus in the sensory ganglion becomes active, it causes a vesicular skin eruption characterized by inflammation, intranuclear inclusion bodies, and giant cell formation. Severe inflammation, hemorrhage, and necrosis occur in the dorsal root ganglia, dorsal horn, and adjacent meninges. Changes in the peripheral nerve include demyelinization, Wallerian degeneration, fibrosis, and cellular infiltration.[98] Noordenbos proposed that pain of postherpetic neuralgia is associated with loss of large afferent fibers with relative preservation of C-fibers.[99] In subsequent studies, however, examination of biopsy and autopsy specimens from patients with or without persistent pain failed to show differences in populations of different fiber types.[98,100] Some specimens showed predominantly large fiber loss, but this was seen in patients with and without postherpetic neuralgia. On the other hand, atrophy of the dorsal horn appears to be a regular autopsy feature in patients who had postherpetic neuralgia at the time of death. Persistence of inflammatory cells has been described in patients with long-standing postherpetic pain.[100]

Because of anecdotal evidence that sympathetic blocks provide lasting pain relief in patients with acute herpes zoster,[101] there has been speculation that intense sympathetic stimulation initiated by the virus is, at least in part, responsible for the pathologic changes that lead to postherpetic neuralgia. Winnie[102] has proposed that the increased sympathetic discharge initiated by the virus produces perineural ischemia that results in loss of large afferent fibers and persistence of small, unmyelinated neurons. There are several problems with the theory, including a lack of evidence that there is a local increase in sympathetic activity or that neural ischemia results from sympathetic discharge. In addition, the Noordenbos theory that pain is associated with small fiber predominance does not appear to be valid, nor is there substantial evidence that early sympathetic blockade reduces the incidence of postherpetic neuralgia.

A variety of treatments have been advocated for managing patients with acute herpes zoster. The goal of management is to control the pain associated with the acute eruption and, if possible, prevent the occurrence of persistent pain, or postherpetic neuralgia. Antiviral agents have been advocated for management of the acute stage of the disease. Acyclovir has been widely used and has been shown to modestly accelerate the rate of cutaneous healing and to reduce the severity of the acute pain, but there is little evidence that it reduces the incidence of postherpetic neuralgia.[103] On the other hand, one of the newer antiviral agents, famcyclovir, does appear to reduce the incidence and severity of postherpetic neuralgia if initiated soon after the eruption begins.[104]

Corticosteroids have enjoyed some popularity for the treatment of the pain of acute herpes zoster. Eaglestein,[105] in a double-blind, controlled study, demonstrated that systemic triamcinolone reduced the duration of acute pain in patients over the age of 60. Several other studies have failed to demonstrate a reduction in the incidence of postherpetic neuralgia. Likewise, subcutaneous steroid infiltration[106] and epidural steroid injection[107] have been shown to reduce the acute pain intensity

and/or duration, but there have been no controlled trials to determine whether they influence the incidence of postherpetic neuralgia. While there is some concern over the possibility that steroids may increase the risk of dissemination of the virus, there is little evidence that this is likely to occur.[95]

Rosenak[108] was the first to report a beneficial effect of local anesthetic blocks on the pain of herpes zoster infection. He found that paravertebral sympathetic blocks or gasserian ganglion blocks with procaine resulted in dramatic relief of pain and rapid drying of vescicles. A number of subsequent uncontrolled studies also attest to the beneficial effect of sympathetic blockade. A single controlled study[109] attests to the ability of sympathetic blocks done early in the acute stage to prevent postherpetic neuralgia. The study contained only 10 patients in each treatment arm, and there have been no subsequent controlled studies to confirm these findings.

There is substantial evidence that local anesthetic blocks are ineffective in the management of postherpetic neuralgia. At best, they provide very temporary relief, often only for the duration of the anesthetic agent. Winnie[102] recently confirmed this observation in a study that showed a very low incidence of lasting benefit from sympathetic blocks instituted more than a few months after the eruption. It is unclear whether the apparently favorable response to blocks instituted early in the course of the disease represents a real benefit from treatment or simply the natural history of the disease in the majority of patients.

The management of postherpetic neuralgia is often frustrating, as some patients respond poorly to nearly every therapy provided. Tricyclic antidepressants provide the best chance of relief with the fewest side-effects, although drowsiness, xerostomia, dysphoria, arrhythmias, and ataxia are potential problems. The onset of analgesia is slow (often requiring 2–3 weeks) and the relief is rarely complete, so many patients fail to realize they are experiencing much relief until they discontinue the drug and the pain returns to its former intensity. The addition of a second drug, such as an anticonvulsant (carbamazepine, valproic acid, phenytoin), may provide some additional benefit, but one must follow patients closely for the possibility of liver dysfunction or bone marrow depression. Gabapentin has been shown to be significantly more effective than placebo for the management of postherpetic neuralgia.[110] The majority of patients required 3600 mg per day. Side effects of gabapentin are usually mild, there are few significant drug interactions, and it does not carry the risk of organ dysfunction seen with older anticonvulsants. Opioids rarely provide dramatic relief, and cause major problems with constipation in older patients. Most studies fail to show much benefit from epidural stimulators. TENS may help in occasional patients, but cause aggravation of pain in patients with severe allodynia and is not beneficial if there is considerable cutaneous sensory loss. Topical capsaicin is occasionally helpful, but can aggravate the pain in some individuals.

PHARMACOLOGIC TREATMENT OF CHRONIC PAIN

The long-term use of systemic opioids in patients who have noncancer pain continues to cause concern for many physicians. While most pain management physicians are comfortable with the use of opioids for patients who do not have a terminal illness, there is much disagreement regarding appropriate dosage, patient selection, and choice of drug. Among primary care practitioners, there remains much resistance to prescribing opioids for noncancer pain for a variety of reasons. These include the following concerns:

1. Addiction will occur.
2. Tolerance will develop, leading to loss of efficacy and increasing drug side effects.

3. Drug regulatory agencies will take action against the prescribing physician.
4. Patients may be diverting (selling) drugs.

The reality is that certain patients experience good pain control over long periods of time with minimal tolerance and few side-effects. Others have pain that is poorly controlled by opioids or have rapid reduction in efficacy requiring substantial dose escalation. While it is difficult to predict response to opioids in a given patient, there are some predictors of poor response. Patients with neuropathic pain are less likely to experience good pain control, and phasic pain (*e.g.,* incident pain) is more difficult to control than constant or tonic pain. Patients with cognitive impairment or high levels of psychological distress are more likely to experience suboptimal pain control from opioids. A history of substance abuse is associated with a high risk of treatment failure and is felt by some physicians to represent a contraindication to opioid use.

The decision to prescribe opioids for patients with chronic pain should be based upon the answers to three questions:

1. Is there a history of significant substance abuse?
2. Is there a good therapeutic effect? The selected medication should provide complete or substantial analgesia. There should be minimal dose escalation over time, and there should be measurable improvement in functional activity.
3. Are there substantial side-effects? These should be minimal or tolerable.

Side effects should be monitored closely. Cognitive impairment is often insidious, and may not be recognized by the patient or family members during treatment, but becomes obvious when the medication is withdrawn. Sedation, nausea, constipation, insomnia, and sexual dysfunction are common problems.

As noted in the section on pain mechanisms, there is substantial theoretical evidence that chronic opioid use may lead to a state of hyperalgesia or sensitization of spinal pain projection systems. Persistent opioid administration may lead to loss of responsiveness to both endogenous and exogenous opioids and to hypersensitivity of systems that respond to noxious stimulation. Therefore, it is reasonable to withdraw and discontinue opioid administration for those patients who have evidence of central facilitation (allodynia hyperalgesia, hyperpathia) and who exhibit poor responsiveness to opioids. Occasionally, such patients experience gradual improvement in pain, generally beginning a few weeks after drug withdrawal. Often, they will experience a reduction in adverse effects, especially cognitive impairment, sedation, constipation, and sexual dysfunction.

Few patients with chronic pain are addicted to opioids. Addiction is defined as compulsive use of a drug or substance resulting in physical, psychological, or social harm to the user, and continued use despite that harm.[111] It may be difficult to recognize addiction in patients with persistent pain. Signs of addiction include:

1. Intense desire for the drug and unfounded concerns over availability.
2. Unsanctioned dose escalation.
3. Use of drug when pain is absent or treatment of non-pain symptoms (anxiety, depression).
4. Aberrant drug-related behaviors.

Some patients, appropriately, become concerned over the threat of drug discontinuation. When the potential loss of therapeutic benefit is anticipated, patients who are not addicted may exhibit anxiety and drug-seeking behavior. Undertreatment of pain may also result in addiction-like behaviors, which subside when pain is adequately treated. This phenomenon has been termed *pseudoaddiction*.[112]

Drug diversion, or sale of drugs for recreational or street use, is difficult to document or to disprove. Occasionally, an acquaintance or a family member will report such activity. Documentation depends upon a negative drug screen. The patient is asked whether he/she has taken the prescribed drug in the past several hours. If the answer is yes, a urine sample is obtained immediately and analyzed for the prescribed drug. If it is absent, diversion is likely.

When opioids are prescribed over long intervals, there should be an agreement, either informal or written, outlining the physician's obligation to continue treatment and the patient's obligation to meet several expectations of behavior. For patients who have previously failed to meet behavioral expectations, a written agreement, or "opioid contract" may be helpful. Under such a contract, the patient agrees to obtain prescriptions from one physician source and to fill prescriptions at one pharmacy, to discontinue use if there is rapid tolerance development, minimal therapeutic effect, substantial side-effects, or failure to achieve improved physical function. The patient agrees to take medications only as prescribed, and is not to request early refills. The patient agrees that no prescription will be issued in the event that drugs are lost, stolen, or accidentally destroyed. The physician, however, should be willing to adjust dosage as needed, within reason, particularly in the early stages of treatment. The patient should agree to unannounced random drug screening and to allow the physician access to all other medical records. The patient understands that violation of this agreement could result in discontinuation of opioid therapy and/or referral to an addiction specialist.

Adjuvant Analgesics

Imipramine was shown to be useful in treating chronic pain in 1960.[113] Since then, the tricyclic antidepressants have come into widespread use in the management of certain chronic pain conditions, particularly neuropathic pain. The most popular explanation of the analgesic property of these drugs is that reuptake inhibition of serotonin and norepinephrine increases the levels of these inhibitory neurotransmitters in the brain stem and spinal cord.

The clinically relevant benefits to be expected from judicious use of these drugs in patients with chronic pain syndromes are normalization of sleep patterns, reduction in anxiety and depression (if present), and reduction of the patient's perception of pain. Although the antidepressant and pain-relieving effects are often delayed in onset, the improvement in sleep patterns provided by these drugs usually occurs promptly, often with the initial dose. Tricyclics suppress rapid eye movement (REM) sleep, and abrupt cessation can be associated with rebound in the form of restless sleep, with excessively vivid and pervasive dreams.

The common side-effects of the tricyclics include the antimuscarinic effects of xerostomia, impaired visual accommodation, urinary retention, and constipation. Antihistaminic effects occur via blockade of both H_1 and H_2 receptors and include sedation and an increase in gastric pH. Orthostatic hypotension is mediated through the blockade of peripheral α_1-adrenergic receptors. Cardiac conduction effects mimic the actions of quinidine but in general are of little clinical relevance, except in the case of overdosage. The lethal potential of these drugs in overdose is substantial, especially when doses exceed 2000 mg of amitriptyline or the equivalent.

Most studies of efficacy of these drugs in pain syndromes are open and are not controlled for placebo effects or for the presence of depression. Since the first double-blind placebo-controlled study by Watson *et al* in 1982,[114] several well-designed studies have been conducted. They studied the effects of gradually increasing doses of amitriptyline in patients suffering from postherpetic neuralgia. After 3 weeks, 16 of 24 patients had obtained good to excellent relief, with doses below the norm for treatment of depression and with no change in a standard psychometric instrument assessing the presence and severity of depression. Getto et al[115] reviewed 24 studies and found 19 to report some degree of benefit. Four double-blind placebo studies with a combined enrollment of 107 subjects yielded a 68% response rate with the active drug, as compared with a 13% response with placebo. Studies of a double-blind placebo crossover design included 140 subjects in five reports and revealed an aggregate response rate of 61%.

Beginning in 1987, Max et al[116,117] published a series of double-blind, placebo-controlled trials that assessed the efficacy of antidepressants in certain painful syndromes. They showed that tricyclic antidepressants had analgesic effects independent of their effects on mood in neuropathic pain states (diabetic neuropathies and postherpetic neuralgia), although not all subjects had a beneficial response.

With the introduction of the serotonin-specific reuptake inhibitor (SSRI) fluoxetine, there was hope that the new class of drugs would provide pain relief at least comparable to the tricyclics. Clinical experience and research into this have yielded mixed results. In 1989, Diamond and Freitag reported their somewhat positive experience with the use of fluoxetine in the treatment of headache.[118] This prompted numerous reports of fluoxetine use in pain, some of which purport to demonstrate some benefit.[119,120] Max compared desipramine, amitriptyline, fluoxetine, and placebo in the treatment of diabetic neuropathy pain and found that, whereas both amitriptyline and desipramine were beneficial, fluoxetine had no more effect than placebo.[121] Paroxetine has, however, been shown to be of benefit in the treatment of diabetic neuropathy pain.[122]

As noted above, the pain-relieving effect of antidepressants has been attributed to the ability to block reuptake of serotonin and norepinephrine. Since serotonin is believed to be an important inhibitory neurotransmitter in descending pain inhibitory pathways, it was anticipated that the SSRIs would be at least as effective as the tricyclics, but with fewer side-effects. This has not generally been the case. It is now postulated that the tricyclic antidepressants may exert their analgesic and antihyperalgesic effects through other mechanisms. These drugs have been shown to bind at NMDA receptors, and can block NMDA-mediated synaptic activity.[123] This property, which may not be shared by many of the SSRIs, may be the principal mechanism of analgesic action.

Another class of agents said to have some efficacy in the treatment of chronic pain syndromes are the anticonvulsants. Unlike the antidepressants and neuroleptics, the pharmacology of this group varies substantially from one drug to another. The older members of this class that have some benefit in pain patients are phenytoin, valproic acid, carbamazepine, and clonazepam. The first three affect sodium, potassium, or calcium flux across the neuronal membrane, while clonazepam is a benzodiazepine and works via the benzodiazepine–GABA–chloride channel receptor complex.

The side-effect profiles of these drugs are also variable, with nausea and ataxia being commonly seen with any of them. Phenytoin can cause vitamin D and K and folate deficiencies, hirsutism, and gingival hyperplasia. Valproic acid use is associated with hepatic enzyme elevations, rare but occasionally fatal hepatic necrosis in children, and significant gastrointestinal effects that can be modified by the use of the enteric coated form of the drug. Carbamazepine can cause clinically a significant decrease in any of the blood elements selectively or can induce pancytopenia. Clonazepam is occasionally associated with disinhibition, leading to hostility and aggression or emotional lability.

Several new anticonvulsants appear to have some efficacy in treating painful conditions, particularly neuropathic pain. Gabapentin has been shown to provide significant pain relief for patients with reflex sympathetic dystrophy,[124] diabetic neuropathy,[125] and postherpetic neuralgia.[110] It has antihyperalgesic

effects in rat mononeuropathy models when administered spinally.[126] While it is a structural analog of GABA, its action does not appear to involve GABA-receptor interaction. Its mechanism of action has not been clearly defined. It has fewer side-effects and drug interaction than most of the older anticonvulsants.

Lamotrigine acts by inhibition of a sodium channel subtype, and has been shown to inhibit glutamate release. While there are a few reports of beneficial effects on neuropathic pain,[127] there are as yet no contolled studies demonstrating efficacy.

Use-dependent sodium channel blocking drugs have a role in the management of neuropathic pain. Systemically administered lidocaine is capable of suppressing spontaneous activity originating from experimentally induced neuromas at blood levels that produce no adverse effects.[128] Intravenous lidocaine and oral mexiletine have analgesic properties in some patients with neuropathic pain.[129] The analgesic effects of lidocaine are generally transient unless a continuous infusion is used. Lidocaine is commonly used to predict response to oral mexiletine, although its prognostic utility has not been well established. Lidocaine is given as a slow intravenous bolus at $1.5 \text{ mg} \cdot \text{kg}^{-1}$ over 5 minutes followed by an infusion of $50 \ \mu g \cdot \text{kg}^{-1} \cdot \text{min}^{-1}$. The infusion is adjusted downward if symptoms of systemic toxicity become evident.

CANCER PAIN

In assessing patients with malignant disease who seek treatment for pain, it is essential to determine the specific site and mechanism of their pain. It is not enough to make a diagnosis of cancer pain. The entire range of acute and chronic pain mechanisms is encountered among patients with malignancy. It is also essential to know the stage of the patient's malignant disease. The approach to a given pain for a terminal patient may vary greatly from the approach to the same type of pain in a patient whose cancer is curable.

It is useful to determine whether the patient's pain is acute or chronic, and whether it is related to tumor progression, therapeutic intervention, or, as is occasionally the case, factors unrelated to the patient's malignant disease (arthritis, herniated disk, etc.). It is also useful to know whether the patient has a history of chronic pain or drug abuse predating the onset of malignant disease. Pain caused by tumor progression can result from compression or infiltration of peripheral nerves, nerve root, or spinal cord; infiltration of bone and soft tissue; obstruction or distension of visceral structures; and vascular occlusion. Surgical intervention may lead to scar pain, neuroma formation, sympathetic dystrophy, and venous or lymphatic obstruction. Chemotherapy may be associated with peripheral neuropathies. Therapy with steroids can cause aseptic bony necrosis or rheumatoid-like symptoms when therapy is withdrawn. Herpes zoster is associated with agents that suppress immune function. Radiation therapy sometimes results in esophagitis, plexopathy and myelopathy, and bone necrosis.

A substantial range of therapeutic options is available to the cancer patient. A major consideration in approaching the patient with severe pain is when to institute a particular modality. It is generally advisable to consider less invasive, lower-risk options initially, progressing to procedures that are more invasive, more painful to perform, and carry a higher risk of complications only when the more benign procedures are ineffective. Occasionally, it is prudent to select a more invasive procedure early in the course of management if it is thought that it will provide the patient maximum comfort or if the patient's pain level has progressed to a crisis state.

Pharmacologic Therapy

The use of oral analgesic agents is the mainstay of treatment for cancer pain. Adequate analgesia can be achieved in the large majority of patients with cancer-related pain if sound pharmacologic principles are employed. Several guidelines are essential to cancer pain management:

1. Use agents appropriate for the nature and severity of the patient's pain. Weaker opioids such as codeine may be adequate for mild to moderate pain. For severe pain, more efficacious agents such as morphine, hydromorphone, or methadone should be employed. Agonist–antagonist agents such as pentazocine and buprenorphine have a ceiling effect on their analgesic efficacy and are generally effective only for mild to moderate pain. Meperidine is a poor drug for repetitive dosing because accumulation of its metabolite normeperidine can cause CNS stimulation manifested as anxiety, tremors, or seizures. Be aware of the oral bioavailability of the drug used. The oral dose of morphine, for instance, is about three times the parenteral dose. When peripheral nociceptive processes are involved (such as bony or soft tissue invasion), the addition of nonsteroidal anti-inflammatory drugs may be very helpful.

2. Use adequate doses. The dose of opioid analgesic should be escalated until satisfactory analgesia occurs (usually the case) or until problematic side-effects occur. The dose required varies tremendously. It is not unusual for cancer patients to require 100–200 mg of oral morphine or its equivalent every 3–4 hours.

3. Maintain steady blood and tissue levels of analgesic. All analgesics should be given by the clock. As-needed administration may result in periods of inadequate relief. The time interval for administration should be consistent with the duration of action of the drug. When possible, use long-acting agents. Methadone, whose plasma half-life is 24–36 hours, can be given twice a day, avoiding the need for nighttime awakening for analgesic administration. Morphine is available in a time-release form that can be administered once or twice a day. Transdermal fentanyl provides prolonged, steady release that achieves fairly constant blood levels.

4. Consider the use of adjuvant drugs. Tricyclic antidepressants are frequently beneficial for postherpetic neuralgia, may be helpful for some patients with other types of neuralgic pain or denervation dysesthesia, and can be effective for treating concomitant depression. Some anticonvulsants may be beneficial for neuralgic pain. Phenothiazines or butyrophenones have been shown to reduce symptoms of nausea, agitation, and pain when used in conjunction with narcotic analgesics. Corticosteroids should be considered for increased intracranial pressure, cord compression, severe bone pain, or pain from liver metastases. Calcitonin is effective in some patients with bone pain.

5. Anticipate and promptly treat side-effects. Constipation, which may become a major problem, occurs in most patients on opiates. Prophylactic management is essential. Nausea is a common opiate side-effect and concomitant administration of antiemetics may be necessary. Respiratory depression is unusual in tolerant patients. When it occurs in opioid-naive patients, it should be treated with small incremental doses of iv naloxone (*e.g.,* 0.05–0.1 mg) until the respiratory rate increases to an acceptable range. Large doses precipitate withdrawal, reverse much of the patient's analgesia, and initiate vomiting.

Patients who are unable to take analgesics orally can often be satisfactorily managed with parenteral opiate administration. Some patients who do not achieve satisfactory analgesia with oral drugs may have adequate control with parenteral agents, possibly because enteric absorption is poor. When the parenteral route is chosen, a constant-infusion technique or infusion plus patient-controlled analgesia (PCA) is usually superior to intermittent intramuscular injections. Many cancer patients have long-term venous access ports for chemotherapy that can be used for narcotic infusion.

When beginning opiate infusions, it is generally prudent to start with a relatively low-dose bolus injection and a modest infusion rate. If analgesia is inadequate after 1–2 hours, a small bolus is repeated and the infusion rate is increased. The process is repeated until the infusion rate is adequate. An alternative, less labor-intensive method is to use a PCA device. Once the daily opiate requirement is established, the patient can be switched to a portable, battery-powered constant-infusion device or portable PCA. When venous access is not available, portable external infusion devices can be used to deliver opiates subcutaneously through a "butterfly" type needle. The infusion site is changed every few days or when soreness occurs. When large doses are required, the use of a concentrated preparation of hydromorphone ($10\ mg \cdot ml^{-1}$) allows for longer intervals between refilling the portable infusion pump and reduces the mass of fluid injected.

Patients may experience diminishing analgesic effects from oral or parenteral opioids either from tolerance development or from increasing noxious stimulation related to tumor spread. A study by Collin et al[130] suggests that increasing dose requirement is nearly always associated with spread of disease. In either event, there may be a rationale for changing from morphine to a more potent drug such as fentanyl or sufentanil. This rationale is related to the concept of intrinsic activity (IA) of analgesics, *i.e.,* the fractional receptor occupancy (FRO) required to produce a given effect. A drug with relatively low IA, such as morphine or meperidine, requires a higher FRO than a drug with a high IA, such as fentanyl or sufentanil. Under conditions of tolerance, some receptors become unresponsive, and a drug with low IA may not be capable of interacting with enough of the remaining receptors to achieve adequate analgesia. Likewise, if the level of noxious stimulation increases, a greater number of receptors must be activated to produce a given analgesic effect, and a drug with a low IA may not interact with sufficient receptors to provide a reasonable analgesic response. Chronic infusion of morphine or meperidine in animals is associated with rapid development of tolerance to subsequent doses of morphine or meperidine, but not fentanyl or sufentanil.[131]

Transdermal fentanyl offers an alternative to parenteral opioids for patients who are unable to take medications orally. It is available in four dosage forms, which deliver 25, 50, 75, or $100\ \mu g \cdot h^{-1}$ of fentanyl. The continuous use of the $100\text{-}\mu g \cdot h^{-1}$ form offers roughly the same analgesia as 360 mg of oral morphine or 60 mg of parenteral morphine per 24 hours. If higher delivery rates are required, multiple patches can be used simultaneously. Several hours are required for analgesia to develop following application of the transdermal patch and for analgesia to dissipate following its removal. An oral transmucosal preparation of fentanyl is available in doses up to 1600 μg. The onset of analgesia is much more rapid with this form of administration, with peak levels occurring at about 20 minutes.

Intraspinal Opioids

Some cancer patients do not achieve satisfactory analgesia with systemic opiates without pushing the doses to the point of marked sedation or confusion. Less conventional methods of opiate administration may be effective for some of these patients. The discovery of spinal cord opiate receptors led to speculation regarding the feasibility of intraspinal administration of opioids. Most experience with chronic intraspinal opioids administration has been with morphine, probably because it has a long duration, allowing bolus as well as continuous administration, and because it has been approved by the FDA for intraspinal use. The use of intraspinal opioids in patients who had not previously been on systemic opioids (*e.g.,* postoperative patients and volunteers) was associated with nausea and vomiting, urinary retention, pruritus, and respiratory depression. As more experience with cancer patients accumulated, it became evident that these problems were, indeed, uncommon in this population, probably because the patients had been on systemic opioids chronically and had become tolerant to these side-effects.

Intraspinal opioids have been chronically administered by both the epidural and IT routes. IT administration has the advantage of allowing use of much lower doses, potentially minimizing systemic side-effects, but carries the risks of cerebrospinal fluid leak, headache, meningitis, and arachnoiditis. With either epidural or IT administration, the drug may be administered as a bolus, by infusion via an external pump, or by infusion via a totally implanted pump.

Percutaneous placement of an epidural catheter followed by bolus administration of opioid constitutes the simplest method of administration. The principal drawback of this technique is the risk of infection, which may spread to the epidural space. Such a technique is useful as a temporary measure to evaluate efficacy of epidural narcotics and is a reasonable method of administration for patients whose life expectancy is relatively short. The simple expedient of tunneling the catheter subcutaneously to the flank decreases the incidence of catheter dislodgement, allows the patient access to the catheter exit site to facilitate dressing changes, and may reduce the risk of epidural infection.

The decision to use an external pump is based on pharmacokinetic, technical, and financial considerations. There is some evidence that lower doses of morphine can be employed when using a continuous infusion. Coombs et al[132] were able to provide good analgesia for a group of cancer pain patients using a mean dose of 2 mg · day^{-1} initially and 6.6 mg · day^{-1} at the end of 12 weeks. Reports of studies that use bolus injection describe much higher daily doses. Bolus injection produces much higher peak cerebrospinal fluid levels,[133] which may predispose to more cephalad migration of the drug. Another advantage to continuous-infusion techniques is the lower incidence of catheter occlusion. Inability to inject is a fairly common problem with bolus injection technique. When an obstructed catheter is removed, it is common to find fibrin material in the lumen. The use of large-bore silicone rubber catheters should minimize that possibility, however. Patients with epidural metastases may have severe pain with bolus injection but tolerate continuous-infusion well. Perhaps the biggest drawback to continuous-infusion techniques is the expense. Portable pumps cost up to several thousand dollars, and the use of implantable systems adds several thousand dollars in additional physician and operating room expenses.

The totally implantable infusion pump is the most elegant, and expensive, drug delivery system. The Infusaid pump is a freon-driven device with a 50-ml, percutaneously filled drug chamber and a constant infusion rate. Pumps with a 2–3 ml · day^{-1} flow rate will run for 15–20 days between refills. Daily dose is adjusted by changing the drug concentration. A separate drug injection septum allows injection directly into the catheter, bypassing the drug chamber. The technique is most appropriate for patients with a relatively long life expectancy (months rather than weeks). Medtronic produces an electronically driven, externally programmable implanted pump that allows variations in rate plus the administration of intermittent bolus injections.

Perhaps the most frustrating problem associated with intraspinal opioid administration is the development of marked resistance or tolerance to the medication. While most patients develop tolerance slowly and to a limited degree, some demonstrate rapid escalation of doses. Woods and Cohen[134] reported a patient who had been on 280 mg of morphine intravenously and 90 mg of methadone orally per day who was initially comfortable on 5 mg · day^{-1} of epidural morphine. However, by the fifth day of epidural morphine administration, the

dose had increased to 7–10 mg · h^{-1}. One of the reported side-effects of such high doses, particularly with high-dose IT morphine, is the paradoxical development of segmental allodynia, which has been reported in patients[135] as well as in animal studies.[136]

Neuraxial administration of nonopioid analgesics, either alone or in combination with opioids, may be effective when opioids alone are ineffective. Limited trials of the α_2-agonist clonidine injected epidurally and intrathecally have proved at least temporarily effective. Animal studies suggest that there is a synergistic interaction between spinally administered α_2-adrenergic agonists and opioids. Eisenach et al[137] found a dose-related analgesic effect from epidural clonidine in a series of nine cancer patients. They reported dose-related decreases in heart rate and blood pressure as well as somnolence. Seven patients were maintained on clonidine plus morphine infusions at home for periods of up to 5 months. These patients reported satisfactory analgesia and less nausea and sedation than they experienced with systemic morphine. There was minimal escalation of either clonidine or morphine during the combined infusions.

The intrathecal administration of baclofen has been used to treat patients with spasticity associated with multiple sclerosis and spinal cord injury. However, baclofen appears to have some potential as a spinal analgesic in patients without increased muscle tone who are resistant or tolerant to opioids. Intrathecal L-baclofen is antinociceptive in several animal models at doses that produce no discernible motor blockade.[138] It has been shown to produce substantial lasting analgesia in opioid-tolerant patients with neuropathic and radiculopathic pain at doses devoid of motor effects.[139]

Another approach to the patient who has become resistant to neuraxial opioids is to use combinations of opioids and dilute local anesthetics. The combined use of these agents makes sense, as the local anesthetic, even at sub-blocking concentrations, can reduce the maximum firing rates of nociceptor fibers, and the opiate reduces the sensitivity of wide dynamic range and nociceptive-specific neurons in the dorsal horn to activation by nociceptors. Hogan et al[140] found that 10 of 16 patients, selected from a total of 1205 cancer admissions, required local anesthetic infusions along with epidural morphine to achieve satisfactory analgesia. Du Pen et al[141] found that 68 of 375 patients (18%) failed to achieve satisfactory analgesia with neuraxial opioids alone. Sixty-one of those 68 patients experienced satisfactory analgesia with the addition of local anesthetics.

Non-neurolytic Nerve Blocks

Myofascial pain is common among cancer patients. It is often associated with bony infiltration, neural compression, or visceral pain. Local anesthetic injections of trigger points may be surprisingly effective. Fluorimethane spray of trigger points combined with gentle stretching of affected muscles can be helpful. TENS is also likely to be of benefit.

Tumor compression of nerve roots, brachial or femoral plexus, or peripheral nerves sometimes responds dramatically to perineural injection of insoluble steroids. Pain relief can be achieved for up to 1 month in many instances. When radicular pain is caused by epidural tumor spread, epidural injections of triamcinolone diacetate are likely to be of benefit. Tumor compression of the brachial plexus may respond to brachial plexus block with a combination of depo steroid and local anesthetic. The interscalene, supraclavicular, infraclavicular, or axillary approaches may all be used, the choice depending on the site of pathology. Femoral plexopathy can be treated with a paravertebral approach (psoas compartment block) to the femoral plexus, again using depo steroids and local anesthetic. Steroid local anesthetic blocks of peripheral nerves that are irritated or compressed by tumor are occasionally beneficial, particularly if they are performed reasonably soon after the onset of pain. Patients with severe neurogenic pain should be warned that if the injections are successful in producing pain relief, they are likely to be left with some numbness, not from the injections, but from the already present neural pathology.

Acute herpes zoster is a relatively common and often debilitating source of pain in patients with malignancy. There is some evidence that local anesthetic blockade of sympathetic fibers, using either paravertebral sympathetic blocks or epidurals, will promptly relieve pain and may shorten the acute phase of the illness.[109] Even if the overall course of the illness is not dramatically affected, patients are usually extremely grateful for any respite from the severe pain associated with this condition.

Occasionally, patients with severe cancer pain are refractory to any opioid intervention. These patients may progress to psychological decompensation without reasonably prompt intervention. The use of continuous-infusion local anesthetic blockade may be the best answer for patients who reach such a crisis. Continuous epidurals with dilute local anesthetics can be performed at any level of the neuraxis. When upper thoracic or cervical approaches are used, close monitoring of blood pressure and respiratory function is necessary.

Neurolytic Blocks

There is a much greater willingness among anesthesiologists to perform neurolytic blocks for terminal cancer patients with pain than for patients with nonmalignant causes of pain. Reluctance to use neurolytic blocks for noncancer pain is certainly justified. The extent and duration of analgesia from neurodestructive procedures is limited by regrowth of axons and development of central pain mechanisms (denervation dysesthesia). While neurolytic blocks can produce dramatic relief for some cancer pain patients, there are some serious potential drawbacks to the technique, and overzealous use of neurodestructive procedures should be avoided.

The principal disadvantage of neurolytic blocks is the inability to precisely control the spread of the destructive agents. Loss of motor function and inability to control bowel or bladder function following neurolysis can be devastating to a patient and will greatly impair the quality of remaining life. The expected analgesia may not always result from destruction of the intended neural structures, even when prognostic local anesthetic blocks have been performed. If CNS mechanisms play a major role in a patient's pain, neurolysis is unlikely to be of benefit. In some cases, tumor progression rapidly produces pain beyond the confines of the block. With the advent of improved methods of cancer therapy, more patients survive well beyond the efficacy of the block. Overall, the incidence of fair to good results following neurolytic blockade is estimated at 50–60%.[142]

Alcohol and phenol are the agents most commonly used for prolonged interruption of neural function. There is relatively little difference in overall efficacy between these agents, but there are major differences in the initial responses. Phenol produces no pain on injection, has an initial anesthetic effect, and takes about 15 minutes to exert its neurolytic effect. Alcohol causes significant pain on injection and produces neurolysis promptly. When used for intrathecal (IT) neurolysis, alcohol is hypobaric, whereas phenol in glycerine, the usual intrathecal preparation, is hyperbaric.

IT neurolysis with small volumes of alcohol or phenol requires careful positioning to place the affected sensory root uppermost (for alcohol) or in the most dependent position (for phenol). In such a way, only the involved sensory roots are affected. Patient movement during or shortly after injection can produce spread of drug to the cord, other dermatomes, or motor roots. Papo and Visca[143] published results in a large series of patients who underwent phenol rhizotomy. They reported good results (pain-free until death) in 40% of 290 patients and fair results (reduced analgesic requirements or temporary complete relief) in 35%. Patients whose pain was localized to sacral dermatomes

had the best results, whereas patients with pain in the upper thoracic area or upper or lower extremities had poor analgesia and more frequent complications. Swerdlow[144] reviewed 13 reports of the results of phenol and alcohol rhizotomies and found good relief of pain in about 60% of patients. In reviewing results on his own patients, he found that analgesia lasted less than 2 months in half the patients and less than 1 month in 25% of patients. Complications lasting longer than a week occurred in 15% of patients.

Patients with severe, localized perineal pain are likely to experience relief with IT blocks with phenol in glycerine. Phenol 7% in glycerine, is injected in 0.25-ml increments up to a maximum of 2 ml, with the patient in the sitting position. Injection is stopped at a lower dose if the patient experiences any lower extremity sensory changes. This treatment is limited to patients who have undergone fecal and urinary diversion procedures.

Celiac plexus block for pain associated with upper abdominal malignancy is the most successful and rewarding of the neurolytic blocks. Thompson et al[145] reported that 94% of 97 patients who underwent celiac plexus block for pain of upper abdominal cancer had good-to-excellent pain relief. Injections were performed with 50 ml of 50% alcohol. Survival from the cancer ranged from 2 days to 14 months. Fourteen patients required repeat injections for recurrent pain. Ten patients experienced transient orthostatic hypotension, and one patient had partial motor loss in one leg.

The classical technique for percutaneous injection of the celiac plexus involves bilateral placement of block needles just anterior to the body of L1 and posterior to the aorta and diaphragmatic crura. Recently, techniques have been described that involve more anterior positioning of the needle tip with computed tomographic assistance so that it lies anterior to the diaphragmatic crura.[146] The injected solution can be seen to spread more anteriorly, surrounding the aorta. There is much less tendency of the injected solution to spread posteriorly to the paravertebral nerve roots or sympathetic chain, minimizing risk of paresis or orthostatic hypotension. Ischia et al,[147] using such a technique, reported 93% success in relieving pain in 28 patients with cancer pain. Similar placement can be achieved with the use of biplane fluoroscopy. Five-inch 22-gauge needles are advanced from both sides at a point 7 cm from the midline, at the lower border of the 12th rib toward the midpoint of the L1 vertebral body, and advanced under anteroposterior fluroscopy until they are just past the lateral border of the body. Under lateral fluoroscopy, the right-sided needle is advanced 1 cm beyond the anterior border of the body. It will probably lie between the aorta and vena cava. The left-sided needle is advanced the same distance, but will usually enter the aorta at this point. If so, it is advanced through the aorta until negative aspiration occurs. Half the total alcohol dose is then injected through each needle (Fig. 55-7). Alternatively, deafferentation of the upper abdominal viscera can be accomplished with the use of splanchnic block. With this technique, the neurolytic agent is injected over the anterolateral surface of the T12 and/or T11 vertebral body (Fig. 55-7). This technique may be more effective than the transcrural approach if there is dense, widespread tumor invasion around the celiac plexus.

Patients with pelvic pain associated with gynecologic, rectal, and genitourinary malignancies may benefit from interruption of pelvic visceral innervation at the level of the superior hypogastric plexus. The technique of needle placement just anterior to the upper portion of the sacrum originally described by Plancarte et al[148] allows for interruption of afferents from the pelvic viscera with minimal risk of somatic blockade. The block is performed by introducing bilateral needles medially and caudally through the space between the L5 spinous process and the upper border of the sacrum under fluoroscopic control. Eight milliliters of phenol introduced through each needle is generally sufficient to provide reduction in pain and opioid requirement[149] (Fig. 55-8). Bladder pain and spasm have been

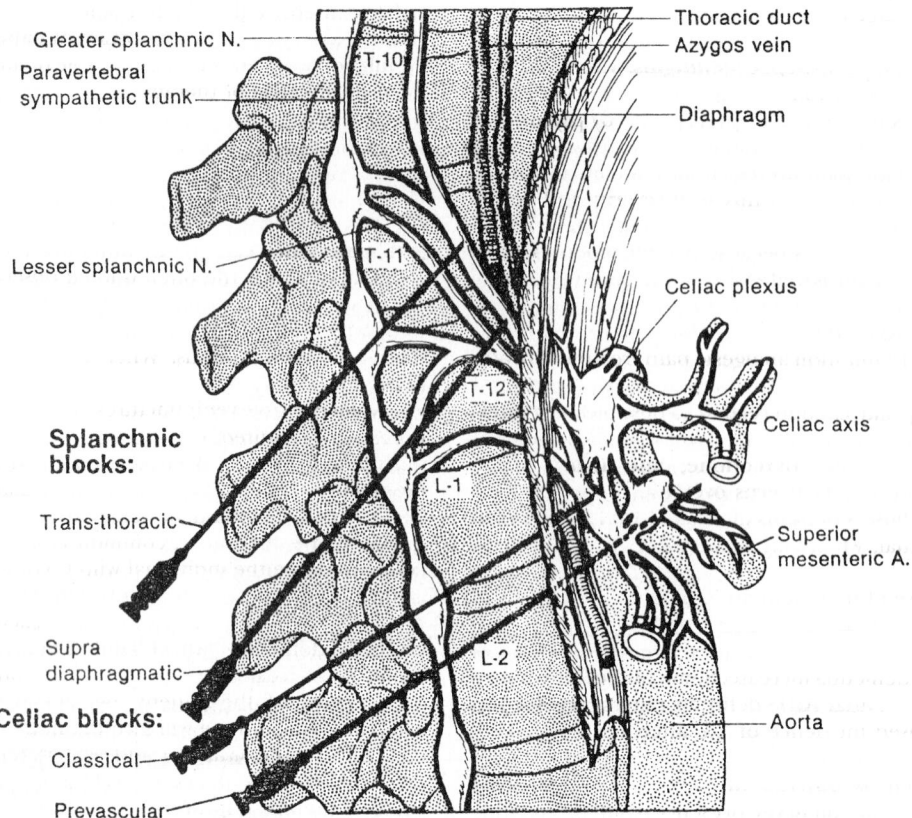

Figure 55-7. Lateral projection showing the splanchnic nerves and celiac plexus in relation to the diaphragm, vertebrae, and aortic vessels. Placement of needles for two approaches to the celiac plexus and two approaches to the splanchnic nerves is shown. (From Abram SE, Boas RA: Sympathetic and visceral nerve blocks. In Benumof JL [ed]: Clinical Procedures in Anesthesia and Intensive Care, p. 787. Philadelphia, JB Lippincott, 1992.)

successfully treated with trans-sacral phenol injections.[150] If blocks are confined to one or two roots, there is little risk of disrupting bladder function.

Other Modes of Therapy

There are a number of therapeutic options that are relatively specific for the type of malignancy one is dealing with. When dealing with tumors that are extremely radiosensitive, radiation therapy is often the most effective form of intervention. If chemotherapeutic options are available, they may provide analgesia

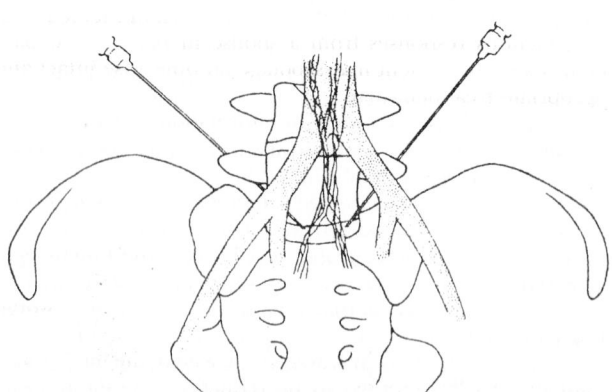

Figure 55-8. Anterior view of the pelvis showing location of the hypogastric plexus and suggested bilateral needle placement. (Reprinted with permission from Plancarte R, Amescua C, Patt RB, Aldrete A: Superior hypogastric plexus block for pelvic cancer pain. Anesthesiology 73:236, 1990.)

through reduction of tumor mass. Pain caused by hormonally sensitive tumors may be best treated by appropriate manipulation of the patient's hormonal environment. Surgical debulking of a large tumor will sometimes relieve pain of obstruction or abdominal distension. Stabilization of an isolated pathologic fracture can be an extremely effective pain-relieving procedure. Certain neurosurgical procedures, such as spinal cord stimulation, cordotomy, or hypophysectomy may afford months of profound relief in certain types of cases. Some patients benefit considerably from psychological interventions such as hypnosis or other cognitive strategies. With the complexity of the disease processes involved with cancer-related pain and the number of pain mechanisms and therapeutic interventions that are possible, it is essential that the full range of medical and behavioral science disciplines be made available to this group of patients.

PAIN IN HIV/AIDS

Knowledge of the syndromes in human immunodeficiency virus (HIV) disease is the fundamental prerequisite for diagnosis of HIV disease pain. HIV disease pain can be divided into three classifications: nociceptive pain, neuropathic pain, and idiopathic pain. The most common pain sources associated with HIV disease–related pain are abdominal pain 26%, peripheral neuropathy 25%, throat pain 20%, HIV disease-related headaches 17%, AZT-induced headache 16%, arthralgia 5%, back pain 5%, and herpes zoster 5%.[151]

Pain in HIV disease varies depending on the stage of HIV disease progression with acute phase evidenced by mononeuritides, brachial plexopathy, and acute demyelinating polyneuropathy, such as Guillain-Barré syndrome. As the disease progresses, pain will be associated with chronic inflammatory demyelinating polyneuropathy, herpes zoster, and mononeuritis multiplex. Late-stage HIV disease pain arises out of sensory polyneuropathy, cytomegalovirus polyradiculopathy, progressive mononeuritis multiplex, aseptic meningitis, lymphomatous meningitis, and nucleoside toxicity.

Pain at any stage is influenced by perception, by psychological, social, and even spiritual anxieties.[152] The psychological sequelae of HIV disease pain are essentially similar to cancer pain, where there is the constant threat of severity and persistence. Optimal HIV disease treatment should incorporate psychological treatment strategies because patient mood, depression, and beliefs about pain as well as the significance (meaning) of pain influence pain perception.

Pharmacologic treatment for HIV disease pain should follow the World Health Organization analgesic pain treatment protocol developed for cancer beginning with acetaminophen and NSAIDs with appropriate caution related to possible drug interaction with acetaminophen and AZT. Weak opioids are next utilized including codeine, oxycodone, and hydrocodone added to acetaminophen. Concerns over use of opioid treatment in substance abusers presents difficulties that require firm limits and contractual, written agreement on the use of narcotic analgesics.

The overall course of treatment and ability of the patient to cooperate in treatment may be compromised by the impact of HIV disease dementia. As the disease progresses, the risks of associated pain and dementia increase. Some studies have found that dementia is the initial AIDS-defining illness, viz. 4% followed by an increased incidence of 7% after a second AIDS-defining illness and a cumulative risk of 25%.[153] Nonpharmacologic treatment such as physical therapy and psychological interventions may be difficult in the presence of apathy, psychomotor retardation, decreased attention span, and short-term memory loss.

Nerve blocks, including injection of local anesthetic or neurolytic agents, are not typically applicable to HIV disease pain. However, temporary relief from pain may facilitate physical therapy and frequently sympathetic or somatic blocks may result in relief of pain that exceeds the actual anesthetic action.

PSYCHOLOGICAL INTERVENTIONS FOR CHRONIC PAIN

Psychological input into the diagnosis and treatment of chronic pain has become an accepted part of any comprehensive team approach to the management of this class of patients. Because the psychological influences on pain experiences are myriad, the regular consultation of a specialist in behavioral medicine is invaluable. In addition to helping to understand some of the psychological influences mentioned earlier, the psychologist has at his or her disposal a number of specific techniques that prove useful as part of a multidisciplinary treatment plan for chronic pain management.

Psychodynamic approaches to the patient in chronic pain are typified by an attempt to understand the patient in terms of personality structure, biologic drives, social contexts, wishes, and expectations. This leads to a psychodynamic formulation that posits a relationship between any or all of these factors and the presenting problem. Therapy is usually done on an individual basis and is aimed at establishing a therapeutic alliance with the patient, providing an interpretation of relevant symptoms, leading the individual to new levels of understanding about the derivation of their symptoms, and enhancing symptom resolution through the patient–therapist relationship, with termination of that relationship as the ultimate goal. To engage in this sort of approach requires a knowledge of fundamental psychoanalytic and therapeutic principles, training in the particulars of psychotherapy with chronic pain patients, and the time to engage in weekly or more frequent sessions with the patient for months to years of therapy. Clearly, this is out of the realm of expertise or desire of most anesthesiologists and is typically

so labor-intensive that it is not practical for many psychologists. In general, a very small proportion of patients in a given clinic population would be either amenable or appropriate to involvement in this style of therapy.

Much more common is the use of cognitive therapies. This group of strategies focuses on the cognitive or thought processes that are found in chronic pain patients. Often the thinking style of an individual has a great deal of effect on how he or she copes with pain. As mentioned earlier, the meaning of the pain experience can greatly influence the suffering. A classic example of this is the often quoted observation by Beecher[154] that injured soldiers on the battlefront in World War II often complained of pain far less than would be expected from the severity of their wounds. When they were safely behind the lines, however, they would complain just as loudly as anyone else when multiple venipunctures or other mildly painful procedures were required, disproving the notion that these people were stoic by nature. Beecher[154] reasoned that the meaning of the pain was making the difference in that a significant injury meant that one would be taken back home and, therefore, would survive the war. A common clinical example in a pain clinic would be the individual who is convinced that he or she cannot cope with a flare-up of pain. Such an individual will frequently think catastrophic thoughts such as "If this pain gets real bad, I don't know what I'll do!" These thoughts can become the focus of treatment and can, with motivation and practice on the part of the patient, be changed to more adaptive thoughts. This in time will give the individual some degree of control over the situation and will prevent him or her from engaging in self-defeating destructive thought patterns. Coping ability is thereby improved.[155]

Behavioral therapies involve efforts to reshape behaviors, rather than the sensory or emotional conditions that underlie them. This is a direct outgrowth of the work of Fordyce et al,[156] who adapted B. F. Skinner's operant model of behavior to the human pain patient. As previously discussed, this model states that behaviors can be cued by certain stimuli and can be modified by conditions that follow the emission of the behavior. Taking this antecedent–behavior–consequence paradigm view of pain behaviors such as limping, groaning, seeking dependence on others, and taking inappropriate analgesics, Fordyce and colleagues imposed strict control on the environment into which the chronic pain patient was placed. No reinforcement of pain behaviors was forthcoming from the staff (extinction) and positive reinforcement for wellness behaviors was instituted. This resulted in a significant decrease in pain behaviors. A critique of this method was that only the behaviors were decreased, but Fordyce et al argue that many patients state that after a largely behavioral treatment program they perceive less pain.[157] The principles of behavior modification extend to the staff of a pain clinic, the patient's workplace, and the home, in that solicitous responses from a spouse in response to pain behaviors by the patient may sabotage an otherwise intact and appropriate treatment plan.

Biofeedback is the providing of information to an individual about bodily functions that are commonly held to be inaccessible to the conscious mind. Commonly used devices measure surface electromyographic activity, temperature, or electrodermal activity. When feedback from these systems is provided, a patient can frequently be taught to control those functions at will. Originally, the logical assumption was made that teaching an individual to reduce muscle tone in a specific muscle would reduce the pain by the mechanism of muscle relaxation. While the outcome is generally that which is expected, the mechanism is not universally accepted to be reduction in muscle tone, leading to decreased activation of muscle nociceptive afferent neurons. The same statement can be made for the other modes of biofeedback. This does not, however, detract from the usefulness of the techniques, and they remain a valuable psychological intervention for some patients.

Numerous strategies have evolved for the induction of a state of relaxation in chronic pain. The theory is that relaxation induces both positive mental and physical changes in the individual that promote a sense of well-being, decrease muscle tone, and enhance coping. Jacobson[158] developed the first standardized approach to relaxation using the progressive contraction and relaxation of muscle groups in an ascending sequence from feet to head. There have been numerous procedures since then that can be learned to induce relaxation. These techniques rely on conscious manipulation of the body to induce a relaxed state, not merely getting comfortable on the couch and propping up one's feet. Benson[159] studied the physiologic concomitants of a relaxed state and found commonalities to the conditions induced by a variety of methods. These included a decrease in sympathetic tone, regularity in respiratory pattern, decreased skeletal muscle tone, and a feeling of well-being. He termed this physiologic pattern the *relaxation response* and postulated that the means of achieving it was unimportant and, in fact, developed a simple and straightforward induction method. This and similar techniques find great applicability to chronic pain patients, especially those with muscular involvement such as myofascial pain syndromes.

Hypnosis has long been used to help alleviate surgical and other acute pains. It has some utility in the chronic pain population as well. For an individual to become hypnotized, several conditions must exist: (1) an ability to concentrate, (2) a belief in the process, and (3) some motivation for the process to ensue. The trance state is thought to be a naturally occurring phenomenon in most people, although there is great variability in the population with regard to frequency and ease of occurrence. Trance state can be defined as an altered state of awareness characterized by extremely focused attention, relaxation, and responsiveness to suggestion. It is thought by most modern practitioners that the hypnotist does not hypnotize the subject but rather facilitates entry into trance by directing and guiding the individual's attention. The use of hypnosis can, in the properly selected individual, be a useful adjunct to therapy of chronic pain. It has found particular utility in the treatment of patients with cancer pain, possibly because these patients are so profoundly motivated. The mechanism of analgesia associated with hypnosis is unclear, but it does not appear to be due to endogenous opiates or to be solely due to placebo effect.

Group therapy, supportive therapy, education, and family therapy are other types of psychological interventions that have utility in the management of chronic pain patients. A skilled practitioner of behavioral medicine will aid the anesthesiologist in the diagnosis, conceptualization, and treatment of patients presenting with chronic pain by selecting evaluation and therapeutic strategies that are tailored to each individual's presentation.

INTERVENTIONAL PAIN MANAGEMENT

Over the past two decades, there has been rapid technological development in the field of pain management. Reliable and sophisticated intraspinal drug delivery devices can provide complex patterns of infusion over long periods of time. Totally implanted spinal cord stimulation devices can now access multiple electrodes simultaneously. Techniques for radiofrequency denervation have been developed for many neurologic structures. Miniaturized endoscopic devices permit more accurate perineural injection of medications within the spinal canal. Systems have been developed for thermocoagulation of annular tears of intervertebral discs and for stabilization of vertebral compression fractures. While these interventional techniques are not appropriate for the majority of patients with chronic pain, they have extended our capability for managing some of the most intractable problems. The following discussion describes a few of these systems.

Intrathecal Drug Delivery Devices

The discovery of opioid receptors and endogenous opioids in the late 1970s[160] led to early experiences with intraspinal opioids in animals[161] and eventually patients with chronic pain.[162] The original research with spinal opioids was fueled by the search for alternatives to irreversible neurodestructive techniques. The advantage of spinal opioid analgesia was thought to lie in the potential for obtaining more potent analgesia and fewer side-effects due to higher drug concentrations at spinal opioid receptors. What made intraspinal opioids suited for continuous administration[163,164] and eventually outpatient use was the selective nature of its action compared to local anesthetics, avoiding sensory, motor, and sympathetic blockade.

The original use of spinal narcotics for continuous drug delivery focused on cancer pain, proving its safety and efficacy in multiple studies.[165,166] A subsequent development was the successful utilization of intrathecal baclofen for the treatment of spasticity and rigidity in patients with spinal cord injuries.[167,168] Utilization of spinal opioids for nonmalignant pain remains controversial but is gaining acceptance.[169] More recent studies in this patient population seem to suggest a lower incidence of tolerance and iatrogenic addiction than first feared.[169]

Opioids administered by the spinal route act preferentially on receptors in the dorsal horn. Pain relief is produced through modulation of incoming A-delta and C-fiber sensory input.[170] In part, opioids also travel rostrally and act on supraspinal opiate receptors.

In selecting patients for chronic intrathecal opioid therapy, one must distinguish between neuropathic and nociceptive pain syndromes. Nociceptive pain is generally opioid-responsive; neuropathic pain, however, may not respond, or may require much larger opioid doses.[171] The latter may respond to the spinal administration of α_2-receptor agonists such as clonidine[172] or local anesthetic/opioid combinations.[173]

Cancer pain is often dynamic, with a mixed nociceptive and neuropathic pain presentation, and may therefore require adjunct therapy. These patients may be candidates for intraspinal opioids if they have proven opioid-responsive pain but have developed either intolerable side-effects or tolerance to systemic opioids. Cost effectiveness of implantable drug delivery systems in this patient population may require a minimum of three months' survival when compared to external infusion systems.[174]

Selection of patients with nonmalignant pain remains difficult, with no clear selection criteria identified. Prior to considering these patients for candidacy, every effort must be made to establish a diagnosis of the pain syndrome at hand. All available surgical and medical alternatives should be explored including trials of long-acting opioids. These should be escalated until side-effects are encountered or inadequate benefit is established. Psychological evaluation and psychometric testing should be considered to investigate the possibility of primary psychological pain states. Contraindications to the placement of implantable infusion devices include, among other things, the presence of sepsis, anticoagulation, severe immune suppression, and drug addiction.

Morphine continues to be the most widely used agent for long-term spinal administration. It remains the only FDA-approved intraspinal analgesic. Its high water solubility and receptor affinity provide for prolonged duration predictability and a widespread distribution throughout the cerebrospinal fluid compartment.[175] Substances with a higher lipid solubility, such as fentanyl, sufentanil, and meperidine, reduce supraspinal effects through limited spread but require accurate catheter placement adjacent to the spinal cord level associated with the specific pain syndrome.[175] Opioid rotation is commonly done in long-term use since tolerance and drug side-effects can develop. Owing to the phenomenon of incomplete cross-tolerance among opioids, a lower dose of a different opioid can often be substituted.

Intrathecally administered baclofen has been very useful for the control of spasticity and rigidity in spinal cord injuries and multiple sclerosis, as first documented by Penn in 1987.[176] Since then, other studies have confirmed the usefulness of baclofen in this setting[168] and in certain central pain states.[177] Baclofen binds to GABA_B receptors, producing inhibition of synaptic transmission leading to a reduction in muscle tone. It is FDA-approved for intrathecal use for patients with spasticity. Recently, intrathecal infusions of baclofen have been shown to provide effective analgesia for patients with chronic pain that is not associated with spasticity or spinal cord injury.[139] It produced sustained benefit in several patients who had become unresponsive to intrathecal morphine.

Efficacy trials are essential to pump implantation. Different methods are in clinical use, ranging from single-shot outpatient drug administration to titration of a continuous epidural or intrathecal infusion in the inpatient setting. Prior oral or systemic opioid needs will determine trial doses of intrathecal drugs. The patient is then observed for analgesic efficacy and drug side-effects. The minimum analgesic response is controversial, but often a minimum of 50% reduction in pain scores and a duration twice the half-life of the agent is sought. Response to placebo injections should be compared to responses to active drug. The development of early side-effects such as intractable pruritus or nausea is often discouraging even though tolerance to them may develop with longer-term administration. Efficacy of intrathecal baclofen for treatment of spasticity is assessed using the Ashworth muscle rigidity/tone scale.

Intrathecal drug delivery systems vary from simple percutaneous catheters (Type I) to totally implantable and programmable infusion pumps (Type VI). Type VI systems have gained in popularity for long-term infusions, both in cancer pain states with long survival times and in nonmalignant pain states. These systems provide for a broad range of delivery rates and modes, and hence flexibility. Refill periods range from weeks to months, depending on drug concentrations and tolerance. FDA approval has been given to Infusaid factory-preset fixed flow rate pumps (Type V) and the Medtronic Synchromed totally programmable pump systems (Type VI).

Examples of postoperative complications include bleeding, infection, seroma formation, and CSF leakage. Infection is usually localized; however, epidural or intrathecal sepsis is disastrous, requiring the removal of all hardware and administration of systemic antibiotics.[179] Long-term complications related to the implanted equipment include catheter disconnects, obstruction, or breakage as well as pump failure among other things. Pump malfunction is uncommon, but errors in refilling and reprogramming have resulted in serious morbidity and mortality.[180]

Spinal Cord Stimulation

The gate control theory, introduced by Melzack and Wall in 1965, provided the theoretical foundation for the use of implanted electrical stimulation. Several years later Shealy[181] was the first to describe what was initially known as dorsal column stimulation and eventually spinal cord stimulation (SCS). Electrical stimulation in proximity of the dorsal columns through epidural lead placement was thought convenient since sensory pathways there are segregated from motor pathways. Initially, however, poor patient selection and technological limitations led to disappointing results. Patient selection improved through work done in the late 1980s and early 1990s.[182] At the same time new technology became available, including the arrival of multichannel leads, dual-lead configurations, totally implantable generators, and expanded programming options. The

specific mechanism of action of SCS remains elusive. Neural and neurochemical changes, perhaps resulting from stimulation in the dorsal roots, dorsal root entry zone, or dorsal columns, have been implicated.[183] The efficacy of spinal cord stimulation is greatest for certain types of ischemic and neuropathic pain syndromes with primarily causalgic and dysesthetic features.[184]

Conditions that have favorably responded to SCS include lumbosacral fibrosis and arachnoiditis,[185] complex regional pain sydromes,[186] and more recently ischemic pain conditions associated with peripheral vascular disease[187] and angina pectoris.[188] Failed back surgery patients with predominantly radicular pain elements have shown response rates of 50–60% at 5 years in recent studies.[189,190] Patients with peripheral vascular disease have also responded favorably with significant limb salvage rates reported.[187,191] Patients with medically refractory angina pectoris who were not candidates for revascularization have experienced pain relief and improvement in cardiac function and stress testing.[188,192]

The most critical issues in patient selection consist of identifying a well founded diagnosis and the presence of specific neuropathic or ischemic pain states. A multidisciplinary approach including a psychological evaluation is recommended. High scores on the Minnesota Multiphasic Personality Inventory's depression scale have been associated with SCS failure.[193] Other contraindications such as the presence of localized infection, systemic sepsis, severe immune suppression, and coagulopathy are similar to other implantable devices.

The two systems in current use are a totally implantable generator system and a system that uses an implantable receiver and external transmitter. Either system is adaptable to multiple leads depending on the need for bilateral extremity stimulation or wider unilateral coverage. Similarly, different electrode configurations exist, varying in number and spacing of electrodes. One can also take advantage of complex programming options to fine-tune or change stimulation patterns.

Prior to permanent placement, a trial stimulation is performed. Generally, temporary percutaneous stimulator leads are used for this purpose. Once an appropriate stimulation pattern is produced, most protocols will require at least a 50% improvement in pain scores. The length of trial screening is controversial, varying from days to weeks.

Lead migration and breakage are common problems with long-term stimulation. Lead migration may produce unwanted paresthesias or diminish benefit in the original area of stimulation. This can sometimes be overcome by reprogramming of the electrode but may require lead replacement. Serious infection, bleeding, and nerve injury are uncommon complications.[189] Generator or transmitter failure is unlikely; however, fully implantable generators will require replacement depending on use.

Radiofrequency Lesioning

Research on the use of radiofrequency (RF) power for use in neurosurgical procedures dates back to work done by Harvey Cushing in the mid-1920s. Clinical use of this technology was first achieved through central nervous system lesions in the 1950s. The technique was further refined in the 1970s by the invention of the RF probe, leading to a variety of new applications.[194] Modern RF thermocoagulation has been used to ablate pain pathways in the spinal cord, dorsal root entry zone, dorsal root ganglion, trigeminal ganglion, sympathetic chain, and peripheral nerves.

An insulated probe with an uninsulated tip is placed in proximity of the target tissue and RF current is allowed to flow from a generator. As the current encounters resistance in the tissue, heat is generated, creating a lesion. Lesion size is directly proportional to tissue temperature at thermal equilibrium between the probe tip and the surrounding tissue. This equilibrium is generally achieved in 1 minute. Prior to lesioning, the target structure must be localized. This is accomplished by electrical stimulation. High frequencies and lower voltages are used to elicit a paresthesia in the desired distribution, while low frequencies and higher voltages are used to assess neuromuscular activity prior to lesioning. Temperatures specific for the target nerve can be chosen, allowing for selective interruption of small unmyelinated fibers, preserving myelinated motor innervation.

Patient selection requires a firm diagnosis verified by prognostic blocks with local anesthetics. RF lesioning is by definition neurodestructive and can be considered only after more conservative options have failed. Patients may require psychological screening and should be aware of all potential adverse sequelae, including neurologic impairment. Thorough knowledge of neuroanatomy and the use of fluoroscopy are mandatory for the pain physician.

The lumbar spine is an area where RF lesioning is often applied. Specific techniques have been developed for pain originating from the facet joints, nerve roots, annulus fibrosis, and sacroiliac joints. Approximately 50–60% of carefully selected patients with mechanical low back pain due to facet arthropathy achieve at least moderate reduction in pain following radiofrequency facet rhizotomy.[195-197] Lesions for discogenic pain are performed at the ramus communicans and intradiscally.[198] Owing to the complexity of disk innervation and disk pathology, this procedure is not nearly as successful. RF dorsal root gangliotomy is in use for the treatment of pain originating from the lumbar spinal nerve.[199] This is reserved for nonsurgical patients after diagnostic sleeve blocks of the segmental nerve have been performed. RF applications for cervical spine pain are primarily oriented toward facet joint denervation. Lesions of the sphenopalatine and trigeminal ganglia[200] have been successfully used for select patients for the treatment of migraine headaches and trigeminal neuralgia respectively. RF neurolysis of the sympathetic chain, though not in widespread use, has been helpful in some patients with Type II complex regional pain syndrome and vasoocclusive disorders.

Patients can experience postoperative pain or dysesthesia for days to weeks after the procedure as a result of low-level heat injuries to tissue. Subsequently, judging the efficacy of the procedure is often difficult in the short term. More permanent nerve injuries and disk infections have been described.[201] Although in clinical use since the 1950s, RF is still a technique used by relatively few clinicians. It is, however, gaining in popularity since a wider range of applications and newer technologies such as pulsed RF are available now. Benefit from RF lesioning is time-limited due to nerve regeneration but the procedure may offer more prolonged analgesia than nerve blocks. Whenever possible, more conservative and less invasive treatment modalities should be entertained prior to RF procedures.

Epiduroscopy

Early experiences with endoscopic visualization of contents of the spinal canal date back to the 1930s.[202] With the development of fiberoptic light source technology in the 1970s, it became possible to develop endoscopes small enough for epidural insertion.[203] In the early 1990s, several flexible fiberoptic systems were developed for direct imaging of epidural contents. These devices eventually featured steerability and multiple channels for irrigation, delivery of medications, and possibly instrumentation. Today's epiduroscopes carry FDA approval for diagnosis of epidural pathology, and direct delivery of normal saline and steroids. The theoretical basis for epiduroscopic injection of steroid lies in investigational data showing poor epidural spread of substances in patients with prior spine surgery.[204] These epidural adhesions are thought to be in part responsible for failed spinal surgery. Lysis of these adhesions appears to offer some

benefit for patients with certain postoperative lumbar radiculopathies.

Epidural access is achieved via the sacral hiatus, while distension of the epidural space is gained through normal saline infusions. Adhesions are then lysed through blunt instrumentation with the endoscope, other instruments introduced through a sideport, or simply through forceful proximity injections of normal saline. The procedure is generally performed under light sedation rather than under anesthesia since a significant increase in epidural pressure due to overdistension may lead to neurologic compromise. Improvement in spread of contrast is often seen following the procedure, but may not correlate with improvement in symptoms.[205] Contraindications to the procedure include coagulopathy, infection, raised intracranial pressure, and severe cerebrovascular disease. While the ultimate role of spinal endoscopy has yet to be established, work is under way to develop instruments that could be used for more definitive therapeutic applications. The current role of the endoscope appears to be limited to diagnosis while outcome studies on its therapeutic value have yet to be conducted.

Intradiscal Electrothermal Therapy

Intradiscal electrothermal therapy involves the percutaneous placement of a heating electrode into the intervertebral disk. The electrode is navigated circumferentially around the inner surface of the disk annulus. By then heating the electrode, annular collagen is denatured and nerve endings innervating the disk are coagulated. The patient target group for this procedure appears to be patients with internal disk disruptions secondary to small contained disk herniations, posterior annular fissures, and degenerated disk with relatively preserved disk height. This group of patients is thought likely to fail conservative therapy while discectomy and fusion surgery for these indications have shown mixed results. MRI evidence of disk disruption and a positive discogram are required for patient selection. Early studies seem to suggest moderate to good short-term results with this new technology. However, long-term efficacy trials and outcome studies have yet to be conducted.

REFERENCES

1. Raja SN, Meyer RA, Campbell JN: Transduction properties of the sensory afferent fibers. In Yaksh TL *et al* (eds): Anesthesia: Biologic Foundations, p 513. Philadelphia, Lippincott-Raven, 1997
2. Klement W, Arndt JO: The role of nociceptors of cutaneous veins in the mediation of cold pain in man. J Physiol (Lond) 449:73, 1992
3. Lynn B: The detection of injury and tissue damage. In Melzack R, Wall PD (eds): Textbook of Pain, p 19. New York, Churchill Livingstone, 1984
4. Freeman MAR, Wyke B: The innervation of the knee joint: An anatomical and histological study of the cat. J Anat 101:505, 1967
5. Tanelian DL, Beuerman RW: Responses of rabbit corneal nociceptors to mechanical and thermal stimulation. Exp Neurol 84:165, 1984
6. Bahr R, Blumberg H, Janig W: Do dichotomizing afferent fibers exist which supply visceral organs as well as somatic structures? Neurosci Lett 24:25, 1981
7. Malliani A: Cardiovascular sympathetic afferent fibers. Rev Physiol Biochem Pharmacol 94:11, 1982
8. Foreman RD: Organization of visceral output. In Yaksh TL *et al* (eds): Anesthesia: Biologic Foundations, p 663. Philadelphia, Lippincott-Raven, 1997
9. Ordway GA, Longhurst JC: Cardiovascular reflexes arising from the gallbladder of the cat. Circ Res 52:26, 1983
10. Cervero F: Afferent nerve activity evoked by natural stimulation of the biliary system in the ferret. Pain 13:137, 1982
11. Light AR, Perl ER: Spinal termination of functionally identified primary afferent neurons with slowly conducting myelinated fibers. J Comp Neurol 168:133, 1979
12. Malmberg AB, Yaksh TL: Hyperalgesia mediated by spinal gluta-

mate or SP receptor blocked by spinal cyclooxygenase inhibition. Science 257:1276, 1992

13. Wilcox GL: Excitatory neurotransmitters and pain. In Bond MR, Charlton JE, Woolf CJ (eds): Proceedings of the Sixth World Congress on Pain, p 97. Amsterdam, Elsevier, 1991

14. Mendell LM: Physiological properties of unmyelinated fibre projections to the spinal cord. Exp Neurol 16:316, 1966

15. Meldrum B, Garthwaite J: Excitatory amino acid neurotoxicity and neurodegenerative disease. Trends Pharmacol Sci 11:379, 1990

16. Coderre TJ, Katz J, Vaccarino AL, Melzack R: Contribution of central neuroplasticity to pathological pain: Review of clinical and experimental evidence. Pain 52:259, 1993

17. Hope PJ, Schaible HG, Jarrott B, Duggan AW: Release and persistence of immunoreactive neurokinin A in the spinal cord is associated with chemical arthritis. Pain 5:S230, 1990

18. Malmberg AB, Yaksh TL: Antinociceptive actions of spinal nonsteroidal anti-inflammatory agents on the formalin test in the rat. J Pharmacol Exp Ther 263:136, 1992

19. Meller ST, Gebhart GF: Nitric oxide (NO) and nociceptive processing in the spinal cord. Pain 52:127, 1993

20. Malmberg AB, Yaksh TL: Spinal nitric oxide synthesis inhibition blocks NMDA-induced thermal hyperalgesia and produces antinociception in the formalin test in rats. Pain 54:291, 1993

21. Coderre TJ: Contribution of protein kinase C to persistent nociception following tissue injury in rats. Neurosci Lett 140:181, 1992

22. Mao J, Price DD, Mayer DJ: Mechanisms of hyperalgesia and morphine tolerance: A current review of their possible interactions. Pain 62:259, 1995

23. Yaksh TL, Elde RP: Factors governing release of methionine enkephalin-like immunoreactivity from mesencephalon and spinal cord of the cat in vivo. J Neurophysiol 46:1056, 1981

24. Van Calker P, Muller M, Hemprecht B: Adenosine regulates via two different types of receptors the accumulation of cAMP in cultured brain cells. J Neurochem 33:999, 1979

25. Daly JW, Bruno RF, Snyder SH: Adenosine receptors in the central nervous system: Relationship to the central action of methylxanthines. Life Sci 28:2083, 1981

26. Yaksh TL, Hammond DL: Peripheral and central substrates involved in the rostrad transmission of nociceptive information. Pain 13:1, 1982

27. Tasker RR: Deafferentation. In Melzack R, Wall PD (eds): Textbook of Pain, p 119. New York, Churchill Livingstone, 1984

28. Willis WD: The origin and destination of pathways involved in pain transmission. In Melzack R, Wall PD (eds): Textbook of Pain, p 88. New York, Churchill Livingstone, 1984

29. Heinricher MM: Organizational characteristics of supraspinally mediated responses to nociceptive inputs. In Yaksh TL et al (eds): Anesthesia: Biologic Foundations, p 643. Philadelphia, Lippincott-Raven, 1997

30. Wall PD, Gutnick M: Ongoing activity in peripheral nerves: The physiology and pharmacology of impulses originating from a neuroma. Exp Neurol 43:580, 1974

31. Blumberg H, Janig W: Discharge pattern of afferent fibers from a neuroma. Pain 20:335, 1984

32. Garry MC, Tanelian DL: Afferent activity in injured afferent nerves. In Yaksh TL et al (eds): Anesthesia: Biologic Foundations, p 531. Philadelphia, Lippincott-Raven, 1997

33. Wall PD, Devor M: Sensory afferent impulses originate from dorsal root ganglia as well as from the periphery in normal and nerve injured rats. Pain 17:321, 1983

34. Blumberg H, Janig W: Changes in vasoconstrictor neurons supplying cat hindlimb following chronic nerve lesions: A model for studying mechanisms of reflex sympathetic dystrophy? J Auton Nerve Syst 7:399, 1983

35. Roberts WJ: A hypothesis on the physiological basis for causalgia and related pains. Pain 24:297, 1986

36. Ramer MS, Thompson SWN, McMahon SB: Causes and consequences of sympathetic basket formation in dorsal root ganglia. Pain 6(suppl):S111, 1999

37. Merskey H: Pain terms: A list with definitions and notes on usage. Pain 6:249, 1979

38. Engel GL: ''Psychogenic'' pain and the pain-prone patient. Am J Med 26:899, 1959

39. Williams JBW (ed): Diagnostic and Statistical Manual of Mental Disorders, 3rd ed. Washington, DC, American Psychiatric Association, 1987

40. Hall RCW, Popkin MK, DeVaul RA et al: Physical illness presenting as psychiatric disease. Arch Gen Psychiatry 35:1315, 1978

41. Haddox JD: Psychological aspects of pain. In Abram SE, Haddox JD, Kettler RE (eds): The Pain Clinic Manual, p 31. Philadelphia, JB Lippincott, 1990

42. Blumer D, Heilbronn M: Chronic pain as a variant of depressive disease—the pain-prone disorder. J Nerv Ment Dis 170:381, 1982

43. Turk DC, Rudy TE, Steig RL: Chronic pain and depression. Pain Management 1:18, 1987

44. Pilowsky I, Chapman CR, Bonica JJ: Pain, depression and illness behavior in a pain clinic population. Pain 4:183, 1977

45. Skinner BF: Science and Human Behavior. New York, Macmillan, 1953

46. Ohnmeiss DD, Vanharanta H, Ekholm J: Degree of disk disruption and lower extremity pain. Spine 22:1600, 1997

47. Brown MF, Hukkanen MVJ, McCarthy ID et al: Sensory and sympathetic innervation of the vertebral endplate in patients with degenerative disk disease. J Bone Joint Surg 79B:147, 1997

48. Dreyer SJ, Dreyfuss PH: Low back pain and the zygapophyseal (facet) joints. Arch Phys Med Rehabil 77:290, 1996

49. Maigne J-Y, Avaliklis A, Pfefer F: Results of sacroiliac joint double block and value of sacroiliac pain provocation tests in 54 patients with low back pain. Spine 21:1889, 1996

50. Kuslich SD, Ulstrom CL, Michael CJ: The tissue origin of low back pain and sciatica: A report of pain response to tissue stimulation during operation on the lumbar spine using local anesthesia. Orthop Clin North Am 22:181, 1991

51. Murphy RW: Nerve roots and spinal nerves in degenerative disc disease. Clin Orthop 129:46, 1977

52. Gertzbein SD, Tile M, Gross A, Falk R: Autoimmunity in degenerative disc disease of the lumbar spine. Orthop Clin North Am 6:67, 1975

53. Marshall LL, Trethwie ER: Chemical irritation of nerve roots in disc prolapse. Lancet 2:230, 1973

54. Saal JS, Franson RC, Dobrow R et al: High levels of phospholipase A_2 activity in lumbar disk herniations. Spine 15:674, 1990

55. Gordon SL, Weinstein JN: A review of basic science issues in low back pain. Phys Med Rehabil Clin North Am 9:323, 1998

56. Lievre JA, Block-Michael H, Attali P: L'injection transsacré: Etude Clinique et Radiologique. Bull Soc Med 73:1110, 1957

57. Benzon HT: Epidural steroid injections for low back pain and lumbosacral radiculopathy. Pain 24:277, 1986

58. Coomes EN: A comparison between epidural anesthesia and bedrest in sciatica. Br Med J 1:20, 1961

59. Swerdlow M, Sayle-Creer W: A study of extradural medication in the relief of the lumbosciatic syndrome. Anaesthesia 25:341, 1970

60. Winnie AP, Hartman JT, Myers HL et al: Pain clinic: II. Intradural and extradural corticosteroids for sciatica. Anesth Analg 51:990, 1972

61. Koes BW, Scholten RJPM, Mens JMA, Bouter LM: Efficacy of epidural steroid injections of low-back pain and sciatica: A systematic review of randomized trials. Pain 63:279, 1995

62. Watts RW, Silagy CA: A meta-analysis on the efficacy of epidural corticosteroids in the treatment of sciatica. Anaesth Intens Care 23:564, 1995

63. Carette S, Leclaire R, Marcoux S et al: Epidural corticosteroids injections for sciatica due to herniated nucleus pulposus. N Engl J Med 336:1634, 1997

64. Abram SE, Hopwood MB: What factors contribute to outcome with lumbar epidural steroids? In Bond MR, Charlton JE, Woolf CJ (eds): Proceedings of the Sixth World Congress on Pain, p 491. Amsterdam, Elsevier, 1991

65. Finneson BE: Low Back Pain. Philadelphia, JB Lippincott, 1973

66. Cicala RS, Turner R, Moran E et al: Methylprednisolone acetate does not cause inflammatory changes in the epidural space. Anesthesiology 72:556, 1990

67. Abram SE, Marsala M, Yaksh TL: Analgesic and neurotoxic effects of intrathecal corticosteroids in rats. Anesthesiology 81:1198, 1994

68. Nelson DA: Dangers from methylprednisolone acetate therapy by intraspinal injection. Arch Neurol 45:804, 1988

69. Kay J, Findling JW, Raff H: Epidural triamcinolone suppresses the pituitary adrenal axis in human subjects. Anesth Analg 79:501, 1994

70. Plumb VJ, Dismukes WE: Chemical meningitis related to intrathecal corticosteroid therapy. South Med J 70:1241, 1977

71. Dougherty JH, Fraser RAR: Complications following intraspinal injection of steroids. J Neurosurg 48:1023, 1978

72. Ryan MD, Taylor TKF: Management of lumbar nerve root pain by intrathecal and epidural injection of depot methylprednisolone acetate. Med J Aust 2:532, 1981
73. Cohen FL: Conus medullaris syndrome following multiple intrathecal corticosteroid injections. Arch Neurol 36:228, 1979
74. Abram SE, Anderson RA: Using a pain questionnaire to predict response to steroid epidurals. Reg Anaesth 5:11, 1980
75. Carrera GF: Lumbar facet joint injection in low back pain and sciatica. Radiology 137:665, 1980
76. Carrera GF, Foley WD, Kozin F et al: CT of sacroiliitis. Am J Radiol 136:41, 1981
77. Travell JG, Simons DG: Myofascial Pain and Dysfunction. Baltimore, Williams & Wilkins, 1983
78. Travell JG, Rinzler SH: The myofascial genesis of pain. Postgrad Med 11:425, 1952
79. Berges PV: Myofascial pain syndromes. Postgrad Med 53:161, 1953
80. Cheshire WP, Abashian SW, Mann JD: Botulinum toxin in the treatment of myofascial pain syndrome. Pain 59:65, 1994
81. Stanton-Hicks M, Janig W, Hassenbusch S et al: Reflex sympathetic dystrophy: Changing concepts and taxonomy. Pain 63:127, 1995
82. Hogan QH, Erickson SJ, Haddox JD, Abram SE: The spread of solutions during stellate ganglion block. Reg Anesth 17:78, 1992
83. Hogan QH, Erickson SJ, Abram SE: Computerized tomography-guided stellate ganglion blockade. Anesthesiology 77:596, 1992
84. Hogan QH, Abram SE: Neural blockade for diagnosis and prognosis. Anesthesiology 86:216, 1997
85. Bonica JJ: Causalgia and other reflex sympathetic dystrophies. In Bonica JJ, Albe-Fessard D (eds): Advances in Pain Research and Therapy, vol 1, p 141. New York, Raven Press, 1979
86. Hannington-Kiff JG: Intravenous regional sympathetic block with guanethidine. Lancet 1:1019, 1974
87. Boneli S, Conoscente F, Movilia PG et al: Regional intravenous guanethidine vs. stellate block in reflex sympathetic dystrophies: A randomized trial. Pain 16:297, 1983
88. Kozin F, Ryan LM, Carrera GF et al: The reflex sympathetic dystrophy syndrome (RSDS): III. Scintigraphic studies, further evidence for the therapeutic efficacy of systemic corticosteroids, and proposed diagnostic criteria. Am J Med 70:23, 1981
89. Poplawski ZJ, Wiley AM, Murray JF: Post-traumatic dystrophy of the extremities. J Bone Joint Surg 65A:642, 1983
90. Abram SE, Asiddao CB, Reynolds AC: Increased skin temperature during transcutaneous electrical stimulation. Anesth Analg 59:22, 1980
91. Stilz RJ, Carron H, Sanders DB: Reflex sympathetic dystrophy in a 6 year old: Successful treatment by transcutaneous nerve stimulation. Anesth Analg 56:438, 1977
92. Spurling RG: Causalgia of the upper extremity: Treatment by dorsal sympathetic ganglionectomy. Arch Neurol Psychiatry 23:784, 1930
93. Mayfield FH: Causalgia. Springfield, Illinois, Charles C Thomas, 1951
94. Boas RS, Hatangdi VS, Richards EG: Lumbar sympathectomy: A percutaneous technique. In Bonica JJ, Albe-Fessard D (eds): Advances in Pain Research and Therapy, vol 1, p 485. New York, Raven Press, 1976
95. Loeser JD: Herpes zoster and postherpetic neuralgia. Pain 25:149, 1986
96. Watson CPN, Watt VR, Chipman M et al: The prognosis with postherpetic neuralgia. Pain 46:195, 1991
97. Rogers RS, Tindall JP: Geriatric herpes zoster. J Am Geriatr Soc 19:495, 1971
98. Zacks SI, Langfitt TW, Elliott FA: Herpetic neuritis, a light and electron microscopic study. Neurology 14:774, 1964;
99. Noordenbos W: Pain, p 182. Amsterdam, Elsevier, 1959.
100. Watson CPN, Deck JH, Morshead C et al: Post-herpetic neuralgia: Further post-mortem studies of cases with and without pain. Pain 44:105, 1991
101. Rosenak S: Procaine injection treatment of herpes zoster. Lancet 2:1056, 1938
102. Winnie AP, Hartwell PW: The relationship between the time of treatment of acute herpes with sympathetic blockade and postherpetic neuralgia: Clinical support for a new theory of the mechanism by which sympathetic blockade provides therapeutic benefit. Reg Anesth 18:277, 1994
103. Whitley RJ, Gnann JW: Acyclovir: A decade later. N Engl J Med 327:782, 1992
104. Tyring S, Barbarash RA, Nahlik JE et al: Famcyclovir for the treat-

ment of acute herpes zoster: A randomized, controlled, double blind trial. Ann Int Med 123:89, 1995
105. Eaglestein WH, Katz R, Brown JA: The effects of early corticosteroid therapy on the skin eruption and pain of herpes zoster. JAMA 211:1681, 1970
106. Epstein E: Herpes zoster and post-zoster neuralgia: Intralesional triamcinolone therapy. Cutis 12:898, 1973
107. Schreuder M: Pain relief in herpes zoster. S Afr Med J 63:820, 1983
108. Rosenak S: Procaine injection treatment of herpes zoster. Lancet 2:1056, 1938
109. Tenicela R, Lovasik D, Eaglestein W: Treatment of herpes zoster with sympathetic blocks. Clin J Pain 1:63, 1985
110. Rowbotham M, Harden N, Stacey B et al: Gabapentin for the treatment of postherpetic neuralgia. JAMA 280:1837, 1998
111. Portenoy RK: Opioid therapy for chronic non-malignant pain: Current status. In Fields HL, Liebeskind JS (eds): Progress in Pain Research and Management, vol 1, p 247. Seattle, IASP Press, 1994
112. Weissman DE, Haddox JD: Opioid pseudoaddiction—an iatrogenic syndrome. Pain 36:363, 1989
113. Paoli F, Darcourt G, Corsa P: Note preliminare sur l'action de l'imipramine dans les etats douloureaux. Rev Neurol 102:503, 1960
114. Watson CP, Evans RS, Reed K et al: Amitriptyline versus placebo in postherpetic neuralgia. Neurology 32:671, 1982
115. Getto CJ, Sorkness CA, Howell T: Antidepressants and chronic nonmalignant pain: A review. J Pain Symptom Management 2:9, 1987
116. Max MB, Culane M, Schafer SC et al: Amitriptyline relieves diabetic neuropathy pain in patients with normal or depressed mood. Neurology 37:589, 1987
117. Max MB, Schafer SC, Culane M et al: Amitriptyline, but not lorazepam, relieves postherpetic neuralgia. Neurology 38:1427, 1988
118. Diamond S, Freitag FG: The use of fluoxetine in the treatment of headache. Clin J Pain 5:200, 1989
119. Camran A, Staumanis J, Chesson A: Fluoxetine prophylaxis of migraine. Headache 32:101, 1991
120. Power-Smith P, Turkington D: Fluoxetine in phantom limb pain. Br J Psychiatry 163:105, 1993
121. Max MB, Lynch SA, Muir J et al: Effects of desipramine, amitriptyline and fluoxetine on pain in diabetic neuropathy. N Engl J Med 326:1250, 1992
122. Sindrup SH, Gram LF, Brsen K et al: The selective serotonin reuptake inhibitor paroxetine is effective in the treatment of diabetic neuropathy symptoms. Pain 42:135, 1990
123. Reynolds IJ, Miller RJ: Tricyclic antidepressants block N-methyl-D-aspartate receptors: Similarities to the action of zinc. Br J Pharmacol 95:95, 1988
124. Mellick GA, Mellicy LB, Mellick LB: Gabapentin in the management of reflex sympathetic dystrophy. J Pain Symptom Management 10:265, 1995
125. Backonja M, Beydoun A, Edwards KR et al: Gabapentin for the symptomatic treatment of painful neuropathy in patients with diabetes mellitus. JAMA 280:1831, 1998
126. Xiao W-H, Bennett GJ: Gabapentin has an antinociceptive effect mediated via a spinal site of acion in a rat model of painful peripheral neuropathy. Pain 2:267, 1996
127. Eisenberg E, Alon N, Ishay A et al: Lamotrigine in the treatment of painful diabetic neuropathy. Eur J Neurol 5:167, 1998
128. Chabal C, Russell LC, Burchiel KJ: The effect of intravenous lidocaine, tocainide, and mexiletine on spontaneously active fibers originating in rat sciatic neuromas. Pain 38:333, 1989
129. Tanelian DL, Brose WG: Neuropathic pain can be relieved by drugs that are use-dependent sodium channel blockers: Lidocaine, carbamazepine, and mexiletine. Anesthesiology 74:949, 1991
130. Collin E, Poulain P, Gauvin-Piquard A et al: Is disease progression the major factor in morphine 'tolerance' in cancer pain treatment? Pain 55:319, 1993
131. Paronis CA, Holtzman SG: Development of tolerance to the analgesic activity of μ agonists after continuous infusion of morphine, meperidine and fentanyl in rats. J Pharmacol Exp Ther 262:1,1992
132. Coombs DW, Saunders RL, Gaylor MS et al: Relief of continuous chronic pain by intraspinal narcotics infusion via an implanted reservoir. JAMA 250:2336, 1983
133. Jorgensen BC, Andersen HB, Engquist A: CSF and plasma morphine after epidural and intrathecal application. Anesthesiology 55:714, 1981
134. Woods WA, Cohen SE: High-dose epidural morphine in a terminally ill patient. Anesthesiology 56:311, 1982

135. Stillman MJ, Moulin DE, Foley KM: Paradoxical pain following high dose spinal morphine. Pain 4:S389, 1987
136. Yaksh TL, Harty GJ: Pharmacology of the allodynia in rats evoked by high dose intrathecal morphine. J Pharmacol Exp Ther 244:501, 1988
137. Eisenach JC, Rauck RL, Buzzanell C et al: Epidural clonidine for intractable cancer pain. Anesthesiology 71:647, 1989
138. Wilson PR, Yaksh TL: Baclofen is antinociceptive in the spinal intrathecal space of animals. Eur J Pharmacol 51:323, 1978
139. Zuniga RE, Schlicht CR, Abram SE: Intrathecal baclofen is analgesic in patients without spasticity. Anesthesiology 92:876, 2000
140. Hogan Q, Haddox JD, Abram SE et al: Epidural opiates for the management of cancer pain. Pain 42:271, 1991
141. Du Pen SL, Kharasch ED, Williams A et al: Chronic epidural bupivacaine-opioid infusion in intractable cancer pain. Pain 49:293, 1992
142. Swerdlow M: Relief of Intractable Pain. Amsterdam, Excerpta Medica, 1974
143. Papo I, Visca A: Phenol subarachnoid rhizotomy for the treatment of cancer pain: A personal account of 290 cases. In Bonica JJ, Ventafridda V (eds): Advances in Pain Research and Therapy, vol 2, p 339. New York, Raven Press, 1979
144. Swerdlow M: Subarachnoid and extradural neurolytic blocks. In Bonica JJ, Ventafridda V (eds): Advances in Pain Research and Therapy, vol 2, p 325. New York, Raven Press, 1979
145. Thompson GE, Moore DC, Bridenbaugh LD et al: Abdominal pain and alcohol celiac plexus nerve block. Anesth Analg 56:1, 1977
146. Singler RC: An improved technique for alcohol neurolysis of the celiac plexus. Anesthesiology 56:137, 1982
147. Ischia S, Luzzani A, Ischia A et al: A new approach to the neurolytic block of the celiac plexus: The transaortic technique. Pain 16:333, 1983
148. Plancarte R, Amescua C, Patt RB, Aldrete A: Superior hypogastric plexus block for pelvic cancer pain. Anesthesiology 73:236, 1990
149. de Leon-Casasola OA, Kent E, Lema MJ: Neurolytic superior hypogastric plexus block for chronic pelvic pain associated with cancer. Pain 54:145, 1993
150. Simon DL, Carron H, Rowlingson JC: Treatment of bladder pain with transsacral nerve block. Anesth Analg 61:46, 1982
151. Bouhassira D, Lefkowitz M, Meynadier J, Serrie A: Origins of pain in HIV/AIDS. In Pain in HIV/AIDS, p 1. Chicago, Addison, 1994
152. O'Neill W, Sherrard S: Pain in human immunodeficiency virus disease: A review. Pain 54:3, 1993
153. McArthur JC, Hoover DR, Bacellar H: Dementia in AIDS patients: Incidence and risk factors. Neurology 43:2245, 1993
154. Beecher HK: The Measurement of Subjective Responses: Quantitative Effects of Drugs. New York, Oxford University Press, 1959
155. Taylor ML: Psychological treatment of chronic pain. In Abram SE, Haddox JD, Kettler RE (eds): The Pain Clinic Manual, p 225. Philadelphia, JB Lippincott, 1990
156. Fordyce WE, Fowler RS, Lehman JF et al: Operant conditioning in the treatment of chronic clinical pain. Arch Phys Med Rehabil 54:399, 1973
157. Fordyce WE, Roberts AH, Sternbach RA: The behavioral management of chronic pain: A response to critics. Pain 22:113, 1985
158. Jacobson E: Progressive Relaxation. Chicago, University of Chicago Press, 1929
159. Benson H: The Relaxation Response. New York, William Morrow, 1975
160. Hughes J, Smith TW, Kosterlitz HW et al: Isolation of two related pentapeptides from brain with potent opiate activity. Nature 258:577, 1975
161. Yaksh TL, Rudy TA: Studies on the direct spinal action of narcotics in the production of analgesia in the rat. J Pharmacol Exp Ther 202:411, 1977
162. Bahar M, Olshwang D, Magora F et al: Epidural morphine in the treatment of pain. Lancet i:527, 1979
163. Onofrio BM, Yaksh TL, Arnold PG: Continuous low dose intrathecal morphine administration in the treatment of chronic pain of malignant origin. Mayo Clin Proc 56:516, 1981
164. Coombs DW, Saunders RL, Gaylor M, Pageau RN: Epidural narcotic infusion: Implantation technique and efficacy. Anesthesiology 56:469, 1982
165. Krames ES, Gershow J, Galssberg A et al: Continuous infusion of spinally administered narcotics for the relief of pain due to malignant disorders. Cancer 56:696, 1985
166. Shetter AG, Hadley MN, Wilkinson E: Administration of intras-

pinal morphine for the treatment of cancer pain. Neurosurgery 18:740, 1986
167. Penn RD, Kroi JS: Long-term intrathecal baclofen infusion for treatment of spasticity. J Neurosurg 66:181, 1987
168. Lazorthes Y, Sallerin-Caute B, Verdie JC et al: Chronic intrathecal baclofen administration for control of severe spasticity. J Neurosurg 72:393, 1990
169. Protenoy RK, Foley KM: Chronic use of opioid analgesics in nonmalignant pain: Report of 38 cases. Pain 25:171, 1986
170. Yaksh TL: Spinal opiates: A review of their effect on spinal function with an emphasis on pain processing. Acta Anaesthesiol Scand 31(suppl):25, 1987
171. Arner S, Meyerson B: Lack of analgesic effect of opioids on neuropathic and idiopathic forms of pain. Pain 33:11, 1988
172. Eisenach JC, Rauck RL, Buzzanell C, Lysack SZ: Epidural clonidine analgesia for intractable cancer pain: Phase I. Anesthesiology 71:647, 1989
173. Nitescu P, Lennart A, Linder L et al: Epidural versus intrathecal morphine-bupivacaine: Assessment of consecutive treatments in advanced cancer pain. J Pain Symptom Management 5:18, 1990
174. Bedder MD, Burchiel JK, Larson A: Cost analysis of two implantable narcotic delivery systems. J Pain Symptom Management 6:638, 1991
175. Krames ES, Schuchard M: Implantable intraspinal infusional analgesia: Management guidelines. Pain Rev 2:243, 1995
176. Penn RD, Kroin JS: Long-term intrathecal baclofen infusion for treatment of spasticity. J Neurosurg 66:181, 1987
177. Herman R, D'Luzansky S, Ippolito R: Intrathecal baclofen suppresses central pain in patients with spinal lesions. Clin J Pain 8:338, 1992
178. Reference deleted
179. Patt RB: Implantable technology for pain control: Identification and management of problems and complications. In Waldman S, Winnie A (eds): Interventional Pain Mangement, p 438. Philadelphia, WB Saunders, 1996
180. Wu C, Patt RB: Accidental overdose of systemic morphine during intended refill of intrathecal infusion device. Anesth Analg 75:130, 1992
181. Shealy C, Mortimer J, Reswik J: Electrical inhibitors of pain by stimulation of the dorsal column. Preliminary clinical reports. Anesth Analg 46:489, 1967
182. North R, Kidd D, Fabarch M et al: Spinal cord stimulators for chronic, intractable pain: Experience over two decades. Neurosurgery 32:384, 1993
183. Campbell JN: Examination of possible mechanisms by which stimulation of the spinal cord in man relieves pain. Appl Neurophysiol 44:181, 1981
184. Tasker RR, de Carvalho GTC, Dolan EJ: Intractable pain of spinal cord origin: Clinical features and implications for surgery. J Neurosurg 77:373, 1992
185. De la Porte C, Siegfried J: Lumbosacral spinal fibrosis (spinal arachnoiditis): Its diagnosis and treatment by spinal cord stimulation. Spine 8:593, 1983
186. Barolat G, Schwartzman R, Woo R: Epidural spinal cord stimulation in the management of reflex sympathetic dystrophy. Stereotact Funct Neurosurgery 53:29, 1989
187. Horsh S, Cleyes L: Epidural spinal cord stimulation in the treatment of severe peripheral artery vascular disease. Ann Vasc Surg 8:468, 1994
188. Houtuast R, Blanksira P, DeJongsle M et al: Effect of spinal cord stimulation on myocardial blood flow assessed by positive emission and tomography in patients with refractory angina. Am J Cardiol 77:462, 1996
189. Turney J, Loeser J, Bell K: Spinal cord stimulation for chronic low back pain: A systematic literature synthesis. Neurosurgery 37:1088, 1995
190. North R, Kidd D, Lee M, Piartodosi S: A prospective randomized study of spinal cord stimulation versus reoperation for failed back surgery syndrome: Initial results. Stereotactic Funct Neurosurgery 74:267, 1994
191. Gersback P, Hasdemir M, Stevens R et al: Discriminative microcirculatory screening of patients with refractory limb ischemia for dorsal column stimulation. J Endovasc Surgery 13:464, 1997
192. Gillian A, Jessurum J, Inge T et al: Sequelae of spinal cord stimulation for refractory angina pectoris. Coronary Artery Dis 8:33, 1997
193. Brandwin MA, Kewman DG: MMPI indicators of treatment re-

sponse to spinal cord stimulation in patients with chronic pain and patients with movement disorders. Psychol Rep 51:1059, 1982

194. Shealy CN: Percutaneous radiofrequency denervation of spinal facets. J Neurosurgery 43:448, 1975

195. North RB, Zahurak M, Kidd D: Radiofrequency lumbar facet denervation: Analysis of prognostic factors. Pain 57:77, 1994

196. Burton CV: Percutaneous radiofrequency facet denervation. Appl Neurophysiol 39:80, 1977

197. Hickey RFJ, Tregonning GD: Denervation of spinal facet joints for treatment of chronic low back pain. N Z Med J 85:96, 1977

198. Sluijter ME: The use of radiofrequency lesions for pain relief in failed back patients. Intl Disability Studies 10:37, 1988

199. Nash TP: Clinical note percutaneous radiofrequency lesioning of dorsal root ganglia for intractable pain. Pain 24:67, 1986

200. Broggi G, Franzini A, Lasio G *et al:* Long-term results of percutane-ous retrogasserian thermorhizotomy for "essential" trigeminal neuralgia. Instituto Neurologico 26:26, 1990

201. Savitz MH: Percutaneous radiofrequency rhizotomy of the lumbar facets: Ten years' experience. Mt Sinai J Med 58:177, 1991

202. Burman MS: Myeloscopy or the direct visualization of the spinal cord. J Bone Joint Surg 13:695, 1931

203. Ooi Y, Satoh Y, Morisaji N: Myeloscopy. Igakuno Ayumi 81:209, 1972

204. Odendaal CL, van Aswgen A: Determining the spread of epidural medication in post laminectomy patients by radionuclide admix-ture (abstract 1487). In Abstracts of the Seventh World Congress on Pain. Paris, Raven Press, 1993

205. Devulder J, Bogaert L, Castille F *et al:* Relevance of epidurography and epidural adhesiolysis in chronic failed back surgery patients. Clin J Pain 11:147, 1995

Clinical Anesthesia (4/e), edited by
Paul G. Barash, Bruce F. Cullen, and
Robert K. Stoelting. Lippincott Williams &
Wilkins, Philadelphia, © 2001.

CHAPTER 56

ICU: CRITICAL CARE

MORRIS BROWN

Critical care medicine is now a clearly recognized specialty of the practice of medicine. It is a multidisciplinary specialty based in the intensive care unit (ICU), with its primary concern being care of the patient with a critical illness. Critical care medicine crosses traditional departmental and specialty lines and requires a physician whose knowledge is broad, involving all aspects of management of the critically ill patient. The core cognitive and procedural skills necessary for the practice of critical care medicine have recently been published.[1]

ANESTHESIOLOGISTS AND CRITICAL CARE MEDICINE

Critical care medicine has always been an integral part of the practice of anesthesiology. Anesthesiologists have been intimately involved, indeed instrumental, in the development of critical care medicine as a specialty. Many consider the practice of operating room anesthesiology the practice of critical care medicine limited to the perioperative period. The anesthesiologist is involved daily with rapid alterations in physiologic status that require prompt recognition and early intervention, the hallmarks of critical care medicine. By virtue of training, experience, competence, and interest, the anesthesiologist brings skills and knowledge that uniquely qualify him or her to care for critically ill patients. This expertise has been recognized by the American Board of Anesthesiology (ABA), which included critical care medicine in its definition of anesthesiology, and by the American Society of Anesthesiologists (ASA), which included critical care medicine in its standards of practice. Further, training in critical care medicine is an integral part of the curriculum for residents in anesthesiology. One year of advanced training in this specialty following completion of residency training is required to be eligible to receive a certificate of special qualifications in critical care medicine by the ABA.

COST AND OUTCOME OF INTENSIVE CARE

The numbers of ICU beds required for an institution vary between 3% and 25% of the total hospital beds, with an average of 12% for major adult and general hospitals. In children's hospitals the amount of special care beds averages more than 23% and may be as high as 46%. Currently, ICU beds constitute 7–8% of all hospital beds. The number of beds required for any institution varies, depending on the patient population served. It appears, however, that with changes in the political climate and the increased preponderance of managed care networks and capitation systems only the very sickest of patients will be admitted to the hospital. Accordingly, there will be a need in the future for more critical care beds and fewer beds for elective admissions.

There is increasing concern about the cost of medical care, especially associated with critical illness. ICU beds are growing at ~6% annually, whereas other beds are closing. ICU care consumes 20% of total hospital charges. In addition, because of the intensity and stress placed on the personnel working in ICUs, the loss of personnel from these areas is disproportionately high. It has been estimated that the annual turnover of nurses from critical care units may be as high as 50%, and it is common not to be able to use all resources because of inadequate staffing.

It is still uncertain whether ICU care decreases patient morbidity and mortality. Reports in the literature are conflicting. Several early studies demonstrated a significant benefit of ICU care when specialty units were reviewed. A reduction in mortality has been reported for coronary ICU patients, burned patients, noncardiac surgical patients, trauma patients, and other selected surgical groups after the introduction of a surgical ICU teaching service and computer-based approach to patient monitoring and therapy. However, these studies and many in the literature have used historical controls. Unfortunately, this does not consider differences in treatment modalities and other factors that may have contributed to the change in morbidity and mortality. Indeed, several studies have failed to show any benefit from hospitalization in critical care units. More carefully designed, rigorously controlled trials are necessary to assess the true efficacy of ICU care.

PATIENT ASSESSMENT SYSTEMS

Because intensive care is so expensive and consumes so many resources, several attempts have been made to develop methods to predict patient outcome. In this way patient care could be optimized by limiting admission to those patients who would benefit from intensive care and withholding or removing therapy from patients who would not. Unfortunately, the systems introduced to assess the severity of illness of patients and their need for intensive care as well as to predict outcome have met with limited success.

Illness severity scoring systems have been devised on an anatomic, therapeutic, and physiologic basis. The Clinical Classification System (CCS) was introduced as a means to assess severity of illness along with a therapeutic intervention scoring system (TISS) to measure the amount of therapy given. The therapeutic intervention scoring system serves as an indirect measure of illness severity, with the greater number of interventions occurring with sicker patients. The CCS, along with TISS, has been used to assist in appropriate use of facilities, to provide information on nurse staffing ratios, and to relate costs to extent of care given in both the adult and pediatric populations. In addition, it was an attempt to compare treatment and outcome in different ICUs, although it has been of limited utility in comparing patients who may be treated by different standards of critical care in different institutions.

The acute physiology and chronic health evaluation (APACHE) system relates the severity of a patient's illness to the degree of physiologic derangement of a series of physiologic measurements. With an assigned weight given to each measurement, it is then possible to assess preadmission health status and probability of survival. It was also proposed to control for case mix, compare outcomes between ICUs, study utilization of ICU resources, and evaluate new therapies. Attempts to simplify the APACHE system resulted in the simplified acute physiologic score (SAPS) and APACHE II.[2,3] Because of concerns of limitations in these systems,[4] APACHE III was developed to refine the selection and weighing of physiologic variables in the system to clarify the distinction between using the system for mortality prediction in groups as opposed to individual patients and to expand the size and diversity of the patient data base.[5] The physiologic stability index (PSI) is an adaptation of the APACHE system for use in the pediatric population.[6] Other scoring systems proposed to aid in the classification of the critically ill and the trauma patient include the mortality prediction model (MPM),[7] computerized intensity intervention scores (CIIS),[8] outcome index (OI),[9] and a new severity characterization of trauma (ASCOT).[10] Unfortunately, to date none of these systems can unequivocally predict outcome or benefit from intensive care.

CENTRAL NERVOUS SYSTEM

Assessment and treatment of critically ill patients with central nervous system (CNS) disorders require a thorough knowledge of cerebral blood flow and metabolism as well as of cerebral pharmacology, neurophysiology, and pathophysiology.

Determinants of Cerebral Blood Flow

Control of cerebral perfusion is essential in maintaining neurologic function in pathologic states. Cerebral blood flow is regulated by intracerebral and extracerebral factors. Intracerebral blood flow regulation is controlled by chemical and metabolic influences, including hydrogen ion concentration, cyclooxygenase, products of phospholipid membrane metabolism, and adenosine. In addition, neurogenic and myogenic components contribute to the regulation of cerebral blood flow.

The extracerebral determinants of blood flow include the arterial partial pressure of carbon dioxide ($Paco_2$) and oxygen (Pao_2), arterial blood pressure, venous blood pressure, and pharmacologic effects of drugs. There is a linear correlation between cerebral blood flow and $Paco_2$ with progressive hypercarbia. Similarly, there is a marked reduction in cerebral blood flow during hypocarbia through a pH-mediated change in arteriolar tone that results in vasoconstriction and reduced intracranial pressure (ICP). Taken to extremes, hypocarbia provides no additional benefit and may be detrimental. Therefore, current recommendations suggest maintaining $Paco_2$ between 25 and 30 mm Hg. However, prolonged hypocarbia is ineffective because cerebrospinal fluid (CSF) bicarbonate adapts to the change in $Paco_2$. Therefore, the long-term value of hyperventilation of the lungs for reducing ICP is offset by the normalization of CSF pH, which occurs in 6 hr.

Arterial oxygenation has a lesser effect on cerebral blood flow than does carbon dioxide. When the Pao_2 falls below 50 mm Hg, cerebral vasodilation and an increase in cerebral blood flow result, which may exacerbate intracranial hypertension. Hyperoxia generally results in small changes in cerebral blood flow until Pao_2 exceeds 300 mm Hg.

Autoregulation

Autoregulation, the ability of the brain to maintain cerebral blood flow constant despite alterations in mean arterial pressure, is functional over a mean arterial pressure range of 50–150 mm Hg. At levels below 50 mm Hg, symptoms of cerebral ischemia may appear. If the upper limit of autoregulation is exceeded, cerebral blood flow increases, which may result in cerebral edema. It is important to note that the autoregulatory curve may be shifted in the presence of chronic hypertension, intracranial tumors, head trauma, and shock states, which render the brain more susceptible to ischemic effects.

Intracranial Pressure Monitoring

ICP can normally range up to 15 mm Hg, and beyond that point any increase in ICP can result in a decrease in cerebral perfusion pressure. Once cerebral perfusion pressure falls below 40–60 mm Hg, ischemic injury to nerve cells may occur. There is a close correlation between clinical outcome and the level of ICP elevation after acute injury. Aggressive treatment of elevated ICP in the ICU is essential. The symptoms associated with increased ICP are variable, although they generally reflect

effects of compression of structures around the tentorial opening. If left untreated, raised ICP leads to global cerebral ischemia, coma, and death.

Continuous monitoring of ICP can be accomplished through a ventriculostomy, a subdural bolt, or an epidural transducer. Advantages and disadvantages of each technique are outlined in Table 56-1. The intraventricular catheter is inserted through a burr hole through the coronal suture. It provides an accurate and reliable reading of ICP as well as allowing withdrawal of CSF for pressure control and culture. Disadvantages of this technique include the necessity of passing through brain tissue to introduce the catheter into the ventricle. This may be difficult when the brain is distorted from trauma and edema. Further, the risk of infection is greatest with this technique as compared with the others. Indeed, positive CSF culture results have been reported in ~9% of patients monitored with intraventricular catheters.[11] The possibility of infection is reduced if catheterization is limited to 3 days and prophylactic antibiotics are administered.

The subarachnoid bolt is a less invasive means of monitoring ICP. This device is inserted into the skull after the dura and arachnoid have been opened. It is easily inserted, does not require penetration of brain tissue, and can be done at the bedside. As with all invasive procedures, insertion of a subarachnoid bolt carries the risk of infection.

The epidural transducer used to monitor ICP is placed between the inner table of the skull and the dura. This device is easy to place and monitors pressures exerted by the CSF and brain on the dura. Although this technique carries little risk of infection, its accuracy and reliability for monitoring ICP are questionable.

Control of Elevated Intracranial Pressure

Treatment of increased ICP is generally recommended when levels exceed 20 mm Hg. Certainly, treatment may be indicated at a lower pressure if evidence of impaired cerebral perfusion is present. Modalities available to treat increased ICP include diuretics and fluid restriction, hyperosmotic agents, hyperventilation of the lungs, corticosteroids, barbiturates, positioning, and removal of CSF.

Once surgically correctable causes of increased ICP have been eliminated, treatment should be initiated with hyperventilation to maintain $Paco_2$ between 25 and 30 mm Hg. Additional measures include drainage of CSF if an intraventricular catheter has been placed and elevation of the head to 30°, which encourages venous drainage from the brain and hence lowers ICP. Mannitol may be added in an attempt to remove brain water. This osmotic agent helps draw water from the tissues because of the transient increase in plasma osmolarity. The onset of action following intravenous (iv) administration of mannitol is 30 min, with a maximum lowering of ICP occurring within 1–2 hr and lasting 6 hr. Diuretics such as furosemide may also be used to lower ICP and are especially useful in patients with increased intravascular volume. Corticosteroids are effective in lowering ICP due to localized cerebral edema surrounding intracranial tumors. Dexamethasone is the most commonly used steroid preparation and generally causes improvement in neurologic status within 12–36 hr of therapy. Barbiturate administration can also assist in lowering ICP by a dose-related reduction in cerebral metabolic oxygen requirement as well as by decreasing cerebral blood volume. Some authors suggest barbiturate coma for cerebral protection in patients with elevated ICP.[12,13]

Fluid and electrolyte abnormalities including hyponatremia, hypokalemia, and hypochloremia with fluid retention are common accompaniments of CNS disease. Other complications include acute respiratory failure, gastrointestinal bleeding, hypertension, cardiac dysrhythmias, and disseminated intravascular coagulation. These related complications must be recognized and treated if they occur.

Table 56-1. TECHNIQUES OF DIRECT INTRACRANIAL PRESSURE MONITORING

ICP Monitor	Advantage	Disadvantage
Ventriculostomy	Very accurate Access to cerebrospinal fluid for pressure control and culture	Must pass through brain tissue Infection
Subarachnoid bolt	Easily performed Bedside procedure	Infection Less accurate
Epidural transducer	Easy to place Little risk of infection	Questionable accuracy and reliability

Seizures

The etiology of a seizure generally depends on the age of the patient and the type of seizure. Young children frequently present with seizures associated with febrile illness. In adolescent and young adults, head trauma is a major cause of focal seizure disorders, whereas generalized seizures tend to be associated with drug or alcohol withdrawal in this age group. Brain tumors are the most common cause of seizures in patients between 30 and 50 years of age, and over 50 years of age cerebrovascular disease is the most common cause of focal or generalized seizure disorders. The initial evaluation of the patient with a seizure consists of ensuring adequate ventilation and perfusion as well as stopping the seizure. A full history and examination must be obtained. It is important to differentiate the kind of seizure to aid in determining the etiology. Treatment is directed at eliminating the cause and suppressing the seizure. Certainly, metabolic disturbances such as hypoglycemia or hypocalcemia should be sought and corrected. Structural brain lesions must be removed. Most seizure disorders are amenable to anticonvulsant medication. However, neurosurgical treatment should be considered if a structural lesion causes recurrent seizures and removal of that lesion and nearby affected brain tissue will make them easier to control or eliminate them entirely. In addition, neurosurgical ablation of epileptogenic foci may be used as a treatment modality.

Central Nervous System Trauma

Head injuries are a significant cause of morbidity and mortality, with more than 2 million injuries causing brain damage yearly. To quantitate the severity of head injury, an objective clinical scale was developed. The Glasgow Coma Scale evaluates motor response, verbal response, and eye opening (Table 56-2). It provides an estimate of the severity of neurologic dysfunction and can predict mortality. Evoked potentials are another means

of assessing prognosis in patients following head injury. The accuracy of evoked potentials is greater than that of clinical observation and ICP measurements. Somatosensory evoked potentials are the most useful and can predict death or a vegetative state in ~90% of patients if they are bilaterally absent.

Any patient who presents with severe head injury should have the airway protected and secured, ventilation and blood pressure stabilized, and attention given to life-threatening noncranial injuries followed by a full neurologic evaluation. As with any head injury, the possibility of cervical spine injury should be considered and the cervical spine should be immobilized until full evaluation is possible. Surgically treatable causes of increased ICP should be sought, including epidural or subdural hematoma and intracerebral hemorrhage. Aggressive surgical intervention may dramatically improve outcome. If, however, there are no surgically treatable lesions found on computed tomographic scan, attention should be directed toward reducing increased ICP. Direct ICP monitoring should be considered. Hypoxia, hyperthermia, hypercarbia, malpositioning of the endotracheal tube, and high mean airway pressures may exacerbate the intracranial hypertension. Persistent elevation of ICP despite conservative therapy generally portends a poor prognosis. Fluid and electrolytes should be monitored closely. Anticonvulsants and prophylaxis to prevent gastrointestinal bleeding are generally administered.

It must be remembered that patients who sustain head trauma have other associated problems. Indeed, medical complications generally dominate the intermediate-term intensive care of head trauma patients. Fluid and electrolyte balance can be a major problem following head injury. Indeed, over half of the patients who have persistent coma develop abnormalities of fluid and electrolyte balance. It is important to monitor serum osmolarity and sodium concentrations because treatment of intracranial hypertension may cause marked alterations in these parameters. Coagulation parameters must also be monitored because disseminated intravascular coagulation may accompany head trauma in 5–10% of cases.

Cerebral Protection

Common causes of acute cerebral injury include anoxic insult, traumatic injury to the brain, and stroke. The mechanism of injury in each case begins with tissue ischemia. Cell death then results from the resultant inflammation, toxicity of excitatory amino acids, and generation of free radicals. Inflammatory mediators such as platelet activating factor (PAF), interleukin-1B (IL-1B), and leukotrienes result in damage to cell membranes, leading to increased intracellular calcium and release of proteases, endonucleases, and phospholipases, which results in cell death. Similarly, excitatory amino acids also cause an increase in intracellular calcium, leading to cell death. Finally, the generation of free radicals damages cell membranes, directly leading to cell death.

Several techniques to promote neuroprotection have been tried to interrupt the pathway to cell death. Therapies for neuroprotection have included hypothermia,[14,15] antagonists of the excitatory amino acids receptors,[16] calcium channel blockers,[17]

Table 56-2. GLASGOW COMA SCALE

Parameter	Response	Score
Eye opening	Spontaneously	4
	To verbal command	3
	To pain	2
	No response	1
Motor response	Obeys verbal command	6
	Localizes pain	5
	Flexion–withdrawal	4
	Decorticate rigidity	3
	Decerebrate rigidity	2
	No response	1
Verbal response	Oriented and converses	5
	Disoriented and converses	4
	Inappropriate words	3
	Incomprehensible sounds	2
	No response	1

corticosteroids,[18] barbiturates, superoxide dismutase,[19] desferoxamine mesylate,[20] antioxidant vitamins, antagonists of PAF, neuronal growth factors, nitric oxide, and gene therapy. Unfortunately, despite being based on sound physiologic principles and promising data in animal models, many of the neuroprotective therapies available today have yielded disappointing results in human trials. It could be that other factors influence outcome, including the timing of the intervention, gender of the patient, and dose/duration of therapy. Further investigation is necessary to determine the most effective means to provide neuroprotection following brain injury.

CARDIOVASCULAR SYSTEM
Cardiogenic Shock

Cardiogenic shock is a syndrome that results directly from severely impaired left ventricular pump function. This may be the result of end-stage cardiac disease or a catastrophic complication of acute myocardial infarction. With improvements in cardiac dysrhythmia monitoring and treatment, cardiogenic shock has emerged as the most common cause of death among patients in coronary care units. Indeed, cardiogenic shock occurs in 10–15% of patients who suffer an acute myocardial infarction. Mortality remains high despite advances in hemodynamic monitoring and newer pharmacologic drugs. Cardiogenic shock, like hypovolemic or septic shock, manifests as inadequate oxygen delivery to tissues, with failure of mitochondrial oxidative metabolism and accumulation of lactic acid. Inadequate organ perfusion in cardiogenic shock is caused by a marked reduction in the quantity of contracting myocardium. The initial insult leads to a decrease in arterial pressure with a resultant decrease in coronary blood flow. This decrease in coronary perfusion pressure further compromises myocardial function, leading to progressive circulatory deterioration. The clinical consequences of the decrease in myocardial contractility manifest as either circulatory insufficiency (forward failure) or circulatory congestion (backward failure).

Typical signs and symptoms of patients in cardiogenic shock include restlessness and mental confusion; the skin is cool, moist, and cyanotic. Peripheral pulses are usually weak and rapid, and arterial blood pressure is decreased. However, shock can occur without severe hypotension, a relatively late indicator of inadequate reflex vasoconstriction. Nonetheless, the syndrome is usually defined by a systolic arterial pressure 80 mm Hg, with a cardiac index of $2 \ L \cdot min^{-1} \cdot m^{-2}$ and an increase in left ventricular end-diastolic pressure or pulmonary capillary wedge pressure (PCWP) to 8 mm Hg.

Because prognosis is poor and mortality is high, close monitoring and early aggressive intervention are essential for successful outcome. Certainly, any patient in shock should have continuous monitoring of arterial pressure and left ventricular filling pressures. Measurement of central venous pressure alone is inadequate and may actually be misleading because it often fails to reliably reflect left ventricular pressures. Close monitoring of urinary output is important because it gives an indication of renal artery perfusion and provides a monitor of the progress of treatment.

Successful treatment of cardiogenic shock depends on early restoration of adequate tissue perfusion to meet metabolic demands. To achieve this goal, initial resuscitation and general supportive measures should be instituted immediately. Specific pharmacologic therapy to maintain adequate blood pressure, cardiac output, and oxygenation should be initiated. Consideration should then be given to mechanical cardiac assist devices or cardiac surgical intervention, including transplantation and implantation of an artificial heart.

Drugs with positive inotropic properties improve the contractile performance of the failing heart. Sympathomimetic amines are potent positive inotropic drugs that exert their effects through action on α- and β-adrenergic receptors. Isoproterenol is rarely used in the treatment of shock. Although it increases contractility, it does so at the expense of an increase in myocardial oxygen consumption and a reduction in coronary perfusion pressure. The net increase in cardiac output seen with this drug may be limited by impairment of cardiac filling resulting from rate and rhythm changes, as well as by decreased venous return to the heart. Epinephrine is a powerful cardiac stimulant. Heart rate is increased, systole is shortened and strengthened, and cardiac work and myocardial oxygen consumption are markedly increased. The hemodynamic effects of epinephrine are dose-dependent, so that in low doses (1–$2 \ \mu g \cdot min^{-1}$) there is primarily β stimulation, intermediate doses (2–$10 \ \mu g \cdot min^{-1}$) result in mixed α and β stimulation, and high doses result primarily in α stimulation. The clinical utility of epinephrine may be limited by its peripheral vascular effects, tachycardia, and dysrhythmias. Norepinephrine is a combined α and β agent, with α properties generally dominant, causing intensive vasoconstriction. It can be useful in raising blood pressure, but the increase in afterload causes a marked increase in myocardial oxygen consumption. Dopamine has been used successfully as a positive inotropic drug with varying effects at different dosage ranges. At low doses the drug has positive chronotropic and inotropic effects, but at higher doses vasoconstriction occurs through an α-mediated response. The dopaminergic properties of the drug, which allow for increased renal blood flow, have proved useful when dopamine is added to more potent inotropic drugs to maximize renal perfusion during borderline low cardiac output states.[21] Dobutamine is a synthetic, sympathomimetic amine with positive inotropic effects without the chronotropic or peripheral vasoconstrictive properties of dopamine. In severe congestive heart failure (CHF) dobutamine improves myocardial contractility, stroke volume, cardiac output, systemic pressures, and perfusion while decreasing ventricular filling pressures. It therefore should be used in patients without profound hypotension. Dopamine and dobutamine may also be used in combination.[22] Dopexamine exerts positive inotropic effects through both direct and indirect mechanisms. It is an agonist for dopaminergic and β II receptors but has little β I and no α-adrenergic effects. It decreases systemic vascular resistance and pulmonary vascular resistance and lowers both left and right ventricular filling pressures while increasing heart rate, stroke volume, and cardiac output.

Recently, two groups of drugs that act primarily through inhibition of phosphodiesterase III have been introduced. These drugs include the bipyridine derivatives amrinone and milrinone and the imidazolones enoximone and piroximone. Amrinone causes a dose-dependent increase in cardiac output while reducing systemic vascular resistance and left ventricular filling pressures. It has been shown to increase cardiac index by 30–100% while decreasing PCWP, systemic vascular resistance (SVR), and pulmonary vascular resistance. Heart rate and blood pressure have generally remained unchanged. Milrinone is ~15 times more potent than amrinone with similar pharmacologic and hemodynamic effects.[23] Milrinone produces no increases in myocardial oxygen consumption, suggesting that cardiac performance increases without increase in myocardial oxygen demand, possibly because its vasodilator action counterbalances the increase in myocardial contractility. Enoximone is structurally different from the bipyridine derivatives but functions also as a phosphodiesterase III inhibitor. It significantly increases cardiac index and decreases SVR and PCWP with minimal increase in heart rate or change in mean arterial pressure. It alters hemodynamics primarily by vasodilation of musculoskeletal and pulmonary vascular beds along with positive inotropism and chronotropism.[24] Piroximone, like enoximone, improves both right and left ventricular function without causing significant changes in heart rate or blood pressure. Myocardial oxygen uptake is not altered and coronary sinus blood flow increases.[25]

Other new agents combining phosphodiesterase inhibition with other actions are currently under investigation.[26]

Mechanical circulatory assist devices, most commonly the intra-aortic balloon pump, have gained widespread clinical use since first introduced by Moulopoulus *et al* in 1962.[27] The balloon pump assist device results in a reduction in myocardial oxygen consumption, and hence myocardial ischemia. In addition, by decreasing left ventricular volume and pressure and augmenting coronary perfusion, there is a positive balance established between myocardial oxygen demand and supply. The intra-aortic balloon pump has been shown in experimental models to improve hemodynamics, augment myocardial perfusion, enhance impaired contractile function, and potentially limit infarct size. Indeed, it has been shown that an increase in coronary blood flow is seen in patients in cardiogenic shock. Unfortunately, although myocardial ischemia is relieved and heart failure lessened in most patients with intra-aortic balloon pump assist, long-term survival has not been established. In recent clinical experience, intra-aortic balloon pumping alone was associated with an overall survival rate of 30% when used in patients with cardiogenic shock. The addition of emergency cardiac surgical revascularization improved survival rates.

Although intra-aortic balloon pumping is generally a simple and relatively safe procedure, serious complications occur in 10% of patients. Complications include aortic and arterial trauma, vascular insufficiency in the catheterized limb distal to the insertion site, infection, embolic phenomena, balloon rupture with gas embolization, and thrombocytopenia. With newer assist devices available and the success of invasive cardiac procedures, temporary assistance may provide support until definitive therapy can be undertaken.

With refractory cardiogenic shock, heart transplantation should be considered. The 1-year survival for heart transplant recipients exceeds 80%, with a 5-year survival of 50–60%.[28] Certainly, surgical approaches should be explored when cardiogenic shock cannot otherwise be managed.

Cardiac Tamponade

The accumulation of fluid or blood in the pericardial space resulting in a fall in cardiac output due to insufficient inflow of blood to the ventricles results in tamponade. The amount of fluid necessary to cause pericardial tamponade is variable, depending on the rapidity of accumulation. Rapid accumulation of as little as 250 ml can result in tamponade, whereas 1000 ml can accumulate slowly in the pericardial space without tamponade. The most common cause of tamponade is blood in the pericardial space following cardiac surgery, trauma, tuberculosis, or tumor. However, other etiologies include acute viral or idiopathic pericarditis, postradiation pericarditis, and renal failure. Clinical manifestations of tamponade include dyspnea, jugular venous distention, and low arterial blood pressure with distant heart sounds. Electrical alternans may be seen on the electrocardiogram (ECG), and distention of the jugular veins on inspiration (Kussmaul's sign) may also be noted. Another finding suggestive of pericardial tamponade is a paradoxical occurrence of 10 mm Hg inspiratory decrease in systolic arterial pressure. Equalization of pulmonary artery wedge, right atrial, right ventricular, and pulmonary artery diastolic pressures with low cardiac output may also be seen.

Treatment of cardiac tamponade must be initiated immediately because pericardiocentesis may be lifesaving. A small catheter advanced over a needle inserted in the pericardial space allows drainage of pericardial fluid and return of cardiac function.

Pulmonary Embolism

Pulmonary embolism is a leading cause of morbidity and mortality in the United States. It has been estimated that pulmonary embolism accounts for more than 50,000 deaths annually, although most pulmonary emboli are nonfatal. The vast majority of pulmonary emboli arise in the deep venous system of the lower extremities. The three primary etiologic factors in the development of deep vein thrombosis and subsequent pulmonary embolism are venous stasis, abnormalities of the vessel wall, and alterations in blood coagulation.

Pulmonary embolism should be suspected in any patient with sudden onset of unexplained dyspnea in association with venous thrombosis. Other symptoms may include substernal chest pain, syncope, cardiac dysrhythmias, worsening of CHF, or sudden worsening of chronic obstructive lung disease. Pleuritic chest pain and hemoptysis may be present, but only when pulmonary infarction has occurred. Physical examination may be remarkably normal. Rales or wheezing may be noted on auscultation of the lungs. A pleural friction rub or effusion may be present if infarction has occurred. Findings on auscultation of the heart may include tachycardia, right ventricular gallop, wide splitting of the second heart sound, or systolic ejection murmur in the pulmonic area.

Laboratory studies may assist with the diagnosis of pulmonary embolism. The ECG is generally normal aside from tachycardia. However, there may be evidence of right axis deviation, tall peaked P waves, or ST-T wave changes consistent with right ventricular strain. Chest x-ray film findings may be subtle. Indeed, a normal chest x-ray film does not exclude the possibility of pulmonary embolism and is a common finding. Arterial blood gases associated with pulmonary embolism generally reveal arterial hypoxemia with hypocapnia and respiratory alkalosis. However, normal arterial blood gas analysis does not exclude the possibility of thromboembolic disease.

The diagnosis of pulmonary embolism can be confirmed by radioisotope-tagged and microaggregated albumin perfusion scan along with a xenon ventilation scan. The definitive diagnosis, however, is with pulmonary angiography, which is the only means for providing anatomic information about the pulmonary vasculature. Heparin administration is the initial treatment of pulmonary thromboembolism. Fibrinolytic agents also have been used to dissolve venous thrombi in the pulmonary vasculature. Surgical therapy with formal thoracotomy and thrombectomy produces uniformly poor results.

Thrombolytic Therapy

Streptokinase (SK), urokinase (UK), and tissue plasminogen activator (tPA) are pharmacologic activators used to accelerate fibrinolysis in patients with massive pulmonary emboli, acute arterial and coronary thrombi, and peripheral venous thrombi. Streptokinase, obtained from the culture of group A β-hemolytic streptococci, is an indirect activator that forms a complex with plasminogen and initiates fibrinolysis. It was the first thrombolytic agent available for clinical use. Urokinase, like tPA, can directly convert plasminogen to plasmin. Urokinase, which is secreted by human kidney cells, was first extracted and purified in 1957. Recombinant tissue plasminogen activator (rtPA, alteplase) peripherally activates plasminogen when it is absorbed to fibrin clots. Anistreptilase (anisoylated plasminogen SK activator complex, APSAC) offered theoretical advantages over SK as did a precursor of UK, single-chain UK plasminogen activator (scuPA). Individual mortality trials of SK, APSAC, and rtPA including risks and benefits of each agent have been well described.[29] In general, studies comparing these agents have shown no significant differences,[30–32] though accelerated-dose rtPA was more efficacious than SK and APSAC.[33,34] Indeed, patients with suspected acute anterior or inferior myocardial infarctions have lower early mortality when treated with streptokinase. In particular, tPA has been used successfully with improved left ventricular function. A variety of newer agents, modifications of tPA, are under evaluation. These newer thrombolytic agents include reteplase (rPA),[35] lenatoplase (nPA),[36] and staphylokinase.[37]

The major complication of fibrinolytic therapy is hemorrhage caused by hypofibrinogenemia and intense systemic fibrinolysis. Therefore, fibrinolytic therapy is not recommended for patients with recent surgery, indwelling cannulas, a history of neurologic lesions, or gastrointestinal bleeding. Indications for fibrinolytic therapy include massive pulmonary emboli, acute peripheral arterial embolism, and extensive iliofemoral thrombophlebitis. The fibrinolysis begins immediately after vascular injury, although clot lysis and vessel recannulation may not be complete for 7–10 days. The Fifth American College of Chest Physicians Consensus Conference on antithrombotic therapy has recently published summary recommendations.[38]

RESPIRATORY SYSTEM

Acute Respiratory Failure

Acute respiratory failure in the critically ill patient is often synonymous with the adult respiratory distress syndrome (ARDS). This is a descriptive term applied to many acute diffuse infiltrative lung lesions with diverse etiology. However, severely diminished lung compliance, refractory hypoxemia, and diffuse radiographic abnormalities are common denominators. Regardless of the initiating event, this form of acute respiratory failure is associated with increased lung water. This type of pulmonary edema, which is associated with relatively normal cardiac function and "leaky" pulmonary capillaries, has been termed high-permeability pulmonary edema. The precise incidence of ARDS is difficult to determine, although it appears to be increasing. One third of adult deaths from shock and trauma following severe injury result from progressive respiratory failure. Although ARDS may be precipitated by many different causes, the resulting clinical syndrome is the same (Table 56-3). The mortality rate remains above 50% despite current supportive therapy and treatment modalities.

Pathophysiology

Following injury to the lung with damage of the alveolar capillary membrane, there is an increased permeability of the capillary endothelium and alveolar epithelium, with leakage of plasma and erythrocytes into the interstitial and alveolar spaces. In addition, there is proliferation of Type II pneumocytes, which probably aid in the restoration of the integrity of the capillary-endothelial lining.

Although platelet aggregation occurs, the major alterations in lung function relate to leukoaggregation on endothelial surfaces. Indeed, bronchoalveolar lavage fluid from patients with ARDS contains an accumulation of neutrophils and leukocyte elastase. These cells release mediators of inflammation such as leukotrienes, thromboxanes, and prostaglandins. These leukoagglutinins are caused by activation of complement factor C5a. Thus, complement activation, a frequent accompaniment of trauma, sepsis, and other predisposing clinical insults, may explain the leukoaggregates commonly found in the lungs of patients with ARDS. With release of toxic oxygen radicals and lysosomal proteases, these aggregated neutrophils damage the endothelial cells by destruction of structural protein and promotion of local inflammatory reactions.

In addition to leukoaggregates, microemboli are commonly found in patients with ARDS at autopsy. Indeed, platelet and coagulation abnormalities have been implicated in the pathogenesis of the syndrome. Trauma, sepsis, and other predisposing conditions can activate the coagulation system, either by release of thromboplastin from soft tissue injury or through complement activation of the coagulation cascade. This results in platelet adhesiveness and aggregation which, along with the generation of fibrin, produce microemboli that are washed into the pulmonary vasculature. These defects have been clearly demonstrated by wedge angiography and correlated with the severity of lung injury.

Clinical Manifestations

Patients may be asymptomatic immediately following insult. The earliest sign is frequently tachypnea followed by dyspnea. Arterial blood gas analysis generally reveals a respiratory alkalosis caused by hyperventilation and mild hypoxemia. At this time, administration of supplementation oxygen frequently improves arterial oxygenation. As the disease progresses, however, hypoxemia cannot be corrected by increasing inspired oxygen concentrations because hypoxemia is the result of right-to-left shunting of blood through collapsed or fluid-filled alveoli. Mechanical ventilatory support with positive airway pressure therapy is then required to maintain adequate oxygenation.

Treatment

Certainly, early recognition and prompt initiation of therapy are essential. The cornerstone of therapy is to ensure adequate tissue oxygenation. An indwelling arterial cannula is useful to monitor arterial blood pressure and allow access for measurement of arterial blood gases and other laboratory values. A pulmonary artery catheter aids immeasurably in optimizing fluid management. A Foley catheter is important to ensure close and accurate measurement of urine output. Bronchial hygiene is an important aspect of the management of these patients. Antibiotics should be used only if evidence of infection is present, and treatment should be guided by the results of cultures and antibiotic sensitivity testing. Prophylactic antibiotics are not indicated and may cause a drug-resistant infection. The use of high-dose corticosteroids in the treatment of ARDS was based on the theoretical advantages of inhibition of complement-induced granulocyte aggregation, disaggregation of neutrophils, and limitation of the increase in lung microvascular permeability. However, prospective double-blind, placebo-controlled trials of methylprednisolone therapy found no difference in mortality.[39]

Fluid management in patients with ARDS presents a clinical dilemma. Fluid is constantly lost through the alveolar capillary membrane into the lung parenchyma, yet adequate circulatory volume is essential to restore the perfusion important in reversal of lung damage. Therefore, it is critical that fluid administration be judicious. It is best guided by the use of a balloon-tipped, flow-directed pulmonary artery catheter. Diuretics and vasoactive agents can be used to maximize tissue oxygen delivery. Fluid replacement with crystalloid or colloid solution remains controversial. Regardless of the choice, meticulous attention must be given to fluid balance.

If adequate oxygenation cannot be maintained with an increased inspired oxygen concentration, mechanical ventilatory support should be instituted. The supportive benefits of positive end-expiratory pressure (PEEP) therapy are well documented. The clinical goals include improvement in arterial oxygenation, decrease in the work of breathing, and improvement in ventilation–perfusion inequality. With diffuse lung injury, PEEP improves functional residual capacity, compliance, and arterial oxygenation. In addition, PEEP decreases shunting, dead space

---

Table 56-3. CONDITIONS ASSOCIATED WITH ADULT RESPIRATORY DISTRESS SYNDROME

Shock	Fat or air embolism
Aspiration	Burns
Sepsis	Drug ingestion
Trauma	Uremia
Pancreatitis	Massive blood transfusion
Head injury	Cardiopulmonary bypass
Radiation of thorax	Drowning

ventilation, and venous admixture. This allows adequate arterial oxygenation with a lower inspired oxygen concentration.

Several criteria have been applied in attempting to define the clinical endpoint for PEEP therapy. Indices used include arterial oxygen tension, alveolar–arterial oxygen gradient, shunt fraction, compliance, and oxygen delivery.[40,41] The usual clinical approach is to increase PEEP in increments of 3–5 cm H_2O and obtain appropriate measurements. Certainly, the optimal PEEP level chosen for any individual must fulfill the oxygenation as well as hemodynamic needs of that patient. The appropriate level depends on the degree of hypoxemia, the type of lung disorder, the functional residual capacity of the lungs, the presence of pre-existing pulmonary disease, lung compliance, the state of hydration, and the status of left ventricular function. Most recent data suggest that lower tidal volumes (6 ml · kg^{-1}) and PEEP adjusted to the beginning of the optimal compliance on the pressure–volume curve may improve prognosis. This "lung protective ventilatory strategy" may avoid volutrauma and shear stress.[42]

Although PEEP therapy is an integral part of the treatment of acute respiratory failure, it causes complex hemodynamic effects. Changes in airway pressure can be anticipated to affect the heart and great vessels within the thorax. Potential adverse effects of PEEP include impaired venous return, decreased ventricular filling, increased pulmonary vascular resistance, interference with subendocardial blood flow, reduced left ventricular afterload, and altered configuration and compliance of the right and left ventricles. In addition to hemodynamic alterations, PEEP may cause interstitial emphysema, pneumothorax, and pneumomediastinum. Other effects of PEEP therapy include changes in ICP, alterations in renal function, and abnormalities in hepatic and gastrointestinal function.

Research on ARDS has emphasized the mechanism of lung injury in the hope of identifying a marker that would facilitate its early recognition. Current investigation is directed at altering the pathogenic sequence of increased alveolar capillary permeability and destruction of pulmonary structure. Therapeutic interventions, including anticoagulation, extracorporeal membrane oxygenation, cyclo-oxygenase inhibitors, oxygen free radical scavenger therapy, antiendotoxin antibody therapy, and prostaglandin E therapy, have not yet proved to be of definite benefit to patients with ARDS and await further prospective, controlled clinical trials.

Inhaled nitric oxide (NO) is a potential therapeutic option in patients with severe ARDS.[43] By decreasing pulmonary hypertension and arterial hypoxemia, inhaled NO (minimal effective inhaled NO concentration for long-term administration is 2–4 ppm) may decrease pulmonary edema, oxygen toxicity, and pulmonary barotrauma, thereby allowing the lungs to heal. A significant unresolved issue is the potential pulmonary toxicity of inhaled NO and its metabolite, nitrogen dioxide. At present, the appropriate role of inhaled NO in the treatment of ARDS remains unknown.

Mechanical Ventilation

Types of Ventilators

There are three kinds of mechanical ventilators. The simplest mechanical ventilators are those that substitute for diaphragmatic function, such as the pneumobelt or rocking bed. These devices have limited utility and are used only in patients with neuromuscular disease and normal lung function. A second kind of mechanical ventilator is the intermittent negative-pressure ventilator. These devices artificially produce a negative extrathoracic pressure during inspiration to substitute for the pleural and airway pressures normally produced by contraction of the respiratory muscles. Examples of this form of mechanical ventilation include the chest cuirass and iron lung. These devices are best suited for patients with respiratory muscle dysfunction and normal lungs.

The third kind of mechanical ventilator, and the one most commonly used today, is the intermittent positive-pressure ventilator. In this system gas is directed under positive airway pressure into the lungs. The major advantages of intermittent positive-pressure ventilation are the ability to ventilate the lungs adequately despite increased airway resistance or decreased lung compliance, patient accessibility, and access for bronchial hygiene. The mean airway pressure is positive with intermittent positive-pressure ventilation, so that venous return is compromised and cardiac performance may be impaired. Most of the positive-pressure ventilators in common clinical use today are volume ventilators that deliver a preset volume to the patient's lungs. Cycling of standard ventilators occurs whenever a certain volume or pressure is reached or at a preset time interval. When PEEP is added to intermittent positive-pressure ventilation, it is called continuous positive-pressure ventilation.

In recent years mechanical ventilators have become sophisticated and complex. The current microprocessor-based new generation of mechanical ventilators is a logical extension of earlier counterparts. The newest generation of adult mechanical ventilators offers more modes of ventilation, intrinsic microprocessors, computer-compatible monitoring or control, and extensive patient data monitoring and collection in a highly versatile and flexible ventilating device. The microprocessor control, in addition, reduces the number of moving components, enhances data management, and allows upgrading or addition of new features with a mere change in software. However, many of the new methods of ventilation available must await the results of rigorously controlled, objective, double-blind, randomized studies. The most common ventilatory modes available today with standard positive-pressure ventilators are controlled-mode ventilation, assist controlled-mode ventilation, and intermittent or synchronized intermittent mandatory ventilation. Newer ventilatory modalities include pressure support ventilation, high-frequency ventilation, extended mandatory minute ventilation, airway pressure release ventilation, pressure control ventilation, pressure control inverse ratio ventilation, and noninvasive positive pressure ventilation (Fig. 56-1).

Controlled Mechanical Ventilation

Controlled mechanical ventilation of the lungs is the oldest mode of intermittent positive-pressure ventilation. The ventilator obligatorily delivers a gas at a preset rate and volume independent of patient effort or response. The patient is unable to alter or influence any portion of the ventilatory cycle. Thus, a patient with an intact ventilatory drive often must be hyperventilated or given sedatives or muscle relaxants to diminish the tendency to breathe asynchronously with the ventilator. In addition, mean airway pressure is highest with this form of intermittent positive-pressure ventilation.

Assist Control Ventilation

Assist control mechanical ventilation, or assist control, is an intermittent positive-pressure ventilation mode in which the patient creates a sub-baseline pressure in the inspiratory limb of the ventilator circuit that triggers the ventilator to deliver a predetermined tidal volume. If the patient's ventilatory rate falls below a preset level, the machine automatically enters the control mode.

Intermittent Mandatory Ventilation

Intermittent mandatory ventilation (IMV) is a mode of intermittent positive-pressure ventilation in which the ventilator delivers a preset volume at a specified interval while also providing a continuous flow of gas for spontaneous ventilation. The patient spontaneously breathes gas with the same temperature, humidity, and oxygen concentration as the ventilator provides while the ventilator delivers a preset tidal volume at predetermined intervals through a parallel ventilatory circuit.

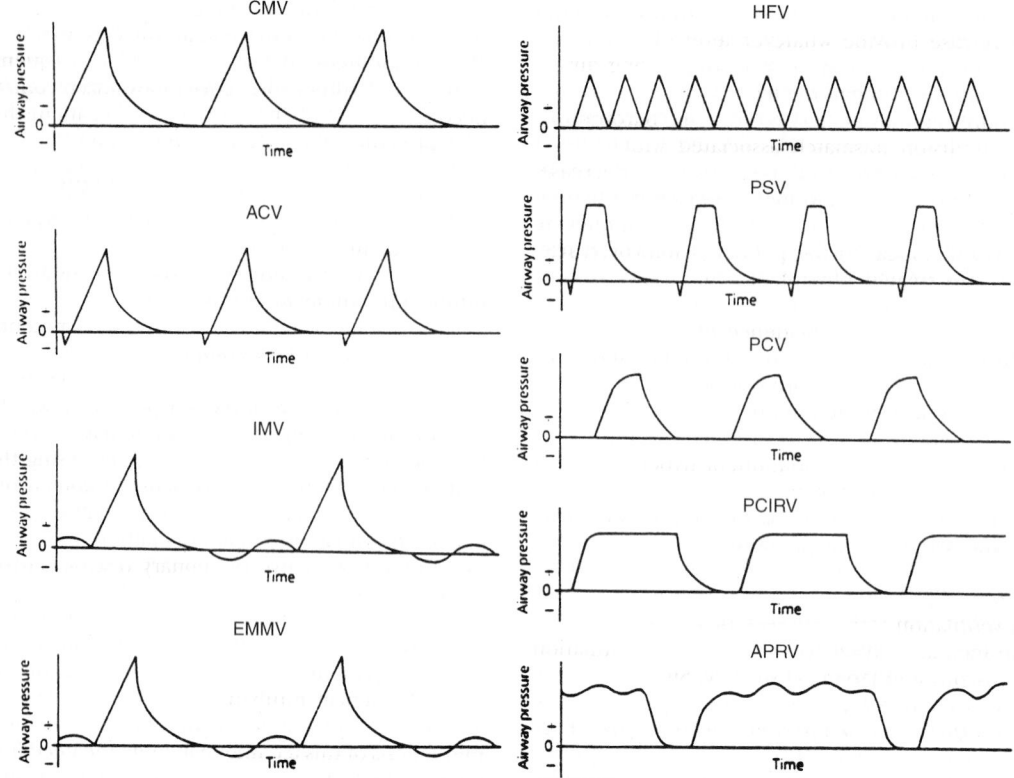

Figure 56-1. Airway pressure waveforms. CMV = controlled mechanical ventilation; ACV = assist control ventilation; IMV = intermittent mandatory ventilation; EMMV = extended mandatory minute ventilation; HFV = high-frequency ventilation; PSV = pressure support ventilation; PCV = pressure control ventilation; PCIRV = pressure control inverse ratio ventilation; APRV = airway pressure release ventilation.

Synchronized Intermittent Mandatory Ventilation

Synchronized intermittent mandatory ventilation (SIMV) is a mode using a combination of assist control with a mechanism and circuitry that allows for independent spontaneous ventilation. In this mode the patient may spontaneously breathe through the circuit, while at a predetermined interval the spontaneous breath is assisted by the machine. Therefore, a positive-pressure breath is always in synchrony with the patient's spontaneous ventilatory pattern. In this system a pressure-sensing device located near the patient's airway detects the initiation of a spontaneous breath; this activates the ventilator or the demand flow device. The major disadvantage of the demand flow system is the delay in providing adequate gas flow, which can result in increased work of breathing.

Pressure Support Ventilation

Pressure support ventilation (PSV) is a form of ventilation that aids normal breathing with a predetermined level of positive airway pressure. PSV is similar to intermittent positive-pressure ventilation but differs in that airway pressure is held constant throughout the inspiratory period. PSV differs from conventional volume-cycled ventilation in that the clinician selects only the inspiratory pressure. The patient controls ventilatory timing and interacts with the delivered pressure to determine the inspiratory flow and tidal volume. The unique waveforms of pressure and flow produced by PSV may have an advantage by providing better support of spontaneous tidal volume and by decreasing the overall work of breathing. The objective of PSV is to increase the patient's spontaneous tidal volume by delivering airway pressure to achieve volumes equal to 10–12 ml · kg^{-1}. PSV may also decrease airway resistance by increasing air flow during inspiration and thereby decrease the work of breathing and delay muscle fatigue. Indeed, the literature suggests that PSV can reduce ventilatory workload, prevent diaphragmatic fatigue,

compensate for the additional work of breathing caused by poorly functioning demand valves and undersized endotracheal tubes, improve patient–ventilator synchrony, and facilitate weaning.[44] Unfortunately, to date there are few clinical studies documenting the efficacy of this ventilatory mode, although theoretical advantages and safety of the mode in appropriately monitored patients support its use. Further studies are required to better evaluate the complex process of ventilatory reflexes and muscle conditioning during mechanical ventilation to fully establish the proper role of PSV.

Extended Mandatory Minute Ventilation

Extended mandatory minute ventilation (EMMV) provides a preset minute volume of gas either from a positive-pressure breath or from spontaneous breathing. The clinician determines the minimal accepted minute volume and selects the appropriate rate and volume. As the patient's ability to breathe spontaneously improves, less assisted ventilation is provided. Application of extended mandatory minute ventilation may enhance the weaning process by encouraging spontaneous breathing and enabling the patient to adjust to short-term changes in oxygen demand. Extended mandatory minute ventilation may also prove useful in tailoring tidal volume and respiratory rate more closely to meet patient needs. It may encourage patients who have become ventilator-dependent to use their respiratory muscles.

Airway Pressure Release Ventilation

Airway pressure release ventilation (APRV) was designed to augment ventilation for those patients with decreased lung compliance. The system is designed to provide alveolar ventilation as an adjunct to continuous positive airway pressure by intermittent and transient release of positive pressure, followed by restoration of pressure back to the continuous positive airway pressure level. The duration and frequency of continuous positive airway pressure release provide whatever level of ventilation is required. Because the peak airway pressure during airway pressure release ventilation equals the level of continuous positive airway pressure, cardiovascular depression, barotrauma, and ventilation–perfusion mismatch associated with conventional forms of ventilatory support may be expected to decrease. Theoretical advantages of airway pressure release ventilation over conventional positive pressure ventilatory techniques include its lower peak and mean airway pressures, improved arterial oxygenation, and smaller physiologic dead space ventilation. These advantages may lead to less depression of cardiac function as well as a decreased incidence of barotrauma. It differs from the inverse inspiratory to expiratory ratio (I:E) ventilation in that with airway pressure release ventilation, the patient breathes in an unrestricted manner during all parts of the ventilatory cycle. In contradistinction, an inverse I:E ratio requires skeletal muscle paralysis, sedation, or hyperventilation because no gas flow is available for spontaneous breathing during mechanical inspiration. Certainly, further study is necessary to better define the role of airway pressure release ventilation.

High-Frequency Ventilation

High-frequency ventilation (HFV) was originally used as a technique to provide adequate oxygenation and alveolar ventilation for rigid bronchoscopy and laryngeal surgery. Since that time, the literature has become replete with clinical applications of high-frequency ventilation. It is important to note that there are several different modalities to provide high-frequency ventilation. These ventilatory modes include high-frequency positive-pressure ventilation, high-frequency jet ventilation, high-frequency flow interrupters, and high-frequency oscillation. The common characteristic of all forms of high-frequency ventilation is ventilation at low tidal volumes (less than dead space) with high rates ($60-3000$ breaths$\cdot$min^{-1}). These systems enhance diffusive transport, minimize bulk transport, and improve intrapulmonary gas distribution. Hazards with high-frequency ventilation include inadequate humidification, barotrauma, necrotizing tracheobronchitis, hepatocellular injury, bronchospasm, and inadequate monitoring capabilities. Thus, although high-frequency ventilation is effective in maintaining pulmonary gas exchange at lower mean airway pressures, its precise role is yet to be determined.

Pressure Control Ventilation

Pressure control ventilation (PCV) is a patient or time-triggered, pressure-limited, time-cycled mode of ventilatory support. It is characterized by a rapid rise to peak pressure afforded by a decelerating inspiratory flow pattern. A pressure-controlled breath can be delivered in intermittent mandatory ventilation or assist mechanical ventilation instead of volume-oriented breaths, or in conjunction with pressure support ventilation. The potential advantage of pressure control ventilation is that because flow rate is geared to reach peak inspiratory pressure quickly, flow will exceed patient demand and therefore will improve patient–ventilator synchrony and decrease the work of breathing. Furthermore, pressure control ventilation might potentially improve distribution of gas within the lung by using the decelerating flow pattern and square wave air pressure pattern. The major disadvantage of pressure control ventilation is that tidal volume varies as compliance and resistance of the airways change.

Pressure Control Inverse Ratio Ventilation

Pressure control inverse ratio ventilation (PCIRV) is a time-triggered, pressure-limited, time-cycled mode of ventilation characterized by a decelerating inspiratory flow pattern, square wave air pressure pattern, and I:E ratio $\geq$ 1:1. The potential advantage of this mode of ventilation is the recruitment of collapsed alveoli by prolonged inspiratory times, which allow

alveolar units with slow time constants to fill. This improves both oxygenation and ventilation. Potential hazards include the development of auto-PEEP and consequent high airway pressures. Further prospective randomized controlled trials are necessary to determine the benefits to patients from the use of pressure control inverse ratio ventilation.

Noninvasive Positive Pressure Ventilation

Noninvasive positive-pressure ventilation (NPPV) provides the delivery of intermittent positive airway pressure through the upper airway and actively assists ventilation without tracheal intubation. This technique is rapidly gaining popularity because of its convenience, lower cost, and the potential significant reduction in morbidity compared with standard invasive positive-pressure ventilation. With the recent development of small, relatively inexpensive, and easily portable ventilators to be used specifically with NPPV using a nasal mask, several investigators have demonstrated successful treatment using this modality in patients with many varieties of acute[45,46] and chronic respiratory failure.[47,48] Most studies report a success rate of $\geq$60% for NPPV in patients with acute respiratory failure caused by exacerbation of chronic obstructive pulmonary disease. Furthermore, substantial reduction in the length of intensive care unit and total hospital stays has been observed. Theoretical advantages of NPPV over traditional modes of ventilatory support include increased patient comfort, reduced need for sedation, avoidance of tracheal intubation and its attendant complications, and maintenance of airway defenses, speech, and swallowing. Limitations of this technique include the need for patient cooperation, the lack of direct access to the airway to provide bronchial hygiene, facial skin ulcers caused by mask pressure, and aerophagia. Proper patient selection for the use of this modality is an integral component for success. The precise mechanism of NPPV has not been fully elucidated. Unlike PPV through an artificial airway, NPPV can be effective only if the patient can cooperate. Patients receiving NPPV must learn to coordinate their breathing efforts with a ventilator, to allow assistance to their spontaneous breath. Properties of the ventilators may also be important in the efficacy of NPPV. The triggering mechanism, for example, may be a critical factor because matching inspiratory airflow with the patient's inspiratory effort helps determine how much assistance a ventilator breath provides.

Several interfaces are available to provide NPPV, including nasal masks, facial masks, and lip seals. Standard nasal continuous positive-pressure masks are commonly selected because of their ease of application and ready availability. Recently, portable pressure-limited systems such as the bilevel positive airway pressure device (BiPAP; Respironic, Inc.) have become popular. These ventilators cycle between two levels of positive airway pressure, with the higher level assisting ventilation during inspiration and the lower level maintaining airway patency during expiration. Typical pressure and volume curves with BiPAP are outlined in Figure 56-1. NPPV clearly represents an important addition to the armamentarium available to manage patients with respiratory failure. However, complications, costs, and eventual outcomes have not been adequately studied. Further evaluation and refinement of the technique may provide a more widely used and valuable modality for selected patients with acute respiratory failure.

Have all the advances in technology and new ventilatory modalities had an impact on the outcome of critically ill patients in the ICU? Clearly, for select patient populations, ventilatory support has improved survival. For example, in the infant respiratory distress syndrome, this has been accomplished by the use of continuous positive airway pressure. Outcome has been similarly affected in patients with neuromuscular paralysis by the use of simple mechanical ventilation. However, despite all the newer ventilatory modalities available, little impact has been made on many other patient groups. The adult form of respiratory distress syndrome has not shown the increase in survival obtained in infants. Further, in patients with multiple organ system failure, including respiratory failure requiring mechanical support, outcome is determined more by the underlying cause than by the technique of mechanical ventilatory support. Despite an increasingly sophisticated array of mechanical support devices and detailed physiologic methodologies for augmenting support, little or no further increment of survival has been demonstrated in patients whose lungs are commonly ventilated with underlying sepsis and multiple organ failure. Certainly, ventilatory support has a place in affecting outcome in critical illness, although newer ventilatory techniques and technology must await further evaluation.

Cystic Fibrosis

Cystic fibrosis (CF) is an inherited multisystem disorder characterized by abnormalities in exocrine gland function. The most common cause of morbidity and mortality in patients with cystic fibrosis is pulmonary dysfunction. Pancreatic dysfunction is also a common accompaniment, as is hepatobiliary and genitourinary disease. The median survival time for patients with cystic fibrosis is about 20 years. However, with improvements in diagnosis and treatment, many patients survive through the third and fourth decades of life.

All levels of the respiratory tract can be involved with cystic fibrosis. Nasal polyposis, sinusitis, and lower respiratory tract disease are common findings in these patients. The common denominator is the alteration in mucus secretion. These patients have large amounts of secretion that predispose them to bacterial pneumonia, particularly with *Pseudomonas aeruginosa*.

Recently, there has been increasing interest in the use of anti-inflammatory medications to decrease airway inflammation and preserve pulmonary function in patients with CF lung disease.[49] Long-term oral corticosteroids,[50] ibuprofen,[51] and inhaled corticosteroids[52] have been shown to have a beneficial effect in slowing the progression of CF. Other agents used to reduce pulmonary inflammation include pentoxifylline,[53] a phosphodiesterase inhibitor, and tyloxapol,[54] a nonionic detergent and antioxidant.

Other organ systems involved with cystic fibrosis include the gastrointestinal and genitourinary systems and the sweat glands. Pancreatic insufficiency leading to protein and fat malabsorption is common, and recurrent pancreatitis may occur. Hepatobiliary disease is common in older patients with chronic cholestasis, inflammation, fibrosis, and even cirrhosis. Extrahepatic disease of the biliary system and abnormalities of the genitourinary tract are also common.

Abnormality in sweat gland function is the most reliable diagnostic test for cystic fibrosis. Examination of sweat of patients with cystic fibrosis reveals elevations of sodium, potassium, and chloride levels. This increase in electrolyte content results from a failure of reabsorption in the sweat duct.

Treatment of patients with cystic fibrosis is primarily directed at the respiratory system. Specifically, treatment has focused on the control of airway infection, secretion mobilization, and reduction of airway inflammation. Since the discovery of the CF gene, research has been directed at methods to correct the basic ion transport defects.[63] Every attempt must be made to increase mechanical drainage and clear secretions with chest physiotherapy and exercise programs. Control of bacterial infection with antibiotic therapy is essential. Bronchodilators should be used to reverse any bronchospastic component of the lung disease. Fluid management and general supportive measures are essential to successful treatment.

RENAL SYSTEM
Acute Renal Failure

Acute renal failure is impairment of the normal homeostatic functions of the kidney resulting in retention of nitrogenous wastes. It is a common problem, occurring in 5% of all hospitalized patients. It is particularly problematic in critically ill patients, in whom the incidence of acute renal failure is significantly higher. Despite advances in understanding the disease process, mortality remains high. Sixty percent of all cases of acute renal failure are related to surgery or trauma. The most common cause is renal ischemia with sepsis, hypovolemic shock, and nephrotoxic agents as major etiologic factors. The site of interference with renal function may be prerenal, renal, or postrenal.

Prerenal Causes

Prerenal causes of acute renal failure result from hypoperfusion of the kidneys, most commonly from extracellular fluid volume contraction. Reduced renal perfusion results from decreased effective circulating volume due to hypovolemia or redistribution of circulating volume. Reduction in cardiac output can also result in prerenal failure because of inadequate perfusion of the kidneys. This may result from primary myocardial disease, valvular heart disease, constrictive pericarditis, or cardiac tamponade. Decreased perfusion of the kidneys may also result from vascular disease of both large and small vessels. Certainly, bilateral renal artery stenosis can cause prerenal azotemia. However, although most prerenal causes of renal failure are accompanied by hypotension, renal artery stenosis is usually associated with hypertension.

Intrinsic Renal Causes

Intrinsic renal causes of acute renal failure can be divided by the component of the kidney most affected, *i.e.*, the glomeruli, blood vessels, and the tubulointerstitial region. Glomerular diseases account for 5–10% of all cases of acute renal failure and may be caused by direct immunologically mediated injury or decreased renal perfusion. Vascular disease can result in intrinsic renal failure primarily caused by either thromboembolic injury or systemic diseases.

Acute tubular necrosis is the most common cause of acute renal failure in critically ill patients and accounts for 75% of the renal causes of kidney failure. The two major causes of acute tubular necrosis are ischemia and nephrotoxins. Renal ischemia is the most common cause of acute renal failure and may be caused by a variety of clinical conditions, including volume depletion, shock, and operations that interrupt the renal circulation. It appears that prostaglandins play an important role in maintaining renal perfusion; therefore, patients taking drugs that inhibit prostaglandin synthesis may be predisposed to renal injury with hypoperfusion.

Nephrotoxic agents may also cause acute tubular necrosis. Categories of toxins include antibiotics, contrast material, anesthetic drugs, heavy metals, and organic solvents. In the past, heavy metals, organic solvents, and glycols were a common cause of acute renal failure. Today, however, aminoglycosides have supplanted them as the major nephrotoxic cause of acute renal failure. All aminoglycosides have nephrotoxic potential. Clinical nephrotoxicity, defined as a decrease in glomerular filtration rate, occurs in 5–25% of patients receiving aminoglycosides. The toxicity of these antibiotics is enhanced by advanced age, pre-existing renal dysfunction, concomitant administration of other nephrotoxic agents, and hypotension. Renal toxicity can also occur with antibiotics other than aminoglycosides, including cephalosporins, penicillins, and amphotericin B.

Toxic acute renal failure associated with the use of radiocontrast media is the second most common cause of nephrotoxic acute tubular necrosis. Patients particularly at risk for radiocontrast-induced renal failure include those with diabetes mellitus, the elderly, and those with pre-existing renal insufficiency. Dehydration compounds the risk in susceptible patients.

Anesthetic-induced nephrotoxicity is generally attributable to fluoride toxicity. Because toxicity results from high free fluoride levels in the plasma, prolonged duration of anesthesia and preexisting renal dysfunction could put patients at risk for nephrotoxicity. Biotransformation of enflurane and sevoflurane may lead to the release of free fluoride, especially when anesthesia is prolonged, or when renal dysfunction is present. However, the usual levels of fluoride required to produce nephrotoxicity (40–50 mM) are rarely exceeded except during dramatically prolonged enflurane or sevoflurane anesthesia. Several common chemotherapeutic drugs can also cause acute tubular necrosis, including cisplatin and high-dose methotrexate. Adequate extracellular fluid volume expansion and concomitant use of diuretics may significantly lessen nephrotoxic effects of cisplatin, and alkalinization of the urine may decrease toxicity of high-dose methotrexate. Rhabdomyolysis has become an important cause of acute renal failure described in association with crush injuries, extensive burns, muscle inflammation, and a variety of settings in which muscle blood flow and metabolism are disturbed or muscle energy production is increased. The toxic effect of myoglobin causes acute tubular necrosis with rhabdomyolysis, just as hemoglobin is the toxic pigment in acute tubular necrosis associated with hemolysis from mismatched blood.

An increasing number of drugs have been associated with acute interstitial nephritis and subsequent acute renal failure. The most common cause of acute interstitial nephritis is an acute drug-induced hypersensitivity reaction. Drugs commonly implicated include β-lactam antibiotics (especially methicillin), nonsteroidal anti-inflammatory drugs, and diuretics. Acute interstitial nephritis is associated with an increased eosinophil count in blood and urine.

Postrenal Causes

Postrenal causes of acute renal failure may be asymptomatic and must be considered in any patient with renal failure. This form of acute deterioration of renal function is often reversible and occurs in up to 10% of patients with decreasing renal function. Obstruction to urine flow may occur at any level from the kidney to the bladder. Ureteral obstruction from calculi, clots, tumor, stricture, retroperitoneal fibrosis, or malignancy may cause ureteral obstruction, whereas bladder tumors or a neurogenic bladder can result in obstruction at the level of the bladder. Urethral obstruction can be caused by prostate disorders, urethral stricture, cervical carcinoma, or meatal stenosis. In most cases of possible obstruction, a combination of a flat abdominal film, renal scan, and ultrasonogram can supply as much information as excretory urography with much less risk. However, if the clinical history is suggestive of obstruction, even if the noninvasive studies are negative, cystoscopy and retrograde pyelography should be considered.

Oliguric Versus Nonoliguric Acute Renal Failure

In the past, acute renal failure was often defined by oliguria, the production of <400 ml · day^{-1} of urine. However, nonoliguric acute renal failure is now recognized as a distinct clinical entity with a more favorable prognosis. Hospitalization time, complications, and mortality are less in nonoliguric patients. Drugs that increase solute excretion, such as mannitol and furosemide, may have the capacity to convert oliguric acute renal failure to the nonoliguric type. Some authors suggest that high doses of iv furosemide be given to attenuate the course of acute renal failure, whereas others claim that furosemide responders simply may have less severe renal impairment. The results are still controversial, and the efficacy of furosemide may depend on its administration in the initiation phase of acute renal failure. Nonetheless, after prerenal and postrenal factors contributing to azotemia have been corrected, a trial of furosemide 2–10 mg · kg^{-1} can be given in an attempt to convert an incipient oliguric renal failure to a nonoliguric state with restoration of blood volume if diuresis ensues.

Urinary Indices

Urine sediment is almost never normal in acute renal failure. A chemical profile of the urine aids immeasurably in assessing the cause of acute renal failure. In prerenal azotemia, tubular function remains relatively intact and sodium and water resorption results. There is an increase in sodium loss in the urine in patients with acute tubular necrosis because tubular function is impaired (Table 56-4). In acute oliguric renal failure, daily increases of blood urea nitrogen and serum creatinine average 10–20 mg · dL^{-1} and 0.5–1 mg · dL^{-1}, respectively. If creatinine is elevated out of proportion to the blood urea nitrogen, it suggests that rhabdomyolysis may be the etiology of acute renal failure. The rapid rise in serum creatinine levels with rhabdomyolysis is attributable to the release of creatine from skeletal muscle; creatine is converted by nonenzymatic hydrolysis to creatinine.

Complications of Acute Renal Failure

Hyponatremia, edema, and pulmonary congestion can occur with oliguric acute renal failure as a result of salt and water overload. In addition, serum potassium concentration may rise because of the decreased elimination of potassium associated with acute renal failure. The usual rate of increase in serum potassium in the noncatabolic, oliguric patient is 0–0.5 mEq · 24 hr^{-1}. If potassium increases at a greater rate, other contributing factors should be sought and treated. Other electrolyte abnormalities present in acute renal failure include hyperphosphatemia, hypocalcemia, and mild hypermagnesemia. These abnormalities must be monitored closely and treated accordingly.

Because the kidneys can no longer eliminate the daily production of nonvolatile acid, there is a daily decrease of 1–2 mEq in plasma bicarbonate levels, with a resultant anion gap metabolic acidosis. Still other complications include anemia, platelet abnormalities, and altered host defenses leading to an increased incidence of infection. Gastrointestinal complications include nausea, vomiting, and, most commonly, gastrointestinal hemorrhage, which occurs in 10–30% of patients.

Treatment

Mortality rates of patients with acute renal failure vary from 30% to 60%. However, if acute renal failure follows surgery or trauma, the mortality may be as high as 70%. The first step in the management of acute renal failure is to exclude remedial causes. Specifically, identification and correction of prerenal and postrenal factors are essential. The treatment of acute renal failure includes diuresis and control of the extracellular fluid volume, treatment of hyperkalemia and acidosis, prophylaxis against infection and gastrointestinal bleeding, nutritional support, and dialysis. Because the prognosis is better with polyuria than with anuria, efforts should be made to produce and maintain a polyuric state. Intake and output must be monitored closely.

Conservative therapy is frequently ineffective for critically ill patients with acute renal failure; therefore, some form of dialytic therapy is usually indicated. The absolute indications for dialysis include symptomatic uremia, development of resistant hyperka-

Table 56-4. DIAGNOSTIC URINARY INDICES

Parameter	Prerenal	Renal
Urinary osmolality (mOsm)	>500	<350
Urine/plasma creatinine	>30	<20
Urine sodium concentration (mEq · l^{-1})	<20	>40
Fractional excretion of sodium (%)	<1	>2
Renal failure index (%)	<1	>2

lemia, severe acidemia or fluid overload not responsive to conservative therapy, and pericarditis. In addition, many advocate maintaining a blood urea nitrogen level of 100 mg · dL^{-1} and a creatinine level 8 mg · dL^{-1}. Inadequate nutrition has recently been recognized as a reason for dialysis. Both hemodialysis and peritoneal dialysis have been used to manage acute renal failure, and survival data are similar. Each method has unique advantages and disadvantages.

Several modifications of hemodialysis have been applied to patients with acute renal failure. These include slow continuous ultrafiltration with intermittent hemodialysis, continuous arteriovenous hemodialysis, and continuous arteriovenous hemofiltration. All of these methods provide excellent hemodynamic stability. Access to blood is obtained either by percutaneous cannulation of the femoral artery and vein or via an arteriovenous shunt. No blood pump is used in this system because blood is driven by the patient's own arterial pressure. In continuous arterial venous hemofiltration, large amounts of ultrafiltrate are removed through a porous filter with the ultrafiltrate replaced by sterile iv fluid. In slow continuous ultrafiltration, much smaller volumes of ultrafiltrate are removed to correct any extracellular fluid volume expansion. However, intermittent dialysis is required to control uremia, hyperkalemia, and acidemia. With continuous arterial venous hemodialysis, dialysate flows through the dialysate compartment at ~20 ml · min^{-1}, which is sufficient to achieve a low, steady-state blood urea nitrogen and creatinine levels. Unfortunately, the various improvements in resuscitative techniques and technical advances in dialytic therapy have not significantly reduced the mortality of acute renal failure.

Hepatorenal Syndrome

Acute renal failure in the presence of severe advanced liver disease in the absence of clinical, laboratory, or anatomic evidence of other causes of renal dysfunction is known as hepatorenal syndrome. It is usually an oliguric form of renal failure with low urinary sodium concentrations. The picture appears similar to that of a prerenal azotemia; however, it occurs in the setting of advanced liver disease. The precise mechanism for the renal failure is unknown. Currently, there is no effective treatment for hepatorenal syndrome.

INFECTIOUS DISEASES
Nosocomial Infections

Advances in technology and the use of a greater number of monitoring devices and therapeutic interventions have led to an increased number of infections. Patients in intensive care units suffer a disproportionate number of nosocomial infections compared with patients in non–critical care areas. These infections result in an increased morbidity, mortality, and cost.[55] Indeed, hospital-acquired infections have emerged as the leading cause of death in most ICUs. These infections are often polymicrobial, involve multiple resistant strains of bacteria, and do not respond to simple therapy. The incidence of nosocomial infections in ICUs is commonly 40–50%, many of which are preventable. The cost implications of prolonged hospitalization and treatment of infection are apparent.

The major determinants of the incidence and outcome of nosocomial infections include patient age, underlying disease, integrity of mucosal and integumentary surfaces, and the status of the immunologic defenses. Common sources of hospital-acquired infections in critically ill patients include the urinary tract, surgical wounds, pneumonia, intravascular devices, and sinusitis. Immunocompromised patients with a deficiency in any of the multifaceted host defenses are particularly prone to these infections and to other unusual infections. In particular, patients with acquired immunodeficiency syndrome commonly present with opportunistic infections caused by viruses, bacteria, parasites, and fungi. These patients invariably die despite transiently effective antimicrobial therapy and current attempts at immune reconstitution.

Selective Decontamination of the Digestive Tract

Selective decontamination of the digestive tract (SDD) has been proposed as a means of reducing the incidence of nosocomial infections in hospitalized patients, particularly those treated in the ICU. This method assumes that many nosocomial infections originate in the digestive tract and that it may be possible to reduce the incidence of such infections by eliminating pathogenic organisms from the digestive tract while leaving normal anaerobic flora intact. This is accomplished through the administration of both oral and parenteral antibiotics. Targeted organisms of selective decontamination include gram-negative aerobic bacilli, gram-positive aerobic cocci, and yeasts. The efficacy of this technique was first demonstrated in multiple trauma patients requiring mechanical ventilation. A dramatic reduction in the rate of infection in patients given antimicrobial decontamination from 81% to 16% was reported.[56] Since that time, several investigators have reported reduction in nosocomial infection rates using SDD.[57,58] However, this has not been the universal experience, and other investigators have shown no change in infection rates.[59,60] Unfortunately, to date, study design flaws have precluded a definitive conclusion on the efficacy of the technique of SDD. Additional large-scale multicenter prospective trials are needed before SDD can be confirmed as an effective method of preventing infection in critically ill patients.

Urinary Tract Infections

Urinary tract infections account for ~40% of hospital-acquired infections. Because most critically ill patients have an indwelling Foley catheter, it is not surprising that the urinary tract is a common source of infection. It is the most common site resulting in gram-negative bacteremia. The urinary tract should be considered a possible source of infection if the patient has bacteriuria and a clinical picture consistent with infection.

Wound Infections

Most surgical wound infections are caused by the introduction of bacteria directly into the tissue at the time of operation. They account for 10% of all infections in postsurgical ICU patients. Wounds should be observed for any signs of infection, and any purulent material should be sampled and sent for Gram stain and culture. Most wound infections are evident 3–7 days after surgical intervention. Wounds infected within 24 hr are generally fulminant infections caused by *Clostridium* or β-hemolytic streptococci. Later surgical wound infections are generally caused by gram-negative bacilli, anaerobic bacteria, and staphylococci. The administration of prophylactic antibiotics has aided immeasurably in reducing the postoperative wound infection rate.

Pneumonia

The most serious complication among hospital-acquired infections is lower respiratory tract infection. Hospital-acquired pneumonia occurs in up to 15% of ICU patients and is the leading cause of mortality in this group. The major organisms causing pneumonia in the critically ill patient population are gram-negative bacilli and *Staphylococcus aureus*. The diagnosis of pneumonia in critically ill patients who are maintained on mechanical ventilatory support can be difficult. Physical examination by itself is not an adequate screening procedure. Bacterial colonization of the upper airway is common and may not reflect lower respiratory tract disease. Nosocomial pneumonia is generally diagnosed by signs and symptoms of infection with bacteriologic verification in addition to a new pulmonary infiltrate that is unchanged by physical therapy. Unfortunately, Gram stain and culture of aspirated material through the endotracheal tube may not be reliable indicators of true lower respiratory tract infection. Antibody coating and quantitative cultures have not significantly improved diagnostic efficacy. Protected brush catheter bronchoscopy has been advocated as an effective adjunct to the diagnosis of pneumonia for patients maintained on mechanical ventilatory support.

Intravascular Devices

With advances in technology and invasive monitoring, intravascular device–related bacteremia has become a common problem, accounting for more than 25,000 cases of bacteremia annually. Contamination of intravascular devices may occur anywhere along the line from the infusate bottle to the skin entry site. Predisposition to intravascular device–related bacteremia is determined by both patient and hospital factors. The patient-related factors generally reflect the severity of underlying disease. Hospital-related factors are more controlled and include the type of catheter, site of insertion, technique of placement, and duration of cannulation. Recommendations for prevention of intravascular device-related infections should be based on the Centers for Disease Control guidelines.[61]

Intra-abdominal Infections

Abdominal infections generally occur in patients who have undergone prior intra-abdominal procedures. Risk factors for infection include prolonged operative time, use of foreign substances, inadequate drainage, presence of devitalized tissue, hematoma formation, and fecal contamination at the time of surgery. Acalculous cholecystitis is another potential etiology of abdominal infection in the postoperative period. Stress ulceration with significant gastrointestinal bleeding and perforation, or perforation due to mechanical causes, such as nasogastric drainage, can result in intra-abdominal infection in the absence of prior surgical intervention. The diagnosis of intra-abdominal infection relies primarily on physical examination with adjunctive radiologic evaluation including computed tomographic scan, ultrasonography, and abdominal roentgenograms.

Sinusitis

One of the recognized complications of nasotracheal intubation is the development of sinusitis. Nosocomial sinusitis accounts for 5% of all nosocomial infections in the critically ill patient population. However, this infection is frequently difficult to diagnose and often goes unrecognized. Patients may present with fever and leukocytosis but with few other signs or symptoms of overt infection. Fewer than half of the patients have purulent nasal drainage. The diagnosis of sinusitis relies on x-ray films of the paranasal sinuses. Unfortunately, these are frequently of suboptimal quality because they are taken in the critical care unit with a portable apparatus. However, if opacification of the sinuses is present or an air-fluid level is noted and aspiration reveals purulent material, the endotracheal tube should be removed and replaced using the oral route along with initiation of antibiotic therapy. Patients generally respond well and rarely require surgical drainage.

Central Nervous System Infections

Nosocomial CNS infections are uncommon in critically ill patients unless there are predisposing conditions such as neurosurgical procedures or CNS trauma. All pyogenic infections of the cranial contents originate either by hematogenous spread or extension from contiguous sites. Acute meningitis is a medical emergency that requires high-level diagnostic and therapeutic skills because it has a significant mortality rate. Patients frequently present with headache, stiff neck, seizures, and altered mental status. To differentiate bacterial meningitis from an aseptic meningitis syndrome, analysis of the CSF is necessary. All febrile patients with lethargy, headache, or confusion of sudden onset, even if only low-grade temperature is present, should be subjected to a lumbar puncture.

Brain abscess has occurred with a constant incidence even with the introduction of broad-spectrum antibiotic coverage. It is associated with a high morbidity and mortality. The most common age of patients for a brain abscess to occur is between 30 and 40 years of age, and it is frequently associated with sinusitis or otitis. Streptococci are the most common etiologic organisms. Treatment is both medical and surgical, with anaerobic antibiotic coverage and surgical drainage. Although mortality has improved, there is still a significant incidence of neurologic residual, primarily seizure disorders.

Fungal Infections

With the use of broad-spectrum antibiotic therapy, organ transplantation, prosthetic cardiac valves, and immunosuppression from neoplasm, transplants, burns, and drugs, there has been an increased incidence of fungal infections. Clinical manifestations range from thrush to disseminated candidiasis. Organs involved with systemic disease include the kidneys, brain, myocardium, and eyes. The hallmark pathologically is diffuse microabscesses with a combined suppurative and granulomatous reaction. The diagnosis of candidemia may be difficult because serum antibodies have been uniformly disappointing and culture results are often negative. Although not all patients with candidemia require antifungal therapy, if treatment is indicated, amphotericin B is the drug of choice.

Sepsis Syndrome/Systemic Inflammatory Response Syndrome

The definition of the sepsis syndrome is based on easily acquired clinical data that can be applied to a broad population of patients. More recently, the term systemic inflammatory response syndrome (SIRS) was developed to describe a clinical response arising from a variety of insults including infection. The clinical evidence of the syndrome is based on a high index of suspicion and does not require confirmation with positive blood cultures or cultures of material from a closed space. Indeed, the sepsis syndrome can be defined in terms of the systemic response to infection expressed as tachycardia, fever or hypothermia, tachypnea, and evidence of inadequate organ perfusion. That is, the systemic response is what differentiates sepsis from simple infection or bacteremia. The object of such a broad definition is to facilitate early recognition and prompt institution of therapeutic interventions.

Sepsis has been estimated to occur in 1 of 100 hospitalized patients in the United States. Although its precise incidence is unknown, it has been estimated that up to 500,000 cases of sepsis occur each year in the United States. When the sepsis syndrome is accompanied by hypotension that is unresponsive to fluid therapy, it is often referred to as septic shock. Shock develops in ~40% of patients with sepsis. The increased survival of immunocompromised patients, those receiving organ transplants, and those with malignancy and inflammatory disease as well as the use of invasive medical devices and procedures has increased the incidence of sepsis.

The clinical response defined as SIRS includes two or more of the following: (1) temperature $>38°C$ or $<36°C$, (2) heart rate >90 beats $\cdot$ min^{-1}, (3) respiratory rate >20 breaths $\cdot$ min^{-1} or P_{CO_2} <32 mm Hg, or (4) white blood cell count

>12.0 × $10^9 \cdot L^{-1}$ or <4.0 × $10^9 \cdot L^{-1}$ or the presence of more than 0.1 immature neutrophils.[62] The primary criteria for the diagnosis of the sepsis syndrome include (a) clinical evidence of infection such as tachycardia, tachypnea, and hyperthermia or hypothermia, and (b) evidence of altered organ perfusion or organ system dysfunction, such as alterations in mental status, arterial hypoxemia, elevated plasma lactate levels, or oliguria (Table 56-5).

The sepsis syndrome can be identified as a systemic manifestation of presumed sepsis. Although the traditional definitions of sepsis (requiring positive blood or closed-space cultures) and of shock are frequently not present, the overall mortality rate is significant and similar to that reported by several investigators in patients with sepsis. The incidence of ARDS is also similar to that of previously published reports with sepsis. Clearly, the sepsis syndrome has a clinically significant morbidity and mortality rate. Progression from the sepsis syndrome to the associated clinical sequelae of septic shock and ARDS may be prevented by intervention at the onset of the sepsis syndrome. Identification and clinical evaluation of the criteria for the sepsis syndrome may demonstrate an appropriate point for evaluating therapeutic interventions. Recently, plasma exchange has been used as salvage therapy in severe infection in an attempt to remove bacterial products and to modulate the host inflammatory response.[63] While initial data suggested a lower mortality and a reduced number of organ failure in the plasma filtration patients, the differences did not reach statistical significance.[64]

Septic Shock

It has been estimated that >300,000 gram-negative bacteremias occur in the United States each year. When bacteremia is caused by gram-negative bacteria, 10–20% may result in a documented period of hemodynamic instability and organ dysfunction. Mortality rates between 20% and 60% are reported for such severe cases, averaging 40% in several prospected trials.[65–67]

Septic shock is the 13th most common cause of death in the United States and is the most common cause of death in medical and surgical intensive units. Statistics compiled by the Centers for Disease Control and Prevention indicate that the incidence of this disease has increased by 137% over the past decade. Both gram-negative and gram-positive bacteria as well as fungi and exogenous microbial components can initiate septic shock. Indeed, it has been extremely difficult to clinically differentiate between gram-positive and gram-negative infections. The gram-negative bacilli have a complex, three-layered cell wall structure. The lipopolysaccharide component of the outermost layer has been of particular interest because of its association with endotoxin properties.

Endotoxin is a complex molecule consisting of an outer core of repetitive sugar moieties, an O-antigen–specific side chain conferring serologic specificity, and an inner core linked to a structure termed lipid A. Endotoxin and other bacterial products activate cell membrane phospholipases to liberate arachidonic acid and initiate synthesis and release of leukotrienes, prostaglandins, and thromboxanes. It is these inflammatory mediators that primarily influence vasomotor tone, microvascular permeability, leukoaggregation, and the aggregation of platelets. Bacterial endotoxin can trigger a cascade of enzymatic processes, which leads to the release of vasoactive kinins, kallikreins in particular. Indeed, the physiologic changes associated with septic shock in humans result from a sophisticated interplay of mediators of cellular function and inflammation. Cytokines including tumor necrosis factor (TNF-α) and interleukins (IL-1, IL-6, and IL-8) influence cardiovascular, hemodynamic, and coagulation mechanisms. The presence of these compounds results in the production of excessive quantities of secondary mediators, which include lipids, peptides, and amines. Examples of secondary mediators include prostaglandin I_2, thromboxane A_2, prostaglandin E_2, platelet-activating factor, bradykinin, angiotensin, vasoactive intestinal peptide, histamine, serotonin, and a variety of complement-derived products. Recently, apoptosis has been shown to be an important mechanism in patients with sepsis, shock, and multiple organ dysfunction.[68] Unfortunately, it remains unclear whether apotosis is beneficial or detrimental to the host. If it is determined to be detrimental, drugs that inhibit caspase-3 may be therapeutically useful.

Monoclonal Antiendotoxin Antibodies

Several strategies have been developed to limit the effects of inflammatory mediators in septic shock. Development of new drugs to treat sepsis has been based in part on the premise that neutralizing bacterial toxins and potentially harmful host mediators could stop or slow this syndrome. Specifically, new therapies have been directed at different elements of the inflammatory cascade including endotoxin, TNF, IL-1, neutrophils, nitric oxide, eicosanoids, platelet activating factor, bradykinin, and leukotrienes. Currently, there are no antiendotoxins in clinical use, although several are under investigation. Antibodies to the O-side chain produce serotype-specific complement-dependent bactericidal activity. However, serotype specificity limits the clinical utility of O-side chain therapies. This led to investigation of antibodies directed at core and lipid A structures of endotoxin because these antibodies might cross-protect against diverse gram-negative bacteria. Core-directed antibodies are the only antiendotoxin therapies studied in clinical trials. Polyclonal core-reactive antiserum or immunoglobulin used to prevent or treat gram-negative sepsis has universally shown essentially no survival benefit.[69–71]

Monoclonal antibodies were developed to produce a more specific antiendotoxin therapy with less risk for transmission of infection. E5, a murine IgM, has been tested in two multicenter randomized placebo-controlled clinical trials to date. Using meta-analysis and combining data from the two trials, it appeared that E5 decreased the time to recovery from organ dysfunction, and improved survival in a subgroup of patients who were not in refractory shock. HA-1A, a human IGM antibody that binds to the lipid A domain of endotoxin, seemed initially to significantly reduce mortality in patients with sepsis and gram-negative bacteremia. However, several subsequent trials revealed a higher mortality rate in patients randomized to receive HA-1A[72] leading to withdrawal of HA-1A from the market in European countries.

Recently, clinical trials have been initiated using neutrophil-derived bactericidal/permeability-increasing protein, high-density lipoproteins, and cationic polypeptides which may neutralize and/or enhance the clearance of endotoxin. To date, however, these antiendotoxin core-directed antibodies have shown little impact on survival in patients with septic shock.

Anticytokine Therapy

Cytokines are peptides that function as cellular signals to regulate the amplitude and duration of the host inflammatory response. Monocytes release TNF and IL-1 in response to bacterial components such as endotoxin. In animal models inhibition of TNF and IL-1 protects against endotoxin or bacteria.[73,74] TNF and IL-1 play protective roles in the immune response to infec-

---

Table 56-5. CLINICAL FEATURES OF THE SEPSIS SYNDROME

Clinical evidence of infection
Hypothermia/hyperthermia
Impaired organ function or evidence of inadequate perfusion
    Altered mentation
    Hypoxemia
    Elevated plasma lactate level
    Oliguria

tion. Both recruit and activate neutrophils, macrophages, and lymphocytes and increase gene expression and release of acute phase proteins and granulocyte colony stimulating factors.[75] To date there have been few clinical trails of anticytokine therapy in humans, but the drugs seem to be effective in the animal model. However, a recent Phase II blinded randomized trial of recombinant human dimeric TNF receptor found no difference in mortality with low-dose anti-TNF compared with placebo; but disturbingly, patients who received medium and high doses had worse outcomes than did patients who received placebo. IL-1 antagonists have primarily been limited to the use of IL-1ra, acute phase cytokines structurally similar to IL-1, that can block the IL-1 receptor site and prevent activation of the target cell by IL-1. Clinical trails with recombinant IL-1ra have yielded conflicting results. This drug is under further investigation at present. Nonetheless, to date, anti-TNF and anti-IL-1 agents have not been shown to improve outcome in the treatment of human sepsis and septic shock and may, in fact, be potentially harmful. Whether it is clinically feasible to inhibit cytokines and limit their harmful effects while preserving their ability to perform necessary beneficial functions is unknown.

Nitric Oxide

NO is a low–molecular-weight, membrane-permeable gas that functions as a neurotransmitter, regulates vascular tone, and inhibits platelet aggregation and leukocyte adhesion.[76-78] At higher concentrations, NO has antitumor and antimicrobial activity. Inhibition of NO production has been proposed as a new approach to treat the hypotension of septic shock. It has been postulated that an increased production of NO during septic shock may lead to several harmful effects. NO may be largely responsible for sepsis-induced hypotension and myocardial depression.[79-81] Further, NO may exert a proinflammatory effect during septic shock by enhancing cytokine release from phagocytic cells. Despite these potential hazards, NO may also have beneficial effects in septic shock. It appears to play a role in maintaining visceral and microvascular blood flow and may serve as a counterregulatory mechanism to maintain perfusion. In addition, its ability to block platelet aggregation and leukocyte adhesion could prevent microvascular stasis and thrombosis. NO synthase inhibitors, indeed, have been used in an attempt to improve survival in septic shock by increasing mean arterial pressure. However, to date, NO synthase inhibitors have not proved beneficial in the treatment of septic shock. In the future, however, NO synthase inhibitors that are highly selective for the induced isoform of the ionized or particular vascular beds may be developed and warrant further investigation.

Hemodynamic alterations in septic shock generally take two forms. Early in shock, the patient may have an increase in cardiac output, vasodilation, decrease in SVR, decrease in central venous pressure, and an increase in stroke volume. As shock progresses, the predominant picture is one of vasoconstriction with an increase in SVR and a decrease in cardiac output, central venous pressure, and stroke volume.

Organ systems involved in septic shock include the cardiac, renal, respiratory, and hematologic systems. Cardiac failure may develop in the setting of sepsis, primarily related to a myocardial depressant factor. Disseminated intravascular coagulation is not uncommon in septic shock. The pathogenesis probably involves the activation of the intrinsic clotting system by Hageman factor leading to activation of kallikrein. This, in turn, activates the potent vasodilator bradykinin, which promotes pooling of blood in peripheral tissues as well as increases in capillary permeability and localized tissue damage. Respiratory failure is probably the most important cause of death in patients with shock. Septic shock is an important cause of ARDS and severe respiratory failure. The kidneys are also target organs in septic shock, with resultant acute renal failure. Oliguria occurs early and probably results from inadequate renal perfusion.

Clinically, gram-negative bacteremia usually begins abruptly with chills, fever, nausea, vomiting, diarrhea, and prostration. When septic shock develops, there is in addition tachycardia, tachypnea, hypotension, cool pale extremities with peripheral cyanosis, mental obtundation, and oliguria.

Laboratory data vary greatly and depend on both the cause and extent of the shock syndrome. There is usually leukocytosis. However, the white blood cell count may be normal or even depressed. Serum bicarbonate is usually low and blood lactate level elevated. Electrolyte pattern may vary considerably, although there is a tendency to hyponatremia and hypochloremia.

Clinical treatment of septic shock is directed at two primary therapeutic goals: (1) rapid reversal of perfusion failure and (2) identification and control of infection. Certainly, every effort should be made to identify the cause of infection. However, treatment must be initiated early if it is to be successful. Indeed, antibiotic therapy should be initiated immediately and not await blood culture results. Early aggressive intervention, including antibiotics, fluid resuscitation, vasoactive drug support, mechanical ventilatory support, and surgical drainage of any infected site, is essential for successful treatment. Surgical drainage of closed space infections is mandatory, and a vigorous search for the infectious site is indicated in all patients.

Fluid resuscitation is the mainstay of treatment of septic shock. The fluid of choice for volume repletion remains controversial. Regardless of the fluid infused, however, it appears that survival can be improved if stroke volume or cardiac output improves in response to fluid challenge. If volume resuscitation and other supportive measures are inadequate in restoring perfusion, vasoactive drug support may be indicated. Because in the low-flow state of hypodynamic septic shock peripheral vascular resistances increase, drugs with predominantly α-adrenergic effects should be avoided. Dopamine and dobutamine have been used successfully in treating septic shock. These drugs have predominantly β-adrenergic effects and result in an increase in cardiac output due to an increase in both contractility and heart rate. Indeed, early data suggested an increased survival with high levels of oxygen delivery and consumption in patients with sepsis. However, a recent randomized controlled trial of the effect of treatment aimed at maximizing oxygen delivery in patients with severe sepsis or septic shock failed to show a reduction in morbidity or mortality.[82] It is also important to maintain urine flow in an attempt to prevent renal failure. Urine output should ideally be kept higher than 30–40 ml · hr^{-1}, with fluid resuscitation and, if necessary, diuretic therapy. Corticosteroids have been advocated in the past as adjunctive therapy to the treatment of septic shock. However, more recent studies suggest that the use of high-dose corticosteroids provides no benefit in the treatment of severe sepsis and septic shock and is no longer recommended. Other areas of active investigation for the treatment of septic shock include high-dose naloxone, prostaglandin E$_1$ anticomplement, C5 antibodies, ibuprofen, indomethacin, and antiserum directed against cachectin.

NUTRITION

Adequate nutrition is essential to replace the nutrients used to meet the energy needs of tissues and to repair tissues being catabolized. In the critically ill or injured patient, nutrition is an essential part of treatment. For patients undergoing surgical procedures, malnutrition is well documented to be a risk factor, and perioperative nutritional support can reduce complications, mortality, morbidity, and length of hospital stay.

Nutritional Assessment

Assessment of nutrition is the first step in ensuring adequate support for the critically ill patient. Adequacy of nutrition can be assessed by anthropomorphic measurements, delayed cutaneous hypersensitivity to several antigens, and laboratory measurements reflecting severe protein and calorie malnutrition. Nitrogen balance is an important measure of nutritional status. The relationship between urea nitrogen excretion and metabolic rate is attributable to the obligatory oxidation of body cell mass that occurs with stress and starvation. Therefore, the extent of hypermetabolism can be predicted from a simple clinical determination of urea nitrogen collected in a timed urine specimen.

Estimation of Energy Requirement

The Harris–Benedict equation derived from indirect calorimetry measurements provides a reasonable estimate of basal caloric requirements (Table 56-6). Basal energy expenditure calculated in this manner correlates well with values obtained by contemporary techniques of continuous expired air analysis. The goal of nutritional support in nondepleted postoperative patients is to prevent excessive loss of lean tissue, whereas in nutritionally depleted patients it is restoration of lean tissue with concomitant restoration of fat reserves. Calculated basal energy needs should be increased by 30% with sepsis. Most of the current literature suggests the majority of critically ill patients require between 25 and 30 $kcal \cdot kg^{-1} \cdot day^{-1}$. However, since most patients respond to overfeeding with retention of water and formation of fat and not protein, a target of providing 80% of the caloric needs in critically ill patients has been described. With the use of growth hormone protein synthesis can be achieved by providing 80% of the necessary calories and utilizing the patient's endogenous fat stores for additional energy. The exceptions to this are burn and trauma patients who may require 40–45 $kcal \cdot kg^{-1} \cdot day^{-1}$ or patients who are calorie-depleted and need increased calories over a longer period of time to increase body fat mass.[83]

Enteral Versus Parenteral Nutrition

The gastrointestinal tract is the route of choice for nutritional supplementation whenever possible. Intragastric feeding requires adequate motility and emptying; a residual greater than 150 ml is a relative contraindication to gastric feeding due to the high risk of aspiration. Small bowel feeding should be initiated under these circumstances. The presence of bowel sounds and the passage of flatus or stool is not necessary to begin postpyloric enteral feeding. There are a variety of commercially available enteral feeding formulas. With near-normal proteolytic and lipolytic activity in the gastrointestinal tract, meal replacement formulas can be used. These formulas are polymeric mixtures containing proteins, fats, and carbohydrates in high–molecular-weight forms. The lactose content is generally low, and fat content represents ~30% of the calories. Elemental diets use amino acids as the nitrogen source and usually contain little fat and no lactose. These diets also have a low viscosity, which makes them particularly useful for infusion through needle catheter jejunostomy tubes. Feeding modules are concentrated sources of one nutrient that can yield a small-volume, high-caloric mixture when added to a formula diet. This is particularly useful for patients on fluid restriction. A continuous-drip infusion

of enteral feedings through a feeding tube is the preferred technique. The most common complication of enteral feedings is diarrhea. Other potential hazards include malpositioning of the feeding tube, hyperglycemia, and abnormalities in liver function tests.

Many disease-specific enteral formulas exist. "Immune-enhancing" preparations including arginine, glutamine, nucleotides, and/or omega-3 fatty acids have been used to reduce infection rates in the treatment of critically ill patients. Pulmonary formulas are designed to reduce CO_2 production and thereby ventilatory demand by providing nutrition high in fat content and low in carbohydrates. Enteral formulas used for patients with hepatic disease contain relatively large amounts of branched-chain amino acids and low quantities of aromatic amino acid. Renal formula used for enteral feeding are low in protein content and are usually calorically dense, containing up to 2 $kcal \cdot ml^{-1}$. They also are significantly lower in potassium, phosphorus, and magnesium content than the usual enteral formula. Other enteral formulations with growth hormone, selenium, vitamin C, vitamin E, and β-carotene are currently under investigation.[83]

When the enteral route is unavailable or provides inadequate intake for the depleted patient, parenteral nutrition support should be undertaken. Contraindications to enteral feeding include diffuse peritonitis, intestinal obstruction, intractable vomiting, paralytic ileus, and severe diarrhea. Certainly, critically ill patients who are hypercatabolic, nutritionally depleted, or have multiple organ system failure should have total parenteral nutrition administered through a central line.

It is important that adequate calories be supplied to critically ill patients, and distribution of calories provided as carbohydrates, fats, and protein is equally important. Historically, caloric requirements for total parenteral nutrition were given primarily as carbohydrates, which has a respiratory quotient of 1, resulting in a large increase in carbon dioxide production and oxygen consumption. Fat emulsions supply essential fatty acids in a concentrated source of calories. Because fat emulsions are oxidized with a respiratory quotient of 0.7, carbon dioxide production and ventilatory requirements are reduced.

Although nutritional support has been shown to improve wound healing, decrease morbidity and mortality, and assist in immunocompetence, many complications have been described. Technical complications relate primarily to insertion of the central venous catheter used for access. Other complications of hyperalimentation include sepsis, metabolic abnormalities, electrolyte disturbances, acid–base disorders, hepatic dysfunction, hypercalcemia and pancreatitis, metabolic bone disease, and fluid overload.

DISORDERS OF COAGULATION

There are three essentials for a normal clotting mechanism: vascular integrity, normal platelet function, and normal coagulation factors. The initial step in normal coagulation is compensatory reduction in intravascular pressure of the severed ends of blood vessels, followed by platelets covering the damaged surfaces. They accumulate at the site, ultimately forming a hemostatic plug. The coagulation cascade is then activated with the formation of fibrin. Two distinct pathways operate to form thrombin, which then converts fibrinogen into fibrin. The intrinsic pathway produces thrombin from factors present only in the plasma, whereas the extrinsic pathway uses extraplasma tissue factors as well as plasma factors. The final step in the normal coagulation scheme is removal of the fibrin and platelet clot by the fibrinolytic system. The end result of the activation of these pathways is the conversion of plasminogen into plasmin, which cleaves both fibrinogen and fibrin. There is an ongoing equilibrium between the activation of the coagulation system and the activation of the fibrinolytic system.

Table 56-6. HARRIS–BENEDICT EQUATIONS FOR ESTIMATION OF BASAL ENERGY EXPENDITURE (BEE)

Female	BEE = 655 + (9.6 × Wt) + (1.8 × Ht) − (4.7 × age)
Male	BEE = 66 + (13.7 × Wt) + (5 × Ht) − (6.8 × age)

Wt = weight in kilograms; Ht = height in centimeters; age = age in years.

Disorders in the coagulation system lead either to bleeding or to thrombosis. Clinical evaluation of disorders of coagulation is based on history, physical examination, and laboratory studies. A history of abnormal bleeding or evidence of bleeding on physical examination may assist in making a definitive diagnosis. Laboratory screening tests for hemostatic profile are essential. Such a profile of test should include a platelet count, bleeding time, prothrombin time, partial thromboplastin time, and review of the peripheral blood smear. The prothrombin time is a measure of the efficiency of thrombin formation by the extrinsic pathway. Abnormalities in the prothrombin time can be caused by absence or impairment of any coagulation factor in the intrinsic or extrinsic clotting system. The partial thromboplastin time is used to assess the efficiency of the intrinsic clotting system. Prolongation of the partial thromboplastin time generally represents deficiency or inhibition of Factors I, II, V, VIII, IX, X, XI, or XII. Qualitative abnormalities in platelets are manifested by prolongation of the bleeding time. If platelet function is intact, bleeding abnormalities usually do not occur unless the platelet count is below 100,000 mm^{-3}.

Disorders of hemostasis in critically ill patients are generally complex and represent multiple acquired deficiencies. Indeed, in most critically ill patients a bleeding disorder is only one manifestation of a complex series of failing organ system interactions. Common acquired deficiencies of hemostasis include disseminated intravascular coagulation, liver disease, vitamin K deficiency, anticoagulants, and massive blood transfusion.

Disseminated Intravascular Coagulation

Disseminated intravascular coagulation is a syndrome and not a primary disease state that reflects severe underlying pathology. The coagulation cascade is activated, resulting in the deposition of small thrombi and emboli throughout the microvasculature. This phase is then followed by secondary fibrinolysis. Repetition of this cycle leads to depletion of coagulation proteins and platelets and the antihemostatic effects of fibrin degradation products. Clinical manifestations of disseminated intravascular coagulation can result in thrombosis or hemorrhage. Most commonly, bleeding is manifest from multiple sites, including venipuncture sites, nasogastric tubes, urinary catheters, or endotracheal tubes. Laboratory manifestations of disseminated intravascular coagulation include thrombocytopenia, hypofibrinogenemia, and prolongation of the prothrombin time. Abnormalities of these indicators confirm disseminated intravascular coagulation. If all are not abnormal, additional studies including partial thromboplastin time, thrombin time, and fibrin degradation products should be ordered. In addition, review of the peripheral smear may reveal a microangiopathic hemolytic anemia from cell trapping and damage within fibrin thrombi.

The treatment of disseminated intravascular coagulation is the treatment of the underlying cause. Some authors have suggested the use of heparin as supportive therapy to reduce thrombin generation and prevent further consumption of clotting proteins until the underlying disease process could be controlled. Although it remains controversial, current recommendations do not support the use of routine heparin therapy, but rather the administration of fresh-frozen plasma and cryoprecipitate to replace depleted clotting factors and of platelet concentrates to correct thrombocytopenia.

An unusual cause of bleeding can result from defects in the fibrinolytic system. Patients with α_2 plasmin inhibitor deficiency, cirrhosis of the liver, or malignancy may develop diffuse bleeding from primary fibrinolysis rather than disseminated intravascular coagulation. Laboratory data reveal relatively normal prothrombin time and partial thromboplastin time with a normal platelet count and a disproportionately low fibrinogen level. Patients with clearly established primary fibrinolysis should receive ε-aminocaproic acid and not heparin. However, if concomitant disseminated intravascular coagulation is suspected, ε-amino-

caproic acid should be avoided because it can cause massive, often fatal thrombosis.

POISONING

Despite preventive health programs and increased public awareness, poisoning remains a common and serious medical problem. Accidental poisonings account for about 5000 deaths per year, with suicides by chemical agents causing an additional 6000 deaths per year. Poisoning is of particular importance in the pediatric population. As many as 2 million children in the United States accidentally swallow toxic material and about 1 ingestion out of 1000 is fatal. However, poisoning is by no means a problem limited to children. One half of all poisoned patients are over the age of 20 years.

The causative agents in poisoning vary with age. Children less than 5 years of age tend to ingest household products, whereas older patients are more likely to choose drugs. Aspirin accounts for 25% of all ingestions and is reported as the most common medicine involved in poisoning.

Prompt recognition and early intervention are essential to the successful treatment of poisoning. The diagnosis of poisoning can be difficult to make because the toxic effects of many agents are nonspecific. Certainly, a high index of suspicion must be maintained when confronted with a patient presenting with seizures, coma, psychosis, acute renal or hepatic insufficiency, or bone marrow depression. However, most poisoning syndromes manifest nonspecific symptoms. Similarly, it is uncommon for the physical examination to show characteristic toxic effects of chemical substances.

Identification of the toxic agent should be attempted in every case of poisoning. Gastric fluid, urine, and blood samples should be sent to the laboratory to screen for possible poisons. Modalities available to identify the offending agents include thin-layer chromatography, gas–liquid chromatography, high-performance liquid chromatography, and spectrometry. Patients poisoned with drugs frequently take more than one agent, which can lead to drug interactions and difficulty in interpreting test results.

Treatment

Treatment of poisoning should not await toxicologic determinations. Supportive care should begin immediately, including the essentials of basic cardiopulmonary support. In addition, symptomatic treatment of neurologic, renal, and hepatic dysfunction is mandatory. Attention should then be directed to minimizing absorption of the poison. For ingested poisons this means prevention of absorption from the gastrointestinal tract by lavage, emetics, and adsorbents such as charcoal. Cathartics generally have no role in treating poisoning.

Attempts should also be made to hasten elimination of absorbed poisons. Techniques available to increase elimination of poisons include diuresis, dialysis, chelation, hemoperfusion, exchange transfusion, and antibodies. Glomerular filtration and dialysis are generally effective only with substances found in plasma water and not protein-bound poisons. Hemoperfusion is most effective if used immediately after ingestion of the poison. Exchange transfusion may be especially useful in small children in whom hemoperfusion may be technically difficult. Antibodies can also be used as a high-affinity adsorbent in the patient's bloodstream to hasten elimination.

Common Poisons

Application of the principles used for the management of acute poisonings can be exemplified by several common agents.

Acetaminophen

This aspirin substitute is a frequent cause of poisoning. Clinical manifestations are generally nonspecific. Patients may initially present with pallor, lethargy, nausea, vomiting, and diaphoresis. Hepatotoxicity may become evident 1–2 days after ingestion and can be fatal. Liver damage results when the normal metabolic pathways become saturated so that an increased fraction of drug is inactivated by the cytochrome P-450 system, glutathione stores are depleted, and the reactive intermediates bind to liver macromolecules. Treatment of acetaminophen intoxication is initiated by induction of emesis or gastric lavage followed by administration of activated charcoal. Attention is next directed toward increasing sulfhydryl donors such as glutathione to allow greater binding of the toxic acetaminophen metabolites and therefore reduce liver damage. Early administration of N-acetyl-cystine can significantly reduce the incidence of acetaminophen-induced hepatotoxicity.

Alcohols

Although the low–molecular-weight alcohols (methanol, ethanol, ethylene glycol, and isopropanol) are relatively weak poisons, the result of their metabolism can be fatal. Ethanol depresses ventilation, decreases myocardial contractility, predisposes to hypothermia, and causes hypoglycemia, especially in children. Although there is no antidote to ethanol and no way to hasten its metabolism, it is readily removed by hemodialysis. However, usually critical care support with assisted ventilation of the lungs suffices in the treatment of ethanol intoxication. It is as important to treat associated illnesses in the patient with an ethanol overdose as it is to support the patient for the effects of the drug poisoning.

Methanol and ethylene glycol poisonings are common, yet frequently undetected. It is important to detect poisoning with these agents early because the metabolites are potent poisons and may lead to irreversible toxicity if they go unrecognized. Methanol is present in windshield washer antifreeze and solvents and in organic synthetic processes, whereas ethylene glycol is the major component in automotive antifreeze and is found in various organic solvents and cosmetics. Treatment of methanol and ethylene glycol poisoning is systemic alkalinization to decrease ocular and renal toxicity followed by hemodialysis to accelerate elimination of the alcohols and their metabolites.

Carbon Monoxide

Carbon monoxide (CO) is a colorless, odorless, tasteless, nonirritating gas produced by the incomplete combustion of carbonaceous material. It is the major cause of death in patients exposed to smoke inhalation from fires. CO is responsible for ~3500 accidental and suicidal deaths per year in the United States. It exerts its toxic effects through tissue hypoxia. The hemoglobin molecule has an affinity for CO that is 200 times greater than its affinity for oxygen. The combination of CO with hemoglobin forms carboxyhemoglobin, which is incapable of carrying oxygen. It also interferes with the release of oxygen from oxyhemoglobin, which decreases the amount of oxygen available to the tissues. In addition, because the rate of dissociation of CO from hemoglobin is extremely low, carboxyhemoglobin produces an acute decrease in blood oxygen content that is not readily reversed. The amount of carboxyhemoglobin present in blood depends on the concentration of CO in the inspired air and on the time of exposure.

Symptoms depend on the amount of carboxyhemoglobin present and the patient's activity level, tissue oxygen demands, and hemoglobin concentration. Exposure to low concentrations of CO causes irritability, altered visual and motor skills, headache, nausea, vomiting, and predisposition to angina pectoris. Severe poisoning may result in seizures, coma, respiratory failure, and death. The classic cherry red color of the skin and mucous membranes of patients with CO poisoning results from the bright red cast of carboxyhemoglobin. However, in patients with severe poisoning, cyanosis may predominate over the cherry red color.

Treatment of CO poisoning is to remove the offending agent and provide a high oxygen-enriched environment. The half-time of CO elimination can be shortened from 4 hr to 40 min by hyperventilation of the lungs with 100% oxygen. Ventilation may require mechanical support. Other treatment modalities include hyperbaric oxygen, transfusion therapy, and diuretics and steroids for the treatment of complicating cerebral edema.

LEGAL AND ETHICAL ISSUES
Brain Death

Brain death is defined as the irreversible cessation of all functions of the entire brain. This clinical definition is confirmed by autopsy studies revealing destruction of the entire brain in both the cerebral hemispheres and the brainstem. The primary insult leads to brain edema with increases in ICP. In the vast majority of brain death cases, the ICP exceeds systolic blood pressure within 12–24 hr. Currently, most states recognize brain death as a sufficient criterion for declaration of death. There have been many definitions offered of brain death. However, the broadly held consensus was reflected in *Defining Death,* a report issued in 1981 by the President's Commission for the Study of Ethical Problems in Medicine and Biomedical and Behavioral Research.[84] In response to a congressional mandate, the commission recommended a statute, the Uniform Determination of Death Act (UDDA), which has become the most widely accepted legal formulation of the standards for determining human death. In addition, it also provided an updated formulation of the medical criteria for applying the standard.[85] Representatives of the American Bar Association, American Medical Association, National Conference of Commissioners on Uniform State Laws, and the Academy of the American Encephalographers Society agreed on the UDDA definition as follows: An individual who has sustained either (1) irreversible cessation of circulatory and respiratory functions, or (2) irreversible cessation of all functions or the entire brain, including the brainstem, is dead. A determination of death must be made in accordance with accepted medical standards. These guidelines are now widely accepted by physicians and hospitals for clinical decision-making. This formulation of brain death is based on a clinical diagnosis with certain preconditions and confirmatory tests.[86,87]

With advances in technology and medical capability, even seemingly clear-cut definitions, such as death, become complex and difficult to translate into law and policy. Indeed, for many years courts were slow to modify the common law definition of death, *i.e.,* cessation of all vital functions including respiration and circulation, to accept the determination of death based on irreversible cessation of all functions of the brain. The most common and familiar criteria for the diagnosis of whole brain death are the Harvard criteria published in 1968[88] by an Ad Hoc Committee of the Harvard Medical School. Tests generally used to determine brain death rely on response to stimuli, the presence of reflexes and spontaneous movements, and the electroencephalogram. There must be no evidence of hypothermia or drugs that depress brain function. The findings must persist over 24 hr. These Harvard criteria are now widely accepted by the medical profession and can be recognized legally as defining death in many states.

Indeed, organ transplantation was a major impetus for focusing public attention on the need to update standards for determining death, even though only ~15% of patients who are declared brain dead become organ donors. A special standard only for organ donors would fail to address the overwhelming majority of comatose ventilator-supported cases. This could create a separate standard of death for donors that could lead to abuse and confusion. Thus, along with the clinical diagnosis, confirmatory tests are generally required and can be dependent on normal function or intracranial blood flow.

Do Not Resuscitate (DNR) Orders

Few areas in clinical medicine generate as much controversy and debate as does the decision to withdraw or withhold treatment of critically ill patients.[89,90] Certainly, the opinion in the Joseph Saikewicz case issued by the Massachusetts Supreme Judicial Court in November 1977 raised much controversy.[91] In this case a guardian was appointed for a profoundly retarded, institutionalized 67-year-old man with acute myeloblastic monocytic leukemia and the court was asked to decide if treatment should be undertaken. It was understood that treatment would be painful and carry potential hazards with very little hope for recovery. The County Probate Court recommended withholding therapy and the Supreme Court affirmed this order. However, the Supreme Court further stated that the decision to withhold or withdraw the life-support measures in a terminally ill, incompetent patient was not within the jurisdiction of any hospital committee or panel, but rather the ultimate decision-making responsibility of the courts. Justice Paul J. Liacos, the author of the Saikewicz decision, offered a different approach to DNR orders when he suggested that they present a case for physician discretion, and that the principles of Saikewicz are inapplicable.[92]

In a subsequent court opinion, in the matter of Dinnerstein, the legality of DNR orders was addressed. In this case, the patient was a 67-year-old woman with Alzheimer's disease, a massive stroke, and left hemiparesis. She was left in a persistent vegetative state, immobile, speechless, unable to swallow without choking, and barely able to cough. The patient's physician recommended no resuscitation in the event of cardiopulmonary arrest and the patient's family concurred. Because of the legal uncertainty surrounding "no code" orders, the physician, hospital, and family asked the court to rule about the legality of the order. The Massachusetts Appeals Court held that a DNR order in these circumstances was lawful and advance judicial approval was not necessary to write such orders. Resuscitation was not "a treatment offering hope of restoration to normal integrated functioning cognitive existence. Attempts to apply resuscitation if successful will do nothing to cure or relieve the illness, which will have brought the patient to the threshold of death."[93] A second Massachusetts case upholding DNR orders involved a 5-month-old infant abandoned at birth who suffered from profound congenital cardiopulmonary disease with little hope of survival. The patient's physician recommended that a DNR order be entered on the patient's medical chart, but the guardian, the Department of Social Services, refused to consent. In this case the Massachusetts Supreme Judicial Court found that a full resuscitation effort would not serve the child's interest and that the child would reject full resuscitation if the child were competent to decide.[94]

The right to reject resuscitative or any lifesaving medical treatment was best outlined in the Karen Ann Quinlan case. The court stated that the constitutional right to privacy encompasses the freedom of the terminally ill but competent individual to decline medical treatment when such treatment will only prolong suffering needlessly and denigrate the quality of life.

In a recent report the Council on Ethical and Judicial Affairs of the American Medical Association outlined the guidelines for the appropriate use of DNR orders.[95] In this report the Council recommended that (1) efforts should be made to resuscitate patients who suffer cardiac or respiratory arrest except when circumstances indicate that administration of cardiopulmonary resuscitation would be futile or not in accord with the desires or best interests of the patient; (2) if a patient is incapable of rendering the decision regarding the use of cardiopulmonary resuscitation, a decision may be made by a surrogate decision maker based on the previously expressed preferences of the patient, or if such preferences are unknown, in accordance with the patient's best interest.

Withholding or withdrawing life-sustaining therapies is becoming more widely accepted. The American Hospital Association has estimated that 70% of patients who die in hospitals have some form of life-sustaining treatment terminated before death. However, perceptions by physicians regarding the legal liability have been slow to change. Indeed, physicians tend to believe that withholding life support is more acceptable than withdrawing it. Indeed, in a recent survey,[96] the majority of health care workers indicated that there is an ethical difference between withdrawing and withholding treatment, despite the unanimity in both law and philosophy that there is no intrinsic moral or legal distinction between the two. However, ICU physicians consider withholding and withdrawal ethically similar and appropriate processes, regard concerns about cost or distributive justice as unimportant in decision making, and consider patient and surrogate wishes paramount in decision making, but view these wishes in the context of their own assessment of prognosis.[97] Finally, despite a contracting health care budget that has sensitized society to the issues of resource allocation, the demand for the health care dollar has continued to expand, creating an inherent conflict between economics and bioethics.[98] This represents but one of the many complex and difficult issues that must be confronted in the care of the critically ill patient.

REFERENCES

1. American College of Critical Care Medicine of the Society of Critical Care Medicine: Guidelines for advanced training for physicians in critical care. Crit Care Med 25(9):1601, 1997
2. LeGall JR, Loirat P, Alperovitch A et al: A simplified acute physiology score for ICU patients. Crit Care Med 12:975, 1984
3. Knaus WA, Draper EA, Wagner DP et al: APACHE II: A severity of disease classification system. Crit Care Med 13:818, 1985
4. Cerra FB, Negro F, Abrams J: APACHE II score does not predict multiple organ failure or mortality in postoperative surgical patients. Arch Surg 125:519, 1990
5. Knaus WA, Wagner DP, Draper EA et al: The APACHE-III prognostic system: Risk prediction of hospital mortality for critically ill hospitalized adults. Chest 100:16, 1991
6. Pollack MM, Yeh TS, Ruttiman VE et al: Development of the physiologic stability index (PSI) for use in critically ill infants and children. Pediatr Res 16:187A, 1982
7. Lemeshow S, Teres D, Pastides H et al: A method for predicting survival and mortality of ICU patients using objectively derived weights. Crit Care Med 13:519, 1985
8. Shabot MM, Leyerle BJ, LoBue M: Automatic extraction of intensity-intervention scores from a computerized surgical intensive care unit flowsheet. Am J Surg 154:72, 1987
9. McFee AS, Gilbert J: The outcome index: A method of quality assurance in the special care area. Presented at the Ninety-Sixth Annual Meeting of the Western Surgical Association. Coronado, California, November 11–13, 1988
10. Champion HR, Copes WS, Sacco WJ et al: A new characterization of injury severity. J Trauma 30:539, 1990
11. Mayball CG, Archer NH, Lamb VA et al: Ventriculostomy-related infections: A prospective epidemiologic study. N Engl J Med 310:553, 1984
12. Rockoff M, Marshall L, Shapiro H: High dose barbiturate therapy in humans: A clinical review of 60 patients. Ann Neurol 6:194, 1979
13. Woodcock J, Ropper AH, Kennedy SK: High dose barbiturates in non-traumatic brain swelling: ICP reduction and effect on outcome. Stroke 13:785, 1982
14. Marion DW, Penrod LE et al: Treatment of traumatic brain injury with moderate hypothermia. N Eng J Med 336:540, 1997
15. Bernard SA, Jones BM et al: Clinical trial of induced hypothermia in comatose survivors of out-of-hospital cardiac arrest. Ann Emerg Med 30:146, 1997
16. Muir KW, Lees KR: Clinical experience with excitatory amino acid antagonist drugs. Stroke 26:506, 1995
17. Kaste M, Fogelholm R et al: A randomized, double-blind, placebo-controlled trial of nimodipine in acute ischemic hemispheric stroke. Stroke 25:1348, 1994

18. Marshall LF, Mass A *et al:* A multicenter trial on the efficacy of using tirilizad mesylate in case of head injury. J Neursurg 89:519, 1998

19. Imaizumi S, Woolworth V *et al:* Liposome-entrapped superoxide dismutase reduces cerebral infarction in cerebral ischemia in rats. Stroke 11:1312, 1990

20. Safar P: Cerebral resuscitation after cardiac arrest: Research initiatives and future directions. Ann Emerg Med 22:324, 1993

21. Schaer GL, Fink MP, Parillo JE: Norepinephrine alone versus norepinephrine plus low-dose dopamine: Enhanced renal blood flow with combination pressor therapy. Crit Care Med 13:492, 1985

22. Richard C, Ricome JL, Rimailho A *et al:* Combined hemodynamic effects of dopamine and dobutamine in cardiogenic shock. Circulation 67:620, 1983

23. Alousi AA, Canter JM, Montenaro MJ *et al:* Cardiotonic activity of milrinone, a new and potent cardiac bipyridine, on the normal and failing heart of experimental animals. J Cardiovasc Pharmacol 5:792, 1983

24. Smith NA, Kates RE, Lebsack C *et al:* Clinical pharmacology of intravenous enoximone: Pharmacodynamics and pharmacokinetics in patients with heart failure. Am Heart J 122:755, 1991

25. Weber KT, Janicki JS, Jain MC: Piroximone (MDL 19, 205) in the treatment of unstable and stable chronic cardiac failure. Am Heart J 114:807, 1987

26. Lubbe WF, Podzuweit T, Opie LH: Potential arrhythmogenic role of cAMP and cytosolic calcium overflow. J Am Coll Cardiol 19:1622, 1992

27. Moulopoulus SD, Topaz S, Kolff WJ: Diastolic balloon pumping with cardon dioxide in the aorta: A mechanical assistance to the failing circulation. Am Heart J 63:669, 1962

28. Schroeder JS, Hunt S: Cardiac transplantation. JAMA 258:3142, 1987

29. Cairns JA, Kennedy JW, Fuster V: Coronary thrombolysis. Chest 114(suppl):634S, 1998

30. International Study Group: In-hospital mortality and clinical course of 20,891 patients with suspected acute myocardial infarction randomized between altepase and streptokinase with or without heparin. Lancet 336:71, 1990

31. ISIS-3 Collaborative Group: ISIS-3: A randomized comparison of streptokinase vs tissue plasminogen activator vs anistreplase and of aspirin plus heparin vs aspirin alone among 41,299 cases of suspected acute myocardial infarction. Lancet 339:753, 1992

32. PRIMI Trial Study Group: Randomized double-blind trial of recombinant pro-urokinase against streptokinase in acute myocardial infarction. Lancet 1:863, 1989

33. The GUSTO Investigators: An international randomized study comparing four thrombolytic strategies for acute myocardial infarction. N Engl J Med 329:673, 1993

34. Cannon CP, McCabe CH, Diver DJ *et al:* Comparison of front-loaded recombinant tissue-type plasminogen activator anistreplase and combination thrombolytic therapy for acute myocardial infarction: Results of the Thrombolysis in Myocardial Infarction (TIMI) 4 trial. J Am Coll Cardiol 24:1602, 1994

35. Global Use of Strategies to Open Occluded Coronary Arteries (GUSTO III) Investigators: A comparison of reteplase with altepase for acute myocardial infarction. N Engl J Med 337:1118, 1997

36. Yui Y, Kawai T, Hosoda S *et al:* Clinical efficacy of SUN9216 (modified tissue plasminogen activator) as compared to altepase in patients with acute myocardial infarction: A multicentre randomized double-blind comparative study. Jpn Pharmacol Ther 25:269, 1997

37. Vanderschueren S, Barrios L, Kerdsinchai P *et al:* A randomized trial of recombinant staphylokinase versus altepase for coronary artery patency in acute myocardial infarction. Circulation 92:2044, 1995

38. Dalen JE, Hirsh J *et al:* American College of Chest Physicians Fifth ACCP Consensus Conference on Antithrombotic Therapy (1998): Summary Recommendations. Chest 114(suppl):439S, 1998

39. Bernard GR, Luce JM, Sprung CL *et al:* High dose corticosteroids in patients with the adult respiratory distress syndrome. N Engl J Med 317:1565, 1987

40. Mathru M: The therapeutic application of positive end-expiratory pressure. Anesth Clin North Am 5:789, 1987

41. Gallagher TJ, Civetta JM, Kirby RR: Terminology update: Optimal PEEP. Crit Care Med 6:323, 1978

42. Amato MBP, Barbas CSV, Medeiros DM *et al:* Effects of a protective-ventilation strategy on mortality in the acute respiratory distress syndrome. N Engl J Med 336:347, 1998

43. Bigatello LM, Hurford WE, Kacmarek RM *et al:* Prolonged inhalation of low concentrations of nitric oxide in patients with severe adult respiratory distress syndrome. Anesthesiology 80:761, 1994

44. Tokioka H, Saito S, Kosaka F: Effects of pressure support ventilation on breathing patterns and respiratory work. Intensive Care Med 15:491, 1989

45. Soo Hoo GW, Santiago S, Williams AJ: Nasal mechanical ventilation for hypercapneic respiratory failure in COPD: Determinants of success (Abstr.) Am Rev Respir Dis 143:A79, 1991

46. Bott J, Carroll MP, Conway JH *et al:* Randomised controlled trial of nasal ventilation in acute ventilatory failure due to chronic obstructive airway disease. Lancet 341:1555, 1993

47. Bach JR, Alba AS: Management of chronic alveolar hypoventilation by nasal ventilation. Chest 97:52, 1990

48. Strumpf DA, Millman RP, Hill NS: The management of chronic hypoventilation. Chest 98:474, 1990

49. Oermann CM, Sockrider MM, Konstan MW: The use of anti-inflammatory medications in cystic fibrosis. Chest 115:1053, 1999

50. Eigen H, Rosenstein BJ: A multicenter study of alternate day prednisone in patients with cystic fibrosis. J Pediatr 126:515, 1995

51. Konstan MW, Byard PJ, Hoppel CL *et al:* Effect of high-dose ibuprofen in patients with cystic fibrosis. N Engl J Med 332:848, 1995

52. Van Haren EHJ, Lammers J-WJ, Festen J *et al:* The effects of the inhaled corticosteroid budesonide on lung function and bronchial hyperresponsiveness in adult patients with cystic fibrosis. Respir Med 89:209, 1995

53. Aronoff SC, Quinn FJ Jr, Carpenter LS *et al:* Effects of pentoxifylline on sputum neutrophil elastase and pulmonary function in patients with cystic fibrosis: Preliminary observations. J Pediatr 125:992, 1994

54. Ghio AJ, Marshall BC, Diaz JL *et al:* Tyloxapol inhibits NF-kB and cytokine release, scavenges HOCL, and reduces viscosity of cystic fibrosis sputum. Am J Respir Crit Care Med 154:783, 1996

55. Weinstein RA: Epidemiology and control of nosocomial infections in adult intensive care units. AM J Med 91(suppl 3B):179S, 1991

56. Stoutenbeek CP, van Saene HKF, Miranda DR *et al:* The effect of selective decontamination of the digestive tract on colonization and infection rate in multiple trauma patients. Intensive Care Med 10:184, 1984

57. Ferrer M, Torres A, Gonzales J *et al:* Utility of selective decontamination in mechanically ventilated patients. Ann Intern Med 120:389, 1994

58. Gastinne H, Wolff M, Delatour F *et al:* A controlled trial in intensive care units of selective decontamination of the digestive tract with nonabsorbable antibiotics. N Engl J Med 326:594, 1992

59. Cockerill FR, Muller SR, Anhalt JP *et al:* Prevention of infection in critically ill patients by selective decontamination of the digestive tract. Ann Intern Med 117:545, 1992

60. Korinek AM, Laisne MJ, Nicolas MH *et al:* Selective decontamination of the digestive tract in neurosurgical intensive care patients: A double-blind, randomized, placebo-controlled study. Crit Care Med 21:1466, 1993

61. Pearson ML: Guideline for prevention of intravascular device-related infections. Part I. Intravascular device-related infections: An overview. The Hospital Infection Control Practices Advisory Committee. Am J Infect Control. 24(4):262, 1996

62. Rangel-Frausto MS, Pittet D, Costigan M *et al:* The natural history of the systemic inflammatory response syndrome (SIRS): A prospective study. JAMA 273:117, 1995

63. Stegmayr BG: Plasmapheresis in severe sepsis or septic shock. Blood Purif 14:94, 1996

64. Reeves JH, Butt WW *et al:* Continuous plasmafiltration in sepsis syndrome. Crit Care Med 27(10):2096, 1999

65. Fisher CJ Jr, Opal SM, Dhainaut J-F *et al:* Influence of an anti-tumor necrosis factor monoclonal antibody on cytokine levels in patients with sepsis. Crit Care Med 21:318, 1993

66. Ziegler EJ, Fisher CJ Jr, Sprung CL *et al:* Treatment of Gram-negative bacteremia in septic shock with HA-1A human monoclonal antibody against endotoxin: A randomized, double-blind, placebo-controlled trial. The HA-1A Sepsis Study Group. N Engl J Med 324:429, 1991

67. Greenman RL, Schein RMH, Martin MA *et al:* A controlled clinical trial of E5 murine monoclonal Igm antibody to endotoxin in the treatment of Gram-negative sepsis. JAMA 266:1097, 1991

68. Hotchkiss RS, Swanson PE *et al:* Apoptotic cell death in patients with sepsis, shock, and multiple organ dysfunction Crit Care Med 27(7):1230, 1999

69. Baumgartner JD: Immunotherapy with antibodies to core lipopolysaccharide: A critical appraisal. Infect Dis Clin North Am 5:915, 1991

70. Intravenous Immunoglobulin Collaborative Study Group: Prophy-

lactic intravenous administration of standard immune globulin as compared with core-lipopolysaccharide immune globulin in patients at high risk of postsurgical infection. N Engl J Med 327:234, 1992

71. J5 Study Group: Treatment of severe infectious purpura in children with human plasma from donors immunized with *Escherichia coli* J5: A prospective double-blind study. J Infect Dis 165:695, 1992

72. Luce JM: Introduction of new technology into critical care practice: A history of HA-1A human monoclonal antibody against endotoxin. Crit Care Med 21:1233, 1993

73. Fischer E, Marano MA, Van Zee KJ *et al:* Interleukin-1 receptor blockade improves survival and hemodynamic performance in *Escherichia coli* septic shock, but fails to alter host responses to sublethal endotoxemia. J Clin Invest 89:1551, 1992

74. Dinarello CA, Thompson RC: Blocking IL-1: Interleukin 1 receptor antagonist *in vivo* and *in vitro.* Immunol Today 12:404, 1991

75. Dinarello CA: The proinflammatory cytokines interleukin-1 and tumor necrosis factor and treatment of septic shock syndrome. J Infect Dis 163:1177, 1991

76. Moncada S, Palmer RM, Higgs EA: Nitric oxide: Physiology, pathophysiology, and pharmacology. Pharmacol Rev 43:109, 1991

77. Radomski MW, Palmer RM, Moncada S: An L-arginine/nitric oxide pathway present in human platelets regulates aggregation. Proc Natl Acad Sci USA 87:5193, 1990

78. Kubes P, Suzuki M, Granger DN: Nitric oxide: An endogenous modulator of leukocyte adhesion. Proc Natl Acad Sci USA 88:4651, 1991

79. Kilbourn RG, Gross SS, Jubran A *et al:* NG-methyl-L-arginine inhibits tumor necrosis factor-induced hypotension: Implications for the involvement of nitric oxide. Proc Natl Acad Sci USA 87:3629, 1990

80. Kilbourn RGD, Jubran A, Gross SS *et al:* Reversal of endotoxin-mediated shock by NG-methyl-L-arginine, an inhibitor of nitric oxide synthesis. Biochem Biophys Res Commun 172:1132, 1990

81. Finkel MS, Oddis CV, Jacob TD *et al:* Negative inotropic effects of cytokines on the heart mediated by nitric oxide. Science 257:387, 1992

82. Alia I, Esteban A, Gordo F *et al:* A randomized and controlled trial of the effect of treatment aimed at maximizing oxygen delivery in patients with severe sepsis or septic shock. Chest 115:453, 1999

83. Chan S, McCowen KC, Blackburn GL: Nutrition management in the ICU. Chest 115:145S, 1999

84. President's Commission for the Study of Ethical Problems in Medicine and Biomedical and Behavioral Research: Defining Death. Washington DC, U.S. Government Printing Office, 1981

85. President's Commission for the Study of Ethical Problems in Medicine and Biomedical and Behavioral Research: Guidelines for the determination of death. JAMA 246:2184, 1981

86. Black PM: Brain death in the intensive care unit. J Intensive Care Med 2:177, 1987

87. Powner DJ: The diagnosis of brain death in the adult patient. J Intensive Care Med 2:181, 1987

88. Ad Hoc Committee of Harvard Medical School: A definition of irreversible coma. JAMA 205:337, 1968

89. Ruark JE, Raffin TA: Initiating and withdrawing life support: Principles and practice in adult medicine. N Engl J Med 318:25, 1988

90. American Thoracic Society Bioethics Task Force: Withholding and withdrawing life-sustaining treatment. Ann Intern Med 115:479, 1991

91. Curran WJ: The Saikewicz decision. N Engl J Med 298:499, 1978

92. Liacos PJ: Dilemma of dying. In Doudera AE, Peters JD (eds): Legal and Ethical Aspects of Treating Critically and Terminally Ill Patients, p 149. Ann Arbor, Michigan, AUPHA Press, 1982

93. In the Matter of Shirley Dinnerstein, 380 N.E. 2d 134 (Mass. App. Ct. 1978)

94. Custody of a Minor, 385 Mass. 697, 434 N.E. 2d 601 (1982)

95. Council on Ethical and Judicial Affairs, American Medical Association: Guidelines for the appropriate use of do-not-resuscitate orders. JAMA 265:4, 1991

96. Solomon MZ, O'Donnell L, Jennings B *et al:* Decisions near the end of life: Professional views on life-sustaining treatments. Am J Public Health 83:14, 1993

97. Luce JM: Withholding and withdrawal of life support: Ethical, legal, and clinical aspects New Horiz 5:30, 1997

98. Weiss SC: Economics, ethics, and end-of-life care. JAMA 282:2076, 1999

Clinical Anesthesia (4/e), edited by
Paul G. Barash, Bruce F. Cullen, and
Robert K. Stoelting. Lippincott Williams &
Wilkins, Philadelphia, © 2001.

CHAPTER 57

CARDIOPULMONARY RESUSCITATION

CHARLES W. OTTO

Treatment of cardiac and respiratory arrest is an integral part of anesthesia practice. The American Board of Anesthesiology indicates in its *Booklet of Information* that the "clinical management and teaching of cardiac and pulmonary resuscitation" are some of the activities that define the specialty of anesthesiology. The cardiopulmonary physiology and pharmacology that form the basis of anesthesia practice are applicable to treating the victim of cardiac arrest. However, there is specialized knowledge relating to blood flow, ventilation, and pharmacology under the conditions of a cardiac arrest that must be understood to maintain leadership of the modern cardiopulmonary resuscitation (CPR) team. This chapter concentrates on those aspects of CPR that are different from the more common circumstances requiring cardiovascular support, *e.g.*, shock and dysrhythmias.

HISTORY

Anesthesiologists have contributed many of the elements of modern CPR and continue to be active investigators and teachers in the field. Discoveries leading to current CPR practice have a long history recorded in many famous works.[1,2] The earliest reference may be the Bible story of Elisha breathing life back into the son of a Shunammite woman (II Kings 4:34). In 1543, Andreas Vesalius described tracheotomy and artificial ventilation.[3] William Harvey's manual manipulation of the heart is well known. Early teaching of resuscitation was organized by the Society for the Recovery of Persons Apparently Drowned, founded in London in 1774. The combined techniques of modern CPR developed primarily from the fortuitous assemblage of innovative clinicians and researchers in Baltimore in the 1950s and early 1960s. Building on the long history of contributions from around the world, these investigators laid the framework for current CPR practice. In the late 1950s, mouth-to-mouth ventilation was established as the only effective means of artificial ventilation.[4-7] The internal defibrillator was developed in 1933[8] but not applied successfully until 1947.[9] It was another decade before general use was made possible by the development of external cross-chest defibrillation.[10,11] Despite these advances, widespread resuscitation from cardiac arrest was not possible until Kouwenhoven *et al* described success with closed-chest cardiac massage in a series of patients.[12] The final major component of modern CPR was added in 1963 when Redding and Pearson described the improved success obtained by administering epinephrine or other vasopressor drugs.[13]

SCOPE OF THE PROBLEM

Cardiovascular disease remains the most common cause of death in the industrialized world. Although cardiovascular mortality has been declining in the United States since the mid-1960s, nearly 50% of all deaths are due to cardiovascular causes.[14] Of the 1 million annual cardiovascular deaths, approximately half are related to coronary artery disease and the majority of these are sudden deaths. Thus, CPR teaching and research tend to focus on myocardial ischemia as the primary cause of cardiac arrest. However, anesthesiologists are more likely than other practitioners to deal with etiologies other than myocardial infarction. Cardiopulmonary resuscitation is symptomatic therapy, aimed at sustaining vital organ function until natural cardiac function is restored. The details of effective resuscitation technique are important. However, search for a remediable cause of the arrest must not be lost in excessive attention to mechanics.

Brain adenosine triphosphate (ATP) is depleted after 4–6 min of no blood flow. It returns nearly to normal within 6 min of starting effective CPR. Studies in animals suggest that good neurologic outcome may be possible from 10–15-min periods of normothermic cardiac arrest if good circulation is promptly restored.[15,16] In clinical practice, the severity of the underlying cardiac disease is the major determining factor in the success or failure of resuscitation attempts. Of those factors under control of the rescuers, poor outcomes are associated with long arrest times before CPR is begun, prolonged ventricular fibrillation without definitive therapy, and inadequate coronary and cerebral perfusion during cardiac massage. Survival from out-of-hospital cardiac arrest is improved when CPR is begun by bystanders.[17] Optimum outcome from ventricular fibrillation is obtained only if ventilation and closed-chest compression are begun within 4 min of arrest and defibrillation applied within 8 min.[18,19] The importance of early defibrillation has been known for some time and it is now being emphasized in CPR practice.[20,21] If the diagnosis of ventricular fibrillation can be established and the equipment is available, defibrillation should take precedence over all other resuscitative measures.

With an effective rapid response emergency medical system, initial resuscitation rates of 40% and survival to hospital discharge of 10–15% are reported after out-of-hospital arrests.[19,21] A better outcome might be expected for in-hospital arrests because of rapid response times and expert personnel. However, overall rates for initial resuscitation and survival to discharge from in-hospital arrest are about 40% and 10%, respectively.[22] Intercurrent illnesses of hospitalized patients reduce the likelihood of survival and the arrest victim is more likely to be elderly, a factor that may reduce survival. Within the hospital, the operating room is the location where CPR has the highest rate of success. Cardiac arrest occurs approximately 7 times for every 10,000 anesthetics.[23] The cause for the arrest is anesthesia-related, ~4.5 times for every 10,000 anesthetics, but mortality from these arrests is only 0.4 per 10,000 anesthetics. Thus, resuscitation is successful ~90% of the time in anesthesia-related cardiac arrests. Outside the operating suite, the best initial resuscitation rates are found in the intensive care unit (ICU), whereas the best survival rates are for patients arresting in the emergency department.[22]

ORGANIZING A SOLUTION

Over the past 30 years, CPR has become widely practiced, facilitated by the efforts of the American Heart Association, the International Red Cross, the European Resuscitation Council, and many other organizations around the world. Specific guidelines for the teaching and practice of CPR are published periodically.[24] These guidelines were developed because numerous individuals with varying levels of expertise (lay public, emergency personnel, nurses, and physicians) need to be trained if CPR is to be effective in saving lives. For training to be effective, a standardized approach is needed (Table 57-1). The organizations also develop and sponsor courses at different levels of

Table 57-1. STANDARD APPROACH TO THE UNCONSCIOUS PATIENT

1. Determine unresponsiveness
2. Activate emergency medical services or team
3. Position victim supine on firm surface
4. Open airway
5. Determine absence of breathing
6. Perform ventilation: 2 breaths
7. Determine absence of pulse
8. Initiate chest compressions
9. Alternate 15 compressions with 2 breaths

complexity for teaching CPR. The two levels of CPR care are referred to as basic life support (BLS) for ventilation and chest compressions without additional equipment and advanced cardiac life support (ACLS) for using all modalities available for resuscitation. Medical personnel need to be well versed in both levels of care. BLS is also appropriate for lay people.

The American Heart Association periodically coordinates a National Conference on CPR and Emergency Cardiac Care during which worldwide experts evaluate the scientific data regarding CPR. The recommendations resulting from the National Conference comprise the most complete compilation of guidelines for CPR practice.[24] International contributions to the most recent Conferences in 1992 and 2000 produce similar CPR practices worldwide. However, no common infrastructure exists that allows adoption of true international guidelines for CPR. The algorithms for approaching the patient with cardiac arrest published in the guidelines are familiar to all physicians and are reproduced throughout this chapter. However, the major purpose of this chapter is not to reiterate the standard approach but to provide the scientific background, where it exists, that led to adoption of the standard approach, to point out areas of continuing controversy, and to suggest areas of possible future development.

ETHICAL ISSUES: DO NOT RESUSCITATE ORDERS IN THE OPERATING ROOM

Institution of cardiopulmonary resuscitation is standard medical care when an individual is found apparently dead. In recent years, terminally ill patients have become increasingly concerned about inappropriate application of life-sustaining procedures, including CPR. Through living wills and other instruments, patients have begun placing limitations on medical treatment, including DNR—do not attempt resuscitation—orders. Such requests are generally accepted, even welcomed, by health care workers. However, the operating room is one area of the hospital where DNR orders continue to cause ethical conflicts between medical personnel and patients.[25,26] There are ethically sound arguments on both sides of the issue as to whether DNR orders should be upheld in the operating room.

The patient's right to limit medical treatment, including refusing CPR, is firmly established in modern medical practice based on the ethical principle of respect for patient autonomy. A terminally ill patient can reject heroic measures such as resuscitation and still choose palliative therapy. If a surgical intervention will ameliorate symptoms or cure a problem that improves quality of life, there is no reason to withhold this treatment. During surgery, the patient reasonably may desire to maintain the DNR status to avoid heroic measures that serve only to prolong death. Operative intervention increases the risk of cardiac arrest, and the patient may not want the burden of surviving in a worse condition than previously. Thus, the time that the DNR order provides the greatest protection against unwanted intervention is during surgery. The possibility of death under anesthesia may be viewed as especially peaceful.

Despite these rather strong arguments for treating a DNR status in the operating room the same way it is treated elsewhere in the hospital, most operating room personnel are at least a little uneasy caring for these patients. Many surgeons require that DNR orders be suspended during the perioperative period or assume that consent to surgery includes such suspension. There are multiple reasons for the reluctance to accept DNR status during surgery and anesthesia. Approximately 75% of cardiac arrests in the operating room are related to a surgical or anesthetic complication and resuscitative attempts are highly successful.[23] Ethically, surgeons and anesthesiologists feel responsible for what happens to patients in the operating room: *primum non nocere* (first, do no harm). Although the physicians are highly diligent in monitoring and managing changes in the patient's status, complications and arrests do occur. Honoring a DNR under these circumstances is frequently viewed as failure to treat a reversible process, and hence tantamount to killing. This is an ethically sound view if the cause of arrest is readily identifiable and easily reversible and treatment is likely to allow the patient to fulfill the objectives of coming to surgery.[25]

Institutionally, these ethical conflicts should be addressed by adoption of clear policies by hospitals.[27] For the individual patient, conflicts can be resolved by communication among the patient, family, and caregivers. A mutual decision can often be reached to suspend or severely limit a DNR order in the perioperative period if the patient understands the special circumstances of perioperative arrest, that interventions are brief and usually successful, and that the physicians support the patient's goals in coming to surgery and values in desiring not to prolong death. Many interventions commonly used in the operating room (mechanical ventilation, vasopressors, antidysrhythmics, blood products) may be considered forms of resuscitation in other situations. The only modalities that are not routine anesthetic care are cardiac massage and defibrillation. Therefore, the specific interventions included in a DNR status must be clarified with specific allowance made for methods necessary to perform anesthesia and surgery.

BASIC LIFE SUPPORT

Basic life support consists of those elements of resuscitation that can be performed without additional equipment: basic airway management, rescue breathing, and manual chest compressions. Common practice is to approach a victim with the airway–breathing–circulation (ABC) sequence, although the circulation–airway–breathing (CAB) sequence has been used in some countries with comparable results. Table 57-1 itemizes the standard approach to an unconscious victim.

Airway Management

The problem of airway obstruction by the tongue in the unconscious patient is familiar to the anesthesiologist. The techniques used for airway maintenance during anesthesia are applicable to the cardiac arrest victim. The primary method recommended to the public is the same "head tilt–chin lift" method commonly employed in the operating room.[28] The head is extended by pressure applied to the brow while the mandible is pulled forward by pressure on the front of the jaw, lifting the tongue away from the posterior pharynx. The "jaw thrust" maneuver (applying pressure behind the rami of the mandible) is an effective alternative. Properly inserted oropharyngeal or nasopharyngeal airways can be useful before intubation, recognizing the danger of inducing vomiting or laryngospasm in the semiconscious victim. Tracheal intubation provides the best airway control, preventing aspiration and allowing the most effective ventilation. Intubation is indicated in any resuscitation lasting more than a few minutes, but it should not be performed until adequate ventilation (preferably with supplemental oxygen) and chest compressions have been established. A number of alternative airways designed for blind placement by individuals who are not skilled laryngoscopists have been described.[24] These include the laryngotracheal mask, pharyngotracheal lumen airway, esophageal obturator airway, esophageal gastric tube airway, and combination esophageal tracheal tube. None ensures airway control as well as an endotracheal tube. When other methods of establishing an airway are unsuccessful, translaryngeal ventilation or tracheotomy by cricothyroid puncture may be necessary.

Foreign Body Airway Obstruction

It is estimated that foreign body airway obstruction accounts for 1% of all sudden deaths (~3900 deaths in the United States in 1989).[24] Airway occlusion by a foreign object must be considered in any victim who suddenly stops breathing and becomes cyanotic and unconscious. It occurs most commonly during eating and is usually due to food, especially meat, impacting in the laryngeal inlet, at the epiglottis or in the vallecula. Sudden death in restaurants from this cause frequently is mistaken for a myocardial infarction, leading to the label "cafe coronary."[29] Poorly chewed pieces of food, poor dentition or dentures, and elevated blood alcohol are the most common factors contributing to choking. The signs of total airway obstruction are the lack of air movement despite respiratory efforts and the inability of the victim to speak or cough. Cyanosis, unconsciousness, and cardiac arrest follow quickly. Partial airway obstruction will result in rasping or wheezing respirations accompanied by coughing. If the victim has good air movement and is able to cough forcefully, no intervention is indicated. However, if the cough weakens or cyanosis develops, the patient must be treated as if there were complete obstruction.

Mothers and friends have been pounding on the backs of choking victims for centuries. In 1974, Heimlich proposed abdominal thrusts as a better method of relieving airway obstruction.[30] In 1976, Guildner et al reported that sternal thrusts were just as effective.[31] Subsequently, there were multiple studies of these maneuvers in experimental animals, anesthetized and awake humans, and even on mathematical models.[32-35] There is general agreement that a normal cough produces higher airway pressures and moves a larger volume of air than any artificial maneuver. Abdominal and sternal thrusts produce modest elevations in airway pressure but can produce high volumes and flows of exhaled air that may result in movement of the impacted obstruction into the pharynx. Back blows produce little flow and volume but result in instantaneous high airway pressures of short duration, considered potentially helpful in dislodging an impacted obstruction. There is no convincing evidence that any one technique is superior to the others. In clinical practice, Redding[34] observed that no maneuver was always successful and that each occasionally was successful when another had failed. To minimize confusion from teaching multiple techniques (especially to the lay public), the American Heart Association has elected to emphasize the abdominal thrust maneuver (with chest thrusts as an alternative for the pregnant and massively obese) and the finger sweep.[24] This recommendation is made on the twofold premise that the abdominal thrust is at least as effective as other techniques and that teaching one method simplifies education.

For the awake victim, abdominal thrusts are applied in the erect position (sitting or standing). The rescuer reaches around the victim from behind, placing the fist of one hand in the epigastrium between the xiphoid and umbilicus. The fist is grasped with the other hand and pressed into the epigastrium with a quick upward thrust. In the unconscious, thrusts are applied by kneeling astride the victim, placing the heel of one hand in the epigastrium and other on top of the first. Care must be taken to ensure that the xiphoid is not pushed into the abdominal contents and that the thrust is in the midline. Sternal thrusts are valuable in the massively obese or in women in advanced pregnancy. In the erect victim, the chest is encircled from behind as in the abdominal maneuver but the fist is placed in the midsternum. For the unconscious, thrusts are applied from the side of the supine victim with a hand position the same as for external cardiac compression. Back blows are applied directly over the thoracic spine between the scapulae. They must be delivered with force. Placing the victim in a head-down position (e.g., leaning over a chair) may help move the obstruction into the pharynx.

Whatever technique is used, each individual maneuver must be delivered as if it will relieve the obstruction. If the first attempt is unsuccessful, repeated attempts should be made because hypoxia-related muscular relaxation may eventually allow success. Complications of thrust maneuvers include laceration of the liver and spleen, gastric rupture, fractured ribs, and regurgitation.

In the unconscious victim, if these maneuvers are unsuccessful, manual dislodgement of the obstruction should be tried. The mouth is opened and the tongue and jaw are grasped between the thumb and fingers and pulled forward. A finger of the other hand is inserted along the buccal mucosa attempting to dislodge the object laterally. Care must be taken not to push the foreign body deeper into the larynx. Direct visualization of the object may also be successful. In the absence of a laryngoscope and Magill forceps, ordinary instruments (such as a tablespoon and ice tongs) may be used.[33] However, blind grasping with instruments is rarely successful and may cause damage to tonsils or other tissue. Finally, if the object cannot be dislodged, a cricothyroidotomy can be life-saving.

Ventilation

The standard approach to the unresponsive victim is to follow opening the airway with ventilation (see Table 57-1). If the airway remains patent, chest compressions cause substantial air exchange. Early studies in anesthetized humans suggested that the airway would not remain open in the unconscious,[6,7] leading to the teaching that airway control and artificial ventilation must accompany chest compressions. However, data from the Belgian CPCR Registry have demonstrated that 14-day survival and neurologic outcome are the same if bystanders initiate full BLS or do only chest compressions. Both lead to substantially better survival than if the bystanders do only mouth-to-mouth ventilation or attempt no CPR.[36,37] Studies in the more controlled setting of the animal laboratory also raise questions about the importance of ventilation during BLS. In a swine model of up to 5 min of untreated fibrillatory cardiac arrest, comparison of 10 min of standard BLS with chest compressions without airway control or ventilation demonstrated that all successfully resuscitated animals in both groups survived for 24 hr and were neurologically normal.[38-41] A separate study using an asphyxial cardiac arrest model found a markedly improved 24-hr outcome when ventilation was added to chest compressions during BLS.[42] These observations suggest that when arrest is witnessed, likely to be of cardiac (rather than respiratory) cause, and intubation will be available within a short time, closed-chest compressions alone may be as efficacious as compressions and mouth-to-mouth ventilation. If these preliminary studies are confirmed, BLS teaching could be considerably simplified, potentially resulting in improved rates of bystander CPR because studies show that many people are reluctant to provide mouth-to-mouth ventilation.[43-45] Currently, airway management and ventilation remain the standard first steps of CPR. Mouth-to-mouth or mouth-to-nose ventilation is the most expeditious and effective method immediately available. Although inspired gas with this method will contain ~4% carbon dioxide and only ~17% oxygen (composition of exhaled air), it is sufficient to maintain viability.

Physiology of Ventilation During CPR

In the absence of an endotracheal tube, the relative impedance of flow into the lungs and stomach will determine the distribution of gas between each compartment during positive-pressure ventilation. Resistance to insufflation of the stomach is usually stated in terms of the static pressure needed to overcome the lower esophageal sphincter. Although there are no measurements during human CPR, opening pressure of the esophagus likely is no higher than it is under anesthesia ($\sim$20 cm H_2O).[46] In experimental animals, lower esophageal sphincter pressure decreases from 28 to 4 mm Hg during 15 min of cardiac arrest without CPR.[47] Resistance in the respiratory system will be determined primarily by lung–thorax compliance except in the rare case of severe bronchospasm. During 15 min of untreated arrest in a swine model, lung–thorax compliance declines by 30%.[47]

Insufflation of air into the stomach during CPR leads to gastric distension, impeding ventilation and increasing the risk of regurgitation and gastric rupture. Avoiding gastric insufflation requires that peak inspiratory airway pressures stay below esophageal opening pressure. Partial airway obstruction by the tongue and pharyngeal tissues is a major cause of increased airway pressure contributing to gastric insufflation during CPR. Meticulous attention to airway management is necessary during rescue breathing. Recommended tidal volumes to cause a noticeable rise in the chest wall in most adults is 0.8–1.2 L. To achieve these tidal volumes with low inspiratory pressures, a slow inspiratory flow rate and long inspiratory time are needed, even with an open airway. Therefore, rescue breaths should be given over 1.5–2 s during a pause in chest compressions.

A useful adjunct for preventing gastric insufflation during positive pressure ventilation without an endotracheal tube is cricoid pressure (Sellick maneuver).[48] Properly applied pressure to the anterior arch of the cricoid causes the cricoid lamina to seal the esophagus and can prevent air from entering the stomach at airway pressures up to 100 cm H_2O.[49] Pressure on the thyroid cartilage is useless. Cricoid pressure should be used during rescue breathing without an endotracheal tube, but this inevitably involves the need for an additional rescuer.

Techniques of Rescue Breathing

While maintaining an open airway with the head tilt–jaw lift technique, the hand on the forehead pinches the nose, the rescuer takes a deep breath and seals the victim's mouth with the lips and exhales, watching for the chest to rise, indicating effective ventilation. For exhalation, the rescuer's mouth is removed from the victim, listening for escaping air and taking a breath. When both hands are being used in the jaw thrust maneuver of opening the airway, the cheek is used to seal the nose. For mouth-to-nose ventilation, the rescuer's lips surround the nose and the victim's lips are held closed. In some patients, the mouth must be allowed to open for exhalation with this technique. On initiation of resuscitation, two consecutive breaths should be given and breathing continued at a rate of 10–12 min^{-1}. During a one-rescuer CPR, a pause for two breaths should be made after each 15 chest compressions. When there are two rescuers, a 1.5–2-s pause after every fifth chest compression will allow a breath to be given. Exhalation can occur during subsequent compressions.

Several adjuncts to ventilation are available. An oropharyngeal airway with mouth guard and external extension mouthpiece has been used, but obtaining a good mouth seal is often difficult. Perhaps the most useful adjunct is a common mask, such as that used for anesthesia. The mask can be applied to the face and held in place with the thumbs and index fingers while the other fingers are used to apply jaw thrust. Breathing into the connector port of the mask provides ventilation. Mouth-to-mask ventilation may be more aesthetic than mouth-to-mouth ventilation and can be just as effective in trained hands. Masks are also available with one-way valves that direct the victim's

exhaled gas away from the rescuer. Masks with integral nipple adapters are useful for providing supplemental oxygen. An oxygen flow of 10 L$\cdot$min^{-1} can raise the inspired concentration to 50%.

The self-inflating resuscitation bag and mask are the most common adjuncts used in rescue vehicles and hospitals. Although these devices have the advantages of noncontact and ability to use supplemental oxygen, they have been shown to be difficult for a single rescuer to apply properly, preventing substantial gas leak while maintaining a patent airway.[50] Tidal volumes with mouth-to-mouth and mouth-to-mask ventilation are often greater than with the resuscitation bag. It is now recommended that if this device is to be used, two individuals manage the airway: one to hold the mask and maintain head position and one to squeeze the bag using both hands.[51] Finally, tracheal intubation provides the best control of ventilation. With a tube in place, breathing can proceed without concern for gastric distension or synchronizing ventilation with chest compressions. Blood flow during CPR slows rapidly when chest compressions are stopped and recovers slowly when they are resumed. Consequently, following intubation, no pause should be made for ventilation and ventilation should be delivered without regard for the compression cycle.

Circulation

Physiology of Circulation During Closed-chest Compression

Two theories of the mechanism of blood flow during closed-chest compression have been suggested.[12,52] They are not mutually exclusive, and which predominates in humans continues to be the subject of controversy.

Cardiac Pump Mechanism. The cardiac pump mechanism was originally proposed by Kouwenhoven et al.[12,53] According to this theory, pressure on the chest compresses the heart between the sternum and the spine. Compression raises the pressure in the ventricular chambers, closing the atrioventricular valves and ejecting blood into the lungs and aorta. During the relaxation phase of closed-chest compression, expansion of the thoracic cage causes a subatmospheric intrathoracic pressure, facilitating blood return. The mitral and tricuspid valves open, allowing blood to fill the ventricles. Pressure in the aorta causes aortic valve closure and coronary artery perfusion. Support for this mechanism comes from echocardiography studies early in CPR demonstrating a reduction in ventricular size and mitral valve closure with chest compression.[54] Additionally, CPR techniques that incorporate direct sternal compressions, compared with techniques that raise intrathoracic pressure without sternal compression, result in better tissue blood flow and 24-hr survival.[55–57]

Thoracic Pump Mechanism. Some early investigators of closed-chest cardiac massage suggested that blood flow may not be due to cardiac compression because there was little difference in iliac arterial and venous pressures or in arterial and right atrial pressures during chest compressions.[58,59] Many practitioners have questioned the ability to depress the sternum enough to compress the heart in very large victims. In 1976, Criley et al[60] reported a patient undergoing cardiac catheterization who simultaneously developed ventricular fibrillation and an episode of cough-hiccups. With every cough-hiccup, a significant arterial pressure was noted. This observation of self-administered "cough CPR" prompted further investigations on the mechanism of blood flow. Taylor et al[61] found that carotid blood flow during prolonged CPR in humans was more dependent on long compression duration than compression rate. Rudikoff et al[62] demonstrated that pressures in all cardiac chambers may be equal during effective closed-chest compression and that carotid blood flow is higher during the first compression following a ventilation. These studies produced the theory of a thoracic pump mechanism for blood flow during closed-chest compressions.[52]

According to this theory, blood flows into the thorax during the relaxation phase of chest compressions in the same manner as that described for the cardiac pump mechanism. During the compression phase, all intrathoracic structures are compressed equally by the rise in intrathoracic pressure caused by sternal depression, forcing blood out of the chest. Backward flow through the venous system is prevented by valves in the subclavian and internal jugular veins and by dynamic compression of the veins at the thoracic outlet by the increased intrathoracic pressure. Thicker, less compressible vessel walls prevent collapse on the arterial side, although arterial collapse will occur if intrathoracic pressure is raised enough.[62] The heart is a passive conduit with the atrioventricular valves remaining open during chest compression. Because there is a significant pressure difference between the carotid artery and jugular vein, blood flow to the head is favored. The lack of valves in the inferior vena cava results in less resistance to backward flow, and pressures in the arteries and veins below the diaphragm are nearly equal. This is consistent with the early observations[58] and with the fact that there is little blood flow to organs below the diaphragm.[63,64]

A number of observations and studies support the concept of the thoracic pump. With the Valsalva maneuver of coughing during ventricular fibrillation, angiographic dye can be seen moving through the left heart and into the aorta without cardiac compression.[65] Raising intrathoracic pressure by abdominal binding or ventilation simultaneous with chest compression increases arterial pressure and carotid blood flow compared with standard CPR.[66,67] Artificial circulation adequate to maintain viability can be accomplished with simultaneous ventilation and inflation of vests surrounding the chest and abdomen in experimental animals.[65]

It seems clear that fluctuations in intrathoracic pressure plays a significant role in blood flow during CPR. It is also likely that compression of the heart occurs under some circumstances. Factors that influence the mechanism probably include the compliance and configuration of the chest wall, size of the heart, force of the sternal compressions, duration of cardiac arrest, and other undiscovered factors. Which mechanism predominates varies from victim to victim and even during the resuscitation of the same victim.

Distribution of Blood Flow During CPR.   Whatever the predominant mechanism, total body blood flow (cardiac output) is reduced to 10–33% of normal during experimental closed-chest cardiac massage. Similar severe reductions in flow are likely during clinical CPR in humans. Nearly all the blood flow is directed to organs above the diaphragm.[63,64] Myocardial perfusion is 20–50% of normal, whereas cerebral perfusion is maintained at 50–90% of normal. Abdominal visceral and lower extremity flow is reduced to 5% of normal. Total flow tends to decrease with time during CPR, but the relative distribution is not altered. Changes in CPR technique and the use of epinephrine may help sustain cardiac output over time.[64] Epinephrine improves flow to the brain and heart while flow to organs below the diaphragm is unchanged or further reduced.

Gas Transport During CPR.   During CPR, measurement of blood gases reveals an arterial respiratory alkalosis and a venous respiratory acidosis with a markedly elevated arteriovenous CO_2 difference.[68] The primary cause of these changes is the severely reduced cardiac output during CPR.

The no-flow state of cardiac arrest and low-flow state of CPR have severe effects on the transport of gases in the blood. To understand these changes, it is important to remember the relationship between the volume content of gas in the blood and the partial pressure of the gas. Molecules of carbon dioxide (CO_2) are produced at the tissue level, transported in the blood, and excreted by the lung. These are measured in volumes of gas, *e.g.*, milliliters of CO_2 produced or excreted and milliliters of $CO_2 \cdot 100$ ml^{-1} of blood. The partial pressure of CO_2 (Pco_2) in the blood is directly related to CO_2 volume content, but is also related to the barometric pressure and influenced by buffers available to combine with CO_2, *e.g.*, bicarbonate and hemoglobin. Thus, the same CO_2 content can result in different Pco_2. Under usual conditions, tissue oxygen (O_2) consumption and CO_2 production are equal to pulmonary O_2 uptake and CO_2 excretion because metabolism, circulation, and ventilation are stable. In unstable conditions, such as CPR, these relationships may not hold.

If ventricular fibrillation occurs in a patient being mechanically ventilated, the cessation of blood flow causes O_2 uptake from the inspired gas to stop and CO_2 excretion in the exhaled gas will rapidly approach zero as the functional residual capacity is washed out by continued ventilation. Because end-tidal CO_2 is a reflection of the CO_2 in the alveolar gas, it will also rapidly approach zero. At the tissue level, continued metabolism depletes meager tissue O_2 stores, resulting in a tissue O_2 deficit and CO_2 excess. Tissue pH will be reduced because of buffering of the excess CO_2. Anaerobic metabolism will contribute more CO_2 and, after many minutes, lactic acid to the acidosis.[69] Because there is no blood flow, these changes in O_2 and CO_2 at the tissue level are not reflected in arterial or venous blood. Blood gases measured during cardiac arrest without CPR are virtually unchanged from prearrest values.[38]

If normal circulation is restored by rapid defibrillation, cellular metabolism returns to normal but the tissue O_2 deficit and CO_2 accumulation remain. More O_2 will move into the tissues from the blood than usually occurs and more CO_2 will diffuse into venous blood. Mixed venous blood will have a lower O_2 content and higher CO_2 content than normal, resulting in increased pulmonary O_2 uptake and CO_2 excretion even though tissue O_2 consumption and CO_2 production may be normal. With constant ventilation, the increase in CO_2 being returned to the lungs causes a temporary rise in alveolar, end-tidal, and arterial CO_2. Within a short time, the excess CO_2 is removed and respiratory physiologic variables return to normal.

During the low-flow state of CPR, excretion of CO_2 (ml $\cdot$ min^{-1} of CO_2 in exhaled gas) is decreased from prearrest levels approximately to the same extent as cardiac output is reduced. This reduced CO_2 excretion is due primarily to shunting of blood flow away from the lower half of the body. The exhaled CO_2 reflects only the metabolism of the part of the body that is being perfused. In the nonperfused areas, CO_2 accumulates during CPR. When normal circulation is restored, the accumulated CO_2 is washed out and a temporary increase in CO_2 excretion is seen.

Although CO_2 excretion is reduced during CPR, the mixed venous partial pressure of CO_2 ($Pvco_2$) usually is increased and pH is decreased.[68,69] Two factors account for this elevation. Buffering acid causes a reduction in serum bicarbonate, so that the same blood CO_2 content results in a higher $Pvco_2$. In addition, the mixed venous CO_2 content is frequently, but not inevitably, elevated. When flow to a tissue is reduced, all the CO_2 produced fails to be removed and CO_2 accumulates, raising the tissue partial pressure of CO_2. This allows more CO_2 to be carried in each aliquot of blood and mixed venous CO_2 content increases. If flow remains constant, a new equilibrium is established where all CO_2 produced in the tissue is removed but at a higher venous CO_2 content and partial pressure. In contrast to the venous blood, arterial CO_2 content and partial pressure ($Paco_2$) usually are reduced during CPR. This reduction accounts for most of the observed increase in arterial–venous CO_2 content difference. Even though venous blood may have an increased CO_2, the marked reduction in cardiac output with maintained ventilation results in very efficient CO_2 removal. These blood gas changes with CPR are identical to those seen with any other low cardiac output (*i.e.*, shock) state.

Decreased pulmonary blood flow during CPR causes many nondependent alveoli not to be perfused. The alveolar gas of these lung units has no CO_2. Consequently, mixed alveolar CO_2 (*i.e.*, end-tidal CO_2) will be very low and correlate poorly with arterial CO_2. However, end-tidal CO_2 does correlate well with cardiac output during CPR. As flow increases, more alveoli become perfused, there is less alveolar deadspace, and end-tidal CO_2 measurements rise.

Technique of Closed-Chest Compression

In an unconscious apneic patient, cardiac arrest must be assumed in the absence of a pulse in a major artery (carotid, femoral, axillary). Because a systolic pressure of ~50 mm Hg is necessary for a palpable pulse, some circulation may remain in the "pulseless" patient with primary respiratory arrest. Opening the airway and ventilation may be sufficient for resuscitation in such circumstances. Therefore, further search for a pulse should always be made following artificial ventilation and before beginning sternal compressions.

Important considerations in performing closed-chest compressions are the position of the rescuer relative to the victim, the position of the rescuer's hands, and the rate and force of compression. The victim must be supine, the head level with the heart, for adequate brain perfusion. The victim must be on a firm surface. The rescuer should stand or kneel next to the victim's side. Compressions are performed most effectively if the rescuer's hips are on the same level, or slightly above the level of, the victim's chest.

Standard technique consists of the rhythmic application of pressure over the lower half of the sternum. The heel of one hand is placed on the lower sternum and the other hand is placed on top of the first. Great care must be taken to avoid pressing the xiphoid into the abdomen, which can lacerate the liver. Even with properly performed CPR, costochondral separation and rib fractures are common. Applying pressure on the ribs by improper hand placement increases these complications and risks puncturing the lung. Pressure on the sternum should be applied through the heel of the hand only, keeping the fingers free of the chest wall. The direction of force must be straight down on the sternum with the arms straight and the elbows locked into position so that the entire weight of the upper body is used to apply force. During relaxation all pressure should be removed from the hands, but they should not lose contact with the chest wall.

The sternum must be depressed 3.5–5.0 cm in the average adult. Occasionally, deeper compressions are necessary to generate a palpable pulse. The duration of compression should be equal to that of relaxation and the compression rate should be 80–100 times · min^{-1}. This rate seems to be optimal for both possible mechanisms of blood flow. The faster rate makes it easier to maintain a 50% compression–relaxation ratio, important in the thoracic pump mechanism.[61] It also requires a rapid, more forceful compression that may be important in the cardiac pump mechanism.[70] A fast rate also allows time to pause for ventilations. With a single rescuer, two ventilations should be given following every 15 compressions. With two rescuers, a 1.5–2.0-sec pause for ventilation should occur every 5 compressions. With an endotracheal tube in place, ventilations at a rate of 12 breaths · min^{-1} should be interposed between compressions without a pause.

Alternative Methods of Circulatory Support

As currently practiced, CPR has limited success, with only ~40% of victims being admitted to hospital and 10% surviving to discharge. Despite the occasional success of prolonged resuscitation, standard CPR will sustain most patients for only 15–30 min. If return of spontaneous circulation has not been achieved in that time, the outcome is dismal. Recognition of these limits and improved understanding of circulatory physiology during CPR have led to several proposals for alternatives to the standard techniques of closed-chest compression. Most, but not all, are based on the thoracic pump mechanism of blood flow. The goals of the new methods are to provide better hemodynamics during CPR and thus improve survival and/

or to extend the duration during which CPR can successfully support viability. Unfortunately, none of the alternatives has proved reliably superior to the standard technique.[71]

Simultaneous Ventilation–Compression CPR and Abdominal Binding. According to the thoracic pump theory, elevation of intrathoracic pressure during chest compression should improve blood flow and pressure.[62] Abdominal binding can improve aortic pressure and carotid blood flow but also may increase traumatic visceral injury during CPR.[67,72,73] The pneumatic anti-shock garment (military antishock trousers [MAST] suit) is another form of abdominal binding that impedes diaphragmatic excursion and elevates intrathoracic pressure during chest compression. Some studies have suggested that ventilation simultaneous with chest compression would raise intrathoracic pressure, aortic pressure, and carotid blood flow.[62,67] Initial studies with these methods were encouraging because the increased aortic pressure suggested better myocardial and cerebral perfusion.[66,67] Subsequent investigations have demonstrated that right atrial pressure and intracranial pressure are elevated as much as, or more than, the arterial pressures.[55,74–76] Thus, no improvement in myocardial or cerebral blood flow is found. Most importantly, survival from cardiac arrest is not improved when these techniques are compared with standard CPR in experimental animals or limited human trials.[57,76,78–80]

Interposed Abdominal Compression CPR. Interposed abdominal compression (IAC) is fundamentally different from abdominal binding. With this technique, an additional rescuer applies abdominal compressions manually during the relaxation phase of chest compression. Abdominal pressure is released when chest compression begins.[81] It has been suggested that the IAC augments aortic pressure and blood flow by counterpulsation on the abdominal aorta or by "priming" the thoracic pump.[82] Studies have been inconsistent in demonstrating improved hemodynamics.[83,84] Animal studies have not shown improved survival with this method.[56] One large randomized trial of out-of-hospital cardiac arrest with IAC CPR found no improvement in survival compared with standard CPR,[85] but a subsequent in-hospital study demonstrated improved outcome.[86] Although this technique remains experimental, investigations of its potential continue.

Pneumatic Vest CPR. Following the description of "cough CPR" and the development of the thoracic pump theory, a pneumatic vest device was developed that would simulate the events of vigorous coughing.[65,87] With the original method, thoracic and abdominal vests containing pneumatic bladders inflate simultaneously with positive-pressure ventilation. Although some survival studies found no improvement in outcome when compared with standard CPR,[57] other animal studies found excellent hemodynamics and the ability to maintain viability for prolonged periods with the method.[88] The technique continues to be investigated with a number of modifications from the original method. One report used a pneumatically powered, single, circumferential thoracic vest system with a pause for ventilation after every fifth compression during 63 human cardiac arrests.[89] In this preliminary study, aortic and coronary perfusion pressure was better with the vest than with standard CPR, but survival was not significantly improved.

High-Impulse CPR. In contrast to the previously described alternative methods, a technique commonly called high-impulse CPR is based on the concept that intrathoracic cardiac and vascular compression are important determinants of blood flow during CPR.[70,90] Relatively short compressions with moderately high force result in blood flow being directly related to rate of compressions. Laboratory investigations of this method found that the optimal rate is 120 compressions per minute to maximize coronary perfusion.[90] Some studies have shown improved survival in animals with this technique,[70] whereas others have found no difference from standard CPR.[57] This method is similar to the standard technique, and many of the studies of this method have influenced standard CPR practice. Emphasis now is placed on ensuring adequate sternal depression and compression rates have been increased to 80–100 min^{-1}.

Active Compression–Decompression CPR. The newest proposed alternative technique developed from the anecdotal report of CPR performed with a plumber's helper applied to the anterior chest wall.[91] This suggested that active decompression of the chest wall might reduce intrathoracic pressure during the relaxation phase of chest compressions, leading to improved venous return, increased stroke volume with compression, and better blood flow. A suction device that can be applied to the chest wall to enable active compression and decompression was developed.[92] Hemodynamic studies in animals and humans with this technique have shown that coronary and cerebral perfusion may be somewhat improved with this method compared with standard CPR, although when epinephrine is used there is no difference between techniques.[92–94] One preliminary in-hospital clinical trial found improved immediate resuscitation but no difference in survival.[95] Two out-of-hospital trials found no difference in immediate resuscitation or survival.[96,97]

Invasive Techniques. In contrast to the closed-chest techniques, two invasive methods have been able to maintain cardiac and cerebral viability during long periods of cardiac arrest. In animal models, open-chest cardiac massage and cardiopulmonary bypass (through the femoral artery and vein using a membrane oxygenator) can provide better hemodynamics and myocardial and cerebral perfusion than closed-chest techniques.[74,98] Preliminary trials of percutaneous cardiopulmonary bypass for refractory human cardiac arrest have been reported.[99–101] Prompt restoration of blood flow and perfusion pressure with cardiopulmonary bypass can provide resuscitation with minimal neurologic deficit after 20 min of fibrillatory cardiac arrest in canines.[15] However, to be effective these techniques must be instituted relatively early (probably within 20–30 min of arrest).[16,102] If open chest massage is begun after 30 min of ineffective closed-chest compressions, there is no better survival even though hemodynamics are improved.[103] The need to apply these maneuvers early in an arrest obviously limits the application. Before invasive procedures play a greater role in modern CPR, a method must be developed to predict, early in resuscitation, which patients will and which will not respond to closed-chest compressions.

Assessing the Adequacy of Circulation During CPR

The adequacy of closed-chest compression is usually judged by palpation of a pulse in the carotid or femoral vessels. The palpable pulse primarily reflects systolic pressure. Cardiac output correlates better with mean pressure and coronary perfusion with diastolic pressure. In the femoral area, the palpable pulse is as likely to be venous as arterial.[104] Despite these shortcomings, palpating the pulse remains the only monitor available during BLS.

Return of spontaneous circulation with an arrested heart is greatly dependent on restoring oxygenated blood flow to the myocardium. In experimental models, a minimum blood flow of 15–20 ml·min^{-1}·100 g^{-1} of myocardium has been shown to be necessary for successful resuscitation.[105] Obtaining such flow depends on closed-chest compressions developing adequate cardiac output and coronary perfusion pressure. Similar to the beating heart, coronary perfusion during CPR occurs primarily in the relaxation phase (diastole) of chest compressions. Crile and Dolley suggested in 1906 that a critical coronary perfusion pressure was necessary for successful resuscitation.[106] This concept has been confirmed in numerous other reports.[64,73,75,105,107–114] During standard CPR, critical myocardial blood flow is associated with aortic diastolic pressure exceeding 40 mm Hg. Because right atrial pressure can be elevated with some techniques, the aortic diastolic pressure minus the right atrial diastolic pressure is a more accurate reflection of coronary perfusion pressure. The critical coronary perfusion pressure is 15–25 mm Hg. When invasive monitoring is available during

CPR, adjustments in chest compression technique and epinephrine should be used to ensure that critical perfusion pressures are exceeded. Damage to the myocardium from underlying disease may preclude survival no matter how effective the CPR efforts. However, vascular pressures below critical levels are associated with poor results even in patients who may be salvageable (Table 57-2).

Although invasive pressure monitoring may be ideal, it is rarely available during CPR. End-tidal CO_2 also has been found to be an excellent noninvasive guide to the adequacy of closed-chest compressions.[115] Carbon dioxide excretion during CPR with an endotracheal tube in place is flow-dependent rather than ventilation-dependent. Because alveolar deadspace is large in low-flow states, end-tidal CO_2 is very low (frequently <10 mm Hg). If blood flow improves with better CPR technique, more alveoli are perfused and end-tidal CO_2 rises (usually to >20 mm Hg with successful CPR). The earliest sign of return of spontaneous circulation frequently is a sudden increase in end-tidal CO_2 to >40 mm Hg. Within a wide range of cardiac outputs during CPR, end-tidal CO_2 correlates well with cardiac output,[116] coronary perfusion pressure,[117] and initial resuscitation.[118,119] End-tidal CO_2 correlates with survival in human CPR and can predict outcome.[120,121] Patients with end-tidal CO_2 < 10 mm Hg will not be resuscitated successfully. In the absence of invasive monitoring, end-tidal CO_2 should be used to judge the effectiveness of chest compressions, whenever possible.[122] Attempts should be made to maximize the measured end-tidal CO_2 by alterations in technique or drug therapy. It should be remembered that sodium bicarbonate administration liberates CO_2 into the blood and causes a temporary increase in end-tidal CO_2. The elevation returns to baseline within 3–5 min of drug administration and end-tidal CO_2 monitoring can again be used for monitoring effectiveness of closed-chest compressions.

ADVANCED CARDIAC LIFE SUPPORT

Advanced cardiac life support (ACLS) encompasses all the cognitive and technical skills that are necessary to restore spontaneous circulatory function when simple support does not result in resuscitation. In addition to BLS skills, it includes use of adjunctive equipment and techniques for assisting ventilation and circulation, electrocardiographic (ECG) monitoring with dysrhythmia recognition and defibrillation, establishment of intravenous (iv) access, and pharmacologic therapy. A number of aspects of ACLS have been discussed in preceding sections. The following sections concentrate on electrical and drug treatment as well as the generalized ACLS algorithms. Figure 57-1 demonstrates the universal algorithm for adult emergency cardiac care.

Defibrillation

Electrical Pattern and Duration of Ventricular Fibrillation

Ventricular fibrillation is the most common electrocardiographic pattern found during cardiac arrest in adults. The only consistently effective treatment is electrical defibrillation. The most important controllable determinant of failure to resusci-

Table 57-2. CRITICAL VARIABLES ASSOCIATED WITH SUCCESSFUL RESUSCITATION

Variable	Amount
Myocardial blood flow (ml·min^{-1}·100 g^{-1})	15–20
Aortic diastolic pressure (mm Hg)	40
Coronary perfusion pressure (mm Hg)	15–25
End-tidal carbon dioxide (mm Hg)	>10

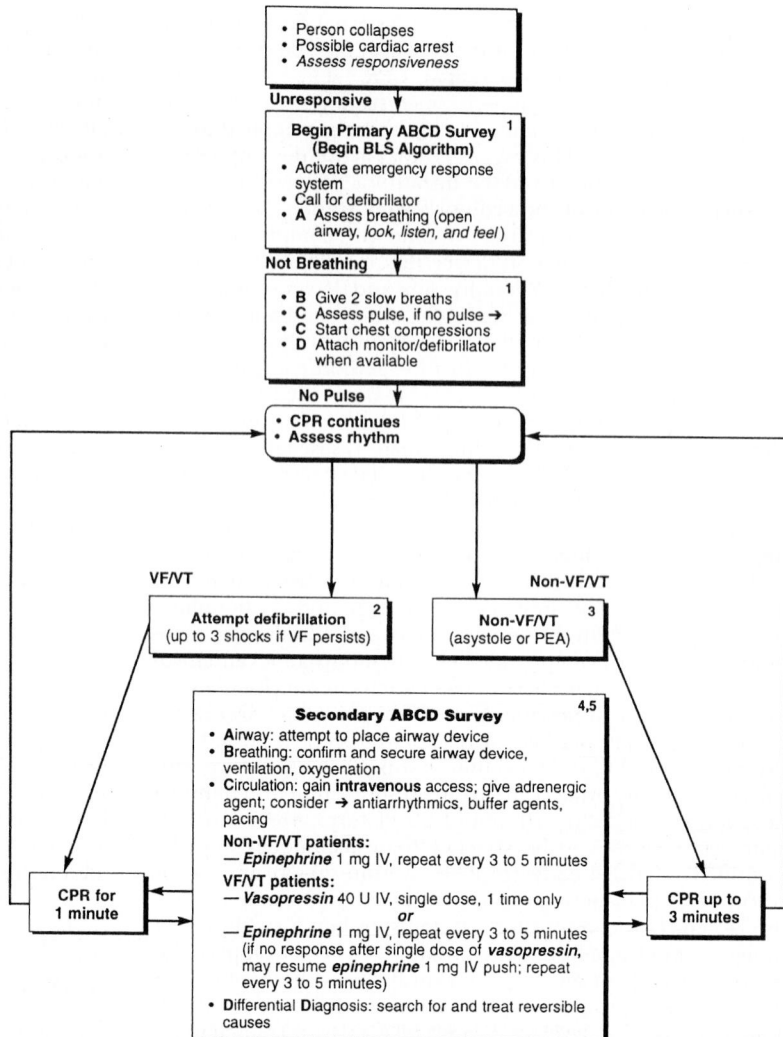

Figure 57-1. Comprehensive emergency cardiac care (ECC) algorithm. (Reprinted with permission from American Heart Association: Guidelines 2000 for cardiopulmonary resuscitation and emergency cardiovascular care: International concensus on science. Circulation 102:I-144, 2000.)

tate a patient with ventricular fibrillation is the duration of fibrillation.[123] Other important factors, such as underlying disease and metabolic status, are largely beyond the control of rescuers. The fibrillating heart has high oxygen consumption, increasing myocardial ischemia and decreasing the time to irreversible cell damage. The longer ventricular fibrillation continues, the more difficult it is to defibrillate and the less likely is successful resuscitation.[102,124] If defibrillation occurs within 1 min of fibrillation, CPR is unnecessary for resuscitation. Initial resuscitation success following out-of-hospital fibrillation and survival to hospital discharge are improved the earlier that defibrillation is accomplished.[18,20,125]

The amplitude (coarseness) of the fibrillatory waves on the ECG may reflect the severity and duration of the myocardial insult and, thus, have prognostic significance.[126] However, the fibrillation amplitude seen on any one ECG lead varies with the orientation of that lead to the vector of the fibrillatory wave.[127] If the lead is oriented at right angles to the fibrillatory wave, a flat line can be seen. For this reason, the trace from a second lead or from a different position of paddle electrodes should always be inspected before a decision is made not to defibrillate.

Coarse (high-voltage) ventricular fibrillation is considered easier to defibrillate than fine (low-voltage) fibrillation. Increasing myocardial ischemia results in less vigorous fibrillation, reduced amplitude electrical activity, and more difficult defibrillation. Low-voltage fibrillation is associated with poor outcome.[126] Catecholamines with β-adrenergic activity increase the vigor of fibrillation and the amplitude of the electrical

activity. Consequently, epinephrine frequently is administered to make it "easier" to defibrillate. However, experimental work has shown that manipulation of the electrical pattern with epinephrine does not influence the success of defibrillation or reduce the energy needed for defibrillation.[124,128] Consequently, defibrillation should not be delayed for epinephrine administration or any other therapy. The algorithm for managing ventricular fibrillation–tachycardia is illustrated in Figure 57-2.

The importance of minimizing the duration of ventricular fibrillation cannot be overemphasized. Conversion of fibrillation to a rhythm capable of restoring spontaneous circulation should be the first priority of any resuscitation attempt. For out-of-hospital arrests, this problem is being addressed by improving the response times of rescue units and teaching less trained individuals to use defibrillators.[18–20] Early defibrillation has been improved recently by the development of automatic external defibrillators that recognize ventricular fibrillation, charge automatically, and give a defibrillatory shock.[129] This device has allowed the introduction of public-access defibrillation because minimally trained individuals can incorporate defibrillation into BLS skills.[21,130] In the hospital setting, defibrillation should be carried out as soon as fibrillation is diagnosed and the equipment is available. The precordial thump, although rarely successful, can be tried while awaiting a defibrillator. It should not be used for the conscious patient with ventricular tachycardia unless a defibrillator is immediately available. It is as likely to induce fibrillation as normal rhythm. Blind defibrillation is recommended in adults if no monitoring is available. This should rarely be necessary because modern defibrillators have built-in monitoring capability using the paddles as electrodes.

Defibrillators: Energy, Current, and Voltage

Defibrillators derive power from a line source of alternating current or an integral battery. The typical defibrillator consists of a variable transformer that allows selection of a variable voltage potential, an AC/DC converter to provide a direct current that is stored in a capacitor, a switch to charge the capacitor, and discharge switches to complete the circuit from capacitor to electrodes. The output current waveform of most clinically used defibrillators is a damped half-sinusoid, although some are designed to deliver trapezoidal or near-square waves. Recently, units with biphasic waveforms have been introduced that may allow effective defibrillation at lower energy.

Defibrillation is accomplished by current passing through a critical mass of myocardium causing simultaneous depolarization of the myofibrils. However, the output of most defibrillators is indicated in energy units (joules or watt-seconds), not current (amperes). The relationships among energy, current, and impedance (resistance) are given by the following equations (standard units are indicated):

$$\text{Energy (joules)} = \text{Power (watts)} \times \text{duration (seconds)} \quad (1)$$

$$\text{Power (watts)} = \text{Potential (volts)} \times \text{current (amperes)} \quad (2)$$

$$\text{Current (amperes)} = \text{Potential (volts)} / \text{resistance (ohms)} \quad (3)$$

$$\text{Current (amperes)} = \{\text{Energy (joules)} / [\text{resistance (ohms)} \times \text{duration (seconds)}]\}^{1/2} \quad (4)$$

From these equations, it can be determined that as the impedance between the paddle electrodes increases, the delivered energy will be reduced. Because internal resistance is low, the primary determinant of delivered energy will be transthoracic impedance. For consistency, the energy level indicated on most commercially available defibrillators is the output when discharged into a 50-ohm load. When transthoracic impedance is higher than that standard, actual delivered energy will be lower. Even at a constant delivered energy, Eq. (4) indicates that delivered current (the critical determinant of defibrillation) will be reduced as impedance increases. At high impedance and relatively low energy levels, current could be too low for defibrillation. Optimal success of defibrillation is obtained by keeping impedance as low as possible.[131]

Transthoracic Impedance

Transthoracic impedance has been measured at 24–109 ohms in patients undergoing cardioversion[132] and at 15–143 ohms in human defibrillation.[133] The major determinants of transthoracic impedance are known and many are under the control of the rescuers. Resistance decreases with increasing electrode size, and studies suggest that optimal paddle size may be 13 cm in diameter.[134,135] Concern has been expressed that a paddle this large may diffuse the current over too great an area for effective defibrillation. The most common paddle size remains 8–10 cm in diameter. The high impedance between metal electrode and skin can be reduced somewhat by use of saline-soaked gauze pads or creams, such as those used for recording ECGs. However, resistance is least when a gel or paste specifically designed to conduct electricity in the defibrillation setting is used.[134,135] Self-adhesive defibrillation/monitor pads also work well when carefully applied. When paste is used, it should be applied liberally to the paddle surface, especially the edges, to prevent burns and obtain the maximum reduction in impedance. In experimental models, transthoracic impedance decreases with successive shocks.[136,137] Although the clinical significance has been questioned,[133] this factor may partially explain why an additional shock of the same energy can cause defibrillation when previous shocks have failed. Transthoracic impedance is slightly, but significantly, higher during inspiration than during exhalation.[138] Air is a poor electrical conductor. Firm paddle pressure of at least 11 kg reduces resistance by improving paddle–skin contact and by expelling air from the lungs.[133]

The average transthoracic impedance in human defibrillation is 70–80 ohms. Resistance is probably of little clinical significance when reasonably proper technique and high energy (300 J) shocks are used. For lower energy shocks, great care should be taken to minimize resistance. Defibrillators have been developed that measure transthoracic impedance prior to the shock by passing a low-voltage current through the chest during the charge cycle.[139,140] This allows the use of low-energy shocks in appropriate patients and identification of victims needing higher energy. Although not widely used, this technology allows current-based defibrillation by adjusting the delivered energy for the measured resistance.[141]

Adverse Effects and Energy Requirements

Repeated defibrillation with high energy in animals can be associated with dysrhythmias, ECG changes suggesting myocardial damage, and morphologic evidence of myocardial necrosis.[142,143] Whether similar injuries occur in humans is less certain. Slight elevations in creatine kinase MB fractions have been

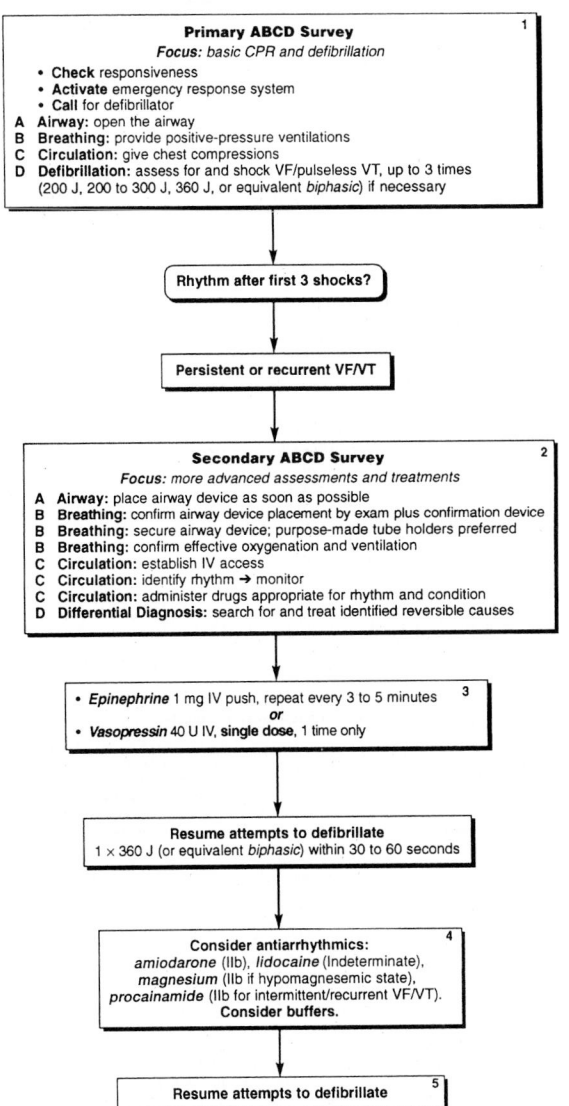

Figure 57-2. Ventricular fibrillation/pulseless VT algorithm. (Reprinted with permission from American Heart Association: Guidelines 2000 for cardiopulmonary resuscitation and emergency cardiovascular care: International concensus on science. Circulation 102:I-147, 2000.)

Table 57-3. ADULT ADVANCED CARDIAC LIFE SUPPORT DRUGS AND DOSES (INTRAVENOUS)

	Dose	Interval	Maximum
Epinephrine	1 mg	Every 3–5 min	None
If dose fails, consider	3–7 mg	Every 3–5 min	None
Amiodarone	300 mg	Repeat in 3–5 min	2 g
Lidocaine	1.5 mg · kg^{-1}	Repeat in 3–5 min	3.0 mg · kg^{-1}
Bretylium tosylate	5 mg · kg^{-1}	Repeat in 5 min	10 mg · kg^{-1}
Atropine	1 mg	Every 3–5 min	0.04 mg · kg^{-1}
Sodium bicarbonate	1 mEq · kg^{-1}	As needed	Check pH

measured in patients following cardioversion with high energies.[144] A higher incidence of atrioventricular block has been observed in patients receiving high-energy shocks than in patients receiving low-energy shock.[145] It seems likely that high-energy shocks, especially if repeated at close intervals, may result in myocardial damage. Therefore, it would be prudent to keep energy levels as low as possible during defibrillation attempts. However, if energy is too low, the delivered current may be insufficient for defibrillation, especially when transthoracic impedance is high.

There is a general relationship between body size and energy requirements for defibrillation. Geddes *et al* observed that the current necessary for defibrillation in animals increased with increasing body mass.[146] Children need less energy than adults, perhaps as low as 0.5 J · kg^{-1},[147] although the recommended dose is 2.0 J · kg^{-1}.[24] However, over the size range of adults, weight variability is not clinically significant and other factors are more important.[148] Multiple studies have demonstrated high rates of successful defibrillation using relatively low levels (160–200 J) of delivered energy.[149–152] Studies of out-of-hospital and in-hospital arrests have demonstrated equal success when using ≤200 J initial energy compared with administering all shocks at energies ≥ 300 J.[145,153] Therefore, current recommendations are to use 200 J for the initial shock followed by a second shock at 200–300 J if the first is unsuccessful. If both fail to defibrillate the patient, additional shocks should be given at 300–360 J (see Fig. 57-2).[24]

Pharmacologic Therapy

This discussion of drug therapy is confined to the use of drugs during CPR attempts to restore spontaneous circulation. The use of drugs to support the circulation when there is mechanical cardiac function is discussed elsewhere (see Chapters 12 and 32). During cardiac arrest, drug therapy is secondary to other interventions. Chest compressions, airway management, ventilation, and defibrillation, if appropriate, should take precedence over medications. Establishing iv access and pharmacologic therapy should come after other interventions are established. The most common drugs and the appropriate adult doses are shown in Table 57-3. Of the drugs given during CPR, only epinephrine is usually acknowledged as being helpful in restoring spontaneous circulation.[154] Asystole and pulseless electrical activity (PEA), also called electromechanical dissociation (EMD), are circumstances in which drugs are most frequently given. The standard algorithms for management of these types of cardiac arrest are shown in Figures 57-3 and 57-4. In addition, the algorithms for the American Heart Association protocols for bradycardia, tachycardia, shock, and synchronized cardioversion are included (Figs. 57-5 to 57-8).

Routes of Administration

The preferred route of administration of all drugs during CPR is intravenous. The most rapid and highest drug levels occur with administration into a central vein. However, peripheral iv administration is also effective. The antecubital and external jugular veins are the sites of first choice for starting an infusion during resuscitation because inserting a central catheter usually necessitates stopping CPR. Because of poor blood flow below the diaphragm during CPR, drugs administered in the lower extremity may be extremely delayed or not reach the sites of action. Even in the upper extremity, drugs may require 1–2 min to reach the central circulation. Onset of action may be speeded if the drug bolus is followed by a 20–30 ml bolus of iv fluid. If iv access cannot be established, the endotracheal tube is an alternative route for administration of epinephrine, lidocaine, and atropine. (Sodium bicarbonate should not be

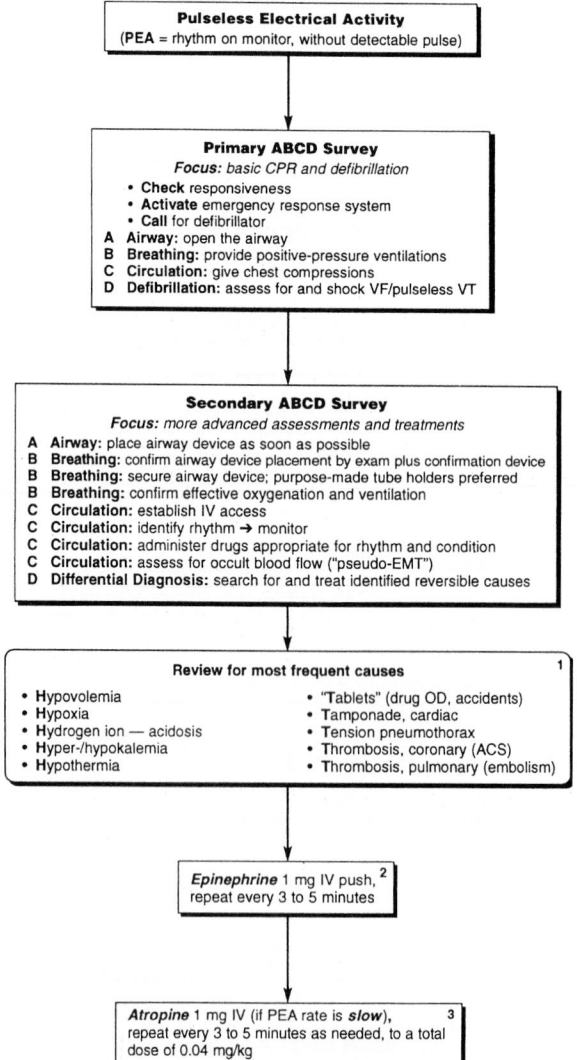

Figure 57-3. Pulseless electrical activity algorithm. (Reprinted with permission from American Heart Association: Guidelines 2000 for cardiopulmonary resuscitation and emergency cardiovascular care: International concensus on science. Circulation 102:I-151, 2000.)

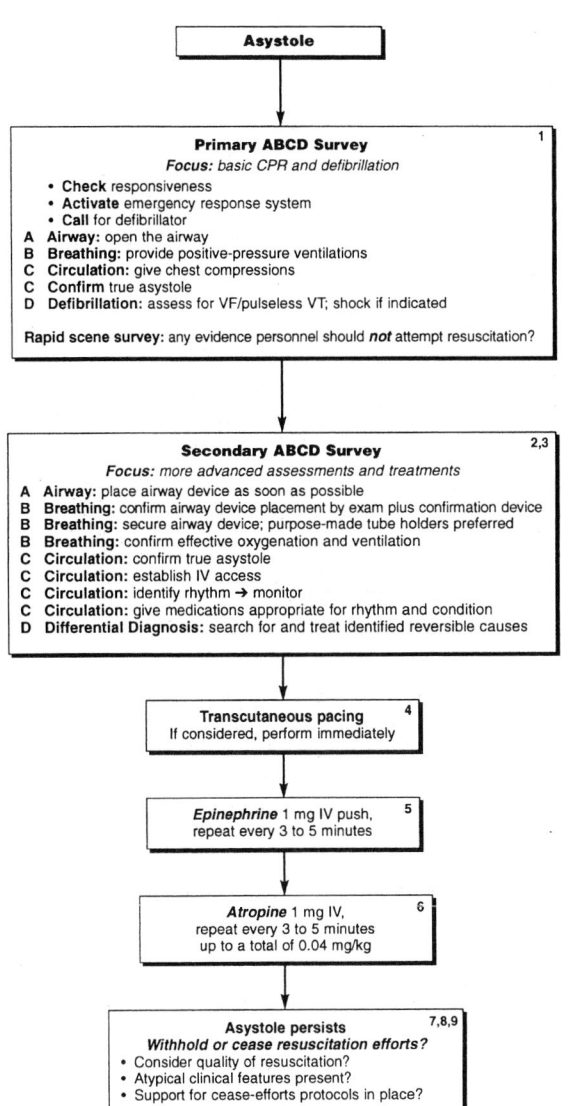

Figure 57-4. Asystole: The silent heart algorithm. (Reprinted with permission from American Heart Association: Guidelines 2000 for cardiopulmonary resuscitation and emergency cardiovascular care: International concensus on science. Circulation 102:I-153, 2000.)

given endotracheally.) The time to effect and drug levels achieved are inconsistent using this route during CPR. Better results may be obtained by administering 5–10 ml volumes. It is unclear whether deep injection is better than simple instillation into the endotracheal tube. Doses 2–2.5 times higher than the recommended iv dose should be administered when this route is used.

Catecholamines and Vasopressors

Mechanism of Action. Epinephrine has been used in resuscitation since the 1890s and has been the vasopressor of choice in modern CPR since the studies of Redding and Pearson in the 1960s.[13,155] Experimental studies have shown that the efficacy of epinephrine lies entirely in its α-adrenergic properties.[111] Peripheral vasoconstriction leads to an increase in aortic diastolic pressure, causing an increase in coronary perfusion pressure and myocardial blood flow.[64,156,157] It is tempting to invoke the β-adrenergic properties of cardiac stimulation to explain the success of epinephrine. However, animal studies have demonstrated that β-adrenergic agonists without α activity (isoproterenol, dobutamine) are no better than placebo. All strong α-adrenergic drugs (epinephrine, phenylephrine, methoxamine, dopamine, norepinephrine), regardless of

β-adrenergic potency, are equally successful in aiding resuscitation, as are strong nonadrenergic vasopressors (vasopressin, endothelin-1).[13,155,158–160] α-Adrenergic blockade precludes resuscitation, whereas β-adrenergic blockade has no effect on the ability to restore spontaneous circulation.[108,109] It is commonly believed that the ability of epinephrine to increase the amplitude of ventricular fibrillation (a β-adrenergic effect) makes defibrillation easier. Animal studies have shown that epinephrine does not improve the success of or reduce the energy necessary for defibrillation.[124,128] Retrospective analysis of out-of-hospital CPR has found no effect of epinephrine on defibrillation success.[126]

The β-adrenergic effects of epinephrine are potentially deleterious during cardiac arrest. In the fibrillating heart, epinephrine increases oxygen consumption and decreases the endocardial–epicardial blood flow ratio, an effect not seen with methoxamine.[161] Myocardial lactate production in the fibrillating heart is unchanged after epinephrine administration during CPR, suggesting that the increased coronary blood flow does not improve the oxygen supply–demand ratio.[162] Large doses of epinephrine increased deaths in swine early after resuscitation due to tachyarrhythmias and hypertension, an effect partially offset by metoprolol treatment.[163,164] Despite these theoretical considerations, survival and neurologic outcome studies have shown no difference when epinephrine is compared with a pure α-agonist (methoxamine or phenylephrine) during CPR in animals[155,165] or humans.[166] Recent animal studies[159,160] and a small randomized clinical trial of out-of-hospital arrests[167] suggest that arginine vasopressin may improve outcome over epinephrine. However, vasopressin causes worse myocardial depression in the early postresuscitation phase than epinephrine.[168] A larger clinical trial of in-hospital arrests did not find a difference in survival when the two drugs were compared. Although epinephrine has never had a rigorous randomized human trial, there is strong animal evidence of its efficacy as well as extensive clinical experience with its use. Epinephrine remains the vasopressor of choice in CPR. It should be administered whenever resuscitation has not occurred after adequate chest compressions and ventilation have been started and defibrillation attempted, if appropriate.

Epinephrine Dose. When added to chest compressions, epinephrine helps develop the critical coronary perfusion pressure necessary to provide enough myocardial blood flow for restoration of spontaneous circulation. With invasive monitoring present during CPR, an arterial diastolic pressure of 40 mm Hg or coronary perfusion pressure of 20 mm Hg must be obtained with good chest compression technique and/or epinephrine therapy (see Table 57-2). In the absence of such monitoring, the dose of epinephrine must be chosen empirically. For many years, the standard iv dose used in animals and humans has been 0.5–1.0 mg. On a weight basis, this dose is ~0.015 mg $\cdot$ kg^{-1} in humans but 0.1 mg $\cdot$ kg^{-1} in animals. In swine the human standard dose of epinephrine (0.02 mg $\cdot$ kg^{-1}) is insufficient to improve coronary perfusion pressure and blood flow, but a high dose (0.2 mg $\cdot$ kg^{-1}) improves hemodynamics to levels compatible with successful resuscitation.[169–171] These animal studies suggest that higher doses of epinephrine in human CPR might improve myocardial and cerebral perfusion and improve success of resuscitation. Support for using higher doses also comes from anecdotal case reports and a series of children (with historical controls) that demonstrated return of spontaneous circulation when large doses (0.1–0.2 mg $\cdot$ kg^{-1}) of epinephrine were given to patients who had failed resuscitation with standard doses.[172,173]

Unfortunately, outcome studies have not conclusively shown that higher doses of epinephrine will improve survival. There are two randomized, blinded animal studies comparing standard and high-dose epinephrine: one with fibrillatory arrest and one with asphyxial arrest.[163,164] In each study, there was no

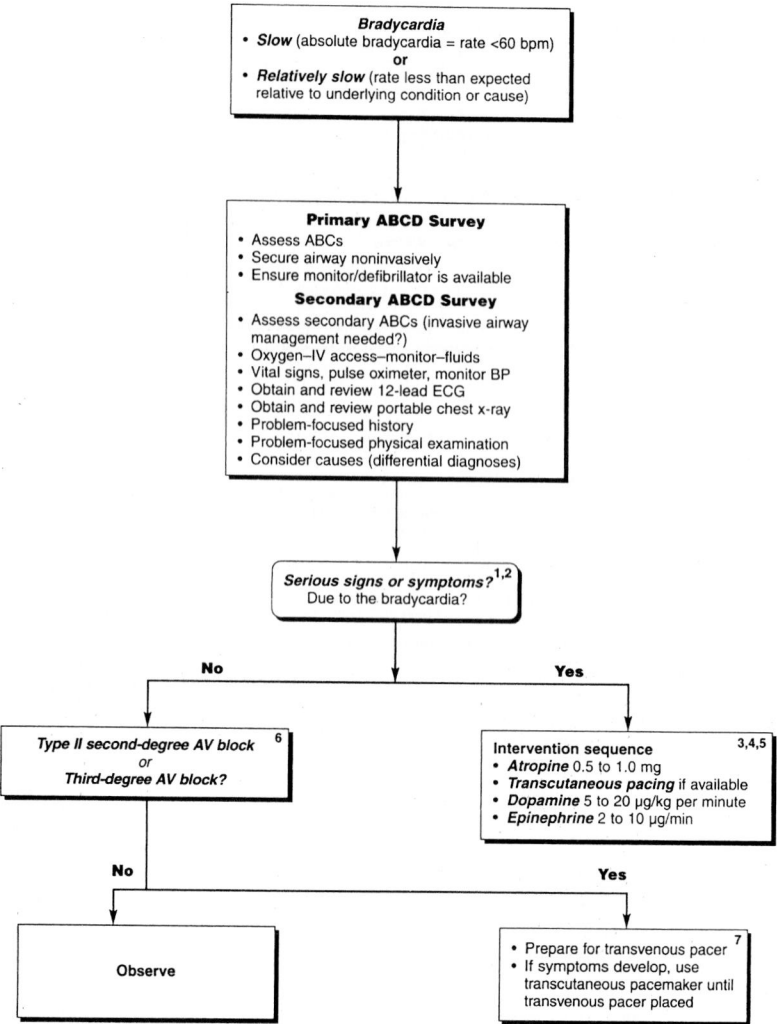

Figure 57-5. Bradycardia algorithm. (Reprinted with permission from American Heart Association: Guidelines 2000 for cardiopulmonary resuscitation and emergency cardiovascular care: International concensus on science. Circulation 102:I-156, 2000.)

difference in 24-hr survival or neurologic outcome, but more animals in the high-dose group died in the early postresuscitation period due to hyperdynamic state. There are several reports of studies comparing standard doses (1–2 mg) to high doses (5–18 mg) of epinephrine in human CPR, totaling approximately 9000 patients.[174-179] All are prospective, randomized, double-blind clinical trials in cardiac arrest victims, primarily out-of-hospital. Some of the studies (and the cumulative data) suggest that there may be an improvement in immediate resuscitation with high-dose epinephrine. None of the studies found improvement in survival to hospital discharge. Retrospective studies of epinephrine dosing have suggested that higher doses may be associated with impaired postresuscitation cardiovascular function and worse neurologic outcome.[180,181] None of the prospective studies found lower survival or worse neurologic outcome with higher epinephrine dosing.

It should be noted that these outcome studies used high-dose epinephrine as initial therapy. High doses apparently are not needed early in most cardiac arrests and could be deleterious under some circumstances. The successful case reports were in patients who had failed conventional treatment. The high doses were given late in prolonged CPR when the vasculature may not be as responsive to catecholamines. Although the use of high-dose epinephrine as rescue therapy when standard doses have failed has not been rigorously studied, this may be its appropriate place in CPR practice. Current recommendations are to give 1 mg iv every 3–5 min in the adult. If this dose seems ineffective, higher doses (3–8 mg) should be considered (see Figs. 57-2 to 57-4).

Amiodarone, Lidocaine, Bretylium

After epinephrine, the most effective drugs during CPR are those that help suppress ectopic ventricular rhythms. Amiodarone, lidocaine, and bretylium are used during cardiac arrest to aid defibrillation when ventricular fibrillation is refractory to electrical countershock therapy or when fibrillation recurs following successful conversion. Lidocaine is primarily an antiectopic agent that depresses automaticity by reducing the slope of Phase 4 depolarization and reducing the heterogeneity of ventricular refractoriness.[182,183] In contrast, bretylium has been called a primary antifibrillatory drug. It reduces the heterogeneity of action potential duration between ischemic and normal myocardium, resulting in less disparity between refractory periods and reducing the chances for re-entry. It does not suppress automaticity or Phase 4 depolarization.[184] Amiodarone is a pharmacologically complex drug with sodium, potassium, calcium, and α- and β-adrenergic blocking properties that is useful for treatment of atrial and ventricular arrhythmias.

When given intravenously, lidocaine has few hemodynamic effects. Conversely, bretylium initially causes release of norepinephrine from adrenergic nerve endings.[184] With a normal circulation, this causes tachycardia, hypertension, and increased contractility. After ~20 min, blockade of the release and reuptake of norepinephrine from the nerve terminal occurs. This effect is maximal 45–60 min following drug administration and can lead to profound hypotension. Amiodarone can cause hypotension and bradycardia when infused too rapidly but less so than bretylium.[185] This can usually be prevented by slowing the rate of drug infusion, or treated with fluids, pressors, chronotropic agents or temporary pacing.

Ventricular fibrillation threshold is reduced by acute ischemia or infarction, an effect partially reversed by both lidocaine and bretylium.[183,186–188] Lidocaine has been reported to raise the defibrillation threshold; *i.e.,* more energy is needed to defibrillate.[188–190] However, peak effect does not occur until 30 min following drug administration and the clinical importance of this effect during CPR is doubtful. Amiodarone also raises the defibrillation threshold.[191] Bretylium either reduces or does not change defibrillation threshold.[188,189,192] These electrophysiologic considerations and anecdotal reports of chemical defibrillation[193] suggest an advantage for bretylium over amiodarone and lidocaine during CPR. However, direct comparison of the drugs in controlled randomized trials during out-of-hospital ventricular fibrillation have failed to demonstrate a difference in resuscitation success or survival.[185,194,195] Consequently, because of the tendency for hypotension from bretylium, it is not recommended as first-line treatment during CPR. Its use should be reserved for fibrilla-

tion refractory to defibrillation, amiodarone and lidocaine, or for recurrent fibrillation uncontrolled by the other drugs. There is one randomized placebo-controlled clinical trial demonstrating improved admission alive to hospital with treatment, suggesting that amiodarone should now be first-line treatment for shock-resistant fibrillation.[196]

When ventricular fibrillation or pulseless ventricular tachycardia is recognized, defibrillation should be attempted as soon as possible (see Fig. 57-2). No antiarrhythmic agent has been shown superior to electrical defibrillation or more effective than placebo in the treatment of ventricular fibrillation. Consequently, defibrillation should not be withheld or delayed to establish iv access or to administer drugs. When ventricular tachycardia or ventricular fibrillation has not responded to or recurred following BLS, epinephrine, and defibrillation, amiodarone should be administered. Amiodarone is usually administered as 150 mg iv over 10 min, followed by 1 mg·min⁻¹ infusion for 6 hours, and 0.5 mg·min⁻¹ thereafter. In cardiac arrest due to pulseless ventricular tachycardia or fibrillation, amiodarone is initially administered as a 300-mg rapid infusion. Supplemental infusions of 150 mg

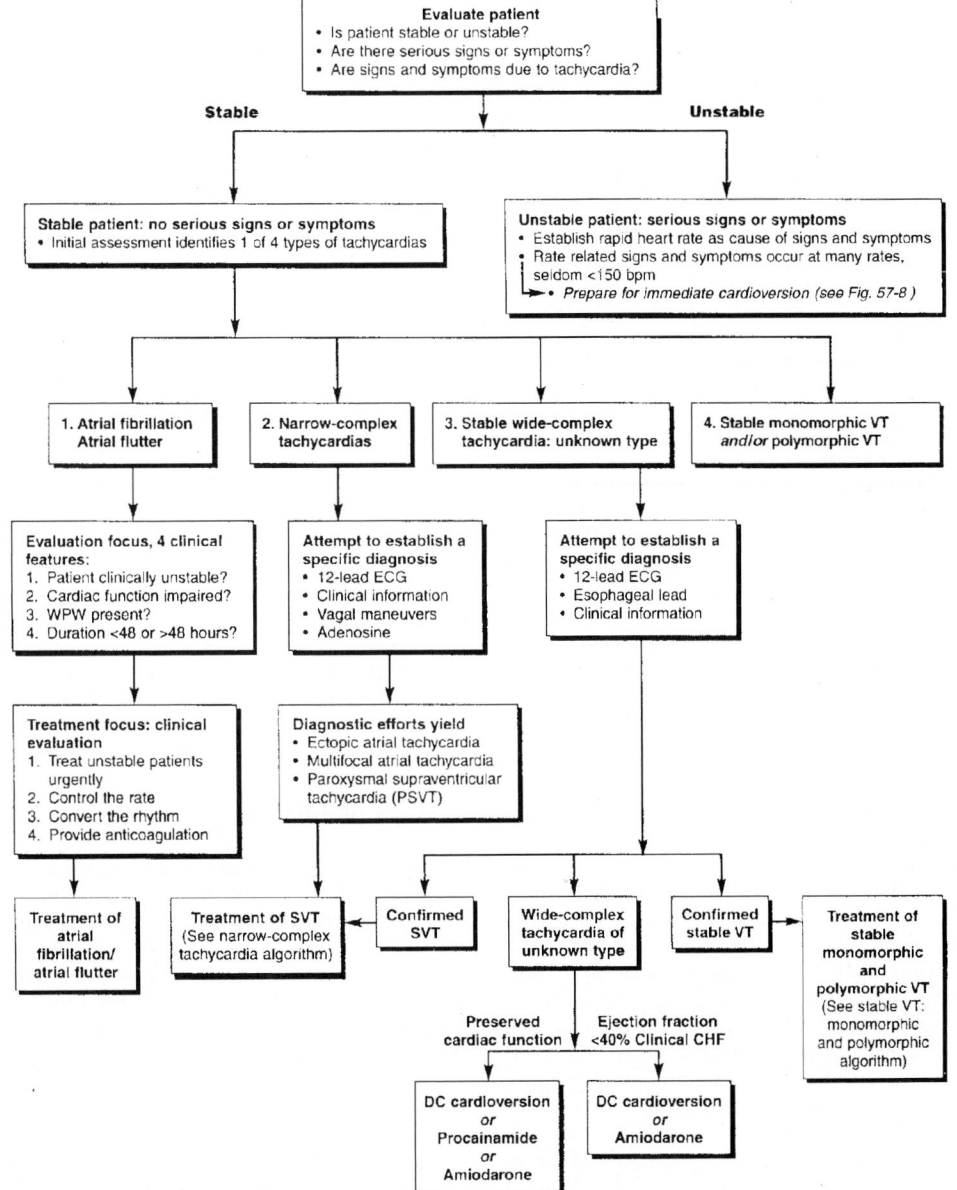

Figure 57-6. The tachycardia overview algorithm. (Reprinted with permission from American Heart Association: Guidelines 2000 for cardiopulmonary resuscitation and emergency cardiovascular care: International consensus on science. Circulation 102:I-159, 2000.)

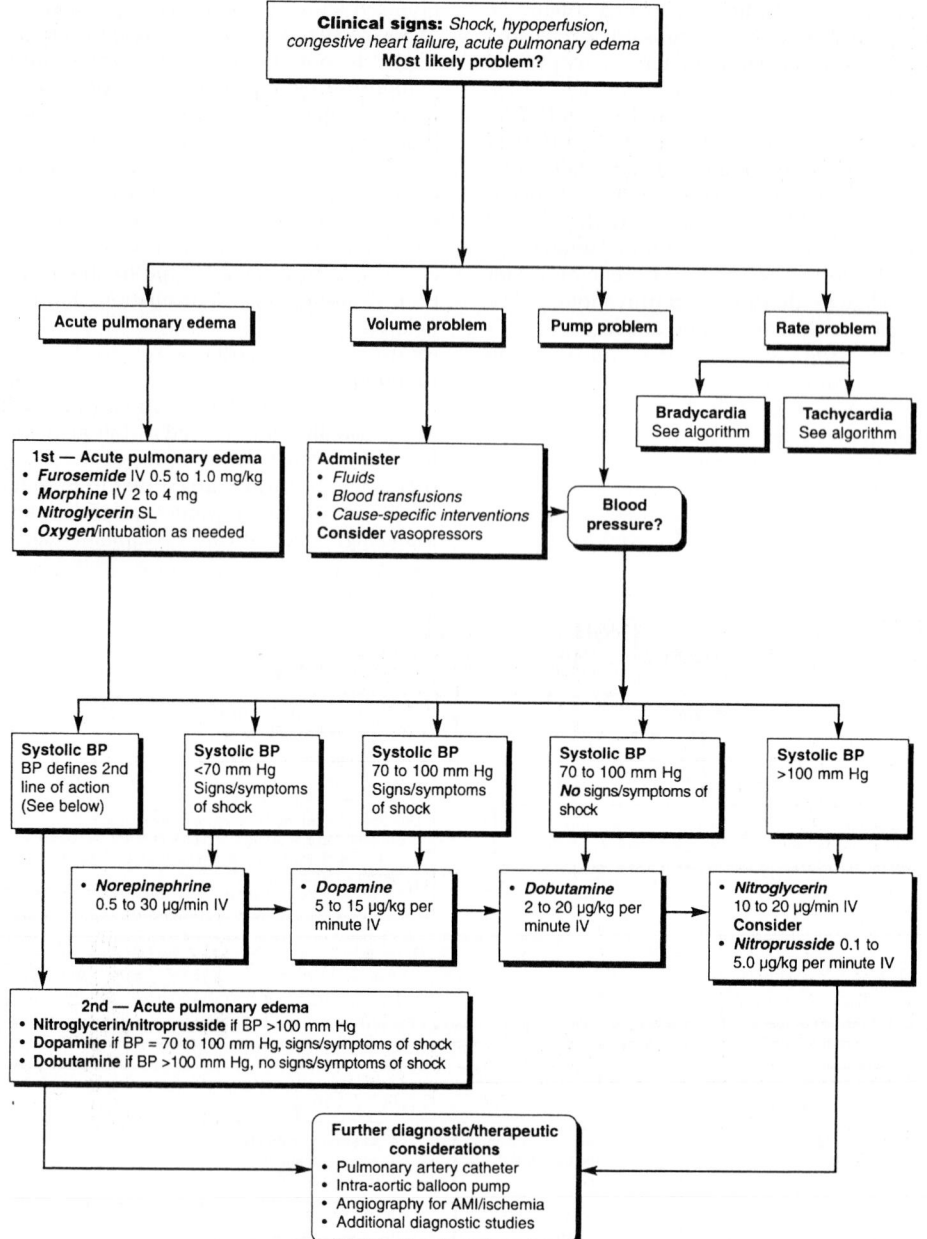

Figure 57-7. The acute pulmonary edema, hypotension, and shock algorithm. (Reprinted with permission from American Heart Association: Guidelines 2000 for cardiopulmonary resuscitation and emergency cardiovascular care: International concensus on science. Circulation 102: I-189, 2000.)

can be repeated as necessary for recurrent or resistant arrhythmias to a maximum total daily dose of 2 g. Lidocaine and bretylium are alternative therapies in refractory fibrillation. To rapidly achieve and maintain therapeutic blood levels of lidocaine during CPR, relatively large doses are necessary. An initial bolus of 1.5 mg · kg^{-1} should be given and additional boluses of 0.5–1.5 mg · kg^{-1} can be given every 5–10 min during CPR up to a total dose of 3 mg · kg^{-1}. Only bolus dosing should be used during CPR, but an infusion of 2–4 mg · min^{-1} can be started after successful resuscitation. If fibrillation persists or recurs after lidocaine therapy, bretylium tosylate can be given in an initial dose of 5 mg · kg^{-1} by iv bolus, followed by electrical defibrillation. If fibrillation persists, the dose can be increased to 10 mg · kg^{-1} and repeated at 5-min intervals for a total dose of 30–35 mg · kg^{-1}. Once the loading dose has been given, the drug can also be given as a continuous infusion at a rate of 1–2 mg · min^{-1}.

Sodium Bicarbonate

Although sodium bicarbonate was used as commonly as epinephrine during CPR in the past, there is little evidence to support its efficacy. Its use during resuscitation is supported by the theoretical considerations that acidosis lowers fibrillation threshold[197] and respiratory acidosis impairs the physiologic response to catecholamines.[198] One older animal study found improved success of resuscitation from prolonged ventricular fibrillation when bicarbonate therapy was added to epinephrine.[155] Most subsequent studies have failed to demonstrate improvement in success of defibrillation or resuscitation with the use of bicarbonate.[199–202] The lack of effect of buffer therapy may be partially explained by the slow onset of metabolic acidosis during cardiac arrest. As measured by blood lactate or base deficit, acidosis does not become severe for 15 or 20 min of cardiac arrest.[68,69,203]

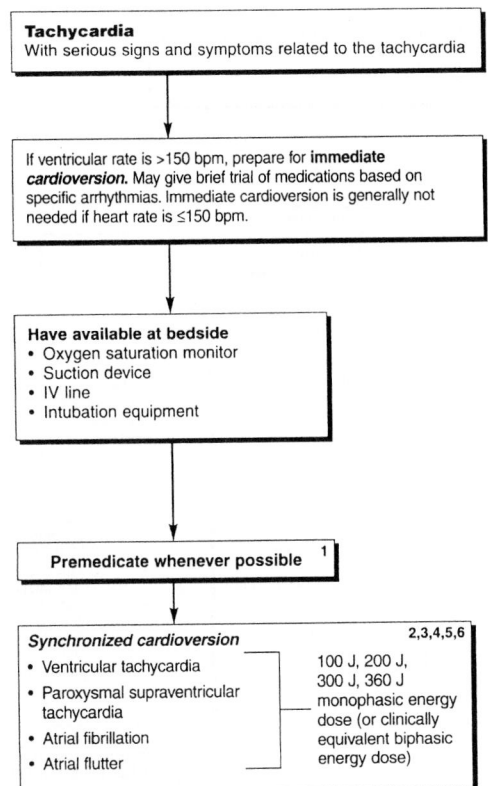

Tachycardia
With serious signs and symptoms related to the tachycardia

↓

If ventricular rate is >150 bpm, prepare for **immediate cardioversion.** May give brief trial of medications based on specific arrhythmias. Immediate cardioversion is generally not needed if heart rate is ≤150 bpm.

↓

Have available at bedside
• Oxygen saturation monitor
• Suction device
• IV line
• Intubation equipment

↓

Premedicate whenever possible   1

↓

Synchronized cardioversion   2,3,4,5,6
• Ventricular tachycardia
• Paroxysmal supraventricular tachycardia
• Atrial fibrillation
• Atrial flutter

100 J, 200 J, 300 J, 360 J monophasic energy dose (or clinically equivalent biphasic energy dose)

Figure 57-8. Synchronized cardioversion algorithm. (Reprinted with permission from American Heart Association: Guidelines 2000 for cardiopulmonary resuscitation and emergency cardiovascular care: International concensus on science. Circulation 102:I-164, 2000.)

In contrast to the lack of evidence that buffer therapy during CPR improves survival, the adverse effects of excessive sodium bicarbonate administration are well documented. In the past, metabolic alkalosis, hypernatremia, and hyperosmolarity were common after administration of bicarbonate during resuscitation attempts.[203,204] These abnormalities are associated with low resuscitation rates and poor outcome. However, if sodium bicarbonate is given judiciously according to standard recommendations, no significant metabolic abnormalities should occur.[205]

Intravenous sodium bicarbonate combines with hydrogen ion to produce carbonic acid which dissociates into CO_2 and water. The P_{CO_2} in blood is temporarily elevated until the excess CO_2 is eliminated through the lungs. Tissue acidosis during CPR is caused primarily by the low blood flow and accumulation of CO_2 in the tissues.[68,69] Therefore, concern has been expressed that the liberation of CO_2 by bicarbonate administration would only worsen the existing problem. This is of particular concern within myocardial cells and the brain. Carbon dioxide readily diffuses across cell membranes and the blood–brain barrier, whereas bicarbonate diffuses much more slowly. Thus, it is possible that sodium bicarbonate administration could result in a paradoxical worsening of intracellular and cerebral acidosis by further raising intracellular and cerebral CO_2 without a balancing increase in bicarbonate. Direct evidence for this effect has not been found. One study demonstrated an elevation in cerebral spinal fluid P_{CO_2} and reduction in pH could occur when very large doses of bicarbonate were given.[206] However, with clinically relevant doses, another study found no changes in spinal fluid acid–base status.[207] Measurement of myocardial intracellular pH during bicarbonate administration also has not detected a worsening in acidosis.[208] Therefore, paradoxical acidosis from sodium bicarbonate therapy remains a concern primarily on theoretical grounds.

Current practice restricts the use of sodium bicarbonate pri-

marily to arrests associated with hyperkalemia, severe preexisting metabolic acidosis, and tricyclic or phenobarbital overdose. It may be considered for use in protracted resuscitation attempts after other modalities have been instituted. When bicarbonate is used during CPR, the usual dose is $1 \text{ mEq} \cdot \text{kg}^{-1}$ initially with additional doses of $0.5 \text{ mEq} \cdot \text{kg}^{-1}$ every 10 min. However, dosing of sodium bicarbonate should be guided by blood gas determination whenever possible.

Atropine

Atropine sulfate enhances sinus node automaticity and atrioventricular conduction by its vagolytic effects. Although evidence for its efficacy is weak, atropine is frequently given during cardiac arrest associated with an ECG pattern of asystole or slow PEA. One animal study found methoxamine preferable to atropine for resuscitation of asphyxia-induced PEA.[209] Two clinical studies reported some success with atropine. Three of eight patients survived in-hospital asystolic arrest following atropine therapy.[210] In out-of-hospital asystolic arrest, atropine treatment was associated with improved resuscitation to hospital admission but not with survival to discharge.[211] Other investigators have observed no response to atropine in asystolic patients[212] or no difference in ECG rhythms or survival with or without atropine.[213]

The predominant cause of asystole and electromechanical dissociation is severe myocardial ischemia. Excessive parasympathetic tone probably contributes little to these rhythms during cardiac arrest in adults. Even in children, it is doubtful that parasympathetic tone plays a significant role during most arrests. Therefore, the most important treatment for asystole and electromechanical dissociation is effective chest compressions, ventilation, and epinephrine to improve coronary perfusion and myocardial oxygenation. However, cardiac arrest with these rhythms has a poor prognosis.[24] Because atropine has few adverse effects, it is recommended in arrest with asystole or PEA and refractory to epinephrine and oxygenation. The dose is 1.0 mg iv, repeated every 3–5 min up to a total of $0.04 \text{ mg} \cdot \text{kg}^{-1}$, which is totally vagolytic.[214,215] Full vagolytic doses may be associated with fixed mydriasis following successful resuscitation confounding neurologic examination. Occasionally, a sinus tachycardia following resuscitation may be due to the use of atropine during CPR.

Calcium

With normal cardiovascular physiology, calcium increases myocardial contractility and enhances ventricular automaticity. Consequently, it has been advocated for years as a treatment for asystole and PEA. It became firmly entrenched as a treatment for these rhythms following an early report by Kay and Blalock of success in four children following open heart surgery.[216] In retrospect, it is likely that these patients were hypocalcemic. Calcium use during CPR was further bolstered by the animal studies of Redding and Pearson showing moderate success with calcium chloride in asphyxial arrest.[13] However, these studies also showed vasopressors to be more successful than calcium. More recent animal studies have not found calcium to influence resuscitation rates or improve electromechanical coupling with pacing.[217] In 1981, Dembo reported dangerously high serum calcium levels (up to $18.2 \text{ mg} \cdot \text{dl}^{-1}$) during CPR and questioned the efficacy of calcium in cardiac arrest.[218] Subsequently, several retrospective studies and prospective clinical trials during out-of-hospital cardiac arrest showed that calcium was no better than placebo in promoting resuscitation and survival from asystole or EMD.[219–224] Consequently, because of potentially deleterious effects, calcium is not recommended during CPR unless specific indications exist. Calcium may prove useful if hyperkalemia, hypocalcemia, or calcium channel blocker toxicity is present. There are no other indications for its use during CPR. When calcium is administered, the chloride salt is recommended because it produces higher and more consistent

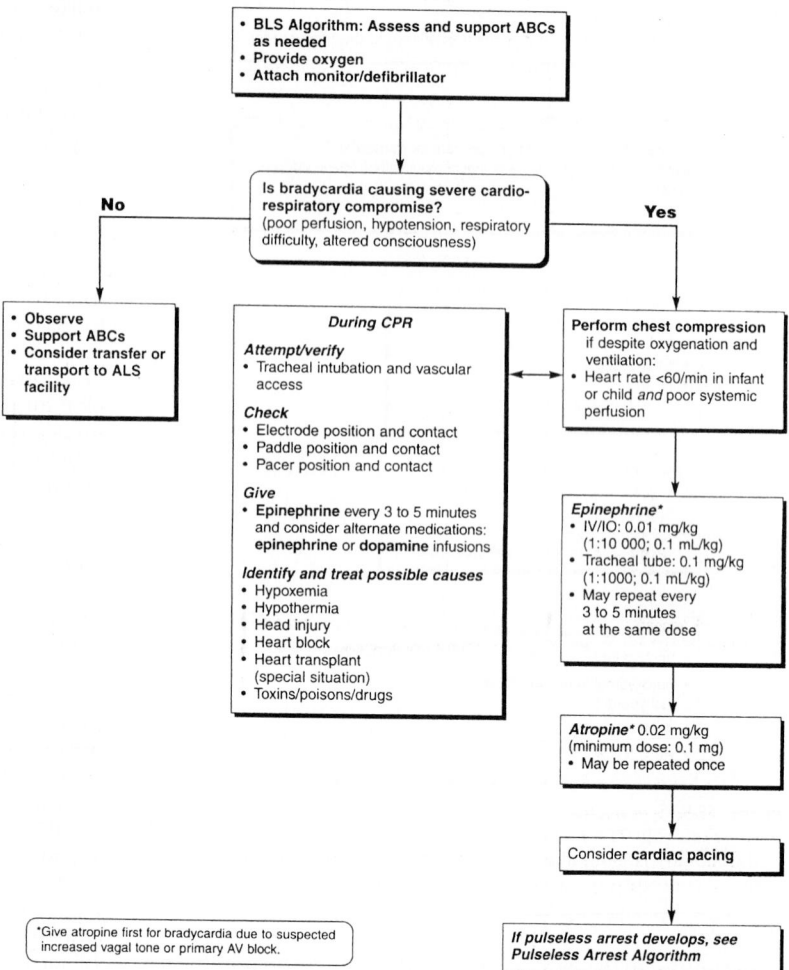

Figure 57-9. PALS (Pediatric Advanced Life Support) bradycardia algorithm. (Reprinted with permission from American Heart Association: Guidelines 2000 for cardiopulmonary resuscitation and emergency cardiovascular care: International concensus on science. Circulation 102:I-313, 2000.)

levels of ionized calcium than other salts. The usual dose is $2-4 \text{ mg} \cdot \text{kg}^{-1}$ of the 10% solution administered slowly intravenously. Calcium gluconate contains one-third as much molecular calcium as does calcium chloride and requires metabolism of gluconate in the liver.

PEDIATRIC CARDIOPULMONARY RESUSCITATION

The principles of CPR discussed previously apply to the child in cardiac arrest. Arrest is less likely to be a sudden event and more likely related to progressive deterioration of respiratory and circulatory function in the pediatric age group. Airway and ventilation problems lead to asystole and PEA as the most common presenting rhythms. However, the consequences of myocardial and cerebral ischemia are the same as for the adult. The basic approach to the arrest victim is the same (see Table 57-1). The specific anatomic and physiologic considerations necessary for the child will be familiar to anesthesiologists. The special circumstance of neonatal resuscitation has been discussed in other chapters.

The problem of airway management in the infant is well known to the anesthesiologist. Effective ventilation is especially critical because respiratory problems are frequently the cause for arrest. Mouth-to-mouth or mouth-to-nose and mouth (for infants) can be used as well as bag-valve mask devices until intubation is possible. Cardiac compression in the infant is provided with two fingers on the midsternum or by encircling the chest with the hands and using the thumbs to provide compression. For the small child, compression can be provided with one hand on the midsternum.

The algorithm for ACLS in the pediatric patient is shown in Figures 57-9 and 57-10. Although defibrillation is less frequently necessary in children, the same principles apply as in the adult. However, the recommended starting energy is $2 \text{ J} \cdot \text{kg}^{-1}$, which is doubled if defibrillation is unsuccessful. Considerations for drug administration are the same as for the adult except that the interosseous route in the anterior tibia provides an additional option in small children. Drug therapy is similar to the adult but plays a larger role because electrical therapy is less often needed (Figs. 57-9 to 57-11).

POSTRESUSCITATION CARE

The major factors contributing to mortality following successful resuscitation are progression of the primary disease and cerebral damage suffered as a result of the arrest. Active management following resuscitation appears to mitigate postischemic brain damage and improve neurologic outcome.[225] Although a significant number of patients have severe neurologic deficits following resuscitation, aggressive brain-oriented support does not seem to increase the proportion surviving in vegetative states. Most severely damaged victims die of multisystem failure within 1–2 weeks.

When flow is restored following a period of global brain ischemia, three stages of cerebral reperfusion are seen in the ensuing 12 hr. Immediately following resuscitation, there are multifocal areas of the brain with no reflow. Within 1 hr there is global hyperemia followed quickly by prolonged global hypoperfusion. Elevation of intracranial pressure is unusual following resuscitation from cardiac arrest. However, severe ischemic injury can lead to cerebral edema and increased intracranial pressure in the ensuing days.

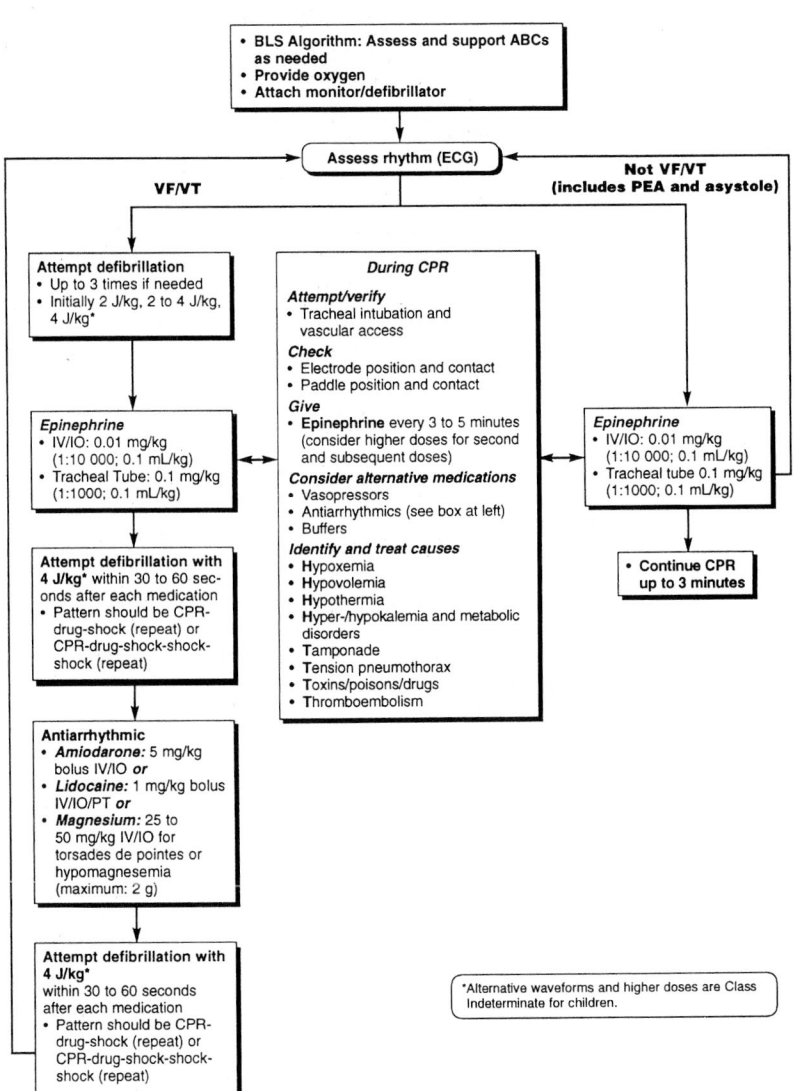

Figure 57-10. PALS pulseless arrest algorithm. (Reprinted with permission from American Heart Association: Guidelines 2000 for cardiopulmonary resuscitation and emergency cardiovascular care: International concensus on science. Circulation 102:I-311, 2000.)

Postresuscitation support is focused on providing stable oxygenation and hemodynamics to minimize any further cerebral insult. A comatose patient should be maintained on mechanical ventilation for several hours to ensure adequate oxygenation and ventilation. Restlessness, coughing, or seizure activity should be aggressively treated with appropriate medications including neuromuscular blockers, if necessary. Arterial Pao_2 should be maintained above 100 mm Hg and hypocapnia ($Paco_2$ < 30 mm Hg) should be avoided. Blood volume should be maintained normal and moderate hemodilution to a hematocrit of 30–35% may be helpful. A brief 5-min period of hypertension to mean arterial pressure of 120–140 mm Hg may help overcome the initial cerebral no reflow. This frequently occurs secondary to the effects of epinephrine given during CPR. Because cerebral autoregulation of blood flow is severely attenuated, both prolonged hypertension and hypotension are associated with a worsened outcome. Therefore, mean arterial pressure should be maintained at 90–110 mm Hg. Hyperglycemia during cerebral ischemia is known to result in increased neurologic damage. Although it is unknown if high serum glucose in the postresuscitation period influences outcome, it seems prudent to control glucose in the 100–250 mg · dl^{-1} range. Mild hypothermia that may occur during cardiac arrest and resuscitation should not be actively treated but induced hypothermia is not currently recommended.

In contrast to general supportive care, specific pharmacologic therapy directed at brain preservation has not been shown to have further benefit. Some animal trials of barbiturates were promising, but a large multicenter trial of thiopental found no improvement in neurologic status when this drug was given following cardiac arrest.[225] Similar results were found with calcium channel blockers. Animal studies were encouraging, but a clinical trial found no improvement in outcome.[226]

Prognosis

For the comatose survivor of CPR, the question of ultimate prognosis is important. One retrospective study demonstrated that the admission neurologic examination of comatose victims is highly correlated with the likelihood of awakening.[227] If there were no pupillary light response and no spontaneous eye movement and if the motor response to pain were absent or extensor posturing, there was only a 5% chance the patient would ever awaken. A companion study demonstrated that the chance of ever awakening fell rapidly in the days following arrest.[228] If the patient was not awake by 4 days following arrest, the chance of ever awakening was 20% and all those awakening had marked neurologic deficits. Most patients who completely recover show rapid improvement in the first 48 hr. There is also a high correlation between severity of neurologic injury and the level of creatine kinase-BB found in the cerebrospinal fluid.[229,230] Peak values of ≥25 IU are associated with severe neurologic damage and are reached 48–72 hr following arrest.

Drug	Dosage (Pediatric)	Remarks
Adenosine	0.1 mg/kg	Rapid IV/IO bolus
	Repeat dose: 0.2 mg/kg	Rapid flush to central circulation
	Maximum single dose: 12 mg	Monitor ECG during dose.
Amiodarone for pulseless VF/VT	5 mg/kg IV/IO	Rapid IV bolus
Amiodarone for perfusing tachycardias	Loading dose: 5 mg/kg IV/IO	IV over 20 to 60 minutes
	Maximum dose: 15 mg/kg per day	Routine use in combination with drugs prolonging QT interval is *not* recommended. Hypotension is most frequent side effect.
Atropine sulfate*	0.02 mg/kg	May give IV, IO or ET.
	Minimum dose: 0.1 mg	Tachycardia and pupil dilation may occur but *not* fixed dilated pupils.
	Maximum single dose: 0.5 mg in child, 1.0 mg in adolescent. May repeat once.	
Calcium chloride 10% = 100 mg/mL (=27.2 mg/mL elemental Ca)	20 mg/kg (0.2 mL/kg) IV/IO	Give slow IV push for hypocalcemia, hypermagnesemia, calcium channel blocker toxicity, preferably via central vein. Monitor heart rate; bradycardia may occur.
Calcium gluconate 10% = 100 mg/mL (=9 mg/mL elemental Ca)	60–100 mg/kg (0.6–1.0 mL/kg) IV/IO	Give slow IV push for hypocalcemia, hypermagnesemia, calcium channel blocker toxicity, preferably via central vein.
Epinephrine for symptomatic bradycardia*	IV/IO: 0.01 mg/kg (1:10 000, 0.1 mL/kg) ET: 0.1 mg/kg (1:1000, 0.1 mL/kg)	Tachyarrhythmias, hypertension may occur.
Epinephrine for pulseless arrest*	First dose:	
	IV/IO: 0.01 mg/kg (1:10 000, 0.1 mL/kg)	
	ET: 0.1 mg/kg (1:1000, 0.1 mL/kg)	
	Subsequent doses: Repeat initial dose or may increase up to 10 times (0.1 mg/kg, 1:1000, 0.1 mL/kg)	
	Administer epinephrine every 3 to 5 minutes.	
	IV/IO/ET doses as high as 0.2 mg/kg of 1:1000 may be effective.	
Glucose (10% or 25% or 50%)	IV/IO: 0.5–1.0 g/kg	For suspected hypoglycemia; avoid hyperglycemia.
	• 1–2 mL/kg 50%	
	• 2–4 mL/kg 25%	
	• 5–10 mL/kg 10%	
Lidocaine*	IV/IO/ET: 1 mg/kg	Rapid bolus
Lidocaine infusion (start after a bolus)	IV/IO: 20–50 µg/kg per minute	1 to 2.5 mL/kg per hour of 120 mg/100 mL solution or use "Rule of 6" (see Table 3)
Magnesium sulfate (500 mg/mL)	IV/IO: 25–50 mg/kg, Maximum dose: 2 g per dose	Rapid IV infusion for torsades or suspected hypomagnesemia; 10- to 20-minute infusion for asthma that responds poorly to β-adrenergic agonists.
Naloxone*	≤5 years or ≤20 kg: 0.1 mg/kg	For total reversal of narcotic effect. Use small repeated doses (0.01 to 0.03 mg/kg) titrated to desired effect.
	>5 years or >20 kg: 2.0 mg	
Procainamide for perfusing tachycardias (100 mg/mL and 500 mg/mL)	Loading dose: 15 mg/kg IV/IO	Infusion over 30 to 60 minutes; routine use in combination with drugs prolonging QT interval is *not* recommended.
Sodium bicarbonate (1 mEq/mL and 0.5 mEq/mL)	IV/IO: 1 mEq/kg per dose	Infuse slowly and only if ventilation is adequate.

IV indicates intravenous; IO, intraosseous; and ET, endotracheal.
*For endotracheal administration use higher doses (2 to 10 times the IV dose); dilute medication with normal saline to a volume of 3 to 5 mL and follow with several positive-pressure ventilations.

Figure 57-11. PALS medications for cardiac arrest and symptomatic arrhythmias. (Reprinted with permission from American Heart Association: Guidelines 2000 for cardiopulmonary resuscitation and emergency cardiovascular care: International concensus on science. Circulation 102:I-308, 2000.)

REFERENCES

1. Wood Library Museum: Resuscitation: An Historical Perspective. Park Ridge, Illinois, Wood Library Museum, 1976
2. Brooks DK: Resuscitation: Care of the Critically Ill. London, Edward Arnold, 1986
3. Vesalius A: *De Humani Corporis.* Basel, Fabrica, 1543
4. Elam JO, Brown ES, Elder JD Jr: Artificial respiration by mouth to mask method: A study of the respiratory gas exchange of paralyzed patients ventilated by operator's expired air. N Engl J Med 250:749, 1954
5. Gordon AS, Frye CS, Gittelson L *et al:* Mouth-to-mouth versus manual artificial respiration for children and adults. JAMA 167:320, 1958
6. Safar P, Escarraga LA, Elam JO: A comparison of the mouth-to-mouth and mouth-to-airway methods of artificial respiration with the chest-pressure arm-lift methods. N Engl J Med 258:671, 1958
7. Safar P: Failure of manual respiration. J Appl Physiol 14:84, 1959
8. Hooker DR, Kouwenhoven WB, Langworthy OR: The effects of alternating current on the heart. Am J Physiol 103:444, 1933
9. Beck CS, Pritchard WH, Feil HS: Ventricular fibrillation of long duration abolished by electric shock. JAMA 135:985, 1947
10. Zoll PM, Linenthal AJ, Gibson W *et al:* Termination of ventricular fibrillation in man by an externally applied electric shock. N Engl J Med 254:727, 1956
11. Kouwenhoven WB, Milnor WR, Knickerbocker GG, Chestnut WR: Closed-chest defibrillation of the heart. Surgery 42:550, 1957
12. Kouwenhoven WB, Jude JR, Knickerbocker GG: Closed-chest cardiac massage. JAMA 173:1064, 1960
13. Redding JS, Pearson JW: Evaluation of drugs for cardiac resuscitation. Anesthesiology 24:203, 1963
14. National Heart Lung and Blood Institute: Morbidity and Mortality Chartbook on Cardiovascular, Lung and Blood Diseases 1990. Bethesda, Maryland, National Heart Lung and Blood Institute, 1990
15. Angelos M, Safar P, Reich H: A comparison of cardiopulmonary resuscitation with cardiopulmonary bypass after prolonged cardiac arrest in dogs: Reperfusion pressures and neurologic recovery. Resuscitation 21:121, 1991

16. Kern KB, Sanders AB, Janas W et al: Limitations of open-chest cardiac massage after prolonged, untreated cardiac arrest in dogs. Ann Emerg Med 20:761, 1991

17. Copley DP, Mantle JA, Rogers WJ et al: Improved outcome for prehospital cardiopulmonary collapse with resuscitation by bystanders. Circulation 56:901, 1977

18. Eisenberg MS, Bergner L, Hallstrom A: Cardiac resuscitation in the community: Importance of rapid provision and implications for program planning. JAMA 241:1905, 1979

19. Weaver WD, Cobb LA, Hallstrom AP et al: Factors influencing survival after out-of-hospital cardiac arrest. J Am Coll Cardiol 7:752, 1986

20. Eisenberg MS, Copass MK, Halstrom AP et al: Treatment of out-of-hospital cardiac arrest with rapid defibrillation by emergency medical technicians. N Engl J Med 302:1379, 1980

21. Weaver WD, Hill D, Fahrenbruch CE et al: Use of the automatic external defibrillator in the management of out-of-hospital cardiac arrest. N Engl J Med 319:661, 1988

22. Taffet BE, Teasdale TA, Luchi RJ: In-hospital cardiopulmonary resuscitation. JAMA 260:2069, 1988

23. Olsson GI, Hallen B: Cardiac arrest during anaesthesia: A computer-aided study of 250,543 anaesthetics. Acta Anaesthesiol Scand 32:653, 1988

24. Emergency Cardiac Care Committee and Subcommittees, American Heart Association: Guidelines for cardiopulmonary resuscitation and emergency cardiac care. JAMA 268:2171, 1992

25. Cohen CB, Cohen PJ: Do-not-resuscitate orders in the operating room. N Engl J Med 325:1879, 1991

26. Walker RM: DNR in the OR: Resuscitation as an operative risk. JAMA 266:2407, 1991

27. Margolis JO, McGrath BJ, Kussin PS, Schwinn DA: Do no resuscitate (DNR) orders during surgery: Ethical foundations for institutional policies in the United States. Anesth Analg 80:806, 1995

28. Guildner CW: Resuscitation. Opening the airway: A comparative study of techniques for opening an airway obstructed by the tongue. JACEP 5:588, 1976

29. Haugen RK: The cafe coronary: Sudden deaths in restaurants. JAMA 186:142, 1963

30. Heimlich HJ: Pop goes the cafe coronary. Emerg Med 6:154, 1974

31. Guildner CW, Williams D, Subtich T: Airway obstructed by foreign material: The Heimlich maneuver. JACEP 5:675, 1976

32. Heimlich HJ, Hoffmann KA, Canestri FR: Food-choking and drowning deaths prevented by external subdiaphragmatic compression: Physiological basis. Ann Thorac Surg 20:188, 1975

33. Gordon AS, Belton MK, Ridolpho PF: Emergency management of foreign body airway obstruction: Comparison of artificial cough techniques, manual extrication maneuvers and simple mechanical devices. In Safar P (ed): Advances in Cardiopulmonary Resuscitation, p 39. New York, Springer-Verlag, 1977

34. Redding JS: The choking controversy: Critique of evidence on the Heimlich maneuver. Crit Care Med 7:475, 1979

35. Day RL, Crelin ES, Dubois AB: Choking: The Heimlich abdominal thrust vs back blows: An approach to measurement of inertial and aerodynamic forces. Pediatrics 70:113, 1982

36. Bossaert L, Van Hoeyweghen R, The Cerebral Resuscitation Study Group: Bystander cardiopulmonary resuscitation (CPR) in out-of-hospital cardiac arrest. Resuscitation 17(suppl):S55, 1989

37. Van Hoeyweghen RJ, Bossaert LL, Mullie A et al: Quality and efficiency of bystander CPR. Resuscitation 26:47, 1993

38. Berg RA, Kern KB, Sanders AB et al: Bystander cardiopulmonary resuscitation: Is ventilation necessary? Circulation 88:1907, 1993

39. Berg RA, Wilcoxson D, Hilwig RW et al: The need for ventilatory support during bystander cardiopulmonary resuscitation. Ann Emerg Med 26:342, 1995

40. Berg RA, Kern KB, Hilwig RW et al: Assisted ventilation does not improve outcome in a porcine model of single-rescuer bystander cardiopulmonary resuscitation. Circulation 95:1635, 1997

41. Berg RA, Kern KB, Hilwig RW et al: Assisted ventilation during 'bystander' CPR in a swine acute myocardial infarction model does not improve outcome. Circulation 96:4364, 1997

42. Berg RA, Hilwig RW, Kern KB et al: Simulate mouth-to-mouth ventilation and chest compressions ('bystander' CPR) improves outcome in a swine model of prehospital pediatric asphyxial cardiac arrest. Crit Care Med 27:1893, 1999

43. Ornato JP, Hallagan LF, McMahan SB et al: Attitudes of BCLS instructors about mouth-to-mouth resuscitation during the AIDS epidemic. Ann Emerg Med 19:151, 1990

44. Brenner BE, Kauffman J: Reluctance of internists and medical nurses to perform mouth-to-mouth resuscitation. Arch Intern Med 153:1763, 1993

45. Locke CJ, Berg RA, Sanders AB et al: Bystander cardiopulmonary resuscitation: Concerns about mouth-to-mouth contact. Arch Intern Med 155:938, 1995

46. Ruben H, Knudsen EJ, Carugati G: Gastric insufflation in relation to airway pressure. Acta Anaesthesiol Scand 5:107, 1961

47. Melker RJ: Recommendation for ventilation during cardiopulmonary resuscitation: Time for change? Crit Care Med 13:882, 1985

48. Sellick BA: Cricoid pressure to control regurgitation of stomach contents during induction of anaesthesia. Lancet 2:404, 1961

49. Salem MR, Wong AY, Fizzotti GF: Efficacy of cricoid pressure in preventing aspiration of gastric contents in paediatric patients. Br J Anaesth 44:401, 1972

50. Harrison RR, Maull KI, Keenan RL, Boyan CP: Mouth-to-mask ventilation: A superior method of rescue breathing. Ann Emerg Med 11:74, 1982

51. Jesudian MCS, Harrison RR, Keenan RL, Maull KI: Bag-valve-mask ventilation; two rescuers are better than one: Preliminary report. Crit Care Med 13:122, 1985

52. Babbs CF: New versus old theories of blood flow during CPR. Crit Care Med 8:191, 1980

53. Jude JR, Kouwenhoven WB, Knickerbocker GG: Cardiac arrest. Report of application of external cardiac massage on 118 patients. JAMA 178:1063, 1961

54. Deshmukh HG, Weil MH, Rackow ED et al: Echocardiographic observations during cardiopulmonary resuscitation: A preliminary report. Crit Care Med 13:904, 1985

55. Luce JM, Ross BK, O'Quinn RJ et al: Regional blood flow during cardiopulmonary resuscitation in dogs using simultaneous and nonsimultaneous compression and ventilation. Circulation 67:258, 1983

56. Kern KB, Carter AB, Showen RL et al: Twenty-four-hour survival in a canine model of cardiac arrest comparing three methods of manual cardiopulmonary resuscitation. J Am Coll Cardiol 7:859, 1986

57. Kern KB, Carter AB, Showen RL et al: Comparison of mechanical techniques of cardiopulmonary resuscitation: Survival and neurologic outcome in dogs. Am J Emerg Med 5:190, 1987

58. Weale FE, Rothwell-Jackson RL: The efficacy of cardiac massage. Lancet 1:990, 1962

59. MacKenzie GJ, Taylor SH, McDonald AH, Donald KW: Haemodynamic effects of external cardiac compression. Lancet 1:1342, 1964

60. Criley JM, Blaufuss AH, Kissel GL: Cough-induced cardiac compression: Self-administered form of cardiopulmonary resuscitation. JAMA 236:1246, 1976

61. Taylor GJ, Tucker WM, Greene HL et al: Importance of prolonged compression during cardiopulmonary resuscitation in man. N Engl J Med 296:1515, 1977

62. Rudikoff MJ, Maughan WL, Effrom M et al: Mechanisms of blood flow during cardiopulmonary resuscitation. Circulation 61:345, 1980

63. Holmes HR, Babbs CF, Voorhees WD et al: Influence of adrenergic drugs upon vital organ perfusion during CPR. Crit Care Med 8:137, 1980

64. Michael JR, Guerci AD, Koehler RC et al: Mechanisms by which epinephrine augments cerebral and myocardial perfusion during cardiopulmonary resuscitation in dogs. Circulation 69:822, 1984

65. Criley JM, Niemann JT, Rosborough JP, Hausknecht M: Modifications of cardiopulmonary resuscitation based on the cough. Circulation 74(suppl 4):42, 1986

66. Chandra N, Rudikoff M, Weisfeldt ML: Simultaneous chest compression and ventilation at high airway pressure during cardiopulmonary resuscitation. Lancet 1:175, 1980

67. Chandra N, Snyder LD, Weisfeldt ML: Abdominal binding during cardiopulmonary resuscitation in man. JAMA 246:351, 1981

68. Weil MH, Rackow EC, Trevino R et al: Difference in acid–base state between venous and arterial blood during cardiopulmonary resuscitation. N Engl J Med 315:153, 1986

69. Weil MH, Grundler W, Yamaguchi M et al: Arterial blood gases fail to reflect acid-base status during cardiopulmonary resuscitation: A preliminary report. Crit Care Med 13:884, 1985

70. Maier GW, Newton JR, Wolfe JA et al: The influence of manual chest compression rate of hemodynamic support during cardiac

massage: High-impulse cardiopulmonary resuscitation. Circulation 74(suppl 4):51, 1986

71. Ewy GA: Alternative approaches to external chest compression. Circulation 74(suppl 4):98, 1986

72. Harris LD, Kirimli B, Safar P: Augmentation of artificial circulation during cardiopulmonary resuscitation. Anesthesiology 28:730, 1967

73. Redding JS: Abdominal compression in cardiopulmonary resuscitation. Anesth Analg 50:668, 1971

74. Bircher N, Safar P, Stewart R: A comparison of standard, MAST-augmented, and open-chest CPR in dogs. A preliminary investigation. Crit Care Med 8:147, 1980

75. Niemann JT, Rosborough JP, Ung S, Criley JM: Coronary perfusion pressure during experimental cardiopulmonary resuscitation. Ann Emerg Med 11:127, 1982

76. Sanders AB, Ewy GA, Alferness CA et al: Failure of one method of simultaneous chest compression, ventilation and abdominal binding during CPR. Crit Care Med 10:509, 1982

77. Niemann JT, Rosborough JP, Criley JM: Continuous external counterpressure during closed-chest resuscitation: A critical appraisal of the military antishock trouser garment and abdominal binder. Circulation 74(suppl 4):102, 1986

78. Niemann JT, Rosborough JP, Ung S, Criley JM: Hemodynamic effects of continuous abdominal binding during cardiac arrest and resuscitation. Am J Cardiol 53:269, 1984

79. Sharff JA, Pantley G, Noel E: Effect of time on regional organ perfusion during two methods of cardiopulmonary resuscitation. Ann Emerg Med 13:649, 1984

80. Kirscher JP, Fine EG, Weisfeld ML et al: Comparison of prehospital conventional and simultaneous compression–ventilation cardiopulmonary resuscitation. Crit Care Med 17:1263, 1989

81. Ohomoto T, Miura I, Konno S: A new method of external cardiac massage to improve diastolic augmentation and prolong survival time. Ann Thorac Surg 21:284, 1976

82. Babbs CF, Tacker WA: Cardiopulmonary resuscitation with interposed abdominal compression. Circulation 74(suppl 4):37, 1986

83. Ralston SH, Babbs CF, Niebauer MJ: Cardiopulmonary resuscitation with interposed abdominal compression in dogs. Anesth Analg 61:645, 1982

84. Voorhees WD, Ralston SH, Babbs CF: Regional blood flow during cardiopulmonary resuscitation with abdominal counterpulsation in dogs. Am J Emerg Med 2:123, 1984

85. Mateer JF, Stueven HA, Thompson BM et al: Pre-hospital IAC-CPR versus standard CPR: Paramedic resuscitation of cardiac arrests. Am J Emerg Med 3:143, 1985

86. Sack JB, Kesselbrenner MB, Bregman D: Survival from in-hospital cardiac arrest with interposed abdominal counterpulsation during cardiopulmonary resuscitation. JAMA 267:379, 1992

87. Niemann JT, Rosborough JP, Criley JM, Niskanen RA: Circulatory support during cardiac arrest using a pneumatic vest and abdominal binder with simultaneous high pressure airway inflation. Ann Emerg Med 13:767, 1984

88. Niemann JT, Rosborough JP, Niskanen RA et al: Mechanical 'cough' cardiopulmonary resuscitation during cardiac arrest in dogs. Am J Cardiol 55:199, 1985

89. Halperin HR, Tsitlik JE, Belfand M et al: A preliminary study of cardiopulmonary resuscitation by circumferential compression of the chest with use of a pneumatic vest. N Engl J Med 329:762, 1993

90. Maier GW, Tyson GS, Olsen CO et al: The physiology of external cardiac massage: High-impulse cardiopulmonary resuscitation. Circulation 70:86, 1984

91. Lurie KG, Lindo C, Chin J: CPR: The P stands for plumber's helper (letter). JAMA 264:1661, 1990

92. Cohen TJ, Tucker KJ, Lurie KG et al: Active compression–decompression. A new method of cardiopulmonary resuscitation. JAMA 267:2916, 1992

93. Linder KH, Pfenniger EG, Lurie KG et al: Effects of active compression–decompression resuscitation on myocardial and cerebral blood flow in pigs. Circulation 88:1254, 1993

94. Shultz JJ, Coffeen P, Sweeney M et al: Evaluation of standard and active compression–decompression CPR in an acute human model of ventricular fibrillation. Circulation 89:684, 1994

95. Cohen TJ, Goldner BG, Maccaro PC et al: A comparison of active compression-decompression cardiopulmonary resuscitation for cardiac arrests occurring in the hospital. N Engl J Med 329:1918, 1993

96. Lurie KG, Shultz JJ, Callaham ML et al: Evaluation of active compression-decompression CPR in victims of out-of-hospital cardiac arrest. JAMA 271:1405, 1994

97. Schwab TM, Callaham ML, Madsen CD et al: A randomized clinical trial of active compression–decompression CPR vs standard CPR in out-of-hospital cardiac arrest in two cities. JAMA 273:1261, 1995

98. DeBehnke DJ, Angelos MG, Leasure JE: Comparison of standard external CPR, open-chest CPR, and cardiopulmonary bypass in a canine myocardial infarct model. Ann Emerg Med 20:754, 1991

99. Reichman RT, Joyo CI, Dembitsky WP et al: Improved patient survival after cardiac arrest using a cardiopulmonary support system. Ann Thorac Surg 49:101, 1990

100. Hartz R, LoCicero J, Sanders JH et al: Clinical experience with portable cardiopulmonary bypass in cardiac arrest patients. Ann Thorac Surg 50:437, 1990

101. Mooney MR, Arom KV, Joyce LD et al: Emergency cardiopulmonary bypass support in patients with cardiac arrest. J Thorac Cardiovasc Surg 101:450, 1991

102. Sanders AB, Kern KB, Atlas M et al: Importance of the duration of inadequate coronary perfusion pressure on resuscitation from cardiac arrest. J Am Coll Cardiol 6:113, 1985

103. Kern KB, Sanders AB, Badylak SF et al: Longterm survival with open-chest cardiac massage after ineffective closed-chest compression in a canine preparation. Circulation 75:498, 1987

104. Coletti RH, Hartjen B, Gozdziewski S et al: Origin of canine femoral pulses during standard CPR. Crit Care Med 11:218, 1983

105. Ralston SH, Voorhees WD, Babbs CF: Intrapulmonary epinephrine during prolonged CPR: Improved regional blood flow and resuscitation in dogs. Ann Emerg Med 13:79, 1984

106. Crile G, Dolley DH: Experimental research into resuscitation of dogs killed by anesthetics and asphyxia. J Exp Med 8:713 , 1906

107. Pearson JW, Redding JS: Influence of peripheral vascular tone on cardiac resuscitation. Anesth Analg 44:746, 1965

108. Yakaitis RW, Otto CW, Blitt CD: Relative importance of alpha and beta adrenergic receptors during resuscitation. Crit Care Med 7:293, 1979

109. Otto CW, Yakaitis RW, Blitt CD: Mechanism of action of epinephrine in resuscitation from asphyxial arrest. Crit Care Med 9:321, 1981

110. Ditchey RV, Winkler JV, Rhodes CA: Relative lack of coronary blood flow during closed-chest resuscitation in dogs. Circulation 66:297, 1982

111. Otto CW, Yakaitis RW: The role of epinephrine in CPR: A reappraisal. Ann Emerg Med 13:840, 1984

112. Sanders AB, Ewy GA, Taft TV: Prognostic and therapeutic importance of the aortic diastolic pressure in resuscitation from cardiac arrest. Crit Care Med 12:871, 1984

113. Niemann JT, Criley JM, Rosborough JP et al: Predictive indices of successful cardiac resuscitation after prolonged arrest and experimental cardiopulmonary resuscitation. Ann Emerg Med 14:521, 1985

114. Paradis NA, Martin GB, Rivers EP et al: Coronary perfusion pressure and the return of spontaneous circulation in human cardiopulmonary resuscitation. JAMA 263:1106, 1990

115. Kalenda Z: The capnogram as a guide to the efficacy of cardiac massage. Resuscitation 6:259, 1978

116. Weil MH, Bisera J, Trevino RP: Cardiac output and end tidal carbon dioxide. Crit Care Med 13:907, 1985

117. Sanders AB, Atlas M, Ewy GA et al: Expired P_{CO_2} as an index of coronary perfusion pressure. Am J Emerg Med 3:147, 1985

118. Sanders AB, Ewy GA, Bragg S et al: Expired P_{CO_2} as a prognostic indicator of successful resuscitation from cardiac arrest. Ann Emerg Med 14:948, 1985

119. Trevino RP, Bisera J, Weil MH et al: End-tidal CO_2 as a guide to successful cardiopulmonary resuscitation: A preliminary report. Crit Care Med 13:910, 1985

120. Sanders AB, Kern KB, Otto CW et al: End-tidal carbon dioxide monitoring during cardiopulmonary resuscitation: A prognostic indicator for survival. JAMA 262:1347, 1989

121. Levine RL, Wayne MA, Miller CC: End-tidal carbon dioxide and outcome of out-of-hospital cardiac arrest. N Engl J Med 337:301, 1997

122. Kern KB, Sanders AB, Raife J et al: A study of chest compression rates during cardiopulmonary resuscitation in humans: The importance of rate-directed compressions. Arch Intern Med 152:145, 1992

123. Kerber RE, Sarnat W: Factors influencing the success of ventricular defibrillation in man. Circulation 60:226, 1979

124. Yakaitis RW, Ewy GA, Otto CW et al: Influence of time and therapy on ventricular defibrillation in dogs. Crit Care Med 8:157, 1980

125. Weaver WD, Copass MD, Bufi D et al: Improved neurologic recovery and survival after early defibrillation. Circulation 69:943, 1984

126. Weaver WD, Cobb LA, Dennis D et al: Amplitude of ventricular fibrillation waveform and outcome after cardiac arrest. Ann Intern Med 102:53, 1985

127. Ewy GA, Dahl CF, Zimmermann M, Otto CW: Ventricular fibrillation masquerading as ventricular standstill. Crit Care Med 9: 841, 1981

128. Otto CW, Yakaitis RW, Ewy GA: Effects of epinephrine on defibrillation in ischemic ventricular fibrillation. Am J Emerg Med 3:285, 1985

129. Cummins RO, Eisenberg MS, Bergner L, Murray JA: Sensitivity, accuracy and safety of an automatic external defibrillator: Report of a field evaluation. Lancet 1:318, 1984

130. Cummins RO, Eisenberg MS, Graves JR et al: Automatic external defibrillators used by emergency medical technicians: A controlled clinical trial. Circulation 72(suppl 3):8, 1985

131. Ewy GA: Electrical therapy for cardiovascular emergencies. Circulation 74(suppl 4):111, 1986

132. Ewy GA, Ewy MD, Silverman J: Determinants of human transthoracic resistance to direct current discharge. Circulation 46(suppl 2):150, 1972

133. Kerber RE, Grayzel J, Hoyt R et al: Transthoracic resistance in human defibrillation: Influence of body weight, chest size, serial shocks, paddle size and paddle contact pressure. Circulation 63:676, 1981

134. Connel PN, Ewy GA, Dahl CF, Ewy MD: Transthoracic impedance to defibrillation discharge: Effect of electrode size and electrode-chest wall interface. J Electrocardiol 6:313, 1973

135. Ewy GA, Taren D: Comparison of paddle electrode pastes used for defibrillation. Heart Lung 6:847, 1977

136. Geddes LA, Tacker WA, Cabler P et al: The decrease in transthoracic impedance during successive ventricular defibrillation trials. Med Instrum 9:179, 1975

137. Dahl CF, Ewy GA, Ewy MD, Thomas ED: Transthoracic impedance to direct current discharge: Effect of repeated countershocks. Med Instrum 10:151, 1976

138. Ewy GA, Hellman DA, McClung S, Taren D: Influence of ventilation phase on transthoracic impedance and defibrillation effectiveness. Crit Care Med 8:164, 1980

139. Kerber RE, Kouba C, Marines J et al: Advance prediction of transthoracic impedance in human defibrillation and cardioversion: Importance of impedance in determining the success of low-energy shocks. Circulation 70:303, 1984

140. Kerber RE, McPherson D, Charbonnier R et al: Automatic impedance-based energy adjustment for defibrillation: Experimental studies. Circulation 71:136, 1985

141. Lerman BB, DeMarco JP, Haines DE: Current-based versus energy-based ventricular defibrillation: a prospective study. J Am Coll Cardiol 12:1259, 1988

142. Dahl CF, Ewy GA, Warner ED, Thomas ED: Myocardial necrosis from direct current countershock. Circulation 50:956, 1974

143. Warner ED, Dahl CF, Ewy GA: Myocardial injury from transthoracic defibrillator countershock. Arch Path 99:55, 1975

144. Ehsani A, Ewy GA, Sobel BE: Effects of electrical countershock on serum creatine phosphokinase (CPK) isoenzyme activity. Am J Cardiol 37:12, 1976

145. Weaver WD, Cobb LA, Copass MK et al: Ventricular defibrillation: A comparative trial using 175-J and 320-J shocks. N Engl J Med 307:1101, 1982

146. Geddes LA, Tacker WA, Rosborough JP et al: Electrical dose for ventricular defibrillation of large and small animals using precordial electrodes. J Clin Invest 53:310, 1974

147. Gutgesell HP, Tacker WA, Geddes LA et al: Energy dose for defibrillation in children. Pediatrics 58:898, 1976

148. Kerber RE, Sarnat W: Factors influencing the success of ventricular defibrillation in man. Circulation 60:226, 1979

149. Pantridge JR, Adgey AAJ, Webb SW, Anderson J: Electrical requirement for ventricular defibrillation. Br Med J 2:313, 1975

150. Adgey AA: Electrical energy requirement for ventricular defibrillation. Br Heart J 40:1197, 1978

151. Crampton JA, Crampton RS, Sipes JN, Cherwek ML: Energy levels and patient weight in ventricular defibrillation. JAMA 242:1380, 1979

152. Gascho JA, Crampton RS, Cherwek ML et al: Determinants of ventricular defibrillation in adults. Circulation 60:231, 1979

153. Kerber RE, Jensen SR, Gascho JA et al: Determinants of defibrillation: Prospective analysis of 183 patients. Am J Cardiol 52:739, 1983

154. Otto CW: Cardiovascular pharmacology II: The use of catecholamines, pressor agents, digitalis, and corticosteroids in CPR and emergency cardiac care. Circulation 74(suppl 4):80, 1986

155. Redding JS, Pearson JW: Resuscitation from ventricular fibrillation (drug therapy). JAMA 203:255, 1968

156. Schleien CL, Dean JM, Koehler RC et al: Effect of epinephrine on cerebral and myocardial perfusion in an infant animal preparation of cardiopulmonary resuscitation. Circulation 73:809, 1986

157. Schleien CL, Koehler RC, Gervais H et al: Organ blood flow and somatosensory-evoked potentials during and after cardiopulmonary resuscitation with epinephrine or phenylephrine. Circulation 79:1332, 1989

158. Otto CW, Yakaitis RW, Redding JS, Blitt CD: Comparison of dopamine, dobutamine, and epinephrine in CPR. Crit Care Med 9:640, 1981

159. Lindner KH, Brinkmann A, Pfenninger EG et al: Effect of vasopressin on hemodynamic variables, organ blood flow, and acid–base status in a pig model of cardiopulmonary resuscitation. Anesth Analg 77:427, 1993

160. Lindner KH, Prengel AW, Pfenniger EG et al: Vasopressin improves vital organ blood flow during closed-chest cardiopulmonary resuscitation in pigs. Circulation 91:215, 1995

161. Livesay JJ, Follette DM, Fey KH et al: Optimizing myocardial supply/demand balance with alpha-adrenergic drugs during cardiopulmonary resuscitation. J Thorac Cardiovasc Surg 76:244, 1978

162. Ditchey RV, Lindenfeld J: Failure of epinephrine to improve the balance between myocardial oxygen supply and demand during closed-chest resuscitation in dogs. Circulation 78:382, 1988

163. Berg RA, Otto CW, Kern KB et al: High dose epinephrine results in greater early mortality following resuscitation from prolonged cardiac arrest in pigs: A prospective, randomized study. Crit Care Med 22:282, 1994

164. Berg RA, Otto CW, Kern KB et al: A randomized, blinded trial of high-dose epinephrine versus standard-dose epinephrine in a swine model of pediatric asphyxial cardiac arrest. Crit Care Med 24:1695, 1996

165. Brillman JC, Sanders AB, Otto CW et al: A comparison of epinephrine and phenylephrine for resuscitation and neurologic outcome of cardiac arrest in dogs. Ann Emerg Med 16:11, 1987

166. Silvast T, Saarnivaara L, Kinnunen A et al: Comparison of adrenaline and phenylephrine in out-of-hospital CPR: A double-blind study. Acta Anaesthesiol Scand 29:610, 1985

167. Lindner KH, Dirks B, Strohmenger HU et al: Randomized comparison of epinephrine and vasopressin in patients with out-of hospital ventricular fibrillation. Lancet 349:535, 1997

168. Prengel AW, Lindner KH, Keller A, Lurie KG: Cardiovascular function during the postresuscitation phase after cardiac arrest in pigs: A comparison of epinephrine versus vasopressin. Crit Care Med 24:2014, 1996

169. Brown CG, Werman HA, Davis EA et al: Comparative effect of graded doses of epinephrine on regional brain blood flow during CPR in a swine model. Ann Emerg Med 15:1138, 1986

170. Brown CG, Werman HA, Davis EA: The effects of graded doses of epinephrine on regional myocardial blood flow during cardiopulmonary resuscitation in swine. Circulation 75:491, 1987

171. Chase PB, Kern KB, Sanders AB et al: Effects of graded doses of epinephrine on both noninvasive and invasive measures of myocardial perfusion and blood flow during cardiopulmonary resuscitation. Crit Care Med 21:413, 1993

172. Koscove EM, Paradis NA: Successful resuscitation from cardiac arrest using high-dose epinephrine therapy: Report of two cases. JAMA 259:3031, 1988

173. Goetting MG, Paradis NA: High-dose epinephrine improves outcome from pediatric cardiac arrest. Ann Emerg Med 20:22, 1991

174. Linder KH, Ahnefeld FW, Prengel AW: Comparison of standard and high-dose adrenaline in the resuscitation of asystole and electromechanical dissociation. Acta Anaesthesiol Scand 35:253, 1991

175. Stiell IB, Hebert PC, Weitzman BN et al: High-dose epinephrine in adult cardiac arrest. N Engl J Med 327:1045, 1992

176. Brown CG, Martin DP, Pepe PE et al: A comparison of standard-dose and high-dose epinephrine in cardiac arrest outside the hospital. N Engl J Med 327:1051, 1992

177. Callaham M, Madsen CD, Barton CW et al: A randomized clinical trial of high-dose epinephrine and norepinephrine vs standard-

dose epinephrine in prehospital cardiac arrest. JAMA 268:2667, 1992

178. Choux C, Gueugniaud P-Y, Barbieux A et al: Standard doses versus repeated high doses of epinephrine in cardiac arrest outside the hospital. Resusciation 29:3, 1995

179. Gueugniaud P-Y, Mols P, Goldstein P et al: A comparison of repeated high doses and repeated standard doses of epinephrine for cardiac arrest outside the hospital. N Engl J Med 339:1595, 1998

180. Rivers EP, Wortsman J, Rady MY et al: The effect of the total cumulative epinephrine dose administered during human CPR on hemodynamic, oxygen transport, and utilization variables in the postresuscitation period. Chest 106:1499, 1994

181. Behringer W, Kittler H, Sterz F et al: Cumulative epinephrine dose during cardiopulmonary resuscitation and neurologic outcome. Ann Intern Med 129:450, 1998

182. Rosen MR, Hoffman BF, Wit AL: Electrophysiology and pharmacology of cardiac arrhythmias: V. Cardiac antiarrhythmic effects of lidocaine. Am Heart J 89:526, 1975

183. Kupersmith J: Electrophysiological and antiarrhythmic effects of lidocaine on canine acute myocardial ischemia. Am Heart J 97:360, 1979

184. Koch-Weser J: Drug therapy: Bretylium. N Engl J Med 300:473, 1979

185. Kowey PR, Levine JH, Herre JM et al: Randomized, double-blind comparison of intravenous amiodarone and bretylium in the treatment of patients with recurrent hemodynamically destabilizing ventricular tachycardia or fibrillation. Circulation 92:3255, 1995

186. Spear JG, Moore EN, Gerstenblith G: Effect of lidocaine on the ventricular fibrillation threshold in the dog during acute ischemia and premature ventricular contractions. Circulation 46:65, 1972

187. Anderson JL: Antifibrillatory versus antiectopic therapy. Am J Cardiol 54:7A, 1984

188. Kerber RE, Pandian NG, Jensen SR et al: Effect of lidocaine and bretylium on energy requirement for transthoracic defibrillation: Experimental studies. J Am Coll Cardiol 7:397, 1986

189. Tacker WA, Niebauer MJ, Babbs CF et al: The effect of newer antiarrhythmic drugs on defibrillation threshold. Crit Care Med 8:177, 1980

190. Dorian P, Fain ES, Daby JM, Winkle RA: Lidocaine causes a reversible, concentration-dependent increase in defibrillation energy requirements. J Am Coll Cardiol 8:327, 1986

191. Zhou L, Chen BP, Kluger J et al: Effects of amiodarone and its active metabolite desethylamiodarone on ventricular defibrillation threshold. J Am Coll Cardiol 31:1672, 1998

192. Koo CC, Allen JD, Pantridge JF: Lack of effect of bretylium tosylate on electrical ventricular defibrillation in a controlled study. Cardiovasc Res 18:762, 1984

193. Sanna G, Arcidiacono R: Chemical ventricular defibrillation of the human heart with bretylium tosylate. Am J Cardiol 32:982, 1973

194. Haynes RE, Chinn TL, Copass MK, Cobb LA: Comparison of bretylium tosylate and lidocaine in management of out of hospital ventricular fibrillation: A randomized clinical trial. Am J Cardiol 48:353, 1981

195. Olson DW, Thompson BM, Darin JC, Milbrath MH: A randomized comparison study of bretylium tosylate and lidocaine in resuscitation of patients from out-of-hospital ventricular fibrillation in a paramedic system. Ann Emerg Med 13:807, 1984

196. Kudenchuk PJ, Cobb LA, Copass MK et al: Amiodarone for resuscitation after out of hospital cardiac arrest due to ventricular fibrillation. N Engl J Med 341:871, 1999

197. Gerst PH, Fleming WH, Malm JR: Increased susceptibility of the heart to ventricular fibrillation during metabolic acidosis. Circulation Res 19:63, 1966

198. Houle DB, Weil MH, Brown EB, Campbell GS: Influence of respiratory acidosis on ECG and pressor response to epinephrine, norepinephrine, and metaraminol. Proc Soc Exp Biol Med 94:561, 1957

199. Minuck M, Sharma GP: Comparison of THAM and sodium bicarbonate in resuscitation of the heart after ventricular fibrillation in dogs. Anesth Analg 56:38, 1977

200. Guerci AD, Chandra N, Johnson E et al: Failure of sodium bicarbonate to improve resuscitation from ventricular fibrillation in dogs. Circulation 74(suppl 4):75, 1986

201. Federiuk CS, Sanders AB, Kern KB et al: The effect of bicarbonate on resuscitation from cardiac arrest. Ann Emerg Med 20:1173, 1991

202. Vukmir RB, Bircher NG, Radovsky A, Safar P: Sodium bicarbonate may improve outcome in dogs with brief or prolonged cardiac arrest. Crit Care Med 23:515, 1995

203. Bishop RL, Weisfeldt ML: Sodium bicarbonate administration during cardiac arrest: Effect on arterial pH, P_{CO_2}, and osmolality. JAMA 235:506, 1976

204. Mattar JA, Weil MH, Shubin H et al: Cardiac arrest in the critically ill: II. Hyperosmolal states following cardiac arrest. Am J Med 56:162, 1974

205. White BC, Tintinalli JE: Effects of sodium bicarbonate administration during cardiopulmonary resuscitation. JACEP 6:187, 1977

206. Berenyi KG, Wolk M, Killip T: Cerebrospinal fluid acidosis complicating therapy of experimental cardiopulmonary resuscitation. Circulation 52:319, 1975

207. Sanders AB, Otto CW, Kern KB et al: Acid–base balance in a canine model of cardiac arrest. Ann Emerg Med 17:667, 1988

208. Kette F, Weil MH, von Planta MS et al: Buffer agents do not reverse intra-myocardial acidosis during cardiac resuscitation. Circulation 81:1660, 1990

209. Redding JS, Haynes RR, Thomas JD: Drug therapy in resuscitation from electromechanical dissociation. Crit Care Med 11:681, 1983

210. Brown DC, Lewis AJ, Criley JM: Asystole and its treatment: the possible role of the parasympathetic nervous system in cardiac arrest. JACEP 8:448, 1979

211. Stueven HA, Tonsfeldt DJ, Thompson BM et al: Atropine in asystole: Human studies. Ann Emerg Med 13:815, 1984

212. Iseri LR, Humphrey SB, Siner EJ: Pre-hospital bradyasystolic cardiac arrest. Ann Intern Med 88:741, 1978

213. Coon GA, Clinton JE, Ruiz E: Use of atropine for brady-asystolic prehospital cardiac arrest. Ann Emerg Med 10:462, 1981

214. Chamberlain DA, Turner P, Sneddon JM: Effects of atropine on heart rate in healthy man. Lancet 2:12, 1967

215. O'Rourke GW, Greene NM: Autonomic blockade and the resting heart rate in man. Am Heart J 80:469, 1970

216. Kay JH, Blalock A: The use of calcium chloride in the treatment of cardiac arrest in patients. Surg Gynecol Obstet 93:97, 1951

217. Nieman JT, Adomian GE, Garner D, Rosborough JP: Endocardial and transcutaneous cardiac pacing, calcium chloride, and epinephrine in post-countershock asystole and bradycardias. Crit Care Med 13:699, 1985

218. Dembo DH: Calcium in advanced life support. Crit Care Med 9:358, 1981

219. Harrison EE, Amey BD: The use of calcium in cardiac resuscitation. Am J Emerg Med 1:267, 1983

220. Harrison EE, Amey BD: Use of calcium in electromechanical dissociation. Ann Emerg Med 13:844, 1984

221. Stueven HA, Thompson BM, Aprahamian C, Darin J: Use of calcium in prehospital cardiac arrest. Ann Emerg Med 12:136, 1983

222. Stueven HA, Thompson BM, Aprahamian C et al: Calcium chloride: Reassessment of use in asystole. Ann Emerg Med 13:820, 1984

223. Stueven HA, Thompson BM, Aprahamian C et al: The effectiveness of calcium chloride in refractory electromechanical dissociation. Ann Emerg Med 14:626, 1985

224. Stueven HA, Thompson BM, Aprahamian C et al: Lack of effectiveness of calcium chloride in refractory asystole. Ann Emerg Med 14:630, 1985

225. Abramson NS, Safar P, Detre KM et al: Randomized clinical study of cardiopulmonary-cerebral resuscitation: Thiopental loading in comatose cardiac arrest survivors. N Engl J Med 314:397, 1986

226. Brain Resuscitation Clinical Trial II Study Group: A randomized clinical study of a calcium-entry blocker (lidoflazine) in the treatment of comatose survivors of cardiac arrest. N Engl J Med 324:1225, 1991

227. Longstreth WT, Diehr P, Inui TS: Prediction of awakening after out-of-hospital cardiac arrest. N Engl J Med 308:1378, 1983

228. Longstreth WT, Inui TS, Cobb LA, Copass MK: Neurologic recovery after out-of-hospital cardiac arrest. Ann Intern Med 98:588, 1983

229. Mullie A, Lust P, Penninck J et al: Monitoring of cerebrospinal fluid enzyme levels in post-ischemic encephalopathy after cardiac arrest. Crit Care Med 9:399, 1981

230. Edgren E, Terent H, Hedstrand U, Ronquist G: Cerebral spinal fluid markers in relation to outcome in patients with global cerebral ischemia. Crit Care Med 11:4, 1983

After this book went into production, new CPR guidelines were published. Here is the full reference for these algorithms: American Heart Association: Guidelines 2000 for Cardiopulmonary Resuscitation and Emergency Cardiovascular Care: International Concensus on Science. Circulation 102(8), 2000.

Clinical Anesthesia (4/e), edited by
Paul G. Barash, Bruce F. Cullen, and
Robert K. Stoelting. Lippincott Williams &
Wilkins, Philadelphia, © 2001.

APPENDIX

ELECTROCARDIOGRAPHY

JAMES R. ZAIDAN AND PAUL G. BARASH

ELECTROCARDIOGRAM

LEAD PLACEMENT

	Electrode	
	Positive	*Negative*
BIPOLAR LEADS		
I	LA	RA
II	LL	RA
III	LL	LA
AUGMENTED UNIPOLAR		
aVR	RA	LA, LL
aVL	LA	RA, LL
aVF	LL	RA, LA

	Position
PRECORDIAL	
V_1	4 ICS–RSB
V_2	4 ICS–LSB
V_3	Midway between V_2 and V_4
V_4	5 ICS–MCL
V_5	5 ICS–AAL
V_6	5 ICS–MAL

THREE-LEAD SYSTEMS

Bipolar Lead System	Electrode Placement	ECG Lead*	Advantage
II	RA R–clavicle LA L–10th rib (midclavicular line) LL Ground	II (II)	Dysrhythmias
MCL 1	RA Ground LA L–clavicle LL V_1	III (V_1)	Dysrhythmias and conduction defects
CS 5	RA R–clavicle LA V_5 LL Ground	I (V_5)	Precordial ischemia
CB 5	RA R–scapula LA V_5 LL Ground	I (V_5)	Precordial ischemia and dysrhythmias

MCL = modified central lead; CB = central back; CS = central subclavian.
*Selected lead on monitor: ( ) = simulated ECG lead.

We wish to thank Dr. Malcom S. Thaler for graciously permitting reproduction of electrocardiographic tracings from his book, *The Only EKG Book You'll Ever Need* (Philadelphia, JB Lippincott, 1988).

THE NORMAL ELECTROCARDIOGRAM—CARDIAC CYCLE

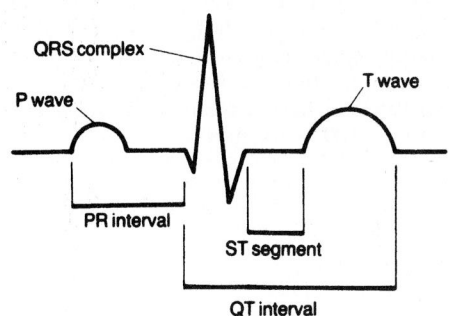

In this section the ECG complex is divided into the atrial (PR interval) and ventricular (QT interval) components.

ASHMAN BEATS

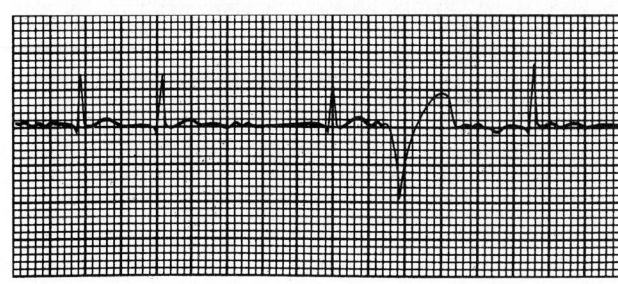

Rate: Variable.

Rhythm: Irregular.

PR interval: P wave may be present if supraventricular premature beat.

QT interval: QRS prolonged (>0.12 s) and altered, revealing bundle-branch pattern, most commonly right bundle. ST segment abnormal.

Note: Ashman beats are often confused with ventricular premature contractions. Ashman beats, usually seen with atrial fibrillation, have no compensatory pause and are a benign ECG finding requiring no treatment.

ATRIAL FIBRILLATION

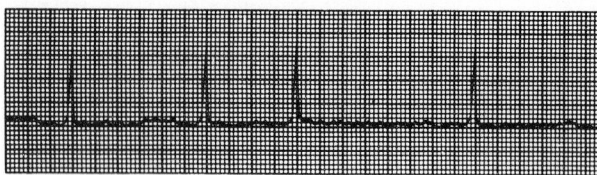

Rate: Variable (~150–200 beats·min⁻¹).

Rhythm: Irregular.

PR interval: No P wave, and PR interval not discernible.

QT interval: QRS normal.

Note: Must be differentiated from atrial flutter: (1) absence of flutter waves and presence of fibrillatory line; (2) flutter usually associated with higher ventricular rates (>150 beats·min⁻¹). Loss of atrial contraction reduces cardiac output (10–20%). Mural atrial thrombi may develop. Considered controlled if ventricular rate <100 beats·min⁻¹.

ATRIAL FLUTTER

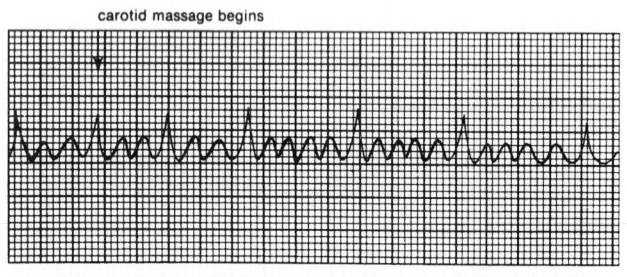

Rate: Rapid, atrial usually regular (250–350 beats·min⁻¹); ventricular usually regular (<100 beats·min⁻¹).

Rhythm: Atrial and ventricular regular.

PR interval: Flutter (F) waves are saw-toothed. PR interval cannot be measured.

QT interval: QRS usually normal; ST segment and T waves are not identifiable.

Note: Carotid massage will slow ventricular response, simplifying recognition of the F waves.

ATRIOVENTRICULAR BLOCK (First-Degree)

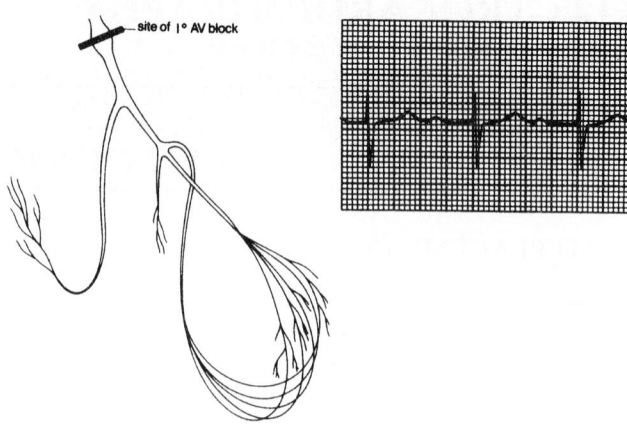

Rate: 60–100 beats·min⁻¹.

Rhythm: Regular.

PR interval: Prolonged (>0.20 s) and constant.

QT interval: Normal.

Note: Usually clinically insignificant; may be early harbinger of drug toxicity.

ATRIOVENTRICULAR BLOCK (Second-Degree), Mobitz Type I/ Wenckebach Block

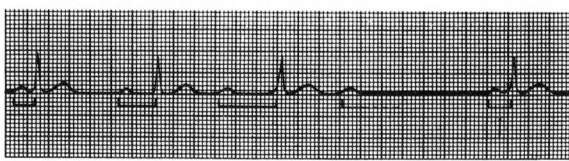

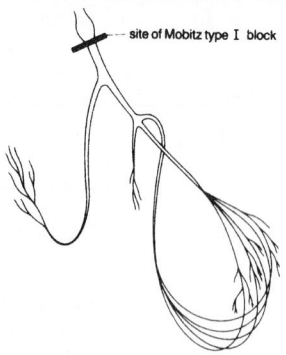

Rate: 60–100 beats·min⁻¹.

Rhythm: Atrial regular; ventricular irregular.

PR interval: P wave normal; PR interval progressively lengthens with each cycle until QRS complex is dropped (dropped beat). PR interval following dropped beat is shorter than normal.

QT interval: QRS complex normal but dropped periodically.

Note: Commonly seen (1) in trained athletes and (2) with drug toxicity.

ATRIOVENTRICULAR BLOCK
(Second-Degree), Mobitz Type II

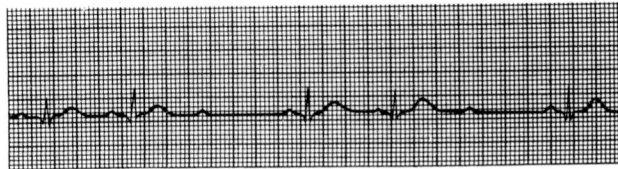

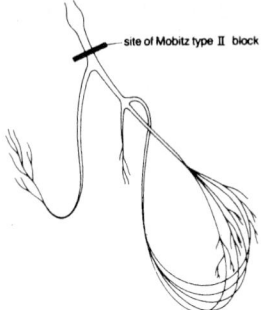

Rate: <100 beats·min⁻¹.

Rhythm: Atrial regular; ventricular regular or irregular.

PR interval: P waves normal, but some are not followed by QRS complex.

QT interval: Normal but may have widened QRS complex if block is at level of bundle branch. ST segment and T wave may be abnormal, depending on location of block.

Note: In contrast to Mobitz type I block, the PR and RR intervals are constant and the dropped QRS occurs without warning. The wider the QRS complex (block lower in the conduction system), the greater the amount of myocardial damage.

ATRIOVENTRICULAR BLOCK
(Third-Degree), Complete Heart Block

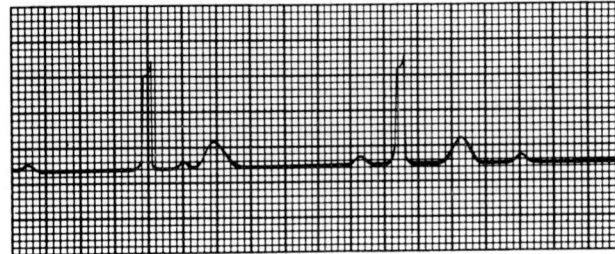

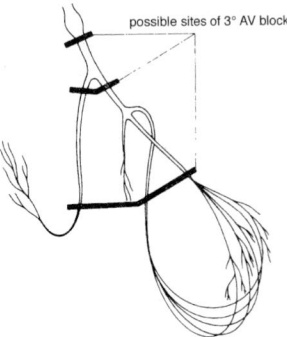

Rate: <45 beats·min⁻¹.

Rhythm: Atrial regular; ventricular regular; no relationship between P wave and QRS complex.

PR interval: Variable because artia and ventricles beat independently.

QT interval: QRS morphology variable, depending on the origin of the ventricular beat in the intrinsic pacemaker system (atrioventricular junctional versus ventricular pacemaker). ST segment and T wave normal.

Note: Immediate treatment with atropine or isoproterenol is required if cardiac output is reduced. Consideration should be given to insertion of a pacemaker. Seen as a complication of mitral valve replacement.

ATRIOVENTRICULAR DISSOCIATION

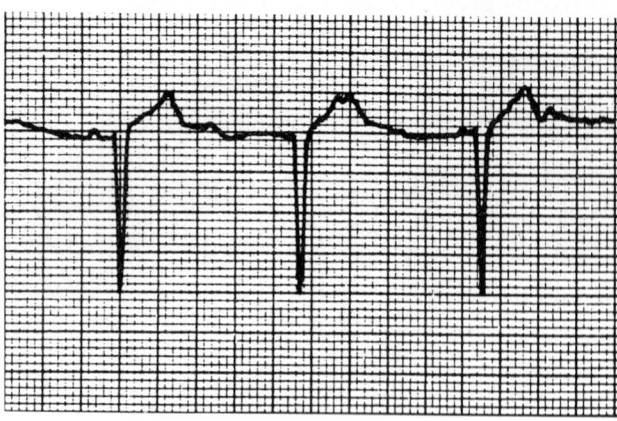

Rate: Variable.

Rhythm: Atrial regular; ventricular regular; ventricular rate faster than atrial rate; no relationship between P wave and QRS complex.

PR interval: Variable because atria and ventricles beat independently.

QT interval: QRS morphology depends on location of ventricular pacemaker. ST segment and T wave abnormal.

Note: Digitalis toxicity can present as atrioventricular dissociation.

BUNDLE-BRANCH BLOCK—RIGHT (RBBB)

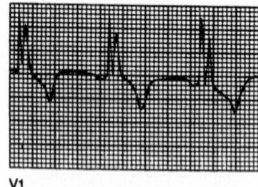

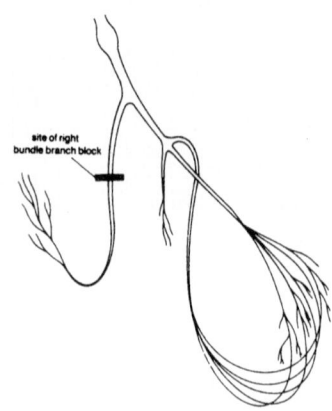

Rate: <100 beats · min^{-1}.

Rhythm: Regular.

PR interval: Normal.

QT interval: Complete RBBB (QRS >0.12 s); incomplete RBBB (QRS = 0.10–0.12 s). Varying patterns of QRS complex; rSR (V_1); RS, wide R with M pattern. ST segment and T wave opposite direction of the R wave.

Note: In the presence of RBBB, Q waves may be seen with a myocardial infarction.

BUNDLE-BRANCH BLOCK—LEFT (LBBB)

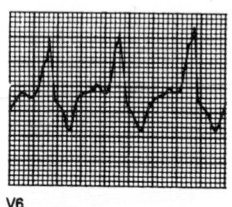

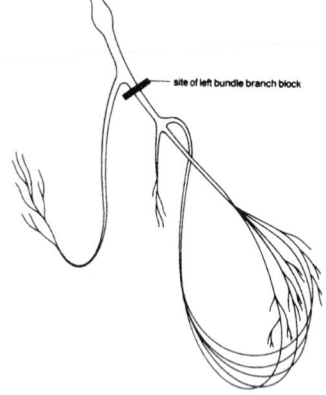

Rate: <100 beats · min^{-1}.

Rhythm: Regular.

PR interval: Normal.

QT interval: Complete LBBB (QRS >0.12 s); incomplete LBBB (QRS = 0.10–0.12 s). Lead V_1 negative rS complex; I, aVL, V_6 wide R wave without Q or S component. ST segment and T wave defection opposite direction of the R wave.

Note: LBBB does not occur in healthy patients and usually indicates serious heart disease with a poorer prognosis. In patients with LBBB, insertion of a pulmonary artery catheter may lead to complete heart block.

ELECTROLYTE DISTURBANCES

	↓ Ca^{2+}	↑ Ca^{2+}	↓ K$^+$	↑ K$^+$
Rate	<100 beats · min^{-1}	<100 beats · min^{-1}	<100 beats · min^{-1}	<100 beats · min^{-1}
Rhythm	Regular	Regular	Regular	Regular
PR interval	Normal	Normal/ increased	Normal	Normal
QT interval	Increased	Decreased	T flat U wave	T peaked QT decreased

Note: ECG changes usually do not correlate with serum calcium. Hypocalcemia rarely causes dysrhythmias in the absence of hypokalemia. In contrast, abnormalities in serum potassium concentration can be diagnosed by ECG.

DIGITALIS EFFECT

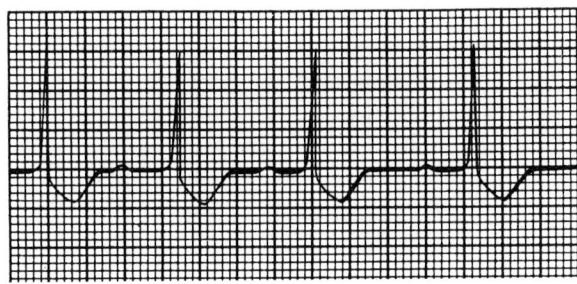

Rate: <100 beats · min^{-1}.

Rhythm: Regular.

PR interval: Normal or prolonged.

QT interval: ST segment sloping ("digitalis effect").

Note: Digitalis toxicity can be the cause of many common dysrhythmias (*e.g.,* premature ventricular contractions, second-degree heart block). Verapamil, quinidine, and amiodarone cause an increase in serum digitalis concentration.

CORONARY ARTERY DISEASE—Ischemia

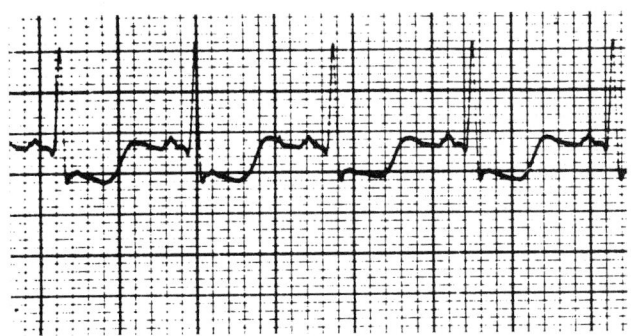

Rate: Variable.

Rhythm: Usually regular, but may show atrial and/or ventricular dysrhythmias.

PR interval: Normal.

QT interval: ST segment depressed; J point depression; T-wave inversion; conduction disturbances. Coronary vasospasm (Prinzmetal) ST segment elevation.

Note: Intraoperative ischemia is usually seen in the presence of "normal" vital signs (*e.g.,* ±20% of preinduction values).

CORONARY ARTERY DISEASE—Myocardial Infarction

Anatomic Site	Leads	ECG Changes	Coronary Artery
Inferior	II, III, aVF	Q, ST, T	Right
Lateral	I, aVL, V$_5$–V$_6$	Q, ST, T	Left circumflex
Anterior	I, aVL, V$_1$–V$_4$	Q, ST, T	Left
Anteroseptal	V$_1$–V$_4$	Q, ST, T	Left anterior descending

SUBENDOCARDIAL MYOCARDIAL INFARCTION (SEMI)

Persistent ST segment depression and/or T-wave inversion in the absence of Q wave. Usually requires additional laboratory data (*e.g.,* isoenzymes) to confirm diagnosis.

TRANSMURAL MYOCARDIAL INFARCTION (TMI)

Q waves seen on ECG useful in confirming diagnosis. Associated with poorer prognosis and more significant hemodynamic impairment; dysrhythmias frequently complicate course.

PAROXYSMAL ATRIAL TACHYCARDIA (PAT)

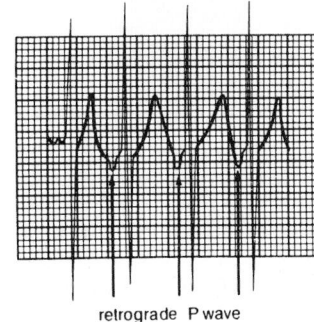
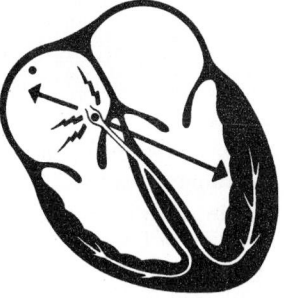

retrograde P wave

Rate: 150–250 beats · min^{-1}.

Rhythm: Regular.

PR interval: Difficult to distinguish because of tachycardia obscuring P wave. P wave may precede, be included in, or follow QRS complex.

QT interval: Normal, but ST segment and T wave may be difficult to distinguish.

Note: Therapy depends on degree of hemodynamic compromise. In contrast to management of PAT in awake patients, synchronized cardoversion rather than pharmacologic treatment is preferred in hemodynamically unstable anesthetized patients.

PREMATURE ATRIAL CONTRACTION (PAC)

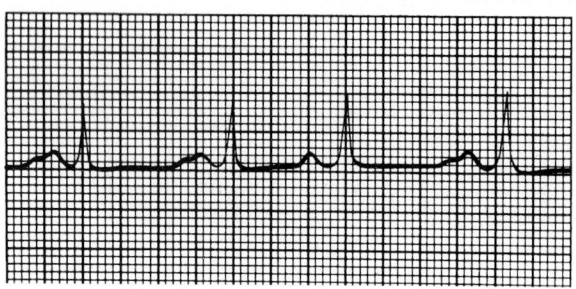

Rate: <100 beats · min⁻¹.

Rhythm: Irregular.

PR interval: P waves may be lost in preceding T waves. PR interval is variable.

QT interval: QRS normal configuration; ST segment and T wave normal.

Note: Nonconducted PAC appearance similar to that of sinus arrest; T waves with PAC may be distorted by inclusion of P wave in the T wave.

SINUS TACHYCARDIA

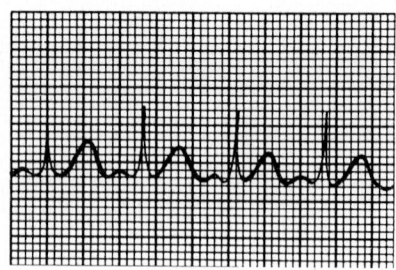

Rate: 100–160 beats · min⁻¹.

Rhythm: Regular.

PR interval: Normal; P wave may be difficult to see.

QT interval: Normal.

Note: Should be differentiated from paroxysmal atrial tachycardia (PAT). With PAT, carotid massage terminates dysrhythmia. Sinus tachycardia may respond to vagal maneuvers but reappears as soon as vagal stimulus is removed.

PREMATURE VENTRICULAR CONTRACTION (PVC)

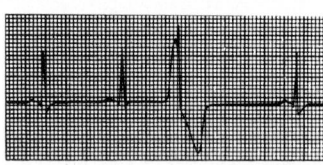

A

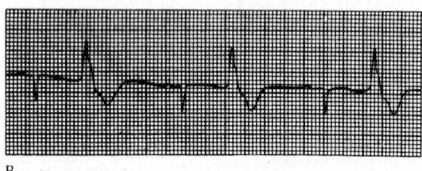

B

Rate: Usually <100 beats · min⁻¹.

Rhythm: Irregular.

PR interval: P wave and PR interval absent; retrograde conduction of P wave can be seen.

QT interval: Wide QRS (>0.12 s); ST segment cannot be evaluated (*e.g.,* ischemia); T wave opposite direction of QRS with compensatory pause (*A*). Bigeminy: every other beat a PVC (*B*); trigeminy: every third beat a PVC. R-on-T occurs when PVC falls in the T wave and can lead to ventricular tachycardia or fibrillation.

Note: If compensatory pause is not seen following an ectopic beat, the complex is most likely supraventricular in origin.

TORSADES DE POINTES

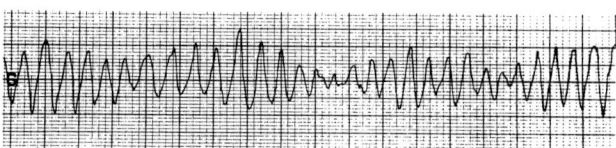

Rate: 150–250 beats · min⁻¹.

Rhythm: No atrial component seen; ventricular rhythm regular or irregular.

PR interval: P wave buried in QRS complex.

QT interval: QRS complexes usually wide and with phasic variation twisting around a central axis (a few complexes point upward then a few point downward). ST segments and T waves difficult to discern.

Note: Type of ventricular tachycardia associated with prolonged QT interval. Seen with electrolyte disturbances (*e.g.,* hypokalemia, hypocalcemia, and hypomagnesemia) and bradycardia. Administering standard antidysrhythmics (lidocaine, proeainamide, etc.) may worsen Torsades de Pointes. Treatment includes increasing heart rate pharmacologically or by pacing.

VENTRICULAR FIBRILLATION

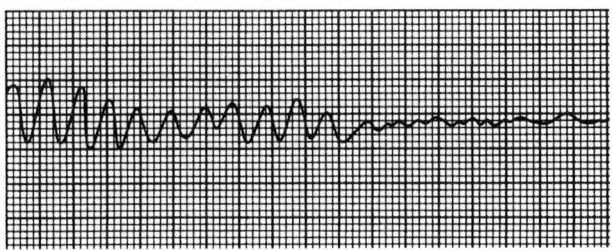

Rate: Absent.

Rhythm: None.

PR interval: Absent.

QT interval: Absent.

Note: "Pseudoventricular fibrillation" may be the result of a monitor malfunction (*e.g.*, ECG lead disconnect). Always check for carotid pulse before instituting therapy.

VENTRICULAR TACHYCARDIA

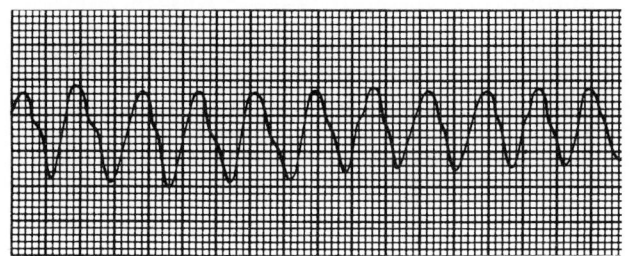

Rate: 100–250 beats · min^{-1}.

Rhythm: No atrial component seen; ventricular rhythm irregular or regular.

PR interval: Absent; retrograde P wave may be seen in QRS complex.

QT interval: Wide, bizarre QRS complex. ST segment and T wave difficult to determine.

Note: In the presence of hemodynamic compromise, immediate DC synchronized cardioversion is required. If the patient is stable, with short bursts of ventricular tachycardia, pharmacologic management is preferred. Should be differentiated from supraventricular tachycardia with aberrancy (SVT-A). Compensatory pause and atrioventricular dissociation suggest a PVC. P waves and SR' (V$_1$) and slowing to vagal stimulus suggest SVT-A.

WOLFF-PARKINSON-WHITE SYNDROME (WPW)

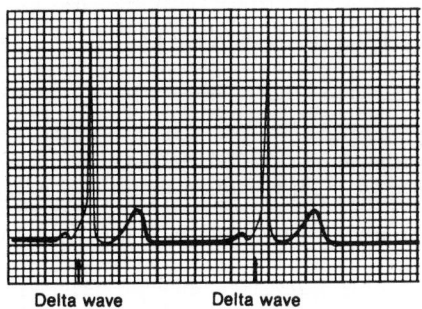

Delta wave   Delta wave

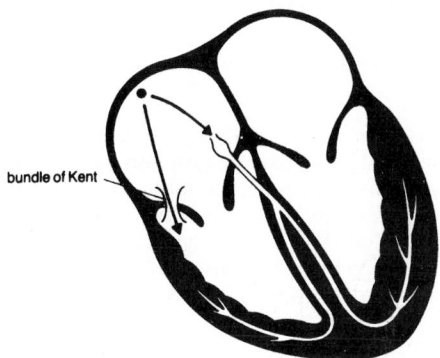

bundle of Kent

Rate: <100 beats · min^{-1}.

Rhythm: Regular.

PR interval: P wave normal; PR interval short (<0.12 s).

QT interval: Duration (>0.10 s) with slurred QRS complex. Type A has delta wave, RBBB, with upright QRS complex V$_1$. Type B has delta wave and downward QRS-V$_1$. ST segment and T wave usually normal.

Note: Digoxin should be avoided in the presence of WPW because it increases conduction through the accessory bypass tract (bundle of Kent) and decreases atrioventricular node conduction; consequently, ventricular fibrillation can occur.

PACEMAKER

PACEMAKER DESIGNATIONS

1 Chamber- Paced	2 Chamber- Sensed	3 Response	4 Program- mability	5 Antitachy- cardia Function
Atrium	Atrium	Inhibit	Programmable (rate/output)	Bursts
Ventricle	Ventricle	Trigger	Multiprogram- mable	Normal rate Competition
Double (A/V)	Double O/None	Double O/None Reverse	Communi- cating O/None	Scanning External

Note: The original pacemaker designation used a three-position code. Subsequently, expanded positions were added (4, 5). For example, the presence of atrial fibrillation may require a pacemaker with the code **VVI**. This designation indicates (1) **V**entricle is paced, (2) **V**entricle is sensed, and the pacemaker is (3) **I**nhibited if a cardiac event is sensed.

EVALUATION OF THE PACEMAKER

1. Ask patient about results of last telephone check.
2. Ask patient about location of pulse generator.
3. Ask patient to exercise muscles in area of generator. Observe for inhibition of pacing.
4. If patient cannot help with 1,2,3, try to obtain ID card.
5. If 4 not possible, assume the patient has VVIR or DDDR, piezoelectric, vibratory-sensing pacemaker.
6. Observe chest x-ray for number and continuity of leads and location of electrodes.
7. Observe ECG for pacemaker dependency, failed capture, undersensing, and ventricular vs. sequential pacing.
8. Apply magnet to check for pacing capture and for rate. If magnet rate is low (≤90 beats · min⁻¹), notify cardiologist.
9. In an emergency, proceed with the surgical procedure. If the intrinsic heart rate is <50–60 beats · min⁻¹ and there are no impulses found on ECG, establish transcutaneous pacing.

Reprinted with permission from Zaidan JR: Pacemakers. In Youngberg JA, Lake CL, Roizeu MF, Wilson KS (eds): Cardiac, Vascular and Thoracic Anesthesia. New York, Churchill Livingstone, 2000.

TREATMENT OF PACEMAKER FAILURE

Rate	Possible Treatment
Adequate to maintain blood pressure	1. Observe, oxygen 2. Atropine 3. Try magnet
Severe bradycardia hypotension	1. Oxygen, airway control 2. Atropine 3. Isoproterenol 4. Try magnet 5. Transcutaneous pacing
No escape rhythm	1. CPR 2. Isoproterenol 3. Try magnet 4. Transcutaneous pacing

Reprinted with permission from Zaidan JR: Pacemakers. In Youngberg JA , Lake CL, Roizeu MF, Wilson KS (eds): Cardiac, Vascular and Thoracic Anesthesia. New York, Churchill Livingstone, 2000.

ATRIAL PACING

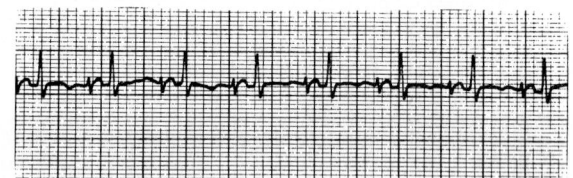

Atrial pacing as demonstrated in this figure is used when the atrial impulse can proceed through the AV node. Examples are sinus bradycardia and junctional rhythms associated with clinically significant decreases in blood pressure.

VENTRICULAR PACING

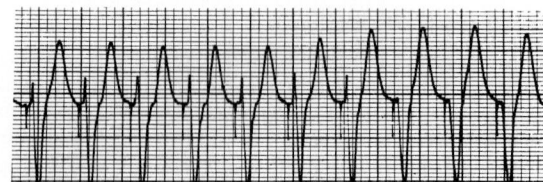

In this tracing ventricular pacing is evident by absence of atrial wave (P wave) and pacemaker spike preceding QRS complex. Ventricular pacing is employed in the presence of bradycardia secondary to AV block or atrial fibrillation.

DDD PACING

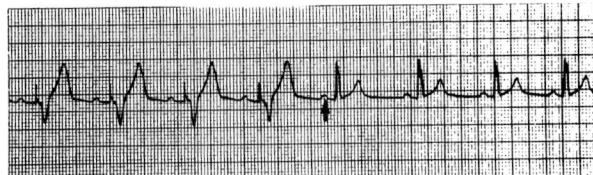

The DDD pacemaker (generator), one of the most commonly used, paces and senses both atrium and ventricle. In the first four beats, the P waves were not followed by a QRS complex within the programmed PR interval. Therefore, a ventricular pacing spike and a ventricular paced beat occurred. In the last four beats (after the arrow), atrial activity proceeded through the AV node in the allotted amount of time; therefore, ventricular pacing was inhibited.

ATRIAL ELECTROGRAM (AEG)

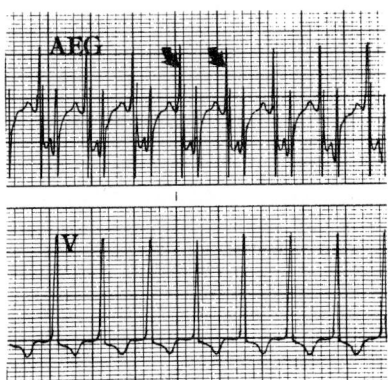

The AEG is useful in differentiating various atrial dysrhythmias. The AEG is obtained from an intracardiac or esophageal lead, if P waves are not clearly seen on the surface ECG. In this trace the V lead does not have obvious P waves; however, the AEG reveals large P waves (arrows) that precede each QRS complex. Locate the QRS on the AEG by matching the R wave on the surface ECG to the AEG. The surface and AEG must be simultaneously recorded.

IMPLANTED CARDIOVERTER-DEFIBRILLATORS

Guidelines for Patient Care

- Preoperative assessment should include those procedures that are standard for patients with heart disease. Evaluate for progression of all types of heart disease.
- Question the patient regarding the number of shocks received in the few days prior to the scheduled surgery. The response will indicate the possibility of requiring therapy during the next few hours.
- Continue antiarrhythmic agents until the time of surgery. Consider discussing with the cardiologist the necessity of the administration of an additional dose of amiodarone should the patient experience an arrhythmia during surgery. If the patient has an arrhythmia, rule out the usual causes, such as hypercarbia, to prevent the arrhythmia from recurring during surgery.
- There is no particular anesthetic technique that is clearly right or wrong for a patient who has an implanted defibrillator.
- Monitoring must include American Society of Anesthesiologists standard monitoring devices. Other monitors should be used as indicated for the individual patient.

- There are no reports concerning the use of a pulmonary arterial catheter in patients who have ICDs. If monitoring with a pulmonary arterial catheter is necessary, discuss the issues of dislodgment of the ICD with the patient and cardiologist. Document your discussions and the logic supporting the necessity for a pulmonary arterial catheter in the chart.
- Patients with transvenous devices are potentially at risk for infection when central lines are inserted without caution for aseptic technique. Consider administering an antibiotic just before inserting central lines. Maintain perfect sterile technique.
- Apply patches for external defibrillation during surgery. Assure that these external patches are as far away as possible from the device.
- Interrogate and reprogram the ICD as soon as possible after surgery.
- Always have the magnet available.

Guidelines for Electrocautery Use

- If the patient has a separately implanted pacemaker, consider programming the pacemaker to asynchronous activity (VOO or DOO) to prevent inhibition while the electrocautery is being used. Pacemaker spikes that occur when a patient's heart rate is greater than an asynchronously programmed pacemaker rate will be counted by the ICD as R waves. The ICD, therefore, could interpret a sinus tachycardia plus pacemaker spikes as a ventricular tachycardia and shock the patient.
- The electrocautery could reprogram the VVI and DDD pacing parameters of the ICD; however, the chance of reprogramming is extremely small. A magnet will not change pacing parameters in patients who require chronic pacing.
- Do not use electrocautery when the device is actively sensing and capable of delivering therapy. Program the ICD to "off." There are no reports of an ICD reprogramming to "monitor plus therapy" once it has been programmed off. Some cardiologists reprogram the ICD to "monitor only" during surgery to record arrhythmias, but the device will then monitor electrocautery signals.
- If a programming device is not available, then use the magnet to change the mode of activity. The CPI device, if it is programmed to respond to the magnet, will have changed to "monitor only" from "monitor plus therapy" once the beeping tone becomes a continuous tone. If charging starts while the surgeon is using the electrocautery, then place the magnet over the generator and the device will discharge into itself, not into the patient. The Medtronic and Intermedics devices suspend monitoring and therapy for as long as the magnet is held over the generator; therefore, if the magnet is on the generator, they will neither sense nor discharge.
- Duration criterion must be met before charging takes place. Additionally, if the patient is in ventricular tachycardia, the ICD reconfirms the arrhythmia before it delivers rapid pacing or shock therapy. These events give the device time to stop the process if an electrocautery signal is sensed as an arrhythmia. Using the electrocautery in short bursts might cause inappropriate sensing; however, sensing will not fulfill the duration criterion, therefore the device will not charge. The ICD could interpret the signal from the electrocautery as ventricular fibrillation even when the activated cautery is not in contact with the patient.
- A bipolar electrocautery has a smaller chance of causing sensing and discharge. A battery-powered electrocautery offers extra safety.
- Do not use the electrocautery within six inches of the device or leads.

- If the ICD begins to charge during the operative procedure, place the magnet over the ICD and keep it in that location. The ICD will discharge into the generator and will stop sensing. It will not stop pacing activity.
- When positioning the external defibrillator patches, assure that they are positioned perpendicular to a plane described by the generator and electrodes.

Adapted from Zaidan JR, Implantable cardioverter-defibrillators. J Cardiothorac Vasc Anesth 13:475, 1999.

INDEX

Page numbers followed by t and f indicate tables and figures, respectively.

Gastroschisis, 1185–1187, 1185–1187f
 antenatal diagnosis of, 1185
 minimal intervention management for, 1186
 perioperative care in, 1186–1187, 1186f
 postoperative care in, 1187
 preoperative care in, 1185–1186
Gastrostomy tube, 1187
Gatch, Elmer, 11
Gatekeepers, 46
Gaussian function. *See* Normal function
General anesthesia. *See also* Inhaled anesthetics
 for ambulatory surgery, 1225, 1226f, 1229–1232
 for bronchoscopy, 834
 for carotid endarterectomy, 943–944
 for cesarean section, 403, 1150
 costs relative to regional techniques, 108
 definition of, 121
 for geriatric patient, 1212
 for labor and vaginal delivery, 1148, 1155, 1155f
 for lower extremity revascularization, 960, 960t, 962
 for microvascular surgery, 1108
 in myasthenia gravis, 844–845
 in obese patient, 1040
 office-based, 1340–1341
 for ophthalmic surgery, 977, 979
 for orthopaedic surgery, 1104
 for radiation therapy, 1333
 for spine surgery, 1112
 for TURP, 1021
General damages, 90
Genetic approach, to study of anesthesia mechanisms, 135–137
Genetic effect, of inhaled anesthetics, 402–403
Genetic test, for malignant hyperthermia, 529
Genitourinary effect
 of morphine, 351
 of postoperative pain, 1408, 1408t
Genitourinary system
 anatomy of, 1005
 innervation of, 1005, 1006f
Gentamicin
 drug interactions, 432
 nephrotoxicity of, 1016
Geriatric patient, 1205–1214
 aging and organ function, 1205–1206, 1206f
 ambulatory surgery in, 1218
 analgesia in, 1211–1213
 anesthetic requirements in, 1211–1213
 autonomic nervous system in, 1211
 body composition in, 1209–1210, 1209f
 cardiovascular function in, 1206–1208
 central nervous system in, 1210–1211
 concepts of aging, 1205
 definition of "geriatric," 1205
 general anesthesia for, 1212
 hepatorenal function in, 1208–1209
 immune function in, 1208–1209
 intravenous anesthetics in, 339
 intravenous hypnotics in, 330
 metabolism in, 1209–1210
 opioids for, 556, 1208
 outcome of surgery in, 1213–1214, 1213f
 perioperative management of, 1213–1214, 1213f
 peripheral nervous system in, 1211, 1211f
 pharmacodynamics in, 1212
 pharmacokinetics in, 1209–1210, 1212
 physical management of, 1214
 postoperative complications in, 1213
 propofol in, 333–334
 pulmonary function in, 1206–1208
German measles. *See* Rubella virus
Gerrard, Geraldine, 21
Gerstmann-Straussler syndrome, 503
GFCI. *See* Ground fault circuit interrupter
GFI. *See* Ground fault interrupter
GFR. *See* Glomerular filtration rate
Gigantism, 768, 1137
Gilbert's disease, 1096
Gilbert's syndrome, 1074t, 1096–1097
Gill, Richard, 20
Gill, Ruth, 20
Gillies, Harold, 16
Gitelman's syndrome, 186t
Glands, adrenergic and cholinergic responses of, 262t
Glasgow Coma Scale, 482, 482t, 777, 777t, 1263–1264, 1263t, 1465, 1465t
Glasgow Outcome Scale, 777
 in subarachnoid hemorrhage, effect of plasma glucose, 175
Glatiramir, for multiple sclerosis, 498
Glaucoma, 971–972
 closed-angle (acute), 971
  postoperative, 985
 congenital, 972
 infantile, 972
 juvenile, 972
 medications for, 311, 975–976
 narrow-angle, 288
 open-angle (chronic), 971
 treatment of, 286, 286t
Glaucoma drainage surgery, 981
Glial cells, 449
Glioma, 762
Global fees, 46
Globe, 969
Glomerular capillary oncotic pressure, 1007
Glomerular capillary pressure, 878, 1007

Glomerular filtrate, 1005
Glomerular filtration, 1005–1007
 effect of fluid infusion on, 171
Glomerular filtration pressure, 1007
Glomerular filtration rate (GFR), 173–174, 878, 1006–1008, 1007f, 1010–1012, 1015
 autoregulation of, 244
 fetal, 1174
 in geriatric patient, 1209
 renal drug clearance and, 244
Glomerulus, 1005, 1007f
 regulation of blood flow to, 1007
 water handling by, 172–173, 173f
Glossopharyngeal nerve (CN IX), 265, 280, 722, 798
Glossopharyngeal nerve blockade, 618, 618f, 723, 834
Glottic stenosis, 768
Glottis, 1175
Gloves, 72–73t, 77
Glucagon, 1134
 actions of, 269t, 306
 in cirrhosis, 1085
 dose of, 306
 effect on denervated heart, 281t
 hemodynamic effects of, 306
 in liver disease, 1091
 receptor-mediated effector mechanisms, 279t
 regulation of hepatic blood flow, 1071
 side effects of, 306
 for sphincter of Oddi spasm, 1061, 1095
 in stress response, 1407
Glucagonoma, 1133
Glucocorticoids, 1125–1129
 actions of, 283
 deficiency of, 181
 excess of. *See* Cushing's syndrome
 physiology of, 1126
Glucocorticoid therapy
 for adrenal insufficiency, 1128
 anti-inflammatory action of, 1126
 exogenous, 1128–1129, 1129f
 for hypercalcemia, 1125
 immunosuppressant action of, 1350–1351, 1351t
 for pituitary surgery, 769
 preparations, 1129t
 side effects and toxicities of, 1367, 1367t
 for thyrotoxicosis, 1121
Gluconeogenesis, 1072, 1126, 1134
Glucose
 blood, 1126
  effect on Glasgow Outcome Scale, 175
  preoperative, 484
 brain metabolism, 745, 748
 cellular uptake of, 1134
 contraindications in neurosurgical patients, 763
 in CSF, 747t
 defects in metabolism of, 542, 542f
 energy source for heart, 873
 homeostasis, 1072
Glucose-insulin-potassium infusion, 1135
Glucose-6-phosphate dehydrogenase (G6PD) deficiency, 504t, 505, 542, 1083
 drugs that produce hemolysis in, 505, 505t
Glucose phosphate isomerase deficiency, 505
Glucuronic acid conjugates, 246
Glutamate, 1436f
 anesthetic effects on, 125
 in chronic pain, 1437
 as neurotransmitter, 744, 748
 in pain modulation, 1404–1406
Glutamate receptor, 329f, 744
 anesthetic effects on, 126–127, 127f, 137f
Glutathione synthetase deficiency, 505
Glutathione *S*-transferase (GST)
 in liver disease, 1074
 liver function tests, 401
Gluteal muscle, myofascial pain involving, 1445
Glutethimide, induction of porphyria by, 541t
Glyburide, drug interactions, 1317
Glyceril trinitrate. *See* Nitroglycerin
Glycerin, effect on intraocular pressure, 973
Glycerol, as systemic ophthalmic drug, 976
Glycine, 553, 553f
 irrigating solution for TURP, 985, 1019–1020, 1019t
 toxicity of, 985
Glycine receptor, anesthetic effects on, 129
Glycocalyx, 217
Glycogen, 1126
Glycogen-glucose-lactate pathway, 542f
Glycogen storage disease, 541–543, 1365
 type I, 542
 type II, 542
 type III, 542
 type IV, 542
 type V, 542
 type VI, 542
 type VII, 542
 type VIII, 542
Glycoprotein IIb/IIIa inhibitors, for peripheral vascular disease, 930
Glycopyrrolate
 actions of, 287–288, 288t
 administration route, 552t
 in Alzheimer's disease, 503
 as antisialagogue, 560, 560t
 for awake intubation, 617
 cardiovascular effects of, 441
 for dental surgery, 1336

dose of, 552t
 drug interactions, 257
 effect on lower esophageal sphincter tone, 1042t
 heart rate and, 560–561, 560t
 for neonatal anesthesia, 1178
 for office-based anesthesia, 1339
 for pediatric patient, 563
 as premedicant, 552t, 557–558, 560–561, 563, 1044
 for prophylaxis against oculocardiac reflex, 974
 sedative effects of, 560t
 side effects of, 288t, 561
 structure of, 288, 288f
 for trauma patient, 1258
Goblet cells, 792
Goiter, 1121, 1121t
Gold
 for rheumatoid arthritis, 509, 509t
 side effects of, 509t
Goldan, Sydney Ormond, 10, 21
Goldenhair's syndrome, 597t
Goldman Cardiac Risk Index, 474–475, 475f
Golgi Mazzoni endings, 1404t
Golgi tendon organ, 797–798
Gonadal dysfunction, in cirrhosis, 1090
Gordth, Torsten, 22
GOS. *See* Glasgow Outcome Scale
Gott shunt, 952
G6PD deficiency. *See* Glucose-6-phosphate dehydrogenase deficiency
G proteins, 255, 277–280, 743, 744–745f, 865, 1407, 1438
 anesthetic effects on, 130
 coupled to opioid receptors, 347
  G_p, 743, 745f
  Gi, 278, 279t, 743, 744f, 864
  Go, 278, 279t
  Gq, 278–279, 278f, 279t, 876f
  Gs, 278, 279t, 306, 743, 744f, 862
GR90291, 1013
Graft-versus-host disease (GVHD)
 in organ transplantation, 208
 transfusion-associated, 208–209
Gran, Sophie, 21
Grand mal seizure, 499–500, 499t
Granisetron, as premedicant, 981
Granulocyte transfusion, 208
Granulomatous disease, 191, 1125
Graves' disease, 1120, 1121t
Gray communicating rami, 264, 265f, 730
Greene needle, 692, 693f
Griffith, Harold, 20
Grounded power system, 146, 147f
Ground fault circuit interrupter (GFCI), 155–156, 155–156f, 162
Ground fault interrupter (GFI), 161
Grounding, 146, 146t
 of electrical power, 146–151, 147–151f
Ground wire, 146–147, 146f, 148–150f, 149, 152, 152f, 155–158, 157f
Group meetings, 34
Groups without walls, 47
Growth hormone, 1137, 1407
GST. *See* Glutathione *S*-transferase
Guanethidine, chemical sympathectomy with, 282
Guanidine, for myasthenic syndrome, 497
Guanylate cyclase, 131, 280f, 876, 876f
Guedel, Arthur, 16–17, 17f, 22
Guidewire-assisted cannulation, 673–674
Guillain-Barré syndrome, 181t, 1387
 anesthesia in, 492t, 497–498
Gum elastic bougie, 629, 630f
Gut, pain perception in, 1436–1437
GVHD. *See* Graft-versus-host disease
Gwathmey, James Tayloe, 11
Gynecoid obesity, 1035
Gynecologic surgery, laparoscopic, 1060
 laryngeal mask airway use in, 603t

Haldol. *See* Haloperidol
Half-time, 249, 252, 256
 context-sensitive. *See* Context-sensitive half-time
 percent of drug removed and, 249, 249t
Hall, Richard, 9
Hallux valgus, 1107t
Halogenated vapors
 effect on hepatic blood flow and oxygen delivery, 1079–1080, 1079f
 hepatitis caused by, 1075–1080
 liver injury other than hepatitis, 1077–1080
 metabolism of, 1076t, 1077
Haloperidol (Haldol)
 actions of, 272, 272t
 antiemetic activity of, 276
 central anticholinergic syndrome and, 289t
 as premedicant, 555
Halothane
 allergic reaction to, 67
 for ambulatory surgery, 1231
 autonomic nervous system effects of, 396–397, 396f
 binding to proteins, 134
 boiling point of, 574
 as bronchodilator, 400, 400f
 cardiac sensitizing action of, 298
 cardiovascular effects of, 395, 409
 cellular effects of, 65
 clinical overview of, 387
 concentration effect, 384f
 contraindications to, 1094